Textbook of

Medical-Surgical Nursing

Lillian Sholtis Brunner

R.N., M.S.N., Sc.D., Litt.D., F.A.A.N.

Vice Chairman (Education and Research):
Board of Trustees; Consultant in Nursing,
Presbyterian–University of Pennsylvania Medical Center,
 Philadelphia, Pennsylvania

Member, Board of Overseers,
School of Nursing, University of Pennsylvania,
Philadelphia, Pennsylvania

Formerly Assistant Professor of Nursing,
Yale University School of Nursing,
New Haven, Connecticut

Doris Smith Suddarth

R.N., B.S.N.E., M.S.N.

Formerly Consultant in Health Occupations, Job Corps Health
 Office,
U.S. Department of Labor, Washington, D.C.

Formerly Coordinator of the Curriculum, Alexandria Hospital
 School of Nursing, Alexandria, Virginia

Brenda G. Bare, R.N., M.S.N.

Director of Medical–Surgical Nursing,
The Alexandria Hospital, Alexandria, Virginia

Mary Jo Boyer, R.N., M.S.N.

Professor of Nursing, Nursing Program Coordinator,
Delaware County Community College, Media, Pennsylvania

Suzanne C. O'Connell Smeltzer, R.N., M.S., Ed.D.

Assistant Professor,
Rutgers University College of Nursing, Newark, New Jersey

With 19 Contributors

Textbook of

Medical–Surgical Nursing

Sixth Edition

J. B. Lippincott Company   *Philadelphia*

London   Mexico City   New York   St. Louis   São Paulo   Sydney

Acquisitions Editor: Diana Intenzo
Developmental Editor: Jeanne H. Wallace
Manuscript Editors: Jeanne Carper and Mary Norris
Indexer: Angela Holt
Design Coordinator: Susan Hess Blaker
Designer: Tracy Baldwin
Cover Designer: Anthony Frizano
Cover Photo: Michael Frankel
Production Manager: Carol A. Florence
Production Editor: Rosanne Hallowell
Production Coordinator: Charlene C. Squibb
Compositor: TAPSCO, Inc.
Text Printer/Binder: The Murray Printing Co., Inc.
Cover Printer: The Lehigh Press, Inc.

Sixth Edition

6 5 4 3 2

Library of Congress Cataloging-in-Publication Data

Textbook of medical–surgical nursing.

   Includes bibliographies and index.
   1. Nursing.   2. Surgical nursing.   I. Brunner,
Lillian Sholtis.   II. Suddarth, Doris Smith.
III. Bare, Brenda G.   IV. Boyer, Mary Jo.   V. Smeltzer,
Suzanne C. O'Connell.   VI. Title: Medical–surgical
nursing.   [DNLM: 1. Nursing Care.   2. Surgical Nursing.
WY 150 T355]
RT41.T46   1988   610.73   87-22669
ISBN 0-397-54641-6

Any medical or nursing procedure or practice described in this book
should be applied by the health care practitioner under appropriate
supervision in accordance with professional standards of care used
with regard to the unique circumstances that apply in each practice
situation. Care has been taken to confirm the accuracy of information
presented and to describe generally accepted practices. However, the
authors, editors, and publisher cannot accept any responsibility for
errors or omissions or for consequences from application of the
information in this book and make no warranty, express or implied,
with respect to the contents of the book.
Every effort has been made to ensure that drug selections and dosages
are in accordance with current recommendations and practice.
Because of ongoing research, changes in government regulations, and
the constant flow of information on drug therapy, reactions, and
interactions, the reader is cautioned to check the package insert for
each drug for indications, dosages, warnings, and precautions,
particularly if the drug is new or infrequently used.

Contributors

Brenda G. Bare, R.N., M.S.N.
Director of Medical–Surgical Nursing, The Alexandria
Hospital, Alexandria, Virginia
*Unit I (Chapters 1–4): Health Maintenance and Health
Needs*
Chapter 24: Assessment of Cardiovascular Function
Chapter 27: Management of the Cardiac Surgery Patient
*Chapter 28: Assessment and Management of Patients
With Vascular Disorders and Problems of Peripheral
Circulation*
*Chapter 29: Assessment and Management of Patients
With Hematologic Disorders*

Elizabeth W. Bayley, R.N., M.S.
Assistant Professor, Burn, Emergency, and Trauma Nursing,
Widener University, Chester, Pennsylvania
Chapter 49: Management of Patients With Burn Injury

Ellen K. Boyda, R.N., M.S., CCRN
Pulmonary Rehabilitation Program Coordinator, Taylor
Hospital, Ridley Park, Pennsylvania
*Unit VI (Chapters 20–23): Problems Affecting Oxygen–
Carbon Dioxide Exchange and Respiration*

Mary Jo Boyer, R.N., M.S.N.
Professor of Nursing, Nursing Program Coordinator,
Delaware County Community College, Media, Pennsylvania
*Unit VIII (Chapters 30–34): Digestive and Gastrointestinal
Problems*
*Chapter 47: Management of Patients With Rheumatic
Disorders*

David B.P. Goodman, M.D., Ph.D.
Professor and Department Chief, Department of Pathology
and Laboratory Medicine, Hospital of the University of
Pennsylvania, Philadelphia, Pennsylvania
Appendix: Diagnostic Studies and Their Meanings

Gail P. Hamilton, R.N.C., M.S.N., D.S.W.
Associate Professor of Nursing, Department of Nursing,
College of Allied Health Professions, Temple University,
Philadelphia, Pennsylvania
Chapter 11: Health Care of the Older Adult

Lois M. Hoskins, R.N., Ph.D.
Dean and Associate Professor of Nursing, School of
Nursing, The Catholic University of America,
Washington, D.C.
Chapter 7: Homeostasis and Pathophysiologic Processes
Chapter 8: Stress and Adaptation

Dorothy B. Liddel, R.N., M.S.N.
Curriculum Coordinator, The Alexandria Hospital School of
Nursing, Alexandria, Virginia
*Unit XV (Chapters 55–58): Musculoskeletal and
Locomotion Problems*

Norma Milligan Metheny, R.N., Ph.D.
Professor and Coordinator, Graduate Medical–Surgical
Nursing Major, St. Louis University, St. Louis, Missouri
*Chapter 9: Fluids and Electrolytes: Balance and
Disturbances*

Rita Nemchik, R.N., M.S.
Director, Center for Continuing Education, University of
Pennsylvania School of Nursing, Philadelphia, Pennsylvania
*Chapter 36: Assessment and Management of Patients
With Diabetes Mellitus*

Kathryn A. Pollon, R.N.C., M.S.N.
Mental Health Specialist, Mt. Vernon Hospital, Alexandria,
Virginia
Chapter 12: Human Response to Illness

Susan A. Rokita, R.N., M.S.
Oncology Clinical Nurse Specialist, The Thomas Jefferson
University Hospital, Philadelphia, Pennsylvania
Chapter 16: Oncology: Nursing the Patient With Cancer

Mona B. Shevlin, M.A., Ph.D.
Licensed Psychologist, Professor, The Catholic University of
America, Washington, D.C.; Director, Counseling Center for
Greater Washington, McLean, Virginia
*Chapter 10: Developmental Concepts of the Adult Life
Phase*

Suzanne C. O'Connell Smeltzer, R.N., M.S., Ed.D.
Assistant Professor, Rutgers University College of Nursing, Newark, New Jersey

Chapter 35: Assessment and Management of Patients With Hepatic and Biliary Disorders
Chapter 37: Assessment and Management of Patients With Endocrine Disorders
Chapter 38: Assessment of Renal and Urinary Function
Chapter 39: Management of Patients With Renal and Urinary Dysfunction
Chapter 40: Management of Patients With Renal and Urinary Disorders

Loretta Spittle, R.N., M.S., CCRN
Director of Critical Care Services, The Fairfax Hospital, Falls Church, Virginia

Chapter 25: Management of Patients With Cardiac Disorders
Chapter 26: Management of Patients With Complications of Cardiac Disorders

Cindy L. Stern, R.N., M.S.N.
Oncology Clinical Nurse Specialist, The Thomas Jefferson University Hospital, Philadelphia, Pennsylvania

Chapter 16: Oncology: Nursing the Patient With Cancer
Chapter 45: The Immune System, Immunopathology, and Immunodeficiency

Contributors to the previous edition whose work appears in the sixth edition are listed below.

Silvia Prodan Lange, R.N., M.N., C.S.
Chapter 12: Human Response to Illness

Margo McCaffery, R.N., M.S., F.A.A.N.
Chapter 15: The Person Experiencing Pain

Diane Deegan McCrann, R.N., M.S.N.
Chapter 5: Clinical Interviewing: The Health History, and selected material on physical assessment, which appears throughout the book

Josephine Messer, R.N., M.S.
Chapter 13: Human Sexuality

Ruth Mrozek, R.N., M.S.
Selected material on documentation of nursing practice in *Chapter 2: The Nursing Process*

Kyriake Valassi, Ph.D.
Selected material on nutritional assessment in *Chapter 6: Physical Assessment and Nutritional Assessment*

Preface

The current revolution in health care profoundly affects nurses in academic and clinical practice settings. It is a challenge that entails commitment to excellence in the educational preparation and professional performance of nurses. In response to these demands, the sixth edition of the *Textbook of Medical–Surgical Nursing* is designed to provide the sound scientific rationale and broad clinical knowledge base that nursing students and practitioners will need. The fund of information is drawn from nursing, the physical, biological, and behavioral sciences, and research. The nursing process is the central, unifying principle of the book and provides the logical framework for its organization. In applying the nursing process to practice, the nurse learns to recognize health–illness problems that can be alleviated by nursing interventions. The planning and implementation of these interventions is based on a thorough understanding of biophysical and psychosocial function and dysfunction in acute and chronic health situations. The effectiveness of the nurse's interventions is measured against expected outcomes established at the outset, reviewed during ongoing assessments, and modified as needed. Therapeutic decisions are, of course, based on individual circumstances.

The perspective of this edition reflects contemporary realities and future possibilities. This approach is evident in the highlighted emphasis on gerontological considerations and in the recognition of changing demands on health care resources. Patients in hospitals, as well as those released to step-down units, extended care facilities, or their own homes, are in the main acutely ill. Because the clinical situations of persons in all of these settings are acute and can change rapidly, health-compromising complications are a major concern. To alert the nurse to problems that may arise, discussions of potential complications and the nurse's role in their assessment and management are strategically placed in the text and in nursing care plans. The object is to encourage sophisticated, creative, and concerted efforts by nurses in various clinical practice settings to identify actual or potential health problems and to plan and initiate individualized care that will continue as the patient returns to his or her previous setting.

The hallmarks of the *Textbook of Medical–Surgical Nursing* are accuracy, accessibility, and practicality. Thus the patient education and home health care sections have been amplifed to reflect the nurse's role in teaching, counseling, and advocacy. The emphasis is on helping patients and their families to have a role in making decisions and to be in control as much as possible. Self-care strategies are stressed, as well as the promotion and maintenance of health. Community-based support groups are identified. Home care of the patient requiring mechanical ventilation is specifically addressed. The new and expanded material that has been added on AIDS and Alzheimer's disease and on many other topics of major importance to nurses reflects current concerns and developments in the field of health care. Nursing care plans and significant tables and charts are presented throughout the book.

As the profession adds to its body of knowledge through more research by nurses, this achievement is given special emphasis. Annotated reviews of pertinent nursing research articles are presented in Nursing Research Profiles that follow clinical units; nursing implications are identified and related to nursing practice and theory. In the bibliographies, each nursing research citation is designated by an asterisk. Bibliographic citations were carefully selected to reflect state-of-the-art knowledge and practice. As an additional aid to research, the bibliographic citations are in the format of the *Index Medicus* and the *MEDLINE* data base.

The style of presentation continues to be eclectic, because this realistic approach allows the student or practitioner to adapt material according to his or her philosophy or theory of nursing. To facilitate understanding of the language of nursing and allied health sciences, definitions are provided for new or less familiar terms as they occur in the text. Since the International System of Units (SI units) is being adopted worldwide for reporting clinical laboratory data, in this edition the conventional laboratory values are followed by the recommended SI units in parentheses. SI units are also included in the appendix of laboratory values at the end of the book.

A flexible approach to gender identification has been maintained in the interest of clarity and readability and in no way reflects a sexist attitude. The use of masculine and feminine gender pronouns is kept to a minimum, but in some instances this literary convention serves to ensure a clearer presentation of the material and preserve the flow of the text.

Thus, the pronoun *he* is used to designate both male and female recipients of care, and *she* is used in referring to both male and female nurses. Persons receiving care are identified as either patients or clients and are always portrayed as individuals whose desire for independence is respected and fostered by nurses.

New technology and exciting changes and trends continue to broaden the scope of medical–surgical nursing. Yesterday's guidelines do not necessarily apply today. A close-working team is required to review the vast amount of literature and to apply the high degree of discrimination needed to select what is most relevant. The senior authors/editors welcome to this edition three nursing colleagues—Brenda G. Bare, Mary Jo Boyer, and Suzanne C. O'C. Smeltzer—who have contributed their specialized expertise and talent.

Through all the changes, the caring values of nursing are the ones that remain constant and make gentle the lives of those whom we are privileged to serve.

Lillian S. Brunner, R.N., M.S.N., Sc.D., Litt.D., F.A.A.N.
Doris S. Suddarth, R.N., B.S.N.E., M.S.N.

Acknowledgments

Judith L. Bachman, R.N., M.S.N.
Assistant Director of Nursing, Presbyterian–University of Pennsylvania Medical Center, Philadelphia, Pennsylvania

Heather Boyd-Monk, S.R.N., R.N., B.S.N.
Assistant Director of Nursing for Education Programs, Wills Eye Hospital, Philadelphia, Pennsylvania

Carol Case, R.N., M.Ed.
Chief: Public Inquiry, National Cancer Institute, Bethesda, Maryland

Tressa A. Cathcart-Silberberg, R.N., M.S.N.
Clinical Nurse Specialist, Assistant Head Nurse, Hospital of the University of Pennsylvania, Philadelphia, Pennsylvania

June Cella, R.N., Ed.D.
Associate Professor, School of Nursing, The Thomas Jefferson University, Philadelphia, Pennsylvania

Jean DeVries, R.N.
Equipment Analyst, Alexandria Hospital, Alexandria, Virginia

Thomas G. Frazier, M.D.
Attending Surgeon, General Surgery, The Bryn Mawr Hospital, Bryn Mawr, Pennsylvania

Karen Javie, R.N., M.S.N.
Vice President for Nursing, Presbyterian–University of Pennsylvania Medical Center, Philadelphia, Pennsylvania

Mary Ellen Kern, R.N., M.S.N.
Clinical Specialist, Critical Care, Presbyterian–University of Pennsylvania Medical Center, Philadelphia, Pennsylvania

Nadine Landis, R.N., M.S.N.
Systems Analyst; Archivist, Hospital of the University of Pennsylvania, Philadelphia, Pennsylvania

Etta J. Liberi, R.N., M.S.N.
Director, School of Practical Nursing, Presbyterian–University of Pennsylvania Medical Center, Philadelphia, Pennsylvania

Kay Martin, R.N., Ed.D.
Director of Nursing Education and Research, Presbyterian–University of Pennsylvania Medical Center, Philadelphia, Pennsylvania

R. Barrett Noone, M.D.
Chief, Service of Plastic Surgery, The Bryn Mawr Hospital, Bryn Mawr, Pennsylvania

Susan R. Pyle, R.N., M.S.N.
Director of Critical Care and Perioperative Nursing, Presbyterian–University of Pennsylvania Medical Center, Philadelphia, Pennsylvania

Ward Rinehart
Associate Director and Editor, *Population Reports*, The Johns Hopkins University, Hopkins Population Center, Baltimore, Maryland

Mel Stills, C.O.
Orthopedic Department, The University of Texas Health Science Center at Dallas, Dallas, Texas

Research/Library

Kathleen M. Ahrens, M.S.
Director, Information Services, Health Sciences Library, Presbyterian–University of Pennsylvania Medical Center, Philadelphia, Pennsylvania

James Cain
Deputy Chief, Public Services Division, National Library of Medicine, Bethesda, Maryland

Ann Campisi
Library Technician, Health Sciences Library, Presbyterian–University of Pennsylvania Medical Center, Philadelphia, Pennsylvania

Catherine A. Dalton, M.S.
Librarian, Crozer-Chester Medical Center Library, Chester, Pennsylvania

Eileen Daget
Librarian, Joseph N. Pew, Jr., Medical Library, The Bryn Mawr Hospital, Bryn Mawr, Pennsylvania

Leslie D. Gundry
Chief Medical Librarian, Joseph N. Pew, Jr., Medical Library, The Bryn Mawr Hospital, Bryn Mawr, Pennsylvania

Elizabeth J. Hamilton, M.L.S.
Medical Librarian, Alexandria Hospital, Alexandria, Virginia

Alexander G. Kulchar
Medical Librarian, Clothier Nurses Library, The Bryn Mawr Hospital, Bryn Mawr, Pennsylvania

Eve-Marie Lacroix
Chief of Public Services Division, National Library of Medicine, Bethesda, Maryland

Katherine M. McCann
Library Technician II, Crozer-Chester Medical Center Library, Chester, Pennsylvania

Alice Makov
Reference User Education, Scott Memorial Library, The Thomas Jefferson University, Philadelphia, Pennsylvania

Reference Librarians and Reference Technicians
National Library of Medicine, Bethesda, Maryland

Ray F. Roedell, Jr., M.L.S., M.A.
Librarian, Health Sciences Library, Presbyterian–University of Pennsylvania Medical Center, Philadelphia, Pennsylvania

Gladys L. Taylor and Staff
Head Monograph Processing Group, Circulation and Control Section, National Library of Medicine, Bethesda, Maryland

Jacqueline van de Kamp
Reference Librarian, National Library of Medicine, Bethesda, Maryland

Research/Art

Michael Harty, M.D.
Emeritus Professor of Anatomy, School of Medicine, University of Pennsylvania, Philadelphia, Pennsylvania

Ernest L. McKenna, Jr., M.D.
Clinical Professor of Otolaryngology, Jefferson Medical College of The Thomas Jefferson University, Philadelphia, Pennsylvania

James Saunders, M.D.
Associate Professor of Otolaryngology, Associate Director, Institute of Neurological Sciences, School of Medicine, University of Pennsylvania, Philadelphia, Pennsylvania

Art

Michael E. Leonard
Baltimore, Maryland

June L. Melloni, Ph.D.
Bethesda, Maryland

Jean E. Wolfe, M.F.A.
Malvern, Pennsylvania

Photography

Glenn Dalby
Takoma Park, Maryland

Leslie A Hoffman, R.N., Ph.D.
University of Pittsburgh School of Nursing, Pittsburgh, Pennsylvania

The authors express special and sincere appreciation to the following who helped to make this sixth edition possible:

Diana Intenzo for her exemplary editorial commitment, understanding of nursing, fantastic memory, and unlimited energy

Jeanne H. Wallace for her gentle caring spirit, meticulous attention to detail, and conscientious devotion to this project

Rosanne Hallowell and *Charlene Squibb* for their skillful guidance of this textbook through the various stages of production

Marsha Bacal and *Susan Hess Blaker* for their creative talent and insight

Richard I. Cordrey, David Barnes, and the sales representatives for their noteworthy competence in the field

Mary Murphy for her many kindnesses, proficiency, and punctuality in handling many details for us

Chairman of the Board *Barton H. Lippincott* for his continuing interest and affirmation through the years

Lastly, but far from least, our devoted husbands, *Mat* and *Hilton,* for their understanding, support, and constant encouragement

Lillian S. Brunner
Doris S. Suddarth

Contents

Unit XVI
Other Acute Problems   *1639*

59 Management of Patients With Infectious Diseases   *1640*

60 Emergency Nursing   *1698*

Appendix: Diagnostic Studies and Their Meaning   *1738*

Index   *1765*

Health Maintenance and Health Needs

Unit I

Chapter 1

Nursing in Today's World: Concepts and Implementation

Nursing Defined

Nursing leaders for decades have been attempting to articulate a universally accepted definition of nursing that identifies the uniqueness of the profession and has meaning for all practitioners of nursing as well as for the members of other professions involved in the delivery of health care. Such a definition has been slow in coming because nursing has lacked a clearly defined body of theoretical knowledge. Historically, nursing practice has been based on tradition. Only in recent years have nurses accepted the challenge to demonstrate that nursing is indeed a profession with its own unique body of knowledge. Nurse theorists are now using scientific methods to describe, explain, and predict nursing practice and its outcomes. As theory development proceeds, it will continue to be refined. The objective of this research is to validate nursing practice and provide society with a definition of nursing that will foster the autonomy of the profession.

Since the time of Florence Nightingale, who wrote in 1858 that the real goal of nursing was "to put the patient in the best condition for nature to act upon him," nursing leaders have defined nursing as both an art and a science. In the earlier years, they tended to emphasize the nursing services that are directed toward the care of the sick. More recently, they have stressed the maintenance and promotion of health as well as the prevention of illness.

One of the classic definitions of nursing, as formulated by Virginia Henderson (1966), delineates the unique function of the nurse as follows:

> to assist the individual, sick or well, in the performance of those activities contributing to health or its recovery (or to peaceful death) that he would perform unaided if he had the necessary strength, will or knowledge. And to do this in such a way as to help him gain independence as rapidly as possible.*

Review of the literature since the time of Henderson's definition of nursing reveals a multitude of attempts at further

---

* Henderson V. The Nature of Nursing. New York, Macmillan, 1966.

defining the unique function of the nurse—unique with regard to the functions of other health care disciplines. Most of these formulations have attempted to define nursing as a profession directed toward meeting both the health and illness needs of "man," who is viewed holistically as having physical, emotional, psychological, intellectual, social, and spiritual needs.

More recently, the American Nurses' Association published *Nursing: A Social Policy Statement* (1980), which provided a description of the social context of nursing and a definition of the nature and scope of nursing practice. Nursing was defined as

- the diagnosis and treatment of human responses to actual or potential health problems.

An illustrative list of human responses that are the focus for nursing intervention was presented as follows:

> Self-care limitations
> Impaired functioning in areas such as rest, sleep, ventilation, circulation, activity, nutrition, elimination, skin, and sexuality
> Pain and discomfort
> Emotional problems related to illness and treatment, life-threatening events, or daily experiences, such as anxiety, loss, loneliness, and grief
> Distortion of symbolic functions, reflected in interpersonal and intellectual processes, such as hallucinations
> Deficiencies in decision making and ability to make personal choices
> Self-image changes required by health status
> Dysfunctional perceptual orientations to health
> Strains related to life processes, such as birth, growth and development, and death
> Problematic affiliative relationships

This definition of the nature and scope of nursing practice clearly reflects a view of man as an integrated whole—a biopsychosocial being. In this holistic concept of health the various aspects of human functioning are seen as interrelated, interdependent, and of equal importance. Nurses have a responsibility to demonstrate and be accountable for their role as defined in the policy statement. They must also comply with the nurse practice act of the state within which they practice and with the guidelines established by the International Council of Nurses (ICN) and the American Nurses' Association (ANA) in their respective codes for nurses.

Yura and Walsh (1983) state that the purposes of nursing are to

> maintain the client's optimal wellness, and, if this state changes, to provide the amount and quality of nursing care the situation demands to direct the client back to wellness. If wellness cannot be achieved, then the nursing process should contribute to the client's quality of life, maximizing the client's resources to achieve the highest quality of living possible for as long as possible.*

* Yura H and Walsh WB. The Nursing Process, 4th ed. East Norwalk, Connecticut, Appleton-Century-Crofts, 1983.

Conceptual Models in Nursing

If nurses are to accomplish the goals of nursing as defined by nursing leaders, nursing must have a body of theoretical knowledge on which to base its practice. Great strides toward "theory building" in nursing have been made in recent years.

In the past, nursing has used theories from various biopsychosocial sciences. Only within the past several decades have nurses made concerted efforts toward identifying a circumscribed body of knowledge that is unique to nursing and that can serve as the theoretical basis for the practice of nursing. Such a theoretical basis, when more fully developed, will consist of scientifically derived general principles that are applied consistently in nursing practice. Nursing theories will provide a guide for viewing nursing holistically and for determining the probable results of nursing actions in advance of their implementation. However, only as theories of nursing evolve and mature and as they are tested and retested will a general theory of nursing develop.

Much of the progress that has been accomplished in the pursuit of a scientific theory of nursing has been in the areas of concept formalization and model construction. Because nursing is a practice-oriented discipline, concepts of nursing have been evolving over the years. However, only in recent years have nurses attempted to articulate these concepts, to propose that they be used as the framework for nursing practice, and to test and validate them. Many concepts that have their foundations in the biopsychosocial sciences have been found to be particularly applicable to nursing and now serve as useful components of frameworks for nursing practice.

Several of the broad concepts that have been used extensively as frameworks for nursing curricula and for nursing practice throughout the country include (1) the wellness–illness continuum, (2) developmental processes throughout the life cycle, and (3) stress adaptation.

The *wellness–illness continuum* provides a means by which the nurse focuses on the patient's positive health attributes and characteristics within the dimensions of his illness or potential illness situation. The individual is recognized as a holistic being who is in interaction with his internal and external environments. With such a focus and view of the individual, the nurse then uses the nursing process to assist the patient to use his attributes in attaining and maintaining the highest level of wellness possible within his physical and psychosocial limitations. Dunn's concept of high-level wellness serves as the basis for this framework for nursing.

The *developmental processes* approach to nursing provides a frame of reference that emphasizes the complexity of variables that are involved in each of the developmental stages of the life cycle. Such a framework provides direction for the nurse in assisting the patient to accomplish his developmental tasks as they are affected by his state of health and wellness. The theories of Havighurst, Erikson, and Piaget serve as the bases for the developmental processes approach to nursing. Havighurst's developmental tasks emphasize the effects of physical and social developmental changes and events on the individual; Erikson's eight stages of human development emphasize the successful completion of psychosocial tasks necessary for attaining and maintaining one's identity; Piaget's stages of cognitive development emphasize development of cognitive abilities and related sensorimotor skills.

The *stress-adaptation framework* emphasizes the role of the nurse in assessing the patient's behavioral responses to the demands of his internal and external environments. Nursing interventions are then directed toward assisting the patient to strive toward adaptive behavior that promotes health and prevents illness. The general adaptation syndrome as described by Selye and the fight-or-flight syndrome as described by Cannon serve as the bases for the stress-adaptation framework.

These broad concepts and other related concepts, while serving as useful frameworks for nursing practice, are not in and of themselves unique to nursing. Therefore, nursing leaders have attempted to develop, more fully, concepts that are inherent within nursing itself and to construct models that describe the relationships between these concepts and their subconcepts. Four such conceptual models of nursing are the *life processes model* developed by Rogers (1970), the *self-care model* as advocated by Orem (1971, 1980, 1985), the *adaptation model* as formulated by Roy (1980), and the *behavioral systems model* developed by Johnson (1980).

These are certainly not the only conceptual models of nursing that have been developed, nor is it our intent to suggest that nurses should subscribe to any one of these models, forsaking other models that may also serve as valuable frameworks for the practice of nursing. However, it is our intent to present these models as examples of contemporary models of nursing, with the hope that they will generate interest, enthusiasm, and inquiry into the present status and future potential of conceptual frameworks of nursing and the state of theory building in nursing.

Life Processes Model

The life processes model of nursing focuses on the wholeness of the human organism in the person who is the recipient of nursing care. It is Rogers's belief that the purpose of the scientific body of knowledge of nursing is to describe, explain, and make predictions about mankind. Such knowledge leads to the evolution of theories that serve to guide nursing practice. Rogers identified fundamental human attributes that constitute the following basic assumptions on which nursing science is built:

1. Man is a unified whole possessing his own integrity and manifesting characteristics that are more than and different from the sum of his parts.
2. Man and the environment are continuously exchanging matter and energy with one another.
3. The life process evolves irreversibly and unidirectionally along the space–time continuum.
4. Pattern and organization identify man and reflect his innovative wholeness.
5. Man is characterized by the capacity for abstraction and imagery, language and thought, and sensation and emotion.

The qualities of the life processes as described in these assumptions include wholeness, openness, unidirectionality, pattern and organization, and sentience and thought. The underlying principles describe man as a dynamic entity who interacts mutually and simultaneously with his environment. The changes that occur during this interaction are irreversible, nonrepeatable, and rhythmical, increasing in complexity and proceeding by the continual repatterning of man and his environment.

- With such a view of man, the goal of nursing becomes that of promoting the person's interaction with his environment in such a way that the maximum state of health that is possible is realized by the utilization of the individual's own energies and potential.

This holistic concept of human functioning serves as the basis for making predictions about nursing intervention. Data gathered for making nursing diagnoses are derived from the total pattern of events that have influenced the extent to which man is achieving his maximum health potential. These data then serve as the basis for the establishment of short-term and long-term health goals for the individual, his family, and society and for the implementation of nursing actions directed toward the achievement of these goals. These nursing actions are aimed at helping the individual to repattern his relationship with himself and his environment so that his maximum health potential can be attained. A conceptual model of nursing such as that proposed by Rogers contributes to the pursuit of a scientific theory of nursing. Testing, retesting, and validation of the model will no doubt serve to further the science of nursing.

Self-Care Model

Orem has developed a concept of nursing that places emphasis on the person's need for self-care—those activities that an individual practices for the purpose of maintaining life, health, and well-being. It is the concern of nursing to provide for and manage the person's self-care actions in an attempt to promote life and health and to assist him to recover from disease and injury or to cope with their effects. The need for nursing exists when an adult is unable to satisfactorily meet his self-care requisites or when a parent is unable to meet these demands for a child.

- Nursing is responsible for assisting the person to overcome those circumstances that interfere with self-care and that cause self-care limitations and deficits.

There are three broad categories of self-care requisites: universal, developmental, and those related to health deviation. *Universal self-care requisites* are those that are required of all individuals to maintain integrated human functioning. *Developmental self-care requisites* are those that occur as a result of developmental processes (*e.g.,* pregnancy) or of conditions that can affect human development (*e.g.,* loss of loved ones). *Health-deviation self-care requisites* are those that occur as a result of disease, injury, disfigurement, disability, or medical diagnoses and treatment and that require that changes be made in the person's routine of self-care depending on the nature and extent of the requisites. Self-care activity is purposeful, deliberate action that is goal directed, self initiated, and self directed and is affected by the person's values and goals. When it is effective it promotes the structural integrity, functioning, and development of the person.

Orem identifies three systems of nursing activities that are designed to meet the individual's self-care requirements, according to the extent to which self-care action is disrupted: the wholly compensatory system, the partly compensatory system, and the supportive-educative (developmental) system. The *wholly compensatory system* is used when the person is unable to assume an active role in his care and the nurse assists him by acting for and doing for him. The *partly compensatory system* is used when the nurse and the patient participate in accomplishing therapeutic self-care actions. The major responsibility for the performance of these actions may be assumed by the nurse or by the patient, depending on the patient's actual or medically prescribed limitations, his knowledge and skills, and his psychological readiness to accomplish such activities. The *supportive-educative system* is used when the patient is capable of performing, or learning to perform, those measures that are necessary to accomplish his self-care requisites but for which he needs assistance in the form of support, guidance, provision of a developmental environment, and teaching.

Thus, as the health status of the patient changes, his needs for nursing activity may demand a change in the nursing system that is appropriate to meet his needs. Such a conceptual model of nursing can serve as a framework for guiding and directing nursing care. Currently, the framework is used within various nursing education and nursing service settings. However, further validation of the concept is necessary for the continuation of nursing's pursuit of a sound theoretical base.

Adaptation Model

The adaptation model of nursing developed by Roy is a systems model that incorporates interactionist concepts. *Adaptation* is defined as the process of change, a universal phenomenon of man. Within the model, man is viewed as a biopsychosocial being who is in constant interaction with his environment—an interaction that requires him to make continual adaptations. The capacity for adaptation depends on the stimuli to which he is exposed and the level of his adaptation. The adaptive level is determined by the effect of three classes of stimuli: (1) focal stimuli, or those with which the person is immediately confronted; (2) contextual stimuli, which include all other stimuli that are present; and (3) residual stimuli, or stimuli that the person has experienced in the past, such as beliefs, attitudes, and traits. Humans have four modes of adaptation: physiologic, self-concept, role function, and interdependence relations. Thus, adaptive or positive responses to stimuli serve to maintain the total integrity of the individual.

- The role of nursing is that of promoting adaptation in all four modes during health and illness by using the four components of the nursing process: assessing, planning, implementing, and evaluating.

During the assessment phase of the nursing process, the person's position on the health–illness continuum is identified and the effectiveness of his ability to cope with the stimuli with which he is confronted is evaluated. The planning phase of the nursing process involves the establishment of goals for changing maladaptive behavior to adaptive behavior. Then, the nursing process is completed by the implementation and

evaluation of a plan of nursing action directed toward promoting adaptation. The adaptation model of nursing is in operation in several schools of nursing and nursing service departments in hospital settings. However, it continues to require further validation as a framework for the practice of nursing.

Behavioral Systems Model

The behavioral systems model for nursing developed by Johnson describes man as a behavioral system that continually strives to maintain balance through adjustments and adaptations to his ever-changing internal and external environments. His behavior is orderly, purposeful, and predictable, and most of the time it is functionally efficient and effective. The behavioral system has seven subsystems (related to affiliation, dependency, ingestion, elimination, sexuality, aggression, and achievement), each of which has a specialized task or function that promotes integrated performance of the system as a whole.

The need for nursing arises when the balance of the system is disturbed or is likely to be disturbed sufficiently to warrant external assistance. Nursing is viewed as an external regulatory force directed toward preventing disturbance in the system and preserving or restoring optimal organization and integration of the patient's behavior. The goal of nursing is to assist the patient to modify his behavioral patterns in such a way that he is able to meet the demands of the elements in his life that cannot be modified.

During the assessment phase of the nursing process, the patient's ability to adapt to his actual or perceived threat without resultant instability is identified. In cases in which instability exists or is expected, an in-depth assessment of the involved subsystems is performed. Identification and validation of dysfunctional behaviors lead to the development of nursing diagnoses. Nursing intervention is then directed toward the promotion of regularity in the patient's behavior so that balance is maintained or attained in each subsystem. The nursing process is completed when expected behavioral outcomes have been measured and the plan of care has been revised as necessary to further promote stability of the behavioral system, adjustment to the situation, and adaptation to stress.

The behavioral systems model has been used in various settings to provide direction for nursing practice, education, and research. However, the empirical and theoretical knowledge base for the model needs further development, and the model requires further testing and validation.

Comments

These are only four of the available models of nursing that can serve as frameworks for nursing practice. Educators throughout the country are using these models, adapting them to meet their own individual needs, following other models of nursing, or developing new models. A curriculum based on a conceptual model provides the student and the graduate with a framework for nursing practice within which the nurse can function while providing nursing care and can be guided in furthering her nursing education experiences. It is our hope that students and graduates who use any of the various nursing models can appropriately incorporate into their own frameworks of nursing practice the information about health, illness, and specific disease entities included in his book. Only with an acute appreciation of the physiologic as well as the psychosocial needs of the individual who has a right to health but who experiences the threat of illness can practitioners of nursing fulfill the expectations that are centered in them by society and by the nursing profession.

Nursing and the Health Care Delivery System

Health Defined

The nursing profession exists to meet the health needs of the people. Hence, as health needs change, so must health care. Unprecedented changes have occurred in the structure of our society, in life styles, and in scientific and technological advances. These changes have altered the pattern of disease and the traditional therapeutic approaches as well as the concept of health care and the expectations that society has of the health professions. Today health is considered more than a basic human right; it has become a matter of public concern, national priority, and political action.

Our health system has traditionally been a disease-oriented system. However, the current trend is to emphasize health and its promotion. Health has been defined by the World Health Organization (WHO) as a "state of complete physical, mental, and social well being and not merely the absence of disease and infirmity."* However, such a definition of health does not allow for any variation in the degrees of wellness or of illness. The concept of a health–illness continuum (as first described by Dunn [1961]) has markedly affected the purposes of the health professions. By viewing health and illness on a graduated continuum, a person is seen as having neither complete health nor complete illness. Instead, a person's state of health is ever changing and has the potential for ranging from high-level wellness to extremely poor health and imminent death. Thus, a person is viewed as simultaneously possessing degrees of both health and illness. A person who has a chronic illness cannot meet the expectations of health as defined by the WHO definition of health. However, according to the health–illness continuum, the person with a chronic illness can attain a high level of wellness if he is successful in meeting his health potential within the limits of his chronic illness.

During the past 50 years, the health problems of the American people have changed significantly. The majority of such problems are no longer infectious and acute but instead are chronic. Almost 50% of the U.S. population have one or more chronic conditions. With this change in the health status of the American people has come an increasing emphasis on health, health promotion, wellness, and self-care. Emphasis has shifted from a focus on cure to a focus on prevention and health maintenance. Health is seen as resulting from a life-style that is oriented toward wellness. The result has been the evolution of a wide range of health promotion techniques and programs, including multiphasic screening, lifetime health monitoring programs, environmental and mental health programs, accident prevention, and nutrition and health education. A growing interest in self-care is evidenced by the myriad of health and medical care publications, conferences, and workshops designed for the lay public. Organized self-care education programs emphasize health promotion, disease prevention, management of illness, self-medication, and use of the professional health care system. In addition, over 500,000 self-help groups exist for the purpose of developing and sharing self-care skills with peers who have common chronic disease or disability problems.

Special efforts are being made by health care professionals to reach and motivate members of various cultural and socioeconomic groups concerning life-style and health practices. The main thrust is to design a health care delivery system that makes comprehensive health care available to all the people at a tolerable cost. Of course, this type of health care has broad political and sociological implications as organizers, consumers, politicians, and health care providers become involved in the planning.

Concept of Promotion of Wellness and Health Maintenance

Members of health care delivery systems need to gain a vision of the concept of wellness, of what society could accomplish if it were freed from the burdens of illness. Each person should be approached in terms of what his potential state of health should and could be. Inherent in this concept is the understanding that health has to be developed, maintained, and cherished by a continuum of effort. After all, it is not a static state of being; instead, it requires that energy be expended toward reaching an ever higher potential.

It was suggested in the early 1970s (Hoffman, 1972) that "the next major advance in the health of this nation will come through health education, not through more doctors or more hospitals or new discoveries. . . . We must persuade the American people that next to genetics the single most important factor in health is life-style. That even more important than environmental pollution is personal pollution." This suggestion still holds true. Stress, improper diet, lack of exercise, smoking, drugs, accidents, and a lack of cleanliness are all related to this concept of how life-style affects health. Health workers, then, should be concerned with changing behavior to promote health. The goal is to motivate people so that they will make improvements in the way they live, in other words, to prompt them toward health behavior changes.

The Health Care Delivery System

The Changing Scene

The health care delivery system is rapidly changing as society's health needs and expectations change. A multitude of societal and legislative factors are significant motivators of the changing patterns of health care. Changes in the population in general are affecting the need for and the delivery of health care.

* Preamble of the Constitution of the World Health Organization.

It is estimated that by the year 2000 there will be over 300 million people in the United States. This population expansion has in part been attributed to improved public health services and improved nutrition. Not only is the population increasing, but the composition of the population also is changing. With the decline in birth rate since the mid 1950s and the increase in life span that has resulted from improved medical care, there are fewer school-age children and more senior citizens. Likewise, the mobility of the population is changing. The advent of sophisticated transportation systems has allowed for extreme mobility. The majority of the population reside in highly congested urban areas. Along with this trend toward urbanization, there has been a steady migration of minority groups to the inner cities and a migration of middle-class persons to suburban areas. Because of such population changes, the need for health care for specific age-groups and for persons within specific geographic localities is altering the effectiveness of the traditional means of providing health care and is necessitating far-reaching changes in the overall health care delivery system.

Technological advances have occurred in greater numbers during the past several decades than in all other epochs of human civilization. This is an era of sophisticated electronic machines, which have revolutionized the labor force by performing many tasks that previously were accomplished by humans. This is also an era of sophisticated communication systems by which most parts of the world are connected. A variety of systems have been devised for storing, retrieving, and disseminating information. Such scientific and technological advances are themselves precipitating rapid change as well as rapid obsolescence.

Public Concern for Quality Care

The general public has become increasingly interested in and knowledgeable about health care and health maintenance. This interest and knowledge have been stimulated by television, newspapers, nonprofessional magazines, and other communications media. The public has become more health conscious and has in general begun to subscribe strongly to the belief that health and health care constitute a basic right, not a privilege for a chosen few. Members of the health care professions have become increasingly aware of the public's beliefs about health and health care. One indication of such awareness is the Patient's Bill of Rights prepared by the American Hospital Association in 1973, which is directed toward the promotion of more effective patient care and patient satisfaction (Chart 1-1).

The National League for Nursing (NLN) has also issued a statement on patients' rights, which "specifies ways in which a respect for patients' rights and a commitment to safeguarding them can be incorporated into nursing education programs and upheld and reinforced by those in nursing service. In many cases, nurses can directly involve themselves in assuring specific rights; in others, they can make their influence felt indirectly" (Chart 1-2).

Awareness of the public's beliefs and concerns about health and health care has also been acknowledged by Congress. Comprehensive health planning legislation was enacted during the 1960s. The National Health Planning and Resources Act of 1974 emphasized the need for planning and providing quality health care for all Americans by means of coordinated health services, manpower, and facilities at the national, state, and local levels. Medically underserved populations were the target for primary care services provided for by this act. However, growing adherence to the philosophy that comprehensive, quality health care should be provided for all citizens prompted governmental concern about spiraling health care costs, wide variations in costs among hospitals, and the increased use of hospital services. These concerns led to the Medicare prospective payment system.

Diagnosis-Related Groups

In 1983, Congress enacted the most significant health legislation since the Medicare program in 1965. The government was no longer able to afford retrospective reimbursement of hospitals. Thus, it approved a prospective payment system for hospital inpatient services. The Diagnosis-Related Groups (DRGs) system of reimbursement was adopted as the rate-setting method used for Medicare payments for hospital services. Hospitals receive payment at a fixed rate for patients in specific DRGs. A payment has been predetermined for over 460 possible diagnostic categories, which cover the majority of disorders of all patients admitted to the hospital. Thus, hospitals receive the same payment for every patient with a given DRG. If the cost of the patient's care is lower than the payment, the hospital gains a profit; if the cost is higher, the hospital incurs a loss. In order to qualify for Medicare reimbursement, hospitals must contract with peer review organizations (PROs) to perform quality and utilization review. The PROs monitor admission patterns, lengths of stay, transfers, and the quality of services, and validate DRG coding. The burden is now on the hospital to reduce costs, utilization, and lengths of stay.

The DRG system provides hospitals with the incentive to cut all unnecessary costs and to discharge patients as quickly as possible. The importance of an effective discharge planning program along with utilization review and quality assurance programs is unquestionable. The impact of all of this on nurses is that they must assume responsibility with other health care team members for maintaining quality care while facing pressures to discharge patients and decrease staffing costs. Combined with this, nurses in hospitals are caring for patients who are older and sicker and demand more nursing services, and nurses in the community are caring for patients who have been discharged earlier and need acute care as well as long-term care.

Alternatives to Traditional Health Care: HMOs and PPOs

In the early 1970s, steadily rising health care costs led to the emergence of new alternative health care delivery systems. The first of these, the health maintenance organization (HMO), provided the first radical change in the provider–insurer relationship and in the traditional fee-for-service system. HMOs provide a means for the delivery of primary health care with emphasis on the adequacy of distribution and the quality of the care provided. They are prepaid group health practice systems designed to deliver comprehensive health care services to a defined group of voluntarily enrolled individuals. HMOs are based on the holistic concept of care—

Chart 1-1
AHA's Patient's Bill of Rights

1. The patient has the right to considerate and respectful care.
2. The patient has the right to obtain from his physician complete current information concerning his diagnosis, treatment, and prognosis in terms the patient can be reasonably expected to understand. When it is not medically advisable to give such information to the patient, the information should be made available to an appropriate person in his behalf. He has the right to know, by name, the physician responsible for coordinating his care.
3. The patient has the right to receive from his physician information necessary to give informed consent prior to the start of any procedure and/or treatment. Except in emergencies, such information for informed consent should include but not necessarily be limited to the specific procedure and/or treatment, the medically significant risks involved, and the probable duration of incapacitation. Where medically significant alternatives for care or treatment exist, or when the patient requests information concerning medical alternatives, the patient has the right to such information. The patient also has the right to know the name of the person responsible for the procedures and/or treatment.
4. The patient has the right to refuse treatment to the extent permitted by law and to be informed of the medical consequences of his action.
5. The patient has the right to every consideration of his privacy concerning his own medical care program. Case discussion, consultation, examination, and treatment are confidential and should be conducted discreetly. Those not directly involved in his care must have the permission of the patient to be present.
6. The patient has the right to expect that all communications and records pertaining to his care should be treated as confidential.
7. The patient has the right to expect that within its capacity a hospital must make reasonable response to the request of a patient for services. The hospital must provide evaluation, service, and/or referral as indicated by the urgency of the case. When medically permissible, a patient may be transferred to another facility only after he has received complete information and explanation concerning the needs for and alternatives to such a transfer. The institution to which the patient is to be transferred must first have accepted the patient for transfer.
8. The patient has the right to obtain information as to any relationship of his hospital to other health care and educational institutions insofar as his care is concerned. The patient has the right to obtain information as to the existence of any professional relationships among individuals, by name, who are treating him.
9. The patient has the right to be advised if the hospital proposes to engage in or perform human experimentation affecting his care or treatment. The patient has the right to refuse to participate in such research projects.
10. The patient has the right to expect reasonable continuity of care. He has the right to know in advance what appointment times and physicians are available and where. The patient has the right to expect that the hospital will provide a mechanism whereby he is informed by his physician or a delegate of the physician of the patient's continuing health care requirements following discharge.
11. The patient has the right to examine and receive an explanation of his bill regardless of source of payment.
12. The patient has the right to know what hospital rules and regulations apply to his conduct as a patient.

(Reprinted with the permission of the American Hospital Association)

providing ambulatory and inpatient facilities that meet the health care needs of the whole person. The goal of HMOs is to give comprehensive health care that is of the best quality and quantity for the money available while eliminating fragmentation and duplication of services. As HMOs have grown they have expanded to include specialist services and programs for Medicare and Medicaid populations.

Studies have shown that HMOs are cost-effective and that the quality of care provided by these health care delivery systems is equal to and possibly superior to the care provided elsewhere in the same communities.

HMOs paved the way and served as the model for the preferred provider organization (PPO), which began in 1980. In contrast to the HMO, the PPO is not a distinct entity. Rather, it is a business arrangement between a group of providers, usually hospitals and physicians, who contract to provide health care to subscribers, usually businesses, for a negotiated fee that usually is discounted. PPOs allow businesses to decrease their expenses for employee health care benefits, and they allow hospitals and physicians to market their services to employers.

The Future

What the future will bring for the health care delivery system is uncertain. However, it is certain that competition for patients and resources will lead to major changes. Market forces are demanding efficiency, cost containment, and innovative systems and patterns of care. Price and service competition for revenue and access to capital will undoubtedly lead to dramatic consolidation of delivery systems.

Chart 1-2
NLN's Statement on Patient's Rights

According to the NLN statement, nurses have a responsibility to uphold the following rights of patients:

- To health care that is accessible and that meets professional standards, regardless of the setting.
- To courteous and individualized health care that is equitable, humane and given without discrimination as to race, color, creed, sex, national origin, source of payment, or ethical or political beliefs.
- To information about their diagnosis, prognosis, and treatment—including alternatives to care and risks involved—in terms they and their families can readily understand, so that they can give their informed consent.
- To informed participation in all decisions concerning their health care.
- To information about the qualifications, names, and titles of personnel responsible for providing their health care.
- To refuse observation by those not directly involved in their care.
- To privacy during interview, examination, and treatment.
- To privacy in communicating and visiting with persons of their choice.

- To refuse treatment, medications, or participation in research and experimentation, without punitive action being taken against them.
- To coordination and continuity of health care.
- To appropriate instruction or education from health care personnel so that they can achieve an optimal level of wellness and an understanding of their basic health needs.
- To confidentiality of all records (except as otherwise provided for by law or third party payer contracts) and all communications, written or oral, between patients and health care providers.
- To access to all health records pertaining to them, and the right to challenge and correct their records for accuracy, and the right to transfer all such records in the case of continuing care.
- To information on the charges for services, including the right to challenge these.
- To be fully informed as to all their rights in all health care settings.

(National League for Nursing. Nursing's Role in Patients' Rights. New York, The League, 1977. Used with permission.)

The Nurse as a Health Care Provider

Professional nursing is adapting to meet changing health needs and expectations. One such adaptation can be noted in the expanded role of the nurse. These expanded roles in nursing have been a response to the need to improve the distribution of health care services and to decrease the cost of medical care. The nurse who functions in an expanded role provides direct care to patients through independent practice, team or interdependent practice, or practice within a health care agency or with a physician. Specialization has evolved within the expanded roles of nursing, a result of the recent explosion of technology.

Nurses now receive advanced education in such specialties as intensive care, coronary care, respiratory care, neonatal intensive care, renal dialysis care, trauma care, and transplant care, to name just a few. With the expanded role of the nurse, various titles have emerged that attempt to specify the functions as well as the educational preparation of nurses. A few of these titles are clinical nurse specialist, nurse practitioner, and independent nurse practitioner.

Clinical nurse specialists are nurses prepared at the master's degree level who are proficient in a selected clinical area of nursing and who use this expertise to provide direct nursing care to patients and consultation services, guidance, and teaching to other nurses.

Nurse practitioners are nurses who have advanced skills in history taking and physical examination, which are used to assess the physical and psychosocial health and illness needs of individuals, families, or groups. The educational preparation for nurse practitioners has shifted from certificate programs to master's degree programs. These nurses have expertise in nursing practice and use a broad range of competencies to plan and implement direct and indirect nursing care with consideration for coordination of care with other health professionals. Most often the nurse practitioner functions in the primary care setting, such as in clinics, schools, and physicians' offices, rather than in the acute care setting.

Independent nurse practitioners have departed from the traditional role of the nurse within the health care delivery system and have developed private practices. The main focus of these nurses is on health maintenance through primary health care that is peripheral to the traditional illness-focused system. These nurses provide services in their offices, in clients' homes, or in nurse-managed clinics or centers, for the purpose of health assessment, counseling, teaching, and making referrals to other health care professionals and agencies. The boundaries of the independent practitioner role are determined by state nurse practice acts.

With the expanded role of the nurse has come a continuing effort by nursing associations to more clearly define the practice of nursing. Nurse practice acts have been amended to give nurses the authority to perform functions that were previously restricted to the practice of medicine. These functions include diagnosis, treatment, performance of invasive procedures, and prescription of medications and treatments. Regulations regarding these functions are stipulated by the board of nursing in each state, which defines the education and experience required and the clinical situations in which a nurse may perform these functions.

In general, initial care, ambulatory health care, and anticipatory guidance are all becoming increasingly important in nursing practice. These expanding roles will enable the nurse to function interdependently with other health care professionals and will help to establish more of a collegial relationship between physician and nurse.

With the advent of DRGs, the role of the nurse in home care service agencies has greatly expanded. Because of early discharge of patients from hospitals, complex care and specialized treatments and procedures are often required. The nurse caring for patients in the home must be skilled in physical assessment of children as well as adult and geriatric patients. In addition, she must have acute care technological skills and the ability to coordinate the services of a variety of health care providers.

Since nursing services are being given outside as well as within the hospital, nurses have a choice of practicing in a multiplicity of health delivery settings: acute medical centers, ambulatory care settings, clinics, urgent care centers, outpatient departments, neighborhood health centers, home health care agencies, independent or group nursing practices, and health maintenance organizations. The expanding scope of nursing practice will require expert skills in interviewing, in observing, in physical assessment and examination, in practicing new clinical techniques, in understanding behavioral patterns, in gathering data, and in solving problems for individuals, families, and groups. In addition, the nurse will be more concerned with decision making and evaluation of the outcomes of care. In order to acquire the necessary clinical expertise, the nurse will be responsible for self-development and continuing education during her professional lifetime.

Roles of the Nurse

The professional nurse in both institutional and community health care settings assumes three roles. These may be defined as the practitioner role, the leadership role, and the research role. However, although each role carries specific responsibilities, various aspects of each role interrelate with one another and are found in all nursing positions. Accomplishment of each of these roles is designed to meet the immediate and future health care and nursing needs of the patients who are the recipients of nursing care.

Practitioner Role

The practitioner role of the nurse involves those actions that the nurse accomplishes when assuming responsibility that is primarily directed toward meeting the health care and nursing needs of individual patients, their families, and significant others. This role is the dominant role of nurses in primary, secondary, and tertiary health care settings. It is a role that can be achieved only through utilization of the nursing process, the fundamental process of all nursing actions.

Because the nursing process serves as the basis of nursing, and because the teaching–learning process is a significant, integral part of the nursing process, Chapters 2 and 3 have been devoted to the study of these two interrelated processes. Careful study of these chapters will enable the nurse to develop expertise in the practitioner role of nursing.

Clinical Ladders. Clinical ladders provide practitioners of nursing an opportunity to advance in clinical practice while at the same time maintaining contact with patients. Clinical expertise is evaluated, recognized, and rewarded. By demonstrating increasing clinical competence, knowledge, and expertise, nurses have the opportunity to advance clinically while continuing to provide direct patient care.

Certification for Practice. Recognition and prestige in nursing practice can also be attained through certification. Certification is voluntary except when required for expanded roles such as nurse anesthetist and nurse midwife. For the most part it is administered by professional nursing organizations and requires varying amounts of experience and education. Certification provides a mechanism for validating nurses' expertise and demonstrating accountability to the public. In 1984 the American Nurses' Association offered certification in 17 generalist and specialist nursing areas.

Leadership Role

The leadership role of the nurse has traditionally been perceived as a specialized role assumed only by those nurses who have titles that suggest leadership and who are the leaders of large groups of nurses, related health care professionals, or patients. However, the definition of nursing leadership developed by Yura, Ozimek, and Walsh (1981) gives a broader scope to the concept and identifies leadership as a role that is inherent within all nursing positions. The leadership role of the nurse involves those actions that the nurse accomplishes when assuming responsibility for affecting the actions of others that are directed toward goal determination and achievement. Nursing leadership is a process that involves four behavioral components: deciding, relating, influencing, and facilitating. Each of these components is directed toward change and the ultimate outcome of goal achievement. Basic to the entire process is communication, the effectiveness of which determines the accomplishment of the process. Thus, the leadership process in nursing can be said to be an interpersonal process in which the nurse as a leader uses interpersonal relations to effect change in the behavior of those to whom she relates.

The leadership role that a nurse assumes may or may not involve a large number of people. The nurse uses the leadership process in a variety of circumstances: when assisting a single patient or his family to make changes in their health-related behaviors, when assisting groups or communities to alter their health practices, and when assisting groups of nurses or other health care professionals to affect the actions of patients, groups of patients, or communities with regard to the achievement of desirable health behaviors. The nurse may even be in a position to use the leadership process for assisting specific sectors of the public or the public in general to alter health-related behaviors through such means as legislation, campaigns, and health-oriented public service programs. Thus, the potential scope of the leadership role of the nurse is vast.

Each nurse assumes a leadership role whether she is focusing her practice on one single patient, groups of nurses or other health care professionals, communities, or the public in general. The role is a significant one that goes hand in hand with and complements the practitioner role of the nurse.

Patient Advocate.   Within an acute care hospital facility, where the nurse is involved in actuating her practitioner role for a single patient or a small group of patients, the role of the nurse as a leader may be rather subtle. She may serve primarily as the patient's advocate, anticipating and meeting the needs that he is unable to meet for himself. She must not only be acutely aware of the patient's needs but be able to communicate his needs to other health care professionals involved in his care and to coordinate the efforts of all of these persons in an effort to promote goal achievement.

Outside the hospital setting the persons served by nurses are more independent and more capable of making decisions about their health and the health behaviors they will strive to achieve. For this reason, the leadership role of the nurse in such a setting may be less subtle than in the hospital setting. The leadership skills are the same as those used within the hospital setting, but they must be adapted to the environmental variables that affect the patient population, specifically those variables that affect their health needs and how they can be met. Environmental variables such as cultural values, attitudes, resources, and the influence of community leaders are just a few of the factors that must be considered by the nurse when attempting to effect changes in the health behaviors of persons within a community.

Research Role

The research role of the nurse has traditionally been assumed only by academicians, nurse scientists, graduate nursing students, and researchers from other disciplines. It has only been recently that nurses in general have recognized the acute need for nursing research. Likewise, nurses have just begun to appreciate the significant contributions that can be made to nursing research by nurses in clinical practice.

The primary task of nursing research is to contribute to the scientific base of nursing practice. Further studies are needed to determine the actual effects of nursing intervention and nursing care. Without such research efforts the science of nursing will not grow and a scientifically based rationale for making changes in nursing practice will not be generated.

It is the responsibility of all nurses to become involved in nursing research—to accept their research role. Nurses who have preparation in research methodology can use their research knowledge and skills to initiate and implement timely studies of nursing. This is not to say that nurses who do not initiate and implement studies of nursing do not play a significant role in nursing research. Every nurse has valuable contributions to make to nursing research and a responsibility to make these contributions. All nurses must constantly be on the alert for nursing problems and important questions about the practice of nursing, which can serve as the basis

for the articulation of researchable problem areas. Those nurses directly involved in giving patient care are often in the best position to identify such problems and questions. Their clinical insights are invaluable. Nurses also have a responsibility to become actively involved in ongoing research studies. This participation may involve facilitating the data collection process, or it may involve the actual collection of data. Interpreting the study to other health care professionals or to patients and their families is often of invaluable assistance to the nurse who is conducting the study.

Above all, nurses must use research findings in their nursing practice. Research for the sake of research is meaningless. Only with the use of research findings in clinical nursing practice will the science of nursing be furthered. Research findings can only be substantiated through utilization and validation. Nurses must be continually aware of studies that are directly related to their own area of clinical practice. The findings of these studies must then be employed in an attempt to improve patient care and to validate the findings themselves. The attitude of every health care agency and every nursing unit within such an agency should be one of interest in the progress of nursing research and of enthusiasm in the implementation of research findings. It must also be remembered that communication of research findings is imperative. When findings of studies are not made available to other nurses, the impact of the findings on nursing practice is diminished.

Thus, research is an inherent part of nursing. The future of nursing science depends on the active involvement of nurses in the implementation and utilization of nursing research. Nurses must cultivate their curiosity about nursing practice and their belief in the worth of the practice of nursing by accepting their research role and responsibility. Only with questioning minds can nurses generate nursing research. The scientific basis of nursing depends on the research efforts of all nurses, practitioners and researchers alike.

The National Center for Nursing Research, legislated in 1985 and established at the National Institutes of Health, represents a triumph for the profession. Its purpose is to promote research pertinent to nursing with a focus on the health needs and well-being of the total person. It is the responsibility of practitioners of nursing to become cognizant of the research generated by the center and incorporate the findings into clinical practice.

The Patient/Client: Consumer and Recipient of Health Care

The term *patient,* which is derived from the Latin verb meaning "to suffer," has traditionally been used to describe those persons who are recipients of nursing care. The connotation commonly attached to the word is one of dependence. For this reason many nurses prefer to use the term *client,* which is derived from the Latin verb meaning "to lean" and which connotes alliance and interdependence. For the purposes of this book the term *patient* will be used throughout, but with appreciation for each nurse's prerogative to choose the term that seems more suitable.

The Patient's Problems

The central figure in health care services is, of course, the patient. The patient who reports to the hospital or health facility with a health problem or problems (increasing numbers of patients have multiple disease disorders) also comes as an individual, a member of a family, and a citizen of the community. Often, he is laden with personal concerns that have been amplified and compounded by the alteration in his health status. Confronting him, perhaps, are problems that he believes are inescapable and insurmountable, problems that demand a solution but are incapable of solution, problems for which he feels solely responsible and that he is reluctant to share. He may be wholly absorbed in problems that are of minor consequence while dismissing others that truly are of paramount importance. One of the nurse's important functions is to help him to sort out his problems, reduce them to their essentials, place them in proper perspective, and cope with them effectively.

Troublesome Symptoms as Problems

From the standpoint of the symptomatic patient, the most important problem confronting him is his major symptom. If he is gasping for breath, his most pressing need is to be relieved of his respiratory distress. Dyspnea is his primary symptom. To evaluate this symptom and to alleviate it effectively, the nurse must correctly understand the pathologic physiology underlying the patient's dyspnea. Is it caused by pulmonary congestion, pneumonia, pleurisy, or asthma? Does the patient have respiratory obstruction? Should he be placed in an orthopneic position or in low Fowler's position, or should he lie flat? Should he be receiving oxygen? Is he in need of tracheal suction? Is endotracheal intubation likely to be required? Should a sedative be administered, or is such medication strictly contraindicated in this patient? Close scrutiny of the patient might convince the nurse that his breathing, although abnormally rapid and deep, is not attended by discomfort and does not involve undue effort. In other words, this particular patient may not be dyspneic but may be hyperpneic. Hyperpnea is a different symptom altogether, and the problems it entails are quite different from those of dyspnea. Is this a case of hysterical hyperventilation or diabetic acidosis? Or has this patient been poisoned? On the appropriate answers to these and a host of other pertinent questions may hinge the correctness of diagnosis, the effectiveness of nursing intervention, and, in many instances, the very survival of the patient.

Every step in the care of the patient represents a team effort, and a key member of the health team charged with this responsibility is the professional nurse. Among the most important of her contributions to this joint effort are her clinical observations. To what extent these observations are significant, informative, and helpful depends on how well the nurse knows and understands symptoms. Confronted with a symptom, the nurse must be able to recognize it as a deviation from the normal. She should also be aware of the patterns of illness in the community and the characteristics of the population being served. The leading causes of death in the United States and hence the most common clinical problems that will be encountered in nursing practice are indicated in Table 1-1.

TABLE 1-1
Death Rates for 15 Leading Causes of Death: United States, 1984

Rank*	Cause of Death†	Death Rate	Percent of Total Deaths
	All causes	866.7	100.0
1	Diseases of heart	324.4	37.4
2	Malignant neoplasms, including neoplasms of lymphatic and hematopoietic tissues	191.6	22.1
3	Cerebrovascular diseases	65.6	7.6
4	Accidents and adverse effects	40.1	4.6
	Motor vehicle accidents	19.6	2.3
	All other accidents and adverse effects	20.4	2.4
5	Chronic obstructive pulmonary diseases and allied conditions	29.8	3.4
6	Pneumonia and influenza	25.0	2.9
7	Diabetes mellitus	15.6	1.8
8	Suicide	12.3	1.4
9	Chronic liver disease and cirrhosis	11.3	1.3
10	Atherosclerosis	10.4	1.2
11	Nephritis, nephrotic syndrome, and nephrosis	8.5	1.0
12	Homicide and legal intervention	8.3	1.0
13	Certain conditions originating in the perinatal period	8.0	0.9
14	Septicemia	6.4	0.7
15	Congenital anomalies	5.6	0.6
	All other causes	103.9	12.0

* Based on a 10% sample of deaths. Rates per 100,000 population.
† Ninth Revision International Classification of Diseases, 1975
(Annual summary of births, marriages, divorces and deaths: United States, 1984. Monthly Vital Statistics Report. National Center for Health Statistics, 1985)

The Patient's Basic Needs

Certain basic needs are common to *all* humans and demand satisfaction accordingly. Such needs are dealt with on the basis of priority, meaning that certain needs are more pressing than others. However, once an essential need is met, a person moves to a need on a higher level. Approaching needs according to priority reflects Maslow's hierarchy of needs, in which human needs may be ranked as follows: physiologic needs; safety and security; belongingness and affection; esteem and self-respect; and self-actualization, which includes self-fulfillment, desire to know and understand, and aesthetic needs.* Lower-level needs always remain, but because there is a reduction in need tension, the person is able to move to higher-level needs. A person's pursuit of higher-level needs indicates that he is moving toward psychological health and well-being. Such a hierarchy of needs is a useful organizational framework for assessment of patients' strengths, limitations, and need for nursing interventions (Fig. 1-1).

Physiologic Needs

Physiologic needs predominate in the motivation of human behavior and drive the mechanisms that maintain *homeostasis*—the constancy of the internal environment of an organism (see Chap. 7). They involve the regulation of respiratory, nutritive, and excretory functions, as well as maintenance of the water content of tissues, adjustments of body temperature, and the operation of numerous protective mechanisms. Also included as physiologic needs are the need for rest and sleep, and the avoidance of pain. Sex is considered a basic motive but is not essential for survival.

These physiologic needs are powerful; unless satisfied, they dominate the conscious mind. For example, if a patient is obliged to restrict his fluid intake for therapeutic reasons, thirst may absorb his thoughts. He may discuss nothing but drinking, complain incessantly of thirst, and repeatedly question his nurse and physician about when fluids will be forthcoming. During this period he is not likely to be too concerned about the aesthetic features of his environment. As soon as his thirst is quenched, he becomes aware of other needs; for example, now he may be disturbed by the absence of privacy.

Safety Needs and Security Needs

If the physiologic needs are satisfied, the concern for safety and security emerges—psychological as well as physical safety. The normal adult is able to protect himself and usually does not feel endangered. He is relatively "safe" from death. His job is "safe." His insurance program and his savings furnish a sense of economic security.

Illness naturally poses a threat. The sick person may be apprehensive in response to the many different persons with unfamiliar functions who enter his room. Diagnostic tests and therapeutic procedures may contribute to his fears. He wants to feel safe and secure. Although he may not express his feelings in these terms, he wants the health team to be aware of his insecurity. To help protect the patient from danger the nurse must know the nature of his illness and be cognizant

* Maslow AH. Motivation and Personality. New York, Harper & Row, 1970.

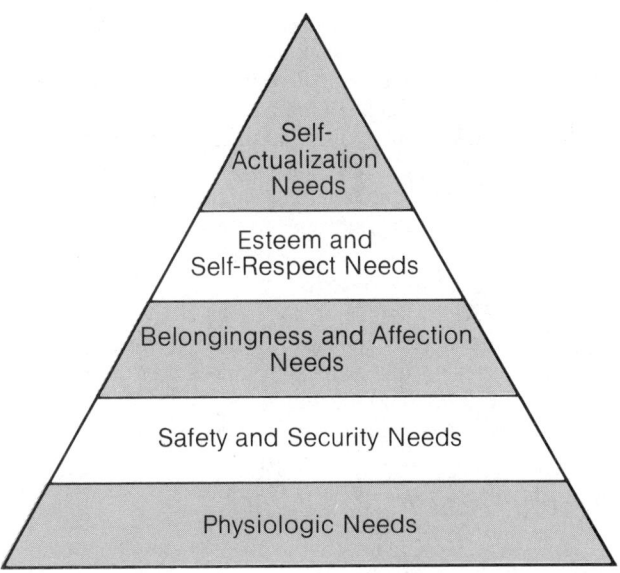

Figure 1-1
This scheme of Maslow's hierarchy of human needs shows how a person moves from basic need fulfillment to higher levels of needs, with the ultimate goal of integrated human functioning and health.

of any possible complications. If complications should occur, she should be able to provide intelligent care. The nurse's role in promoting the psychological safety of the patient is discussed in Chapter 12.

Need for Belongingness and Affection

Once the patient's physiologic and safety needs have been satisfied, his need for belongingness and affection will become apparent. Every person, sick or well, desires the companionship and recognition of others. A sick person wants and needs his family or, in their absence, friends. Thus, any signs of friendliness are usually appreciated. The wise nurse is constantly aware of this need and of its importance in relation to the patient's morale. One way to achieve this end is to help the family members feel that they have a definite contribution to make to the patient's recovery. Assessment and interpretation of the patient's behavior are essential for identification of indicators of his unmet need for belongingness and affection. He may be quiet, uncomplaining, and eager to please. Or, he may demand attention by constantly making requests, asking questions, and being generally disruptive. By accurately interpreting such behaviors, the nurse can intervene in ways that will promote the patient's feeling of acceptance and belonging. Mutual goal setting is important in assuring the patient and his family that they are important members of the health care team.

Need for Esteem and Self-Respect

Man is by nature a social being, abhorring isolation. Illness removes him from his relatively convivial world and transplants him into a strange environment, an environment that is entirely unsought and unfamiliar, one in which he feels incompetent and alone. Previously an actively contributing member of society, he now must accept a position of dependency. This patient needs to preserve his self-esteem. He needs to be recognized as an individual, a distinct personality. The professional nurse, imbued with the concept of the individual worth and dignity of man, sees to it that this need is fulfilled. She takes time to listen to the patient. To the extent that he desires it and opportunity permits, she joins him in conversation. She exhibits interest in all matters that seem important to him; her attentiveness, thoughtfulness, and kindliness convey that he is held in esteem and that his needs and problems are recognized.

Unmet esteem and self-respect needs are exhibited by feelings of dependency and lack of confidence, competence, and ability. Patient education that focuses on the patient's acquisition of skills and knowledge is helpful in increasing the patient's self-esteem and self-respect.

Need for Self-Actualization

Maslow estimated that only about 1% of the adult population ever reach the level of self-actualization. Self-actualization may not be possible for persons in poverty-stricken or emotionally deprived environments. Additionally, many people are satisfied with meeting lower-level needs and do not strive for self-actualization.

Need for Self-Fulfillment. Once the patient's physiologic needs have been compensated and he is feeling secure, esteemed, and wanted, his creative impulses may now emerge. During the course of a short hospital stay this need is not likely to be frustrated. However, the patient with a long-term illness must be assured an opportunity to express himself creatively and to feel useful.

Need to Know and Understand. The need to know and understand is a strong drive. The intelligent person seeks information, organizes it, analyzes it, and searches for its meaning. In general, patients want to know what is in store for them, and they are thwarted by explanations that are too brief or vague. Many patients know a surprising amount about the bodily functions. However, while some of their information may be factual, some of it is likely to be erroneous, and correction or clarification is usually necessary. Instruction is the responsibility of the nurse, and the teaching of patients is one of the most important functions of her profession. To teach correctly and effectively the nurse must have a thorough knowledge of the subject, be skilled in communication, and be cognizant of the basic mechanisms of learning. The explanations, while simple for the sake of comprehension, at the same time must be meaningful if they are to be accepted. The patient's physical and emotional status, his intelligence, his experience as a patient, and his awareness of the situation, as well as the urgency of his need to know and understand must be given consideration. The nurse must also consider the possible implications of her intended remarks and guard with equal care against inaccuracies on her part and misunderstandings on the part of the patient.

Aesthetic Needs. Aesthetic needs vary in importance from person to person, but for all patients the most salutary environment is one that is orderly and one in which there is beauty. The patient with highly developed aesthetic sensibilities will be distressed by unpleasant sights, sounds, odors, and disarray. He may crave flowers, books, or music—amenities that, when supplied, add immeasurably to his well-being.

Comments

In concluding this discussion, it may be pointed out that most of the needs of the average individual, ill or well, can be satisfied only in part. Moreover, the nurse, whose responsibility and privilege it is to help the patient meet his needs and resolve his problems, must recognize the fact that some problems can be neither eliminated nor solved. In relation to the patient with such a problem, the nurse's role is to help him to make a mature, objective, and compensatory adjustment to its continued existence or to its imperfect solution, if this solution is the best that can be achieved.

Approach to the Patient

In the process of searching for ways of fulfilling patient needs, nursing has devised various methods of approaching the patient. During the 1950s and 1960s the concept of team nursing came to the fore. In recent years, however, questions have been raised concerning the effectiveness of team nursing, and a different approach in the form of primary nursing has been advocated and implemented in many hospital settings. Some studies have shown that primary nursing, when compared with team nursing, significantly increases the quality of patient care and is more cost-effective. However, more research is needed to substantiate these findings.

Primary Nursing

Primary nursing, not to be confused with primary health care, which deals with first-contact general health care, refers to comprehensive, individualized care that is provided with continuity. Individualized total care is provided to the patient by the same nurse from the time of the patient's admission until his discharge. This type of nursing care eliminates the fragmented care that has typified team nursing and serves to accomplish a goal for which nurses have recognized a need for years: it allows the nurse to once again give direct patient care rather than manage and supervise the functions of others who care for the patient. In essence, it allows the nurse the opportunity to implement her practitioner role and her leadership role within the framework of rendering direct patient care.

The focus of primary nursing is the patient. The primary nurse accepts total 24-hour responsibility for quality nursing care for the patient. This nursing care is directed toward meeting his total, individualized nursing needs—his biopsychosocial needs. The primary nurse is responsible and accountable for involving the patient and his family directly in all facets of his care. The primary nurse has autonomy that allows her to make decisions with the patient and his family concerning his care. Thus she is a facilitator of family-centered as well as patient-centered nursing care. All communications with other members of the health team regarding the patient and his health care are made by the primary nurse. This allows the nurse to provide for continuity of care and to promote collaborative efforts directed toward the assurance of quality care. It provides the other health care professionals with the opportunity to communicate directly with the nurse who is responsible for the patient's care.

Ideally, the number of patients for whom the nurse acts as the primary nurse is limited to three or four. However, this number may range from one to ten depending on the extent of the nursing needs of the patients. The nurse meets the patient as soon as possible after his admission to the health care facility. This allows her to begin to establish a relationship with the patient, which will continue until discharge and, in some cases, after discharge. It allows the patient to identify with the nurse who will be responsible for his care on a continuous basis. Each day that the primary nurse works she cares for the patient. She is aware of problems and needs as they arise, and she assumes responsibility for securing the means to solve the problems and meet the needs. Prior to the patient's discharge to another health care facility or to his home, the primary nurse assumes the responsibility for making the appropriate referrals and for ensuring that all relevant information is provided to those persons who will be involved in his care. Throughout the entire admission the nurse continually strives to involve the patient's family in his care and in the preparations that are made for his discharge.

During the times when the primary nurse is not scheduled to work, she is assisted by an associate nurse, or co-nurse. This associate nurse implements the nursing care plan and provides feedback to the primary nurse that is invaluable in evaluation of the care plan. However, it remains the responsibility of the primary nurse to make sure that the patient's needs are met and that continuity of care is not lost when she is not present to render the care herself.

Within the concept of primary nursing, the head nurse (or patient care supervisor) functions as a consultant for the primary nurses, and she strives toward providing opportunities for these nurses to continually improve their clinical expertise. The head nurse initiates the nurse–patient relationship by assigning the primary nurse to her designated patients. This is done with knowledge of the primary nurse's capabilities and her particular areas of nursing expertise. The head nurse then serves as a resource person for the primary nurse when she is confronted with patient problems or needs that she is unable to resolve. Periodic evaluation of the primary nurse's performance is the responsibility of the head nurse. Frequent interaction with the primary nurse and her patients gives the head nurse much information that can be used positively in assisting the primary nurse to use her capabilities to their utmost and to make strides toward overcoming her limitations. The head nurse may also function as a primary nurse for a small group of patients. By assuming such responsibility, she is allowed to use her clinical expertise in giving direct patient care and to serve as a role model for the primary nurses.

Nursing students, practical nurses, and nursing assistants function within the primary nursing framework. The responsibility for maintaining continuity of total individualized nursing care remains with the primary nurse. However, when direct patient care is not given by the primary nurse, other members of the health care team assume this responsibility. They implement the plan of care developed by the primary nurse and consult with the primary nurse when changes in the plan of care seem warranted. In such instances the primary nurse serves as a valuable consultant and teacher for associate nurses and other personnel. Nursing care conferences provide a means for the exchange of information. In these conferences the quality of care rendered to the patient is the focus, and continuity of individualized total patient care is the goal.

Primary nursing has been designed to increase the accountability and responsibility of the nurse to the patient. Studies conducted at selected hospitals that have implemented primary nursing reveal that primary nurses recognize greater enrichment from their jobs because of the high degree of autonomy, identity, significance, and variety afforded them by the primary nursing system of delivering care.

The long-term survival of primary nursing as it is currently implemented is in doubt. As cost containment measures accelerate, staffing ratios of patients to nurses are increasing. Many nursing service departments and agencies are meeting the increased workload demands by making modifications in their approach to primary nursing or by reverting to team or functional systems for delivering care. Regardless of the system used, it is the responsibility of individual nurses and groups of nurses to ensure that quality of care is not jeopardized.

Summary

Throughout this chapter, the evolution of the profession of nursing has been explored. Many references have been made to the significance of nurses as members of the health care team. Over the years nurses have strived to change their role from one of subservience to other members of the health care team, particularly the physician, to one that is collegial. As nursing practitioners and researchers make advances in the area of concept formalization and theory building, the unique competencies of the profession of nursing become more clearly articulated. It becomes increasingly more evident that nursing provides certain health care services that are unique to this profession. However, nursing continues to recognize the importance of collaboration with other health care disciplines in meeting all of the health care needs of patients.

Bibliography

Books

American Nurses' Association. Issues In Professional Nursing Practice. Kansas City, Missouri, ANA, 1984.

Birmingham JJ. Home Care Planning Based on DRGs: Functional Health Pattern Model. Philadelphia, JB Lippincott, 1986.

Chinn P and Jacobs MK. Theory and Nursing: A Systematic Approach. St Louis, CV Mosby, 1983.

Curtin LL and Zurlage MA. DRGs: The Reorganization of Health. Chicago, S-N Publications, 1984.

Duldt BW and Giffin K. Theoretical Perspectives for Nursing. Boston, Little, Brown & Co, 1985.

Dunn HL. High-Level Wellness. Arlington, Virginia, RW Beatty, 1961.

Ellis JR and Hartley CL. Nursing in Today's World: Challenges, Issues, and Trends. Philadelphia, JB Lippincott, 1984.

Fitzpatrick JJ and Whall AL. Conceptual Models of Nursing: Analysis and Application. Bowie, Maryland, Robert J. Brady, 1983.

George JB. Nursing Theories. The Base For Professional Nursing Practice. Englewood Cliffs, New Jersey, Prentice-Hall, 1985.

Grippando GM. Nursing Perspectives & Issues. Albany, New York, Delmar Publishers, 1986.

Henderson V. The Nature of Nursing. New York, Macmillan, 1966.

Johnson DE. The behavioral system model in nursing. In Riehl JP and Roy C (eds). Conceptual Models for Nursing Practice. New York, Appleton-Century-Crofts, 1980.

King IM. A Theory for Nursing: Systems, Concepts, Process. New York, John Wiley & Sons, 1981.

Leddy S and Pepper JM. Conceptual Bases of Professional Nursing. Philadelphia, JB Lippincott, 1985.

Maslow AH. Motivation and Personality. New York, Harper & Brothers, 1970.

McClelland E, Kelly K, Buckwalter KC. Continuity of Care: Advancing the Concept of Discharge Planning. Orlando, Grune & Stratton, 1985.

Meleis AI. Theoretical Nursing: Development and Progress. Philadelphia, JB Lippincott, 1985.

Moloney MM. Professionalization of Nursing: Current Issues and Trends. Philadelphia, JB Lippincott, 1986.

Neuman B. The Neuman Systems Model: Application to Nursing Education and Practice. Norwalk, Connecticut, Appleton-Century-Crofts, 1982.

Nightingale F. Notes on Nursing: What It Is, and What It Is Not. New York, D Appleton, 1860.

Norris CM. Concept Clarification in Nursing. Rockville, Maryland, Aspen Systems Corporation, 1982.

Nursing. A Social Policy Statement. Kansas City, Missouri, American Nurses' Association, 1980.

Orem DE. Nursing: Concepts of Practice. New York, McGraw-Hill, 1985.

Riehl JP and Roy C. Conceptual Models for Nursing Practice. New York, Appleton-Century-Crofts, 1980.

Stevens BJ. Nursing Theory: Analysis, Application, Evaluation. Boston, Little, Brown, & Co, 1984.

Styles MM. On Nursing: Toward a New Endowment. St Louis, CV Mosby, 1982.

Torres G. Theoretical Foundations of Nursing. Norwalk, Connecticut, Appleton-Century-Crofts, 1986.

Yura H, Ozimek D, and Walsh MB. Nursing Leadership: Theory and Process. New York, Appleton-Century-Crofts, 1981.

Articles

(Asterisks indicate nursing research articles.)

Theories and Concepts of Nursing

Adam E. Frontiers of nursing in the 21st century: Development of models and theories on the concept of nursing. J Adv Nurs 1983 Jan; 8(1): 41–45.

Avant KC and Walker LO. The practicing nurse and conceptual frameworks. Matern Child Nurs J 1984 Mar/Apr; 9(2):87–88, 90.

Brooks JA. Evaluation of a definition of nursing. Adv Nurs Sci 1983 July; 5(4):51–85.

Condon EH. Caring: its importance and recognition. Virginia Nurse 1984 Spring; 52(1):21–23.

Cronenwett LR. Helping and nursing models. Nurs Res 1983 Nov/Dec; 32(6):342–343.

Cunningham SG. The Neuman systems model applied to a rehabilitation setting. Rehabil Nurs 1983 July/Aug; 8(4):20–22.

*Davis-Sharts J. An empirical test of Maslow's theory of need hierarchy using hologeistic comparison by statistical sampling. Adv Nurs Sci 1986 Oct; 9(1):58–72.

*Floyd JA. Research using Rogers' conceptual system: Development of a testable theorem. Adv Nurs Sci 1983 Jan; 5(2):37–48.

Hall BA. Toward an understanding of stability in nursing phenomena. Adv Nurs Sci 1983 Apr; 5(3):15–20.

*Harper DC. Application of Orem's theoretical constructs to self-care medication behaviors in the elderly. Adv Nurs Sci 1984 Apr; 6(3): 29–45.

Herrington JV and Houston S. Using Orem's theory: A plan for all seasons. Nurs Health Care 1984 Jan; 5(1):45–47.

Johnson M. Some aspects of the relation between theory and research in nursing. J Adv Nurs 1983 Jan; 8(1):21–28.

Melnyk KAM. The process of theory analysis: An examination of the nursing theory of Dorothea E. Orem. Nurs Res 1983 May/June; 32(3):170–174.

Moscovitz AO. Orem's theory as applied to psychiatric nursing. Perspect Psychiatr Care 1984 Jan/Mar; 22(1):36–38.

*Nicoll LH, Meyer PA, and Abraham IL. Critique: External comparison of conceptual nursing models. Adv Nurs Sci 1985 Jul; 7(4):1–9.

Perry PD and Sutcliffe SA. Conceptual frameworks for clinical practice. J Neurosurg Nurs 1982 Dec; 14(6):318–321.

Runtz SE and Urtel JG. Evaluating your practice via a nursing model. Nurse Pract 1983 Mar; 8(3):30–40.

Schmieding NJ. Putting Orlando's theory into practice. Am J Nurs 1984 June; 84(6):759–761.

*Silva MC. Research testing nursing theory: State of the art. Adv Nurs Sci 1986 Oct; 9(1):1–11.

*Suppe F and Jacox AK. Philosophy of science and the development of nursing theory. Ann Rev Nurs Res 1985; 3:241–267.

Roles of Nurses

Ahrens W and Norris B. Expanded roles in critical care: Nurse practitioner or clinical specialist? Dimens Crit Care Nurs 1983 Mar/Apr; 2(2): 98–101.

Ambiguities limit the role of nurse practitioners and physician assistants. Am J Public Health 1984 Jan; 74(1):6–7.

Blickfeldt MP. What is wrong with nursing's image. Focus Crit Care 1984 Apr; 11(2):55–57.

Calkin JD. A model for advanced nursing practice. J Nurs Adm 1984 Jan; 14(1):24–30.

Clayton GM. The clinical nurse specialist as leader. Top Clin Nurs 1984 Apr; 6(1):17–27.

Diers D and Molde S. Nurses in primary care: The new gatekeepers? Am J Nurs 1983 May; 83(5):742–745.

Edlund BJ and Hodges LC. Preparing and using the clinical nurse specialist. Nurs Clin North Am 1983 Sept; 18(3):499–507.

Garvey JL and Rottet S. Expanding the hospital nursing role: An administrative account. J Nurs Adm 1982 Dec; 12(12):30–35.

Gikow F et al. The continuing care nurse. Nurs Outlook 1985 July/Aug; 33(4):195–197.

Lang NM. Nurse-managed centers: Will they survive? Am J Nurs 1983 Sept; 83(9):1290–1293.

Morath J. Putting leaders, consultants and teachers on the line. Nurs Manage 1983 Jan; 14(1):50–52.

Munroe D et al. Prescribing patterns of the nurse practitioners. Am J Nurs 1982 Oct; 82(10):1538–1542.

Nurses eligible for direct payment in 13 states. Am Nurse 1983 June; 15(1):1.

Ropka ME and Fay FC. Clinical nurse specialist—alive and well? Am J Nurs 1984 May; 84(5):661–664.

Selby TL. Nurse-managed centers show their potential. Am Nurse 1984 May; 16(5):10, 19.

Shaw EA. The emerging role of the critical care nurse. Focus Crit Care 1984 Feb; 11(1):13–17.

Sultz HA et al. A decade of change for nurse practitioners. Nurs Outlook 1983 May/June; 31(3):137–140, 141, 188.

Sultz HA et al. Nurse practitioners: A decade of change: II. Nurs Outlook 1983 July/Aug; 31(4):216–219.

Sultz HA et al. Nurse practitioners: A decade of change: III. Nurs Outlook 1983 Sept/Oct; 31(5):266–269.

Wiemerslage D. The expanded role of the nurse. Crit Care Update 1983 Sept; 10(9):50–51.

Practitioner

Gassert C, Holt C, and Pope K. Building a ladder. Am J Nurs 1982 Oct; 82(10):1527–1530.

Guidelines for developing clinical ladders. AORN J 1983 May; 37(6): 1209–1222.

Huey FL. Looking at ladders. Am J Nurs 1982 Oct; 82(10):1520–1526.

Leadership

Larsen J. Leadership, nurses and the 1980s. J Adv Nurs 1983 Sept; 8(5): 429–435.

Lawrence SA and Lawrence RM. Leadership—what it is and how to teach it. J Nurs Ed 1984 Apr; 23(4):173–174.

Smith HL and Mitry NW. Nursing leadership: A buffering perspective. Nurs Admin Q 1984 Spring; 8(3):43–52.

Research

Batra C. Motivating nurses to do nursing research. Nurs Health Care 1983 Jan; 4(1):18–22.

Brown JS, Tanner CA, and Padrick KP. Nursing's search for scientific knowledge. Nurs Res 1984 Jan/Feb; 33(1):26–32.

Fawcett J. Another look at utilization of nursing research. Image 1984 Spring; 16(2):59–62.

Fawcett J. Hallmarks of success in nursing research. Adv Nurs Sci 1984 Oct; 7(1):1–11.

Fleming JW. Selecting a clinical nursing problem for research. Image 1984 Spring; 16(2):62–64.

Haughey BP. Considerations in applying research findings to practice. Dimens Crit Care Nurs 1984 Sept/Oct; 3(5):288–292.

Hindshaw AS. The image of nursing research: Issues and strategies. Commun Nurs Res 1983 Summer; 16:1–13.

Loanzon P. Clinical research and nursing in the intensive care unit. Heart Lung 1983 Sept; 12(5):480–484

Stetler CB. Nurses and research: Responsibility and involvement. Natl Intraven Ther Assoc 1983 May/June; 6(3):207–212.

Primary Nursing

Campbell SD. Primary nursing: It works in long-term care. J Gerontol Nurs 1986 Dec; 11(12):12–16.

McLennon M. Nursing care delivery systems: What is the most effective means of assigning patients for nursing care? Nurs Leadership 1983 Sept; 6(3):72–77.

Primary care nursing promotes professional autonomy. AORN J 1984 June; 39(7):1268–1269.

*Sellick KJ, Russell S, and Beckmann JL. Primary nursing: An evaluation of its effects on patient perception of care and staff satisfaction. Int J Nurs Stud 1983; 20(4):265–273.

*Shukla RK and Turner WE. Patients perception of care under primary and team nursing. Res Nurs Health 1984 June; 7(2):93–99.

Diagnosis-Related Groups

Hamilton JM. Nursing and DRGs: Proactive responses to prospective reimbursement. Nurs Health Care 1984 Mar; 5(3):155–159.

Henderson DP and Sullivan TV. Diagnosis-related groups: Effects on nursing. JEN 1984 Mar/Apr; 10(2):117–118.

How DRGs work in a hospital: Issues and answers for providers. Am J Nurs 1983 Nov; 83(11):1608–1609, 1621.

Joel LA. DRGs: The state of the art and reimbursement for nursing services. Nurs Health Care 1983 Dec; 4(10):560–563.

Lee AA. How DRGs will affect your hospital—and you. RN 1984 May; 47(5):71–81.

Lee A and Sandroff R. 1984 and beyond: What's ahead for nursing. RN 1984 Jan; 47(1):26–29.

Mundinger M. DRGs: A glass half full for nursing. Nurs Outlook 1985 Nov/Dec; 33(6):265.

Piper LR. Accounting for nursing functions in DRGs. Nurs Manage 1983 Nov; 14(11):46–48.

Scott SJ. The Medicare prospective payment system. Am J Occup Ther 1984 May; 38(5):330–334.

Shaffer FA. A nursing perspective of the DRG world: I. Nurs Health Care 1984 Jan; 5(1):48–51.

Shaffer FA. Nursing: Gearing up for DRGs: II: Management strategies. Nurs Health Care 1984 Feb; 5(2):93–99.

Taylor MB. The effect of DRGs on home health care. Nurs Outlook 1985 Nov/Dec; 38(6):288–289.

Thompson JD and Diers D. DRGs and nursing intensity. Nurs Health Care 1985 Oct; 6(8):435–439.

Trandel-Korenchuk DM and Trandel-Korenchuk KM. Medicine, DRGs and nursing practice. Nurs Adm Q 1984 Summer; 8(4):85–87.

HMOs and PPOs

Benezra N. Alternative care: The increasing clout of HMOs. Med Lab Observ 1983 Jan; 15(1):53–58.

Coleman JR, Dayani EC, and Simms E. Nursing careers in the emerging systems. Nurs Manage 1984 Jan; 15(1):19–27.

Collins JB and McDonald J. Health care for Medicare beneficiaries: The HMO option. Nursing Econ 1984 July/Aug; 2(4):259–265.

Davy JD. Preferred provider organizations. Am J Occup Ther 1984 May; 38(5):327–329.

The Nursing Process

The nursing process has been accepted as the essence of nursing. It is a deliberate, problem-solving approach to meeting the health care and nursing needs of patients. Although the steps of the nursing process have been delineated in various ways by many nursing leaders, the commonalities found in all definitions are assessment, planning, implementation, and evaluation. These fundamental components can be used to define the nursing process as follows:

1. Systematic assessment of the patient to determine his state of wellness, identify any actual or potential health problems, and establish nursing diagnoses.
2. Development of a plan of care to assist the patient in resolving the nursing diagnoses.
3. Implementation of the plan of care or supervision of the implementation of the plan of care by others.
4. Evaluation of the effectiveness of the plan of care in resolving the nursing diagnoses and meeting all needs for care.

- Thus, the nursing process is a data-collecting, decision-making process that incorporates evaluation and subsequent modification as feedback mechanisms that promote the ultimate resolution of the patient's nursing diagnoses.

Division of the nursing process into four distinct components or steps serves to emphasize the critical nursing actions that must be accomplished when the nurse assumes responsibility for resolving the patient's nursing diagnoses. However, the nurse must remember that the divisions are artificial and that the process as a whole is cyclic, the steps being interrelated, interdependent, and recurrent (Fig. 2-1).

Assessment

The assessment component of the nursing process begins with the nurse's first encounter with the patient. It involves the systematic collection of data about the patient's health status, analysis of the data to determine his actual and po-

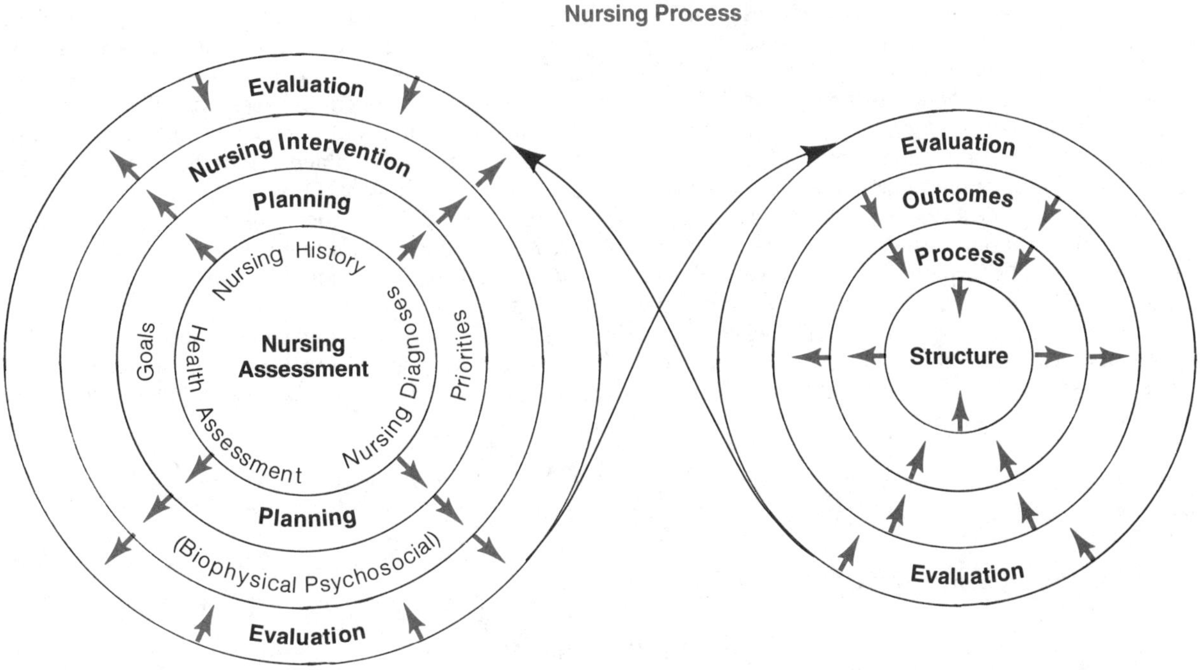

Nursing Process

Figure 2-1

The nursing process is depicted schematically in the circle on the left. Starting from the innermost circle, nursing assessment, the process moves outward through the taking of the nursing history, the making of nursing diagnoses, planning, the setting of goals and priorities, and actual nursing intervention, and arrives at the ongoing process of evaluation. To show the consistent role of evaluation, the right circle indicates a gearlike activity: (1) structure—the organizational pattern within which the nursing process takes place and which involves personnel, environment, and facilities; (2) process—the providing of care, including the interaction that takes place between the patient recipient and the care provider; and (3) the final outcome—the condition of the patient/client following this process.

tential health needs, and use of the data to formulate nursing diagnoses.

- The nursing diagnoses then become the basis for the nursing care plan.

Sensitive and continuous nursing assessment by means of the nursing history and the health assessment is essential to maintain an awareness of the patient's needs and the effectiveness of the nursing care that he receives.

Nursing History

The nursing history is carried out for the purpose of determining the patient's state of wellness or illness and is best accomplished as part of a planned interview. The interview is a dialogue between the patient and the nurse and is a very personal experience. Interviewing is a process that requires wisdom, judgment, tact, and experience. It involves the sensitive direction of a conversation with a patient in order to obtain information about him. The nurse's approach to the patient will largely determine the amount and quality of information that is received. Achieving a relationship of mutual trust and respect requires the ability to communicate a sincere interest in the patient. The patient should be made as comfortable as possible and afforded privacy for the interview.

The skills involved in interviewing a patient include the following:

1. Listening and questioning
2. Observing and interpreting
3. Synthesizing
4. Incorporating what is learned into a plan of care

To learn about a patient, one must talk little and listen a lot. Listen to the patient with "hearing ears." What is he saying? Because an ill person is so suggestible, do not put words in his mouth. Let him tell his story in his own way. Although many topics may be brought up, look for the main area of concern. Give the patient time, without interruptions, to tell why he is seeking help. Be attentive not only to his verbal expression but also to his nonverbal behavior, which may be exhibited in such subtle forms as gestures, posture, and facial expressions. Anxiety is present in almost every patient; it may be well concealed, but it is there. Anticipate the patient's anxieties and try to relieve them during the interview. All inquiries should be relevant. The patient has the right to expect something from each interview. He should especially be made to feel that he is being understood.

The use of a nursing history guide may help the nurse to obtain pertinent information and to facilitate the course of the interview. A variety of nursing history guides have been developed by individual nurses and committees of nurses. Many health care agencies have developed guides that are specifically directed toward obtaining the information that is most essential for their particular patients. Guides that are standard for a particular health care agency tend to reflect the agency's specific philosophy and concept of man, nursing, and health. These nursing history guides are just that—guides. They are designed to guide the interview but must be adapted to the individual responses, problems, and needs of the patient. As the nurse gains expertise in conducting a nursing history, she should strive toward developing her own format, one that allows for adaptability and flexibility while still obtaining the essential information. This essential information must reflect an assessment of the total patient with regard to

his basic human needs and his state of wellness or illness. A variety of models can serve as the framework for the assessment of basic needs. Functional health patterns (Gordon, 1982), Maslow's hierarchy of needs, and Erikson's eight stages of man are examples of frameworks that provide bases for the assessment of the total needs of the client—his physical, psychological, emotional, intellectual, developmental, social, cultural, and spiritual needs. The questions in Chart 2-1 are offered as guidelines for interviewing, but the questions actually asked are determined by the reaction of the individual patient.

In some instances it may be appropriate for the patient to fill out the nursing history form. If this technique of history taking is used, it remains the responsibility of the nurse to

Chart 2-1
Suggestions for Interviewing Patients

Current Health Status

Nursing Focus: At the beginning of the interview, focus on what is most troublesome to the patient.

- What brought you to the hospital?
- What is causing you the most discomfort?
- When did the symptoms appear?
- What did you do when you noticed these symptoms?
- Does anything seem to relieve these symptoms?
- Do you believe you are getting better or worse? (the directional trend: improvement or deterioration)
- How do you feel now?
- What do you know about your illness or condition?
- What do you do for yourself at home when you are sick?
- How has the illness affected your way of life? For how long?
- What factors aggravate or help your condition?
- Are you taking any medications?
- Do you have any allergies? (food, drugs)
- What is your greatest concern?
- What have you been told about the treatment or tests that have been planned for you?
- Who or what has been your chief source of information?

Past Health History

Nursing Focus: Learn about the patient's background and experience in order to determine his needs.*

- Would you tell me a little about yourself, your family, your way of life?
- What types of things do you do to try to stay healthy?
- How do you usually react to being ill?
- Whom do you usually turn to for help?
- What type of work do you do? If someone else is the provider, what type of work does he do?
- Has your illness interfered with your work?
- How do you like to be treated when you are ill?
- What activities, hobbies, and forms of recreation do you enjoy?

Nursing Needs

Nursing Focus: Ascertain what can be done to support the patient and help him to make the best use of his resources. What are his strengths? limitations?

- What would you like to be able to do to help yourself get better?
- What kinds of help do you need?
- Who do you think could provide this help?
- What aspects of your life are being disrupted by your illness?
- How do you think your illness will affect your family?
- What do you think will be the hardest part of the situation?
- What are your food preferences? dislikes?
- What are your sleeping habits?
  Regular retiring time?
  Do you like a night light?
  How many pillows do you use?
- What are your elimination habits (bowel and urinary)?
- Do you have any limitations of seeing? hearing? walking?
- Would it be helpful to have a family member or friend stay with you?
- What annoys you most about being in the hospital?
- What do you miss the most in the hospital?
- How long do you think you will stay?
- What do you not understand as well as you would like to?
- What could the nursing staff do that would be most helpful for you?

* Social, cultural, developmental, and educational levels, and the patient's readiness to learn can be assessed throughout the interview.

verify and clarify the information provided by the patient and to seek any additional information that is necessary to identify the patient's nursing needs. Throughout the interview the nurse has the opportunity to interact with the patient not only for the purpose of data collection but also for the purpose of conveying interest, support, and understanding to the patient. For a more detailed discussion of the concepts and techniques of clinical interviewing, see Chapter 5.

The Health Assessment

The health assessment of the patient may be carried out prior to, during, or following the nursing history, depending on the patient's physical and emotional state, his response to his illness and hospitalization, and the immediate priorities of his illness situation.

The purpose of the health assessment is to identify those parameters of physical, psychological, and emotional functioning that indicate that a nursing need exists. It requires the use of the senses of sight, hearing, touch, and smell as well as the appropriate interview skills and techniques. Physical examination techniques as well as techniques and strategies for assessing behaviors and role changes are used.

The physical examination is designed to determine the patient's physical alterations and limitations and also to determine his assets, which may serve to compensate for his limitations.

- To accomplish the purposes of the physical examination, the nurse must be skilled in the techniques of inspection, palpation, percussion, and auscultation; she must also have a sound basic knowledge of anatomy and physiology and of the symptomatology of the disease process with which the patient presents.

Because the physical examination is such an important part of the health assessment component of the nursing process, and because it involves specific technical skills that must be learned and continuously refined, Chapter 6 is devoted to the study of the basic techniques of the physical examination. Significant observations that should be made with specific clinical conditions appear in the chapters in which the conditions are discussed. Careful study is required because the nurse must learn to observe with "seeing" eyes, hear with "hearing" ears, feel with "feeling" hands, and interpret the findings of the examination.

At the completion of the nursing history and the health assessment the patient should be told how the data will be used, the conclusions that will be drawn, and the fact that he and his family or significant others will be involved in developing the plan for his care. By the termination of the assessment, he should know who his nurse is and how he can communicate with her.

Other Components of the Data Base

Following the nursing history and the health assessment, the nurse seeks additional relevant information from the patient's family or significant others, from other members of the health team, and from the patient's health record or chart. Depending on the patient's immediate illness needs, this information may have been obtained prior to the nursing history and the health assessment. Whatever the sequence of events, the nurse uses all available sources of pertinent data to complete the nursing assessment. It is imperative that she study the patient's health record to determine the problem that caused the patient to seek help.

A tentative medical diagnosis has usually been formulated by the physician on the patient's admission to the hospital. It is absolutely essential to understand the pathophysiological processes underlying this diagnosis. "Therapeutic conversation" is no substitute for knowing the effects of altered physiology, rationale of treatment, and potential complications. This knowledge helps the nurse to anticipate problems that may evolve, to formulate a nursing approach to their solution, and to participate with other members of the health care team in providing coordinated health care.

Recording the Data Base

After completion of the nursing history and health assessment, the information obtained must be recorded. It is recorded in the patient's permanent record as a part of his problem-oriented health record.

The problem-oriented health record provides a systematic method of organizing all the information needed to diagnose the patient's needs and to meet these needs. The scientific method of problem solving is used. The components of the record are the data base, the patient problem list, the patient progress notes, and the discharge summary. The record provides a means of communication between the members of the health care team and facilitates coordinated planning and continuity of care. The record fulfills other functions as well:

- It serves as the business and legal record for the hospital and for the professional staff responsible for the patient's care.
- It serves as a basis for evaluating the quality of care as well as for reviewing the effective use of patient care health practices.
- It provides data useful in research, education, and short- and long-range planning.

The information that is recorded first on the patient's record is the *data base,* which is a compilation of all of the data obtained on each patient at the time of his entry into the health care system. It consists of the nursing history and health assessment as well as the history and physical examination obtained by the physician and patient profiles from other sources, such as the social worker, pharmacist, nutritionist, dentist, physical therapist, and respiratory therapist. It also includes laboratory and radiologic data and any other data or profiles from other members of the health care team involved in the patient's care. The form and content of the data base are predetermined by the agency. Although many disciplines may participate in collecting different parts of the information, all of the data should be placed together in the same section of the health record. When all disciplines are not using the problem-oriented system, it is not always possible to achieve an integrated data base. In this case the nursing department should determine what information is needed about all patients and seek to avoid duplication as much as possible.

Experience with the problem-oriented record system has shown that definite time limits need to be established by the agency so that the patient's problems are identified as soon after admission as possible. Many agencies set 8 to 24 hours as the time limit for recording the data base. An example of a nursing data base is found on page 23.

Nursing Diagnosis

The assessment component of the nursing process is concluded with the formulation of the nursing diagnoses. As soon as possible after the completion of the nursing history and the health assessment, the nurse organizes, analyzes, synthesizes, and summarizes the data collected and determines the patient's need for nursing care.

- Those actual or potential health problems that are amenable to resolution by nursing actions are identified as *nursing diagnoses.*

Nursing, unlike medicine, does not yet have a standard taxonomy of diagnostic labels that convey the same meaning to all nurses. Until recent years, the nursing literature has contained little substantive work on the classification of nursing diagnoses. The 1970s brought a surge of professional activity aimed at making nursing diagnosis a function for which the nurse is held legally responsible and accountable. A large number of nurse practice acts were revised to include nursing diagnosis as a nursing function. Nursing diagnosis was included in the American Nurses' Association Standards of Nursing Practice (1973) and in the standards developed by many nursing specialty organizations.

The National Conferences on the Classification of Nursing Diagnoses held in the 1970s and 1980s have provided an impetus for the identification and classification of nursing diagnoses according to symptomatology. At the fifth conference, held in 1982, a major step was taken toward coordinating the work of developing nursing diagnoses—a new organization, the North American Nursing Diagnosis Association (NANDA), was created. The diagnostic categories identified by the conference groups are gaining general acceptance by nurses but require further validation and expansion. They are not yet complete or mutually exclusive. More research is needed to determine the predictive and prognostic attributes of the diagnostic labels. It is hoped that in the future, nursing diagnosis will attain its potential of decreasing the ambiguity about the nurse's role so that a more clearly defined scope of nursing practice will evolve. A list of accepted nursing diagnoses from the seventh Conference on the Classification of Nursing Diagnoses is shown in Chart 2-2.

In spite of the need for research on the diagnostic process itself and on the diagnostic nomenclature, the term *nursing diagnosis* will be used in sections of this book where we have applied the nursing process to specific illness conditions. Both nurses and nursing students have a unique opportunity to use currently accepted nursing diagnoses and to develop additional diagnoses that describe actual or potential health problems that are amenable to nursing care. Only through clinical use and research of nursing diagnostic labels can these labels be validated and expanded.

When developing the nursing diagnoses for a particular patient, the nurse must first identify the commonalities among the assessment data collected. These common features lead to the categorization of related data that reveal the existence of a problem and the need for nursing intervention. *The patient's nursing problem is then defined as the nursing diagnosis.*

It must be remembered that nursing diagnoses are *not* medical diagnoses; they are *not* medical treatments prescribed by the physician; they are *not* diagnostic studies; they are *not* the equipment used to implement medical therapy; and they are *not* the problems that the nurse experiences while caring for the patient. They *are* the patient's actual or potential health problems that are amenable to resolution by nursing actions. Nursing diagnoses that are succinctly stated in terms of the specific problems of the patient will guide the nurse in the development of the nursing care plan.

In order to give additional meaning to the diagnosis, the characteristics and the etiology of the problem must be identified and included as a part of the diagnosis. Consider this clinical example:

> Assessment of a patient with a medical diagnosis of diabetes mellitus reveals that the patient does not adhere to his dietary regimen. He has the financial means necessary for purchasing the foods included in his diet, he has the home facilities required for preparing his foods, and he expresses a sincere desire to comply with his diet. However, he does not understand the food exchange system that is necessary for meal planning.

For this patient, the nursing diagnosis of "nonadherence" would give little guidance to the nurse in establishing a plan of care to meet the patient's needs. However, a more specific diagnosis of "nonadherence to dietary regimen related to lack of understanding of the diabetic exchange system" provides the nurse with information about the characteristics and cause of the problem. With such a diagnosis, the nurse is then ready to record the diagnosis and plan nursing care measures directed toward resolution of the problem.

Recording the Nursing Diagnoses

The patient's nursing diagnoses should be recorded on the nursing care plan as well as in the patient problem list. The patient problem list serves as the "index" or "table of contents" to the record. A *problem* is defined as anything that concerns the patient, endangers his health, requires management, and concerns any member of the health care team.

If all professionals are using the problem-oriented system then they all contribute to the same problem list. The problems are numbered and used by all concerned for writing progress notes.

Planning

Once the nursing diagnoses have been identified, the planning component of the nursing process is developed. This phase involves the following:

1. The assignment of priorities to the nursing diagnoses
2. The specification of immediate, intermediate, and long-term goals of nursing action
3. The identification of specific nursing interventions appropriate for attaining the goals

Nursing Assessment

Rm # 2065-B

Walker, Susan
Hx # 094460
F   45   Barnes
Acct # 731861   2/15/88

NURSING DATA BASE

GENERAL ADMISSION INFORMATION

DATE: 2/15/88   TIME: 1:00 p.m.

BASELINE DATA: Height: 5'3" Weight: 165 Temp.: 37°C Pulse: 96 Resp.: 20 BP:Ra: 162/112 La: 160/112

PROSTHESES OR ASSISTIVE DEVICES: Contact Lens

DIET AT HOME: Low sodium, low cholesterol, 1500 calories —"not sticking to it"

ALLERGIES: none   SIGNATURE: B. Smith, R.N.

PATIENT/FAMILY ASSESSMENT

REASON FOR HOSPITALIZATION OR ADMITTING PROBLEM: Evaluation of hypertension + initiation of therapy

DURATION OF THIS PROBLEM: 3 months

OBSERVATION OF PATIENT'S CONDITION:
   Gastrointestinal status: Normal
   Neurologic status: Alert; oriented to time, place, + person; no sensory deficits
   Respiratory status: quiet + unlabored
   Skin condition: intact; well cared for; slight edema of ankles + feet —"Always puffy at night"

CONCURRENT CONDITIONS: none

PREVIOUS EXPERIENCE WITH HOSPITALIZATIONS: normal deliveries in 1970 + 1972

MEDICATION: Aspirin occasionally for headache

REACTION TO ALLERGIES: —

PATTERNS:
   HYGIENE: shower every A.M.
   REST/SLEEP: 6 hrs./night : 12MN – 6 A.M
   MEALS/DIET: Appetite good; "Eats on the run—fixes things that are quick + easy"
   ACTIVITY STATUS: Independent ADL; activity as tolerated
   ELIMINATION—BOWEL: daily
             BLADDER: 4-5 times/day; no changes noted recently
   MENSTRUAL HISTORY: LMP 2/5/88

HEALTH HAZARD APPRAISAL: yearly physical exam; BSE q month; no smoking

LIFE-STYLE: Real Estate Agent past 2 yrs. —"hectic schedule; work all hours of day + night"
       Lives c̄ husband + 2 daughters

TYPICAL DAY PROFILE: Depends on number of clients—unpredictable; difficult to plan ahead;
             activities c̄ daughters at least 4 nights/week

MENTAL/EMOTIONAL STATUS:
       calm; "have to slow down + get my blood pressure under control"

SAFETY APPRAISAL: no problems

DISCHARGE PLANNING: Anticipated LOS 3 days; will be followed in physician's office;
       will need follow-up evaluation of dietary adherence

INFORMANT: Patient

                    SIGNATURE: B. Smith, R.N.

(Based on form used by Presbyterian-University Hospital Nursing Service Department, Pittsburgh, PA)

Chart 2-2
Accepted Nursing Diagnoses from the Seventh Conference on the Classification of Nursing Diagnoses

Activity Intolerance
Activity Intolerance, Potential
* Adjustment, Impaired
Airway Clearance, Ineffective
Anxiety
* Body Temperature, Potential Alteration in
Bowel Elimination, Alteration in: Constipation
Bowel Elimination, Alteration in: Diarrhea
Bowel Elimination, Alteration in: Incontinence
Breathing Pattern, Ineffective
Cardiac Output, Alteration in: Decreased
Comfort, Alteration in: Pain
* Comfort, Alteration in: Chronic Pain
Communication, Impaired: Verbal
Coping, Family: Potential for Growth
Coping, Ineffective Family: Compromised
Coping, Ineffective Family: Disabling
Coping, Ineffective Individual
Diversional Activity, Deficit
Family Process, Alteration in
Fear
Fluid Volume, Alteration in: Excess
Fluid Volume Deficit, Actual
Fluid Volume Deficit, Potential
Gas Exchange, Impaired
Grieving, Anticipatory
Grieving, Dysfunctional
* Growth and Development, Altered
Health Maintenance, Alteration in
Home Maintenance Management, Impaired
* Hopelessness
* Hyperthermia
* Hypothermia
* Incontinence, Functional
* Incontinence, Reflex
* Incontinence, Stress
* Incontinence, Total
* Infection, Potential for
Injury, Potential for:
   Poisoning
   Suffocation
   Trauma
Knowledge Deficit (specify)
Mobility, Impaired Physical
Noncompliance (specify)
Nutrition, Alteration in: Less than Body Requirements
Nutrition, Alteration in: More than Body Requirements
Nutrition, Alteration in: Potential for More than Body Requirements

Oral Mucous Membrane, Alteration in
Parenting, Alteration in: Actual
Parenting, Alteration in: Potential
* Post Trauma Response
Powerlessness
Rape Trauma Syndrome
Self-Care Deficit:
   Feeding
   Bathing/hygiene
   Dressing/grooming
   Toileting
Self-Concept, Disturbance in:
   Body image
   Self-esteem
   Role performance
   Personal identity
Sensory-Perceptual Alteration
   Visual
   Auditory
   Kinesthetic
   Gustatory
   Tactile
   Olfactory
Sexual Dysfunction
* Sexuality Patterns, Altered
Skin Integrity, Impairment of: Actual
Skin Integrity, Impairment of: Potential
Sleep Pattern Disturbance
* Social Interaction, Impaired
Social Isolation
Spiritual Distress (distress of the human spirit)
* Swallowing, Impaired
* Thermoregulation, Ineffective
Thought Processes, Alteration in
* Tissue Integrity, Impaired
Tissue Perfusion, Alteration in:
   Cerebral
   Cardiopulmonary
   Renal
   Gastrointestinal
   Peripheral
* Unilateral Neglect
Urinary Elimination, Alteration in Patterns of
* Urinary Retention
Violence, Potential for:
   Self-directed
   Directed at others

   * Diagnoses accepted in 1986.

4. The identification of interdependent interventions
5. The specification of expected outcomes
6. The documentation of the nursing diagnoses, goals, nursing interventions, and expected outcomes on the nursing care plan

Also, during this phase of the nursing process it is the responsibility of the nurse to communicate to the appropriate persons any assessment data indicative of health needs that can best be met by other members of the health care team.

Setting Priorities

The assignment of priorities to the nursing diagnoses should be a joint effort by the nurse and the patient or his family members. Any disagreement about the priorities should be resolved in a way that is mutually acceptable. Consideration must be given to the urgency of the problems, the most critical problems receiving the highest priorities. Maslow's hierarchy of needs provides a useful framework for the determination of priority problems. The use of this hierarchy requires that high priorities be given to physical needs. Subsequent to the resolution of physical needs, priorities are reassigned according to the urgency of needs at other levels of the hierarchy (see pp. 12–14).

Establishing Goals for Nursing Action

After the priorities of the nursing diagnoses have been established, the immediate, intermediate, and long-term goals and the nursing actions appropriate for attainment of the goals are identified. The patient and his family should be included in the establishment of the goals of the nursing actions. The immediate goals are those that can be reached in a short period of time. The intermediate and long-term goals require a longer period of time for their accomplishment and usually involve prevention of complications and further health problems, health education, and rehabilitation. For example, goals for an uncontrolled diabetic patient with a nursing diagnosis of "nonadherence to dietary regimen related to lack of understanding of the diabetic exchange system" may be stated as follows:

Immediate goal:	Oral intake and tolerance of 1500-calorie diabetic diet spaced in three meals and one snack
Intermediate goal:	Planning of meals for 1 week based on diabetic exchange system
Long-term goal:	Adherence to prescribed diabetic diet

The patient and his family should be included whenever possible in the decisions about the nursing interventions to meet the goals. Involvement of the patient and his family in the planning of nursing interventions promotes their cooperation in the implementation of nursing care. The identification of appropriate nursing interventions and their related goals depends on the nurse's recognition of the strengths and potential of the patient and his family; her understanding of the pathophysiologic alterations that he experiences; and her sensitivity to his emotional, psychological, and intellectual response to his illness state. Likewise, the nurse's knowledge of nursing, her clinical experience, and her awareness of available supporting resources influence the validity of the nursing interventions that she identifies as appropriate for resolving the patient's nursing diagnoses.

Establishing Expected Outcomes

Expected outcomes of the nursing interventions should be stated in terms of the patient's behaviors. They should be realistic and measurable. Standard outcome criteria established by the health care agency for the target population applicable to the patient should be used whenever possible. However, it may be necessary to adapt these outcome criteria so that they are realistic in terms of the specific patient's potential for resolution of his problems. The critical time period within which the outcomes should be demonstrated by the patient are also identified.

- The outcomes that define the expected behavior of the patient will serve as the basis for evaluation of the effectiveness of the nursing interventions.
- The critical time periods provide a time frame for determining the effectiveness of the nursing interventions and the existence of a need for additional or altered nursing care.

Team Planning

Ideally, the accomplishment of all aspects of the planning phase of the nursing process is a group effort. The nurse collaborates with other members of the nursing team, with the patient and his family, and with appropriate resource persons from the health care agency and community agencies.

In planning with other members of the nursing team, the nurse recognizes that each team member has a role that is supported and respected. The physician initiates the medical regimen and is a valuable counselor, teacher, and resource person. A nurse clinical-specialist, when available, can make a significant contribution.

Because the plan revolves around a patient, he should have a part in it. The ultimate goal is to help the patient help himself. This means that the patient is accepted as a worthy individual and his right to self-determination is respected. Since the plan is oriented in terms of the patient's goals and capabilities, he has every right to express his feelings and voice his opinions about his care. He should be kept informed about his current health status (when feasible), any change in plans, the roles of health care personnel, and the resources available to him.

It is also important to remember that the patient is part of a family. The family members have needs that arise from the patient's illness. They may be included in the planning by questioning them about the patient's reactions and informing them about the nursing care plan and the expected results of treatment. The family may also make pertinent observations and offer effective suggestions.

Another aspect of care planning takes into account the fact that the patient comes from the community. Community agencies have an interest in the patient and are involved in planning. This means that the nurse must be aware of the community services that may be offered a patient following discharge from the hospital. These agencies can be informed of the goal to be reached, and decisions can then be made regarding the type of services that will be needed. Many communities have a directory listing all community resources available. These include community health and visiting nursing services, homemaking services, meals on wheels, and social and recreational services. A knowledge of these resources and the method of referral is of inestimable value in helping to cope with long-term health needs.

Because discharge from the hospital has been accelerated with the advent of Diagnosis-Related Groups, many patients are leaving the hospital with complex needs, many of which require advanced technologies. For this reason, discharge planning must begin when the patient is first admitted to the hospital so that appropriate home health care services are available to him and his family when he is ready for discharge. It is imperative that this discharge planning is accomplished by multidisciplinary efforts.

Formulating the Nursing Care Plan

The entire planning phase of the nursing process culminates in the formulation of the patient's nursing care plan by the professional nurse. The nursing care plan serves to communicate the following information to all members of the nursing team.

1. The nursing diagnoses and their priorities
2. The goals of the nursing interventions
3. The nursing interventions, which are expressed in the form of nursing orders
4. The expected outcomes, which identify the expected behavioral responses for the patient
5. The critical time period within which each outcome must be met

The information incorporated into the nursing care plan should be written in a concise, systematic manner that facilitates its use by all nursing personnel. Space must be provided in the care plan for documentation of the patient's response to the nursing interventions—the outcomes. It must be remembered that the care plan is subject to change as the patient's problems change, as the priorities of the problems shift, as resolution of problems occurs, and as additional information about the patient's state of health is collected. As the nursing interventions are implemented, the patient's responses are evaluated and documented, and the care plan is changed accordingly. A well-developed, continuously updated nursing care plan is the patient's greatest assurance that his nursing diagnoses will be resolved and that his basic needs will be met (see pp. 28–29).

Implementation

The implementation phase of the nursing process follows the formulation of the nursing care plan. Implementation refers to carrying out the proposed plan of care. The nurse assumes responsibility for the implementation but includes the patient and his family and other members of the nursing team and the health care team as appropriate. The activities of all persons involved in implementation are coordinated by the nurse.

- The nursing care plan serves as the basis for implementation.
- The immediate, intermediate, and long-term goals are used as a focus for the implementation of the designed nursing interventions.
- While implementing nursing care, the nurse continually assesses the patient and his response to the nursing care.
- Alterations are made in the care plan as the patient's condition, problems, and responses change and as reassignment of priorities is required.

Implementation includes all of the nursing interventions that are directed toward resolution of the patient's nursing diagnoses and meeting his health needs. Some of these needs have already been discussed (pp. 12–14). Needs specific to certain conditions are presented in the chapter in which the particular condition is discussed.

General Categories of Nursing Interventions

Included among nursing interventions are hygienic care; promotion of physical and psychological comfort; support of respiratory and elimination functions; facilitation of the ingestion of food, fluids, and nutrients; environmental management; health teaching; promotion of a therapeutic relationship; and a host of therapeutic nursing activities. The nurse uses judgment and decision-making skills in the selection of nursing interventions that are based on physiologic principles.

Knowledge of physiology must be constantly sought, integrated, and applied. Consider this clinical example:

A patient who 3 days previously had a cholecystectomy and is allowed to ambulate as tolerated is complaining of abdominal pain. He states that he "feels full," has not had a bowel movement, and has no appetite. Bowel sounds are present. The self-directing nurse, using nursing judgments based on an understanding of pathophysiology, will encourage measures that promote ambulation. She will also explain to the patient the positive effects of mobility on peristalsis and the negative effects of analgesics on peristalsis. Follow-up evaluation will then indicate whether the problem has been resolved or if further nursing interventions are needed.

- All nursing interventions are patient focused and goal directed. They are based on scientific principles and are implemented with compassion, confidence, and a willingness to understand the patient's problems.

Many nursing actions are independent. Others are interdependent, such as carrying out physicians' prescriptions for medications and therapies and collaborating with other health care team members to accomplish specific expected outcomes. Such interdependent functioning is just that—interdependent. Requests from other health care team members should not be followed blindly but should be assessed critically and questioned as necessary.

Delegating Nursing Actions

The nurse may delegate certain specific actions to other members of the nursing team. When delegating, the nurse must know the capabilities and limitations of the members of the nursing team, select the most appropriate person to implement the actions, and supervise the performance of the actions. The nursing team member should be provided with all of the information that she needs to perform the actions in such a way that the patient remains the focus of the actions at all times.

Many members of the nursing team and the health care team may become involved in the patient's care. In order to provide for coordination and continuity of care, information about the patient's response to his care and any changes that must be made in the plan of care must be communicated verbally and in writing to the appropriate persons. Continual updating of the care plan is of paramount importance in ensuring coordination and continuity.

Recording Outcomes

The implementation phase of the nursing process is concluded when the nursing interventions have been completed and the patient's responses to them have been recorded. Recordings should be made concisely, precisely, and objectively. The recordings should:

- Be related to the nursing diagnoses
- Describe the nursing interventions and the patient's responses to the interventions
- Include any additional pertinent data

Only with accurate recording can evaluation be carried out. Documentation of information provides the basis for the measurement of the patient's behavioral response to the nursing interventions—his accomplishment of the defined outcome criteria.

Patient Progress Notes. The progress notes are written in a format that not only relates them clearly and unmistakably to the numbered problem—in the case of nursing, to the nursing diagnosis—but also uses the scientific method of problem solving on a day-by-day basis (see p. 30). Progress notes are written in a narrative form, using the acronym "SOAPIE."

- S   Subjective data (symptoms that the patient describes)
- O   Objective data (signs that the professional observes)
- A   Assessment (the professional's conclusion about the subjective and objective data)
- P   Plan (immediate or future, including patient education)
- I   Intervention (nursing action done to, for, or with the patient)
- E   Evaluation (patient outcome of nursing process)

Flow sheets are used to follow or monitor a problem that does not lend itself to a single note or requires that multiple parameters be observed and recorded more often than every 6 hours or four times a day, or they may be used for the documentation of nursing and patient activities, such as treatments and daily care.

- The progress notes are the most critical part of the problem-oriented system. They are the mechanism that provides a minute-by-minute ongoing assessment of the patient's problem. The progress notes can detect faulty understanding and poor decisions made by the health care provider. They do not improve care, but they can identify inadequate logic in seconds. Progress notes provide the feedback on problem identification and the plans formulated. If all professionals are recording on integrated progress notes, the patient has a greater chance of receiving continuity of care.

The progress notes always begin with the date, time, and problem number and title, and they continue, using the following format.

Subjective Data. The subjective or symptomatic data are obtained from the patient's or family's point of view. When recording subjective data, consider the following: onset (date, time, type), intensity, quality, location, radiation, number of episodes, time of day of episodes, sources of relief (rest, position, medication), precipitating factors, factors that make the problem worse, other associated symptoms existing at the same time, overall course, and the degree to which the symptoms have affected the patient's life-style.

Objective Data. These include actual clinical observations or laboratory findings appropriate to the problem. When recording objective data, always include the following: location, size, shape, color, temperature, moisture, and consistency. Also, note the presence or absence of swelling, movement, weakness, and associated pain with movement or touch. Many nurses record their nursing actions in this section; others add their immediate interventions to the plan component of the progress notes.

Assessment. This is the portion of the progress notes that deals directly with the subjective and objective data just collected and that presents the health care provider's conclusion, based on that information. If both are consistent with the problem statement, little needs to be said here. One way of considering assessment in relation to patient progress or regress will be a comparison with the previous documentation, using such terms as "improved," "worse," or "deteriorating," or "same" or "stable." If the problem is a new one, the subjective and objective data should support a new assessment of what is going on with the patient. If the problem statement and the subjective and objective data are not consistent, one can quickly assess the logic or accuracy of the information recorded.

Assessment occurs when the provider records his thinking and conclusions at his level of understanding.

Plan. The original or initial plan, if well thought out and developed, will continue to be followed or will be modified as new information is obtained. The plan will always consider the three areas described earlier: the need for more information, management and treatment, and patient and family education.

Intervention and Evaluation. Nurses use the same problem-oriented procedure to document their practice. However, there are two components that many nurses have added in order to comply with the requirements of the nursing process and of some regulatory agencies for documenting nursing

(Text continues on p. 30)

Example of an Individualized Nursing Care Plan

Mrs. Susan Walker, a 45-year-old real estate agent, was admitted to the nursing unit from her physician's office. A routine physical examination 3 months previously had revealed essential hypertension with BP 170/110 and decreased urine creatinine clearance. During the subsequent 3 months the blood pressure elevation did not respond to diet therapy. Mrs. Walker admitted that she had not been successful in adhering to the low sodium, low cholesterol, weight reduction diet that had been prescribed for her. She stated "my life is just too busy—I work all hours of the day and night and usually eat on the run." She indicated that in addition to her work she and her husband share the responsibility for raising their two teenage daughters. She drinks five to seven cups of coffee daily and drinks alcohol only at social occasions. Admission physical examination revealed BP 162/112, P 96, R 20, T 37°C, height 5′3″, weight 165 lbs., and slight edema of the ankles and feet. Mrs. Walker stated that her feet are "always puffy at night." A brief hospitalization was planned for thorough evaluation and initiation of therapy. The physician's regimen on admission included activity as desired; Lasix, 40 mg bid; monitor vital signs every 4 hours while awake; diet regimen: 1500 calories, 1 gm sodium, low cholesterol.

Nursing Diagnoses
1. Alteration in blood pressure related to increased peripheral resistance and aggravated by stress, obesity, and caffeine
2. Emotional stress related to role responsibilities at work and home
3. Potential nonadherence to therapeutic regimen

Goals
Immediate: Gradual decrease in blood pressure
Intermediate: Initiation of life-style alterations to decrease stress
Long-term: Alteration of life-style to reduce emotional and environmental stressors
         Adherence to therapeutic regimen

Nursing Interventions	Expected Outcomes	Critical Times*	Outcomes
Monitor BP lying, sitting, and standing every 4 hr	Experiences no further increase in BP	24 hr	BP range of 162/112–138/98 since admission No variation greater than 5 mm Hg in systolic or diastolic pressures with position changes No variation between right and left arms
	Maintains BP at less than 162/112	Prior to discharge	Maximum BP from 24 hr after admission to time of discharge: 138/98
Monitor fluid status: I&O	Urinary output adequate in relation to oral intake	24 hr	Intake: 1850 ml Output: 1685 ml
Peripheral edema	No evidence of peripheral edema	48 hr	Minimal edema of feet late in evening
Promote atmosphere conducive to physical & mental rest: Encourage alternation of rest and activity	Alternates periods of rest and activity	24 hr	Rests in bed 1 hr in morning and 2 hr in afternoon; disconnects phone during rest periods Awake at intervals during night: 8 hr of uninterrupted sleep at night after initiation of 30 mg Dalmane at bedtime

(continued)

Nursing Interventions	Expected Outcomes	Critical Times*	Outcomes
Encourage limitation of visitors and interactions that are stress producing	Limits visitors to family in the evenings	24 hr	Husband and daughters visit 2 hr in evening; calm and relaxed after visits
	Avoids stress-producing interactions	24 hr	Husband and daughters aware of need to decrease stress: they consult with patient about regular family activities
Assist patient to alter life-style to decrease stress:			
Discuss relationship between emotional stress and physiologic functioning	Describes stress as a precursor to alteration in physiological functioning	48 hr	Accurately described relationship between stress and hypertension
Encourage patient to identify stress-producing stimuli	Identifies life-style factors that produce stress	48 hr	Identified the following stressors: Self-imposed demands of job: inability to refer clients to other agents Excessive involvement in daughters' school and recreational activities
Encourage patient to identify adjustments necessary to reduce stress	Identifies life-style adjustments necessary to reduce stress	48 hr	Verbalized that her income is not a necessity for the family; plans to make more referrals Identified need to decrease work hours to maximum of 6 hr per day
	Discusses life-style adjustments with family	48 hr	Consulted with husband and daughters; will alternate with husband in attending daughters' activities; all family members supportive
Encourage patient to identify obesity, nicotine, and caffeine as stressors and aggravators of hypertension	Identifies harmful effects of obesity and caffeine	48 hr	Accurately described effects of obesity and caffeine on blood pressure
	Makes plans for losing weight	Prior to admission	Plans to go to Weight Watchers; has had success with their program in the past
	Makes plans for decreasing caffeine intake	48 hr	Drinks 1 cup of coffee for breakfast; uses decaffeinated coffee at mid morning, lunch, and dinner; expressed satisfaction with this plan
Promote adherence to therapeutic regimen	(See teaching plan, p. 39)		

* These times have not been standardized but are individualized according to the patient's needs.

Patient Progress Notes

Date	Time	Problem	Progress Notes
2/15/88	5pm	#2: Emotional Stress R/T Role Responsibilities @ Work + Home	S: "I hope I'm able to go home in 3 days; my family needs me + I need to get back to work."
			O: Anxious $\bar{p}$ phone call from husband. Pacing in room; requested coffee. BP 160/110, P 100, R 28
			A: Emotional stress increased when faced $\bar{c}$ responsibilities of work + home.
			P: 1) Encourage periods of rest. 2) Discuss $\bar{c}$ husband the necessity of decreasing stress – producing interactions $\bar{c}$ wife. 3) Be available to let patient verbalize feelings. 4) Begin to work $\bar{c}$ relaxation techniques + use distractive activities.
			I: 1) Encouraged patient to rest in room + work on needlework. 2) Discussed $\bar{c}$ husband the need to decrease stress – producing interactions.
			E: Patient resting in room 1 hr. later; visibly less anxious; BP 142/102
			L. Jones, R.N.

Each Progress Note consists of the number and title of problem as stated on the Problem List and any or all of the following components.

S — Subjective Data (Symptoms)
O — Objective Data (Measurable Signs)
A — Assessment (Conclusion)
P — Plan — Immediate or Future
I — Intervention — Nursing Action
E — Evaluation — Effectiveness of Intervention

(Based on form used by Presbyterian-University Hospital Nursing Service Department, Pittsburgh, PA)

practice. These components are labeled *I*, for the nursing intervention that was carried out immediately (*e.g.*, raise the head of the bed, perform postural drainage) and *E*, for evaluation of the nursing intervention (was it effective or ineffective?) as documented according to patient outcomes. Sometimes the evaluation will appear in the next progress note because more time is needed to observe the patient's response to the nursing intervention.

One can see that when the plan is incorporated in the patient progress notes, it readily becomes a permanent part

of the legal record, and the Kardex system reverts to being a tool to facilitate the implementation of the plan.

Points to keep in mind when writing problem-oriented progress notes are summarized in Chart 2-3.

Evaluation

Evaluation is the final component of the nursing process and is directed toward determining the patient's response to the

Chart 2-3
Writing Problem-Oriented Progress Notes

Reminders to Consider Before Writing Problem-Oriented Progress Notes

1. Have the patient's problem list in front of you or open to the problem list on the patient's health record.
2. Think about your patient in light of each problem listed in the active column. Are there any new problems to be added or considered as a result of your observations or interactions with the patient today?
3. Read the immediately preceding notes so that you will not unnecessarily repeat information already recorded and so that you will be aware of plans that are in progress.
4. Decide which are the most important problems for you to discuss; always consider life-threatening or major problems first (*e.g.*, although a myocardial infarction may be a very threatening problem, if it is relatively stable or has recently been discussed, the patient's acute anxiety may be a more pertinent topic; it may have a significant impact on his survival).
5. A follow-up note on data-base information or on your plans identified in previous notes may be appropriate if the data are now available, or you might want to comment on the effectiveness or ineffectiveness of your plan (*e.g.*, vital signs, weight, response to nursing measures).
6. Always begin your note with the date, time, problem number, and title. List the subjective or objective data, using the factors suggested in this chapter. Record both follow-up data and any new information you have gathered.

7. Write an assessment for each problem considered, stating your thoughts at the level at which you actually understand the information. If you want to write about specific observations or responses to medications or treatments with which you have had little experience, look them up first; you may find valuable information that will help all members of the health care team, or you might learn that your idea does not logically follow from the data you have available.
8. Review the plan for each problem listed, or initiate a new plan if you have identified a new problem. Always consider the following three factors:
   a. The *need for more information,* such as specific observations that might help clarify the problem
   b. *Nursing intervention,* such as specific nursing measures you can order or initiate to resolve the problem (*e.g.*, have patient turn, cough, and take deep breaths every hour for 24 hours)
   c. *Patient or family teaching:* what you have told or plan to tell the patient and his family about this problem to increase their understanding of the management
9. Write a progress note when there is something pertinent to say, such as when there has been a change. Some days several notes for the day or for the shift may be indicated, whereas on other days *no* notes will be appropriate for some problems.

Some Don'ts *When Recording on the Progress Notes*

DON'T include comments on nonproblem item (*e.g.*, bed baths, h.s. care given, doing well).

DON'T write about things that have already been discussed unless you disagree with the data listed or the conclusions drawn. Be sure to defend your position with exact literature references if you do disagree.

DON'T include comments on normal physiologic functions unless they are pertinent to a particular problem (*e.g.*, the daily bowel movements should be kept on a routine care flow sheet unless you are discussing a patient who has diarrhea or who has a previously identified problem, such as constipation).

DON'T use the progress notes to record routine tests done or care given (these can be checked off on the Kardex care plan or considered recorded when the laboratory or x-ray reports come back).

---

nursing interventions and the extent to which the goals have been achieved. The nursing care plan provides the basis for evaluation; the nursing diagnoses, goals, nursing interventions, and expected outcomes provide the specific guidelines that dictate the focus of the evaluation.

Evaluation will answer the following questions:

- Were the nursing diagnoses accurate?
- Did the patient reach the expected outcomes?
- Did the patient attain the expected outcomes within the critical time periods?
- Have the patient's nursing diagnoses been resolved?
- Have the patient's nursing needs been met?

- Should the nursing interventions be retained, altered, or discontinued?
- Have new problems evolved for which nursing interventions have not been planned or implemented?
- What factors influenced the achievement or lack of achievement of the goals?
- Do priorities need to be reassigned?
- Should changes be made in the goals and expected outcomes?

Objective data that answer these questions must be collected from all available sources (*i.e.*, patient, family or significant others, nursing and other health care team members).

Chart 2-4
Steps of the Nursing Process

Assessment

1. Conduct the nursing history.
2. Perform the health assessment.
3. Interview the patient's family or significant others.
4. Study the health record.
5. Formulate the nursing diagnoses:
   a. Organize, analyze, synthesize, and summarize the collected data.
   b. Identify the patient's nursing problems.
   c. Identify the defining characteristics of the nursing problems.
   d. Identify the etiology of the nursing problems.
   e. State nursing diagnoses concisely and precisely.

Planning

1. Assign priority to the nursing diagnoses.
2. Specify the goals.
   a. Develop immediate, intermediate, and long-term goals.
   b. State the goals in realistic and measurable terms.
3. Identify nursing interventions appropriate for goal attainment.
4. Establish expected outcomes.
   a. Make sure that the outcomes are realistic and measurable.
   b. Identify critical times for the attainment of outcomes.
5. Develop the written nursing care plan.
   a. Include nursing diagnoses, goals, nursing interventions, expected outcomes, and critical times.
   b. Write all entries precisely, concisely, and systematically.
   c. Keep the plan current and flexible to meet the patient's changing problems and needs.
6. Involve the patient, his family or significant others, nursing team members, and other health team members in all aspects of planning.

Implementation

1. Put the nursing care plan into action.
2. Coordinate the activities of the patient, his family or significant others, nursing team members, and other health team members.
3. Record the patient's responses to the nursing actions.

Evaluation

1. Collect objective data.
2. Compare the patient's behavioral outcomes with the expected outcomes. Determine the extent to which the goals were achieved.
3. Include the patient, his family or significant others, nursing team members, and other health care team members in the evaluation.
4. Identify alterations that need to be made in the nursing diagnoses, goals, nursing interventions, and expected outcomes.
5. Continue all steps of the nursing process: assessing, planning, implementing, evaluating.

These data should be available in the patient's record and should be substantiated by direct observation of the patient.

Quality Assurance

Evaluation has traditionally been the most neglected component of the nursing process. However, during the past decade the increased emphasis placed on professional accountability and the advent of quality assurance programs have tended to focus much attention on evaluation. Quality assurance programs are now required for reimbursement of services and for JCAH (Joint Commission on Accreditation of Hospitals) accreditation of hospitals.

- The concept of quality assurance refers to the accountability of the health professions to society for the quality, quantity, and costs of the health services provided.

The impetus for the establishment of quality assurance programs by the health professions was provided by the enactment of the Social Security Amendments of 1972, which provided for the creation of professional standards review organizations (PSROs) as a system for evaluating the quality of health care delivered. Since the advent of diagnosis-related groups (DRGs), hospitals must contract with peer review organizations (PROs) to perform quality and utilization review. The PROs monitor admission patterns, lengths of stay, transfers, and the quality of services and also validate DRG coding.

Nursing has accepted its responsibility for implementation of peer review and thus for accountability for the quality of the nursing care provided. Nurses have recognized their accountability to their patients, their employing institutions, their colleagues and subordinates, other members of the health care team, and the nursing profession.

Quality assurance programs in nursing are viewed as evaluation systems with three components: structure, process, and outcome (see Fig. 2-1).

- The *structural dimension* focuses on the organization within which nursing care is provided.

- The *process dimension* focuses on the actual performance of the tasks, functions, and activities of nursing care.
- The *outcome dimension* focuses on patient welfare, the end results of the care provided to the patient.

The purpose of quality assurance programs is to assure the consumer of excellence of nursing care through objective and continuous measurement of the structure, process, and outcome components against preestablished nursing standards.

Evaluation of structure, process, and outcome are all important and are interrelated, each influencing the other. However, outcomes that provide clinical evidence of the results of care are the ultimate validators of the care rendered. Outcomes focus the attention of the practitioner on the response of the patient to the care that he received. The aim of quality assurance in nursing is to provide a means of improving nursing care where deficits exist.

Outcome Criteria

Goals for accountability and quality assurance in nursing are being realized. The American Nurses' Association has developed basic standards that provide a general model for nursing practice by which the quality of nursing practice may be evaluated. Record keeping has been revised to provide a problem-oriented approach to documentation of data. The problem-oriented record focuses attention on the patient and his problems and allows for the systematic documentation of data by various health care team members. The use of outcome criteria as validators of the nursing process has become an accepted trend. Nurses in various health care settings have developed outcome criteria for specific patient populations. Likewise, the American Nurses' Association has developed outcome criteria that have served as guidelines and as prototypes for criteria used in various health care agencies. The nursing audit has become an accepted method for comparing results of the actual nursing performance with the established criteria. Nursing audit may involve concurrent review or retrospective review of the patient's record. While the patient is in a health care agency, there can be a concurrent review of the patient's record by a nursing group to evaluate whether or not quality care has been given. This provides the opportunity to make changes. There can be a retrospective review of the patient's record (after he leaves the health care agency), which provides another method of evaluation. However, this method of evaluation does not provide an opportunity to make changes for the specific patient who is evaluated.

All methods used to accomplish the evaluation component of the nursing process are directly related to the nursing care plan. Evaluation of the patient's response to nursing interventions is accomplished by comparing the patient's behavioral outcomes with the established outcome criteria. This information then serves as a basis for modification of the nursing care plan.

Evaluation should include self-assessment by the nurse. This can be done through courses of study, programmed learning, reading professional literature, and so on. Concurrently, the nurse reviews her own nursing care. She studies the patient's care plan to decide how many correct decisions were made in nursing assessment, planning, and implementation, as compared with ineffective decisions, and how effective the nursing care is, as measured by valid outcome criteria.

However, it is not enough to evaluate only the effectiveness of the nursing care. An important phase of evaluation is "What should be done to improve the nursing care?" Other nursing interventions may have to be tried. Goals may have to be redesigned. Priorities may have to be reassigned. Outcome criteria may have to be made more realistic. There must be a continuous and thorough scrutiny of the care provided. Then changes are made, plans are altered, and a course of action initiated that will be most supportive to the patient.

Thus, the steps of the nursing process are cyclic and recurrent. Each step is ongoing and is related to all other steps. Continuous evaluation provides the means for maintaining the viability of the entire nursing process and for demonstrating accountability for the quality of nursing care rendered.

For an overall view of the steps of the nursing process, see Chart 2-4.

Bibliography

Books

Alfaro R. Application of the Nursing Process: A Step-by-Step Guide. Philadelphia, JB Lippincott, 1986.

Atkinson LD and Murray ME. Understanding the Nursing Process: New York, Macmillan, 1983.

Carnevali DL. Nursing Care Planning: Diagnosis and Management. Philadelphia, JB Lippincott, 1983.

Carpenito LJ. Handbook of Nursing Diagnosis, 2nd ed. Philadelphia, JB Lippincott, 1987.

Carpenito LJ. Nursing Diagnosis: Application to Clinical Practice, 2nd ed. Philadelphia, JB Lippincott, 1987.

Duke University Hospital Nursing Services. Guidelines for Nursing Care: Process and Outcome. Philadelphia, JB Lippincott, 1983.

Erikson EH. Childhood and Society. New York, WW Norton, 1963.

Gordon M. Manual of Nursing Diagnosis. New York, McGraw-Hill, 1982.

Mayers MG. A Systematic Approach to the Nursing Care Plan. Norwalk, Connecticut, Appleton-Century-Crofts, 1983.

Yura H and Walsh MB. The Nursing Process, 4th ed. Norwalk, Connecticut, Appleton-Century-Crofts, 1983.

Articles

(Asterisks indicate nursing research articles.)

Baer CL. Nursing diagnosis: A futuristic process for nursing practice. Top Clin Nurs 1984 Jan; 5(4):89–97.

Barnard KE. Nursing diagnosis: A descriptive method. Matern Child Nurs J 1983, May/June; 8(3):223.

Barnum BJ. Holistic nursing and nursing process. Holist Nurs Pract 1987 May; 1(3):1–6.

Brooks ER. The starting point. Nurs Manage 1983 June; 14(6):35–37.

Buchanan VR. Efficient nursing care planning. Crit Care Nurs 1984 Mar/Apr; 4(2):14–15.

Bulechek GM and McCloskey JC. Nursing interventions: What they are and how to choose them. Holist Nurs Pract 1987 May; 1(3):36–44.

Carnevali DL. Nursing diagnosis: An evolutionary view. Top Clin Nurs 1984 Jan; 5(4):10–20.

Carpenito LJ. Is the problem a nursing diagnosis? AJN 1984 Nov; 84(11):1418–1419.

Clark SR. Nursing diagnosis: Its application in an ambulatory care setting. Top Clin Nurs 1984 Jan; 5(4):68–77.

Davidson SB. Nursing diagnosis: Its application in the acute-care setting. Top Clin Nurs 1984 Jan; 5(4):50–56.

DeGasperis M. Implementing nursing diagnosis in the critical care setting. Dimens Crit Care Nurs 1983 Jan/Feb; 2(1):44–49.

Donnelly GF. The promise of nursing process: An evaluation. Holist Nurs Pract 1987 May; 1(3):1–6.

Fadden TC and Seiser GK. Nursing diagnosis: A matter of form. Am J Nurs 1984 Apr; 84(4):470–473.

Fraher JE. Nursing diagnoses and care plans in critical care. Crit Care Nurs 1983 Nov/Dec; 3(6):94–98.

Gebbie KM. Nursing diagnosis: What is it and why does it exist? Top Clin Nurs 1984 Jan; 5(4):1–9.

Gerrity PL. Perception in nursing: The value of intuition. Holist Nurs Pract 1987 May; 1(3):63–71.

*Gordon M. Nursing diagnosis. Ann Rev Nurs Res 1985; 3:127–146.

Groah L and Reed EA. Your responsibility in documenting care. AORN J 1983 May; 37(6):1174–1188.

Guzzetta CE and Dossey BM. Nursing diagnosis: Framework, process, and problems. Heart Lung 1983 May; 12(3):281–291.

Hagey RS and McDonough P. The problem of professional labeling. Nurs Outlook 1984 May/June; 32(3):151–157.

Henderson V. Nursing process—a critique. Holist Nurs Pract 1987 May; 1(3):7–18.

Hudson MF. Safeguard your elderly patient's health through accurate physical assessment. Nursing '83 1983 Nov; 13(11):58–64.

King IM. Effectiveness of nursing care: Use of a goal-oriented nursing record in end-stage renal disease. AANNT J 1984 Apr; 11(2):11–17.

Lissesand KM and Korff S. Nursing process evaluation: A quality assurance tool. Nurs Admin Q 1983 Spring; 7(3):9–14.

*Meisenhelder JB. Self-esteem: A closer look at clinical interventions. Int J Nurs Studies 1985; 22(2):127–135.

Neel CJ. Make nursing diagnoses work for you—every day. Nursing '86 1986 May; 16(5):56–57.

Parker SO. A conceptual model for outcome assessment. Nurs Pract 1983 Jan; 8(1):41–45.

Patient-oriented QA activities. QRB 1984 Jan; 10(1):19–25.

Peterson M. Time and nursing process. Holist Nurs Pract 1987 May; 1(3):72–80.

Prose GJG, Gianni N, and Scharf L. Nursing process: One more time. Nurs Manage 1983 Nov; 14(11):32–34.

Putzier DJ and Padrick KP. Nursing diagnosis: A component of nursing process and decision making. Top Clin Nurs 1984 Jan; 5(4):21–29.

Rick PL. Make the most of your charting time. Nursing '83 1983 Mar; 13(3):36–39.

*Roberts SL. The future marriage between diagnosis-related groups and nursing diagnosis-related groups. Crit Care Nurs Q 1987 Mar; 9(4):70–81.

Rutkowski B. How DRGs are changing your charging. Nursing '85 1985 Oct; 15(10):49–51.

*Shea HL. A conceptual framework to study the use of nursing care plans. Int J Nurs Stud 1986; 23(2):147–157.

Smeltzer CH. Organizing the search for excellence. Nurs Manage 1983 June; 14(6):19–21.

Tanner CA and Hughes AG. Nursing diagnosis: Issues in clinical practice research. Top Clin Nurs 1984 Jan; 5(4):30–38.

Warren JJ. Accountability and nursing diagnosis. J Nurs Adm 1983 Oct; 13(10):24–37.

Westfall UE. Nursing diagnosis: Its use in quality assurance. Top Clin Nurs 1984 Jan; 5(4):78–88.

Wiemerslage D. Legal guidelines for documentation. Crit Care Update 1983 June; 10(6):22–23.

Yoder ME. Nursing diagnosis: applications in perioperative practice. AORN J 1984 Aug; 40(2):183–188.

Young CE. Intuition and nursing process. Holist Nurs Pract 1987 May; 1(3):52–62.

Young MS and Lucas CM. Nursing diagnosis: Common problems in implementation. Top Clin Nurs 1984 Jan; 5(4):68–77.

Chapter 3

Patient Education/ Health Teaching

Health Education Today

Health promotion and self-care are concepts that have become a part of the American way of life. Inherent within them is the concept of health education. One of the greatest challenges facing members of the nursing profession today is that of meeting the health education needs of the American public. In this respect, nurses are becoming increasingly sensitive to and conscious of their role as teachers. Health education is considered to be an independent function of nursing practice and a primary responsibility of the nursing profession. Teaching, as a function of nursing, is included in many state nurse practice acts as well as in the American Nurses' Association Standards of Nursing Practice.

- Health education is an essential component of nursing care and is directed toward promotion, maintenance, and restoration of health and toward adaptation to residual effects of illness.

The emphasis placed on the need for health education during recent years perhaps stems in part from the belief of many health care leaders that the American public has the right to expect and receive comprehensive health care, including health education. It also reflects the emergence of a better informed American public, who are asking more significant questions about health, health care, and the services offered by the health care delivery system. Because of the emphasis that the American culture places on health and the responsibility of each individual for the maintenance and promotion of his own health, it is the obligation of the members of the health care delivery system and, specifically, of nurses to make health education available to the American public.

One of the largest groups of people in need of health education today are persons with chronic illnesses. As the life span of our population continues to increase, the number of people in this category will also increase. It is the belief of many health care leaders that persons with chronic illness are entitled to as much health care information as they can handle in order that they may actively participate in and assume responsibility for much of their own care. Health education can aid the individual in adapting to his illness, in cooperating with his prescribed therapy, and in learning to solve problems when confronted with new situations. Health education can prevent rehospitalization for the same condition, which is a frequent result when a person does not understand how to care for his chronic condition.

- The goal of health education is teaching people to live life to its healthiest—that is, to strive toward achieving one's maximum health potential.

Every contact that a nurse has with a patient, whether he is ill or not, should be considered an opportunity for patient teaching. It is the patient's right to decide whether or not he will learn, but it is the nurse's responsibility to present him with the information that he needs to make the decision and to motivate him to appreciate the need for learning.

Many health care agencies are directing their educational efforts not only toward their patient populations but also toward the community in general. A wide variety of health promotion programs are offered either free of charge or for a minimal fee. It is not unusual for health care agencies to offer programs that promote weight reduction, smoking cessation, and exercise, as well as prenatal classes, classes for grandparents, baby-sitter classes, and classes for adults with aging parents. Many of these classes are presented by nurses who have expertise in health promotion.

Adherence to the Therapeutic Regimen

Inherent within the area of patient teaching is the concern for the promotion of the patient's adherence to his therapeutic regimen. The term *compliance* is often used to describe this behavior. However, this term suggests that the patient's role is passive. The term *adherence* implies that the patient assumes an active role in altering his health behaviors.

Adherence to a therapeutic regimen requires that the patient make one or more changes in his life-style. The patient may need to take medications, adhere to a diet, restrict his activities, observe himself for signs and symptoms of illness, practice specific hygienic measures, seek periodic evaluation of his health status, and attend to a host of other therapeutic and preventive measures. The fact that many patients do not adhere to their prescribed regimens cannot be ignored or minimized. The rates of patient adherence to therapeutic and preventive regimens are generally very low, especially when the regimens are complex or of long duration. The characteristics of nonadherent patients and their reasons for not adhering to their prescribed therapy have been the subjects of many studies. For the most part, the findings have been inconclusive. No one factor has been found to be the predominant cause of nonadherence. Instead, it seems that a wide range of variables interacting with one another influence the degree of adherence.

The factors influencing adherence include the following:

- Demographic variables, such as age, sex, race, socioeconomic status, and education
- Illness variables, such as the severity of the illness and the relief of symptoms afforded by the therapy

- Therapeutic regimen variables, such as the complexity of the regimen and uncomfortable side-effects
- Psychosocial variables, such as intelligence, attitudes toward health professionals, acceptance or denial of illness, religious or cultural beliefs, and the costs involved in actuating the regimen.

Knowledge alone concerning health and health promotion and illness and illness prevention has not been found to be a sufficient stimulus to motivate total adherence. However, it has been found that some degree of adherence in some patients is obviously enhanced by the use of teaching programs and by methods directed toward stimulating motivation to adhere to a regimen. The problem of nonadherence to therapeutic regimens is a substantial one that needs to be remedied to assist patients to participate in self-care and to achieve their maximum health potential.

Written contracts between patients and nurses have been found to promote motivation toward adherence for some patients. Contracting is based on the principles of positive reinforcement and behavior modification. Small, easily attainable goals are used to help the patient shape his behavior and then move to more complex goals.

The role of the nurse in teaching and directing patients toward adherence behavior is a significant one. It is the responsibility of the nurse to assess all variables that may have an effect on the patient's adherence and to use this information when developing and implementing the patient's teaching plan.

Gerontological Considerations

The problem of nonadherence to therapeutic regimens is a particularly significant problem among the elderly. Elderly persons frequently have one or more chronic illnesses that are periodically complicated by acute episodes and managed with numerous medications. Besides these problems they also often present with other variables that affect adherence to therapeutic regimens, such as increased sensitivity to drugs and their side-effects, difficulty in adjusting to change and stress, financial constraints to costly therapies, forgetfulness, inadequate support systems, lifetime habits of self-medication with over-the-counter drugs, visual impairments, hearing impairments, and mobility limitations.

To promote adherence to therapeutic regimens by the elderly, time and effort must be taken to assess all variables that may affect this health behavior. In addition, the patient's strengths as well as limitations must be assessed so that his strengths can be capitalized on to minimize his limitations. Above all, continuous coordinated care must be provided to him. Otherwise, the efforts of one health care professional may be negated by the efforts of another.

The Nature of Teaching and Learning

When learning is defined as the acquiring of knowledge, attitudes, or skills, and teaching is defined as helping another person to learn, it becomes evident that the teaching–learning process is an active one. It requires the active involvement of both the teacher and the learner in the effort to reach the desired outcome—change in behavior. The teacher does not give knowledge to the learner but instead serves as a facilitator of learning. In general, there is a lack of knowledge about how learning occurs and is affected by teaching. No single theory of learning suffices to explain how learning occurs. However, some specific principles of learning and some guidelines for teaching have been identified.

Learning Readiness

There are many variables, both internal and external, that affect the learner and the learning situation. One of the most significant of these factors is the learner's readiness to learn—his physical, emotional, and experiential readiness to learn.

Physical readiness is of vital importance because until a patient is physically capable of learning, attempts at teaching and learning may be both futile and frustrating. A patient who is experiencing acute pain is unable to focus his attention away from the pain long enough to concentrate on learning. Likewise, a patient who is short of breath will concentrate his energies on breathing rather than on learning.

- Maslow's hierarchy of needs is helpful in considering the concept of physical readiness for learning.

Emotional readiness involves the patient's motivation to learn. Until the person has begun to accept his illness or to accept the fact that illness is a threat to him, he may not be motivated to learn. If his therapeutic regimen is not acceptable to him or is in conflict with his life-style, he may consciously avoid learning. Until he recognizes the need to learn and his own ability to learn, teaching efforts may be thwarted. However, it is not always wise to wait for the patient to become emotionally ready to learn—this time may never come unless efforts are made by the nurse to stimulate the patient's motivation to learn. Illness and the threat of illness are usually accompanied by anxiety and stress. The nurse who recognizes the patient's reactions to his illness or threatened illness can use simple explanations and instructions to alleviate his anxieties and to further motivate him to learn. It must be remembered that since learning involves changes in behavior, it normally produces mild anxiety. Such anxiety is often a useful motivating factor.

- Emotional readiness can be promoted by creating a warm, accepting, positive atmosphere and by establishing realistic learning goals with the patient so that he can realize success and a feeling of accomplishment, which in themselves are motivators of learning.

Feedback about progress also serves to motivate learning. Such feedback should be presented in the form of positive reinforcement when the patient is successful and in the form of constructive criticism when he is unsuccessful.

Experiential readiness to learn refers to the patient's past experiences that enable him to learn what is being taught. Previous educational experiences and life experiences in general are significant determinants of the patient's approach to learning. A person who has had little or no formal education may not be able to understand the instructional materials presented to him—although this is not always true. The person

who has experienced difficulty in learning in the past may be hesitant to make new attempts to learn. Many behaviors required for meeting one's maximum health potential require a rather extensive background of knowledge, physical skills, and attitudes. If the person does not have this background on which to build, learning may be very difficult and very slow for him. For example, until a patient understands the basics of normal nutrition he may not be able to understand the restrictions of a special diet. Also, a person who is not future oriented will be unable to appreciate many aspects of preventive health teaching. And a person who does not view the desired learning as meaningful to himself and his life-style will reject teaching efforts.

Thus, experiential readiness is closely related to emotional readiness, since motivation tends to be stimulated by one's appreciation for the need to learn and by those learning tasks that are familiar, interesting, and meaningful.

- Prior to initiating a teaching–learning program, the nurse must assess the patient's physical and emotional readiness to learn as well as his level of attainment of those behaviors that are prerequisites to learning what is being taught. This information then becomes the basis for the goals to be established, goals that in themselves can motivate the patient to learn.
- Involvement of the patient in the establishment of goals that are mutually acceptable to him and to the nurse serves the purpose of encouraging the patient to be actively involved in the learning process and to share the responsibility for his learning progress.

The Learning Atmosphere

Although a teacher is not always necessary, most patients who are attempting to learn new or altered health behaviors will need the services of a nurse-teacher at least part of the time. The interpersonal interaction between the patient and the nurse who is attempting to meet the patient's learning needs may be formal or informal, depending on the method and techniques of teaching that are found to be most appropriate for the individual patient.

The nurse facilitates learning by manipulating those external variables that affect the patient's learning. For example, the physical environment should be such that it is conducive to learning. That is, the room temperature, lighting, noise levels, and so on should be appropriate to the learning situation. Also, the time selected for teaching should be suited to the patient's needs. Scheduling a teaching session at a time of day when the patient is fatigued, when he is anticipating diagnostic or therapeutic procedures about which he is anxious, or when he has visitors does not provide a conducive learning environment. Timing of teaching may also be determined by visits of the family members, if they are to be included in the teaching plan.

Teaching Techniques

The nurse also facilitates learning by selecting teaching techniques and methods that are most appropriate to meet the individual patient's needs.

The *lecture or explanation* method of teaching is commonly used but should always be accompanied by discussion.

The discussion is important, since it affords the patient an opportunity to express his feelings and concerns, to ask questions, and to receive clarification of any misinformation or misunderstandings that he may have.

Group teaching is appropriate for some patients because it allows them not only to receive the information that is needed but also to experience security through being a member of a group. Patients with similar problems or learning needs have the opportunity to identify with each other and thus to gain moral support and encouragement. However, it must be remembered that all patients do not relate well in groups and therefore may not benefit from such experiences. It must also be remembered that if group teaching is used, assessment and follow-up of each individual patient is imperative to ensure that each patient gains the knowledge and skills that he needs.

Demonstration and practice are often essential ingredients of the patient's teaching program, especially when skills are to be learned. The nurse first demonstrates the skill to the patient and then allows him ample opportunity to practice the skill. When special equipment is necessary to perform the skill, such as insulin syringes, colostomy bags, dressings, and the like, it is important that the nurse provide the patient with the same equipment that he will be using after he leaves the hospital. Learning to perform a skill with one kind of equipment and then having to change to a different kind of equipment is more than can be expected of most patients.

Teaching aids are available to supplement the abilities of the nurse to help the patient to learn. These include books, pamphlets, pictures, films, slides, tapes, models, and programmed instruction. Such teaching aids are invaluable when used appropriately. It is the responsibility of the nurse to review all such aids before presenting them to patients to be sure that they are designed to meet the individual patient's learning needs.

Reinforcement and follow-up are also important factors to consider, since learning takes time. The patient must be allowed ample time to learn and to have his learning reinforced. A single teaching session is never adequate. Follow-up sessions are imperative to promote the patient's confidence in his ability to follow through with what he has learned. Such sessions also give the nurse the opportunity to evaluate the patient's progress and to plan for additional teaching sessions as required. It is also important to realize that the patient may not be able to transfer what he has learned in the hospital to his home setting. Thus, arrangements for follow-up after discharge are often essential for ensuring that the full benefits of the hospital teaching program have been realized.

The Nursing Process in Patient Teaching

The teaching–learning process is an integral part of the nursing process. With a focus on learning and with regard for the principles of teaching and learning, the steps of the nursing process—assessment, planning, implementation, and evaluation—are used for the purpose of meeting the teaching and learning needs of the patient and his family.

Assessment

Assessment in the teaching–learning process is comparable to that component of the nursing process. It is directed toward the systematic collection of data about the patient's learning needs and readiness to learn and about the family's learning needs. All internal and external variables that affect the patient's readiness to learn are assessed. A learning assessment guide may be helpful in obtaining pertinent information about the patient's need to learn and his readiness to learn. Some of the learning assessment guides available are very general and are directed toward the assessment of general health information. Others are specific to common medication regimens or disease processes. An example is the *Diabetes Mellitus Assessment Guides* published by the American Diabetes Association, North Carolina affiliate, Inc. These assessment guides are designed for the assessment of the diabetic's learning needs with regard to all aspects of the diabetic regimen. Such guides serve to facilitate the assessment but must be adapted to the individual responses, problems, and needs of the patient. As soon as possible after completing the assessment, the nurse organizes, analyzes, synthesizes, and summarizes the data collected and determines the patient's need for teaching. Nursing diagnoses that specifically relate to the patient's learning needs are then succinctly stated and serve to guide the nurse in the development of the teaching plan.

Planning

Once the nursing diagnoses related to the patient's need for learning have been identified, the planning component of the teaching–learning process follows. This plan follows the same sequence used in the nursing process:

1. Assigning priorities to the diagnoses
2. Specifying the immediate, intermediate, and long-term goals of learning
3. Identifying specific teaching strategies appropriate for attaining the goals
4. Specifying the expected outcomes
5. Documenting the diagnoses, goals, teaching strategies, and expected outcomes on the teaching plan

As in the nursing process, the assignment of priorities to the diagnoses should be a joint effort by the nurse and the patient or his family members. Consideration must be given to the urgency of the patient's learning needs, the most critical needs receiving the highest priority.

After the priorities of the diagnoses have been established, the immediate, intermediate, and long-term goals and the teaching strategies appropriate for attaining the goals are identified. Studies have indicated that teaching is most effective when the patient's goals and the nurse's goals are in agreement. Goal-directed learning should begin with the establishment of goals that are appropriate to the situation and that are realistic in terms of the patient's ability to achieve them. Goals should be individualized according to the needs of the patient, specifically the needs perceived by the patient, and must be acceptable to the nurse, the patient, and the family. Involving the patient and his family in goal establish-

Chart 3-1
Example of a Teaching Plan*

Assessment of Mrs. Walker's teaching and learning needs revealed the following:

Basic knowledge about the relationship between stress and physiologic functioning
Life-style conducive to excessive stress
Irregularity of meals
Previous nonadherence to dietary regimen
Inadequate knowledge about diet restrictions

Nursing Diagnosis

Potential nonadherence to dietary regimen related to knowledge deficit and life-style

Goals

Immediate: Demonstrates knowledge of dietary regimen
Intermediate: Adheres to the dietary regimen
Long-term: Alters life-style to reduce emotional and environmental stressors

Teaching Strategies	Expected Outcomes	Critical Times†	Outcomes
Provide consultation with dietitian			
Reinforce instructions given by dietitian regarding: 1500-calorie diet	Explains purposes of diet restrictions in relation to own condition	24 hr	Related explanation accurately.
1-gm sodium diet Low cholesterol diet	Identifies ways in which her diet can be compatible with family's diet	48 hr	Planned meals for family for 1 week that included modifications compatible with dietary restrictions
			Identified need to plan schedule to accommodate regularity of meals
			Called Weight Watchers and made plans to begin in 1 week
Discuss necessity for life-style alterations with patient and husband	Decreases daily and weekend work hours Plans for daily periods of rest and relaxation	During and after hospitalization	Patient and husband working together to begin life-style alterations that will promote stress reduction; daughters included in plans
	Shares, with husband, responsibilities related to daughters' activities		Patient and husband developed schedule of daily and weekend activities, incorporating plans for designated periods of rest and relaxation; aware of desirability of flexibility of schedule
Notify physician's office nurse of patient's need for reinforcement of teaching plan	Demonstrates adherence to dietary regimen	First physician visit after discharge	

* For background information, see Example of an Individualized Nursing Care Plan, pp. 28–29.
† These times have not been standardized but are individualized according to the patient's needs.

Chart 3-2
A Guide to Patient Teaching

Assessment

1. Assess the patient's readiness for health education.
   a. What are his health beliefs and behaviors?
   b. What psychosocial adaptation is he making?
   c. Is he ready to learn?
      Is he able to learn these behaviors?
      What additional information about him is needed?
      What are his expectations?
      What does he want to learn?
2. Formulate the nursing diagnoses that relate to the patient's learning needs.
   a. Organize, analyze, synthesize, and summarize the collected data.
   b. Identify the patient's learning needs, their characteristics, and etiology.
   c. State nursing diagnoses concisely and precisely.

Planning

1. Assign priority to the nursing diagnoses that relate to the patient's learning needs.
2. Specify the immediate, intermediate, and long-term nurse–patient established learning goals.
3. Identify teaching strategies appropriate for goal attainment.
4. Establish expected outcomes.
5. Develop the written teaching plan.
   a. Include diagnoses, goals, teaching strategies, and expected outcomes.
   b. Put the information to be taught in logical sequence.
   c. Write down the key points.
   d. Select appropriate teaching aids.
   e. Keep the plan current and flexible to meet the patient's changing learning needs.
6. Involve the patient, his family or significant others, nursing team members, and other health care team members in all aspects of planning.

Implementation

1. Put the teaching plan into action.
2. Know the material to be presented.
3. Use language the patient can understand.
4. Use appropriate teaching aids.
5. Use the same equipment that the patient will use after discharge.
6. Encourage the patient to actively participate in learning.
7. Record the patient's responses to the teaching actions.
8. Give feedback.

Evaluation

1. Collect objective data.
   a. Observe the patient.
   b. Ask questions to determine if he understands.
   c. Use rating scales, checklists, anecdotal notes, and written tests when appropriate.
2. Compare the patient's behavioral responses with the expected outcomes. Determine the extent to which the goals were achieved.
3. Include the patient, his family or significant others, nursing team members, and other health care team members in the evaluation.
4. Identify alterations that need to be made in the teaching plan.
5. Make referrals to appropriate sources or agencies for reinforcement of learning after discharge.
6. Continue all steps of the teaching process: assessing, planning, implementing, evaluating.

ment and subsequent planning of teaching strategies promotes their cooperation in the implementation of the teaching plan.

Expected outcomes of the teaching strategies are stated in terms of the patient's behaviors. Every effort is made to develop outcomes that are realistic and measurable. The critical time periods within which the outcomes should be demonstrated by the patient are also identified. The outcomes and the critical time periods will serve as a basis for evaluation of the effectiveness of the teaching strategies.

During the planning phase, the nurse gives consideration to the sequence in which the subject matter will be presented to the patient when each of the teaching strategies is implemented. An outline is often helpful for arranging subject matter and for ensuring that all necessary information is included. Also during this time, the nurse selects and secures the appropriate teaching aids to be used in implementing the teaching strategies.

The entire planning phase of the teaching–learning process is concluded with the formulation of the patient's teaching plan by the nurse. This teaching plan communicates the following information to all members of the nursing team.

1. The nursing diagnoses that specifically relate to the patient's learning needs and the priorities of these diagnoses
2. The goals of the teaching strategies
3. The teaching strategies, which are expressed in the form of teaching orders
4. The expected outcomes, which identify the expected behavioral responses for the patient
5. The critical time period within which each outcome must be met
6. The patient's behavioral responses (must be documented on the teaching plan)

The same rules that apply to writing and revising the nursing care plan apply to the teaching plan. (For a sample teaching plan, see Chart 3-1. Note that it is not different from but is simply a continuation of the nursing care plan.)

Implementation

The implementation phase of the teaching–learning process follows the formulation of the teaching plan. The patient, his family, and other members of the nursing team and the health care team are included in the implementation. The activities of all of these persons are coordinated by the nurse, and the teaching plan serves as the basis for implementation.

- It is important to remain flexible during the implementation phase of the teaching–learning process and to continuously assess the patient's responses to the teaching strategies and to make alterations in the teaching plan as necessary.

It is highly desirable that the nurse use her creativity to the fullest to promote and sustain the patient's motivation to learn; she should anticipate teaching needs that may arise after the patient's discharge from the hospital that are not foreseen by the patient while he is still in the hospital. Then, and only then, can she assist the patient in transferring knowledge from the hospital to his home. The implementation phase is concluded when the teaching strategies have been completed and when the patient's responses to the actions have been recorded. This record serves as the basis for the evaluation of the patient's accomplishment of the defined expected outcomes.

Evaluation

Evaluation is the final component of the teaching–learning process and is directed toward the determination of the patient's response to the teaching strategies and the extent to which the goals have been achieved. Evaluation for the teaching–learning process will answer the same question as that used for the nursing process but with specific regard to teaching and learning. An important phase in evaluation remains: "What should be done to improve the teaching?" Answers to this question will dictate changes that must be made in the teaching plan.

It should never be assumed that an individual has learned because he has been taught. Learning does not automatically follow teaching. A variety of measurement techniques can be used to measure changes in behavior that give evidence of learning. These include direct observation of behavior, using rating scales, checklists, or anecdotal notes to document the behaviors, and indirect measures, such as oral questioning and written tests. Measurement of actual behavior (direct measurement) is the most accurate and appropriate technique in many patient teaching situations. However, it should be supplemented with indirect measurements whenever possible. When more than one measurement technique is employed, the reliability of the resultant data is enhanced since each individual measurement technique carries with it a potential source of error.

The use of measurement techniques is only the beginning of evaluation. It is followed by the interpretation of the data and the making of value judgments about learning and teaching. Such evaluation should be done periodically throughout the teaching–learning program, at its conclusion, and at varying periods subsequent to the program. Evaluation of learning after hospitalization is highly desirable but is not always feasible in terms of time, economics, and nursing personnel required for such evaluation. However, coordination of efforts and sharing of information between hospital-based and community-based nursing personnel serves to facilitate such post-hospital evaluation.

It should always be remembered that evaluation is not the end step in the teaching–learning process. The information gathered during evaluation should be used to redirect teaching actions with the goal of improving the patient's responses and outcomes that result from the teaching actions.

As in the nursing process, the steps of the teaching–learning process are cyclic and recurrent. Each step is ongoing and is related to all other steps. Continuous evaluation provides the means for maintaining the viability of the entire teaching–learning process and for demonstrating accountability for the quality of the teaching provided.

Chart 3-2 is intended to assist in the nurse's utilization of the teaching–learning process.

Bibliography

Books

Rankin SH and Duffy KL. Patient Education: Issues, Principles, and Guidelines. Philadelphia, JB Lippincott, 1983.

Redman BK. The Process of Patient Education. St Louis, CV Mosby, 1984.

Articles

Baer CL. Compliance: The challenge of the future. Top Clin Nurs 1986 Jan; 7(4):77–85.

Ballard NR. Promoting compliance in rehabilitation of a patient with a myocardial infarction. Top Clin Nurs 1986 Jan; 7(4):57–64.

Bille DA. Process-oriented patient education. Dimens Crit Care Nurs 1983 Mar/Apr; 2(2):108–115.

Brunner NA. Principles of teaching and learning. Orthop Nurs 1983 July/Aug; 2(4):22–23.

Burckhardt CS. Ethical issues in compliance. Top Clin Nurs 1986 Jan; 7(4):9–16.

Clark SR. Compliance and health behaviors. Top Clin Nurs 1986 Jan; 7(4):39–46.

Corkadel L and McGlashan R. A practical approach to patient teaching. J Contin Educ Nurs 1983 Jan/Feb; 14(1):9–15.

Cushing M. Legal lessons on patient teaching. Am J Nurs 1984 June; 84(6):721–722.

Davidson SB. Using compliance research in clinical practice. Top Clin Nurs 1986 Jan; 7(4):65–76.

Edel MK. Noncompliance: An appropriate nursing diagnosis? Nurs Outlook 1985 July/Aug; 33(4):183–185.

Fedder DO. Drug use in the elderly: Issues of noncompliance. Drug Intell Clin Pharm 1984 Feb; 18:158–162.

Ford D and Griffin J. Closed-circuit TV. Nurs Manage 1983 Jan; 14(1):19–21.

Levin LS. Prospective payment and the educational component. Patient Educ Couns 1984; 6(2):66–68.

Lewis SJ. Teaching patient groups. Nurs Manage 1984 May; 15(5):49–56.

Loughrey L. Dealing with the illiterate patient . . . you can't read him like a book. Nursing '83 1983 Jan; 13(1):65–67.

Lucas CM. Compliance and illness responses. Top Clin Nurs 1986 Jan; 7(4):47–56.

McCord MA. Compliance: Self care or compromise? Top Clin Nurs 1986 Jan; 7(4):1–8.

Padrick KP. Compliance: Myths and motivators. Top Clin Nurs 1986 Jan; 7(4):17–22.

Rankin SH and Duffy KL. 15 problems in patient education and their solutions. Nursing '84 1984 Apr; 14(4):67–81.

Rice NC. Guidelines for patient education. Physician Assist 1983 Sept; 7(9):55–56.

Rutkowski BC. The nurse: Also an educator, patient advocate, and counselor. Nurs Clin North Am 1982 Sept; 17(3):455–466.

Stanton MP. Patient education in the hospital health-care setting. Patient Educ Couns 1983; 5(1):14–22.

Steckel SB. Predicting, measuring, implementing and following up on patient compliance. Nurs Clin North Am 1982 Sept; 17(3):491–497.

Tarcinale MA. Adult learning principles—basis for educating the burn nurse. J Burn Care Rehabil 1983 Jan/Feb; 4(1):19–23.

Trekas J. It takes 2 to achieve compliance. Nursing '84 1984 Sept; 14(9):58–59.

Ward DB. Why patient teaching fails. RN 1986 Jan; 49(1):45–47.

Westfall UE. Methods for assessing compliance. Top Clin Nurs 1986 Jan; 7(4):23–30.

Young MS. Strategies for improving compliance. Top Clin Nurs 1986 Jan; 7(4):31–38.

Chapter 4

Health Promotion

In recent years there has been a virtual explosion of health promotion activities. Health care professionals who have traditionally focused on the curing of disease are turning their attention to prevention. Their focus is on improvement of health by altering life-style and by modifying factors that predispose to undesirable alterations in health.

The concept of health promotion has evolved from a changing definition of health and from an awareness that wellness exists on a continuum that extends from premature death at one extreme to optimal health at the other extreme. The definition of health as the mere absence of disease or as the quality of a person's physiologic functioning is no longer accepted. Today, *health* is regarded as a composite of physical, psychological, emotional, social, and spiritual functioning that allows the person to carry out his roles and responsibilities and to move toward self-fulfillment in a variety of situations. Health is viewed as a dynamic, ever-changing condition, the status of which is measured in terms of how well the person uses his skills and abilities to strive toward functioning at his optimum potential at any given point in time. The ideal health status is one in which the person is successful in achieving his full potential regardless of any disabilities he may have.

The concept of wellness expands on the idea of health. *Wellness* is a process with many possible levels or degrees. It involves a conscious and deliberate approach toward maximizing one's health. Wellness does not just happen—it requires planning and conscious commitment. It is the result of life-style behaviors that are designed for the purpose of attaining one's highest potential for well-being. Wellness is not the same for every person. The person with a chronic illness or disability can have the same or a greater level of wellness as a person without such an illness or disability. The key to wellness is whether or not the person is functioning at his highest potential within the limitations over which he has no control.

A significant amount of research has shown that people, by virtue of what they do or what they fail to do, influence their own health. Today, many of the major causes of illnesses are chronic diseases that have been closely related to life-style behaviors (*e.g.,* heart disease, lung and colon cancer, chronic obstructive pulmonary diseases, hypertension, cirrhosis, and peptic ulcers). Thus, a person's health status to a large extent reflects his style of living.

Health promotion can be defined as activities that, by accentuating the positive, assist the person to develop those resources that will maintain or enhance his well-being and improve the quality of his life. It refers to the activities that a person does for himself in the absence of symptoms in an attempt to remain healthy and that do not need the assistance of a member of the health care team. The purpose of health promotion is to focus on the person's potential for wellness and to encourage him to alter his personal habits, life-style, and environment in ways that will enable him to enhance his health and well-being. Health promotion is an active process, that is, it is not something that can be prescribed or dictated. It is up to the individual to decide for himself whether he will make the changes that will help him to enhance his own health status and attain a higher level of wellness. Choices must be made, and only the person himself can make these choices.

A variety of health appraisal tools have been developed to facilitate the health promotion process. These tools generally are used to collect information about the person's health habits and life-style and related information such as age, sex, race, past health history, and family health history. The information is then used to determine the strengths and limitations of the individual's life-style and health habits, providing a basis for counseling him in making choices about his health behaviors.

The concepts of health, wellness, and health promotion have been extensively addressed in the lay literature and news media as well as in professional journals. The result has been a public outcry for health information and a tremendous response by health care professionals and agencies to provide this information. Health promotion programs that were once limited to hospital settings have now moved into the community in settings such as schools, churches, business, and industry. The topic of health is of interest to virtually every individual and every group.

Health Promotion Principles

Health promotion as a concept and as an active process is built on the principles of self-responsibility, nutritional awareness, stress reduction and management, and physical fitness.

Self-Responsibility

Self-responsibility is the key to successful health promotion. It involves the recognition that the individual, and only the individual, has control over his life. He and only he can make those choices that determine whether his life-style is one that promotes health. As more people are recognizing the significant effect that life-style behaviors have on health, they are assuming responsibility for avoiding high-risk behaviors such as smoking, abusing alcohol and drugs, overeating, driving while intoxicated, and other unhealthy practices. They are also assuming responsibility for developing practices that have been found to be positive influences in promoting health, such as engaging in regular exercise, wearing a seat belt, and following a balanced diet.

A variety of different techniques have been used to try to encourage people to accept responsibility for promoting their health. These have ranged from extensive educational programs to reward systems and contracts. Studies have not shown any one technique to be superior to any other. Instead, it seems that self-responsibility for health promotion is very individualized and depends on the person's desires and inner motivations. Health promotion programs are important tools for offering encouragement to the individual to assume responsibility for his health and to develop behaviors that positively affect health.

Nutrition

Nutrition as a component of health promotion has received more attention and publicity than any other. There is a vast array of books and magazine articles that address the topics of special diets, natural foods, and the hazards of certain substances such as sugar, salt, cholesterol, and food additives. Good nutrition has been suggested as the single most significant factor in determining health status and longevity.

Nutritional awareness involves an understanding of the importance of a properly balanced diet that supplies all of the essential nutrients and an understanding of the relationship between diet and disease. A diet that promotes health is thought to be one that substitutes natural foods for processed and refined ones and that reduces intake of sugar, salt, fat, caffeine, alcohol, and food additives and preservatives.

Chapter 6 of this text, Physical Assessment and Nutritional Assessment, contains detailed information on the assessment of the individual's nutritional status. Physical signs indicating nutritional status, anthropometric measurements, assessment of food intake (food record, 24-hour recall), the basic four food groups, recommended daily dietary allowances, and ideal-weight tables are covered in the text and in tables.

Stress Management

Stress management and stress reduction have become important aspects of health promotion as studies have shown the deleterious effects of stress on health and a cause-and-effect relationship between stress and infectious diseases, traffic accidents, and some chronic illnesses. Stress is a part of the American way of life. It has become inevitable in our high-tech, urban society in which self-imposed demands for productivity have become excessive. Thus, more and more emphasis is placed on encouraging people to manage their stress appropriately and to reduce stress that is counterproductive. Techniques such as relaxation training, exercise, and modification of stress-producing situations are often included in health promotion programs that deal with stress. The reader is referred to Chapter 8, Stress and Adaptation, for further information on stress management, including health risk appraisal and stress reduction methods such as biofeedback and the relaxation response.

Exercise

Physical fitness is another important component of health promotion. The relationship between health and physical fitness has been studied closely. It has been found that a regular exercise program can promote health by improving functioning of the circulatory system and the lungs, decreasing cholesterol and low density lipoproteins, lowering body weight by increasing calorie expenditure, delaying degenerative changes such as osteoporosis, and improving flexibility and overall muscle strength and endurance. Despite these benefits, exercise can be harmful if it is not started gradually and increased slowly in accordance with the individual's response. An exercise program should be designed specifically for the individual, with consideration given to age, physical condition, and any known cardiovascular risk factors. An appropriate exercise program can have a significant positive effect on the individual's performance capacity, appearance, and general state of health.

Health Promotion Throughout the Life Span

Health promotion as a concept and a process is not limited to any particular age-group. Instead, it extends throughout the life span. Studies have shown that the health of a child can be affected, either positively or negatively, by the health practices of the mother during the prenatal period. Thus, health promotion starts before birth and extends through childhood, adulthood, and old age.

Childhood

For many years health screening has been an important aspect of childhood health care. The goal has been to detect health problems at an early age so that they can be remedied and the child's health status can be improved. Today, health promotion goes beyond the mere screening of children for disabilities. Extensive efforts are made to promote positive health practices at a very young age. Since health habits and practices are in the formative stages during the years of childhood, children are more susceptible to influences that promote positive health attitudes than they are in the adult years. For this reason more and more programs are being offered to school-age children to help them to develop good health habits. The emphasis is not so much on the negative results of such practices as smoking, alcohol and drug abuse, and poor nutrition as on values training, building of self-esteem, and wellness life-style practices. The programs are designed to appeal to the particular age-group, with emphasis on learning experiences that are fun and interesting.

Young and Middle-Aged Adults

Health promotion for young and middle-aged adults has received more emphasis than for any other age-group. These groups, as a whole, are fascinated by health and health promotion. They have responded positively and enthusiastically to studies that show how life-style practices affect health. Those who are highly motivated are self-sufficient in changing their life-styles in ways that are believed to enhance health and wellness. More often than not, however, adults who wish to improve their health turn to health promotion programs to assist them in making the desired changes in their life-styles. They respond in overwhelming numbers to programs

that focus on such topics as general wellness, smoking cessation, exercise, physical conditioning, weight control, and stress management. Because of the nationwide emphasis on health during the reproductive years, young adults actively seek out programs that address prenatal health, parenting, family planning, and women's health issues. Programs that provide health screening such as those that screen for cancer, hypertension, diabetes, and hearing impairments are quite popular with adults. Programs that deal with health promotion for people with specific chronic illnesses such as cancer, diabetes, heart disease, and pulmonary disease are also popular. It is becoming more and more evident that chronic disease does not preclude health and wellness but that positive health attitudes and practices can promote optimal health for persons who must live with the limitations imposed by the chronic nature of their illnesses.

Because a person's motivation does not always suffice to encourage him to strive toward optimal health, health promotion programs are being offered in a variety of settings. For many adults, it is too much to expect that they will spend excessive time after a day at work traveling to an inconvenient place to exercise, learn about health risks, or perhaps join a smoking cessation group. Thus, health promotion programs have subscribed to the outreach approach. Although many programs are still available in centrally located health care agencies, more and more are becoming available in neighborhood settings. Common sites are elementary schools, high schools, community colleges, recreation centers, and churches. Health fairs are common in civic centers and shopping malls. The outreach idea for health promotion programs has served to meet the needs of many adults who otherwise would not avail themselves of opportunities to strive toward a healthier life-style.

Health promotion has also entered the realm of business and industry. Employers are becoming increasingly concerned about the rising costs of health care to treat illnesses that are related to life-style behaviors. They are also concerned about increased absenteeism and lost productivity. For these reasons many businesses are instituting health promotion programs in the workplace. Some employ health promotion specialists to develop and implement the program for them, while others purchase packaged programs that have already been developed by health care agencies or private health promotion corporations. The programs that are offered at the workplace usually include employee health screening and counseling, physical fitness, nutritional awareness, work safety, and stress management and reduction. Efforts are made to promote a safe and healthy work environment. Many large businesses provide exercise facilities for their employees and offer their health promotion programs to retirees. If employers can show cost-containment benefits from such programs, their dollars will be considered well spent, and more businesses will provide health promotion programs as a benefit of employment.

Elderly Adults

Health promotion is as important for the elderly as it is for other age-groups. Despite the fact that 80% of people over the age of 65 have one or more chronic illnesses and about 50% of the aged population have activity limitations, the elderly as a group have been found to experience significant gains from health promotion. Studies have shown that the elderly are very health conscious and that many of them are willing to adopt practices that will improve their health and well-being. Although their chronic illnesses and disabilities cannot be eliminated, these adults can benefit from activities that help them to achieve an optimal level of health.

Activities directed toward health promotion for the elderly are the same as those for other age-groups: physical fitness and exercise, nutrition, safety, and stress management and reduction. Physical fitness and exercise have not enjoyed as much popularity among the elderly as they have among younger people, but they are slowly catching on. Studies have shown that more than half of all people over the age of 65 do not exercise on a regular basis. However, this figure is slowly decreasing because the elderly are becoming more aware of the benefits of exercise for them, such as improved cardiovascular function, increased ventilatory capacity, reduced body fat, and enhanced muscle strength, endurance, and flexibility. Exercise programs for the elderly, as for other people, are based on each person's physical abilities. They are begun slowly and, when appropriate, with medical advice. Programs that meet the needs of older people confined to wheelchairs or beds are not uncommon.

The importance of adequate nutrition for the elderly is paramount. Nutritional deficiencies are common among the elderly and have been found to cause depression, confusion, headache, fatigue, and irritability. There is a significant need for nutritional counseling that does not simply stress those foods that are to be avoided but that presents information about what constitutes a healthy diet. Consideration must be given to physiologic factors such as impaired senses of taste or smell and dental health. Nutritional deficiencies can sometimes be easily remedied with properly fitting dentures. Psychosocial variables such as income, cultural influences, and food habits must be considered also.

The safety aspect of health promotion is as important, if not more important, for the elderly as for younger people. The elderly are particularly prone to injuries resulting from falls and automobile accidents. In many cases falls could be prevented if the person's home environment were altered to include appropriate safety features. Many older people can benefit from knowing that their visual acuity is impaired at night because of decreased ability of the eye to adapt to the darkness. In such cases the use of nightlights and the restriction of automobile driving to the daytime hours can help to prevent accidents. Encouragement of the elderly to use seat belts in automobiles is also important, since only 10% of elderly people report that they use seat belts on a regular basis. Proper use of drugs is another aspect of safety that is important for the elderly, who are heavy consumers of medications. They often do not take drugs as prescribed and mix prescription with nonprescription drugs. Community programs directed toward health promotion for the elderly are beginning to focus on the various aspects of safety that are particularly important to this age-group.

Finally, stress management and reduction is not reserved for younger age-groups but must be considered equally important for the elderly. The stresses confronted by the elderly are varied and can include difficulty coping with retirement, financial insecurity, health problems, unwanted change of residence, loss of a spouse, and feelings of helplessness and despair. Some strides have been made in helping people plan for their later years in an attempt to decrease these stresses.

It seems that health promotion that starts during the young and middle years and that focuses on making plans for the later years is more successful than are efforts directed toward stress reduction after the elderly person is already faced with stress-provoking situations that seem insurmountable. Many businesses offer pre-retirement programs designed to help their employees prepare for the life-style changes that accompany retirement. As the population of older Americans continues to increase, more and more of these programs are needed. Health care and community groups are also recognizing this need and are beginning to offer such programs. The focus of these programs is the idea that aging is not synonymous with illness and uselessness, and that focusing on wellness while growing old can promote control over one's health and state of well-being.

Many health promotion programs have been developed to meet the needs of older Americans. Many of these began within the Department of Health and Human Services. Both public and private organizations have been responsive to this initiative, and more programs that serve the elderly are emerging. Many of these are offered by health care agencies, churches, recreational centers, senior citizen residences, and a variety of other organizations.

Health Promotion Programs

Considering the fact that health promotion encompasses the entire life span and is applicable to both sexes, to people of all socioeconomic and cultural backgrounds, and to people who have no health problems as well as those with chronic illnesses and disabilities, the numbers and types of health promotion programs that have been developed are extensive. These can be categorized as health screening, wellness, safety, disease management, and various others. Examples of each of these categories of programs are presented in Chart 4-1. The formats for these programs vary from lectures to workshops, support groups, health fairs, and computer-assisted programs. The settings vary depending on the needs of the target group. Some are presented in schools, churches, businesses, day-care centers, recreational centers, and shopping malls. As the health promotion movement continues to grow, more and more programs and activities will move out of the health care agencies into the community where larger numbers of people can be reached and served.

Future Trends

With the current progress that is being made in health promotion, future trends can be anticipated. It is expected that the government and employers will become more aggressive in their efforts to decrease health care costs. More emphasis will be placed on health promotion in the workplace. Insurance policies will offer incentives for wellness. The government will increase the regulations on the health care industry, requiring health promotion and wellness programs as a way of controlling costs.

Two specific groups who will have a significant impact on health promotion are children and the elderly. It is ex-

Chart 4-1
Health Promotion Programs

Health Screening

Cancer
Diabetes
Growth and development
Heart disease
Hypertension
Self-examination (breasts, testes)
Speech and hearing

Wellness

Aerobic exercise
Aging
Alcohol abuse prevention
Cancer prevention
Childbirth preparation
Drug abuse prevention
Exercise
General wellness
Heart disease prevention
Mental health
Nutrition
Physical fitness and conditioning
Planning for retirement
Prenatal classes
Smoking cessation
Stress reduction and management
Stroke prevention
Weight control and management
Women's health issues

Safety

Accident prevention
Child safety
First aid
Infant safety
Medication use
Poison prevention
Sports injury prevention

Disease Management

Alcohol abuse
Arthritis
Cancer
Diabetes
Drug abuse
Heart disease
Hypertension
Pain
Pulmonary disease

Miscellaneous

Babysitter classes
Cardiopulmonary resuscitation (CPR)
Family planning
Grandparenting
Parenting
Sibling classes

pected that a large proportion of health promotion programs will be aimed at school-age children, particularly those between the ages of 8 and 12. The purpose of this is to promote good health practices at an age when children are most susceptible to such influences. In the long run, it is believed that this will pay off by increasing the health of future generations and thus controlling the monies that are spent on medical care.

It is anticipated that the growing population of older people will provide a major market for health promotion programs. The number of Americans over the age of 65 is expected to increase to about 20% of the population by the middle of the 21st century. This generation of senior citizens is expected to be more self-sufficient, more responsible for their own health, and more demanding of means to promote their health and wellness. They are a prime target group for health promotion programs and activities.

Health promotion is certainly not the only answer to the health problems that exist in this country, but it is one answer. Without it, the health problems of this nation will not be solved. It is one opportunity to be used to strive toward meeting the health needs of individuals and of our society in general.

Bibliography

Books

Creek SF and Mettler M. A Healthy Old Age: A Sourcebook for Health Promotion with Older Adults. New York, Haworth Press, 1984.

Edelman C and Mandle CL. Health Promotion Throughout the Lifespan. St Louis, CV Mosby, 1986.

Ewles L and Simnett I. Promoting Health: A Practical Guide to Health Education. New York, John Wiley & Sons, 1985.

Greene WH and Simons-Morton BG. Introduction to Health Education. New York, Macmillan, 1984.

Murray RB and Zentner JP. Nursing Assessment and Health Promotion Through the Life Span. Englewood Cliffs, New Jersey, Prentice-Hall, 1985.

O'Donnell MP and Ainsworth TH. Health Promotion in the Workplace. New York, John Wiley & Sons, 1984.

Articles

(Asterisks indicate nursing research articles.)

Ardell DB. The history and future of wellness. Health Values 1985 Nov/Dec; 9(6):37–56.

Bragg C and Hughes GH. Understanding and managing patients who smoke. Fam Community Health 1984 May; 7(1):12–21.

Branden JE. Health promotion and wellness in rehabilitative services. J Rehabil 1985 Oct/Dec; 51(4):54–58.

Brown-Bryant R. The issue of women's health: A matter of record. Fam Community Health 1985 Feb; 7(4):53–65.

Butnarescu G. Women's health: An investment in the future. Issues Health Care Women 1983 Mar/June; 4(2/3):93–105.

Carlyon WH. Disease prevention/health promotion—bridging the gap to wellness. Health Values 1984 May/June; 8(3):27–30.

Carter GF. Health is a status. Health Educ 1984 Jan/Feb; 15(1):33–35.

Chalmers K and Farrell P. Nursing interventions for health promotion. Nurs Pract 1983 Nov/Dec; 8(10):62, 64.

Clark SR. Compliance and health behaviors. Top Clin Nurs 1986 Jan; 7(4):39–46.

Fiorello J. Creating health for a new age. Home Healthcare Nurse 1984 Mar/Apr; 2(2):18–32.

Flynn JB and Giffin PA. Health promotion in acute care settings. Nurs Clin North Am 1984 June; 19(2):239–250.

Frachel RR. Health hazard appraisal: Personal and professional implications. J Nurs Educ 1984 June; 23(6):265–267.

Fretz WS. Maintaining wellness: Yours and theirs. Nurs Clin North Am 1984 June; 19(2):263–269.

Grasser C and Craft BJG. The patient's approach to wellness. Nurs Clin North Am 1984 June; 19(2):207–218.

Greenberg JS. Health and wellness: A conceptual differentiation. J Sch Health 1985 Dec; 55(10):403–406.

Hall BA and Allen JD. Sharpening nursing's focus by focusing on health. Nurs Health Care 1986 June; 7(6):315–320.

Haskell WL and Superko R. Designing an exercise plan for optimal health. Fam Community Health 1984 May; 7(1):72–88.

Hataway H, Raines JL, and Weinsier RL. Nutrition: Its ever-increasing role. Fam Community Health 1984 May; 7(1):22–37.

Hataway J and Bragg C. Cancer: What is prevention? Fam Community Health 1984 May; 7(1):59–71.

Heckler MM. Health promotion for older Americans. Public Health Rep 1985 Mar/Apr; 100(2):225–230.

Herman JA. Exploding aging myths through retirement counseling. J Gerontol Nurs 1984 Apr; 10(4):31–33.

Hettler B. Wellness: Encouraging a lifetime pursuit of excellence. Health Values 1984 July/Aug; 8(4):13–17.

Hyner GC and Melby CL. Health risk appraisals: Use and misuse. Fam Community Health 1985 Feb; 7(4):13–25.

Jordan-Marsh M, Gilbert J, Ford JD, and Kleeman C. Life-style intervention: A conceptual framework. Patient Educ Couns 1984; 6(1):29–38.

Kee CC. A case for health promotion with the elderly. Nurs Clin North Am 1984 June; 19(2):251–262.

*Killeen ML. Taking risks with health. West J Nurs Res 1985 Feb; 7(1):116–124.

Kirkpatrick SL. Nurses: Leaders in wellness. Occup Health Nurs 1985 Sept; 33(9):450–452.

Kolanowski A and Gunter LM. What are the health practices of retired career women? J Gerontol Nurs 1985 Dec; 11(12):22–30.

Kulys R and Meyer R. Good health: Whose responsibility? Soc Work Health Care 1985 Fall; 11(1):63–84.

*Laffrey SC. Development of a health conception scale. Res Nurs Health 1986; 9:107–113.

Laffrey SC. Health promotion: Relevance for nursing. Top Clin Nurs 1985 July; 7(2):29–38.

McClary CL et al. Wellness: The mode in the new paradigm. Health Values 1985 Nov/Dec; 9(6):8–12.

McCracken-Knights A. Look beyond your clients' answers: Are the elderly as healthy as they say? J Gerontol Nurs 1985 May; 11(3):20–22.

Moore PV and Williamson GC. Health promotion: Evolution of a concept. Nurs Clin North Am 1984 June; 19(2):195–206.

Oberman A. Components of health promotion. Fam Community Health 1984 May; 7(1):1–11.

O'Connell JK and Price JH. Ethical theories for promoting health through behavioral change. J Sch Health 1983 Oct; 53(8):476–479.

*Pender NJ. Health promotion and illness prevention. Annu Rev Nurs Res 1984; 2:83–105.

*Pender NJ and Pender AR. Attitudes, subjective norms, and intentions to engage in health behaviors. Nurs Res 1986 Jan/Feb; 35(1):15–18.

Post S. Changing attitudes in health promotion. Can Nurse 1986 Feb; 82(2):34–37.

Robinson TC. Health promotion, disease prevention: An allied health initiative. J Allied Health 1984 Nov; 13(4):243–251.

Shultz CM. Life-style assessment: A tool for practice. Nurs Clin North Am 1984 June; 19(2):271–281.

Tatro S and Gleit CJ. A wellness model for nursing: Promoting high level wellness in any setting through independent nursing functions. Nurs Leadership 1983 Mar; 6(1):5–9.

Washington WN. An interactive model for wellness: A systems approach. Fam Community Health 1985 Feb; 7(4):44–52.

Webster JA. The wellness model: Feeling good about yourself. AORN J 1985 Apr; 41(4):713–718.

Weiner H. An integrative model of health, illness, and disease. Health Soc Work 1984 Fall; 9(4):253–259.

Weisensee MG. Evaluation of health promotion. Occup Health Nurs 1985 Jan; 33(1):9–14.

Yoder LE, Jones SL, and Jones PK. The association between health care behavior and attitudes. Health Values 1985 July/Aug; 9(4):24–31.

Zajac DL. Women's health: Problems and options: An overview. Issues Health Care Women 1983 Nov/Dec; 4(6):287–310.

Health Assessment of
the Client/Patient

Unit II

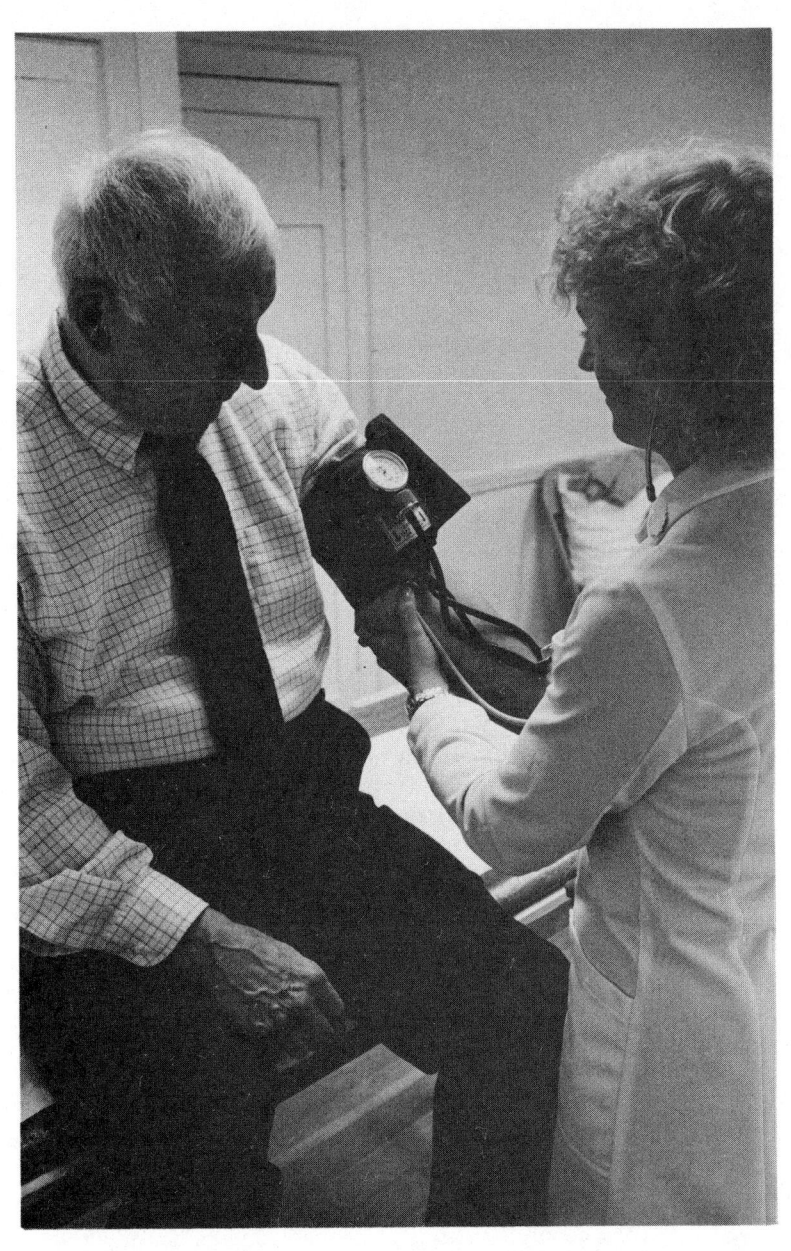

Chapter 5

Clinical Interviewing: The Health History

The clinical interview is one of the most important facets of the nurse–patient relationship. It is through this process that the quality of the relationship is established, information sufficient to provide a thorough assessment of the patient's health status is obtained, and the foundation for nursing diagnoses is made. Behaviors appropriate to the interview and the techniques required to elicit appropriate information are not part of our everyday social lives. These behaviors and techniques must be learned. Interviewing skills require careful development and are refined through experience.

The Role of the Nurse

The role of the nurse in the provision of health care is a dynamically changing one. The scope of nursing practice now includes not only those functions for which the nurse has traditionally been prepared but also a breadth of activities once reserved for physicians and other members of the health care team. In order to facilitate the nursing process, nurses are now employing skills that include gathering the patient data base and performing a physical examination. The concept that only the physician diagnoses patient problems and plans appropriate interventions has also changed.

Intrinsic to the concept of the health care team is the interdependence of health professionals, including physicians, nurses, nutritionists, social workers, and others, each maximizing his or her skills in contributing to the resolution of patient problems. Traditionally, nursing assessments and nursing histories have been present in a variety of styles, lengths, and focuses. Institutions and agencies developed tools that addressed their particular philosophies and concerns, and these tools often appeared in the patient's record as isolated data sheets. Rarely were such assessments reviewed by physicians and other members of the health care team and incorporated into a total plan of care.

The Health History

Throughout the nursing assessment, and particularly in the nursing history, interest is centered on the patient's psychosocial and cultural patterns. The interpersonal and physical environments, as well as the patient's life-style and activities of daily living, are explored in depth. Currently, however, many nurses are responsible for gathering a data base that includes a detailed history of the patient's current health problems, his past medical history, his family history, and a review of body systems. These areas, which constitute the focus of a medical history, were previously explored by the physician. The inclusion of these categories within the context of the nursing history has resulted in a total health profile that focuses on health as well as illness and is more appropriately called a health history, rather than a medical or a nursing history. The format of the health history is a combination of the traditional medical history and the nursing assessment. Both the review of systems and patient profile are expanded to include individual and family relationships, life-style patterns, health practices, and coping strategies. These components of the health history are the backbone of the nursing assessment and can easily be adapted to address the philosophy of nursing at a particular institution or agency and the needs of a particular patient population.

The consolidation of the medical history format and the nursing history format within one health history avoids a duplication of information, minimizes efforts on the part of the patient to provide this information, and encourages collaborative effort between the nurse and physician, who may choose to share in the collection and interpretation of the data base.

In order to contribute significantly to the health history, it is necessary for the nurse to be cognizant of (1) ethical considerations in data collection, (2) communication skills and techniques of the interviewing process, and (3) the content of the health history.

Ethical Considerations in Data Collection

Whenever information is elicited from a person, that person has the right to know why the information is sought and how it will be used. For this reason, the nurse not only identifies herself and her role but also explains in detail what a health history is, how the information is elicited, and how it will be used.

It is important that the patient be fully informed of all aspects of the data collection process and that his decision to participate be freely made. A private setting for the interview promotes an atmosphere of trust between the patient and the nurse and encourages open, honest communication.

Following the interview, the nurse selectively records data that is pertinent to the patient's health status on the health history form. Isolated personal facts or highly sensitive information (arrest record, illegal drug use) are not initially entered in the health record but are discussed with the head nurse, supervisor, or physician. Occasionally, a patient will share very confidential matters with the nurse, and the responsibility for the disposition of such information is best shared.

When the interview is completed and the data recorded, the written record is secured from the public and from those health professionals not directly involved in the care of the patient. This is another method of ensuring confidentiality and maintaining a high standard of nursing care and professional conduct.

Basic Guidelines for the Interviewer

- The interviewer approaches the patient as a unique individual. The interviewer puts the patient at ease and provides for his comfort.

The person who seeks health care for a specific problem is almost invariably anxious. He does not fully understand the significance of his symptoms. Anxiety is compounded by fears related to potential disruption of the person's life-style and perhaps by apprehension about the costs of health care. Given this set of circumstances, the person feels helpless, for he perceives that the outcome with respect to both his health and his economic well-being lies in the hands of others.

To minimize the patient's anxieties, the nurse introduces herself to the patient, defines her role on the health care team, and explains what the health history is. The nurse further explains that the health history will be used to identify areas of concern to the patient and the nurse regarding his health status. The patient is reassured that all the information shared is confidential and that only health professionals directly involved in his care will have access to that information.

The nurse ensures a private setting for the interview. If visitors are present, they are asked, firmly but politely, to leave, since the patient may find it difficult to communicate when visitors (even close relatives) are present. If, on the other hand, the patient expresses a desire to have a family member present during the interview, this is acceptable and may generate additional information that the patient might otherwise forget or be unable to share. Distractions, such as those caused by radios or television sets, are excluded from the environment.

The interview is conducted with due consideration for the patient's comfort and self-respect. Before beginning, the nurse sees that the person is comfortable. If the interview is taking place in a hospital room, the nurse askes the patient if he would like another pillow or would prefer to be seated in a chair rather than in bed. The patient who is short of breath may be more comfortable in a sitting position than he would be if supine. If the patient is in pain or in urgent need of going to the bathroom, his discomfort is attended to before the interview begins.

- The interviewer permits the individual to express himself fully.

The goal of the clinical interview is to obtain all of the facts that will ultimately influence both the nursing diagnoses and the plan of care. When pursuing this objective, one constantly strives to assert the least amount of authority necessary to obtain information in the time allotted. This is best achieved in an atmosphere that encourages spontaneity on the part of the patient. Such spontaneity is influenced by the physical setting and by the behavior of the nurse. Even the simple act of the nurse's sitting during the interview conveys an important message to the patient.

It is therefore the nurse's role to facilitate spontaneous behavior and an unrestricted description of the problem as the patient perceives it. Nonverbal communication on the part of the nurse is a critical element in promoting full expression by the patient. The nurse may actively encourage the patient to elaborate or continue by a nod of the head or by repeating the last few words if the patient appears hesitant. A puzzled look will encourage the patient to clarify apparent inconsistencies in the story.

Questions posed are frequently open ended. "How can we help you?" "Tell me about it." "How did it feel?" are all appropriate questions. "Was it a sharp pain?" "Did it happen only on weekdays?" are inappropriate questions. Such questions presume the answer. Although one certainly wishes to obtain this information, it is sought in a more open-ended way. Otherwise, the patient attempts to "help" the nurse by providing the answer he thinks the nurse wants to hear.

However, the use of open-ended questions is not a useful technique to be employed throughout the entire interview. In order to refine the details that are important to the analysis of symptoms, some degree of direct questioning is necessary. Such questions provide the patient with options for his response. For example, the question "Does the pain have any relationship to meals?" gives the person the option of answering yes or no. Similarly, the question "Does the pain come before the meal, during the meal, or after the meal?" gives the person the opportunity to select from among several options. This more direct line of questioning is deferred until later in the interview when the patient has had an opportunity to express himself as fully as possible and his urge to "help" the nurse has been submerged by a well-developed sense of trust and confidence.

It is not assumed that the approach to every patient will be the same. Clearly, the nurse will have to be more directive with certain patients. The sophistication that allows modulation of the interview technique comes only with experience.

- The interviewer uses a health history form to guide the interview and adjusts the sequence of questions to coincide with the flow of conversation.

The health history form is a tool designed to assist the nurse in the collection of data relevant to the patient's health status. For this reason, the form is not memorized or rigidly adhered to at the expense of the individual. For example, if the person is sharing information about a particular problem and the nurse interrupts to ask direct questions about occupation, education, or family relationships, the flow of information may be broken and important facts overlooked.

It is also essential to "listen" to the patient as he answers the questions. Brief note taking during the interview is acceptable, but when overdone it is highly distracting to the person being interviewed. It also limits eye contact and conveys an impersonal message.

- The interviewer demonstrates an understanding of the nature and intensity of the patient's problem.

The interviewing process does not consist entirely of questions and answers. The manner in which the nurse responds nonverbally to the patient and her ability to listen convey a genuine willingness to understand the meaning of the patient's concerns. Such behavior is often very reassuring, and thus the mode of the interview moves from inquiring to therapeutic.

When the patient becomes silent during the interview, he may be emotionally overcome or may be attempting to formulate an accurate description of events. Such silences need not be intruded on by the nurse. Tearful episodes are also not interrupted, and the urge to tell the patient that matters are going to be all right or to provide similar verbal reassurances is resisted. Things may not be all right, and the reassurance may appear false. Moreover, the nurse has much to learn by exploring the patient's fears and anxieties. Sometimes open-ended statements, such as "You look sad," or "You seem frightened," will encourage the person to elaborate on his feelings and at the same time convey the nurse's empathy.

The nurse also makes every attempt to convey an understanding of and a respect for the patient's beliefs and attitudes. This is done in spite of the fact that such beliefs and attitudes may differ sharply from those held by the nurse. There is no place in the interview for a comment such as "You don't really believe that, do you?" If the person does not believe it, it is unlikely that he would state it candidly to the health professional conducting the interview. A nonjudgmental attitude is especially necessary when dealing with matters related to sexuality, drug and alcohol use, and cultural patterns.

- The interviewer takes into account the person's cultural background.

Cultural attitudes about family relationships and the role of women are accepted at face value, just as attitudes toward pain, illness, and hospitalization are accepted. These beliefs and attitudes are derived from personal experiences, which vary according to the person's cultural background.

- The interviewer is aware of his or her own feelings and attitudes.

Patient behavior that the nurse might find offensive in herself, her family, or her friends may arouse hostility, anger, anxiety, or even, at times, revulsion. The professional cannot allow this to be conveyed to the patient. Quite unconsciously, the nurse might convey irritation, boredom, or disbelief. Similarly, the nurse may be acutely uncomfortable when dealing with people who have certain kinds of illnesses, because of her own fears. The nurse's own ethical and moral sense may make it difficult to develop relationships with alcoholic or drug-dependent patients. It is a frequent failing of health professionals to view self-inflicted illness with disdain, hostility, and anger. Feelings are intensified when the patient is acutely intoxicated, and the nurse may return hostility for hostility. The first step in dealing effectively with such patients is to understand the inner compulsions that cause the interviewer to reject the patient.

- The interviewer is attuned to nonverbal communication and learns to recognize gestures that convey defensiveness, hostility, confidence, impatience, and so on.

The nurse learns to respond to body language the same way she responds to the spoken word. Much has been written about body language, and a quick perusal of an illustrated book on this subject is highly informative. Frequently, the body language and the patient's verbal expression are at variance. Often, this is obvious—as when the patient describes a seemingly happy event yet appears to be on the verge of tears. The interviewer might respond to such inconsistencies by drawing them to the patient's attention.

- The interviewer communicates in a manner that is consistent with the individual's level of understanding.

It is important for the nurse to take into consideration the patient's educational background. The nurse is an intelligent person selected from the population for advanced education by virtue of capacities and opportunities not possessed by a large segment of the population. Her use of the English language is sophisticated, and she also possesses a health care vocabulary that is foreign to the majority of the population. Realizing this, she takes care to phrase questions in such a way that they are easily understood by the patient; in counseling, she uses as few technical terms as possible. If the patient does not understand the language being used, it is unlikely that he will interrupt for clarification, largely out of fear that he will appear ignorant. Careful questioning may reveal the level of the patient's understanding of an issue that has just been discussed.

A second factor influencing the patient's level of understanding is cultural background. The Puerto Rican mother, for example, has a different perception of personal health than does a mother born and raised in an American suburb. Pregnancy is not something for which she would seek care and attention until labor begins. Thus, she would not understand the need for prenatal care as advocated by health professionals. In addition, a woman from a culture in which obesity is a way of life and admired by men would not understand the need for diet and weight control. Similarly, Asian women, not accustomed to complaining of pain, even when it is severe, would not appreciate the advantages of taking analgesics. All such differences in outlook must be taken into account when dealing with members of other cultures.

Even differences in the life experiences of those who are well educated and from the same cultural background must be considered. An only child of an urban or suburban family may be less able to deal with the problems of being a mother than a woman from a rural society who was reared in a family of eight children and participated in rearing younger siblings.

- The interviewer terminates the interview in an appropriate manner that summarizes the information obtained and ensures that the patient has understood major points discussed.

Before ending the interview, the nurse inquires whether the patient has any questions. The nurse specifically searches for areas of misunderstanding by briefly summarizing the patient's responses. This give the patient the opportunity to correct misinformation and also to add facts that he may have forgotten to mention earlier.

Content of the Interview

When the patient is seen for the first time by the health team (except in the emergency care situation), the first requisite is to obtain a *data base*. The nurse may be responsible for all or a part of that data base, but in either case she must be familiar with all of its facets. The data base contains the following components:

1. Biographical data
2. Informant
3. Chief complaint
4. History of present illness (or present health concern)
5. Past medical history
6. Review of systems
7. Family history
8. Patient profile
9. Physical examination
10. Radiologic and laboratory information
11. Problem formulation (medical and nursing diagnoses)

Biographical Data

Biographical or introductory identifying information helps to put much of the history in context. This information includes the name, address, age, sex, marital status, occupation, and ethnic origins of the patient. Some people prefer a full patient profile at this juncture, but most believe a full profile to be inappropriate until the interviewer has obtained the trust and confidence of the patient. Moreover, a patient in pain, or with an equally urgent problem for which he seeks attention, is unlikely to put a great deal of confidence in an interviewer who is more concerned with the details of his marital status than with quickly addressing the problem for which the patient seeks help.

The Informant

The informant may not always be the patient, as is the case if the patient is a child or an elderly person or is unconscious, in a coma, or suffering a severe psychiatric disturbance. The interviewer assesses the reliability of the informant and the usefulness of the information provided. For example, hysterical or depressed patients are unlikely to provide a reliable data base, while patients who abuse drugs and alcohol are likely to use denial as part of their operating mechanism. It is reasonable for the interviewer to make such judgments (based on the context of the entire interview) and to incorporate them in the record.

Chief Complaint

The chief complaint is the issue that brings the patient to seek help. Questions such as "What brings you to the clinic today?" or "Why have you been admitted to the hospital?" usually elicit the chief complaint. Frequently, the patient appears without a specific complaint, seeking an ongoing relationship with a health care team or requesting a "checkup." If this is the case, it is noted in lieu of a chief complaint. Once the patient has expressed his concern, his exact words are recorded in quotation marks. However, a statement such as "Doctor Smith sent me" is not a chief complaint. Although such information can be included as part of the introductory patient profile, the patient should be asked why he sought Dr. Smith's attention, and this reason should be entered as the chief complaint. If the patient has been admitted for a special purpose, it is so stated (*e.g.*, "for cholecystectomy").

Frequently, the patient will have more than one problem and, therefore, more than one complaint. These are listed in terms of the patient's priorities and then explored as separate entities, if they represent separate problems, or as a single present illness if they are multiple manifestations of one cohesive problem.

History of Present Illness (HPI)

Exploration of the facts related to a present illness frequently requires substantial knowledge of the pathophysiology and natural history of disease. If one does not know, for example, the manifestations of an acute myocardial infarction, it is difficult to subtly extract information that will ultimately lead to the diagnosis. The history of any illness is the single most important factor in enabling the health professional to arrive at a diagnosis. The physical examination is helpful but usually reveals manifestations that are an expected consequence of the story that has unfolded. Occasionally, laboratory and radiologic information can be singularly helpful; only rarely do they establish the diagnosis. On the other hand, judicious selection of laboratory and radiologic inquiry demands a careful history.

The "present illness" may well be but one episode in a sequence that is contained within a single disease process. An episode of insulin shock, for example, is only one of an ordered series of occurrences that define the natural history of diabetes. In such an instance, the entire course of the diabetic illness is unfolded in order to put the current complaint in context. Although the episode of insulin shock gains prominence in the delineation of the story, the description of it is obtained in the context of the natural history of the disease and communicated to the record in a similar manner. After all the facts have been obtained from the patient, the details of the present illness, or health concern, from onset until the time of contact with the health care team, are constructed. These facts are recorded in *chronological order,* beginning with, for example, "The patient was in good health until. . . ." or "The patient first experienced nausea 2 months prior to admission 1/4/88."

The history of the present illness is a compact, complete story, rather than a statement of numerous disconnected facts. It includes such information as the date and manner (sudden, gradual) of the onset of the problem, the setting in which the problem developed (at home, at work, after an argument), manifestations of the problem, and the course of the illness or problem. The course of the illness or problem includes self-treatment, medical interventions, progress and effects of treatment, and the patient's perceptions of the cause or meaning of the problem.

Specific symptoms (pain, headache, fever, change in bowel habits) are delineated in detail. Critical to the analysis of a symptom is its location and radiation (if pain), quality, severity, and duration. The interviewer also pursues the persistence or intermittence of the symptom, factors that aggravate or alleviate it, and any associated manifestations that the patient may be aware of.

Associated manifestations are symptoms that occur simultaneously with the chief complaint. The presence or absence of associated symptoms may shed light on the origin or extent of the patient's problem, as well as on the diagnosis. These symptoms are referred to as significant positive or negative findings and are derived from a review of systems directly related to the chief complaint. For instance, if the patient is complaining of a vague symptom, such as fatigue or weight loss, all body systems are reviewed and included in the history of the present illness. If, on the other hand, the patient's chief complaint is chest pain, only the cardiopulmonary and gastrointestinal systems would be included in the history of the present illness. In either situation, both positive and negative findings are recorded.

Past Health History

A detailed summary of the patient's past health history is a valuable component of the data base. After obtaining a statement about the patient's general health in the past, the nurse proceeds in an orderly fashion to inquire about the patient's immunization status and any known allergies to drugs or other substances. The dates of immunization, along with the type of allergy and adverse reactions, are recorded. The patient is asked to provide information about his last physical examination, chest x-ray film, electrocardiogram (ECG), eye examination, hearing examination, dental checkup, and Papanicolaou smear (if female). The patient is then interviewed about previous illnesses. Negative as well as positive responses are recorded. Dates, or the age of the patient at the time of illness, as well as the names of the physician and hospital, the diagnosis, and the treatment are also recorded. A history of the following areas is elicited:

- Childhood illness—rubeola, rubella, polio, whooping cough, mumps, chickenpox, scarlet fever, rheumatic fever, strep throat
- Adult illnesses
- Psychiatric illnesses
- Injuries—burns, fractures, head injuries
- Hospitalizations
- Operations
- Current medications—prescription, over-the-counter, home remedies

If a particular hospitalization or major medical intervention is related to the present illness, it need not be repeated; rather, the nurse makes a reference such as "see history of present illness" or "see HPI" on the data sheet.

Family History

The age and health status, or the age and cause of death, of first-order relatives (parents, siblings, spouse, children) and second-order relatives (grandparents, cousins) are elicited to identify diseases that may be hereditary, communicable, or possibly environmental. The nurse specifically inquires about such conditions as cancer, hypertension, heart disease, diabetes, epilepsy, mental illness, tuberculosis, kidney disease, arthritis, allergies, asthma, alcoholism, and obesity. One of the easiest methods of recording such data is by using the family tree (Fig. 5-1).

Review of Systems

The review of systems includes a complete inventory of major body organ systems in terms of the presence or absence of symptoms past or present. It serves as a check and balance to prevent the interviewer from overlooking any relevant data. Negative as well as positive responses are recorded. If the patient responds positively, that symptom is analyzed according to the process outlined under History of Present Ill-

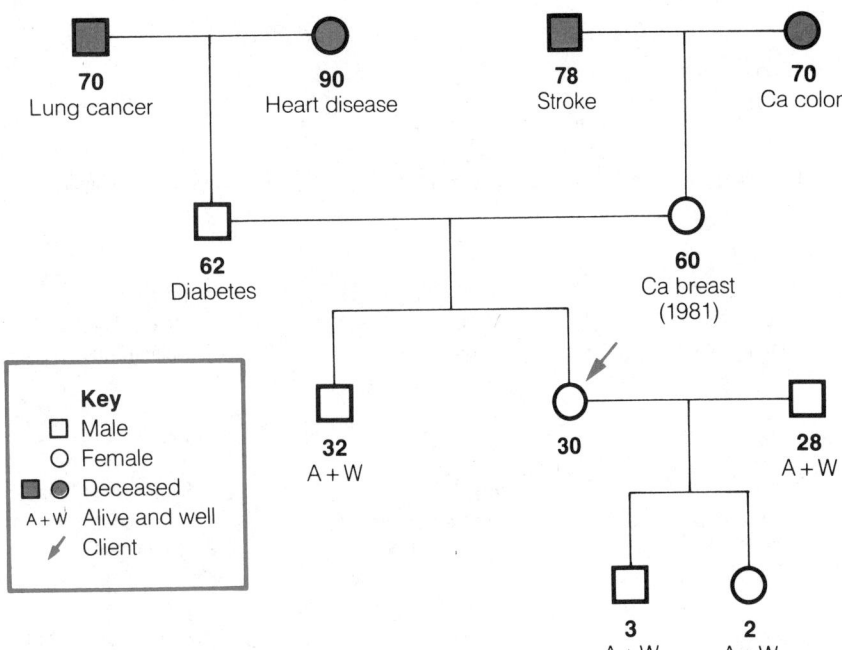

Figure 5-1
Sample recording of family history as a "family tree." Grandparents, parents, siblings, spouse, and children are identified.

Key
☐ Male
○ Female
■ ● Deceased
A + W Alive and well
⚡ Client

ness. Illnesses that have been previously described in the history of the present illness or the past medical history need not be repeated. Reference is made to the appropriate location of relevant information. The system review includes an overview of general health as well as symptoms related to each body system. A review of systems can be organized in a formal checklist, which becomes a part of the health history. Some of these forms are commercially available, and others are prepared by health care teams in a manner appropriate to link goals and functions. One asset of the checklist process is that it is easily audited and less subject to error than is relying on the memory of the interviewer, who must obtain detailed information relevant to each organ system. One such format is outlined in Chart 5-1.

Patient Profile

The patient profile is an amplification of the biographical data elicited at the beginning of the interview. A complete composite, or profile, of the patient is critical to an analysis of his problem, his capacity to deal with the problem, and the health care team's capacity to provide assistance.

The information elicited at this point in the interview is highly personal and subjective. During this stage, the nurse encourages the patient's open and uninhibited expression of feelings, values, and personal experiences. Usually, the nurse begins with general open-ended questions and then moves to direct questioning when specific facts are needed. The patient is often less anxious when the interview progresses from information that is less personal (birthplace, occupation, education) to information that is more personal (sexuality, body image, coping abilities).

A general patient profile consists of six content areas:

1. Past development
2. Education and occupation
3. Environment (physical, spiritual, interpersonal)
4. Life-style (patterns and habits)

5. Self-concept
6. Stress response

The patient profile is outlined in Chart 5-2.

Past Development.   The patient profile begins with a brief life history. Questions about the patient's place of birth and places where he has lived in the past help him to focus on the earlier years of his life. Personal experiences during childhood or adolescence that have special significance to the patient may be elicited by asking, "Was there anything that you experienced as a child or adolescent that would be helpful for me to know about?" The interviewer's intent is to encourage the patient to make a quick review of his earlier life, highlighting an event or circumstance of particular significance. Sometimes the person will not be able to recall anything that he believes is meaningful to share with the nurse. On the other hand, he may take the opportunity to share information such as a personal achievement, a failure, a developmental crisis, an instance of physical or emotional abuse, or a valued loss.

Education and Occupation.   Questions related to economic status and educational preparation can be threatening to the patient and are approached indirectly through a focus on his current occupation. If the patient is employed, a statement such as "Tell me about your job" often elicits information about his role, job tasks, and satisfaction with the position. It may be necessary to interject direct questions about past employment and career goals if the person does not initially provide this information.

Asking the person what kind of educational requirements were necessary to attain his present job is a more sensitive approach to educational background than asking whether he graduated from high school. It is rarely necessary to know the actual numerical value of the person's salary; the information needed is whether his income is sufficient to meet his expenses and support the life-style to which he is accustomed. Questions such as "Do you have any financial concerns at this time?" or "Sometimes there just doesn't seem

Chart 5-1
Review of Systems

Positive responses are circled and described in detail. Negative responses are underlined to indicate the absence of the symptom.

General

Usual weight
Weight change
Appetite change
Night sweats

Weakness
Fatigue
Fever

Skin

Rash
Color change
Dryness
Nail changes

Pruritus
Growths or masses
Hair changes

Head

Headache
Trauma

Dizziness

Eyes

Vision (near and far)
Glasses or contacts
Photophobia
Diplopia

Blurring
Pain
Infection
Itching

Ears

Hearing
Pain
Infection
Excessive cerumen

Hygiene practices
Tinnitus
Vertigo

Nose and Sinuses

Discharge
Allergies
Obstruction

Epistaxis
Pain
Frequent colds

Mouth and Throat

Sore throats
Difficulty swallowing
Taste
Gums
Dentition

Dentures or partial plate
Hoarseness
Lesions (lips, tongue, mucosa)
Hygiene practices

Neck

Stiffness
Swelling
Pain

Limited motion
"Swollen glands"
Thyroid disease

Breasts

Pain
Swelling
Self-examination practices

Nipple discharge
Dimpling

Respiratory

Cough
Shortness of breath
Hemoptysis
Wheezing

Sputum (color, quantity)
Asthma
Recurrent upper respiratory tract infection

Cardiovascular

Shortness of breath
Dyspnea on exertion
Orthopnea
Chest pain
Palpitations
Paroxysmal nocturnal dyspnea

Phlebitis
Coldness or numbness of extremities
Edema
Varicosities
Claudication

Gastrointestinal

Anorexia
Nausea
Vomiting
Indigestion
Diarrhea
Pain
Constipation

Hematemesis
Melena
Jaundice
Food intolerance
Change in bowel pattern
Hemorrhoids

Genitourinary

Nocturia
Incontinence
Infection
Urgency

Dysuria
Dribbling
Frequency
Hematuria

Genitoreproductive

Female

Menses (menarche, cycle, duration, amount, cramps, intermittent bleeding, last menstrual period [LMP])
Number of pregnancies, live births, abortions (G__P__Ab__)
If menopausal: age of menses cessation, symptoms of menopause, postmenopausal bleeding
Vaginal discharge
Dyspareunia
Contraception
Pruritus
Social (sexually transmitted) disease

Male

Pain
Discharge
Swelling

Sores
Social (sexually transmitted) disease
Contraception practices

(continued)

Chart 5-1 *Review of Systems* (continued)

Musculoskeletal

Muscular pain or cramps
Pain, swelling, or redness
   of joints

Back pain or history of injury
Limitation of movement
Ability to perform ADL

Endocrine

Heat or cold intolerance
Excessive sweating
Changes in hair pattern

Excessive thirst, hunger,
   or urination

Neurologic

Syncope
Seizures
Paralysis
Weakness
Dizziness
Vertigo

Numbness or tingling
Problems with speech or gait
Tremors
Memory loss
Loss of sensation

Hematologic

Blood transfusions
Anemia

Easy bruising or bleeding

---

to be enough money to make ends meet. Are you finding this true?'' may be helpful. Inquiry about the person's insurance coverage and plans for health care payment are also appropriate.

Environment. The person's physical environment and its potential hazards, his spiritual awareness, and his cultural background, interpersonal relationships, and support system are included in the concept of environment.

Physical Environment. The type of housing (apartment, duplex, single family) in which the person lives, its location, and information related to safety and comfort within the person's home and neighborhood is elicited. The nurse attempts to identify environmental hazards, such as isolation, inadequate protection, potential fire risks, pollution (noise, air, water), and inadequate sanitation facilities.

Spiritual Environment. To be thoughtful or contemplative about one's existence, to accept challenges in one's life, and to seek and find answers to personal questions is to be ''spiritual.'' For many persons, this spirituality is expressed through identification with a particular religion. Like cultural influences, spiritual values and beliefs direct a person's behavior and his approach to health problems and the health care system in general. A person's spirituality is often challenged during the experience of an illness or a developmental crisis. The patient may experience considerable turmoil about the meaning of this problem or crisis in his life. He is challenged to new perceptions and spiritual growth, and he may find this difficult. A brief spiritual assessment by the nurse is important; it focuses on three areas:

1. The extent to which religion is a part of the person's life
2. Religious beliefs related to the person's perception of health and illness
3. Religious practices

The following questions can be used in a spiritual assessment:

- Is religion or God important to you?
  If yes, in what way?
  If no, what is the most important thing in your life?
- Are there any religious practices that are important to you?
- Do you have any spiritual concerns because of your present health problem?

Interpersonal Environment. Cultural influences, relationships with family and friends, and the presence or absence of a suport system are all a part of the inter-personal environment.

Ethnic Background. The beliefs and practices that have been shared from generation to generation are known as cultural or ethnic patterns. They are expressed through language, dress, dietary choices, and role behaviors, in perceptions of health and illness, and in health-related behaviors. The influence of these beliefs and customs on the patient's experience with a health problem and his relationship with the health care team cannot be underestimated. For this reason, a patient's ethnic identity (cultural and social) as well as his racial identity (biological) are determined. The following questions may assist the nurse in obtaining relevant information:

- Where did your parents or ancestors come from? When?
- What language do you speak at home?
- Are there certain customs or values that are important to you?
- Is there anything special you do to keep in good health?
- Do you have any specific practices for treating illness?

Family Relationships and Support System. An assessment of family structure (members, ages, roles), patterns of communication, and the presence or absence of a support system is an integral part of the patient profile. Although the traditional ''family'' is recognized as a mother, father, and children, it is important to keep in mind that there are many different types of living arrangements within our society. ''Family'' may be interpreted to mean two or more people bound by emotional ties or commitments. Such an open definition of ''family'' encompasses the couple who live together but are not married, the college student whose dormitory companions provide a ''family'' structure, and the single person who lives alone but has significant relationships and a support system.

Life-Style. The life-style section of the patient profile provides the nurse the opportunity to gain information about health-related behaviors. These behaviors include patterns of sleep, exercise, nutrition, and recreation, as well as personal habits of smoking and the use of alcohol and caffeine. Most people have little difficulty sharing particulars about their sleeping patterns or recreational choices. On the other hand,

Chart 5-2
Patient Profile

Past Development

Place of birth
Places lived
Significant childhood/adolescent experiences

Education and Occupation

Jobs held in past
Current position/job
Length of time at position
Educational preparation
Work satisfaction and career goals
Financial resources
Insurance coverage

Environment

Physical

Living arrangements (type of housing, neighborhood, presence
    of hazards)

Spiritual

Extent to which religion is a part of individual's life
Religious beliefs related to perception of health and illness
Religious practices

Interpersonal

Ethnic background (language spoken, customs and values held,
    folk practices used to maintain health or to cure illness)
Family relationships (family structure, roles, communication
    patterns, support system)
Friendships (quality of relationship)

Life-style

Patterns

Sleep (time individual retires, hours per night, comfort mea-
    sures, awakens rested?)
Exercise (type, frequency, time spent)
Nutrition (24-hour diet recall, idiosyncrasies, restrictions)
Recreation (type of activity, time spent)

Caffeine (coffee, tea, cola, chocolate)—kind, amount
Smoking (cigarette, pipe, cigar, marijuana)—kind, amount per
    day, number of years, desire to quit
Alcohol—kind, amount, pattern over past year

Self-concept

View of self in present
View of self in future
Body image (level of satisfaction, concerns)
Sexuality—Perception of self as a man or woman
Quality of sexual relationships
Concerns related to sexuality or sexual functioning

Stress Response

Major concerns or problems at present
Past experiences with similar problems
Past coping patterns and outcomes
Present coping strategies and anticipated outcomes
Individual's expectations of family/friends and health care team
    in problem resolution

---

many people are quite sensitive to questions about their smoking and alcohol use. The person may fear the nurse's scrutiny and thus may minimize the extent of his habit. For this reason, the nurse may be able to elicit more information by asking "What kind of alcohol do you enjoy drinking at a party?" rather than "Do you drink?" Describing the person as a "social drinker" is vague and not recommended. Instead, the nurse identifies specifically the type of alcohol and the amount ingested per day or per week (*e.g.,* 1 pint whiskey daily for 2 years).

When the nurse suspects that alcohol abuse may be a problem, additional information may be obtained by asking "Has anyone ever said that drinking might be causing a problem for you?" or "Have you ever considered cutting down your alcohol intake?" In a similar fashion, the nurse elicits information related to smoking and caffeine consumption.

Self-Concept.   The self-concept is a product of relevant experiences with others and is the result of others' reactions to the "self." It is the impression one has of oneself, the product of years of input and interpretation by the individual. Sometimes the interviewer can assess a person's self-concept

by asking him about his view of the present ("How do you feel about your life in general?") and his outlook for the future ("What will your life be like in the future?" or "How do you see yourself in a few years?").

Health concerns may threaten the way a person perceives himself. His body image, the mental picture he has of himself, is vulnerable during normal developmental crises (adolescence, pregnancy, aging) and also as a result of certain medical and surgical interventions. Simply being hospitalized can alter a person's perception of himself. Suddenly he sees himself as weak, helpless, and impotent. Surgical alterations such as a colostomy or a mastectomy pose an even greater threat to body image. It is therefore important for the nurse to be aware of the person's perceptions of himself and his body. The following questions may elicit useful information:

- What do you like most about yourself?
- What would you change about yourself if you could?
- Do you have any particular concerns about your body?

Sexuality.   No area of assessment is more personal than a sexual history. Because of anxiety on the part of the interviewer, this area of the patient profile is often overlooked or inadequately assessed. A lack of knowledge related to sexuality combined with anxiety about her own sexuality may hinder the nurse's effectiveness. The nurse may be perplexed about how or when to elicit this information in a sensitive way.

Sexual assessment can be approached at the end of the interview along with the interpersonal or life-style assessment, or it can be a part of the genitourinary history within the review of systems. The nurse may find it easier to approach a discussion of sexuality following a discussion of menstruation, for instance. A similar discussion with the male patient would follow questions related to the urinary system.

It is advisable to begin the assessment with a general question that takes into consideration the developmental stage of the person and the presence or absence of intimate relationships. For instance, when discussing sexuality with an adolescent, one or two of the following questions may be helpful:

- Do you have a special friend, a close relationship right now? Tell me about this closeness.
- Some teenagers are interested in having a sexual relationship at this age . . . how do you feel about that?

Such questions may lead to a discussion of concerns related to sexual expression, to the quality of a relationship, or to questions about contraception.

Whether the person is young or old, the nurse determines whether he is sexually active before exploring issues related to sexual identity, contraception, or the quality of the sexual relationship. The nurse is careful to avoid making assumptions related to fidelity, heterosexuality, or sexual practices. Questions are worded in such a way that the person feels free to discuss his sexuality as a single person or as a homosexual. Direct questions are usually less threatening when prefaced with such statements as "Most people feel that . . ." or "Many people worry about . . ." This suggests the normalcy of such feelings or behavior and encourages the person to share information that he might otherwise leave out because he believes that his behavior or feelings are objectionable or different.

The needs of the patient direct the flow of the interview at all times. If the patient is abrupt with his responses and indicates that he does not wish to carry the discussion any further, the nurse proceeds to another part of the data collection. By introducing the subject of sexuality, however, the nurse has indicated to the person that a discussion of sexual concerns is acceptable and that she will be approachable in the future. (See also Chap. 13, Human Sexuality.)

Stress Response. Every person handles a stressful event in a manner that is intended to eliminate or minimize the stress. Each individual's adaptive ability hinges on his capacity to cope effectively with the stressful situation. Exploring past coping patterns, as well as perceptions of current stresses and anticipated outcomes, assists the nurse in identifying the person's overall ability to handle stress. It is especially important to identify expectations that the person may have of his family, friends, and the health care team in helping him resolve his problems.

As was previously mentioned, the patient profile section of the data base constitutes the major component of the nursing assessment and represents the nursing profession's strongest contribution to the data base. The education of the nurse and the focus of nursing practice clearly demonstrate this. The extent of the patient profile is usually determined by the patient's needs and the philosophy of nursing at a particular institution or agency. For all patients, however, a general assessment of the categories outlined provides a significant composite profile of the patient. Such a profile is appropriate whether the health problem is acute or chronic and whether the setting is inpatient or outpatient.

Health concerns that usually are not complex (earache, tonsillectomy) and can be resolved in a short period of time usually do not require the depth or detail that is required when one is confronted with a person who is experiencing a major illness or health concern. Additional assessments that go beyond the general patient profile may be employed when the patient's health problems are acute and complex or when the illness is chronic. Specific interviewing tools have been developed by nurses to address areas of family assessment, spiritual assessment, sexuality assessment, and psychological assessment. The reader is referred to articles and books listed in the bibliography for additional learning.

The Remainder of the Data Base

Following the health history, a physical examination is performed. The basic techniques and skills required for performing the physical examination are presented in Chapter 6. Special observations and assessments that must be made in specific clinical situations are described in the chapters in which these conditions are discussed. Based on the information elicited from the history and the physical examination, radiologic and laboratory tests may be indicated and prescribed. Problem identification, the formulation of nursing diagnoses, and the development of nursing care plans are discussed in Chapter 2, The Nursing Process.

Summary

The process of eliciting a health history is a highly complex one that requires new knowledge and understanding, clinical laboratory learning, and reinforcement in the practice setting. There is no one way to approach a patient or to elicit a health history. The nurse is encouraged to develop a style of interviewing that complements her personality and a health history format that is flexible, to accommodate the practice setting and the patient's needs. The health history format and interviewing techniques outlined in this chapter are presented as guidelines for the nurse in her acquisition of the initial components of the data base.

Bibliography

Books

Bernstein L and Bernstein RS. Interviewing: A Guide for Health Professionals, 3rd ed. New York, Appleton-Century-Crofts, 1980.

Brown MS and Hudak C. Student Manual of Physical Examination, 2nd ed. Philadelphia, JB Lippincott, 1984.

Enelow A. Interviewing and Patient Care. New York, Oxford University Press, 1986.

Hillman RS et al. Clinical Skills: Interviewing, History Taking and Physical Diagnosis. New York, McGraw-Hill, 1981.

Kneedler JA and Dodge GH. Perioperative Patient Care, pp 41–51. Boston, Blackwell Scientific, 1983.

Malasanos L et al. Health Assessment, 3rd ed. St. Louis, CV Mosby, 1985.

Rudy EB and Gray VR. Handbook of Health Assessment. Bowie, Maryland, Robert J. Brady, 1981.

Sherman JL Jr and Fields SK. Guide to Patient Evaluation. Garden City, New York, Medical Examination, 1982.

Articles

Aker JG. Communicating effectively: The preoperative interview. AANA J 1985 Feb; 53(1):54–59.

Barth RT et al. Learning to interview: The quality of training opportunities. Clin Superv 1984 Spring; 2(1):3–14.

Bates B and Hoekelman RA. Interviewing and the health history. In Bates B. A Guide to Physical Examination, 4th ed, pp 1–27. Philadelphia, JB Lippincott, 1987.

Bray KA. The interviewing process. Crit Care Nurs 1984 May/June; 4(3): 65–67.

Collecting and documenting patient data. Nursing '84 1984 Mar; 14(3): 26, 28.

Jones DA and Lepley MK. Establishing a data base. In Jones DA (ed). Health Assessment Manual, pp 1–26. New York, McGraw Hill, 1986. (includes interviewing techniques)

Mengel A. Getting the most from patient interviews. Nursing '82 1982 Nov; 12(11):46–49.

Steel K. History taking from elderly patients. Hosp Pract 1985 May 30; 20(5A):70–71.

Wolf S. The fine art of taking a history (editorial). Hosp Pract 1985 Sept 30; 20(9A):6–9.

Chapter 6

Physical Assessment and Nutritional Assessment

Physical assessment, or the physical examination, is an integral part of the nursing assessment. The basic techniques and tools typically used in performing a physical examination are described in this chapter. The detailed discussion required for the thorough examination of specific systems, including special maneuvers, are found in appropriate chapters throughout the book. Because the patient's nutritional status is an important element of his total health profile, a section on nutritional assessment is included in this chapter.

The Physical Assessment

The physical examination is usually performed following the health history. In order to facilitate this portion of the data collection process, the examiner performs the assessments in a well-lighted, warm area. The patient is undressed and draped appropriately so that only the area to be examined is exposed. The physical and psychological comfort of the patient are considered at all times. For this reason, procedures and their rationale are fully explained. If a particular maneuver may cause discomfort, an explanation of what to expect precedes that part of the examination. The examiner's hands are washed prior to and immediately following the examination. Fingernails are kept short to avoid injuring the patient.

The key to obtaining appropriate data in the least possible amount of time is an organized and systematic examination. Such an approach refines physical assessment skills and encourages cooperation and trust on the part of the patient.

The patient's health history provides the examiner with a complete health profile that guides all aspects of the physical examination. It helps to focus on body organs and systems that are of particular concern to the patient.

The complete physical examination is usually envisioned in a logical head-to-toe sequence, as follows:

- Skin
- Head and neck
- Thorax and lungs
- Breast
- Cardiovascular system

- Abdomen
- Rectum
- Genitalia
- Neurologic system
- Musculoskeletal system

In actual practice, all relevant organ systems are tested in the course of the physical examination, but not necessarily in the sequence described. For example, when the face is examined, it is appropriate at the same time to check for facial asymmetry and, thus, for the integrity of the seventh cranial nerve; one does not return to this point later, as part of a "neurologic" examination. When systems are combined in this manner, the patient is spared the sequence of sitting up, lying down, sitting up, and so forth, which would be, to say the least, exhausting.

A "complete" physical examination is not a "routine." Many of the elements fall in the category of "subroutines," which are selectively addressed as a function of the patient's particular problem. If, for example, a healthy 20-year-old college student reports for an examination in order to satisfy a requirement to play basketball, and reports no history of neurologic abnormality, the requirements for an adequate survey of the neurologic system are minimal. Conversely, a complaint of transient numbness and diplopia elicits from the examiner a quite complete neurologic investigation. Similarly, a person with pleuritic chest pain receives a much more intensive examination of the chest than the person with, for instance, leg cramps.

The process of physical examination is a thoughtful one. Attempts to elicit physical findings are based on all the information available at the time the examination is conducted. In general, it is the patient's health history that directs the examiner in efforts to obtain additional data for a complete patient profile.

The process of learning physical examination requires memorization, skill repetition, and reinforcement in a clinical setting. Only after basic physical assessment techniques are mastered and integrated into a complete examination, can the examiner "tailor" the routine screening examination to include thorough assessments of a particular system, including special maneuvers.

The basic tools of the physical examination are the human senses of vision, hearing, touch, and smell. These human tools may be augmented by special man-made tools (*e.g.,* stethoscope, ophthalmoscope) to permit a better definition of visual and acoustic details, but these man-made tools should be recognized only as extensions of the human senses. It is sometimes implied that such tools are sophisticated devices requiring superhuman intelligence for their use; in fact, they are simple instruments that anyone can learn to use well. Sophistication comes with the interpretation of what is seen and heard.

The Process of Physical Examination

Four fundamental processes are employed in the examination of the patient: *inspection, palpation, percussion,* and *auscultation.*

Inspection

The first fundamental process is inspection. The power to observe is one that must be cultivated. General inspection is carried out at the first moment of contact with the patient. The examiner introduces herself to the patient and perhaps shakes hands with him, and they exchange the first words of communication. Many impressions register in this exchange, and numerous valuable observations can be made. The patient is old or young (how old? how young? does his appearance correspond to his/her stated age?); the patient is thin or fat; the patient is anxious or depressed; the patient's body structure is normal or perhaps deformed in some way (what way? how different from normal?).

It is essential to pay attention to the details of observation. Vague general statements, which are often used, are a poor substitute for specific descriptions based on careful observation:

1. *The patient looks sick.* In what way does the patient look sick? Is he pale, is his skin clammy; is he grimacing in pain; is he dyspneic; is the skin jaundiced or cyanotic; does he have edema? What specific physical features or behavioral manifestations convey that he is "sick"?

2. *The patient appears chronically ill.* In what way does the patient appear chronically ill? Does he appear to have lost weight? Patients who lose weight secondary to malignancy or other muscle-wasting disease appear different from those who are merely thin. The distribution of their weight loss takes a different form. Does the skin have the appearance of chronic illness? That is, is it pale, or does it give the appearance of dehydration or loss of subcutaneous tissue? These are important observations that health professionals frequently fail to note on the record.

Among general observations that should be noted in the initial examination of the patient are posture and stature, body movements, nutrition, speech pattern, and body temperature.

Posture and Stature. The posture that a patient assumes can often reveal much about his illness. Patients with the dyspnea of cardiac disease prefer to sit and may complain of "smothering" if forced to lie down for even brief periods of time. Persons with emphysema not only sit upright but also assume a posture that is quite characteristic. They thrust their arms forward and laterally onto the edge of the bed (tripod position) in order to place accessory muscles of respiration at an optimum mechanical advantage for respiratory assistance. Patients with abdominal pain due to peritonitis prefer to lie perfectly still. Even slight jarring of the bed by the examiner will incite agonizing accentuation of pain. On the other hand, patients with abdominal pain due to renal or biliary colic are exceedingly restless. They may writhe in bed or even get up and pace the room. Patients with meningeal irritation associated with headache cannot bend the head or flex the knees without aggravating their pain.

Body Movements. Abnormalities of body movement may be of two general kinds: generalized discontinuity of voluntary or involuntary movement and asymmetry of movement. In the former category are included tremors of a wide variety, some of which may occur at rest (Parkinson's disease), while others are incited only on voluntary movement (cerebellar ataxia). Other tremors may exist both during rest and activity (delirium tremens of the alcoholic, thyrotoxicosis). Some voluntary or involuntary movements are fine, others quite coarse. At the extreme are the convulsive movements of epilepsy or tetanus and the gross choreiform movements of patients with rheumatic fever or Huntington's disease.

Asymmetry of movement is seen in patients with disease of the central nervous system (CNS), principally in those who have had cerebral vascular accidents. The patient may manifest drooping of one side of the face or be incapable of normal movement of the right or left upper and lower extremities. Strength is impaired on the involved side, and the patient walks with a foot-dragging gait.

Nutrition. States of nutrition are important to note. Obesity may be generalized as a function of excessive intake of calories or may be specifically localized to the trunk in patients with endocrine disorders (Cushing's disease) or those who have been taking steroid drugs for long periods of time. Loss of weight may be generalized as a function of caloric deprivation or may be reflected more strikingly in loss of muscle mass in patients whose diseases interfere with protein building. A detailed discussion of nutritional assessment is presented later in this chapter.

Speech Pattern. Speech may be slurred owing to CNS disease or because of incapacity to articulate owing to damage to cranial nerves. Damage to the recurrent laryngeal nerve will produce hoarseness, as will those diseases that produce edema or swelling of the vocal cords. Speech may be halting or interrupted in flow in some CNS disorders (multiple sclerosis).

Body Temperature. The recording of body temperature is a part of every physical examination. Fever is an increase in body temperature above normal. A normal oral temperature for most persons is an average of 37.0°C (98.6°F). It should be recognized that there is some variation that is still within the range of normal. Some persons are quite normal at 36.6°C (98°F) and others at 37.3°C (99° F). Children playing hard during summer months quite regularly run temperatures as high as 37.7°C (100°F), and occasionally higher, but this should subside quite promptly with rest. Moreover, it should be recognized that there is a normal diurnal variation of a degree or two in body temperature throughout the day. Most persons achieve their low early in the morning. Body temperature rises during the day to 37.3°C (99°F) or 37.5°C (99.5°F) and then subsides through the night.

Palpation

Palpation is a vital part of the physical examination. Many structures of the body, although not visible, are accessible by the hand and may, in a way, be "felt." Examples include blood vessels, lymph nodes, the thyroid, the organs of the abdomen and pelvis, and the rectum. It should be noted that in examining the abdomen, auscultation is performed *before* palpation and percussion to avoid altering bowel sounds.

Sounds generated within the body, if within specified frequency ranges, also may be "felt." Thus, certain murmurs generated in the heart or within blood vessels (thrills) may be detected. Thrills cause a sensation to the hand much like the purring of a cat. Voice sounds are transmitted along the bronchi to the periphery of the lung. These may be perceived by touch and will be altered by certain disease states within the lung. The phenomenon is called *tactile fremitus* and is useful in assessing diseases of the chest.

Percussion

The technique of percussion translates the application of physical force into sound. It is a difficult art to perfect but one capable of yielding much information about disease processes in the chest and abdomen. The principle is to set the chest wall or abdominal wall into vibration by striking it with a firm object. The sound produced is reflective of the density of the underlying structure. Certain densities produce sounds that can be identified as percussion notes. These sounds, listed in a sequence that proceeds from the least to the most dense, are called *tympany, hyperresonance, resonance, dullness,* and *flatness.* The pitch of the sound progresses through a series, from lowest for tympany to highest for flatness; the duration of the sound ranges from long to short.

Tympany is the drumlike sound produced by percussing the air-filled stomach. *Resonance* is the sound elicited over air-filled lungs. *Hyperresonance* is audible while percussing over inflated lung tissue of the patient with emphysema. Percussion of the liver produces a dull sound, while percussion of the thigh results in flatness.

The procedure (for right-handed persons; hands should be reversed if the examiner is left-handed) is conducted as follows (Fig. 6-1): Place the distal phalanx of the left middle finger firmly against the chest wall. The other fingers should be held away from the chest wall, since any pressure they

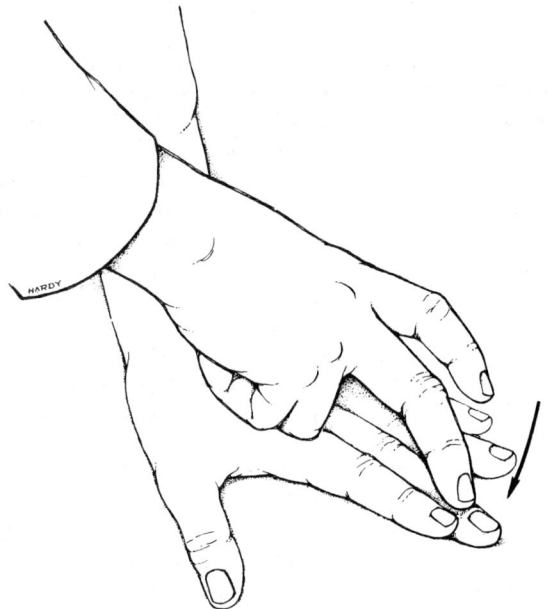

Figure 6-1
Percussion technique. The middle finger of the right hand strikes the terminal phalanx of the middle finger of the left hand. Care should be taken that only the terminal part of the middle finger of the left hand is in contact with the area to be percussed. The middle finger of the right hand should be held rigidly. It is properly a wrist action, and the intensity and clarity of the note will be a function of the quickness with which it is performed.

might exert against the thorax would tend to mute or dampen the sound produced. The right hand now becomes the striking object. The middle finger of the right hand is used to strike the terminal phalanx of the middle finger of the left hand just behind the nail bed. If done sharply, a brief resonant tone will be produced. The motion of the right hand should be dominantly a wrist action. The forearm itself should be held steady. The clarity of the sound produced is dependent on the brevity of the action. The intensity is a function of the force used.

Percussion gives one the capacity to assess such normal anatomical details as the degree to which the diaphragm descends during inspiration. The sound over lung tissue is normally resonant; the sound over the diaphragm is dull. One may percuss the border of the heart. One may determine the level of pleural effusion or the location of pneumonic consolidation or atelectasis of a lobe of the lung. Further application of the technique is discussed under examination of the thorax and abdomen.

Auscultation

Sound is produced within the body either by the movement of air through hollow structures or by the forces set up by the movement of columns of fluid that set solid structures in motion. Examples of clinically important acoustical phenomena include the movement of air through the trachea and bronchi (breath sounds), the movement of air past functioning vocal cords (spoken voice), the movement of air through the intestines (bowel sounds), the movement of blood through vascular structures that provide critical resistance to flow (murmurs), and the impedance to flowing blood provided by closed valves and the heart wall (heart sounds). Physiologic sounds may be normal (*e.g.*, first and second heart sounds) or pathologic (*e.g.*, murmurs in diastole produced in the heart, or crackles in the lung). Some normal sounds may be distorted by pathology of structures through which the sound must travel (*e.g.*, changes in the character of breath sounds as they travel through the consolidated lung of the patient with lobar pneumonia).

Sound produced within the body, if of sufficient amplitude, will set in vibration all structures between the origin of the sound and the body surface. Sound vibration emanating from the body surface may be captured directly by the examiner's ear, or more appropriately, by the stethoscope, an instrument devised as an extension of the human ear.

Although the stethoscope does not have the capacity to amplify sound, it does channel it, thereby making physiologic sound more readily available for our critical evaluation. Two end-pieces are available for the stethoscope: the *bell* and the *diaphragm*. Many stethoscopes come with both pieces built into a single head. Alternating between the pieces becomes a matter of turning the head of the stethoscope or flipping a switch. The bell is a small disc mounted on a conical base; it is attached to a larger disc, the diaphragm. The bell is better suited for the transmission of very low frequency sounds. It is important to place the bell so that the entire surface of the disc rests lightly on the skin surface, to avoid flattening the skin and reducing audible vibratory sensations. The diaphragm, the larger disc, is more appropriately constructed

for the reception of high-frequency sounds. It is placed firmly against the skin for optimal transmission of sound.

The head of the stethoscope is held between the index and middle fingers to provide a firm contact with the skin surface. Care is taken to avoid touching the tubing or rubbing other surfaces (hair, clothing) during auscultation. This minimizes extraneous noises that could confuse the examiner. The earpieces of the stethoscope should fit snugly into the ear canals, and the tubing should not be more than 20 cm in length. Dual tubing transmits sound more faithfully than single tubing.

Sound produced by the body has the features of sound produced in any other manner; that is, it is characterized by intensity, frequency, and quality. The *intensity,* or loudness, associated with physiologic sound is low. Rarely may sounds of the body, except for speech, be heard without direct application of the ear or the stethoscope to the body surface. With respect to *frequency,* or pitch, it may be said that physiologic sound is in reality "noise," in that most sounds consist of a frequency spectrum as opposed to single-frequency sounds that we associate with music or the tuning fork. The frequency spectrum may be quite low, yielding a rumbling noise, or comparatively high, producing a harsh or blowing sound. The third feature of sound is *quality*. This relates to overtones and is the characteristic of sound that allows one to differentiate sound produced by the piano from that produced by the violin. Sound quality enables the examiner to distinguish between the musical quality of high-pitched wheezing (sibilant rhonchi) and the low-pitched rumbling of a diastolic murmur.

Special applications of the fundamental processes of inspection, palpation, percussion, and auscultation with respect to specific organ systems and parts of the body are discussed in appropriate chapters throughout this book.

The Nutritional Assessment

Nutrition plays an important role in maintaining health and preventing disease. When illness or injury occurs, nutrition is an essential factor in promoting healing and reinforcing resistance to infection. Assessment of the person's nutritional status provides information on obesity, undernutrition, weight loss, malnutrition, deficiencies in specific nutrients, metabolic abnormalities, the effects of medications on nutrition, and special problems of the hospitalized patient.

Certain signs and symptoms that suggest possible nutritional deficiency are easy to note because they are specific. However, there are physical signs that have no relation to poor diet and that must be carefully distinguished from nutritional deficiencies. Some of the physical signs may be the result of other factors, such as poor hygiene or exposure to the sun or, possibly, systemic disorders. A physical sign that suggests a nutritional abnormality should be considered a clue rather than a diagnosis and as such should be pursued further. For example, certain signs that may appear to indicate nutritional deficiency may actually reflect other conditions, such as endocrine disorders, infectious disease, or disorders affecting digestion and absorption capacity or the excretion or storage of nutrients in the body.

Nutritional status can be determined by one or more of the following methods:

- Medical and clinical examination
- Anthropometric measurements
- Biochemical tests
- Dietary intake

Clinical Examination

The state of nutrition is reflected in a person's appearance. Although the most obvious physical sign of good nutrition is a normal body weight with respect to height, body frame, and age, other tissues can serve as indicators of nutritional status; these include the hair, skin, teeth, gums, mucous membranes, mouth and tongue, skeletal muscles, abdomen, lower extremities, and thyroid gland (Table 6-1).

Anthropometric Measurements

The most common anthropometric measurements include height, weight, and the circumferences of the upper arm and arm muscle. When anthropometric measurements are gathered as part of data collection, standardized equipment and procedures are used, as well as standard measurement guides. Although such measurements focus on undernutrition, they also detect obesity. See Table 6-2 for ideal adult weight. Measurement of skinfold thickness and arm and muscle circumference is described under Assessment of the Hospitalized Patient, later in this chapter (see Table 6-6).

Biochemical Assessment

Biochemical assessment reflects both the tissue level of a given nutrient and any abnormality of metabolism in the uti-

TABLE 6-1
Physical Signs Indicative of Nutritional Status

Body Area	Signs of Good Nutrition	Signs of Poor Nutrition
Hair	Shiny, lustrous; firm, healthy scalp	Dull and dry, brittle, depigmented, easily plucked
Face	Skin color uniform; healthy appearance	Skin dark over cheeks and under eyes, skin flaky, face swollen
Eyes	Bright, clear, moist	Eye membranes pale, dry (xerophthalmia); Bitot's spots, increased vascularity, cornea soft (keratomalacia)
Lips	Good color (pink), smooth	Swollen and puffy (cheilosis), angular lesion at corners of mouth (angular fissures)
Tongue	Deep red in appearance; surface papillae present	Smooth appearance, swollen, beefy red, sores, atrophic papillae
Teeth	Straight, no crowding, no cavities, bright	Cavities, mottled appearance (fluorosis), malpositioned
Gums	Firm, good color (pink)	Spongy, bleed easily, marginal redness, recession
Glands	No enlargement of the thyroid	Thyroid enlargement (simple goiter)
Skin	Smooth, good color, moist	Rough, dry, flaky, swollen, pale, pigmented; lack of fat under skin
Nails	Firm, pink	Spoon shaped, ridged
Skeleton	Good posture, no malformation	Poor posture, beading of ribs, bowed legs or knock knees
Muscles	Well developed, firm	Flaccid, poor tone, wasted, underdeveloped
Extremities	No tenderness	Weak and tender; presence of edema
Abdomen	Flat	Swollen
Nervous system	Normal reflexes	Decrease in or loss of ankle and knee reflexes

TABLE 6-2
Ideal Weights Derived From Life Insurance Statistics

1983 Metropolitan Height and Weight Tables*

Men Height Feet	Inches	Small Frame	Medium Frame	Large Frame	Women Height Feet	Inches	Small Frame	Medium Frame	Large Frame
5	2	128–134	131–141	138–150	4	10	102–111	109–121	118–131
5	3	130–136	133–143	140–153	4	11	103–113	111–123	120–134
5	4	132–138	135–145	142–156	5	0	104–115	113–126	122–137
5	5	134–140	137–148	144–160	5	1	106–118	115–129	125–140
5	6	136–142	139–151	146–164	5	2	108–121	118–132	128–143
5	7	138–145	142–154	149–168	5	3	111–124	121–135	131–147
5	8	140–148	145–157	152–172	5	4	114–127	124–138	134–151
5	9	142–151	148–160	155–176	5	5	117–130	127–141	137–155
5	10	144–154	151–163	158–180	5	6	120–133	130–144	140–159
5	11	146–157	154–166	161–184	5	7	123–136	133–147	143–163
6	0	149–160	157–170	164–188	5	8	126–139	136–150	146–167
6	1	152–164	160–174	168–192	5	9	129–142	139–153	149–170
6	2	155–168	164–178	172–197	5	10	132–145	142–156	152–173
6	3	158–172	167–182	176–202	5	11	135–148	145–159	155–176
6	4	162–176	171–187	181–207	6	0	138–151	148–162	158–179

To Make an Approximation of Your Frame Size . . .

Extend your arm and bend the forearm upward at a 90°
angle. Keep fingers straight and turn the inside of your wrist
toward your body. If you have a caliper, use it to measure the
space between the two prominent bones on *either side* of your
elbow. Without a caliper, place thumb and index finger of
your other hand on these two bones. Measure the space
between your fingers against a ruler or tape measure.
Compare it with these tables that list elbow measurements for
medium-framed men and women. Measurements lower than
those listed indicate you have a small frame. Higher
measurements indicate a large frame.

Men Height in 1″ Heels	Elbow Breadth	Women Height in 1″ Heels	Elbow Breadth
5′2″–5′3″	2½″–2⅞″	4′10″–4′11″	2¼″–2½″
5′4″–5′7″	2⅝″–2⅞″	5′0″–5′3″	2¼″–2½″
5′8″–5′11″	2¾″–3″	5′4″–5′7″	2⅜″–2⅝″
6′0″–6′3″	2¾″–3⅛″	5′8″–5′11″	2⅜″–2⅝″
6′4″	2⅞″–3¼″	6′0″	2½″–2¾″

* Weights at ages 25–59 based on lowest mortality. Weight in pounds according to frame (in indoor clothing weighing 5 lbs. for men and 3 lbs. for women; shoes with 1″ heels).

(Revised Height–Weight Tables derived from life-insurance statistics prepared by the Metropolitan Life Insurance Company: men and women. Copyright 1983, Metropolitan Life Insurance Company.)

lization of nutrients. These determinations are made from
blood studies (serum protein, serum albumin and globulin,
hemoglobin, serum vitamin A, carotene, and vitamin C) and
from urine studies (creatinine, thiamine, riboflavin, niacin,
and iodine). Some of these tests, while reflecting recent intake
of the elements detected, can also identify suboptimum levels
when there are no clinical symptoms of deficiency. (See Table
6-7 for a suggested guide for the interpretation of blood data.)

Assessment of Food Intake

The appraisal of food intake considers quantity and quality
of diet and also frequency of consumption of certain food
items in order to determine current or customary intake of
nutrients. Commonly used methods of determining individual
consumption include the food record and intake estimation
by recall. These methods are discussed with the patient and
explained during the taking of the diet history.

Food Record. The food record is used most often in
nutritional status studies. The person is asked to keep a record
of food actually consumed over a period of time, varying
from 3 to 7 days. Some instructions are given for accuracy
in estimating and describing the specific foods consumed.
This method appears to be fairly accurate, depending on the
subject's integrity and ability to estimate quantity of food.

24-Hour Recall. The 24-hour recall method is, as the
name implies, recall of food intake over a 24-hour period.
The subject is asked by the interviewer to recall all food eaten
during the previous day and to estimate the quantities of the
food consumed. Information obtained by this method is not
always representative of usual intake. For this reason, at the
end of the interview the subject is asked if the previous day's
food intake was a typical one. To obtain supplementary information about the typical diet, the interviewer should also
ask how frequently foods from certain food groups are eaten.

The dietary and biochemical data for most nutrients provide more information than the clinical examination. The clinical examination is not sensitive enough to detect subclinical deficiencies unless such deficiencies become so advanced that overt signs develop. A low dietary intake of nutrients over a period of time may lead to low biochemical levels and, without nutritional intervention, may result in characteristic and observable signs and symptoms.

Conducting the Interview

As was indicated in the chapter on interviewing techniques, it is important that the interviewer establish a rapport with the patient in order to promote respect and trust. The success of the interviewer in eliciting pertinent information for dietary assessment depends on the quality of communication established at the outset.

In the initial stages of the interview, the interviewer should introduce and explain the purpose of the interview. The rest of the session should be conducted in a nondirective and exploratory way, allowing the respondent to express his feelings and thoughts. At the same time, the respondent should be encouraged to respond specifically to the questions asked.

The manner in which a question is asked will influence the extent to which the respondent will cooperate. To this end, the interviewer should accept a reply to a question without expressing disapproval, either directly by comment or indirectly by facial expression. For example, if the respondent says, 'We eat rattlesnake meat as an appetizer," the reviewer should not express amazement or disgust by making faces or saying anything negative.

Sometimes a series of questions is necessary in order to elicit the information needed. Consider the following exchange:

Interviewer: "What time did you get out of bed yesterday?"

Respondent: "I got up at six o'clock in the morning to prepare breakfast for my husband, and I had a cup of coffee with him."

Interviewer: "Did you put anything in your coffee?"

Respondent: "Only a teaspoon of sugar, nothing else."

Interviewer: "Did you have anything else with your coffee?"

Respondent: "No, not at that time. I had breakfast later, around eight o'clock in the morning."

When attempting to elicit information about the kind and quantity of food eaten at a particular time, the interviewer should not ask a suggestive question, such as "Did you put sugar or cream in your coffee?" Also, assumptions should not be made about the size of servings. Instead, questions should be phrased so that quantities are more clearly determined. For example, to help determine indirectly the size of one hamburger eaten, the following question may be asked: "How many hamburgers were prepared out of the pound of ground meat you said you bought?" Another approach to determining quantities is to use food models of known sizes in estimating portions of meat, cake, or pie or to record quantities in common measurements, such as cups or spoonfuls, (or according to the size of containers, when discussing intake of bottled beverages).

In recording a particular combination dish, such as "Spanish rice" or "stew," ask for the ingredients in the recipe, recording the largest quantities first. Note whether the ingredients were raw or cooked and the number of servings provided by the recipe. When the client has finished listing the foods for the recall questionnaire, it may be helpful to read the list of foods back and ask if anything was forgotten, such as fruit, cake, candy, between-meal snacks, or cocktails.

Additional information obtained during the interview should include methods of preparing food, sources available for food (donated foods, food stamps), food buying practices, vitamin and mineral supplements, and income range.

Evaluating the Dietary Information

Once the dietary information has been obtained, the diet must be evaluated for its nutritive value. The first method is to use acceptable food composition tables, like those issued by the Department of Agriculture. The diet is then calculated in terms of grams and milligrams of specific nutrients. The total nutritive value is then compared with the Recommended Dietary Allowances, or RDAs, (Table 6-3), and the nutritional evaluation is expressed in terms of percentage of adequacy for each nutrient.

A second method of evaluation is to compare the diet data with recommendations based on foods selected from various food groups for various age levels, such as the "Basic Four Food Groups" or "The Guide to Good Eating" (Table 6-4).

The choice of a method for dietary evaluation depends on the purpose of the assessment. If the health counselor is interested in knowing about the intake of specific nutrients, such as vitamin A, iron, or calcium, then the food record method would be the one to use. The food intake would be analyzed by consulting an official publication listing foods according to composition and nutrient content. This analysis would then be compared with the RDAs (Table 6-3) and the nutrient intake evaluated in terms of percentage of adequacy in reference to that standard.

Interpreting the 24-Hour Recall Form. An example of a 24-hour recall form is detailed in Table 6-5. This sample contains dietary information about Mrs. Brown, a 25-year-old housewife, indicating the different kinds of food she consumed, the times during the day when she consumed them, and the quantities she consumed, as measured in household units. The questionnaire indicates that Mrs. Brown's diet is adequate with respect to the bread and cereal group and foods rich in vitamin A, low in food sources of calcium and vitamin C, and only slightly lacking in servings of protein foods. On the other hand, Mrs. Brown's 24-hour recall record shows an excessive intake of high-calorie foods from the miscellaneous food group. This food consumption practice is reflected in her weight, which is 19% over acceptable normal standards—enough to characterize her as obese.

A plan of action for nutritional care should be based on the results of the dietary assessment and the client's profile. Two main objectives derived from the nutritional assessment and evaluation are

- Appropriate food selection for a balanced diet
- Appropriate food intake for weight control

TABLE 6-3
Food and Nutrition Board, National Academy of Sciences–National Research Council Recommended Daily Dietary Allowances,[a] Revised 1980

	Age (years)	Weight (kg)	Weight (lb)	Height (cm)	Height (in)	Protein (g)	Vitamin A (µg RE)[b]	Vitamin D (µg)[c]	Vitamin E (mg α-TE)[d]	Vitamin C (mg)	Thiamin (mg)	Riboflavin (mg)	Niacin (mg NE)[e]	Vitamin B6 (mg)	Folacin (µg)[f]	Vitamin B12 (µg)	Calcium (mg)	Phosphorus (mg)	Magnesium (mg)	Iron (mg)	Zinc (mg)	Iodine (µg)
Infants	0.0–0.5	6	13	60	24	kg × 2.2	420	10	3	35	0.3	0.4	6	0.3	30	0.5[g]	360	240	50	10	3	40
	0.5–1.0	9	20	71	28	kg × 2.0	400	10	4	35	0.5	0.6	8	0.6	45	1.5	540	360	70	15	5	50
Children	1–3	13	29	90	35	23	400	10	5	45	0.7	0.8	9	0.9	100	2.0	800	800	150	15	10	70
	4–6	20	44	112	44	30	500	10	6	45	0.9	1.0	11	1.3	200	2.5	800	800	200	10	10	90
	7–10	28	62	132	52	34	700	10	7	45	1.2	1.4	16	1.6	300	3.0	800	800	250	10	10	120
Males	11–14	45	99	157	62	45	1000	10	8	50	1.4	1.6	18	1.8	400	3.0	1200	1200	350	18	15	150
	15–18	66	145	176	69	56	1000	10	10	60	1.4	1.7	18	2.0	400	3.0	1200	1200	400	18	15	150
	19–22	70	154	177	70	56	1000	7.5	10	60	1.5	1.7	19	2.2	400	3.0	800	800	350	10	15	150
	23–50	70	154	178	70	56	1000	5	10	60	1.4	1.6	18	2.2	400	3.0	800	800	350	10	15	150
	51+	70	154	178	70	56	1000	5	10	60	1.2	1.4	16	2.2	400	3.0	800	800	350	10	15	150
Females	11–14	46	101	157	62	46	800	10	8	50	1.1	1.3	15	1.8	400	3.0	1200	1200	300	18	15	150
	15–18	55	120	163	64	46	800	10	8	60	1.1	1.3	14	2.0	400	3.0	1200	1200	300	18	15	150
	19–22	55	120	163	64	44	800	7.5	8	60	1.1	1.3	14	2.0	400	3.0	800	800	300	18	15	150
	23–50	55	120	163	64	44	800	5	8	60	1.0	1.2	13	2.0	400	3.0	800	800	300	18	15	150
	51+	55	120	163	64	44	800	5	8	60	1.0	1.2	13	2.0	400	3.0	800	800	300	10	15	150
Pregnant						+30	+200	+5	+2	+20	+0.4	+0.3	+2	+0.6	+400	+1.0	+400	+400	+150	[h]	+5	+25
Lactating						+20	+400	+5	+3	+40	+0.5	+0.5	+5	+0.5	+100	+1.0	+400	+400	+150	[h]	+10	+50

[a] The allowances are intended to provide for individual variations among most normal persons as they live in the United States under usual environmental stresses. Diets should be based on a variety of common foods in order to provide other nutrients for which human requirements have been less well defined.

[b] Retinol equivalents. 1 retinol equivalent = 1 µg retinol or 6 µg β-carotene.

[c] As cholecalciferol. 10 µg cholecalciferol = 400 IU of vitamin D.

[d] α-tocopherol equivalents. 1 mg d-α-tocopherol = 1 α-TE.

[e] 1 NE (niacin equivalent) is equal to 1 mg of niacin or 60 mg of dietary tryptophan.

[f] The folacin allowances refer to dietary sources as determined by Lactobacillus casei assay after treatment with enzymes (conjugases) to make polyglutamyl forms of the vitamin available to the test organism.

[g] The recommended dietary allowance for vitamin B12 in infants is based on average concentration of the vitamin in human milk. The allowances after weaning are based on energy intake (as recommended by the American Academy of Pediatrics) and consideration of other factors, such as intestinal absorption.

[h] The increased requirement during pregnancy cannot be met by the iron content of habitual American diets nor by the existing iron stores of many women; therefore, the use of 30 mg to 60 mg of supplemental iron is recommended. Iron needs during lactation are not substantially different from those of nonpregnant women, but continued supplementation of the mother for 2 to 3 months after parturition is advisable in order to replenish stores depleted by pregnancy.

TABLE 6-4
Basic Four Food Groups: The Daily Guide to Good Eating

Food Groups	Recommended Amounts	
Milk Group	*8-ounce cups:*	
Milk, cottage cheese, ice cream, yogurt	Children under 9	2 to 3 cups
	Children 9–12	3 to 4 cups
	Adolescents	4 or more cups
	Adults	2 or more cups
	Pregnant women	3 or more cups
	Nursing mothers	4 or more cups
Meat Group	2- to 3-ounce serving; cooked, without bone; 2 servings total	
Lean beef, veal, pork, lamb, poultry, fish		
Alternatives:		
Dried beans, peas, lentils	1-cup serving, cooked	
Peanut butter	4-tablespoons serving	
Eggs	2	
Vegetables, Fruits	½-cup serving, 1 piece fruit; 4 servings total	
Dark green or yellow	1 serving, vitamin A rich	
Citrus fruit or vegetable	1 serving, vitamin C rich—or 2 servings of a fair source	
Other vegetables and fruits	2 or more servings	
Breads and Cereals	4 servings total	
Bread, rolls, biscuits, muffins	1 slice or small piece	
Ready-to-eat cereals	1-ounce serving	
Cooked cereal, cornmeal, grits, macaroni, noodles, rice, spaghetti	½- to ¾-cup serving, cooked	
Miscellaneous Group		
Cream, bacon, butter, margarine, shortening, oil, salad dressing, olives, jam, jelly, sugar, candy, cake, pie, carbonated beverages, relishes, alcoholic beverages, snack foods, pretzels, potato chips, etc.	Provide mostly calories for the day's total intake	

Nutritional Assessment of the Hospitalized Patient

Many disease conditions produce metabolic alterations that result in *negative nitrogen balance*. When these conditions are coupled with anorexia, they can lead to malnutrition. It is known that malnutrition interferes with wound healing, increases susceptibility to infection, and contributes to prolonged bed confinement in the hospital population.

Butterworth cites several examples of nutritional neglect in hospitals. He points out that iatrogenic malnutrition has become a significant factor in determining the outcome of illness in many patients. Among the undesirable practices affecting the nutritional health of hospital patients are the following:

- Prolonged use of glucose and saline IV therapy
- Withholding of meals because of diagnostic tests
- Use of tube feedings in inadequate amounts and of uncertain composition
- Failure to recognize increased nutritional needs resulting from injury or illness

Many drugs also influence the nutritional status of patients. Some of these medications may have a specific appetite-depressant effect, may irritate the mucosa, or may cause nausea and vomiting. Others may influence bacterial flora in the intestine or directly affect nutrient absorption, so that secondary malnutrition results.

The body in starvation may convert protein to glucose for energy; the result is persistent loss of muscle tissue. One sensitive indicator of the body's gain or loss of protein is its *nitrogen balance*. An adult is said to be in *nitrogen equilibrium* when the nitrogen intake (from food) equals the nitrogen output (in urine, feces, and perspiration); it is a sign of health. A positive nitrogen balance exists when nitrogen intake exceeds nitrogen output and indicates tissue growth, such as

TABLE 6-5
24-Hour Recall Questionnaire for Adults

Name: *Mrs. Brown*	Date of recall: *3/4*	Day of recall: *Tuesday*	
Age: *24 Years*	Male _____	Female __✓__	Occupation: *Housewife*
Height (in): *64*	Weight (lb): *148*	Ideal weight (lb): *124*	% of ideal: *119%*

Ingestion Period	Kinds of Foods and Description	Amount in Household Units	Frequency of Consumption of Various Foods	Times per Day-Week-Month ×D	×W	×M
6:00 AM	Coffee	1 cup	Milk, whole		4	
	Sugar	1 tsp	Milk, skim			
	Cream	2 tbsp	Yogurt		3	
8:00 AM	Cornflakes	1 cup	Cheese		3	
	Milk, whole	½ cup	Ice cream		5	
			Beef		4	
12:00 NOON	Sandwich		Pork			1
	Bread, white	2 slices	Lamb			1
	Peanut butter	2 tbsp	Fish		1	
	Apple	1 small	Poultry		3	
	Coffee	1 cup	Eggs		5	
	Sugar	1 tsp	Cream	3		
	Cream	2 tbsp	Butter		3	
3:00 PM	Coca-Cola, regular	1 (12-ounce can)	Margarine	3		
	Almond Joy bar	1½ ounces	Oil	1		
			Salad dressings	1		
6:30 PM	Fried filet of sole	3 ounces	Vegetables			
	Green beans	½ cup	Green-yellow	1		
	Boiled potato	1 medium	Citrus fruits		3	
	Lettuce salad	1 cup	Legumes			
	French dressing	2 tbsp	Beans		1	
	Muffin	1 small	Chick peas			1
	Coffee	1 cup	Lentils			
	Sugar	1 tsp	Potatoes	1		
	Cream	2 tbsp	Breads	3		
10:30 PM	Chocolate cake (8″ diam.)	¹⁄₁₆ cake	Pastas		4	
	Coca-Cola, regular	1 (12-ounce can)	Rice			
			Cakes	1		
			Pies		4	
			Candy bars	1		
			Jams-jellies		5	
			Sugar	3		
			Alcoholic beverage			
			Carbonated beverage	3		
			Coffee, tea	3		
			Snack foods	1		
			Vitamin supplement			
			Mineral supplement			

occurs during pregnancy, childhood, recovery from surgery, and rebuilding of wasted tissue. Negative nitrogen balance indicates that tissue is breaking down faster than it is being replaced. It can be brought about by fever, surgery, burns, and other debilitating diseases, as well as by starvation. For instance, each gram of nitrogen loss in excess of intake represents the depletion of 6.25 gm of protein or 25 gm of muscle tissue. Therefore, a negative nitrogen balance of 10 gm/day for 10 days could mean the wasting of 2.5 kg (5.5 pounds) of muscle tissue.

The hospital may have a metabolic nutrition support unit, managed by a physician working with a specially trained team consisting of a pharmacist, a nurse, and a dietitian. The following parameters are used in nutritional assessment of the hospitalized patient:

1. Anthropometric measurement
    Weight/height
    Triceps skinfold thickness
    Mid-arm and arm muscle circumferences

2. Biochemical measurements
   Albumin
   Transferrin
   Total lymphocyte count
   Creatinine/height index
   Urinary tests (sodium, potassium, urea, creatinine)

Weight loss is an extremely important measurement since it reflects inadequate calorie intake. In the semistarved patient, weight loss indicates an increased loss of protein from the body cell mass. With respect to *anthropometric measurements* for protein calorie malnutrition, the best available indicators are triceps skinfold thickness (Fig. 6-2), which indicates fat stores, and muscle circumference (Fig. 6-3), which indicates the state of muscle protein (Table 6-6).

Lower serum albumin and *transferrin* levels are useful measures of visceral protein deficits in adults and are expressed as percentages of normal values (Table 6-7). Both are indicators of the degree of malnutrition. Serial measurements of these are used to assess the results of nutritional therapy.

Reduced amounts of *leukocytes* in hospitalized patients who become acutely malnourished as a result of stress and low-calorie feeding are associated with impairment of cellular immunity.

Information about *electrolyte balance* provides an assessment of kidney function as a metabolic response to infused electrolytes. The creatinine/height index calculated over a 24-hour period assesses the metabolically active tissue and indicates the degree of protein depletion, comparing expected body mass for height and actual body cell mass.

The nurse is in a position to take part in nutrition screening by devising her own nutrition record as a tool, if the hospital does not have a separate screening form. Such a brief assessment guide can help to identify patients who need more intensive nutritional evaluation. The findings can then be communicated to the dietitian and the rest of the team for further assessment and for clinical nutrition intervention.

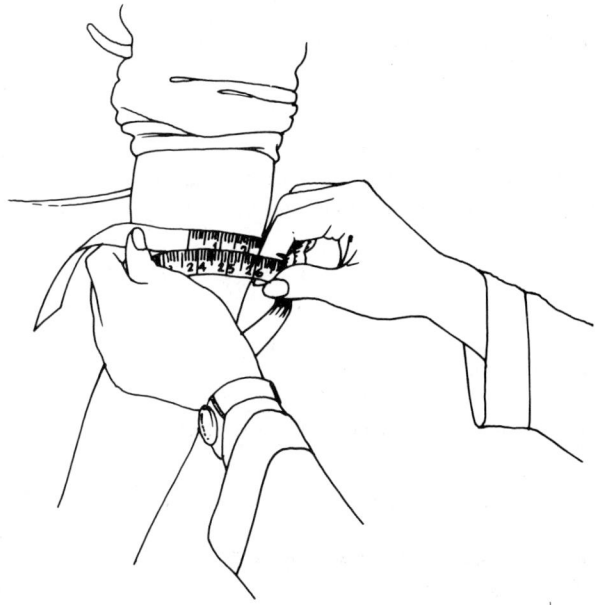

Figure 6-3
Measurement of arm muscle circumference.

Diagnostic Categories of Malnutrition

After the data for nutritional assessment have been collected, determination of the category of malnutrition that applies to the individual patient becomes the first consideration in order to plan an effective regimen for nutritional support of the hospitalized patient. Table 6-8 indicates nutritional status classification.

Gerontological Considerations

Without a doubt, disease affecting any part of the gastrointestinal tract can be expected to alter nutritional requirements

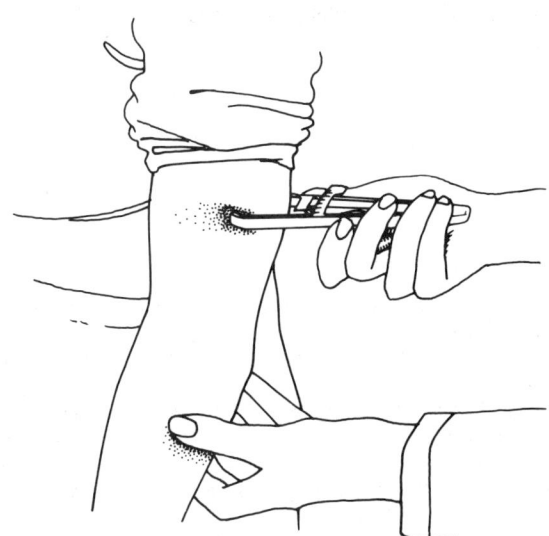

Figure 6-2
Skinfold calipers for measurement of skinfold thickness.

TABLE 6-6
Anthropometric Measurements: Standard Values at Various Deficiency Levels

	(mm) *Standard*	*90% Standard*	*80% Standard*	*70% Standard*	*60% Standard*
Triceps Skinfold (Adult)					
Male	12.5	11.3	10.0	8.8	7.5
Female	16.5	14.9	13.2	11.6	9.9
Arm Circumference (Adult)					
Male	29.3	26.3	23.4	20.5	17.6
Female	28.5	25.7	22.8	20.0	17.1
Muscle Circumference (Adult)					
Male	25.3	22.8	20.2	17.7	15.2
Female	23.2	20.9	18.6	16.2	13.9

(Adapted from Butterworth CE and Blackburn GL. Hospital malnutrition. Nutr Today 1975 Mar/Apr; 10[2]:11–12.)

TABLE 6-7
Suggested Guide to Interpretation of Blood Data*

	Deficient	Low	Acceptable	High
Total plasma protein: gm/dl	<6.0	6.0–6.4	6.5–6.9	≥7.0
Serum albumin (electrophoretic method): gm/dl	<2.80	2.80–3.51	3.52–4.24	≥4.25
Serum globulin (percent of serum protein):				
α_1			4–7	
α_2			9–11	
β			11–15	
γ			12–16	
Hemoglobin, gm/dl:				
Men	<12.0	12.0–13.9	14.0–14.9	≥15.0
Women (nonpregnant, nonlactating; ≥13 years)	<10.0	10.0–10.9	11.0–14.4	≥14.5
Children (3–12 years)	<10.0	10.0–10.9	11.0–12.4	≥12.5
Hematocrit (PCV), percent:				
Men	<36	36–41	42–44	≥45
Women (nonpregnant, nonlactating; ≥13 years)	<30	30–37	38–42	≥43
Children (3–12 years)	<30.0	30.0–33.9	34.0–36.9	≥37.0
Plasma ascorbic acid: mg/dl	<0.10	0.10–0.19	0.20–0.39	≥0.40
Plasma vitamin A: μg/dl	<10	10–19	20–49	≥50
Plasma carotene: μg/dl	3	20–39	40–99	≥100
Red cell riboflavin: μg/dl—red blood cells	<10.0	10.0–14.9	15.0–19.9	≥20

* Except for the particulates in blood, serum levels of nutrients in children do not differ appreciably beyond infancy from those of adults. Similarly, with the exception of hemoglobin and hematocrit, the serum levels of blood constituents in women of childbearing age are comparable to those of men.

(Interdepartmental Committee on Nutrition for National Defense: Manual for Nutrition Surveys, 2nd ed.)

and patient status. The goal of diet therapy in the elderly is to maintain nutrition and replace nutrient losses within the framework of the patient's condition and environment. This takes patience and imagination.

Elderly persons often take excessive and inappropriate medications. The number of adverse reactions increases proportionately with the number of prescribed and over-the-counter drugs taken. Age-related physiologic and pathophysiologic changes may alter the metabolism and elimination of many drugs. Consequently, drugs can influence food intake by producing side-effects such as nausea, vomiting, and decreased appetite. They may alter nutrient metabolism by interfering with distribution, utilization, and storing of nutrients.

Furthermore, in the elderly, nutritional problems often occur or are precipitated by such infectious illnesses as pneumonia, urinary tract infections, pyodermas, and herpes zoster. Like malnutrition, acute and chronic diseases may affect the metabolism and utilization of nutrients, which already are altered owing to the aging process. The goal obviously is to prevent infections or to shorten such illnesses by prescribing antibiotics and using available vaccines.

Bibliography

Books

Physical Assessment

Barry PO. Psychosocial Nursing Assessment and Intervention. Philadelphia, JB Lippincott, 1984.
Bates B. A Guide to Physical Examination, 4th ed. Philadelphia, JB Lippincott, 1987.
Block GJ and Nolan JW. Health Assessment for Professional Nursing: A Developmental Approach, 2nd ed. Norwalk, Connecticut, Appleton-Century-Crofts, 1986.
Brown MS. Student Manual of Physical Examination, 2nd ed. Philadelphia, JB Lippincott, 1985.
Carcio HN. Manual of Health Assessment. Boston, Little, Brown & Co, 1985.
Grimes J and Iannopollo E. Health Assessment in Nursing Practice. Monterey, California, Wadsworth Health Sciences Division, 1982.

TABLE 6-8
Nutritional Status Classification

Standards		Mild	Moderate	Severe
Albumin (gm/dl)		3.5–3.0	<3.0–2.5	<2.5
Transferrin (gm/dl)		200–180	<180–160	<160
Lymphocyte count		1800–1500	<1500–900	<900
Triceps skinfold	% deficit			
Mid-arm circum.	% deficit	>5%–15%	>15%–30%	>30%
Arm muscle circum.	% deficit			

(Adapted from Kaminski MV and Winborn AL: Nutritional Assessment Guide. Midwest Nutrition, Education and Research Foundation Inc, 1978.)

Jones DA, Lepley MK, and Baker BA. Health Assessment Across the Life Span. New York, McGraw-Hill, 1984.

Malasanos L et al. Health Assessment, 3rd ed. St Louis, CV Mosby, 1985.

Weed L. Medical Records, Medical Education and Patient Care. Cleveland, Case Western Reserve University Press, 1968.

Nutritional Assessment

Anderson CE and Coursin DB (eds). Nutritional Support of Medical Practice. New York, Harper & Row, 1983.

Cerra FB. Pocket Manual of Surgical Nutrition. St Louis, CV Mosby, 1984.

Krause MV and Mahon LK. Food Nutrition and Diet Therapy. Philadelphia, WB Saunders, 1984.

Suitor CJW and Crowley MF. Nutrition, 2nd ed. Philadelphia, JB Lippincott, 1984.

Articles

Documentation

Beyond data gathering: Twelve functions of the medical history (editorial). Hosp Pract 1985 Mar 30; 20(3A):11–12.

Gawlinski A and Rasmussen S. Improving documentation through the use of change theory. Focus Crit Care 1984 Dec; 11(6):12–17.

Hnott ES and Davis D. Triage problem oriented documentation reflects quality care. Point of View (Ethicon) 1984; 21(2):10–11.

Kiely MA. Guidelines for systems-oriented charting and reporting. Crit Care Nurs 1984 May/June; 4(3):62–64.

Lichtenstein MJ and Schaffner W. Assessing activities of daily living. Hosp Pract 1985 May 30; 20(5A):8–9.

McGrath A. Second thoughts on annual physicals. Forbes 1985 Sept 23; 194–195.

Ninos M and Makohon R. Functional assessment of the patient. Geriatr Nurs 1985 May/June; 6(3):139–142.

Nowack DH. Beyond data gathering: Twelve functions of the medical history. Hosp Pract 1985 Mar 31; 20(3A):11–12

Rutkowski B. How DRGs are changing your charting. Nursing '85 1985 Oct; 15(10):49–51.

Steel K. History taking from elderly patients. Hosp Pract 1985 May 30; 20(5A):70–71.

Torre CT. Assessing the adolescent. Top Clin Nurs 1986 Apr; 8(1):11–12.

Wolf S. The fine art of taking a history. Hosp Pract 1985 Sept 30; 20(9A):6–9.

Physical Assessment

Bower FN and Patterson J. A theory-based nursing assessment of the aged. Top Clin Nurs 1986 Apr; 8(1):27–32.

Gender AR. Development of a comprehensive nursing history and physical assessment program in a rehabilitation setting. Rehabil Nurs 1983 Sep/Oct; 8(5):17–21.

Nutritional Assessment

Baker JP et al. Nutritional assessment: A comparison of clinical judgment and objective measurements. N Engl J Med 1982 Apr 22; 306(16):969–972.

Butterworth CE Jr and Blackburn GL. Hospital malnutrition. Nutr Today 1975 Mar/Apr; 10(2):8–18.

Cockran D and Kaminski MV. Current concepts in nutritional assessment. Nutr Support Services 1986 May; 6(5):14–15.

Hall CA. Nutritional assessment. N Engl J Med 1982 Sept 16; 307(12):754.

Hinson LR. Nutritional assessment and management of the hospitalized patient. Crit Care Nurs 1985 Feb; 5(2):53–57.

Laffrey SC. Normal and overweight adults: Perceived weight and health behavior characteristics. Nurs Res 1986 May/June; 35(6):173–177.

Lipschitz DA. Protein–calorie malnutrition in the hospitalized elderly. Med Clin North Am 1982 Sept; 9(3):531–543.

McLaren DS and Meguid MM. Nutritional assessment at the crossroads. JPEN 1983 June; 7(6):575–579.

Morgan J. Nutritional assessment of critically ill patients. Focus Crit Care 1984 June; 11(3):28–34.

Morowitz HJ. Ecology and the great cold cereal rip-off. Hosp Pract 1985 Mar 15; 20(3):30–31.

Orme JF and Clemmer TP. Nutrition in the critical care unit. Med Clin North Am 1983 Nov; 67(6):1295–1302.

Seltzer MH et al. Instant nutritional assessment: Absolute weight loss and surgical mortality. JPEN 1982 May/June; 6(3):218–221.

Superko HR, Haskell WL, and Wood PD. Modification of plasma cholesterol through exercise. Postgrad Med 1985 Oct; 78(5):64–75.

Vitale JJ. Nutrition and the elderly. Postgrad Med 1985 Oct; 78(5):93–102.

Vitamin supplements. Med Lett 1985 Aug 2; 27(693):66–67.

Warnould J and Lundholm K. Clinical significance of preoperative nutritional status in 215 non-cancer patients. Ann Surg 1984 Mar; 199(3):299–305.

Biophysical and Psychosocial Concepts Related to Health and Illness

Unit III

Homeostasis and Pathophysiologic Processes

When the body is threatened or suffers an injury, its response may involve functional and structural changes; these changes may be adaptive or maladaptive. The defense mechanisms that the body can mount will determine the difference between adaptation and maladaptation, health and disease. Physiology is the study of the functional activities of the living organism and its parts. *Patho*physiology is the study of *disordered* function of the body. *Mechanisms* are patterns of action performed by different parts of the body to serve a common goal. These mechanisms may be compensatory to restore a lost balance, such as hyperpnea to correct an oxygen deficit and lactic acid excess following running. Or, they may be pathophysiologic, such as failure of the heart, leading to sodium and water retention and high venous pressure, which contribute to further disorder. These mechanisms give rise to signs that may be observed by the nurse or symptoms that may be related by the patient. Based on these observations and a knowledge of the physiologic processes involved, the nurse can determine the existence of a problem and plan her course of action to treat it.

Dynamic Balance: The Steady State

Physiologic mechanisms must be understood in the context of the body as a whole. Man, as a living system, has both an internal and an external environment. Information and matter are continuously exchanged from one environment to the other. Within the body itself, each organ, tissue, and cell is also a system or subsystem of the whole, each with its own internal and external environment, each exchanging information and matter (Fig. 7-1). The goal of the interaction of the body's subsystems is to produce a dynamic balance or steady state, so that all are in harmony with each other, just as man, as an individual, seeks harmony with those with whom he interacts. For a better understanding of the concept of

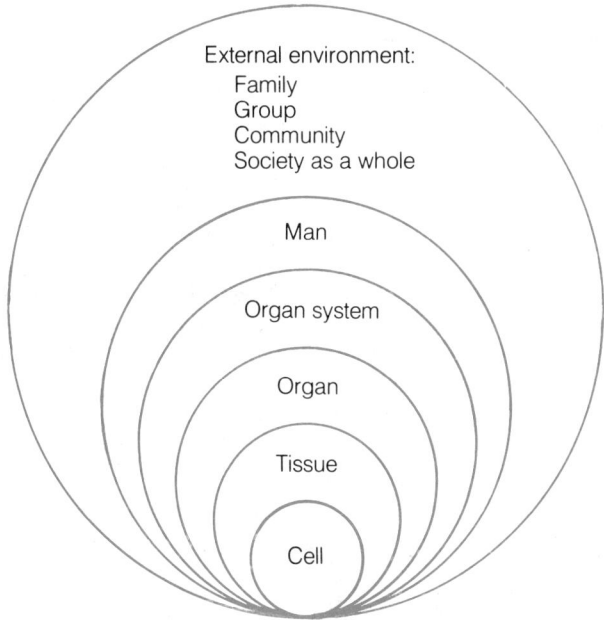

Figure 7-1
Constellation of systems. Each system is a subsystem of the larger system (suprasystem) of which it is a part. In this figure the cell is the smallest system, being a subsystem of all other systems.

steady state, the development of the principles of internal constancy, homeostasis, and adaptation will be described.

Internal Constancy, Homeostasis, and Adaptation

Claude Bernard, a French physiologist in the 19th century, developed the biological principle that for a "free life" there must be a *constancy* or "fixity of the internal milieu," despite changes in the external environment. The internal milieu he addressed was the fluid that bathes the cells, and the constancy was maintained by physiologic and biochemical processes; his principle implied a static process.

Later, Walter B. Cannon coined the term *homeostasis* to describe this constancy; his term introduced a change process into the concept of constancy. Cannon enlarged on Bernard's work by emphasizing the importance of involuntary neural control of the physiochemical responses to stimuli.

Dubos (1965) took the change or dynamic nature of responses one step further: he stated that there are two complementary concepts, homeostasis and adaptation, both necessary for a successful life. Homeostasis refers to the "necessary adjustments that the body can make rapidly" to maintain its internal composition "within limits precisely defined for each organism." This means that "absolute constancy" is "only a concept of the ideal": there are acceptable ranges of response to stimuli, and the organism chooses among them. *Adaptation,* on the other hand, refers to the responses the individual makes to function adequately under "changed conditions of the environment." Dubos was pri-

marily concerned with man's survival in and adaptation to a changing physical world.

Maintenance of the Steady State

With the application of the theory of general systems to the behavioral sciences, the terms *steady state* or *dynamic equilibrium,* which will be used here, describe this condition of internal consistency and harmony with the external environment. The maintenance of the steady state, which is necessary for a condition of health, is under the control of the body's regulatory processes, both voluntary and involuntary. In response to either internal or external stimuli, compensatory mechanisms are put into operation. These mechanisms are adaptive as long as they can maintain a steady state. If the compensatory response is not adequate, a threat to the steady state exists, function will become disordered, and pathophysiologic mechanisms will become operative. The pathophysiologic mechanisms can lead to disease, and they are also active during disease. *Disease* is a threat to the steady state and is defined as any process or event that promotes a change in the internal environment that results in loss or disruption of cell function and thus limits man's freedom to act in the external world.

An analogy can be made to the pendulum of a clock. As it swings to and fro, maintaining correct time, it is in dynamic balance, or a steady state. Someone tips the clock, and the pendulum swings a bit to one side but is still able to maintain reasonably accurate time. The clock is tipped more; now the pendulum swings more to one side than the other, and with each swing the pendulum's own weight increases the erratic movement. The clock's functional ability to provide accurate time is damaged and, if nothing intervenes, may be destroyed altogether.

Nursing Implications

It is important for the nurse to realize that the optimal point of intervention to promote health is during the stage when the individual's own compensatory processes are still functioning. It is therefore imperative to be able to relate the presenting signs and symptoms to the physiology they represent. This makes it possible to identify the individual's position on the continuum of function, from health and compensation to pathophysiology and disease. Thus, if a middle-aged woman presented for a checkup and was found to be overweight, with a blood pressure of 130/85 mm Hg, the nurse would most likely counsel her with respect to diet and activity. She would encourage weight loss; question her intake of salt, which affects her fluid balance, and her intake of caffeine, for its stimulant effect; and discuss ways to decrease the stress in her life. The ultimate goal of her activities would be to control her blood pressure and prevent hypertension.

Another reason for becoming well versed in symptomatology and physiology is that there are many diseases, too numerous to memorize. However, the number of physiologic processes is limited. Having a knowledge of these processes makes it possible to detect the abnormalities or the degree of risk involved and to intervene effectively.

Pathophysiologic Processes at the Cellular Level

The processes described may occur at all levels of the biological organism. (They also occur in society and populations, but in this chapter we will focus on the physiology of the individual.) If the cell is considered the smallest unit or subsystem (tissues being aggregates of cells, organs aggregates of tissues, etc.), the processes of health and disease, adaptation and maladaptation may all occur at the cellular level. Indeed, pathologic processes are described at the subcellular or molecular level. The cell may then be described as existing on a continuum of function and structure, from the normal cell, to the adapted cell, to the injured or diseased cell, to the dead cell (Fig. 7-2).

Nature of Changes

Changes from one state to another may occur rapidly and may not be readily detectable, because each state does not have distinct or discrete boundaries, and disease represents an extension and distortion of normal processes. For example, tanning of the skin is an adaptive, morphologic response to exposure to the rays of the sun. If the exposure is continued, however, sunburn and injury may occur, and some cells may die, as is evidenced by "peeling."

Earliest changes occur at the molecular or subcellular level and are not easily detectable. Not until steady state functions or structures are altered do changes become apparent. With cell injury some changes may be reversible, whereas others are lethal and lead to death. Also, the adapted state is generally at a lower functional level, in that it is maintained by the use of additional energy or reserves or by a morphologic change of tissue cells into a less specific, or less differentiated, cell type.

Responses to Stimuli/Stressors

Different cells and tissues respond to stimuli with different patterns and rates of response, some being more vulnerable to one type of stimulus or stressor than another. Thus, cardiac muscle cells respond to hypoxia (inadequate oxygenation) more quickly than smooth muscle cells. The cell involved, its ability to adapt, and its physiologic state are determinants of the response.

Other determinants of the response are the type or nature of the stressor, its duration, and its severity. For example, a drug tolerance to regular small amounts of a barbiturate may develop, but one large dose may result in unconsciousness and death.

Nursing Implications

Organs are capable of a wide range of activity: the heart rate can change from 60 to 150 beats/min, the volume of air breathed can vary from 0.3 to 150 liters/min; thus, the ability of the body to compensate and adapt to differing environmental conditions is remarkable. When injury does occur, it may be reversible up to a point; earliest morphologic changes may be regarded as "fingerprints of disease; when the damage is slight the prints can be erased" (Boyd & Sheldon, 1984). For the health of the patient, it is imperative to detect these early changes.

Control of the Steady State: Control Systems

The concept of the cell on a continuum of function and structure (illustrated in Figure 7-2) includes the relationship of the "normal cell" and the "adapted cell" to compensatory mechanisms. These mechanisms include the adjustment processes that are continuously occurring in the body to maintain the dynamic balance, or steady state. These processes involve neural and hormonal mechanisms, and control is achieved through negative feedback.

Negative Feedback Process

Through the process of negative feedback, deviations from a predetermined set point or range of adaptability are detected, and these trigger a response in which the action offsets the deviation. Blood pressure, acid–base balance, blood glucose level, body temperature, and fluid and electrolyte balance are examples of parameters regulated through such compensatory mechanisms. Each of these parameters has a range for optimal function. If there is either an excess or a deficiency, negative feedback will trigger activity to cause a return to the optimal level.

A familiar illustration of the negative feedback process in a simple control system is the control of room temperature. The door is opened and a cold draft reduces room temperature, which is detected by a thermometer and relayed to a thermostat. The thermostat compares this temperature with

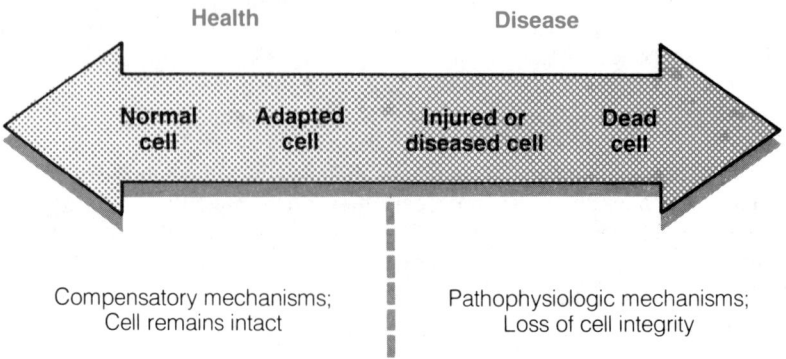

Figure 7-2
The cell on a continuum of function and structure. Changes in the cell are not as easily discerned as the diagram depicts. The point at which compensation is lost and pathophysiology begins is not clearly defined.

a preset reference point. Detecting that the room is cooler, it sends a message to the furnace to fire up, with the effect of heating the room air. The new temperature is fed into the thermostat, and if it is equal to the reference point, the furnace is signaled to shut off. This is *negative feedback,* which is a series of actions in which the goal is to counter the influence of an initiating stimulus or disturbance. It does not change the disturbance, only its effect. In this case, the door was not closed, but its cooling effect was offset by the heating action of the furnace.

Organs of Homeostasis or Adjustment. Most of the human body's control systems are integrated at the level of the brain in the nervous and endocrine systems. Control activities involve detecting deviations from the predetermined reference point and stimulating compensatory responses in the muscles and glands of the body. The major organs affected are the heart, lungs, kidneys, liver, gastrointestinal tract, and skin. When stimulated, these organs alter the rate of their activity or the amount of secretions they produce. They have been called the organs of homeostasis or adjustment.

Local Responses: Feedback Loops. In addition to the responses controlled by the above system, there are local responses that consist of small feedback loops in a group of cells or tissues. The cells detect a change in their immediate environment and initiate an action to counteract its effect. For example, the accumulation of lactic acid in an exercised muscle will stimulate dilation of blood vessels in the area to increase blood flow and improve the delivery of oxygen and removal of waste products.

The net result of the activities of the control system through feedback loops is a dynamic equilibrium, a steady state achieved by the continuous, variable action of the organs of adjustment along with continuous small exchanges of chemical substances between cells, interstitial fluid, and blood throughout the body. For example, an increase in the carbon dioxide concentration of the extracellular fluid leads to increased pulmonary ventilation, which in turn decreases the carbon dioxide level. The increased carbon dioxide raises the hydrogen ion concentration of the blood. This is detected by chemosensitive receptors in the respiratory control center of the medulla. This stimulates an increase in the rate of discharge of the inspiratory neurons, which innervates the diaphragm and intercostal muscles and increases the rate of respiration. Excess carbon dioxide is exhaled, the hydrogen ion concentration returns to normal, and the chemically sensitive neurons are no longer stimulated.

Positive Feedback. Before closing this discussion, another type of feedback, positive feedback, should be mentioned. Positive feedback perpetuates the chain of events set in motion by the original disturbance. Compensation does not occur, and the system becomes more out of balance; disorder and disintegration occur. (There are some exceptions to this: blood clotting in humans, for example, is an important positive feedback mechanism.)

Cellular Adaptation and Injury

Cells are complex units dynamically responding to the changing demands and stresses of daily life. They possess a maintenance function and a specialized function: the mainte-

nance function refers to the activities the cell must perform with respect to itself; specialized functions are those that the cell performs in relation to the tissues and organs of which it is a part. Individual cells may cease to function without posing a threat to the organism; however, as the dead cells multiply, the specialized functions are altered and the individual's health is threatened.

Common Adaptations

Cells can adapt to environmental stress by structural and functional changes. A number of these adaptations are common and include hypertrophy, atrophy, hyperplasia, and metaplasia (Table 7-1).

Hypertrophy and Atrophy. Hypertrophy and atrophy lead to changes in the size of cells and hence the size of the organs they form. Compensatory hypertrophy resulting in an enlarged muscle mass commonly occurs in skeletal and cardiac muscle under prolonged, increased workloads. Atrophy can be the consequence of a disease but is more readily associated with aging. There is a decrease in cell and organ size that affects, principally, skeletal muscle, secondary sex organs, the heart, and the brain.

Hyperplasia. Hyperplasia is an increase in the number of new cells in an organ or tissue; as cells multiply, volume increases. It is a mitotic response, but it is reversible when the stimulus is removed. This distinguishes it from neoplasia or malignant growth, which continues after the stimulus is removed. Hyperplasia may occur in response to a body loss or may be hormonally induced.

Metaplasia. Metaplasia is a cell transformation in which a highly specialized cell changes to a less specialized cell. This serves a protective function, because the less specialized cell is more resistant to the stress that stimulated the change. In smokers, the ciliated columnar epithelium lining the bronchi is replaced by squamous epithelium. The squamous cells can survive; however, loss of the cilia and protective mucus can have damaging consequences.

Thus, the adaptations afford the survival of the organism. They reflect changes in the normal cell in response to stress. If the stress continues, the function of the adapted cell may succumb and cell injury will occur.

Injury

Injury is defined as a disorder in steady-state regulation; any stressor that alters the ability of the cell or system to maintain the optimal balance of its adjustment processes will lead to injury. Structural and functional damage then occurs, which may be reversible, permitting recovery, or irreversible, leading to death. Homeostatic adjustments are concerned with the small, minute-by-minute changes within the body's systems. With adaptive changes, compensation occurs and a steady state is achieved, although it may be at new levels; with injury, steady-state regulation is lost and pathophysiology ensues.

Causes of disorder and injury in the system (cell, tissue, organ, body) may arise from the external or internal environment of the system (Fig. 7-3). Causes may include the following: physical agents, chemical agents, infectious agents,

TABLE 7-1
Cellular Adaptation

Change	Stimulus	Example
Hypertrophy		
Increase in cell size, leading to increase in organ size	Increased workload	Leg muscles of runner Arm muscles of tennis player Cardiac muscle in person with hypertension
Atrophy		
Shrinkage in size of cell, leading to decrease in organ size	Decrease in: 1. Use 2. Blood supply 3. Nutrition 4. Hormonal stimulation 5. Innervation	Secondary sex organs in aging person Extremity immobilized in plaster cast
Hyperplasia		
Increase in number of new cells (increase in mitosis)	Hormonal influence Tissue removal or destruction	Breast changes of a girl in puberty or of a pregnant woman Regeneration of liver cells New red blood cells in blood loss
Metaplasia		
Transformation of one adult cell type to another (reversible)	Stress applied to highly specialized cell	Changes in epithelial cells lining bronchi in response to smoke irritation (cells become less specialized)

immune mechanisms, genetic defects, hypoxia, and nutritional imbalance.

The most common causes are hypoxia, chemical injury, and infectious agents. An additional factor is that the presence of one injury makes the system more susceptible to another; for example, inadequate oxygenation and nutritional deficiencies make the system vulnerable to infection. These agents act at the cellular level by damaging or destroying the following:

- The integrity of the cell membrane, necessary for ionic balance
- The cell's ability to transform energy (aerobic respiration, production of adenosine triphosphate [ATP])
- The cell's ability to synthesize enzymes and other necessary proteins
- The cell's ability to grow and reproduce (genetic integrity)

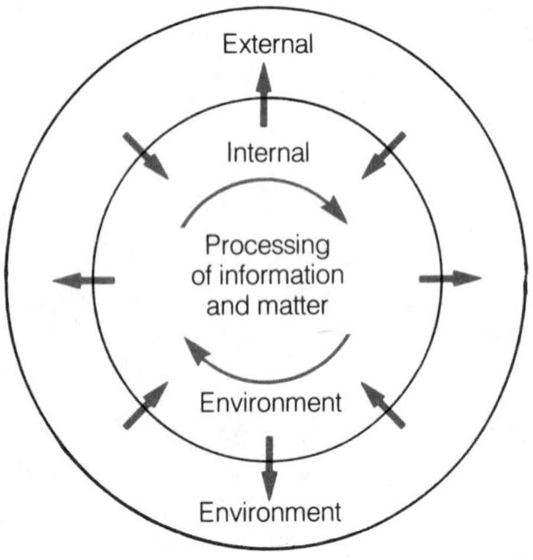

Hypoxia

Inadequate cellular oxygenation, hypoxia, interferes with the cell's ability to transform energy. Hypoxia may be caused by a decrease in blood supply to an area; by a decrease in the oxygen-carrying capacity of the blood (decreased hemoglobin); by a ventilation–perfusion or respiratory problem, reducing the amount of oxygen available in the blood; or by a problem in the cell's enzyme system, making it unable to use the oxygen delivered to it. The usual cause is *ischemia*, or deficient blood supply. This is commonly seen in myocardial cell injury, in which arterial blood flow is decreased because of atherosclerosis. Intravascular clots (thrombi, emboli) interfering with blood supply are the common causes of cerebrovascular accidents. The length of time different tissues can survive without oxygen varies: brain cells may succumb in 3 to 6 minutes (sources vary). If the condition leading to hypoxia is slowly progressive, collateral circulation to the

Figure 7-3
Influences leading to disorder may arise from the internal environment and the external environment of the system. Excesses or deficits of information and matter may occur or there may be faulty regulation of processing.

area may develop; however, this mechanism is not highly reliable.

Nutritional Imbalance

Nutritional imbalance refers to a relative or absolute deficiency or excess of one or more essential nutrients. This may be manifested as undernutrition, in which there is an inadequate consumption of food or calories, or in overnutrition, in which there is a caloric excess. Caloric excess to the point of obesity, in which the person is 20% or more above his ideal weight, overloads cells in the body with lipids. By requiring more energy to maintain the extra tissue, obesity places a strain on the body and has been associated with the production of disease, especially pulmonary and cardiovascular disease.

Specific deficiencies arise when an essential nutrient is deficient or when there is a disproportion of nutrients. Protein deficiencies and avitaminosis are examples.

An energy deficit leading to cell injury can occur when there is insufficient glucose or insufficient oxygen to transform the glucose into energy. A lack of insulin may also prevent glucose from entering the cell from the blood. This is the problem in diabetes mellitus, which represents a metabolic disorder, leading to nutritional deficiency.

Diabetes Mellitus. The exact cause of diabetes mellitus is unknown; however, in most cases, it is probably inherited. It most likely involves a combination of the causative factors of injury: genetic defect, diet, and, possibly, destruction of the insulin-producing pancreatic islet cells by a virus. In any event, when there is a lack of insulin, a series of pathophys-

iologic events occur (Fig. 7-4). Insulin is necessary to transport glucose into the cell. If it is absent, the food eaten is converted to glucose, and the blood sugar level rises; because the glucose cannot get into the cell, the body excretes it. Because this hypertonic glucose load must be diluted, fluid is pulled into the circulation from the body. Excessive urination, which occurs to flush out the sugar, leads to excessive thirst. Because the body is literally not being fed, the satiety center sends a hunger signal. At the same time, fatigue and weakness are experienced, and eventually the body looks to its own tissue stores of proteins and fats for energy, and weight loss occurs. The major symptoms are polydipsia (excessive thirst), polyuria (excessive urination), and polyphagia (excessive hunger).

Physical Agents

Physical agents, including extremes of temperature, radiation, electrical shock, and mechanical trauma, may cause injury to the cells or the entire body. The duration of exposure and the intensity of the stressor determine the severity of damage.

Extremes of High Temperature. When temperatures are elevated, irrespective of cause, hypermetabolism occurs: the respiratory rate, heart rate, and basal metabolic rate increase. Eventually, the high temperature causes coagulation of cell proteins, and the cells die. With fever induced by infections the hypothalamic thermostat may be reset at a higher temperature. Thus, the person responds to external heat and cold with a new setpoint of perhaps 40°C (104°F), just as he did with the normal setpoint of 37°C (98.6°F). When the fever breaks, the thermostat returns to normal. With fever from heat stroke, the function of the thermoreg-

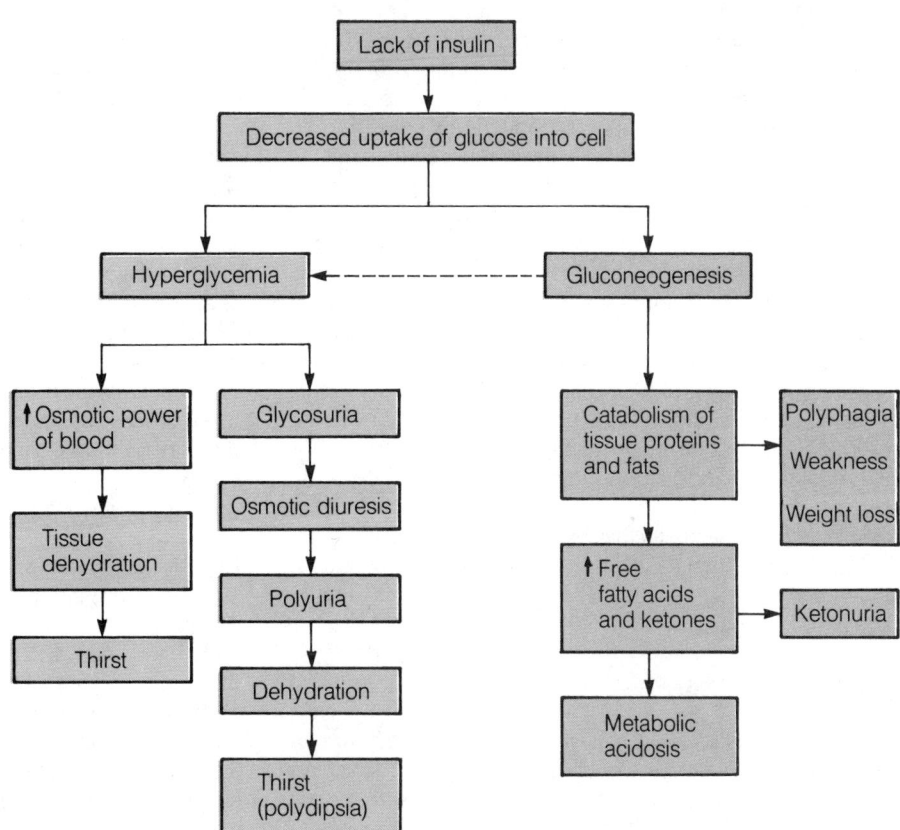

Figure 7-4
Pathophysiology of diabetes mellitus.

ulatory center breaks down, and temperature soars. It is imperative that the body be cooled rapidly or minor brain damage may occur.

The local response to thermal injury is similar. There is an increase in metabolic activity, and, as heat increases, protein is coagulated, enzyme systems are destroyed, and, in the extreme, charring or carbonization occurs. Burns of the epithelium are classified as partial-thickness burns if epithelializing elements remain to support healing; full-thickness burns lack such elements and must be grafted for healing. The amount of body surface involved determines the prognosis for the patient. If severe, the entire body system becomes involved, and hypermetabolism will develop as a pathophysiologic response.

Extremes of Low Temperature. Extremes of low temperature or cold cause vasoconstriction; blood flow becomes sluggish, and clots may form, leading to ischemic damage in the involved tissues. With still lower temperatures, ice crystals may form, and the cells may burst.

Radiation. Radiant energy may be used for diagnosis and treatment of diseases. In excessive amounts, it causes injury by its ionizing action. Electrical shock may produce burns as a result of the heat generated when electric current travels through the body. It may also stimulate nerves abnormally; for example, fibrillation of the heart may occur.

Mechanical Trauma. Mechanical trauma can result in wounds that disrupt the cells and tissues of the body. The severity of the wound, the blood loss, and the nerve damage are significant factors in the outcome.

Chemical Agents

Chemical injuries may be caused by known poisons, such as lye, which has a corrosive action on epithelial tissue, or by heavy metals, such as mercury, arsenic, and lead, each with its own specific destructive action. Many other chemicals may be toxic in certain amounts, in certain people, and in certain tissues; these include compounds of extrinsic and intrinsic origin. Too much hydrochloric acid can damage the stomach lining; large amounts of glucose can cause osmotic shifts, affecting the fluid and electrolyte balance; and too much insulin can cause hypoglycemia and lead to coma. Drugs, including those prescribed by the physician, may cause chemical poisoning. Some individuals are less tolerant of drugs than others and manifest toxic reactions at customary dosages. Aging tends to decrease tolerance to drugs. Polypharmacy, the taking of many drugs at one time, also occurs in the aging population. It is a problem because of the unpredictable effects of the resulting drug combinations.

Alcohol (ethanol) is a chemical irritant. In the body, alcohol is broken down into acetaldehyde, which has a direct toxic effect on liver cells that leads to a variety of liver abnormalities, including cirrhosis in susceptible individuals. Disordered liver cell function leads to complications in other organs of the body.

Infectious Agents

Biological agents known to cause disease in humans are viruses, bacteria, rickettsiae, mycoplasmas, fungi, protozoa, and nematodes. The severity of the infectious disease depends on the number of microorganisms entering the body, their virulence, and the host's defenses, such as health, age, and immune defenses. Some bacteria, such as those in tetanus and diphtheria, produce exotoxins that circulate and create cell damage; some, such as the gram-negative bacteria, produce endotoxins when they are killed; and others, such as the tubercle bacillus, induce an immune reaction. Viruses, as the smallest living organisms, survive as parasites of the living cells they invade. Viruses infect specific cells; through a complex mechanism, they replicate within the cells they invade, and then burst out to invade other cells and continue to replicate. An immune response is mounted by the body to eliminate the viruses, and the cells harboring the viruses can be injured in the process.

Typically, an inflammatory response and immune reaction are the pathophysiologic responses of the body to the presence of infection.

Immune Mechanisms

The immune system is an exceedingly complex system; its purpose is to defend the body from invasion by any foreign object or foreign cell type, such as cancerous cells. This is a steady-state mechanism, but like other adjustment processes, it can become disordered, and cell injury occurs. Basically, the immune response detects foreign bodies or distinguishes nonself from self and destroys nonself entities. The entrance of an antigen (foreign body) into the body evokes the production of antibodies that attack and destroy the antigen (antigen–antibody reaction). The immune system can be hypoactive or hyperactive. When it is hypoactive, immunodeficiency diseases occur; when it is hyperactive, hypersensitivity disorders arise. In hypersensitivity disorders, the antigen reacts with the cells of immunity (lymphocytes, macrophages, neutrophils, antibodies, or complement) in such a way that "self" or normal cells are injured.

For example, a person with seasonal allergic rhinitis due to pollen hyperreacts to the foreign protein by producing a sensitivity (Fig. 7-5). IgE, the immunoglobulin normally produced as an antibody against such an allergen, is produced in excessive amounts. This antibody attaches to the skin surfaces of the nasal mucosa. When the foreign protein, pollen, is inhaled again, an antigen–antibody reaction occurs at the site. Histamine and other irritating chemical substances are released and cell injury occurs, as is indicated by copious secretions, edema of the mucosa, sneezing because of secretions, and local itching. Basically, the immune response is the process of inflammation described below amplified by the participation of antibodies and sensitized lymphocytes.

Genetic Disorders

Genetic defects as causes of disease are of intense interest as more environmental pollutants are formed and their effects on our genetic structure are studied. Over 2300 inherited traits have been described in humans (Purtilo, 1978). Many of these produce mutations that have no recognizable effect, such as lack of a single enzyme; others contribute to more gross congenital abnormalities, such as Down's syndrome. Sickle cell disease, the hemophilias, and phenylketonuria are examples of diseases arising from genetic defects.

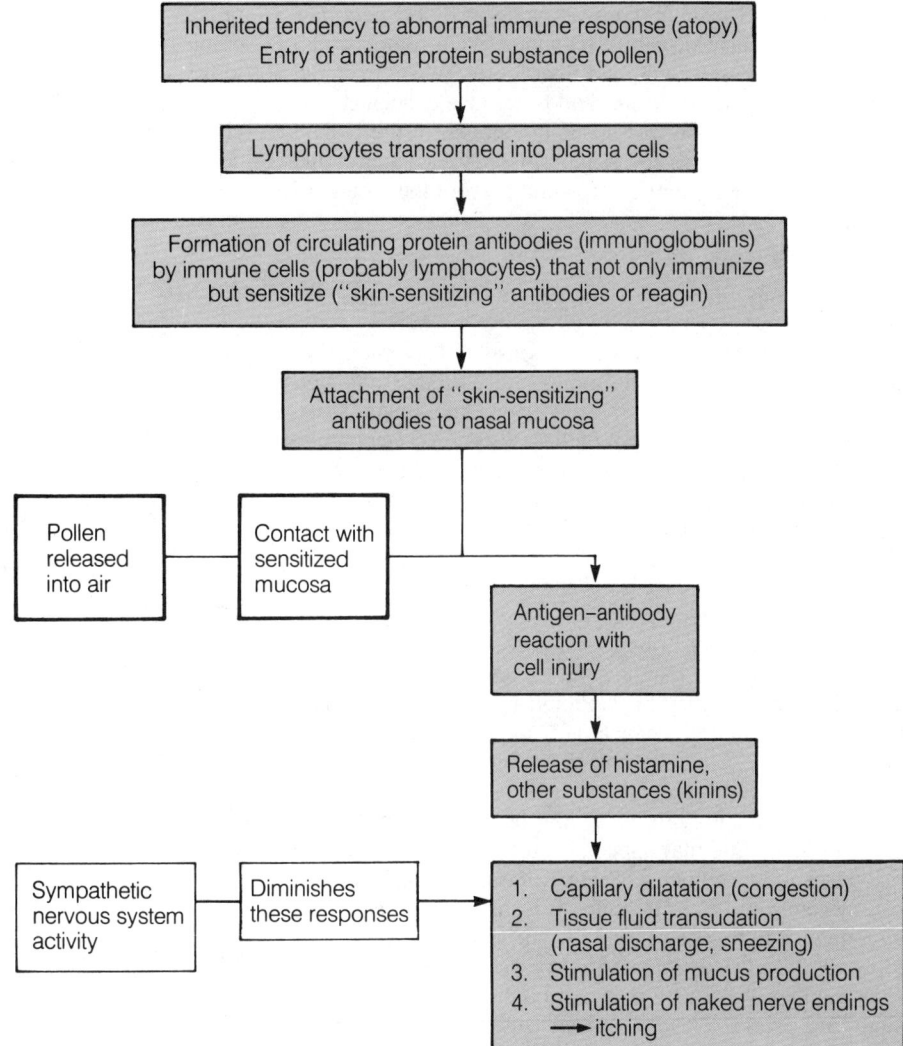

Figure 7-5
Pathophysiology of seasonal
allergic rhinitis owing to pollen.

Response to Injury: Inflammation

Cells or tissues of the body may be injured or killed by any of the agents (physical, chemical, infectious) just described. When this happens there is a naturally occurring response in the healthy tissues adjacent to the site of injury. This is called the *inflammatory response*, or *inflammation*. It is a defensive reaction whose intent is to neutralize, control, and/or eliminate the offending agent and to prepare the site for repair. It is a nonspecific response (not dependent on a particular cause) meant to serve a protective function. For example, inflammation may be observed at the site of a bee sting, a sore throat, a surgical incision, and a burn. Inflammation also occurs in more serious cell injury events such as strokes and heart attacks.

It is important to distinguish between inflammation and infection. An infectious agent is only one of several agents that may trigger an inflammatory response. An infection exists when the infectious agent is living, growing, and multiplying in the tissues and is able to overcome the body's normal defenses.

Regardless of the cause, there is a general sequence of events that can be described as the local inflammatory response. This sequence involves changes in the microcirculation in the area of the injury that include vasodilation, increased vascular permeability, and leukocytic cellular infiltration. As these changes take place, *five cardinal signs of inflammation* are produced: redness, heat, swelling, pain, and loss of function.

A transient vasoconstriction that occurs immediately after injury is followed by vasodilation and an increased rate of blood flow through the microcirculation. Local heat and redness result. Next, vascular permeability increases, and plasma fluids (including proteins and solutes) leak into the inflamed tissues, producing swelling. The pain produced is attributed to the pressure of fluids (swelling) on nerve endings and possibly to direct irritation of nerve endings by chemical mediators released at the site. Bradykinin is one of the chemical mediators suspected of causing pain. Loss of function is most likely related to the pain and swelling, but the exact mechanism has not been explained.

As the blood flow increases and fluid leaks into the surrounding tissues, the formed elements (red blood cells, white blood cells, and platelets) are left and the blood becomes more viscous and sluggish. Leukocytes (white blood cells) collect in the vessels, exit, and migrate to the site of injury to engulf offending organisms and to remove cellular debris in a process called phagocytosis. Fibrinogen in the leaked plasma fluid coagulates, forming fibrin for clot formation that serves to wall off the injured area and prevent the spread of infection.

Chemical Mediators

Injury initiates the inflammatory response, but chemical substances released at the site induce the vascular changes. Foremost among these are histamine and the kinins. Histamine is present in many tissues of the body but is concentrated in mast cells. It is released when injury occurs and is responsible for the early changes in vasodilation and vascular permeability. Kinins increase vasodilation and vascular permeability; they also attract neutrophils to the area. Prostaglandins, another group of chemical substances, are also suspected of causing increased permeability.

The process described is complex. Although it has phases, once started they may all be occurring at the same time. The process may be modified by different variables, the most important of which are (1) the nature and intensity of the injury, (2) the site and tissue affected, and (3) the resistance of the host.

The inflammatory response may be confined to the site, and only local signs may appear. On the other hand, systemic responses may also occur. Fever is the most common sign of a systemic response to injury. It is most likely caused by endogenous pyrogens released from neutrophils and macrophages (specialized forms of leukocytes). These substances reset the hypothalamic thermostat controlling body temperature and produce fever. Leukocytosis, an increase in the synthesis and release of neutrophils from bone marrow, may occur. Constitutional symptoms may develop, including malaise, loss of appetite, aching, and weakness.

Types of Inflammation

Inflammation is categorized primarily by duration and the type of exudate produced. It may be acute, subacute, or chronic. A typical case of *acute inflammation* is characterized by the local vascular and exudative changes described above and usually lasts for less than 2 weeks. An acute inflammatory response is immediate, and it serves a protective function. When the injurious agent is removed, the inflammation subsides, and healing takes place with the return of normal or near-normal structure and function.

Chronic inflammation develops when the injurious agent persists and the acute response is perpetuated. Symptoms may appear for many months or years. Chronic inflammation may also begin insidiously and never have an acute phase. The chronic response does not serve a beneficial and protective function but, on the contrary, is debilitating and may produce long-lasting effects in the person. As the inflammation becomes chronic, changes occur at the site of injury and the nature of the exudate becomes proliferative. There is a continuing cycle of cellular infiltration, necrosis, and fi-

brosis (repair and breakdown go on side by side). Considerable scarring may occur, resulting in permanent damage to tissues.

Subacute inflammation falls in between acute and chronic inflammation. There are elements of the active exudative phase of the acute response, and simultaneously there is also some repair occurring as in the chronic response. The term is not widely used.

Repair

The reparative process begins at approximately the same time as the injury and is indeed interwoven with inflammation. Healing proceeds after the inflammatory debris is removed. Healing may be by *regeneration,* in which there is gradual repair of the defect by proliferation of cells of the same type as those destroyed. Or, it may be by *replacement* with cells of another type, usually connective tissue, resulting in scar formation.

Healing by Regeneration. The ability of cells to regenerate depends on whether they are labile, stable, or permanent. *Labile* cells include those that multiply constantly to replace cells worn out by normal physiologic processes; these include epithelial cells of the skin and those lining the gastrointestinal tract. *Permanent* cells include neurons—the nerve cell bodies, not their axons. Destruction of a neuron is a permanent loss, but axons may regenerate. If normal activity is to return, tissue regeneration must occur in a functional pattern, especially in the growth of several axons. *Stable* cells have a latent ability to regenerate. Under normal physiologic processes, they are not shed and do not need replacement, but if they are damaged or destroyed, they are able to regenerate. These include functional cells of the kidney, liver, pancreas, and other glands of the body.

Healing by Replacement. Healing may be by primary intention or secondary intention. In *primary intention healing,* the wound is clean and dry and the edges are approximated, such as may occur in a surgical wound. Little scar formation occurs, and the wound is usually healed in a week. In *secondary intention healing,* the wound or defect is larger and gaping and has more necrotic material. The wound fills from the bottom upward with granulation tissue. The process of repair takes longer and results in more scar formation with loss of specialized function. Persons who have recovered from myocardial infarcts will have abnormal electrocardiographic tracings because the electrical signal cannot be conducted through the connective tissue that replaces the defect.

As has been stated many times in this chapter, the condition of the host, the environment, and the nature and severity of the injury affect the process and outcome, in this case, the process of inflammation and repair.

Cell Death

Any of the injuries discussed can lead to death of the cell. Essentially, the cell membrane becomes impaired, resulting in a nonrestricted flow of ions. Sodium and calcium enter the cell, followed by water, which leads to edema, and energy transformation ceases. Nerve impulses are no longer transmitted; muscles no longer contract. As the cells rupture, lysosomal enzymes escape that destroy tissues; cell death and necrosis occur.

A Representative Pathophysiologic Process: Hypertensive Heart Disease

Hypertensive heart disease is presented here as a representative pathophysiologic process. Unfortunately, words and figures can only dimly portray the patient's condition, moment by moment or day by day in acute illness, or week by week in chronic illness. The influence of physiologic changes, of social adjustments between patient and health care personnel or family, of unknown or expressed concern and anxiety, and of the patient's total life experience in the development and course of disease is well recognized by the health care team. These variables cannot be inserted into a flow diagram, yet they may be major factors governing the course of the disease.

Mechanisms of Blood Pressure Regulation

A brief summary of selected mechanisms for regulating blood pressure will facilitate the understanding of hypertensive heart disease. The regulation of arterial pressure involves complex nervous and hormonal controls that interrelate to affect the cardiac output and peripheral resistance. This relationship is expressed in the following equation:

mean arterial pressure

= cardiac output (CO) × total peripheral resistance (TPR)

Cardiac output is determined by the stroke volume and the heart rate. Peripheral resistance is determined by the diameter of the arterioles. If the diameter is decreased (vasoconstriction), peripheral resistance increases; if the diameter is increased (vasodilation), peripheral resistance decreases.

Primary regulation of arterial pressure is effected by the baroreceptors in the carotid sinus and aortic arch, which relay impulses to the sympathetic nervous centers in the medulla. These impulses act to inhibit the stimulation of the sympathetic nervous system. When the arterial pressure is increased, the baroreceptor endings are stretched. They fire, inhibiting the sympathetic center. This reduces the discharge of the sympathetic center, with the result that the heart rate is decreased, the arterioles dilate, and the arterial pressure returns to its former level. The reverse happens with a fall in arterial pressure. The baroreceptors control only temporary changes in blood pressure.

One other mechanism, which has a longer-term effect, will be described. Renin, produced by the kidneys when their blood flow is decreased, leads to the formation of angiotensin I, which converts to angiotensin II. Angiotensin II elevates the blood pressure by direct constriction of arterioles. It also indirectly stimulates the release of aldosterone, which leads to renal retention of sodium and water. The latter increases the extracellular fluid volume, which in turn increases the flow returned to the heart, thereby raising the stroke volume

and cardiac output. The kidneys also have an intrinsic mechanism to increase sodium and water retention.

When a *persistent* disturbance occurs that causes arteriolar constriction, total peripheral resistance is increased and the mean arterial pressure rises. In the face of the persistent disturbance, cardiac output must increase to maintain balance in the system (see equation). This is necessary to overcome the peripheral resistance, so that delivery of oxygen and nutrients to the cells and removal of cellular waste products will be maintained. To increase the cardiac output, the sympathetic nervous system stimulates the heart to beat faster; it also increases the stroke volume by causing a selective vasoconstriction in peripheral organs that returns more blood to the heart. With chronic hypertension, the baroreceptors are reset at a higher level, and they respond as though the new level were normal.

Initially, this mechanism is compensatory. This adaptive mechanism, however, exacts a toll by creating an increased workload for the heart. At the same time, degenerative changes take place in the arterioles that are subjected to continuous high pressure. These changes occur in organs throughout the body, including the heart, which may contribute to a depleted blood supply in the myocardium. To eject blood, the heart must exert enough force to overcome the pressure reflected back to the aortic inlet. In response to this workload, the muscle of the left ventricle hypertrophies. Eventually, it dilates, and the heart becomes enlarged. These two structural changes are adaptive; they improve the stroke volume delivered by the heart. At rest, these compensatory mechanisms may be effective, but on exertion, the heart cannot meet the demands of the body; the patient is easily fatigued and becomes short of breath.

The point at which compensation ends and injury and failure begin is not continuous or discrete. With the increased demands, there are changes in the distribution of blood flow that result in a reduced flow to the kidneys. This stimulates the renin–angiotensin–aldosterone mechanism. This mechanism, once compensatory, now aggravates the failing heart by increasing the extracellular fluid volume and the peripheral resistance. The heart becomes engorged with blood that it cannot pump out, and left ventricular heart failure occurs. Failure of the left ventricle has both forward and backward effects. The forward effects are due to low output, which decreases the perfusion of tissues of the body. The decreased perfusion activates sodium and water retention mechanisms in the kidneys and glands, giving positive feedback to the failing heart. The backward effects are due to the decreased emptying of the left ventricle, which raises the end-diastolic pressure. This rise in pressure is reflected back into the left atrium and the pulmonary veins, and congestion occurs in the pulmonary capillaries. Gas exchange is disrupted, and fluid exudes from the capillaries into the alveolar spaces, leading to pulmonary edema. Crackles (rales) will be heard when the lungs are auscultated; severe dyspnea and orthopnea will be present; coughing will occur; and, with pulmonary edema, pink, frothy sputum may be present. Eventually, this backward progression will affect the right side of the heart and lead to right-sided heart failure accompanied by congestion in the veins and organs drained by the venae cavae. The system is in total failure, and death is imminent.

The initial disturbance that caused the increased peripheral resistance may be unknown, as is the case in primary or essential hypertension, although a number of agents have been postulated as being contributory. The pathologic mechanism was hypoxia owing to failure of the blood transportation system. In the latter stages, oxygen saturation of the blood was also decreased by the pulmonary edema.

Nursing Implications

In the assessment of the patient who seeks health care, objective signs will be the primary indicators of the physiologic processes that are occurring. Are the heart rate, respiratory rate, and temperature normal? If not, is any change only a temporary one? Are there other indicators of steady-state deviation? What is the blood pressure, height, and weight? Are there any problems in movement or sensation? Does the patient demonstrate any problems in orientation or memory? Are there obvious lesions or deformities? Further signs of internal processes are indicated in laboratory data, including electrolytes, blood urea nitrogen [BUN], blood sugar, and urinalysis. In making a nursing diagnosis, it is necessary to coordinate the symptoms or complaints expressed by the patient with the physical signs present.

Specific problems and their nursing treatment are addressed in greater depth in other chapters. It has been reiterated many times in this chapter that the state of the host and the environment are two of the three predictors of the health outcome in all situations. These two are directly related to the health patterns of the individual. The nurse has a significant role and responsibility in identifying the health patterns of the patient treated. If those patterns are not achieving balance for the patient physiologically, psychologically, and socially, the nurse is obligated—with the assistance and agreement of the patient—to seek ways to achieve balance. This chapter is physiologically oriented; in that context, the nutrition–metabolism pattern, elimination pattern, activity–exercise pattern, and sleep–rest pattern would be specifically analyzed. However, the way one copes with stress, the way one relates to others, and the values and goals held are interwoven in those "physiologic" patterns. Who you eat with, when you eat, and how much money you have for food are directly related to what you eat and how much. To evaluate the patient's health patterns and to intervene if a problem exists requires a total assessment of the patient.

Bibliography

Books

Boyd W, Sheldon H. Boyd's Introduction to the Study of Disease. Philadelphia. Lea & Febiger, 1984.

Bullock BL and Philbrook P. Pathophysiology: Adaptations and Alterations in Function. Boston, Little, Brown & Co, 1984.

Dubos R. Man Adapting. New Haven, Yale University Press, 1965.

Frohlich ED (ed). Pathophysiology, Altered Regulatory Mechanisms in Disease. Philadephia, JB Lippincott, 1984.

Groer MW and Shekleton ME. Basic Pathophysiology, A Conceptual Approach. St Louis, CV Mosby, 1983.

Guyton AC. Textbook of Medical Physiology. Philadelphia, WB Saunders, 1986.

Harrison TR, Braunwald E et al (eds). Harrison's Principles of Internal Medicine, 11th edition. New York, McGraw-Hill, 1987.

Kissane JM. Anderson's Pathology (2 vols). St Louis, CV Mosby, 1985.

Porth C. Pathophysiology: Concepts of Altered Health States, 2nd ed. Philadelphia, JB Lippincott, 1986.

Price SA and Wilson LM. Pathophysiology, Clinical Concepts of Disease Processes. New York, McGraw-Hill, 1986.

Robbins SL, Angell M, and Kumar V. Basic Pathology. Philadelphia, WB Saunders, 1981.

Robbins SL, Cotran RS, and Kumar V. Pathologic Basis of Disease. Philadelphia, WB Saunders, 1984.

Vander AJ, Sherman JH, and Luciano DS. Human Physiology: The Mechanisms of Body Function. New York, McGraw-Hill, 1985.

Articles

Adams A. External barriers to infection. Nurs Clin North Am 1985 Mar; 20(1):145–149.

Cohen JJ. Stress and the human immune response: A critical review. J Burn Care Rehabil 1985 Mar/Apr; 6(2):167–173.

Chandra S et al. Nutritional regulation of the immune responses: Basic considerations and practical applications. J Burn Care Rehabil 1985 Mar/Apr; 6(2):174–178.

Fouad FM et al. Pathophysiology and treatment of hypertension. Appl Cardiol 1984 Nov/Dec; 12(6):17–21.

Gurevich I. The competent internal immune system. Nurs Clin North Am 1985 Mar; 20(1):151–161.

Gurevich I and Tafuro P. Nursing measures for the prevention of infection in the compromised host. Nurs Clin North Am 1985 Mar; 20(1): 257–261.

Mennies JH et al. An overview of adult allergic disorders. Nurs Pract 1985 June; 10(6):16, 19–20, 22–23.

Pathophysiology of congestive heart failure. Hosp Med 1984 Sept; 20(9): 31.

Chapter 8

Stress and Adaptation

Stress is a term that is difficult to define: it is used loosely and means different things to different people. Some use it to describe an *upset feeling* or response; others use it to describe the *source* or *stimulus* for their feeling upset. It has even been suggested that the term is so confusing it should be done away with. Historically, Cannon, in 1936, described the "fight or flight" response that prepared the individual to cope with immediate danger. Selye (1956), who is sometimes called the "father of stress," stated that "stress is essentially the rate of wear and tear in the body." Later (1976), he spoke of stress as being a "nonspecific response," meaning that regardless of the stimulus producing the stress, the physiologic response of the body was always the same. More recent research has demonstrated that the body does have different patterns of response to different threats, most likely related to how emotionally aroused the person becomes (Mason, 1975). These researchers have concentrated on the physiologic reactions of the body in response to stress.

Psychologists have been more concerned with predisposing factors and with the mental processes involved in stress. Engel (1960), studying psychosomatic illness, defined psychological stress as referring to

> all processes, whether originating in the external environment or within the person, which impose a demand or requirement upon the organism, the resolution or handling of which necessitates work or activity of the mental apparatus before any other system is involved or activated*

Lazarus and Folkman (1984) have developed a theory of stress that emphasizes a "transaction" between the individual and the environment.

Thus, study in the field of stress has been pursued by researchers in different disciplines. Biologists have concentrated on physiology, while psychologists and sociologists have focused on the psychological and social aspects of stress. Each group has come up with a different approach or theory related to stress.

---

* Engle G. Health and disease. Perspect Biol 1960 Summer; 3(4): 459–485.

Nursing, as an applied science, uses these theories in developing its own approach to the diagnosis and treatment of stress. For example, nurse scientists such as Shaver (1985) and Sutterley and Donnelly (1981) have provided models that link the environment, the mind, and the body; they provide a holistic approach. Neuman's theory of nursing focuses on the client's reaction to stress and adaptation, while Roy's theory emphasizes the adaptive system of the person (Marriner, 1986).

The use of a holistic framework grew from the view that the body, mind, and spirit of a person are an integral unit. An individual's characteristic behavior patterns reflect this unity. Although the particular behavior patterns of an individual can be assessed, it must be realized that they reflect the whole person. This is a basic concept in nursing.

The move to holistic health care is recent, having received its impetus in this century largely from investigations in psychosomatic medicine. From ancient times, the mind, body, and spirit were considered separate entities; physicians or "bleeders" and "bile examiners" treated the body; the mind was treated by magicians and occult scientists, and the clergy tended the spirit. It was attractive to attribute disease to a single cause, which, it was thought, could be eradicated. The interrelation of the multitude of factors producing the necessary and sufficient conditions for illness to develop was not a prime consideration. Studies in psychosomatic illness have revealed the interaction between mind and body in all aspects of health and illness. Increasingly, it is being realized that emotional stress may contribute to physiologic illness and that physiologic illness contributes to psychological stress. Indeed, as one experiences joy or sadness, physiologic changes occur as part of that same event.

The process of stress, the adaptive responses to stress, some of the maladaptive outcomes, and the nursing implications associated with the process are described in this chapter. The focus is on the individual. To provide a background, some definitions, descriptions, and assumptions are necessary.

Stress and Adaptation Defined

Stress

Stress is a state produced by a change in the environment that is perceived as challenging, threatening, or damaging to the person's dynamic equilibrium. There is an actual or perceived imbalance in the person's capability to meet the demands of the new situation. The change or stimulus that evokes this state is the *stressor*. The nature of the stressor is variable: an event or change that will produce stress in one person will be neutral for another, and an event that may produce stress at one time and place for one person may not do so for the same person at another time and place. A person appraises and copes with changing situations. The desired goal is adaptation, or adjustment to the change, so that the person is again in equilibrium and has the energy and ability to meet new external demands.

Adaptation

Adaptation is a constant, ongoing process that occurs along the time continuum, beginning with birth and ending with death. Also existing along this lifetime continuum are the dimensions of health and illness. Health and illness are relative concepts. As a person traverses the life continuum, he encounters stressors that challenge his ability to meet his needs and maintain equilibrium. Successful positive adaptation to these stressors represents health; illness is an unsuccessful or maladaptive outcome. According to Dubos (1965), "Health in the case of human beings means more than a state in which the organism has become physically suited to the surrounding physiochemical conditions through passive mechanisms; it demands that the personality be able to express itself creatively." Dubos described human life as the interplay of three classes of determinants: the universal characteristics of man's nature, "which are inscribed in his flesh and bone"; the conditions of any given situation; and man's ability to make choices and control his own actions.

Because both stress and adaptation may exist at different levels of a system, it is possible to study them at cell, tissue, and organ levels. The biologist's study is mainly concerned with subcellular components or with subsystems of the total body. Stress and adaptation may also be studied in individuals, families, groups, and societies; thus, the sociologist speaks of the adaptation of groups, in the sense that their organization is modified to meet the requirements of the social and physical environment in which they exist. Adaptation is a continuous process of seeking harmony in an environment. The desired end goals of adaptation for any system are growth and reproduction. A major nursing objective is to support and promote the efforts of each patient to achieve a healthy adaptation.

Stressors: The Sources of Stress

Each person operates at a certain level, or within a range, that may be considered his adaptation level. A certain amount of change is encountered regularly: it is expected, it contributes to growth, and it enhances life. This healthy state can be upset by a number of stressors. This leads to imbalance in the person's physiologic or psychological state, or both, resulting in responses that, if prolonged or severe, may lead to illness. Sources of stress may be broadly categorized into physiologic stressors and psychosocial stressors.

Physiologic Stressors. The following agents may be considered as primarily physiologic stressors: chemical agents (drugs, poisons, alcohol), physical agents (heat, cold, radiation, electrical shock, trauma), infectious agents (viruses, bacteria, fungi), faulty immune mechanisms, genetic disorders, nutritional imbalance, and hypoxia. All stressors have both a general effect and a specific effect. The specific effect of these agents and the pathophysiology they incur are the subjects of another chapter and thus are not described further here. The general effect is the subject of the stress response in this chapter.

Psychosocial Stressors. The list of sources of psychosocial stress is extensive and for convenience can be broken down into three groups: (1) day-to-day stressors, or commonly occurring frustrations; (2) major complex occurrences that may involve large groups, even entire nations; and (3) stressors that fall in-between, that occur less frequently and involve fewer people. The first group, the day-to-day stressors, includes such common occurrences as getting caught in a traffic jam, running out of ribbon on the typewriter, having an argument with a spouse or roommate, and feeling lonely. These experiences vary in effect; for example, a rainstorm while one is vacationing at the beach will most likely evoke a more negative response than it might at another time. These less dramatic, frustrating, and irritating events, called "daily hassles," have been shown to affect health more strongly than major life events.

Some stressors influence not only the individual but also larger groups, possibly even entire nations of people. These include events of history such as terrorism, war, and rape, which are threatening situations brought into the living room through live news coverage and dramatization by the mass media. The changes occurring in society, such as demographic, economic, and technological changes, are stressors. The stress produced is sometimes an effect not only of the change but also of the rapidity of the change.

The third group of stressors has been studied most frequently and deals with relatively infrequently occurring situations that directly affect the individual. This category includes the influence of life events, such as death, birth, marriage, divorce, and retirement. It includes the psychosocial crises described by Erikson as occurring in the life-cycle stages of the human experience. More enduring chronic stressors have also been placed in this category. The latter may include having a permanent functional disability or the burden associated with providing long-term care to a frail elderly parent.

Relating life events to illness has been a major focus of psychosocial studies and can be traced to Adolph Meyer, who in the 1930s used "life charts" of his patients from which he observed a linkage between illnesses and critical life events. Harold Wolff, following this line of research, concluded that people under constant stress had a high incidence of psychosomatic disease. More recently, Holmes and Rahe (1967) have developed life events scales that assign numerical values to typical life events. They call these *life-change units*. By checking off the number of recent events and deriving a total score, the likelihood of illness can be predicted. The items reflect events that require a change in the person's life pattern; the variable of change is important because it requires adjustment. The Recent Life Changes Questionnaire (RLCQ) contains 118 items related to events such as death, birth, marriage, divorce, promotions, demotions, serious arguments, and vacations. The events listed include both desirable and undesirable happenings.

Stressors can also be categorized according to their duration. They may be acute, time-limited stressors, such as awaiting surgery or a final examination. They may be stressor sequences consisting of a series of events over a period of time that result from some initiating event such as job loss or divorce. They may be chronic and intermittent (hassles fall into this category), or they may be chronic enduring sources of stress that persist over time.

The sources of stress may be discrete events, or they may be the presence of relatively continuous problems. Pearlin and associates (1981) have presented an explanation for how these two major sources of stress, eventful experiences and chronic strain, operate to produce stress. This is done in two ways. A seemingly unimportant event may occur that triggers a reaction; the event "functions to bring into focus the unfavorable implications of life problems, and it is the new meaning of old problems that creates distress." In the second way, life events and life strains come together and create new strains or intensify preexisting strains that then evoke stress. In addition to life events and life strains, there is another step in the etiology of stress that involves self-concept, particularly mastery and self-esteem. Mastery is concerned with the sense of control a person has over his own life, and self-esteem refers to a sense of self-worth. When noxious strains persist, unaltered by the person's efforts, and control is threatened or lost, the self-concept becomes vulnerable. The combination of life events, persistent life strains, and the diminished self-concept leads to stress.

Summary. Stressors create a change in a person's equilibrium. Each person has a range of adaptability. Changes occurring within this range produce demands that fall within his existing capability. Changes falling outside this range lead to disequilibrium and require readjustment; such readjustment may lead to a new adaptation level, increasing the person's repertoire of adaptive responses. The stress precipitated will depend on the number of life events or changes occurring simultaneously, the magnitude of the changes, and the nature of the changes.

The Stress Response

Perception of the stressor is coordinated by structures of the brain and may be a conscious or unconscious process. Initially, following perception, there is a *global response*, a generalized state of anxiety involving psychoneuroendocrine activation. A *more specific response* develops as the person has more time to appraise the stressor and the resources available to cope with it. Anxiety will change from a diffuse reaction to a specific emotion: joy–sadness, fear–anger, acceptance–distrust, surprise–anticipation; the endocrine responses will become more specific. In all, there will be a more defined pattern of emotional and physiologic responses. Perception and response are intertwined and occur simultaneously; they cannot be singled out, except for the purposes of discussion as presented here. The stress response has both physiologic and emotional components, and manifestations of these are demonstrated in a person's behaviors: signs, symptoms, and self-reports. As the person copes with the situation, reappraisal will occur. Coping and reappraisal will become a circular activity providing feedback to the perception of the situation. If the person is successful in his activity, adaptive outcomes will occur; if unsuccessful, a pattern of maladaptive responses to specific situations may develop, or one of the so-called diseases of adaptation may occur. This is also a period when the person is particularly vulnerable to other stressors. The sequence of processes described is diagrammed in Figure 8-1.

Perception of Stress: Mind–Body Reaction

Psychosocial research has been concerned with the input side of stress: What kinds of life events are stressful, and what resources does the person have for coping with the stress situation? Physiologic research has dealt with the output side. What neurophysiologic responses occur in stress? How do the two get together? This is not known, but it is speculated that it is the emotional arousal or psychological impact of noxious or stressful agents that leads to the neuroendocrine responses. Lazarus states that it is the cognitive appraisal that

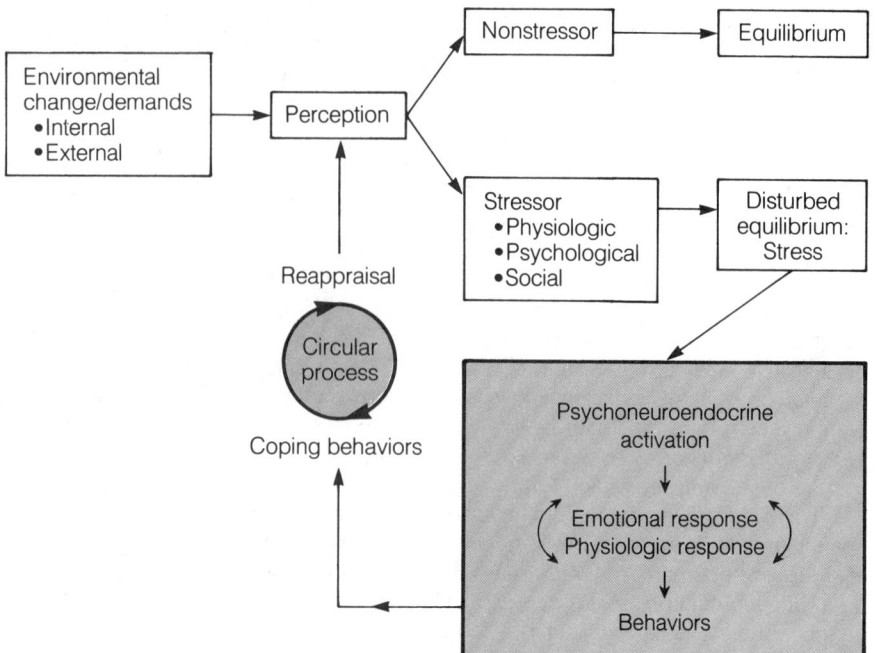

Figure 8-1
The stress process. When an environmental change is perceived by the brain as stressful, psychoneuroendocrine activation occurs, which elicits emotional and physiologic responses in the individual. These are manifested in objective and subjective behaviors. As the individual copes, using his own resources and social supports, reappraisal will recur again and again, providing feedback to the perception of the situation.

sets the whole train of events in motion, including the emotional reaction, the physiologic changes, and the coping activity.

Appraisal and Coping. Appraisal and coping are important processes to be considered in the stress response. In Lazarus's theory, appraisal is a cognitive process through which an event is evaluated with respect to what is at stake (primary appraisal) and what coping resources and options are available (secondary appraisal). During primary appraisal, the situation may be identified as either nonstressful or stressful. If nonstressful, the situation is irrelevant or benign-positive. A stressful situation may be one of three kinds: (1) those in which harm or loss has occurred; (2) those that are threatening, in that harm or loss is anticipated; and (3) those that are challenging, in that some opportunity or gain is anticipated. The degree of stress is determined by a comparison of what is at stake and what resources the person has for coping with it (a sort of risk–benefit analysis). Reappraisal also occurs and refers to a changed appraisal based on new information.

There is an emotional response as an outcome of the appraisal process. Negative emotions such as fear, anger, and resentment accompany harm/loss appraisals, while positive emotions such as excitement and eagerness accompany challenge. To illustrate this concept, an unexpected quiz in the classroom might be judged as threatening by the unprepared student, and fear, anger, and resentment might be felt. These emotions might be expressed by outward hostile behavior or comments.

Coping, according to Lazarus, consists of the cognitive and behavioral efforts made to manage the specific external or internal demands that tax a person's resources. Coping can be emotion focused or problem focused. Coping that is emotion focused seeks to make the person feel better by lessening the emotional distress felt. Problem-focused coping aims to manage the problem causing the distress. Both types of coping usually occur in a stressful situation.

The ability to cope effectively is influenced by a person's resources. These include such internal capabilities as the person's health and energy, his problem-solving skills, and his social skills. Having a sense of control or power in a situation is also important. Important external resources include money and the services and materials that money can buy. The most valuable external resource is social support (discussed in a subsequent section).

Interpretation of Stimuli by the Brain

The perception of stress involves taking in a sensation and giving meaning to it; this occurs in the brain. The brain has been compared to an international casino visited by people from all over the world. Each person comes to the casino with his own currency; to gamble, he must change it into the currency of the casino. In a similar fashion, all sensations, internal and external, coming into the brain must be converted into electrochemical impulses that are the "currency of the brain." Different stimuli are registered in different areas of the brain in different patterns, and the brain interprets these patterns and responds to them. In this way, it controls and regulates the activities of the body.

A model to explain the functional organization of the brain for the interpretation of stimuli is presented in Figure 8-2. This may be considered a communication and control hierarchy for the pituitary–adrenal system. There are three functional levels: interpretation of basic drive or need states occurs at the lowest level; emotions are interpreted at the intermediate level; and cognitions are interpreted at the highest level.

The hypothalamus sits in the center of the brain, surrounded by the limbic system and the cerebral hemispheres. It integrates autonomic mechanisms that maintain the chemical constancy of the internal environment of the body. With the limbic system, the hypothalamus also regulates emotional and instinctual behavior. The hypothalamus is made up of a

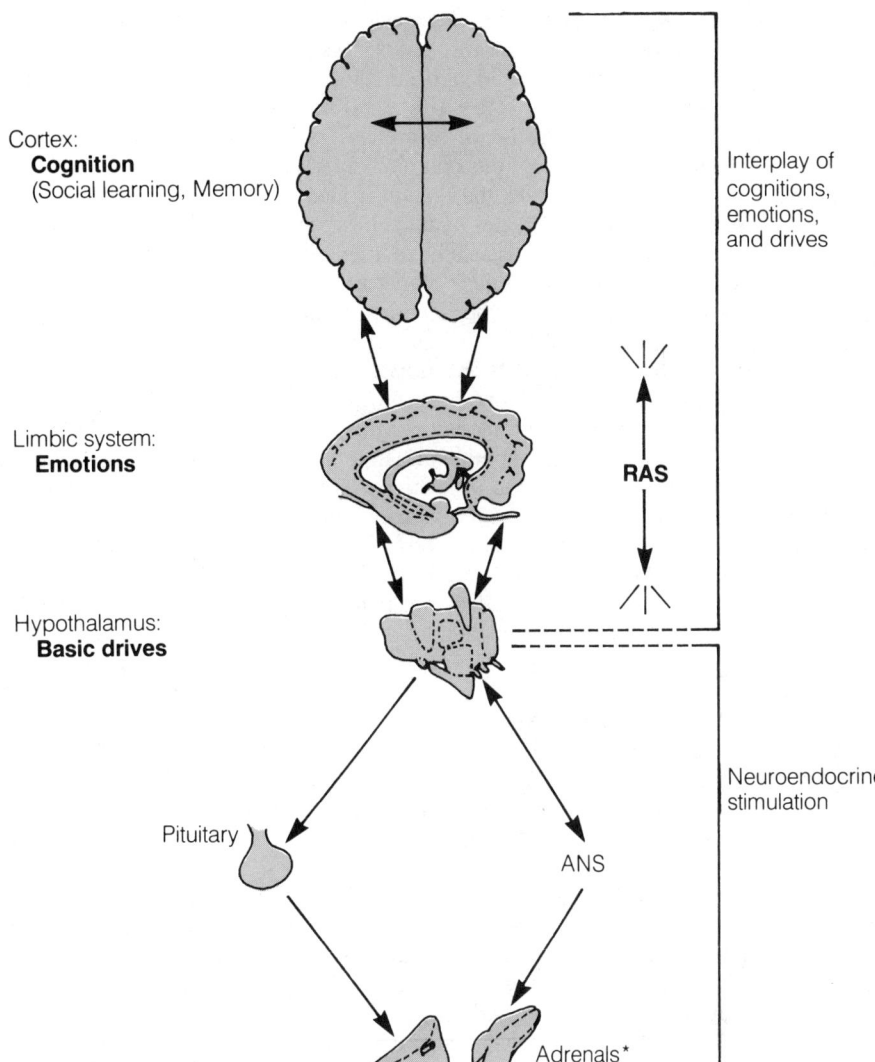

Cortex:
Cognition
(Social learning, Memory)

Limbic system:
Emotions

Hypothalamus:
Basic drives

Pituitary

ANS

Adrenals*

RAS

Interplay of
cognitions,
emotions,
and drives

Neuroendocrine
stimulation

Figure 8-2
Functional organization of the brain.
In the process of appraisal of
environmental change, different
levels of the brain are involved. The
highest level, the cortex, has evolved
more than the other two levels and
can exert control over emotional
states and basic drives. The reticular-
activating system (RAS) is a network
of cells that forms a two-way
communication system extending
from the brain stem into the
midbrain and limbic system. The
lower half of the diagram depicts the
response, neuroendocrine
stimulation (hypothalamus controls
pituitary, autonomic nervous system
[ANS]).

   *Other glands are also affected by
pituitary hormones; however, the adrenal
glands play a greater role in stress.

number of nuclei, and the limbic system contains the amyg-
dala, hippocampus, and septal nuclei, along with other structures. Research supports the concept that these structures
each respond differently to stimuli, and each has its characteristic response. The cerebral hemispheres are concerned
with cognitive functions: thought processes, learning, and
memory. The limbic system has connections with both the
cerebral hemispheres and the brain stem. In addition, the
reticular activating system (RAS), which is a network of cells
that forms a two-way communication system, extends from
the brain stem into the midbrain and limbic system. This network controls the alert or "waking" state of the body; it sends
signals that are relayed up to the cortex and relays signals
from the cortex downward. Its signals are capable of modifying ongoing input and processing.

   In the process of appraising environmental change to
determine whether a stressor is present, cognition, emotion,
and drive states interact. Emotions are complex and are described as having both mental and physical components: there
is the feeling itself, or affect; there is an awareness of the
feeling and possibly its cause, or cognition; there is an urge
to take action; and there are physical changes. The cognitive

appraisal of the potential stressor contributes to the type of
emotional response and its intensity.

   Whatever the outcome of the primary appraisal, the response is integrated in the hypothalamus. Either there is no
stressor and the hypothalamus continues to maintain a steady
state, or there is a stressor and the hypothalamus activates
the sympathetic and pituitary adrenal responses.

Physiologic Response

Neural and neuroendocrine pathways under the control of
the hypothalamus are activated in the stress response. First,
there is a sympathetic nervous system discharge followed by
a sympathetic-adrenal-medullary discharge, and finally if the
stress persists, the hypothalamic-pituitary system is activated.

   Sympathetic Nervous System Response. The sympathetic nervous system response is rapid and short-lived. Norepinephrine is released at nerve endings in direct contact
with their respective end organs to cause an increase in function of the vital organs and a state of general body arousal.
The heart rate is increased. Peripheral vasoconstriction occurs, raising the blood pressure. Blood is also shunted away

from abdominal organs. The purpose of these activities is to provide better perfusion of vital organs (brain, heart, skeletal muscles). Blood glucose is increased and supplies more readily available energy. The pupils are dilated, and mental activity is increased; a greater sense of awareness exists. Constriction of the blood vessels of the skin limits bleeding in the event of trauma. Subjectively, the person is likely to experience cold feet, clammy skin and hands, chills, palpitations, and a knot in the stomach. Typically, the person appears tense, with the muscles of the neck, upper back, and shoulders tightened; respirations may be rapid and shallow, with the diaphragm tense.

Sympathetic-Adrenal-Medullary Response. In addition to its direct effect on major end organs, the sympathetic nervous system (SNS) stimulates the medulla of the adrenal gland to release the hormones epinephrine and norepinephrine into the bloodstream. The action of these hormones is similar to that of the SNS and has the effect of sustaining and prolonging its actions. Epinephrine and norepinephrine together also stimulate the nervous system and produce metabolic effects that increase the blood sugar and stimulate the metabolic rate. The effect of the sympathetic and adrenal-medullary responses is summarized in Table 8-1. This effect is called the "fight or flight" reaction.

Hypothalamic-Pituitary Response. The longest-acting phase of the physiologic response, which is more likely to occur in persistent stress, involves the hypothalamic-pituitary pathway. The hypothalamus secretes corticotropin-releasing factor, which stimulates the anterior pituitary to produce adrenocorticotropic hormone (ACTH). ACTH in turn stimulates the adrenal cortex to produce glucocorticoids, primarily cortisol. Cortisol stimulates protein catabolism, releasing amino acids; stimulates liver uptake of amino acids and their conversion to glucose (gluconeogenesis); and inhibits glucose uptake (anti-insulin action) by many body cells but not those of the brain and heart. These cortisol-induced metabolic effects provide the body with a ready source of energy during a stressful situation. There are some important implications

to this effect: a person with diabetes under stress, such as an infection, will need more insulin than usual; any patient who is under stress (illness, surgery, prolonged psychological stress) will catabolize body protein and need supplements; and children subjected to severe stress will have retarded growth.

The glucocorticoids also depress the immune system. When they are present in high concentrations there is a reduction in the inflammatory response to injury or infection. The steps of the inflammatory process are inhibited, lymphocytes are destroyed in lymphoid tissues, and antibody production is decreased. As a result, the ability of the person to resist infections is reduced. This effect can also be used to advantage pharmacologically in the prescription of cortisol to treat the inflammatory and allergic responses in arthritis, asthma, and transplant resection.

The relationship of stress to the immune response is a subject of new fields of study called behavioral immunology, psychoneuroimmunology, and neuroimmunomodulation. Studies of animals have shown that extreme psychological stress can have a profound effect on immune competence. Studies in humans have not been as conclusive (partially because of problems in experimental design and control), but investigators believe that the mind influences immune responses with consequences that can be harmful to the host (Cohen, 1985).

The action of the catecholamines (epinephrine and norepinephrine) and cortisol are most important in the general response to stress. Other hormones that are also released are antidiuretic hormone (ADH) from the posterior pituitary and aldosterone from the adrenal cortex. ADH and aldosterone promote sodium and water retention, which is an adaptive mechanism in the event of hemorrhage or loss of fluids through excessive perspiration. ADH has also been shown to influence learning and so may facilitate coping in new and threatening situations. Growth hormone and glucagon are secreted and stimulate the uptake of amino acids by cells helping to mobilize energy resources. The secretion of other

TABLE 8-1
Sympathetic-Adrenal-Medullary Response

Effect	Goal	Mechanism
↑Heart rate ↑Blood pressure	Better perfusion of vital organs	Increased cardiac output due to increased myocardial contractility and heart rate; also, increased venous return (peripheral vasoconstriction)
↑Blood glucose	Increased available energy	Increased liver and muscle glycogen breakdown; also, increased breakdown of adipose tissue triglycerides
↑Mental activity	Alert state	
Dilated pupils	Increased awareness	
↑Tension of skeletal muscles	Preparedness for activity, decreased fatigue	Excitation of muscles; also, increase in amount of blood shunted to the muscles from the abdominal viscera
↑Ventilation (may be rapid and shallow)	Provision of oxygen for energy	
↑Coagulability of blood	Prevention of hemorrhage in event of trauma	Vasoconstriction of surface vessels

hormones is also affected, but their adaptive function is less clear.

The production of endorphin, an endogenous opiate, is also increased during stress and enhances the threshold for toleration of painful stimuli. It may also affect mood. It has been implicated in the so-called "high" that long-distance runners experience.

Summary. The initial components of the physiologic response to stress, the sympathetic response, and the sympathetic-adrenal-medullary response occur in practically all stressful situations. The observable behaviors (*e.g.,* blood pressure, pulse) may vary, but the essential neuroendocrine response is the same. With the onset of the more chronic phase, there is a great deal of variability. The hypothalamic-pituitary-adrenal-cortical response will be activated in most cases, but the total pattern of the endocrine response will vary with the nature, duration, and severity of the chronic stressor. With continued exposure to the same stressor, the response will be attenuated.

Social Support: Influence on Stress

The nature of social support and its influence on coping has been studied extensively, and it has been demonstrated to be an effective moderator of life stress. Cobb (1976) defined social support as information belonging to one or more of three classes. The first class of information leads the subject to believe that he is cared for and loved. This appears most often in a relationship between two people in which mutual trust and attachment are expressed by helping one another meet their needs. Such expressions, sometimes called *emotional support*, are most commonly thought of in the marital relationship, but also occur between a nurse and patient.

The second class of information leads the subject to believe that he is esteemed and valued. This is most effective when it is announced in public and thus demonstrates the favorable position the individual has in the group. It elevates his sense of self-worth; this is called *esteem support*.

The third class of information leads the subject to believe that he belongs to a network of communication and mutual obligation. Information is shared by the members of the network, they all know what it is, and they are all aware that it is shared. This information is of two types. One is communications, which are "the essence of history"—what is going on, who is affected, and so forth. Another communication in this category is the knowledge that goods and services are available to the members on demand; for example, a person can call on a close friend in an emergency. Cobb emphasized that social support encourages independent behavior; it does not lead to dependency.

Social support begins in utero; it is fostered through maternal and paternal attachment behavior and develops through family, peer, and community relationships as the person grows. A number of sociological and family theories attest to the production of stress and illness when the family structure is disrupted so that there is no stable hierarchy or authority, territorial limits are not well defined, and strong attachment behavior is lacking.

Social support facilitates the coping behaviors of a person; however, this is conditional on the nature of the social support. People can have extensive relationships and interact frequently, but the necessary support comes only when there is a deep level of involvement and concern, not when people merely touch the surface of each others' lives. The critical qualities within the network are the exchange of intimate communications and the presence of solidarity and trust. Recognizing the value of social support theory to nursing, Brandt and Weinert (1981) and Norbeck and associates (1981) have developed questionnaires to identify the social support used by patients.

Selye and the General Adaptation Syndrome

Because of his profound influence on the scientific development of the study of stress and the manner in which he has popularized the concept, it is important to understand Hans Selye's theory. In 1936, Selye first described a syndrome consisting of enlargement of the adrenal cortex; shrinkage of the thymus, spleen, lymph nodes, and other lymphatic structures; and the appearance of deep, bleeding ulcers in the stomach and duodenum. He identified this as a "nonspecific response" to diverse, noxious stimuli. From this beginning, he developed a theory of adaptation to biological stress, which he named the General Adaptation Syndrome (GAS).

Phases of the GAS. The GAS has three phases: alarm, resistance, and exhaustion. During the acute phase, or alarm reaction, the sympathetic fight or flight response is activated with release of adrenal medullary hormones, and the ACTH–adrenal cortical response begins. The alarm reaction is defensive and anti-inflammatory but self-limited. Because it is impossible to live in a continuous state of alarm (death would ensue), the person moves into the second stage, resistance. During this stage, adaptation to the noxious stressor occurs. Cortisol activity is still increased. If exposure to the stressor is prolonged, exhaustion sets in, and endocrine activity increases, producing deleterious effects on the body systems (especially circulatory, digestive, and immune) that can lead to death. Stages one and two of this syndrome are repeated, in different degrees, throughout life as the person encounters stressors.

Selye also compared the GAS with the life process. During childhood, the first stage, there have been few encounters with stress to promote the development of adaptive functioning, and the child is vulnerable. During the next stage, adulthood, the person has encountered a number of life's stressful events and has developed a resistance or adaptation. In the final stage, senility, the accumulation of life's stressors and the wear and tear on the organism again deplete the person's ability to adapt, resistance falls, and eventually death ensues.

Local Adaptation Syndrome. According to Selye's theory, there is also a local adaptation syndrome (LAS). The syndrome includes the inflammatory response and repair processes that occur at the local site of tissue injury. The LAS occurs in small, topical injuries, such as bee stings; in the case of emotional arousal, the cerebral cortex is involved. "Even if the target area is not a small area but instead the cerebral cortex, the general metabolism, or the reticuloendothelial system, there is a primary topical response" (Selye, 1976b). Depending on the severity of the injury, stimuli are sent to the nervous system to elicit the hypothalamic-pituitary-adrenocortical response; this results in the GAS or systemic stress response. Cortical hormones are released and then superimpose their effect on the LAS.

Selye emphasized that stress is the nonspecific response common to all stressors, regardless of whether they are physiologic, psychological, or social. The fact that different demands are interpreted by different people as stressors is explained by the many conditioning factors in each person's environment. Conditioning factors also account for differences in the tolerance of different persons for stress. Some may develop diseases of adaptation, such as hypertension and migraine headaches, while others appear to be unaffected.

Recent Views. In his early research, Selye used extremes of physical stressors. With newer hormone detection techniques, a variety of stressors of differing intensities have been used, and multihormonal patterns of response are being detected. These studies indicate that there are different patterns of response to different stimuli, *stimulus specificity*, and that each person develops a characteristic pattern of autonomic response that carries over from one type of stress to another, *individual response specificity*. It has been suggested that the nonspecific response is not elicited by a diverse number of stimuli but rather by one factor, emotional arousal, and that it is the degree of the arousal that affects the intensity of the hormonal response and thus the manifestations displayed by the individual.

Maladaptive Responses

The mechanisms identified by Cannon and Selye serve as adaptations to meet threatening situations. These can be both beneficial and harmful. Dubos (1965) stated that these are traits retained from the human evolutionary past that "no longer fit the needs of life in civilized societies." The fight or flight response, for example, is an anticipatory response that mobilized the bodily resources of our ancestors to deal with predators and other harsh exigencies of the environment. This same mobilization comes into play in response to emotional stimuli unrelated to danger.

> Whatever the life situation, whether it corresponds to an actual physical danger or merely to an emotional crisis, the nature and intensity of the anticipatory changes the symbol elicits in the body have remained much the same in modern man as they were in his Paleolithic ancestor.*

When the body has been prepared physiologically to act and does not do so, the result is likely to be frustrating and injurious to the person's health. For example, consider the father waiting outside the delivery room for his wife to deliver

---

* Dubos R. Man Adapting, p 30. New Haven, Yale University Press, 1965.

their first baby. He may be as exhausted at the end of labor as the mother. Anxiety prepared him for "fight or flight"; when he could not do either, conflict developed, frustration appeared, tension became obvious, and pacing, perspiration, and other behaviors occurred that used up as much energy as the physical labor. In this case, the father was rewarded; in instances in which that might not be true, the conflict and frustration would be intensified.

The fight or flight and rage responses stimulate sympathetic adrenal-medullary activity. In instances in which this is prolonged or excessive, a state of chronic arousal develops, leading to high blood pressure, arteriosclerotic changes, and cardiovascular disease. When the production of the adrenal cortical hormone is prolonged or excessive, behavior patterns of withdrawal and depression are seen. In addition, the immune response is decreased, and infections and tumors may develop. Two behavior patterns have been observed and correlated with the two extremes in endocrine activity just described: excessive dominance and excessive subordination.

Risk-Inducing Coping Processes

Coping itself can add to social, psychological, and physiologic malfunction that increases the risk of illness. One way in which it does this is by direct damage to tissues. For example, the use of alcohol or drugs to alleviate stress may create liver damage; social relationships and psychological welfare may also be affected. Coping by smoking may create lung damage. Overeating or undereating may have serious nutritional effects; psychosocial welfare may also be harmed. All of these increase the vulnerability of the body to further disease.

A second way in which coping increases the risk of illness is more indirect and can best be understood through an example. Type A people are driving, competitive, and achievement-oriented. The pattern they have developed reflects a socialization process that emphasizes the Protestant work ethic. Mobilization of type A behavior requires the increased output of catecholamines, the adrenal-medullary hormones. One might say the life of a type A person is a series of fight or flight responses.

A third way in which coping can increase health risk is called palliative. This is typified by the woman who feels a lump in her breast but denies its seriousness and delays seeking medical attention. The intention of palliative coping methods is to control the threat to life, but in the end they increase the risk of developing more severe illnesses because of their delaying action.

Ego defenses are "basically a coping srategy to deal with conflicts over a particular emotion." For example, if you are angry with someone, rather than create a scene that may lead to threats and retaliation, which would endanger your self-concept, you are likely to pick a less dangerous scapegoat or possibly work the anger out in physical exercise. Ego defenses imply an unconscious aspect in that usually the behavior is not the result of a deliberate thinking process, although some of it may be. Continual internal conflict and repression of emotions can lead to psychopathology.

Indices of Stress

Laboratory measurements of indicators of stress have significantly improved since the early experiments in the field and

---

Chart 8-1
Indices of Stress

General irritability, hyperexcitation, or depression
Dryness of the throat and mouth
Overpowering urge to cry or run and hide
Easily fatigued, loss of interest
"Floating anxiety"—do not know exactly why or what
Easily startled
Stuttering or other speech difficulties
Hypermotility: pacing, moving about, cannot sit still
Gastrointestinal signs and symptoms: "butterflies" in the stomach, diarrhea, vomiting
Change in menstrual cycle
Loss of or excessive appetite
Increased use of legally prescribed drugs, such as tranquilizers or psychic energizers
Accident proneness
Disturbed behavior

Pounding of the heart
Impulsive behavior, emotional instability
Inability to concentrate
Feelings of unreality, weakness, or dizziness
Tension, alertness
Trembling, nervous tics
Nervous laughter
Grinding of teeth
Insomnia
Perspiring
Increased frequency of urination
Muscle tension and migraine headaches
Pain in the neck or lower back
Increased smoking
Alcohol and drug addiction
Nightmares

(Based on Selye H. Stress in Health and Disease. Woburn, Butterworths, 1976. Reprinted by permission of the publisher.)

---

are daily adding to the understanding of this complex process. Among the measures, blood and urine analyses can be used to demonstrate changes in hormonal levels and hormonal breakdown products. Reliable measures of stress include blood levels of catecholamines, corticoids, ACTH, and a drop in eosinophils. The blood creatine/creatinine ratio and elevations of cholesterol and free fatty acids can also be measured. Immunoglobulin assays may be done. (With the growth of neuroimmunology, improved laboratory measures should be developed.)

The electroencephalogram may be used to measure brain activity. Galvanic skin resistance, which measures the electrical conductivity of the skin, may be done. This is primarily a measure of sweat excretion, which rises in stress, and is typically used in lie detector tests. Rises in blood pressure and heart rate can also be measured.

In addition to these measurable signs, there are a number of other indices of stress that may be observed by others or by the person himself; they are listed in Chart 8-1. Over time, each person tends to develop a characteristic pattern of behavior in stress that is a warning that the system is out of balance. Researchers have developed many questionnaires to identify the *state* of stress in people and also the tendency toward stress, a *trait* of the personality.

Diseases of Adaptation: Maladaptation

The autonomic and endocrine responses to stress serve an adaptive function; their purpose is to restore equilibrium in the individual. They may last minutes, hours, or days; the disturbance they cause is reversible. However, when we speak of "diseases of adaptation," we mean diseases in which the stress response plays the predominant etiologic role and irreversible pathology may be present. The preceding discussion has identified the mechanisms contributing to the for-

mation of these diseases. Other chapters of the book discuss individual diseases in greater detail.

Selye (1976a) gives the following comprehensive list of disorders:

> High blood pressure, diseases of the heart and blood vessels, diseases of the kidney, eclampsia, rheumatic and rheumatoid arthritis, inflammatory diseases of the skin and eyes, infections, allergic and hypersensitivity diseases, nervous and mental diseases, sexual derangements, digestive diseases, metabolic diseases, cancer, and diseases of resistance in general.*

Some are due to an "excess of defensive, others to an overabundance of submissive bodily reactions." It is important to retain the holistic concept in considering the multiple factors involved in these diseases. Emotional arousal may lead to the neuroendocrine responses. A pattern of positive feedback may develop that continues to stimulate the production of hormones, the bodily responses feed the emotional arousal, and a vicious cycle ensues. Other regulatory mechanisms, which have been on the periphery, become involved and contribute to further disturbances.

Summary

Stress, like beauty, is in the eye of the beholder. Each person perceives and reacts to situations and change differently depending on his personal characteristics, abilities, and experiences, his external support systems, and characteristics of the stressor itself. The stress response produced may be elicited by real, potential, or imagined threats, leading to varied and multiple patterns of hormonal discharge. The goal is to

* Selye H. The Stress of Life, pp 169, 170. New York, McGraw-Hill, 1976.

mobilize the person's energy resources to cope with the stressor and to promote adaptive outcomes.

Stress Management

Stress or the potential for stress is ubiquitous: it can be everywhere and anywhere at once. Throughout this book, health problems will be identified that carry with them the potential for stress. Anxiety is the usual emotion accompanying stress. In the presence of anxiety, the customary activities of daily living may be disrupted; for example, sleep disturbance may be present and eating patterns altered. Coping patterns may be ineffective, thought processes impaired, and role relationships may suffer. It is obvious that many nursing diagnoses are possible.

Major factors that influence the development and impact of stress have been identified as the person's inner capabilities, his external resources, and the nature of the stressor itself. These are considered in discussing methods that nurses might use for reducing and controlling stress, not only in their patients but also in themselves. The need to prevent illness, improve the quality of life, and decrease the cost of health care makes efforts to promote health even more significant. The decrease of stress is an important goal.

Health Risk Appraisal

Health risk appraisal is an activity designed to promote health by examining the personal habits of the patient and recommending changes where health risk is indicated. Health risk questionnaires estimate the likelihood that a person with a given set of characteristics will become ill within a given time span. It is reasoned that if the patient is provided with this information, he will alter his activities (*e.g.,* stop smoking, have periodic screening examinations) to improve his health status. Questionnaires typically collect the following types of information:

1. Demographic data: age, sex, race, ethnic background
2. Personal and family history of certain diseases
3. Life-style factors

   * Eating, sleeping, exercise, smoking, drinking, and driving habits
   * Stressors on the job
   * Role relationships and associated stressors

4. Physical measurements

   * Blood pressure
   * Height, weight
   * Laboratory analyses of blood and urine

5. Membership or nonmembership in a high-risk group, such as a family with a history of cancer

The personal data are compared with average population risk data, and the risk factors are identified and weighted. From this analysis the person's chronological age and risk age are determined, and a list of the person's major health hazards are identified. If the person makes suggested changes, further comparisons with population data can estimate how many years will be added to his life span (compliance age).

Research so far has not demonstrated that providing people with such information ensures that they will change their habits (Doerr & Hutchins, 1981; Goetz & McTyre, 1981).

Nursing Implications

Although the collection of data bases like the one just described is a common part of taking a nursing history, the controlled analysis of risk is not customary. The development of a *nursing* data base that supplies the essential information for making decisions about patient care is a necessity.

Health risk appraisal and patient education to improve health behavior are activities that nurses can perform to prevent health problems and reduce stress. In patients who *already* have health problems, there will be some degree of stress, and the nurse can *anticipate* changes based on the stress response. For example, the postsurgical patient will have fluid and electrolyte changes corresponding to the general neuroendocrine response. It should be mentioned that this response has a snowballing effect. Although it does not primarily affect the kidney, the vasoconstriction induced as part of the stress response may decrease the flow of blood to the kidney, which stimulates the renin–angiotensin mechanism, leading to an increase in aldosterone with sodium and water retention. Psychosocially, if the person typically withdraws and becomes nonexpressive in stress situations, that same behavior may be expected here.

Coping Behaviors

It should be remembered that a person is in constant interaction with his environment, both internal and external. This implies that change is constant and necessary for optimal psychosocial and physiologic growth. Responding to change requires adaptive energy; the important issue is to regulate the use of energy so that there is an adequate store. This then becomes an issue of regulating one's own actions to reduce stress.

The functions of coping were listed earlier, as follows:

* *Emotion-focused:* directed at lessening emotional distress; include such strategies as avoidance, minimizing, distancing, selective attention
* *Problem-focused:* directed to management of the problem; include such strategies as defining the problem, finding alternative solutions, weighing them, and acting

Two commonly prescribed nursing interventions, the provision of sensory information and preoperative teaching (Christman & Kirchhoff, 1985; Felton, 1985), have the goal of improving the patient's coping ability. Major nursing research using these interventions has been conducted by Leventhal and Johnson (1983). They have tested the theory that people acquire a sense of control over events when they are given information that makes it possible for them to form a mental image of them. If people were provided with a description of the sensations they could expect to feel (*e.g.,* pulling, burning, pressure), if the routine of the procedure were described to them, and if they were given instructions in coping behaviors (deep breathing, coughing, turning, exercises) they would experience less distress and have better outcomes (less pain, better mood, fewer analgesics needed, more rapid recovery). In their work, the researchers have tested these techniques alone and in combination in different short-term and long-term threatening situations (diagnostic examinations and surgery). The outcomes have been complex and illustrate that individual differences in the perception of stress and its management must be taken into consideration.

Among their findings, Leventhal and Johnson discovered that the combination of sensory information and postoperative exercise instruction was not consistently effective. If the instruction provided the patient with a way of coping when he previously had none, it was more likely to be effective. If he already had an effective coping strategy, any new ones could be considered conflicting. In some instances, attempting to use the new strategy rather than relying on existing strategies was thought to delay recovery, particularly after the patient went home. Specific coping strategies were usually more effective in short-term than in long-term events. Individual differences were found to be significant.

The importance of this research lies in helping the nurse to decide who will benefit from the information provided, the goal to be achieved, and the specific outcome criteria to be used in evaluating the information.

Through health appraisals, nurses may identify patient stressors. However, stress control requires self-care and motivation, and therefore the patient must actively and willingly participate in appraising, identifying, and managing his sources of stress. At the same time, sources of strength should be identified and capitalized on. This helps to improve the self-esteem of the patient and reinforces positive behavior patterns.

Stress-Reduction Methods

Numerous methods for reducing stress are available and being publicized. The important point to be remembered is that just as each person develops a particular pattern of stress response, so will each person have his preferred method of stress reduction. Bulechek and McCloskey (1985) described three nursing interventions for stress management: relaxation training, cognitive reappraisal, and music therapy. Sutterley and Donnelly (1981) identified six categories of activities for the self-regulation of stress including nutrition; exercise, physical activity, and recreation; muscle control and kinesiology; meditation and creative imagery; communication and time management; and group process and support systems.

Proper nutrition, adequate rest, and regular exercise improve one's well-being and help develop resistance to stressors. Regular exercise assists in weight control, decreases a sense of fatigue and monotony, and increases the exercise tolerance for some patients with angina pectoris and peripheral arterial disease. Some studies indicate that it may prevent heart attacks, and it may help to prevent premature atherosclerosis. The need for outside and diversionary activities for everyone has become a fact of life.

Biofeedback. The purpose of biofeedback is to gain some degree of mental control over the autonomic nervous system and possibly decrease blood pressure, control heart rate, and prevent disorders such as migraine headache and hyperactive stomach. Some form of electronic instrumentation is used to monitor a biological function, such as measuring skin conductance with the galvanic skin responder. This information is amplified and sent back to the person, who then tries consciously to alter the machine in some way. For example, by relaxing and decreasing the sweating of his palms, the person attempts to alter the tone of the machine. The activity that produces an altered tone in the machine alters the biological functioning. Through practice and reinforcement, the person learns how to control the activity without the machine. Some people suffering from migraine headaches have developed a technique of "thinking their hands hot," and theoretically have directed the blood flow from the head to the hands. The long-term efficacy of such techniques is still being tested.

Relaxation Response. The "relaxation response" is a calming state opposite to the arousal state of stress. Four elements are necessary to produce the relaxation response: a quiet environment, a comfortable position, a passive attitude, and a mental device or object, such as a word, sound, or phrase to occupy the mind and keep out thoughts. For example, the word "one" could be repeated silently or audibly. By sitting quietly and practicing relaxation 15 to 20 minutes once or twice a day, a person should be able to achieve positive results in lowering stress levels. Other techniques, such as meditation and yoga, also produce the relaxation response. Still others use the sound of pleasant music or a mountain stream in conjunction with relaxation techniques to help achieve the desired state. Progressive relaxation is a technique in which muscle groups are alternately tensed and relaxed in a systematic fashion so that the person can compare the two effects, and ends with a period of complete relaxation.

Other techniques, such as massage, may be used; the effectiveness of slow-stroke back massage in patients with high emotional and physiologic arousal has been demonstrated. Relaxation training might be used in the following nursing diagnoses: Anxiety, Sleep disturbance, Ineffective breathing pattern, Ineffective coping, and Alteration in comfort: Pain.

It is important for the nurse to determine what type of stress reduction activities work best and to encourage their regular use.

Social Support. The importance of social support as a mediating resource in stress has already been identified. To reinforce that information, the function of social networks includes the following:

- The maintenance of positive social identity
- The provision of emotional support
- The provision of material aid and tangible services
- Access to information
- Access to new social contacts and new social roles

The emotion—anxiety, fear, guilt—that accompanies stress is unpleasant, and it may continue to grow in a spiraling fashion without intervention. Emotional support from family and significant others provides a person with love and a sense of sharing the burden. Being able to talk with someone and express one's feelings openly may help one to gain mastery of the situation. Nurses can provide this source of support; however, it is important to identify the patient's social support system and encourage its use. People who are loners, or isolated, or who withdraw in times of stress have a high risk of coping failure.

Anxiety may also distort a person's ability to process information. Perception is narrowed, thoughts may be unclear, and reality may be distorted. For a time, this cognitive blurring is adaptive and allows the person to tolerate a threat, perhaps some bad news. However, reality must be faced for the longer run. It helps to seek information and advice from others who can assist with analyzing the threat and developing a strategy to manage it. Again, this use of others helps the person to maintain mastery of a situation and to keep his self-esteem.

There is a growing awareness in the public of the need for support groups. Groups have been formed by parents of children with leukemia, ostomates, mastectomy patients (Reach to Recovery) and other cancer victims, and persons with other serious diseases. There are groups for single parents, Alcoholics Anonymous and spouses of alcoholics, drug addiction groups, and child abuse groups meet for mutual support. Professional, civic, and religious support groups are active in the community. Being a member of a group with similar problems has a releasing effect on the person that promotes freedom of expression and exchange of ideas. There are also encounter groups, assertiveness training programs, and consciousness raising groups to help people modify their usual behavior.

Human evolution has led to a brain that possesses neural networks characterized by a plasticity that permits behavior to be modified. This flexibility allows people to make choices and thereby exert some control over the strategies they select for survival. The nurse can play a significant role in influencing those choices.

Bibliography

Books

Asterita MF. The Physiology of Stress. New York, Human Sciences Press, 1985.

Bulechek GM and McCloskey JC. Nursing Interventions: Treatments for Nursing Diagnoses. Philadelphia, WB Saunders, 1985.

Dubos R. Man Adapting. New Haven, Connecticut, John Wiley & Sons, 1965.

Groer MW and Shekleton ME. Basic Pathophysiology, A Conceptual Approach. St Louis, CV Mosby, 1983.

Guyton AC. Textbook of Medical Physiology. Philadelphia, WB Saunders, 1986.

Lazarus RS and Folkman S. Stress, Appraisal, and Coping. New York, Springer, 1984.

Marriner A (ed). Nursing Theorists and Their Work. St Louis, CV Mosby, 1986.

Milsum JH. Health, Stress, and Illness, a Systems Approach. New York, Praeger, 1984.

Moberg GP (ed). Animal Stress. Bethesda, Maryland, American Psychological Association, 1985.

Pelletier KR. Mind as Healer, Mind as Slayer. New York, Dell, 1977.

Restak RM. The Brain. New York, Bantam Books, 1984.

Riehl JP and Roy C (eds). Conceptual Models for Nursing Practice. New York, Appleton-Century-Crofts, 1980.

Selye H. The Stress of Life. New York, McGraw-Hill, 1976a.

Selye H. Stress in Health and Disease. Boston, Butterworths, 1976b.

Selye H (ed). Selye's Guide to Stress Research, vol I. New York, Van Nostrand Reinhold, 1980.

Sutterley DC and Donnelly GF (eds). Coping with Stress. Rockville, Maryland, Aspen Systems Corporation, 1981.

Vander AJ, Sherman JH, and Luciano DS. Human Physiology: The Mechanisms of Body Function. New York, McGraw-Hill, 1985.

Wolf SW and Goodell H. Harold G. Wolff's Stress and Disease, 2nd ed. Springfield, Illinois, Charles C Thomas, 1968.

Wooldridge PJ, Schmitt MH, Skipper JK, and Leonard RC (eds). Behavioral Science & Nursing Theory. St Louis, CV Mosby, 1983.

Articles

(Asterisks indicate nursing research articles.)

Axelrod J and Reisine TD. Stress hormones: Their interaction and regulation. Science 1984 May 4; 224(4648):452–459.

Berglas S. Special section: Stress and coping. J Pers Soc Psychol 1984 Apr; 46(4):837–949.

Blue CL, Brubaker KM, Papazian KR, and Riester CM. Sister Callista Roy: Adaptation model. In Marriner A (ed). Nursing Theorists and Their Work. St Louis, CV Mosby, 1986.

*Brandt P and Weinert C. The PRQ—a social support measure. Nurs Res. 1981 Sept/Oct; 30(5):277–280.

Chiriboga DA. Social stressors as antecedents of change. J Gerontol 1984 Jul; 39(4):468–477.

Christman NJ and Kirchhoff KT. Preparatory sensory information. In Bulechek GM and McCloskey JC (eds). Nursing Interventions: Treatments for Nursing Diagnoses. Philadelphia, WB Saunders, 1985.

Cobb S. Social support as a moderator of life stress. Psycho Med 1976 Sept/Oct; 38(5):300–314.

Cohen JJ. Stress and the human immune response: A critical review. J Burn Care Rehabil 1985 Mar/Apr; 6(2):167–173.

*Doerr BT and Hutchins EB. Health risk appraisal: Process, problems and prospects for nursing research and practice. Nurs Res 1981 Sept/Oct; 30(5):299–307.

Felton G. Preoperative teaching. In Bulechek GM and McCloskey JC (eds). Nursing Interventions: Treatments for Nursing Diagnoses. Philadelphia, WB Saunders, 1985.

*Goetz AA and McTyre RB. Health risk appraisal: Some methodologic considerations. Nurs Res 1981 Sept/Oct; 30(5):307–313.

Hermiz ME and Meininger M. Betty Neuman: systems model. In Marriner A (ed). Nursing Theorists and Their Work. St Louis, CV Mosby, 1986.

Holmes TH and Rahe RH. The social readjustment rating scale. J Psychosom Res 1967 Aug; 11(2):213–218.

*Leventhal H and Johnson JE. Laboratory and field experimentation: development of a theory of self-regulation. In Wooldridge PJ, Schmitt MH, Skipper JK, and Leonard RC (eds). Behavioral Science and Nursing Theory. St Louis, CV Mosby, 1983.

Marx JL. The immune system "belongs to the body." Science 1985 Mar 8; 227(4691):1190–1192.

Mason JW. A historical view of the stress field: I. J Hum Stress 1975 Mar; 1(1):6–12.

Mason JW. A historical view of the stress field: II. J Hum Stress 1975 June; 1(2):22–36.

*Norbeck JS, Lindsey AM, and Carrieri VL. The development of an instrument to measure social support. Nurs Res 1981 Sept/Oct; 30(5): 264–269.

*Panzarine S. Coping: conceptual and methodological issues. ANS 1985 July; 7(4):49–57.

Pearlin LI, Lieberman MA, Menaghan EG, and Mullan JT. The stress response. J Health Soc Behav 1981 Dec; 22(4):337–356.

*Rice VH, Caldwell M, Butler S, and Robinson J. Relaxation training and response to cardiac catheterization. Nurs Res 1986 Jan/Feb; 35(1): 39–44.

*Rock DL, Green KE, Wise BK, and Rock RD. Social support and social network scales: A psychometric review. Res Nurs Health 1984 Dec; 7(4):325–332.

*Scott DW, Oberst MT, and Bookbinder MI. Stress-coping response to genitourinary carcinoma in men. Nurs Res 1984 Nov/Dec; 33(6): 325–329.

Shaver JF. A biopsychosocial view of human health. Nurs Outlook 1985 July/Aug; 33(4):186–191.

Viney LL and Westbrook MT. Coping with chronic illness: Strategy preferences and associated emotional reactions. J Chron Dis 1984; 37(6):489–502.

Wallace LM. Psychological preparation as a method of reducing the stress of surgery. J Hum Stress 1984 Summer; 10(2):63–77.

Chapter 9

Fluids and Electrolytes: Balance and Disturbances

Glossary

Acidosis — an acid–base disturbance characterized by increased hydrogen ion concentration (decreased *p*H); may be due to increased production of acids or loss of base.

Alkalosis — an acid–base disturbance characterized by decreased hydrogen ion concentration (increased *p*H); may be due to loss of acids or increased production of base.

Diffusion — passive movement of particles from an area of high concentration to one of lower concentration.

Osmosis — movement of fluid through a semipermeable membrane from an area of low concentration to an area of high concentration of particles to equalize the concentration on both sides of the membrane.

Hydrostatic pressure — force exerted by a fluid against the walls of the container (in the body, the pressure of fluid against the walls of the blood vessels results from the weight of the fluid itself and the force resulting from cardiac contraction).

Osmolality — number of dissolved particles contained in a specific unit or volume of fluid (*i.e.*, 1 liter).

Isotonic solution — solution in which the *number* of dissolved particles is equal to the number of particles dissolved in normal body fluids.

Hypotonic solution — one with fewer dissolved particles than another solution (*i.e.*, fewer than the number of particles in normal body fluids).

Hypertonic solution — one with more dissolved particles than another solution (*i.e.*, more than the number of particles in normal body fluids).

Fundamental Concepts

Amount and Composition of Body Fluids

Factors that influence the amount of body fluid in humans are age, sex, and body fat content. As a general rule, younger people have a higher percentage of body fluid than do older people, and men have proportionately more body fluid than do women (Table 9-1). Obese people have less fluid than thin people since fat cells contain little water.

The typical adult is approximately 60% fluid (water and electrolytes) by weight. Approximately two thirds of the body fluid in adults exists in the intracellular space (primarily in the skeletal muscle mass). The remaining one third is found in the extracellular space, between the cells and in the plasma.

Electrolytes

Electrolytes in body fluids are active chemicals (anions and cations) that unite in varying combinations. Therefore, electrolyte concentration in the body is expressed in terms of milliequivalents (mEq) per liter, a measure of chemical activity, rather than in terms of milligrams (mg), a unit of weight. More specifically, a milliequivalent is defined as being equivalent to the electrochemical activity of 1 mg of hydrogen.

TABLE 9-1

Approximate Values of Total Body Fluid as a Percentage of Body Weight in Relation to Age and Sex

Age		Total Body Fluid (% body weight)
Full-term newborn		70%–80%
1 year		64%
Puberty to 39 years	Men:	60%
	Women:	52%
40 to 60 years	Men:	55%
	Women:	47%
More than 60 years	Men:	52%
	Women:	46%

(Metheny N. Quick Reference to Fluid Balance. Philadelphia, JB Lippincott, 1984.)

TABLE 9-2

Plasma Electrolytes

Electrolytes	mEq/liter
Cations	
Sodium (Na^+)	142
Potassium (K^+)	5
Calcium (Ca^{2+})	5
Magnesium (Mg^{2+})	2
Total cations	154
Anions	
Chloride (Cl^-)	103
Bicarbonate (HCO_3^-)	26
Phosphate (HPO_4^{2-})	2
Sulfate (SO_4^{2-})	1
Organic acids	5
Proteinate	17
Total anions	154

(Metheny N. Fluid and Electrolyte Balance: Nursing Considerations. Philadelphia, JB Lippincott, 1987.)

Electrolyte concentrations in intracellular fluid (ICF) differ from those in extracellular fluid (ECF). Because special techniques are required to measure electrolyte concentrations in the ICF, it is customary to measure the electrolytes in the most accessible portion of body fluids, namely, the plasma.

Sodium ions in the ECF far outnumber other extracellular cations (Table 9-2). About 90% of the ECF osmolality is determined by the sodium concentration. As a result, sodium is important in the regulation of body fluid volume. Retention of sodium is associated with fluid retention; conversely, excessive sodium loss is usually associated with decreased body fluid volume.

As shown in Table 9-3, the major electrolytes in the ICF are potassium and phosphate. Since the ECF can tolerate only small potassium concentrations (approximately 5 mEq/liter), release of large stores of intracellular potassium by trauma can be extremely dangerous. The body expends a great deal of energy maintaining the extracellular preponderance of sodium and the intracellular preponderance of potassium. It does so by means of cell hydrostatic pressure (the pressure exerted by the fluid on the walls of the blood vessel) at both the arterial and the venous ends of the vessel and by the osmotic pressure exerted by the protein of plasma. Direction of fluid movement depends on the differences in these two opposing forces. The ECF transports other substances, such as enzymes and hormones. It also carries blood components, such as red and white blood cells, throughout the body.

Regulation of Body Fluid Compartments

Osmosis. When two different solutions are separated by a membrane impermeable to the dissolved substances, a shift of water occurs through the membrane from the region of low solute concentration to the region of high solute con-

TABLE 9-3

Approximation of Major Electrolyte Content in Cellular Fluid

Electrolytes	mEq/liter
Cations	
Potassium (K$^+$)	150
Magnesium (Mg^{2+})	40
Sodium (Na$^+$)	10
Total cations	200
Anions	
Phosphates } Sulfates	150
Bicarbonate (HCO$_3^-$)	10
Proteinate	40
Total anions	200

(Metheny N. Fluid and Electrolyte Balance: Nursing Considerations. Philadelphia, JB Lippincott, 1987.)

centration until the solutions are of equal concentration (Fig. 9-1). The magnitude of this force depends on the *number* of particles dissolved in the solutions and not on their weights. The number of dissolved particles contained in a unit of water determines the osmolality of a solution.

Diffusion. Diffusion is defined as the natural tendency of a substance to move from an area of higher concentration to one of lower concentration. It occurs through the random movement of ions and molecules. An example of diffusion is the exchange of oxygen and carbon dioxide between the pulmonary capillaries and alveoli.

Filtration. Hydrostatic pressure in the capillaries tends to filter fluid out of the vascular compartment into the interstitial fluid. An example of filtration is the passage of water and electrolytes from the arterial capillary bed to the interstitial fluid; in this instance, the hydrostatic pressure is furnished by the pumping action of the heart.

Sodium–Potassium Pump. As stated earlier, sodium concentration is greater in ECF than in ICF; because of this, there is a tendency for sodium to enter the cell by diffusion. This tendency is offset by the sodium–potassium pump, which is located in the cell membrane and actively moves sodium

from the cell into the ECF. Conversely, the high intracellular potassium concentration is maintained by pumping of potassium into the cell. By definition, active transport implies that energy expenditure must take place for the movement to occur against a concentration gradient.

Routes of Gains and Losses

Water and electrolytes are gained in various ways. In health, one gains fluids by drinking and eating. In some types of illness, fluids may be gained by the parenteral route (intravenously or subcutaneously) or by means of an enteral feeding tube in the stomach or intestine. When fluid balance is critical, all routes of gain and all routes of loss must be recorded and the volumes compared. Organs of fluid loss include the kidneys, skin, lungs, and gastrointestinal tract.

Kidneys. The usual urine volume in the adult is between 1 and 2 liters each day. A general rule is that the output is approximately 1 ml of urine per kilogram of body weight per hour (1 ml/kg/hr) in all age-groups.

Skin. Sensible perspiration refers to visible water and electrolyte loss through the skin by way of sweating. The chief solutes in sweat are sodium chloride and potassium. Actual sweat losses can vary from 0 to 1000 ml or more every hour, depending on the environmental temperature. Continuous water loss by evaporation (approximately 600 ml/day) occurs through the skin as insensible perspiration, a nonvisible form of water loss. Fever greatly increases insensible water loss through the lungs and the skin, as does loss of the natural skin barrier through major burns.

Lungs. The lungs normally eliminate water vapor (insensible loss) at a rate of 300 to 400 ml every day. The loss is much greater with increased respiratory rate or depth, or both.

Gastrointestinal Tract. The usual loss through the gastrointestinal tract is only 100 to 200 ml every day even though approximately 8 liters of fluid circulate through the gastrointestinal system every 24 hours (called the "gastrointestinal circulation"). Since the bulk of fluid is reabsorbed in the small intestine, it is obvious that large losses can be incurred from the gastrointestinal tract if diarrhea or fistulas occur.

In healthy persons the 24-hour average intake and output of water are approximately equal (Table 9-4).

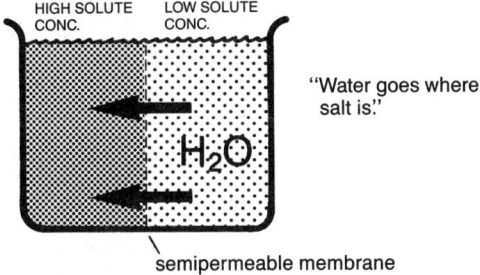

Figure 9-1
Osmosis. ("Water goes where salt is.") (Metheny N. Fluid and Electrolyte Balance: Nursing Considerations. Philadelphia, JB Lippincott, 1987.)

TABLE 9-4

Average Intake and Output in an Adult for a 24-Hour Period

Intake		Output	
Oral liquids	1300 ml	Urine	1500 ml
Water in food	1000 ml	Stool	200 ml
Water produced by			
metabolism	300 ml	*Insensible*	
Total	2600 ml	Lungs	300 ml
		Skin	600 ml
		Total	2600 ml

(Metheny N. Fluid and Electrolyte Balance: Nursing Considerations. Philadelphia, JB Lippincott, 1987.)

Homeostatic Mechanisms

The body is equipped with remarkable homeostatic mechanisms to keep the composition and volume of body fluid within narrow limits of normal. Organs involved in homeostasis include the kidneys, lungs, heart, adrenal glands, parathyroid glands, and pituitary mechanism.

Kidneys. Vital to the regulation of fluid and electrolyte balance, the kidneys normally filter 170 liters of plasma every day in the adult, while excreting only 1.5 liters of urine. They act both autonomously and in response to blood-borne messengers, such as aldosterone and antidiuretic hormone (ADH). Major functions of the kidneys in fluid balance homeostasis include the following:

- Regulation of ECF volume and osmolality by selective retention and excretion of body fluids
- Regulation of electrolyte levels in the ECF by selective retention of needed substances and excretion of unneeded substances
- Regulation of pH of ECF by excretion or retention of hydrogen ions
- Excretion of metabolic wastes and toxic substances

Given the above facts, it is readily apparent that renal failure will result in multiple fluid and electrolyte problems.

Heart and Blood Vessels. The pumping action of the heart circulates blood through the kidneys under sufficient pressure for urine to form. Failure of this pumping action interferes with renal perfusion and thus with water and electrolyte regulation.

Lungs. The lungs are also vital in maintaining homeostasis. The lungs remove approximately 300 ml of water daily through exhalation in the normal adult. Abnormal conditions such as hyperpnea or continuous coughing increase this loss; mechanical ventilation with excessive moisture decreases it. The lungs also have a major role in maintenance of acid–base balance, which is discussed later in this chapter.

Pituitary Gland. The hypothalamus manufactures a substance known as antidiuretic hormone (ADH), which is stored in the posterior pituitary gland and released as needed. Sometimes referred to as the "water conserving hormone," ADH makes the body retain water. Functions of ADH include maintenance of osmotic pressure of the cells by controlling renal water retention or excretion, and control of blood volume (Fig. 9-2).

Adrenal Glands. Aldosterone, a mineralocorticoid secreted by the zona glomerulosa (outer zone) of the adrenal cortex, has a profound effect on fluid balance. Increased secretion of aldosterone causes sodium retention (and thus water retention) and potassium loss. Conversely, a decreased secretion of aldosterone causes sodium and water loss and potassium retention. Cortisol, another adrenocortical hormone, has only a fraction of the mineralocorticoid potency of aldosterone. However, when secreted in large quantities, it can also produce sodium and fluid retention and potassium deficit.

Parathyroid Glands. The parathyroid glands, embedded in the corners of the thyroid gland, regulate calcium and phosphate balance by means of parathyroid hormone (PTH). PTH influences bone resorption, calcium absorption from

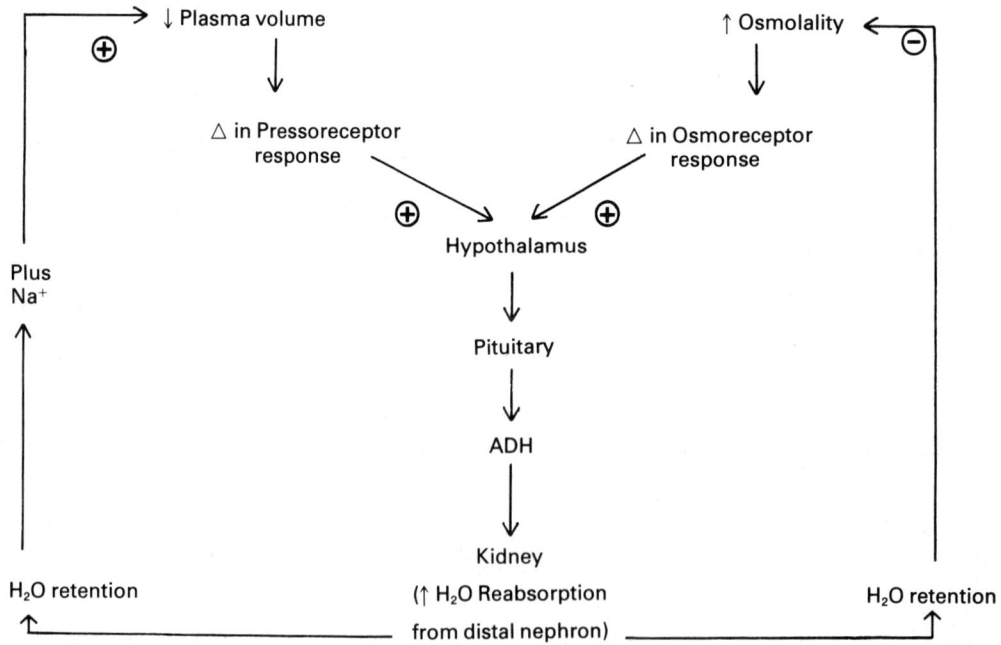

Figure 9-2

ADH-induced water retention. The major stimulus for ADH secretion is increased serum osmolality. A secondary stimulus is a severe decrease in extracellular volume. (Rokosky JS and Shaver J. Fluid and electrolyte balance. In Underhill SL et al. Cardiac Nursing, p 90. Philadelphia, JB Lippincott, 1982.)

the intestines, and calcium reabsorption from the renal tubules.

Fluid Volume Disturbances

Fluid Volume Deficit

Definition and Etiology

Fluid volume deficit (FVD) results when water and electrolytes are lost in the same proportion as they exist in normal body fluids, so that the ratio of serum electrolytes to water remains the same. It should not be confused with the term *dehydration,* which refers to loss of water alone with increased serum sodium levels. FVD may occur alone or in combination with other imbalances. Unless other imbalances are present concurrently, serum electrolyte levels remain essentially unchanged.

FVD results from loss of body fluids and occurs more rapidly when coupled with decreased fluid intake. It is possible to develop FVD on the basis of inadequate intake alone if the decreased intake is prolonged. Causes of FVD include abnormal fluid losses, such as resulting from vomiting, diarrhea, gastrointestinal suction, and sweating, and decreased intake, as in the presence of nausea or inability to gain access to fluids. Third-space fluid shifts or the movement of fluid from the vascular system to other body spaces (*i.e.,* with edema formation in burns or ascites with liver dysfunction) also produces FVD.

Clinical Manifestations

FVD can develop rapidly and can be mild, moderate, or severe, depending on the degree of fluid loss. Important characteristics of FVD include acute weight loss, decreased skin turgor, oliguria, concentrated urine, postural hypotension, and a weak, rapid pulse.

Diagnostic Evaluation

Laboratory data useful in evaluating fluid volume status include the blood urea nitrogen (BUN) level and its relationship with the serum creatinine concentration. A volume-depleted patient has a BUN elevated out of proportion to the serum creatinine level (>10:1). Also, the hematocrit level is greater than normal as the red blood cells become suspended in a decreased plasma volume. Normal values for these tests are listed in Table 9-5.

Management

In planning correction of fluid loss for the patient with FVD, usual maintenance requirements and other factors (such as fever) that can influence fluid needs are considered. When the deficit is not severe, the oral route is preferred, provided the patient is able to drink. However, when fluid losses are acute or severe, the intravenous route is required. Isotonic electrolyte solutions (such as lactated Ringer's or 0.9% sodium chloride) are frequently used to treat the hypotensive patient with FVD since such fluids expand plasma volume. As soon as the patient becomes normotensive, a hypotonic electrolyte solution (such as 0.45% sodium chloride) is often used to provide both electrolytes and free water for renal excretion of metabolic wastes. These, and additional fluids, are summarized in Table 9-8.

If the patient with severe FVD is oliguric, it must be determined whether the depressed renal function is the result of reduced renal blood flow secondary to FVD (prerenal azotemia) or, more seriously, to acute tubular necrosis due to prolonged FVD. The therapeutic test used in this situation is referred to as a fluid challenge test. Prompt treatment of FVD is imperative to prevent renal damage.

▶ Nursing Process
The Patient with Fluid Volume Deficit

▷ Assessment

To assess for the presence of FVD, fluid intake and output are measured and evaluated at least at 8-hour intervals; sometimes, hourly measurements are indicated. As FVD is developing, body fluid losses exceed fluid intake. This loss may be in the form of polyuria, diarrhea, vomiting, and so on. Later, after FVD has fully developed, the kidneys attempt to conserve needed body fluids, leading to a urinary output less than 30 ml/hr in an adult; urine in this instance is concentrated and represents a healthy renal response. Daily body weight measurements are monitored, keeping in mind that an acute weight loss of 0.5 kg (1 pound) represents a fluid loss of approximately 500 ml. (One liter of fluid weighs approximately 1 kg, or 2.2 pounds.)

The vital signs are closely monitored. The nurse should be particularly alert for a weak rapid pulse and postural hypotension (*i.e.,* a drop in the systolic pressure greater than 10 mm Hg when changed from a lying to a sitting position). A decrease in body temperature often accompanies fluid volume deficit, unless there is a concurrent infection.

Skin and tongue turgor are monitored on a regular basis. In a normal person, pinched skin will immediately fall back to its normal position when released. This elastic property, referred to as turgor, is partially dependent on interstitial fluid volume. In a person with FVD, the skin flattens more slowly after the pinch is released; when the FVD is severe, the skin may remain elevated for many seconds. Tissue turgor is best measured by pinching the skin over the sternum, inner aspects of the thighs, or forehead. The skin turgor test is not as valid in elderly people as in younger people since skin elasticity is affected by age. Evaluation of tongue turgor, which is not affected by age may be more valid than evaluation of skin turgor. In a normal person, the tongue has one longitudinal furrow. In the person with FVD there are additional longitudinal furrows and the tongue is smaller, owing to fluid loss. The degree of oral mucous membrane moisture is also assessed; a dry mouth may indicate either FVD or mouth breathing.

Urinary concentration is monitored; when available, a urinometer should be used to measure urinary specific gravity

TABLE 9-5
Laboratory Tests Used to Evaluate Fluid, Electrolyte, and Acid–Base Status

Test	Usual Reference Range	SI Units
Serum sodium	135–145 mEq/liter	135–145 mmol/L
Serum potassium	3.5–5.5 mEq/liter	3.5–5.5 mmol/L
Serum calcium	8.5–10.5 mg/dl (approximately 50% in ionized form)	2.1–2.6 mmol/L
Serum magnesium	1.5–2.5 mEq/liter	0.80–1.2 mmol/L
Serum phosphorus	2.5–4.5 mEq/liter	0.80–1.5 mmol/L
Serum chloride	100–106 mEq/liter	100–106 mmol/L
Carbon dioxide content	24–30 mEq/liter	24–30 mmol/L
Serum osmolality	280–295 mOsm/kg	280–295 nmol/L
Blood urea nitrogen (BUN)	10–20 mg/dl	3.5–7 mmol/L of urea
Serum creatinine	0.7–1.5 mg/dl	60–130 μmol/L
BUN: Creatinine ratio	10:1	
Hematocrit	Male: 44–52%	Volume fraction: 0.44–0.52
	Female: 39–47%	Volume fraction: 0.39–0.47
Serum glucose	70–110 mg/dl	3.9–6.1 mmol/L
Serum albumin	3.5–5.5 gm/dl	3.5–5.5 g/L
Arterial blood gases		
pH	7.35–7.45	7.35–7.45
$PaCO_2$	38–42 mm Hg	38–42 mm Hg
HCO_3^-	22–26 mEq/liter	22–26 mmol/L
Urinary sodium	80–180 mEq/day	80–180 mmol/d
Urinary potassium	40–80 mEq/day	40–80 mmol/d
Urinary chloride	110–250 mEq/day	110–250 mmol/d
Urinary specific gravity	1.003–1.035	1.003–1.035
Urine osmolality		
Extreme range:	50–1400 mOsm/liter	50–1400 mmol/kg
Typical urine:	500–800 mOsm/liter	500–800 mmol/kg
Urinary pH	4.5–8.0	4.5–8.0
Typical urine:	<6.6	<6.6

(SG). In a volume-depleted patient, the urinary SG should be above 1.020 (indicating healthy renal conservation of fluid).

Severe volume depletion eventually affects the sensorium by decreasing cerebral perfusion. Decreased peripheral perfusion can result in cold extremities. In patients with relatively normal cardiopulmonary function, a low central venous pressure is indicative of hypovolemia. Patients with acute cardiopulmonary decompensation require more extensive hemodynamic monitoring with a device that measures pressures in both sides of the heart.

▷ Nursing Diagnosis

The nursing assessment and identification of patients at risk for this disturbance lead to a nursing diagnosis of fluid volume deficit. For example, in a patient with volume depletion secondary to uncontrolled diabetes mellitus, the diagnosis may be stated as fluid volume deficit related to osmotic diuresis.

▷ Planning and Implementation

▷ Goals: A major goal is, of course, prevention of this common disturbance. Once the imbalance has developed,

the goal is to correct the abnormal fluid volume status before renal damage results. More precise nursing goals vary with the cause of FVD and individual patient characteristics.

Nursing Interventions

Prevention of FVD. In order to prevent FVD, one must be aware of patients at risk and take measures to minimize fluid losses. For example, if the patient has diarrhea, measures should be implemented to control the diarrhea while replacing fluids. These may include the administration of antidiarrheal medications and small volumes of oral fluids at frequent intervals.

Correction of FVD. When possible, oral fluids are given to help correct FVD, keeping in mind the patient's likes and dislikes. Also, the type of fluid the patient has lost is considered and attempts are made to select fluids most likely to replace the lost electrolytes. If the patient is reluctant to drink because of oral discomfort, frequent mouth care is given and fluids that are nonirritating to the mucosa are provided. It is often helpful to offer small volumes of fluids at frequent intervals rather than a large volume all at once. If nausea is present, antiemetics may be needed before oral fluid replacement can be tolerated.

If the patient is unable to eat and drink, the physician may consider an alternative route (enteral or parenteral) for fluid intake. This intervention is important to prevent renal damage related to prolonged FVD.

▷ *Evaluation*

▷ *Expected Outcomes*

1. Patient exhibits normal turgor of skin and tongue
2. Excretes increased amount of urine with normal specific gravity
3. Exhibits return of pulse and blood pressure to normal
4. Exhibits clear sensorium; is oriented to time, person, and place
5. Drinks fluids as prescribed
6. Exhibits absence of precipitating risk factors (*e.g.*, excessive fluid loss, decreased fluid intake)

Fluid Volume Excess

Definition and Etiology

Fluid volume excess (FVE) refers to an isotonic expansion of the ECF caused by the abnormal retention of water and sodium in approximately the same proportions in which they normally exist in the ECF. It is always secondary to an increase in the total body sodium content, which, in turn, leads to an increase in total body water. Because there is isotonic retention of body substances, the serum sodium concentration remains essentially normal.

FVE may be caused by simple fluid overloading or by diminished function of the homeostatic mechanisms responsible for regulating fluid balance. Etiologic factors can include congestive heart failure, renal failure, and cirrhosis of the liver. Overzealous administration of sodium-containing fluids to persons with impaired regulatory mechanisms particularly predisposes to serious fluid volume excess. Excessive ingestion of table salt (sodium chloride) or other sodium salts also predisposes to fluid overload.

Clinical Manifestations

The clinical manifestations of FVE stem from expansion of the ECF compartment and include edema, distended veins, increased venous pressure, bounding pulse, and crackles.

Diagnostic Evaluation

Laboratory data useful in the diagnosis of FVE include the BUN and hematocrit levels. In the presence of FVE, both of these values may be decreased owing to plasma dilution. Other causes for abnormalities in these values include low protein intake and anemia.

Management

Management of FVE is directed at the causative factors. Symptomatic treatment consists of administration of diuretics, restriction of fluids, or both. When the fluid excess is related to excessive administration of sodium-containing fluids, discontinuing the infusion may be all that is needed. Since treatment almost always involves sodium restriction in the diet, concepts related to sodium-restricted diets are discussed below.

Sodium-Restricted Diets. An average daily diet not restricted in sodium contains 6 to 15 gm of salt, whereas low-sodium diets can range from a mild restriction to as low as 250 mg of sodium per day, depending on the patient's needs. A mild sodium-restricted diet allows only light salting of food (about half the amount as usual) in cooking and at the table, and no addition of salt to commercially prepared foods that are already seasoned. Of course, foods high in sodium must be avoided. Since about half of ingested sodium is in the form of seasoning, use of substitute seasonings plays a major role in decreasing sodium intake. Lemon juice, onion, and garlic are excellent substitute flavoring agents; however, some patients prefer salt substitutes. Most salt substitutes contain potassium and should be used cautiously by those patients taking potassium-sparing diuretics (*e.g.*, spironolactone, triamterene and amiloride). They should not be used at all in patients with conditions associated with potassium retention, such as advanced renal disease. Salt substitutes containing ammonium chloride can be harmful to patients with liver damage.

In certain communities, the drinking water may contain too much sodium for a sodium-restricted diet. Depending on its source, water may contain as little as 1 mg or more than 1500 mg per quart. It may be necessary for patients to use distilled water when the local water supply is very high in sodium. Also, patients on sodium-restricted diets should be cautioned to avoid "water softeners" that add sodium to water in exchange for other ions, such as calcium.

▶ *Nursing Process*
The Patient with Fluid Volume Excess

▷ *Assessment*

To assess for FVE, the fluid intake and output are measured at regular intervals for indication of excessive fluid retention. The patient is weighed daily, and acute weight gain is noted. (Remember that an acute weight gain of 0.9 kg (2 pounds) represents a gain of approximately 1 liter of fluid.)

It is important to assess breath sounds at regular intervals in at-risk patients, particularly when parenteral fluids are being administered. The nurse monitors the degree of edema in the most dependent parts of the body, such as the feet and ankles in ambulatory patients and the sacral region in bedridden patients. The degree of pitting edema is assessed and the extent of peripheral edema is measured with a tape marked in millimeters.

▷ *Nursing Diagnosis*

Based on the nursing assessment and identification of the patient at risk for this disturbance, the nursing diagnosis is fluid volume excess. For example, in a patient with congestive heart failure, the nursing diagnosis might be stated as follows:

fluid volume excess related to compromised regulatory mechanism (cardiac failure).

▷ *Planning and Implementation*

▷ *Goals:* A major goal is the prevention of FVE in patients at risk. If prevention is not possible, the presence of FVE must be detected early so that therapeutic interventions can be implemented before the condition becomes severe. Specific goals vary with individual patients and their clinical conditions.

Nursing Interventions

Prevention of FVE. Specific interventions vary somewhat with the underlying pathologic condition and the degree of FVE. However, most patients require sodium-restricted diets in some form. Therefore, adherence to the prescribed diet is encouraged. The patient is instructed to avoid "over-the-counter" drugs without first checking with the health care provider since these substances may contain sodium. When fluid retention persists despite adherence to a prescribed diet, one should consider hidden sources of sodium, such as the water supply or use of water softeners.

Detection and Control of FVE. Detection of FVE is of primary importance before the condition becomes critical. Interventions include providing rest, sodium restriction, close monitoring of parenteral fluid therapy, and administration of appropriate medications. Some patients benefit from regular rest periods since bed rest favors diuresis of edema fluid. Sodium and fluid restriction should be instituted as indicated. Since most patients with FVE require diuretics, the patient's response to these drugs is monitored. The rate of parenteral fluids and the patient's response to the fluids are also closely monitored. If dyspnea or orthopnea is present, the patient is placed in semi-Fowler's position to favor lung expansion. The patient is turned and positioned at regular intervals since edematous tissue is more prone to skin breakdown than normal tissue.

Since conditions predisposing to FVE are likely to be chronic, the patient is taught how to monitor his own response to therapy by recording and evaluating fluid intake and output and body weight changes. The importance of adherence to the medical regimen is emphasized.

▷ *Evaluation*

▷ *Expected Outcomes*

1. Patient exhibits absence of edema and normal skin turgor
2. Excretes increased amount of urine
3. Demonstrates return of body weight to normal
4. Demonstrates no distention of jugular veins
5. Adheres to diet with prescribed sodium intake
6. States rationale for dietary prescription
7. Exhibits normal breath sounds without adventitious sounds (crackles, rhonchi, wheezes)
8. Maintains bed rest when prescribed
9. Exhibits absence of precipitating risk factors (*e.g.,* fluid overload, high sodium intake)

Gerontological Considerations

The percentage of elderly persons is increasing in our society. The aged have special nursing care needs because of their propensity for developing fluid and electrolyte problems. Fluid balance in the elderly is often marginal at best because of certain physiologic changes associated with the aging process. Some of these changes include reduction in total body water (associated with increased body fat content and decreased muscle mass), reduction in renal function resulting in decreased ability to concentrate urine, decreased cardiovascular and respiratory function, and disturbances in hormonal regulatory functions. Although these changes are viewed as normal in the aging process, they must be considered when the elderly person becomes ill since they predispose to fluid and electrolyte imbalances.

Assessment of the elderly client should be modified somewhat from that of younger adults. For example, skin turgor is less valid as an assessment tool in the elderly since their skin has lost some of its elasticity; therefore, other assessment measures, such as slowness in filling of veins of the hands and feet, become more important in detecting fluid volume deficit. When skin turgor is tested in the elderly, it is best tested over the forehead or the sternum since alterations in skin elasticity are less marked in these areas. As in any patient, skin turgor should be monitored serially to detect subtle changes.

The nurse should perform a functional assessment of the aged person's ability to determine his need for and to obtain adequate food and fluid intake. For example, is the client mentally clear? Is he able to ambulate and use his arms and hands to reach fluids and foods? Is he able to swallow? All of these questions have direct bearing on how the client will be able to manage his own need for fluids and foods. The nurse must, of course, provide for the patient when he is unable to provide for himself.

Sodium Imbalances

Disturbances in sodium balance occur frequently in clinical practice and can develop under simple and complex circumstances. Prior to discussion of disruptions in sodium balance, important facts about the role of sodium in physiologic activities are reviewed.

Functions of Sodium

Sodium is the most abundant electrolyte in the ECF; its concentration ranges from 135 to 145 mEq/liter (SI: 135–145 mmol/L). Because of this, it is the primary determinant of ECF concentration. The fact that sodium does not easily cross the cell-wall membrane, plus its dominance in quantity, accounts for its primary role in controlling water distribution throughout the body. In addition, sodium is the primary regulator of ECF volume. A loss or gain of sodium is usually accompanied by a loss or gain of water. Sodium also functions in the establishment of the electrochemical state necessary for muscle contraction and the transmission of nerve impulses.

Sodium Deficit (Hyponatremia)

Definition and Etiology

Hyponatremia refers to a serum sodium level that is below normal (less than 135 mEq/liter) (SI: 135 mmol/L). It may be due to an excessive loss of sodium or an excessive gain of water; in either event, it results in a relatively greater concentration of water than of sodium. This imbalance should not be confused with FVD, which refers to an isotonic or equivalent loss of sodium and water, resulting in an essentially normal serum sodium level. A hyponatremic state can, however, be superimposed on an existing FVD or FVE.

Sodium may be lost by way of vomiting, diarrhea, fistulas, or sweating, or it may be associated with diuretics, particularly in combination with a low-salt diet. A deficiency of aldosterone, as occurs in adrenal insufficiency, also predisposes the patient to sodium deficiency.

Water may be gained abnormally by the excessive parenteral administration of dextrose and water solutions, particularly during periods of stress. It may also be gained by compulsive water drinking (psychogenic polydipsia).

A special type of hyponatremia associated with excessive antidiuretic hormone (ADH) activity is referred to as the syndrome of inappropriate ADH secretion (SIADH). The basic physiologic disturbances in SIADH are excessive ADH activity, with water retention and dilutional hyponatremia, and inappropriate urinary excretion of sodium in the presence of hyponatremia. SIADH can be the result of either sustained secretion of ADH by the hypothalamus or production of an ADH-like substance from a tumor (aberrant ADH production). Conditions associated with SIADH include oat-cell lung tumors, head injuries, endocrine and pulmonary disorders, and use of drugs such as pitocin, cyclophosphamide, vincristine, thioridazine, and amitriptyline.

Clinical Manifestations

Clinical manifestations of hyponatremia depend on the cause, magnitude, and rapidity of onset. Although nausea and abdominal cramping occur, most of the symptoms are neuropsychiatric and are probably related to the cellular swelling and cerebral edema associated with hyponatremia. As the extracellular sodium level decreases, the cellular fluid becomes relatively more concentrated and "pulls" water into the cells (Fig. 9-3). In general, those patients having acute decline in serum sodium levels have more severe symptoms and higher mortality rates than do those with more slowly developing hyponatremia.

Features of hyponatremia associated with sodium loss and water gain include anorexia, muscle cramps, and a feeling of exhaustion. When the serum sodium level drops below 115 mEq/liter (SI: 115 mmol/L), signs of increasing intracranial pressure, such as lethargy, confusion, muscular twitching, focal weakness, hemiparesis, papilledema, and convulsions, may occur.

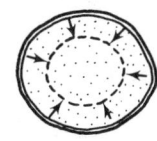

Explains why hyponatremic patients may develop brain swelling

Explains why hypernatremic patients may develop brain contraction

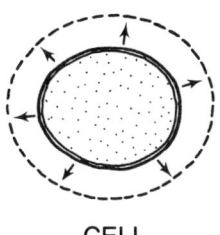

CELL

Hyponatremia:
Na less than 130 mEq/liter

CELL

Hypernatremia:
Na greater than 150 mEq/liter

Figure 9-3
Effect of extracellular sodium levels on cell size. (Metheny N. Fluid and Electrolyte Balance: Nursing Considerations. Philadelphia, JB Lippincott, 1987.)

Diagnostic Evaluation

Regardless of the cause of hyponatremia, the serum sodium level is less than 135 mEq/liter; it may be quite low, such as 100 mEq/liter (SI: 100 mmol/L) or less, in SIADH. When hyponatremia is due primarily to sodium loss, the urinary sodium content is less than 10 mEq/liter (SI: 10 mmol/L) and the specific gravity is low, such as 1.002 to 1.004. However, when hyponatremia is due to SIADH, the urinary sodium content is greater than 20 mEq/liter and the urinary specific gravity is usually greater than 1.012. Although the patient with SIADH gains water abnormally and thus gains body weight, there is no peripheral edema; instead, the edema is inside the cells. This phenomenon is sometimes manifested as "fingerprinting" when the finger is pressed over a bony prominence, such as the sternum.

Management

The obvious treatment for hyponatremia is careful administration of sodium. This may be accomplished orally, by nasogastric tube, or parenterally. For patients who are able to eat and drink, sodium replacement is easily accomplished since sodium is plentiful in a normal diet. For those unable to take sodium orally, lactated Ringer's solution or isotonic saline (0.9% sodium chloride) may be prescribed. See Table 9-8 in the section Parenteral Fluid Therapy at the end of this chapter. The usual daily sodium requirement in adults is approximately 100 mEq, provided there are no abnormal losses.

When hyponatremia is present in a patient with normovolemia or hypervolemia, the treatment of choice is water restriction. This is far safer than sodium administration and is usually quite effective. However, when neurologic symptoms are present, it may be necessary to administer small volumes of a hypertonic sodium solution, such as 3% or 5% sodium chloride. Incorrect use of these fluids is extremely dangerous; this is understandable when one considers that a liter of 3% sodium chloride solution contains 513 mEq of sodium and a liter of 5% sodium chloride solution contains 855 mEq of sodium. Grossly hypertonic sodium solutions (3% and 5% sodium chloride) should be administered only in intensive care settings under close observation since only small volumes are needed to elevate the serum sodium level from a dangerously low value. These fluids are administered slowly, in small volumes, while the patient is monitored closely for fluid overload.

▶ Nursing Process
The Patient with Sodium Deficit

▷ Assessment

It is important to identify patients at risk for hyponatremia so that they can be monitored. Early detection and treatment of this disorder are necessary to prevent serious consequences. For patients at risk, the nurse monitors fluid intake and output as well as daily body weight. Abnormal losses of sodium and/or gains of water are noted. Gastrointestinal manifestations, such as anorexia, nausea, vomiting, and abdominal cramping, are also noted. One is particularly alert for central nervous system changes, such as lethargy, confusion, muscular twitching, and convulsions. In general, more severe neurologic signs are associated with very low sodium levels that have fallen rapidly owing to water overloading. It is most important to monitor serum sodium levels closely in patients at risk for hyponatremia. When indicated, urinary sodium levels and specific gravity are also monitored.

▷ Nursing Diagnosis

The nursing assessment data and the presence of clinical manifestations associated with hyponatremia in a patient at risk lead to the appropriate nursing diagnosis. For example, in a patient with diarrhea who drinks large amounts of tap water to relieve thirst, the diagnosis might be stated as follows: alteration in sodium balance (hyponatremia) related to excessive sodium loss and water gain. Once the etiologic factors have been identified, therapeutic measures are taken to deal with the disturbance. Some of the nursing interventions for this imbalance are independent (such as increasing dietary sodium or limiting free water intake, as tolerated). Often, however, the nursing interventions are meshed with those of other disciplines, such as the safe parenteral administration of fluids containing sodium.

▷ Planning and Implementation

▷ *Goals:* A major goal is the early detection of hyponatremia so that interventions can be implemented before the condition becomes severe. Once hyponatremia has developed, the goal is a safe return of the serum sodium level to normal. How quickly this can be accomplished depends on a number of variables, such as the cause and severity of the imbalance.

Nursing Interventions

Early Detection and Control of Hyponatremia. One should be aware of patients at risk for hyponatremia and initiate measures to detect the disturbance before it becomes severe. For patients suffering abnormal losses of sodium, yet able to consume a general diet, foods and fluids with a high sodium content are encouraged and provided. For example, broth made with one beef cube contains approximately 900 mg of sodium, and 8 ounces of tomato juice contains approximately 700 mg of sodium.

It is important to be familiar with the sodium content of parenteral fluids. See Table 9-8 under Parenteral Fluid Therapy at the end of this chapter. When administering fluids to patients with cardiovascular disease, one should monitor the patient for signs of circulatory overload, such as crackles with auscultation of the lungs. As was stated earlier, extreme care is essential when administering grossly hypertonic sodium fluids (such as 3% or 5% sodium chloride), since these fluids can be lethal if they are infused carelessly.

For patients taking lithium, one should be alert for lithium toxicity when sodium is lost by an abnormal route. In such instances, supplemental salt and fluid are administered. Because diuretics promote sodium loss, patients taking lithium are instructed not to use diuretics unless under close medical supervision. For all patients on lithium therapy, an adequate salt intake should be ensured.

Excess water supplements are avoided in patients receiving isotonic or hypotonic tube feedings, particularly if routes of abnormal sodium loss are present or water is being abnormally retained (as in SIADH). Actual fluid needs are determined by evaluating the intake and output, urinary specific gravity, and serum sodium levels.

Safe Return of Serum Sodium Level to Normal. When the primary problem is water retention, it is safer to restrict fluid intake than to administer sodium. Administration of sodium to a patient with normovolemia or hypervolemia predisposes to fluid volume overload. As was stated previously, patients with cardiovascular disease receiving fluids containing sodium should be monitored very closely for signs of circulatory overload, such as crackles. In severe hyponatremia, the aim of therapy is to elevate the serum sodium level only enough to alleviate neurologic signs. For example, it has been recommended that the serum sodium concentration be raised to a level no higher than 125 mEq/liter (SI: 125 mmol/L) with hypertonic saline.

▷ Evaluation

▷ *Expected Outcomes*

1. Patient is oriented to time, place, and person
2. Reports decreased muscle cramping and muscle twitching
3. Exhibits normal strength of upper and lower extremities
4. Reports decreased level of fatigue, exhaustion, and lethargy
5. Achieves normal body weight
6. Excretes normal urine volume with normal concentration and specific gravity
7. Demonstrates no seizure activity
8. Consumes food and fluids within prescribed fluid and sodium intake
9. Exhibits absence of precipitating risk factors (*e.g.,* gastrointestinal loss of sodium, diuretic therapy, excessive intake of electrolyte-free fluid)

Sodium Excess (Hypernatremia)

Definition and Etiology

Hypernatremia refers to a greater than normal serum sodium level, that is, a serum level greater than 145 mEq/liter (SI: 145 mmol/L). It can be caused by a gain of sodium in excess of water or by a loss of water in excess of sodium. It can occur in patients with normal fluid volume or in those with FVD or FVE.

A common cause of hypernatremia is deprivation of water in unconscious patients, who are unable to perceive or respond to thirst. Most often affected are very old, very young, and cognitively impaired patients who are unable to communicate their thirst. Administration of hypertonic tube feedings without adequate water supplements leads to hypernatremia, as does watery diarrhea and greatly increased insensible water loss (as in hyperventilation or denuding effects of burns). Diabetes insipidus leads to hypernatremia if the patient does not experience, or cannot respond to, thirst or if fluids are excessively restricted. Less common are heat-stroke, drowning in sea water (which contains a sodium concentration of approximately 500 mEq/liter), accidental introduction of hypertonic saline into the maternal circulation during therapeutic abortion, and malfunction of either hemodialysis or peritoneal dialysis proportioning systems.

Clinical Manifestations

The clinical manifestations of hypernatremia are primarily neurologic and are presumably the consequence of cellular dehydration. Hypernatremia results in a relatively concentrated ECF, causing water to be pulled from the cells (see Fig. 9-3). Clinically, these changes may be manifested by restlessness and weakness in moderate hypernatremia and by disorientation, delusions, and hallucinations in severe hypernatremia. If hypernatremia is severe, permanent brain damage can occur (especially in children). Brain damage is apparently due to subarachnoid hemorrhages that result from brain contraction.

A primary characteristic of hypernatremia is thirst. Thirst is so strong a defender of serum sodium levels in normal people that hypernatremia never occurs unless the person is unconscious or is denied access to water; unfortunately, ill people may have an impaired thirst mechanism. Other signs include dry, swollen tongue and sticky mucous membranes. A mild elevation in body temperature may occur, but on correction of the hypernatremia the body temperature should return to normal.

Diagnostic Evaluation

In hypernatremia the serum sodium level is greater than 145 mEq/liter (SI: 145 mmol/L) and the serum osmolality is greater than 295 mOsm/kg (SI: 295 mmol/L). The urinary specific gravity is greater than 1.015 as the kidneys attempt to conserve water (provided the water loss is from a route other than the kidneys).

Management

Treatment of hypernatremia consists of a *gradual* lowering of the serum sodium level by the infusion of a hypotonic electrolyte solution (such as 0.3% sodium chloride). A hypotonic sodium solution is considered safer than 5% dextrose in water by many clinicians because it allows a gradual reduction in the serum sodium level and thus decreases the risk of cerebral edema. A rapid reduction in the serum sodium level temporarily decreases the plasma osmolality below that of the fluid in the brain tissue, causing dangerous cerebral edema.

The exact rate at which serum sodium levels should be reduced is not agreed on. As a general rule, the serum sodium level is reduced at a rate no faster than 2 mEq/liter/hr in order to allow sufficient time for readjustment through diffusion across fluid compartments.

▶ Nursing Process
The Patient with Sodium Excess

▷ Assessment

Fluid losses and gains are carefully monitored in patients at risk for hypernatremia. One should look for abnormal losses of water or low water intake and for large gains of sodium, as might occur with ingestion of proprietary drugs with a high sodium content (such as Alka-Seltzer). Also, it is important to obtain a drug history since some prescription drugs may have a high sodium content.

The presence of thirst or an elevated body temperature is noted and evaluated in relation to other clinical signs. The patient is monitored for changes in behavior, such as restlessness, disorientation, and lethargy.

▷ Nursing Diagnosis

The nursing assessment and identification of the presence of clinical manifestations associated with hypernatremia in patients at risk for this disorder should lead to the appropriate nursing diagnosis. For example, in an elderly patient receiving a hyperosmolar tube feeding solution with no additional water, the nursing diagnosis might be alteration in sodium balance (hypernatremia) related to hypertonic tube feeding and inadequate water supplementation.

▷ Planning and Implementation

▷ *Goals:* A major goal is to prevent hypernatremia in patients at risk. Once hypernatremia has developed, the primary goal is to return the serum sodium level to normal gradually, thus avoiding further cerebral changes.

Nursing Interventions

Prevention of Hypernatremia. The nurse attempts to prevent hypernatremia by offering fluids at regular intervals, particularly in debilitated patients unable to perceive or respond to thirst. If fluid intake remains inadequate, the nurse consults with the physician to plan an alternate route for intake, either by tube feedings or by the parenteral route. If tube feedings are used, sufficient water should be given to keep the serum sodium and blood urea nitrogen levels within normal limits. As a general rule, the higher the osmolality of the tube feeding, the greater is the need for water supplementation.

For patients with diabetes insipidus, it is important to ensure adequate water intake. If the patient is alert and has an intact thirst mechanism, merely providing access to water may be sufficient. However, if the patient has a decreased level of consciousness, or other disability interfering with adequate fluid intake, parenteral fluid replacement may be prescribed. This therapy in patients with neurologic disorders, particularly in the early postoperative period, can be anticipated.

Safe Correction of Hypernatremia. When hypernatremia is present and parenteral fluids are necessary for its management, the nurse monitors the patient's response to the fluids by reviewing serial serum sodium levels and by observing for changes in neurologic signs. With a gradual decrease in the serum sodium level, the neurologic signs should improve. As stated in the section on management, too rapid reduction in the serum sodium level renders the plasma temporarily hypo-osmotic to the fluid in the brain tissue, causing dangerous cerebral edema.

▷ *Evaluation*

▷ *Expected Outcomes*

1. Patient is oriented to time, place, and person
2. Exhibits absence of delusions, hallucinations, and restlessness
3. Reports normal thirst
4. Exhibits moist skin and mucous membranes
5. Demonstrates normal body temperature
6. Excretes normal urinary volume with normal specific gravity
7. Consumes adequate fluid and adheres to low-sodium diet
8. States rationale for adequate fluid intake and sodium restriction
9. Reports decreased lethargy
10. Exhibits normal serum and urinary sodium levels
11. Exhibits absence of precipitating risk factors (*e.g.*, excessive fluid restriction, ingestion of hypertonic tube feedings, excess fluid loss from diabetes insipidus)

Potassium Imbalances

Disturbances in potassium balance are common since they are associated with a number of disease and injury states. Unfortunately, they may also be induced by medications such as diuretics, laxatives, and certain antibiotics, as well as by therapies such as hyperalimentation and chemotherapy. It is helpful to review some pertinent facts about potassium before proceeding to a discussion of hypokalemia and hyperkalemia.

Functions of Potassium

Potassium is the major intracellular electrolyte; in fact, 98% of the body's potassium is inside the cells. The remaining 2% is in the ECF; it is this 2% that is all important in neuromuscular function. Potassium influences both skeletal and cardiac muscle activity. For example, alterations in its concentration change myocardial irritability and rhythm. Potassium is constantly moving in and out of cells according to the body's needs, under the influence of the sodium–potassium pump. The normal serum potassium concentration ranges from 3.5 to 5.5 mEq/liter (SI: 3.5 to 5.5 mmol/L), and even minor variations are significant. Normal renal function is necessary for maintenance of potassium balance since 80% of the potassium is excreted daily from the body by way of the kidneys. The other 20% is lost through the bowel and sweat glands.

Potassium Deficit (Hypokalemia)

Definition and Etiology

Hypokalemia refers to a below normal serum potassium concentration. It usually indicates a real deficit in total potassium stores; however, it may occur in patients with normal potassium stores when alkalosis is present since alkalosis causes a temporary shift of serum potassium into the cells. (See pp. 122, 123 for a discussion of alkalosis.)

As stated earlier, hypokalemia is a common imbalance. Gastrointestinal loss of potassium is probably the most common cause of potassium depletion. Vomiting and gastric suction frequently lead to hypokalemia, partly because of actual potassium loss in gastric fluid but largely because of increased renal potassium loss associated with metabolic alkalosis. Relatively large amounts of potassium are contained in intestinal fluids; for example, diarrheal fluid may contain as much as 30 mEq/liter. Therefore, potassium deficit occurs frequently with diarrhea, prolonged intestinal suction, recent ileostomy, and villous adenoma (a tumor of the intestinal tract characterized by excretion of potassium-rich mucus).

Alterations in acid–base balance have a significant effect on potassium distribution. The mechanism involves shifts of hydrogen ions and potassium ions between the cells and ECF. Hypokalemia can cause alkalosis, and alkalosis can cause hypokalemia. For example, hydrogen ions move out of the cells in alkalotic states to help correct the high *p*H, and potassium ions move in to maintain electroneutrality. (See pp. 120, 123 for a discussion of acid–base balance).

Hyperaldosteronism increases renal potassium wasting and can lead to severe potassium depletion. Primary hyperaldosteronism is seen in patients with adrenal adenomas. Secondary hyperaldosteronism occurs in patients with cirrhosis, nephrotic syndrome, congestive heart failure, and malignant hypertension. Potassium-losing diuretics, such as furosemide, the thiazides, and ethacrynic acid, can certainly induce hypokalemia, particularly when given in large doses to patients with poor potassium intake. Other medications that can lead to hypokalemia include steroids, sodium penicillin, carbenicillin, and amphotericin B.

Entry of potassium into skeletal muscle and hepatic cells

is promoted by insulin. Thus, patients with persistent insulin hypersecretion may experience hypokalemia; this is often seen in patients receiving high-carbohydrate parenteral fluids (as in hyperalimentation).

Patients unable or unwilling to eat a normal diet for a prolonged period are candidates for hypokalemia. This may occur in debilitated elderly people, alcoholics, and patients with anorexia nervosa. In addition to poor intake, people with bulimia frequently suffer increased potassium loss through self-induced vomiting and laxative and diuretic abuse.

Clinical Manifestations

Potassium deficiency can result in widespread derangements in physiologic function. Most important, severe hypokalemia can result in death through cardiac or respiratory arrest. Clinical signs rarely develop before the serum potassium level has fallen below 3 mEq/liter (SI: 3 mmol/L) unless the rate of fall has been rapid. Manifestations of hypokalemia include fatigue, anorexia, nausea, vomiting, muscle weakness, decreased bowel motility, paresthesias, dysrhythmias, and increased sensitivity to digitalis. If prolonged, hypokalemia can lead to impaired renal concentrating ability, causing dilute urine, polyuria, nocturia, and polydipsia.

Diagnostic Evaluation

In hypokalemia the serum potassium concentration is less than the lower limit of normal. Electrocardiographic changes can include flat T waves and ST segment depression (Fig. 9-4). Hypokalemia increases sensitivity to digitalis, predisposing to digitalis toxicity at lower digitalis levels. Metabolic alkalosis is frequently associated with hypokalemia. This is discussed further in the section on acid–base disturbances.

Management

The best treatment of hypokalemia is prevention. Potassium loss must be corrected daily; administration of 40 to 60 mEq/day of potassium is adequate in the adult if there are no abnormal losses of potassium. For patients at risk, a diet containing sufficient potassium should be provided; dietary intake of potassium in the average adult is 50 to 100 mEq/day. Foods high in potassium include raisins, bananas, apricots, oranges, avocados, beans, and potatoes. When dietary intake is inadequate for any reason, the physician may prescribe potassium supplements. Many salt substitutes contain 50 to 60 mEq

of potassium per teaspoon and may be all the patient needs to supplement potassium intake.

When oral administration of potassium is not feasible, the intravenous route is indicated. In fact, the intravenous route is mandatory for patients with severe hypokalemia (such as a serum level of 2 mEq/liter). Although potassium chloride is usually used to correct potassium deficits, the physician may prescribe potassium acetate or potassium phosphate.

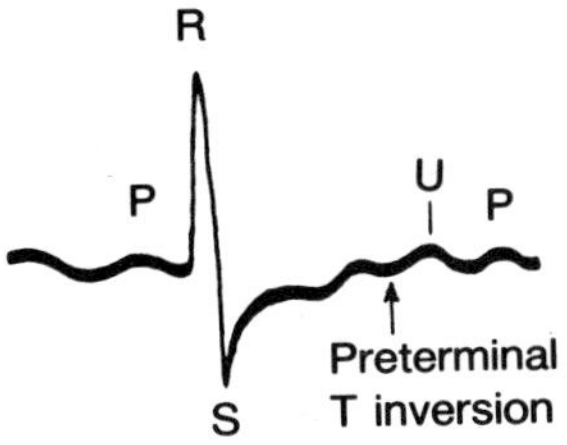

▶ Nursing Process
The Patient with Potassium Deficit

▷ Assessment

Since hypokalemia can be life threatening, it is important to monitor for its early presence in patients at risk. The presence of fatigue, anorexia, muscle weakness, decreased bowel motility, paresthesias, or dysrhythmias should prompt one to examine the serum potassium concentration. When available, electrocardiograms may provide useful information. Patients receiving digitalis are at risk for potassium deficiency and should be monitored closely for signs of digitalis toxicity since hypokalemia potentiates the action of digitalis. In fact, physicians usually prefer to keep the serum potassium level greater than 3.5 mEq/liter (SI: 3.5 mmol/L) in digitalized patients.

▷ Nursing Diagnosis

The nursing assessment data and identification of patients at risk for this disturbance lead to the appropriate nursing diagnosis. For example, in a patient with diarrhea, the diagnosis might be stated as follows: alteration in potassium imbalance (hypokalemia) related to excessive potassium loss in diarrheal fluid. Once the etiologic factors have been identified, therapeutic measures are taken to deal with the imbalance.

▷   *Goals:* A major goal is, of course, the prevention of hypokalemia. Once it has developed, the goal of nursing management is to help correct the condition safely before serious derangements in cardiac or respiratory function occur.

Nursing Interventions

Prevention of Hypokalemia. Measures are taken to prevent hypokalemia when possible. Prevention may take the form of encouraging extra potassium intake for the patient at risk (when the diet allows). See Table 9-6 for a list of high-potassium foods. When hypokalemia is due to abuse of laxatives or diuretics, patient education may help alleviate the problem. Part of the nursing history and assessment should be directed at identifying problems amenable to prevention through education.

Safe Correction of Hypokalemia. Great care should be exercised when administering potassium intravenously. Concentrated potassium solutions are *never* administered without first diluting them as directed by the manufacturer. The usual concentration is 40 mEq/liter of infusion solution, with 80 mEq/liter as the maximum desired concentration. In general, concentrations greater than 60 mEq/liter are not

Figure 9-4
Electrocardiogram in hypokalemia. Note increased height of U wave.

TABLE 9-6
Some High-Potassium Foods

Food	Potassium (mEq, approximate)
Apricots, raw, 3 medium	8.0
Bananas, raw, 1 medium	11.6
Orange, navel, raw, 1 medium	6.4
Beans, white, cooked,	10.7
Potato, baked, 1 medium	12.9

(Adapted from Pennington J and Church H. Bowes and Church's Food Values of Portions Commonly Used, 14th ed. Philadelphia, JB Lippincott, 1985.)

given in peripheral veins since venous pain and sclerosis may occur. For routine maintenance needs, potassium is administered at a rate no faster than 10 mEq/hr, suitably diluted.

In critical situations, more concentrated solutions (such as 20 mEq/dl) may be administered through a central line. Even in extreme hypokalemia, it is recommended that potassium be administered no faster than 20 to 40 mEq/hr (suitably diluted); in such a situation, the patient should be monitored by electrocardiogram (ECG) and observed closely for other signs, such as changes in muscle strength.

Potassium should be administered only after adequate urine flow has been established. A decrease in urine volume to less than 20 ml/hr for 2 consecutive hours is an indication to stop potassium infusion until the situation is evaluated. Potassium is primarily excreted by the kidneys; therefore, when oliguria is present, administration of potassium can cause the serum potassium concentration to rise to dangerous levels.

▷ *Evaluation*

▷ *Expected Outcomes*

1. Patient exhibits normal cardiac function with regular pulse rate, normal electrocardiogram, and absence of dysrhythmias
2. Demonstrates normal muscle strength of upper and lower extremities
3. Exhibits normal bowel sounds and gastrointestinal function
4. Reports decreased level of fatigue
5. Reports normal appetite without nausea or vomiting
6. Consumes prescribed foods high in potassium and potassium supplements
7. Excretes adequate urine volume
8. Exhibits absence of precipitating risk factors (*e.g.*, diarrhea, vomiting, laxative and diuretic abuse)

Potassium Excess (Hyperkalemia)

Definition and Etiology

Hyperkalemia refers to a greater than normal serum potassium concentration. It seldom occurs in patients with normal renal function. Like hypokalemia, it is often due to iatrogenic (treatment-induced) causes. Although less common than hypokalemia, it is usually more dangerous since cardiac arrest is more frequently associated with high serum potassium levels.

Before considering real causes of hyperkalemia, one must be aware that there are a number of causes of factitious ("pseudo") hyperkalemia. The most common are the use of a tight tourniquet around an exercising extremity while drawing the blood sample and hemolysis of the sample before analysis. Other causes include marked leukocytosis or thrombocytosis and drawing blood above a site where potassium is infusing. Failure to be aware of factitious causes of hyperkalemia can result in aggressive treatment of nonexistent hyperkalemia, resulting in serious lowering of serum potassium levels. Thus, measurements of grossly elevated levels should be corroborated.

The major cause of hyperkalemia is decreased renal excretion of potassium. Thus, significant hyperkalemia is commonly seen in untreated patients with renal failure, particularly when potassium is being liberated from cells during infectious processes or exogenous sources of potassium are excessive, as in diet or medications. A deficiency of adrenal steroids causes sodium loss and potassium retention; thus, hypoaldosteronism and Addison's disease predispose to hyperkalemia.

Although a high intake of potassium can cause severe hyperkalemia in patients with impaired renal function, the disorder rarely occurs in normal people. However, for all patients, improper use of potassium supplements predisposes to hyperkalemia, especially when salt substitutes are used. It should be remembered that not all patients receiving potassium-losing diuretics require potassium supplements. Certainly those patients receiving potassium-conserving diuretics should not receive supplements. Potassium supplements are extremely dangerous when patients have impaired renal function and thus decreased ability to excrete potassium. Even more dangerous is the intravenous administration of potassium to such patients since serum levels can rise very quickly. Aged blood should not be given to patients with impaired renal function because the serum concentration of stored blood increases as storage time increases, a result of red blood cell deterioration. It is possible to exceed the renal tolerance of *any* patient with rapid intravenous potassium administration, as well as when large amounts of oral potassium supplements are ingested.

In the presence of acidosis, potassium leaks out of the cells into the ECF. This occurs as hydrogen ions enter the cells, a process that buffers the *p*H of the ECF. (See pp. 122, 123 for further discussion of acidosis.) An elevated extracellular potassium level should be anticipated when extensive tissue trauma has occurred, as in burns, crushing injuries, or severe infections. Similarly, it can occur with lysis of malignant cells after chemotherapy.

Clinical Manifestations

By far the most clinically important effect of hyperkalemia is its effect on the myocardium. Cardiac effects of an elevated serum potassium level are usually not significant below a concentration of 7 mEq/liter (SI: 7 mmol/L), but they are almost always present when the level is 8 mEq/liter (SI: 8

mmol/L) or greater. As the plasma potassium concentration is increased, disturbances in cardiac conduction occur. The earliest changes, often occurring at a serum potassium level greater than 6 mEq/liter (SI: 6 mmol/L), are peaked narrow T waves and a shortened QT interval. If the serum potassium level continues to rise, the PR interval becomes prolonged and is followed by disappearance of the P waves. Finally, there is decomposition and prolongation of the QRS complex (Fig. 9-5). Ventricular dysrhythmias and cardiac arrest may occur at any point in this progression.

Severe hyperkalemia causes muscle weakness and even paralysis, related to a depolarization block in muscle. Similarly, ventricular conduction is slowed. Although hyperkalemia has marked effects on the peripheral neuromuscular system, it has little effect on the central nervous system. Rapidly ascending muscular weakness leading to flaccid quadriplegia has been reported in patients with very high serum potassium levels. Paralysis of respiratory muscles and those required for phonation can also occur.

Gastrointestinal manifestations, such as nausea, intermittent intestinal colic, and diarrhea, usually occur in hyperkalemic patients.

Diagnostic Evaluation

Serum potassium levels and electrocardiographic changes are crucial to the diagnosis of hyperkalemia. See the discussion of clinical manifestations.

Management

In nonacute situations, restriction of dietary potassium and potassium-containing medications may suffice. For example, eliminating the use of potassium-containing salt substitutes in the patient taking a potassium-conserving diuretic may be all that is needed to deal with mild hyperkalemia. Prevention of serious hyperkalemia by the administration of cation-exchange resins (such as Kayexalate) may be necessary in renal patients.

Emergency Measures. In emergency situations, it may be necessary to administer calcium gluconate intravenously. Within minutes after administration, calcium antagonizes the action of hyperkalemia on the heart. The ECG should be continuously monitored during administration; the appearance of bradycardia is an indication to stop the infusion. The myocardial protective effects of calcium are transient, lasting about 30 minutes. Extra caution is required if the patient has been digitalized, since parenteral administration of calcium sensitizes the heart to digitalis and may precipitate digitalis toxicity.

Intravenous administration of sodium bicarbonate may be necessary to alkalinize the plasma and cause a temporary shift of potassium into the cells. Also, sodium bicarbonate furnishes sodium to antagonize the cardiac effects of potassium. Effects of this therapy begin within 30 to 60 minutes and may persist for hours; however, they are only temporary.

Intravenous administration of regular insulin and hypertonic dextrose causes a temporary shift of potassium into the cells. Glucose and insulin therapy has an onset of action within 30 minutes and lasts for several hours.

The above stopgap measures only temporarily protect the patient from hyperkalemia. If the hyperkalemic condition is not transient, actual removal of potassium from the body is required; this may be accomplished by way of cation-exchange resins, peritoneal dialysis, or hemodialysis.

▶ Nursing Process
The Patient with Potassium Excess

▷ Assessment

Patients at risk for potassium excess should be identified so they can be monitored closely for signs of hyperkalemia. (See the section dealing with etiologic factors.) The nurse observes for signs of muscular weakness and dysrhythmias. The presence of paresthesias is noted, as are gastrointestinal symptoms such as nausea and intestinal colic. For patients at risk, serum potassium levels are measured periodically.

It is important to remember that elevated serum potassium levels may be erroneous; thus, grossly abnormal levels should be corroborated. To avoid false reports of hyperkalemia, prolonged use of a tourniquet while drawing the blood sample is avoided and the patient is cautioned not to exercise the extremity immediately prior to drawing of the sample. The blood sample is taken to the laboratory as soon as possible since hemolysis of the sample results in a falsely elevated serum potassium level.

▷ Nursing Diagnosis

The nursing assessment data are used to identify the patient at risk for this disturbance and nursing diagnoses are made. For example, in a patient with oliguric renal failure, the nursing diagnosis might be stated as alteration in potassium balance (hyperkalemia) related to decreased potassium excretion.

▷ Planning and Implementation

▷ *Goals:* A major goal in the care of patients at risk for hyperkalemia is prevention of the disorder. If the imbalance cannot be prevented, it must be detected early so that therapeutic interventions can be undertaken to safely restore potassium balance and prevent life-threatening effects such as cardiac arrest.

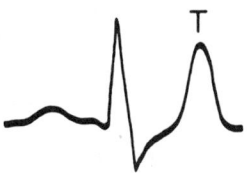

Figure 9-5
Electrocardiogram in hyperkalemia, showing widening QRS complex, decreased amplitude of P wave, and peaked T wave.

Nursing Interventions

Prevention of Hyperkalemia. Measures are taken to prevent hyperkalemia in patients at risk, when possible, by encouraging the patient to adhere to the prescribed potassium restriction. Foods high in potassium to be avoided include coffee, cocoa, tea, dried fruits, dried beans, and whole grain breads. Milk and eggs also contain substantial amounts of potassium. Conversely, foods with minimal potassium content include butter, margarine, cranberry juice or sauce, ginger ale, gumdrops or jellybeans, lollypops, root beer, sugar, and honey.

Safe Restoration of Potassium Balance. As stated earlier, it is possible to exceed the tolerance for potassium in any person if the substance is administered rapidly by the intravenous route. Therefore, great care should be taken to monitor potassium solutions closely, paying careful attention to the solution's concentration and rate of administration. When adding potassium to parenteral solutions, the added potassium is mixed with the fluid by inverting the bottle several times. Potassium chloride should *never* be added to a hanging bottle since it might result in the potassium being administered as a bolus (potassium chloride is heavy and settles to the bottom of the container).

It is important to caution patients to use salt substitutes sparingly if they are taking other supplementary forms of potassium or potassium-conserving diuretics. Also, potassium-conserving diuretics (such as spironolactone, triamterene, and amiloride), potassium supplements, and salt substitutes should not be administered to patients with renal dysfunction.

▷ *Evaluation*

▷ *Expected Outcomes*

1. Patient exhibits normal cardiac function with normal pulse rate and no dysrhythmias on ECG
2. Excretes adequate urine volume
3. Exhibits normal thoracic excursion and normal respiratory function
4. Reports normal gastrointestinal function without diarrhea or abdominal cramping
5. Consumes foods low in potassium and avoids use of salt substitutes
6. States rationale for low-potassium diet
7. Exhibits normal serum potassium level
8. Exhibits absence of precipitating risk factors (*e.g.*, decreased renal function, excessive intake of potassium, extensive tissue trauma as in burns or crushing injuries)

Calcium Imbalances

Because many factors affect calcium regulation, both hypocalcemia and hypercalcemia are relatively common disturbances. To facilitate understanding of calcium disturbances, it is helpful to review factors affecting calcium balance.

Functions of Calcium

Over 99% of the body's calcium is concentrated in the skeletal system, where it is a major component of strong durable bones and teeth. About 1% of skeletal calcium is rapidly exchangeable with blood calcium; the rest is more stable and only slowly exchanged. The small amount of calcium located outside the bone circulates in the serum, partly bound to protein and partly ionized. Calcium helps hold body cells together. In addition, calcium exerts a sedative action on nerve cells and thus plays a major role in the transmission of nerve impulses. It helps regulate muscle contraction and relaxation, including normal heartbeat. Calcium is instrumental in activating enzymes that stimulate many essential chemical reactions in the body and also plays a role in blood coagulation.

The normal total serum calcium level is 8.5 to 10.5 mg/dl (SI: 2.1–2.6 mmol/L). About 50% of the serum calcium exists in an ionized form that is physiologically active and important for neuromuscular activity. The remainder of serum calcium exists bound to serum proteins, primarily albumin.

Calcium Deficit (Hypocalcemia)

Definition and Etiology

Hypocalcemia refers to a lower than normal serum concentration of calcium, which occurs in a variety of clinical situations. A patient, however, may have a total body calcium deficit (as in osteoporosis) and maintain a normal serum calcium level.

A number of factors can cause hypocalcemia. Primary hypoparathyroidism results in this disturbance, as does surgical hypoparathyroidism. The latter is far more common. Not only is it associated with thyroid and parathyroid operations, but it can also occur after radical neck dissection and is most likely in the first 24 to 48 hours after surgery. Transient hypocalcemia can occur with massive administration of citrated blood (as in exchange transfusions in newborns), since citrate can combine with ionized calcium and temporarily remove it from the circulation.

Inflammation of the pancreas causes release of proteolytic and lipolytic enzymes; it is thought that calcium ions combine with the fatty acids released by lipolysis, forming soaps. As a result of this process, hypocalcemia is common in pancreatitis. It has also been suggested that hypocalcemia might be related to excessive secretion of glucagon from the inflamed pancreas, resulting in increased secretion of calcitonin (a hormone that lowers serum calcium).

Hypocalcemia is common in patients with renal failure because these patients frequently have elevated serum phosphate levels. Hyperphosphatemia usually causes a reciprocal drop in the serum calcium level. Other causes of hypocalcemia can include inadequate vitamin D consumption, magnesium deficiency, medullary thyroid carcinoma, low serum albumin levels, and alkalosis. Drugs predisposing to hypocalcemia can include aluminum-containing antacids, aminoglycosides, caffeine, cisplatin, corticosteroids, mithramycin, phosphates, isoniazid, and loop diuretics.

A condition referred to as osteoporosis is associated with prolonged low intake of calcium and represents a total body calcium deficit, even though serum calcium levels are usually normal. This disease strikes millions of Americans, mostly women. It is characterized by loss of bone mass, causing bones to become porous and brittle and, therefore, susceptible to fracture. (See Chap. 58.)

Clinical Manifestations

Tetany is the most characteristic manifestation of hypocalcemia. Tetany refers to the entire symptom complex induced by increased neural excitability. These symptoms are due to spontaneous discharges of both sensory and motor fibers in peripheral nerves. Sensations of tingling may occur in the tips of the fingers, around the mouth, and, less commonly, in the feet. Spasms of the muscles of the extremities and face may occur. Pain may develop as a result of these spasms.

Trousseau's sign (Fig. 9-6) can be elicited by inflating a blood pressure cuff on the upper arm to about 20 mm Hg above systolic pressure; within 2 to 5 minutes carpal spasm will occur as ischemia of the ulnar nerve develops. Chvostek's sign consists of twitching of muscles supplied by the facial nerve when the nerve is tapped about 2 cm anterior to the earlobe, just below the zygomatic arch.

Seizures may result because hypocalcemia increases irritability of the central nervous system as well as of the peripheral nerves. Other changes associated with hypocalcemia include an increased QT interval and mental changes such as emotional depression, impairment of memory, confusion, delirium, and even hallucinations. Chronic hypocalcemia in children can retard growth and lower the IQ.

Diagnostic Evaluation

When evaluating serum calcium levels, one must consider several other variables, such as serum protein levels and arterial *p*H. Clinically, it is important to correlate the serum calcium concentration with the serum albumin level. Each fall (or rise) of the serum albumin level by 1 gm/dl (beyond the normal range of 4 to 5 gm/dl)(SI: 40 to 50 g/L) is associated with a fall (or rise) of serum calcium concentration of approximately 0.8 mg/dl (SI: 0.2 mmol/L). For example, if a person with a total serum calcium level of 10 mg/dl, and a serum albumin value of 4 gm/dl, develops a decrease in serum albumin level to 3 gm/dl, the serum calcium value will drop to 9.2 mg/dl. Because of this, clinicians will often ignore a low serum calcium level in the presence of a similarly low serum albumin level. The ionized calcium level is usually normal in patients with reduced total serum calcium levels and concomitant hypoalbuminemia. When the arterial *p*H increases (alkalosis), more calcium becomes bound to protein. As a result, the ionized portion decreases. Symptoms of hypocalcemia often occur in the presence of alkalosis. Acidosis (low *p*H) has the opposite effect, that is, less calcium is bound to protein and thus more exists in the ionized form. Rarely will signs of hypocalcemia develop in the presence of acidosis, even when the total serum calcium level is lower than normal.

Ideally, the laboratory should measure the ionized level. However, in most laboratories only the total calcium level is reported; thus, concentration of the ionized fraction must be estimated by simultaneous measurement of serum protein level and arterial *p*H.

Management

Acute symptomatic hypocalcemia is a medical emergency, requiring prompt intravenous administration of calcium. Parenteral calcium salts include calcium gluconate, calcium chloride, and calcium gluceptate. Although calcium chloride produces a significantly higher ionized calcium than an equimolar amount of calcium gluconate, it is not used as often since it is more irritating and can cause sloughing of tissue if allowed to infiltrate. Too rapid intravenous administration of calcium can induce cardiac arrest, preceded by bradycardia. Intravenous calcium administration is particularly dangerous in digitalized patients since calcium ions exert an effect similar to that of digitalis and can cause digitalis toxicity with adverse cardiac effects.

Nursing Interventions

It is important to observe for hypocalcemia in patients at risk. One should be prepared to take seizure precautions when hypocalcemia is severe. The condition of the airway is closely monitored since laryngeal stridor can occur. Safety precau-

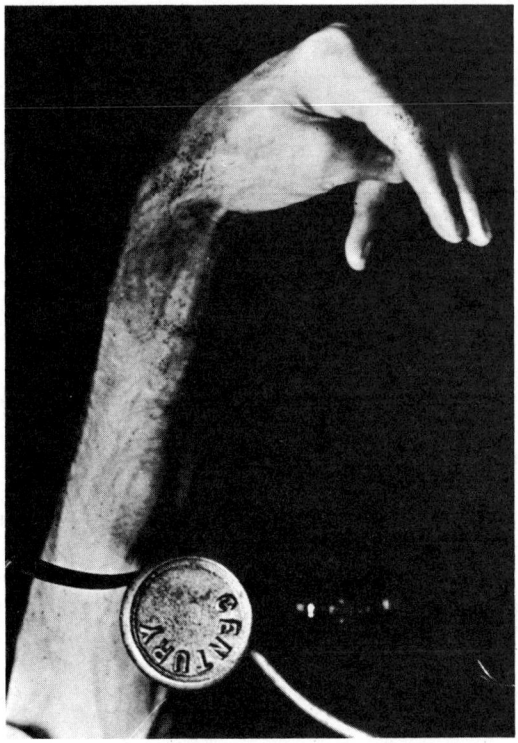

Figure 9-6
Trousseau's sign. Carpopedal spasm with hypocalcemia. (Ezrin C, Godden JO, Volpe R and Wilson R. Systematic Endocrinology, 2nd ed, p 1510. Hagerstown, Maryland, Harper & Row, 1979.)

tions are taken, as indicated, if confusion is present. Persons at high risk for osteoporosis are instructed about the need for adequate dietary calcium intake; if not consumed in the diet, calcium supplements should be considered. Also, the value of regular exercise in decreasing bone loss should be emphasized.

Calcium Excess (Hypercalcemia)

Definition and Etiology

Hypercalcemia refers to an excess of calcium in the plasma. It is a dangerous imbalance when severe; in fact, hypercalcemic crisis has a mortality as high as 50% if not treated promptly.

The most common causes of hypercalcemia are malignant neoplastic diseases and hyperparathyroidism. Malignant tumors can produce hypercalcemia by a variety of mechanisms. The excessive parathyroid hormone secretion associated with hyperparathyroidism causes increased bony release of calcium and increased intestinal and renal absorption of calcium.

Bone mineral is lost during immobilization, sometimes causing elevation of total (and especially ionized) calcium in the bloodstream. Symptomatic hypercalcemia from immobilization, however, is rare; when it does occur it is virtually limited to persons with high calcium turnover rates (such as adolescents during a growth spurt). Most cases of hypercalcemia secondary to immobility occur after severe or multiple fractures or after extensive traumatic paralysis.

Thiazide diuretics may cause a slight elevation in serum calcium levels since they potentiate the action of parathyroid hormone on the kidneys, reducing urinary calcium excretion. The milk-alkali syndrome can occur in patients with peptic ulcer treated for a prolonged period with milk and alkaline antacids, particularly calcium carbonate.

Clinical Manifestations

As a rule, the symptoms of hypercalcemia are proportional to the degree of elevation of the serum calcium level. Hypercalcemia reduces neuromuscular excitability since it acts as a sedative at the myoneural junction. Symptoms such as muscular weakness, incoordination, anorexia, and constipation may be due to decreased tone in smooth and striated muscle.

Anorexia, nausea, vomiting, and constipation are common symptoms of hypercalcemia. Abdominal pain may also be present and at times may be so severe as to be mistaken for an acute abdominal emergency. Abdominal distention and ileus may complicate severe hypercalcemic crisis. Severe thirst may occur, secondary to the polyuria caused by the high solute (calcium) load. Patients with chronic hypercalcemia may develop symptoms similar to those of peptic ulcer since hypercalcemia increases the secretion of acid and pepsin by the stomach.

Mental confusion, impairment of memory, slurred speech, lethargy, acute psychotic behavior, or coma may occur. The more severe symptoms tend to appear when the serum calcium level is approximately 16 mg/dl or above.

However, some patients may become profoundly disturbed with serum calcium levels of only 12 mg/dl.

Polyuria due to disturbed renal tubular function produced by hypercalcemia may be present. Cardiac standstill can occur when the serum calcium is about 18 mg/dl. The inotropic effect of digitalis is enhanced by calcium; therefore, digitalis toxicity is aggravated by hypercalcemia.

Hypercalcemic crisis refers to an acute rise in the serum calcium level to 17 mg/dl or higher. Severe thirst and polyuria are characteristically present. Other findings may include muscular weakness, intractable nausea, abdominal cramps, obstipation (very severe constipation) or diarrhea, peptic ulcer symptoms, and bone pain. Lethargy, mental confusion, and coma may also occur. This condition is very dangerous and may result in cardiac arrest.

Diagnostic Evaluation

The serum calcium level is greater than 10.5 mg/dl (SI: 2.6 mmol/L). Cardiovascular changes may include a variety of dysrhythmias and shortening of the QT interval.

Management

Therapeutic aims in hypercalcemia include decreasing the serum calcium level and reversing the process causing hypercalcemia. General measures include administering fluids to dilute serum calcium and promote its renal excretion, mobilizing the patient, and dietary calcium restriction. Administration of 0.45% sodium chloride or 0.9% sodium chloride solutions intravenously dilutes the serum calcium level and increases urinary calcium excretion by inhibiting tubular reabsorption of calcium. Furosemide (Lasix) is often used in conjunction with saline administration; in addition to causing diuresis, furosemide increases calcium excretion. Calcitonin can be used to lower the serum calcium level and is particularly useful for patients with heart disease or renal failure who cannot tolerate large sodium loads.

For patients with malignant disease, treatment is directed at controlling the condition by surgery, chemotherapy, or radiation therapy. Corticosteroids may be used to decrease bone turnover and tubular reabsorption for patients with sarcoidosis, myelomas, lymphomas, and leukemias; patients with solid tumors are less responsive. Mithramycin, a cytotoxic antibiotic, inhibits bone resorption and thus lowers the serum calcium levels. This drug must be used cautiously since it has significant side-effects, including thrombocytopenia, nephrotoxicity, and hepatotoxicity. Inorganic phosphate salts can be given orally or by nasogastric tube (in the form of Phospho-Soda or Neutra-Phos), rectally (as retention Fleet enemas), or intravenously. Intravenous phosphate therapy is used with extreme caution in the treatment of hypercalcemia since it can cause severe calcification in various tissues, including the vein through which it is given.

Nursing Interventions

It is important to monitor for the occurrence of hypercalcemia in patients at risk for this disorder. Initiation of interventions, such as increasing patient mobility and encouraging fluids, can help prevent hypercalcemia, or at least minimize its severity. Hospitalized patients at risk for hypercalcemia are allowed to ambulate as soon as possible; outpatients are told the importance of frequent ambulation. When encouraging oral fluids, the nurse considers the patient's likes and dislikes. Sodium-containing fluids should be given, unless contraindicated by other conditions, since sodium favors calcium excretion. Patients at home are encouraged to drink 3 to 4 quarts of fluid daily, if possible. Adequate bulk should be provided in the diet to offset the tendency for constipation. Safety precautions are taken, as necessary, when mental symptoms of hypercalcemia are present. The patient and family are informed that these mental changes are reversible with treatment.

Magnesium Imbalances

Functions of Magnesium

Next to potassium, magnesium is the most abundant intracellular cation. It acts as an activator for many intracellular enzyme systems and plays a role in both carbohydrate and protein metabolism. Magnesium balance is important in neuromuscular function. Since magnesium acts directly on the myoneural junction, variations in its serum concentration affect neuromuscular irritability and contractility. For example, an excess of magnesium diminishes excitability of the muscle cells while a deficit increases neuromuscular irritability and contractility. Magnesium produces its sedative effect at the neuromuscular junction, probably by inhibiting the release of the neurotransmitter acetylcholine. It also increases the stimulus threshold in nerve fibers.

Magnesium exerts effects on the cardiovascular system, acting peripherally to produce vasodilatation. Magnesium is thought to have a direct effect on peripheral arteries and arterioles, which results in a decreased total peripheral resistance.

Magnesium Deficit (Hypomagnesemia)

Definition and Etiology

Hypomagnesemia refers to a below normal serum magnesium concentration. The normal serum magnesium level is 1.5 to 2.5 mEq/liter (or 1.8 to 3.0 mg/dl; SI: 0.75 to 1.25 mmol/L). Approximately one third of serum magnesium is bound to protein; the remaining two thirds exists as free cations (Mg^{2+}). Like calcium, it is the ionized fraction that is primarily involved in neuromuscular activity and other physiologic processes.

Hypomagnesemia is a common imbalance in critically ill patients, yet it is frequently overlooked. Magnesium deficit also occurs in less acutely ill patients, such as those experiencing withdrawal from alcohol and those receiving nourishment after a period of starvation, as in tube feedings or total parenteral nutrition.

An important route for magnesium loss is the gastrointestinal tract. Losses may take the form of drainage from nasogastric suction, diarrhea, or fistulas. Since fluid from the lower gastrointestinal tract is richer in magnesium (10 to 14 mEq/liter) than is fluid from the upper tract (1 to 2 mEq/liter), losses from diarrhea and intestinal fistulas are more likely to induce magnesium deficit than are those from gastric suction. Although magnesium losses are relatively small in nasogastric suction, hypomagnesemia will occur if losses are prolonged and parenteral fluids are magnesium free. Because the distal small bowel is the major site of magnesium absorption, any disruption in small bowel function, as in intestinal resection or inflammatory bowel disease, can lead to hypomagnesemia.

Alcoholism is currently the most common cause of symptomatic hypomagnesemia in the United States. It is particularly troublesome during treatment of alcohol withdrawal. Because of this, it is recommended that the serum magnesium level be measured every 2 or 3 days in hospitalized patients going through withdrawal from alcohol. While the serum magnesium level may be normal on admission, it can fall as a result of metabolic changes associated with therapy, such as the intracellular shift of magnesium associated with intravenous glucose administration.

During nutritional repletion, the major cellular electrolytes are taken from the serum and deposited in newly synthesized cells. Thus, if the enteral or parenteral feeding formula is deficient in magnesium content, serious hypomagnesemia will occur. Because of this, serum levels of these primarily intracellular ions should be measured at regular intervals during the administration of total parenteral nutrition and even during enteral feedings, especially to patients who have undergone a period of starvation.

Other causes of hypomagnesemia include the administration of gentamicin and cisplatin and the rapid administration of citrated blood, especially to patients with renal or hepatic disease. Magnesium deficiency is often seen in patients with diabetic ketoacidosis; it is primarily the result of increased renal excretion of magnesium during osmotic diuresis and shifting of magnesium into the cells with insulin therapy.

Clinical Manifestations

Clinical manifestations of hypomagnesemia are largely confined to the neuromuscular system. Some of the effects are due directly to the low serum magnesium level; others are due to secondary changes in potassium and calcium metabolism. Symptoms do not usually occur until the serum magnesium level is less than 1 mEq/liter (SI: 0.5 mmol/L).

Among the neuromuscular changes are hyperexcitability with muscular weakness, tremors, and athetoid movements (slow, involuntary twisting and writhing movements). Others include tetany, generalized tonic-clonic or focal seizures, layngeal stridor, and positive Chvostek's and Trousseau's signs (see discussion on p. 115).

Magnesium deficiency predisposes to cardiac dysrhythmias, such as premature ventricular contractions, supraventricular tachycardia, and ventricular fibrillation. Increased susceptibility to digitalis toxicity is associated with low serum magnesium levels. This is an important consideration since patients receiving digoxin are also likely to be on diuretic therapy, predisposing to renal loss of magnesium.

Hypomagnesemia may be accompanied by marked alterations in mood. Apathy, depression, apprehension, or extreme agitation have been noted, as well as ataxia, vertigo, and a confusional state. At times, delirium and frank psychoses may occur, as may auditory or visual hallucinations.

Diagnostic Evaluation

On laboratory analysis, the serum magnesium level is less than 1.5 mEq/liter or 1.8 mg/dl (SI: 0.75 mmol/L).

Management

Mild magnesium deficiency can be corrected by diet alone. Principal dietary sources of magnesium are green vegetables, nuts and legumes, and fruits such as bananas, grapefruits, and oranges. Magnesium is also plentiful in peanut butter and chocolate. When necessary, magnesium salts can be given orally to replace continuous excessive losses. Patients receiving total parenteral nutrition require magnesium in the solution to prevent the development of hypomagnesemia.

Overt symptoms of hypomagnesemia are treated with parenteral administration of magnesium. Magnesium sulfate is the most commonly used magnesium salt. Serial magnesium concentrations can be used to regulate the dosage.

Nursing Interventions

The nurse should be aware of patients at risk for hypomagnesemia and observe for its presence. Patients on digitalis are monitored closely since a deficit of magnesium predisposes to digitalis toxicity. When hypomagnesemia is severe, one should be prepared to take seizure precautions. Other safety precautions are instituted, as indicated, if confusion is present.

Since difficulty in swallowing may occur in magnesium-depleted patients, the ability to swallow should be tested with water before oral medications or foods are offered. Dysphagia is probably related to the athetoid or choreiform (rapid, involuntary and irregular jerky movements) movements associated with magnesium deficit.

When magnesium deficit is due to abuse of diuretics or laxatives, patient education may help alleviate the problem. For patients on a general diet who are experiencing abnormal magnesium losses, the intake of magnesium-rich foods (*e.g.,* green vegetables, nuts and legumes, bananas and oranges) is encouraged.

Magnesium Excess (Hypermagnesemia)

Definition and Etiology

Hypermagnesemia refers to a greater than normal serum concentration of magnesium. A serum magnesium level can appear falsely elevated when blood specimens are allowed to hemolyze or are drawn from an extremity with an excessively tight tourniquet.

By far the most common cause of hypermagnesemia is renal failure. In fact, most patients with advanced renal failure have at least a modest elevation in serum magnesium levels. This condition is aggravated when such patients are given magnesium to control convulsions or inadvertently receive one of the many commercial antacids that contain magnesium salts. Patients with renal failure may also receive an exogenous magnesium load during hemodialysis, either because of inadvertent use of hard water or an error in manufacture of the concentrate used for preparing the dialysate.

Hypermagnesemia can occur in a patient with untreated diabetic ketoacidosis when catabolism causes release of cellular magnesium that cannot be excreted because of profound fluid volume depletion and resulting oliguria. An excess of magnesium can also result from excessive magnesium administration.

Clinical Manifestations

Acute elevation of the serum magnesium level depresses the central nervous system as well as the peripheral neuromuscular junction. At mildly elevated levels, there is a tendency for lowered blood pressure because of peripheral vasodilatation. Facial flushing and hypotension may occur, as well as sensations of warmth. At higher elevations, lethargy, dysarthria, and drowsiness can appear. Deep tendon reflexes are lost, and muscular weakness and paralysis may supervene. The respiratory center is depressed when serum magnesium levels exceed 10 mEq/liter. Coma and cardiac arrest can occur when the serum magnesium level is greatly elevated.

Diagnostic Evaluation

On laboratory analysis, the serum magnesium level is greater than 2.5 mEq/liter or 3.0 mg/dl (SI: 1.25 mmol/L).

Management

The best treatment for hypermagnesemia is prevention. This can be accomplished by avoiding magnesium administration to patients with renal failure and by careful vigilance when magnesium salts are administered to seriously ill patients. In the presence of severe hypermagnesemia, all parenteral and oral magnesium salts are discontinued. When respiratory depression or defective cardiac conduction is present, emergency measures such as ventilatory support and intravenous administration of calcium are indicated. Hemodialysis with a magnesium-free dialysate is an effective treatment that should produce a safe serum magnesium level within hours.

Nursing Interventions

Patients at risk for hypermagnesemia are identified and assessed. When hypermagnesemia is suspected, the nurse should monitor the vital signs, noting the presence of hypotension and shallow respirations, and check for decreased patellar reflexes and changes in the level of consciousness. Care should be taken to avoid giving magnesium-containing medications to patients with renal failure or compromised renal function. Similarly, one should caution patients with renal failure to check with their health care providers before taking over-the-counter medications. Care should also be used when magnesium fluids are administered parenterally.

Phosphorus Imbalances

Functions of Phosphorus

Phosphorus is a critical constituent of all the body's tissues. It is essential to the function of muscle, red blood cells, and the nervous system and to the intermediary metabolism of carbohydrate, protein, and fat. The normal serum phosphorus level ranges between 2.5 to 4.5 mg/dl (SI: 0.8 to 1.5 mmol/L) and may be as high as 6 mg/dl (SI: 1.94 mmol/L) in infants and children. Serum phosphorus levels are presumably greater in children because of the high rate of skeletal growth.

Phosphorus Deficit (Hypophosphatemia)

Definition and Etiology

Hypophosphatemia is defined as a below normal serum concentration of inorganic phosphorus. Although it often indicates phosphorus deficiency, it may occur under a variety of circumstances in which total body phosphorus stores are normal. Conversely, phosphorus deficiency refers to an abnormally low content of phosphorus in lean tissues and may exist in the absence of hypophosphatemia.

Hypophosphatemia may occur during the administration of calories in normally required amounts to patients with severe protein-calorie malnutrition. It is most apt to occur with overzealous refeeding with simple carbohydrates. This syndrome can be induced in anyone with severe protein–calorie malnutrition (such as patients with anorexia nervosa, or alcoholism, or elderly debilitated patients unable to eat).

Marked hypophosphatemia may develop in malnourished patients receiving total parenteral nutrition if correction of phosphorus loss is inadequate. Other causes of hypophosphatemia include prolonged intense hyperventilation, alcohol withdrawal, poor dietary intake, diabetic ketoacidosis, and major thermal burns.

Clinical Manifestations

Most of the signs and symptoms of phosphorus deficiency appear to result from deficiency of adenosine triphosphate (ATP), of 2,3-diphosphoglycerate (DPG), or of both. The former impairs cellular energy resources, and the latter impairs oxygen delivery to tissues.

A wide range of neurologic symptoms may occur, such as irritability, apprehension, weakness, numbness, paresthesias, confusion, seizures, and coma. Low levels of 2,3-DPG may reduce the delivery of oxygen to peripheral tissues, resulting in tissue anoxia.

It is thought that hypophosphatemia predisposes to infection. In laboratory animals, hypophosphatemia has been noted to produce depression of the chemotactic, phagocytic, and bacterial activity of granulocytes.

Muscle damage may develop as the ATP level in the muscle tissue declines. This is manifested clinically by muscle weakness, muscle pain, and, at times, acute rhabdomyolysis (disintegration of striated muscle). Weakness of respiratory muscles may greatly impair ventilation. Also, hypophosphatemia may predispose to an insulin-resistant state, and thus hyperglycemia.

Diagnostic Evaluation

On laboratory analysis, the serum phosphorus level will be less than 2.5 mg/dl (SI: 0.80 mmol/L) in adults. It is important to remember that glucose administration causes a slight decrease in the serum phosphorus level.

Management

As in any electrolyte imbalance, the best treatment is prevention. In patients at risk for hypophosphatemia, serum phosphate levels should be closely monitored and correction initiated before deficits become severe. Adequate amounts of phosphorus should be added to hyperalimentation solutions, and attention should also be paid to phosphorus levels in enteral feeding solutions.

Severe hypophosphatemia is dangerous and requires prompt attention. Aggressive intravenous phosphorus repair is usually limited to patients with serum phosphorus levels below 1 mg/dl (SI: 0.3 mmol/L). Possible dangers of intravenous administration of phosphorus include hypocalcemia and metastatic calcification from hyperphosphatemia. In less acute situations, oral phosphorus replacement is satisfactory.

Nursing Interventions

The nurse should identify patients at risk for hypophosphatemia and monitor for its presence. Since malnourished patients receiving hyperalimentation are at risk when calories are introduced too aggressively, prevention can take the form of gradual introduction of the feeding solution to avoid rapid shifts of phosphorus into the cells.

For patients with documented hypophosphatemia, careful attention should be paid to preventing infection since hypophosphatemia may produce changes in the granulocytes. For patients requiring correction of phosphorus losses, frequent monitoring of the serum phosphorus levels is indicated to augment clinical assessment.

Phosphorus Excess (Hyperphosphatemia)

Definition and Etiology

Hyperphosphatemia refers to a serum phosphorus level greater than normal. A variety of conditions can lead to this imbalance.

The most common cause of hyperphosphatemia is decreased renal phosphorus excretion in renal failure. Other causes include chemotherapy for neoplastic disease, high phosphate intake, profound muscle necrosis, and increased phosphorus absorption.

Clinical Manifestations

An elevated serum phosphorus level causes little in the way of symptoms. The most important long-term consequence is soft tissue calcification, which occurs mainly in patients with reduced glomerular filtration rates; the most important short-term consequence is tetany. High levels of serum inorganic phosphorus are harmful because they promote precipitation of calcium phosphate in nonosseous sites. Because of the reciprocal relationship between phosphorus and calcium, a high serum phosphorus level tends to cause a low calcium concentration in the serum. Tetany can result and can present as sensations of tingling in the tips of the fingers and around the mouth.

Diagnostic Evaluation

On laboratory analysis, the serum phosphorus level is greater than 4.5 mg/dl (SI: 1.5 mmol/L) in adults. Serum phosphorus levels are normally higher in children, presumably because of the high rate of skeletal growth.

Management

When possible, treatment is directed at the underlying disorder. For example, hyperphosphatemia related to tumor cell lysis might be lessened by prior administration of allopurinol to prevent urate nephropathy. For patients with renal failure, measures to decrease the serum phosphate level are indicated; these include the administration of phosphate-binding gels, dietary phosphate restriction, and dialysis.

Nursing Interventions

The nurse should be aware of patients at risk for hyperphosphatemia and monitor for its presence. When a low-phosphorus diet is prescribed, the patient is instructed to avoid foods high in phosphorus content. Such foods include hard cheese; cream; nuts; whole grain cereals; dried fruits; dried vegetables; special meats, such as kidneys, sardines, and sweetbreads; and desserts made with milk. When appropriate, the nurse instructs the patient to avoid phosphate-containing substances, such as phosphate-containing laxatives and enemas.

Summary of Fluid and Electrolyte Imbalances

Major fluid and electrolyte imbalances are summarized in Table 9-7.

Acid-Base Disturbances

Regulation of Acid-Base Balance

There are four types of acid–base imbalances: metabolic acidosis and alkalosis and respiratory acidosis and alkalosis. The causes, characteristics, and management of each of these disorders are discussed here.

Remarkable homeostatic mechanisms exist to maintain plasma pH, an indicator of hydrogen ion (H^+) concentration, within the narrow normal range of 7.35 to 7.45. These consist of chemical buffering mechanisms, the kidneys, and the lungs. In review, pH is defined as H^+ concentration; the more hydrogen ions, the more acidic is the solution. The pH range compatible with life (6.8 to 7.8) represents a tenfold difference in hydrogen ion concentration in plasma.

Chemical Buffers

Chemical buffers are substances that prevent major changes in the pH of body fluids by removing or releasing hydrogen ions; they can act quickly to prevent excessive changes in hydrogen ion concentration. The body's major buffer system is the bicarbonate–carbonic acid (HCO_3^-–H_2CO_3) buffer system. Normally, there are 20 parts of bicarbonate to one part of carbonic acid. If this ratio is upset, the pH will change. It is the ratio that is important in maintaining pH, not absolute values. One must remember that carbon dioxide (CO_2) is a potential acid; when CO_2 is dissolved in water, it becomes carbonic acid ($CO_2 + H_2O = H_2CO_3$). Thus, when carbon dioxide is increased, the carbonic acid content is also increased and vice versa. If either bicarbonate or carbonic acid is increased or decreased so that the 20:1 ratio is no longer maintained, acid–base imbalance results.

Other less important buffer systems in the ECF include the inorganic phosphates and the plasma proteins. Intracellular buffers include proteins, organic and inorganic phosphates, and, in red blood cells, hemoglobin.

Kidneys

The kidneys regulate the bicarbonate level in ECF; they are able to regenerate bicarbonate ions as well as reabsorb them from the renal tubular cells. In the presence of respiratory acidosis, and most cases of metabolic acidosis, the kidneys excrete hydrogen ions and conserve bicarbonate ions to help restore balance. In the presence of respiratory and metabolic alkalosis, the kidneys retain hydrogen ions and excrete bicarbonate ions to help restore balance. The kidneys obviously cannot compensate for the metabolic acidosis created by renal failure. Renal compensation for imbalances is relatively slow (a matter of hours or days).

Lungs

The lungs, under the control of the medulla, control the carbon dioxide, and thus carbonic acid content of ECF. They do so by adjusting ventilation in response to the amount of carbon dioxide in the blood. A rise in the partial pressure of carbon dioxide in arterial blood ($PaCO_2$) is a powerful stimulant to respiration. Of course, the partial pressure of oxygen in arterial blood (PaO_2) also influences respiration. However, its effect is not as marked as that produced by the $PaCO_2$.

In the presence of metabolic acidosis, the respiratory rate is increased, causing greater elimination of carbon dioxide (to reduce the acid load). In the presence of metabolic alkalosis, the respiratory rate is decreased, causing carbon dioxide to be retained (to increase the acid load).

TABLE 9-7
Summary of Major Fluid and Electrolyte Imbalances

Imbalance	Causes	Clinical Signs and Symptoms
Fluid volume deficit	Loss of water and electrolytes, as in vomiting, diarrhea, fistulas, gastrointestinal suction, and third-space fluid shifts; and decreased intake, as in anorexia, nausea, and inability to gain access to fluid	Acute weight loss, decreased skin and tongue turgor, oliguria, concentrated urine, weak rapid pulse, and low central venous pressure
Fluid volume excess	Compromised regulatory mechanisms, such as renal failure, congestive heart failure, and cirrhosis; and overzealous administration of sodium-containing fluids	Acute weight gain, edema, distended veins, crackles, and elevated central venous pressure
Sodium deficit (hyponatremia)	Loss of sodium, as in use of diuretics, loss of gastrointestinal fluids, and adrenal insufficiency; Gain of water, as in excessive administration of D_5W and excessive water supplements for patients receiving hypotonic tube feedings; disease states associated with SIADH such as head trauma and oat cell lung tumor; and pharmacologic agents associated with water retention such as oxytocin and certain tranquilizers	Anorexia, nausea and vomiting, lethargy, confusion, muscle cramps, muscular twitching, seizures, papilledema, serum sodium < 135 mEq/liter (SI: 145 mmol/L)
Sodium excess (hypernatremia)	Water deprivation in patients unable to drink at will, hypertonic tube feedings without adequate water supplements, diabetes insipidus, heatstroke, hyperventilation, and watery diarrhea	Thirst, elevated body temperature, swollen dry tongue and sticky mucous membranes, hallucinations, lethargy, irritability, focal or grand mal seizures, serum sodium > 145 mEq/liter (SI: 145 mmol/L)
Potassium deficit (hypokalemia)	Diarrhea, vomiting, gastric suction, steroid administration, hyperaldosteronism, carbenicillin, amphotericin B, bulemia, and osmotic diuresis	Fatigue, anorexia, nausea and vomiting, muscle weakness, decreased bowel motility, dysrhythmias, paresthesias, and serum potassium < 3.5 mEq/liter (SI: 3.5 mmol/L), and flat T waves on ECG
Potassium excess (hyperkalemia)	Pseudohyperkalemia (as in hemolysis of blood sample), oliguric renal failure, use of potassium-conserving diuretics in patients with renal insufficiency, acidosis	Vague muscular weakness, bradycardia, dysrhythmias, flaccid paralysis, paresthesias, intestinal colic, tall tented T waves on ECG, serum potassium > 5.8 mEq/liter (SI: 5.8 mmol/L)
Calcium deficit (hypocalcemia)	Hypoparathyroidism, surgical hypoparathyroidism (may follow thyroid surgery or radical neck dissection), malabsorption, pancreatitis, and alkalosis	Numbness, tingling of fingers, toes, and circumoral region; Trousseau's sign; Chvostek's sign; convulsions; and serum calcium < 8.6 mg/dl (SI: 2.2 mmol/L) or ionized calcium < 50%
Calcium excess (hypercalcemia)	Hyperparathyroidism, malignant neoplastic disease, prolonged immobilization, and overuse of calcium supplements	Muscular weakness, constipation, anorexia, nausea and vomiting, polyuria and polydipsia, neurotic behavior, cardiac dysrhythmias, and serum calcium >10.5 mg/dl (SI: 2.6 mmol/L)
Magnesium deficit (hypomagnesemia)	Chronic alcoholism, malabsorptive disorders, diabetic ketoacidosis, refeeding after starvation, and certain pharmacologic agents (such as gentamicin and cisplatin)	Neuromuscular irritability, dysrhythmias, disorientation, serum magnesemia <1.5 mEq/liter (SI: <0.75 mmol/L)
Magnesium excess (hypermagnesemia)	Renal failure (particularly when magnesium-containing medications are administered), adrenal insufficiency, excessive magnesium administration	Flushing, hypotension, drowsiness, hypoactive reflexes, depressed respirations, cardiac arrest, and coma, and serum Mg > 2.5 mEq/L (SI: 1.25 mmol/L)
Phosphorus deficit (hypophosphatemia)	Refeeding after starvation, alcohol withdrawal, diabetic ketoacidosis, respiratory alkalosis	Paresthesias, muscle weakness, muscle pain and tenderness, mental changes, cardiomyopathy, respiratory failure
Phosphorus excess (hyperphosphatemia)	Renal failure, excessive intake of phosphorus (as in phosphorus supplements and phosphate-containing laxatives)	Short-term consequences (symptoms of tetany, such as tingling of fingertips, and around mouth); long-term consequences (precipitation of calcium phosphate in nonosseous sites)

Metabolic Acidosis (Base Bicarbonate Deficit)

Definition and Etiology

Metabolic acidosis is a clinical disturbance characterized by a low *p*H (increased hydrogen concentration) and a low plasma bicarbonate concentration. It can be produced by a gain of hydrogen ion or a loss of bicarbonate. It can be divided clinically into two forms according to the values of the serum anion gap (AG): high anion gap acidosis and normal anion gap acidosis. Anion gap refers to the difference of anions (negatively charged electrolytes) and cations (electrolytes with a positive charge). The anion gap can be calculated by subtracting the sum of the serum chloride and bicarbonate concentrations (anions, or negatively charged electrolytes) from the serum sodium level (a cation, or positively charged electrolyte): $AG = Na^+ - (Cl^- + HCO_3^-)$. There are some unmeasured anions in the serum, such as sulfates, ketones, and lactic acid, that normally account for less than 16 mEq/liter of the anion production. An anion gap greater than 16 mEq suggests excessive accumulation of unmeasured anions.

High anion gap acidosis results from excessive accumulation of fixed acid. It occurs in ketoacidosis, lactic acidosis, late phase of salicylate poisoning, uremia, methanol or ethylene glycol toxicity, and ketoacidosis with starvation. In all of these instances, abnormally high levels of anions flood the system, increasing the anion gap above normal limits.

Normal anion gap acidosis results from direct loss of bicarbonate, as in diarrhea and intestinal fistulas, or from excessive gain of chloride, as in the administration of large quantities of isotonic saline or ammonium chloride.

Clinical Manifestations

Signs and symptoms of metabolic acidosis vary with the severity of metabolic acidosis. They may include headache, confusion, drowsiness, increased respiratory rate and depth, nausea, and vomiting. Peripheral vasodilatation and decreased cardiac output occur when the *p*H falls below 7.

Diagnostic Evaluation

Arterial blood gas measurements are valuable in the diagnosis of metabolic acidosis. Expected blood gas changes include a low bicarbonate level (less than 22 mEq/liter) and a low *p*H (less than 7.35). Hyperkalemia may accompany metabolic acidosis, as a result of shift of potassium out of the cells. Hyperventilation decreases the carbon dioxide level as a compensatory action. As stated previously, calculation of the anion gap is helpful in determining the cause of metabolic acidosis.

Management

Treatment is directed at correcting the metabolic defect. If the cause of the problem is excessive intake of chloride, treatment is obviously elimination of the source of the chloride. When necessary, bicarbonate is administered.

Metabolic Alkalosis (Base Bicarbonate Excess)

Definition and Etiology

Metabolic alkalosis is a clinical disturbance characterized by a high *p*H (decreased hydrogen ion concentration) and a high plasma bicarbonate concentration. It can be produced by a gain of bicarbonate or a loss of hydrogen ions.

Probably the most common cause of metabolic alkalosis is vomiting or gastric suction with loss of hydrogen and chloride ions; it is particularly a problem in pyloric stenosis since only gastric fluid is lost in this disorder. Gastric fluid has an acid *p*H (usually 1 to 3); therefore, loss of this highly acidic fluid increases alkalinity of body fluids. Other situations predisposing to metabolic alkalosis include those associated with loss of potassium, such as potassium-losing diuretics (*e.g.*, thiazides, furosemide, and ethacrynic acid) and excessive adrenalcorticoid hormones (as in hyperaldosteronism and Cushing's syndrome). Hypokalemia produces alkalosis in two ways: (1) in the presence of hypokalemia, the kidneys conserve potassium and thus hydrogen ion excretion is increased, and (2) cellular potassium moves out of the cells into the ECF in an attempt to maintain near-normal serum levels (as potassium ions (K^+) leave the cells, hydrogen ions must enter to maintain electroneutrality). Excessive alkali ingestion, as of bicarbonate-containing antacids or sodium bicarbonate during cardiopulmonary resuscitation, can also cause metabolic alkalosis.

Clinical Manifestations

Alkalosis is primarily manifested by symptoms related to decreased calcium ionization, such as tingling of the fingers and toes, dizziness, and hypertonic muscles. The ionized fraction of serum calcium decreases in the presence of alkalosis as more calcium combines with serum proteins. Since it is the ionized fraction of calcium that influences neuromuscular activity, it is understandable why symptoms of hypocalcemia are often the predominant symptoms of alkalosis. Respirations are depressed as a compensatory action by the lungs.

Diagnostic Evaluation

Evaluation of arterial blood gases reveals a *p*H greater than 7.45 and a serum bicarbonate concentration greater than 26 mEq/liter. The partial pressure of carbon dioxide will increase as the lungs attempt to compensate for the excess bicarbonate by retaining carbon dioxide. This hypoventilation is more pronounced in semiconscious, unconscious, or debilitated patients than in alert patients. The former may develop marked hypoxemia as a result of hypoventilation. Hypokalemia may accompany metabolic alkalosis.

Management

Treatment is aimed at reversal of the underlying disorder. Sufficient chloride must be supplied for the kidney to absorb sodium with chloride (allowing the excretion of excess bicarbonate). Treatment also includes restoration of normal fluid volume by administration of sodium chloride fluids (because continued volume depletion serves to maintain the alkalosis).

Respiratory Acidosis (Carbonic Acid Excess)

Definition and Etiology

Respiratory acidosis is a clinical disorder in which the *p*H is less than 7.35 and the $PaCO_2$ is greater than 42 mm Hg. It may be either acute or chronic.

Respiratory acidosis is always due to inadequate excretion of carbon dioxide with inadequate ventilation, resulting in elevated plasma carbon dioxide levels and thus elevated carbonic acid levels. In addition to an elevated $PaCO_2$, hypoventilation usually causes a decrease in PaO_2. Acute respiratory acidosis occurs in emergency situations, such as acute pulmonary edema, aspiration of a foreign object, atelectasis, pneumothorax, overdosage of sedatives, and severe pneumonia. Chronic respiratory acidosis is associated with chronic disorders such as emphysema, bronchiectasis, and bronchial asthma.

Clinical Manifestations

Clinical signs are variable in acute and chronic respiratory acidosis. Sudden hypercapnia (elevated $PaCO_2$) can cause increased pulse and respiratory rate, increased blood pressure, mental cloudiness, and feeling of fullness in the head. An elevated $PaCO_2$ causes cerebrovascular vasodilatation and increased cerebral blood flow, particularly when it is higher than 60 mm Hg. Ventricular fibrillation may be the first sign of respiratory acidosis in anesthetized patients.

The patient with chronic respiratory acidosis may complain of weakness, dull headache, and symptoms of the underlying disease process. Patients with chronic obstructive pulmonary disease who gradually accumulate carbon dioxide over a prolonged period (days to months) may not develop symptoms of hypercapnia because compensatory renal changes have had time to occur.

▷ *When the $PaCO_2$ is chronically above 50 mm Hg, the respiratory center becomes relatively insensitive to carbon dioxide as a respiratory stimulant, leaving hypoxemia as the major drive for respiration. Excessive oxygen administration removes the stimulus of hypoxemia, and the patient develops "carbon dioxide narcosis" unless the situation is quickly reversed.*

Diagnostic Evaluation

Arterial blood gas evaluation reveals a *p*H less than 7.35 and a $PaCO_2$ greater than 42 mm Hg in acute respiratory acidosis. When compensation (renal retention of bicarbonate) has fully occurred, the arterial *p*H may be within the lower limits of normal.

Management

Treatment is directed at improving ventilation; exact measures vary with the cause of inadequate ventilation. Pharmacologic agents are used as indicated. For example, bronchodilators help reduce bronchial spasm; antibiotics are used for respiratory infections. Pulmonary hygiene measures are employed, when necessary, to rid the respiratory tract of mucus and purulent drainage. Adequate hydration (2 to 3 liters/day) is indicated to keep the mucous membranes moist and thereby facilitate removal of secretions. Supplemental oxygen is used as necessary. A mechanical ventilator, used cautiously, may improve pulmonary ventilation. Overzealous use of a mechanical ventilator may cause such rapid excretion of carbon dioxide that the kidneys will be unable to eliminate excess bicarbonate with sufficient rapidity to prevent alkalosis and convulsions. For this reason, the elevated $PaCO_2$ must be decreased slowly.

Respiratory Alkalosis (Carbonic Acid Deficit)

Definition and Etiology

Respiratory alkalosis is a clinical condition in which the arterial *p*H is greater than 7.45 and the $PaCO_2$ is less than 38 mm Hg. As with respiratory acidosis, acute and chronic conditions can occur in respiratory alkalosis.

Respiratory alkalosis is always due to hyperventilation, which causes excessive "blowing off" of carbon dioxide and, hence, a decrease in plasma carbonic acid content. Causes can include extreme anxiety, hypoxemia, the early phase of salicylate intoxication, gram-negative bacteremia, and excessive ventilation by mechanical ventilators.

Diagnostic Evaluation

Analysis of arterial blood gases is needed to diagnose respiratory alkalosis. In the acute state, the *p*H is elevated above normal as a result of a low $PaCO_2$ and a normal bicarbonate level. (The kidneys cannot alter the bicarbonate level quickly.) In the compensated state, the kidneys have had sufficient time to lower the bicarbonate level to a suitable level.

Clinical Manifestations

Clinical signs consist of lightheadedness due to vasoconstriction and decreased cerebral blood flow, inability to concentrate, numbness and tingling due to decreased calcium ionization, tinnitus, and at times loss of consciousness.

Management

Treatment depends on the underlying cause of respiratory alkalosis. If due to anxiety, the patient should be made aware that the abnormal breathing pattern is responsible for the symptoms. Instructing the patient to breathe more slowly to cause accumulation of CO_2 or to breathe into a closed system (such as a paper bag) is helpful. Usually a sedative is required to relieve hyperventilation in very anxious patients. Treatment for other causes of respiratory alkalosis is directed at correcting the underlying problem.

Systematic Assessment of Arterial Blood Gases

A systematic approach to the analysis of acid–base disturbances helps to clarify acid–base concepts (Chart 9-1).

Parenteral Fluid Therapy

Purpose

The choice of an intravenous solution depends on the specific purpose for which it is intended. Generally, intravenous fluids are administered to achieve one or more of the following goals:

- To provide water, electrolytes, and nutrients to meet daily requirements
- To replace water and correct electrolyte deficits
- To provide a medium for intravenous drug administration

Intravenous solutions contain dextrose or electrolytes mixed in various proportions with water. Pure or "free" water can never be administered intravenously because it rapidly enters red blood cells and causes them to burst.

Types of Intravenous Solutions

Solutions are often categorized as isotonic, hypotonic, or hypertonic, according to whether their total osmolality is the same as, less than, or greater than that of blood.

Some common water and electrolyte solutions are listed in Table 9-8 with comments about their use. Electrolyte so-

---

Chart 9-1
Systematic Assessment of Arterial Blood Gases

The following steps are recommended to evaluate arterial blood gas values. They are based on the assumption that the average values are

$pH = 7.4$
$PaCO_2 = 40$ mm Hg
$HCO_3^- = 24$ mEq/liter

1. First, look at the pH. It can be high, low, or normal:

   $pH > 7.4$ (alkalosis)
   $pH < 7.4$ (acidosis)
   $pH = 7.4$ (normal)

2. The next step is to determine the primary cause of the disturbance. This is done by evaluating the $PaCO_2$ and HCO_3^- in relation to the pH:

   $pH > 7.4$ (alkalosis):

   a. If the $PaCO_2$ is <40 mm Hg, the primary disturbance is respiratory alkalosis.
   b. If the HCO_3^- is >24 mEq/liter, the primary disturbance is metabolic alkalosis.

   $pH < 7.4$ (acidosis):

   a. If the $PaCO_2$ is >40 mm Hg, the primary disturbance is respiratory acidosis.
   b. If the HCO_3 is <24 mEq/liter, the primary disturbance is metabolic acidosis.

3. The next step involves determining if compensation has begun. This is done by looking at the value other than the primary disorder. If it is moving in the same direction as the primary value, compensation is underway. Consider the following blood gases:

   a. pH 7.20 $PaCO_2 = 60$ mm Hg $HCO_3^- = 23$ mEq/liter
   b. pH 7.40 $PaCO_2 = 60$ mm Hg $HCO_3^- = 37$ mEq/liter

   In "a", respiratory acidosis is present. Note that the CO_2 level is high, while the bicarbonate is normal (uncompensated respiratory acidosis).
   In set "b", the CO_2 is still high, but the HCO_3^- has risen, allowing the pH to return to a normal level (compensated respiratory acidosis).

(Adapted from Metheny N. Fluid and Electrolyte Balance: Nursing Considerations. Philadelphia, JB Lippincott, 1987.)

TABLE 9-8
Selected Water and Electrolyte Solutions

Solution	Comments
0.9% NaCl (Isotonic saline) Na$^+$ 154 mEq/liter Cl$^-$ 154 mEq/liter (308 mOsm/kg) Also available with varying concentrations of dextrose (the most frequently used is a 5% dextrose concentration)	• An isotonic solution that expands the extracellular fluid volume, used in hypovolemic states • Supplies an excess of Na$^+$ and Cl$^-$; can cause fluid volume excess and hyperchloremic acidosis if used in excessive volumes, particularly in patients with compromised renal function • Not desirable as a routine maintenance solution since it provides only Na$^+$ and Cl$^-$ (and these are provided in excessive amounts) • Sometimes used to correct mild Na$^+$ deficit • When mixed with 5% dextrose, the resulting solution becomes hypertonic in relation to plasma and, in addition to the above described electrolytes, provides 170 calories per liter
0.45% NaCl (half-strength saline) Na$^+$ 77 mEq/liter Cl$^-$ 77 mEq/liter (159 mOsm/kg) Also available with varying concentrations of dextrose (the most common is a 5% concentration)	• A hypotonic solution that provides Na$^+$, Cl$^-$, and free water • Free water is desirable to aid the kidneys in elimination of solute • Lacking in electrolytes other than Na$^+$ and Cl$^-$ • When mixed with 5% dextrose, the solution becomes slightly hypertonic to plasma and in addition to the above-described electrolytes provides 170 calories
Lactated Ringer's solution (Hartmann's solution) Na$^+$ 130 mEq/liter K$^+$ 4 mEq/liter Ca^{2+} 3 mEq/liter Cl$^-$ 109 mEq/liter Lactate (metabolized to bicarbonate) 28 mEq/liter (274 mOsm/kg) Also available with varying concentrations of dextrose (the most common is 5% dextrose)	• An isotonic solution that contains multiple electrolytes in roughly the same concentration as found in plasma (note that solution is lacking in Mg^{2+}) • Used in the treatment of hypovolemia, burns, and fluid lost as bile or diarrhea • Does not supply free water for renal excretory purposes; excessive use without provision for free water (as with D$_5$W or hypotonic electrolyte solutions) can cause elevation of the serum sodium level in persons not deficient in sodium • When mixed with 5% dextrose, the resulting solution becomes hypertonic to plasma and provides 170 calories per liter. Of course, the electrolyte concentration remains constant.
5% dextrose in water (D$_5$W) No electrolytes 50 gm of dextrose	• An isotonic solution that supplies 170 calories per liter and free water to aid in renal excretion of solutes • Should not be used in excessive volumes in the early postoperative period (when ADH secretion is increased due to stress reaction) • Should not be used solely in treatment of fluid volume deficit since it dilutes plasma electrolyte concentrations.
3% NaCl (hypertonic saline) Na$^+$ 513 mEq/liter Cl$^-$ 513 mEq/liter (1026 mOsm/kg)	• Grossly hypertonic solution used only in critical situations to treat hyponatremia

(Adapted from Metheny N. Fluid and Electrolyte Balance: Nursing Considerations. Philadelphia, JB Lippincott, 1987.)

lutions are considered isotonic if the total electrolyte content (anions plus cations) approximate 310 mEq/liter. They are considered hypotonic if the total electrolyte content is less than 250 mEq/liter and hypertonic if the total electrolyte content exceeds 375 mEq/liter. The nurse must also consider a solution's osmolality, keeping in mind that the osmolality of plasma is approximately 300 mOsm/liter (SI: 300 mmol/L). For example, a 10% dextrose solution has an approximate osmolality of 505 mOsm/liter.

When administering parenteral fluids, it is important to monitor the patient's response to the fluids. One should con-sider the fluid volume, the content of the fluid, and the patient's clinical status.

Isotonic Fluids

Fluids that are classified as isotonic have a total osmolality close to that of ECF and do not cause red blood cells to shrink or swell. The composition of these fluids may or may not approximate that of ECF, however.

A solution of 5% dextrose in water has a serum osmolality of 252 mOsm/liter. Once administered, the glucose is rapidly metabolized, and this initially isotonic solution then disperses as a hypotonic fluid, one third extracellular and two thirds intracellular. Therefore, 5% dextrose in water is mainly used to supply water and to correct an increased serum osmolality. One liter of 5% dextrose in water provides less than 200 kcal and is a minor source of calories for the body's daily requirements.

Normal saline (0.9% sodium chloride) has a total osmolality of 308 mOsm/liter. Because the osmolality is entirely contributed by electrolytes, the solution remains within the extracellular compartment. For this reason, normal saline is often used to treat an extracellular volume deficit. Although referred to as normal, it contains only sodium and chloride and does not actually simulate ECF.

Several other solutions contain ions in addition to sodium and chloride and are somewhat more similar to ECF in composition. Ringer's solution contains potassium and calcium in addition to sodium chloride. Lactated Ringer's solution contains bicarbonate precursors as well. These solutions are marketed, with slight variations, under a variety of different trade names.

Hypotonic Fluids

One purpose of hypotonic solutions is to replace cellular fluid, because it is hypotonic as compared with plasma. Another is to provide free water for excretion of body wastes. At times, hypotonic sodium solutions are used to treat hypernatremia and other hyperosmolar conditions. Half-strength saline (0.45% sodium chloride) is frequently used. Multiple-electrolyte solutions are also available.

Hypertonic Fluids

When 5% dextrose is added to normal saline or Ringer's solution, the total osmolality exceeds that of ECF. The dextrose is quickly metabolized, however, and only the isotonic solution remains. Therefore, any effect on the intracellular compartment is temporary: Similarly, 5% dextrose is usually added to hypotonic multiple-electrolyte solutions. Once the dextrose is metabolized, these solutions disperse as hypotonic fluids.

Higher concentrations of dextrose, such as 50% dextrose in water, are given to help meet calorie requirements. These solutions are strongly hypertonic and must be administered into central veins so that they can be diluted by rapid blood flow.

Saline solutions are also available in osmolar concentrations greater than that of ECF. These solutions draw water from the intracellular compartment to the extracellular compartment and cause cells to shrink. If given rapidly or in quantity, they may cause an extracellular volume excess and precipitate pulmonary edema. As a result, these solutions are given cautiously and usually only when the serum osmolality has decreased to dangerously low levels.

Other Substances Given Intravenously

When someone's gastrointestinal tract cannot accept food, nutritional requirements are often met intravenously. Parenteral administration may include high concentrations of glucose, protein, or fat to meet nutritional requirements.

Many drugs are also delivered intravenously, either by infusion or directly into the vein. Because intravenous medications circulate rapidly, administration by this route is potentially very hazardous. Administration rates and recommended dilutions for individual drugs are available in specialized texts pertaining to intravenous medications.

Nursing Management of Intravenous Therapy

Venipuncture

The ability to gain access to the venous system is an expected nursing skill in many settings. Components of this responsibility include knowledgeable selection of venipuncture site and type of cannula, and proficiency in the technique of vein entry.

Before proceeding with venipuncture, decisions must be made as to the most appropriate location and type of cannula for a particular patient. Factors influencing these choices include the type of solution to be administered, the expected length of intravenous therapy, the patient's general condition, and the availability of veins. The skill of the person initiating the infusion is also an important consideration.

Choice of Site. Many sites can be used for intravenous therapy, but ease of access and potential hazards vary among them. Veins of the extremities are designated as peripheral locations and are ordinarily the only sites used by nurses. Because they are relatively safe and easy to enter, upper extremity veins are most commonly used. Veins of the arm and hand are shown in Figure 9-7. Leg veins should rarely, if ever, be used, because of the high risk of thromboembolism. Central veins frequently cannulated by physicians include the subclavian and internal jugular veins. It is possible to enter these larger vessels even when peripheral sites have collapsed, and they allow administration of high-osmolar solutions. However, hazards are much greater, including, for example, inadvertent entry into an artery or the pleural space.

Ideally, both arms and hands should be carefully inspected before a specific venipuncture site is chosen. A location should be selected that does not interfere with mobility. For this reason, the antecubital fossa is avoided, except as a last resort. The most distal site of the arm or hand is generally used first so that subsequent IVs can be moved progressively upward. The vein chosen should be palpated for elasticity and absence of hard knots that may indicate thromboses.

Venipuncture Devices. Three main types of cannulas are available: steel scalp vein needles, indwelling plastic catheters inserted over a steel needle, and indwelling plastic catheters inserted through a steel needle. Scalp vein or butterfly needles are short steel needles with plastic wing handles. These are easy to insert but, because they are small and nonpliable, infiltrate easily (Fig. 9-8). Depending on the brand, short plastic catheters inserted over steel needles are called a variety of names, such as Saf-T-Cath (Deseret Pharmaceutical Inc), Longdwel (Becton-Dickinson Company), and Angiocath (Inspiron/Bard Company). Insertion requires the additional step of advancing the catheter into the vein following

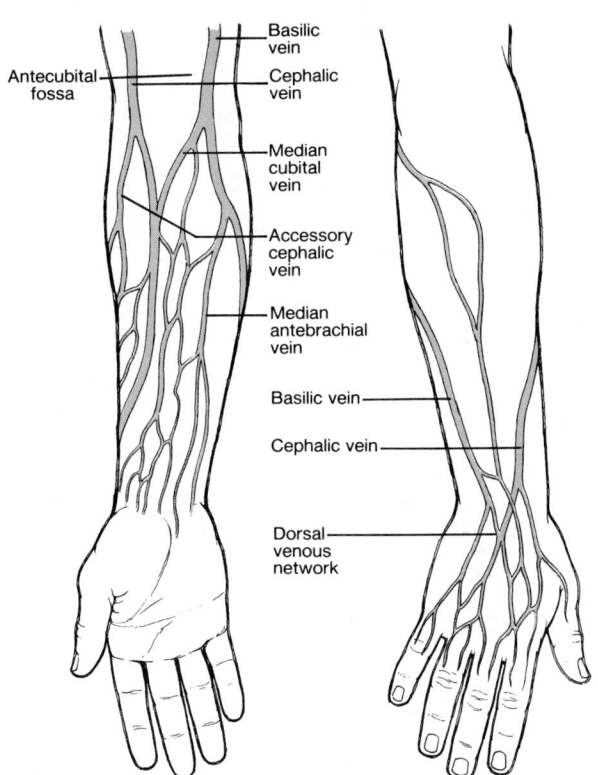

Figure 9-7
Sites of selection for the insertion of intravenous needles for the parenteral administration of fluids or for blood transfusion.

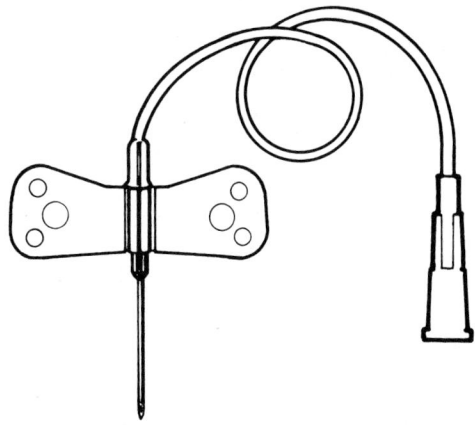

Figure 9-8
Scalp-vein needle: Winged infusion set. (Metheny NM. Fluid and Electrolyte Balance, p 127. Philadelphia, JB Lippincott, 1987.)

venipuncture (Fig. 9-9). Because they are less likely to infiltrate, these devices are frequently preferred over scalp vein needles. Plastic catheters inserted through a hollow needle are usually called intracatheters. They are available in long lengths and are well suited for placement in central locations. Because insertion requires threading the catheter through the vein for a relatively long distance, these are the most difficult catheters to place (Fig. 9-10).

Informing the Patient. Except in emergency situations, a patient should be prepared in advance for having an intravenous infusion. A brief description of the venipuncture

process, information about the expected length of infusion, and restrictions on activities are important topics. An opportunity should also be given for the patient to verbalize concerns. For example, some patients believe they will die if small bubbles in the tubing enter their veins. After acknowledging this fear, the nurse can explain that usually only relatively large quantities of air administered rapidly are fatal.

Preparation of Site. Because infection is the major complication of intravenous therapy, strict asepsis is essential during venipuncture. In addition to hand washing and the use of sterile materials, careful preparation of the site is important. The insertion site should be scrubbed with an iodine-containing agent for 60 seconds, working from the center of the field to the periphery. The solution is allowed to remain on the skin for 2 minutes, then removed with alcohol pledgets. For patients allergic to iodine, vigorous swabbing with alcohol is substituted.

Vein Entry. Guidelines and a suggested sequence for venipuncture are presented in Chart 9-2. For veins that are very small or particularly fragile, modifications in this technique may be necessary. Alternative methods can be found in journal articles or in specialized textbooks of intravenous therapy.

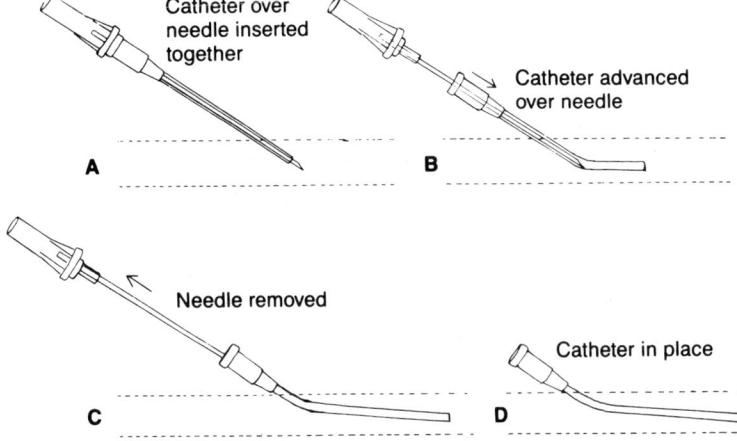

Figure 9-9
Insertion of catheter over a needle. (Kaye W. Intravenous techniques. In Textbook of Advanced Cardiac Life Support, Chap XII, pp 1–12. Dallas, American Heart Association, 1981. Reprinted by permission of the American Heart Association, Inc.)

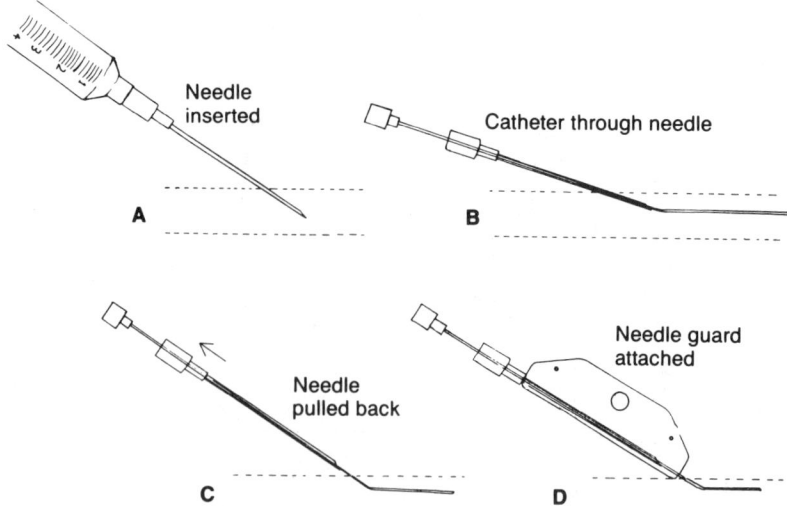

Figure 9-10
Insertion of catheter through a needle. (Kaye W. Intravenous techniques. In Textbook of Advanced Cardiac Life Support, Chap XII, pp 1–12. Dallas, American Heart Association, 1981. Reprinted by permission of the American Heart Association, Inc.)

Monitoring Intravenous Therapy

Maintenance of an existing intravenous infusion is a nursing responsibility that demands knowledge of the solutions being administered and principles of flow. In addition, patients must be assessed carefully for both local and systemic complications.

Factors Affecting the Flow of Intravenous Fluids

The flow of an intravenous infusion is subject to the same principles that govern fluid movement in general.

- *Flow is directly proportional to the height of the liquid column.* Raising the height of the infusion container will sometimes improve a sluggish flow.
- *Flow is directly proportional to the diameter of the tubing.* The clamp on IV tubing regulates the flow by changing the tubing diameter. In addition, the flow will be faster through cannulas of large gauge, as opposed to those of small gauge.
- *Flow is inversely proportional to the length of the tubing.* Adding extension tubing to an IV line will decrease the flow.
- *Flow is inversely proportional to the viscosity of a fluid.* Viscous intravenous solutions, like blood, require a larger cannula than do water or saline solutions.

Monitoring the Flow

Because so many factors influence the flow, a solution does not necessarily continue to run at the speed originally set. Therefore, intravenous infusions must be monitored frequently to ascertain that the fluid is flowing at the intended rate. The IV flask or bag should be marked with tape to indicate at a glance whether the correct amount has infused. The flow rate should be calculated when the solution is originally hung, then rechecked at least hourly. To calculate the flow rate, the number of drops delivered per milliliter must be ascertained. This number varies with equipment and is usually printed on the solution set packaging. A formula that can be used to calculate the drop rate follows:

$$\frac{\text{gtt/ml of given set}}{60 \text{ (min in hour)}} \times \text{total hourly volume} = \text{gtt/min}$$

A variety of infusion pumps are available to assist in intravenous fluid delivery. These pumps are particularly useful when potent medications, such as heparin, are being infused. They do not, however, eliminate the need for frequent monitoring of the infusion.

Discontinuing an Infusion

The removal of an intravenous cannula is associated with two possible dangers: hemorrhage and catheter embolism. To prevent excessive bleeding, a dry, sterile sponge should be held over the site as the cannula is removed. Firm pressure should then be applied until all bleeding has stopped. If a plastic IV catheter is severed, it can travel to the right ventricle and block the blood flow. To prevent this complication during cannula removal, the type and length of the cannula should be ascertained before the IV is discontinued. Plastic catheters should be withdrawn carefully and their length measured to make certain that no fragment has broken off.

Complications Associated with Parenteral Fluid Therapy

Unfortunately, intravenous therapy predisposes to numerous hazards; these include both local and systemic complications. Systemic complications occur less frequently but are often more serious than local complications and include circulatory overload, air embolism, febrile reaction, and infection.

Systemic Complications

Overloading the circulatory system with excessive intravenous fluids will cause increased blood pressure and central venous pressure and even severe dyspnea and cyanosis. This is par-

Chart 9-2
Guidelines for Starting an Intravenous Infusion

Nursing Action

Preparation

1. Verify order for IV therapy, check solution label, and identify patient.
2. Explain procedure to patient.

3. Wash hands.
4. Choose site.

5. Choose IV cannula.

6. Connect infusion flask or bag and tubing, and run solution through tubing to remove air; cover end of tubing.
7. Raise bed to comfortable working height and position for patient; adjust lighting.

Procedure

1. Apply tourniquet 5 to 15 cm (2–6 inches) above injection site; check for radial pulse below tourniquet.

2. Prepare site by scrubbing with iodine-containing solution for 60 seconds in circular motion, moving outward from injection site; allow 2 minutes to dry, then wipe off with alcohol pledget. (If the patient is allergic to iodine, scrub with 70% alcohol.)
3. With hand not holding needle, steady extremity and use finger or thumb to pull skin taut over vessel.
4. Holding needle bevel up and at 45-degree angle, pierce skin to reach but not penetrate vein.
5. Decrease angle of needle until nearly parallel with skin, then enter vein either directly above or from the side.
6. If backflow of blood is visible, straighten angle and advance needle.
   Additional steps for catheter inserted over needle:
   a. Advance needle 0.6 cm (¼ inch) after successful venipuncture.
   b. Hold needle hub, and slide catheter over the needle into the vein. *Never* reinsert needle into a plastic catheter or pull the catheter back into the needle.

   c. Remove needle, while pressing lightly on the skin over the catheter tip; hold catheter hub in place.
7. Release tourniquet, and attach infusion tubing; open clamp enough to allow drip.
8. Slip a sterile 2 × 2 inch gauze pad under the catheter hub.
9. Anchor needle firmly in place with a tape.

10. Apply antimicrobial ointment over site and cover with Band-aid or sterile gauze; tape in place, but do not encircle limb.
11. Tape a small loop of IV tubing onto dressing.

12. Label dressing with type and length of cannula, date, and initials.
13. Calculate drop rate, and regulate flow of infusion.

14. Document site, cannula type, and time in chart.

Rationale

1. Serious errors can be avoided by careful checking.

2. Knowledge increases both patient comfort and cooperation.
3. Asepsis is essential to prevent infection.
4. Careful site selection will increase likelihood of successful venipuncture and preservation of vein.
5. Length and gauge of cannula should be appropriate for both site and purpose of infusion.
6. Equipment must be attached immediately following successful venipuncture to prevent clotting.
7. Proper positioning will increase likelihood of success and provide comfort for patient.

1. The tourniquet distends the vein and makes it easier to enter; it should never be tight enough to occlude arterial flow.
2. Strict asepsis and careful site preparation is essential to prevent infection.

3. Applying traction to the vein helps to stabilize it.

4. Bevel-up position usually produces less trauma to skin and vein.
5. Two-stage procedure decreases chance of thrusting needle through posterior wall of vein as skin is entered.
6. Backflow may not occur if vein is small; this position decreases chance of puncturing posterior wall of vein.

   a. Advancing the needle slightly makes certain the plastic catheter has entered the vein.
   b. Reinsertion of the needle or pulling the catheter back can sever the catheter, causing catheter embolism.

   c. Slight pressure prevents bleeding before tubing is attached.
7. Infusion must be attached promptly to prevent clotting in cannula.
8. The gauze acts as a sterile field.

9. A stable needle is less likely to become dislodged or to irritate the vein.
10. Antimicrobial ointments somewhat decrease risk of infection; tape encircling extremity can act as tourniquet.

11. The loop decreases the chance of inadvertent cannula removal if the tubing is pulled.
12. Labeling facilitates assessment and safe discontinuation.
13. Infusion must be regulated carefully to prevent overinfusion or underinfusion
14. Documentation is essential to facilitate care and for legal purposes.

ticularly likely to occur in patients with cardiac disease and is referred to as *circulatory overload.*

The danger of *air embolism* is always present, even though it does not occur frequently. It is most often associated with cannulation of central veins. The presence of air embolism may be manifested by dyspnea and cyanosis, hypotension, weak rapid pulse, and loss of consciousness. The amount of air necessary to induce death in humans is not known. Some sources state that as little as 10 ml of air may be fatal in seriously ill patients. Apparently, the rate of entry is as important as the actual volume of air.

The presence of pyrogenic substances in either the infusion solution or the administration setup can induce a *febrile reaction.* With such a reaction, one might observe an abrupt temperature elevation shortly after the infusion is started, backache, headache, general malaise, and, if severe, vascular collapse.

Infection ranges in severity from local involvement of the insertion site to systemic dissemination of organisms through the bloodstream. Measures to prevent infection are essential at the time of insertion and throughout the entire period of infusion. Some of these include the following:

- Careful hand washing before every contact with any part of the infusion system or patient
- Examination of flasks or bags for cracks, leaks, or cloudiness, which may indicate a contaminated solution
- Strict asepsis
- Firm anchoring of the IV cannula to prevent to-and-fro motion
- Daily IV site inspection and replacement of sterile dressing (application of an antimicrobial ointment to the insertion site probably confers a slight additional benefit)
- Removal of the IV cannula at the first sign of local inflammation
- Replacement of the IV cannula every 48 hours
- Replacement of the IV cannula inserted during emergency conditions (with questionable asepsis) as soon as possible
- Replacement of the flask or bag every 24 hours and the entire administration set at least every 48 hours, and every 24 hours when blood or lipid products are being infused

Local Complications

Local complications of intravenous therapy include infiltration, phlebitis, and thrombophlebitis.

Dislodging of a needle and local infiltration of the solution into subcutaneous tissues is not uncommon. *Infiltration* is characterized by edema at the site of the injection, pain and discomfort in the area of infiltration, and significant decrease in the flow rate. When the solution is particularly irritating, sloughing of tissue may result. Close monitoring of the insertion site is necessary to detect infiltration before it becomes severe. Infiltration is easily recognized if the insertion area is larger than an identical region in the opposite extremity. However, infiltration is not always so obvious. A common misconception is that a backflow of blood into the tubing proves that the cannula is properly placed within the vein. However, if the catheter tip has pierced the wall of the vessel, intravenous fluid will seep into tissues as well as flow into the vein. A more reliable means of confirming infiltration is

to apply a tourniquet above or proximal to the infusion site and tighten it enough to restrict venous flow. If the infusion continues to drip despite the venous obstruction, infiltration is present.

Phlebitis is defined as inflammation of a vein and is evidenced by heat, redness, and swelling at the injection site. The incidence of phlebitis increases with the length of time the intravenous line is in place. *Thrombophlebitis* refers to the presence of a clot plus inflammation in the vein. It is evidenced by localized heat, redness, swelling, and hardness of the vein.

Summary

The administration of intravenous fluids is frequently managed by nurses. Although it is a common and extremely important form of treatment, intravenous therapy is associated with several serious hazards. These potential risks include infection, embolism, and fluid and electrolyte imbalances. By the use of aseptic technique during every contact with the apparatus, application of principles of flow, and frequent patient assessment, the nurse can reduce the likelihood of any of these complications.

Bibliography

Books

Doenges M, Jeffries M, and Moorhouse M. Nursing Care Plans: Nursing Diagnoses in Planning Patient Care. Philadelphia, FA Davis, 1984.

Goldberger E. A Primer of Water, Electrolyte & Acid–Base Syndromes, 7th ed. Philadelphia, Lea & Febiger, 1986.

Kim M, McFarland G, and McLane A. A Pocket Guide to Nursing Diagnoses. St Louis, CV Mosby, 1984.

Kokko JP and Tannen RL. Fluids and Electrolytes. Philadelphia, WB Saunders, 1986.

Lamb J. Laboratory Tests for Clinical Nursing. Bowie, Maryland, Robert J Brady, 1984.

Leaf A and Cotran R. Renal Pathophysiology, 3rd ed. New York, Oxford University Press, 1985.

Metheny N. Fluid and Electrolyte Balance: Nursing Considerations. Philadelphia, JB Lippincott, 1987.

Pennington J and Church H. Bowes and Church's Food Values of Portions Commonly Used, 14th ed. Philadelphia, JB Lippincott, 1985.

Pestano C. Fluids and Electrolytes in the Surgical Patient, 3rd ed. Baltimore, Williams & Wilkins, 1985.

Rose B. Clinical Physiology of Acid–Base & Electrolyte Disorders, 2nd ed. New York, McGraw-Hill, 1984.

Scherer J. Lippincott's Nurses' Drug Manual. Philadelphia, JB Lippincott, 1985.

Schrier R. Renal and Electrolyte Disorders, 3rd ed. Boston, Little, Brown, & Co, 1986.

Shapiro B. Clinical Application of Respiratory Care, 3rd ed. Chicago, Year Book Medical Publishers, 1985.

Toledo-Pereyra L. The Pancreas-Principles of Medical and Surgical Practice. New York, John Wiley & Sons, 1985.

Articles

(Asterisks indicate nursing research articles.)

Adams M and Condon R. Fluid and electrolyte therapy. In Condon R and Nyhus L (eds). Manual of Surgical Therapeutics, 6th ed. Boston, Little, Brown, & Co, 1985.

Adler S. Electrolyte abnormalities: classify sodium and potassium imbalances to speed therapy. Consultant 1985 Mar 15; 25(5):76–80.

Barkin J et al. Hypercalcemia associated with cancer of prostate without bony metastases. Urology 1984 Oct; 24(4):368–371.

Batuman V et al. Renal and electrolyte effects of total parenteral nutrition. JPEN 1984 Sept/Oct; 8(5):546–551.

Bidani A. Electrolyte and acid–base disorders. Med Clin North Am 1986 Sept; 70(5):1013–1036.

Boineau F and Lewy J. Parenteral fluid therapy for infants and children. In Rakel R (ed). Conn's Current Therapy. Philadelphia, WB Saunders, 1986.

Burman R and Berkowitz HS. IV bolus: effective, but potentially hazardous. Crit Care Nurs 1986 Jan/Feb; 6(1):22–27.

Burnakis T et al. Combined therapy with captopril and potassium supplementation: a potential for hyperkalemia. Arch Intern Med 1984 Dec; 144(12):2371–2372.

Delmez J. Fluid and electrolyte disturbances. In Campbell J and Frisse M (eds). Manual of Medical Therapeutics, 24th ed. Boston, Little, Brown, & Co, 1983.

DeRubertis FR. Hypercalcemia and hypocalcemia. Top Emerg Med 1984 Jan; 5(4):64–78.

*Drew D and Shumann D. Homogeneity of potassium chloride in small volume intravenous containers. Nurs Res 1986 Dec; 35(6):325–329.

Epstein Y et al. Fluid balance in hot climates: sweating, water intake, and prevention of dehydration. Public Health Rev 1985; 13(1/2):115–137.

Evans RA. Hypercalcaemia—what does it signify? Drugs 1986; 31(1):64–74.

Finberg L. Oral electrolyte/glucose solutions. J Pediatr 1984 Dec; 105(6):939–940.

Gaz RD and Wang C. Management of asymptomatic hyperparathyroidism. Am J Surg 1984 Apr; 147(4):498–502.

Gleit C et al. The role of calcium and estrogen in osteoporosis. Orthop Nurs 1985 May/June; 4(3):13–18.

Goldman J et al. Vitamin D and hypercalcemia (letter). JAMA 1985 Oct 4; 254(13):1719.

Goldstein C et al. Syndrome of inappropriate antidiuretic hormone secretion in advanced age (letter). Ann Intern Med 1985 Apr; 102(4):563.

Gould R et al. Potentially fatal cardiac dysrhythmia and hyperkalemic periodic paralysis. Neurology 1985 Aug; 35(8):1208–1212.

Greenburg A. Common emergencies of acid–base balance. Topics Emerg Med 1984 Jan; 5(4):1–16.

Hakki A-H et al. A simple formula for monitoring parenteral infusion. Crit Care Nurs 1986 May/June; 6(3):57–62.

Havestadt C et al. Electrolytes and ventricular arrhythmias. Magnesium 1985; 4(1):29–33.

Huerta B et al. Potassium imbalance in the coronary unit. Heart Lung 1985 Mar; 14(2):193–195.

Jamieson M. Hyponatremia. Br Med J (Clin Res) 1985 June 8; 290(6483):1723–1728.

Johnson D. Fluid and electrolyte dysfunction in alcoholism. Crit Care Q 1986 Mar; 8(4):53–64.

Kingston M et al. Treatment of severe hypophosphatemia. Crit Care Med 1985 Jan; 13(1):16–18.

Knochel J. Hypokalemia. Adv Intern Med 1984; 30:317–335.

Kromhout D et al. Potassium, calcium, alcohol intake and blood pressure: the Zutphen study. Am J Clin Nutr 1985 June; 41(6):1299–1304.

Lorch V et al. Treatment of hyperkalemia with exchange transfusion. Transfusion 1985 July/Aug; 25(4):390–391.

Mascaro J. Managing I.V. therapy in the home. Nursing '86 1986 May; 16(5):50–51.

McCarron DA and Morris CD. Calcium, parathyroid hormone, and hypertension. Adv Nephrol 1985; 14:479–501.

McFadden EA, Zaloga GP, and Chernow B. Hypocalcemia: A medical emergency. Am J Nurs 1983 Feb; 83(2):225–230.

McGovern B. Hypokalemia and cardiac arrhythmias. Anesthesiology 1985 Aug; 63(2):927–929.

Nanji A. Symptomatic hypercalcemia precipitated by magnesium therapy. Postgrad Med J 1985 Jan; 61(711):47–48.

Nelson R and Miller H. Keeping air out of I.V. lines. Nursing '86 1986 Mar; 16(3):57–59.

Nieman GF. Current concepts of lung-fluid balance. Respir Care 1985 Dec; 30(12):1062–1076.

Otrakji J. Disorders of potassium metabolism. Top Emerg Med 1983 July; 5(2):53–57.

Pfister S and Bullas JB. Interpreting arterial blood gas values. Crit Care Nurs 1986 July/Aug; 6(4):9–14.

Recker R et al. The effect of milk supplements: bone metabolism and calcium balance. Am J Clin Nutr 1985 Feb; 4(2):254–263.

Romanski SO. Interpreting ABGs. Nursing '86 1986 Sept; 16(9):58–63.

Scholten D. Electrolytes and plasma volume regulation in hypovolemic shock. Am J Emerg Med 1984 Jan; 2(1):86–91.

Schrier R. Treatment of hyponatremia. N Engl J Med 1985 Apr 25; 312(17):1121–1123.

Sneid D. Hypercalcemia. Top Emerg Med 1983 July; 5(2):8–17.

Stanaszek W. Current approaches to management of potassium deficiency. Drug Intell Clin Pharm 1985 Mar; 19(3):176–183.

Stuhler-Schlag MK. Pre and postoperative fluids and electrolytes. Today's OR Nurse 1982 Sept; 4(7):11–15, 66–67.

Thomas AG. Disorders of sodium metabolism. Top Emerg Med 1983 July; 5(2):46–52.

Todd B. Can osteoporosis be treated? Geriatr Nurs 1985 Nov/Dec; 6(6):359–360.

Verbalis JG and Robinson AG. Hypernatremia and hyponatremia. Top Emerg Med 1984 Jan; 5(4):79–89.

Zucker AR and Chernow B. Diabetes insipidus and the syndrome of inappropriate antidiuretic hormone release. Crit Care Q 1983 Dec; 6(3):63–74.

Chapter 10

Developmental Concepts of the Adult Life Phase

During the past 75 years, the major efforts in research, theory building, and life stage development have been focused on and devoted to childhood, adolescence, and old age. The time of early adulthood, encompassing the chronological ages of 18 to 35, and the time of middle adulthood, ages 36 to 60, until recently have been relatively uncharted and unexplored aspects of the life span. The main development attributed to this period in life consists of simultaneous processes of change and continuity. This chapter focuses on an overview of early, middle, and late adulthood, stressing aspects of developmental changes, transitions, and tasks, as well as themes and variations of human life.

Stages of Adulthood

Books, monographs, and reports treating the concerns of early and middle adulthood began to appear in 1976. These efforts in research, theory building, and life stage development focused on the divisions of adulthood and the major question of what it means to be an adult. The divisions of adulthood, as developed by theoreticians, have been subdivided into approximately 11 stages, as shown in Chart 10-1.

Note that there are overlapping age dates in the various stages; this is due both to differences in theories about stage development and to the difficulty involved in applying specific age classifications to all people.

The major question of what it means to be an adult is divided into several subquestions:

- What are the things that I can expect in my development?
- Is what is happening to me normal?
- Will there be order in my life throughout the adult years as there was during childhood and adolescence?
- How will I adjust to the losses and changes in my personal identity?

The issues and essential problems of adult life, as well as the sources of its disappointments, joys, griefs, and fulfillment, are all topics of research and investigation.

Interest in adult development was originally prompted by the increasing number of people entering this period of life. However, although interest was intensifying, there was also reluctance to explore this phase of life because of anxiety and the fear that deliberate and organized scrutiny would uncover many negative factors. Dread of the process of change, unfulfilled expectations, decline, and decay were ever present.

Early Adulthood Transition (17–22 Years)

The myth that "now that you are 21 you have all the attributes for success" is scary to many young adults. Although young adults are biologically and legally adults at 21, they receive conflicting messages from society. "You're only young once," heard simultaneously with "You should be getting on with your life," can produce confusion, indecision, impulsiveness, and sometimes irrational and destructive behavior patterns. Most people in early adulthood are fearful of leaving the pre-adult world. People in this age-group have been instructed to believe that they must separate from their parents financially, socially, and psychologically and learn to become independent. Yet, during this period of life, most young adults believe that they will always belong to their parents and that their parents will support them financially, psychologically, and socially, no matter what happens. They believe in their parents' world.

Parents are the bulwark of young adults. Many people in their late teens and early 20s think that only their parents will keep them safe and that their parents represent the only "true" family they will ever have. Often, marriage at this time is a means of breaking away from the parents and gaining greater independence; however, in many cases such marriages result in greater dependence and are likely to fail. Marrying to get away from one's parents is one of the most common unstated reasons for marriage and one of the poorest foundations for its success.

At this time also, the young adult must pull away from adolescent peers and give up hero worship of teachers and adulation of significant others. The relinquishment of these once important experiences and the changes that result may produce a sense of loss, feelings of anxiety, and fear about one's personal future.

Entering the Adult World (22–28 Years)

The chronological age period of 22 to 28, although described as relatively tranquil in comparison to early adulthood transition, is marked by many confrontations with reality and the collapse of childhood myths. This is a period described as "postponement." Young people are postponing traditional social responsibility and allowing themselves personal space.

Confronting Childhood Myths. In childhood, it was sufficient to tell adults in authority that one had tried, even if the effort was unsuccessful. The child received positive reinforcement for just making the effort. In adulthood, one must learn that trying is not enough and that it will not suffice to make excuses for one's efforts. Positive reinforcement will not be forthcoming for merely trying. Rewards will be given solely for meeting the standard of what the "prudent man," in whatever state of life, would do.

The adult in this period of life must discard the fallacious thinking that if one does all the right things, one will automatically be rewarded. The person must realize that following

Chart 10-1
Stages of Adulthood

1. Early adulthood transition	17 to 22 years
2. Entering the adult world	22 to 28 years
3. Age 30 transition	28 to 33 years
4. Settling down period	33 to 40 years
5. Mid-life transition	35 to 45 years
6. Entering middle adulthood	45 to 50 years
7. Age 50 transition	48 to 55 years
8. Culmination of middle adulthood	55 to 60 years
9. Late adulthood transition	60 to 65 years
10. Late adulthood	65 to 80 years
11. Late late adulthood	80+ years

the activity patterns of one's parents does not guarantee success, and that one should not expect or anticipate parental intervention when one's projects are faltering. The idea that parents will always be available to rescue the young adult fosters increasing dependence, which precludes growth toward adult maturity.

One of the most difficult myths to dispel is the belief that there is only one right way to do things. Black-and-white thinking must be shaded with gray in order to begin successful interaction in the adult world. The realization that fair treatment of others does not guarantee fairness in return is not easily accepted by this age-group. The idea that a rational approach toward and commitment to important life events will ensure the results that one wants must be abandoned. These beliefs, adopted in childhood and reinforced in adolescence, must be challenged and rethought in adulthood.

Rejecting one of the major premises of our society, that working hard will always bring success, is extremely difficult for the young adult, who has grown up hearing this prescription for succeeding in life. On the personal level, the young adult needs to realize that reliance on self and self-direction must supplant the expectation that his or her spouse or children will provide personal fulfillment. Failure to relinquish this expectation often leads to highly disturbed situations.

Establishing Relationships. The transition into early adulthood has two unique dimensions that must be noted. The first is that during this period many people establish a relationship with a mentor, an older and more experienced person who assists the young person in entering his or her chosen field of work. Initially, the mentor is superior to the young person, but gradually the relationship becomes equalized. Eventually, young adults give up their mentors in much the same way they gave up their parents.

The second relationship is formed with a special man or woman who brings out the young person's affectionate, romantic, and sexual feelings and simultaneously serves as a critic, guide, and sponsor as the person works toward his or her goals. This special person fulfills a transitional role by helping the young adult to move from dependency on father and mother toward autonomous independence.

Finding Oneself. In addition to the task of confronting childhood myths about how life is managed, this period requires extensive exploration of life structures and the making of tentative commitments that can be modified if necessary. It is a time for broadening one's experience and approaching life with a sense of adventure. However, later in this period some hard life choices must be faced. The person must consider whether or not to marry, whether to seek a job or a career, and how to establish goals to be pursued. During this period, both men and women confront the conflict inherent in trying to meet the contradictory demands of marriage and work. Premature commitments in one or both of these areas are often questioned at this time.

Age 30 Transition (28–33 Years)

The hallmark of the age 30 transition for many people is the growing awareness that if a change is to be made, it must be made soon; otherwise, one will be riveted to commitments made in the 20s, and future possibilities for desired change will be ruled out. This stage of aging is often characterized by a period of depression, which is usually alleviated when the person develops a different perspective of the world and its inhabitants. It can also be identified as a period of discovery (or rediscovery) of suppressed feelings, interests, aptitudes, talents, and goals that have been ignored or deeply hidden. A realistic understanding of one's strengths, abilities, and liabilities is a formidable task to be undertaken at this time. If the task is successfully completed, the person becomes aware both of the contradictory feelings competing within himself and of similar feelings that originate in the outside world.

In the age 30 transition, there is a greater sense of urgency. Life is more serious, more restrictive, and more real. For many people, the age of 30 provides a long-awaited second chance to construct a more satisfactory life structure.

Settling Down (33–40 Years)

The transitional period of the late 20s and early 30s is usually followed by a calmer period characterized as "settling down." Settling down is interpreted as that period in life when one takes a hard look at what is really important, becomes serious about a few major goals, and begins to build a life structure around the determined choices. Selecting and purchasing a home at this time fulfills the need of many people to establish roots and become more home oriented. The need to establish a niche is further extended by a focus on childrearing, which often results in a decline in marital satisfaction. By this time, the romanticism of marriage has lapsed into daily routine.

Consolidating One's Position. In the world of work, advancement becomes a major task. Conflict often occurs because the young person must challenge senior people in the establishment, the very people who have the power to grant or deny the bid for advancement. In this vulnerable position, the young adult often feels both oppressed by others and restrained by internal conflicts and inhibitions. Despite these difficulties, this is a period of extending and attempting to solidify one's position in the work force and at home.

Mid-Life Transition (35–45 Years)

The adage that life begins at 40 was heralded as a great positive statement of life; however, many adults secretly believe that life ends at 40 and that this age marks the end of a fulfilling, exciting, and self-directed life. Stereotypes of being 40 only add to internal confusion, because in the 40s individual differences are becoming more significant. Many people go through difficult changes in the 40s that are often compared with the changes of adolescence (labeled "middlescence"). Some people experience mild self-questioning. The true feelings of dread about entering middle age have kept this stage of life a well-guarded secret. The mid-life transition is a bridge between early and middle adulthood. It is a point in time when one begins to count the years that are left, rather than all those that are yet to come.

Reappraising the Past. The initial task of this transitional phase is to reappraise the past. The awareness of one's mortality is uppermost in the consciousness. One is confronted with a limited amount of time remaining and a desire to use that time wisely. This is a time when the person's previous life structure comes seriously into question, and answers must be found to questions that assume a new importance:

- How satisfactory is my present life structure—how meaningful to myself, how meaningful to the world?
- How shall that life structure be changed to provide a better basis for the future?

Discarding Illusions. One of the profound discoveries made at this time is the extent to which one's life has been based on illusion. A formidable task that must be undertaken is the process of "de-illusionment"—dealing with the recognition that many long-held and cherished assumptions about oneself and the world are not true. Although one may have been indulged in childhood to encourage imaginative development, as an adult, one is expected to be more realistic and practical. Dispensing with illusions is considered desirable and is anticipated as a natural step in attaining maturity. At the same time, it is also the process through which a person is stripped of most of his cherished values, beliefs, and opinions about life and people. The result may be feelings either of irreparable loss or of being liberated so that one may develop more flexible values, beliefs, and opinions. One may be able to look at oneself and others in a more genuine, less idealized manner.

Adapting to Change. As time passes in this life phase, a major task is to modify the life structure of the 30s transition so that it will become appropriate to middle adulthood. External changes at this time, such as distance in the marital relationship (sometimes better, sometimes worse), children grown and leaving home, and parents dead or dependent, have a specific impact on the role expectations of the person as a spouse, family member, son, or daughter.

Changes in a person's position in the work force have a profound impact. As the character of work alters, the person must change with the innovations or be left behind. World events, social movements, and economic conditions affect each person according to age and period of development.

The internal changes in a person's life structure are significant at this juncture. It is quite common to revise one's social outlook, personal values and goals, and career objectives. Many people describe a feeling of "internal slippage" at this time.

Coming to Terms with Mortality and Creative/Destructive Forces. The mid-life transition activates one's awareness of death and destruction. The person becomes aware of his mortality as well as of the actual and impending death of significant others; he also realizes that significant persons in his life have acted destructively toward him with both good and bad intentions in mind. He, in turn, has inflicted irrevocable hurt on parents, spouse, lovers, children, friends, and colleagues with the same mixed motivation. In middle adulthood, one becomes painfully aware of the ability to be simultaneously creative and destructive while working toward control of these powerful forces.

Achieving Individualization. At mid-life, people must come to terms with the synchronous existence of masculine and feminine parts of the self. A man must integrate his powerful need for attachment to others with his antithetical but equally important need for separateness. A woman must integrate her new-found need for separateness and achievement with her lesser need for attachment. As the individualization process occurs, the person becomes a more differentiated and complex human; most important, he develops effective boundaries that link him to the external world with a more satisfying interaction process.

Entering Middle Adulthood (45–50 Years)

Mature adulthood is not a period of stability and certainty, but rather one of change. The changes that occur during this stage of life have no absolute chronological or sequential order, although certain events are biologically, psychologically, and socially determined or expected. The impact of these changes, which often include new sets of relationships, new expectations, and altered or modified evaluations of self, inevitably involves the adult in transitions or turning points. The events of adult life entail either role gains or role losses. Getting married, having a child, acquiring a new home, obtaining a job, and receiving a promotion are usually perceived as role gains. Becoming separated, getting a divorce, being chronically ill, retiring from work, going through menopause, and being widowed are perceived as role losses.

The main themes of adulthood include stress, stock-taking and *locus of control,* shifts in time perspective, changes in biological and psychological functioning, generational roles, sex role reversal, and the evolution of careers and activities.

Stress. The primary source of stress for middle-aged men is their work. For middle-aged women, stress is often a result of their concern for their husbands' work and health; their own health and physical appearance and the events in the lives of their children are a secondary cause.

Stock-Taking, Locus of Control. Although adults of any age may go through the process of reassessment, the stock-taking of middle age is characterized by a focus on the inner self, a concern with self-development, and a reexamination and reevaluation of competency. The period of "middlescence" often causes people to see their children as capable of getting more enjoyment from sex, love, and life in general than they can; moreover, at the same time, they are aware that their children view them as being on the decline. For some middle-aged people, the position of being "caught between two generations" intensifies a sense of loss and a fear of aging; it also confirms the feeling that they are no longer masters of their fates and their environments.

People inclined toward this view may be described as having an *external locus of control,* in that they feel like puppets on a string, controlled by other people, impersonal social forces, or fate. On the other hand, people with an *internal locus of control* perceive themselves as having power over their own destinies. These are the people who view middle adulthood as a period of maximum capacity that underscores their ability to handle a highly complex environment and more challenging self-goals. For these people, stock-taking produces a renewed sense of self as they triumph over difficulties and develop new coping skills. For others, however, it is a time of feeling trapped, anxious, or panic-stricken by life events. Many of these people become immobilized and are unable to act, thus sinking into deeper depression.

Shift in Time Perspective. One of the most startling events in middle age is a shift in time perspective; one starts thinking in terms of the time left to live, rather than the time lived since birth. This awareness of mortality appears to be somewhat more important to men than to women. Men become more conscious of their loss of strength and vitality, more preoccupied with their health, and more fearful that time is running out. Women become more concerned with the health of the significant people in their lives, particularly their spouses. Women may "rehearse for widowhood" by fantasizing about being on their own. However, like men, they become overwhelmingly aware that they have little time left.

The shift in time perspective brings a confrontation with death that is now a personal reality rather than something that happens to other people. An awareness that life in middle age is not progressing as smoothly as was expected may lead middle-aged adults to believe they are abnormal. They often do not realize that other adults experience the same self-doubts, feelings of helplessness, lost hopes, and sense of inadequacy that they are experiencing.

Changes in Biological Functioning. Although biological decline for most people ordinarily occurs gradually, several minute changes often bring about a major qualitative drop in bodily function by the early 40s. It is necessary to exercise extreme caution when making generalizations about physical changes during the adult years—not only about when they will happen, but whether they will, in fact, occur at all. There is no physical change that can be predicted to happen to all adults. It should be noted that the ages discussed are averages and not absolutes. People deviate widely from these averages at both ends. Some people die of "old age" in their 40s, whereas others live to be well over 100.

Generally, one has reached maximum strength by age 30. After this point in life, there is a slight but steady loss of strength through the adult years. The points of experienced weakness occur more in the back and leg muscles and less in the arm muscles. These weaknesses can be halted by individualized exercise that is undertaken on a regular basis.

The loss of physical attributes takes its greatest toll on people who derive their feelings of worth from their bodies. People who value themselves for their strength or beautiful bodies exhibit psychological patterns of aging as soon as their bodies begin to age significantly. An overemphasis on physical development and beauty in childhood and adolescence can boomerang in maturity and later adult years.

Changes in health during adulthood are not all negative. Middle age does not necessarily bring poor health. Many people live all their adult years without ever being sick or incapacitated in any way. In general, adults can expect fewer acute illnesses, fewer accidents, and more chronic illness.

Sensory Acuity. In the area of the senses, the process of aging starts in infancy. Visual acuity for most people is best at about 20, remains relatively constant to 40, and then, barring gross organic difficulties, begins a slow decline. Hearing, like sight, seems to be at its peak at about 20; from about 20 on, a gradual loss occurs that affects high tones more than low tones and, after age 55, more men than women. Furthermore, after 50 there is a higher incidence of loss of ability to distinguish the finer nuances of taste, although the four basic tastes of sweet, sour, salt, and bitter remain constant. There also appears to be a sharp decrease in the sense of touch after 45.

In the area of sensitivity to pain, there is marked disagreement. Some theorists believe that sensitivity to pain tends to remain steady to approximately age 50 and then declines for different parts of the body, occasioning an increase in pain tolerance. Other theorists believe that the consciousness of pain increases after 50, making older people victims of wide pain sensitivity. The one sense that seems to retain a high level of effectiveness is balance, which is at its best between 40 and 50.

Physical Appearance and Health. One's physical appearance and physical health are probably the most important factors in determining how one approaches everyday life. The influence of physical appearance on physical health can be seen in the attention a person pays to nutrition, exercise, and relaxation. Although there is a minimal amount of physical change throughout early adulthood, middle age is often characterized by dramatic changes in appearance. Probably the most obvious change perceived by others is weight gain. Redistribution of body fat makes the body structure look like a diamond—narrow at both ends and heavy in the middle. The thinning and color change of hair are also noticeable physical changes. Many men in their 40s begin to experience hairline recession, reduced hair growth, and ultimate baldness. By the 50s, both women and men are at least gray, if not white-haired. Women begin to experience some hair growth on their upper lips and chins at this time also.

For both men and women, the skin loses elasticity and becomes coarser and darker on the face, arms, and hands. Wrinkles and looseness of the skin also appear. The lower part of the face changes because of alterations in teeth, bone, muscles, and connective tissues. The voice loses timbre and quality and becomes more high-pitched. The physical movements of the body become less graceful owing to joint stiffening and loss of resiliency in the muscles. The cumulative effects of these changes make it painful for the middle-aged adult to look at himself in a mirror.

Psychological Functioning. In the area of psychological functioning, the middle-aged adult recognizes that of all age-groups, his is the most powerful. Despite the fact that society is oriented toward youth, it is controlled by the middle-aged. They are the norm-bearers and the policy makers. Furthermore, middle age is generally a period of heightened sensitivity to one's position in a highly complex and confusing social environment. Assessing and reassessing oneself is a major and continual theme throughout this period of life.

Psychologically, the rewards associated with middle age are not as easily discerned as those of early adulthood and old age. In early adulthood, chronological aging (*i.e.*, getting older) means becoming increasingly eligible for adult rewards, such as more status, power, and attractivness, whereas ad-

vanced old age means receiving rewards for simply surviving; each additional year lived brings a mark of distinction. The middle-aged rely more on the functioning of their bodies, career status, and family cycles to determine their identities than on chronological age. Since changes in these aspects of their lives are not synchronized or predictable, the middle-aged often experience intense conflict and confusion.

Relating to Other Generations. One of the major psychological stresses is the distance the middle-aged experience from both the younger and the older generations. In general, the distance from the young is much greater; younger people can neither understand nor relate to the middle-aged because they lack the necessary life experience. The particular historical events of living create a bond between people who have lived through them together and a distance from those who have not. Although there is also a certain degree of distance between the middle-aged and the elderly, the sense of proximity and identification with them is more intense, because those who are older have experienced what it is like to be middle-aged. There is often a tendency to blur the differences between the middle-aged and the older generation.

Although most middle-aged people have either become or are in the process of becoming aware of the finiteness of time, very few express a desire to be young again. Rather, they wish to have again the vigor and appearance of youth while enjoying the authority and autonomy they have acquired.

A special task of the middle-aged adult is to become more conscious of both the child and the older person within himself and others. Attention to this task allows him to transcend, at least in some degree, the barriers that tend to separate the generations. It is important because one of the major enrichments in life is learning how to be successful in relating in a fully human way to people of all ages.

Relationships between generations are important in all societies. Although most people are aware of profound differences between generations, one can concentrate on increasing positive interaction between them. At each stage of development, people carry within themselves aspects of every generation. However, it is difficult for the child and the adolescent to visualize the "older self" and to develop empathy for persons who are more than 10 years older than they are.

The concept of generation is, for the most part, poorly understood. Members of a given generation are classified at the same age level by contrasting them to both younger and older generations. As years pass, a young adult develops a sense of moving from one generation to the next and of establishing new relationships with the other generations in his world. During adulthood, other persons are roughly the same age if they are not more than 6 or 7 years older or younger. Thus, one's own generation covers a span of some 12 to 15 years. A half generation includes an age spread of from 8 to 15 years in either direction. An older person in a generational relationship maintains an implicit claim to greater authority in the relationship and is often viewed as an older sibling. As the age difference increases to 20 years and beyond, a full generation is marked, and the older person in the relationship carries a parental role. When the age difference is 40 years or more, there is a distance of two generations, and the older person is often viewed as a symbolic grandparent.

A new and troubling change in generational status begins in the late 30s and is usually well established by the middle 40s. People in their 40s are usually regarded by people in their 20s as a full generation removed and as part of the "establishment." Furthermore, the people in their 40s are often perceived as parental figures and, at a deeper level, as becoming "old," losing their place in society, and having lost their capacity for youthful adventures. More frightening to these people is the growing realization that they are leaving the youthful generation and entering the vaguest and most poorly defined of all generations—"the middle-aged."

Generativity vs. Stagnation. The theory of the life cycle developed by Erik Erikson encompasses stages from early childhood to late adulthood. The stage that has the most relevance to the middle-aged is that of "generativity versus stagnation." Generativity means the ability to develop authority in younger persons and to establish mutuality with them. It also means offering leadership to younger people while simultaneously treating them as adults and encouraging them to develop greater independence and personal authority. Stagnation refers to the sense of not growing, that is, being static and bogged down in a life that is full of heavy obligations and devoid of self-fulfillment.

The middle-aged person, if generative, is becoming a senior member of the adult world and must learn to relate to persons in their 30s as junior but fully adult members who will succeed him in a few years. He must also be able to relate to people in their 20s as neophytes going through their initial formative period within the adult world.

A formidable but necessary task to be accomplished by the person in middle adulthood is to experience, endure, and fight against stagnation. Stagnation is not purely negative and should not be totally avoided. It is necessary to do battle with stagnation in order to recognize that one's own vulnerability is a source of wisdom that increases one's capacity for sympathy and compassion for others.

Sex Role Reversal. Sex role reversal is a phenomenon in which women become more assertive, more autonomous, more oriented toward achievement in the work place, and more personally active, while men become more nurturant, more emotional, more home and family oriented, and more passive. The process of becoming more androgynous tends to be actualized during middle age. It involves allowing the development of *all* the male and female qualities in a person that have been socially identified as male or female. As sexual role stereotypes dissipate and drop away, people can become more truly human.

Evaluating Past Achievements and Setting New Goals. Each segment of a person's life is variously mirrored in the relationship of the person to work, family, individual self, social self, life plans, and goals. In general, life has been divided into two halves, with the dividing point at about age 40. By age 40, one has had an opportunity to build a personal life and, ideally, to realize the rewards of youthful endeavors. For most people, the 40s are a period of reexamination. Questions about what has been accomplished, what is yet to be done, and the value of the person's life to the society as well as to others and to himself are posed. The reexamination culminates in coming to terms with the disparity between what a person is and what he had hoped to become.

Irrespective of what answers surface to these profound questions of living, a person must move forward. If one has not been successful in achieving early life goals, this reality must be accepted, and goals to rebuild one's life must be formulated. If one has achieved according to or in excess of expectations of early life goals, the meaning and value of one's success must be considered. A few people may be satisfied with their present lives and may wish to continue as they are for the remainder of the life span. However, despite their satisfactory situations, there will be changes that cannot be anticipated at this point. Many more people experience feelings of entrapment and meaninglessness when they realize that the attainment of their early adulthood goals has not provided the satisfaction they had hoped for. The lives of many people are relatively satisfactory in some respects and disappointing or destructive in others. Whatever the life condition at 40, each person must go through the process of sorting things out, coming to terms with personal limitations, reformulating goals, and moving forward through the life span.

Culminating Events. Events of marked significance may occur in the late 30s and early 40s: promotion, demotion, firing, establishing a family unit, divorce, personal health breakdown, illness or death of significant others, loss of financial base, acquisition of considerable wealth, and lack of recognition or accolades from the society. Any of these may serve as a culminating event. A culminating event represents a form of success or failure, necessitating movement forward or backward on the path of life. How the person deals with a culminating event dictates chances for the future.

The culminating event frequently makes one aware of the period of mid-life transition. If the precipitating event occurred at another stage of life, it would have different meanings and implications. During middle adulthood, the culminating event must be integrated with life reappraisal. One must look at the event as a factor in the possibilities for a better or worse life in the future. The successful handling of culminating events demands continuous self-renewal and creative involvement in one's own life, as well as in the lives of others.

One of the most important services rendered by members of the helping professions is to assure people who are struggling with the "crises" of middle age and aging that they are not alone in what they are feeling and that the process of handling culminating events is not outside the range of normal experience.

Age 50 Transition (48–55 Years)

At every point in adult life, crossing the threshold into the next stage represents a loss of youth, diminishing vitality, and, finally, a threat to life itself. Many people use the term "the big O" in referring to the transitions of the 20s, 30s, 40s, 50s, 60s, 70s, 80s, 90s, and 100s (*e.g.*, "the big four-O"). The age 50 transition is considered to include the ages of 48 to 55. This is a time to continue working on the tasks of the mid-life transition while anticipating and planning for the building of a second middle adult structure that will be the medium for completing middle adulthood.

One of the difficult aspects of the age 50 transition is the realization that one is neither young nor old but rather suspended in the middle. At 50, one cannot ignore the graying hair, the wrinkling skin, and the frequent pains, aches, and strained muscles occasioned by activities that in previous years would have caused only minimal physical stress.

One of the worst feelings at this period of transition is the contemplation of long and continuing years of a meaningless existence—a time when youthful passions have ceased, there is little opportunity for creative tasks, and one's contributions to society are minimal. This period evokes strong feelings of self-doubt that intensify as the person realizes he is moving toward being old and begins to fear disintegration, despair, and eventual death. There is often an inner voice that says, "There is little time left to enjoy life— the end is nearly here."

Achieving Immortality. Two of the major tasks in the 50s are defining the ultimate value of life and how one is going to achieve a form of immortality. Successfully resolving these basic needs of life can help to ease the strong feelings of self-doubt, meaninglessness, and despair that so many people experience when entering this period of life. For most people, dealing with a form of immortality translates into a personal decision about the legacy they can or will bequeathe to future generations.

Many people place the highest value on having and raising children and maintaining familial relationships, viewing these accomplishments as their most precious gifts to generations to come. Children take the places of their parents in the adult world. Whatever rewards, accomplishments, and satisfactions children receive are also regarded as gifts of the parents. Parents generally feel that parts of them will live on in their children.

Another way of confronting mortality is to bequeathe one's material possessions to charities and worthy causes. People often make sizable contributions to religious groups, colleges, unions, professional organizations, and community projects. These groups reflect continuance and enduring value. The giver's munificence is often accompanied by a pervasive need to guarantee personal immortality by means of a name registered or engraved on a worship bench or plaque.

The legacy of professional and artistic people to future generations can take the form of an enduring product, such as a book, statue, painting, or poem; or perhaps their work will contribute to improved health and better and more comprehensive education for future generations. Whatever the means of attempting to guarantee immortality, be it material possessions, creative products or enterprises, or influences on others, the process must be recognized and implemented for success in the transition of the 50s.

Culmination of Middle Adulthood (55–60 Years)

The end of middle adulthood occurs at approximately 55 to 60 years of age. This period has often been compared to the settling down period of early adulthood. The task of this period is completing middle adulthood and becoming ready for late adulthood. For most people, the decade of the 50s can be a period of great fulfillment if they can resolve the young/old conflict. This conflict suggests that one is both young and old at every age; moreover, the human starts becoming old at birth, yet often remains young in certain respects during old age.

The serenity of ending middle adulthood is achieved when one accepts that there are clearly advantages as well as disadvantages in growing older, just as there were in being young. At this time, the mature adult realizes that when he was young he was lively, growing, heroic, and full of potential, but at the same time impulsive, lacking in experience and wisdom, and imperfectly developed. While growing old, he can still be lively and full of potential as well as wise, psychologically and socially powerful, and accomplished.

At the culmination of middle adulthood, one should have struck a balance with the young/old continuum. Once the balance is struck, one can have a solid structure on which to base the use of considerable energy, imagination, and motivation for change. Middle adulthood is the core of the life cycle and the period of intense preparation for what is to come.

Late Adulthood Transition (60–65 Years)

We describe the period of late adulthood transition as the period from ages 60 to 65. It is often marked by the recognition and experience of physical decline. The fact that one becomes more forgetful, takes longer to complete tasks, and has more difficulty getting the body to move heralds the passage from middle to old age. Even if one is in relatively good health and remains physically active, he is constantly reminded of the tentativeness of his condition. Reminders of serious illness and death occur with increasing frequency in the experiences of family and friends. As one approaches 60, it seems that all traces of youth, even the last vestiges remaining from middle age, are about to vanish, leaving only the undetermined vagaries of old age. Not all these aspects of physical and mental change happen to all people, but all are likely to experience some changes and be affected by them.

A major task of the 60s is to maintain youthfulness in a new form appropriate to late adulthood. The process of termination and the modification of the earlier life must take place. As they enter this period, many people have not yet internalized the fact that they will become old; they are aware that old age comes to all people, but somehow believe that this applies to everyone except them. The 60 transition signals the culmination of the strivings of middle age. One must begin to relinquish the role occupied in the center stage of one's world, reduce the heavy responsibilities of middle adulthood, and learn to live in a different relationship with one's society. The gradual loss of recognition, power, and authority can become traumatic.

Probably one of the most difficult changes to accept is the movement of one's generation out of the limelight into a position of subservience. To allow one's children to assume the power and authority of the family is necessary but difficult to accept. In the world of business, similar transitions are also taking place. An older person who has a great deal of authority and the power to make decisions must make way for the middle adult generation, who need to acquire the ultimate power and responsibility. If he tries to hold on to formal authority after 70, he is "out of sync" with his own generation and in conflict with the generation of middle adulthood.

Retirement from formal work endeavors does not mean the end of one's worth; instead, it is an opportunity to continue in valued work that stems from one's own creative energies rather than from societal pressures and financial need. At this point, a person who is in the young/old category has a series of options regarding the form of retirement available: *early retirement,* an option that requires sound financial planning and a secure economic base; *gradual retirement,* an option that allows a slow phasing out of a major career or shifting to a new, less demanding career or job; *traditional retirement,* an option that provides for the cessation of work in the marketplace at age 65; *late retirement,* an option that provides for the cessation of work at the now-legal age of 70; and the final option of *nonretirement,* which is to continue work until death. These several options are now available to more and more people. The "work" a retired person chooses may encompass play or, in other words, involve him in his own determined interests for financial gain or personal satisfaction. At this time of life, one should be relatively free from pressures of society and should be able to choose the activities, be they work, play, or a combination of both, that meet one's needs. Thus, the older person should be able to fulfill one of the primary developmental tasks of late adulthood—achieving a balance of involvement with society and self.

Late Adulthood (65–80 Years)

Late adulthood ushers in a period of decline as well as an opportunity for development. This is the period of life when many people must begin the process of rehearsal for or the actual experience of widowhood. Needs that have been met in marriage are no longer met. For many, this period of life is filled with loneliness, since widowhood is both a personal and a social loss. The social role of husband or wife, head of household or homemaker, no longer applies.

In late adulthood, chronic disease processes become more common. Also, sociogenic aging, that is, aging caused by social expectations, comes to the fore. If we act old, we physically decline, fulfilling our own prophecy. A further complication of sociogenic aging is hypokinetic disease, disease that occurs as a result of too little physical movement. Thus, one's attitude and expectations can influence biological aging.

The person entering late adulthood senses that he has most probably completed the major part, if not all, of his life work. Whatever he was to do for society has been done, and his choice of a way to guarantee immortality has been made. At this time, the ultimate appraisal of life must be achieved. Finding meaning and value in life as a whole is necessary to avoid bitterness and despair in the final years. In striving to attain personal integrity, the person can come to terms with his own view of death. It is necessary for most people to realize that whatever values and expectations they had held dear are not likely to be fully realized. Each person must reconcile the imperfections and elements of destruction in his life. Making peace with oneself and with those who are perceived as having injured one is a necessary task of late adulthood. Most people at this stage of life continue to hold strong convictions but are more realistic about how these convictions can be carried out in daily life.

Late Late Adulthood (80 Years and Older)

Late late adulthood, the last period of life, encompasses ages 80 and beyond. People who survive beyond 80 generally ex-perience a myriad of infirmities and at least one chronic condition. At this point, signs of aging are more evident than any signs of growth. The scope of life tends to be narrowed, and the individual focuses intently on a few significant relationships—the place where he lives, immediate bodily concerns, and personal comforts. The person has to fight diligently to avoid the feeling that life has no meaning or, worse, that he is simply being tolerated.

All other phases of the life cycle have focused on the development of strategies for a new beginning—a new basis for living. This era focuses on strategies to learn how to die. One approach is disengagement, in which the older person progressively withdraws from society, ceases caring about things and people, and becomes increasingly self-concerned. The second approach follows the activity theory, in which the older person engages in a high level of physical activity and social integration, and follows a controlled nutrition regimen, all of which result in a healthy and involved late, late adulthood. To continue to live effectively, one must make peace with dying. If one can maintain a personal vitality, engagement in social life will continue. Most important, people at this stage of life can serve as models of wisdom, hope, integrity, and personal nobility. At this time, one reaches an ultimate involvement with self—an awareness that the final task of life is accepting and loving oneself and being ready to move on to the next stage, which is death.

Bibliography

Books

Allen VL and Villert E van de (eds). Role Transitions: Explorations and Expectations. New York, Guilford Press, 1983.

Colarruso CA and Nemiroff RA. Adult Development: A New Dimension in Psychodynamic Theory and Practice. New York, Plenum Press, 1981.

Bowd J. Stratification Among the Aged. Monterey, California, Brooks-Cole, 1980.

George LK. Role Transitions in Later Life. Monterey, California, Brooks-Cole, 1980.

Henig R. How A Woman Ages. New York, Ballantine Books, 1985.

Hughes FP. Human Development Across the Life Span. St Paul, West Publishing, 1985.

Hultsch DF and Deutsch F. Adult Development and Aging: A Life-Span Perspective. New York, McGraw-Hill, 1981.

Kimmel DC. Adulthood and Aging: An Interdisciplinary Developmental View. 2nd ed., New York, John Wiley & Sons, 1980.

Levinson DJ et al. The Seasons of a Man's Life. New York, Ballantine Books, 1979.

Marshall VW. Last Chapters: A Sociology of Aging and Dying. Monterey, California, Brooks-Cole, 1980.

Myerhoff B. Number Our Days. New York, Simon & Schuster, 1980.

Okun BF. Working With Adults: Individual Family and Career Development. Monterey, California, Brooks-Cole, 1984.

Pesmen C. How A Man Ages. New York, Ballantine Books, 1984.

Rogers D (ed). Issues in Life-Span Human Development. Monterey, California, Brooks-Cole, 1980.

Schale KW. Adult Development and Aging. New York, Guilford Press, 1983.

Sheehy G. Pathfinders. New York, Bantam Books, 1982.

Troll LE. Early and Middle Adulthood: The Best is Yet to Be—Maybe. Monterey, California, Brooks-Cole, 1975.

Van Hoose W and Worth MR. Counseling Adults: A Developmental Approach. Monterey, California, Brooks-Cole, 1982.

Walsh PB. Growing Through Time: An Introduction to Adult Development. Monterey, California, Brooks-Cole, 1983.

Whitbourne SK. Adult Development, 2nd ed. New York, Praeger, 1986.

Articles

(Asterisks indicate nursing research articles.)

Apolito A. Middle-age crisis: A preventive approach. J Med Soc NJ 1981 Aug; 78(9):603–605.

*Beard MT. Trust, life events, and risk factors among adults. ANS 1982 Jul; 4(4):26–43.

Bengston VL and Treas J. Intergenerational relations and mental health. In Birren JE and Sloan RM (eds). Handbook of Mental Health and Aging, pp 400–408. Englewood Cliffs, New Jersey, Prentice Hall, 1980.

Brock AM and O'Sullivan P. From wife to widow: Role transition in the elderly. J Psychosoc Nurs Ment Health Serv 1985 Dec; 23(12): 6–12.

*Broom BL. Concensus about the marital relationship during transition to parenthood. Nurs Res 1984 Jul–Aug; 33(4):223–228.

Dohrenwend BS. Social status and responsibility for stressful life events. Issues Ment Health Nurs 1985; 7(1–4):105–127.

Elwell F and Maltbie-Crannell AD. The impact of role loss upon coping resources and life satisfaction of the elderly. J Gerontol 1981 Mar; 36(2):223–232.

Gould RL. The phases of adult life: a study in developmental psychology. Am J Psychiatry 1972 Nov; 129(5):521–531.

Holahan CJ and Moos RH. Life stress and health: personality, coping and family support in stress resistance. J Pers Soc Psychol 1985 Sept; 49(3):730–747.

Holahan CK, Holahan CJ, and Belk SS. Adjustment in aging: the roles of life stress, hassles and self-efficacy. Health Psychol 1984; 3(4):315–328.

Lakey B and Heller K. Response biases and the relation between negative life events and psychological symptoms. J Pers Soc Psychol 1985 Dec; 49(6):1662–1668.

Lowenthal MF and Weiss L. Intimacy and crises in adulthood. Counseling Psychologist 1976; 6(1):10–15.

*McBride AB. The experience of being a parent. Ann Rev Nurs Res 1984; 2:63–81.

*Mercer RT. The relationship of developmental variables to maternal behavior. Res Nurs Health 1986 Mar; 9(1):25–33.

Neugarten GL. Adult personality: Toward a psychology of the life cycle, pp 137–147. In Neugarten BL (ed). Middle Age and Aging. Chicago, University of Chicago Press, 1968.

Neugarten BL. The awareness of middle age. In Neugarten BL (ed). Middle Age and Aging, pp 93–98. Chicago, University of Chicago Press, 1968.

Neugarten BL. Adaptation and the life cycle. Counseling Psychologist 1976; 6(1):16–20.

*Norbeck JS. Modification of life event questionnaires for use with female respondents. Res Nurs Health 1984 Mar; 7(1):51–71.

Portnoi VA. The natural history of retirement: Mainly good news. JAMA 1981 May; 245(17):1752–1754.

Richman J. Sex differences in social adjustment: Effects of sex role socialization and role stress. J Nerv Ment Dis 1984 Sept; 172(9):539–545.

*Reed PG. Implications of the life-span developmental framework for well-being in adulthood and aging. ANS 1983 Oct; 6(1):18–25.

Rosenfeld JP. Benevolent disinheritance: The kindest cut. Psychology Today 1980 May; 13(12)48–49.

Rotter JB. Generalized expectancies for internal versus external control of reinforcement. Psychol Monogr 1966; 80(#1, whole No. 609): 1–28.

Shainess N. Menopause: Midlife crisis or milestone-marker? J Am Med Wom Assoc 1982 Apr; 37(4):87–90.

*Spotts SJ. Love: Crisis and consolation for the middlescent woman. ANS 1981 Jan; 3(2):87–94.

*Stevenson JS. Adulthood: A promising focus for future research. Ann Rev Nurs Res 1986; 1:55–74.

Streff MD. Examining family growth and development: a theoretical model. ANS 1981 July; 3(4):61–69.

*Taft LB. Self-esteem in later life: A nursing perspective. ANS 1985 Oct; 8(1):77–84.

*Woods NF. Self-care practices among young adult married women. Res Nurs Health 1985 Sep; 8(3):227–233.

Chapter 11

Health Care of the Older Adult

The Study of Aging

Aging, the normal process of time-related change, begins with birth and continues throughout life. Old age is the final phase of the life span.

The older population is growing faster than the rest of the population and will continue to do so for the next 50 years. With increased quantity of life, as indicated by increasing life expectancy, the helping professions must focus on improving the quality of life for elderly persons. Regular mental, social, and physical activities should be available. Community-based support services provide essential help to the elderly to enable them to remain in a familiar setting with meaning and dignity.

Geriatrics, the study of old age, includes the physiology, pathology, diagnosis, and treatment of the diseases of older adults. The broader field of *gerontology*, the study of the aging process, includes the biological, psychological, and sociological sciences. Because old age is a normal occurrence within the life span that encompasses all experiences of life, it cannot be limited to one discipline. Insight and optimal care of elderly persons can best be provided through a cooperative effort. The *interdisciplinary team,* made up of specialists from many fields, can combine expertise and resources in contributing knowledge and research to provide insight into all aspects of the aging process.

Gerontological or gerontic nursing is the field of nursing that specializes in care of the elderly. Standards of gerontological nursing practice were originally developed in 1969 and revised in 1976 by the American Nurses' Association. The nurse gerontologist can be either a specialist or a generalist offering comprehensive nursing care to the older person. The basic nursing process of assessment, planning, implementation, and evaluation is used in combination with a specialized knowledge of aging. Gerontological nursing can be provided in acute, chronic, or community settings. Emphasis of care is placed on promoting, maintaining, and restoring independence and health. Strengths of older adults are identified and used to help them maximize independence.

Old Age Defined

The definition of old age varies with the frame of reference. A parent of 35 years may be considered old by the child of 10 years and young by his parents of 65 years. The active person of age 65 may consider 75 years as the beginning of old age.

With the adoption of the retirement age of 65 years through Social Security legislation in the 1930s, American society accepted 65 years as the beginning of old age. This represents the chronological definition of old age and is used by society. Functional and physiologic age differs with the individual and therefore cannot be standardized. Functionally, a professional basketball player is old at the age of 35, although he may be in superb physical health and physiologically young. Gerontologists have attempted to allow for individual differences by using the classification of young-old for 65 to 74 years and old-old for 75 years and beyond.

Life Span vs. Life Expectancy

Life span is the maximum number of years a person can live under the best of conditions in the absence of disease. The longest verified life span is about 113 years. There has been little change in the life span in recorded history. *Life expectancy* is the average number of years that a person can be expected to live. In the 20th century, life expectancy from birth has risen dramatically from an average of 48 years (1900) to 74.7 years (1985), with women (78.1 years) living about 7 years longer than men (71.2 years). Early in this century, increases in life expectancy were attributed to the decreased death rates of infants and young people. Since 1970, however, increases in life expectancy are due to decreased mortality among the middle-aged and elderly population (Fig. 11-1). The difference in life expectancy at birth between whites and blacks was 4.5 years in 1984.

It is predicted that in future years more people will live longer. The health professions are challenged to make these added years healthy and productive ones.

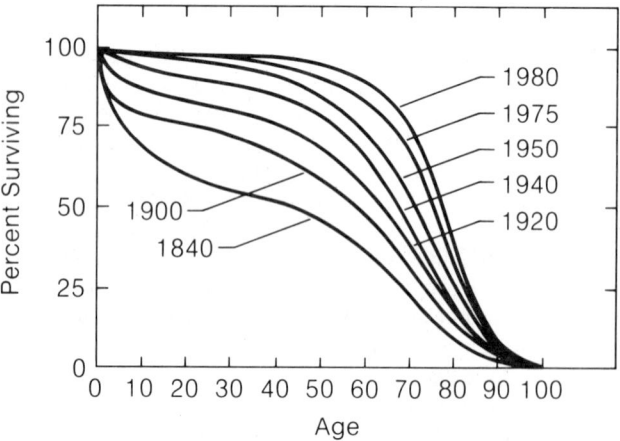

Figure 11-1
Life expectancy in the United States: the increasingly rectangular survival curve. (US Bureau of Health Statistics. In Fries VF and Crapo LM. Vitality and Aging. San Francisco, WH Freeman, 1981.)

Profile of an Aging American

The older population in America has been increasing steadily in proportion and numbers. Since 1900, the total population of persons 65 years and older has tripled (4.1% in 1900 to 11.9% in 1984). In 1984 there were 28 million Americans over age 65; presently one in nine persons is over 65 years (Fig. 11-2). By the year 2000, one in eight will be over 65 years. Those 75 and older, the fastest growing segment of the population, will place greater demands on the health care system.

For the majority of those 65 and older, Social Security is the single largest source of income. Although there is a growing perception that the elderly are well off financially, they are more likely to be poor than other adults in our society. Economic status varies considerably within the older age-group. Some older people have substantial resources, while many others have incomes that are either below or barely above the poverty level. About 3.3 million elderly persons (12.4%) were below the poverty level in 1984. (The 1984 poverty level was defined as $6282 for an older couple or $4979 for a single person.) Older consumers spent proportionately more of their incomes on housing, food, transportation, and health care than their younger counterparts.

Psychosocial Aspects of Aging

The study of the psychosocial development of older adults is relatively new. Gerontologists are attempting to understand the complex process of successful aging. Psychological adjustment is believed to be related to successful completion of developmental tasks as identified by Erikson, Havighurst, and others.

The societal position of the elderly is determined by culture. Although attitudes toward old people differ in ethnic subcultures of America, a subtle theme of ageism predominates. *Ageism* is a prejudice against a distinct group of people who are defined by age boundaries. *Stereotypes*, simplified and often untrue beliefs, reinforce society's negative image of the aged person. Elderly people make up an extremely heterogeneous group, yet negative stereotypes are attributed to all of them.

It is believed that this prejudice is based on fear of aging and the inability of many to confront their own aging process. Retirement and perceived nonproductivity are also responsible for negative feelings. The younger working person may see the older person as one who is not contributing to society and who is actually draining economic resources. This negative image is so common in American society that the elderly themselves believe it. Stereotypes call for certain behaviors, and the elderly may adopt these expected roles. Thus negative stereotypes are reinforced.

Health professionals may be instrumental in perpetuating a negative image. Nurses who care for sick old people see many problems that they may generalize to the entire elderly community. Only by understanding the aging process and respecting each person as an individual can the myths of aging be dispelled. If aged persons are treated with dignity and encouraged to make decisions and maintain independence, the quality of their lives should improve.

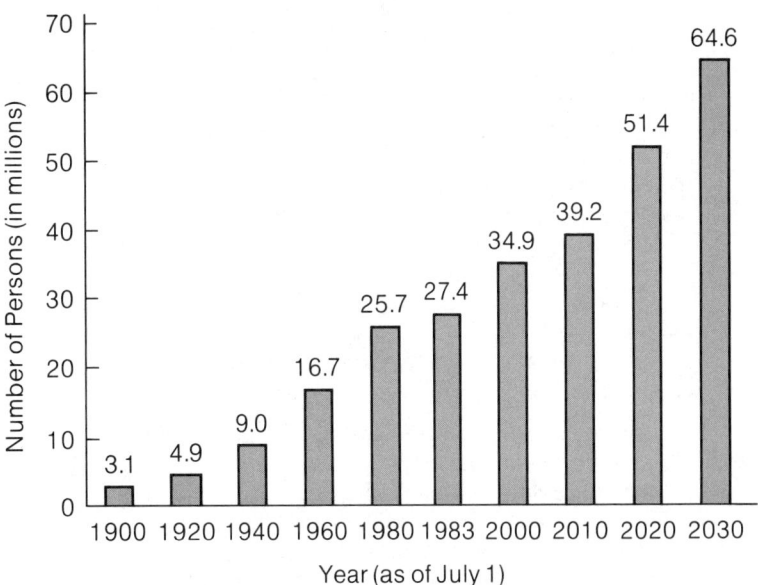

Figure 11-2
Number of persons over age 65 in the United States: 1900 to 2030. Note: Increments in years on horizontal scale are uneven. (Based on data from US Bureau of Census. In Profile of Older Americans: 1984, prepared by the Program Resources Department, American Association of Retired Persons [AARP] and the Administration on Aging [AoA], US Department of Health and Human Services.)

Developmental Theories

Erikson developed the concept of eight stages of human life, with each stage representing crucial turning points in the life span stretching from birth to death. He delineated the one major developmental task of old age as ego integrity versus despair. *Ego integrity* suggests an acceptance of one's lifestyle and a belief that choices made were the best that could be made at a particular time. One is still in control of one's life, a life of dignity. Despair, the opposite, implies that the older person feels dissatisfied and disappointed with this life. If given another chance, the person would live life differently.

Havighurst lists developmental tasks that occur during a lifetime. A person who completes the tasks successfully will feel contentment. The tasks of aging persons include adjusting to decreases in physical strength and health, retirement, reduced income, and death of a spouse; establishing affiliation with one's age-group; adopting and adapting to social roles in a flexible way; and establishing satisfactory physical living arrangements.

Combining the concepts of Erikson and Havighurst, the following achievements and adaptations are recommended for the aged person: (1) maintain feelings of self-worth; (2) resolve old conflicts; (3) adjust to loss of power roles; (4) adjust to the deaths of significant others; (5) adapt to environmental changes; and (6) maintain an optimal level of wellness.

Sociological Theories of Aging

Aged persons are influenced in their behavior and life-style by society. Gerontologists have proposed the following theories of aging to understand and predict the successful adjustments of elderly people.

The *disengagement theory* suggests that by withdrawing from society at the same time that society is withdrawing its support from his age-group, the elderly person achieves high morale and life satisfaction. This theory has been refuted by research findings showing that engaged, active persons achieve higher life satisfaction than disengaged, more passive people.

The *activity theory* proposes that life satisfaction in normal aging involves maintaining the active life-style of middle age. This theory reflects the majority thinking of middle class America. It assumes that the older person will find satisfying replacements for activities.

The *continuity theory* proposes that successful adjustment to old age rests with the ability of the person to continue life patterns across a lifetime. A person who adjusted well in earlier life will continue to do so in later life.

Cognitive Aspects of Aging

Intelligence

Stereotypes suggest that older people experience slow thinking processes, forgetfulness, confusion, and senility. Many people erroneously believe that it is difficult, if not impossible, to introduce new learning to an older adult.

Intelligence tests measure the ability to accomplish intellectual tasks such as forming concepts, solving problems, acquiring information, and reasoning. When intelligence test scores from people of all ages are compared (cross-sectional testing), test scores for older adults show a progressive decline beginning in midlife. Because older persons are slower in their responses and need more time to react, their scores may not reflect their actual ability. The presence of disease, predisease conditions, and stress may also negatively affect intellectual functioning.

Research studies as well as demonstrations of creativity by older adults show that creativity is found in all persons regardless of age. Creative performance in older adults is best manifested within a society that will provide stimulating opportunities and reward risk taking.

Learning and Memory

The ability to learn and remember is generally affected by the aging process. However, many older persons are able to continue to learn. The process by which older adults learn is facilitated when the nurse

- Uses visual, auditory, and other sensory cues
- Encourages the learners to wear their glasses and hearing aids
- Provides glare-free lighting
- Provides a quiet, nondistracting environment
- Sets short-term goals with input from the learning group
- Keeps teaching periods short
- Paces learning tasks according to the stamina of the group
- Encourages verbal participation from the learners
- Reinforces successful learning in a positive manner

Memory is a complex process that involves acquiring, storing, and retrieving or remembering information. Sensory losses, distractions, and disinterest interfere with acquiring information; age-related changes in the brain affect storing and remembering. Many older people are able to recall episodes from many years past with clarity and precision. These selected events were probably of great importance and recalled to memory many times.

Normal Physiologic Aging

Primary (Normal) vs. Secondary (Pathologic) Aging

Primary aging refers to the changes caused by the normal aging process and is characterized by being universal, progressive, decremental (gradually less), and intrinsic (from within the person). Universality is the major criterion that distinguishes primary (normal) aging from secondary (pathologic) aging. Using the above characteristics, the nurse can distinguish normal from pathologic aging. Secondary (pathologic) aging results from influences outside of the person. Illness and disease, air pollution, and sunlight are all examples of environmental factors that may hasten the aging process. The nurse can be instrumental in eliminating or retarding secondary aging processes.

Structural Changes of Aging

Advanced age is accompanied by cellular and extracellular changes in structure that negatively affect body function and appearance. Postmitotic cells, primarily found in the nervous system, musculo-skeletal system, and heart, are incapable of reproduction. These cells gradually die and contribute to a slow loss of lean muscle mass. The remaining cells must repair themselves, replacing intracellular elements on a regular basis. Aging postmitotic cells accumulate a pigment known as lipofuscin, indicating that the process of intracellular repair is incomplete. Mitotic cells have the ability to reproduce themselves and are found in the other body systems.

Collagen and elastin, two essential components of the intercellular connective tissue matrix, demonstrate significant age-related changes. Collagen fibers become more dense. Thickening and denseness result in stiffness and impaired diffusion of nutrients and wastes. Elastin, a major component

of elastic fibers, becomes fragmented and calcified. This contributes to reduced tissue elasticity. Denseness, stiffness, and loss of tissue elasticity have a profound influence on the functioning of the cardiovascular system.

A redistribution of major body components occurs in later life. Fat-free body tissues, which comprise the lean body mass (skeletal muscles and nerves), progressively diminish with age. Fat (adipose tissue) is redistributed from subcutaneous tissues and the extremities to the trunk. There is a higher proportion of fat in the aged body, and intracellular fluid volume decreases. Extracellular water and plasma fluid remain the same.

Age-Related Body System Changes: Health Promotion

The well-being of an aged person depends on physical, mental, social, and environmental factors. A total assessment includes an evaluation of all major body systems, social and mental status, and the ability of the person to function independently despite the presence of a chronic illness. (See Table 11-1 for nursing assessment and interventions for age-related changes in body systems.)

Cardiovascular Changes

Heart disease is the leading cause of death for all age-groups including the elderly (Fig. 11-3). The mortality rate from cardiovascular disease also increases with age. The normal structural changes of aging that occur in the heart and vascular system reduce their ability to function efficiently. The heart valves become thicker and stiffer, and the heart and arteries lose their elasticity. Arteries become distended and tortuous. Calcium and fat deposits accumulate within their walls.

Although function is maintained under normal circumstances, the cardiovascular system has less reserve and its ability to respond to stress is reduced. Under conditions of stress in the elderly, the ability of the heart to deliver its maximal cardiac output (heart rate × stroke volume) is diminished.

With greater arterial rigidity, systolic blood pressure increases. Diastolic pressure rises to maintain blood flow against increased peripheral resistance. Hypertension has been shown to be a prominent risk factor at all ages for cardiovascular disease. Older people with a blood pressure reading of less than 140/90 mm Hg live longer than those with higher readings. A diagnosis of hypertension is based on an average of blood pressure readings taken at different times. In older people, the diagnosis of hypertension is classified in two ways: (1) isolated systolic hypertension in which the systolic reading exceeds 160 mm Hg with the diastolic measurement less than 90 mm Hg, and (2) typical hypertension in which the diastolic pressure is greater than 90 mm Hg and the systolic pressure is greater than 160 mm Hg.

Cardiovascular malfunction may become exaggerated and interfere with normal activities of daily living. The normal changes of aging, genetic factors, and life-style may contribute to major disorders that include cardiac dysrhythmias, congestive heart failure, coronary artery disease, arterioscle-

TABLE 11-1
Body Systems: Normal Changes in Functional Status with Nursing Recommendations

Normal Changes in Functional Status	Subjective and Objective Assessment	Health Promotion/Nursing Recommendations
Cardiovascular System		
Decreased cardiac output; diminished ability to respond to stress; heart rate and stroke volume do not increase with maximum demand; slower heart recovery rate; increased blood pressure	Complaints of fatigue with increased activity Increased heart rate recovery time Normal BP < 140/90 mm Hg	Exercise regularly; pace activities; avoid smoking; eat a low-fat, low-salt diet; participate in stress reduction activities; check blood pressure regularly
Respiratory System		
Increase in residual lung volume; decrease in vital capacity; decreased gas exchange and diffusing capacity; decreased cough efficiency	Fatigue and breathlessness with sustained activity; impaired healing of tissues due to decreased oxygenation; difficulty coughing up secretions	Exercise regularly; avoid smoking; take adequate fluids to liquefy secretions; receive yearly influenza immunization; avoid exposure to upper respiratory tract infections.
Integumentary System		
Decreased protection against trauma and solar exposure; decreased protection against temperature extremes; diminished secretion of natural oils and perspiration	Skin appears thin and wrinkled; complaints of injuries, bruises, and sunburn; complaints of intolerance to heat; bone structure is prominent; dry skin	Avoid solar exposure (clothing, sunscreen, stay indoors); dress appropriately for temperature; maintain a safe indoor temperature; bathe only 1–2 times weekly; lubricate skin.
Reproductive System		
Female: Vaginal narrowing and decreased elasticity; decreased vaginal secretions Male: Decreased size of penis and testes Male and female: Slower sexual response	Female: Painful intercourse; vaginal bleeding following intercourse; vaginal itching and irritation; delayed orgasm Male: Delayed erection and achievement of orgasm	May require a prescription for estrogen/antibiotic cream; use a lubricant with intercourse; seek health/sexual counseling if needed.
Genitourinary System		
Male and female: Bladder capacity decreases; delayed sensation to void Male: Benign prostatic hypertrophy Female: Relaxed perineal muscles	Urinary retention Difficulty voiding Urgency, frequency and incontinence of urine	Seek regular medical supervision; have ready access to toilet; wear easily manipulated clothing; drink adequate fluids; practice pelvic floor muscle exercises Maintain perineal hygiene; skin clean and dry; absorbent pads; water resistant skin cream; clean underclothes.
Gastrointestinal System		
Decreased salivation; difficulty swallowing food Delayed esophageal and gastric emptying Reduced gastrointestinal motility	Complaints of dry mouth Complaints of fullness, heartburn, and indigestion Complaints of constipation, flatulence, and abdominal discomfort	Use ice chips, mouthwash; brush, floss, and massage gums daily; receive regular dental care. Eat small frequent meals; sit up and avoid heavy activity after eating; limit antacids. Eat a high-fiber, low-fat diet; limit laxatives; toilet regularly; drink adequate fluids.
Musculoskeletal System		
Loss of bone density Loss of muscle strength and size Degenerated joint cartilage	Height loss; prone to fractures; kyphosis; complaints of back pain. Loss of strength, flexibility, and endurance. Complaints of joint pain.	Exercise regularly; eat a high-calcium diet; limit phosphorus intake. Estrogens and calcium supplements may be prescribed.

(continued)

TABLE 11-1 (continued)

Normal Changes in Functional Status	Subjective and Objective Assessment	Health Promotion/Nursing Recommendations
Nervous System		
Reduced speed in nerve conduction; increased confusion with physical illness and loss of environmental cues; reduced cerebral circulation (becomes faint, loses balance)	Person is slower to respond and react; learning takes longer; becomes confused with hospital admission; complaints of faintness; frequent falls	Pace teaching. With hospitalization, encourage visitors; enhance sensory stimulation; with sudden confusion, look for cause. Encourage slow rising from a resting position; encourage use of a cane.
Special Senses		
Vision: Diminished ability to focus on close objects; inability to tolerate glare; difficulty adjusting to changes of light intensity; decreased ability to distinguish colors.	Holds objects far away from face; complaints of glare; complaints of poor night vision; confuses colors	Wear eyeglasses; use sunglasses outdoors; use adequate indoor lighting with area lights and nightlights. Use large-print books; avoid night driving; use contrasting colors for color coding;
Hearing: Decreased ability to hear high frequency sounds.	Gives inappropriate responses; asks people to repeat words; strains forward to hear	Recommend a hearing examination; reduce background noise; face person; enunciate clearly; speak with a low pitched voice; use nonverbal cues.
Taste and smell: Decreased ability to taste and smell.	Uses excessive sugar and salt	Encourage use of lemon, spices, herbs.

rosis, hypertension, intermittent claudication, and cerebrovascular accidents.

Promotion of Cardiovascular Health. A program of regular exercise, avoidance of smoking, weight control, a nutritious low-fat diet, and relief of stress help the older person to maintain independence, maximize productivity, improve the quality of life and minimize pathologic disease processes. The nurse encourages the older person to pace activities according to tolerance. Medications and blood pressure are monitored regularly. The nurse must be alert for adverse responses to medication, including orthostatic hypotension, electrolyte imbalance, confusion, and depression. To avoid faintness and possible falls caused by orthostatic hypotension, the older person should be counseled to rise slowly from a lying to a sitting and then to a standing position.

Respiratory Changes

Age-related changes in the respiratory system that affect lung capacity and function include the following possibilities: an increase in the anteroposterior chest diameter; osteoporotic collapse of vertebrae resulting in kyphosis; calcification of the costal cartilages and reduced mobility of the ribs; diminished efficiency of the respiratory muscles; an increase in lung rigidity; and a decrease in alveolar surface area. The increased rigidity or loss of elastic recoil results in an increase in residual lung volume and a decrease in vital capacity. Gas exchange and diffusing capacity are diminished.

Decreased cough efficiency, reduced ciliary activity, and increased dead space make the older person more vulnerable to respiratory infections. Although older adults have sufficient respiratory function to carry out activities of daily living, there is a diminished ventilatory capacity. This results in a decreased

tolerance for sustained exercise and a need for short rest periods during prolonged activity.

Promotion of Respiratory Health. To prevent acute and chronic respiratory problems, the nurse encourages the older person to

- Exercise regularly to maintain general fitness and muscle tone
- Stop smoking and avoid smoke-filled areas
- Drink adequate amounts of fluids to liquefy secretions
- Receive an annual influenza immunization
- Avoid exposure to upper respiratory tract infections

Integumentary Changes

The functions of the skin include protection, temperature regulation, sensation, and excretion. With advanced age, intrinsic and extrinsic changes occur that affect function and appearance. The epidermis and dermis become thinner. There are fewer elastic fibers; collagen becomes stiffer. Subcutaneous fat diminishes, particularly in the extremities. A loss of capillaries in the skin results in a decreased blood supply. These changes result in a loss of resiliency and a wrinkling and sagging of the skin. Hair pigmentation decreases and hair becomes gray. The skin becomes drier and susceptible to irritations because of decreased activities of the sebaceous and sweat glands. Spotty and irregular distribution of pigment occurs, particularly in areas that have previously been exposed to sunlight. These changes in the integument reduce tolerance to extremes of temperature and solar exposure. Skin dryness makes the person susceptible to itching and skin irritation.

Promotion of Integumentary Health. The following preventive measures are encouraged:

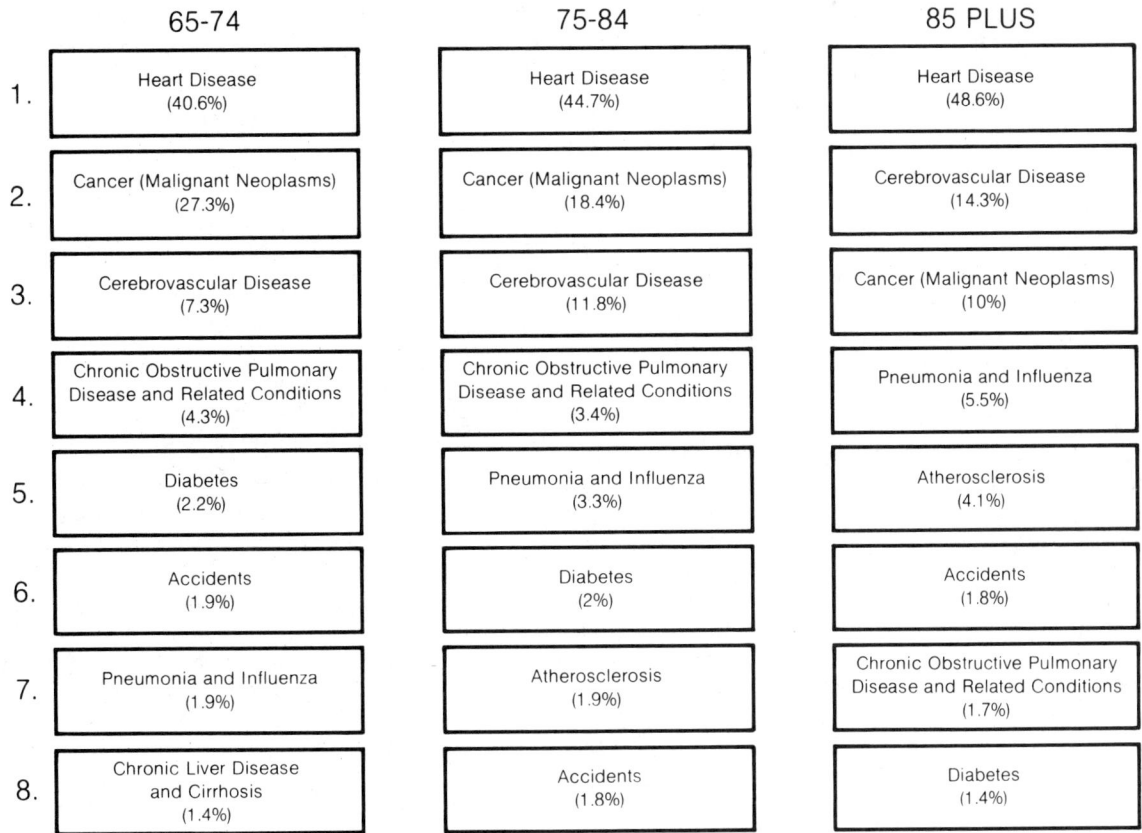

65-74

1. Heart Disease (40.6%)
2. Cancer (Malignant Neoplasms) (27.3%)
3. Cerebrovascular Disease (7.3%)
4. Chronic Obstructive Pulmonary Disease and Related Conditions (4.3%)
5. Diabetes (2.2%)
6. Accidents (1.9%)
7. Pneumonia and Influenza (1.9%)
8. Chronic Liver Disease and Cirrhosis (1.4%)

75-84

1. Heart Disease (44.7%)
2. Cancer (Malignant Neoplasms) (18.4%)
3. Cerebrovascular Disease (11.8%)
4. Chronic Obstructive Pulmonary Disease and Related Conditions (3.4%)
5. Pneumonia and Influenza (3.3%)
6. Diabetes (2%)
7. Atherosclerosis (1.9%)
8. Accidents (1.8%)

85 PLUS

1. Heart Disease (48.6%)
2. Cerebrovascular Disease (14.3%)
3. Cancer (Malignant Neoplasms) (10%)
4. Pneumonia and Influenza (5.5%)
5. Atherosclerosis (4.1%)
6. Accidents (1.8%)
7. Chronic Obstructive Pulmonary Disease and Related Conditions (1.7%)
8. Diabetes (1.4%)

Figure 11-3
Eight leading causes of death in the United States by age-group: 1980. (National Center for Health Statistics: Advance report, final mortality statistics, 1980. Monthly Vital Statistics Report, Vol. 32, No. 4, Supplement DHHS Pub. No. [PHS] 83-1120. Hyattsville, Maryland, Public Health Service, August 1983.)

- Avoid solar exposure (use sunscreens and protective clothing).
- Avoid the heat of summer (stay indoors at midday and wear appropriate clothing).
- Dress warmly and maintain adequate warmth in winter.
- Bathe totally only once or twice weekly and use sponge baths in between.
- Apply oil or lotion to the skin immediately after bathing while the skin is still moist.

Reproductive Changes

Ovarian production of estrogen and progesterone ceases with menopause. Changes occurring in the female reproductive system include thinning of the vaginal wall with a narrowing in size and a loss of elasticity; decreased vaginal secretions resulting in vaginal dryness, itching, and decreased acidity; involution (atrophy) of the uterus and ovaries; and decreased perineal muscle tone resulting in stress incontinence and urgency. These changes contribute to bleeding and painful intercourse. The penis and testes decrease in size in the older male. Levels of androgens diminish.

Promotion of Sexual Health. Sexual desires and activity decline, but do not disappear. Neither should they be discouraged. Society often erroneously views older people as asexual. The nurse can explain that sexual activity varies individually and is related to sexual behavior at an earlier age. To replace reduced vaginal secretions and reduce trauma, a water-soluble lubricant may be required. A couple may wish to see a sexual counselor.

Genitourinary System Changes

The genitourinary system continues to function adequately although there is a loss in kidney mass due primarily to loss of nephrons. Changes in kidney function include decreased filtration rate, diminished tubular function with less efficiency in resorbing and concentrating the urine, and a slower restoration of acid–base balance in response to stress. The ureters, bladder, and urethra lose muscle tone. The bladder capacity decreases, and the older person may be unable to empty the bladder completely. Retention of urine increases the risk of infections. Frequency, urgency, and incontinence are also common problems. Women may have decreased perineal muscle tone, resulting in stress incontinence and urgency. Benign prostatic hypertrophy is a common finding in older men. Enlargement of the prostate causes chronic urinary retention, frequency, and incontinence.

Health Promotion for the Genitourinary System.
Adequate consumption of fluids is necessary to prevent bladder infections and to maintain fluid balance. Problems of urinary incontinence and frequency can be reduced if the older person

- Has ready access to toilet facilities
- Voids regularly
- Practices pelvic floor exercises

These exercises, first described by Kegel, can be highly useful in reducing the symptoms of urinary stress incontinence. Because achievement of better muscle control takes several months to accomplish, the nurse encourages the patient to persist regularly with the exercises. The patient is first taught to tense, then relax, the perineal, anal, and abdominal muscles as if to stop diarrhea. Second, the muscles surrounding the urethra and vagina are tightened. These two exercises should be alternated and repeated ten times, four to six times a day. They can be practiced while standing, sitting, or lying down. The nurse can suggest incorporating the exercises into other daily activities, since they go undetected by others. These exercises are also recommended for men with dribbling incontinence related to prostatic surgery. The nurse instructs the patient to tighten the rectal sphincter until the penis retracts. Frequent repetition produces the desired muscle tone.

Gastrointestinal Changes

The function of the gastrointestinal tract usually remains adequate throughout life. Nevertheless, many older people suffer from discomforts that are related to the sluggish passage of food or delayed motility. About half the population have lost all their teeth by the age of 60. Although this is not an inevitable consequence of aging, periodontal disease leading to dental decay and loss of teeth occurs commonly. Salivary flow diminishes, and the older person may experience a dry mouth.

Peristalsis in the esophagus is less efficient in the elderly. In addition, the gastroesophageal sphincter may fail to relax, leading to delayed esophageal emptying and dilation of the lower esophagus. Major complaints often center on feelings of fullness, heartburn, and indigestion. Gastric motility may decrease, resulting in delayed emptying of stomach contents. Diminished secretion of acid and pepsin reduce the absorption of iron, calcium, and vitamin B_{12}.

Small intestinal absorption of nutrients appears to be diminished but is adequate throughout life. The function of the liver, gallbladder, and pancreas is generally maintained, although there exist some inefficiencies in absorption and tolerance to fat. The incidence of gallstones and common bile duct stones increases progressively with advanced years. Abdominal surgery in persons 60 years and older is done more frequently for gallbladder disease than for any other disorder.

Constipation is high on the list of complaints of aged persons. When mild, the symptoms involve abdominal discomfort and flatulence. However, more serious consequences include fecal impaction that contributes to diarrhea around the impaction, fecal incontinence, and obstruction. Predisposing factors for constipation include lack of dietary bulk, prolonged use of laxatives, ignoring the urge to defecate, side-effects of medications, emotional problems, inactivity, insufficient fluid intake, and excessive dietary fat.

Health Promotion for the Gastrointestinal System.
The nurse can teach that correct oral hygiene includes

- Regular toothbrushing and flossing
- Massage of gums and tongue with a soft brush
- Regular dental care
- Ice chips or a mouthwash for a dry mouth

Upper gastrointestinal discomfort due to delayed esophageal emptying can create significant distress. Teaching includes encouraging the older person to

- East small amounts of food frequently
- Sit up after meals
- Avoid heavy activity following a meal
- Use antacids with care and supervision
- See a physician if the distress continues

Nutritional Health. The social, psychological, and physiologic functions of eating influence the dietary habits of the aged person. Decreased physical activity and a slower metabolic rate reduce the number of calories needed by the older adult to maintain an ideal weight. Although fewer calories are desirable, the older person continues to require the same nutrients. Apathy, immobility, depression, loneliness, poverty, inadequate knowledge, lack of oral health, and lack of taste discrimination contribute to undesirable eating habits. Wasted, empty calories are found primarily in foods that are high in fats, cholesterol, and sugar.

The nurse encourages a diet low in sodium and saturated fats, with an emphasis on vegetables, fruits, and fish. The older adult requires a variety of foods to maintain balanced nutrition. Fats, particularly saturated fats, should be avoided because they are high in calories and contribute to atherosclerosis. There is an association between obesity and cardiovascular disease. No more than 20% to 25% of dietary calories should be consumed by fat intake. Sodium reduction has been shown to reduce levels of hypertension.

Protein intake should remain the same in later adulthood. Dried beans and peas are inexpensive and excellent sources of protein and fiber. Red meats, whole milk, eggs, and cheese should be replaced by chicken, fish, and low-fat dairy products to provide adequate protein and reduce fat intake.

Carbohydrates, a major source of energy, should supply the diet with 55% to 60% of the daily calories. Simple sugars should be avoided and complex carbohydrates encouraged. Potatoes, whole grains, brown rice, and fruit provide the person with minerals, vitamins, and fiber; eating these foods should be encouraged, even though they are more difficult to prepare and chew. Commercially processed foods often have a low nutritional and high-sodium content in proportion to the number of calories they contain.

Insufficient consumption of water leads to dehydration and constipation, common problems for aged persons. Adequate fluid balance is necessary to maintain peristalsis and urinary functions. Secretions will be less viscous and more plentiful. Eight glasses of water are recommended daily unless contraindicated by a medical condition.

Musculoskeletal Changes

A gradual, progressive decrease in bone mass begins before the age of 40 years. Excessive loss of bone density results in *osteoporosis* (see Chap. 58). This condition is more apparent in postmenopausal women and is associated with inactivity, inadequate calcium intake, and loss of estrogens. Its incidence is higher in northern Europeans and other whites, and in Chinese and Japanese. Bone resorption occurs, and there is danger of fracture, especially in the vertebrae, shoulders, wrists, femoral necks, femurs, and tibias. A loss of height occurs in later life. This shortening of the trunk is due to osteoporotic changes of the spine, kyphosis (rounding of the shoulders), and flexion of the hips and knees. These changes have a negative effect on mobility, balance, and internal organ function.

The muscles, composed of postmitotic cells, diminish in size and lose strength, flexibility, and endurance with decreased activity and advanced age. Back pain is common. Beginning in middle age, the cartilage of joints shows progressive deterioration. Degenerative joint disease is found in all older persons past the age of 70.

Health Promotion for Bones. The demineralization that occurs in osteoporosis is accelerated by the loss of estrogens, and a low-calcium, high-phosphorus diet. The nurse can recommend:

- A high calcium intake (dairy products and dark green vegetables are excellent sources, as are soups and broths made from soup bones cooked with added vinegar to leach calcium from the bone)
- A low-phosphorus diet (a calcium–phosphorus ratio of 1:1 is ideal; avoid red meats, cola drinks, and processed foods that are low in calcium and high in phosphorus)
- Exercise (the pull of muscle insertions on the long bones strengthens them and retards calcium resorption)

Calcium supplements, vitamin D, fluoride, and estrogens are often prescribed for the person who is at high risk of having or who already has osteoporosis. Although osteoporosis cannot be reversed, the disease process can be prevented or arrested.

Health Promotion for Musculoskeletal Function. A program of regular exercise can be lifelong or can begin in later life. The axiom "use it or lose it" is very relevant when considering the physical capacity of aged persons. A major barrier to exercise is societal attitude in general and a negative attitude of older people themselves; old people are considered to be frail and physically unfit. Many elderly people believe that they need less exercise, that vigorous exercise has many risks, and that they have limited ability to perform exercise. They tend to stay indoors and often lack motivation to initiate or maintain physical activity. The nurse plays an important role by encouraging and challenging older adults to participate in a regular exercise program. Research shows that exercise enhances cardiovascular and respiratory efficiency. Regular exercise increases the strength and speed of heart contractions and improves oxygen uptake by cardiac and skeletal muscles. Exercise has been shown to reduce fatigue, increase energy, and reduce cardiovascular risk factors. Muscle endurance, strength, and flexibility, all outcomes of regular exercise, help to promote independence and psychological well-being. Aerobic exercises are the foundation of programs of cardiovascular endurance conditioning. Basic principles of judgment should be followed by the elderly person. A physical examination by a physician is necessary prior to initiating an exercise program. The program is based on current health status and past activity, with a warm-up and cool-down period before and after exercise. The older person should perform exercises in moderation and use short rest periods to avoid undue fatigue. Swimming and brisk walking are often recommended because they are managed easily and usually enjoyed by the older person.

Nervous System Changes

The structure and function of the nervous system diminish with advanced age. However, in the absence of pathologic changes, the older person functions adequately because brain reserve is ample. A progressive loss in brain mass is attributed to loss of nerve cells that are not replaced. The nerve cells accumulate lipofuscin pigment, which has an uncertain effect on function. Accompanying the nervous system changes are a significant reduction of cerebral blood flow and use of oxygen. Mental deficits are associated with low blood flow, but some persons with low blood flow may show normal cognitive function. Nerve conduction slows significantly in later life, and therefore older persons take a longer time to respond and react.

Health Promotion for the Nervous System. A slowed reaction time places the older person at risk for accidents and injury. The nurse advises the person to allow a longer time to respond to a stimulus. Mental function is threatened by physical or emotional stress. A sudden onset of confusion may be the first symptom of a physical condition such as pneumonia, fecal impaction, drug interactions, or dehydration. The nurse paces the teaching session according to the person's learning ability.

Sensory Changes

The sensory organs of sight, hearing, taste, touch, and smell allow each person to communicate with the environment. Messages received from the surroundings keep the person oriented, interested, and contented. Sensory losses with old age affect all sensory organs and threaten this interaction. This is a time of life when the older person is less able to perform physically and is sedentary. Sensory losses can be devastating to the person who cannot see to read or watch television, who cannot hear conversation well enough to communicate, or who cannot discriminate taste well enough to enjoy food.

Sensory Losses vs. Sensory Deprivation. The diminishing function of the sensory organs results in sensory losses that can often be helped by appliances such as glasses or hearing aids. Sensory deprivation is the absence of stimuli in the environment or the inability to interpret existing stimuli (perhaps as a result of a sensory loss). This deprivation can lead to boredom, confusion, irritability, disorientation, and anxiety. Meaningful sensory stimulation offered to the older person is often helpful in correcting this problem. Although all old people have sensory losses and as a result are at high risk of sensory deprivation, they do not all suffer from sensory deprivation. One sense can substitute for another in observing and interpreting stimuli. The nurse can enhance sensory stimulation in the environment with colors, pictures, textures, tastes, smells, and sounds. The stimuli are most meaningful when they are interpreted to the older person and if they are changed often. The confused person responds well to touching and to familiar songs.

Vision

New cells form around the outside edge of the lens and create an accumulation of older cells. The lens becomes yellow, rigid, and cloudy. Thus, only the outer portion of the lens is elastic enough to change shape (accommodate) and focus at near and far distances. As the loss of lens flexibility progresses, the near point of focus gets farther away. This condition, *presbyopia*, usually begins in the 40s. Reading glasses for magnifying objects are required. In addition, the yellowing, cloudy lens causes light to scatter and therefore makes the older person susceptible to glare. The ability to discern blue from green declines. The pupil dilates slowly and less completely because of increased stiffness of the muscles of the iris. The older person takes longer to adjust when going to and from dark and light environments.

Health Promotion. The nurse can help the older person compensate for visual losses by encouraging him to:

- Use adequate lighting
- Avoid the glare of shiny surfaces and direct sunlight
- Avoid abrupt changes from dark to light
- Use vision aids such as eyeglasses or a magnifying glass
- Use large print
- Use highly contrasting colors
- Avoid combinations of blue and green

Hearing

Loss of the ability to hear high-frequency tones occurs in mid-life. This age-related hearing loss, called presbycusis, is attributed to irreversible inner ear changes. Older persons are often unable to follow conversation because tones of high-frequency consonants (letters *f, s, th; ch, sh; b, t, p;*) all sound alike. Unable to communicate, they feel isolated and withdraw from social events. When hearing difficulties are suspected, ears and hearing should be checked. Wax buildup or other correctable problems may be responsible for major hearing difficulties. A properly prescribed and fitted hearing aid is useful in reducing hearing deficits.

Health Promotion. Hearing loss may cause the older person to respond inappropriately and to avoid social interaction. This behavior may be interpreted as confused or "senile." When speaking to a hearing impaired person, the nurse should:

- Speak using a low tone of voice
- Reduce background sound
- Face the person when speaking
- Enunciate words clearly
- Speak at a moderate pace
- Use gestures along with speech

Touching

The sense of touch offers the most intimate of messages and is easiest to interpret. When other senses diminish, touching can reduce feelings of isolation and give a sense of well-being. Although sensory receptors dull with age, they do not disappear. Older persons are eager to touch and be touched. Reduced mobility and fewer social contacts often diminish such opportunities. The nurse can enhance touching contact by offering back rubs, foot massages, and hand pats. Companion animals are becoming popular in nursing homes with residents and staff. These pets offer many older persons love,

warmth, and touching stimulation that vastly improves their quality of life.

Taste and Smell

The four basic tastes are sweet, sour, salty, and bitter. Of these, sweet tastes are particularly dulled in older persons. This explains why they tend to use sweets excessively. Blunted taste may contribute to preference for salty, highly seasoned foods. The nurse encourages the use of herbs, onions, garlic, and lemon, unless restricted, and discourages the use of salt.

Mental Health Disorders

Mental health disorders are a major problem and threat to older adults and their families. It is estimated that as many as 15%–20% of the elderly have a mental or psychiatric disorder that is significant enough to require evaluation and treatment. The major portion of these disorders can be helped with medications and psychological counseling. (For mental status assessment see Chart 11-1.)

Mental health disorders are loosely classified as functional (psychogenic) and organic. The functional or psychogenic disorders often originate prior to old age. They are caused by biochemical, genetic, and psychosocial factors and respond well to medication and psychotherapeutic counseling. Organic mental disorders are accompanied by abnormal mental and behavioral functioning and pathologic changes of the brain. Four to six percent of persons over 65 and 20% of persons over 80 have an organic mental disorder.

Age-Related Stress and Coping Mechanisms

Coping patterns and the ability to adapt to stress are developed over the course of a lifetime. In youth or mid-life, the recovery from grief or stress can be hastened by options that are made available by an active life-style. For example, a young widow may find happiness in a new marriage. A job loss can be replaced by a new opportunity. In later life, the coping mechanisms are consistent with those of earlier life. A flexible, well-functioning person will probably continue as such. However, the same options may not be available to aged persons. Losses may accumulate within a short period of time and be overwhelming. The older person will have fewer choices and diminished resources to deal with stress. Common stressors of old age include normal aging changes that impair physical function, activities, and appearance; disabilities of chronic illness; social and environmental losses of income, roles, and activities; and the death of significant others.

Functional Disorders

Depression is the most common functional disorder. Signs of depression include sadness, low energy, diminished memory and concentration, sleeping disturbances, appetite disturbances, withdrawal, irritability, alcohol abuse, expressed

Chart 11-1
Mental Status Assessment

The mental status assessment is a narrative report that should incorporate observations from each of the following parameters with detailed descriptions where indicated.

Column 1 parameters require simple descriptions.
Column 2 parameters require active interventional testing.

Column 1

Appearance

- neat
- untidy
- appropriate
- clean
- healthy
- apparent age

Attitude

- cooperative
- hostile
- suspicious
- fearful
- evasive

Activity Level

- restless
- slow
- appropriate
- threatening
- repetitive movement

Mood

- appropriate
- apathetic
- sad (crying)
- happy
- mood swing

Communication

- nonverbal (facial expression, body language)
- speech patterns
- word selection
- articulation of words
- flight of ideas
- rambling

Attention and Concentration

- distracted
- normal

Column 2

Orientation

- time (today's date)
- place (where are we?)
- person (what is your name?)

Remote Memory

- birthdate
- stories from childhood
- current U.S. president
- last U.S. president

Recent Memory

- what did you eat for lunch? (verify)

Retention Memory

- repeat the names of 3 items that you list (immediately and in 5 minutes)

General Intellect

- name 5 cities
- simple math ($3 \times 8 =$?)

Attention and Concentration

- serial 7s ($100 - 7$ and continue)

Abstract Reasoning

- ask to explain "Don't cry over spilt milk" or "A stitch in time."

Judgment

- ask "What would you do with a stamped, addressed letter that you find on the sidewalk?"
- or "Why are criminals put into prison?"

feelings of helplessness and hopelessness, apathy, impaired attention span, and expression of suicidal wishes.

Many depressed persons are thought to be confused or suffering from an organic mental disease. Depression is often treatable and reversible through use of antidepressant medications and counseling. Suicide attempts are a potential threat when depression exists. The suicide rate in older white men is higher than in any other age-group.

Other functional disorders include hypochondriasis and paranoia. *Hypochondriasis* is characterized by a preoccupation with body functioning and an overconcern with physical complaints. Loneliness, isolation, and sensory impairments may make the older person feel threatened and mistrustful of others, resulting in *paranoia.*

Organic Mental Disorders

Organic brain syndrome is a general term that refers to a group of mental symptoms found in specific organic mental disorders. The five major symptoms are loss of memory, loss of intellect, loss of judgment, impairment of orientation, and lability of affect (excessive or shallow emotional response). Two of the most commonly occurring syndromes characterized by some or all of these are delirium (usually acute) and dementia (usually chronic).

Delirium

Delirium, often called acute brain syndrome, begins with confusion and progresses to disorientation and change in the level of consciousness. The onset is rapid and often occurs in a hospital or other unfamiliar setting.

The brain dysfunction is secondary to any number of causes, including physical illness, drug or alcohol toxicity, dehydration, fecal impaction, malnutrition, infection, head trauma, lack of environmental cues, and sensory deprivation or overload. Older adults are particularly vulnerable to symptoms of delirium because of their marginal biological reserve and the high number of medications that they take.

The major manifestation in delirium is disturbance in the level of consciousness, which may range from stupor to excessive activity. Thinking is disorganized, and the attention span is characteristically fleeting. Hallucinations, delusions, fear, anxiety, and paranoia may be evident. The course of this syndrome is short, usually lasting less than a week and no more than a month. If the symptoms go unrecognized and the underlying cause is not treated, permanent irreversible brain damage or death will follow.

Therapeutic interventions vary, depending on the reason for the symptoms. Because drug interactions and toxicity are often implicated, it is desirable that unessential medications be withdrawn. To improve orientation and provide familiar environmental cues, the nurse encourages family members or friends to touch and talk to the patient. With a newly admitted patient, the nurse questions the family carefully about his prior cognitive state. Ongoing mental status assessments using this baseline will be helpful in evaluating responses to treatment.

Dementia

Dementia (senile dementia, chronic brain syndrome) is a syndrome rather than a distinct disease entity. It is usually progressive and irreversible and is not a part of normal aging. It is characterized by a general decline in cognitive abilities that may include losses of memory, abstract reasoning, judgment, and impulse control, as well as changes in personality. It is usually subtle in onset and often progresses slowly until the symptoms are very obvious and profoundly devastating. The three most common dementias are Alzheimer's disease, multi-infarct dementia, and a mixed Alzheimer's disease and multi-infarct dementia.

Alzheimer's Disease

Alzheimer's disease is sometimes called primary degenerative dementia or senile dementia of the Alzheimer's type (SDAT). It accounts for at least 50% of all the dementias suffered by the elderly. It is a progressive, irreversible, degenerative neurologic disease of uknown origin that begins insidiously. Alzheimer's disease is not found only in old people. Its onet can begin in the 40s and 50s, and it is then called *presenile dementia.* However, the highest incidence is among persons 65 years and older with increasing incidence after age 70. The life expectancy following the diagnosis varies from 6 to 20 years. Presenile dementia often has a more rapid course, but regardless of time of onset, both conditions are considered to be clinically and pathologically identical.

Pathophysiology. The etiology of the disease is unknown, but there are specific neuropathologic and biochemical changes. These include neurofibrillary tangles (a tangled mass of nonfunctioning neurons) and senile or neuritic plaques (deposits of protein and altered cell structures on the interneuronal junctions). This neuronal damage occurs primarily in the cerebral cortex and results in decreased brain size. These changes are found to a lesser extent in normal brain tissue of older adults. Cells principally affected by this disease are the ones that use the neurotransmitter acetylcholine. Biochemically, the enzyme active in producing acetylcholine is decreased. Acetylcholine is specifically involved in memory processing.

Diagnostic Evaluation. There has been a major research effort to develop a specific diagnostic test for Alzheimer's disease. However, at present the diagnosis is one of exclusion and is confirmed by autopsy. Clinical symptoms, electroencephalography (EEG), computed tomography (CT scan), magnetic resonance imaging (MRI), and examination of the blood and cerebrospinal fluid may all refute or support a diagnosis. The electroencephalographic changes are not always specific. The CT and MRI scans are very useful for excluding hematoma, brain tumor, stroke, and atrophy but are not reliable in making the diagnosis of Alzheimer's disease. Infections and chemical abnormalities can be excluded by examination of the blood and cerebrospinal fluid, but findings are not specific enough to make the diagnosis.

Clinical Manifestations. Symptoms of Alzheimer's disease are highly variable. Early in the disease, forgetfulness and subtle memory loss occur, but the victim has adequate cognitive function to hide the loss. Social skills and behavior patterns remain intact; problems are difficult to detect on casual observation. With further progression of the disease there is an inability to conceal the deficits. Forgetfulness is manifested in many daily actions. The victim may lose his way in a familiar environment. He may repeat the same stories because he forgets that he told them. Reasoning and reality orientation by caretakers increase the patient's anxiety without increasing function, because this is also forgotten.

Conversation becomes difficult because the victim forgets what he was about to say or may not be able to remember words. Ability to formulate concepts and think abstractly disappears. The person can interpret a proverb only in concrete terms. The victim is often unable to appreciate the consequences of his actions and will therefore exhibit impulsive behavior. For example, on a hot day he may decide to wade in the city fountain fully clothed. He will have difficulty with everyday activities such as working simple appliances and handling money.

Personality changes are usually negative. The patient may become depressed, suspicious, paranoid, hostile, and even combative. Progression of the disease intensifies the symptoms. Speaking skills deteriorate to nonsense syllables; agitation and physical activity increase. A voracious appetite often develops because of the high activity level. The patient may wander at night for hours. Eventually he will need help in all areas of personal care including toileting and eating; dysphagia occurs and incontinence develops. The terminal stage may last for months. The patient is usually immobile and requires total care. Occasionally the person may recognize family or caretakers. Death occurs as a result of a complicating condition such as pneumonia, malnutrition, or dehydration.

Nursing Considerations. Interventions by the nurse are aimed at maintaining optimal cognitive function, promoting physical safety, reducing anxiety and agitation, improving communication, promoting independence in self-care activities, providing for the patient's needs for socialization and intimacy, maintaining adequate nutrition, managing sleep pattern disturbances, and supporting and educating family caregivers.

Support of Cognitive Function. As the patient's cognitive ability declines, the nurse provides a calm, predictable environment that helps him interpret his surroundings and activities. Environmental stimuli are limited and a regular routine is followed. The nurse's quiet, pleasant manner, clear and simple explanations, and the use of memory aids and cues help to minimize confusion and disorientation and give the patient a sense of security. A prominently displayed clock and calendar will enhance orientation to time. Color coding the doorway will help the patient who has difficulty locating his room.

Promoting Physical Safety. A safe home environment will allow the patient to move about as freely as possible and relieve the family of constant worry about his safety. To prevent falls and other accidents, all obvious hazards are removed. Night lights, a call light, and a low bed with half bedrails are used at bedtime. The nurse or family monitors the patient's intake of medications and food. Smoking is allowed only with supervision. A hazard-free environment allows the patient maximum independence and a sense of autonomy. Because of the patient's short attention span and forgetfulness, wandering behavior indoors can often be directed with gentle persuasion and distraction. Restraints are avoided because they may increase agitation. Doors leading from the house must be secured. Outside the home all activities must be supervised to protect the patient. The patient should wear an identification bracelet or neck chain in case he becomes separated from the caregiver.

Reducing Anxiety and Agitation. Despite profound cognitive losses, there will be times when the patient is aware of his rapidly diminishing abilities. He will need constant emotional support to reinforce a positive self-image. When loss of skills occurs, the nurse adjusts goals to the patient's declining ability.

The nurse appreciates the importance of recreation and encourages the patient to enjoy simple activities. Realistic goals that provide satisfaction are appropriate. Hobbies and activities (walking, exercise, socializing) can improve the quality of life.

The nurse actively tries to keep the environment simple, familiar, and noise free. Excitement and confusion can be upsetting and may precipitate a combative, agitated state known as a catastrophic reaction (overreaction to excessive stimulation). During such a reaction the patient responds by screaming, crying, or becoming abusive (physical or verbal assault). This is his way of expressing his inability to deal with the environment. When this occurs, the nurse remains calm and unhurried. Measures such as listening to music, stroking, rocking, or distraction may quiet the patient. Frequently he forgets what triggered the reaction. Structuring activities is also helpful for this patient. Familiarity with his predicted responses to certain stressors helps the nurse avert similar situations.

Improving Communication. To promote the patient's interpretation of messages, the nurse remains unhurried and reduces noise and distractions. Clear, easy-to-understand sentences are used to convey messages because the meaning of words is frequently forgotten or there is difficulty with organizing and expressing a thought. Lists and simple written instructions can serve as reminders to the patient and are often helpful.

Sometimes the patient can point to an object or use nonverbal language to communicate. Touching stimuli such as a hug or a hand pat are usually interpreted as signs of affection, concern, and security.

Promoting Independence in Self-Care Activities. Pathophysiological changes in the cerebral cortex make it difficult for a patient with a self-care deficit to achieve physical independence. Efforts are directed toward helping him maintain independent functioning for as long as possible. One suggestion is to simplify daily activities by organizing them into short, achievable steps so that the patient can experience a sense of accomplishment. Frequently the occupational therapist is able to suggest ways to simplify tasks or recommend adaptive equipment. Direct patient supervision is sometimes necessary.

Maintaining personal dignity and autonomy are important for this patient. He is encouraged to make choices when appropriate and to participate in self-care activities as much as he can.

Providing for Socialization and Intimacy Needs. Socializing with old friends can be comforting. The nurse and family should encourage visits, letters, and phone calls. Visits should be brief and nonstressful; two to three visitors at one time is recommended.

The confused, lonely person may find stimulation, comfort, and contentment in the purring or licking softness of a pet. The nonjudgmental friendliness of an animal can be helpful. Care of the pet by the patient can provide satisfying activity and an outlet for energy.

Alzheimer's disease does not eliminate the need for intimacy. The patient and his spouse may or may not continue to enjoy sexual activity. The nurse encourages the spouse to talk about any sexual concerns and suggests sexual counseling if necessary. Simple expressions of love, such as touching and holding, are often meaningful for this couple.

Inappropriate sexual behaviors seldom occur, but when

they do they can cause extreme embarrassment to family members. For example, the patient may undress in a public place on a hot day or may masturbate publicly. The use of gentle distraction is recommended.

Promoting Adequate Nutrition. Mealtime can be a pleasant social occasion, or it can become a time of upset and distress. Mealtime should be kept simple and calm without confrontations. The patient will prefer familiar foods that look appetizing and taste good. To avoid "playing," the nurse offers one dish at a time. Food is cut into small pieces to prevent choking. Liquids may be easier to swallow if they are converted to gelatin. Hot food and beverages are served warm; the nurse monitors the temperature to prevent burns.

When lack of coordination interferes with self-feeding, adaptive equipment is helpful. Some patients may do well eating with their fingers. If this is the case, an apron or a smock, rather than a bib, is used to protect clothing. As deficits progress, it may be necessary to feed the patient. Forgetfulness, disinterest, dental problems, incoordination, overstimulation, and choking can all provide barriers to good nutrition.

Promoting Balanced Activity and Rest. Many Alzheimer's disease patients exhibit sleep disturbances and wandering behavior. These behaviors are most likely to occur when the patient is bored, restless, agitated, or disoriented, particularly in a new setting and frequently at night. The patient who wanders outside of the house is often unable to find his way home and is at risk of accident and injury. Family members and neighbors are frequently asked to search for the patient.

All Alzheimer's patients should wear some form of visible identification (bracelet or neck chain) at all times. Although the patient is allowed to walk around in a protected environment, his access to the outdoors should be blocked. If his sleep is disturbed or he is unable to go to sleep, music, warm milk, or a back rub may help him relax. During the day he is given sufficient opportunity to participate in exercise activities, since a regular pattern of activity and rest will enhance nighttime sleep. Long periods of daytime sleeping are discouraged.

Support and Education of Family Caregivers. The emotional burden placed on the family of a patient with Alzheimer's disease is enormous. The physical health of the patient is usually excellent, and the mental degeneration is gradual. Because the diagnosis is not specific, the family may cling to the hope that the diagnosis is incorrect and that the patient will improve if he tries harder. Aggression and hostility exhibited by the victim are often misunderstood by the caregiver or family, who feel unappreciated, frustrated, and angry. Feelings of guilt, nervousness, and worry contribute to caregiver fatigue, depression, and family dysfunction.

The multiple needs of family caregivers have been addressed by the Alzheimer Disease and Related Disorders Association (ADRDA). This national organization with more than 100 local chapters is a coalition of family members and professionals sharing the goals of family support and service, education, research, and advocacy. Family support groups, respite care, and adult day care are available through the ADRDA.

The nurse must be sensitive to the highly emotional issues that the family is confronting. Support and education of the caregivers are essential components of care. The family can contact the ADRDA or comparable group to meet with others experiencing similar problems. (See Nursing Care Plan 11-1, Care of the Patient With Alzheimer's Disease, pp. 156–162.)

Multi-Infarct Dementia

Multi-infarct dementia (MID) is an organic mental disorder second to Alzheimer's disease in incidence. It is characterized by an uneven, downward decline in mental function. About 15% of the cases of dementia are attributed to this disease.

Cerebral damage occurs when blood supply to the brain is disrupted. Infarction, the death of brain tissue, occurs with striking rapidity. Multiple small cerebral infarctions, clinically manifested as small strokes, result in multi-infarct dementia. Instead of displaying the progressively downhill course of Alzheimer's disease, the progress of multi-infarct dementia is uneven. Every small infarct is followed by some recovery and a plateau until the next infarction occurs. Often the patient has a history of hypertension. The age at onset is between 50 and 70 years, and the condition occurs more frequently in men than in women.

Dizziness, headaches, and decreased mental and physical vigor are early signs of the disease. In more than half the cases, the disease appears acutely as sudden confusion. This is followed by gradual, spotty memory loss. The patient may hallucinate and display symptoms of delirium. Speech disturbances may be present.

MID is sometimes confused with Alzheimer's disease, paranoia, or delirium because of its unpredictable clinical course. The diagnosis can sometimes be even more difficult because the victim may be suffering from both Alzheimer's disease and MID. Early treatment of hypertension and vascular disease may prevent progression of the disease. With progression, manifestations of the decline are similar to the signs discussed under Alzheimer's disease.

Drugs and the Elderly

Elderly people use more drugs than any other age-group, averaging more than 13 prescriptions and renewals a year. One of every four prescriptions is dispensed to a person over 65. As a result, the aged are more likely to have adverse drug reactions and interactions than younger people. One study reported that 59% of the elderly outpatient population with chronic illness made errors in self-administration of prescribed medications, and 25% committed potentially serious errors.

Physiologic Considerations

There is great variability in the absorption, distribution, metabolism, and excretion of drugs in older patients owing in part to a reduced capacity of the liver and kidneys to metabolize and excrete the drugs and to lowered levels of circulatory and nervous system efficiency in coping with the effect of certain drugs. Many drugs and their metabolites are excreted by the kidney. However, in the elderly patient, both glomerular and tubular functions are reduced. See Table 11-2 for the effect of aging on pharmacologic response.

(Text continues on p. 162)

TABLE 11-2
The Effects of Aging on Pharmacologic Response

Commonly Used Drugs	Actions and Nursing Implications
Digitalis Glycosides	
Digoxin Digitoxin	A reduction in kidney function allows an increase in the plasma concentration and possible toxicity. Lower dosages are often indicated.
Diuretics	

Thiazides
  Chlorothiazide (Diuril)
  Hydrochlorothiazide
    (Hydrodiuril, Esidrix)
Loop diuretics
  Furosemide (Lasix)
	Drug effects at usual therapeutic dosages are often accentuated. Dehydration, electrolyte disturbances (particularly hypokalemia), and impaired mental function may result.

Antihypertensive Drugs	Age-related impaired baroreceptor responses, decreased venous tone (varicose veins), and reduced cardiovascular and autonomic nervous system responses create a high potential for postural hypotension with usual dosages.
Rauwolfia Alkaloids	
Reserpine (Serpasil)	*Rauwolfia* alkaloids may induce mental depression.
Anticoagulants	
Heparin Warfarin (Coumadin)	Elderly women have shown an increased incidence of bleeding complications with usual therapeutic dosages of heparin. There is a greater risk of bleeding with usual doses of warfarin in the elderly due to (1) greater inhibition of vitamin K synthesis at usual doses and (2) reduced protein binding and therefore increased amounts of circulating free drug.
Narcotic Analgesics	
Morphine sulfate Meperidine hydrochloride (Demerol)	Enhanced effects are due to a higher pain threshold and greater sensitivity. Lower dosages are often sufficient.
Sedatives and Hypnotics	
Barbiturates Benzodiazepines (Librium) Diazepam (Valium)	Sensitivity is heightened and adverse reactions are increased. These drugs remain in the body longer due to slower liver metabolism, reduced renal excretion, and increased tissue uptake. Smaller doses are usually sufficient.
Antipsychotic Drugs	

Phenothiazides (Mellaril,
  Thorazine, Prolixin,
  Compazine)
Butyrophenones (Haldol)
	Increased sensitivity to the effects of these drugs and slow excretion place elderly persons at a high risk for serious adverse effects such as parkinsonism and tardive dyskinesia. Because of the significant potential for toxicity, these drugs should be given cautiously and only to those persons exhibiting severe symptoms of agitation and psychosis.

Care of the Patient With Alzheimer's Disease

Nursing Interventions	*Rationale*	*Expected Outcomes*

Nursing Diagnosis: Alterations in thought processes related to confusion and disorientation

Goal: Maintenance of optimal cognitive functions

1. Reduce environmental confusion.
  a. Approach patient in a pleasant, calm way.
  b. Be predictable in your manner and conversation.
  c. Keep the environment simple and pleasing.
  d. Maintain a regular daily schedule.
  e. Devise memory aids as needed (lists, reminding notes, labels on items, pictures, diagrams).
2. Increase environmental cues.
 	
  a. Identify yourself when interacting with the patient.
  b. Address patient by name.
  c. Offer environmental cues for orientation to time, place, and person (Pictures, photos, clock, calendar with crossed-off days, color-coded halls and doors.)
  d. Provide hourglass timer if unable to tell time on clock.
  e. Interpret environmental stimulation as part of the conversation.
	1. Simple and limited stimuli will facilitate interpretation and reduce distortion of input.
	  b. Predictable behavior is less threatening.
	
	  e. Memory aids will assist the patient to remember.
	
	2. Environmental cues will enhance orientation to time, place, and person by filling memory gaps and serving as reminders.
	  a. As memory loss increases, this may be required with every encounter.
		• Maintains optimal memory function.
		• Shows a reduction in confused behavior.
		• Demonstrates an awareness of environmental stimuli.
		• Verbalizes a sense of security and protection.
		
		• Demonstrates optimal orientation to time, place, and person.

Nursing Diagnosis: Potential for injury related to impulsive behavior and confusion

Goal: Maintenance of physical safety

1. Control the environment.
  a. Remove obvious hazards.
  b. Reduce injury potential from bedtime falls.
    (1) Use only half bedrails.
    (2) Keep bed in low position.
    (3) Use night lights.
    (4) Have accessible call light.
  c. Monitor medication regimen.
  d. Permit smoking only with supervision.
  e. Monitor food temperature.
  f. Supervise all activities outside the home.
	1. A hazard-free environment will reduce the risk of injury and free the family from constant worry. Outside the home, everything is assumed to be a hazard.	• Complies with safety procedures.
		• Moves freely and independently around the home.

(continued)

Nursing Interventions	*Rationale*	*Expected Outcomes*

Nursing Diagnosis: Potential for injury related to impulsive behavior and confusion

Goal: Maintenance of physical safety

2. Permit maximum independence and freedom.		• Verbalizes a sense of security and contentment.
a. Allow freedom in the "safe" environment.	a. This will give the patient a sense of autonomy.	
b. Avoid use of restraints.	b. Restraints may increase agitation.	
c. When wandering, distract rather than force.	c. Force will increase anxiety. Distraction is facilitated by immediate memory loss.	
d. Keep identification tag on patient.	d. A name and phone number will facilitate a safe return when the patient wanders away.	

Nursing Diagnosis: Anxiety related to cognitive losses and reduction in self concept

Goal: Maintenance of an optimal level of psychological functioning

1. Reduce anxiety-provoking situations in daily routine.		
a. Keep reality orientation non-threatening.	a-c. Constant corrections will increase anxiety and may result in a highly agitated, angry, and combative state known as a catastrophic reaction.	• Shows fewer episodes of catastrophic reactions.
b. Be patient with forgetfulness.		• Demonstrates a lower level of anxiety.
c. Accept harmless eccentric behavior.		
d. Maintain a daily, regular routine.	d-e. Simple, structured stimuli are easiest to interpret.	
e. Keep stimuli simple.		
f. Distract rather than confront unacceptable behavior.	f-g. Often forgets immediately and becomes involved in new activity.	
g. When the patient demonstrates a negative attitude in interacting, leave patient and return in a short time.		
h. Avoid situations that have upset patient in the past.		
i. Reassure following a catastrophic reaction.		
j. Do not try to reason with the patient.	j. Unable to conduct abstract thinking.	
2. Enhance the quality of life.	2. Goals are minute-by-minute. The patient has the capacity to enjoy and experience happiness.	• Seeks out the companionship of others.
a. Offer multiple opportunities for fulfillment. (music, pets, walks, exercise, old hobbies, simple chores.)		• Participates in activities willingly; verbalizes contentment.
b. Provide comfort and security.		
3. Encourage positive feelings of self.	3. Acceptance will give support. This person is in the process of grieving over his profound losses.	• Shows a greater level of self assurance in difficult situations.
a. Treat the patient as a person with feelings.		
b. Openly discuss his feelings of anxiety and offer encouragement.		
c. Praise appropriately.		

(continued)

Nursing Interventions	*Rationale*	*Expected Outcomes*

Nursing Diagnosis: Anxiety related to cognitive losses and reduction in self concept

Goal: Maintenance of an optimal level of psychological functioning

d. Do not infantilize (treat as a child) by using baby talk or child terms.	d. Infantilization increases the anxiety.	
e. When skills are lost, do not try to retrain.	e. Deterioration of the cognitive processes makes losses of skills inevitable.	

Nursing Diagnosis: Impaired verbal communication related to cognitive losses

Goal: Attainment of an optimal exchange of ideas between the patient and others

1. Implement strategies to promote the patient's interpretation of messages. a. Be calm, pleasant, and unhurried. b. Keep verbal messages short and simple. c. Avoid decision-making situations. d. Use nonverbal messages along with words. e. Be consistent in conversation. f. Avoid competing noises and distractions. g. Avoid complex issues.	a-g. Simple, short messages are easiest to interpret.	• Shows an improved ability to understand messages. • Shows an improved ability to express himself verbally. • Uses alternate methods of communication (writing, nonverbal).
h. Write down simple instructions and lists. i. Observe patient's expression for signs that he understands. j. Talk to the patient even if he gives little response.	h. Alternate methods for communication often are successful. i. A good listener must be responsive to feedback. j. The patient may not be indicating how much he understands of the conversation.	
2. Develop strategies to improve the patient's ability to express messages. a. Supply forgotten words when possible. b. Guess the message and confirm with the patient. c. Ignore mistakes. d. Allow adequate time for conversation. e. Encourage short, simple sentences. f. Ask "yes–no" questions. g. Provide alternative methods for communication (pointing, describing, pictures). h. Acknowledge the frustration that the patient is experiencing.	2. This will allow the patient to express his needs and feelings. Feelings of isolation are reduced. a-b. Active helpful listening can minimize frustrations when the patient needs help communicating his message. d-f. An unhurried attitude will enhance communication. g. Certain methods may be more successful than others.	• Shows fewer frustrations when communicating.

(continued)

Nursing Interventions	*Rationale*	*Expected Outcomes*

Nursing Diagnosis: Self-care deficits related to inability to bathe, dress, toilet, and maintain self

Goal: Maintenance of maximum independence in activities of daily living

1. Develop strategies to facilitate daily performance of activities
  a. Provide adaptive devices.
  b. Maintain a regular daily schedule at a time convenient with the patient.
  c. Keep the environment simple and pleasant.
  d. Keep instructions simple and divide tasks into small parts.
  e. Monitor function of body systems.
	a-d. A regular schedule, adaptive equipment, and simple tasks will reduce confusion, enhance ability to care for self, and ensure safety.
	
	e. Supervision will promote optimal function and detect early problems.
		• Performs activities of daily living at expected optimal level.

2. Provide specific safeguards of safety in bathing.
  a. Monitor bath water temperature.
 	
  b. Encourage use of safety devices (*e.g.,* handrails, rubber mats).
	a. The patient is unreliable in adjusting bath temperature.
	
	b. Impulsive behavior increases a risk of accidents.
		• Demonstrates the ability to use adaptive equipment.
		• Uses safety measures to prevent injury.

3. Allow patient autonomy and dignity while providing needed care.
  a. Encourage patient to make choices of selection (*e.g.,* clothing, foods, schedule).
  b. Provide adequate privacy.
	3. Encouraging autonomy will enhance a sense of dignity and well-being.	• Verbalizes an awareness of dignity and autonomy.

4. Provide specific measures to encourage continency.
  a. Provide accessibility to the bathroom. If needed, color code the door of bathroom.
  b. Use clothing that opens easily.
 	
  c. Maintain toileting schedule (every 2 hours, after meals).
  d. Encourage adequate fluids, fiber, and activity for regular bowel elimination.
  e. Recommend restricting fluids in evening hours.
	a. Visual stimuli can reinforce recognition.
	
	b. This facilitates continence when haste is necessary.
	c-d. These help to maintain normal elimination.
	
	e. Excessive fluids in the evening may interfere with the sleep-activity routine.	

(continued)

Nursing Interventions	*Rationale*	*Expected Outcomes*

Nursing Diagnosis: Alterations in family process related to care of an ill family member

Goal: Attainment of family adaptation and harmony

1. Initiate and enhance family knowledge of disease. a. Teach family about Alzheimer's disease. b. Encourage family members to read *The 36-Hour Day* and ask questions.	1. If the family understands the disease, they will be better prepared to help the patient and adjust their style of living to his needs.	The family will: • provide appropriate care and support to the patient. • discuss feelings and frustrations with the nurse. • seek appropriate help from community agencies. • join a self-help group.
2. Acknowledge the emotional impact of the disease on the family system. a. Elicit family reaction to patient's illness. b. Encourage family to talk about their worry, guilt, anger, and frustrations. c. Encourage use of stress-reduction techniques. d. Encourage family to share concerns and feelings with patient.	2. This illness has profound effects on the family. They will be frightened, frustrated, angry, guilty, and feel helpless.	
3. Initiate referrals to obtain community help. a. Assist the family in contacting community agencies to receive such support services as respite care, adult day care, visiting nurse services, and social work services. b. Encourage the family to contact Alzheimer's Disease and Related Disorders Association (ADRDA) and participate in a self-help group.	a. Community services will provide respite care, suggestions for home management, financial advice, and nursing. These will help the family cope and manage this family crisis in the best possible way. b. A support group will help the family better understand how others are dealing with similar problems.	

Nursing Diagnosis: Impaired social interaction related to cognitive impairment

Goal: Enhancement of socialization and fulfillment of intimacy needs

1. Encourage social encounters with family and friends. Encourage family and friends to: a. Use touching to maintain contact with patient.	a. Tactile stimulation is easiest to interpret.	• Participates in social events with family and friends. • Increases touching behavior. • Verbalizes or demonstrates contentment when socializing and interacting with others.
b. Touch, hug, and demonstrate affection. c. Share feelings honestly and openly with patient.	b-c. The patient continues to need love and affection.	

(continued)

Nursing Interventions	*Rationale*	*Expected Outcomes*

Nursing Diagnosis: Impaired social interaction related to cognitive impairment

Goal: Enhancement of socialization and fulfillment of intimacy needs

d. React objectively to negative responses.	d-e. Positive interactions are best maintained if the family overlooks negative encounters.	
e. Accept patient despite negative interactions.		
f. Limit numbers of visitors to 1 or 2 at a time.	f. Fewer visitors will help maintain simple stimuli and avoid a catastrophic reaction.	
g. Provide a companion animal if possible and appropriate.	g. Pets provide loving acceptance and opportunities for touching, and are a catalyst to socialization.	
2. Provide opportunities for meeting intimacy needs and sexual expression:	2. Intimacy and sexual expression will provide a sense of contentment and fulfillment to the patient.	• Engages in sexual activity or intimate behavior with spouse.
a. Encourage expressions of intimacy and tenderness with spouse.		• Meets sexual needs privately in an acceptable manner.
b. Encourage a sexual relationship with spouse if interests exists.		
c. Provide privacy if patient masturbates or exposes self.		

Nursing Diagnosis: Alterations in nutrition related to confusion and imbalance of intake/activity

Goal: Maintenance of an optimal level of nutrition

1. Monitor food intake and observe food habits.	1. Encouragement and reminders to eat will help patient eat adequately and regularly.	• Eats a balanced diet and drinks needed fluids.
a. Note weight loss or gain.		
b. Encourage adequate fluid intake.		
c. Provide regular mealtime schedule.		
2. Maintain a favorable environment for eating.		
a. Allow patient optimal independence.	a. Finger foods, adaptive equipment, and a large apron will facilitate independence if lack of coordination interferes with the patient's ability to use utensils.	• Demonstrates enjoyment and maximum independence at mealtime.
b. Maintain a calm pleasant environment.	b-d. If mealtime is pleasant, with favorite and familiar foods, the patient will eat well with enjoyment.	
c. Offer a menu choice.		
d. Offer familiar foods.		
3. Promote regular mouth care.	3. Healthy teeth and properly fitted dentures are important for maintaining nutritional health. A reminder may be necessary if patient forgets.	• Teeth and gums are brushed regularly.
a. Encourage care of gums and teeth after meals.		
b. Encourage the patient's participation with care.		

(continued)

Nursing Interventions	*Rationale*	*Expected Outcomes*

Nursing Diagnosis: Sleep pattern disturbances related to anxiety, confusion, and activity/rest imbalance

Goal: Maintenance of a balance of sleep and activity

1. Reduce night-time distractions. a. Identify and reduce discomforts such as noise and anxiety. b. Avoid disturbing patient during the night for procedures or medications.	1. A nonstimulating environment will decrease confusion and minimize hyperactive behavior.	• Establishes rest and sleep patterns on a regular schedule. • Reduces wandering behaviors at night.
2. Take measures to increase safety. a. Provide nightlights. b. Block accessibility to the outdoors. c. Distract, monitor, and confine patient to a safe area. d. Provide patient with identification bracelet.	2. These will enhance the patient's safety if he wanders at night.	• Verbalizes a feeling of safety and comfort at bedtime.
3. Enhance comfort if awake at night. a. Avoid the use of restraints. b. Provide comfort measures when awake at night (warm milk, bath, backrub, soft music, rocking, caressing pet).	3. A pleasant, nonrestrictive environment will enhance return to sleep, minimize anxiety, and increase the patient's sense of well-being.	
4. Design a balanced schedule of activity/sleep. a. Increase daytime wakefulness and encourage short rests rather than long naps. b. Encourage regular exercise and activity programs.	4. Daily activity and regular exercise reduce agitation and produce a calming effect.	• Establishes activity patterns on a regular schedule.

(Text continued from p. 154)

- Those administering medications to the elderly must be aware of the commonly used drugs that are removed from the body primarily by *renal excretion*. Drugs that the kidneys excrete remain in the elderly person for a longer time. Drug dosages often must be reduced. Overdosage and drug toxicity at usual therapeutic dosages may result.
- At the same time, it is important to realize that a decline in *cardiac output* may decrease the delivery rate to the target organ or storage tissue.
- Changes in the *gastrointestinal system* may also affect drug therapy. In some elderly patients, a reduced number of mucosal cells and a slowing of gastric motility can prevent the drug from reaching therapeutic plasma and tissue concentrations, and delayed gastric emptying has undesirable effects on drugs that are acid labile or metabolized by the stomach mucosa. Alterations in intestinal motility and activity thus change the drug's contact time with the absorptive surface of the mucosa.
- As a result of a slowing *metabolism*, the drug levels may increase in the tissues and plasma, leading to a prolongation of drug action.

Because some or all of the organ systems may be marginally operational, older patients may show paradoxical or unusual responses to drugs and may develop toxic reactions and complications. In addition, the elderly have multiple medical problems requiring drug treatment.

In any drug regimen for the elderly, one must bear in mind that drugs are capable of altering the patient's nutritional status, which may already be compromised by a marginal diet and chronic disease and its treatment. Drugs can depress the appetite, cause nausea, irritate the stomach, and decrease absorption of nutrients, in addition to altering the electrolyte balance and the carbohydrate and fat metabolism. A few examples of drugs that are capable of altering the nutritional status are the antacids (produce thiamine deficiency), cathartics (diminish absorption), corticosteroids (lower serum calcium by reducing its absorption), aspirin (associated with folate deficiency), and phenothiazines and tricyclic depressants (increase food intake and weight gain).

Possible Drug Side-Effects

The drugs commonly used by elderly people are capable of producing potentially serious problems.

- Since sedatives and hypnotics can lead to confusion, delusion, hallucinations, falls, habituation, agitation, and altered behavior, such drugs should be given in smaller doses. Caution should also be taken when opiates are administered since they act as respiratory depressants.
- Before a prescribed opiate is given, the respiratory rate should be counted; if the rate drops below 14 per minute, the drug should be withheld. Because of the addicting nature of these drugs, no opiate should be given for longer than 72 hours unless specifically prescribed.
- The side-effects of commonly used pain relievers must be taken into account when older patients are concerned. Although salicylates are well tolerated, they can produce salicylism, electrolyte depletion, and possibly serious bleeding from prolonged prothrombin time. Phenacetin, a frequently used over-the-counter pain reliever, may be nephrotoxic and habit-forming.
- If tranquilizers are used for older patients, it is important to note that some (the phenothiazines) can cause hypotension, cerebral depression, and worsening of the agitated state. The minor tranquilizers meprobamate and chlordiazepoxide are useful in alleviating symptoms of anxiety in the ambulatory patient and in calming agitation. However, these drugs have a narrow therapeutic range, so that they may worsen the agitation and produce uninhibited aggressive states in some patients.
- Central nervous system stimulants may be prescribed with the hope of relieving depression, apathy, and lethargy. However, these drugs are given in small dosages since they have a tendency to exaggerate confusion and paranoia in some patients who have a chronic brain disorder. The tricyclic antidepressants may cause cardiac tachyarrhythmias and conduction disturbances.
- Since the heart conduction system, in general, is less effective in older patients, even small doses of digitalis can cause dysrhythmias and gastrointestinal and mental symptoms. Digitalis is also not as well tolerated because of less effective kidney function, a decrease in myocardial potassium, and a reduction in body weight. As a result, supplementary potassium and careful dosage maintenance of digitalis are required. Digitalis toxicity and cardiac dysrhythmias are enhanced by the depletion of intracellular potassium. Patients taking digitalis preparations in combination with non-potassium-sparing diuretics are at high risk of hypokalemia and digitalis toxicity. Digitalis blood levels must be monitored regularly; correction of potassium loss with diet and supplements is necessary. The most common signs of digitalis toxicity are fatigue, visual disturbances, muscle weakness, nausea, and anorexia.

With self-administered medication, it is important to consider possible sensory and memory losses as well as decreased manual dexterity. To help the client manage his medications and improve patient compliance, the nurse can:

- Explain the action, side-effects, and dosage of each medication
- Write out the drug schedule
- Encourage use of standard containers rather than safety lids
- Destroy old unused medications
- Periodically review the medication schedule
- Discourage the use of over-the-counter drugs without consulting a health professional.

Throughout the teaching process, the nurse can ask questions of the client and request return demonstrations to be sure learning has occurred.

The patient often feels that unless a drug has been prescribed, adequate treatment has not been given. As with other age-groups, this type of thinking must be corrected. The concept that health maintenance includes proper nutrition, a daily program of activity, and periodic health checkups is reinforced. Drugs are no substitute for caring persons and sound health practices.

In taking medication, if the person sips water first and takes several more swallows with the pill, it will go down more easily. Capsules will dissolve better if the water is room temperature rather than iced. If a patient has a history of suicide threats or attempts, the nurse must be sure that the medication (pill or capsule) is actually swallowed and not retained between the cheeks and the gums or teeth.

The Older Person in the Community

Ninety-five percent of the elderly live in the community; seventy-two per cent own their own homes. In 1984, in the 65 and older age-group, half as many women as men were married (40% of women, 78% of men). The majority of women over age 65 are widowed. This difference in marital status is due to several factors: women have a longer life expectancy than men, women tend to marry older men, and women remain widowed while men often remarry.

Family

Planning for care and understanding the psychosocial aspects of the older person are done within the context of the family. When dependency needs occur, the spouse assumes the role of primary caregiver. In the absence of the surviving spouse, a child usually assumes caregiver responsibilities and eventually may need help in providing care and support. A widely held myth within American society is that adult children and their aged parents are socially alienated. Furthermore, many believe that adult children abandon their parents when health and other dependency problems arise. Extensive reseach refutes these beliefs. Of the 80% of the elderly who have living children, three fourths have at least one child living within 30 minutes of their home, and they see each other at least once a week.

Social attitudes and cultural values have been formulated that prescribe an "etiquette of filial behavior." These rules and social expectations dictate that adult children should provide services, financial support, and the burden of care for their aged parents. Children of the aged are aware of these expectations and are profoundly influenced by their implications. Most people want to do the "right" thing and conform to the norms society has placed on human behavior.

Regardless of the amount of responsibility and love the adult child exhibits toward the dependent aged parents, strains will develop if care continues over a period of time. Research exploring the relationship between aged parents and their adult children shows that with poor health of the parent, the quality of the parent–child relationship declines. Under certain circumstances of high risk, strains in intergenerational relationships can result in elder abuse. *Elder abuse* is an active or passive act or behavior that is harmful to the elderly person. Such behavior includes physical violence, personal neglect, mental anguish, financial exploitation, violation of rights, denial of health care, and self-inflicted abuse. Before elder abuse occurs, when strains are evident, the nurse takes preventive action. Interdisciplinary team members can be enlisted to help the caregiver develop self-awareness, increased insight, and understanding of the aging process. At the same time, community resources may be useful for both the aged person and the caregiver. Independence of the elderly person should be encouraged and supported.

The Home Environment

Safety and Comfort. Accidents rank sixth as a cause of death for older people. Two of every 100 deaths in the elderly population can be attributed to accidents. *Falls,* the major cause of accidents in the elderly, are often nonfatal but threaten health and the quality of life. Normal and pathologic consequences of aging that contribute to increased falls include visual changes such as the loss of depth perception, susceptibility to glare, loss of visual acuity, and difficulty in light accommodation; neurologic changes, including loss of balance, loss of position sense, and delayed reaction time; cardiovascular changes, resulting in cerebral hypoxia and postural hypotension; cognitive changes, including confusion, loss of judgment, and impulsive behavior; and musculoskeletal changes, including altered posture and decreased muscle strength. Many drugs, drug interactions, and alcohol use precipitate falls by causing drowsiness, incoordination, and postural hypotension.

There are life-style and environmental changes that the nurse can encourage the older adult and his family to adopt. Adequate lighting with minimal glare and shadow calls for small area lamps, indirect lighting, sheer curtains to diffuse direct sunlight, dull rather than shiny surfaces, and night lights. Sharply contrasting colors can be used to mark the edges of stairs. Grab-bars by the tub and toilet are useful. Canes are excellent deterrents to falls, particularly outdoors where many hazards exist. Loose clothing, improperly fitting shoes, scatter rugs, small objects, and pets create hazards and increase the risk of accidents. A person will function best in familiar settings if furniture and objects remain unchanged. When the older person enters a new environment, he should be watched carefully, assisted often, and urged to use a cane because the potential for accidents is greater in unfamiliar spaces.

Personal Space. The older person needs a place of his own, a very special location that can offer him security, comfort, and privacy. This important "charted territory" can be a house, a room, or part of a room. It will contain treasures and mementos from a lifetime. The nurse can help the older person to maintain his own space. If he is moved, he will adjust more easily if he can establish a new area of privacy. Clutter is understandable if the space is small and the items are many. These articles can be touched, thought about, and enjoyed regularly to enhance the quality of life.

Chronic Illness and Common Disturbances of Well-Being

Fatigue. There is a well-circulated myth that older people should "take it easy" and avoid vigorous activity. Many of the elderly, therefore, may expect to feel tired and adopt an inactive role. Activity, however, is a desired state in older adults. Normal fatigue following strenuous or sustained exercise is expected with the aging process. A short rest usually restores vigor.

General chronic fatigue is not normal and may be a consequence of oversedation. Fatigue may be an indicator of depression or a symptom of physical illness such as anemia or heart disease.

Headaches. Most headaches are caused by incorrect posture and muscle strain around the head and neck. Heat, ice, massage, and exercise are used to relieve the symptoms. Serious organic disease such as brain tumor or hematoma may be the underlying cause and needs to be ruled out. The patient should be encouraged to seek medical advice if headaches persist.

Back Pain. The common complaint of back pain can accompany a number of chronic problems requiring medical attention. Back pain may be a sign of osteoporosis; accompanying vertebral fractures may press on the spinal nerves, causing severe pain that radiates to the legs (sciatica). Other, less common causes of back pain include metastatic cancer and infection. Muscle spasms responsible for much of the discomfort can be relieved by heat, ice, and rest. When acute back pain subsides, recurrence can be prevented by initiating a low back muscle exercise program.

Sleep Disturbances. Drowsiness is often due to boredom, habit, depression, or organic disease. Sleep patterns change with advanced age. Levels 3 and 4 of the sleep cycle are the stages of deepest sleep when arousal is most difficult. These levels of deepest sleep occur with less frequency in later life. Many brief arousals are predominant in the sleep of older persons. This increased wakefulness, although brief, may create an impression of sleeplessness or insomnia. Daytime napping and inactivity contribute to reduced sleep at night. Arthritis, muscle aches, nocturia, or sleep apnea may cause interruption in sleep.

A positive and reassuring attitude is necessary when the nurse counsels older adults about sleep. Quiet activity and reading are fine alternatives if sleep does not come. Symptoms are dealt with individually and sedatives discouraged. Some people find a warm bath and a glass of milk at bedtime helpful.

Heartburn and Indigestion. Heartburn occurs as a result of a reflux of stomach acid into the esophagus. Common causes include overeating, an incompetent lower esophageal sphincter, hiatal hernia, side-effects of medications, and organic disease.

The nurse can advise the older person to chew his food carefully, eat small meals, avoid heavy spices, and sit rather than recline after eating. Medical evaluation is necessary if this symptom persists.

Dyspnea. A normal decline in pulmonary function may be responsible for shortness of breath following physical exertion. Obesity, anemia, smoking, lung disease, respiratory infections, and heart disease are all causes of increased breathlessness. Because fever may not occur with respiratory infection in the older adult, increased respirations followed by increased pulse rate often are the first observable signs of acute illness.

Foot Problems. The feet of the older person should be given particular attention. Diminished subcutaneous fat reduces the protective padding and makes the skin more vulnerable to injury. Diminished blood supply as a result of circulatory impairment puts the older person at high risk for foot infections and subsequent complications. Ingrown toenails, corns, and calluses all cause discomfort and may lead to infection and tissue necrosis. Toenails often are thick and difficult to cut.

If the older person is unable to care for his toenails, the nurse can provide nail care. The feet are soaked in warm water and dried thoroughly. Debris around the cuticles and between the toes is removed with a soft towel. The nails are cut straight across beyond the nail grooves. Sharp edges are blunted with an emery board. Lotion is applied regularly. For the diabetic, only a podiatrist or other specially trained person should cut the nails.

Community Programs and Services

Hospital and health services are used more by the elderly than by other age-groups in the population. In 1984, the elderly (12% of the population) accounted for 31% of total personal health care expenditures. Chronic rather than acute disease is the major cause of illness. Over 80% of people age 65 and older have at least one chronic condition; multiple conditions are common. With advancing age, disabilities resulting from these chronic illnesses create the need for help with basic activities of daily living. Twenty-two percent of the elderly are limited to a point where they can no longer carry on regular daily activities. Community programs provide help beyond the capabilities of informal supports. Such valuable services as health care at home or in an adult day care center, opportunities for socialization, transportation, and home-delivered meals often keep the older person in the community and postpone or possibly eliminate the need for a nursing home.

Medicare and Medicaid

Medicare is a federal social insurance program designed to provide health care for elderly persons who are entitled to social security benefits. It has two parts; part A is hospital insurance and part B is medical insurance. All entitled persons receive part A, which provides limited coverage for hospital and post-hospital nursing home care and unlimited visits for home health care. Part B is a voluntary program that costs a small additional monthly premium. Part B pays for limited outpatient medical services and doctor's visits. Major items

not covered by either part include nonskilled home nursing care, ongoing nursing home care, prescription drugs, eyeglasses, and dental care. Medicare pays about 45% of the health costs of older people.

Medicaid is a health assistance program financed by state funds and matching federal grants. This program varies from state to state and is available only to the poor. It is the major source of public funding that provides nursing home care for the poor elderly. This program covers all the basic medical services and often covers such items as medications, eyeglasses, and dental care. Eligibility requirements prevent many low income people from receiving financial support for health care.

Home Care

The older adult usually prefers to live independently, even if he has difficulty getting around the home. This may be against the wishes of his adult children. If the older person is capable of accepting responsibility for the personal risk involved and other persons are not endangered, the adult children should not interfere with this decision. There are many community supports that help the older person maintain independence. Informal sources of help such as family, friends, the mailcarrier, church members, and neighbors can all keep an informal watch. Area agencies on aging (AAAs) perform many community services, including telephone reassurance, friendly visitors, home repair services, and home-delivered meals. Homemaker and chore services can be obtained on an hourly rate through AAAs or the local community nursing services. If the person is financially unable to pay, these services are subsidized through local and state funds. Nursing care and rehabilitation services requiring the expertise of a registered nurse and appropriate health professionals are paid by Medicare.

There are other community support services available to help the older person outside his home. Senior centers have social and health promotion activities; some provide a nutritious noontime meal. Adult day care facilities offer daily nursing care and social opportunities. Family members can carry on daily activities while the older person is at the day care center.

Ethical and Legal Issues

The nurse as an advocate can help the older person to plan for disability and death. A legal will and the advice of a competent attorney regarding financial and personal issues can preserve future stability. The older person is sometimes unable to take responsibility for legal, financial, or personal matters because of physical and mental incapacity. Legally, there are a number of ways that this is handled. It is best if arrangements and choices are made by the older person.

In the event of severe illness, with no reasonable expectation of recovery, the older person may not want to have his life extended by "heroic measures." Those who want to avoid technological interventions can draw up a *living will*. This document is given to the physician and incorporated into the medical record. Many states have enacted legislation to accept such a document. The nurse can help the person keep this document current and encourage discussion with the physician.

The Older Adult in an Acute Care Setting: Altered Responses to Illness

Pain and Fever

Altered physical, emotional, and systemic reactions to disease are attributed to age-related changes in the older person. Useful and reliable physical indicators of illness in the young and middle-aged person cannot be relied on for the diagnoses of potential life-threatening problems in the older adult. The response to pain in the older person may be altered owing to reduced acuity of touch, decreased speed of response, and diminished processing of sensory data. Research has demonstrated the absence of chest pain in 81% of older adults experiencing a myocardial infarction. Hiatal hernia or upper gastrointestinal tract distress are often responsible for chest pain in the elderly. Acute abdominal conditions such as mesenteric infarction and appendicitis often go unrecognized in elders because of atypical signs and an absence of pain.

Fever, with pneumonia or urinary tract infection, may be absent or delayed in the older person. Elevations in temperature rarely exceed 39.5°C (103°F). The nurse must be alert to more subtle signs of infection: mental confusion, increased respirations, tachycardia, changed facial appearance and color.

Emotional Impact

The emotional component of illness in older people may differ from that of younger people. Many elderly people equate good health with the absence of old age. "You are as old as you feel" is a belief of many. An illness that requires hospitalization or a change in life-style is an imminent threat to well-being. Admission to the hospital is often feared and actively avoided. Economic concerns and fear of becoming a burden to the family often lead to high anxiety in an older person. The nurse must recognize the implications of fear, anxiety, and dependency in the elderly patient. Autonomy and independent decision making are encouraged. A positive and confident demeanor of the nurse and the family help lift the mental outlook of the patient. In addition to anxiety and fear, older people are at high risk of disorientation, confusion, change in levels of consciousness, and other symptoms of delirium when they are admitted to the hospital.

Systemic Impact

The systemic impact of illness on the aged person has far-reaching effects. The decline in organ function that occurs in every system of the aging body eventually forces one or more body systems to function at full capacity. Illness places new demands on body systems that have little or no reserve to meet this crisis. Homeostasis, the ability of the body to maintain an internal balance of function and chemical composition, is jeopardized. The old person may be unable to respond effectively to an acute illness, or, if he has a chronic health condition, he may be unable to sustain appropriate responses over a long period of time. Furthermore, the older person's ability to respond to definitive treatment is impaired.

The Older Adult in a Protected Environment

Many housing communities for older people will perform routine maintenance and provide opportunities for socialization and recreation. Easier access to shopping and health care may convince the person that a new location will solve many residential problems. When preparation time is sufficient and money, energy, and health are adequate, a move to a new home can be a positive life experience.

Retirement communities have living quarters of apartments, condominiums, and houses that are developed specifically for the older person. An independent life-style is enhanced with social and recreational events. Health services are not provided. *Life care (continuing care) communities* offer all the features of retirement communities plus health care and skilled nursing care units. When entering such a community, the resident must be capable of independent living.

Although only 5% of the elderly population live in nursing homes, the percentage ranges from 2% for persons aged 65 to 74 years to 23% for persons 85 and older. Nursing homes offer a variety of health and personnel services that include skilled nursing care and rehabilitation. They do not provide acute care. Medicare will pay nursing home costs only for a limited number of days, and Medicare does not pay for personal care. The cost of nursing home care comes out of the family's funds. When money and all assets are totally depleted, the costs will be paid by Medicaid.

Often, a decision for a nursing home placement is made by the family without consulting the older person. Research indicates that successful adjustment to the nursing home is enhanced if the older person participates in the decision-making process. The nurse and social worker as advocates can emphasize this point and encourage a family decision that includes the client. When this occurs, the client selects the home of his choice and will enter with a positive mental attitude and a feeling of control. If the client wants to remain in his home, he may be able to manage with the help of community supports. Decisions made "for your own good" by the family may, in fact, not be. Placement of a person in a nursing home against his wishes should be made as a last resort when no other alternative is available.

Bibliography

Books

Beaver ML. Human Service Practice with the Elderly. Englewood Cliffs, New Jersey, Prentice-Hall, 1983.

Brubaker TH (ed). Family Relationships in Later Life. Beverly Hills, California, Sage Publications, 1983.

Burnside IM. Working With the Elderly: Group Process & Techniques, 2nd ed. Monterey, California, Wadsworth Health Sciences Division, 1984.

Butler RN and Lewis MI. Aging and Mental Health, 3rd ed. St Louis, CV Mosby, 1982.

Carcio HN. Manual of Health Assessment. Boston, Little, Brown, & Co, 1985.

Carnevali DL and Patrick M. Nursing Management for the Elderly, 2nd ed. Philadelphia, JB Lippincott, 1986.

Carotenuto R and Bullock J. Physical Assessment of the Gerontologic Client. Philadelphia, FA Davis, 1980.

Conrad KA and Bressler R (eds). Drug Therapy for the Elderly. St Louis, CV Mosby, 1982.

Dychtwald K. Wellness and Health Promotion for the Elderly. Rockville, Maryland, Aspen Publishers, 1986.

Ebersole P and Hess P. Toward Healthy Aging: Human Needs and Nursing Response, 2nd ed. St Louis, CV Mosby, 1985.

Erikson EH. Childhood and Society, 2nd ed. New York, WW Norton, 1963.

Ewles L and Simnett I. Promoting Health: A Practical Guide to Health Education. New York, John Wiley & Sons, 1985.

Gioiella EC and Bevil CW. Nursing Care of the Aging Client. Norwalk, Connecticut, Appleton-Century-Crofts, 1985.

Gress LD and Bahr RT Sr. The Aging Person: A Holistic Perspective. St Louis, CV Mosby, 1984.

Havighurst R. Developmental Tasks and Education, 3rd ed. New York, David McKay, 1972.

Hendricks J and Hendricks CD. Aging in Mass Society, 3rd ed. Boston, Little, Brown, & Co, 1986.

Hickey T. Health and Aging. Monterey, California, Brooks/Cole, 1980.

Hogstel MO (ed). Home Nursing Care for the Elderly. Bowie, Maryland, Robert J. Brady, 1985.

Kapp MB and Bigot A. Geriatrics and the Law. New York, Springer, 1985.

Kenney RA. Physiology of Aging. Chicago, Year Book Medical Publishers, 1982.

Mace NL and Rabins PV. The 36-Hour Day. Baltimore, Johns Hopkins Press, 1981.

Murray RB and Zentner JP. Nursing Assessment & Health Promotion Through the Life Span, 3rd ed. Englewood Cliffs, New Jersey, Prentice-Hall, 1985.

Oppeneer JE and Vervoren TM. Gerontological Pharmacology. St Louis, CV Mosby, 1983.

Pagliaro LA and Pagliaro AM (eds). Pharmacologic Aspects of Aging. St Louis, CV Mosby, 1983.

Rossman I (ed). Clinical Geriatrics, 3rd ed. Philadelphia, JB Lippincott, 1986.

Schuster CS and Ashburn SS. The Process of Human Development: A Holistic Life-Span Approach, 2nd ed. Boston, Little, Brown, & Co, 1986.

Schwartz AN et al. Aging and Life, 2nd ed. New York, Holt, Rinehart, & Winston, 1984.

US Bureau of the Census, Current Population Reports, Series P-23, No 128. America in Transition: An Aging Society. Washington, DC, US Government Printing Office, 1983.

US Senate Special Committee on Aging. Aging America: Trends and Projections 1984. Washington, DC, Department of Health and Human Services, 1984.

US Senate Special Committee on Aging. Aging America: Trends and Projections 1985-6. Washington, DC, Department of Health and Human Services, 1986.

Vestal RE. Drug Treatment in the Elderly. Sydney, ADIS Health Science Press, 1984.

Whanger AD and Myers AC. Mental Health Assessment and Therapeutic Intervention with Older Adults. Rockville, Maryland, Aspen Publishers, 1984.

Yurick AG et al. The Aged Person and the Nursing Process, 2nd ed. Norwalk, Connecticut, Appleton-Century-Crofts, 1984.

Articles

(Asterisks indicate nursing research articles.)

*Adams M. Aging: Gerontological nursing research. Annu Rev Nurs Res 1986; 4:77–103.

Andreasen MEK. Make a safe environment by design. J Gerontol Nurs 1985 June; 11(6):18–22.

Arluke A and Levin J. Another stereotype: Old age as a second childhood. Aging 1984 Aug/Sept; No. 346:7–11.

Aronson MK and Yatzkan ES. Coping with Alzheimer's disease through support groups. Aging 1984; No. 347:3–9.

Berkman B and Abrams RD. Factors related to hospital readmission of elderly cardiac patients. Soc Work 1986 Mar/Apr; 31(2):99–103.

Bookin D and Dunkle RE. Elder abuse: Issues for the practitioner. Soc Casework 1985 Jan; 66(1):3–12.

Braunstein C and Schlenker R. The impact of change in Medicare payment for acute care. Geriatr Nurs 1985 Sept/Oct; 6(5):266–270.

Brody E. Parent care as a normative family stress. Gerontologist 1985 Feb; 25(1):19–29.

*Burbank P. Psychosocial theories of aging: A critical evaluation. ANS 1986 Oct; 9(1):73–86.

Calabrese J et al. Nursing home keeps limbs moving. Aging 1985; No. 350:18–21.

Cieplik C. Prospective payment, diagnosis-related groups, and elder care. Geriatr Nurs 1985 Sept/Oct; 6(5):261–263.

Erickson R. Companion animals and the elderly. Geriatr Nurs 1985 Mar/Apr; 6(2):92–96.

Gaffney J. Toward a less restrictive environment. Geriatr Nurs 1986 Mar/Apr; 7(2):94–95.

Genevay B. Intimacy as we age. Generations 1986 Summer; 10(4):12–15.

Goldenberg B and Chiverton P. Assessing behavior: The nurse's mental status exam. Geriatr Nurs 1984 Mar/Apr; 5(2):94–98.

Gray-Vickrey M. Education to prevent falls. Geriatr Nurs 1984 May/June; 5(3):179–183.

Hall G et al. Sheltered freedom—An Alzheimer's unit in an ICF. Geriatr Nurs 1986 May/June; 7(3):132–137.

Hallal JC. Osteoporotic fractures exact a toll. J Gerontol Nurs 1985 Aug; 11(8):13–19.

Hamner ML and Lalor LJ. The aged patient in the critical care setting. Focus Crit Care 1983 Dec; 10(6):23–29.

Hayter J. Modifying the environment to help older persons. Nurs Health Care 1983 May; 4(5):265–269.

Hepburn K. Training the caregivers. Generations 1984 Winter; 9(2):58–59.

Hollinger LM. Communicating with the elderly. J Gerontol Nurs 1986 Mar; 12(3):9–13.

Hussar DA. Drug interactions. Nursing '86 1986 Aug; 16(8):34–39.

Johnson-Pawlson J and Koshes R. Exercise is for everyone. Geriatr Nurs 1985 Nov/Dec; 6(6):322–325.

Kahan J et al. Decreasing the burden in families caring for a relative with a dementing illness. J Am Geriatr Soc 1985 Oct; 33(10):664–670.

Kannel WB. Nutritional contributors to cardiovascular disease in the elderly. J Am Geriatr Soc 1986 Jan; 34(1):27–36.

Kee CC. A care for health promotion with the elderly. Nurs Clin North Am 1984 June; 19(2):251–263.

Kelly CH (ed). The living will—where it stands. Geriatr Nurs 1985 Jan/Feb; 6(1):18–20.

*Kim KK. Response time and health care learning of elderly patients. Res Nurs Health 1986 Sep; 9(3):233–239.

Lantz JM. In search of agents for self-care. J Gerontol Nurs 1985 July; 11(7):10–14.

*Laschinger SJ. The relationship of social support to health in elderly people. West J Nurs Res 1984 Summer; 6(3):341–350.

Lund C and Sheafor ML. Is your patient about to fall? J Gerontol Nurs 1985 Apr; 11(4):37–41.

Martinson I. Gerontology comes of age. J Gerontol Nurs 1984 July; 10(7): 8–17.

Mitchell CA. Generalized chronic fatigue in the elderly: Assessment and intervention. J Gerontol Nurs 1986 Apr; 12(4):19–23.

Mohs RC et al. A medical overview of Alzheimer's disease. Pride Institute J Long-Term Home Health Care 1984 Fall; 3(4):11–22.

Morscheck P. Introduction: An overview of Alzheimer's disease and long-term care. Pride Institute J Long Term Home Health Care 1984 Fall; 3(4):4–10.

Morse JM. The patient who falls and falls again: Defining the aged at risk. J Gerontol Nurs 1985 Nov; 11(11):15–18.

Oktay JS. Maintaining independent living for the impaired elderly: The role of community support groups. Aging 1985; No. 349:14–18.

Ory MG. Health promotion strategies for the aged. J Gerontol Nurs 1984 Oct; 10(10):31–37.

Pajk M. Alzheimer's disease inpatient care. Am J Nurs 1984 Feb; 84(2): 217–232.

Pardini A. Exercise, vitality and aging. Aging 1984 Apr/May; 19–29.

Picariello G. A guide for teaching elders. Geriatr Nurs 1986 Jan/Feb; 7(1):38–39.

Record longevity maintained. Stat Bull 1986 July/Sept; 67(3):25–29.

Resnick B. Constipation common but preventable. Geriatr Nurs 1985 July/Aug; 6(4):213–215.

Reynolds CF III. Sleep problems. Drugs aren't always the answer. Generations 1986 Spring; 10(3):24–26.

Rice JA and Taylor S. Assessing the market for long-term care services. Health Care Finan Manage 1984 Feb; 32–44.

Ross V and Robinson B. Dizziness: Causes, prevention, and management. Geriatr Nurs 1984 Sept/Oct; 5(7):291–304.

Rozovski SJ. Nutrition for older Americans. Aging 1984 Apr/May; No. 344:49–64.

Schaefer SC. Modifying the environment. Geriatr Nurs 1985 May/June; 6(3):157–159.

Schlenker R and Braunstein C. Case mix and Medicaid payment. Geriatr Nurs 1985 Sept/Oct; 6(5):275–277.

Schmidt MD. Meet the health care needs of older adults by using a chronic care model. J Gerontol Nurs 1985 Sept; 11(9):30–34.

Schwab M Sr et al. Relieving the anxiety and fear in dementia. J Gerontol Nurs 1985 May; 11(5):8–15.

Shanas E. Social myth as hypothesis: The case of the family relations of old people. Gerontologist 1979; 19(1):3–9.

Stoedefalke KG. Motivating and sustaining the older adult in an exercise program. Top Geriatr Rehabil 1985 Oct; 1(1):78–83.

*Taft LB. Self-esteem in later life: A nursing perspective. Adv Nurs Sci 1985 Oct; 8(1):77–84.

Taylor MB. The effect of DRGs on home health care. Nurs Outlook 1985 Nov/Dec; 33(6):288–289.

Thompson LW and Gallagher D. Depression and its treatment in the elderly. Aging 1985; No. 348:14–18.

Troll LE. Parents and children in later life. Generations 1986 Summer; 10(4):23–25.

Wasow M. Support groups for family caregivers of patients with Alzheimer's disease. Soc Work 1986 Mar/Apr; 31(2):93–97.

Weisberg J. Raising the self-esteem of mentally impaired nursing home residents. Soc Work 1983 Mar/Apr; 28(2):163–164.

Wetle T. Long-term care: A taxonomy of issues. Generations 1985 Winter; 10(2):30–34.

Williams L. Alzheimer's: The need for caring. J Gerontol Nurs 1986 Feb; 12(2):21–28.

*Wolanin MO. Clinical geriatric nursing research. Annu Rev Nurs Res 1986; 1:77–99.

Agencies

Governmental

Health and Human Services, Human Development Services, Administration on Aging, North Building, 330 Independence Avenue, SW, Washington, DC 20201; (202) 245–0641.

National Institute of Mental Health, Mental Disorders of the Aging Research Branch, Room 11C-03, 5600 Fishers Lane, Rockville, MD 20857; (301) 443–1185.

National Institute on Aging, N.I.A. Information Center, 2209 Distribution Circle, Silver Spring, MD 20910; (301) 496-3455.

Special Committee on Aging, US Senate SD-G33, Washington, DC 20510; (202) 224-5364.

Voluntary

Alzheimer's Disease and Related Disorders Association (ADRDA), 70 East Lake Street, Chicago, IL 60601-5997; (312) 853-3060 or (800) 621-0379; in Illinois only (800) 572-6037.

American Association for International Aging, Suite 1028, 1511 K Street, NW, Washington, DC 20005; (202) 638-6815.

American Association of Retired Persons (AARP), 1909 K Street, NW, Washington, DC 20049; (202) 728–4891.

American Geriatrics Society, 770 Lexington Ave., Ste. 400, New York, NY 10021; (212) 308-1414.

American Health Care Association, 1200 Fifteenth Street, NW, Washington, DC 20005; (202) 833-2050.

Children of Aging Parents (CAPS), 2761 Trenton Rd, Levittown, PA 19056; (215) 547–1070.

Council on Gerontological Nursing, American Nurses' Association, 2420 Pershing Road, Kansas City, MO 64108; (816) 474-5720.

Gerontological Society of America, 1411 K Street, Suite 300, Washington, DC 20005; (202) 393-1411.

Gray Panthers, 311 S. Juniper St., Philadelphia, PA 19107; (215) 545-6555.

Hospice Association of America, 214 Massachusetts Ave., NE, Suite 240, Washington, DC 20002; (202) 547-5263.

National Association for Home Care, 519 C Street, NE, Stanton Park, Washington, DC 20002; (202) 547-7424.

National Council on the Aging, Inc., 600 Maryland Ave., SW, West Wing 100, Washington, DC 20024; (202) 479-1200.

National Foundation for Long-Term Health Care, 1200 15th Street, NW, Washington, DC 20005; (202) 659-3148.

National Health Law Program, 2025 M Street, NW, Suite 400, Washington, DC 20036; (202) 887–5310.

Chapter 12

Human Response to Illness

Most people do not expect to get sick or have life-altering accidents. One of the most prominent hopes among Americans is that they and their families will have long and healthy lives. Yet, at any point along the life continuum they may be faced with difficult and painful changes in their health status. Everyone eventually dies.

The experience of illness precipitates many stressful feelings and reactions. These include frustration, anxiety, anger, denial, shame, grief, and uncertainty. Patients and their families have to adapt to the demands of the different stages of illness. Painful and disturbing symptoms lead to diagnostic tests and medical treatment. There are often dreaded questions about prognosis, body changes, and the reactions of others. Hospitalization is a major stress. Although necessary and often life-saving, it plunges people into an unfamiliar and often frightening environment, where they feel vulnerable and out of control. Acute illness calls for immediate action; chronic illness involves intricate changes in life-style with an uncertain future.

Sick people are often sensitive and vulnerable. Their whole lives are changed, at least temporarily. They struggle with the resurgence of past experiences as they cope with the present reality and the anticipated future. Issues of mortality, dependency, trust, and identity are raised.

The nurse is a central figure in the patient's immediate life. Through sensitive understanding and intelligent action she provides many opportunities for patients to maintain basic security, self-esteem, and integrity. She helps patients and families to cope with the crisis of illness.

Serious illness or injury is always more than just physical pain and inconvenience. A person's life goals, family, work and income, mobility, body image, and life-style may be drastically altered. Whether the changes are temporary or permanent, the situation may develop into a crisis for the person—a crisis that affects family, friends, and professional helpers. Emotional demands on the nurse are often continuous and draining. Without proper understanding and coping skills, the cumulative effect may be overwhelming and may lead to professional and personal problems.

To be of optimal help to patients, families, staff, and themselves, the nurse needs to know the following:

- The usual stages of illness and various emotional responses
- The major tasks of adapting to significant illness or injury
- The typical coping strategies used by patients and families
- The psychological and social factors that help or hinder coping
- Her own reactions to the various stresses and how to deal with them

Stages of Illness

The transition from health to illness is a complex and highly individualized experience. In addition to restoring physiologic balance, the two main tasks are (1) to modify the body image, concept of self, and relations to other people and work, and (2) to readjust realistically to the limitations imposed by the condition. The two tasks begin in the setting in which the person is being treated for the health problem.

In the cycle of health and illness, most people go through three stages: (1) the transition from health to illness, (2) the period of "accepted" illness, and (3) convalescence. The duration and quality of the experience vary with differences in personality, the specific disorder, and the changes made in the person's life.

First Stage

The development of symptoms usually is accompanied by unpleasant sensations, loss of vigor and stamina, and a decrease in the ability to function. Certain symptoms, such as chest pain, indigestion, and headache, may increase in frequency and intensity. Anxiety is often present and is handled with the person's usual coping mechanisms. To ward off the prospect of sickness, one person may plunge into activity, keeping late hours with extra work and social activities. Another may become passive and withdrawn, hoping that the vague symptoms will go away. A person may put off seeking medical care for fear of the diagnosis, especially if something serious is suspected, such as cancer. Anxiety, guilt, shame, and denial are prominent during this initial period.

If the symptoms persist, the person seeks medical attention. He may have ambivalent feelings toward examination and diagnostic tests, which are reflected in canceled or missed appointments. He may not follow initial recommendations or take prescribed medication. Some patients go from physician to physician, hoping to learn "what's really the matter" or that a previous diagnosis was inaccurate.

When a person experiences a sudden catastrophe, such as heart attack or stroke, he is instantly shifted from health to illness. His immediate concern is that help will not arrive in time or that the medical strangers on whom he is suddenly so dependent will not be competent. Families experience similar fears but have no time to consider alternatives. Apprehension is expressed through excessive demands, denial that the problem exists, refusal to cooperate or accept the proposed treatment, withdrawal, and suspicion of the motives and methods of those trying to help. To offset this reaction, it is helpful to contact close relatives, significant others, and the person's own physician, if possible. Calm explanation of

the necessary procedures and demonstration of technical skill will convey to patients that they are being cared for adequately.

When patients and families are experiencing shock, disbelief, and denial of the condition, the nurse helps by listening. In a noncritical way, she does not support the denial but accepts the need to cope with the situation in this way at the present time. She establishes herself as a professional person who wants to understand and help. She orients patients to the immediate environment and answers questions to the best of her ability.

Second Stage

The second stage is a shift to the period of accepted illness. The patient recognizes and admits that he is sick and in need of help from others, especially from the medical and nursing staffs. Temporarily, he adopts the patient role. This includes abdication from usual responsibilities and cooperation in the task of getting well. In this stage, patients become preoccupied with themselves, their symptoms, and their treatment; interest in current events and even concern about family and friends may be quite limited. Increased dependency accompanies preoccupation with somatic concerns. This behavior is often described as regressive, since it is a return to earlier forms of acting, feeling, and relating to others.

A certain amount of regression is necessary so that patients can allow themselves to rest in bed, eat specified diets, sleep, and let their bodies heal. People who normally resist being dependent may find this very difficult. They are so threatened that they continue to deny their condition in part or refuse prescribed treatment. They push themselves beyond their physical limits and discontinue treatment prematurely. The other extreme of dependency problems is seen in patients who receive so much gratification from dependency that they attempt to continue it indefinitely; the terms *hospitalitis* and *secondary gain* refer to this.

When acutely ill, patients need a great deal of help from others. Nursing students are often unduly concerned that patients will become too dependent on them. There must be a realistic evaluation of the stage of illness, the patient's need for dependency, and the need for a trusting, caring person. The nurse who cares for the same patients over long periods of time should evaluate her own needs for having others dependent on her. The nurse can help patients move through the stages of illness, so that they become autonomous and able to care for themselves again.

During the stage of accepted illness, the patient may express anger, guilt, and resentment. He may be very critical of care and medical management, attacking the very people he depends on. The most helpful nursing approach is to view this reaction as the person's attempt to deal with the situation. The nurse tries to understand how patients and families feel. She encourages the expression of feelings without passing judgment, moralizing, or arguing. Labeling the feeling (*i.e.*, "This must be difficult to believe," or "You must be feeling a loss of control") will encourage patients to verbalize fears.

When sick, patients often feel helpless and hopeless. The nursing staff assumes responsibility for the care of patients and are alert to individual differences and needs. They provide opportunities for the patient to make decisions and assume responsibility whenever indicated. As the patient improves and becomes more assured of the staff's availability, interest, and competence, he is less anxious and more able to relinquish dependency. During this period, the patient may be experiencing an acute sense of loss. The clinical picture is depression with sadness, hopelessness, and anger. He may be mourning the loss of health and vigor, the loss of a body part or function, or changes anticipated in job and family. He may be moving into the emotional reactions to dying (see Dying and Death discussion, at the end of this chapter.)

Third Stage

The third stage is the convalescent or restitution period. The return of health and physical strength often precedes the patient's feeling and acting "well." Just as a lag usually occurs in the initial stage between the appearance of physical symptoms and the emotional acceptance of illness, a reverse lag occurs in recovery. Getting well implies giving up a dependent, regressive position and resuming adult responsibilities and normal relations with others. Although some people are reluctant to give up the patient role, most are motivated toward health but are afraid or hesitant to try out new skills. This is particularly true if the illness and treatment require major changes in work and family relations.

The nurse helps patients in this stage by assuming a role analogous to that of an adequate parent of a teenager. She gradually relaxes protection and offers guidance, advice, and encouragement to progress. She quietly retires to the sidelines, ready to reassure but encouraging experimentation with new skills. She steps in only when gross errors in judgment occur. The patient senses the confidence of the nurse and is reassured by it, especially if ideal or perfect results are not expected.

During the convalescent stage, the nurse can stimulate the patient to renew his interest in the world, communicate better with family, and make plans for the future. For example, there are support groups for people who have had strokes, mastectomies, and other conditions. A member of one of these groups may be called in to talk to the patient both before and after an operation, to convey hope and to give realistic, firsthand information on coping with their common disability. At first, the patient may be overwhelmed by anxiety or grief and unable to use these services. During convalescence, he is reminded and encouraged to avail himself of this help. It is important to keep individual differences in mind because some patients do not want to affiliate with such groups. The connotation of being different, especially with a stigmatized condition, may be too painful to admit publicly.

Adapting to Illness

Just what is it that patients and families have to cope with when they become sick? The major tasks have been identified by Moos (1984) as follows:

- Dealing with the discomfort, incapacitation, and symptoms of the illness or injury
- Managing the stress of treatment procedures and hospitalization

- Developing and maintaining adequate relationships with the medical, nursing, and other caretaking staff
- Preserving a satisfactory self-image and maintaining a sense of competence and mastery
- Balancing the disturbing feelings aroused by illness and treatment
- Maintaining relationships with family and friends despite a changed role identity
- Preparing for an uncertain future in which further loss, death, or recovery are possibilities

These adaptive tasks often occur simultaneously or recur at different stages of the illness.

The stages of transition from health to illness and back to health are most clearly defined when a person has an acute condition that responds favorably to treatment. A similar series of steps takes place in adapting to a chronic condition. The stages are disbelief, developing awareness, reorganization, and resolution. In a successful adaptation to a chronic illness, the person can comfortably or resignedly regard himself as having a specific condition. He acknowledges and copes with the necessary changes in his life imposed by the condition. Although he may have gone through periods of despair, anger, and self-depreciation, he is able to regard himself as a worthwhile person who happens to need help in some form and degree.

Adaptation to chronic illness is a lengthy and continuous process. The extent of adaptation required depends on the type of illness, the degree of disability, and the patient's unique personality. Some chronic illnesses are relatively stable, with few changes; others have acute remissions and slow degeneration; some are terminal. Unpredictability is a hallmark of chronic illness, in terms of symptoms, effectiveness of treatment, hopes for future remissions and medical breakthroughs, and the reactions of others. Patients are often torn between living within their limitations and pushing for more.

Basic Emotional Needs

Everyone has the same basic emotional needs. These have been variously categorized as the need for love, trust, autonomy, identity, self-esteem, recognition, and security, and are summarized by Schutz (1966) as the interpersonal need for inclusion, control, and affection. The nonrealization of a need leads to undesired feelings and behaviors. Feelings such as anxiety, anger, loneliness, and self-doubt are raised.

The interpersonal needs for inclusion, control, and affection are expressed in group as well as one-to-one situations. This is seen in relationships among patients on a ward or unit and within their families. The needs are present in staff relationships and often make the difference in the morale of a unit as well as in how well it is run.

These needs are overlapping and continuous. Inclusion is primarily related to the formation of a relationship, while control and affection are demonstrated within the relationship. Inclusion is feeling "in" or "out"; control is "top" or "bottom"; and affection is "remote" or "close." Generally, people establish equilibrium between themselves and others in these three areas. Sickness with hospitalization disturbs this equilibrium, giving rise to a wide variety of new stresses.

Need for Inclusion

The need for inclusion is defined behaviorally as the need to establish and maintain satisfactory relationships with people with respect to association and interaction. It refers to the establishment and maintenance of a feeling of mutual interest in others. The need for inclusion is the need to feel that the self is significant and worthwhile. Inclusion behavior refers to association between individuals and is indicated by such words as "associate," "interact," "belong," "join," and "communicate." Lack of inclusion is connoted by words such as "excluded," "ignored," "withdrawn," "aloof," or "isolated." The need to be included is shown by the desire to attract attention and interest. The "demanding" patient who frequently signals and monopolizes the staff with extensive conversation may simply be indicating strong needs for inclusion. The nurse who feels personally slighted when a patient ignores her attempts at polite conversation or treats her like a servant rather than a professional person may be demonstrating her own inclusion needs.

The desire for prestige and status is a part of inclusion needs; the individual needs people to pay attention to him, know who he is, and distinguish him from others. Identity is closely related to inclusion. One is known as a distinct individual, who therefore deserves attention. The height of inclusion is to be understood, which implies that someone is interested enough to seek and discover a person's particular characteristics, likes, and dislikes.

When a person enters a hospital situation, his first crisis involves inclusion needs. Will the staff know who he is? Will he be treated like a person and not just another case—"Room 111" or "the new cardiac"? Many routines of hospital admission strip the patient of outward signs of prestige and status. His clothes and belongings, even his dentures, may be taken away. He receives a uniform and, often humiliating, a hospital gown. He may be bombarded by a series of questions relating to the most intimate details of his life. He is expected to join the patient "group" but may be given little explanation or few guidelines about what to do. When it is necessary to place a patient in isolation, attention should be given to his inclusion needs—the nurse becomes a vital link in satisfying them.

Other ways to help a patient with his inclusion needs include giving him a thorough and considerate orientation to his physical surroundings. The nurse can inquire about the patient's questions and expectations related to treatment. She can give some guidelines about the scope of her professional responsibility, explaining that she will be available to help in a variety of ways.

The patient who is withdrawn and avoids association with others may have unmet inclusion needs. He may not talk to his roommates or the nurse and may spend long periods sleeping or with the curtains pulled. A certain amount of regression and isolation is often a necessary part of adaptation to illness and recovery, but extremes over a period of time are significant. Underneath an apparent indifference to others may lie a basic anxiety in relation to people. The patient's worse fear may be that others will ignore him and show no interest in him, although the fear is disguised with a lack of interest in others and a seeming independence. Patients who feel abandoned and isolated from their families

and friends, who believe that they are so changed now as to be unacceptable, or who feel rejected and ignored by the medical and nursing staff may give up the struggle. On the other hand, such patients may get lifesaving reassurance and support from the nurse who continues to include them in the human race and communicates her recognition of their individuality and worth.

Part of the decision of where to place a patient is based on the need for inclusion. Will he do better in a room with three other people? How close to the nursing station should he be? Patients who are together for long periods of time, such as in an orthopedic ward or a rehabilitation facility, demonstrate a particularly wide variety of inclusion needs.

Need for Control

The second major need is control. This is the need to establish and maintain a satisfactory relation to others with regard to power, decision making, and authority. It has to do with the feeling of mutual respect for the competence and responsibility of oneself and others. Control needs are suggested by such words as "dominance," "influence," "boss," "rebellion," "submission," "leader," "noncooperation," and "follower." Control represents assumption of power over others and therefore over one's own future, whereas *being* controlled means giving up responsibility for oneself.

When a person comes to a hospital, he struggles with his need for control. In addition to the problems of inclusion, he may find other people making decisions for him that he would ordinarily make for himself—when to get up, what to eat, and when to go to the toilet. The rules of the hospital may take away his usual decision-making capacity. An extreme example of control behavior is the person who completely gives up or abdicates his own responsibility. He is a clinging, helpless patient who seeks direction from everyone about what to do and how to do it. This reinforces his conviction that he is incompetent, irresponsible, and powerless. Behind these beliefs often lie anxiety, hostility, and a lack of trust in others as well as oneself. Nursing interventions that help the patient to assume responsibility early for making decisions about his own care contribute to restoring control.

The other extreme in control behavior is reflected in actions of constant rebellion and domination. Although the patient's overt behavior may be that of a strong, competent, responsible person, his underlying feelings may be those of uncertainty in his own power. He takes every opportunity to disprove these fears and therefore has a great deal of difficulty in accepting the need for dependency in such matters as bed rest or following "doctor's orders." Nurses also need to examine their own needs for power and control in relation to patients, co-workers, and physicians.

Need for Affection

The third major need is that of affection. This represents the need to establish with another person a give-and-take relationship based on mutual liking. Affection is suggested by such words as "love," "like," "emotionally close," "personal," "friendship," and "intimacy." Lack of affecton is connoted by "hate," "dislike," and "emotionally distant." The need for affection is usually met by family members, spouses, and close friends. When a person is separated from these sources by illness or hospitalization, the need for affection may not be satisfied. Being emotionally close to another generally results in confiding to that person one's innermost anxieties, wishes, and feelings. In the hospital setting, the patient may turn to the nurse to share these things, especially if the family member is unavailable or too anxious to listen. One difference between a social and a professional relationship is that the former implies mutual need satisfaction, the latter, exclusive attention to the patient's needs. However, the need for affection in both patient and nurse must be considered, particularly when the relationship continues over a period of time.

Self-Image and Body Image

The person has a mental and social picture of himself that is based on multiple experiences in the past, present, and anticipated future. Serious illness and injury abruptly interfere with that self-concept. Adaptation to the changes imposed by illness can affect the person's sense of identity. People often rate themselves as courageous or cowardly in terms of how they handle pain; crying may be a sign of weakness to them. A major disability can be viewed as a limitation to be challenged. Some people regard themselves as cripples, which emphasizes the disability and is stigmatizing. An important aspect of the total self-image that is often affected by physical illness is body image.

Concept of Body Image

The concept of body image is useful in understanding the many complex reactions of people to changes in health status. Body image may be considered as the total, constantly changing and evolving perception of one's physical self as separate and distinct from all others. This perception is based on inner sensations and functionings as well as on information derived from the external environment. Society prescribes norms of physical appearance and behavior. The perception of body image operates on both conscious and unconscious levels.

Integration of experiences with use of the body takes place over a long period of time. The formative years of childhood are particularly significant in laying down the basic body image and its relation to the personality. While a child is being held, fondled, fed, played with, and toilet-trained, he gradually accumulates related concepts pertaining to ability to use his physical body, pride, and sense of identity. Through sensory impressions, mobility, and touch he experiences pleasure, pain, shame, failure, or pride of accomplishment as he tests his boundaries and abilities. As the small child becomes aware of his separation from others, he grows increasingly conscious of his own body, its relation to others, and his ability to control his muscles in the acts of locomotion, bowel and bladder retention and release, motor coordination, and speech. During this period, he begins to master these abilities, and thus acquires pride and self-esteem. If he is not able to gain this mastery, because of loss of self-control and parental overcontrol, he may develop basic attitudes that lead him to regard his body as inadequate, worthless, and shame-

ful. Illness, with enforced dependency and lack of body control, reactivates in people of all ages many of these early conflicts and perceptions of body image. Feeling ashamed of a disfigurement or deformity stems from early feelings of smallness, weakness, and ugliness as compared to others. The prominent sociocultural values of youth, physical attractiveness, health, and wholeness are incorporated early and reinforced throughout life.

Threats to Body Image. Threats to the body image, and hence to self-esteem, are recognizable in many nursing situations. Feelings of shame, inadequacy, and guilt may be precipitated, depending on the patient's definition of the situation. Violation of modesty and invasion of privacy cause anxiety and embarrassment. Exposure of the body during physical examinations and such treatments as enemas and catheterizations may be upsetting, even though expected as part of the therapeutic regimen. Disturbances in usual elimination processes and the need for using a bedpan or talking about bowel and bladder habits threatens self-esteem. This is a major problem for people requiring the type of surgery that produces such drastic changes as a colostomy or ileostomy.

Major changes in the body image are brought about by amputation of any part or by surgery on the face, hands, and reproductive organs—areas particularly related to identity and self-esteem. Other parts of the body may have unconscious symbolic meanings for a person and may cause unexpected reactions to relatively minor external changes.

Besides the sudden changes in body structure and functioning that occur through accident or surgical intervention, subtle changes occur in progressive diseases such as arthritis, obesity, and multiple sclerosis. Even normal changes in the body, such as occur in puberty and pregnancy, pose a problem of altering the body image. During adolescence there is a sensitive, often painful awareness of the body and its many changes. Complexion, weight, and development of primary and secondary sexual characteristics are closely linked to feelings of worth and sexual desirability.

Changes in the body image may result from such side-effects of medication as development of a moon face, changes in the secondary sex characteristics, and growth of facial hair. The reaction of the body to radiation treatment may further threaten the body image, as may changes in skin color, such as occurs in jaundice.

Changes in medical technology require that nurses meet the challenge of new and different approaches to helping people. A person with chronic kidney damage extends his body image to include the "artificial kidney." Organ transplants are another development that raises questions about body image. What does it mean to a person to have another person's heart beating in his chest? What would it be like to have parts of your own body live on after you are clinically dead?

Nursing Implications. The first step in understanding the concept of body image is to become more aware of one's own attitude toward health, illness, mutilation, disfigurement, and changes in body functioning. Anxiety, revulsion, disgust, and pity are often automatic responses to abnormal body appearance and functioning. To help patients who have these conditions, nurses must come to terms with their own feelings. A patient has a right to expect that nurses will be knowledgeable about his condition, impartial toward it, willing to help him, and concerned about him. A patient often uses the nurse's reactions as a test of whether he is still a worthwhile person in spite of his altered appearance or functioning.

The nurse needs to learn what alteration in the body can mean to the individual patient and what adjustments it will require. Both the patient and his family should be considered, because ideally the adjustment that takes place is mutual. In formulating the nursing care plan for a particular patient, it is useful to include the ability of the family to help the patient cope with changes, orientation to reality, specific problems in coping and methods of coping, and nursing care. The nurse needs to determine how she can support the family and the steps she will take in response to the patient's positive moves. She can anticipate grief, mourning, and anger as reactions to changes in body appearance and functioning. The need for hope and steps toward full rehabilitation must be supported.

Social Adjustments. Even after the patient has begun to alter his body image and feels worthwhile and accepted in the hospital setting, he is faced with adjusting to society. Many conditions of altered appearance and functioning are stigmatizing. Because of their close proximity to illness, nurses may lose sight of the fact that being disfigured or incapacitated still evokes negative responses and rejection by most of the population. Any such stigma implies that the person is not quite normal—that he is a disabled person, rather than a person having a specific disability. The tendency to stereotype denies the person's individuality. A person with an obvious physical disability has a major problem in handling tensions in interpersonal situations. He may be subjected to curiosity and stares. He may be asked intrusive questions about his condition or treated as if he were completely helpless.

If the condition is not readily visible, learning to exercise information control may help one to avoid being stigmatized. For instance, wearing a prosthesis for a mastectomy can keep one's radical surgery from becoming common knowledge. Talking about one's health status, body functioning, and difficulties in adjustment is appropriate with health personnel and close family and friends. With other people, excessive dwelling on these topics may lead to rejection and ostracism.

A person making necessary adjustments to alterations in his body is often faced with physical and social insecurity. A physically normal person has a general idea of how high the bus steps are and is able to read from a menu. However, the person with a physical impairment may have to make constant and vigilant adaptations to his physical world. The person who uses a wheelchair must find a restroom large enough to maneuver in; one with diabetes must calculate his allowed intake at a cocktail party; a person with crutches may find a revolving door almost impossible to manage. Adaptation requires energy, ingenuity, and persistence. Sometimes a person limits his living space and activities in order to provide more predictable situations. Although this arrangement may be safer, it also limits a person's full participation in life.

Reactions of others toward a person with a disability are ambiguous and conflicting. Acceptance and rejection, sympathy and pity, trust and fear, curiosity and revulsion, valuation and devaluation face him in countless interpersonal situations. He is often unsure of where he stands, particularly with strangers. He is also often unsure of himself, because the process of adaptation and self-acceptance is a shifting one.

Emotional Reactions to Illness and Treatment

Many disturbing feelings are aroused by acute and chronic illness and the treatment they require. Some emotional reactions commonly experienced by patients and their families are anxiety, anger, grief, hope, shame, guilt, courage, pride, despair, love, depression, helplessness, envy, loneliness, and faith. Nursing staff members also experience these feelings. How they are experienced and expressed depends on the basic personality, the perception of the situation, and the amount of support from others. There is no right or wrong way to feel about serious illness. Nurses can anticipate patterns and help patients and families express feelings in a constructive way.

Anxiety

Anxiety is a normal reaction to stress and threat. It is an emotional reaction to the perception of danger, real or imagined, that is experienced physiologically, psychologically, and behaviorally. Anxiety and fear are often used synonymously; however, fear generally refers to a specific threat, anxiety to a nonspecific one. A person experiencing anxiety may feel uneasy and apprehensive and may have a vague sense of dread. Feelings of helplessness and inadequacy may be present along with a sense of alienation and insecurity. The intensity of these feelings may range from mild to severe enough to cause panic, and the intensity may be increased or diminished by interpersonal means.

Anxiety can be viewed as a process that includes the following steps: (1) an expectation exists; (2) the expectation is not met; (3) internal tension occurs; (4) relief behaviors are manifested; and (5) relief is experienced (Fig. 12-1). A typical example is that of a student taking an examination.

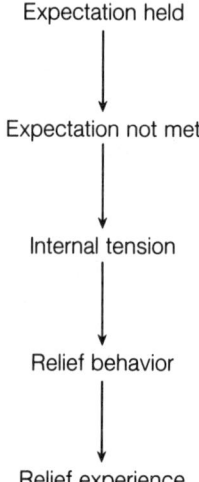

Expectation held

↓

Expectation not met

↓

Internal tension

↓

Relief behavior

↓

Relief experience

Figure 12-1
Operational definition of the anxiety process model. (Adapted from Anxiety: Concept and Manifestations [videocassette], 1977. Reproduced with permission from American Journal of Nursing.)

The student's expectation is that he will pass the examination. This expectation is not met when he learns that he has failed. His internal tension rises and he experiences increased perspiration, palpitations, and abdominal discomfort. Relief behaviors are manifested, such as gum chewing, crying, or making an appointment to talk with the instructor. He experiences relief when he meets with the instructor and together they develop a structured study plan for him.

The anxiety process model can be used to facilitate nursing interventions. When a relief behavior is identified, the nurse can assist the patient to correlate the behavior with the increase in anxiety. Once this is accomplished, the nurse and the patient can explore what expectation was held and what occurred that prevented that expectation from being met. In doing this, the nurse helps the patient examine and handle future anxiety-producing situations in a healthier manner.

Anxiety is caused by a threat to the functioning of the organism—either to physical survival or to the integrity of the psychosocial self (self-image). Often, the threat affects both of these areas: a person who is anxious because of acute pain may also be anxious in response to his feelings about his levels of courage and dependency. Illness and hospitalization include the following anxiety-precipitating threats: general threat to life, health, and body integrity; exposure and embarrassment; discomfort from pain, cold, fatigue, and changes in diet; deprivation of sexual satisfaction; restriction of movement; isolation; interruption or loss of one's means of livelihood, precipitation of a financial crisis; dislike, rejection, or ridicule from others as the result of the condition; inconsistent and unpredictable behavior of the authority figures on whom one's welfare depends; frustration of goals and expectations; confusion and uncertainty about the present and the future; separation from family and friends.

Physiologic reactions to anxiety are primarily reactions of the autonomic nervous system and are defensive. They include increases in pulse and respiratory rates; shifts in blood pressure and temperature; relaxation of the smooth muscles in the bladder and bowel; cold, clammy skin; increased perspiration; dilated pupils; and dry mouth. The bodily responses to mild anxiety initially promote learning and the ability to function, but as the reaction increases in severity, learning decreases, perception is reduced or distorted, and the ability to concentrate is greatly diminished (Fig. 12-2). Nurses must be able to evaluate the level of anxiety in a patient so that they can be effective in reducing it. An extremely anxious person is suffering and is very uncomfortable. He has difficulty giving or receiving information of any kind. He learns little about health matters and magnifies or distorts what he hears.

Characteristic manifestations of anxiety reflect a person's individuality. They include withdrawal, muteness, hyperactivity, swearing, talking and joking excessively, striking out verbally or physically, fantasizing, complaining, and crying. The specific means of coping with anxiety, whether successful or not, vary with individuals and with the situation. One disadvantage of enforced immobility and isolation is that a person who is used to active approaches in handling anxiety is deprived of his usual means of coping and so must develop alternative channels.

Nursing Interventions. Nursing intervention in anxiety has four aspects:

1. The nurse recognizes that the patient is anxious. She is aware of situations that can potentially precipitate anxiety and is alerted to physiologic, emotional, and behavioral clues.
2. The nurse verbally encourages the patient to recognize and express his feelings of anxiety.
3. If the source of the anxiety is external, such as poor orientation to the ward or disturbing noises and sights, the nurse takes steps to change these conditions or, if this is impossible, helps the patient to understand and cope with his reactions. She encourages the patient to share his immediate experience by open-ended statements, such as "Tell me what happened," "What was

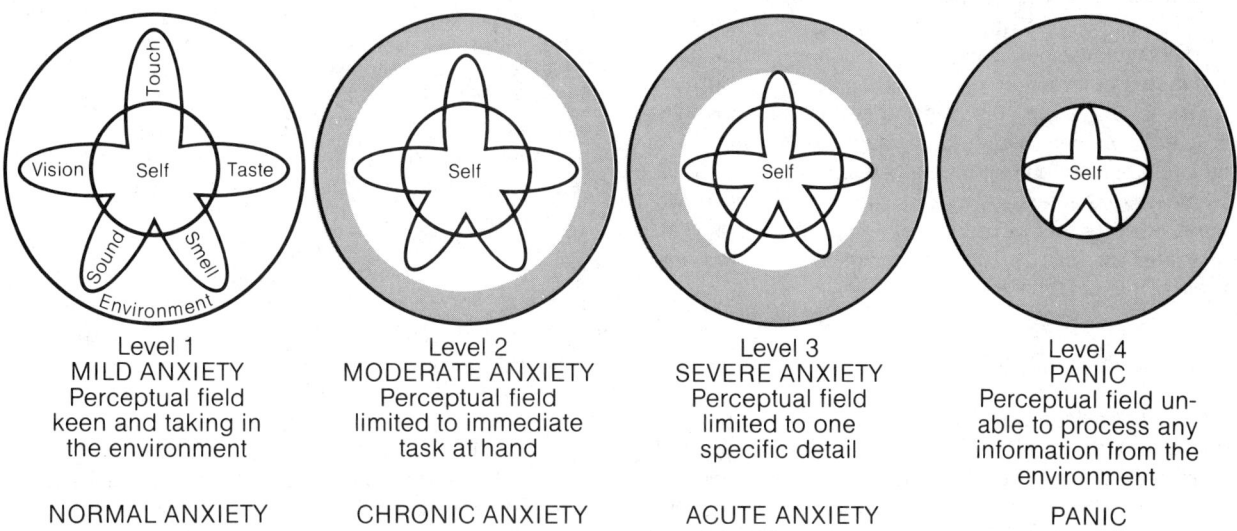

Level 1	Level 2	Level 3	Level 4
MILD ANXIETY	MODERATE ANXIETY	SEVERE ANXIETY	PANIC
Perceptual field keen and taking in the environment	Perceptual field limited to immediate task at hand	Perceptual field limited to one specific detail	Perceptual field unable to process any information from the environment
NORMAL ANXIETY	CHRONIC ANXIETY	ACUTE ANXIETY	PANIC

Figure 12-2

Levels of anxiety and the perceptual field. Shaded area indicates amount of environmental stimuli not attended to. (Haber J et al. Comprehensive Psychiatric Nursing. New York, McGraw-Hill, 1982.)

going on?'' or ''What did you expect to happen?'' Patients often need help in describing their reactions and thoughts. To ask initially, ''Why are you anxious?'' may or may not elicit the information. The person may be too afraid or unsure to tell you, he may not know why he is anxious, or he may resent the inquisition.

4. The nurse helps the patient to cope with what is now a specific threat. The patient may be helped to reevaluate the situation and his reaction to it. Many times just the sharing of a feeling reduces its intensity. The nurse asks the patient what he usually does to handle anxious feelings and helps him to use similar or other means. The physical presence of the nurse may help, as well as the appropriate use of touch, physical care, and tone of voice.

The apprehension of patients recovering from surgery may be demonstrated by their anxiety about whether the operation was a success and whether they will survive the bewildering, painful, often uncertain postoperative period. The expert physical nursing care given in the recovery room or intensive care unit must take into consideration the patient's fears resulting from isolation; the weird noises and equipment attached to all parts of the body; the blinking, beeping monitor signaling the body's functioning; and the periods of disorientation and loss of physical and emotional control. In this tense situation the nurse must be constantly aware of her own behavioral manifestations of anxiety.

Illness and its treatment precipitate anxiety. For many people, early conflicts are revived. There is often a great deal of uncertainty about the future. Nurses sometimes are powerless to decrease the patient's anxiety at all, but they can avoid adding to it. For some patients, the thought of getting well and leaving the hospital produces anxiety. The nurses can be helpful to these people by encouraging them to mobilize their strengths and by encouraging decision making and the reacquisition of responsibility.

Nursing in almost all areas is a professon that deals continually with anxiety. The intimate association with life, death, and all the stages in between arouses within the nurse conscious and unconscious fears about her own vulnerability. Recognition, achievement, and attention are all important; she must be able to say that she did all that was possible. There are emotional ''high-risk'' situations in nursing, such as the intensive care unit and the emergency department, in which the nurse's understanding and management of her own anxiety as well as that of patients and their families is vital. See Nursing Care Plan 12-1 for an example of a nursing care plan for the patient with anxiety.

Anger and Hostility

In addition to anxiety, expressions of anger are common in nursing situations. Conflict, frustration, and loss of control often precipitate aggression, a complex reaction of feelings and behavior that varies in intensity, duration, and expression. Words such as ''irritated,'' ''sullen,'' ''unfriendly,'' ''hostile,'' ''assertive,'' ''belligerent,'' ''defiant,'' ''uncooperative,'' ''resentful,'' ''enraged,'' ''furious,'' and ''indignant'' describe various forms of aggressiveness. Anger, the general term for this emotion, is one way of handling anxiety, particularly in response to real or perceived threat, insult, or injury. To be

a patient means to be sick, helpless, controlled by others, and assaulted—however therapeutically—by needles, catheters, enemas, and surgical procedures. Being told to wait for medication angers many patients who are in pain. Being awakened in the middle of the night to cough and take deep breaths taxes anyone's patience. Hospital rules such as lights out and restrictions on visitors may arouse feelings of anger. When a patient is new to the hospital or clinic, he is often uncertain and anxious about his diagnosis, treatment, and prognosis; as a defense, he may flare up at the nurse or withdraw in sullen noncommunicativeness. Expressions of anger may decrease markedly as the element of the unknown is reduced and the patient becomes more familiar with his surroundings, the personnel, and the treatment program. On the other hand, anger may increase if the threat grows and the patient's needs are not met adequately. Allowing the patient choices provides for control by the patient and often helps reduce feelings of anger and frustration.

A person who has been angry, unhappy, and chronically dissatisfied with himself and others brings this behavior with him to the clinical setting. He may be argumentative, demanding, unappreciative, sarcastic, and unwilling to go along with nursing care. Extreme overfriendliness, ingratiation, and refusal to make any decision concerning one's care are also expressions of aggression. Occasionally, a patient is aggressive to the point of violence—throwing his dinner tray, shouting, cursing, doing or threatening to do physical harm. Nonverbal expressions of anger—glaring eyes, clenched fist, a sneer— can be nearly as eloquent. A patient's regressive behavior may produce avoidance by the nurse, thus increasing feelings of distrust in the patient. The nurse then needs to make a conscious effort not to act on her feelings of avoidance but to be even more supportive to the patient.

Aggressive behavior that is ascribable to a toxic condition is acceptable; the patient can be excused because he was delirious or ''not in his right mind.'' The continuously hostile patient who is fully conscious and in control is much harder to understand and deal with. The expression of anger in the clinical situation may reflect the person's best manner of coping with perceived threats. Anger may be an attempt to relieve feelings of helplessness and dependency. In other situations, anger is part of the grief process or emergence from apathy and depression. A patient's anger may vanish when someone helps him to identify what is frustrating or threatening him and to take steps toward successfully dealing with the threat.

It is not unusual for people to displace feelings of anger, that is, to express them toward someone or something other than the original frustrator. When one believes oneself to be in a vulnerable position, it may not be safe to express dissatisfaction and anger directly. Therefore, one takes it out on somebody less likely to retaliate or less vitally important to one's emotional and physical well-being. A patient may be very angry with his physician but afraid to complain for fear that he will receive less attention. Instead, he bawls out the nurse and later insists that she contact his doctor. Or, the nurse and the physician may have a covert misunderstanding; she finds herself snapping at the aides and being irritable with the patients. Generally, direct expressions of anger are not socially acceptable, and outbursts are followed by guilt, shame, and profuse apologies. Moreover, because of cultural and socioeconomic differences in the expression of anger,

(Text continues on p. 179)

Care of the Patient With Anxiety

Mr. Robert Faltz, a 35-year-old truck driver, was admitted to the nursing unit from his physician's office. Mr. Faltz had sought medical attention for a "lump" in his right leg. Following admission, a biopsy was performed and osteosarcoma was diagnosed. Surgery was scheduled for the third day following admission and the only decision to be made was whether the leg was to be amputated above or below the knee. Miss Sloan, the primary nurse, entered Mr. Faltz's room to begin preoperative teaching. His vital signs were as follows: BP 140/90, P 96, R 26, T 37.2°C (99°F). His speech was rapid, and it was difficult to follow what he was saying. He had difficulty concentrating on information presented by Miss Sloan. He chain-smoked, tossed from side to side in the bed, and continuously readjusted the bed covers. He complained of his "heart pounding" and "pain where they took the biopsy."

Nursing Diagnoses
1. Anxiety related to crisis situation and impending surgery
2. Pain related to surgical removal of tissue

Goals
1. Use of effective methods to cope with and lessen anxiety
2. Relief of pain

Nursing Interventions	Expected Outcomes	Critical Times*	Outcomes
1. Establish relationship built on trust.			
a. Introduce self.	a. Acknowledges presence of nurse	24 hr	• Called primary nurse by name.
b. Obtain patient's perception of problem.	b. Verbalizes events leading to hospitalization and feelings about anticipated surgery and recovery	24 hr	• On admission, reconstructed events leading to hospitalization and events that followed; described feelings as "I don't know what will happen now"; unable to identify fears.
c. Provide consistency in care and in approach to patient.	c-d. Exhibits behavior indicative of trust	48 hr	• One day after admission, expressed fears of unknown and anger at the situation; fearful about job security; fearful of spread of cancer.
d. Accept patient as an individual			
e. Provide preoperative instructions in clear, simple manner.	e. Focuses on preoperative instructions	48 hr	• Verbalized that talking is helpful; asked when nurse will return; body posture relaxed.
			• Provided accurate feedback of instructions.
2. Assist patient to identify anxious feelings.			
a. Encourage patient to verbalize feelings of anxiety.	a. Verbalizes feelings of anxiety	24 hr	• Expressed anxiety about surgery, learning to walk, expenses of treatment, returning to job.
b. Remain with patient when appropriate.	b. Anxiety decreases	24 hr	• Restlessness and smoking decreased.

(continued)

Nursing Interventions	Expected Outcomes	Critical Times*	Outcomes
c. Assist to identify events that increase anxiety.	c. Identifies events that increase anxiety	48 hr	• Identified the following as increasing anxiety: hurried atmosphere, pain in leg when analgesic wears off, early morning hours.
d. Discusses relationship between increased anxiety and physiologic function.	d. Identifies increased anxiety as a precursor to altered physiologic function	48 hr	• Accurately described relationship between anxiety and heart palpitations; reported fewer incidents of palpitations.
e. Discusses relationship between increased anxiety and behavior patterns.	e. Identifies increased anxiety as a precursor to alterations in behavior	48 hr	• Identified motor activity and chain smoking as consequences of increased anxiety.
f. Note time and occasion of increased restlessness.	f. Decrease in restlessness	24 hr	• Restlessness decreased; less adjustment of bed covers; able to process preoperative instructions; speech remains rapid at times.
g. Promote use of effective coping measures to decrease anxiety.	g. Identifies effective coping mechanisms.	48 hr	• Identified the following as effective in decreasing anxiety: listening to music, visiting with family, reading magazines.
h. Teach relaxation techniques.	h. Uses relaxation techniques to decrease anxiety	48 hr	• Practiced relaxation techniques when feeling anxious; stated that relaxation techniques decreased feelings of anxiety.
i. Encourage patient to use support systems.	i. Uses support of wife	48 hr	• Discussed impending surgery and fears about future with wife.
3. Relieve pain and discomfort and promote healing.			
a. Administer analgesics as prescribed.	a. Experiences relief from pain	24 hr	• Denied pain 30 minutes after analgesic administered; analgesic changed to acetaminophen (Tylenol) 48 hr after admission.
b. Observe for side-effects of analgesic.	b. Absence of side-effects	48 hr	• No evidence of side-effects.
c. Assess for signs and symptoms of complications: TPR, BP q4h.	c. Vital signs normal	24 hr	• Elevation of vital signs continues 24 hr after admission: T 37.4°C, P 90–100, R 22–26, BP 130/86–146/90.
d. Observe dressing at site of biopsy for amount, color, odor of drainage.	d. Absence of drainage on dressing	24 hr	• Dressing dry and intact.

* These times have not been standardized but are individualized according to the patient's needs.

the nurse may be bewildered, insulted, and overwhelmed by behavior considered normal by another person.

The usual social responses to anger are counterattack, withdrawal, and avoidance of the situation. A nurse's initial reaction to an angry patient is to treat him as she would in social circumstances. Many times this is not appropriate from the therapeutic standpoint. The professional nursing responsibility is to try to help this person, even with and in spite of his anger. The nurse does this by first recognizing her own responses to angry behavior. It is not unusual for a nurse to experience feelings of irritation and annoyance. She may be frightened, embarrassed, and hurt. When a patient lashes out verbally, she may feel inadequate and guilty, even if she has acted appropriately. She may feel helpless or immobilized to the extent that she dreads caring for the patient and begins to avoid him whenever possible. This kind of behavior may heighten the patient's frustration by leaving him isolated, helpless, and unable to depend on the nursing staff to meet his physical and emotional needs. Thus, a vicious circle is established.

Nursing Interventions. Therapeutic responses to angry patients are based on the attempt to understand the person and his situation. The nurse is aware of her own reaction to the patient and attempts to help him sort out the issues involved. She enables the patient to maintain his dignity, pride, and self-esteem so that his situation can be accepted as reality. She sets limits on his behavior so that he does not hurt himself or others and helps him to find more appropriate means of expressing his feelings. Although she may feel angry or frightened in reaction to the behavior, she uses her feelings for further problem solving, instead of giving way to retaliation or withdrawal. Helpful questions in arriving at a nursing care plan for patients who are angry and hostile include the following: When does the patient get angry and how does he show it? Does his anger interfere with his receiving the care he needs? Why does his behavior bother me? How do I react? Does he get angry with other people too? Is there someone who does get along with him? What does that person do that is different? Does the patient's hostility serve a useful purpose? How much of this behavior reflects his usual way of reacting to people? How much is he willing to change? What realistic goals shall we work toward? Are there any other resources—physician, family, psychiatric nursing consultant, psychiatrist, occupational therapist, or other patients—that we could call in? If the patient stops expressing anger, will he develop more destructive patterns?

Learning to work therapeutically with angry, hostile patients is a challenging and rewarding part of nursing. Patients who disguise temporary fear and shame with anger appreciate the nurse who stands by them in the crisis without condemnation, rejection, or retaliation. Patients who have made a lifelong adjustment by means of hostile attack are also grateful, although they may never express it directly, to the nurse who refuses to be alienated and who applies herself to understanding and caring for them. Nursing Care Plan 12-2 is an example of a nursing care plan for the patient with anger and hostility.

Grief and Mourning

Grief is a complex of emotional responses to the anticipated or actual loss of someone or something valued. The loss may be that of a relative or friend, a part of the body, a job, health, or life. Feelings of anxiety, helplessness, hopelessness, guilt, anger, depression, remorse, sadness, and loneliness are part of grief. Mourning refers to the processes that follow the loss and ultimately result in overcoming the grief. Grief and mourning involve social responses that are best dealt with by the inclusion of others. There are many cultural factors involved in the specific way in which grief and mourning take place, from the extremes of stoic appearance to elaborate and ritualistic weeping, keening, and public display.

The intensity of grief and mourning depends on the significance and extent of the loss to the person. It is generally greater if the loss, especially through death, comes suddenly. If the survivor has been particularly dependent on the deceased person, or if in any way he was responsible for the death, grief is intensified. A person who is very sensitive to separation as a result of early separations may be deeply affected. Ambivalence (mixed feelings) is present in all significant relationships. If the ambivalence is marked, grief may be particularly intense. Guilt and irrational ideas about the causation of the death may prevent a person from facing himself and mourning effectively.

The stages of mourning are similar to the stages of adaptation to illness—shock and disbelief, awareness, and restitution. On recognition of a loss, people often experience a sinking feeling, tightness in the throat, loss of appetite, fatigue, tension, and acute anxiety. The sensorium is altered, and there is a feeling of unreality and distance from people. There is a preoccupation with the deceased or lost object and a state of readiness for its return. Feelings of guilt may be present, and there may be soul-searching and remorse about things that could have been done differently. The grieving person's relationships with other people lack warmth and are characterized by irritation and the desire not to be bothered. He is likely to withdraw from activities, neglect personal care, or be restlessly and purposelessly busy. He may develop symptoms similar to those of the deceased person. Sometimes the shock of the loss is accepted intellectually and the person goes through the motions of making arrangements and caring for others. His emotional reaction is cut off in his attempt to protect himself from the pain of the loss.

In the stage of developing awareness, the person experiences pain, anguish, emptiness, and acute sadness. Crying or the desire to cry is common and often elicits support from others. Many people cannot allow themselves to cry in public and need privacy to handle their grief.

In the stage of restitution, the physical reality of the loss is emphasized. In the case of death, the funeral makes this fact unavoidable. In the case of an amputation, the sight of the stump and the first attempt at using a prosthesis underline the reality. The mourner begins a long process of coping with the absence of the loved person or object. There may be repetitive talk about the person or object and there is a tendency to idealize, so that only pleasant memories are reinforced. Gradually, this assists in the task of achieving emotional detachment. As dependence on the lost object decreases, the person begins to develop new interests and invests energy in other people. He is able to remember the relationship more realistically, with its good and bad aspects, and can talk about it without emotional dependence on the memory of the relationship.

Nursing Interventions. Nursing interventions to help

Care of the Patient With Anger and Hostility

Following an above-the-knee amputation of the right leg, Miss Sloan entered Mr. Faltz's room. He became angry, sarcastic, and demanding. He complained that "no one has been in to check on me and I could have died—then all you nurses would be in trouble." He demanded that she "take care of me just like the doctor said" and then told her to leave the room and "send someone else who knows what they're doing."

Nursing Diagnosis
1. Ineffective coping:
   a. Verbal abuse related to feelings of helplessness
   b. Uncooperative behavior related to feelings of loss of control

Goals
1. Restoration of appropriate communication
2. Verbalization of feelings
3. Participation in therapeutic regimen

Nursing Interventions	Expected Outcomes	Critical Time* (postop)	Outcome
1. Promote appropriate communications.			
a. Establish relationship built on trust (see Nursing Care Plan 12-1).			
b. Remain calm; do not take verbal abuse personally.	b. Communicates within normal limits of volume	24 hr	• Voice raised only occasionally at 24 hr.
c. Set and keep limits; withdraw attention as needed.	c. Communicates appropriately	48 hr	• Requests, observations, questions expressed verbally in an appropriate manner.
d. Encourage patient to express feelings.	d. Verbalizes feelings of anger, fear, frustration, and loss of control	48 hr	• Verbalized frustration, fear, anger, and loss of control; expressed fear and concern over loss of leg and effect on employment.
e. Do not argue with patient.	e. Verbalizes how anger affects his verbal communication	48 hr	• Apologized for shouting and belittling behavior; verbalized ways in which he used anger to avoid dealing with changes in body image.

(continued)

patients and families with the experience of grief and mourning include anticipating reactions to loss, supporting the usual coping mechanisms, and allowing the expression of feelings. The nurse provides privacy and availability. When a body part or function is lost, the nurse designs specific nursing care and controls the environment to prevent additional loss of self-esteem. The presence and willingness of nurses to participate in the painful experiences that accompany grief help to prevent feelings of total abandonment. By being aware of the usual patterns of grief and mourning, nurses can recognize maladaptive patterns and help evaluate the need for other types of therapeutic intervention, such as psychotherapy. Nursing Care Plan 12-3 is an example of a nursing care plan for the patient experiencing grief and mourning.

Hope

Hope is a complex human experience that has a relationship to health. It is a mixture of feelings and thoughts that center on the fundamental belief that there are solutions to significant human needs and problems. Most people have hoped for and expected a long and healthy life for themselves and sig-

Nursing Interventions	Expected Outcomes	Critical Time* (postop)	Outcome
2. Promote verbalization of feelings.			
a. Encourage patient to express feelings about dependency.	a. Verbalizes feelings about dependency	24 hr	• Described feeling dependent on nursing staff for satisfaction of basic needs.
b. Allow patient to make as many choices as possible.	b. Maintains as much control as possible	24 hr	• Established own schedule for ADL and dressing changes; consulted with physical therapist and chose time for therapy.
c. Involve patient in goal establishment.	c. Verbalizes goals and expectations	48 hr	• Identified realistic expectations for therapy, discharge, and rehabilitation; established goal for job retraining as a truck dispatcher.
d. Discuss feelings of loss of control and helplessness.	d. Verbalizes feelings of loss of control and helplessness	48 hr	• Identified changes that had occurred since hospital admission; expressed his perception of the effect of these changes on life-style; identified need to regain control and to learn to care for self.
3. Promote participation in therapeutic regimen.			
a. Emphasize strengths and potential.	a. Identifies own strengths and potentials	72 hr	• Identified age, physical condition and stamina, and work record as strengths; expressed desire to talk to employer about job retraining.
b. Encourage involvement in self-care.	b. Accomplishes self-care activities	72 hr	• After establishing schedule for ADLs, began active participation in own care; self-sufficient in ADL by 72 hr; has begun talking about caring for self at home; is interested in learning to care for stump.

* These times have not been standardized but are individualized according to the patient's needs.

nificant others. Serious illness and injury raise questions of vulnerability and uncertainty about the future.

The purpose of hope is to ward off despair, which is characterized by mental anguish, disorganization, helplessness, and hopelessness. Loss of hope leads to giving-up behavior that leads to physical and emotional disequilibrium. Death may result from the loss of the will to live or through suicide. Hope is a catalyst that activates the motivational system. It is reinforced by other people who give support and encouragement to continue the struggle. When patients see "the light at the end of the tunnel," they can persist in moving toward future goals of improved functioning. Even with patients who are dying, hope for relief of suffering and meaningful living in the present are important aspects that can be reinforced with nursing care.

Nursing Interventions. To help patients and families maintain or restore hope, nurses contribute to a hopeful atmosphere that comes from themselves, other staff members, patients, and the physical environment. This is possible if individuals have faced and explored their views of the meaning of life, illness, and death. Feelings of hope, hopelessness, and helplessness are found in all nursing situations. Even while

Care of the Patient Experiencing Grief and Mourning

As Mr. Faltz's residual limb began to heal and his rehabilitative therapy began, he verbalized feelings of loss and fear regarding his career and job. He told Miss Sloan, "You know—maybe I just bumped my leg. If I had gone to the doctor the first day I noticed the lump, maybe he wouldn't have had to amputate." When alone, Mr. Faltz was observed staring off at a blank wall. He told his wife he had a "sinking feeling" and that he "couldn't help but think about the lost leg."

Nursing Diagnosis
1. Anticipatory grieving related to expected consequences of loss of extremity

Goals
1. Acceptance of loss
2. Alteration of life-style to incorporate loss

Nursing Interventions	*Expected Outcomes*	*Critical Time* (postop)*	*Outcomes*
Encourage patient to identify meaning of loss.			
a. Establish relationship built on trust (see Nursing Care Plan 12-1).			
b. Encourage expression of feelings about loss.	b. Identifies feelings about loss	48 hr	• Cried and talked about loss of right leg.
c. Encourage to identify effects of loss.	c. Identifies effects of loss on life-style	72 hr	• Talked about decreased mobility; identified need to modify car and truck so he can drive.
d. Assist in decreasing depressive symptoms.	d. Experiences decrease in symptoms of depression	4 days	• Reported increase in appetite and extended periods of uninterrupted sleep; fewer periods of crying; increased ability to concentrate while reading a book; participating in ADL and physical therapy.
e. Facilitate movement through the stages of grieving	e. Resolves loss	5 days	• Talked positively about rehabilitation; expressed interest in joining amputee support group; described family support system.
f. Assist in altering life-style	f. Identifies necessary life-style changes	4 days	• Identified ways to remain in trucking industry by exploring different jobs within company; identified necessary modifications to be made on car.

* These times have not been standardized but are individualized according to the patient's needs.

helping others with these feelings, nurses must deal with similar shifts in their own experience of hope. If they feel hopeless, they talk about feelings with others to get encouragement and a clearer picture of the reality of the situation. When hopes for the recovery of a patient are disappointed, staff members, along with families, feel bewildered, angry, and grief stricken. Nursing Care Plan 12-4 is an example of a nursing care plan to assist the patient in restoring hope.

Role Changes

When people get sick, their role identities change. This affects the ways in which others interact with them and relate to them; relationships with family and friends must be reestablished and maintained.

Some of the most important role changes are those that take place in the family when parents are no longer able to carry out their usual activities with their children. There may be role reversals, with children caring for their parents. In the usual life cycle, aging parents become increasingly dependent on their middle-aged children for help and direction; serious illness makes this even more evident.

Role changes in terms of occupational functioning may be drastically altered. When physicians and nurses become patients, they often find it very difficult to accept the patient role; staff members also have difficulty seeing them in a new light. This is true of persons who are considered "VIPs." They may demand and get deferential treatment, which at times is detrimental to their best interests as well as disruptive to the unit. Many people base their sense of self-worth on the ability to work and be productive. If forced to convalesce or retire because of illness, some people tend to feel lost and bereft of important links with others. Vocational rehabilitation is an important part of health planning for patients who must make major alterations.

A difficult role for a patient to deal with and others to react to is that of a terminally ill patient, a dying person. For many people, this is an unfamiliar and frightening aspect of life. They do not know what is expected of them, what to talk about, and how to carry on in light of the poor prognosis. Health professionals may withdraw from patients once it is clear that they are not going to recover. Nurses play an important part in helping patients and families go through this period.

Persons with chronic illness struggle with the role of being impaired. They want to be as normal as possible, yet sometimes the conditions of illness interfere with this to a large degree. They must continually make decisions about how to act and what to tell others. This is especially true in social situations; some people simply withdraw and cut themselves off from others, which leads to loneliness and depression.

Coping Strategies

Patients, families, and staff strive to adapt to serious illness in many ways. These coping skills are generally the approaches that were used in other difficult periods. Moos (1984) described these as coping skills that can be learned and practiced. Although divided into seven categories, the skills are often used in different combinations and vary in appropriateness and helpfulness. At different stages of illness, one or more of the coping skills may predominate.

Denial

Denial involves denying or minimizing the seriousness of the crisis, as well as isolating or dissociating feelings connected with the condition. This approach downplays the symptoms as evidence of illness or disregards the seriousness of the diagnosis. The first reaction to loss is shock and disbelief. Denial or numbing of feelings gives one time to absorb the meaning and protects one from being overwhelmed by feelings. Denial and isolation are ego defense mechanisms that protect against anxiety by distorting reality. Generally, the increase or persistence of symptoms forces the person to abandon the denial in time.

As a coping skill, denying or minimizing the problem helps to maintain psychological equilibrium. It can be harmful when it leads to such things as missing appointments, signing out of the hospital, and refusing appropriate treatment. Inappropriate cheerfulness and lack of concern about symptoms may indicate denial. If anxiety, depression, and anger are not expressed in situations where they are expected, the patient may be using denial for self-protection. However, sometimes patients act this way to protect others. This happens when patients are aware they are dying but perceive that the family would be more comfortable if the mutual deception was continued. They may be able to talk about fears and feelings with the staff, thereby lessening isolation.

Denial mechanisms operate in families as they try to protect themselves from recognizing the severity of the situation. Even when imminent death is discussed, the family may deny this is possible and act (or fail to act) accordingly.

Nursing Interventions. In dealing with denial of illness as a nursing problem, nurses assess the extent to which the denial is harmful and the ways in which it is beneficial. Generally, the defense of denial is not challenged directly, because such action tends to reinforce the position or leaves the person without necessary ego protection. The nurse does not support or encourage the denial and remains available. The nurse's use of gentle exploring questions may help the patient's acceptance of reality. When patients can relinquish denial, they need help in dealing with the difficult aspects of reality that they were attempting to ward off.

Denial is a coping skill that nurses use to handle their own feelings about illness, radical surgery, and death. Along with other health professionals, they may need this defense to keep working in high-risk areas. When nurses can talk about their feelings with others, they develop more realistic ways of dealing with the stresses and thus are better equipped to help patients and families face their difficult problems.

Seeking Information

The coping skill of seeking information involves (1) seeking relevant information that can relieve anxiety caused by misconceptions and uncertainty, and (2) using one's intellectual resources effectively. Patients and families are often relieved by information about the illness, its treatment, and the course the illness is expected to take. This provides a framework in which plans can be made and effective action taken. Patients and their families are encouarged by hearing about successful treatment of others with the same condition. Worrying is decreased when correct facts and clarification of misconceptions and fears are supplied. Giving a time dimension in which certain reactions are anticipated helps to decrease feelings of helplessness. Informed patients are better able to participate in their own treatment.

Requesting Emotional Support

Being able to request reassurance and emotional support from family, friends, and medical/nursing staff while maintaining a sense of personal competence is important. Patients are often frightened and anxious. They may feel very much alone. A valuable coping skill is being able to reach out for or receive the concern of others. This maintains hope through encour-

Assisting the Patient in Restoring Hope

Mr. Faltz made progress in learning to walk with crutches and was measured for his prosthesis. He looked forward to his therapy sessions and worked hard during these sessions. He spoke to Miss Sloan about his plans after discharge: "Of course I'll have to continue with therapy for a while and the amputee group will be helpful. My wife is supportive of the changes we'll have to make in our life. Things really do look hopeful."

Nursing Diagnoses
1. Disturbance in self-concept: Self-esteem, body image, role performance
2. Potential nonadherence to therapeutic regimen

Goals
1. Improvement in self-concept
2. Resumption of independent life-style
3. Adherence to therapeutic regimen

Nursing Interventions	Expected Outcomes	Critical Time* (postop)	Outcomes
1. Increase self-esteem.			
a. Give positive feedback for progress made in self-care and ambulation.	a. Accomplishes crutch walking	1 week	• Safely ambulates with crutches on flat surface and stairs.
b. Help patient identify strengths and potentials.	b. Identifies strengths and potentials	1 week	• Made a list of physical activities he will be able to continue; identified supports within family and community; verbalized self-determination as an inner strength.
c. Give positive feedback for progress made in accepting change in body image.	c. Describes feelings about how body has changed	1 week	• Verbalized sadness related to loss of leg and put into perspective the effect of this loss on self and family; stated that he is looking forward to using prosthesis and becoming independent.

(continued)

agement. Whether limitations are temporary or permanent, people need to have a sense of mastery over other functions.

Patients can be encouraged by other people with similar conditions. Support groups for patients and families are helpful in encouraging the expression of feelings, sharing practical problems, and passing along effective ways of coping. Patients are reassured by being told that their cooperation with the health team is helpful in fighting together against the difficult illness.

Sometimes, physicians and nurses use shaming and guilt-provoking tactics to get patients to adhere to treatment programs. These are generally ineffective and lead to the patient's being all the more demoralized or seeking health treatment elsewhere.

Learning Self-Care

Learning illness-related procedures confirms personal ability and effectiveness. People can learn to care for themselves even in the aftermath of catastrophic illness and injury. Helplessness is decreased because the sense of pride in accomplishments helps to restore or maintain self-esteem. Family members can often learn how to help a loved one during acute as well as chronic illness. Being able to do something often relieves anxiety and guilt. Patient teaching is an important aspect of nursing care.

Setting Concrete, Limited Goals

The overall tasks of adaptation to serious illness seem overwhelming, yet they can be done. Breaking down the components into small, manageable goals will eventually lead to greater risks and success. Motivation is maintained. The feelings of helplessness are decreased as patients experience the impact of action on outcome. Instead of just worrying about results and the future, the person takes action that is effective. Principles of learning are important in accomplishing the eventual long-term goals.

Nursing Interventions	Expected Outcomes	Critical Time* (postop)	Outcomes
2. Encourage efforts toward successfully altering lifestyle.	2. Makes necessary arrangements for promoting mobility	1 week	• Enrolled in driving school to learn to drive manually equipped car, to begin after discharge. • Made appointment with car dealer to discuss purchase of manually equipped car. • Contacted Department of Motor Vehicles regarding handicapped license plates.
3. Encourage adherence to therapeutic regimen. a. Encourage participation in discharge planning.	a. Participates in making plans for discharge	1 week	• Attended discharge planning conference; consulted with physical therapist and established schedule for outpatient appointments.
b. Provide patient with discharge instructions.	b. Exercises according to plan Carries out residual limb care daily Reports problems with residual limb, prosthesis Keeps appointments with physician, physical therapist, prosthetist	Following discharge	

* These times have not been standardized but are individualized according to the patient's needs.

Rehearsing Alternative Outcomes

There are usually multiple alternatives in most situations. Recognizing this helps a person to feel less trapped and helpless. This is accomplished through mental preparation and discussion with others. Exploring options with the nurse and one's family helps to expand the reality base on which to make decisions. Anticipatory planning reduces helplessness by rehearsing "what will happen if. . . ."

This coping skill is often used in conjunction with information seeking. It helps to decrease anxiety by preparing for the future. Recalling how one has been able to manage other difficulties bolsters confidence.

When there is a choice of several treatment modalities, talking over the alternatives is a vital part of including the patient in self-determination. Health professionals do not always know what is best. They can give information based on knowledge and past experience; the patient and family are left with the final decision. Patients may have def-inite ideas about what they want done in the final stages of life.

Rehearsing skill is very important for patients with altered body parts and functions. They may need to rehearse what to do in a variety of social situations. They use the staff as sounding boards. Groups of patients and other individuals may be helped by role-playing situations.

Finding Meaning in Illness

Illness is a human experience. Many people have found that serious illness was a turning point in their lives. This may reflect either a spiritual orientation or a philosophical approach to life. Patients find encouragement in the belief that their suffering may have some meaning or be helpful to others. They may participate in research projects or training programs to this end. Sensitive, poignant accounts of illness have been written by patients, families, and health professionals that convey hope and inspiration. Plays, movies, and television dramas have made it possible for millions of people to share in some of the finest moments of human caring, courage, and compassion.

Families may be brought together by illness in a painful but very meaningful way. People experience a sense of their basic worth as well as that of others. Many survivors of serious illness interviewed by Smith (1979) reported that they had experienced a change in values and priorities, greater concern for others, and a heightened appreciation for the beauty of nature. After serious illness, people may find meaning in helping others through support groups or political action or by entering one of the health professions.

Factors That Help or Hinder Coping

Serious physical illness is a potential life crisis for the patient and family. Crisis is that state in which the person feels that obstacles to important life goals are insurmountable and that the usual means of problem solving are not sufficient. New approaches are needed. Successful mastery leads to greater self-integration, understanding, and trust in others.

Stressors that disturb equilibrium are divided into biological and psychosocial stressors. These are most often intertwined, since one system affects the other. The *biological stressors* include illness and injury. Not only is the degree of impairment important but so is the meaning of the condition to the individual. Lack of sleep, poor nutrition, dehydration, drugs, and pain are biological stressors that hinder coping with ongoing and new difficulties.

Psychosocial stressors include interpersonal problems with family and significant others, occupational situations, finances, living circumstances, and legal problems. The person's maturational age, especially childhood, adolescence, and aging, specifically affects the impact of illness. Sometimes, psychosocial issues drop away in importance in the face of acute illness and possible death. In many instances, the coping abilities are stretched even more as new problems are created by the illness.

The *personal characteristics* of an individual include age, intelligence, basic personality style, religious and philosophical beliefs, and previous experiences in coping with difficulties, especially prior illness. These affect the person's perception of the illness and his resources for handling the problems.

Social and situational supports affect the way in which a person copes with illness. There are primarily interpersonal supports—people to whom the distressed person turns. Close friends and understanding family members may be vital to maximal recovery. Isolated persons or patients whose family ties are chaotic and disturbed will be under even greater stress with illness. The professional health team is part of the support system. Because nurses are so close and necessary to the ongoing care of patients, they become vital supports during the uncertainty of illness and treatment. They are sensitive to the patient's need for additional help and are instrumental in arranging for this support from family, clergy, other patients, psychiatric and psychological therapists, and social service agencies.

The *physical environment* may help or hinder coping. The problems of sensory overload, sensory deprivation, and isolation, along with the unfamiliar and frightening aspects of the hospital, all contribute to problems of adjustment. Sometimes, although little can be done about these problems,

just recognizing that they cause stress can be reassuring to patients and families.

The patient's *basic coping mechanisms* may be altered because of the circumstances of the illness. Pain, fatigue, and immobility interfere with action methods of tension release. Important persons to whom the patient usually turns may not be available, and impaired mobility may restrict his ability to visit them. Generally, the families of seriously ill patients are also very anxious, which leaves them less able to respond to their loved one. An intensification of usual coping patterns may be seen in disturbed communication, behavior, and ways of interacting with others. Common patterns of disturbed behavior resulting from efforts to cope include excessive withdrawal, making demands, disorientation, depression, and manipulative behavior. Changes in a patient's perceptual field as the intensity of anxiety increases to a state of panic are illustrated in Figure 12-2.

Assessing Psychosocial Needs

Nurses encounter sick people at many stages of illness and treatment. They often see only a small part of the picture. When dealing with acute illness, they see patients and families in the crisis situation without knowing much about what preceded or followed the condition. Strauss (1984) regards sick persons as having at least three biographies that have meaning in their illness; they are (1) the person's chronological experience with the illness, (2) treatment experiences with prior medical aid (legitimate or not), and (3) the social biography of the person's life history with family, friends, work colleagues, and strangers. Staff members often know very little about these biographies, although they may affect treatment and recovery in definite ways.

Psychosocial History

A psychosocial history is the organized assessment of the important events of a person's life; it is sometimes referred to as a *case history*. The psychosocial history is a specific biography of a person from before birth (heritage and heredity) through the important developmental stages to the present. The anticipated future is also part of the material. The psychosocial history touches on the turning points—the important milestones. Significant illnesses, physical and mental, experienced by the patient and family members have an important impact on the immediate situation.

The specific psychosocial history is obtained through initial interviewing and from additional contacts. Nurses should be familiar with the elements of a psychosocial assessment. It describes patients in the context of their lives and identifies major problems and assets. Nurses can obtain and use this information while they are providing other nursing care for patients. The nurse talks with patients in a goal-directed way to determine areas in which help is needed. For those patients too ill or young, the nurse may gather these data from family members and significant others.

In many instances, these are action interviews. The contacts continue over the period of illness; the time spent corresponds to the needs of the patient. Critically ill patients will not be able to communicate much more than immediate needs. It is not necessary to get all this information at one time. As the nurse–patient relationship develops, patients feel more confident in talking about matters of serious concern to them. This is particularly true if the listener is interested, compassionate, and nonjudgmental. Nurses also talk with and assess the psychosocial needs of the family members. In the uncertainty and stress of illness, many persons want and need to talk with their professional helpers.

Mental Status Examination

In addition to the psychosocial history, nurses pay attention to the current mental status of the patient. The mental status examination assesses the ways in which a person is thinking, feeling, and acting. It is both a descriptive inventory of behavior and a method of organizing and recording observations of behavior. Problems are identified, and working diagnoses determine the treatment plan. Many of the aspects of the mental status examination are expressed in ongoing speech and behavior. Specific questions are necessary during a formal examination or when clarification, update, or additional information is needed. Patients with serious physical illness often show dramatic shifts in mental status when recovering from surgery, when delirious, or when experiencing changes in body temperature or reactions to medication. The patient with a history of mental illness may decompensate during the stress of illness. Confusion may escalate to extreme behavior unless it is recognized and treated along with the medical condition. Families may need reassurance about the changes in the psychological state of their loved ones.

Aspects of Communication

Acute and chronic physical illness pose many problems to patients and their families. Nurses communicate with them to (1) identify health needs, (2) clarify misconceptions, and (3) help them verbalize fears and other reactions. Anxiety is lessened or channeled through sharing. Nurses are concerned with the impact of illness on the person's life. They are aware of the need to provide privacy while talking with the patient about his conditions in order to help him.

The basic nurse–patient relationship takes into account the physician, the family, other patients, the rest of the health team, and society at large. The relationship is established and maintained by the communication process—a complex, dynamic exchange of verbal and nonverbal messages.

Communication is based on mutually intelligible symbols. To be understood, a person must have a knowledge of himself and his needs, an ability to speak the language and express himself clearly, and a familiarity with the usual conventions of the situation. To understand others, he must be able to observe and evaluate behavior. To make oneself understandable and to understand others is vital to the establishment of relationships. The patient whose English is inept or who speaks a foreign language, or whose ability to express himself is markedly impaired through physical or psychological causes, poses a challenge to the nurse.

The process of communication may be considered to consist of four segments: (1) *I* (2) *am communicating something* (3) *to you* (4) *in this situation.* Breakdowns in communication can be pinpointed by identifying the segment in which the interference is taking place.

The sender of the message, the *I*, is affected by such factors as age, sex, socioeconomic status, marital status, occupation, intelligence, physical condition (especially as related to the nervous system and the organs of communication), personality, and current emotional status.

The message, *am communicating something,* consists of both verbal and nonverbal elements that may be complementary or incongruous. The patient who says, "Oh, I'm fine. Nothing is the matter," while restlessly moving about, wringing his hands, and sighing, frequently illustrates the latter.

The receiver of the communication, *to you,* is influenced by the same factors as the sender with respect to behavior. The ability to hear or "read" a patient's behavior depends largely on the ability to listen openly and sensitively. The presence of stereotypes, misconceptions, and anxiety may prevent the nurse from correctly identifying the message from a particular patient.

The context of the communication, *in this situation,* refers to the sociocultural status of the patient, the context of illness, the social order of the hospital, and immediate environmental aspects. The importance of understanding the cultural background and the values of patients has gained recognition in all areas of nursing. When patients enter the hospital world, they may be overwhelmed and bewildered by the change in their status and role. The nurse plays a vital part in orienting patients to their new position. She also needs to acquaint them with the scope of her professional services. Many people do not know that the nurse is prepared and eager to help with a wide variety of health needs. In addition to performing the traditional services related to physical needs, she offers help as a health teacher, a rehabilitation worker, a communications link with other professional services, and, in some instances, a psychotherapeutic counselor.

A person in the first stages of adapting to illness, who is taking the defensive measure of denying his illness, does not seek or welcome accurate information about his condition or treatment. A nurse who attempts to do effective health teaching will find her efforts of little avail at this time. The behavior of the patient, the questions he asks or avoids, and his reactions to the changes in his health status all give clues to his readiness and needs. In turn, the patient is also very sensitive to the reactions of the medical and nursing staff and seeks to interpret nonverbal messages with regard to his prognosis, especially when it is not favorable.

The expressive function of the nurse involves helping the patient to maintain equilibrium and motivation and supporting his attempts to cope with the experience of illness and treatment, by providing direct gratifications that reduce his tension level. The provision of physical comfort and care is combined with such interpersonal activities as explaining, reassuring, understanding, protecting, and simply being with the patient. When a patient is acutely ill, communication generally takes place on a primitive, chiefly nonverbal level. A touch, a soft but reassuring tone of voice, and the presence of the nurse may convey to the patient that he is not alone and that he is being cared for. When it is anticipated that a patient will experience a direct interference with communication patterns as a result of treatment, it is vital to set up a system of communication in advance. One patient reported: "The worst part about my laryngectomy was that I couldn't tell anyone what I needed—but the magic slate helped."

An important part of the development of interpersonal and communication tools is the nurse's understanding of herself, her interpersonal needs, and her usual patterns of communication. As she becomes more aware of her own needs, she is better able to identify those of her patients and to know when her own perceptions and reactions are preventing her from accurately assessing the situation. This is particularly true when the patient's behavior is frustrating, puzzling, hostile, or demanding. The nurse must be able to evaluate her own responses so that she does not retaliate with anger or rejection. The situations that lead to feelings of helplessness and hopelessness must be talked about and shared so that the nurse can maintain her own equilibrium and give optimal nursing care to patients with incurable, repulsive, or terminal conditions. The nurse's awareness of her own need for approval and recognition plays an important part in her reactions to patient behavior and to the behavior of co-workers, supervisors, and the medical staff.

Reactions of Nurses to Illness

Nurses have many personal emotional reactions to patients and families in the crisis of physical illness. Some common responses are frustration, anxiety, anger, hope, guilt, compassion, helplessness, love, hopelessness, disgust, envy, and pride. These are stimulated by the combination of the personal characteristics of the nurse, the professional tasks and obligations involved, and the intricacies of the patient's illness and personality. Nurses not only react emotionally to patients and families but also have important emotional interactions with other members of the health team. Illness in a patient may evoke emotional responses based on personal experiences or the experiences of close family members.

Nurses are faced with difficulties in adjusting to the many changes in the health status of their patients. This is particularly true with "difficult" patients, those who are not responding to treatment, and dying patients. A high-risk factor is involved in working in settings such as the emergency unit, intensive care unit, premature nursery, and medical units, where a high percentage of patients die. Nurses have to struggle with conflicts between the idealism instilled in nursing school and the reality of the usual work situation. Even when they recognize psychosocial needs, many nurses feel overwhelmed in helping patients—there is "no time." Yet, the ultimate recovery and maximal functioning of patients with serious illnesses depend on their ability to deal with multifaceted problems. Sensitive attention to the emotional needs of patients and families helps make hospitalization and treatment smoother, enhances health teaching, and contributes to the quality of life.

It is important for nurses to be aware of their emotional reactions to clinical situations so that they do not become overstressed and unable to cope. When this happens, they experience the phenomenon known as "burnout," which results in personal distress, in indifference to the suffering of others, and often in the decision to leave the job or profession. Nurses who are aware of their many reactions are better able to help others.

"Problem Patients"

Many patients cope with the difficult and often frightening tasks of adaptation to illness. Some inspire with their courage and dignity. Others simply do the best they can in the immediate situation and over the long period in which they convalesce and learn to live with a chronic illness.

Some patients stand out as not dealing with their illness and treatment in the usual expected ways. They may be called "difficult," "management problems," or, in exasperation, "impossible" or "crocks." These labels indicate the breakdown of usually effective coping patterns in both the staff and the patient. The staff need to talk together about the situation. Consultation is often indicated—with a psychiatrist, a consultation-liaison team, or a psychiatric nursing clinical specialist. These persons can help by clarifying the factors, suggesting alternative approaches, giving reassurance to the staff and patient, providing short-term psychotherapy, and evaluating the need for psychoactive drugs. The principle underlying these approaches is that problem patients are patients with problems.

Problems With Cognition, Affect, and Behavior

According to Groves (1982) problems of patients can be classified in three groups, although there is often overlap. These groups are as follows:

1. *Problems of cognition*—delirium, denial, psychosis, failure to process information
2. *Problems of affect*—anxiety, hostility, depression, apathy
3. *Problems of behavior*—noncompliance, withdrawal, dependency, aggressiveness, manipulation

Cognition refers to the ways in which people process information—their ways of thinking, and hence of responding. Perception, memory, understanding, and judgment are involved. Medical–surgical problems often affect these processes. This is seen particularly in *delirium* and *dementia*. The therapeutic approach consists largely in recognizing the nature of the impairment. When the source is identified, steps can be taken, such as clarifying the medical treatment, changing the environment, and readjusting the medication regimen.

Disturbances of affect (emotions) become problems in a medical-surgical situation when they are overwhelming or inappropriate. Disturbed behavior may result as an exacerbation of a previous mental illness or in response to the immediate situation, illness, or treatment. Excessive anxiety comes from many sources. The therapeutic approach consists in recognizing the causes of the disturbed feelings and helping to restore control. This is done by talking with patients and families about the situation, making necessary changes, and prescribing medication if needed.

Disturbed behavior is directly related to disturbed cognition and overwhelming affects. Severe depression is very distressing to the patient and interferes with healing. It can also precede suicidal behavior. Misinterpretation of the environment leads to panic and aggressive behavior. Patients signal their unmet needs by such behavior as signing out of the hospital, refusing medical treatment, using drugs and alcohol on the unit, and inappropriate sexual behavior.

Extreme dependency leads to difficult patient–staff interactions. This is shown through clinging, demanding behavior in which the patient begs for reassurance yet is unrelieved by it. There may be ongoing demands for services and for pain medication beyond the expected need. Dependent patients are often manipulative and play staff members off against one another. They show anger and hostility both directly and covertly. Nurses feel frustrated, angry, and hopeless in working with these patients.

Nursing Interventions. The therapeutic approach to patients showing disturbed behavior begins with an assessment of the situation from the standpoint of both the staff and the patient. Clear communication is vital. Necessary limits are spelled out. Generally, long-standing personality styles and defenses are not challenged in the midst of a physical illness. The staff members are encouraged to meet needs as much as possible and to allow the patient to exert interpersonal control and distance without being punished or abandoned. During the crisis of illness, psychoactive medication, such as tranquilizers and antianxiety agents, can be used to help patients manage disturbed feelings and behavior.

A way of understanding and dealing with problem behavior is through learning theory. Behavior that is learned and continued is behavior that is reinforced (rewarded). There is a system of rewards and punishments (even if not acknowledged) in all social systems, including that of the hospital. Patients bring their learned behavior patterns and react to the new interpersonal environment accordingly.

If patients' behaviors tag them as "difficult," nurses should study the situation to identify (1) what constitutes the maladaptive behavior and how this interferes with care, progress, and rehabilitation; (2) how and by whom the behavior is reinforced; and (3) how the environment and reinforcers can be changed so that the behavior changes. This is the approach to behavior modification. Nurses should examine their own behavior to see if they are inadvertently playing a part in continuing the situation. Nursing behavior can influence patient behavior in either positive or negative directions. Positive reinforcers include spending time, smiling, showing interest in the conversation, providing food, giving medication as needed, giving backrubs, and granting extra privileges.

Psychophysiologic Interactions

Knowledge about the relationship between emotions and physical reactions is increasing. This is a highly complex and little understood matter that the mass media have simplified to the point at which the words "psychophysiologic," "psychosomatic," "neurotic," "imaginary," "faking," "malingering," "psychogenic," and "somatopsychic" are used loosely and create confusion.

Anxiety is experienced as both emotional and physiologic reactions. Many people seek treatment for symptoms that are due to chronic, continued anxiety. The anxiety may represent a reaction to reality factors in the present, such as a job or a marriage, or to long-standing conflicts over sexuality, dependency, aggression, and other factors.

Psychophysiologic Illness. Anxiety reactions in which the symptoms center around one organ system are described in the nomenclature as psychophysiologic reactions having autonomic and visceral responses (*e.g.*, "psychophysiologic reaction, cardiovascular," if the symptoms are predominantly cardiac in nature). Any organ system can be affected. When actual structural changes do occur, the condition is described as a psychophysiologic illness that has resulted from a combination of emotional and physiologic factors. Common conditions that are generally considered to involve psychophys-

iologic factors are peptic ulcer, chronic ulcerative colitis, hyperthyroidism, bronchial asthma, essential hypertension, and neurodermatitis. The frequency and severity of these illnesses point to the need for greater understanding of the relationship between mind and body.

Hypochondriasis. Another manifestation of underlying emotional conflict that expresses itself in physical symptoms is hypochondriasis. A hypochondriacal patient may be totally absorbed in his body and its functioning and presents endless complaints and reports. Hypochondriasis may be used as a means of attempting to meet long-standing dependency needs. The nurse must evaluate her reactions to such a patient's complaints and demands. Frustration and anger are common responses to this type of patient. The hardworking nurse often resents someone who avoids adult responsibility so easily. Expressing this anger directly to the patient is not helpful, since he is struggling to maintain some kind of equilibrium. Not recognizing her own anger could result in the nurse's avoiding the patient and not caring for his realistic needs. If the nurse attempts to meet all of the patient's unsatisfied dependency needs, she soon finds that the patient is insatiable. Finding a reasonable middle ground is a challenge in working with these patients. Very little is known about successful nursing approaches to hypochondriacal patients. Excessive preoccupation with one's body, accompanied by unusual ideation, may be a sign of more severe emotional disorders, such as psychotic depression or schizophrenia. Through proper assessment of needs and evaluation of behavior, the nurse may help plan for more appropriate treatment.

Conversion Reactions. Another group of physical reactions that have an emotional basis are conversion reactions. Conversion is an ego defense mechanism in which anxiety is eliminated or reduced by the production of a physical symptom. This symptom may be directly related to the emotional conflict; the hand that would strike out is paralyzed; the eyes that would look at the forbidden become blind. In most instances, the conflict and the symbolic meaning of the symptom are complex, disguised, and difficult to unravel. These patients come into a medical–surgical setting for differential diagnosis. A conversion reaction may develop after an organic illness has occurred, which tends to prolong the secondary gains of dependency and security.

Generally, the symptoms of converson reactions simulate disturbances in the voluntary nervous system or in the organs of the special senses. Disturbances of sensation and motion are the most common. Sensation changes include anesthesia, paresthesia, and pain. Loss of hearing and sight are much more common than loss of the other special senses. Disturbances of motion include paralysis, usually of the extremities or speech mechanism, and uncontrolled movements, such as tics and nonorganic convulsions. If the symptom is diagnosed as a conversion reaction, the treatment is generally best directed by a psychiatrist. The nurse can help greatly by accurately observing the patient's behavior, including his reaction to other people. She must keep in mind that symptom formation in a person with a conversion reaction occurs on an unconscious level—the patient is not faking, and his symptoms are not imaginary. This is his way of coping with situations at the present time; with professional help he may be able to find more adequate ways of doing so.

Disturbances in Orientation. Disturbances in orientation occur frequently in patients on medical–surgical services. Acute brain syndrome, which may be a reaction to anesthesia, infection, surgical or metabolic disturbances, overdose of drugs or alcohol, or assault of the brain, as in head injury, often produce delirium. *Delirium* is a state of altered consciousness or awareness manifested by disorientation and confusion. It is induced by interference with the metabolic processes of the brain and is generally acute in onset and reversible. The first signs are restlessness, anxiety, and suspicion, which quickly mount to agitation, excitement, and confusion. The patient often begins to hallucinate and experience delusions. These distortions of reality are extremely frightening, and the desperate behavior of the person experiencing them necessitates skilled nursing action. Patients recovering from cardiac surgery, in particular, often become delirious. It is necessary to reduce the terror and extreme anxiety of these patients not only for emotional reasons but also to prevent overloading the body with more stress.

Nursing care for a delirious patient includes continual reorientation, a calm voice, and adequate lighting through the night. If possible, the same nurses should attend the patient much of the time, since they repeatedly demonstrate by familiar words and action that he is safe and cared for. It often helps to tell the patient that you know he is very frightened but that the things he is experiencing are a reaction to his illness that will go away. Hallucinations caused by organic processes are often vivid and threatening. Along with visual hallucinations, the patient may experience tactile hallucinations in which he feels he is being touched or bugs are crawling on him.

Acute brain syndrome is treated by alleviating the causative agents, and the nurse must be aware that proper hydration, nutrition, and medication are directed toward this end. Restraints may be necessary to keep the patient in bed, but they may also frighten and irritate him. The nurse must be aware of his distortion of reality and poor judgment in order to protect him from injuring himself or others. Patients have walked out of unprotected windows while delirious.

Following an episode of delirium, a person may experience anxiety and shame over his behavior when not in full control. He may fear that he has acted inappropriately, hurt someone, or said vulgar or obscene things. He may be afraid of having told confidences and secrets about himself. If the patient gives evidence of such concern, the nurse can encourage him to talk about his fears and then reassure him that his behavior was understandable in the situation and that his confidence will not be betrayed. This is a potentially shameful situation in which the rights, dignity, and privacy of the patient must be protected.

Chronic brain syndrome may result from damage to brain tissue sustained by the causes of acute brain syndrome; from long-term infections such as syphilis; from heavy metal intoxication; from circulatory disturbances such as cerebral arteriosclerosis; from convulsive disorders; from disturbances of growth, metabolism, or nutrition; from intracranial neoplasm; from prenatal factors; and from diseases of unknown etiology, such as multiple sclerosis. The behavior common to people with these conditions is decribed as *dementia,* and it represents chronic, irreversible brain damage with deterioration of intellectual capacities due to structural changes. Both delirium and dementia are characterized by loss of abilities—defects in memory, orientation (of time, place, and person), and judgment. In planning nursing care and long-term treatment, the patient's strengths must be evaluated

along with his limitations. Environmental manipulation and simplification may help him to live his life to the fullest.

Dying and Death

The style in which a person dies is individual, just as his life was. One of the major problems in understanding death is that, in our culture, it is a taboo and unfamiliar experience. Dying usually takes place in hospitals or nursing homes rather than as part of the life cycle at home. Death is a strange new experience that does not affect most people until their adults years. Many nursing students come into contact with death for the first time during the medical–surgical clinical experience.

For most people, just the thought of death is frightening and even impossible. Regardless of religious beliefs, it is difficult to imagine oneself not existing in the world. Nurses are deeply committed to life and health. The dying patient is a direct contradiction to that commitment. Sometimes the medical and nursing staff react to dying patients as if they represent a failure of their skill and care. Although nothing can be done to reverse the ultimate process, dying patients and their families can be helped during the final days.

People face death in many ways. According to Kübler-Ross (1969), the emotional responses of a person facing death can be traced through five stages: denial and isolation, anger, bargaining, depression, and acceptance. These five stages do not always occur in sequence; they may be mixed or overlapping. Patients and their families move back and forth through the experience and may be at different stages at a given time.

Denial and Isolation

Recognition and acceptance of the fact that death is to be faced shortly is difficult; the common reaction is to insulate oneself until other defenses are marshaled. Denial permits hope to exist. Often, patients are ready to accept the fact that they are dying, but the family continues to express denial. This delays communication of concerns. Denial and isolation are interrupted when the patient begins to think about unfinished business—personal affairs, finances, arrangements for spouse, children, and others.

Anger

The next emotion expressed is anger. The question, "Why me?" does not require an answer, but the patient is helped if the nurse is present to offer support and to listen. The behavior of patients in this stage is difficult because nothing can be done that seems to please. Nurses can expect this expression of anger and should not take it personally. Patients often want to express their sense of outrage and helplessness. When feelings have been vented, they are able to move on.

Bargaining

Bargaining is a phase of coping during which the dying person attempts to negotiate a trade. Usually, it involves a deal with God, the physician, or the nurse: "If I can live long enough to attend my son's wedding, I'll be ready to die." If at all possible, patients should be granted their requests.

Depression

The full impact of the inevitable is apparent to patients in this stage. Defense mechanisms are no longer effective; sadness and anguish are felt and expressed. By crying they also elicit the support of loved ones and nurses. The resolution of this phase leads quietly into the final stage.

Acceptance

This is a time of relative peace. The patient seems to want to review the past and contemplate the unknown future. Often, patients do not talk a great deal but want others nearby. If pain is relieved, the person who has accepted death often wants to be comforted by having contact with those who are meaningful.

Nursing Interventions

To give maximal help to the dying, nurses should examine their own feelings about death. An underlying principle in nursing is that patients are individuals to be treated with respect and dignity regardless of their background or condition. However, studies have shown that social values determine reactions to the dying person. Such factors as age, attractiveness, socioeconomic status, and former accomplishments affect whether the patient is cared for or abandoned while dying. Many times, nurses become the most important link with life for dying patients. They promote physical comfort and emotional support. It is an emotional strain to attend people who are dying. Nurses assigned to areas in which death is a common occurrence need to share their feelings and reactions with others, to obtain needed support.

Bibliography

Books

Aguilera DC and Messick JM. Crisis Intervention: Theory and Methodology, 5th ed. St Louis, CV Mosby, 1986.

Barry P. Psychosocial Nursing Assessment and Intervention. Philadelphia, JB Lippincott, 1984.

Brallier L. Successfully Managing Stress. Los Altos, California, Natl Nurs Rev, 1982.

Burgess AW. Psychiatric Nursing in the Hospital and the Community, 4th ed. Englewood Cliffs, New Jersey, Prentice-Hall, 1985.

Clayton PJ and Barrett JE (eds). Treatment of Depression. New York, Raven Press, 1983.

Friedman M. Family Nursing Theory and Assessment, 2nd ed. Norwalk, Connecticut, Appleton-Century-Crofts, 1986.

Fritz P et al. Interpersonal Communication in Nursing. Norwalk, Connecticut, Appleton-Century-Crofts, 1984.

Gallon RL. The Psychosomatic Approach to Illness. New York, Elsevier Biomedical, 1982.

Haber J et al. Comprehensive Psychiatric Nursing. New York, McGraw-Hill, 1982.

Hawes C and Joseph D. Basic Concepts of Helping. Norwalk, Connecticut, Appleton-Century-Crofts, 1986.

Infante MS (ed). Crisis Theory: A Framework for Nursing Practice. Reston, Virginia, Reston Publishing Co, 1982.

Janosik EH and Phipps LB. Life Cycle Group Work in Nursing. Monterey, California, Wadsworth Health Services Division, 1982.

Kenner CV, Suzetta CE, and Dassey BM. Critical Care Nursing: Body-Mind-Spirit, 2nd ed. Boston, Little, Brown, & Co, 1985.

Kriegh H and Perka J. Psychiatric and Mental Health Nursing. Reston, Virginia, Reston Publishing Co, 1983.

Kübler-Ross E. On Death and Dying. New York, Macmillan, 1969.

Lambert V and Lambert C. Psychosocial Care of the Physically Ill, 2nd ed. Englewood Cliffs, New Jersey, Prentice-Hall, 1985.

Lipp MR. Respectful Treatment: The Human Side of Medical Care, 2nd ed. New York, Harper & Row, 1986.

McCann/Flynn JB and Heffron PB. Nursing From Concept to Practice. Bowie, Maryland, Robert J. Brady, 1984.

Miller JF. Coping with Chronic Illness: Overcoming Powerlessness. Philadelphia, FA Davis, 1983.

Millon I et al (eds). Handbook of Clinical Health Psychology. New York, Plenum Press, 1982.

Millman H (ed). Therapies for Adults: Depressive, Anxiety and Personality Disorders. San Francisco, Jossey-Bass, 1982.

Moos R(ed). Coping with Physical Illness, vol. 2. New York, Plenum Medical Book Co, 1984.

Morce N and Robins P. The 36-Hour Day. Baltimore, Johns Hopkins University Press, 1981.

Norris CM (ed). Concept Clarification in Nursing. Rockville, Maryland, Aspen Systems, 1982.

Purtila R. Health Professional/Patient Interaction, 3rd ed. Philadelphia, WB Saunders, 1984.

Roberts S. Behavioral Concepts and the Critically Ill Patient, 2nd ed. Englewood Cliffs, New Jersey, Prentice-Hall, 1986.

Schultz W. The Interpersonal Underworld. Palo Alto, Science and Behavior Books, 1966.

Selzer R. Letters to a Young Doctor. New York, Simon & Schuster, 1982.

Simons RC. Understanding Human Behavior in Health and Illness, 3rd ed. Baltimore, Williams & Wilkins, 1985.

Strauss A. Chronic Illness and the Quality of Life, 2nd ed. St Louis, CV Mosby, 1984.

Wilkes E. The Dying Patient: The Medical Management of Incurable and Terminal Illness. Ridgewood, New Jersey, George A. Boyden & Son, 1982.

Williams JM and Mark G. The Psychological Treatment of Depression. New York, Free Press, 1984.

Wilson HS and Kneisl CR. Psychiatric Nursing, 2nd ed. Menlo Park, California, Addison-Wesley, 1983.

Woods NF. Human Sexuality in Health and Illness, 3rd ed. St Louis, CV Mosby, 1984.

Articles

(Asterisks indicate nursing research articles.)

Anger/Anxiety

*Anxiety in surgical patients and families. AORN J 1984 July; 40(1):131–137.

Beatty J et al. Anger generated by unmet expectations. MCN 1985 Sept/Oct; 10(5):324–327.

Bushman P. Anger in the clinical setting. MCN 1985 Sept/Oct; 10(5):314–316.

Chansky ER. Reducing patients' anxieties: Techniques for dealing with crisis. AORN J 1984 Sept; 40(3):375–377.

Duer-Hefele J et al. Managing intractable anger. MCN 1985 Sept/Oct; 10(5):328–332.

Dult B. Helping nurses to cope with the anger/dismay syndrome. Nurs Outlook 1982 Mar; 30(3):168–174.

Dunne K et al. Anger: Normal, appropriate and justifiable. MCN 1985 Sept/Oct; 10(5):317–319.

Flannery RB. Major life events and daily hassles in predicting health status: Methodological inquiry. J Clin Psychol 1986 May; 42(3):485–487.

Galub Z et al. The ripple effect of anger. MCN Sept/Oct 1985; 10(5):333–337.

Gomez EA et al. Anxiety as a human emotion: Some basic conceptual models. Nurs Forum 1984; 21(1):38–42.

Hewitt D. Don't forget your preop patient's fear. RN 1984 Oct; 47(10): 63–68.

Lindgren K et al. Avoidance of anger. MCN 1985 Sept/Oct; 10(5):320–323.

Magni G et al. Anxiety, hostility, and blood pressure variation during heart surgery. Psychomatics 1986 May; 27(5):362–365, 369.

Richardson J et al. In the face of anger. Nursing '84 1984 Feb; 14(2): 66–71.

Body Image/Self-Concept

*Champion VL et al. Assessment of relationship between self concept and body image using multivariate techniques. Issues Ment Health Nurs 1982 Apr; 4(4):229–315.

Grumbaun J. Helping your patient build a sturdier body image . . . damaged by disease, trauma, or surgery. RN 1985 Oct; 48(10):51–55.

Jemmott JB et al. Judging health status: Effects of perceived prevalence and personal relevance. J Pers Soc Psychol 1986 May; 50(5):899–905.

*Morris CA. Self-concept as altered by the diagnosis of cancer. Nurs Clin North Am 1985 Dec; 20(4):611–630.

*Norris J et al. Self esteem disturbance . . . Nursing diagnoses. Nurs Clin North Am 1985 Dec; 20(4):745–761.

Communication

Adams R et al. Communication: say what you mean! Hosp Top 1983 May/June 61(3):13–21.

Auvil CA. The sounds of silence. Am J Nurs 1984 Aug; 84(8):1072.

Brackopp DY. What is NLP? Am J Nurs 1983 July; 83(7):1012–1014.

Communication and counseling: Modern nursing roles. Regan Rep Nurs Law 1913 Feb; 23(9):1.

Communications: Doctor–nurse–patient triangle. Regan Rep Nurs Law 1983 Jan; 23(8):1.

Forsyth DM. Looking good to communicate better with patients. Nursing '83 1983 July; 13(7):34–37.

Greenlaw J. The deadly toll of communication failure. RN 1982 Nov; 45(11):81–82, 84.

Harris RD. Overcoming communication blocks. Hosp Top 1983 July/Aug; 61(4):19–20, 23.

*McFarland GK et al. Impaired communication: A descriptive study. Nurs Clin North Am 1985 Dec; 20(4):775–785.

Morgan RH. Breaking through the sound barrier. Nursing '83 1983 Feb; 13(2):112,114.

Rich P. Make the most of charting. Nursing '83 1983 Mar; 13(3):34–39.

Talento B et al. Improving interviewing techniques. Nurs Outlook 1983 July/Aug; 31(4):234–235.

Weist JK et al. The hospitalized alcoholic: Hospital dialogues. Am J Nurs 1982 Dec; 82(12):1874–1877.

Coping

*Beard MT. Life events, method of coping, and interpersonal trust: Implications for nursing actions. Issues Ment Health Nurs 1982 Jan/Mar; 4(1):25–49.

Clarke M. Stress and coping constructs for nursing. J Adv Nurs 1984 Jan; 9(1):3–13.

Craig HM et al. Adaptation in chronic illness: An eclectic model for nursing. J Adv Nurs 1983 Sept; 8(5):397–404.

Fritz WS. Maintaining wellness: Yours and theirs. Nurs Clin North Am 1984 June; 19(2):263–269.

Hamm BH et al. Teaching the client to cope through guided imagery. J Community Health Nurs 1984; 1(1):39–45.

Ostechega G et al. Providing "safe conduct": Helping your patient cope with cancer. Nursing '84 1984 Apr; 14(4):42–47.

Robinson KM. Concepts of stress for nursing. Issues Ment Health Nurs 1982 July/Sept; 4(3):167–176.

Smith DW. Survivors of serious illness. Am J Nurs 1979 Mar; 79(3):441–446.

Soffer RS. Coping mechanisms of the chronically ill during family separation. Home Health Care Nurs 1983 Nov–Dec; 1(2):52–55.

Culture

Brink PJ. Value orientations as an assessment tool in cultural diversity. Nurs Res 1984 July/Aug; 33(4):198–203.

Kubricht D and Clark JA. Foreign patients: A system of providing care. Nurs Outlook 1982; 67(1):55–57.

La Fargue JP. Mediating between two views of illness. Top Clin Nurs 1985 Oct; 7(3):70–77.

Tripps-Reimer T et al. Cultural assessment: Content and process. Nurs Outlook 1984 Mar/Apr 32(2):78–82.

Death/Grief

Benoliel JQ. Nursing research on death, dying, and terminal illness: Development, present state, and prospects. Ann Rev Nurs Res 1986; 1:101–130.

Cowles KV. Life, death, and personhood. Nurs Outlook 1984 May/June; 32(3):168–172.

Dealing with your feelings about death. Nursing '84 1984 Aug; 14(8):68.

*Demi AS et al. Research on nursing practice: Bereavement. Annu Rev Nurs Res 1986; 4:105–123.

Franks LC et al. When a patient dies . . . grief—the patient's, the family's and your own. RN 1984 Feb; 47(2):24–30.

Fulton R et al. Loss, social changes, and the prospects of mourning. Death Educ 1982 Summer; 6(2):137–153.

Kastenbaum R. New fantasies in the American death system. Death Educ 1982 Summer; 6(2):155–166.

Kellar MH. What is it like to be dying? Nursing '83 1983 Sept; 13(9):65–67.

*Kirschling JM et al. Nursing and the terminally ill: Beliefs, attitudes, and perceptions of practitioners. Issues Ment Health Nurs 1982; 4(4):275–286.

Martacchia BC. Grief and bereavement: Healing through hurt . . . loss through death. Nurs Clin North Am 1985 June; 20(2):327–341.

*Miles MS. Emotional symptoms and physical health in bereaved parents. Nurs Res 1985 Mar/Apr; 34(2):76–81.

Neki JS. Grief . . . different cultures have developed different ways of dealing with it. World Health 1982 Nov; 20–23.

Norton MA. Daring to care . . . for a dying patient. Am J Nurs 1985 Oct; 85(1):1098–1099.

Page MS. Saying goodbye. Am J Nurs 1985 Oct; 85(10):1112–1113.

*Pender NJ et al. Attitudes: Subjective norms, and intentions to engage in health behaviors. Nurs Res 1986 Jan/Feb; 35(1):15–18.

Poster EC et al. When the patient dies: Dealing with the family's anger. Dimens Crit Care Nur 1984 Nov/Dec; 3(6):372–377.

Probert W. Ethics and the law of dying. Death Educ 1984; 8(1):70–76.

Ronere R. Thoughts while dying. Nursing '84 1984 Nov; 14(11):67–68.

Zack MV. Loneliness: A concept relevant to the care of dying persons. Nurs Clin North Am 1985 June; 20(2):403–414.

Depression

Laurent CL. Hidden depression. Am J Nurs 1985 May; 85(5):534.

Manderino MA et al. Mobilizing depressed clients. J Psychosoc Nurs Ment Health Serv 1986 May; 24(5):23–28.

Rabin PL. What is depression? Nephrol Nurse 1983 Jan/Feb; 5(1):20–22.

Hope

Dufault K. Hope: Its spheres and dimensions. Nurs Clin North Am 1985 June; 20(2):379–391.

McGee R. F. Hope: A factor influencing crisis resolution. ANS 1984 July; 6(4):34–44.

Miller JF. Inspiring hope. Am J Nurs 1985 Jan; 85(1):22–25.

Richardson K. Hope and flexibility: Your keys to helping OBS patients. Nursing '82 1982 June; 12(6):65–69.

Taylor P et al. Holding our hope to your dying patient. Nursing '82 1982 Feb; 12(2):42–45.

Problem Patients

Assey JL et al. Who is the seductive patient? Am J Nurs 1983 Apr; 83(4): 530–532.

Barash DA. Defusing the violent patient—before he explodes. RN 1984 Mar; 47(3):34–37.

Francis B. The turning point. Nursing '86 1986 Feb; 16(2):65.

Law CP. One of our patients is missing! RN 1983 Dec; 46(12):48–49.

Luna ML. The patient who complains. Nursing '84 1984 Nov; 4(1):46–49.

Maagdenberg AM. The "violent" patient. Am J Nurs 1983 Mar; 83(3):402–403.

Meer J. Loneliness. Psychology Today. 1985 July; 19(7):28–33.

*Munns DC. A validation of the defining characteristics of the nursing diagnosis "potential for violence." Nurs Clin North Am 1985 Dec; 20(4):711–722.

Psychosocial Aspects of Illness

Bayer LN et al. Psychosocial aspects of nutritional support. Nurs Clin North Am 1983 Mar; 18(1):119–128.

Benoliel JQ. Loss and terminal illness. Nurs Clin North Am 1985 Jan; 20(2):439–448.

Bergman R. Understanding the patient in all his human needs. J Adv Nurs 1983 May; 8(3):185–190.

Clark B. What to do when your patient lets slip his grip on reality. Nursing '84 1984 July; 14(7):50–56.

Dolan MB. By the rules . . . twenty years of rheumatoid arthritis. Am J Nurs 1983 May; 83(5):815, 819.

*Dracups KA and Melsis AI. Compliance: An interactionist approach. Nurs Res 1982 Jan/Feb; 31(1):31–36.

Fitzsimon V. When the older patient's apathetic. Nursing '82 1982 Apr; 12(4):53–57.

*Frank-Stromberg M et al. Ambulatory cancer patients' perception of the physical and psychosocial changes in their lives since the diagnosis of cancer. Cancer Nurs 1984 Apr; 7(2):117–130.

*Frank-Stromberg M et al. Psychological impact of the "cancer" diagnosis. Oncol Nurs Forum 1984 May/June; 11(3):16–22.

Groves C et al. Nursing grand rounds: I.C.U. psychosis; helping your patient return to reality. Nursing '82 1982 Jan; 12(1):58–63.

Hagan IJ. Bring help and hope to the patient with Hodgkin's disease. Nursing '83 1983 Aug; 13(8):58–64.

Hansen AC. There's a person within. RN 1984 Apr; 47(4):31–32.

*Krouse HJ and Krouse JH. Cancer as crisis: The critical elements of adjustment. Nurs Res 1982 Mar/Apr; 31(2):96–101.

Krumm S. Psychosocial adaptation of the adult with cancer. Nurs Clin North Am 1982 Dec; 17(4):729–737.

Locke AM et al. Managing psychological disturbances in critical care. Dimens Crit Care Nurs 1983 Sept/Oct; 2(5):314–320.

McHugh MK. Psychosocial aspects of cancer: A review. Top Clin Nurs 1985 Apr; 7(1):1–9.

*Mishel M. The measurement of uncertainty in illness. Nurs Res 1982 Sept/Oct; 30(5):258–263.

Richardson B. A tool for assessing the real world of diabetic noncompliance. Nursing '82 1982 Jan; 12(1):68–73.

Roberts CS. Symposium on patient compliance: Identifying the real patient problems. Nurs Clin North Am 1982 Sept; 17(3):481–489.

*Scott DW. Anxiety, critical thinking and information processing during and after breast biopsy. Nurs Res 1983 Jan/Feb; 32(1):24–28.

*Snyder M. Effect of relaxation on psychosocial functioning in persons with epilepsy. J Neurosurg Nurs 1983 Aug; 15(4):250–254.

*Sparachine J et al. Psychological correlates of blood pressure: A closer examination of hostility, anxiety, and engagement. Nurs Res 1982 May/June; 31(3):143–149.

Stanites MA and Regan J. Noncompliance: an unacceptable diagnosis? Am J Nurs 1982 June; 82(6):941–942.

Stanton GM. Spinal cord injury: Psychological adaptation. J Neurosurg Nurs 1983 Oct; 15(5):306–309.

Wright LK. Life-threatening illness. J Psychosoc Nurs Ment Health Serv 1985 Sept; 23(9):6–11.

Psychosocial Support

Anderson ML. Nursing intervention: What did you do that helped? Perspect Psychiatr Care 1983 Jan/Mar; 21(1):4–8.

Gault P. Plan for a patchwork of problems when your patient is elderly. Nursing '82 1982 Jan; 12(1):50–54.

*Grerszciwski SA. The relationship of weight loss, locus of control, and social support. Nurs Res 1983 Jan/Feb; 32(1):43–47.

Hein EC and Leanith MB. Providing emotional support to patients. Nursing '82 1982 June; 12(6):127–129.

Johnson SH. 10 ways to help the family of a critically ill patient. Nursing '86 1986 Jan; 16(1):50–53.

McHugh MK et al. Preparatory information: What helps and why. Am J Nurs 1982 May; 82(5):780–782.

Osterlund H. Humor, a serious approach to patient care. Nursing '83 1983 Dec; 13(12):46–47.

Schoenhoper SO. Support as legitimate nursing action. Nurs Outlook 1984 July/Aug; 32(4):218–219.

Self-care

Caporal-Katz B. Health, self-care and power: Shifting the balance. Top Clin Nurs 1983 Oct; 5(3):31–41.

Sloan MR et al. How to get your patient involved in his care? Use a contract. Nursing '82 1982 Dec; 12(12):48–49.

Stress

*Baldee KS et al. Stress identification and coping patterns in patients on hemodialysis Nurs Res 1982 Mar/Apr; 31(2):107–112.

Dones AJ. Stress. Am J Nurs 1984 Mar; 84(3):365–368.

*Gilliss CL. Reducing family stress during and after coronary artery bypass surgery. Nurs Clin North Am 1984 Mar; 19(1):103–112.

Maier SF et al. Stress and health: Exploring the links. Psychology Today 1985 Aug; 19(8):44–49.

Shaver JF. A biopsychosocial view of human health. Nurs Outlook 1985 July/Aug; 33(4):186–191.

*Woods NF et al. Major life events, daily stressors, and perimenstrual symptoms. Nurs Res 1985 Sept/Oct; 34(5):263–267.

Touch

Bledsoe A. The importance of touch in nursing care. Imprint 1984 Nov; 31(4):58–59.

Clark PE et al. Therapeutic touch: Is there a scientific basis for the practice? Nurs Res 1984 Jan/Feb; 33(1):37–41.

Fanslow CA. Therapeutic touch: A healing modality throughout life. Top Clin Nurs 1983 July; 5(2):72–79.

Kopac CA. Sensory loss in the aged: The role of the nurse and the family. Nurs Clin North Am 1983 June; 18(2):373–384.

McAuliffe K et al. I care . . . reaching patients through touch. Nursing '84 1984 Apr; 14(4):58–59.

*Randolph GL. Therapeutic and physical touch: Physiological response to stressful stimuli. Nurs Res 1984 Jan/Feb; 33(1):33–36.

Raucheisen ML. Therapeutic touch: Maybe there's something to it after all. RN 1984 Dec; 47(12):49–51.

Videocassettes

American Journal of Nursing Educational Services Division:
    Anxiety Concepts and Manifestations, 1981.
    Creative Listening Part 2, 1981.
    Crisis Intervention: Theory and Application, 1975.
    Depressed Client, 1977.
    Manipulative Client, 1977.
    Psychosocial Assessment Part I and II, 1975.
    Suspicious Client, 1977.
    Therapeutic Relationship, 1981.
    Therapeutic Silence Part I, 1981.
    Withdrawn Client, 1977.

Chapter 13

Human Sexuality

The Delivery of Sexual Health Care

To deliver sexual health care effectively, the nurse must balance rational scientific data with a humanistic client-centered approach. Three elements help the nurse separate her sexual self from that of the patient: an adequate knowledge base, critical sexual self-assessment, and a person-centered approach.

An Adequate Knowledge Base.   Acquisition of knowledge about sexuality is a lifelong process. In the past decade, sexuality has been redefined in a holistic perspective and has become recognized as an important component of the total person interacting with the environment. In order to distinguish between healthy and unhealthy responses, the nurse must have an understanding of psychosexual development, sexual growth and reproduction, variations in sexual behavior, sexual responses in health and illness, and the impact of life events on sexuality.

Sexual Self-Awareness.   A critical sexual self-assessment is a desensitization process leading to a greater self-awareness. It includes an acknowledgment of one's own sexuality, as well as an understanding and acceptance of personal attitudes, values, and beliefs. Attitudes stem from religious teachings, cultural mores, familial beliefs, myths, and social taboos; they may interfere with the acquisition of knowledge, objective listening, and proper patient management.

A variety of tools can be used for a critical sexual self-assessment. Attitude questionnaires listing issues (*e.g.*, contraception, abortion), behaviors (*e.g.*, masturbation, homosexuality), and life-styles (*e.g.*, open marriage, cohabitation, and personal reactions) can provide the nurse with insight for determining personal attitudes and identifying strengths and limitations in sexual aspects of clinical practice.

Once an attitude is acknowledged, it can be further clarified through introspection, peer group discussions, value clarification exercises, and role playing. A log book with care plans and process recordings can reveal the inability to intervene appropriately owing to conflict. Conflicts may arise from the care of a person whose behavior, attitudes, and values differ from that of the nurse.

Person-Centered Approach. A person-centered approach is appropriate for dealing with sexual problems to ensure recognition of individual differences and to help patients in making their own informed choices. Acceptance of the sexual assessment, sex education, anticipatory guidance, and sexual counseling are based on the individual's perception of sexuality.

Caution and tolerance, as well as effective communication, are necessary to adapt the nursing process to sexual health care. The nurse and the patient may experience varying degrees of comfort when discussing sexuality.

The Role of the Nurse

The role of the nurse in the delivery of sexual health care is to provide a therapeutic environment conducive to sexual health. When acting as a sex educator and counselor, the nurse can assist the patient to acquire knowledge, validate normalcy, and prepare for changes in sexuality throughout the life cycle, in both health and illness. The nurse using the nursing process is able to carry out a meaningful assessment, identify problem areas, plan, implement, coordinate referral sources, and evaluate effectiveness of care.

Sexual Development

Sexual development begins at conception. The woman's egg carries the X chromosome, and the male's sperm carries either an X or a Y chromosome. Thus, the sperm determines the sex of the offspring. X paired with X equals a female embryo; when X is paired with Y in the presence of androgens, a male embryo develops. All embryos are female until the sixth week of life, when androgens stimulate male sexual development in the XY fetus. Deviations in early sexual development can occur from chromosomal error or hormonal disturbances. After birth, sexual development is influenced by the behavior of other people through the socialization process.

Basic to our development as sexual humans is our personal sense of maleness or femaleness and the way we perceive and express it. To provide clarity and consistency, several related terms are defined.

Biological sex is defined as the basic anatomical and reproductive differences between males and females. The components are chromosomal differentiation, hormonal secretions, differentiation of internal sex organs, and external genitalia.

Gender is a behavioral term, a psychological phenomenon. The two components are biological sex and gender identity.

Gender identity refers to the degree to which an individual perceives being a male or a female. To a great extent, this perception is culturally determined. The core of juvenile gender identity is established by 18 months. At the time of puberty, hormonal influences on pubertal morphology, eroticism, and body image lead to the development of adult gender identity. Gender identity becomes relatively immutable by the end of adolescence (Money and Ehrhardt, 1972).

Gender role refers to the way in which a person expresses gender identity. It is learned behavior through imitation of the same-sex parent and complementation of the opposite-sex parent. It is influenced by the complex interaction of parental rewards and punishments. Gender role continues to be defined throughout the life cycle.

Traditionally, in our Western culture, masculinity and femininity referred to restrictive sex-role stereotyped behavior. "Masculine" was defined in terms of strong, aggressive, logical, and independent characteristics. "Feminine" was defined in terms of weak, submissive, dependent, and emotional characteristics. Gender roles have changed for both women and men over the past two decades. Gender is now viewed on a continuum, so that having characteristics traditionally identified as male traits does not necessarily make a person less feminine, and vice versa. The term *androgenous* (unisex) refers to both masculine and feminine characteristics, providing more options for individuals and ultimately greater equality between sexes (Bem, 1974).

Sexual preference refers to choice of sexual partner: heterosexual (opposite sex), homosexual (same sex), bisexual (both sexes).

In order to provide anticipatory guidance throughout the life cycle, the nurse should be familiar with psychosexual development: developmental tasks, sexual growth, sexual behaviors, and common sexual concerns, problems, and areas of intervention.

Table 13-1 is a summary of psychosexual development that should be used only as a guideline for obtaining assessment data. The framework used has been provided by Erikson; however, in all cases, individual differences should be considered (Erikson, 1963).

Human Sexual Response Patterns

The findings of Masters and Johnson indicated that the human sexual response could be described as a cycle with four stages (Masters & Johnson, 1966). These stages follow a consistent pattern of progression, from excitement to plateau, then to orgasm and resolution. Two basic physiologic responses are responsible for the sexual response cycle: vasocongestion and myotonia.

Vasocongestion is the filling of blood vessels of the genitals and specific body regions, causing enlargement and color changes. *Myotonia* is increased muscle tension, voluntary and involuntary. Both are a result of sexual stimulation, begin during excitement, become more pronounced and reach a peak at orgasm, and subside during resolution.

Sexual desire preceding excitement is controlled by the limbic system in the brain and is greatly influenced by the hormone testosterone. Therefore, anything that inhibits testosterone production may inhibit sexual desire. Stress causes a decrease in testosterone levels; consequently, a person who perceives a threat, pain, or fear is not likely to experience sexual desire (Kaplan, 1974).

Excitement

Sexual excitement may be triggered by external stimuli (visual, auditory, tactile, and olfactory) or by internal stimuli (fantasy and memory).

(Text continues on p. 200)

TABLE 13-1
Summary of Stages of Psychosexual Development and Related Nursing Intervention

Developmental Tasks	Sexual Growth	Sexual Behaviors	Sexual Concerns and Problems	Intervention
Developmental Stage: Infancy (0–18 months)				
Developmental Crisis: Trust vs. Mistrust				
Develops a need for affection and to return affection	Sensitivity to a warm, loving environment	Cuddling, hugging, kissing	Touch deprivation	Reinforce the importance of close physical contact and related problems.
	Oral sensitivity, lips, tongue, mouth (oral stage)	Sucking	Oral deprivation (early weaning)	Explain the significance of early weaning and related problems: thumb sucking, emotional difficulty.
Begins to interpret expectations of significant others	Genital sensitivity; erectile potential in males; orgasmic potential in males and females	Stimulation of genitals by self or others; erections in males; primitive orgasms	Parental concern Parental fear	Clarify parental attitudes and beliefs toward self. Explain the primitive nature of the response: higher brain centers not well developed. Reinforce that behavior is normal and cannot harm the infant.
Develops a communication system	Feels good/bad about body parts and functions	Labels body parts based on parental values, voice inflections	Body image	Stress the importance of relating to infant's body in a positive way.
Establishes separateness and becomes social; can differentiate between strange and familiar people	Distinguish between self and others Reinforcement of gender identity	Begins to show maleness or femaleness Identifies with same sex parent	Blurred identity, restrictive sex role, stereotyping, coding (pink for girls, blue for boys), limiting play objects	Infant needs close contact with a person to develop gender identity. Sex-role stereotyping can be avoided by focusing on the infant as an individual.
Developmental Stage: Toddler (18 months–3 years)				
Developmental Crisis: Autonomy vs. Shame, Doubt				
Begins to demonstrate toilet training	Learns control of bowel and bladder (anal stage)	Sensual pleasure derived from elimination	Strict toilet training	Relate problems identified with strict toilet training: compulsive behavior, castration anxiety. Provide alternative methods of toilet training.
Begins to participate as a family member	Development of core of gender identity	Imitates behavior of parent of same sex	Anxiety about acceptable behavior for males and females	Avoid sex role stereotyping by providing options: dress, playthings, focus on individual child.
Communicates with others outside family	Learns differences between male and female bodies	Shows an interest in bodies of other children	Parental concern	Clarify attitudes, values, and beliefs.
	Establishes concept of body image	Labels body parts and may ask questions	Poor self-image; may view sexual organs as "dirty"	Provide vocabulary that emphasizes acceptance of body: genitals, reproduction, elimination.
Develops autonomous behavior	Genital sensitivity Erection potential Orgasmic potential	Sensual, erotic behaviors; masturbation patterns of self-pleasure, toys, objects	Parental concern	Emphasize normal part of sexual development. Clarify values, attitudes and beliefs.

(continued)

TABLE 13-1 *(continued)*

Developmental Tasks	Sexual Growth	Sexual Behaviors	Sexual Concerns and Problems	Intervention
Developmental Stage: Preschool (4–6 years) *Developmental Crisis: Initiative vs. Guilt*				
Participates actively as a family member	Oedipal attachment to opposite sex parent: complementation— learns what to expect from opposite parent; identification with same sex parent; learns sex roles	Physically affectionate; interested in parents' bodies; fantasizes about parents; may dress in parents' clothing	Excessive attachment to parent; seductive behavior of parent toward child; hostility of same sex parent	Provide alternatives for seductive parent in a nonthreatening manner. Refer parents to parenting class (avoid confusing messages for child). Sexual variations may be related to seductive parent. Refer for counseling.
Responds to expectations of others; begins to understand and establish a sense of morality	Sexual curiosity; penis and clitoris become chief areas of erotic pleasure (phallic stage); capacity to perceive sexual odors	Self-play increases; "plays doctor," touches and sees other children's bodies; asks questions about genitals, reproduction	Parental concern; child may learn to suppress sexual feelings and behavior in order to be accepted by others.	Overreaction leads to guilt; anticipate sexual curiosity; stress importance of answering questions in a nonjudgmental manner. Use penis, vagina as appropriate terminology.
Developmental Stage: School Age (6–12 years) *Developmental Crisis: Industry vs. Inferiority*				
Decreases dependency on family for total love and support; begins to understand peer relationships	Close contact with same sex peers; development of friendships	Homosexual experiences part of same sex relationships; also, sex play with opposite sex common	Parental overreaction; guilty child	Reassure parents that this is a normal part of psychosexual growth and development. Validate normalcy.
	Curiosity about sex (no latency)	Discussion of sex with peers	Confusing or frightening information	Clarify myths, giving accurate information about reproduction.
	Orgasm potential (males and females); some girls begin menarche	Mutual masturbation, self-stimulation	Fear owing to lack of information	
Acknowledges body changes	Increasing self-awareness; interest in body growth	Comparison of body growth with peers	Concerns over body growth	Elicit sexual history in a comfortable, confidential manner: What do you know about having babies? When you have questions about sex, who do you ask? Do you have questions about sex? Have you noticed changes in your body? How do you feel about changes in your body?
Relates to social, religious, or familial values, attitudes, and beliefs	Learns internal sexual value system; learns self-control	Learns to be secretive; may use slang for shock value	Testing behavior limits; obsessive, antisocial behavior; repression	Refer for counseling, family therapy. Attempts by parents to restrict may lead to low self-esteem. No limits delay internal value-system formation.

(continued)

TABLE 13-1 *(continued)*

Developmental Tasks	Sexual Growth	Sexual Behaviors	Sexual Concerns and Problems	Intervention
Developmental Stage: School Age (6–12 years) *Developmental Crisis: Industry vs. Inferiority*				
	Understands concepts of masculinity and femininity	Continues to define sex role in activities inside and outside family	Strict sex-role stereotyping by parents: male may be discouraged from developing "female" skills; females may be discouraged from sports activities	Provide alternatives to limitations of sex-role stereotyping. Focus on preferences of the individual child.
Developmental Stage: Early Adolescence (12–15 years) and Late Adolescence (15–18 years) *Developmental Crisis: Identity Formation vs. Identity Diffusion*				
Acknowledges and accepts physical changes and body image	Female: menarche; development of breasts; distribution of fat to hips and thighs; increased size of uterus; pubic hair growth Male: ejaculation; testicular enlargement; growth of pubic hair and facial hair; voice change and nocturnal emissions	Comparison of body changes with same sex peers; sexual fantasies related to body	Anxiety over change in body image; embarrassment	Discuss relationship of body image and sexual growth and how these changes perceived by the individual are a reflection of self-image. Adolescents have the pain and pleasure of observing the whole process.
Develops close peer relationships with both sexes; develops deep personal relationship with opposite sex	Learns intimacy, heterosexual relationships; develops "crushes"	Heterosexual encounters: kissing, petting, mutual masturbation; heterosexual fantasies. One half of teenagers will have intercourse.	Performance; orgasm; virginity; anxiety.	Provide direct and confidential approach in eliciting sexual history: Are you sexually active? Frequency? How do you feel about it? Provide birth control counseling. STD risk-reduction counseling, Pap testing, BSE, TSE.
			Compulsive, mechanical masturbation	May represent escape from another problem; provide sex counseling
Attains a male or female role	Increased awareness of sexual feelings integrated in self	Males group together in sports; females group together	Sexual variations may surface: homosexuality, transsexuality, bisexuality	Provide role clarification: What do you think it means to be a man or a woman? Validate normalcy. Refer to sex counseling if problems exist.
Seeks more of a peer relationship with parents	Express feelings about sexual self	Responds to parental limitations	Parental concern, communication breakdown; guilt	Communication is essential. Parents fail to take "crush" seriously. Problems related to double standard may surface. Restrictive limitations impede development.

(continued)

TABLE 13-1 *(continued)*

Developmental Tasks	Sexual Growth	Sexual Behaviors	Sexual Concerns and Problems	Intervention
Developmental Stage: Young Adult (20–45 years) *Developmental Crisis: Intimacy vs. Self-Isolation*				
Stabilizes self-image	Acceptance of one's body; pregnancy	Comfortable nude with intimate others	Male: anxiety over penis size Female: anxiety over breast size. Both: self-consciousness; shame	Stress the fact that size of breasts or penis has little to do with sexual gratification. Negative body image may interfere with the establishment of sexual relationships.
Establishes sexual behavior patterns	Mature concept of sexual self; gender role continues to be defined; sexual orientation and sexual life-style established	Heterosexual adjustment—bisexuality, homosexuality, celibacy, masturbation, cohabitation, monogamy, marriage, extramarital sex	Ambivalence to gender role, identity, sexual orientation, "homosexual panic," feelings of being trapped by sex orientation	Elicit sexual history: How do you feel about gender identity, role, and orientation? Explore feelings about sex partner. Regardless of expression, intimacy vs. isolation should be evaluated. Validate normalcy.
	Learns to give and receive pleasure	Experimentation with different forms of sexual expression	Boredom; fear of experimentation; inability to communicate sexual needs to partner; lack of information	Explain sexual response cycle. Discuss patterns of sexual behavior. Identify areas of concern. Possible referrals.
Determines desire for having family; protects reproductive integrity	Makes decisions about childbearing	Reproduction control; maintains integrity of sex organs; Pap screening, BSE, TSE-STD risk-reducing behaviors	Unwanted pregnancy; fear of physical exam—pelvic; lack of information about STDs or birth control	Elicit sexual history and birth control method, and provide alternatives. Explore feelings about childbearing, STD counseling, and risk reduction.
Formulates life philosophy and develops ethical standards	Develops sexual value system	Behavior reflects individual values, attitudes, and beliefs.	Sexual needs are not met owing to strict, inflexible beliefs.	Values clarification is needed: absolutistic—sexuality for reproduction; hedonistic—pleasure; relativistic—acts judged on the basis of their effects.
Developmental Stage: Middle Age (45–65 years) *Developmental Crisis: Generativity vs. Self-Absorption/Stagnation*				
Acknowledges and accepts physical and emotional changes	Declining hormonal production: menopause—vaginal atrophy and loss of vaginal mucosa; vasomotor symptoms—hot flashes, irritability, fatigue, external genitalia, and breast tissue changes; male climacteric—slower to attain erection, sustained shorter, and ejaculatory force lessens	Focus on quality of sexual encounter vs. quantity; frequency may decline; intercourse expression of love and trust; reaffirmation of self-concept	Anxiety about losing youthfulness, vitality, sex appeal, and fear of loss of partner; may stop sexual activity owing to dyspareunia caused by lack of vaginal secretions; self-image crisis; depression and denial; male concern: losing vigor and virility.	Give anticipatory guidance. Explain changes in sexual response with aging. Postmenopausal women: recommend vaginal lubricant. Regular sexual activity will increase capacity for sexual performance.

(continued)

TABLE 13-1 *(continued)*

Developmental Tasks	Sexual Growth	Sexual Behaviors	Sexual Concerns and Problems	Intervention
Developmental Stage: Middle Age (45–65 years) *Developmental Crisis: Generativity vs. Self-Absorption/Stagnation*				
Adjusts to independence of grown children	Adjusts to "empty nest"; redefines sex roles	Spends time reestablishing primary relationship; develops and cultivates new joint activities; relinquishes control of children	Attempts to continue to control offspring	Focus on maintenance of relationship with spouse or intimate other.
Developmental Stage: Later Maturity (65+) *Developmental Crisis: Ego Integrity vs. Despair*				
Continues close, loving relationship with spouse	Accepts slowed sexual response cycle; development of alternative ways to achieve sexual satisfaction	Adjusts sexual activities; appropriate time may be AM, when less fatigued; oral or manual stimulation; fantasy; emphasis on sensual touching, holding, kissing	Conforms to prevailing societal myth of sex for procreation; lack of information; rigid stereotyped image of what older person should be	Sexual need for intimacy and sexual expression does not change with age. Explain physical changes in sexual response with aging.
Copes with illness or death of spouse or friend	Learns new social patterns; develops alternative ways to achieve sexual satisfaction	Cohabitation; homosexual or lesbian relationship; masturbation; heterosexual relationship; remarriage	Guilt; anxiety; depression; isolation; avoidance of sex altogether	Elicit sexual history: Are you sexually active? Assess sexual patterns and satisfaction. Values clarification needed. Give patient permission for sexual behavior.
Maintains an interdependent relationship with children	Maintaining control of developing relationships	Continues to meet sexual needs	Lack of privacy in environment; children's reactions; anxiety, jealousy, anger	Assist client in maintaining independence. Some grown children fear exploitation of parents. Some are "will watchers." Recommend premarital legal planning.

Female Response. In women, the first sign of excitement begins with vaginal lubrication owing to transudation of fluid from engorged vessels through the vaginal wall. The inner two thirds of the vagina lengthen and widen; the walls become dark purple and smooth. The uterus begins to be pulled upward in the lower abdomen. Labia majora become thin and flattened in a nulliparous woman. In a multiparous woman, the labia majora swell with blood, double in size, and hang, owing to increased vascularization occurring with pregnancy. The labia minora swell and become engorged with blood, eventually serving to lengthen the vagina.

The nipples become erect owing to involuntary contraction of muscle fibers in the areola. Venous blood trapped in the breasts causes an increase in size. The clitoris enlarges as it fills with blood. This process of tumescence is very similar to penile enlargement, although it occurs not nearly as quickly as it does in the penis.

In older women, the clitoris maintains its high degree of sensitivity. The vagina's ability to expand decreases. The walls become thin and smooth; consequently, there is less protection for the bladder and urethra during intercourse, predisposing the aging female to cystitis. Lubrication may be slower in developing or may be diminished, causing *dyspareunia* (painful intercourse). Water-soluble lubricant will help alleviate this symptom.

Male Response. During the exitement phase, the penis becomes tumescent (erect); this process takes from several seconds to several minutes. The scrotum tenses and thickens; at the same time, the testes elevate toward the perineum as the muscles associated with the spermatic cords contract.

In both men (25%) and women (74%), a skin flush causing a maculopapular sex flush owing to superficial vasocongestive reaction in skin occurs late in excitement or early in plateau. The blood pressure and heart rate begin to accelerate.

Older men experience a slowing of the sexual response. If an older man is slow to reach erection, he can stimulate his partner and continue to maintain high levels of excitement. Erection takes two to three times longer in men over 50 years of age, and full erection may not be attained until orgasm. In both older men and women, vasocongestive and myotonic responses diminish, causing associated color changes to be less apparent.

Plateau

The length of plateau depends on the effectiveness of the stimulation, the age of the person, and the desire to attain orgasm. If there are any negative stimuli perceived by males or females, resolution can occur without orgasm. During plateau, muscular tension, heart rate, and blood pressure increase.

Female Response. The outer third of the vagina becomes distended and shortened, with the engorged labia minora forming the orgasmic platform. The clitoris retracts under the clitoral hood but maintains a high degree of sensitivity. The Bartholin's glands secrete a small amount of mucoid substance.

In older women, the engorgement of labia and ballooning of the vagina is decreased, but constriction responses assisting in the formation of the orgasmic platform continue.

Male Response. The penis increases in diameter, and the glans may darken. The testes elevate tightly against the perineum and increase in size owing to vasocongestion. Pre-ejaculatory fluid is secreted from the Cowper's glands.

In both men and women, myotonia increases, resulting in voluntary and involuntary contractions of arms, legs, neck, rectum, and buttocks. Carpopedal spasms of hands and feet may occur. Women may contract pubococcygeal muscles (Kegel exercises) to enhance sexual pleasure.

In older men, testicular elevation and scrotum changes diminish. Ejaculatory control increases; however, if erection is partially lost, there may be difficulty in attaining a full erection again, and resolution may occur without orgasm.

Orgasmic Phase

During orgasm, vasocongestion and myotonia reach a peak and are released during involuntary contractions throughout the body. Both male and female orgasms may be described as occurring in stages.

Female Response. Female orgasm begins with intense sensual awareness of the clitoris and pelvis. In the second stage, there is a suffusion of warmth generating from the pelvic area throughout the entire body. In the third and final stage, involuntary rhythmic contractions of the orgasmic platform and the uterus occur, causing a throbbing sensation.

The female orgasmic response is highly variable from individual to individual, as well as from orgasm to orgasm in the same woman. Recent research has indicated that some women ejaculate. The Grafenberg spot, a dime-sized area on the anterior surface of the vaginal wall, secretes a prostatic-like fluid during orgasm with stimulation (Addiego, 1981).

Multiple orgasms occur when sexual tensions do not fall below the plateau phase and stimulation is continued.

Status orgasmus occurs when orgasmic levels can be maintained from 20 seconds to a minute.

Male Response. Male orgasmic response is described in two stages. In the first stage, the prostate seminal vesicles and ampullae contract rhythmically, expelling seminal fluid into the prostatic portion of the urethra and causing a feeling of ejaculatory inevitability.

In the second stage, semen flows into the distended urethral meatus by a series of rhythmic contractions. The male is aware of urethral contractions, as well as fluid volume.

In both males and females, there are generalized muscular contractions of face, thighs, buttocks, and anal sphincter. Vital signs reach their peak: respiration—40/min; heart rate—110 to 180 beats/min; blood pressure increases —30 to 100 mm Hg systolic, 20 to 50 mm Hg diastolic.

The orgasm decreases in duration in the older man and woman. In women, the number of contractions of both the orgasmic platform and the uterus decrease. In men, a single-stage expulsion of seminal fluid occurs, and ejaculatory emission and force decrease.

Resolution

Resolution is characterized by the release of muscular tension and the return of organs to the unstimulated state. There is a physiologic retreat through plateau and excitement that can take from 10 to 15 minutes. If orgasm has not been achieved, resolution may take all day; however, this causes no harm to the individual. Superimposed on the resolution phase for the male is a mandatory refractory period in which the man cannot attain another erection.

In both the aging man and woman, resolution occurs more rapidly. In the aging man, the mandatory refractory period is lengthened.

Deviations From Health and Effects on Sexuality

Deviations from sexual health occur as a result of the complex interaction between the individual and the environment. A holistic approach requires that biological, psychological, and environmental variables be evaluated to achieve an accurate assessment of a person's level of sexual health.

Kaplan estimates that 3% to 20% of sexual dysfunction or inadequate sexual response is due to purely organic etiology (Kaplan, 1974). Biological variables include anatomical or physiologic disruptions that inhibit any or all of the phases of the human sexual response cycle. The desire phase (libido) of the human sexual response is affected by pain, fatigue, and depression, as well as damage to higher brain centers, specifically the limbic cortex. Any condition that alters the necessary hormonal environment (*i.e.*, blood-level androgens) will influence sexual desire.

Myotonia and vasocongestion may be impaired by disease or trauma that affects the autonomic nervous system and the cardiovascular system. Trauma, surgery, and acute and chronic illness all affect the human sexual response, either directly or indirectly.

Medications prescribed as part of the therapeutic regimen can affect sexual desire, vasocongestion, and myotonia by interfering with hormonal, neurologic, or circulatory mechanisms.

The majority of sexual dysfunctions are due to psychological etiology. These include both intrapersonal and interpersonal factors. Intrapersonal factors include development, thought content and process, mood and affect, and body image. Interpersonal variables include communication, patterns of sexual expression, physical attraction to the sex partner, and conflicts with the sex partner (values, attitudes and beliefs, sex role, and preference). Problems arising from psychological variables can be precipitated by illness or can occur in healthy people. They affect the human sexual response by decreasing libido and inhibiting myotonia or vasocongestion, together or separately.

Environmental variables having a negative effect on sexual functioning can arise from life-style changes, life cycle changes, or life events. The hospitalized, institutionalized, or socially isolated person may have difficulty in meeting sexual needs. An older adult living with grown children in an environment shared with grandchildren may have limits placed on healthy sexual expression.

Death of a spouse or divorce may force an older adult to develop new patterns of sexual expression. Failure to adapt may cause a person to repress, avoid, or withdraw from sex altogether.

The combination of physical, psychological, and environmental variables is seen in patients in the health care setting. The therapeutic intervention is based on the identification of problems arising from the interaction of these variables.

Sexual Assessment

A sexual assessment is initiated by collecting subjective and objective data. Essential information from medical and sexual histories, physical examination, and laboratory findings all make significant contributions to the data base.

Sexual History

The sexual history is a tool that enables the nurse to discuss sexual matters openly and gives the patient permission to express sexual concerns to an informed professional. This information can be obtained in conjunction with the medical history after the obstetrical or genitourinary history is completed. By incorporating the sexual history into the general medical history, the nurse is able to move from areas of lesser sensitivity to areas of greater sensitivity after establishing initial rapport.

The interviewing style should be nonjudgmental. If the patient perceives negative verbal or nonverbal communication, sensitive information is likely to be withheld. Language used during the interview should be appropriate to the person's age and background. Ambiguity should be avoided by not using euphemisms, which are inaccurate and imprecise and will inevitably lead to confusion (*i.e.*, a couple can make love without having intercourse, can have intercourse without

sleeping together, and can sleep together without making love). Open-ended questions may be preferable as discussion starters. For example, when interviewing an adolescent, "How did you learn about masturbation?" is more appropriate than "Do you masturbate?"

Patients may experience considerable anxiety, guilt, and embarrassment during the sexual assessment. Therefore, the environment in which the interview takes place is extremely important. Comfort and privacy *without* interruption, as well as verbal and nonverbal assurances of confidentiality, are essential to establishing and maintaining rapport. Relevant assessment data for the adult include the areas listed in Chart 13-1.

The sexual history of the adult can be initiated by the general open-ended question, "Are you sexually active?" If the answer is no, the nurse should explore

- Sexual experiences in the past and why they were discontinued
- Level of satisfaction with the present status

The person may be satisfied with the present status but still may have concerns about sexual attitudes or behaviors of family and friends. An invitation to ask questions about any aspect of sexuality is appropriate at this time. The nurse may provide anticipatory guidance or information related to the patient's developmental stage. Also, information about medications and illnesses and their effects on sexual functioning should be explored.

If the patient is sexually active, and if the setting and situation are appropriate, the nurse may explore six areas:

1. Variety and frequency of sexual activity (includes choice of sex partner and degree of sex drive)
2. Current satisfaction with present sexual functioning (which includes sufficient stimulation and lubrication for women, the ability to obtain an erection and control ejaculation in men, and the ability of either party to have a satisfying orgasm without pain)
3. Partner function and satisfaction (which include all aspects of sexual and social compatibility)
4. Marital or relationship history
5. The effects of life events (*i.e.*, rape, death of spouse, aging, medication, illness, contraception) on sexual functioning
6. The need for information about sexual concerns

A more detailed history is required when the patient identifies a problem. This should include information about the following:

1. Early sexual development (*i.e.*, parental, peer, and religious influences on values, attitudes, and beliefs)
2. Adolescent sexual development and experiences (*i.e.*, puberty, masturbation, nocturnal emissions, menstruation, first intercourse, and sexual fantasies)
3. Premarital and postmarital sexual history (*i.e.*, dating, nonmarital sexual relationships, sexual techniques used, frequency of nonmarital sex, and frequency of marital sex and any changes)
4. History of the present problem (*i.e.*, onset, duration, severity, contributing factors and alleviating factors)

This information should be recorded in the patient's own words (Leiblum and Rosen, 1980).

Sexual history taking becomes a dynamic process in

Chart 13-1
Components of the Sexual Assessment

A. Identification Data

Age	Marital status		
Date of birth	Income		
Education	Employment	Past development	Ethnic background
		Urban or rural background	Family
B. Chief Complaint		Church	Current life situation

C. Past Medical History

General health	Psychiatric illness	Genitourinary history
Adult medical illness	Injuries	
Surgical procedures	Hospitalizations	
Current medications		

D. Habits:

Diet	Exercise
Use of alcohol/drugs	Sleep

which there is an exchange of information between the person and the nurse. It provides the opportunity to clarify myths and explore areas of concern that the person may not have had permission to discuss in the past.

Physical Examination

Similarly, the physical examination affords the nurse an opportunity to provide role modeling and sex education, thus creating a therapeutic milieu.

During the physical assessment, a woman can be taught breast self-examination (BSE), Kegel exercises, purpose of Papanicolaou (Pap) screening, effective contraception, and behaviors that reduce the risk of contracting sexually transmitted disease. A man can be taught testicular self-examination (TSE), sexually transmitted disease risk reduction, contraception, and breast examination.

The attitude of the practitioner doing the physical examination is of the utmost importance. Concerned practitioners may make the process of the physical examination a wholesome, positive experience, taking care to afford comfort and privacy and explaining all procedures with sensitivity.

Persons at risk for sexual problems are those who are unaware of the effects of life cycle changes on sexuality, particularly at adolescence and middle age; those who have communication or behavioral problems; those who experience traumatic life events (*i.e.,* rape, death of a spouse); those who have changes in self-image (*i.e.,* surgery); those who have anatomical or physiologic disruptions (*i.e.,* trauma); those who are taking pharmacologic agents that affect sexuality; and those who have changes in life-style (*i.e.,* hospitalized person).

Annon describes a four-level treatment model for sexual therapy that can be adapted to nursing practice (1974):

1. The first level is *permission* and basically involves validating normalcy. Receiving permission for thoughts, fantasies, sexual behavior, and so on may prevent a person from developing a significant problem and can also relieve guilt. This is primarily preventive intervention.
2. *Limited information* is the second level and provides information specific to the person's needs. It can be preventive or therapeutic. An example is provision of anticipatory guidance to the adolescent to dispel misinformation and myths regarding sexually transmittable disease. The foregoing could then be reinforced by teaching sexually transmitted disease (STD) risk-reduction behaviors.
3. The third level of intervention is giving *specific suggestions* or a description of a therapeutic technique. The specific suggestion of using a water-soluble lubricant for a postmenopausal woman with atrophic vaginitis is an appropriate nursing intervention.
4. Occasionally in clinical practice, the nurse identifies a person who may require *intensive therapy,* as in the case of someone who has behavior or communication problems resulting in a sexual dysfunction. The nurse can identify referral sources by contacting the American Association of Sex Educators, Counselors and Therapists (AASECT), Washington DC, for the names of qualified professionals in the area.

Interventions for Specific Health Problems Affecting Sexuality

Body Image Changes and Sexuality

In understanding the effects of illness on sexuality, one must understand the effects of illness on body image, common coping mechanisms, and the influence of the specific pathologic process on the human sexual response.

Body image, which is the self-perception of the body, begins in early childhood and continues to evolve throughout the life span. It is interwoven with sexual identity, sexual role, and patterns of sexual functioning.

In our society, we see idealized standards of the perfect body and face for men and women. A high value is placed on physical appearance. Conflict arises when self-image does not conform with idealized image. When there is a loss or disfigurement of body structure or function, self-perception, environmental interaction, and interpersonal relationships change.

Moving from levels of health to illness can threaten a person's sense of normalcy, causing lowered self-esteem, a negative self-image, and insecurity. The result can be disturbances of mood and affect. Depression is commonly seen in people with changes in body image and is recognized as part of the grieving process. Dependency occurring as an adjustment to the sick role can be accompanied by feelings of powerlessness and loss of control, influencing sexual adequacy. Prolonged denial or guilt can prevent a person from revising his self-image to a more positive one.

Performance anxiety occurs when a person perceives the body change as having a negative impact on sexual role, identity, or functioning. Traditional male and female stereotyped roles may be incompatible with altered body structure or function. Traditional patterns of sexual functioning may no longer be possible. Myths, misinformation, and negative attitudes and values can prohibit a person from finding new sexual expression, a change often required for those with altered body structure or function.

The severity of the reaction to altered body image is also influenced by the visibility of the affected part, the meaning or symbolism attached to it, and the person's perception of the way others view the change. Usually, the more visible the part, the more severe the emotional reactions. If the body part is strongly correlated with sexual identity, the impact on self-image may be profound. A person who perceives the sexual partner as reacting to the altered body image with disgust may fear rejection. The result may be avoidance of sex, withdrawal, and self-imposed isolation.

The relationship between sexual partners is the most important factor in sexual functioning after illness. In a marital relationship, an unexplained decrease in sexual activity owing to illness, lack of communication, or negative body image usually results in conflict, frustration, and irritability. The sexual partner may withdraw affection for fear that sexual intercourse may harm the patient. Anger and hostility can occur if this is not communicated.

Assessment of patients with body image changes includes evaluating the effects on self-concept and self-esteem; the impact on sex role, sexual identity, sexual functioning, and sexual relationships; and the person's coping mechanisms.

General goals of intervention include allowing the patient to ventilate negative feelings, clarifying misinformation and myths with the patient and spouse separately and together, encouraging recognition of sexual attributes and capabilities, and widening sexual repertoire through permission and education.

Two major conditions that cause changes in self-image are myocardial infarction and mastectomy.

Myocardial Infarction

The patient who has a myocardial infarction (MI) is at risk for sexual dysfunction because of perceived body image changes. Fear of sudden death, fear of impotence, feelings of emasculation, increased dependency on the sick role, and decreased general activity may prevent a patient from returning to pre-infarct levels of sexual functioning.

The actual incidence of sudden death during intercourse post-MI is very low, although it is slightly higher with an unfamiliar partner in a stressful environment (*e.g.*, extramarital affair). The body's energy expenditure during intercourse is equated to that required to walk up two flights of stairs. Depending on the extent of cardiac damage, most post-MI patients can resume normal sexual activity after exercise tolerance is assessed and results are evaluated—usually in 8 to 12 weeks.

Assessment factors include the usual or preferred type, time, and frequency of sexual activity; alcohol and food consumption associated with sexual activity; previous occurrences of angina; previous symptoms of fatigue; sleeplessness associated with sexual activity; and prescribed medications.

Sexual counseling as a part of cardiac rehabilitation has a significant impact on the frequency and quality of subsequent sexual functioning. After the fear of death has passed, a patient may act out sexually toward the nurse. This situation can be used as an opportunity to begin sexual education and counseling. Permission begins by acknowledging the behavior as normal.

Conjugal counseling is necessary to clarify myths and misinformation. Information about the normal sexual response cycle, extent of cardiac damage, and effects on intercourse should be included in the teaching plan.

The environment in which intercourse is initiated should be familiar, avoiding extremes of temperature. Food and alcoholic beverages should not be consumed for at least 3 hours prior to intercourse.

If angina is a concern, a nitroglycerin tablet may be taken before intercourse. The patient's lowered level of activity and assertiveness can be supplemented, for example, by foreplay.

The patient can be informed of self-assessment factors or warning signs to stop intercourse until a physician is consulted. These include angina during or after intercourse, prolonged palpitations 15 minutes after intercourse, sleeplessness or fatigue the following day, and elevated heart rate and respirations that continue 20 minutes after intercourse.

Medications frequently prescribed for the cardiac patient include antihypertensives, antidepressants, tranquilizers, hypnotics, and ganglionic blocking agents. These may cause a decrease in sex drive or libido and impair vasocongestion and myotonia. The patient should be informed of these side-effects.

The patient who experiences sexual dysfunction following an MI (erectile dysfunction, premature ejaculation, orgasmic dysfunction) should be referred for further evaluation. Sexual dysfunction may be a result of impaired vasocongestion due to cardiovascular assault, prescribed medications, anxiety, depression, fear of failure, or fatigue.

Mastectomy

To many women, breasts are a symbol of femininity and are equated with sexual attractiveness and desirability. The reality of cancer, fear of death, change in body image, and fear of rejection create multiple adjustment problems for a woman undergoing a mastectomy. Denial, depression, and anger are experienced as part of the grieving process. Guilt may also be experienced if the woman views the mastectomy as punishment for sexual activity that she believes is excessive or inappropriate, such as engaging in an extramarital affair. The spouse may also experience guilt if he believes that he may have caused damage to the breast during sexual activity. The quality of the marital relationship before the mastectomy influences the subsequent postoperative relationship.

Supportive sexual counseling and enhancement of communication between partners during hospitalization can have a positive effect on postoperative sexual functioning.

Misinformation and myths can be clarified in preoperative counseling. Permission is given when the nurse validates that the woman's concerns are normal. Reassurance that the mastectomy will not affect the capacity for sexual responsiveness is vital. Assessment factors include the marital relationship, the perceived effect of body image change on sex role and identity, the importance of the breast in sexual arousal during foreplay, the identification of support systems, the ability of the woman to express her sexual needs and concerns, and the sexual history. Using a person-centered approach, the nurse should identify whether the spouse should be included in the initial assessment. If not, counseling the spouse separately is recommended.

In the immediate postoperative period, the spouse may be present, providing additional support. He should also be actively involved in postoperative care to prevent delaying confrontation or prolonged denial. Communication, touching, holding, and caressing should be encouraged early in the postoperative period.

The woman and spouse may fear wound disruption. They should be informed that with proper positioning, intercourse usually can be resumed in 1 week. Male superior and side-by-side positions are usually more comfortable. The use of a prosthesis during sexual activity is discouraged to increase comfort and enhance self-acceptance.

Positive role modeling and additional support can be obtained by referral to "Reach to Recovery." It may also dispel the myth that the mutilation is unique.

A woman who does not have a male partner may feel sexually unattractive and experience low self-esteem similar to that experienced by the married woman. However, she may lack the additional support system available to the married woman. It is especially important that this woman move through the stages of denial and establish a positive self-image early in rehabilitation to avoid feelings of abandonment when she goes home.

Specific suggestions to enhance positive body image include looking in the mirror nude to desensitize reactions and explore feelings about altered body image. This reduces the conflict of imagined body image and real body image. Sensate focus exercises or pleasuring exercises can enhance the establishment of a positive body image. Water play with a shower massage is a nonthreatening, self-pleasuring exercise that can increase sensory discrimination. Touching is also an important part of sensate focus.

Asking the client to draw a picture of herself may assist her in venting feelings of altered body image. The nurse can then provide feedback and stress positive aspects of body and sexual functioning.

Breast self-examination should be taught to the mastectomy patient. Because there is a three times greater chance of developing cancer in the other breast, early detection can decrease the risk of mortality.

Health Problems Affecting Sexuality

Spinal Cord Injuries

Adolescents and young adults are frequently the victims of spinal cord accidents and represent a challenge to the delivery of sexual health care. The majority of these patients are male. The injury and consequential changes in self-esteem, self-image, sexual functioning, and interpersonal relationships pose a serious threat to a person's physical and psychological well-being. Sexual rehabilitation begins when the threat of death is no longer perceived by the person during hospitalization. It is essential that patients with spinal cord injuries receive information about sexual functioning before going home.

The two variables in planning sexual rehabilitation include the level of the injury and the number of fibers severed (complete or incomplete lesion). Patients with upper motor neuron lesions usually exhibit increased spasticity, hyperreflexia, and reflexogenic erections. Those with lower motor neuron lesions exhibit flaccidity and hyporeflexia. Psychogenic erections are possible but are seen less frequently.

Reflexogenic erections can be stimulated by genital manipulation or a full bladder and occur during rapid eye movement sleep in healthy males. The stimulus is transmitted from the penis to the sacral area of the cord by way of sympathetic nerves to the pelvis. Women experience reflexogenic vaginal lubrication and pelvic engorgement from the stimulation of perineal structures.

Psychogenic erections are initiated in the higher brain centers and travel by way of thoracolumbar sympathetic nerves to the genitalia. Psychogenic erections are more common in lower motor neuron lesions because impulses pass down and leave the cord above the level of the injury. The reflex arc is interrupted, and reflexogenic erections are improbable with complete lower motor neuron lesions. The effects on the human sexual response in complete upper motor neuron lesions and lower motor lesions are outlined in Table 13-2. It is essential that the patient have realistic expectations about the ability to meet his or her sexual needs.

The following assessment factors provided by Comarr and Gunderson (1975) can be used in distinguishing complete or incomplete upper motor neuron lesions from complete or incomplete lower motor neuron lesions after spinal shock subsides:

- *Complete upper motor neuron lesion (UMNL):* No sensation or voluntary control of external rectal sphincter; evidence of external rectal sphincter tone and a positive bulbocavernosus reflex
- *Incomplete upper motor neuron lesion:* Positive light touch sensation or partially diminished responses to pinprick; the loss of voluntary control of external rectal sphincter; external rectal sphincter tone and a positive bulbocavernosus reflex
- *Complete lower motor neuron lesion (LMNL):* No sensation or voluntary control or tone of the external rectal sphincter and no bulbocavernosus reflex
- *Incomplete lower motor neuron lesion:* Partial sensation; no voluntary control of external rectal sphincter; no sphincter tone or bulbocavernosus reflex

Persons who have incomplete lesions will experience less neurologic deficit and have a greater chance of successful

TABLE 13-2
Complete Lesions and Effects on Human Sexual Response

Phase of Human Sexual Response	Upper Motor Neuron (C1, T12)	Lower Motor Neuron (T12, S4)
Excitement (psychogenic)	No psychogenic erection No vaginal lubrication Other manifestation activated by fibers above the lesion; change in BP, respirations, pulse Breast changes, sex flush	Psychogenic erection Vaginal lubrication Visual, auditory, olfactory, stimuli; dreams, memory fantasy
Plateau (reflexogenic)	Reflexogenic erection caused by stroking penis, catheter change, full bladder (When lesion is T5 to T6, erection is absent, possibly owing to vascular insufficiency of cord.) Reflexogenic vaginal lubrication and pelvic engorgement with perineal stimulation.	No reflex response Reflexes are interrupted
Orgasm	Ejaculation: rare Orgasms can occur as purely cerebral events	Ejaculation and orgasm occur more frequently Ejaculatory force varies

(Adapted from Geiger RC. Neurophysiology of sexual response in spinal cord injury. In Bullard D and Knight V. Sexuality and Physical Disability. St. Louis, CV Mosby, 1981.)

coitus. Individual differences must be considered and should influence the approach to sexual rehabilitation.

A patient with a spinal cord injury may be troubled by many myths regarding his sexuality and sexual functioning after the injury. Counseling begins with validating his concerns as normal and giving information to dispel myths and misinformation. Cultural, religious, and social taboos associated with anal intercourse or oral sex should be discussed. Conjugal counseling is recommended; if the patient objects, the spouse can be counseled separately.

Several principles related to the human sexual response in spinal cord injuries should be incorporated into the teaching plan. Sexual excitement occurring from thoughts, fantasies, or tactile stimulation in areas above the level of the lesion does not result in any genital response, and, conversely, reflexogenic genital responses occur without cognitive awareness.

Even though erections are more frequent in complete upper motor lesions, they may not produce sexual satisfaction. Orgasm, however, may occur as a purely cerebral event without either genital stimulation or manifestation of physical components of the human sexual response. Imagery, autosuggestion, and erotic visual material can enhance the possibility of achieving a "phantom orgasm."

Areas available for tactile stimulation are dependent on the level of the injury. Even though people with upper motor neuron lesions manifest similar erectile ability, a larger area is sensitive to tactile stimulation in lower-level injuries. Frequently, areas such as the neck, ears, and breasts, which may previously have been insensitive, become highly sensitive with increased stimulation. Areas of tactile hypersensitivity at the level of the lesion can induce profound sexual pleasure for the person with a spinal cord injury.

Infertility in the male is a common sequel to spinal cord injuries. Fertility in the female is usually not affected. The sensory level of the uterus is at T6, and if the injury is at that level, sensation of labor will be absent.

Problems in meeting sexual needs can arise from the absence of a partner, from an inability to engage in traditional sexual patterns, from sexual inexperience before the injury, and from the perception of oneself as asexual.

Sexual assertiveness training can help alleviate some of these problems. Confidence and skillful communication are essential in establishing a new sexual relationship or altering a familiar one.

A person with spinal cord injury can be encouraged to widen his sexual repertoire with new patterns of sexual functioning. Areas of hypersensitivity may be discovered through different approaches to stimulation. Enhanced communication will assist in expressing what feels good.

An indwelling catheter can be taped in place and left in during intercourse. Spasticity in clients with UMNL can be reduced by administering antispasmodics before intercourse, even though there may be a resultant decrease in sensation.

Even with the most profound disability, patients are capable of expressing their sexuality and with education and training are able to achieve high levels of sexual satisfaction. Sexual rehabilitation depends on self-confidence, a willing sex partner, and a sensitive, knowledgeable health care team.

Diabetes Mellitus

Diabetes mellitus is a common health problem that causes erectile dysfunction in one half of all diabetic men and orgasmic dysfunction in one third of all diabetic women. In both men and women, there is usually no decrease in sexual desire. There is no clear-cut relationship between control and sexual dysfunction. However, transient impotence can occasionally be reversed with diabetic control. Additional dysfunctions that are seen less frequently are retrograde ejaculation and premature ejaculation in males, and dyspareunia in female diabetics with vaginitis, commonly caused by *Candida albicans*.

The etiology is complex; contributing factors include diabetic neuropathy, microangiopathies of chronic diabetes, decreased androgens, decreased pituitary gonadotropins, testicular atrophy, and candidal vaginitis.

Psychogenic factors include adaptation to a chronic illness, dependency, depression, and low self-esteem, leading to performance anxiety.

The onset of sexual dysfunction usually occurs early in men but can occur years after the diagnosis. The onset of sexual dysfunction in women usually occurs 4 to 6 years after the diagnosis (Green, 1979). In both men and women, organic dysfunctions develop gradually, whereas the onset of psychogenic dysfunctions is usually abrupt and can be related to a specific time, event, or person. The absence of a reflexogenic erection without significant change in libido rules out psychogenic etiology.

Fertility problems seen in diabetic men are caused by retrograde ejaculation, ejaculatory dysfunction, and decreased sperm count and volume.

Although usually not infertile, women with diabetes have a higher number of stillborns, spontaneous abortions, and infants with high birth weight. Ovarian malformations occur in some women with diabetes.

Assessment factors include sexual history, detailed physical examination, present coping mechanisms, laboratory tests to determine if there is a fertility or control problem, and the existing marital relationship.

Counseling begins with the sexual history. At this time, myths and misinformation should be dispelled and guilt alleviated if it is present, as is frequently the case. For those who are married, conjugal counseling is recommended. Information about genetic transmission and the impact of the disease on fertility and sexual functioning may be discussed. Techniques to overcome intromission difficulties and to enhance stimulation may be explored if the couple is receptive.

For women with dyspareunia, a water-soluble lubricant can be suggested. In addition, any existing candidal infection should be treated. Women with diabetes could be counseled on wearing cotton underpants, avoiding pantyhose, and inserting plain yogurt in the vagina as an aid to maintaining an acid *p*H to prevent recurrent infections.

The diabetic client who experiences sexual dysfunction due to psychogenic etiology and who identifies the need for assistance with the problem may be referred for sexual therapy.

Hypertension

Hypertension alone has no documented negative effect on the human sexual response, and no restrictions on sexual activity are necessary.

The silent noncompliance with the therapeutic regimen seen in those who are hypersensitive is frequently attributed to drug-induced sexual dysfunction. Antihypertensive agents produce vasodilation and decreased cardiac output by acting on the sympathetic nervous system either peripherally or centrally. The effects on the human sexual response include decreased libido, erectile difficulty, retrograde ejaculation, and reduced orgasmic intensity. Several antihypertensives block ovulation and suppress menstruation, causing infertility in females.

A detailed sexual history and physical examination are necessary to determine if the sexual dysfunction is due to the antihypertensive medication, other medication, other organic etiology (*e.g.*, diabetes), or psychological factors. If the onset is related specifically to an increase in dosage or changes of medication with no apparent psychogenic etiology or organic pathology, the dysfunction is likely to be due to medication (Tables 13-3 and 13-4).

A person experiencing sexual dysfunction as a result of antihypertensives should be counseled that the problem is reversible and that alternative medications are available. It is necessary to point out that adverse reactions on the human sexual response are highly individual.

Stress management techniques, such as deep relaxation, yoga, cardiovascular exercise, and compliance with the therapeutic diet, may decrease the necessity of high doses of antihypertensives and can enhance the sexual response.

Sexual Disorders

Sexual Dysfunction Due to Psychogenic Etiology

The human sexual response is controlled by the autonomic nervous system with sympathetic and parasympathetic subsystems. Under stress and anxiety, the sympathetic system overpowers the parasympathetic system, making the relaxation required for the sexual response impossible. Vaso-

TABLE 13-3
Possible Effects of Antihypertensive Drugs on Sexual Response

Antihypertensive Drug	Possible Adverse Effects On Human Sexual Response
Clonidine (Catapres)	Impotence and retrograde ejaculation in men; orgasmic dysfunction in women
Guanethidine (Ismelin)	Erectile dysfunction; ejaculatory dysfunction in men; orgasmic dysfunction in both men and women
Mecamylamine (Inversine); Trimethaphan camsylate (Arfonad)	Erectile and ejaculatory dysfunction
Methyldopa (Aldomet)	Inhibited libido; erectile and ejaculatory dysfunction
Phenoxybenzamine (Dibenzyline)	Ejaculatory dysfunction
Propranolol (Inderal)	Impotence when given in large doses
Reserpine (Serpasil)	Inhibited libido; ejaculatory dysfunction. In women: blocks ovulation; infertility; pseudopregnancy; lactation

TABLE 13-4
Commonly Prescribed Medications That Have Adverse Effects on the Human Sexual Response

Drug	Probable Mechanism of Action
Antidepressants Amitriptyline (Elavil) Desipramine (Norpramin, Pertofrane) Imipramine (Tofranil) Nortriptyline (Aventyl) Pargyline (Eutonyl) Phenelzine sulfate (Nardil) Protriptyline (Vivactil) Tranylcypromine sulfate (Parnate)	Central depression; peripheral blockade of nervous innervation of sex glands
Antihistamines Chlorpheniramine maleate (Chlor-Trimeton) Diphenhydramine (Benadryl) Promethazine (Phenergan)	Blockade of parasympathetic nervous innervation of sex glands
Antispasmodics Glycopyrrolate (Robinul) Hexocyclium methylsulfate (Tral) Methantheline bromide (Banthine) Poldine (Nacton)	Ganglionic blockage of nervous innervation of sex glands
Sedatives and Tranquilizers Benperidol Chlordiazepoxide (Librium) Chlorpromazine (Thorazine) Chlorprothixene (Taractan) Diazepam (Valium) Mesoridazine (Serentil) Methaqualone (Quaalude) Phenoxybenzamine (Dibenzyline) Prochlorperazine (Compazine) Thioridazine (Mellaril)	Central sedation; blockage of autonomic innervation of sex glands; suppression of hypothalamic and pituitary function; tranquilization and relaxation
Ethyl Alcohol	Central depression; suppression of motor activity, diuresis; release of inhibitions; relaxation
Barbiturates	Central depression; suppression of motor activity; hypnosis
Narcotics and Psychoactive Drugs Amphetamines Cocaine	Central depression; decreased libido; impaired potency
Sex-Hormone Preparations Cyproterone acetate Methandrostenolone (Dianabol) Nandrolone phenpropionate (Durabolin) Norethandrolone (Nilevar)	Antiandrogenic effects on sexual function; loss of libido; decreased potency

(Adapted from Woods JS. Drug effects on human sexual behavior. In Woods NF. Human Sexuality in Health and Illness, 3rd ed. St Louis, CV Mosby, 1984.)

congestion and myotonia may be inhibited together or separately. This type of dysfunction results in inadequate sexual responses.

Masters and Johnson (1966) estimated that 50% of all couples may require some assistance with sexual dysfunctions. The etiology is complex. Chart 13-2 summarizes some of the psychological causes of sexual dysfunction.

Sexual dysfunctions are categorized as primary or secondary. An individual who has never experienced an adequate response suffers from a *primary dysfunction. Secondary sexual dysfunction* occurs when an adequate sexual response was achieved at least once in the past. The onset of the dysfunction may be related to a specific time, event, or person.

There are a variety of individual responses within each

Chart 13-2
Psychological Causes of Sexual Dysfunction

Predisposing Factors

Restrictive upbringing
Disturbed family relationships
Inadequate sexual information
Traumatic early sexual experiences
Early insecurity in psychosexual role

Precipitants

Childbirth
Discord in the general relationship
Infidelity
Unreasonable expectations
Dysfunction in the partner
Random failure
Reaction to organic factors
Aging
Depression and anxiety
Traumatic sexual experience

Maintaining Factors

Performance anxiety
Anticipation of failure
Guilt
Loss of attraction between partners
Poor communication between partners
Discord in the general relationship
Fear of intimacy
Impaired self-image
Inadequate sexual information; sexual myths
Restricted foreplay
Psychiatric disorder

(Hawton K. Sex Therapy: A Practical Guide. New York, Oxford University Press, 1985.)

dysfunction. They can be viewed on a continuum, depending on the frequency and severity of the inadequate response.

Male Sexual Dysfunctions

Erectile dysfunction occurs when the vasocongestion aspects of the sexual response are impaired. Varying responses include the complete inability to attain an erection, a partial erection, or a firm extravaginal erection. The presence of a reflexogenic erection rules out organic etiology.

Premature ejaculation occurs when a man is unable to voluntarily control the ejaculatory reflex and, once aroused, reaches orgasm before or shortly after intromission. It is the most common dysfunction in men.

Retarded ejaculation is the involuntary inhibition of the ejaculatory reflex. The varying responses include occasional ejaculation, ejaculation through self-stimulation, or the complete inability to ejaculate under any circumstances.

Female Sexual Dysfunction

Orgasmic dysfunction occurs when involuntary control of the orgasmic reflex leads to the inability to achieve orgasm (similar to retarded ejaculation). Varying responses include the complete inability to achieve orgasm under any circumstances and achievement of orgasm through self- or partner stimulation. The latter response is termed *coital orgasmic inadequacy,* and controversy currently exists about whether it is actually a dysfunction.

Sexual therapy is recommended. Organic etiology is ruled out by laboratory tests and a complete physical examination. The prognosis with therapy varies with the severity of the problem and its underlying etiology. When there is deep-rooted conflict or guilt, psychoanalysis or long-term psychotherapy may be necessary.

Inhibited Sexual Desire

Disorders of sexual desire differ from other sexual dysfunctions in that clients have deeper and more intense anxiety, hostility, and defense patterns (Kaplan, 1979). The result is impairment of libido. Organic etiology includes depression, stress, medications, illness, and low testosterone levels.

Sexual aversion is the fear of sexual activity, leading to avoidance. The phobia may be accompanied by vaso-sympathetic responses (diaphoresis, nausea, diarrhea, and palpitations).

Disorders of sexual desire require psychotherapy; the prognosis with brief intensive sexual therapy is poor.

The nurse who identifies a person who is at risk for sexual dysfunction can use the nursing process and plan sex education and counseling to dispel misinformation, myths, and negative attitudes and beliefs.

An explanation of the human sexual response and the need for relaxation, freedom from guilt and anxiety, and the validation of normalcy are preventive nursing interventions for all clients.

When a patient who is dysfunctional is identified, the nurse employs a person-centered approach to determine whether the person is seeking help for the problem. If so, the person can be referred for sexual therapy. Follow-up on the success of therapy will evaluate the person's satisfaction with the therapist, therapy, alleviation of the dysfunction, and enhancement of the sexual relationship.

Bibliography

Books

Annon JS. Behavioral Treatment of Sexual Problems, Vol I, Brief Therapy. Honolulu, Enabling Systems, Inc., 1974.

Bancroft J. Human Sexuality and Its Problems. New York, Churchill Livingstone, 1983.

Chilman CS. Adolescent Sexuality in a Changing American Society. New York, John Wiley & Sons, 1983.

Erikson EH. Childhood and Society, 2nd ed. New York, WW Norton, 1963.

Farber M. Human Sexuality: Psychosexual Effects of Disease. New York, Macmillan, 1985.

Green R. Human Sexuality: A Health Practitioner's Text, 2nd ed. Baltimore, Williams & Wilkins, 1979.

Hawton K. Sex Therapy: A Practical Guide. New York, Oxford University Press, 1985.

Hogan R. Human Sexuality: A Nursing Perspective. New York, Appleton-Century-Crofts, 1985.

Johnson WR and Kempton W. Sex Education and Counseling of Special Groups. Springfield, Illinois, Charles C Thomas, 1981.

Kaplan HS. Disorders of Sexual Desire. New York, Simon & Schuster, 1979.

Kaplan HS. The New Sex Therapy. New York, Brunner-Mazel, 1974.

Kerfoot KM and Buckwalter KC. Sexual Counseling. In Bulecheck GM and McCloskey JC (eds). Nursing Interventions: Treatments for Nursing Diagnoses, pp 127–138. Philadelphia, WB Saunders, 1985.

Kinsey AC, Pomeroy WB, and Martin CW. Sexual Behavior in the Human Male. Philadelphia, WB Saunders, 1948.

Kolodny R, Masters W, and Johnson V. Textbook of Human Sexuality for Nurses. Boston, Little, Brown, & Co, 1979.

Lions EM. Human Sexuality in Nursing Process. New York, John Wiley & Sons, 1982.

Masters W and Johnson V. Human Sexual Response. Boston, Little, Brown, & Co, 1966.

McCary J. McCary's Human Sexuality, 3rd ed. New York, D. Van Nostrand, 1982.

Money J and Ehrhardt A. Man, Woman, Boy and Girl. Baltimore, Johns Hopkins, 1972.

Simons RC. Understanding Human Behavior in Health and Illness, 3rd ed. Baltimore, Williams & Wilkins, 1985.

Smith PB and Mumford DM. Adolescent Reproductive Health: A Handbook for the Health Professionals. New York, Gardner Press, 1985.

Tallmer M (ed). Sexuality and Life-Threatening Illness. Springfield, Illinois, Charles C Thomas, 1984.

Webb C. Sexuality, Nursing and Health. New York, John Wiley & Sons, 1985.

Weg RB (ed). Sexuality in Later Years. New York, Academic Press, 1983.

Woods N. Human Sexuality in Health and Illness, 3rd ed. St Louis, CV Mosby, 1984.

Articles

Adolescence and Sex

Brooks B. Sexually abused children and adolescent identity development. Am J Psychother 1985 July; 39(3):401–410.

Eisen M and Zellman GL. The role of health belief attitudes, sex education, and demographics in predicting adolescents' sexual knowledge. Health Educ Q 1986 Spring; 13(1):9–22.

Furstenberg FF Jr, Moore KA, and Peterson JL. Sex education and sexual experience among adolescents. Am J Public Health 1985 Nov; 75(11):1331–1332.

Howe CL. Developmental theory and adolescent sexual behavior. Nurse Pract 1986 Feb; 11(2):65, 68, 71.

Pestrak VA and Martin D. Cognitive development and aspects of adolescent sexuality. Adolescence 1985 Winter; 20(8):981–987.

Smith EA, Udry JR, and Morris NM. Pubertal development and friends: A biosocial explanation of adolescent sexual behavior. J Health Soc Behav 1985 Sept; 26(3):183–192.

Aging and Sexuality

Hobson KG. The effects of aging on sexuality. Health Soc Work 1984 Winter; 9(1):25–35.

Steinke EE and Bergen MB. Sexuality and aging. J Gerontol Nurs 1986 June; 12(6):6–10.

Walbroehl GS. Sexuality: Advising the older patient. Compr Ther 1986 May; 12(3):35–38.

Assessment

Conte HR. Multivariate assessment of sexual dysfunction. J Consult Clin Psychol 1986 Apr; 54(2):149–157.

Hammond DC. Screening for sexual dysfunction. Clin Obstet Gynecol 1984 Sept; 27(3):732–737.

Hoon PW. Physiologic assessment of sexual response in women: The unfulfilled promise. Clin Obstet Gynecol 1984 Sept; 27(3):767–780.

Stoudemire A, Techman T, and Graham SD Jr. Sexual assessment of the urologic oncology patient. Psychosomatics 1985 May; 26(5):405–408, 410.

Waterhouse J and Metcalfe MC. Development of the sexual adjustment questionnaire, Oncol Nurs Forum 1986 May/June; 13(3):53–59.

Watters WW et al. An assessment approach to couples with sexual problems. Can J Psychiatry 1985 Feb; 30(1):2–11.

White EJ. Appraising the need for altered sexuality information. Rehabil Nurs 1986 May/June; 11(3):6–9.

Cancer and Sexuality

Anderson BL et al. Sexual dysfunction and signs of gynecologic cancer. Cancer 1986 May 1; 57(9):1880–1886.

MacElveen-Hoehn P and McCorkle R. Understanding sexuality in progressive cancer. Semin Oncol Nurs 1985 Feb; 1(1):56–62.

Schwarz-Appelbaum J et al. Nursing care plans: Sexuality and treatment of breast cancer. Oncol Nurs Forum 1984 Nov/Dec; 11(6):16–24.

Walbroehl GS. Sexuality in cancer patients. Am Fam Physician 1985 Jan; 31(1):153–158.

Yarbro CH et al (eds). Sexuality and cancer. Semin Oncol Nurs 1985 Feb; 1(1):1–75.

Diabetes

Hollander P. The need to address sexual dysfunction in diabetes. Postgrad Med 1986 Apr; 79(5):15–16, 18.

House WC and Pendleton, L. Sexual dysfunction in diabetes. Postgrad Med 1986 Apr; 79(5):227–235.

Jensen SB. Sexual dysfunction in insulin-treated diabetics: A six-year follow-up study of 101 patients. Arch Sex Behav 1986 Aug; 15(4):271–283.

Dysfunction

Avery-Clark C. Sexual dysfunction and disorder patterns of working and nonworking wives. J Sex Marital Ther 1986 Summer; 12(2):93–107.

Barlow DH. Causes of sexual dysfunction: The role of anxiety and cognitive interference. J Consult Psychol 1986 Apr; 54(2):140–148.

Bernstein J, Potts N, and Mattox JH. Assessment of psychological dysfunction associated with infertility. JOGN 1985 Nov/Dec; 14 (suppl 6):63s–66s.

Hesford A. Sexual dysfunction in women. Nurs Times 1986 Apr 2–8; 82(14):49–51.

LoPiccolo J and Stock WE. Treatment of sexual dysfunction. J Consul Clin Psychol 1986 Apr; 54(2):158–167.

Newton W and Keith LG. Role of sexual behavior in the development of pelvic inflammatory disease. J Reprod Med 1985 Feb; 30(2):82–88.

Pariser SF, Levine SB, and Gardner MC. Clinical sexuality. Reprod Med 1983; 3:1–222.

Steege JF. Dyspareunia and vaginismus. Clin Obstet Gynecol 1984 Sept; 27(3):750–759.

Human Sexuality

Addiego F et al. Female ejaculation: A case study. J Sex Res 1981 Feb; 17(1):13–21.

Bem S. The measurement of psychological androgyny. J Consul Clin Psychol 1974 Apr; 42(4):155–162.

Chinn PL (ed). Sexuality and sex roles. ANS 1985 Apr; 7(3):1–86.

Comarr A and Gunderson B. Sexual function in traumatic paraplegia and quadriplegia. Am J Nurs 1975 Feb; 75:(2):250–255.

Greener D and Reagan P. Sexuality: Knowledge and attitudes of student nurse-midwives. J Nurse Midwife 1986 Jan/Feb; 31(1):30–37.

Lieblum S and Rosen R. Guidelines for taking a sexual history. Unpublished paper presented at course on human sexuality. Department of Psychiatry, CMDNJ, Rutgers Medical School, New Jersey, Jan 1980.

Rosenbaum J and Monaghan ML. A sexuality workshop: Increasing sexual self-awareness. Can J Psychiatr Nurs 1986 Apr; 27(2):8–10.

Semmens JP and Semmens EC. Sexual function and the menopause. Clin Obstet Gynecol 1984 Sept; 27(3):717–723.

Weisberg M. Physiology of female sexual function. Clin Obstet Gynecol 1984 Sept; 27(3):697–705.

Myocardial Infarction; Hypertension

Baggs J. Nursing diagnosis: Potential sexual dysfunction after myocardial infarction. Dimens Crit Care Nurs 1986 May/June; 5(3):178–181.

MacKey FG. Sexuality in coronary artery disease: A problem-oriented approach. Postgrad Med 1986 July; 80(1):58–60, 63–64, 67–69 passim.

Smith PJ and Talbert RL. Sexual dysfunction with antihypertensive and antipsychotic agents. Clin Pharm 1986 May; 5(5):378–384.

Spinal Cord Injury

Comarr AE. Sexuality and fertility among spinal cord and/or corda equina injuries. J Am Paraplegia Soc 1985 Oct; 8(4):67–75.

Persaud DH. Assessing sexual function of the adult with traumatic quadriplegia. J Neurosci Nurs 1986 Feb; 18(1):11–12.

Agencies

American Association of Sex Educators, Counselors, and Therapists, 11 Dupont Circle, NW, Suite 220, Washington, DC 20036.

Sex Information and Education Council of the US (SIECUS), 80 Fifth Avenue Suite 801, New York, New York 10011.

Concepts and
Challenges in
Patient Management

Unit IV

Chapter 14

Principles and Practices of Rehabilitation

Philosophy of Rehabilitation

It is never how high one rises that determines one's merit, but rather how far one has come, considering his difficulties.

—Archibald Rutledge

Rehabilitation is a dynamic, active program that enables an ill and disabled person to achieve his greatest possible level of physical, psychological, mental, social, and economic functioning. How close he comes to achieving this goal determines the degree to which he becomes a socially and economically independent member of society. Modern rehabilitation is a process whereby a patient adjusts to a disability by learning how to integrate all of his resources and to concentrate more on existing abilities than on the permanent disabilities he must live with. Genuine adjustment is in great part an inner process, because it involves reorientation of the patient's values.

The economic advantage of rehabilitation is readily apparent; instead of receiving welfare aid, the person is rehabilitated into employment. Instead of being dependent on society, he contributes to it. The effect on the person is to change him from a hopeless dependent to an active, self-sufficient citizen. But it is even more important that the person is helped to develop a satisfying way of life that preserves his individuality. He gains inner strength from his own resources that makes it possible for him to partake of the joys and meet the problems of life in a meaningful way.

The trend in rehabilitation is to include not only the physically, mentally, and emotionally handicapped (including those suffering from cancer) but also the aged and those who are disadvantaged because of poverty or social deprivation. Because the aging population is increasing and advances in technology are saving the lives of the seriously ill and disabled, more people will require rehabilitation services in the future.

Rehabilitation begins during the first contact with the patient. The emphasis is on restoring the patient to independence or helping him regain his pre-illness/predisability level of function in as short a period as possible.

In the health care setting, the patient and his problems are assessed, mutual goals are set, and a program is set up to enable him to achieve self-sufficiency up to the level of his capabilities and desires. His abilities are stressed rather than his disabilities. Since each patient has a different level of capability, the program is individualized. The ultimate goal is to obtain optimal function in his daily routine—that is, the activities of daily living. Rehabilitation goals must be realistic, taking into consideration the patient's ability (the most important factor) and then his disability. Through such a program, the patient is motivated and helped to attain social interdependence and vocational reintegration when possible.

The Rehabilitation Team

Rehabilitation is a creative process that requires a team of people working together and contributing specialized services for a common goal. The team members represent a variety of disciplines, with each health professional making a unique contribution. They meet in group sessions at frequent intervals to evaluate the patient's progress and collaborate in a dynamic process of modifying goals and enhancing functional performance.

The *patient* is the key member of the rehabilitation team because he is the one who determines the final outcome. He participates in goal setting and in learning and working on his rehabilitation program, so that he can eventually control his own life.

The *patient's family* is incorporated into the team, giving ongoing support and participating in problem solving and care.

The *rehabilitation nurse* is responsible for developing a patient care plan directed toward defined patient goals and for coordinating the actions of other team members toward these goals. Additional goals include the prevention of complications and the restoration and maintenance of optimal physical and psychosocial health. The nurse establishes a sustained supporting relationship with the patient and applies the nursing process in skin care, positioning, transfer techniques, bladder and bowel management, nutrition, psychosocial support, and patient and family education. In accordance with the American Nurses' Association Standards of Rehabilitation Nursing Practice, the functions of rehabilitation nursing may be listed as follows:

- Collecting data on the health status of the patient
- Developing a nursing diagnosis (identifying the problems, limitations, and methods of adaptation to health problems)
- Developing goals for nursing care (the end state toward which nursing action is directed)
- Prescribing action to meet the goals (*e.g.,* priority setting, alternative interventions)
- Implementing the nursing care plan
- Evaluating the nursing care plan in terms of stated goals
- Reassessing and reordering priorities and setting new goals; revising the plan of care*

The *physician* has the responsibility of making the medical diagnosis so that therapy can be directed toward realistic

* Adapted from the American Nurses' Association Division of Medical-Surgical Nursing Practice and the Association of Rehabilitation Nurses: Standards of Rehabilitation Nursing Practice. Kansas City, ANA, 1977.

goals. Part of this responsibility includes directing the patient's therapeutic program.

The *physiatrist* is a physician-specialist in physical medicine and rehabilitation who is responsible for testing the patient's physical functioning, determining the potential functional goal, prescribing treatment, especially for disorders of neuromuscular and musculoskeletal function, and supervising the rehabilitation program.

The *psychologist* assesses the patient's cognitive, perceptual, and behavioral impairments, as well as his motivation, values, and attitudes toward the disability. He also works with the family to help them cope with the problems that have arisen as a result of the patient's condition. The psychologist also helps to ease the stress of staff members involved in patient care.

The *physical therapist* teaches and supervises the patient through a prescribed exercise program designed to strengthen weak muscles and prevent deformities. The physical therapist also teaches new ways of locomotion, transportation, and daily activities.

The *occupational therapist* assists the disabled person in adaptating to challenges of daily living and interacting successfully with the environment. Practical projects are devised to improve the patient's coordination and strength. The occupational therapist recommends adaptive equipment and teaches energy conservation and work simplification.

The *social worker* assesses the patient's social environment (life-style, coping patterns, resources, support system) and socioeconomic status and assists the patient and his family in adjusting to the home and community. The social worker advises on financial matters and disability benefits.

The *vocational counselor* tests the patient to determine his interests and aptitudes so that vocational training can be instituted. He also helps plan job modifications and advises the patient of employment opportunities.

The *rehabilitation engineer* uses science and technology in designing and constructing devices that help severely and multiply disabled persons to function despite their disabilities. The rehabilitation engineer may also design and fabricate orthoses and prostheses.

The *sex counselor* is trained to diagnose and treat sexual dysfunctions of disabled persons. This role may be assumed by the social worker, nurse, psychologist, or other prepared health professional.

Other team members may include an orthotist, prosthetist, and speech-language pathologist.

An estimated 5% to 10% of the population in the United States need some type of rehabilitation service. Approximately 42 million persons in this country have some limitation of activity. Many older people, whose numbers are increasing, have disabling conditions requiring rehabilitation services. Every patient, regardless of his problem or diagnosis, has the right to rehabilitation services.

Rehabilitation is an integral part of nursing. *It should begin with the initial contact with the patient.* Every major illness carries with it the threat of disability. If the patient is hospitalized with a burn and develops a contracture deformity, his recovery time will be greatly delayed. Disabilities are not static but tend to become worse, and some complications of inactivity can give the patient more pain and discomfort than the initial injury or disease.

Although not all health care facilities have departments

of physical medicine and rehabilitation, *the principles of rehabilitation are basic to the care of all patients,* and the discussion that follows points out how the nurse applies them. Other aspects of rehabilitation are discussed under the appropriate clinical conditions throughout the book.

Psychological Implications of a Disability

A physical disability often has a deep psychological significance to the patient. It has a direct impact on the patient's body image and can cause a state of conflict. Physically, a part of his body has deteriorated. He may have the shattering realization that he can do less than he did formerly. His shape and posture may have changed, as may his state of mind. Even his position in society may be altered, as well as his social interaction with others. He perceives himself as a second-class citizen, a devalued person. In short, he feels that he is different.

Disability may mean hardship or even tragedy to the individual, depending on his premorbid personality, occupation, cultural background, and social status, and on the support he receives from significant others.

A person usually goes through a series of emotional reactions to a newly acquired disability. The first reaction may be confusion, disorganization, and denial. The patient is in a state of conflict and has to cope with problems of forced dependence, loss of self-esteem, and feelings that his personal and family integrity are threatened. The patient may refuse to accept his new limitations and at times has an unjustified overconfidence in speedy recovery. His false hopes lead him to hear only what he wants to hear. He is likely to be self-centered and even childlike in his demands. The mechanism of denial is useful up to a certain point, but eventually the reality of the situation must be accepted.

The patient may progress to a stage of grief and depression in which he appears to mourn for his lost function or missing body part. (Depression may also be caused by sensory deprivation and restricted environmental stimulation.) There may be behavioral changes, particularly regression. This stage of grief appears to be a necessary phase in adapting to the disability. Mourning is part of the process of working through the meaning of the losses and is part of the emotional work of rehabilitation. Therefore, the patient should not merely be encouraged blithely to "cheer up." Such an approach can evoke extreme hostility and provoke behavior that will result in a "problem patient." Listening to the patient talk about his loss is important for healing.

The patient may go through a stage of anger in which he projects blame on others. This behavior frequently alienates the family and health care personnel, who may either capitulate to his demands or withdraw from him.

Following the stages of depression, grief, and anger, there is generally a period of adaptation and adjustment. In time, the patient becomes more familiar with his condition and is able to tolerate it better. As he revises his body image and modifies his former picture of himself, he redirects his energies toward coping with his physical functioning.

He is able to accept a degree of dependency and not resent being "waited on." He begins to realize that hope-lessness is futile and knows that he must adapt to the permanent aspects of the disability and modify his goals.

The acceptance of the limitations imposed by the disability and the total investment of the patient in his rehabilitation program is basic to adjustment. It is from this point in rehabilitation that the patient begins to look ahead and develop realistic goals for his future.

At the same time, it is important to realize that not every patient will progress in orderly fashion through the stages of grieving. Many frequently fluctuate between acceptance and grief, so that angry outbursts and depression may continue long after the usual period of mourning has supposedly passed. Each new situation (going home, starting vocational rehabilitation, entering a new relationship) reminds the patient anew of his limitations, his changed body image, and the reality of the permanence of his situation. Thus, even though the disabled person makes progress and increases his independence, he must continually deal with the grief process and the need to grow throughout his life.

At the other end of the spectrum are those patients who do not accept their disability but instead waste emotional energy in rebelling futilely against unalterable damage. Or, there are those patients who ignore the disability and refuse to put forth any effort to adapt to everyday living. Still others may overreact and build a false reputation for being "cheerful and courageous." Although "ignoring" may seem healthy, often it involves a total rejection of the disability, which keeps the patient from doing the things that will be helpful to him. When a person fails to react at the appropriate time, it may indicate that he is not coping adequately. These patients may require assistance from either a psychologist or a psychiatrist.

Diagnostic Evaluation

A team of health professionals (see The Rehabilitation Team) is required to evaluate the patient's physical condition and assess his cognitive, emotional, social, and psychological functioning. The clinical examination also includes a history, physical examination, and evaluation of functional abilities. Functional ability depends on good joint motion, muscle strength, and an intact neurologic system. Disabilities most likely to produce loss of function are those involving the musculoskeletal, neurologic, and cardiovascular systems. In addition, secondary problems related to the disability, such as muscle atrophy and deconditioning, and the residual strengths unaffected by the disease or disability are assessed.

There are numerous indexes and scales to evaluate the rehabilitation needs of patients with regard to functional performance. The PULSES profile has six components evaluating independence in self-care and mobility:

P   Physical condition; health/illness status
U   Upper extremity functions; self-care activities such as eating, dressing
L   Lower extremity functions; mobility functions that depend on lower extremity functioning (transfers, ambulation, climbing stairs)
S   Sensory function; relates to vision, hearing, speech
E   Excretory function; control of bladder and bowel
S   Social and mental status; social and financial support network

Each of the above is scored on a scale from 1 (least dependency) to 4 (greatest dependency). A periodic reevaluation of functional status will direct attention to changes that can be evaluated and treated. The therapeutic plan is revised as the patient's condition improves so that the goals and direction of treatment are consistent and progressive.

Nursing Assessment and Management

The nurse's responsibility is to find out how the patient and his family perceive his change in body function or structure. No two people react in the same way to a disability. Notice the patient's grooming and affect. Can he make eye contact? Does he refer to his disability or seem to ignore it? Listen and help the patient identify his feelings toward his disability, treatment, and those involved in his rehabilitation. A patient who has difficulty expressing his emotions may be helped with a statement such as "I wonder how you are coping with _____."

The nursing assessment also focuses on the functional effects of the patient's disability or disease with particular attention paid to self-care and mobility. Assessment of functioning is best done by watching the patient perform an activity (eating, dressing) and noting the degree of independence/dependence, the time taken, and the amount of assistance required. Notice the patient's coordination and endurance, as this alerts to the potential for falls. The community health nurse is particularly concerned about how the patient manages his environment in the home setting.

In general, the rehabilitation goals of the patient and nurse are to facilitate independence ultimately in the home and community settings where possible.

The nurse continues to work with the patient, always emphasizing his assets and remaining strengths, while at the same time listening to him, encouraging him, and sharing in his triumphs as he progresses in the program. The patient is praised for efforts to improve his self-concept and self-care abilities (using positive self-talk, grooming). The nurse helps the patient to identify his strengths and past successes and develop new goals. Participation in the ongoing rehabilitation regimen, achieving satisfactory experiences, and engaging in social activities will be helpful in renewing a positive self-concept. It is through the support and inspiration of the members of the rehabilitation team that the patient becomes all that he is capable of being.

Gerontological Considerations

In restoring the older person to his fullest functional capacity, the nursing assessment focuses not only on information about pathologic processes and disability but also on how the impairment is affecting his ability to move about, communicate, live at home, and engage in social activities. Geriatric rehabilitation is directed toward maintenance of well-being and support of independent living for as long as possible. Fear of dependency is the greatest anxiety of the aged. Doing even simple activities is very important to the frail elderly. In goal setting find out what short-term goals are important. Health care personnel need to believe in the older person's ability to make progress.

The rehabilitation management and interventions are similar to those of the young: treatment of underlying disease or disability, prevention of secondary disabilities, restoration of physical and mental capabilities, and adaptation in managing persisting disability. High priority is given to performing standing exercises, maintenance of balance, and walking. Certain modifications have to be made when there is multiple pathology along with lessened physiologic reserve, impairments of mobility and balance, as well as mental status changes. Extra time will be needed to learn to manage the components of the program. The very old require a more extensive support system.

Principles and Practices of Rehabilitation Nursing

The most common complications that threaten a patient with a prolonged illness or disability are contractures, pressure sores, and bladder and bowel problems.

Contractures result when muscles are not used or joints are not put through their full range of motion. A contracture is actually a shortening of the muscle, which leads to deformity. Contractures increase the energy expenditure for movement, produce pain, and limit joint mobility. They are prevented by continuing assessment, passive and active exercise of all joints, particularly those affected by the patient's disability, and proper positioning.

When tissues do not receive adequate nourishment, circulation, and exercise, they tend to deteriorate and atrophy. Initiating deliberate and proper measures can combat and prevent tissue damage and pressure sores.

Bladder and bowel difficulties may result from disease, injury, or shock. In many patients, refunctioning can be accomplished through individualized teaching and persistent attention to the establishment of regular function.

The major goals of the nurse in rehabilitation are as follows:

1. To prevent deformities and complications
2. To motivate, teach, and support the patient (and his family) during the daily activities of living, which include self-care
3. To refer the patient for proper follow-up care and supervision.

Each of these categories will now be discussed in more detail.

Prevention of Deformities and Complications

Positioning

Deformities and complications of illness or injury can often be prevented by proper positioning in bed, frequent changes of position, and exercise. Turning and positioning the patient correctly can relieve pressure on a body area, prevent contractures, stimulate circulation, help prevent edema, and promote lung expansion and drainage of respiratory secretions.

Assuming and maintaining correct body alignment while in bed is essential regardless of the position selected. The nurse observes the patient's position during every patient contact. While carrying out other nursing activities, the nurse suggests and helps the patient to make changes that will place him in alignment. The nurse observes the appearance of the body parts in the positions that the patient commonly assumes. The most common positions that a patient assumes in bed are the dorsal, or supine; the side-lying, or lateral; and the prone positions. The essential principles of body alignment applied in maintaining these positions are as follows:

Dorsal or Supine Position
1. The head is in line with the spine, both laterally and anteroposteriorly.
2. The trunk is positioned so that flexion of the hips is minimized.
3. The arms are flexed at the elbow with the hands resting against the lateral abdomen.
4. The legs are extended with a small, firm support under the popliteal area.
5. The heels are suspended in a space between the mattress and the footboard.
6. The toes are pointed straight up.
7. Trochanter rolls are placed under the greater trochanters in the hip joint areas.

Side-Lying or Lateral Position
1. The head is in line with the spine.
2. The body is in alignment and is not twisted.
3. The uppermost hip joint is slightly forward and supported in a position of slight abduction by a pillow.
4. A pillow supports the arm, which is flexed at both the elbow and the shoulder joints.

Prone Position (on Abdomen)
1. The head is turned laterally and is in alignment with the rest of the body.
2. The arms are abducted and externally rotated at the shoulder joint; the elbows are flexed.
3. A small, flat support is placed under the pelvis, extending from the level of the umbilicus to the upper third of the thigh.
4. The lower extremities remain in a neutral position.
5. The toes are suspended over the edge of the mattress.

Therapeutic Exercises

Exercise involves the function of muscles, nerves, bones, and joints as well as the cardiovascular and respiratory systems. *Return to function is dependent on the strength of the musculature that controls the joints.* The therapeutic exercises are prescribed by the physician and performed with the assistance and guidance of a physical therapist or nurse.

Before a therapeutic exercise program is started, a functional evaluation is made by the physical therapist or physiatrist, or by both. Included are posture assessment, goniometric measurements (use of a protractor for measurement of joint motion), manual muscle testing, range of motion testing, and flexibility and endurance testing. A neurologic assessment for motor weakness and change in sensation may be indicated.

The nurse reviews the results of these procedures and provides additional data on the activities that cause and influence the patient's symptoms. The nurse observes the patient's activities throughout the day (and night) to determine how the patient moves and his willingness to move. Important also is the nurse's assessment of how the patient perceives his symptoms and his coping methods.

Patient Education. The patient should have a clear understanding of what the prescribed exercise is to accomplish. Providing written instructions setting forth the frequency, duration, and number of repetitions as well as simple line drawings of the exercise will help transfer this learning to the home setting.

Exercise, when correctly done, assists in (1) maintaining and building muscle strength, (2) maintaining joint function, (3) preventing deformity, (4) stimulating circulation, (5) building strength and endurance, and (6) promoting relaxation. Exercise is also valuable in helping restore the motivation and well-being of the patient. There are five types of exercise: passive, active assistive, active, resistive, and isometric. The description, purpose, and action of each of these exercises are summarized in Table 14-1 (p. 222).

Range of Motion Exercises

Range of motion is the movement of a joint through its full range in all appropriate planes (see Chart 14-1). Usually, range of motion testing is done by the physician or physical therapist to determine the movement that exists at the joint areas. Testing helps set positive and realistic goals. Standardized testing procedures may be used. Goniometric measurements can be made to obtain a baseline of range of motion and flexibility.

Each joint of the body has a normal range of motion. In many musculoskeletal and neurologic conditions, the joints may lose their normal range, stiffen, and produce a permanent disability. If the range of motion is limited, the functions of the joint and of the muscle that moves the joint are impaired. In order to prevent painful deformities, range of motion activities are carried out when permitted, to either maintain or increase the maximal motion of a joint and to prevent deterioration.

These exercises should begin as soon as the patient's clinical condition allows. The range of motion exercises are planned for the individual to accommodate the wide variation in the degrees of motion that persons of varying body build and age-groups can attain.

Technique. The patient must be in a comfortable position, lying supine with his arms to the side and his knees extended. Good body posture is to be maintained in each position assumed during the exercise. The bed should be high enough to permit the nurse to reach and move the part to be exercised. Unless prescribed otherwise, a joint should be moved through its range of motion about three times, at least once a day. The extremity is held at the joint, and the joint is moved smoothly, slowly, and gently through its range. If the joint is painful, as in arthritis, the extremity may be supported in the muscular area. A joint should not be moved beyond its free range of motion. Therefore, the motion should be stopped at the point of pain. When muscle spasm is pres-

Chart 14-1
Range of Motion

CERVICAL SPINE

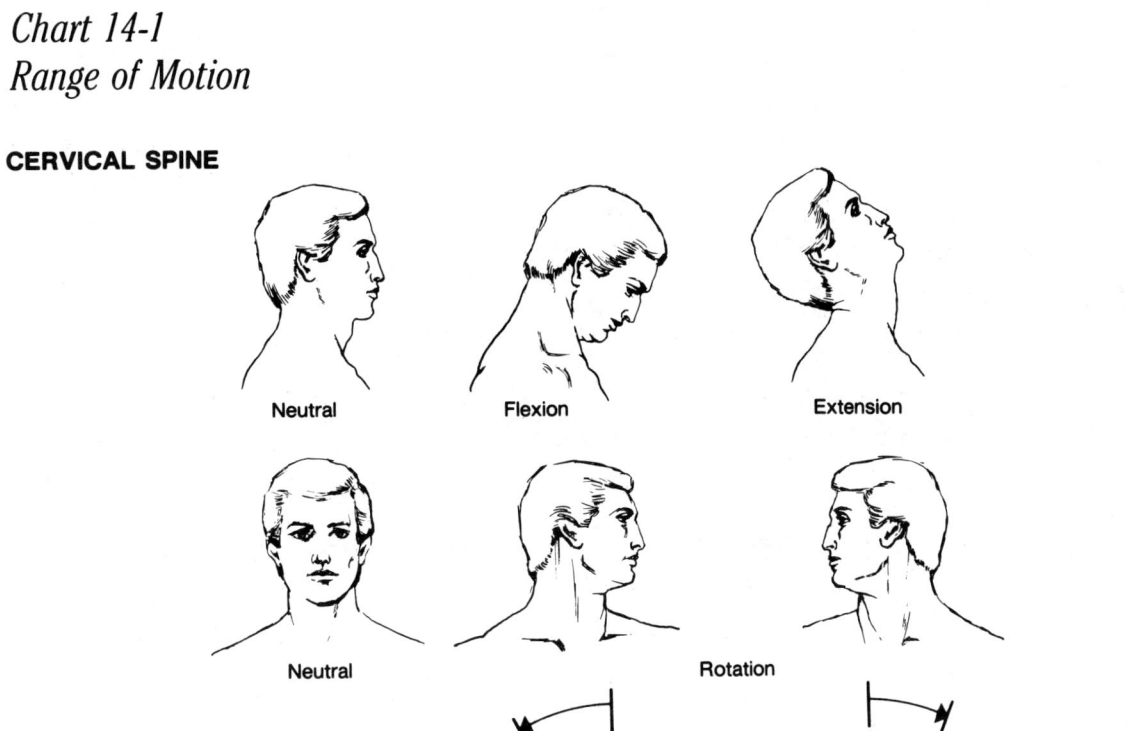

Neutral   Flexion   Extension

Neutral   Rotation

Neutral   Lateral bend

(continued)

ent, the joint should be moved slowly and to the point of resistance. Then a gentle, steady pressure is exerted until the muscle relaxes.

When range of motion exercises are performed, consideration must be given to the bones above and below the joint to be moved. For example, when the elbow is taken through its range of motion, the humerus must be stabilized while the radius and the ulna are moved through their range of motion in the elbow joint. (Refer to Charts 14-1 and 14-2 for joint motion and a pictorial review of range of motion exercises. See Chart 14-3 for definitions of terms.)

Preventing External Rotation of the Hip

Patients who are in bed for periods of time may develop external rotation deformity of the hip. The hip is a ball-and-socket joint and has a tendency to rotate outward when the patient lies on his back. A trochanter roll extending from the crest of the ilium to the midthigh will prevent this deformity (Fig. 14-1, p. 226). With correct placement, the trochanter roll serves as a mechanical wedge under the projection of the greater trochanter.

Preventing Footdrop (Plantar Flexion)

Footdrop is a deformity in which the foot is plantar flexed (the ankle bends in the direction of the sole of the foot). If the condition continues without correction, the patient will not be able to hold the foot in a normal position and will walk on his toes without touching the ground with the heel of his foot. The deformity is caused by contracture of both the gastrocnemius and the soleus muscles. It may also be produced by loss of flexibility of the Achilles tendon.

- Prolonged bed rest, lack of exercise, incorrect positioning in bed, and the weight of the bedding, forcing the toes into plantar flexion, are factors that contribute to footdrop.

To prevent this crippling deformity, a footboard or pillows are used to keep the feet at right angles to the legs when the patient is in a supine position. The feet are positioned so that both plantar surfaces are firmly against the footboard or pillows. A trochanter roll(s) is used to maintain the leg(s) in a neutral position. The patient is encouraged to flex and then to extend (curl and stretch) his feet and toes frequently. The

(Text continues on p. 222)

Chart 14-1 *(continued)*

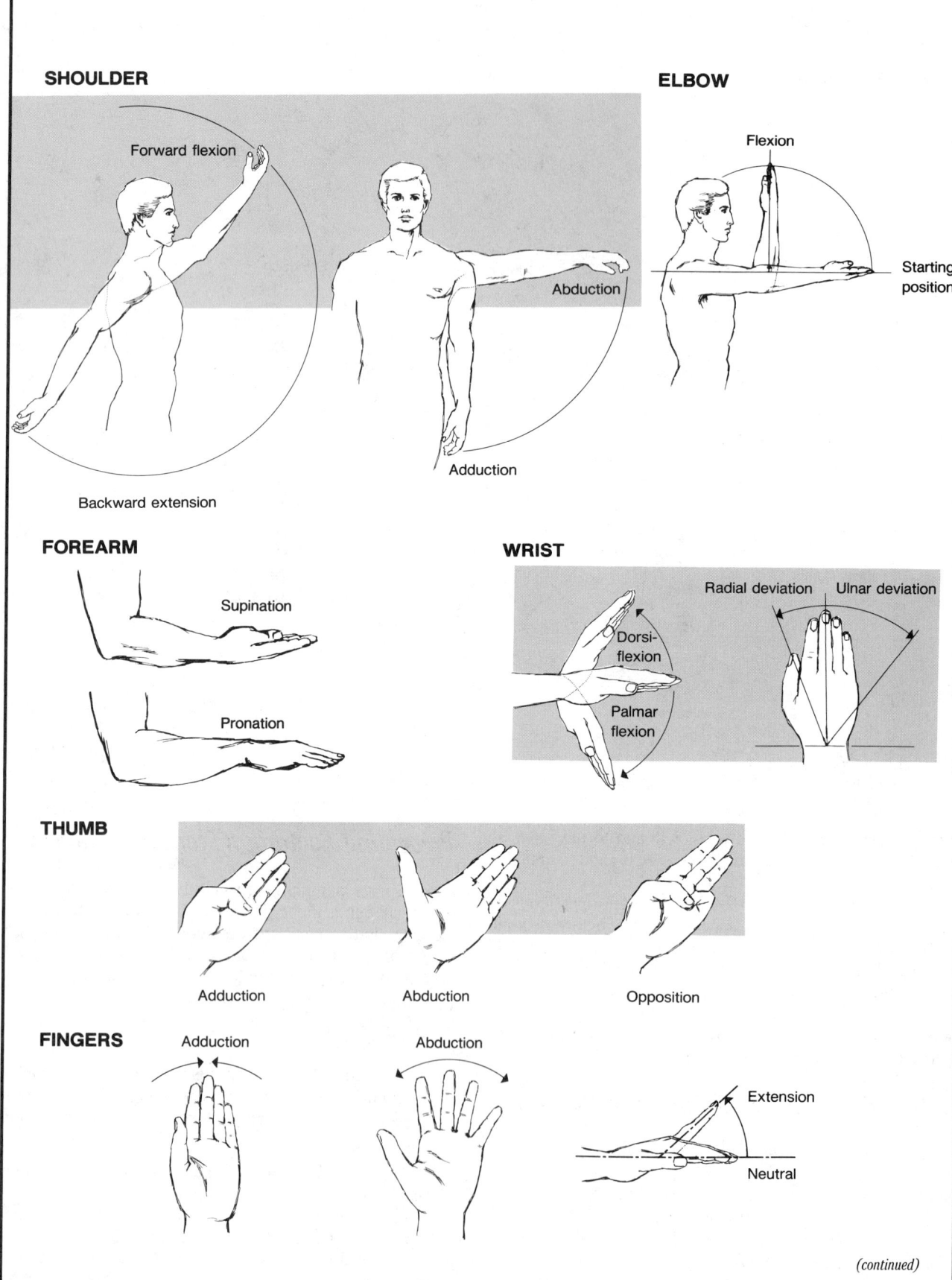

SHOULDER

Forward flexion

Abduction

Adduction

Backward extension

ELBOW

Flexion

Starting position

FOREARM

Supination

Pronation

WRIST

Radial deviation   Ulnar deviation

Dorsi-flexion

Palmar flexion

THUMB

Adduction

Abduction

Opposition

FINGERS

Adduction

Abduction

Extension

Neutral

(continued)

Chart 14-1 (continued)

HIP

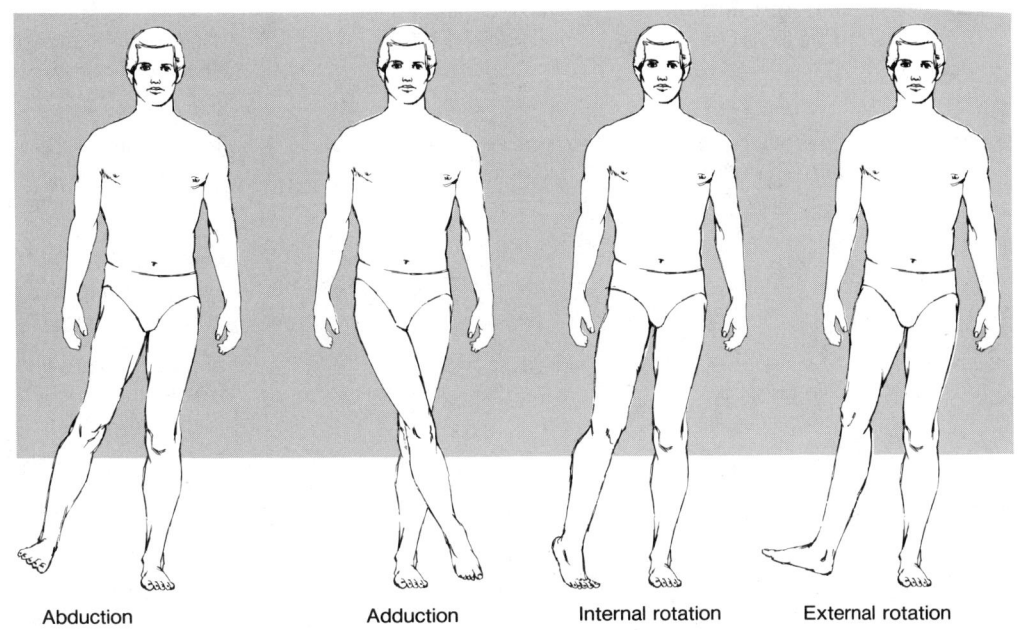

Abduction   Adduction   Internal rotation   External rotation

KNEE

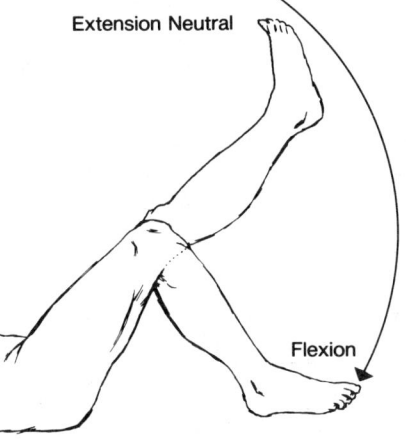

Extension Neutral

Flexion

ANKLE

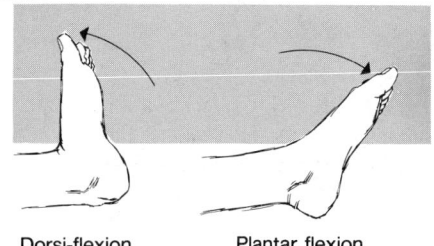

Dorsi-flexion   Plantar flexion

TOES

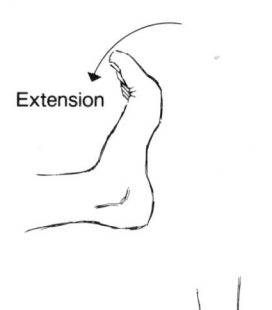

Extension   Flexion

FOOT

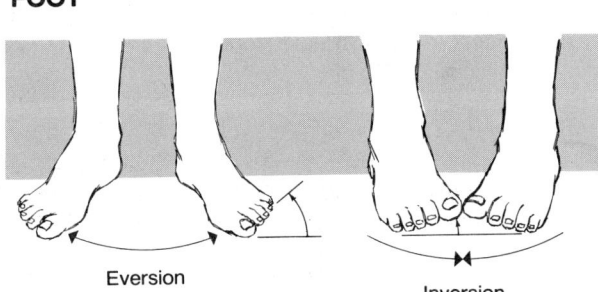

Eversion   Inversion

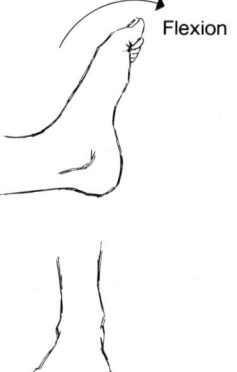

Adduction   Abduction

TABLE 14-1
Therapeutic Exercises

Exercise	Description	Purposes	Action
Passive	An exercise carried out by the therapist or the nurse without assistance from the patient	To retain as much joint range of motion as possible, to maintain circulation	Stabilize the proximal joint, and support the distal part. Move the joint smoothly, slowly, and gently through its full range of motion. Avoid producing pain.
Active assistive	An exercise carried out by the patient with the assistance of the therapist or the nurse	To encourage normal muscle function	Support the distal part, and encourage the patient to take the joint actively through its range of motion. Give no more assistance than is necessary to accomplish the action. Short periods of activity should be followed by adequate rest periods.
Active	An exercise accomplished by the patient without assistance, activities include turning from side to side and from back to abdomen and moving up and down in bed	To increase muscle strength	When possible, active exercise should be done against gravity. The joint is moved through full range of motion without assistance. (Make sure that the patient does not substitute another joint movement for the one intended.)
Resistive	An active exercise carried out by the patient working against resistance produced by either manual or mechanical means	To provide resistance in order to increase muscle power	The patient moves the joint through its range of motion while the therapist resists slightly at first and then with progressively increasing resistance. Sandbags and weights can be used and are applied at the distal point of the involved joint. The movements should be done smoothly.
Isometric or muscle setting	Alternately contracting and relaxing a muscle while keeping the part in a fixed position; this exercise is performed by the patient	To maintain strength when a joint is immobilized	Contract or tighten the muscle as much as possible without moving the joint, hold for several seconds, then "let go" and relax. Breathe deeply.

ankles should be moved clockwise and counterclockwise in a rotary motion several times each hour.

Preventing and Treating Pressure Sores

Etiology and Pathogenesis

Pressure sores (bedsores, decubitus ulcers) are localized areas of infarcted soft tissues that occur when pressure greater than normal capillary pressure (32 mm Hg) is applied to the skin for a prolonged period of time. Pressure is exerted on the skin and subcutaneous tissues by the objects on which they rest, such as a mattress, chair seat, or cast. There is compression of the small nutrient vessels of the skin and underlying tissues, which results in tissue anoxia or ischemia. The cutaneous tissues become broken or destroyed, leading to progressive destruction of underlying soft tissue. Once the skin breaks, an ulcer may form, which may be painful and very slow to heal. Invasion by a profusion of microorganisms (streptococci, staphylococci, *Pseudomonas aeruginosa*,

Escherichia coli, Proteus species) and secondary infections are difficult to avoid. There emanates from the lesion an obnoxious-smelling discharge, which is the product of bacterial invasion and tissue breakdown. The lesion, if large enough, permits a continuous loss of serum, which may deplete the circulating blood and the entire body of essential protein constituents. Also, when the ulcer is infected, it may extend deep into the fascia, muscle, and bone, and multiple large sinus tracts may radiate from it. Thus, systemic infection can easily develop, especially from bloodstream invasion by gram-negative bacilli.

Pressure sores also develop from shearing forces, friction, and moisture. Shearing force is created by the interplay of two other forces: gravitational forces that pull the patient's body toward the foot of the bed and resting forces created by friction taking place on the skin surface. Shearing forces permit pulling on tissues, stretching and injuring tissues and blood vessels. Friction also occurs when the patient is handled improperly. Spasticity increases vulnerability to shearing and friction. Moisture from perspiration, urine, and feces can produce maceration of the skin, which is another risk factor.

(Text continues on p. 226)

Chart 14-2
Range of Motion Exercises

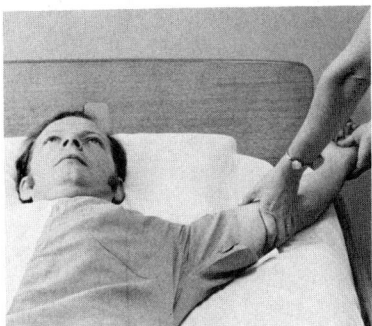

Abduction of shoulder. Move arm from side of body to above the head. Then return arm to side of body or neutral position (adduction).

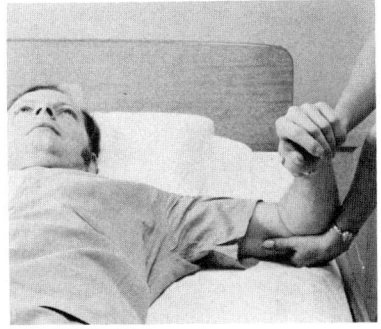

Internal rotation of shoulder. With arm at shoulder height, elbow bent at a 90-degree angle, and palm toward feet, turn upper arm until palm and forearm face backward.

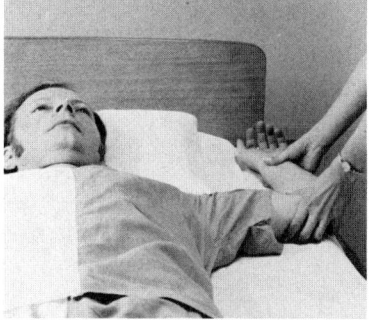

External rotation of shoulder. With arm at shoulder height, elbow bent at a 90-degree angle, and palm toward feet, turn upper arm until the palm and forearm face forward.

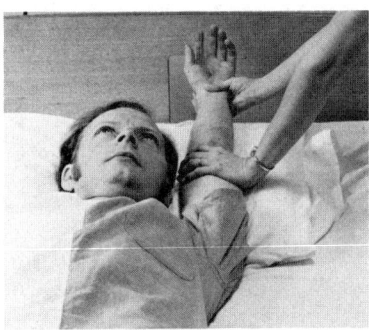

Forward flexion of shoulder. Move arm forward and upward until it is alongside of head.

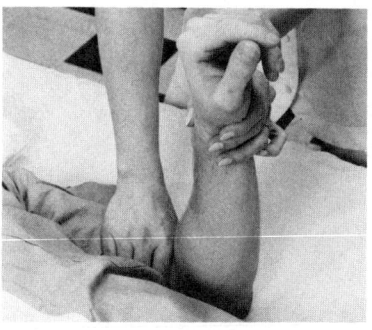

Pronation of forearm. With elbow at waist and bent at 90-degree angle, turn hand so that palm is facing down.

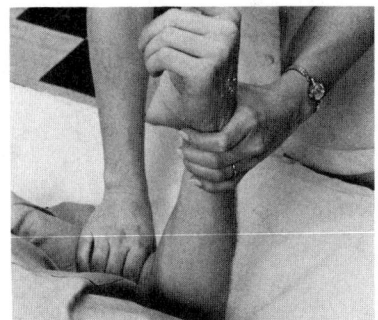

Supination of forearm. With elbow at waist and arm bent at 90-degree angle, turn hand so that palm is facing up.

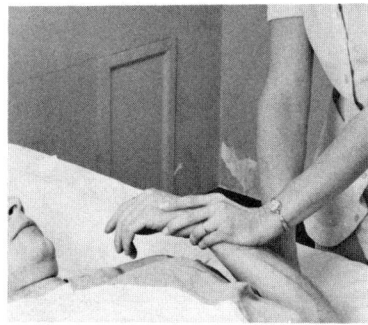

Flexion of elbow. Bend elbow, bringing forearm and hand toward shoulder. Then return forearm and hand to neutral position (arm straight).

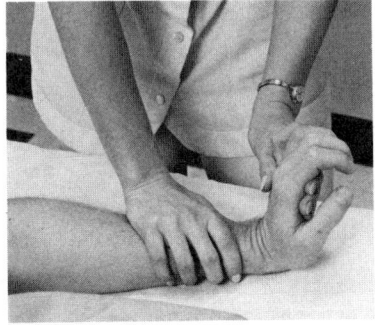

Wrist extension.

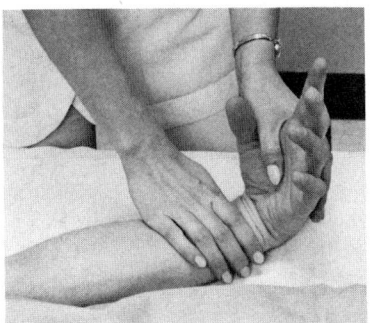

Flexion of wrist. Bend wrist so that palm is toward forearm. Straighten to a neutral position.

(continued)

Chart 14-2 *(continued)*

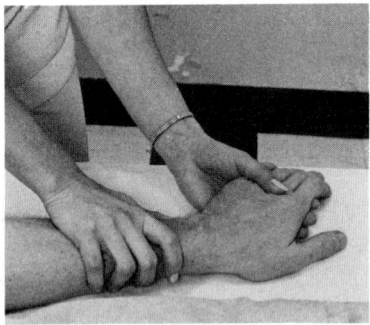

Ulnar deviation. Move hand sideways so that the side of hand on which little finger is located moves toward forearm.

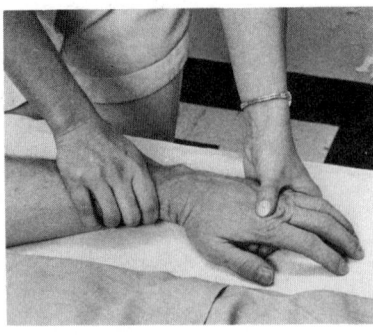

Radial deviation. Move hand sideways so that side of hand on which thumb is located moves toward forearm.

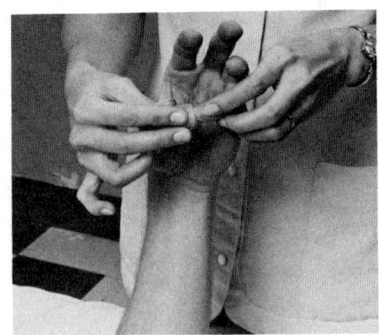

Thumb opposition. Move thumb out and around to touch little finger.

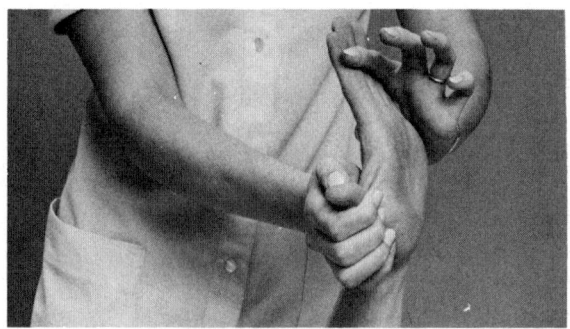

Extension of fingers.

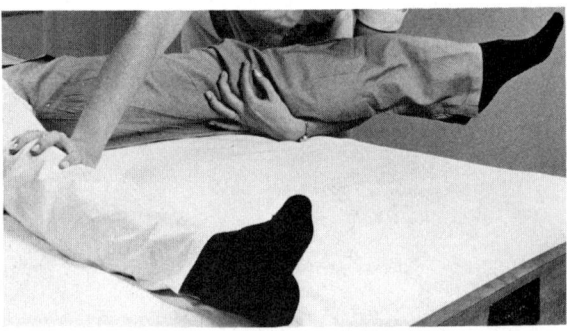

Abduction-adduction of hip. Move leg outward from the body as far as possible. Return leg from abducted position to neutral position and across the other leg as far as possible.

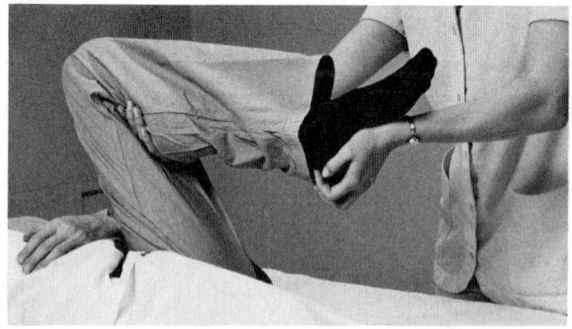

Flexion of hip and flexion of knee. Bend hip by moving the leg forward as far as possible. Return leg from the flexed position to the neutral position.

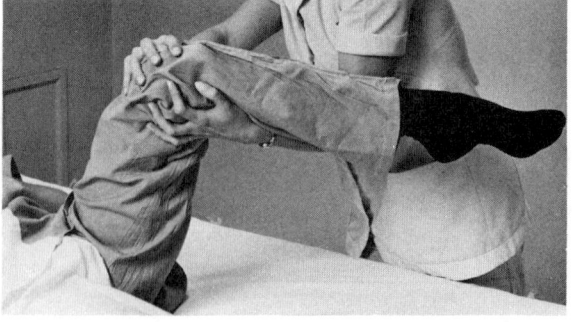

Internal-external rotation of hip. Turn leg in an inward motion so that toes point in. Turn leg in an outward motion so that toes point out.

(continued)

Chart 14-2 (continued)

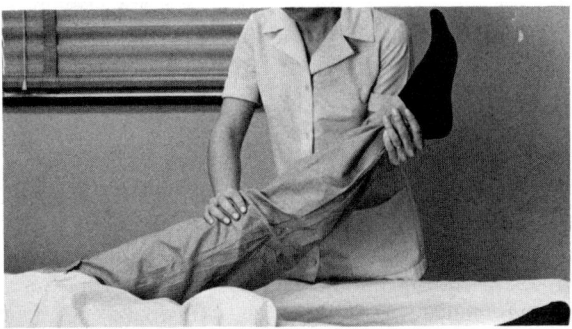

To stretch hamstring muscles, straighten leg and then raise the leg.

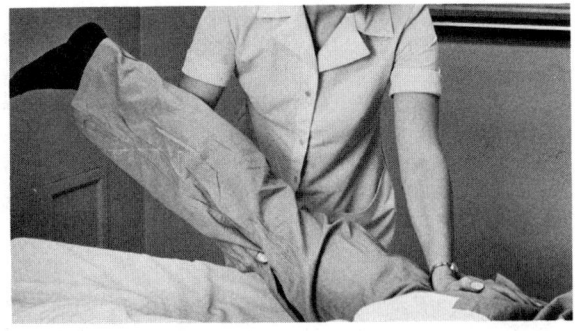

Hyperextension of hip. Place the patient in a prone position, and move leg backward from the body as far as possible.

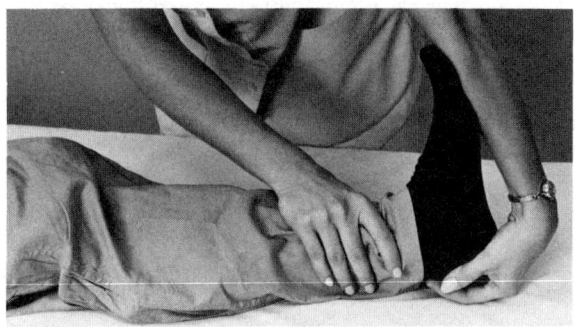

Dorsiflexion of foot. Move foot up and toward the leg. Then move foot down and away from the leg (plantar flexion).

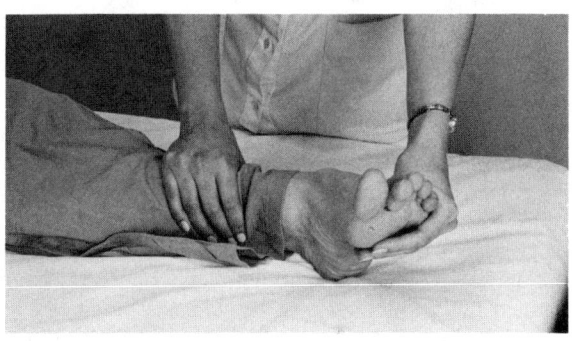

Inversion and eversion of foot. Move foot so that sole is facing outward (eversion). Then move foot so that sole is facing inward (inversion).

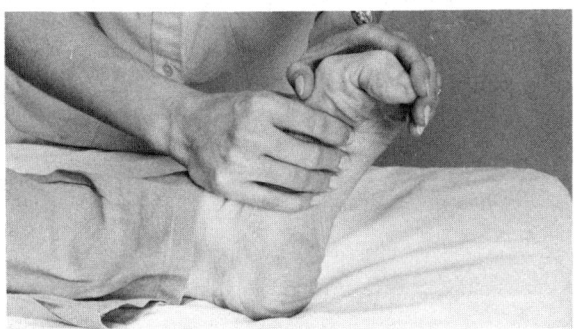

Flexion of toes. Bend the toes toward the ball of foot.

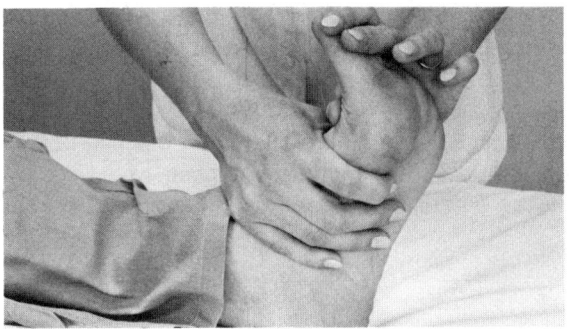

Extension of toes. Straighten toes and pull them toward the leg as far as possible.

Chart 14-3
Definitions

Abduction—movement away from the midline of the body

Adduction—movement toward the midline of the body

Flexion—bending of a joint so that the angle of the joint diminishes

Extension—the return movement from flexion; the joint angle is increased

Inversion—movement that turns the sole of the foot inward

Eversion—movement that turns the sole of the foot outward

Dorsiflexion—movement that flexes or bends the foot toward the leg

Plantar flexion—movement that flexes or bends the foot in the direction of the sole

Pronation—rotation of the forearm so that the palm of the hand is down

Supination—rotation of the forearm so that the palm of the hand is up

Rotation—turning or movement of a part around its axis

    Internal: turning inward, toward the center

    External: turning outward, away from the center

In patients with neurologic dysfunction who have motor paralysis and associated muscular atrophy, reduction of padding between the overlying skin and the underlying bone occurs and leads to pressure sores. Paralyzed patients tend to lie in one position, with the body weight concentrated on small areas of skin. This high pressure collapses blood vessels and impedes blood flow, causing a pressure sore to form in a very short time. If the patient has suffered sensory loss, he will not be aware of pain and pressure and will not be aware that the skin is breaking down.

Other factors contribute to the development of pressure sores. Anemia, whether caused by hemorrhage, nutritional deficiency, or infection, decreases the blood's oxygen-carrying ability and predisposes to ulcer formation. Patients with nutritional deficiencies have negative nitrogen, phosphorus, sulfur, and calcium balances, which will produce wasting of tissue and loss of weight. All patients should be screened on admission for susceptibility to pressure sores.

Other metabolic disorders can also contribute to low protein levels. Persons with malabsorption syndrome may develop protein deficiency and severe anemia because of

failure to absorb folic acid. Persons with diabetes may have poor quality of tissue, which is easily injured. Many people have hidden vitamin C deficiencies. (Vitamin C is needed for fibroblast functioning and collagen formation.) In all of these conditions there is evidence of protein depletion, in the form of a low serum albumin level, which diminishes tissue vitality.

Another cause of pressure sores is edema, which impairs circulation and interferes with the supply of nutrients to the cells.

Pressure Sites

If one bears in mind that the weight-bearing prominences are covered only by skin and small amounts of subcutaneous fat, it is easily seen that the majority of pressure sores are located at such sites: the sacrum and coccygeal areas, greater trochanter, and ischial tuberosities, especially in persons who sit for prolonged periods (Fig. 14-2). Other bony promontories that are susceptible to pressure sore development are the knees, medial condyle of the tibia, fibular head, malleoli, heels, and elbows.

Gerontological Considerations

The aging skin has diminished epidermal thickness, dermal collagen, and tissue elasticity, making the skin of the elderly more susceptible to damage. An estimated 35% of the institutionalized elderly may be afflicted with pressure sores at any given time. The major factors producing pressure sores are summarized in Chart 14-4.

▶ ## Nursing Process
The Patient at Risk for Pressure Sores

▷ ### Assessment

In assessing the patient at potential risk for skin breakdown, determine the patient's status in the following areas: physical condition, mental condition, mobility/activity level, bladder and bowel control, and circulatory status.

- Inspect each pressure site for erythema.
- Press on the area. Look for blanching.
- Note how long reactive hyperemia persists following removal of pressure.
- Palpate for warmth. Is skin temperature increased?
- Inspect for dry skin, moist skin, or a break in the skin.
- Palpate peripheral pulses to evaluate circulatory status.
- Evaluate the nutritional status.

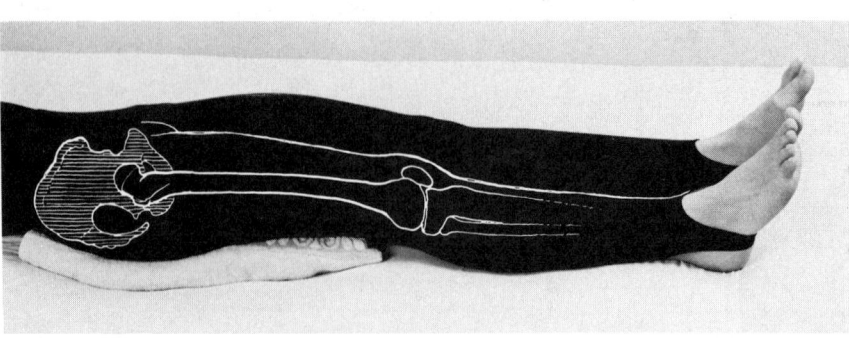

Figure 14-1
Placement of trochanter roll. The hip is a ball-and-socket joint and has a tendency to rotate outward when the patient lies on his back. The proper placement of a trochanter roll helps prevent external rotation of the hip.

Chart 14-4
Risk Factors for Development of Pressure Sores

Prolonged pressure
Shearing forces, friction, trauma
Immobility, compromised mobility
Loss of protective reflexes, motor or sensory deficit/loss
Malnutrition, hypoproteinemia, vitamin deficiencies, anemia
Incontinence
Skin dryness, excessive skin moisture, maceration
Edema, poor skin perfusion
Infection
Advancing age, debilitation
Equipment: traction, casts, restraints, improper bedding and
    seats

- Check the patient's record for hematocrit, hemoglobin, and blood chemistry values (serum albumin) for assessment of protein intake.
- What other health problems are present?
- What medications are being taken?
- Does the patient smoke?
- Are there any restrictive devices? Casts?
- In the aging patient, look for loss of appetite, dehydration, onset of confusion, slumping in the chair, onset of incontinence, and other signs of illness.

▷ Nursing Diagnosis

Based on the nursing assessment data, the patient's major nursing diagnosis is potential alteration in skin integrity related to pressure.

▷ Planning and Implementation

▷ *Goals:* The major goals of the patient may include (1) relief or removal of pressure, (2) avoidance of shearing and

friction, (3) maintenance of clean and healthy skin, and (4) promotion of nutrition.

Nursing Interventions

Relief or Removal of Pressure. The patient needs frequent changes of position and the avoidance of positions that result in excessive pressure. Such measures will prevent prolonged blocking of blood flow, which interferes with skin nutrition. Shifting the weight of the patient lets the blood flow back to the ischemic areas and helps tissue to recover from pressure.

- Thus, the patient should be turned at 1-hour or 2-hour intervals.

He should be positioned on all four sides (laterally, prone, dorsally) in sequence unless contraindicated. In addition to regular turning, there should be small shifts of body weight, such as repositioning an ankle, elbow, or shoulder. The skin is inspected at each position change and checked for temperature elevation. If redness or heat is noted, keep pressure off the area.

In the aging patient small shifts of body weight are effective. Placing a small rolled towel or sheepskin under a shoulder or hip will allow a return of blood to the skin on which the patient is sitting or lying. Move the towel or sheepskin around the patient's pressure points in a clockwise fashion. Of course all other preventive measures should be used.

Another way to relieve pressure over bony prominences is the bridging technique accomplished through the correct positioning of pillows. Just as a bridge is supported on pillars to allow traffic to move underneath, so can the body be supported by pillows to allow for space between bony prominences and the mattress. For the feet and extremities, a footboard or pillows will support the bedding and thus reduce pressure. To protect the heels, 2.5 cm (1 inch) of foam rubber may be placed between a well laundered soft sheet and the mattress.

A variety of pressure relief systems are available, including mattresses and beds. These are designed to provide support for specific body areas or for distributing pressure evenly and uniformly.

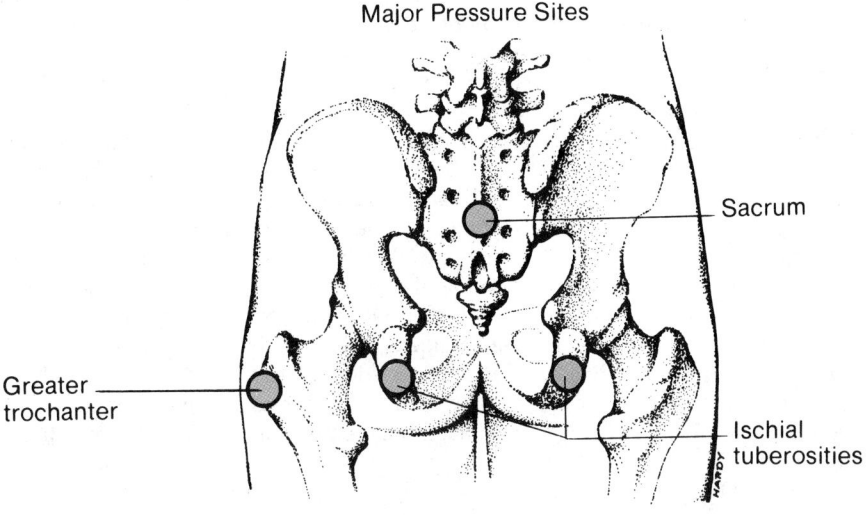

Major Pressure Sites

Figure 14-2
Areas of major pressure sites where pressure sores can develop.

An alternating pressure pad mattress may be used in conditions in which the patient cannot turn. The alternating inflation and deflation of the pad produces constriction followed by dilatation of the superficial blood vessels of the skin. By such action, pressure on any one part is reduced and the blood supply is increased.

A polyurethane foam mattress (egg-crate mattress) distributes pressure evenly by bringing more of the patient's body surface in contact with the supporting surface.

The use of the flotation mattress, or water bed, has been advocated for the prevention (and treatment) of pressure sores. As the patient's body sinks into the fluid, additional surface becomes available for weight bearing, thereby further decreasing body weight per unit area. (Pascal's law states that the weight of the body floating on a fluid system is evenly distributed over the entire supporting surface.) Thus, the body weight is lightened and there is less pressure on the body parts. However, shearing forces can be built up on the water bed as the patient's body is suspended on the plastic covering over the surface of the water.

Other beds in current use are the air-fluidized bed (Cliniton), low-air-loss bed (Mediscus), and the kinetic bed (Roto-Rest).

For patients susceptible to pressure on bony prominences, a variety of pads and supportive devices are available that can be placed on top of the mattress. The gel-type flotation pad reduces pressure because the material is similar in consistency to human adipose tissue and "gives" with the patient's weight. Soft, moisture-absorbing padding is also useful because the softness and resilience of padding provides even distribution of pressure and the dissipation and absorption of moisture, along with freedom from wrinkles and friction. Bony prominences may be protected by inserting pieces of gel pads, sheepskin padding, or soft foam rubber beneath the sacrum, the trochanters, heels, elbows, scapulae, and the back of the head when there is pressure on these sites.

Patients sitting in wheelchairs for prolonged periods should have wheelchair cushions fitted and adjusted on an individualized basis, using pressure measurement techniques as a guide to selection and fitting. The aim is to redistribute pressure away from areas at risk for developing sores. However, no cushion is able to eliminate excessive pressure. The patient should be reminded to shift his weight frequently and raise himself up for a few seconds every half hour while sitting in a chair (Fig. 14-3).

Avoidance of Shearing Forces and Friction. A shearing force is applied when the patient is pulled up in bed, is allowed to slump in bed or a chair, or moves up in bed by digging his heels or elbows into the mattress. To prevent this the patient is lifted, not dragged, up in bed or on a chair. Raising the head of the bed by even a few centimeters increases the shearing force over the sacral area. Thus the semi-reclining posture for the patient at risk is avoided. Protect the patient from sliding down by using a well-padded footboard and placing extra protection on the heels. Large sheepskin pads are thought to have sheer-resistant properties, help distribute pressure over a greater surface area, absorb moisture, allow for air circulation, and reduce friction. The patient should not be placed on a poorly ventilated mattress that is covered with plastic or some other impermeable material.

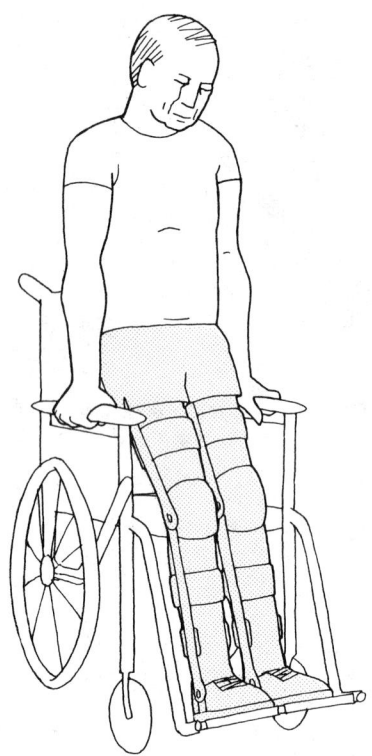

Figure 14-3
Wheelchair push-up to prevent ischial pressure sores. These push-ups should become an automatic routine (every 30 minutes) for the person with paraplegia. He should stay up, out of contact with the seat, for 60 seconds. The wheel is kept in the locked position during the exercise. (Adapted from Hirschberg GG, Lewis L, and Vaughan P. Rehabilitation: A Manual for the Care of the Disabled and Elderly, 2nd ed. Philadelphia, JB Lippincott, 1976.)

Maintenance of Clean and Healthy Skin. Maceration of the skin by continuous moisture must be prevented by meticulous hygienic measures. The skin should be washed with a mild soap and water and blotted dry with a soft towel. The skin is then lubricated with a bland lotion or a thin layer of silicone cream to keep it soft and pliable. It is desirable that the patient participate in caring for his skin. He should be encouraged to inspect it at frequent intervals for evidence of pressure. He should be taught to use a mirror and inspect posterior areas if he is paraplegic or has other neuromuscular disorders. He should massage and stroke lightly around bony prominences because this promotes venous return, reduces edema, and increases vascular tone. Foreign bodies are kept out of the bed because they serve to irritate the skin. Foundation sheets are tightly stretched to prevent wrinkles.

Since the stimulation of circulation relieves tissue ischemia, the forerunner of pressure sores, the patient is encouraged to keep active. Active and passive exercises increase muscular, skin, and vascular tone. The patient is ambulated whenever possible because the level of mobility is an important criterion for prognosis and treatment. (Activity also stimulates the metabolic processes and helps to improve morale.) Gentle skin massage with lotion is useful as another means of stimulating the blood flow in the skin, but only if tissue damage is not present. Circulation is also aided by turning the patient. Turn or, if this is not possible, tilt the patient toward one side and then the other. The use of a rocking bed and a tilt table also aids in stimulating circulation.

Promotion of Nutrition. The patient's nutritional status must be adequate and a positive nitrogen balance must be maintained. Pressure sores develop more quickly and are more resistant to treatment in patients suffering from nutritional disorders. A high protein diet with protein supplements may be helpful. Iron preparations and whole blood transfusions may be necessary to raise the hemoglobin level above 12 gm/dl (SI: 1.86 mmol/L) so that tissue oxygen levels will be maintained within acceptable limits. (The hemoglobin level is a critical criterion for the development of pressure sores). Ascorbic acid (vitamin C) is necessary for tissue vitality and healing.

▷ *Evaluation*

▷ *Expected Outcomes*

Patient prevents pressure sores from occurring.

1. Avoids pressure
   a. Changes position every 1 to 2 hours
   b. Changes from supine to side-lying to prone positions
   c. Sleeps in prone position as much as possible
   d. Uses trapeze to raise self off bed at 30-minute intervals while awake
   e. Raises self from seat/wheelchair every 30 minutes
   f. Uses warning system (sensor or timing device) as a reminder to relieve pressure
2. Avoids shearing forces and friction
   a. Avoids semi-reclining posture
   b. Uses sheepskin pad/heel protectors when appropriate
3. Maintains clean and healthy skin
   a. Monitors self for signs and symptoms of skin reddening and changes in skin temperature
   b. Uses hand mirror to inspect hard-to-see areas
   c. Keeps skin in good condition
4. Attains/maintains adequate nutritional intake
   a. Verbalizes the importance of protein and vitamin C in diet
   b. Selects foods high in protein and vitamin C
   c. Hemoglobin level is maintained at an acceptable level.

Management of a Patient With Pressure Sores

Clinical Manifestations. The first sign of a potential pressure sore is the appearance of erythema (redness) of the skin, which will blanch on pressure. Skin temperature is increased because of vasodilation. The redness progresses to a dusky, cyanotic blue-gray appearance, which is the result of skin capillary occlusion and subcutaneous weakening. Blistering and a break in the skin occur, and the early stages of necrosis follow. With necrosis there is venous sludging

and thrombosis and edema with cellular extravasation and infiltration. Pathologic changes occur in muscle fibers.

A skin lesion may represent only the "tip of the iceberg," since a small surface sore may overlie a large undermining defect below. This process may involve deeper soft tissues, bursae, muscles, tendons, and even bone or joints. If the ulcer is of long standing and has repeatedly broken down and healed, secondary induration (hardening of tissue) develops and the blood supply to the area is compromised by underlying scar tissue. Deep pockets of infection are often present. These may be covered by a dark crust, which also impedes healing.

The complications of pressure sores, which may be life threatening, are sepsis, osteomyelitis, pyarthrosis (pus formation within a joint cavity), and joint disarticulation (separation at the joint).

The goals of management are elimination of local pressure, restoration of circulation and cellular function, and promotion of wound healing.

Elimination of Pressure. First, local pressure must be eliminated. The ulcer will not heal until all pressure is removed. The patient must not lie or sit on the ulcer, even for a few minutes. If the lesion is on the posterior surface, the patient will need to spend more time in the prone and/or side-lying positions. A turning schedule is written in the nursing care plan, and the position options are individualized.

Restoration of Circulation and Cellular Function. In addition to relief of pressure, which permits immediate recirculation and tissue oxygenation, fluid and electrolyte abnormalities are corrected. These wounds leak body fluids and protein, placing the patient in a catabolic state and predisposing him to the serious problems of secondary infection, hypoproteinemia, and vitamin deficiencies. Protein deficiency must be corrected in order to heal the pressure sore. Carbohydrates are necessary to "spare" protein and provide an energy source as well as resistance to infection. Wound healing is also dependent on collagen. In turn, ascorbic acid (vitamin C) is necessary for collagen formation. Trace elements, especially zinc, are necessary for wound healing.

Wound Cleansing and Removal of Necrotic Tissue. Wound cleansing and dressing changes produce patient anxiety in anticipation of pain. Important nursing interventions are explanations of the procedure and administration of appropriate analgesia when appropriate.

The ulcer must be cleansed to clear up sepsis and stimulate the regeneration of epithelium. It is debrided of necrotic material because devitalized tissue favors bacterial growth, delays granulation, and inhibits healing. If an eschar covers the ulcer, it is removed to ensure a clean wound base because an eschar does not permit free drainage.

Debridement may be done by sharp debridement (scalpel, scissors, forceps), by enzyme action, or by mechanical means (flushing and mechanical removal of dead tissue). Proteolytic enzymes (preparations containing collagenase, fibrinolysin, desoxyribonuclease, streptokinase) may be applied to help dissolve the necrotic tissue that is inaccessible to excision. This has a cleansing effect on the ulcer. Cultures are obtained of the material deep in the ulcer to determine the resident flora. Usually in the hospitalized patient there is a mixture of gram-positive and gram-negative bacteria.

Numerous agents may be used to cleanse and flush the

Erythema - redness

wound. After the ulcer is clean, some form of topical therapy may be prescribed. The large variety of agents available is evidence that the best therapeutic modality for pressure sores has not been found.

Local infection may be treated with a local disinfectant. Local disinfection is stopped when newly formed granulation around the ulcer appears. New granulation tissue must be protected from reinfection, drying, and damage to tissue during subsequent dressing changes. A moist dressing may be prescribed to maintain hydration. Other dressings in current use are wet-to-dry dressings or absorbent dressings, depending on the nature of the wound. Dampening the dressing just before removal will ease the pain. A semi-occlusive or permeable dressing over a clean wound keeps the wound environment moist, allowing migration of epidermal cells over the moist skin surface.

Surgical intervention is necessary when the ulcer is extensive, when potential complications (such as fistulas) exist, and if the patient is not responding to treatment. Surgical procedures include incision and drainage, skin grafting, bone resection, skin flaps, and myocutaneous flaps.

Patient Education and Home Health Care. Recurrence of pressure sores should be anticipated, and continuing assessment must be made for them in the home setting. The patient's tolerance for sitting/lying on the area is built up *slowly;* the time that pressure is allowed is increased in 5- to 15-minute increments. Instruct the patient to increase his mobility and to follow the regimen of turning, weight shifting, and repositioning. Give the patient written instructions on skin care, diet, and the signs and symptoms of recurrence. A physical therapy referral may be made to help supervise mobility and exercise.

Supporting the Patient in Daily Self-Care: Activities of Daily Living

Activities of daily living (ADL) are those self-care activities that must be accomplished each day in order for the patient to care for his own needs and the demands of daily life. ADL include personal hygiene, dressing, eating, toileting, getting in and out of bed (transfers), using a wheelchair, ambulating (when possible), and performing manual tasks. Indeed, the ability to perform ADL is the key to reentry to home and the community.

Assessment

Before initiating an ADL program, the nurse performs an assessment to learn about the patient's medical condition, his functional capacity (whether he can sit or stand; his posture, ease of movement), and his therapeutic goals, as well as the details of his care. It is also wise to learn about the patient's family background in order to know how much support the family can give.

An important component of the assessment is determining exactly what the patient can do by watching him perform an activity. The ADL sheet is an information sheet for those who are taking care of the patient. The data on it serve to inform each member of the rehabilitation team what activities the patient can perform. It also serves as an index of progress, which in itself is a source of motivation and a morale builder. For example, after it has been determined that the patient can bathe himself, this information is noted on the ADL sheet. The nurse who is responsible for the patient reviews this sheet at morning care time and notes what the patient is capable of doing and what activities he is learning. Thus, the patient does not regress because all members of the rehabilitation team are working toward the same goal.

The ADL sheet is a guide to the assessment of the patient's functions. These activities are key goals. If the patient can sit up and raise his hands to his head, he probably can begin to bathe himself.

The goal of the patient is to care for himself in his daily routine without depending on others. Nursing interventions include teaching, supporting and supervising the patient while he performs these activities.

An ADL program is started as soon as the rehabilitation process starts. The longer a muscle is in disuse, the weaker and more atrophied it becomes. The patient must learn that he will lose what he does not use.

In order to effectively teach a person methods of self-care, he must be motivated. "I'd rather do it myself" is a good concept for the patient to develop. The nurse teaches and guides, but the patient must do the work. Since there are individual differences in all persons, self-care techniques need to be flexible and adapted to the patient's needs and mode of living. It is important to remember that there is usually more than one way to accomplish self-care. Since many patients do not perform these commonplace activities easily, a great deal of common sense and a little ingenuity are frequently called for. Often a simple maneuver requires concentration and the exertion of considerable effort.

Guidelines for Teaching the Activities of Daily Living

1. Define the goal of the activity; understand the purpose.
2. Ascertain what methods can be used to accomplish the task. (Example: There are several ways of putting on a given garment.)
3. Identify the motions necessary for the accomplishment of the activity.
4. Encourage the patient to exercise the muscles necessary to perform the motions involved in the activity.
5. Select activities that encourage gross functional movements of the upper and lower extremities (*e.g.*, bathing, holding larger objects).
6. Gradually include activities that use finer motions (*e.g.*, buttoning clothes, eating with a spoon).
7. Extend the period of activity as much and as fast as the patient can tolerate.
8. Perform and practice the activity in a real-life situation.
9. Encourage the patient to perform every activity up to his maximal capabilities within the framework of his disability.
10. Support the patient by giving justifiable praise for effort put forth and for acts accomplished.

If a person is severely disabled, having a personal attendant can save energy and make more time for employment or social interaction opportunities. It may be necessary to accept dependency in some areas of daily living in order to accomplish independence in other areas.

Using Assistive Devices (Self-Help Devices)

Assistive devices (self-help devices) include equipment that can help a person carry out his daily activities (Fig. 14-4). These may be devised by the patient, nurse, or family or purchased ready made. If the patient has difficulty in performing the activity, an adaptation will have to be made. Often, a new method can be learned. If the patient cannot quite reach his head, perhaps he will be able to touch his head by leaning forward. Or, if the method cannot be changed, adaptive equipment (self-help devices) may be used—such as those devised by adding a long handle to a comb, "building up" the handle of a spoon, or making similar modifications. Equipment such as an automatic toothbrush has been found to improve the oral hygiene of those having limited movements of the hands, wrists, and arms. Velcro fastening is easier to manage than buttons or zippers in clothing. Be alert to "gadgets" coming on the market that may be useful to the handicapped. There are mobility aids and systems for those with paralysis or cerebral palsy; educational aids; occupational and vocational tools; personal aids; and writing, typewriting, and communication aids that have been designed and are in use. There is also a wide selection of electronic assistive devices that help severely disabled persons to function with less dependence on others. These allow a task to be completed faster and with less fatigue. Electronic devices in use include visual and mobility aids for the blind, aids for persons with hearing and tactile impairments, aids for those with communicative disorders, and manipulation and mobility aids.

The Abledata System is a computerized listing of commercially available aids and equipment for disabled persons.

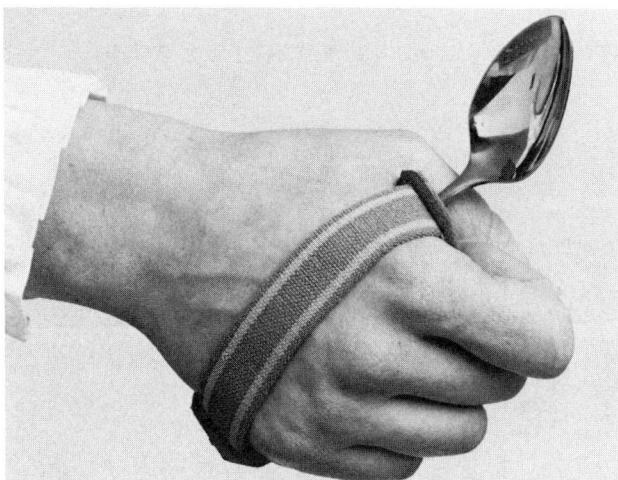

Figure 14-4
The universal ADL cuff is helpful for persons with limited use of the hands. Eating utensils, toothbrush, comb, or other essentials can be inserted in the cuff.

This is part of the services offered by the National Rehabilitation Information Center.*

Assisting the Patient with Ambulation

Assessment

Preparation for ambulation begins with maintaining joint range of motion, preventing contractures, and achieving bed mobility. Muscle strengthening exercises are started while the patient is still in bed. As soon as he can tolerate it, the patient is assisted to sit up on the side of the bed and taught to transfer from the bed to the chair (if this is necessary) and then to walk.

During these activities, assessment focuses on the patient's abilities, the extent of his disability, and his residual capacity for physiologic adaptation. The nurse observes for signs and symptoms of fatigue and orthostatic hypotension and for pallor, diaphoresis, nausea, and tachycardia. If these occur, the activity should be stopped and the patient encouraged to rest.

Use of the Tilt Table

Weight bearing on the long bones is essential for normal physiologic functioning. In order to prevent complications of inactivity, the upright position with weight-bearing on the long bones is desirable at the earliest possible time. This position prevents decalcification of the bones, thus aiding in the maintenance of normal acid–base balance and the prevention of renal calculi; it also stimulates circulation to the lower extremities.

Some disabilities, such as spinal cord injuries, orthostatic hypotension, brain damage, and those requiring extended periods in the recumbent position, prevent patients from assuming an upright position by the usual methods. In such instances, a tilt table can be of tremendous use. A tilt table is a board or table that can be tilted gradually from a horizontal to a vertical position, permitting the patient to assume an upright position. It helps the patient with his weight-bearing activities and standing balance, prevents disuse syndrome, and conditions the vascular system. Before the patient is placed on a table, a compression leotard or a snug-fitting abdominal binder and elastic bandages are applied from the toes to the groin. Compression on the abdomen prevents pooling of blood in the splanchnic (visceral) area and subsequent postural hypotension and inadequate cerebral circulation. Compression applied to the legs restricts the vascular walls of the blood vessels and prevents blood from pooling in the legs and edema from developing.

Tilting the patient from a supine to an upright position causes a decrease in the systolic blood pressure. For this reason, a blood pressure cuff is applied before the table is

* National Rehabilitation Information Center, 4407 Eighth Street, NE, Washington, DC 20017, Toll-free telephone number: 800-346-2742

tilted. The table should be tilted gradually, and someone should stay with the patient throughout this process. If the patient feels dizzy and his blood pressure drops, return him to a flat position. Observe for pallor, diaphoresis, tachycardia, and nausea. These are the signs and symptoms of insufficient cerebral circulation. The tilt of the table is increased by 5- to 10-degree increments. The angle of the tilt is determined by the patient's tolerance and the desired amount of weight-bearing. Be careful that the patient does not stand too long, especially if he cannot move his extremities. Prolonged standing may cause pressure ulceration on the bottom of the feet. The feet should be protected with a pair of properly fitted shoes.

Transfer Activities

A *transfer* is the movement of the patient from one piece of furniture or equipment to another (*i.e.*, from bed to chair or bed to wheelchair).

As soon as the patient is permitted out of bed, transfer activities are started. While still confined to his bed, it is important that the patient practice "push-up" exercises to strengthen the arm and shoulder extensors. It is desirable that the patient be able to raise and move his body in different directions by means of these push-up exercises. A simple, effective procedure follows:

1. Have the patient sit upright in bed.
2. Place a book under each hand.

3. Instruct the patient to push down on the book and thus raise his body weight.

Since the nurse is so frequently concerned with getting weak and incapacitated patients out of bed, it is important to be familiar with the techniques of moving the patient to the edge of the bed, sitting him on the edge of the bed, and assisting him to stand. The steps in each of these maneuvers are listed in Chart 14-5.

Before the patient is taught to transfer, he is evaluated to determine his ability to transfer from one area to another. Always have the patient move toward his stronger side. The nurse demonstrates the technique of transfer, and the patient then is ready to practice and perform this activity (Fig. 14-5).

Use of a Transfer or Sliding Board. If the muscles that the patient uses to lift himself off the bed are not strong enough to overcome the resistance of body weight, a polished lightweight board may be used to bridge the gap between the bed and the chair, and the patient slides across on it. This board (or bench) also may be used to transfer the patient from the chair to the toilet or the bathtub.

- Place one end of the transfer board under the patient's buttocks and the other end on the surface to which the transfer is being made (*i.e.*, the chair).
- Instruct the patient to push up with his hands to shift the buttocks and then to slide across the board to the other surface. There are other methods of transferring from the bed to the wheelchair when the patient in unable to

Chart 14-5
Assisting the Patient Out of Bed

Technique for Moving the Patient to the Edge of the Bed

- Move head and shoulders of patient toward the edge of the bed.
- Move feet and legs to the edge of the bed (The patient is now in a crescent position, which gives good range of motion to the lateral trunk muscles.)
- Place both arms well under the patient's hips (Before the next maneuver, you should tighten [set] the muscles of your back and abdomen.)
- Straighten your back while moving the patient toward you.

Technique for Sitting Patient on the Edge of the Bed

- Place arm and hand under shoulders of the patient.
- Instruct the patient to push his elbow into the bed while you lift his shoulders with one arm and swing his legs over the edge of the bed with the other. (Gravity pulls the legs downward, which aids in raising the patient's trunk.)

Technique for Assisting Patient to Stand

- Place patient's feet well under him.
- Face the patient while firmly grasping each side of his rib cage with your hands.
- Push your knee against one knee of the patient.
- Rock the patient forward as he comes to a standing position. (Your knee is pushed against the patient's knee as he comes to the standing position.)
- Ensure that the patient's knees are "locked" (full extension) while he is standing. (Locking the knees of the patient is a safety measure for those who are weak or have been in bed for a period of time.)
- Give the patient *enough time* to balance himself.
- Pivot the patient to position him to sit in the chair.

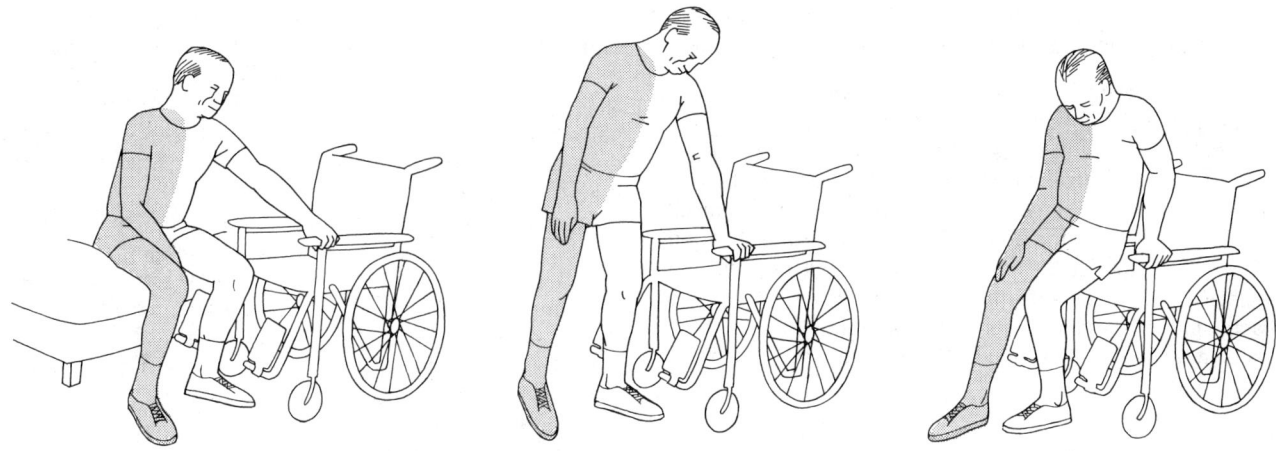

A. Weight-bearing transfer from bed to chair. The patient stands up, pivots until his back is opposite the new seat, and sits down.

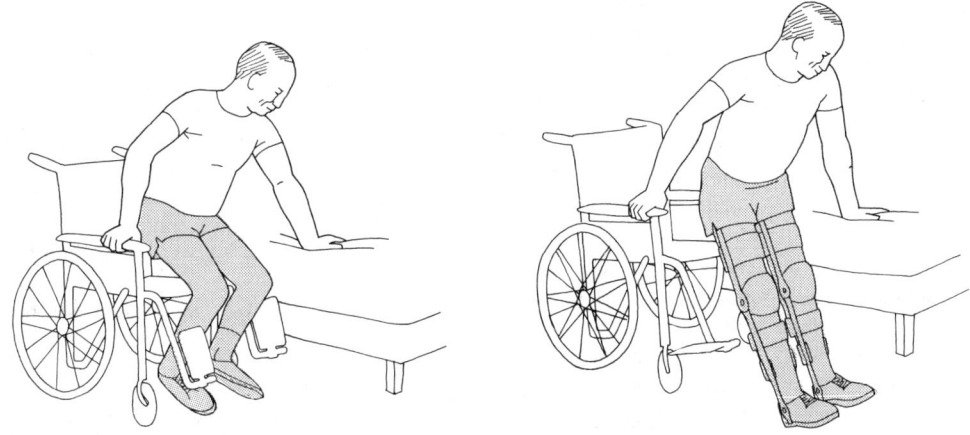

B. (*Left*) Non-weight-bearing transfer from chair to bed. (*Right*) With legs braced.

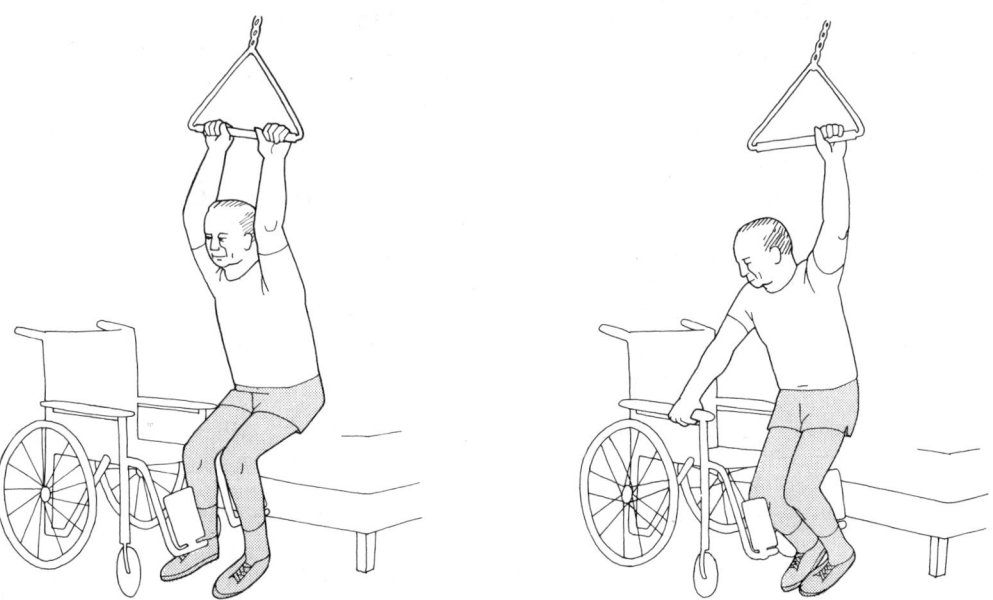

C. (*Left*) Non-weight-bearing transfer, pull-up method (*Right*). Non-weight-bearing transfer, combined method.

Figure 14-5
Methods of transferring the patient from the bed to a wheelchair. The wheelchair is in a locked position. Shaded areas indicate non-weightbearing body parts.

stand. Figure 14-5 shows the weight-bearing and non-weight-bearing transfers.

Patient Education for Transfers at Home. In the home setting, getting in and out of bed and performing chair, toilet, and tub transfers for persons with weak musculature and loss of hip, knee, and ankle motion are difficult. A rope attached to the headboard of the bed helps the patient to pull himself toward the center of the bed, and the use of a rope attached to the footboard facilitates getting in and out of bed. The height of a chair can be raised with hollowed-out blocks placed under the chair legs or with cushions on the seat. Bars can be attached to the wall near the toilet and tub to provide leverage and stability.

Preparation for Ambulation

Regaining the ability to walk is a prime morale builder. To be prepared for ambulation—whether with brace, walker, cane, or crutches—the patient must be strengthened and conditioned. *Exercise is the foundation of preparation.* By performing mat and parallel-bar exercises, the patient develops balance and coordination and strengthens his muscles. The following are preconditioning exercises that the nurse can teach and supervise:

To strengthen the muscles needed for ambulation, *quadriceps setting* is used. The quadriceps muscles also guard the knee joint. Strengthening these muscles acts as a deterrent to flexion contractures for instability of the knee. The patient contracts the quadriceps muscle while attempting to push the popliteal area against the mattress and at the same time raising the heel. He maintains the muscle contracture until the count of five and relaxes for the count of five. The exercise is repeated 10 to 15 times hourly. In *gluteal setting,* he contracts or "pinches" the buttocks together until the count of five, relaxes for the count of five, and repeats.

To strengthen the muscles of the upper extremities, which are used for handling the cane, crutches, or walker employed in early ambulation, *sit-ups* are helpful. While in a sitting position, the patient raises his body from the chair by pushing his hands against the chair seat (or mattress). He also should be encouraged to do *push-ups* while in a prone position. Teach him to *raise his arms* above his head and lower them in a slow, rhythmical manner while holding traction weights, gradually increasing the poundage of the weights. He can *strengthen his hands* by crumpling newspaper and squeezing a rubber ball. *Pull-ups* on a trapeze, while lifting the body, is another effective conditioner.

If the patient has difficulty standing, parallel bars can be used to provide stability. After standing balance is achieved, he can practice shifting his weight from side to side, lifting one leg while supporting his weight with the other, and then walking.

Mobility Aids

Crutch Walking

In the treatment of various forms of arthritis and of most fractures of the lower extremity, and after operations on the

leg—especially after amputation—crutches provide a support and balance and a convenient method of getting from one place to another. Since crutch walking is not an inherited skill, it must be taught, and this learning process must begin early. Crutch walking requires a high energy expenditure and considerable cardiovascular stress. Older persons with reduced exercise capacity, arm strength, and problems with balance due to age and multiple diseases may be unable to meet the energy demands of crutch walking.

One of the first prerequisites is to develop power in the shoulder girdle and upper extremity muscles, which will bear the patient's weight while he is crutch walking. Exercise to increase the strength and coordination of these muscle groups should be started before the patient is ambulating and then should progress to balancing exercises between parallel bars.

The following muscle groups are important for crutch walking (Fig. 14-6, *A*):

- Shoulder depressors—to stabilize the upper extremity and prevent shoulder hiking
- Shoulder adductors—to hold the crutch top against the chest wall
- Arm flexors, extensors, and abductors (at the shoulder)—to move crutches forward, backward, and sideward
- Forearm extensors—to prevent flexion or buckling; important in raising the body for swinging gait
- Wrist extensors—to enable weight-bearing on hand pieces
- Finger and thumb flexors—to grasp the hand piece

Of equal importance is psychological preparation, which can be developed long before the physical need is present. The individual needs of each patient must be considered and the methods of approach directed to them. The patient's age, interests, and future intentions, as well as his prognosis, are essential factors.

Measurement for Crutches. Adjustable crutches are practical because the disease may cause changes in the muscles and the joints, or because the patient may improve and progress to a different crutch base and gait.

To measure a standing patient for crutches, position the patient against the wall with the feet slightly apart and away from the wall. Mark 5 cm (2 inches) out to the side from the tip of the toe. Measure 15 cm (6 inches) straight ahead from the first mark and mark this point. Measure from 5 cm (2 inches) below the axilla to the second mark. This measurement is the approximate crutch length.

If the patient has to be measured while lying down, measure from the anterior fold of the axilla to the sole of the foot, and then add 5 cm (2 inches). Another method is to determine the height of the patient and subtract 40 cm (16 inches).

The hand piece should allow 20 to 30 degrees of flexion at the elbow. The wrist should be extended and the hand dorsiflexed. The patient should wear shoes that fit well and have firm soles. The crutches should be fitted with large rubber suction tips before measuring.

The maintenance of an erect posture is essential to crutch walking. Before trying to use crutches, the patient should learn to stand by a chair on the unaffected leg in order to achieve balance. The nurse explains and demonstrates to the patient how he should manipulate his crutches before he attempts to do so.

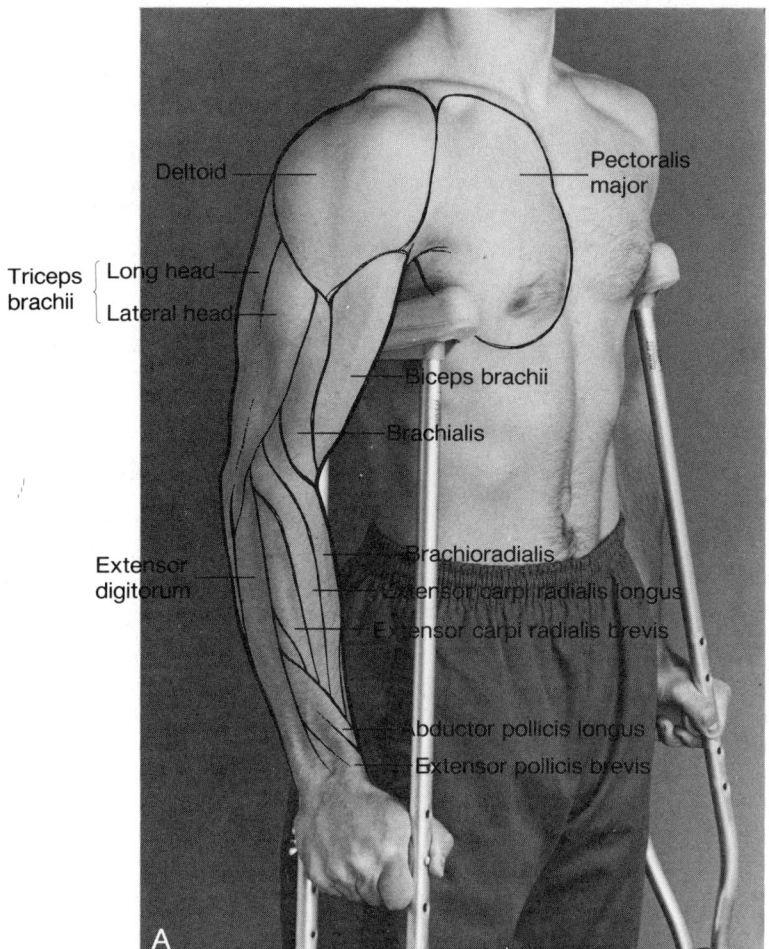
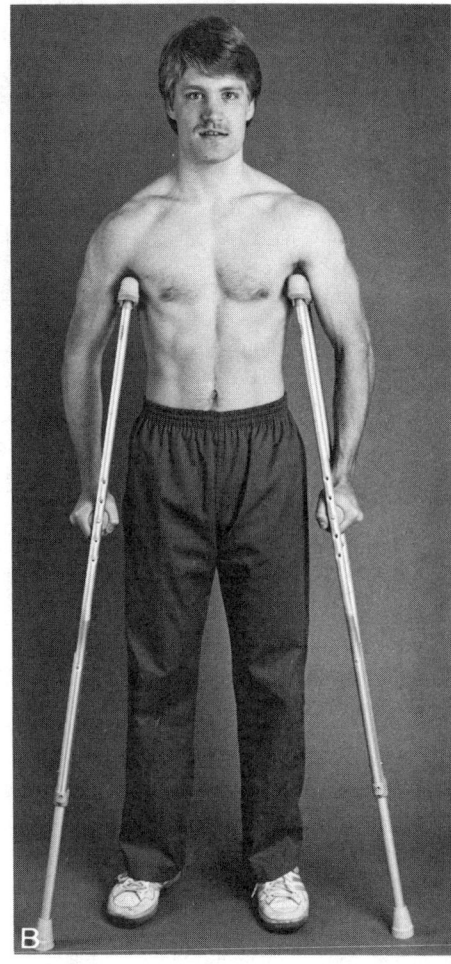

Figure 14-6
Crutch walking. (*A*) Muscle groups important for crutch walking. (*B*) The tripod position
for the basic crutch stance.

Crutch Stance. The *tripod position* is the basic crutch
stance. The crutches rest approximately 20 cm to 25 cm
(8–10 inches) in front and to the side of the patient's toes.
This gives the strongest and most balanced support (see Fig.
14-6, *B*). Since, to provide stability, a greater height requires
a broader base, a taller patient needs a wider base and a
shorter patient a narrower base.

The patient must be taught to support his weight on the
hand piece. If the weight is borne on the axilla, the pressure
of the crutch can damage the brachial plexus nerves and
produce "crutch paralysis." A foam-rubber pad on the underarm piece will relieve pressure on the upper arm and the
thoracic cage.

Ability to shift body weight is the next step. The crutch
gait selected depends on the nature of the patient's disability.
The nurse must know how much (if any) weight can be placed
on the affected side and whether the crutches are being used
for balance and support.

Crutch Gaits. The selection of the crutch gait depends
on the type and severity of the disability and on the patient's
physical condition, arm and trunk strength, and body balance.
The patient should be taught two gaits so that he may change
from one to another. Shifting crutch gaits relieves fatigue since
each gait requires the use of a different combination of mus-

cles. (If a muscle is forced to contract steadily without relaxing, the circulation of the blood to the part is reduced.) A
faster gait can be used for making speed, whereas a slower
one is used in crowded places.

All gaits begin in the tripod position. The more common
gaits are the 4-point, the 2-point, the 3-point, and the swinging-
to and swinging-through gaits. The sequence of movements
for each of these gaits is listed in Chart 14-6.

The patient should not practice crutch walking for too
long, especially if he has been in bed for a prolonged period.
Such signs as sweating or shortness of breath should be indications that the lesson on crutches should be stopped and
the patient permitted to rest or go back to bed.

Other Crutch-Maneuvering Techniques. Before a
patient is sent home on crutches, it is important to ascertain
whether he can dress himself and whether he can get in and
out of chairs, on and off the toilet, in and out of doors, up
and down stairs and ramps, and in and out of a car, taxi, or
public conveyance.

The following procedures are taught to the patient.

To Sit in a Chair
1. Grasp the crutches at the hand pieces for control.
2. Bend forward slightly while assuming a sitting position.

Chart 14-6
Gaits for Crutch Walking

4-Point Gait

This gait can be used when supported weight-bearing is permitted for both legs. It is safe and gives maximal balance because there are always three points of contact with the floor; thus, it is slow because it requires constant shifting of weight.

Sequence
1. Right crutch
2. Left foot
3. Left crutch
4. Right foot

2-Point Gait

This gait is faster since there are only two points of contact with the floor at one time.

Sequence
1. Advance right crutch and left foot.
2. Simultaneously shift weight and advance left crutch and right foot.

3-Point Gait

This is a faster gait but requires more strength and balance. The patient must be able to support his entire body weight on his arms.

Sequence
1. Advance the weaker leg and both crutches simultaneously.
2. While putting most of the body weight on the crutches, advance the stronger lower extremity.

Swing-Crutch Gaits

Swing-To Gait

Sequence
1. Bear weight on good leg.
2. Advance both crutches forward simultaneously.
3. While leaning forward, swing the body to a position that is even with the crutches.

Swing-Through Gait

Sequence
1. Advance both crutches forward.
2. Lift both legs off ground and swing forward, landing in advance of the crutches.
3. Bring crutches forward again, rapidly, to prevent being caught off balance.

To Stand Up
1. Move forward to the edge of the chair with the strong leg slightly under the seat.
2. Place both crutches in the hand on the side of the affected extremity.
3. Push down on the hand piece while raising the body to a standing position.

To Go Down Stairs
1. Walk forward as far as possible on the step.
2. Advance crutches to the lower step. The weaker leg is advanced first and then the stronger one. In this way, the stronger extremity shares the work of raising and lowering the body weight with the patient's arms.

To Go Up Stairs
1. Advance the stronger leg first up to the next step.
2. Then advance the crutches and the weaker extremity. (Strong leg goes up first and comes down last.) A memory device for the patients is "up with the good; down with the bad."

Use of a Walker

A walker provides more support than a cane or crutches for the patient who has poor balance and cannot use crutches. It gives stability but it does not permit a natural reciprocal walking pattern. Teach the following sequence:

1. Lift the walker, placing it in front of you while leaning your body slightly forward.
2. Take a step or two into the walker.
3. Lift the walker and place it is front of you again.

Ambulation with a Cane

A cane is used to help the patient walk with greater balance and support and with less fatigue. It also relieves the pressure on weight-bearing joints and prevents undue pressure and use of the unaffected extremity. To fit the patient for a cane, have him flex his elbow at a 30-degree angle and hold the cane 15 cm (6 inches) lateral to the base of his fifth toe. Adjust the cane so that the handle is approximately level with the greater trochanter. An adjustable aluminum cane fitted with a gently flaring tip that has flexible and concentric rings gives optimum stability, functions as a shock absorber, and enables the patient to walk with greater speed and less fatigue.

Cane–Foot Sequence
1. Hold the cane in the hand opposite to the affected extremity (*i.e.*, the cane should be used on the good side. In normal walking, the opposite leg and arm move together; thus, holding the cane opposite the involved side widens the base of support and reduces stress on the involved extremity.)

2. Advance the cane at the same time the affected leg is moved forward.
3. Keep the cane fairly close to the body to prevent leaning, and bear down on the cane when the unaffected extremity begins the swing phase.
4. If for some reason the patient is unable to use the cane in the opposite hand, the cane may be carried on the same side and advanced when the affected leg is advanced.

To Go Up and Down Stairs Using the Cane–Foot Sequence
1. Step up on the unaffected extremity.
2. Then place the cane and affected extremity up on the step.
3. Reverse this procedure for descending steps. (Strong leg goes up first and comes down last).

Supporting the Patient with an Orthotic or a Prosthetic Appliance

Orthotic Devices

An *orthosis* is an external appliance used to provide support and alignment, prevent or correct deformities, and improve the function of the body. It includes braces, splints, collars, corsets, supports, or calipers that may be designed and produced by an orthotist. An orthosis may be static (no moving parts) or dynamic (with moving parts). Static orthoses are used to stabilize joints and prevent contractures, while dynamic orthoses are flexible and used to improve functioning by assisting weak muscles.

The field of orthotics has enlarged to include equipment such as wheelchairs and environmental control systems (devices and systems to improve the quality of life for the severely disabled).

Patient Education.   The nurse reinforces the orthotist's instructions concerning care of the skin under an orthotic device because skin problems/pressure sores may develop if the device is applied too tightly. Teach the patient to examine the orthosis periodically to see that it has not slipped out of position or become distorted and that the padding distributes the pressure evenly.

Prosthetic Devices

A *prosthesis** is a replacement for a missing part of the body (*e.g.,* extremity, joint, eye, breast, tooth). A *prosthetist* is a limb maker or a maker of other prostheses. He is responsible for fabricating the prosthesis, fitting it, and training the patient to use the device. The training may be also carried out under the supervision of an occupational therapist with prosthetic expertise.

Nursing Interventions.   The nurse performs an essential function in the preprosthetic phase of the patient's care by helping him to develop an attitude of realistic hopefulness and by preventing deformities, so that the time between the

----

* Specific prostheses are described later in this book when the clinical conditions calling for them are discussed (*e.g.,* extremity prostheses for the amputee and a breast prosthesis for the patient who has had a radical mastectomy). Information concerning prosthetic and orthopedic appliances may be obtained also from The American Orthotic and Prosthetic Association, 717 Pendleton Street, Alexandria, VA 22314.

----

healing of the tissues and the fitting of the prosthesis is kept to a minimum. In the amputation of an extremity, the physical therapist (or the nurse) is responsible for bandaging the stump (or the residual extremity) correctly, so that proper shrinkage and shaping occur and the patient can be fitted more effectively with a prosthesis.

Coping With Fatigue

Because it is uncomfortable and tiring to live with a physical disability, the disabled are vulnerable to fatigue. Physical disabilities have to be faced daily, and frustration brings weariness to mind and body. The fear of falling may be always present, and mobility often remains a minute-by-minute challenge fraught with difficulties. Walking with crutches or braces requires a high expenditure of energy.

The following may be useful in teaching patients how to reduce their energy output, thus conserving their strength to achieve a meaningful life-style.

Have well-defined goals and priorities.
- Keep priorities in order; eliminate nonessential activities.
- Plan and pace your activities.
   Plan each day.
   Distribute heavy work load throughout week.
   Organize work; have equipment within easy reach.
   Keep work in front of you.
- Rest before undertaking difficult tasks.
- Stop before fatigue sets in.
- Continue with exercise conditioning program to strengthen muscles.

Control your environment.
- Try to be well organized.
- Place possessions in same place, so that they can be found with minimum of effort.
- Place equipment in box/basket (personal care, crafts, work).
- Use energy conservation and work simplification techniques.
- Use adaptive equipment, self-help aids, labor-saving devices.
- Take safety precautions.

Take control of your life.
- Face the reality of your disability.
- Emphasize areas of strength.
- Remain outward looking.
- Seek inventive ways to tackle problems.
- Maintain and improve general health.
- Plan for recreation.

Helping to Overcome Elimination Problems

Urinary and bowel incontinence are frequent problems in the disabled patient. Bladder and bowel control are important functions of the body and are influenced by prescribed social behavior. Incontinence curtails a person's independence, causing embarrassment, isolation, and often institutionalization of the elderly. It occurs in up to 15% of the community-based elderly population, while almost half of nursing home residents are either bowel or bladder incontinent or both.

Bladder Training

In order to treat urinary incontinence, its etiology and pattern must be evaluated. The causes of incontinence are complex. It may be caused by obvious urologic problems (urinary tract infection, detrusor instability, bladder outlet obstruction), or by congenital or acquired neurologic disease.

Urodynamic testing (p. 1005) gives clues to the pathophysiologic features of the patient's incontinence. Neurologic incontinence (disorders caused by partial or complete disturbance of the neurologic control of the bladder) and its management are discussed on pp. 1014–1015.

Biofeedback, through which the patient can learn to contract urinary (and anal) sphincters, has shown promise in the management of urinary incontinence. If the patient has uncontrolled incontinence, the nurse may facilitate the patient's adjustment by teaching self-catheterization when feasible.

Once reversible causes are identified and treated, an individual incontinence pattern is determined by keeping a voiding record to record the number and timing of incontinence episodes and associated circumstances such as coughing or lifting. An hourly voiding record is kept for at least 48 hours; it shows whether the patient is wet or dry so that his voiding habits are visualized. The record is studied to determine whether incontinence is transient (from confusion, infection, certain drugs, restricted mobility) or established and of long-term duration.

The nursing assessment also includes evaluating the mobility and energy levels of the patient. Determine whether the patient is taking diuretics (which increase urinary output) or sedatives (which decrease alertness).

The patient's goal is to achieve control of voiding. Incontinence should not be regarded as inevitable in any patient, since bladder training is an alternative in most instances. The selection of the method of bladder management depends on the cause. The key to successful urinary control is conditioning of the body and includes

- Sufficient fluid intake (2500 to 3000 ml/day)
- Establishment of regular time to void (*i.e.*, a habit pattern)

The voiding record is analyzed so that a voiding/toileting schedule can be formulated. This schedule is set up with definite times indicated for the patient to try to empty his bladder using either the toilet or commode when possible. The interval between voidings in the early phase of the training period is fairly short (1½ to 2 hours), but as the patient's bladder capacity increases, the interval is lengthened. A suggested procedure is to give a measured amount of fluid every 2 hours. After drinking, the patient waits for 30 minutes and then attempts to void. He gradually lengthens the period between voiding times. (It is best to give larger amounts of fluid during the day and to withhold fluids after 5 PM.)

The patient is encouraged to hold his urine until the specified voiding time. Usually, there is a relationship between drinking, eating, exercising, and voiding, and the alert patient soon can determine his own intake schedule. Have the patient keep a written voiding schedule, which will give a continuous record of the time and amounts of fluid ingested and the time and amount of each voiding. Regularity is the key to success. To assist in the act of voiding, the patient should either stand or sit with the thighs flexed and the feet and the back supported. Increasing intra-abdominal pressure by massage over the bladder or by leaning forward while sitting will help to initiate evacuation of the bladder.

Gerontological Considerations

Study the voiding record of the confused elderly person and take him to the bathroom before involuntary voiding occurs. Create an environment that keeps sensory monotony to a minimum. Orient the patient to time and place. Extend his social environment beyond the confines of his room and try to increase the number of his social contacts. An alarm clock may be set at regular intervals throughout the day and several times during the night to remind the patient to void. The patient must approve of the program and have a firm desire to establish control. It may take several weeks to accomplish this end. An optimistic attitude and positive feedback for even slight gains are necessary. It is also important to encourage the patient to continue with self-care and the exercise and occupational therapy programs—boredom and frustration can lead to incontinence. Encourage the patient to make decisions and do meaningful tasks. Have the patient wear his own clothing, since this enhances his self-esteem and dignity and is a strong deterrent to regressive behavior. The use of a diaper at any time is discouraged, because its psychological effect is one of regression rather than progression.

Bowel Training

A bowel training program incorporates regularity, timing, nutrition and fluids, and correct positioning to take advantage of the patient's natural reflexes and establish a predictable time for defecation. The goals of a bowel training program are to develop regular bowel habits and to prevent fecal incontinence, fecal impaction, and irregularity.

The patient's signs and symptoms associated with defecation, which may include constipation, diarrhea, irregularity, incontinence or impaction, are evaluated. A record of his defecation pattern is kept to analyze his bowel cycle, which can vary from 24 to 48 to 72 hours.

The patient's goal is to achieve bowel control. The bowel program is individualized, making certain that the patient takes responsibility for this important facet of rehabilitation.

- The first essential step in bowel training that requires reflex assistance is the establishment of regularity, a specific and definite time for bowel evacuation.

Any attempts at evacuation should be made within 15 minutes of the same time daily. An active aid to bowel evacuation is the stimulation of peristalsis and the gastrocolic and duodenocolic reflexes. Therefore, the patient should establish his bowel evacuation time after a regularly scheduled meal. One of the best times is after breakfast. However, if the patient has a previously established habit pattern, it should be followed.

Physical activity and exercise are important aids to peristaltic activity and bowel movement. Unless contraindicated by other existing conditions, the diet should include adequate intake of fiber-containing foods (vegetables, fruit, bran, cereals) to prevent hard stools and stimulate peristalsis, and a fluid intake between 2 liters and 4 liters (2.1 to 4.2 quarts) daily. Prune juice or fig juice (120 ml) taken 30 minutes before a meal once daily is helpful when constipation is a problem.

The reflex habit should be established by regularity early in the course of the patient's illness. It may be aided by mechanical means. About 30 minutes before the scheduled bowel time, a glycerin suppository is inserted into the rectum in order to stimulate the anorectal reflex (Digital stimulation with a lubricated gloved finger will induce reflex contraction also). Suppository inserters or anal dilators are available for patients with inadequate hand strength and control.

After the scheduled interval, the patient is encouraged to attempt to have a bowel movement. If at all possible, he should assume the normal position for defecation, which allows gravity to assist in stool elimination. Instruct him to bear down and to contract his abdominal muscles. If necessary, he can lean forward to increase intra-abdominal pressure. The patient may be taught to apply pressure to the abdominal wall and to massage the abdomen from right to left to facilitate movement of feces in the lower tract.

After this routine is well established, mechanical stimulation with the suppository probably will not be necessary, and in a few weeks the patient will be having regular daily bowel movements.

Sexuality and the Disabled

There is a growing recognition of the sexual rights and problems of the disabled. Sexual health is a vital element in total rehabilitation. Physical disability does not necessarily lead to sexual disability. Sexuality involves not only biological sexual activity but also the person's concept of his masculinity or her femininity and the way he or she reacts to others and is perceived by them. It takes many forms: caring, reaching out, sharing, and emotional intimacy.

Sexual matters are considered to be in the very private realm, and the patient is apt to be reticent about discussing his feelings. The professional person is focusing so intently on the rehabilitation of the patient (*i.e.,* helping him to gain independence) that there is a tendency to forget that sexuality is part of the patient's personality. Recognizing and dealing with sexual concerns is basic in establishing feelings of self-worth, which are essential to total rehabilitation. Professional personnel, family members, and the community must deal with the reality that disabled persons are sexual humans with needs for social affiliation and sexual intimacy.

Problems faced by the disabled include limited access to information about sexuality, lack of opportunity to form friendships and loving relationships, impaired self-image and low self-esteem, and lack of social skills.

The sex-related concerns of the patient must be identified through an individual approach. Allow the patient to talk about his anxieties related to sex. The disabled person may need further sex education, communication, social, and assertiveness skills to develop relationships in general. The specialized services of a sex counselor are available to help those with specific sexual needs or conflicts. Classes, books, and movies are useful.

The reader is referred to Chapter 13 and the bibliography at the end of the chapter for additional reading on this subject.

Patient Education and Home Health Care

An important goal of rehabilitation is to assist the person to return to his own environment after learning to manage his disability. A referral system maintains continuity of care when the patient is transferred to his home or an extended care facility. The plan for discharge is formulated when the patient is first admitted to the hospital, and discharge plans are made with the patient's functional potential in mind.

The patient's support system (family, friends) is assessed and every effort is made for successful home placement. The family will need to know as much about the patient's condition and care as possible so that they will not fear his return home. Their attitude toward the patient, his disability, and his return home should be assessed.

The community health nurse visits the patient in the hospital, interviews the patient and family, reviews the ADL sheet, and gains first-hand knowledge of the activities the patient can perform. This helps ensure continuity of management and that the patient does not "lose ground" and maintains the independence gained while in the hospital. It may be necessary to help the family purchase, improvise, or borrow needed equipment such as safety rails, a tub bench, or raised toilet seat or commode. Ramps may have to be built or doorways widened to achieve full access. Plan with the patient ways and methods of coping with problems that may arise. A skills checklist can be developed to make certain that the family is proficient in assisting the patient with certain tasks. Family members are taught how to use equipment and are given a copy of the manufacturer's instruction booklet, the names of resource persons, and lists of supplies and where these may be obtained. A written summary of the care plan is included in family teaching.

A network of support services and communication systems may be required to enhance opportunities for independent living. The nurse uses collaborative, coordination, and administration skills to pull the network of care together. The nurse also provides skilled care, initiates additional referrals when indicated, and serves as the patient's advocate and counselor when obstacles are encountered. She continues to reinforce the teaching that has been done and helps the patient to set and achieve attainable goals. The degree to which he adapts to his home and community environment depends on the confidence and self-esteem developed during his rehabilitation program and on the acceptance, support, and reactions of his family, employer, and community members.

Not all families can be expected to carry on the arduous programs of exercise and physical training that a patient may need or have the resources or stability to care for a severely disabled member. Even a stable family may be overwhelmed by the physical, emotional, economic, and energy drains of disabling disease. The family may require family therapy to allow them to discuss and explore their feelings and attitudes (rejection, aversion, avoidance) toward the disabled family member.

If the patient is transferred to an extended care facility, his ADL sheet goes with him to orient the staff to activities that he can perform independently. The staff continue to encourage the family to visit, to be involved, and to take the patient home on weekends and holidays if possible.

There is a growing trend toward independent living by severely disabled people, either independently or in groups that share resources. Skill training in attendant management, financial management, and mobility are necessary for the severely disabled person to achieve personal self-determination. The goal is integration into the community, living and working in the community with accessible housing, employment, public buildings, transportation, and recreation.

The Rehabilitation Services Administration provides services whereby disabled persons or those disadvantaged by advanced age or other conditions obtain the help they need to engage in gainful employment. These services are provided by state agencies and include diagnostic, medical, surgical, psychiatric, and hospital services, and assistance in securing prosthetic appliances. There is a counseling, training, placement, and follow-up service available to help the patient select and attain a vocational objective.

Bibliography

Books

American Academy of Orthopaedic Surgeons. Atlas of Orthotics, 2nd ed. St. Louis, CV Mosby, 1985.

Basmajian JV and Kirby RL (eds). Medical Rehabilitation. Baltimore, Williams & Wilkins, 1984.

Dagher FJ (ed). Cutaneous Wounds. Mt. Kisco, New York, Futura, 1985.

Dietz JH Jr. Rehabilitation Oncology. New York, John Wiley & Sons, 1981.

Eisenberg MG, Sutkin LC, and Jansen MA. Chronic Illness and Disability Through the Life Span: Effects on Self and Family. New York, Springer, 1984.

Halstead LS and Grabois M. Medical Rehabilitation. New York, Raven Press, 1985.

Henderson G and Bryan WV. Psychosocial Aspects of Disability. Springfield, Illinois, Charles C Thomas, 1984.

Hopkins HL and Smith HD. Willard and Spackman's Occupational Therapy. Philadelphia, JB Lippincott, 1983.

Kamenetz HL. Dictionary of Rehabilitation Medicine. New York, Springer, 1983.

Kaplan PE. The Practice of Physical Medicine. Springfield, Illinois, Charles C Thomas, 1984.

Kisner C and Colby LA. Therapeutic Exercise: Foundations and Techniques. Philadelphia, FA Davis, 1985.

Kottke FJ, Stillwell GK, and Lehmann JF. Krussen's Handbook of Physical Medicine and Rehabilitation, 3rd ed. Philadelphia, WB Saunders, 1982.

Krueger DW. Emotional Rehabilitation of Physical Trauma and Disability. New York, SP Medical & Scientific Books, 1984.

Krueger DW. Rehabilitation Psychology. Rockville, Maryland, Aspen Systems Corporation, 1984.

Lee BY. Chronic Ulcers of the Skin. New York, McGraw-Hill, 1985.

Marinelli RP and Dell Orto AE. The Psychological and Social Impact of Physical Disability. New York, Springer, 1984.

Norback J and Weitz P. Sourcebook of Aid for the Mentally and Physically Handicapped. New York, Van Nostrand Reinhold, 1983.

Okamoto GA and Phillips TJ. Physical Medicine and Rehabilitation. Philadelphia, WB Saunders, 1984.

O'Neill GW and Gardner R Jr. Behavioral Principles in Medical Rehabilitation. Springfield, Illinois, Charles C Thomas, 1983.

Rule WR. Lifestyle Counseling for Adjustment to Disability. Rockville, Maryland, Aspen Systems Corporation, 1984.

Ruskin AP. Current Therapy in Physiatry. Philadelphia, WB Saunders, 1984.

Saxon SV and Etten MJ. Psychosocial Rehabilitative Programs for Older Adults. Springfield, Illinois, Charles C Thomas, 1984.

Stewart W. Counselling in Rehabilitation. London, Croom Helm, 1985.

Trombly CA. Occupational Therapy for Physical Dysfunction, 2nd ed. Baltimore, Williams & Wilkins, 1983.

Webster JG et al (eds). Electronic Devices for Rehabilitation. London, Chapman and Hall, 1985.

Wehman P, Renzaglia A, and Bates P. Functional Living Skills for Moderately and Severely Handicapped Individuals. Austin, Texas, PRO-ED, 1985.

Williams TF. Rehabilitation in the Aging. New York, Raven Press, 1984.

Sexuality and Rehabilitation

Bullard DG and Knight SE. Sexuality and Physical Disability. St Louis, CV Mosby, 1981.

Farber M (ed). Human Sexuality: Psychosexual Effects of Disease. New York, Macmillan, 1985.

Halstead LS. Sexuality and disability. In Drueger DW (ed). Emotional Rehabilitation of Physical Trauma and Disability, pp 235–252. New York, SP Medical and Scientific Books, 1984.

Hogan RM. Human Sexuality: A Nursing Perspective. Norwalk, Connecticut, Appleton-Century-Crofts, 1985.

Sexuality and disability (Part VI). In Marinelli RP and Dell Orto AE. The Psychological and Social Impact of Physical Disability, pp 205–246. New York, Springer, 1984.

Tallmer M et al. Sexuality and Life-Threatening Illness. Springfield, Illinois, Charles C Thomas, 1984.

Woods NW. Human Sexuality in Health and Illness, 3rd ed. St Louis, CV Mosby, 1984.

Journal

Sexuality and Disability, published quarterly by: Human Science Press, 75 Fifth Avenue, New York, New York 10011.

Articles

(Asterisks indicate nursing research articles.)

Assessment

Keith RA. Functional assessment measures in medical rehabilitation: Current status. Arch Phys Med Rehabil 1984 Feb; 65(2):74–78.

Moskowitz E. PULSES profile in retrospect. Arch Phys Med Rehabil 1985 Sept; 66(9):647–648.

Wiens AG. Rehabilitation assessment—a nursing perspective. Rehabil Nurse 1985 Mar/Apr; 10(2):25–27.

Management of Elimination Problems

Autrey D, Lauzon F, and Holliday P. The voiding record, an aid to decrease incontinence. Geriatr Nurs 1984 Jan/Feb; 5(1):22–25.

Burgio KL, Whitehead WE, and Engel BT. Urinary incontinence in the elderly. Ann Intern Med 1985 Oct; 103(4):507–515.

Burton JR. Managing urinary incontinence—a common geriatric problem. Geriatrics 1984 Oct; 39(10):46–51.

Clinical Practice Committee. Guidelines for nursing care of patients with alteration in elimination. Oncol Nurs Forum 1984 Jan/Feb; 11(1): 108–112.

Dugan JS. Winning the battle against incontinence. Nursing '84 1984 June; 14(6):59.

McCormick KA and Burgio KL. Incontinence: An update on nursing care measures. J Gerontol Nurs 1984 Oct; 10(10):16–23.

Ouslander JG and Fowler E. Management of urinary incontinence in Veterans Administration nursing homes. J Am Geriatr Soc 1985 Jan; 33(1):33–40.

Resnick NM and Yalla SV. Current concepts: Management of urinary incontinence in the elderly. N Engl J Med 1985 Sept 26; 313(13): 800–805.

Snustad DG and Rosenthal T. Urinary incontinence in the elderly. Am Fam Physician 1985 Nov; 32(5):182–196.

Voith AM. A conceptual framework for nursing diagnoses: Alterations in elimination. Rehabil Nurse 1986 Jan; 11(1):18–21.

Voith AM and Smith DA. Validation of the nursing diagnosis of urinary retention. Nurs Clin North Am 1985 Dec; 20(4):723–729.

Philosophy of Rehabilitation

Dudas S. Rehabilitation concepts of nursing. J Enterostomal Ther 1984 Jan/Feb; 11(1):6–15.

Soric R, Hilbert L, and Tepperman PS. Rehabilitation medicine: Its time has come. Postgrad Med 1985 June; 77(8):13–18.

Symington DC. The goals of rehabilitation. Arch Phys Med Rehabil 1984 Aug; 65(8):427–430.

Watson PG. Components of rehabilitation: Nursing practice advancement. Rehabil Nurse 1985 Sept/Oct; 10(5):28–31, 34.

Young C, Saelinger D, and Moore P. A conceptual framework for rehabilitation nursing. Rehabil Nurse 1984 Mar/Apr; 9(2):17–19.

Pressure Sores: Prevention and Management

Beaver MJ. Mediscus low air-loss beds and the prevention of decubitus ulcers. Crit Care Nurse 1986 Sept–Oct; 6(5):32–39.

Brown MM et al. Nursing innovation for prevention of decubitus ulcers in long-term care facilities. Plast Surg Nurs 1985 Summer; 5(2):57–64.

Byrne N and Feld M. Preventing and treating decubitus ulcers. Nursing '84 1984 Apr; 14(4):55–57.

DeLisa JA and Mikulik MA. Pressure ulcers: What to do if preventive management fails. Postgrad Med 1985 May; 77(6):209–212, 218–220.

*Kurzuk-Howard G, Simpson L and Palmieri A. Decubitus ulcer care: A comparative study. West J Nurs Res 1985; 7(1):58–79.

Lucke K and Jarlsberg C. How is the air-fluidized bed best used? Am J Nurs 1985 Dec; 85(12):1338, 1340.

Merbitz CT et al. Wheelchair push-ups: Measuring relief frequency. Arch Phys Med Rehabil 1985 July; 66(7):433–438.

Messner RL. Targets for infection: Institutionalized elderly. Can Nurse 1985 Sept; 81(8):24–26.

Phipps M et al. Staging care for pressure sores. Am J Nurs 1984 Aug; 84(8):999–1003.

Seiler WO and Stähelin HB. Decubitus ulcers: Preventive techniques for the elderly patient. Geriatrics 1985 July; 40(7):53–60.

Seiler WO and Stähelin HB. Decubitus ulcers: Treatment through five therapeutic principles. Geriatrics 1985 July; 40(9):30–42.

Seiler WO and Stähelin HB. Recent findings on decubitus ulcer pathology: Implications for care. Geriatrics 1986 Jan; 41(1):47–57.

Shanon ML. Five famous fallacies about pressure sores. Nursing '84 1984 Oct; 14(10):34–41.

Sklar CG. Pressure ulcer management in the neurologically impaired patient. J Neurosurg Nurs 1985 Feb; 17(1):30–36.

Stephens SJ. Creative approaches to pressure sore problems. Orthop Nurs 1985 July/Aug; 4(4):40–44.

Sugarman B. Infection and pressure sores. Arch Phys Med Rehabil 1985 Mar; 66(3):177–179.

*Tooman T and Patterson J. Decubitus ulcer warfare: Product vs. process. Geriatr Nurs 1984 May/June; 5(3):166–167.

*Whitney JD, Fellows BH, and Larson E. Do mattresses make a difference? J Gerontol Nurs 1984 Sept; 10(9):20–25.

Yarkony GM et al. Pressure sore management: Efficacy of a moisture reactive occlusive dressing. Arch Phys Med Rehabil 1984 Oct; 65(10):597–600.

Principles and Practices of Rehabilitation Nursing

Balsmeyer B. Locus of control and use of strategies to promote self-care. J Community Health Nurs 1984; 1(3):171–179.

Bruno J. Some considerations and guidelines for crutch walking. Clin Podiatry 1984 Aug; 1(2):291–294.

*Creason NS et al. Validating the nursing diagnosis of impaired physical mobility. Nurs Clin North Am 1985 Dec; 20(4):669–683.

Davis AE. Focus on rehabilitation in the acute care setting: The role of the neuro/clinical nurse specialist. J Neurosurg Nurs 1985 Aug; 17(4):244–246.

Dell Orto AE. Coping with the enormity of illness and disability. Rehabil Lit 1984 Jan/Feb; 45(1-2):22–23.

Elliott FC. A nursing protocol for anxiety following catastrophic injury. Rehabil Nurse 1983 May/June; 8(3):18–20, 38.

Harris M. Helping the person with an altered self-image. Geriatr Nurs 1986 Mar/Apr; 7(2):90–92.

Hochberger JM. Family-centered care in rehabilitation. Rehabil Nurs 1985 Jan/Feb; 10(1):13–14.

Liang MH et al. Management of functional disability in homebound patients. J Fam Pract 1983 Sept; 17(3):429–435.

Myers JE. Rehabilitation of older people. Ann Rev Rehabil 1985; 4:1–54.

Palmer S et al. Psychosocial services in rehabilitation medicine: An interdisciplinary approach. Arch Phys Med Rehabil 1985 Oct; 66(10):690–692.

Reeder JM. Help your disabled patient be more independent. Nursing '84 1984 Nov; 14(11):43.

Staros A. Rehabilitation engineering and the growth of prosthetics/orthotics practice. Int Rehabil Med 1984; 6(2):79–84.

Stewart T and Shields CR. Grief in chronic illness: Assessment and management. Arch Phys Med Rehabil 1985 July; 66(7):447–450.

Agencies

A selected list of agencies and organizations, both governmental and voluntary, that work with or for patient needing rehabilitation services is listed in the Directory of National Information Services on Handicapping Conditions and Related Services, 4th ed, 1986, which can be obtained from the Superintendent of Documents, U.S. Government Printing Office, Washington, D.C. 20402. This directory contains abstracts and services of organizations and federal agencies offering services, information, and resources to handicapped individuals.

Chapter 15

The Person Experiencing Pain

Pain disables and distresses more people than any single disease entity. It is probably the most common and compelling reason why a person seeks health care. Most medical–surgical problems are associated with pain, resulting either from the disease process, diagnostic tests, or treatment modalities.

Ironically, little is known about pain. *Algology*—the study of pain—is a new science. Most experts consider pain a mysterious phenomenon that defies precise definition. At the very least, it appears to have three components: (1) a stimulus, physical or mental; (2) a bodily sensation of hurting; and (3) the reaction of the person experiencing it.

The nurse spends more time with the patient with pain than any other member of the health care team and therefore has the opportunity to make a significant contribution toward increasing the patient's comfort and relieving pain. The physician must seek to verify the patient's complaint of pain by establishing the cause and treating it. The nurse, in addition to collaborating with the physician toward this goal, also makes a major contribution to palliative pain relief—relief of pain that does not necessarily involve curing the cause of the pain.

In clinical practice, when direct care is given to a patient with pain, it is essential that the nurse adopt the patient's point of view about his pain. A cardinal rule in the care of patients with pain is that *all pain is real*, regardless of its cause—even when the cause remains unknown. Therefore, the nurse's verification of pain is based simply on the patient's indication that it exists.

Within this context, *the nursing definition of pain may be stated as whatever bodily hurt the patient says he has, existing whenever he says it does*. This definition encompasses two important points that are ultimately relevant to assessment, intervention, and evaluation.

First, the nurse believes the patient when he indicates that he has pain. It is important to avoid making the erroneous judgment that the patient does not have pain because no physical origin can be identified. Although some painful sensations are initiated by or sustained by the patient's mental or psychological state, he actually feels a sensation of pain; he does not merely think or imagine that he has pain. Furthermore, painful states initiated by psychological states, such as anxiety, are usually accompanied by physical changes, such as decreased blood flow or muscle tension. Most painful sensations are the result of two sets of stimuli: physical and mental or emotional. Therefore, the assessment of pain involves obtaining information about the physical *and* mental or emotional causes of pain. Nursing intervention involves attempting to reduce or relieve both sources of pain.

The second point to keep in mind is that what the patient "says" about his pain need not be limited to verbal statements. Some patients cannot or will not verbalize. Therefore, the nurse is also responsible for observing the many nonverbal behaviors that indicate the presence of the pain sensation and all that the patient experiences in relation to his pain.

Some patients deny pain, and they pose a different assessment problem. Although it is important to believe the patient who admits he has pain, it is equally important to be alert to patients who deny pain when they do in fact "hurt." A very common reason is fear of becoming addicted to narcotics. If the nurse suspects pain in a patient who denies it, she should explore with the patient her reason for suspecting pain, such as the fact that the disorder or procedure is usually painful, or that he grimaces when he moves, or avoids any movement. The nurse should also explore with the patient any reason that may cause him to deny pain, such as fear of addiction or further treatment.

Nursing Assessment

Assessment of the patient experiencing pain involves

- Recognizing whether the pain is acute or chronic
- Identifying the phases of the experience
- Observing the patient's behavioral responses
- Identifying the factors that influence the pain and the patient's response to it

A thorough assessment is of the utmost importance. To help the patient with his pain, the nurse must know that pain is occurring and how it is affecting the patient. This is not always obvious. The patient may try to hide his pain, or there may be a language barrier. Or, the patient may exhibit minimal responses to pain and, therefore, may appear not to experience pain.

Differences Between Acute and Chronic Pain

Pain specialists agree that there are two types of pain—acute and chronic. The differences between acute and chronic pain have implications for both assessment and intervention.

The terms *acute* and *chronic* are classifications of pain, based on the duration of pain. Quite simply, acute pain is of brief duration and chronic pain is prolonged. Acute does not necessarily mean severe; acute pain may range in intensity from mild to severe.

Acute Pain. Acute pain, which is a very common daily occurrence, is usually defined as an episode of pain that lasts from a split second to about 6 months. Generally, it serves the purpose of warning the patient that some degree of damage has occurred within the body that requires some form of treatment or intervention. Usually organic disease or injury is present, although healing may also be accompanied by acute pain. As the healing process progresses, the pain subsides and gradually disappears.

Injuries or diseases that cause acute pain may require treatment or may heal spontaneously. For example, a prick of the finger may heal rapidly, the pain subsiding quickly, perhaps within a few minutes. In the case of a more drastic condition, such as appendicitis, surgery may be necessary. In these cases, the pain decreases with healing of the injury or surgical trauma.

Chronic Pain. Chronic pain is sometimes defined as pain that lasts for 6 months or longer, although six months is a rather arbitrary period of time for differentiating between acute and chronic pain. An episode of pain may assume the characteristics of chronic pain long before 6 months have elapsed, or some types of pain may remain primarily acute in nature for longer than 6 months. Nevertheless, after 6 months, the majority of pain experiences are accompanied by problems associated with chronic pain. Chronic pain serves no useful purpose, and if it persists, the pain itself may become the major disorder.

The following are four common types of chronic pain, that is, prolonged pain experiences: (1) recurrent acute pain, (2) pain with obvious ongoing peripheral pathology, (3) chronic benign pain that may have peripheral or central pathology, and (4) chronic intractable benign pain syndrome.

Recurrent acute pain is intermittent pain. The patient has fairly well-defined episodes of pain interspersed with pain-free intervals. Because these episodes may recur over a period of years, recurrent acute pain is sometimes considered a type of chronic pain. Examples of recurrent acute pain are migraine headaches, sickle cell crises, and exacerbations of rheumatoid arthritis.

Pain with ongoing peripheral pathology may be of limited or unlimited duration. An example of time-limited pain with obvious ongoing peripheral pathology is the pain related to cancer. The pain may be of limited duration because the patient is eventually relieved after months of painful treatments, or the patient lives only a few months. In either case, the pain does not last for an extended period. An example of pain with ongoing peripheral pathology and unlimited duration is pain associated with degenerative arthritis.

Chronic benign pain (CBP) may be due to peripheral or central (brain and spinal cord) pathology. The pathology is often unclear, but it is not life threatening, as in cancer. (Benign means nonmalignant). An example of CBP with central pathology is post-stroke syndrome following a brain infarct. Tic douloureux is an example of central and peripheral pathology. Low back pain, a very common example of CBP, may be due to peripheral pathology, such as ischemic muscles, or central pathology, such as emotions causing muscle tension. As long as the patient functions well in daily life in spite of his pain, he usually remains classified in this category of CBP.

Chronic intractable benign pain syndrome (CIBPS) has the same characteristics as CBP, but the patient copes poorly. For example, the patient with low back pain may begin to use his pain to avoid dealing with marital or employment problems. Eventually, he may cope poorly with his job or marriage.

Phases of the Pain Experience

The patient may experience any or all of the three phases of a pain experience:

1. The anticipation of pain
2. The sensation of pain
3. The aftermath of pain

Each of these phases must be assessed because each requires nursing intervention, not just the phase during which pain is sensed. Even the patient who has relatively persistent and chronic pain may experience modified forms of these phases as the pain waxes and wanes in intensity.

The anticipation or fear of pain is sometimes more difficult for the patient to bear than the actual sensation of pain. The anticipation phase affects the patient's response to the sensation of pain.

Of the three phases, the most frequently overlooked is probably the aftermath. However, close observation may reveal any number of behavioral responses indicating such feelings as fear, embarrassment, or guilt. These feelings may last from hours to months following the cessation of the pain sensation.

Behavioral Responses

The patient's responses during any of the three phases of pain experience may be any one or a combination of possible reactions. These may include physiologic manifestations, verbal statements, vocal behaviors, facial expressions, body movements, physical contact with others, or alterations in response to the surrounding environment. These behaviors vary greatly from one person to another and may differ within the same person from one time to the next.

The nurse observes the patient's behavioral response to identify the following:

- The phase of pain the patient is experiencing (*i.e.*, anticipation, sensation, or aftermath).
- The intensity of the patient's pain. Whenever possible, it is helpful to ask the patient to rate his pain on a verbal or numerical scale (*e.g.*, none, slight, moderate, severe, or very severe; or 0 to 10: 0 = no pain, 10 = worst possible pain).
- The patient's tolerance for this particular painful sensation. Pain tolerance may be defined as the maximum intensity or duration of pain the person is willing to endure.
- Characteristics of the painful sensation. These include location (see Figure 15-1 for areas to which pain in various organs may be referred), duration, rhythmicity (periods of waxing and waning of the intensity or existence of pain), and quality (*e.g.*, pricking, burning, aching).
- Effects of pain on activities of daily living (*e.g.*, sleep, appetite, concentration, interactions with others, and physical movement). Acute pain is usually associated with anxiety, chronic pain with depression.
- What the patient believes will help him with his pain. Many patients have definite ideas about what will increase or decrease the intensity of their pain or what will make it more tolerable.
- The patient's concern about his pain. This may include a wide variety of items, such as financial burdens, prognosis, interference with role performance, and body image changes.

Adaptation of Responses to Pain

Assessment of physiologic and behavioral indications of pain sometimes is difficult, if not impossible, during periods of adaptation. During this time, observable clues to the existence and nature of pain may be absent or minimal. An understanding of adaptation in contrast to the acute pain model will help one avoid the mistaken conclusion that a patient has no pain simply because "he doesn't act as though he has pain" (Fig. 15-2).

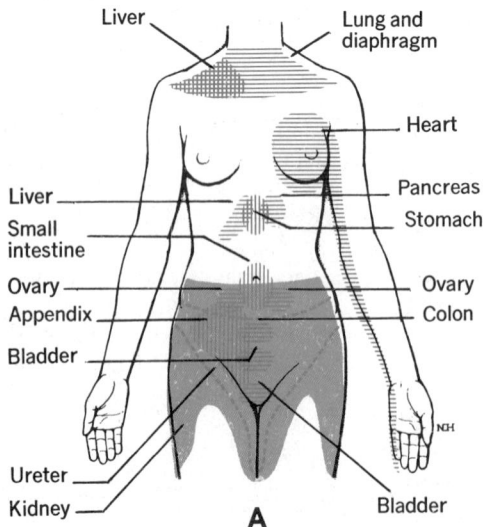
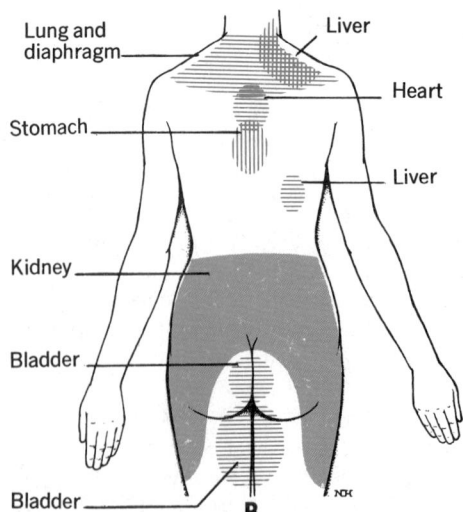

Figure 15-1
Referred pain. (*A*) Anterior view. (*B*) Posterior view. (Chaffee EE and Lytle IM. Basic Physiology and Anatomy, 4th ed. Philadelphia, JB Lippincott, 1980.)

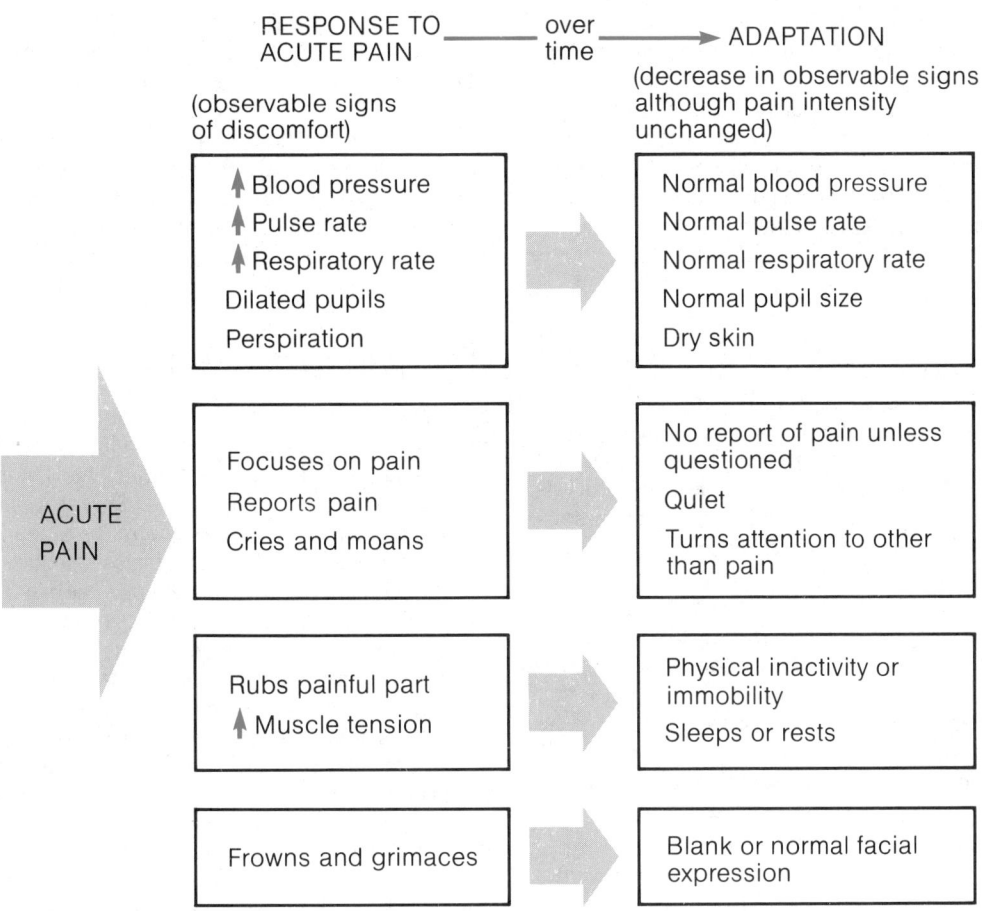

Figure 15-2
Adaptation to acute pain.

Without realizing it, most members of the health care team are familiar only with the acute pain model. It is not unusual for the nurse or physician to doubt the statement of a calm patient who says, "I have severe pain in my right leg." One mistakenly tends to expect *all* patients with pain to exhibit some behavioral or physiologic responses associated with acute pain, including increased pulse and respiratory rates and the occurrence of pallor and perspiration. The patient in acute pain may also cry, moan, frown, immobilize a body part, clench his fist, or withdraw.

The responses a particular patient makes to the sudden onset of acute pain may not be the ones he makes when pain lasts more than a few minutes or when it becomes chronic. Because the body is unable to sustain an intense physiologic reaction to pain for weeks or years, or even several hours, a patient usually responds differently to acute and chronic pain.

Other behavioral manifestations of pain may also change drastically. The fatigue of being in pain may leave the patient too exhausted to moan or cry. He may sleep even with severe pain. Or, the patient may appear relaxed and involved in activities because he has become a master of the art of distracting himself from pain. It is unfortunate when the patient who has succeeded in minimizing the effect of chronic pain on his life is then doubted by others.

Regardless of the type of adjustment made by the patient with chronic pain, pain over an extended period of time often produces behaviors typical of a disability. To some extent,

the patient may be unable to continue the activities and interpersonal relationships he engaged in before pain began. This may range from merely having to curtail his participation in some vigorous sport to being unable to take care of his personal needs, such as undressing.

Assessing the Harmful Effects of Pain

Special emphasis should be placed on assessing the harmful effects of pain. Frequently, the initial effect of a painful sensation is that of a helpful warning signal. Pain warns us that injury has occurred and that efforts must be taken to treat the injury or prevent further injury. After this initial warning signal, the existence of pain becomes a distressing and often harmful experience. Prolonged or chronic pain may prevent rehabilitation from an illness, or the pain itself may become a disability. Prolonged pain may result eventually in depression, persistent fatigue due to the inability to sleep well, weight gain or loss, problems with concentration, job loss, and divorce or other interpersonal problems.

Acute pain may result in problems that delay recovery from the acute illness associated with the pain. Acute pain may disturb the amount and quality of sleep, decrease appetite, reduce fluid intake, and cause nausea and vomiting. For years, rest and nutrition have been recognized as important factors in recovery from illness. When pain interferes with sleep and nutritional intake, the patient is deprived of natural resources for getting well. In addition, the nausea, vomiting, or decreased fluid intake is a potential threat to fluid and electrolyte balance.

Assessing the existence of pain, its nature, and its distressing and harmful effects requires that the nurse ask specific questions and make careful observations. Global, nonspecific questions are not sufficient because patients tend to give incomplete and inaccurate reports of their pain experience unless the nurse asks for details.

Assessment Tools

The initial assessment of pain may be accomplished using the assessment tool in Figure 15-3. If the location of pain is difficult to identify, the drawings in Figure 15-4 may also be used. Once completed, these forms may become a part of the health record. As the nurse gains experience in the assessment of pain, it may be necessary to expand the assessment tool. Chart 15-1 provides guidelines for assessment of the patient with pain.

To the extent possible, the information on the assessment tool should come from the patient. The health record and the patient's family may supplement the information obtained from the patient. However, it is important to remember that only the patient can feel the sensation of pain. Therefore, he is the only one who can rate it. Any verbal or numerical scale can be used as long the same scale is used with that patient each time. The scale suggested on the assessment tool is 0 to 10 (0 = no pain, 10 = worst possible pain).

Preexisting Factors Influencing the Pain Experience

All aspects of the patient's pain experience are subject to the influence of a large number of factors. These factors may increase or decrease the perceived intensity of pain, increase or decrease the patient's tolerance for pain, and elicit one particular set of behavioral responses rather than other possible reactions.

Some are situational, arising from the immediate circumstances. Others, discussed here, were already a part of the patient's physical and emotional makeup prior to the onset of pain. This section focuses on only a few of these preexisting factors that both influence the patient's pain experience *and* interfere with the nurse's understanding of it.

Neurophysiologic Mechanisms of Pain

Specific neuroanatomic structures are involved in the transformation of a stimulus into a sensation perceived as painful by the patient. Unfortunately, this fact leads to the erroneous impression that there is a direct and predictable relationship between a stimulus and the occurrence of pain. As a result, the nurse may expect all patients exposed to the same stimulus (*e.g.*, appendectomy) to experience the same intensity of pain. This is *not* true. Comparable lesions in different patients do not produce the same sensations of pain. A nurse who does not realize this may believe that the patient has pain when he does not or that he has no pain or only slight pain when he is actually experiencing severe pain.

There is lack of agreement about the neurologic mechanisms that underlie a sensation of pain. Currently, the three theories most frequently considered are (1) the specificity theory, (2) the pattern theory, and (3) the gate control theory. These theories are not mutually exclusive, and none is considered entirely accurate or comprehensive. However, each makes a contribution to our understanding of what causes a person to perceive pain following a specific stimulus.

The gate control theory provides a particularly helpful basis for beginning to appreciate the individuality of the pain

---

NAME _____ **DATE** _____

LOCATION: Describe or point to area of pain. _____

_____

QUALITY: What words best describe your pain? _____

_____

INTENSITY: Rate your pain on a scale of 0 (no pain) to 10 (worst pain possible)

      At present _____   1 hour after medication _____

      Worst it gets _____   Best it gets _____

ONSET: When did pain begin? _____   What time of day does it occur? _____

      How often does it occur? _____   How long does it last? _____

EFFECT OF PAIN: What relieves the pain? _____

      What makes the pain worse? _____

      What other problems/symptoms occur with the pain? _____

      How does the pain affect your life and your activities? _____

PLAN:

_____

Figure 15-3
Pain assessment tool.

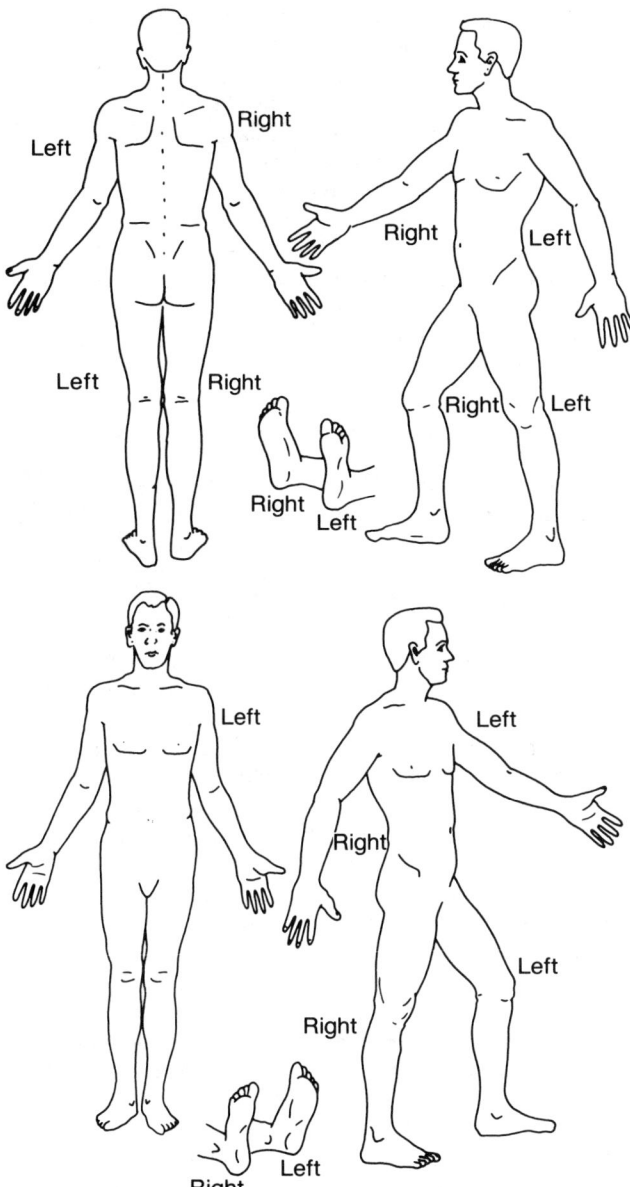

Figure 15-4
Pain assessment. The location of pain is noted and recorded on the figures as appropriate. (Melzack R [ed]. Pain Measurement and Assessment, p 216. New York, Raven Press, 1983.)

Chart 15-1
Guidelines for Assessment of the Patient With Pain

A. Assess the patient's behavioral responses to the pain experience.
   1. Identify whether the pain is acute or chronic.
   2. Identify the phase or phases (anticipation, presence, aftermath) the patient experiences.
   3. During each phase of the pain experience, observe all of the patient's behavioral responses, using the following as a guide:
     a. Physiologic manifestations
     b. Verbal statements
     c. Vocal behaviors
     d. Facial expressions
     e. Body movements
     f. Physical contact with others
     g. Alterations in response to the surrounding environment
     h. Adaptation of physiologic or behavioral responses
   4. Use the patient's behavioral responses to determine the following:
     a. Severity of pain
     b. Tolerance for pain
     c. Characteristics such as location, duration, rhythmicity, and quality
     d. Harmful effects of pain on recovery
     e. What the patient believes will help him with his pain
     f. The patient's concerns about his pain
     g. Any pattern in the patient's behaviors (*i.e.,* behaviors the patient tends to exhibit repeatedly)
B. Assess factors that influence each of the following:
   1. The presence of each phase of the pain experience
   2. The nature of the painful sensation(s)
   3. The patient's behavioral responses, including his concerns and beliefs
C. Identify the phases of the patient's pain experience and the nature of the pain sensation(s), and identify those factors that influence the existence of the phases of the pain experience and the nature of the pain sensation(s).
D. Describe the patient's behavioral responses to each phase of the pain experience, and identify those factors that help to explain why the patient behaves as he does.

---

experience. It suggests that the existence and intensity of pain are dependent on various neurologic activities that include the transmission of signals from the cortex and thalamus. These structures send signals that involve the individual's memories and feelings as well as cultural influences.

Endorphins and Enkephalins

The term *endorphin* is a combination of two words: *endog*enous and mo*rphin*e. It means morphine within. Recently, it has been discovered that the human body manufactures its own supply of endorphins and enkephalins, another mor-

phine-like substance. (*Endorphin* and *enkephalin* are sometimes used interchangeably.) When the body releases these substances, one effect is pain relief.

Endorphins and enkephalins are peptides that are found in heavy concentrations in the central nervous system. These substances relieve pain by the same mechanism as morphine and other narcotics. They are thought to inhibit impulses that would be felt as painful by blocking their transmission in the brain and spinal cord.

The fact that these substances exist in the body has several possible implications in clinical practice. First, it helps explain why different people feel different amounts of pain from comparable stimuli. There are individual differences in endorphin levels as well as certain situational factors, such as anxiety, that influence endorphin levels. Obviously, people with more endorphin feel less pain, and those with less endorphin feel more pain.

Second, certain techniques may relieve pain at least in part because they cause the release of endorphins. Studies have suggested that placebos, acupuncture, and transcutaneous electric nerve stimulation may cause the release of endorphins.

Third, other methods of pain relief, such as mental imagery, may help the patient release his own endorphins.

Cultural Influences

Early in childhood a person begins to learn what those around him expect and accept with respect to painful experiences. For example, the person may learn that an injury sustained during a sports activity is not expected to hurt as much as a comparable injury caused by an unexpected accident. Or, he may learn that the latter warrants a greater expression of pain than the former. From all of his experiences with stimuli he begins to learn from others what stimuli are supposed to be painful and what kind of behavioral responses he should make. The people in his culture teach him this by their behavior toward him. They may ignore, punish, or praise him, depending on his behavior and their beliefs. Since these beliefs vary from one culture to another, it is apparent that patients reporting the same intensity of pain will not necessarily respond to it in the same ways.

Each person learns his own culture's expectations about pain throughout his life. Once these expectations are internalized, they are rarely altered by exposure to the opposing values of other cultures. Consequently, a person tends to grow up believing that his perceptions of and reactions to pain are the only correct and normal ones.

Consider what may happen when a nurse from one culture cares for a patient with pain who comes from another culture. The expectations of the nurse's culture may include avoiding expressions of pain, such as crying and moaning; seeking immediate relief from pain; giving complete descriptions of the pain; and having confidence in the health professions. This nurse may tend to ignore or be skeptical of the patient whose cultural experiences have taught him to moan and complain about pain, to refuse pain relief measures that do not cure the cause of the pain, to use adjectives like "unbearable" in describing his pain, and to be somewhat distrustful of the physician's ability. A patient with still another cultural background may behave differently, or he may behave similarly but for different reasons.

Many other attitudes and behaviors—a patient's preference for having visitors or being alone or his attitude toward his diagnosis—may vary from one culture to another. Recognizing the values of one's own culture and learning how these values differ from those of other cultures help the nurse overcome the tendency to evaluate behavior on the basis of her own cultural expectations. A nurse who appreciates cultural differences will have greater understanding of what the patient is experiencing. Assessment is far more accurate when it takes into account the wide range of possible attitudes and behavioral responses, and measures for pain relief are more effective when the nurse is able to respond to the patient's particular beliefs and values.

It is important to avoid stereotyping a patient and his pain experience and reaction according to his cultural group. Each patient's personal experiences vary. It is more productive to use information about the patient's cultural background to identify those questions that the nurse must ask about every patient. For example, determining whether a patient wants to be alone with his pain, and why, is far more helpful in planning individualized care than assuming that his preferences will always correspond to those of his sociocultural group.

Past Experience With Pain

It is tempting to expect that a person who has had multiple or prolonged experiences with pain will be less anxious and more tolerant of pain than a person who has not experienced much pain. Occasionally, this may be observed, but for the majority of patients, the reverse is true.

Probably the more experience the patient has with pain, the more frightened he will be about subsequent painful events. He may also tend to be less willing to tolerate pain, that is, to want relief from the pain sooner and at lower levels of intensity. This is understandable if we realize that most patients with pain receive unsatisfactory or inadequate pain relief from time to time. Thus, the patient with repeated pain experiences may learn to fear the escalation of pain and the possibility that he will not receive relief. Furthermore, once a patient experiences severe pain, he knows just how bad pain can become. On the other hand, the patient who has never experienced severe pain actually does not know what to be afraid of.

Sometimes the effect of past experience with pain is a result of an accumulation of many separate painful events throughout the patient's life. For other patients, past painful experiences may have been more or less constant, as in prolonged or chronic and persistent pain. The patient who feels pain for months or years may suffer additional effects from this type of past experience and his personality may undergo a change. He may become quite irritable, withdrawn, and depressed, and others may find him unpleasant to be around.

The undesirable effects that may result from past experiences point to the need for the nurse to be aware of all of the patient's experiences with pain. If the patient's pain is relieved promptly and adequately, he may be less fearful of future pain and more able to tolerate it.

Gerontological Considerations

Assessment of pain in the elderly may be difficult because of physiologic, psychological, and social characteristics found in the aged. Older persons may experience reduced sensory perception and increased pain threshold because of degeneration of neurons in the dorsal column of the spinal cord. As a result, they may incur injury without being aware of it or may experience a painful condition in an atypical way. Acute pain may not be as sharply perceived in the elderly, although chronic pain may be more intense. The pain response and pattern may be different from those usually seen in younger patients, or the pain may be referred far from the site of injury or disease.

Although pain is one of the major reasons that many of the elderly seek health care, others are reluctant to seek help even if in severe pain because they think of pain as a problem expected in old age. Others fail to seek care because they fear that the pain may indicate a serious illness or they fear loss of control. The elderly person deals with pain according to his life-style, personality, and cultural background. Many elderly people are very fearful of addiction and as a result will not admit that they are in pain or ask for pain medication.

Contrary to the views of the elderly as well as many health care providers, pain in the elderly is often *more* significant than in younger persons. For example, the onset of persistent headache in the elderly may be a symptom of serious intracranial bleeding.

Nursing Interventions

Basic Care Plan

Once information about the patient is organized, it provides a basis for designing individualized nursing care. *First, the nurse plans to alter factors that influence the nature of the pain sensation and factors that increase the intensity of the patient's behavioral responses to the pain experience.* Of course, some influencing factors cannot or should not be altered. For example, if a painful sensation is being caused by pressure from an inoperable malignancy, it is not possible to alter this factor because the tumor cannot be removed. However, in some cases, positioning, drug therapy, or irradiation may decrease the pressure. The influence of the patient's cultural expectations usually cannot be altered, and no attempt should be made to do so.

Since it may not be possible or desirable to alter some of the patient's responses to his pain experience, *the second part of the nurse's plan of care includes determining appropriate responses to the patient's behaviors and attitudes about pain.* For example, the patient's cultural and personal experiences may have taught him that the preferred and natural response to pain experiences is not to share his feelings and sensations with anyone. Another patient may feel quite the opposite, wanting to describe his feelings and pain in detail. Appropriate and helpful nursing approaches to these two patients will differ markedly.

After examining what can be done to assist the particular patient with his pain experience, *the third phase of the nurse's plan is to select appropriate goals for nursing intervention.* Whenever possible, these goals are shared with the patient. For a few patients, the goal may be total elimination of the painful sensation. For most patients, this is rarely realistic. Other goals may include a decrease in intensity, duration, or frequency of pain and a decrease in the detrimental effects of pain on the patient. For example, pain may decrease appetite or interfere with sleep and thereby retard recovery from an acute illness. Thus, goals may be a good night's sleep and increased intake of nourishing food. Prolonged pain may decrease the quality of life by interfering with work or interpersonal relationships. Thus, a goal may be to decrease time off from work or increase the quality of interpersonal relationships.

These goals may be accomplished by pharmacologic or nonpharmacologic, noninvasive means. In the acute stages of illness, the patient may be a less active participant in pain relief measures, but when the patient has the mental and physical energy, he may learn self-management techniques for pain relief, such as relaxation or imagery. Hence, as the patient progresses through the stages of recovery, a goal may be to decrease reliance on medication for pain relief and increase the patient's use of self-management and noninvasive pain relief measures.

Managing Anxiety Related to Pain

It is well known that anxiety may have a profound influence on the sensation and response to pain. Therefore, anxiety related to the three phases of the pain experience—anticipation, sensation of pain, and aftermath—will be discussed in some detail.

Anticipation Phase. During the anticipation phase of the pain experience, it may be desirable for the patient to have a moderate amount of anxiety about the impending pain so that he will be motivated to find methods of coping with it. It is not unusual for this patient to worry about his anticipated pain some of the time but not all of the time. Usually, this useful level of anxiety results from informing the patient about when his pain will occur, its locations, and the intensity and duration of pain that are expected. The nurse then channels this anxiety into helping the patient learn a variety of pain relief measures (see pp. 250–254).

During the anticipatory phase of pain, teaching the patient about the nature of the impending painful experience and what he can do to obtain relief usually minimizes the anxiety he will have when he actually feels the pain sensation. With this approach, the patient knows that he can do something about the pain when it occurs. Hence, anticipation of pain is less likely to increase anxiety as much as it would if the patient had no knowledge of what to do about the pain. Learning about pain relief measures may give the patient a sense of control over sensations of pain, since he views pain as less threatening.

One of two extremes of reaction sometimes occurs when a patient is taught about a future painful event: intense anxiety or no anxiety. Anxiety-reducing techniques that may be effective with patients who appear to be highly anxious include focusing the patient's attention on a specific problem or eliminating a source of anxiety; for instance, by helping an anxious relative to become less anxious. Administering tranquilizing drugs, if prescribed, or using desensitization, a form of behavior therapy, may be necessary in cases of extreme anxiety.

Desensitization presents information to the patient in a sequence progressing from least to most frightening information. Working with the patient, family, and other members of the health care team, the nurse first constructs a hierarchy of stimuli that are frightening to the patient. She then provides a relaxing and pleasurable environment for the patient, begins talking with him about the least frightening stimulus, and progresses up the hierarchy until the patient shows signs of anxiety. At this point, she reverts to a less frightening stimulus. This process is repeated at intervals until the patient's anxiety about the most frightening stimulus decreases to a moderate level. Occasionally, it may be necessary to postpone a painful event if these measures are not effective in reducing the patient's anxiety to a moderate level.

The person who shows little or no anxiety about impending pain may know from his past experiences that he has a high tolerance for pain. But some patients who show low anxiety or no anxiety are denying the fact that they may have pain. When pain actually occurs, these patients tend to be quite anxious and to have considerable difficulty in coping with pain. What can be done to assist these patients prior to the painful event is largely unknown. We do not yet know with certainty whether it is better to continue to give them information or to give them no information. When giving the patient specific information about pain does not result in moderate anxiety, further information probably should be brief, essential, and general. Emphasis should be placed on pain relief measures.

When the nurse suspects that the patient's lack of anxiety reflects an effort to deny information he receives about pain, she explores with the patient whether he wants more information about either pain or its relief. It appears that his decision should be respected. However, the patient should be closely observed for a marked increase in anxiety as the time approaches for the painful event to occur. The previous suggestions regarding interactions with patients with moderate and severe anxiety can then be employed, depending on the level of anxiety noted.

At times, the nurse may be tempted not to tell a patient that he may experience pain or that the pain may be much greater than he seems to think. She may reason that such knowledge will make him anxious. Indeed, she may be correct. The prospect of pain usually arouses some anxiety in the patient. However, if the patient is to learn ways of coping with pain, he must first know that pain may occur. Failure to forewarn the patient of pain is probably a mistake *unless* one of the following conditions exists: (1) previous experience shows that forewarning this patient produces such a high level of uncontrollable anxiety that the patient is unable to take positive steps toward learning to handle his pain; (2) the patient specifically requests that he not be forewarned, and this request has been thoroughly explored with the patient; or (3) previous experience shows that teaching this patient about pain and its relief impedes his coping mechanism of denial and that he has no other effective mechanism for coping with stress.

What the nurse tells the patient about the pain relief measures available and their effectiveness may also be relevant to the anxiety component of the patient's pain experience. The nurse may prevent an increase in anxiety by explaining briefly to the patient the general type of pain relief he can expect from each pain relief measure. For example, if the patient expects distraction or medication to eliminate his pain totally, his anxiety may increase when this does not happen. These pain relief measures along with many others frequently do not eliminate the pain completely or even reduce its intensity. Instead they tend to increase the patient's tolerance for pain or render pain much less bothersome to the patient.

The Sensation of Pain. During the time when pain sensations are felt by the patient, it is desirable to reduce the patient's anxiety to as low a level as possible. When the patient is anxious about his pain, there is a tendency for him to perceive a greater intensity of pain or to be less tolerant of the pain. This in turn produces greater anxiety. Thus, a spiraling process is initiated in which the patient becomes more anxious and experiences greater pain or becomes progressively less tolerant of pain.

Obviously, it is important to interrupt this process as soon as possible. Low levels of anxiety or pain are easier to reduce or control than are higher levels. Consequently, *pain relief measures should be utilized before pain becomes severe.* Many patients believe that they should not request pain relief measures until pain approaches or exceeds the maximum level they are able to tolerate. Therefore, it is important to explain to all patients that pain relief or control is more successful if pain relief measures are used before pain becomes unbearable.

Anxiety during the anticipatory and sensation phases of the pain experience may be managed effectively by establishing a relationship with the patient with pain and by patient teaching (see Nurse–Patient Relationship and Teaching). Almost all nursing interventions for pain relief contribute in some way toward utilizing anxiety or decreasing anxiety.

Aftermath. During the aftermath phase of pain, when the pain sensation subsides, it is hoped that the patient's anxiety also will subside. When this does not happen, certain techniques may help the patient to integrate the pain experience (see Table 15-1).

For many patients, the experience of pain continues after the sensation of pain ceases or subsides. Some patients continue to fear pain simply because they do not know that there is no longer any danger that pain will occur. Conveying to the patient that the noxious stimuli have been removed or decreased helps prevent him from anxiously expecting pain to continue or to occur again shortly.

Most patients do not simply forget about a painful experience as soon as pain is no longer felt or anticipated. The patient may be disturbed about his behavior during the pain experience or he may be concerned about how others view his responses. He may have unclear and somewhat frightening ideas about the cause of his pain or the treatment for it. His general sense of personal safety and control may be shaken by his having felt more intense pain than he had ever imagined was possible. The patient who is relieved of chronic pain actually may experience an identity crisis, fearing what he will be like without his pain. In the aftermath phase, the patient also may suddenly begin trembling or perspiring. He may have nausea, vomiting, or chills. Some patients have nightmares about a painful experience for weeks and months after it is over. Obviously, the care of the patient with pain, especially the management of anxiety, extends beyond the anticipation and sensation phases of pain into this aftermath phase to help him cope with these reactions.

Noninvasive Pain Relief Measures

Because of the lack of knowledge or time, many patients and health team members tend to regard analgesics as the major method of pain relief. However, there are many nursing activities that can be used to assist the patient with his pain experience. Various categories of such nursing activities are outlined in Table 15-1.

The purpose of the table is to introduce the nurse to the variety of nursing activities that may be used to help patients with their pain experiences. This brief synopsis is intended to introduce these measures. For help in acquiring additional knowledge, the nurse is referred to more complete sources

TABLE 15-1
Nursing Activities to Assist the Patient With His Pain Experience

Category of Nursing Activity	*Explanation*	*Example of Nursing Activity*
1. Establishing a relationship with the patient with pain	Interacting with the patient as a total person, believing what he says he experiences, and respecting his reactions and attitudes regarding pain (see text)	Telling the patient you believe what he says about his pain experience
2. Teaching the patient about pain and its relief	Using a variety of the patient's sensory modalities for the purpose of conveying to him information about his pain experience (see text)	Explaining the quality and location of impending pain by applying pressure and pulling the skin in the area where the patient will have an incision
3. Using the patient–group situation	Using the principles of small group functioning to teach the patient and his family about the patient's pain experience	The nurse, two female patients with arthritis, and their husbands discussing modifications in homemaking activities following discharge from the hospital
4. Managing other people who come in contact with the patient	Assisting other people to reach their maximum potential for helping the patient with his pain experience	Talking alone with a patient's wife who shows marked anxiety in the presence of her husband when he complains of his undiagnosed abdominal pain
5. Using cutaneous stimulation	Using various qualities, locations, durations, and intensities of stimuli in contact with the skin (see text)	Applying a hand-held vibrator to the scalp and back of the neck to relieve headache
6. Providing distraction from pain	Obtaining the patient's response to and participation in stimuli through the major sensory modalities (see text)	Helping the patient to use chant with breathing during a painful dressing change
7. Promoting relaxation	Using a variety of techniques to assist the patient to avoid fatigue and to achieve skeletal muscle relaxation	Helping the patient learn to use slow, rhythmic breathing
8. Using guided imagery	Assisting the patient to imagine a pleasant event as a substitute for the pain experience or to imagine a means of ridding his body of the pain (see text)	Helping the patient imagine that he is ridding himself of pain as he exhales slowly
9. Administering pharmacologic agents	Giving medications with pain-relieving potential to the patient and explaining the effects; assisting the physician in determining the patient's need for analgesics (see text)	Administering analgesics on a preventive basis
10. Decreasing noxious stimuli	Using a variety of techniques to reduce the transmission of pain signals to the cortex of the brain	Splinting an abdominal incision during coughing and deep breathing
11. Using the assistance of professionals	Assisting the patient, his family, and his physician to identify the need for additional help in dealing with pain; assisting the patient and his family to obtain this help and to use it to their best advantage	Suggesting to the patient that his clergyman may be able to counsel him about his concern (reduce his anxiety) that his pain is punishment for a sin
12. Being with the patient	Identifying and responding to the patient who would benefit from the mere presence of the nurse or someone else	Getting a hospital volunteer to sit at the bedside of the patient who does not want to be alone with his pain experience

(continued)

TABLE 15-1 *(continued)*

Category of Nursing Activity	Explanation	Example of Nursing Activity
13. Conveying that the source of noxious stimuli has been removed or decreased	Conveying to the patient, when appropriate, that something has been done to diminish or eliminate a cause of his pain (see text)	Telling the patient that the needle for his lumbar puncture has just been removed and all that remains is to cleanse his back
14. Assisting with the assimilation of the painful experience	Identifying the patient's need for and assisting him with the intellectual and emotional incorporation of a painful experience (see text)	Discussing with the patient what sensations he felt and what he was thinking while experiencing his myocardial infarction on the previous day

(Adapted from McCaffery M. Nursing Management of the Patient with Pain, 2nd ed. Philadelphia, JB Lippincott)

of information (see Bibliography). Through reading and practice, the nurse may easily learn to use these activities with patients.

Some of the noninvasive nursing activities listed in Table 15-1 will be discussed here in more detail. "Noninvasive" simply means that no physical or bodily intrusion is involved. Noninvasive methods of pain relief entail very low risks, compared with analgesics. Although noninvasive pain relief measures are not necessarily a substitute for analgesics, for brief episodes of pain lasting only seconds or minutes, a noninvasive technique may be all that is necessary or appropriate. In other instances, especially when there is severe pain that lasts for hours or days, the use of some noninvasive techniques along with medications may be the most effective way to relieve pain.

Nurse–Patient Relationship and Teaching

The two pain relief measures basic to all others are the nurse–patient relationship and patient teaching about pain and its relief. These activities may reduce pain in the absence of any other pain relief measures. Certainly, each may enhance the effectiveness of all other pain relief measures used with the patient. Certain aspects of the relationship and teaching serve to reduce the patient's anxiety about pain, and, as was indicated earlier, reducing anxiety commonly results in pain relief, either by decreasing the intensity of pain or by rendering the pain more tolerable to the patient.

Trust is an important aspect of the nurse–patient relationship. Conveying to the patient that his complaints about his pain are believed can help reduce his anxiety. Some patients spend considerable time and energy trying to convince others that they have pain. The presence of pain may be doubted by others because no cause can be found for it or because the person's behavior is not "typical" of what the health care team expects. To say to a patient, "I know you have pain (or discomfort); I only want to understand it better," often will set the patient's mind at rest. Occasionally, a patient who has feared that no one will believe him will become tearful with gratitude and relief when he knows that he can trust the nurse and that she believes him.

Whenever she encounters a patient with pain, the nurse must convey to the patient that she cares about helping him obtain pain relief. The patient may not know where to turn for help in relieving the pain; it is seldom that anyone on the health care team is explicitly responsible for providing pain relief. However, when the nurse says very simply, "Let me know when you begin to hurt so I can help you do something about it," she conveys to the patient that she cares and assumes responsibility for helping with his pain.

The nurse also provides information, through patient teaching, about how pain can be controlled. The patient needs to know, for example, that pain should be reported in the early stages. When the patient waits too long before reporting it, the pain may be intense and his anxiety may be very high. It is much easier to prevent severe pain and panic than to relieve them once they occur.

Cutaneous Stimulation

According to the gate control theory, stimulation of large-diameter nerve fibers in the skin may reduce the intensity of pain. Skin stimulation may also cause the release of endorphins. Such skin stimulation can be accomplished in a variety of ways. In devising methods of cutaneous stimulation for pain relief, the nurse considers which quality of stimulation is to be used and the location, duration, and intensity of stimulation. The approach is one of trial and error, but common sense often is an effective guide.

Various qualitites of cutaneous stimulation are easily available at low cost. Although some form of cutaneous stimulation is usually acceptable, consultation with the patient's physician may be necessary for some and other forms may be contraindicated because of the patient's condition. Different types of skin sensations may be elicited when the following measures are applied: pressure, vibration, heat, cold, bathing, lotion, menthol cream, and transcutaneous electric nerve stimulation (TENS). Although TENS is not as readily available as the other measures, it has proven to be very helpful in both acute and chronic pain relief, and its use is becoming more widespread. It consists of a battery-operated unit with electrodes that are applied to the skin to produce a tingling, vibrating, or buzzing sensation in the area of pain (Fig. 15-5.)

Local application of cold to a painful part is an underused but often highly effective method of relieving pain. Compared with local applications of heat, cold relieves pain faster and has a longer carryover effect. Contrary to popular belief, cold does not necessarily cause muscle contraction but slows the conduction of impulses that maintain muscle tone and may

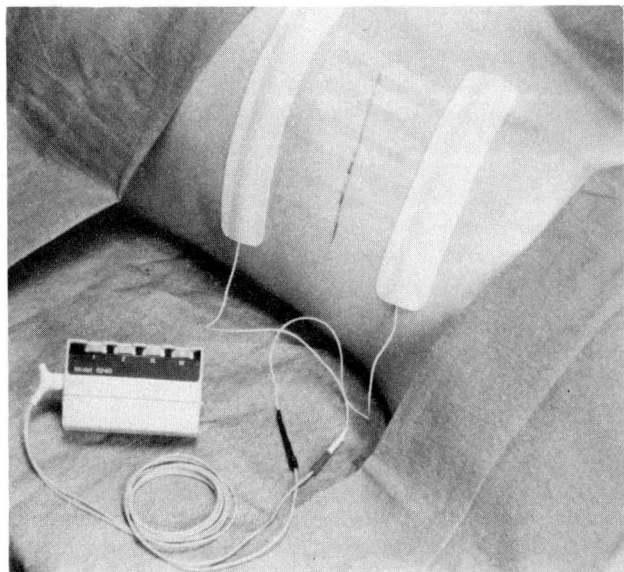

Figure 15-5
Transcutaneous electric nerve stimulation (TENS) being used for relief of incisional pain postoperatively. (Courtesy of Health Care Specialties Division/3M, St. Paul, Minnesota.)

cause muscle relaxation. Therefore, cold is not only indicated to decrease bleeding and swelling of a new injury but also may be continued for pain relief.

When cutaneous stimulation is employed, it is applied to different areas of the body. Usually, stimulating the skin on or near the pain site is effective. In other instances, direct stimulation over the pain site must be avoided because it elicits more pain. If stimulation of the skin near the pain site is ineffective or painful, the side of the body opposite the painful area may be stimulated for pain relief. This is called *contralateral stimulation.* For example, the pain of "tennis elbow" on the left side may be relieved as well or better by applying menthol cream to the right elbow rather than the left. This is especially helpful to remember when the site of pain is difficult to stimulate directly, such as when a thick cast has been applied over a painful area or when the entire extremity is injured or burned.

The appropriate intensity of stimulation to be applied is generally moderate. Mild stimulation tends to be ticklish or annoying, whereas intense stimulation may cause pain.

In general, the duration of cutaneous stimulation indicated and the intervals between its applications vary considerably. Some patients experience pain relief for hours or days following cutaneous stimulation. Others obtain relief only while stimulation is being applied. For these patients, use of a menthol cream or a TENS unit is an efficient means of providing continuous stimulation without hampering activity. It takes only a few minutes to apply, but the stimulation lasts for hours. The TENS unit may be worn 24 hours a day.

Distraction

Distraction, or focusing the patient's attention away from his painful sensations, may be an effective method of pain relief.

It may decrease the perceived intensity of pain, but usually it increases tolerance for pain, making pain less bothersome. Pain tends to draw attention to itself; but if the person is less aware of pain or pays less attention to it, he will be less bothered by pain and more tolerant of it.

There are many degrees and types of distraction, ranging from simply preventing monotony to the use of highly complicated physical and mental activity. When environmental stimuli are deficient in amount, patterning, or variation, the person's centrally regulated thresholds for sensation tend to be lowered. This allows the person to use more of the available input, and he becomes more sensitive to input such as pain and other sensations.

If the patient with pain is experiencing some form of sensory restriction, pain relief may result when the nurse provides environmental stimuli. This is a mild form of distraction that focuses the patient's attention away from his painful sensations. The distraction may involve minimizing strange noises, making brief but frequent visits to the patient, bringing him a snack, or teaching him physical exercises appropriate to his condition. The latter is a particularly effective method of reducing the effects of sensory restriction.

More deliberate and intense forms of sensory stimulation may be necessary to distract the patient from brief episodes of increased pain, such as pain from bone marrow aspiration or wound debridement, or longer periods of moderate to severe intensities of pain. Some patients are able to use distraction for hours.

The value of distraction techniques for pain relief is frequently misunderstood by the health care team. A common misconception is that the patient who can be distracted from his pain does not have as much pain as he wants others to believe. For example, the nurse may erroneously assume that the patient cannot have pain if he is laughing and talking with visitors. However, distraction is a powerful method of pain relief. Doubting the patient's pain because he uses distraction effectively may result in the patient's discarding this effective way to cope with pain.

The effectiveness of distraction depends on the degree to which the patient is able to receive and create sensory input other than pain. As a rule, pain relief is increased in direct relation to the patient's active participation, the number of sensory modalities used, and the patient's interest in the stimuli. Therefore, seeing, hearing, and keeping a box score of a baseball game will distract the patient from his pain more than would only one or two of these activities. If the patient prefers baseball to football, stimuli related to baseball will distract him from pain more than stimuli associated with football.

Increasing the complexity of the distractor as pain increases will be effective in pain relief, however, only up to a certain level of pain intensity. With severe pain, the patient may be unable to concentrate well enough to engage in highly complicated mental or physical activities.

Many patients devise their own distraction strategies. The patient may hum, mentally calculate math problems, or choose an absorbing television program. The nurse may support these efforts and assist the patient to elaborate on them.

Under conditions of brief, severe pain, it may be effective to teach the patient a distraction strategy. A technique that may be taught quickly, even to patients who are debilitated, fatigued, sedated, or in severe pain, is to combine rhythmic rubbing with visual concentration. The patient is asked to open his eyes, stare at a specific spot on the wall or ceiling, and rub a part of his body. The rubbing may be done initially by the nurse. Then the nurse may take the patient's hand and guide him in doing the rubbing. Rubbing with a firm, circular motion on bare skin seems to be effective. The rubbing and staring involve a steady source of sensory input through visual and tactile-kinesthetic modalities along with a focus of rhythm. If this is not distracting enough, the patient can be instructed to add another activity, such as breathing in and out slowly. The patient may chant silently to himself, "Breathe in slowly, breathe out slowly." Sensory input through several modalities combined with rhythm and a focus on breathing are common characteristics of successful distraction techniques.

Another distraction technique that is very useful with patients who are fatigued or sedated, or when pain lasts longer than several minutes, is "active listening." The patient may use a tape recorder with an earphone or headset, select a cassette of fast music, and listen to the music, while keeping time by tapping his finger or nodding his head. For visual input, he can focus on an object or close his eyes and imagine something about the music, such as dancing to the music. When the pain increases, the patient can increase the volume; when pain decreases, he decreases the volume. For example, a burned patient undergoing a painful dressing change might use this method of distraction to make the painful experience more tolerable.

Relaxation

Skeletal muscle relaxation may reduce the intensity of pain or increase pain tolerance. It can also be combined with other pain relief measures, such as analgesics or a heating pad, to enhance their effectiveness. Many people learn relaxation techniques for the purpose of dealing with life stresses. Community agencies offer adult education programs in transcendental meditation, yoga, hypnosis, music therapy, and a variety of other potentially relaxing activities. If a patient already knows a technique for relaxing, the nurse may need only suggest that he use it to reduce or to prevent increased pain.

Almost all patients with chronic pain need to learn some method of relaxing and to employ it on a regular basis several times a day. Regular periods of relaxation are needed to combat the fatigue and muscle tension that occur with chronic pain and decrease pain tolerance or increase the intensity of the pain.

A simple relaxation technique for patients with acute or chronic pain consists of abdominal breathing at a slow, rhythmic rate. The patient may close his eyes and breathe slowly and comfortably (not too deeply) at about 6 to 9 breaths per minute. The patient can maintain a constant rhythm by counting silently and slowly to himself as he inhales ("in, 2, 3") and as he exhales ("out, 2, 3"). The patient concludes this relaxation technique by taking another deep breath. When the nurse is teaching this technique to the patient, it is helpful to count out loud for him at first. Initially the patient may benefit from keeping his eyes open as the nurse breathes in coordination with him.

Slow, rhythmic breathing may also be used as a distraction technique. However, it may require practice before the patient becomes skillful in using it.

A quick and easy method of helping the tense patient with severe pain to relax is to give the following instructions: "Clench your fists; breathe in deeply and hold it a moment. As you breathe out, feel yourself go limp. Now start yawning."

Guided Imagery

Therapeutic guided imagery may be defined as the use of one's imagination in an especially designed manner to achieve a specific positive effect. In this instance, the effects desired are relaxation and pain relief. Imagery of various types is capable of altering body functions over which we seem to have no direct or conscious control. Most people have experienced this in the form of increased cardiac rate (pounding heart) or perspiration when a distressing mental image comes to mind just before falling asleep. Although images of this sort seem to provoke a stresss response, certain other images seem to evoke relaxation responses or pain relief. A considerable amount of the nurse's time is usually required to teach and explain the technique of guided imagery. The patient, too, must invest time and energy in practicing it. For these reasons, guided imagery most often is taught to patients with chronic pain, although it is effective with acute pain as well. To learn to use guided imagery, the patient must be able to concentrate, use his imagination, and follow directions. It is not advisable to try to teach it when the patient is fatigued, sedated, or in severe pain. One simple form of therapeutic guided imagery for relaxation and pain relief consists of combining the slow rhythmic breathing described as a relaxation technique with a mental image of relaxation and comfort. With eyes closed, the patient imagines that each time he exhales slowly he is breathing out muscle tension and discomfort, leaving behind a relaxed and comfortable body. Each time he inhales, he can imagine that the air sends healing energy to the area of discomfort. Each time he exhales, he can imagine that the air floats away from his body, carrying with it the pain and tension. It enters the body again immediately, in a purified state, and can be circulated to the area of discomfort again.

Usually, the patient is asked to practice guided imagery for about 5 minutes, three times a day. Several days of practice may elapse before the patient finds that he can reduce the intensity of pain through this technique. Pain relief can continue for hours after the imagery is used. Most patients begin to experience the relaxing effects of guided imagery the first time they try it.

Medications for Pain Relief

Whether pain is acute or chronic, certain guidelines are useful when medications are indicated for the relief of pain. Usually, medications are most effective when a preventive approach is used and when the dose and interval between doses is individualized to meet the patient's needs. The only safe and effective way to administer narcotics is to observe the patient's response.

Preventive Approach

Using a preventive approach to pain relief means that medications (analgesics in particular) are given before the pain occurs, if it can be predicted, or at least before it reaches a severe intensity. If the patient's pain is expected to occur daily for a great portion of the 24-hour period, a regular schedule around the clock may be indicated. Even if the analgesic is prescribed "as needed" or "prn," the nurse can administer the analgesic on a preventive basis before it is needed as long as the prescribed interval between doses is observed. This is preferable to the usual approach to a prn request, which may require that the patient have intense pain before requesting and receiving his medication.

A preventive approach has many advantages. It usually takes a smaller dose to alleviate mild pain or prevent the occurrence of pain than it does to relieve severe pain. Thus, a preventive approach may result in a lower total 24-hour dose. This helps prevent tolerance to analgesics and decreases the severity of side-effects such as sedation and constipation. Furthermore, pain relief can be more complete with a preventive approach. For example, there need not be any peaks of severe pain and the patient spends less time in pain. On a prn approach to pain relief, the patient usually experiences pain, obtains his analgesic, and waits for it to take effect. Within a 24-hour period, this may result in his spending a total of several hours in pain.

Better pain control achieved with a preventive approach may reduce the likelihood of the patient's craving the drug. Some health care team members seem to feel that the frugal use of narcotics will help prevent addiction in the patient with acute pain. However, there is no basis for this belief. Certainly, a patient who is in pain and has his analgesic withheld is more likely to crave the medication than the patient whose pain is relieved before it becomes distressing to him.

Individualized Doses

Individualizing the dose and the interval between doses is necessary because patients metabolize and absorb medications at different rates and because adjustments are required for varying intensities of pain. It should not be surprising that a certain dosage of a narcotic given at specified intervals would be effective for one patient but totally inappropriate for another. However, too often analgesics, especially narcotics, are prescribed and given in a very standardized, inflexible manner. The nurse must remember that there are no magic numbers for milligrams or for hours between doses. For example, when a patient metabolizes 100 mg of meperidine (Demerol) intramuscularly (IM) in 2 hours, it should be understood that this is a well-documented physiologic phenomenon, not a drug abuse problem.

Because of the fear of promoting addiction or causing respiratory depression, there is a trend toward underusing narcotics in the treatment of acute pain or prolonged pain in the terminally ill. The result is much needless suffering. Even prolonged administration of a narcotic is associated with less than 3% incidence of addiction. Furthermore, small doses are not necessarily safe doses. Patients receiving 25 mg to 50 mg of meperidine IM have experienced life-threatening respiratory depression, while other patients have not exhibited any sedation or respiratory depression after 200 mg of meperidine IM.

Therefore, it is mandatory for purposes of safety and pain relief that the effects of narcotics be observed, especially when a narcotic is given for the first time to a patient or when

a change is made in dosage or frequency. A simple way to make these observations is to maintain a flow sheet, noting time and date, pain rating (scale of 0–10), the pain relief measure, side-effects, and patient activity. At regular intervals, such as every hour following an IM injection, the patient is asked to rate his pain on a scale of 0 to 10. Respiratory rate is also noted, along with other physiologic changes of concern. For example, when a postoperative patient is given the first dose of meperidine, 75 mg IM, a pain rating and respiratory rate, along with other relevant physiologic parameters, should be noted. If 1 hour later the pain rating has not decreased, the patient is reasonably alert, and the respiratory status, blood pressure, and pulse rate are satisfactory, some change in analgesia is indicated. The meperidine dose is safe for this patient but does not relieve the pain. Another dose of meperidine may be indicated.

Gerontological Considerations

Physiologic changes in the elderly make it important to administer analgesics with caution. Drug interactions are more of a possibility in the elderly because of the higher incidence of chronic illness and increased use of prescription and over-the-counter drugs. Before administering narcotic and nonnarcotic analgesics to the elderly, it is important to obtain a careful drug history to identify potential harmful drug interactions.

Absorption and metabolism of drugs are altered in the elderly patient because of decreased liver, renal, and gastrointestinal function. In addition, changes in body weight, protein stores, and distribution of body fluid alter the distribution of drugs in the body. As a result, drugs are not metabolized as quickly and blood levels of the drug remain higher for a longer period of time. The patient is more sensitive to drugs and is at increased risk of drug toxicity.

Narcotic and nonnarcotic analgesics can be given effectively to the elderly but must be used cautiously because of increased susceptibility to depression of the nervous system and respiratory system. Meperidine must be used with particular caution because decreased binding of the drug by plasma proteins results in blood concentrations of the drug twice those found in younger patients. Because the elderly are generally more sensitive to analgesics, it is advisable to begin with a smaller dose of a nonnarcotic analgesic first, increasing the dose slowly, and adding additional drugs carefully. Frequent monitoring is necessary for safe, effective pain relief.

Routes of Administration for Moderate to Severe Pain

The route of administration of analgesics selected is based on the patient's condition and desired effect of the drug. For moderate to severe pain, the most common routes of administration of a narcotic are the intramuscular or subcutaneous routes. Parenteral administration of the medication produces more rapid analgesic effects than oral administration, but these effects are of shorter duration. Intravenous or rectal routes of administration may also be indicated if the patient is not permitted any oral intake or is vomiting. Postoperative pain, for example, has been effectively relieved with rectal suppositories of 10 mg of oxymorphone (Numorphan; two suppositories, totaling 10 mg, provide analgesia equivalent to that of 10 mg of morphine intramuscularly or 75 mg of meperidine intramuscularly). The rectal route may be indicated for patients with bleeding problems, such as hemophilia.

Intravenous narcotics may be administered by "push" (or "slow push," *e.g.,* over a 5- to 10-minute period) or by continuous drip using an infusion pump. The latter provides a more steady level of analgesia and is indicated when pain is to be controlled over a 24-hour period, such as postoperatively for the first day or so, or in a patient with prolonged cancer pain who cannot take medication by mouth. Preliminary studies show that the majority of patients do not absorb meperidine IM well during the first 8 hours postoperatively and that the intravenous (IV) route may be much safer and more effective in relieving pain. The amount of narcotic administered intravenously is calculated carefully to relieve pain without producing respiratory depression and other side-effects.

If the patient can take medication by mouth, this route is preferred to all others since it is easy, noninvasive, and not painful, as are injections. Severe pain can be relieved with oral narcotics *if* the doses are high enough. Certainly, patients with prolonged pain should receive analgesics orally rather than by injection if at all possible. Many narcotics can be given effectively by mouth for severe pain. However, to be effective, dosage must be altered because of differences in absorption of drugs given by different routes. Oral doses of narcotics that are equal to 10 mg of morphine or 75 mg of meperidine given intramuscularly are 10 to 20 mg of methadone; 30 to 60 mg of morphine; and 4 to 8 mg of hydromorphone (Dilaudid). In terminally ill patients with prolonged pain, doses may gradually become much higher owing to increased pain or tolerance to analgesia. In the majority of these patients, the higher doses provide additional pain relief (*i.e.,* there is no ceiling on the analgesia of the powerful narcotics) and the higher doses are not lethal (the patient is tolerant to respiratory depression and sedation as well as analgesia). If the patient's medication is changed from a parenteral dose to an oral narcotic at a dose that is not equivalent in strength (equianalgesic), the lesser dose of oral narcotic may result in a withdrawal reaction and the reappearance of pain and anxiety.

New Routes and Approaches to Pain Management

Recent attention to the problem of acute and chronic pain has led to the development of new methods of pain relief. Newer methods of delivering analgesics include intraspinal infusion and patient-controlled analgesia.

Intraspinal Infusion of Analgesics.   Intraspinal infusion of narcotics or local anesthetic agents has been effective in pain control in postoperative patients as well as those with chronic pain unrelieved by usual methods of pain relief. A catheter is inserted by the physician into the subarachnoid or epidural space in the thoracic or lumbar region for administration of narcotics or local anesthetics. Repeated infusion of these agents through the catheter results in pain relief without many of the side-effects of systemic analgesia, including sedation.

If analgesics are needed for a longer period of time or if the patient has chronic, terminal disease, the catheter may be tunneled through the subcutaneous tissue and the inlet or port is placed under the skin in the abdominal region. The narcotic analgesic is injected through the skin into the outlet or port and catheter, which delivers the medication directly into the subarachnoid or epidural space. This method may require injection of the narcotic several times a day to maintain an adequate level of pain relief.

In those patients who are likely to require more frequent doses or continuous infusions of narcotics to keep them pain free, an implantable infusion device may be used to administer the narcotic continuously. The dose of narcotic is administered at a small, constant dose at a preset rate into the epidural or subarachnoid space. The infusion device has a reservoir that stores the medication for slow release and needs to be refilled once every 1 or 2 months depending on the patient's needs. This eliminates the need for repeated injections through the skin and reduces the number of trips to the hospital for frequent injections.

Very small doses of narcotic analgesics can be administered by these methods to block pain pathways with little effect on pulse, respiration, or blood pressure. The shortcomings of intramuscular administration of narcotic analgesia, such as delay in pain relief and need for frequent injections, are eliminated. Adverse side-effects such as respiratory depression and sedation are reduced because of the small doses given by these methods. However, the patient must be monitored very closely when the loading dose of the medication is given, to detect respiratory depression. Delayed onset of respiratory depression has been reported with use of intraspinal analgesia; therefore, the patient must be monitored and narcotic antagonists such as naloxone (Narcan) should be available for administration to reverse respiratory depression if it occurs.

Patient-Controlled Analgesia.   Patient-controlled analgesia has been used effectively with postoperative patients. This method of pain management allows the patient to control his own intravenous medication within a predetermined time and dose using an automated and preloaded pump system. This results in a more consistent level of analgesia with few side-effects. Although the drug is under the patient's control within safety limits to prevent inadvertently administering an overdose, the amount of medication administered by the patient has not been greater than in traditional methods of pain relief. Pulmonary complications have been less frequent and patients have been more alert with this system.

Drug Preferences

With both acute and chronic pain, it is wise to use aspirin, acetaminophen (*e.g.,* Tylenol, Datril), or the more potent nonsteroidal anti-inflammatory drugs (NSAIDs), such as ibuprofen (Motrin), to the extent possible. These drugs provide nonnarcotic analgesia without the unpleasant sedation and constipation that so often accompany narcotics. Furthermore, when narcotics are necessary, it is logical to give the nonnarcotic analgesic concurrently because the effect decreases the dosage of narcotic needed. Also, aspirin, acetaminophen, and NSAIDs produce analgesia by action at the peripheral nervous system level to relieve pain, whereas narcotics act primarily at the central nervous system level.

Chronic pain is often accompanied by depression. Therefore, the use of tricyclic antidepressants may be considered. These drugs have a sedative effect and may be given at bedtime; therefore, they assist in relieving sleep disturbances, a common problem in depression and chronic pain. Because these drugs have an analgesic effect after 10 days of regular administration, the patient may receive an added benefit of nonnarcotic analgesia.

Probably the most commonly prescribed injectable narcotic is meperidine. However, there are several indications that this practice should be reevaluated. Meperidine is short acting and very irritating to the tissues; therefore, adequate pain control may require frequent (every 2 to 3 hours) injections of an irritating substance. Furthermore, meperidine is more toxic than was previously recognized. Neuropsychiatric effects, such as disorientation, bizarre feelings, and hallucinations, are relatively intense with parenteral meperidine. Accumulation of the metabolite normeperidine, as a result of multiple doses of meperidine, especially in patients with renal failure, can result in excitatory effects, such as twitching, irritability, and seizures. These problems have not been observed with morphine, which is an acceptable alternative to meperidine.

Another potential problem is the common practice of giving so-called potentiators with narcotics. Those most frequently prescribed for parenteral administration are promethazine (Phenergan) and hydroxyzine (Vistaril). Studies and clinical practice have shown that promethazine is highly sedating; it is not a potentiator of narcotic analgesia but instead is a potentiator of respiratory depression and hypotension, and it may even increase the perceived intensity of pain. Hydroxyzine, by contrast, may have some analgesic properties but is extremely irritating and painful when given intramuscularly. It must be given by the Z-track method (see p. 675). There probably are no potentiators of narcotic analgesia. Most of the time analgesia is best achieved with drugs known to be analgesics—the narcotics and nonnarcotics. However, potentiators may have some use in decreasing the nausea that often occurs with pain and meperidine.

Patient Education and Home Health Care

Acute Pain.   The patient who has experienced acute pain as a result of injury, illness, procedure, or surgery often fears its recurrence once he is discharged from the hospital. Fear and anticipation of pain are further increased because nurses, physicians, and pain relief are less available to the patient for control of pain in the home. The patient may leave the hospital with the expectation that the pain will not recur and is very frightened if it returns unexpectedly or persists longer than expected. In preparation for hospital discharge, the patient and family members receive instruction and guidance about what type of pain or discomfort to expect, how long that discomfort is expected to last, and when the pain or discomfort signals a problem that should be reported. Additionally, they are prepared for home care by guidance about medication to be used in case of pain as well as its side-effects. The patient is reminded that those pain relief strategies

that were effective in the hospital can be used at home. The nurse gives support and reassurance to the patient and family that pain can be successfully managed at home.

Chronic Pain.   Inadequate control of pain in the outpatient is a common cause of readmission to the hospital. If chronic pain was the primary reason for the patient's initial hospitalization, the anxiety and fear of the patient and family are multiplied when the patient is about to return home. The patient and family are instructed in the techniques of pain assessment and administration of pain medications. These instructions are given verbally and in writing, and opportunities are provided for the patient and family member to practice administration of the medication until they are comfortable and confident with the procedure. They are instructed how to monitor respiratory status and to recognize central nervous system depression and other side-effects of narcotic and nonnarcotic analgesics. If the medications cause other predictable effects such as constipation, the patient and family are instructed about its treatment and prevention so that pain relief is not interrupted to resolve the problem.

If the patient is to receive analgesics at home by intramuscular or subcutaneous injection or intravenous or intraspinal infusions, a referral to a community health nurse is indicated. The community health nurse visits the patient in the home after discharge to assess the patient, to determine if the patient and family are carrying out the pain management program effectively, and if indicated, to evaluate the injection or infusion technique used by the patient and family for accuracy and safety. If the patient has an implanted infusion pump in place, the nurse examines the condition of the pump or injection site and may refill the reservoir with medication as prescribed by the physician or supervise family members in the procedure. The community health nurse assesses the patient for changes in his need for analgesic medications. She assists the patient and family in altering the medication dose in collaboration with the patient's physician. She supports and encourages the patient and family members to use noninvasive pain management techniques to supplement analgesic therapy. These efforts enable the patient to obtain adequate pain relief while remaining in his own home and with his family.

Pain Centers and Pain Clinics

Pain clinics have been established in the United States to help patients with chronic pain.* They use a multidisciplinary approach and offer a variety of perspectives on the relief of pain. Therapy may include biofeedback, acupuncture, nerve blocks, hypnosis, autogenic training, group therapy, medication, physical therapy, nutritional counseling, and many others. Not all pain centers offer the same approaches to pain

---

* For information on obtaining directories of pain clinics, listing the locations of and services offered by pain clinics, write: Committee on Pain Therapy, American Society of Anesthesiologists, 515 Busse Hwy., Park Ridge, IL 60068 or Medical World News, 1221 Avenue of the Americas, New York, NY 10020.

For assistance in locating hospice programs throughout the United States, write: National Hospice Organization, 1311 Dolly Madison Blvd., McLean, VA 22101.

Care of the Patient With Pain

Nursing Interventions	Rationale	Expected Outcomes

Nursing Diagnosis: Alteration in comfort: pain

Goal: Relief of pain or decrease in intensity of pain

Nursing Interventions	Rationale	Expected Outcomes
1. Assure patient that you know pain is real and will assist him in dealing with it	1. Fear that pain will not be accepted as real increases tension and anxiety and decreases pain tolerance	• Reports relief that pain is accepted as real and that he will receive assistance in pain relief
2. Use pain assessment scale to identify intensity of pain and discomfort	2. Provides baseline for assessing changes in pain level and evaluating interventions	• Reports lower intensity of pain and discomfort after interventions used
3. Assess and record pain and its characteristics: location, quality, frequency, duration	3. Assists in evaluation of pain and pain relief and identifying multiple sources types of pain	• Reports less disruption from pain and discomfort following use of intervention
4. Administer analgesics to promote optimum pain relief within limits of physician's prescription	4. Analgesics are more effective when administered early in pain cycle.	• Accepts pain medication as prescribed
5. Assess patient's behavioral responses to pain and pain experience	5. Provides additional source of information about patient's pain	• Exhibits decreased physical and behavioral signs of pain and discomfort in *acute pain* (no grimacing, crying, is aware of surroundings, participates in events and activities)
6. Identify and encourage strategies of pain relief that patient has used successfully in previous pain experiences	6. Encourages success of pain relief strategies familiar to and accepted by patient	• Identifies effective pain relief strategies
7. Teach patient new strategies to relieve pain and discomfort: • distraction • imagery • relaxation • cutaneous stimulation	7. Increases number of options and strategies available to patient	• Demonstrates use of new strategies to relieve pain and reports their effectiveness

(continued)

relief. Some clinics or centers treat the patient on an outpatient basis, whereas others admit the patient to a pain control unit.

When the patient is not able to obtain satisfactory pain relief, the physician may refer him to a pain center for evaluation and treatment. Unfortunately, there are not enough pain centers to care for all the patients with chronic pain. The waiting lists at such clinics often are quite long.

Hospice programs have been developed in many areas to give care and symptomatic relief to the dying patient. Pain control is one of their primary goals. Again, there are not enough of these agencies to care for all of the patients who need them.

Evaluating the Effectiveness of Pain Relief Measures

To determine objectively the effectiveness of nursing activities designed to help the patient with his pain experience, the patient's behavioral responses prior to intervention are compared with those that follow intervention. After the nurse intervenes, she once again assesses the patient's behavioral responses, much as she did in her initial assessment. This assessment is repeated at appropriate intervals following the intervention.

The *comparison* of these assessments reveals the effectiveness of the pain relief measures. This provides a basis for continuing or modifying nursing intervention. (See Nursing Care Plan 15-1.)

The expected outcome of nursing intervention for pain relief is usually one or more of the following possibilities, each having many possible manifestations:

1. Achieves pain relief or decreased intensity of pain
   a. Rates pain at a lower intensity (on a scale of 0–10) following intervention
   b. Rates pain at a lower intensity for longer periods of time
2. Uses coping strategies effectively
   a. Is alert and pain free enough to engage in activities important to recovery (*e.g.*, drinking fluids, coughing, ambulating)

Nursing Interventions	*Rationale*	*Expected Outcomes*

Nursing Diagnosis: Potential ineffective coping related to anticipation and stress of pain

Goal: Increased effectiveness of coping

1. Assess patient's coping strategies and factors that produce ineffective coping	1. Provides baseline for assessing interventions and allows patient and health care provider to identify factors that have hampered effective coping	• Identifies effective and ineffective coping strategies • Demonstrates use of effective strategies • Avoids destructive coping strategies (smoking, aggression, abuse of alcohol and drugs)
2. Teach patient appropriate and safe ways to use analgesics	2. Provides patient with alternate and safe coping strategies	• Explains safe and appropriate use of analgesics • Uses analgesics safely and appropriately • States side-effects of analgesics and adequate pain relief • Exhibits absence of side-effects of analgesics and adequate pain relief • Reports decreasing reliance on analgesics • Reports pain relief with less potent analgesics
3. Assist patient to identify and use effective coping strategies	3. Previous reliance on ineffective or less effective coping strategies indicates the need for assistance in identifying effective ones	• Verbally acknowledges need for new, more effective coping strategies
4. Assist patient to plan and participate in activities	4. Provides distraction for patient and assists patient, who may have decreased all participation in activities, to become involved	• Participates in family, social, and work activities • Exhibits awareness of events and environment • Reports ability to sleep and rest • Reports less preoccupation with pain • Converses about topics other than own pain experience • Reports that life-style is appropriate and acceptable to him

b. Sleeps all night
c. Increases the amount of time spent out of bed
d. Increases the amount of time spent at work
e. Says the pain does not bother him as much as it did prior to intervention
f. Says he pays less attention to the pain
g. Spends less time talking about pain

Bibliography

Books

Aronoff GM. Evaluation and Treatment of Chronic Pain. Baltimore, Urban & Schwarzenberg, 1985.

Bellissimo A and Tunks E. Chronic Pain: The Psychotherapeutic Spectrum. New York, Praeger, 1984.

Benedetti C, Chapman CR, and Moricca G. Recent Advances in the Management of Pain: Advances in Pain Research and Therapy, vol 7. New York, Raven Press, 1984.

Bromm B. Pain Measurement in Man: Neurophysiological Correlates of Pain. New York, Elsevier, 1984.

Fields HL, Dubner R, and Cervero F. Proceedings of the Fourth World Congress on Pain: Advances in Pain Research and Therapy, vol 9. New York, Raven Press, 1985.

Gildenberg PL and DeVaul RA. The Chronic Pain Patient: Evaluation and Management: Pain and Headache, Vol 7. New York, S Karger, 1985.

Goldberg IK, Kurscher AH, and Malitz S. Pain, Anxiety, and Grief. New York, Columbia University Press, 1986.

Holzman AD and Turk DC. Pain Management: A Handbook of Psychological Treatment Approaches. New York, Pergamon Press, 1986.

Kotarba JA. Chronic Pain—Its Social Dimensions. Beverly Hills, California, Sage, 1983.

Meinhart NT and McCaffery M. Pain: A Nursing Approach to Assessment and Analysis. New York, Appleton-Century-Crofts, 1983.

Melzack R. Pain Measurement and Assessment. New York, Raven Press, 1983.

Smith G and Covino BG. Acute Pain. Boston, Butterworth & Co, 1985.

Stimmel B. Pain, Analgesia, and Addiction: The Pharmacologic Treatment of Pain. New York, Raven Press, 1983.

Swerdlow H. Relief of Intractable Pain: Monographs in Anaesthesiology, vol 13. New York, Elsevier, 1983.

Turk DC, Meichenbaum D, and Genest M. Pain and Behavioral Medicine: A Cognitive-Behavioral Perspective. New York, Guilford Press, 1983.

Vestal RE. Drug Treatment in the Elderly. Boston, ADIS Health Science Press, 1984.

Wall PD and Melzack R. Textbook of Pain. New York, Churchill Livingstone, 1984.

Articles

(Asterisks indicate nursing research articles.)

Ahles TA, Blanchard EB, and Ruckdeschel JC. The multidimensional nature of cancer-related pain. Pain 1983 Nov; 17(3):277–288.

Ahles TA, Ruckdeschel JC, and Blanchard EB. Cancer-related pain: I. Prevalence in an outpatient setting as a function of stage of disease and type of cancer. J Psychosom Res 1984; 28(2):115–119.

Ahles TA, Ruckdeschel JC, and Blanchard EB. Cancer-related pain: II. Assessment with visual analogue scales. J Psychosom Res 1984; 28(2):121–124.

Alberico JG. Breaking the chronic pain cycle. Am J Nurs 1984 Oct; 84(10):1222–1225.

Bailey CJ et al. Epidural morphine infusion. AORN J 1984 May; 39(6):997–1008.

Bullngham RES. Optimum management of postoperative pain. Pain 1985 Apr; 29(4):376–386.

Chapman CR et al. Pain measurement: An overview. Pain 1984 May; 22(1):1–31.

Citron ML et al. Safety and efficacy of continuous intravenous morphine for severe cancer pain. Am J Med 1984 Aug 77(2):199–204.

Copolov DL and Helme RD. Enkephalins and endorphins: Clinical, pharmacological and therapeutic implications. Drugs 1983 Dec; 26(6):503–519.

Copp LA. Pain coping model and typology. Image: J Nurs Sch 1985 Summer; 17(3):69–71.

Cuschieri RJ et al. Postoperative pain and pulmonary complications: Comparison of three analgesic regimes. Br J Surg 1985 June; 72(6):495–498.

Digregorio GJ and Koin SH. Adjuvant drug therapy for pain. Am Fam Physician 1986 Apr; 33(4):227–232.

Dolphin NW. Neuroanatomy and neurophysiology of pain: Nursing implications. Int J Nurs Stud 1983; 20(4):255–263.

Escobar PL. Management of chronic pain. Nurs Prac 1985 Jan; 10(1):24–25, 29–30, 32.

*Faherty BS and Grier MR. Analgesic medication for elderly people post-surgery. Nurs Res 1984 Nov/Dec; 36(6):369–372.

Farrell J. Orthopedic pain: What does it mean? Am J Nurs 1984 Apr; 84(4):466–469.

Foley KM. The treatment of cancer pain. N Engl J Med 1985 July 11; 313(2):84–95.

*Geden E et al. Self-report and psychophysiological effects of five pain-coping strategies. Nurs Res 1984 Sept-Oct; 33(5):260–265.

Goldberg-Sklar C. Chronic pain management: A Research Focus. J Neurosurg Nurs 1984 Feb; 16(1):10–14.

Gourlay GK and Cousins MJ. Strong analgesics in severe pain. Drugs 1984 July; 28(1):79–81.

Grinde JW, Grina R, and Gellatly T. Pain management by epidural analgesia: The challenge for nursing. Heart Lung 1984 Mar; 13(2):105–110.

Health and Public Policy Committee. American College of Physicians. Drug therapy for severe chronic pain in terminal illness (Position Statement) Ann Intern Med 1983 Dec; 99(6):870–873.

*Horowitz BF, Fitzpatrick JJ, and Flaherty GG. Relaxation techniques for pain relief after open heart surgery. Dimens Crit Care Nurs 1984 Nov/Dec; 3(6):323–325.

Jacobsen L. Intrathecal and extradural narcotics. Adv Pain Res Ther 1984; 7:199–236.

James EC and Gellatly TA. Pain management by epidural analgesia. Heart Lung 1984 Mar; 13(2):103–104.

Johnson JA and Repp EC. Nonpharmacologic pain management in arthritis. Nurs Clin North Am 1984 Dec; 19(4):583–591.

Kibbee E. Burn pain management. Crit Care Q 1985 Mar; 7(4):54–62.

Krames ES et al. Continuous infusion of spinally administered narcotics for the relief of pain due to malignant disorders. Cancer 1985 Aug 1; 56(3):696–702.

Kumar K and Wyant GM. Deep brain stimulation for alleviating chronic intractable pain. Can J Surg 1985 Jan; 28(1):20–22.

Lamy PP. Pain management, drugs and the elderly. J Am Health Care Assoc 1984 July; 10(4):32–36.

Leib RA and Hurtig JB. Epidural and intrathecal narcotics for pain management. Heart Lung 1985 Mar; 14(2):164–174.

Malone BT, Beye R, and Walker J. Management of pain in the terminally ill by administration of epidural narcotics. Cancer 1985 Jan 15; 55(2):438–440.

Mayock J. Towards pain relief. Nurs Mirror 1985 Jan 16; 160(3):40–41.

McCaffery M. Pain in the critical care patient. Dimens Crit Care Nurs 1984 Nov/Dec; 3(6):323–325.

McGivney WT and Crooks GM. The care of patients with severe chronic pain in terminal illness. JAMA 1984 Mar 2; 251(9):1182–1188.

*McGuire DB. Assessment of pain in cancer inpatients using the McGill pain questionnaire. Oncol Nurs Forum 1984 Nov/Dec; 11(6):32–37.

*McGuire DB. The measurement of clinical pain. Nurs Res 1984 May/June; 33(3):152–156.

McGuire L and Wright A. Continuous narcotic infusion: It's not just for cancer patients. Nursing '84 1984 Dec; 14(12):50–55.

Michaels PJ, Adams DB, and McBride P. Chronic Pain. J Fam Pract 1983 Oct; 17(4):591–610.

Miller TW and Jay LL. Cognitive-behavioral and pharmaceutical approaches to sensory pain management. Top Clin Nurs 1985 Jan; 6(4):34–43.

Moore DE and Blacker HM. How effective is TENS for chronic pain. Am J Nurs 1983 Aug; 83(8):1175–1177.

Moseley JR. Alterations in comfort. Top Clin Nurs 1985 June; 20(2):427–438.

Pageau MG, Mroz WT, and Coombs DW. New analgesic therapy relieves cancer pain without oversedation. Nursing '85 1985 Apr; 15(4):46–49.

Payne R and Foley KM. Advances in the management of cancer pain. Cancer Treat Rep 1984 Jan; 69(1):173–183.

Payne R and Foley KM (eds). Cancer pain (symposium). Med Clin North Am Mar 1987; 71(2):153–348.

Pearce S. A review of cognitive-behavioural methods for the treatment of chronic pain. J Psychosom Res 1983; 27(5):431–440.

Portnoy RK. Continuous infusion of opioids. Am J Nurs 1986 Mar; 86(3):318, 322.

Rahr V. Giving intrathecal drugs. Am J Nurs 1986 July; 86(7):829–831.

Reading AE. Pain measurement and experience. J Psychosom Res 1983; 27(5):415–420.

Skevington SM. Social cognitions, personality and chronic pain. J Psychosom Res 1983; 27(5):421–428.

Smith KA. Teaching family members intrathecal morphine administration. J Neurosurg Nurs 1986 Apr; 18(2):95–97.

Smith S. Drugs and pain. Nurs Times 1985 Jan 30; 81(5):36–37.

Spiegel D. The use of hypnosis in controlling cancer pain. CA 1985 July-Aug; 35(4):221–231.

Sriwatanakul L et al. Analysis of narcotic analgesic usage in the treatment of postoperative pain. JAMA 1983 Aug 19; 250(7):926–929.

Stimmel B. Under-prescription/over-prescription: Narcotic as metaphor. Bull NY Acad Med 1985 Oct; 61(8):742–752.

Talbert RL. Pharmacotherapeutic modification of the stress response: Analgesics. Crit Care Q 1985 Mar; 7(4):27–40.

*Taylor AG, Skelton JA, and Butcher J. Duration of pain condition and physical pathology as determinants of nurses' assessments of patients in pain. Nurs Res 1984 Jan/Feb; 33(1):4–8.

Taylor AG et al. How effective is TENS for acute pain? Am J Nurs 1983 Aug; 83(8):1171–1174.

Torda TA. Management of acute and postoperative pain. Int Anesthesiol Clin 1983 Winter; 21(4):27–46.

Turk DC, Wack JT, and Kerns RD. An empirical examination of the "pain-behavior" construct. J Behav Med 1985 June; 8(2):119–130.

Wachter-Shikora N. The elderly patient in pain and the acute care setting. Nurs Clin North Am 1983 June; 18(2):395–401.

Wallenstein SL. Measurement of pain and analgesia in cancer patients. Cancer 1984 May 15(suppl); 53(10):2260–2264.

Warfield CA. Intraspinal narcotics: A new method of pain management. AORN J 1985 May; 41(5):910–914.

Wells N. Responses to acute pain and the nursing implications. J Adv Nursing 1984 Jan; 9(1):51–58.

Williams AE. Deep brain stimulation—A contemporary methodology for chronic pain. J Neurosurg Nurs 1984 Feb; 16(1):1–9.

Wyant GM. Chronic pain: Principles and treatment. Drugs 1983 Sept; 26(3):262–267.

Zaloga GP, Hostinsky C, and Chernow B. Endogenous opioid peptides: Critical care implications. Heart Lung 1984 July; 13(4):421–430.

Agencies

National Committee on the Treatment of Intractable Pain, P.O. Box 9553, Friendship Station, Washington, DC 20016.

Committee on Pain Therapy, American Society of Anesthesiologists, 515 Busse Highway, Park Ridge, Illinois 60068.

National Hospice Organization, 1311 Dolly Madison Boulevard, McLean, VA 22101.

Oncology: Nursing the Patient With Cancer

Cancer nursing is an area of practice that covers all age-groups and nursing specialties and is carried out in a variety of health care settings, including the home, community, acute care institutions, and rehabilitation centers. The field or specialty of cancer nursing, or oncology nursing, has paralled the development of medical oncology and the major therapeutic advances that have occurred in the care of the person with cancer.

The scope, responsibilities, and goals of cancer nursing are as diverse and complex as those of any nursing specialty. There is a special challenge inherent in caring for people with cancer because the word *cancer* is often equated with pain and death in our society. In order to meet this challenge, the nurse must first identify her own reactions to cancer and realistically set goals that can be attained.

The nurse must be equipped to support the patient and his family through a wide range of physical, emotional, social, cultural, and spiritual upheavals. In order to accomplish the desired outcomes, the nurse provides realistic support to those in her care, using standards of practice and the nursing process as the basis of her care. The major areas of responsibility for the nurse caring for the patient with cancer are listed in Chart 16-1.

Epidemiology of Cancer

Incidence.   Cancers affect every age-group; however, most cancers occur in people over 65 years of age. Overall, men experience a higher incidence of cancer than do women. At least 930,000 Americans are diagnosed each year with a cancer affecting one of various body sites (Fig. 16-1). Cancer incidence is higher in the industrialized nations of the world and in the industrial sectors of more developed countries.

Mortality Rates.   Cancers are second only to cardiovascular disease as a leading cause of death in the United States. Each year more than 472,000 Americans die of a malignant process. In the United States, in order of frequency, the leading causes of cancer deaths include cancers of the lung, colorectal area, and prostate in men and cancers of the lung, breast, and colorectal area in women. Relative 5-year survival rates in 1986 are 37% for black Americans and 50% for white Americans.

Chart 16-1
Responsibilities of the Nurse Caring for the Patient with Cancer and His Family

- Support the idea that cancer is a chronic illness that has acute exacerbations rather than one that is solely synonymous with death and suffering.
- Assess own level of knowledge relative to the pathophysiology of the disease process.
- Make use of current research findings and practices in the care of the patient with cancer and his family.
- Identify persons at high risk for the development of cancer.
- Participate in primary and secondary prevention efforts.
- Assess the nursing care needs of the person with cancer.
- Assess the learning needs, desires, and capabilities of the person with cancer.
- Identify nursing problems of the person and his family.

- Assess the social support networks available to the person.
- Plan appropriate interventions with the person and his family.
- Assist the person to identify his strengths and limitations.
- Assist the person to design short-term and long-term goals for care.
- Implement a nursing plan that interfaces with the medical care regimen and that is consistent with the established goals.
- Collaborate with members of a multidisciplinary team to foster continuity of care.
- Evaluate the goals and resultant outcomes of care with the patient, his family, and the members of the multidisciplinary team.
- Reassess and redesign the direction of the care as determined by the evaluation.

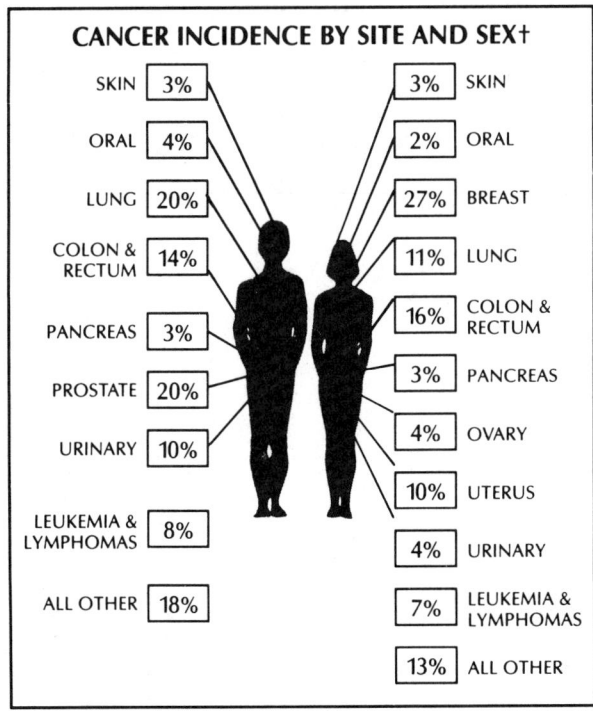

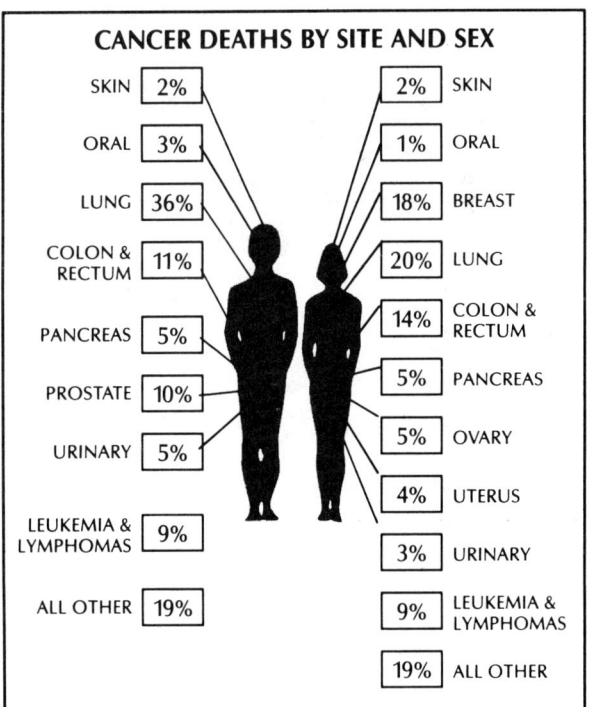

†Excluding non-melanoma skin cancer and carcinoma in situ.

Figure 16-1
Cancer statistics for 1987. The estimates of the incidence of cancer are based on data from the National Cancer Institute's Surveillance Epidemiology and End Results (SEER) program (1977–1981). Nonmelanoma skin cancer and carcinoma *in situ* have not been included in the statistics. The incidence of nonmelanoma skin cancer is estimated to be more than 400,000. (Cancer Facts & Figures–1987. New York, American Cancer Society, 1987.)

Pathophysiology of the Malignant Process

Cancer is a disease process that begins when abnormal cells arise from normal body cells as a result of some poorly understood mechanism of change. As the disease progresses, these abnormal cells proliferate, still within a local area. However, a stage is then reached in which the cells acquire invasive characteristics, and changes occur in surrounding tissues. The cells infiltrate these tissues and gain access to lymph and blood vessels by which they are transported to form *metastases* (cancer spread) in other parts of the body.

Although the disease process can be described in the general terms used above, cancer is not a single disease with a single cause; rather it is a group of distinct diseases with different causes, manifestations, treatments, and prognoses.

Benign vs. Malignant Proliferative Patterns

During the life span, various body tissues normally experience periods of rapid or proliferative growth that must be distin-

guished from malignant growth activity. There are several patterns of cell growth, designated by the terms *hyperplasia, metaplasia, dysplasia, anaplasia,* and *neoplasia,* that may be described as follows.

Hyperplasia. Hyperplasia, an increase in the number of cells of a tissue, is a common proliferative process during periods of rapid body growth (*e.g.,* fetal and adolescent growth and development) and during epithelial and bone marrow regeneration. It is a normal cellular response when a physiologic demand exists and an abnormal response when growth exceeds the physiologic demand.

Metaplasia. Metaplasia occurs when one type of mature cell is converted to another type by means of an outside stimulus that affects the parent stem cell. Chronic irritation or inflammation, vitamin deficiency, and chemical exposure may be factors leading to metaplasia. Metaplastic changes may be reversible or may progress to dysplasia.

Dysplasia. Dysplasia is bizarre cell growth resulting in cells that differ in size, shape, or arrangement from other cells of the same type of tissue. Dysplasia can occur from chemicals, radiation, or chronic inflammation or irritation. It can be reversible or can precede irreversible neoplastic change.

Anaplasia. Anaplasia is a lower degree of differentiation of dysplastic cells. (*Differentiation* refers to the extent

TABLE 16-1

Names of Selected Benign and Malignant Tumors According to Tissue Types

Tissue Type	Benign	Malignant
Epithelial Tumors		
Surface	Papilloma	Squamous cell carcinoma
Glandular	Adenoma	Adenocarcinoma
Connective Tissue Tumors		
Fibrous	Fibroma	Fibrosarcoma
Adipose	Lipoma	Liposarcoma
Cartilage	Chondroma	Chondrosarcoma
Bone	Osteoma	Osteosarcoma
Blood vessels	Hemangioma	Hemangiosarcoma
Lymph vessels	Lymphangioma	Lymphangiosarcoma
Muscle Tumors		
Smooth	Leiomyoma	Leiomyosarcoma
Striated	Rhabdomyoma	Rhabdomyosarcoma
Nerve Cell Tumors		
Nerve cell	Neuroma	
Glial tissue		Glioma
Nerve sheaths	Neurilemmoma	Neurilemic sarcoma
Hematologic Tumors		
Granulocytic		Myelocytic leukemia
Erythrocytic		Erythroleukemia
Plasma cells		Multiple myeloma
Lymphoid		Lymphocytic leukemia

(Porth CM. Pathophysiology: Concepts of Altered Health States, 2nd ed. Philadelphia, JB Lippincott, 1986.)

TABLE 16-2
Characteristics of Benign and Malignant Neoplasms

Characteristics	Benign	Malignant
Cell characteristics	Cells resemble normal cells of the tissue from which the tumor originated	Cells often bear little resemblance to the normal cells of the tissue from which they arose; there is both anaplasia and pleomorphism
Mode of growth	Tumor grows by expansion and does not infiltrate the surrounding tissues; encapsulated	Grows at the periphery and sends out processes that infiltrate and destroy the surrounding tissues
Rate of growth	Rate of growth is usually slow	Rate of growth is usually relatively rapid and is dependent on level of differentiation; the more anaplastic the tumor the more rapid the rate of growth
Metastasis	Does not spread by metastasis	Gains access to the blood and lymph channels and metastasizes to other areas of the body
Recurrence	Does not recur when removed	Tends to recur when removed
General effects	Is usually a localized phenomenon that does not cause generalized effects unless by location it interferes with vital functions	Often causes generalized effects such as anemia, weakness, and weight loss
Destruction of tissue	Does not usually cause tissue damage unless location interferes with blood flow	Often causes extensive tissue damage as the tumor outgrows its blood supply or encroaches on blood flow to the area; may also produce substances that cause cell damage
Ability to cause death	Does not usually cause death unless its location interferes with vital functions	Will usually cause death unless growth can be controlled

(Porth CM. Pathophysiology: Concepts of Altered Health States, 2nd ed. Philadelphia, JB Lippincott, 1986.)

to which the cells differ from their cells of origin and to their degree of maturity.) Anaplastic cells are poorly differentiated, irregularly shaped, or disorganized with respect to growth and arrangement. Anaplastic cells lack normal cellular characteristics and are nearly always malignant.

Neoplasia. Neoplasia, described as uncontrolled cell growth that follows no physiologic demand, can be either benign or malignant. Benign and malignant neoplastic growths are classified and named by tissue of origin (Table 16-1).

Benign and malignant cells differ in many cellular growth characteristics, as summarized in Table 16-2. The degree of anaplasia (lack of differentiation of cells) ultimately determines the malignant potential.

Malignant Cell Characteristics

Despite their individual differences, all cancer cells share some common cellular characteristics. Nuclei of cancer cells are often large and irregularly shaped (pleomorphism). Nucleoli, structures within the nucleus that house ribonucleic acid (RNA), are larger and more numerous in malignant cells, perhaps due to increased RNA synthesis. Chromosomal abnormalities and fragility of chromosomes are commonly found on analysis of cancer cells. Mitosis (cell division) occurs more frequently in malignant cells than in normal cells. Additionally, cancer cells have altered amounts of cyclic adenosine monophosphate (AMP) and cyclic guanosine monophosphate (GMP). These substances, which are the building blocks of nucleic acids, facilitate the utilization of nutrients and the

synthesis of RNA. As a result, cell growth and division are promoted.

Invasion and Metastasis. Malignancies have the ability to spread or transfer cancerous cells from one organ or body part to another by invasion and metastasis. *Invasion* involves the growth of the primary tumor into the surrounding host tissues. The process of invasion occurs in several ways. Mechanical pressure exerted by rapidly proliferating neoplasms may force fingerlike projections of tumor cells into surrounding tissue. Malignant cells may break off from the primary tumor and invade adjacent structures. Malignant cells are thought to possess specific destructive enzymes (lysosomal hydrolases or collagenases) that destroy surrounding tissue and facilitate invasion by malignant cells. The mechanical pressure of a rapidly growing tumor may enhance this process.

Metastasis is the dissemination of malignant cells from the primary tumor to distant sites by direct spread of tumor cells to body cavities or through lymphatic and hematogenous circulation. Tumors growing in or penetrating body cavities may shed cells or emboli that travel within the body cavity and "seed" the surfaces of other organs. This can occur in ovarian cancer when malignant cells enter the peritoneal cavity and seed peritoneal surfaces of abdominal organs such as the liver or pancreas.

The most common mechanism of metastasis is transport of tumor cells through the lymphatic circulation. Tumor emboli enter the lymph channels by way of the interstitial fluid that communicates with lymphatic fluid. In addition, malignant cells may penetrate lymphatic vessels by invasion. After entering the lymphatic circulation, malignant cells either become lodged in the lymph nodes or pass between lymphatic and venous circulation. Tumors arising in areas of the body with rapid and extensive lymphatic circulation have a high risk of metastasis through lymphatic channels. Breast tumors frequently metastasize in this manner through axillary, clavicular, and thoracic lymph channels.

Hematogenous spread, or dissemination through the bloodstream, of malignant cells is less common than spread by other means. Few malignant cells are able to survive the turbulent nature of arterial circulation. In addition, the structure of most arteries and arterioles is far too secure to permit malignant invasion. Malignant cells do have the ability to induce the growth of new capillaries from the host tissue in order to meet their needs for nutrients and oxygen. This process is referred to as *angiogenesis*. It is through this vascular network that tumor emboli may enter the systemic circulation and travel to distant sites. Large tumor emboli that become trapped in the microcirculation of distant sites serve as the origin of growth for metastasis.

Metastasis from the primary tumor to other sites is not a random process. Since the late 1800s, investigators have recognized the tendency for malignancies of specific cell classifications to spread, or metastasize, to specific organs. Several theories have been generated to explain how and why metastasis occurs. Investigators are focusing their attention on the following factors in metastasis: organ vascularity, immune defenses at the tissue level, surface recognition factors on tumor cells, and differing behavioral characteristics among cells within one tumor.

Carcinogenesis

Malignant transformation is thought to be at least a two-step cellular process. In the first or *initiation* step, initiators such as chemicals, physical factors, and biological agents escape normal enzymatic mechanisms and cause alterations in the genetic structure of the cellular deoxyribonucleic acid (DNA). These alterations are irreversible but usually are not of significance to cells until the second step of carcinogenesis occurs—*promotion*. During this step, repeated exposure to promoting agents causes the expression of abnormal or mutant genetic information. Once this genetic expression occurs in cells, they begin to produce mutant cell populations that are different from their original cellular ancestors. Those agents that initiate or promote cellular transformation are referred to as *carcinogens*.

Etiologies

Certain categories of agents or factors have been implicated in the carcinogenic process. These include viruses, physical agents, chemical agents, genetic or familial factors, dietary factors, and hormonal agents.

Viruses. Viral causation in human cancers is very difficult to ascertain because isolation of viruses is very difficult. Infectious etiologies are considered when clusters of specific cancers are noted. Viruses are thought to incorporate themselves in the genetic structure of cells, thus altering future generations of that cell population—perhaps leading to a cancer. For example, the Epstein-Barr virus is highly suspect as a causative agent in Burkitt's lymphoma and nasopharyn-

geal cancers. Herpes simplex type II virus, cytomegalovirus, and papillomavirus have all been associated with dysplasia and malignancy of the uterine cervix; the hepatitis B virus has been implicated in hepatocellular carcinoma.

Physical Agents. Physical factors associated with carcinogenesis include exposure to sunlight or to radiation and chronic irritation or inflammation.

Excessive exposure to the ultraviolet radiation of the sun, especially in fair-skinned, blue- or green-eyed people, increases the risk of skin cancers. Exposure to ionizing radiation can occur with repeated diagnostic radiographic procedures or radiation therapy and from exposure to radioactive materials at atomic bomb test sites or nuclear power plants. Those exposed to extensive radiation have a higher incidence of leukemia and cancers of the lung, bone, thyroid, and other tissues.

Chronic irritation or inflammation is thought to damage cells, leading to abnormal cell differentiation. Cell mutations secondary to chronic irritation or inflammation are associated with lip cancers among pipe-smokers. Oral cancers are associated with prolonged tobacco use or ill-fitting dentures. Melanomas are associated with chronically irritated moles, colorectal cancers with ulcerative colitis, and liver cancers with cirrhosis.

Chemical Agents. Many chemical substances found in the workplace have proven to be carcinogens or co-carcinogens in the cancer process. The extensive list of suspected chemical substances continues to grow. Currently, approximately 80% of all cancers are thought to be environmentally related. Most hazardous chemicals produce their toxic effects by altering DNA structure in body sites distant from chemical exposure. The liver and kidneys are the organ systems most often affected, presumably owing to their roles in detoxification of chemicals.

Genetic and Familial Factors. Genetic factors also play a role in cancer cell development. If DNA damage occurs in cell populations where chromosomal patterns are abnormal, mutant cell populations may develop. Abnormal chromosomal patterns and cancer have been associated with extra chromosomes, too few chromosomes, or translocated chromosomes. Specific cancers with underlying genetic abnormalities include Burkitt's lymphoma, chronic myelogenous leukemia, meningiomas, acute leukemias, retinoblastomas, and skin cancers.

Some adult and childhood cancers display familial predisposition. These cancers tend to occur at an early age and at multiple sites in one organ or pair of organs. Cancers associated with familial inheritance include retinoblastomas, nephroblastomas, pheochromocytomas, malignant neurofibromatosis, leukemias, and breast, endometrial, colorectal, stomach, prostate, and lung cancers.

Dietary Factors. Dietary factors are thought to be related to 40% to 60% of all environmental cancers. Dietary substances can be either proactive (protective) or carcinogenic/co-carcinogenic. The risk of cancer increases over long-term ingestion of carcinogens/co-carcinogens or chronic absence of proactive substances in the diet.

Hormonal Agents. Tumor growth may be promoted by disturbances in hormonal balance, by either the body's own (endogenous) hormone production or administration of exogenous hormones. Cancers of the breast, prostate, and uterus are considered to be dependent on endogenous hormonal levels for growth. Administration of oral contraceptives and diethylstilbestrol (DES) has been associated with hepatocellular carcinomas and vaginal carcinomas, respectively.

The Role of the Immune System

The development of cancer is closely linked to failure of the normal immune system. The increased incidence of malignancies in organ transplant recipients who receive immunosuppressive therapy to prevent rejection of the transplanted organ supports this belief. In addition, patients receiving long-term chemotherapy to treat a malignancy are also at increased risk for the development of a second malignancy.

Malignant cells undergo many changes in structure and function. As a result, new surface antigens are formed on cell membranes. These antigens are capable of stimulating the cellular and humoral immune responses. The T lymphocyte, the soldier of the cellular immune response, is responsible for the recognition of tumor cell antigens. When tumor antigens are recognized by T lymphocytes, other T lymphocytes toxic to the tumor cells are stimulated, proliferate, and are released into the circulation. In addition to possessing these cytotoxic properties, T lymphocytes are capable of stimulating other components of the immune system to rid the body of malignant cells. Certain *lymphokines,* which are substances produced by lymphocytes, are capable of killing or damaging various types of malignant cells. Other lymphokines are able to mobilize other cells such as macrophages that disrupt cancer cells. *Interferon,* a substance produced by the body in response to viral infection, also possesses some antitumor characteristics. Antibodies, produced by B lymphocytes of the humoral immune response, also defend against malignant cells.

How is it, then, that malignant cells are able to survive and proliferate despite the immune system defense mechanisms? There are several suggestions for how tumor cells can overcome an apparently intact immune system. If the body fails to recognize the malignant cell as different from "self," the immune response may fail to be stimulated. The failure of the immune system to respond promptly to the malignant cells allows the tumor to grow to a size that is too large to be managed by normal immune mechanisms.

The tumor cells may actually suppress the patient's immune defenses. Tumor antigens may combine with the antibodies produced by the person and hide or mask themselves from normal immune defense mechanisms. Tumors are also capable of producing substances that impair usual immune defenses. These substances not only promote growth of the tumor but also increase the patient's susceptibility to infection by a variety of pathogenic organisms. As a result of prolonged contact with a tumor antigen, the patient's body may be depleted of the specific lymphocytes and no longer be able to mount an appropriate immune response.

Abnormal concentrations of host suppressor T lymphocytes may play a role in the development of malignancies. Suppressor T lymphocytes normally assist in the regulation of antibody production and diminish immune responses when they are no longer required. Studies have demonstrated that low levels of serum antibodies and high levels of suppressor cells have been found in patients with multiple myeloma, a malignancy associated with hypogammaglobulinemia (low

amounts of serum antibodies). Carcinogens such as viruses or certain chemicals, including chemotherapeutic agents, may weaken the immune system and ultimately enhance tumor growth. Finally, altered immune mechanisms associated with the aging process may allow malignant cells to overcome normal immune defenses.

Detection and Prevention of Cancer

Nurses as well as physicians have traditionally been involved with tertiary prevention, the care and rehabilitation of the patient after cancer has been diagnosed and treated. However, in the past 20 years the American Cancer Society, the National Cancer Institute, clinicians, and researchers have placed greater emphasis on primary and secondary prevention of cancer. *Primary prevention* is concerned with reducing the risk or preventing the development of cancer in healthy people. *Secondary prevention* involves detection and screening efforts in order to achieve early diagnosis and prompt intervention to halt the cancerous process.

Nurses in all settings have an important role in cancer prevention. To participate in prevention of cancer, nurses must acquire the knowledge and skills necessary to provide the community with cancer prevention education about health-related behaviors, risk factors associated with the development of cancer, and screening and detection methods. Epidemiologic and laboratory studies have shown that dietary habits, sun exposure, tobacco use, and alcohol consumption can greatly influence the risk of developing cancer. Nurses also need teaching and counseling skills to foster client participation in cancer prevention programs and to promote healthy lifestyles.

Public awareness about health promotion can be increased in a variety of ways. Health education and health maintenance programs are sponsored by community organizations such as churches, senior citizen groups, and parent–teacher associations. Primary prevention programs may focus on the hazards of tobacco or the importance of nutrition. Secondary prevention programs may include breast and testicular self-examination and Papanicolaou tests. The American Cancer Society has developed a public education program, "Taking Control," which integrates diet, exercise, and general health habit tips that people can follow to reduce their risk of developing cancer (Table 16-3). Nurses in acute care settings can identify risks for patients and families and incorporate teaching and counseling in discharge planning.

Screening of cancers for which there is a high incidence rate or in which early diagnosis plays a major role in improved survival rates is usually the focus of early detection efforts. Examples of these types of cancer include breast, colorectal, cervical, endometrial, testicular, skin, and oropharyngeal cancers.

Diagnosis of Cancer

The diagnosis of cancer is based on the assessment of physiological and functional changes as well as on the results of

TABLE 16-3
Ten Steps of Cancer Prevention

Action	Rationale
Protective Factors	
1. Increase consumption of fresh vegetables (especially those of the cabbage family).	Increase fiber intake; increase intake of vitamins.
2. Increase fiber intake.	High-fiber diets reduce risk of developing certain cancers (cancer of breast, prostate, and colon).
3. Increase intake of vitamin A.	Reduces risk of cancers (esophagus, larynx, and lung).
4. Increase intake of foods rich in vitamin C.	Citrus fruits and vegetables rich in vitamin C may protect against cancer of the stomach and esophagus.
5. Practice weight control.	Obesity is linked to cancers of the uterus, gallbladder, breast, and colon.
Risk Factors	
6. Reduce the amount of dietary fat.	A high-fat diet increases risk of developing breast, colon, and prostate cancers.
7. Cut down on salt-cured, smoked, and nitrate-cured foods.	Moderation in consumption of these foods is recommended since they have been linked to cancers of the esophagus and stomach.
8. Stop cigarette smoking.	Smokers are at risk for lung cancer.
9. Reduce alcohol intake.	Drinking large amounts of alcohol increases the risk of liver cancer. Heavy drinkers who smoke are at greater risk for cancers of the mouth, throat, larynx, and esophagus.
10. Avoid overexposure to the sun.	Overexposure to the sun increases the risk of skin cancer. Protective clothing or use of a sunscreen reduces the risk.

(Modified from the Taking Control Program of the American Cancer Society.)

the diagnostic evaluation. Patients with suspected cancer undergo extensive diagnostic testing to determine the presence of tumor and the extent of disease, to identify possible spread (metastasis) or invasion of other body tissues, to evaluate the function of involved as well as uninvolved body systems and organs, and to obtain tissue and cells for analysis of the cancer, including its stage and grade. A patient undergoing extensive testing is usually fearful of the procedures themselves and anxious about the possible results of the testing. The patient and his family require information about the tests to be performed and the patient's role in the testing procedures. The nurse provides opportunities for the patient and family to verbalize their fears about the test results. She supports the patient and family throughout the period of diagnostic testing and reinforces and clarifies information conveyed to them by the physician. She also encourages the patient and family members to communicate and share their concerns and to discuss their questions with each other.

Staging and Grading.   A complete diagnostic evaluation includes identifying the stage and grade of malignancy. This must be accomplished prior to the initiation of treatment to provide for and maintain a systematic and consistent approach to diagnosis, treatment, and evaluation of interventions. Treatment options and prognosis are determined on the basis of staging and grading. This approach facilitates the exchange of information about similar types of cancer and their associated survival and response rates. Ultimately, these classifications can assist in ongoing cancer research.

Staging determines the size of the tumor and the existence of metastasis. Several systems exist for classifying the anatomic extent of disease. The *TNM system*, developed from the work of the International Union Against Cancer (IUCC) and the American Joint Committee for Cancer Staging and End Stage Reporting (AJCCS) is most frequently used in describing malignancies such as breast, lung, or ovarian cancer. In this system the *T* refers to the extent of the primary tumor, *N* refers to lymph node involvement, and *M* refers to the extent of metastasis (Chart 16-2).

Grading refers to the classification of the tumor cells. Grading systems seek to define the origin of tissue of the tumor and the degree to which the tumor cells retain the functional and histologic characteristics of the tissue of origin. Tumors that closely resemble the tissue of origin in structure and function are said to be *well differentiated*. Tumors that do not clearly resemble the tissue of origin in structure or function are graded as *poorly differentiated*. These tumors tend to be more virulent and less responsive to treatment than well-differentiated tumors.

Management of Cancer

Treatment options offered to cancer patients should be based on realistic and achievable goals for each specific type of cancer. The range of possible treatment goals may include

Chart 16-2
TNM Classification System

T* subclasses

Tx—tumor cannot be adequately assessed
T0—no evidence of primary tumor
TIS—carcinoma *in situ*
T1, T2, T3, T4—progressive increase in tumor size and involvement

N† subclasses

Nx—regional lymph nodes cannot be assessed clinically
N0—regional lymph nodes demonstrably abnormal
N1, N2, N3, N4—increasing degrees of demonstrable abnormality of regional lymph nodes

M‡ subclasses

Mx—not assessed
M0—no (known) distant metastasis
M1—distant metastasis present, specify site(s)

Histopathology

G1—well-differentiated grade
G2—moderately well-differentiated grade
G3, G4—poorly to very poorly differentiated grade

* T = Primary tumor.
† N = Regional lymph nodes.
‡ M = Distant metastasis.
(American Joint Committee on Cancer: Manual for Staging of Cancer. Chicago, American Joint Committee.)

complete eradication of malignant disease (*cure*), prolonged survival with the presence of malignancy (*control*), or relief of symptoms associated with the cancerous disease process (*palliation*). It is imperative that the health care team, the patient, and the patient's family have a clear understanding of the treatment options and goals. Open communication and support are vital as the patient and his family periodically reassess treatment plans and goals when complications of therapy develop or disease progression occurs.

Multiple modalities are often employed in cancer treatment. A variety of therapies, including surgery, radiation therapy, chemotherapy, and immunotherapy may be employed at various times during the course of treatment. An understanding of the principles of each and how they interrelate is important in understanding the rationale and goals of treatment.

Surgery

Surgical removal of the entire cancer remains the best and most frequently used modality of treatment. However, the surgical approach may be selected for a variety of reasons. Surgery may be selected as the primary method of treatment, or it may be diagnostic, prophylactic, palliative, or reconstructive.

Surgery as Primary Treatment. When surgery is used as the primary approach in the treatment of cancer, the goal is to remove the entire tumor (or as much as is feasible, a procedure often called *debulking*) and any involved surrounding tissue, including regional lymph nodes. Contrary to the design of surgical therapy in the past, the goal is not to excise all possible tumor cells. It is now recognized that the growth and dissemination of cancer cells have often produced distant micrometastases by the time the patient seeks treatment. Therefore, attempting to remove wide margins of tissue in the hopes of "getting all the cancer cells" is often not

realistic. This reality substantiates the need for a coordinated multidisciplinary approach to cancer therapy. Once the surgery has been completed, one or more additional modalities may be chosen to increase the likelihood of cancer cell destruction. There are, however, cancers that when treated surgically in the very early stages are considered to be curable (*e.g.*, skin cancers, testicular cancers).

Diagnostic Surgery. Diagnostic surgery is usually performed to obtain a biopsy (excision of a piece of tissue from a suspicious growth) in order to analyze the tissues and cells of the suspected malignancy. The three most common biopsy methods are the excisional, incisional, and needle methods. The *excisional method* is most frequently used for biopsies of the skin, the upper respiratory tract, and the upper and lower portions of the gastrointestinal tract, in which removal of the entire tumor is often possible. This approach not only provides the pathologist with the entire specimen but also decreases the chance of cellular seeding of the tumor. The *incisional method* is used if the tumor mass is too large to be removed. It is imperative that the biopsy be representative of the tumor mass so that the pathologist can provide an accurate diagnosis. Both of these approaches are often endoscopic procedures. Surgical incision is often required to determine the anatomic extent or stage of the tumor.

Needle biopsy is used to sample suspicious masses that are easily accessible, such as some growths in the breasts, lung, liver, and kidney. The procedure is fast, relatively inexpensive, and easy to perform. In general, the patient experiences minimal and temporary physical discomfort. In addition, the degree to which the surrounding tissue is disturbed is kept to a minimum, thus decreasing the likelihood of disseminating cancer cells (seeding). There is, however, a chance that even the most skilled physician will obtain a biopsy from such a small area that a full description of the cellular types is not possible.

The choice of biopsy to be performed takes into account many factors. Of greatest importance is the type of treatment anticipated if a diagnosis of cancer is confirmed. The surgical area includes the site of biopsy so that any cells that might have been dislodged during the procedure are excised at the time of surgery. In addition, the condition of the patient is considered. Assessment of nutritional, respiratory, renal, and hepatic systems is essential in determining the most appropriate method of treatment. If the biopsy requires general anesthesia, and subsequent surgery is likely, the effects of total anesthesia on the patient are considered. The patient and his family are given an opportunity to discuss the available options before definitive plans are made. The nurse, as the patient's advocate, serves as a liaison between the patient and the physician in order to facilitate this process. Time should be set aside to minimize interruptions. Time for questions and for "thinking through" all that has been discussed should be provided.

Prophylactic Surgery. Prophylactic surgery involves the removal of lesions that are apt to develop into cancer, such as small tumors (polyps) that often grow in the colon. Recently, more aggressive surgical procedures have been performed as prophylactic measures. The two most common are colectomies and mastectomies in persons who are at a significantly high risk owing to personal and family history. Since the long-term physiological and psychological effects are not currently known, these therapeutic approaches are offered selectively to patients. Preoperative information and counseling, as well as long term follow up, should be available.

Palliative Surgery. When cure of the cancer is not possible, the goal of treatment is to provide the patient with as much comfort as possible and a satisfying and productive life for as long as is possible. Whether the period of time is extremely short or lengthy, the major goal is a high quality of life—with "quality" defined by the patient and his family.

Palliative surgery is performed in an attempt to relieve complications of cancer, such as ulcerations, obstructions, hemorrhage, pain, or infection. This type of surgery includes nerve blocks and cordotomies designed to relieve intractable pain; tumor resection, to relieve obstruction that may occur if a segment of bowel is obstructed (this may result in ostomies, depending on the extent of invasion); and simple mastectomies for ulcerative breast disease. The nurse provides appropriate counseling and referrals for patients and their families. Radiation therapy is frequently used to shrink the tumor, slow its growth, and relieve pain. In addition, various chemotherapeutic and hormonal regimens can be prescribed. Finally, surgical removal of hormone-producing glands that might enhance tumor growth is often performed. These glands include the pituitary, adrenals, ovaries, and testes.

Reconstructive Surgery. Reconstructive surgery may follow curative or radical surgery and is carried out in an attempt to produce a better return of function or a better cosmetic effect. It may be done in one operation or in stages. Presurgery counseling and evaluation are recommended. The surgeon who is to perform the reconstructive surgery is often called in preoperatively. For example, the woman who is to have breast reconstruction done may see the surgeon before hospitalization for a mastectomy. This approach provides the woman something positive to focus on, at a time when thoughts of mutilation and death may be paramount. The physician performing the reconstructive surgery also benefits from seeing the way the woman's breasts appear normally and from establishing rapport with her. The nurse must be cognizant of the woman's sexual needs and the impact that an altered body image may have on her sexuality. Providing the woman and her family with opportunities to discuss these issues is imperative. The needs of the individual must be accurately assessed and validated in each situation for any type of reconstructive surgery.

Nursing Considerations

The patient undergoing surgery for the diagnosis or treatment of cancer is often anxious about the surgical procedure, possible findings, postoperative limitations, changes in normal body functions, and prognosis. The patient and family require time and assistance to deal with the possible changes and outcomes. At the same time, the patient requires expert medical and nursing management in the preoperative and postoperative phases of surgery and illness. The nurse who is asked about the results of diagnostic testing and surgical procedures is guided in her response by the information conveyed to the patient and family by the physician. She may be asked by the patient and family to explain and clarify information that was provided by the physician at a time when their level of anxiety kept them from understanding the information and its implications. It is important for the nurse to communicate frequently with the physician and other health care team members to be certain that a consistent approach is used. Plans for discharge and follow-up care and treatment are initiated as early as possible in order to ensure continuity of care from hospital to home or from a cancer referral center to the patient's local hospital and health care provider.

Radiation Therapy

Radiation therapy is the use of ionizing radiation to interrupt cellular growth. Approximately 50% of patients with cancer receive a form of irradiation at some point in their course of treatment. This treatment modality may be chosen when the treatment goal is curative, such as in Hodgkin's disease, testicular seminomas, localized cancers of the head and neck, and cancers of the uterine cervix. Radiation therapy may also be used to control malignant disease when a tumor cannot be removed surgically or when local nodal metastasis is present, or prophylactically to prevent leukemic infiltration to the brain or spinal cord. Palliative irradiation is frequently used to relieve the symptoms of metastatic disease especially when it has spread to brain, bone, or soft tissue.

Two types of ionizing radiation exist: electromagnetic rays (x-rays and gamma rays) and heavier particulate radiation (electrons, protons, neutrons, alpha particles, and beta particles). Either type can lead to tissue disruption by ionization. The most harmful tissue disruption is the alteration of the DNA molecule within the cells of the tissue. Ionizing radiation causes breakage among the strands of the DNA helix, leading to cell death. Cell regulatory mechanisms are disturbed by radiation, shortening the life span of the cell.

Cells are most vulnerable to the disruptive effects of radiation during DNA synthesis and mitosis (S and M phases of the cell cycle, respectively). Therefore, those body tissues that undergo frequent cell division are most sensitive to radiation therapy. These tissues include bone marrow, lymphatic tissue, epithelium of the gastrointestinal tract, and gonads.

Those tissues that are slower growing or at rest are relatively radioresistant; they include muscle, cartilage, and connective tissues. A *radiosensitive tumor* is one that can be destroyed by a dose of radiation that still allows for normal cell regeneration in the tissue. Tumors that are well oxygenated also seem to be more sensitive to radiation; therefore, radiation therapy might be enhanced if oxygen concentrations to tumors could be increased. In addition, if the radiation could be delivered at a time when most tumor cells were in either the S or M phases, the number of cancer cells destroyed ("cell kill") would be increased.

Radiation is delivered to tumor sites by either external or internal mechanisms. If external radiation therapy is used, one of several methods of delivery may be chosen, depending on the depth of the tumor to be radiated. *Orthovoltage* machines deliver the maximum radiation dose to superficial lesions such as lesions of the skin and breast, while *megavoltage* machines (cobalt-60 units) deliver radiation dose to deeper body structures and spare the skin from possible adverse effects. Other radiation therapy machines, *linear accelerators* (Fig. 16-2), deliver their dosage to deeper structures without harming the skin and also create less scattering of radiation within the body tissues.

Internal radiation implants are used to deliver a high dose of radiation to a localized area. The specific radioisotope for implantation is selected on the basis of its *half-life*, which is the time it takes for half of its radioactivity to decay. This internal radiation can be implanted by way of needles, seeds, beads, or catheters. With internal radiation therapy, as the distance from the radiation source increases, the dosage delivered to the patient decreases. This allows for sparing of tissue away from the local area. Patients receiving internal radiation emit radiation while the implant is in place. Principles of time, distance, and shielding must be used in planning care for these patients to minimize exposure of personnel to radiation.

Radiation Dosage. The radiation dosage is dependent on the sensitivity of the target tissues to radiation and the tumor size. The *lethal tumor dose* is defined as that dose that will eradicate 95% of the tumor. The total radiation dose is delivered over several weeks to allow repair of healthy tissue and to achieve a greater cell kill by increasing the availability of a greater number of cells in the S or M phases of the cell cycle. Repeated radiation treatments over a period of time (fractionated doses) also allow time for the periphery of the tumor to be repeatedly reoxygenated, since tumors shrink from the outside inward. This increases the radiosensitivity of the tumor, thus increasing tumor cell death.

Toxicity. Toxicity of radiation therapy is usually localized to the region being irradiated. Local reactions occur when normal cells in the treatment area are also destroyed and cellular regeneration falls behind cellular death. Body tissues most frequently affected are those that normally proliferate rapidly; they include the skin, the epithelial lining of the gastrointestinal system, and the bone marrow. Alteration in skin integrity is a common effect and can include alopecia, erythema, and shedding of skin (desquamation). Once treatments have been completed, reepithelialization occurs. Alterations in oral mucosal membranes secondary to radiation therapy include stomatitis, dryness of the mouth (xerostomia), and decreased salivation. The entire gastrointestinal mucosal membranes may be involved, and esophageal irritation with

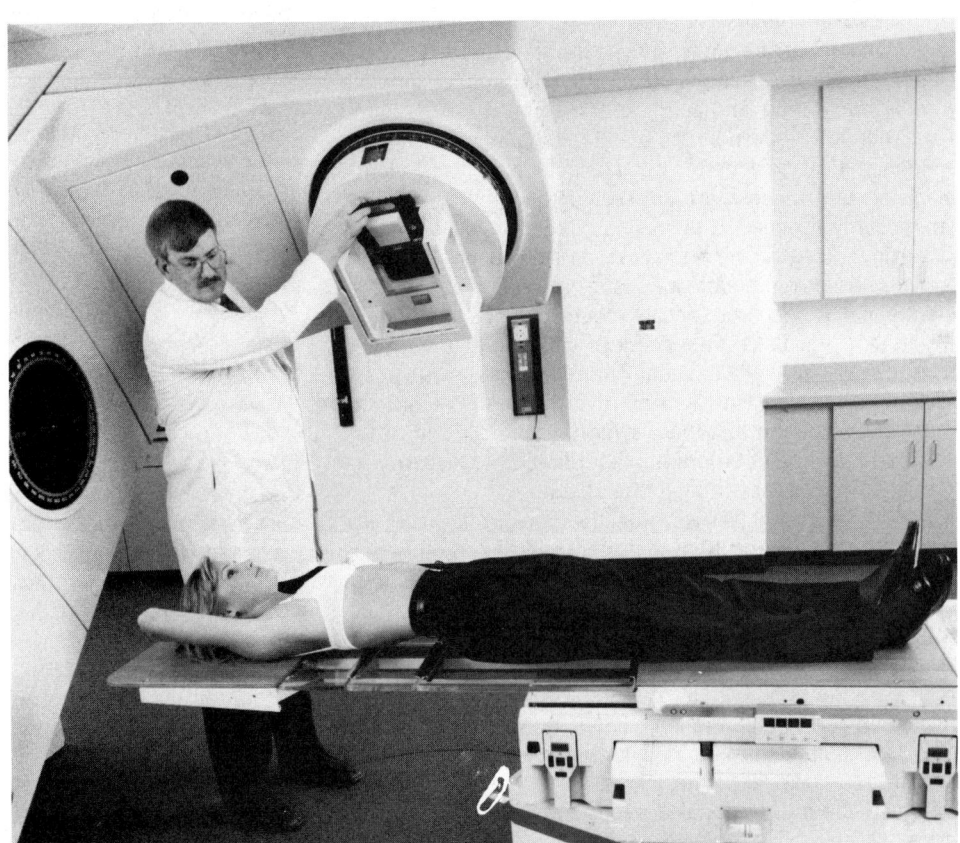

Figure 16-2
Mevatron, a linear electron accelerator used for radiotherapy. (Courtesy of Siemens Medical Laboratories, Inc.)

chest pain and dysphagia may result. Anorexia, nausea, vomiting, and diarrhea may occur if the stomach or colon is in the irradiated field. Symptoms subside and gastrointestinal reepithelialization occurs once treatments are complete. Bone marrow cells proliferate rapidly, and if bone marrow producing sites are included in the field of irradiation, anemia, leukopenia, and thrombocytopenia may result. Patients are then at increased risk of infection and bleeding until blood cell counts return to normal.

Certain systemic side-effects are also commonly experienced by patients receiving radiation therapy. These manifestations, which are generalized, include fatigue, malaise, headache, nausea, and vomiting. This syndrome may be secondary to substances released on the breakdown of tumor cells. The effects are temporary and subside with the cessation of treatments.

Late effects of radiation therapy may also occur in various body tissues. These effects are chronic, usually display fibrotic changes secondary to a decreased vascular supply, and are irreversible.

Nursing Considerations

The patient who is receiving radiation therapy and his family often have questions and concerns about its safety. The nurse is often in a position to answer questions and allay fears about its effects on others, on the tumor, and on the patient's normal tissues and organs. The actual procedure for delivering the radiation is explained, along with a description of the equipment to be used, the duration of the procedure (often minutes only), the possible need for immobilization of the patient during the procedure, and the absence of new sensations during the procedure. If the patient receives radiation therapy by means of a radioactive implant, he will require explanations about limitation of visitors and health care personnel and other radiation precautions. He also needs to understand his role before, during, and after the procedure.

Attention is given by the nurse to the patient's skin, nutritional status, and general feeling of well-being. The patient's skin and oral mucosa are assessed frequently for changes (particularly if radiation therapy is directed to these areas). The skin is protected from irritation, and the patient is advised to avoid using ointments, lotions, or powders on the area. Gentle oral hygiene is essential to remove debris and prevent irritation. If the patient experiences systemic changes such as weakness and fatigue, he may need assistance with activities of daily living and personal hygiene. Additionally, the nurse's explanation that these symptoms are a result of the treatment, and do not represent deterioration or disease progression is often reassuring to the patient.

When a patient has a radioactive implant in place, the nurse also takes precautions to protect herself and other personnel as well as the patient from the effects of radiation. Generally, the patient is either on bed rest or restricted to his room while the radioactive implant is in place. Specific instructions are frequently provided by the radiation safety officer from the radiology department and usually include the maximum amount of time to be spent in the patient's room, shielding equipment to be used, and special precautions and actions to be taken if the implant is dislodged. The patient is informed about the rationale for these precautions so that he does not feel unduly isolated.

Chemotherapy

Chemotherapy is the use of antineoplastic drugs to promote tumor cell death by interfering with cellular functions and reproduction. It is used primarily to treat systemic disease rather than lesions that are localized and amenable to surgery or irradiation. Chemotherapy may be combined with surgery or radiation therapy, or both, to reduce tumor size preoperatively, to destroy remaining tumor cells postoperatively, or to treat some forms of leukemia. Goals of chemotherapy (cure, control, palliation) must be realistic because they will define the drugs to be used and the aggressiveness of the treatment chosen.

Each time a tumor is exposed to a chemotherapeutic agent, a percentage of tumor cells (20% to 99%, depending on dosage) is destroyed. Repeated doses of drugs are necessary over a prolonged period in order to achieve regression of the tumor. Eradication of 100% of the tumor is nearly impossible, but a goal of chemotherapy is to eradicate enough of the tumor so that the remaining tumor cells can be destroyed by the body's immune system.

Actively proliferating cells within a tumor (growth fraction) are the most sensitive to chemotherapeutic agents. Nondividing cells capable of future proliferation are the least sensitive to antineoplastic drugs and consequently are potentially dangerous. However, they must be destroyed in order to eradicate a malignancy completely. Repeated cycles of chemotherapy are used to enhance tumor cell kill by destroying these nondividing cells as they are signaled into active proliferation. These effects are related to the phases of the reproductive cycle of the cell—the cell cycle. Reproduction of both healthy and malignant cells follows the cell cycle pattern (Fig. 16-3). The *cell cycle time* is the time required for one tissue cell to divide and reproduce into two identical daughter cells. The cell cycle of any cell has four distinct phases, each with a vital underlying function: (1) G_1 phase—RNA and protein synthesis occurs; (2) S phase—DNA synthesis occurs; (3) G_2 phase—premitotic phase, DNA synthesis complete; and (4) mitosis—cell division occurs. The G_0 phase, the resting or dormant phase of cells, can occur after mitosis and during the G_1 phase. In the G_0 phase are those dangerous cells that are not actively dividing but have the future potential for replication. The administration of certain chemotherapeutic agents (as well as of some other forms of therapy) is coordinated with the cell cycle.

Classification of Chemotherapeutic Agents

Certain chemotherapeutic agents (cell cycle specific drugs) destroy cells in specific phases of the cell cycle. Most cell cycle specific drugs affect cells in the S phase by interfering with DNA and RNA synthesis. Others, such as the *Vinca* or plant alkaloids, are specific to the M phase where they halt mitotic spindle formation.

Those chemotherapeutic agents that act independently of the cell cycle phases are termed *cell cycle nonspecific drugs*. These agents usually have a prolonged effect on cells, leading to cellular damage or death. Many treatment plans combine cell cycle specific and cell cycle nonspecific drugs in order to increase the number of vulnerable tumor cells killed during a treatment period.

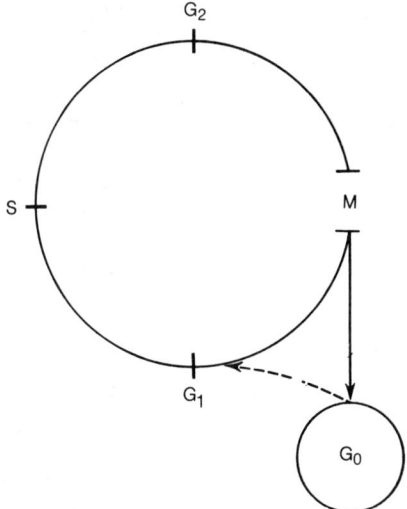

Figure 16-3
Phases of the cell cycle. The cycle represents the interval between the midpoint of mitosis to the subsequent end point in mitosis in one daughter cell or both. G_1 is the postmitotic phase during which RNA and protein synthesis is increased and cell growth occurs. G_0 is the resting or dormant phase of the cell cycle. The S phase represents synthesis of nucleic acids with chromosome replication in preparation for cell mitosis. During G_2, RNA and protein synthesis occurs as in G_1. (Porth CM. Pathophysiology: Concepts of Altered Health States, 2nd ed. Philadelphia, JB Lippincott, 1986.)

Chemotherapeutic agents are also classified according to various chemical groups, each with a different mechanism of action. These include the alkylating agents, nitrosoureas, antimetabolites, antitumor antibiotics, plant alkaloids, hormonal agents, and miscellaneous agents. The classification, mechanism of action, common drugs, cell cycle specificity, and common side-effects of antineoplastic agents are listed in Table 16-4. Chemotherapeutic agents from each category may be used in order to enhance the tumor cell kill during therapy.

Investigational Drugs and Clinical Trials. Investigational antineoplastic drugs undergo thorough trials to test their toxicities and effectiveness. Before new chemotherapeutic agents are approved for clinical use in the treatment of cancer, they are subjected to rigorous and often lengthy evaluation to identify beneficial effects, side-effects, and safety.

Administration of Chemotherapeutic Agents

Routes of Administration. Chemotherapeutic drugs may be administered by topical, oral, intravenous, intramuscular, subcutaneous, arterial, intracavitary, and intrathecal routes. The route of administration is usually dependent on the type of drug, the required dose, and the type and extent of tumor being treated.

Dosage. Dosage of antineoplastic agents is based primarily on the patient's total body surface area, previous response to chemotherapy or radiation therapy, and physical status.

Extravasation. Special care must be taken whenever intravenous vesicant agents are administered. *Vesicant drugs* are those agents that, if deposited into the subcutaneous tissue (extravasated), cause tissue necrosis and damage to underlying tendons, nerves, and blood vessels. Although the complete mechanism of tissue destruction is unclear, it is known that the *p*H of many antineoplastic drugs is responsible for the severe inflammatory reaction. Sloughing and ulceration of tissue may be so severe that skin grafting may be necessary. The full extent of tissue damage may take several weeks to become apparent. Drugs classified as vesicant agents include dactinomycin, daunorubicin, doxorubicin (Adriamycin), nitrogen mustard, mithramycin, mitomycin, vinblastine, vincristine, and vindesine.

Only specially trained physicians and nurses should be involved in the administration of vesicants to prevent extravasation. Careful selection of peripheral veins, skilled venipuncture, and careful drug administration are essential. Indications of extravasation during drug administration include loss of blood return from the intravenous device; resistance to intravenous fluid flow; and swelling, pain, or redness at the site. If extravasation is suspected, the drug administration should be stopped immediately and ice applied to the site (except for *Vinca* alkaloid extravasation). The physician may aspirate any infiltrated drug from the tissues and inject a neutralizing solution into the area to reduce damage. Recommendations and guidelines for management of vesicant extravasation have been issued by individual drug manufacturers, pharmacies, and the Oncology Nursing Society, and differ from one drug to the next.

When frequent, prolonged administration of vesicant antineoplastic agents is anticipated, right atrial Silastic catheters or venous access devices may be inserted. These devices promote safety during drug administration and reduce problems with access to the circulatory system.

Toxicity

Toxicity associated with chemotherapy can be acute or chronic. Cells with rapid growth rates (*e.g.*, epithelium, bone marrow, hair follicles) are more susceptible to damage from these agents. Various body systems may be affected by these drugs and are discussed in the following paragraphs.

Gastrointestinal System. Nausea and vomiting are the most common side-effects of chemotherapy and may persist for up to 24 hours following drug administration. Stimulation of nausea and vomiting occurs by (1) irritation of the gastrointestinal tract, (2) stimulation of the chemoreceptor trigger zone of the medulla, (3) stimulation of the true vomiting center of the brain, (4) anticipatory stimulation, and (5) a combination of factors. Use of phenothiazines, sedatives, and steroids, alone or in combination, is often effective in minimizing nausea and vomiting. Relaxation techniques and imagery can also help to decrease stimuli contributing to symptoms. Alterations in the patient's diet may reduce the frequency or severity of these symptoms.

Although the epithelium that lines the oral cavity quickly renews itself, its rapid rate of proliferation makes it susceptible to the effects of chemotherapy. As a result, stomatitis and anorexia are common. The entire gastrointestinal tract is susceptible to mucositis (inflammation of the mucosal lining),

TABLE 16-4
Classification of Antineoplastic Agents

Category	Mechanism of Action	Common Drugs	Cell-Cycle Specificity	Common Side-Effects
Alkylating agents	Alter DNA structure by • Misreading of DNA code • Breaks in DNA molecule • Cross-linking of DNA strands	Nitrogen mustard Cyclophosphamide Melphalan Chlorambucil Thiotepa Cisplatin Busulfan	Cell-cycle nonspecific	Bone marrow suppression, nausea, vomiting, cystitis (cyclophosphamide) stomatitis, alopecia, gonadal suppression
Nitrosoureas	Similar to alkylating agents; cross blood–brain barrier	Carmustine (BCNU) Lomustine (CCNU) Semustine (methyl CCNU) Streptozocin	Cell-cycle nonspecific	Delayed and cumulative myelosuppression, especially thrombocytopenia; nausea, vomiting
Antimetabolites	Interfere with the biosynthesis of metabolites/nucleic acids necessary for RNA and DNA synthesis	Cytarabine 5-fluorouracil Methotrexate (MTX) Hydroxyurea 6-Mercaptopurine 6-Thioguanine 5-Azacytadine	Cell-cycle specific (S phase)	Nausea, vomiting, diarrhea, myelosuppression, proctitis, stomatitis, renal toxicity (MTX), hepatotoxicity.
Antitumor antibiotics	Interfere with DNA synthesis by binding DNA; prevent RNA synthesis	Dactinomycin Bleomycin Daunorubicin Mithramycin Mitomycin Doxorubicin (Adriamycin)	Cell-cycle nonspecific	Bone marrow suppression, nausea, vomiting, alopecia, anorexia, cardiac toxicity (Daunorubicin Doxorubicin)
Plant alkaloids	Cause metaphase arrest by inhibiting mitotic tubular formation (spindle); inhibit DNA and protein synthesis	Vincristine (VCR) Vinblastine Vindesine VP-16 VM-26	Cell-cycle specific (M phase)	Bone marrow suppression (mild with VCR), neuropathies (VCR), stomatitis
Hormonal agents	Bind to hormone receptor sites that alter cellular growth; block binding of estrogens to receptor sites (antiestrogens); inhibit RNA synthesis	Androgens Estrogens Antiestrogens Progesterone Steroids	Cell-cycle nonspecific	Hypercalcemia, jaundice, increased appetite, masculinization, feminization, sodium and fluid retention, nausea, vomiting, hot flashes
Miscellaneous agents	Unknown; too complex to categorize	Asparaginase Procarbazine M-AMSA Hexamethylmelamine Dacarbazine (DTIC) Mitoxantrone Methyl-GAG	?	Anorexia, nausea, vomiting, myelosuppression, hepatotoxicity, anaphylaxis, hypotension, altered glucose metabolism

with diarrhea a common result. Antimetabolites and antitumor antibiotics are the major culprits in mucositis and other gastrointestinal symptoms.

Hematopoietic System. Most chemotherapeutic agents depress bone marrow function (myelosuppression), resulting in decreased production of blood cells. Myelosuppression decreases the number of white blood cells or leukocytes (leukopenia), red blood cells (anemia), and platelets or thrombocytes (thrombocytopenia) and increases the risk of infection and bleeding. Depression of these cells is the usual reason for limiting the dose of the chemotherapeutic drugs. Frequent monitoring of blood cell counts is essential, and the patient must be protected from infection and injury, particularly while the blood cell counts are depressed.

Renal System. Chemotherapeutic agents can be harmful to the kidneys owing to direct effects of the drugs during their excretion and to the accumulation of end products following cell lysis. Cisplatin, methotrexate, and mitomycin are particularly toxic to the kidneys. Rapid cell lysis following chemotherapy results in increased urinary excretion of uric acid, which can lead to renal damage. Monitoring of blood urea nitrogen (BUN), serum creatinine, and creatinine clearance is essential. Adequate fluid hydration, alkalinization of the urine to prevent formation of uric acid crystals, and the use of allopurinol are frequently indicated to prevent these side-effects.

Cardiopulmonary System. Antitumor antibiotics (daunorubicin and doxorubicin) are known to cause irreversible cumulative cardiac toxicities, especially when total dosage reaches 550 mg/m^2. Cardiac ejection fraction, electrocardiographic (ECG) tracings, and signs of congestive heart failure must be monitored closely. Bleomycin and busulfan are known for their cumulative toxic effects on lung function. Pulmonary fibrosis can be a long-term effect of prolonged dosage with these drugs. Therefore, the patient is monitored closely for changes in pulmonary function.

Reproductive System. Testicular and ovarian function can be affected by chemotherapeutic agents, resulting in possible sterility. Reproductive ability may return following chemotherapy; however, reproductive cells may have been damaged during treatment and result in chromosomal abnormalities in offspring. Therefore, banking of sperm is recommended for men prior to the initiation of treatments. Patients and significant others are informed about potential changes in reproduction resulting from chemotherapy.

Neurologic System. The plant alkaloids, especially vincristine, can cause neurologic damage with repeated doses. Peripheral neuropathies, loss of deep tendon reflexes, and paralytic ileus may occur. These side-effects are usually reversible and disappear after completion of chemotherapy.

Nursing Considerations

The nurse has an important role in assessing and managing many of the problems experienced by the patient undergoing chemotherapy. Because of their systemic effects on normal as well as malignant cells, these problems are often widespread, affecting many body systems. Anorexia, nausea, vomiting, altered taste, and diarrhea put the patient at risk for nutritional and fluid and electrolyte disturbances. Changes in the mucosa of the gastrointestinal tract may lead to irritation of the oral cavity and intestinal tract, further threatening the patient's nutritional status. Therefore, it is important for the nurse to assess the patient's nutritional and fluid and electrolyte status frequently and to use creative ways to encourage an adequate fluid and dietary intake. Suppression of the bone marrow and immune system is an expected consequence of chemotherapy and frequently serves as a guide in determining appropriate chemotherapy dosage. However, this effect also increases the risk of anemia, infection, and bleeding disorders. Therefore, nursing assessment and care focus on identifying and modifying factors that further increase the patient's risk.

Asepsis and gentle handling are indicated to prevent infection and trauma. Laboratory test results, particularly blood cell counts, are monitored closely. Untoward changes in blood test results and the occurrence of signs of infection and bleeding are reported promptly to the patient's physician. The patient and family members are instructed about measures to prevent these problems at home. (See Nursing Care Plan 16-1 for detailed nursing care.)

Local effects of the chemotherapeutic agent are also of concern. The patient is observed closely during its administration because of the risk and consequences of extravasation (particularly of vesicant agents or those that may produce tissue necrosis if deposited in the subcutaneous tissues). Local difficulties or problems with administration of chemotherapeutic agents are brought to the attention of the physician promptly so that corrective measures can be taken immediately.

Nurses involved in handling chemotherapeutic agents may be exposed to low doses of the drugs by direct contact, inhalation, and ingestion. Personnel repeatedly exposed to cytotoxic drugs have demonstrated mutagenic activity in their urine. Although not all mutagens are carcinogenic, they do have the ability to produce permanent inheritable changes in the genetic material of cells. Although long-term studies of nurses handling chemotherapeutic agents have not been conducted, it is known that chemotherapeutic agents are associated with secondary formation of cancers and chromosome abnormalities. Nausea, vomiting, dizziness, alopecia, and nasal mucosal ulcerations have been reported in health care personnel who have handled chemotherapeutic agents. Because of known and potential hazards associated with handling chemotherapy, the Occupational Safety and Health Administration (OSHA), hospitals, and other health care agencies have developed specific precautions for those involved in preparation and administration of chemotherapy. When followed, these precautions greatly minimize the risk of exposure.

Hyperthermia

Hyperthermia (thermal therapy), the generation of temperatures greater than physiologic fever range (>106.70°F or 41.5°C), has been used for many years to elicit tumoricidal effects in human cancers. Research suggests that malignant cells are more sensitive than normal cells to the harmful effects of high temperatures for several reasons. Malignant cells lack enzymes for repair of DNA and cell membranes that are damaged by elevated temperatures. These cells are deficient in enzymes that generate adenosine triphosphate (ATP), which are necessary for a normal cellular response to the increased metabolic demands that occur with hyperthermia. Most tumor cells lack an adequate blood supply to provide needed oxygen during periods of increased cellular demand, such as during hyperthermia. Cancerous tumors lack blood vessels of adequate size for dissipation of heat. Research also suggests that the body's immune system may be indirectly stimulated when hyperthermia is used.

Hyperthermia is most effective when used in combination with radiation therapy or chemotherapy. Hyperthermia and radiation therapy are thought to work well together because hypoxic tumor cells and cells in the S phase of the cell cycle

(Text continues on p. 286)

Nursing Care Plan 16-1

Care of the Patient With Cancer

Nursing Interventions	Rationale	Expected Outcomes

Nursing Diagnosis: Potential for infection related to altered immunologic response

Goal: Prevention of infection

1. Assess patient for evidence of infection:
   a. Check vital signs every 4 hours.
   b. Monitor WBC count and differential WBC count each day.
   c. Inspect all sites that may serve as entry ports for pathogens (intravenous sites, wounds, skin folds, bony prominences, perineum and oral cavity).
2. Report fever ≥ 101°F (38.3°C), chills, diaphoresis, swelling, heat, pain, erythema, exudate on any body surfaces.
3. Report change in respiratory or mental status, urinary frequency or burning, malaise, myalgias, arthralgias, rash, or diarrhea.
4. Obtain cultures and sensitivities as indicated prior to initiation of antimicrobial treatment (wound exudate, sputum, urine, stool, blood).

5. Initiate measures to minimize infection.
   a. Discuss with patient and family
      (1) Placing patient in private room if absolute WBC count < 1000/cu mm
      (2) Importance of patient avoiding contact with persons having known or recent infection.
   b. Instruct all personnel in careful hand washing before and after entering room.
   c. Avoid rectal or vaginal procedures (rectal temperatures, examinations, suppositories; vaginal tampons).

   d. Use stool softeners to prevent constipation and straining.
   e. Assist patient in practice of meticulous personal hygiene.

1. Signs and symptoms of infection may be diminished in the immunocompromised host. Prompt recognition of infection and subsequent initiation of therapy will reduce morbidity and mortality associated with infection.

4. These tests will identify organism and indicate most appropriate antimicrobial therapy. Use of inappropriate antibiotics will enhance proliferation of additional flora and encourage growth of antibiotic-resistant organisms.

   (1) Exposure to infection is reduced.

   b. Hands are significant source of contamination.

   c. Incidence of rectal, perianal abscesses and subsequent systemic infection is high. Manipulation may cause disruption of membrane integrity and enhance progression of infection.

- Demonstrates normal temperature and vital signs.
- Exhibits absence of signs of inflammation: local edema, erythema, pain, and warmth.
- Exhibits normal breath sounds on auscultation.
- Takes deep breaths and coughs every 2 hours to prevent respiratory dysfunction and infection.

- Exhibits absence of pathologic bacteria on cultures.

- Patient avoids contact with others with infections.
- Patient avoids crowds.
- All personnel wash hands after each voiding and bowel movement.
- Excoriation and trauma of skin is avoided.
- Trauma to mucous membranes is avoided (avoidance of rectal temperatures, suppositories, vaginal tampons, perianal area trauma).
- Patient uses recommended procedures and techniques if participating in management of invasive lines or catheters.

(continued)

Nursing Interventions	*Rationale*	*Expected Outcomes*

Nursing Diagnosis: Potential for infection related to altered immunologic response

Goal: Prevention of infection

f. Avoid fresh fruits, raw meat, fish, and vegetables if absolute WBC count < 1000/cu mm; also remove fresh flowers and potted plants.	f. Fresh fruits and vegetables harbor bacteria not removed by ordinary washing. Flowers and potted plants are also sources of organisms.	
g. Change drinking water, denture cleaning fluids, and respiratory equipment containing water daily.	g. Stagnant water is a source of infection.	
6. Assess intravenous sites every day for evidence of infection:	6. Nosocomial staphylococcal septicemia is closely associated with intravenous catheters.	• Exhibits no signs of septicemia or septic shock
a. Change intravenous sites every other day.	a. Incidence of infection is increased when catheter is in place <72 hr.	• Exhibits normal vital signs, cardiac output, and arterial pressures when monitored
b. Cleanse skin with povidone-iodine prior to arterial puncture or venipuncture.	b. Povidone-iodine is effective against many gram-positive and gram-negative pathogens.	
c. Change central venous catheter dressings every other day.		
d. Change all solutions and infusion sets every 24 h.	d. Once introduced into the system, microorganisms are capable of growing in infusion sets despite replacement of bottle and high flow rates.	
7. Avoid intramuscular injections.	7. Risk of skin abcesses is reduced.	
8. Avoid insertion of urinary catheters; if necessary use strict aseptic technique.	8. Rates of infection *greatly* increase following urinary catheterization.	

Nursing Diagnosis: Potential for injury related to bleeding problems

Goal: Prevention of injury and bleeding

1. Assess for potential for bleeding: monitor platelet count.	1. Mild risk: 50,000–100,000/cu mm (SI: 0.05–0.1×10^{12}/L) Moderate risk: 20,000–50,000/cu mm (SI: 0.02–0.05×10^{12}/L) Severe risk: less than 20,000/cu mm (SI: 0.02×10^{12}/L)	
2. Assess for bleeding: a. Petechiae or ecchymosis	a. Indicates injury to microcirculation and larger vessels.	• Signs and symptoms of bleeding are identified. • Patient exhibits no blood in feces, urine, or emesis.
b. Decrease in Hgb/Hct	b. Indicates blood loss.	• Patient exhibits no bleeding of gums or of injection or venipuncture sites.
c. Prolonged bleeding from invasive procedures, venipunctures, minor cuts or scratches		• Patient exhibits no ecchymosis (bruising).
d. Frank or occult blood in any body excretion, emesis, sputum		
e. Bleeding from any body orifice		
f. Altered mental status	f. Indicates neurologic involvement.	

(continued)

Nursing Interventions	Rationale	Expected Outcomes

Nursing Diagnosis: Potential for injury related to bleeding problems

Goal: Prevention of injury and bleeding

3. Instruct patient and family about ways to minimize bleeding:
  a. Use soft toothbrush or toothette for mouth care.
  b. Avoid commercial mouthwashes.
 	
  c. Use electric razor for shaving.
  d. Use emery board for nail care.
  e. Avoid foods that are difficult to chew.
	a. Prevents trauma to oral tissues.
	
	b. Contains high alcohol content that will dry oral tissues.
	c. Prevents trauma to skin.
	
	e. Prevents oral tissue trauma.
		• Patient and family identify ways to prevent bleeding.
		• Patient uses recommended measures to reduce risk of bleeding (uses soft toothbrush, shaves with electric razor only).

4. Initiate measures to minimize injury related to bleeding.
  a. Draw all blood for lab work with one daily venipuncture.
  b. Avoid taking temperature rectally or administering suppositories and enemas.
  c. Avoid intramuscular injections; use smallest needle possible.
  d. Apply direct pressure to injections and venipuncture sites for at least 5 minutes.
  e. Lubricate lips with petrolatum.
  f. Avoid bladder catheterizations; use smallest catheter if necessary.
  g. Maintain fluid intake of at least 3 liters/24 hr unless contraindicated.
  h. Use stool softeners or increase bulk in diet.
  i. Avoid medications that will interfere with clotting (*e.g.,* alcohol, aspirin).
	a. Minimizes trauma.
	
	b. Prevents trauma to rectal mucosa.
	
	c. Prevents intramuscular bleeding.
	
	e. Prevents skin from drying.
	f. Prevents trauma to urethra.
	
	g. Hydration helps to prevent skin drying.
	
	h. Prevents constipation and straining that may injure rectal tissue.
	i. Minimizes risk of bleeding.
		• Exhibits normal vital signs.
		• Reports that environmental hazards have been reduced or removed.
		
		• Consumes adequate fluid.
		
		• Reports absence of constipation.

3. When platelet count is less than 20,000/cu mm, institute the following:
  a. Bed rest with padded side rails.
  b. Avoidance of strenous activity.
 	
  c. Platelet transfusions as prescribed; administer prescribed diphenhydramine hydrochloride (Benadryl) or hydrocortisone sodium succinate (Solu-Cortef) to prevent reaction to platelet transfusion.
	3. Platelet count of less than 20,000/cu mm is associated with increased risk of spontaneous bleeding.
	
	b. Increases intracranial pressure and risk of cerebral hemorrhage.
	c. Allergic reactions to blood products are associated with antigen–antibody reaction that causes platelet destruction.
		• Exhibits normal mental status and absence of signs of intracranial bleeding.
		
		• Avoids medications that interfere with clotting (aspirin).

(continued)

Nursing Interventions	*Rationale*	*Expected Outcomes*

Nursing Diagnosis: Alteration in skin integrity: erythematous/wet desquamation skin reactions

Goal: Maintenance of skin integrity

1. In erythematous areas,
  a. Avoid the use of soaps, cosmetics, perfumes, powders, lotions and ointments, deodorants.
  b. Use only lukewarm water in bathing the area.
  c. Avoid rubbing or scratching the area.
  d. Avoid shaving the area with a straight-edge razor.
  e. Avoid applying hot water bottles, heating pads, ice, and adhesive tape to the area.
  f. Avoid exposing the area to sunlight or cold weather.
  g. Avoid tight clothing in the area. Use cotton clothing.
  h. Apply vitamin A&D ointment to the area.
	1. Care to the affected areas must focus on preventing further skin irritation, drying, and damage.
	
	g. Allows air circulation to affected area.
	h. Aids healing.
		• Avoids use of soaps, powders, and other cosmetics on site of radiation therapy.
		• States rationale for special care of skin.
		• Exhibits minimal change in skin.
		• Avoids trauma to affected skin region (avoids shaving, constricting and irritating clothing, extremes of temperature, and use of adhesive tape).
		• Reports changes in skin promptly.

2. If wet desquamation occurs,
  a. Do not disrupt any blisters that have formed.
  b. Avoid frequent washing of the area.
  c. Notify physician of blistering.
  d. Use *prescribed* creams or ointments.
  e. If area weeps, apply a thin layer of gauze dressing.
	2. Open weeping areas are susceptible to bacterial infection. Care must be taken to prevent introduction of pathogens.
	
	d. Decreases irritation and inflammation of the area.
	e. Enhances drying.
		• Demonstrates proper care of blistered or open areas.
		• Exhibits absence of infection of blistered and opened areas.

Nursing Diagnosis: Impairment of oral mucous membranes: stomatitis

Goal: Maintenance of intact oral mucous membranes

1. Assess oral cavity daily.
 	
2. Instruct patient to report oral burning, pain, areas of redness, open lesions on the lips, pain associated with swallowing or decreased tolerance to temperature extremes of food.
3. Encourage and assist in oral hygiene regimens.
Preventive
  a. Avoid commercial mouthwashes.
 	
  b. Brush with soft toothbrush; use nonabrasive toothpaste after meals and bedtime; floss every 24 hr.
	
	2. Identification of initial stages of stomatitis will facilitate prompt interventions including modification of treatment as prescribed by physician.
	
	a. Alcohol content of mouthwashes will dry oral tissues and potentiate breakdown.
	b. Limits trauma and removes debris.
		• States rationale for frequent oral assessment and hygiene.
		• Identifies signs and symptoms of stomatitis to report to nurse or physician.
		
		• Participates in recommended oral hygiene regimen:
		  Avoids mouthwashes with alcohol.
		  Brushes teeth and mouth with soft bristle toothbrush.
		  Uses lubricant to keep lips soft and nonirritated.
		  Avoids hard to chew, spicy, and hot foods.

(continued)

Nursing Interventions	Rationale	Expected Outcomes

Nursing Diagnosis: Impairment of oral mucous membranes: stomatitis

Goal: Maintenance of intact oral mucous membranes

Mild Stomatitis (generalized erythema, limited ulcerations, small white patches: *Candida*)

c. Use normal saline mouthrinses every 2 hr while awake; every 6 hr at night.

d. Use soft toothbrush or toothette.

e. Remove dentures except for meals.

f. Use lip lubricant.

g. Avoid foods that are spicy or hard to chew and those with extremes of temperature.

Severe stomatitis (confluent ulcerations with bleeding and white patches covering more than 25% of oral mucosa)

h. Obtain cultures and sensitivities of areas of infection.

i. Assess ability to chew and swallow; assess gag reflex.

j. Oral rinses as prescribed or place patient on side and irrigate mouth; have suction available (may combine in solution saline, anti-*Candida* agent such as Mycostatin and topical anesthetic agent as described below).

k. Remove dentures.

l. Use toothette or gauze soaked with solution for cleansing.

m. Use lip lubricant.

n. Provide liquid or pureed diet.

o. Monitor for dehydration.

4. Minimize discomfort.

a. Consult physician for use of topical anesthetic such as dyclonine and diphenhydramine or viscous lidocaine.

b. Administer systemic analgesics as prescribed.

c. Perform mouth care as described.

---

c. Oxidizing action assists in removing debris, thick secretions, and bacteria.

d. Minimizes trauma.

e. Minimizes friction and discomfort.

g. Limits trauma, promotes comfort.

h. Assists in identifying need for antimicrobial therapy.

i. Patient may be in danger of aspiration.

j. Facilitates cleansing, provides for safety and comfort.

l. Limits trauma, promotes comfort.

o. Decreased oral intake and ulcerations potentiate fluid deficits.

a. Alleviates pain and increases sense of well-being; promotes participation in oral hygiene and nutritional intake.

c. Facilitates healing.

- Exhibits clean, intact oral mucosa.
- Exhibits no ulcerations or infections of oral cavity.
- Reports absent or decreased oral pain.
- Reports no difficulty swallowing.
- Exhibits healing (reepithelialization) of oral mucosa within 5 to 7 days if mild stomatitis has developed.
- Exhibits healing of oral tissues within 10 to 14 days if severe stomatitis has developed.
- Exhibits no bleeding or ulcerations of oral mucosa.
- Consumes adequate fluid and food intake.
- Exhibits absence of dehydration and weight loss.

(continued)

Nursing Interventions	*Rationale*	*Expected Outcomes*

Nursing Diagnosis: Alteration in tissue integrity: alopecia

Goal: Maintenance of tissue integrity; coping with hair loss

1. Discuss potential hair loss and re-growth with patient and family.	1. Provides information so patient and family can begin to prepare cognitively and emotionally for loss.	• Identifies alopecia as potential side-effect of treatment.
2. Explore potential impact of hair loss on self-image, interpersonal relationships, and sexuality.	2. Facilitates coping.	• Identifies positive and negative feelings and threats to self-image.
		• Verbalizes meaning that hair and possible hair loss have for him.
3. Prevent or minimize hair loss through the following:		• States rationale for modifications in hair care and treatment.
a. Scalp hypothermia	a. Decreases hair follicle uptake of chemotherapy (not used for patients with leukemia or lymphoma because tumor cells may be present in blood vessels or scalp tissue).	• Uses mild shampoo and conditioner and shampoos hair only when necessary.
		• Avoids hair dryers, curlers, sprays and other stresses on hair and scalp.
b. Cutting long hair prior to treatment.	b. Minimizes hair loss due to the weight and pulling on hair.	
c. Avoiding excessive shampooing.		
d. Using mild shampoo and conditioner, gently pat dry.		
e. Avoiding use of electric curlers, curling irons, dryers, clips, barrettes, and hair sprays.		
f. Avoiding excessive combing or brushing; use of wide-toothed comb.		
4. Prevent trauma to scalp.		
a. Lubricate scalp with vitamin A&D ointment to decrease itching	a. Assists in maintaining skin integrity.	• Wears hat or scarf over hair when exposed to sun.
b. Have patient use sunscreen or wear hat when in the sun.	b. Prevents ultraviolet light exposure.	
5. Suggest ways to assist in coping with hair loss:		
a. Purchase wig prior to hair loss.	a. Wig that closely resembles hair color and style is more easily selected if hair loss has not begun.	• Takes steps to deal with possible hair loss before it occurs; purchases wig or hair replacement.
b. If hair loss is present, take photograph to wig shop to assist in selection.	b. Facilitates adjustment.	• Maintains hygiene and grooming.
c. Begin to wear wig prior to hair loss.		• Interacts and socializes with others.
d. Contact the American Cancer Society for donated wigs, or store that specializes in this product.		
e. Wear hat, scarf, or turban.	e. Conceals loss.	
f. Wear accessories that are attractive and stylish.	f. Redirects attention.	

(continued)

Nursing Interventions	*Rationale*	*Expected Outcomes*

Nursing Diagnosis: Alteration in tissue integrity: alopecia

Goal: Maintenance of tissue integrity, coping with hair loss

6. Encourage patient to wear own clothes, retain social contacts, bring items of interest or special meaning to hospital room.	6. Assists in maintaining personal identity.	
7. Explain that hair growth usually begins again once therapy is completed.	7. Reassures patient that hair loss is usually temporary.	• States that hair loss and necessity of wig are temporary.

Nursing Diagnosis: Alteration in nutrition, less than body requirements, related to nausea/vomiting

Goal: Fewer episodes of nausea/vomiting prior to, during, and following chemotherapy administration

1. Adjust diet prior to and following drug administration according to patient preference and tolerance.	1. Each patient responds differently to food after chemotherapy. A diet containing foods that relieve the patient's nausea or vomiting is most helpful.	• Reports decrease in nausea. • Reports decrease in incidence of vomiting. • Consumes adequate fluid and food when nausea subsides.
2. Prevent unpleasant sights, odors, and sounds in the environment.	2. Unpleasant sensations can stimulate the nausea/vomiting center.	
3. Use distraction, relaxation techniques, and imagery prior to, during, and after chemotherapy.	3. Decreases anxiety, which can contribute to nausea/vomiting. Psychological conditioning may also be decreased.	• Demonstrates use of distraction, relaxation, and imagery when indicated.
4. Administer prescribed antiemetics, sedatives, and steroids as prescribed.	4. Combination drug therapy attempts to reduce nausea/vomiting through control of the various triggering pathways.	
5. Ensure adequate fluid hydration prior to, during, and following drug administration; assess intake and output.	5. Adequate fluid volume will dilute drug levels, decreasing stimulation of vomiting receptors.	• Exhibits normal skin turgor and moist mucous membranes • Reports no additional weight loss
6. Provide frequent oral hygiene.		
7. Provide pain relief measures, if necessary.	7. Increased comfort will increase physical tolerance of symptoms.	

Nursing Diagnosis: Alteration in nutrition: less than body requirements, related to anorexia/cachexia/malabsorption

Goal: Maintenance of nutritional status and of weight within 10% of pretreatment weight

1. Avoid unpleasant sights, odors, sounds in the environment during mealtime.	1. Anorexia can be stimulated or increased with noxious stimuli.	• Exhibits weight loss no greater than 10% of pretreatment weight. • Reports decreasing anorexia and increased interest in eating.
2. Provide foods preferred and well tolerated by the patient, preferably high-calorie/high-protein foods. Respect ethnic food preferences.	2. Foods preferred, well tolerated, and high in calories and protein will maintain nutritional status during periods of increased metabolic demand.	• Demonstrates normal skin turgor. • Identifies rationale for dietary modifications. • Participates in calorie counts and diet histories.

(continued)

Nursing Interventions	*Rationale*	*Expected Outcomes*

Nursing Diagnosis: Alteration in nutrition: less than body requirements, related to anorexia/cachexia/malabsorption

Goal: Maintenance of nutritional status and of weight within 10% of pretreatment weight

Nursing Interventions	*Rationale*	*Expected Outcomes*
3. Provide adequate fluid intake, but limit fluids at mealtime.	3. Fluid levels are necessary to eliminate waste products and prevent dehydration. Increased fluid levels with meals can lead to early satiety.	• Uses appropriate relaxation and imagery before meals. • Exhibits laboratory and clinical findings indicative of adequate nutritional intake: normal serum protein and transferrin levels, normal serum iron levels, normal hemoglobin, hematocrit and lymphocyte levels, normal urinary creatinine levels.
4. Provide smaller, more frequent meals.	4. Smaller feedings given more frequently are more easily tolerated since early satiety does not develop.	
5. Provide relaxed, quiet environment during mealtime with increased social interaction as desired.	5. A quiet environment promotes relaxation. Social interaction at mealtime increases appetite.	
6. If possible, serve wine at mealtime with foods.	6. Wine often stimulates appetite and adds calories.	
7. Offer cold foods, if desired.	7. Cold, high-protein foods are often more tolerable and less odorous than hot foods.	
8. Provide nutritional supplements, high-protein foods between meals.	8. Supplements/snacks add protein and calories to meet nutritional requirements.	• Consumes diet high in required nutrients
9. Provide frequent oral hygiene.	9. Oral hygiene measures stimulate appetite and increase saliva production.	• Carries out oral hygiene before meals.
10. Provide pain relief measures.	10. Pain increases anorexia.	• Reports that pain does not interfere with meals.
11. Provide control of nausea/vomiting.	11. Nausea/vomiting increases anorexia.	• Reports decreasing episodes of nausea and vomiting.
12. Increase activity level as tolerated.	12. Increased activity enhances appetite and appropriately utilizes nutrients.	• Participates in increasing levels of activity.
13. Decrease anxiety by encouraging verbalization of fears, concerns; use of relaxation techniques; imagery at mealtime.	13. Relief of anxiety may increase appetite.	
14. Position patient properly at mealtime.	14. Proper body position and alignment is necessary to aid chewing and swallowing.	
15. Provide enteral tube feedings of commercial liquid diets, elemental diets or blenderized foods via Silastic feeding tubes as prescribed.	15. Tube feedings may be necessary in the severely debilitated patient who has a functioning gastrointestinal system.	• States rationale for use of tube feedings and/or hyperalimentation.
16. Provide parenteral hyperalimentation with lipid supplements as prescribed.	16. Parenteral hyperalimentation with supplemental fats supplies needed amounts of calories and proteins to meet nutritional demands, especially in the nonfunctional gastrointestinal system.	• Participates in management of tube feedings and/or hyperalimentation.

(continued)

Nursing Interventions	*Rationale*	*Expected Outcomes*

Nursing Diagnosis: Activity intolerance: fatigue

Goal: Increased activity tolerance and decreased fatigue level

1. Provide several rest periods during the day, especially prior to and after physical exertion.	1. During rest, energy is conserved and levels are replenished. Several shorter rest periods may be more beneficial than one longer rest period.	• Reports decreasing levels of fatigue. • Increases participation in activities gradually. • Rests when fatigued.
2. Increase total hours of nighttime sleep.	2. Sleep helps to restore body energy levels.	• Reports restful sleep.
3. Rearrange daily schedule and organize activities to conserve energy expenditure.	3. Reorganization of activities can reduce energy losses and reduce stressors.	
4. Allow/ask for others' assistance with necessary chores such as housework, child care, shopping, cooking.		• Requests assistance with activities appropriately.
5. Encourage reduced job workload, if possible, by reducing number of hours worked per week.	5. Reducing workload will decrease physical and psychological stress and increase periods of rest/relaxation.	• Reports adequate energy to participate in activities important to him (visiting with family, hobbies, etc.).
6. Provide adequate protein and calorie intake.	6. Protein and calorie depletion decreases activity tolerance.	• Consumes diet with recommended protein and caloric intake.
7. Encourage use of relaxation techniques, mental imagery.	7. Promotion of relaxation and psychological rest will decrease physical fatigue.	• Uses relaxation exercises and imagery to decrease anxiety and promote rest.
8. Encourage participation in planned exercise programs.	8. Proper exercise programs will increase endurance and stamina.	• Participates in planned exercise program gradually. • Reports no breathlessness during activities.
9. Administer blood products as prescribed.	9. Lowered hemoglobin and hematocrit will predispose patient to fatigue due to decreased oxygen availability.	• Exhibits acceptable hemoglobin and hematocrit levels.

Nursing Diagnosis: Alteration in comfort: pain and discomfort

Goal: Relief of pain and discomfort

1. Assess pain and discomfort characteristics: location, quality, frequency, duration, etc.	1. Provides baseline for assessing changes in pain level and evaluation of interventions.	• Reports decreased level of pain and discomfort.
2. Assure patient that you know that pain is real and will assist him in reducing it.	2. Fear that pain will not be considered real increases anxiety and reduces pain tolerance.	• Reports less disruption from pain and discomfort.
3. Assess other factors contributing to patient's pain: fear, fatigue, anger, *etc.*	3. Provides basis for dealing with other factors that decrease patient's ability to tolerate pain and increase pain level.	• Explains how fatigue, fear, *etc.* contribute to severity of his pain and discomfort.
4. Administer analgesics to promote optimum pain relief within limits of physician's prescription.	4. Analgesics tend to be more effective when administered early in pain cycle.	• Accepts pain medication as prescribed.

(continued)

Nursing Interventions	*Rationale*	*Expected Outcomes*

Nursing Diagnosis: Alteration in comfort: pain and discomfort

Goal: Relief of pain and discomfort

5. Assess patient's behavioral responses to pain and pain experience.	5. Provides additional information about patient's pain.	• Exhibits decreased physical and behavioral signs of pain and discomfort in *acute pain* (no grimacing, crying, moaning; displays interest in surroundings and activities around him).
6. Collaborate with patient, physician, and other healthcare team members when changes in pain management are necessary.	6. New methods of administration of analgesia must be acceptable to patient, physician, and healthcare team to be effective; patient's participation decreases his sense of powerlessness.	• Takes an active role in administration of analgesia.
7. Encourage strategies of pain relief that patient has used successfully in previous pain experience.	7. Encourages success of pain relief strategies accepted by patient and family.	
8. Teach patient new strategies to relieve pain and discomfort: distraction, imagery, relaxation, cutaneous stimulation, etc.	8. Increases number of options and strategies available to patient.	• Identifies additional effective pain relief strategies.
		• Uses alternative pain relief strategies appropriately.
		• Reports effective use of new pain relief strategies and decrease in pain intensity.
		• Reports that decreased level of pain permits participation in other activities and events.

Nursing Diagnosis: Grieving related to anticipatory loss; altered role functioning

Goal: Progression through grieving process appropriately

1. Encourage verbalization of fears/concerns/questions regarding disease, treatment, and future implications.	1. An increased and accurate knowledge base will decrease anxiety and dispel misconceptions.	• The patient and family will progress through the phases of grief as evidenced by increased verbalization and expression of grief.
2. Encourage active participation of patient and/or family in care and treatment decisions.	2. Active participation will maintain patient independence and control.	• The patient and family will identify resources available to aid coping strategies during grieving.
3. Visit family frequently to establish/maintain relationships and physical closeness.	3. Frequent contacts will promote trust and security and reduce feelings of fear and isolation.	• The patient and family use resources and supports appropriately.
		• The patient and family discuss the future openly with each other.
4. Allow for ventilation of negative feelings including projected anger and hostility within acceptable limits.	4. This allows for emotional expression without destruction of self-esteem.	• The patient and family discuss concerns and feelings openly with each other.
5. Allow for periods of crying and expression of sadness.	5. These feelings are necessary for separation and detachment to occur.	• The patient and family use nonverbal expressions of concern for each other.
6. Involve clergy as desired by the patient and family.	6. This facilitates the grief process and spiritual care.	

(continued)

Nursing Interventions	Rationale	Expected Outcomes

Nursing Diagnosis: Grieving related to anticipatory loss; altered role functioning

Goal: Progression through grieving process appropriately

Nursing Interventions	Rationale	Expected Outcomes
7. Advise professional counseling as indicated for patient and/or family to alleviate pathologic grieving.	7. This facilitates the grief process.	
8. Allow for progression through the grieving process at the individual pace of the patient and family.	8. Grief work is variable. Not every person uses every phase of the grief process, and the time spent in dealing with each phase varies with every person. To complete grief work, this variability must be allowed.	

Nursing Diagnosis: Altered body image and self-esteem related to changes in appearance, function, and roles

Goal: Improved body image and self-esteem

Nursing Interventions	Rationale	Expected Outcomes
1. Assess patient's feelings about body image and level of self esteem.	1. Provides baseline assessment for evaluating changes and assessing effectiveness of interventions.	• Identifies concerns of importance.
2. Identify potential threats to patient's self-esteem (*e.g.,* altered appearance, decreased sexual function, hair loss, decreased energy, role changes). Validate concerns with patient.	2. Anticipates changes and permits patient to identify importance of these areas to the patient.	
3. Encourage continued participation in activities and decision-making.	3. Encourages/permits continued control of events and self.	• Takes active role in activities. • Maintains previous role in decision-making.
4. Encourage patient to verbalize concerns.	4. Identifying concerns is an important step in coping with them.	• Verbalizes feelings/reaction to losses or threatened losses.
5. Individualize care for the patient.	5. Prevents or reduces depersonalization and emphasizes patient's self-worth.	• Participates in self-care activities.
6. Assist patient in self-care when fatigue, lethargy, nausea, vomiting, and other symptoms prevent independence.	6. Physical well-being improves self-esteem.	• Permits others to assist in care when he/she is unable to be independent.
7. Assist patient in selecting and using cosmetics, scarves, hair pieces, and clothing that increase his sense of attractiveness.	7. Promotes positive body image.	• Exhibits interest in appearance and uses aids (cosmetics, scarves, etc.) appropriately.
8. Encourage patient and partner to share concerns about altered sexuality/sexual function and to explore alternatives to their usual sexual expression.	8. Provides opportunity for expressing concern, affection, and acceptance.	• Participation with others in conversations and social events and activities. • Verbalizes concern about sexual partner. • Explores alternative ways of expressing concern and affection.

are more heat sensitive than radiosensitive; the addition of heat damages tumor cells so that they are unable to repair themselves after radiation therapy damage. Hyperthermia is thought to alter cellular membrane permeability when used with chemotherapy, allowing for an increased uptake of the chemotherapeutic drug. Also, hyperthermia is thought to inhibit cellular repair processes, enhancing tumor death.

Heat can be produced with the use of radiowaves, ultrasound, microwaves, magnetic waves, hot water baths, or even hot wax immersions. Hyperthermia may be local or regional, or it may include the whole body. Local or regional hyperthermia may be delivered to a cancerous extremity (for malignant melanoma) by regional perfusion, in which the affected extremity is isolated by a tourniquet and an extracorporeal circulator heats the blood flowing through the affected part. Chemotherapeutic agents such as melphalan may also be heated and instilled into the regionally circulating blood. Local or regional hyperthermia may also include infusion of heated solutions into cancerous body organs. Whole body hyperthermia to treat disseminated disease may be achieved by extracorporeal circulation, immersion of patients in heated water or paraffin, or enclosure in heated suits.

Side-effects of hyperthermia treatments include skin burns and tissue damage, fatigue, hypotension, peripheral neuropathies, thrombophlebitis, nausea, vomiting, diarrhea, and electrolyte imbalances. Resistance to hyperthermia may develop during the treatment because cells adapt to repeated thermal insult. Research into the efficacy of hyperthermia, its delivery, and its side-effects is continuing.

Nursing Considerations

Although hyperthermia has been used for many years, many patients and their families are unfamiliar with this treatment for cancer. Consequently, they will need explanations about the procedure, its goals, and its effects. The patient is assessed for side-effects, and efforts are made to reduce their occurrence and severity.

Biological Response Modifiers

Biological response modifiers (BRMs) are agents or methods of treatment that have the ability to alter the immunologic relationship between the tumor and the cancer patient (host) to provide a therapeutic benefit. Although the mechanisms of action vary with each type of BRM, the goal is destruction or cessation of the malignant growth. Over the years we have come to understand the role of the body's natural immune defenses against cancer. The basis of BRM treatment lies in the restoration, stimulation, or augmentation of those natural immune defenses.

Some of the early investigations of the stimulation of the immune system involved nonspecific agents such as bacille Calmette-Guérin (BCG) and *Corynebacterium parvum* (*C. parvum*). These agents serve as antigens that stimulate an immune response when injected into the patient. It is hoped that the stimulated immune system will then be able to eradicate malignant growths. Extensive animal and human investigations with BCG have yielded some promising results, especially in the treatment of malignant melanoma, bladder cancer, and colorectal cancer. However, the exact role of these agents requires further investigation.

Interferons are another example of BRMs with both antiviral and antitumor properties. When stimulated, all nucleated cells are capable of producing these glycoproteins, which are classified according to their biological and chemical properties: α-interferons are produced by leukocytes, β-interferons are produced by fibroblasts, and γ-interferons are produced by lymphocytes.

Although the exact antitumor effects of interferons have not been thoroughly established, it is thought that they either stimulate the immune system or assist in prevention of tumor growth. Interferons enhance both lymphocyte and antibody production. They also facilitate the cytolytic role of macrophages and natural killer cells. Additionally, interferons are able to inhibit cell multiplication by increasing the duration of various phases of the cell cycle. The effects of interferons have been demonstrated in hairy cell leukemia, non-Hodgkin's lymphoma, renal cell carcinoma, melanoma, and Kaposi's sarcoma. Further efforts are underway to investigate the role of interferons in cancer treatment.

Monoclonal antibodies are another type of BRM; they became available through recent technological advances that enabled investigators to grow and produce specific antibodies for specific malignant cells. The production of monoclonal antibodies involves injecting tumor cells into mice and harvesting the antibodies produced by the immune systems of the mice. The antibodies are then infused into the cancer patient. Preliminary investigations of monoclonal antibody therapy for leukemia and lymphoma have been disappointing; however, initial reports of its use in treatment of solid tumors have been more promising. The feasibility of combining monoclonal antibodies and chemotherapeutic agents in hopes of improving the effectiveness of these agents is under investigation.

Lymphokines and *cytokines*, cell products of lymphocytes with known biological roles in the normal immune response, are also the focus of current research efforts. The most widely publicized agent is interleukin-2 (IL-2), which is known to stimulate the production and activation of T lymphocytes. Its role in the treatment of acquired immunodeficiency syndrome (AIDS) is under investigation.

Nursing Considerations

Patients receiving BRM therapy have many of the same needs as other cancer patients undergoing more conventional therapies. However, for many patients who have failed to respond to standard treatment modalities, BRM therapy may be viewed as a "last chance" effort. Consequently, it is essential that the nurse assess the need for education, support, and guidance for both the patient and family, and assist in planning and evaluating patient care. Nurses need to be familiar with each agent given and the potential adverse effects. Because of the investigational nature of these agents, the nurse will be administering them in a research setting. Accurate observations and careful documentation are essential components of the data collection process.

Unproven Methods

Forty-five percent of all cancer patients currently survive at least 5 years from the time of diagnosis and are potentially "cured" of their disease. However, those patients who do not receive desired results from treatment are susceptible targets for deceptive practices and quackery. Fear, ignorance, desperation, and family pressures are major factors that motivate patients to seek unproven methods of cancer treatment. Unfortunately, such unconventional therapies may interfere with conventional approaches, cause increased financial burdens, and increase morbidity among cancer patients.

Most unproven cancer treatments can be categorized as machines and devices, drugs and biologicals, metabolic and dietary regimens, or mystical and spiritual approaches.

Machines and Devices. Electrical gadgets and devices are commonly reputed to cure cancers. Most are operated by persons with questionable training who report incredulous success stories. Such machines are often decorated with elaborate lights and dials and produce vibrations or other sensations of currents or energy.

Drugs and Biologicals. Medicinal agents, herbs, vaccines, enzymes, and sera have been frequent components of fraudulent cancer therapy. These agents have included oral and external medications derived from weeds, flowers, and herbs and the blood and urine of patients and animals.

Metabolic and Dietary Regimens. Metabolic and dietary regimens emphasize the ingestion of only natural substances in order to purify the body and retard cancerous growth. These regimens include the grape diet, the carrot juice diet, coffee colonic irrigations, and raw liver intake. Laetrile (Vitamin B_{17}, amygdalin), one of the best-known forms of cancer quackery, was advocated as an agent to kill tumor cells by releasing cyanide, which is especially toxic to malignant cells. The National Cancer Institute, in response to public demand, investigated the effects of laetrile and reported no therapeutic benefits with its use. Many toxic effects (cyanide poisoning, fever, rash, headache, vomiting, diarrhea, and hypotension) were reported. Macrobiotic diets have also been advocated as cancer treatment to reestablish balance between the major forces in the universe, yin and yang. Persons adhering to macrobiotic diets tend to develop vitamin, mineral, and protein deficiencies; experience additional weight loss due to decreased calorie intake; and achieve no therapeutic benefits from the dietary manipulation.

Mystical and Spiritual Approaches. Mystical or spiritual approaches to cancer therapy include such techniques as psychic surgery, faith healing, "laying on of hands," and invocation of mystical universal powers to kill cancerous growths. These techniques are difficult to disclaim since they are based on faith.

Nursing Considerations

A trusting relationship, supportive care, and promotion of hope in the patient and his family are the most effective means of protecting them from fraudulent therapy and questionable claims of cancer cures. Truthful responses given in a nonjudgmental manner to questions and inquiries about unproven methods of cancer treatments may alleviate the fear and guilt on the part of the patient and family that they are not "doing everything" to obtain a cure. Characteristics common to fraudulent therapy may be shared with patients and their family so that they are informed and cautious in evaluating other forms of "therapy" (See Chart 16-3).

Nursing Care of the Patient With Cancer

The outlook for patients with cancer has greatly improved because of scientific and technological advances. However, as a result of the underlying malignancy or various treatment

---

Chart 16-3
Common Characteristics Associated With Practitioners of Fraudulent Therapy

- They tend to be isolated from established scientific facilities or associates.
- They do not use regular channels of communication (current, reputable scientific journals) for reporting scientific information. Physicians of this type tend to publish articles in journals that are not read by cancer specialists.
- They claim that prejudice of organized medicine hinders their efforts.
- They are prone to challenge established theories and attack prominent scientists with bitter criticism.
- They are quick to cite examples of physicians and scientists of the past who were forced to fight the rigid dogma of their day.
- They are often inclined to use complex jargon and unusual phraseology to embellish their writing.
- Their records are scanty or nonexistent.
- They often discourage, or even refuse, consultation with reputable physicians. If a scientific evaluation of their methods is made, they generally decline to accept the results, claiming that the "medical trust" is against them.

- Their method of treatment is often secret and is available only from them. Or, the mode of administration depends on special judgment that can be learned only from them.
- They discount biopsy verification in cancer diagnosis, sometimes by saying that it "spreads" the cancer. They may accept patients who have already been cured of cancer by orthodox means but fear they have not.
- They may use proven drugs or other methods of treatment as adjuvants to the unproven therapy, and if a favorable effect on cancer is shown, claim that it is the result of their unproven remedy.
- They may have multiple unusual degrees such as N.D. (Doctor of Naturopathy), Ph.N. (Philosopher of Naturopathy), or Ms.D. (Doctor of Metaphysics). These degrees may have been received from correspondence schools.
- Their chief supporters tend to be prominent statesmen, actors, writers, lawyers, even members of state or national legislatures—persons not trained or experienced in the natural history of cancer, the care of patients with cancer, or in scientific methodology.

(Unproven Methods of Cancer Management. New York, American Cancer Society, 1982.)

modalities, the patient with cancer may confront or experience a variety of secondary problems. Regardless of the type of cancer, treatment used, or prognosis, many patients with cancer are susceptible to these problems and complications. An important role of the nurse on the oncology team is to assess the patient for these problems and complications.

▶ Nursing Process
The Patient With Cancer

▷ Assessment

At all stages of cancer, the patient is assessed for those factors that predispose the patient to *infection and bleeding problems*. These factors include suppression of bone marrow and blood cell production by chemotherapy, radiation therapy, or the malignancy itself. The nurse monitors laboratory studies, particularly the complete blood cell count and blood coagulation studies, to detect early changes in white blood cells, red blood cells, and platelets. Common sites of infection and bleeding, such as the patient's pharynx, skin, perianal area, urinary tract, and respiratory tract, are assessed frequently. However, it is important to keep in mind that the typical signs of infection (fever, swelling, redness, drainage, and pain) may be absent in the immunosuppressed patient. The patient is monitored for sepsis, particularly if invasive catheters or infusion lines are in place.

The functions of the white blood cells are often impaired in cancer patients. A decrease in circulating white blood cells (WBCs) is referred to as *leukopenia* or *granulocytopenia*. There are three types of white blood cells: neutrophils, basophils, and eosinophils. The neutrophils, totaling 60% to 70% of all the body's white blood cells, play a major role in combating infection through phagocytosis. Both the total WBC count and concentration of neutrophils are important in determining the patient's ability to fight infection. A differential count supplies the relative numbers of the various types of WBCs and permits tabulation of polymorphonuclear neutrophils (mature neutrophils, reported as "polys," "PMNs," or "segs") and immature forms of neutrophils (reported as bands, metamyelocytes, and "stabs"). These numbers are compiled and reported as the absolute neutrophil count. The risk of infection rises as the absolute neutrophil count decreases.

The cancer patient is also closely monitored for signs of bleeding; the most common sites include the skin and mucous membranes, the intestinal, urinary, and respiratory tracts, and the brain. Gross bleeding as well as oozing at injection sites, bruising (ecchymosis), and changes in mental status that may indicate intracranial bleeding are monitored and reported.

Skin and tissue integrity is at risk in cancer patients because of the effects of chemotherapy, radiation therapy, surgery, and invasive procedures for diagnosis and therapy. As part of the assessment, the nurse identifies which of these predisposing factors are present and assesses the patient for other risk factors including nutritional deficits, bowel and bladder incontinence, immobility, immunosuppression, and changes related to aging. Skin lesions or ulceration secondary to the tumor are noted. Alterations in tissue integrity throughout the gastrointestinal tract are particularly bothersome to the patient. The oral mucous membranes and the appearance of lesions are noted, as is their effect on the patient's nutritional status and level of comfort. Hair loss (alopecia) is another form of tissue disruption common to cancer patients who receive radiation therapy or chemotherapy. In addition to noting its loss, the nurse also assesses the meaning of hair and hair loss to the patient and his family.

Assessment of the patient's *nutritional status* is an important part of the nurse's role. Alterations in nutritional status and weight loss may be secondary to the effects of a local tumor, systemic disease, treatment-related side-effects, or the emotional status of the patient. The patient's weight and calorie intake are monitored daily. Other information obtained through assessment includes diet history, frequency and duration of episodes of anorexia, changes in appetite, situations and foods that aggravate or relieve the anorexia, and medication history. Difficulty in chewing or swallowing is determined and the occurrence of nausea, vomiting, or diarrhea is noted. Clinical and laboratory data useful in assessing the patient's nutritional status include anthropometric measurements (triceps skin fold and mid upper arm circumference) serum protein levels (albumin and transferrin), lymphocyte count, hemoglobin levels, hematocrit, urinary creatinine levels, and serum iron levels.

Pain and discomfort in cancer may be related to the tumor or malignancy itself, to pressure exerted by the tumor, to diagnostic testing procedures, or to many of the cancer treatments that may be used. As in any other situation involving pain, the experience of cancer pain is affected by both physical and psychosocial influences. In addition to assessing the source and site of pain, the nurse also assesses those factors that increase the patient's perception of pain, such as fear and apprehension, fatigue, anger, and social isolation. Assessment scales for pain (see Chap. 15) are useful in assessing the patient's pain level before use of pain relieving treatments and in evaluating the patient's response to them.

Assessment of the cancer patient is not limited to the physiological changes that may occur in the course of the disease but also focuses on the patient's *psychological and mental status* as he and his family face this life-threatening experience, unpleasant diagnostic tests and treatment modalities, and progression of disease. The patient's mood and emotional reaction to the results of diagnostic testing and prognosis are assessed. His progression through stages of grief is assessed, as is his communication about his diagnosis and prognosis with his family.

Cancer patients are forced to cope with many *assaults to body image* throughout the course of disease and treatment. Entry into the health care system is often accompanied by depersonalization. Threats to self-concept are enormous as patients face the realization of illness, possible disability, and death. Many cancer patients are forced to alter their lifestyles to accommodate treatments or as a direct result of disease pathology. Priorities and value systems are often forced to change when body image is threatened and physical characteristics become less important. Disfiguring surgery, hair loss, cachexia, skin changes, altered communication patterns, and sexual dysfunction are some of the devastating results of cancer and its treatment that may threaten the patient's self-esteem and body image. During assessment, these potential threats are identified, as is the patient's ability to cope with these changes.

▷ *Nursing Diagnoses*

Based on the assessment data, nursing diagnoses of the patient with cancer may include the following:

- Potential for infection related to altered immunologic response
- Potential for injury related to bleeding disorder
- Alterations in tissue integrity related to the effects of treatment and disease
- Alterations in nutrition: less than body requirements related to anorexia and gastrointestinal changes
- Alterations in comfort: pain related to disease and treatment effects
- Grieving related to anticipated loss and altered role function
- Disturbance in self-concept: altered body image related to changes in appearance and role functions

▷ *Planning and Implementation*

▷ *Goals:*   The major goals of the patient may include prevention of infection, prevention of injury related to bleeding disorder, maintenance of tissue integrity, maintenance of nutrition, relief of pain, progression through grieving process appropriately, and improved body image.

Nursing Interventions

Prevention of Infection.   Despite advances in the care of patients with cancer, infection remains the leading cause of death. Defense against infection is compromised in many different ways. Skin and mucous membrane integrity, the body's first line of defense, is challenged by multiple invasive diagnostic and therapeutic procedures, adverse effects of irradiation and chemotherapy, and the detrimental effects of immobility. Impaired nutrition resulting from anorexia, nausea, vomiting, diarrhea, and the underlying malignant process can alter the body's ability to combat invading organisms. Medications such as antibiotics disturb the balance of normal flora, allowing the overgrowth of pathogenic organisms. Other medications can also alter the immune response (see Chap. 45). Cancer itself may be immunosuppressive. Malignancies such as leukemia and lymphoma are often associated with defects in cellular and humoral immunity. Advanced cancer can lead to tumor obstruction of hollow viscera, blood, and lymphatic vessels, creating a favorable environment for proliferation of pathogenic organisms. In some patients, tumor cells infiltrate bone marrow and prevent normal production of white blood cells. Most often, however, a decrease in white blood cells is a result of bone marrow suppression following chemotherapy or irradiation.

Infections in the myelosuppressed or immunosuppressed patient are most often nosocomial, a result of organisms that have become part of the patient's resident flora after being acquired from the hospital environment. The most threatening pathogens are the gram-negative bacilli such as *Pseudomonas aeruginosa* and *Escherichia coli*. Gram-positive bacilli such as *Staphylococcus aureus* and fungal organisms such as *Candida albicans* can also contribute to serious infection.

Fever is probably the most important sign of infection in the immunocompromised patient. Although fever may be related to a variety of noninfectious conditions including the underlying malignancy, any temperature elevation of 101°F (38.3°C) or above is reported and dealt with promptly. Antibiotic agents may be prescribed to treat infections after results of cultures and sensitivities of wound drainage, exudate, sputum, urine, stool, or blood specimens are obtained. An important component of the nurse's role is to administer these medications promptly according to the prescribed schedule to achieve adequate blood levels of the medication. Strict asepsis is essential when handling intravenous lines, catheters, and other invasive equipment. The patient is protected from exposure to others with active infections and is strongly advised to avoid crowds. Handwashing and appropriate hygiene are necessary to reduce exposure to potentially harmful bacteria and to eliminate environmental sources of contamination. The patient is also encouraged to cough and take deep breaths frequently to prevent atelectasis and other potential respiratory problems.

Assessment of the patient for infection and inflammation is frequent and continues throughout the course of disease. Septicemia and septic shock are life-threatening complications that must be prevented or detected early in their course. The patient and family members are instructed about signs of septicemia, preventive actions, and actions to take if infection or septicemia occurs.

Prevention of Injury Related to Bleeding Disorder. A decrease in the number of circulating platelets (thrombocytopenia) is the most common cause of bleeding in the patient with cancer. Thrombocytopenia is often a result of bone marrow depression following certain types of chemotherapy and radiation therapy. Tumor infiltration of bone marrow can also impair the normal production of platelets. In some cases, platelet destruction is associated with an enlarged spleen (hypersplenism) and abnormal antibody function that occur with leukemia and lymphoma.

Platelets are essential for normal blood clotting and coagulation (hemostasis). *Thrombocytopenia* is defined as a platelet count less than 100,000/cu mm (SI: 0.1×10^{12}/L). When the count falls to 20,000 to 50,000/cu mm (SI: 0.02 to 0.05×10^{12}/L), the risk for bleeding increases. Counts less than 20,000/cu mm (SI: 0.02×10^{12}/L) are associated with an increased risk for spontaneous bleeding. In addition to monitoring laboratory values, the nurse continues to assess the patient for evidence of bleeding. The nurse also takes steps to prevent trauma and minimize the risk of bleeding by replacing the patient's hard-bristled toothbrush with a soft-bristled one, by using an electric razor rather than a safety or straight-edge razor, and by avoiding unnecessary invasive procedures (*e.g.*, rectal temperatures, catheterization). The patient and family are assisted in identifying and removing environmental hazards that may lead to falls or other trauma. Soft foods, increased fluid intake, and stool softeners, if prescribed, may be indicated to reduce trauma to the gastrointestinal tract. The joints and extremities are handled and moved gently to minimize the risk of spontaneous bleeding.

Maintenance of Tissue Integrity.   The person with cancer is at risk for the development of a variety of skin and mucous membrane impairments. The nurse in all health settings is in an ideal position to assess and assist the patient and family in the management of these problems. Some of the most frequently encountered disturbances include skin and tissue reactions to radiation therapy, stomatitis, alopecia, and metastatic skin lesions.

The patient who is experiencing skin and tissue reactions to radiation therapy requires careful skin care to prevent further skin irritation, drying, and damage. The skin over the affected area is handled gently; rubbing and use of hot or cold water, soaps, powders, lotions, and cosmetics are avoided. Trauma to the area is prevented by use of loosely fitting clothes that do not constrict, irritate, or rub the affected area. If blistering occurs, care is taken not to disrupt the blisters to reduce the risk of introducing bacteria. Aseptic wound care is indicated to minimize the risk of infection and sepsis.

Stomatitis. Stomatitis is a common problem in cancer patients as a result of chemotherapy or radiation therapy. It is an inflammatory response of the oral tissues that may progress from mild erythema and edema to painful ulcerations, bleeding, and secondary infection. This condition most often develops within 5 to 14 days of the administration of certain chemotherapeutic agents such as doxorubicin and 5-fluorouracil. It may also occur with irradiation to the head and neck area. In very severe cases of stomatitis, chemotherapy may be temporarily halted until resolution of inflammation.

As a result of normal everyday wear and tear, the epithelial cells that line the oral cavity have a very rapid turnover or routinely slough off. Chemotherapy and irradiation interfere with the body's ability to replace those cells. An inflammatory response develops as denuded areas appear in the oral cavity. Myelosuppression as a result of the underlying malignancy or treatment predisposes the patient to oral bleeding and infection. Pain associated with ulcerated oral tissues can significantly interfere with nutritional intake and willingness to maintain oral hygiene. Soft-bristled toothbrushes and nonabrasive toothpaste prevent or reduce the trauma to the oral mucosa. Restriction of foods that are difficult to chew, too hot, or spicy may further reduce trauma and promote comfort. The patient's lips are lubricated to keep them soft. Topical antifungal agents and anesthetics may be prescribed to promote healing and minimize patient discomfort. The patient who experiences severe pain and discomfort with stomatitis will require encouragement and assistance to use these prescribed agents and to maintain an adequate fluid and food intake.

Alopecia. The temporary or permanent thinning or complete loss of hair, referred to as *alopecia,* is a potential adverse effect of certain forms of radiation therapy and several chemotherapeutic agents. The extent of alopecia depends on the dose and duration of therapy. These treatment modalities cause alopecia by damaging stem cells and hair follicles. As a result, the hair is brittle and may fall out or break off at the surface of the scalp. Loss of other body hair is less frequent.

Many health professionals view hair loss as a minor problem when compared with the potential life-threatening consequences of the underlying malignancy. However, for many patients, hair loss poses a major threat to body image, arousing feelings of anxiety, sadness, anger, rejection, ridicule, and isolation. To patients and families, hair loss can serve as a constant reminder of cancer, interfering with coping abilities, interpersonal relationships, and sexuality. The nurse's role is to provide information about alopecia and to assist the patient and family in coping with hair loss and changes in body image. The patient is encouraged to acquire a wig or hairpiece before hair loss so that the replacement matches the patient's own hair. Use of attractive scarves and hats may make the patient feel more attractive. It is frequently of some comfort to patients that the hair usually begins to grow again after completion of the chemotherapy; however, the color and texture of the new hair may differ.

Malignant Skin Lesions. Skin lesions may occur with local extension or tumor embolization into the epithelium and its surrounding lymph and blood vessels. Secondary growth of cancer cells into the skin may be characterized as erythematous areas progressing to wounds involving tissue necrosis and infection. The most extensive lesions are friable, purulent, and malodorous. In addition, these lesions are a source of considerable pain and discomfort. Although this type of wound is most often associated with breast cancer, it can also accompany lymphoma, leukemia, melanoma, and cancers of the head and neck, lung, uterus, kidney, colon, and bladder. The development of severe skin lesions is usually considered to be a very poor prognostic sign for expected length of survival.

Ulcerating skin lesions usually indicate the presence of widely disseminated disease. Therefore, eradication of the problem is usually not feasible. The management of these lesions becomes a nursing priority. Nursing care includes careful assessment, cleansing, reduction of superficial bacterial flora, control of bleeding, reduction of odor, and protection against pain and further trauma to the skin. The patient and family will require assistance and guidance to care for these skin lesions at home. Referral to a community health nurse is indicated to provide assistance and evaluation of wound care at home.

Maintenance of Nutritional Status. Most cancer patients experience some degree of weight loss during their illness. Anorexia, malabsorption, and cachexia are examples of nutritional problems commonly seen in cancer patients.

Anorexia. There are many theories about the etiology of anorexia in the cancer patient. Alterations in taste manifested by increased salty, sour, and metallic tastes and altered responses to sweet and bitter tastes lead to decreased appetite, decreased intake, and protein–calorie malnutrition in the cancer patient. Taste alterations may be due to deficiencies of minerals such as zinc, increases in circulating amino acids, and the administration of chemotherapeutic agents. Individuals undergoing radiation therapy to the head and neck may experience "mouth blindness," which is a severe impairment of taste. Alterations in the sense of smell also alter taste, which is a common experience of patients with head and neck cancers. Anorexia may be related to early satiety and a sense of fullness secondary to decreased digestive enzymes, abnormalities of glucose and triglyceride metabolism, and prolonged stimulation of gastric volume receptors. Psychological distress such as fear, pain, depression, and isolation throughout illness may have a negative impact on appetite. Conditioned food aversions due to past experiences with nausea, vomiting, and treatment modalities may also contribute to anorexia.

Malabsorption. Many cancer patients are unable to absorb nutrients from the gastrointestinal system secondary to tumor activity and cancer treatment. Tumors may impair enzyme production; create fistulas; secrete hormones and enzymes such as gastrin, which leads to increased gastrointestinal irritation, peptic ulcer disease, and decreased fat digestion; and interfere with protein digestion. Chemotherapy and irradiation can irritate and damage mucosal cells of the bowel, inhibiting absorption. Radiation therapy can cause sclerosis of the blood vessels in the bowel and fibrotic changes in the gastrointestinal tissue. Surgical intervention may change peristaltic patterns, alter gastrointestinal secretions, and reduce the absorptive surfaces of the gastrointestinal mucosa, all leading to malabsorption.

Cachexia. Cachexia (wasting syndrome) is common in the cancer patient, especially in advanced disease states. Cancer cachexia is related to inadequate nutritional intake along with increasing metabolic demand, increased energy expenditure due to anaerobic metabolism of the tumor, impaired glucose metabolism, competition of the tumor cells for nutrients, altered lipid metabolism, and failure of appetite.

Creative dietary modification to overcome the factors contributing to anorexia must be carried out for each patient. Family members are included in the dietary plan of care to maintain consistency and aid compliance. Factors contributing to the patient's anorexia (unpleasant sights and odors) are eliminated. The patient's preferences as well as his physiologic and metabolic requirements are considered in selecting foods. Small, frequent meals are provided with additional supplements between meals. Oral hygiene and pain relief measures are offered before mealtime to make meals more pleasant.

Interventions to relieve malabsorptive states may include enzyme and vitamin replacement, changes in feeding schedule, use of elemental diets, and measures to relieve diarrhea. If malabsorption is severe, hyperalimentation may be necessary via a right atrial Silastic catheter, such as a Hickman or a Broviac catheter (see Fig. 32-11). These catheters are surgically placed and are maintained for long-term venous access. In order to prevent infection, these catheters are tunneled under the skin through the subcutaneous tissue before entering the superior vena cava and the right atrium. A Dacron cuff located just under the skin at the exit site anchors the catheter and prevents entry of bacteria. Maintenance of the catheter requires heparinization to prevent clotting and dressing changes at the exit site to prevent infection. Specific procedures for catheter care will vary among health care institutions. General nursing interventions include flushes with small doses of heparin in normal saline, infused every 24 to 48 hours or after each use of the catheter. The dressings are changed three times a week, and the exit site is assessed for redness, swelling, discharge, pain, or protrusion of the Dacron cuff. The site should be cleansed aseptically with alcohol followed by povidone-iodine (Betadine). An anti-infective topical agent is applied to the site, and an occlusive gauze or transparent dressing is applied. The infusion cap at the end of the catheter is changed weekly to prevent infection. Patient education is essential for prevention and management of potential complications including catheter breakage, air emboli, and infection.

Interventions to reduce cachexia usually do not prolong survival but improve the quality of life. Creative dietary therapies, enteral (tube) feedings, or hyperalimentation may be chosen to deliver nourishment. Nursing care is also directed toward prevention of trauma, infection, and other complications that increase metabolic demands.

Relief of Pain. It is estimated that 60% to 96% of all individuals with progressive malignant disease experience pain. Although patients with cancer may have acute pain, their pain is more frequently characterized as chronic. (For a complete discussion of pain, see Chap. 15.) As in other situations involving pain, the experience of cancer pain is influenced by both physical and psychosocial factors.

Malignancies can cause pain in a variety of ways. Bone destruction as a result of tumor invasion is one of the most devastating sources of pain. Bone involvement is seen commonly in multiple myeloma and cancers of the breast and prostate. Infiltration or compression of nerves can cause pain that is described as sharp and burning. Vertebral metastasis involving spinal nerves may occur with breast and lung cancer. Tumors causing lymphatic or venous obstruction may lead to a dull, throbbing type of pain. This is often associated with lymphoma or Kaposi's sarcoma. Ischemic pain results from any tumor that occludes arterial circulation. Obstruction of hollow viscera is often associated with colon cancer. Patients with abdominal obstruction often complain of pain that is dull and poorly localized. Finally, tumors invading skin or mucous membranes may cause pain associated with inflammation, ulceration, infection, and tissue necrosis; this is common in patients with progressive head and neck malignancies and Kaposi's sarcoma.

Pain is also associated with various cancer treatment modalities. Acute pain is linked with trauma that results from surgical procedures. Tissue necrosis, peripheral neuropathies, and stomatitis are potential sources of pain that may occur with certain chemotherapeutic agents. Radiation therapy can cause inflammation of the skin or irradiated organs.

In today's society, most people expect pain to pass quickly, and in fact it usually does. However, although it is controllable, cancer pain is often irreversible and not quickly resolved. For many patients, pain is a signal of continued tumor progression and impending death. As anticipation and anxiety about the pain increase, the patient's perception of the pain is heightened producing fear and additional pain. Chronic cancer pain, then, can be best described as a cycle progressing from pain to anxiety to fear and back to pain again.

Pain tolerance, the point past which pain can no longer be tolerated, varies among patients. Pain tolerance is decreased by fatigue, anxiety, fear of death, anger, powerlessness, social isolation, changes in role identity, loss of independence, and past experiences. Tolerance to pain is enhanced by adequate rest and sleep, diversion, mood elevation, empathy, antidepressants, antianxiety agents, and analgesics.

Successful management of cancer pain is based on a thorough and precise pain assessment that examines physical, psychosocial, environmental, and spiritual factors. A multidisciplinary team effort is essential to determine the most optimal approach for pain management. Prevention and reduction of pain serve to lessen anxiety and break the previously described pain cycle. This can be accomplished best by administering analgesics on a regularly scheduled basis as prescribed and not as needed (prn). A variety of pharmacologic and nonpharmacologic approaches offer the best methods of providing for cancer pain management. No reasonable approaches, even those that may be somewhat invasive, should be overlooked because of a poor or terminal prognosis. Improving the quality of life is as valuable as preventing a painful death.

Progression through the Grieving Process. Because there are so many kinds of cancer (over 100), the diagnosis of cancer need not indicate a fatal outcome. Many forms of cancer are curable; many others achieve "cure" status if they are treated early. Despite these facts, many patients and their families view cancer as a fatal disease that is inevitably accompanied by pain, suffering, debility, and emaciation. Grieving is a normal response to these fears and to the losses anticipated or experienced by the patient with cancer. These may include loss of health, normal sensations, body image, social interaction, sexuality, and intimacy. The patient, his family, and friends may grieve the loss of quality time to spend with others, the loss of a future and unfulfilled plans, and the loss of control over one's own body and emotional reactions.

The patient and his family who have just been informed by their physician about the diagnosis of cancer frequently respond with shock, numbness, and disbelief. It is often during this stage that the patient and family are called on to make important initial decisions about treatment and require the support of the physician, nurse, and other health care team members to make these decisions. An important role of the nurse is to answer the questions of the patient and family and clarify information provided by the physician. In addition to assessing the response of the patient and family to the diagnosis and planned treatment, the nurse assists them in framing their questions and concerns, identifying resources and support persons (*e.g.,* clergy, counselor), and communicating and sharing their concerns with each other.

As the patient and family progress through the grieving process, they may express feelings of anger, frustration, and depression. During this time, the nurse encourages the patient and family to verbalize their feelings in an atmosphere of trust and support. She continues to assess their reactions and provides assistance and support as they confront and learn to deal with new problems.

If the patient enters the terminal phase of disease, it may become obvious that the patient and family members are at different stages of the grieving process. Therefore, the nurse assists the patient and family at these different stages to come to grips with their reactions and feelings. Physical support, including holding the patient's hand or just being present at his bedside, frequently contributes to his feelings of trust and peace of mind. Maintaining contact with the surviving family members after death of the cancer patient may help them to progress through the process of grieving and to work through their feelings of loss.

Improved Body Image and Self-Esteem. A positive approach is essential when caring for the patient with an altered body image. Independence and continued participation in self-care and decision making are encouraged to help the patient retain control and a sense of self-worth. The patient is encouraged to express his feelings about threats to his body image. Assistance is provided to enable the patient to assume those tasks and participate in those activities of most importance and interest to him. The nurse serves as a good listener and counselor to the patient as well as to the family. Referral to a support group for cancer patients, their families, or both often provides additional assistance in coping with the changes resulting from cancer or its treatment.

The patient who is experiencing alterations in sexuality and sexual function is encouraged to share and discuss his concerns openly with his partner. Alternative forms of sexual expression are explored with the patient and partner to promote positive self-worth and acceptance. The nurse who identifies serious physiologic, psychological, or communication difficulties related to sexuality or sexual function is in a key position to assist the patient and partner to seek further counseling if necessary.

▷ *Evaluation*

▷ *Expected Outcomes*
(See Nursing Care Plan 16-1 for specific outcomes.)

1. Patient experiences no infection or inflammation
2. Exhibits no bleeding
3. Maintains adequate tissue (skin and mucous membrane) integrity
4. Maintains adequate nutritional status
5. Achieves relief of pain and discomfort
6. Progresses through grieving process
7. Exhibits improved body image and self-esteem

Rehabilitation

The diagnosis of cancer may be accompanied by emotional turmoil and changes in life-style or daily habits. However, with advances in diagnosis and treatment, survival rates are improving. Many patients, including those who receive primary surgical treatment and adjuvant chemotherapy or irradiation, are returning to work and their usual activities of daily living. These patients may encounter a variety of problems, including coping with changes in functional abilities and attitudes of employers, co-workers, and families.

Nurses play an important role in the rehabilitation of the cancer patient. Assessment of body image changes as a result of disfiguring treatments is necessary in order to facilitate the patient's adjustment to changes in appearance or functional abilities. The nurse can refer the patient and family to a variety of support groups sponsored by the American Cancer Society, such as those for people who have had laryngectomies or mastectomies. Nurses also collaborate with physical and occupational therapists in improving the patient's abilities and use of prosthetic devices.

Some patients return to work and continue to receive either chemotherapy or radiation therapy for extended periods of time. These people may experience transient problems such as lethargy, easy fatigue, anorexia, nausea, or vomiting. Nurses assess for the existence of these problems and assist the patient in identifying strategies for coping with them. For patients with gastrointestinal disturbances following chemotherapy, altering work hours or receiving treatments in the evenings may prove to be helpful. Nurses collaborate with dietitians to help patients plan meals that will be tolerable and meet nutritional requirements.

Discrimination against recovering cancer patients has been demonstrated in several forms. Often employers lack the understanding of the variability that exists in the diagnosis of cancer in terms of functional capacity and prognosis. As a result, employers may be hesitant to hire or continue employment of people with cancer, especially if continued treatment regimens might require adjustments in work schedules. Attitudes of co-workers can become a problem when related to communication impairments such as those experienced by some head and neck cancer patients. Finally, employers, co-workers, and families may continue to view the person as being "sick" despite ongoing recovery or completion of treatment.

Nurses can participate in efforts to educate employers and the public in general to ensure that the rights of patients with cancer are maintained. Whenever possible, nurses assist patients and families to resume preexisting roles. Nurses can encourage patients to regain the highest level of independence possible. In addition, the patient may be directed to vocational rehabilitation services of the American Cancer Society or other agencies. The diagnosis of cancer need not be a "death sentence." Many people can resume active roles in life.

Gerontological Considerations

Oncology nurses are working with increasing numbers of elderly patients. Approximately 55% of all cancers occur after 65 years of age. Common malignancies in the elderly include multiple myeloma, non-Hodgkin's lymphoma, oropharyngeal cancers, and cancers of the bladder, breast, colon, lung, and prostate.

It is important for oncology nurses working with this population to understand the normal physiologic changes that occur with aging. These changes include decreased skin elasticity; decreased skeletal mass, structure, and strength; decreased organ function and structure; impaired immune system mechanisms; alterations in neurologic function; and altered drug absorption, distribution, metabolism, and elimination. These changes ultimately influence the elderly patient's ability to tolerate treatment for cancer. In addition, many elderly patients have other chronic diseases that may also limit tolerance of treatment.

Potential toxicities associated with chemotherapeutic agents such as cisplatin may be enhanced by a decline in renal blood flow and creatinine clearance normally associated with the aging process. Cardiac toxicities associated with chemotherapy with doxorubicin may be more pronounced in the elderly patient who already has a decreased cardiac output as a result of normal physiologic aging.

The elderly person receiving radiation therapy may have a delayed recovery of normal tissues as a result of the changes in tissue repair associated with aging. The potential adverse effects involving the bone marrow, gastrointestinal tract, and skin may be enhanced, leading to an increased incidence and severity of myelosuppression, skin impairments, anorexia, nausea, vomiting, and diarrhea.

The older patient is often slower to recover from surgical interventions. Decreased tissue healing capacity and pulmonary and cardiovascular functioning may increase the risk of the patient developing postoperative complications such as atelectasis, pneumonia, and wound infections.

The nurse must be aware of the increased risk of complications following cancer treatment in the elderly and carefully assess for signs and symptoms of adverse effects. In addition, the elderly patient is instructed to report all symptoms to the physician. It is not uncommon for the elderly patient to delay reporting symptoms, attributing them to "old age." Many elderly persons do not want to report illness for fear of loss of independence, role functions, and financial security. The nurse acts as a patient advocate, encouraging independence and providing support when indicated.

Care of the Patient With Advanced Cancer

The patient with advanced cancer is likely to experience many of the problems previously described, but all to a greater degree. Symptoms of gastrointestinal disturbances, nutritional problems, weight loss, and cachexia make him more susceptible to skin breakdown, fluid and electrolyte problems, and infection. Although not all cancer patients experience pain, those who do often fear that it will not be adequately treated. Although treatment at this stage of illness is likely to be palliative rather than curative, prevention and appropriate management of problems can improve the quality of the patient's life considerably. For example, use of analgesia on a regular basis at set intervals rather than on an "as needed" basis frequently breaks the cycle of tension and anxiety associated with waiting until pain becomes severe and pain relief is inadequate once the analgesic is given. Working with the patient and family as well as other health care providers on a pain management program based on the patient's individual requirements frequently increases his comfort and sense of control. In addition, the dose of narcotic analgesic required is often reduced as pain becomes more manageable and other medications (*e.g.*, sedatives, tranquilizers, muscle relaxants) are added to assist in relieving pain.

The patient may be a candidate for radiation therapy or surgical intervention to relieve severe pain. The consequences of these procedures (*e.g.*, percutaneous nerve block, cordotomy) are explained to the patient and family, and measures are taken to prevent complications resulting from altered sensation, immobility, and changes in bowel and bladder function.

With the appearance of each new symptom, the patient often experiences dread and fear that the disease is progressing. However, one cannot assume that all symptoms are related to the cancer. The new symptoms and problems are evaluated and treated aggressively if possible to increase the patient's comfort and improve the quality of life.

Weakness, immobility, fatigue, and inactivity often occur in the advanced stages of cancer as a result of the tumor itself, treatment, inadequate nutritional intake, or dyspnea. The nurse works with the patient to set realistic goals and to provide rest balanced with planned activities and exercise. She assists the patient in identifying less energy-consuming methods of accomplishing tasks and activities that he values the most.

Efforts are made throughout the course of the disease to provide the patient with as much control and independence as he wants, but with assurance that support and assistance will be provided. Additionally, the health care team works with the patient and family to ascertain and adhere to the patient's wishes about treatment methods and care as he approaches the terminal phase of illness and death.

Hospice

For many years society was unable to appropriately cope with patients in the most advanced stages of cancer, and patients were left in acute care settings to die rather than at home or in facilities specifically designed to manage the needs of patients with terminal disease. The needs of these persons do not require advanced technology or sophisticated equipment but are best managed by a comprehensive multidisciplinary program that focuses on symptom relief and psychosocial and spiritual support for the patient and family when cure and remission are no longer possible. The concept of hospice, which originated in Great Britain, best addresses these needs. Most importantly, the unit of care is the family, not just the patient. Hospice may take on several forms: free-standing hospices, hospital-based programs, and community or home-based programs.

Because of high costs associated with maintaining free-standing hospices, care is often provided by coordinating hospital-based and community services. Although physicians, social workers, clergy, dietitians, physical therapists, and volunteers are involved in patient care, nurses are most often the coordinators of all hospice activities. It is essential that community-based nurses possess great skill in the assessment and management of pain, nutrition, bowel dysfunction, and skin impairments. Community health nurses are also actively involved in bereavement counseling. Through collaboration with other support disciplines, nurses often assist patients and families to cope with changes in role identity, family structure, grief, and loss. In many instances, family support for survivors continues for a period of approximately 1 year.

Oncologic Emergencies

In addition to assessment and management of the previously described problems experienced by the patient with cancer, the nurse also has an important role in the prompt detection of complications of cancer and its treatment that are considered oncologic emergencies. As a result of the underlying malignancy, its metastasis, or the effects of treatment, the oncology patient is at risk for the development of a unique group of acute conditions requiring immediate medical or surgical intervention. Common oncologic emergencies include superior vena cava syndrome, spinal cord compression, hypercalcemia, pericardial effusion, disseminated intravascular coagulation, and the syndrome of inappropriate secretion of antidiuretic hormone.

Superior Vena Cava Syndrome

The superior vena cava is the major site of venous drainage from the head, neck, arms, and upper thorax. Positioned within the rigid compartment of the mediastinum, it is closely surrounded by major structures, including the heart, lungs, vertebral bodies, and esophagus. Consequently, compression of the superior vena cava by tumor or enlarged lymph nodes can result in markedly impaired venous drainage of the head, neck, arms, and thorax. In the vast majority of patients, the superior vena cava syndrome occurs with lung cancer, but it can also occur with lymphoma and metastasis from other sites.

The clinical manifestations of impaired venous drainage usually develop gradually over a period of 3 to 4 weeks, but they may also appear suddenly. Progressive shortness of breath, dyspnea, cough, and facial swelling are common. Edema of the neck, arms, hands, and thorax may develop with associated sensations of skin tightness and difficulty swallowing. The jugular, temporal, and arm veins may be engorged and distended. Dilated thoracic vessels often cause prominent venous patterns visible on the chest wall. Continued venous obstruction may lead to increased intracranial pressure, associated visual disturbances, headache, and altered mental status. If untreated, the superior vena cava syndrome may lead to cerebral anoxia, laryngeal edema, bronchial obstruction, and death.

Management. Prompt diagnosis and treatment are essential in managing this syndrome. Radiation therapy is the treatment of choice to decrease the tumor size and alleviate symptoms. Chemotherapy is used when the tumor is known to be responsive (lymphoma or small cell lung cancer). Other supportive measures such as oxygen therapy and diuretics may be used.

Nursing Interventions. Nursing care includes identifying patients at risk for developing superior vena cava syndrome. Clinical manifestations detected by the nursing assessment are reported to the physician and investigated promptly. Continued assessment of the patient's cardiopulmonary and neurologic status is essential. As a result of increasing difficulty in breathing and progressive edema, many patients become anxious and fearful of suffocating. Nursing care is directed toward facilitating breathing by positioning, promoting comfort, and reducing anxiety. Minimizing the patient's energy expenditure by energy conservation techniques may minimize shortness of breath. In addition, the patient's fluid volume status is monitored and fluids are administered cautiously to minimize edema.

Spinal Cord Compression

Malignancies such as breast, lung, kidney, and prostate cancers, myeloma, and lymphoma that metastasize to the spine may cause spinal cord compression. Most lesions develop in the space between the periosteum of the vertebrae and the dura of the spinal cord (extradural), leading to destruction of the vertebral bodies and epidural tissue. Less commonly, tumors develop in the spinal cord itself.

Spinal cord compression is characterized by pain that may be constant and exacerbated by movement, coughing, sneezing, or the Valsalva maneuver. The location and characteristics of the pain depend on the area of involvement of the spinal cord. Neurologic dysfunction develops when cord compression is prolonged or severe and may include motor and sensory deficit. Sensory deficits generally begin as loss of pinprick sensation, progressing to decreased vibratory sense and finally to loss of position sense. The sense of touch usually remains intact even when motor dysfunction is advanced. Motor loss (weakness and ataxia) is often present at the time of diagnosis. Progression of compression ultimately leads to flaccid paralysis. The occurrence of other dysfunctions such as urinary and fecal incontinence is dependent on the level of the lesion compressing the cord. Compression of upper motor neurons above S2 can lead to bladder-overflow incontinence. Cord compression at levels S3, S4, and S5 can result in flaccid sphincter tone and bowel incontinence.

Prompt neurologic assessment is essential if sensory and motor function is to be maintained or restored. Although a variety of diagnostic procedures may assist in identifying the compressing lesion, the myelogram is considered the most accurate means of localizing the site of compression. Once the diagnosis is established, medical intervention is quickly initiated because symptoms can progress within a relatively short period of time.

Management. Radiation therapy is most commonly used to reduce tumor size and halt disease progression. In most cases surgical decompression is not used unless the symptoms progress despite irradiation or the patient has previously received a maximum amount of radiation to the area of the cord involved. Surgery may be indicated when the tumor involved in known to be insensitive or nonresponsive to radiation therapy. Steroids are often given in addition to radiation therapy to decrease the edema and inflammation at the site of compression. Recovery of neurologic function is influenced by promptness of diagnosis and treatment. Despite treatment, patients who develop complete paralysis usually do not regain neurologic function.

Nursing Interventions. Nursing interventions include ongoing assessment of neurologic function in order to identify existing and progressing dysfunction. Most patients will require both pharmacologic and nonpharmacologic measures to control pain. Because of pain and decreased functional abilities associated with spinal cord compression, patients are often at risk for the hazards of immobility such as skin breakdown, urinary stasis, thrombophlebitis, and decreased clearance of pulmonary secretions. Nursing measures are directed toward prevention of these problems and maintenance of muscle tone through range of motion exercises. For patients with bladder or bowel incontinence, intermittent urinary catheterization and bowel training programs are essential. Additionally, the patient and family will require assistance in coping with pain and alterations in body functioning, lifestyles, roles, and level of independence.

Hypercalcemia

Hypercalcemia is a potentially life-threatening complication that is characterized by abnormal calcium metabolism resulting in serum calcium levels in excess of 11 mg/dl (SI: 2.74 mmol/L) of blood. The skeletal system serves as the storage site for approximately 99% of all the calcium in the body. Hypercalcemia associated with cancer occurs when the release of calcium from the bones is more than the kidneys can excrete or the bones can reabsorb. (See Chapter 9, *Fluid and Electrolytes: Balance and Disturbance,* for a discussion of normal calcium metabolism.) Hypercalcemia is commonly seen in patients with multiple myeloma, and breast, squamous cell lung, and prostatic cancer. Less commonly, it develops in patients with leukemia, lymphoma, or renal cancer.

The underlying cause of hypercalcemia in the cancer patient varies. Approximately 70% of all cancer patients with hypercalcemia have metastatic bone disease. In this situation, direct invasion of the bone by tumor cells causes bone destruction and subsequent release of calcium. Hypercalcemia may also be caused by the production of *osteoclast-activating factor* and prostaglandins. These substances, produced by cancer cells, stimulate the breakdown of bone and the release of calcium. Hypercalcemia may also be caused by tumors that produce parathyroid-like substances and promote release of calcium from bones.

Management. The manifestations of hypercalcemia and its medical management are discussed in Chapter 9.

Nursing Interventions. Nursing care begins with identification of patients at risk for hypercalcemia. Careful nursing assessment will assist in identifying the signs and symptoms of hypercalcemia. Patients at risk are encouraged to maintain adequate fluid intake of 2 to 3 liters of fluid per day unless contraindicated by existing renal or cardiac disease. The importance of mobility must be emphasized in order to prevent demineralization and breakdown of bones. Patients with alterations in mental status and mobility as a result of hypercalcemia will require additional nursing measures to prevent the hazards of immobility and promote safety.

Pericardial Effusion/Cardiac Tamponade

Cardiac tamponade is a cardiovascular disorder that occurs when fluid accumulates in the pericardial space and compresses the heart, impairing cardiac filling during diastole. Neoplastic disease or its treatment is the most common cause of cardiac tamponade. Pericardial disease secondary to neoplastic growth usually occurs by direct invasion from adjacent thoracic tumors (lung and breast cancers) or metastasis to the pericardium (lymphomas, leukemias, and melanomas). Fluid produced by the invasive tumor, metastatic lesion, or pericardial tissue in response to the malignant processes accumulates in the pericardial space, increases pressure on the myocardium, and impedes expansion of the ventricles. As ventricular volume and cardiac output fall the cardiac pump fails and circulatory collapse develops. Radiation therapy of 4000 rad or more to the mediastinal area has also been implicated in pericardial fibrosis, pericarditis, and resultant cardiac tamponade, which may occur months or even years after the cessation of radiation therapy.

Pericardial disease and cardiac tamponade may occur gradually or very rapidly. Gradual fluid accumulation allows the parietal (outer) layer of the pericardial space to stretch and compensate for the increased pressure. Therefore, large fluid volumes may accumulate before symptoms appear. However, when fluid accumulates rapidly, the pericardial pressures rise quickly and compensatory stretching cannot occur. Increased central venous pressures (CVP) and jugular distention develop. Distention of neck veins during inspiration (Kussmaul's sign) is suggestive of pericardial disease. Pulsus paradoxus (a decrease in systolic blood pressure of more than 10 mm Hg during inspiration with strengthening of the pulse on expiration) may be detected in moderate cardiac tamponade. Heart sounds diminish, and increased areas of cardiac dullness may be percussed. As cardiac output decreases, compensatory tachycardia and systemic vascular resistance occur. As tamponade progresses, the systolic blood pressure continues to fall and the diastolic pressure rises in compensatory effort, creating a narrow pulse pressure. Shortness of breath and tachypnea may also develop. Weakness, diaphoresis, lethargy, and altered consciousness due to decreased cerebral perfusion may result. Circulatory collapse with cardiac arrest is imminent if untreated.

ECG tracings during pericardial effusion usually reveal nonspecific T-wave changes with reduced QRS voltage. Electrical alternans (QRS complexes that alternate in size) is common with tamponade. The chest x-ray film is not usually diagnostic with small-volume pericardial effusions. However, with larger effusions, a "water-bottle" heart appearance (obliteration of vessel contour and cardiac chambers) becomes apparent on x-ray. Echocardiography and computed tomography are valuable in the diagnosis of cardiac tamponade and evaluation of the effectiveness of treatment.

Management. The usual treatment of cardiac tamponade is *pericardiocentesis* (the aspiration of the pericardial fluid by a large-bore needle inserted into the pericardial space). Unfortunately, the benefits of pericardiocentesis in malignant effusions are only temporary, and fluid accumulation frequently recurs. Pericardial windows are often surgically created as a palliative measure to drain pericardial effusions into the pleural space. Catheters may also be placed in the pericardial space and sclerosing agents (such as tetracycline) may be injected to prevent effusive reaccumulation. In mild effusions, prednisone and diuretics may be prescribed with careful monitoring of patient status.

Nursing Interventions. Nursing assessment includes frequent monitoring of vital signs; assessment for pulsus paradoxus; monitoring of ECG tracings; assessment of heart and lung sounds, neck vein filling, level of consciousness, respiratory status, and skin color and temperature; accurate monitoring of intake and output; and laboratory studies such as arterial blood gases and electrolytes.

Appropriate nursing actions may include elevation of the head of the patient's bed; minimization of physical activity to reduce oxygen requirements; supplemental oxygen as prescribed; frequent oral hygiene; turning, and encouraging the patient to cough and take deep breaths every 2 hours; reorientation, if needed; supportive measures; maintenance of patent intravenous access; and appropriate patient education.

Disseminated Intravascular Coagulation

Disseminated intravascular coagulation (DIC, consumption coagulation) is the abnormal activation of both the coagulation and fibrinolytic mechanisms, resulting in the consumption of coagulation factors and platelets. DIC can occur with any malignant process; however, it is most commonly associated with cancers of the lung, gastrointestinal system, and prostate, and melanoma and the leukemias. Certain chemotherapeutic agents are also thought to precipitate DIC. These drugs include vincristine, methotrexate, 6-mercaptopurine, prednisone, and L-asparaginase. Certain disease processes commonly seen in the cancer patient may also initiate DIC, including sepsis, hepatic failure, and anaphylaxis.

Clot formation is initiated by triggering of the intrinsic or extrinsic mechanisms of normal coagulation. Malignant tumors stimulate the intrinsic coagulation pathway during metastasis when endothelial injury occurs. The extrinsic coagulation pathway is also activated by the release of thromboplastin (or thromboplastin-like substances) from tumor cells. Once activated, the clotting cascade continues to consume clotting factors and platelets and forms fibrin clots in the microvasculature. These clots place the patient at high risk for thrombus formation, infarction, and bleeding. The last stage of the clotting cascade, fibrinolysis, also continues to occur at an abnormally high rate in DIC. Fibrinolysis, or clot dissolution, breaks down clots that have formed and places the patient at an even higher danger of hemorrhage.

Laboratory results indicative of DIC include prolonged prothrombin time (PT or Protime) and partial thromboplastin time (PTT), decreased platelet counts and fibrinogen levels, and increased fibrin split products (FSP). Bleeding from multiple body sites is commonly found in patients with DIC. Clinical symptoms of this syndrome are varied and depend on the organ system involved in thrombus/infarct or bleeding episodes.

Management. Treatment of DIC centers on control of the underlying disease process. Supportive measures with antithrombinolytic agents such as heparin or antithrombin III are often employed to decrease stimulation of the coagulation pathways. Transfusion with fresh frozen plasma or cryoprecipitates (which contain clotting factors and fibrinogen) may be used in conjunction with heparin therapy but is rarely effective when used alone. Antifibrinolytic agents such as ε-aminocaproic acid are controversial forms of therapy and are associated with high incidence of thrombus formation.

Nursing Interventions. Indicated nursing assessments for the patient experiencing DIC include monitoring of vital signs; accurate intake and output measurements; assessment of skin color and temperature; assessment of lung, heart, and bowel sounds; assessment of level of consciousness; assessment of headache, visual disturbances, chest pain, decreased urinary output, and abdominal tenderness; assessments of all body orifices, tube insertion sites, incisions, and bodily excretions for bleeding; and monitoring of indicated laboratory test results.

Appropriate nursing interventions involve the minimization of physical activity to decrease risk of injury and oxygen requirements; increasing pressure to all venipuncture sites; minimization of invasive procedures; maintenance of adequate oral hygiene; assisting the patient to turn, cough, and take deep breaths every 2 hours; reorientation, if needed; maintenance of a safe environment; and appropriate patient education and supportive measures.

Syndrome of Inappropriate Secretion of Antidiuretic Hormone

The syndrome of inappropriate secretion of antidiuretic hormone (SIADH) is characterized by continuous, uncontrolled release of antidiuretic hormone (ADH). This leads to increased extracellular fluid volume with decreased osmolality, water intoxication, hyponatremia, increased urine osmolality, and increased excretion of urinary sodium. The most common cause of SIADH is malignancy; it occurs most often in patients with cancers of the lung, pancreas, duodenum, brain, esophagus, colon, ovary, larynx, prostate, and nasopharynx and Hodgkin's disease, thymomas, and lymphosarcomas. Two antineoplastic drugs, vincristine and cyclophosphamide, also stimulate ADH secretion leading to SIADH. Certain processes commonly seen in the cancer patient such as pain, stress, trauma, and hemorrhage are also associated with SIADH.

The ADH produced, stored, and released by tumor cells is identical to ADH normally produced by the posterior pituitary gland. When ADH is produced, the distal renal tubules and collecting ducts of the kidney conserve and reabsorb water. In SIADH, the posterior pituitary becomes unresponsive to the normal feedback mechanisms and water conservation continues despite decreasing serum osmolality and increasing urine osmolality. With continued absorption of fluid, circulatory volume increases, and sodium is actively excreted by the kidneys in compensation. If the serum sodium levels fall below 120 mEq/liter (SI: 120 mmol/L), patients usually display symptoms of hyponatremia, which include personality changes, irritability, nausea, anorexia, vomiting, weight gain, lethargy, and confusion. If serum sodium levels continue to fall below 110 mEq/liter, seizure, coma, and death may result. Edema is rarely seen with SIADH.

Laboratory findings indicative of SIADH include (1) serum hyponatremia, (2) increased urine osmolality, and (3) increased urinary sodium. Decreased BUN, creatinine, and serum albumin levels secondary to dilution may also occur. Abnormal results of water load tests would also indicate the presence of SIADH.

Management. Treatment of SIADH depends on the severity of symptoms. With mild symptoms, fluids are limited to 500 to 1000 ml/day to increase the serum sodium level and decrease fluid overload. When neurologic symptoms are severe, parenteral sodium replacement and diuretic therapy are indicated. Electrolytes are monitored carefully during treatment since secondary magnesium, potassium, and calcium imbalances may occur.

Following control of the symptoms of SIADH, the underlying malignancy is treated. If water excess continues despite oncologic treatment, pharmacologic intervention (demeclocycline, urea, and furosemide) may be indicated to control symptoms.

Nursing Interventions. Nursing assessment of the patient with SIADH includes accurate measurement of intake and output and assessment of level of consciousness, lung and heart sounds, vital signs, daily weight, and urine specific gravity. The patient is also assessed for nausea, vomiting, anorexia, edema, fatigue, and lethargy. The nurse monitors laboratory test results, including serum electrolytes, osmolality, BUN, creatinine, and urinary sodium and osmolality.

Indicated nursing interventions involve minimization of activity; appropriate oral hygiene measures; maintenance of environmental safety measures; reorientation, if necessary; fluid restriction, if necessary; and appropriate patient education and supportive measures.

Bibliography

Books

American Cancer Society. American Cancer Society Special Report: Nutrition and Cancer: Cause and Prevention. New York, American Cancer Society, 1984.

American Cancer Society. Unproven Methods of Cancer Management. New York, American Cancer Society, 1982.

Beyers M, Werner J, and Durburg S (eds). Complete Guide to Cancer Nursing. Oradell, New Jersey, Medical Economics, 1984.

Billings JA. Outpatient Management of Advanced Cancer: Symptom Control, Support, and Hospice-in-the-Home. Philadelphia, JB Lippincott, 1985.

Brager BL and Yasko JM. Care of the Client Receiving Chemotherapy. Reston, Virginia, Reston Publishing Co, 1984.

Carrieri VK, Lindsey AM, and West CM (eds). Pathophysiological Phenomena in Nursing. Philadelphia, WB Saunders, 1986.

Cassileth BR and Cassileth PA (eds). Clinical Care of the Terminal Cancer Patient. Philadelphia, Lea & Febiger, 1982.

Chernecky CC and Ramsey PW. Critical Care Nursing of the Client With Cancer. Norwalk, Connecticut, Appleton-Century-Crofts, 1984.

Corr CA and Corr DM (eds). Hospice Care: Principles and Practice. New York, Springer, 1983.

del Regato JA and Spjut HJ. Cancer: Diagnosis, Treatment and Prognosis. St Louis, CV Mosby, 1984.

Devita V, Hellman S, and Rosenberg S (eds). Cancer: Principles and Practice of Oncology, 2nd ed. Philadelphia, JB Lippincott, 1985.

Donovan MI and Girton SE. Cancer Care Nursing. Norwalk, Connecticut, Appleton-Century-Crofts, 1984.

Griffiths MJ, Murray KH, and Russo PC. Oncology Nursing: Pathophysiology, Assessment and Intervention. New York, Macmillan, 1984.

Hafen BQ and Frandsen KJ. Faces of Death. Englewood, Colorado, Morton, 1983.

Johnson BL and Grose J. Handbook of Oncology Nursing. New York, John Wiley & Sons, 1985.

Knobf MKT, Fischer DS, and Welch-McCaffrey D (eds). Cancer Chemotherapy, Treatment and Care. Boston, GK Hall, 1984.

McCaffery M. Nursing Management of the Patient With Pain, 3rd ed. Philadelphia, JB Lippincott, 1983.

McCorkle R and Hongladarom G. Issues and Topics in Cancer Nursing. Norwalk, Connecticut, Appleton-Century-Crofts, 1986.

McIntire SN and Cioppa AL (eds). Cancer Nursing: A Developmental Approach. New York, John Wiley & Sons, 1984.

McNally JC, Stair JC, and Somerville ET (eds). Guidelines for Cancer Nursing Practice. Orlando, Florida, Grune & Stratton, 1985.

Meinhart NJ and McCaffery M. Pain: A Nursing Approach to Assessment and Analysis. Norwalk, Connecticut, Appleton-Century-Crofts, 1983.

Oncology Nursing Society. Cancer Chemotherapy: Guidelines and Recommendations for Nursing Education and Practice. Pittsburgh, Oncology Nursing Society, 1984.

Page HS and Asire AJ. Cancer Rates and Risks. Bethesda, Maryland, U.S. Department of Health and Human Services, National Institutes of Health, 1985.

Piper BF. Pathophysiological Phenomena in Nursing. Philadelphia, WB Saunders, 1986.

Porth C. Pathophysiology: Concepts of Altered Health States, 2nd ed. Philadelphia, JB Lippincott, 1986.

U.S. Department of Health and Human Services. Cancer Rates and Risks, 3rd ed. Public Health Services, National Institutes of Health, 1985.

Vredevo DL et al (eds). Concepts of Oncology Nursing. Englewood Cliffs, New Jersey, Prentice-Hall, 1981.

Wall PD and Melzack R. Textbook of Pain. New York, Churchill Livingstone, 1984.

Yasko JM. Guidelines for Cancer Care: Symptom Management. Reston, Virginia, Prentice-Hall, 1983.

Articles

(Asterisks indicate nursing research articles.)

General

Amenta MO. Hospice in the United States: Multiple and varied programs. Nurs Clin North Am 1985 June; 20(2):269–279.

Ash CR. Cancer care for the elderly: A need for emphasis. Cancer Nurs 1986 Oct; 9(5):229.

Benoliel JQ. Loss and terminal illness. Nurs Clin North Am 1985 June; 20(2):439–448.

Christensen S and Harding M. Integrating theories of crisis intervention into hospice home care teaching. Nurs Clin North Am 1985 June; 20(2):449–455.

Cunningham CAP. Putting the patient in control. Am J Nurs 1985 June; 85(6):676–677.

Dellefield ME. Caring for the elderly patient with cancer. Oncol Nurs Forum 1986 May/June; 13(3):19–27.

*Driever MJ and McCorkle R. Patient concerns at 3 and 6 months post-diagnosis (cancer). Cancer Nurs 1984 June; 7(3):235–241.

Ellerhorst-Ryan JM. Troubleshooting the venous access system. Am J Nurs 1985 July; 85(7):795.

Ellison SA. Geriatric oncology: A development approach. Cancer Nurs 1985 Sept; 8(suppl 1):28–32.

Gruca JK. Oncology rehabilitation. Rehabil Nurs 1984 May/June; 9(3): 27–30.

*Itano J et al. Compliance of cancer patients to therapy. West J Nurs Res 1983 Winter; 5(1):5–16.

Martocchio BC. Grief and bereavement: Healing through hurt. Nurs Clin North Am 1985 June; 20(2):327–341.

Maxwell MB. Dyspnea in advanced cancer. Am J Nurs 1985 June; 85(6): 672–677.

Mellette SJ. The cancer patient at work. CA 1985 Nov/Dec; 35(6):360–373.

Morris CA. Self-concept as altered by the diagnosis of cancer. Nurs Clin North Am 1985 Dec; 20(4):611–630.

Moseley JR. Alterations in comfort. Nurs Clin North Am 1985 June; 20(2): 427–438.

*Padilla GV and Grant MM. Quality of life as a cancer nursing outcome variable. ANS 1985 Oct; 8(1):45–60.

Saunders JM and McCorkle R. Models of care for persons with progressive cancer. Nurs Clin North Am 1985 June; 20(2):365–377.

Watson S and Hickey P. Cancer surgery: Help for the family in waiting. Am J Nurs 1984 May; 84(5):604–607.

Wilkes G, Vannicola P, and Starck P. Long-term venous access. Am J Nurs 1985 July; 85(7):793, 794, 796.

Woods ME and Kowalski JD. Symposium on oncologic nursing practice. Nurs Clin North Am 1982 Dec; 17(4):539–783.

Cancer Process/Epidemiology

Burkitt DP. Etiology and prevention of colorectal cancer. Hosp Pract 1984 Feb; 19(2):67–77.

Fraser MC and Tucker MA. Host susceptibility factors in cancer etiology. Semin Oncol Nurs 1986 Aug; 2(3):170–175.

Gallo RC. The virus cancer story. Hosp Pract 1983 June; 18(6):79–89.

Jamison DS. Hereditary predisposition to cancer: Opportunity for early detection and intervention. Semin Oncol Nurs 1986 Aug; 2(3):176–183.

Konicki AM. Physical and psychological effects of DES on exposed offspring. Cancer Nurs 1985 Aug; 2(3):161–169.

Kupchella CE. Environmental factors in cancer etiology. Semin Oncol Nurs 1986 Aug; 2(3):161–169.

Loescher LJ and Sauer KA. Vitamin therapy for advanced cancer. Oncol Nurs Forum 1984 Nov/Dec; 11(6):38–45.

Lowenfele AB and Anderson ME. Diet and cancer. Cancer 1977 Apr; 39(4):1809–1814.

Olsen SJ and Love RR. A new direction in preventive oncology: Chemoprevention. Semin Oncol Nurs 1986 Aug; 2(3):211–221.

Pollack ES. Tracking cancer trends: Incidence and survival. Hosp Pract 1984 Aug; 19(8):99–116.

Rensberger B. Cancer: The new synthesis: Cause. Science '84 1984 Sept; 5(7):28–33.

Scanlon EF. The process of metastasis. Cancer 1985 Mar; 55(6):1163–1166.

Schirrmacher V. Cancer metastasis: Experimental approaches, theoretical concepts and impacts for treatment strategies. Adv Cancer Res 1985; 43:1–73.

Senie RT. Assessment of carcinogenesis through epidemiologic and experimental investigations. Semin Oncol Nurs 1986 Aug; 2(3):154–160.

Silverberg E and Lubera J. Cancer statistics, 1986. CA 1986 Jan/Feb; 36(1):9–25.

Weisburger JH. Mechanisms of action of diet as a carcinogen. Cancer 1979 May; 43(5):1987–1995.

Cancer Detection and Prevention

Baker L. Breast cancer detection demonstration projects: Five-year summary report. CA 1982 July/Aug; 32(4):194–225.

Faulkenberry JE. Cancer prevention and detection: Colorectal cancer. Cancer Nurs 1984 Oct; 7(5):415–424.

Gianella A. Teaching cancer prevention and detection. Cancer Nurs 1985 Sept; 8(suppl 1):9–12.

Glasel M. Cancer prevention: The role of the nurse in primary and secondary cancer prevention. Cancer Nurs 1985 Sept; 8(suppl 1):5–8.

Love RR and Olsen SJ. An agenda for cancer prevention in nursing practice. Cancer Nurs 1985 Dec; 8(6):329–338.

Miller DG. Principles of early detection of cancer. Cancer 1981 Mar; 47(suppl 5):1142–1145.

Nash JA. Cancer prevention and detection: Breast cancer. Cancer Nurs 1984 Apr; 7(2):163–176.

Sandella JA. Cancer prevention and detection. Cancer Nurs 1985 Feb; 8(1):63–74.

Stromberg MF. The role of the nurse in cancer detection and screening. Semin Oncol Nurs 1986 Aug; 2(3):191–199.

Stromberg MF et al. Carcinogens: Are some risks acceptable? Am J Nurs 1986 July; 86(7):815–817.

White LN. Cancer prevention and detection: From twenty to sixty-five years of age. Oncol Nurs Forum 1986 Mar/Apr; 13(2):59–64.

Chemotherapy and Radiation Therapy

Butler MC. Families' responses to chemotherapy by an ambulatory infusion pump. Nurs Clin North Am 1984 Mar; 19(1):139–144.

Cline BW. Prevention of chemotherapy-induced alopecia: A review of the literature. Cancer Nurs 1984 June; 7(3):221–228.

Derby CE. Alternate methods of chemotherapy administration. Can Nurse 1985 Oct; 81(9):44–45.

*Dodd MJ. Measuring informational intervention for chemotherapy knowledge and self-care behavior. Res Nurs Health 1984 Mar; 7(1): 43–50.

Engelking CH and Steele NE. A model for pretreatment nursing assessment of patients receiving cancer chemotherapy. Cancer Nurs 1984 June; 7(3):203–212.

Gross J. Clinical research in cancer chemotherapy. Oncol Nurs Forum 1986 Jan/Feb; 13(1):59–65.

Hassey KM. Demystifying care of patients with radioactive implants. Am J Nurs 1985 July; 85(7):788–792.

Hospital hazards: Cancer drugs. Am J Nurs 1983 May; 83(5):758–762.

Hughes CB. Giving cancer drugs IV: Some guidelines. Am J Nurs 1986 Jan; 86(1):34–38.

Longman AJ and Rogers BP. Altered cell growth in cancer and the nursing implications. Cancer Nurs 1984 Oct; 7(5):405–412.

Lyndon J. Nephrotoxicity of cancer treatment. Oncol Nurs Forum 1986 Mar/Apr; 13(2):68–77.

Rahr V. Giving intrathecal drugs. Am J Nurs 1986 July; 86(7):829–831.

Redd WH. Control of nausea and vomiting in chemotherapy patients. Postgrad Med 1984 Apr; 75(5):105–113.

Schaffner A. Safety precautions in home chemotherapy. Am J Nurs 1984 Mar; 84(3):346–347.

Thomson L. Side-effects of radiotherapy. Nurs Times 1980 May; 76(20): 877–881.

Trester AK. Nursing management of patients receiving cancer chemotherapy. Cancer Nurs 1982 June; 5(3):201–210.

Varricchio CG. The patient in radiation therapy. Am J Nurs 1981 Feb; 81(2):334–337.

von Roemeling R et al. Chemotherapy via implanted infusion pump: New perspectives for delivery of long-term continuous treatment. Oncol Nurs Forum 1986 Mar/Apr; 13(2):17–24.

Biological Response Modifiers

DiJulio JE and Bedigiam JS. Hybridoma monoclonal antibody treatment of T-cell lymphomas: Clinical experience and nursing management. Oncol Nurs Forum 1983 Spring; 10(2):22–27.

Mayer D and Smalley RV. Interferon: Current status. Oncol Nurs Forum 1983 Fall; 10(4):14–19.

Moldawer NP and Murray JL. The clinical uses of monoclonal antibodies in cancer research. Cancer Nurs 1985 Aug; 8(4):207–213.

Morrin BM. Cancer immunology. Heart Lung 1980 July/Aug; 9(4):636–639.

Scogna DM and Schoenberger CS. Biological response modifiers: An overview and nursing implications. Oncol Nurs Forum 1982 Winter; 9(1):45–49.

Suppers VJ and McClamrock EA. Biologicals in cancer treatment: Future effects on nursing practice. Oncol Nurs Forum 1985 May/June; 12(3):27–32.

Oncologic Emergencies

Ali KM et al. Critical cardiopulmonary problems in the cancer patient. Cancer Bull 1984 May/June; 36(3):128–134.

Baldwin P. Epidural spinal cord compression secondary to metastatic disease: A review of the literature. Cancer Nurs 1983 Dec; 6(6): 441–446.

Borenstein M (ed). Emergency oncology. Topics Emerg Med 1986 July; 8(2):1–81.

Concilus EM and Bohachick PA. Cancer: Pericardial effusion and tamponade. Cancer Nurs 1984 Oct; 7(5):391–397.

Coward DD. Cancer-induced hypercalcemia. Cancer Nurs 1986 June; 9(3):125–132.

Cunningham SG. Fluid and electrolyte disturbances associated with cancer and its treatment. Nurs Clin North Am 1982 Dec; 17(4):579–591.

Flier J and Moore MJ. The hypercalcemia of cancer: Clinical implications and pathogenic mechanisms. N Engl J Med 1984 June 28; 310(20): 1718–1725.

Glover DJ and Glick JH. Managing oncologic emergencies involving structural dysfunction. CA 1985 July/Aug; 35(4):238–251.

Griffin JP. Nursing care of the critically ill cancer patient with cardiopulmonary failure. Crit Care Q 1986 June; 9(1):35–48.

Kalin S and Tintinalli JE. Emergency evaluation of the cancer patient. Ann Emerg Med 1984 Sept; 13(9):723–729.

Kirchner CW and Reheis CE. Two serious complications of neoplasia: Sepsis and disseminated intravascular coagulation. Nurs Clin North Am 1982 Dec; 17(4):595–605.

Klein PW. Neurologic emergencies in oncology. Semin Oncol Nurs 1985 Nov; 1(4):278–284.

Moore JM. Metabolic emergencies. In Johnson BL and Gross J (eds). Handbook of Oncology Nursing, 459–483. New York, John Wiley & Sons, 1985.

Morse LK et al. Early detection to avert the crisis of superior vena cava syndrome. Cancer Nurs 1985 Aug; 8(4):228–232.

Pursley P. Acute cardiac tamponade. Am J Nurs 1983 Oct; 83(10):1414–1418.

Rooney A and Haviley C. Nursing management of disseminated intravascular coagulation. Oncol Nurs Forum 1985 Jan/Feb; 12(1):15–22.

Siegrist CW and Jones JA. Disseminated intravascular coagulopathy and nursing implications. Semin Oncol Nurs 1985 Nov; 1(4):237–243.

Valentine AM and Stewart JA. Oncologic emergencies. Am J Nurs 1983 Sept; 83(9):1282–1285.

Pain

Alberico JG. Breaking the chronic pain cycle. Am J Nurs 1984 Oct; 84(10): 1222–1225.

Austin C et al. Hospice home care pain management: Four critical variables. Cancer Nurs 1986 Apr; 9(8):58–65.

Coyle N. Symptom management: Pain—an overview of current concepts. Cancer Nurs 1985 Sept; 8(suppl 1):44–49.

Coyle N et al. Continuous subcutaneous infusions of opiates in cancer patients with pain. Oncol Nurs Forum 1986 July/Aug; 13(4):53–57.

Donovan M. Cancer pain: You can help. Nurs Clin North Am 1982 Dec; 17(4):713–728.

Foley KM. Treatment of cancer pain. N Engl J Med 1985 July 11; 313(2): 84–94.

Hauck SL. Pain: Problem for the patient with cancer. Cancer Nurs 1986 Apr; 9(2):66–76.

Levy MH. Pain management in advanced cancer. Semin Oncol 1985 Dec; 12(4):394–410.

McGivney WT and Crooks GM. The care of patients with severe pain in terminal illness. JAMA 1984 Mar 2; 251(9):1182–1188.

Paice JA. Intrathecal morphine infusions for intractable cancer pain: A new use for implanted pumps. Oncol Nurs Forum 1986 May/June; 13(8):41–47.

Payne R and Foley KM (eds). Cancer pain (symposium). Med Clin North Am Mar 1987; 71(2):153–348.

Portnoy RK. Continuous infusion of opioids. Am J Nurs 1986 Mar; 86(3): 318, 322.

Psychological Concerns

Adams J and Guido G. The adolescent coping with cancer. Dimens Crit Care Nurs 1984 Mar/Apr; 3(2):70–75.

Benoliel JQ. Loss and terminal illness. Nurs Clin North Am 1985 June; 20(2):439–448.

Fountain MJ. Psychosocial support for the patient experiencing cancer. Orthop Nurs 1985 Sept/Oct; 4(5):33–35.

Heinrich RL and Schag CC. A behavioral medicine approach to coping with cancer: A case report. Cancer Nurs 1984 June; 7(3):243–247.

Hickey SS. Enabling hope. Cancer Nurs 1986 June; 9(3):133–137.

Krumm S. Psychosocial adaptation of the adult with cancer. Nurs Clin North Am 1982 Dec; 17(4):729–737.

Martocchio BC. Family coping: Helping families help themselves. Semin Oncol Nurs 1985 Nov; 1(4):292–297.

Martocchio BC. Grief and bereavement. Nurs Clin North Am 1985 June; 20(2):327–341.

Pepper CB. The roles of care and love and hope between nurse and patient in cancer survival. Cancer Nurs 1985 Sept; 8(suppl 1):50–53.

Thorne S. The family cancer experience. Cancer Nurs 1985 Oct; 8(5): 285–291.

Unproven Methods

American Society for Clinical Oncology. Ineffective cancer therapy: A guide for the lay person. J Clin Oncol 1983 Feb; 1(2):154–163.

Arnold C. The macrobiotic diet: A question of nutrition. Oncol Nurs Forum 1984 May/June; 11(3):50–53.

Howard-Ruben J and Miller NJ. Unproven methods of cancer management: I: Current status and implications for patient care. Oncol Nurs Forum 1983 Fall; 10(4):46–52.

Howard-Ruben J and Miller NJ. Unproven methods of cancer management: II: Current status and implications for patient care. Oncol Nurs Forum 1984 Jan/Feb; 11(1):67–73.

Skin Integrity

Baxley KO et al. Alopecia: Effect on cancer patients' body image. Cancer Nurs 1984 Dec; 9(6):499–503.

Beck S. Impact of systemic oral care protocol on stomatitis after chemotherapy. Cancer Nurs 1979 June; 2(3):185–199.

Daeffler R. Oral hygiene measures for patients with cancer: I. Cancer Nurs 1980 Oct; 3(5):347–356.

Daeffler R. Oral hygiene measures for patients with cancer: II. Cancer Nurs 1980 Dec; 3(6):427–432.

Daeffler R. Oral hygiene measures for patients with cancer: III. Cancer Nurs 1981 Feb; 4(1):29–34.

Didonato K. Standards of clinical nursing practice: Alopecia. Cancer Nurs 1985 Feb; 8(1):76–77.

Foltz AT. Nursing care of ulcerating metastatic lesions. Oncol Nurs Forum 1980 Spring; 7(2):8–13.

Hyperthermia

Bull JMC. Whole body hyperthermia as an anticancer agent. CA 1982 Mar/Apr; 32(2):123–128.

Loescher LJ and Leigh S. Isolated regional limb hyperthermia perfusion as treatment for melanoma. Cancer Nurs 1984 Dec; 7(6):461–467.

Moore C. Hyperthermia: A modern experiment in cancer treatment. Oncol Nurs Forum 1984 Mar/Apr; 11(2):31–35.

Storm FK and Morton DL. Localized hyperthermia in the treatment of cancer. CA 1983 Jan/Feb; 33(1):44–56.

Nutrition

Bayer LM, Bauers CM, and Kapp SR. Psychosocial aspects of nutritional support. Nurs Clin North Am 1983 Mar; 18(1):119–128.

Forlaw L. The critically ill patient: Nutritional implications. Nurs Clin North Am 1983 Mar; 18(1):111–117.

Goodman MS and Wickham R. Venous access devices: An overview. Oncol Nurs Forum 1984 Sept/Oct; 11(5):16–23.

Knox L. Nutrition and cancer. Nurs Clin North Am 1983 Mar; 18(1):97–109.

Lym LL and Gallagher-Allred CR. Nutrition and the cancer patient: A cooperative effort by nursing and dietetics to overcome problems. Cancer Nurs 1984 Dec; 7(6):469–474.

Infection

Adams A. External barriers to infection. Nurs Clin North Am 1985 Mar; 20(1):145–149.

Brandt B. A nursing protocol for the client with neutropenia. Oncol Nurs Forum 1984 Mar/Apr; 1(2):24–27.

Carlson AC. Infection prophylaxis in the patient with cancer. Oncol Nurs Forum 1985 May/June; 12(3):56–64.

Crane LR, Emmer DR, and Graguras A. Prevention of infection on the oncology unit. Nurs Clin North Am 1980 Dec; 15(4):843–849.

Cunha BA. Significance of fever in the compromised host. Nurs Clin North Am 1985 Mar; 20(1):163–169.

Ellerhost-Ryan JM. Complications of the myeloproliferative system: Infection and sepsis. Semin Oncol Nurs 1985 Nov; 1(4):244–250.

Fox LS. Granulocytopenia in the adult cancer patient. Cancer Nurs 1981 Dec; 4(6):459–463.

Gurevich I and Tafuro P. The compromised host: Deficit-specific infection and the spectrum of prevention. Cancer Nurs 1986 Oct; 9(5):263–275.

Gurevich I and Tafuro P. Nursing measures for the prevention of infection in the compromised host. Nurs Clin North Am 1985 Mar; 20(1):257–260.

Jones P and Bodey GP. Infection in the critically ill cancer patient. Cancer Bull 1984; 36(3):143–147.

McCormick RD. Infections in patients with solid tumors. Nurs Clin North Am 1985 Mar; 20(1):199–205.

Newman KA. The leukemias. Nurs Clin North Am 1985 Mar; 20(1):227–234.

Pike AW. Antiseptic use in wound management. Crit Care Nurse 1983 Nov/Dec; 3(6):87–93.

Reheis CE. Neutropenia: Causes, complications, treatment, and resulting nursing care. Nurs Clin North Am 1985 Mar; 20(1):219–225.

Ristuccia AM. Hematologic effects of cancer chemotherapy. Nurs Clin North Am 1985 Mar; 20(1):235–239.

Ristuccia P. Microbiologic aspects of infection in the compromised host. Nurs Clin North Am 1985 Mar; 20(1):171–179.

Terry BA. Hodgkin's disease and non-Hodgkin's lymphoma. Nurs Clin North Am 1985 Mar; 20(1):207–217.

Patient/Family Resources

American Cancer Society, 90 Park Avenue, New York, New York 10016.

Burning N. Coping with Chemotherapy. New York, Doubleday, 1985.

Fiore NA. The Road Back to Health: Coping with the Emotional Side of Cancer. Toronto, Canada, Bantam Books, 1984.

Holleb AI (ed). The American Cancer Society Cancer Book: Prevention, Detection, Diagnosis, Treatment, Rehabilitation, Cure. New York, Doubleday, 1986.

National Cancer Institute, Office of Cancer Communications, Bethesda, Maryland 20892. Cancer Information Service: 1-800-4-CANCER.

Oncology Nursing Society, 3111 Banksville Road, Pittsburgh, Pennsylvania 15216.

Salsbury KH and Johnson EL. The Indispensable Cancer Handbook. New York, Seaview Books, 1981.

Support Groups: Check your local area.

International Association of Laryngectomies and the Lost Cord
Make Today Count
Reach to Recovery (mastectomy patients)
American Cancer Society Ostomy Rehabilitation Program
We Can Do, PO Box 731, Arcadia, California 91006 (ATT: Norman Cousins).

Perioperative Management of the Surgical Patient

Unit V

The person with a diagnosis that requires surgical intervention usually undergoes an operation during which anesthesia is used. Anesthesia may also be used in certain nonsurgical procedures, such as closed reduction of a dislocation or fracture. Most surgical procedures are performed in a hospital operating room, although many simpler procedures that do not require hospitalization are carried out in surgicenters.

Recent technological advances have led to more complex procedures, such as those requiring microsurgical techniques or the use of lasers, more sophisticated bypass equipment, and highly sensitive monitoring devices. More daring surgery involves the transplantation of human organs or the implantation of mechanical devices. Concomitant advances have also been made in the development of anesthetic agents, pharmaceutical preparations, and nutritional supplements and in the establishment of more extensive and refined rehabilitation procedures. These technological advances have focused attention on the essential ''hi-tech, hi-touch'' role of nursing personnel.

At the same time, the manner of delivering and paying for health care has changed, resulting in shorter hospital stays and cost containment measures. As a result, many people scheduled for surgery undergo diagnostic and preoperative preparation before entering the hospital. They also leave the

---

Examples of Nursing Activities in the Perioperative Role

Preoperative Phase

Preoperative Assessment

Home/Clinic
1. Initiates initial preoperative assessment
2. Plans teaching methods appropriate to patient's needs
3. Involves family in interview

Surgical Unit
1. Completes preoperative assessment
2. Coordinates patient teaching with other nursing staff
3. Explains phases in perioperative period and expectations
4. Develops a plan of care

Surgical Site
1. Assesses patient's level of consciousness
2. Reviews chart
3. Identifies patient
4. Verifies surgical site

Planning

Determines a plan of care

Psychological Support

1. Tells patient what is happening
2. Determines psychological status
3. Gives prior warning of noxious stimuli
4. Communicates patient's emotional status to other appropriate members of the health care team

Intraoperative Phase

Maintenance of Safety

1. Assures that the sponge, needle, and instrument counts are correct
2. Positions the patient
   a. Functional alignment
   b. Exposure of surgical site
   c. Maintenance of position throughout procedure
3. Applies grounding device to patient
4. Provides physical support

Physiological Monitoring

1. Calculates effects on patient of excessive fluid loss
2. Distinguishes normal from abnormal cardiopulmonary data
3. Reports changes in patient's pulse, respirations, temperature, and blood pressure

Psychological Monitoring (Prior to Induction and If Patient Is Conscious)

1. Provides emotional support to patient
2. Stands near/touches patient during procedures/induction
3. Continues to assess patient's emotional status
4. Communicates patient's emotional status to other appropriate members of the health care team

Nursing Management

1. Provides physical safety for the patient
2. Maintains aseptic, controlled environment
3. Effectively manages human resources

Postoperative Phase

Communication of Intraoperative Information

1. Gives patient's name
2. States type of surgery performed
3. Provides contributing intraoperative factors, *i.e.*, drain, catheters
4. States physical limitations
5. States impairments resulting from surgery
6. Reports patient's preoperative level of consciousness
7. Communicates necessary equipment needs

Postoperative Evaluation

Recovery Area
Determines patient's immediate response to surgical intervention

Surgical Unit
1. Evaluates effectiveness of nursing care in the OR
2. Determines patient's level of satisfaction with care given during perioperative period
3. Evaluates products used on patient in the OR
4. Determines patient's psychological status
5. Assists with discharge planning

Home/Clinic
1. Seeks patient's perception of surgery in terms of the effects of anesthetic agents, impact on body image, distortion, immobilization
2. Determines family's perception of surgery

hospital sooner, increasing the need for home care teaching and preparation for self-care.

Ambulatory or "same-day" surgery requires the nurse to have a solid knowledge of all aspects of surgical patient care. No longer are preoperative and postoperative nursing knowledge sufficient; complete care must include intraoperative nursing competency. This unit focuses on the nursing process in its perioperative approach as well as its applicability to involvement in short procedures. The basic principles remain the same.

Perioperative Nursing

Perioperative nursing is the term used to describe the wide variety of nursing functions associated with the patient's surgical experience. The word "perioperative" is an encompassing term that incorporates the three phases of the surgical experience—preoperative, intraoperative, and postoperative. Each of these phases begins and ends at a particular time in the sequence of events that constitute the surgical experience, and each includes a wide range of behaviors and nursing activities that the nurse performs using the nursing process as reflected in the standards of practice (see the chart on p. 338).

The *preoperative phase* of the perioperative nursing role begins when the decision for surgical intervention is made and ends with the transfer of the patient to the operating room table. The scope of nursing activities during this time can be as broad as establishing a baseline assessment of the patient in the clinical setting or at home, carrying out a preoperative interview, and preparing the patient for the anesthetic he is to receive and the surgery he is to undergo. Or it may be as limited as doing a preoperative patient assessment in the holding area or surgical suite.

The nursing functions included in the *intraoperative phase* begin when the patient is admitted or transferred to the surgery department and end when he is admitted to the recovery area. In this phase, the scope of nursing activity can be as broad as starting the IV, administering IV medications, carrying out the full scope of physiologic monitoring throughout a surgical procedure, and providing for the patient's safety. Or it can be as limited as holding the patient's hand during general anesthesia induction, acting in the role of scrub nurse, or assisting in positioning the patient on the operating room table using basic principles of body alignment.

The *postoperative phase* begins with the admission of the patient to the recovery area and ends with a follow-up evaluation in the clinical setting or at home. The scope of nursing activities during this period may be as broad as assessing the postoperative status of the patient in terms of the effects of the anesthetic agents and the impact of surgery on body image or role function, as well as evaluating the family's perception of the surgery. Or it can be as limited as communicating pertinent information about the patient's surgery to personnel in the recovery area or surgical nursing unit.

Each phase is reviewed in more detail in this unit. Where pertinent and possible, the nursing process of assessment, planning, intervention, and evaluation is described. (This is also outlined in Chart 18-5, pp 338–339.)

Gerontological Overview

Surgery imposes physical and psychological stress, but advances in evaluation techniques, surgical procedures, anesthetic techniques, and monitoring capabilities allow older patients to tolerate elective surgery surprisingly well. The principle to be kept in mind during preoperative evaluation, surgery, and postoperative care is that the aged patient has *less physiologic reserve* (the ability of an organ to return to normal after a disturbance in its equilibrium) than the younger patient. The special requirements for optimum results following surgery on an elderly patient include (1) skillfull preoperative evaluation and treatment, (2) experienced and careful anesthesia and surgery, and (3) meticulous and competent postoperative management. The hazards of surgery for the aged are proportional to the number and severity of coexisting diseases and the nature and duration of the operative procedure.

Chapter 17

Preoperative Nursing Management

Surgical Indications and Classifications

Surgery may be performed for a variety of reasons. It may be *diagnostic*, such as when a biopsy is obtained or an exploratory laparotomy performed; it may be *curative*, such as when a tumor mass is excised or an inflamed appendix removed; it may be *reparative*, such as when multiple wounds must be mended; it may be *reconstructive* or *cosmetic*, such as when a harelip is repaired or a face lift done; and it may be *palliative*, such as when pain must be relieved or a problem corrected—for example, when a gastrostomy is performed to compensate for the inability to swallow food.

Surgery may also be classified according to the degree of urgency involved, using the terms *emergency, urgent, required, elective,* and *optional.* These terms are defined in Table 17-1, and examples of the types of surgery involved are provided.

Nursing Process Overview

▷ Assessment

As is indicated in the pages that follow, assessment of the surgical patient involves evaluation of a wide range of physical and psychological factors. Many parameters are taken into account in the overall assessment of the patient, and a variety of patient problems or nursing diagnoses can be anticipated or identified on the basis of the data gathered. Detailed discussions of the psychosocial assessment and the physical examination of the surgical patient follow this section.

▷ Nursing Diagnoses

Based on the assessment data, major preoperative nursing diagnoses of the surgical patient may include

- Anxiety related to the surgical experience (anesthesia, pain) and the outcome of surgery

TABLE 17-1
Categories of Contemplated Surgery Based on Urgency

Classification	Indications for Surgery	Examples
I. *Emergency*—Requires immediate attention; may be life-threatening	Without delay	Severe bleeding Bladder or intestinal obstruction Fractured skull Gunshot/stab wounds Extensive burns
II. *Urgent*—Requires prompt attention	Within 24–30 hr	Acute gallbladder infection Kidney or ureteral stones
III. *Required*—Patient needs to have operation.	Plan within a few weeks or months.	Prostatic hyperplasia without bladder obstruction Thyroid problems Eye cataracts
IV. *Elective*—Patient should be operated upon.	Failure to have surgery not catastrophic.	Repair of scars Simple hernia Vaginal repair
V. *Optional*—Decision rests with patient.	Personal preference	Cosmetic surgery

- Knowledge deficit regarding preoperative procedures and protocols and postoperative expectations

▷ *Planning and Implementation*

▷ *Goals:* The surgical patient's major goals may include (1) relief of preoperative anxiety and (2) increased knowledge of preoperative preparations and postoperative expectations.

Nursing Interventions

Reduction of Preoperative Anxiety. Specific nursing interventions are discussed in detail under Psychosocial Nursing Assessment and Interventions.

Patient Education. Specific nursing interventions are discussed in detail under Preoperative Patient Education. See also Preoperative Nursing Interventions and Immediate Preoperative Nursing Interventions.

▷ *Evaluation*

▷ *Expected Outcomes*
1. Patient's anxiety is relieved.
   a. Verbalizes relief about hospital bills and other costs after talking with social worker
   b. Tells mate he is looking forward to having problem corrected
   c. Queries anesthesiologist about concerns related to types of anesthesia and induction
   d. Verbalizes an understanding of the preanesthetic medication and general anesthesia
   e. Queries staff about last-minute concerns
   f. Requests visit with member of clergy
   g. Relaxes quietly after being visited by health team members

2. Patient learns about and prepares for surgical intervention.
   a. Participates willingly in preoperative preparation
   b. Describes kind of exercises he is expected to do postoperatively
   c. Reviews information about postoperative care
   d. Accepts preanesthetic medication
   e. Remains in bed; tells nurse why side rails are in place
   f. Relaxes and closes eyes during transportation to operating unit

Psychosocial Nursing Assessment and Interventions

Any surgical procedure is always preceded by some type of emotional reaction in a patient, whether it is obvious or hidden, normal or abnormal. For example, preoperative anxiety is an anticipatory response to an experience that the patient may view as a threat to his customary role in life, body integrity, or even life itself. It is known that a mind that is not at peace directly influences the functioning of the body. Therefore, it is imperative to know what anxieties the patient is experiencing.

By taking a careful *nursing history*, the nurse will elicit patient concerns that can have a direct bearing on the course of the surgical experience. Undoubtedly, a patient facing surgery is beset by fears: fears of the unknown, of death, of anesthesia, of cancer. Add to worries about the possible loss of a job, the need to support a family, or the possibility of permanent incapacity and one can get a sense of the enormous emotional strain created by the prospect of surgery. Consequently, the nurse needs to be tolerant and understanding.

The extent of the patient's reaction is based on many factors, including the discomforts and sacrifices he anticipates—whether physical, financial, psychological, spiritual, or social—and the surgical outcome he imagines. Will the operation improve his present condition? Will he be disabled? Is this just a temporary measure in a chronic condition?

An important part of the social assessment is to determine the role of the patient's family or persons who are meaningful to him. The value and reliability of all available support systems is also determined. Other pertinent findings are the usual function level and typical daily activities of the patient, information which may assist in his care and future rehabilitation plans.

Fear is expressed in different ways by different people. For example, fear may be expressed indirectly by the patient who asks a lot of questions, repeating them constantly even though answers were given previously. For another person, the reaction may be withdrawal—deliberately avoiding communication, perhaps by concentrating on a book. Still others may talk incessantly about trivialities. Often such behavior ends abruptly as the patient turns to the nurse and says, "I guess you can tell I'm a bit nervous about my operation." The need to keep the outlet of communication open is never greater than at this time. To belittle the patient's fears by saying, "Oh, there's nothing to be afraid of," immediately closes the door and causes the patient to lapse into less effective means of coping with his worries.

Such breakdowns in satisfactory interrelations may leave the patient upset, bewildered, and even unable to follow simple directions. Often in the course of conversation something that was mentioned by a nurse or a physician becomes exaggerated out of all proportion to its importance. For example, if an operation is postponed because of a filled schedule, the patient who is merely told that "something has come up" may begin to worry that the reason for the delay is a deterioration in his condition.

A preoperative patient may experience a number of fears. *Fear of anesthesia* was justified years ago, when little was known about the control and the effect of anesthetic agents. But with refined methods, tested drugs, and skilled anesthesiologists, the hazards are minimized. The ease with which a patient accepts an anesthetic today is attributed to the adequacy of the physical and mental preparation he receives. The price of poor preparation is a difficult period of induction, followed by an unpleasant emergence from the anesthetic agent. The nurse in daily association with each patient can do much to dispel false conceptions and misinformation. When the anesthesiologist and the operating room nurse visit the patient the day before surgery, real confidence is established, and the patient accepts the anesthetic more readily and is less fearful because the number of unknowns has been reduced.

Often the fear of the anesthetic is secondary to the *fear of pain or of death.* Will I feel the knife? What if the anesthesia wears off? The patient needs reassurance that the anesthesiologist will be in constant attendance to take care of these problems. Some surgeons will not operate on a patient who is convinced that he will die. This is a real fear, and it cannot be dismissed lightly. Good rapport between patient and nurse, together with tact on the nurse's part, may bring the patient to a realization that his fear is magnified. It will help him

greatly if those responsible for his care build up his confidence.

The *fear of the unknown* is the worst of all. This fear stems partly from a belief on the patient's part that he is not being told "everything" about his diagnosis or his illness. The more understanding one has of the probabilities for the future, the better is the adjustment. The nurse can do much to allay the patient's anxieties and induce a certain peace of mind. A patient frequently expresses fears and misgivings to the nurse but hides them from the surgeon. In such circumstances the nurse communicates these evidences of anxiety privately to the surgeon.

The patient who has had a previous positive experience with surgery may feel less apprehensive. However, an earlier negative experience can aggravate the person's fear. The nurse can help the patient to view the impending operation as a new and unique situation, not a repetition of the past.

The *fear of destruction of body image* occurs frequently because in many instances surgery has become more radical. Also, there is greater emphasis today on youth, the body beautiful, and more revealing clothing, as is demonstrated by magazine and television advertising. Consequently any surgical encroachment on the body, including the scar of a surgical incision, is viewed with distress by many patients.

Fear of separation from a loved one, from familiar support systems, and from former activities can also create anxieties.

In addition to the above fears, the average patient has many other worries. He may have financial problems, family responsibilities, and employment obligations, and he may fear a poor prognosis or the probability of a handicap in the future. These problems can be investigated by the nurse. If the difficulty is of such a nature that a medical social worker can give assistance, the aid of such a person is enlisted. If the worry stems from fear of what the prognosis is likely to be, the physician is informed.

When some of these fears have been expressed, brought to light, and examined in their proper perspective, it is possible and even essential to get the patient to reveal what the operation means to him. Have him express his thoughts about the importance and the meaning of this surgery for the immediate future as well as the more distant future. Most fears are manifestations of concern over losing control over one's person, either physically or socially. The patient may be concerned about losing some of his independence, his integrity, and his control over his effectiveness in coping with his environment. The nurse may be in a position to elicit these concerns from the patient. The importance of adequate lines of communication between surgeon and nurse as they work together to prepare the patient for surgery must be emphasized here.

Psychological preparation for subsequent stress includes permitting the patient some degree of worrying. This is more desirable than having little or no anticipatory fear. Moderately fear-arousing information allows the patient to increase his tolerance for stress by developing effective ways of coping with his problems. Absence of worry will deprive the patient of the motivation to prepare psychologically for a stressful experience, with the result that when a crisis develops he will have a low tolerance for stress.

The significance of *spiritual therapy* must not be forgotten. Regardless of the religious affiliation of the patient, the nurse recognizes that faith in a Higher Power can be as therapeutic as medication. Every attempt must be made to help the patient obtain the spiritual help that he requests. This may be accomplished by participating in prayer, by reading passages from the Scriptures, or by calling a member of the clergy. Faith has great sustaining power; thus, the beliefs of each individual patient should be respected and supported.

The interval of time preparatory to surgery in some instances may become very extended. *Cognitive control* in the form of *recreation and diversion* can be provided by such activities as reading, listening to the radio, watching television, engaging in handcrafts and games, and so forth. The nurse can arrange for people with similar interests to meet. Many times patients can help one another.

Perhaps the most valuable facility at the disposal of the nurse is the ability to *listen* to the patient, especially during the nursing history. By engaging in conversation and using the principles of tactful interviewing, the nurse can acquire invaluable bits of information. An unhurried, understanding, and kind nurse invites confidence on the part of the patient.

Every patient should be treated as an individual who has fears and hopes quite distinct from the fears or hopes of the next person. Understanding and helping one patient may require an approach completely different from that used with another. Providing time to answer questions and offering psychological support will ensure a smoother postoperative course. The patient will sleep better, recall fewer fearful images, need less anesthetic and pain medication, recover more rapidly, and be discharged from the hospital sooner.

Denial of Anxiety. The preceding discussion of preoperative anxiety emphasizes the most common problems of the patient facing an operation. The opposite reaction, denying anxiety, can also provide obstacles to effective treatment, as in the case of a person who notices abnormal signs or symptoms but puts off seeking treatment. Denial is a reaction noted in many persons when they are suddenly confronted with potentially shocking information. Usually this reaction does not last longer than a few days or a few weeks, but nevertheless such denial and delay may have serious consequences. The nurse's responsibility in this area extends to all members of the community. She should encourage anyone with a questionable abnormal physical finding to have it checked as soon as possiible by a knowledgeable person in the health care field.

General Physical Assessment

Before treatment is initiated, a *nursing history* is taken and the patient is given a *physical examination,* during which vital signs are noted and a data base is established for future comparisons. Many diagnostic tests may be performed, such as blood analyses, roentgenographic studies, endoscopies, tissue biopsies, and stool and urine studies. In all of these tests the nurse is in a position to help the patient understand the need for the diagnostic studies. There is also an opportunity during the physical examination to note significant physical findings, such as a rash or pressure sores, that may be contributing to the patient's condition.

These preliminary contacts with the staff during the nursing history, physical examination, and diagnostic tests provide the patient with opportunities to ask questions and to get acquainted with those who will be caring for him. In their efforts to establish rapport with the patient, the physician and nurse must respect the patient's feelings and needs.

Nutritional Status

Nutritional needs are determined by measuring the patient's height and weight, triceps skin fold, upper arm circumference, serum protein levels, and nitrogen balance. These measurements are discussed in detail in the nutritional assessment section of Chapter 6.

Proteins and Vitamins. Replacement of deficits is especially important with respect to protein and calorie malnutrition, since protein is essential for tissue repair. Protein deficiency may result from anorexia concomitant with the aging process, chronic debilitating illness, cancer, or frequent vomiting. Or, it may be caused by poor food habits and a diet in which meats and eggs are almost absent. Protein may also be lost in severe burns and through draining abscesses or wounds.

Protein replacement is a slow process and may take several days or weeks. The replacement may be accomplished by means of (1) a diet high in protein (meat, milk, eggs, and cheese), carbohydrates, and calories, but low in fat; (2) supplementary liquid feedings, such as milk enriched with skim milk powder; or (3) protein hydrolysates given orally or by infusion. Hypertonic parenteral therapy may be given through a polyethylene tubing placed percutaneously in a large vein, such as the subclavian (using a cutdown). (See Parenteral Hyperalimentation Therapy in Chapter 32.)

Vitamins are required for specific purposes. Thiamine (vitamin B_1) is necessary for oxidizing carbohydrates and maintaining normal gastrointestinal function. A deficiency in vitamin B_1 is noted in chronic gastrointestinal and liver diseases. Ascorbic acid (vitamin C) is required for wound healing and synthesis of collagen. Vitamin K is necessary for blood clotting and prothrombin production. These vitamins may be given orally or parenterally.

Loss of body fluids results in electrolyte imbalances. The replacement of these fluids is discussed in Chapter 9. The nurse records all intake and output and keeps a daily record of the patient's weight. Periodic evaluations are made to note the patient's progress and readiness for surgery. Dental caries and poor mouth hygiene may contribute to general debilitation and should be corrected (Chap. 30).

A nursing goal and challenge is to encourage the patient to eat by serving attractive and palatable meals made up of small, manageable servings. Patients on parenteral/enteral therapy or receiving gastrostomy feedings or infusions may need diversion and encouragement. The method of giving fluids depends on the type of replacement therapy. If a nasogastric tube is being used, liquids will be taken more readily if the patient is in a sitting position. If gastrostomy feedings are used, an upright or Fowler's position is effective.

Dehydration, hypovolemia, and electrolyte imbalances are common and should be carefully substantiated. The degree of severity is often difficult to determine. When a patient is being prepared for surgery, often additional time is needed to replace deficits in order to get him in the best possible condition.

Obesity. If the patient is overweight and if preoperative time permits, physicians will insist that a prescribed and systematic program of weight reduction be undertaken to lessen the surgical risk. Obesity greatly increases the seriousness of complications. During surgery, fatty tissues are not highly resistant to infection and the surgeon faces increased technical and mechanical problems; therefore, dehiscence (wound separation) and wound infections are more common. The obese patient is difficult to care for because of his weight; he breathes poorly when lying on his side and thus is subject to hypoventilation and postoperative pulmonary complications, distention, and phlebitis. In addition, cardiovascular, endocrine, hepatic, and biliary diseases are more common in obese patients. It has been estimated that for each 30 pounds of excess weight, about 25 additional miles of blood vessels are needed. The increased demands on the heart are obvious.

Addiction to Narcotics, Drugs, or Alcohol. People who have an addiction to drugs or alcohol frequently attempt to hide the habit. Often a variety of infections and trauma sites on the body can be noted. This situation calls for meticulous attention, patience, and a degree of skepticism on the part of the nurse who is assessing the patient.

The acutely intoxicated person is susceptible to injury. If surgery is required, local or regional block anesthesia is used for minor surgery; for more extensive injury, surgery is postponed if possible. Otherwise, the stomach must be intubated and aspirated before general anesthesia is administered in order to prevent vomiting and aspiration.

The person with a history of chronic alcoholism often suffers from malnutrition and other systemic problems that increase the surgical risk. In view of this, delirium tremens may be anticipated on the second or third day postoperatively; it is associated with a significant mortality rate.

Respiratory Status

The goal for potential surgical patients is to have optimum respiratory function. All patients are urged to stop smoking 4 to 6 weeks before an operation; those undergoing upper abdominal and chest surgery are taught breathing exercises and how to use an incentive spirometer.

Since it is necessary to maintain adequate ventilation during all phases of surgical treatment, surgery is usually contraindicated when the patient has a respiratory infection. Respiratory difficulties increase the possibility of atelectasis, bronchopneumonia, and respiratory failure when anesthetics are superimposed. Patients with pulmonary problems are evaluated by testing pulmonary function and determining blood gas values to note the extent of respiratory insufficiency. Antibiotics may be given for infections.

Cardiovascular Status

The goal in preparing any patient for surgery is to have a well-functioning cardiovascular system to meet the oxygen, fluid, and nutritional needs throughout the perioperative period.

Since the margin of safety is lessened when a patient exhibits signs of cardiovascular disease, this condition demands greater than usual diligence during all phases of management and care. Depending on the severity of symptoms, surgery may be deferred until maximal benefits have been obtained from medical treatment. At times surgical treatment can be modified to meet the likely tolerance of the patient. For example, in an obese patient with acute obstructive cholecystitis and possible diabetes and coronary artery disease, simple gallbladder drainage with removal of calculi may be done rather than a more extensive operation.

Of particular significance in the patient with cardiovascular disease is the necessity to avoid sudden changes of position, prolonged immobilization, hypotension or hypoxia, and overloading of the body with fluids or blood.

Hepatic and Renal Function

The goal is to have maximum functioning of the liver and urinary systems so that drugs, anesthetic agents, and body waste and toxins are adequately removed from the body.

The *liver* is important in the biotransformation of anesthetic compounds. Therefore, any disease of the liver has an effect on anesthetic intake. Because acute liver disease is associated with a high surgical death rate, preoperative improvement in liver function is desired. Careful assessment is made using various liver function tests (see Chap. 35).

The *kidney* is involved in the excretion of anesthetic drugs and their metabolites. Acid–base and water metabolism are also important considerations in anesthetic administration. Surgery is contraindicated when a patient has acute nephritis, acute renal insufficiency with oliguria or anuria, or other acute renal problems, unless the surgery is a lifesaving measure or is necessary to improve urinary function, as in an obstructive uropathy.

Endocrine Function

In uncontrolled diabetes the chief life-threatening hazard is that of hypoglycemia, which may develop during anesthesia or postoperatively. It results from inadequate intake of carbohydrates or from insulin overdosage. Other hazards that threaten but occur less rapidly are acidosis and glucosuria. In general, the surgical risk of the patient with controlled diabetes is not greater than that of the nondiabetic patient (see Chap. 37).

Immunologic Function

An important nursing goal is to determine the presence of an allergy history, including previous allergic reactions. Particularly significant is the notation of sensitivities to certain drugs and past adverse reactions to these medications. Obtain a list of offending agents and document how the allergy was manifested. Also, ask about blood transfusion reactions in the past. Record any affirmative response. Current pharmacotherapy also is recorded. A history of bronchial asthma is reported to the anesthesiologist.

Immunosuppression is now common with steroid therapy, renal transplantation, cancer radiotherapy, and chemotherapy. The mildest symptoms or slightest temperature elevation need to be investigated. Because these patients will not tolerate breaks in technique, great care is taken in practicing meticulous asepsis.

Prior Drug Therapy

Attention is given to the history of drug usage by the patient. Potent medications have an effect on physiologic functions; interactions of such drugs with anesthetic agents have caused serious problems, such as arterial hypotension and circulatory collapse or depression.

The potential effects of prior drug therapy are evaluated by the anesthesiologist, who considers the length of time the patient has used the drugs, his condition, and the nature of the proposed surgery. Drugs that cause particular concern are the following:

Adrenal steroids—It is not advisable to discontinue corticosteroids before surgery. Because the sudden termination of therapy may cause cardiovascular collapse if steroid therapy has been used for a chronic problem over a period of time, it is usually advisable to give a "burst" of high-dose steroid immediately before and after surgery.

Diuretics—In particular, the thiazide drugs may cause excessive respiratory depression during anesthesia; this results from an electrolyte imbalance.

Phenothiazines—These drugs may increase the hypotensive action of anesthetics.

Antidepressants—In particular, monoamine oxidase (MAO) inhibitors increase the hypotensive effects of anesthetics.

Tranquilizers—Barbiturates, diazepam, and chlordiazepoxide are medications that can cause anxiety, tension, and even seizures if withdrawn suddenly.

Insulin—Interaction between anesthetics and insulin must be considered when a diabetic patient is undergoing surgery.

Antibiotics—"Mycin" drugs such as neomycin, kanamycin, and, less frequently, streptomycin may present problems; when these drugs are combined with a curariform muscle relaxant, nerve transmission is interrupted and apnea due to respiratory paralysis may result. For the reasons cited, it is imperative that the patient's drug history be assessed by the nurse and anesthesiologist.

Gerontological Considerations

An older person facing an operation usually has a combination of medical problems in addition to the specific one for which surgery is indicated. Elderly people frequently do not report symptoms, perhaps because they fear that a serious illness may be diagnosed or because they accept such symptoms as part of growing old. A high level of awareness of subtle clues will alert the nurse to underlying problems.

In general, the elderly are considered poorer surgical risks than younger patients. Cardiac reserves are lower, renal and hepatic function are depressed, and gastrointestinal activity is likely to be reduced. Dehydration, constipation, and malnutrition may be evident.

Sensory limitations such as dimming vision, impaired hearing, and reduced sensitivity of touch are often the reasons for accidents, injuries, and burns. Therefore the nurse must be alert to maintaining a safe environment. Arthritis is common in older persons and may affect mobility, making it difficult for the patient to turn from one side to the other without discomfort. Protective measures include adequate padding for tender areas, moving the patient slowly, protecting bony prominences against prolonged pressure, and providing gentle massage to promote adequate circulation.

The condition of the mouth is important to assess because of the frequent presence of dental caries, dentures, and partial plates. Such findings are particularly significant to the anesthesiologist.

The loss of sweat glands leads to dry, itchy skin. Such fragile skin is easily abraded, so added precautions are taken in moving an elderly person. The loss of subcutaneous fat makes older people less resistant to temperature changes. A lightweight cotton blanket is a desirable cover when an elderly patient is moved to and from the operating room.

The elderly person has had innumerable experiences in his lifetime. He has been exposed to personal illness and life-threatening illnesses of friends and family. Consequently he has fears about his own future that may not be obvious but nonetheless are there. Taking time to talk with him may bring forth his fears and make possible the relaxation and acceptance he needs.

Risk Factor Summary

The optimum goal is to have as many positive factors as possible. Every attempt is made to stabilize those conditions that otherwise hinder a smooth recovery. When balance is lost in favor of negative factors, the risks increase, as do postoperative complications (see Chart 17-1).

Informed Consent

In order to attain the right to operate, it is necessary for the surgeon to obtain a voluntary and informed consent from the patient. Such written permission protects the patient against unsanctioned surgery and protects the surgeon against claims of an unauthorized operation. In the best interests of all parties concerned, sound medicolegal principles are followed.

The nurse's responsibility is to ensure that an *informed* consent has been obtained voluntarily from an informed and comprehending person. (See Table 17-2, Criteria for Valid Informed Consent.)

Before the patient signs the permit, the surgeon should inform him in clear and simple terms what a reasonable person would want to be told and what the surgery will entail. The surgeon should also inform the patient of possible risks, complications, disfigurement, disability, and removal of body parts, as well as what to expect in the early and late postoperative periods.

Informed consent is obtained when

- The procedure is invasive, such as a surgical incision, a cystoscopy, or paracentesis
- Anesthesia is used
- A nonsurgical procedure is done in which there is more than slight risk to the patient, such as an arteriogram
- A procedure is done that involves radiation, cobalt therapy, and the like

The patient may sign his own permit for operation if he is of age and mentally capable. If he is a minor or is unconscious or incompetent, permission must be obtained from a responsible family member. If he is an emancipated minor

Chart 17-1
Risk Factors for Any Surgical Procedure

Systemic Factors
Hypovolemia
Dehydration or electrolyte imbalance
Nutritional deficits
Extremes of age
Extremes of weight
Infection and sepsis
Toxic conditions
Immunologic abnormalities

Pulmonary Disease

Renal Disease

Pregnancy—because of
Diminished maternal physiologic reserve
Fetal susceptibility to disease

Cardiovascular Disease
Coronary artery disease
Cardiac failure
Dysrhythmias
Hypertension
Prosthetic heart valve
Thromboembolism
Hemorrhagic diathesis
Cerebrovascular disease

Endocrine Dysfunction
Diabetes mellitus
Adrenal corticosteroid conditions
Thyroid malfunction

Hepatic Disease

(married or independently earning his own living), he may sign his own permit. Bear in mind that state regulations and agency policy must be followed. In an emergency, it may be necessary for the surgeon to operate as a lifesaving measure without the patient's informed consent. However, every effort should be made to contact the patient's family. In such a situation, contact can be made by telephone or telegram.

When the patient has doubts and has not had the opportunity to investigate alternative treatments, he is entitled to a second opinion. No patient should be forced to sign an operative permit. Refusing to have an operation is a person's privilege. However, such information must be documented and relayed to the surgeon so that other arrangements can be made; for instance, additional explanations may be offered to the patient and family, or the operation may be rescheduled at a more suitable time.

The consent process can be improved by providing audiovisual materials to supplement discussion, by ensuring that

TABLE 17-2
Criteria for Valid Informed Consent

Component	Comments
Consent voluntarily given	Valid consent must be freely given, without coercion.
Incompetent subject	Legal definition: individuals who are *not* autonomous and cannot give or withhold consent (*e.g.*, individuals who are mentally retarded, mentally ill, or comatose)
Informed subject	Consent form should be in writing (although law does not require written documentation). It should contain the following: Explanation of procedure and its risks Description of benefits An offer to answer questions about procedure Instructions that the patient may withdraw A statement informing the subject if the protocol differs from customary consent
Subject able to comprehend	Information must be written and delivered in language understandable to the patient. Questions must be answered to facilitate comprehension if material is confusing.

(Adapted from Douglas S and Larson E. There's more to informed consent than information. *Focus on Critical Care* 1986 April; 13(2):44)

the language of the consent form is understandable and by using other strategies and resources as needed to help the patient understand.

- The informed consent is placed in a prominent place on the patient's chart and accompanies the patient to the operating room.

Preoperative Patient Education

The value of preoperative instruction to the patient has long been recognized. Each patient should be taught as an individual, in terms of his anxieties, needs, and hopes. The background information of one patient is usually very different from that of the next patient. Once these differences are recognized and particular needs are assessed, a program of instruction can be planned and then implemented at the proper time. If the patient is taught essential information several days before he needs it, he may not remember what he was told. If he is instructed too close to the time of surgery, he may not be in prime learning condition because of the effect of the preanesthetic medication.

If instruction is offered at a time when the patient is most receptive and can participate in the learning process, the chances are that he will retain more of the information. In actuality, instruction is spaced over a period of time to allow the patient to assimilate information and to ask questions as they arise. Frequently, teaching sessions are combined with various preparation procedures to allow for an easy flow of information. In essence, the nurse must make a judgment about how much the patient wants and needs to know. In some instances, too much explanation can be worse than not enough.

Limiting teaching to a description of the various steps of a procedure is not as helpful as telling the patient what sensations he will experience. For example, telling the patient that preoperative medication will relax him before the operation is not as effective as informing him that the medication will make him feel lightheaded and sleepy. Once he knows what to expect, he will anticipate these reactions and thus attain a higher degree of relaxation than might otherwise be expected.

Deep Breathing, Coughing, and Relaxation Skills

One goal of preoperative nursing care is to show the patient how to promote lung ventilation and blood oxygenation following general anesthesia. This is done by demonstrating to the patient how to take a deep, slow breath (maximal sustained inspiration, MSI) and how to exhale slowly. The patient is placed in a sitting position to provide maximum lung expansion. After practicing deep breathing several times, he is instructed to breathe deeply, exhale through the mouth, take a short breath, and cough from deep in the lungs (see Chart 17-2, *A* and *B*). In addition to enhancing respiration, these exercises make the patient more relaxed.

If there is to be a thoracic or abdominal incision, the nurse can demonstrate how the incision line can be splinted so that pressure is minimized and pain is controlled. The patient should put the palms of both hands together, interlacing the fingers snugly. Placing the hands across the incisional site acts as an effective splint when coughing. Of course the patient needs to know that medications will be given to control pain.

The goal in promoting coughing is to mobilize secretions so that they can be removed. When a deep breath is taken before coughing, the cough reflex is stimulated. If coughing is not encouraged, hypostatic pneumonia and other lung complications may occur.

Turning and Active Body Movement

The goals of promoting deliberate body movement postoperatively are to have the patient improve his circulation, to prevent venous stasis, and to contribute to optimal respiratory exchange.

The patient is shown how to turn from side to side and how to assume the lateral position. This position will be used postoperatively (even before the patient is conscious) and assumed every second hour.

Exercises of the extremities include extension and flexion of the knee and hip joints (similar to bicycle-riding while lying on the side). The foot is rotated as though tracing the largest possible circle with the great toe (see Chart 17-2, *C* and *D*). The elbow and shoulder are also put through the range of motion. At first the patient will be assisted and reminded to do these exercises, but later is encouraged to do them himself.

The nurse is reminded to use proper body mechanics and to instruct the patient to do the same. When he is placed in any position, the body is to be maintained in proper alignment. Muscle tone is maintained so that ambulation will be made easier.

Pain Control and Medications

The patient is told that he will receive a preanesthetic medication to help him relax and perhaps feel sleepy. He is also informed that it may make him thirsty. Postoperatively, he can expect medications to keep him comfortable but not to prevent him from regaining activity and maintaining an adequate air exchange.

Prophylactic antibiotics may be prescribed in specific instances. Frequently, the cephalosporins are chosen because these agents have a low toxicity and wide spectrum of action.

Cognitive Control

Useful techniques for relieving tension, overcoming anxiety, and achieving relaxation are the following:

Imagery—Ask the patient to concentrate on a happy experience during his last vacation.

Distraction—Suggest that the patient think of and recite several nursery rhymes.

Optimistic self-recitation—"I know all will go well."

Other Information

The patient feels more at ease when he knows at what point postoperatively he can expect a visit from family or friends.

Chart 17-2
Preoperative Patient Instruction

A. Diaphragmatic Breathing

Diaphragmatic breathing refers to a flattening of the dome of the diaphragm during inspiration with resulting enlargement of the upper abdomen as air rushes in. During expiration, the abdominal muscles contract.

1. Practice in the same position you would assume in bed following surgery: a semi-Fowler's position, propped in bed with the back and shoulders well supported with pillows.
2. With the hands in a loose-fist position, allow the hands to rest lightly on the front of the lower ribs—fingernails against lower chest to feel the movement (Fig. 17-1).
3. Breathe out gently and fully as the ribs sink down and inward toward midline.
4. Then take a deep breath through your nose and mouth, letting the abdomen rise as the lungs fill with air.
5. Hold this breath for a count of five.
6. Exhale and let out *all* the air through the nose and mouth.
7. Repeat 15 times with a short rest after each group of five.
8. Practice this twice a day preoperatively.

B. Coughing

1. Lean forward slightly from a sitting position in bed, interlace the fingers together, and place the hands across the incisional site to act as a splint when coughing (Fig. 17-2).
2. Breathe with the diaphragm as described in *A*.
3. With the mouth slightly open, breathe in fully.
4. "Hack" out sharply for three short breaths.
5. Then, keeping the mouth open, take in a quick deep breath and immediately give a strong cough once or twice. This will help clear secretions from the chest. It may cause some discomfort but will not harm incision.

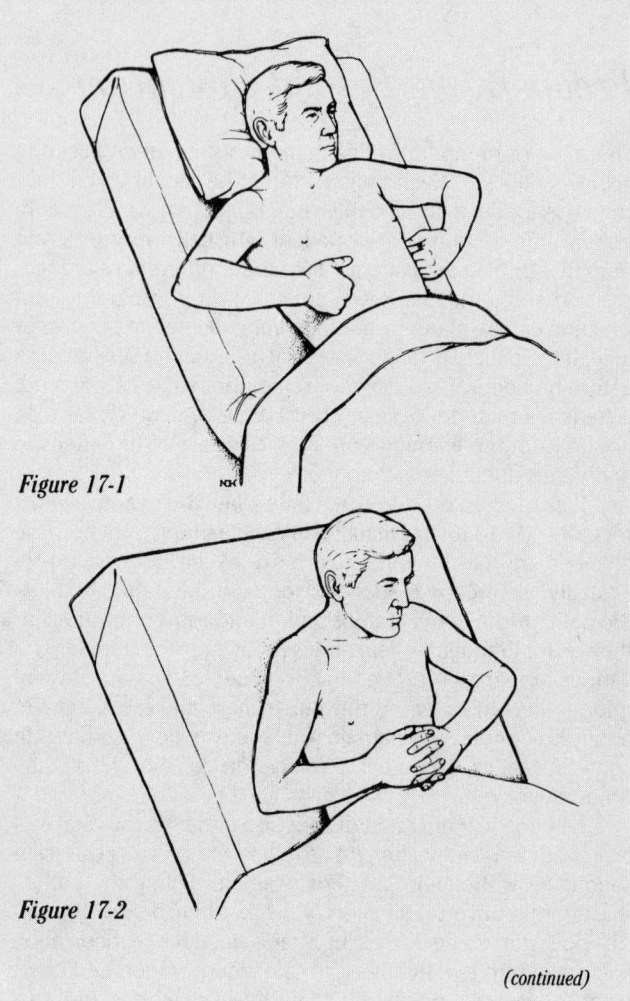

Figure 17-1

Figure 17-2

(continued)

It helps him to know that the family will be kept informed about the acute phases of the surgical experience. He also appreciates knowing that a spiritual adviser of his preference will be available if he so desires.

If the patient knows beforehand that he will be on assisted breathing and that drainage tubes will be in place along with any special equipment required, he is more likely to accept these accoutrements postoperatively without too much concern.

Preoperative Nursing Interventions

Nutrition and Fluids

When the operation is scheduled for the morning, the meal on the preceding evening may be an ordinary light diet. In dehydrated patients, and especially in older ones, fluids by mouth often are encouraged before an operation. In addition, fluids may be administered by vein, as prescribed, especially in patients to whom fluids cannot be given by mouth. If the operation is scheduled to take place after noon and does not involve any part of the gastrointestinal tract, the patient may be given a soft diet for breakfast. Most often, oral intake of food or water is withheld 8 to 10 hours before the operation.

The goal in withholding food before surgery is to prevent aspiration. Aspiration occurs when food or fluid is regurgitated from the stomach and inhaled into the pulmonary system. Such inhaled material acts as a foreign substance, is irritating, and causes an inflammatory reaction, and at the same time interferes with and even intercepts adequate air exchange. Aspiration is a serious problem, as is reflected in a high mortality rate (60%–70%) when it occurs. Thus, to prevent aspiration, food and fluid intake is restricted for 8 to 10 hours preoperatively. If obstruction is suspected, a nasogastric tube is positioned.

Chart 17-2 *(continued)*

C. Leg Exercises

1. Lie in a semi-Fowler's position and perform the following simple exercises to improve circulation.
2. Bend the knee and raise the foot—hold it a few seconds, then extend the leg and lower it to the bed (Fig. 17-3).
3. Do this about five times with one leg, then repeat with the other leg.
4. Then trace circles with the feet by bending them down, in toward each other, up, and then out (Fig. 17-4).
5. Repeat these five times.

D. Turning to the Side

1. Turn on your side with the uppermost leg flexed most and supported on a pillow.
2. Grasp the side rail as an aid to maneuver to the side.
3. Practice diaphragmatic breathing and coughing while on your side.

E. Getting Out of Bed

1. Turn on your side.
2. Push yourself up with one hand as you swing your legs out of bed.

F. Using the Urinal (For Male Patient)

When in bed for a period of time, have the nurse explain the method for using the urinal in bed.

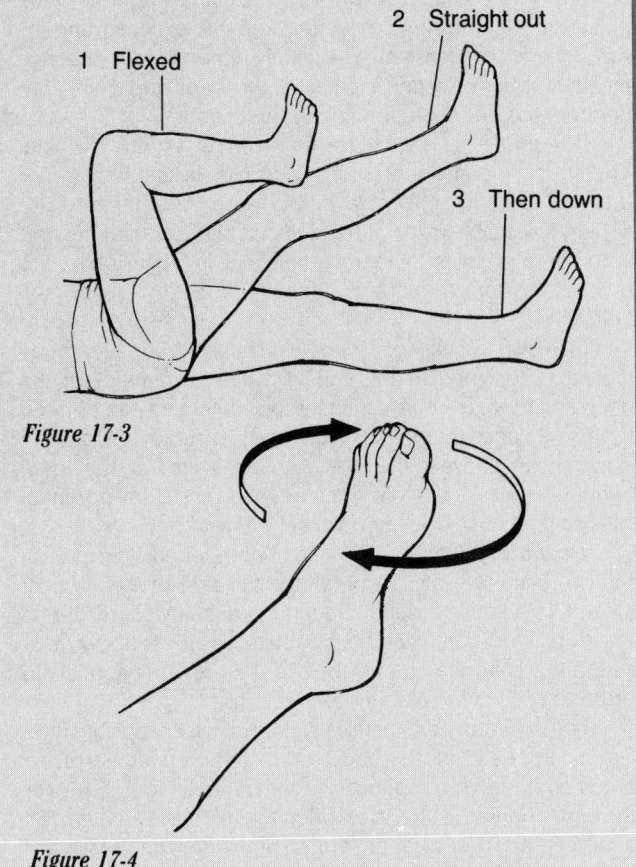

Figure 17-3

Figure 17-4

Intestinal Preparation

A warm cleansing enema or laxatives may be given the evening before an operation and may be repeated if ineffectual. This is to prevent defecation during anesthesia or to prevent accidental surgical trauma during abdominal surgery. Unless the condition of the patient presents some contraindication, the toilet, and not the bedpan, is used in evacuating the enema. In addition, antibiotics may be prescribed to reduce intestinal flora.

Preoperative Skin Preparation

When there is time, such as in surgery of a nonemergency nature, the patient may use a soap containing a detergent-germicide to cleanse the skin area for several days before surgery in order to reduce the number of skin organisms.

Prior to surgery, the patient should take a warm, relaxing bath or shower, using povidone-iodine (Betadine) soap. Although it is preferable that this be done on the day of surgery, the time schedule may require that the shower be taken the night before. The purpose for recommending that the cleansing shower be taken as close to surgery as possible is to reduce the risk of skin contamination of the surgical wound. A shampoo the day before the operation is advisable unless the condition of the patient does not make it feasible.

It is preferred that the skin at and around the operative site NOT be shaved. However, the use of a depilatory to remove skin hair is acceptable. If the hair on the skin is shaved, the skin may be injured by the razor and become a portal of entry for bacteria; this injured tissue may act as a substrate for bacterial growth. In addition, *the longer the interval between the shave and the operation, the higher the rate of postoperative wound infection.* Skin that is well cleansed but unshaven is less often implicated in wound infections than shaved skin. Some surgeons prefer that hair be removed in and around the operative site. One approach is to use electrical clippers to remove hair to within 1 mm to 2 mm of the skin; in this way, skin is not abraded.

If agency protocol or the surgeon requires that the skin be shaved, the patient is told about the shaving procedure, placed in a comfortable position, and not exposed unduly. Any adhesive or grease may be readily removed with a sponge moistened in benzene or ether, if the odor and cold temperature are not objectionable to the patient.

The *goal* is to remove the hair without injuring the skin. There are several options. One is to use an electric clipper that can be thoroughly cleaned after use. Another is to use a sharp disposable razor with a recessed blade. A third method is to use a scissors to remove hair that is 3 mm or longer in length. A fourth option is to use a depilatory cream (see below).

Skin shaving may be done by a special "prep" team, by the nurse assigned to the patient, or by a member of the operating room team. An antimicrobial detergent can be used to raise a lather that makes hair easier to remove. Hold the skin taut and shave in the direction of hair growth. Use long, continuous strokes. Avoid scratches and report any potential sites of infection. Document all actions and findings.

Depilatory Cream. Chemical compounds (creams to remove hair) are safe for preparing the skin of the surgical patient. If there is question about the possibility of an allergic reaction, a test patch can be tried first. As an economy measure, long hairs may be cut before the cream is applied in order to reduce the amount of cream used.

The depilatory cream usually comes in a collapsible tube and is expressed on the body surface. The cream is spread in a smooth layer of about 1.25 cm (½ inch) in depth over the entire operative site. A wooden tongue blade or a gloved hand can be used to apply the cream. After the cream has been allowed to remain on the skin for 10 minutes, it is scraped off gently with the tongue blade or multiple moistened gauze sponges. When all cream and hair have been removed, the skin is then washed with soap and water and patted dry.

There are several advantages in using a depilatory cream for preoperative skin preparation. The end result is a clean, smooth, and intact skin. Scrapes, abrasions, cuts, and inadequate hair removal are eliminated. It is more comfortable for the patient, since he is less apprehensive and often finds this method relaxing. There is even the possibility of the patient's preparing himself in selected operative procedures. Depilatory creams are more effective and safer for use on uncooperative or agitated patients. This method is no more expensive than other methods. A disadvantage is that a few patients have had some transient skin reactions if depilatory cream is used near the rectal and scrotal areas.

Immediate Preoperative Nursing Interventions

The nurse clothes the patient in the regulation short gown, leaving it untied and open in the back. If the patient has long hair it is plaited in two braids, any hairpins are removed, and the head and the hair are entirely covered with a disposable paper cap. The mouth must be inspected and dentures or plates, chewing gum, and so forth removed. If left in the mouth, these items could easily fall to the back of the throat during induction of anesthesia and cause respiratory obstruction.

Jewelry is not to be worn to the operating room; even wedding rings should be taken off. If a patient has any real objection to the removal of a ring, a narrow tape may be tied to the ring and then fastened securely around the patient's wrist. All articles of value, including dentures and prosthetic devices, are labeled clearly with the patient's name and stored in a safe place according to local agency policy.

When the gastrointestinal tract is to be operated on, a small prepackaged (Fleet's) enema may be requested until returns are clear. Otherwise, cathartics are often prescribed. Routine tap water enemas are usually not suggested because of the possibility of creating an electrolyte imbalance.

All patients (except those with urologic problems) should void immediately before going to the operating room to maintain continence during low abdominal surgery and to make abdominal organs more accessible. Catheterization should not be resorted to, except in an emergency or when it is desirable to have an indwelling catheter in place to ensure an empty bladder. In this instance, such a catheter would be connected to a closed drainage system. The urine voided is measured, and the amount and the time of voiding are recorded on the preoperative check slip.

Preanesthetic Medication: Pharmacokinetics

A complete drug history on every patient scheduled for surgery is imperative because of possible problems of drug interaction. The history should include all the medications the patient has been taking or has taken within the past 2 months. Note should be taken of drug hypersensitivity, drug dosage, and the conditions for which drugs were prescribed.

As with other management modalities, medication is prescribed on an individual basis to meet the needs of the particular patient.

Barbiturates/Tranquilizers. For sedation, barbiturates are commonly used—mainly pentobarbital (Nembutal) and secobarbital (Seconal Sodium)—as are hypnotics such as benzodiazepines (flurazepam, diazepam). However, it is worth noting that studies have shown that the reassuring visit of the anesthesiologist and operating room nurse prior to the operation has a more calming effect than the barbiturates. Nonetheless, the night before surgery a hypnotic is usually given to allay insomnia.

Opiates. Drugs such as morphine and meperidine (Demerol) may be prescribed before an operation to reduce the amount of general anesthetic required. These drugs can also be used to produce analgesia in patients who have pain before the operation. At the same time it is important to realize that analgesic doses may depress respiration and the cough reflex and present an increased risk of respiratory acidosis and aspiration pneumonitis. Full doses may cause hypotension, nausea, vomiting, constipation, and abdominal distention.

Anticholinergics. Anticholinergic drugs may be prescribed to reduce respiratory tract secretions and to prevent or treat severe reflex slowing of the heart during anesthesia. They are given also to counteract secretions that are anticipated with anesthetic induction and intubation. Atropine is frequently prescribed; however, it must be used with caution in patients with glaucoma, thyrotoxicosis, prostatic hyperplasia, or some forms of heart disease.

Because the belladonna alkaloids (atropine and scopolamine) have varying effects on pulse rate, as well as other shortcomings, a quaternary ammonium compound, glycopyrrolate (Robinul), is often used. It is an anticholinergic drug that is twice as potent an antisialogogue (reducing secretions) and acts three times as long.

Other Preanesthetic Drugs. Other drugs used as preanesthetic medication are droperidol, fentanyl, or a combination of these. They should not be used with sedatives since they may cause respiratory or circulatory depression and may potentiate depressants.

Prophylactic antibiotics are administered when bacterial contamination is expected, or for the patient with a clean wound where a prosthetic device is being inserted.

Timing of Administration of Drugs. Because preanesthetic medications should be given from 45 to 75 minutes before anesthesia is begun, it is most important that the nurse give this medication precisely at the prescribed time; otherwise, its effect will have worn off, or it will not have begun to act when anesthesia is started.

After the preanesthetic medication is given, the patient is kept in bed because he will begin to feel lightheaded and drowsy. (If the patient is unattended, the side rails are placed in position.) If he receives atropine or glycopyrrolate (Robinul), he may be told it will make his mouth dry. During this time, the nurse observes the patient for any untoward reaction to the medications. His environment is kept quiet to assist in relaxing him.

Very frequently, operations are delayed or schedules changed, and it becomes impossible to request that a medication be given at a specific time. In these situations the preoperative medication is prescribed "on call from operating room." Although this is far from ideal and should be avoided whenever possible, the nurse can help by having the medication ready to give and by administering it as soon as the patient is called for. It usually takes 15 to 20 minutes to get a patient ready for the operating room. If the nurse gives the medication before attending to the other details of preparing the patient, he will have at least partial benefit from the preoperative medication and will have a smoother and more pleasant anesthetic and operative course.

Preoperative Record

A preoperative check list is shown in Figure 17-5. The completed chart accompanies the patient to the operating room. The informed consent is also attached, as are all laboratory reports and nurses' records. Any unusual last-minute observations that may have a bearing on the anesthesia or surgery are to be put at the front of the chart in a prominent place.

Transportation to the Presurgical Suite

The patient is transferred to the holding area or presurgical suite in bed or on a previously prepared stretcher about 30 to 60 minutes before the anesthetic is to be given. The stretcher should be as comfortable as possible, with a suffi-

cient number of blankets to ensure against chilling from drafty corridors. A small pillow at the head is usually acceptable. The top covers of the stretcher should be long enough to tuck in around the patient at both feet and shoulders. Preferably, the nurse who has cared for the patient up to this time should accompany him to the operating room. An attendant always remains with the patient in the holding area until relieved by one of the anesthesiologists. The chart is given to the anesthesiologist or an operating room nurse; it never is left with the patient.

It is desirable to have the patient brought directly to a preoperative holding room or induction room, where he is greeted by name and made to feel that he is in safe hands. The area must be quiet if the preoperative medication is to have maximal effect. The patient should not hear undesirable sounds or conversations that might be misinterpreted or exaggerated.

It is important that someone be with the preoperative patient at all times. Even though he has had preoperative medication, appears to be dozing, and seems to be secure on the stretcher with a strap in place, he should not be left alone.

It is assumed that preoperative preparation has covered every contingency before the patient comes to the operating room. However, as the patient waits with eyes closed, he is often reviewing some personal thoughts; a question or concern about a particular thing may occur to him and may assume an exaggerated importance. Someone should be available to answer or attempt to find the answer to his question.

Reassurance is given not only verbally but also by facial expression, manner, and a touch or warm grasp of the hand. It is important for the patient to have the security of seeing a familiar face—the nurse who helped to prepare him before he was sent to the operating unit, or the anesthesiologist who visited with him the day before and discussed anesthetic management.

Helping the Family Cope

Most hospitals have a special waiting room where the family can wait while the patient is having surgery. This room may be equipped with comfortable chairs, television, telephones, and facilities for light refreshment. Volunteers may remain with the family, serve them coffee, boost their morale, and even keep them informed of the patient's progress. After surgery, the surgeon may meet the family here, join them for coffee, and report his findings.

The family never should judge the seriousness of an operation by the length of time the patient is in the operating room. He may be in surgery much longer than the actual operating time for several reasons:

- It is customary to send for the patient some time in advance of the actual operating time.
- Anesthesiologists often make additional preparations that may take from ½ to 1 hour.
- Occasionally the surgeon takes longer than expected with the preceding case, which delays the time of beginning the next operation.
- After surgery the patient is taken to the recovery room to ensure satisfactory emergence from the anesthetic.

PREOPERATIVE CHECK LIST

1. Patient's name: _____ Date: _____ Height: _____ Weight: _____
   Identification band present: _____

2. Informed Consent signed: _____ Special permits signed: _____
   (Ex: Sterilization)

3. History & Physical Examination report present: _____ Date: _____

4. Laboratory records present: _____
   CBC: _____ Hb: _____ Urinalysis: _____ Hct: _____

5. | Item | Present | Removed |
   |---|---|---|
   | a. Natural teeth | _____ | _____ |
   | Dentures: upper, lower, partial | _____ | _____ |
   | Bridge, fixed; crown | _____ | _____ |
   | b. Contact lenses | _____ | _____ |
   | c. Other prostheses—type: _____ | _____ | _____ |
   | d. Jewelry: | | |
   | Wedding band (taped/tied) | _____ | _____ |
   | Rings | _____ | _____ |
   | Earrings: pierced, clip-on | _____ | _____ |
   | Neck chains | _____ | _____ |
   | e. Make-up | _____ | _____ |
   | Nail polish | _____ | _____ |

6. Clothing
a. Clean patient gown	_____	_____
b. Cap	_____	_____
c. Sanitary pad, *etc.*	_____	_____

7. Family instructed where to wait? _____

8. Valuables secured? _____

9. Blood available? _____ Ordered? _____ Where? _____

10. Preanesthetic medication given: _____ _____
                                 Signature   Time

11. Voided: _____ Amount: _____ Time: _____ Catheter: _____
    Mouth care given: _____

12. Vital signs: Temperature: _____ Pulse: _____ Resp: _____ Blood Press: _____

13. Special problems/precautions: (Allergies, deafness, *etc.*): _____

14. Area of skin preparation: _____

15. _____ Date: _____ Time: _____
         Signature: Nurse releasing patient

Figure 17-5
Preoperative check list.

Those waiting to see the patient after the operation should be forewarned that the patient may be returned to his room with a variety of equipment in place, including blood transfusion lines, suction bottles, nasal tube, airway and oxygen lines, tracheostomy tube, monitoring equipment, and the like. Family members need to know how they can support the patient preoperatively and in the recovery room. If the prognosis for the patient is more negative than positive, it is not the prerogative of the nurse to relay this information to the family, even when the odds appear in the patient's favor.

Bibliography

See Bibliography at end of Chapter 19.

Intraoperative Nursing and Anesthesia

The center of attention and activity in the operating room is the patient who is undergoing a surgical procedure for the repair, correction, or relief of a physical problem. The immediate concern from the time the patient arrives in the operating room through the period when the anesthesia is being administered is the psychological reactions of the patient.

Throughout the surgical experience, the nurse functions as the patient's chief advocate. The "caring" and concern of nursing management extends from the time when the patient is prepared for and instructed about the forthcoming operation, through the immediate preoperative period, into the operative phase and the recovery from anesthesia, and on through convalescence. Throughout this continuum, *priority is given to the patient, his safety, his understanding of the care he is receiving, and the biophysical and psychosocial needs he is experiencing.* Because the operation is usually a unique experience in the patient's life, he needs the security of knowing that someone is protecting his best interests at this time, especially when he is unable to make decisions for himself.

A preoperative visit the day before (or the day of) surgery by the operating room nurse as well as the anesthesiologist has been documented as effective in smoothing the transition of the patient from the hospital unit to the operating room. Time is provided for the patient to become acquainted with what he will experience in the operating room; he is encouraged to ask questions. Later, meeting "familiar faces" when he is transported to the OR provides another psychological comfort.

When a patient arrives in the operating room, essentially three different groups are preparing for his care: (1) the anesthesiologist and those assistants who administer the anesthetic agent and place the patient in the proper position on the operating table; (2) the surgeon and those assistants who scrub and perform the operation; and (3) the intraoperative nurses who manage the operating room, are responsible for the safety and well-being of the patient, coordinate the many activities of the operating personnel, and also provide care by performing "scrub nurse" and circulating activities during the operation.

A recent addition has been made to the personnel of the operating room. *RN First Assistant (RNFA)* is a recently created role that has been approved by the Association of Operating Room Nurses. This role has been endorsed by the American College of Surgeons, and the approval of all State Boards of Nurse Examiners is being sought. The RNFA practices under the direct supervision of the surgeon; responsibilities may include tissue handling, providing exposure at the operative field, using instruments, suturing, and providing hemostasis. Specific requirements must be met to qualify for this expanded role.

During the course of the operation, information about the patient must be shared by the anesthesiologist, the nurse, and the surgeon, in order to assure optimum patient care. In addition, any pertinent developments, such as undue hemorrhage, unexpected findings, fluid and electrolyte problems, shock, or respiratory difficulties, that are related to patient care in the recovery room must be noted and documented.

Intraoperative Nursing Functions

Frequently, nursing functions in the operating room are described in terms of "circulating" and "scrub" activities.

The *circulating nurse* manages the operating room and protects the safety and health needs of the patient by controlling the activities and state of the environment and ensuring cleanliness, proper temperature, humidity, and lighting, safety of equipment, and availability of supplies and materials. It is also the responsibility of the circulating nurse to observe and check the patient throughout the operative procedure to ensure that his needs are provided for and his rights upheld. It is necessary also to coordinate the activities of related personnel (laboratory, x-ray, medical, and so on) and to monitor aseptic practices in order to avoid breakdowns in technique.

Scrub activities include "scrubbing" for the operation (see Charts 18-1 through 18-4); setting up the sterile tables; preparing sutures, ligatures, and special equipment; assisting the surgeon and the surgical assistants during the operation by anticipating the required instruments, sponges, drains, and other equipment; and keeping to a minimum the time the patient is under anesthesia and the time the wound is open. Toward the end of the operation, equipment and materials must be checked to ensure that all needles, sponges, and instruments are accounted for. In addition, specimens must be labeled and sent to the laboratory. The entire process requires a thorough understanding of the principles of asepsis, anatomy, and tissue care; an awareness of the objectives of the surgery; the knowledge and skill to anticipate needs and work as a skilled member of a team; and the ability to handle any emergency situation in the operating room.

Principles of Health and Operating Room Attire

Good health is essential for any person in the operating room. Colds, sore throats, and infected fingers are sources of pathogenic organisms and must be reported. A series of wound infections in postoperative patients was traced in one instance to a mild throat infection in an operating room nurse. Therefore, the importance of reporting any seemingly slight ailment without delay can be readily understood.

Clothing.   Street clothes are never worn in the operating room. Only approved, clean, operating room attire is permitted. Likewise, OR attire is not worn out of the operating room. Written policies describe the practice that all persons are required to follow. Dressing rooms are located near the operating suite and are reached from an outer corridor. Clothing is changed in the dressing room before entering and upon leaving the operating room.

Close-fitting cotton dresses, pants suits, and jumpsuits are available in a variety of styles. When pants are worn, the ankles should have close-fitting cuffs (drawstring or knitted) to contain organisms shed from the perineum and legs. Shirts and waist drawstrings should be tucked inside the pants to prevent any accidental contact with sterile areas and again to contain skin sheddings. Garments that are visibly wet or soiled should be changed. Fresh OR attire is put on each time the person enters the operating room; when this clothing is removed, it is bagged and sent to the laundry.

Mask.   Masks are worn at all times in the operating room for the purpose of minimizing airborne contamination. Droplets containing microorganisms from the oropharynx and nasopharynx must be contained and filtered. Therefore, the mask must not leak air and should cover the nose and mouth completely. At the same time, it should not interfere with breathing, speech, or vision, and must be compact and comfortable. Forced expiration, such as that produced by talking, laughing, sneezing, and coughing, should be avoided, since it deposits additional organisms on the mask. Many effective disposable masks are available that have high filtration efficiency: 95+%. Tests prove their superiority over gauze masks. Masks are changed at a minimum between patients and are not to be worn outside the surgery department.

Since the mask loses much of its effectiveness when it becomes moistened, it is changed between operations and more often if necessary. The mask is either on or off; it must not be allowed to hang around the neck. When the mask is removed, only the strings are handled in order to prevent contamination of the hands. Mask strings are tied snugly; top strings are tied at the back of the head, and bottom strings are tied at the back of the neck.

Headgear.   Headgear should completely cover the hair (head and neckline including beard), so that single strands of hair, bobbypins, clips, or particles of dandruff or dust do not fall on sterile fields. The styles of headgear available are disposable, lint-free, and clothlike.

Shoes.   Shoes should be comfortable and supportive; clogs, tennis shoes, sandals, and boots are not permitted because they are unsafe and difficult to clean. Shoes are covered with disposable or canvas shoe covers. Conductive covers establish an electrical ground for the wearer. The black strips provided with some conductive shoe covers should be placed inside the shoe in contact with the sole of the foot. Shoe covers are worn one time only and are removed upon leaving the restricted area. Conductometers are usually located at the entrance to the operating room area.

Principles of Perioperative Asepsis

As indicated earlier, in all phases of the surgical experience the main priority for all personnel is prevention of patient

Chart 18-1
Guidelines: "Scrubbing" for an Operation

Action	*Rationale*
1. The nails are kept short and free of nail polish; special attention is given to the subungual space (beneath nail) with a sterile nail cleaner early in the scrub.	1. Scrubbing can cause nail polish to chip and peel; this would produce nicks in which microbes could breed.
2. A soft but firm-bristled brush or one of the numerous polyurethane disposable sponges that are impregnated with soap is used for scrubbing.	2. The brush or special sponge facilitates removal of dead skin, soil, and resident organisms.
3. There are many acceptable antiseptic detergents, such as the iodophors.	3. Broad-spectrum antimicrobial solution is preferred where gram-negative nosocomial infections predominate.
4. Hands and arms must be well lathered and rinsed frequently. No chemical agent can be relied upon as a substitute for conscientious mechanical cleansing of the skin.	4. Microbes are removed by two actions: a. Physical mechanical separation b. Chemical antisepsis from action of antimicrobial solution
5. The duration of the scrub may be determined by setting a time limit for the conscientious scrubbing of one part after another in a prescribed manner, or by counting a certain number of strokes per part. A practical, reliable, and effective procedure should be followed. Because the moisture and warmth present under surgical gloves provide an ideal growing medium for bacteria, it is essential that a prescribed scrub be done between operations.	5. Individual conscientious attention to detail is important. Agency policy is followed.
6. Following the scrub, hands and arms are rinsed thoroughly; soap and brush are left in sink or discarded in appropriate container. The elbow or the knee is used to turn the water off. Hands are held higher than the elbows and away from the body.	6. Holding hands higher than the elbows and away from the body allows water to run off at the elbow and prevents contaminated water (from above the elbow) from running down to the scrubbed hands.
7. When drying hands, care is taken to prevent the towel from touching the scrub dress or suit. One hand and then the arm are dried with a towel, proceeding from fingertips to elbow; the other hand and arm are dried in similar fashion using a dry segment of the towel.	7. Proceeding from the fingertips to the elbow will prevent above-elbow sources of contamination from affecting scrubbed hands and lower arms.

(With advancing technology, an automatic hand washing system has been developed that uses a nonabsorbent, nonirritating system of pressurized water, air, and surfactant at sufficient pressure to remove bacteria from the skin in a matter of seconds without antiseptics or scrubbing. Scientific Growth, Inc, Phoenix, Arizona)

complications, which includes protection of the patient from infection. Inherent in this goal is strict adherence to the principles of asepsis.

The successful practice of aseptic surgery requires the strict observance of rigorous standards for *preoperative* sterilization of surgical materials and of precautions against infection, both *during* the course of the operation and *after* the operation, when the wound must be guarded until such time as it is healed.

To provide the best possible conditions for performing a surgical operation, the operating room is placed in a section of the hospital where it is free from such hazards as contaminating particles, dust, other pollutants, radiation, and noise. Strict building codes must be set and adhered to in the selection of materials for construction and in determining room size and air circulation patterns. Electrical hazards, conductivity checks, emergency exit clearances, and storage of equipment and anesthetic gases are checked periodically by

the state and the Joint Commission for the Accreditation of Hospitals.

In surgical practice, asepsis prevents the contamination of surgical wounds. Although postoperative wound infection may be caused by natural skin flora or a previously existing infection, it is the responsibility of the personnel in the operating room to use aseptic principles to minimize this risk. These principles are described and illustrated in detail in the pages that follow, in terms of the various protocols and practices to be carried out.

Protocols

Preoperative

Prior to the operation, all surgical material must be sterilized; this includes any instruments, needles, sutures, dressings,

(Text continues on p. 325)

Chart 18-2
Gowning

After the hands and arms are scrubbed using an antiseptic detergent, a sterile gown and gloves are put on. These are worn to allow the wearer to participate in or observe the surgical operation while maintaining a state of asepsis in as practical a way as possible.

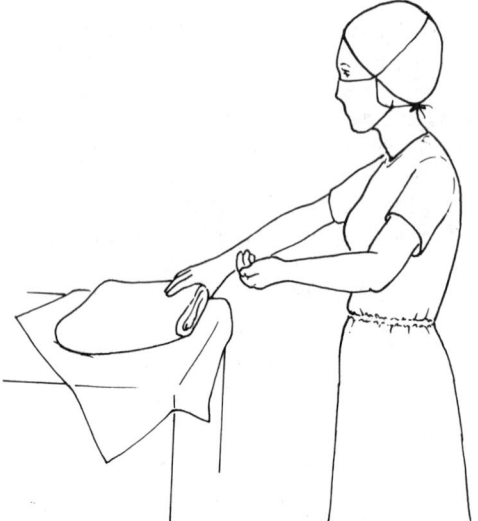

1. The sterile gown may be obtained from an open pack, or it may be handed by someone already scrubbed.

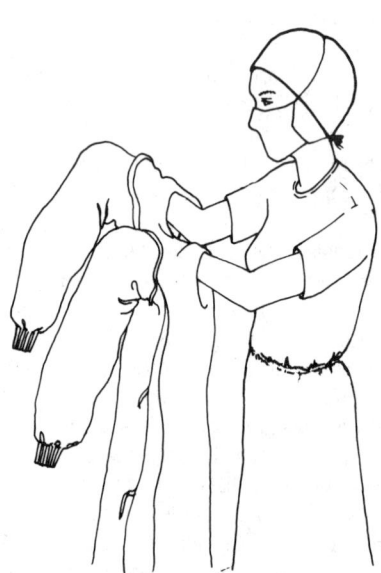

2. Since gowns are folded inside out (to eliminate the need to touch the outside of the garment), the gown can be held by the neckband and allowed to unfold from the extended hands. As the gown unfolds, the armholes should face the wearer. The hands are held upward and slipped into the armholes—but only as far as the sleeve cuff.

3. The circulating nurse can assist by reaching inside the gown and pulling the sleeves over the hands. (Sleeves are pulled to the hands, not over them, when the "closed glove technique" is to be used. See page 323.)

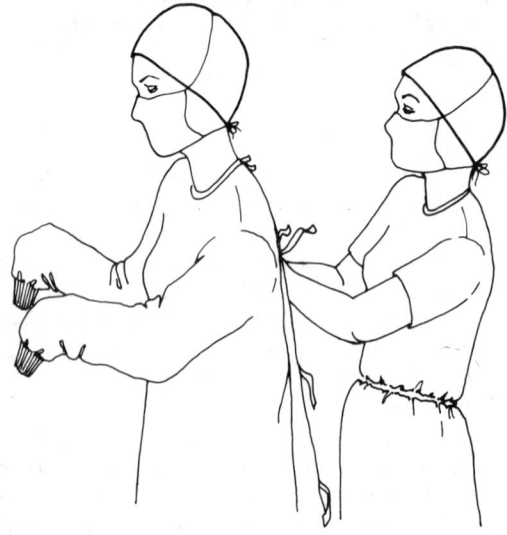

4. To secure the gown, the tapes at the back are tied. If the gown has tapes at the waist, the circulating nurse reaches for the ends of the tapes without touching the gown, draws the tapes back, and ties them. (Gowns may be fastened with Velcro, which eliminates the need for tapes.)

Note: A gown is sterile only as long as it is dry and not torn. If it is wet from perspiration or from any other cause, if must be considered contaminated.

Chart 18-3
Putting on Sterile Gloves: Closed Method

When the gown is donned, the hands are slid into the sleeve only as far as the cuff seam, which is then grasped by the thumb and index finger through the fabric.

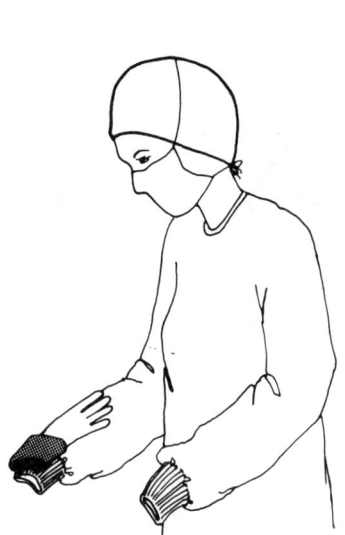

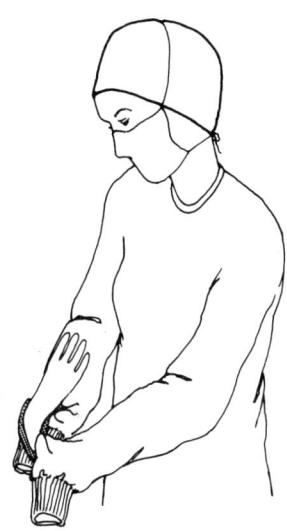

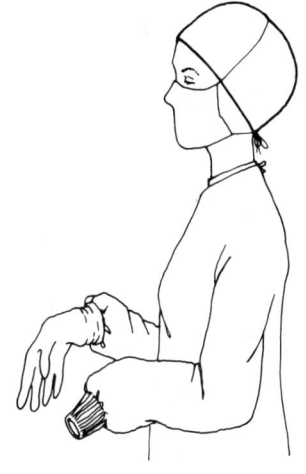

1. One glove is grasped (while the hand is still inside the sleeve) and placed thumbside down on the palmside of the other arm, with glove fingers pointing toward the shoulder. (Glove cuff lies over gown cuff.)*

2. The wrist edge of the glove that is against the sleeve is grasped with the finger that holds the seam, and the uppermost glove wrist edge is grasped with the sleeve-covered fingers of the other hand.

3. The glove wrist is pulled over the gown cuff, care being taken not to fold the gown cuff back or to expose the fingers inside it.

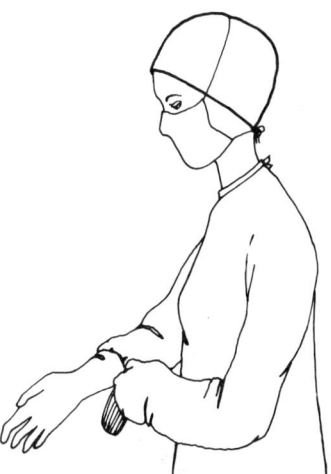

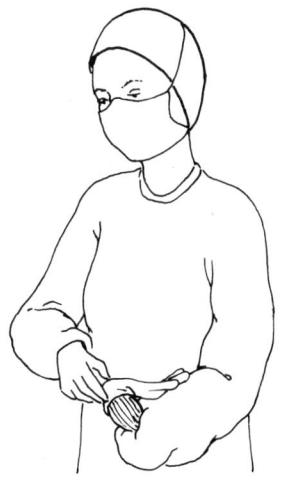

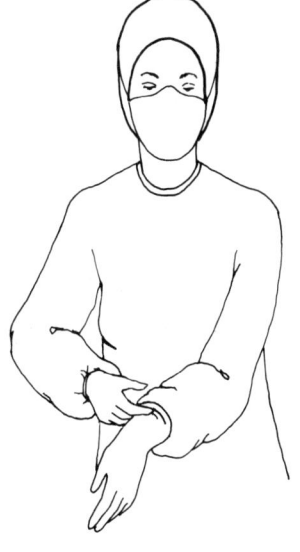

4. As cuff is drawn onto the wrist, the fingers are directed into cots in the glove, and the glove is adjusted to the hand.

5. The second glove is put on in the same manner, using the newly gloved hand to hold the glove.

* Shaded or crosshatched areas of the glove (representing the inside of glove) are considered unsterile.

Chart 18-4
Putting on Sterile Gloves: Open Method

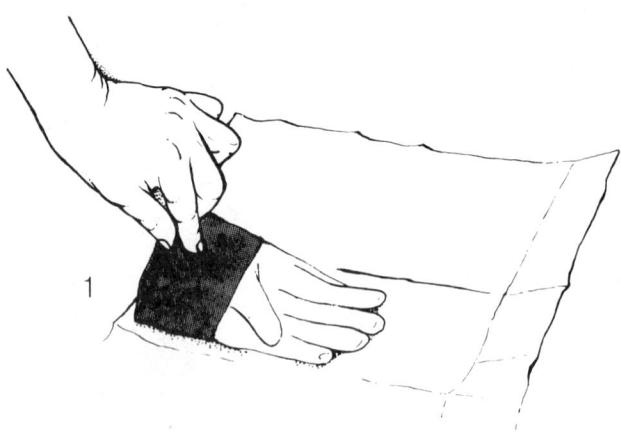

1. When the right glove is put on first, the cuff is grasped on the inside by the left hand.

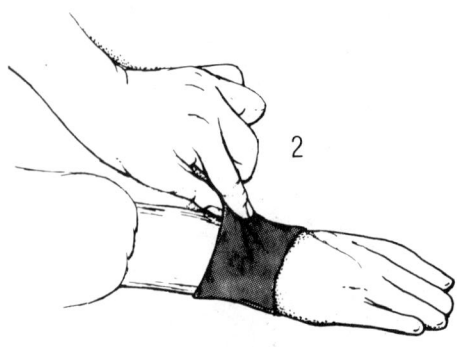

2. The right hand is inserted into the glove, which is then pulled into place with the left hand (the cuff is left in a turned-down position). The grasp is then released.

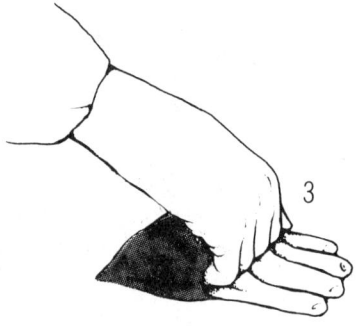

3. Now the right gloved hand can pick up the left glove by inserting the fingers under its cuff. (The outside is the sterile side.)

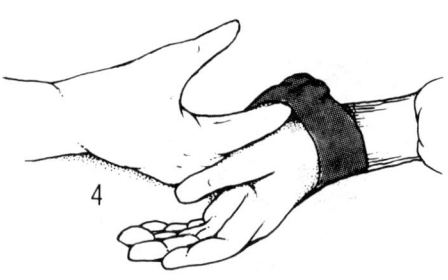

4. The left hand is inserted into the left glove and the glove is pulled into place. The cuff is left in a turned-down position.

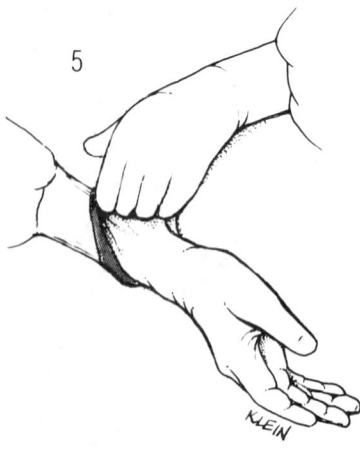

5. After folding the gown cuff snugly to the wrist, and while holding this fold in place with the sterile right gloved thumb, the fingers can safely pull the sterile glove cuff over the gown cuff.

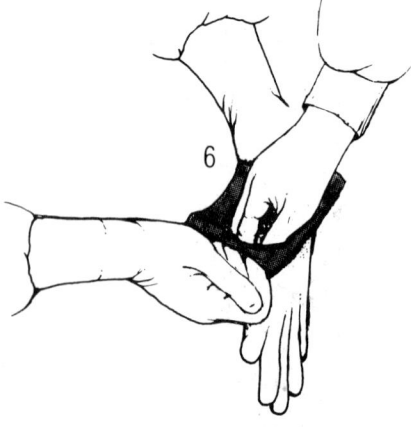

Another method: The scrub nurse holds the glove open for the person donning the gloves. The glove is held with the thumb facing the recipient. The top of the glove is spread wide so that the hand can be thrust into the glove without touching the person holding the glove. The glove cuff is pulled up over the gown cuff.

gloves, covers, and the like that may come in contact with the wound and exposed tissues. In addition, the surgeon, surgical assistants, and nurses must prepare themselves by scrubbing their hands and arms with soap and water ("scrubbing") and donning long-sleeved, sterile gowns and gloves. Head and hair are covered with a cap, and a mask is worn over the nose and mouth to minimize the possibility of bacteria from the upper respiratory tract entering the wound. The patient's skin, over an area considerably larger than that requiring exposure during the course of the operation, also requires meticulous cleansing followed by the application of an antiseptic agent. The rest of the patient's body is covered with sterile drapes.

Intraoperative

During the operation, none of the personnel who have scrubbed touches anything that has not been sterilized. Nonscrubbed personnel refrain from touching or contaminating anything that is sterile.

Postoperative

After the operation, the wound is protected from possible contamination by means of sterile dressings and by the use of sterile saline and antiseptics when the wound is cleansed and the dressings changed. Particular care is taken to protect the unhealed wound from coming in contact with anything that is not sterile. In wounds that become infected, it may be necessary to remove and destroy microorganisms that are already in the tissues by removing or "débriding" devitalized tissues. To prevent subsequent infection from without, rigid aseptic technique must be followed during the course of treatment.

When infection has already developed in tissues, antimicrobials specific for the offending organism are prescribed, and heat is applied or drainage established to assist the body in eliminating the offending organisms.

Environmental Controls

In addition to the above protocols, the implementation of aseptic principles requires meticulous housekeeping in the operating room. Floors and horizontal surfaces are cleaned frequently with detergent soap and water or detergent germicide, and sterilizing equipment is inspected regularly to assure optimum operation and performance. Prepackaged sterilized linens, drapes, and solutions are used; instruments are cleaned and sterilized in a unit close to the operating room. Peel-apart, individually wrapped sterile items are used when additional individual items are needed.

Many operating rooms are equipped with laminar air flow systems that filter out a high percentage of dust and bacteria. Originally designed for spacecraft, these systems use high-efficiency particulate air (HEPA) filters to remove more than 99% of airborne particles measuring 0.3 microns or more. Laminar flow also changes air more effectively—about 200 times an hour, as compared with air conditioning, which exchanges air 12 times per hour.

Unfortunately, in spite of all these precautions, postoperative wound infections may occasionally occur during an operation, appearing days or weeks later in the form of an incisional infection or abscess.

- Constant surveillance and conscientiousness in carrying out aseptic practices must be stressed continually, because errors and misjudgments can occur as a result of human failure.

Basic Rules of Surgical Asepsis

General
- Sterile surfaces or articles may touch other sterile surfaces or articles and remain sterile; unsterile contact at any point renders a sterile area contaminated.
- If there is any doubt about the sterility of an article or area, it is considered unsterile.
- Whatever is sterile for one patient (an opened sterile tray or tables with sterile supplies) can be used for this patient only. Unused sterile supplies must be discarded or resterilized if they are to be used again.

Personnel
- Scrubbed personnel remain in the area of the operation; if a scrubbed person leaves the room, that person's sterile status is lost. To return to the operation, this person is required to go through the procedure of scrubbing, gowning, and gloving.
- Only a small part of a scrubbed person's body is considered sterile: from front waist to the shoulder area; forearms and gloves. Therefore, the gloved hands must be kept in front and above the waistline.
- In some clinics, a special wraparound gown is worn, which extends the sterile area.
- The "circulator" and any unscrubbed personnel remain on the periphery of the surgical operating area at a safe distance in order not to contaminate any sterile area.

Draping
- During draping of a table or patient, the sterile drape is held well above the surface to be covered and is positioned from front to back.
- Only the top of the patient or table that is draped is considered sterile; drapes hanging over the edge are not regarded as sterile.
- Sterile drapes are to be kept in position by the use of clips or adherent material; drapes are not to be moved during the operation. A tear or puncture of the drape permitting access to an unsterile surface underneath renders the area unsterile. Such a drape must be replaced.

Delivery of Sterile Supplies
- Packages are wrapped or sealed in such a way that they can be opened easily without risk of contaminating contents.
- Sterile supplies, including solutions, are delivered to a sterile field or handed to a "scrubbed" person in such a way that sterility of the object or fluid remains intact.
- Edges of wrappers covering sterile supplies or outer lips of bottles or flasks containing sterile solutions are not considered sterile.
- The unsterile arm of the "circulator" must not extend over a sterile area. Sterile articles are to be dropped at a reasonable distance from the edge of the sterile area.

Fluids

- Sterile fluids are poured from a point high enough to prevent accidental touching of the sterile receiving cup or basin, but not so high as to produce splashing (this may cause fluid to touch an unsterile surface and then flow back into the receptacle, causing contamination).

The Patient Undergoing Anesthesia

The Patient and the Anesthesiologist

An *anesthesiologist* is specifically trained in the art and the science of anesthesiology. After consulting with the surgeon, he usually selects the anesthesia and deals with any technical problems relating to the administration of the anesthetic agent and supervision of the patient's condition during the operation.

An *anesthetist* is a qualified nurse, dentist, physician, or anesthesia assistant who administers anesthetics. The majority of anesthetists are nurses who have graduated from an accredited nurse anesthesia program and have passed certification by the American Association of Nurse Anesthetists to become certified registered nurse anesthetists (CRNA).

The surgical patient usually is interested in and concerned about the anesthesia that he is to receive. He has heard friends or relatives discuss the subject on the basis of personal experience or hearsay, and not infrequently has formed opinions as to the merits or demerits of various methods in use. Therefore, it is helpful for the anesthesiologist to visit the patient in his room before the operation and to point out that the purpose of the visit is to allay any fears that may exist in the patient's mind. Choice of anesthetic agent is discussed and the patient has an opportunity to disclose idiosyncrasies as well as medications he is currently taking that may affect the choice of an agent (see p. 311).

During this essential visit, the anesthesiologist determines the condition of the patient's cardiovascular system and lungs and inquires about any preexisting pulmonary infections and the extent to which the patient smokes. The patient's general physical condition must also be ascertained because it may affect the management of anesthesia (Table.18-1).

The preoperative visit from the anesthesiologist and the surgical (OR) nurse builds confidence and enables the patient to recognize a familiar face as he is being wheeled into the operating suite. Uncertainty and anxiety are relieved to a certain degree, and a smoother course can be anticipated.

In the anesthetizing room the patient is transferred to the operating table and a last-minute check of his condition is made; blood pressure, pulse, and respiratory rates in particular are noted. Induction of the anesthetic is usually done in the operating room.

During the course of surgery, the anesthesiologist monitors the patient's blood pressure, pulse, and respirations as well as the electrocardiogram, tidal volume, blood gas levels, blood pH, alveolar gas concentrations, and body temperature. Monitoring by electroencephalograph may be required in some instances. Anesthetic levels in the body can also be determined; a mass spectrometer is able to provide instant readouts of the critical concentration levels on strategically located display terminals.

After surgery when the patient is recovering from the anesthetic, the mass spectrometer can reveal the concentration of gaseous anesthetic still remaining in the patient. When he breathes on his own, the device assesses his ability to

TABLE 18-1
Classification of Physical Status for Anesthesia Prior to Surgery

Classification	Description	Example
1. Good	No organic disease, no systemic disturbance	Uncomplicated hernias, fractures
2. Fair	Mild to moderate systemic disturbance	Mild cardiac (I and II), mild diabetes
3. Poor	Severe systemic disturbance	Poorly controlled diabetes, pulmonary complications, moderate cardiac (III)
4. Serious	Systemic disease threatening life	Severe renal disease, severe cardiac disease (IV), decompensation
5. Moribund	Little chance of survival but submitting to operation in desperation	Massive pulmonary embolus, ruptured abdominal aneurysm with profound shock
E. Emergency	Any of the above when surgery is done in an emergency situation	Hitherto uncomplicated hernia that is now strangulated and associated with nausea and vomiting; designation 1(E) If classification is 3 and an emergency the designation is 3(E)

(American Society of Anesthesiology, Inc. Codes for the Collection and Tabulation of Data Relating to Anesthesia, Inhalation Therapy and Therapeutic Diagnostic Blocks.)

breathe unassisted and indicates the need for mechanical assistance.

Gerontological Considerations

Elderly patients face higher risks from anesthesia and surgery than younger persons. However, with new research findings potential hazards are lowered. Increasing numbers of older patients are being operated on, and certain findings are becoming obvious. An older person *needs less* anesthetic agent to produce anesthesia, and it *takes longer* to eliminate anesthetic drugs. One reason this is true is that as people age the amount of fatty tissue steadily increases, from about 20%–30% at age 20 to 35%–45% at ages 60–70. Those anesthetic agents that have an affinity for fatty tissue will concentrate in body fat and the brain.

In addition, there is a shrinkage of body tissues that are made up predominantly of water and those with a very rich blood supply, such as skeletal muscle, liver, and kidney. Reduction in size of the liver means that the rate at which it can inactivate many anesthetics slows down.

With aging, the heart and blood vessels decrease in their ability to respond to stress. Brain cells are reduced. The function of kidney cells is decreased, which means that waste products and anesthetics are not excreted as readily as in a younger person.

Excessive or over-rapid infusions may cause pulmonary edema. Blood pressure that takes a sudden or prolonged drop may lead to circulatory insufficiency, which in turn may cause cerebral ischemia, thrombosis, embolism, infarction, and anoxemia. Consequently, continuous and careful monitoring with rapid interventions when needed are essential for those in the older age group.

Types of Anesthesia

Anesthesia is a state of narcosis, analgesia, relaxation, and reflex loss. Inhalation anesthesia is the most popular because of its controllability. The intake and elimination of the agent is in large measure affected by pulmonary ventilation. Greater depth or plane of anesthesia requires greater concentration of the agent and vice versa.

Anesthetics are divided into two classes according to whether they suspend sensation (1) in the whole body (general anesthesia) or (2) in parts of the body (local, regional, epidural, or spinal anesthesia).

General anesthesia can be obtained by inhalation or by intravenous or rectal techniques.

Volatile liquid anesthetics produce anesthesia when their vapors are inhaled. Included in this group are halothane, enflurane, and isoflurane. All are given with oxygen, and usually with nitrous oxide as well (Table 18-2).

Gas anesthetics are administered by inhalation, always in combination with oxygen. This group of anesthetics includes nitrous oxide (Table 18-3).

The substances, when inhaled, enter the blood through the pulmonary capillaries and, when in sufficient concentration, act on the cerebral centers to produce loss of consciousness and of sensation. When administration of the anesthetic is discontinued, the vapor or gas is eliminated by way of the lungs.

Physiologic and Physical Factors

General anesthetics produce anesthesia because they are delivered to the brain at high partial pressure. Relatively large amounts of anesthetic must be given during induction and the early maintenance phases because the anesthetic is recirculated and deposited in body tissues. As these depots become saturated, smaller amounts of the anesthetic agent are required to maintain anesthesia because equilibrium or near equilibrium has been achieved between brain, blood, and other tissues. It is apparent that anything that diminishes peripheral blood flow, such as vasoconstriction or a condition of shock, may cause only small amounts of anesthetic to be required. Conversely, when peripheral blood flow is unusually high, as in the muscularly active or apprehensive patient, the brain receives a smaller quantity of anesthetic, with the result that induction is slower and larger than usual quantities of anesthetic are required.

Methods of Administration. Liquid anesthetics may be giving by mixing the vapors with oxygen or nitrous oxide–oxygen and then having the patient inhale the mixture. The vapor is conducted to the patient by a tube and a mask.

The endotracheal technique for administering anesthetics consists of introducing a soft rubber or plastic tube into the trachea by means of a flexible fiberoptic endoscope, either by exposing the larynx with a laryngoscope or by passing the tube "blindly." It may be inserted through either nose or mouth (Fig. 18-1, p. 330). When in place, the breathing tube seals the lungs off from the esophagoscope, so if a patient vomits, none of the stomach contents enter the lungs.

Stages of Inhalation Anesthesia

Anesthesia generally is described as consisting of four stages, each of which presents a definite group of signs and symptoms. These stages are usually seen best when ether is the anesthetic used. When narcotics and neuromuscular blockers (relaxants) are given, several of the stages are absent.

Stage I: Beginning Anesthesia. As the patient breathes in the anesthetic mixture, a feeling of warmth steals over his body, dizziness occurs, and a feeling of detachment develops. He experiences a ringing, roaring, or buzzing in the ears and, though still conscious, is aware that he is unable to move his extremities easily. During this stage noises are exaggerated; even low voices or minor sounds appear distressingly loud and unreal. For this reason, unnecessary noise or motion must be prevented when anesthesia is started.

Stage II: Excitement. The excitement stage—characterized variously by struggling, shouting, talking, singing, laughing, or even crying—frequently may be avoided by judicious suggestion before anesthesia is begun and by the smooth and rapid administration of the anesthetic. The pupils become dilated but contract if exposed to light; the pulse rate is rapid and respiration irregular.

Because of the uncontrolled movements of the patient during this stage, the anesthesiologist always should be attended by someone ready to help restrain the patient. A strap is in place across the thighs of the patient, and the hands are

TABLE 18-2
Volatile Liquids as Agents of General Anesthesia

Agent	Administration	Advantages	Disadvantages	Implications
Diethyl ether	Open-drop; inhalation	Excellent relaxant Wide margin of safety Inexpensive Relatively nontoxic Used for all types of surgery	Explosive Slow induction: 10 minutes Long recovery; not eliminated for approximately 8 hours Irritating to skin, eyes May cause metabolic acidosis Causes nausea and vomiting Flammable	Protect eyes by keeping them closed. Expect nausea and vomiting—turn head to side to prevent aspiration of vomitus. Practice safeguards in view of flammability.
Halothane (Fluothane)	Inhalation; special vaporizer	Not explosive or flammable Induction rapid and smooth Useful in almost every type of surgery Low incidence of postoperative nausea and vomiting	Requires skillful administration to prevent overdosage May cause liver damage May produce hypotension Requires special vaporizer for administration	In addition to observation of pulse and respiration postoperatively, it is important that blood pressure be determined frequently.
Methoxyflurane (Penthrane)	Inhalation; special vaporizer	Nonflammable Seldom causes postoperative nausea and vomiting Analgesic action continues several hours after surgery Excellent muscle relaxation	Requires skillful administration Renal damage may occur Unpleasant odor	Prolonged postoperative depressant action calls for careful observation by recovery room personnel.
Enflurane (Ethrane)	Inhalation	Rapid induction and recovery Potent analgesic Nonflammable and nonexplosive	Respiratory depression may develop rapidly along with EEG abnormalities Not compatible with epinephrine	Observe for possible respiratory depression. Administration with epinephrine may cause ventricular fibrillation.
Isoflurane (Forane)	Inhalation	Rapid induction and recovery Muscle relaxants are markedly potentiated	This is a profound respiratory depressant.	Respiration must be monitored closely and supported when necessary.

fixed to an intravenous armboard. Also, the patient lies on a conduction strap for the purpose of avoiding burns during use of diathermy, ECG leads, and the like. The patient should not be touched except for purposes of restraint, and under no circumstances should there be palpation of the operative site.

Stage III: Surgical Anesthesia. Surgical anesthesia is reached by continued administration of the vapor or gas. The patient is unconscious, lying quietly on the table. The pupils are small but retain contractile power on exposure to light. Respiration is regular, pulse rate is about normal and of good volume, and the skin is pink or slightly flushed. By proper administration of the anesthetic, this stage may be maintained for hours in one of several planes (1, 2, 3, 4), depending upon the depth of anesthesia needed.

Stage IV: Danger. The danger stage is reached when too much anesthesia has been given. Respiration becomes shallow, the pulse weak and thready; the pupils become widely dilated and no longer contract when exposed to light.

Cyanosis develops and, unless prompt action is taken, death follows rapidly. If this stage should develop, the anesthetic is discontinued immediately and artificial respiration is given. Stimulants, although rarely used, may be administered for circulation if an overdosage of anesthetic has been given. Narcotic antagonists can be used if these agents are at fault.

During smooth administration of an anesthetic there is, of course, no sharp division between the various stages. The patient passes gradually from one stage to another, and it is only by close observation of the signs exhibited by the patient that an anesthesiologist can control the situation. The condition of the pupils, the blood pressure, and the respiratory and cardiac rates are probably the most reliable guides to the patient's condition.

Other Physiologic Changes

The administration of an anesthetic is attended by other physiologic activities that have not been mentioned. A few

TABLE 18-3
Gases as Agents of General Anesthesia

Agent	Administration	Advantages	Disadvantages	Implications
Nitrous oxide (N_2O)	Inhalation (semiclosed method)	Induction and recovery rapid Nonflammable Useful with oxygen for short procedures Useful with other agents for all types of surgery	Poor relaxant Weak anesthetic May produce hypoxia	Most useful in conjunction with other agents. Observe precautions with "other agents."
Cyclopropane (C_3H_6)	Inhalation (closed method)	Good relaxant Useful for all types of surgery Rapid induction and emergence Wide margin of safety Pleasant	Explosive Powerful depressant; therefore should be administered skillfully Frequently produces disturbances in heart rhythm May cause bronchospasm and acidosis	Employ precautions against explosions. Because cyclopropane may be followed by hypotension, it is important to observe blood pressure postoperatively.

anesthetics may produce hypersecretion of mucus and saliva. This may be minimized by the preoperative administration of atropine. Vomiting or regurgitation may occur, especially when the patient comes to the operating room with a full stomach. If gagging occurs, the patient's head is turned to the side, the head of the table is lowered, and a basin is provided to collect the vomitus. Suction apparatus is always available.

During anesthesia the patient's temperature may fall, and therefore every precaution must be taken against chilling. Warm, cotton blankets should be available (see Hypothermia). Glucose metabolism is much reduced, and as a result acidosis may develop.

In addition to the dangers of the anesthetic itself, the anesthesiologist must guard against asphyxia. This may be caused by foreign bodies in the mouth, spasm of the vocal cords, relaxing of the tongue, or aspiration of vomitus, saliva, or blood. These complications are avoided by the use of an endotracheal tube with an inflated cuff.

Neuromuscular Blockers (Muscle Relaxants)

Neuromuscular blockers are agents that block transmission of nerve impulses at the neuromuscular junction of skeletal muscles. Goals in using muscle relaxants are to relax muscles in abdominal and thoracic surgery, relax eye muscles in certain kinds of eye surgery, facilitate endotracheal intubation, treat laryngospasm, and assist in mechanical ventilation.

Purified curare was the first widely used muscle relaxant; tubocurarine was isolated as the active principle. After that, succinylcholine was introduced because it acts more rapidly than curare. Several other agents have since been added (Table 18-4). The ideal muscle relaxant should

- Be nondepolarizing, with an onset time and duration of action similar to that of succinylcholine but without its problems

- Have a duration of action between those of succinylcholine and pancuronium
- Lack cumulative and cardiovascular effects
- Be metabolized and not dependent upon the kidneys for its elimination

Intravenous Barbiturate Anesthesia

General anesthesia also can be produced by the intravenous injection of various substances, such as thiopental (Table 18-5). A short-acting barbiturate, thiopental sodium (Pentothal) is the anesthetic most commonly used for this purpose. This substance leads to unconsciousness within 30 seconds.

Advantages.   The onset of anesthesia is pleasant; there is none of the buzzing, roaring, or dizziness known to follow administration of an inhalation anesthetic. For this reason, induction of anesthesia with an intravenous agent is preferred by patients who have experienced various methods. The duration of action is brief, and the patient awakens with little nausea or vomiting. Thiopental often is given with other anesthetic agents in prolonged procedures.

Intravenous anesthesia has the advantage of being non-explosive, of requiring little equipment, and of being easy to administer. The low incidence of postoperative nausea and vomiting makes the method useful in eye surgery, in which retching endangers vision in the operated eye. It is useful for short procedures, but is used less often for abdominal surgery. It is not indicated for children, who have small veins and who are more susceptible to respiratory obstruction. The reasons in both instances are apparent.

Disadvantages.   Thiopental is a powerful depressant of breathing, and its chief danger lies in this characteristic. It should be administered by skilled anesthesiologists and nurse anesthetists, and only when some method of giving oxygen is available immediately should trouble arise. Sneezing, coughing, and laryngospasm are sometimes noted.

Intranasal intubation

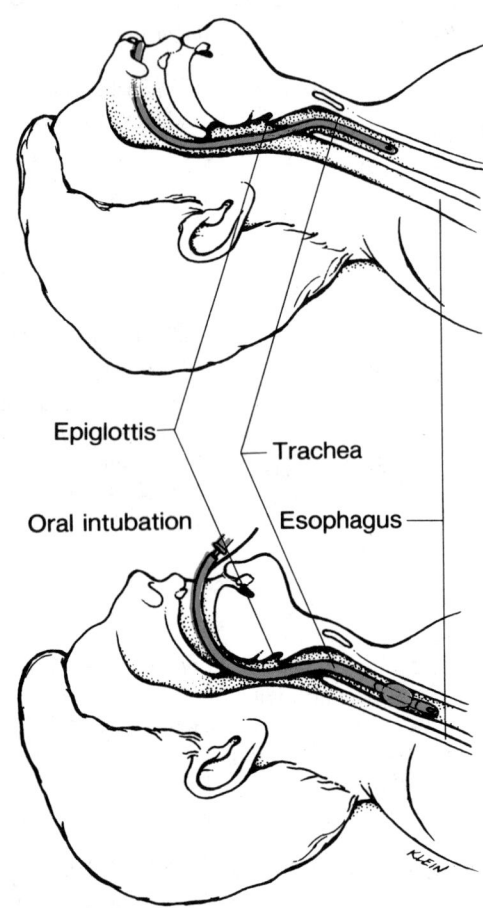

Figure 18-1
Endotracheal anesthesia. (*Top*) Nasal endotracheal catheter in proper position. (*Bottom*) Oral endotracheal intubation; tube in position with cuff inflated. For both methods, the head is tilted back to permit the airway to be open.

Spinal Anesthesia

It must never be forgotten that the patient under spinal, regional, or local anesthesia is awake and aware of his surroundings. Careless conversation, unnecessary noise, unpleasant odors—all are noticed by the patient on the operating table and reflect discredit on the operating room staff. Quiet must be insisted upon. The diagnosis must not be made aloud if the patient is not to be made aware of it at this time.

Anesthesia of the lower extremities, the abdomen, and even the chest may be induced by the introduction of anesthetic drugs into the subarachnoid space. A spinal puncture is made, with sterile precautions, and the drug is injected in solution through the needle. As soon as the injection has been made, the patient is placed on his back. If a relatively high level of block is sought, the head and the shoulders are lowered, depending on the height of anesthesia desired. The spread of the anesthetic agent and the level of anesthesia

depend on the amount of fluid injected, the rapidity with which it is injected, the positioning of the patient after the injection, and the specific gravity of the agent. If the specific gravity of the agent is greater than cerebrospinal fluid (CSF), that is, if the agent is *hyperbaric,* the drug moves to the dependent position of the subarachnoid space; if *hypobaric,* the drug moves away from the dependent portion. These boundaries can obviously be controlled by the anesthesiologist.

In a few minutes anesthesia and paralysis appear, first of the toes and the perineum and then gradually of the legs and the abdomen. The drugs generally used are procaine, tetracaine (Pontocaine), and lidocaine (Xylocaine) (Table 18-6).

Nausea, vomiting, and pain may occur during surgery under spinal anesthesia. As a rule, these reactions result from traction on various structures, particularly those within the abdominal cavity. Such reactions may be avoided by the simultaneous intravenous administration of a weak solution of thiopental and inhalation of nitrous oxide.

When the anesthetic drug reaches the upper thoracic and cervical cord in high concentration, a temporary respiratory paralysis, partial or complete, may occur. This complication is treated by maintaining artificial respiration until the effects of the drug on the respiratory nerves have worn off.

Headache may occur as a postoperative complication. Several factors are involved in the incidence of headache: the size of the spinal needle used, the leakage of fluid from the subarachnoid space through the puncture site, and the degree of the patient's hydration. Measures that increase cerebrospinal pressure are helpful in relieving headache. These include keeping the patient flat and quiet, providing body hydration, applying a tight abdominal binder, and injecting fluid into the epidural space.

Nursing Assessment After Spinal Anesthesia.   In addition to taking the blood pressure, the nurse observes these patients closely and records the time when motion and sensation return in the legs and the toes. When there is complete return of sensation in the toes (in response to pinprick), the patient may be considered to have recovered from the effects of the spinal drug.

"Serial" or Continuous Spinal Anesthesia.   The tip of a plastic catheter may be left in the subarachnoid space during operation, so that more anesthestic may be injected as needed. Greater control of dosage is afforded by this technique. However, there is greater potential for postanesthetic headache because of the large-gauge needle used.

Epidural or Peridural Anesthesia.   Epidural or peridural anesthesia is obtained by the injection of a local anesthetic into the spinal canal in the space surrounding the dura mater. Interest in this approach has increased because of a desire to find a method of anesthesia without undesirable neurologic sequelae, notably headache, that occasionally result from subarachnoid injection.

Advantages of epidural anesthesia appear to be the absence of neurologic complications and slightly less disturbance of blood pressure. One disadvantage lies in the greater technical problem of introducing the anesthetic into the epidural rather than the subarachnoid space. Another is that the level of anesthesia is less controllable.

TABLE 18-4
Muscle Relaxants

Muscle Relaxant	Action	Advantages	Disadvantages	Uses and Comments
Tubocurarine chloride (Tubarine)	Peaks at 30–60 min	50%–70% excreted unchanged in 3–6 hr	Histaminelike reaction Hypotension Increased airway resistance Skin erythema	Contraindicated with history of allergy, asthma
Gallamine (Flaxedil)	$\frac{1}{5}$ as potent as curare Lasts 25% shorter than curare Blocks vagal ganglia in heart	All excreted unchanged	Tachycardia	Used well with cyclopropane or halothane
Pancuronium bromide (Pavulon)	Similar to curare but 5 times more potent Duration, 60–85 min	Safe; stable Good muscle relaxant Reversible by neostigmine and atropine		Excellent for situations requiring complete relaxation Avoid with myasthenia gravis or renal disease. Avoid with patients sensitive to bromide.
Vecuronium bromide (Norcuron)	Blocks depolarization	Facilitates endotracheal intubation; good muscle relaxant	Prolonged dose-related apnea	Related to Pavulon Well tolerated in patients with renal failure

Depolarizing Neuromuscular Blocking Agents

These mimic the action of acetylcholine at the neuromuscular junction.
Acetylcholine is discharged almost immediately upon release → repolarization of muscle takes place. When depolarizing neuromuscular blocking agents are used, skeletal muscle depolarizes.

Muscle Relaxant	Action	Advantages	Disadvantages	Uses and Comments
Succinylcholine (Anectine; Sucostrin)	Onset is rapid: 3–5 min	Ideal for endotracheal intubation, fracture reduction; treatment of laryngospasm	Contraindicated for patients with low pseudocholinesterase On second IV injection, bradycardia and various dysrhythmias May cause fasciculations of the muscles—pain	Treat laryngospasm Treat toxic reaction to local anesthetic drugs Treat status asthmaticus
Decamethonium bromide (Syncurine)	Onset: 30–40 sec Duration: 15–20 min	Excreted unchanged by kidney	Some fasciculation of muscle: jaw masseter muscles; posterior calf muscles Difficult to reverse its action	Produces depolarization of endplate region

Regional Anesthesia

Regional anesthesia is a form of local anesthesia in which an anesthetic agent is injected into or around nerves so that the area supplied by these nerves is anesthetized. The effect depends on the type of nerve involved. Motor fibers are the largest and have the thickest myelin sheath. Sympathetic fibers are the smallest and have a minimal covering. Sensory fibers are intermediary. Thus, a local anesthetic blocks motor nerves least readily and sympathetic nerves most readily. An anesthetic cannot be regarded as having "worn off" until all three systems (motor, sensory, and autonomic) are no longer affected by the anesthetic.

There are many types of regional anesthesia depending on the various nerve groups that are injected.

Brachial Plexus Block. A brachial plexus block produces anesthesia of the arm.

Paravertebral Anesthesia. Paravertebral anesthesia pro-

TABLE 18-5
Intravenous Anesthetic Agents

Agent	Administration	Advantages	Disadvantages	Implications
Barbiturates				
Thiopental sodium (Pentothal)	Intravenous injection (or rectal)	Rapid induction Nonexplosive Requires little equipment Low incidence of postoperative nausea and vomiting	Powerful depressant of breathing Poor relaxant Sometimes produces coughing, sneezing, and laryngospasm Not useful for children because of small veins	Requires intelligent and close observation because of potency and rapidity of drug action.
Narcotics				
Meperidine hydrochloride (Demerol)	Intravenously Subcutaneously Intramuscularly	Prompt onset Because of spasmolytic effect, it is drug of choice for surgery of bile duct, distal colon, and rectum; easily detoxified and excreted	May slow rate of respirations Adverse reactions: dizziness, nausea, and vomiting	In some patients, histamine may be released; treatment is diphenhydramine (Benadryl).
Morphine (high doses)	Intravenously	Not a myocardial depressant	Can depress arterial blood pressure by decreasing systemic vascular resistance Does not provide good amnesia Does not give adequate muscular relaxation	Orthostatic hypotension may occur after morphine.

Neuroleptanalgesics

The term *neuroleptanalgesic* refers to a combination of a short-acting synthetic narcotic agent (fentanyl) and a butyrophenone (droperidol). Patient becomes very drowsy; responds to voice command, although analgesia is profound. Of significance: The combination produces peripheral vasodilation followed by a decrease in arterial blood pressure. If administered rapidly, it may cause skeletal muscular rigidity and possibly respiratory impairment.

Agent	Administration	Advantages	Disadvantages	Implications
Fentanyl (Sublimaze; related chemically to meperidine)	Intravenously	75–100 times more potent than morphine and about 25% of duration of morphine (IV) Little effect on cardiovascular system	In very high dosage, an alpha-adrenergic blocking effect Respiratory depression	Short duration of action is due to its more rapid redistribution and more active metabolism by liver than other narcotics.
Sufentanil		Onset, extremely rapid		Duration only about one-third that of fentanyl

Dissociative Agents

When under dissociative analgesia, the patient appears to be not asleep or anesthetized, but rather dissociated from the surroundings.

Agent	Administration	Advantages	Disadvantages	Implications
Ketamine (Ketalar; Ketaject)	Intravenously Also, intramuscularly	Rapid induction and short action; often used to supplement nitrous oxide Useful where hypotension may be hazardous; can be	May cause elevated blood pressure and depressed repirations Patient may experience hallucinations	Avoid verbal, visual, or tactile stimulation since this may trigger psychic aberration. Droperidol or diazepam (see p. 333) may eliminate such psychic emergence phenomena.

(continued)

TABLE 18-5 *(continued)*

Agent	Administration	Advantages	Disadvantages	Implications
		administered as analgesic or anesthetic	Vomiting and aspiration may occur	Observe for signs of respiratory depression. Keep resuscitative equipment nearby.
Tranquilizers				
Benzodiazepines: Diazepam (Valium) Chlordiazepoxide (Librium)	Intravenously Orally Intramuscularly	Preoperative sedation Intraoperative tranquilization during regional anesthesia Production of hypnosis during anesthetic induction	Absorbed unpredictably when given intramuscularly	IV administration may produce thrombophlebitis (central vein therefore is preferred).
Droperidol (Inapsine)	Intravenously	Long duration of action	Weak antihistaminic action and alpha-adrenergic blocking action; inhibition of basic ganglionic dopaminergic pathways—may lead to extrapyramidal rigidity resembling parkinsonism	Major tranquilizer Keep IV fluids and vasopressors available for hypotension.

duces anesthesia of the nerves supplying the chest, abdominal wall, and extremities.

Transsacral (Caudal) Block. A transsacral block produces anesthesia of the perineum and, occasionally, the lower abdomen.

Local Infiltration Anesthesia

Infiltration anesthesia is the injection of a solution containing the local anesthetic into the tissues through which the incision is to pass. Often it is combined with a local regional block by injection of nerves immediately supplying that area. Local anesthesia is popular for several reasons:

- It is simple, economical, and nonexplosive. The amount of equipment is minimal. Postoperative care is lessened.
- Undesirable effects of general anesthesia are avoided.
- It is ideal for short and superficial operations.

In operations on the abdominal viscera, complete anesthesia is not obtained by infiltration or local block of the anterior abdominal wall, because the viscera are supplied by nerves that have not been affected by the anesthetic. For this reason, a separate injection must be made into the region of the splanchnic nerves, which supply the abdominal organs, except those of the pelvis. This injection may be made from the back (posterior splanchnic anesthesia), or anteriorly, after the abdomen is opened.

Local anesthesia is often administered in combination with epinephrine. Epinephrine causes constriction of blood vessels, which prevents rapid absorption of the anesthetic drug and thus prolongs its local action; absorption into the bloodstream, which could cause convulsions, is also prevented.

Different types of local anesthetic agents are listed in Table 18-7.

TABLE 18-6
Spinal Anesthetic Agents

Agent	Advantages of Spinal Anesthesia (Includes All Agents)	Disadvantages of Spinal Anesthesia (Includes All Agents)
Procaine (Novocain) Tetracaine (Pontocaine) Xylocaine (Lidocaine)	Easily administered by a physician Inexpensive Minimum of equipment required Rapid onset Excellent muscular relaxation	Blood pressure may fall rapidly unless watched carefully and treated with such drugs as ephedrine. If the spinal anesthesia ascends to the chest, there may be respiratory difficulties. Occasionally postoperative complications occur, such as headache or, rarely, meningitis or paralysis.

TABLE 18-7
Local Anesthetic Agents

Agent	Administration and Action	Advantages	Disadvantages	Implications and Use
Amides				
Lidocaine (Xylocaine) and mepivacaine (Carbocaine)	Topical or injection	Rapid Longer duration of action (compared with procaine) Free from local irritative effect	Occasional idiosyncrasy	Useful topically for cystoscopy Injected for use in dental work and surgery Watch for untoward reactions—drowsiness, depressed respiration.
Bupivacaine (Marcaine)	Infiltration Peripheral nerve block Epidural	Duration is 2–3 times longer than lidocaine or mepivacaine	Use cautiously in persons with known drug allergies or sensitivities.	A period of analgesia persists after return of sensation; therefore, need for strong analgesics is reduced.
Etidocaine (Duranest)	Infiltration Block			Greater potency and longer action than lidocaine
Esters				
Procaine (Novocain)	Subcutaneously, intramuscularly, intravenously, or spinal	Low toxicity Inexpensive	Some idiosyncrasies Skin rash Poor stability	Watch for reaction: BP, bradycardia, weak pulse. Usually given with epinephrine, causing vasoconstriction, thereby slowing absorption and prolonging nerve-deadening effect
Tetracaine (Pontocaine)	Topical Infiltration Nerve block	Same as procaine	Same as procaine	More than 10 times as potent as procaine Usually given with epinephrine

Contraindications.   Local anesthesia is the anesthesia of choice in any operation in which it can be used. However, it is contraindicated for operations upon highly nervous, apprehensive patients. The emotional trauma experienced by these patients during local anesthesia may be harmful. A patient who begs to be put to sleep rarely does well under local anesthesia.

For some kinds of operations, local anesthesia is impractical because of the number of injections and the amount of anesthetic required—in breast reconstruction, for example.

Technique.   The technique for the introduction of local infiltration requires few materials. The following are all that are needed:

- Solution of local anesthetic in various concentrations (0.5%–2%)
- Sterile container
- Sterile syringes and needles to fit
- Sterile sponges and drape

The skin is prepared as for any operation, and a small-gauge needle is used to inject a little of the anesthetic into the skin layers. This produces blanching or a wheal. The anesthetic then is carried ahead of the needle in the skin until an area as long as the proposed incision is anesthetized. A larger, longer needle then is used to infiltrate deeper tissues with the anesthetic. The action of the drug is almost immediate, so the operation may begin as soon as the injection is finished. Anesthesia lasts anywhere from 45 minutes to 3 hours, depending on the anesthetic and the use of epinephrine.

Patient Position on Operating Table

The position in which the patient is placed on the operating table depends on the operation to be performed as well as on the physical condition of the patient (Fig. 18-2). Factors to consider include the following:

- The patient should be in as comfortable a position as possible, whether asleep or awake.
- The operative area must be adequately exposed.
- Circulation should not be obstructed by an awkward position or undue pressure on a part.
- There should be no interference with the patient's respiration as a result of pressure of the arms on the chest or constriction of the neck or chest caused by a gown.

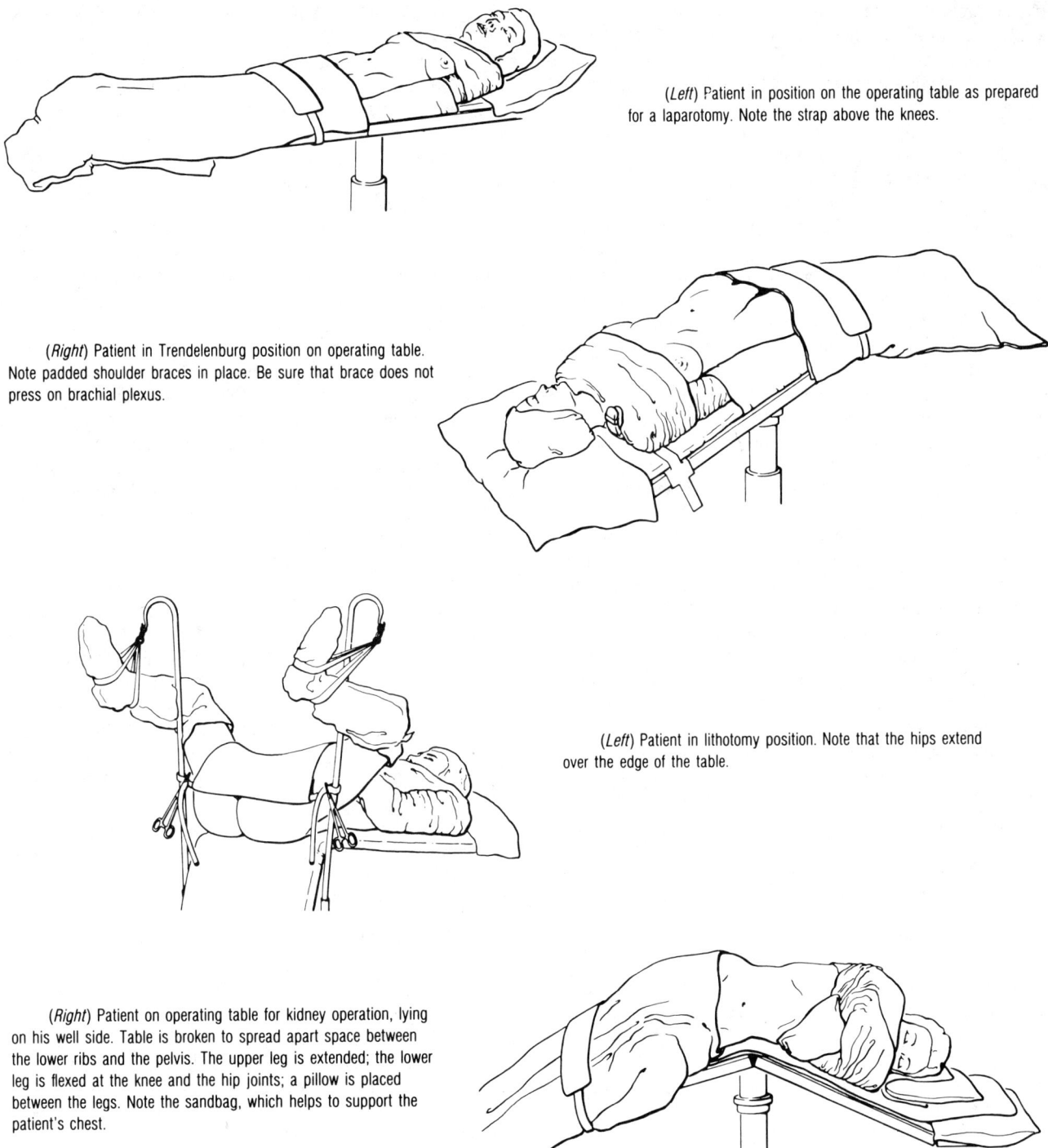

(*Left*) Patient in position on the operating table as prepared for a laparotomy. Note the strap above the knees.

(*Right*) Patient in Trendelenburg position on operating table. Note padded shoulder braces in place. Be sure that brace does not press on brachial plexus.

(*Left*) Patient in lithotomy position. Note that the hips extend over the edge of the table.

(*Right*) Patient on operating table for kidney operation, lying on his well side. Table is broken to spread apart space between the lower ribs and the pelvis. The upper leg is extended; the lower leg is flexed at the knee and the hip joints; a pillow is placed between the legs. Note the sandbag, which helps to support the patient's chest.

Figure 18-2
Positions on the operating table. Adjacent captions call attention to safety and comfort features. Of course all surgical patients would wear a cap to completely cover the hair.

- Nerves must be protected from undue pressure. Improper positioning of the arms, hands, legs, or feet may cause serious injury or paralysis. Shoulder braces must be well padded to prevent irreparable nerve injury, especially when the Trendelenburg position is necessary.

- Concerns for the patient as an individual must be prac-

ticed, particularly with the very thin, the elderly, or the obese patient.

- Every patient needs *gentle* restraint before induction, in case of excitement.

Dorsal Recumbent Position. The usual position is flat on the back; one arm is at the side of the table, with the hand placed palm down; the other is carefully positioned on an armboard for intravenous infusion (see Fig. 18-2). This position is used for most abdominal operations, except for those upon the gallbladder and the pelvis, and for the operations described below.

Trendelenburg Position. The Trendelenburg position usually is employed for operations on the lower abdomen and the pelvis in order to obtain good exposure by displacing the intestines into the upper abdomen. In this position the head and body are lowered so that the plane of the body meets the horizontal at an angle. The knees are flexed by "breaking" the table, and the patient is held in position by padded shoulder braces (Fig. 18-2).

Lithotomy Position. In the lithotomy position the patient is lying on his back with the legs and thighs flexed at right angles. The position is maintained by placing the feet in stirrups. Nearly all perineal, rectal, and vaginal operations require this posture (see Fig. 18-2).

For Kidney Operations. The patient is placed on his well side in Sims's position with an air pillow 12.5 cm to 15 cm (5 or 6 inches) thick under the loin, or he is placed on a table with a kidney or back lift (see Fig. 18-2).

For Chest and Abdominothoracic Operations. The position varies with the operation to be performed. The surgeon and the anesthesiologist place the patient on the operating table in the desired position.

Operations on the Neck. Neck operations—for example, those involving the thyroid—are performed with the patient on his back, the neck extended somewhat by a pillow beneath the shoulders, and the head and chest elevated in order to reduce venous pressure.

Operations on the Skull and the Brain. Such procedures demand special positions and apparatus, usually adjusted by the surgeon.

Artificial Hypotension During the Operation

There are times during surgery when it is desirable to lower blood pressure in order to reduce bleeding at the operative site, since this allows for more rapid surgery with less blood loss. In operations such as brain surgery, radical neck dissection, and radical pelvic surgery, artificially induced hypotension has been used.

Deliberate hypotension is accomplished by inhalation or intravenous injection of drugs that affect the sympathetic nervous system and peripheral smooth muscle. Halothane is the inhalational anesthetic agent commonly used. This anesthetic is supplemented with other measures to lower blood pressure, such as a head-up position, positive pressure applied to the airway, and administration of a ganglionic blocking drug such as pentolinium (Ansolysen) or sodium nitroprusside.

Hypothermia

Hypothermia is the state of body core temperature lowered below physiologic normal limits. *Normothermia* is 36.6°–

37.5°C (98.0°–99.5°F). Inadvertent hypothermia may be experienced by the surgical patient as a result of a low temperature in the OR, infusion of cold fluids, inspiration of cold gases, open body wounds or cavities, decreased muscle activity, advanced age, or the pharmaceutical agents used (vasodilators, phenothiazines, general anesthetics).

Treatment. Prevention of hypothermia is a first consideration; if it occurs, minimizing or reversing the physiological process is the goal.

Environmental temperature should be set at 25.0°–26.6°C (78.0°–80°F). Intravenous and irrigating fluids are warmed to 37°C (98.6F). Wet gowns and drapes are removed promptly and replaced with dry materials, because wet linens conduct heat loss. Whatever methods are employed to rewarm the patient, warming must be done gradually and not rapidly. Conscientious monitoring of the parameters (core temperature, urinary output, ECG, blood pressure, arterial blood gases, and serum electrolytes) is required.

Attention to hypothermia management extends into the postoperative period to prevent significant nitrogen loss and catabolism. Treatment includes oxygen administration, adequate hydration (fluids without lactate, electrolytes) and proper nutrition.

Gerontological Considerations. Recent reports indicate that heat loss in older patients in the operating room can be prevented by covering the head of the patient during anesthesia. According to Biddle and Biddle, an ordinary disposable plastic packaging bag applied after the patient is anesthetized and removed before consciousness is regained can be effective and inexpensive. Also the operating room temperature should be maintained at 26.6°C (80°F). Antiseptic solutions used in the initial preparation of the skin before the application of drapes should be comfortably warm, not cold.

Malignant Hyperthermia During General Anesthesia

Malignant hyperthermia is a pharmacogenic syndrome that is chemically induced by anesthetic agents.

Etiology and Pathophysiology. During anesthesia, potent agents such as inhalation anesthetics (halothane, enflurane) and relaxants (succinylcholine) may trigger the symptoms of malignant hyperthermia. Such drugs as sympathomimetics (epinephrine), theophylline, aminophylline, anticholinergics (atropine), and cardiac glycosides (digitalis) can also induce or intensify such a reaction. The process is also enhanced by stress.

The pathophysiology is related to muscle cell activity. Muscle cells are composed of inner fluid (sarcoplasm) and an outer surrounding membrane. Calcium, an essential factor in the process of muscle contraction, is normally stored in sacs in the sarcoplasm. When nerve impulses stimulate the muscle, the sacs release calcium, allowing contraction to occur. A pumping mechanism returns calcium to the sacs so that relaxation can take place. In malignant hyperthermia this process is disrupted. Calcium ions are not reabsorbed and they accumulate, causing clinical symptoms of hypermetabolism, which in turn increases muscle contraction (rigidity),

TABLE 18-8
Pharmacologic Agents Used in Treating Malignant Hyperthermia

Generic (Trade) Name Usual Dose in MH	Action	Nursing Responsibilities
Dantrolene Sodium (Dantrium)	Direct skeletal muscle relaxant Reduces release of calcium from sarcoplasmic reticulum, thus decreasing muscle contraction	Monitor ECG, temperature, BP, central venous pressure, serum potassium. Observe for infiltration to surrounding tissues. Maintain intravenous infusion until symptoms decrease. Mix with distilled water without bacteriostatic agents.
Sodium Bicarbonate	Increases blood pH by buffering excess hydrogen ion concentration	Assess electrolytes. Monitor arterial blood gas values.
Regular Insulin (Regular Iletin)	Increases glucose uptake into liver to meet hypermetabolic demands of body Forces potassium into cells	Observe for hypoglycemia.
Dextrose 50%	Increases movement of potassium from extracellular fluid back into cell	Monitor urine and blood glucose levels. Infuse via central venous catheter. Assess electrolytes.
Furosemide (Lasix)	Potent diuretic Enhances excretion of myoglobins, potassium, sodium, and magnesium	Monitor for hypotension. Observe urinary output. Assess BUN and creatinine. Assess electrolytes. Observe for dehydration. Weigh patient every day. Administer potassium supplements.
Mannitol (Osmitrol)	Osmotic diuretic for excretion of excess fluid load Increases urinary output to prevent renal failure	Monitor input and output. Weigh patient every day. Assess electrolytes. Maintain catheter patency.
Procainamide Hydrochloride	Antiarrhythmic Decreases cardiac muscle excitability and slows conduction velocity	Monitor for hypotension. Monitor ECG, cardiac output. Check urine pH for drug toxicity.
Hydrocortisone Sodium Succinate (Solu-Cortef)	Given for its mineralocorticoid effect of potassium excretion and increased glomerular filtration rate Affects calcium absorption from gastrointestinal tract Used to reduce cerebral edema	Weigh patient every day. Do not use with salicylates. Monitor blood pressure. Observe for gastrointestinal bleeding. Assess electrolytes.
Heparin Sodium (Hepathrom)	Anticoagulant to treat disseminated intravascular coagulation	Observe for bleeding. Monitor coagulation status. Check stool/urine for occult blood.

(After Caine R, Molla K, and Reynolds R. Malignant hyperthermia: A critical care challenge. DCCN 1986 May/June; 5 [3]:148.)

Chart 18-5
The Nursing Process

Assessment

A. Use data from patient and the patient record to identify variables that can affect care and that serve as guidelines for developing an individualized plan of patient care.
  1. Identify patient.
  2. Validate necessary data with patient per department policy.
  3. Review patient record for:
     a. Correct informed surgical consent
     b. Completed records for health history and physical examination
     c. Results of diagnostic studies
     d. Nursing history and nursing assessment
     e. Preoperative Check List
  4. Complete immediate preoperative nursing assessment.
     a. Physiologic status (*e.g.,* health–illness level, level of consciousness, etc.)
     b. Psychosocial status (*e.g.,* expressions of concern, anxiety level, verbal communication problems, coping mechanisms, etc.)
     c. Physical status (*e.g.,* operative site, skin condition and effectiveness of preparation, shave or depilatory; immobile joints, etc.)

Planning

A. Interpret common variables and incorporate them into the plan of care.
  1. Age, size, sex, surgical procedure, type of anesthesia planned, surgeon, anesthesiologist, and team members
  2. Availability of necessary equipment specific to procedure and surgeon
  3. Need for nonroutine drugs, blood, instruments, etc.

  4. Readiness of room for patient; completeness of physical setup; completeness of instrument, suture, and dressing setups.
B. Identify aspects of the operating room environment that may negatively affect the patient.
  1. Physical
     a. Room temperature and humidity
     b. Electrical hazards
     c. Potential contaminants (dust, blood, and discharge stains on floor or furniture; uncovered hair, faulty personnel attire, jewelry worn by personnel, "dirty" footwear)
     d. Unnecessary traffic
  2. Psychosocial
     a. Noise
     b. Lack of recognition as a person
     c. Sense of abandonment—unchaperoned in waiting area
     d. Social "chit-chat"

Intervention

A. Provide nursing care based on priority of patient needs.
  1. Set up and maintain suction in working order.
  2. Set up invasive monitoring equipment.
  3. Assist with line insertion (arterial, Swan–Ganz, CVP, IV)
  4. Initiate appropriate physical comfort measures for patient.
  5. Position patient correctly for anesthesia and surgical procedures; maintain functional body alignment.
  6. Follow steps in surgical procedure.
     a. Scrub/circulate competently.

(continued)

hyperthermia, and damage to the central nervous system. Persons susceptible to malignant hyperthermia include those having a history of muscle abnormality: bulky, strong muscles, hernia, and musculoskeletal problems such as scoliosis. Malignant hyperthermia affects more males than females and more children than adults.

Clinical Manifestations. The first symptoms of malignant hyperthermia are related to musculoskeletal and cardiovascular activity: tachycardia, tetanylike movements, rigidity, diaphoresis, and tachypnea. Other manifestations are ventricular dysrhythmia, hypertension, cyanosis, decreased level of consciousness, and temperature elevation. Late symptoms are anuria, renal failure, left heart failure, pulmonary edema, and central nervous system damage.

Management. Early recognition of symptoms by the critical care nurse and the prompt discontinuance of anesthesia are imperative. It is also necessary to monitor all vital signs, arterial blood gases, electrolytes, and the ECG. Goals of treatment are to decrease metabolism, reverse metabolic and respiratory acidosis, correct dysrhythmias, decrease body temperature, provide oxygen and nutrition to tissues, and correct electrolyte imbalance.

As soon as the medical diagnosis is made, anesthesia and surgery are halted and the patient is hyperventilated with 100% oxygen. Pharmacotherapy is initiated as described in Table 18-8 (p. 337); note the nursing responsibilities. Continued monitoring of all parameters is necessary to evaluate the patient's progress. For the high temperature elevation, it

Chart 18-5 *(continued)*

Intervention

    b. Respond to needs of patient by anticipating what supplies and equipment are required before they are requested.

    c. Assume role of RN First Assistant as required.

  7. Follow established procedures—for example (not all-inclusive):

    a. Care and use of blood and blood products

    b. Care and handling of specimens, tissue, and cultures

    c. Antiseptic skin preparation

    d. Donning gown—self; holding gown for surgeon

    e. Open and closed gloving

    f. Counts; sponge, instrument, needle, special

    g. Septic case technique

    h. Urinary catheter management

    i. Drainage/dressing management

  8. Communicate adverse situations to surgeon, anesthesiologist, or charge nurse, or act appropriately to control or reverse the situation.

  9. Use supplies judiciously for cost-effectiveness.

  10. Assist the surgeon and anesthesiologist in implementing their plans of care.

B. Act as the patient's advocate.

  1. Provide physical privacy.

  2. Maintain confidentiality.

  3. Act to provide physical safety and comfort.

C. Inform patient regarding his intraoperative experience.

  1. Describe any sensory stimulation he will experience.

  2. Use common, basic communication skills to reduce anxiety in the patient—for example (list not all-inclusive):

    a. Touch

    b. Eye contact

    c. Assuring the patient you will be with him in the operating room

    d. Realistic verbal reassurance

D. Coordinate activities of significant others involved in patient care (list not all-inclusive)

  1. X-ray, laboratory, recovery or intensive care unit, surgical floor

  2. Technicians—cast, laboratory, etc.

  3. Pharmacist

  4. Ancillary operating room personnel and nonprofessional staff

E. Operate and troubleshoot for all equipment commonly used in the operating room and assigned specialty service (including autoclaves).

F. Participate in patient care conferences.

G. Document all observations and appropriate actions on the required forms, including patient's record.

H. Communicate, orally and in writing, with the recovery room and outpatient surgical nursing staff (as pertinent) regarding the health status of the patient on transfer from the operating room.

Evaluation

A. Evaluate the condition of the patient immediately prior to his discharge from the operating room—for example:

  1. Respiratory condition: breathing easily (on his own or assisted)

  2. Skin condition: color good; absence of abrasions, burns, bruises

  3. Functioning of invasive tubing: IV, drains, catheters, nasogastric—no kinks or obstruction, functioning normally, etc.

  4. Grounding pad site: good condition

  5. Dressings: adequate for drainage, fastened securely, not too tight, etc.

B. Participate in the identification of unsafe patient care practices and intervene appropriately.

C. Participate in evaluating the safety of the environment—for example; equipment, cleanliness, etc.

D. Report and document any adverse behavior or problem.

E. Demonstrate understanding of principles of asepsis and technical nursing practices.

F. Accept legal responsibilities inherent in perioperative nursing.

(Adapted from procedure and practices at Memorial Hospital Medical Center of Long Beach, California)

---

may be necessary to administer iced saline solutions intravenously, or iced saline lavages of stomach, bladder, and rectum. A hypothermia blanket may also be effective.

Dantrolene sodium is the prescribed medication of choice in treating this patient and may even be used prophylactically in susceptible patients. It is a skeletal muscle relaxant.

Although the condition happens infrequently, enough is now known about the problem that, if it does occur, it can be identified. It is imperative that the nurse recognize the problem, have the appropriate medication and equipment available, and know the protocol to follow. This information may be life-saving should malignant hyperthermia occur.

Intraoperative Nursing: The Nursing Process

The nursing process as applied to intraoperative nursing is summarized in Chart 18-5.

Bibliography

See Bibliography for unit following Chapter 19.

Chapter 19

Postoperative Nursing Management

The nursing process continues in the postoperative period and is directed toward the reestablishment of the patient's physiologic equilibrium and the prevention of pain and complications. Careful assessment and immediate intervention will assist the patient in planning a return to normal function as quickly, safely, and comfortably as possible.

Considerable effort is expended on *anticipation* and *prevention* of difficulties in the postoperative period. The nursing care of the patient after operation is second in importance only to the operation itself.

Transferring the Patient to the Recovery Room

The patient is moved from the operating table to the bed or the stretcher with the least possible delay and exposure. The site of the surgical incision is kept in mind every time a newly operated patient is moved. Many wounds are closed under considerable tension, and every effort is made to prevent further strain on the sutures. Thus, in nephrectomy the patient is not allowed to lie on the affected side because of the possibility of obstructing drains in the wound.

Serious arterial hypotension may occur when a patient is moved from one position to another, such as from a lithotomy position to a horizontal position, from a lateral to a supine position, or from a prone to a supine position. Even moving the anesthetized patient to the stretcher can precipitate this problem. Thus, the patient must be moved *slowly* and *carefully*.

As soon as the patient is placed on the stretcher or bed, he is covered with lightweight blankets that have been arranged previously on the stretcher. The wet and soiled gown is removed and a dry gown applied. On the stretcher the patient is held with straps above the knees and the elbows. The straps serve the double purpose of securing the blankets and restraining the patient, should he pass through a stage of excitement as he recovers from the anesthetic. Side rails are raised to protect against falls.

Transfer of the postoperative patient from the OR to the

recovery room is the responsibility of the anesthesiologist, with a member of the surgical team in attendance. Additional assistance may be provided by a nurse assigned to this particular patient. Transfer of the patient is done expeditiously, with special attention paid in transit to comfort, safety, and general condition. Tubes and drainage equipment are handled carefully for optimum function.

Postanesthesia Recovery Room (PARR)

The post-anesthesia recovery room (PARR) is a unit usually located adjacent to the operating rooms. Patients who are still under anesthesia or recovering from it are placed in this unit for easy access to (1) nurses who are especially prepared in caring for the immediate postoperative patient, (2) anesthesiologists and surgeons, and (3) monitors and special equipment, medications, and replacement fluids. In this setting, the newly operated patient is given the best care available by those best qualified to give it.

The room should be quiet, clean, and free of unnecessary equipment. It should also have (1) walls and ceiling painted in soft, pleasing colors; (2) indirect lighting; (3) soundproof ceiling; (4) equipment that controls or eliminates noise (*e.g.*, synthetic emesis basins, rubber bumpers on beds and tables); and (5) isolated quarters (glass encased) for noisy patients. These features are of real value to the patient psychologically.

Equipment includes every type of breathing aid: oxygen, laryngoscopes, tracheotomy sets, bronchial instruments, catheters, mechanical ventilators, and suction equipment. Another necessity is equipment for meeting circulatory needs, such as blood pressure apparatus, parenteral equipment, universal donor blood, plasma expanders, intravenous trays and cutdown trays, cardiac arrest equipment, defibrillator, venous catheters, and tourniquets. Surgical dressing materials, narcotics, and emergency drugs are available, as well as catheterization sets and drainage equipment. Monitoring devices may be at hand to provide an accurate and instant appraisal of the patient's condition.

The recovery bed is one that affords easy access to the patient, is safe and easily movable, can readily be placed in shock position, and possesses features that facilitate care, such as intravenous poles, side guards, wheel brakes, and chart storage rack.

Room temperature should be 20°C to 22.2°C (68°F–70°F), and the room should have good ventilation.

A patient remains in this unit until he has fully recovered from the anesthetic agent, that is, until he has a stable blood pressure, good air passage, and a reasonable degree of consciousness. Criteria to determine the degree of recovery are provided in detail on p. 344.

Goals are to care for the patient until he has recovered from the effects of anesthesia (*i.e.*, until return of motor and sensory functions), vital signs are stable, there is no evidence of hemorrhage, and he is oriented. If a problem arises, the proximity to the operating room, surgeon, and anesthesiologist provides assurance of immediate expert assistance. The patient who responds positively progresses to the point of being released from the PAR to his unit. This status is described later using a scoring guide.

Immediate Postoperative Assessment

The recovery room nurse who receives the patient reviews the following with the anesthesiologist:

1. Medical diagnosis and type of surgery performed
2. Patient's age and general condition: airway patency, vital signs, blood pressure
3. Anesthetic and other medications used: narcotics, muscle relaxant, antibiotics, and the like
4. Any untoward problems that occurred in the operating room that might influence postoperative care (*e.g.*, extensive hemorrhage, shock, cardiac arrest)
5. Pathology encountered (if malignancy, whether the patient or family has been informed)
6. Fluid administered, blood loss and replacement
7. Any tubing, drains, catheters, or other supportive aids
8. Specific information about which the surgeon or anesthesiologist wishes to be notified

This joint preliminary assessment of the patient includes an evaluation of pulse volume and regularity, depth and nature of respirations, skin color, level of consciousness, and even ability of the patient to respond to commands. The operative site is checked for evidence of hemorrhage or drainage and for tubing that needs to be connected to a drainage receptacle.

It is also essential for the nurse to know anything pertinent in the preoperative history that may be significant at this time (*e.g.*, patient is hard of hearing, epileptic, diabetic, allergic to certain medications). This information may have been acquired in a preoperative visit with the patient.

Nursing Interventions

Vital signs are checked and general physical assessment of the patient is done at least every 15 minutes. In the order of priority, respiratory function and patency of the airway are always evaluated first, followed by assessment of cardiovascular function (including vital signs), the condition of the surgical site, and function of the central nervous system.

- *The chief goal is to maintain pulmonary ventilation and thus prevent hypoxemia* (reduced O_2 in blood) *and hypercapnia* (excess CO_2 in blood). *These can occur if the airway is obstructed and ventilation is reduced* (hypoventilation).

Shock can be avoided largely by the timely administration of intravenous fluids and blood, and appropriate drugs as prescribed.

Respiratory Considerations. Respiratory difficulties are treated as they arise or, better, the patient is treated so that such problems do not arise. Patients under local anesthesia or nitrous oxide usually are "awake" within a few minutes of leaving the operating room. However, patients who have experienced prolonged anesthesia usually are completely unconscious, with all muscles relaxed. This relaxation extends to the muscles of the pharynx; therefore, when the patient lies on his back the lower jaw and the tongue fall backward, and the air passages close more or less completely (Fig. 19-1, *A*). Signs of this difficulty include choking, noisy and irregular respirations, and within minutes, a blue duskiness (cyanosis) of the skin.

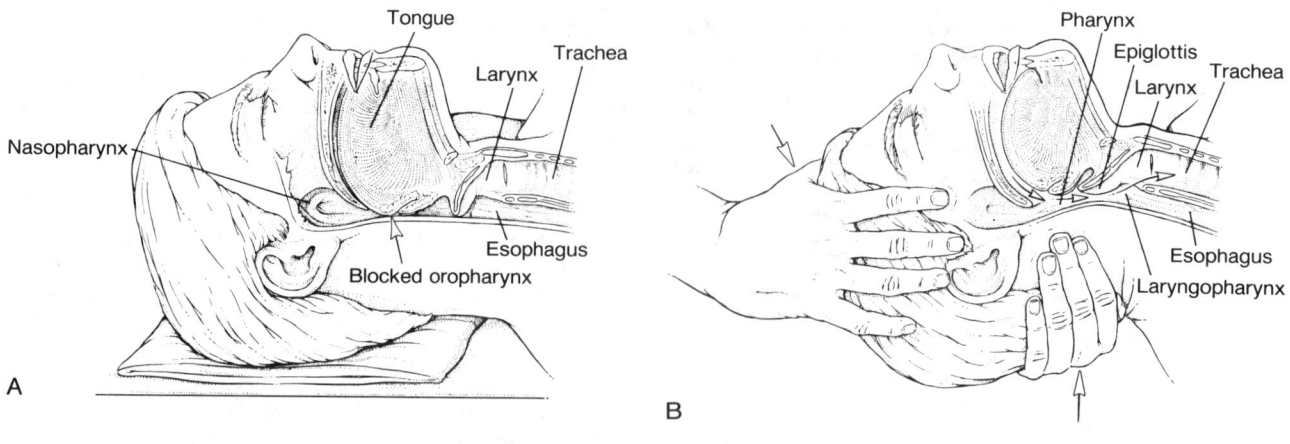

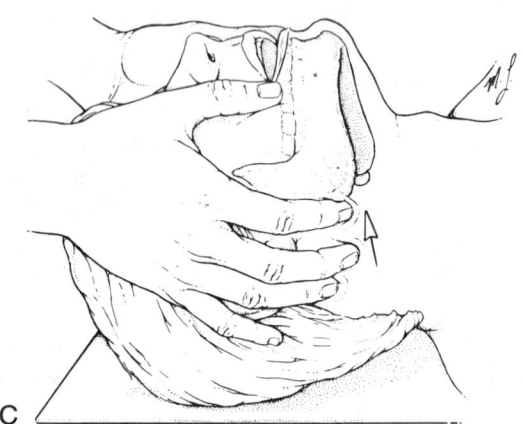

Figure 19-1
(*A*) A hypopharyngeal obstruction occurs when the flexing of the neck permits the chin to drop toward the chest; obstruction almost always happens when the head is in the midposition. (*B*) Tilting the head back to stretch the anterior neck structure will cause the base of the tongue to be lifted off the posterior pharyngeal wall. Note the direction of the areas to indicate the pressure of hands. (*C*) Opening the mouth is necessary to correct valvelike obstruction of the nasal passage during expiration which occurs in about 30% of unconscious patients. Open the patient's mouth (separate lips and teeth) and move the lower jaw forward so that the lower teeth are in front of the upper teeth. To regain backward lilt of the neck, lift with both hands at the ascending rami of the mandible.

- The only sure way of knowing whether a patient is breathing or not is to place the palm of the hand over the patient's nose and mouth in order to feel the exhaled breath. Movements of the thorax and the diaphragm do not necessarily mean that a patient is breathing.
- The treatment of hypopharyngeal obstruction involves tilting the head back and pushing forward on the angle of the lower jaw, as if to push the lower teeth in front of the upper teeth (Fig. 19-1 *B*, *C*). This maneuver pulls the tongue forward and opens the air passages. At times it may be necessary to grasp the tongue between layers of gauze and pull it forward for a time. This maneuver prevents respiratory obstruction and is continued when necessary until the patient has regained reflex functions sufficiently to carry on normal respiration.

Often the anesthesiologist leaves a hard rubber or plastic airway in the mouth (Fig. 19-2) that is used to maintain a patent airway. Such a device should not be removed until signs, such as gagging, indicate that reflex action is returning.

Occasionally, a patient may be brought to the recovery room with an endotracheal tube (ET tube) still in place and may require continued mechanical ventilation. The nurse will then assist in the preparation of the respirator and in the weaning and extubation procedures.

Clearing Secretions from the Airway. Not infrequently, respiratory difficulty is produced by an excessive secretion of mucus. Turning the patient on one side allows the collected fluid to escape from the side of the mouth. If the patient's teeth are clenched, the mouth may be opened manually. The nurse places a thumb against the patient's lower teeth and the index finger against the upper teeth. The mouth is opened by crossing the thumb and index finger to obtain better leverage. If the teeth are tightly clenched, the nurse inserts the tip of the index finger behind the last molar and pries the mouth open. If vomiting occurs, the head is turned to the side and the vomitus collected in the emesis basin. The face is wiped with gauze or paper wipes. The nature and amount of the vomitus are recorded.

Mucus or vomitus obstructing the pharynx or the trachea should be aspirated with a pharyngeal suction tip or a nasal catheter introduced into the nasopharynx or the oropharynx. Wall suction or suction machines are available for this purpose. The catheter can be passed into the nasopharynx or the oropharynx safely to a distance of 15 to 20 cm (6–8 inches) if secretions are obtained at this level.

If frequent aspiration of the nasopharynx and oropharynx is indicated, a clean aspirating catheter is used and a basin of water kept nearby to flush and clean the catheter. Caution is necessary in suctioning the throat of a patient who has had a tonsillectomy, since the operative area may become irritated, causing bleeding and added discomfort.

Positioning. Until the patient regains consciousness, the bed is kept flat. Unless contraindicated, the unconscious patient is positioned on one side with a pillow at the back and with chin extended to minimize any danger of aspiration. Knees are flexed and a pillow positioned between the legs to reduce strain on abdominal sutures.

Psychological Support. The function of the recovery room nurse is not limited to bedside procedures, safety mea-

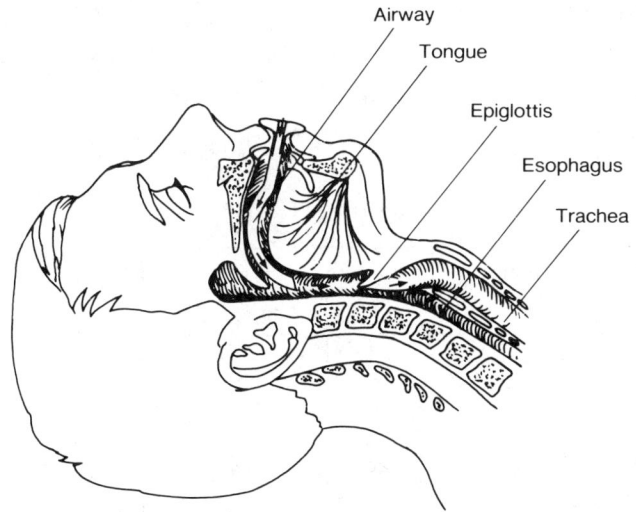

Airway
Tongue
Epiglottis
Esophagus
Trachea

Figure 19-2
Diagrammatic view showing a method by which an "airway" prevents respiratory difficulty after anesthesia. The "airway" passes over the base of the tongue and delivers air into the pharynx in the region of the epiglottis. Patients are often brought from the operating room with an "airway" in place. This should remain in place until the patient recovers sufficiently to breathe normally. Usually, as the patient regains consciousness, the airway causes irritation; then it should be removed.

sures, and the relief of pain; an understanding of the significance of psychological support is also important. If the nurse has never seen the patient before, a definite handicap is immediately presented. The nurse who knows the patient and accompanies him through the immediate preoperative and operative experiences is in a unique position to offer valuable support. In the absence of such continuous care by one nurse, pertinent nurses' notes on the chart help the recovery room nurse to recognize the particular needs of each individual patient.

Postanesthesia Recovery Room Criteria and Scoring Guide

Usually the following criteria are included in determining the patient's readiness to be discharged from the postanesthesia recovery room:

- Uncompromised pulmonary exchange
- Stable vital signs, including blood pressure
- Orientation to place, events, time
- Urine output not less than 30 ml/hr
- Nausea/vomiting under control; pain minimal

Many hospitals use a scoring system to determine the patient's general condition and readiness to be released from the recovery room. As the patient progresses through the recovery period, his physical signs are observed and evaluated by means of a scoring system based on a set of objective criteria. This evaluation guide, a modification of the Apgar scoring system used for evaluating newborns, makes possible a more objective assessment of the patient's physical condition in the recovery area.

The patient's score is taken at stated intervals, such as every 15 or 30 minutes, and totaled on the official scorecard (Fig. 19-3). A patient with a total score of less than 7 must remain in the recovery room until his condition improves or he is transferred to an intensive care area.

Transfer to Unit

Baseline data on the patient's condition are relayed to the receiving nurse by the nurse from the recovery room. The criteria listed above have been met, and the scoring chart tally (see Fig. 19-3) confirms the patient's responsiveness. Pertinent data are reassessed in the new unit. Specific instructions and postoperative requests are reviewed. The goals of the patient are recognized and nursing interventions are continued and documented, with particular attention given to each patient according to his individual needs.

Patient's Reception and Care on the Clinical Unit

The patient's unit is readied by assembling any equipment that is necessary to meet his specific needs: intravenous pole, drainage receptacle holder, emesis basin, tissues. When the call comes to the unit from the PARR, any additional items that might be needed are mentioned.

Usually the surgeon speaks to the family following the operation and relates the general condition of the patient and what to expect when the patient arrives on the unit. The receiving nurse needs to know what the surgeon said so that consistency of information is retained.

▶ Nursing Process
Caring for the Postoperative Patient

▷ Assessment

The unit nurse receives information from the PARR nurse about the patient's status. When the patient arrives, the nurse does an initial assessment and proceeds with any immediate nursing interventions. Usually the question, "How are you feeling?" provides information about the patient's discomforts as well as the level of mental alertness. Often the physical transfer adds some temporary discomfort. With current anesthetic agents and medications, it is less common for the patient to be nauseated; however, an emesis basin is kept nearby.

Immediate assessment of the surgical patient upon returning to the clinical unit consists of the following:

- *Respiratory:* Airway patency; depth, rate, and character; nature of breath sounds
- *Circulatory:* Vital signs including blood pressure; skin condition
- *Neurologic:* Level of responsiveness
- *Drainage:* Presence; need to connect tubes to a specific drainage system
- *Comfort:* Type of pain and location; nausea or vomiting; position change required

POSTANESTHESIA RECOVERY ROOM
Scoring

Patient: _____

Room: _____

Date: _____

Final Score: _____

Surgeon: _____

R.R. Nurse: _____

Area of Assessment	Point Score	Upon Admission	After 1 hr	After 2 hr	After 3 hr
Respiration:					
• Ability to breathe deeply and cough	2				
• Limited respiratory effort (dyspnea or splinting)	1				
• No spontaneous effort	0				
Circulation: Systolic arterial pressure					
• 20% of preanesthetic level	2				
• 20-50% of preanesthetic level	1				
• 50% + of preanesthetic level	0				
Consciousness Level:					
• Verbally responds to questions/ oriented to location	2				
• Aroused when called by name	1				
• Failure to respond to command	0				
Color:					
• Normal skin color and appearance	2				
• Altered skin color: pale, dusky, blotchy, jaundiced	1				
• Frank cyanosis	0				
Muscle Activity: Moves spontaneously or on command:					
• Ability to move all extremities	2				
• Ability to move 2 extremities	1				
• Unable to control |any| extremity	0				
Totals:					

Required for Discharge from Recovery Room: 7-8 points

Time of Release _____

Signature of Nurse _____

Figure 19-3
Postanesthesia recovery room scoring chart. This may be used in the day surgery unit also.

- *Psychological:* Nature of patient's questions; need for rest/sleep; disturbance by noise, visitors; availability of call bell
- *Safety:* Need for side rails; drainage tubes unobstructed; IV sites properly splinted, if necessary
- *Equipment:* Checked for proper functioning

Respiratory Assessment.   Upon admission to the clinical unit, the patient is observed for patency of the airway. The quality of respirations is noted, such as depth, rate, and sound. Often, because of medications given for pain, respirations are slow. Shallow and rapid respirations may be due to pain, constricting dressings, gastric dilatation, or obesity. Noisy breathing may be due to obstruction by secretions or perhaps the tongue has relaxed (see p. 341). Lung auscultation with accurate documentation can be used as a baseline for later comparisons. Crackles may indicate secretions that should be mobilized.

Circulatory Assessment.   The basic consideration in assessing cardiovascular function is monitoring the patient for signs of shock and hemorrhage. The chief guides are the patient's appearance and determinations of pulse, respiration, blood pressure, temperature, central venous pressure (CVP), and blood gas. CVP and blood gas values are monitored if the patient's condition requires such assessment. The pulse and respiration are noted at frequent intervals for the first 2 hours, and every ½ hour for the next 2 hours. Thereafter, they may be taken less frequently if they remain stable. The blood pressure is taken as often as indicated.

- A temperature over 37.7°C (100°F) or under 36.1°C (97°F), respirations over 30 or under 16, and a falling systolic blood pressure under 90 are usually considered reportable at once. However, the patient's preoperative or baseline blood pressure should be known in order to make effective postoperative comparisons.
- A blood pressure that shows a downward trend of 5 mm Hg at each reading should also alert the nurse to a problem.

The general condition of the patient is assessed and recorded, including whether color is good or cyanotic, skin is cold and clammy or warm and moist, or there is excessive mucus in the throat and in the nostrils.

▷ Nursing Diagnoses

Based on the assessment data, major nursing diagnoses might include entries such as the following:

- Ineffective airway clearance related to depressant effects of medications and anesthetic agent
- Alteration in comfort: Pain and other postoperative discomforts
- Potential for injury related to postanesthesia status
- Alteration in tissue perfusion, systemic, secondary to hypovolemia, peripheral blood pooling, and possibly vasoconstriction
- Potential fluid volume deficit
- Alteration in nutrition: Less than body requirement
- Alteration in pattern of urinary elimination: Retention related to decreased activity, effects of drugs, and reduced intake of fluids
- Alteration in bowel elimination: Constipation related to

decreased gastric and intestinal motility during intraoperative period
- Impaired skin integrity related to the surgical incision and drainage exits
- Potential for infection: Wound related to susceptibility to bacterial invasion
- Impaired physical mobility related to depressant effects of anesthesia, decreased activity tolerance, and activity restriction required by therapeutic plan
- Anxiety related to postoperative experience, possible changes in life-style, and alteration in self-concept

▷ Planning and Implementation

▷ *Goals.*   The major goals of the patient may include optimum respiratory function, relief of pain and postoperative discomforts (nausea and vomiting, abdominal distention, hiccups), freedom from injury, maintenance of normal body temperature, maintenance of adequate tissue perfusion, maintenance of nutritional balance, return of normal urinary function, resumption of usual pattern of bowel elimination, maintenance of skin integrity and avoidance of infection, restoration of mobility within limitations of postoperative and rehabilitative plan, and abatement of anxiety and achievement of psychosocial well-being.

Nursing Interventions

Ensuring Optimum Respiratory Function

Measures to maintain a patent airway are carried out as described earlier in this chapter.

Promoting Lung Expansion.   To encourage lung expansion and exchange of gas, a variety of measures may be followed. For example, having the patient yawn or take sustained maximal inspirations (SMI) will create a negative intrathoracic pressure of minus 40 mm Hg and will expand lung volume to total capacity. During this maneuver, right atrial and pulmonary artery pressures decrease, while venous return and cardiac output (CO) increase.

At least every 2 hours the patient is turned and encouraged to take deep breaths. Coughing is also encouraged to dislodge mucus plugs. Careful splinting of abdominal or thoracic incision sites helps the patient to overcome the fear that the exertion of coughing might cause the wound to break open. Collaborative interventions include the administration of pain medications to permit more effective coughing and the administration of oxygen as prescribed to prevent or relieve hypoxemia or hypoxia. (It is important to remember that coughing is contraindicated in patients who have a head injury or have undergone head surgery, because of increasing intracranial pressure; in eye surgery patients, because of increasing intraocular pressure; and in plastic surgery patients, because of increasing tension on delicate tissues.)

Incentive Spirometry.   Incentive spirometry is a method by which the patient performs SMI and at the same time sees the results of his efforts as registered on the spirometer equipment. Such motivation encourages the patient to continue to take deep breaths in order to maximize voluntary lung expansion. The patient needs to be taught how to use the device for maximum effectiveness.

An example of this type of equipment is a deep-breathing

exerciser that shows the patient how well he is inhaling (Fig. 19-4). A goal is established toward which the patient works. First he exhales; then he places his lips around the mouthpiece and slowly inhales, trying to drive the piston on the device to a marked goal. Such a device offers several advantages:

(1) the patient is encouraged to participate actively in his own treatment; (2) since the device is preset and prescribed, it assures that the maneuver will be physiologically appropriate and repeated; and (3) it is a cost-effective way of preventing complications.

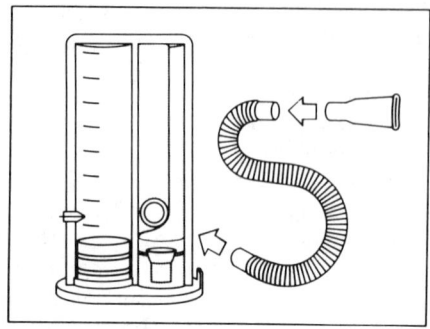

Remove components from package and attach mouthpiece to one end of tubing. Attach remaining free end of tubing to stem on front side of exerciser.

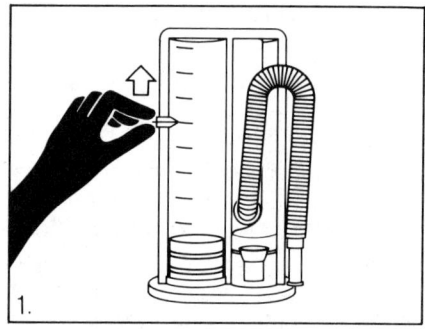

1. Slide the pointer of unit to prescribed volume level. Hold or stand exerciser in an upright position.

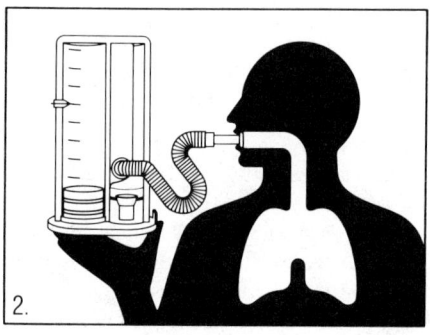

2. Exhale normally. Then place lips tightly around mouthpiece.

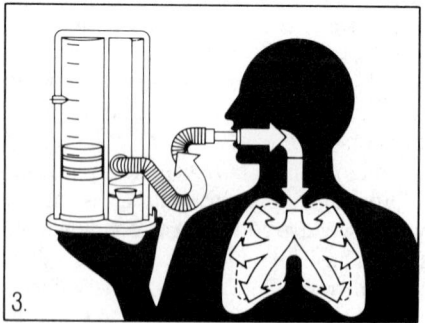

3. Inhale slowly, to raise the piston in the chamber.

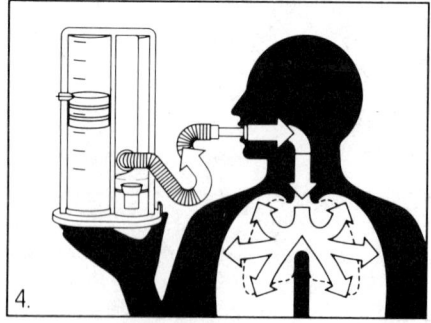

4. Continue inhaling and try to raise piston to prescribed level. Top of piston indicates level attained.

Figure 19-4
Volumetric Incentive Deep Breathing Exerciser (Voldyne). Follow instructions below each illustration. When inhalation is complete, remove mouthpiece, hold breath as prescribed, and exhale normally. Allow piston to return to bottom of chamber, rest, and repeat exercise. (Follow text for additional directives.)

▷ *Evaluation: Expected Outcomes*

The patient maintains optimum respiratory function.

- Performs deep-breathing exercises
- Displays clear breath sounds
- Uses incentive spirometer when necessary and as directed
- Maintains normal arterial blood gas values
- Exhibits normal chest x-rays
- Turns from one position to another as instructed
- Coughs effectively to clear secretions
- Exercises and ambulates every second hour
- Avoids persons with upper respiratory infections

Relief of Pain and Postoperative Discomforts

Relief of Pain. Many psychological factors (motivational, affective, cognitive, and emotional) influence the patient's total pain experience. Recent findings have led to a better understanding of how perception, learning, personality, ethnic and cultural factors, and even environment can affect anxiety, depression, and pain. The degree and severity of postoperative pain depends on the physiological and psychological makeup of the person, the subsequent tolerance level, the incision site, the nature of the operation, the extent of surgical trauma, the type of anesthetic agent and how it was administered. The preoperative preparation received by the patient (including information about what to expect as well as reassurance and psychological support) is a significant factor in decreasing anxiety, apprehension, and even the pain experienced in the postoperative period.

With regard to the need for narcotics, about one third of patients complain of severe pain, one third of moderate pain, and one third of little or no pain. These statistics do not mean that the patients in the last group have no pain; rather, they appear to activate psychodynamic mechanisms that impair the registering of pain ("gate closing" theory and impaired nociceptive transmission). It is interesting to note that one third of patients will receive relief from a placebo.

Morphine or meperidine hydrochloride (Demerol) often is prescribed for pain and immediate postoperative restlessness. The time of administration frequently is left to the judgment of the nurse, but one should realize that pain in the first 24 hours after an operation requires relief by narcotics, and these drugs should not be denied when the patient is in pain.

For thoracic and major abdominal surgery, morphine given by epidural infusion is effective. Relief of pain by this method permits the patient to breathe deeply without pain, which reduces postoperative lung complications. Complete pain relief in the operative region is seldom attainable for a few weeks, depending upon the site and nature of surgery; however, changing the patient's position, using diversionary methods, applying cool washcloths to the face, and rubbing the back with a soothing lotion may be useful in assuaging general discomfort temporarily and rendering the medication more effective when it is given. In addition, the extremities may be stroked very lightly with alcohol or lotion. *The legs should never be rubbed vigorously;* to do so may dislodge a thrombus and result in embolism and death.

Studies of the effectiveness of transcutaneous electrical nerve stimulation (TENS) in controlling pain show that patients using TENS have an easier time handling pain, reflected in less frequent requests for analgesics.

Relief of Restlessness. Restlessness is a postoperative symptom that is not to be passed over lightly. The most common cause probably is general discomfort from the operation owing to the patient's lying in one position on the operating table, the surgeon's handling of tissues, and the body's reaction to recovering from the anesthetic. These discomforts may be relieved by giving the prescribed postoperative sedation and changing the patient's position frequently. At the same time, the nurse assesses other possible contributing causes, such as tight, drainage-soaked bandages. Reinforcing or changing the dressing completely will make the patient more comfortable. Urinary output is noted and the patient is observed for urinary retention. Overdistention of the bladder is to be avoided. If possible, the patient should be helped to assume as normal a position as possible for voiding. Various techniques are tried to encourage voiding before resorting to catheterization.

Relief of Nausea and Vomiting. With the advent of other anesthetic agents and antiemetic drugs, vomiting has become a less common postoperative phenomenon, although inadequate ventilation during anesthesia can increase the incidence of vomiting. Also, the vomiting that occurs as the patient comes out of anesthesia is frequently an attempt to relieve the stomach of the mucus and saliva swallowed during the anesthetic period.

Other causes of postoperative vomiting include an accumulation of fluid in the stomach, inflation of the stomach, and the ingestion of food and fluid before peristalsis returns. Psychological factors also may play a role; the patient who expects to vomit postoperatively usually will. Thus, helpful preoperative instruction can reduce the probability of vomiting after surgery.

After surgery, simple symptomatic therapy is usually all that is required. Many authorities believe that most antiemetic drugs (usually derivatives of phenothiazine) promote more undesirable effects, such as hypotension and respiratory depression. If a medication is required, short-acting barbiturates are often prescribed. Droperidol (Inapsine) may be prescribed for intravenous or intramuscular use to produce tranquilization and reduce the incidence of nausea and vomiting. The drug may be given preoperatively and during surgery; its effects carry over into the postoperative period.

- Following the slightest indication of nausea, the patient is turned completely on one side to increase mouth drainage.
- The most important nursing intervention required when vomiting occurs is to prevent aspiration of vomitus, which can cause asphyxiation and death (see p. 500).

After the airway is removed, the patient is usually turned to the side-lying position to provide effective drainage from the throat and to help prevent the tongue from slipping backwards and irritating the pharynx or possibly obstructing the airway. If the patient is in a prone position, such as is generally used for children following tonsillectomy, adequate mouth drainage is provided by the position itself. However, to facilitate breathing, a pillow may be placed under the abdomen to permit the chest to expand.

When vomiting is likely because of the nature of surgery, a nasogastric tube is passed beforehand and remains in place throughout the operative procedure and the immediate postoperative period.

Vomiting requires no special treatment beyond rinsing out the mouth and withholding fluids for a few hours. The main danger, as already indicated, is from aspiration of the vomitus. Thus, precautions are necessary even before the patient begins to vomit.

In an emergency situation, a patient may be brought to the operating room with food in his stomach. Some anesthesiologists administer preoperative oral antacids to counteract the acid-aspiration syndrome. Otherwise, if acid from the vomitus is inhaled into the lungs it causes an asthmalike attack, with severe bronchial spasms and wheezing. Patients can subsequently develop pneumonitis and pulmonary edema and become extremely hypoxic.

Increasing medical attention is being paid to silent regurgitation of gastric contents because it occurs more frequently than was previously realized. The importance of *pH* in the etiology of acid aspiration is being studied, as is the value of administering an H_2-receptor antagonist such as cimetidine preoperatively.

Relief of Abdominal Distention.   Postoperative distention of the abdomen results from the accumulation of gas in the intestinal tract. Manipulation of the abdominal organs during the operation may produce a loss of normal peristalsis for 24 to 48 hours, depending on the type and the extent of surgery. Even though nothing is given by mouth, swallowed air and gastrointestinal secretions enter the stomach and the intestines; if not propelled by peristaltic activity they collect in the intestinal coils, producing distention and causing the patient to complain of fullness or pain in the abdomen. Most often the gas collects in the colon; hence, a rectal tube or catheter may give relief (Fig. 19-5).

After major abdominal surgery, distention may be avoided by having the patient turn frequently, exercise, and, when permissible, ambulate. Distention may be anticipated preoperatively and therefore a nasogastric tube may be inserted prior to surgery. Swallowing of air (often done by patients as part of an anxiety reaction) provides most of the gas

that produces distention. The nasogastric tube may be retained until full peristaltic activity (passage of flatus) has resumed.

Another nursing action to relieve distention is as follows. Because of the anatomic structure of the colon, a gas bubble will move from the lower right side upward to the hepatic flexure, and then proceed to the left splenic flexure and down the left side to the rectum. Gas movement can be facilitated by having the patient lie on the back with legs extended and a pillow placed under the knees. The right leg is slowly flexed at the knee, and the knee is pulled toward the abdomen. The patient holds the knee on the abdomen for 10 seconds before slowly lowering and extending the leg. After 3 or 4 deep breaths, the exercise is repeated with the other leg. After doing this 3 or 4 times, the patient rests. This may be repeated several times. With this exercise gas has a tendency to be moved and expelled. Another method that is often helpful is to gently massage the abdomen in the same direction as gas moves in the colon.

Relief of Hiccups.   *Hiccup* is produced by intermittent spasms of the diaphragm and is manifested by a coarse sound (an audible "hic"), a result of the vibration of the closed vocal cords as the air rushes suddenly into the lungs. The cause of the diaphragmatic spasm may be any irritation of the phrenic nerve from its center in the spinal cord to its terminal ramifications on the undersurface of the diaphragm. This irritation may be (1) direct—such as stimulation of the nerve itself by a distended stomach, peritonitis or subdiaphragmatic abscess, abdominal distention, pleurisy, or tumors in the chest pressing on the nerves; (2) indirect—such as from toxemia or uremia that stimulates the center; or (3) reflexive—such as irritation from a drainage tube, exposure to cold, drinking very hot or very cold fluids, or obstruction of the intestines.

Hiccup occurs occasionally after abdominal operations. Often it occurs in mild transitory attacks that cease spontaneously or with very simple treatment. When hiccups persist,

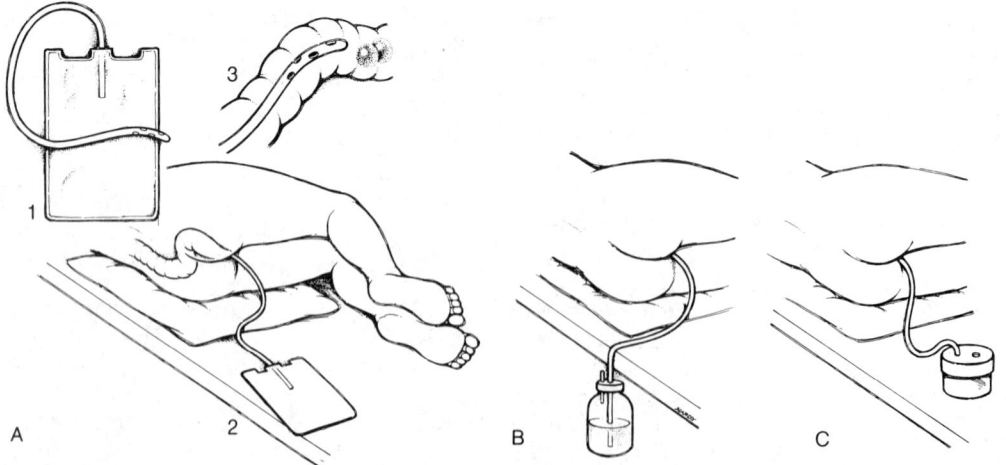

Figure 19-5
Relief of abdominal distention. (*A*) 1—Rectal tube or catheter attached to plastic bag; 2—tube/catheter in place, patient lying on left side; 3—enlargement of lower colon showing gas bubbles that will be tapped by rectal tube/catheter. (*B*) Tubing or catheter connected to a water bottle with vent. (*C*) Tubing or catheter connected to a plastic receptacle.

they may produce considerable distress and serious effects, such as vomiting, acid–base and fluid imbalance, malnutrition, exhaustion, and possibly wound dehiscence.

The multitude of remedies suggested for the relief of this condition is proof that no one treatment is effective in every situation. The best remedy is to eliminate causes, such as not administering fluids that are too hot or too cold. Probably the most efficient of the older and simpler remedies is to hold the breath while taking large swallows of water. Prescription of phenothiazine drugs has been helpful on occasion. Another method is finger pressure on the eyeballs, applied through closed lids for several minutes. Induced vomiting has helped in some instances. If these are not successful, more drastic medical measures may need to be tried.

Freedom from Injury. A patient coming out of anesthesia may display restless behavior. If at all possible he should not be restrained, but he must be protected from injuring himself or interfering with IV therapy, tubes, and monitoring equipment. Analgesics and sedatives are administered as prescribed. Attention is given to possible causes of discomfort that can affect subconscious cognition, such as dressings that are too tight, pressure on a nerve due to improper positioning, irritating drainage, leakage of IV fluids, a hot water bag that is too hot, and so forth. Through careful monitoring as the patient emerges from the anesthetic, the nurse can detect problems before they can cause injury. This helps to prevent subsequent litigation, since the nurse can be held liable for patient injuries due to negligence.

▷ *Evaluation: Expected Outcomes*
The patient experiences relief of pain and postoperative discomforts.

- Indicates that pain is much relieved
- Splints incision site when coughing to prevent pain
- Participates in diversionary measures (*e.g.*, conversation, television)
- Reports absence of nausea; no vomiting
- Is free of abdominal distress/gas pains
- Demonstrates the absence of hiccups
- Avoids injury
- Accepts side rails in "up" position when required
- Is free from injury related to faulty position, falling, other hazards
- Attains normal sensorium

Maintenance of Adequate Tissue Perfusion

The patient is monitored for any signs and symptoms suggesting diminished tissue perfusion: a decreasing blood pressure, rapid or labored respirations, resting pulse greater than 100 beats per minute, restlessness, slow responses, cold, clammy, pale, or cyanotic skin, diminished or absent peripheral pulses, urine output less than 30 ml/hr. Any such signs and symptoms are reported.

Measures are initiated to maintain adequate tissue perfusion. Room temperature is kept comfortable and the patient is provided with sufficient clothing and blankets to prevent chilling, which causes vasoconstriction. The effects of fluid and blood replacement therapy are monitored. Activities are initiated to stimulate circulation, such as leg exercises learned preoperatively; the patient is encouraged to turn and change position slowly, and to avoid positions that compromise ve-

nous return such as a raised knee gatch or pillow under the knees, sitting for long periods, and dangling legs with pressure in back of the knees. The patient is assisted in getting out of bed and walking if prescribed; antiembolic hose are applied if prescribed but removed about 1 hour out of every 8 and the legs lightly stroked.

The patient is observed for evidence of electrolyte imbalance: weakness, lassitude, nausea, vomiting, irritability, and possibly neuromuscular abnormalities. Monitoring of mental status, skin color, and temperature is continued, and the presence and quality of peripheral pulses are noted. Signs of decreasing tissue perfusion are reported. The obese patient, it should be remembered, perspires profusely and thus loses fluid and salt much more rapidly than the patient who is of normal weight.

- *Signs of hypovolemia:* Decreased blood pressure, tachycardia, reduced urinary output, CVP less than 4 cm H_2O
- *Signs of hypervolemia:* Increased blood pressure, CVP greater than 15 cm H_2O, crackles in lung bases (wet), an S_3 gallop

Maintenance of Adequate Fluid Volume. A considerable loss of body fluids occurs with surgery as a result of increased perspiration, increased mucus secretion in the lungs, and loss of blood. To combat the loss of fluids, solutions are given intravenously for the first few hours after operation. Even though an adequate amount of fluid is taken by this method, often it does not relieve thirst. Thirst is also a troublesome symptom after many general anesthetics, and even after local anesthesia. It stems largely from the dryness of the mouth and the pharynx caused by the inhibition of mucus secretion after the usual preoperative medication of atropine. Many patients operated on under local anesthesia complain of thirst during the operation.

Because a sticky, dry mouth demands moisture, fluids may be given to most patients as soon as the postoperative nausea and vomiting have passed. Sips of hot tea with lemon juice helps to dissolve the mucus better than cold water. As soon as the patient can take water by mouth in sufficient quantities, parenteral administration is discontinued.

Maintenance of Normal Body Temperature. Patients who have been anesthetized are susceptible to chills and drafts. If the patient had undergone prolonged exposure to cold in the OR and received large amounts of intravenous infusions, monitor for potential hypothermia. Report signs of hypothermia to the physician. Maintain comfortable room temperature and provide blankets as needed to prevent chilling.

▷ *Evaluation: Expected Outcomes*
The patient maintains adequate tissue perfusion.

- Increases fluid intake gradually
- Maintains fluid balance; relieves thirst
- Voids adequately without use of catheter
- Displays no symptoms of hypovolemia
- Maintains normal body temperature

Maintenance of Nutritional Balance

Following surgery, the more rapidly the patient can accept his usual diet, the more quickly will his normal gastrointestinal function resume. The best way for the postoperative patient to take food is by mouth. This stimulates digestive juices and promotes gastric function and intestinal peristalsis. Exercise in bed or early ambulation also assists the digestive process and prevents such problems as distention "gas pains" and constipation. Chewing of food prevents parotitis (inflammation of the parotid glands), a formerly common postoperative problem that occurred in dehydrated patients who also practiced poor mouth hygiene.

The return to a normal dietary pattern should proceed at the pace set by the individual patient. Of course, the nature of surgery and the type of anesthesia directly affect the rate of return. Once the patient has completely recovered from the effects of anesthesia and is no longer nauseated, steps may be taken to restore a normal diet.

Liquids are usually the first substances desired and tolerated by the patient after operation. Water, fruit juices, and tea with lemon and sugar may be given in increasing amounts if vomiting does not occur. The fluids administered should be cool, not ice cold or tepid. Since fluids supply relatively few calories and are tolerated well, gelatin, junket, custard, and even buttered toast, milk, and creamed soups may be added gradually. As soon as the patient tolerates soft foods well, solid food may be given.

A well-balanced diet is provided and includes foods that have been selected and preferred by the patient. Usually it takes 2 to 3 days for appetite to return, so attractive trays are a therapeutic consideration.

- When surgery has been done on the gastrointestinal tract, fluids and food are not given until peristalsis returns.

The nurse can determine when peristaltic bowel sounds return by listening to the abdomen with a stethoscope. The presence of bowel sounds is reported so that the proper diet modification can be prescribed.

Usually, a nasogastric or gastrointestinal tube is in place for the first 24 to 48 hours following gastrointestinal surgery. Such decompression tubes remove flatus and secretions. Attention is given to the maintenance of proper fluid and electrolyte balance, and an attempt is made with parenteral fluids and perhaps even hyperalimentation to achieve this nutritional level (see Chap. 32).

When nothing is given by mouth postoperatively, conscientious mouth hygiene is required. A clean, refreshed mouth encourages eating and diminishes nausea. Weighing the patient daily provides an indication of level of progress.

▷ *Evaluation: Expected Outcomes*
The patient maintains nutritional balance.

- Resumes normal dietary patterns as appropriate
- Gains weight to recover the amount lost during the previous week
- Shows evidence of increased motility and absence of ileus

Return of Normal Urinary Function

The length of time a patient may be permitted to go without voiding after operation varies considerably with the type of operation performed.

- Generally, every effort must be made to avoid the use of a catheter.

All known methods to aid the patient in voiding should be tried—letting water run, applying heat to perineum. A patient should never be given a cold bedpan. When a patient complains of not being able to use the bedpan, it may be permissible to use a commode rather than resort to catheterization. Male patients are often permitted to sit up or stand beside the bed, but safeguards should be taken to prevent falling or fainting.

- All urine, whether voided or catheterized, must be measured and the amount noted on the nurse's record.
- An intake and output chart is kept on all patients following urologic or complex operative procedures and on all aged persons.
- A urine output of less than 30 ml for each of 2 consecutive hours is reported.

▷ *Evaluation: Expected Outcomes*
Normal urinary function returns.

- Voids adequately without use of a catheter
- Demonstrates absence of frequent small amounts in voiding (indicative of retention)
- Assumes responsibility for adequate intake of fluids

Resumption of Usual Pattern of Bowel Elimination

Preoperative bowel preparation, immobility, intestinal manipulation during surgery, and reduced oral intake can all affect bowel function. Increased fluid intake and early ambulation can facilitate the return of bowel sounds and peristalsis. Abdominal auscultation using a stethoscope assists the nurse in determining the presence of bowel sounds; if sounds are heard, the patient's diet is gradually increased.

Paralytic ileus is a complication that may occur after intestinal or abdominal surgery. It is characterized by the absence of bowel sounds (no peristalsis) and discomfort and distention of the abdomen (denoted by increased abdominal girth). The condition may even result in reverse peristalsis, which causes nausea and vomiting, and possibly the vomiting of fecal material. Usually a nasogastric tube is inserted as prescribed; preparation for intravenous hyperalimentation may be in order.

Constipation. The causes of constipation after operation may be minor or serious. Irritation and trauma to the bowel at the time of the operation may inhibit intestinal movement for several days, but usually peristaltic function returns after the third day, following the combined effect of early ambulation, perhaps a simple enema, and an increase in diet. Local inflammation, peritonitis, or abscess may cause constipation, in which case treatment of the causal condition is indicated.

- Constipation has been described as a constant symptom of complete intestinal obstruction.

It must be borne in mind, also, that many people are constipated habitually and often give a history of having taken some form of laxative drug every day for years. Attempts should be made to correct their bowel habits as soon as is practical. However, in some instances, especially with elderly patients, these attempts may not be feasible. Enemas usually are effective in evacuating the lower bowel.

- Cathartic drugs should not be given unless prescribed by the physician.

▷ *Evaluation: Expected Outcomes*

The patient resumes normal bowel function.

- Exhibits normal and effective bowel sounds on auscultation
- Is free of abdominal distress, gas pains, and constipation
- Is able to demonstrate former usual bowel elimination process

Avoidance of Infection and Maintenance of Skin Integrity

Between 10% and 15% of surgical patients will develop nosocomial (hospital-acquired) infections. Most of these will be in one of four anatomical sites: surgical wound, urinary tract, bloodstream, or respiratory tract. The infections occur for several reasons:

- Intact skin and mucous membranes have been invaded by tubes and catheters, by the disease process, or by the surgical operation.
- The effects of anesthesia and surgery reduce the resistance of the body.
- The patient environment is made up of many persons who have complicating and often chronic medical problems; consequently, the patient may be exposed to infection.
- The organisms that are found in hospital infections are widespread and resistant: *e.g., Staphylococcus aureus, Escherichia coli, Serratia marcescens, Pseudomonas, Klebsiella pneumoniae,* and *Proteus.*
- Poor hand washing practices and careless techniques are used.

When postoperative infections occur, healing is delayed, convalescence is prolonged, functional recovery may be impaired, and death may occur. These complications impose serious burdens on the patient, the family, other patients (cross-contamination and consequent cross-infections), hospital staff (the increased patient care and hospitalization required), and society as a whole (increased hospitalization, insurance costs, loss of manpower, and so on).

Each hospital must make an all-out effort to control infections by an intensive education program that reaches every employee. Usually an active infection control committee (including an epidemiologist) can be effective in establishing policies and procedures and monitoring practice.

Effective infection control is carried out postoperatively by encouraging the patient to cough, by frequent turning, and by deep breathing. These measures will prevent secretions from being retained and possibly causing atelectasis, lung congestion, and pneumonia. Use of sterile equipment (needles, cannulae, dressings), including equipment for respiratory management, will prevent transmission of pathogenic organisms. Antibiotics may be prescribed prophylactically by the physician when infected areas are encountered, and antimicrobials may be prescribed for specific identified organisms in established infections. *The nurse plays a key role in infection control by practicing flawless technique and by conscientiously monitoring and instructing others.*

- *Conscientious hand washing is essential for every person who comes in contact with patients and moves from one patient to the next.*

Dressings are inspected periodically to detect signs of undue hemorrhage or abnormal drainage. When incisions are on the anterior part of the body, the posterior area is checked for signs of bleeding, since gravity enables seepage to accumulate in an area quite removed from the incision. Dressings should be reinforced if necessary, and the time noted on the nurses' record. (Dressings and care of the incision are discussed in detail on p. 356.)

Judicious control of upper respiratory infections and skin lesions must be practiced. A most common cause of infections is contamination related to intravenous infusions (see p. 130 for methods of control).

▷ *Evaluation: Expected Outcomes*

The patient avoids infection and maintains skin integrity following the normal healing process.

- Shows evidence of minimal or no wound drainage
- Has no skin breakdown or infection
- Can identify initial symptoms of hematoma, injury, and infection
- Applies cocoa butter or other soothing ointments as prescribed
- Is afebrile with normal white blood cell count

Restoration of Mobility

Hampered by dressings, splints, or drainage apparatus, the patient frequently is unable to shift position. Lying constantly in the same position may lead to pressure sores or hypostatic pneumonia, to mention only two of the more serious resulting complications.

- The helpless patient must be turned from side to side at least every 2 hours, and his position must be changed as soon as he becomes uncomfortable.

Positioning.　Following surgery, the patient may be placed in a variety of positions (depending on the nature of the operation) to promote comfort and ease pain.

Supine Position.　The patient lies on his back without elevation of the head. In most cases this is the position in which the patient is placed immediately after operation. Bed covers should not restrict the movement of the patient's toes and feet.

Lateral Position.　The patient lies on either side with the upper arm forward. The underleg is slightly flexed, while the upper leg is flexed at the thigh and the knee. The head is supported on a pillow, and a second pillow is placed longitudinally between the legs. This position is used when it is desirable to have the patient change position frequently, to aid in the drainage of cavities, such as chest and abdomen, and to prevent postoperative pulmonary, respiratory, and circulatory complications.

Fowler's Position.　Of all the positions prescribed for a patient, perhaps the most common, as well as the most difficult to maintain, is Fowler's position. The difficulty in most instances lies in trying to make the patient fit the bed rather than having the bed conform to the needs of the patient. The patient's trunk is raised to form an angle of from 60° to 70° with the horizontal plane. This is a comfortable sitting position. Patients with abdominal drainage usually are put in Fowler's position as soon as they have recovered consciousness, but great caution must be observed in raising the bed.

· It is not unusual for a patient to feel faint after the head of the bed is raised; for this reason, a close watch must be kept on pulse rate and color. If the patient complains of any dizziness, the bed must be slowly lowered. If the dizziness ends, the head of the bed may be raised within 1 to 2 hours.

The nurse must determine whether the patient is in correct position and comfortable. Often, very short people are most uncomfortable in the ordinary hospital bed and must be supported by pillows. It is advisable to place a support against the feet to prevent the patient from slipping down in bed, to prevent foot drop, and to make the patient feel more secure.

It is the nurse's responsibility to see that the Fowler's position is maintained at all times. No matter how correctly placed or how well supported by pillows, the patient will slip down in the course of time. Thus it will be necessary to move the patient up in bed frequently and to readjust the pillows.

Ambulation. Most surgical patients are encouraged to be out of bed as soon as it is safe. This is determined by the stability of a patient's cardiovascular and neuromuscular systems, his usual level of physical activity, and the nature of the surgery performed. Following spinal anesthesia, minor surgery, and same-day surgery, the patient is ambulating the same day.

· The advantage of early ambulation is that it reduces postoperative complications such as atelectasis, hypostatic pneumonia, gastrointestinal discomfort, and circulatory problems.

Atelectasis and hypostatic pneumonia are relatively infrequent when the patient is ambulatory, since ambulation increases respiratory exchange and aids in preventing stasis of bronchial secretions within the lung. Ambulation also reduces the possibility of postoperative abdominal distention because it helps to increase the tone of the gastrointestinal tract and the abdominal wall.

Thrombophlebitis or phlebothrombosis occurs less frequently because ambulation, by increasing the rate of circulation in the extremities, prevents stasis of venous blood. Clinical as well as experimental evidence shows that the rate of healing in abdominal wounds is more rapid when ambulation is started early, and the occurrence of postoperative evisceration in a series of cases actually was less frequent when patients were allowed to be out of bed soon after operation. Statistics also indicate that pain is decreased when early ambulation is allowed. Comparative records show that the pulse rate and the temperature return to normal sooner when the patient attempts to regain normal preoperative activity as quickly as possible. Finally, there are the further advantages to the patient of a shorter stay in the hospital, with the consequent lower expense.

However, early ambulation should not be overdone. The condition of the patient must be the deciding factor, and a progression of steps must be followed in getting the patient out of bed.

1. First of all, with nursing support and encouragement, and with safety as the main concern, the patient moves gradually from the lying position to the sitting position until any evidence of dizziness has passed.

This position can be obtained by raising the head of the bed.

2. Then the patient may be placed completely upright and turned so that both legs hang over the edge of the bed.
3. After this preparation, the patient may be helped to stand beside the bed.

When accustomed to the upright position, the patient may start to walk. *The nurse should be at the patient's side to give physical support and encouragement.* Care must be taken not to tire the patient, and the extent of the first few periods of ambulation will vary with the type of operation and the patient's physical condition and age.

Bed Exercises. When early ambulation is not feasible because of circumstances already mentioned, bed exercises may achieve the same desirable results to some extent. General exercises should begin as soon after operation as possible—preferably within the first 24 hours—and are carried out under supervision to ensure their adequacy. These exercises are done to promote circulation and prevent the development of contractures and other deformities as well as to permit the patient the fullest return of physiologic functions. Such exercises include the following:

· Deep-breathing exercises for complete lung expansion.
· Arm exercises through full range of motion, with specific attention to abduction and external rotation of the shoulder.
· Hand and finger exercises.
· Foot exercises to prevent foot drop and toe deformities and to aid in maintaining good circulation. A plastic ball under the covers may be a help in reminding the patient to exercise leg muscles. Grasping the ball with the toes contracts calf muscles, stimulates circulation, and reduces venous stasis.
· Exercises to prepare the patient for ambulation activities.
· Abdominal and gluteal contraction exercises.

▷ *Evaluation: Expected Outcomes*

The patient resumes mobility within the limitations of the postoperative and rehabilitation plan.

· Resumes mobility; alternates periods of rest and activity
· Increases ambulation progressively
· Resumes normal activities within prescribed time frame
· Performs activities related to self-care
· Participates in a rehabilitation program (when pertinent)

Abatement of Anxiety and Achievement of Psychosocial Well-Being

Almost all postoperative surgical patients need psychological support during the immediate postoperative period. When the patient's condition permits, a close member of his family may see him for a few moments. Thus the family is reassured and the patient feels more secure.

The questions posed by an awakening patient often indicate his deep feelings and thoughts. Perhaps he shows concern about the outcome of the operation or about the future—whatever the patient's expression, the nurse should be in a position to answer queries reassuringly without going into a discussion of details. The immediate postoperative period is not the time for discussion of operative findings or prognosis. On the other hand, these questions ought not to be dismissed lightly because they may offer clues that suggest the method to select in directing future treatment and rehabilitation.

As the patient moves through the early postoperative phases, measures are implemented to provide feelings of stability. This is accomplished by assuring the patient that a nurse is available at all times to talk with him, to reinforce the explanations of the physician, and to correct any misconceptions he may have. He is instructed in relaxing techniques and diversional activities. Significant others are included in instructional sessions to assist the patient when he leaves the hospital. Projections are made about his adjustment and needs when he leaves the hospital. The nurse encourages the patient to verbalize his concerns about the recovery phase and his increasing assumption of his own care.

▷ *Evaluation: Expected Outcomes*
The patient attains/maintains psychosocial well-being.

- Participates in self-care activities
- Takes time for grooming
- Talks positively about future plans
- Ask questions about resuming sexual relations
- Expresses happiness in seeing friends and family

Documentation and Reporting of Data

Determining the significance of the signs and symptoms noted in assessing the patient is a matter of judgment. When viewed in isolation one sign may be of little importance, but in the broader context it may be the missing link in a very important total evaluation.

There are a few general rules that may be of some assistance in guiding the nurse to make accurate value judgments. Of course, any severe symptom always is important.

- Any apparently slight symptom that tends to recur repeatedly or to increase in severity should be regarded as significant—for example, hiccups may or may not be of importance, depending on their duration.
- A symptom may be of no consequence in itself but when associated with other definite changes may foretell danger. For example, a repeated sigh means nothing, but when accompanied by increasing restlessness, pallor, and a rising pulse rate, it becomes one of the clinical signs of dangerous hemorrhage.
- Any steadily progressive change for the worse in the general condition of the patient, even with no outstanding symptoms evident, is of the gravest importance.
- The patient's complaints and statements never should be passed over without investigation.

Recording information accurately and concisely not only informs all medical and nursing personnel of the patient's condition, but also satisfies medicolegal requirements.

If a physician is to be notified for any reason, all necessary information should be at hand before the telephone is picked up, including the latest vital signs and monitor readings. It is also advisable to take the patient's chart, including nursing records, to the telephone in order to refer to them should questions arise.

Gerontological Considerations

Transfer of the elderly patient from the operating room table to the bed is done *slowly* and *gently* while monitoring the effects of this action on blood pressure, observing facial expression (if the patient is awake), and watching for evidence of hypoxia. Special attention is given to keeping the patient warm, since body temperature in the elderly is labile. Position is changed frequently not only for comfort, because lying in one position can be painful, but to stimulate respirations and circulation.

Immediate postoperative care for the older adult is the same as that for any surgical patient, but additional support is given if there is impaired function of the cardiovascular, pulmonary, or renal systems.

With invasive monitoring, it is possible to detect cardiopulmonary deficit before obvious signs and symptoms are apparent. Because of monitoring and better individualized preoperative preparation, many older adults are tolerating surgery and recovering well.

Confusion is one of the most common experiences of an older postoperative patient. This is aggravated by social isolation, restraints, and sensory deprivation. It is important to recognize that nighttime confusion can be reduced by frequent nursing attention and caution in use of drugs, especially narcotic analgesics and sedatives.

Early mobilization is instituted to prevent pneumonia, the most frequent respiratory complication in the elderly. Keeping the patient active also prevents atelectasis, irritation of pressure areas, deep venous thrombosis, and undue weakness. Sitting positions that promote venous stasis in the lower extremities are to be avoided. *Ambulation means that the patient walks, not sits in a chair.* Adequate assistance is required to prevent bumping into things and falling.

Urinary incontinence can be prevented by providing easy access to the call bell, the commode, and the bathroom. Early ambulation and familiarity with the room help the patient to become self-sufficient sooner. Postoperative distention, reduced peristalsis, and fecal impaction can be prevented by promoting adequate hydration and activity.

During the early postoperative days the patient may complain of sore muscles. This is common and usually due to maintaining confined positions during the operation. Massaging aching parts *gently* and providing support with pillows can ease the discomfort.

Fluids and electrolytes are monitored to avoid the extremes of fluid overload and dehydration. The nurse compares previous documentation with current records to note changes in fluid balance and weight. It may be necessary to recommend physical therapy and intensive rehabilitation for patients undergoing prolonged convalescence.

Encouragement and positive thinking are always offered. The nurse gently challenges the older adult to recognize that participation in all activities can enhance recovery and prevent complications.

Care of the Wound

A *wound* may be described as a disruption in the continuity of cells; it follows, then, that *wound healing* is the restoration of that continuity.

When wounds occur, a variety of effects may result: (1) immediate loss of all or part of organ functioning, (2) sympathetic stress response, (3) hemorrhage and blood clotting, (4) bacterial contamination, and (5) death of cells. Careful asepsis is the most important factor in keeping these effects to a minimum and promoting the successful care of wounds.

Wound Classification

Wounds may be classified in two different ways: according to the manner in which they were made, and according to the likelihood and degree of wound contamination at the time of surgery.

Mechanism of Injury.   Wounds may be described as incised, contused, lacerated, or puncture.

- *Incised wounds* are made by a clean cut with a sharp instrument—for example, those made by the surgeon in every operation. Clean wounds (those made aseptically) are usually closed by sutures after all bleeding vessels have been ligated carefully.
- *Contused wounds* are made by blunt force and are characterized by considerable injury of the soft parts, hemorrhage, and swelling.
- *Lacerated wounds* are those with jagged, irregular edges, such as would be made by glass or barbed wire.
- *Puncture wounds* result in small openings in the skin— for example, those made by bullets or knife stabs.

Degree of Contamination.   Wounds may be described as clean, clean-contaminated, contaminated, or dirty or infected.*

- *Clean wounds* are uninfected surgical wounds in which there is no inflammation and the respiratory, alimentary, genital, or uninfected urinary tracts are not entered. Clean wounds are primarily closed; if necessary, they are drained with closed drainage. The relative probability of wound infection is 1% to 5%.
- *Clean-contaminated wounds* are surgical wounds in which the respiratory, alimentary, genital, or urinary tract is entered under controlled conditions; there is no unusual contamination. The relative probability of wound infection is 3% to 11%.
- *Contaminated wounds* include open, fresh, accidental wounds, and operations with major breaks in aseptic technique or gross spillage from the gastrointestinal tract; in this category are also incisions in which there is acute, nonpurulent inflammation. The relative probability of wound infection is 10% to 17%.
- *Dirty or infected wounds* are those in which the organisms that caused postoperative infection were present in the operative field before surgery. These include old traumatic wounds with retained devitalized tissue and those that involve existing clinical infections or perforated viscera. The relative probability of wound infection is over 27%. (See Wound Sepsis, p. 361.)

Treatment.   *Prophylactic antibiotics* are administered when bacterial contamination is expected, or for the patient

* (Centers for Disease Control: Guidelines for Prevention of Surgical Wound Infection. Washington, DC, U.S. Department of Health and Human Services, 1985.)

with a clean wound in which a prosthetic device is being inserted.

When wounds are potentially infected, they cannot be closed until every effort has been made to remove all devitalized and infected tissue. Therefore, a formal operation is performed for the purpose of cutting out the infected and devitalized tissue. This operation is called *debridement.* Often a small drain is inserted before the wound is sutured to prevent lymph and blood from collecting and retarding the healing process.

Physiology of Wound Healing

Various continuous and overlapping cellular processes contribute to the restoration of a wound: cell regeneration, cell proliferation, and collagen production. The response of tissue to injury goes through several phases: inflammatory, proliferative, and maturation (Table 19-1). See also Chapter 7.

Inflammatory Phase.   Vascular and cellular responses occur immediately when tissue is cut or injured. Vasoconstriction of vessels occurs with a deposition of a fibrinoplatelet clot in an attempt to control bleeding. This lasts from 5 to 10 minutes and is followed by vasodilatation of the venules. Microcirculation loses its tonus because norepinephrine is destroyed by the intracellular enzymes. Also, histamine and serotonin are released, which act directly on microcirculation.

When there is damage to microcirculation, blood elements such as antibodies, plasma proteins, electrolytes, complement, and water permeate the vascular space for 2 to 3 days, causing edema, warmth, redness, and pain.

Polymorphonuclear granulocytes and erythrocytes are the first leukocytes to appear. If there is no infection they decline in numbers; monocytes that transform to macrophages engulf the debris and transport it from the area. Antigen-antibodies also appear.

Basal cells at wound edges undergo mitosis, and the resulting daughter cells migrate. With this activity proteolytic enzymes are secreted, which dissolve the base of blood clots. The gap between both sides of the wound is progressively filled, and the sides eventually meet in 24 to 48 hours. At this point, cell migration is replaced by cell mitosis.

Proliferative Phase.   Fibroblasts multiply and form a lattice framework for migrating cells. Epithelial cells form buds at the edges of the wound; these buds develop into

TABLE 19-1
Phases of Wound Healing

Phase	Also Referred to As	Length of Time
Inflammatory	Lag Exudative	1–4 days
Proliferative	Fibroblastic Connective tissue	5–20 days
Maturation	Differentiation Resorptive Remodeling Plateau	21 days to months and even years

capillaries, the nutritional source for the new granulation tissue.

Collagen is the primary component of replaced connective tissue. Fibroblasts initiate the synthesis of collagen and mucopolysaccharides. In a 2- to 4-week period, amino acid chains collect into fibers of increasing length and diameter; these become a well-structured pattern of packed bundles. The synthesis of collagen causes capillaries to reduce in number. Thereafter, collagen decreases in an attempt to balance the amount of collagen that is destroyed. Such synthesis and lysis result in increased tensile strength. However, after 2 weeks the wound has only 3% to 5% of the original skin strength. By the end of a month only 35% to 59% of wound strength has been reached. Never more than 70% to 80% of strength is regained.

Many vitamins, particularly vitamin C, aid in the metabolic process involved in wound healing.

Maturation Phase. At this time (3 weeks after injury) fibroblasts begin to leave the wound. The scar appears large, but collagen fibrils reorganize into tighter positions. This, along with dehydration, reduces the scar but increases its strength. Such tissue maturation continues and reaches maximum strength in 10 or 12 weeks, but it never reaches the original strength of the prewound tissue.

Forms of Healing

In the surgical management of wound healing, wounds are described as healing by first, second, or third intention.

Healing by First Intention (Primary Union). Wounds made aseptically, with a minimum of tissue destruction and properly coapted, as with sutures, heal with very little tissue reaction "by first intention" (Fig. 19-6). When wounds heal by first intention, granulation tissue is not visible and scar formation is minimal.

Healing by Second Intention (Granulation). In wounds in which pus formation (suppuration) has occurred or in which the edges have not been approximated, the process of repair is less simple and is delayed. When an abscess is incised it collapses partly, but the dead and the dying cells forming its walls are still being released into the cavity. For this reason, rubber tubes, rubber tissue, or gauze packing often is inserted into the abscess pocket to allow the pus to escape easily. Gradually the necrotic material disintegrates and escapes, and the abscess cavity fills with a red, soft, sensitive tissue that bleeds very easily. It is composed of minute, thin-walled capillaries growing off from the parent vessels, each bud surrounded by cells that later form connective tissue. These buds, called *granulations,* enlarge until they fill the area left by the destroyed tissue (see Fig. 19-6). The cells surrounding the capillaries change their round shape; they become long and thin, intertwining with each other to form a *scar* or *cicatrix.* Healing is complete when skin cells (epithelium) grow over these granulations. This method of repair is called *healing by granulation,* and it takes place whenever pus is formed or when loss of tissue has occurred for any reason.

Healing by Third Intention (Secondary Suture). If a deep wound either has not been sutured early or breaks down and then is resutured later, two apposing granulation surfaces are brought together. This results in a deeper and wider scar (see Fig. 19-6).

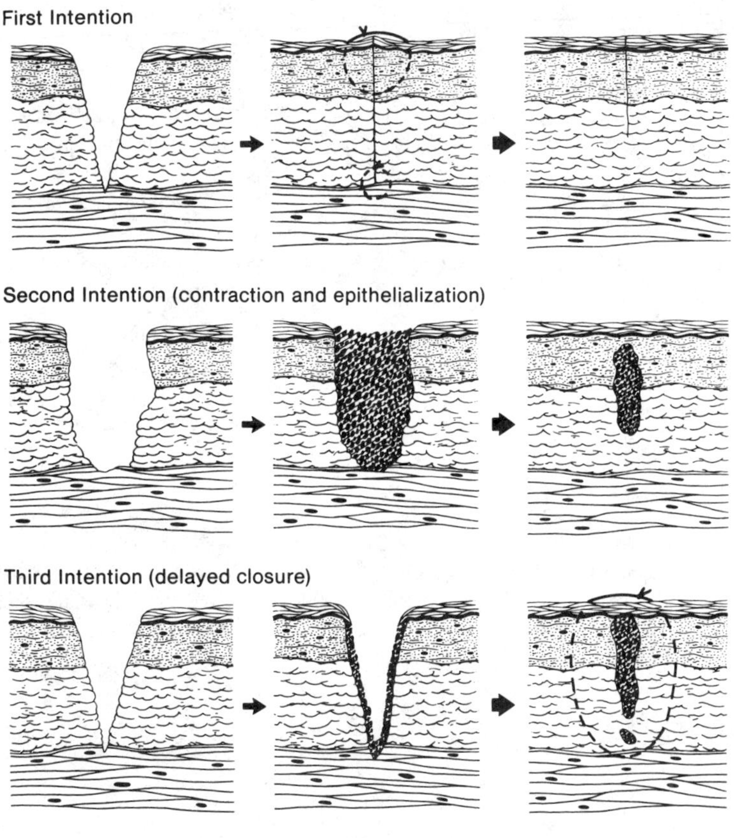

First Intention

Second Intention (contraction and epithelialization)

Third Intention (delayed closure)

Figure 19-6
Classification of wound healing. *First intention*—A clean incision is made with primary closure; there is minimal scarring. *Second intention* (contraction and epithelialization)—The wound is left open to granulate in with resultant large scab and abnormal dermal–epidermal junction. *Third intention* (delayed closure)—The wound is left open and closed secondarily when there is no evidence of infection. (Hardy JD. Hardy's Textbook of Surgery, p 109. Philadelphia, JB Lippincott, 1983.)

Nursing Management and Its Effect on Wound Healing

As a wound moves through the phases of healing, many elements, such as adequate nutrition, cleanliness, rest, and position, determine how quickly the process occurs. These factors are influenced by nursing interventions. Specific nursing assessments and interventions that address these factors and help to promote wound healing are presented in Chart 19-1. Methods for reducing the incidence of wound infection are described in Chart 19-2.

Dressings

The Purposes of an Effective Dressing

A dressing is applied to a wound for one or more of the following reasons: (1) to provide a proper environment for wound healing; (2) to absorb drainage; (3) to splint or immobilize the wound; (4) to protect the wound and new epithelial tissue from mechanical injury; (5) to replace the old dressing, in order to prevent adherence of the old dressing to the wound as ingrowth of new tissue occurs; (6) to protect

Chart 19-1
Factors Affecting Wound Healing

Factors	Rationale	Nursing Assessment/Interventions
Age of Patient	The older the patient, the less resilient the tissues	Handle all tissues gently.
Handling of Tissues	Rough handling causes injury and delayed healing.	Handle tissues carefully and evenly.
Hemorrhage	Accumulation of blood creates dead spaces as well as dead cells that must be removed. The area becomes a culture medium for infection.	Monitor vital signs. Observe incision site for evidence of bleeding.
Hypovolemia	Insufficient blood volume leads to vasoconstriction and reduced oxygen and nutrients available for wound healing.	Monitor for volume deficit (circulatory impairment). Correct by fluid replacement as prescribed.
Local Factors Edema	Constricts blood supply by exerting increased interstitial pressure on vessels	Elevate part; apply cool compresses.
Inadequate Dressing Technique Too Small	Permits bacterial invasion and contamination	Follow guidelines for proper dressing technique, p. 358.
Too Tight	Reduces blood supply carrying nutrients and oxygen	
Nutritional Deficits	Insulin secretion may be inhibited, causing blood glucose to rise. Protein-calorie depletion may occur.	Monitor blood glucose levels. Administer vitamins A & C supplements as prescribed. Correct deficits: this may require parenteral nutritional therapy.
Foreign Bodies	Foreign bodies adversely affect healing.	Keep wounds free of dressing threads, talcum, and starch from gloves.
Oxygen Deficit Tissue-Oxygenation Insufficient Growth of Microorganisms	Inadequate oxygen may be due to inadequate lung and cardiovascular function as well as localized vasoconstriction.	Encourage deep breathing, turning, controlled coughing. Monitor portable and other closed drainage systems for proper functioning.

(continued)

the wound from bacterial contamination and soiling by feces, vomitus, and urine; (7) to promote hemostasis, as in a pressure dressing; (8) to maintain proper moisture conditions at the wound surface; and (9) to provide mental and physical comfort for the patient.

Some surgeons prefer to eliminate dressings during the immediate postoperative period whenever feasible. Examples of circumstances in which dressings are not necessary are facial lacerations, pedicle flaps (see skin grafts, p. 1281), or skin grafts on a smooth surface.

When the initial dressing on a clean, dry incision is removed, often it is not replaced. Generally, initial dressings on clean, dry incisions are left in place until the wound edges are sealed and the wound is healing (usually 24 hours for most wounds).

The apparent advantages of not using any dressings include the following: (1) it eliminates the conditions necessary for growth of organisms (warmth, moisture, and darkness); (2) it allows for better observation and early detection of wound difficulties; (3) it facilitates bathing; (4) it tends to minimize the operative procedure; (5) it avoids adhesive-tape reaction; (6) it appears to be more comfortable for the patient and facilitates his activity; and (7) it is economical.

In spite of the advantages of not using a dressing, most

Chart 19-1 *(continued)*

Factors	Rationale	Nursing Assessment/Interventions
Drainage Collection	Malfunctioning drainage	Institute measures to remove accumulated secretions.
Drugs: Steroids	May mask presence of infection by impairing normal inflammatory response to injury	Be aware of action/effect of medications patient is receiving.
Anticoagulants	May cause hemorrhage	
Broad-Spectrum/Specific Antibiotics	Effective if given immediately before surgery for specific pathology or bacterial contamination If given after wound is closed, ineffective because of intravascular coagulation	
Patient Overactivity	Prevents wound edges from approximating Resting favors healing.	Utilize measures to keep wound edges approximated: taping, bandaging, splints. Encourage rest.
Systemic Disorders Hemorrhagic Shock Acidosis Hypoxia Renal Failure Hepatic Disease Sepsis	These are depressants of cell function that directly affect wound healing.	Be familiar with the nature of the specific disorder. Administer prescribed treatment. Cultures may be requested to determine proper antibiotic.
Immunosuppressive Therapy	Patient is more vulnerable to bacterial/viral invasion; defense mechanisms are reduced.	Provide maximum protection to prevent infection. Restrict visitors with colds; institute mandatory hand-washing of all attendants.
Wound Stressors Vomiting Valsalva Maneuver Heavy Coughing Straining	Produce tension on wounds, particularly of the torso	Encourage frequent turning, ambulation, and antiemetic medications.

Chart 19-2
Effective Methods of Lowering Incidence of Wound Infection

GOALS: Reduce risks that inhibit wound healing.
Lower incidence of wound infections.

Interventions	*Rationale*
Preoperative	
Shorter preoperative hospitalization	Reduces exposure of patient to nosocomial infections.
Treatment of coexistent infections	Infections, such as respiratory, can initiate pulmonary complications.
Avoid shaving of hair; if necessary, remove hair with clippers or depilatories rather than a razor.	The fewer nicks and cuts in the skin, the less opportunity for infection.
If shaving is requested, it is to be done immediately before the operation.	The longer the time between shaving and the operation, the greater the incidence of infection.
Thorough cleansing of operative site—Betadine shower the evening before and repeated preoperative cleansing with antiseptic detergents	Resident bacteria and skin contaminants are reduced to a minimum.
Prophylactic antibiotics	
Intraoperative	
Cleanse operative site thoroughly to remove superficial flora, soil, and debris.	To reduce risk of contaminating the wound with patient's skin flora.
Flawless aseptic technique.	Any breaks in technique can initiate infection by introducing contaminants.
Powder or talcum washed off sterile gloves	Foreign particles in a wound, such as talcum or starch, will adversely affect the healing process.
Bleeding controlled with meticulous hemostasis.	A clean wound heals without infection.
Drains eliminated in clean wounds	Drains are associated with higher wound infection rates.
Closure delayed in contaminated wounds	Permits healing from base of wound to exterior—otherwise, pocket or infection may develop.

---

surgeons prefer to apply a dressing at the time of operation and a second dressing between 4 and 6 days later, after the removal of sutures. Stitches (black silk, nylon, or fine wire) or metal skin clips used to approximate the skin edges are of little value after the sixth or seventh day and are therefore removed. The dressings are purely protective from a functional point of view, and they give the patient a sense of security that is not present if wounds are treated without dressings.

The suture line is gently cleansed and swabbed at prescribed intervals until drainage ceases. When sutures are removed (before the 7th day), center sutures are removed first and replaced with steristrips to keep the tender incision line reinforced (Fig. 19-7). Thereafter, the incision line may be swabbed with tincture of benzoin for protection until complete healing has taken place.

Gas- and vapor-permeable dressings that are impermeable to liquids and bacteria are available (Op-site, Tegaderm, Bioclusive). These dressings, which resemble clear plastic film, are made of polyurethane film that is coated on one side with a hypoallergenic, water-resistant adhesive. Being highly elastic, they conform easily to body contours. They are used most commonly as coverings for arterial and venous catheter sites, pressure ulcers, skin around stomas and fistulas, skin graft donor sites, and surgical wounds. Their chief ad-

vantages are that the wound is visible so infection can be detected early and treated promptly, and patients can bathe with these dressings in place.

Odor-absorbent dressings consisting of carbon granules embedded in foam matrix are also available. Another specialty dressing provides a pouch that collects excess fluid from the wound and permits its evaporation.

Surgical Dressings—Nursing Interventions

Although all initial postoperative dressings are done by the surgeon with the nurse as assistant, subsequent applications may be done by the nurse. The condition of surgical dressings and wounds is documented as carefully as is any medication or treatment.

Preparation of the Patient. The patient is told that the dressing is to be changed and that it is a simple procedure associated with little discomfort. The dressing change is scheduled for a suitable time. *Dressings should not be done at mealtime.* If the patient is in an open unit, the curtains are drawn to ensure privacy and to accommodate the patient's sense of modesty. In this regard, the patient should not be exposed unduly. When the dressing has a foul odor or the patient is unusually squeamish, it is better to take the patient

Figure 19-7
Removing stitches. (*A*) With the hemostat or forceps, lift the stitch upward and away from the skin surface. This permits the blades of the scissors to slide under the stitch (*B*) and cut it near the skin. (*C*) Using the hemostat, pull the freed stitch up and out.

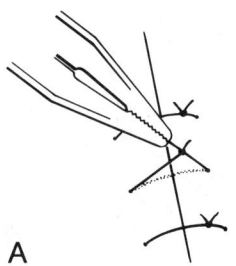 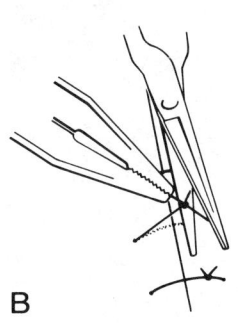 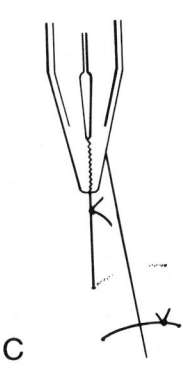

A   B   C

to the treatment room, away from other patients. At no time should the incision be referred to as a "scar," since for some patients the term has ugly or undesirable connotations.

Removal of Adhesive Dressings. The adhesive is removed by pulling it parallel with the skin surface and in the direction of hair growth, rather than at right angles (Fig. 19-8). Nonirritating solvents available in aerosol containers aid in removing adhesive tapes painlessly and quickly.

The old dressing and the pledgets used in cleaning the wound are removed by means of a forceps and are then deposited in a waterproof bag for easy disposal by burning. Such dressings are never touched by ungloved hands because of the danger of transmitting pathogenic organisms. After instruments are used in the changing of dressings they are placed in a bag or covered receptacle, not on surfaces where contamination of clean areas is possible. Disposable instruments are discarded in the proper receptacle.

A Simple Dressing. The routine dressing requires cotton balls, dressings, and perhaps a solution container, along with such instruments as a scissors, forceps, hemostat, and

**Loosen all ends of tape.
Gently pull toward wound.**

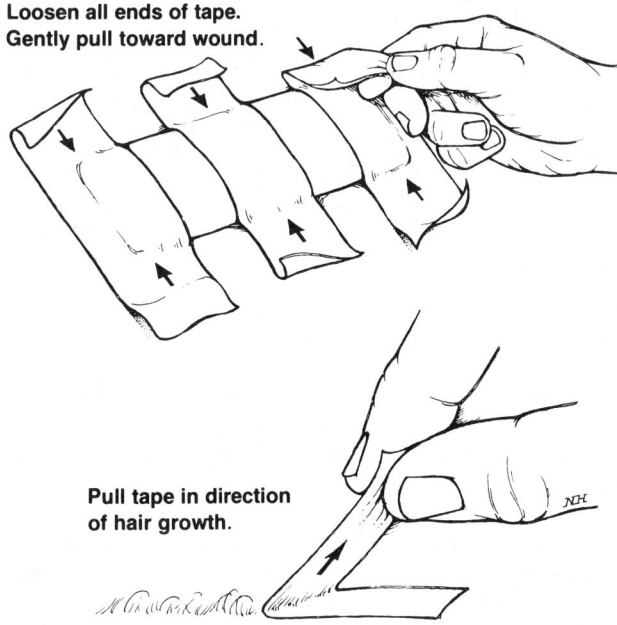

**Pull tape in direction
of hair growth.**

Figure 19-8
Removing adhesive tape.

possibly a probe. When the tray has been properly opened, the person changing the dressing grasps a cotton ball with a forceps and holds it over the emesis basin as the assistant pours a small quantity of the desired antiseptic. After the wound and surrounding skin are cleansed with an antiseptic, the sutures are removed and a new dressing is applied.

- *All wound dressings are changed only with sterile gloves.*
- *If there is any doubt about the sterility of an instrument or a dressing, it is considered unsterile.*
- *In no circumstances should the nurse touch soiled dressings with ungloved hands.*

Tape is used to keep dressings in place. A variety of tapes are available for patients who are sensitive to the rubber base in adhesive tape. Many tapes are porous and thus permit ventilation and prevent maceration. Tension sutures are allowed to remain in place for a longer period of time in some instances.

The Dressing of Draining Wounds. The risk of wound infection is reduced if there is adequate drainage. The wound needs to drain freely to release accumulated blood (clots), body fluids, pus, and necrotic material which otherwise collect in the wound and provide a rich growth medium for microorganisms. If a wound is draining, the skin is not completely closed, so that a pathway exists for microorganisms to enter and cause infection. Therefore, closed drainage is preferred to open drainage.

The drainage from an infected wound frequently proves to be irritating to the surrounding skin. Often this situation can be avoided by the use of a protective ointment or dressing. Petrolatum gauze and zinc oxide ointment are effective preparations.

Portable Wound Suction. The principle involved in portable wound suction is the use of gentle, constant suction to effect drainage of serosanguineous fluid and to collapse the skin flaps against the underlying tissue. The *Hemovac* apparatus is a spring diaphragm evacuator for closed suction equipped with multiple small, perforated, inert polyethylene tubes. The tubes are inserted in the drainage areas in the operating room, and the wound is completely closed (Fig. 19-9). The *Surgivac* is a bellows-shaped evacuator for thicker drainage. These devices come in different sizes. *Redi-Vacette* is flat and canteen-shaped.

Portable suction has several advantages: it is silent, saves space, is disposable, is light in weight and permits the patient to ambulate, and is inexpensive.

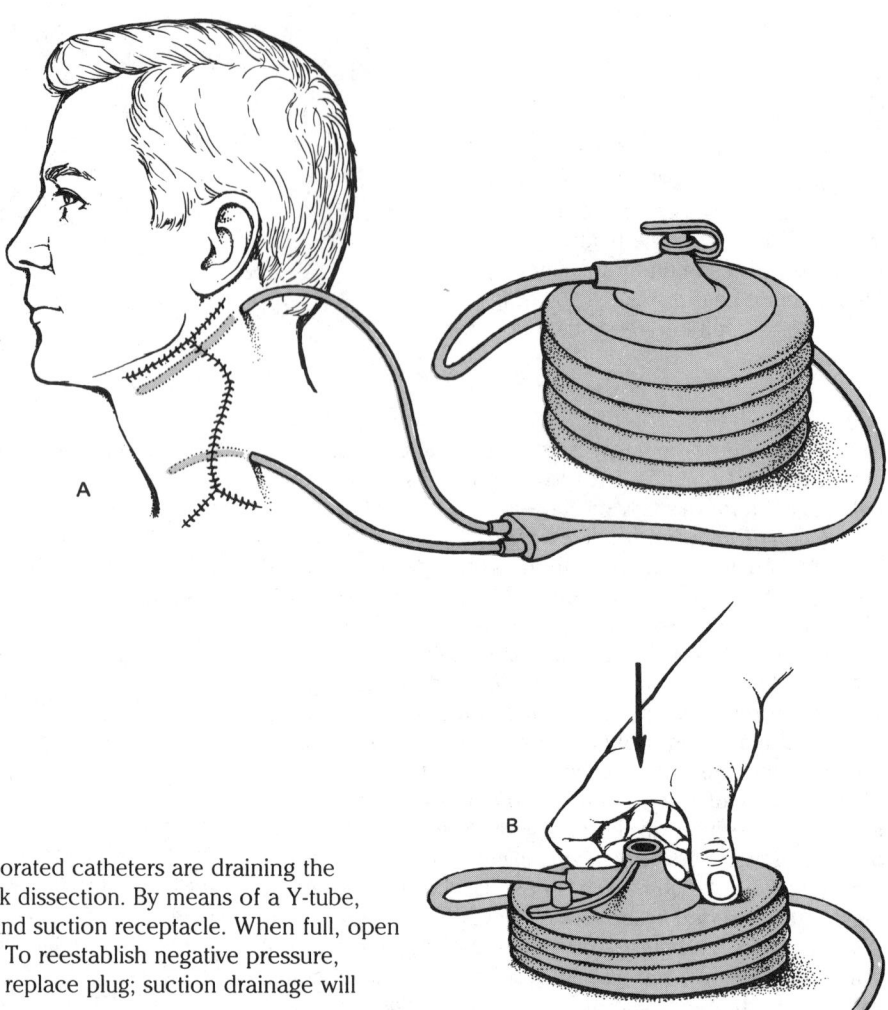

Figure 19-9
Portable wound suction. (*A*) Two perforated catheters are draining the incisional area following a radical neck dissection. By means of a Y-tube, drainage is drawn into a portable wound suction receptacle. When full, open top plug of receptacle and empty. (*B*) To reestablish negative pressure, compress receptacle as indicated and replace plug; suction drainage will resume.

The Completion of a Dressing.   Dressings are held in place with tape that comes in many types and widths. If the patient is sensitive to adhesive material, hypoallergenic tape should be used.

The correct way to apply tape is to place the tape at the center of the dressing and then press the tape down on both sides, applying tension evenly away from the midline (Fig. 19-10). Unfortunately, the wrong method of applying tape is more common—fixing one end of the tape to the skin and then pulling it tight over the dressing, often wrinkling and pulling the skin in the process. The resulting continuous and forceful traction produces a shearing effect, causing the epidermal layer to slip sideways and become prematurely separated from the deeper dermal layers.

A commercial silicone aerosol is available that can be sprayed over the adhesive used to hold dressings in place; the silicone waterproofs the dressing so that the patient can bathe or swim, and isolates the area from contamination. The spray is odorless, colorless, nonstaining, noninflammatory, heat stable, and hypoallergenic.

Elastic adhesive bandage (Elastoplast, Microfoam-3M) is preferable for holding dressings in place over mobile areas, such as the neck or the extremities, or where pressure is required. When the dressing is completed, the soiled dressings are wrapped in a waterproof bag and deposited in a covered utility can to await removal for final disposal.

Patient Education.   While changing the dressing, the nurse has an opportunity to teach the patient how to care for the wound when he is discharged from the hospital. Information on self-care activities is summarized in Chart 19-3.

Wound Complications

Hematoma (Hemorrhage)

The nurse should know the location of the patient's incision so that the dressings may be inspected for hemorrhage at intervals during the first 24 hours after operation. Any undue amount of bleeding is reported. At times concealed bleeding occurs in the wound, beneath the skin. This hemorrhage usually stops spontaneously but results in clot formation within the wound. If the clot is small, it will be absorbed and need not be treated. When the clot is large, the wound usually bulges somewhat, and healing will be delayed unless it is removed. After several stitches are removed, the clot is evacuated, after which the wound is packed lightly with gauze.

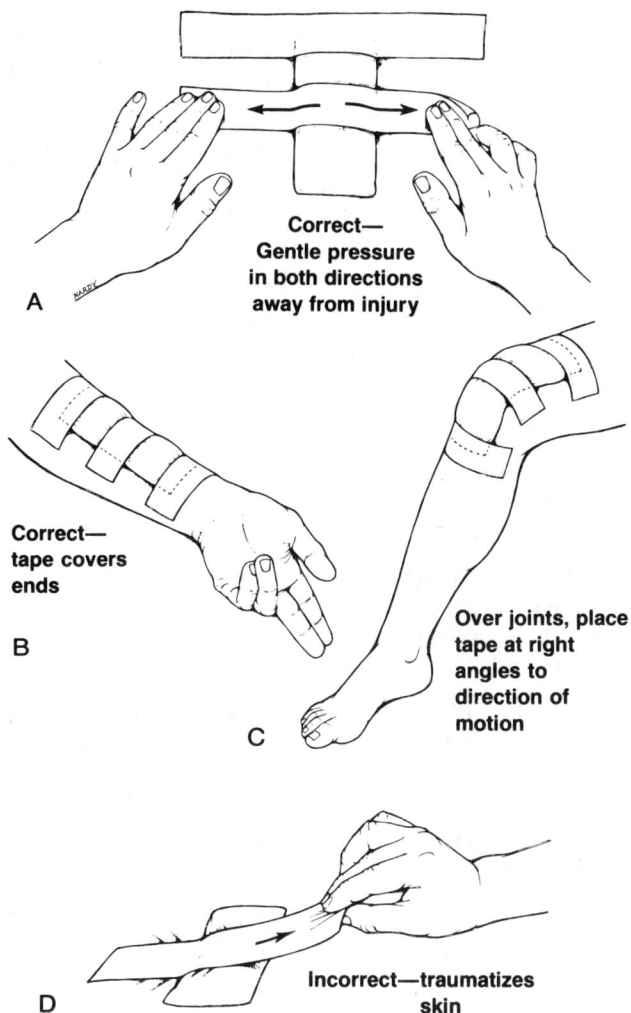

A — Correct—
Gentle pressure
in both directions
away from injury

B — Correct—
tape covers
ends

C — Over joints, place
tape at right
angles to
direction of
motion

D — Incorrect—traumatizes
skin

Figure 19-10
Application of tape. Views *A*, *B*, and *C* illustrate the correct method of application. The method shown in *D* is incorrect. (*A*) Note that pressure is applied evenly and directed away from the incision, whereas in *D*, incorrect, the tape is pulling against the skin and exerting pressure over the wound. (*B*) The proper way to cover the ends of a dressing for additional protection of the wound. (*C*) The correct way to position a dressing over a joint for maximum comfort and effectiveness.

Healing occurs usually by granulation, or a secondary closure may be performed.

Infection (Wound Sepsis)

Of nosocomial infections in hospitals, surgical wound infections are the second most frequent. Risk factors for wound infections are listed in Chart 19-4.

Staphylococcus aureus accounts for many postoperative wound infections. Other infections may result from *Escherichia coli, Proteus vulgaris, Aerobacter aerogenes, Pseudomonas aeruginosa,* and other organisms (see Nosocomial Infections, Chap. 59). The most important area of prevention lies in meticulous wound management and surgical technique.

In addition, housekeeping cleanliness and environmental disinfection are important. When the inflammatory process occurs, it usually causes symptoms in 36 to 48 hours. The patient's pulse rate and temperature increase, the white blood cell count (WBC) elevates, and the wound usually becomes somewhat tender with incisional pain, and becomes swollen and warm. At times, when the infection is deep, there may be no local signs.

When a diagnosis of wound infection is made in a postoperative wound, the surgeon usually removes one suture or more and, under aseptic precautions, separates the wound edges with a pair of blunt scissors or a hemostat. Once the infection is opened, a drain of rubber or gauze is inserted.

Cellulitis is a bacterial infection that spreads into tissue planes. All the manifestations of inflammation are evident; streptococcus is frequently the responsible organism. Systemic antibiotics are usually effective. If an extremity is the focus of the infection, elevation will reduce dependent edema and the application of heat will promote local blood supply. Rest will decrease muscular contractions which would force offending organisms into the circulatory system.

Abscess is a localized bacterial infection characterized by a collection of pus (bacteria, necrotic tissue, and white blood cells). Usually a "point" develops which is tender. Because the area is under pressure, there is a tendency for the infection to seed bacteria which may invade adjacent tissues (cellulitis) or vascular spaces (bacteremia, sepsis). Treatment is surgical drainage or excision. A goal is to prevent a recurrence of an infection if the wound is closed too soon. Rest, elevation of the part, and heat are helpful; antibiotics are not given unless there is evidence of regional or systemic spread.

Lymphangitis is a spread of infection from a cellulitis or abscess to the lymphatic system. This is treated by rest and antibiotics.

Disruption, Evisceration, and Dehiscence

The complications of disruption, evisceration, and dehiscence are especially serious when they involve abdominal wounds. These complications result from sutures giving way, from infection, and, more frequently, after marked distention or cough. They may also occur because of increasing age and the presence of pulmonary or cardiovascular disease in abdominal surgical patients.

The earliest sign is usually a gush of serosanguineous peritoneal fluid from the wound. The rupture of the wound may occur suddenly. When a lower abdominal wound is disrupted, coils of intestine may push out of the abdomen. Such a catastrophe causes considerable pain and often is associated with vomiting. Frequently the patient says that "something gave way." When the wound edges part slowly, the intestines may protrude gradually or not at all, and the presenting symptom may be the sudden drainage of a large amount of peritoneal fluid into the dressings.

- When disruption of a wound occurs, the surgeon is notified at once. The protruding coils of intestine should be covered with sterile dressings moistened with sterile saline.

An abdominal binder, properly applied, is an excellent prophylactic measure against an evisceration of this kind,

Chart 19-3
Patient Education: Wound Care

Until Sutures Are Removed

1. Keep the wound dry and clean.
   a. If there is no dressing, ask your nurse or physician if you can bathe or shower.
   b. If a dressing or splint is in place, do not remove it unless it is wet or soiled.
   c. If wet or soiled, change it yourself if you have been taught*; otherwise call your nurse or physician for guidance.
   *d. If you have been taught, instruction might be as follows:
      (1) Cleanse area *gently* with 70% isopropyl alcohol once or twice daily.
      (2) Cover with a sterile Telfa pad or gauze square—sufficiently large to cover wound.
      (3) Apply hypoallergenic Dermacel or paper tape (adhesive is not preferred because it is difficult to remove without possible injury to incision site).
2. Report immediately if any of these signs of infection occur!
   a. Redness, marked swelling (beyond 2.5 cm (½ inch) from incision site), tenderness, increased warmth around wound
   b. Red streaks in skin near wound
   c. Pus or discharge, foul odor
   d. Chills or fever (over 37.7°C or 100°F)
3. If soreness or pain is discomforting, apply a dry cool pack (containing ice or cold water) or take prescribed acetaminophen tablets (2) every 4–6 hours. Avoid aspirin without direction or instruction since bleeding may be enhanced with its use.

4. Swelling following surgery is common. To help reduce swelling, elevate the injured part to above the level of the heart.
   a. Hand or arm
      (1) Sleep—elevate arm on pillow at side.
      (2) Sitting—place cushion or pillow on adjacent table.
      (3) Standing—rest affected hand on opposite shoulder; support elbow with unaffected hand.
   b. Leg or foot
      (1) Sitting—place a pillow on a facing chair; provide support underneath the knee.
      (2) Lying—place a pillow under injured leg.

After Sutures Are Removed

Although the wound appears to be healed when stitches are removed, it is still tender and will continue to heal and strengthen for several weeks.

1. Follow directives of physician or nurse as to extent of activity.
2. Keep suture line clean; do not rub vigorously; pat dry. Wound may look red and be slightly elevated. This is normal.
3. Massage around wound gently using a bland baby oil, petrolatum, or moisterizing cream (twice a day).
4. Report to the health care person if after 8 weeks the site continues to be red, thick, painful to pressure. (This may be due to excessive collagen formation and should be checked.)

---

and often it is used along with the primary dressing, especially for operations on patients with weak or pendulous abdominal walls, or when rupture of a wound has occurred. Vitamin deficiency or lowered serum protein or chloride may require correction.

Keloid

Not infrequently in an otherwise normal wound, the scar develops a tendency to excessive growth. Sometimes the entire scar is affected; at other times the condition is segmented. This keloid tendency is unexplainable, unpredictable, and unavoidable in some people.

Much investigation has been done into prevention and cure. Careful closure of the wound, complete hemostasis, pressure support without undue tension on the suture lines—all are reputed to combat this distressing wound complication.

Postoperative Complications

The danger inherent in surgery involves not only the risk of the operative procedure, but also the very definite hazard of postoperative complications that may prolong convalescence or even adversely affect the surgical outcome. The nurse plays an important part in the prevention of these complications and in their early treatment, should they arise. The signs and symptoms of the more common postoperative complications are discussed below. In each instance the most effective method of prevention and the usual treatment are emphasized.

It should constantly be borne in mind that attention must be paid to the patient as an individual as well as to his particular surgical condition.

Shock

One of the most serious postoperative complications is shock, which may be described as inadequate cellular oxygenation accompanied by inability to excrete waste products of metabolism. Shock can occur in association with many kinds of major illness, such as hemorrhage, trauma, burns, infection, and heart disease, and results from a failure of three aspects of circulation: the heart pump, peripheral resistance, and blood volume. Thus, while there are many kinds of shock, the basic definition centers on an inadequate blood flow to

Chart 19-4
Risk Factors Contributing to Wound Sepsis

Local

Wound contamination
Foreign body
Faulty suturing technique
Devitalized tissue
Hematoma
"Dead" space

General

Debilitation
   Dehydration
   Malnutrition
   Anemia
Advanced age
Extreme obesity
Shock
Length of preoperative hospitalization
Length of operation
Associated diseases (*i.e.*, diabetes mellitus)

vital organs or the inability of the tissues of these organs to utilize oxygen and other nutrients.

Pathophysiology

Catecholamines (epinephrine and norepinephrine) are elevated during shock and appear to be the dominant hormones in response to severe shock. Their effect is to constrict arterioles in the skin, subcutaneous tissue, and kidneys; they dilate arterioles of skeletal muscles and liver. Heart output is increased by increasing heart rates and increasing myocardial contractility. The great veins are constricted, thereby increasing venous return. Shock stimulates corticotropin (ACTH) release from the pituitary and thereby increases plasma levels of glucocorticoids. Mineralocorticoids are elevated mostly because of increased activity in the renin–angiotensin systems. Glucagon is released and antidiuretic hormone (ADH) is released. Endorphins are released in conjunction with the release of corticotropin. Endorphins act like opiates, which may contribute to low blood pressure.

The effect of high levels of epinephrine, cortisol, and glucagon and lower levels of insulin (insulin does rise, but not as greatly as the antagonists) stimulates catabolism. There is decreased oxygen utilization owing to decreased cardiac output and insulin insufficiency. See Figure 19-11 in Chart 19-5 for microcirculatory changes in shock.

Classification

Shock may be classified as hypovolemic (oligemic), cardiogenic, neurogenic, or septic. The differences are noted as each is described.

Hypovolemic Shock. Hypovolemic shock is caused by decreased fluid volume owing to loss of blood or plasma, or even fluid losses from prolonged vomiting or diarrhea. Fluid volume is frequently decreased after surgery for a number of reasons. At times more blood is lost at operation than is realized. In addition, the handling of body tissues may cause local trauma and loss of blood and plasma from the circulation, thereby creating a decrease in the circulating blood volume. Hypovolemic shock is characterized by a fall in venous pressure, a rise in peripheral resistance, and tachycardia. For additional symptoms see Table 19-2.

Cardiogenic Shock. Cardiogenic shock results from cardiac failure or an interference with heart function (poor heart-pump function, causing diminished cardiac output), as in myocardial infarction, dysrhythmias, tamponade, pulmonary embolism, advanced (late) hypovolemia, or epidural and general anesthesia. The signs are increased pressure in the venous bed and an increase in peripheral resistance.

Neurogenic Shock. Neurogenic shock occurs as a result of a failure of arterial resistance (such as may be caused by spinal anesthesia, quadriplegia). It is characterized by a fall in blood pressure owing to pooling of blood in dilated capacitance vessels (those with the ability to change volume capacity). Heart activity increases and thus maintains a normal output (stroke volume); this helps to fill the dilated vascular system as it attempts to preserve perfusion pressure.

Septic Shock. Septic shock results most frequently from gram-negative septicemia (infection, peritonitis, and the like). At first the patient exhibits a fever, a rapid, strong pulse, rapid respirations, and normal or slightly decreased blood pressure. Skin is flushed, warm, and dry. However, if infection continues untreated, hypovolemic shock develops. These two phases may be referred to as hyperdynamic septic shock (the former) and hypodynamic shock (the latter, which is similar to hypovolemic shock). Hypovolemia develops along with depressed cardiac function. (See also Chap. 25.)

Clinical Manifestations

Even though shock can result from widely differing causes (trauma, systemic infection, or cardiac dysfunction), clinical manifestations are generally similar.

- The classic signs of shock are pallor; cool, moist skin; rapid breathing; ischemia of the eyelids, lips, gums, and tongue; a rapid, weak, thready pulse; decreasing pulse pressure; and usually a low blood pressure and concentrated urine. See Table 19-2 for progression of symptoms in relation to severity.

Diagnostic Assessment

Before treatment can be instituted promptly and intelligently, the *goal* in initial assessment is to determine the cause of volume loss and the status of the airway. The initial assessment includes the following:

1. Respirations. Hyperventilation is an early sign of septic shock.

2. Skin. A cold, pale, moist skin indicates vasoconstriction with increased arteriolar resistance and is suggestive of hypovolemic shock. Warm, red skin indicates a decrease in arteriolar resistance and may be seen in septic and neurogenic shock.

Chart 19-5
Pathophysiology of Shock

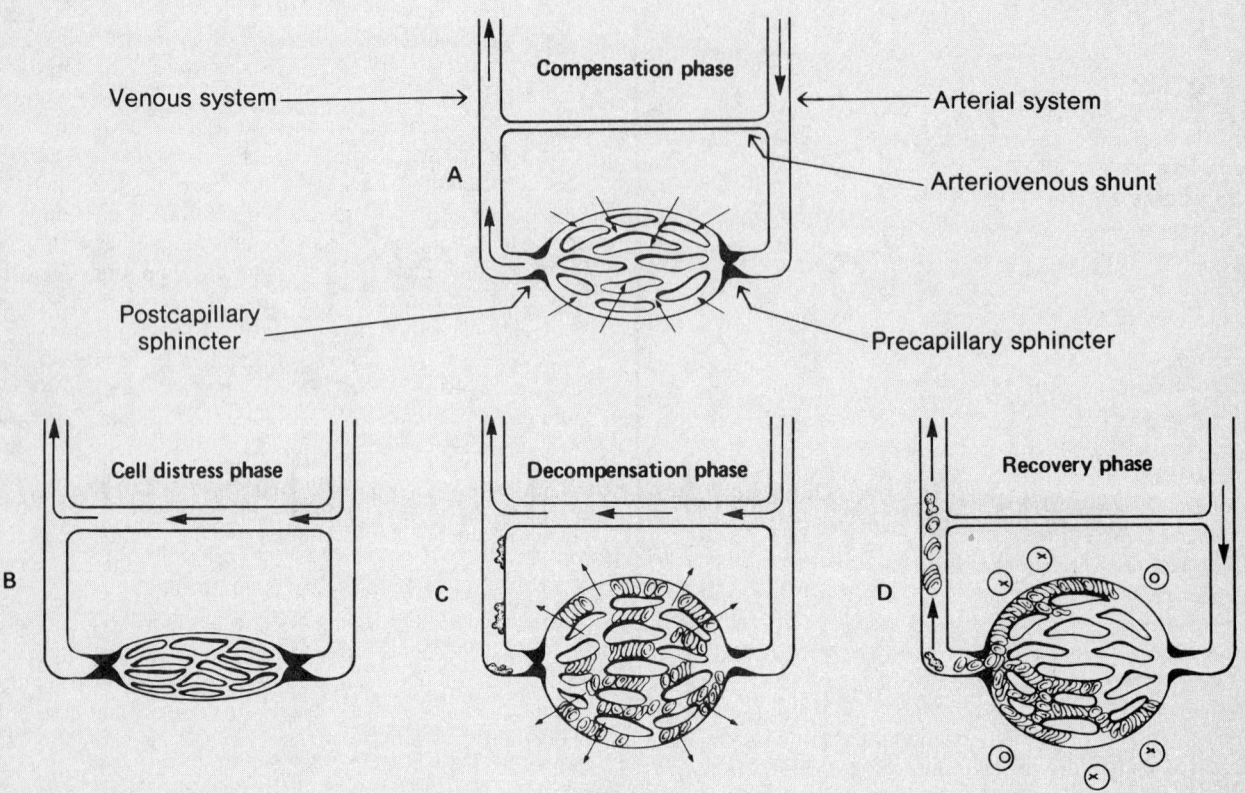

Figure 19-11
Microcirculatory changes in shock. (*A*) Compensation phase. (*B*) Cell distress
phase. (*C*) Decompensation phase. (*D*) Recovery phase. (Dunphy JE and Way LW.
Current Diagnosis and Treatment. Los Altos, California, Lange Medical Publishers.)

When the body sustains an insult, such as hemorrhage, extensive burns, or heart failure, a compensatory reaction occurs.
The adrenal cortex releases catecholamines to constrict arterioles and venules in the major organs of the body (kidneys, liver,
intestines, *etc.*) so that more blood is diverted to the brain and
heart.

Pathophysiologic Consequences of Shock

The greatest impact of all types of shock is exerted on the microcirculation (arterioles, capillaries, venules—microvasculature), which reacts to shock in a series of steps. The first phase
involves a response to the hypovolemia, as is seen in the contraction of the precapillary arteriole sphincters (Fig. 19-11*A*).
This causes capillary pressure to fall, with the result that fluid
moves into the vascular spaces and increases the blood volume.
By such compensatory action, blood volume returns to normal
and the precapillary sphincters relax. However, if shock is more
prolonged, recovery is prevented and the next phase, cell distress, is entered (Fig. 19-11*B*). In this phase, arteriovenous

shunts open and divert arterial flow directly back into the venous system. Meanwhile, the cells in the bypassed segment of
microcirculation rely on anaerobic metabolism for energy. Glucose and oxygen are reduced markedly for the cells, and waste
products such as lactate increase. Histamine is released and the
postcapillary sphincter closes. Capillary flow is slowed considerably and the bed constricts with very few capillaries remaining
open. In the decompensation phase (Fig. 19-11*C*), just before
the death of the cell, acidosis (decreasing serum *p*H) causes
the precapillary sphincter to open. Fluid and protein are lost in
the interstitial space and the capillary expands with agglutinated
red blood cells (sludge). White cells and platelets gather in the
venules where acidosis is most profound. Arteriovenous circulation continues to supply essential oxygen to the vital areas of
heart and brain. In the recovery phase (Fig. 19-11*D*), if the
blood volume is restored during the decompensation phase
while the effects on microcirculation are still reversible, badly
damaged cells can be repaired. Cell aggregates can be filtered
out by the lungs and into the systemic circulation. However, if
there is an overabundance of dead cells, secondary morbidity
results.

TABLE 19-2
Classification and Symptoms of Hypovolemic Shock

	Mild	Moderate	Severe
Percent of Blood Volume Loss	Up to 20%	20% to 40%	40% or more
Decreased Perfusion	Skin, fat, skeletal muscle, bone	Liver, intestine, kidneys	Brain, heart
Pulse	Rapid	Rapid—weaker, thready	Very rapid—irregular
Respirations	Deep and rapid	Shallow and rapid	Even more shallow and rapid
Blood Pressure	120/80	60–90 mm Hg systolic	Under 60 mm Hg systolic
Skin	Cool, pale	Cold, pale, moist	Cold, clammy, cyanotic lips and nails
Urinary Output	Above 50 ml/hr	10–25 ml/hr	10 ml or less/hr → anuria
Level of Consciousness	Anxious but oriented and alert	Restless, mentally "fuzzy," vertigo	Lethargic → comatose

3. Pulse and Blood Pressure. Alone, pulse and blood pressure may not be reliable guides to the severity of shock, but their progressive pattern is significant. That is, if each 10-minute interval shows a rise in pulse and a rise followed by a fall in blood pressure, then such signs are indicative of shock. A pulse of 80/min and a blood pressure of 120/80 are normal. When systolic pressure is between 90 mm Hg and 60 mm Hg (in the normotensive person), shock is well advanced. (For the hypertensive person, 30 mm Hg below the baseline systolic pressure is a sign of shock.) With a more rapid pulse rate, the amplitude is weaker and thready in hypovolemic and cardiogenic shock. Dysrhythmia may be noted in cardiogenic shock.

4. Urinary Output. Because the output of urine is one of the most valuable indices of adequacy of vital organ perfusion, an indwelling catheter is recommended for any patient susceptible to shock. A drop in renal artery pressure and flow produces renal artery vasoconstriction and results in decreased glomerular filtration and decreased urine output. Normal urine flow is 50 ml/hr. An output of 30 ml/hr or less (oliguria or anuria) is suggestive of cardiac failure or inadequate volume replacement.

5. Central Venous Pressure. Central venous pressure (CVP) is the pressure within the right atrium or in the great veins within the thorax. It is a valuable guide to vascular volume replacement when other parameters are also considered: vital signs, cardiopulmonary status, and the like. Average CVP is 5 to 12 cm water. Several readings are taken to determine the range; a reading near zero may indicate hypovolemia (if patient improves with rapid IV infusion, the patient was hypovolemic). Readings over 15 cm water may suggest hypervolemia, vasoconstriction, or congestive heart failure. Pulmonary artery pressure (PAP) and pulmonary capillary wedge pressure (PWP) are more accurate indications of the pumping ability of the left side of the heart. (See Chap. 24.)

6. Arterial Blood Gases. The partial pressures of oxygen (Po_2) and carbon dioxide (Pco_2) are useful indices in providing therapy. An arterial oxygen tension below 60 mm Hg indicates a marginal respiratory reserve. A Pco_2 over 45 mm Hg indicates serious hypoventilation. In shock, Pco_2 is usually within normal limits.

7. Serum Lactate. In shock there is a closer correlation between arterial blood lactate levels and survival. The higher the lactate level, the greater the oxygen need.

8. Hematocrit. Hematocrit is useful in determining the type of fluid to use in replacement. (Such a study must be repeated, since a few hours are required to reflect correctly the amount of blood loss.) If the hematocrit is over 55, plasma and saline are given. If the hematocrit is 20 or lower, blood is needed. The maximal oxygen-carrying capacity is best when the hematocrit is between 35 and 45.

9. Levels of Consciousness. Consciousness levels may range from alert in mild shock to mental cloudiness in moderate shock. As the condition worsens, the patient becomes lethargic and reacts only to noxious stimuli. Irreversible shock is noted when the patient fails to react to stimuli.

Management and Nursing Interventions

Prevention. The best treatment for shock is prophylaxis. This consists of adequate preparation of the patient, mental as well as physical, and anticipation of any complication that may arise during or after operation. Special equipment for the treatment of shock must be on hand. The proper type of anesthesia should be chosen after careful consideration of the patient and the disease. Blood and blood substitute should be available if indicated. Blood loss should be accurately measured or intelligently estimated.

- If the amount of blood loss exceeds 500 ml (especially if it is rapid), replacement is usually indicated.

Obviously, the individual patient and the particular circumstances must be considered in determining replacement therapy. An older, malnourished person is more likely to require this therapy than a patient whose health is generally good.

Operative trauma should be kept at a minimum as the first step in avoiding shock. After operation, factors that may promote shock are to be prevented. Pain is controlled by making the patient as comfortable as possible and by using narcotics judiciously. Exposure is avoided, and lightweight, unheated covers are used to prevent vasodilation. In the recovery room the patient can be watched and cared for by nurses trained especially in the recovery of patients from anesthesia. In addition, a quiet room helps to reduce mental trauma. Any moving of the patient is done gently. He is placed in the supine position to facilitate circulation. Monitoring of vital signs is continued until the patient's recovery indicates that shock is unlikely.

Treatment.   (See also Emergency Treatment of Shock, Chap. 60.) The patient is kept warm, but overheating is avoided to prevent cutaneous vessels from dilating and depriving vital organs of blood. An infusion of Ringer's lactated solution is started. The patient is placed flat in bed with legs elevated as in Figure 19-12. (Avoid the Trendelenburg position.) The patient's respiratory and circulatory status is monitored constantly: respiration, pulse, blood pressure, skin, urinary output, level of consciousness, central venous pressure (CVP), pulmonary artery pressure (PAP), pulmonary capillary wedge pressure (PWP), and cardiac output (CO).

- *The basic approach to the treatment of shock is to determine its cause and correct it if possible.*

1. *Ensure adequacy of airway.* When the patient is ventilating adequately, blood gas determinations are made to determine adequacy of pulmonary function, and the patient is given oxygen by intubation or nasal cannula.
2. *Restore blood/fluid volume.* The kind of fluid and blood replacement depends upon the kind and

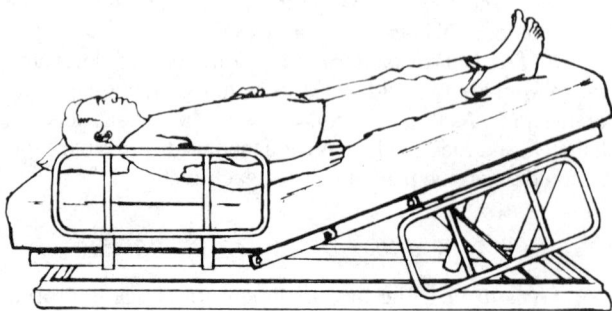

Figure 19-12
Proper positioning of the patient who shows signs of shock. The lower extremities are elevated to an angle of approximately 20 degrees; knees are straight, trunk is horizontal, and head is slightly elevated.

amount lost as well as the condition of the patient. Fluids are administered intravenously immediately; when the nature of loss is determined, fluid replacement is modified accordingly. Of the total blood volume, under normal conditions 20% is in the capillaries, 10% in the arterial system, and the balance in the veins and heart. In shock there is dilatation of the capillary beds, so a considerable volume of blood can be accommodated.

Two kinds of fluids are used: crystalloids and colloids. *Crystalloids* are electrolyte solutions that diffuse into interstitial spaces. An example is lactated Ringer's injection, a buffering solution in which lactate is metabolized and excess hydrogen ions are neutralized.

Three parts of crystalloids are lost to extravascular space for every one part that remains in the vascular system. This means that for every 2000 ml given, 500 ml increase the vascular volume. For hemorrhagic shock, crystalloids are given initially to lower blood viscosity and aid in microcirculation.

Colloids are blood, artificial blood, blood substitutes, plasma, serum albumin, and plasma substitutes, such as dextran; these remain in the intravascular compartment. Blood of the same type as the patient's should be administered in preference to the generally used O-Rh-negative blood. Burn shock requires large amounts of colloid replacement.

3. *Drug Therapy:* (cardiotonics, diuretics, vasoactive medications.) Vasodilators are prescribed to reduce peripheral resistance, which in turn decreases the work of the heart and increases cardiac output and tissue perfusion. The drug frequently used is sodium nitroprusside (Nipride), which stimulates myocardial contractility and lowers peripheral resistance. Some clinics advocate the use of steroids, while others use combinations of pharmacotherapeutic agents. Some authorities believe that hypovolemic shock should not be treated with vasoactive drugs. Their effect is to increase vascular resistance and decrease tissue perfusion, thus aggravating the effects of shock.

Currently, a miniature computerized pump that can be bolted on an IV support pole can carefully calculate the amount of sodium nitroprusside that should be given. Also available are monitors that measure the patient's blood pressure every 10 seconds and automatically adjust the drug dosage if there are any changes.

Nursing Interventions.   The nurse assists the physician in carrying out the treatment modalities just described. When vasodilators are prescribed, the patient's blood pressure requires constant monitoring. The patient is kept flat during the administration of these drugs. If the systolic blood pressure continues to fall, the drug is stopped and fluids are increased.

The following nursing measures are carried out:

1. *Psychological support is provided and the patient's energy expenditure is reduced.* Rest is promoted for the patient and his reactions to treatment are assessed. Support and reassurance are offered to relieve apprehension. Sedatives are administered cautiously as prescribed for pain, so that circulation is not further depressed. The patient is kept warm, because

hypothermia decreases tissue oxygenation. Hypothermia also affects peripheral circulation. The patient is turned every 2 hours and deep breathing is encouraged to promote optimum cardiopulmonary function.

2. *Complications are prevented.* All parameters are observed and the patient is monitored closely in the 24-hour period following onset of shock, since complications may develop. Peripheral and pulmonary edema due to fluid overload is the most common complication, resulting from administering fluids faster than the body can accommodate them.

3. *All observations and actions are documented.*

Hemorrhage

Classification

Hermorrhage is classified as (1) *primary,* when it occurs at the time of the operation; (2) *intermediary,* when it occurs within the first few hours after an operation, because of the return of blood pressure to its normal level and the consequent washing out of the insecure clots from untied vessels; and (3) *secondary,* when it occurs some time after the operation, as a result of the slipping of a ligature because of infection, insecure tying, or erosion of a vessel by a drainage tube.

A further classification frequently is made according to the kind of vessel that is bleeding. *Capillary* hemorrhage is characterized by a slow, general ooze; *venous* hemorrhage bubbles out quickly and is dark in color; *arterial* hemorrhage is bright in color and appears in spurts with each heartbeat.

When the hemorrhage is on the surface and can be seen, it is spoken of as *evident;* when it cannot be seen, as in the peritoneal cavity, it is spoken of as *concealed.*

Clinical Manifestations

Hemorrhage presents a more or less well-defined syndrome, depending on the amount of blood lost and the rapidity of its escape. The patient is apprehensive and restless, moves continually, and is thirsty; the skin is cold, moist, and pale. The pulse rate increases, the temperature falls, and respirations are rapid and deep, often of the gasping type spoken of as "air hunger." As the hemorrhage progresses, cardiac output decreases, arterial and venous blood pressure and the hemoglobin of the blood fall rapidly, the lips and the conjunctivae become pallid, spots appear before the eyes, a ringing is heard in the ears, and the patient grows weaker but remains conscious until near death.

Management

Often the signs of hemorrhage after an operation are masked by the effects of the anesthetic or shock; therefore, the initial treatment of the patient is in a general way almost identical to that described for shock. (See previous section on shock.) Place the patient in shock position (see Fig. 19-12) and administer sedation or narcotic as prescribed to keep the patient quiet. The wound always should be inspected to find the site of the bleeding if possible. A sterile gauze pad and a snug bandage are indicated, as well as elevation of the part, arm, or leg.

- Giving a transfusion of blood and determining the cause of hemorrhage are the most logical therapeutic measures.
- In giving fluids by vein in cases of hemorrhage, remember that too large a quantity of fluid or too rapid administration may raise the blood pressure enough to start the bleeding again, unless the hemorrhage has been well controlled.

Deep Venous Thrombosis

Deep venous thrombosis (DVT) is a thrombosis of deep rather than superficial veins. Two serious complications are pulmonary embolism and postphlebitic syndrome (see p. 369).

Incidence

Postoperatively, those at greatest risk for deep venous thrombosis have been identified as follows*:

- Orthopedic patients having hip surgery, knee reconstruction, and elective lower extremity surgery
- Urologic patients having transvesical prostatectomy, and older patients having urologic surgery
- General surgical patients over age 40, obese, with malignancy, or having had prior DVT or pulmonary embolism, or those having extensive complicated surgical procedures
- Gynecology (and obstetric) patients over age 40 with added risk factors (varicose veins, previous venous thrombosis, infection, malignancy, obesity)
- Neurosurgical patients, similar to other surgical high risk groups (In stroke, for example, the risk of DVT in the paralyzed leg is as high as 75%.)

Pathophysiology

A mild to severe inflammation of the vein occurs in association with a clotting of blood. The complication may result from a number of causes, including injury to the vein by tight straps or leg-holders at the time of operation, pressure from a blanket-roll under the knees, concentration of blood by loss of fluid or dehydration, or, more commonly, the slowing of the blood flow in the extremity owing to a lowered metabolism and depression of the circulation after operation. It is probable that several of these factors act together to produce thrombosis. The left leg is affected more frequently.

Clinical Manifestations

The first symptom of deep vein thrombosis may be a pain or a cramp in the calf (Fig. 19-13). Pressure there gives pain, and a day or so later a painful swelling of the entire leg occurs, often associated with a slight fever and sometimes with chills and perspiration. The swelling is due to a soft edema that pits easily on pressure. There is marked tenderness over the anteromedial surface of the thigh.

A milder form of the same disease is termed *phlebothrombosis,* to indicate intravascular clotting without marked

* Consensus Development Conference Statement: Prevention of Venous Thrombosis and Pulmonary Embolism. Bethesda, Maryland, National Institutes of Health, March, 1986.

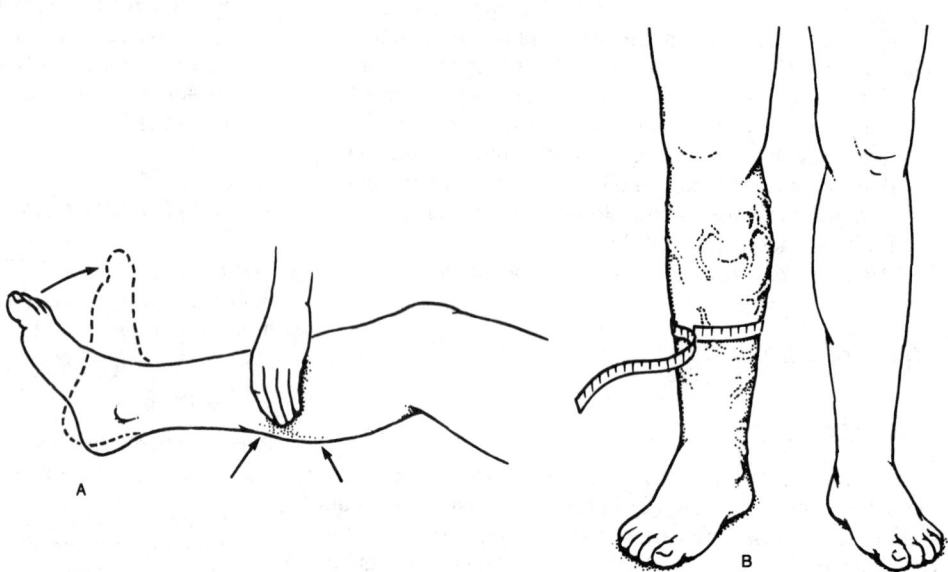

Figure 19-13
Assessment of signs and symptoms of phlebothrombosis. (*A*) With the knee flexed, the patient may complain of pain in the calf on dorsiflexion of foot (Homans's sign)—this was considered an unmistakable sign of early and subclinical thrombosis; it may or may not be present. Gentle compression reveals tenderness of the calf muscles (note arrow). (*B*) The affected leg may swell; veins are more prominent and may be palpated easily. (Brunner LS and Suddarth DS. The Lippincott Manual of Nursing Practice, 4th ed. Philadelphia, JB Lippincott, 1986.)

inflammation of the vein. The clotting occurs usually in the veins of the calf, often with few symptoms except slight soreness of the calf. The danger from this type of thrombosis is that the clot may be dislodged, producing an embolus. It is believed that most pulmonary emboli arise from this source (see Fig. 19-13).

Medical and Nursing Management

The treatments of thrombophlebitis and deep venous thrombosis may be considered as (1) preventive and (2) active.

Prevention. Efforts directed toward preventing the formation of a thrombus include such measures as leg exercises that can be taught before surgery (see Chap. 17, Chart 17-2). If the patient recognizes their significance in preventing circulatory complications, he will often initiate his own exercises. To avoid thrombus formation, leg straps should not be fastened in the recovery room, particularly with stretchers that are equipped with side rails. The straps are not only restrictive, but can constrict and impair circulation.

The use of low-dose heparin until the patient is ambulatory is becoming increasingly common. This is given in prescribed units subcutaneously. Dextran 40 or Dextran 70 is comparable in effectiveness but is more expensive. Low-dose warfarin is another possible anticoagulant. External pneumatic compression and gradient elastic stockings can be used alone or in combination with low-dose heparin. Dehydroergotamine has also been used with low-dose heparin; some claim that it is more efficacious, but the potential risks of vasoconstriction and its contraindications must be recognized. Aspirin has not been shown to be beneficial.

No one method is ideal, but prophylactic use tailored to meet individual needs can be effective in markedly reducing what otherwise can be a very serious and potentially lethal complication.

In addition to the nursing measures cited above, it is important to avoid the use of blanket-rolls, pillow-rolls, or any form of elevation that can constrict vessels under the knees. Even the practice of "dangling" (having the patient sit on the edge of the bed with legs hanging over the side) can be dangerous and is not recommended because pressure under the knees can impede circulation.

Active Treatment. Some surgeons believe that ligation of the femoral veins is an important therapeutic method. The rationale behind this method of therapy is to prevent pulmonary embolism by eliminating the cause (thrombi that could become detached from femoral veins and circulate in the blood).

Anticoagulant therapy has taken a prominent place in the treatment of phlebitis and phlebothrombosis. Heparin, given intravenously by the drip method or subcutaneously, reduces the coagulability of the blood rapidly and is used most often when an immediate effect is desired. Repeated checks of the coagulation time of the blood are necessary to control its administration. Dicumarol (or a drug with a similar action) is used for the same purpose. It is given by mouth and does not become effective for about 24 hours. Daily dosage is controlled by daily estimations of the prothrombin time of the blood (see also p. 652).

Encasing the legs from toes to groin with elastic stockings has been used as an active treatment of phlebitis and thrombosis. These stockings prevent swelling and stagnation of venous blood in the legs and do much to relieve pain in the phlebitic extremity. However, to be effective, elastic stockings must be used in combination with leg elevation and leg exercises. Early ambulation is helpful, but the nurse also needs to be aware of the problem that can result when a patient with a protuberant abdomen walks a few steps and then sits with legs dependent; namely, the pressure of the abdomen can obstruct venous flow. Several research studies have questioned the value of elastic stockings, suggesting an actual danger when they are not applied correctly. Some clinics now do not advocate the use of elastic stockings for any surgical patient.

Pulmonary Embolism

An *embolus* is a foreign body in the bloodstream, formed by a blood clot that becomes dislodged from its original site and is carried along in the blood.

When the clot is carried to the heart it is forced by the blood into the pulmonary artery, where it plugs the main artery or one of its branches. The symptoms produced may be among the most sudden and startling in surgical practice. A patient experiencing an apparently normal convalescence suddenly cries out with sharp, stabbing pains in the chest and becomes breathless, cyanotic, and anxious. The pupils dilate, cold perspiration appears, the pulse becomes rapid, irregular, and then imperceptible, and death usually results. If death does not occur within 30 minutes there is a chance of recovery.

Fortunately, pulmonary embolism is usually a less dramatic event than that described above and may be heralded by no more than mild dyspnea, dysrhythmia, or seemingly innocent chest pain. Alertness on the part of the nurse is necessary to detect these subtle emboli in order that early treatment may be initiated and further embolization avoided.

- One of the many reasons for getting the patient out of bed as soon after surgery as possible is to avoid a pulmonary embolism.

(See pp. 488–492 for full discussion of pulmonary embolus.)

Respiratory Complications

Respiratory complications are among the most frequent and serious problems that confront the surgical team. (See Chart 19-6.)

Experience has shown that such complications may be avoided in large measure by careful preoperative observation and teaching and by taking every precaution during and after the operation. It is well known that patients who have some respiratory disease before operation are more apt to develop serious complications after operation. Therefore, only emergency operations are performed when acute disease of the respiratory tract exists. The nurse reports any symptom, such as cough, sneezing, inflamed conjunctivae, and nasal discharge, to the surgeon and anesthesiologist before the operation.

During and immediately after the operation every effort should be made to prevent chilling. Aspiration of the nasopharynx in the recovery room removes secretions that would otherwise cause respiratory problems in the postoperative period. Occasionally, when secretions form that cannot be coughed up by the patient, aspiration of secretions may be carried out through a bronchoscope. In very debilitated patients in whom retained secretions are a complicating factor, a tracheostomy may be performed so that aspiration of the trachea is done directly through the tube as necessary.

Respiratory complications are described briefly here and in more detail in Chapters 22 and 23.

Atelectasis. When the mucus plug closes one of the bronchi entirely, there is a collapse of the pulmonary tissue

---

> ## Chart 19-6
> ## *Risk Factors Affecting Postoperative Pulmonary Complications*
>
> Type of surgery—Greater incidence following all forms of abdominal surgery when compared with peripheral surgery
> Location of incision—The closer the incision to the diaphragm, the higher the incidence of pulmonary complications
> Preoperative respiratory problems
> Age—Greater risk over age 40 than under age 40
> Sepsis
> Obesity—Weight greater than 110% of ideal body weight
> Prolonged bed rest
> Duration of operation—Over 3 hours
> Aspiration
> Dehydration
> Malnutrition
> Hypotension and shock

beyond, and a massive atelectasis is said to result. (See p. 414.)

Bronchitis. Bronchitis may appear at any time after operation, usually within the first 5 to 6 days. The symptoms vary according to the disease. A simple bronchitis is characterized by a cough that produces considerable mucopus, but without marked temperature or pulse elevation.

Bronchopneumonia. Bronchopneumonia is perhaps the second most frequent pulmonary complication. Along with a productive cough, there may be considerable temperature elevation and an increase in the pulse and the respiratory rates.

Lobar Pneumonia. Lobar pneumonia is a less frequent complication after operation. Usually, it begins with a chill, followed by high temperature, pulse, and respiration. There may be little or no cough, but the respiratory embarrassment, the flushed cheeks, and the evident illness of the patient make a combination of clinical signs that is distinctive. The disease runs its usual course with the added complication of the operative wound.

Hypostatic Pulmonary Congestion. Hypostatic pulmonary congestion is a condition that may develop in elderly or very weak patients. Its cause is a weakened heart and vascular system that permit a stagnation of secretions at the base of both lungs. It occurs most frequently in elderly patients who are not mobilized effectively. The symptoms often are not marked for a time—perhaps a slight elevation of temperature, pulse, and respiratory rate and a slight cough. However, physical examination reveals dullness and crackles at the base of the lungs. If the condition goes untreated the outcome may be fatal.

Pleurisy. Pleurisy is not an uncommon occurrence after operation. Its chief symptom is an acute, knifelike pain in the chest on the affected side that is particularly excruciating when the patient takes a deep breath. There usually is some slight temperature and pulse rise, and respirations are rapid and more shallow than normal.

Management

A most effective method of treating *bronchitis* is the inhalation of cool mist or steam, which may be administered by electric vaporizers as prescribed. The apparatus must be kept filled with water, and precautions are taken to prevent the patient from being burned.

In *lobar pneumonia* and *bronchopneumonia,* the patient is encouraged to take fluids; expectorant and antibiotic drugs also are given as prescribed. Distention is watched for and prevented, if possible, so as to avoid added respiratory or cardiac embarrassment.

For *pleurisy,* analgesics may be prescribed, or the physician may do a procaine intercostal block to provide symptomatic relief. A search is made to detect any possible underlying disease (pneumonia, infarction).

Pleurisy with effusion may result secondary to a primary pleurisy. In these patients aspiration of the pleural space is frequently necessary.

Many times the pulmonary complication of *hypostatic pulmonary congestion* becomes more serious than the original surgical condition, in which case the prime objective of therapeutic management is to treat the hypostatic pneumonia.

Because of reduced aeration in many of the pulmonary complications, which means that less oxygen reaches the blood, many clinics employ oxygen therapy in treatment. Principles and management are presented on pages 424–426.

Superinfections. Superinfections can occur when antimicrobial agents change the bacterial flora of the respiratory tract. Susceptible bacteria are killed and resistant bacteria multiply. These infections must be treated aggressively.

Nursing Interventions. Awareness of the many possible respiratory complications enables the nurse to initiate the preventive measures cited in the previous discussion (pp. 313, 345). Timely recognition of signs and symptoms allows the nurse to direct efforts toward combating specific respiratory difficulties. Not only is the first postoperative day one of concern, but the first postoperative week of the patient's recovery requires close observation and careful management. The early signs of elevations in temperature, pulse, and respiration rate are significant. Chest pain, dyspnea, and cough may or may not accompany these elevations; however, the patient may seem to be restless and apprehensive. Such indications are important and should be reported and documented.

Measures to Promote the Full Aeration of the Lungs. The prophylactic treatment of respiratory complications includes measures to promote full aeration of the lungs. The nurse instructs the patient to take at least 10 deep inhalations every hour. Frequently the patient uses an incentive spirometer in an effort to expand the lungs fully (see p. 345 for fuller discussion). Turning the patient from side to side sometimes results in coughing, with expulsion of a mucus plug and increased aeration of the lungs.

The increased metabolism, more complete pulmonary aeration, and general improvement of all body functions incidental to getting the patient up out of bed for ambulation is one of the best prophylactic measures for pulmonary complications. When the wound or other condition permits, the patient is usually allowed to get up on the first or second day after operation, and frequently on the day of surgery. This practice is especially valuable in preventing pulmonary complications in older patients.

Urinary Retention

Urinary retention may follow any operation, but it occurs most frequently after operations on the rectum, the anus, and the vagina, and after herniorrhaphies and operations on the lower abdomen. The cause is thought to be a spasm of the bladder sphincter.

Nursing Interventions. Quite often patients are unable to void while lying in bed, but when allowed to sit or stand up they do so without difficulty. When standing or sitting does not interfere with the operative result, male patients may be allowed to stand by the side of the bed and female patients to sit on the edge of the bed with their feet on a chair or a stool. However, some patients cannot be permitted this activity, and other means of encouraging urination must be tried. Some people cannot void with another person in the room. These patients should be left alone for a time after being provided with a warm bedpan or urinal.

Frequently the sound or sight of running water relaxes the spasm of the bladder sphincter. Using a bedpan containing warm water or irrigating the perineum with warm water frequently initiates urination for female patients. A small, warm enema often is of value in such a situation. If the retention of urine continues for some hours and the patient complains of considerable pain in the lower abdomen, the bladder frequently can be palpated and seen in outline distending the lower anterior abdominal wall.

When all conservative measures have failed, catheterization becomes necessary. If the patient has voided just before operation, this procedure may be delayed for 12 to 18 hours. There are two reasons for wishing to avoid catheterization: (1) there is the possibility of infecting the bladder and producing a cystitis, and (2) experience has shown that once a patient has been catheterized, often subsequent catheterizations are needed.

Many patients exhibit a palpable bladder, with lower abdominal discomfort, and still void small amounts of urine at frequent intervals. The alert nurse does not mistake this for normal functioning of the bladder. This voiding of 30 to 60 ml (1–2 oz) of urine at intervals of 15 to 30 minutes is, rather, a sign of an overdistended bladder, the very distention being sufficient to allow the escape of small amounts of urine at intervals. The condition usually is spoken of as the "overflow of retention." A catheter usually relieves the patient by draining from 600 to 900 ml (20–30 oz) of urine from the bladder. No more than 1000 ml of urine are removed at a time. "Incontinence of retention" may be evidenced by a constant dribble of urine while the bladder remains overdistended. Because distention injures the bladder, catheterization is indicated. There may be a psychic element in urinary retention.

At times the surgeon may anticipate voiding difficulties following extensive surgery, and an indwelling catheter is inserted before the patient emerges from anesthesia. Usually, the surgeon desires to be notified if an amount less than 30 ml of urine per hour is collected in the calibrated receptacle.

Gastrointestinal Complications

Nutritional Considerations

Surgery of the gastrointestinal tract frequently disrupts the normal physiologic processes of digestion and absorption. Complications arising from this disruption may take several forms, depending on the location and extent of surgery. For example, oral surgery may present problems of chewing and swallowing, requiring that diet be modified to accommodate the difficulty. Other surgical procedures, such as gastrectomy, small bowel resection, ileostomy, colostomy, and the like, have a more drastic effect on the gastrointestinal system and require more extensive dietary considerations, as indicated in Table 19-3.

Intestinal Obstruction

Intestinal obstruction is a complication that may follow abdominal operations. It occurs most often after operations on the lower abdomen and the pelvis, and especially after operations in which drainage has been necessary. The symptoms usually appear between the third and fifth days but may occur at any time, even years after the operation. The cause is some obstruction of the intestinal current—frequently a loop of intestine that has become kinked from inflammatory adhesions or is involved with peritonitis or generalized irritation of the peritoneal surface.

Usually there is no temperature or pulse elevation. At first the pains are localized, a point which should be noted by the nurse because the localization of the early pains represents in a general way the loop of intestine that is just above the obstruction.

Usually the patient continues to have abdominal pains, with shorter and shorter intervals between waves of pain. When a stethoscope is placed on the abdomen, sounds may be heard that give evidence of extremely active intestinal movements, especially during an attack of pain. The intestinal contents, being unable to move forward, distend the intestinal coils, are carried backward to the stomach, and are vomited. Thus, vomiting and increasing distention gradually become

TABLE 19-3
Dietary Support of Common Complications in Surgical Treatment

Procedure	*Complications*	*Dietary Support*
Radical oropharyngeal surgery	Difficulty in mastication and swallowing	*Diet:* Liquid consistency—tube feedings. Fluid by mouth: Fruit juices as tolerated. Coffee, tea, gelatin, ice cream
Gastrectomy	*Small pouch:* "Dumping syndrome" Epigastric fullness, distention; pallor, sweating, tachycardia, hypotension, diarrhea	Low-carbohydrate. Moderate-fat. High-protein. Small, frequent feedings. Periodic injections of vitamin B_{12}
Small bowel resection	Poor absorption. Weight loss (absorptive capacity improves with time)	*Immediate support after surgery:* Long-term parenteral nutrition. *Later:* oral intake of high protein, high-calorie, low-fat diet. Medium-chain triglycerides
Ileostomy Colostomy	Initial loss of water and electrolytes	Daily replacement of electrolytes, full liquid diet, high in protein
Bypass surgery	For relief of pain and obstruction. Malabsorption syndrome. Maldigestion, diarrhea	Feedings by natural route. High-protein, high-vitamin C. Adequate vitamins and minerals

(Valassi K. Nutritional management of cancer patients in a variety of therapeutic regimens. Arch Phys Med Rehab, Vol 58.)

more prominent symptoms. Hiccup often precedes the vomiting in many patients. Defecation does not occur, and enemas return nearly clear, showing that a very small amount of the intestinal contents has reached the large bowel. Unless the obstruction is relieved, the patient continues to vomit, distention becomes more pronounced, the pulse becomes rapid, and the end is death.

Management.   Sometimes the distention of the intestine above the obstruction can be prevented by the use of constant-suction drainage with a nasoenteral or simple nasogastric tube, in which case the inflammatory reaction of the bowel at the site of the obstruction may subside and the obstruction is relieved. However, at times it is necessary to relieve the obstruction surgically. Intravenous infusions of prescribed solutions usually are given as well. (See the section on intestinal obstruction for a more complete discussion of the treatment and postoperative care, pp. 828–829.)

Postoperative Psychosis

Postoperative psychosis (mental aberrations) may be physiological or psychological in origin. Cerebral anoxia, thromboembolism, and fluid–electrolyte imbalances are recognized physical factors in postoperative central nervous system impairment and stress. Emotional factors such as fear, pain, and disorientation can contribute to postoperative depression and anxiety.

Older patients are most susceptible to psychological disturbances, particularly those with cerebrovascular atherosclerosis. Usually they manage fairly well until they have been subjected to the anesthetic and operation. Postoperatively they may become very disturbed and disoriented. Disfiguring surgery and operations for cancer also predispose to intense emotional problems. Dressings that obscure vision or confinement in a body cast can result in behavioral changes because of the reduced sensory input.

A high incidence of psychotic sequelae appears to occur in patients who have had open-heart surgery. Several factors seem significantly related to neurologic damage: age (the older, the more likely), length of extracorporeal circulation (the longer, the greater the likelihood), mean arterial pressure of less than 50 mm Hg during perfusion, and the possibility of air emboli. Even the sensory overload of the intensive care unit is believed to contribute to postcardiotomy delirium.

Nursing Intervention: Preoperative and Postoperative.   The patient should be thoroughly informed before the operation about what to expect after surgery. Opportunities need to be provided for the patient to express thoughts and fears; misinformation can be corrected and reassurance provided. High-risk patients as described above may require special attention and support. More judicious use of narcotics can also reduce confusion and disorientation.

Orienting the patient to time, day, and place can help him to accept unfamiliar surroundings. Studies have indicated that thorough preoperative briefing of both patient and family can usually counteract many of the potential postoperative psychological stresses. In addition, a positive attitude conveyed by all personnel who come in contact with the patient will foster positive feelings in the patient.

For overt psychosis, the patient may require major tranquilizers and consultation and therapy with mental health professionals. Since postoperative psychosis does occur, it is helpful when discussing this with patients to indicate that it is transient. A patient with illusions or hallucinations is often reassured to know that these aberrations are occasionally experienced and do not reflect on his sanity.

The patient's room should be lighted to reduce the incidence of visual hallucinations. It is desirable to have a family member stay with the patient as much as possible, since the presence of another person has a reassuring and quieting effect.

Restraint.   In the postoperative care of patients with psychological disturbances, it is prudent for the nurse to explain the necessity for the patient's remaining in bed. Often, patients prefer to get out of bed to void or to get a drink of water rather than bother the nurse. This may lead to serious complications that a brief explanation can prevent. However, some patients, especially older patients and those who are disoriented, may find it impossible to grasp. For such patients, the simplest form of restraint is the use of beds with side rails or side protection. This permits patients to move about in bed but prevents them from getting out of bed easily and injuring themselves.

To protect both patient and nurse, it often becomes necessary to apply some form of restraint in cases of delirium. The psychological effect of being restrained can be severe; therefore, any form of restraint is applied *only as a last resort.* All other means of quieting the patient are tried first. If possible, he should be isolated from other patients. Any potentially harmful article in the vicinity is removed.

When restraints are used, the patient should be in a comfortable and natural position, and care is taken that the part is not so constricted as to interfere with the circulation. Restraint to the chest is avoided, if possible. The appearance of cyanosis of the hand or foot indicates that the appliance is too tight. The appliances are padded carefully and placed so as to prevent chafing or pressure sores. The skin underneath them is inspected frequently, bathed carefully, and massaged at least every 2 to 3 hours. Even though restraints are applied, the patient is never left unwatched. Any patient requiring restraint should have constant and careful nursing attention. Consideration is given to respecting the patient as a person. He is experiencing changes in body image and self-esteem, and needs understanding and support.

Delirium

Postoperative delirium occurs occasionally in several groups of patients. The most common types of delirium are toxic, traumatic, and alcoholic (delirium tremens).

Toxic Delirium.   Toxic delirium occurs in conjunction with the signs and symptoms of a general toxemia. The patient with toxic delirium is very ill, usually with a high temperature and pulse rate. The face is flushed, and the eyes are bright and roving. The patient moves incessantly, often attempting to get out of bed and disarranging the bedcothes continually. A marked degree of mental confusion is present. These states are seen most often in patients with general peritonitis or other septic conditions.

In such patients, elimination is promoted by encouraging the intake of fluids and the causative condition is treated by antimicrobial therapy. At times, however, the outcome is death.

Traumatic Delirium. Traumatic delirium is a mental state resulting from sudden trauma of any sort, especially in highly nervous people. The malady may take the form of wild, maniacal excitement, simple confusion with hallucinations and delusions, or depression. Sedative drugs (chloral hydrate, paraldehyde, and morphine) are used in treatment. Usually, the state begins and ends suddenly.

Delirium Tremens. Individuals who have used alcohol habitually over a long period of time are poor surgical risks. Not only is their resistance lower than normal, but the effects of alcohol have most likely damaged practically every organ. In addition, these patients take anesthesia poorly.

After operation, the alcoholic patient may do well for a few days, but the prolonged abstinence from alcohol causes him to become restless, nervous, and irritated easily by little things. Facial expression may change entirely. Sleep is poor and often disturbed by unreal dreams. When approached by the doctor or the nurse, the patient appears to wake suddenly, asks "Who are you?" and, when told where he is, appears to be fairly normal for a short time. These symptoms should be watched for in patients who have been alcoholics; by active treatment at this stage, the more violent delirium may be avoided.

Active delirium tremens may come on suddenly or gradually. After a period of restless, nervous semidelirium, the patient finally loses entire control of mental functions and "horrors reign supreme." His mind is a chaos of ever-changing ideas. He talks incessantly and tries to get out of bed to get away from the hallucinations of fear and persecution that torment him continually. If attempts are made to restrain him, he may fight maniacally and often injures himself and others. In this stage the patient is obviously sick. He is sleepless, perspires freely, and displays a marked tremor in the extremities. Finally, after many hours of torture, the patient becomes stuporous.

Medical and Nursing Management. When possible, the treatment of patients with delirium tremens should begin 2 or 3 days before operation with an increased fluid intake to encourage elimination from the kidneys, the bowels, and the skin. These measures should be continued after operation, especially if any of the early signs of the condition develop. Sedative drugs or tranquilizers should be given to keep the patient quiet. The chief cause of the symptoms in patients with chronic alcoholism has been shown to be a depletion of the carbohydrate stores of the body and an inadequate ingestion of vitamins. Therefore, glucose is given intravenously and vitamins are administered in concentrated form by mouth and by injection.

Ambulatory Surgery

Ambulatory surgery (same-day surgery, in-and-out surgery, outpatient surgery) is the product of advances in surgery practice and anesthesia techniques that permit the patient to return home on the day of the operation. Many surgical experiences that previously included several days of hospitalization can now be completed in the space of a day.

The preoperative phase is usually initiated in the physician's office. Diagnostic evaluation, laboratory studies, complete assessment, and preoperative interview are followed by preoperative planning and instruction plus a subsequent phone call for final checking with the patient to ensure that the whole procedure is understood. The patient's chart is continually developed, and the business office is contacted to handle its phase of the total record.

The preoperative phone call is designed to remind the patient not to drink after 12 midnight of the day before surgery; he may brush his teeth but is told not to swallow any fluids. The patient is told to wear comfortable cloths (*e.g.,* sweat suit), flat shoes, and no jewelry, to bring his medications along, and what time to arrive at the clinic.

Advantages of Ambulatory Surgery
- It is cost-effective to the patient, hospital, insurance carriers, and government agencies.
- There is less psychological stress for the patient.
- Hospital-acquired infections are prevented or reduced in incidence.
- Recovery is more rapid; the patient is more in charge.

Types of Procedures Handled as Ambulatory Surgery

Ambulatory procedures are usually of short duration, from 15 to 90 minutes, in which minimal bleeding and minor physiological disturbance are anticipated, as in the following examples:

General surgery—hernia repair, vasectomy, excision of small lumps or tumors
Gynecology—dilatation and curettage (D & C), tubal ligation, pregnancy termination, cervical diagnostic laparoscopy, biopsy, and conization
Dermatology—excision of warts and condylomata
Ophthalmology—cataract extraction, minor eye operations
Ear, nose, and throat—myringotomy, adenoidectomy, nasal polypectomy, oral surgery
Cardiac surgery—cardioversion, insertion and replacement of pacemakers
Orthopedic surgery—carpal tunnel surgery, ganglionectomy

Patient Selection

The patient should be in stable medical condition and be free of infection. It may be more practical for the person with a mild systemic disease to have a surgical procedure in this short-term facility than to be exposed to the greater risk of hospitalization. Usually age is not a factor; however, premature infants are usually not considered because of potential problems. It is desirable that the patient be psychologically willing to accept this mode of treatment.

Patient Assessment and Preoperative Preparation

Within 7 days before surgery, the history, physical examination, and laboratory studies should be completed. Written instructions usually present in detail the procedures to follow relative to abstaining from food and fluid; what to bring and what not to bring; what information may be requested by the anesthesiologist.

The nurse administers the preanesthetic medication and checks the vital signs. After voiding, the patient is accompanied to the anesthesia unit. It has been observed that when the patient receives *heated* humidified inspired gas during anesthesia induction and delivery, the recovery time is reduced by one third.

Recovery Room

The patient remains in the recovery unit until recovered sufficiently from the anesthetic to go home, accompanied safely by a responsible person. At this time the patient demonstrates a stable circulation, absence of bleeding, no nausea or vomiting, and no excessive pain. Postoperative orders, necessary prescriptions, and an information sheet are given. The usual recommended recovery time is 24 to 48 hours of "taking it easy." During this time the patient is not to drive a vehicle, drink alcoholic beverages, or perform tasks that require much skill or fine fingerwork. Fluids may be drunk as desired, and smaller than normal amounts eaten at mealtime. The patient is cautioned not to make important decisions at this time because the medications, anesthesia, and surgery may prevent his thinking as clearly as usual.

Bibliography

Books

Altemeier WA et al. Manual on Control of Infection in Surgical Patients. Philadelphia, JB Lippincott, 1984.

AORN Standards and Recommended Practices for Perioperative Nursing. Denver, The Association of Operating Room Nurses, 1986.

Atkinson L. Berry and Kohn's Introduction to Operating Room Technique. New York, McGraw-Hill, 1986.

Barret J and Nyhus LM. Treatment of Shock, 2nd ed. Philadelphia, Lea & Febiger, 1986.

Cameron J. Current Surgical Therapy, 2nd ed. St Louis, CV Mosby, 1986.

Committee on Pre- and Postoperative Care. Manual of Preoperative and Postoperative Care, 3rd ed. Philadelphia, WB Saunders, 1983.

Cordner, JW. Logic of Operating Room Nursing, 3rd ed. Oradell, New Jersey, Med Econ Books, 1984.

Cowley RA and Trump BE. Pathophysiology of Shock, Anoxia, and Ischeia. Baltimore, Williams & Wilkins, 1982

Deitel M (ed). Nutrition in Clinical Surgery, 2nd ed. Baltimore, Williams & Wilkins, 1985.

Dripps RD, Eckenhoff JE and Vandam LD. Introduction to Anesthesia, 6th ed. Philadelphia, WB Saunders, 1982.

Etheredge EE. Management Techniques in Surgery. New York, John Wiley & Sons, 1986.

Frost AME. Recovery Room Practice. St Louis, CV Mosby, 1985.

Garner JS. Guidelines for Prevention of Surgical Wound Infections. Atlanta, Centers for Disease Control, 1985.

Groah L. Operating Room Nursing: The Perioperative Role. Reston, Virginia, Reston Publishing Company, 1983.

Gruendemann BJ and Meeker MH. Alexander's Care of the Patient in Surgery, 8th ed. St Louis, CV Mosby, 1987.

Kirkwood EK. Guidelines for Preparing and Sterilizing Wrapped Packs. Erie, Pennsylvania, American Sterilizer Company, 1983.

Kneedler JA and Dodge GH. Perioperative Patient Care. Boston, Blackwell Scientific, 1983.

Liechty RD. Synopsis of Surgery, 5th ed. St Louis, CV Mosby, 1985.

Luczun ME. Postanesthesia Nursing. St Louis, CV Mosby, 1984.

Perry AG and Potter PA. Shock—Comprehensive Nursing Management. St Louis, CV Mosby, 1983.

Ratz J. Lasers in Cutaneous Medicine and Surgery. New York, Year Book Medical Publishers, 1986.

Ravitch M (ed). Current Problems in Surgery 1985. New York, Year Book Medical Publishers, 1985.

Rothrock J. RN First Assistant: An Expanded Perioperative Nursing Role. Philadelphia, JB Lippincott, 1987.

Sabiston D (ed). Textbook of Surgery, 13th ed. Philadelphia, WB Saunders, 1986.

Schrock TR (ed). Handbook of Surgery. Greenbrae, California, Jones Medical Publishers, 1985.

Schwartz S et al. Principles of Surgery. New York, McGraw-Hill, 1984.

Seymour G. Medical Assessment of the Elderly Surgical Patient. Hagerstown, Aspen Systems, 1986.

Zollinger RM and Zollinger RM Jr. Atlas of Surgical Operations, 5th ed. New York, Macmillan, 1983.

Articles

(Asterisks indicate nursing research articles.)

Perioperative Nursing

Barness SK and Long CS. Perioperative nursing. AORN J 1984 Mar; 39(4): 609–615.

Botsford J. Implementing outcome standards. AORN J. 1984 Oct; 40(4): 572–575, 578–580.

Dowdell DM. Theory has a place in OR nursing. Today's OR Nurse 1985 Apr; 8(4):9.

Durrence C et al. Potential drug interactions in surgical patients. Am J Hosp Pharm 1985 July; 42(7):1553–1556.

Garner JS and Favero MS. CDC guidelines for handwashing and hospital environmental controls. Today's OR Nurse 1986 Apr; 8(4):26–37.

Georges JM. Ethical issues in perioperative nursing practice. PNQ 1986 June; 2(2):13–19.

Glover SF. Perioperative nursing—vital to holistic care. Today's OR Nurse 1985 Aug; 7(8):18–23.

Hercules P, Kneedler JA, and Roth RA. Perioperative nursing competencies: The model. AORN J 1986 Jan; 43(1):229–235.

Mackie R, Peddie R, and Pendleton R. Perioperative care plan guides. AORN J 1984 Aug; 40(2):192–205.

Packard S, Polifrani ED, and Kramer M. Nursing education: Perioperative and community health nursing combined. AORN J 1985 Dec; 42(6): 888–890, 892–893.

Rabinow J. Avoiding legal risks in the OR. Nurs Life 1985 Nov/Dec; 5(6): 24–26.

Reeder JM and Kapsar PP. Perioperative nursing competencies: The process and study. AORN J 1986 Jan; 43(1):220–222, 224–247.

Tollerud L et al. A model for perioperative nursing practice. AORN J 1985 Jan; 41(1):188–194.

Webster JA. Planning your wellness: Personalized strategies for the perioperative nurse. PNQ 1986 Mar; 2(1):11–19.

Yoder ME. Nursing diagnosis: Applications in perioperative practice. AORN J 1984 Aug; 40(2):183–188.

Preoperative Nursing

Alverson E. The preoperative interview. AORN J 1987 May; 45(5):1158–1164.

Antimicrobial prophylaxis for surgery. The Med Letter 1985 Dec 20; 27(703):105–108.

Blackwood S. Back to basics—the preoperative examination. Am J Nurs 1986 Jan; 86(1):39–44.

*Hathaway D. Effect of preoperative teaching on postoperative pain: A replication and explanation. Int J Nurs Stud 1985; 22(3):267–280.

*Mogan J, Walls N, and Robertson E. Effects of preoperative teaching on postoperative pain: A replication and explanation. Int J Nurs Stud 1985; 22(3):267–280.

Peterson KL. Perioperative vascular monitoring. CCQ 1985 Sept; 8(2): 1–8.

Reilly JJ Jr and Gerhardt AL. Modern surgical nutrition. Current Prob Surg 1985 Oct; 22(10):4–81.

Stuhler–Schlag MK. Pre- and postoperative fluids and electrolytes. Today's OR Nurse 1982 Sept; 4(7):11–15, 66–67.

Warfield CA and Stein JM. The use of systemic analgesics. Hosp Pract 1982 July; 17(7):88a–88s.

*Wong J and Wong S. A randomized controlled trial of a new approach to preoperative teaching and patient compliance. Int J Nurs Stud 1985; 22(2):105–115.

OR Documentation

Sabatino K, Arnold A, and Rhinehart C. Standards for OR nurse's notes. Point of View (Ethicon) 1984; 21(2):12–13.

Terrion J. Documentation of nursing care in the operating room. Point of View (Ethicon) 1984; 21(2):10–11.

Informed Consent

*Cassidy VR and Oddi LF. Legal and ethical aspects of informed consent: A nursing research perspective. J Prof Nurs 1986 Nov/Dec; 2(6): 343–349.

Davis AJ. Informed consent: How much information is enough? Nurs Out 1985 Jan/Feb; 33(1):40–42.

Douglas S and Larson E. There's more to informed consent than information. Focus on Crit Care 1986 Apr; 13(2):43–47.

Falvo DR. Informed consent. In Falvo D (ed). Effective Patient Education: A Guide to Increased Compliance. Rockville, Maryland, Aspen Systems, 1985.

Fay MF. Informed consent: A confusing concept. Today's OR Nurse 1986 July; 8(7):6–10.

Hogue E. Informed consent. Nursing '86 1986 June; 16(6):47–48.

Northrop CE. The ins and outs of informed consent. Nursing '85 1985 Jan; 15(1):9.

President's Commission for the Study of Ethical Problems in Medicine and Biomedical Behavioral Research, Making Health Care Decisions. Vol 1: Report. Washington DC, US Government Printing Office, Oct 1982, Library of Congress #82-600637.

*Silva MC and Sorrell JM. Factors influencing comprehension of information for informed consent: Ethical implications for nursing research. Int J Nurs Stud 1984; 21(4):233–240.

Stanley B et al. The elderly patient and informed consent. JAMA 1984 Sept 14; 252(10):1302–1306.

Taylor S and Hobaugh R. The role of the critical care nurse in developing informed consent. DCCN 1986 Mar/Apr; 5(2):98–105.

Weaver JP. The problem with the operative permit. Surg Gynecol Obstet 1984 Dec; 159(6):579–580.

Weikel C. Informed consent: An ethical dilemma. Today's OR Nurse 1987 Jan; 9(1):10–15.

Whalen ER. Informed consent: The opinions of critical care nurses. Heart Lung 1984 Nov; 13(6):662–666.

Psychological Preparation

Brennan PE. Preoperative visits–controlling the stress. Today's OR Nurse 1982 Dec; 4(10):9–13.

Chansky ER. Reducing patient's anxieties. AORN J 1984 Sept; 40(3): 375–377.

*Devine EC and Cook TD. A meta-analytic analysis of effects of psychoeducational interventions on length of postsurgical stay. Nurs Res 1983 Sept/Oct; 32(5):267–274.

Hamer BA. Managing OR patients' fears. Today's OR Nurse 1985 May; 7(5):28–30.

*Johnson JE, Christman NJ and Stitt C. Personal control interventions: Short- and long-term effects on surgical patients. Res Nurs Health 1985 Jun; 8(2):131–146.

McNeal P and Duncan ML. Assessing patients in the holding area. Today's OR Nurse 1985 Mar; 7(3):16–19.

Mumford E et al. The effects of psychological intervention in recovery

from surgery and heart attacks: An analysis of the literature. Am J Pub Health 1982 Feb; 72(2):141–151.

Wallace LM. Psychological preparation as a method of reducing the stress of surgery. J Human Stress 1984 Summer; 10(2):62.

Ziemer MM. Effects of information on postsurgical coping. Nurs Res 1983 Sept/Oct; 32(5):282–287.

Nutrition

Palmer PV. Malnutrition (reversing the trend in the surgical patient). AORN J 1984 Sept; 40(3):347–352.

Reilly JJ Jr and Gerhardt AL. Modern surgical nutrition. Current Prob in Surg 1985 Oct; 22(10):4–81.

Skin Preparation

Geelhoed GW and Sharpe K. The rationale and ritual of preoperative skin preparation. Contemp Surg 1983 Sept; 23(3):31–36.

Geelhoed GW, Sharpe K, and Simon GL. A comparative study of surgical skin preparation methods. Surg Gynecol Obstet 1983 Sept; 157(3): 265–268.

Rathbrun AM, Holland LA, and Geelhoed GW. Preoperative skin decontamination. AORN J 1986 July; 44(1):62–65.

One-Day Surgery

Recommended practices: Monitoring the patient receiving local anesthesia. AORN J 1984 May; 39(6):1080–1088.

*Streiff LD. Can clients understand our instructions? IMAGE: J Nurs Scholarship 1986 Summer; 18(2):48–52.

Wicklund S. Special report: Drug management and elective surgery. Nurses' Drug Alert 1983 Jan; 7(1):4–5.

Intraoperative Nursing

Personnel/Communications

AORN approves guidelines for RN first assistants. Am J Nurs 1984 June; 84(6):818–820.

AORN official statement on RN first assistants. AORN J 1984 Sept; 40(3): 441–443.

Hanson RL and Nelson AH. OR personnel functions. AORN J 1985 Sept; 43(3):376–387.

Koerner M, Gatch G, and Taylor C. Communicating in the OR. AORN J 1984 Dec; 40(6):858–866.

Leske JS and McKnight EA. First assisting for RNs. AORN J 1985 Aug; 42(2):185–192.

Patterson RE and Daake JW. First assisting. Today's OR Nurse 1985 Dec; 7(12):10–16.

Scrubbing/Handwashing

Brockhurt G. Face masks and wedding rings. Lancet 1983 July 16; 2(8342): 157.

*Jacobson G et al. Handwashing: Ring-wearing and number of microorganisms. Nurs Res 1985 May/June; 34(3):186–187.

*Kabara J and Brady M. Contamination of bar soaps under "in-use" conditions. J Environ Pathol Toxicol Oncol 1983 Apr; 5(4):1–14.

Anesthesia and Surgery

Biddle CJ and Biddle WL. A plastic head cover to reduce surgical heat loss. Geriatr Nurs 1985 Jan/Feb; 6(1):39–41.

*Boucher BA, Witt WO, and Foster TS. The postoperative adverse effects of inhalational anesthetics. Heart Lung 1986 Jan; 15(1):63–69.

Gupta BS, Wolf KW, and Postlethwait RW. Effect of lubrication on frictional properties of sutures. Surg Gynecol Obstet 1985 Nov; 161(5): 416–417.

*Kasal SE. Infractions in aseptic techniques: A research study. AORN J 1985 Mar; 41(3):611–620.

Midazolam. Med Lett Drugs Ther 1986 Aug; 28(719):73–74.

Miner D. Patient positioning. AORN J 1987 May; 45(5):1117–1127.

Moss V and Schweiner M. Hypnosis and the surgical patient. AORN J 1985 Sept; 42(3):389–400.

Pierce EC. Anesthesiology. JAMA 1985 Oct 25; 254(16):2317–2318.

Sufentanil—a new opioid anesthetic. The Med Letter 1984 Nov 23; 26(675):106.

Winter PM and Miller JN. Anesthesiology. Scient Amer 1985 Apr; 252(4): 124–131, 146.

Wlody GS. Isoflurane. AORN J 1984 Oct; 40(4):568–571.

Hypothermia and Malignant Hyperthermia

Biddle C. Hypothermia: Implications for the critical care nurse. Crit Care Nurs 1985 Mar/Apr; 5(2):34–37.

Biddle CA and Biddle WL. A plastic head cover to reduce surgical heat loss. Geriatr Nurs 1985 Jan/Feb; 6(1):39–41.

Caine R, Molla K, and Reynolds R. Malignant hyperthermia: A critical care challenge. DCCN 1986 May/June; 5(3):144–154.

Fallacaro M, Fallacaro N, and Radel TJ. Inadvertent hypothermia. AORN J 1986 July; 44(1):54–61.

Greany D and Brown MM. Malignant hyperthermia. Focus on Crit Care 1986 Apr; 13(2):52–57.

Mavity CB. OR crisis! Malignant hyperthermia. Today's OR Nurse 1985 Jan; 7(1):8–11.

Rosenberg H. Malignant hyperthermia. Hosp Pract 1985 Mar 15; 20(3): 139–149.

Welch TC. Hypothermia. Today's OR Nurse 1985 Apr; 8(4):20–22.

Sterilization

Sparks BJ. Product sterilization (radiation). AORN J 1984 Sept; 40(3): 389–390.

Postoperative Nursing

Recovery Room

Consensus Conference. Prevention of venous thrombosis and pulmonary embolism. JAMA 1986 Aug 8; 256(6):744–749.

General

Fahey VA. Life-threatening pulmonary embolism. Crit Care Quart 1985 Sept; 8(2):81–87.

Fernsebner B, Baum PL, and Bartlett C. Surgical prevention of pulmonary emboli. AORN J 1984 Jan; 39(1):56–64.

Fraulini KE and Murphy P. R.E.A.C.T.—A new system for measuring postanesthesia recovery. Nursing '84 1984 Apr; 14(4):101–102.

Montanari J. Documenting your postoperative assessment findings. Nursing '85 1985 Aug; 15(8):31–35.

Rice V. The clinical continuum of septic shock. Crit Care Nurs 1984 Sept/Oct; 4(5):88–109.

Robinson JA. Septic shock in cardiopulmonary patients. Hosp Med 1983 June; 19(6):117–138.

*Rose SEM and MacKay RC. Postoperative stress: Do nurses accurately assess their patients? J Psychosoc Nurs Ment Health. 1986 Apr; 24(4):16–22.

Stevenson CK. Take no chances with fat embolism. Nursing '85 1985 June; 85(6):58–63.

Sutterley DC. Stress management: Grazing the clinical turf. Holistic Nurs Pract 1986 Nov; 1(1):36–53.

Vaughn JB and Nemcek MA. Postoperative flatulence: Causes and remedies. Today's OR Nurse 1986 Oct; 8(10):19–23.

Woodruff ML. Pulmonary thromboembolism: Risk factors, pathophysiology, and management. Crit Care Nurs 1984 July/Aug; 4(4):52–63.

Pain

Bailey CJ et al. Epidural morphine infusion. AORN J 1984 May; 39(6): 997–1008.

Bonica J. Postoperative pain—Part 1 (Symposium). Contemp Surg 1982 Jan; 20(1):83–137.

Cramer C. Morphine epidural anesthesia. J Post Anesth Nurs 1986 May; 1(2):129–131.

*Faherty BS and Grier MR. Analgesic medication for elderly people postsurgery. Nurs Res 1984 Nov/Dec; 36(6):369–372.

Managing intractable pain with methadone. Nursing '85 1985 May; 85(5): 33–37.

McCaffery M. Newer uses of NSAIDS. Am J Nurs 1985 July; 85(7):781–782.

Nichols RR. Simple remedies for postoperative gas pain. RN 1986 Feb; 42–44.

Ross SEM and MacKay RC. Postoperative stress. J Psychosoc Nurs 1986 Apr; 24(4):16–22.

Wounds

Alexander JW (ed). Bacteriologic comparison of closed suction and Penrose drainage. Am J Surg 1984 Nov; 148(5):699.

Baron MC. The skin and wound healing. Top Clin Nurs 1983 July; 5(2): 11–22.

Bassan M et al. Near-fatal systemic oxygen embolism due to wound irrigation with hydrogen peroxide. Postgrad Med 1982 July; 58(681): 448–450.

Becker L and Palenesar RF. Nosocomial infections: Using CDC guidelines for tracking infections. AORN J 1986 Jan; 43(1):274–276.

Birdsall C. What suction pressure should I use? Am J Nurs 1985 Aug; 85(8):866.

Boucek RJ. Factors affecting wound healing. Otolaryngol Clin North Am 1984 May; 17(2):243–264.

Bradley SJ et al. Controlled drainage of severe intra-abdominal sepsis. Arch Surg 1985 May; 120(5):629–631.

Brozenec S. Caring for the postoperative patient with an abdominal drain. Nursing '85 1985 Apr; 15(4):55–57.

Ducey DY. The phases of wound healing and wound irrigation. Point of View (Ethicon) 1983; 20(4):4–7.

Edlich RF et al. Evaluation of a new improved surgical drainage system. Am J Surg 1985 Feb; 149(2):295–298.

Jasinkowski NL and Cullum JL. Human amniotic membrane (as a wound dressing). AORN J 1984 Apr; 39(5):894–899.

Mancusi–Ungaro HR Jr and Rappaport NH. Preventing wound infection. Am Fam Physician 1986 Apr; 33(4):147–153.

Montanari J. Wound dehiscence. Nursing '86 1986 Feb; 16(2):33.

Neuberger GB and Reckling JB. A new look at wound care. Nursing '85 1985 Feb; 15(2):34–41.

Ramirez OM et al. Optimal wound healing under Op-Site dressing. Plast Reconstr Surg 1984 Mar; 73(3):474–475.

Raves JJ, Slifkin M, and Diamond DL. A bacteriologic study comparing closed suction and simple conduit drainage. Am J Surg 1984 Nov; 148(5):618–620.

Sondak VK and Morton DL. A simple, inexpensive technique for clearing obstructed closed suction drainage catheters. Surg Gynecol Obstet 1985 Dec; 161(6):594–596.

Starting a wound on its way to healing. Patient Care 1984 Mar 15; 18(5): 101–126.

Transparent wound dressings. The Med Letter 1983 Nov 11; 25(64):104.

When wound healing problems arise. Patient Care 1984 Aug 15; 18(14): 190–226.

Wound care: Taking a drain check. Am J Nurs 1984 Aug; 84(8):1039–1041.

Infection

Baker RJ et al. A prospective double-blind comparison of piperacillin, cephalothin, and cefoxitin in the prevention of postoperative infections in patients undergoing intra-abdominal operations. Surg Gynecol Obstet 1985 Nov; 161(5):409–415.

Broughton RA. Rapid diagnosis of infections. Postgrad Med 1985 Feb 15; 77(3):201–210.

Fry DE and Polk HC Jr. Infection in the surgical patient: Prevention and treatment. Drug Ther 1982 Aug; 82(8):19–28.

Garner JS (revised by). Guidelines for prevention of surgical wound infections. USDHHS 1985 (Atlanta).

Gary JP. JCAH Policies on infection control. AORN J 1984 May; 39(6): 1056–1057.

Gordon M. A career in infection control. Imprint 1984 Feb/Mar; 31(1): 22–27.

Hammond WP IV. Infections in the compromised host (Part 1). Hosp Med 1983 Oct; 19(10):40–52.

Jones I. You can drive back infection—if you know where to make your stand. Nursing '85 1985 Apr; 15(4):50–52.

Masci JR. Infectious problems in surgical patients. Resident and Staff Physician 1986 Feb; 32(2):86–95.

*McCarthy DO. The adaptive value of fever during infection. Crit Care Nurs Currents (Ross) 1985; 3(1):1–5.

Nichols RL. Postoperative wound infection. N Engl J Med 1982 Dec 30; 307(27):1701–1702.

Olson M, O'Connor M, and Schwartz ML. Surgical wound infections: A 5-year prospective study of 20,193 wounds at the Minneapolis VA Medical Center. Ann Surg 1984 Mar; 199(3):253–259.

Stotts NA. Predicting pressure ulcers in a surgical population. Heart Lung 1986 May; 15(3):315–316.

Troxler SH and Nichols RL. Surgical wound infections. Today's OR Nurse 1987 Mar; 9(3):16–22.

Ambulatory Surgery

Ambulatory surgery. AORN J 1984 Apr; 39(5):770–771.

Growth of same-day surgery demands patient education. Same-day Surg 1985 Jan; 9(1):1–3.

McCartney BJ. Implementing wellness philosophy in an ambulatory surgery center. Periop Nurs Q 1985 Mar; 1(1):63–67.

Poland V. Strategies for ambulatory surgery. AORN J 1984 June; 39(7): 1245–1253.

Spielman FJ. Ambulatory surgery. Med Times 1983 Sept; 111(9):62–66.

*Streiff LD. Can clients understand our instructions? IMAGE; J Nurs Scholarship 1986 Summer; 18(2):48–52.

Turcotte MA and Irish EM. Innovations and excellence: quality ambulatory surgery. Periop Nurs Q 1985 Sept; 1(3):62–69.

Agencies

American Society of Anesthesiologist, 500 North Michigan Avenue, Chicago IL 60611.

Association of Operating Room Nurses, Inc., 10170 E. Mississippi Avenue, Denver CO 80231.

American Society of Postanesthesia Nurses, P.O. Box 11083, Richmond VA 23230.

Malignant Hyperthermia Association of the United States (MHAUS), 163 Waverly Street, Arlington MA 02174.

Nursing Research Profile for Unit V

Perioperative Nursing

Overview

Recent nursing research in perioperative nursing covers a number of areas: the effect of preoperative teaching on postoperative recovery; the meaning of an informed consent, including ethical implications; and infractions in aseptic techniques. In the latter area, the study of skin disinfection continues as attempts are made to reduce microbacterial contaminants. Some studies address the effectiveness of bar soap as compared with that of liquid soaps.

Another area of research is the psychological analysis of stress management for both staff and patients. This continues to be studied, particularly in the light of staff reduction to reduce costs.

Preoperative Patient Teaching

Several investigators chose to search for more effective preoperative teaching techniques that would reduce postoperative discomfort and minimize complications.

▷ *Wong J and Wong S. A randomized controlled trial of a new approach to pre-operative teaching and patient compliance. Int J Nurs Stud 1985; 22(2):105–115.*

Wong and Wong measured patient compliance with prescribed postsurgical activities in relation to preoperative teaching, using the variables of accuracy, regularity, and willingness of the patient. Their findings suggest that patient compliance improved when teaching methods incorporated basic principles of educational and behavioral psychology. These principles include patient readiness, effectiveness of teaching methods, repetition, reinforcing learning, and active participation of the patient.

Nursing Implications. Merely reviewing a preoperative teaching plan with a patient does not ensure postoperative effectiveness. The use of well-known principles of learning (repeating information, being sure the patient is in a receptive mood to learn, and providing reinforcement) is essential in helping the patient to learn and to use what he has learned. Complimenting the patient when he remembers to do what he has been taught encourages him to continue the practice.

▷ *Mogan J, Wells N and Robertson E. Effects of preoperative teaching on post-operative pain: A replication and expansion. Int J Nurs Stud 1985 22(3):267–280.*

The effectiveness of brief relaxation training in managing postoperative pain was studied as it affected certain measurable entities: vital signs, anxiety, analgesic use, and patient report of incisional pain/distress. Relaxation techniques were taught the evening before surgery and included such directives as, "Close your eyes. Let your mind recall a pleasant memory. Relax and let the tension dissolve." "Let your lower jaw drop slightly—let your lips go soft—breathe slowly and rhythmically." Subjects were requested to practice several techniques before surgery and were provided with written instructions. Following a structured procedure that included a "blind" group for comparison, observation of key points, and documentation, the investigators included comparisons for two groups of patients, one group having cholecystectomy and the other hysterectomy. The distress of painful sensations was significantly lower for the experimental group. Other variables were not altered. Patients with hysterectomy appeared to benefit more from relaxation training.

Nursing Implications. The teaching of relaxation techniques certainly reduces the distress of painful sensations. Aspects not altered by relaxation training were vital signs, analgesic consumption, and self-reported pain sensation. Incorporation of relaxation techniques is an important addition to the preoperative teaching session by the nurse.

▷ *Rice VH and Johnson JE. Preadmission self-instruction booklet, postadmission exercise performance, and teaching time. Nurs Res 1984 May/Jun; 33(3): 147–151.*

Rice and Johnson studied patients' mastering of exercise behaviors preoperatively for use postoperatively, and addressed the following questions: Was preadmission instruction more effective in producing subsequent mastery of the exercises (1) when specific instructions were given, (2) when nonspecific instruction was given, or (3) when there was no preadmission information? After studying 130 presurgical cholecystectomy and herniorrhaphy patients, results showed that patients receiving specific exercise instruction performed significantly better than those receiving nonspecific exercise instruction. Both groups required much less teaching time after admission than the group that had no preadmission instruction.

Nursing Implications. Patients can learn exercise behaviors prior to hospital admission. This reduces the amount of time spent teaching patients after admission; the time saved can be devoted to meeting other needs: providing support, correcting misinformation, and individualizing subsequent planning.

Additional Studies

Devine EC and Cook TD. A meta-analytic analysis of effects of psychoeducational interventions on length of postsurgical stay. Nurs Res 1983 Sept/Oct; 32(5):267–274.

Hathaway D. Effect of preoperative instruction on postoperative outcomes: A meta-analysis. Nurs Res 1986 Sept/Oct; 35(5):269–274.

Streiff LD. Can clients understand our instructions? IMAGE: Jour Nurs Scholarship 1986 Summer; 18(2):48–52.

Scrubbing/Handwashing

Research continues in the area of more effective methods of reducing microbacterial presence on skin surfaces; this applies to preparing the patient's skin for an operation and also to scrubbing procedures used by members of the surgical team.

▷ *Rathburn AM, Holland LA and Geelhoed GW. Preoperative skin decontamination. AORN J 1986 July; 44(1):62–65.*

The goal of preoperative skin decontamination is to promote optimal postoperative healing of the surgical wound in a cost-effective manner. The antiseptic should have broad-spectrum antibacterial action, be nontoxic, and provide long-acting protection. The Rathburn study reviews three methods: (1) conventional 5-minute iodophor scrub followed by an io-

dophor paint; (2) a 5-minute iodophor scrub followed by a 1-minute alcohol wipe and application of an antimicrobial drape; and (3) a 1-minute alcohol wipe followed by application of an antimicrobial drape.

The two groups using the alcohol wipe had the most effective bacterial reduction immediately following skin preparation. At wound closure, group 2 had the lowest bacterial count overall.

Nursing Implications. For surgical preparation of a patient's skin, the use of an alcohol wipe and application of antimicrobial film produces the most effective bactericidal results, takes less time, and is less costly.

▷ *Jacobson G et al. Handwashing: Ring-wearing and number of microorganisms. Nurs Res 1985 May/June; 34(3):186–188.*

Questions continue to be raised about proper and effective protocol related to ring wearing by those normally required to use rigorous hand washing or scrubbing in high-risk areas such as the operating room. Generally, a vigorous hand scrub using running water and soap with particular attention to nail cleansing is recommended.

Conditions were set to compare scrubs with multiple rings and no rings (with one exception of a subject wearing a single plain wedding band). A standardized hand washing procedure was used. Results: Wearing rings while washing hands left a greater number of microorganisms on the hands, but thorough hand washing reduced the number to a count similar to that obtained when rings are not worn.

Nursing Implications. Although the study revealed that there was no significant difference in the number of microorganisms grown on bacteriological plates whether rings were worn or not, this study is predicated on a vigorous standardized hand washing procedure generally followed in the operating room. Shortening the procedure or not washing hands thoroughly in patient contact areas may result in greater numbers of microorganisms on the nurse's hands when wearing rings.

Additional Studies

Kabara J and Brady M. Contamination of bar soaps under "in-use" conditions. J Environ Pathol Toxicol Oncol 1983 Apr; 5(4):1–14.

Postoperative Pain

The traditional method of reducing postoperative pain is to administer narcotics or analgesics. On occasion these agents may not be as effective as desired, may cause unwanted side-effects, and frequently cause a physiological depression. Other ways of reducing or eliminating pain and discomfort continue to be sought.

▷ *Taylor AG et al. How effective is TENS for acute pain? Am J Nurs 1983 Aug; 83(8):1171–1174.*

The effectiveness of transcutaneous electrical nerve stimulation (TENS) in controlling acute pain was compared with that of narcotics and non-narcotic analgesics. Three groups of postabdominal surgical patients were studied and designated as functional TENS (FT), sham TENS (ST), and narcotic analgesic group. Patients on TENS were told that if relief was not obtained in 30 minutes, they could have pain medication.

Results indicated that both TENS groups experienced

greater pain relief than the narcotic group and therefore required less medication. The sham group, authors explained, may have reacted to the placebo effect, which stimulates the release of enkephalins (endogenous opiates). The psychological effect of the patient's reacting to "something being done for my pain" may also have affected the results of the sham group.

Nursing Implications.   Functional TENS is an effective method of relieving acute postoperative pain. In addition, it has been demonstrated that bowel sounds return sooner in patients using TENS and that these patients ambulate faster than those who receive narcotic analgesics. Cost-effectiveness was not explored in this study.

▷   *Locsin AC. The effect of music on the pain of selected post-operative patients. J Adv Nurs 1981 Jan; 6(1): 19–25.*

The goal of Locsen's study was to determine whether listening to music made a difference in the perception of pain in women having abdominal incisions. (The women chose the music they preferred.) An overt pain reaction rating scale was devised by the author to describe gradations of manifestations of pain. Additional variables noted were blood pressure, pulse rate, respiratory rate, and analgesics received. There were significant differences in musculoskeletal, verbal, and physiologic autonomic pain reactions during the first 48 hours and the women used less pain-relief medication. Respiratory rates were not affected.

Nursing Implications.   Music decreases overt pain reaction during the first 48 hours postoperatively. Since it relieves or alleviates pain to a certain extent, it is useful to introduce this modality in the first 48 hours postoperative.

Additional Studies

Faherty BS and Grier MR. Analgesic medication for elderly people post-surgery. Nurs Res 1984 Nov/Dec; 33(6):369–372.

Postoperative Grief

Although planned preoperative teaching results in improved patient behaviors postoperatively, additional measures can be used to improve psychosocial reaction to an operation recently experienced. The grieving process is frequently observed when a body part is removed. The stages of grief are experienced in progression before the loss is assimilated and accepted. In other surgical operations, diversionary techniques may be effective. The following study provides an example of how the effects of surgery can be accepted more comfortably.

▷   *Kelly MP. Loss and grief reactions as responses to surgery. Jour Adv Nurs 1985 Nov; 10(6):517–525.*

Kelly presents autobiographical material of a patient who has had major surgery (panproctocolectomy and ileostomy). Various stages of experience are described: dependence prior to the operation, isolation from the social world postoperatively, and later grief over loss. A theoretical analysis by the patient of the psychological and emotional processes is described and analyzed based on theoretical models. Although the patient's conclusions appear unexceptional, there are nursing implications.

Nursing Implications.   A hospital setting probably is not the best place for counseling a grieving patient because activities and procedures are organized around "rapid intervention and immediate results," so that the patient's physical dependence takes priority over his psychological needs. There should be more emphasis on awareness of the patient's psychosocial needs, since his physical dependency may be the prime manifestation of an underlying problem. Such a problem may account for delayed recovery.

Other Perioperative Nursing Research Studies

Boucher BA, Witt WO and Foster TS. The postoperative adverse effects of inhalational anesthetics. Heart Lung 1986 Jan; 15(1):63–69.

Kasal SE. Infractions in aseptic techniques: A research study. AORN J 1985 Mar; 41(3):611–620.

McCarthy DO. The adaptive value of fever during infection. Crit Care Nurs Currents (Ross) 1985; 3(1):1–5.

Rose SEM and MacKay RC. Postoperative stress: Do nurses accurately assess their patients? J Psychosoc Nurs Ment Health 1986 Apr; 24(4): 16–22.

Stotts NA. Predicting pressure ulcers in a surgical population. Heart Lung 1986 May; 15(3):315–316.

Sutterly DC. Stress management: Grazing the clinical turf. Holistic Nurs Pract 1986 Nov; 1(1):36–53.

Problems Affecting Oxygen–Carbon Dioxide Exchange and Respiration

Unit VI

Chapter 20

Management of Patients With Conditions of the Upper Respiratory Airway

Anatomy of the Upper Respiratory Airway

Nose

The external, visible portion of the nose and the internal portion are separated into right and left nasal cavities by a narrow vertical divider, the septum. The anterior *nares* (nostrils) are the outside openings of the nasal cavities. The posterior nares (*choanae*) open into the nasopharynx. Projecting from the lateral walls of the interior nasal cavities are three turbinate bones (also called *conchae*). The nasal cavities are lined with a highly vascular ciliated mucous membrane called the *nasal mucosa*. Mucus secreted continuously by goblet cells covers the surface of the nasal mucosa and is moved back to the nasopharynx by the action of the cilia. The paranasal sinuses, which are cavities within the surrounding facial bones, drain into the interior nasal cavities. The nose filters, humidifies, and warms the air as it is inhaled into the lungs, and is also responsible for olfaction (smell), a function that diminishes with age.

Paranasal Sinuses

The paranasal sinuses include the frontal sinuses, located in the lower forehead between and above the eyes; the ethmoidal group of sinuses, both anterior and posterior, extending along the roof of the nostrils; the sphenoidal sinuses, opening at the rear; and, located on either side of the nose, the maxillary sinuses. The same type of ciliated epithelium that lines the nasal passages also lines these paranasal sinuses.

A prominent function of the sinuses is to help give resonance and timbre to speech. One notes how "nasal" the voice is when a person has a head cold and sinusitis.

Turbinate Bones (Conchae)

The turbinate bones, or conchae (the name suggested by their shell-like appearance), are adapted by shape and position to increase the mucous membrane surface of the nasal pas-

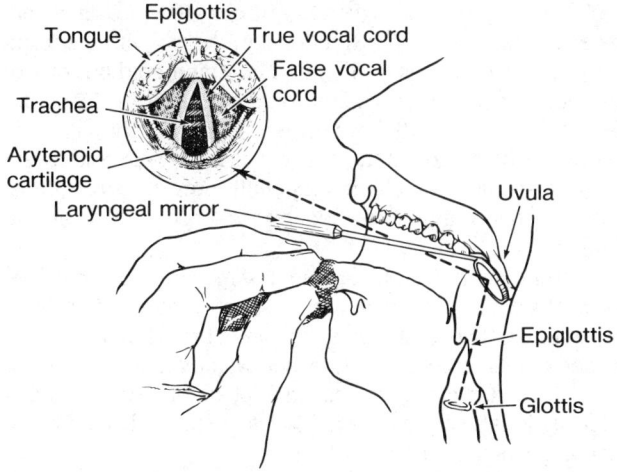

Figure 20-1
Normal laryngeal anatomy and indirect laryngoscopy.
(Wolcott MW. Ambulatory Surgery. Philadelphia, JB
Lippincott, 1988.)

sages and to slightly obstruct the current of air flowing through
them. The sense organs of smell are located in the olfactory
membrane, which covers the roof of the nose and the superior
turbinate bones.

The current of air entering the anterior nostrils is deflected upward to the roof of the nose and follows a circuitous
route before it reaches the nasopharynx. On its way, it comes
into contact with a large surface of moist, warm mucous
membrane that catches practically all of the dust and germs
in the inhaled air. This air is moistened and warmed to body
temperature and brought into contact with sensitive nerves.
Some of these nerves detect odors, and others provoke
sneezing to expel irritating dust.

Pharynx

The pharynx, or throat, is limited below by the larynx and
the upper end of the esophagus. Its upper extension is the
nasopharynx, into which open the posterior nostrils and the
auditory (eustachian) tubes from the middle ears. The nose
and the nasopharynx are lined with the same type of ciliated
epithelium as that which lines the trachea and bronchial tree;
but the pharynx, which serves as both a respiratory and an
alimentary passage, is lined with squamous (flat-celled) epithelium.

Tonsils and Adenoids

The faucial or palatine tonsils are two almond-shaped bodies,
one on each side of the oropharynx. The adenoids, or pharyngeal tonsils, are located in the roof of the nasopharynx.
The tonsils and the adenoids constitute only two of a ring of
similar masses of lymphoid tissue that completely encircles
the throat. These organs are important links in the chain of
lymph nodes guarding the body from invasion by organisms
entering the nose and the throat.

Larynx

The larynx is a cartilaginous epithelium-lined structure that
is the transition between the upper airway and the lower

airway (see Fig. 20-1). The major function of the larynx is to
permit vocalization. It also protects the lower airway from
foreign substances and facilitates coughing. It is frequently
referred to as the voice box and consists of the following:

- *Epiglottis*—a valve flap of cartilage that covers the
  opening to the larynx during swallowing
- *Glottis*—the opening between the vocal cords in the
  larynx
- *Thyroid cartilage*—part of it forms the "Adam's apple,"
  the largest cartilage in the trachea
- *Cricoid cartilage*—the only complete cartilaginous ring
  in the larynx (located below the thyroid cartilage)
- *Arytenoid cartilages*—used in vocal cord movement with
  the thyroid cartilage
- *Vocal cords*—ligaments controlled by muscular movements that produce vocal sounds; they are mounted in
  the lumen of the larynx

Assessment of the Upper Respiratory Airway

The Nose and Sinuses

The nose and sinuses are examined by inspection and palpation. For a routine examination, only a simple light source,
such as a penlight, is necessary. A more thorough examination
requires the use of a nasal speculum.

The external nose is inspected for lesions, asymmetry,
or inflammation. The patient is then instructed to tilt his head
backward while the examiner gently pushes the tip of the
nose upward to examine the internal structures of the nose.
The mucosa is inspected for color, swelling, exudate, or
bleeding. The nasal mucosa is normally more red than the
oral mucosa but may appear swollen and hyperemic in the
presence of the common cold. Allergic rhinitis, on the other
hand, is suspected when the mucosa appears pale and
swollen.

The septum is inspected for deviation, perforation, or
bleeding. A slight degree of septal deviation is present in
most people. Actual displacement of the cartilage into either
vestibule may produce nasal obstruction, but such deviation
is usually asymptomatic.

With the patient's head tilted back, the examiner attempts
to visualize the inferior and middle turbinates. In chronic rhinitis, nasal polyps may develop between the inferior and middle turbinates and are distinguished by their gray appearance.
Unlike the turbinates, they are gelatinous and freely movable.

The frontal and maxillary sinuses are palpated for tenderness. Using the thumbs, the examiner applies gentle pressure in an upward fashion at the supraorbital ridges (frontal
sinuses) and in the cheek area adjacent to the nose (maxillary
sinuses). Tenderness in either area suggests inflammation.

The Pharynx

A tongue blade, which is often used to depress the tongue
for adequate visualization of the pharynx, is not always necessary. The patient is instructed to open his mouth wide and
take a deep breath. Often this will flatten the posterior tongue

and briefly expose a full view of the anterior and posterior pillars, tonsils, uvula, and posterior pharynx. These structures are inspected for color, symmetry, and evidence of exudate, ulceration, or enlargement. If a tongue blade is used to visualize the pharynx, it is pressed firmly beyond the midpoint of the tongue. Proper placement avoids a gagging response and minimizes the patient's aversion to future oral examinations.

The Trachea

The position and mobility of the trachea are usually noted by direct palpation. This is done by placing the thumb and index finger of one hand on either side of the trachea just above the sternal notch. The trachea is highly sensitive, and palpating too firmly may incite a coughing or gagging response. The trachea is normally midline as it enters the thoracic inlet behind the sternum but may be deviated by masses in the neck or mediastinum. Pleural or pulmonary disorders, such as a significant pneumothorax, may result in displacement of the trachea.

Upper Airway Infections

Upper airway infections are common conditions that affect most people on occasion. Some of these conditions are acute, with symptoms that last several days; others are chronic, with symptoms that last a long time or occur repeatedly. Seldom do patients with these conditions require hospitalization; however, the nurse may encounter these infections in patients hospitalized for other reasons or in other nurse–client settings. Thus it is important to recognize the signs and symptoms and give useful approaches to care.

Common Cold

The phrase "common cold" is usually used when referring to symptoms of an upper respiratory tract infection. Colds are highly contagious since patients shed virus for about 2 days before the symptoms appear and during the first part of their symptomatic phase. Colds prevail among 15% of the work population at any time during the winter and account for almost half of all work absences and one fourth of the total time lost from work.

Three waves of colds appear yearly in the United States—in the fall just after the opening of school, in mid-winter, and in spring. Immunity after recovery is variable and depends on many factors, including natural host resistance and the specific causative virus.

Clinical Manifestations. The signs and symptoms of a cold are nasal discharge and obstruction, sore throat, sneezing, malaise, fever, chills, and often headache and muscle aching. As the cold progresses, cough usually appears. Most specifically, the term *cold* refers to an afebrile, infectious, acute inflammation of the mucous membranes of the nasal cavity. More broadly, the word refers to an acute upper respiratory tract infection, whereas terms such as *rhinitis, pharyngitis, laryngitis,* and *chest cold* distinguish the sites of the major symptoms.

The symptoms last 5 days to 2 weeks. If there is significant fever or more severe constitutional problems with the respiratory symptoms, it is no longer a common cold but one of the other acute upper respiratory tract infections. Many different viruses (over 100) are known to produce the signs and symptoms of the common cold, and about 10% of colds seem to be associated simultaneously with more than one virus. Also, allergic conditions affecting the nose can mimic the symptoms of a cold.

Management. Management of the common cold consists of adequate fluid intake, rest, prevention of chilling, aqueous nasal decongestants, vitamin C, bronchodilators, and expectorants as needed. Warm salt water gargles soothe the sore throat, and aspirin or acetaminophen relieves the general constitutional symptoms. Antibiotics are not indicated in the uncomplicated common cold.

Using disposable tissues and discarding them hygienically, covering the mouth when coughing, and avoiding crowds are important measures to prevent the spread of an upper respiratory airway infection.

Herpes Simplex Infection

The herpes simplex virus (HSV-1) most commonly produces the familiar *herpes labialis* (cold sore, fever blister, or canker). Small vesicles, single or clustered, may erupt on the lips, the tongue, the cheeks, and the pharynx. These soon rupture, forming sore, shallow ulcers that are covered with a gray membrane.

Herpes virus infections appear often in association with other febrile infections, such as streptococcal pneumonia, meningococcal meningitis, and malaria. The virus remains latent in cells of the lips or nose and is activated by febrile illnesses.

Management. The herpes virus does not respond well to many chemotherapeutic agents. However, acyclovir has been useful in some newly diagnosed cases. In addition, antiviral agents that may be of use in the future include cytarabine and vidarabine taken systemically or hydrocortisone acetate (Orabase) topically. Analgesics and codeine are helpful in relieving pain and discomfort. Topical anesthetics, such as lidocaine (Xylocaine) or dyclonine (Dyclone), give a measure of relief for oral pain. Applications of drying lotions or liquids may help to dry the lesions.

Sinusitis

The sinuses are involved in a high proportion of upper respiratory tract infections. If their openings into the nasal passages are clear, the infections resolve promptly. However, if their drainage is obstructed by a deflected septum or by hypertrophied turbinates, spurs, or polyps, sinusitis may persist as a smoldering secondary infection or flare up into an acute suppurative process.

Acute Sinusitis

Clinical Manifestations. Acute sinusitis may be localized in one sinus or may involve several (Fig. 20-2). If all are involved, the condition is called *pansinusitis*. The most

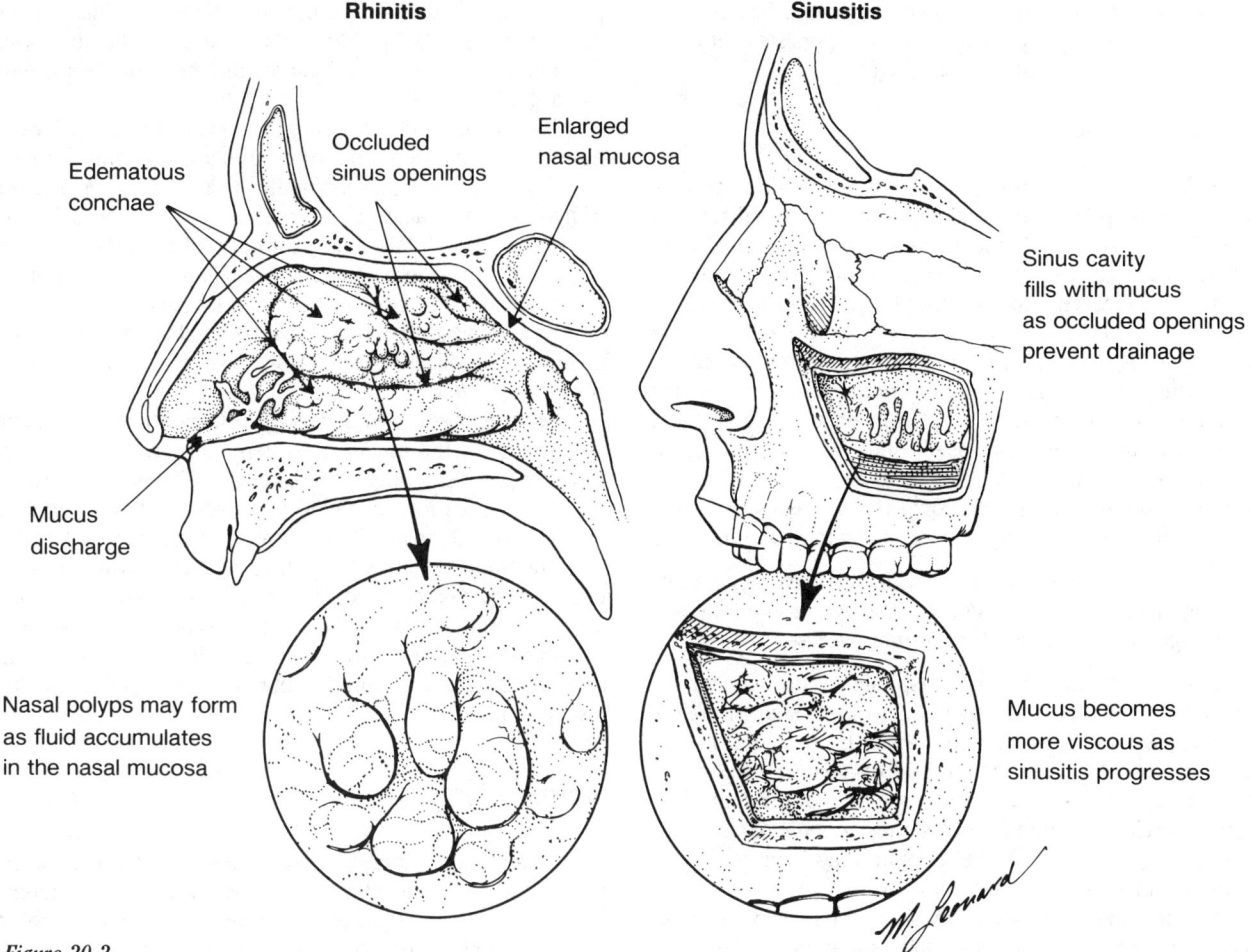

Rhinitis

Edematous conchae

Occluded sinus openings

Enlarged nasal mucosa

Mucus discharge

Nasal polyps may form as fluid accumulates in the nasal mucosa

Sinusitis

Sinus cavity fills with mucus as occluded openings prevent drainage

Mucus becomes more viscous as sinusitis progresses

M. Leonard

Figure 20-2
Rhinitis and sinusitis.

prominent symptom of acute sinusitis is pain. Since the location of the pain is diagnostically important, it is noted and documented by the nurse. In *frontal sinusitis*, the patient complains of frontal headache; in *ethmoidal sinusitis*, the pain is usually in or about the eyes; in *maxillary sinusitis*, pain may be referred to the brow but usually is lateral to the nose and sometimes is accompanied by aching of the upper teeth of the corresponding side; in *sphenoidal sinusitis*, occipital headache may result. Aside from being located in a specific area, pain also may be referred, for example, to the forehead. Nasal congestion and discharge are usually, but not necessarily, present. The patient feels generally miserable, quite apart from pain. Fever, if present at all, is usually mild. This may be the case even in the presence of an acute suppurative infection, or "empyema," of a sinus. *Hemophilus influenzae* is the most common type of bacteria cultured from the sinus; there is low correlation between nasal and sinus cultures.

- The most dangerous variety of sinusitis is empyema of a frontal sinus, because it may rupture posteriorly, producing a brain abscess.

A careful history and diagnostic assessment is done to rule out other local or systemic disorders, such as tumor, fistula, allergy, and viral infections.

Management. The goals of treatment of acute sinusitis are relief of pain, shrinkage of the nasal mucosa, and control of infection. Relief of pain is achieved by administering prescribed codeine, meperidine hydrochloride (Demerol), or acetaminophen with codeine. Bed rest is recommended, as well as the establishment of free drainage of the sinuses. No single antibiotic is effective against all the possible pathogens. If prescribed, the antibiotics used include ampicillin or amoxicillin, cefaclor (Ceclor), and trimethoprim-sulfamethoxazole (Bactrim, Septra). If allergy is suspected as a basis of the inflammatory process, one of the antihistaminic agents in oral form may be beneficial. Caution is necessary because antihistamines increase the viscosity of secretions and may hinder rather than promote sinus drainage.

Nursing Interventions. Hot wet packs applied to the face over the involved sinus area four times a day will hasten resolution of the infection. Relief is also obtained by nasal instillations or sprays of phenylephrine (Neo-Synephrine, 0.25%) or by oral decongestants. Depending on the type of infecting organism and the extent of the infection, the nurse instructs the patient to apply local therapy of this sort at intervals of 1 to 4 hours until drainage is established. The nurse teaches the patient the early signs of a sinus infection and recommends preventive measures:

- Avoid allergens if allergies are suspected.
- Maintain general health so that the body's resistance is not lowered (eat properly, get plenty of rest and exercise).

- Avoid others with upper respiratory tract infections.
- Notify physician if pain in sinus areas persists or if nasal discharge is present and discolored.

Chronic Sinusitis

Clinical Manifestations. Chronic sinusitis is usually manifested by persistent nasal obstruction due to discharge and edema of the nasal mucous membrane. The patient experiences cough, because of the constant dripping of the discharge backward into the nasopharynx, and headaches, which are apt to be most pronounced on awakening in the morning. Fatigue is also common, as is nasal stuffiness.

Management. Treatment of chronic sinusitis includes measures to facilitate drainage, antibacterial therapy, and antiallergic measures. Increased humidity, steam inhalations, increased fluid intake, and local heat applications will assist in promoting drainage. Local use of vasoconstricting drugs in the form of sprays or nose drops may be tried.

- Overuse or prolonged use of vasoconstrictive nasal drugs may aggravate rhinitis and sinusitis by causing rebound congestion, which leads to further overuse.

Because of the danger of aspiration and subsequent pneumonia, oily nose drops are to be avoided. Sterile Ringer's solution used with a nasal douche can be obtained in any drugstore and is a soothing method of cleansing the nose. Structural deformities that obstruct the ostia of the sinus may require surgical attention: polyps may require excision or cauterization, and a deflected septum may have to be removed or a narrowed ostium widened.

For drainage of the maxillary sinus, the incision is made along the upper gum line above the canine teeth (Caldwell-Luc operation). To drain the frontal sinus, an incision is made through the inner third of the eyebrow. Another surgical approach is an incision made above the brow line. After the entire sinus is explored, diseased tissue is removed and the sinus is obliterated with abdominal fat.

Some victims of severe chronic sinusitis obtain relief only by moving to a dry climate.

Rhinitis

Pathophysiology. Rhinitis is an inflammatory lesion involving the mucous membrane of the nose. It is sometimes a manifestation of allergy (see p. 1207), in which instance the condition is referred to as "allergic rhinitis." Usually, however, rhinitis is due to an infection. The most common variety of infection causing viral rhinitis is the common cold. Rhinitis also is encountered with regularity in the early stages of measles and other specific viral infections. Bacterial rhinitis is usually caused by a gram-positive bacterium and is characterized by a purulent nasal discharge. The infection is often secondary to a viral upper respiratory tract infection. If untreated, rhinitis can lead to sinusitis, otitis media, bronchitis, and pneumonia.

In acute rhinitis, the nasal mucous membrane becomes congested, swollen, and edematous for a short period of time and then quickly returns to normal. After repeated attacks, however, particularly in cases that originate as a result of chronic sinusitis, this swelling becomes obstinate and the patient has a chronic inflammation. Patients with this problem say that they are "subject to colds." The fact is that, excluding the recurring attacks of allergic rhinitis, their attacks are acute exacerbations of the same "cold."

If continued, chronic rhinitis leads to the deposition of abnormally large amounts of connective tissue in the nasal mucous membrane, which greatly thickens it and, in addition to hypertrophy, causes the formation of spurs and polyps on the nasal septum. Wasting or atrophy of the mucous membrane, the cartilage, and the bones lining the nasal passages eventually may occur, and these passages become large, empty caverns. An abundant exudate builds up on the walls, giving off a disagreeable odor. This condition is called *atrophic rhinitis*.

Management and Nursing Interventions. In acute viral rhinitis, symptomatic treatment includes topical or systemic vasoconstricting medications to relieve nasal obstruction, analgesics for headache, and rest to alleviate general discomfort. Adults are advised to avoid crowds.

The nurse cautions the patient against blowing his nose too frequently or too hard. He should blow his nose by opening his mouth slightly and blowing through both nostrils to equalize the pressure. Physical therapy, medications, and surgery are used to treat rhinitis, but response to therapy is often disappointing.

Acute Pharyngitis

Assessment and Clinical Manifestations. Acute pharyngitis, which is caused by several viruses and bacteria, is a febrile inflammation of the throat. The pharyngeal membrane becomes fiery red; the lymphoid follicles of the throat and the tonsils become swollen and flecked with exudate; and the cervical lymph nodes may become tender and enlarged. Uncomplicated viral infections usually subside promptly, within 3 to 10 days after the onset. However, pharyngitis caused by more virulent bacteria, such as group A streptococcus or hemolytic *Staphylococcus aureus*, is a more severe illness during the acute stage and far more important because of the incidence of dangerous complications. These complications include sinusitis, otitis media, mastoiditis, cervical adenitis, rheumatic fever, and nephritis. A throat culture is the chief means of determining the causative organism, and after it is obtained proper therapy can be prescribed. If one member of a family has a streptococcal infection, all other family members should have throat cultures done. If the cultures are positive, treatment with penicillin is preferred.

Management. If a bacterial etiology is suspected or demonstrated, treatment may include the administration of antimicrobial agents. For group A streptococcus, penicillin is the drug of choice. For those patients who are sensitive to penicillin and resistent to tetracycline (one fifth of group A streptococci and most *Staphylococcus aureus* organisms are resistant to tetracycline), erythromycin is the drug of choice. Antibiotics are administered for at least 10 days for an optimal rate of eradication of group A streptococcus from the oropharynx.

A liquid or soft diet is provided during the acute stage of the disease, depending on the patient's appetite and the degree of discomfort caused by swallowing. Occasionally, the throat is so sore that liquids cannot be taken in adequate amounts by mouth; in this situation, fluids are administered intravenously. Otherwise, the patient is encouraged to drink to the limit of tolerance, with the minimum intake during the febrile stage exceeding, if possible, 2500 ml each day. Often, the patient can achieve this goal more easily if the rationale of therapy is explained to him. His personal tastes (in liquids) should be considered and indulged when possible.

Nursing Interventions. The patient is kept in bed during the febrile stage of illness. When he is ambulatory he needs periods of rest. Secretion precautions must be observed to prevent the spread of infection. The skin is examined once or twice daily for possible rash, because acute pharyngitis may precede some other communicable disease.

Aside from throat cultures, it may be necessary to secure nasal swabbings and blood cultures for further laboratory investigation to determine the nature of the causative organism (Fig. 20-3).

Warm saline gargles or irrigations are employed, depending on the severity of the lesion and the degree of pain. Recognizing that the benefits of this treatment depend on

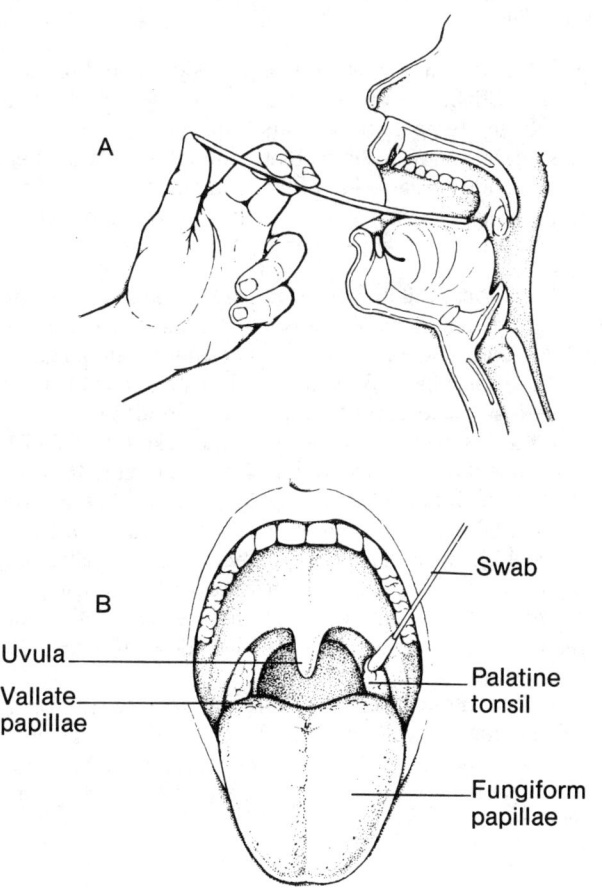

A

B
Uvula
Vallate papillae
Swab
Palatine tonsil
Fungiform papillae

Figure 20-3
Taking a throat culture. When obtaining a throat culture from a patient who "gags," it is helpful to have him close his eyes. Since anticipation is lessened, the culture can be obtained with only a slight gag. (*A*) Grasp the tongue blade so that the thumb pushes the end upward (as a fulcrum) while the fingers push the middle section downward. (*B*) Vigorously rub a cotton or Dacron swab over each tonsilar area and the posterior pharynx.

the degree of heat that is applied, the nurse ensures that the temperature of the solution is sufficiently high to be effective, that is, approaching the limits of tolerance, which vary with each patient and are usually between 105°F to 110°F (40.6°C to 43.3°C). A properly performed throat irrigation is an effective means of reducing spasm in the pharyngeal muscles and relieving soreness of the throat. However, unless the purpose of the procedure and its technique are understood clearly by the patient, the results may be less than satisfactory. If throat irrigation is a new experience for the patient, the nurse should explain the procedure and its purpose before beginning.

Symptomatic relief in patients with severe sore throat also may be afforded by applying an ice collar and administering analgesic drugs, as prescribed; for example, aspirin or acetaminophen can be given at 3- to 6-hour intervals and, if required, codeine sulfate is administered three or four times daily. Antitussive medication, in the form of codeine or hydrocodone bitartrate (Hycodan), may be required to control a persistent and painful cough that often accompanies acute pharyngitis. One of the barbiturates, for example, pentobarbital (Nembutal), may be administered as prescribed for the patient to promote sleep at bedtime.

Mouth care may add greatly to the patient's comfort and may prevent the development of fissures of the lips and inflammation about the mouth when bacterial infection is present.

Patient Education and Home Health Care. Resumption of activity is permitted gradually. Unusually conservative management is indicated in patients with hemolytic *Streptococcus* infection in view of the possible development of complications such as nephritis and rheumatic fever, which may have their onset 2 or 3 weeks after the pharyngitis has subsided. Local extension of an apparently quiescent pharyngitis may develop in the form of sinusitis, otitis media, mastoiditis, or cervical adenitis. Daily assessment of morning and evening temperatures is continued until convalescence is complete. The patient or his family are advised that a full course of therapy is necessary and what symptoms to watch for that may indicate possible complications.

Chronic Pharyngitis

Chronic pharyngitis is common in adults who work in dusty surroundings, use the voice to excess, and suffer from chronic cough. Its incidence also is high among habitual users of alcohol and tobacco.

Three types of chronic pharyngitis are recognized: (1) hypertrophic, characterized by general thickening and congestion of the pharyngeal mucous membrane; (2) atrophic, probably a late stage of type 1 (the membrane is thin, whitish, glistening, and, at times, wrinkled); and (3) chronic granular ("clergyman's sore throat"), with numerous swollen lymph follicles on the pharyngeal wall.

Clinical Manifestations and Management. Patients with chronic pharyngitis complain of a constant sense of irritation or fullness in the throat; of mucus, which collects in the throat and can be expelled by coughing; and of difficulty in swallowing. The treatment of chronic pharyngitis consists of avoiding alcohol, tobacco, and other irritants; resting the voice; and correcting any upper respiratory, pulmonary, or cardiac condition that might be responsible for a chronic cough.

Nasal congestion may be relieved by nasal instillations or sprays containing ephedrine sulfate, phenylephrine hydrochloride (Neo-Synephrine), or tuaminoheptane sulfate (Tuamine) in saline. If there is a history of allergy, one of the antihistaminic drugs, such as tripelennamine (Pyribenzamine), is administered orally every 4 to 6 hours. The attendant malaise is controlled effectively by aspirin or acetaminophen. Contact with others should be avoided, at least until the fever has subsided completely, in order to prevent the infection from spreading. (See also Chap. 59.)

Tonsillitis and Adenoiditis

The tonsils are composed of lymphatic tissue and are situated on each side of the oropharynx. They frequently serve as the site of acute infection. Chronic tonsillitis is less common and may be mistaken for other disorders such as allergy, asthma, and sinusitis.

The adenoids consist of an abnormally large lymphoid tissue mass near the center of the posterior wall of the nasopharynx. Infection of the adenoids frequently accompanies acute tonsillitis.

Clinical Manifestations. The symptoms of tonsillitis include sore throat, fever, snoring, and difficulty in swallowing. Adenoid hypertrophy may cause mouth-breathing, earache, draining ears, frequent head colds, bronchitis, fetid breath, voice impairment, and noisy respiration. Unusually enlarged adenoids may cause nasal obstruction. Extension of infection to the middle ears by way of the auditory (eustachian) tubes may result in acute otitis media, the potential complications of which include spontaneous rupture of the eardrums and further extension into the mastoid cells, causing acute mastoiditis. The infection may also reside in the middle ear as a chronic, low-grade, smoldering process that eventually may cause permanent deafness.

Diagnostic Evaluation. A thorough physical examination is performed, and a careful history is obtained to rule out related or systemic conditions. A culture of the organisms at the tonsillar site is done to determine the presence of bacterial infection. In adenoiditis, if there are recurrent episodes of suppurative otitis media that are causing a hearing loss, it is important for the patient to have a comprehensive audiometric examination (see p. 1372).

Tonsillectomy and Adenoidectomy

Appropriate antibiotic therapy is initiated for both tonsillectomy and adenoidectomy. Tonsillectomy is usually not done unless medical treatment is unsuccessful and there is severe hypertrophy or peritonsillar abscess that occludes the pharynx, making swallowing difficult and endangering the airway. Enlargement of the tonsils is rarely an indication for their removal; most children have normally large tonsils, which decrease in size with age. Despite the continuing debate over the effectiveness of many tonsillectomies, the operation is still the most common nondiagnostic surgical procedure done in the United States.

Tonsillectomy or adenoidectomy is done only if the patient has had any of the following: repeated bouts of tonsillitis;

hypertrophy of the tonsils and adenoids that could cause obstruction; repeated attacks of purulent otitis media; suspected hearing loss due to serous otitis media that has occurred in association with enlarged tonsils and adenoids; and some other conditions, such as an exacerbation of asthma or rheumatic fever. Laser surgery has been tried, but it prolongs anesthesia and causes other laser-related complications; therefore, in this situation laser surgery must be used judiciously.

Postoperative Nursing Interventions. Continuous nursing observation is required in the immediate postoperative and recovery period because of the significant risk of hemorrhage. After the operation, the most comfortable position is prone with the head turned to the side to allow for drainage from the mouth and pharynx. The oral airway is not removed until the patient demonstrates that his swallowing reflex has returned. An ice collar is applied to the neck, and a basin and tissues are provided for the expectoration of blood and mucus.

Bleeding may be bright red if the patient expectorates blood at once. Often, however, the blood is swallowed and immediately becomes brown owing to the action of the acid gastric juice.

- If the patient vomits large amounts of altered blood or spits bright blood at frequent intervals, or if the pulse rate and temperature rise and the patient is restless, the surgeon is notified immediately and the following items are made available in order to examine the surgical area for a bleeding site: a light, a head mirror, gauze, curved hemostats, and a waste basin.

Occasionally, it may be necessary to suture or ligate the bleeding vessel. In such cases the patient is taken to the operating room and placed under anesthesia. After ligation, continuous nursing observation and postoperative care are required, as in the initial postoperative period.

If there is no bleeding, water and cracked ice are given to the patient as soon as desired. He is instructed to refrain from too much talking and coughing, because this can produce throat pain. Alkaline mouthwashes are useful in coping with the thick mucus that may be present after a tonsillectomy. A liquid or semiliquid diet is given for several days; acid juices (orange, apple, or lemon), which may cause burning when swallowed, are avoided. Sherbet, gelatin desserts, and junkets are acceptable foods.

Patient Education and Home Health Care. On returning home, the patient needs to get plenty of rest, eat soft foods, drink fluids, and resume activity gradually. Any bleeding is reported to the physician; delayed hemorrhage may occur up to a week after surgery.

Peritonsillar Abscess

Peritonsillar abscess develops above the tonsil in the tissues of the anterior pillar and soft palate. As a rule, it is secondary to a tonsillar infection.

Clinical Manifestations. The usual symptoms of an infection are present, together with such local symptoms as difficulty in swallowing (dysphagia), thickening of the voice, drooling, and local pain. An examination shows marked swelling of the soft palate, often to the extent of half-occluding the orifice from the mouth into the pharynx.

Management. Antibiotics (usually penicillin) are extremely effective in the control of the infection in peritonsillar abscess. If antibiotics are given early in the course of the disease, the abscess may be aborted and incision avoided. If antibiotics are not given until later, the abscess must be drained, but improvement in the inflammatory reaction is rapid.

The abscess is evacuated as soon as possible. The mucous membrane over the swelling is first sprayed with a topical anesthetic and then injected with a local anesthetic; after a small incision has been made, the points of a blunt hemostat are forced into the abscess pocket and opened as they are withdrawn. This operation is performed best with the patient in the sitting position, since this will make it easier for him to expectorate the pus and blood that accumulate in the pharynx. Almost immediate relief is experienced.

Some laryngologists advocate bilateral tonsillectomy for acute peritonsillar abscess; they claim that this is necessary to prevent recurrences and eliminate unsuspected asymptomatic pockets of infection.

Nursing Interventions. A considerable measure of relief may be obtained by throat irrigations or the frequent use of mouthwashes or gargles, using saline or alkaline solutions at a temperature of 105°F to 110°F (40.6°C to 43.3°C). The nurse instructs the patient to gargle at intervals of 1 or 2 hours for 24 to 36 hours.

Laryngitis

Inflammation of the larynx often occurs as a result of voice abuse or as a part of an upper respiratory tract infection. It may also be caused by an isolated infection involving only the vocal cords.

The cause of this inflammation is almost always a virus. Bacterial invasion may be secondary. Laryngitis is usually associated with acute rhinitis or nasopharyngitis. The onset of infection may be associated with exposure to sudden temperature changes, dietary deficiencies, malnutrition, and lack of immunity. Laryngitis is common in winter and is readily transmitted.

Clinical Manifestations and Diagnostic Evaluation. Acute laryngitis is manifested by hoarseness or complete loss of the voice (aphonia) and by severe cough, whereas chronic laryngitis, which is marked by persistent hoarseness, may follow repeated attacks of acute laryngitis. It is sometimes a complication of chronic sinusitis and chronic bronchitis. The condition also may be induced by the frequent inhalation of irritating gases, the excessive use of tobacco or alcohol, or the habitual overuse of the voice, as in the case of public speakers. Laryngoscopic examination of the patient with chronic laryngitis is indicated in order to eliminate the possibility of tuberculosis or tumor of the larynx.

Management. For acute laryngitis, the treatment is abstinence from talking and smoking, bed rest, and cool steam or aerosol therapy. If the laryngitis is part of a more extensive respiratory infection owing to a bacterial organism or if it is severe, appropriate antibacterial chemotherapy is instituted. The majority of patients recover with conservative treatment;

however, the disease tends to be more severe in elderly patients and may be complicated by pneumonia.

For chronic laryngitis, the treatment of the condition is rest of the voice, elimination of any primary respiratory tract infection that may be present, and restriction of smoking. Recently, the use of topical steroid preparations, such as beclomethasone dipropionate (Vanceril) inhalation, has been advocated. These preparations have no systemic or long-lasting effects and may reduce local inflammatory reactions. A well-humidified environment is important, and expectorant drugs are helpful in thinning laryngeal secretions during acute episodes. A daily fluid intake of 3 liters is also necessary to thin secretions.

Nursing Process Overview for Upper Airway Infection

▷ Assessment

The nurse obtains a complete history of the patient's problem. Signs and symptoms may include headache, sore throat, pain around the eyes and on either side of the nose, difficulty in swallowing, cough, hoarseness, fever, stuffiness, and generalized discomfort and fatigue. The nurse determines onset of the symptoms, what precipitated them, what relieves them, if anything, and what aggravates them. A history of allergy and the existence of a concomitant illness are identified.

On inspection, the nurse looks for swelling, lesions, or asymmetry of the nose as well as for any bleeding or discharge. The nasal mucosa is inspected for abnormal findings such as a reddened color, swelling, or exudate, and nasal polyps, which may develop in chronic rhintis, are searched for.

The frontal and maxillary sinuses are palpated for tenderness, which suggests inflammation. The throat is observed by having the patient open his mouth wide and take a deep breath. The tonsils and pharynx are inspected for the abnormal findings of reddened color, asymmetry, or evidence of drainage, ulceration, or enlargement.

The trachea is palpated for midline position in the neck, and any lumps or deformities are identified. The neck lymph nodes are also palpated for associated enlargement.

▷ Nursing Diagnoses

Based on all the assessment data, the patient's major nursing diagnoses may include the following:

- Ineffective airway clearance related to excessive secretions secondary to an inflammatory process
- Alteration in comfort, soreness, or pain related to upper airway irritation secondary to an infection
- Fluid volume deficit related to increased fluid loss secondary to diaphoresis associated with a fever

▷ Planning and Implementation

▷ *Goals:* The major goals for the patient may include maintenance of a patent airway, improvement in comfort, absence of fluid volume deficit, and knowledge of how to prevent upper airway infections.

Nursing Interventions

Airway Clearance. An accumulation of secretions can block the airway in many patients with an upper airway infection. Changes in the respiratory pattern result, and the work of breathing required to get beyond the blockage is increased. There are several measures that can be employed to loosen thick secretions or to keep the secretions moist so that they can be easily expectorated. Increasing fluid intake provides systemic hydration, which is an effective expectorant. Humidifying the environment by room vaporizers or steam inhalations also loosens secretions and reduces inflammation of the mucous membranes. The patient is instructed about the best position to assume for facilitating drainage. This will depend on the location of the infection or inflammation. For example, drainage for sinusitis or rhinitis is achieved in the upright position. In some conditions, topical or systemic vasoconstricting medications are administered as prescribed to relieve nasal or throat congestion.

Comfort Measures. Upper respiratory tract infections usually produce localized discomfort. In sinusitis, pain may occur in the area of the sinuses or the patient may experience a headache. In pharyngitis, laryngitis, or tonsillitis, a sore throat occurs. The nurse can help to relieve this discomfort by administering analgesics such as acetaminophen, codeine, or meperidine as prescribed by a physician. Topical anesthetics provide symptomatic relief for herpes simplex blisters and sore throats. Hot packs help relieve the congestion of sinusitis and promote drainage. Warm water gargles or irrigations relieve the pain of a sore throat. An ice collar is applied in the immediate postoperative period following a tonsillectomy and adenoidectomy to reduce swelling and decrease bleeding. Encouraging the patient to rest will help relieve the generalized discomfort or fever that accompanies many upper airway conditions (especially rhinitis, pharyngitis, and laryngitis). The nurse instructs the patient in general oral and nasal hygiene techniques to help relieve localized discomfort and to prevent the spread of infection.

Fluid Intake. In upper airway infections, the work of breathing and the respiratory rate increase as inflammation and secretions develop. This in turn increases insensible fluid loss. An associated fever increases the metabolic rate, which results in diaphoresis and increased fluid loss. The patient is encouraged to drink 2 to 3 liters of water per day during his upper airway infection, unless contraindicated, to thin secretions and promote drainage.

Patient Education. The prevention of most upper airway infections is difficult because there are many potential causes. The responsible pathogen usually cannot be identified, and vaccines are unavailable except in rare instances. Allergies, pathologic conditions of the septum and the turbinates, emotional problems, and various systemic illnesses may be predisposing factors in isolated cases.

The nurse instructs the patient about the following hygienic measures, which support the body's defenses and reduce susceptibility to respiratory infections:

- Practice good health measures—nutritious diet, appropriate exercise, adequate rest and sleep.
- Avoid excesses in alcohol and smoking.

- Correct air dryness by proper home humidification, especially during cold weather.
- Avoid air contaminants (dust, chemicals) when possible.
- Avoid unnecessary chilling of the skin, especially the feet; chilling lowers resistance.
- Obtain influenza vaccination if advised by a physician. This is usually recommended for the elderly and those with chronic illness.
- Avoid crowds during flu season.
- Maintain adequate dental hygiene.

▷ *Evaluation*

▷ *Expected Outcomes*

1. Patient maintains a patent airway by managing secretions.
   a. Reports decreased congestion.
   b. Uses room humidifier or vaporizer.
   c. Assumes best position to facilitate drainage of secretions for the condition.
   d. Verbalizes familiarity with use of vasoconstricting medications (oral or nasal spray) to relieve nasal congestion.
2. Patient is comfortable.
   a. States the use of analgesics helps relieve localized pain or headache.
   b. Demonstrates the application of hot packs for sinusitis, warm water gargles or irrigations for a sore throat, and an ice collar following a tonsillectomy and adenoidectomy.
   c. Verbalizes an understanding of the need for rest at this time.
   d. Demonstrates adequate oral hygiene.
3. Patient maintains an adequate fluid balance.
   a. States rationale for drinking plenty of fluids.
   b. Demonstrates no significant weight loss.
   c. Is not dehydrated.
4. Patient knows how to prevent upper airway infections.
   a. Eats a balanced diet daily.
   b. Does not smoke.
   c. Avoids enclosed areas polluted with smoke.
   d. Stays away from crowded areas during the flu season (shopping malls, crowded restaurants, movie theaters).
   e. Contacts physician/clinic to receive a flu shot.
   f. Uses room humidifiers when necessary.
   g. Wears protective clothing (hat, scarf, gloves, boots) to keep warm and avoid chilling.

Obstruction and Trauma of the Upper Respiratory Airway

Epistaxis (Nosebleed)

Pathophysiology. A hemorrhage from the nose, referred to as *epistaxis*, is caused by the rupture of tiny, distended vessels in the mucous membrane of any area of the nose. Rarely does epistaxis originate in the densely vascular tissue over the turbinates. Most commonly, the site is the anterior septum, where three major blood vessels enter the nasal cavity: (1) the anterior ethmoidal artery on the forward part of the roof, (2) the sphenopalatine artery in the posterosuperior region, and (3) the internal maxillary branches (the plexus of veins located at the back of the lateral wall under the inferior turbinate).

Epistaxis results from injury or disease, although the usual cause of small nosebleeds is "picking" of the nose. Other local causes are deviated septum, perforated septum, cancer, and trauma. Epistaxis also occurs as a sign of acute rheumatic fever, acute sinusitis, arterial hypertension, and hemorrhagic diseases.

Management and Nursing Interventions. In providing emergency nursing care, the nurse must remember that cessation of bleeding is aided by having the patient sit upright and by promoting vasoconstriction in the nasal mucous membrane. The patient should breathe through his mouth, refrain from talking, and compress the soft outer portion of the nose against the midline septum for 5 or 10 minutes continuously. A medical protocol may advise saturating a piece of cotton with a local vasoconstricting drug such as phenylephrine hydrochloride (Neo-Synephrine) and then inserting the cotton into the nostril.

The patient is instructed not to blow his nose during or after a nosebleed. Tissues and an emesis basis are provided into which he can expectorate any blood that collects in the nasopharynx. Should these measures fail, the problem is reported to the physician, who may control the epistaxis by applying aqueous epinephrine 1:1000 to a cotton pledget, inserting it in the nostril near the bleeding source, and applying pressure. The physician may then cauterize the site (if the bleeding point is visible) using an electric cautery (after injection of a local anesthetic) or a chemical agent such as a silver nitrate stick, a chromic acid bead, or trichloroacetic acid. If pain is present, a narcotic analgesic may be prescribed.

A major nursing goal is identifying the bleeding site; however, sometimes only the general bleeding area can be determined. A light source whose rays are parallel to the line of vision, such as a concave head mirror, is used to view deep, narrow spaces of the nasal cavity. If bleeding is occurring from the posterior regions, drug-moistened cotton pledgets may be inserted into the nostril to reduce the blood flow and improve the view. Suction can remove excess blood and clots from the field of inspection. The search should shift from the anteroinferior quadrant to the anterosuperior, then to the posterosuperior, and finally to the posteroinferior area. The field is kept clear by using suction and by shifting the cotton tampons. However, only about 60% of the total nasal cavity can actually be seen.

When the origin of the bleeding cannot be found, the physician will prescribe that the nose be sprayed with a topical anesthetic and a decongestant and then packed with gauze impregnated with petrolatum. A postnasal packing may be inserted with a balloon-inflated catheter or by the methods shown in Figure 20-4. Pressure is increased by moistening

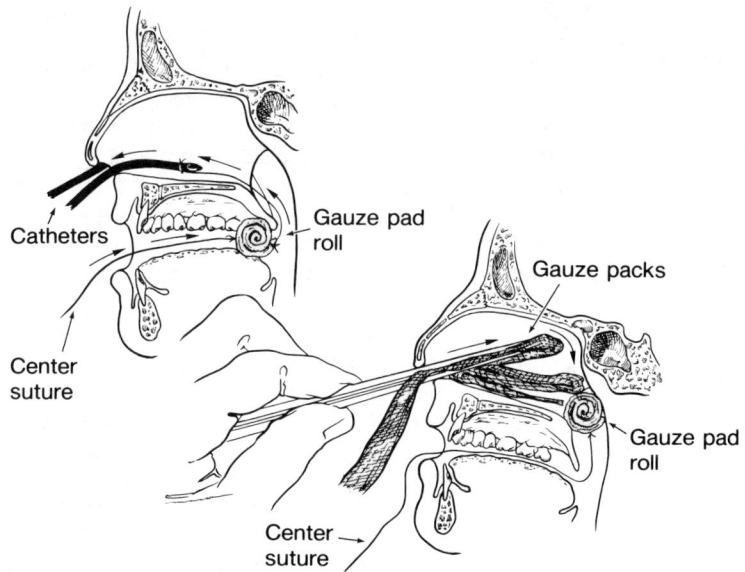

Figure 20-4
Anterior and posterior nasal packing. A red rubber catheter is directed through each anterior naris into the posterior pharynx, where the catheters are grasped with a clamp and brought out through the mouth. A heavy silk suture attached to the posterior pack of rolled 4 × 4 gauze pad is then tied to the end of each catheter. The catheters are then pulled out through the nose to advance the pack into the nasopharynx, while a finger of the opposite hand directs the pack around and above the soft palate. The pack is then secured anteriorly to the nose by tying the silk suture over dental rolls at the nares. The other end of the silk suture coming from the mouth is taped to the cheek to use as a traction stitch for later removal of the pack. Anterior packing of petrolatum gauze is then layered in front of the posterior pack. (Wolcott MW. Ambulatory Surgery. Philadelphia, JB Lippincott, 1981.)

the gauze. The packing is kept in place for 48 hours or up to 5 or 6 days if necessary.

Nasal Obstruction

The passage of air through the nostrils is frequently obstructed by a deflection of the nasal septum, hypertrophy of the turbinate bones, or the pressure of polyps, which are grapelike swellings that arise from the mucous membrane of the sinuses, especially the ethmoids. This obstruction also may lead to a condition of chronic infection of the nose and result in frequent attacks of nasopharyngitis. Very frequently, the infection extends to the sinuses of the nose (mucus-lined cavities filled with air that drain normally into the nose). When sinusitis develops and the drainage from these cavities is obstructed by deformity or swelling within the nose, pain is experienced in the region of the affected sinus.

Management.   The treatment of nasal obstruction requires the removal of the obstruction, followed by measures to overcome whatever chronic infection exists. In many patients the underlying nasal allergy requires treatment. At times it is necessary to drain the nasal sinuses by a radical operation. The operations performed depend on the type of nasal obstruction found. Usually, they are performed using local anesthesia.

If a deflection of the septum is the cause of the obstruction, the surgeon makes an incision into the mucous membrane and, after raising it from the bone, removes the deflected bone and cartilage with bone forceps. The mucosa then is allowed to fall back in place and is held there by tight packing. Generally, the packing used is soaked in liquid petrolatum to facilitate its removal in 24 to 36 hours. This operation is called a *submucous resection* or septoplasty.

Nasal polyps are removed by clipping them at their base with a wire snare. Hypertrophied turbinates may be treated by astringent applications to shrink them close to the side of the nose.

After these procedures, the head of the bed is elevated to promote drainage and to help in alleviating the patient's discomfort owing to edema. Frequent oral hygiene care is given because the patient breathes through his mouth.

Fractures of the Nose

The location of the nose makes it susceptible to injury by a wide variety of causes. In fact, the nose sustains fractures more frequently than any other bone in the body. Fractures of the nose usually result from direct trauma. As a rule, no serious consequences result, but the deformity that may follow often gives rise to obstruction of the nasal air passages and to facial disfigurement.

Assessment and Clinical Manifestations.   The nose should be examined internally to rule out the possibility that the injury may be complicated by a fracture of the nasal septum and submucosal septal hematoma. If a hematoma develops and is not drained, it may eventually become an abscess with a dissolution of the septal cartilage. The familiar saddle deformity of the nose results.

Immediately after the injury there is usually considerable bleeding from the nose externally and internally into the pharynx. There is marked swelling of the soft tissues adjacent to the nose and, frequently, a definite deformity. Because of this swelling and bleeding, an accurate diagnosis can only be made after the swelling has subsided.

Diagnostic Evaluation.   If there is clear fluid draining from either nostril, it suggests a fracture of the cribriform plate with leakage of cerebrospinal fluid. Since cerebrospinal fluid contains sugar, it can readily be differentiated from nasal mucus by using a dipstick (Dextrostix). Usually, careful inspection or palpation will reveal any deviations of the bone or disruptions of the nasal cartilages. An x-ray film may help to determine displacement of the fractured bones and help rule out extension of the fracture into the skull.

Management.   As a rule, the bleeding is controlled with the use of cold compresses. With the application of local anesthesia to the nose or with intravenous anesthesia, it is usually possible to bring displaced fragments into alignment and then hold them by intranasal packing or external splints. In reducing the fracture it is important to re-form the nasal passages and to realign the bones so as to prevent a disfiguring deformity. After reduction the swelling that occurs may be decreased by the application of ice compresses with the patient in the sitting position.

Laryngeal Obstruction

Edema of the larynx is a serious, often fatal, condition. The larynx is a stiff box that will not stretch, and the space within it between the vocal cords (glottis), through which the air must pass, is narrow. Swelling of the laryngeal mucous membrane, therefore, may close this orifice tightly, leading to suffocation. Edema of the glottis occurs rarely in patients with acute laryngitis, occasionally in patients with urticaria, and more frequently in severe inflammations of the throat—for example, erysipelas and scarlet fever. It is an occasional cause of death in severe anaphylaxis (angioneurotic edema).

When caused by an allergic reaction, treatment includes the self-administration of subcutaneous epinephrine or an adrenal corticosteroid and the application of an ice pack to the neck.

Foreign bodies frequently are aspirated into the pharynx, the larynx, or the trachea and cause a twofold problem. First they obstruct the air passages and cause difficulty in breathing, which may lead to asphyxia; later they may be drawn farther down, entering the bronchi or one of their branches and causing symptoms of irritation, such as a croupy cough, blood or mucous expectoration, and paroxysms of dyspnea. The physical signs and x-ray films confirm the diagnosis.

In emergencies, when the signs of asphyxia are evident, immediate treatment is necessary. Frequently, if the foreign body has lodged in the pharynx and can be visualized, it is dislodged by the finger. If the obstruction is in the larynx or the trachea, the abdominal thrust (Heimlich) maneuver is tried. If all efforts are unsuccessful, an immediate tracheotomy is necessary.

- To perform the abdominal thrust maneuver, stand behind the person who is choking and place both arms around his waist, with one hand grasping the other fist. Then quickly and forcefully apply pressure against the victim's diaphragm, pressing slightly upward, just below the ribs.

The pressure will compress the lungs and expel the aspirated object. Do this repeatedly until the object is expelled.

Cancer of the Larynx

Cancer of the larynx is potentially curable if detected early. It represents 3% to 5% of all cancers and occurs about eight times more frequently in men than in women and most commonly in men 50 to 65 years of age.

Each year in the United States, approximately 11,700 new cases are discovered and 3,800 persons with cancer of the larynx will die. Factors that contribute to laryngeal cancer are irritants such as cigarette smoke and alcohol (and their combined effects), vocal straining, chronic laryngitis, industrial exposure, nutritional deficiencies, and family predisposition.

Clinical Manifestations. A malignant growth may occur on the vocal cords (intrinsic) or on another part of the larynx (extrinsic). Hoarseness is noted early in the patient with intrinsic cancer since accurate approximation of the cords during phonation is interrupted by the presence of the tumor. Affected voice sounds are not early signs of extrinsic or supraglottic cancer; however, the patient may complain of pain and burning in the throat when drinking hot liquids and citrus juices. Later a lump may be felt in the neck. Subsequently, too, dysphagia, dyspnea, hoarseness, and foul breath are noticed. Enlarged cervical nodes, weight loss, general debility, and the discomfort of pain radiating to the ear may be suggestive of metastasis.

Diagnostic Evaluation. Direct laryngoscopic examination may be necessary if the larynx cannot be completely visualized; it is also used for biopsy of the tumor. The growth may involve any of the three areas (glottis, supraglottis, or subglottis) and varies in appearance. The precise involvement is determined since this affects the treatment. Since many of these lesions are submucosal, biopsy may necessitate that an incision be performed with microlaryngeal techniques or laser to transect the mucosa and reach the tumor.

Mobility of the vocal cords is assessed; if normal movement is limited, the growth may affect muscle, other tissue, and even the airway. The lymph nodes of the neck and the thyroid gland are palpated to determine spread of the malignancy.

Computed tomography and laryngography are effective in determining the extent of tumor growth.

Management

Treatment varies with the extent of the malignancy. Precise determination of the exact location and involvement of the malignancy is done by indirect and direct laryngoscopy, biopsy, and radiography before radiation therapy or surgery is prescribed.

If surgery is to be performed, thorough mouth hygiene prior to the procedure is imperative. Antibiotics may be prescribed to reduce the possibility of infection. In men, preoperative shaving includes the beard and the hair on the neck and the chest down to the nipple line.

Radiation Therapy. Good results have been produced by radiation therapy in patients in whom only one cord was affected and was normally mobile (*i.e.*, moved with phonation). In addition, these patients retain a practically normal voice. A few may develop chondritis or stenosis; a small number may later require laryngectomy.

Partial Laryngectomy (Laryngofissure, Thyrotomy). A partial laryngectomy is recommended in the early stages, especially in intrinsic cancer of the larynx (limited to the vocal cords), and has a cure rate of more than 80%. In this operation, the thyroid cartilage of the larynx is split in the midline of the neck, and the portion of the vocal cord that is involved with tumor growth is removed. Sometimes a tracheostomy tube (see p. 432) is left in the trachea when the wound is closed; it is usually removed after a few days.

Supraglottic (Horizontal) Laryngectomy. A supraglottic laryngectomy is used in the management of certain extrinsic tumors. After adequate resection, sufficient normal larynx is left so that the cords remain intact and their function is maintained. During surgery a radical neck dissection is also done on the involved side. Postoperatively, the patient may experience some difficulty in swallowing for the first 2 weeks. The chief advantage of this operation, of course, is that it preserves the voice. The major problem is that there may be local recurrence; therefore, patients have to be selected carefully.

Total Laryngectomy. For extrinsic cancer of the larynx (extension beyond the vocal cords), the entire larynx is removed; this includes the thyroid cartilage, the vocal cords, and the epiglottis. Many surgeons recommend that a neck dissection be performed on the same side as the lesion even though no lymph nodes are palpable. The rationale for this approach is that as many as 35% of patients have had metastases to the cervical lymph nodes. Obviously, the problem is more complex when a lesion involves midline structures or both vocal cords. With or without neck dissection, a total laryngectomy requires a permanent tracheal stoma (Fig. 20-5). This is done to prevent aspiration of food and fluid into the lower respiratory tract, since the larynx that provides the protective sphincter is no longer present.

Total Laryngectomy With Laryngoplasty. In this delicate three-stage procedure (Assai operation), a dermal tube is fashioned from the upper end of the trachea into the hypopharynx. By closing the permanent tracheostomy opening with his finger, the patient can exhale air up through the dermal tube and into the pharyngeal cavity. The sound produced is transformed into speech that is almost normal and far superior to esophageal speech.

▶ Nursing Process
The Patient Undergoing Laryngectomy

▷ Assessment

The nurse needs to assess the patient for the following symptoms: hoarseness, sore throat, dyspnea, dysphagia, or pain and burning in the throat. The patient's neck is palpated for swelling.

If treatment includes surgery, it is important for the nurse to know the nature of the surgery in order to plan appropriate care. For example, some patients experience loss of speech.

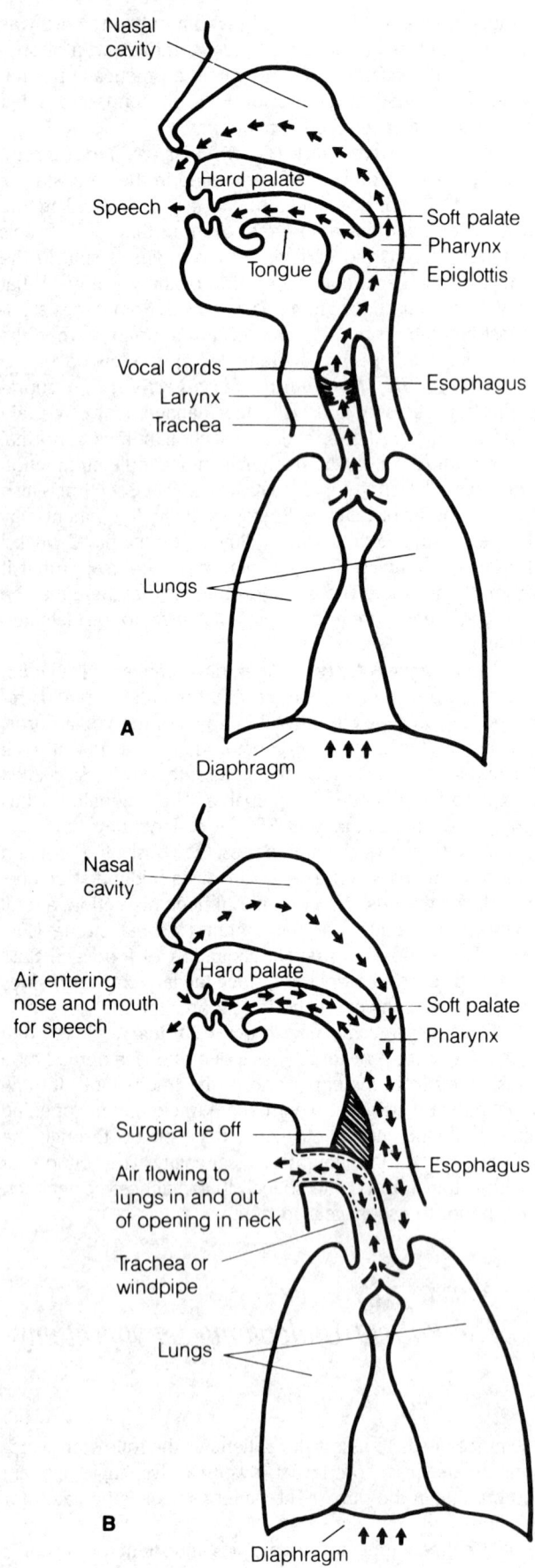

Once the nurse has determined that speech will be lost, a preoperative evaluation by the speech-language pathologist is indicated.

In addition, the nurse needs to determine the psychological preparedness of the patient. The idea of cancer is terrifying to most people; this is compounded by the potential for permanent loss of speech. The nurse needs to evaluate the patient's coping methods in order to develop an effective approach to supporting him both preoperatively and postoperatively.

▷ Nursing Diagnoses

Based on all the assessment data the patient's major nursing diagnoses may include the following:

· Knowledge deficit about the surgical procedure and postoperative course
· Anxiety and depression related to the diagnosis of cancer
· Ineffective airway clearance related to surgical alterations in the airway
· Impaired verbal communication related to impaired ability to speak words
· Inadequate nutrition related to swallowing difficulties
· Potential for nonadherence to rehabilitation program and home maintenance management

▷ Planning and Implementation

▷ *Goals:* The major goals for the patient may include attainment of an adequate level of knowledge, reduction in anxiety and depression, attainment of a patent airway (patient is able to handle own secretions), improvement in communication by use of alternative methods, attainment of an optimal level of nutrition, and adherence to rehabilitation program and home care.

Preoperative Nursing Interventions

Patient Education. The diagnosis of cancer of the larynx is associated with preconceived notions and fears. Many categorize it with other "cancers" and assume the worst. Others assume that loss of speech and disfigurement are inevitable with this condition. Once the physician explains the diagnosis to the patient, the nurse clarifies any misconceptions by identifying where the larynx is, what it does, and what the particular procedure will be. The patient's role in the postoperative and rehabilitative period is explained (see below).

Measures to Reduce Anxiety and Depression. Since surgery of the larynx is done most commonly for a tumor that may be malignant, the patient has many questions: Will the surgeon be able to remove all of the tumor? Is it cancer? Will I die? Will I choke? Will I ever speak again? Therefore, the psychological preparation of the patient is as important

Figure 20-5
Direction of the air flow before (*A*) and after (*B*) total laryngectomy. (Courtesy of American Cancer Society.)

as the physical preparation. If the patient is going to have a complete laryngectomy, he should know that he will lose his natural voice completely and that, with training, there are ways in which he can carry on a fairly normal conversation. (He will not be able to sing, laugh, or whistle.) Until he receives this training, the patient needs to know that the nurse can be reached by using the call light and that he can communicate in the immediate postoperative phase by writing. The nurse answers questions about the nature of the surgery and tells the patient that he will lose his ability to vocalize speech. He is reassured that much can be done for him through a rehabilitation program.

The patient is given the opportunity to verbalize his feelings and share his perceptions. Any misconceptions he might have about his condition are resolved. He is given complete but concise answers to his questions. During the postoperative period, someone who has had a laryngectomy should visit him. This visit should help him realize that there are people willing to help him cope with his situation.

Postoperative Nursing Interventions

Airway Maintenance. Respiratory effectiveness is promoted by positioning the patient in the semi-Fowler's to Fowler's position following recovery from anesthesia. The patient is observed for restlessness, labored breathing, apprehension, and increased pulse rate, since these suggest respiratory or circulatory problems. Medications that depress respirations are to be avoided. Like other surgical patients, the laryngectomy patient needs to be turned and reminded to cough and take deep breaths; suctioning may be necessary. Early ambulation, also, aids in preventing atelectasis and pneumonia. If a laryngofissure has been performed, a tracheostomy tube will be in place for 2 or 3 days (see p. 433). Then the nurse may have to administer enteral feedings through a nasogastric tube. Intravenous therapy is monitored concurrently with the tube feedings. Oral intake is begun, when prescribed, with ice chips and clear fluids. Patient tolerance is evaluated. There is a gradual resumption of the use of the voice (2 to 3 days).

If a total laryngectomy was performed, a laryngectomy tube will most likely be in place. (In some instances a laryngectomy tube is not used, in others it is used temporarily, and in many it is used permanently.) The laryngectomy tube (which is shorter than a tracheostomy tube but has a larger diameter) is the only airway the patient has. The care of this tube is the same as for a tracheostomy tube (see p. 433).

The stoma is kept clean by daily cleansing with saline solution or prescribed solution; antibiotic ointment (of a non-oil base), as prescribed, may then be applied around the stoma and suture line.

Wound drains may be in place to assist in removal of fluid and air from the dead space. Portable suction may also be used. Drainage is observed, measured, and recorded; when drainage amounts to less than 50 to 60 ml/day, the physician is alerted and the drains usually are removed.

The laryngectomy tube may be removed when the stoma is well healed, usually within 3 to 6 weeks after the operation. Until that time, the patient will need to be taught how to clean and change the laryngectomy tube (see p. 396) and how

to clear his airway of secretions. Through the postoperative period, the nurse must be alert for the possible serious complication of rupture of the carotid artery, particularly if wound infection is present. Should this occur, she would apply direct pressure over the artery, summon assistance, and provide psychological support to the patient until the vessel can be ligated.

Nutrition. Nutrition is maintained initially by means of a nasogastric catheter or a tube passed through a cervical pharyngostomy. The physician places the nasogastric tube postoperatively. After that, the nurse can remove and pass the tube because there is no danger of its getting into the trachea since the trachea now bypasses the pharynx and upper airway. Tube feedings are given 2 to 3 days postoperatively depending on the patient's nutritional needs. After that, the tube is usually removed. The nurse explains to the patient that he will start with thick fluids such as custard and Jello, which are easy to swallow. He is also instructed to avoid sweet foods, which increase salivation and suppress the appetite. Solid foods are introduced as tolerated. In addition, the patient is instructed to rinse his mouth with warm water or mouthwash and to brush his teeth frequently.

Communication and Speech Rehabilitation. Since a "magic slate" is often used for communication, it is well to remember which hand the patient uses for writing so that the opposite arm can be used for intravenous infusions. When notes are the means of communication, they should be destroyed to ensure the patient's privacy. If the patient is not able to write, flash cards can be used.

Another method of communication is esophageal speech. This can be taught once the patient begins oral feedings or 1 week postoperatively. The patient first develops his ability to belch. An hour after he has eaten, the nurse reminds him to belch. This is practiced repeatedly. Later this conscious action is transformed into simple explosions of air from the esophagus for speech purposes. From here the speech-language pathologist works with him in an attempt to make his speech intelligible and as close to normal as possible.

If esophageal speech is not successful, or until the technique is mastered, an electric larynx may be used for communication. This apparatus projects sound into the oral cavity. When words are formed by the mouth (articulated), the sound from the electric larynx becomes words that can be heard. The voice that is produced is obviously not the patient's normal voice, but he is able to communicate with relative ease.

Another form of communication that will help the patient be better understood is called tracheoesophageal puncture (TEP). In this method the voice is restored by diverting air, which travels from the lungs through a puncture in the posterior wall of the trachea, into the esophagus, and out of the mouth. Once the puncture is surgically created and has healed, a voice prosthesis (Blom-Singer) is fitted over the puncture site. The prosthesis is removed and cleaned when there is mucus buildup in order to prevent airway obstruction. The patient is given lessons in voice production by the speech-language pathologist, but the speech is produced just as before by moving the tongue and lips to form the sound into words.

Other alternatives or interim methods of communication include a call bell, sign language, lip reading, and computer aids.

The International Association of Laryngectomees is a voluntary organization that sponsors "Lost Chord" or "New Voice" clubs to encourage and give opportunities for laryngectomized persons to learn to speak again.

Patient Education. The following areas are addressed.

Tracheostomy and Stomal Care. The nurse conveys optimism to the patient, assuring him that he will be able to carry on most of his preoperative activities. The patient needs specific information about what to expect from his tracheostomy. He will frequently cough up rather large amounts of mucus through this opening. Because air passes directly into the trachea without being warmed and moistened by the upper respiratory mucosa, the tracheobronchial tree compensates by secreting excessive amounts of mucus. Therefore, the patient will have frequent coughing episodes and may be somewhat troubled by the brassy sounding, mucus-producing cough. However, he should be assured that these problems diminish in time as the tracheobronchial mucosa adapts to the patient's altered physiology.

When the patient coughs, the orifice should be wiped clean and cleared of mucus. In addition, the skin around the stoma should be washed twice daily. If crusting occurs, the skin around the stoma is lubricated with a non-oil base ointment (prescribed by the physician) and the crusts removed with sterile tweezers. It may be necessary that a bib be worn in front of the tracheostomy to keep the mucus from soiling the clothing. The bib may be a simple gauze dressing taped over the neck or one made of other porous fabric.

One of the most important factors in decreasing cough and mucus production as well as crusting around the stoma is to provide adequate humidification of the environment. Mechanical humidifiers and aerosol generators (nebulizers) are excellent sources of humidification and are absolutely essential for the patient's comfort. Some system of humidification should be set up in the home before the patient is discharged from the hospital. An air-conditioned atmosphere may be distressing to the newly laryngectomized patient, since the air may be too cool or too dry and thus too irritating.

Changes in Taste and Smell. The patient can expect to have a diminished sense of taste and smell for a period after the operation. Because he is breathing directly into the trachea, air is not passing through the nose to the olfactory end organs. Because taste and smell are so closely connected, his taste sensations are altered. However, in time the patient usually accommodates to this problem and his olfactory sensation adapts to meet his needs.

Hygienic and Recreational Measures. Special precautions need to be taken in a shower to prevent water from entering the stoma. Wearing a loose-fitting plastic bib or simply holding one's hand over the opening is effective. However, swimming is not recommended, because the patient with a laryngectomy can drown without getting his face wet. Barbers and beauticians need to be cautioned so that hair sprays, loose hair, and powder do not get near the stoma, since they could cause blockage, irritation, and possibly infection.

Recreation and exercise are important. Golf, bowling, bridge, spectator activities, and walking can be enjoyed safely. Moderation in order to prevent fatigue is important because, when tired, the laryngectomee has more difficulty speaking with his new voice. At such times he can easily become discouraged and depressed.

Follow-up and Emergency Care. The nurse encourages the laryngectomee to visit his physician regularly for physical examinations and for advice concerning any problems relating to his convalescent program. He should also carry proper identification, such as a card, to alert a first-aider to the special requirements of resuscitation should this need arise. On the back of the card can be included the name of a responsible person to notify in the event of emergency.

▷ *Evaluation*

▷ *Expected Outcomes*

1. The patient acquires an adequate level of knowledge.
   a. Verbalizes an understanding of his specific surgical procedure.
   b. States his role in his own care.
   c. Performs self-care adequately.
2. The patient experiences less anxiety and depression.
   a. Describes the reason for his surgery and desires to work with staff.
   b. Verbalizes confidence that health care personnel will give him the care he needs.
   c. Develops a sense of hope about his condition.
   d. Expresses that he is comfortable with the support group (Fig. 20-6).
   e. Meets with someone from the "Lost Chord" or "New Voice" club.
3. The patient maintains a clear airway and handles own secretions.
   a. Demonstrates practical and correct technique involved in cleaning and changing the laryngectomy tube.
   b. Demonstrates how to raise secretions from stoma or tube by coughing or by suctioning.
   c. Is afebrile and eupneic (normal respiratory rate); has normal breath sounds.
   d. Relates the significance of good hygienic measures in keeping mouth and stoma clean.
   e. Covers stoma opening securely when shaving or showering.
4. The patient acquires effective communication techniques.
   a. Uses a "magic slate" until whispering is permitted.
   b. Is comfortable with alternative communication techniques when voice is not audible: call bell, flash cards, sign language, lip reading, computer aids.
   c. Verbalizes how the vocal problem can be improved with adherence to the therapeutic plan, eventually mastering his very own program, whether it is "belch" speech or artificial larynx.
   d. Communicates with family using newly learned speech techniques.
   e. Practices the directives of the speech-language pathologist.
5. The patient maintains balanced nutrition.
   a. Verbalizes need to drink viscous fluids when experiencing swallowing difficulties.
   b. Avoids sweet foods.
   c. Tolerates solid foods.
   d. Rinses mouth and brushes teeth frequently.

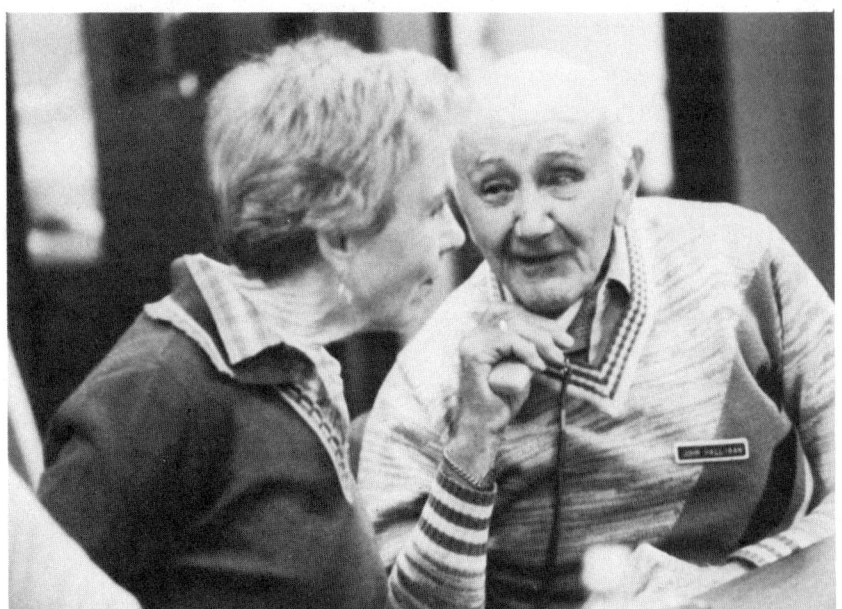

Figure 20-6
During recovery, a former laryngectomee may visit the "new" laryngectomee. This caller will use esophageal speech and answer questions written by the patient. Such contact with a former patient has been very effective in encouraging the new patient when he needs it most. (Courtesy of American Cancer Society, New Jersey Division, Inc., Middlesex County Unit, and Larynx Visitation Program.)

6. The patient adheres to rehabilitation and home care program.
   a. No longer smokes.
   b. Practices recommended speech therapy in addition to keeping appointments with speech-language pathologist.
   c. Demonstrates understanding of hygienic principles when caring for stoma and laryngectomy tube (if present).
   d. Involves spouse with his care activities.
   e. Plans how to increase the humidity in his home.
   f. Covers stomal opening securely when shaving or showering.
   g. Verbalizes understanding of symptoms that require medical attention.
   h. Makes follow-up appointments with appropriate health care personnel.
   i. Carries a card indicating procedures to follow in the event of an emergency, including who to contact for assistance.

Bibliography

Books

Ballenger JJ. Diseases of the Nose, Throat, Ear, Head and Neck, 13th ed. Philadelphia, Lea & Febiger, 1985.

Baum G and Wolinsky E. Textbook of Pulmonary Disease, 2nd ed. Boston, Little, Brown, & Co, 1983.

DeVita VT Jr, Hellman S, and Rosenberg SA. Cancer—Principles and Practices of Oncology, 2nd ed. Philadelphia, JB Lippincott, 1985.

Donovan M and Girton S. Cancer Care Nursing. Norwalk, Connecticut, Appleton-Century-Crofts, 1984.

Glauser F (ed). Signs and Symptoms in Pulmonary Medicine. Philadelphia, JB Lippincott, 1983.

Lucente FE and Sobol SM. Essentials of Otolaryngology. New York, Raven Press, 1983.

McNally JC et al (eds). Guidelines for Cancer Nursing Practice. Orlando, Florida, Grune & Stratton, 1985.

Raffensperger E, Zusy ML and Marchesseau HLC. Clinical Nursing Handbook. Philadelphia, JB Lippincott, 1986.

Rakel RE (ed). Conn's Current Therapy. Philadelphia, WB Saunders, 1985.

Traver G (ed). Respiratory Nursing: The Science and the Art. New York, John Wiley & Sons, 1982.

Articles

Upper Airway Infections

Davis RK and Simpson GT III. Safety with the carbon dioxide laser. Otolaryngol Clin North Am 1983 Nov; 16(4):801–812.

Fuller E. Helping patients pick cold remedies. Patient Care 1985 Sept 15; 19(15):24–30, 37–38, 40–44.

Gillette RD. Pharyngitis: Reevaluating diagnosis and treatment. Consultant 1985 Apr; 25(7):59–66.

Kimmelman CP and Ali GHA. Vasomotor rhinitis. Otolaryngol Clin North Am 1986 Feb; 19(1):65–71.

Platt AF Jr. Bacterial pharyngitis in adults (protocol). Physician Assist 1985 May; 9(5):171–172, 176–171, 181.

Stool SE. Diagnosis and treatment of sinusitis. Am Fam Physician 1985 Dec; 32(6):101–107.

Telian SA. Sore throat and antibiotics. Otolaryngol Clin North Am 1986 Feb; 19(1):103–109.

Travis HR. Vitamin C and the common cold revisited. Health Educ 1984 Jan/Feb; 15(1):13–15.

Obstruction and Trauma of the Upper Respiratory Airway

Colton JJ and Beckhuis GJ. Management of nasal fractures. Otolaryngol Clin North Am 1986 Feb; 19(1):73–85.

Kimmitt TP et al. Pharyngeal emergencies. Top Emerg Med 1984 Oct; 6(3):66–81.

Silfen EZ et al. Nasal emergencies. Top Emerg Med 1984 Oct; 6(3):40–47.

Cancer of the Larynx

Harris LL and Kraege J. After T-E puncture: Relearning to speak. Am J Nurs 1986 Jan; 86(1):55–58.

Kaplan MJ et al. Glottic carcinoma. Cancer 1984 June 15; 53(12):2641–2647.

Koop CE. Smoking and cancer. Hosp Pract 1984 June; 19(6):107–111, 117–120, 125–126.

Levine HL and Tubbs R. Nonsquamous neoplasms of the larynx. Otolaryngol Clin North Am 1986 Aug; 19(3):475–487.

McCormick GP et al. Artificial speech devices. Am J Nurs 1982 Jan; 82(1):122–132.

Patry-Lahey R. Helping a laryngectomy patient go home. Nursing '85 1985 Mar; 15(3):63–64.

Pilcher L. Carbon dioxide lasers in laryngeal surgery. AORN J 1981 June; 33(7):1402–1407.

Riches KG. Postoperative nursing care of laryngectomy patients and pharyngeal diverticulae. NAT News 1984 May; 21(5):18–21.

Romm S. Cancer of the larynx: Current concepts of diagnosis and treatment. Surg Clin North Am 1986 Feb; 66(1):109–118.

Silverberg BS and Lubera J. Cancer statistics, 1986. CA 1986 Jan/Feb; 36(1):9–25.

Wetmore SJ et al. Long-term results of the Blom-Singer speech rehabilitation procedure. Arch Otolaryngol 1985 Feb; 111(2):106–109.

Agency

Lost Chord Club, American Cancer Society, Inc., 90 Park Ave, Dept. N85, New York, NY 10016.

Chapter 21

Assessment of Respiratory Function

Physiologic Overview

The cells of the body derive the energy they need from the oxidation of carbohydrates, fats, and proteins. For this process, as for any type of combustion, oxygen is required. Certain vital tissues, such as those of the brain and the heart, cannot survive for long without a continuing supply of oxygen. As a result of oxidation in the body tissues, carbon dioxide is produced and must be removed from the cells to prevent buildup of acid waste products.

Oxygen is supplied to cells and carbon dioxide is removed from cells by way of the circulating blood. Cells are in close contact with capillaries, whose thin walls permit easy passage or exchange of oxygen and carbon dioxide. Oxygen diffuses from the capillary, through the capillary wall to the interstitial fluid, and then through the membrane of tissue cells, where it can be used by mitochondria for cellular respiration. The movement of carbon dioxide also occurs by diffusion and proceeds in the opposite direction, from cell to blood.

After these tissue capillary exchanges, blood enters the systemic veins (where it is called *venous blood*) and travels to the lung circulation. The oxygen concentration in blood within the lung capillaries is lower than it is in the lung gas spaces, which are called *alveoli*. As a result, oxygen diffuses from the alveoli to the blood. Carbon dioxide, whose concentration in the blood is higher than in the alveoli, diffuses from the blood into the alveoli. Movement of fresh air in and out of the airways (called *ventilation*) continually replenishes the oxygen and removes the carbon dioxide from the air spaces in the lung. This whole process of gas exchange between the atmospheric air and the blood and between the blood and the cells of the body is called *respiration*.

Anatomy of the Lung

The lungs are elastic structures enclosed in the thorax, which is an airtight chamber with distensible walls. Ventilation involves movements of the walls of the thorax and of its floor, the diaphragm. The effect of these movements is alternately to increase and decrease the capacity of the chest. When the capacity of the chest is increased, air enters through the trachea, because of the lowered pressure within, and inflates the lungs. When the chest wall and diaphragm return to their previous positions, the elastic lungs recoil and force the air out through the bronchi and trachea.

The outer surfaces of the lungs are enclosed by a smooth, slippery membrane, the *pleura*, which also extends to cover the interior wall of the thorax and the superior surface of the diaphragm. The pleura is termed *parietal pleura* where it lines the thorax and *visceral pleura* where it covers the lungs. Between the two pleural surfaces is a small amount of fluid that lubricates the surfaces and allows them to slide freely during ventilation.

The *mediastinum* is the wall that divides the thoracic cavity into two halves. It is composed of two layers of pleura between which lie all of the thoracic structures except the lungs.

Each lung is divided into lobes. The left lung consists of upper and lower lobes, whereas the right lung has upper, middle, and lower lobes. Each lobe is further subdivided into two to five segments separated by fissures, which are extensions of the pleura. A schematic diagram of the airways and the lobes of the lungs is shown in Figure 21-1.

There are several divisions of the bronchi within each lobe of the lung. First are the lobar bronchi (three in the right lung and two in the left lung). Lobar bronchi divide into segmental bronchi (10 on the right and 8 on the left), which are

the structures identified when choosing the most effective postural drainage position for a given patient. Segmental bronchi then divide into subsegmental bronchi. These bronchi are surrounded by connective tissue that contains arteries, lymphatics, and nerves. The subsegmental bronchi then branch into *bronchioles*, which have no cartilage in their walls. Their patency depends entirely on the elastic recoil of the smooth muscle that surrounds it and on the alveolar pressure. The bronchioles contain submucosal glands, which produce mucus that forms an uninterrupted covering for the inside lining of the airway. The bronchi and bronchioles are also lined with cells whose surfaces are covered with short "hairs" called *cilia*. These cilia create a constant whipping motion that serves to propel mucus and foreign substances away from the lung toward the larynx.

The bronchioles then branch into *terminal bronchioles*, which do not have mucus glands or cilia. Terminal bronchioles then become *respiratory bronchioles*, which are considered to be the transition passageways between the conducting airways and the gas exchange airways. Up to this point the conducting airways contain about 150 ml of air caught in the tracheobronchial tree that does not participate in gas exchange. The respiratory bronchioles then lead into alveolar ducts and alveolar sacs and then alveoli. Oxygen and carbon dioxide exchange takes place in the alveoli.

The lung is made up of about 300 million alveoli, which are arranged in clusters of 15 to 20. So numerous are these

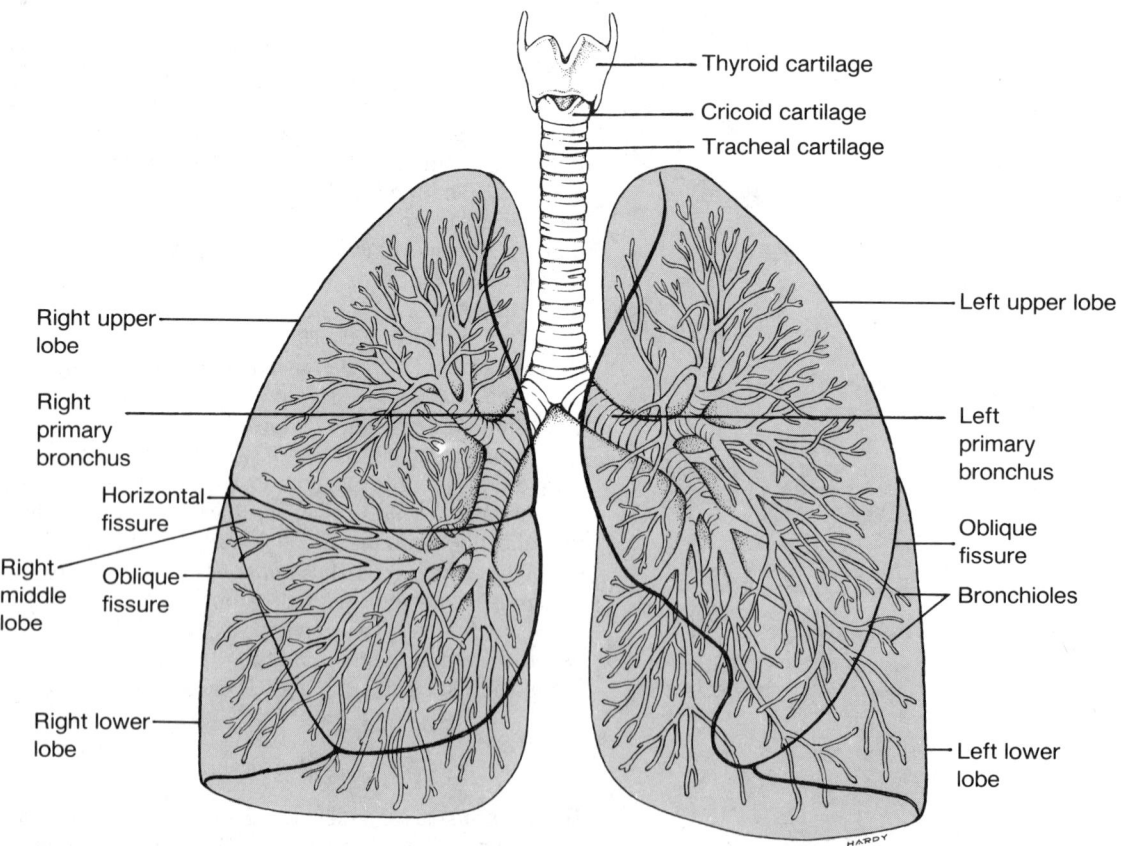

Figure 21-1
Larynx, trachea, and bronchial tree (anterior view). (Chaffee EE and Greisheimer EM. Basic Physiology and Anatomy. Philadelphia, JB Lippincott.)

alveoli that if their surfaces were united to form one sheet it would cover an area the size of a tennis court (or 70 square meters).

There are three types of alveolar cells. Type I alveolar cells are epithelial cells that form the alveolar walls. Type II alveolar cells, metabolically active cells, secrete *surfactant,* which is a phospholipid that lines the inner surface of the alveoli. Type III, alveoli cell macrophages, are large phagocytic cells that ingest foreign matter (*e.g.,* mucus, bacteria) and act as an important defense mechanism.

Mechanics of Ventilation

During inspiration, air flows from the environment into the trachea, bronchi, bronchioles, and alveoli. During expiration, alveolar gas travels the same route in reverse.

The physical factors that govern air flow in and out of the lungs are collectively referred to as the mechanics of ventilation. Air flows from a region of higher pressure to a region of lower pressure. During inspiration, contraction of the diaphragm and other muscles of respiration enlarges the thoracic cavity and thereby lowers the pressure inside the thorax to a level below that of atmospheric pressure. Therefore, air is drawn through the trachea and bronchi into the alveoli.

During normal expiration, the muscles of respiration relax and the thoracic cavity decreases in size. The alveolar pressure now exceeds atmospheric pressure, and air flows from the lungs into the atmosphere.

Resistance is determined chiefly by the radius of the airway through which the air is flowing. Any process that changes bronchial diameter will therefore affect airway resistance and alter the rate of air flow for a given pressure gradient during respiration. Common factors that may alter bronchial diameter include contraction of bronchial smooth muscle, as in asthma; thickening of bronchial mucosa, as in chronic bronchitis; or obstruction of the airway due to mucus, a tumor, or a foreign body. Loss of lung elasticity, such as is seen in emphysema, may also alter bronchial diameter since the lung connective tissue encircles the airways and helps to keep them open during both inspiration and expiration. With increased resistance, greater than normal respiratory effort is required by the patient to achieve normal levels of ventilation.

The pressure gradient between the thoracic cavity and the atmosphere causes air flow in and out of the lungs and also stretches the lung tissue itself. The pressure required to stretch the lung is determined by the properties of its elastic tissue. A measure of how easily lungs can be stretched is called *lung compliance*. Compliance is usually measured under static conditions.

A compliant lung (high compliance) distends easily when pressure is applied, whereas a noncompliant lung (low compliance) requires greater than normal pressure to distend it. The major factors that determine lung compliance are connective tissue (collagen and elastin) and the surface tension in the alveoli. The surface tension at the surface of the alveoli is normally maintained at a low level by the presence of the alveolar lining material (lung surfactant). Increased connective tissue or increased alveolar surface tension results in low compliance. In adult respiratory distress syndrome there is a surfactant deficiency and the lungs are stiff (low compliance). In pulmonary fibrosis, connective tissue proliferates and

compliance is decreased. Lungs with low compliance require a greater than normal energy expenditure to achieve normal levels of ventilation.

The mechanics of ventilation can be measured to evaluate lung function (Fig. 21-2). Included in these measurements are

- *Inspiratory reserve volume (IRV)*—the maximum volume of air that can be inhaled after a normal inhalation.
- *Tidal volume (V_T)*—the volume of air normally inhaled or exhaled.
- *Expiratory reserve volume (ERV)*—the maximum volume of air that can be exhaled after a normal exhalation.
- *Residual volume (RV)*—the volume of air remaining in the lungs after a maximum exhalation.
- *Total lung capacity (TLC)*—the volume of air in the lungs after a maximum inhalation.
- *Functional residual capacity*—the volume of air in the lungs at resting and exhalation.

Several additional useful measurements include

- *Vital capacity (VC)*—the maximum volume of air that is exhaled after a full inspiration (includes inspiratory reserve volume, tidal volume, and expiratory reserve volume).
- *Forced vital capacity (FVC)*—same as vital capacity except that it is achieved by forceful expiration.
- *Maximum voluntary ventilation (MVV)*—the volume of air exhaled per minute while breathing fast and deep.
- *Minute ventilation ($\dot{V}_E$)*—the volume of air exhaled in 1 minute.
- *Flow volume curves*—a single breath test that measures most of the above volumes and tends to be more accurate than the traditional volume–time curves of pulmonary function studies. (See Table 21-1.)

In healthy upright lungs, ventilation is greatest in the lower regions of the lung and decreases toward the apices. In addition to this regional inequality of ventilation, there is uneven ventilation among alveoli, permitting air to be distributed more evenly between them.

Diffusion and Perfusion

Diffusion is the process by which oxygen and carbon dioxide are exchanged at the air–blood interface. The alveolar-capillary membrane is ideal for diffusion because of its large surface area and thin membrane. In healthy lungs oxygen and carbon dioxide travel across the alveolar-capillary membrane without difficulty.

Pulmonary perfusion is the actual blood flow through the pulmonary circulation. The blood is pumped into the lungs by the right ventricle through the pulmonary artery. The pulmonary artery divides into the right and left branches to supply both lungs. These two branches divide further to supply all parts of each lung. The pulmonary circulation is considered a low pressure system since the systolic blood pressure in the pulmonary artery is 20 to 30 mm Hg and the diastolic pressure is 5 to 15 mm Hg. Because it is low, the pulmonary vasculature normally can vary its resistance to accommodate the blood flow it receives. However, when a person is in an erect position, the pulmonary artery pressure is not great enough to supply blood to the apex of the lung against the

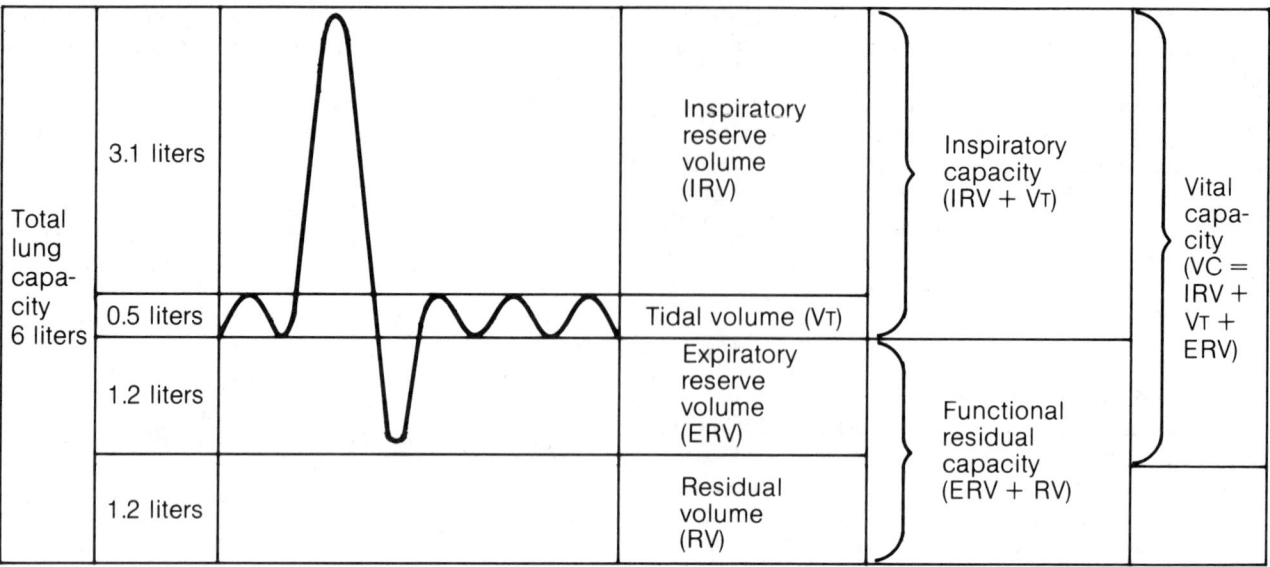

Total lung capacity 6 liters	3.1 liters	Inspiratory reserve volume (IRV)	Inspiratory capacity (IRV + VT)	Vital capacity (VC = IRV + VT + ERV)
	0.5 liters	Tidal volume (VT)		
	1.2 liters	Expiratory reserve volume (ERV)	Functional residual capacity (ERV + RV)	
	1.2 liters	Residual volume (RV)		

Figure 21-2

Respiratory volumes and capacities: Normal spirogram of relative volumes in the lung. Inspiratory reserve volume (IRV)—maximum volume of air inhaled after a normal inhalation; tidal volume (VT)—volume of air normally inhaled or exhaled; expiratory reserve volume (ERV)—maximum volume of air exhaled after a normal exhalation; residual volume (RV)—volume of air remaining in the lungs after a maximum expiration; total lung capacity (TLC)—volume of air in the lungs after a maximum inhalation. These volumes change in disease states. They are useful in evaluating lung mechanics.

force of gravity. Thus, when a person is erect, the lung may be considered to be divided into three sections: an upper part with poor blood supply, a lower part with maximum blood supply, and the section in between the two with an intermediate supply of blood. When a person turns to one side, more blood passes to the dependent lung.

Perfusion is also influenced by alveolar pressure. The pulmonary capillaries are sandwiched between adjacent alveoli. If the alveolar pressure is sufficiently high, the capillaries will be squeezed. Depending on the pressure, some capillaries will be completely collapsed whereas others will be narrowed.

Pulmonary artery pressure, gravity, and alveolar pressure determine the patterns of perfusion. In lung disease these factors vary and the perfusion of the lung may become very abnormal.

Shunting

Normally about 2% of the blood pumped by the right ventricle does not perfuse the alveolar capillaries. This blood, which cannot participate in gas exchange with alveolar gas, is called *shunted blood*. It drains into the left side of the heart through the bronchial, pleural, and thebesian veins. In some pathologic states of the heart and great vessels (ventricular septal defect, patent ductus arteriosus) and lung diseases (pulmonary edema, atelectasis) the amount of blood shunted exceeds the normal 2%.

The shunted blood, which contains the same amount of oxygen as venous blood, mixes with the blood returning from the alveoli to produce arterial blood. The oxygen content of the arterial blood depends on both the oxygen content and the volume of each fraction. Severe hypoxia results when the

amount of blood shunted exceeds 20%. The hypoxia is not significantly improved by breathing even 100% oxygen because the oxygen does not come in contact with the shunted blood.

Distribution of Ventilation and Perfusion

Ventilation is the flow of gas in and out of the lung, and *perfusion* is the filling of the pulmonary capillaries with blood. The pulmonary arterial pressure, gravity, and alveolar pressure lead to uneven perfusion of the lung. The main factors leading to uneven distribution of ventilation of the lung include patency of the airways, local changes in compliance within the lung, and gravity.

Any factor that reduces the airway caliber (mucosal edema, inflammation, secretion, bronchospasm) will raise the resistance to air flow and decrease the ventilation of the corresponding alveoli. Similarly, any area in which the local compliance has decreased (*i.e.*, that portion of the lung has become more stiff) will receive less ventilation than the surrounding more expandable portions of the lung.

The effect of gravity on ventilation is complex. Because of the consistency of the lung, its weight is distributed within the chest cavity in such a manner that the intrapleural pressure is less negative at the bottom (-2.5 cm H_2O) than at the top of the lung (-10 cm H_2O) when a person is in the erect position. However, the pressure within the airways is the same in all parts of the lung; consequently, the alveoli at the apex are larger than the alveoli at the base of the lung. When one applies these facts to the pressure–volume relationship of the lung, it becomes clear why, in the early phase of inspiration, more of the tidal volume is distributed to the basal region of

TABLE 21-1
Pulmonary Function Tests

Description	Term Used	Symbol	Remarks
The maximum volume of air exhaled from the point of maximum inspiration	Vital capacity	VC	Slow vital capacity may be normal or reduced in COPD patients.
Vital capacity performed with a maximally forced expiratory effort	Forced vital capacity	FVC	Forced vital capacity is often reduced in COPD owing to air trapping.
Volume of air exhaled in the specified time during the performance of forced vital capacity	Forced expiratory volume (qualified by subscript indicating the time interval in seconds)	FEVt, usually FEV_1	A valuable clue to the severity of the expiratory airway obstruction.
FEVt expressed as a percentage of the forced vital capacity	Ratio of timed forced expiratory volume to forced vital capacity	FEVt/FVC%, usually FEV_1/FVC%	Another way of expressing the presence or absence of airway obstruction.
Mean forced expiratory flow between 200 and 1200 ml of the FVC	Forced expiratory flow	$FEF_{200-1200}$	Formerly called maximum expiratory flow rate (MEFR). An indicator of large airway obstruction.
Mean forced expiratory flow during the middle half of the FVC	Forced mid-expiratory flow	$FEF_{25\%-75\%}$	Formerly called maximum and mid-expiratory flow rate. Slowed in small airway obstruction.
Mean forced expiratory flow during the terminal portion of the FVC	Forced end-expiratory flow	$FEF_{75\%-85\%}$	Slowed in obstruction of smallest airways.
Volume of air expired in a specified period during repetitive maximal effort	Maximal voluntary ventilation	MVV	Formerly called maximum breathing capacity. An important factor in exercise tolerance.

COPD = Chronic obstructive pulmonary disease.
(Chronic Obstructive Pulmonary Disease, 8th ed. New York, American Lung Association, 1985.)

the lung. The basal region of the erect lung, therefore, receives more blood and air than the apex.

Matching of Ventilation and Perfusion. For optimum gas exchange the perfusion of each alveolus must be matched by optimum ventilation. In addition to the pressure–volume relationship of the lung, there are other mechanisms, such as changes in caliber of airways or capillaries, that ensure that ventilation and perfusion are properly matched in the normal lung.

Mismatching of ventilation and perfusion leads to hypoxia. It appears to be the main cause of hypoxia following thoracic or abdominal surgery and most types of respiratory failure. Its effects can be similar to those of shunts, or 100% oxygen can eliminate hypoxia, depending on the type of ventilation–perfusion mismatch.

Partial Pressure

Partial pressure is the pressure exerted by each type of gas in a mixture of gases. The partial pressure of a gas is proportional to the concentration of that gas in the mixture. The total pressure exerted by the gaseous mixture is equal to the sum of the partial pressures.

The air we breathe is a gaseous mixture consisting mainly of nitrogen (78.62%) and oxygen (20.84%), with traces of carbon dioxide (0.04%), water vapor (0.05%), helium, argon, and so on. The atmospheric pressure at sea level is about 760 torr (torr = mm Hg). Based on these facts the partial pressure of nitrogen and oxygen can be calculated. Partial pressure of nitrogen is 79% of 760 (.79 × 760) = 600 torr, and that of oxygen is 21% of 760 (.21 × 760) = 160 torr.

The following is a reference list of expressions related to partial pressure:

P = pressure
PO_2—partial pressure of oxygen
PCO_2—partial pressure of carbon dioxide
PAO_2—partial pressure of alveolar oxygen
$PACO_2$—partial pressure of alveolar carbon dioxide
PaO_2—partial pressure of arterial oxygen
$PaCO_2$—partial pressure of arterial carbon dioxide
PvO_2—partial pressure of venous oxygen
$PvCO_2$—partial pressure of venous carbon dioxide
P_{50}—partial pressure of oxygen when the hemoglobin is 50% saturated

Once the air enters the trachea it becomes fully saturated with water vapor, which displaces some of the gases in order that the air pressure within the lung may remain equal with the air pressure outside (760 torr). Water vapor exerts a pressure of 47 torr when it fully saturates a mixture of gases at the body temperature of 37°C (98.6°F). Nitrogen and oxygen are therefore now responsible for the remaining 713 torr (760 − 47) pressure. Once this mixture enters the alveoli, it is further diluted by carbon dioxide. In the alveoli, the water vapor continues to exert a pressure of 47 torr. The remaining 713 torr pressure is now exerted as follows: nitrogen, 569 torr (74.9%); oxygen, 104 torr (13.6%), and carbon dioxide, 40 torr (5.3%).

When a gas is exposed to a liquid, the gas will dissolve in the liquid until an equilibrium is reached. The dissolved gas also exerts a partial pressure. At equilibrium, the partial pressure of the gas in the liquid is the same as the partial pressure of the gas in the gaseous mixture. Oxygenation of venous blood in the lung illustrates this point. In the lung, venous blood and alveolar oxygen are separated by a very thin alveolar membrane. Oxygen diffuses across this membrane to dissolve in the blood until the partial pressure of oxygen in the blood is the same as that in the alveoli (104 torr). However, since carbon dioxide is manufactured in the cells, venous blood contains carbon dioxide at a higher partial pressure than that in the alveolar gas. In the lung, carbon dioxide diffuses out of venous blood into the alveolar gas. At equilibrium, the partial pressure of carbon dioxide in the blood and in alveolar gas is the same (40 torr).

The entire sequence of changes in partial pressure readings (in torr) may be summarized as follows:

	Atmospheric Air	Tracheal Air	Alveolar Air
P_{H_2O}	3.7	47.0	47.0
P_{N_2}	597.0	563.4	569.0
P_{O_2}	159.0	149.3	104.0
P_{CO_2}	0.3	0.3	40.0
Total	760.0	760.0	760.0

Oxygen Transport

Oxygen and carbon dioxide are carried simultaneously by virtue of their abilities to dissolve in blood or to combine with some of the elements of blood. Oxygen is carried in the blood in two forms: (1) as physically dissolved oxygen in the plasma and (2) in combination with the hemoglobin of the red blood cells. Each 100 ml of normal (P_{O_2} = 100) arterial blood carries 0.3 ml of oxygen physically dissolved in the plasma and 19 ml of oxygen in combination with hemoglobin. Note that the volume of oxygen carried by hemoglobin is considerably greater than that carried in physical solution.

The volume of oxygen physically dissolved in the plasma varies directly with the PaO_2. The higher the PaO_2, the greater the oxygen dissolved. For example, it is found that at a PaO_2 of 10 mm Hg, 0.03 ml of oxygen is dissolved in 100 ml of plasma. At 20 mm Hg, twice this amount is dissolved in plasma and at 100 mm Hg, ten times this amount is dissolved. Therefore, the amount of dissolved oxygen is directly proportional to the partial pressure, and this is true no matter how high the oxygen pressure rises. For example, in a hyperbaric chamber in which a subject is breathing oxygen at 3 atmo-

spheres, the PaO_2 would be 2000 mm Hg. The dissolved oxygen would be 6 ml of oxygen per 100 ml of blood.

The volume of oxygen that combines with hemoglobin also depends on PaO_2, but only up to a PaO_2 of about 150 mm Hg. Above this PaO_2, hemoglobin is 100% saturated, by which it is meant that hemoglobin will not combine with any additional oxygen. When hemoglobin is 100% saturated, 1 gm of hemoglobin will combine with 1.34 ml of oxygen. Therefore, in a person with 14 gm/dl of hemoglobin, each 100 ml of blood will contain about 19 ml of oxygen associated with hemoglobin. If the PaO_2 is less than 150 mm Hg, the percentage of hemoglobin saturated with oxygen is lower. For example, at a PaO_2 of 100 mm Hg (normal value) saturation is 97%, and at a PaO_2 of 40 mm Hg, the saturation is 70%.

The oxygen dissociation curve of hemoglobin (Fig. 21-3) shows the relationship between the partial pressure of oxygen and the percentage saturation of the hemoglobin more clearly (SaO_2). The unusual shape of the oxygen dissociation curve is a distinct advantage to the patient for two reasons:

1. If the arterial PO_2 decreases from 100 to 80 mm Hg as a result of lung disease or heart disease, the hemoglobin of the arterial blood will still be almost maximally

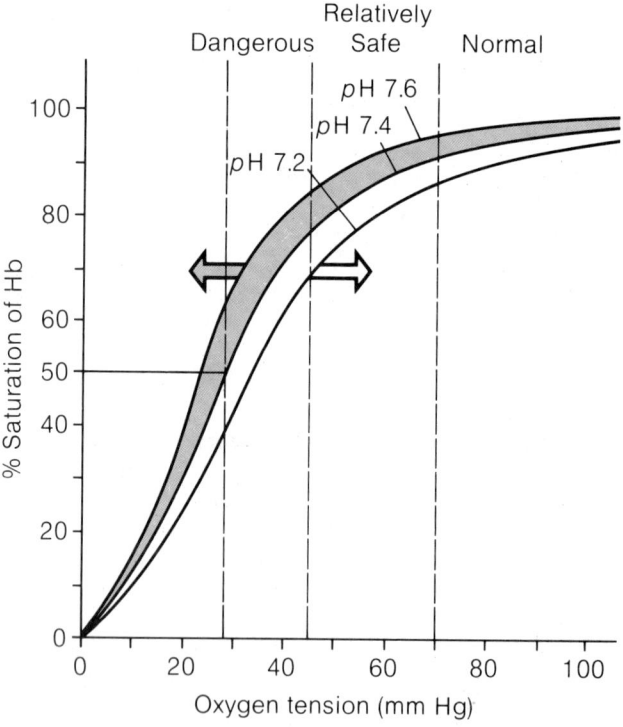

Figure 21-3
Oxygen–hemoglobin dissociation curve. The oxygen can attach to the hemoglobin more easily (higher SaO_2 per PO_2) but has more trouble coming off the hemoglobin at the tissues (less tissue oxygenation). Decreased oxygen affinity (shift to the right) means that it is more difficult for the oxygen to attach to the hemoglobin (lower SaO_2 per PO_2), but it can come off at the tissues more easily. P_{50} is normally 27 mm Hg. A shift to the right gives a higher P_{50}, and a shift to the left gives a lower P_{50}.

saturated (94%) and the tissues will not suffer from anoxia.

2. When the arterial blood passes into tissue capillaries and is exposed to the tissue tension of oxygen (about 40 mm Hg), hemoglobin gives up large quantities of oxygen for use by the tissues.

Oxygen Dissociation Curve

The oxygen dissociation curve indicates the methods used by the body to release oxygen to the tissues so that the oxygen obtained from the lungs is stored and then released to the tissues in amounts sufficient for their needs. The oxygen dissociation curve in Figure 21-3 is marked to show three levels of sufficiency: (1) normal levels—PaO_2 above 70 mm Hg; (2) relatively safe levels—PaO_2 45 to 70 mm Hg; and (3) dangerous levels—PaO_2 below 40 mm Hg.

Figure 21-3 shows that at a normal pH of 7.40, the steep part of the curve is between a PaO_2 of 40 mm Hg (75% hemoglobin saturation) and 20 mm Hg (33% hemoglobin saturation). P_{50} refers to the oxygen tension (27 mm Hg) at 50% hemoglobin saturation. When we talk about changes in PaO_2 and saturation, we talk about changes in P_{50}.

The oxygen–hemoglobin dissociation curve will shift to either the right or the left, depending on the presence of the following: CO_2, hydrogen ion concentration (acidity), temperature and 2,3-diphosphoglycerate.

A rise in these factors will shift the curve to the right, so that more oxygen is then released to the tissues at the same PaO_2. A reduction in these factors will cause the curve to shift to the left, making the bond between oxygen and hemoglobin stronger, so that less oxygen is given up to the tissues at the same PaO_2. In Figure 21-3, the normal (middle) curve shows that 75% saturation occurs at a PaO_2 of 40 mm Hg. If the curve shifts to the right, the same saturation (75%) occurs at the higher PaO_2 of 57 mm Hg. If the curve shifts to the left, 75% saturation occurs at a PaO_2 of 25 mm Hg.

Clinical Significance. With a normal hemoglobin of 15 gm/dl (2.3 mmol/L) and a PaO_2 level of 40 mm Hg (oxygen saturation 75%), there is adequate oxygen available for the tissues but there is no reserve. With a catastrophe (*e.g.*, bronchospasm, aspiration, hypotension, or cardiac dysrhythmias), which reduces the intake of oxygen from the lungs, tissue hypoxia would result. The normal value of PaO_2 is 80 to 100 mm Hg (95%–98% saturation). With this level of oxygenation, there is a 15% margin of excess oxygen available to the tissues.

An important consideration in the transport of oxygen is the cardiac output, which determines the amount of oxygen delivered to the body. If the cardiac output is normal (5 liters/min), the amount of oxygen delivered to the body per minute will be normal. If cardiac output falls, the amount of oxygen delivered to the tissues will also fall. This is why cardiac output measurements are so important. Not all of the oxygen delivered to the body is used up. In fact, only 250 ml of oxygen is used up per minute. The rest of the oxygen returns to the right side of the heart, and the PO_2 of venous blood drops to about 40 mm Hg.

Carbon Dioxide Transport

Simultaneously with the diffusion of oxygen from the blood into the tissues, carbon dioxide diffuses in the opposite direction (*e.g.*, from tissue cells to blood) and is transported to the lung for excretion. The amount of carbon dioxide in transit is one of the major determinants of the acid–base balance of the body. Normally, only 6% of the venous carbon dioxide is removed and enough remains in the arterial side to exert a pressure of 40 mm Hg. Most of the carbon dioxide (90%) enters the red blood cells, and the small portion (5%) that remains dissolved in the plasma (PCO_2) is the critical factor that will determine carbon dioxide movement in or out of the blood.

In summarizing respiratory gas transport, it is important to emphasize that the many processes described do not take place in intermittent stages but occur rapidly, simultaneously, and continuously.

Neurocontrol of Ventilation

The rhythmicity of breathing is controlled by respiratory centers located in the brain. The inspiratory and expiratory centers located in the medulla oblongata control the rate and depth of ventilation to meet the body's metabolic demands. The *apneustic center* in the lower pons possibly stimulates the inspiratory medullary center to promote deep, prolonged inspirations. In the upper pons is the *pneumotaxic center,* which possibly stimulates the expiratory medullary center.

There are several groups of receptor sites that assist in the brain's control of respiratory function. The *central chemoreceptors* are located in the medulla and respond to chemical changes in the cerebrospinal fluid, which are in turn due to chemical changes in the blood. They respond to an increase or decrease in the pH and convey a message to the lungs to change the depth and then the rate of ventilation to correct the imbalance. The *peripheral chemoreceptors* are located in the aortic arch and the carotid arteries and respond first to changes in PaO_2, then to $PaCO_2$ and pH. The *Hering-Breuer reflex* is brought about by stretch receptors located in the alveoli. This reflex is stimulated when the lungs are distended and inhibits inspiration so that the lungs do not become overdistended. There are also *proprioceptors* in muscles and joints that respond to body movements such as exercise, causing an increase in ventilation. Thus, range of motion exercises in an immobile patient will stimulate breathing. *Baroreceptors,* also located in the aortic and carotid bodies, respond to an increase or decrease in arterial blood pressure and cause a reflex hypoventilation or hyperventilation.

Assessment of Patients with Pulmonary Disease

History

The nursing history incorporates the physical findings and often indicates why the patient has certain signs and symptoms. The chief complaint usually relates to one of the following: dyspnea, pain, shortness of breath, the accumulation of mucus, wheezing, hemoptysis, swelling of the ankles and feet, cough, and general fatigue/weakness. In addition to identifying the chief reason why the patient is seeking health care, it is important to determine when the chief complaint started, how long it lasted, if it was relieved at any time, and how relief was obtained. Information on precipitating factors, duration, severity, and associated factors or symptoms is collected. In a respiratory history, factors that may contribute to the patient's lung condition are assessed:

- Smoking (the single most important factor that contributes to lung disease)
- Previous personal or family history of lung disease
- Occupational history
- Allergens and environmental pollutants
- Hobbies

Psychosocial factors that may affect the patient's life are evaluated and include anxiety, role changes, family relationships, financial problems, and employment/unemployment. What are the patient's coping mechanisms? Is he reacting to problems in his life with anxiety, anger, hostility, dependency, withdrawal, isolation, avoidance, noncompliance, acceptance, or denial? Finally, what are the support systems the patient uses to deal with the illness? Are supportive family members, friends, or community resources available?

Physical Assessment

If a patient has a known or suspected pulmonary condition, respiratory function needs to be assessed. Assessment of the thorax and lungs employs the skills of inspection, palpation, percussion, and auscultation. When these techniques are properly performed and the results logically interpreted, much can be learned that will help the nurse develop a care plan.

Critical to nursing practice is the capacity to communicate what has been assessed to others, either in writing or orally. Therefore it becomes necessary to develop a common language. It is inefficient to draw a picture of the thorax each time we wish to display the location of critical findings. Rather, it is customary to refer to distance from known anatomical landmarks or from imaginary lines in common usage.

With respect to the thorax, location is defined both horizontally and vertically. Horizontal reference is made in terms of the rib or the intercostal space overlying the examiner's fingers (Fig. 21-4). On the anterior surface, identifying the specific rib is facilitated by locating the angle at which the manubrium joins the body of the sternum in the midline. The second rib joins the sternum at this prominent landmark. Other ribs may be identified by counting down from the second rib. The intercostal spaces are referred to in terms of the rib immediately above the intercostal space. Thus, the fifth intercostal space is the space below the fifth rib. It is in this intercostal space that the male nipple and the impulse of the heart may be seen in normal persons.

Location of ribs on the posterior surface of the thorax is more difficult. The first step is to identify the spinous process. This is accomplished by finding the most prominent of the spinous processes, the seventh cervical vertebra (*vertebra prominens*). When the neck is slightly flexed, the seventh cervical spinous process stands out. Other vertebrae are then identified by counting down.

To identify thoracic findings in terms of vertical location, reference is made to several imaginary lines (Fig. 21-5). The *midsternal line* is drawn down through the center of the sternum. The *midclavicular line* is an imaginary line drawn from the middle of the clavicle. The point of maximum impulse of the heart most generally lies along this line on the left thorax. When the arm is abducted from the body at 90

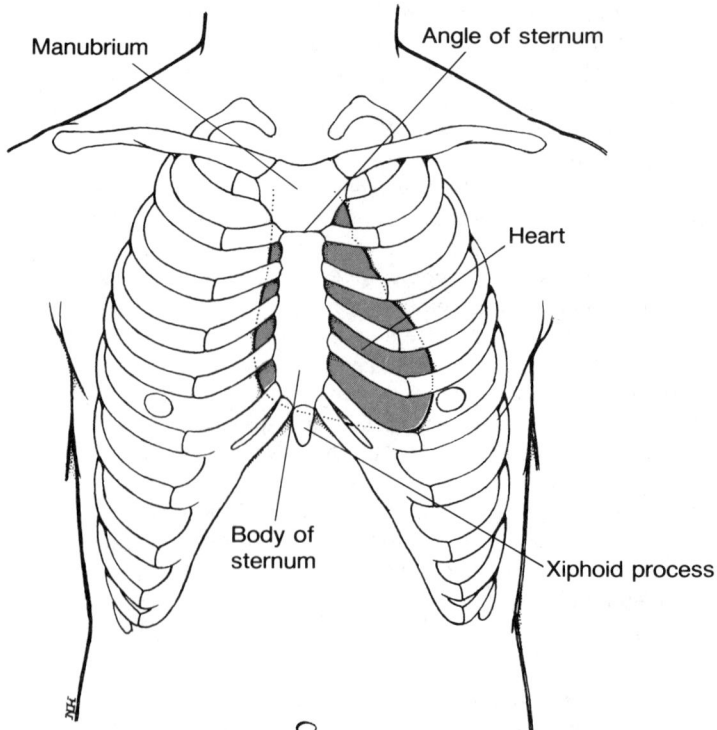

Figure 21-4
Topography of the anterior thorax.

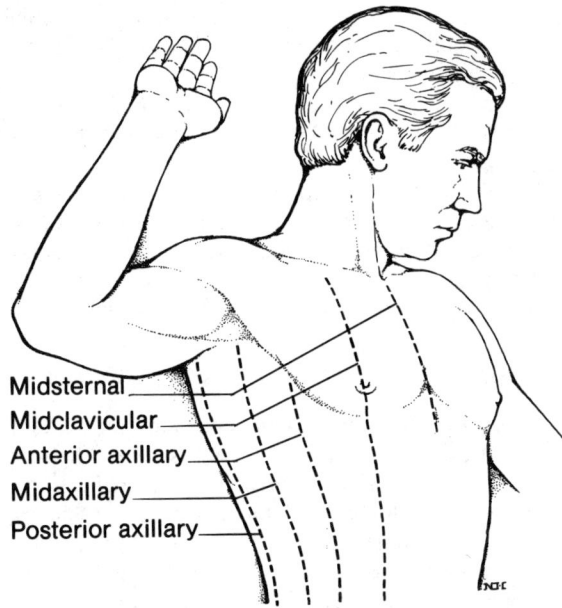

Figure 21-5
Topographical lines of the chest. Imaginary "longitudinal
lines" permit verbal reference to the location of
abnormalities over the chest wall.

degrees, imaginary vertical lines may be drawn from the anterior axillary fold, from the middle of the axilla, and from the posterior axillary fold. These lines are called, respectively, the *anterior axillary line,* the *midaxillary line,* and the *posterior axillary line.* A line drawn vertically through the superior and inferior poles of the scapula is called the *scapular line,* and a line drawn down the center of the vertebral column is called the *vertebral line.*

It is apparent that the examiner can easily be understood when referring to a heart sound in the sixth left intercostal space at the anterior axillary line. Similarly, one may describe an area of dullness extending from the vertebral to the scapular line between the seventh and tenth ribs on the right without equivocation or confusion.

Topographically, the lobes of the lung may be located on the surface of the chest wall in the following manner (Fig. 21-6). The line between the upper and lower lobes on the left begins at the fourth thoracic spinous process posteriorly, proceeds around to cross the fifth rib in the midaxillary line, and meets the sixth rib at the sternum. This line on the right divides the right middle lobe from the right lower lobe. The line dividing the right upper lobe from the middle lobe is an incomplete one that begins at the fifth rib in the midaxillary line, where it intersects the line between the upper and lower lobes and traverses horizontally to the sternum. Thus, the upper lobes are dominant on the anterior surface of the thorax

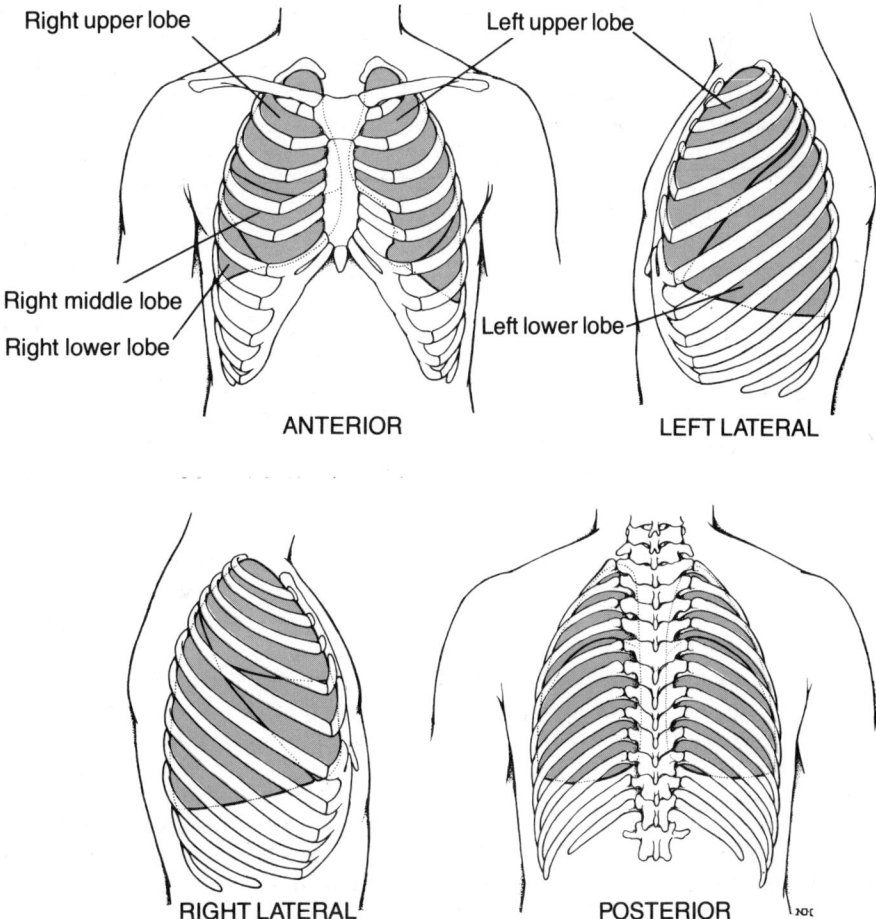

Figure 21-6
Topographical relationship of
the ribs to the lobes of the lung.

and the lower lobes are dominant on the posterior surface. There is no presentation of the middle lobe on the posterior surface of the chest.

Inspection of the Thorax

Inspection of the thorax reveals much about musculoskeletal structure, nutrition, and the status of the respiratory system. The skin over the thorax is observed for color and turgor and for evidence of loss of subcutaneous tissue. The musculature of the thorax may reflect recent weight loss. Asymmetry, if present, is noted.

Breathing Patterns.   The manner in which the patient breathes is of particular importance. Normally, the ribs articulate with the spine at a 45-degree angle. The act of breathing elevates the ribs, thrusting the sternum forward and up. The intercostal spaces widen, and the angle that the ribs make with the spine more nearly approaches 60 degrees. Patients with emphysema have excessive residual volume; that is, they cannot expel the usual volume of air from the lungs during expiration. Because of the large residual volume, the ribs make a less acute angle with the spine, and the sternum is thrust forward excessively, even during expiration. This has the effect of *increasing the anteroposterior diameter* of the thorax.

Normally, the anteroposterior diameter, in proportion to the lateral diameter, is 1:2. In the patient with emphysema the ribs are more widely spaced and the intercostal spaces tend to bulge on expiration. As a result of overinflation of the lungs, not only is the capacity of the thorax to expand limited, but the diaphragm is also depressed, limiting vertical filling. Consequently, the patient must bring into play accessory muscles of respiration, such as the sternocleidomastoids. The appearance of the patient with advanced emphysema is thus quite characteristic and allows the observer to diagnose the disease easily, even from a distance.

Observation of the rate and depth of respiration is also important. In the adult, the normal respiratory rate is 12 to 18 breaths per minute; it is regular in depth and rhythm. An increase in the rate of respiration is called *tachypnea;* an increase in depth is called *hyperpnea.* An increase in both rate and depth that results in a lowered arterial P_{CO_2} is referred to as *hyperventilation.* At the extreme of hyperventilation is the marked increase in rate and depth, associated with severe acidosis of diabetic or renal origin, that is called *Kussmaul* respiration. In the critically ill patient, alternating episodes of apnea (cessation of breathing) and hyperpnea may occur on a continuum. This cyclic phenomenon is referred to as *Cheyne-Stokes breathing.*

The inspiratory phase of respiration is the only one requiring energy in normal physiology. Expiration is passive. Inspiration occupies the first third of the respiratory cycle, expiration the latter two thirds. With rapid breathing, inspiration and expiration are nearly equal.

In thin persons, it is quite normal to note a slight retraction of the intercostal spaces during quiet breathing. Bulging during expiration implies obstruction of expiratory air flow, as in emphysema. Marked retraction on inspiration, particularly if asymmetrical, implies blockage of a branch of the respiratory tree. Asymmetrical bulging of the intercostal spaces, on one side or the other, is created by an increase in pressure within the hemithorax. This may be a result of air trapped under pressure within the pleural cavity where it does not belong (pneumothorax) or the pressure of fluid within the pleural space (pleural effusion).

The severe pain associated with pleurisy causes intercostal muscle spasm and a "lag" in respiration on the involved side.

Certain patterns of respiration are characteristic of specific disease states. Although the nurse need not recognize the specific pattern or be acquainted with the association of a certain pattern with a disease state, she is expected to be able to describe abnormal patterns of rhythmicity.

Palpation of the Thorax

Following inspection, the thorax is palpated for tenderness, masses, lesions, respiratory excursion, and vocal fremitus. If the patient has reported an area of pain, or if lesions are apparent, direct palpation with the fingertips (for skin lesions and subcutaneous masses) or with the ball of the hand (for deeper masses or generalized flank or rib discomfort) is done.

Respiratory Excursion.   Respiratory excursion is an estimation of thoracic expansion and may reveal significant information about the symmetry of breathing. Differences in expansion are more readily detectable on the anterior thorax, where a fuller range of motion occurs during respiration. The examiner's thumbs are placed along each costal margin, below the xiphoid process, while the hands rest along the lateral rib cage. Sliding the thumbs medially about 2.5 cm (1 inch) raises a small skin fold between the thumbs. The patient is instructed to inhale deeply while the examiner observes the movement of the thumbs during inspiration and expiration. This movement is normally symmetrical. A posterior assessment is done by placing the thumbs adjacent to the spinal column at the level of the tenth ribs. The hands lightly grasp the lateral rib cage. Again, a medial motion of the thumbs raises a skin fold, and the patient is instructed to take a full inspiration and expiration. The examiner observes for normal flattening of the skin fold and feels the symmetrical movement of the thorax. Respiratory lag or impairment is often the result of pleurisy, fractured ribs, or trauma to the chest wall.

Tactile Fremitus.   Sound generated by the larynx travels distally along the bronchial tree to set the chest wall in resonant motion. This is especially true of consonant sounds. The capacity to *feel* sound on the chest well is called *vocal* or *tactile fremitus.*

There is a wide variation in normal fremitus. It is obviously influenced by the thickness of the chest wall, most especially if that thickness is muscular, although the increase in subcutaneous tissue associated with obesity has some influence. Lower-pitched sounds travel better through the normal lung and incite the chest wall to greater vibration. Thus, fremitus is more pronounced in men than in women because of the deeper male voice.

Normally, fremitus is most pronounced where the large bronchi are closest to the chest wall and least palpable as the examiner progresses from the major bronchi to the distant lung fields. Therefore, it is most palpable in the upper thorax anteriorly and posteriorly. To elicit tactile fremitus, the examiner instructs the patient to repeat the words "ninety-nine" or "one, two, three" with each movement of the examiner's hands. The vibrations are perceived by placing the palmar surfaces of the fingers and hands, or the ulnar aspect of the extended hands, on the thorax. To facilitate comparison, only one hand is used as the examiner moves in sequence down the thorax. Corresponding areas of the thorax are compared (Fig. 21-7). Bony areas are not tested.

The physics of sound transmission through the lung requires explanation. Air does not conduct sound well; solid substance (tissue) does, provided that it has elasticity and is not conglomerated into a nonresonant mass. Thus, an increase in solid tissue per unit volume of lung will enhance fremitus. An increase in air per unit volume of lung will impede sound. Patients with emphysema will exhibit almost no tactile fremitus. A patient with consolidation of a lobe of the lung owing to pneumonia will have an increase in tactile fremitus over the distribution of the projection of that lobe on the surface of the chest wall. Air in the pleural space will not conduct sound.

Percussion of the Thorax

Percussion sets the chest wall and underlying structures in motion, producing audible and tactile vibrations. The examiner uses percussion to determine whether underlying tissues are filled with air, fluid, or solid material. One also uses this technique to estimate the size and location of certain structures within the thorax (diaphragm, heart, liver).

The examination is usually initiated with percussion of the posterior thorax. Ideally, the patient is in a sitting position with his head flexed forward and his arms crossed on his lap. This position separates the scapulae widely and exposes more lung area for assessment. The procedure is as follows: Percuss

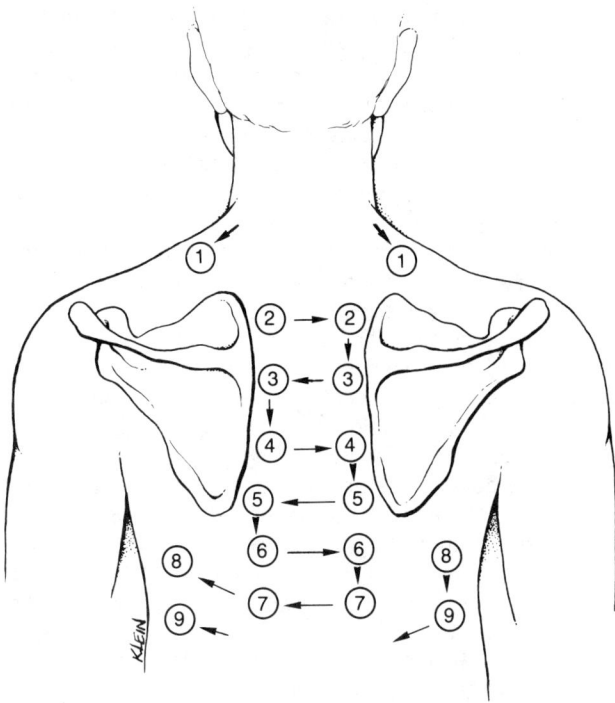

Figure 21-8
Percussion of the posterior thorax. With the patient in a sitting position, symmetrical areas of the lungs are percussed at 5-cm intervals. This progression starts at the apex of each lung and concludes with percussion of each lateral chest wall. (Adapted from Bates B. A Guide to Physical Examination, 3rd ed, p 142. Philadelphia, JB Lippincott, 1983.)

across each shoulder top, locating the 5-cm width of resonance overlying the lung apices (Fig. 21-8). Proceed down the posterior thorax, percussing symmetrical areas at 5- to 6-cm (2 to 2½ inches) intervals. It is important to parallel the middle finger firmly against the chest wall between the intercostal spaces prior to striking it with the middle finger of the opposite hand. Percussion over the scapulae or rib surfaces yields a dull sound and only confuses findings. Percussion over the anterior chest is performed with the patient in an upright position with shoulders arched backward and arms at the side. The examiner begins in the supraclavicular area and proceeds downward, from intercostal space to intercostal space. In the female patient, it is often necessary to displace the breasts for an adequate examination. Dullness noted to the left of the sternum between the third and fifth intercostal spaces is the heart and is a normal finding. Similarly, there is a normal span of liver dullness in the right thorax from the fifth intercostal space to the right costal margin at the midclavicular line.

The lateral walls are examined by having the patient alternately raise an arm and rest the hand on his head while the examiner percusses from the axilla down to the costal margin. The anterior and lateral thorax are examined with the patient in a supine position. If the patient is too ill or is unable to sit up, percussion of the posterior thorax is done with the patient rolled on his side.

Indication of Disease. Dullness over the lung is a

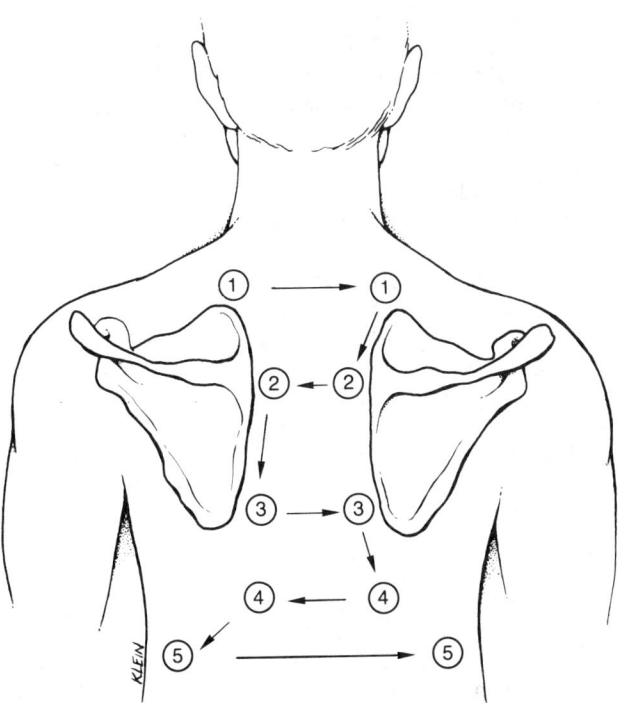

Figure 21-7
Palpation: Tactile fremitus. Numbers and arrows indicate sequence of examination. (Adapted from Bates B. A Guide to Physical Examination, 3rd ed, p 138. Philadelphia, JB Lippincott, 1983.)

function of increased density of the lung and is seen in those circumstances that lead to an increased transmission of sound (*i.e.*, consolidation and compression atelectasis). On the other hand, pleural effusion and obstructive atelectasis, although they do not conduct sound, are nevertheless detected by dullness on percussion. Pneumothorax produces a tympanic, or drumlike sound, whereas emphysema is perceived as hyperresonant.

Diaphragmatic Excursion. The normal resonance of the lung stops at the diaphragm, where it becomes dull. The position of the diaphragm is different during inspiration than it is during expiration. For assessment of size and position, the patient is instructed to take a deep breath and hold it while the maximum descent of the diaphragm is percussed. This is done along the midscapular lines bilaterally. The point at which the percussion note changes from resonance to dullness is noted. If desired, this point can be marked with a pen. The patient is then instructed to exhale fully and hold it while the examiner again percusses downward to the dullness of the diaphragm. This location is marked. The distance between the two markings indicates the range of motion of the diaphragm.

Maximum excursion of the diaphragm may amount to as much as 8 to 10 cm (3 to 4 inches) in healthy, tall, young men. For most persons, it is usually 5 to 7 cm (2 to 2¾ inches). The diaphragm is 2 cm (¾ inch) or so higher on the right than on the left. This is because of the spatial relationships of the heart and the liver above and below the left and right segments of the diaphragm respectively. A decreased diaphragmatic excursion may be apparent in patients with pleurisy and emphysema. An increase in intra-abdominal pressure, such as occurs in pregnancy or ascites, may account for a diaphragm that is positioned high in the thorax.

Auscultation of the Thorax

Auscultation is useful in assessing the flow of air through the bronchial tree and in evaluating the presence of fluid or solid obstruction in the lung structures. To determine the condition of the lungs, the examiner auscultates for normal breath sounds, adventitious sounds, and voice sounds.

A thorough examination includes auscultation of the anterior, posterior, and lateral thorax and is performed as follows. The diaphragm of the stethoscope is placed firmly against the chest wall as the patient breathes slowly and deeply through his mouth. Corresponding areas of the chest are auscultated in a systematic fashion from the apices to the bases and along the midaxillary lines. The sequence of auscultation and the positioning of the patient are similar to those used for percussion. It is often necessary to listen to two full inspirations and expirations at each anatomical location to ensure valid interpretation of the sound heard. Deep breathing may result in symptoms of hyperventilation (*e.g.*, lightheadedness) and can be avoided by having the patient rest and breathe normally once or twice during the examination.

Breath Sounds. Normal breath sounds are distinguished by their location over a specific area of the lung and are identified as *vesicular* and *bronchial* (tubular) breath sounds. Vesicular sounds are audible as quiet, low-pitched sounds that have a long inspiratory phase and a short expiratory phase. They are heard normally throughout the entire lung field, except over the upper sternum and between the

scapulae, where they are replaced with bronchial breath sounds. Bronchial breath sounds are usually louder and higher pitched than vesicular sounds. In comparison, the expiratory phase is longer than the inspiratory phase. Bronchial sounds audible elsewhere in the lung are an indication of pathology and necessitate physician consultation.

The quality and intensity of breath sounds are determined during auscultation. When air flow is decreased by bronchial obstruction (atelectasis) or when fluid (pleural effusion) or tissue (obesity) separates the air passages from the stethoscope, breath sounds are diminished or absent. For example, the breath sounds of the patient with emphysema are faint and often completely absent.

When heard, the expiratory phase is prolonged and may exhibit a high-pitched whistling tone called *wheezing*. This same sound is also heard in asthma and in any process associated with marked bronchoconstriction.

Adventitious Sounds. The presence of an abnormal condition that affects the bronchial tree and alveoli may produce additional or adventitious sounds. The terminology used to describe these abnormal sounds is changing. For this reason, verbal and written communication regarding the presence of adventitious sounds is sometimes confusing. The current view is as follows.

Adventitious sounds are divided into two categories: discrete, noncontinuous sounds and continuous musical sounds. The duration of the sound is the important distinction to make in identifying the sound as noncontinuous or continuous. *Crackles* (rales) are discrete, noncontinuous sounds that result from delayed reopening of deflated airways. *Fine crackles* are usually audible at the end of inspiration and originate from the alveoli. Their sound can be re-created by rubbing several pieces of hair next to one's ear. *Coarse crackles* have a gross, moist sound. They are produced in the large bronchi and are audible in early to mid-inspiration. Crackles may or may not be cleared by coughing. Crackles are a reflection of underlying inflammation or congestion and are often present in such conditions as pneumonia, bronchitis, congestive heart failure, and pulmonary fibrosis.

Wheezes (rhonchi) are continuous musical sounds that are longer in duration than crackles. They may be audible during inspiration, expiration, or both. These sounds result from the passage of air through narrowed or partially obstructed passages. Obstruction is often due to the presence of secretions or swelling, and hence wheezes may clear with coughing. Wheezes originate in the smaller bronchi and bronchioles; they are high pitched and whistling. Rhonchi originate in the larger bronchi or trachea and are lower pitched and sonorous. They are heard in patients with increased secretions. Wheezes are commonly heard in patients with asthma and emphysema.

Inflammation of pleural surfaces induces a crackling, grating sound that is usually heard in both inspiration and expiration. The sound is called a *friction rub*. It seems to be quite "close" to the ear and is enhanced by applying pressure with the head of the stethoscope. The sound is imitated by rubbing the thumb and index finger together near the ear. The grating sound of a friction rub is not altered by coughing. If audible only during inspiration, it may be difficult to distinguish from crackles, which may be multiple and so frequent that a continuous sound is perceived.

Voice Sounds. The sound heard through the stethoscope as the patient vocalizes is known as *vocal resonance*. The vibrations produced in the larynx are transmitted to the chest wall as they pass through the bronchi and alveolar tissue. During the process the sounds are diminished in intensity and altered so that syllables are not distinguishable. The spoken voice is usually assessed by having the patient repeat the phrase "ninety-nine" while the examiner listens with the stethoscope in corresponding areas of the chest from the apices to the bases.

If the vocal resonance is increased in intensity and clarity, *bronchophony* is said to be present. *Egophony* is best appreciated by having the patient repeat the letter "e." The distortion produced by consolidation transforms the sound into a clearly heard "a" rather than "e."

Bronchophony and egophony have precisely the same connotation as bronchial breathing and an increase in tactile fremitus. Where one abnormality is detected, so should the others be. A change in tactile fremitus is more subtle and can be missed, but bronchial breathing and bronchophony present loudly and clearly to the examiner.

A very subtle finding, heard only in the presence of rather dense consolidation, is the phenomenon of *whispered pectoriloquy*. Transmission of high-frequency components of sound is so enhanced that even whispered words are heard, a circumstance not noted in normal physiology. The implication is the same as that of bronchophony.

A routine assessment of the thorax and lungs includes the following: inspection of the thorax and respirations, percussion of the posterior thorax, and auscultation of the thorax for breath sounds and the presence of adventitious sounds. Unless some facet of the history or a prior observation in the physical assessment leads the nurse to pursue additional information about respiratory status, palpation for fremitus and auscultation of voice sounds are omitted.

Assessment of Respiratory Signs and Symptoms

The major signs and symptoms of respiratory disease are dyspnea, cough, sputum production, chest pain, wheezing, clubbing of the fingers, hemoptysis, and cyanosis. These clinical manifestations are related to the duration and severity of the disease.

Dyspnea

Dyspnea (difficult or labored breathing) is a symptom common to many pulmonary and heart conditions, particularly when there is increased lung rigidity and airway resistance. The right ventricle of the heart will ultimately be affected by lung disease since it must pump blood through the lungs. Sudden dyspnea in a healthy person may indicate pneumothorax (air in the pleural cavity). Sudden shortness of breath in an ill patient or after surgery may denote pulmonary embolism. *Orthopnea* (inability to breathe except in an upright position) is characteristic of cardiogenic pulmonary congestion. Shortness of breath with an expiratory wheeze is seen in chronic obstructive pulmonary disease (asthma, bronchitis, emphysema). Noisy breathing may result from a narrowing of the airway or localized obstruction of a major bronchus

by a tumor or foreign body. The presence of both inspiratory and expiratory wheezing usually signifies asthma, if the patient is not in congestive heart failure. Shortness of breath is quite commonly related to tension and anxiety. In general, the acute diseases of the lungs produce a more severe grade of dyspnea than do the chronic diseases. The circumstances that produce the patient's dyspnea must be determined. How much exertion triggers shortness of breath? Is there an associated cough? Is dyspnea related to other symptoms? What was the mode of onset: sudden or gradual? At what time of day or night is it obvious? Is it worse when the patient is flat in bed? Does it occur at rest? with exercise? walking? (how far?) climbing stairs? running?

The management of dyspnea depends on the success with which its cause can be alleviated. Relief of the symptom is sometimes achieved by placing the patient at rest with his head elevated and, in severe cases, by administering oxygen.

Cough

Cough results from irritation of the mucous membranes anywhere in the respiratory tract. The stimulus producing a cough may arise from an infectious process or from an airborne irritant, such as smoke, smog, dust, or a gas. "The cough reflex is the watchdog of the lungs" and is the patient's chief protection against the accumulation of secretions in the bronchi and bronchioles.

On the other hand, the presence of cough may indicate serious pulmonary disease. Of equal importance is the type of cough. A dry, irritative cough is characteristic of upper respiratory tract infection of viral etiology. Laryngotracheitis causes an irritative, high-pitched cough. Tracheal lesions produce a brassy cough. A severe or *changing* cough may indicate bronchogenic carcinoma. Pleuritic chest pain accompanying coughing may indicate pleural or chest wall (musculoskeletal) involvement.

The character of the cough is then evaluated. Is it dry? hacking? brassy? wheezing? loose? severe? Note the time of coughing. Coughing at night may herald the onset of left-sided heart failure or bronchial asthma. A cough in the morning with sputum production is indicative of bronchitis. A cough that worsens when the patient is supine may indicate a postnasal drip (sinusitis). Coughing after food intake may indicate aspirated material in the tracheobronchial tree. A cough of recent onset is usually from an acute infectious process.

Sputum Production

A patient who coughs long enough will almost invariably produce sputum. Violent coughing causes bronchial spasm, obstruction, and further irritation of the bronchi and may result in syncope. A severe, repeated, or uncontrolled cough that is nonproductive is potentially harmful. Sputum production is the reaction of the lungs to any constantly recurring irritant. It may also be associated with a nasal discharge. If there is a profuse amount of purulent sputum (thick yellow or green) or a change in color of the sputum, the patient probably has a bacterial infection. Rusty sputum indicates the presence of bacterial pneumonia, if the patient has not received antibiotics. A thin, mucoid sputum frequently results from viral bronchitis. A gradual increase of sputum over period of time may reveal the presence of chronic bronchitis or bronchiectasis. Pink-tinged mucoid sputum is suggestive of a lung tumor, whereas profuse, frothy, pink material, often welling up into the throat, may indicate pulmonary edema. Malodorous sputum and bad breath point to the presence of lung abscess, bronchiectasis, or an infection caused by fusospirochetal or other anaerobic organisms.

If the sputum is too thick to raise, it is necessary to decrease its viscosity by increasing its water content through adequate hydration (drinking water) and inhalation of aerosolized solutions. These may be delivered via any type of nebulizer. Methods of assisting the patient to cough productively are discussed on page 446.

Smoking is definitely contraindicated since it interferes with ciliary action, increases bronchial secretions, causes inflammation and hyperplasia of the mucous membranes, and reduces production of surfactant. Thus, bronchial drainage is impaired. If smoking is stopped, sputum volume will decrease and resistance to bronchial infections will improve.

The patient's appetite may be depressed because of the odor of the sputum and the taste it leaves in the mouth. Adequate mouth hygiene, proper environment, and wise selection of food will stimulate appetite. After the patient's mouth is carefully cleansed and rinsed, sputum cups and emesis basins should be removed before the next meal arrives. Serving citrus juices at the beginning of the meal will make the mouth feel better and will help to make the patient more receptive to the rest of the meal.

Chest Pain

Chest pain associated with pulmonary conditions may be sharp, stabbing, and intermittent or dull, aching, and persistent. The pain usually is felt on the side where the pathologic process is located, but it may be referred elsewhere, for example, to the neck, the back, or the abdomen. Chest pain is experienced by many patients with pneumonia, pulmonary embolism with lung infarction, and pleurisy, and is a late symptom of bronchogenic carcinoma. In carcinoma the pain may be dull and persistent because of invasion into the chest wall, mediastinum, or spine.

Lung disease does not always produce thoracic pain since the lungs and the visceral pleural covering lack sensory nerves and are insensitive to pain stimuli. But the parietal pleura has a rich supply of sensory nerves that are stimulated by inflammation and stretching of the membrane. Pleuritic pain due to irritation of the parietal pleura is sharp and seems to "catch" on inspiration; patients say it is "like the stabbing of a knife." They are more comfortable when they lie on the affected side, a posture that tends to "splint" the chest wall, restrict the expansions and contractions of the lung, and reduce the friction between the injured or diseased pleurae on that side. Pain associated with cough may be lessened by manual splinting of the rib cage (p. 446).

The quality, intensity, and radiation of pain are assessed and factors that precipitate it are searched for. Whether there is a relationship between pain and the patient's posture should be determined. Also, the inspiratory and expiratory phase of respiration and its effect on pain are evaluated.

Analgesic medications are effective in relieving chest pain, but care must be taken not to depress the respiratory center or a productive cough. For relief of extreme pain, a regional anesthetic block is done by injecting procaine along the intercostal nerves that supply the painful area.

Wheezing

Wheezing is often the major finding in a patient with bronchoconstriction or airway narrowing. It is heard with or without a stethoscope, depending on its location. Wheezing is a high-pitched, musical sound heard mainly on expiration. (See p. 410 for assessment.)

Clubbing of the Fingers

Clubbing of the fingers as a sign of lung disease is found in patients with chronic hypoxic conditions, chronic lung infections (bronchiectasis), and malignancies of the lung. This finding may be initially manifested as sponginess of the nailbed and loss of the nailbed angle.

Hemoptysis

Hemoptysis (expectoration of blood from the respiratory tract) is a symptom of pulmonary or cardiac disorders. It varies from blood-stained sputum to a large, sudden hemorrhage and always merits investigation. The most common causes are (1) pulmonary infection (bronchitis, bronchiectasis, tuberculosis), (2) carcinoma of the lung, (3) abnormalities of the heart or blood vessels, (4) pulmonary artery–vein abnormalities, and (5) pulmonary emboli and infarction. The onset of hemoptysis is usually sudden and may be intermittent or continuous. Several investigations are usually done to determine the cause: blood examination, chest angiography, chest radiography, and bronchoscopy. A careful history and physical examination are necessary to establish a diagnosis of the underlying disease, irrespective of whether the bleeding produced involved a fleck of blood in the sputum or a massive hemorrhage. The amount of blood produced is not always indicative of the seriousness of the cause.

First it is important to determine where the blood is coming from. Has it come from the gums, nasopharynx, lungs, or stomach? The nurse may be the only witness to the episode. The following points should be borne in mind in making and recording observations. In patients whose bloody sputum originates from the nose or the nasopharynx, expectoration is usually preceded by considerable sniffing and blood may appear in the nares. Blood from the lung is usually bright red, frothy, and mixed with sputum. Initial symptoms include a tickling sensation in the throat, a salty taste, a burning or bubbling sensation in the chest, and perhaps chest pain, in which case the patient tends to splint the bleeding side. The term *hemoptysis* is reserved for the coughing up of blood arising from a pulmonary hemorrhage. This blood has an alkaline pH (greater than 7.0).

In contrast, if the hemorrhage is in the stomach, the blood is vomited (*hematemesis*) rather than coughed up. Blood that has been in contact with gastric juice is sometimes so dark that it is referred to as "coffeeground" material. This blood has an acid pH (less than 7.0).

Cyanosis

Cyanosis, a bluish coloring of the skin, is a very late indicator of *hypoxia*. In order for cyanosis to appear, there must be at least 5 gm/dl (0.77 mmol/L) of unoxygenated hemoglobin. A patient whose hemoglobin is 15 gm/dl (2.3 mmol/L) will not demonstrate cyanosis until 5 gm/dl (0.77 mmol/L) of that hemoglobin becomes unoxygenated, resulting in an effective circulating hemoglobin of two thirds of the normal level. This determines cyanosis even if the hemoglobin level is low or high (the anemic patient will rarely manifest cyanosis, and the polycythemic patient will look cyanotic even if adequately oxygenated). Therefore the presence of cyanosis is *not* a reliable sign.

Assessment of cyanosis is affected by room lighting, skin color, and depth of the vessels from the surface of the skin. In the presence of a pulmonary condition, *central cyanosis* is looked for by observing the color of the tongue and lips. This indicates a decrease in oxygen tension in the blood. *Peripheral cyanosis* results from decreased blood flow to a certain area of the body, as in vasoconstriction of the nailbeds or ear lobes from cold weather, and does not necessarily indicate a central systemic problem.

Assessment of Breathing Ability

Tests of the patient's breathing ability are easily assessed at the bedside by measuring the respiratory rate, tidal volume, minute ventilation, vital capacity, inspiratory force, and compliance. These tests are particularly important for patients at risk of developing pulmonary complications, including those who have undergone chest or abdominal surgery, have experienced prolonged anesthesia, have preexisting pulmonary disease, or are elderly.

Patients whose chest expansion is limited by external restrictions such as obesity or abdominal distention and who are unable to breathe deeply because of postoperative pain or sedation produce low tidal volumes. Ventilation at low tidal volumes without sigh inflations can produce alveolar collapse or atelectasis. The functional residual capacity falls, lung compliance is reduced, and the patient must breathe faster to maintain the same degree of tissue oxygenation. These events can be exaggerated in patients who have preexisting pulmonary diseases and in elderly patients whose airways are less compliant owing to earlier closure of small airways during the expiratory cycle.

Respiratory Rate

The normal adult who is resting comfortably breathes at 12 to 18 breaths per minute. Except for occasional sighs, the breathing is reasonably regular.

- *Bradypnea*, or slow breathing, is associated with raised intracranial pressure, brain injury, and drug overdose.
- *Tachypnea*, or rapid breathing, is commonly seen in pneumonia, pulmonary edema, metabolic acidosis, septicemia, and rib fracture.

Tidal Volume

The volume of each breath is referred to as the tidal volume. The simplest instrument commonly used to measure volumes at the bedside is known as the Wright respirometer (Fig. 21-9).

If the patient is breathing via an endotracheal tube or tracheostomy, the respirometer is directly attached to it and

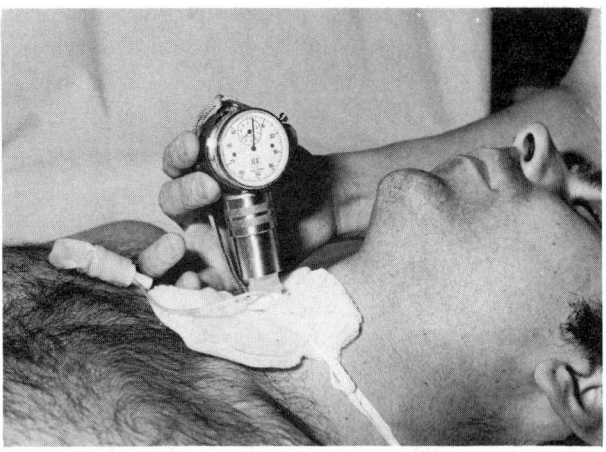

Figure 21-9
Wright respirometer connected to a tracheostomy tube with the cuff inflated. The small dial measures the tidal volume and vital capacity. The large dial measures the minute volume.

the exhaled volume is obtained from the dial. In others, the respirometer is attached to a face mask, which is placed to cover the nose and mouth so that it is airtight, and the exhaled volume is measured as before. Hand-held electronic respirometers that provide digital readouts of lung volumes are also available.

The tidal volume may vary from breath to breath. To make the measurement reliable, the volumes of several breaths are measured, and the range of tidal volumes together with the average tidal volume are noted. The normal tidal volume is 5 to 8 ml per kilogram of body weight.

Minute Ventilation

Tidal volume and respiratory rates alone are unreliable indicators of the adequacy of ventilation because both can vary widely from breath to breath. Together, however, the tidal volume and respiratory rate are important because they determine the minute ventilation, which is useful in the detection of respiratory failure. Minute ventilation ($\dot{V}_E$) is the volume of air expired per minute. It is equal to the product of the tidal volume (V_T) and respiratory rate or frequency (f) according to the following equation:

$$\dot{V}_E = V_T \times f$$

In practice, the minute ventilation is not calculated but is measured directly using a respirometer. Minute ventilation may be decreased by a variety of conditions, including those that

- Limit neurologic impulses transmitted from the brain to the respiratory muscles, such as spinal cord trauma, cerebrovascular accidents, tumors, myasthenia gravis, Guillain-Barré syndrome, polio, and drug overdose.
- Depress respiratory centers in the medulla, as with anesthesia and narcotic sedative overdose
- Affect the lungs by
    Limiting thoracic movement: kyphoscoliosis
    Limiting lung movement: pleural effusion, pneumothorax

Reducing functional lung tissue: chronic pulmonary diseases, severe pulmonary edema

When the minute ventilation falls, the amount of alveolar ventilation reaching the lungs must also decrease, and the $PaCO_2$ increases.

- Remember, do not rely on visual inspection of the rate and depth of a patient's respiratory excursions to determine the adequacy of ventilation. Respiratory excursions may appear normal or exaggerated, but the patient may actually be moving only enough air to ventilate his dead space.

Vital Capacity

Vital capacity is measured by having the patient inspire maximally and exhale fully through a respirometer. The normal value depends on age, sex, body build, and weight.

- Most patients can generate a vital capacity twice their predicted tidal volume. If the vital capacity is less than 10 ml per kilogram of body weight, the patient will be too weak to sustain spontaneous ventilation and respiratory assistance will be required.

When the vital capacity is exhaled at a maximum flow rate, the forced vital capacity (FVC) is measured. Most patients can exhale at least 75% of their vital capacity in 1 second (forced expiratory volume in 1 second, or FEV_1) and almost all of it in 3 seconds (FEV_3). A reduction in the FEV_1 suggests abnormal pulmonary air flow. If a patient's FEV_1 and FVC are proportionally reduced, his maximum lung expansion is restricted in some way. If the reduction in FEV_1 greatly exceeds the reduction in FVC, the patient may have some degree of airway obstruction.

Inspiratory Force

Inspiratory force evaluates the effort a patient is making during inspiration. It does not require patient cooperation and hence is useful in the unconscious patient. The equipment needed for this measurement includes (1) a manometer that measures negative pressure and (2) adapters for connection to an anesthetic mask or a cuffed endotracheal tube. The manometer is attached and the airway is completely occluded (Fig. 21-10). This is continued for 10 to 20 seconds while the inspiratory efforts of the patient are registered on the manometer. The normal inspiratory pressure is −100 cm H_2O. If the negative pressure registered after 15 seconds of occluding the airway is less than −25 cm H_2O, mechanical ventilation is usually required, because the patient lacks sufficient muscle strength for deep breathing or effective coughing.

Compliance

Compliance is the distensibility or stretchability of the lung. The healthy lung is usually said to be compliant. Compliance is calculated at the patient's bedside by measuring the tidal volume and airway pressure during inspiration. It can also be measured in the pulmonary laboratory using special instruments. When a patient is mechanically ventilated, his ease of breathing is quickly and easily estimated by measuring his compliance. This is accomplished by dividing the tidal volume

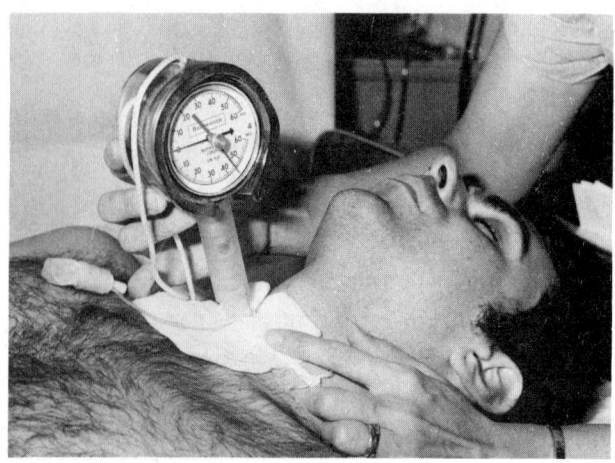

Figure 21-10
Measurement of inspiratory force. The inspiratory force manometer is connected to the tracheostomy tube. The tracheostomy cuff should be inflated. The hole in the connector between the tracheostomy and manometer is plugged so that the airway is obstructed on inspiration. Negative inspiratory force is reflected at −45 cm H_2O pressure. The patient is allowed to breathe between measurements by unplugging the hole.

delivered to the patient by the static pressure measured minus the PEEP value.

For example, if the tidal volume is 450 ml and the pressure is 15 cm H_2O, compliance is estimated to be $450 \div 15$ or 0.30/cm H_2O. If 20 cm H_2O is later required to deliver the same tidal volume, compliance has decreased ($450 \div 20$ = 0.225 liters/cm H_2O).

If the pressure measurement is made while air is flowing into the lungs, it reflects changes in air flow resistance as well as lung and chest wall compliance (lung stiffness) and is termed *dynamic compliance*. Low compliance is a characteristic finding in pneumothorax, hemothorax, pleural effusion, pulmonary edema, atelectasis, and most acute illnesses of the lung. Compliance is useful in assessing the progress of the disease in adult respiratory distress syndrome.

- In general, a rapid reduction in static compliance suggests a pneumothorax. A gradual compliance reduction suggests progressive decreases in lung and chest wall compliance from conditions that restrict lung expansion, such as pleural effusion or atelectasis. A rapid reduction in dynamic compliance suggests air flow resistance, such as with accumulated secretions.

Atelectasis

Atelectasis refers to the collapse of an alveoli or a lobule or larger lung unit (Fig. 21-11). It may be caused by obstruction of a bronchus, the effect of which is to impede the passage of air to and from the alveoli communicating with it. The alveolar air thus trapped soon becomes absorbed into the bloodstream, and, all external communication having been blocked, its replacement from the outside air is impossible. The net result is that the portion of lung so isolated becomes

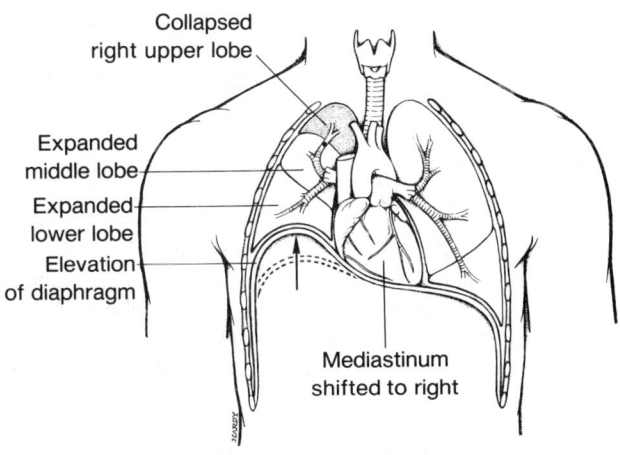

Figure 21-11
Atelectasis.

airless: it shrinks in size, causing the remainder of the lung to overexpand. Bronchial obstruction capable of causing atelectasis may follow inhalation of a foreign body. It may result from a plug of thick exudate that is not, or cannot be, expelled by coughing. Also, the supine position, splinting of respiratory function due to pain, respiratory depression from narcotics and relaxants, and abdominal distention increase the potential of airway closure. Atelectasis resulting from bronchial obstruction by secretions is the usual mechanism that produces the "massive collapse" occasionally observed postoperatively and in debilitated bedridden patients. In these patients there is likely to be long, continued respiratory depression, together with inadequate depth of respiratory excursion and perhaps unusually profuse or poorly expectorated bronchial secretions. Tumors of the bronchi often make their presence known first by an atelectasis resulting from their obstructive growth.

Atelectasis may result from pressure on the lung tissue, which restricts normal lung expansion on inspiration. Such pressure may be produced by a variety of causes: fluid accumulation within the thorax (pleural effusion), air in the pleural space (pneumothorax), an extremely large heart, a pericardium distended with fluid (pericardial effusion), tumor growth within the thorax, or an elevated diaphragm that is displaced upward as the result of abdominal pressure. Under such circumstances there is crowding of the intrathoracic contents, and since the spongy lung tissue is most compressible, the lung collapses without resistance. Where it is compressed it becomes airless, or atelectatic, and the efficiency of pulmonary function is reduced accordingly. Atelectasis caused by pressure is encountered most often in patients with pleural effusion due to cardiac failure or pleural infection.

Assessment. If lung collapse occurs suddenly, and if sufficient lung tissue is involved, the following may be anticipated: marked dyspnea, cyanosis, prostration, and pleural pain, which usually is referred to the lower chest. Fever commonly occurs. Tachycardia and dyspnea are unusually prominent. The patient characteristically sits bolt upright in bed, appears anxious and cyanotic, and has difficulty in breathing. The chest wall on the affected side moves little, if at all, whereas on the opposite side the excursion appears excessive. Lungs that have collapsed because of the obstruction of a bronchus should be reexpanded as rapidly as possible to avoid the common complications of pneumonia or lung abscess.

Management. The goal is to improve ventilation and remove secretions. If atelectasis has resulted from a pleural effusion or pressure pneumothorax, the fluid or air may be removed by needle aspiration. If bronchial obstruction is the cause, it must be removed in order to permit air to enter the lung again. If respiratory care measures fail to remove the obstruction, a bronchoscopy is done. It may be necessary to use endotracheal intubation and mechanical ventilation for a few days.

Nursing Interventions. Methods to relieve bronchial obstruction include aspirating secretions, encouraging the patient to cough, and using an aerosol nebulizer, followed by postural drainage and chest percussion. The patient should be turned frequently in an effort to stimulate coughing. If possible, he is assisted out of bed and walked to aid in mobilizing and in expelling secretions.

All stuporous, debilitated, and sedated patients are turned frequently in bed, a procedure that affords increased respiratory excursion on the uppermost side. Encouragement of coughing and deep breathing (at least every 2 hours) is important in preventing and treating atelectasis. The use of incentive spirometry or voluntary deep breathing enhances large-volume inhalation; this emphasis on inspiration is necessary to decrease the potential for airway closure. Judicious use of nasopharyngeal and nasotracheal suction is also helpful in stimulating patients to cough, thereby removing tenacious secretions.

Diagnostic Assessment of Respiratory Function

Aside from the general physical examination of the chest, which was discussed earlier in the chapter, a wide range of diagnostic studies, described in the following pages, may be conducted in patients with respiratory conditions.

Radiographic Examinations of the Chest

Normal pulmonary tissue is radiolucent; therefore, densities produced by tumors, foreign bodies, and other pathologic conditions can be detected by means of radiographic examination. A chest x-ray film may reveal an extensive pathologic process in the lungs in the absence of symptoms. The routine chest x-ray film consists of two views—the posteroanterior projection and the lateral projection. Chest films are usually taken after full inspiration (deep breath) since the lungs are best demonstrated when they are well aerated. Also, the diaphragm is at its lowest level and the largest expanse of lung is visible. Chest films taken on expiration may accentuate an otherwise unnoticed pneumothorax or obstruction of a major artery.

Tomography (Planigraphy). Tomography provides films of sections of the lungs at different planes within the thorax. It gives detailed analysis of pulmonary parenchyma and mediastinum and is valuable in demonstrating the presence of solid lesions, calcification or cavitation within a lesion, and the surrounding vascular patterns.

Computed Tomography. Computed tomography is an imaging method in which the lungs are scanned in successive layers by a narrow-beam x-ray. A computer printout may be obtained of the absorption values of the tissues in the plane that is being scanned. It has the capability to demonstrate the chest in cross sections and to distinguish small differences in tissue density, thus demonstrating lesions that cannot be detected by conventional radiology. It may be used to define pulmonary nodules and small tumors adjacent to pleural surfaces that are not visible on routine chest films, and to demonstrate mediastinal abnormalities and hilar adenopathy, which are difficult to visualize with other techniques.

Positron Emission Tomography. Positron emission tomography (PET) uses high-energy physics and sophisticated computer techniques to study the way cells function in a living person. The patient inhales or is injected with a short-lived radioactive version of an element that occurs naturally in the body (oxygen, nitrogen, carbon, fluorine). The radio-isotopic emits subatomic particles called *positrons* (a positively charged electron). When a positron encounters an electron, which is does just after emission, both are destroyed and two gamma rays are released. These burst of energy are recorded by the PET scanner, and its computer determines where in the body the radioactive material is located. PET is particularly useful for quantitative measurements of regional pulmonary perfusion and for studying ventilation–perfusion relationships.

Fluoroscopy. Fluoroscopy is helpful in evaluating a lesion that has been previously identified on an x-ray film, to see if it is pulsatile. It is also useful in the study of pulmonary dynamics (the motion of pulmonary structures; diaphragmatic motion) and in detecting regional variations in ventilation.

Barium Swallow. A barium swallow outlines the esophagus and reveals displacement of the esophagus and encroachment on its lumen by cardiac, pulmonary, and mediastinal abnormalities.

Bronchography. A bronchogram provides an outline of the bronchial tree or selected areas after a radiopaque medium that coats the bronchial mucosa has been instilled directly into the trachea, bronchi, and the entire bronchial tree. This is a diagnostic test for any disease that alters the caliber or patency of the bronchial tree or causes displacement there. It reveals anomalies of the bronchial tree and is important in the diagnosis of bronchiectasis, since involved segments cannot always be outlined by other methods.

The procedure must be carried out while the patient is in a fasting state to reduce the possibility of aspiration of gastric contents. Preoperative medication may include atropine to decrease secretions and vagally mediated reflex bradycardia, and diazepam (Valium) for sedation.

A topical anesthetic is sprayed into the nose and then in the mouth and posterior pharynx to prevent gagging and coughing when the tube is passed. The contrast medium is instilled by dripping it over the glottis, by slowly injecting it through a tube in the trachea, or by injecting it through a needle inserted percutaneously into the trachea below the glottis.

Nursing Interventions. Bronchograms cause some discomfort to the patient, and the nurse should support the patient and provide relief where appropriate. After such a procedure, food and fluids are withheld until the patient demonstrates he has a cough reflex. Once the cough reflex has returned, the patient is encouraged to cough and clear the bronchial tree. Postural drainage may be required. A slight temperature elevation is common following this procedure.

Angiographic Studies of the Pulmonary Vessels

Angiographic studies include pulmonary angiography, angiocardiography, aortography, bronchial arteriography, superior vena cava angiography, and azygography. Pulmonary angiography is most commonly used to investigate thromboembolic disease of the lungs and congenital abnormalities of the pulmonary vascular tree and to detect abnormal vasculature arising from tumors.

Pulmonary angiography is the rapid injection of a radiopaque medium into the vasculature of the lungs for radiographic study of pulmonary vessels. It can be performed by venous injection into one or both arms (simultaneously) or femoral vein, through a needle or catheter; by introducing a catheter into the main pulmonary artery or its branches; or by introducing a catheter into the great veins or heart proximal to the pulmonary artery.

Endoscopic Procedures

Bronchoscopy. Bronchoscopy is the direct inspection and examination of the larynx, trachea, and bronchi through either a flexible fiberoptic bronchoscope or a rigid bronchoscope. In current practice the fiberoptic scope is used more frequently.

The *diagnostic purposes* of bronchoscopy are (1) to examine tissues or collected secretions; (2) to determine the location and extent of the pathologic process and to obtain a tissue sample for diagnosis (by biting forceps, curettage, or brush biopsy); (3) to determine whether a tumor can be resected surgically; and (4) to diagnose bleeding sites (source of hemoptysis).

Therapeutically, bronchoscopy is used to (1) remove foreign bodies from the tracheobronchial tree, (2) remove secretions obstructing the tracheobronchial tree when the patient is unable to clear them, (3) provide postoperative treatment in atelectasis, and (4) destroy and excise lesions.

The *fiberoptic bronchoscope* is a thin, flexible bronchoscope that can be directed into the segmental bronchi (Fig. 21-12). Because of its smaller size, flexibility, and excellent optical system, it allows increased visualization of the peripheral airways and is ideal for diagnosing pulmonary lesions. Cytologic examinations can be performed without surgical intervention. Fiberoptic bronchoscopy is better tolerated by patients than rigid bronchoscopy, allows biopsy of previously inaccessible tumors, is safer to use in the very ill patient, and can be performed at the bedside or through endotracheal or tracheostomy tubes of patients on ventilators in whom it is desirable to ensure airway patency. Fiberoptic bronchoscopy allows direct intubation of the right upper lobe, which is impossible with the rigid bronchoscope.

The *rigid bronchoscope* is a hollow metallic tube with a light at its end; it is used mainly for the removal of foreign bodies, for suctioning thick secretions, or investigating the source of massive hemoptysis, or for endobronchial surgical procedures.

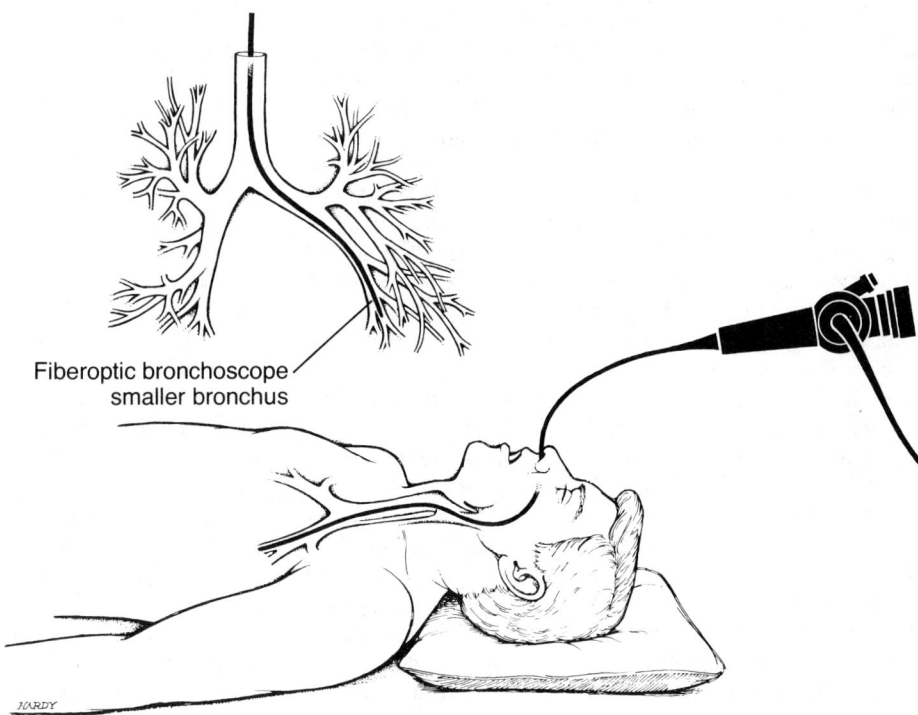

Figure 21-12
Fiberoptic bronchoscopy.

Possible complications of bronchoscopy include reaction to the local anesthetic, infection, aspiration, bronchospasm, hypoxemia, pneumothorax, bleeding, and perforation.

Nursing Interventions. An informed consent is obtained before the procedure. Food and fluids are withheld for 6 hours before the test to reduce the risk of aspiration when reflexes are blocked. The patient is told what to expect, in order to reduce fear and correct misapprehensions. Preoperative medications (usually atropine and a sedative or narcotic) are given as prescribed to inhibit vagal stimulation (thereby guarding against bradycardia, dysrhythmias, hypotension), suppress the cough reflex, sedate the patient, and relieve anxiety.

- *Caution:* Sedation given to patients with respiratory insufficiency may precipitate respiratory arrest.

Contact lenses, dentures, and other prostheses are removed. The examination is usually done under local anesthesia, but general anesthesia may be given, especially if the rigid bronchoscope is used.

If local anesthesia is used, the nurse may assist the physician as he sprays the pharynx with a topical anesthetic such as lidocaine (Xylocaine). The solution is dropped on the epiglottis and vocal cords and into the trachea to reduce the cough reflex and pain. Diazepam (Valium) may be administered as prescribed, intravenously for additional sedation and for amnesia.

Following the procedure, the patient is given nothing by mouth until the cough reflex returns, since the preoperative sedation and local anesthesia impair the protective laryngeal reflex and swallowing for several hours. Once the patient demonstrates that he can cough, cracked ice and eventually fluids may be given. The nurse watches for confusion and lethargy in the elderly, possibly due to large doses of lidocaine given during the procedure. Difficulty in breathing is looked

for and reported promptly. The patient is observed for evidence of cyanosis, hypotension, tachycardia, dysrhythmias, hemoptysis, and dyspnea.

Esophagoscopy. Esophagoscopy is the viewing of the interior of the esophagus through a lighted tube. It is used in removing foreign bodies; in inspecting lesions of the esophagus, such as ulcers, diverticuli, and tumors; and often in making a positive diagnosis by removing small bits of tissue for microscopic examination (biopsy). The care before and after the procedure is the same as for bronchoscopy.

Thoracoscopy. Thoracoscopy (pleuroscopy) is a diagnostic procedure in which the pleural cavity is examined with an endoscope. A small incision is made into the pleural cavity in an intercostal space, with the location depending on clinical and radiologic findings. After aspiration of fluid present in the pleural cavity, the fiberoptic mediastinoscope is inserted into the pleural cavity and an inspection is made of its surface. Lesions can be biopsied under direct vision. Following the procedure, a chest tube is inserted and the pleural cavity is drained by underwater-seal drainage.

Mediastinoscopy. See page 422.

Sputum Studies

Sputum is obtained for study to identify pathogenic organisms and determine whether malignant cells are present. It may also be used to assess for hypersensitivity states (in which there is an increase of eosinophils). Periodic sputum examinations may be necessary for patients receiving antibiotics, steroids, and immunosuppressive drugs for prolonged periods, since these agents give rise to opportunistic infections. In general, sputum cultures are used in diagnosis, for drug sensitivity testing, and as a guide in treatment. Sputum can be obtained by expectoration. If the patient cannot raise the sputum spontaneously, he can often be induced to cough deeply by breathing an irritating aerosol of supersaturated saline, propylene glycol, or some other agent delivered with an ultrasonic nebulizer. Other methods of collecting sputum specimens include endotracheal aspiration (p. 433), bronchoscopic removal (p. 416), bronchial brushing (p. 421), transtracheal aspiration (p. 418), and gastric aspiration, usually for tuberculosis organisms (Chap. 31). Generally, the deepest specimens are obtained in the early morning.

The patient is instructed to clear his nose and throat and rinse his mouth in order to decrease contamination of the sputum. He then takes a few deep breaths; coughs (rather than spits), using his diaphragm; and expectorates into a sterile container.

The specimen is sent to the laboratory immediately; allowing it to stand for several hours in a warm room will result in the overgrowth of contaminant organisms and may make culture more difficult (especially for *Mycobacterium tuberculosis.*)

Often a qualitative study is done to determine whether the secretions are saliva, mucus, or pus. Usually, they separate into layers that are seen readily when a conical, glass container is used. A yellow-green color of the material expectorated usually implies infection (*i.e.*, bronchitis or pneumonia).

For quantitative studies, the patient is given a special container in which to expectorate. This is weighed at the end of 24 hours, and the amount and the character of the contents are described and recorded. Such a specimen is disposed of by wrapping it in paper and sending it to the incinerator. To prevent odors, all sputum containers are covered. Malodorous discarded mouth wipes are removed, and good room ventilation is ensured. Of course, frequent oral hygiene is a nursing priority for these patients.

Transtracheal aspiration of sputum is accomplished by transtracheal puncture through the cricothyroid membrane and by the introduction of a fine catheter through the needle into the trachea (Fig. 21-13). The needle is withdrawn, leaving the catheter in place. Sterile saline (2 to 5 ml) is injected into the catheter to loosen secretions and induce coughing. Then material is aspirated back through the catheter into a syringe. The contents of the syringe are expressed into a sterile culture tube. The catheter is withdrawn, and pressure is applied over the puncture site for 5 to 10 minutes to minimize bleeding and subcutaneous emphysema.

This technique is also used to promote coughing and sputum production in thoracotomy patients and in those patients with an absent cough reflex. In this instance, the catheter is left in place for periodic instillation of saline to induce coughing.

Transtracheal aspiration bypasses the oropharynx and thus avoids specimen contamination by mouth flora, particularly anaerobes. It is of special value to the immunocompromised patient with pneumonia who does not produce sputum.

The patient is observed for several hours following the procedure. Possible complications include intratracheal bleeding, hypoxemia, cardiac dysrhythmias, pneumomediastinum, subcutaneous emphysema, and infection.

Thoracentesis

A thin layer of pleural fluid normally remains in the pleural space. A sample of this fluid can be obtained by thoracentesis or by tube thoracotomy. Thoracentesis is the aspiration

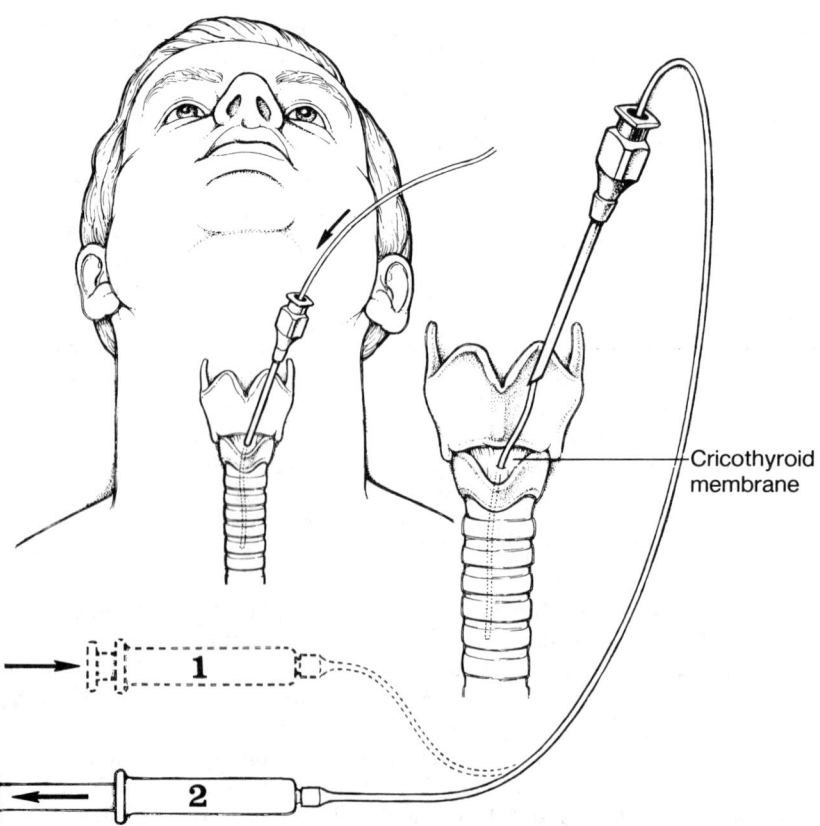

Figure 21-13
Transtracheal aspiration. After the catheter is positioned into the trachea, the needle is withdrawn, leaving the catheter in place. Sterile saline (2 ml–5 ml) is injected into the catheter (1) to loosen secretions and induce coughing. Then the material is aspirated back through the catheter into a syringe (2).

Cricothyroid membrane

of pleural fluid for diagnostic or therapeutic purposes (Fig. 21-14).

Frequently, a needle biopsy of the pleura is taken at the same time. Guidelines for assisting the patient undergoing a thoracentesis are presented in Chart 21-1. Studies of pleural fluid include Gram stain culture and sensitivity, acid-fast staining and culture, differential cell count, cytology, *p*H, specific gravity, total protein, and lactic dehydrogenase.

Pleural Biopsy

Pleural biopsy is accomplished by needle biopsy of the pleura or by pleuroscopy, which is a visual exploration of the pleural space through a fiberoptic bronchoscope inserted into the pleural space. Pleural biopsy is done when there is pleural exudate of undetermined etiology and when there is need for pathologic tissue staining or tissue culture for tuberculosis and fungi.

Pulmonary Function Tests

Pulmonary function tests are done to detect abnormalities in respiratory function and to determine the extent of the abnormality. Such tests include measurements of lung volumes, ventilatory function, diffusing capacity, gas exchange, lung compliance, airway resistance, and distribution of gases in the lung.

The newer tests include more sophisticated measurements. Pulmonary function tests are useful in following the course of a patient with established respiratory disease and assessing response to therapy. They are useful as screening tests in potentially hazardous industries, such as coal mining and those that involve exposure to asbestos and other noxious fumes, dusts, or gases. Preoperatively, they are useful for patients scheduled for thoracic and upper abdominal surgery, patients with a history of smoking and cough, obese patients, patients over 35 years of age, and patients with pulmonary disease.

Pulmonary function tests require some type of spirometer that has a volume-collecting device attached to a recorder that demonstrates volume and time simultaneously. Pulmonary function testing is moving in the direction of comput-

erization; some systems measure multiple parameters. Smaller hospitals, by using a data transmitter, can send test information to a larger medical facility's computer for analysis.

A number of function tests are carried out since no single measurement can be done to evaluate pulmonary function. Usually, test results are interpreted on the basis of degree of deviation from normal, taking into consideration the patient's height, weight, age, and sex. Normal values have been established on nomograms, which are available in manufacturer's handbooks or with pulmonary function equipment.

Since there is a wide range of normal values, pulmonary function tests may not detect early localized changes. The patient with respiratory symptoms (dyspnea, wheezing, cough, sputum production) should undergo a complete diagnostic evaluation, even though the results of pulmonary function tests are "normal."

The most frequently used pulmonary function tests are described in Table 21-1.

Arterial Blood Gas Studies

Measurements of blood *p*H and of arterial oxygen and carbon dioxide tensions are made when managing patients with respiratory problems and in adjusting oxygen therapy as needed. The arterial oxygen tension (PaO_2) indicates the degree of oxygenation of the blood, and the arterial carbon dioxide tension ($PaCO_2$) indicates adequacy of alveolar ventilation. Arterial blood gas studies aid in assessing the degree to which the lungs are able to provide adequate oxygen and remove carbon dioxide and the degree to which the kidneys are able to reabsorb or excrete bicarbonate ions to maintain normal body *p*H. Serial blood gas analysis is also a sensitive indicator of whether the lung has been damaged following chest trauma. Arterial blood gases are obtained through an arterial puncture at the radial, brachial, or femoral artery (Figure 21-15).

Radioisotope Diagnostic Procedures (Lung Scan)

A *perfusion lung scan* is done by injecting a radiopharmaceutical (technetium) into a peripheral vein and then taking

Figure 21-14
Positioning the patient for a thoracentesis. The nurse assists the patient to one of three positions, and offers comfort and support throughout the procedure. (*A*) Sitting on the edge of the bed with his head and arms on and over the bed table. (*B*) Straddling a chair with his arms and head resting on the back of the chair. (*C*) Lying on his unaffected side with the bed elevated 30 to 45 degrees. (Brunner LS, Suddarth DS: The Lippincott Manual of Nursing Practice, 4th ed. Philadelphia, JB Lippincott, 1986.)

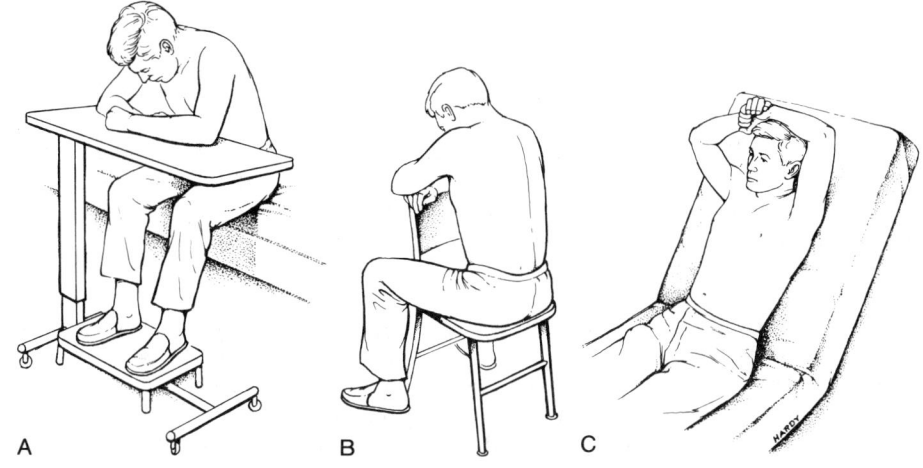

A   B   C

Chart 21-1
Guidelines for Assisting the Patient Having a Thoracentesis

A thoracentesis (aspiration of fluid or air from the pleural space) is done on patients with various clinical problems. It may be a diagnostic or therapeutic procedure for
1. Removal of fluid and air from the pleural cavity
2. Diagnostic aspiration of pleural fluid
3. Pleural biopsy
4. Instillation of medication into pleural space

The responsibilities of the nurse in relation to the patient having a thoracentesis and the rationale for her participation are summarized below:

Nursing Activities	*Amplification/Rationale*
1. Ascertain in advance whether chest x-ray films have been prescribed and completed and the consent form has been signed.	1. Posteroanterior and lateral chest x-ray films are used to localize fluid and air in the pleural cavity and to aid in determining the puncture site. Ultrasound scanning is done when fluid is loculated (pocket of pleural fluid) to help select the best site for needle aspiration.
2. Determine whether the patient is allergic to the local anesthetic agent to be used. Give sedation if prescribed.	
3. Inform the patient about the procedure and indicate how he can be helpful. Explain the following: a. The nature of the procedure b. The importance of remaining immobile c. Pressure sensations to be experienced d. That no discomfort is anticipated after the procedure	3. An explanation helps to orient the patient to the procedure, assists him to mobilize his resources, and gives him an opportunity to ask questions and verbalize anxiety.
4. Make the patient comfortable with adequate supports (see Fig. 21-14). If possible, place him upright and in one of the following positions: a. Sitting on the edge of the bed with the feet supported and his arms and head on a padded over-the-bed table b. Straddling a chair with his arms and head resting on the back of the chair c. Lying on his unaffected side with the bed elevated 30 to 45 degrees if he is unable to assume a sitting position	4. The upright position facilitates the removal of fluid that usually localizes at the base of the chest. A position of comfort helps the patient to relax.
5. Support and reassure the patient during the procedure. a. Prepare the patient for cold sensation of skin germicide solution and of pressure sensation from infiltration of local anesthetic agent. b. Encourage the patient to refrain from coughing.	5. Sudden and unexpected movement by the patient can cause trauma to the visceral pleura with resultant trauma to the lung.

(continued)

a scan of the chest and body to detect radiation. The isotope particles pass through the right side of the heart and are distributed into the lungs in amounts proportional to the regional blood flow, making it possible to trace and measure the blood perfusion through the lung. This procedure is used clinically to measure the integrity of the pulmonary vessels relative to blood flow and to evaluate blood flow abnormalities as seen in pulmonary emboli. The nurse informs the patient that the imaging time is 20 to 40 minutes, that he will lie under the camera, and that a mask will be fitted over his nose and mouth during the test.

A *ventilation scan* is done after the perfusion scan. The patient takes a deep breath of a mixture of oxygen and radioactive gas (xenon, krypton), which diffuses throughout the lungs. A scan is done to detect ventilation abnormalities, especially in patients who have regional differences in ventilation (*e.g.*, emphysema).

The *gallium scan* is a radioisotope lung scan used to detect inflammatory conditions of the lungs.

When the chest x-ray film is inconclusive or reveals pulmonary density (indicating an infiltrate or lesion), it is desirable to examine lung tissue to establish the nature of the lesion. There are several nonoperative lung biopsy techniques that are being used because they yield accurate information with low mor-

Chart 21-1 *(continued)*

6. Expose the entire chest. The site for aspiration is determined from chest x-ray films and by percussion. If fluid is in the pleural cavity, the thoracentesis site is determined by the chest x-ray films, ultrasound scanning, and physical findings, with attention to site of maximal dullness on percussion.

7. The procedure is done under aseptic conditions. After the skin is cleansed, a local anesthetic is injected slowly with a small-caliber needle into the intercostal space by the physician.

8. The physician advances the thoracentesis needle with the syringe attached. When the pleural space is reached, suction may be applied with the syringe.

   a. A 20-ml syringe with a three-way adapter (stopcock) is attached to the needle (one end of the adapter is attached to the needle and the other to the tubing leading to a receptacle that receives the fluid being aspirated).

   b. If a considerable quantity of fluid is removed, the needle is held in place on the chest wall with a small hemostat.

9. After the needle is withdrawn, pressure is applied over the puncture site and a small, sterile dressing is fixed in place.

10. The patient is placed on bed rest. A chest x-ray film is obtained following thoracentesis.

11. Record the total amount of fluid withdrawn and the nature of the fluid, its color, and its viscosity. If requested, prepare samples of fluid for laboratory evaluation. A small amount of heparin may be needed for several of the specimen containers in order to prevent coagulation. A specimen container with formalin may be needed if a pleural biopsy is to be obtained.

12. Evaluate the patient at intervals for increasing respiratory rate; faintness; vertigo; tightness in chest; uncontrollable cough; blood-tinged, frothy mucus; a rapid pulse, and signs of hypoxemia.

6. If air is in the pleural cavity, the thoracentesis site is usually in the second or third intercostal space in the midclavicular line. Air rises in the thorax because the density of the air is much less than the density of liquid.

7. An intradermal wheal is raised slowly; rapid injection causes pain. The parietal pleura is very sensitive and should be well infiltrated with anesthetic before the thoracentesis needle is passed through it. To minimize intercostal artery laceration, the needle is inserted into the intercostal space just above the lower rib.

   a. When a large quantity of fluid is withdrawn, a three-way adapter serves to keep air from entering the pleural cavity.

   b. The hemostat steadies the needle on the chest wall. Sudden pleuritic chest pain or shoulder pain may indicate that the visceral or diaphragmatic pleurae are being irritated by the needle point.

10. A chest x-ray film verifies that there is no pneumothorax.

11. The fluid may be clear, serous, bloody, purulent, etc.

12. Pneumothorax, tension pneumothorax, subcutaneous emphysema, or pyrogenic infection may result from a thoracentesis. Pulmonary edema or cardiac distress can be produced by a sudden shift in mediastinal contents when large amounts of fluid are aspirated.

bidity: (1) transcatheter bronchial brushing, (2) percutaneous (through the skin) needle biopsy, or (3) transbronchial lung biopsy.

In *transcatheter bronchial brushing* a fiberoptic bronchoscope is introduced into the bronchus under fluoroscopic monitoring. A small brush is attached to the end of a flexible wire, which is inserted through the fiberscope. Under direct vision, the area under suspicion is brushed back and forth, causing cells to slough off and adhere to the brush. The catheter may be irrigated with saline to secure material for additional studies. The brush is removed from the bronchoscope and a microscopic slide is made. Sometimes the brush is cut off and sent to the laboratory for pathologic tests.

This procedure is useful for cytologic evaluations of lung lesions and for the identification of pathogenic organisms (*Nocardia, Aspergillus, Pneumocystis carinii*, and other pathogens). It is especially useful in the immunologically compromised patient.

Nursing support for this procedure includes reinforcing the patient's understanding and seeing that the consent form has been signed. Following the procedure, the patient may have a mild sore throat and transient hemoptysis. Fluids and food are withheld for several hours following the procedure. Possible complications include anesthetic reactions, laryngospasm, hemoptysis, and, rarely, pneumothorax.

Another method of bronchial brushing involves the introduction of the catheter through the transcricothyroid membrane by needle puncture. Following this procedure the

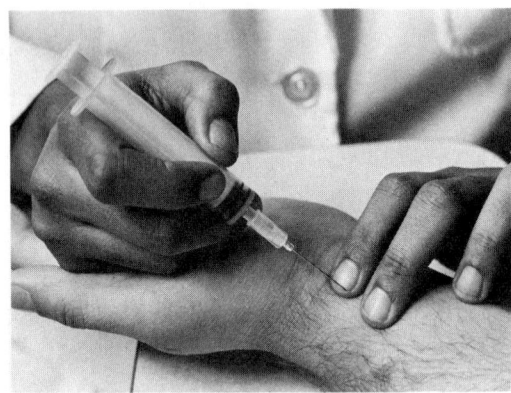

Figure 21-15
Technique of arterial puncture for blood gas analysis.

patient is instructed to hold his thumb over the puncture site while coughing to prevent air from leaking into the surrounding tissues.

Percutaneous needle biopsy may be accomplished with a cutting needle or by aspiration with a spinal-type needle that provides a tissue specimen for histologic study. A *transbronchial lung biopsy* uses cutting forceps introduced by fiberoptic bronchoscope. This study is indicated when a lung lesion is suspected and routine sputum samples and bronchoscopic washings are negative.

A narcotic analgesic may be given before the procedure. The skin over the biopsy site is cleansed and anesthetized, and a small incision is made. The biopsy needle is inserted through the skin into the pleura while the patient holds his breath in midexpiration. With fluoroscopic monitoring, the surgeon guides the needle into the periphery of the lesion and obtains a tissue sample from the mass. Possible complications include pneumothorax, pulmonary hemorrhage, and empyema.

Lymph Node Biopsy

The scalene lymph nodes are enmeshed in the deep cervical pad of fat overlying the scalenus anterior muscle. They drain the lungs and mediastinum and may show histologic changes owing to intrathoracic disease. When these nodes are palpable on physical examination, a biopsy may be in order. A biopsy of these nodes may be done to detect lymph node spread of pulmonary disease and to establish a diagnosis or prognosis in such diseases as Hodgkin's disease, sarcoidosis, fungal disease, tuberculosis, and carcinoma.

Mediastinoscopy is the endoscopic examination of the mediastinum for exploration and biopsy of mediastinal lymph nodes that drain the lungs, without requiring a thoracotomy. Biopsy is usually done through a suprasternal incision. Mediastinoscopy is carried out to detect mediastinal involvement of pulmonary malignancy and to obtain tissue for diagnostic studies of other conditions (*e.g.*, sarcoidosis).

An *anterior mediastinotomy* is thought to provide better exposure and diagnostic possibilities than a mediastinoscopy. An incision is made in the area of the second or third costal cartilage. The mediastinum is explored, and biopsies are done

on any lymph nodes found. Chest tube drainage is required after the procedure. This diagnostic modality is particularly valuable to determine whether a pulmonary lesion is resectable.

Laser Detection

Currently, the laser is used in the dectection and photoradiation of early bronchogenic carcinoma. Two or three days after the intravenous injection of a hematoporphyrin derivative, the violet light of an argon or krypton laser can be used to detect early bronchogenic carcinoma.

Bibliography

Books

Andres R et al. Principles of Geriatric Medicine. New York, McGraw-Hill, 1985.

Baum GL and Wolinsky E (eds). Textbook of Pulmonary Diseases, 3rd ed. Boston, Little, Brown, & Co, 1983.

Borg N et al (eds). Core Curriculum for Critical Care Nursing, 2nd ed. Philadelphia, WB Saunders, 1981.

Boyda EK. Respiratiry Problems. Oradell, New Jersey, Medical Economics, 1985.

Burton GG and Hodgkin JE (eds). Respiratory Care: A Guide to Clinical Practice, 2nd ed. Philadelphia, JB Lippincott, 1984.

Fishman AP. Pulmonary Diseases and Disorders, vol. 1. New York, McGraw-Hill, 1980.

Guyton AC. Textbook of Medical Physiology, 7th ed. Philadelphia, WB Saunders, 1986.

Harper R. A Guide to Respiratory Care. Philadelphia, JB Lippincott, 1981.

Krupp MA and Chatton MJ (eds). Current Medical Diagnosis and Treatment, 1984. Los Altos, California, Lange Medical Publications, 1984.

Porth CM. Pathophysiology: Concepts of Altered Health States. Philadelphia, JB Lippincott, 1986.

Shapiro BA et al. Clinical Application of Respiratory Care, 3rd ed. Chicago, Year Book Medical Publishers, 1985.

Wade JF. Respiratory Nursing Care: Physiology and Technique, 3rd ed. St Louis, CV Mosby, 1981.

Articles

(Asterisks indicate nursing research articles.)

Altose MD. Assessment and management of breathlessness. Chest 1985 Aug; 88(suppl 2):77S–83S.

Assessing chest pain and cough. Am J Nurs 1984 Jan; 84(1):101, 150.

Barbee RA. The medical history in pulmonary disease. Respir Care 1984 Jan; 29(1):68–75.

*Carrieri VK et al. The sensation of dyspnea: A review. Heart Lung 1984 July; 13(4):436–447.

*Carrieri VK and Janson-Bjerklie S. Strategies patients use to manage the sensation of dyspnea. West J Nurs Res 1986 Aug; 8(3):284–305.

Chadha TS et al. Noninvasive monitoring of breathing pattern. Respir Ther 1985 May/June; 15(3):27–28, 30, 35–36.

Dean E. Effect of body position on pulmonary function. Phys Ther 1985 May; 65(5):613–618.

Dennison R. Cardiopulmonary assessment: How to do it better in 15 easy steps. Nursing '86 1986 Apr; 16(4):34–40.

Donham JA. Rales and rhonchi: Why do we use these terms? Focus Crit Care 1984 Oct; 11(5):20–22.

*Grosmaire EK. Use of patient positioning to improve PaO_2: A review. Heart Lung 1983 Nov; 12(6):650–653.

Herman J. Issues in computerized spirometry. Respir Ther 1984 Sept/Oct; 14(5):52, 56–57.

Keely BR. Ventilation–perfusion balance. Dimens Crit Care Nurs 1984 May/June; 3(3):140–146.

McLoud TC (ed). Symposium on chest radiology. Clin Chest Med 1984 June; 5(2):211–378.

Mecca R. Airway resistance. Curr Rev Nurs Anesth 1984; 6(23):178–184.

Mecca R. The physiology and physics of ventilation: I. Static lung volume. Curr Rev Nurs Anesth 1983; 6(14):107–112.

Mecca R. The physiology and physics of ventilation: II. Mechanics of ventilation. Curr Rev Nurs Anesth 1984; 6(15):115–120.

Ramachandram PR et al. History of ventilation during bronchoscopy. Respir Technol 1984; 20(2):12–15.

Siefkin AD. Dyspnea: Evaluating elderly patients who can't breathe. Consultant 1985 June; 25(9):53–56, 63–66.

Smith CE. Breath sounds. Nursing Life 1986 July/Aug; 6(4):33–42.

Smith FB. Role of pulmonary surfactant in adult lung diseases. Curr Rev Respir Ther 1985; 7(9):67–72.

Tyler ML. The respiratory effects of body positioning and immobilization. Respir Care 1984 May; 29(5):472–483.

Zena MJ et al. Dyspnea: The heart or the lungs? Chest 1984 Jan; 85(1):59–64.

Agencies

Governmental

National Heart, Lung and Blood Institute, National Institutes of Health, Bethesda, Maryland 20892.

Voluntary

American Association for Respiratory Care, 7411 Hines Place, Suite 101, Dallas, Texas 75235

American Lung Association, 1740 Broadway, New York, New York 10019.

American Thoracic Society, 1740 Broadway, New York, New York 10019.

Chapter 22

Respiratory Care Modalities

The Patient Requiring Specific Management of Respiratory Conditions

A wide variety of treatment modalities are used when caring for patients with different types of respiratory conditions. The most common are oxygen therapy, nebulizer therapy, hyperinflation maneuvers, and chest physiotherapy (postural drainage, percussion and vibration, breathing exercises, and physical conditioning).

Oxygen Therapy

Oxygen therapy is the administration of oxygen at a concentration of pressure greater than that found in the environmental atmosphere. It is particularly useful in the treatment of hypoxemic states that result in inadequate transport of oxygen by the blood. The goal in oxygen therapy is to treat the hypoxemia while decreasing the work of breathing and the stress on the myocardium. Oxygen transport to the tissues depends on factors such as cardiac output, arterial oxygen content, adequate concentration of hemoglobin, and metabolic requirements. All of these must be considered when oxygen therapy is considered. (Respiratory physiology and oxygen transport are discussed in Chapter 21.)

Assessment.   A change in the patient's respiration may be evidence of the need for oxygen therapy. The clinical signs of *hypoxemia* (a decrease in the arterial oxygen tension in the blood) include changes in mental status (progressing through impaired judgment, agitation, disorientation, confusion, lethargy, and coma), dyspnea, increase in blood pressure, changes in heart rate, dysrhythmias, cyanosis (late sign), diaphoresis, and cool extremities. Hypoxemia usually leads to *hypoxia,* which is a decrease in oxygen supply to the tissues. Hypoxia, if severe enough, can be life-threatening.

The signs and symptoms of the need for oxygen may depend on how suddenly this need develops. With rapidly developing hypoxia there are changes in the central nervous system since the higher centers are more sensitive to oxygen deprivation. The clinical picture may resemble that of drunkenness, with the patient exhibiting signs of incoordination and impaired judgment. Long-standing hypoxia (as seen in chronic obstructive pulmonary disease [COPD] and chronic congestive heart failure) may produce fatigue, drowsiness, apathy, inattentiveness, and delayed reaction time. The need for oxygen is assessed by arterial blood gas analysis (p. 419) as well as by clinical evaluation.

Types and Treatment of Hypoxia. There are four types of hypoxia: hypoxic hypoxia, anemic hypoxia, stagnant hypoxia, and histotoxic hypoxia.

Hypoxic hypoxia occurs when a decrease in the oxygen level in the blood results in decreased oxygen diffusion into the tissues. This is caused by hypoventilation, high altitude, and diffusion defects, and it is corrected by increasing alveolar ventilation and providing supplemental oxygen.

Anemic hypoxia is present when a decrease in the effective hemoglobin concentration causes a decrease in the oxygen carrying capacity of the blood to the tissues. It is caused by anemia, and is corrected by giving whole blood or packed cells.

Stagnant hypoxia occurs when there is a decrease in cardiac function (cardiac output) and the blood is not adequately pumped to the tissues. This is caused by bradycardia, hypotension, and cardiac arrest. Therapy includes hydration, cardiac stimulants, vasopressors, and resuscitation.

Histotoxic hypoxia exists when a toxic substance blocks the release or use of oxygen at the tissue level resulting in rapid anoxia and death, as in cyanide poisoning.

Clinical Considerations. Oxygen is administered with care, and its effects on each patient are carefully assessed. Oxygen is a drug and except in emergency situations is prescribed by a physician.

In general in patients with respiratory conditions, oxygen therapy is given only to raise the PaO_2 to 60 to 80 mm Hg. At this level the blood is 80% to 90% (0.80–0.90) saturated, and higher PaO_2 values will not add further significant amounts of oxygen to the red blood cells or plasma. Instead of helping, increased amounts of oxygen may possibly suppress ventilation in certain types of pulmonary patients.

Excessive oxygen may produce toxic effects on the lungs and central nervous system or may result in depression of ventilation. For example, in patients with COPD, the stimulus for respiration is a decrease in blood oxygen rather than an elevation in carbon dioxide levels. Thus, sudden administration of a high concentration of oxygen will remove the respiratory drive that has been created largely by the patient's chronic low oxygen tension. This can cause a progressive increase in $PaCO_2$, ultimately leading to death from carbon dioxide narcosis and acidosis (see p. 123).

When oxygen is administered by any method, the patient is assessed frequently for signs of oxygen need: mental aberration, disturbed consciousness, abnormal color, perspiration (diaphoresis), changes in blood pressure, and increasing heart rate (tachycardia) and respiratory rate (tachypnea).

Other precautions to be taken when administering oxygen involve the careful handling of the equipment. Since oxygen supports combustion there is always a danger of fire when oxygen is used. "No smoking" signs must be posted when oxygen is in use. Oxygen therapy equipment is also a potential source of bacterial cross-infection and thus the tub-

ing is changed frequently depending on infection control policy and the type of oxygen delivery equipment.

Hazards of Oxygen Therapy

Oxygen is a drug and can cause serious side-effects, such as oxygen-induced hypoventilation (prevented by giving low-flow oxygen rates of 1–2 liters/min) and atelectasis. Perhaps the most serious and insidious hazard is oxygen toxicity, which is caused by too high a concentration of oxygen for an extended period of time. The pathophysiology of oxygen toxicity is not fully understood, but is related to a destruction and decrease of surfactant, the formation of a hyaline membrane lining the lung, and the development of pulmonary edema that is not cardiac in origin. Signs and symptoms of oxygen toxicity include substernal distress, paresthesias in the extremities, dyspnea, anorexia, flaring of the nares, restlessness, fatigue, malaise, and progressive respiratory difficulty. Prevention of oxygen toxicity is achieved by using oxygen according to prescription. If high concentrations of oxygen are necessary, the duration of administration is kept to a minimum and reduced as soon as possible.

Methods of Oxygen Administration

Oxygen is dispensed from a cylinder or from a piped-in system. A reduction gauge is necessary to reduce the pressure to a working level, and a flowmeter regulates the control of oxygen in liters per minute. Oxygen is moistened by passing it through a humidification system to prevent the mucous membranes of the respiratory tree from becoming dry.

There are many different oxygen devices; all will deliver oxygen if used as prescribed and if proper installation is maintained (Table 22-1). The amount of oxygen delivered is expressed as a percentage concentration (as in 70%). The appropriate form of oxygen therapy is best determined by arterial blood gas levels, which indicate the patient's oxygenation status.

The *nasal cannula* is used when the patient requires a low-to-medium concentration of oxygen for which precise accuracy is not essential. This method is relatively simple and allows the patient to move about in bed, talk, cough, and eat without interruption of oxygen flow. Flow rates in excess of 6 to 8 liters/min may lead to air swallowing and cause irritation to the nasal and pharyngeal mucosa.

The *oropharyngeal catheter* is rarely used, but may be prescribed for short-term therapy to administer low to moderate concentrations of oxygen. This method can lead to irritation of the nasal mucosa. When oxygen is administered nasally (cannula or catheter), the percentage of oxygen reaching the lungs varies with the depth and rate of respirations.

Simple masks are used for low to moderate concentrations of oxygen, whereas *partial or nonrebreathing masks* are used for moderate to high concentrations of oxygen. Although popular, these masks cannot be used for controlled oxygen concentrations and must be adjusted for proper fit. They should not press tightly against the skin and cut off circulation; adjustable elastic bands are provided to ensure comfort and security. Bags on partial and nonrebreather masks must remain inflated during both inspiration and ex-

TABLE 22-1
Oxygen Administration Devices

Device	Suggested Flow Rate (liters/min)	O_2 Percentage Setting	Advantages	Disadvantages
Cannula	1–2 3–5 6	23–30 30–40 42	Lightweight, comfortable, inexpensive, continuous use with meals and activity	Nasal mucosal drying, variable FiO_2
Catheter	1–6	23–42	Inexpensive	Variable FiO_2, requires frequent change (q8h), gastric distention
Mask, simple	6–8	40–60	Simple to use, inexpensive	Poor fitting, variable FiO_2, must remove to eat
Mask, partial rebreather	8–11	50–75	Moderate O_2 concentration	Warm, poor fitting, must remove to eat
Mask, nonrebreather	12	80–100	High O_2 concentration	Poor fitting
Mask, Venturi	4–6 6–8	24, 26, 28 30, 35, 40	Precise FiO_2, additional humidity available	Must remove to eat
Mask, aerosol	8–10	30–100	Good humidity, accurate FiO_2	Uncomfortable for some
Tracheostomy collar	8–10	30–100	Good humidity, comfortable, fairly accurate FiO_2	
T-piece, Briggs	8–10	30–100	Same as tracheostomy collar	Heavy with tubing
Face tent	8–10	30–100	Good humidity, fairly accurate FiO_2	Bulky and cumbersome

piration. This is accomplished by adjusting the liter flow so the bag does not collapse on inspiration.

The *Venturi mask* is the most reliable and accurate method for delivering precise oxygen concentration. The mask is constructed in such a way as to allow a constant flow of room air blended with a fixed flow of oxygen. It is used primarily for patients with COPD. The Venturi mask employs the principle of air entrainment (trapping in the air like a vacuum), which provides a high air flow with controlled oxygen enrichment. Excess gas leaves the mask through the perforated cuff, carrying with it the exhaled carbon dioxide. This method allows inhalation of a constant oxygen concentration regardless of the depth or rate of respiration.

The mask should fit snugly enough to prevent oxygen flow into the eyes, and the patient's skin is checked for irritation. The mask must be removed in order that the patient may eat, drink, and take medications.

Aerosol masks, tracheostomy collars, and *face tents* are used with aerosol devices (nebulizers) that can be adjusted for oxygen concentrations in ranges from 27% to 100% (0.27–1.00). If the gas mixture flow falls below patient demand, room air will be pulled in, diluting the concentration. The aerosol mist must be constantly available for the patient during the entire inspiratory phase.

Home Health Care. At times oxygen must be administered to the patient at home. The patient or family should be instructed in the methods for administering oxygen and should be informed that oxygen is available in gas, liquid,

and concentrated forms. The gas and liquid forms come in portable devices so that the patient can leave his home while receiving oxygen therapy. Humidity must be provided while oxygen is used (except with portable devices) in order to counteract the dry, irritating effects of compressed oxygen on the airway.

Intermittent Positive Pressure Breathing

Intermittent positive pressure breathing (IPPB) is the breathing of air or oxygen (or a combination of both) at a pressure higher than atmospheric pressure to produce air flow into the lungs during inhalation. IPPB is applied by a mechanical device that inflates the lungs through positive pressure, dispersing a prescribed medication. When the patient inhales, the machine delivers a positive pressure breath; after a preset pressure is reached on the machine, the machine cycles off and there is passive exhalation. The IPPB machine may be powered by electricity or gas and may be connected with a mouthpiece, mask, or tracheostomy adapter.

In recent years there has been controversy over the effectiveness of IPPB therapy. There is no clear evidence of its value in routine use.

Indications. IPPB is typically used in COPD, acute pulmonary edema, drug overdose, and restrictive lung disorders, and to prevent postoperative atelectasis. It is intended to mobilize secretions, increase ventilation, bronchodilate mechanically, decrease the work of breathing, and reduce cardiac output. Its primary indication is to deliver medications deep in the lower respiratory tract in patients who cannot take deep breaths on their own.

Hazards. IPPB can cause pneumothorax, mucosal drying, increased intracranial pressure, hemoptysis, gastric distention, vomiting with possible aspiration, psychological dependency (especially with long-term use, as in COPD), hyperventilation, excessive oxygen (due to uncontrolled oxygen–air dilution), and cardiovascular problems.

Mini-nebulizer Therapy

The mini-nebulizer is a hand-held apparatus that disperses a liquid (medication) into microscopic particles and delivers it to the lungs as the patient inhales. The mini-nebulizer is usually air-driven by means of a compressor through connecting tubing. In some instances, the nebulizer is oxygen-driven rather than air-driven. To be effective, a visible mist must be available for the patient to inhale.

Indications. The indications for use of a mini-nebulizer are similar to the indications for IPPB except that the patient must be able to generate a deep breath without the aid of the positive pressure machine. Diaphragmatic breathing is helpful as a technique to prepare for the proper use of the mini-nebulizer. Mini-nebulizers are frequently used in patients with COPD to dispense inhaled medications and are commonly used at home on a long-term basis.

Nursing Considerations. The patient breathes through his mouth, taking slow, deep breaths. The nurse instructs him to hold his breath for a few seconds at the end of inspiration to increase intrapleural pressure and reopen collapsed alveoli, thereby increasing functional residual capacity. The patient is encouraged to cough and to evaluate his progress with the therapy. He is instructed in proper cleaning and storing of the equipment if it is to be used at home.

Incentive Spirometry (Sustained Maximum Inspiration)

The incentive spirometer gives visual feedback to guide the patient to inhale slowly and deeply to maximize lung inflation (Fig. 22-1). The patient is placed in a sitting or semi-Fowler's position, since the diaphragmatic excursion is greater with this posture. However, this treatment may be done with the patient in any position. The tidal volume of the spirometer is set according to the manufacturer's instructions. The purpose of the device is to measure a gradually increasing inhaled volume as the patient takes deeper and deeper breaths. The patient takes a deep breath from the mouthpiece, pauses at peak inflation, then relaxes and exhales. To avoid fatigue he should take several normal breaths before attempting another with the incentive spirometer. The volume is periodically increased as tolerated.

Indications. Incentive spirometry is used postoperatively to prevent or treat atelectasis, resulting in shunting. As prophylaxis, incentive spirometry may be more effective than IPPB since it encourages a maximal inspiratory effort.

Nursing Considerations. Nursing management of the patient using incentive spirometry includes the following:

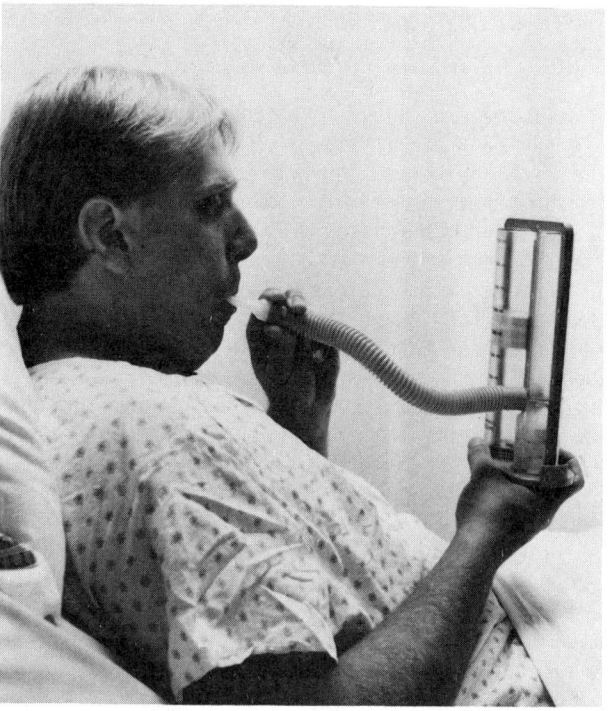

Figure 22-1
An incentive spirometer designed to encourage sustained maximum inspiration for patients who are predisposed to atelectasis. (Courtesy of Photography Department, Montefiore Hospital, Pittsburgh, Pennsylvania. Brunner LS, Suddarth DS: The Lippincott Manual of Nursing Practice, 4th ed, p 208. Philadelphia, JB Lippincott, 1986.)

- Explaining the reason for therapy
- Positioning the patient in semi-Fowler's or an upright position (although any position is acceptable)
- Teaching the patient to use diaphragmatic breathing (p. 430)
- Instructing the patient to hold his breath at the end of inspiration (for 3 seconds), then to exhale slowly
- Encouraging coughing during and after each session
- Helping the patient splint the incision while coughing postoperatively
- Setting a reasonable volume goal (in order not to discourage the patient)
- Placing the machine within the patient's reach
- Beginning therapy immediately postoperatively (atelectasis can start within 1 hour after hypoventilation begins)
- Encouraging approximately 10 breaths per hour while awake
- Recording effectiveness and number of breaths achieved every 2 hours

Chest Physiotherapy

Chest physiotherapy includes postural drainage, chest percussion and vibration, breathing exercises/breathing retraining, and effective coughing. The goals of chest physiotherapy are removal of bronchial secretions, improved ventilation, and increased efficiency of the respiratory musculature.

Postural Drainage (Segmented Bronchial Drainage)

Postural drainage is the use of specific positions so the force of gravity can assist in the removal of bronchial secretions. The secretions drain from the affected bronchioles into the bronchi and trachea and are removed by means of coughing or suctioning. It is used to prevent or relieve bronchial obstruction due to secretions.

Because the patient is usually in an upright position, secretions are likely to accumulate in the lower part of the lung. When postural drainage is used, the patient is positioned sequentially in different postures (Fig. 22-2), so that the force of gravity helps to drain secretions from the smaller bronchial airways to the main bronchi and trachea. The secretions are then removed by coughing. Inhalation of prescribed bronchodilators before postural drainage assists in draining the bronchial tree.

Postural drainage exercises can be directed at any of the segments (bilateral) of the lung. The lower and middle lobe bronchi empty more effectively when the head is down; the upper lobe bronchi empty more effectively when the head is up. Frequently, the patient is placed in five positions, one for drainage of each lobe: head down, prone, right and left lateral, and sitting upright.

Nursing Interventions.   The nurse should be aware of the patient's diagnosis as well as the lung lobes or segments involved, the cardiac status, and any structural deformities of the chest wall and spine. To determine the area(s) needing drainage and the effectiveness of treatment, the chest is auscultated before and after the procedure. This gives immediate feedback on the effectiveness of treatment.

Postural drainage is usually done two to four times daily, before meals (to prevent nausea, vomiting, and aspiration) and at bedtime. If prescribed, bronchodilators, water, or saline may be nebulized and inhaled before postural drainage to dilate the bronchial tubes, reduce bronchospasm, decrease thickness of mucus and sputum, and combat edema of the bronchial walls. The patient is made as comfortable as possible in each position, and an emesis basin, sputum cup, and paper tissues are provided. The patient is instructed to remain in each position for 10 to 15 minutes and to breathe in slowly through his nose and then breathe out slowly through pursed lips to help keep airways open so that secretions can be drained while the various positions are assumed. If he cannot tolerate the position, he is helped to assume a modified posture. When the patient changes position, he is instructed to cough and remove secretions as follows:

1. Assume a sitting position and bend slightly forward because the upright position permits a stronger cough.
2. Keep the knees and hips flexed to promote relaxation and lessen the strain on the abdominal muscles while coughing.
3. Inhale slowly through the nose and exhale through pursed lips several times.
4. Cough twice during each exhalation while contracting (pulling in) the abdomen sharply with each cough.
5. Splint incision, using pillow support, if necessary.

The secretions may need to be suctioned mechanically if the patient is unable to cough. It may also be necessary to use chest percussion and vibration to loosen bronchial secretions and mucus plugs that adhere to the bronchioles and bronchi and to propel sputum in the direction of gravity drainage.

Following the procedure, the amount, color, viscosity, and character of the ejected sputum is noted; the patient's color and pulse are evaluated the first few times the exercises are performed. It may be necessary to administer oxygen during postural drainage.

If the sputum is foul smelling, postural drainage is carried out in a room away from other patients and deodorizers are used. After the procedure the patient may find it refreshing to brush his teeth and use a mouthwash before resting in bed.

Chest Percussion and Vibration

To aid in the loosening and removal of thicker secretions, the chest may be tapped (percussion) and vibrated by the therapist or nurse. Percussion and vibration help to dislodge mucus adhering to the bronchioles and bronchi.

Percussion is carried out by cupping the hands and lightly striking the chest wall over the lung segment to be drained in a rhythmical fashion. The wrists are alternately flexed and extended so that the chest is cupped or clapped in a painless manner (Fig. 22-3). A linen towel may be placed over the segment of the chest that is being cupped to prevent skin irritation and redness from direct contact. Percussion, alternating with vibration, is maintained for 3 to 5 minutes for each position. The patient uses diaphragmatic breathing during this procedure to promote relaxation (see Breathing Retraining, p. 429). As a precaution, percussion over the sternum, spine, liver, kidneys, spleen, or breasts (in females) is avoided. Percussion is done cautiously in the elderly because of their increased incidence of osteoporosis and risk of rib fracture.

Vibration is the technique of applying manual compression and tremor to the chest wall during the exhalation phase of respiration (see Fig. 22-3). This maneuver helps to increase the velocity of the expired tidal volume from the small airways, thus freeing the mucus. After three or four vibrations the patient is encouraged to cough, using his abdominal muscles. (Contracting the abdominal muscles increases the effectiveness of the cough.) A scheduled program of coughing and clearing sputum, together with hydration, will reduce sputum in the majority of patients. The number of times the percussion and vibration cycle is repeated depends on the patient's tolerance and clinical response. Breath sounds are evaluated after the procedures.

Nursing Considerations

When performing chest physiotherapy it is important to make sure the patient is comfortable, is not wearing restrictive clothing, and has not just eaten a meal. The uppermost areas of the lung are treated first. Medication is given for pain as prescribed before percussion and vibration, the incision is splinted, and pillows are used for support as needed. The positions are varied, but focus is placed on the affected area(s). On completion of the treatment, the therapist returns the patient to a comfortable position. He is never positioned so that he cannot move. The treatment is stopped if any of the following untoward symptoms develop: increased pain, increased shortness of breath, weakness, light-headedness, or hemoptysis. Therapy ends when the patient has normal respirations, can mobilize secretions, and has normal breath sounds, and when the chest film is normal.

Patient Education and Home Health Care

Chest physiotherapy is frequently indicated at home for patients with COPD, bronchiectasis, and cystic fibrosis. The techniques are the same as described above, but gravity drainage is achieved by placing the hips over a stack of mag-

azines, newspapers, or pillows (unless a hospital bed is available). The patient or family is instructed in the positions and the techniques of percussion and vibration, so that therapy can be continued throughout the day.

Breathing Retraining

Breathing retraining consists of exercises and breathing practices designed and carried out to achieve a more efficient

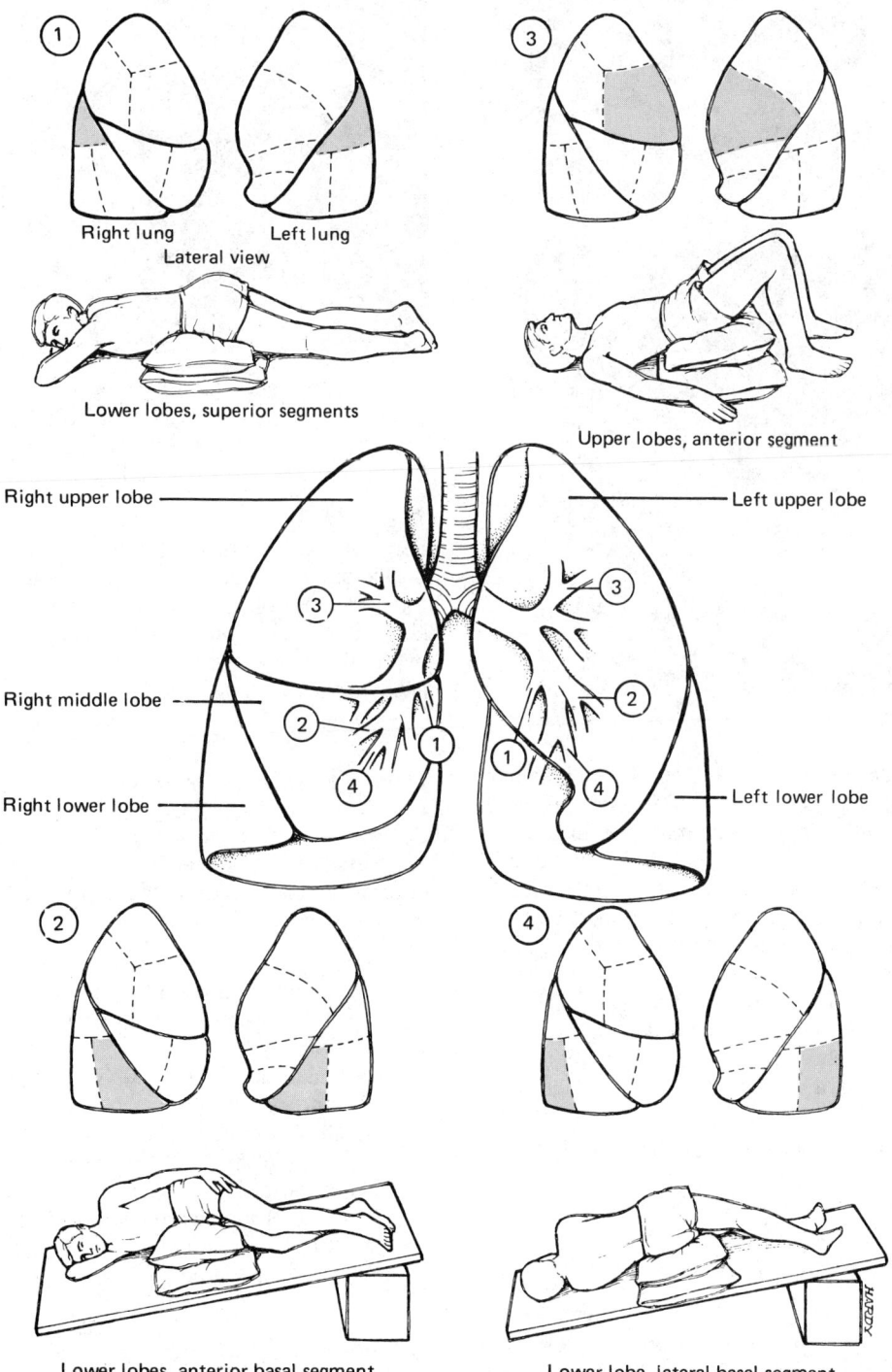

Figure 22-2
Anatomic segments of the lung with four postural drainage positions. The numbers relate the position to the corresponding anatomic segment of the lung.

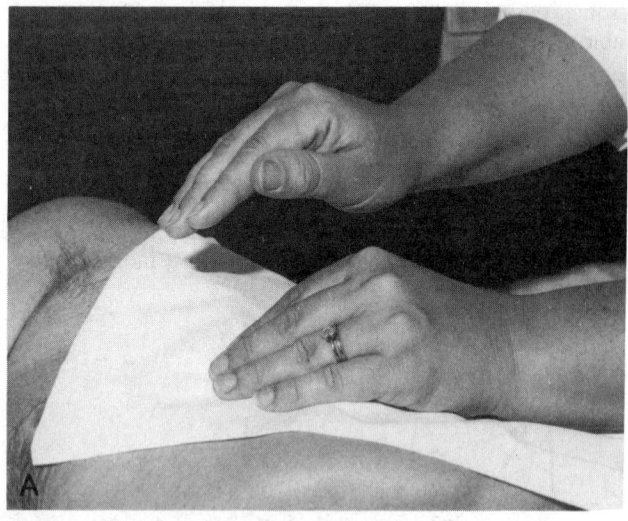

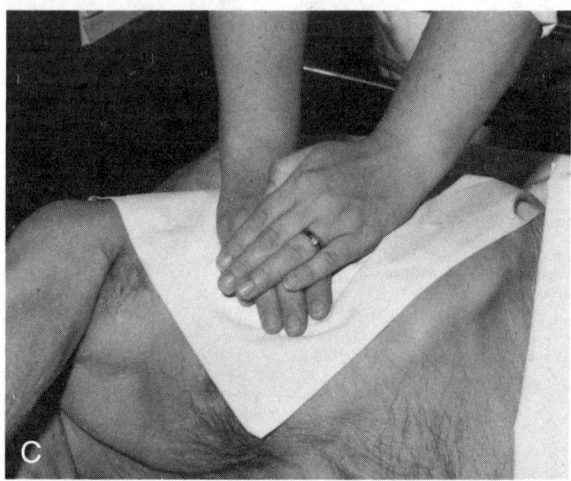

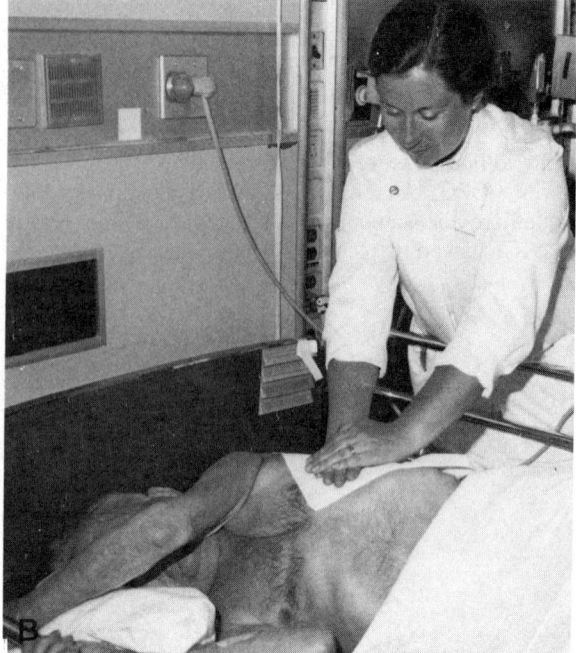

Figure 22-3
Percussion and vibration. (*A*) Proper hand positioning for percussion. (*B*) Proper technique for vibration. Note that the wrists and elbows are kept stiff and the vibrating motion is produced by the shoulder muscles. (*C*) Proper hand position for vibration.

and controlled ventilation, to decrease the work of breathing, and to correct respiratory deficits. These exercises promote maximum alveolar inflation; promote muscle relaxation; relieve anxiety; eliminate useless, uncoordinated patterns of respiratory muscle activity; slow the respiratory rate; and decrease the work of breathing. Slow, relaxed, and rhythmic breathing also helps to control the anxiety that is present when the patient is dyspneic.

Breathing exercises may be practiced in several positions, since air distribution and pulmonary circulation vary according to the position of the chest. Many patients will require additional oxygen, using a low flow method, while doing breathing exercises. Emphysema-like changes in the lung occur as part of the natural aging process of the lung; therefore, breathing exercises are taught to all elderly hospitalized patients regardless of whether they have primary lung disease.

Patient Education and Home Health Care

The patient is told to breath slowly and rhythmically in a relaxed manner in order to permit more complete exhalation and emptying of the lungs. He is instructed to always inhale through the nose since this filters, humidifies, and warms the air. If the patient becomes short of breath, he should concentrate on breathing slowly and rhythmically.

Diaphragmatic Breathing

The *goal* of diaphragmatic breathing is to use and strengthen the diaphragm during breathing. Diaphragmatic breathing can become automatic with sufficient practice and concentration.
   The patient is instructed to

1. Place one hand on the stomach (just below the ribs) and the other hand on the middle of the chest. This increases awareness of the diaphragm and its function in breathing.
2. Breathe in slowly and deeply through the nose, letting the abdomen protrude as far as it will.
3. Breathe out through pursed lips while tightening (contracting) the abdominal muscles. Press firmly inward and upward on the abdomen while breathing out.
4. Repeat for 1 minute; follow by a rest period of 2 minutes. Work up to 5 minutes, several times a day (before meals and at bedtime).

Pursed Lip Breathing

Pursed lip breathing, which improves oxygen transport, helps to induce a slow, deep breathing pattern and assists the patient to control his breathing, even during periods of physical stress.

This type of breathing helps prevent alveolar collapse owing to loss of lung elasticity in emphysema.

The *goal* of pursed lip breathing is to train the muscles of expiration so as to prolong exhalation and increase airway pressure during expiration, thus lessening the amount of airway trapping and resistance.

The patient is instructed as follows:

1. Inhale through the nose while counting to 3, and exhale slowly and evenly against pursed lips while tightening the abdominal muscles. (Pursing the lips increases intratracheal pressure; exhaling through the mouth offers less resistance to expired air.)
2. Count to 7 while prolonging expiration through pursed lips.
3. Sit in a chair and fold arms over the abdomen:
   - Inhale through the nose (count to 3). Exhale slowly through pursed lips while bending forward. Count to 7.
4. While walking:
   - Inhale while walking two steps.
   - Exhale through pursed lips while walking four or five steps.

The above steps may also be performed while practicing diaphragmatic breathing.

Segmental Breathing

Segmental breathing is more difficult to accomplish since it focuses on an area where increased muscular effort and expansion are needed. It is achieved by placing a hand over the affected area or segment of the lung. The patient is then asked to use pursed lip breathing while slight hand pressure is applied to the chest wall. The patient should try to move that hand and that particular area of the lung while breathing. This should be practiced for 3 to 5 minutes, then focus is put on another lung segment, if applicable.

The Patient Requiring Airway Management

Adequate ventilation is dependent on free movement of air through the upper and lower airways. In many conditions the airway becomes narrowed or blocked as a result of a disease process, bronchoconstriction (narrowing of airway by contraction of muscle fibers), a foreign body, or secretions. Maintaining a patent (open) airway is achieved through meticulous airway management, whether in an emergency situation, such as airway obstruction, or in long-term management, as in caring for a patient with an endotracheal or a tracheostomy tube.

Emergency Management of Upper Airway Obstruction

Upper airway obstruction is caused by food particles, vomitus, blood clots, or any other particle that enters and obstructs the larynx or trachea. It may also occur from enlargement of tissue in the wall of the airway, as in epiglottitis, laryngeal edema, laryngeal carcinoma, or peritonsillar abscess, or from thick secretions. Collapse of the walls of the airway as occurs in retrosternal goiter, enlarged mediastinal lymph nodes, hematoma around the upper airway, and thoracic aneurysm may also result in upper airway obstruction. Finally, the unconscious or comatose patient is at risk of obstructing the upper airway because he loses the protective reflexes (cough and swallowing) and the tone of the pharyngeal muscles, causing the tongue to fall back and block the airway.

The patient is observed for the following signs of upper airway obstruction:

- Inspiration causing indrawing of parts of the upper chest, sternum, and intercostal spaces.
- Exhalation that is characterized by a jerky protrusion and prolonged, somewhat sustained contraction of the abdominal muscles, followed by a brief relaxation before another contraction.
- Seesaw movement of the chest and abdomen (combination of the above). As the inspiratory muscles contract, an inward thoracic depression results while relaxed abdominal muscles are jerkily pushed up. Exhalation is produced by a labored and prolonged abdominal muscle contraction, causing a jerky upward push of the thorax.
- Tracheal tug or indrawing of the suprasternal notch.

As soon as an upper airway obstruction is identified the following emergency measures are taken:

- The mouth is opened to see if the tongue has fallen back or if there are secretions, blood clots, or any particles obstructing the airway. Secretions are suctioned, and any particulate matter in the pharynx is removed immediately with forceps or by suctioning.
- Extension of the head is the simplest way of relieving upper airway obstruction caused by the tongue's falling back. The head is extended at the atlanto-occipital joint. This increases the distance between the chin and the cervical spine, which puts the muscles that support the tongue under tension and pulls the tongue forward.
- If simple extension of the head is not adequate to clear the airway, the mandible is forced forward. This maneuver is designed to put further tension on the musculature that supports the tongue. It is best achieved by the head-tilt/chin-lift method. The nurse stands beside the patient and uses two fingers of one hand to lift up the jaw by pulling up on the chin. At the same time, her opposite hand pushes down on the forehead to tilt the head backward (Fig. 22-4).
- If this maneuver is not adequate and partial airway obstruction still exists, then endotracheal intubation is done. Unconsciousness and loss of protective airway reflexes require endotracheal intubation to maintain a patent airway and prevent aspiration.
- If assisted ventilation is required, a resuscitator bag and mask are used initially prior to intubation and mechanical ventilation. The mask is sealed onto the patient's face by pressing the mask with the left thumb on the bridge of the nose while the index finger presses around the lips. At the same time the rest of the fingers of the left hand pull on the chin and the angle of the mandible to

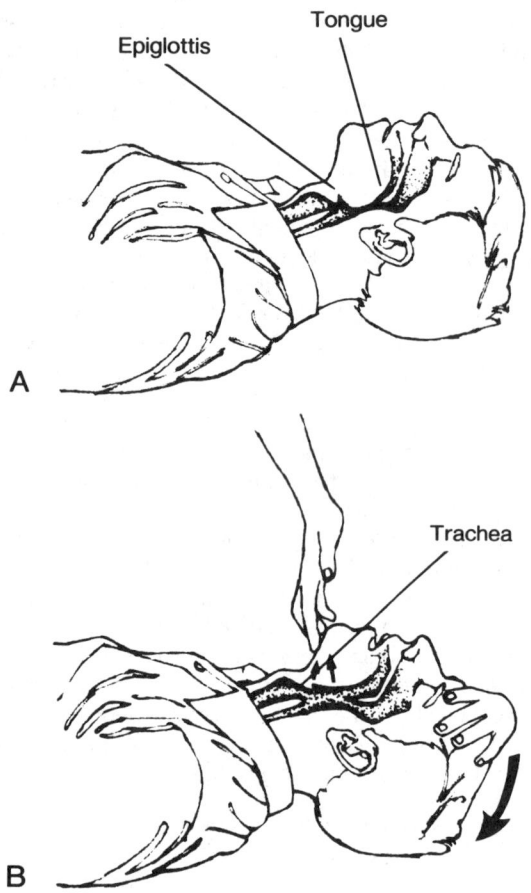

Figure 22-4
Opening the airway. (A) Airway obstruction caused by the tongue and epiglottis. (B). Relieving the obstruction by using the head-tilt/chin-lift method. (Standards and Guidelines for Cardiopulmonary Resuscitation and Emergency Cardiac Care. 1986 June 6;255[21]:2916. Reprinted by permission of JAMA.)

maintain the head in extension (Fig. 22-5). The right hand inflates the lungs by periodically squeezing the bag to its full volume.

A self-inflating or resuscitation bag is also used after the patient is intubated. The bag is squeezed in the same manner to its full volume, but head extension is not necessary because the upper airway is bypassed by the tube and thus always open. Ventilation through a self-inflating bag is accomplished by one person and is used not only for emergency ventilation but also during suctioning, ventilator maintenance, and ambulation of the patient on a ventilator.

Endotracheal Intubation

Endotracheal intubation refers to the passing of a tube through the mouth or nose into the trachea. It is done to provide an airway when the patient is having respiratory difficulty that cannot be treated by simpler methods. It is the method of choice in emergency care. Endotracheal intubation is used as a means of providing an airway for patients who cannot

maintain an adequate airway on their own (comatose patients, those with upper airway obstruction), and it provides an excellent means for suctioning secretions from the pulmonary tree.

An endotracheal tube usually is passed with the aid of a laryngoscope by medical personnel who are specifically trained in this technique. Once the tube is inserted, a cuff around the tube is inflated to prevent leakage around the outer part of the tube and to minimize the possibility of subsequent aspiration. Suctioning of the tracheobronchial secretions is done through the tube. Warm, humidified oxygen can be introduced through the tube, or the tube may be connected to ventilatory support. Endotracheal intubation may be used for up to 2 to 3 weeks. Then a tracheostomy is considered.

As in any other treatment modality there are disadvantages associated with endotracheal or tracheostomy tubes. For one thing, the tube causes discomfort. In addition, the cough reflex is depressed because closure of the glottis is hindered, and this prevents the generation of the high intrathoracic airway pressure necessary to produce an expulsive cough. Secretions tend to become thicker because the warming and humidifying effect of the upper respiratory tract has been bypassed. The swallowing reflexes, composed of the glottic, pharyngeal, and laryngeal reflexes, are depressed because of prolonged disuse and the mechanical trauma of the endotracheal or tracheostomy tube. Ulceration and stricture of the larynx or trachea may develop. Finally, the patient is not able to talk.

For nursing management of the patient with endotracheal intubation, see Chart 22-1.

Tracheostomy

A tracheotomy is an operation in which an opening is made into the trachea. When an indwelling tube is inserted into the

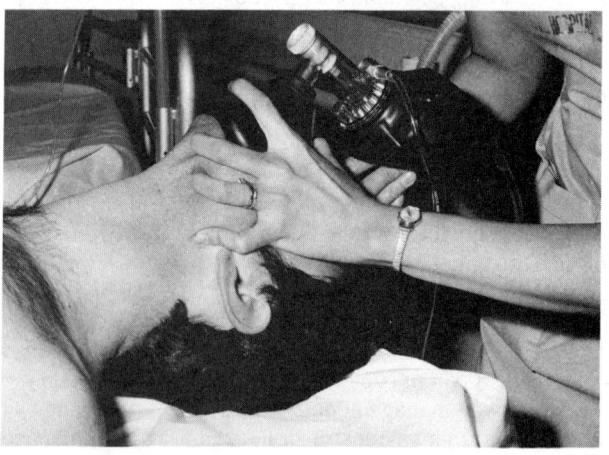

Figure 22-5
Bag and mask ventilation. The head is extended and the mask is sealed to the face by pressing the left thumb on the bridge of the nose and the index finger on the chin. The remaining three fingers pull the chin and mandible upward to maintain the head in extension. The right hand then squeezes the bag. Bag and mask ventilation should be performed only by specially trained and authorized personnel.

Chart 22-1
Nursing Management of the Patient With an Endotracheal Tube

1. Check symmetry of chest expansion
   a. Auscultate breath sounds of anterior and posterior chest bilaterally.
   b. Do this immediately and then every 30 minutes to 1 hour.
2. Ensure high humidity.
   • A visible mist should be seen from the T-piece
3. Administer oxygen concentration as prescribed by physician.
4. Secure the tube to the patient's face with tape and mark the proximal end for position maintenance.
   a. Cut proximal end of tube if it is longer than 7.5 cm (3 inches) to prevent kinking.
   b. An oral airway or mouth bite should be in place to stabilize the tube and prevent the patient from biting on the tube.
5. Use sterile suction technique and airway care to prevent iatrogenic contamination and infection.
6. "Sigh" or hyperinflate the patient every hour to open up atelectatic alveoli.
   a. A self-inflating bag is used if the patient is on a T-piece or pressure-controlled ventilator.
   b. Volume ventilators have built-in sigh mechanisms.

7. Give oral hygiene and suction the oropharynx whenever necessary.
8. To extubate the patient (remove the tube):
   a. Have self-inflating bag and mask ready in case ventilatory assistance is required immediately after extubation.
   b. Suction the tracheobronchial tree and oropharynx, then deflate the cuff.
   c. Give oxygen for a few breaths, then insert suction catheter inside tube.
   d. Have the patient inhale, and at peak remove the tube, suctioning the airway through the tube as it is pulled out.

Care of Patient Following Removal of the Endotracheal Tube

1. Give heated humidity and oxygen by way of face mask.
2. Monitor respiratory rate and quality of chest excursions. Note stridor, color change, and change in mental alertness or personality.
3. Give coughing and deep-breathing exercises for the next few days.

---

trachea, the term *tracheostomy* is used. A tracheostomy may be either temporary or permanent.

A tracheostomy is done to bypass an upper airway obstruction, to remove tracheobronchial secretions, to permit the use of mechanical ventilation, to prevent aspiration of oral or gastric secretions in the unconscious or paralyzed patient (by closing off the trachea from the esophagus), and to replace an endotracheal tube. There are many disease processes and emergency conditions that make a tracheostomy necessary.

The procedure is usually done in the operating room or in an intensive care unit, where the patient's ventillation can be well controlled. An opening is made in the second and third tracheal rings. After the trachea is exposed, a cuffed tracheostomy tube of an appropriate size is inserted (Fig. 22-6A). The cuff is an inflatable attachment to a tracheostomy or endotracheal tube that is designed to seal off the tracheal lumen for mechanical ventilation.

The tracheostomy tube is held in place by tapes fastened around the patient's neck. Usually, a square of sterile gauze is placed between the tube and the skin to absorb drainage and prevent infection (Fig. 22-6B).

Complications. Complications may occur early or late in the course of tracheostomy tube management. They may even occur years after the tube has been removed. Immediately after the tracheostomy is performed there may be bleeding, pneumothorax, air embolism, aspiration, subcutaneous or mediastinal emphysema, recurrent laryngeal nerve damage, or posterior tracheal wall penetration. Long-term complications include airway obstruction due to accumulation of secretions or protrusion of the cuff over the opening of

the tube, infection, rupture of the innominate artery, dysphagia, tracheoesophageal fistula, tracheal dilation, or tracheal ischemia and necrosis. Problems that may arise after the tube is removed include tracheal stenosis and vocal cord paralysis (secondary to laryngeal nerve damage).

Postoperative Nursing Interventions. The patient requires continuous monitoring and assessment. The newly made opening must be kept patent by proper suctioning of secretions (see p. 434). After the vital signs are stable, the patient is placed in a semi-Fowler's position to facilitate ventilation, promote drainage, minimize edema, and prevent strain on the suture lines. Analgesic and sedative drugs are given with caution since it is undesirable to depress the cough reflex.

Another objective of nursing care is to alleviate the apprehension of the patient. He needs reassurance, since he may have a real fear that he will asphyxiate while he is asleep. Since the patient cannot speak, paper and pencil or a "magic slate" is kept within his reach so that he has a means of communication. A tap bell or other signaling device should be available.

Tracheal Suctioning (Tracheostomy or Endotracheal Tube)

When a tracheostomy or an endotracheal tube is present, it is necessary to suction the patient's secretions, since his own cough mechanism is not as effective. Tracheal suctioning is performed every 1 to 2 hours or whenever secretions are present. Unnecessary suctioning can initiate bronchospasm and cause mechanical trauma to the tracheal mucosa.

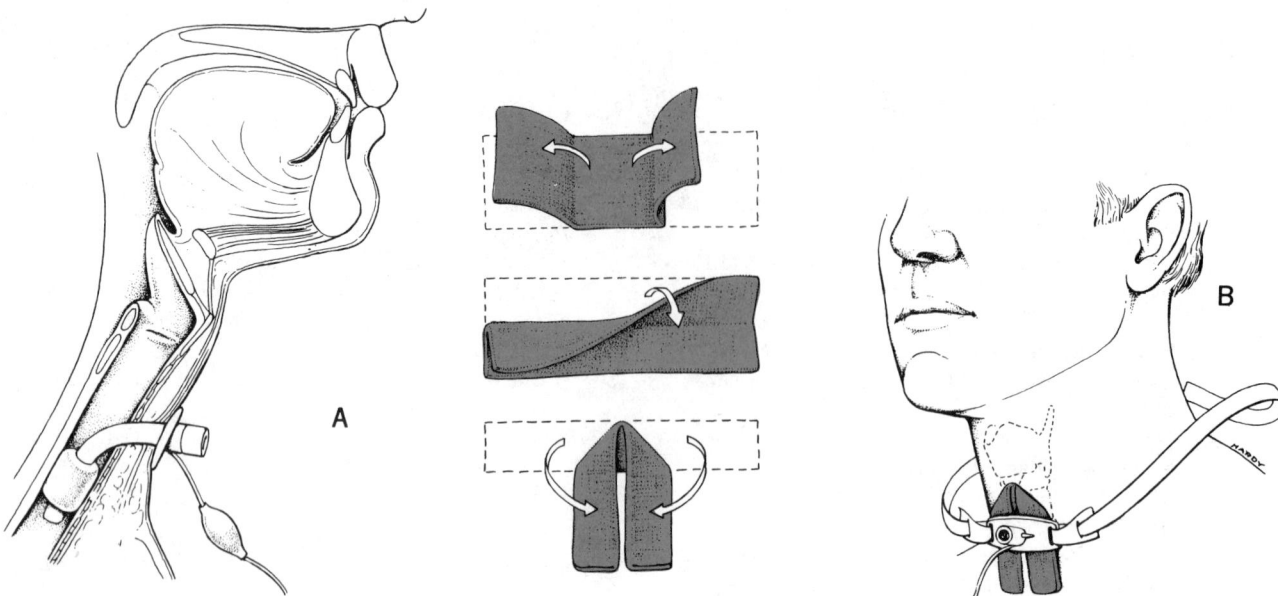

Figure 22-6
Tracheostomy tube dressing and tape changes. Drawing *A* shows how the cuff of the tracheostomy tube fits smoothly within the tracheal wall. Pressure should be great enough to ensure a snug fit but not so great as to produce a stenosis. Illustration *B* shows how to unfold a 3 × 3-inch gauze square and refold it so that it need not be cut (cut frayed threads could be aspirated) and yet will provide a comfortable neck pad. Use tracheostomy gauze sponges with slits already made and oversewn if available. These are changed as often as necessary. Note the manner in which the neck twill tapes are fastened to the openings in the neck plate of the tracheostomy tube; this eliminates a knot, which may create pressure on the neck. Twill tape ends should be tied to the side of the neck rather than in back. (A knot at the back would not be comfortable to lie on.)

All equipment that comes into direct contact with the patient's airway must be sterile in order to prevent overwhelming pulmonary and systemic infections. The following equipment is used:

- Suction catheters
- Gloves
- 5-ml to 10-ml syringe
- Normal saline poured in a cup for irrigation
- The patient's own self-inflating bag (hand resuscitator) with supplemental oxygen (the bag should be changed daily to reduce infection)
- Suction machine

The steps in the tracheal suctioning procedure are as follows:

- Explain the procedure to the patient before beginning and reassure him during suctioning, since he may be apprehensive about choking and about his inability to communicate.
- Begin by washing hands thoroughly.
- Turn on suction source (pressure should not exceed 120 mm Hg).
- Open suction catheter kit.
- Fill basin with sterile normal saline.
- Put on sterile gloves.
- Pick up suction catheter in gloved hand and connect to suction.

- Instill 3 to 5 ml normal saline into tube if secretions are thick.
- Hyperinflate/hyperoxygenate the patient's lungs for several deep breaths with a self-inflating bag.
- Insert catheter at least as far as the end of the tube without applying suction.
- Apply suction while withdrawing catheter, rotating catheter gently 360 degrees (no longer than 10 to 15 seconds, because patient can become hypoxic and develop dysrhythmias, which can lead to cardiac arrest).
- Reoxygenate and inflate the patient's lungs for several breaths.
- Repeat previous three steps until airway is clear.
- Rinse catheter in basin with sterile normal saline between suction attempts if necessary.
- Suction oropharyngeal cavity after completing tracheal suctioning.
- Rinse suction tubing.
- Discard catheter, gloves, and basin.

Cuff Management. As a general rule, the cuff on a tracheostomy tube should be deflated. It is inflated in the following situations: continuous mechanical ventilation, during and after eating or during and 1 hour after a tube feeding, during IPPB treatments, when the patient is unable to handle oral secretions, and when there is increased risk of aspiration (*e.g.*, when the patient is unconscious or has continuous tube feedings).

The key to minimizing many tracheostomy tube complications is the proper management of the cuff of the tracheostomy or endotracheal tube. Proper inflation of the cuff is important to prevent excessive pressure from being exerted on the tracheal wall. The goal is to keep the pressure in the cuff below capillary perfusion pressure (approximately 25 cm H_2O). The cuff is inflated until a seal (or contact with the tracheal wall) is established. The volume of air needed to inflate the cuff should be documented, but it is not as important as the cuff measurement. The optimal cuff pressure is 15 to 25 cm H_2O.

The steps for inflating the cuff and for measuring cuff pressure include the following:

- Deflate cuff completely.
- Connect pressure gauge and 10-ml syringe to a three-way stopcock.
- Inject 1 ml of air at a time into the cuff during inspiration (positive pressure phase), using a self-inflating bag or a ventilator.
- Listen for air (a gurgling sound) by placing the stethoscope on one side of the neck. If gurgling is present or air can be felt coming out of the mouth, then inject more air into the cuff.
- Seal the airway with the cuff. A seal is created when the gurgling disappears, no air leaks from the mouth, or the conscious patient cannot make a sound.
- Note and record the volume and pressure required to seal the cuff.
- Remove the pressure gauge; the cuff will remain inflated because of the one-way valve on the external port of the tube.

Tracheostomy Care.   The care of the patient with a tracheostomy tube is summarized in Chart 22-2.

The Patient Requiring Mechanical Ventilation

A mechanical ventilator is a positive/negative pressure breathing device that can maintain respirations automatically for long periods of time. Caring for a patient on mechanical ventilation has become an integral part of nursing care in critical care units, on general medical–surgical units, in extended care facilities, and even in the home. Nurses, physicians, and respiratory therapists must understand each patient's specific pulmonary needs and work together to set realistic goals. Understanding the principles of mechanical ventilation and the care of a patient on a ventilator are necessary for achieving these goals.

Indications for Mechanical Ventilation

If a patient is experiencing a continuous decrease in oxygenation (PaO_2) an increase in arterial carbon dioxide levels ($PaCO_2$), and a persistence of acidosis (a decreased *p*H), then mechanical ventilation may be necessary. Conditions such as postoperative thoracic or abdominal surgery, drug overdose, neuromuscular diseases, inhalation injury, COPD,

multiple trauma, shock, multisystem failure, and coma may all lead to respiratory failure and the need for mechanical ventilation. The criteria for mechanical ventilation (Chart 22-3, p. 438) are guidelines for making the decision to place a patient on a ventilator. A patient with apnea that is not reversible is also a candidate for mechanical ventilation.

Classification of Ventilators

There are several types of mechanical ventilators. Ventilators are classified according to the manner in which they support ventilation. The two general categories are negative pressure and positive pressure ventilators. Positive pressure ventilators are also classified by their controlling or cycling feature such as volume-cycled, pressure-cycled, and time-cycled ventilators.

Negative Pressure Ventilators

Negative pressure ventilators exert a negative pressure on the external chest and the underlying lung to expand it during inspiration. Air then flows into the lung, filling its volume. Physiologically, this type of assisted ventilation is similar to spontaneous ventilation. It is used mainly in respiratory failure associated with neuromuscular conditions such as poliomyelitis, muscular dystrophy, multiple sclerosis, and myasthenia gravis. Negative pressure ventilators are simple to use and do not require intubation of the airway. Consequently, they are especially adaptable for home use. There are several types of negative pressure ventilators: iron lung, portalung, body wrap, and chest cuirass.

Drinker Respirator Tank (Iron Lung).   The iron lung is a negative pressure chamber used for ventilation. It was used extensively during polio epidemics in the past and is currently used by polio survivors and other neuromuscularly impaired patients. It is efficient and reliable and does not require intubation. However, it is cumbersome to use, not very portable, and not always effective in the presence of diseased lungs.

Body Wrap (Pneumowrap).   The body wrap ventilators (also called a "raincoat" or "poncho") require a rigid cage and a nylon wrap to create a negative pressure chamber around the thorax and abdomen. They are easy to fit and are quite portable. However, musculoskeletal pain is often a problem and leaks develop that decrease the effectiveness of these devices.

Chest Cuirass (Tortoise Shell).   The chest cuirass uses a rigid shell placed on the chest to create a chamber for negative pressure ventilation. Its advantage over other negative pressure ventilators is that it can be used by a patient in a wheelchair. Incorrect fit and persistent back pain are common problems.

Positive Pressure Ventilators

Positive pressure ventilators inflate the lungs by exerting positive pressure on the airway, thus forcing the alveoli to expand during inspiration. Expiration occurs passively. For continuous use, endotracheal intubation or tracheostomy is necessary. These ventilators are widely used in the hospital setting and are increasingly used in the home in patients with primary

Chart 22-2
Care of the Patient With a Tracheostomy

Tracheostomy Care	Rationale
Tracheostomy Cuff	
1. Cuffed tube (air injected into cuff) is required during prolonged mechanical ventilation.	The purpose of a cuffed tube is to prevent air from leaking during positive pressure ventilation and to prevent tracheal aspiration of gastric contents. An adequate seal is indicated by the disappearance of any air leakage from the mouth or tracheostomy or disappearance of the harsh, gurgling sound of air coming from the throat.
2. Low-pressure cuff	Low-pressure cuffs exert minimal pressure on the tracheal mucosa and thus reduce the danger of tracheal ulceration and stricture.
3. Indications for cuff inflation	Mechanical ventilation
	During and 1 hour after eating (or tube feeding)
	During IPPB treatments
	Inability to handle oral secretions
	Increased risk of aspiration (such as unconsciousness)
Tracheostomy Tube and Skin Care	The tracheostomy dressing is changed as needed to keep the skin clean and dry. Do not allow moist or soiled dressings to remain on the skin.
1. Wash hands.	
2. Explain procedure to patient.	A patient with a tracheostomy is apprehensive and requires continuing assurance and support.
3. Remove twill tapes (if soiled) by untying.	
4. Hold tube in place and replace tape immediately.	Tracheostomy tube can be dislodged by movement or forceful cough. It is difficult to reinsert the tracheostomy tube. Airway catastrophe may occur if the tracheostomy tube is dislodged.
5. Clean tracheostomy area with water and prescribed solution.	
6. Place clean twill tapes in position to secure tracheostomy tube. Insert one end of tape through the side opening of the outer cannula. Wrap it around the patient's neck and thread it through the opposite opening of the outer cannula. Bring both ends around so that they meet on one side of the neck. Secure with a knot.	This will provide a double thickness of tape around the neck.

(continued)

lung disease. There are three types of positive pressure ventilators.

Pressure-Cycled Ventilators. The pressure-cycled ventilator is a positive pressure ventilator in which the inspiratory pressure to be reached with each inspiration is controlled. The ventilator cycles on, delivers a flow of air until a certain predetermined pressure is reached, and then cycles off. The major limitation with this type of ventilator is that the volume of air or oxygen can vary as the patient's airway resistance or compliance changes. The result is an inconsistency in the amount of tidal volume delivered and a possible compromise of ventilation. Consequently, in adults, pressure-cycled ventilators are only intended for short-term use in the recovery room.

Time-Cycled Ventilators. Time-cycled ventilators terminate or control inspiration after a preset time. The volume of air the patient receives is regulated by the length of inspiration and the flow rate of the air. Most ventilators have a rate control that determines the respiratory rate, but pure time-cycling is rarely used for adults. These ventilators are used in newborns and infants.

Volume-Cycled Ventilators. Volume-cycled ventilators are the most commonly used positive pressure ventilators. With this type of ventilator, the volume of air to be delivered with each inspiration is controlled. Once this preset volume is delivered to the patient, the ventilator cycles off and exhalation occurs passively. From breath to breath, the volume of air delivered by the ventilator is constant, assuring consistent, adequate breaths. Volume ventilators are intended for long-term use, for patients with primary pulmonary disease, or for patients with an impaired bellows mechanism (such as occurs in neuromuscular disease).

Chart 22-2 *(continued)*

Tracheostomy Care	*Rationale*
7. Remove soiled dressing and discard.	
8. Put on sterile gloves.	
9. Cleanse wound with sterile applicators moistened with prescribed solution.	
10. Cleanse entire flange of tracheostomy tube with sterile applicator moistened with prescribed solution. Do not allow solution to enter tracheostomy. Rinse with sterile water.	Fluid entering the tracheostomy will irritate the respiratory tract.
11. Use neosporin or povidone-iodine ointment on the edge of the tracheostomy wound.	
12. Use sterile tracheostomy dressing from the wrappers, and fit securely under the twill tapes and flange of tracheostomy tube so that the incision is covered (see Fig. 22-6*B*).	Dressings that will shred are not used around a tracheostomy because of the danger that pieces of material, lint, or thread may get into the tube, and eventually into the trachea, causing obstruction or abscess formation. Special dressings that do not have a tendency to shred are used.

Changing of Tracheostomy Tube

1. Varies from 3 to 5 days	Frequency depends on amount of crust and thickened secretions adhering to the tracheostomy tube.
2. Only a skilled physician should change a fresh tracheostomy.	Because airway problems can develop, original stomal tract may be hard to find.
3. A nurse can change the tracheostomy tube if a patent stomal tract has developed.	
4. Have resuscitation equipment, spare tracheostomy tube, and hemostat ready.	Equipment is needed in case airway problems develop while changing tube.
5. Procedure:	
a. Suction tracheostomy and laryngo-oropharynx.	
b. Cut off twill ties.	
c. Remove tracheostomy tube after deflating cuff.	
d. Insert new tracheostomy tube with obturator following the curvature of the tube until it is set in place.	
e. Remove obturator, inflate cuff, tie twill ties.	
f. Apply tracheostomy dressing.	

Features and Settings of Volume Ventilators

Numerous features are used in the management of the patient on a mechanical ventilator. The features and settings of a volume ventilator are presented in Chart 22-4.

Adjustment on the Ventilator. The ventilator is adjusted so that the patient is comfortable and "in phase" with the machine (Fig. 22-7). Minimal alteration of the normal cardiovascular and pulmonary dynamics is desired. If the volume ventilator is adjusted appropriately, the patient's arterial blood gas levels will be satisfactory and auscultation of the chest will indicate bilateral lung expansion. To determine how to achieve adequate mechanical ventilation for each patient, the following guidelines are recommended as initial ventilator settings for the patient:

1. Set the machine to deliver tidal volume required (10 to 15 ml/kg).
2. Adjust the machine to deliver 100% inspired oxygen or whatever is necessary to maintain normal PaO_2 (70 to 100 mm Hg, or 9.31 to 13.30 kPa[a]).
3. Record peak inspiratory pressure.
4. Adjust inspiratory-expiratory ratio. Within the above criteria, make a setting that will provide satisfactory blood gases, with adequate tidal volume and inspiratory-expiratory ratio at the minimum airway pressure.
5. Adjust sensitivity so that the patient can trigger the machine with a minimum effort. Adjust the rate to provide normal Pco_2 (38 to 42 mm Hg, or 5.50 to 5.58 kPa[a]).

Chart 22-3
Criteria for Mechanical Ventilation

$PaO_2 < 50$ mm Hg with $FIO_2 > 0.60$
$PaO_2 > 50$ mm Hg with $pH < 7.25$
Vital capacity < two times tidal volume
Negative inspiratory force < 25 cm H_2O
Respiratory rate > 35

Sensitivity is not set if the patient's respirations are controlled.

6. Record minute volume and measure Pco_2, pH, and Po_2 after 20 minutes of continuous ventilation at 100% inspired O_2 concentration. Estimate inspired O_2 concentration required to maintain Po_2 between 70 and 100 mm Hg (9.31 to 13.30 kPa[a]).

7. Adjust fraction of inspired oxygen (FIO_2) according to results of arterial blood gases on 100% (1.00) inspired oxygen. Appropriate FIO_2 level should periodically be assessed and adjusted.

8. Add mechanical dead space if required to maintain normal $PaCO_2$ when large tidal volumes are used.

9. Use 100% (1.00) FIO_2 setting to follow progress of pulmonary status. A true physiologic shunt can be estimated from the arterial blood gases and an FIO_2 of 100% (1.00) by calculating the alveolar arterial oxygen content difference.

10. Rule out the possibility of an impending catastrophe whenever a patient is out of phase with the ventilator. The "out of phase" patient may have hypoxemia, air leak, obstruction, or inadequate flow rate, minute volume, or inspiratory-expiratory ratios.

Care of the Mechanically Ventilated Patient

▷ Assessment

The nurse has a vital role in assessing the patient's status and the functioning of the ventilator. In assessing the patient, the nurse evaluates the following:

- Vital signs
- Evidence of hypoxia (restlessness, anxiety, tachycardia, increased respiratory rate, cyanosis)
- Respiratory rate and pattern
- Breath sounds
- Neurologic status
- Tidal volume, minute ventilation, forced vital capacity
- Nutritional status
- Suctioning needs
- Psychological status
- Patient's inspiratory effort and synchrony with the ventilator

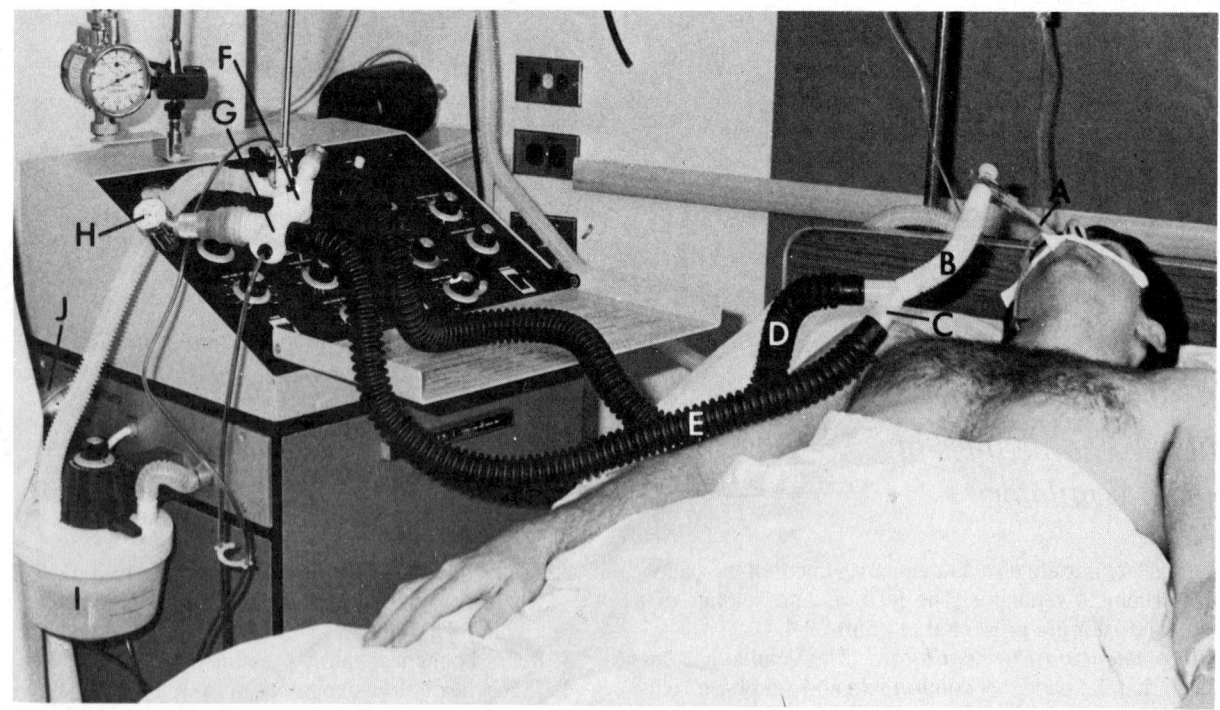

Figure 22-7
Patient on MA1 mechanical ventilator. Lettered items are as follows: (*A*) Endotracheal tube. (*B*) Mechanical dead space. (*C*) Y-piece. (*D*) Inspiratory hose. (*E*) Expiratory hose. (*F*) Inspiratory valve. (*G*) Expiratory valve. (*H*) Wright respirometer. (*I*) Cascade humidifier. (*J*) Knob for positive end-expiratory pressure (PEEP).

Chart 22-4
Features and Settings of a Volume Ventilator

A volume-controlled ventilator (MAI, Bear, Servo) will deliver set tidal volume with varying pressures.

Fraction of Inspired Oxygen (F$_{IO_2}$)

The concentration of oxygen delivered is dependent on patient need, as determined by the physician and evaluated by arterial blood gas levels.

Tidal Volume (V$_T$)

10–15 ml/kg body weight

Respiratory Rate

12–16/min

Sensitivity Setting

- Increased sensitivity indicates that very low negative pressure is required to trigger the machine.
- Do not allow the patient to generate more than −2 cm H$_2$O to trigger the ventilator.

Type of Ventilation

Controlled. The machine ventilates the patient according to set tidal volumes and respiratory rate. The patient usually requires medication with morphine or pancuronium.

Assist/control. The patient triggers the machine. If the patient fails, the machine will deliver a controlled breath at a minimum rate already set.

Inspiration to Exhalation Ratio

- Should be 1:3, 1:2, or more (1 second of inspiration to 3 seconds of exhalation, *etc.*)
- Inspiration should never be longer than exhalation, because venous return to the right side of the heart occurs on exhalation. Prolonged inspiration prevents venous return and may cause hypotension.
- Patients with obstructive pulmonary disease need longer exhalation time to keep the bronchi open and allow exit of more air.

Minute Volume (V$_T$)

Tidal volume × respiratory rate/min.
Normal = 6–8 liters/min.

Airway Pressure

Normal = 15–20 cm/H$_2$O, but varies.
Low airway pressure is seen with air leak.
High airway pressure is seen in
- Increased secretions
- Airway obstruction
- Bronchospasms
- Pulmonary edema
- Pneumothorax
- Flail chest
- Patient out of phase with respirator

Sigh

- The lungs are hyperinflated periodically to open collapsed alveoli.
- The sigh is given by machine or manual hand-bag ventilation.
- Sigh volume is 2 times tidal volume every 5–10 minutes.

Mechanical Dead Space

Refers to the volume of tubing from endotracheal or tracheostomy tube connector to the Y-piece.

Purpose:
- To rebreathe exhaled CO$_2$.
- Serves as a pliable connector from tracheostomy tube to Y-piece; thus prevents discomfort when patient moves.

Caution: The volume of mechanical dead space should not be larger than one third of the set tidal volume, especially at 21% of F$_{IO_2}$, because hypoxic oxygen concentrations may result owing to exhaled CO$_2$ dilution. Should not be used to correct metabolic alkalosis.

Flow Rate

Slow
- Opens up more alveoli because of a more even air flow distribution within the respiratory tract.
- If flow rate is too slow it will prolong inspiration and may hinder venous return.

High
- Shortens inspiratory time.
- Preferential flow of gases to alveoli with least resistance and may not open atelectatic alveoli at all.

Expiratory Retard
- Used only when prescribed by physician.
- Keeps the terminal bronchioles patent, preventing early closure on exhalation; thus, more air can be exhaled.

Humidity and Temperature
- Heated humidity is provided for all intubated and tracheotomized patients to avoid thick and viscid secretions
- Daily clinical evaluation of the viscosity of the patient's secretions provides a guideline for the effectiveness of humidification and nebulization.

Positive-End-Expiratory Pressure
- A positive pressure of 5 cm, 10 cm, or 15 cm H$_2$O is maintained at the end of exhalation instead of a normal 0 cm H$_2$O pressure.
- Increases functional residual capacity and improves oxygenation.

Synchronization of Patient With Ventilator
- Inspiratory and expiratory time of the patient and respirator should be synchronized.
- Asynchrony (out of phase) with ventilator will result in altered cardiopulmonary hemodynamics and will cause dysrhythmias, hypotension, and increased airway pressure.

Assessment of Cardiac Function. Alterations in cardiac output may occur as a result of positive pressure ventilation. The positive intrathoracic pressure during inspiration compresses the heart and great vessels, thereby reducing venous return and cardiac output. This is usually corrected during exhalation when the positive pressure is off. To evaluate cardiac function, the nurse assesses vital signs, cardiac output (if a pulmonary artery line is inserted), and urinary output. She also looks for signs of decreased tissue oxygenation (restlessness, apprehension, confusion, tachycardia, tachypnea, increased work of breathing, pale or cyanotic skin, or shock).

Assessment of Equipment. The ventilator also needs to be assessed to make sure that it is functioning properly and that the settings are appropriate. Even though the nurse may not be primarily responsible for adjusting the settings on the ventilator or measuring ventilator parameters (usually the responsibility of the respiratory therapist), she is responsible for the patient and therefore needs to evaluate how the ventilator affects the patient. In monitoring the ventilator, the nurse should note the following:

- Type of ventilator (volume-cycled, pressure-cycled, negative pressure)
- Controlling mode (control, assist/control, intermittent mandatory ventilation)
- Tidal volume and rate settings
- FiO_2 (fraction of inspired oxygen) setting
- Inspiratory pressure reached and pressure limit
- Sigh settings
- Presence of water in the tubing, disconnection, or kinking of the tubing
- Humidification (humidifier filled with water)
- Alarms (functioning properly)
- PEEP (positive end-expiratory pressure) level, if applicable

▷ Nursing Diagnoses

Based on the assessment data, the patient's major nursing diagnoses may include

- Ineffective airway clearance related to increased mucus production associated with continuous positive pressure mechanical ventilation
- Potential for injury/infection related to endotracheal intubation or tracheostomy
- Impaired physical mobility related to ventilator dependency
- Impaired verbal communication related to endotracheal tube attachment to ventilator
- Ineffective individual coping and powerlessness related to ventilator dependency

▷ Planning and Implementation

▷ *Goals:* The major goals of the patient may include the following:

- Reduction of mucus accumulation
- Absence of injury/infection
- Attainment of optimum mobility
- Adjustment to nonverbal methods of communication
- Acquisition of successful coping measures

▷ Nursing Interventions

Nursing care of the mechanically ventilated patient requires unique technical and interpersonal skills. Nursing interventions are similar whether the patient is in an intensive care unit, a medical-surgical unit, or an extended care facility. The frequency of administering the care and the stability of the patient are the factors that vary from unit to unit.

Airway Management. Continuous positive pressure ventilation increases the production of secretions regardless of the patient's underlying condition. The nurse must identify the presence of secretions by lung auscultation every 2 to 4 hours. Measures to clear the airway of secretions include suctioning, chest physiotherapy, frequent position changes, and ambulation as soon as possible. The sigh mechanism on the ventilator is adjusted to deliver at least 8 to 10 sighs per hour at two times the tidal volume if the patient is not on IMV. Periodic sighing prevents atelectasis and the further retention of secretions. Humidification by way of the ventilator is to be maintained to help liquefy secretions so they are more easily raised. Bronchodilators, either intravenous or inhaled, are administered as prescribed to dilate the bronchial tubes so that secretions are more easily mobilized.

Prevention of Injury and Infection. Airway management also involves maintenance of the endotracheal or tracheostomy tube. The ventilator tubing is positioned so there is minimal pulling or distortion of the tube in the trachea. Cuff pressure is monitored every 8 hours to keep the pressure under 25 cmH_2O. The presence of a cuff leak is evaluated at the same time. Tracheostomy care is performed every 4 hours to prevent the increased risk of infection. Oral hygiene is given every 8 hours because the oral cavity is a primary source of contamination of the lungs in the intubated and compromised patient.

Promotion of Optimal Level of Mobility. The patient's mobility is limited because of his attachment to the ventilator. If his condition is stable, he should get out of bed and to a chair as soon as possible. Ambulation is also encouraged when indicated. A manual self-inflating bag with oxygen is used to ventilate the patient while he is walking. Mobility and muscle activity are beneficial because they stimulate respirations and improve morale.

If the patient is not able to get out of bed or walk, then active or passive range of motion exercises are performed every 8 hours to prevent muscle atrophy, contractures, and venous stasis.

Promotion of Optimal Communication. Alternative methods of communication must be developed for the patient on a ventilator. The nurse assesses the patient's communication abilities:

- Is his hand strong and available for writing? (If he is right-handed, the intravenous line is placed in his left hand)
- Is his mouth unobstructed by tube for mouthing words?
- Is the patient conscious and able to communicate?

Once the patient's limitations are known, the nurse offers several appropriate communication approaches:

- Lip reading (use single key words)
- Pad and pencil or "magic slate"
- Communication board
- Gesturing
- Electric larynx

- Ventri-voice (electronic voice synthesizer powered by a gas source)

The patient must be helped to find the communication method best suited for him. Some methods may be frustrating to the patient and they need to be identified and minimized. A speech-language pathologist will assist in determining the most appropriate method for the patient.

Promotion of Coping Ability. Dependence on a ventilator is frightening to both the patient and his family and will disrupt even the most stable families. The patient and his family are helped to verbalize their feelings about the ventilator, the patient's condition, and the environment in general. Explaining procedures every time they are performed will help to reduce anxiety and familiarize the patient with hospital routines. To restore a sense of control, the patient is encouraged to participate in decisions about his care, schedules, and treatment when possible. There is a tendency to become withdrawn or depressed during mechanical ventilation, especially if it is prolonged. Consequently, the patient is encouraged about his progress when appropriate. Diversion is provided by watching television, playing music, or taking a walk (if appropriate). Stress-reduction techniques (a back rub, relaxation measures) help release tension and enable the patient to deal with his anxieties and fears about his condition and his dependence on the ventilator.

▷ *Evaluation*

▷ *Expected Outcomes*

1. Patient manages ventilation with minimal mucus accumulation.
   a. Tolerates frequent suctioning.
   b. Assists with position changes.
   c. Attempts to ambulate within limitations of equipment and condition.
2. Is free of injury/infection.
   a. Assists with oral care if possible.
   b. Tolerates tracheostomy care every 4 hours.
3. Is mobile within limits of ability.
   a. Gets out of bed to chair as soon as possible.
   b. Walks around room as tolerated.
   c. Performs range-of-motion exercises every 6 to 8 hours.
4. Communicates effectively.
   a. Writes messages as necessary.
   b. Is able to use gestures to communicate.
5. Copes effectively.
   a. Verbalizes fears and concerns about his condition and the equipment.
   b. Participates in decision making when possible.
   c. Uses stress-reduction techniques when necessary.
   d. Seeks support groups when needed.

Factors Causing the Patient to "Fight" the Ventilator

The patient is in synchrony with the ventilator when thoracic expansion coincides with the inspiratory phase of the machine and exhalation occurs passively. The patient "fights" the ventilator when he is out of phase with the machine. This is manifested when the patient attempts to breathe in during the ventilator's mechanical expiratory phase or when there is jerky and increased abdominal muscle effort.

The following factors contribute to this problem: increased secretions, low FIO_2, hypercarbia, inadequate minute volume, and pulmonary edema. These problems must be corrected before the prescribed sedation or muscle relaxant is given to the patient. Otherwise, the basic problem is masked and the patient's condition will continue to deteriorate.

Life-threatening problems, of course, require immediate correction. Such conditions as airway obstruction, tension pneumothorax, hemothorax, flail chest, and cardiac tamponade could occur or be the presenting problem and must be managed quickly (see Chest Trauma, p. 496). Thus, the nurse is constantly monitoring the patient for these difficulties and is prepared to act.

Problems with Mechanical Ventilation

Because of the seriousness of the patient's condition and the highly complex and technical nature of mechanical ventilation, a number of problems can arise. Such situations as inadequate alveolar ventilation, an air leak in the system, a cuff leak, obstruction or resistance to air flow, condensation in the ventilator tubing, "fighting" the ventilator, secretions, bronchospasm, and atelectasis all need to be identified and corrected. Frequently encountered ventilator problems are listed with probable causes and solutions in Table 22-2.

Weaning the Patient From the Ventilator

Weaning the patient from his dependence on the ventilator takes place in four stages. The patient is gradually weaned from the (1) ventilator, (2) cuff, (3) tube, and (4) oxygen. Weaning from mechanical ventilation is done at the earliest possible time consistent with patient safety. It is essential that the decision be made from a physiological rather than from a mechanical viewpoint. A total understanding of the patient's clinical status is required in making this decision.

Weaning is started when the patient is recovering from the acute stage of his medical and surgical problems and when the cause of respiratory failure is sufficiently reversed.

The objective measurements of the patient's ventilatory capacities include the following:

1. An ability to generate a minimum vital capacity of 15 ml/kg of body weight or a vital capacity twice as large as the predicted normal resting tidal volume. The minimum required volume is usually in the range of 1000 ml in a normal adult.
2. An inspiratory force of at least −20 cm H_2O pressure
3. A PaO_2 of greater than 60% (0.6) with an FIO_2 of less than 0.5
4. Vital signs that are stable

When the decision has been made that the patient has adequate ventilatory capacity, baseline measurements are noted: (1) vital capacity, (2) inspiratory force, (3) respiratory rate, (4) resting tidal volume, (5) minute ventilation (frequency times total volume, or f × VT), (6) arterial blood gases, and (7) FIO_2. It is important to follow the trend of these values as the weaning progresses, rather than to rely on isolated measurements.

The patient's endotracheal or tracheostomy tube is then attached to a large-bore tubing (called a T-piece), which is connected to an aerosol and oxygen source. The patient

TABLE 22-2
Causes and Solutions of Ventilator Problems

Problem	Cause	Solution
Increase in pressure or volume	Coughing or plugged airway tube	Suction airway for secretions, etc.
	Patient "fighting" ventilator	Adjust sensitivity.
		Manually ventilate patient—check for bronchospasm.
		Check blood gases.
		Sedate only if necessary.
	Tubing kinked	Check tubing; reposition patient if necessary.
	Pneumothorax	Manually ventilate patient; notify physician.
	Decrease in compliance due to atelectasis or bronchospasm	Clear secretions.
Decrease in pressure or loss of volume	Increase in compliance	None
	Leak in ventilator or tubing; cuff on tube/ humidifier not tight	Correct leak.
Change in inspiratory to expiratory	Flow rate setting	Adjust setting.
	Any changes in ventilator	Adjust.
Change in oxygen delivered	Gas supply decreased	Correct.
	Oxygen blender malfunction	Correct.
	Inaccurate reading	Check and calibrate O_2 analyzer.
Any changes in ventilation	Possible change in ventilator settings	Always *assess patient first*, then check ventilator tubing *while ventilating patient* manually.

breathes spontaneously with the aid of the humidified oxygen. During the weaning process, the patient is maintained on the same or higher oxygen concentration than when he is on the ventilator.

Adequate psychological preparation is necessary before and during the weaning process. The patient needs to know what is expected of him during the procedure. He is frightened by having responsibility for his own breathing again and needs the reassurance that he is improving and is well enough to handle spontaneous breathing. The nurse explains what will happen during weaning and what his role in the procedure will be. She emphasizes that someone will be with him or near him at all times and allows time to answer any of his questions simply and concisely. A properly prepared patient can reduce the weaning time.

While the patient is on the T-piece, the baseline measurements mentioned above are closely monitored. The frequency of these measurements depends on the patient's clinical progress. The second set of arterial blood gases is drawn 20 minutes after the patient has been on spontaneous ventilation at a constant FIO_2. (It takes 15 to 20 minutes for alveolar arterial equilibration to take place.) The patient is observed for signs of hypoxemia or increasing fatigue as manifested by the following: (1) bradycardia, premature ventricular contractions (PVCs), or any sign of increasing cardiac irritability; (2) restlessness; (3) a respiratory rate greater than 35/min; and (4) labored respiration. Fatigue or exhaustion is initially manifested by an increased respiratory rate associated with a gradual reduction in tidal volume. Later there is a slowing of the respiratory rate.

The appearance of signs of exhaustion and hypoxemia correlated with a deterioration of the above measurements suggest the need for ventilatory support. The patient is placed back on the ventilator each time signs of fatigue or deterioration develop.

Patients who have had short-term ventilatory assistance usually can be extubated within 2 or 3 hours of weaning and allowed spontaneous ventilation by means of a mask with humidified oxygen. Patients who have had prolonged ventilatory assistance usually require more gradual weaning, which may take several days. They are weaned primarily during the day and placed back on the ventilator at night to sleep.

Intermittent Mandatory Ventilation.   Some patients are difficult to wean from mechanical ventilation. An intermittent mandatory ventilation (IMV) device incorporated into the respirator will allow the patient to breathe spontaneously as desired but also delivers a mandatory hyperinflation at regular intervals. IMV is indicated if the patient satisfies all the criteria for weaning but cannot sustain adequate spontaneous ventilation for long periods of time. On initiation of IMV the machine is set at a slower rate but at a larger tidal volume than the patient's spontaneous respiratory activity. It then can be adjusted to maintain satisfactory arterial blood gases.

Following initiation of IMV, serial determinations of the following are made and recorded: (1) respiratory rate, (2) minute volume (VE), (3) tidal volume (VT) of patient and machine, (4) FIO_2, and (5) arterial blood gas values.

If there is no deterioration in these parameters, and as the patient's tidal volume improves, the rate of the ventilator is progressively decreased and the patient is allowed to rely more on spontaneous respiration until weaning is complete.

Successful weaning from the ventilator is followed by intensive pulmonary care. The following are continued: (1) oxygen therapy, (2) arterial blood gas evaluation, (3) nebulizer therapy, (4) chest physiotherapy, and (5) adequate hydration and humidification. These patients still have minimum pulmonary function and need vigorous supportive therapy before their respiratory status returns to normal.

Weaning From the Cuff. While the patient is on the ventilator, the cuff is kept inflated to avoid aspiration and prevent an air leak, and thus allow adequate chest expansion.

Once the patient is removed from the ventilator, the cuff is deflated to allow air to flow around the cuff from the upper airway. The cuff remains inflated when there is a risk of aspiration (as in the unconscious or neck surgery patient). A cuffed tube remains in the patient initially so that the patient can be placed back on mechanical ventilation should an emergency arise. When the patient is stable, the cuffed tube can be replaced by a cuffless tube in preparation for total removal of the tube.

Weaning From the Tube. The tracheostomy or endotracheal tube can be removed if the following criteria are present: (1) spontaneous ventilation is adequate; (2) the pharyngeal and laryngeal gag reflexes are active; (3) the patient is maintaining an adequate airway and can swallow, move his jaw, or clench his teeth; and (4) voluntary cough is effective in bringing up secretions. If these are ineffective, the tracheostomy tube is needed so that tracheobronchial secretions can be suctioned.

Before the patient is weaned from the tracheostomy tube, he is given a trial of mouth- or nose-breathing. This is accomplished by (1) changing to a smaller size tube to reduce the resistance to air flow and plugging the tracheostomy (deflate the cuff) at the same time; (2) switching to a cuffless tracheostomy tube; (3) changing to a fenestrated tube (one with an opening or window in the bend of the tube), which permits air to flow around and through the tube to the upper airway; (4) changing to a tracheostomy button; or (5) removing the tracheostomy tube completely.

Weaning From Oxygen. The patient has been weaned from the ventilator, cuff, and tube. His respiratory function has been checked, and oxygen has been given according to the result of the blood gas determinations. The FiO_2 is then gradually reduced until the Po_2 is in the 70 to 100 mm Hg range (9.31 to 13.30 kPaª) while the patient is breathing room air. If the Po_2 is less than 70 mm Hg (9.31 kPaª) on room air, supplementary oxygen is recommended.

Mechanical Ventilation in the Home

Under certain physiological, psychological, or economic conditions, it is possible that the patient may not be completely weaned from the ventilator, from the tube, or from oxygen before leaving the hospital. Patients are being discharged to extended-care facilities or home on mechanical ventilators, with tracheostomy tubes, or on oxygen therapy. Patients on home ventilator care usually have neuromuscular conditions or COPD.

Mechanical ventilation in the home (or an extended-care facility) is occurring because of a number of influences:

1. Early diagnosis and treatment of pulmonary disorders has resulted in increased patient longevity.

2. Committed health care members are willing to offer supportive and rehabilitative care to the patient at home.
3. Socioeconomic stresses demand reductions in costs placed on the health care industry.
4. Concerned family members are willing to give necessary support care.
5. Recent technological advances have made ventilators simple, portable, versatile, compact, and safe for use by the homebound patient and his caregivers.

Caring for the patient with mechanical ventilator support at home can be accomplished quite successfully. Multiple factors are considered in order for this endeavor to work. The family must emotionally, educationally, and physically be able to assume the role of primary caregiver. A home care team consisting of physician, respiratory therapist, nurse, social service or home care agency, and equipment supplier needs to be available. The home itself is evaluated to determine if it is adequate for the safe operation of all electrical equipment. A summary of the basic assessment criteria needed for successful home care is presented in Chart 22-5.

Once the decision is made to initiate mechanical ventilation at home, the patient and his family are prepared for home care. Home health teaching includes information about the ventilator, suctioning, tracheostomy care, signs of pulmonary infection, cuff inflation and deflation, and assessment of vital signs. Family instruction begins in the hospital and continues in the home. Nursing responsibilities include evaluating the patient's and the family's understanding of the information presented.

Once the patient is at home, the community health nurse is involved in monitoring and evaluating the adaptation of the patient and family to the home environment. The adequacy of ventilation and oxygenation are assessed, as is airway patency. The nurse needs to solve any unique adaptation problems the patient may have. She listens to the patient's and the family's anxieties and frustrations and offers support and encouragement where appropriate. She helps identify and contact appropriate community resources that may assist in home management of the patient with mechanical ventilation.

The technical aspects of the ventilator are managed by vendor follow-up. A respiratory therapist is usually assigned to the patient and makes frequent visits to evaluate the patient and perform a maintenance check of the ventilator.

Transportation services are identified to determine the procedure for providing patient transportation in an emergency. These arrangements need to be made before an emergency arises because of the uniqueness of the situation.

The family is taught cardiopulmonary resuscitation, including mouth-to-tracheostomy tube (instead of mouth-to-mouth) breathing. Handling a power failure is also explained. This involves the conversion of most ventilators from an electrical power source to a battery power source. Conversion is automatic in most types of home ventilators and lasts approximately 1 hour. The family is also instructed in the manual self-inflation technique should it be necessary.

Ultimately the patient/family responsibilities at home include the following:

Patient Care
· Monitor vital signs as directed.
· Observe physical signs such as color, secretions, breathing pattern, and state of consciousness.

Chart 22-5
Summary of Assessment Criteria for Successful Home Ventilator Care

1. The family members and professional staff are competent, dependable, and willing to spend the time required for proper training.
2. The patient is willing to go home.
3. The family understands the diagnosis and prognosis.
4. There is evidence of acute underlying pulmonary abnormalities.
5. The patient's clinical pulmonary status is stable.
6. The family is aware of the financial responsibilities.
7. A psychological consultation is made before the patient is discharged.
8. The home environment is conducive to accepting the patient.
9. The electrical facilities are adequate to operate all equipment safely.
10. The patient environment is controlled, preventing drafts in cold weather and ensuring proper ventilation in warm weather.
11. Equipment cleaning and storage space is available.

(Adapted from O'Ryan JA and Burns DG. Pulmonary Rehabilitation: From Hospital to Home. Chicago, Year Book Medical Publishers, 1984.)

- Perform physical care such as suctioning, postural drainage, and ambulation.
- Observe the tidal volume and pressure manometer regularly. Intervene when they are abnormal (*i.e.,* suction if airway pressure increases).
- Provide a communication method for the patient (*e.g.,* pad and pencil, electric larynx, Venti-voice).

Ventilator Care
- Check the ventilator settings twice each day and whenever the patient is removed from the ventilator.
- Adjust the volume and pressure alarms if needed.
- Fill humidifier as needed and check its level three times a day.
- Empty water in tubing as needed.

Ventilator Maintenance
- Use a clean humidifier when circuitry is changed.
- Keep exterior clean and free of any objects.
- Change external circuitry once a week or more.
- Report malfunction or strange noises right away.

Providing the opportunity for ventilator-dependent patients and their families to return home to live in familiar surroundings can be a rich, rewarding experience for all. The technical ability now exists to accomplish this. The ultimate goal for the patient on home ventilator therapy is to enhance life, not simply to support or prolong life.

The Patient Undergoing Thoracic Surgery

Assessment and management are particularly important in the patient undergoing thoracic surgery. Thoracic operations are done for a wide variety of reasons; in addition, the patient may have obstructive pulmonary disease with compromised breathing. Preoperative management is important because there may be a narrower margin of safety in chest operations.

Fortunately, the lungs have a large functional reserve. Newer techniques of anesthesia, respiratory therapy, skillful surgery, and intensive postoperative care have made possible more extensive thoracic surgery.

The objectives of preoperative care are to ascertain the patient's functional reserve to determine if he can survive the operation, and to ensure the optimal condition of the patient for surgery.

Diagnostic Evaluation

A number of preoperative tests are done to determine the preoperative status of the patient and to assess his physical assets and liabilities. The initial investigation starts with the history and physical examination—the foundation of preoperative evaluation. The general appearance of the patient, his behavior, and his mental alertness will indicate whether a significant surgical risk is involved.

The decision to perform any pulmonary resection is based on the patient's cardiovascular status and pulmonary reserve. Pulmonary function studies (especially lung volume and vital capacity) are done to determine whether the contemplated resection will leave sufficient functioning lung tissue. Arterial blood gas values are assessed to provide a more complete picture of the functional capacity of the lung. Exercise tolerance tests have predictive value. Such tests are especially important to determine whether the patient who is a candidate for pneumonectomy can tolerate whole lung removal.

Preoperative studies are done to provide a baseline for comparison during the postoperative period and to reveal any unsuspected abnormalities. These studies include chest radiography, electrocardiography (for arteriosclerotic heart disease, conduction defects), determination of blood urea nitrogen and serum creatinine (renal function), glucose tolerance or blood sugar (diabetes), assessment of blood electrolytes, serum protein studies, blood volume determinations, and complete blood cell count.

Operative Procedures

Lobectomy. When the pathology is limited to one area of a lung, a lobectomy (removal of a lobe of a lung) is per-

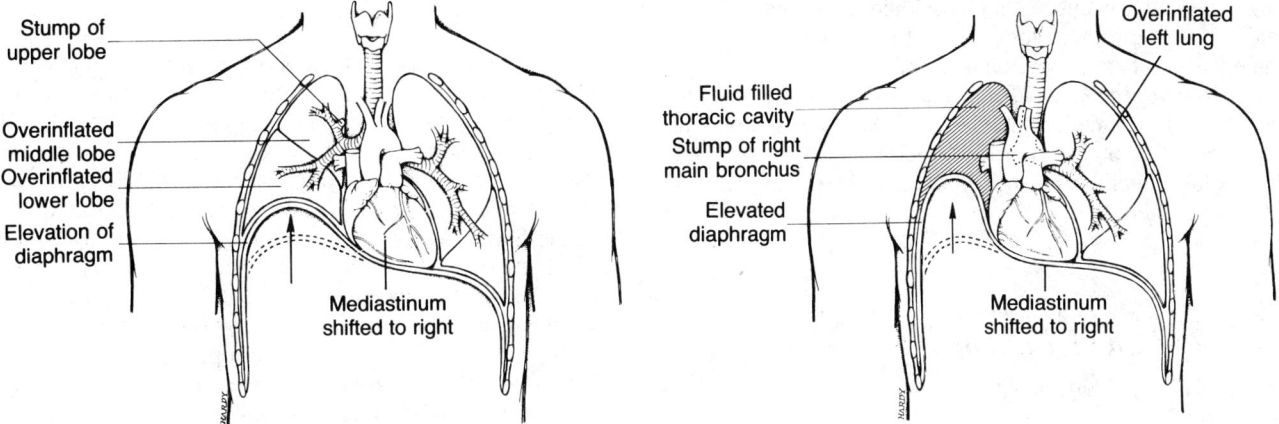

Figure 22-8
Operative procedures. (*Left*) Lobectomy. (*Right*) Pneumonectomy.

formed. This operation, which is more common than pneumonectomy, may be carried out for bronchogenic carcinoma, giant emphysematous blebs or bullae, benign tumors, metastatic malignant tumors, bronchiectasis, and fungus infections (Fig. 22-8).

A thoracotomy incision is used, its exact location depending on the lobe to be resected. When the pleura is entered, the involved lung collapses and the lobar vessels and the bronchus are ligated and divided. After the lobe is removed, the remaining lobes of the lung are reexpanded. Usually, two chest catheters are inserted for drainage (Fig. 22-9).

The upper tube is for the removal of air; the lower one is for drainage of fluid. Sometimes, only one catheter is needed. The chest tube is connected to a chest drainage apparatus for several days.

Pneumonectomy. The removal of an entire lung (pneumonectomy) is done chiefly for cancer when the lesion cannot be removed by a lesser procedure. It also may be performed for lung abscesses, bronchiectasis, or extensive unilateral tuberculosis. The removal of the right lung is more dangerous than the removal of the left since the right lung has a larger vascular bed and its removal imposes a greater physiological burden.

A posterolateral or anterolateral thoracotomy incision is made, sometimes with resection of a rib. The pulmonary artery and the pulmonary veins are ligated and severed.

The main bronchus is divided and the lung removed. The bronchial stump is stapled, and usually no drains are used because the accumulation of fluid in the empty hemithorax is the desired end result.

Segmentectomy (Segmental Resection). Some lesions are located in only one segment of the lung. Bronchopulmonary segments are subdivisions of the lung that function as individual units (see Fig. 22-2). They are held together by delicate connective tissue; disease processes may be limited to a single segment. Care is used to preserve as much healthy and functional lung tissue as possible, especially in patients who already have a limited cardiorespiratory reserve. Single segments can be removed from any lobe, but the right middle lobe, since it has only two small segments, invariably is removed entirely. On the left side, corresponding to a middle lobe, is a "lingular" segment of the upper lobe. This can be

removed as a single segment or by *lingulectomy*. This segment is frequently involved in bronchiectasis.

Wedge Resection. A wedge resection of a small, well-circumscribed lesion may be done without regard for the location of the intersegmental planes. The pleural cavity usu-

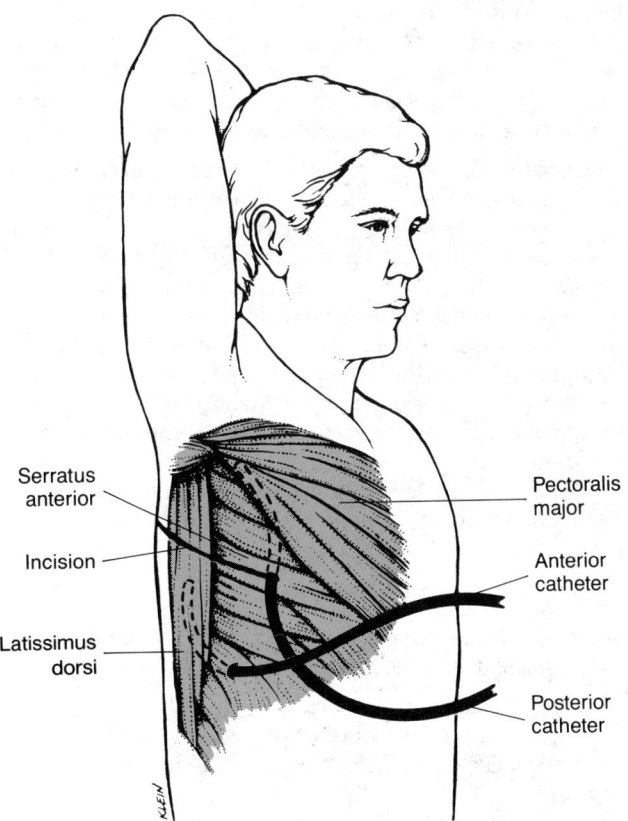

Figure 22-9
Postoperative drainage of the chest. The upper drainage tube is used for the escape of air from leaks in the resected lung. The tip is anchored in the parietal pleura near the apex and brought out through the anterior end of the incision. The lower tube is usually for serosanguineous drainage.

ally is drained because of the possibility of an air or blood leak. This procedure is done for random lung biopsy and for the excision of small peripheral nodules.

Bronchoplastic or Sleeve Resection. Bronchoplastic resection is a procedure in which only one lobar bronchus together with a part of the right or left bronchus is excised. The distal bronchus is reanastomosed to the proximal bronchus or trachea.

▶ Nursing Process
The Patient Undergoing Thoracic Surgery

Preoperative Management

▷ Assessment

Chest auscultation gives an estimate of the intensity of breath sounds in the different regions of the lungs (see Chap. 21). When the chest is auscultated, it is important to note whether breath sounds are normal, indicating a free flow of air in and out of the lungs. (In the patient with emphysema, the breath sounds may be markedly decreased or even absent on auscultation.) Crackles, wheezes, and hyperresonance are noted, along with decreased diaphragmatic motion. Unilateral diminished breath sounds and rhonchi can be the result of occlusion of the bronchi by mucus plugs. Evidence of retained secretions is evaluated during auscultation by asking the patient to cough. Any signs of rhonchi or wheezing are noted. The nursing assessment includes the following:

- What signs and symptoms are present—cough, expectoration (amount), hemoptysis, chest pain, dyspnea?
- What is the smoking history? How long has the patient been smoking? How much is he currently smoking?
- What is the patient's cardiopulmonary tolerance while resting, eating, bathing, walking?
- What is his breathing pattern? How much exertion is required to produce dyspnea?
- What is the physiologic age of the patient—for example, general appearance, mental alertness, behavior, degree of nutrition?
- What other medical conditions exist—allergies, *etc*?
- What are his personal preferences and dislikes?

▷ Nursing Diagnoses

Based on the assessment data, the patient's major preoperative nursing diagnoses may include the following:

- Impaired gas exchange related to lung impairment
- Ineffective airway clearance related to lung impairment
- Knowledge deficit about the surgical procedure and self-care
- Anxiety related to diagnosis and surgical procedure

▷ Planning and Implementation

▷ *Goals:* The major goals for the patient may include improvement of gas exchange, improvement in airway clearance, acquisition of knowledge about the surgical procedure and self-care, and relief of anxiety.

Nursing Interventions

Improvement of Gas Exchange. An important preoperative goal is to improve alveoli ventilation, thereby enhancing gas exchange. The nurse assists in the delivery of care, which includes avoidance of bronchial irritants, especially cigarette smoking; drinking of more fluids and use of humidification to loosen secretions; administration of bronchodilators as prescribed to relieve bronchospasm; and instruction in diaghragmatic breathing for more effective ventilation. Incentive spirometry is initiated preoperatively to teach the patient the technique so postoperatively he will be able to perform the maneuver without problems.

Improvement of Airway Clearance. The underlying lung condition is often associated with increased respiratory secretions. Preoperatively, the airways are cleared of secretions to reduce the possibility of postoperative atelectasis or infection. This is accomplished through humidification, postural drainage, and chest percussion following the administration of bronchodilators, if prescribed. The volume of sputum is measured daily in patients who expectorate large amounts of secretions. Such measurements are carried out to determine if the amount is decreasing. Antibiotics are administered as prescribed for infection, which may be causing the excessive secretions.

Understanding of the Surgical Procedure and Self-Care Techniques. The patient is informed of what to expect in the postoperative period, that is, the possible presence of chest tube(s) and drainage bottles, the usual postoperative administration of oxygen to facilitate breathing, and the possible use of a ventilator. The importance of frequent turning to promote drainage of lung secretions is explained. Instruction in the use of incentive spirometry begins preoperatively to familiarize the patient with its correct use. Diaphragmatic and pursed lip breathing are taught and should be practiced at this time.

Since a coughing schedule will be necessary in the postoperative period to bring up secretions, the patient should be instructed in the technique of coughing and warned that the coughing routine may prove to be uncomfortable. He is taught to splint his incision with his hands, a pillow, or a folded towel.

The patient is taught coughing and huffing techniques as follows:

Coughing Technique
1. Sit upright with knees flexed and body bent slightly forward.
2. Splint the incisional area with firm hand pressure or support it with a pillow or rolled blanket while coughing. (The nurse can initially demonstrate this by using her hands.)
3. Take three deep breaths followed by a deep inspiration (inhaling slowly and evenly through the nose).
4. Contract (pull in) the abdominal muscles and cough twice forcefully, with mouth open and tongue out.
5. If unable to sit, lie on one side with hips and knees flexed.

Huffing Technique
''Huffing'' is the expulsion of air through an open glottis and may be helpful for the patient with diminished expiratory flow rates or for the patient in severe pain who refuses to

cough. This type of forceful exhalation stimulates pulmonary expansion and assists in alveolar inflation.

1. Take a deep diaphragmatic breath and exhale forcefully against your hand. Exhale forcefully in a quick, distinct pant, or "huff."
2. Practice doing small "huffs" and progress to one strong "huff" during exhalation.

Relief of Anxiety. Patients are admitted only 1 or 2 days prior to surgery, which does not provide much time for the nurse to talk with the patient. To effectively use the time before surgery, the nurse listens to the patient to evaluate how he feels about his illness and proposed treatment. She also determines his motivation to return to normal function. He may reveal significant reactions: the fear of hemorrhage because of bloody sputum, the discomfort of a chronic cough and chest pain, or the fear of death because of dyspnea and tumor.

The nurse helps the patient overcome many of his fears and mobilize his intellectual functions to cope with the stress of surgery. This is done by correcting any false impressions, by offering reassurance about the capability of the surgical team, by reassuring the patient that his incision will "hold," and by dealing honestly with questions about pain and discomfort and their treatment. The management and control of pain begins before surgery when the patient is informed that he can overcome many postoperative problems by following certain routines related to deep breathing, coughing, turning, and moving.

▷ *Evaluation*

▷ *Expected Outcomes*

1. Patient improves gas exchange.
   a. Stops smoking.
   b. Avoids bronchial irritants.
   c. Demonstrates diaphragmatic breathing.
   d. Uses incentive spirometer correctly.
2. Improves airway clearance.
   a. Verbalizes importance of measures to improve airway clearance (humidification, postural drainage, chest percussion, bronchodilators).
   b. Collects sputum so that it can be measured.
3. Attains knowledge of surgery and care.
   a. Verbalizes what to expect in postoperative period, especially the presence of chest tubes.
   b. Demonstrates effective breathing, coughing, and splinting techniques.
4. Improves ability to cope.
   a. Verbalizes that misconceptions have been clarified.
   b. Expresses confidence in the capability of the hospital staff.
   c. Demonstrates techniques to help control pain such as deep breathing, coughing, turning, and moving.

Postoperative Management

Potential Complications

Complications following thoracic surgery are always a possibility and are identified and managed early. Pulmonary edema due to overinfusion of intravenous fluids is a real danger. The early symptoms are dyspnea, crackles, bubbling sounds in the chest, cyanosis, and pink, frothy sputum. This constitutes an emergency and is reported immediately. In addition, the patient is monitored at regular intervals for signs of hemorrhage, mediastinal shift, bronchopulmonary fistula, infection, shock, atelectasis, pneumothorax, dysrhythmias, pleural effusion, and gastric distention.

Chest Drainage

A crucial intervention for improving gas exchange and breathing is the proper management of chest drainage. Following thoracic surgery, chest tubes and a closed drainage system are used to reexpand the involved lung and to remove excess air and fluid (or blood).

The normal breathing mechanism operates on the principle of negative pressure (the pressure in the chest cavity is lower than the pressure of the atmosphere, causing air to move into the lungs during inspiration). Whenever the chest is opened, from any cause, there is a loss of negative pressure, which can result in the collapse of the lung. The collection of air, fluid, or other substances in the chest can compromise cardiopulmonary function and even cause collapse of the lung. Pathologic substances that collect in the pleural space include fibrin, or clotted blood; liquids (serous fluids, blood, pus, chyle); and gases (air from the lung, tracheobronchial tree, or esophagus).

Surgical incision of the chest wall almost always causes some degree of pneumothorax. Air and fluid collect in the intrapleural space, restricting lung expansion and reducing air exchange. It is necessary to keep the pleural space evacuated postoperatively and to maintain negative pressure within this potential space. Therefore, during or immediately after thoracic surgery, chest catheters are positioned strategically in the pleural space (see Fig. 22-9), sutured to the skin, and connected to some type of drainage apparatus in order to remove the residual air and drainage fluid from the pleural or mediastinal space. This results in the reexpansion of remaining lung tissue.

A chest drainage system must be capable of removing whatever collects in the pleural space so that a normal pleural space and normal cardiopulmonary function may be restored and maintained. There are many types of commercial chest drainage systems in use, most of which use the water-seal principle. The chest catheter is attached to a bottle, using a one-way valve principle. Water acts as a seal and permits air and fluid to drain from the chest, but air cannot reenter the submerged tip of the tube. The care of the patient with water-seal chest drainage is discussed in Chart 22-6.

Chest drainage can be categorized into three types of mechanical systems (Fig. 22-10, p. 450).

Single-Bottle Water-Seal System. The end of the drainage tube from the patient's chest is covered by a layer of water, which permits drainage of air and fluid from the pleural space but does not allow air to move back into the chest. Functionally, drainage depends on gravity, on the mechanics of respiration, and, if desired, on suction by the addition of *controlled* vacuum.

The tube from the patient extends approximately 2.5 cm (1 inch) below the level of the water in the container. There is a vent for the escape of any air that might be leaking from the lung. The water level fluctuates as the patient breathes; it goes up when the patient inhales and down when the patient exhales. At the end of the drainage tube, bubbling may or may not be visible. Bubbling can mean either persistent leak-

Chart 22-6
Guidelines to the Nurse's Role in the Management of the Patient With Water-Seal Chest Drainage*

An intrapleural drainage tube is used after most intrathoracic procedures. One or more chest catheters are held in the pleural space by suture to the chest wall and are attached to a drainage system. The purposes are

1. To remove solids, liquids, and gas from the pleural space or thoracic cavity and the mediastinal space
2. To bring about reexpansion of the lung and restore normal cardiorespiratory function after surgery, trauma, or medical conditions by establishing negative pressure in the pleural cavity

Procedure

Nursing Action	*Rationale/Amplification*
1. Fill the water-seal chamber with sterile water to the level equaling 2 cm H_2O	Water-seal drainage provides for the escape of air and fluid into a drainage bottle. The water acts as a seal and keeps the air from being drawn back into the pleural space.
2. If suction is used, fill the suction control chamber with sterile water to the 20-cm level or as prescribed.	The water level will determine the degree of suction applied.
3. Attach the drainage catheter from the pleural space (the patient) to the tubing coming from the collection chamber of the water seal system. Tape securely.	In disposable units, the system is a closed system, with the only connection being the one to the patient catheter.
4. If suction is used, connect the suction control chamber tubing to the suction unit. Turn on suction unit and increase pressure until bubbling appears in the suction control chamber.	The degree of suction is determined by the amount of water in the suction control chamber and *is not* dependent on the rate of bubbling nor the pressure gauge setting on the suction unit.
5. Mark the original fluid level with tape on the outside of the drainage unit. Mark hourly/daily increments (date and time) at the drainage level.	This marking will show the amount of fluid loss and how fast fluid is collecting in the drainage bottle. It serves as a basis for blood replacement, if the fluid is blood. Grossly bloody drainage will appear in the bottle in the immediate postoperative period and if excessive may require reoperation. Drainage usually declines progressively in the first 24 hours.
6. Ensure that the tubing is not looping or interfering with the movements of the patient.	Kinking, looping, or pressure on the drainage tubing can produce back-pressure, and may thus possibly force drainage back into the pleural space or impede drainage from the pleural space.
7. Encourage the patient to assume a position of comfort. Encourage good body alignment. When the patient is in the lateral position, place a rolled towel under the tubing to protect it from the weight of the patient's body. Encourage the patient to change position frequently.	The patient's position should be changed frequently to promote drainage, and the body should be kept in good alignment to prevent postural deformities and contractures. Proper positioning helps breathing and promotes better air exchange. Pain medication may be needed to enhance comfort and deep breathing.
8. Put the arm and shoulder of the affected side through range of motion exercises several times daily. Some pain medication may be necessary.	Exercise helps to avoid ankylosis of the shoulder and assists in lessening postoperative pain and discomfort.

* There are commerical disposable chest drainage devices available that use the water-seal principle, and these guidelines refer to their use.

(continued)

age of air from the lung or other tissues or a leak in the system.

Two-Bottle System. The two-bottle system consists of the same water-seal chamber plus a fluid collection bottle. Drainage is similar to that of a single unit, except that when pleural fluid drains, the underwater seal system is not affected by the volume of drainage.

Effective drainage depends on gravity or on the amount of suction added to the system. When vacuum (suction) is added to the system from a vacuum source, such as wall

Chart 22-6 *(continued)*

Nursing Action	*Rationale/Amplification*
9. "Milk" the tubing in the direction of the drainage chamber every 2 hours.	"Milking" the tubing prevents it from becoming plugged with clots and fibrin. Constant attention to maintaining the patency of the tube facilitates prompt expansion of the lung and minimizes complications.
10. Make sure there is fluctuation ("tidaling") of the fluid level in the water-seal chamber.	Fluctuation of the water level in the tube shows that there is effective communication between the pleural cavity and the drainage bottle, provides a valuable indication of the patency of the drainage system, and is a gauge of intrapleural pressure.

11. Fluctuations of fluid in the tubing will stop when
  a. The lung has reexpanded
  b. The tubing is obstructed by blood clots or fibrin, or kinking
  c. A dependent loop develops
  d. Suction motor or wall suction is not working properly	

12. Watch for leaks of air in the drainage system as indicated by constant bubbling in the water-seal chamber.
  a. Report excessive bubbling in the water-seal chamber immediately.
  b. "Milking" of chest tubes in patients with air leaks should only be done if requested by the surgeon.
	Leaking and trapping of air in the pleural space can result in tension pneumothorax.

13. Observe and report immediately signs of rapid, shallow breathing; cyanosis; pressure in the chest; subcutaneous emphysema; symptoms of hemorrhage; significant changes in color or vital signs.	Many clinical conditions may cause these signs and symptoms, including tension pneumothorax, mediastinal shift, hemorrhage, severe incisional pain, pulmonary embolus, and cardiac tamponade. Surgical intervention may be necessary.
14. Encourage the patient to breathe deeply and cough at frequent intervals. If there are signs of incisional pain, adequate pain medication is indicated.	Deep breathing and coughing help to raise the intrapleural pressure, which allows emptying of any accumulation in the pleural space and removes secretions from the tracheobronchial tree, so that the lung expands and atelectasis is prevented.
15. If the patient has to be transported to another area, place the drainage system below the chest level, if he is lying on a stretcher. If the tube becomes disconnected, cut off the contaminated tips of the chest tube and tubing, insert a sterile connector in the chest tube and tubing, and reattach to the drainage system. Otherwise, do not clamp chest tube during transport.	The drainage apparatus must be kept at a level lower than the patient's chest to prevent backflow of fluid into the pleural space.

16. When assisting the surgeon in removing the tube:
  a. Instruct the patient to perform the Valsalva maneuver (forcible exhalation against a closed glottis, holding one's breath).
  b. The chest tube is clamped and quickly removed.
  c. Simultaneously, a small bandage is applied and made airtight with petrolatum gauze covered by a 4 × 4-inch gauze pad and thoroughly covered and sealed with adhesive tape.
	The chest tube is removed as directed when the lung is reexpanded (usually 24 hours to several days). During removal of the tube the chief priorities are prevention of entrance of air into the pleural cavity as the tube is withdrawn and prevention of infection.

suction, the connection is made at the vent stem of the underwater-seal bottle. The amount of suction applied to the system is regulated by the wall gauge.

Three-Bottle System.   The three-bottle system is similar in all respects to the two-bottle system, except for the addition of a third bottle to control the amount of suction applied. The amount of suction is determined by the depth to which the tip of the venting glass tube is submerged. (For example, submersion to 10 cm below the surface of the water will equal 10 cm of water suction applied to the patient.)

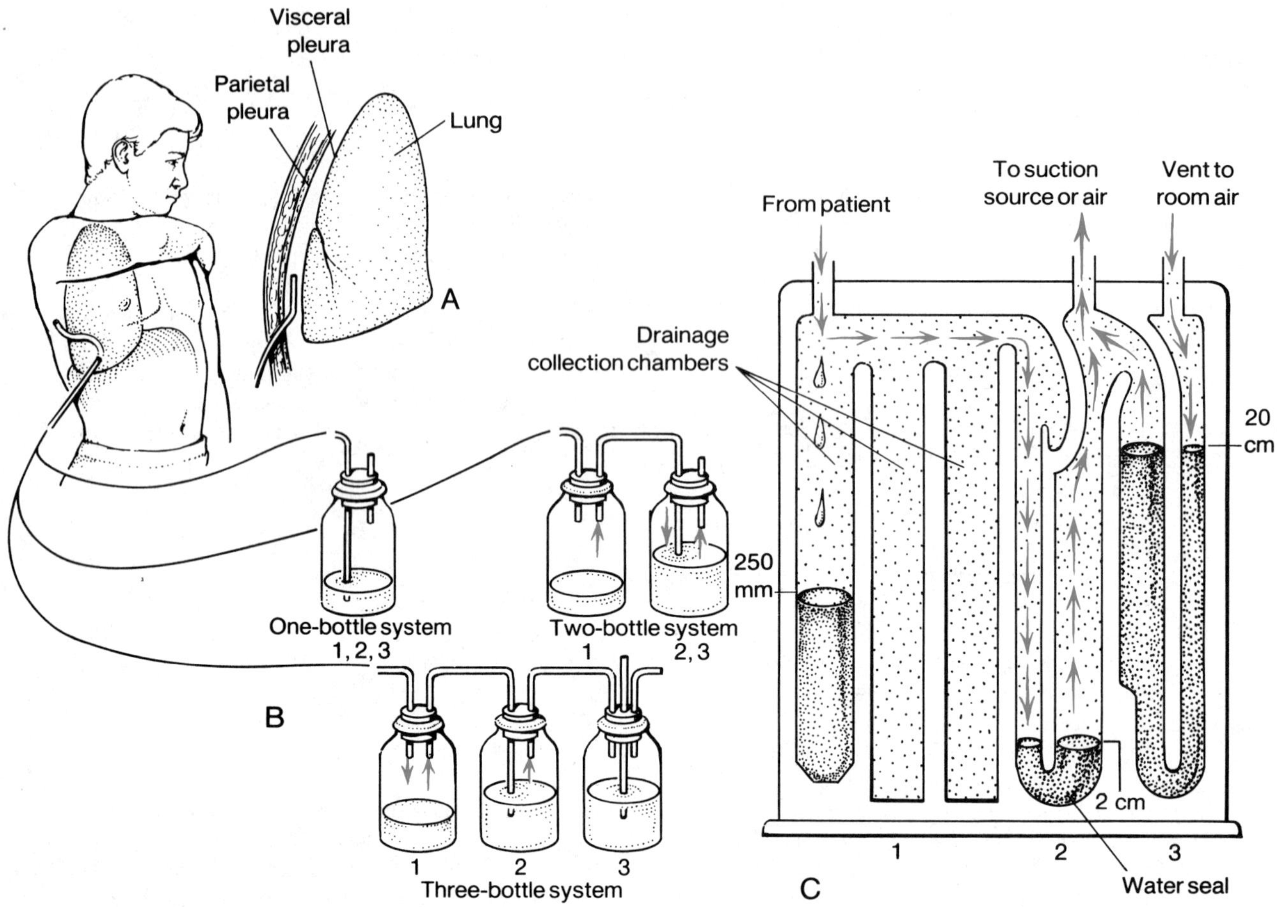

Figure 22-10
Chest drainage system. (*A*) Strategic placement of a chest catheter in the pleural space.
(*B*) Three types of mechanical drainage systems. (*C*) A Pleur-Evac operating system:
(1) the collection chamber, (2) the water seal chamber, and (3) the suction control
chamber. The Pleur-Evac is a single unit with all three bottles identified as chambers.

In the three-bottle system (as in the other two), drainage depends on gravity or the amount of suction applied. The amount of suction in this system is controlled by the manometer bottle. The mechanical suction motor or wall suction creates and maintains a negative pressure throughout the entire closed drainage system.

The third bottle regulates the amount of vacuum in the system. This depends on the depth to which the tube is submerged—the usual depth is 20 cm (7.6 inches).

When the vacuum in the system becomes greater than the depth to which the tube is submerged, outside air is sucked into the system. This results in constant bubbling in the manometer (or pressure-regulator) bottle, which indicates that the system is functioning properly.

- *Note:* When the motor is off or the wall vacuum is turned off, the drainage system should be open to the atmosphere so that intrapleural air can escape from the system. This can be done by detaching the tubing from the suction port to provide a vent.

In the commercially available systems, all three bottles are contained in a single unit and are identified as "chambers." These systems are safer because they are self-contained, unbreakable, and disposable, and have no connections (except to the chest catheter) that may become loose. Nursing care is easier to provide, and their convenience encourages easier and earlier ambulation for the patient.

▷ *Assessment*

The character and depth of the respiration and the patient's color serve as important criteria in evaluating whether the lungs are being adequately expanded. The heart rate and rhythm are monitored by auscultation and electrocardiography, since major dysrhythmic episodes are common after thoracic and cardiac surgery. Dysrhythmias can occur at any time but frequently are seen between the second and sixth postoperative days. The rate of occurrence of dysrhythmias increases with patients over 50 years of age and with those undergoing pneumonectomy or esophageal surgery.

An arterial line is maintained to facilitate frequent monitoring of blood gases, serum electrolytes, hemoglobin and hematocrit values, and arterial pressure. Central venous pressure is monitored for the early recognition of hypovolemia.

▷ Nursing Diagnoses

Based on the assessment data, the patient's major postoperative nursing diagnoses may include

- Impaired gas exchange related to lung impairment and surgery
- Ineffective airway clearance related to lung impairment and anesthesia
- Alteration in comfort, pain, related to incision, drainage tubes, and the surgical procedure
- Impaired physical mobility of the upper extremities related to thoracic surgery
- Fluid volume deficit related to the surgical procedure
- Knowledge deficit of care procedures at home

▷ Planning and Implementation

▷ *Goals:* The major goals for the patient may include improvement of gas exchange and breathing, improvement of airway clearance, relief of pain and discomfort, mobility and shoulder exercises, maintenance of adequate fluid volume, and understanding of self-care procedures.

Nursing Interventions

Improvement of Gas Exchange and Breathing. Gas exchange is determined by evaluating oxygenation and ventilation. In the immediate postoperative period, this is achieved by measuring the blood pressure, pulse, and respirations every 15 minutes for the first 1 to 2 hours, then less frequently as the patient's condition stabilizes.

The diaphragmatic and pursed lip breathing taught preoperatively should be practiced every 2 hours to expand alveoli and prevent atelectasis. Another technique to improve ventilation is sustained maximal inspiratory (SMI) therapy or incentive spirometry (p. 427). This technique optimizes lung inflation, improves the cough mechanism, and provides for early assessment of acute pulmonary changes.

When the patient is oriented and his blood pressure stabilized, the head of the bed is elevated 30 to 40 degrees during the immediate postoperative period. This facilitates ventilation and helps residual air to rise in the upper portion of pleural space, where it can be removed through the upper chest tube.

The surgeon is consulted about individual patient positioning. The patient with limited respiratory reserve may not be able to turn on the unoperated side, since this limits ventilation of the operated side. The position is varied from horizontal to semi-upright, since remaining in one position tends to promote the retention of secretions in the dependent portion of the lungs. Following a pneumonectomy, the operated side should be dependent so that fluid in the pleural space remains below the level of the bronchial stump.

Turning Procedure

1. Instruct the patient to bend his knees and use his feet to push.
2. Have the patient shift his hips and shoulders to the opposite side of the bed while pushing with his feet.
3. Bring the patient's arm over his chest, pointing it in the

direction toward which he is being turned and have him grasp the side rail with his hand.
4. Turn patient in "log roll" fashion to prevent twisting at the waist and possible pulling of the incision, which could be painful.

Improvement of Airway Clearance. Secretions become a real problem in the thoracotomy patient postoperatively. Trauma to the tracheobronchial tree during operation, diminished lung ventilation, and diminished cough reflex all result in the accumulation of excessive secretions. If the secretions are not managed or removed, airway obstruction will occur, which causes air in the alveoli distal to the obstruction to become absorbed and the lung to collapse. Atelectasis, pneumonia, and respiratory failure may result.

There are a few techniques that are used to maintain a patent airway. First, secretions are suctioned from the tracheobronchial tree before the endotracheal tube is removed (this begins in the recovery room). Secretions continue to be removed by suctioning until the patient can cough up secretions effectively. Nasoendotracheal suctioning is difficult to perform and is learned under expert clinical supervision.

Technique for Endotracheal Suctioning
(Sterile technique is to be used.)

1. Place the patient in a sitting or semi-Fowler's position. Attach the sterile catheter to tubing that has been connected to a suction device.
2. Oxygenate the patient several minutes before each suctioning procedure.
3. Give the patient a gauze square, and instruct him to grasp and pull his tongue outward; this tilts the epiglottis forward. If the patient cannot comply, have another person do this.
4. Pass a lubricated (with water-soluble gel) catheter through the nostril to the pharynx. Check the position of the tip of the catheter; it should be in the lower pharynx.
5. Instruct the patient to take a deep breath. This opens the epiglottis and helps the catheter to move in the direction of the negative pressure generated by inspiration.
6. Advance the catheter into the trachea only during inspiration.
7. Apply suction intermittently by closing the open end of the "Y" or "T" catheter with the finger and slowly rotating the catheter between the thumb and forefinger.
8. Avoid prolonging suction more than 10 seconds, since bradycardia or cardiac arrest may ensue in patients with borderline oxygenation.
9. While the catheter is being withdrawn, apply gentle suction to clear the tracheal walls of secretions.
10. Oxygenate for several minutes before a second passage of the catheter (if a second aspiration is necessary). Check the pulse rate.

Another measure that is used in maintaining a patent airway is the coughing technique. The patient is encouraged to cough effectively, since ineffective coughing will result in exhaustion and retention of secretions. To be effective, the cough is to be low pitched, deep, and controlled. Since it is difficult to cough in a supine position, the patient is helped to a sitting position on the edge of the bed, with his feet resting on a chair. Coughing is carried out at least every hour (as described on p. 446) during the first 24 hours and when necessary thereafter. If audible crackles are present, it may be necessary to use chest percussion with the cough routine until the lungs are clear. Aerosol therapy is helpful in humidifying and mobilizing secretions so that they can be readily coughed up. To lessen incisional pain during coughing, the nurse supports the incision firmly over the operated side and against the opposite chest (Fig. 22-11).

After helping the patient to cough, the nurse should listen to both lungs, anteriorly and posteriorly, to determine whether there are any changes in breath sounds, since diminished sounds may indicate collapsed or hypoventilated alveoli.

The final technique for maintaining a patent airway is chest physiotherapy. If a patient is identified as being at high risk of developing postoperative pulmonary complications, then chest physiotherapy is started immediately (perhaps even preoperatively). The techniques of postural drainage, vibra-

tion, and percussion help to loosen and mobilize the secretions so that they can be coughed up or suctioned (see p. 451).

Relief of Pain and Discomfort. Pain following a thoracotomy may be severe, depending on the type of incision and the patient's reaction to and ability to cope with pain. Deep inspiration is very painful following thoracotomy. Pain can lead to postoperative complications if it reduces the patient's ability to breathe deeply and cough and if it further limits chest excursions so that effective ventilation is decreased. Immediately after the surgical procedure and before the incision is closed, the surgeon may perform a nerve block with a long-acting local anesthetic, which can reduce postoperative pain. Small, intravenous doses of a narcotic are given as prescribed and are titrated to relieve pain while still allowing the patient to cooperate in deep breathing, coughing, and mobilization efforts. However, it is important to avoid depressing the respiratory system with too much narcotic, since the patient should not be so somnolent that he does not cough.

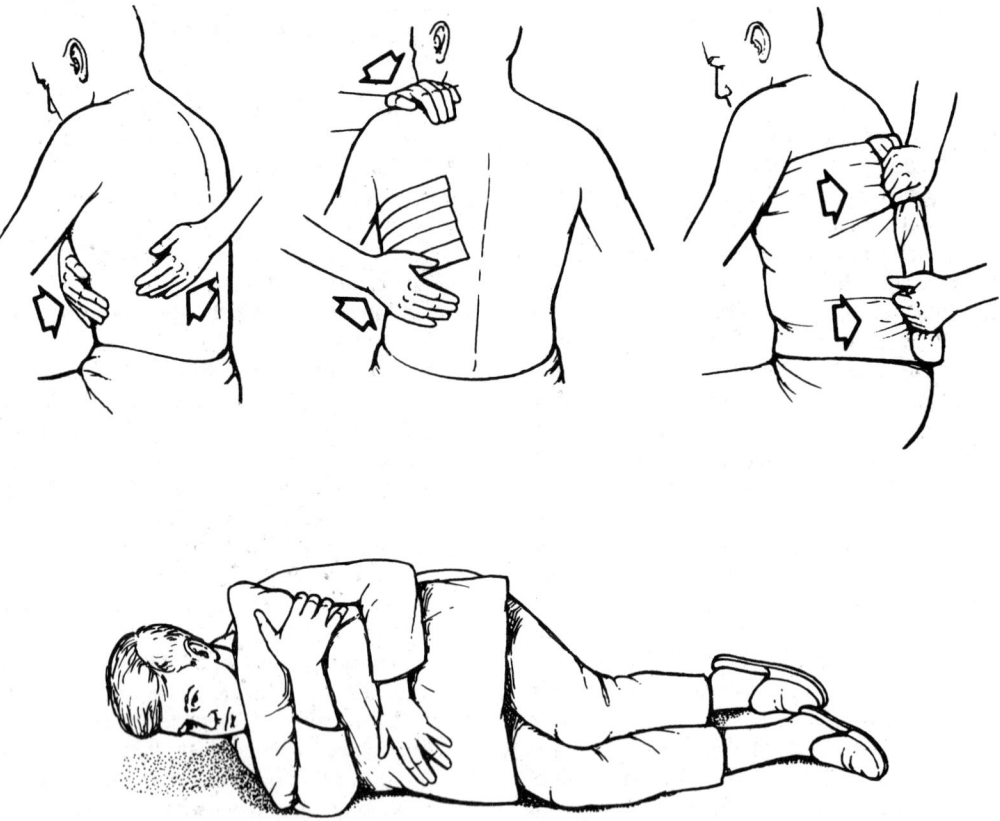

Figure 22-11

Techniques for support of incision while patient with thoracic surgery coughs. (*Top left*) The nurse's hands should support the chest incision anteriorly and posteriorly. The patient is instructed to take several deep breaths, inhale, and then cough forcibly. (*Top middle*) With one hand, the nurse exerts downward pressure on the shoulder of the affected side while firmly supporting beneath the wound with the other hand. The patient is instructed to take several deep breaths, inhale, and then cough forcibly. (*Top right*) The nurse can wrap a towel or sheet around the patient's chest and hold the ends together, pulling slightly as the patient coughs, releasing as he takes deep breaths. (*Bottom*) The patient can be taught to hold a pillow firmly against his incision while coughing. This can be done while lying down or sitting in an upright position.

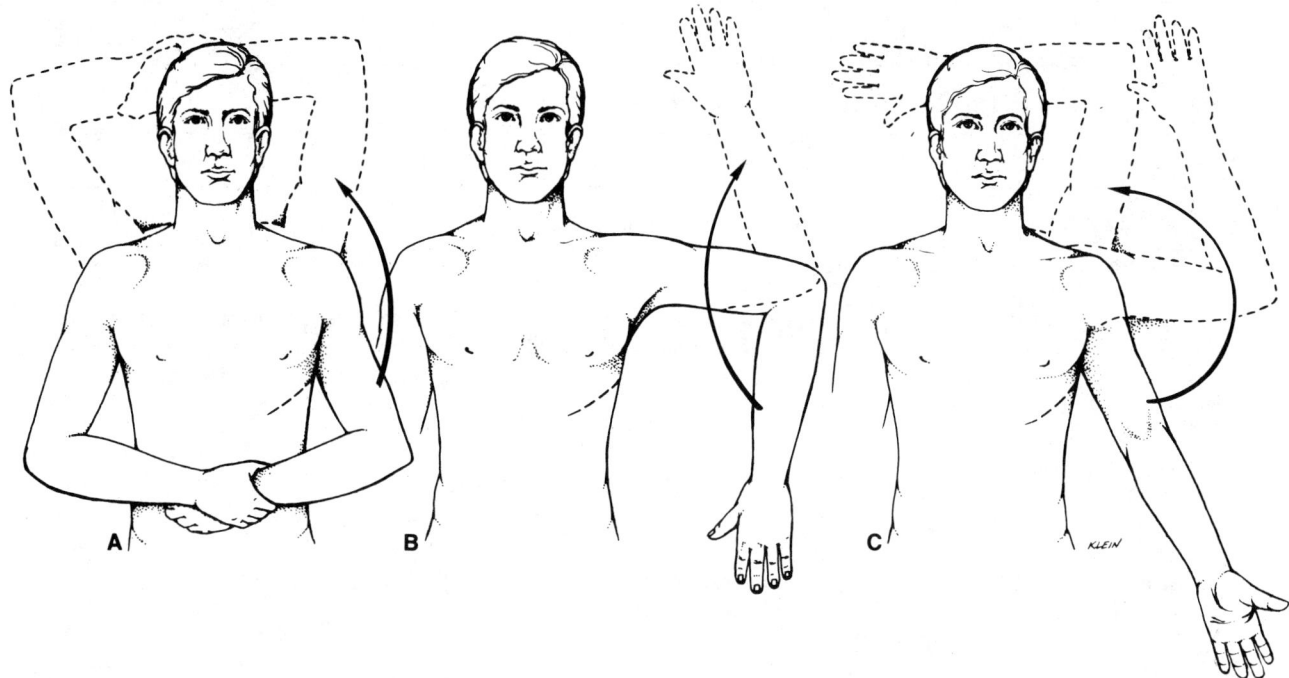

Figure 22-12
Arm and shoulder exercises are done following thoracic surgery to restore movement, prevent painful stiffening of the shoulder, and improve muscle power. (*A*) Hold hand of the affected side with the other hand, palms facing in. Raise the arms forward, upward, and then overhead, while taking a deep breath. Exhale while lowering the arms. Repeat five times. (*B*) Raise arm sideward, upward, and downward in a waving motion. (*C*) Place arm at side. Raise arm sideward, upward, and over the head. Repeat five times. Both exercises can also be done while lying in bed.

- *Note:* Do not confuse the restlessness of hypoxia with restlessness due to pain. Dyspnea, restlessness, increasing respiratory rate, increasing blood pressure, and tachycardia are warning signs of impending respiratory insufficiency.

Mobility and Shoulder Exercises. When the physician determines that the patient is ready for activity, he may get out of bed. Often this occurs on the evening of the day of surgery. Although this may be painful initially, the earlier the patient moves, the sooner the pain will subside. In addition to getting out of bed, arm and shoulder exercises are started (Fig. 22-12) to restore movement and prevent painful stiffening of the affected arm and shoulder. Specific skeletal exercises designed to restore function following thoracic surgery are described in Table 22-3.

(Text continues on p. 457)

TABLE 22-3
Skeletal Exercises Designed to Restore Function Following Thoracic Surgery

Muscle Affected by Thoracotomy	Function	Activities to Restore Function
Trapezius	Promotes arm extension, abduction, and reach extension	Extend the arm up and back, out to the side and back, down at the side and back.
Rhomboideus major	Adducts and slightly elevates scapula	Place hands in small of back. Push elbows as far back as possible.
Latissimus dorsi	Depresses the shoulder	Sit erect in an armchair: place the hands on the arms of the chair directly opposite either side of the body. Press down on hands, consciously pulling the abdomen in and stretching up from the waist. Inhale while raising the body until the elbows are extended completely. Hold this position a moment, and begin exhaling while lowering the body slowly to the original position.
Serratus anterior	Rotates scapula and fixes it against the rib cage	Reach over head and "push" in an upward and outward motion.

Care of the Patient Following Thoracotomy

Nursing Interventions	*Rationale*	*Expected Outcomes*

Nursing Diagnosis: Impaired gas exchange related to lung impairment and surgery

Goal: Improvement of gas exchange and breathing

1. Monitor pulmonary status as directed and as needed:
  a. Auscultate breath sounds.
  b. Check rate depth and pattern of respirations.
  c. Evaluate patient's color for cyanosis.
  d. Assess blood gases for signs of hypoxemia or CO_2 retention.
	1. Changes in pulmonary status indicate improvement or onset of complications.	• Lungs are clear on auscultation.
		• Respiratory rate is within normal range with no episodes of dyspnea.

2. Take and record blood pressure, apical pulse, and temperature every 2–4 hours, central venous pressure (if used) every 2 hours.	2. Aid in evaluating effect of surgery on cardiac status.	• Vital signs are stable.
3. Monitor continuous electrocardiogram for pattern and dysrhythmias.	3. Dysrhythmias are more frequently seen after thoracic surgery (especially atrial fibrillation and atrial flutter). A patient with total pneumonectomy is especially prone to cardiac irregularity.	• Dysrhythmias are not present or are under control.
4. Elevate head of bed 30 to 40 degrees when patient is oriented and hemodynamic status is stable.	4. Maximum lung excursion is achieved when patient is as close to upright as possible.	
5. Encourage deep breathing exercises (see section Breathing Retraining, p. 429) and effective use of incentive spirometer (sustained maximal inspiration).	5. Helps to achieve maximal lung inflation and to open closed airways.	• Demonstrates deep, controlled, effective breathing to allow maximal lung expansion. • Uses incentive spirometer every 2 hours while awake.
6. Encourage and promote an effective cough routine to be performed every 1 to 2 hours.	6. Coughing is necessary to remove retained secretions, which will be difficult to move from operative side.	• Demonstrates deep, effective coughing technique.

7. Assess and monitor the water-seal system*:
  a. Assess for leaks and patency as needed.
  b. Monitor amount and character of drainage and document every 2 hours. Notify physician if drainage is 150 ml/hr or greater.
  c. See Chart 22-4 for summary of nurse's role in management of water-seal drainage.
	7. System is used to eliminate any residual air or fluid following thoracotomy.	• Lungs are expanded to capacity (evidenced by chest film).

* A patient with a pneumonectomy usually does not have water-seal chest drainage, since it is desirable that the pleural space fill with an effusion, which eventually obliterates this space. Some surgeons do use a "modified" water-seal system.

(continued)

Nursing Interventions	Rationale	Expected Outcomes

Nursing Diagnosis: Ineffective airway clearance related to lung impairment and anesthesia

Goals: Improvement of airway clearance
Achievement of a patent airway

Nursing Interventions	Rationale	Expected Outcomes
1. Maintain an open airway.	1. Provides for adequate ventilation and gas exchange.	• Airway is patent.
2. Perform endotracheal suctioning until patient is able to raise secretions effectively.	2. Endotracheal secretions are present in excessive amounts in post-thoracotomy patients owing to trauma to the tracheobronchial tree during surgery, diminished lung ventilation, and cough reflex.	
3. Encourage deep breathing and coughing exercises. Assist in splinting the incision during coughing.	3. Helps to achieve maximal lung inflation and to open closed airways. Coughing is painful; incision needs to be supported.	• Coughs effectively. • Splints incision while coughing.
4. Monitor amount, viscosity, color, and odor of sputum. Notify physician if sputum is excessive or contains bright red blood.	4. Changes in sputum suggest presence of infection or change in pulmonary status. Colorless sputum is not unusual; opacification or coloring of sputum may indicate dehydration or infection.	• Sputum is clear or colorless.
5. Administer humidification and mini-nebulizer therapy as prescribed.	5. Secretions must be moistened and thinned if they are to be raised from the chest with the least amount of effort.	
6. Perform postural drainage, percussion, and vibration as prescribed. Do not percuss or vibrate directly over operative site.	6. Chest physiotherapy uses gravity to help remove secretions from the lung.	
7. Auscultate both sides of chest to determine changes in breath sounds.	7. Indications for tracheal aspirations are determined by chest auscultation.	• Lungs are clear on auscultation.

Nursing Diagnosis: Alteration in comfort, pain, related to incision and surgical procedure

Goal: Relief of pain and discomfort

Nursing Interventions	Rationale	Expected Outcomes
1. Evaluate location, character, quality and degree of pain. Administer pain medication as prescribed and as needed. • Watch for respiratory effect of narcotic or analgesic. Is patient too somnolent to cough? Are respirations depressed?	1. Pain limits chest excursions and thereby decreases ventilation.	• Asks for pain medication, but verbalizes he expects some discomfort while deep breathing and coughing.
2. Maintain care postoperatively in positioning the thoracotomy patient: a. Place patient in semi-Fowler's position. b. Patients with limited respiratory reserve may not be able to turn on unoperated side. c. Assist or turn patient every 2 hours.	2. If patient is comfortable and free of pain, he will be less likely to splint his chest while breathing. A semi-Fowler's position permits residual air to rise to upper portion of pleural space and be removed via the upper chest catheter.	• Verbalizes that he is comfortable and in no acute distress.

(continued)

Nursing Interventions	*Rationale*	*Expected Outcomes*

Nursing Diagnosis: Alteration in comfort, pain, related to incision and surgical procedure

Goal: Relief of pain and discomfort

3. Assess incision area every 8 hours for signs of infection: redness, heat, induration, swelling, separation, and drainage.		• No signs of incisional infection evident.

Impaired physical mobility of the upper extremities related to thoracic surgery

Absence of disability of the affected shoulder and arm

Assist patient with normal range of motion and function of shoulder and trunk. a. Teach breathing exercises to mobilize thorax. b. Encourage skeletal exercises to promote abduction and mobilization of shoulder (see Fig. 22-7 and Table 22-3). c. Ambulate as soon as pulmonary and circulatory systems are compensated (usually by evening of surgery). d. Encourage progressive activities according to development of fatigue.	Necessary to regain normal mobility of arm and shoulder and to speed recovery and minimize discomfort.	• Demonstrates arm and shoulder exercises and verbalizes intent to perform them on discharge.

Nursing Diagnosis: Fluid volume deficit related to the surgical procedure

Goal: Maintenance of adequate fluid volume

1. Monitor and record hourly intake and output. Patient should excrete at least 30 ml of urine hourly after surgery. 2. Administer blood and parenteral fluids as prescribed to restore and maintain fluid volume.	1. Fluid management may be altered before, during, and after surgery, and patient's response to and need for fluid management must be assessed. 2. Pulmonary edema owing to transfusion overload is an ever-present threat; following pneumonectomy, the pulmonary vascular system has been greatly reduced.	• Patient is adequately hydrated.

Nursing Diagnosis: Knowledge deficit of care procedures at home

Goal: Ability to carry out care procedures at home

1. Encourage patient to practice arm and shoulder exercises five times daily at home. 2. Instruct patient to practice assuming a functionally erect position in front of a full-length mirror.	1. Exercise accelerates recovery of muscle function and reduces long-term pain and discomfort. 2. Practice will help restore normal posture.	• Demonstrates arm and shoulder exercises. • Verbalizes need to try to assume an erect posture.

(continued)

Nursing Interventions	*Rationale*	*Expected Outcomes*

Nursing Diagnosis: Knowledge deficit of care procedures at home

Goal: Ability to carry out care procedures at home

3. Instruct patient in following aspects of home care:		• Verbalizes the importance of relieving discomfort, alternating walking and rest, practicing breathing exercises, avoiding heavy lifting, avoiding undue fatigue, avoiding bronchial irritants, preventing colds or lung infections, getting flu vaccine, keeping follow-up visits, and stopping smoking.
a. Relieve intercostal pain by local heat or oral analgesia.	a. Some soreness may persist for several weeks.	
b. Alternate activities with frequent rest periods.	b. Weakness and fatigability are common for the first 3 weeks.	
c. Practice the breathing exercises at home.	c. Effective breathing is necessary to prevent splinting of affected side, which may lead to atelectasis.	
d. Avoid heavy lifting until complete healing has occurred.	d. Chest muscles may be weaker than normal for 3 to 6 months.	
e. Avoid undue fatigue, increased shortness of breath, or chest pain.	e. Undue stress may prolong the healing process.	
f. Avoid bronchial irritants.	f. The lung's resistance is lowered and more susceptible to irritant substances.	
g. Prevent colds or lung infection.	g. The lung is more susceptible during the recovery phase.	
h. Get annual influenza vaccine.	h. Vaccination helps prevent flu.	
i. Keep follow-up appointment with physician.		
j. Stop smoking!	j. Smoking will slow healing process and make lung susceptible to infection and other complications.	

Fluid Volume and Nutritional Considerations. During the operation or immediately after, the patient may receive a blood transfusion, followed by an intravenous infusion to "keep the vein open" until the blood volume can be reassessed. The rate of administration is slow (10 ml/hr), especially when there is evidence of limited cardiopulmonary reserve and when the pulmonary vascular bed has been greatly reduced, as in pneumonectomy.

A liquid diet is provided as soon as there is evidence of bowel sounds. The patient is progressed to a full diet as soon as possible. Well-balanced meals are crucial to the recovery and maintenance of lung function.

Patient Education and Home Care Considerations. Because large shoulder girdle muscles are transected during a thoracotomy, the arm and shoulder must be mobilized by full range of motion of the shoulder. This is accomplished by teaching the patient exercises necessary to improve function and encouraging him to continue them on discharge. He is taught to extend his arm (stretch and reach) and then reach behind his head, and to do these exercises five times daily (see Fig. 22-12 and Table 22-3). This accelerates recovery of muscle function affected by incision, pain, and "splinting," and reduces long-term pain and discomfort and particularly the development of adhesions. All joints should be stretched and flexed. The patient is encouraged to assume a functional erect position to restore normal posture (preferably in front of a full-length mirror).

In addition to the arm and shoulder exercises, the patient is instructed in the following on discharge:

1. Relieve intercostal pain that may occur by using local heat and oral analgesia.
2. Alternate walking and other activities with frequent rest periods. Be aware that weakness and fatigue are common for the first 3 weeks.
3. Practice breathing exercises for the first few weeks at home.
4. Avoid lifting more than 20 pounds until complete healing has taken place; the chest muscles may be weaker than normal for 3 to 6 months following surgery.
5. Walk at a moderate pace, and gradually extend walking time and distance. Be persistent.
6. Stop any activity immediately that causes undue fatigue, increased shortness of breath, or chest pain.
7. Avoid bronchial irritants (smoke, fumes, air pollution, aerosol sprays).

8. Prevent colds or lung infections.
9. Get an annual influenza vaccine. Also discuss vaccination against pneumonia with the physician.
10. Report for follow-up care by the surgeon or clinic as necessary.
11. Stop smoking!

▷ *Evaluation*

▷ *Expected Outcomes*

1. Improves gas exchange.
   a. Demonstrates diaphragmatic and pursed lip breathing.
   b. Uses incentive spirometer hourly while awake.
   c. Verbalizes absence of dyspnea.
2. Improves airway clearance.
   a. Is free of infection.
   b. Demonstrates deep, controlled coughing.
   c. Verbalizes importance of humidity for keeping secretions moist.
3. Is relieved of pain and discomfort.
   a. Verbalizes that pain is diminishing.
   b. Splints incision during coughing.
4. Improves mobility of shoulder and arm; demonstrates arm and shoulder exercises to relieve stiffening.
5. Maintains adequate fluid intake.
   a. Drinks 6 to 8 glasses of water a day.
   b. Eats well-balanced meals.
6. Adheres to therapeutic program and home care.
   a. Demonstrates arm and shoulder exercises and the importance of practicing them five times a day.
   b. Verbalizes the importance of alternating walking and rest, practicing breathing exercises, avoiding heavy lifting, relieving intercostal pain, avoiding bronchial irritants, preventing colds or lung infections, getting flu and pneumonia vaccines, keeping follow-up appointment, and stopping smoking.

For a detailed plan of nursing care for the patient who has had a thoracotomy, see Nursing Care Plan 22-1 (pp. 454–457).

Bibliography

Books

Bell CW et al. Home Care and Rehabilitation in Respiratory Medicine. Philadelphia, JB Lippincott, 1984.

Bone RC and Eubanks DH. Comprehensive Respiratory Care: A Learning System. St Louis, CV Mosby, 1985.

Borg N et al (eds). Core Curriculum for Critical Care Nursing, 2nd ed. Philadelphia, WB Saunders, 1981.

Boyda EK. Respiratory Problems. Oradell, New Jersey, Medical Economics, 1985.

Burton GG and Hodgkin JE (eds). Respiratory Care—A Guide to Clinical Practice, 2nd ed. Philadelphia, JB Lippincott, 1984.

Carpenito LJ. Nursing Diagnosis—Application to Clinical Practice. Philadelphia, JB Lippincott, 1983.

Fishman AP. Pulmonary Diseases and Disorders, vol 1. New York, McGraw-Hill, 1980.

Harper R. A Guide to Respiratory Care. Philadelphia, JB Lippincott, 1981.

Hodgkin JE et al (eds). Pulmonary Rehabilitation: Guidelines to Success. Boston, Butterworth, 1984.

Holloway NM. Nursing the Critically Ill Adult. Menlo Park, California, Addison-Wesley, 1984.

Johanson BC et al. Standards For Critical Care. St Louis, CV Mosby, 1981.

Kirby RR, Smith RA, and Desautels DA. Mechanical Ventilation. New York, Churchill Livingstone, 1985.

Luce JM, Tyler M, and Pierson DJ. Intensive Respiratory Care. Philadelphia, WB Saunders, 1984.

O'Ryan JA and Burns DG. Pulmonary Rehabilitation: From Hospital to Home. Chicago, Year Book Medical Publishers, 1984.

Roberts SL. Behavioral Concepts and the Critically Ill Patient, 2nd ed. Norwalk, Connecticut, Appleton-Century Crofts, 1986.

Roberts SL. Physiological Concepts and the Critically Ill Patient. Englewood Cliffs, New Jersey, Prentice-Hall, 1985.

Spearman CB, Sheldon RL, and Egan DF. Egans' Fundamentals of Respiratory Therapy, 4th ed. St Louis, CV Mosby, 1982.

Articles

(Asterisks indicate nursing research articles.)

Therapeutics

Castillo R et al. Chest physical therapy: Comparative efficacy of preoperative and postoperative in the elderly. Arch Phys Med Rehabil 1985 June; 66(6):376–379.

Clanton TL et al. Inspiratory muscle conditioning using a threshold loading device. Chest 1985 Jan; 87(1):62–66.

Fanta CH, Leith DE, Brown R. Maximal shortening of inspiratory muscles: Effect of training. J Appl Physiol 1983 June; 54(6):1618–1623.

Fulmer JD and Snider L. American College of Chest Physicians/National Heart, Lung and Blood Institute National Conference on Oxygen Therapy. Heart Lung 1984 Sept; 13(5):550–562.

Gramse CA. CPT: Make the most of this hands-on technique. Nurs '85 1985 Jan; 15(1):32C, 32F–G.

Kirilloff LH et al. Does chest physical therapy work? Chest 1985 Sept; 88(3):436–444.

Mohsenifar Z. Mechanical ventilation and conventional chest physiotherapy in outpatients with stable chronic obstructive lung disease. Chest 1985 Apr; 87(4):483–485.

Performing postural draining. Patient Care 1984 Nov 30; 18(20):114, 119–120.

Airway Management

*Ackerman MH. The use of bolus normal saline instillations in artificial airways: Is it useful or necessary? Heart Lung 1985 Sept; 14(5):505–506.

Artificial airways: Which one's right for your patient? Nurs '85 1985 May; 15(5):8X, 8BB.

*Barnes CA and Kirchoff KT. Minimizing hypoxemia due to endotracheal suctioning: A review of the literature. Heart Lung 1986 Mar; 15(2):164–178.

*Baun MM. Physiological determinants of a clinically successful method of endotracheal suction. West J Nurs Res 1984 Spring; 6(2):214–225.

Bernhard WN et al. Intracuff pressures in endotracheal and tracheostomy tubes. Chest 1985 Jan; 87(6):720–725.

Birdsell C. What suction pressure should I use? Am J Nurs 1985 Aug; 85(8):866.

Demers RR. Management of the airway in the perioperative period. Respir Care 1984 May; 29(5):529–539.

*Goodnough SKC. The effects of oxygen and hyperinflation on arterial oxygen tension after endotracheal suctioning. Heart Lung 1985 Jan; 14(1):11–17.

*Harris RB et al. Clean vs. sterile tracheotomy care and level of pulmonary infection. Nurs Res 1984 Mar/Apr; 33(2):80–85.

Kacmarek RM. The art of artificial airways. Emerg Med 1984 Oct 15; 16(17):30–35, 38–40, 45.

Oerann MH et al. Patient sensations following a tracheostomy: A discussion. Crit Care Q 1983 Sept; 6(2):53–58.

Pfister S and Bullas J. Caring for a patient with an endotracheal tube. Crit Care Nurs 1984 Jan/Feb; 4(1):29, 56–58, 60–61.

*Riegal BA. Review and critique of the literature on preoxygenation for endotracheal suctioning. Heart Lung 1985 Sept; 14(5):507–518.

Mechanical Ventilation

Chalikian J and Weaner TE. Mechanical ventilation: Where it's at; where it's going. Am J Nurs 1984 Nov; 84(11):1372–1379.

Cronin LR and Carrizosa AA. The computer as a communication device for ventilator and tracheostomy patients in the intensive care unit. Crit Care Nurs 1984 Jan/Feb; 4(1):72–76.

Gruden M. High-frequency ventilation: An overview. Crit Care Nurs 1985 Jan/Feb; 5(1):36–40.

*Hagarty E. Weaning your COPD patient from the ventilator. Nurs Res 1984 July; 47(8):36–40.

Herrold RK. The drug connection. Am J Nurs 1984 Nov; 84(11):1389–1391.

Hess D. Bedside monitoring of the patient on a ventilator. Crit Care Q 1983 Sept; 6(2):23–32.

Irwin MM and Openbrier DR. A delicate balance: Strategies for feeding ventilated COPD patients. Am J Nurs 1985 Mar; 85(3):274–280.

Janowski MJ. Accidental disconnections from breathing systems. Am J Nurs 1984 Feb; 84(2):241–244.

*Kopacz MA and Moriarty-Wright R. Multidisciplinary approach for the patient on a home ventilator. Heart Lung 1984 May; 13(3):255–262.

Landis K and Smith S. The mechanically ventilated patient: A comprehensive nursing care plan. Crit Care Q 1983 Sept; 6(2):43–52.

Mizuki JA. There's no place like home. Am J Nurs 1984 May; 84(5):646–648.

Teaming up to send end-stage COPD patient home. Nurs '84 1984 Jan; 14(1):65–68, 71.

Votava KM et al. Home care of patients dependent on mechanical ventilation: Home care policy development and goal setting using outcome criteria for quality assurance. Home Health Care Nurs 1985 Mar/Apr; 3(2):18–25.

Zori SJ. Mechanical ventilation: Bringing the patient into focus. Am J Nurs 1984 Nov; 84(11):1384–1388.

Thoracic Surgery

Boysen PG. Assessment for lung resection. Respir Care 1984 May; 29(4):506–515.

Burkhart C. Pneumonectomy. Am J Nurs 1983 Nov; 83(11):1562–1565.

Castillo R and Haas A. Chest physical therapy: Comparative efficacy of preoperative and postoperative in the elderly. Arch Phys Med Rehabil 1985 June; 66(6):376–379.

Hodgkin JE. Preoperative assessment of respiratory function. Respir Care 1984 May; 29(5):496–505.

Hughes JM. Postoperative pulmonary care: Past, present, and future. Crit Care Q 1983 Sept; 6(2):67–71.

Luce JM. Clinical risk factors for postoperative pulmonary complications. Respir Care 1984 May; 29(5):484–495.

O'Donahue WJ. National survey of usage of lung expansion modalities for the prevention and treatment of postoperative atelectasis following abdominal and thoracic surgery. Chest 1985 Jan; 87(1):78–80.

Stock MC et al. Prevention of postoperative pulmonary complications with CPAP, incentive spirometry, and conservative therapy. Chest 1985 Feb; 87(2):151–157.

Thompson PA. Postoperative respiratory distress: Life or death? J Pract Nurs 1983 Nov/Dec; 33(9):19–22.

Unger M (ed). Symposium on laser technique. Clin Chest Med 1985 June; 6(2):177–296.

Agencies

Governmental

National Heart, Lung and Blood Institute, National Institutes of Health, Bethesda, Maryland 20892.

Voluntary

American Association for Respiratory Care, 7411 Hines Place, Suite 101, Dallas, Texas 75235.

American Lung Association, 1740 Broadway, New York, New York 10019.

American Thoracic Society, 1740 Broadway, New York, New York 10019.

Chapter 23

Respiratory Infections

Acute Tracheobronchitis

Acute tracheobronchitis is an acute inflammation of the mucous membranes of the trachea and the bronchial tree that often follows infections of the upper respiratory tract. A patient with a viral infection has a lessened resistance and can readily develop a secondary bacterial infection. Thus, the adequate treatment of upper respiratory tract infections is one of the major factors in the prevention of acute bronchitis. Aside from infection, inhalation of physical and chemical irritants, gases, or other air contaminants can also cause acute bronchial irritations.

Clinical Manifestations.   The signs and symptoms of acute tracheobronchitis result from the mucopurulent sputum that is secreted by the inflamed mucosa of the bronchi. Initially, the patient has a dry, irritating cough and expectorates a scanty amount of mucoid sputum. He complains of sternal soreness from coughing and has fever, headache, and general malaise. As the infection progresses, the sputum is more profuse and purulent and the cough becomes looser.

Examination and culture of the sputum is essential to identify the specific causative organism. Although *Streptococcus pneumoniae* and *Haemophilus influenzae* often cause this infection, tracheobronchitis is the most common clinical syndrome that results from infection from *Mycoplasma pneumoniae.*

Management.   The treatment is largely symptomatic. The patient is placed on bed rest. Moist heat to the chest will relieve the soreness and pain. Cool vapor therapy or steam inhalations are beneficial in relieving the laryngeal and tracheal irritation. Increasing the vapor pressure (moisture content) in the air will reduce irritation.

Cough depressants are not given or are prescribed only with caution when the cough is productive. Antihistamines may be excessively drying, making secretions more difficult to expectorate. An expectorant such as potassium iodide may be prescribed and the fluid intake increased to ''thin'' the viscous and tenacious secretions. Antibiotic treatment is indicated when the sputum becomes purulent.

Nursing Interventions. The nurse's observations are important in determining the therapeutic plan because care of the patient is largely symptomatic.

A primary nursing function is to caution the patient against overexertion, which can induce a relapse or extension of the infection. The elderly patient can easily develop bronchopneumonia from acute tracheobronchitis if adequate care is not given. The patient is turned often and placed in a sitting position at frequent intervals to facilitate effective coughing and prevent retention of mucopurulent sputum. An adequate time is allowed for convalescence after the acute infection subsides to avoid recurrence.

Pneumonia

Pneumonia is an inflammatory process of the lung substance that is commonly caused by infectious agents. Pneumonia is the most common infectious cause of death in the United States. It is classified according to its causative agent, if known: for example, it may be a *bacterial, viral, fungal, parasitic,* or *lipid* pneumonia. There is also a *chemical* pneumonia, such as that seen after ingestion of kerosene or inhalation of irritating gases. *Radiation pneumonitis* may follow radiation therapy for breast or lung cancer and usually occurs 6 weeks or more after completion of radiation therapy. *Aspiration pneumonia* is discussed on page 500.

If a substantial portion of one or more lobes is involved, the disease is referred to as *lobar pneumonia. Bronchopneumonia* implies that the pneumonic process is distributed in patchy fashion, having originated in one or more localized areas within the bronchi and extended to the adjacent surrounding lung parenchyma. Of these two types, bronchopneumonia is more common that lobar pneumonia.

In general, patients with bacterial pneumonia usually have acute or chronic underlying disease that impairs host defenses. More often, pneumonia arises from endogenous flora of the patient whose resistance has been altered or from aspiration of mouth flora. Although most viral infections occur in previously healthy persons, when bacterial pneumonia occurs in a healthy person there is usually a history of preceding viral illness. In recent years there has been an increase in the number of patients who have deficient defenses against infections: those on corticosteroids or other immunosuppressive drugs, those on broad-spectrum antimicrobials, those with acquired immunodeficiency syndrome (AIDS), and those requiring the use of life-support technology. These patients who have suppressed immune systems often acquire pneumonia from organisms of low virulence. In addition, there are increasing numbers of patients with impaired defenses who develop hospital-acquired pneumonia from gram-negative bacilli (*Klebsiella, Pseudomonas, Escherichia coli,* Enterobacteriaceae, *Proteus, Serratia*). Also, gram-positive cocci, anaerobes, mycobacteria, nocardial species, and viral, chlamydial, fungal, and parasitic agents can cause pneumonia. Commonly encountered pneumonias and their clinical features, treatment, and complications are presented in Table 23-1.

Prevention and Risk Factors

The nurse should be acquainted with the factors and circumstances that commonly predispose the person to pneumonia in order to identify the patient at high risk and to engage in anticipatory and preventive nursing.

- Any condition producing mucus or bronchial obstruction and interfering with normal drainage of the lung (cancer, chronic obstructive pulmonary disease [COPD]) renders the patient susceptible to pneumonia.
- Immunosuppressed patients are at risk.
- People who smoke are at risk because cigarette smoke disrupts both mucociliary and macrophage activity.
- Any patient who is permitted to lie passively in bed for prolonged periods, relatively immobile and breathing shallowly, is highly vulnerable to the risk of bronchopneumonia.
- Any person who has a depressed cough reflex (owing to drugs or weakness), has aspirated foreign material into the lungs during a period of unconsciousness (head injury, anesthesia), or has an abnormal swallowing mechanism is very likely to develop bronchopneumonia.
- Any hospitalized patient on a nothing-by-mouth regimen or who is receiving antibiotics has increased pharyngeal colonization or organisms and is at risk. In very ill persons, the oropharynx is likely to be colonized by gram-negative bacteria.
- People who are intoxicated frequently are particularly susceptible to this infection, since alcohol suppresses the body's reflexes, white cell mobilization, and tracheobronchial ciliary motion.
- Any person scheduled to receive a sedative is observed for respiratory rate and depth before the drug is given; if respiratory depression is apparent, the drug should not be administered. Respiratory depression predisposes to the pooling of bronchial secretions and subsequent development of pneumonia.
- An important preventive measure is the frequent suctioning of secretions in patients who are unconscious or have poor cough and gag reflexes; this reduces the likelihood that secretions will be aspirated or accumulate in the lungs and induce bronchopneumonia.
- Elderly people are especially vulnerable to pneumonia. Postoperative pneumonia should be anticipated in the elderly and forestalled by frequent mobilization, effective coughing, and breathing exercises.
- Anyone receiving treatment with respiratory therapy equipment can develop pneumonia if the equipment has not been properly cleaned.

Pneumonia has been known to be more prevalent with certain underlying disorders such as congestive heart failure, diabetes, alcoholism, and COPD. Certain diseases have also been associated with specific pathogens. For example, staphylococcal pneumonia has been noted after epidemics of influenza, and patients with COPD are at increased risk of developing pneumonia caused by pneumococci or *Haemophilus influenzae*.

Cystic fibrosis is associated with respiratory infection with *Pseudomonas* and *Staphylococcus. Pneumocystis carinii* pneumonia has been associated with AIDS. Pneumonias oc-

(Text continues on p. 464)

TABLE 23-1
Commonly Encountered Pneumonias

Type	Organism Responsible	Manifestations
Bacterial Pneumonias		
Streptococcal pneumonia	*Streptococcus pneumoniae*	May be history of previous respiratory infection
		Sudden onset, with shaking and chills
		Rapidly rising fever; tachypnea
		Cough, with expectoration of rusty or green (purulent) sputum
		Pleuritic pain aggravated by cough
		Chest dull to percussion; crackles, bronchial breath sounds
		Confusion may be only presenting feature in elderly
Staphylococcal pneumonia	*Staphylococcus aureus*	Often prior history of viral infection
		Insidious development of cough, with expectoration of yellow, blood-streaked mucus
		Onset may be sudden if patient is outside hospital
		Fever
		Pleuritic chest pain
		Pulse varies; may be slow in proportion to temperature
Klebsiella pneumonia	*Klebsiella pneumoniae* (Friedländer's bacillus— encapsulated gram-negative aerobic bacillus)	Onset sudden with high fever, chills, pleuritic pain, hemoptysis
		Dyspnea, cyanosis
		Dark brown-red gelatinous sputum expectorated
		Profound prostration and toxicity
Pseudomonas pneumonia	*Pseudomonas aeruginosa*	Apprehension; confusion
		Cyanosis; bradycardia
		Reversal of diurnal temperature curve
Legionnaires' disease	*Legionella pneumophila*	Prodromal period of abdominal pain and diarrhea
		High fever, chills, cough, chest pain, tachypnea
Pittsburgh pneumonia agent (PPA)	*Legionella micdadei*	Fever, myalgias, nonproductive cough, dyspnea; pleuritic pain may occur. Patchy alveolar infiltrates on chest film
Mycoplasma pneumonia	*Mycoplasma pneumoniae*	Gradual onset; severe headache; irritating, hacking cough producing scanty, mucoid sputum
		Anorexia; malaise
		Fever; nasal congestion; sore throat

Clinical Features	Treatment	Complications
Herpes simplex lesions often present on face or lips Usually involves one or more lobes	Penicillin G Alternate drug therapy; erythromycin, clindamycin, cephalosporins, other penicillins, trimethoprim-sulfamethoxazole	Shock Pleural effusion Superinfections Pericarditis Otitis media
Frequently seen in hospital setting Staphylococcal pneumonia is a necrotizing infection Treatment must be vigorous and prolonged owing to disease's tendency to destroy the lungs Organism may develop rapid drug resistance Prolonged convalescence expected	Nafcillin, methicillin, clindamycin, vancomycin, cephalothin	Effusion/pneumothorax Lung abscess Empyema Meningitis
Tends to attack chronically ill, debilitated, alcoholic, and elderly men or those with chronic obstructive pulmonary disease Tissue necrosis occurs rapidly in lungs with cavity formation in some patients May be rapidly fulminating, progressing to fatal outcome High mortality rate	Gentamicin, cefazolin, tobramycin	Multiple lung abscesses with cyst formation Persistent cough with expectoration remains for prolonged period Empyema Pericarditis
Usually acquired in the hospital Susceptible persons: those with preexisting lung disease, cancer (particularly leukemia); those with homograft transplants, burns; debilitated persons; patients receiving prolonged courses of antibiotics and treatment such as tracheostomy, suctioning Respiratory equipment may be contaminated with these organisms	Gentamicin, carbenicillin, tobramycin	Has capacity to invade blood vessel walls, causing hemorrhage and lung infarction High fatality rate
Peak incidence in persons over 50 who are cigarette smokers and have underlying diseases that increase susceptibility to infection	Erythromycin	Respiratory failure
May be hospital-acquired Generally seen in immunocompromised patient	Erythromycin, rifampin, trimethoprim-sulfamethoxazole	Involves multiple lobes; bilateral consolidation common High mortality rate; clinical recovery slow
Occurs most commonly in children and young adults as well as in older adults in community hospital setting Rise in serum complement-fixing antibodies to the organism	Erythromycin, tetracycline	Persisting cough, meningoencephalitis, polyneuritis, monoarticular arthritis, pericarditis, myocarditis

(continued)

TABLE 23-1 *(continued)*

Type	Organism Responsible	Manifestations
Nonbacterial Pneumonias		
Viral pneumonia	Influenza viruses	Cough
	Parainfluenza viruses	Constitutional symptoms may be pronounced (severe headache, anorexia, fever, and myalgia)
	Respiratory syncytial viruses	
	Adenovirus	
	Varicella, rubella, rubeola, herpes simplex, cytomegalovirus, Epstein-Barr virus	
Pneumocystis carinii pneumonia	*Pneumocystis carinii*	Insidious onset
		Increasing dyspnea and nonproductive cough
		Tachypnea; progresses rapidly to intercostal retraction, nasal flaring, and cyanosis
		Lowering of arterial oxygen tension
		Chest film will reveal diffuse, bilateral interstitial pneumonia
Fungal pneumonia	*Aspergillus fumigatas*	Hectic fever, productive cough, chest pain, hemoptysis
		Chest film reveals broad range of abnormalities from infiltration to consolidation, cavitation, and empyema

curring in hospitalized patients often involve organisms not usually found in the nonhospitalized population, including enteric gram-negative bacilli and *Staphylococcus aureus.*

Bacterial Pneumonia

Pneumonia caused by *Streptococcus pneumoniae* is the most common bacterial pneumonia and is most prevalent during the winter and spring, when upper respiratory tract infections are most frequent. It may occur as a lobar or bronchopneumonic form in patients of any age. A history of recent respiratory illness can often be elicited.

Streptococcus pneumoniae is a gram-positive, capsulated, nonmotile coccus that resides naturally in the upper respiratory tract. It is commonly referred to as the pneumococcus.

Pathophysiology. The altered physiology occurring with the pneumonic process is a ventilation problem. The pneumococci gain access to the alveoli where an inflammatory reaction occurs that produces an exudate that pours into the air spaces. White blood cells, mostly neutrophils, also migrate into the alveoli, so that the lung segment assumes a more solid structure as the air-containing spaces become filled. Areas of the lung are not adequately ventilated because of secretions, mucosal edema, and bronchospasm. These conditions cause partial occlusion of the bronchi or alveoli, producing a drop in the alveolar oxygen tension. Venous blood coming into the lungs passes through the underventi-

lated area and goes out of the lung to the left side of the heart without being oxygenated. In essence, the blood is shunted from the right to the left side of the heart. This mixing of oxygenated and unoxygenated blood eventually results in arterial hypoxemia.

Clinical Manifestations. Classic bacterial (or pneumococcal) pneumonia usually starts with a sudden onset of shaking chills, rapidly rising fever (39.5°C to 40.5°C [101°F to 105°F]) and stabbing chest pain that is aggravated by respiration and coughing. The patient is severely ill with marked tachypnea (25 to 45/min) accompanied by respiratory grunting, nasal flaring, and the use of accessory muscles of respiration. He often lies on his affected side in an attempt to splint his chest. The pulse is rapid and bounding. It usually increases about 10 beats/min for every degree of Celsius temperature elevation. A pulse temperature deficit (*i.e.,* a relative bradycardia for the amount of fever) should suggest viral infection, *Mycoplasma* infection, or infection with *Legionella* species. The cheeks are flushed, the eyes bright, and the lips and nail beds cyanotic. The patient prefers to be propped up in bed because of his cough, which is short, painful, and incessant. He perspires profusely. The sputum is purulent and sometimes blood tinged or rusty.

Other signs occur in patients who suffer from a condition such as cancer or those who are undergoing treatment with immunosuppressants, which lower their resistance to infection and to organisms heretofore not considered serious pathogens. Such patients present with fever, crackles, and physical

Clinical Features	Treatment	Complications
In majority of patients influenza begins as an acute coryza; others have bronchitis, pleurisy, etc., while still others develop gastrointestinal symptoms Risk of developing influenza related to crowding and close contact of groups of people	Treat symptomatically Does not respond to treatment with presently available antimicrobials Prophylactic vaccination recommended for high-risk persons (over 55, chronic cardiac or pulmonary disease, diabetes and other metabolic disorders)	May develop a superimposed bacterial infection Bronchopneumonia Pericarditis, endocarditis
Usually seen in host whose resistance is compromised; seen also in male homosexual population Organism invades lungs of patients who have suppressed immune system (from cancer, leukemia) or following immunosuppressive therapy for cancer, organ transplant, or collagen disease Frequently associated with concurrent infection by viruses, (cytomegalovirus) bacteria, and fungi	Pentamidine methanesulfonate	Patients are critically ill Prognosis guarded, since it usually is a complication of a severe underlying disorder
Neutropenic person most susceptible May develop *Aspergillus* as a superinfection	Amphotericin B; ketoconazole	High fatality rate Invades blood vessels and destroys lung tissue by direct invasion and vascular infarction

signs of lobar consolidation (tactile and vocal fremitus, egophony, bronchial breathing, and percussion dullness).

In older patients or those with COPD, the symptoms may develop insidiously. Purulent sputum may be the only sign of pneumonia in these patients. It is difficult to detect subtle changes in their conditions since they already have seriously compromised pulmonary function.

Diagnostic Evaluation. The diagnosis is made by history (particularly of recent respiratory tract infection), physical examination, chest film, blood culture (bloodstream invasion, called *bacteremia,* occurs frequently), and sputum examination.

- In order to get an adequate sample of sputum, the patient rinses his mouth with water to minimize contamination by normal oral flora. He is told to breathe deeply several times and then to cough deeply and expectorate the raised sputum into a sterile container.

Sputum may also be obtained by transtracheal aspiration (p. 418) or fiberoptic bronchoscopy (p. 416) in patients who cannot raise sputum or those who are obtunded, have abnormal host defense mechanisms, or have developed pneumonia after antimicrobial therapy or while hospitalized.

Management. The treatment of pneumonia depends largely on giving the appropriate antibiotic as determined by the results of the Gram stain. Penicillin G is clearly the antibiotic of choice for infection with *S. pneumoniae.* Other effective drugs include erythromycin, clindamycin, the cephalosporins, other penicillins, and trimethoprim-sulfamethoxazole.

The patient is placed on bed rest until infection shows signs of clearing. He is observed carefully and continually until his clinical condition improves.

The patient who is hypoxemic is given oxygen. Arterial blood gas analysis is done to determine the need for oxygen and to evaluate oxygen effectiveness. A high concentration of oxygen is to be avoided in patients with COPD since it may worsen alveolar ventilation by removing the patient's only remaining ventilatory drive and lead to respiratory decompensation. Respiratory support measures such as endotracheal intubation, high inspiratory oxygen concentrations, mechanical ventilation, and positive end-expiratory pressure (PEEP) may be required for some patients. These treatment modalities are discussed in Chapter 22.

▶ *Nursing Process*
The Patient With Pneumonia

▷ *Assessment*

The presence of a fever in any hospitalized patient should alert the nurse to the possibility of the development of bacterial pneumonia. Use of assessment skills will further identify the clinical manifestations of pain; tachypnea; use of accessory muscles; rapid, bounding pulse; coughing; and purulent sputum. The nurse determines the severity, location, and cause of the chest pain as well as what relieves it. Any changes in temperature, amount and color of secretions, frequency and severity of the cough, and degree of tachypnea or shortness of breath are also monitored. Consolidation is assessed by evaluating breath sounds (bronchial breathing and rhonchi), fremitus, egophony, and the results of percussion (dullness in the chest area).

The elderly patient is assessed for unusual behavior, alterations in mental status, prostration, and congestive heart failure. A restless, excited delirium may be exhibited, especially in patients with alcoholism.

The potential complications of bacterial pneumonia are routinely evaluated so that intervention can begin early.

Complications. Lethal complications may develop during the first few days of antibiotic treatment. The patient is observed for continuing or recurring fever. Inadequate lung drainage or insufficient blood supply to the involved lung may reduce the amount of antibiotic agent reaching the invading organism. Resistant or recurring fever may be due to drug allergy (assess for rash), drug resistance or slow response of the susceptible organism, superinfection, infected pleural effusion, or pneumonia caused by unusual organisms (such as *Pneumocystis carinii* or fungi). Failure of the pneumonia to resolve raises the suspicion of underlying carcinoma of the bronchus.

Patients should respond to treatment within 24 to 48 hours after antibiotic therapy is initiated. Complications of pneumonia include sustained *hypotension and shock* (especially in gram-negative bacterial disease in the elderly). These complications are encountered chiefly in patients who have received no specific treatment, have been treated too little or too late, have received chemotherapy to which the infecting organism is resistant, or are suffering from a preexisting disease that complicates the pneumonia.

To combat peripheral collapse and maintain arterial blood pressure, the physician prescribes a vasopressor agent to be given intravenously in the form of a constant infusion and at a rate that is readjusted constantly in accordance with the pressure response. Corticosteroid drugs may be administered parenterally to combat shock and toxicity in patients with pneumonia who are extremely ill and in apparent danger of succumbing to the infection.

Atelectasis (from obstruction of bronchus by accumulated secretions) may occur at any stage of acute pneumonia. Pleural effusion (p. 471) also is fairly common and may signal the beginning of empyema. A diagnostic thoracentesis is usually necessary to evaluate an effusion. A chest tube may be required to control pleural infection by establishing proper drainage of the empyema.

Delirium is another possible complication and is considered a medical emergency when it occurs. It may be caused by hypoxia, meningitis, or the delirium tremens of alcoholism. The patient with delirium is given oxygen, adequate hydration, and mild sedation and is observed constantly. Congestive heart failure, cardiac dysrhythmias, pericarditis, and myocarditis are also complications of pneumonia.

Superinfection is an important complication that may occur with the administration of very large amounts of penicillin or with the use of combinations of antibiotics. If the patient improves and the fever diminishes after initial antibiotic therapy but subsequently there is a rise in temperature with increasing cough and evidence of spread of pneumonia, then a superinfection has occurred. Antibiotics are changed appropriately or, in some cases, discontinued entirely.

The influenza vaccine is recommended yearly to all patients at risk (the elderly, cardiac and pulmonary disease patients), since pneumonia is a complication of influenza. The pneumococcal vaccine is also recommended for the same high-risk group, as well as for patients who have had a splenectomy and those with sickel cell disease and alcoholism. The vaccine provides specific prevention against pneumonia that is caused by major organisms.

▷ *Nursing Diagnoses*

Based on the assessment data, the patient's major nursing diagnoses may include

- Ineffective airway clearance related to copious tracheobronchial secretions
- Activity intolerance related to altered respiratory function
- Potential fluid volume deficit related to fever and dyspnea
- Knowledge deficit about the treatment regimen and preventive health measures

▷ *Planning and Implementation*

▷ *Goals:* The major goals for the patient may include improvement of airway patency, obtaining enough rest to conserve energy, maintenance of proper fluid intake, and an understanding of the treatment protocol and preventive measures.

Nursing Interventions

Improvement of Airway Patency. Retained secretions interfere with gas exchange and may cause slow resolution of the disease. A high level of fluid intake (2 to 3 liters/day) is encouraged, since adequate hydration thins and loosens pulmonary secretions and also replaces fluid losses owing to fever, diaphoresis, dehydration, and dyspnea. The air is humidified in order to loosen secretions and improve ventilation. A high-humidity face mask (using either compressed air or oxygen) delivers warm, humidified air to the tracheobronchial tree and liquefies secretions. The patient is encouraged to cough in the manner described for the postoperative patient (p. 446).

Chest physiotherapy is extremely important in loosening and mobilizing secretions. The patient is placed in the proper position to drain the involved lung, and then the chest is vibrated and percussed. After the lung has drained for 10 to 20 minutes (depending on tolerance), the patient is encouraged to breathe deeply and cough. If he is too weak to cough effectively, the mucus may have to be removed by nasotracheal suctioning or by bronchoscopic aspiration as determined by the physician.

If oxygen is prescribed, the nurse provides the necessary method of oxygen administration and monitors the effectiveness of the oxygen concentration by assessing for the clinical manifestations of hypoxia.

Rest and Energy Conservation. The patient is encouraged to rest and remain in bed to avoid overexertion and possible exacerbation of symptoms. He is placed in a comfortable position for resting and breathing (*e.g.*, semi-Fowler's) and encouraged to change position frequently.

If sedatives or tranquilizers are prescribed, the patient's sensorium is evaluated first. Restlessness, confusion, and aggression may be due to cerebral hypoxemia, in which case sedatives are contraindicated.

Proper Fluid Intake. The patient's respiratory rate increases because of dyspnea and fever. With an increased rate there is an increase in insensible fluid loss during exhalation. The patient can quickly become dehydrated. Therefore, fluids are encouraged (at least 2 liters/day). Frequently, a patient who is dyspneic is anorexic and will only take fluids. Fluids, then, are beneficial for volume replacement as well as nutrition.

Patient Education and Home Health Care. After the fever subsides, the patient may gradually increase his activities. Fatigue, weakness, and depression may be prolonged after pneumonia. Breathing exercises to clear the lungs and promote full lung expansion are encouraged. The patient is instructed to return to the clinic or physician's office for follow-up chest films.

The nurse explains to the patient that it is wise to stop cigarette smoking since it destroys tracheobronchial ciliary action, which is the first line of defense of the lungs. Smoking also irritates the mucous cells of the bronchi and inhibits the function of alveolar macrophage (scavenger) cells. The patient is instructed to avoid fatigue, sudden changes in temperature, and excessive alcohol intake, which lowers resistance to pneumonia. The nurse reviews with the patient the principles of adequate nutrition and rest, since one episode of pneumonia may make him susceptible to recurring respiratory tract infections. He is encouraged to obtain influenza vaccine at the prescribed times, because influenza increases susceptibility to secondary bacterial pneumonia, especially that caused by *Staphylococcus, Haemophilus influenzae,* and *Streptococcus pneumoniae.* The patient is also encouraged to seek medical advice about receiving vaccine against *S. pneumoniae* (Pneumovax). The care plan for the patient with bacterial pneumonia is found in Nursing Care Plan 23-1.

▷ *Evaluation*

▷ *Expected Outcomes*

1. Patient improves airway patency.
   a. Maintains an arterial blood gas oxygen tension of 60 mm Hg or above.
   b. Has a normal temperature.
   c. Exhibits normal breath sounds.
   d. Demonstrates effective coughing technique.
   e. Adheres to humidification measures.
2. Attains proper amount of rest.
   a. Remains in bed while symptomatic.
   b. Avoids the recumbent position.
   c. Shows no signs of restlessness, confusion, or aggression.
3. Achieves an adequate fluid intake.
   a. Verbalizes the importance of drinking at least 2 liters of fluid per day.
   b. Has sufficient skin turgor.
4. Understands treatment protocol and prevention aspects.

   a. Is aware of factors that contribute to development of pneumonia.
   b. Talks of joining a support group to stop smoking.
   c. Makes an appointment at clinic for follow-up chest film and influenza and pneumococcal vaccine.
   d. Verbalizes that he will cope with fatigue by rest, alternating with increasing activity.

Atypical Pneumonia Syndromes

Pneumonias associated with mycoplasmas, psittacosis, Q fever, Legionnaires' disease, and viruses are included in the atypical pneumonia syndromes (Table 23-1).

Mycoplasma pneumoniae is the most common cause of primary atypical pneumonia. Mycoplasmas are small organisms surrounded by a triple-layered membrane without a cell wall. The organisms grow on a special culture medium but differ from viruses. Mycoplasma pneumonia occurs most frequently in older children and young adults.

It is probably spread by infected respiratory droplets, through person-to-person contact. Patients can be tested for mycoplasma antibodies.

The inflammatory infiltrate is primarily interstitial rather than alveolar. It spreads throughout the entire respiratory tract, including the bronchioles. Generally, it has the characteristics of a bronchopneumonia. Earache and bullous myringitis are common.

Clinical Manifestations. Usually, the patient has had an upper respiratory tract infection, and the onset of his pneumonic symptoms is gradual. The predominant symptoms are a harassing and nonproductive cough, a feeling of tightness in the chest, and generalized aching and prostration, along with tracheal pain when coughing. After a few days, mucoid or mucopurulent sputum is expectorated. The patient complains of headache that is aggravated by the cough.

Nursing Interventions. The goal of nursing care is to promote the patient's rest and comfort and to encourage the proper intake of prescribed drugs. *Mycoplasma* pneumonia responds to erythromycin and tetracycline. Other atypical pneumonias are viral in origin, and most do not respond to antimicrobials. Warm, moist inhalations are helpful in relieving bronchial irritation. The nursing care and treatment (with the exception of antimicrobial therapy) is the same as that given to the patient who has bacterial pneumonia (pp. 466–467).

Lung Abscess

Pathogenesis. A lung abscess is a localized lesion in the lung containing pus and necrotic (dead) tissue that collapses and forms cavities, or pockets, in the lung. It may occur from aspiration of vomitus or infected material (nasotracheal secretions, blood) from the upper respiratory tract. After aspiration, pneumonitis develops and the area of pneumonia cavitates because the microorganisms have necrotizing potential; hence a lung abscess may develop very rapidly. A lung abscess may also occur secondary to bronchial obstruction due to a tumor. Infection or necrosis within the tumor mass results in the accumulation of secretions. Or, it may be a sequela of necrotizing pneumonias, tuberculosis, pulmonary embolism, chest trauma, or bronchial neoplasm.

In the initial stages the cavity in the lung may or may not

Nursing Care Plan 23-1

Care of the Patient With Bacterial Pneumonia

Nursing Interventions	Rationale	Expected Outcomes

Nursing Diagnosis: Ineffective airway clearance related to tracheobronchial secretions

Goal: Improvement of airway patency

1. Assist the patient to cough productively:
  a. Splint the patient's chest while coughing.
  b. Give codeine as prescribed.
  c. Humidify air to loosen secretions and improve ventilation. Encourage increased fluid intake.
	1. Depression of the cough reflex may produce retention of pulmonary secretions and lead to atelectasis. Elderly patients have a diminished cough reflex and may require vigorous measures (suctioning, bronchoscopy) for removal of secretions. Adequate hydration thins mucus and serves as an effective expectorant.	• Demonstrates effective coughing techniques.
		• Verbalizes importance of drinking plenty of fluids.

2. Perform postural drainage, percussion, and vibration to mobilize secretions.	2. Postural drainage uses gravity to remove secretions from the lung.	• Airway is clear of secretions.

3. Use measures to reduce pleuritic pain:
  a. Apply heat and cold as directed.
  b. Assist with intercostal nerve block with procaine when indicated.
  c. Use analgesics with caution to prevent depression of cough reflex and central nervous system respiratory drive when prescribed.
  d. Treat dry cough and laryngospasm with aerosol therapy.
	3. Pain and cough result from pleuritic invasion by pneumococci. The discomfort of pleuritic pain can interfere with the mechanics of ventilation and effective airway clearance.	• Verbalizes minimal pleuritic pain and knows methods to reduce it.

4. Administer prescribed antibiotic at correct time intervals.
  a. Penicillin is usually the drug of choice. Erythromycin or clindamycin can be given if patient is allergic to penicillin.
  b. Observe patient for nausea, vomiting, diarrhea, anal pruritus, rash, and soft tissue reactions.
	4. The therapy of pneumonia depends on laboratory identification of the agent causing the infection and on the drainage of purulent secretions. Pneumococci are highly susceptible to the action of penicillin.	• Verbalizes importance of taking antibiotics at prescribed intervals and knows side-effects.

(continued)

communicate with a bronchus; eventually, however, it becomes surrounded, or "encapsulated," by a wall of fibrous tissue, except at one or two points where the necrotic process extends until it reaches the lumen of some bronchus or the pleural space and thus establishes a communication with the respiratory tract, the pleural cavity, or both. In the first instance, its purulent contents are evacuated continuously in the form of sputum, whereas if a pleural exit is accessible, empyema (collection of pus in the pleural cavity) results; if both types of communication are furnished, the problem becomes one of *bronchopleural fistula.*

Clinical Manifestations. The majority of patients have a cough that produces a small amount of sputum, a low-grade fever, and malaise. In time the sputum becomes copious and often foul smelling and at time contains blood. This occurs frequently when the abscess extends into the bronchus and begins to drain. The patient may complain of a pleuritic type of chest pain. Sometimes the onset is acute, with chills, high fever, cough, and malaise.

Diagnostic Evaluation. Physical examination may reveal an area of consolidation and pleural thickening, dullness to percussion, and suppressed breath sounds. Confirmation of the diagnosis is made by chest films, sputum culture, and direct visualization with fiberoptic bronchoscopy, which is

Nursing Interventions	*Rationale*	*Expected Outcomes*

Nursing Diagnosis: Ineffective airway clearance related to tracheobronchial secretions

Goal: Improvement of airway patency

5. Give oxygen as prescribed for dyspnea, circulatory disturbance, hypoxemia, or delirium. Monitor arterial blood gases to determine oxygen need and evaluate oxygen effectiveness.	5. Restlessness, confusion, and aggressiveness may be due to cerebral hypoxia.	• Arterial oxygen tension is 60 mm Hg.
6. Monitor the patient's response to therapy. a. Check temperature, pulse, respiration, and blood pressure every 4 hours and more frequently if indicated. Watch for continuing and recurring fever from drug allergy, drug resistance or slow response to therapy, inadequate/ inappropriate antimicrobial therapy, superinfection, or failure of pneumonia to resolve. b. Auscultate chest for crackles, signs of consolidation, or pleural effusion.	6. Lethal complications may develop during the early period of antimicrobial treatment. The temperature curve provides an index of the patient's response to therapy. Hypotension occurring early in the course of the illness may indicate hypoxia or bacteremia. Salicylates are given with caution since they produce a drop in temperature and thus interfere with evaluation of the temperature curve.	• Temperature is normal • Pulse and respiration are within normal limits. • Is normotensive. • Breath sounds are normal.

Nursing Diagnosis: Activity intolerance related to altered respiratory function

Goal: Rest to conserve energy

1. Encourage patient to rest as much as possible	1. Rest decreases the work of the lungs and facilitates ventilation.	• Remains in bed as needed.
2. Assist patient to assume a comfortable position and to change position frequently.	2. A comfortable position promotes rest. Semi-Fowler's position is desirable if patient is dyspneic. Changing positions frequently prevents pooling of secretions in the lungs.	• Assumes best position for adequate breathing.

(continued)

necessary to rule out the possibility of tumor or a foreign body in the lung.

Usually, sputum specimens are obtained by transtracheal aspiration since an expectorated sputum specimen will be contaminated by the indigenous flora of the mouth and gingivae. Several species of bacteria are often present in a lung abscess. The most common cause is the anaerobic bacteria that normally colonize the upper airway.

Management. The goals of management of a lung abscess are prevention, eradication of the infection, and establishment of adequate drainage. The following measures will reduce the risk of suppurative lung disease:

1. Patients who must have teeth extracted while their gums and teeth are infected may be given appropriate antibiotic therapy before any dental manipulations.
2. The patient is instructed to maintain adequate dental and oral hygiene, since anaerobic bacteria play a role in the pathogenesis of lung abscess.
3. Appropriate antimicrobial therapy is given to patients with pneumonia.

Bronchoscopy is indicated if inhalation of foreign material is suspected. A patient with impaired cough reflexes and loss of glottis closure or one who has swallowing difficulties is

Nursing Interventions	*Rationale*	*Expected Outcomes*

Nursing Diagnosis: Activity intolerance related to altered respiratory function

Goal: Rest to conserve energy

3. Evaluate sensorium before sedatives or tranquilizers are given.	3. Restlessness, confusion, and aggression may indicate cerebral hypoxemia. If this is present, sedatives are inappropriate.	• Evidences a calm affect.

Nursing Diagnosis: Potential fluid volume deficit related to fever and dyspnea

Goal: Achieves an adequate fluid intake

Give patient 2 to 3 liters of fluid per day.	Fever and tachypnea cause an increase in insensible volume loss. Patient may become dehydrated. A poor appetite during bacterial pneumonia increases the need for increased fluid intake.	• Verbalizes the importance of drinking 2 to 3 liters of fluid per day. • Is adequately hydrated.

Nursing Diagnosis: Knowledge deficit about the treatment protocol and methods of prevention

Goal: Acquisition of knowledge about the treatment protocol and preventive aspects

1. Teach the patient about preventive measures: a. Avoid smoking b. Keep up natural resistance (adequate rest and nutrition and proper exercise). c. Obtain influenza vaccine and pneumococcal vaccine at prescribed times. d. Avoid overfatigue, chilling, and excessive alcohol intake, which lower resistance to pneumonia. e. Report any signs and symptoms of a respiratory tract infection to a physician. f. Have follow-up examinations after discharge from the hospital.	1. Cigarette smoking destroys tracheobronchial cilial action, stimulates mucosal cells, causes increased mucus production, and inhibits alveolar scavenger cells (macrophages). Susceptibility to recurring respiratory infections increases after initial exposure. Colds and upper respiratory tract infections may lead to bacterial invasion of the respiratory tract. Pneumonia frequently coexists with other pathologic pulmonary conditions, namely, cancer of the lung.	• Is aware of factors that contribute to development of pneumonia. • Verbalizes need to stop smoking. • Makes an appointment for a follow-up chest film and influenza and pneumococcal vaccination. • Verbalizes that he will cope with fatigue by alternating rest periods with increasing activity.

apt to aspirate foreign material and hence develop lung abscess. Other patients at risk are those with an altered state of consciousness from anesthesia, central nervous system disorders (seizures, stroke), drug addiction, alcoholism, or esophageal disease, as well as patients being fed by nasogastric tube.

Antimicrobial therapy depends on the results of sputum culture and sensitivity and is given for an extended period of time. Penicillin G is still the treatment of choice in most cases and often supplemented by metronidazole (Flagyl) or clindamycin (Cleocin) if the patient is seriously ill. High intravenous doses are generally required, because the antibiotic must penetrate necrotic tissue and abscess fluid.

Adequate drainage of the lung abscess is achieved through postural drainage aided by percussion, effective coughing, and breathing exercises. Sometimes bronchoscopy is needed to drain the abscess.

A high-protein, high-calorie diet is necessary since chronic infection is associated with a catabolic state, which requires calories and protein to facilitate healing.

After the patient shows signs of improvement as demonstrated by normal temperature, lowering of white blood cell count, and improvement in the chest film (resolution of surrounding infiltrate, reduction in the size of the cavity, and absence of fluid), the antibiotic is administered orally rather than intravenously. If treatment is stopped too soon, a relapse may occur. The duration of antibiotic therapy may be from 6 to 16 weeks.

Surgical intervention is indicated only when medical therapy has been proved inadequate by failure of the cavity to resolve, by a continuing septic condition, or when major hemoptysis occurs. Pulmonary resection (lobectomy) is the procedure usually performed when there is a thick-walled abscess with purulent drainage. If the patient cannot tolerate thoracic surgery, tube thoracotomy is done. (See p. 444 for care of the patient undergoing thoracic surgery.)

Nursing Interventions. The nurse administers the antibiotic and intravenous therapy as directed and monitors the patient for any adverse effects. Chest physiotherapy is initiated as prescribed to drain the abscess. The patient is taught deep breathing and coughing exercises to help expand the lungs. To ensure proper nutritional intake, a diet high in protein and calories is encouraged. Emotional support is provided because the abscess may take a long time to resolve.

Patient Education and Home Health Care. If surgery has been necessary, the patient will most likely return home before the wound closes entirely. It will be necessary to teach him or a caregiver how to change the dressings as needed to prevent skin excoriation and an offensive odor. Deep breathing and coughing exercises are to be practiced every 2 hours during the day. Postural drainage and percussion techniques are taught to a caregiver so that lung secretions can be removed. Counseling is provided for attaining and maintaining an optimal state of nutrition.

Pleural Conditions

Pleurisy

Pleurisy (pleuritis) refers to inflammation of both the visceral and parietal pleurae. When these inflamed membranes rub together during respiration (particularly inspiration), the result is severe, sharp, "knifelike" pain. The pain may become minimal or absent when the breath is held, or it may be localized or radiate to the shoulder or abdomen. Later, as pleural fluid develops, the pain lessens. In the early dry period, the pleural friction rub can be heard with the stethoscope, only to disappear later as fluid appears to separate the roughened pleural surfaces.

Pleurisy may develop with pneumonia or upper respiratory tract infection, tuberculosis, collagen disease, after trauma to the chest or pulmonary infarction or embolism, in primary and metastatic cancer, in the viral disease known as epidemic pleurodynia, and after thoracotomy.

Careful radiographic and sputum examinations and thoracentesis with pleural fluid examination and possibly pleural biopsy are indicated in order to discover the underlying condition.

Management. The objective of treatment is to discover the underlying condition causing the pleurisy. As the underlying disease is treated (pneumonia, infarction) the pleuritic inflammation usually resolves. At the same time it is necessary to watch for signs of pleural effusion, such as shortness of breath, pain, and decreased local excursion of the chest wall.

Prescribed analgesics and applications of heat or cold will provide symptomatic relief. Indomethacin, an anti-inflammatory drug, may give pain relief while allowing the patient to cough effectively. If the pain is severe, a procaine intercostal block may be required.

Nursing Interventions. Since this patient has real pain on inspiration, the nurse can offer suggestions to enhance comfort, such as turning frequently on the affected side in order to splint the chest wall; this will lessen the stretch of the pleura. She can also teach the patient to use his hands to splint the rib cage while coughing. Since pain on breathing produces anxiety, the patient will require support and understanding.

Pleural Effusion

Pleural effusion, a collection of fluid in the pleural space, is rarely a primary disease process but is usually secondary to other diseases. Normally, the pleural space may contain a small amount of fluid (5 to 15 ml) acting as a lubricant that allows the visceral and parietal surfaces to move without friction.

In certain intrathoracic and systemic diseases, fluid may accumulate in the pleural space to a point where it becomes clinically evident, and it is almost always of pathologic significance. The effusion can be a relatively clear fluid, which may be a transudate or an exudate, or it can be blood, pus, or chyle. A *transudate* (filtrates of plasma that move across intact capillary walls) occurs when factors influencing formation and reabsorption of pleural fluid are altered, usually by imbalances in hydrostatic or oncotic pressures. A transudate indicates that a condition such as ascites or a systemic disease such as congestive heart failure or renal failure underlies the fluid accumulation. An *exudate* (extravasation of fluid into tissues/cavity) usually results from inflammation by bacterial products or tumors involving the pleural surfaces. In general, the differentiation is made on the basis of protein content and lactic dehydrogenase activity. Pleural effusion may be a complication of tuberculosis, pneumonia, congestive heart failure, pulmonary viral infections, and neoplastic tumors. In fact, 50% of patients with cancer of the lung develop pleural effusion. In approximately one in four patients, pleural effusion is secondary to carcinoma.

Clinical Manifestations. Usually, the clinical manifestations are those caused by the underlying disease; pneumonia will cause fever, chills, and pleuritic chest pain, whereas a malignant effusion may result in dyspnea and coughing. A large quantity of pleural effusion will cause shortness of breath with dullness or flatness to percussion over areas of fluid with minimal or absence of breath sounds. Egophony ("E" to "A" changes) will be present above the effusion (see p. 411). Confirmation of the presence of fluid is obtained by chest film, ultrasound, physical examination, and thoracentesis. Tests made of pleural fluid include bacterial cultures, Gram stain, acid-fast bacillus stain (for tuberculosis), red cell count, white cell count, chemistry studies (glucose, amylase, lactic dehydrogenase, protein), and *p*H.

Management. The objectives of treatment are to discover the underlying cause to prevent fluid collection from recurring, and to relieve discomfort and dyspnea. Specific treatment is directed to the underlying cause (*e.g.*, congestive heart failure, cirrhosis).

Thoracentesis is done to remove fluid, to collect a specimen for analysis, and to relieve dyspnea. However, if the underlying cause is a malignancy, the effusion may recur within a few days or weeks. Repeated thoracenteses result in pain, depletion of protein and electrolytes, and sometimes pneumothorax. In this event the patient may be treated with chest tube drainage connected to a water-seal drainage system or suction to evacuate the pleural space and reexpand the lung. Sometimes tetracycline, radioactive isotopes, or cytotoxic or other chemically irritating drugs are instilled in the pleural space to obliterate the pleural space and prevent further accumulation of fluid. After drug instillation, the chest tube is clamped and the patient is assisted to assume various positions to ensure uniform drug distribution and to maximize drug contact with the pleural surfaces. The tube is unclamped as prescribed, and chest drainage is usually continued several days longer to prevent reaccumulation of fluid and to facilitate obliteration of the pleural space by formation of adhesions between the visceral and parietal pleurae. Other modalities of treatment for malignant pleural effusions include radiation of the chest wall, surgical pleurectomy, and diuretic therapy.

If the pleural fluid is an exudate, more extensive diagnostic procedures are done in order to determine the cause. Therapy for pleural disease is then instituted.

Nursing Interventions. The nurse's role in the care of the patient with a pleural effusion involves implementing the medical regimen. The nurse prepares and positions the patient and offers support throughout the procedure. Because the pleura is involved, there will be considerable pain; therefore, the patient is assisted to assume positions that are the least painful and pain medication is administered as prescribed and as needed. If a chest tube drainage and water-seal system is used, the nurse is responsible for monitoring the system's function and recording the amount of drainage every 8 hours. Nursing care related to the underlying cause of the pleural effusion will be specific to that condition.

Empyema

Empyema is a collection of pus in the pleural cavity. At first the pleural fluid is thin, with a low leukocyte count, but frequently it progresses to a fibropurulent stage and finally to a stage where it encloses the lung within a thick exudative membrane.

In most instances an empyema is associated with an underlying pulmonary infection. Organisms may invade the pleural space by direct extension or as the result of the rupture of a lung abscess. An empyema may also follow thoracic surgery or penetrating wounds of the chest. The character of the exudate varies according to the infecting organism.

Clinical Manifestations. The patient has fever, pleural pain, dyspnea, anorexia, and weight loss. Chest auscultation reveals the absence of breath sounds, and there is flatness to chest percussion as well as decreased fremitus (vocal vibration felt by palpation). If the patient has received antibiotic therapy, the clinical manifestations may be altered. The diagnosis is established on the basis of chest films and thoracentesis.

Management. The objectives of treatment are to drain the pleural cavity and to achieve full expansion of the lung. This is accomplished by adequate drainage and by appropriate antibiotics selected on the basis of the causative organism. Large doses of the drug are usually given.

Drainage of the pleural fluid or pus depends on the stage of the disease and is accomplished by:

- Needle aspiration (thoracentesis) if the fluid is not too thick
- Closed-chest drainage using a large-diameter intercostal tube attached to water-seal drainage (p. 448)
- Open drainage by means of rib resection to remove the thickened pleura, pus, and debris and to resect the underlying diseased pulmonary tissue

If the inflammation has been of long-standing, an exudate can form over the lung and interfere with its normal expansion. This will have to be removed surgically (decortication). The drainage tube is left in place until the pus-filled space is obliterated completely. The complete obliteration of the pleural space is checked radiographically, and the patient should be aware that this process may take a long time.

Nursing Interventions. Resolution of an empyema is a prolonged process. The nurse helps the patient cope with the condition and instructs him in breathing exercises (pursed lip and diaphragmatic breathing), which help to restore normal respiratory function. The nurse also provides care specific to the method of drainage of the pleural fluid, such as needle aspiration, closed chest drainage, or rib resection and drainage. (See nursing management following a thoracotomy, p. 447).

Chronic Obstructive Pulmonary Disease

Chronic obstructive pulmonary disease (COPD) is the most common cause of death and disability due to lung disease in the United States. COPD is a broad classification that includes a group of conditions associated with chronic obstruction of air flow entering or leaving the lungs. *Airway obstruction* is diffuse airway narrowing, causing increased resistance to air flow. Included in the COPD category are chronic bronchitis, bronchiectasis, emphysema, and asthma. Basically, the person with COPD has (1) excessive secretion of mucus within the airways not due to specific causes (bronchitis or bronchiectasis), (2) an increase in the size of the air spaces distal to the terminal bronchioles with loss of alveolar walls and elastic recoil of the lungs (emphysema), and (3) narrowing of the bronchial airways that varies in severity (asthma). As a result there is a subsequent derangement of airway dynamics—for example, loss of elasticity and obstruction of air flow. There is often an overlap of these conditions.

Studies support the theory that COPD is a disease of genetic and environmental interaction; cigarette smoking and air pollution contribute to its development, which may occur over a 20- to 30-year span. It appears to begin fairly early in life and is a slowly progressive disorder that is present many years before the onset of clinical symptoms and impairment of pulmonary function.

▶ Nursing Process
The Patient With COPD

▷ Assessment

The nurse's observations, history, and recording should yield an understanding of the patient and his disease. Data collection involves obtaining information about current symptoms as well as previous disease manifestations. The following is a list of questions that a nurse can use as a guide to obtain a clear history of the disease process:

- How long has the patient had respiratory difficulty?
- What are the pulse and the respiratory rates?
- Are the respirations even?
- Does the patient contract his abdominal muscles during inspiration?
- Does the patient have prolonged expiration?
- Are the accessory muscles of respiration used?
- Does exertion increase the dyspnea? What type of exertion?
- What are the limits to his exercise tolerance?
- Is cyanosis evident?
- Are the patient's neck veins engorged?
- Does the patient have peripheral edema?
- Is he coughing?
- What is the color, amount, and consistency of the sputum?
- What is the status of the patient's sensorium?
- Is there increasing stupor? apprehension?
- At what times during the day does he complain most of fatigue and shortness of breath?
- Have his habits of eating or sleeping been affected?
- What does he know about the disease and his condition?

▷ Nursing Diagnoses

Based on all the assessment data, the patient's major nursing diagnoses may include the following:

- Impaired gas exchange related to ventilation–perfusion inequality
- Ineffective airway clearance related to bronchoconstriction, increased mucus production, ineffective cough, and bronchopulmonary infection
- Ineffective breathing pattern related to shortness of breath, mucus, bronchoconstriction and airway irritants
- Self-care deficit related to fatigue secondary to increased work of breathing and insufficient ventilation and oxygenation
- Activity intolerance due to fatigue, hypoxemia, and ineffective breathing patterns
- Ineffective individual coping related to less socialization, anxiety, depression, lower activity level, and the inability to work
- Knowledge deficit of self-care procedures to be performed at home

▷ Planning and Implementation

▷ *Goals:* The major goals for the patient may include improvement in gas exchange, achievement of airway clearance, improvement in breathing pattern, independence in self-care activities, improvement in activity tolerance, improvement in coping ability, and adherence to therapeutic program and home care.

Nursing Interventions

Improvement in Gas Exchange. Bronchospasm, which is present in many forms of pulmonary disease, causes reduction in the caliber of the small bronchi, resulting in stasis of secretions and infection. Bronchospasm is detected when wheezes are heard on auscultation with a stethoscope. Increased mucus production along with decreased mucociliary action contributes to further reduction in the caliber of the bronchi and results in decreased air flow and decreased gas exchange, which is aggravated by the loss of lung elasticity.

These changes in the airway demand that the nurse frequently assess the level of dyspnea and hypoxia in the patient. If bronchodilators are prescribed, the nurse must properly administer the medications and be alert for potential side-effects. The relief of bronchospasm is confirmed by measuring improvement in expiratory flow rates and assessing whether the patient has a reduction in dyspnea.

Aerosol therapy helps loosen secretions so that they can be removed. Inhaled bronchodilators are often added to the nebulizer to provide direct bronchodilator action on the airways, thereby improving gas exchange. Nebulizer treatments should be given before meals to improve lung ventilation and thus reduce the fatigue that accompanies eating. Following inhalation of nebulized bronchodilators, the patient is advised to inhale moisture to further liquefy secretions. Then expulsive coughing or postural drainage will aid him in expectorating secretions. The patient is helped to do this in a manner that it will not be exhausting to him.

Oxygen is prescribed by the physician when hypoxemia is present. The nurse must monitor the effectiveness of the oxygen therapy and ensure that the patient is compliant in his use of the oxygen delivery device. The nurse instructs him in the proper use of oxygen and cautions that smoking with or near oxygen is extremely dangerous. In some cases, the patient may be discharged home with oxygen. Oxygen can be supplied to the home by compressed gas, liquid, or concentrator systems. Portable oxygen systems are available that allow the patient to work and travel. Patient education includes reassuring the patient that oxygen is not "addicting" and explaining the precautions involved in using oxygen (no smoking) and the necessity of having regular measurements of arterial blood gases.

Continuous oxygen therapy has been demonstrated to prolong life for those with a PaO_2 of 55 mm Hg (7.31 kPa^a) or less on room air. Intermittent oxygen use has little value in the patient with COPD, except during an intensive exercise program or in the form of nocturnal therapy.

Removal of Bronchial Secretions. A major goal in the treatment of COPD is to diminish the quantity and tenacity of sputum in order to improve pulmonary ventilation and gas exchange. All pulmonary irritants must be eliminated, particularly cigarette smoking, which is the most persistent source of pulmonary irritation. A high fluid intake (6 to 8 glasses) daily is encouraged to liquefy secretions. An added reason for encouraging fluid intake is the tendency for the patient to breathe through his mouth, which accelerates water loss.

Inhaling nebulized water is also helpful since it humidifies the bronchial tree, adding water to the sputum and decreasing its viscosity, so that evacuation of sputum is facilitated.

Postural drainage with percussion and vibration uses gravity to help raise secretions so that they can be coughed out or suctioned easily. When used in conjunction with bronchodilators and nebulizer therapy or an intermittent positive pressure breathing (IPPB) treatment, postural drainage should follow either of these therapies because drainage is facilitated after the tracheobronchial tree is dilated. The patient is instructed in effective breathing and coughing to help raise the secretions. Postural drainage is usually carried out when the patient wakes up, to remove secretions that have accumulated overnight, and before he retires, to promote sleep. The frequency of these measures throughout the day will be dictated by the patient's needs.

Prevention of Bronchopulmonary Infection. Bronchopulmonary infections must be controlled to diminish inflammatory edema and to permit recovery of normal ciliary action. Minor respiratory infections that are of no consequence to the person with normal lungs can produce fatal disturbances of pulmonary function in the person with COPD. The cough associated with bronchial infection introduces a vicious cycle with further trauma and damage to the lungs, further progression of symptoms, increased bronchospasm, and further increase in susceptibility to bronchial infection. Infection compromises lung function and is a common cause of respiratory failure.

In COPD, infection does not manifest itself in the same way as it does elsewhere in the body. The patient is instructed to report to the physician immediately if the sputum becomes discolored, since purulent expectoration or a change in the character, color, or amount of the sputum is evidence of infection. He should be taught that any worsening of his symptoms (increased tightness of the chest, increase in dyspnea, and fatigue) is also suggestive of infection and must be reported. Viral infections are hazardous to these patients because they are so often followed by infections caused by *Streptococcus pneumoniae*, *Haemophilus influenzae*, and so on.

Patients with COPD are prone to respiratory infections and should be immunized against influenza and *S. pneumoniae*. During highly polluted or heavily pollinated days (in the spring) these persons should avoid outdoor exposure since it may increase bronchospasm. Outdoor periods of high temperatures associated with high humidities should also be avoided.

Breathing Exercises and Retraining. Most people with COPD breathe shallowly from the upper chest in a rapid and inefficient manner. This type of upper chest breathing can be changed to diaphragmatic breathing with practice. Training in diaphragmatic breathing reduces the respiratory rate, increases alveolar ventilation, and sometimes causes a reduction of functional residual capacity. (See p. 430 for technique.)

Pursed-lip breathing slows expiration, prevents collapse of lung units, and helps the patient to control the rate and depth of respiration and to relax, which enables him to gain control of his dyspnea and feelings of panic.

A patient with COPD has definite periods of the day when his exercise tolerance is decreased. This is especially true on arising in the morning, because bronchial secretions and edema collect in the lungs during the night while he is lying on his back. He often will be unable to shave or wash. Activities requiring the arms to be supported above the level of the thorax may produce distress. These activities may be tolerated better after the patient has been up and moving around for an hour or more. Because of these limitations, the patient has the right to participate in planning his care with the nurse and in determining the best time for bathing and shaving. A hot beverage on arising, along with diaphragmatic breathing, will assist him to expectorate and will shorten the period of disability experienced on arising.

Another period of increased disability occurs immediately after meals, particularly the evening meal. Fatigue from the day's activities coupled with abdominal distention limits his exercise tolerance. The patient's chief complaint at this time is fatigue or dyspnea.

Once the patient has learned diaphragmatic breathing, an inspiratory muscle trainer may be employed to help strengthen the muscles used in breathing. This device requires that the patient breathe against a resistance. The resistance is gradually increased and the muscles become better conditioned. Conditioning of the respiratory muscles takes a long time, and the patient is instructed to continue practicing at home.

Self-Care Activities. As gas exchange, airway clearance, and the breathing pattern improve, the patient is encouraged to assume some of his own care. He is taught to try to coordinate diaphragmatic breathing with activities such as walking, bathing, bending, or climbing stairs. He should begin to bathe himself, dress himself, and take short walks, resting as needed to avoid fatigue and excessive dyspnea. The inspiratory muscle trainer is used for 10 to 15 minutes every day and the patient urged to initiate this technique on his own. Fluids should be readily available, and the patient should begin to drink without encouragement. If the patient will be using postural drainage at home, he is instructed and supervised by the nurse prior to discharge.

Physical Conditioning. Physical conditioning techniques include breathing and general physical conditioning exercises intended to conserve and increase pulmonary ventilation. There is a close relationship between physical fitness and respiratory fitness. Graded exercises and physical conditioning programs employing treadmills, stationary bicycles, and measured level walks have been shown to improve symptoms and to increase work capacity and exercise tolerance. It is useful for the patient to have a physical activity that he can do on a regular sustained basis. A lightweight portable oxygen system is available for the ambulatory patient who requires oxygen therapy during physical activity to improve hypoxia. This type of rehabilitation improves the quality of life.

Coping Measures. Any factor that interferes with normal breathing quite naturally induces anxiety, depression, and changes in behavior. Many patients find the slightest exertion exhausting. Constant shortness of breath and fatigue may render the patient irritable and apprehensive to the point of panic. His enforced inactivity (and reversal of family roles owing to loss of employment), the frustration of having to work to breathe, and the realization that he faces a prolonged, unrelenting disease may cause the patient to react with anger, depression, and demanding behavior. Sexual ability may be compromised, which also diminishes self-esteem.

It is important for the nurse and other health care personnel to adopt a cautiously hopeful and encouraging attitude and keep the patient active up to his level of symptom tolerance. Emphasis should be on controlling his symptoms and increasing self-esteem and sense of mastery and of well-being. Supportive medical and nursing care, ongoing patient teaching, exercise conditioning, and possibly group therapy sessions help to relieve somewhat an almost overwhelming burden.

The patient should also be directed to support groups conducted by the American Lung Association, to pulmonary rehabilitation programs where available, to smoking cessation programs (if still smoking), and to senior citizens' groups for social interaction. These groups will help to improve the patient's knowledge of his condition, his ability to cope with his disease, and his sense of self-worth.

Patient Education and Home Health Care. To help the patient with COPD live better, it is essential that he be educated about his disease process. One of the major teaching factors is helping the patient accept realistic short-term and long-range goals. If he is severely disabled, the objective of treatment is to preserve his present pulmonary function and relieve his symptoms as much as possible. If his disease is mild, the objective is to increase his exercise tolerance and prevent further loss of pulmonary function. The patient has to be told what to expect. He and those caring for him need patience to achieve these goals.

The patient is instructed to avoid extremes of heat and cold. Heat increases the body temperature, thereby raising the oxygen requirements of the body; cold tends to promote bronchospasm. High altitudes aggravate the hypoxia. Bronchospasm may also be initiated by air pollutants such as fumes, smoke, dust, and even talcum, lint, and aerosol sprays.

Protection of the lung is basic for the preservation of lung function. Patients with COPD should be informed unequivocally that, for them, smoking is dangerous. Cigarette smoking depresses the activity of scavenger cells and affects the ciliary cleansing mechanism of the respiratory tract, the function of which is to keep the breathing passages free of inhaled irritants, bacteria, and other foreign matter. This is one of the major defense mechanisms of the body. When this cleansing mechanism is damaged by smoking, air flow is obstructed and air becomes trapped behind the obstructed airway. The air sacs greatly distend and the lung capacity is diminished. Cigarette smoking also irritates the goblet cells and mucous glands, causing an increased accumulation of mucus. The mucus accumulation produces more irritation, infection, and damage to the lung capacity. Frequently, the patient is unaware of what is happening until he notices that extra physical effort produces respiratory distress. At this point the damage may be irreversible. Therefore, patients with COPD should definitely refrain from smoking. There is a wide variety of smoking control strategies, including *prevention, cessation,* and behavior modification. (Unfortunately, not all patients are capable of stopping smoking completely.)

Patients with COPD should restrict themselves to a life of moderate activity, ideally in a climate with minimal shifts in temperature and humidity. Stress situations that might trigger a coughing episode or emotional disturbance should be avoided.

Patients should be directed to community resources such as pulmonary rehabilitation programs, smoking cessation programs, and other programs to help improve their ability to cope with their chronic condition and their therapeutic regimen and to give them a sense of worth, hope, and well-being.

▷ *Evaluation*

▷ *Expected Outcomes*

1. Patient improves gas exchange.
   a. Verbalizes need for bronchodilators and for taking them on schedule.
   b. Demonstrates ability to use and clean respiratory therapy equipment.
   c. Uses oxygen equipment appropriately.
   d. Evidences stable arterial blood gas values (but not necessarily normal due to chronic changes in gas exchange capability of the lung).
2. Achieves airway clearance.
   a. States that 6 to 8 glasses of fluids per day are needed.
   b. Understands that pollens, fumes, gases, dusts, and extremes of temperature and humidity are respiratory irritants to be avoided.
   c. Stops smoking or agrees to attend a smoking cessation program.
   d. Performs postural drainage correctly and reports that caregiver can do percussion/vibration.
   e. Coughs less.
   f. Knows signs of early infection and need to notify physician at earliest sign of infection.
   g. Is free of infection on discharge.
   h. Verbalizes need to stay away from crowds and people with colds during the flu season.
   i. Plans to discuss flu and pneumonia vaccines with his physician to help prevent infection.
3. Improves breathing pattern.
   a. Practices pursed-lip and diaphragmatic breathing and uses them during activity and when short of breath.
   b. Uses inspiratory muscle trainer for 10 minutes daily.
   c. Shows signs of decreased respiratory effort.
4. Performs self-care activities.
   a. Paces activities of daily living with alternate rest periods to reduce fatigue and dyspnea.
   b. Uses controlled breathing while bathing, bending to tie shoes, and so on.
   c. Knows about energy conservation.
5. Achieves activity tolerance.
   a. Performs activities with less shortness of breath.
   b. Verbalizes need to exercise daily and demonstrates an exercise plan to be carried out at home.
   c. Walks and gradually increases walking time and distance to improve physical conditioning.
6. Acquires effective coping mechanisms.
   a. Verbalizes activities or methods to ease shortness of breath.
   b. Plans on joining a support group.
   c. Participates in a pulmonary rehabilitation program.
7. Adheres to therapeutic program.
   a. Is able to list those factors that improve his condition as well as those that make his condition worse.

b. Verbalizes the need to preserve existing lung function by adhering to treatment and rehabilitation program.

Chronic Bronchitis

Clinical Manifestations and Pathophysiology.   The defining characteristic of chronic bronchitis is a productive cough that lasts for 3 months a year for 2 successive years. In chronic bronchitis, excessive mucus secretion and dyspnea are associated with recurring infections of the lower respiratory tract and often with reduced ability to ventilate the lungs. The patient's major problem is the protracted and abundant production of inflammatory exudate that fills and obstructs the bronchioles and is responsible for a persistent, productive cough and shortness of breath. This constant irritation causes hypertrophy of mucus-secreting glands, goblet cell hyperplasia, and increased mucus production, leading to bronchial plugging and bronchial narrowing. Alveoli adjacent to the bronchioles may become damaged and fibrosed. Further bronchial narrowing follows as a result of these fibrotic changes in the airways. In time, irreversible lung changes may occur, with resultant emphysema or bronchiectasis.

A wide range of viral, bacterial, and mycoplasmal infections can produce acute episodes of bronchitis. Bronchitis is encountered in people who smoke heavily or are exposed to air pollutants that produce abnormal secretion of mucus and impair ciliary function. Hereditary factors and reaction to allergens also play a part in its development. Exacerbations of chronic bronchitis are most likely to occur during the winter. The inhalation of cold air produces bronchospasm in sensitive persons. Progressive bronchitis will almost invariably result in COPD.

Preventive Measures.   Because of the disabling nature of chronic bronchitis, every effort is directed toward its prevention. An important feature is the avoidance of respiratory irritants (particularly tobacco smoke). People who are prone to respiratory tract infections should be immunized against common viral agents with vaccines for influenza and for *Streptococcus pneumoniae*. All patients with acute upper respiratory tract infections should receive proper treatment, including antibiotic therapy based on cultures and sensitivity studies at the first sign of purulent sputum.

Management.   The main objectives of treatment are to maintain the patency of the peripheral bronchial tree, to facilitate removal of bronchial exudates, and to prevent disability. Changes in the sputum pattern (nature, color, amount, thickness) and in the cough pattern are important signs to note. Recurrent bacterial infections are treated with antibiotic therapy after the completion of culture and sensitivity studies.

To facilitate the removal of bronchial exudates, bronchodilators are prescribed to relieve bronchospasm and reduce airway obstruction; thus, gas distribution and alveolar ventilation are improved. Postural drainage and chest percussion following treatments are usually helpful. Water (given orally or parenterally if bronchospasm is severe) is an important part of therapy, since proper hydration helps the patient cough up secretions. Steroid therapy may be used when the patient fails to respond to more conservative measures, but its use is still controversial. When there is an underlying bronchiectasis, postural drainage is most important. The patient must stop smoking because smoke inhalation causes bronchoconstriction, paralysis of ciliary activity, and inactivation of surfactant. Smokers are also more susceptible to bronchial infection.

For nursing management and patient education, see Nursing Process: The Patient With COPD, pages 473–476.

Bronchiectasis

Bronchiectasis is a chronic dilatation of the bronchi and bronchioles. Bronchial dilatation may be caused by a variety of conditions, including pulmonary infections and obstruction of the bronchus, aspiration of foreign bodies, vomitus, or material from the upper respiratory tract, and extrinsic pressure from tumors, dilated blood vessels, and enlarged lymph nodes. A person may be predisposed to bronchiectasis as a result of respiratory infection in early childhood, measles, influenza, tuberculosis, and IgA deficiency. Following surgery, bronchiectasis may develop when the patient's cough is ineffective, with the result that mucus obstructs the bronchus and leads to atelectasis.

Pathophysiology.   The infection damages the bronchial wall, causing loss of its supporting structure and producing thick sputum that may ultimately obstruct the bronchi. The walls become permanently distended by severe coughing. The infection extends to the peribronchial tissues, so that in the case of saccular bronchiectasis, each dilated tube virtually amounts to a lung abscess, the exudate of which drains freely through the bronchus. The lower lobes are most frequently involved.

The retention of secretions and obstruction ultimately lead to collapse of the distally situated lung (atelectasis). Inflammatory scarring or fibrosis replaces functioning lung tissue. In time the patient develops respiratory insufficiency with reduced vital capacity, decreased ventilation, and an increased ratio of residual volume to total lung capacity. There is impaired mixing of inspired gas (ventilation–perfusion imbalance) and hypoxemia.

Clinical Manifestations.   Characteristic symptoms of bronchiectasis include chronic cough and the production of purulent sputum in copious amounts. The sputum has a characteristic quality of a "layering out" into three layers on standing: a frothy top layer, a middle clear layer, and a dense particulate bottom layer. A high percentage of patients with this disease experience hemoptysis. Clubbing of the fingers is also very common. The patient is likely to be subject to repeated episodes of pulmonary infection.

Many persons with bronchiectasis are not readily diagnosed because their symptoms are mistaken for those of simple chronic bronchitis. A definite clue is offered by the prolonged history of productive cough, with sputum consistently negative for tubercle bacilli. The diagnosis is established on the basis of bronchography (p. 416) and bronchoscopy (p. 416). These procedures give proof of the presence or absence of bronchial dilatation.

Preventive Measures.   All respiratory infections should be promptly treated. Bronchial secretions can be removed (by expectorants, postural drainage, therapeutic bronchoscopy) in order to prevent bronchiectasis. If a child has a prolonged cough and fever, the family should be urged to seek medical treatment. Unconscious persons should be turned (prone position to lateral) to drain all bronchial segments. The educational programs concerning immunization should be continued to prevent pertussis and measles (which may lead to bronchiectasis) so that these severe viral infections will not occur. All patients should be vaccinated against influenza and pneumococcal pneumonia.

Management. The objectives of treatment are to prevent and control infection and to promote bronchial drainage to rid the affected portion of the lung(s) of excessive secretions. Infection is controlled with antibiotic therapy guided by results of sensitivity studies on organisms cultured from sputum. Patients may be put on a year-round regimen of antibiotics, alternating types of drugs at intervals. Some clinicians use antibiotics throughout the winter or when acute upper respiratory tract infections occur.

Postural drainage of the bronchial tubes underlies all treatment considerations because draining the bronchiectatic areas by gravity reduces the amount of secretions and the degree of infection. (Sometimes mucopurulent sputum must be removed by bronchoscopy.) The affected chest area may be percussed or "cupped" to assist in raising secretions.

The patient is started out with short periods of postural drainage and the time is increased steadily. Bronchodilators may be given to persons who also have obstructive airway disease. Patients with bronchiectasis almost always have associated bronchitis. β-Sympathomimetics may be used for bronchodilation and to increase the mucociliary transport of secretions.

To make sputum expectoration easier, the water content of the sputum is increased by aerosolized nebulizer treatments and by an increase in oral fluid intake. A face tent is ideal for providing extra humidification for aerosols. The patient should not smoke since this impairs bronchial drainage by paralyzing ciliary action, increasing bronchial secretions, and causing inflammation of the mucous membranes, resulting in hyperplasia of the mucous glands.

Surgical intervention may be indicated for the patient who continues to expectorate fairly large amounts of sputum and experience repeated bouts of pneumonia and hemoptysis in spite of a successful treatment regimen, provided the disease involves only one or two areas of the lung that can be removed without producing respiratory insufficiency. The goal of surgical treatment is to conserve normal pulmonary tissue and avoid infectious complications.

All diseased tissue is removed provided that the postoperative lung function will be adequate. It may be necessary to remove a segment of a lobe (segmental resection), a lobe (lobectomy), or an entire lung (pneumonectomy). *Segmental resection* is the removal of an anatomical subdivision of a pulmonary lobe. The chief advantage is that only diseased tissue is removed, with greater conservation of healthy lung tissue. Bronchography aids in the delineation of the segment. The operation is preceded by a period of preparation, which is exceedingly important. The objective is to obtain a dry (as dry as possible) tracheobronchial tree in order to prevent complications (atelectasis, pneumonia, bronchopleural fistula, and empyema). This is accomplished by means of postural drainage or, if the abscess is suitably situated, by direct suction through a bronchoscope. A course of antibacterial therapy may be started.

Following the operation, the care is the same as for any chest surgical patient, as is discussed on pages 444 to 458.

Patient Education. The patient is taught diaphragmatic breathing and postural drainage exercises. He is encouraged to have regular dental care and to avoid all pulmonary irritants (cigarette smoke, noxious fumes). He should monitor his sputum and report any change in its character or quantity. A decrease in sputum production is as significant as is an increase. An important preventive aspect is immunization against influenza and pneumococcal pneumonia. Other aspects of health teaching are included under COPD on pages 473–475.

Pulmonary Emphysema

Pulmonary emphysema is a complex and destructive lung disease characterized by destruction of the alveoli, enlargement of air spaces, and loss of airway support by the lung parenchyma. It appears to be the end stage of a process that has slowly progressed for many years. In fact, by the time the patient develops symptoms, pulmonary function is often irreversibly impaired. Along with chronic obstructive bronchitis, it is a major cause of disability under Social Security and is the *most common respiratory cause of death* in the United States.

Cigarette smoking is the major cause of emphysema. However, in a small percentage of patients there is a familial predisposition to emphysema associated with a plasma protein abnormality, a deficiency of α_1-antitrypsin. The genetically susceptible person is sensitive to environmental influences (smoking, air pollution, infectious agents, allergens) and, in time, develops chronic obstructive symptoms. It is imperative that the carriers of this genetic defect be identified to permit genetic counseling and that the environmental factors be modified to delay or prevent overt symptoms of disease.

Pathophysiology. In emphysema the major site of obstruction is the airways which become plugged with mucus and narrowed from inflammation. In later stages the obstruction is caused by loss of the supporting tissues of the airway (elasticity of the lung), which causes the bronchioles to collapse during expiration. The smaller air passages dilate and the alveoli fuse together, resulting in a loss of normal lung elasticity and an increase in dead space. The alveolus is the site in the lung where venous blood and inhaled air complete the process of gas exchange. In order for gas exchange to be effective, the alveoli must be adequately ventilated with air. Interference with alveolar ventilation may occur if there is bronchial obstruction or uneven expansion of the lungs with poor air distribution.

The person with emphysema has a chronic obstruction (marked increase in airway resistance) to the inflow and outflow of air from the lungs. The lungs are in a state of chronic hyperexpansion. In order to get air into and out of the lungs, negative pressure is required during inspiration and an adequate level of positive pressure must be attained and maintained during expiration. The rest position is one of inflation. Instead of being an involuntary passive act, expiration becomes a muscular active act. The patient becomes increasingly short of breath, the chest becomes rigid, and the ribs are fixed at their joints. The "barrel chest" of many of these patients is due to loss of lung elasticity in the presence of the continued tendency of the chest wall to expand (Fig. 23-1).

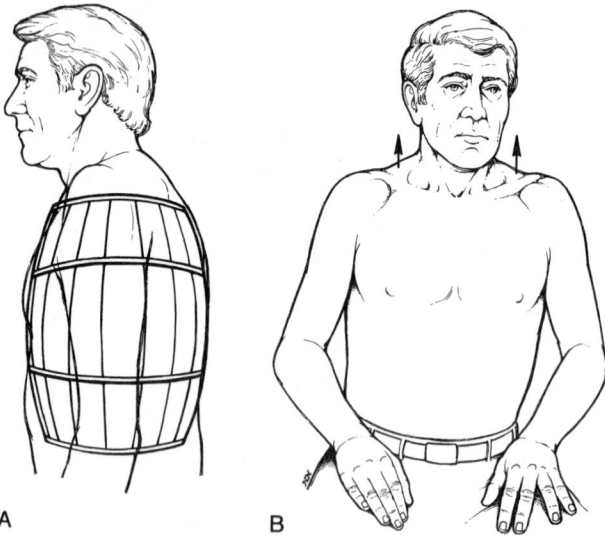

Figure 23-1
Comparison of typical findings in the patient with pulmonary emphysema. (*A*) The common "barrel chest" condition of the patient with emphysema, showing characteristic increase of anteroposterior diameter. (*B*) Another posture of the patient with emphysema, showing elevation of shoulder girdle and retraction of the supraclavicular fossae on inspiration.

In some instances the barrel chest is due to kyphosis. Some patients bend forward to breathe, using the accessory muscles of respiration. There is also retraction of the supraclavicular fossae on inspiration (see Fig. 23-1*B*). In advanced disease there is also contraction of the abdominal muscles on inspiration. There is a progressive reduction of the vital capacity. Full deflation becomes increasingly difficult and finally impossible. The total vital capacity may be normal, but the 1-second vital capacity is low. The patient moves air more slowly and inefficiently and has to work hard to do it. Alveolar integrity begins to break down. As the walls of the alveoli are destroyed (a process accelerated by recurrent infections), the alveolar-capillary surface area continually decreases. In late stages of the disease there is interference with carbon dioxide elimination and the increased carbon dioxide tension in arterial blood (called *hypercapnia*) causes respiratory acidosis. There is also impairment of oyxgen diffusion resulting in hypoxemia.

As the alveolar walls continue to rupture, the pulmonary capillary bed is reduced. The pulmonary blood flow is increased and the right ventricle is forced to maintain a higher blood pressure in the pulmonary artery. Thus, right-sided heart failure (cor pulmonale) is one of the complications of emphysema. The presence of leg edema (dependent edema), distended neck veins, or pain in the region of the liver suggests the development of cardiac failure.

Secretions are increased and retained, since the person is unable to make a forceful cough to expel them. Chronic and acute infections thus take hold in the emphysematous lungs, adding to the air transfer problem.

Classification.   There are two main pathologic types of emphysema, which are classified on the basis of the kind of changes taking place in the lung: (1) panlobular (panacinar) and (2) centrilobular (centriacinar).

In the *panilobular (panacinar) type,* there is destruction of the respiratory bronchiole, alveolar duct, and alveoli. All air spaces within the lobule are more or less enlarged. This patient typically has a hyperinflated chest and marked dyspnea on exertion. Sometimes he is referred to as a "pink puffer." This patient remains "pink," or well-oxygenated, until the disease becomes terminal.

In the *centrilobular (centriacinar) form,* the pathologic changes take place mainly in the center of the secondary lobule while the peripheral portions of the acinus are preserved. Frequently, there is a derangement of ventilation–perfusion ratios, producing chronic hypoxia, hypercapnia, and polycythemia. This leads to cyanosis, peripheral edema, and respiratory failure. The patient may be called a "blue bloater." In addition to the management outlined below, the blue bloater usually receives diuretic therapy for edema. Both types of emphysema very often occur in the same patient.

Clinical Manifestations.   Dyspnea is the presenting symptom in emphysema and has an insidious onset. The patient usually has a history of cigarette smoking and a long history of chronic cough, wheezing, and increasing shortness of breath, especially with respiratory infection. In time even the slightest exertion, such as bending over to tie his shoelaces, produces dyspnea and fatigue (exertional dyspnea). The emphysematous lung is not contracted on expiration, and the bronchioles are not effectively emptied of their secretions.

The patient readily develops inflammatory reactions and infections owing to the pooling of these secretions. After these infections, the patient experiences a prolonged wheezing expiration. Anorexia, weight loss, and weakness are common complaints.

Diagnostic Evaluation.   The patient's symptoms and the clinical findings on physical examination provide the initial clues to the patient's problem. Other aids in diagnosis include chest films, pulmonary function tests (particularly spirometry), and blood gas studies (to assess ventilatory function and pulmonary gas exchange).

Management.   The major objectives of treatment are to improve the quality of life, to slow the progression of the disease process, and to treat the obstructed airways to relieve hypoxia. The therapeutic approach includes (1) treatment measures designed to improve ventilation and decrease the work of breathing, (2) prevention and prompt treatment of infection, (3) the use of physical therapy techniques to conserve and increase pulmonary ventilation, (4) maintenance of proper environmental conditions to facilitate breathing, (5) supportive and psychological care, and (6) an ongoing program of patient education and rehabilitation.

Bronchodilators.   Bronchodilators are prescribed to dilate the airways, because they combat both bronchial mucosal edema and muscular spasm and help in reducing airway obstruction and improving gas exchange. These drugs include the β-adrenergic agonists (metaproterenol, isoproterenol) and the methylxanthines (theophylline, aminophylline), which produce bronchial dilatation by different mechanisms. Bronchodilator drugs may be administered orally, subcutaneously, intravenously, rectally, or via nebulization (conversion into a spray). Nebulized drugs may be delivered by pressurized aerosols, hand-bulb nebulizers, pump-driven nebulizers, or IPPB. Bronchodilators may produce unwanted side-effects, which include tachycardia, cardiac dysrhythmias, and central nervous system excitation. The methylxanthines may also produce gastrointestinal disturbances such as nausea and vomiting. Since side-effects are common, the drug dosage is carefully adjusted for each patient in accordance with his tolerance and clinical response.

Aerosol Therapy. Aerosolization (the process of dispensing particles in a fine mist) of saline bronchodilators and mucolytics is frequently used to aid in bronchodilatation. The particle size in the aerosol mist must be small enough to allow the medication to be deposited deep within the tracheobronchial tree.

Nebulized aerosols relieve bronchospasm, decrease mucosal edema, and liquefy bronchial secretions. This facilitates the process of bronchial clearance, helps to control the inflammatory process, and improves ventilatory function. Hand-bulb nebulizers and metered-dose aerosol devices give the patient quick relief. Electrically powered nebulizers and air-powered nebulizers are useful if the patient has more marked ventilatory impairment. The improvement of the oxygen saturation of the arterial blood and the reduction of its carbon dioxide content assists in relieving the patient's hypoxia and gives considerable relief from constant respiratory fatigue. Nebulizer treatments driven with oxygen must be given with extreme caution in patients who have chronically elevated carbon dioxide tensions and are breathing on hypoxic stimuli. There is a trend away from the use of IPPB, especially in the home-care setting.

Superimposed Infection. Patients with emphysema are susceptible to lung infections and must be treated at the earliest signs of infection. The physician usually prescribes antimicrobial therapy with tetracyclines, ampicillin (Amcill), amoxicillin (Amoxil), or trimethoprim-sulfamethoxazole (Bactrim). An antimicrobial regimen is helpful in treating recurrent episodes of purulent bronchitis and appears to shorten the course of fever and cough. Steroids may be prescribed in selected patients with severe disease.

Removal of Secretions. Removal of secretions is achieved through chest physiotherapy to facilitate drainage of accumulated secretions and tracheal suctioning when the patient is unable to cough up his secretions (see Chap. 22). Bronchoscopic removal of secretions may be occasionally necessary for the patient who is unable to cough and raise sputum. For the patient who develops acute respiratory failure (p. 500), endotracheal intubation or tracheostomy may be indicated to permit more effective suctioning of secretions, to prevent mucus plugging, and to provide ventilatory assistance.

Oxygenation. Alterations in the level of oxygen in the arterial blood results in hypoxemia in patients with severe emphysema. When present, low concentrations of oxygen are administered during acute episodes to correct the hypoxemia. The amount and duration of oxygen is determined by the periodic measurement of arterial blood gas. For certain patients with advanced emphysema, *continuous low-flow oxygen* is used for hypoxemia with cor pulmonale and secondary erythrocytosis that cannot be corrected by conventional methods. This modality of treatment may alleviate the patient's symptoms and improve his quality of life and usually involves long-term home use of oxygen (see Nursing Care Plan 23-2, pp. 484–487).

Asthma

Asthma is an intermittent, reversible, obstructive airway disease characterized by increased responsiveness of the trachea and bronchi to various stimuli. This results in narrowing of the airways, causing dyspnea. This narrowing of the airway changes in degree, either spontaneously or because of therapy. Asthma differs from other obstructive lung diseases in that is is a *reversible process*, and patients may exhibit no symptoms for a prolonged period of time. When asthma and bronchitis occur together, the obstruction is compounded and is called *chronic asthmatic bronchitis*.

Asthma can begin at any age; about half of the cases develop in childhood and another third before age 40. Approximately 17% of all Americans have had asthma at some time in their lives. Although asthma is rarely fatal, it affects school attendance, occupational choices, physical activity, and many other aspects of life.

Asthma is often characterized as extrinsic (allergic), intrinsic (idiopathic or nonallergic), or mixed (both factors):

Extrinsic asthma is caused by a known allergen or allergens (*e.g.,* dust, pollens, animals, dander, food). Patients with extrinsic asthma usually have a family history of allergies and a past medical history of eczema or allergic rhinitis. Exposure to the allergen triggers an asthmatic attack. Children with extrinsic asthma often outgrow the condition by adolescence.

Intrinsic asthma is not related to specific allergens. Factors such as a common cold, respiratory tract infections, exercise, emotions, and environmental pollutants may trigger an attack. Aspirin or other nonsteroidal anti-inflammatory drugs may also be a factor. The attacks of intrinsic asthma become more severe and frequent with time and can progress to chronic bronchitis and emphysema. Some patients will develop mixed asthma.

Mixed asthma is the most common form of asthma. It has characteristics of both the extrinsic and the intrinsic forms.

Pathophysiology. Asthma is a reversible diffuse airway obstruction. The obstruction is caused by one or more of three developments: (1) contraction of muscles surrounding the bronchi, which narrows the airway; (2) swelling of membranes that line the bronchi; and (3) filling of the bronchi with thick mucus (Fig. 23-2). In addition, there is bronchial muscle enlargement, mucous gland enlargement, thick, tenacious sputum, and hyperinflation or air trapping in the alveoli. The exact mechanism for these changes is not known, but most of what is known involves the immunologic system and the autonomic nervous system.

Some persons with asthma develop exaggerated IgE responses to their environments. This means that abnormally large amounts of IgE are produced in response to certain antigens and allergens. The IgE antibodies then attach to mast cells, which are found in the lung. Reexposure to the antigen results in the antigen's binding to the antibody. This causes the release of mast cell products (called mediators) such as histamine, bradykinin, and prostaglandins and of the slow-reacting substance of anaphylaxis (SRS-A). The release of

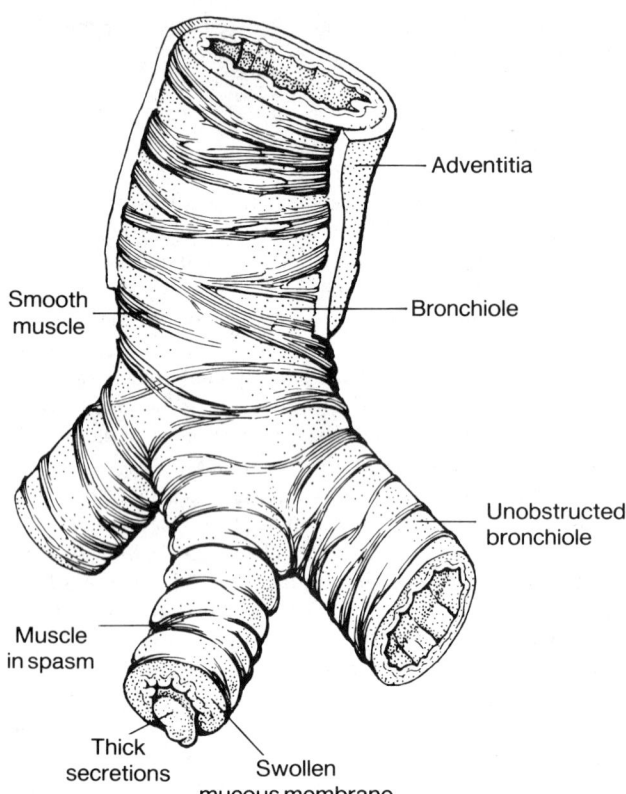

Figure 23-2
Obstruction of a bronchiole in asthma.

Adventitia

Bronchiole

Smooth muscle

Unobstructed bronchiole

Muscle in spasm

Thick secretions

Swollen mucous membrane

these mediators in the lung tissue affects the smooth muscle and glands of the airway, causing bronchospasm, mucous membrane swelling, and excessive mucus production.

The autonomic nervous system innervates the lung. Bronchial muscle tone is regulated by vagal nerve impulses via the parasympathetic system. In intrinsic asthma, when the nerve endings in the airway are stimulated by such factors as infection, exercise, cold, smoking, emotions, and pollutants, an increased amount of acetylcholine is released. This can directly cause bronchoconstriction as well as stimulate the production of the chemical mediators discussed above. A proposed theory is that persons with asthma have a low tolerance for parasympathetic responses.

In addition, α- and β-adrenergic receptors of the sympathetic nervous system are located in the bronchi. When the α-adrenergic receptors are stimulated, bronchoconstriction occurs; bronchodilation occurs when the β-adrenergic receptors are stimulated. The balance between α- and β-receptors is controlled primarily by cyclic adenosine monophosphate (cAMP). Alpha-receptor stimulation results in a decrease in cyclic AMP, which leads to an increase in mast cell release of chemical mediators and bronchoconstriction. Beta-receptor stimulation results in increased levels of cyclic AMP, which inhibits release of chemical mediators and causes bronchodilation. A proposed theory is that β-adrenergic blockade occurs in persons with asthma. Consequently, asthmatics are prone to an increased release of chemical mediators and constriction of smooth muscle.

Clinical Manifestations. It is interesting to note that cough may be the only symptom in some patients with asthma.

In others, in addition to contraction of smooth muscles, there is edema of the bronchial mucosa and production of excess mucus.

The asthmatic attack starts suddenly with coughing and a sensation of tightness in the chest. Then slow, laborious, wheezy breathing begins. Expiration is always much more strenuous and prolonged than inspiration, which forces the patient to sit upright and use every accessory muscle of respiration. Obstructed air flow creates the sensation of dyspnea. The person becomes blue from hypoxia and breaks out into a profuse sweat; the pulse is weak; the extremities are cold; and there may be fever, and, occasionally, pain, nausea, vomiting, and diarrhea. The cough at first is tight and dry, but it soon becomes more violent; a distinctive sputum of thin mucus containing small, round, gelatinous masses is coughed up with much difficulty. The attack may last from one-half hour to several hours. Under certain circumstances, the attack may subside spontaneously, but this should not be counted on. Such attacks are rarely fatal. However, occasionally "status asthmaticus" occurs, in which therapeutic measures fail and the patient has repeated attacks or continuous asthma. This condition is life-threatening (see p. 482).

Related Reactions. Allergic reactions related to asthma include eczema (present at some time during life in 75% of patients with asthma), urticaria, and angioneurotic edema (present in 50% of patients). Emotional stress may bring on an attack in those who are susceptible, just as any other organ system in the body may be stimulated by psychic factors. However, rarely are emotions the sole cause of asthma.

Diagnostic Evaluation. A clear history of hypersensitivity (at home or at work) to some known substance that may be inhaled or ingested, such as a pollen, a particular type of food, feathers, animal hair, or face powder, or a history suggesting the probability of such a sensitivity is very important in determining the type and cause of asthma present in any given patient. The close association of the attacks with allergic rhinitis, together with the discovery, during the attack, of marked pallor and swelling of the nasal mucous membrane, aids in establishing the case as one of extrinsic allergic asthma (Table 23-2). The finding of an abnormally high count of eosinophilic cells in the blood or the sputum tends to confirm this diagnostic impression. Blood gas evaluation and simple spirometry are useful in evaluating gas exchange and providing baseline data that assist in identifying dangerous hypoxemia and respiratory acidosis.

Physical exertion may induce acute bronchospasm in most patients with asthma. The key factor appears to be heat loss from the respiratory tract induced by hyperventilation. Inhalation of cold air during exercise rapidly increases bronchoconstriction, whereas warm, humid air does not.

With more industries releasing chemical irritants in the work place or into the environment, the asthmogenic result is increasingly apparent. Common air pollutants can depress pulmonary function. People exposed to grains and wood dusts often show symptoms of respiratory irritation and allergic reaction. Certain drugs, such as aspirin, indomethacin, and related anti-inflammatory agents, may trigger asthmatic attacks.

However, "all that wheezes is not asthma," and it is important to be able to rule out congestive cardiac failure or bronchial obstruction due to a foreign body or a tumor as the underlying cause or precipitating factor that may explain

TABLE 23-2
Comparison of Extrinsic and Intrinsic Asthma

Extrinsic (Allergic)	Intrinsic (Infectious)
Age at Onset	
3 to 35	Under 3, over 35 or 40
Symptoms	
Season or perennial, frequently pollen and mold related	Worse in winter, exacerbated by cold air, air pollution, and primarily by infection
Mucus	
Clear and foamy	Thick and white or discolored
Family History of Atopy	
Positive	No greater than in general population
Skin Tests	
Positive and correlating	Negative or positive noncorrelating
Serum IgE	
High or normal	Normal
Response to Therapy	
Good response to immunotherapy and bronchodilators	Poor response to bronchodilators; no response to immunotherapy

(Patterson R [ed]. Allergic Diseases, 3rd ed. Philadelphia, JB Lippincott, 1985.)

the attack. Hence, in every case of doubtful origin, there is the necessity for careful radiologic and, often, bronchoscopic examination.

In patients who do not have obvious clinical manifestations, testing in a pulmonary function laboratory can usually provide objective evidence of airway obstruction. An office spirometer is less expensive, as is a peak flowmeter, in determining the presence of asthma. The peak expiratory flow rate (PEFR) measures the maximum flow at the outset of forced expiration.

Often a diagnosis is confirmed by instructing the patient to inhale a trial aerosol bronchodilator (during a coughing episode). If the wheezing is caused by bronchitis, the cough is not relieved; if the underlying cause is asthma, the cough is relieved. An even more effective diagnostic aid is the monitoring of PEFRs. Since this is a simple test, the patient can be instructed to monitor his own flow rates. It has been found that patients are far more accurate in assessing their own PEFR than are health care providers. In addition, patients are quite accurate in judging whether the obstruction is better or worse from day to day. Symptoms such as cough and chest tightness must also be evaluated.

Prevention. In every patient with recurrent asthma, evidence should be sought that might implicate a foreign protein to which the patient is hypersensitive and which might precipitate the attacks. If attacks occur chiefly at night, when the patient is in bed, skin tests are conducted with material from the mattress and pillows. If the test results are positive, then a mattress and pillow made from other materials are substituted. If attacks appear to be associated with the presence of a particular species of animal, such as a horse or a cat, similar skin tests are made with an antigen composed of hair or skin scrapings from the animal concerned. The examiner should search for foci of bacterial infection (*e.g.*, of chronically infected sinuses or teeth) because their eradication may be strikingly beneficial in certain patients. A seasonal incidence of attacks in a patient suggests an airborne allergen as the chief etiologic agent. In such cases, therapy may be attempted with pollen extracts. Air conditioning offers possibilities in the prevention of attacks, depending on the extent to which the patient can restrict his life to air-conditioned rooms during the pollen season. A complete change of climatic environment to a locality with different flora during that period is the most satisfactory solution, when feasible.

Exercise-induced asthma (EIA) can be prevented by inspiring air at 37°C (body temperature) and 100% relative humidity. Covering the nose and mouth with a mask necessitates rebreathing expired air that has been warmed and moistened by its passage through the respiratory tract. A simple face mask is an inexpensive, practical method for asthmatic ball players, runners, and skiers.

Associated Psychotherapeutic Modalities. It is important to remember that asthmatic attacks, once started, may indicate that the patient will be susceptible to repeated attacks. In some patients, attacks may be induced by suggestion alone. Good general physical and mental health is most important.

Complications of Asthma. The acute asthmatic attack per se is seldom serious; however, death occasionally occurs as a result of respiratory exhaustion, which is particularly possible if sedatives are administered too freely.

Complications of asthma include a ruptured bleb, causing pneumothorax; mediastinal or subcutaneous emphysema; chronic and recurrent acute bronchitis; bronchiectasis; pulmonary hypertension; and hypertrophy of the right side of the heart with right-sided heart failure (pulmonary heart disease). Chronic hypoxia due to these complications leads to symptoms and personality changes.

Medication to dilate the bronchioles is used in both prevention and treatment of asthma. Categories of bronchodilators usually prescribed include the xanthine derivatives aminophylline (Amoline) and theophylline (Theo-Dur); the sympathomimetics epinephrine (Adrenalin), terbutaline sulfate (Brethine), and isoetharine hydrochloride (Bronkosol); and steroids, which moderate the inflammatory response. Cromolyn sodium (Aarane), an inhaled medication that is not a bronchodilator but prevents the release of chemical mediators of anaphylaxis, is also used to prevent attacks.

In an acute attack, the sympathetic drugs and the theophyllines are used. Epinephrine (Adrenalin) is given initially subcutaneously and repeated in 15 to 30 minutes if there is no improvement in the bronchospasm. If this does not help, intravenous aminophylline is started. Status asthmaticus does not respond readily to the theophyllines and sympathomimetics. Administration of intravenous corticosteroids is necessary. In patients with chronic asthma or frequent attacks, continuous therapy is indicated. The same combination of medications is prescribed; sometimes oral steroids are added.

Sedatives or tranquilizers are administered to calm the anxious patient who is not in danger of developing respiratory failure. Antibiotics are prescribed if an infection occurs. Patients with extrinsic (allergic) asthma may undergo treatment to reduce their sensitivity to the allergens.

Airway obstruction, particularly during acute episodes, often results in hypoxemia, requiring the administration of oxygen and the monitoring of arterial blood gases. The administration of fluids is also important because persons with asthma are frequently dehydrated from diaphoresis and the insensible fluid loss of hyperventilation.

Breathing exercises along with postural drainage and aerosol therapy are prescribed in order to aid in removing retained secretions. IPPB is not advocated for acute asthma attacks. If the patient's condition worsens to the point of acute respiratory failure, intubation and mechanical ventilation will be necessary.

Status Asthmaticus

Status asthmaticus is severe asthma that is unresponsive to conventional therapy with epinephrine and theophylline and lasts longer than 24 hours. A vicious self-perpetuating cycle may occur as a result of infection, anxiety, overuse of tranquilizers, nebulizer abuse, dehydration, increased β-adrenergic block, and nonspecific irritants. An acute episode may sometimes be precipitated by hypersensitivity to aspirin.

Pathophysiology. A combination of factors, including constriction of the bronchiolar smooth muscle, swelling of bronchial mucosa, and thickened (inspissated) secretions, contribute to one pathologic problem—a decrease in the diameter of the bronchi. Another problem is the ventilation–perfusion abnormality that results from hypoxemia and respiratory acidosis or alkalosis.

There is a reduced PaO_2 and an initial respiratory alkalosis with a decreased $PaCO_2$ and an increased pH. As the severity of status asthmaticus increases, the $PaCO_2$ increases and the pH falls, reflecting respiratory acidosis.

Clinical Manifestations. Breathing is labored, with a greater effort made on exhalation. The neck veins and even the face veins become engorged. Expelled air escapes with a wheeze; however, the amount of wheezing does not correlate with the severity of the attack. With greater obstruction, the wheeze may disappear.

Diagnostic Evaluation. The rising P_{CO_2} suggests progressive pulmonary failure and requires aggressive drug intervention and other therapeutic measures to prevent death from respiratory failure. Therefore, blood gas determinations are an important guide to the severity of the condition and offer a reliable method of checking the patient's response to therapy.

Management. Treatment is best given in a pulmonary intensive care unit where clinical management is in the hands of the allergist, pulmonary disease specialist, and anesthesiologist, as well as a nurse clinician. Frequent serum electrolyte determinations are made to guide proper electrolyte therapy. Aminophylline is administered intravenously or at 6-

hour intervals until adequate theophylline levels in the blood serum are reached.

To treat dyspnea, cyanosis, and hypoxemia, oxygen therapy is initiated on low-flow humidified oxygen, either by Venturi mask or nasal catheter. The amount is determined following blood gas determinations. The PaO_2 is kept between 65 and 85 mm Hg (8.64 to 11.30 kPa[a]).

Corticosteroids are also prescribed to restore bronchial reactivity. Mucolytic agents, such as acetylcysteine (Mucomyst), are effective after bronchodilation has occurred. Cough suppressants and sedatives are avoided. If symptoms suggest the presence of an infection, antibiotics are given. The drugs of choice (if the patient is not sensitive to them) are tetracycline, cephalothin, and ampicillin. Appropriate agents are determined following Gram-stain sputum studies. Epinephrine may be administered every 4 hours subcutaneously for acute dyspnea; however, little or no effect is noted in the first 24 hours.

Nursing Interventions. Signs of dehydration are assessed by checking skin turgor. Fluid intake is essential to combat dehydration, to loosen secretions, and to facilitate expectoration. Intravenous fluids are administered as prescribed up to 3000 to 4000 ml/day.

Constant monitoring of the patient by the nurse is important for the first 12 to 24 hours, or until status asthmaticus is halted. When it is necessary to question the patient, the nurse should try to phrase the questions so that he can answer in only one or two words. The room should be quiet and free of respiratory irritants, including flowers and cigarette smoke. The patient should have a nonallergenic pillow.

Mechanical assistance for breathing may be required when maximum medical therapy fails. Volume-cycled respirators are preferable to pressure-cycled ventilators, because large tidal volumes are necessary to overcome airway resistance. During mechanical ventilation, the patient's cardiac function and blood gas values must be carefully monitored to avoid such complications as heart failure and pneumothorax.

Patient Education and Home Health Care. Patient education is an important part of post-hospital care if recurrences are to be kept to a minimum. Bronchodilators may be required on an "around-the-clock" basis. Certain medications can be increased when asthmatic attacks occur. Adequate hydration must be maintained at home to keep secretions from thickening. The patient needs to recognize that infection is to be avoided, since it can trigger an attack.

In some clinics, patients are being instructed in self-care protocols designed with goals of (1) aborting severe attacks and (2) giving the patient with asthma a measure of independence. Included in this regimen is the administration of theophylline with a long-acting oral preparation. This is regulated within the narrow therapeutic ratio with careful instructions on the hazards of overuse. The patient gets a hand-held metered-dose inhaler that uses a β_2-selective adrenergic, such as metaproterenol or albuterol. This also is used within prescribed limitations. Should these bronchodilators fail, the patient is further instructed on beginning a corticosteroid drug (short, high dose), usually prednisone, at a prescribed dosage. He notifies the physician or nurse clinician of his progress.

Nursing Care Plan 23-2 provides a detailed review of the care of the patient with COPD (see pp. 484–487).

Pulmonary Hypertension

Pulmonary hypertension is a condition that is not clinically evident until late in its disease progression. Pulmonary hypertension exists when the pulmonary arterial pressure exceeds 30 mm Hg systolic, 10 mm Hg diastolic, and 15 mm Hg mean pressure. These pressures, however, cannot be measured indirectly as can systemic blood pressure but must be measured during right-sided heart catheterization. In the absence of these measurements, clinical recognition becomes the only indicator for the presence of pulmonary hypertension. There are two forms of pulmonary hypertension: primary (or idiopathic) and secondary. *Primary pulmonary hypertension* is of unknown cause and is rare. It occurs most often in women between 20 and 40 years of age and is usually fatal within 7 years of diagnosis. *Secondary pulmonary hypertension* is more common and results from existing cardiac or pulmonary disease. Its prognosis depends on the severity of the underlying disorder and the changes in the pulmonary vascular bed. The most common cause of pulmonary hypertension is pulmonary artery vasoconstriction due to hypoxia from COPD (Chart 23-1).

Pathophysiology. Normally, the pulmonary vascular bed can handle whatever the right ventricle delivers. It has a low resistance to blood flow and compensates for increased blood volume by opening unused vessels in the pulmonary circulation. However, if the pulmonary vascular bed is destroyed or obstructed, as in pulmonary hypertension, the ability to handle whatever flow or volume of blood it receives is lost and the increased blood flow then increases the pulmonary arterial pressures. As the pulmonary arterial pressure increases, the pulmonary vascular resistance also increases. Both pulmonary artery vasoconstriction (as in hypoxia or hypercapnia) and a reduction of the pulmonary vascular bed (which occurs with pulmonary emboli) result in an increase in pulmonary vascular resistance and pressure. This increased work load affects right ventricular function. The myocardium ultimately is unable to meet the increasing demands imposed on it, leading to right ventricular hypertrophy (dilation) and failure (cor pulmonale).

Clinical Manifestations. The signs and symptoms are usually associated with the underlying cardiac or pulmonary disorder. Increasing dyspnea on exertion is the most common symptom; chest pain occurs in 30% to 60% of those affected. Other signs and symptoms include weakness; fatigability; syncope; signs of right-sided heart failure (peripheral edema, ascites, distended neck veins, liver engorgement, crackles, heart murmur); electrocardiographic changes showing right ventricular hypertrophy, right axis deviation, tall peaked P waves in inferior leads, and decreased PaO_2 (hypoxemia).

Diagnostic Evaluation. Cardiac catheterization of the right side of the heart will reveal elevated pulmonary arterial pressures. Pulmonary angiography will detect defects in pulmonary vasculature such as pulmonary emboli. Pulmonary function studies will reveal an increased residual volume and total lung capacity and a decreased forced expiratory volume in 1 second (FEV_1) in obstructive pulmonary diseases and a decreased vital capacity and total lung capacity in restrictive lung diseases.

Management. The objective of treatment is to manage the underlying cardiac or pulmonary condition. Since hypoxia is the most common cause of pulmonary vasoconstriction leading to increased pulmonary vascular resistance and pulmonary hypertension, oxygen therapy is the major component of management. In acute conditions, appropriate oxygen therapy (see Table 22-1) will reverse the vasoconstriction and reduce the pulmonary hypertension in a relatively short time. In more chronic, progressive conditions, continuous oxygen therapy may be necessary to slow down the pro-

(Text continues on p. 487)

Chart 23-1
Causes of Pulmonary Hypertension

Primary or Idiopathic

Altered immune mechanisms
Silent pulmonary emboli
Raynaud's phenomenon
Oral contraceptives
Sickle cell disease
Collagen diseases

Secondary

Pulmonary Vasoconstriction Due to Hypoxia
COPD
Kyphoscoliosis
Obesity
Smoke inhalation
High altitude
Neuromuscular disorders
Diffuse interstitial pneumonia

Reduction of the Pulmonary Vascular Bed (Must Impair 50% to 75% of the Vascular Bed)

Pulmonary emboli
Vasculitis
Widespread interstitial lung disease (sarcoidosis, sclerosis)
Tumor emboli

Primary Cardiac Disease

Congenital (patent ductus, atrial septal defect, ventricular septal defect)
Acquired (rheumatic valvular disease, mitral stenosis, myxoma, left ventricular failure)

Nursing Care Plan 23-2

Care of the Patient With Chronic Obstructive Pulmonary Disease

Nursing Interventions	*Rationale*	*Expected Outcomes*

Nursing Diagnosis: Impaired gas exchange related to ventilation–perfusion inequality

Goal: Improvement in gas exchange

1. Administer bronchodilators as directed:
  a. Can be given orally, intravenously, rectally, or via nebulization
  b. If giving oral or intravenous bronchodilators and nebulizer or IPPB treatments with bronchodilators, give at alternate times so effects of medication will be enhanced.
  c. Observe for side-effects: tachycardia, dysrhythmias, central nervous system excitation, nausea, and vomiting.
	1. Bronchodilators dilate the airways and help to combat bronchial mucosa edema and muscular spasm. Since side-effects are common, the drug dosage is carefully adjusted for each patient, in accordance with his tolerance and clinical response.	• Verbalizes need for bronchodilators and for taking them on schedule.
		• Evidences minimal side-effects; heart rate near normal, absence of dysrhythmias, normal mentation.

2. Assess effectiveness of mini-nebulizer or IPPB treatments.
  a. Look for decreased shortness of breath, decreased wheezing or crackles, secretions loosened, decreased anxiety.
  b. Ensure that treatment is given before meals to avoid nausea and to reduce fatigue that accompanies eating.
	2. Combining medication with aerosolized bronchodilators is typically used to control bronchoconstriction. Improper administration of the treatment will render it ineffective. Aerosolization facilitates bronchial clearance, helps control the inflammatory process, and improves ventilatory function.	• Reports a decrease in dyspnea.
		• Shows an improved expiratory flow rate.
		• Demonstrates ability to use and clean respiratory therapy equipment where applicable.

3. Instruct and encourage patient in diaphragmatic breathing and effective coughing.	3. These techniques improve ventilation by opening airways and clearing the airways of sputum. Gas exchange is improved.	• Demonstrates diaphragmatic breathing and coughing.

4. Administer oxygen by the method prescribed.
  a. Explain importance to patient.
  b. Evaluate effectiveness; look for signs of hypoxia. Notify physician if restlessness, anxiety, somnolence, cyanosis, or tachycardia is present.
  c. Analyze arterial blood gases as prescribed. When arterial puncture is performed and a blood sample is obtained, hold puncture site for 5 minutes to prevent arterial blood leakage.
  d. Explain that no smoking is permitted by patient or visitors while oxygen is in use.
	4. Oxygen will correct the hypoxemia. Careful observation of the liter flow or the percentage administered and its effect on the patient is needed. If the patient has chronic CO_2 retention, then hypoxia is his stimulus to breathe. Too much oxygen could suppress the hypoxic drive and death would occur. These patients need low-flow oxygen rates of 1 to 2 liters/min. Periodic arterial blood gases help evaluate adequacy of oxygenation.	• Uses oxygen equipment appropriately where indicated.
		• Evidences normal arterial blood gases

(continued)

Nursing Interventions	*Rationale*	*Expected Outcomes*

Nursing Diagnosis: Ineffective airway clearance related to bronchoconstriction, increased mucus production, ineffective cough, and bronchopulmonary infection

Goal: Achievement of airway clearance

1. Give patient 6 to 8 glasses of fluids/day unless cor pulmonale is present.	1. Systemic hydration keeps secretions moist and easier to raise. Fluids will not be handled well by the heart if right-sided heart failure is present.	• Verbalizes need to drink 6 to 8 glasses of fluids/day.
2. Teach and encourage the use of diaphragmatic breathing and coughing techniques.	2. These techniques will help to improve ventilation and to produce secretions without causing breathlessness and fatigue.	• Demonstrates diaphragmatic breathing and coughing.
3. Assist in administering nebulizer or IPPB treatments.	3. These treatments add water to the bronchial tree and to the sputum, decreasing its viscosity, so that evacuation of secretions is facilitated.	
4. Perform postural drainage with percussion and vibration in the morning and at night as prescribed.	4. Uses gravity to help raise secretions so they can be more easily coughed up or suctioned.	• Performs postural drainage correctly. • Coughs less.
5. Instruct patient to avoid bronchial irritants such as cigarette smoke, aerosols, extremes of temperature, and fumes.	5. Bronchial irritants cause bronchoconstriction and increased mucus production, which then interferes with airway clearance.	• Does not smoke. • Verbalizes that pollens, fumes, gases, dusts, and extremes of temperature and humidity are irritants to be avoided.
6. Teach early signs of infection that are to be reported to the physician immediately: a. Increased sputum b. Change in color of sputum c. Increased thickness of sputum d. Increased shortness of breath or tightness in chest or fatigue e. Increased coughing	6. Minor respiratory infections that are of no consequence to the person with normal lungs can produce fatal disturbances in the lungs of the person with emphysema. Early recognition becomes crucial.	• Knows signs of early infection. • Is free of infection on discharge (no fever, no change in sputum, lessening of dyspnea. • Verbalizes need to notify physician at the earliest sign of infection.
7. Administer antibiotics as ordered.		
8. Encourage patient to be immunized against influenza and *Streptococcus pneumoniae*.	8. People with respiratory conditions are prone to respiratory infections and are encouraged to be immunized.	• Verbalizes need to stay away from crowds or people with colds in flu season. • Plans to discuss flu and pneumonia vaccines with physician to help prevent infection.

Nursing Diagnosis: Ineffective breathing pattern related to shortness of breath, mucus, bronchoconstriction, and airway irritants

Goal: Improvement in breathing pattern

1. Teach patient diaphragmatic and pursed lip breathing.	1. Helps patient control the rate and depth of respirations. With these techniques, patient will breathe more efficiently and effectively.	• Practices pursed-lip and diaphragmatic breathing and uses them when short of breath and with activity.
2. Encourage alternating activity with rest periods. Let patient make some decisions (bath, shaving) about his care based on his tolerance level.	2. Pacing activities will conserve patient's lung capacity and permit him to do activities without excessive distress.	• Shows signs of decreased respiratory effort by pacing activities.
3. Teach the use of an inspiratory muscle trainer.	3. Strengthens and conditions the respiratory muscles.	• Uses inspiratory muscle trainer for 10 minutes every day.

(continued)

Nursing Interventions	*Rationale*	*Expected Outcomes*

Nursing Diagnosis: Self-care deficits related to fatigue secondary to increased work of breathing and insufficient ventilation and oxygenation

Goal: Independence in self-care activities

1. Teach patient to coordinate diaphragmatic breathing with activity (*e.g.,* walking, bending).	1. This will allow him to be more active and to avoid excessive fatigue or dyspnea during activity.	• Uses controlled breathing while bathing, bending, and walking. • Paces activities of daily living to alternate with rest periods to reduce fatigue and dyspnea.
2. Encourage patient to begin to bathe himself, dress himself, walk, and drink fluids. Discuss energy conservation measures.	2. As condition resolves, patient will be able to do more but needs to be encouraged or he may become dependent.	• Knows about energy conservation. • Can perform the same self-care activities he was doing prior to admission.
3. Teach postural drainage if appropriate.	3. Encourages patient to get involved in his own care. Builds self-esteem and prepares him to manage at home.	• Performs postural drainage correctly.

Nursing Diagnosis: Activity intolerance due to fatigue, hypoxemia, and ineffective breathing patterns

Goal: Improvement in activity tolerance

Support patient in establishing a regular regimen of exercise using treadmill and exercycle walking.
   a. Assess the patient's current level of functioning and develop exercise plan from there.
   b. Suggest consultation with a physical therapist to determine an exercise program specific to the patient's capability. Have portable oxygen units available in case oxygen is needed during exercise.
	Muscles that are deconditioned consume more oxygen and place an additional burden on the lungs. Through regular, graded exercise, these muscle groups become more conditioned, and the patient can do more without getting as short of breath. The less people do, the less they can do or emotionally feel like doing. Graded exercise breaks this cycle of debilitation.	• Performs activities with less shortness of breath.
		 • Verbalizes need to exercise daily and demonstrates an exercise plan to be carried out at home.
		 • Walks and gradually increases walking time and distance to improve physical condition.

Nursing Diagnosis: Ineffective individual coping related to less socialization, anxiety, depression, lower activity level, and the inability to work

Goal: Attainment of an optimal level of coping

1. Adopt a hopeful and encouraging attitude toward patient.	1. Giving the patient a sense of hope will give him something to work toward; rather than a defeated, hopeless attitude.	
2. Encourage activity to level of symptom tolerance.	2. Activity reduces tension and decreases degree of dyspnea as patient becomes conditioned.	• Discusses activities or methods that can be performed to ease shortness of breath.
3. Teach relaxation technique or provide a relaxation tape for patient to listen to.	3. Relaxation reduces stress and anxiety and helps patient to cope with disability.	• Uses relaxation techniques appropriately.

(continued)

Nursing Interventions	*Rationale*	*Expected Outcomes*

Nursing Diagnosis: Ineffective individual coping related to less socialization, anxiety, depression, lower activity level, and the inability to work

Goal: Attainment of an optimal level of coping

4. Enroll patient in pulmonary rehabilitation program where available.	4. Pulmonary rehabilitation programs have demonstrated a subjective improvement in a patient's status and self-esteem as well as increased exercise tolerance and decreased hospitalizations.	• Expresses interest in a pulmonary rehabilitation program.
5. Suggest vocational conseling to explore alternative avenues of employment (if applicable).	5. Work modification may need to be made and appropriate resources used to achieve this goal.	• Explores resources available for work modification.

Nursing Diagnosis: Potential for nonadherence to recommended care procedures at home

Goal: Adherence to therapeutic program and home care

1. Help patient accept realistic short- and long-term goals. • Teach the patient about his disease and his care.	1. Patient needs to see that there is a method and plan for his care in which he plays a major role. He has to be told what to expect. Teaching him about his condition is one of the most important aspects of his care; it will prepare him to live and cope with his condition and improve his quality of life.	• Understands his disease and what affects his condition. • Verbalizes that he must preserve existing lung function by adhering to his program.
2. Discuss the need to stop smoking and teach methods to do so.	2. Cigarette smoking causes definite damage to the lung and diminishes the lungs' protective mechanisms. Air flow is obstructed and lung capacity is reduced.	• Stops smoking or enrolls in a smoking cessation program.

gression of the disease. In the presence of cor pulmonale, treatment should include fluid restriction, digitalis to improve cardiac function, rest, and diuretics to decrease fluid accumulation. In primary pulmonary hypertension, vasodilators have been administered with variable success.

Nursing Interventions. The major nursing goals are to identify those patients who are at high risk of developing pulmonary hypertension (*i.e.*, those with COPD, pulmonary emboli, congenital heart disease, and mitral valve disease); to be alert for signs and symptoms; and to administer oxygen therapy appropriately.

Pulmonary Heart Disease (Cor Pulmonale)

Cor pulmonale is a condition in which the right ventricle enlarges (with or without failure) as a result of diseases that affect the structure or function of the lung or its vasculature.

Any disease that affects the lungs and has associated hypoxemia may result in cor pulmonale. The most frequent cause is COPD in which changes in the airway and retained secretions reduce alveolar ventilation. Other causes are conditions that restrict or compromise ventilatory function, leading to hypoxia or acidosis (deformities of the thoracic cage, massive obesity) or conditions that reduce the pulmonary vascular bed (primary idiopathic pulmonary arterial hypertension, pulmonary embolus). Certain disorders of the nervous system, respiratory muscles, chest wall, and pulmonary arterial tree may be responsible for cor pulmonale.

Pathophysiology. Pulmonary disease can produce a chain of events that will in time produce hypertrophy and failure of the right ventricle. Any condition that deprives the lungs of oxygen can cause hypoxemia (decreased arterial oxygen tension) and hypercapnia (increased carbon dioxide in the blood), resulting in ventilatory insufficiency. Airway hypoxia and hypercapnia cause pulmonary arterial vasoconstriction. There may be associated reduction of the pulmonary vascular bed, as in emphysema or pulmonary emboli. The result is increased resistance in the pulmonary circuit, with a subsequent rise in pulmonary blood pressure (pulmonary hypertension). One sees pulmonary arterial mean pressures of 45 mm Hg or more in cor pulmonale. Right ventricular hypertrophy may then result and be followed by right ventricular failure. In short, cor pulmonale results from pulmonary hypertension that causes the right side of the heart to enlarge because of the increased work required to pump blood against high resistance through the pulmonary vascular system.

Clinical Manifestations.   Usually, the symptoms of cor pulmonale are those of underlying lung disease. COPD produces shortness of breath and cough. As the right ventricle fails, the patient develops edema of the feet and legs, distended neck veins, an enlarged, palpable liver, pleural effusion, ascites, and a heart murmur. Headache, confusion, and somnolence may be manifested as a result of carbon dioxide narcosis.

Management.   The objectives of treatment are to improve the patient's ventilation and to treat both the underlying lung disease and the manifestations of heart disease. In COPD the airways have to be opened to improve gas exchange. With improved oxygen transport, the reactive pulmonary hypertension that leads to cor pulmonale is relieved. In short, the lung must be treated first. Oxygen is given to reduce pulmonary arterial pressure and pulmonary vascular resistance. Although the ideal number of hours per day of oxygen therapy is under study, better survival and greater reduction in pulmonary vascular resistance have been reported with continuous (24 hours/day) oxygen therapy for patients with severe hypoxia. Substantial patient improvement may require 4 to 6 weeks of oxygen therapy. This is usually carried out at home. Assessment of arterial blood gases is necessary to determine adequacy of alveolar ventilation and to monitor low-flow oxygen.

Additional measures include bronchial hygiene and the administration of bronchodilators and chest physical therapy to improve ventilation. If the patient is in respiratory failure, endotracheal intubation and mechanical ventilation may be necessary. If the patient is in heart failure, the improvement of hypoxemia and hypercapnia will be necessary to improve cardiac action and output. In addition, he is placed on bed rest, and sodium restriction and diuretic therapy are employed judiciously to reduce peripheral edema (to lower pulmonary arterial pressure through a decrease in total blood volume) and the circulatory load on the right side of the heart. Digitalis may be given if the patient has coincident left ventricular failure, a supraventricular arrhythmia, or right ventricular failure that does not respond to other therapy to relieve pulmonary hypertension. It is given with extreme caution, since pulmonary heart disease appears to enhance susceptibility to digitalis toxicity.

Electrocardiographic monitoring is done when necessary, since there is a high incidence of dysrhythmias in these patients. Respiratory infection must be treated, since it commonly precipitates pulmonary heart disease. The patient's prognosis depends on whether the hypertensive process is reversible. (The management of the patient with respiratory failure is discussed on p. 502).

Patient Education and Home Health Care.   Because management of pulmonary heart disease is related to treating the underlying cause, it is often a long-term process. Consequently, most of the care and monitoring is done in the home. The patient is told to avoid those things that irritate the airway if he has COPD. If continuous oxygen is administered, the patient and his family are instructed in its use. Most important, the patient is urged to stop smoking! Nutrition counseling is necessary if he is on a sodium-restricted diet or is taking diuretics. The family is counseled that restlessness, depression, and irritable or angry behavior may be encountered with hypoxemia or hypercapnia and should decrease as the arterial blood gas values improve.

Pulmonary Embolism

Pulmonary embolism refers to the obstruction of one or more pulmonary arteries by a thrombus (or thrombi) that originates somewhere in the venous system or in the right side of the heart, becomes dislodged, and is carried to the lung. An infarction of lung tissue caused by interruption of the lung's blood supply results in 10% of embolic episodes. Pulmonary embolism is a common disorder and is often associated with advanced age, postoperative states, and prolonged immobility. It may occur in an apparently healthy person. Persons who are at risk of developing a pulmonary embolus are listed in Chart 23-2.

The majority of thrombi originate in the deep veins or the legs. Other sources include the pelvic veins and the right atrium of the heart. Stasis, or slowing of blood flow, owing to damage to the blood vessel wall (particularly the endothelial lining) and changes in the blood coagulation mechanism, are factors favoring formation of venous thrombi.

Pathophysiology.   Following a massive embolic obstruction of the pulmonary arteries, there is an increase in alveolar dead space since the area, although continuing to be ventilated, receives little or no blood flow. In addition, a number of vasoactive and bronchoconstrictive substances are released from the clot. These substances compound the ventilation–perfusion imbalance, causing venous admixture and shunting.

The hemodynamic consequences are increased pulmonary vascular resistance due to reduction in the size of the pulmonary vascular bed, a consequent increase in pulmonary arterial pressure, and, in turn, an increase in right ventricular work to maintain pulmonary blood flow. When the work requirements of the right ventricle exceed its capacity, right ventricular failure occurs. When this happens there is a decrease in cardiac output followed by a drop in systemic blood pressure and the development of shock.

Clinical Manifestations.   The symptoms of pulmonary embolism depend on the size of the thrombus and the area of the pulmonary artery occluded. Dyspnea is the one symptom that is usually consistently present with pulmonary embolism. A massive embolism occluding the bifurcation of the pulmonary artery can produce pronounced dyspnea, sudden substernal pain, rapid and weak pulse, shock, syncope, and sudden death.

If one or more branches of the right or left pulmonary arteries are obstructed, the patient experiences dyspnea, mild substernal pain, anxiety, weakness, and tachycardia. Usually, these symptoms are the result of pulmonary infarction. There may also be fever, cough, and hemoptysis. The patient's respiratory rate is accelerated out of proportion to the degree of fever and tachycardia. If the terminal pulmonary arteries

> ## Chart 23-2
> ## Pulmonary Embolism: Risk Factors
>
> The following events and conditions predispose to thrombophlebitis and pulmonary embolism.
>
> **Venous Stasis** (slowing of blood flow in veins)
>
> Prolonged immobilization
> Prolonged periods of sitting/traveling
> Varicose veins
>
> **Hypercoagulability** (owing to release of tissue thromboplastin following injury/surgery)
>
> Injury
> Tumor
> Increased platelet count (polycythemia, splenectomy)
>
> **Venous Endothelial Disease**
>
> Thrombophlebitis
> Vascular disease
> Foreign bodies (IV/central venous catheters)
>
> **Certain Disease States** (combination of stasis, coagulation alterations, and venous injury)
>
> Heart disease (especially congestive heart failure)
> Trauma (especially fracture of hip, pelvis, spine, lower extremities)
> Postoperative state/postpartum period
> Diabetes
> Chronic obstructive pulmonary disease
> Previous pulmonary embolism
>
> **Other Predisposing Conditions**
>
> Advanced age
> Obesity
> Pregnancy
> Oral contraceptive use
> History of preceding thrombophlebitis
> Constrictive clothing

are occluded, a pleuritic type of pain develops, together with cough and hemoptysis. Multiple small emboli can lodge in the terminal pulmonary arterioles, producing multiple small infarctions. The clinical picture may simulate that of bronchopneumonia or heart failure. In some instances, the disease presents in an atypical fashion with few signs and symptoms, while in other instances it mimics various cardiopulmonary disorders.

Diagnostic Evaluation. The chest film will reveal subtle or nonspecific changes. Pleural effusion, which is evidenced radiographically by locally increased radiolucency and enlargement of the central pulmonary arteries, may contribute to the diagnosis. An electrocardiogram may show characteristic but nonspecific changes and needs to be compared with a previous electrocardiogram in order to correlate changes with the suspected embolism. Auscultation of the lungs reveals decreased breath sounds and wheezing in the affected area along with crackles if there is associated atelectasis in the same area as the embolus. Auscultation of the heart will demonstrate a loud pulmonary second sound and a third heart sound, which may indicate the presence of pulmonary hypertension and right-sided heart failure. Arterial blood gas analysis will show hypoxemia, and pulmonary function studies will be abnormal but nonspecific to pulmonary embolism. A perfusion lung scan coupled with a ventilation lung scan will confirm the presence of emboli when the ventilation scan is normal in an area where there is a defect in the perfusion scan (indicating areas of diminished or absent blood flow). If lung scanning is not definitive, then pulmonary angiography will usually confirm the diagnosis of pulmonary emboli. A phlebogram may be done to detect "silent" thrombi in the legs.

An ultrasound procedure has yielded a high percentage of correct diagnoses. This test consists of three parts, each focusing on a separate clinical sign. In the first part of the test, ultrasound transmission is directed at the lung. A lung

with pulmonary embolus, pneumonia, or atelectasis reflects fewer ultrasound waves; therefore, more waves pass through in comparison to the normal lung. Such a finding rules out COPD and congestive heart failure. The energy from ultrasound waves is absorbed more readily by a pulmonary embolus and atelectasis. In the second part of the test, if energy loss is significantly high, a pulmonary embolus is suspected and pneumonia can be ruled out. In the third part, pulsed Doppler ultrasound is used to monitor blood flow in the affected area of the lung. Diminished blood flow indicates a pulmonary embolus and atelectasis is ruled out.

Preventive Measures. A liberal fluid intake is encouraged because dehydration predisposes to thrombus formation. Suppression of platelet function by pharmacologic agents (aspirin, dipyridamole) is being used to prevent platelet aggregation to reduce the likelihood of thromboembolism.

The American Heart Association recommends that patients who are over 40 and hemostatically competent, and who are undergoing major elective abdominothoracic surgery, be given low doses of heparin to diminish postoperative deep thrombus and pulmonary embolism. The heparin is given subcutaneously 2 hours before surgery and continued every 12 hours until the patient is discharged., Low-dose heparin is thought to enhance the activity of antithrombin III, a major plasma inhibitor of clotting factor X. (This regimen is not recommended for patients who are experiencing an active thrombotic process or those undergoing major orthopedic surgery, open prostatectomy, or operations on the eye or brain.)

Emergency Interventions. *Massive pulmonary embolism is a true medical emergency; the patient's condition tends to deteriorate rapidly.* The immediate objective of treatment is to stabilize the cardiorespiratory system. The majority of patients who die of massive pulmonary embolism do so in the *first 2 hours* following the embolic event. Emergency management consists of the following:

- Nasal oxygen is administered immediately to relieve hypoxemia, respiratory distress, and cyanosis.
- An infusion is started to open an intravenous route for drugs/fluids that will be needed.
- Pulmonary angiography, hemodynamic measurements, arterial blood gas determinations, and perfusion lung scans are carried out. A sudden rise in pulmonary resistance increases the work of the right ventricle, which can cause acute right-sided heart failure with cardiogenic shock.
- If the patient has suffered massive embolism and is hypotensive, an indwelling urethral catheter is inserted to monitor urinary volume.
- Hypotension is treated by a slow infusion of isoproterenol (has a dilating effect on pulmonary vessels and bronchi) or dopamine.
- The electrocardiogram is monitored continuously for right ventricular failure, which may have a rapid onset.
- Sodium bicarbonate may be administered to correct metabolic acidosis. Digitalis glycosides, intravenous diuretics, and antiarrhythmic agents are given when appropriate.
- Blood is drawn for serum electrolytes, blood urea nitrogen, complete blood count, and hematocrit.
- If clinical assessment and arterial blood gases indicate the need, the patient is placed on a volume-controlled ventilator.
- Small doses of intravenous morphine are given to relieve the patient's anxiety, to alleviate chest discomfort, to help him accept the discomfort of the endotracheal tube, and to ease his adaptation to the mechanical ventilator.

Management

The alteration in respiratory function is due to a reduction in the size of the pulmonary vascular bed caused by the pulmonary embolus. To correct or treat this alteration, drug therapy is initially administered to remove the thrombus/embolus and restore the pulmonary circulation to normal and then to prevent recurrence.

The consensus is changing in the management of pulmonary embolism. Although anticoagulant therapy (heparin, warfarin sodium) has traditionally been the primary method of management of acute deep vein thrombosis and pulmonary embolism, thrombolytic therapy (urokinase, streptokinase) is now widely used to dissolve thrombi in the deep veins and in the pulmonary circulation. This thrombolytic therapy results in a more rapid resolution of the thrombi/emboli. It restores more normal hemodynamic functioning of the pulmonary circulation, resulting in a reduction of pulmonary hypertension. On a long-term basis, thrombolytic therapy prevents permanent damage to the pulmonary vascular bed. Bleeding, however, is a significant side-effect. Consequently, thrombolytic agents are advocated only for patients with thrombi affecting the popliteal vein or deep veins of the thigh and pelvis, and for patients with massive pulmonary emboli affecting a significant area of blood flow to the lung.

Before the thrombolytic infusion, a thrombin time (TT), activated partial thromboplastin time (APTT), prothrombin time (PT), hematocrit values, and platelet counts are obtained. During therapy all but absolutely essential invasive procedures are avoided, with the exception of careful venipuncture with a No. 22-gauge or 23-gauge needle for therapeutic monitoring. If necessary, fresh whole blood, packed red cells, cryoprecipitate, or frozen plasma is given to replace blood loss and reverse the bleeding tendency.

After completion of the thrombolytic infusion (which varies in duration according to the agent used and condition being treated) the patient is placed on anticoagulants. Anticoagulation slows or stops the underlying thrombotic process, thus preventing recurrence. Heparin is given and controlled according to standard procedures and is followed by warfarin sodium.

Other measures are initiated to support the patient's respiratory and vascular status. Oxygen therapy is administered to correct the hypoxia and to relieve the pulmonary vascular vasoconstriction and reduce the pulmonary hypertension. Elastic stockings are used to compress the superficial venous system and increase the velocity of deep venous blood by redirecting the blood through the deep veins. Venous stasis is then reduced. However, simple leg elevation (above the level of the heart) with flexion at the knees also increases venous flow. Some authorities believe elastic stockings are unnecessary if the patient's legs are elevated.

Surgical Intervention. If the patient has persistent hypotension, shock, and respiratory distress; if pulmonary artery pressure is greatly elevated; and if angiograms reveal obstruction of a large part of the pulmonary vasculature, embolectomy may be indicated. This requires a thoracotomy with cardiopulmonary bypass technique.

Another surgical technique used when pulmonary emboli recur, despite adequate medical therapy (or if the patient is intolerant of anticoagulant therapy), is an interruption of the inferior vena cava. This method prevents dislodged thrombi from being swept into the lungs while at the same time permitting adequate blood flow. This can be done by total ligation or the use of Teflon clips applied to the vena cava to divide the caval lumen into small channels without occluding caval blood flow. The use of transvenous devices that occlude or filter the blood through the inferior vena cava is a fairly safe procedure for the prevention of recurrent pulmonary embolism. One such technique is the insertion of a prosthetic umbrella device through a cervical incision in the internal jugular vein (Fig. 23-3). The device is advanced through the superior vena cava and the right atrium into the inferior vena cava where it is brought into an open position. The perforated umbrella permits the passage of blood but prevents the passage of large thrombi.

Transvenous catheter embolectomy is a technique in which a vacuum-cupped catheter is introduced transvenously into the affected pulmonary artery. Suction is applied to the end of the embolus, and the embolus is aspirated into the cup. The surgeon maintains suction to hold the embolus within the cup, and the entire catheter is withdrawn through the right side of the heart and out the femoral venotomy. An inferior caval filter is often inserted at the same time to protect against a recurrence.

Nursing Assessment

The nurse examines each susceptible patient for a positive Homan's sign, which may or may not indicate impending thrombosis of the leg veins (see Chap. 28). Testing proceeds as follows:

1. Position the patient on his back.
2. Lift the leg and dorsiflex the foot.
3. Note if there is pain in the calf during this maneuver (positive Homan's sign); it may indicate deep venous thrombosis.
4. Conduct another clinical assessment by tapping on the anterior tibial crest to see if this elicits pain.
5. Apply a blood pressure cuff around the patient's calf and inflate it. Pain on inflation of the cuff (80 to 100 mm Hg) is significant, as is tenderness along the course of a vein, pain in the calf or foot area, or edema in the ankle or calf area. It is best to compare both extremities.
6. Look for swelling and palpable veins. Clinical evidence of phlebitis in one leg does not necessarily indicate that this is the site of the embolus; the other leg, even though normal on examination, may be the site.

The nurse's key role is to try to prevent the occurrence of pulmonary embolism in all patients and to identify those who are at high risk. (See Chart 23-2). The nurse must have a high degree of suspicion for pulmonary embolism in any patient, but particularly those with conditions predisposing to slowing of venous return. Such conditions include trauma to the pelvis (especially surgical) and lower extremities (especially hip fractures), obesity, history of thromboembolic disease, varicose veins, pregnancy, congestive heart failure, myocardial infarction, oral contraceptive use, and malignant disease; also, postoperative patients and the elderly often have a slower venous return.

Nursing Interventions

The nurse must be alert for the potential complication of shock or right ventricular failure subsequent to the effect of the pulmonary embolus on the cardiovascular system. Nursing activities for management of shock are found on pages 365–367.

Prevention of thrombus formation is a major nursing responsibility. Ambulation and active and passive leg exercises are encouraged to prevent venous stasis in patients on bed rest. When the legs are moved in a "pumping" exercise, the leg muscles help to increase venous flow. The patient is advised to avoid prolonged sitting, immobility, or constricting clothing. He is *not* permitted to "dangle" his legs and feet in a dependent position while sitting on the edge of the bed. His feet should be on the floor or on a chair and he should avoid crossing his legs. Intravenous catheters (for parenteral therapy or measurements of central venous pressure) should not be left in the veins for prolonged periods of time.

The nurse is responsible for monitoring thrombolytic and anticoagulant therapy. Thrombolytic therapy (streptokinase) causes lysis of deep vein thrombi and pulmonary emboli, promoting resolution. During thrombolytic infusion, the patient remains on bed rest, vital signs are assessed every 3 to 4 hours, and invasive procedures are limited. The PT or APTT is performed 3 to 4 hours after starting the thrombolytic infusion to confirm activation of the fibrinolytic systems. Because of the prolonged clotting time, only essential arterial

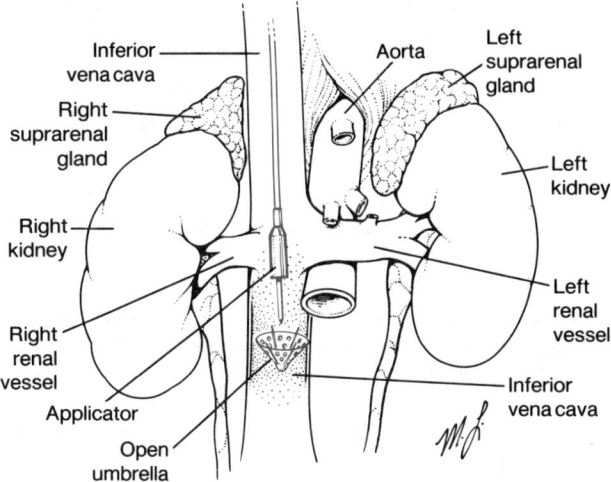

Figure 23-3
Insertion of umbrella filter in inferior vena cava to prevent pulmonary embolism. Filter (compressed within an applicator catheter) is inserted through an incision in the right internal jugular vein. The applicator is withdrawn when the filter fixes itself to the wall of the inferior vena cava after ejection from the applicator.

blood gas studies are performed on the upper extremities, with digital compression of the puncture site for at least 30 minutes. The infusion is immediately discontinued if uncontrolled bleeding occurs. (See Chap. 28 for nursing management for anticoagulant therapy.)

When chest pain is present, it is usually pleuritic. The patient should be in semi-Fowler's position to allow for maximum ease in breathing and distribution of air. Narcotic analgesics are administered as prescribed for severe pain.

Careful attention is given to the proper use of oxygen. It is important to make sure that the patient understands the need for continuous oxygen therapy. The nurse assesses the patient frequently for signs of hypoxia as a means of evaluating the effectiveness of the oxygen therapy. Nebulizer therapy, incentive spirometry, and/or postural drainage are administered if there is an accumulation of secretions complicating the pulmonary embolism.

Coping With Anxiety. After the patient's condition stabilizes, he is encouraged to express his feelings about this condition. His questions are answered concisely and accurately. His therapy is explained and he is told how he can help by early recognition of untoward effects. The nurse reassures him of the competency of the health care personnel. On discharge, the patient is instructed how to prevent recurrence and what signs and symptoms should alert him to seek medical attention.

Postoperative Nursing Care. If surgery was performed, the patient's pulmonary arterial pressure and urinary output are measured. The insertion site of the arterial catheter is checked for hematoma formation and infection. An adequate blood pressure must be maintained to ensure perfusion of the vital organs. To prevent peripheral venous stasis and lower extremity edema, the foot of the bed is elevated. Isometric exercises, elastic stockings, and walking are encouraged when the patient is permitted out of bed. Sitting is discouraged, since hip flexion causes compression of the large veins in the legs.

Patient Education and Home Health Care.   The following patient instructions are intended to help prevent recurrences:

- When taking anticoagulants, look for bruising and bleeding and try to protect yourself from bumping into objects that can cause bruising.
- Use a toothbrush with soft bristles.
- Do not take aspirin or antihistamine drugs while receiving warfarin sodium (Coumadin). Always check with your physician before taking any medication, including over-the-counter medications.
- Continue to wear antiembolism stockings as long as directed.
- Avoid laxatives, since they affect vitamin K absorption.
- Avoid sitting with your legs crossed or sitting for prolonged periods.
- When traveling, change your position regularly, walk occasionally, and do active exercises of the legs and ankles while sitting. Drink plenty of liquids while traveling to avoid hemoconcentration owing to fluid loss.
- Report dark, tarry stools to your physician/clinic immediately.
- Wear an identification bracelet (or carry a card) stating that anticoagulants are being taken.

Breathing Disorders During Sleep

Respiratory abnormalities can occur during sleep. Some patients who have adequate blood oxygenation while awake develop hypoxemia while sleeping. *Apnea* is the cessation of air flow at the nose and mouth for more than 10 seconds. *Sleep apnea syndrome,* which is evaluated in a sleep laboratory, is present when there are at least 30 apneic episodes during both rapid eye movement sleep and nonrapid eye movement sleep during 7 hours of nocturnal sleep. Oxygen desaturation is usually evident in apneic episodes.

Sleep apnea is classified into three types: (1) *central*—simultaneous cessation of both air flow and respiratory movements; (2) *obstructive*—lack of air flow due to pharyngeal occlusion; and (3) *mixed*—a combination of central and obstructive apnea within one apneic episode.

The patient, usually male, snores loudly, stops breathing up to 10 seconds or more, and then awakens abruptly with a loud snort as his blood oxygen level drops. He may have more than ten apneic episodes per hour to several hundred per night. This can seriously tax the heart and lungs. Increasing age and obesity correlate positively with alterations in breathing and nocturnal oxygen desaturation. Other symptoms include excessive daytime sleepiness, morning headache, sore throat, and complaints by the bed partner that the patient snores loudly or is unusually restless during sleep.

Management is based on whether complications of life-threatening dysrhythmias, chronic cardiovascular effects, memory loss, and intellectual impairment are present. If obese, the patient is placed on a weight-reduction program.

(Most patients with obstructive apnea are obese.) Tricyclic antidepressants, respiratory stimulants, and tracheostomy to bypass the obstruction may be modalities of treatment according to the problems of the individual patient. Nocturnal oxygen is beneficial for relieving hypoxemia in some patients. Pacemaker stimulation of the phrenic nerves may be helpful in patients with central sleep apnea.

Sarcoidosis

Sarcoidosis is a systemic granulomatous disease of unknown cause. It may involve almost any organ or tissue but most commonly involves the lungs, lymph nodes, liver, spleen, skin, eyes, phalangeal bones, and parotid glands. The onset usually occurs between the third or fourth decade. Sarcoidosis is fairly common worldwide.

Patients with sarcoidosis may have a number of immunologic abnormalities. The first clinical manifestations are usually thoracic, with hilar gland enlargement. The clinical picture includes shortness of breath, cough, vague chest pain, and congestion. The chest film may show hilar adenopathy and disseminated miliary and nodular lesions in the lungs. The granulomas may disappear or gradually convert to fibrous tissue. Extrathoracic involvement includes uveitis, joint pain, fever, and granulomatous lesions of the skin, liver, spleen, kidney, and central nervous system. With multiple organ system involvement, the patient experiences fatigue, fever, anorexia, weight loss, and joint pain.

The diagnosis is confirmed by biopsy of the skin and lymph nodes, which reveal noncaseating granulomas. Pulmonary function tests are abnormal if there is restriction of lung function.

There is no specific treatment, since the natural course of the disease is toward resolution. Corticosteroid therapy may benefit some patients because of its anti-inflammatory effect, which relieves symptoms and improves organ function. It is useful for patients with ocular and myocardial involvement, extensive pulmonary disease with compromise of pulmonary function, and hypercalcemia. Isoniazid may be given to patients with positive tuberculin tests.

Occupational Lung Diseases

Diseases of the lungs can occur in a variety of occupations as a result of exposure to organic or inorganic (mineral) dusts and noxious gases (fumes and aerosols). The effect of inhaling these materials depends on the composition of the inhaled substance, its antigenic (precipitating an immune response) or irritating properties, the dose inhaled, the length of time inhaled, and the host's response (a person's susceptibility to the irritant). There are a growing number of occupational lung diseases owing to new and untested industrial substances and chemicals (presumed to be harmless). The problem may be compounded by smoking, which appears to have a synergistic effect on occupational lung disease and may increase the risk of lung cancers in people exposed to asbestos.

Preventive Measures and Health Maintenance

First, every effort is made to reduce the exposure of the worker to industrial products. The work environment must be ventilated properly to remove the noxious agent from the worker's breathing zone. Dust control can prevent many of the pneumoconioses and includes ventilation, spraying an area with water to control release of dust, and effective and frequent floor cleaning. Air samples need to be monitored. Toxic substances should be enclosed to reduce their concentration in the air. Workers must wear protective devices (face masks, hoods, industrial respirators) to provide a safe air supply when in a toxic atmosphere. Every employee should be carefully screened and followed, especially the worker at high risk for developing occupational lung disease (hypersensitivity states, asthma). There is a risk of developing serious smoking-related illness (cancer) in industries in which there are unsafe levels of certain gases, dusts, fumes, fluids, and other toxic substances. Ongoing educational programs to teach the worker to bear responsibility for his own health, including smoking cessation and influenza vaccination, have a major role in the prevention of occupational lung disease. The responsibility for implementation of these controls inevitably falls on the federal or state governments, as exemplified by the Coal Mine Health and Safety Act of 1969, the Occupational Safety and Health Act of 1970, and the Federal Mine Safety and Health Amendment Act of 1977. The workplace is currently monitored by the Mining Safety and Health Administration (MSHA) of the Department of Labor and the National Coal Workers' Health Surveillance Program of the National Institute for Occupational Safety and Health (NIOSH).

The Pneumoconioses

Pneumoconiosis refers to a nonneoplastic alteration of the lung resulting from exposure to inorganic dust (*e.g.*, "dusty lung"). The most common pneumoconioses are silicosis, asbestosis, and coalworker's pneumoconiosis.

Silicosis. Silicosis is a chronic pulmonary disease caused by inhalation of silica dust (silicon dioxide particles). Since the earth's crust is composed of silica and silicates, exposure is encountered in almost any form of mining (*i.e.*, coal, tin, copper, silver, gold, uranium mining), quarrying (slate, sandstone), or tunneling operations. Stonecutting, the manufacture of abrasives and pottery, and foundry work are other occupations presenting exposure hazards. When the silica particles, which have fibrogenic properties, are inhaled, nodular lesions are produced throughout the lungs. With the passage of time and exposure, the nodules enlarge and coalesce. Dense masses form in the upper portion of the lungs, resulting in loss of pulmonary parenchymal volume. Restrictive lung disease (inability of the lungs to expand fully) and obstructive lung disease from secondary emphysema result. Cavity formation is likely to be the result of superimposed tuberculosis. Exposure of 10 to 20 years is usually required before the disease develops and shortness of breath is manifested. Fibrotic destruction of pulmonary tissue can lead to emphysema, pulmonary hypertension, and cor pulmonale.

There is no specific treatment, and therapy is directed at the complications of silicosis. Preventive measures must be directed at protecting workers from inhaling silica dust. With cavitary lesions or advanced fibrosis, many physicians treat the patient for tuberculosis, even when cultures are negative.

Asbestosis. Asbestosis is a disease characterized by diffuse pulmonary fibrosis due to the inhalation of asbestos dust. The use of asbestos is almost indispensable in modern industry and there are thousands of applications for its use. Exposure occurs in numerous occupations, including asbestos mining and manufacturing, demolition work, and roofing. Materials such as shingles, cement, vinyl asbestos tile, fireproof paint and clothing, brake linings, and filters all contain asbestos. The risk appears to lie in the manufacture, cutting, and demolition of asbestos-containing materials.

The asbestos fibers are inhaled and enter the alveoli, which, in time, are eventually obliterated by fibrous tissue that surrounds the asbestos particles. There is fibrous pleural thickening and pleural plaque formation. The altered physiologic pattern is that of restrictive lung disease with decrease in lung volume, diminished gas transfer, and hypoxemia. The patient has progressive dyspnea, mild to moderate chest pain, anorexia, and weight loss. Cor pulmonale and respiratory failure occur as the disease progresses. A significant proportion of workers exposed to asbestos dust die of lung cancer, especially those who smoke. In addition to lung cancer and asbestosis, exposure to asbestos can produce nonmalignant pleural disease, diffuse malignant mesothelioma, and possibly neoplasms of other tissues. Avoidance, in general, is essential and *asbestos workers should stop smoking*.

There is no effective treatment for asbestosis. Management is directed at intercurrent infection and coexisting lung disease. In patients with severe gas transport abnormalities, continuous oxygen therapy may improve exercise tolerance.

Coal Worker's Pneumoconiosis. *Coal worker's pneumoconiosis* ("black lung") includes a variety of respiratory diseases found in coal workers in which there is an accumulation of coal dust in the lungs causing a tissue reaction to its presence. Coal miners are exposed to dusts that are mixtures of coal, kaolin, mica, and silica. The first physiologic reaction to the deposition of coal dust in the alveoli and respiratory bronchioles is an increase of macrophages that engulf (by phagocytosis) the particles and transport them to the terminal bronchioles where they are removed by mucociliary clearance. In time, the clearance mechanisms are unable to handle the excessive dust load and the macrophages aggregate in the respiratory bronchioles and alveoli. Fibroblasts appear and a network of reticulin is laid down surrounding the dust-laden macrophages. The respiratory bronchioles and the alveoli become clogged with coal dust, dying macrophages, and fibroblasts, which leads to the formation of the coal macule, the primary lesion of the disorder. (Macules appear as blackish dots on the lungs.) As the macules enlarge, there is a dilation of the weakening bronchiole with subsequent development of a focal emphysema.

The patient with complicated coal worker's pneumoconiosis has massive lesions of dense fibrotic tissue containing black material. These masses eventually destroy blood vessels and the bronchi of the affected lobe. The patient develops dyspnea, cough, and sputum production with expectoration of varying amounts of black fluid (melanoptosis), particularly if he is a smoker. Eventually cor pulmonale and respiratory failure result. The treatment is symptomatic. (See also treatment of emphysema, p. 477).

Tumors of the Chest

A chest tumor may be *primary,* arising within the lung or the mediastinum, or it may represent a *metastasis* from a primary tumor site elsewhere. Metastatic tumors of the lungs occur frequently, since the bloodstream transports free cancer cells from primary cancers elsewhere in the body. Such tumors grow in and between the alveoli and the bronchi, which they push apart in their growth. This process may occur over a long period of time, causing few or no symptoms.

Primary tumors of the lung may be benign or malignant. Most arise from the bronchial epithelium. Bronchial adenomas are slow growing, usually benign tumors, but they are very vascular and therefore produce symptoms of bleeding and bronchial obstruction. Bronchogenic carcinoma is a malignant tumor arising from the bronchus. Such a tumor is epidermoid, usually located in the larger bronchi, or is an adenocarcinoma, arising farther out in the lung. There are also several intermediate or undifferentiated types of lung cancer, identifiable by cell type.

Lung Cancer (Bronchogenic Carcinoma)

Lung cancer is the number one cancer killer among men in the United States. It is increasing at a greater rate in women than it is in men and now exceeds breast cancer as the most common cause of cancer death. The survival rate is low, for in approximately 70% of patients, the disease has spread to regional lymphatics and other sites at the time of diagnosis.

It has been suggested that carcinoma tends to arise at sites of previous scarring (tuberculosis, fibrosis) in the lung.

Classification and Staging. The four major cell types of lung cancer (which differ significantly) are epidermoid (squamous cell) carcinoma, small cell (oat cell) carcinoma, adenocarcinoma, and large cell (undifferentiated) carcinoma. The World Health Organization's classification of lung tumors by histologic type is shown in Chart 23-3. Many tumors contain more than one cell type. The different cell types display different biological behavior and have prognostic significance. Therefore, different approaches to treatment may be indicated by the cell type.

The stage of the tumor refers to the anatomical extent of the tumor, spread to the regional lymph nodes, and metastatic spread. Staging is accomplished by tissue diagnosis, lymph node biopsy, and mediastinoscopy. It is important in determining whether tumor resection should be attempted. Prognosis appears most favorable for epidermoid and adenocarcinoma, whereas undifferentiated small cell (oat cell) tumors have a poor prognosis.

Risk Factors. Bronchogenic cancer is ten times more common in cigarette smokers than in nonsmokers, with the prevalence being related to the length of time and the intensity of smoking. Epidermoid carcinoma, involving the larger bronchi, is thought to be almost entirely associated with heavy (1 pack or more per day) cigarette smoking. Few cases of this type of cancer have been reported in nonsmokers. For reasons unknown, the incidence of adenocarcinoma is rising faster than that of other types.

Adenocarcinoma of the peripheral bronchi is not associated with any known cause and occurs equally in smokers and nonsmokers. Another risk factor is occupational exposure

---

Chart 23-3
Histopathologic Types of Lung Tumors

I. Epidermoid carcinomas (squamous cell)
II. Small cell anaplastic carcinomas
   A. Fusiform cell type
   B. Polygonal cell type
   C. Lymphocyte-like ("oat-cell") type
   D. Others
III. Adenocarcinomas
   A. Bronchogenic
      1. Acinar ⎤ with or without
      2. Papillary ⎦ mucin formation
   B. Bronchioloalveolar
IV. Large cell carcinomas
   A. Solid tumors with mucin-like content
   B. Solid tumors without mucin-like content
   C. Giant cell carcinomas
   D. "Clear" cell carcinomas
V. Combined epidermoid and adenocarcinomas
VI. Carcinoid tumors

VII. Bronchial gland tumors
   A. Cylindromas
   B. Mucoepidermoid tumors
   C. Others
VIII. Papillary tumors of the surface epithelium
   A. Epidermoid
   B. Epidermoid with goblet cells
   C. Others
IX. "Mixed" tumors and carcinosarcomas
   A. "Mixed" tumors
   B. Carcinosarcomas of embryonal type ("blastomas")
   C. Other carcinosarcomas
X. Sarcomas
XI. Unclassified
XII. Mesotheliomas
   A. Localized
   B. Diffuse
XIII. Melanomas

(Kreyberg L, Leibow AA, and Vehlinger EA. Histological Typing of Lung Tumors. Geneva, World Health Organization.)

to asbestos, radioactive dusts, arsenic, and certain plastics alone or in combination with tobacco smoke. It is reported that the risk of lung cancer is 92 times greater for people exposed to tobacco smoke and asbestos dust. People at high risk who insist on continuing to smoke should have regular chest films and sputum examinations in order to increase their chances that lung cancer will be detected while it is still treatable.

Clinical Manifestations. Tumors of the bronchopulmonary system may affect the lining of the respiratory tract, lung parenchyma, pleura, or chest wall. The disease begins insidiously (over several decades) and often is asymptomatic until late in its course. The signs and symptoms depend on the location and size of the tumor, the degree of obstruction, and the existence of metastases to regional or distant sites.

The most frequent symptom is cough, probaby from irritation by the tumor mass. It is frequently ignored as a "cigarette cough." Starting as a hacking, nonproductive cough, it later progresses to a point where it produces a thick, purulent sputum as secondary infection occurs.

- Thus, a cough that changes in character should arouse suspicion of lung cancer.

A wheeze in the chest (occurs when a bronchus becomes partially obstructed by the tumor) is noted in about 20% of patients. The expectoration of blood-tinged sputum is common, particularly in the morning, and is due to sputum becoming streaked with blood as it passes over the ulcerated tumor surface. In some patients, recurring fever owing to a persisting infection in an area of pneumonitis distal from the tumor is the early symptom. In fact, cancer of the lung should be suspected in persons with repeated unresolved upper respiratory tract infections. Pain is a late manifestation and is often found to be related to bone metastasis. If the tumor spreads to adjacent structures and regional lymph nodes, the patient may present with chest pain and tightness, hoarseness (involvement of recurrent laryngeal nerve), dysphagia, head and neck edema, and symptoms of pleural or pericardial effusion. The most common sites of metastases are lymph nodes, bone, brain, contralateral lung, and adrenal glands. General symptoms of weakness, anorexia, weight loss, and anemia appear late.

Diagnostic Evaluation. If the patient with pulmonary symptoms is a heavy smoker, cancer of the lung is suspected. Chest radiography is done to search for pulmonary density, a solitary peripheral nodule (coin lesion), atelectasis, and infection. Cytologic examination of fresh sputum obtained by cough or saline washings from a suspected bronchus is done to search for malignant cells. Bronchoscopy with a flexible fiberoptic instrument allows a detailed study of the bronchial segments and identification of the source of malignant cells and of the probable extent of anticipated surgery. Fluorescent bronchofibroscopy is used to detect small, early bronchogenic cancers. Systemically injected hematoporphyrin is absorbed by malignant cells and presents a red fluorescent glow when examined under illumination by violet light.

Lung scans are part of the diagnostic workup. A bone scan or bone marrow study is done for detection of bone metastasis, and liver scanning is used to verify metastatic spread to the liver. Detection of central nervous system metastases is accomplished by brain scanning, computed tomography, and other neurologic diagnostic procedures. Mediastinoscopy may be used to evaluate tumor spread to hilar lymph nodes of the right lung, and mediastinotomy gives access to the hilar lymphatics of the left lung.

Before surgery, the patient is evaluated to determine whether the tumor is resectable and whether he can tolerate the physiologic impairment resulting from such surgery. Pulmonary function tests combined with split-function perfusion scans are done to determine if the patient will have adequate pulmonary reserve following the procedure. The patient's ability to move air (vital capacity, FEV_1) is important since the ability to generate an effective cough is imperative in the postoperative period.

Management

The objective of management is to provide the maximum likelihood of cure. The treatment depends on the cell type, the stage of the disease (anatomical event), and the physiologic status (particularly cardiac and pulmonary status) of the patient. In general, treatment may involve surgery, radiation therapy, chemotherapy, and immunotherapy, used separately or in combination.

Surgery. Surgical resection is the preferred method for patients with localized tumors with no evidence of metastatic spread and whose cardiopulmonary function is adequate. (Usually, surgery for small cell cancer of the lung is not advisable because this is a rapidly growing tumor that metastasizes early and widely.) Unfortunately, in a large number of patients with bronchogenic cancer the lesion is inoperable at the time of diagnosis. The usual operation for small, apparently curable tumor of the lung is lobectomy (removal of a lobe of the lung). An entire lung may be removed (pneumonectomy) in combination with other surgical procedures, such as resection of involved mediastinal lymph nodes. Before surgery, the cardiopulmonary reserve of the patient must be determined. (See pp. 444–458 for the preoperative and postoperative management of the patient undergoing chest surgery.)

Radiation Therapy. Radiation therapy may cure a small percentage of patients. It is useful in controlling radioresponsive neoplasms that cannot be resected. The small cell and epidermoid tumors are usually radiation sensitive. It may be used as palliative treatment to decrease tumor size and relieve pressure on vital structures. It can control symptoms of spinal cord metastasis and superior vena cava compression. Also, prophylactic brain irradiation is used on certain patients to kill microscopic metastases to the brain. Respite may be obtained from cough, chest pain, dyspnea, hemoptysis, and bone and liver pain. Relief of symptoms may last from a few weeks to many months and is important in improving the quality of the remaining period of life.

With radiation therapy there is usually toxicity to normal tissue within the irradiation field. Complications of radiation therapy include esophagitis, pneumonitis, and radiation lung fibrosis, which may impair ventilatory and diffusion capacity with a significant reduction in pulmonary reserve. Irradiation can also affect the heart in a variety of ways.

Attention is paid to the patient's nutrition and psychological outlook. The patient should be monitored for signs of anemia and infection. (See pp. 270–272 for management of the patient receiving radiation therapy.)

Chemotherapy. At the present time chemotherapy is used to manipulate tumor growth patterns, to treat patients with distant metastases, or with small cell cancer of the lung, and in combination with surgery or radiation therapy. Combinations of two or more drugs may be more beneficial than single-dose regimens. A large number of drugs are reported to have some activity against lung cancer. Various combinations of doxorubicin hydrochloride (Adriamycin), cyclosphosphamide (Cytoxan), vincristine (Oncovin), and cisplatin (Platinol) are used. An effective drug in small-cell lung cancer is VP-16. It is currently used in combination with cisplatin. The choice depends on the growth of the tumor cell and the specificity of the drug for cell cycle phase. These agents are toxic and have a narrow margin of safety. Chemotherapy may provide palliation, especially of pain, but does not cure and rarely prolongs life. It is valuable in reducing pressure symptoms of lung cancer and in treating brain, spinal cord, and pericardial metastasis. (See pp. 272–275 for chemotherapy for the patient with cancer.)

Nursing Interventions

Nursing care of the patient with lung cancer is similar to that of any cancer patient (see Chap. 16). Special attention is focused on the respiratory manifestations of the disease. Airway management is needed to maintain airway patency through the removal of secretions or exudate. As the tumor enlarges, there may be compression on a bronchus or involvement of a large area of lung tissue, resulting in an impaired breathing pattern and poor gas exchange. Deep breathing and coughing, aerosol therapy, oxygen therapy, and mechanical ventilation may be necessary when there is respiratory impairment.

The psychological aspects of nursing the patient with lung cancer are extremely important.

Tumors of the Mediastinum

Most mediastinal tumors are adjacent to vital structures and have an unpredictable manner of growth. They include neurogenic tumors, thymic tumors, and mesodermal and endocrine tumors. Thymic tumors have the highest percentage of malignancy.

Cysts of the mediastinum usually are small when benign. Dermoid cysts occasionally develop, and these may ulcerate into the air passages.

Clinical Manifestations. Nearly all the symptoms of mediastinal tumors are due to the pressure of the mass against important intrathoracic organs. Among these pressure symptoms are chest pain; bulging of the chest wall; orthopnea (an early sign owing to pressure against the trachea, a main bronchus, the recurrent laryngeal nerve, or the lung); cardiac palpitation, anginal attacks, and various other circulatory disturbances; cyanosis; superior vena caval syndromes (*i.e.*, swelling of the face, the neck, and the upper extremities) and the marked distention of the veins of the neck and the chest wall (evidence of the closure of large veins of the mediastinum by extravascular compression or intravascular invasion); and dysphagia owing to pressure against the esophagus.

Diagnostic Evaluation. Chest films are of great value in the diagnosis of mediastinal tumors and cysts. Lateral and oblique films and tomography are used to localize the tumor.

CT scans are used to detect occult thymomas as well as to define a mass lesion.

The biopsy of an enlarged lymph node removed from above the clavicle or one removed during mediastinoscopy may reveal the diagnosis. Blood studies are of value in excluding leukemia, and sputum examinations aid in ruling out tuberculosis.

Management. Many mediastinal tumors are benign and operable. The location of the tumor in the mediastinum will dictate the type of incision. Most incisions are median sternotomies. The care is the same as for any patient who is undergoing thoracic surgery (pp. 444–458). The major complications, although infrequent, include hemorrhage, phrenic or recurrent laryngeal nerve injury, and infection. If the tumor is malignant and infiltrating, radiation therapy and chemotherapy are the therapeutic modalities used when complete surgical removal is not feasible.

Chest Trauma

Injuries to the chest may cause minor or serious disturbances of cardiorespiratory function, depending on which part of the complex mechanism is involved. Thus, a fall against the side of a bathtub may fracture one or two ribs with painful but rather slight disturbance of respiratory function, whereas an automobile accident in which the driver of the car is thrown against the steering wheel may crush the chest, causing cardiac and lung injuries that may be rapidly fatal. In the United States approximately 25% of trauma-related deaths are caused by thoracic injuries alone, and in an additional 50%, chest trauma is a major factor leading to death. *There is frequent association of other injuries, most commonly major fractures, cerebrocranial injuries, and abdominal trauma.* In high-speed accidents there is an abrupt application of a shearing force to the intrathoracic structures as the person rapidly decelerates (a fast-stop situation). This compresses all of the structures within the rib cage, especially the lungs. Other causes of trauma to the chest are falls, crushing injuries, blows to the chest, and knife and gunshot wounds.

The most serious consequences of chest trauma are acute respiratory failure from damage to the chest wall, airways, diaphragm, and lungs and shock due to large vessel and extrathoracic injuries. Frequently, acute respiratory failure and shock are encountered in combination, a particularly lethal situation.

Chest injuries may be caused by *nonpenetrating (blunt) trauma,* which does not penetrate but injures by force, and by *penetrating injuries.* Both types of injuries can cause serious respiratory and hemodynamic dysfunction.

Immediate Assessment and Management. In the treatment of injuries to the chest, efforts are made to correct disturbances of cardiorespiratory function caused by the trauma. The first requirement is to evaluate the patency of the airway by assessing for signs of obstruction, sternal retraction, stridor, wheezing, and cyanosis. Agitation, irrational behavior, and hostility are signs of decreased oxygen delivery to the cerebral cortex. To restore and maintain cardiopulmonary function, an adequate airway is created and ventilation is ensured. (This includes stabilizing and reestablishing chest wall integrity, correcting open pneumothorax, decompressing pneumothorax/hemothorax, and eliminating cardiac tamponade.) Hypovolemia and low cardiac output are corrected. These treatment efforts, along with the control of hemorrhage, are usually carried out simultaneously by the emergency department team. The patient is completely undressed to avoid missing additional injuries. The entire chest is first inspected and palpated. Many injuries involving the chest have associated head and abdominal injuries that require care. Ongoing assessment is essential to see if the patient is responding to treatment or to detect early signs of a deteriorating condition.

Principles of management are essentially those pertaining to care of the posoperative thoracic patient (see pages 447–458).

Rib Fractures

Rib fractures are the most common chest injury and should be taken seriously, since they may result in underlying lung contusion. Such injuries are of special concern in middle-aged and elderly patients who may already have seriously reduced vital capacity. The fifth to the ninth ribs are the ribs most commonly broken. If the rib fragments are driven inward, the jagged edges of the rib(s) may lacerate the lung, spleen, or liver as well as cause hemothorax, pneumothorax, or hemopneumothorax.

If the patient is conscious, he will experience severe pain, tenderness, and muscle spasm over the area of fracture, which is aggravated by coughing, deep breathing, and motion. To reduce the pain the patient will breathe in a shallow manner and will avoid sighs, deep breaths, coughing, and moving. This results in diminished ventilation, collapse of unaerated alveoli (atelectasis), pneumonitis, and hypoxemia. Respiratory insufficiency and failure can be the outcome of such a cycle. Following blunt chest trauma, serial analysis of arterial blood gases is a sensitive indicator to determine whether the lung has been injured.

Management. If there are no complications (pneumothorax, hemothorax), the objective is to relieve the pain so that the patient can breathe effectively. Sedation may be given to relieve pain and allow deep breathing and coughing. Using the nurse's hands to support the injured area (or by wrapping a towel around the chest), the patient is encouraged to breathe deeply and cough. Relief of pain can also be achieved by blocking the intercostal nerves that transmit painful sensations from the affected area. Nerve block also abolishes muscle splinting, which limits respiratory excursion. Injections of the intercostal nerve(s) may be made at the lower border of the rib in the region of the intercostal nerve. If necessary, narcotic analgesics are used in small, titrated doses and with caution because of their tendency to suppress the cough and depress respiration. Usually, the pain abates in 5 to 7 days and discomfort can be controlled with non-narcotic analgesia. Most rib fractures heal in 3 to 6 weeks.

Flail Chest

Flail chest is the loss of stability of the chest wall with subsequent respiratory impairment. It is usually the result of multiple rib or sternal fractures. When this happens one portion of the chest wall no longer has a bony connection with the rest of the rib cage. It is usually accompanied by a severe degree of respiratory distress.

During inspiration, as the chest expands, the detached part of the chest (flail segment) will show a paradoxical movement in that it is pulled inward during inspiration. On expiration, since the intrathoracic pressure will exceed atmospheric pressure, the flail segment will bulge outward, impairing the patient's ability to exhale. This paradoxical action results in increased dead space ventilation, retained airway secretions, increased lung resistance and decreased compliance, and reduction in alveolar ventilation. Lung contusion and atelectasis frequently accompany flail chest. As a result, blood oxygen content decreases and carbon dioxide content increases, producing respiratory acidosis. Often, hypotension, inadequate tissue perfusion, and metabolic acidosis follow as cardiac output decreases by the paradoxical motion of the mediastinum.

Management. Several modes of therapy are available, depending on the degree of respiratory dysfunction. If only a small segment of the chest is involved, the objectives are to clear the airway (coughing, deep breaths, gentle suctioning) in order to aid in the expansion of the lung, and to relieve pain by intercostal nerve blocks, high thoracic epidural blocks, or careful use of intravenous narcotics.

For mild to moderate flail chest injuries, some clinicians advocate treating the underlying pulmonary contusion with fluid restriction, diuretics, corticosteroids, and albumin while relieving chest pain and by employing pulmonary physiotherapy, combined with close and continuing patient monitoring.

When a severe flail is encountered, endotracheal intubation and mechanical ventilation with a volume-cycled ventilator and sometimes positive end-expiratory pressure is used to splint the chest wall (internal pneumatic stabilization) and to correct abnormalities in gas exchange. This helps to treat the underlying pulmonary contusion, serves to stabilize the thoracic cage for healing of fractures, and improves alveolar ventilation and intrathoracic volume by decreasing the work of breathing. However, this treatment modality requires long-term endotracheal intubation and ventilator support.

Hemothorax and Pneumothorax

Severe chest injuries usually are accompanied by the collection of blood in the chest cavity (hemothorax) because of torn intercostal vessels, lacerations of the lungs, or the escape of air from the injured lung into the pleural cavity (pneumothorax). Often, both blood and air are found in the chest cavity (hemopneumothorax). The lung on that side of the chest is compressed, which interferes with its normal function.

The seriousness of the problem depends on the amount and rate of thoracic bleeding. Needle aspiration (thoracentesis) or chest tube drainage of the blood or air allows decompression of the pleural cavity so that the lung is able to reexpand and again perform its function in respiration. Operative intervention is carried out if bleeding continues at a rate greater than 300 ml/hr for 3 to 4 hours, if the rate of bleeding increases, or if it is not possible to evacuate the blood within the pleural space.

Management. A large-diameter intercostal tube (catheter) is usually inserted in the second intercostal space or in the fifth space in the axilla. This usually brings about prompt and effective decompression of the pleural cavity (drainage of blood/air). If there is an excessive amount of bleeding from the chest tube in a relatively short period of time, autotransfusion may be employed. This technique takes the patient's own blood that is drained from the chest, filters it, and then transfuses it back into the patient's vascular system.

Tension Pneumothorax

In some patients, air may be drawn into the pleural space from the lacerated lung or through a small hole in the chest wall. In either case, the air that enters the chest cavity with each inspiration is trapped there: it cannot be expelled through the air passage or small hole in the chest wall.

A tension (pressure) thus is built up within the pleural space, which produces a collapse of the lung and may even push the heart and the great vessels toward the unaffected side of the chest. This not only interferes with respiration but also disrupts circulatory function, because with increased intrathoracic pressure, venous return to the heart is compromised, causing decreased cardiac output and impairment of peripheral circulation. Diminished cardiac output leads to cardiac arrest. The clinical picture is one of air hunger, agitation, hypotension, and cyanosis.

- *Relief of tension pneumothorax must be looked on as an emergency measure.*

Management. Immediate thoracentesis is done to relieve the positive pressure or "tension" within the chest. If the lung expands and there is no continuing leakage from the lung, further drainage may be unnecessary. If the lung is still leaking, as evidenced by the reaccumulation of an inexhaustible volume of air during the thoracentesis, then constant egress of this air must be provided by a large-bore chest tube with water-seal drainage.

In an emergency situation a tension pneumothorax can be quickly converted to a simple pneumothorax by insertion of a large-bore needle into the pleural space, which relieves the pressure and vents the intrathoracic air to the outside. Then a chest tube can be inserted and connected to suction in order to remove the remaining air and fluid and reexpand the lung.

Penetrating Wounds of the Chest

Open Pneumothorax

Open pneumothorax implies an opening in the chest wall large enough to allow air to pass freely in and out of the thoracic cavity with each attempted respiration. Since the rush of air through the hole in the chest wall produces a sucking sound, such injuries are termed *sucking wounds* of the chest. In such patients not only is the lung collapsed, but the structures of the mediastinum (heart and great vessels) are also pushed toward the uninjured side with each inspiration and in the opposite direction with expiration. This is termed *mediastinal flutter*, and it produces serious circulatory embarrassment.

Management. Open pneumothorax calls for emergency interventions.

- *Stopping the flow of air through the opening in the chest wall is a lifesaving measure.*

In such an emergency, anything may be used that is large enough to fill the hole—a towel, a handkerchief, or the heel of the hand. If the patient is conscious, tell him to inhale and strain against a closed glottis. This action assists in the reexpansion of the lung and the ejection of the air from the thorax. In the hospital, the opening is plugged by sealing it with gauze impregnated with petrolatum. A pressure dressing is applied by circumferential strapping. Usually, a chest tube connected to water-seal drainage is inserted to permit egress of air and fluid. Antibiotics are usually prescribed to combat infection from contamination.

Stab Wounds

Stab wounds are a common cause of penetrating wounds of the chest, most of which are caused by knives and switchblades, and are frequently associated with alcohol or substance abuse. The appearance of the external wound may be very deceptive, since pneumothorax, hemothorax, and cardiac tamponade along with severe and continuing hemorrhage can occur from any small wound, even one caused by an icepick.

Management. The objective of immediate management is to restore and maintain cardiopulmonary function. After an adequate airway is ensured and ventilation is corrected, the patient is examined for shock and intrathoracic and intra-abdominal injuries. The patient is undressed completely so that additional injuries will not be missed. There is a high risk for associated intra-abdominal injuries with stab wounds below the level of the fifth anterior intercostal space. Death can result from exsanguinating hemorrhage or intra-abdominal sepsis.

After the status of the peripheral pulses is assessed, an intravenous line is secured. Blood is withdrawn for chemistries, typing, and cross-matching. Simultaneously, a central venous pressure line is established. An indwelling catheter is inserted to monitor urinary volume and to collect a urine sample for laboratory study.

Shock is treated simultaneously with colloid solutions, crystalloids, blood, or vasopressors as indicated by the condition of the patient. Chest films are taken, and other diagnostic procedures are carried out (esophagogram, flat plate of the abdomen, arteriogram) as dictated by the needs of the patient.

A chest tube is inserted in the pleural space in most patients with penetrating wounds of the chest in order to achieve rapid and continuing reexpansion of the lungs. Frequently, this will cause a complete evacuation of hemothorax and will decrease the incidence of clotted hemothorax. The chest tube allows early recognition of continuing intrathoracic bleeding, which will make surgical exploration necessary.

If the patient has a penetrating wound of the heart and great vessels, the esophagus, and the tracheobronchial tree, surgical intervention is required. Associated intra-abdominal wounds also necessitate abdominal exploration.

Pulmonary Contusion

Pulmonary contusion is damage to the lung parenchyma that results in leakage of blood and fluid. It may occur any time when there is rapid compression and decompression of the chest wall (*e.g.*, a steering wheel injury or the blast effect from gunshot wounds).

Pathophysiology. The primary pathologic defect is the abnormal accumulation of fluid in the interstitial and intra-alveolar spaces. It is thought that injury to the lung parenchyma and its capillary network results in a serum protein and plasma leak. The extravascular serum protein exerts an osmotic pressure that enhances loss of fluid from the capillaries. Blood, edema, and cellular debris (from cellular response to injury) enter the lung and accumulate in the bronchioles and alveolar surface, where they interfere with the efficiency of gas exchange. There is an increase in pulmonary vascular resistance and pulmonary artery pressure. The patient experiences systemic hypoxia and carbon dioxide retention. Occasionally, a contused lung occurs on the other side of the point of body impact. This is called a *contrecoup contusion*.

Clinical Manifestations. Pulmonary contusion may be mild, moderate, or severe. The efficiency of gas exchange is determined by arterial blood gas measurements. The chest films will reveal pulmonary infiltration. The patient experiences tachypnea, tachycardia, crackles on auscultation, increased work of breathing, pleuritic chest pain, and copious secretions that are sometimes bloody or blood-tinged.

Management. In mild cases of pulmonary contusion, ultrasonic mist nebulization is used to keep the secretions fluid. Postural drainage, physiotherapy, and sterile endotracheal suctioning are used to remove the secretions. Pain is managed by intercostal nerve blocks or by narcotics. Usually, antimicrobial therapy is given, since a damaged lung is susceptible to infection. Oxygen by mask or cannula is usually given for 24 to 36 hours. Fluids are restricted because the injury is thought to be due to an abnormal collection of fluid in the interstices of the lung.

If moderate lung contusion is encountered, in addition to the above symptoms, the patient will have a large amount of mucus, serum, and frank blood in the tracheobronchial tree. He coughs constantly but is unable to clear his secretions. This patient usually requires intubation with a cuffed endotracheal tube and is placed on a ventilator with low-concentration oxygen and positive end-expiratory pressure to maintain the pressure and keep the lungs inflated. Diuretics may be given to reduce edema. A nasogastric tube is passed to relieve gastrointestinal distention. Metabolic acidosis is corrected with intravenous sodium bicarbonate. Frequent cultures are made of tracheobronchial secretions.

A patient with severe pulmonary contusion presents with the signs and symptoms of adult respiratory distress syndrome (ARDS), which include rapid respirations, tachycardia, cyanosis, agitation, combativeness, and continuous and productive coughing of mucoid, frothy, and bloody secretions. This patient is treated vigorously with endotracheal intubation and ventilatory support, plasma or albumin (to maintain normal oncotic pressure to prevent leakage out of pulmonary capillaries), diuretics, fluid restriction, and perhaps the prophylactic administration of antimicrobials. Whole blood or fresh, frozen plasma may be used to treat hypovolemia.

The complications of pulmonary contusion are infections, especially pneumonia in the contused segment, since the extravasation of fluid and blood into the alveolar and interstitial spaces is an excellent culture medium.

Cardiac Tamponade

Cardiac tamponade is the compression of the heart as a result of fluid within the pericardial sac. It is usually caused by blunt or penetrating trauma to the chest. (A penetrating wound of the heart is associated with a high mortality rate.) Cardiac tamponade may also follow diagnostic cardiac catheterization, angiographic procedures, and pacemaker insertion, which can produce perforations of the heart and great vessels. Pericardial effusion may also develop from metastases to the pericardium from malignant tumors of the breast and lung as well as from lymphomas and leukemias, uremia, and high-dose radiation to the chest.

Pathophysiology. If the fluid formation is slow, the pericardium will distend without producing noticeable clinical symptoms until enough fluid develops to raise the intrapericardial pressure. A rapidly developing effusion interferes with ventricular filling and causes impairment of circulation. Thus, there is a reduced cardiac output and insufficient venous return to the heart. Circulatory collapse can result.

Clinical Manifestations. The clinical manifestations depend on the speed of fluid accumulation. Important signs to watch for are a falling blood pressure, rising venous pressure (distended neck veins), and distant (muffled) heart sounds from impaired diastolic filling of the heart. Pulsus paradoxus (systolic blood pressure drops and fluctuates with respiration) may occur early in the development of cardiac tamponade. The patient may be anxious, confused, and restless and may have dyspnea, tachypnea, and precordial pain. The central venous pressure is elevated. However, the venous pressure may be low or normal if a large amount of blood has been lost as a result of associated injuries.

Management. The treatment of cardiac tamponade is thoracotomy for penetrating cardiac injuries where cardiorrhaphy (suturing the heart muscle) is done to stop hemorrhage, relieve tamponade, and repair associated lacerations and lesions. (See the care of the patient undergoing heart surgery [Chap. 27] and of the patient undergoing chest surgery [Chap. 22]). Pericardiocentesis (needle aspiration of fluid from the pericardium, Chap. 26) may be performed to "buy time" before the patient is taken to surgery. This decompression of the pericardial sac permits effective heart action to be resumed.

Subcutaneous Emphysema

When the lung or the air passages are injured, air may enter the tissue planes and pass for some distance under the skin (*e.g.*, neck, chest). The tissues give a crackling sensation when palpated, and the subcutaneous air produces an alarming appearance as face, neck, body, and scrotum become misshapen by subcutaneous air. Fortunately, subcutaneous emphysema is of itself not a serious complication. The subcutaneous air is spontaneously absorbed, if the underlying air leak is treated or stops spontaneously. Giving the patient inhalations of high concentrations of oxygen will promote the reabsorption of subcutaneous air by washing nitrogen from the blood and improving its diffusion from the subcutaneous tissues back into the circulation. In severe cases, when there is widespread subcutaneous emphysema, a tracheostomy is indicated to ensure patency of the airway.

The Clinical Problem of Aspiration

Aspiration (inhalation) of stomach contents is a serious complication that may cause death. It can occur when there is loss of protective airway reflexes, such as is seen in patients who are unconscious from drugs, alcohol, stroke, or cardiac arrest, or in instances when a nonfunctioning nasogastric tube allows the gastric contents to drain around the tube and cause silent aspiration.

Massive inhalation of gastric contents, if untreated, will, in a period of several hours, result in the clinical syndrome of tachycardia, dyspnea, cyanosis and hypertension followed by hypotension, and finally death. The primary factors responsible for morbidity and mortality after aspiration of gastric contents are the volume of aspirated gastric contents and their character. A full stomach contains solid particles of food. If these are aspirated, the problem then becomes one of mechanical blockage of the airways and secondary infection. A fasting stomach contains acidic gastric juice, which, if aspirated, may prove destructive to the alveoli and capillaries. The presence of fecal contamination (more likely seen in intestinal obstruction) will increase the likelihood of mortality because the endotoxins produced by intestinal organisms may be absorbed systemically, or the thick proteinaceous material found in the intestinal contents may obstruct the airway, leading to atelectasis and secondary bacterial invasion.

Chemical pneumonitis may develop from aspiration and result in destruction of alveolar-capillary endothelial cells, with a consequent outpouring of protein-rich fluids into the interstitial and intra-alveolar spaces. This results in loss of surfactant, which in turn causes early closure of the airway. Finally, the impaired exchange of oxygen and carbon dioxide causes respiratory failure.

It is essential to remember the following:

- *Massive aspiration is fatal.*
- *Small, localized aspiration from regurgitation can cause pneumonia and respiratory distress.*
- *Silent regurgitation often takes place unobserved and may be more common than we think.*

Preventive Measures

When Reflexes Are Lacking.   Aspiration is likely to occur if the patient cannot adequately coordinate his protective glottic, laryngeal, and cough reflexes. This hazard is increased if the patient has a distended abdomen, is in a supine position, and has his upper extremities immobilized by intravenous infusions or hand restraints. A normal person, when vomiting, can take care of his airway by sitting up or turning on his side and coordinating his breathing, coughing, gag, and glottic reflexes. If these reflexes are active, an oral airway should

not be inserted. If an airway is in place, it should be pulled out the moment the patient gags on it so as not to stimulate the pharyngeal gag reflex and promote vomiting and aspiration. Catheter suction of oral secretions should be executed with minimal pharyngeal stimulation yet at the same time should be effective.

During Tube Feeding.   The patient who is receiving tube feedings should be positioned upright during the feeding and for 30 minutes thereafter to allow the stomach to partially empty. Small volumes given under low pressure will help to prevent aspiration.

With Delayed Emptying Time of Stomach.   A full stomach may cause aspiration because of increased intragastric or extragastric pressure. The following clinical situations cause delayed emptying time of the stomach and may contribute to aspiration: intestinal obstruction; increased gastric secretions during anxiety, stress, or pain; or abdominal distention because of ileus, ascites, peritonitis, drugs, severe illness, or vaginal delivery.

Following Prolonged Endotracheal Intubation.   Prolonged endotracheal intubation or tracheostomy can depress the laryngeal and glottic reflexes because of disuse. Patients with prolonged tracheostomies are encouraged to phonate and exercise their laryngeal muscles. The pharynx is suctioned before deflating the cuff to prevent aspiration of regurgitated material. It is important to remember that improperly administered IPPB treatments by mask can distend the stomach and promote aspiration.

Acute Respiratory Failure

Respiratory failure exists whenever the exchange of oxygen for carbon dioxide in the lungs cannot keep up with the rate of oxygen consumption and carbon dioxide production in the cells of the body. This results in a fall in arterial oxygen tension (hypoxemia) and a rise in arterial carbon dioxide tension (hypercapnia).

One must distinguish between acute respiratory failure and acute exacerbation of chronic respiratory failure. Acute respiratory failure is the respiratory failure appearing in the patient whose lung was structurally and functionally normal before the onset of the present illness. *Chronic respiratory failure* is the respiratory failure seen in patients with chronic lung diseases such as chronic bronchitis, emphysema, and black lung disease (coal miner's disease). These patients develop a tolerance to the gradually worsening hypoxia and hypercapnia. Following acute respiratory failure, the lung usually returns to its original state. In chronic respiratory failure the structural damage is irreversible. The principles of management of these two conditions are different; this discussion will be confined to acute respiratory failure.

Causes of acute respiratory failure are numerous and may be subdivided into various categories. One major group includes those diseases in which respiratory failure results from inadequate ventilation: the lung itself remains structurally normal in the early stages. One of the most important causes of inadequate ventilation is upper airway obstruction. Its etiology, diagnosis, and management are discussed on page 431.

Central nervous system depression will also result in inadequate ventilation. The respiratory center, which controls every breath, lies in the lower part of the brain stem (pons and medulla). Drug overdose, anesthesia, head injury, stroke, brain tumors, encephalitis, meningitis, hypoxia, and hypercapnia are all capable of depressing the respiratory center. In these patients, respiration becomes slow and shallow. Respiratory arrest may occur in severe cases.

The impulses arising in the respiratory center travel in nerves that extend from the brain stem down the spinal cord to receptors in the muscles of respiration. Any disease of the nerves, spinal cord, muscles, or neuromuscular junction involved in respiration will seriously affect ventilation. Polyneuritis, myasthenia gravis, damage to the cervical segment of the spinal cord, and poliomyelitis are examples of such diseases.

Respiratory failure owing to inadequate ventilation is looked for in the immediate postoperative period, especially following major thoracic or upper abdominal surgery. The reasons for respiratory failure during this period are numerous. The effects of anesthetic drugs (morphine, pentobarbital) are long lasting. They depress respiration by their own effects or by enhancing the effects of narcotic analgesics. Pain in the thoracic and abdominal area interferes with deep breathing and coughing. Muscle relaxants are frequently used during anesthesia. Some patients may have difficulty in breaking down or excreting these drugs, so that their effects last longer than usual, making patients weak in the postoperative period. Ventilation–perfusion abnormality also accounts for respiratory failure following major abdominal and thoracic operations.

Pleural effusion, hemothorax, and pneumothorax are a group of conditions that interfere with ventilation by preventing expansion of the lung. They are usually produced by an underlying lung disease or pleural disease.

Trauma resulting from motor vehicle accidents is a very common cause of acute respiratory failure. In this type of accident, head injury, unconsciousness, and bleeding from the nose and mouth lead to upper airway obstruction and respiratory depression. Hemothorax, pneumothorax, and rib fractures may occur and may be responsible for inadequate ventilation. Flail chest may also occur and may lead to respiratory failure.

There are many acute diseases of the lung that may lead to acute respiratory failure. Of these diseases, pneumonia is perhaps the most common. It is usually caused by viral or bacterial activity. Chemical pneumonitis is pneumonia produced by the inhalation of irritant fumes or the aspiration of acidic gastric material. Bronchial asthma, atelectasis, pulmonary embolism, and pulmonary edema are some other conditions that cause acute respiratory failure.

Adult Respiratory Distress Syndrome

Most patients in acute respiratory failure get better with the proper management of airway ventilation and oxygenation. However, a small group of patients do not respond to this treatment. They become severely hypoxic (PaO_2 of 50 mm Hg or below) in spite of adequate ventilation with 100% oxygen. These symptoms are caused by widespread injury to the alveolar-capillary bed. Adult respiratory distress syndrome (ARDS) is the name given to this clinical picture.

ARDS frequently results from pneumonia or shock. The pneumonia is usually caused by a virus but may be caused by microorganisms such as bacteria, rickettsia, or leptospira. Chemical pneumonitis, which follows inhalation of noxious fumes or aspiration of acidic gastric material, accounts for some patients having pneumonia. Shock is usually due to blood loss but may be caused by septicemia.

Motor vehicle accidents or gunshot injuries account for the incidence of shock owing to blood loss. However, blood loss occurring during childbirth, ruptured aortic aneurysm, ruptured esophageal varices, peptic ulceration, and major surgery may also lead to shock. ARDS may also follow near drowning, massive fat embolism, acute pancreatitis, massive blood transfusions, and extracorporeal circulation for open-heart surgery.

Pathophysiology

The arterial oxygen tension (PaO_2) is low (usually around 50 mm Hg) even when the patient is breathing 100% (1.00) oxygen. In other words, the alveolar to arterial oxygen gradient $P(A - a)O_2$, is widened. Severe hypoxia is the result of extensive shunting in the lungs. The functional residual capacity (FRC) is markedly diminished. When the FRC falls below the closing capacity, small airways close and the air in the corresponding alveoli is absorbed, leading to atelectasis. Oxygen cannot reach the alveolar capillaries, and the blood passing through these capillaries constitutes shunted blood.

Pulmonary edema (fluid in the alveoli) and interstitial edema (fluid in the lung substance) are also seen and contribute to hypoxia. As a result of all of these changes, the lung becomes more stiff (low compliance).

ARDS used to be associated with high mortality. The use of positive end-expiratory pressure has increased the survival rate.

Clinical Manifestations

The clinical features of the syndrome include initial severe illness with no pulmonary component, followed by a latent period in which pulmonary abnormalities are minimal. There is a subsequent period of progressive respiratory distress with dyspnea and hypoxia. The x-ray will show bilateral involvement of the lungs leading to pulmonary edema.

In spite of the different causes, the clinical picture, pathophysiology, and pathology are similar. ARDS appears 6 to 48 hours after the onset of the illness. The patient develops respiratory distress; the rate of breathing increases (tachypnea) and may reach 40 breaths per minute. Each breath is shallow and labored (dyspnea) and may be associated with grunting. Retraction of the intercostal and suprasternal areas is seen during inspiration. Widening of the alae nasi and contractions of the accessory muscles of respiration are other signs of respiratory distress.

Cyanosis appears and fails to respond to oxygen therapy. Evidence of cerebral hypoxia, such as anxiety, confusion, irritability, lack of cooperation, drowsiness, and mental obtundation may appear. Hypoxia of the heart will result in tachycardia, dysrhythmias, and hypotension.

Auscultatory findings are minimal in the early stages, but later bronchial breathing may be heard. In the early stages chest x-ray may show patchy alveolar infiltrates in both lungs, which later become more diffuse.

Management

The principles of management of acute respiratory failure are the following:

1. Treat the cause.
2. Maintain a patent airway.
3. Provide adequate ventilation.
4. Provide optimum oxygen.
5. Carry out chest physiotherapy.

Treatment of the cause may involve evacuating the pleural cavity, giving antibiotic treatment for infection, reversing effects of drugs or accelerating their excretion, and decreasing raised intracranial pressures. Diseases such as bronchial asthma and pulmonary edema require specific therapy. In some illnesses, such as polyneuritis and poliomyelitis, one has to wait for the illness to resolve.

To maintain a patent airway it may be necessary to intubate the patient or to do a tracheostomy. Once the airway is clear, adequacy of ventilation is assessed by measuring the respiratory rate, tidal volume, vital capacity, inspiratory force, arterial carbon dioxide tension ($PaCO_2$), and oxygen tension (PaO_2). Depending on the results, the patient is allowed to breathe spontaneously or is helped by a ventilator (Table 23-3) and by being monitored in the intensive care unit.

The arterial oxygen tension (PaO_2) will show the degree of oxygenation.

Administration of Oxygen. The concentration of oxygen in air is 21%. Another way of expressing the same fact is to say that the fraction of inspired oxygen (FiO_2) is 0.21. The FiO_2 may be increased by the addition of oxygen to inspired air. The oxygen must always be humidified to prevent drying of the upper airway or secretions in the airway. Nasal prongs, nasal catheters, or face masks are commonly used to administer oxygen to the spontaneously breathing patient.

If the patient has an endotracheal tube or a tracheostomy, a T-bar (Briggs adapter) is used for the administration of oxygen. Since the upper airway is bypassed in these patients, the inspired air must be humidified.

The percentage of oxygen inspired by the patient depends on (1) the diluter valve setting of the nebulizer, (2) the output of the nebulizer, (3) the reservoir tube on the expiratory limb, and (4) the inspiratory effort of the patient.

The diluter valve setting puts an upper limit on the inspired oxygen concentration. This concentration may be reduced by air pulled in via the expiratory limb during the inspiratory effort of the patient. By increasing the nebulizer outflow and by using a reservoir tube on the expiratory limb, air dilution may be reduced or completely eliminated.

Humidification. The air we breathe contains water in the form of vapor. This is referred to as humidity. The amount of water vapor present in the air at any time varies with the weather conditions and greatly influences our comfort. A given volume of air at a given temperature cannot contain more than a certain amount of water vapor, and when it contains the maximum amount of water vapor, it is said to be 100% (1.00) saturated.

If the temperature of this sample of air is raised, more water vapor will have to be added to it to saturate it to 100%. Whatever the temperature and percentage saturation of the air we breathe, it is rendered 100% saturated at body temperature when it passes through the nose and reaches the lower part of the trachea.

The oxygen that is commercially available is totally devoid of water vapor (100% dry), and humidifiers are required to provide the water vapor that will make oxygen breathing comfortable and prevent drying up of the respiratory tract and the secretions therein. If the patient is using his own airway, a simple humidifier is used that will add some water vapor to the oxygen and allow the patient's airway to saturate it to 100%. A simple humidifier is formed by bubbling oxygen through water. Its efficiency is increased by various methods that make the bubbles very small. Many disposable simple humidifiers are available that produce 80% to 100% saturated

TABLE 23-3
Indications for Respiratory Support

Parameter	Assessment Criteria	Acceptable Range	Chest Physiotherapy, Oxygen, Close Monitoring	Endotracheal Intubation, Tracheostomy, Ventilation
Muscle power	Respiratory rate per minute	12–25	25–35	>35
	Vital capacity in ml/kg (ideal body weight)	70–30	30–15	<15
	Inspiratory force in negative cm H_2O	100–50	50–25	<25
Oxygenation	Alveolar to arterial O_2 tension gradient in mm Hg*	50–200	200–350	>400
	PaO_2 mm Hg	100–75 air	200–70 (on mask O_2)	<65
Ventilation	$PaCO_2$ mm Hg	35–45	45–60	>60†

* After 15 minutes of 100% O_2.
† Except in chronic hypercapnia.

Recognition of Respiratory Complications: Table 23-3 shows objective, practical guidelines used in the bedside evaluation of the patient's respiratory status. (The trend of change in values is of utmost importance.) The third column refers to the values of normal acceptable range. The fourth column lists borderline values where chest physiotherapy, oxygen, and close monitoring are essential. The fifth column lists values that indicate the necessity of intubation, tracheostomy, or ventilation.

(Adapted from Pontoppidan H. Treatment of respiratory failure in nonthoracic trauma. J Trauma 8:940.)

oxygen at room temperature (100% saturated oxygen at room temperature becomes 37% saturated at body temperature unless more water vapor is added).

A patient breathing via an endotracheal tube or a fresh tracheostomy must be provided with 100% saturated air at body temperature. This may be achieved by heating the water in the humidifier to a temperature above that of the body and letting the humidified oxygen cool to body temperature as it passes through the delivery tube. Many mechanical ventilators use this technique.

Alternatively, a nebulizer may be used to provide humidity. A nebulizer produces small particles of water, some of which evaporate to produce water vapor. Suspension of small particles of gas is referred to as an *aerosol*. There are several types of nebulizers. The Puritan nebulizer is capable of delivering aerosol for a long period. It also traps air that dilutes the oxygen. By adjusting a valve on the nebulizer, it is possible to set the nebulizer to deliver 40%, 60%, 70%, or 100% oxygen. Because of air entrapment, when the nebulizer is set at 40% and 10 liters of 100% oxygen per minute are run through, 40 liters per minute of 40% oxygen with water particles are delivered by the nebulizer.

Positive End-Expiratory Pressure. Positive end-expiratory pressure (PEEP) means the airway pressure remains higher than atmospheric pressure at the end of expiration. Normally, during spontaneous breathing or during mechanical ventilation, at the end of expiration the airway pressure equals the atmospheric pressure (zero end-expiratory pressure). The airway pressure is measured in centimeters of water (cm H_2O). The usual range of PEEP used is 5 to 15 cm H_2O. However, higher PEEP values (20 to 35 cm H_2O) are also used.

PEEP may be applied to a patient on a mechanical ventilator. Such a patient would have positive airway pressure during inspiration and expiration and at the end of expiration. The term *continuous positive pressure ventilation* (CPPV) is sometimes used to describe this situation. When PEEP is applied to a patient who is breathing spontaneously (via his own airway, an endotracheal tube, or a tracheostomy), it is called CPAP (continuous positive airway pressure).

However, PEEP can be regulated so that a spontaneously breathing patient on PEEP will have zero airway pressure during the inspiratory phase. The term *CPAP* cannot strictly be applied to this method. The term *sPEEP* (spontaneous PEEP) has been used by some to describe the situation.

When PEEP is applied, the FRC is increased, so that small airway closure is prevented. PEEP also splints the airways. With PEEP, shunting is decreased and compliance is improved. The end result is improved oxygenation, as is demonstrated by the decrease in the alveolar to arterial oxygen tension gradient $P(A - a)O_2$. With improved oxygenation the FiO_2 may be reduced to less toxic levels.

PEEP may produce some undesirable results. A fall in cardiac output may be seen when more than 5 cm of H_2O PEEP is used.

- The amount of oxygen carried to the tissues per minute (oxygen flux) depends as much on the cardiac output as on the degrees of oxygenation. Care must be taken not to compromise oxygen flux by decreasing the cardiac output.

Other complications reported with PEEP include pneumothorax, pneumomediastinum, and interstitial emphysema.

Nursing Interventions

The patient in acute respiratory failure is seriously ill and requires close monitoring because his condition could quickly change to a life-threatening situation. Most of the respiratory modalities discussed in Chapter 22 will be used in this situation (oxygen administration, mini-nebulizer therapy, chest physiotherapy, endotracheal intubation or tracheostomy, suctioning, tracheostomy care and ventilator management). Frequent assessment of the patient's status is necessary to evaluate the effectiveness of the management program.

In addition to implementing the medical plan of care, the nurse observes other needs of the patient. If the patient is not being mechanically ventilated, he is placed in semi-Fowler's or high-Fowler's position to allow maximum excursion of the thorax. He is supported in whatever position he feels most comfortable, using pillows, blankets, or an overbed table. If fluids are not restricted, fluid intake is encouraged to correct fluid loss that occurs during rapid breathing and to loosen secretions. The patient will be extremely anxious because of the hypoxemia and dyspnea. The nurse should reassure him of the ability and concern of the health care team, explain all procedures, and deliver care in a calm, patient manner. It is important to reduce the patient's anxiety because its manifestations prevent rest and increase oxygen expenditure. Rest is essential to conserve oxygen use, thereby reducing the oxygen need.

If the patient is on PEEP, there are several unique nursing considerations. PEEP is an unnatural pattern of breathing and will feel strange to the patient. He is reassured about his status and encouraged to work with the ventilator. If the PEEP level is not maintained, pancuronium (Pavulon) or another neuromuscular blocker may be administered. In this situation, the patient loses motor function but retains sensation. He will feel paralyzed and be unable to breathe, talk, or blink. The nurse must be sure the patient is not disconnected from the ventilator. Neuromuscular blockers paralyze the respiratory muscles so the patient does not resist the ventilator and PEEP. This means that the patient will be apneic if removed or disconnected from the ventilator. Consequently, the nurse ensures that the patient is closely monitored at all times. When he is removed from the ventilator for suctioning or measurements, it is done quickly to minimize the time without ventilation. He may also experience discomfort or pain and be unable to communicate it. He will appear unconscious, yet be awake and able to hear. He is reassured that what he is experiencing is a result of the medicine and is temporary. The nurse must anticipate his needs regarding pain and comfort. She checks his position to ensure that he is comfortable and talks to him and not about him while in his presence. Complete eye care is important because of the patient's inability to blink and the risk of corneal abrasions.

Bibliography

Books

Andres R et al. Principles of Geratric Medicine. New York, McGraw-Hill, 1985.

Baum GL and Wolinsky E (eds). Textbook of Pulmonary Diseases, 3rd ed. Boston, Little, Brown & Co, 1983.

Bell CW et al. Home Care and Rehabilitation in Respiratory Medicine. Philadelphia, JB Lippincott, 1984.

Borg N et al (eds). Core Curriculum for Critical Care Nursing, 2nd ed. Philadelphia, WB Saunders, 1981.

Boyda EK. Respiratory Problems. Oradell, New Jersey, Medical Economics, 1985.

Brenner BE. Comprehensive Management of Respiratory Emergencies. Rockville, Maryland, Aspen, 1985.

Burton GG and Hodgkin JE (eds). Respiratory Care—A Guide to Clinical Practice, 2nd ed. Philadelphia, JB Lippincott, 1984.

Carpenito LJ. Nursing Diagnosis: Application to Clinical Practice. Philadelphia, JB Lippincott, 1983.

Fishman AP. Pulmonary Diseases and Disorders. New York, McGraw-Hill, 1981.

Harper RA. A Guide to Respiratory Care. Philadelphia, JB Lippincott, 1981.

Hodgkin JE et al (eds). Pulmonary Rehabilitation: Guidelines to Success. Boston, Butterworth, 1984.

Johanson BC et al. Standards for Critical Care. St Louis, CV Mosby, 1981.

Kneisel CR (ed). Wadsworth's Review of Nursing. Monterey, California, Wadsworth, 1985.

Krupp MA and Chatton MJ (eds). Current Medical Diagnosis and Treatment 1984. Los Altos, California, Lange Medical Publications, 1984.

Mandell JL, Douglas RG, and Bennett JE (eds). Principles and Practices of Infectious Diseases, 2nd ed. New York, John Wiley & Sons, 1985.

O'Ryan JA and Burns DG. Pulmonary Rehabilitation: From Hospital to Home. Chicago, Year Book Medical Publishers, 1984.

Petty TL. Pulmonary Rehabilitation: Basics of RD. New York, American Thoracic Society, 1975.

Petty TL and Nett L. Living Life with Emphysema. Philadelphia, Lea & Febiger, 1984.

Shapiro BA et al. Clinical Application of Respiratory Care, 3rd ed. Chicago, Year Book Medical Publishers, 1985.

Shayevitz MB and Shayevitz BR. Living Well with Emphysema and Bronchitis: A Handbook for Everyone with Chronic Obstructive Pulmonary Disease. New York, Doubleday, 1985.

Shayevitz MB and Shayevitz BR. The Lung: Research Accomplishments and Frontiers. New York, American Lung Association, 1986.

Wade JF. Respiratory Nursing Care: Physiology and Technique, 3rd ed. St Louis, CV Mosby, 1981.

Articles

(Asterisks indicate nursing research articles.)

Pulmonary Infections

Belshe RB. Viral respiratory disease in the intensive care unit. Heart Lung 1986 May; 15(3):222–225.

Gleckman RA. Community-acquired pneumonia in the geriatric patient. Hosp Pract 1985 Mar 30; 20(3):57–60.

Kent JM. The new flu and pneumococcal vaccines. Patient Care 1984 Aug 15; 18(14):62–65, 68–70, 72.

Ristuccia P. Microbiologic aspects of infection in the compromised host. Nurs Clin North Am 1985 Mar; 20(1):171–179.

Stratton CW. Bacterial pneumonias: An overview with emphasis on pathogenesis diagnosis, and treatment. Heart Lung 1986 May; 15(3):226–243.

Tafuro P. Approach to hospital-acquired pneumonias. Heart Lung 1984 Sept; 13(5):482–485.

Todd B. Preventing influenza and pneumonia. Geriatr Nurs 1984 Nov/Dec; 5(8):399–401.

Wilson J and Pfister S. Caring for a patient with pneumococcal pneumonia. Crit Care Nurs 1984 Sept/Oct; 4(5):50, 52–54.

Chronic Obstructive Pulmonary Disease

Aguis L et al. The role of the practice nurse in management of asthma. Nurs '84 1984 Aug; 2(28):815–819.

Alexander MR et al. Therapy of chronic obstructive airways disease. Drug Intell Clin Pharm 1984 Apr; 18(4):279–291.

Anthonisen NR. Long-term oxygen therapy. Ann Intern Med 1983 Oct; 99(4):519.

Ballenger MJ. Asthma. Emergency 1984 Nov; 16(11):62–65.

Berman LB and Sutton JR. Exercise for the pulmonary patient. J Cardiopul Rehabil 1986 Feb 20; 6(2):52–61.

Blair GP and Light RW. Treatment of chronic obstructive pulmonary disease with corticosteroids. Chest 1984 Oct; 86(4):524–528.

Braum SR et al. The prevalence and determinants of nutritional changes in chronic obstructive pulmonary disease. Chest 1984 Oct; 86(4):558–563.

Brodoff AS. Diagnosing COPD earlier. Patient Care 1984 May 15; 18(9):128–132, 134–135, 138.

Brodoff AS. Helping the COPD patient help himself. Patient Care 1984 June 15; 18(11):177–180, 183–184.

Bukantz SC. Acute severe asthma–the late phase reaction and the continuing challenge. Hosp Pract 1986 Nov 15; 21(11):10–16.

*Carrieri VK and Janson-Bjerklie S. Strategies patients use to manage the sensation of dyspnea. West J Nurs Res 1986 Aug; 8(3):289–305.

Cherniack RM. Comprehensive approach to asthma. Chest 1985 Jan; 87(Suppl 1):94S–97S.

Curgian LM. Nutrition in chronic respiratory disease. Rehabil Nurs 1985 July/Aug; 10(4):22–23.

Daly WJ. COPD—Assessing functional status. Hosp Pract 1985 Mar 30; 20(3):73–77, 82–85, 89–93.

DeVito AJ. Rehabilitation of patients with chronic obstructive pulmonary disease. Rehabil Nurs 1985 Mar/Apr; 10(2):12–15.

*Esquibel KP et al. A proposal for an educational program to assist asthmatic students in reaching their full potential. J Prof Nurs 1985 Jan/Feb; 9(1):55–63.

Exercise, diet and COPD. Patient Care 1984 Nov 30; 18(20):123, 125, 129.

Farr RS. One definition of asthma . . . hyperactive airways. Chest 1985 Jan; 87(Suppl 1):20S–21S.

Fernandez E. Update on the pharmacologic approach to asthma: Xanthine and adrenergic bronchodilators. Respir Ther 1984 July/Aug; 14(4):42–44, 48, 50.

Giovanni R. Chronic ventilator care: From hospital to home. Respir Ther 1984 July/Aug; 14(4):29–30, 32–33.

Halcomb R. Promoting self-help in pulmonary patient education. Respir Ther 1984 May/June; 14(3):49–50, 52, 54.

Harris PL. A guide to prescribing pulmonary rehabilitation. Primary Care 1985 June; 12(2):253–266.

Higgins M. Epidemiology of COPD: State of the art. Chest 1984 June; 85(Suppl 6):3S–8S.

Hudson LD. Management of COPD: State of the art. Chest 1984 June; 85(Suppl 6):76S–81S.

*Janson-Bjerklie S et al. Emotionally triggered asthma as a predictor of airway response to suggestion. Res Nurs Health 1986 June; 9(2):163–170.

Kattan M. Emergency management of acute asthma. Hosp Pract 1986 Nov 15; 21(11):81–88.

Kelly K et al. Living with COPD: Caribbean cruise opens new worlds to patients. AART Times 1985 Dec; 9(12):18–21.

*Kim MJ. Respiratory muscle training: Implications for patient care. Heart Lung 1984 July; 13(4):333–340.

Kirilloff L and Tibbals S. Drugs for asthma: A complete guide. Am J Nurs 1983 Jan; 83(1):55–61.

Konig P. Spacer devices used with metered-dose inhalers: Breakthrough or gimmick? Chest 1985 Aug; 88(2):276–284.

Mitler LG. Exercise-induced asthma. Hosp Med 1986 Mar; 22(Suppl 3):101–102, 104–105, 108, 112.

Montenegro HD. Complications of mechanical ventilation. Respir Ther 1984 Sept/Oct; 14(5):20, 22–24, 26–27.

Murciano D et al. Effects of theophylline on diaphragmatic strength and fatigue in patients with chronic obstructive pulmonary disease. N Engl J Med 1984 Aug 9; 311(6):343-353.

Petty TL. Pulmonary rehabilitation: Better living with new techniques. Respir Care 1985 Feb; 30(2):98-107.

Phillipson EA et al. Breathing during sleep in chronic obstructive pulmonary disease: State of the art. Chest 1984 June; 85(Suppl 6): 24S-30S.

Rifas E. Teaching patients to manage acute asthma. Nurs '83 1983 Apr; 13(4):77-82.

Rogers RM et al. Nutrition and COPD: State of the art minireview. Chest 1984 June; 85(Suppl 6):63S-66S.

Rochester DD. The respiratory muscles in COPD: State of the art. Chest 1984 June; 85(Suppl 6):47S-50S.

*Shenkman B. Factors contributing to attrition rates in a pulmonary rehabilitation program. Heart Lung 1985 Jan; 14(1):53-58.

Snider GL (ed). Symposium on emphysema. Clin Chest Med 1983 Sept; 4(3):327-482.

Snider GL. Distinguishing among asthma, chronic bronchitis, and emphysema. Chest 1985 Jan; 87(Suppl 1):35S-39S.

Summers WR. Status asthmaticus. Chest 1985 Jan; 87(Suppl 1):87S-94S.

Warren B. Is your patient's job or home killing him? Nurs '85 1985 Mar; 15(3):64Q, 64T, 64X.

Your role in C.O.P.D. Nurs '85 1985 Feb; 15(2):32C, 32F, 32J.

Zwillich CW. Asthma therapy: An update. Respir Ther 1986 Mar/Apr; 16(2):13-14, 16-17.

Pulmonary Vascular Disorders

*Burke CM and Morris AJ. Perfusion scans and pulmonary angiography. Heart Lung 1986 July; 15(4):357-360.

Cooke DH. Focusing on pulmonary embolism. Emerg Med 1985 May 15; 17(9):86-89, 92, 97.

D'Alonzo GE, Bowes JS, and Dantzker DR. Differentiation of patients with primary and thromboembolic pulmonary hypertension. Chest 1984 Apr; 85(4):457-461.

Fernsebner B and Baum P. Teaching the patient having a vena caval filter. AORN J 1984 Jan; 39(1):65-76.

Fernsebner B et al. Surgical prevention of pulmonary emboli: Vena caval interruption. AORN J 1984 Jan; 39(1):56-64.

Fishman AJ, Moser KM, and Fedullo PF. Perfusion lung scans vs pulmonary angiography in evaluation of suspected primary pulmonary hypertension. Chest 1983 Dec; 84(6):679-683.

Goldhaber S. Pulmonary embolism: Diagnostic and therapeutic options. Consultant 1986 Feb; 26(2):124-128, 133, 136-137.

*Hurewitz AN and Bergofsky EH. Pathogenic mechanisms in chronic pulmonary hypertension. Heart Lung 1986 July; 15(4):327-335.

Peterson RT and Goldman AL. Pulmonary embolism. Primary Care 1985 June; 12(2):383-396.

Rounds S and Hill NS. Pulmonary hypertensive diseases. Chest 1984 Mar; 85(3):397-405.

Viamonte M. What's new in pulmonary embolism? Appl Radiol 1984 July/Aug; 13(4):105-107.

Vicari RM and Messer JV. Cor pulmonale: Often overlooked, always a therapeutic challenge. Consultant 1986 Jan; 26(1):186-192, 197, 200.

Williams MH. Pulmonary embolism. Emerg Med 1984 Feb 29; 16(4): 135-136, 138-140.

Wollschlager CM and Khan FA. Secondary pulmonary hypertension: Clinical features. Heart Lung 1986 July; 15(4):336-340.

Woodruff ML. Pulmonary thromboembolism: Risk factors, pathophysiology, and management. Crit Care Nurs 1984 July/Aug; 4(4):52-60.

Occupational Lung Diseases

Cassingham B. The silent epidemic: Asbestosis and related diseases. Occup Health Nurs 1985 July; 33(7):360-362.

Krokosky NJ. Black lung and silicosis. Am J Nurs 1985 Aug; 85(8):883-886.

Shaman D. Silicosis: The occupational disease that shouldn't exist. Am Lung Assoc Bull 1983 Mar/Apr; 69(2):6-12.

Weill H. Asbestos-associated diseases: Science, public policy, and litigation. Chest 1983 Nov; 84(5):601-608.

Lung Cancer

Arabian A and Spagnolo SV. Laser therapy in patients with primary lung cancer. Chest 1984 Oct; 86(4):519-523.

Cooper ET. A pilot study on effects of the diagnosis of lung cancer on family relationships. Cancer Nurs 1984 Aug; 7(4):301-308.

Falconer EG. Present management of lung cancer. Med Ed 1984; 801-804.

Faulkenberry JE. Programmed instruction: Cancer prevention and detection: Lung cancer. Cancer Nurs 1985 Jan; 8(3):185-194.

Gelb AF and Epstein JD. Laser in treatment of lung cancer. Chest 1984 Nov; 86(4):662-666.

Hande KR and Des Prez RM. Current perspectives in small cell lung cancer. Chest 1985 May; 85(5):669-677.

Koop CE. Smoking and cancer. Hosp Pract 1984 June; 19(6):107-111.

Matthay RA. Symposium on recent advances in lung cancer. Clin Chest Med 1982 May; 3(2):217-452.

Matthews JI and Blanton HM. Lung cancer: An update. Primary Care 1985 June; 12(2):267-281.

Mier JW. Management of metastatic cancer of the lung. Hosp Formulary 1983 Sept; 18(9):856-862.

Rosetti AC. Nursing care of patients treated with intrapleural tetracycline for control of malignant pleural effusion. Cancer Nurs 1985 Apr; 8(2):103-109.

Tockman MS. Update on lung cancer. Hosp Med 1985 Apr; 21(4):85-85, 90-92, 94-98.

Varricchio CG and Jassak PF. Acute pulmonary disorders associated with cancer. Semin Oncol Nurs 1985 Nov; 1(4):269-277.

Trauma

Branson RD et al. Synchronous independent lung ventilation in the treatment of unilateral pulmonary contusion: A report of two cases. Respir Care 1984 Apr; 29(4):361-367.

Carroll PF. Action STAT! Tension pneumothorax. Nurs '85 1985 Sept; 15(9):41.

Ozgen G et al. Chest injuries in civilian life and their treatment. Chest 1984 Jan; 85(1):89-92.

Rhodes M. Update on chest trauma. Crit Care Q 1983 Sept; 6(2):59-66.

Sonnesso G. When your patient has a tracheobronchial injury. Nurs '86 1986 Mar; 16(3):64E, 64G.

Tanamelin BR. Respiratory management of the trauma patient. Top Emerg Med 1984 Apr; 6(1):25-34.

Acute Respiratory Failure and ARDS

Bernard GR and Bradley RB. Adult respiratory distress syndrome: Diagnosis and management. Heart Lung 1986 May; 15(3):250-255.

Bone RC. The adult respiratory distress syndrome: Treatment in the next decade. Respir Care 1984 Mar; 29(3):249-262.

Boucher BA and Foster TS. The adult respiratory distress syndrome. Drug Intell Clin Pharm 1984 Nov; 18(11):862-868.

Brandstetter RD. The adult respiratory distress syndrome—1986. Heart Lung 1986 Mar; 15(2):155-165.

Concepcion I. Ventilatory support in ARDS. Respir Ther 1984 Jan/Feb; 14(1):53-58.

Craig KC, Pierson DJ, and Carrico CJ. The clinical application of positive end-expiratory pressure (PEEP) in the adult respiratory distress syndrome (ARDS). Respir Care 1985 Mar; 30(3):184-201.

Domigan-Wentz J. The CPAP mask: A "comfortable" approach to ARDS. Am J Nurs 1985 July; 85(8):813-815.

Grossman J. Insight into adult respiratory distress syndrome. Respir Ther 1984 Mar/Apr; 14:21–26.

Halevy A et al. Long-term evaluation of patients following the adult respiratory distress syndrome. Respir Care 1984 Feb; 29(2):132–137.

Katz JA. PEEP and CPAP in perioperative respiratory care. Respir Care 1984 June; 29(6):614–624.

Miscellaneous

Boylan CT. Clinical approach to a diagnostic dilemma. Consultant 1985 Jan 15; 25(1):41–43, 46–47.

Cherniack NS. Breathing disorders during sleep. Hosp Pract 1986 Feb 15; 21(2):81–86, 88–89, 93–97.

Hurley EJ. Lung abscess. Hosp Med 1983 Dec; 19(12):79–81, 84–88, 98, 100.

Kotagel S et al. Geriatric sleep disorders: Overview of sleep apnea and its prevalence in the elderly. Consultant 1985 Feb; 25(3):86–87, 90, 92–93.

Kryger MH. Symposium on sleep disorders. Clin Chest Med 1985 Dec; 6(4):553–718.

Light RW. Postoperative pleural effusion: Pathophysiology, clinical importance, and principles of management. Respir Care 1984 May; 29(5):540–549.

Marini JJ. Postoperative atelectasis: Pathophysiology, clinical importance and principles of management. Respir Care 1984 May; 29(5):516–528.

Thawley SE (ed). Symposium on sleep apnea disorders. Med Clin North Am 1985 Nov; 69(6):1121–1358.

Agencies

American Cancer Society, 90 Park Avenue, New York, NY 10016.

American Lung Association, 1740 Broadway, New York, NY 10019.

International Association of Laryngectomees, c/o American Cancer Society, 777 Third Avenue, New York, New York 10017.

Nursing Research Profile for Unit VI

Respiratory Nursing

Overview

Most of the nursing research studies in chronic respiratory problems are in the area of dyspnea management for patients with chronic obstructive pulmonary disease. Studies have indicated that nurse-managed pulmonary rehabilitation programs and specific respiratory muscle exercise training programs have significantly helped patients improve the quality of their lives by increasing their ability to manage their activities of daily living. Recent research is exploring the impact of a significant other on the patient's coping abilities and reduced reporting of symptoms.

Nurses are also searching for improved methods of performing endotracheal suctioning and tracheostomy care to eliminate the occurrence of infection, and of decreasing the severity of hypoxemia. Most of the research studies review implications for family management, because many pulmonary disorders are of a chronic nature.

Dyspnea Management and Respiratory Muscle Exercise

▷ *Martin LL. Respiratory muscle function: A clinical study. Heart Lung 1984 July; 13(4):346–348.*

The aim of Martin's study was to demonstrate that health maintenance measures could be more successful for persons with chronic obstructive pumonary disease (COPD) if respiratory muscle strength could be improved. The hypothesis was based on the assumption that exercise intolerance or difficulty in performing activities of daily living can result from respiratory muscle weakness.

The limited sample (N = 13) was divided into group A (N = 7) and group B (N = 6). All subjects were chosen from an outpatient education and exercise program designed for persons with stable COPD. Group A performed incentive spirometry and were referred to as the exercise group; group B did no exercise and served as the control group. The incentive spirometer was used to force the patient to achieve maximum inspiration, thus causing an increase in transdiaphragmatic pressure from the resting state. Those in group A performed sustained maximal inspiration, holding the ball against the inner cylinder of the spirometer for 1 second, 20 times, twice a day, for 5 days a week. Maximal inspiratory and maximal expiratory pressure readings were done for all subjects prior to the use of incentive spirometry.

After 5 weeks, inspiratory and expiratory muscle strengths were measured again. Results of the study indicated that the maximum inspiratory pressure significantly increased for the exercise group as compared with the baseline reading but did not significantly change for the nonexercise group. The maximum expiratory pressure showed a significant mean increase. Some subjects were able to increase their inspiratory muscle strength by 80% to 100% and their expiratory muscle strength by 53% to 62%.

Nursing Implications. An exercise protocol that includes the use of incentive spirometry may increase inspiratory muscle strength. Persons with severe COPD may find a respiratory muscle exercise program beneficial. They may be able to improve their ability to be self-sufficient and increase their independence in performing activities of daily living.

▷ *Janson-Bjerklie S, Carrieri V and Hudes M. The sensations of pulmonary dyspnea. Nurs Res 1986 May/June; 35(3):154–159.*

The authors studied patient sensations of dyspnea across pulmonary disease groups (emphysema-bronchitis, asthma, vascular disease, and restrictive disease) and looked for common dyspnea predictors, prodromal indicators, and physical and emotional reactions. A convenience sample of 68 subjects who had documented pulmonary disease and experienced shortness of breath was chosen. The group included 29 men and 39 women with a mean age of 54.34 years. A semistructured interview tool was used to obtain information about emotional sensations experienced during an attack of dyspnea. The Dyspnea Visual Analog Scale (DVAS) was used to estimate the amount of usual and worst dyspnea noted. The Asthma Symptom Checklist and the Bronchitis–Emphysema Symptom Checklist were also used to identify other symptoms not mentioned during the interview. The Profile of Mood States and the Norbeck Social Support Questionnaire were used to measure personal and situational variables.

Results indicated that half of the group (N = 34) perceived their symptom of dyspnea as a major problem; 13 felt it caused a moderate amount of concern and 20 viewed it as a minor problem. The mean grade of breathlessness on the Grade of Breathlessness Scale was 3.24 (±1.67), with significant differences across disease groups noted by analysis of variance. The Grade of Breathlessness Scale uses a range of 0 (no shortness of breath) to 5 (too breathless to leave home).

The highest usual dyspnea intensity scores were 55 for vascular subjects and 25.3 for asthmatic subjects. However, the asthmatic subjects had the highest worst dyspnea scores (87.83), followed by 82.6 for the vascular subjects. Across pulmonary groups, the women rated their usual dyspnea (38.5) significantly higher than the men (27.8). All groups showed few differences in their descriptions of precipitating factors. The majority of subjects (66%) had no sense that an attack was approaching, while 34% recognized some indicator. As many as 21% felt that they were not always aware that they were experiencing shortness of breath until someone told them so. Most (97%) described the sensation with the words, "I feel short of breath," and 85% said the experience was similar to being unable to move air or not get enough air. The most common emotions associated with the sensation were panic (24%), frustration (15%), worry (12%), anxiety (10%), anger (8%), and fear of death (7%).

The researchers concluded that most persons with dyspnea described their sensation using the words "suffocation," "tightness," and "congestion." Dyspnea did not usually occur alone but was frequently accompanied by nausea, fatigue, headache, and pain. Emotional responses occurred with dyspnea, their severity directly correlated with the acuity of the dyspnea. A person's disease group, gender, and social support network were variables that significantly related to the experience of dyspnea.

Nursing Implications. The sensations of dyspnea across a given pulmonary disease category appear to be similar. The frequency and intensity of the sensation have the most impact on the severity of the problem. Asthmatic subjects had the lowest mean score of intensity, and persons with vascular disease with pulmonary hypertension scored the highest. Therefore, nursing care plans for the vascular disease group would reflect their greater need for nursing intervention for pulmonary management. Women seemed to be more sensitive to the severity of the sensation than men. These conclusions are important when planning care for patients with pulmonary disease and anticipating the severity of symptoms based on the variables of gender, disease group, and support system.

▷ *Carrieri VK and Janson-Bjerklie S. The sensation of dyspnea: A review. Heart Lung 1984 July; 13(4):436–445.*

The authors reviewed current research about the sensation of dyspnea and suggested a framework for nurses to use when managing patients who experience this symptom. Dyspnea was defined as a subjective sensation of labored breathing that can only be completely understood and described by the patient himself.

Approaches to researching the mechanisms, measurement, and management of dyspnea were reviewed. Recognizing that no one theory existed to explain the mechanism of dyspnea, the authors listed the four most common categories cited as possible causes: (1) stimulation of afferent intrapulmonary receptors; (2) central nervous system sensitivity to ventilation changes; (3) decreased ventilatory ability; and (4) neural receptor stimulation in the intercostals, diaphragm, and skeletal joints. Physiological and psychological correlates that influenced dyspnea were also identified and explained.

Various experimental methods to induce dyspnea were mentioned (breath-holding, vagal nerve block, chest wall block, chest strapping, CO_2 inhalation); no one method clearly demonstrated a cause-and-effect correlation. Fletcher's scale, an instrument used for measuring dyspnea, was explained and illustrated. The scale grades the severity of the patient's shortness of breath using a range of 0 to 3. Although rating scales provide baseline assessment data for future reference, their retrospective nature is seen as a disadvantage. Another instrument reviewed and recommended was the Visual Analog Scales, which can be used to rate the severity and patterns of symptoms in patients who are critically ill and cannot undergo physical endurance testing.

In reviewing the literature, the researchers concluded that nurse-managed pulmonary rehabilitation programs have been most successful in improving exercise tolerance and subsequently improving the quality of a person's life. Nursing research studies have documented increases in walking distances and exercise tolerance when graded exercise regimens were used. Teaching patients pursed-lip and diaphragmatic breathing techniques has helped slow the respiratory rate and decrease airway collapse during periods of dyspnea. Inspiratory muscle training has also shown improved exercise endurance and performance. Measures to control anxiety (meditation, relaxation) were found successful in reducing the symptoms associated with dyspnea.

The researchers also found that patients discovered their own coping strategies that were successful in reducing the sensations of dyspnea. Two major strategies identified were organizing activities to decrease energy expenditure and choosing a significant other for support. Also important was whether the patient had sufficient money, time, and energy to cope with the limitations of the condition.

Nursing Implications. The debilitating effects of dyspnea can be controlled by encouraging patient participation in pulmonary rehabilitation and exercise programs. Patients can also be taught how to control the anxiety associated with the sensation and can be encouraged to seek a social support person. Nursing plans of care should be specific so that the individual can improve his quality of life and participate in activities of daily living to the best of his ability.

▷ *Parkosewich JA. Sleep-disordered breathing: A common problem in chronic obstructive pulmonary disease. Crit Care Nurs 1986 Nov/Dec; 6(6):60–64.*

The effects of noctural arterial oxygen desaturation caused by sleep-disordered breathing (SDB) were studied in patients diagnosed with COPD. Nocturnal desaturation can cause transient hypoxemia, which can have serious and irreversible implications.

Sleep-disordered breathing refers to alterations in normal respiratory function during periods of sleep. Apnea and hypopnea are examples of SDB. These periods occur in many persons and usually during REM sleep. However, when a person with COPD experiences such an episode, there is an associated significant decrease in oxygen saturation, even with a small decrease in oxygen tension. This occurs because patients with COPD usually have a decreased alveolar oxygen tension. In addition, COPD patients do not have the same use of their accessory muscles during REM sleep that they have while awake and thus have difficulty maintaining the same levels of tidal volume.

The author noted a significant correlation between nocturnal desaturation and pulmonary artery pressure increases, especially during REM sleep. This suggests that transient episodes of pulmonary artery hypertension during REM sleep may lead to cor pulmonale in high-risk groups. Other authors suggest that nocturnal desaturation may lead to episodes of myocardial ischemia and increased incidence of dysrhythmias. Medical intervention includes nocturnal low-flow oxygen to reduce hypoxemia and pulmonary hypertension caused by hypopnea.

Nursing Implications. It is important to identify the COPD patient who is at risk by obtaining a complete nursing history. Patients with COPD who experience sleep-disturbed breathing have an increased incidence of hypoxemia resulting from ineffective nocturnal ventilation due to inadequate sleep and rest. Data about sleep patterns must be collected and analyzed.

▷ *Carrieri VK and Janson-Bjerklie S. Strategies patients use to manage the sensation of dyspnea. West J Nurs Res 1986 Aug; 8(3):284–305.*

Coping strategies used for managing dyspnea were studied in a group limited to subjects diagnosed with emphysema. The study also sought to determine whether the findings were applicable to other chronic pulmonary disorders. The stress and coping paradigm developed by R. S. Lazarus (1980) was chosen as the framework for the study. Dyspnea was identified as the stressor influencing the relationship between the patient and the environment. The individual's ability to appraise the situation and use coping strategies was measured. *Coping*

was defined as the ability to handle acute episodes of stress, whereas *adaptive changes* referred to long-term adjustments.

The purpose of the study was to describe coping strategies used by patients with emphysema and determine whether the strategies were learned from others or personally chosen to meet individual needs. The reseachers also wanted to know whether there was a relationship between the perceived severity of the dyspnea and the type of coping strategy used.

The study design was descriptive and exploratory. A questionnaire and structured interview were developed to obtain information about the types of coping strategies used. Sample characteristics were tabulated by having subjects complete the American Thoracic Society (ATS) Respiratory Questionnaire. Two instruments measured the severity of dyspnea: the American Thoracic Society Grade of Breathlessness Scale (GBS) and the Visual Analogue Scales (VAS).

Of 68 subjects, 59% had high grades of dyspnea using the 0–5 GBS, with the highest mean score (3.59) recorded for the emphysema–bronchitis group. The total group mean score was 3.24. Using the VAS instrument, the asthmatic group had the highest mean worst dyspnea score. The results of the interview yielded 38 categories of strategies, with some patients using as many as 23 different ones. The mean number of strategies used for the entire group was 13 ± 5 (SD). Again, the asthmatics used the greatest number. The strategies used by the subjects were organized into three groups: problem-focused, emotion-focused, and mixed.

Problem-focused coping strategies were identified as position and motion changes (keeping still, leaning forward over the back of a chair); breathing strategies (pursed-lip or diaphragmatic breathing); physically distancing themselves from the aggravating factor; and self-selected treatments (self-adjustment of medications). Emotion-focused coping strategies consisted of self-isolation and tension reduction (relaxation techniques). Mixed strategies consisted of support groups and diversional activities.

Long-term problem-focused coping strategies consisted of modifications in grooming and clothing (slip-on shoes, loose clothing), weight reduction through dieting, planned modification in activities of daily living, transfer of home responsibilities to a family member, and manipulation of the social and physical environment to prevent stressors that would precipitate an attack. Long-term emotion-focused coping strategies consisted of adopting a positive attitude, although 25% of the subjects felt that they were socially or geographically isolated because of having to modify their activities. Long-term mixed coping strategies included close family relationships and formal participation in a support group. Thirteen subjects (19%) learned coping strategies from formal sources.

Nursing Implications. Most patients with significant attacks of dyspnea must modify their activities of daily living and use self-taught coping strategies that are similar across all pulmonary disease groups. Therefore, a nursing care plan for a patient experiencing dyspnea should include a complete assessment of his normal adaptive strategies, his support systems, and the limitations of his environment. The patient should be encouraged to practice breathing exercises and identify a family member or significant other who can help him with his activities of daily living. The feasibility of having him participate in a formal support group should be explored.

Tracheostomy Care

▷ *Harris RB and Hyman RB. Clean vs sterile tracheotomy care and level of pulmonary infection. Nurs Res 1984 Mar/Apr; 33(2):80–85.*

Three approaches to tracheotomy suctioning and cleaning (clean, sterile, and mixed) were studied to determine whether use of the clean technique was as safe and effective as use of the sterile technique, as measured by the occurrence of postoperative pulmonary infection. The study was conducted at 10 clinical sites using a sample of 209 subjects. A "weighted level of pulmonary infection" tool, developed by the nurse researchers, separated clinical and laboratory measurements of infection and weighed each variable according to its level of objectivity (higher weights had higher infection predictability). A cumulative score indicated the presence of a pulmonary infection.

The study indicated a statistically significant difference in the occurrence of postoperative pulmonary infection when the results of clean and sterile techniques were compared. A higher infection rate occurred with the use of sterile technique and was attributed to failure to maintain a sterile field. Individual variations during performance of the sterile technique led to contamination. However, those who used clean technique were able to remember the steps of the procedure and followed directions appropriately. The study needs to be duplicated to see if the conclusions would be similar.

Nursing Implications. The results of this study have significant implications for patient education, especially for those patients who must care for themselves at home. If clean technique is as effective or more effective than sterile technique, then nurses can recommend the use of clean technique when patients and families are to care for a tracheotomy. In addition, when sterile technique is necessary, nurses need to be extra cautious in maintaining strict aseptic technique because research studies have shown that strict asepsis is not always used as directed.

Endotracheal Suctioning

▷ *Goodnough SKC. The effects of oxygen and hyperinflation on arterial oxygen tension after endotracheal suctioning. Heart Lung 1985 Jan; 14(1):11–17.*

This study explored the frequency of hypoxemia after endotracheal suctioning even when the fraction of inspired oxygen (FIO_2) was increased before or after the suctioning procedure. Previous studies had shown a decrease in PaO_2 for as long as 5 minutes after suctioning when hyperinflation and increased FIO_2 were used. This study attempted to separate the effects of increased FIO_2 and hyperinflation as presuctioning interventions from the postsuctioning effects, and to extend the final PaO_2 reading to 10 minutes after suctioning.

The study was conducted on 28 subjects in intensive care units 4 to 6 hours after cardiac surgery. Two medical centers were used to obtain the necessary number of subjects. Each patient met certain criteria: $FIO_2 \leq 0.8$; peak inspiratory pressure ≤ 50 cm H_2O; an absence of positive end-expiratory pressure; a $PaO_2 \geq 80$ mm Hg; a functional arterial line; stable arterial blood pressure with systolic blood pressure ≥ 90 mm Hg; and an absence of acute dysrhythmias.

Endotracheal suctioning lasted an average of 8 seconds and was performed with 14 Fr catheters using a wall-mounted suction apparatus that delivered a peak pressure of 140 mm Hg. Hyperinflation was delivered at 150% of the patient's baseline tidal volume at a rate necessary to maintain the baseline minute volume. The FIO_2 was increased to 1.0 on the ventilator for 1 minute. All blood samples were drawn from indwelling arterial lines. The baseline PaO_2, the control for the study, was drawn immediately after suctioning but before postsuctioning administration of increased FIO_2 and/or hyperinflation. Additional blood samples were drawn at 5- and 10-minute intervals to reflect the PaO_2 after suctioning and the residual effects of postsuctioning interventions. Four sequences for suctioning were used for each patient, including the following combinations: (1) increased FIO_2 before suctioning and hyperinflation after suctioning; (2) increased FIO_2 before and after suctioning; (3) hyperinflation before and after suctioning; and (4) increased FIO_2 and hyperinflation before and after suctioning. Analysis of variance was used for any differences between procedures. Mean and standard deviations were reported with a $p < 0.01$. The results indicated a significant difference in PaO_2 among the procedures and among the time periods, and a significant interaction of procedure with time.

The study showed that presuctioning hyperinflation did not protect the majority (75%) of the subjects from a decrease in PaO_2 immediately after suctioning. However, preoxygenation protected 75% of the subjects from a decrease in PaO_2 after endotracheal suctioning. Preoxygenation combined with hyperinflation protected 96% of the sample from a decrease in PaO_2. All postsuctioning interventions successfully prevented a decrease in PaO_2 or restored a decreased PaO_2 to control levels at the 5- and 10-minute intervals. The researchers concluded that 1 minute of 100% oxygen administered with hyperinflation of 150% of the patient's tidal volume at a rate to maintain the baseline minute volume provides protection against a decrease in PaO_2 when used before and after endotracheal suctioning.

Nursing Implications. This study has obvious implications for nursing practice: (1) Hyperinflation with 100% oxygen should be administered for 1 minute before and after suctioning to protect cardiac patients from hypoxemia; and (2) vital signs should be monitored during the endotracheal procedure because hyperinflation can cause arterial blood pressure alterations and changes in heart rate.

Additional Studies

Douglas S and Larson EL. The effect of a positive end-expiratory pressure adapter on oxygenation during endotracheal suctioning. Heart Lung 1985 Jul; 14(4):396–400.

Hayter J. Sleep behaviors of older persons. Nurs Res 1983 Jul/Aug; 32(4): 242–246.

Kim MJ. Respiratory muscle training: Implications for patient care. Heart Lung 1984 July; 13(4):333–338.

Norbeck JS, Lindsey AM and Carrieri VL. The development of an instrument to measure social support. Nurs Res 1981 Sept/Oct; 30(5): 264–269.

Norbeck JS, Lindsey AM and Carrieri VL. Further development of the Norbeck Social Support Questionnaire: Normative data and validity testing. Nurs Res 1983 Jan/Feb; 32(1):4–9.

Sexton DL and Munro BH. Impact of a husband's chronic illness (COPD) on the spouse's life. Res Nurs Health 1985 Mar; 8(1):83–90.

Cardiovascular, Circulatory, and Hematologic Problems

Unit VII

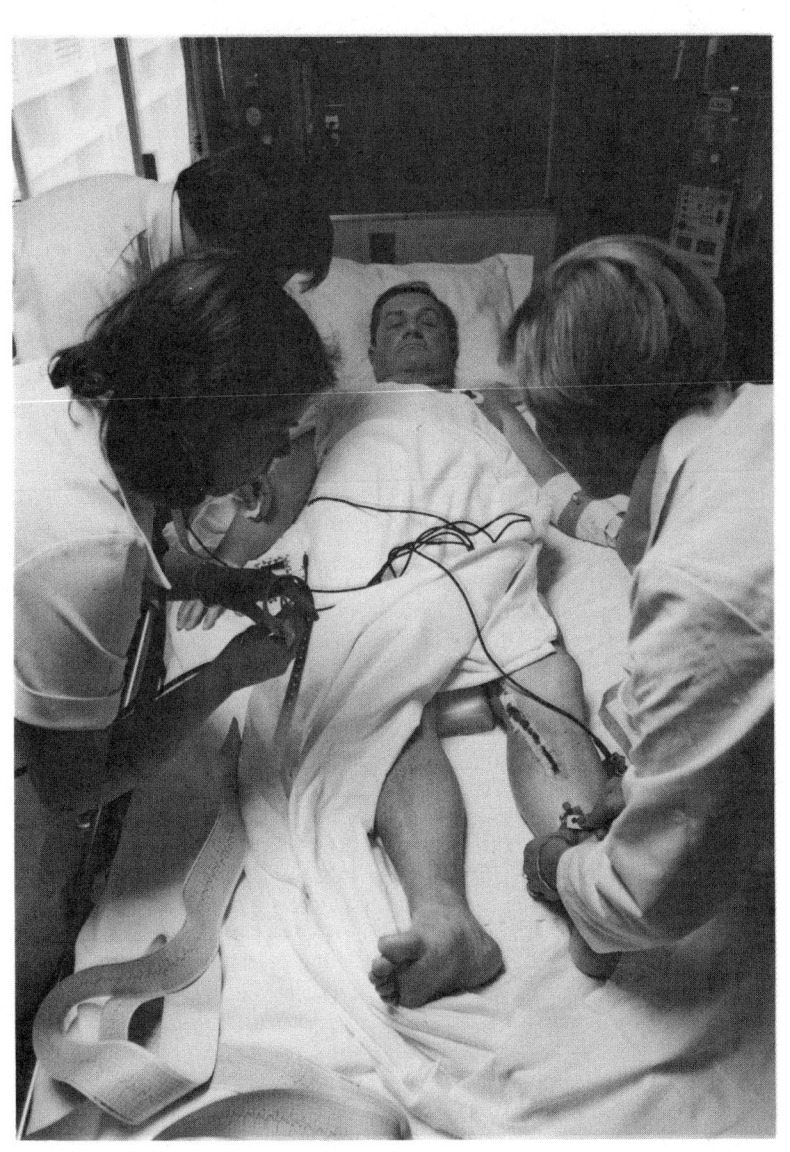

Chapter 24

Assessment of Cardiovascular Function

Nursing assessment of a patient with heart disease includes taking a history, performing a physical examination, and monitoring tests of cardiac functioning. Sound knowledge of cardiac anatomy, physiology, and pathophysiology is necessary for developing assessment skills, defining nursing diagnoses, planning nursing care, and understanding the purposes of diagnostic tests.

Physiologic Overview

The heart is a hollow, muscular organ located in the center of the thorax where it occupies the space between the lungs and rests upon the diaphragm. It weighs approximately 300 gm (10.6 oz), although heart weight and size are influenced by age, sex, body weight, frequency of physical exercise, and heart disease. The function of the heart is to pump blood to the tissues, supplying them with oxygen and other nutrients and at the same time removing carbon dioxide and other waste products of metabolism. There are actually two pumps within this organ, located on the right and left sides of the heart. The output of the right heart is distributed entirely to the lungs via the pulmonary artery, and the output of the left heart is distributed to the remainder of the body via the aorta. These two pumps eject blood simultaneously at approximately the same rate of output.

The pumping action of the heart is accomplished by the rhythmical contraction and relaxation of its muscular wall. During contraction of the muscle (*systole*), the chambers inside the heart become smaller as the blood is ejected. During relaxation of the muscles of the heart wall (*diastole*), the heart chambers fill with blood in preparation for the subsequent ejection. A normal adult heart beats approximately 60 to 80 times per minute, ejects approximately 70 ml from each side per beat, and has a total output of approximately 5 liters/min.

Cardiac Anatomy

The space in the middle of the chest between the two lungs is called the *mediastinum*. The bulk of the mediastinal space is occupied by the heart, which is encased in a thin, fibrous sac called the *pericardium*. The pericardium is not essential for the proper functioning of the heart, but serves as an envelope to protect its surface. The space between the surface of the heart and the pericardial lining is filled with a very small amount of fluid, which lubricates the surface and tends to reduce friction during cardiac muscle contraction.

Heart Chambers. The right and left sides of the heart are each composed of two chambers, an *atrium* (pl. atria) and a *ventricle*. The common wall between the right and left chambers is called the *septum*. The ventricles are the chambers that eject blood into the arteries. The functions of the atria are to receive incoming blood from the veins and to act as temporary storage reservoirs for subsequent emptying into the ventricles. The relationship of the four chambers of the heart is shown in Figure 24-1.

The atria and ventricles are easily distinguished by the greater thickness of the muscle that forms the ventricular wall. The left ventricle ejects blood against high systemic pressure, whereas the right ventricle ejects blood against the low-resistance pulmonary vasculature. Therefore, because of the increased work of the left heart, the left ventricular wall is about 2½ times as thick (approximately 1 cm) as the right ventricular wall.

Because of the rotation of the heart within the chest cavity, the right ventricle lies anteriorly (just beneath the sternum) and the left ventricle is situated posteriorly. The left ventricle is responsible for the apex beat or the *point of maximum impulse (PMI)*, usually apparent on the left side of the chest wall.

Heart Valves. Heart valves permit blood to flow in only one direction through the heart. Valves, which are composed of thin leaflets of fibrous tissue, open and close passively in response to pressure changes and blood movement. There are two types of valves: *atrioventricular* and *semilunar*.

Atrioventricular Valves. Valves separating the atria from the ventricles are termed atrioventricular valves. The *tricuspid*

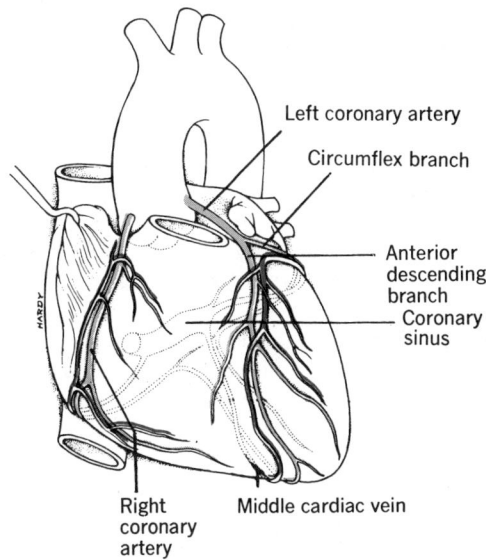

Figure 24-2
Diagram of the coronary arteries arising from the aorta and encircling the heart. The coronary sinus and some of the coronary veins also are shown. (Chaffee EE and Greisheimer EM. Basic Physiology and Anatomy. Philadelphia, JB Lippincott.)

valve, so named because it is composed of three cusps, or leaflets, separates the right atrium from the right ventricle. The *mitral* or *bicuspid valve* (two cusps) lies between the left atrium and left ventricle.

Semilunar Valves. Semilunar valves are situated between each ventricle and its corresponding artery. The valve between the right ventricle and the pulmonary artery is called the *pulmonic valve;* the valve between the left ventricle and the aorta is called the *aortic valve*. Both of the semilunar valves are normally composed of three cusps. There are no valves between the large veins and the atria.

Papillary Muscles and Chordae Tendineae. Normally, when the ventricles contract, ventricular pressure tends to push the atrioventricular valve leaflets upward into the atrial cavity. If enough pressure were to be exerted on the valves, blood would be ejected backward from the ventricles to the atria. Papillary muscles and chordae tendineae are responsible for maintaining unidirectional blood flow through the atrioventricular valves (from the ventricle to the respective artery). Papillary muscles are muscle bundles that are located on the sides of the ventricular walls. Chordae tendineae are fibrous bands extending from the papillary muscles to the edges of the valve leaflets, acting to tether the free edges of the valves to the ventricular wall. Contraction of the papillary muscles causes the chordae tendineae to become taut. This keeps the valve leaflets closed during systole, preventing backflow of blood. Papillary muscles and chordae tendineae are not necessary for proper functioning of the semilunar valves.

Coronary Arteries. The heart muscle is metabolically active in that its requirements for oxygen and nutrients are large and continuous. These required substances are supplied to the heart muscle by blood flowing in the coronary arteries (see Fig. 24-2). The heart, with large metabolic requirements, uses approximately one half of the oxygen delivered through

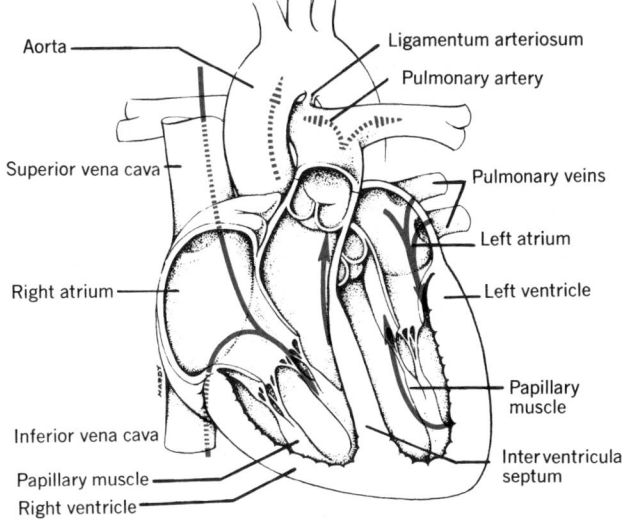

Figure 24-1
Interior of the heart. Arrows indicate the direction of blood flow. (Chaffee EE and Greisheimer EM. Basic Physiology and Anatomy. Philadelphia, JB Lippincott.)

the coronary arteries; in contrast, other organs use, on the average, only one quarter of the oxygen delivered to them. The coronary arteries arise from the aorta near its origin at the left ventricle. The wall of the left side of the heart is supplied in large part through the left main coronary artery, which divides into several large branches that run down (left anterior descending coronary artery) and across the left side of the myocardium (circumflex artery). The right heart wall is supplied similarly from a separate right coronary artery. Unlike other arteries, the coronary arteries are perfused during diastole.

Cardiac Muscle. The specialized muscle tissue composing the wall of the heart is called cardiac muscle. Microscopically, cardiac muscle resembles striated (skeletal) muscle, which is under conscious control. However, heart muscle is not under conscious control and in that sense resembles smooth (involuntary) muscle. The cardiac muscle fibers are arranged in an interconnected manner (called a *syncytium*) so that they can contract and relax in coordination. The sequential pattern of contraction and relaxation of individual muscle fibers ensures the rhythmic behavior of the heart muscle as a whole and enables it to function as a pump. The heart muscle itself is called the *myocardium*. The segment of cells on the inner surface of this muscle, which is in contact with the blood, is called the *endocardium*, and the portion of cells on the outer surface of the heart is called the *epicardium*.

Conduction System of the Heart

Specialized cells of the conduction system generate and conduct electrical impulses to myocardial cells, resulting in myocardial contraction. Cardiac muscle cells have an inherent rhythmicity, which is illustrated by the fact that a segment of myocardium removed from the rest of the heart will continue to contract rhythmically if maintained under the proper conditions. The heart rate is determined by the group of myocardial cells with the fastest intrinsic rate. These specialized cells, located at the junction of the superior vena cava and the right atrium, are known as the *sinoatrial (SA) node* and function as the pacemaker for the entire myocardium (see Fig. 24-3). The SA node initiates approximately 60 to 100 impulses per minute in a resting normal heart but can change its rate in response to the needs of the body. The electrical signal initiated by the SA node is conducted along the myocardial cells of the atrium to the *atrioventricular (AV) junction.* The AV junction (located in the right atrial wall near the tricuspid valve) is another group of specialized muscle cells similar to the SA node, but with an intrinsic rate of about 40 to 60 impulses per minute. The AV junction coordinates the incoming electrical impulses from the atria and relays an electrical impulse to the ventricles. This impulse is conducted away from the AV junction through a bundle of specialized muscle fibers (the *bundle of His*) that travel in the septum separating the left and right ventricles. The His bundle divides into right and left bundle branches, which terminate in fibers called *Purkinje fibers*. The right bundle fans out into the right ventricular muscle. The left bundle divides again into the left anterior and left posterior bundle branches, which fan out into the left ventricular muscle. Further spread of depolariza-

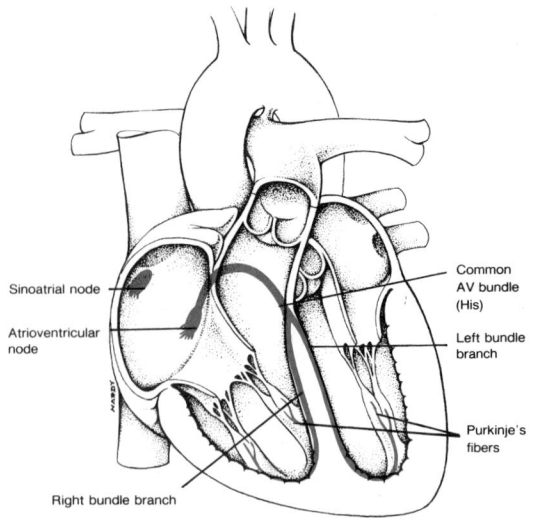

Figure 24-3
Conduction system. Diagram shows relationships of the sinoatrial node, the atrioventricular node, the common atrioventricular bundle and its branches. (Chaffee EE and Greisheimer EM. Basic Physiology and Anatomy. Philadelphia, JB Lippincott.)

tion through the rest of the myocardium takes place by conduction through the muscle fibers themselves.

If the SA node malfunctions, the AV node generally takes over the pacemaker function of the heart. Should both the SA and AV nodes fail in their pacemaker function, the myocardium will continue to beat at a rate of less than 40 beats per minute, the intrinsic pacemaker rate of the electrical impulse of the ventricular myocardial cells.

Cardiac Physiology

Electromechanical Coupling

In the normal cardiac muscle cell, an electrical difference (voltage) exists between the inside and the outside of the cell across its membrane. The inside of the cell is negative relative to the outside of the cell. When the magnitude of this difference is reduced (the inside of the cell becomes less negative), *depolarization* has occurred and contraction of muscle cell results. A cardiac muscle cell is normally depolarized when a neighboring cell is depolarized (although it can also be depolarized by external electrical stimulation). Sufficient depolarization of a single specialized conduction system cell will therefore result in depolarization and contraction of the entire myocardium. *Repolarization* occurs as the cell returns to its baseline state (becomes more negative), and corresponds to relaxation of myocardial muscle.

During depolarization the permeability of the cell membranes to certain ions (sodium, chloride, calcium, potassium) changes. One of those changes results in an increased permeability to calcium, allowing for uptake of calcium into the cell. This increase in intracellular calcium concentration leads to shortening of the muscle fibers and development of tension (contraction). After a short period, the membrane voltage returns to its original value, the calcium that had accumulated in its interior is removed, and the cell relaxes. This interaction between changes in membrane voltage and muscle contraction is called *electromechanical coupling.*

Cardiac muscle, unlike skeletal or smooth muscle, has a prolonged refractory period during which it cannot be restimulated to contract. This protects the heart from sustained contraction (*tetany*), which would result in sudden cardiac death.

Normal electromechanical coupling and contraction of the heart are dependent on the composition of the interstitial fluid surrounding the heart muscle cells. The composition of this fluid is in turn influenced by the composition of the blood. A change in blood calcium concentration may therefore alter contraction of the heart muscle fibers. A change in blood potassium concentration is also important, because potassium affects the normal electrical voltage of the cell.

Cardiac Hemodynamics

What determines the direction of blood flow from the heart through the circulation and then back to the heart? The important principle is that fluid will flow from a region of higher pressure to a region of lower pressure. The pressures that are responsible for blood flow in the normal circulation are generated by contraction of the ventricular muscle. When the muscle contracts, blood is forced from the ventricle into the aorta during the period of time when left ventricular pressure exceeds aortic pressure. When these two pressures become equal, the aortic valve closes and output from the left ventricle ceases. The blood that has entered the aorta increases the pressure in that vessel. This provides a pressure gradient to force blood progressively through the arteries and capillaries and into the veins. The blood returns to the right atrium because pressure in this chamber is lower than pressure in the veins. Similarly, a gradient of pressure is responsible for blood flow from the pulmonary artery through the lung and back to the left atrium. The pressure gradients within the pulmonary circulation are considerably lower than those in the systemic circulation because the resistance to flow in the pulmonary vessels is lower.

Cardiac Cycle. Let us consider the pressure changes that occur in the chambers of the heart during the cardiac cycle, beginning with *diastole* when the ventricles are relaxed (Fig. 24-4). During diastole the atrioventricular valves are open, and blood returning from the veins flows into the atrium and then into the ventricle. Toward the end of this diastolic period, the atrial muscle contracts in response to a signal initiated by the SA node. The contraction raises the pressure inside the atrium and forces an increment of blood into the ventricle. This blood augments the volume of the ventricles by an additional 10%. At this point, the ventricles themselves begin to contract (*systole*) in response to propagation of the electrical impulse that began in the SA node some milliseconds previously. During systole, the pressure inside the ventricle rapidly rises, forcing the AV valves to close. The consequence of this action is that no further filling of the ventricle from the atrium can occur, and blood ejected from the ventricle cannot flow back to the atrium. The rapid rise of pressure inside the ventricles forces the pulmonic and aortic valves to open, and blood is ejected into the pulmonary artery and

aorta, respectively. The exit of blood is at first rapid, and then, as the pressures in each ventricle and its corresponding artery approach equalization, the flow of blood gradually decreases. At the cessation of systole, the ventricular muscle relaxes and the pressure within the chamber rapidly decreases. This decrease in pressure creates a tendency for blood to come back from the artery into the ventricle, which forces the semilunar valves to close. Simultaneously, as the pressure within the ventricle drops to below atrial pressure, the AV valves open, the ventricles begin to fill, and the entire sequence is repeated. It is important to note that the mechanical events related to filling and ejection by the heart are closely coupled to the corresponding electrical events that cause cardiac contraction and relaxation. When interpreting Figure 24-4, it is necessary to realize that the electrical events (ECG) precede the mechanical events (pressures).

The events just described lead to the repetitive rise and fall of pressures inside the ventricles. The maximum pressure reached is called *systolic pressure* and the minimum pressure *diastolic pressure.*

Cardiac Output

Cardiac output is the amount of blood pumped by either of the ventricles during a given period of time. The cardiac output of a typical adult is normally about 5 liters/min but varies greatly, depending on the metabolic needs of the body. Cardiac output equals the stroke volume times the heart rate. *Stroke volume* is the amount of blood ejected per heartbeat. Cardiac output can be affected, therefore, by changes in either stroke volume or heart rate. The resting heart rate of an average adult is approximately 72 beats/min and the average stroke volume is about 70 ml/beat.

Control of Heart Rate. Since the function of the heart is to supply blood to all tissues of the body, its output must vary as the metabolic needs of the tissues themselves change. For example, during exercise the total cardiac output may increase fourfold, to 20 liters/min. This increase is normally accomplished by approximately doubling both the heart rate and the stroke volume. Changes in heart rate are accomplished by reflex controls mediated by the autonomic nervous system, including its sympathetic and parasympathetic divisions. The parasympathetic nerves, which travel to the heart through the vagus nerve, can slow the cardiac rate, whereas sympathetic nerves increase it. These nerves exert their effect on heart rate through their action on the SA node to either decrease or increase its rate of intrinsic depolarization. The balance between these two reflex control systems normally determines the heart rate. The heart rate is also stimulated by an increased level of circulating catecholamines (secreted by the adrenal gland) and by the presence of excess thyroid hormone, which produces a catecholamine-like effect.

Control of Stroke Volume. Stroke volume is primarily determined by three factors: (1) intrinsic contractility of the cardiac muscle, (2) the degree of stretch of the cardiac muscle prior to its contraction, and (3) the pressure against which the heart muscle has to eject blood during contraction.

Intrinsic contractility is a term used to denote the force that can be generated by the contracting myocardium under any given condition. It is increased by circulating catecholamines, sympathetic neuronal activity, and certain drugs (such

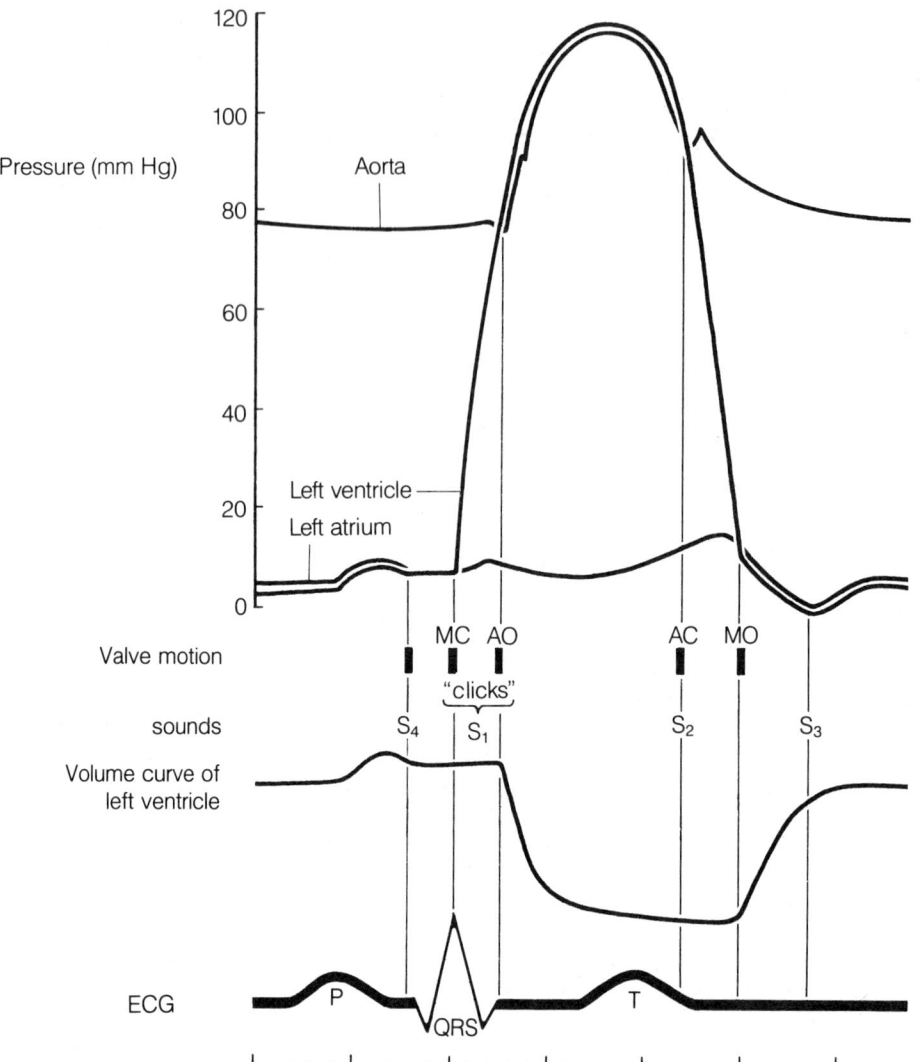

Figure 24-4
Events in the cardiac cycle. Three pressure curves are displayed: aortic, left ventricular, and left atrial. Electrocardiographic events precede the mechanical events. Valve closure and opening are indicated, as is the relationship of the cardiac sounds to these events.

as digitalis). It is depressed by hypoxemia and acidosis. Increased contractility results in increased stroke volume.

The precontraction length of the ventricular muscle fibers is determined by the volume of blood within the ventricle at the end of diastole. This volume, the ventricular end-diastolic volume, is called *preload*. The larger the preload, the greater will be the stroke volume, until a point is reached when the muscle is so stretched it can no longer contract. The relationship between increased stroke volume and increased ventricular end-diastolic volume for a given intrinsic contractility is called *Starling's Law of the Heart*, which is based on the fact that a greater initial length leads to a greater degree of shortening of cardiac muscle. This results from increased interaction between thick and thin filaments of the sarcomeres (similar to that discussed more fully in the chapter on skeletal muscle physiology).

The pressure against which the left ventricle ejects blood is the pressure in the aorta; right ventricular ejection works against the pressure in the pulmonary artery. The greater these pressures, the greater will be the tension in the ventricular wall during contraction. This tension is called *afterload*. Increased afterload leads to decreased stroke volume.

The heart can achieve a greatly increased stroke volume,

as during exercise, by increasing preload (through increased venous return), by increasing contractility (through sympathetic nervous discharge), and by decreasing afterload (through peripheral vasodilatation with decreased aortic pressure).

The fraction of the end-diastolic volume that is ejected with each stroke is called the *ejection fraction*. With each stroke, 0.56 to 0.78 of the end-diastolic volume is ejected by the normal heart. The ejection fraction can be used as an index of myocardial contractility; it is decreased if contractility is depressed.

Gerontological Considerations

Atherosclerosis of the coronary arteries and the resultant effects on the heart have long been associated with the aging process. However, recent investigations show little evidence that age is the precipitating factor. Current evidence indicates that the cardiac changes once attributed to aging can be minimized by modifying life-style and personal habits, that is, by following a low-sodium, low-fat diet, not smoking, and exercising regularly.

Studies have shown that the normal aging heart is able to provide an adequate cardiac output under ordinary circumstances, but may have limited functional ability to respond to situations that cause physical or emotional stress. In the elderly person who has decreased activity, the left ventricle may become smaller in response to the decreased workload demand. Aging also results in decreased elasticity and widening of the aorta, thickening and rigidity of the cardiac valves, and increased connective tissue in the SA and AV nodes and bundle branches. These changes lead to decreased myocardial contractility, increased left ventricular ejection time, and delayed conduction. Thus, stressful physical and emotional conditions, especially those that occur suddenly, may have adverse effects on the aged person. The heart is unable to respond to such conditions with an adequate increase in rate, and more time is required for the heart rate to return to basal levels after even a minimal increase. In some patients heart failure may be precipitated.

Nursing History

Cardiac patients who are acutely ill require a different initial nursing history than do cardiac patients with stable or chronic problems. A patient experiencing an acute myocardial infarction requires immediate, and possibly life-saving, medical and nursing interventions—for example, relief of chest discomfort or prevention of dysrhythmias—rather than an extensive interview. For this patient, a few well-chosen questions about chest discomfort, associated symptoms (such as shortness of breath or palpitations), drug allergies, and smoking history should be asked at the same time one is assessing heart rate, rhythm, and blood pressure, and starting an intra-venous line. When the patient is more stable, a more extensive history should be obtained.

When caring for an acutely ill cardiac patient, one first must focus on assessment of the heart and cardiac output. Patients with atherosclerotic coronary artery disease commonly experience chest discomfort (angina pectoris or myocardial infarction); shortness of breath, fatigue, and reduced urine output (left ventricular failure with decreased cardiac output); palpitations and dizziness (dysrhythmias due to ischemia, aneurysm, stress, or electrolyte imbalance); edema and weight gain (right ventricular failure); and postural hypotension with dizziness and light-headedness (saline depletion from diuretic therapy). Patients with valvular disease may have symptoms of heart failure, dysrhythmias, and chest discomfort.

Not all chest discomfort is related to myocardial ischemia. Guidelines are useful in differentiating the chest discomfort of serious, life-threatening conditions from that of conditions less serious or that would be treated in a different manner. Table 24-1 summarizes characteristics of the pain associated with angina pectoris, myocardial infarction, and pericarditis. Figure 24-5 illustrates the pain patterns both in these conditions and in noncardiac conditions. However, there are four important points to remember when evaluating chest discomfort:

- There is little correlation between the severity of the chest discomfort and the gravity of its cause.
- There is poor correlation between the location of chest discomfort and its source.
- The patient may have more than one clinical problem occurring simultaneously.
- In a patient with a history of atherosclerotic coronary artery disease, assume that the chest discomfort is secondary to ischemia until proven otherwise.

TABLE 24-1
Characteristics of Pain Associated With Angina Pectoris, Myocardial Infarction, and Pericarditis

Location and Radiation	*Character and Duration*	*Precipitating Events*
Angina Pectoris		
Substernal or retrosternal pain spreading across chest	*Pressure*; squeezing, heavy discomfort	Usually related to exertion, emotion, eating, cold
May radiate to *inside* of either arm or to both arms, neck, or jaws	Usually subsides within 1–10 min	
Myocardial Infarction		
Substernal or over precordium	Crushing, viselike, gripping	Occurs spontaneously
May spread widely throughout chest. Painful disability of shoulders and hands may be present.	More severe and prolonged than angina	Unrelated to emotion, exercise
	May be associated with dizziness, perspiration, and nausea	
	15%–25% may be silent	
Pericarditis		
Substernal or to left of sternum	Sharp, intermittent pain; made worse by swallowing, coughing, *rotation of trunk*	Often severe and sudden in onset. Pain increases with inspiration and motion of trunk.
May be felt in epigastrium		
May be referred to neck, arms, back		

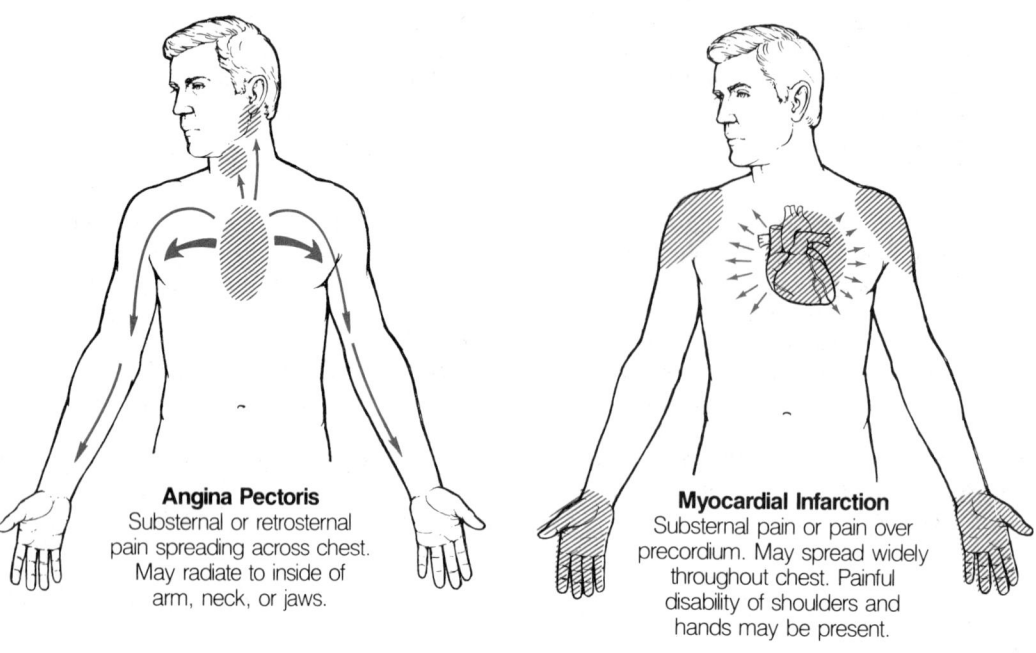

Angina Pectoris
Substernal or retrosternal pain spreading across chest. May radiate to inside of arm, neck, or jaws.

Myocardial Infarction
Substernal pain or pain over precordium. May spread widely throughout chest. Painful disability of shoulders and hands may be present.

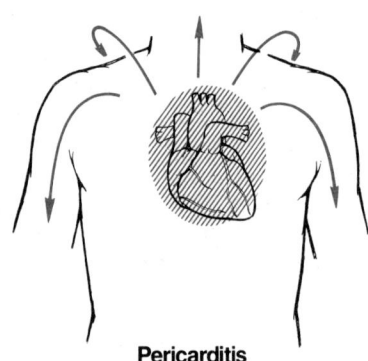

Pericarditis
Substernal pain or pain to the left of sternum. May be felt in epigastrium and may be referred to neck, arms, and back.

Pain of Pulmonary Origin
Pain arises from inferior portion of pleura. May be referred to costal margins or upper abdomen. Patient may be able to localize the pain.

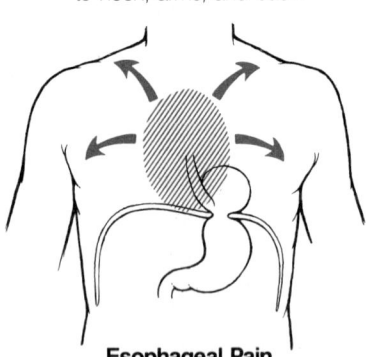

Esophageal Pain
(Hiatus Hernia, Reflux Esophagitis)
Substernal pain. May be projected around chest to shoulders.

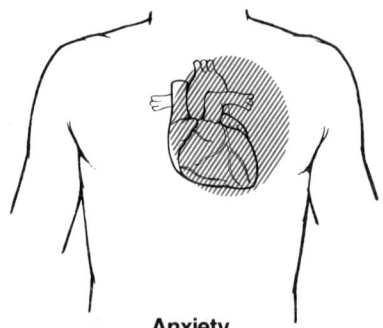

Anxiety
Pain over left chest. May be variable. Does not radiate. Assess for hyperventilation, sighing respiration, palpitations. Patient may complain of numbness and tingling of hands and mouth.

Figure 24-5
Assessment of chest pain.

To facilitate the gathering of subjective information for a cardiovascular nursing history, the patient should be questioned as indicated below. However, it is important to phrase the questions according to the appropriateness of the situation and to pursue areas where further clarification is necessary.

Breathing
- Are you ever short of breath?
- When do you become short of breath?
- How do you make your breathing better?
- What makes it worse?
- How long has breathing been a problem?
- What activities are necessary for you to do that you are no longer able to do because of your breathing?
- Are you on any medication to improve your breathing?
- Does any medication you are taking affect your breathing?
- What time of day do you prefer to take your medication?

Circulation
- Describe the discomfort that you have in your chest.*
- Does the pain spread to your arms, neck, jaw, or back?
- Is there anything that seems to cause the pain?
- How long does the pain usually last?
- Have you gained or lost any weight recently?
- Have you noticed any swelling of your hands, feet, or legs (or sacrum, if bedridden)?
- Do you ever feel dizzy or light-headed?
    What seems to cause this?
- Have you noticed any changes in your energy level? Tired? Fatigued?
- Do you ever feel as if your heart is racing or skipping beats? or pounding?
- Have you had problems with your blood pressure?
- Do you have headaches?
    What seems to cause them?
- Have you noticed that your hands or feet get unusually cold?
    When does this seem to happen?

Urination
- Is the amount of your urine output normal for you?
- Do you ever get up at night to use the bathroom? How many times? When did you notice the change?
- Do you take a diuretic? When do you take it?

Mentation
- Do you think as fast as you used to? As clearly?
- Do you laugh or cry more easily than before?
- When did you notice the change?
- Are you taking any medication that might affect your thinking?

When the patient's condition permits, other functional areas should also be assessed.

Information obtained in the nursing history is needed in order to plan individualized care while the patient is hospitalized, to aid in discharge planning, and to provide appropriate teaching. Knowing how the patient perceives the effects

* Because patients do not always admit to having chest "pain," word equivalents of pain should be used when eliciting the quality of discomfort. Common descriptions used by patients include strangling, constriction, tightness, aching, squeezing, pressing, heaviness, expanding sensation, choking in throat, indigestion, and burning.

of the disease process on activities of daily living will help to identify specific aims for cardiac rehabilitation or strategies for modifying certain activities to be devised. Since dietary modification (reduction of sodium, saturated fat, or caloric intake) will probably be prescribed, the history should include the following: food preferences (including cultural or ethnic); eating habits (canned or commercially prepared foods versus fresh foods, and restaurant cooking versus home cooking); who shops for groceries; and who prepares the meals. Knowledge of the patient's financial status assists the nurse in advocating an affordable therapeutic regimen—for example, avoiding an expensive combination of drugs or expensive sustained-release medications when drugs that are as effective and less costly are available. Knowing if any risk factors for coronary artery disease exist will enable the nurse to help the patient modify behaviors that may be contributing to the progression of heart disease. Refer to Chapter 5 for a more complete description of the nursing history.

Risk Factors in Coronary Artery Disease

The presence of coronary artery disease is associated with one or more characteristic findings known as risk factors. Risk factors have been determined on the basis of systematic observations of relationships between certain characteristics and the subsequent development of coronary artery disease. Current research is finding physiological explanations for these relationships.

Effective patient teaching requires a knowledge base for recognizing the risk factors, for interpretating the data from studies that identify risk factors, and for making effective explanations about the significance of the risk factors and how they can be modified. However, there is not complete agreement about the importance or the effectiveness of modifying risk factors in patients with known coronary artery disease.

Risk factors for atherosclerosis tend to make an individual more prone to developing coronary heart disease. These risk factors are classified according to whether or not they can be modified by changing an element of life-style or a personal habit. Nonmodifiable risk factors include the following:

- Positive family history
- Increasing age
- Sex (males greater than females)

Modifiable risk factors include the following:

- Hyperlipidemia
- Elevated blood pressure
- Elevated blood sugar (diabetes mellitus)
- Obesity
- Physical inactivity
- Stress
- Use of oral contraceptives

Assessment of these risk factors is an important and necessary part of cardiovascular assessment. Detailed discussion of these risk factors is presented in Chapter 25.

Physical Assessment

Assessment of physical findings should confirm data obtained in the nursing history. Baseline information is obtained on admission. Until the examiner becomes skilled in physical assessment, the initial findings should be validated by an experienced clinician. For the acutely ill cardiac patient, physical examination is performed with routine vital signs (every 4 hours, or more frequently if indicated). Because nurses spend 24 hours a day with the patient, they are in the best position to identify any changes that may occur. It is to the patient's benefit to detect changes early, before serious complications develop. Any changes observed in the assessment are reported to the physician and noted in detail in the chart.

A cardiac physical assessment should include an evaluation of the following:

- Patient appearance
- The heart as a pump
- Filling volumes and pressures
- Cardiac output
- Compensatory mechanisms

Factors that reflect decreased contractility and efficiency of the heart as a pump are reduced pulse pressure, cardiac enlargement, and the presence of murmurs and gallop rhythms.

Filling volumes and pressures are estimated by the degree of jugular vein distention (JVD) and the presence or absence of congestion in the lungs, peripheral edema, and postural changes in blood pressure.

Cardiac output is reflected by heart rate, pulse pressure, peripheral vascular resistance, urine output, and central nervous system manifestations.

Examples of compensatory mechanisms that help maintain cardiac output are increased filling volumes and elevated heart rate.

The order of examination proceeds logically from head to toe, and with practice can be done in approximately 10 minutes: (1) general appearance, (2) blood pressure, (3) pulse, (4) hands, (5) head and neck, (6) heart, (7) lungs, (8) abdomen, and (9) feet and legs.

General Appearance

Observe the patient's level of distress. Level of consciousness should be noted and described. Appropriateness of thought content, reflecting the adequacy of cerebral perfusion, is particularly important to evaluate. Family members who are most familiar with the patient can be helpful in alerting the examiner to subtle behavioral changes. The nurse should also take note of the patient's anxiety level and should know how anxiety affects the cardiovascular system. The nurse attempts to put the anxious patient at ease.

Examination of Blood Pressure

Blood pressure occurs as a cyclic phenomenon and is measured in millimeters of mercury (mm Hg). The peak of the cycle is called the *systolic pressure;* the low point of the cycle is called the *diastolic pressure.* Blood pressure is usually expressed as the ratio of the systolic pressure over the diastolic pressure, with normal values measuring 120/80 mm Hg.

The difference between the systolic and the diastolic pressures is called the *pulse pressure.* Normally, this amounts to 40 mm Hg. An increase in blood pressure is called *hypertension;* a decrease is called *hypotension.* When only the systolic pressure is elevated (*systolic hypertension*), a widening of the pulse pressure results. This happens in atherosclerosis (hardening of the arteries) and in thyrotoxicosis. Elevation of the diastolic pressure is always associated with elevation of the systolic pressure, and the circumstance represents true hypertension. An increase in the diastolic pressure to 95 mm Hg gives rise to concern, particularly in younger patients; an increase in excess of 95 mm Hg in the diastolic pressure constitutes true hypertension and requires investigation and control.

The blood pressure is measured by the use of the sphygmomanometer and the stethoscope. The sphygmomanometer consists of an inflatable cuff and a pressure gauge that communicates with the hollow portion of the cuff. The device is calibrated in such a manner that the pressure read on the manometer is quite comparable to the pressure in millimeters of mercury that is being transmitted to the brachial artery. The cuff is wrapped tightly around the upper arm and is inflated by a bulb. Pressure on the cuff is increased until the radial pulse disappears. The disappearance of the radial pulse signifies that systolic blood pressure has been exceeded and the brachial artery is occluded. The cuff is then inflated 20 to 30 mm Hg above the point at which radial pulsation disappears. If one now slowly lowers the pressure within the cuff by deflating the bulb, there will come a point at which a pulse will again become discernible in the radial artery. This is the systolic blood pressure. At the same time, a sound is produced within the brachial artery just below the cuff and is audible with the stethoscope. This sound (*Korotkoff sound*) coincides with each pulse beat and will continue to emanate from the brachial artery until the pressure in the cuff has been reduced below diastolic pressure. At that point, the sound ceases. In actual practice, the sound more often becomes muffled (changes character) as diastolic pressure is reached and then disappears at 10 to 20 mm Hg below normal diastolic pressure. One is interested in the point at which the sound becomes muffled. If there is any doubt, the blood pressure may be recorded as a tripartite pressure (120/80/60), to imply that the sound became muffled at 80 mm Hg and disappeared at 60 mm Hg.

Accurate recording of the blood pressure depends upon attention to several critical details. The cuff is firmly wrapped around the arm, and the cuff bladder is centered over the brachial artery. The stethoscope is placed directly over the brachial artery, just below the crease of the elbow, the point at which the brachial artery emerges from the two heads of the biceps muscle. If the cuff is too large for the arm, as with a child, the magnitude of pressure will be underestimated; that is, the pressure obtained will be substantially below true pressure. If the arm is excessively large, as with many obese persons, the level of pressure will be overestimated; that is, the patient will appear to be hypertensive when the pressure is, in fact, normal (Fig. 24-6). Special cuffs are manufactured for obese persons and for children.

Blood pressure in hypertensive persons is usually measured while the patient is lying down, sitting, and then standing. It is measured in both the right and the left arms. Unless there is disease of the vasculature, a difference of no more than 5 mm Hg should be found.

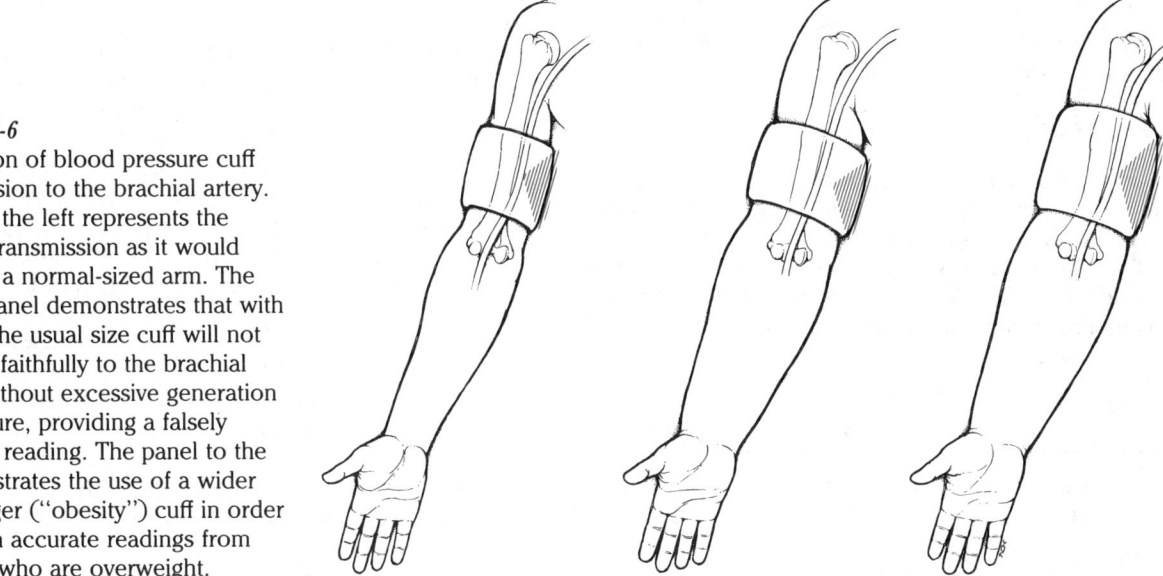

Figure 24-6
Illustration of blood pressure cuff transmission to the brachial artery. Panel to the left represents the normal transmission as it would occur in a normal-sized arm. The center panel demonstrates that with obesity the usual size cuff will not transmit faithfully to the brachial artery without excessive generation of pressure, providing a falsely elevated reading. The panel to the right illustrates the use of a wider and longer ("obesity") cuff in order to obtain accurate readings from persons who are overweight.

Blood pressure can also be measured in the lower extremities using an extra-wide cuff.

Remember the following points when measuring blood pressure:

- Cuff size must be appropriate for the patient.
- Patient's arm should be at heart level.
- Initial recordings are made on both arms, and subsequent measurements are taken on the arm with the highest pressure.
- Position of the patient and site of blood pressure measurement (*e.g.*, RA for right arm) are recorded.
- Presence of auscultatory gap (the difference between the true systolic pressure and the audible systolic pressure) is considered, especially in a patient with high blood pressure. To avoid obtaining falsely low systolic blood pressures, palpate prior to auscultating the systolic pressure.

Pulse Pressure. Pulse pressure (difference between systolic and diastolic pressures) reflects stroke volume, ejection velocity, and systemic vascular resistance. Use pulse pressure as a noninvasive indicator of the patient's ability to maintain cardiac output. If the pulse pressure in the cardiac patient falls below 30 mm Hg, further assessment of the patient's cardiovascular status may be indicated.

Postural Blood Pressure Changes. Postural (orthostatic) hypotension occurs when the blood pressure drops after an upright posture is assumed; it is usually accompanied by dizziness, light-headedness, or syncope. Although there are many causes of postural hypotension, the three most commonly seen in the cardiac patient are saline depletion, inadequate vasoconstrictor mechanisms, and autonomic insufficiency. Postural changes in blood pressure, along with appropriate history, can help the clinician differentiate between these causes. Remember the following points when assessing postural blood pressure changes:

- Position the patient supine and as flat as symptoms permit for 10 minutes prior to the initial blood pressure and heart rate measurement.

- Always check supine measurements before checking upright measurements.
- Always record both heart rate and blood pressure at each postural change (lying down, sitting, standing).
- Do not remove the blood pressure cuff between position changes, but do check to see that it is still correctly placed.
- Assess postural blood pressure changes with the patient sitting on the edge of the bed with feet dangling and, if necessary, with the patient standing at the side of the bed.
- Wait 1 to 3 minutes after each postural change before recording blood pressure and heart rate.
- Be alert for any signs or symptoms of patient distress and, if necessary, return the patient to bed prior to test completion.
- Record any signs or symptoms that accompany the postural change.

Normal postural responses are increased heart rate (to offset reduced stroke volume and maintain cardiac output), a slight to a 15-mm Hg drop in systolic pressure, and a slight drop to an increase of 5 to 10 mm Hg in diastolic pressure.

Saline depletion should be suspected (in the presence of a history of saline loss, *e.g.,* diuretic therapy) when, in response to sitting or standing, the heart rate increases and *either* the systolic pressure decreases by 15 mm Hg *or* the diastolic blood pressure drops by 10 mm Hg. It is difficult to differentiate saline depletion from inadequate vasoconstrictor mechanisms by postural changes in vital signs alone. With saline depletion, reflexes to maintain cardiac output (increased heart rate and peripheral vasoconstriction) function correctly but, because of lost extracellular fluid volume, the blood pressure falls. With inadequate vasoconstrictor mechanisms, the heart rate again responds appropriately but, because of diminished peripheral vasoconstriction, the blood pressure drops. The following is an example of a postural blood pressure recording showing either saline depletion or inadequate vasoconstrictor mechanisms:

	Blood Pressure	*Heart Rate*
Lying down	120/70	70
Sitting	100/55	90
Standing	98/52	94

In autonomic insufficiency, the heart rate is unable to increase to compensate for the gravitational effects of upright posture. Peripheral vasoconstriction may be absent or diminished. The presence of autonomic insufficiency does not rule out concurrent saline depletion. The following is an example of autonomic insufficiency as demonstrated by postural blood pressure changes:

	Blood Pressure	*Heart Rate*
Lying down	150/90	60
Sitting	100/60	60

Examination of the Pulse

In examining the pulse, one is interested not only in the obvious information to be determined from rate and rhythm, but in the configuration of the pulse wave and in the quality of the vessel itself.

The normal pulse *rate* varies from a low of 50 in healthy, athletic, young adults to rates well in excess of 100 following exercise or during times of excitement. Anxiety frequently elevates the pulse rate during the physical examination. If the rate is higher than expected, it is appropriate to reassess it near the end of the physical examination, at a time when the examiner has established better rapport with the patient.

Equally important in assessing the pulse is notation of the *rhythm*. Minor variations in the regularity of the pulse are normal. The pulse rate, particularly in young people, increases during inspiration and slows during expiration. This is called *sinus dysrhythmia*.

If the pulse rhythm is irregular, the pulse should be counted apically and radially (simultaneously, by two nurses) for a full minute, and any discrepancy between contractions heard and pulses felt should be noted. Disturbances of rhythm (dysrhythmias) often result in a "pulse deficit," a difference between the apical rate (heart rate heard at the apex of the heart) and the peripheral rate. Pulse deficits commonly occur with atrial fibrillation, atrial flutter, premature ventricular contractions, and varying degrees of heart block.

An understanding of the complexity of dysrhythmias that may be encountered during the examination requires a sophisticated knowledge of cardiac electrophysiology, knowledge usually possessed by the nurse who specializes in cardiovascular nursing.

The *quality*, or amplitude, of the pulse can be described as normal, diminished, or absent. Some authorities suggest a numerical classification based on a 0 to 4 scale:

> 0—absence of pulsation
> +1—marked impairment of pulsation
> +2—moderate impairment of pulsation
> +3—slight impairment of pulsation
> +4—normal pulsation

Numerical classification is quite subjective; thus, in written communication it is helpful to specify the scale range (*e.g.*, radial +4/+4).

The configuration, or contour, of the pulse frequently conveys important information. In stenosis of the aortic valve, the pulse pressure is narrow and the pulse appears to be feeble. When insufficiency of the aortic valve is present, the rise of the pulse wave is abrupt and its fall is precipitous, a "collapsing" pulse. The true configuration of the pulse is best appreciated by palpating over the carotid artery rather than the distal radial artery, since the dramatic characteristics of the pulse wave may be distorted or damped by transmission to smaller vessels.

The condition of the vessel wall is of vital concern, especially in older patients. The pulse rate is usually determined by placing the tips of the index and middle fingers over the radial artery. Once rate and rhythm have been determined, the quality of the vessel itself can be assessed. Does it appear to be thickened? Is it tortuous? In order to properly assess the vessel, one must do more than simply compress it. It is necessary to slide the fingers along the vessel and compare its feel with the feel of the normal vessels.

Arterial pulses are commonly palpated at points where the arteries are near the skin surface and easily compressible against bones or firm musculature. Pulses are detected over the temporal, carotid, brachial, radial, femoral, popliteal, dorsalis pedis, and posterior tibial arteries. For convenience, the radial artery is usually selected for determination of pulse.

Two or three fingertips compress the artery against the distal radius, and the rate, rhythm, quality, contour, and condition of the vessel wall are determined. Similarly, all arterial pulses are located and evaluated as a part of a thorough cardiovascular assessment. A reliable assessment of the pulses of the lower extremities depends on accurate identification of the artery location and careful technique (see Fig. 28-2). Firm finger pressure can easily obliterate the dorsalis pedis and posterior tibial pulses and confuse the examiner. Light palpation is essential. In approximately 10% of the population the dorsalis pedis arteries are not palpable. In such circumstances both are usually absent together, and the posterior tibial arteries alone provide adequate blood supply to the feet.

Hands

In the cardiac patient, the following are the most important findings to note:

- Peripheral cyanosis implies decreased flow rate of blood in the periphery, allowing more time for the hemoglobin molecule to become desaturated. This may occur normally with the peripheral vasoconstriction associated with a cold environment, or pathologically in conditions that reduce blood flow, for example, cardiogenic shock.
- Pallor can denote anemia or an increased systemic vascular resistance.
- Capillary refill time provides the basis for an estimate of the rate of peripheral blood flow. Normally, reperfusion occurs almost instantaneously. More sluggish reperfusion indicates a slower peripheral flow rate, for example, as in heart failure.
- Hand temperature and moistness are controlled by the autonomic nervous system. Normally, hands are warm

and dry. Under stress, they may be cool and moist. In cardiogenic shock, hands become cold and clammy due to stimulation of the sympathetic nervous system and resulting vasoconstriction.
- Edema decreases skin mobility.
- Dehydration and aging reduce skin turgor.
- Clubbing of the fingers and toes implies chronic hemoglobin desaturation, as in congenital heart disease.

Head and Neck

When examining the head of a cardiac patient, one needs to be concerned primarily with checking the lips and earlobes for cyanosis. In cyanosis, hemoglobin does not become fully saturated with oxygen and a bluish color occurs.

A gross estimate of right heart function can be made by observing the pulsations of the jugular veins of the neck. This enables estimation of central venous pressure, which reflects right atrial or right ventricular end-diastolic pressure (the pressure immediately preceding right ventricular contraction).

Jugular vein distention (JVD) is caused by increased filling volume and pressure on the right side of the heart. Measure jugular vein pressure (JVP) as follows:

- Begin with the patient supine, with the head of the table or bed elevated 15 to 30 degrees.
- The patient's head is turned slightly away from the side of the neck that is being examined.
- Identify the external jugular vein.
- Locate the pulsations of the internal jugular vein. (Distinguish these pulsations from those of the adjacent carotid artery.)
- Identify the highest point at which the internal jugular vein pulsations can be seen.
- Using a centimeter ruler, measure the vertical distance between this point and the sternal angle. (See Fig. 24-7.)
- Record the distance in centimeters and indicate the angle at which the patient was lying, *e.g.,* "The internal jugular vein pulse is 5 cm above the sternal angle, with the head elevated to 45°."

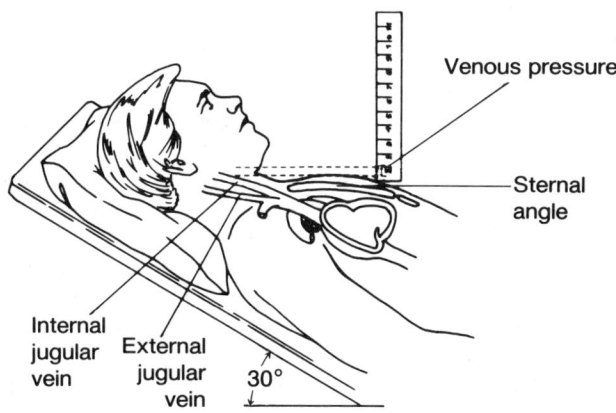

Figure 24-7
An assessment of jugular venous pressure. The highest point at which jugular vein pulsations can be seen is noted. The vertical distance between this point and the sternal angle is measured and recorded as centimeters "above or below" the sternal angle.

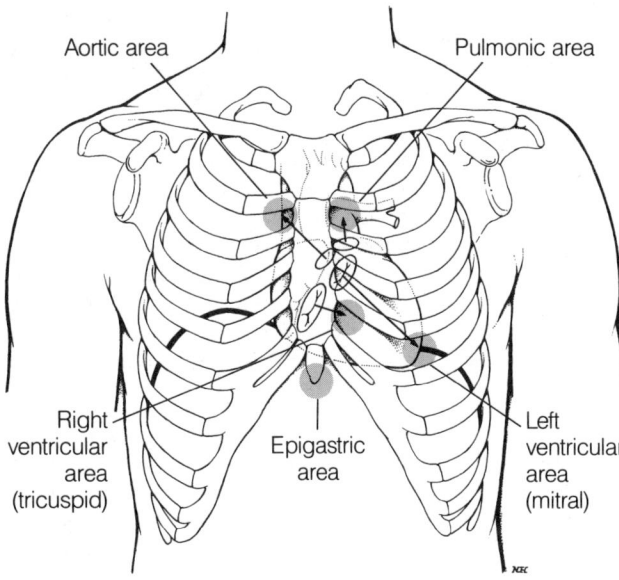

Figure 24-8
Topographical anatomy of the heart as it projects upon the thoracic wall.

- Measurements greater than 3 cm to 4 cm above the sternal angle are considered elevated.

When visualization of the internal jugular veins is difficult, observe the pulsations of the external jugular veins. These are more superficial and visible just above the clavicles adjacent to the sternomastoid muscles. They are frequently distended while the patient lies supine on the examining table or bed. As the patient's head is elevated, the distention of the veins will disappear. The veins are not normally apparent once the angle that the patient makes with the examining table exceeds 30 degrees.

Obvious distention of the veins with the patient's head elevated 45 to 90 degrees implies an abnormal increase in the volume of the venous system. This is associated with right-sided cardiac failure or, less commonly, with obstruction to flow in the superior vena cava.

Inspection and Palpation of the Heart

Inspection and palpation of the chest wall are concentrated in five areas (see Fig. 24-8):

1. *Aortic area*—second intercostal space to the right of the sternum
2. *Pulmonary area*—second intercostal space to the left of the sternum
3. *Right ventricular or tricuspid area*—fourth and fifth intercostal spaces to the left of the sternum
4. *Left ventricular or apical area*—fifth intercostal space to the left and right of the sternum
5. *Epigastric area*

For the examination, the patient is supine, with head slightly elevated. Oblique lighting is used to assist the examiner in identifying subtle pulsation. In a systematic fashion, each area of the precordium is inspected and then palpated. There is a normal impulse that is discrete and well localized directly over the apex of the heart; it may be observed in young persons and in older persons who are thin. This is called the *apical impulse* or *point of maximal impulse* (PMI) and is normally located in the left fifth intercostal space in the midclavicular line.

The apical impulse can often be palpated. It is normally felt as a light pulsation, 1 cm to 2 cm in diameter. It is felt at the onset of the first heart sound and lasts only half of systole. The palm of the hand is used initially to locate the apical impulse, and the finger pads are used to describe its size and quality. If the apical impulse is broad and forceful, it is often referred to as a *left ventricular heave or lift*. It is so named because it appears to "lift" the hand from the chest wall during palpation.

- *Abnormal point of maximal impulse (PMI)*. Left ventricular enlargement from left ventricular failure is evident if the PMI is below the 5th intercostal space or lateral to the midclavicular line. When palpated, the PMI should be felt in only one intercostal space. If palpated in two or more adjacent intercostal spaces, left ventricular enlargement can be diagnosed. If two distinctly separate areas with paradoxical movement are seen, a ventricular aneurysm should be suspected.

Murmurs, when they are exceptionally loud, may also be palpated and are felt by the palm of the hand as a "purring" sensation. This phenomenon is called a *thrill* and is always indicative of significant pathology within the heart. Thrills also may be palpated over vessels when there is significant substantial obstruction to blood flow, and will occur over the carotid arteries in the presence of narrowing (or stenosis) of the aortic valve.

Percussion of the Heart

In the normal patient, only the left border of the heart is located by percussion. It extends from the sternum to the midclavicular line in the third to fifth intercostal space. The right border lies under the right margin of the sternum, but the sternum is a sounding board and does not permit definition of the border. Enlargement of the heart to either the left or right can usually be noted. In many persons who have very thick chests, are obese, or have emphysema, the heart may lie sufficiently far beneath the thoracic surface so that not even its left border can be noted unless the heart is enlarged.

Unless the examiner detects a displaced apical impulse and suspects cardiac enlargement, percussion is omitted.

Auscultation of the Heart

Heart Sounds.   The normal heart sounds are produced primarily by closure of the heart valves. The first heart sound, S_1, coincides with closure of the AV valves and is a normal sound. The major component of this sound is the vibration

of the leaflets of the mitral and tricuspid valves as they close, although vibration of the myocardial wall may also contribute. S_1 is heard loudest at the apex of the heart. The second heart sound, S_2, also normal, occurs upon closure of the aortic and pulmonic valves. Although these two valves close almost simultaneously, the pulmonic valve usually lags slightly behind. Therefore, under certain circumstances, the two components of the second sound may be heard separately (split S_2). S_2 is heard loudest at the base of the heart.

The time between S_1 and S_2 corresponds to systole. This is normally shorter than the time between S_2 and S_1 (diastole). As the heart rate increases, diastole shortens (see Fig. 24-9). In normal physiology, the periods of systole and diastole are silent. Pathology of the ventricle, however, can give rise to transient sounds in systole and diastole that are called *gallops*, *snaps*, or *clicks*. Significant pathologic narrowing of the valve orifices at times when they should be open, or residual gapping of valves at times when they should be closed, gives rise to prolonged sounds that are called *murmurs*. Proper identification of normal and abnormal sounds over the precordium is a sophisticated and challenging process, but one with which the nurse can become familiar.

Auscultatory Valve Areas.   Events occurring at each of the four valves are uniquely reflected at specific locations on the chest wall (see Fig. 24-8). These locations do not correspond to the anatomical location of the valve within the chest. Rather, they are reflective of the patterns of radiation of heart sounds toward the chest wall. Sound in vessels through which blood is flowing is always reflected downstream. Events of the mitral valve are usually heard best in the fifth intercostal space at the midclavicular line. This is called the *mitral valve area*. Events occurring at the tricuspid valve are heard best in the fourth intercostal space just to the left of the sternum. This is called the *tricuspid valve area*. The *aortic valve area* is located in the second intercostal space to the right of the sternum, and the *pulmonic valve area* is located in the second intercostal space to the left of the sternum.

First Heart Sound.   The *first heart sound* (S_1) is created by the simultaneous closure of the mitral and tricuspid valves. Although heard over the entire precordium, it is heard best in the mitral area. It is increased in intensity when the valve leaflets are made rigid by calcium in rheumatic heart disease and in any circumstance in which ventricular contraction intervenes at a time when the valve is caught wide open. The latter circumstance will occur, for example, when a premature ventricular contraction interrupts the normal cardiac cycle. The first heart sound varies in intensity from beat to beat when atrial contraction is not synchronous with ventricular contraction. This is because the valve may be fully or partially closed on one beat and quite widely patent on the subsequent one as a function of irregular atrial activity. The first heart sound is easily identifiable and serves as the point of reference for the remainder of the cardiac cycle (see Fig. 24-4).

Second Heart Sound.   The *second heart sound* (S_2) is

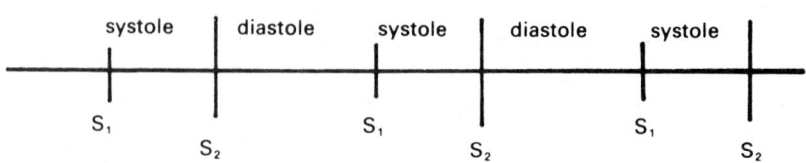

Figure 24-9
The normal heart sounds.

produced by the closure of the aortic and pulmonic valves. It is quite usual for these valves to close separately, the aortic valve first, followed by the pulmonic valve, and for the resultant sounds to be clearly distinguished as a "split" second sound. It is even more usual for this split to be accentuated on inspiration and to disappear on expiration as a function of respiratory influence on right ventricular ejection (augmenting it on inspiration, inhibiting it on expiration). The aortic component of the second sound is heard clearly in both the aortic and pulmonic areas, and is heard less clearly at the apex. The pulmonic component of the second sound, if present, may only be heard over the pulmonic area. Thus, one may hear a "single" second heart sound in the aortic area and a split second heart sound in the pulmonic area.

Gallop Sounds. Impedance to diastolic filling of the ventricle in certain disease states may give rise to transient vibrations in diastole that are much akin to, although usually softer than, the first and second heart sounds. Heart sounds then come in triplets and have the acoustical effect of a galloping horse; they are therefore called *gallops*. This may occur early in diastole, during the rapid-filling phase of the cardiac cycle, or at the time of atrial contraction. A gallop sound occurring during rapid ventricular filling is called a *third heart sound* (S_3) and represents a normal finding in children and young adults. Such a sound is heard in patients who have myocardial disease or in those who are in congestive heart failure and whose ventricles fail to eject all of their blood during systole.

Gallop sounds heard during atrial contraction are called *fourth heart sounds* (S_4). An S_4 is often heard when the ventricle is hypertrophied and therefore resistant to filling. Such a circumstance may be associated with coronary artery disease, hypertension, or aortic stenosis. On rare occasions all four heart sounds are heard within a single cardiac cycle, giving rise to what is called a *quadruple rhythm*.

Gallop sounds are very low-frequency sounds and may only be heard with the bell of the stethoscope placed very lightly against the chest. They are heard best at the apex, although occasionally, when emanating from the right ventricle, they may be heard to the left of the sternum.

Snaps and Clicks. Stenosis of the mitral valve owing to rheumatic heart disease gives rise to an unusual sound very early in diastole that is high-pitched and best heard along the left sternal border. The sound is caused by high pressure in the left atrium, abruptly displacing a rigid mitral valve. The sound is called an *opening snap*. It occurs too long after the second sound to be mistaken for a split second sound and too early in diastole to be mistaken for a gallop. It is almost always associated with the murmur of mitral stenosis and is specific for that disease.

In an analogous manner, stenosis of the aortic valve gives rise to a short, high-pitched sound immediately after the first heart sound that is called an *ejection click*. This is due to very high pressure within the ventricle, displacing a rigid and calcified aortic valve.

Murmurs. Murmurs are created by the turbulent flow of blood past a critically narrowed valve, by the regurgitant flow of blood through a valve that has failed to close properly, by the flow of blood through a congenital defect within the wall of the ventricle or between the aorta and the pulmonary artery, or by increased flow through a normal structure. Murmurs are characterized and consequently identified by several characteristics, including *timing* in the cardiac cycle, *location* on the chest wall, *intensity, pitch, quality,* and *pattern of radiation*.

The *timing* of the murmur in the cardiac cycle is vital. First, the observer determines whether the murmur is occurring in systole or in diastole. Does it begin simultaneously with the first heart sound, or is there some delay between the sound and the beginning of a systolic murmur? Does the murmur run up to (or through) the second heart sound, or is there again delay between the end of the murmur and the occurrence of the second heart sound? Are diastolic murmurs continuous, or do they die out in mid- or late diastole?

Location of the murmur is critical. The diastolic murmur of *mitral stenosis* is heard only at the apex (mitral area) and may indeed be confined to only a few centimeters of the chest wall. The murmurs of *aortic and pulmonic stenosis*, although usually widely heard, are nevertheless heard best over their respective valve areas. The murmur of *aortic insufficiency* is heard best along the left sternal border, between the third and fourth interspace. (The murmur of aortic insufficiency may not be heard at all in the aortic area. This is because the "forward" direction of blood flow for regurgitation at the aortic valve is in the reverse direction.)

The *intensity* of murmurs is conventionally graded from I through VI. It is sometimes difficult to hear a grade I murmur. A grade II cardiac murmur should be easily perceived. Murmurs of grades IV or louder are usually associated with thrills that may be palpated on the surface of the chest wall. A grade VI murmur can often be heard with the stethoscope off the chest. A murmur may vary in intensity from its inception to its conclusion. This is very characteristic of certain valvular disorders. The murmur of aortic stenosis, for example, begins sometime after the first heart sound, increases in intensity to midsystole, and then decreases in intensity, stopping prior to the second heart sound. The sound configuration is referred to as "diamond" in shape, and the murmur is referred to as an *ejection murmur* (see Fig. 24-10). The midsystolic increase in intensity is characteristic of murmurs that result from ejection through either the aortic or the pulmonic valve. The mur-

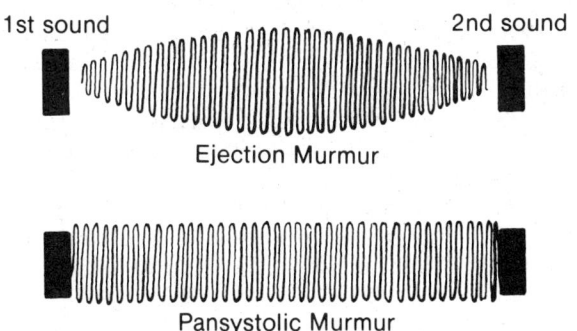

1st sound   2nd sound

Ejection Murmur

Pansystolic Murmur

Figure 24-10
Differentiation between ejection murmurs generated at the pulmonic and aortic valves and pansystolic murmurs generated at the mitral and tricuspid valves. Ejection murmurs begin after the first sound, peak in midsystole, and generally conclude before the second sound. Pansystolic murmurs are of equivalent intensity throughout systole, beginning with the first sound and ending with the second sound.

mur of mitral insufficiency and the murmur of a ventricular septal defect are, on the other hand, constant in intensity throughout systole. Moreover, they begin simultaneously with the first heart sound and end simultaneously with the second heart sound. They are referred to as *holosystolic* or *pansystolic murmurs.*

In the patient with coronary artery disease, the murmur most frequently heard is the holosystolic murmur (cardiac murmur that extends through systole) of mitral regurgitation. Backflow of blood from the left ventricle through the mitral valve occurs if the papillary muscles become ischemic and are no longer able to contract properly. This murmur is loudest at the apex, and may be heard with the diaphragm of the stethoscope.

The next important quality of a murmur is its *pitch.* The murmur of mitral stenosis is a low, rumbling sound, often heard only with the bell placed lightly on the chest wall. By contrast, the murmur of aortic insufficiency is a very high-pitched murmur, occasionally "whistling" in character, heard best with the diaphragm. Other murmurs, especially the murmur of aortic stenosis, contain the full spectrum of sound frequency, a characteristic that makes the murmur appear to be very harsh in quality.

The last feature of concern is *radiation* of the murmur. The murmur of mitral insufficiency, best heard at the apex (mitral area), radiates into the axilla. This, of course, reflects the "downstream" nature of its transmission. The murmur of aortic stenosis will, for analogous reasons, radiate into the carotid arteries in the neck. The murmur of pulmonic stenosis, which may sound identical to that of aortic stenosis, will not radiate into the neck; rather, it may radiate into the left shoulder or into the back.

Friction Rub. In pericarditis, a harsh grating sound that can be heard in both systole and diastole is called a *friction rub.* It is caused by the abrasion of the pericardial surfaces during the cardiac cycle. This may be confused with a murmur; care should be taken to identify the sound when appropriate and to distinguish it from murmurs that may be heard in both systole and diastole. A pericardial friction rub can be heard best using the diaphragm of the stethoscope, with the patient sitting up and leaning forward.

Procedure for Auscultation. For auscultation, the patient remains supine and the examining room is as quiet as possible. The right-handed examiner is positioned at the right side of the patient, the left-handed examiner at the left side. Again, a systematic examination is the cornerstone of a thorough assessment.

Using the diaphragm of the stethoscope, the examiner starts at the apical area and progresses upward along the left sternal border to the pulmonic and aortic areas. If desired,

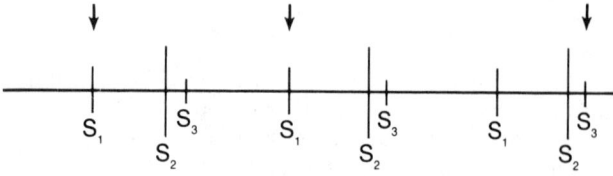

S_3 gallop immediately following the S_2

Figure 24-11
An S_3 gallop is heard immediately following the S_2.

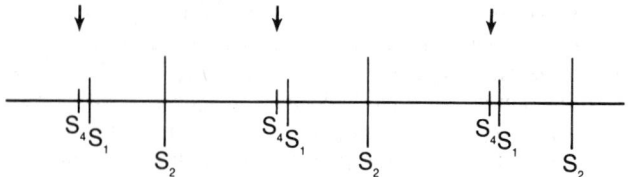

S_4 gallop immediately preceding the S_1

Figure 24-12
An S_4 gallop is heard immediately preceding the S_1.

the examiner may choose to begin the examination at the aortic and pulmonic areas and progress downward to the apex of the heart. Initially, S_1 is identified and evaluated with respect to its intensity and splitting. It is normally loudest in the apical area and may be split in the tricuspid area. Next, S_2 is identified and its intensity noted. It is loudest in the aortic and pulmonic areas. A physiologic splitting of S_2 is usually audible in the pulmonic area and is accentuated by inspiration. This splitting sound may be perceived as two distinct but close sounds or as one sound that appears flattened or slightly prolonged.

After concentrating on S_1 and S_2, (see Fig. 24-9) the examiner listens for extra sounds in systole and then in diastole. Sometimes it is useful to ask oneself the following questions: Do I hear snapping or clicking sounds? Do I hear any high-pitched blowing sounds? Is this sound in systole, or diastole, or both? Diastolic filling sounds (S_3 or S_4 gallops) (see Figs. 24-11 and 24-12) are low-frequency sounds and are best auscultated with the bell of the stethoscope placed lightly and completely against the chest. The examiner again proceeds "inch by inch" along the precordium, listening carefully for these sounds. An S_3 sound and mitral murmurs are heard best with the patient lying on the left side and the stethoscope in the apical area.

If an abnormality is heard, the entire chest surface is reexamined to determine the exact location of the sound and its radiation. Murmurs are described fully by their timing, location, intensity, pitch, quality, and radiation. Once the characteristics of each phase of the cycle have been determined, the relationship of one to another, and the synthesis of events within the cardiac cycle, may be summarized.

Interpretation of Cardiac Sounds

The interpretation of cardiac sounds requires intimate knowledge of cardiac physiology and the pathophysiology of cardiac diseases. However, there are different levels of performance at which the nurse may be expected to function. The first level of function is simply the recognition that what one is hearing is not normal. There may be a third heart sound; there may be a murmur in systole or diastole; there may be a pericardial friction rub over the midsternum; the second heart sound may be widely split. These findings are to be brought to the attention of a physician and acted upon accordingly. This level of function is useful in screening. It is the kind of activity involved in doing school physicals on normal children or in performing routine physical examinations of patients.

The second level of function employs pattern recognition. The nurse correctly observes the findings and is capable of recognizing the constellation of sounds and the diagnostic significance of common ones. This is the role in which the nurse practitioner has recently been placed.

At its most sophisticated level, cardiac diagnosis can be interpretive. Highly skilled nurses can differentiate among dysrhythmias and respond accordingly. They can determine the significance of the appearance and disappearance of gallops during treatment of patients who have had myocardial infarctions or who are in heart failure. This is the role in which the coronary care nurse and the cardiovascular nurse specialist have been cast. They function with a team of professionals for whom the fine details of cardiovascular diagnosis have become highly tuned, shared skills.

Lungs

Respiratory assessment is described in Chapter 21. Findings frequently exhibited by cardiac patients include the following:

- *Tachypnea*. Rapid, shallow breathing may be noted in patients who have heart failure or pain, or who are extremely anxious.
- *Cheyne-Stokes respirations*. Patients in severe left ventricular failure may exhibit Cheyne-Stokes breathing. Of particular importance is the duration of the apneic period.
- *Hemoptysis*. Pink, frothy sputum is indicative of acute pulmonary edema.
- *Cough*. A dry, hacking cough from irritation of small airways is common in patients with pulmonary congestion from heart failure.
- *Crackles*. Heart failure, or atelectasis associated with bed rest, splinting from ischemic pain, or the effects of pain medication and sedatives, often results in the development of crackles. Typically, crackles are first noted at the bases (because of gravity's effect on fluid accumulation and decreased ventilation of basilar tissue) but may progress to all portions of the lung fields.
- *Wheezes*. Compression of the small airways by interstitial pulmonary edema may cause wheezing. Beta-blocking agents, such as propranolol, may precipitate airway narrowing, especially in patients with underlying pulmonary disease.

Abdomen

For the cardiac patient, two components of the abdominal examination are frequently performed.

- *Determination of liver size*. Liver engorgement occurs because of decreased venous return secondary to right ventricular failure. The liver will be enlarged, firm, nontender, and smooth. Hepatojugular reflux may be demonstrated by pressing firmly over the liver for 30 to 60 seconds and noting a 1-cm rise in JVD.
- *Assessment of bladder distention*. Urine output is an important indicator of cardiac output. In a patient who has not voided or who is unable to void, always assess for bladder distention prior to initiating other measures.

Feet and Legs

Many patients with heart disease have associated peripheral vascular disease, or peripheral edema secondary to right ventricular failure. Therefore, adequacy of peripheral arterial circulation and venous return should be assessed in all cardiac patients. In addition, thrombophlebitis is a complication associated with bed rest and requires careful monitoring. Refer to Chapter 28 for a complete description of these techniques.

Summary

Physical examination of the cardiovascular system is complex and may be time-consuming. What constitutes a competent and sufficiently thorough examination in the absence of cardiac symptoms? The blood pressure and the pulses should certainly be assessed. Blood pressure may indeed be the most important observation that is made in the examination of any patient, since hypertension is exceedingly common in the population and amenable to adequate control. Inspection of the anterior thorax is easily accomplished, and an apical impulse, if present, should be noted. Percussion of the cardiac border in normal persons is not usually rewarding and only yields valuable information when cardiac hypertrophy is anticipated. The heart is auscultated with care in the four principal areas. Any variation from normal mandates further evaluation by a physician.

Diagnostic Tests and Procedures

Diagnostic tests and procedures are used to confirm data obtained by interview and examination. Some tests are easy to interpret, while others must be interpreted by expert clinicians. All require that basic explanations be given to patients. Some necessitate special orders prior to the test and special monitoring by the nurse following the procedure.

Laboratory Tests

Laboratory tests may be requested for a variety of reasons: to assist in the diagnosis of acute myocardial infarction (angina pectoris cannot be confirmed by either blood or urine studies); to measure abnormalities in blood chemistries that could affect the prognosis of a cardiac patient; to assess the degree of the inflammatory process; to screen for risk factors associated with the presence of atherosclerotic coronary artery disease; to determine baseline values prior to therapeutic intervention; to assess drug levels; and to screen generally for any abnormalities. Laboratory studies relating specifically to the cardiac patient are summarized. Because many different methods of measurement are used, refer to individual health care agencies for their normal laboratory values.

Cardiac Enzymes and Isoenzymes

Acute myocardial infarction can be confirmed by the presence of abnormally high levels of enzymes or isoenzymes in the serum. Enzymes are released from cells when the cells are injured and their walls break down and die. Most of these enzymes are nonspecific in relation to the particular organ that has been damaged. Certain isoenzymes, however, come only from myocardial cells and are released when the cells are damaged by hypoxia resulting from ischemia or infarction. The isoenzymes leak into the interstitial spaces of the myocardium and are carried into the general circulation by the lymph system and the coronary circulation. Because different enzymes are released into the blood at varying periods following myocardial infarction, it is crucial to time the drawing of blood in relation to the time of onset of chest discomfort. If blood is drawn too early, enzymes may not yet be elevated; if it is drawn too late, enzymes may already have returned to baseline. (See Table 25-2 for the time course of cardiac enzymes.) Enzymes used in the diagnosis of acute myocardial infarction are creatine kinase (CK) and its isoenzyme CK-MB, and lactic dehydrogenase (LDH) and its isoenzymes.

The enzymes are evaluated as a part of the patient's total diagnostic profile, including history, symptoms, and ECG.

Blood Chemistries

Serum Electrolytes. Serum electrolytes can affect the prognosis of a patient with acute myocardial infarction or any cardiac condition. Serum sodium reflects relative water balance. Calcium is necessary for blood coagulability and neuromuscular activity. Hypocalcemia and hypercalcemia can cause ECG changes and dysrhythmias.

Serum potassium is an indicator of renal function and may be decreased by diuretic agents that are often used to treat congestive heart failure. A decrease in potassium causes cardiac irritability and predisposes the patient receiving a digitalis preparation to digitalis toxicity and to the development of dysrhythmias. Elevated serum potassium has a myocardial depressant effect and a ventricular irritability effect. Hypokalemia and hyperkalemia can each lead to ventricular fibrillation or cardiac standstill.

Blood Urea Nitrogen. Blood urea nitrogen (BUN) is an end product of protein metabolism and is excreted by the kidneys. In the cardiac patient, elevated BUN could reflect reduced renal perfusion (due to decreased cardiac output) or saline depletion (due to diuretic therapy).

Glucose. Serum glucose is important to measure because many cardiac patients also have diabetes mellitus. Serum glucose may be mildly elevated in stressful situations when mobilization of endogenous epinephrine results in conversion of liver glycogen to glucose.

Blood Lipids and Lipoproteins. Cholesterol and triglyceride levels may be measured to evaluate a person's risk of developing atherosclerotic disease. The patient should be fasting prior to the test. Stress may alter the results.

Measurement of lipoproteins is also useful in evaluating risk, especially if there is a positive family history of heart disease or to diagnose a specific lipoprotein abnormality. Decreased levels of high-density lipoprotein (HDL) and elevated levels of low-density lipoprotein (LDL) increase the risk of development of atherosclerotic coronary artery disease.

Chest X-Ray and Fluoroscopy

A chest x-ray is usually requested to determine the size, contour, and position of the heart. It reveals cardiac and pericardial calcifications and demonstrates physiologic alterations in the pulmonary circulation. It does not aid in the diagnosis of acute myocardial infarction, but can confirm the presence of some complications, *e.g.*, congestive heart failure. Correct placement of heart catheters, such as pacemakers and pulmonary artery catheters, is also confirmed by chest x-ray.

Fluoroscopy provides visual observation of the heart on a luminescent x-ray screen. It shows heart and vascular pulsations and is useful in the assessment of unusual cardiac contours. Fluoroscopy is a useful tool for the placement and positioning of intravenous pacemaking electrodes and for guiding the catheter in cardiac catheterization.

Electrocardiography

The *electrocardiogram (ECG)* is a visual representation of the electrical activity of the heart as reflected by changes in electrical potential at the skin surface. The ECG is recorded as a tracing on a strip of paper or appears on the screen of an oscilloscope. In order to facilitate the interpretation of the ECG, data about the patient's age, sex, blood pressure, height, weight, symptoms, and medications (especially digitalis and antidysrhythmic drugs) should be noted on the ECG requisition. Electrocardiography is particularly useful in the evaluation of conditions that interfere with normal heart functions, such as disturbances of rate or rhythm, disorders of conduction, enlargement of heart chambers, presence of a myocardial infarction, and electrolyte imbalances.

The standard ECG consists of 12 leads. Information regarding the electrical activity of the heart is obtained by placing electrodes on the skin surface at standardized anatomical positions. The various electrode positions that may be monitored are referred to as leads. For example, lead 1 measures the electrical activity between the left arm and the right arm. For a complete 12-lead ECG, the heart is viewed from each of 12 different anatomical positions.

Procedure for Obtaining an Electrocardiogram

To obtain an ECG, electrodes are placed on the patient as shown in Figure 24-13. With the electrodes in these positions, the first six leads can be obtained. To ensure good contact between skin and electrode, the electrodes are placed on a flat surface just above the wrists and ankles, and electrode paste or an alcohol sponge is placed under each electrode. The extremity straps are adjusted firmly to hold the electrodes in place. These straps should not pinch the patient's skin or be so tight as to decrease circulation distal to the strap. The lead selected on the machine is then turned on to record each of the six leads. Next, the six V leads are obtained by moving the chest leads in the six precordial positions. A lead selector switch is turned to "V" to record each of these leads. The arm and leg electrodes must be attached to the patient in order to obtain the V leads. There are some ECG machines that record three or six leads simultaneously.

Each ECG should include the following identifying information:

1. Patient name and identification number
2. Location, date, and time of the recording
3. Patient age, sex, and cardiac medications
4. Race, body build (weight and height measurements), blood pressure, tentative clinical diagnosis, clinical status, and noncardiac medications such as phenothiazines
5. Any unusual position of the patient during the record-

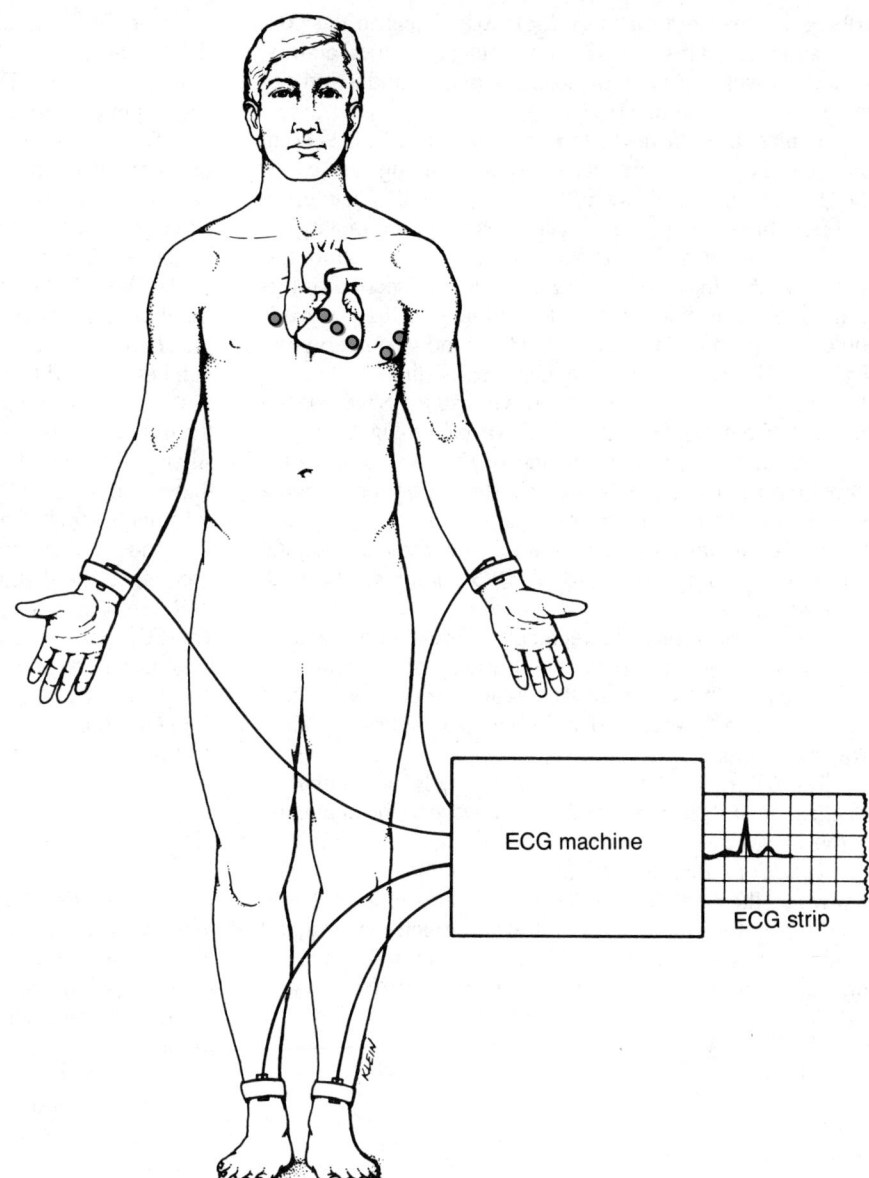

Figure 24-13
Twelve-lead ECG-electrode
placement.

ing, or the presence of thoracic deformities, amputation, respiratory distress, or muscle tremor

Electrocardiographic Variations

In addition to the standard 12-lead ECG, the ECG can be used in other ways. One lead of the ECG can be continuously monitored on an oscilloscope (a fluorescent screen). The waveform from this lead can be written out to provide a permanent record. Continuous ECG monitoring is especially useful in the cardiac care unit to detect dysrhythmias.

One lead of the ECG can be monitored by a small tape recorder (Holter Recorder) and recorded on a continuous (1–24 hours) magnetic tape recording. The patient can then be monitored day or night to detect dysrhythmias or evidence of myocardial ischemia during activities of daily living. The tape recorder weighs approximately 2 pounds and can be carried over the shoulder. The patient keeps a diary of activity,

noting the time of any symptoms, experiences, or unusual activities performed. The tape recording is then examined (using a specialized instrument called a scanner), analyzed, and interpreted. Evidence obtained in this way is helpful in diagnosing dysrhythmias and myocardial ischemia and in evaluating therapy such as antidysrhythmic and antianginal drugs or pacemaker function.

The ECG can also be transmitted by telemetry (telephone lines), thus freeing the patient from a cable connected to the oscilloscope. The ECG signal can then be monitored miles away.

Analysis of the ECG

When analyzed accurately, the ECG offers important information about the electrical activity of the myocardium. ECG waveforms are printed on graph paper. Time or rate is measured on the horizontal axis of the graph, and amplitude or voltage is measured on the vertical axis. Because the conduction system of the heart is responsible for electrical activity, the ECG waveforms are representative of the conduction system's function (see p. 514).

Waves, Complexes, and Intervals.   The ECG is composed of several components or waves, including the P wave, the QRS complex, the T wave, the ST segment, the PR interval, and possibly a U wave (usually indicates an abnormality).

The *P wave* represents atrial muscle depolarization. It is normally 2.5 mm or less in height and is 0.11 second or less in duration. The first negative deflection after the P wave is the Q wave, which is less than 0.03 second in duration and less than 25% of the R wave amplitude; the first positive deflection after the P wave is the R wave; and the S wave is the first negative deflection after the R wave (see Fig. 24-14).

The *QRS complex* (beginning of Q wave to end of S wave) represents ventricular muscle depolarization. When a wave is less than 5 mm vertically, small letters (q, r, s) are used; when a wave is greater than 5 mm vertically, capital letters (Q, R, S) are used. Not all QRS complexes have all three waveforms.

The *T wave* represents ventricular muscle repolarization. It follows the QRS complex and is usually of the same deflection as the QRS complex. If a U wave is seen, it will follow the T wave. The presence of a U wave may indicate an electrolyte abnormality.

The *ST segment*, which represents early ventricular repolarization, lasts from the end of the S wave to the beginning of the T wave.

The *PR interval* is measured from the beginning of the P wave to the beginning of the R wave and represents the time required for the impulse to travel through the atria and conduction system to the Purkinje fibers. In adults, the PR interval normally ranges from 0.12 second to 0.20 second in duration.

The QRS complex is measured from the beginning of the Q wave, or the R wave if no Q wave is present, to the end of the S wave. The QRS complex is normally 0.04 to 0.10 second in duration.

The *QT interval*, which represents electrical systole, is measured from the beginning of the Q wave, or R wave if no Q wave is present, to the end of the T wave. The QT interval varies with heart rate, is usually less than half the RR interval (measured from the beginning of one R wave to the beginning of the next R wave), and is usually 0.32 to 0.40 second in duration if the heart rate is 65 to 95.

Determination of Heart Rate From ECG.   Heart rate can be obtained from the ECG strip by several methods. The first, and most accurate, if the rhythm is regular, is to count the number of 0.04-second intervals (0.04 second equals one small box) between two R waves, and then divide 1500 by that number. (There are 1500 0.04-second interval boxes in a 1-minute strip) See Fig. 24-15, *A*.

The second method for computing heart rate, especially used when the rhythm is irregular, is to count the number of R–R intervals in 6 seconds and multiply that number by 10. The ECG paper is usually marked at 3-second intervals (15 large boxes, horizontally) by a vertical line at the top of the paper (see Fig. 24-15, *B*). The R–R intervals are counted rather than QRS complexes, because a computed heart rate based on the latter might be inaccurately high.

Abnormal Findings

Myocardial Ischemia and Injury.   Myocardial ischemia causes the T wave to be larger and inverted owing to altered late repolarization. Possibly, the ischemic region remains depolarized, whereas adjacent areas have returned to the resting state. The change is seen in the leads closest to the involved surface of the heart. Ischemia also causes ST segment changes. If there is epicardial myocardial injury, the injured cells depolarize normally but repolarize more rapidly than do normal cells; thus, the ST segment is elevated. If the myocardial injury is on the endocardial surface, then the ST segment is depressed (1 mm or more) in the leads where the positive electrode faces the area of injury. With injury, the ST segment depression is horizontal or slopes downward and is 0.08 second in duration.

Myocardial Infarction.   Myocardial infarction usually causes abnormal Q waves within 1 to 3 days, because of both the absence of depolarization current from necrotic tissue and opposing currents from other parts of the heart. An abnormal Q wave is 0.04 second or longer in duration and is, in depth, 25% of the R wave (provided the R wave itself exceeds 5 mm). Old transmural MI is usually indicated by significant Q waves without ST segment and T wave changes or by reduced voltage of the R wave. In some patients, Q waves disappear. With a transmural MI (involving all three layers of the heart), injury and ischemic changes are also present (see Fig. 24-16). The ST segment elevation lasts a few days to 2 weeks. The T wave becomes large and symmetric for 24 hours, and then inverts within 1 to 3 days for 1 to 2 weeks. During recovery from an MI, the ST segment often is first to return to normal (1–6 weeks), followed by the T wave (weeks to months). Q wave alterations are usually permanent.

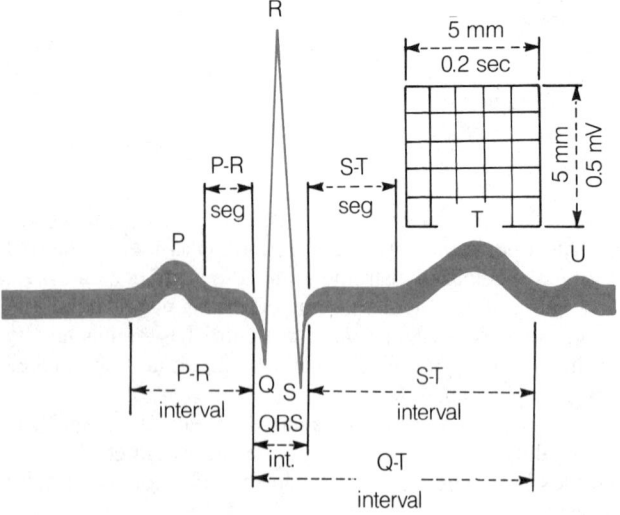

Figure 24-14
Commonly measured complex components. The PR interval is measured from the beginning of the P wave to the beginning of the QRS; the QRS is measured from the beginning of the Q wave to the end of the S wave; the QT interval is measured from the beginning of the Q wave to the end of the T wave.

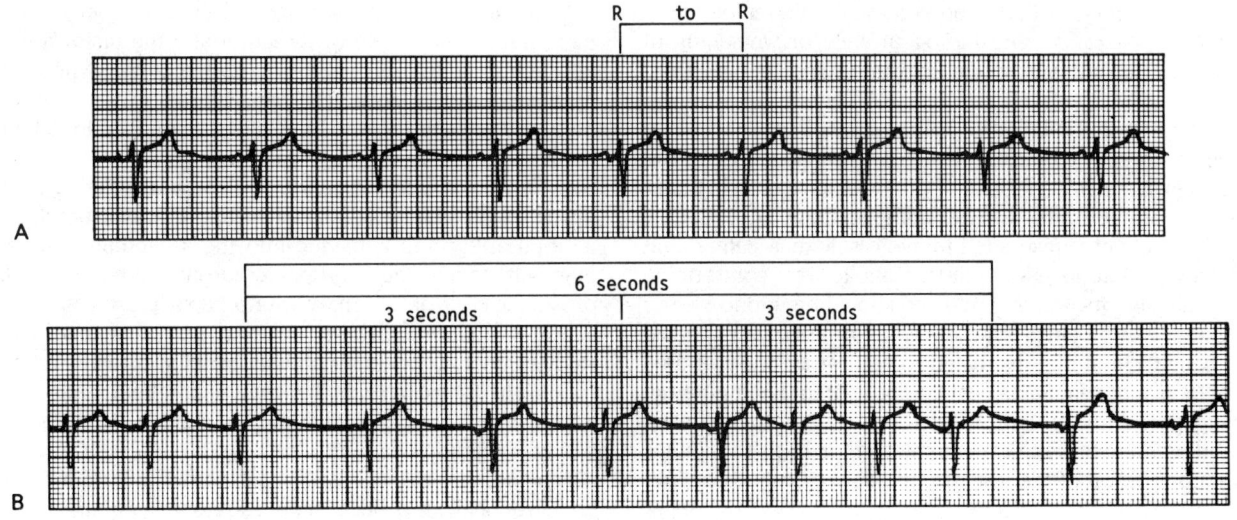

Figure 24-15
(*A*) Heart rate determination for a regular rhythm. There are approximately 25 little boxes between two R waves. 1500 divided by this number equals 60. The heart rate is 60. There are five large boxes between R waves, thus the rate is approximately 60.
(*B*) Heart rate determination if the rhythm is irregular. There are approximately seven RR intervals in 6 seconds. Seven times 10 equals 70. The heart rate is 70. (Underhill SL et al. Cardiac Nursing, p 201, Philadelphia, JB Lippincott, 1982.)

Exercise Stress Testing

Exercise stress testing is a noninvasive means of assessing certain aspects of cardiac function. By evaluating cardiac action during physical stress, the heart's response to an increased demand for oxygen can be determined. The test is used for the following purposes: to assist in diagnosing the cause of chest pain, to screen for ischemic heart disease, to determine the functional capacity of the heart after an MI or after surgery, to assess the effectiveness of antianginal or antidysrhythmia drug therapy, to identify dysrhythmias that occur during physical exercise, and to aid in the development of a physical fitness program.

Exercise stress testing may be done by having the patient walk on a treadmill, pedal a stationary bicycle, or climb a set of stairs. The patient is exercised by increasing walking speed and the incline of the treadmill or by increasing the load against which the bicycle is pedaled. ECG electrodes are applied to the patient, and tracings are made before, during,

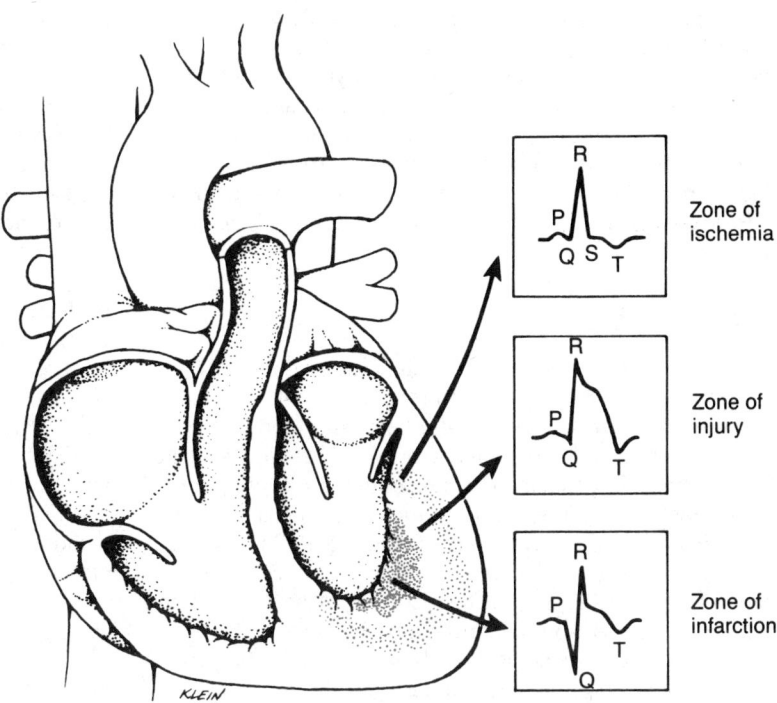

Figure 24-16
Effects of ischemia, injury, and infarction on ECG recording. Ischemia causes inversion of T wave because of altered repolarization. Cardiac muscle injury causes elevation of the ST segment. Infarction causes Q or Q–S waves because of the absence of depolarization current from the dead tissue and opposing currents from other parts of the heart.

and after exercise testing. Blood pressure, skin temperature, physical appearance, and the occurrence or worsening of chest pain are monitored closely during and following the test.

The test is continued until the patient's predetermined target heart rate is reached, but it is terminated early if the patient experiences chest pain, extreme fatigue, drop in blood pressure or pulse rate, or other complications.

The patient is instructed to avoid smoking, eating, and drinking for 4 hours prior to the test and to wear comfortable shoes suitable for walking. Women should be told to wear a brassiere that provides adequate support. Following the test the patient should be instructed to rest for a period of time and to avoid stimulants, eating, or extreme temperature changes (*i.e.*, hot or cold showers, going out into the cold). Blood pressure and ECG are monitored for 10 to 15 minutes after completion of the test, or until they return to baseline.

Vectorcardiography

Vectorcardiography, which is similar to electrocardiography, presents a three-dimensional view of the electrical forces of the heart: horizontal or transverse, frontal, and left sagittal or lateral planes. This diagnostic modality amplifies understanding of the ECG and gives more accurate diagnostic information in certain areas of cardiac diagnosis, *e.g.*, ventricular hypertrophy, conduction disturbances, and myocardial infarction. The patient should be assured that the test is similar to an ECG and that it is safe and painless.

Cardiac Catheterization

Cardiac catheterization is an invasive diagnostic procedure in which one or more catheters are introduced into the heart and selected blood vessels in order to measure pressures in the various heart chambers and to determine oxygen saturation of the blood by sampling specimens. By far the most common use of cardiac catheterization is to assess the patient's need and readiness for coronary bypass surgery (see Chap. 27). During cardiac catheterization the patient is monitored electrocardiographically by means of an oscilloscope. Because the introduction of the catheter into the heart can induce potentially fatal dysrhythmias, resuscitative equipment should be readily available when the procedure is being performed.

Angiography

Cardiac catheterization is usually done in tandem with angiography, a technique of injecting a contrast medium into the vascular system to outline the heart and blood vessels. When a particular heart chamber or blood vessel is singled out for study, the procedure becomes *selective angiography*. Angiography makes use of *cineangiograms*, a series of rapidly changing films or movies on an intensified fluoroscopic screen that records the passage of the contrast medium through the vascular site(s). The recording of the information allows for comparison of information over time.

Four of the more common sites for selective angiography are the aorta, the coronary arteries, and the right and left hearts.

Aortography. An aortogram is a form of angiography that outlines the lumen of the aorta and the major arteries arising from it. In *thoracic aortography* a contrast medium is used to study the aortic arch and its major branches. The translumbar or retrograde brachial or femoral approach may be used.

Coronary Arteriography. In coronary arteriography a radiopaque catheter is introduced into the right brachial or femoral artery and is passed into the ascending aorta and manipulated into the appropriate coronary artery under fluoroscopic control. Coronary arteriography is used as an evaluation tool before coronary artery surgery. It is also used to study suspected congenital anomalies of the coronary arteries.

Right-Heart Catheterization. Right-heart catheterization involves passing a radiopaque catheter from an antecubital or femoral vein into the right atrium, right ventricle, and pulmonary vasculature. This is carried out under direct visualization with a fluoroscope. Pressures within the right atrium are measured and recorded, and blood samples are removed for measurement of the hematocrit and oxygen saturation. The catheter is then passed through the tricuspid valve, and similar tests are performed on the blood within the right ventricle. Finally, the catheter is introduced into the pulmonary artery (through the pulmonic valve) and as far as possible beyond that point, where "capillary" samples are obtained and "capillary" pressures (also known as wedge pressures) are recorded. Then the catheter is withdrawn.

Right-heart catheterization is considered a relatively safe procedure. Complications, when they do occur, include cardiac dysrhythmias, venous spasm, infection of the cutdown site, cardiac perforation, and, rarely, cardiac arrest.

Left-Heart Catheterization. Left-heart catheterization is usually done by retrograde catheterization of the left ventricle or by transseptal catheterization of the left atrium. In the retrograde technique, the catheter is inserted under direct vision into the right brachial artery (arteriotomy) and advanced under fluoroscopic control down into the ascending aorta and into the left ventricle; or the catheter may be introduced percutaneously by puncture of the femoral artery.

In the transseptal approach, the catheter is passed from the right femoral vein (percutaneously or by saphenous vein cutdown) into the right atrium. A long needle is passed up through the catheter and is used to puncture the septum separating the right and left atria. The needle is withdrawn and the catheter is advanced under fluoroscopic control into the left ventricle. In both of these techniques the patient is monitored by electrocardiogram.

Left-heart catheterization is most often performed to evaluate the function of the left ventricular muscle and the mitral and aortic valves or the patency of the coronary arteries. It is used to evaluate patients before and after cardiac surgery. Usually, the right side of the heart is catheterized before the left side is done. Complications include dysrhythmias, myocardial infarction, perforation of the heart or great vessels, and systemic embolization.

Following the catheterization, the catheter is slowly withdrawn, the artery is repaired, and the cutdown site is closed and bandaged.

Nursing Interventions

Precatheterization nursing responsibilities include the following:

- Prepare the patient to fast prior to the procedure.
- Prepare the patient for the expected duration of the procedure; indicate that it will involve lying on a hard table for about 2 hours.
- Prepare the patient to experience certain sensations during the catheterization. Knowing what to expect can help the patient cope with the experience.

   An occasional thudding sensation (palpitation) may be felt in the chest because of extra systoles that almost always occur, particularly when the catheter tip touches the myocardium.

   When contrast medium is injected into the right heart (during angiography), there may be a strong desire to cough.

   The injection of contrast medium into either side of the heart may produce a feeling of heat, particularly in the head, which leaves in a minute or less.

- Encourage the patient to express fears and anxieties. Provide teaching and reassurance to reduce apprehension.

Postcatheterization nursing interventions include the following:

- Watch the puncture (or cutdown) sites for hematoma formation, and check the peripheral pulses in the affected extremity (dorsalis pedis and posterior tibial pulses in the lower extremity, radial pulse in the upper extremity) every 15 minutes for 1 to 2 hours, and then every 1 to 2 hours until stable.
- Evaluate extremity temperature and color and any patient complaints of pain, numbness, or tingling sensations in the affected extremity to determine signs of arterial insufficiency. Report changes promptly.
- Watch for dysrhythmias by observing the cardiac monitor or by listening to the apical heart rate and evaluating the pulse for rhythm changes.
- If protocol requires, see that the patient remains in bed with little movement of the involved extremity until the following morning.
- Report any complaint of chest discomfort immediately.
- Discomfort at the site is not unexpected. Administer pain medication as prescribed.

Echocardiography

Echocardiography is a noninvasive ultrasound test used to examine the size, shape, and motion of cardiac structures.

High-frequency sound waves are sent into the heart through the chest wall and are recorded as they return. The ultrasound is generated by a hand-held transducer (a device that converts one form of energy to another form of energy) applied to the front of the chest. The transducer picks up the echoes, converts them to electrical impulses, and transmits them to the echocardiography machine for display on an oscilloscope and for recording on a videotape. This is the same sonar principle by which submarines detect ships. An ECG is recorded simultaneously to time events within the cardiac cycle. Echocardiography is a safe method that gives information similar in many respects to the data obtained with angiocardiography. It is especially useful in the diagnosis and differentiation of heart murmurs. An echocardiogram can show whether the heart is dilated, the walls or septum are thickened, or pericardial effusion is present. It has also been used to study the motion of prosthetic heart valves.

The patient should be assured that the test is safe and painless. He should know that he will be expected to change positions several times during the procedure, to breathe slowly, and periodically to hold his breath.

Phonocardiography

Phonocardiography is the graphic recording of heart sounds and pulse waves and their relation to time. It helps the observer to identify, accurately time, and differentiate among various sounds and murmurs. It is used to aid in the precise timing of cardiac events and in the diagnosis of valvular and other cardiac disorders.

Microphones containing miniature transducers are placed on the patient's chest at the apex and base of the heart. The transducers pick up heart sounds, amplify them, convert them to electrical impulses, and transmit them to a recorder which produces a waveform graph of the sounds.

The patient should be assured that the procedure is safe and painless. He should know that he will be expected to remain still and quiet during the test except when asked to change positions, to breathe slowly, or hold his breath.

Radioisotope Studies

Radioisotope studies are useful for detecting myocardial infarction and decreased myocardial blood flow, and for evaluating left ventricular function. The radioisotopes are injected intravenously, and scans are done using a gamma scintillation camera.

Myocardial Infarction Imaging. Technetium pyrophosphate (^{99m}TC-PYP) is taken up in areas of the heart where there is damaged myocardial tissue, forming a *hot spot* on a scan made with a scintillation camera. Hot spots appear within 12 hours of infarction, are most evident 48 to 72 hours after infarction, and usually disappear within 1 week unless there is continuing myocardial damage.

The patient is assured that the scan involves less radiation exposure than a chest x-ray and is told to remain motionless during the scan.

Myocardial Blood Flow Evaluation. Thallium-201 is used to evaluate blood flow through vessels that are too small to visualize with coronary arteriography. Thallium concentrates in normal myocardial tissue but not in ischemic or necrotic tissues.

Often this test is paired with an exercise stress test to compare changes in myocardial perfusion during exercise and at rest. In this technique, "cold spots" correlating with lack of myocardial perfusion correlate with infarcted areas. The patient should be assured that there is no known radiation danger from Thallium.

Blood Pool Scanning. The technique of gated cardiac blood pool scanning utilizes a computer to analyze left ventricular function. By determining the difference between the amount of the radioactive tracer technetium pyrophosphate (^{99m}Tc-PYP) in the end-diastolic volume and the amount in the end-systolic volume, the ejection fraction can be calculated. This test can also be used to assess the differences in left ventricular function during rest and exercise.

In *multiple-gated acquisition* (MUGA) *scanning,* the scintillation camera records 14 to 64 points of one single cardiac cycle. The sequential pictures are studied to evaluate ventricular wall motion and to determine the ejection fraction.

The patient is assured that there is no known radiation danger, and is told to remain motionless during the scan.

Hemodynamic Monitoring

Central Venous Pressure Monitoring

Central venous pressure (CVP) is the pressure within the right atrium or in the great veins within the thorax. It represents the filling pressure of the right ventricle and indicates the ability of the right side of the heart to manage a fluid load. It serves as a guide to fluid replacement in seriously ill patients and is a measurement of effective circulating blood volume.

CVP reflects right ventricular failure. Most right ventricular failure is secondary to left ventricular failure. Therefore, an elevated CVP can be a *late* sign of left ventricular failure.

CVP is a dynamic or changing measurement. The change in CVP correlated with the patient's clinical status is a more useful indication of adequacy of venous blood volume and alterations of cardiovascular function than is a single measurement of CVP. A lowered CVP indicates that the patient is hypovolemic, and this is verified when a rapid intravenous infusion causes the patient to improve. A rising CVP may be due to either hypervolemia or poor cardiac contractility.

The CVP site should be prepared by shaving and cleansing with an antiseptic solution. A local anesthetic may be used. The catheter is threaded through the external jugular, antecubital, or femoral vein into the vena cava just above or within the right atrium. Once the CVP catheter is inserted, antiseptic ointment and a dry, sterile dressing are applied. The dressing, intravenous bag, manometer, and tubing are changed every 24 hours.

CVP is measured by the height of a column of water in a manometer. When measuring CVP, it is crucial that the zero mark on the manometer be placed at the phlebostatic axis. When this position is located, an ink mark is made on the chest to indicate the location. If the phlebostatic axis is used, CVP can be measured correctly with the patient supine at any backrest position. Normal CVP is 4 cm to 10 cm of water. The most common complications of CVP monitoring are infection and air embolism.

Pulmonary Artery and Pulmonary Artery Wedge Pressure Monitoring

Pulmonary artery pressures reflect left-sided heart pressures and therefore are more useful in assessing left ventricular failure than is CVP. Pulmonary artery pressures are monitored only in cardiac care units or other intensive care units and not on general medical–surgical units.

A balloon-tipped, flow-directed catheter is inserted into a large vein that leads into the superior vena cava and right atrium. The balloon is inflated, and the catheter is carried rapidly by the flow of blood through the tricuspid valve, into the right ventricle, through the pulmonic valve, and into a branch of the pulmonary artery. When the catheter reaches a small pulmonary artery, the balloon is deflated and the catheter is secured with sutures.

Pulmonary artery systolic and diastolic pressures are obtained via a transducer and blood pressure monitor. Normal pulmonary artery pressure is 25/9 mm Hg, with a mean pressure of 15 mm Hg. When the balloon is inflated, the catheter is "wedged" in the pulmonary artery. Pressures transmitted to the catheter reflect left ventricular end-diastolic pressure. At end-diastole, when the mitral valve is open, pulmonary artery wedge pressure is the same as the pressure in the left atrium and the left ventricle, *unless* the patient has mitral valve disease or pulmonary hypertension. Pulmonary artery wedge pressure is a mean pressure and is normally 4.5 mm Hg to 13 mm Hg.

Catheter site care is the same as that for a CVP catheter. The catheter flush solution is heparinized normal saline, delivered in small amounts using a pressure bag and flush device. As in measuring CVP, it is essential to place the transducer at the phlebostatic axis to ensure accurate readings. Measurement of cardiac output can also be obtained by using a pulmonary artery catheter. Complications of pulmonary artery monitoring include infection, pulmonary artery rupture, pulmonary thromboembolism, pulmonary infarction, catheter kinking, dysrhythmias, and air embolism.

Systemic Intra-arterial Monitoring

Intra-arterial monitoring is used to obtain direct and continuous blood pressures in critically ill patients with severe high blood pressure or hypotension. Arterial catheters are also useful when obtaining arterial blood gases and serial blood samples. Intra-arterial monitoring is restricted to critical care units.

Once an arterial site is selected (radial, brachial, femoral, or dorsalis pedis), collateral circulation to the area must be confirmed prior to catheter placement. This can be done by either the *Allen test* or the ultrasonic *Doppler test.* (If no collateral circulation existed, and the cannulated artery became occluded, ischemia and infarction of the area distal to the cannulated site could occur.) Site preparation and care are the same as for CVP catheters. The catheter flush solution is the same as for pulmonary artery catheters. A transducer is attached, and pressures are obtained in mm Hg. Complications include local obstruction with distal ischemia, external hemorrhage, massive ecchymosis, dissection, air embolism, blood loss, pain, arteriospasm, and infection.

Bibliography

Books

Andreoli KG et al. Comprehensive Cardiac Care. St Louis, CV Mosby, 1983.

Bates B. A Guide to Physical Examination, 4th ed. Philadelphia, JB Lippincott, 1987.

Braunwald E. Heart Disease. Philadelphia, WB Saunders, 1984.

Connor WE and Bristow JD. Coronary Heart Disease: Prevention, Complications, and Treatment. Philadelphia, JB Lippincott, 1985.

Conover MB. Understanding Electrocardiography. St Louis, CV Mosby, 1984.

Fishback FT. Manual of Laboratory Tests. Philadelphia, JB Lippincott, 1984.

Grossman W. Cardiac Catheterization and Angiography. Philadelphia, Lea & Febiger, 1986.

Guzzetta CE and Dossey BM. Cardiovascular Nursing. St Louis, CV Mosby, 1984.

Horwitz LD and Groves BM. Signs and Symptoms in Cardiology. Philadelphia, JB Lippincott, 1985.

Hurst JW et al. The Heart. New York, McGraw-Hill, 1985.

Perloff JA. Physical Examination of the Heart and Circulation. Philadelphia, WB Saunders, 1982.

Sadler D. Nursing for Cardiovascular Health. Norwalk, Connecticut, Appleton-Century-Crofts, 1984.

Underhill SL et al. Cardiac Nursing. Philadelphia, JB Lippincott, 1982.

Vinsant MO and Spence MI. Commonsense Approach to Coronary Care. St Louis, CV Mosby, 1985.

Articles

Antman EM. Ambulatory ECG monitoring: Clinical applications of Holter recording. Consultant 1985 Mar 30; 25(6):96–105.

Antman E and Cohn PF. Coronary artery disease: Clinical versus angiographic findings. Hosp Med 1983 Apr; 19(4):173–210.

Armstrong F and Finesilver C. Cardiac catheterization. Crit Care Update 1983 Apr; 10(4):7–13.

Assessing neck vessels. Nursing 83 1983 Aug; 13(8):32F, 32P.

Balloon flotation catheters today: What they tell you, why they're vital, RN 1983 Sept; 46(9):36–41.

Balloon flotation catheters today: New protocols for the Swan-Ganz. RN 1983 Oct; 46(10):54–59.

Boyd AD and Boyd KD. Complications of use of flow-directed pulmonary artery catheters. CVP 1983 Nov; 11(6):28, 30, 34–35.

Brenner ZR and Wood KM. Cardiac radionuclide imaging: Patient education. DCCN 1984 May–June; 3(3):172–183.

Bruya MA et al. Nursing decisionmaking in critical care: Traditional versus invasive blood pressure monitoring. Nurs Adm Q 1985 Summer; 9(4):19–31.

Chrzanowski A. Cardiac catheterization and coronary angiography. Occup Health Nurs 1984 Feb; 32(2):81–85.

Dennis JW and Greisler HP. Noninvasive cardiac monitoring. Nurs Clin North Am 1987 Mar; 22(1):111–120.

Dennison AD. Visual clues to cardiac diagnosis . . . external skin signs. Emerg Med 1984 Nov 15; 16(9):98–112.

Dodek A. When echocardiography provides the final diagnosis. Chest 1984 May; 85(5):678–682.

Erickson BA. Detecting abnormal heart sounds. Nursing 86 1986 Jan; 16(1):58–64.

Ewy GA. Answers to questions on bedside cardiovascular evaluation. Hosp Med 1984 Mar; 20(3):39, 42–64.

Francis K. Coronary risk evaluation. Phys Ther 1985 July; 65(7):1099–1109.

Funk M. Preparing the patient for a MUGA study. Crit Care Nurse 1983 Sept–Oct; 3(5):57–61.

Gould KL and Goldstein RA. Cardiovascular imaging: Metabolic and functional. Hosp Pract 1984 Jan; 19(1):115–139.

Haughey CW. Preparing your patient for echocardiography. Nursing 84 1984 May; 14(5):68–71.

Hudson-Civetta J. Intravascular catheters: Current guidelines for care and maintenance. Heart Lung 1983 Sept; 12(5):466–476.

Hurst JM. Invasive hemodynamic monitoring: An overview. JEN 1984 Jan–Feb; 10(1):11–22.

Irwin S. Clinical manifestations and assessment of ischemic heart disease. Phys Ther 1985 Dec; 65(12):1806–1811.

Kutcher KL. Cardiac electrophysiologic mapping techniques. Focus Crit Care 1985 Aug; 12(4):26–30.

Lem V. A nurse-supervised exercise stress testing laboratory. Heart Lung 1985 May; 14(3):280–284.

Marpole DGF. Coronary angiography: When and why it might be needed, post MI. Consultant 1983 Mar; 23(3):224–235.

Matthay RA. Cardiovascular function in the intensive care unit: Invasive and noninvasive monitoring. Respir Care 1985 June; 30(6):432–455.

Measuring your patient's PAWP. Nursing 83 1983 Feb; 13(2):72–73.

Miller PG. Assessing C.V.P. Nursing 85 1985 Sept; 15(9):44–46.

Moses B. Nuclear cardiology. Occup Health Nurs 1984 Feb; 32(2):72–74.

Murray MA. Chest pain, dyspnea, confusion: When should you sound the alarm? RN 1983 Jan; 46(1):67–74.

Newell JD et al. Diagnostic capabilities of current imaging techniques. Consultant 1984 May; 24(5):91–105.

Roderick B. How to manage CVP lines. RN 1985 Aug; 48(8):22–24.

Ryan AM. What cardiac enzymes tell you about acute MI. RN 1984 Mar; 47(3):46–49.

Santolla A. A new closed system for arterial lines. RN 1983 June; 46(6):49–52.

Saul L. Heart sounds and common murmurs. Am J Nurs 1983 Dec; 83(12):1679–1689.

Shaver JA. Role of auscultation in cardiac diagnosis. Hosp Med 1984 May; 20(5):59–84.

Sheffield LT. Clinical use of exercise test results. Hosp Med 1985 May; 21(5):233–237, 241–243, 247.

Smalling RW and Gould KL. Cardiovascular imaging: Ischemia and reperfusion. Hosp Pract 1984 Mar; 19(3):163–185.

Spangler RA. Update on pulmonary artery catheterization. Nursing 85 1985 Aug; 15(8):42–45.

Stefadouros MA. Noninvasive diagnosis. Emerg Med 1983 Jan 1; 15(1):54, 58–65.

Taylor DL. Assessing heart sounds. Nursing 85 1985 Jan; 15(1):57–58.

Vaughan P. Bedside assessment of the myocardial infarction patient. Crit Care Nurse 1984 Mar–Apr; 4(2):60–77.

Ventura B. What you need to know about cardiac catheterization. RN 1984 Sept; 47(9):24–30.

Winters WL. Imaging techniques in patients with acute myocardial infarction. Heart Lung 1985 May; 14(3):259–264.

Yacone L. Cardiac diagnostic studies: Nuclear scanning and cardiac catheterization. RN 1984 May; 47(2):129–130.

Chapter 25

Management of Patients With Cardiac Disorders

Coronary Artery Disease

Coronary Atherosclerosis

The most common heart disorder in the United States is coronary atherosclerosis, a form of arteriosclerosis. This pathologic condition of the coronary arteries is characterized by an abnormal accumulation of lipid substances and fibrous tissue in the vessel wall that leads to changes in arterial structure and function and reduction of blood flow to the myocardium. Causes of atherosclerotic heart disease probably involve alterations in lipid metabolism, blood coagulation, and the biophysical and biochemical properties of the arterial walls.

Pathophysiology. The functional lesion of atherosclerosis is called the *atheroma*. Atherosclerosis begins when the waxy cholesterol atheroma, which looks like pearly gray mounds of tissue, becomes deposited on the intima of the major arteries. These deposits interfere with the absorption of nutrients by the endothelial cells that compose the vessel lining, and obstruct blood flow by protruding into the lumen of the vessel (Fig. 25-1). The vascular endothelium in involved areas becomes necrotic and then scarred, further compromising the lumen and impeding the flow of blood. At sites such as these, where the lumen is narrowed and the wall rough, there is a great tendency for clots to form, which explains the fact that intravascular coagulation, followed by thromboembolic disease, is among the most important complications of atherosclerosis.

Our knowledge of atherogenesis is limited. Several theories are propounded, but as yet none has been conclusively substantiated. Among suspected mechanisms are thrombus formation on the surface of the plaque followed by fibrous organization of the thrombus, hemorrhage into a plaque, and continuing lipid accumulation. If the fibrous cap of the plaque ruptures, the lipid debris is swept into the bloodstream and obstruction of the arteries and capillaries distal to the ruptured plaque results.

The coronary arteries are particularly susceptible to the effects of atherosclerosis. They twist and turn as they supply

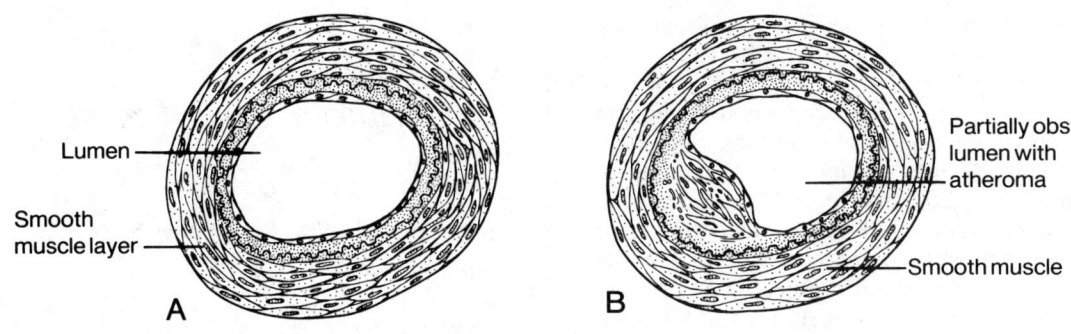

Figure 25-1
Cross-sections of a normal and an atherosclerotic artery. (*A*) Cross-section of normal artery showing patent lumen. (*B*) Cross-section of artery showing atheroma and diminished patency of artery lumen.

the heart, thereby creating angles and nooks ripe for atheroma development (Fig. 25-2).

Clinical Manifestations. Coronary atherosclerosis produces symptoms and complications as a result of the narrowing of the arterial lumen and obstruction of blood flow to the myocardium. This impediment to blood flow is progressive, and the inadequate blood supply (ischemia) that results deprives the muscle cells of the blood components they need for their survival. Varying degrees of cell damage are produced by ischemia. The major manifestation of ischemia of the myocardium is chest pain. *Angina pectoris* refers to recurrent chest pain that is not accompanied by irreversible damage to myocardial cells. More severe ischemia with cell damage is termed *myocardial infarction*. Irreversibly damaged myocardium undergoes degeneration and is replaced by scar tissue. If the damage to the myocardium is extensive, the heart may eventually fail, that is, it may be unable to support the body's needs for blood by providing an adequate cardiac output.

Other clinical manifestations of coronary artery disease may be ECG changes, ventricular aneurysms, dysrhythmias, and sudden death.

Risk Factors and Prevention of Atherosclerotic Heart Disease

Epidemiologic studies and observations reveal that there are risk factors for atherosclerosis that tend to make a person more prone to develop coronary heart disease. A risk factor may be modifiable or nonmodifiable. A *modifiable risk factor* is one over which an individual may exercise control by changing a life-style or personal habit; a *nonmodifiable risk factor* is a consequence of genetics over which an individual has no control. (See Chart 25-1.) A risk factor may operate independently or in tandem with other risk factors. The more risk factors a person has, the greater is the likelihood of developing coronary artery disease. Persons at risk should have periodic medical examinations, modify their life-styles, and alter their dietary habits.

Four modifiable risk factors—cigarette smoking, elevated blood pressure, hyperlipidemia, and behavior patterns—have received major attention. The two risk factors cited as major causes of coronary artery disease (CAD) and its consequent complications are cigarette smoking and hypertension.

Cigarette Smoking. Cigarette smoking contributes to the development and severity of coronary artery disease in two ways. First, the inhalation of smoke increases the blood carbon monoxide (CO) level. Hemoglobin, the oxygen-car-

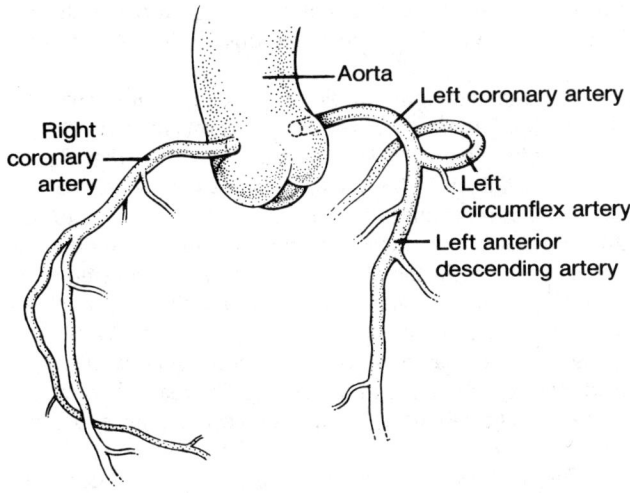

Figure 25-2
Angles of the coronary arteries. The many angles and curves of the coronary arteries contribute to the vessels' susceptibility to the development of atheromatous plaques.

Chart 25-1
Risk Factors for Atherosclerosis

Nonmodifiable Risk Factors	Modifiable Risk Factors
Positive family history	Hyperlipidemia
Increasing age	Elevated blood pressure
Sex—Occurs three times more often in men than in women	Cigarette smoking
	Elevated blood sugar (diabetes mellitus)
Race—Higher incidence in blacks than in whites	Obesity
	Physical inactivity
	Stress
	Use of oral contraceptives

rying component of blood, combines more readily with CO than with O_2. Thus, the oxygen being supplied to the heart is severely limited, which makes the heart work harder to produce the same amount of energy. Second, nicotinic acid in tobacco products causes arteries to constrict, which compromises blood flow and subsequent oxygenation. A person with increased risk for CAD is encouraged to stop smoking.

Elevated Blood Pressure.   Elevated blood pressure is the most insidious of all risk factors because it is asymptomatic until disease is well advanced. An elevated blood pressure creates a very high pressure gradient against which the left ventricle must pump. The continued high pressure forces the myocardial oxygen demands to exceed the supply. This initiates the vicious cycle of pain associated with coronary artery disease.

Early detection of high blood pressure and compliance with a therapeutic regimen can prevent the serious consequences associated with untreated elevated blood pressure.

Hyperlipidemia.   The association of elevated blood lipids (fats) with coronary artery disease has been established through epidemiologic studies. *Lipids* are a mixed group of biochemical substances that may be manufactured by the body or derived from metabolism of ingested substances. An *endogenous lipid* is one produced by the normal metabolic functions of the body; an example of an endogenous fat is sterol. An *exogenous lipid* is one derived from a source external to the body; an example of an exogenous fat is an egg.

Lipids have the common property of being more soluble in fat or organic solvents than in water. In the blood, the principal lipids are cholesterol, triglycerides, and phospholipids. To render them suitable for transport in the blood, the lipids are attached to a variety of proteins; the resulting product is called a *lipoprotein*. The lipoproteins are described clinically by their respective densities (see Chart 25-2).

There are five types of hyperlipidemias. Table 25-1 describes the five types, the associated lipoprotein abnormality, and the potential clinical outcomes of elevated levels. Determining the underlying lipid abnormality by blood studies is essential before suggesting dietary control.

Cholesterol and triglycerides are the lipids most frequently associated with coronary heart disease.

For clinical purposes, hyperlipidemia may be suspected if the *fasting* blood cholesterol or triglyceride levels are elevated.

Hyperlipidemia may be primary or secondary. *Primary* hyperlipidemia is generally a hereditary disorder and is the rarest of the phenotypes. The *secondary* type occurs as a manifestation of numerous other diseases, including hypothyroidism, nephrotic syndrome, diabetes mellitus, and alcoholism. Therapy consists in treating the basic disorder.

For some individuals, the control of fat consumption is an important factor in preventive nutrition. Dietary fat may be regulated by changing the total amount or the type of fat in the diet, or both. Assisting the patient to modify dietary fat intake through effective counseling requires an understanding of the differences between saturated and polyunsaturated fatty acids, cholesterol, medium-chain triglycerides, and various other fractions as well as of their functions in the human body.

No single diet or drug will be effective in all conditions in lowering the particular elevated lipid abnormality, but in

---

Chart 25-2
Composition of Lipids Present in Plasma

α-Lipoproteins—High-Density Lipoproteins (HDL)

Protein	35%–60%*
Phospholipid	34%–44%
Cholesterol	20%–28%
Triglyceride	17%

β-Lipoproteins—Low-Density Lipoproteins (LDL)

Protein	20%–25%
Phospholipid	25%
Cholesterol	46%*
Triglyceride	14%

Very-Low-Density Lipoproteins (VLDL)

Protein	10%
Phospholipid	20%
Cholesterol	5%
Triglyceride	65%*

Chylomicrons (Nonmigrating)

Protein	2%
Phospholipid	6%–9%
Cholesterol	2%
Triglyceride	85%–95%*

* The highest component in each type of lipid

---

most people with such an abnormality the level can be brought within the upper average range.

The compositions of the various types of lipids are indicated in Chart 25-2. The α-lipoproteins (high-density, or HDL) are highest in protein, and the β-lipoproteins (low-density, or LDL) are highest in cholesterol. The very-low-density lipoproteins (VLDL) and chylomicrons are higher in triglycerides.

For patients in whom diet alone cannot normalize the specific lipid, there are several medications that have a synergistic effect when taken with the prescribed diet. These agents are shown to be biochemically effective, in that elevated lipoprotein concentration tends to return toward normal and manifestations of the abnormalities, such as xanthomas (yellow papules in the skin caused by lipid deposits), may disappear. Drug treatment also varies with the type of hyperlipidemia. The drugs used are usually grouped into two types: those that decrease lipoprotein synthesis, such as nicotinic acid and clofibrate, and those that increase lipoprotein breakdown (catabolism), such as cholestyramine, sitosterol, and D-thyroxine.

The usefulness of diet and drugs in reversing coronary artery disease is still under investigation. A major factor influencing the thoughts of researchers is that, because lipids are manufactured within the body, in certain cases dietary control may have no influence on serum lipid levels. Despite

TABLE 25-1
Primary Hyperlipidemias and Associated Clinical Features

Phenotype	Dominant Lipids	Dominant Lipoproteins	Clinical Features of Elevated Levels
I (rare)	Triglycerides	Chylomicron	Xanthoma Enlarged liver Pancreatitis
II (common)	Cholesterol	Beta	Premature atherosclerosis Xanthoma
III (uncommon)	Cholesterol Triglycerides	Floating beta	Premature atherosclerosis Xanthoma
IV (uncommon)	Triglycerides	Prebeta	Glucose intolerance Hyperuricemia Premature atherosclerosis
V (uncommon)	Triglycerides	Chylomicron Prebeta	Xanthoma Enlarged liver Pancreatitis Glucose intolerance Hyperuricemia Premature atherosclerosis

controversy due to such questions, however, it is now broadly accepted that preventive nutrition can have a significant impact on coronary artery disease.

Behavior Patterns of Coronary-Prone Persons. It is believed that stress and certain behaviors contribute to the pathogenesis of coronary (atherosclerotic) heart disease. Psychobiological and epidemiologic studies have investigated behaviors that characterize people who are prone to coronary artery disease: competitive striving for achievement, exaggerated sense of time urgency, aggressiveness, and hostility. A person who manifests these behaviors is classified as type A coronary-prone. It appears that, in addition to reducing other risk factors (smoking, dietary fats), such a person should make some effort to alter life-style and long-term habit patterns.

The type A behavior pattern has been widely accepted as a risk factor for coronary heart disease. Contemporary research indicates that it may not be as significant as was once thought, but there is not yet conclusive evidence of its precise role.

Gerontological Considerations

Atherosclerotic coronary artery disease is not a function of aging. The longer a person survives without coronary artery disease, the less likely it is that the disease will develop. Aging does, however, produce changes in the integrity of the lining of the walls of arteries (arteriosclerosis), thus impeding blood flow and tissue nutrition. These changes are often sufficient to diminish oxygenation and increase myocardial oxygen consumption (MVo_2). The result can be debilitating angina pectoris and eventually congestive heart failure.

Angina Pectoris
Definition, Etiology, and Pathophysiology

Angina pectoris is a clinical syndrome characterized by paroxysms of pain or a feeling of pressure in the anterior chest. The cause is considered to be insufficient coronary blood flow, resulting in inadequate oxygen supply of the myocardium; in other words, myocardial oxygen demands exceed supply.

Angina is usually caused by atherosclerotic heart disease, and almost invariably is associated with a significant obstruction of a major coronary artery. (The characteristics of the various types of angina are listed in Chart 25-3.)

Any number of factors can produce anginal pain. Physical exertion can precipitate an attack by increasing myocardial oxygen demands. Exposure to cold or even the drinking of iced beverages can cause vasoconstriction and an elevated blood pressure, with increased oxygen demand. Eating a heavy meal increases the blood flow to the mesenteric area and places a heavier demand on the heart. Stress and any emotion-provoking situation causing the release of adrenalin and increased blood pressure may accelerate the heart rate. If blood flow from the left ventricle is obstructed, as in aortic stenosis, the oxygen needs of the myocardium are drastically increased.

Clinical Manifestations

Ischemia of the heart muscle produces *pain*, varying in severity from upper substernal pressure to agonizing pain that is accompanied by severe apprehension and a feeling of im-

Chart 25-3
Types of Angina

Unstable Angina
(Preinfarction Angina; Crescendo Angina)

Progressive increase in frequency, intensity, and duration of anginal attacks

Increasing danger of myocardial infarction within 3 to 18 months

Chronic Stable Angina

Predictable, consistent, rarely occurs while at rest

Nocturnal Angina

Pain occurs at night usually during sleep; may be relieved by sitting upright.

Commonly due to left ventricular failure

Angina Decubitis

Angina while lying down

Intractable or Refractory Angina

Severe incapacitating angina

Prinzmetal's Angina (Variant: Resting)

Spontaneous type of anginal pain accompanied by ST-segment elevation in ECG

Thought to be due to coronary artery spasm

Associated with high risk of infarction

---

pending death. The pain is usually felt deep in the chest behind the upper or middle third of the sternum (retrosternal). Although the pain frequently is localized, it may radiate to the neck, jaw, shoulders, and inner aspects of the upper extremities. The patient often experiences a tightness, a choking or strangling sensation that has a viselike, insistent quality. A feeling of weakness or numbness in the arms, wrists, and hands may accompany the pain. Along with the physical pain, the patient also has a sense of impending death, an apprehension so characteristic of angina that if it occurs alone, as it sometimes does, it is sufficient for diagnosis.

Gerontological Considerations

The elderly person who experiences angina may not exhibit the typical pain profile because of changes in neuroreceptors. Pain is often manifested in the elderly as weakness or fainting. When exposed to cold temperatures, elderly persons may experience anginal symptoms more quickly because they have less subcutaneous fat to provide insulation. They should be encouraged to dress with extra clothing and advised to recognize feelings of weakness as an indication that they should rest or take prescribed medications.

Diagnostic Evaluation

The diagnosis of angina is often made by an evaluation of the clinical manifestations of pain and the patient's history. In certain types of angina, ECG changes are helpful in making a differential diagnosis of the angina. The patient's response to exertion or stress may also be tested by means of electrocardiographic monitoring while the patient exercises on a bicycle or treadmill.

Medical Management

The objectives of medical management of angina are to decrease the oxygen demands of the myocardium and to increase the oxygen supply. Medically these objectives are met through pharmacologic therapy and risk factor control. Surgically the objectives are met by revascularization of the blood

supply to the myocardium, through coronary artery bypass surgery or percutaneous transluminal angioplasty (see Chap. 27). Frequently a combination of medical and surgical therapies is employed.

Pharmacologic Therapy: Nitroglycerin. The nitrates are still the mainstay of treatment for angina pectoris. Nitroglycerin is given to reduce myocardial oxygen consumption, which decreases ischemia and relieves anginal pain. Nitroglycerin is a vasoactive drug that acts to dilate both the veins and the arteries and thus has an effect on the peripheral circulation. Dilation of the veins causes venous pooling of blood throughout the body. As a result, less blood is returned to the heart and there is a reduction in filling pressure (preload). Nitrates also relax the systemic arteriolar bed and thus cause a fall in blood pressure (decrease afterload). These effects decrease myocardial oxygen requirements, bringing about a more favorable balance between supply and demand.

Nitroglycerin taken sublingually or in the buccal pouch alleviates the pain of ischemia within 3 minutes.

- The patient should be instructed to keep the tongue still and to avoid swallowing saliva until the nitroglycerin tablet is dissolved. If the pain is severe, the tablet can be crushed between the teeth to hasten sublingual absorption.
- As a precaution, the patient should carry the medication at all times in a securely capped dark glass bottle, not in a metal or plastic pillbox.

Nitroglycerin is volatile and is inactivated by heat, moisture, air, light, and time. If the nitroglycerin is fresh, the patient will feel a burning sensation under the tongue and often a feeling of fullness or throbbing in the head. The nitroglycerin supply should be renewed every 6 months.

Instead of using a fixed dosage, the patient regulates drug usage, taking the smallest dose that relieves pain. The drug should be taken in anticipation of any activity that may produce pain. Because nitroglycerin will increase the patient's tolerance for exercise and stress when taken prophylactically (*e.g.*, before exercise, stair-climbing, and sexual intercourse), it is best that it be taken *before* the pain develops.

- The patient should note how long it takes for the nitroglycerin to relieve the discomfort. If the pain lasts more than 20 or 30 minutes after the nitroglycerin has been taken, an impending myocardial infarction may be suspected.

Side-effects of nitroglycerin include flushing, throbbing headache, hypotension, and tachycardia. The use of long-acting nitrate preparations is controversial. Isosorbide dinitrate appears to be effective for up to 2 hours if taken sublingually but has an uncertain effect if taken orally.

Topical Nitroglycerin Ointment. Nitroglycerin is also available in a lanolin-petrolatum base. In this form it is applied to the skin to protect against anginal pain and promote its relief. It is especially useful when patients experience nocturnal angina or are involved in periods of extended activity (*e.g.*, golfing) because it has a prolonged effect of up to 24 hours. The dose is usually increased until headache or an excessive effect on blood pressure or heart rate occurs, and then is reduced to the largest dose that does not produce these side-effects. Instructions for application accompany the various products.

Beta-Adrenergic Blockers. If the patient continues to have chest pain despite treatment with nitroglycerin and modification of life-style, the beta-adrenergic blocking agent propranolol hydrochloride (Inderal) is given. This drug appears to reduce myocardial oxygen consumption by blocking the sympathetic impulses to the heart. The result is a reduction in heart rate, blood pressure, and myocardial contractility that establishes a more favorable balance between myocardial oxygen needs and the amount of oxygen available. This helps to control chest pain and allows the patient to work or exercise. Propranolol may be given with sublingual isosorbide dinitrate for anti-anginal and anti-ischemia prophylaxis. Propranolol is cleared by the liver at varying rates, depending on the individual patient. It is usually given at 6-hour intervals. Side-effects include musculoskeletal weakness, hypotension, bradycardia, and mental depression.

When propranolol is started, blood pressure and heart rate should be taken (while the patient is in an upright position) 2 hours after the medication has been administered. If the blood pressure drops significantly, a vasopressor may be needed. If severe bradycardia occurs, atropine is the antidote of choice. It is also important to remember that propranolol can precipitate congestive heart failure and asthma.

- Caution the patient not to stop taking propranolol abruptly, because there is evidence that angina may worsen and myocardial infarction may develop if this drug is abruptly discontinued.

Calcium Ion Antagonists. The calcium blockers, or antagonists, possess properties that have profound effects on myocardial oxygen demands and supply, hence their value in the treatment of angina. Physiologically, the calcium ion performs at the cellular level to influence contraction of all types of muscle tissue and plays a role in the electrical stimulation of the heart.

Calcium ion antagonists increase myocardial oxygen supply by dilating the smooth muscle wall of the coronary arterioles, and decrease myocardial oxygen demands by reducing systemic arterial pressure and thus the work load of the left ventricle.

The two calcium antagonists most commonly used are nifedipine and verapamil. The vasodilating effects of these agents, particularly on the coronary circulation, have made them valuable in angina that results from coronary vasospasm (*Prinzmetal's angina*). Calcium blockers should be used with great caution in individuals with heart failure because they block the calcium that supports contractility. Hypotension may occur after IV administration. Other side-effects that may occur are constipation, gastric intolerance, dizziness, or headache associated with dizziness.

Calcium ion antagonists are usually given every 4 to 6 hours. Therapeutic doses vary from one person to another.

Risk Factor Control. Several other measures may be necessary in order to decrease the oxygen demands of the myocardium. It is important that the patient stop smoking, because smoking produces tachycardia and raises the blood pressure, thus increasing the work of the heart. Obese persons should lose weight to reduce cardiac work.

Physical conditioning should be encouraged because it increases exercise capacity and produces a lower heart rate and blood pressure in response to a given exercise. (See page 547 for rehabilitation of the heart patient.)

Surgical Management

Angina pectoris may persist for many years in a stable form with brief attacks. However, it is a serious disease. In the unstable stage the episodes of chest pain become more frequent and intense, occurring without apparent provocation. When symptoms cannot be controlled despite an adequate trial of drug therapy, some form of surgical revascularization is considered that can correct the basic problem by bringing a new blood supply to the ischemic myocardium (see page 600).

Percutaneous Transluminal Angioplasty. Interventional radiology has made possible a procedure for the revascularization of the coronary arteries that is less invasive than bypass surgery. The procedure is referred to as *percutaneous transluminal angioplasty*. A balloon-tipped catheter is inserted into the coronary artery and is rapidly inflated and deflated. The purpose of this procedure is to compress the atheroma into the intimal lining of the artery, thereby increasing blood flow in the artery.

Patients eligible for this procedure have atherosclerotic disease, preferably affecting only one vessel, have had angina for less than 1 year, and are candidates for surgical revascularization. Because of these rigid criteria, the population that the procedure may benefit is severely limited.

Myocardial infarction is a major complication of this procedure. For this reason it is recommended that this procedure be performed only if a cardiovascular surgical team is on standby.

▶ Nursing Process
The Patient With Angina Pectoris

▷ Assessment

In the hospital the nurse should observe and record all facets of the patient's activities, with particular regard for those that have been found to precede and precipitate attacks of anginal pain.

> When do attacks tend to occur?
> Following a meal?
> After engaging in certain activities?
> After physical activities in general?
> After visits from members of the family or others?
> How does the patient describe the pain?
> Is the onset of pain gradual or sudden?
> How long does it last—seconds? minutes? hours?
> Is the pain steady and unwavering in quality?
> Is the discomfort accompanied by other symptoms, such as excessive perspiration, light-headedness, nausea, palpitation, shortness of breath?
> How many minutes after taking nitroglycerin does the pain last?
> What is the mode of abatement?

The answers to these questions, ascertained from observation, can form a basis for designing a logical program of prevention.

When sensing that an attack is imminent, a patient should cease all movement in order to reduce to a minimum the oxygen requirements of the ischemic myocardium. This is done with the hope that oxygen needs can be met by the limited supply available at the moment and the impending attack can thus be averted.

▷ *Nursing Diagnoses*

Based on the assessment data, major nursing diagnoses for the patient may include the following:

- Pain related to myocardial ischemia
- Anxiety related to fear of death
- Deficit in knowledge of underlying nature of disease and methods for avoiding complications
- Potential nonadherence to therapeutic regimen related to nonacceptance of necessary life-style changes

▷ *Planning and Implementation*

▷ *Goals:* The major goals of the patient include prevention of pain, reduction of anxiety, awareness of the underlying nature of the disorder and understanding of the prescribed care, and adherence to the self-care program.

Nursing Interventions

Prevention of Pain. The patient must understand the symptom complex and the need to avoid activities known to cause anginal pain, such as sudden exertion, walking against the wind, exposure to cold, emotional excitement, and so forth. The patient must learn to change, modify, or adapt to these stresses.

There are patients whose attacks occur predominantly in the morning. This idiosyncrasy obviously calls for a change in the schedule of daily activities. As a first step, the patient should plan to rise earlier each morning in order to shave, wash, and dress in a more leisurely fashion. Ideally, this unhurried pace should be maintained throughout the entire day, so that scheduled tasks and commitments are handled without haste or a sense of pressure. Any patient with angina pectoris

should be instructed to initiate all movements with deliberation, avoid exposure to cold, avoid tobacco, eat regularly but lightly, and maintain a proper weight. Use of over-the-counter drugs should be discouraged, especially diet pills, nasal decongestants, or other drugs containing agents that will increase heart rate and blood pressure.

Reduction of Anxiety. This patient has a strong fear of death. Staying with the patient is important as a step to minimize it. Plan nursing care so that time away from the bedside is kept to a minimum, because this fear of death is often alleviated by the physical presence of another person. Provide essential information about the illness, and explain why it is important to follow prescribed directives.

Understanding of the Illness and Ways to Avoid Complications. The education of the patient with angina is designed to acquaint him with the basic nature of his illness and to furnish him with the facts he needs if he is to reorganize his living habits in a way that will reduce the frequency and severity of anginal attacks; delay the progress of the underlying disease, if possible; and help protect him from other complications. The factors outlined in Chart 25-4 are important in the education of the patient with angina pectoris.

Adherence to the Self-Care Program. The self-care program is prepared in cooperation with the patient and his significant other (see Chart 25-4). Activities should be planned so as to minimize the occurrence of episodes of angina. The patient should understand that any pain unrelieved by his usual methods should be treated at the closest emergency center.

▷ *Evaluation*

▷ *Expected Outcomes*

1. Is relieved of pain (see Chart 25-4 on patient education)
2. Reduces anxiety
   a. Understands the illness and purpose of treatment
   b. Adheres to medical regimen
   c. Knows to seek medical assistance if pain persists or changes in quality
   d. Avoids being alone during painful episodes
3. Understands ways to avoid complications and demonstrates freedom from complications
   a. Describes the process of angina
   b. Explains reasons for measures to prevent complications
   c. Exhibits normal ECG and level of cardiac enzymes
   d. Is free of signs and symptoms of acute myocardial infarction
4. Adheres to self-care program
   a. Demonstrates an understanding of pharmacological therapy
   b. Daily habits reflect modification of life-style (see Chart 25-4).

Myocardial Infarction
Definition, Etiology, and Pathophysiology

Myocardial infarction refers to the process by which myocardial tissue is destroyed in regions of the heart that are deprived of an adequate blood supply because of a reduced

Chart 25-4
Patient Education for the Person With Angina

Goal: To improve the quality of life and promote health

Expected Outcomes

I. Patient prevents an episode of anginal pain.
  A. Uses moderation in all activities of life
    1. Participates in a normal daily program of activities that do not produce chest discomfort, shortness of breath, and undue fatigue
    2. Exercises before work, after work, or before meals
    3. Avoids exercises requiring sudden bursts of activity, avoids all isometric exercise
    4. Avoids activities that require heavy effort
    5. Alternates activity with periods of rest. Some fatigue is normal and temporary.
  B. Avoids situations that are emotionally stressful
  C. Avoids overeating
    1. Eats smaller portions
    2. Avoids excessive caffeine intake (coffee, cola drinks), which can increase the heart rate and produce angina
    3. Refrains from engaging in physical exercise for 2 hours after meals
    4. Does not use "diet pills," nasal decongestants, or any over-the-counter medications that can increase the heart rate
  D. Stops smoking, since smoking increases the heart rate, blood pressure, and blood carbon monoxide levels
  E. Avoids cold weather, if possible
    1. Wears scarf over nose/mouth during very cold weather to warm the air
    2. Walks more slowly in cold weather
    3. Dresses warmly in winter
  F. Follows general principles of good hygienic living

II. Patient copes with an attack of anginal pain.
  A. Carries nitroglycerin at all times
    1. Keeps nitroglycerin in a tightly capped, dark-colored glass bottle
    2. Discards the cotton filler/packing
    3. Avoids opening the bottle unnecessarily
    4. Tries to avoid carrying supply right next to body
    5. Discards tablets after 5 months
    6. If tablets are fresh, they should cause a burning sensation when placed under the tongue.
  B. Places nitroglycerin under the tongue at first sign of chest discomfort
    1. Does not swallow saliva until the tablet has dissolved
    2. Stops and rests until all pain subsides
    3. States the significance of using the upright position to potentiate the effects of nitroglycerin
    4. Usually, another nitroglycerin tablet may be taken in 3 to 5 minutes if pain relief is not obtained. If pain persists, patient calls the physician. If the anginal discomfort is unrelieved by the usual number of nitroglycerin tablets, or if it recurs after a short interval, goes to the nearest emergency facility.
  C. Takes nitroglycerin prophylactically to avoid pain known to occur with certain activities (stair-climbing, sexual intercourse)
  D. Is alert for the side-effects of nitroglycerin: headache, flushing, and dizziness

coronary blood flow. The cause of the reduced blood flow is either a critical narrowing of a coronary artery owing to atherosclerosis or a complete occlusion of an artery owing to embolus or thrombus. Decreased coronary blood flow may also result from shock and hemorrhage. In this situation, there is a profound imbalance between myocardial oxygen supply and demand.

"Coronary occlusion," "heart attack," and "myocardial infarction" are all used synonymously, but the preferred term is myocardial infarction. In the United States, well over a million of these attacks occur annually.

The pathophysiology of atherosclerotic heart disease and risk factors for it are discussed in the opening pages of this chapter.

Clinical Manifestations

The patient with myocardial infarction is usually male, is over 40, and has atherosclerosis of the coronary vessels, often with arterial hypertension. Attacks also occur in women and in younger men in their early 30s or even 20s. Women who take oral contraceptives and also smoke are at very high risk. Overall, however, the rate of myocardial infarction is greater in men than in women at all ages.

In a typical patient, the pain starts suddenly, usually over the lower sternal region and the upper abdomen, and is continuous, but it may increase steadily in severity until it becomes almost unbearable. It is a heavy, viselike pain, which may radiate to the shoulders and down the arms, usually the left arm. Unlike the pain of true angina, it begins spontaneously (not following effort, emotional upset, and the like), persists for hours or days, and is relieved neither by rest nor by nitroglycerin. The pulse may become very rapid, irregular, and feeble, even imperceptible.

Gerontological Considerations

The elderly patient may not experience the typical viselike pain associated with myocardial infarction because of the diminished responses of neurotransmitters that occur in the aging process. Often the pain is atypical, such as jaw pain, or fainting may be experienced.

The arteriosclerosis that accompanies aging may compromise tissue perfusion because of increased peripheral vascular resistance. Because elderly patients may have a well-established collateral circulation of the myocardium, they are often spared the lethal complications associated with myocardial infarction.

Diagnostic Evaluation

The person with a severe occlusion may be in shock, appearing ashen and becoming cold and clammy. Vomiting is common. In a few hours body temperature rises, blood pressure falls to an unusually low point, and the leukocyte count rises to 15,000 or 20,000 cu mm. Changes may be seen in the electrocardiogram within 2 to 12 hours (but may take as long as 72 to 96 hours). These changes reveal not only the presence but also the location of the infarct. Serum enzymes and isoenzymes are elevated and can be correlated with the patient's clinical course. Even if the ECG is normal, elevation of serum enzymes reveals that caution is indicated in the management of this person.

Diagnosis is generally based on patient history, ECG, and serial enzyme studies. Prognosis depends on the severity of coronary artery obstruction and hence the extent of myocardial damage.

Serum Enzymes and Isoenzymes. Serial enzyme studies include the following.

Creatine Kinase and Its Isoenzymes. Creatine kinase (CK, with its isoenzyme CK-MB) is regarded as the most sensitive and reliable indicator of all cardiac enzymes. There are three CK isoenzymes; CK-MM (skeletal muscle), CK-MB (heart muscle), and CK-BB (brain tissue). CK-MB is the cardiac-specific isoenzyme; *i.e.*, CK-MB is found only in cardiac cells and therefore rises only when there has been damage to these cells. CK-MB is the most specific index for the diagnosis of acute myocardial infarction. It is always increased in cases of severe angina pectoris, coronary insufficiency, and AMI.

Lactic Dehydrogenase and Its Isoenzymes. Lactic dehydrogenase (LDH) is not as reliable an indicator of acute myocardial damage as CK. However, because it peaks later and is elevated longer than other cardiac enzymes, LDH is useful for diagnosis in patients who may have sustained acute myocardial infarction but have delayed admission to the hospital. There are five LDH isoenzymes, but only two (LDH_1 and LDH_2) are important in the diagnosis of acute myocardial infarction. Both LDH_1 and LDH_2 predominate in the heart, kidney, and brain, but normally the percentage of LDH_2 compared to LDH_1 is greater. When the percentage of LDH_1 exceeds that of LDH_2, the pattern is said to have "flipped," indicating acute myocardial infarction.

Table 25-2 shows the time courses of cardiac enzymes.

Medical Management

Generally, medical management of myocardial infarction includes relief of pain, prevention of ventricular fibrillation and other lethal dysrhythmias, prescription for rest and exercise, dietary modifications, and the prevention and management of anxiety.

The most critical period for the patient with a myocardial infarction is the first 48 hours following the attack. The area of infarction can increase in size for several hours or days

TABLE 25-2
Time Course of Cardiac Enzymes Following Acute Myocardial Infarction

Enzyme	Onset	Peak	Return to Normal
CK	3–6 hr	12–24 hr	3–5 days
CK-MB	2–4 hr	12–20 hr	48–72 hr
LDH	24 hr	48–72 hr	7–10 days
LDH_1	4 hr	48 hr	10 days
LDH_2	4 hr	48 hr	10 days

after the onset of the attack. Cardiogenic shock and ventricular fibrillation are common causes of sudden death during this time period.

Thrombolytic Therapy. The goal of management is to minimize myocardial damage and thus reduce the probability of complications. Important in reducing the size of the infarction is the administration of thrombolytic agents. The purpose of these drugs is to dissolve any thrombus which may have formed in a coronary artery, minimizing the occlusion and hence the infarction size. Critical to the effectiveness of these agents is the early administration of the drug after the onset of chest pain.

Two antithrombolytic agents have proven to be valuable in thrombolysis: streptokinase and tissue-type plasminogen activator (t-PA).

Streptokinase. Streptokinase acts systemically on the body's hemostatic function. Although this drug has demonstrated effectiveness in clot lysis, the potential for systemic hemorrhage has made its use less than desirable. Streptokinase entails a risk of allergic reactions and has proven to be maximally effective only when injected directly into the coronary arteries. Intracoronary administration requires a cardiac catheterization facility, a highly skilled physician, and a cardiothoracic surgery standby team.

Tissue-Type Plasminogen Activator (t-PA). Tissue-type plasminogen activator, in contrast, has a specificity of function in the body's hemostatic function, so the risk of systemic bleeding is reduced. The enzyme t-PA is a naturally occurring enzyme, so allergic reactions are minimized. Finally, studies thus far indicate that intracoronary and intravenous administration of t-PA are equally effective.

These drugs are only effective if administered within 6 hours of the onset of chest pain, before transmural tissue necrosis occurs; the population of patients that this treatment benefits is thus limited. Coronary artery bypass surgery remains the viable alternative for revascularization of the myocardium in those persons for whom clot lysis is ineffective or unacceptable treatment. (See Chap. 27 for a detailed discussion of bypass surgery.)

Nursing Implications of Thrombolytic Therapy

The nursing management of the patient receiving thrombolytic therapy is directed toward anticipation of the complications associated with administration of the drug and immediate intervention if complications occur.

The complications associated with streptokinase administration include systemic bleeding, dysrhythmias produced by coronary artery reperfusion, allergic reactions, and a recurrent thrombosis. Anxiety, which often accompanies the administration of a potentially dangerous drug, can be expected.

Before administration of streptokinase is begun, the nurse conducts a baseline cardiovascular assessment and determines any contraindications to streptokinase therapy. During therapy, the patient's cardiac rhythm is assessed by ECG monitor so that if any new dysrhythmias are produced by reperfusion of a previously obstructed artery, early dysrhythmia management can be implemented. The potential for systemic bleeding can be minimized by monitoring coagulation study results, such as partial thromboplastin time (PTT). Patients who have had surgery in the recent past may not be candidates for this therapy because of the hazard of bleeding.

The complications associated with administration of tissue-type plasminogen activator (t-PA) are minimal compared to those associated with streptokinase. t-PA acts directly on the clot and thus does not harbor the risk of systemic bleeding. Reperfusion dysrhythmias are as likely to occur as with streptokinase, thus necessitating monitoring of cardiac rhythm. Coagulation study results and the patient's response to concomitant anticoagulation therapy are monitored.

The nurse must remember at all times that thrombolytic therapy, whether streptokinase or t-PA, is superimposed upon a patient who is experiencing or recovering from myocardial infarction. Thus, the patient must be continuously observed for complications of his primary illness.

Because of the aggressive nature of the therapies required to minimize myocardial damage, the patient suspected of having a myocardial infarction is managed in a coronary or intensive care unit.

Intensive and coronary care units are equipped with continuous-monitoring equipment, which facilitates monitoring of dysrhythmias and other hemodynamic parameters. The patient is connected to a variety of monitoring devices. Nurses and physicians with special preparation and skills are assigned to care for these patients.

▶ *Nursing Process*
The Patient With
Myocardial Infarction

▷ *Assessment*

One of the most important aspects of care of the patient with a myocardial infarction is the nursing assessment. This serves to establish a baseline of information on the present status of the patient, so that any deviations may be noted immediately. The nursing assessment is orderly and inclusive and has as its objectives identification of the needs of the cardiac patient and determining their priority.

Systematic assessment of the patient includes a careful history, particularly as it relates to the description of symptoms: chest pain, dyspnea, palpitations, faintness (syncope),

or sweating (diaphoresis). Each symptom must be evaluated with regard to time, duration, and precipitating and relieving factors.

In addition, a precise and complete physical assessment is critical to the observations for complications. A systematic method is used and should include the following:

1. *Level of Consciousness.* The patient's orientation to time, place, and person is very important to determine. Often changes in sensorium are produced by drug therapies or impending cardiogenic shock. An altered sensorium can mean that the heart is not perfusing the cerebral circulation satisfactorily.
2. *Heart Size.* The size of the heart may be assessed by identifying its location through palpation. The apical beat, often referred to as the point of maximum impulse (PMI), is normally found at the fifth intercostal space in the midclavicular line (see Fig. 25-3). A shift of the heart to the left and downward may indicate left ventricular enlargement.
3. *Heart Sounds.* Auscultation is the method used to identify the normal heart sounds. A stethoscope of good quality and proper fit is essential for the interpretation of heart sounds. The chest piece must have a bell to pick up low-pitched sound and should possess a diaphragm for the auscultation of high-pitched sounds. When using the bell of the stethoscope, apply it to the skin lightly; when using the diaphragm, apply it firmly.

    The first heart sound (S_1), heard best over the base of the heart and indicating the beginning of systole, should be identified first. The second sound (S_2), heard best at the base and indicating the beginning of diastole, is identified next (Fig. 25-4).

    Abnormal sounds are noted. These include the third heart sound (S_3), known as ventricular gallop, and the fourth heart sound (S_4), known as an atrial or presystolic gallop. S_1 and S_2 together sound like the syllables LUB DUB. S_1 (LUB) is louder at the apex, and

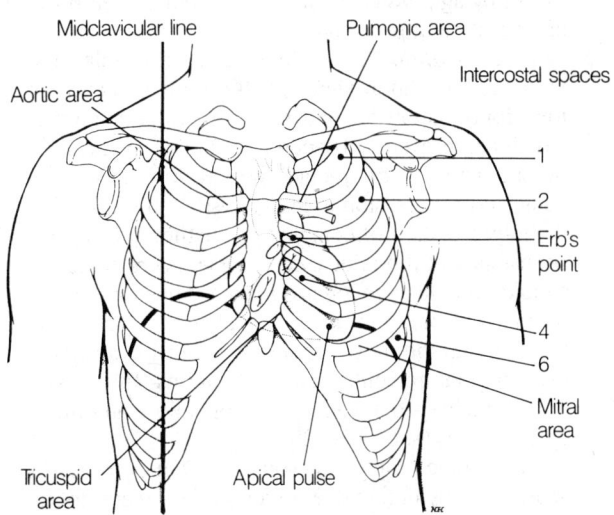

Figure 25-3
The apex beat, often referred to as the point of maximum impulse (PMI), is normally found at the fifth intercostal space in the midclavicular line.

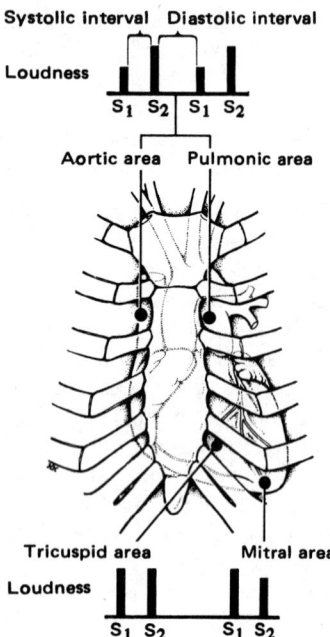

Figure 25-4
Identification of first and second heart sounds.

S_2 (DUB) louder at the base. The S_3 sound follows closely after S_2 in a cadence similar to that of the word *Ken-tuck-y* (S_1-S_2-S_3). The S_4 sound precedes the S_1 in the cadence of the word Ten-nes-see (S_4-S_1-S_2). Other sounds, that is, murmurs, created by blood flowing around an obstruction or flowing backward through an incompetent value, are also noted.

The nurse listens frequently after a myocardial infarction for the development of an S_3. The sound of the S_3 is produced when the blood in the ventricles hits against the noncompliant walls of a damaged myocardium. An S_3 is the earliest sign of impending left ventricular failure. Early detection of an S_3 followed by aggressive medical management can prevent life-threatening pulmonary edema.

4. *Cardiac Rhythm.* The incidence of dysrhythmias after an acute MI is approximately 90%. Early detection allows for initiation of antidysrhythmia drug therapy, which can prevent subsequent reduction in cardiac output, hypotension, reduction of perfusion to vital organs, and progression to lethal dysrhythmias. While the interpretation of complex dysrhythmias is the responsibility of the critical care nurse, every nurse should be able to recognize normal sinus rhythm and deviations from the normal. It is also important to be familiar with the most commonly occurring dysrhythmias: premature ventricular contractions (PVCs), ventricular tachycardia, ventricular fibrillation, and brady-dysrhythmias (see Chap. 26).

A cardiac monitor is used to continuously assess heart rate, rhythm, and conduction. These are documented every 4 hours and prior to the administration of medications that have cardiovascular effects. A 12-lead ECG is taken when any marked change in rhythm occurs. This assists in the diagnosis of dysrhythmias, conduction disturbances, and any further myocardial damage.

5. *Peripheral Pulses.* Rate, rhythm, and volume of pulses are assessed. Cardiovascular disorders will be reflected here. For example, a rapid, regular, but weak pulse may indicate reduced cardiac output. A slow pulse may indicate heart block. An irregular pulse indicates cardiac dysrhythmias. Diminished or absent pulses may indicate that the left ventricle has distributed a thrombus to the periphery. The femoral arteries are shown statistically to be a frequent site of peripheral arterial emboli.

6. *Fluid Volume Status.* Urinary output is important, especially in relation to intake. An early sign of cardiogenic shock is diminished or no urinary output. The nurse should observe for edema. In the patient who is on bedrest, the sacrum should be observed for edema.

7. *Pulse Pressure.* Careful attention is given to pulse pressure measurements. Pulse pressure is the numerical difference between the systolic and diastolic pressures. A narrowing pulse pressure is often seen after a myocardial infarction. Stroke volume may be inferred from the pulse pressure; that is, *stroke volume* is the amount of blood ejected with each ventricular contraction. Since effective ventricular contraction is a function of systole and diastole, the quantitative difference between these two hemodynamic parameters reflects the stroke volume.

8. *Bowel Sounds.* An assessment of bowel motility is important in monitoring for mesenteric artery thrombosis. A reduction of blood supply will cause infarction of the bowel, a potentially fatal complication.

9. *Lung Sounds.* Auscultation of the lung fields at frequent intervals is essential in assessing for signs of ventricular failure. Hearing an S_3 is almost predictable of crackles in the lung bases.

▷ *Nursing Diagnoses*

Based on the clinical manifestations, nursing history, and the diagnostic assessment data, the patient's major nursing diagnoses may include the following:

- Altered comfort, chest pain related to reduced coronary blood flow
- Potential alteration in breathing patterns related to fluid overload
- Potential alteration in tissue perfusion related to decreased cardiac output
- Anxiety related to fear of death
- Potential nonadherence to self-care program related to denial of diagnosis of myocardial infarction

▷ *Planning and Implementation*

▷ *Goals:* The major goals of the patient include relief of chest pain, absence of respiratory difficulties, maintenance/attainment of adequate tissue perfusion, reduction of anxiety, and adherence to the self-care program.

Nursing Interventions

Relief of Chest Pain. The most expedient and appropriate method to relieve chest pain associated with myocardial infarction is the intravenous administration of an analgesic agent, as prescribed by the physician. The drug of choice is morphine sulfate. Two important criteria are met by the administration of this drug intravenously rather than intramuscularly: a more rapid absorption is assured, and the serum enzyme levels are not falsely skewed as they would be by injection into a muscle. An additional benefit of morphine is the euphoric effect it produces, which is helpful in the management of anxiety. Morphine is also an effective preload and afterload reducer and thus serves to reduce myocardial workload. It accomplishes reduction in preload by causing vasodilation of the vascular smooth muscle, thus pooling the blood in the periphery. Arterial blood pressure is reduced concomitantly, which minimizes afterload. Because morphine is given intravenously and takes effect rapidly, the nurse monitors the patient closely for hypotension, respiratory depression, and decreased mental acuity.

Administration of oxygen should occur in tandem with analgesia to assure maximal relief of pain. Inhalation of oxygen even in low doses raises the circulating level of oxygen and reduces pain associated with low levels of circulating oxygen.

Vigorous assessment of all vital signs should take place as long as the patient is experiencing pain. Physical rest, in bed with the backrest elevated or in a cardiac chair, will assist in decreasing chest discomfort and dyspnea. The head-up position is beneficial for the following reasons: (1) tidal volume is improved because there is reduced pressure from abdominal contents on the diaphragm, and thus oxygen exchange is improved; (2) drainage of the upper lobes of the lungs is improved; and (3) venous return to the heart is reduced, which reduces the work of the heart.

Absence of Respiratory Difficulties. Regular and vigorous assessment of respiratory function can help the nurse detect early signs of complications associated with the lungs. Scrupulous attention to fluid volume status will prevent overloading the heart and hence the lungs. Encouraging the patient to breathe deeply and change position frequently will prevent stagnation of fluid in the lung bases.

Maintenance/Attainment of Adequate Tissue Perfusion. Keeping the patient on bed or chair rest is particularly helpful in reducing myocardial oxygen consumption (MVO_2). Checking skin temperature and peripheral pulses with frequency is important to the maintenance of adequate tissue perfusion. Oxygen can be administered to enrich the supply of circulating oxygen.

Reduction of Anxiety. Developing a trusting and caring relationship with such patients is critical in reducing their anxiety. Provide frequent and private opportunities for them to share their concerns and fears. Create an atmosphere of acceptance of their fears, and help them to know that their feelings are both realistic and normal.

Adherence to a Self-Care Program. The most effective way to increase the probability of adherence to a self-care regimen is adequate education about the disease process. Working with patients in the development of plans streamlined to meet their specific needs further enhances potential for adherence (see Chart 25-5).

▷ *Evaluation*

▷ *Expected Outcomes*

1. Patient experiences relief of pain.
2. Shows no signs of respiratory difficulties.
3. Maintains adequate tissue perfusion.
4. Anxiety is reduced.
5. Adheres to self-care program.

Care of the patient with an uncomplicated MI is summarized in Nursing Care Plan 25-1 (pp. 550–553).

Cardiac Rehabilitation

Once an acute myocardial infarction has been diagnosed and the patient progresses to symptom-free status, an active rehabilitation program is provided.

The goals of rehabilitation for the patient with myocardial infarction are to extend and improve the quality of life. The immediate objectives are to return the patient as rapidly as possible to a normal or near-normal life-style. This includes training the patient for physical activity, educating both patient and family, and initiating psychosocial and vocational counseling when necessary.

Cardiac rehabilitation actually begins as soon as the acute episode occurs. During this stage the nurse can assist the patient toward the realization of his goal of independence, even when he is on strict bed rest. This is achieved by directing his thinking toward the time when he will be active again. The goal here is not to change the patient's life-style but to make necessary modifications. It is best to avoid focusing on what the patient should not do. Instead, he should be encouraged to develop short-term and long-range goals based on his needs. It is important to explain the nature of the disease, answer questions honestly, and reassure the patient that most persons return to a useful economic life and resume their usual activities. These positive approaches help to keep the patient from becoming a cardiac invalid.

There is a divergence of opinion about the amount of activity in which a patient may participate following a myocardial infarction. Complications commonly occur early during convalescence. Physiological resolution of the infarction continues to occur over time and varies among individuals. Scar formation over the infarcted area is seen at the beginning of the third week, and the necrotic debris is resolved by the fourth week. Thus, there is an area of ischemia in some patients for varying lengths of time, which affects their exercise prescriptions.

Physical Conditioning. Physical conditioning or exercise training is done to improve cardiac efficiency and enhance the patient's ability to perform work at reduced heart and blood pressure rates. This will reduce the oxygen requirements of the heart and enable the patient to perform more physical activity before developing symptoms of myocardial ischemia (*e.g.*, chest pain, ECG changes). Physical conditioning may be divided into the acute phase, convalescent phase (up to 8 weeks), and maintenance phase (lifelong).

As soon as the patient is *stable* and the physician permits, the arms are put through range of motion exercises. Active motion of the muscles of the shoulder girdle helps to prevent anterior chest wall pain, which may be interpreted as being cardiac in origin. Once asymptomatic, the patient may be able to sit in a chair for 20 to 30 minutes several times a day. Encourage the patient to participate in self-care activities as soon as possible. Early mobilization under supervision is usually permitted after an uncomplicated myocardial infarction. Mobilization begins with walking and progresses to stairclimbing. Prolonged immobilization has a deconditioning effect and also contributes to anxiety and depression.

Chart 25-5
Self-Care for the Patient With a Myocardial Infarction

A patient who has had an MI should learn to regulate activity according to personal responses to each situation.

Goal: To improve the quality of life and promote health

Expected Outcomes

I. Patient modifies activities during convalescence so that complete recovery is realized.
   A. Myocardial healing starts early but is not complete for varying periods, usually 6 to 8 weeks.
   B. A myocardial infarction usually requires some modification of life-style; adaptation to a heart attack is an ongoing process.
      1. Patient avoids any activity that produces chest pain, dyspnea, or undue fatigue.
      2. Avoids extremes of heat and cold and walking against the wind
      3. Loses weight as directed
      4. Stops smoking
      5. Alternates activity with rest periods. Some fatigue is normal and expected during convalescence.
      6. Uses personal strengths to compensate for limitations
      7. Eats 3 or 4 meals daily, each containing the same amount of food
         a. Avoids large meals and hurrying while eating
         b. Restricts caffeine-containing beverages, because caffeine can affect heart rate, rhythm, and blood pressure
         c. Complies with prescribed diet, modifying calories, fat, and sodium as prescribed
      8. Makes every effort to adhere to medical regimen, especially in taking medications
      9. Pursues a pleasurable hobby that affords release of tension

II. Patient undertakes an *orderly* program of increasing activity and exercise for long-term rehabilitation.
   A. Engages in a regimen of physical conditioning with a gradual increase in activity levels
      1. Walks daily, increasing distance and time as prescribed
      2. Monitors pulse during physical activity until the maximal level of activity is attained
      3. Avoids activities that tense the muscles: isometric exercise, weight-lifting, any activity that requires sudden bursts of energy
      4. Avoids physical exercise immediately after a meal
      5. Exercises before work, after work, or before retiring
      6. Shortens work hours when first returning to work
   B. Participates in a *daily* program of exercise that develops into a program of regular exercise for a lifetime
   C. Notifies physician when the following symptoms occur:
      1. Chest pressure or pain not relieved in 15 minutes by nitroglycerin (and reports to nearest emergency facility)
      2. Shortness of breath
      3. Fainting
      4. Slow or rapid heartbeat
      5. Swelling of feet and ankles

- Watch the patient closely and carefully during physical activity for chest pain, dyspnea, weakness, fatigue, and an increase in heart rate of more than 20 beats from baseline or more than 120 beats per minute.
- Watch also for a fall in systolic blood pressure, the development of a dysrhythmia, and ECG changes. If these occur, the activity is stopped immediately and the patient's clinical status is reevaluated.

Isometric exercises are contraindicated because they may impose stress on the left ventricle by raising the blood pressure while at the same time decreasing coronary perfusion. The performance of the Valsalva maneuver (straining) is to be avoided.

A treadmill test with ECG monitoring is done to help in developing guidelines for the design of an appropriate exercise program for the patient. Submaximal testing is done before the patient leaves the hospital, and maximal testing before return to work. The patient who demonstrates low functional capacity with ischemic ST segment depression and premature ventricular beats will need a different activity program than the patient who has good functional capacity with no significant ECG abnormalities. The level of the patient's physical activity before infarction is also considered.

In general, the activity is increased in distance and speed. The cardiovascular benefits of exercise depend on whether or not the patient can exercise long enough to reach and maintain the prescribed pulse rate for a period of 15 minutes.

Several months after myocardial infarction the maintenance phase begins. As a result of physical training, the patient may participate in activities that promote endurance—jogging, running, swimming, cycling. These appear to be useful for heart and lung conditioning. In general, the best type of exercise consists of rhythmic and repetitive movements (calisthenics, walking, running) that require maximal or submaximal effort. Short bursts of intensive effort are to be avoided because they produce a marked rise in blood pressure.

Sexual Activity. Many patients fear that sexual activity will be harmful to their heart condition and will precipitate chest pain.

If the patient can walk vigorously around the block or climb a flight of stairs without symptoms, sexual activity may usually be resumed. Some modifications may be necessary—that is, intercourse after a night's sleep and followed by a rest period, or the use of more passive positions to decrease cardiac work load. Sexual relations should be avoided after drinking alcohol or ingesting a large meal, if the situation produces anxiety, or if abnormal symptoms develop and persist.

Infectious Diseases of the Heart

The endocardium is the endothelial layer of tissue that lines the heart's cavities and covers the flaps of its valves. Of the diseases that affect it, the majority represent various types and stages of inflammation (*i.e., endocarditis* or its aftermath). They include (1) rheumatic endocarditis, one of the many complications of acute rheumatic fever; (2) infective endocarditis, produced by direct bacterial invasion of the endocardium, particularly that portion covering the valve leaflets; and (3) chronic valvular heart disease, based on structural deformities of the heart valves, whether of congenital origin or acquired as a result of either rheumatic or bacterial endocarditis in the past.

When an area of endocardium becomes inflamed, a fibrin clot, called a *vegetation,* may form. In time this clot becomes converted into a mass of scar tissue. The scarred endocardium becomes thickened, stiffened, contracted, and deformed. A fringe of vegetations ranging along the free margins of the valve flaps, marking the site of earlier erosions, represents the basic lesion of endocarditis and is the forerunner of chronic valvular heart disease.

Two functional disorders of the valves may result from these pathologic changes: stenosis or regurgitation. In stenosis the valvular opening becomes narrowed and does not permit the passage of normal amounts of blood. Regurgitation results from the valves' shriveling and producing a wider opening. The valve leaflets can no longer perform their function of closing to prevent a backflow of blood.

Rheumatic Endocarditis

Pathophysiology.   Rheumatic fever is a sequel to a Group A streptococcal infection. It is considered a preventable disease. The most prominent symptom of rheumatic fever is polyarthritis, but the most serious damage occurs in the heart, where every structural component is likely to be the site of an inflammatory reaction. The heart damage and the joint lesions are not infectious in origin, in the sense that these tissues are not invaded and directly damaged by destructive organisms; rather, they represent a sensitivity phenomenon occurring in response to the *hemolytic streptococcus.* Blood leukocytes accumulate in the affected tissues and form nodules, which eventually are replaced by scars. The myocardium is certain to be involved in this inflammatory process; that is, *rheumatic myocarditis* develops, which temporarily weakens the contractile power of the heart. The pericardium likewise

is affected; that is, *rheumatic pericarditis* also occurs during the acute illness. These myocardial and pericardial complications usually are without serious sequelae; on the other hand, the effects of *rheumatic endocarditis* are permanent and often crippling.

Clinical Manifestations.   Rheumatic endocarditis anatomically manifests itself first by tiny translucent vegetations, which resemble beads about the size of the head of a pin, arranged in a row along the free margins of the valve flaps. These tiny beads look harmless enough and may disappear without injuring the valve flaps, but more often they have serious effects. They are the starting point of a process that gradually thickens the flaps, rendering them just a little shorter, just a little thicker than normal, just a little shriveled along their edges—enough to prevent them from closing the orifice of the valve perfectly. The result is leakage, a condition called *valvular regurgitation.* The most common type of valvular regurgitation is mitral regurgitation.

In other patients, the inflamed margins of the valve flaps become adherent, resulting in *valvular stenosis,* a narrowed or "stenotic" valvular orifice. A small percentage of patients with rheumatic fever become critically ill with intractable heart failure, serious dysrhythmias, and rheumatic pneumonia. These patients should be treated in an intensive care unit.

Most patients recover with gratifying speed and their recovery ostensibly is complete. However, although free of symptoms, the patient is left with certain permanent residuals that often lead gradually to progressive valvular deformities. The extent of cardiac damage, or even its existence, may not have been apparent in clinical examinations during the acute phase of the disease. Eventually, however, the heart murmurs that are characteristic of valvular stenosis, regurgitation, or both, become audible on auscultation and, in some patients, even detectable as "thrills" on palpation. The myocardium usually can compensate for these valvular defects very well for a time, despite its increased burden. As long as it can do so, the patient remains in apparent good health. However, sooner or later it fails to compensate—and decompensation, when it occurs, is signaled by the manifestations of congestive heart failure, as described on page 581.

Management.   The objectives of management are to observe for and control congestive heart failure and pericarditis (which may be life-threatening), and to give symptomatic relief to other manifestations.

Patients with rheumatic endocarditis should be confined to bed as long as they are febrile and have signs of active carditis. They should remain quiet thereafter until the erythrocyte sedimentation rate (a fair though nonspecific index of rheumatic activity) returns to normal. Salicylates are prescribed in large doses to suppress rheumatic activity by controlling toxic manifestations, lessening constitutional symptoms, and improving the well-being of the patient. Corticosteroid therapy is given to the very ill person with carditis. However, treatment has no effect on valvular deformities that may occur.

The patient with rheumatic endocarditis, whose valve function is faulty but whose disease is quiescent, does not require therapy as long as the heart pumps effectively. Nevertheless, the danger exists of recurrent attacks of acute rheumatic fever, of bacterial endocarditis, of embolism from vegetations or mural thrombi in the heart, and of eventual cardiac failure. (The relation between valvular disease and congestive

(Text continues on p. 554)

Care of the Patient With an Uncomplicated Myocardial Infarction

Nursing Interventions	*Rationale*	*Expected Outcomes*

Nursing Diagnosis: Chest pain related to reduced coronary blood flow

Goal: Relief of chest pain

1. Initially assess, document, and report to the physician the following:

   a. The patient's description of chest discomfort, including location, radiation, duration of pain, and factors that affect it
   b. The effect of chest discomfort on cardiovascular hemodynamic perfusion—to the heart, to the brain, to the kidneys, and to the skin

1. These data assist in determining the cause and effect of the chest discomfort and provide a baseline to which post-therapy symptoms can be compared.

   a. There are many conditions associated with chest discomfort. There are characteristic clinical findings of ischemic pain.
   b. Myocardial infarction decreases myocardial contractility and ventricular compliance, and may produce dysrhythmias by promoting reentry and increased automaticity. Cardiac output is reduced, resulting in reduced blood pressure and decreased organ perfusion. The heart rate may increase as a compensatory mechanism to maintain cardiac output.

- Patient reports relief of chest discomfort within 15 to 30 minutes.
- Appears comfortable:
  Seems restful
  Respiratory rate, cardiac rate, and blood pressure return to prediscomfort level.
  Skin warm and dry
- Effects of chest discomfort on cardiovascular hemodynamics detected to maintain within normal limits:
  Heart rate, rhythm, and conduction
  Blood pressure
  Mentation
  Urine output
  Serum BUN and creatinine
  Skin color, temperature, and moisture

2. Obtain a 12-lead ECG recording during pain, as prescribed, to determine extension of infarction.

2. An ECG during pain may be useful in the diagnosis of an extension of myocardial ischemia, injury, and infarction, and of variant angina.

3. Administer oxygen as prescribed

3. Oxygen may increase the oxygen supply to the myocardium if actual oxygen saturation is less than normal.

4. Administer narcotic or analgesic medications as prescribed and evaluate the patient's response continuously.

4. Narcotics are useful in alleviating chest discomfort, decreasing anxiety, and increasing sense of well-being. The side-effects of these medications can be dangerous, and the patient's status must be assessed.

5. Ensure physical rest; use of the bedside commode with assistance; backrest elevated to comfort; full liquid diet as tolerated; arms supported during upper extremity activity; use of stool softener to prevent straining at stool. Teach patient to exhale with physical movement to avoid a Valsalva maneuver, and to practice the relaxation response. Visitor privileges are individualized, based on patient response. Provide a restful environment, and allay fears and anxiety by being supportive, calm, and competent.

5. Physical rest reduces myocardial oxygen consumption. Fear and anxiety precipitate the stress response; this results in increased levels of endogenous catecholamines, which increase myocardial oxygen consumption. Also, with increased epinephrine the pain threshold is decreased and pain increases the myocardial oxygen consumption.

(continued)

Nursing Interventions	*Rationale*	*Expected Outcomes*

Nursing Diagnosis: Chest pain related to reduced coronary blood flow

Goal: Relief of chest pain

6. Promote the patient's physical comfort by providing individualized basic nursing care.	6. Physical comfort promotes the patient's sense of well-being and reduces anxiety.	

Nursing Diagnosis: Potential alteration in breathing patterns related to fluid overload

Goal: Absence of respiratory difficulties

1. Initially and every 4 hours, and with chest discomfort, assess, document, and report to the physician abnormal heart sounds (particularly S_3 and S_4 gallops and the holosystolic murmur of left ventricular papillary muscle dysfunction), abnormal breath sounds (particularly crackles), and patient intolerance to specific activities.	1. These data are useful in diagnosing left ventricular failure. Diastolic filling sounds (S_3-S_4 gallop) result from decreased left ventricular compliance associated with myocardial infarction. Papillary muscle dysfunction (from infarction of the papillary muscle) can result in mitral regurgitation and a reduction in stroke volume, leading to left ventricular failure. The presence of crackles (usually at the lung bases) may indicate pulmonary congestion from increased left heart pressures. The association of symptoms and activity can be used as a guide for activity prescription and a basis for patient teaching.	• Patient does not complain of shortness of breath, dyspnea on exertion, orthopnea, or paroxysmal nocturnal dyspnea.
		• Respiratory rate remains less than 20 breaths/min with physical activity and 16 breaths/min with rest.
		• Skin color is normal.
		• PaO_2 and $PaCO_2$ are within normal range.
		• Heart rate is less than 100 beats/min with blood pressure within this patient's normal limits.
		• Chest film normal.
		• Patient reports relief of chest discomfort within 15 to 30 minutes.
		• Appears comfortable:
		   Seems restful
		   Respiratory rate, cardiac rate, and blood pressure return to prediscomfort level.
		   Skin warm and dry

2. Ensure physical rest; use of the bedside commode with assistance; backrest elevated for comfort; full liquid diet as tolerated; arms supported during upper extremity activity; use of stool softener to prevent straining at stool. Teach patient to exhale with physical movement to avoid a Valsalva maneuver, and to practice the relaxation response. Visitor privileges are individualized, based on patient response. Provide a restful environment, and allay fears and anxiety by being supportive, calm, and competent.	2. Physical rest reduces myocardial oxygen consumption. Fear and anxiety precipitate the stress response; this results in increased levels of endogenous catecholamines, which increase myocardial oxygen consumption. Also, with increased epinephrine the pain threshold is decreased and pain increases the myocardial oxygen consumption.	
3. Promote the patient's physical comfort by providing individualized basic nursing care.	3. Physical comfort promotes the patient's sense of well-being and reduces anxiety.	
4. Full liquid diet for 24 hours as prescribed	4. Digestion requires increased cardiac output, which increases the myocardial oxygen consumption. Full liquid diet facilitates digestion because the need to chew has been eliminated, thus requiring less cardiac demand than eating a regular diet.	

(continued)

Nursing Interventions	*Rationale*	*Expected Outcomes*

Nursing Diagnosis: Potential alteration in breathing patterns related to fluid overload

Goal: Absence of respiratory difficulties

5. Teach patient:
   a. To adhere to the diet prescribed (for example, explain low-sodium, low-calorie)

   b. To adhere to activity prescription

a. Low-sodium diet may reduce extracellular volume, thus reducing preload and afterload, and thus myocardial oxygen consumption. In the obese patient, weight reduction may decrease cardiac work and improve tidal volume.

b. The activity prescription is determined individually to maintain the heart rate and blood pressure within safe limits.

Nursing Diagnosis: Potential inadequate tissue perfusion related to decreased cardiac output

Goal: Maintenance/attainment of adequate tissue perfusion

1. Initially and every 4 hours, and with chest discomfort, assess, document and report to the physician the following:
   a. Hypotension
   b. Tachycardia and other dysrhythmia
   c. Fatigability
   d. Mentation changes (use family input)
   e. Reduced urine output (less than 250 ml per 8 hours)
   f. Cool, moist, cyanotic extremities

1. These data are useful in determining a low cardiac output state. An ECG with pain may be useful in the diagnosis of an extension of myocardial ischemia, injury, and infarction, and of variant angina.

- Blood pressure remains within the patient's normal range.
- Ideally, normal sinus rhythm without dysrhythmia is maintained, or patient's baseline rhythm is maintained between 60 and 100 beats/min without further dysrhythmia.
- No complaints of fatigue with prescribed activity
- Patient remains fully alert and oriented and without personality change.
- Appears comfortable
  a. Seems restful
  b. Respiratory rate, cardiac rate, and blood pressure return to prediscomfort level
  c. Skin warm and dry
- Urine output is greater than 40 ml/hr.
- Extremities remain warm and dry with normal color.

2. Ensure physical rest; use of the bedside commode with assistance; backrest elevated to comfort; full liquid diet as tolerated; arms supported during upper extremity activity; use of stool softener to prevent straining at stool. Teach patient to exhale with physical movement to avoid a Valsalva maneuver, and to practice the relaxation response. Visitor privileges are individualized, based on patient response. Provide a restful environment, and allay fears and anxiety by being supportive, calm, and competent.

2. Physical rest reduces myocardial oxygen consumption. Fear and anxiety precipitate the stress response; this results in increased levels of endogenous catecholamines, which increase myocardial oxygen consumption. Also, with increased epinephrine the pain threshold is decreased and pain increases the myocardial oxygen consumption.

(continued)

Nursing Interventions	*Rationale*	*Expected Outcomes*

Nursing Diagnosis: Potential inadequate tissue perfusion related to decreased cardiac output

Goal: Maintenance/attainment of adequate tissue perfusion

3. Promote the patient's physical comfort by providing individualized basic nursing care.	3. Physical comfort promotes the patient's sense of well-being and reduces anxiety.	

Nursing Diagnosis: Anxiety related to fear of death

Goal: Reduction of anxiety

1. Assess, document, and report to the physician the patient's and family's level of anxiety and coping mechanisms.	1. These data provide information about the psychological well-being and a baseline so that post-therapy symptoms can be compared. Causes of anxiety are variable and individual, and may include acute illness, hospitalization, pain, disruption of activities of daily living at home and at work, changes in role and self-image owing to chronic illness, and lack of financial support. Because anxious family members can transmit anxiety to the patient, the nurse must also reduce the family's fear and anxiety.	• Patient reports less anxiety. • Patient and family discuss their anxieties and fears about death. • Patient and family appear less anxious. • Patient appears restful, respiratory rate less than 16/min, heart rate less than 100/min without ectopic beats, blood pressure within patient's normal limits, skin warm and dry. • Patient participates actively in a progressive rehabilitation program. • Practices stress-reduction techniques
2. Assess the need for spiritual counseling and refer as appropriate.	2. If a patient finds support in a religion, religious counseling may assist in reducing anxiety and fear.	

3. Allow patient (and family) to express anxiety and fear:
  a. By showing a genuine interest and concern
  b. By providing a conducive atmosphere
  c. By facilitating communication (listening, reflecting, guiding)
  d. By answering questions
	3. Unresolved anxiety (the stress response) increases myocardial oxygen consumption.	

4. Use of flexible visiting hours allows the presence of a supportive family to assist in reducing the patient's level of anxiety.	4. The presence of supportive family members may reduce both patient's and family's anxiety.	
5. Encourage active participation in a hospital cardiac rehabilitation program	5. Prescribed cardiac rehabilitation may help to eliminate fear of death, may reduce anxiety, and may enhance feelings of well-being.	
6. Teach stress reduction techniques	6. Stress reduction may help to reduce myocardial oxygen consumption and may enhance feelings of well-being.	

Nursing Diagnosis: Potential nonadherence to self-care program related to denial of diagnosis of myocardial infarction

Goal: Adherence to the home health-care program

(See Chart 25-5, p. 548.)

(Adapted from Underhill SL et al. Cardiac Nursing. Philadelphia, JB Lippincott, 1982.)

failure is discussed on p. 581 and the treatment of heart failure on p. 583.)

Prevention. The prevention of rheumatic fever is accomplished by (1) prevention of streptococcal infections, especially in susceptible persons, and (2) early and adequate treatment of streptococcal infections in all persons.

Persons who present a well-documented history of rheumatic fever (or chorea) or who show evidence of rheumatic heart disease should be given continuous prophylaxis with penicillin (or other suitable antibiotic) indefinitely. Such patients must recognize and should accept the fact that they are "rheumatic fever patients," and as such can lead a normal life only if willing to submit to certain limitations and inconveniences. In relation to this facet of patient education, the nurse is in a position to play a very important role.

A first-line approach in preventing initial attacks of rheumatic fever is to recognize streptococcal infections, treat them adequately, and control epidemics in the community. Every nurse should be familiar with the symptoms and signs of streptococcal pharyngitis (see Chart 25-6). *A throat culture is the only method by which accuracy of the diagnosis can be determined.*

Infective Endocarditis

Infective endocarditis (bacterial endocarditis) is an infection of the valves and endothelial surface of the heart caused by direct invasion of bacteria or other organisms and leading to deformity of the valve leaflets. It may be acute, subacute, or chronic. Acute endocarditis usually occurs on normal valves. Causative microorganisms include bacteria (streptococci, enterococci, pneumococci, staphylococci), fungi, and rickettsiae. The subacute form is usually caused by *Streptococcus viridans*.

Etiology. Infective subacute endocarditis usually develops in patients who have a history of valvular heart disease.

Chart 25-6
Prevention of Rheumatic Heart Disease

Rheumatic fever is a preventable disease. By eradication of rheumatic fever, the great cardiac crippler—*rheumatic heart disease*—would be virtually eliminated. Through the use of penicillin therapy in patients with streptococcal infections, almost all primary attacks of rheumatic fever can be prevented. The symptoms and signs of streptococcal pharyngitis are the following:
- Fever (38.9°C to 40°C, or 101°F to 104°F)
- Chilliness
- Sore throat (sudden in onset)
- Diffuse redness of throat with exudate on oropharynx (may not appear until after the first day)
- Enlarged and tender lymph nodes
- Abdominal pain (more common in children)
- Acute sinusitis and acute otitis media (may be due to streptococcus)

At great risk are patients with rheumatic heart disease or mitral valve prolapse and individuals who have had prosthetic-valve surgery.

Hospital-acquired endocarditis occurs most often in patients with debilitating disease, those with indwelling catheters, and those on prolonged intravenous or antibiotic therapy. Patients on immunosuppressive drugs or steroids may develop fungal endocarditis. Therefore, infective endocarditis often accompanies medical and surgical therapy. It is more common in older persons, probably due to decreased immunologic responses to infection, metabolic alterations arising from changes in the aging body, and increased instrumentation, especially in genitourinary disease. There is a high incidence of staphylococcal endocarditis among drug addicts, the disease occurring for the most part on normal valves.

Clinical Manifestations. The onset of infective endocarditis usually is insidious. The signs and symptoms develop from destruction of heart valves, from embolization of fragments of vegetations, and from toxicity of the infection.

The general manifestations, which may be mistaken for influenza, include vague complaints of malaise, anorexia, weight loss, cough, and back and joint pain. Fever is intermittent and may be absent in patients who are receiving antibiotics or corticosteroids or in those who are elderly or have congestive heart failure or uremia. Splinter hemorrhages (linear and hemorrhagic streaks) may be noted under the fingernails and toenails, and petechiae may appear in the conjunctiva and mucous membranes. Hemorrhages with pale centers (Roth's spots) that may be seen in the fundi of the eyes are caused by emboli in the nerve fiber layer of the eye. Osler's nodes (painful, raised, tender, red lesions on the pads of fingers and toes) may occur and are thought to be secondary to acute vasculitis from an immunologic reaction. Janeway's lesions, hemorrhagic macular areas found on the palms or soles, are now thought to be a hypersensitivity reaction or a deposit of immune complex.

The cardiac manifestations include heart murmurs, which may be absent initially. Changing murmurs may be encountered in the acute form and indicate valvular damage due to vegetations or to perforation of the valve or of the chordae tendinae. Heart enlargement or evidences of congestive heart failure are also seen.

The central nervous system manifestations include headache, transient cerebral ischemia, focal neurologic lesions, and strokes, which may be caused by emboli involving the cerebral arteries.

Embolization may be a presenting symptom occurring at any time and involving other organ systems. The embolic phenomena may be manifested in the lung (recurrent pneumonia; pulmonary abscesses), kidney (hematuria; renal failure), spleen (left upper quadrant pain), heart (myocardial infarction, brain (stroke), or peripheral vessels.

Management. The objective of treatment is total eradication of the invading organism by adequate doses of an appropriate antimicrobial. The causative organism can be isolated through serial blood cultures. It is treated with a bactericidal (capable of destroying bacteria) agent or other appropriate drug based on proven sensitivity to the causative agent. The antibiotic is usually given parenterally in a continuous intravenous infusion for a period of 4 to 6 weeks; thus it is important to note on the nursing care plan the date on which the intravenous needle or cannula was inserted. Bactericidal serum levels of the selected antibiotic are monitored by titering it against the causative organism. If the serum does not demonstrate bactericidal activity, increased dosages of the antibiotic are given or a different antibiotic is tried. There are numerous antimicrobial regimens currently in use, but penicillin is usually the drug of choice. Blood cultures are taken periodically to monitor the course of therapy.

Treatment with amphotericin B and surgery with valve replacement are usually required for the patient with fungal endocarditis.

Evaluation of Therapy.   The patient's temperature is monitored at regular intervals, because the course of fever is one indication of the effectiveness of treatment. However, febrile reactions may also occur as a result of drug therapy. After adequate antimicrobial therapy is initiated, bacteria usually disappear. The patient should demonstrate an improved sense of well-being, better appetite, and decreased lethargy. During this time, patients require a great deal of psychosocial support, especially because they feel well but find themselves confined to the hospital with restrictive IV therapy.

Complications.   Even if the patient responds to the antimicrobial therapy, endocarditis can be very destructive to the heart and other organs. Congestive heart failure and cerebral vascular catastrophes may occur before, during, or after therapy. Valve stenosis or regurgitation, myocardial erosion, and mycotic aneurysms are some potential heart complications. Many other organ complications can result from septic or nonseptic emboli, immunologic responses, or hemodynamic deterioration.

Surgery.   The advent of surgical valve replacement has favorably changed the prognosis of patients with severely damaged heart valves. Usually, valve excision and replacement are required for (1) patients who develop congestive heart failure as a result of aortic or mitral valve involvement in spite of adequate medical treatment; (2) patients who have more than one serious systemic embolic episode; and (3) persons with uncontrolled infection, recurrent infection, or fungal endocarditis. A large number of patients who have prosthetic valve endocarditis (infected prostheses) will require valve replacement.

Prevention.   Infective endocarditis occurs most often in persons with structural abnormalities of the heart and great vessels, especially valvular heart disease. Any procedure that is associated with transient bacteremia may cause bacteria to lodge on damaged or abnormal valves. *Persons at risk are patients with structural abnormalities of the heart and great vessels, those with prosthetic heart valves, and patients with most types of congenital heart disease, rheumatic or other acquired valvular heart disease, and idiopathic hypertrophic or subaortic stenosis.*

Antibiotic prophylaxis (usually penicillin, penicillin plus streptomycin, or penicillin plus gentamicin) is recommended for persons at risk who undergo the following procedures and circumstances*:

All dental procedures likely to induce gingival bleeding (not simple adjustment of orthodontic appliances or shedding of deciduous teeth)

Tonsillectomy and/or adenoidectomy
Surgical procedures or biopsy involving respiratory mucosa
Bronchoscopy, especially with a rigid bronchoscope
Incision and drainage of infected tissue
Genitourinary and gastrointestinal procedures

Myocarditis

Acute myocarditis is an inflammatory process involving the myocardium. The heart is a muscle, hence its efficiency depends on the health of the individual muscle fibers. When the muscle fibers are healthy, the heart can function well in spite of severe valvular injuries; when the muscle fibers are poor, life is in jeopardy.

Pathophysiology.   Myocarditis usually results from an infectious process, particularly of viral, bacterial, mycotic, parasitic, protozoal, or spirochetal origin, or it may be produced by hypersensitivity states such as rheumatic fever. Therefore, myocarditis may be seen in patients with acute systemic infections, those receiving immunosuppressive therapy, or those with infective endocarditis.

Myocarditis can cause heart dilatation, mural thrombi, infiltration of circulating blood cells around the coronary vessels and between the muscle fibers, and degeneration of the muscle fibers themselves.

Clinical Manifestations.   The symptoms of acute myocarditis depend on the type of infection, the degree of myocardial damage, and the capacity of the myocardium to recover. Symptoms may be mild or absent. The patient may complain of fatigue and dyspnea, palpitations, and occasional precordial discomfort. Clinical examination may reveal cardiac enlargement, faint heart sounds, gallop rhythm, and a systolic murmur. A pericardial friction rub may be heard if the patient has associated pericarditis. Pulsus alternans (a pulse in which there is a regular alternation of weak and strong beats) may be present. Fever and tachycardia are frequently seen and evidences of congestive heart failure usually develop.

Management.   The patient is given specific treatment for the underlying cause, if it is known (*e.g.*, penicillin for hemolytic streptococci), and is placed on bed rest to decrease cardiac work, that is, to reduce the heart rate, stroke volume, blood pressure, and heart contractility. Bed rest also helps to decrease residual myocardial damage and the complications of myocarditis. The treatment is essentially the same as that used for congestive heart failure (see p. 583). The pulse, heart sounds, and temperature are evaluated to determine whether the disease is subsiding and whether congestive heart failure has occurred. If a dysrhythmia occurs, the patient should be placed in a unit with continuous cardiac monitoring so that personnel and equipment are readily available if a life-threatening dysrhythmia occurs.

When there is evidence of congestive heart failure, digitalis is given to slow the heart rate and augment myocardial contractility.

- Patients with myocarditis are sensitive to digitalis. There must be continuing nursing surveillance to assess the patient for digitalis toxicity (evidenced by dysrhythmia, anorexia, nausea, vomiting, bradycardia, headache, malaise).

---

* From Statement Prepared by the Committee on Prevention of Rheumatic Fever and Bacterial Endocarditis of the American Heart Association. Circulation 1984 Dec; 70:1123A–1127A.

Elastic stockings and passive and active exercises should be used, because embolization from venous thrombosis and mural thrombi can occur.

Patient Education. The prevention of infectious diseases by means of appropriate immunizations and early treatment appears to be important in decreasing the incidence of myocarditis. Following a bout of myocarditis, there is usually some residual heart enlargement. Physical activity is increased slowly, and the patient is instructed to report any symptoms that occur with increasing activity, such as a rapidly beating heart. Competitive sports and alcohol must be avoided.

Pericarditis

Definition and Etiology

Pericarditis refers to an inflammation of the pericardium, the membranous sac enveloping the heart. It may be a primary illness or may develop in the course of a variety of medical and surgical diseases. The following are some of the causes underlying or associated with pericarditis:

1. Idiopathic or nonspecific causes
2. Infection
   a. Bacterial (*e.g.*, streptococcus, staphylococcus, meningococcus, gonococcus)
   b. Viral (*e.g.*, coxsackie, influenza)
   c. Mycotic (fungal) (*e.g.*, rickettsia, parasite)
3. Disorders of connective tissue—systemic lupus erythematosus, rheumatic fever, rheumatoid arthritis, polyarteritis
4. Hypersensitivity states—immune reactions, drug reactions, serum sickness
5. Diseases of adjacent structures—myocardial infarction, dissecting aneurysm, pleural and pulmonary disease (pneumonia)
6. Neoplastic disease
   a. Secondary to metastasis from lung cancer, breast cancer
   b. Leukemia
   c. Following radiation
   d. Primary (mesothelioma)
7. Trauma—chest injury, cardiac surgery, during cardiac catheterization, pacemaker implantation
8. Association with renal disorders (uremia)

Clinical Manifestations

The characteristic symptom of pericarditis is *pain* and the characteristic sign is a *friction rub*. Pain is almost always present in acute pericarditis and is most common over the precordium. The pain may be felt beneath the clavicle and in the neck and left scapular region. Pericardial pain is aggravated by breathing, turning in bed, and twisting the body; it is relieved by sitting up. In fact, the patient prefers to adopt a forward-leaning or a sitting posture. Dyspnea may occur as the result of restriction of the heart contraction, which leads to a decreased cardiac output. The patient may appear extremely ill. Pericarditis *per se* often gives rise to no signs other than fever and the production of a friction rub.

Diagnostic Evaluation

Diagnosis is most often made on the presentation of signs and symptoms. The ECG may be helpful in confirming the diagnosis.

Management

The objectives of management are to determine the cause, to administer therapy for the specific cause (when known), and to be on the alert for *cardiac tamponade* (compression of the heart from fluid in the pericardial sac; see Chap. 26). The patient is placed on bed rest when cardiac output is impaired, until the fever, chest pain, and friction rub have disappeared.

Meperidine or morphine may be given for pain relief during the acute phase. Salicylates relieve pain and hasten reabsorption of fluid in the patient with rheumatic pericarditis. Corticosteroids are sometimes given to control symptoms, hasten resolution of the inflammatory process in the pericardium, and prevent recurring pericardial effusion.

• Be alert to the possibility of cardiac tamponade. Use nursing assessment skills to anticipate and identify the triad of symptoms—falling arterial pressure, rising venous pressure, and distant heart sounds.

Patients with infections of the pericardium are treated with the antimicrobial agent of choice based on identification and sensitivity tests. The pericarditis of rheumatic fever may respond to penicillin. Isoniazid, ethambutol, rifampin, and streptomycin in various combinations are used in the treatment of tuberculosis that produces pericarditis. Amphotericin B is used in fungal pericarditis, and adrenal steroids are used in disseminated lupus erythematosus.

As the patient's condition improves, activity may be increased gradually. However, if pain, fever, or friction rub reappear, bed rest must be resumed.

▶ Nursing Process
The Patient With Pericarditis

▷ Assessment

Pain is the primary distress of the patient with pericarditis. The pain of pericarditis is assessed by observation and by evaluation while having the patient vary positions in bed.

While observing the patient, try to discover whether or not the pain is influenced by respiratory movements, with or without the actual passage of air; by flexion, extension, or rotation of the spine, including the neck; by movements of the shoulders and arms; by coughing; or by swallowing. Recognizing these relationships may be very helpful in establishing a diagnosis.

A pericardial friction rub occurs when the pericardial surfaces lose their lubricating fluid because of inflammation. The rub is audible on auscultation and is synchronous with the heartbeat. A pericardial friction rub is diagnostic of pericarditis and should be searched for diligently.

• Place the diaphragm of the stethoscope tightly against the thorax and listen at the left sternal edge in the fourth intercostal space. This is where the pericardium comes into contact with the left chest wall. A pericardial friction rub has a scratching or leathery sound. The rub is louder at the end of expiration and may be heard best while the patient is sitting.

If there is difficulty in distinguishing a pericardial friction rub from a pleural friction rub, ask the patient to hold his breath. A pericardial friction rub will be continuous.

Monitor the patient's temperature frequently. Pericarditis will cause an abrupt onset of fever in a patient who has been afebrile.

▷ *Nursing Diagnoses*

Based on the assessment data, major nursing diagnoses of the patient may include the following:

- Pain related to inflammation of the pericardium
- Potential development of decreased cardiac output related to restriction of cardiac contraction

▷ *Planning and Implementation*

▷ *Goals:* The major goals of the patient may include relief of pain and maintenance/attainment of cardiac output.

Nursing Interventions

Relief of Pain. Relief of pain is achieved by having this patient remain on bed rest or chair rest, whichever is more comfortable. Because the posture the patient assumes to relieve the pain is that of sitting upright and leaning forward, chair rest may be more comfortable. As the chest pain and friction rub abate, activities of daily living may be resumed gradually.

If the patient is receiving medications for the pericarditis, such as analgesics, antibiotics, or steroids, monitor and record the patient's responses.

If chest pain and the friction rub should recur, have the patient resume bed rest.

Maintenance/Attainment of Adequate Cardiac Output. If the patient does not respond to medical management, fluid may develop or accumulate between the pericardial linings or in the sac. This condition is called *pericardial effusion* (see Chap. 26). Fluid in the pericardial sac can cause constriction of the myocardium and interrupt its ability to pump. Thus, the cardiac output will decline with each contraction. Failure to identify the onset of this problem can lead to cardiac tamponade and the possibility of sudden death.

Early signs and symptoms of this event to watch for are those that indicate a falling arterial pressure. Usually the systolic pressure falls while the diastolic remains stable; hence the pulse pressure narrows. Heart sounds may progress from being distant to being imperceptible. Neck vein distention and other signs of rising central venous pressure are observed. These signs and symptoms occur because, as the fluid-filled pericardial sac compresses the myocardium, blood continues to return to the heart from the periphery but cannot be pumped back into the circulation.

The physician must be notified immediately. The nurse should probably prepare for a pericardiocentesis (see Chap. 26). The nurse stays with the patient and continues to assess and record signs and symptoms until the physician arrives to prescribe more definite therapy.

▷ *Evaluation*

▷ *Expected Outcomes*

1. Patient is free of pain.
   a. Performs activities of daily living comfortably.
   b. Temperature returns to patient's normal range.
   c. Pericardial friction rub is absent.
2. Maintains/attains adequate cardiac output.
   a. Blood pressure remains in patient's normal range.
   b. Heart sounds are of good volume and can be auscultated.
   c. Neck veins are not distended.

Chronic Constrictive Pericarditis

Chronic constrictive pericarditis is a condition in which chronic inflammatory thickening of the pericardium compresses the heart and prevents it from expanding to normal size. The major hemodynamic deficit results from a restriction of ventricular filling.

Often the adherent pericardium becomes calcified. The heart action is greatly restricted by this tough, unyielding enclosure, and edema, ascites, and hepatic enlargement result. The fixation of the heart to the pericardium may produce a retraction of the chest wall with every beat.

Chronic restrictive pericarditis is caused by long-standing pyogenic infections, postviral infections, tuberculosis, or hemopericardium.

The signs and symptoms are predominantly those of congestive heart failure (see p. 581), but dyspnea on effort is the most prominent symptom. Chronic atrial fibrillation is commonly present.

Surgical removal of the tough encasing pericardium (pericardiectomy) is the only treatment of any benefit. The objective of the operation is to release both ventricles from the constrictive and restrictive inflammation. (See Chap. 27 for care of the patient after cardiac surgery.)

Acquired Valvular Diseases of the Heart

The function of normal heart valves is to maintain the forward flow of blood from the atria to the ventricles and from the ventricles to the great vessels. Valvular damage may interfere with valvular function by stenosis (narrowing) of the valve or by impaired closure that allows backward leakage of blood (valvular insufficiency, regurgitation, or incompetence).

Acquired valvular heart disease often is a result of previous rheumatic carditis that has damaged one or more of the heart valves. The mitral valve is involved most frequently, followed by the aortic, tricuspid, and pulmonic valves. If the heart muscle remains strong, the circulatory apparatus can adjust itself efficiently even though a valve is injured badly. The details of such adjustment, called *compensatory changes,* include modifications in the rate and character of the heartbeat, changes in the blood, hypertrophy of the myocardium, redistribution of the blood in the body, and so forth. All of these changes reduce the unfavorable impact of the valve defect.

Mitral Valve Prolapse Syndrome

The mitral valve prolapse syndrome is a dysfunction of the mitral valve leaflets that renders the mitral valve incompetent and results in valvular regurgitation. This syndrome may produce no symptoms or it may progress rapidly and result in sudden death. In recent years the syndrome has been diagnosed more frequently, ostensibly as a result of improved diagnostic methods. Many individuals have the syndrome but no symptoms. Often the symptoms are first identified during a physical examination of the heart, which reveals an extra heart sound referred to as a *mitral click*. The presence of a click indicates early valvular incompetence with disruption of normal blood flow. The mitral click may deteriorate into a murmur over a period of time as the valve leaflets become progressively dysfunctional. Concomitant with the progression of the murmur may be signs and symptoms of heart failure as mitral regurgitation ensues.

Medical management is directed at controlling the associated symptoms. Some persons experience worrisome dysrhythmias and require antidysrhythmic agents. Others experience mild heart failure and require therapy (see p. 583 for a discussion of heart failure). In advanced stages, mitral valve replacement may be necessary.

It is important to educate patients with this syndrome about the need for prophylactic antibiotic therapy before undergoing invasive procedures that may introduce infectious agents systemically (*e.g.*, dental work, GU/GI procedures, IV therapy). If in doubt, patients are advised to consult their physician.

Mitral Stenosis

Mitral stenosis is the progressive thickening and contracture of the mitral valve cusps, which causes narrowing of the orifice and progressive obstruction to blood flow. It is by far the most common of the late cardiac lesions produced by rheumatic fever and is considered the typical lesion.

Pathophysiology. In this disorder, acute rheumatic endocarditis has "glued" the mitral valve flaps (*commissures*) together and, by shortening the chordae tendineae, has pulled the flap edges down almost to the tips of the papillary muscles, greatly narrowing the mitral orifice. Normally, three fingers should pass easily through this orifice, but in cases of marked stenosis a lead pencil will hardly fit through it. The left ventricle is not affected, but the left atrium has great difficulty in emptying itself through the narrow orifice into the ventricle. Therefore, it dilates and hypertrophies. Because no valve protects the pulmonary veins from a backward flow from this atrium, pulmonary circulation becomes markedly congested. As a result of the abnormally high pulmonary arterial pressure that must be maintained by the right ventricle, it is subjected to an unfunctional strain and eventually fails.

Clinical Manifestations. Patients with mitral stenosis are likely to show progressive fatigue as a result of low cardiac output, hemoptysis and dyspnea on exertion due to pulmonary venous hypertension, cough, and repeated respiratory infections.

The pulse is weak and often irregular because of atrial fibrillation caused by the atrium's dilation and hypertrophy. These render the atrium electrically unstable, resulting in a permanent atrial dysrhythmia. Diagnostic aids for the cardiologist are phonocardiography, echocardiography, and cardiac catheterization with angiography to verify the severity of the mitral stenosis.

Management. Antibiotic therapy is instituted to prevent rheumatic recurrences, while developing congestive heart failure is treated with digitalis, sodium restriction, and limitation of activity. Surgical intervention consists of a valvotomy to rupture the fused commissures of the mitral valve or replacement of the mitral valve with a prosthetic valve (see p. 597).

Mitral Insufficiency (Regurgitation)

Mitral insufficiency results when incompetence and distortion of the mitral valve prevent the free margins from coming into apposition during systole. The chordae tendineae may become shortened, preventing complete closure of the leaflets. Valvular movement is more restricted than in mitral stenosis. In about half of the patients, mitral regurgitation is caused by chronic rheumatic heart disease.

Pathophysiology. Shortening or tearing of one or both of the mitral valve flaps prevents the perfect closure of the mitral orifice, while the powerful left ventricle is forcing the blood into the aorta. Then, at each beat the left ventricle forces some of the blood back into its atrium. Because this blood is added to the blood that is beginning to flow into this chamber from the lungs, the left atrium must dilate and hypertrophy. This backward flow of blood from the ventricle also checks the current of blood flowing under low pressure from the lungs. As a result the lungs become congested, which throws an extra strain on the right ventricle. Therefore, the result of even a slight mitral leak always involves both lungs and the right ventricle.

Clinical Manifestations. Palpitation of the heart, shortness of breath on exertion, and cough due to chronic passive pulmonary congestion are common symptoms. The pulse may be regular and of good volume, but frequently it becomes irregular as a result of either extrasystoles or fibrillation, which may persist indefinitely.

Management. Management is the same as that for congestive heart failure (see p. 583). Surgical intervention consists of mitral valve replacement.

Aortic Valve Stenosis

Aortic valve stenosis is the narrowing of the orifice between the left ventricle and the aorta. In adults the stenosis may be congenital, or it may be a result of rheumatic fever or cusp calcification of unknown cause. There is progressive narrowing of the valve orifice over a period of several years to several decades.

Pathophysiology. The obstruction to the aortic outflow places a pressure load on the left ventricle, which shows the strain by a thickening of the muscle wall. The heart muscle increases in size (hypertrophy) in response to all degrees of obstruction, but heart failure occurs when obstruction is severe.

The flaps of the aortic valve fuse and partially close the opening between the heart and the aorta. The left ventricle overcomes this obstruction to circulation by contracting more slowly but with greater energy than normal, forcibly squeezing the blood through the very small orifice. The heart's compensatory mechanisms begin to fail and clinical signs develop.

Clinical Manifestations. In moderate to severe cases of aortic stenosis the patient first experiences exertional dyspnea, which is a manifestation of left ventricular decompensation with pulmonary congestion. Other signs are dizziness and fainting because of reduced volume of blood going to the brain. Angina pectoris is a frequent symptom that results from the increased oxygen demands imposed by the increased work of the left ventricle and by myocardial hypertrophy. Blood pressure may be low, and often there is a low pulse pressure because of diminished blood flow.

On physical examination, a loud, rough systolic murmur may be heard over the aortic area. The sound to listen for is a systolic crescendo–decrescendo murmur, which may radiate into the carotid arteries and to the left ventricular apex. The murmur is low-pitched, rough, rasping, and vibrating. If one rests the hand over the base of the heart, a vibration is felt that is the most intense of all cardiac thrills and resembles the purring of a cat. The purring sound is related to the turbulence caused by the blood flow across a narrowed valve orifice. The evidence of left ventricular hypertrophy may be seen on a 12-lead ECG.

Left-heart catheterization is necessary in order to accurately measure the severity of this valvular abnormality. Pressure tracings are taken from the left ventricle and the base of the aorta. The systolic pressure in the left ventricle is considerably higher than that in the aorta during systole.

Management. A significant risk of sudden death exists for those patients who are treated medically without surgical repair. The uncorrected condition can lead to irreversible heart failure which is intractable to medical therapies. Studies have shown that the average life expectancy is 3 to 4 years from the onset of syncope, 2 to 3 years from the onset of angina, and 18 months to 2 years from the onset of dyspnea and heart failure.

Because the aortic valve cusps fuse and the leaflets become rigid, scarred and, in advanced disease, calcified, it is necessary to repair and restore function through surgery (aortic valve replacement). See Chap. 27 for care of the patient undergoing cardiac surgery.

Aortic Insufficiency (Incompetence; Regurgitation)

Aortic insufficiency is caused by inflammatory lesions that deform the flaps of the aortic valve, preventing them from completely sealing the aortic orifice during diastole and thus allowing a backflow of blood from the aorta into the left ventricle. This valvular defect may follow endocarditis of the rheumatic or bacterial type or may be due to congenital abnormalities or diseases that cause dilatation or tearing of the ascending aorta (syphilitic disease, rheumatoid spondylitis, dissecting aneurysm).

Pathophysiology. Because of the leak in the aortic valve during diastole, some of the blood in the aorta, always under high pressure, hisses back into the left ventricle, which must handle both the blood normally delivered by the left atrium into the ventricle through the mitral orifice and that returning from the aorta. The left ventricle dilates to accommodate this increased volume, hypertrophies in order to expel it, and does so with more than normal force, thus raising systolic blood pressure. By another reflex, the cardiovascular system tends to become accommodated: the peripheral arterioles become relaxed, so peripheral resistance is lessened and diastolic pressure greatly lowered.

Clinical Manifestations. The disease develops insidiously, and the earliest manifestation is awareness of the increased force of the heartbeat. There may be marked arterial pulsations that are visible or palpable over the precordium. Arterial pulsation in the neck will also be marked, the head sometimes bobbing in synchrony with the heartbeat. This is a result of the increased force and volume of the blood ejected from the hypertrophied left ventricle. Exertional dyspnea and easy fatigability follow. Signs and symptoms of left ventricular failure (orthopnea, paroxysmal nocturnal dyspnea) occur with moderate to severe regurgitation.

The pulse pressure (the difference between systolic and diastolic pressures) is considerably widened in these patients. One of the characteristic signs of the disease is the manner in which the pulse strikes the palpating finger with quick, sharp strokes and then suddenly collapses (water-hammer pulse). The nature of the pulse wave is quite unmistakable, since it rises rapidly to a peak and collapses quickly.

Diagnostic Evaluation. The diagnostic method used is cineangiography, in which an opaque medium is injected into the root of the aorta, usually by way of a catheter passed from the femoral artery. In aortic regurgitation, the opaque liquid can be seen passing into the left ventricle from the aorta.

Compensation may remain excellent for a long time, but when the left ventricle dilates because of weakness, a rapid downhill course is initiated.

Management. A major priority is the prevention of infection of the already deformed aortic leaflets. Antimicrobial prophylaxis is used for all dental procedures, any form of instrumentation, and all surgical procedures involving the genitourinary tract, the lower intestinal tract, the gallbladder, and the drainage of infected material.

Aortic valve replacement is the treatment of choice, but the optimal time for valve replacement remains controversial. (Management of the patient undergoing cardiac surgery is discussed in Chap. 27.)

Tricuspid Lesions

Tricuspid stenosis is the restriction of the tricuspid valve orifice as the result of commissural fusion and fibrosis usually following rheumatic fever. It is commonly associated with diseases of the mitral valve.

Tricuspid insufficiency allows the regurgitation of blood from the right ventricle into the right atrium during ventricular systole.

Clinical Manifestations. The symptoms of tricuspid regurgitation are marked. At each beat the right ventricle forces blood in two directions: through the pulmonary valve (the normal direction), and back through the leaking tricuspid valve into the right atrium. The flow of venous blood from the systemic circulation is impeded, causing signs of general cyanosis and overfilling of all the veins of the body.

A pulse wave similar to that sent by the left ventricle throughout the arterial tree may be transmitted into the larger veins. Therefore, the liver, now swollen to perhaps two or three times its normal size, pulsates. The walls of the stomach, intestines, kidneys, and other abdominal organs, because they are turgid with venous blood, cannot function well and produce symptoms of chronic passive congestion. The legs and the dependent portions of the body become edematous. Fluid collects in the abdominal cavity (ascites) and in the pleural cavities (hydrothorax). If the heart responds to medical or surgical therapy, circulation improves, the congestion of the various organs is relieved, and all symptoms may abate.

Management. The treatment consists of surgical treatment of associated mitral valve disease, tricuspid valvuloplasty, or tricuspid valve replacement.

Cardiomyopathies

Definition, Etiology, and Pathophysiology

Myopathy is a disease of muscle. The cardiomyopathies are a group of diseases that affect the structure and function of the myocardium. They are considered to be primary or secondary according to their etiology. The term *primary cardiomyopathy* is used if the condition is of unknown etiology; *secondary cardiomyopathy* indicates that the myocardial involvement results from a systemic disorder such as excessive alcohol intake, infections, metabolic diseases, immune diseases, toxic response, pregnancy, and hypertension.

When the cardiomyopathies are categorized by pathological, physiological, and clinical signs, they are defined as (1) dilated cardiomyopathy, or sometimes congestive cardiomyopathy; (2) hypertrophic cardiomyopathy; and (3) restrictive cardiomyopathy.

Regardless of the category and the etiology, these diseases lead to severe heart failure and often death.

Dilated or *congestive cardiomyopathy* is the most commonly occurring form of the cardiomyopathies. It is distinguished by a dilated and enlarged ventricular cavity along with decreasing muscle wall thickness, left atrial enlargement, and stasis of blood in the ventricle. Microscopic examination of the muscle tissue reveals a diminishing of the contractile elements of the muscle fibers. Excessive alcohol intake is often implicated in this type of cardiomyopathy.

Hypertrophic cardiomyopathy occurs less frequently and is most often associated with idiopathic hypertrophic subaortic stenosis (IHSS). In hypertrophic cardiomyopathies the heart muscle actually increases in mass weight, especially along the septum. The septal size increase may produce obstruction to the flow of blood from the atria to the ventricles; hence, this category is divided further into obstructive and nonobstructive types. Nonobstructive hypertrophic cardiomyopathy is usually associated with hypertension.

The last and least frequently occurring category is *restrictive cardiomyopathy.* This form is seen less frequently than all other forms and is characterized by an impairment of ventricular stretch and hence volume. Restrictive cardiomyopathy can be associated with amyloidosis and other such infiltrative diseases.

Regardless of the distinguishing features, the pathophysiology of cardiomyopathy is a series of progressive events which culminates in impaired pumping of the left ventricle. As the stroke volume becomes less and less, the sympathetic system is stimulated, resulting in increased systemic vascular resistance. As in the pathophysiology of heart failure from any cause, the left ventricle enlarges to accommodate the demands and eventually fails. Failure of the right ventricle usually accompanies this process (see Fig. 25-5).

Clinical Manifestations

The cardiomyopathies may occur at any age and affect both men and women. Most persons with cardiomyopathy present initially with signs and symptoms of heart failure. Dyspnea on exertion, paroxysmal nocturnal dyspnea, cough, and easy fatigability are early symptoms. A physical examination usually indicates systemic venous congestion, jugular vein distention, pitting edema of dependent body parts, hepatic engorgement, and tachycardia.

Diagnostic Evaluation

Diagnosis of cardiomyopathy is usually made from findings revealed by patient history and by ruling out other causes of the failure, such as myocardial infarction. There is no specific test which is best for diagnosing cardiomyopathy. The ECG will demonstrate changes consistent with left ventricular hypertrophy. The echocardiogram is probably one of the most helpful diagnostic tools in that the functioning of the left ventricle can be observed easily. Cardiac catheterization is sometimes used to rule out coronary artery disease as a causative factor.

Medical Management

Medical management is directed toward correcting the heart failure. When heart failure has progressed beyond being medically responsive, heart transplant is the patient's only hope for survival. (See Chap. 27.)

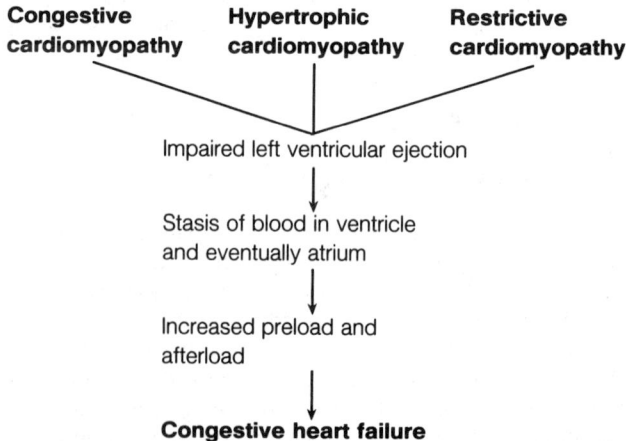

Figure 25-5
Cardiomyopathy and the development of congestive heart failure.

▶ *Nursing Process*
The Patient With Cardiomyopathy

▷ *Assessment*

The nursing assessment for the patient with cardiomyopathy begins with a detailed history of the presenting signs and symptoms. Because of the chronic nature of this problem, a careful psychosocial history is also important. The patient's family support system should be identified very early and involved in the management of the patient.

The physical assessment should be directed toward signs and symptoms of congestive heart failure. A careful evaluation of fluid volume status, vital signs (including calculation of pulse pressure), and auscultation for an S_3 are all extremely important in a baseline assessment. The physician may want to place the patient on a cardiac monitor; however, when the diagnosis is made and dysrhythmia is not a significant problem, the patient may not need to be monitored. The acuteness of the heart failure will determine whether or not the patient needs to be in a critical care environment.

▷ *Nursing Diagnoses*

Based on the assessment data, major nursing diagnoses for the patient may include the following:

- Potential alteration in breathing pattern related to myocardial failure
- Activity intolerance related to excessive fluid volume
- Anxiety related to the disease process
- Potential nonadherence to the self-care program

▷ *Planning and Implementation*

▷ *Goals:* The major goals of the patient include absence of respiratory difficulties, increased activity tolerance, reduction of anxiety, and adherence to a self-care program.

Nursing Interventions

Absence of Respiratory Difficulties. Because many of the patient's signs and symptoms are corrected by pharmacological agents, attention to the timeliness of administration of prescribed medications is vitally important. Careful documentation of the patient's response is critical.

Supporting respiratory exchange with oxygen by way of nasal prongs is indicated.

The patient may be more comfortable if allowed to rest at the bedside in a chair. This position will be helpful in pooling venous blood in the periphery and reducing preload. Helping the patient to keep warm and to change position frequently will stimulate circulation and reduce the possibility of skin breakdown. Maintaining an environment free of dust, lint, flowers, and such will also support easier respiratory exchange.

Increased Activity Tolerance. Planning nursing care so that the patient participates frequently in activities of short duration is important. Allowing the patient to accomplish a goal, no matter how small, will also enhance his sense of well-being. For example, working with the patient to deter-mine what part of the bath can be completed without aid, and then providing a period of rest before the nurse completes the bath, will help the patient conserve energy which is in short supply. Minimize or abolish activities that deplete the patient's energy.

Reduction of Anxiety. Provide the patient with appropriate information about his signs and symptoms. Assist him to accomplish certain activities for himself. Provide an atmosphere in which he feels free to verbalize his fears, and let him know that his concerns are legitimate. If the patient is facing death or awaiting transplant surgery, allow him all the time he requires to discuss his concerns. Spiritual support may be indicated for the patient and his significant others.

Adherence to a Self-Care Program. It is particularly important for the patient with cardiomyopathy to learn what self-care activities are necessary and how to perform them at home. An optimum health status is very desirable should the patient be a candidate for a heart transplant. Satisfactory improvement can be obtained by meticulous attention to a medication program, which usually consists of several different medications to maintain a state free of cardiac failure.

The nurse can be integral to the process as patients review life-style and work to incorporate the above therapeutic activities with minimal intrusion. Helping patients to accept their disease status will facilitate their adherence to a self-care program at home.

Establishing trust is vital to the relationship with these chronically ill and debilitated patients. Providing realistic hope helps reduce their anxiety while awaiting a donor heart when transplant is an acceptable treatment modality.

When a patient can no longer be helped by any therapeutic technique, allowing the patient and significant others the freedom to begin the grieving process is vitally important.

▷ *Evaluation*

▷ *Expected Outcomes*

1. Patient demonstrates improved respiratory function:
   a. Respiratory rate is within normal limits.
   b. Blood gases are normal.
2. Increases actvity tolerance.
   a. Carries out activities of daily living, *e.g.*, brushes teeth, feeds self.
   b. Transfers self from chair to bed.
3. Experiences reduction of anxiety.
   a. Discusses prognosis freely.
4. Adheres to a program of self-care.
   a. Takes medications according to prescribed schedule.
   b. Modifies life-style to accommodate activity limitations.
   c. Identifies signs and symptoms to be reported to the health-care professional.

Bibliography

Books

Abels L. Critical Care Nursing. St Louis, CV Mosby, 1986.
Andreoli K et al. Comprehensive Cardiac Care. St Louis, CV Mosby, 1984.

Basta L. Cardiovascular Disease—Essentials of Primary Care. New York Medical Examination Publishing, 1983.

Beamish RE, Singal PK, and Dhalla N. Stress and Heart Disease. Boston, Martinus Nijhoff, 1984.

Berman N. Geriatric Cardiology. Lexington, The Collamore Press, 1982.

Bigger JT. A Primer on Calcium Ion Antagonists. Whippany, New Jersey, Knoll Pharmaceutical Co, 1981.

Braunwald E. Heart Disease: A Textbook of Cardiovascular Disease. Philadelphia, WB Saunders, 1984.

Chernow B. The Pharmacologic Approach to the Critically Ill Patient. Baltimore, Williams & Wilkins, 1983.

Coodley EL (ed). Geriatric Heart Disease. Littleton, PSG Publishing, 1985.

Cornett SJ and Watson JE. Cardiac Rehabilitation—An Interdisciplinary Team Approach. New York, John Wiley & Sons, 1984.

Das Gupta D. Principles and Practice of Acute Cardiac Care. Chicago, Year Book Medical Publishers, 1984.

Douglas MK and Shinn JA. Advances in Cardiovascular Nursing. Rockville, Maryland, Aspen Systems, 1985.

Feldman EB (ed). Nutrition and Heart Disease. New York, Churchill Livingstone, 1983.

Guzetta EC and Dossey BM. Cardiovascular Nursing: Bodymind Tapestry. St Louis, CV Mosby, 1984.

Hojnacki, LH and Halfman–Franey M. Handbook of Cardiac Rehabilitation for Nurses and Other Health Professionals. Reston, Virginia, Prentice-Hall, 1985.

Holloway N. Nursing the Critically Ill Adult. Menlo Park, California, Addison-Wesley, 1984.

Hurst JW (ed). The Heart. New York, McGraw-Hill, 1982.

King SB and Douglas SJ. Coronary Arteriography and Angioplasty. New York, McGraw-Hill, 1985.

Kloner R. The Guide to Cardiology. New York, John Wiley & Sons, 1984.

Meltzer LE, Pinneo R, and Kitchell JR. Intensive Coronary Care: A Manual for Nurses. Bowie, Maryland, Prentice-Hall, 1983.

Messerli FH. Cardiovascular Disease in the Elderly. Boston, Martinus Nijhoff, 1984.

Nursing Photobook: Giving Cardiac Care. Springhouse, Pennsylvania, Springhouse Corporation, 1983.

Price S and Wilson L. Pathophysiology—Clinical Concepts of Disease Process. New York, McGraw-Hill, 1986.

Sadler D. Nursing for Cardiovascular Health. Norwalk, Appleton-Century-Crofts, 1984.

Sanderson RG and Kurth CL. The Cardiac Patient—A Comprehensive Approach. Philadelphia, WB Saunders, 1983.

Silver MD. Cardiovascular Pathology, Vol 1. New York, Churchill Livingstone, 1983.

Silver MD. Cardiovascular Pathology, Vol 2. New York, Churchill Livingstone, 1983.

Underhill SL et al. Cardiac Nursing. Philadelphia, JB Lippincott, 1982.

Warren JV and Lewis RP. Diagnostic Procedures in Cardiology. Chicago, Year Book Medical Publishers, 1985.

Wells SJ (ed). Manual of Cardiovascular Assessment. Reston, Virginia, Reston Publishing Co, 1983.

Woods SL. Cardiovascular Critical Care Nursing. New York, Churchill Livingstone, 1983.

Yee BH and Zorb SL. Cardiac Critical Care Nursing. Boston, Little, Brown, & Co, 1986.

Yurick et al. The Aged Person and the Nursing Process. Norwalk, Appleton-Century-Crofts, 1984.

Articles

(Asterisks indicate nursing research articles.)

Coronary Artery Disease

Ackley E and Valentine S. Smoking cessation by patients with coronary artery disease. Focus Crit Care 1985 April; 12(2):50–55.

Casdorph HR. Abnormal lipid values and family history of heart disease: Prevention management. JAMA 1985 Feb 22; 253(8):1185.

Cholesterol and Your Heart (pamphlet). American Heart Association, 1984.

Consensus Conference. Lowering cholesterol to prevent heart disease. JAMA 1985 Apr 12; 253(14):2080–2086.

Coronary risk factor statement for the American public. American Heart Association, Dallas, Texas, 1985.

Gilliss CL. Events leading to the treatment of coronary artery disease: Implications for nursing care. Heart Lung 1984 July; 14(4):350–356.

Hallad J. Caffeine: Is it hazardous to your patient's health? Nursing '86 1986 April; 86(4):423–425.

Heart Facts 1986 (pamphlet). American Heart Association, 1985.

Hennekens C and Burning J. Smoking and coronary heart disease in women. JAMA 1985 May 24; 253(20):3003–3004.

Kannel WB. Nutritional contributors to cardiovascular disease in the elderly. J Am Geriatric Soc 1986 Jan; 34(1):27–36.

Pinneo R. Living with coronary artery disease. The nurse's role. Nurs Clin North Am 1984 Sept; 19(3):459–467.

Sex and Heart Disease (pamphlet). American Heart Association, 1983.

Shea S. Family history: A risk factor for coronary heart disease? Primary Cardiology 1985 Dec; 11(2):109–116.

Smoking and Heart Disease (pamphlet). American Heart Association, 1981.

Angina

Boden WE, Korr KS, and Bough EW. Nifedipine-induced hypotension and myocardial ischemia in refractory angina pectoris. JAMA 1985 Feb 22; 253(8):1131–1135.

Conti R. Unstable angina before and after infarction: Thoughts on pathogenesis and therapeutic strategies. Heart Lung 1986 July; 15(4):361–367.

Foley J and Brown G. Nursing management of the patient with coronary artery spasm. Cardiovasc Nurs 1984 Sept/Oct; 5(5):25–29.

Glasbrenner K. Calcium channel antagonists. JAMA 1985 Apr 19; 253(15):2179–2180.

Goldsmith M. Recombinant plasminogen agent continues to show promise. JAMA 1985 Feb; 253(17):2555–2557.

Kafla KR et al. Antianginal agents. Part 1: Ischemic heart disease and the role of nitrates. Hosp Formul 1985 Nov; 20(11):1144–1153.

Kupersmith J and Slater W. Calcium channel blockers: Pharmacologic basis for therapeutic properties. Hosp Formul 1985 Feb; 20(2):184–195.

Loan T. Nursing interaction with patients undergoing coronary angioplasty. Heart Lung 1986 July; 16(4):368–375.

Mullin SM. Percutaneous transluminal angioplasty (PTCA). Occ Health Nurs 1984 Feb; 32(2):75–77.

Prolonging the protection after unstable angina. Emergency Medicine 1986 Feb 28; 18(4):65–66.

Renlund DG and Gerstenblith G. Angina: Current approaches to diagnosis, drug therapy, and surgical referral. Geriatrics 1986 Jan; 41(1):35–45.

Sipperly ME. Thrombolytic therapy update. Crit Care Nurse 1985 Nov/Dec; 5(6):30–57.

Strauss E and Rudy E. Tissue-plasminogen activator: A new drug in reperfusion therapy. Crit Care Nurse 1986 May/Jun; 6(3):30–42.

Touboukian JE. Calcium channel blocking agents: Physiologic basis of nursing intervention. Heart Lung 1985 July; 14(4):342–349.

Wescott BL and Yee SC. Intravenous fibrinolytic therapy in a community hospital. Focus Crit Care 1986 Feb; 13(1):33–37.

Myocardial Infarction

Alpert JS. Cardiovascular diseases. JAMA 1985 Oct 25; 254(16):2264–2267.

Bayer et al. Changing presentation of myocardial infarction with increasing old age. J Am Geriatr Soc 1986 Apr; 34(4):263–266.

Becker S. Monitoring the patient with acute myocardial infarction. Crit Care Update 1983 Sept; 10(9):18–26.

Burggraf V and Donlon B. Assessing the elderly, Part 1. Am J Nurs 1985 Sept; 85(9):974–984.

Burggraf V and Donlon B. Assessing the elderly, Part 2. Am J Nurs 1985 Oct; 85(10):1103–1111.

Burke LJ et al. Nursing diagnosis indicators and intervention in an out-patient cardiac rehabilitation program. Heart Lung 1986 Jan; 15(1): 70–76.

Dennison R. Cardiopulmonary assessment. Nursing '86 1986 Apr; 16(4): 58–63.

Forshee T. Track down the what, where, when, and how of chest pain. Nursing '86 1986 May; 16(5):34–41.

Gloag D. Rehabilitation of patients with cardiac conditions. Br Med J 1985 Feb; 290(28):618–620.

*Hentinen M. Need for instruction and support of the wives of patients with myocardial infarction. J Adv Nurs 1983 Nov; 8(6):510–524.

Holm E et al. The cardiac patient and exercise: A sociobehavioral analysis. Heart Lung 1985 Nov; 14(6):586–593.

Lewis VC. Monitoring the patient with acute myocardial infarction. Nurs Clin North Am 1987 Mar; 22(1):15–32.

*McMahon M et al. Life situations, health benefits, and medical regimen adherence of patients with myocardial infarction. Heart Lung 1986 Jan; 15(1):82–86.

*Mickus D. Activities of daily living in women after myocardial infarction. Heart Lung 1986 July; 15(4):376–381.

Stanley M. Cardiovascular physiology in the elderly. Crit Care Nurse 1985 Nov/Dec; 5(6):69–71.

Taylor DL. Assessing heart sounds. Nursing '85 1985 Jan; 15(1):51–53.

Vaughn P. Bedside assessment of the myocardial infarction patient. Crit Care Nurse 1984 Mar/Apr; 4(2):60–77.

Webb C. Myocardial infarction. Geriatrics 1986 Jan; 41(1):89–100.

Weisfeldt M. The aging heart. Hosp Prac 1985 Feb 15; 20(2):115–130.

Yacone L. Acute M.I.: The first crucial hours. RN 1986 Jan; 49(1):20–27.

Yacone L. Acute M.I.: The road to recovery. RN 1986 Feb; 49(6):45–51.

Infectious/Valvular

Cash J and Grissett G. Mitral valve prolapse syndrome. Focus Crit Care 1985 Dec; 12(6):54–57.

Dean G. Mitral valve prolapse. Hosp Prac 1985 Sept 15; 20(9):75–83.

Guntheroth WG. Infective endocarditis: The role of dental procedures. Primary Cardiology 1986 May; 12(5):19–26.

Kotler MN et al. Severity of nonrheumatic mitral regurgitation. Primary Cardiology 1985 Feb; 11(2):66–76.

Leonard JJ and Shaver JA. Acute mitral insufficiency. Hosp Practice 1985 May 30; 20(5):75–96.

Morrow A. Hypertrophic subaortic stenosis. J Thorac Cardiovasc Surg 1978 Oct; 76(4):423–430.

Statement prepared by the Committee on Prevention of Rheumatic Fever and Bacterial Endocarditis of the American Heart Association. Circulation 1984 Dec; 70(6).

Weinstein L. A case of modern infective endocarditis. Hosp Prac 1985 May 15; 20(5):86A–86JJ.

Cardiomyopathy

Bullas J. Understanding hypertrophic cardiomyopathy. Crit Care Nurse 1984 May; 4(3):102–106.

Cardin S and Clark S. A nursing diagnosis approach to the patient awaiting cardiac transplantation. Heart Lung 1985 Sept; 15(5):499–504.

Child J. Echocardiographic evaluation of cardiomyopathies. Appl Rad 1984 March/April; 13(2):103, 105, 108.

Figulla HR and Kreuzer H. Biopsy findings and prognosis for congestive cardiomyopathy. Cardiology Board Review 1985 Dec; 2(6):71–76.

Oakley C. Clinical decisions in the cardiomyopathies. Hosp Pract 1985 October 15; 20(10):41–60.

Painvin GA et al. Cardiac transplantation: Indications, procurement, operation, and management. Heart Lung 1984 Sept; 14(5):484–489.

Sanzobrino B and Lemberg L. The cardiomyopathies. Heart Lung 1986 July; 15(4):416–419.

Topol EJ and Traill T. Hypertrophic cardiomyopathy with normal systolic function in the elderly. Cardiology Board Review 1985 Sep/Oct; 2(5):83–95.

Wingate S. Dilated cardiomyopathy, Part 1. Focus Crit Care 1984 Aug; 11(4):49–56.

Wingate S. Dilated cardiomyopathy, Part 2. Focus Crit Care 1984 Oct; 11(5):59–68.

Agencies

Governmental

National Heart, Lung, and Blood Institute; National Institutes of Health, Building 31, Room 5A52, Bethesda, Maryland 20892.

Voluntary

American Heart Association, 7220 Greenville Avenue, Dallas, Texas 75231.

Coronary Club, 3659 Green Road, Cleveland, Ohio 44122.

Heartlife, P.O. Box 54305, Atlanta, Georgia 30308.

Chapter 26

Management of Patients With Complications of Cardiac Disorders

Cardiac Complications: Overview

The complications of cardiac diseases are responsible for many deaths from heart disease. The most common complications are dysrhythmias, acute pulmonary edema, cardiac failure, cardiogenic shock, thromboembolic episodes, and myocardial rupture. The goals of medical and nursing management of patients with heart disease are the prevention of complications and the early identification of signs and symptoms that signal the onset of a complication.

Dysrhythmias are the most common complication of cardiac disease. They may vary in severity from a benign premature beat to a malignant and fatal ventricular fibrillation. Mobile intensive care units, new drug therapies, and increasingly sophisticated pacemakers have all contributed to improvement in the control of compromising dysrhythmias.

Cardiac failure, which covers a spectrum of complications from acute pulmonary edema to cardiogenic shock, remains a leading cause of cardiac morbidity and mortality. The factor of greatest importance in cardiac failure is the extent of myocardial fiber damage. The severity of failure will be directly proportional to the extent of damaged muscle mass.

Though not as common because of more aggressive activity programs for patients with heart disease, thromboembolic episodes still occur. The cerebral, renal, femoral, mesenteric, and pulmonary arteries are most often affected.

Myocardial rupture, too, is rare. It presents itself often enough, however, that observing for signs and symptoms in the high-risk patient population is critical.

All complications of cardiac diseases can result in cardiac arrest. Cardiopulmonary resuscitation is the treatment of choice and is a skill that is essential for all health-care workers.

The best resource in the prevention of complications is nursing care that involves early recognition and reporting of cardinal signs and symptoms of the various complications.

Dysrhythmias

A dysrhythmia is a disorder of the heartbeat that may include a disturbance of rate, rhythm, or both. Dysrhythmias are derangements of the heart's conduction system and not of heart structure. Dysrhythmias are identified by analyzing ECG waveforms. They are named according to the site of impulse origin and the mechanism of conduction involved. For example, a dysrhythmia that originates in the sinus node (SA node) and is slow in rate is called sinus bradycardia. There are four possible sites of origin, as indicated in Chart 26-1. Note also the possible altered conduction mechanisms that can occur.

Properties of Cardiac Muscle

The cardiac muscle possesses the physiological properties of excitability, automaticity, conductivity, and contractility.

Excitability is the ability of a myocardial cell to respond to a stimulus; *automaticity* allows a cell to reach a threshold potential and generate an impulse without being stimulated by another source. *Conductivity* refers to the ability of the muscle to move an impulse from cell to cell. *Contractility* allows the muscle to shorten when stimulated.

When all of these properties are functioning without deviations, the heart muscle is stimulated by impulses originating in the sinus node; hence, *the sinus node is referred to as the heart's pacemaker*. If disequilibrium occurs in one of the heart's basic properties, a dysrhythmia may result. The disequilibrium can be caused by normal activity such as exercise or by a pathologic occurrence such as a myocardial infarction. In myocardial infarction, because reduced oxygenation to the myocardium can increase excitability, the myocardium has an increased response to stimuli. This is an example of one of the most common causes of a dysrhythmia.

Normal Conduction Pathway. Once an impulse originates in the sinus node, a normal electrical pathway is followed. The impulse travels from the sinus node through the atria to the AV node or junction, which also includes the bundle of His. The impulse is delayed in time at the AV node to allow the ventricles to fill with blood. From the AV node the impulse travels very quickly through the bundle branches, terminating in the Purkinje fibers of the ventricular walls to initiate systole. The cycle begins again. It is important to remember that an electrical stimulus is followed by a mechanical event of the heart (see Chap. 24).

Autonomic Nervous System. The heart is under the control of the autonomic nervous system, which consists of sympathetic and parasympathetic fibers. The *sympathetic* system is also referred to as *adrenergic*, a word derived from the root word adrenalin. Thus, stimulation of the sympathetic system accelerates heart rate, raises blood pressure, and enhances the force of myocardial contraction. *Parasympathetic* stimulation, conversely, slows the heart rate, lowers blood pressure, and reduces the force of contraction.

Manipulation of the autonomic nervous system forms the foundation for much of the drug therapy in dysrhythmia control, *e.g.*, β-adrenergic blockers.

Dysrhythmias Originating in the Sinus Node

Sinus Bradycardia

Sinus bradycardia may be due to vagal stimulation, digitalis intoxication, increased intracranial pressure, or MI. It is also seen in highly trained athletes, in persons in severe pain, in persons under medication (propranolol, reserpine, methyldopa), in hypoendocrine states (myxedema, Addison's disease, panhypopituitarism), in anorexia nervosa, in hypothermia, and after surgical damage to the SA node.

The following are characteristics of this dysrhythmia (Fig. 26-1):

Rate: 40 to 60 beats per minute.
P waves: Precede each QRS complex; PR interval normal
QRS complex: Usually normal
Conduction: Usually normal
Rhythm: Regular

All characteristics of sinus bradycardia are the same as those of normal sinus rhythm, except for the rate. If slow heart rate is causing significant hemodynamic changes with resultant syncope, angina, or ectopic dysrhythmias, then treatment is directed toward increasing the heart rate. If the decrease in heart rate is due to vagal stimulation such as bearing down at stool or vomiting, attempts are made to prevent further vagal stimulation. If the patient has digitalis intoxication, then digitalis is withheld. The drug of choice in treating sinus bradycardia is atropine. Atropine blocks vagal stimulation, thus allowing a normal rate to occur.

Sinus Tachycardia

Sinus tachycardia may be caused by fever, acute blood loss, anemia, shock, exercise, congestive heart failure (CHF), pain, hypermetabolic states, anxiety, or sympathomimetic or parasympatholytic drugs. The ECG pattern is as follows (Fig. 26-2):

Rate: 100 to 180 beats per minute
P waves: Precede each QRS complex; may be buried in the preceding T wave; PR interval normal
QRS complex: Usually has a normal interval
Conduction: Usually normal
Rhythm: Regular

All aspects of sinus tachycardia are the same as those of normal sinus rhythm, except for the rate.

Carotid sinus pressure may be effective in slowing the rate temporarily, and thereby help to rule out other dysrhyth-

---

Chart 26-1
Identification of Dysrhythmias by Site of Origin

Sites of Origin	*Mechanisms of Conduction*
Sinus node	Bradycardia
Atria	Tachycardia
AV node or junction	Flutter
Ventricles	Fibrillation
	Premature beats
	Heart blocks

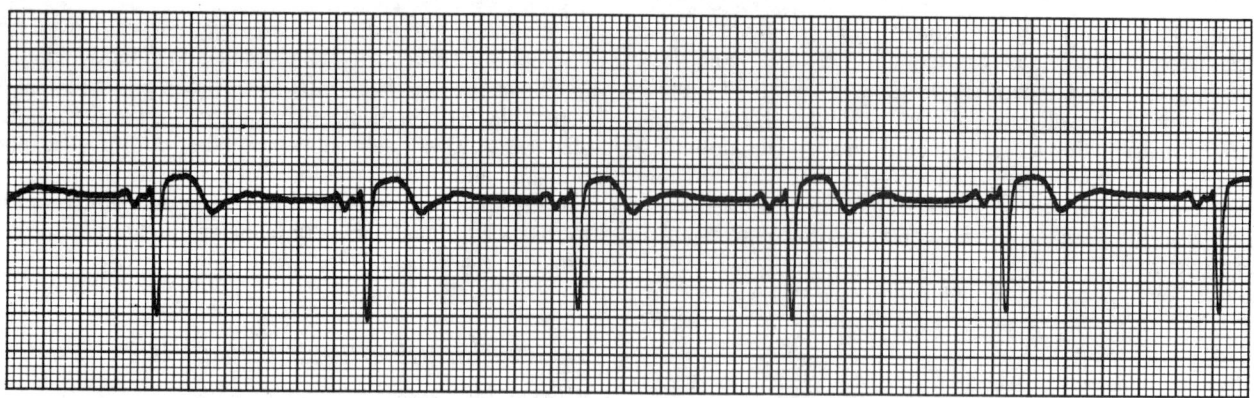

Figure 26-1
Sinus bradycardia.

mias. As heart rate increases, diastolic filling time decreases, resulting in reduced cardiac output and subsequent symptoms of syncope, fainting, and low blood pressure. If the rapid rate persists and the heart is unable to compensate for the decreased ventricular filling, the patient may develop acute pulmonary edema.

Treatment of sinus tachycardia is usually directed at abolishing the cause. Propranolol (Inderal) may be used if rapid reduction of rate is necessary. Propranolol blocks the effect of adrenergic fibers, thus slowing the rate.

Dysrhythmias Originating in the Atrial Muscle

Premature Atrial Contractions

Premature atrial contractions (PACs) may be due to atrial muscle irritability caused by caffeine; alcohol; nicotine; stretched atrial myocardium as in congestive heart failure (CHF); stress or anxiety; hypokalemia; atrial ischemia, injury, or infarction; and hypermetabolic states.

Premature atrial contractions have the following characteristics (Fig. 26-3):

Rate: 60 to 100 beats per minute.
P waves: Usually have a configuration different from that of the P waves that originate in the SA node. Another site in the atria has become irritable (enhanced automaticity) and fires before the normal firing time of the SA node. PR interval may vary from the PR intervals of impulses originating in the SA node.
QRS complex: May be normal, aberrant, or absent. If the ventricles have completed their repolarization phase, they can respond to this early stimulus from the atria.
Conduction: Usually normal.
Rhythm: Regular, except when the PACs occur. The P wave will be early in the cycle and usually will not have a complete compensatory pause. (Time between the preceding complex and the following complex is less than the time for two R–R intervals.)

Premature atrial contractions are frequently seen in normal hearts. The patient may say that the heart "skipped a beat." A pulse deficit (the difference between apical and radial pulse rate) may exist. If PACs are infrequent, no treatment is necessary. If they are frequent (more than 6 per min-

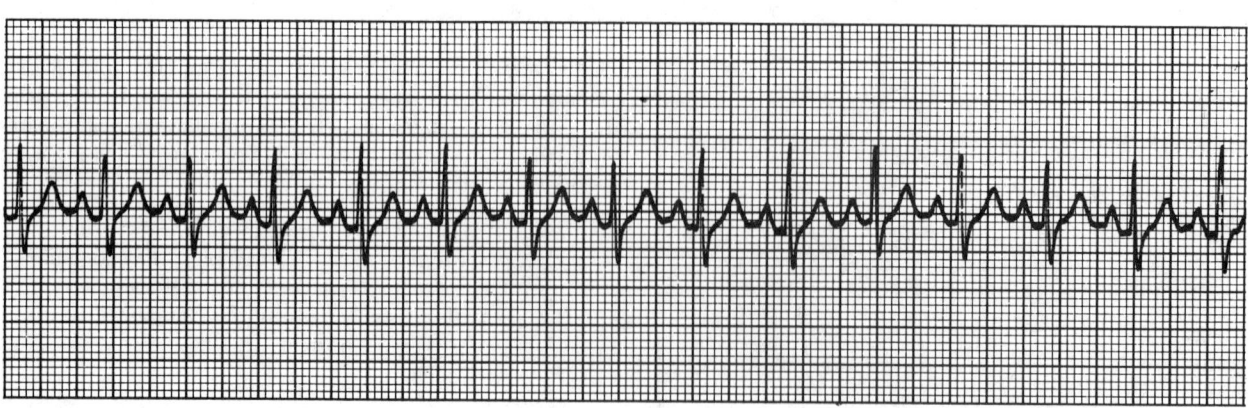

Figure 26-2
Sinus tachycardia.

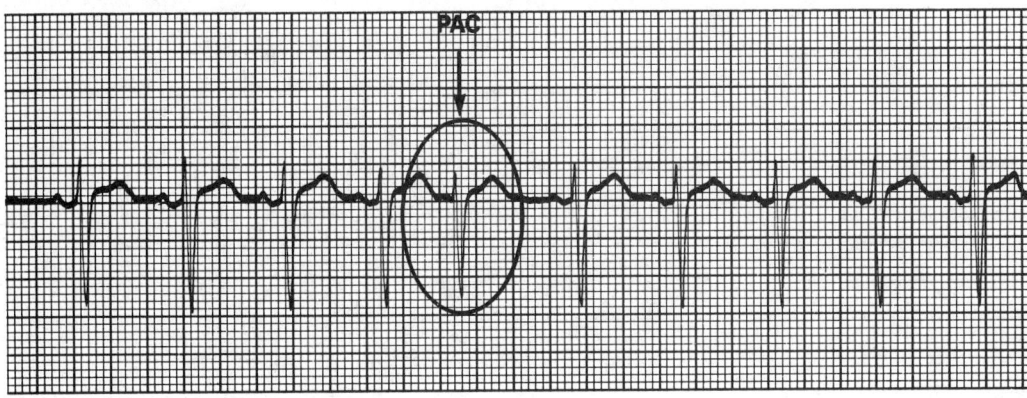

Figure 26-3
Premature atrial contraction.

ute) or occur during atrial repolarization, this may herald more serious dysrhythmias such as atrial fibrillation. Again, treatment is directed toward the cause.

Paroxysmal Atrial Tachycardia

Paroxysmal atrial tachycardia is characterized by abrupt onset and abrupt cessation. Rhythm may be triggered by emotions, tobacco, caffeine, fatigue, sympathomimetic drugs, or alcohol. Paroxysmal atrial tachycardia is not usually associated with organic heart disease. The rapid rate may produce angina due to decreased coronary artery filling. Cardiac output is reduced and heart failure may occur. The patient frequently does not tolerate this rhythm for long periods.

Paroxysmal atrial tachycardia is characterized by the following (Fig. 26-4):

Rate: 150 to 250 beats per minute
P waves: Ectopic and distorted as compared to normal P wave; may be found in the preceding T wave; PR interval shortened (less than 0.12 second)
QRS complex: Usually normal, but may be distorted if aberrant conduction is present
Conduction: Usually normal
Rhythm: Regular

The patient may not be aware of paroxysmal atrial tachycardia. Treatment is directed toward eliminating the cause and decreasing the heart rate. Morphine sedation may slow the rate without further treatment. Carotid sinus pressure usually slows the rate or stops the attack and is usually more effective after digitalis or vasopressors. The use of vasopressors has a reflex effect on the carotid sinus by elevating the blood pressure and thus slowing the heart rate. Short-acting digitalis preparations may be used. Propranolol may be tried if digitalis is unsuccessful. Quinidine may be effective, or the calcium channel blocker verapamil (Calan) can be used. Cardioversion may be necessary if the patient does not tolerate the fast heart rate.

Atrial Fibrillation

Atrial fibrillation (disorganized and uncoordinated twitching of atrial musculature) is usually associated with atherosclerotic heart disease, rheumatic heart disease, CHF, thyrotoxicosis, cor pulmonale, or congenital heart disease.

Atrial fibrillation (Fig. 26-5) is characterized by the following:

Rate: An atrial rate of 350 to 600 beats per minute; ventricular response usually 120 to 200 beats per minute.

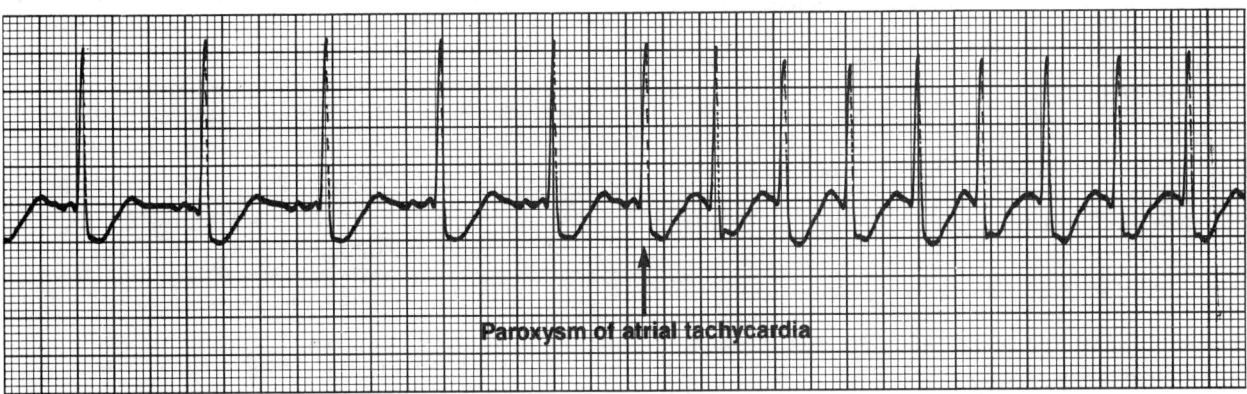

Figure 26-4
Paroxysmal atrial tachycardia.

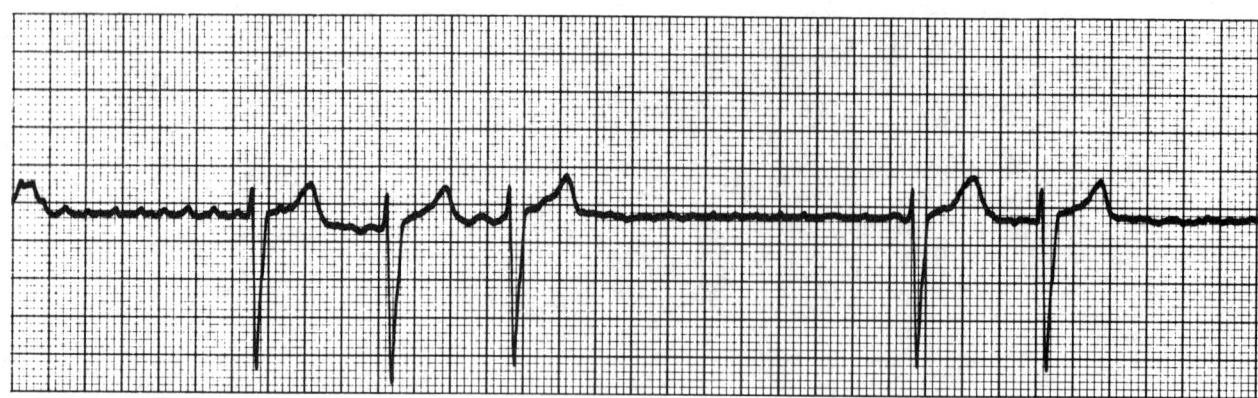

Figure 26-5
Atrial fibrillation.

P waves: No discernible P waves; irregular undulation, termed fibrillary or "f" waves, is seen; PR interval cannot be measured.
QRS complex: Usually normal.
Conduction: Usually normal through the ventricles. Characterized by an irregular ventricular response, because the AV node is incapable of responding to the rapid atrial rate. Impulses that are transmitted cause the ventricles to respond irregularly.
Rhythm: Irregular and usually rapid, unless controlled. Irregularity of rhythm is due to concealed conduction within the AV node.

A rapid ventricular response reduces the time for ventricular filling and hence the stroke volume. The atrial kick, which is 25% to 30% of the cardiac output, is also lost. Congestive heart failure frequently follows. There is usually a *pulse deficit,* the numerical difference between apical and radial pulse rates.

Treatment is directed toward eliminating the cause, decreasing the atrial irritability, and decreasing the rate of the ventricular response. In patients with chronic atrial fibrillation, anticoagulant therapy may be used to prevent thromboemboli from forming in the atria.

At times a mixture of atrial flutter and atrial fibrillation is seen, sometimes called atrial flutter-fibrillation or coarse atrial fibrillation. Such a dysrhythmia is best classified as atrial fibrillation when the criteria for atrial flutter are not satisfied.

Drugs of choice to treat atrial fibrillation are similar to those used in the treatment of paroxysmal atrial tachycardia (PAT). A digitalis preparation is used to slow the heart rate, and an antidysrhythmic such as quinidine is used to correct the dysrhythmia.

Dysrhythmias Originating in the Ventricular Muscle

Premature Ventricular Contractions

Premature ventricular contractions (PVCs) are the result of increased automaticity of the ventricular muscle cells. PVCs can be due to digitalis intoxication, hypoxia, hypokalemia, fever, acidosis, exercise, or increased circulating catecholamines.

Infrequent PVCs are not serious in themselves. Usually, the patient feels a palpitating sensation but has no other complaints. However, the concern lies in the fact that these premature contractions may lead to more serious ventricular dysrhythmias.

In the patient with acute MI, PVCs are considered serious precursors of ventricular tachycardia and ventricular fibrillation when they (1) occur in increasing number, more than 6 per minute; (2) are multifocal or originate from several areas in the heart; (3) occur in pairs or triplets; and (4) occur in the vulnerable phase of conduction. The T wave represents the period when the heart is most likely to respond to any stray beat and be excited in a dysrhythmic manner. This phase of T wave conduction is said to be the vulnerable phase.

PVCs (Fig. 26-6) have the following characteristics:

Rate: 60 to 100 beats per minute.
P waves: Will not be present because impulse originates in the ventricles.
QRS complex: Usually wide and bizarre. Usually longer than 0.10 second in duration. May have the same focus in the ventricle, or may have a wide variety of configurations if occurring from multiple foci in the ventricles.
Conduction: Occasionally retrograde through the junctional tissue and atria.
Rhythm: Irregular when the premature beat occurs.

In order to decrease the myocardial irritability, the cause must be determined and, if possible, corrected. An antidysrhythmic drug may be used for immediate and possibly long-term therapy. The drug most commonly used in acute care is lidocaine; for long-term therapy procainamide (Pronestyl) or quinidine may be effective.

Ventricular Bigeminy

Ventricular bigeminy is frequently associated with digitalis excess, coronary artery disease, acute MI, and CHF. The term *bigeminy* refers to a condition in which every other beat is premature.

Ventricular bigeminy (Fig. 26-7) has the following characteristics:

Rate: May occur at any heart rate, but rate is usually less than 90 beats per minute.

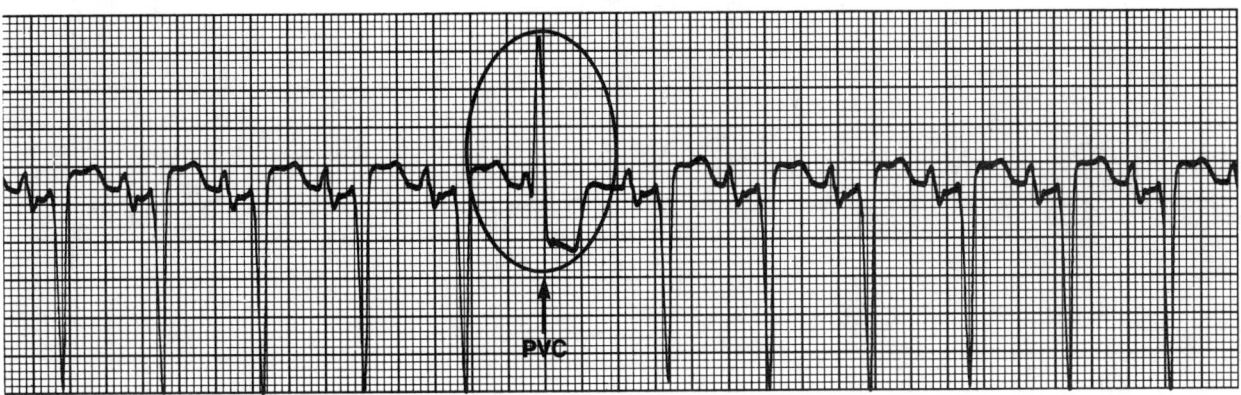

Figure 26-6
Premature ventricular contraction.

P waves: The same as described for PVCs; may be hidden within the QRS complex.

QRS complex: Every other beat is a PVC with a wide, bizarre QRS complex and a complete compensatory pause.

Conduction: The sinus beats are conducted from the sinus node in a normal fashion, but alternating PVCs start in the ventricles and may have retrograde conduction through the junctional tissue and atria.

Rhythm: Irregular.

If the ectopic beats occur every third beat, this is termed *trigeminy;* every fourth beat, *quadrigeminy.*

The treatment for ventricular bigeminy is the same as for PVCs. Since the underlying cause of ventricular bigeminy is frequently digitalis toxicity, this should be ruled out or treated if present. Ventricular bigeminy caused by digitalis toxicity is treated with phenytoin (Dilantin).

Ventricular Tachycardia

This dysrhythmia is caused by increased myocardial irritability, as are PVCs. It is usually associated with coronary artery disease, atherosclerotic heart disease, and rheumatic heart disease, and may precede ventricular fibrillation. Ventricular tachycardia is extremely dangerous and should be considered an emergency. The patient is generally aware of this rapid rhythm and is quite anxious. Accelerated ventricular rhythm and ventricular tachycardia have the following characteristics (Fig. 26-8):

Rate: 150 to 200 beats per minute.

P waves: Usually buried in the QRS complex; if seen, they do not necessarily fall in the normal pattern with the QRS. The ventricular contractions are dissociated from the atrial contractions.

QRS complex: Have the same configurations as those of a PVC—wide and bizarre, with T waves in the opposite direction. A ventricular beat may fuse with a normal QRS, resulting in a fusion beat.

Conduction: Originates in the ventricle, with possible retrograde conduction to the junctional tissue and atria.

Rhythm: Usually regular, but irregular ventricular tachycardia is also seen.

The patient's tolerance or lack of tolerance for this rapid rhythm will dictate the therapy to be given. The cause of the myocardial irritability must be determined and corrected, if possible. Antidysrhythmic drugs may be used. Cardioversion may be indicated if the reduction in cardiac output is marked.

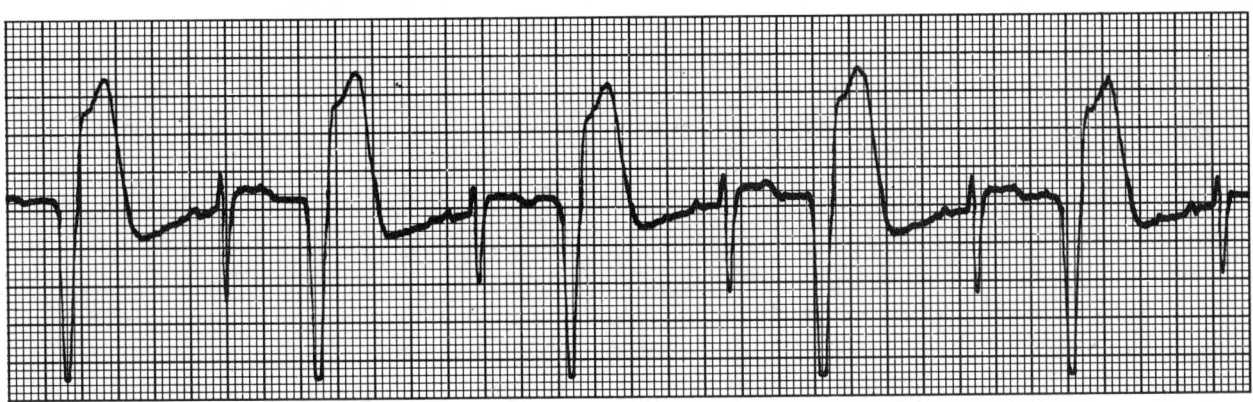

Figure 26-7
Ventricular bigeminy.

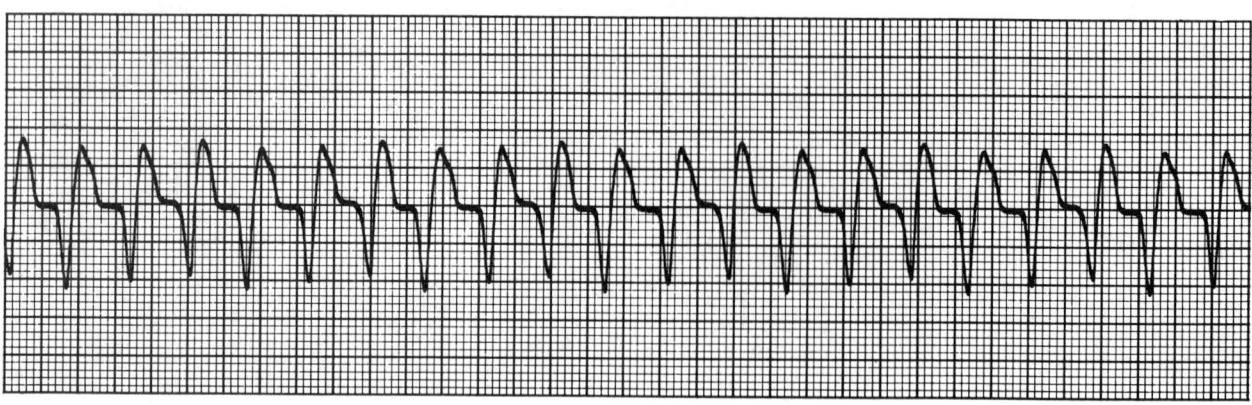

Figure 26-8
Ventricular tachycardia.

Ventricular Fibrillation

Ventricular fibrillation is rapid, ineffective quivering of the ventricles. With this dysrhythmia there is no audible heart beat, no palpable pulse, and no respiration. This pattern is so grossly irregular it can hardly be mistaken for another type of dysrhythmia.

Ventricular fibrillation (Fig. 26-9) has the following characteristics:

Rate: Rapid, uncoordinated, ineffective.
P waves: Not seen.
QRS complex: Rapid, irregular undulation without specific pattern (multifocal). The ventricles have only a quivering motion.
Conduction: Foci are located in the ventricles, but so many foci are firing at one time that there is no organized conduction; no ventricular contractions occur.
Rhythm: Extremely irregular and uncoordinated, without specific pattern.

Immediate treatment is defibrillation.

Ventricular Asystole

In ventricular asystole there are no QRS complexes. There is no heartbeat, no palpable pulse, and no respiration. Without immediate treatment ventricular asystole is fatal.

Ventricular asystole (Fig. 26-10) has the following characteristics:

Rate: None.
P waves: May be visible, but they do not conduct through the AV node and ventricles.
QRS complex: None.
Conduction: Possibly, through the atria only.
Rhythm: None.

Cardiopulmonary resuscitation (CPR) is necessary to keep the patient alive. To decrease any vagal stimuli, 0.5 mg of atropine should be administered intravenously. Epinephrine (intracardiac) should be administered and repeated at 5-minute intervals. Sodium bicarbonate should be given intravenously. Insertion of a transthoracic or transvenous pacemaker may be necessary.

Conduction Abnormalities

First-Degree AV Block

First-degree AV block is usually associated with organic heart disease or may be due to the effect of digitalis. It is seen frequently in patients with inferior MIs.

First-degree heart block has the following characteristics (Fig. 26-11):

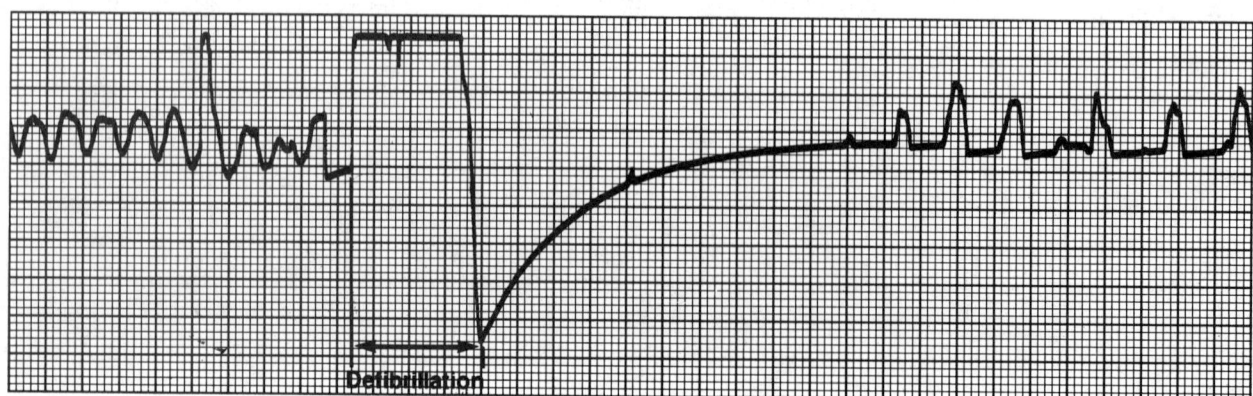

Figure 26-9
Ventricular fibrillation with defibrillation.

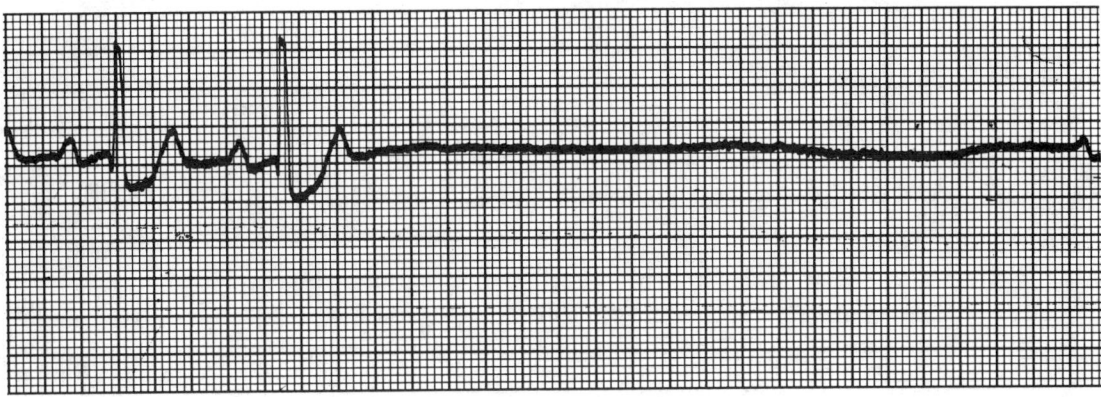

Figure 26-10
Ventricular asystole.

Rate: Variable, usually 60 to 100 beats per minute.
P waves: Precede each QRS complex. The PR interval is greater than 0.20 second in duration.
QRS complex: Follows each P wave; usually normal.
Conduction: Delayed conduction, usually anywhere between the junctional tissue and the Purkinje network, produces a prolonged PR interval. Ventricular conduction is usually normal.
Rhythm: Usually regular.

This dysrhythmia is important because it may lead to more serious forms of heart block. It is often a warning signal. The patient should be monitored closely for any advancing block.

Second-Degree AV Block—Mobitz Type II

Second-degree AV block, Mobitz type II, is also caused by organic heart disease, by MIs and by digitalis intoxication. This type of block results in a reduced heart rate and usually a reduced cardiac output. (Cardiac output is the product of stroke volume and heart rate.)

Second-degree heart block has the following characteristics (Fig. 26-12):

Rate: 30 to 55 beats per minute. The atrial rate may be two, three, or four times faster than the ventricular rate.

P waves: There are two, three, or four P waves for each QRS complex. The PR interval of the conducted beat is usually normal in duration.
QRS complex: Usually normal.
Conduction: One or more of the impulses are not conducted through the ventricles.
Rhythm: Usually slow and regular. When an irregularity is seen, it is due to the fact that the block is varying from 2:1 to 3:1 or to some other combination.

Treatment is directed toward increasing the heart rate to maintain a normal cardiac output. Digitalis intoxication should be ruled out and myocardial depressant drugs withheld.

Third-Degree AV Block

Third-degree AV block (complete heart block) is also associated with organic heart disease, digitalis intoxication, and MI. The heart rate may be markedly decreased, resulting in a decrease in perfusion to vital organs, such as the brain, heart, kidneys, lungs, and skin.

Complete block—third-degree AV block—has the following characteristics (Fig. 26-13):

Origin: Impulses originate in the SA node, but are not conducted to the Purkinje fibers. They are completely blocked. An escape rhythm from either the

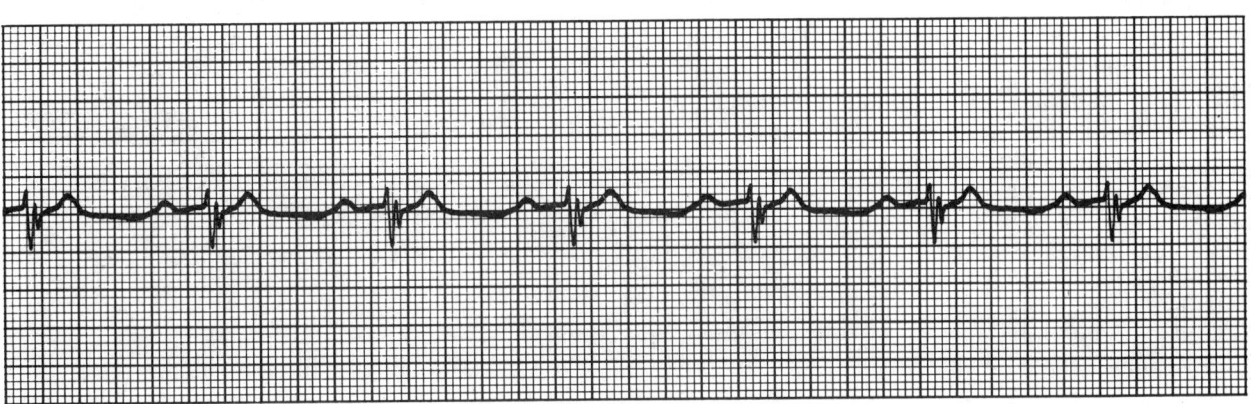

Figure 26-11
First-degree heart block.

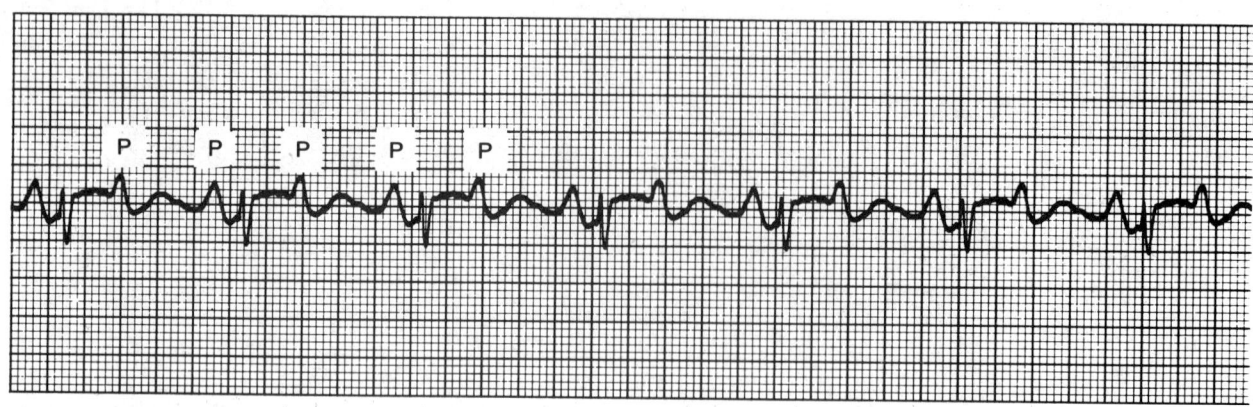

Figure 26-12
Second-degree heart block.

junctional or the ventricular area therefore takes over as the pacemaker.

Rate: Atrial rate 60 to 100 beats per minute; ventricular rate 40 to 60 beats per minute if the escape rhythm originated in the junction, 20 to 40 beats per minute if the escape rhythm originated in the ventricle.

P waves: The P waves originating from the SA node are seen regularly throughout the rhythm, but they have no association with the QRS complexes.

QRS complex: If the escape rhythm originated in the junction, the QRS complexes have a normal supraventricular configuration, but have no association with the P waves. QRS complexes occur regularly. If the escape rhythm originated in the ventricle, the QRS complex is longer than 0.10 second in duration, and is usually broad and slurred. These QRS complexes have the same configuration as the QRS complex of a PVC.

Conduction: The SA node is firing, and P waves can be seen. They are all blocked and not conducted to the ventricles. Escape rhythms originating in the junction are usually conducted normally through the ventricles. Escape rhythms from the ventricles are ectopic with aberrant configuration.

Rhythm: Usually slow but regular.

Treatment is directed toward increasing perfusion to vital organs. The insertion of a temporary transvenous pacemaker is the acceptable treatment. A permanent pacemaker may be necessary if the block is persistent.

Medical Management

Dysrhythmias are most commonly treated with drug therapy. In situations where drugs alone are not adequate, certain adjunctive mechanical therapies are available. The most common are elective cardioversion, defibrillation, and pacemakers.

Cardioversion

Cardioversion is the use of electricity to terminate dysrhythmias that have QRS complexes. It is usually an elective procedure. The patient is alert, and informed consent is obtained. The patient is usually given diazepam (Valium) intravenously prior to cardioversion to promote anesthesia, and is usually intubated after being anesthetized. The amount of voltage used varies from 25 to 400 watt-seconds. Digoxin is usually withheld for 48 hours prior to cardioversion to prevent postcardioversion dysrhythmias.

The synchronizer is turned on. The defibrillator is synchronized with a cardiac monitor so that an electrical impulse is discharged during ventricular depolarization (the QRS complex). If not synchronized, the defibrillator could dis-

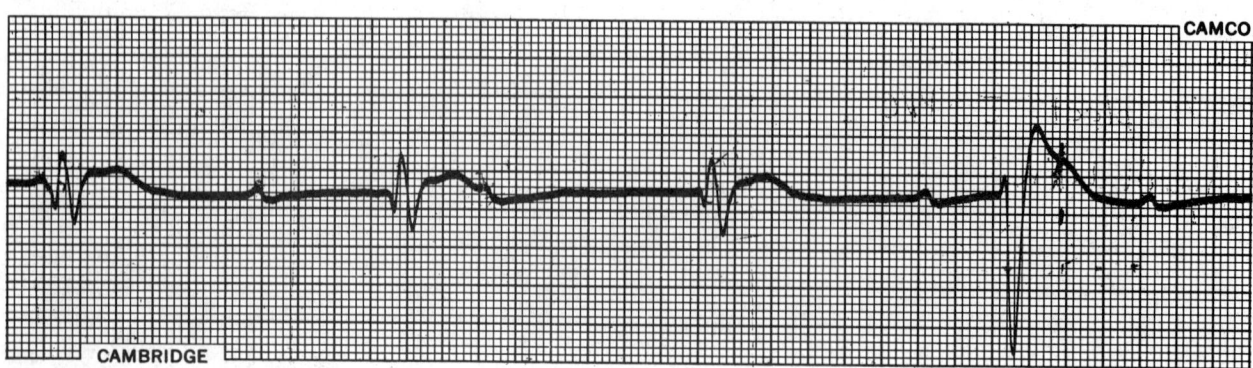

Figure 26-13
Third-degree AV block.

charge during the vulnerable period (T wave), resulting in ventricular tachycardia or fibrillation. The synchronizer switch is therefore turned on in advance so that the unit discharges immediately after the onset of the next QRS complex.

If ventricular fibrillation occurs after cardioversion, the defibrillator must be recharged immediately, the synchronizer turned off, and defibrillation repeated. After use, the defibrillator should be turned off to prevent accidental discharge of the paddles. Oxygen flow should be stopped during cardioversion if possible, to avoid the hazard of fire.

Indications of a successful response are conversion to sinus rhythm, strong peripheral pulses, and adequate blood pressure. Airway patency should be maintained, and the patient's state of consciousness assessed. Vital signs should be obtained at least every 15 minutes for 1 hour, every 30 minutes for 2 hours, and then every 4 hours. ECG monitoring is required during and after cardioversion; therefore, these patients are in a critical care environment.

Defibrillation

Defibrillation is asynchronous cardioversion that is used in an emergency situation. Its use is usually confined to the treatment of ventricular fibrillation when there is no organized cardiac rhythm. Defibrillation completely depolarizes all the myocardial cells at once, allowing the sinus node to recapture its role as the pacemaker. The electrical voltage required to defibrillate the heart is much greater than that usually required for cardioversions. For defibrillation to be successful an electrical arc must be created, which is managed by maintaining good contact between the machine paddles and the skin. The following are some key points to remember in assisting with defibrillation or cardioversion:

- Use a good conducting agent between the skin and the paddles, such as saline pads or electrode paste.
- Position the paddles so as to create an effective arc (see Figure 26-14).
- Exert 20 to 25 pounds of pressure on each paddle to ensure good skin contact.
- Practice safety by being certain no one is touching the bed or patient when the paddles are discharged.

If defibrillation has been unsuccessful, cardiopulmonary resuscitation is started immediately. Epinephrine may be used if the fibrillation is fine. Epinephrine may make the fibrillation coarser and thus easier to convert with defibrillation. Sodium bicarbonate is given to reverse the acidosis caused by lack of respiratory exchange. Epinephrine and sodium bicarbonate are incompatible when mixed together and must be given separately. Blood pressure is supported, using vasopressors. At no time during the resuscitation should the external cardiac massage and the assisted ventilation be stopped for longer than 5 seconds.

Pacemaker Therapy
Definition and Indications for Use

A pacemaker is an electronic device that provides repetitive electrical stimuli to the heart muscle for the control of heart rate. It initiates and maintains the heart rate when the natural pacemakers of the heart are unable to do so. Pacemakers are generally used when a patient has a dysrhythmia, or the

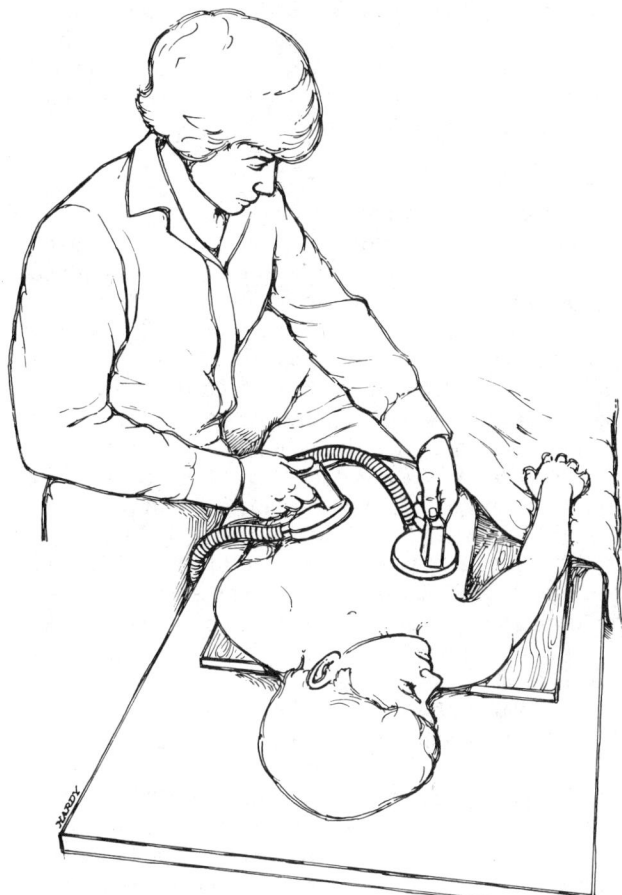

Figure 26-14
One method of paddle placement in cardioversion.

forerunner of a dysrhythmia that causes failure of cardiac output. Pacemakers are most commonly used as part of the treatment in complete heart block following myocardial infarction. A pacemaker can also be used to control tachydysrhythmias that otherwise do not respond to drug therapy. Temporary pacing may also be done following open heart surgery.

Pacemaker Design

Pacemakers consist of two component parts: (1) the electronic pulse generator, which contains the circuitry and batteries that generate the electrical signal; and (2) the pacemaker electrodes (also called leads or wires), which transmit the pacemaker impulses to the heart. The stimuli from the pacemaker travel through a flexible catheter electrode that is threaded through a vein into the right ventricle or introduced by direct penetration of the chest wall. The pulse generator is usually implanted in a subcutaneous pocket in the pectoral or axillary region. Sometimes an abdominal site is selected.

Pacemaker generators are insulated to protect against body moisture and warmth. The pulse generator (or pacemaker) contains its own supply of power, which is provided by battery cells. The main power sources in current use are mercury-zinc batteries (lasting 3 to 4 years), lithium cell units (lasting up to 10 years), and a nuclear-powered pacemaker (^{238}plutonium source) that lasts 20 years to a lifetime. There are also pacemakers that can be recharged externally. Since pacemakers rely on batteries, battery exhaustion (with the exception of nuclear-power and rechargeable batteries) is inevitable. Therefore, the generator that contains the batteries must be replaced periodically.

Types of Pacemakers

The most commonly used pacemaker is the *demand* (synchronous; noncompetitive) pacemaker, which is set for a specific rate and stimulates the heart when normal ventricular depolarization does not occur. It functions only when the natural heart rate goes below a certain level. The *fixed rate* pacemaker (asynchronous; competitive) stimulates the ventricle at a preset constant rate that is independent of the patient's rhythm. It is used infrequently, usually in patients with complete and unvarying heart block.

Temporary Pacemaker Systems. Temporary pacing is usually an emergency procedure and permits the observation of the effects of pacing on heart function so that the optimum pacing rate for the patient can be selected before a permanent pacemaker is implanted. It is used in patients who have suffered myocardial infarction complicated by heart block, in patients with cardiac arrest with bradycardia and asystole, or in selected postoperative cardiac surgery patients. Temporary pacing may be done for hours, days, or weeks and is continued until the patient improves or a permanent pacemaker is implanted.

Temporary pacing may be carried out either by an endocardial (transvenous) approach or by the transthoracic approach to the myocardium. The transvenous electrode is passed under fluoroscopic guidance through any peripheral vein (antecubital, brachial, jugular, subclavian, femoral) and the catheter tip is positioned in the apex of the right ventricle. The most common complication occurring during pacemaker insertion is ventricular dysrhythmia. Cardiac perforation occurs rarely. A defibrillator should be immediately available.

Permanent Pacemaker Systems. For permanent pacing, the endocardial lead is passed transvenously into the right ventricle, and the pulse generator is implanted within the body underneath the skin below the right or left pectoral region or below the clavicle (Fig. 26–15). This is termed an endocardial or transvenous implant. This procedure is usually done under local anesthesia. Another method of permanent pacing is the implantation of the pulse generator in the abdominal wall. The electrode is passed transthoracically to the myocardium, where it is sutured in place. For this method, termed an epicardial or myocardial implant, a thoracotomy is required to provide access to the heart.

Atrioventricular Pacemakers (Physiological Pacing). Pacemaker technology, through the development of atrioventricular (AV) pacemakers, has fostered the growth of safe and effective pacemaker therapy for many complex cardiac problems. AV pacemakers are considered highly desirable because they can be programmed to mimic the patient's own intrinsic cardiac function; hence they are referred to as *physiological pacemakers*.

Because of the sophistication of these AV pacemakers, a universal code has been adopted to provide a means of safer communication about their function. The coding is referred to as the *ICHD code* because it is sanctioned by the Inter-Society Commission for Heart Disease. The complete

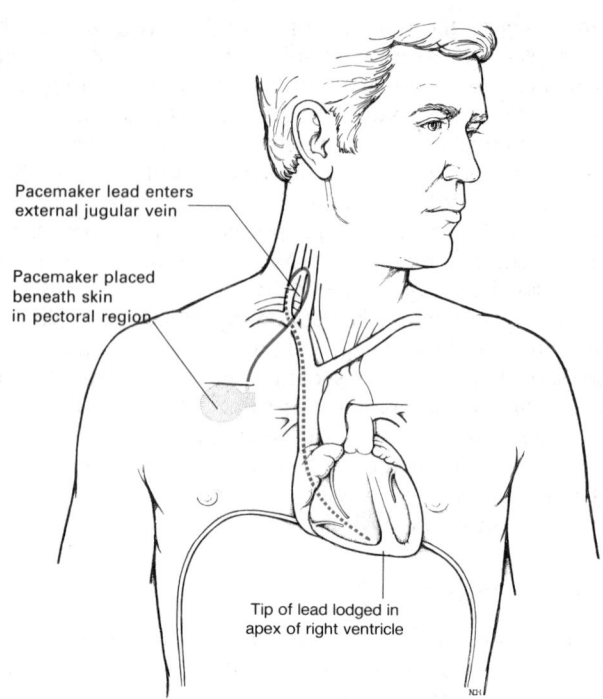

Figure 26-15
Implanted transvenous pacing electrode and pacemaker generator.

Labels on figure:
- Pacemaker lead enters external jugular vein
- Pacemaker placed beneath skin in pectoral region
- Tip of lead lodged in apex of right ventricle

code consists of five letters, but only three are used in common parlance. The *first letter* of the code always describes the chamber(s) being paced, that is, the chamber containing the pacing electrode. The possible letter characters for this code are A (atrium), V (ventricle), or D (dual, meaning both A and V). The *second letter* describes the chamber(s) being sensed by the pacemaker generator. Information sensed is dispatched to the generator for interpretation and action by the generator. The possible letter characters here are once again A (atrium), V (ventricle), and D (dual). The *third letter* of the code always describes the type of response exhibited by the pacemaker. There are five characters used to describe this response, but of the five only two are in common use: I (inhibitory) and T (triggered). Inhibitory response means that the response of the pacemaker is controlled by the activity of the patient's own heart. That is, the pacemaker will not function when the patient's heart beats. In contrast, triggered response means that the pacemaker will trigger a response based on intrinsic heart activity.

An example of an ICHD-coded pacemaker is DVI:

D—Both the atrium and the ventricle have a pacing electrode in place.
V—The pacemaker is sensing the activity of the ventricle only.
I—The pacemaker's stimulating effect is being inhibited by the activity of the patient's ventricle.

Complications. Complications associated with pacemakers relate to (1) their presence within the body, and (2) improper functioning. The following complications may arise from the presence of the pacemaker:

- Local infection (sepsis or hematoma formation) may occur at the site of venous cutdown or subcutaneous pacemaker placement.
- Dysrhythmias—ventricular ectopic activity may follow irritation of the ventricular wall by the electrode. (Pacemakers can produce baffling dysrhythmias.)
- Perforation of the myocardium or right ventricle by the catheter may occur.
- High ventricular threshold may cause abrupt loss of pacing.

Pacemaker malfunction can arise from failure in one or more components of the pacing system. The majority of pulse generator failures are from depletion of the power supply (*i.e.*, battery failure). The patient should be informed that the battery cells are sealed in the pulse generator. When it is time for a battery change, a new incision is made over the old incision. The old pulse generator is removed, and the new unit is connected to the existing leads and reimplanted in the already existing pocket. This is usually done under local anesthesia. Other complications include fracture (breakage) or dislocation of the electrodes and electronic failure.

These complications are manifested by abrupt changes in heart rate and rhythm. Their visibility as symptoms will depend on the patient's level of dependency on the pacemaker. The diagnosis of these complications is made by ECG analysis. Manipulation of the electrode(s) or replacement of the pacemaker generator may be necessary.

Pacemaker Surveillance. Pacemaker clinics have been established to monitor patients and to test pulse generators for warnings of impending pacemaker system failure. Testing of pacemaker pulse amplitude and duration and analysis of pulse contour require amplification equipment. With special equipment, lead fracture and insulation disruption can be detected. A 12-lead ECG is done during each patient visit to the clinic.

Another method of follow-up is evaluation by transtelephone monitoring of the transmission of the generator's pulse rate. By means of special equipment, the sound tone of the patient's pacemaker is transmitted over the telephone to a receiving system at a pacemaker clinic. The sounds are converted into an electronic signal and permanently recorded on an ECG strip. The pacemaker rate and other data concerning pacemaker function are obtained and evaluated by a cardiologist or a cardiovascular surgeon. This simplifies the diagnosis of a failing generator, provides reassurance, and improves the management of the person who is physically remote from pacemaker testing facilities.

Pacemaker Developments.

External and Long-Range Recharging. There is now available an electronic pacemaker with a battery that can be recharged externally. Like other pacemakers, the device is implanted under the skin in the chest wall or in the abdomen. Its lead wires (one enclosed inside the other) are threaded through a vein so that one end is in the heart and the other attached to a battery. To recharge the battery the patient dons a light-weight canvas shoulder harness and attaches the charger unit to it over the location of the implanted battery. The charger is linked to a small console that is plugged into an ordinary electric socket. When the unit is turned on, an electromagnetic field is generated that rejuvenates the power

cell in the battery through the skin. Recharging the battery takes only about 90 minutes at home each week.

Nuclear-Powered Pacemakers. Nuclear-powered pacemakers are now being implanted in patients in selected centers in the United States. The nuclear heart pacer is designed to operate for at least 15 to 20 years. The design of the pacemaker's nuclear power source is based on the principle of thermoelectricity—the direct conversion of heat to electrical energy. When certain metals are joined together, they form a thermocouple that, when heated at one end, will generate an electrical current. The pacemaker's thermocouple is composed of a copper and nickel alloy and a nickel and chromium alloy drawn into wire strands and woven into a glass tape. The heat developed by the decay of the radioisotope nuclear fuel (plutonium-238) is used to heat the wires at one end. The electrical current, as in conventional pacemakers, is fed into a pulse generator that supplies the pacing pulses to the heart via conventional wire electrodes. The radiation exposure to the patient from the nuclear fuel is considered to be within acceptable levels.

▶ *Nursing Process*
The Patient With a Pacemaker

▷ *Assessment*

Following the insertion of either a temporary or a permanent pacemaker, the patient is monitored by electrocardiogram. The pacemaker rate may vary as much as 5 beats above or below the preset pacemaker rate. An intravenous line is kept open to provide a readily accessible vein for drug administration, as prescribed, in the event of a dysrhythmia and for fluids to combat dehydration.

The incision site where the pulse generator is implanted (or the entry site for the pacing electrode if the pacemaker is temporary) is watched for evidence of bleeding, hematoma formation, or infection.

Infection is a major threat to the patient who has received a new pacemaker. The insertion site is observed primarily for swelling, unusual tenderness, and increased heat. The patient may complain of continuous throbbing or pain. Any unusual drainage is reported to the physician.

All electrical equipment used in the vicinity of the patient is grounded with three-pronged plugs inserted into a proper outlet. Improperly grounded equipment can generate leakage currents capable of producing ventricular fibrillation. A biomedical engineer, electrician, or other qualified person should make certain that the patient is in an electrically safe environment.

The nurse observes for potential sources of electrical hazards. No metal parts of the output terminal or pacemaker wires should be exposed. All such bare metal should be scrupulously covered with nonconductive tape to prevent accidental ventricular fibrillation from stray currents, which might reach the heart if exposed metal parts were to come in contact with a metal conductor, such as a bedrail. Aberrant current sources (from malfunctioning equipment) can travel over the surface of a damp skin and can also cause ventricular fibrillation. *The patient must be placed in an electrically safe environment.*

Complications. In the initial hours following the insertion of either a temporary or a permanent pacemaker, the most common complication is dislodgement of the pacing electrode. The identification of this complication is made by examination of the ECG pattern; the relationship between the pacing spike and the patient's QRS becomes asynchronous (Fig. 26-16).

The nurse can help to avoid this complication by minimizing the patient's activities. If a temporary electrode is in place, the extremity used can be immobilized. The ECG is monitored very carefully for the presence of a pacing spike. Because of the importance of such monitoring, this patient is ideally in an intensive care unit.

Data about the model of pacemaker, date and time of its insertion, location of the pulse generator, stimulation threshold, and pacer rate should be noted on the patient's record. This information is important for solving any unusual dysrhythmia problem.

▷ *Nursing Diagnoses*

Based on assessment data, major nursing diagnoses of the patient may include the following:

- Potential for infection related to catheter or generator insertion
- Knowledge deficit regarding self-care program

▷ *Planning and Implementation*

▷ *Goals:* The major goals of the patient may include (1) absence of infection and (2) adherence to a self-care program.

Nursing Interventions

Prevention of Infection. The wound site is inspected daily for redness, edema, pain, or any unusual bleeding. The physician does the initial dressing change and the nurse inspects and changes the dressing each day thereafter. Changes are reported to the physician.

Adherence to the Self-Care Program. Because of the nature of the need for a pacemaker, most patients are very compliant with the home health-care program. See Chart 26-2 for details of patient education.

▷ *Evaluation*

▷ *Expected Outcomes*

1. Patient is free of infection.
   a. Temperature normal
   b. WBCs within normal range (5,000–10,000/cu mm)
   c. Exhibits no redness or swelling of pacemaker insertion site.
2. Adheres to a self-care program.
   a. Responds appropriately when queried about the signs and symptoms of infection
   b. Knows when to seek medical attention (as demonstrated in responses to signs and symptoms)
   c. See Chart 26-2.

Acute Pulmonary Edema

Definition, Etiology, and Pathophysiology

Pulmonary edema is the abnormal accumulation of fluid in the lungs, either in the interstitial spaces or in the alveoli.

Pulmonary edema represents the ultimate stage of pulmonary congestion, in which fluid has leaked through the capillary walls and is permeating the airways, giving rise to dyspnea of dramatic severity. Pulmonary congestion occurs when the pulmonary vascular bed has received more blood from the right ventricle than the left can accommodate and remove. The slightest imbalance between inflow on the right side and outflow on the left side of the heart may have drastic consequences. For example, if with each heartbeat the right ventricle pumps out just one more drop of blood than the left, within the space of only 3 hours the pulmonary blood volume will have expanded 500 ml!

Noncardiac pulmonary edema has a wide variety of causes: toxic inhalants, drug overdose, neurogenic pulmonary edema. Clinical management is directed toward reducing pulmonary blood flow and pulmonary arterial pressure.

The most common cause of pulmonary edema is cardiac

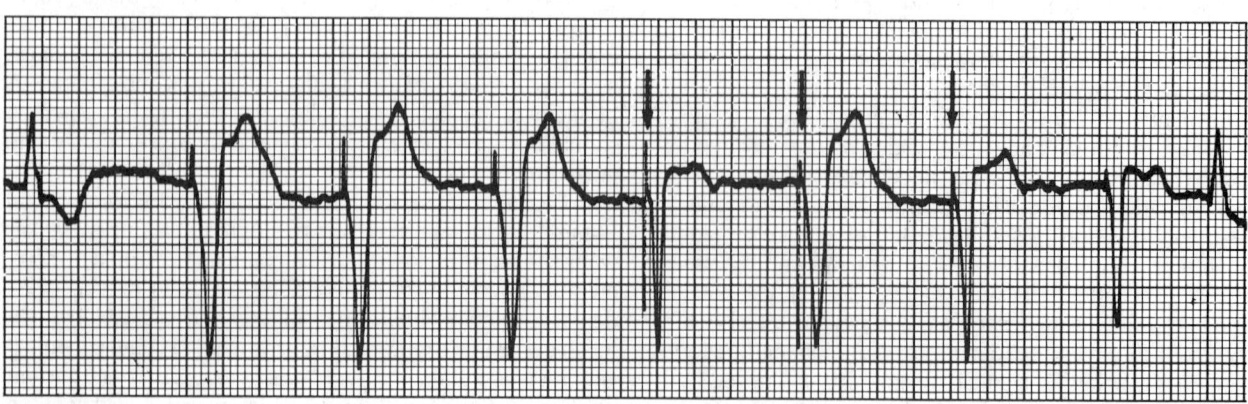

Figure 26-16
Synchronized pacemaker rhythm. Arrows indicate presence of sensed pacing spike.

Chart 26-2
Patient Education: The Patient With a Pacemaker

1. Report to physician/pacemaker clinic periodically as prescribed, so that the rate of the pacemaker and its function can be checked. This is especially important during the first month after implantation.
   a. Adhere to weekly monitoring schedule during the first month after implantation.
   b. Check pulse daily. Report *immediately* any sudden slowing or increasing of the pulse rate. This may indicate pacemaker malfunction.
   c. Resume weekly monitoring when battery depletion is anticipated. (The time for reimplantation depends on the type in use.)
2. Wear loose-fitting clothing around the area of the pacemaker.
   a. Understand the reason for the slight bulge over the pacemaker implant.
   b. Notify physician if the area becomes reddened or painful.
   c. Avoid trauma to the area of the pacemaker generator.

3. Study the manufacturer's instructions and become familiar with pacemaker.
4. Physical activity does not usually have to be curtailed, with the exception of heavy contact sports.
5. Carry an identification card/bracelet indicating physician's name, type and model number of pacemaker, manufacturer's name, pacemaker rate, and hospital where pacemaker was inserted.
6. Avoid being close to microwave ovens, arc welders and large electrical generators, and electric cautery and diathermy equipment (although at this time electrical interference is not a major problem).
7. Show identification card and request scanning by a hand scanner when going through weapons detector at airport.
8. Remember that hospitalization is necessary periodically for battery changes/pacemaker unit replacement.

---

disease—atherosclerotic, hypertensive, valvular, myopathic. Most patients with pulmonary edema have chronic heart disease of a type that imposes a strain on the left ventricle, such as arterial hypertension or aortic valve disease. The edema is particularly likely to arise from the damage to the heart muscle caused by acute MI. The development of pulmonary edema signifies that cardiac function has become grossly inadequate. There is an elevated left ventricular end-diastolic pressure and a rise in pulmonary venous pressure. This produces an increase in hydrostatic pressure, which results in transudation of fluid. Impaired lymphatic drainage contributes to the accumulation of fluid in the lung tissues.

The pulmonary capillaries, engorged with an excess of blood that the left ventricle is incapable of pumping, no longer are able to retain their contents. Fluid, first serous and later bloody, escapes into the adjacent alveoli through the communicating bronchioles and bronchi. It then mixes with air and, churned by respiratory agitation, is expelled from the mouth and nostrils, producing the ominous "death rattle." Because of the fluid buildup, the lungs become stiff and cannot expand, and air cannot enter. The result is severe hypoxia.

Death from pulmonary edema is by no means inevitable. If appropriate measures are taken promptly, attacks can be aborted and patients can survive this complication to benefit from measures directed against its recurrence. Fortunately, pulmonary edema usually does not develop precipitously but is preceded by the premonitory symptoms of pulmonary congestion.

Clinical Manifestations

The typical attack of pulmonary edema occurs at night after the patient has been lying down for a few hours. Recumbency increases the venous return to the heart and favors the resorption of edema fluid from the legs. The circulating blood becomes diluted, and its volume expands. The venous pressure mounts and the right atrium fills with increasing rapidity. There is a corresponding increase in the right ventricular output, which eventually surpasses the output from the left ventricle. The pulmonary vessels become engorged with blood and proceed to leak. Meanwhile, the patient has become increasingly restless, anxious, and unable to sleep.

There is a sudden onset of breathlessness and a sense of suffocation. The patient's hands become cold and moist, the nail beds become cyanotic, and the skin color turns gray. In addition, the pulse is weak and rapid and the neck veins are distended. There is incessant coughing, which produces increasing quantities of mucoid sputum. As the pulmonary edema progresses, anxiety develops into near panic and the patient becomes confused, then stuporous. Breathing is noisy and moist, and the patient, nearly suffocated by the blood-tinged, frothy fluid now pouring into his bronchi and trachea, is literally drowning in his own secretions. The situation demands immediate action.

Diagnostic Evaluation

The diagnosis is made upon evaluation of the clinical manifestations resulting from pulmonary congestion. In complex cases, a pulmonary artery catheter may be inserted to facilitate the retrieval of hemodynamic data essential to the diagnosis and treatment (described later in this chapter in Chart 26-4).

Management

The goals of medical management for the patient with acute pulmonary edema are to reduce total circulating volume and to improve respiratory exchange. These goals are accomplished through a combination of oxygen and drug therapies and nursing support.

Oxygenation. Oxygen is administered in concentrations adequate to relieve hypoxia and dyspnea.

If signs of hypoxemia persist, oxygen may be delivered by intermittent or continuous positive pressure. If respiratory failure occurs despite optimal management, endotracheal intubation and mechanical ventilation are required. The use of positive end-expiratory pressure (PEEP) is effective in reducing venous return, lowering pulmonary capillary pressure, and improving oxygenation. Oxygenation is monitored by measurement of arterial blood gases.

Pharmacologic Therapy: Morphine. Morphine is given intravenously in small doses to reduce anxiety and dyspnea and to decrease peripheral resistance so that blood can be redistributed from the pulmonary circulation to the periphery. This action decreases pressure in the pulmonary capillaries and decreases transudation of fluid. The decrease in rate of respirations resulting from morphine is also beneficial.

- Morphine may not be given if pulmonary edema is caused by cerebral vascular accident or if chronic pulmonary disease or cardiogenic shock is present.
- Watch for excessive respiratory depression and have a morphine antagonist (naloxone hydrochloride [Narcan]) available.

Diuretics. Either furosemide (Lasix) or ethacrynic acid (Edecrin) may be given intravenously to produce a rapid diuretic effect. In addition, furosemide causes vasodilatation and peripheral venous pooling, with a subsequent reduction in venous return that occurs even before the diuretic effect. Thus dyspnea is rapidly relieved and pulmonary congestion is decreased. Because a large volume of urine will accumulate within minutes after administration of a potent diuretic, an indwelling catheter may be required.

- Watch for falling blood pressure, increasing heart rate, and decreasing urinary output; these indicate that the total circulation is not tolerating diuresis.
- Patients with prostatic hypertrophy must be watched for signs of urinary retention (Table 26-1).

Digitalis. To improve the contractile force of the heart, thus increasing the output of the left ventricle, the patient may be given a rapid-acting digitalis preparation. The improved cardiac contractility will increase cardiac output, enhance diuresis, and reduce diastolic pressure. Thus pulmonary capillary pressure and the transudation of fluid into the alveoli will be reduced.

- Digitalis must be given with extreme caution to patients with acute myocardial infarction, because these patients are sensitive to digitalis and may develop toxic dysrhythmias.
- The serum potassium level is measured at intervals because diuresis may have produced hypokalemia. The effect of digitalis in the presence of hypokalemia is enhanced, so digitalis toxicity may occur.
- If the patient has been on digitalis, the drug is usually withheld until the possibility of digitalis intoxication is ruled out (Chart 26-3).

Aminophylline. When the patient is wheezing and bronchospasm appears to play a significant role, aminophylline may be given to relax bronchospasm.

- Give aminophylline by way of continuous intravenous drip in dosages based on body weight.

Rotating Tourniquets. The application of rotating tourniquets on the extremities decreases venous return and right ventricular output, which aids in reducing preload. Rotating tourniquets are used as an adjunct to pharmacologic therapy. (Fig. 26-17.)

Tourniquets should be used with caution and only in the most extreme situations. Serious thromboembolic consequences can result from the application of tourniquets. The trapping of blood in the periphery contributes to stagnation of blood and creates an environment conducive to clot formation. The benefit derived from the application of rotating tourniquets must be carefully weighed against the risk of injury (*risk:benefit ratio*).

If the physician chooses to use either tourniquets or automatic inflating cuffs, the following steps are taken:

- Tell the patient the purpose of the treatment and that the skin of the extremities may become discolored.
- Take an initial blood pressure reading to serve as a baseline for future comparisons.
- Mark the peripheral pulses, if time permits.
- If tourniquets are used (instead of cuffs), they are positioned over a small towel as high as possible on three extremities. The arterial pulse should not be occluded. One extremity should be free of a tourniquet during each time interval. (A tourniquet is not placed on an extremity in which an IV line is inserted.)
- Release one tourniquet every 15 minutes; then apply a tourniquet to the previously free extremity. The venous outflow in any one extremity may be occluded for 45 minutes and unoccluded for 15 minutes. However, tourniquets may have to be rotated at 5-minute intervals on elderly patients or those with poor circulation in order to prevent gangrene and other complications.
- Rotate the tourniquets in a consistent clockwise pattern.
- Monitor the blood pressure every few minutes, since the use of tourniquets may precipitate hypotension in some patients.
- When the patient's symptoms have been relieved, discontinue the use of the tourniquets by removing them one at a time at 15-minute intervals. Simultaneous removal of all tourniquets could precipitate a recurrence of pulmonary edema.
- Examine each extremity after the tourniquet is removed for color, warmth, and the presence of a palpable pulse.

Phlebotomy. If the patient's condition is refractory to management, it is sometimes helpful to reduce the venous return to the heart by withdrawing 250 ml to 500 ml of blood from a peripheral vein (a phlebotomy or venesection). Phlebotomy is especially valuable when pulmonary edema has followed overtransfusion or administration of excessive intravenous fluid.

The resulting decrease in venous return is accompanied by a corresponding decline in the right ventricular output. Accordingly, the pulmonary artery pressure drops, the pulmonary vessels become less congested, and the lung capillaries, no longer congested, reabsorb the fluid that has escaped. The edema clears; the immediate danger has passed.

Positioning. Proper positioning can help reduce venous return to the heart.

TABLE 26-1
Commonly Used Diuretics

Definition: Diuretics are agents that increase the rate of urine flow.

Action: Dependent upon functionally active kidneys; most diuretics decrease the reabsorption of electrolytes (principally sodium) by the kidneys, promoting water loss as a secondary action. In the treatment of hypertension, the naturetic (sodium excretion) effect is probably the action of importance. In edema states, the salt and water actions are both important.

Special Precaution: Some diuretics may produce electrolyte depletion, including potassium loss, which causes weakness and induces cardiac dysrhythmias. Vigorous diuresis can produce hypovolemia.

Dosage Determination: (1) Patient's daily weight; (2) clinical signs and symptoms; (3) state of renal function

Diuretic	*Action*	*Nursing Implications*
Thiazides and Related Drugs		
Examples: Chlorothiazide (Diuril) Hydrochlorothiazide (HydroDIURIL, Esidrix, Oretic) Methyclothiazide (Enduron) Polythiazide (Renese) Chlorthalidone (Hygroton) Quinethazone (Hydromox)	Increases renal excretion of sodium (naturesis), potassium, chloride, bicarbonate (alkaline urine), with accompanying "osmotic" water loss Used principally in states of edema and hypertension Most widely used for prolonged administration	Monitor for electrolyte depletion: hyponatremia, hypokalemia, hypochloremic alkalosis Watch for signs and symptoms of electrolyte imbalance, dizziness, lightheadedness. Adverse reactions may occur, manifested by gastrointestinal, central nervous system, hematologic, and cardiovascular signs and symptoms. Supplementary potassium is usually given with these diuretics.
Potassium-Sparing Diuretics		
Spironolactone (Aldactone)	Inhibits action of aldosterone in distal tubule and reduces reabsorption of sodium and chloride Gives gradual diuretic effect Used in treatment of cirrhosis and edema when other diuretics are toxic or ineffective	Monitor for electrolyte depletion. Usually used in combination with thiazide diuretic Watch for side-effects—skin rash, gynecomastia.
Triamterene (Dyrenium)	Inhibits reabsorption of sodium ions in exchange for potassium and hydrogen ions in distal tubule	Usually used as an adjunct to thiazide therapy May cause elevation in blood uric acid Watch for nausea, vomiting, diarrhea, weakness, headache, and skin rash.
Potent Diuretics		
Furosemide (Lasix) Ethacrynic Acid (Edecrin)	Usually reserved for patients who do not respond to classical thiazide diuretics Blocks the reabsorption of sodium and water in proximal renal tubule and interferes with reabsorption of sodium in ascending limb of loop of Henle and in the most proximal portion of the distal tubule Associated with sodium, potassium, chloride, and hydrogen ion loss (acid urine) Has an almost immediate action (within 5 minutes) when given IV	Monitor for electrolyte depletion: may produce *profound diuresis* with hyponatremia, hypokalemia, hypochloremic alkalosis, and circulatory collapse. Potent and rapid-acting Especially useful in acute pulmonary edema Watch for nausea, vomiting, diarrhea, skin rash, pruritus, blurring of vision, postural hypotension, vertigo, hearing loss. Furosemide is chemically related to sulfonamides; consider cross allergies. Administer early in the day to avoid nocturia and consequent loss of sleep. Some patients may benefit from taking diuretics at bedtime to avoid PND (paroxysmal nocturnal dyspnea).

Chart 26-3
Digitalis and Cardiac Glycoside Preparations

Actions of Digitalis

Increases force of myocardial contractions
- Increases cardiac output by enhancing force of contraction of ventricle
- Slows heart rate
- Decreases heart size
- Decreases venous pressure
- Promotes diuresis
- Slows the ventricular rate in the setting of supraventricular dysrhythmias

Clinical Uses

- Congestive heart failure
- Atrial fibrillation; atrial flutter
- Supraventricular tachydysrhythmias
- Before cardiac surgery

Preparations

The choice of drug depends on the speed of onset desired, duration of action required, and individual patient response. The recommended dosage varies considerably.

Oral	*Parenteral*
Digitalis	Ouabain
Digoxin (Lanoxin)	Digoxin (Lanoxin)

Nursing Considerations and Actions

Special Precaution: The incidence of digitalis toxicity is high. Toxic effects do not always appear in a predictable manner.
- Watch for toxic effects: dysrhythmias (most important toxic effect), anorexia, nausea, vomiting, bradycardia, headache, malaise.
- Assess clinical response of patient by relief of symptoms (dyspnea, orthopnea, crackles, hepatomegaly, peripheral edema).
- Elderly patients may tolerate digitalis therapy poorly; assess for bradycardia, impaired renal function.
- Monitor serum potassium levels in patients receiving digitalis, especially those receiving both digitalis and diuretics. There is a predisposition to dysrhythmias if a potassium imbalance is not detected and corrected.
- Assess for symptoms of electrolyte depletion in patients taking digitalis: lassitude, apathy, mental confusion, anorexia, decreasing urinary output, azotemia.
- The following factors may increase sensitivity to digitalis: myocardial infarction, potassium depletion, kidney or hepatic disease, diuretic therapy, diarrhea, loss of appetite, advancing age, hypoxia and hypercapnia in pulmonary disease, acidosis, alkalosis.
- Check apical rate prior to each dose. A rate of 60 or above with no dysrhythmias is desirable. Check with the patient's physician regarding specific guidelines for each individual patient.

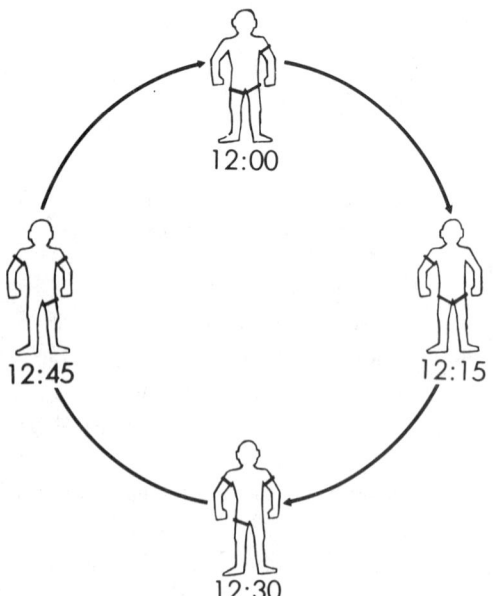

Figure 26-17
One method of rotating tourniquets. This illustration shows a clockwise pattern.

- Place the patient upright, with legs and feet down, preferably with legs dangling over the side of the bed. This has the immediate effect of decreasing venous return, lowering the output of the right ventricle, and decongesting the lungs, *e.g.,* reducing preload.
- If unable to sit with lower extremities dependent, the patient may be placed in an upright position in bed.

Psychological Support.   Extreme fear and anxiety are cardinal features of pulmonary edema. These emotions, which are self-perpetuating, make the condition more severe. Reassuring the patient and providing skillful anticipatory nursing are integral parts of the therapy. Because this patient experiences a sense of impending doom, it is essential that the nurse stay close. Touching the patient offers a sense of concrete reality. Nursing care should be organized to maximize the nurse's presence at the bedside. Offer the patient frequent information about what is being done to treat the condition and what the patient's responses to the treatment mean.

Prevention

Like most complications, pulmonary edema is easier to prevent than to treat. To recognize it in its early stages, when the presenting symptoms and signs are solely those of pulmonary congestion, the nurse should auscultate the lung fields daily on susceptible patients. A dry, hacking cough and the presence of a third heart sound (S_3) are often the earliest indications of pulmonary congestion. The S_3 is best heard at the apex with the patient lying in the left lateral decubitus position.

In an early stage, the situation may be corrected by relatively simple measures. These include (1) placing the patient in an upright position with the feet and legs dependent, (2) eliminating overexertion and emotional stress to reduce the left ventricular load, and (3) administering morphine to reduce anxiety, dyspnea, and preload.

The long-range approach to the prevention of pulmonary edema must be directed at its precursor, pulmonary congestion. See measures to prevent congestive heart failure (p. 588) and the various facets of patient teaching (p. 589).

In addition to these measures, it may be wise for the patient to sleep with the head of the bed elevated on 25-cm (10-inch) blocks. It is especially important to take extreme precautions when giving infusions and transfusions to cardiac patients and elderly persons.

- In order to prevent circulatory overloading, which could precipitate acute pulmonary edema, intravenous fluids are given at a slower rate, with the patient positioned upright in bed and kept under close nursing surveillance.
- Intravenous control devices are used to restrict the volume of fluid that can be delivered.

Surgical treatment may be necessary to eliminate or to minimize valvular defects that limit the flow of blood into or out of the left ventricle, because such defects impair the cardiac output and predispose the patient to the development of pulmonary congestion and edema.

Cardiac Failure

Definition, Etiology, and Pathophysiology

Cardiac failure, often referred to as congestive heart failure, is the inability of the heart to pump sufficient blood to meet the needs of the tissues for oxygen and nutrients. The term *congestive heart failure* is most commonly used when reference is made specifically to left-sided and right-sided failure.

The underlying mechanism of cardiac failure involves impairment of the contractile properties of the heart, which leads to a lower than normal cardiac output. The concept of cardiac output is best explained by the equation CO = HR $\times$ SV, where cardiac output (CO) is a function of heart rate (HR) times stroke volume (SV).

Heart rate is a function of the autonomic nervous system. When cardiac output falls, the sympathetic nervous system accelerates the heart rate to maintain adequate cardiac output. When this compensatory mechanism fails to maintain adequate tissue perfusion, the properties of stroke volume compensate.

In cardiac failure in which the primary problem is damaged and inhibited myocardial muscle fibers, stroke volume is impaired. *Stroke volume,* the amount of blood pumped with each contraction, is dependent upon three factors: preload, contractility, and afterload.

Preload is synonymous with Starling's Law of the Heart, in which the amount of blood filling the heart is directly proportional to pressure created by the length of the stretch of the myocardial fibers. *Contractility* refers to an alteration in the force of contraction that occurs at the cellular level and is unrelated to changes in myocardial fiber length. *Afterload* refers to the amount of pressure the ventricle must create in order to pump blood across the pressure gradient created by the semilunar valves. In cardiac failure, any one or more of these three factors may be altered such that cardiac output is impaired. The relative ease of determining hemodynamic measurements via invasive monitoring procedures has greatly facilitated differential diagnosis and pharmacologic manipulation of the problem.

Cardiac failure most commonly occurs with disorders of cardiac muscle that result in decreased contractile properties of the heart. Common underlying conditions that lead to disordered muscle function include coronary atherosclerosis, arterial hypertension, and inflammatory or degenerative muscle disease.

Coronary atherosclerosis leads to myocardial dysfunction by interfering with the normal supply of blood to cardiac muscle. Hypoxia, acidosis (due to accumulation of lactic acid), and nutrient deprivation of heart muscle result. Myocardial infarction (death of myocardial cells) frequently precedes the development of overt cardiac failure.

Systemic or pulmonary hypertension (increased afterload) increases the work requirement of the heart, and this in turn leads to hypertrophy of myocardial muscle fibers. This effect (*i.e.,* myocardial hypertrophy) can be considered a compensatory mechanism because it increases the contractility of the heart. However, for reasons that are not clear, the hypertrophied cardiac muscle does not function normally, and cardiac failure may eventually result.

Cardiac failure associated with inflammatory and degenerative diseases of the myocardium is due to direct damage to myocardial fibers, with a resultant decrease in contractility.

Cardiac failure may occur as a result of heart disease that only secondarily affects the myocardium. The mechanisms involved include impediment to flow of blood through the heart (*e.g.,* stenosis of a semilunar valve), inability of the heart to fill with blood (*e.g.,* pericardial tamponade, constrictive pericarditis, or stenosis of AV valves), or abnormal emptying of the heart (*e.g.,* insufficiency of AV valves). Sudden increase in afterload due to elevated systemic blood pressure ("malignant" hypertension) may result in cardiac failure in the absence of myocardial hypertrophy.

A number of systemic factors can contribute to the development and severity of cardiac failure. Increased metabolic rate (*e.g.,* fever, thyrotoxicosis), hypoxia, and anemia require an increased cardiac output to satisfy systemic oxygen demand. Hypoxia or anemia also may decrease the supply of oxygen to the myocardium. Acidosis (respiratory or metabolic) and electrolyte abnormalities may decrease myocardial contractility. Cardiac dysrhythmias, which may be present independently or secondary to cardiac failure, decrease the efficiency of overall myocardial function.

Clinical Manifestations

The dominant feature in cardiac failure is increased intravascular volume. Congestion of tissues results from increased arterial and venous pressures due to decreased cardiac output in the failing heart. Increased pulmonary venous pressure can lead to passage of fluid from pulmonary capillaries to the alveoli (pulmonary edema), manifested by cough and shortness of breath. Increased systemic venous pressure can result in generalized peripheral edema and weight gain.

The diminished cardiac output of cardiac failure has widespread manifestations because of diminished tissue and end-organ perfusion. Some commonly encountered effects related to low perfusion are dizziness, confusion, fatigue, exercise or heat intolerance, cool extremities, and oliguria. Renal perfusion pressure falls, which results in the release of renin from the kidney, which in turn leads to aldosterone secretion, sodium and fluid retention, and increased intravascular volume.

Left-Sided and Right-Sided Cardiac Failure

The left and right ventricles can fail separately. Left ventricular failure most often precedes right ventricular failure. Pure left ventricular failure is synonymous with acute pulmonary edema. Because the outputs of the ventricles are coupled, failure of either ventricle may lead to decreased tissue perfusion. The congestive manifestations, however, may differ according to whether left or right ventricular failure exists.

Left-Sided Cardiac Failure. Pulmonary congestion predominates when the left ventricle fails, because the left ventricle is unable to adequately pump the blood coming to it from the lungs. The increased pressure in the pulmonary circulation causes fluid to be forced into the pulmonary tissues. The clinical manifestations that ensue include dyspnea, cough, fatigability, tachycardia with an S_3 heart sound, and anxiety and restlessness.

Dyspnea results from the accumulation of fluid in the alveoli, which impairs gas exchange. Dyspnea may occur even at rest or may be precipitated by minimal to moderate exertion. *Orthopnea*, difficulty in breathing when lying flat, may be present. The patient who experiences orthopnea will not lie flat, but instead will use pillows to prop himself up in bed or will sit in a chair, even to sleep. Some patients experience orthopnea only at night, a condition known as *paroxysmal nocturnal dyspnea*. This occurs when the patient, who has been sitting for a long period with his feet and legs in a dependent position, returns to bed. After several hours the fluid that accumulated in the dependent extremities begins to be reabsorbed, and the impaired left ventricle is unable to adequately empty the increased volume. As a result, the pressure in the pulmonary circulation increases and causes further shifting of fluid into the alveoli.

The cough associated with left ventricular failure may be dry and nonproductive but is most often moist. Large quantities of frothy sputum, which is sometimes blood-tinged, may be produced.

Fatigability results from the low cardiac output that deprives tissues of normal circulation and decreases the removal of catabolic waste products. It is also a result of the increased energy expended for breathing and the insomnia that results from respiratory distress and coughing.

Restlessness and anxiety result from the impaired oxygenation of tissues, the stress associated with respiratory difficulty, and the knowledge that the heart is not functioning properly. As anxiety increases, so does dyspnea, which in turn further enhances the anxiety, creating a vicious cycle.

Right-Sided Cardiac Failure. When the right ventricle fails, congestion of the viscera and the peripheral tissues predominates. This is because the right side of the heart is unable to adequately empty its blood volume and thus cannot accommodate all of the blood that normally returns to it from the venous circulation. The clinical manifestations that ensue include edema of the lower extremities (dependent edema), which is usually pitting edema, weight gain, hepatomegaly, distended neck veins, fluid in the abdominal cavity, anorexia and nausea, nocturia, and weakness.

The dependent edema begins in the feet and ankles and can gradually progress up the legs and thighs and eventually into the external genitalia and lower trunk. Sacral edema is not uncommon for patients who are on bed rest, since the sacral area is dependent. *Pitting edema*, edema in which pits remain after even slight compression with the fingertips, is obvious only after retention of at least 4.5 kg (10 lb) of fluid.

Venous engorgement of the liver leads to hepatomegaly and tenderness in the right upper abdominal quadrant. As this process progresses, pressure within the portal vessels can become great enough to cause fluid to be forced into the abdominal cavity, a condition known as *ascites*. This collection of fluid in the abdominal cavity can cause pressure on the diaphragm and thus precipitate respiratory distress. Anorexia and nausea result from the venous engorgement and venous stasis within the abdominal organs.

Nocturia occurs because renal perfusion is promoted by periods of recumbency. Diuresis results, and is most common at night because cardiac output is improved with physical rest. The weakness that accompanies right-sided failure is due to the reduced cardiac output, impaired circulation, and inadequate removal of catabolic waste products from the tissues.

Diagnostic Evaluation

The diagnosis is made by evaluation of the clinical manifestations of pulmonary and systemic congestion. Of extreme value in the determination of effective stroke volume is the use of the pulmonary artery catheter. This catheter may be inserted at the bedside. The catheter's technology has expanded to include a multilumen apparatus that allows one catheter to make more than one hemodynamic measurement. The catheter enters the right atrium via the superior vena cava. A balloon is then inflated, allowing the catheter to follow the blood flow through the tricuspid valve, through the right ventricle, through the pulmonic valve, and into the main pulmonary artery. Waveform and pressure readings are noted during insertion to identify location of the catheter within the heart. The balloon is deflated once the catheter is in the pulmonary artery and properly secured (see Fig. 26-18).

Actual measurements of preload, afterload, and cardiac output can be obtained. There are lumina at various intervals along the catheter. One lumen is attached to the proximal port of the catheter and lies at the level of the right atrium. Because preload is the amount of venous return to the heart and is therefore equal to the central venous pressure measurement, measuring the pressure at the proximal port yields an accurate preload and hence CVP measurement. The tip of the catheter rests in the pulmonary artery where left ventricular pressure measurements are made. The balloon is inflated and flows into a small pulmonary capillary, occluding

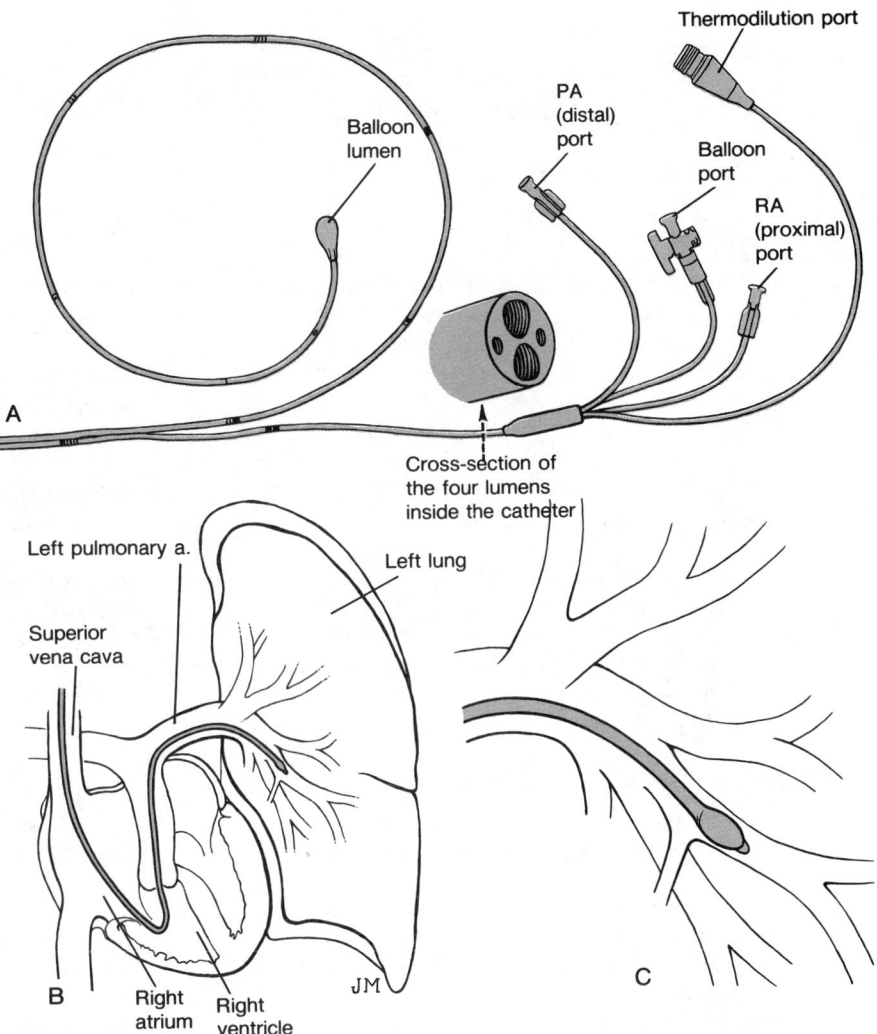

Figure 26-18
(*A*) The multilumen pulmonary artery catheter. (*B*) Location of the catheter within the heart. The catheter enters the right atrium via the superior vena cava. The balloon is then inflated, allowing the catheter to follow the blood flow through the tricuspid valve, through the right ventricle, through the pulmonic valve, and into the main pulmonary artery. Waveform and pressure readings are noted during insertion to identify location of the catheter within the heart. The balloon is deflated once the catheter is in the pulmonary artery and properly secured. (*C*) Pulmonary capillary wedge pressure (PWP). The catheter floats into a distal branch of the pulmonary artery when the balloon is inflated, and becomes "wedged." The wedged catheter occludes blood flow from behind, and the tip of the lumen records pressures in front of the catheter. The balloon is then deflated, allowing the catheter to float back into the main pulmonary artery. (Brunner LS and Suddarth DS. The Lippincott Manual of Nursing Practice, 4th ed. Philadelphia, JB Lippincott, 1986.)

or wedging the capillary. A pressure measurement is made which is the left ventricular end-diastolic pressure or afterload, the resistance against which the left ventricle must pump. Cardiac output is measured via a thermodilution lumen connected to a computer.

Measurements of the various pressures are made at intervals prescribed by the physician, and drug therapy is adjusted based on the readings.

The nursing management of the patient who has a hemodynamic catheter is highly specialized and is ideally conducted in an intensive care environment. The guidelines for managing a patient with a hemodynamic catheter are summarized in Chart 26-4.

Medical Management

The basic objectives in the treatment of patients with cardiac failure are the following:

1. To promote rest in order to reduce the work load on the heart
2. To increase the force and efficiency of myocardial contraction through the action of pharmacologic agents

3. To eliminate the excessive accumulation of body water by means of diuretic therapy, diet, and rest

Pharmacologic Therapy

Cardiac glycosides (digitalis), diuretics, and vasodilators form the basis of the pharmacologic treatment of cardiac failure. Chart 26-3 summarizes the major cardiac glycosides, along with their actions and the nursing surveillance required when these drugs are administered.

Digitalis. Digitalis increases the force of myocardial contraction and slows the heart rate. Several effects are produced: an increase in cardiac output; a decrease in heart size, venous pressure, and blood volume; and diuresis, which relieves edema. The effect of a given dose of digitalis depends on the state of the myocardium, electrolyte and fluid balance, and renal and hepatic function.

A loading dose of digitalis may be given to induce the full therapeutic effect of the drug. This is usually done in the treatment of more severe forms of cardiac failure. Otherwise, the digitalis is started without a loading dose. A maintenance dose is given and continued daily. In either case, the patient is observed closely and given a daily dose just adequate to replace the amount of drug that is destroyed or excreted, in

(Text continues on p. 586)

Chart 26-4
Guidelines: Hemodynamic Monitoring: Multi-lumen Pulmonary Artery Catheter

Nursing Action	*Rationale/Amplification*

Preparatory Phase

1. Explain procedure to patient and family/significant other.

2. Check vital signs and apply ECG electrodes.
3. Place patient in a position of comfort, this is the baseline position.

4. Set up equipment according to manufacturer's directives:
   a. The pulmonary artery catheter requires a transducer; recording, amplifying, and flush systems.

   b. The pressure equipment is calibrated and flushed according to manufacturer's directives.
   c. The balloon is inflated with air and then deflated or it is inflated with air under sterile water or saline to test for leakage (bubbles).
5. Shave and prepare the skin over insertion site.

1. Tell the patient that it is normal to feel the catheter moving through the vein.

3. Note the angle of elevation if patient cannot lie flat, as subsequent pressure readings are taken from this baseline position to ensure consistency.
4.
   a. Monitoring systems may vary greatly. The complexity of equipment requires an understanding of the equipment in use.
   b. Flushing of the catheter system ensures patency and eliminates air bubbles.
   c. Testing is done to ensure that the balloon is intact.

Performance Phase (by the Physician)

1. The pulmonary artery catheter is inserted through the internal jugular, subclavian, or any easily accessible vein by either percutaneous puncture or venotomy.
2. The catheter is advanced to the superior vena cava. Oscillations of the pressure waveforms will indicate when the tip of the catheter is within the heart. The patient may be asked to cough.
3. When the catheter is in the superior vena cava, it is inflated with air and advanced gently.
4. The inflated balloon at the tip of the catheter will be guided by the flowing stream of blood through the right atrium and tricuspid valve into the right ventricle. From this position it finds its way into the main pulmonary artery, carried by blood flow. The catheter tip pressures are recorded continuously by specific pressure waveforms as the catheter advances through the various chambers of the heart.
5. The flowing blood will continue to direct the catheter more distally into the pulmonary tree. When the catheter reaches a pulmonary vessel that is approximately the same size or slightly smaller in diameter than the inflated balloon, it cannot be advanced any further. This is the wedge position, called pulmonary capillary wedge pressure (PCWP) or pulmonary artery wedge pressure (PAWP).
6. The pressure is recorded with the balloon wedged in the pulmonary vascular bed. A mean capillary wedge pressure between 14 and 18 mm Hg appears to indicate optimal left ventricular function.

1. The internal jugular vein establishes a short route into the central venous system.

2. Catheter placement may be determined by characteristic waveforms and changes. Coughing will produce deflections in the pressure tracing when the catheter tip is in the heart.
3. The amount of air to be used is indicated on the catheter.

4. Watch ECG monitor for signs of ventricular irritability as catheter enters the right ventricle. Report any signs of dysrhythmia to the physician.

5. With the catheter in the wedge position, the balloon blocks the flow of blood from the right side of the heart toward the lungs. The resulting capillary wedge pressure is equal to the mean left atrial pressure.

6. Wedge pressure reading provides information about the level of pulmonary congestion and is closely related to left atrial pressure and to left ventricular end-diastolic pressure (in the absence of mitral valve disease). This is a valuable parameter of cardiac function. Filling pressures less than 8 to 10 mm Hg in an acutely injured heart are often associated with reduction in cardiac output, hypotension, and tachycardia. A pressure greater than 18 mm Hg indicates pulmonary congestion.

(continued)

Chart 26-4 *(continued)*

Nursing Action	*Rationale/Amplification*
7. The balloon is deflated, causing the catheter to retract spontaneously into a larger pulmonary artery. This gives a continuous pulmonary artery systolic, diastolic, and mean pressure.	7. The normal systolic pulmonary pressure range is 15 to 25 mm Hg, and the diastolic pulmonary pressure range is 8 to 12 mm Hg. The normal mean pulmonary artery pressure (average pressure in pulmonary artery throughout the entire cardiac cycle) ranges from 10 to 20 mm Hg.
8. The catheter is sutured in place.	8. An antibiotic ointment may be placed around the site and covered with a sterile dressing.
9. The patency of the catheter is maintained with low-flow continuous irrigation.	9. A chest x-ray to confirm catheter position and as a baseline for future reference is obtained after Swan-Ganz catheter insertion.

To Obtain a Wedge Pressure Reading

1. Close off the microdrip.	1. The transducer converts the pressure wave into an electronic wave that is displayed on a screen.
2. Inflate the balloon slowly until the contour of the pulmonary arterial pressure changes to that of pulmonary wedge pressure. As soon as a wedge pattern is observed, no more air is introduced. Do not introduce more air into balloon than specified.	2. *Caution: Do not allow catheter to remain in the wedge position when patient is unattended or when not directly making the measurement. Segmental lung infarction may occur if the catheter balloon is left inflated for long periods.*
3. Deflate the balloon as soon as the pressure reading is obtained.	

To Obtain a Central Venous Pressure Reading

1. Turn the stopcock so that the CVP port is connected to the transducer.	1. Confirm the waveform to be that of the right atrium.
2. The pressure recorded is the central venous pressure.	2. Flush the tubing to ensure patency and return the stopcock to the continuous drip position.

Follow-Up Phase

1. Inspect the insertion site daily. Look for signs of infection, swelling, and bleeding.	1. A foreign body (catheter) in the vascular system increases the risk of sepsis.
2. Record data and time of dressing change and IV tubing change.	
3. If a peripheral vessel access site is used, assess the extremity for color, temperature, capillary filling, and sensation.	3. Ischemia (with possible loss of digits) may occur from inadequate arterial flow.
4. Evaluate pulse.	
5. Assess for complications: pulmonary embolism, dysrhythmias, heart block, damage to tricuspid valve, intracardiac knotting of catheter, thrombophlebitis, infection, balloon rupture, rupture of pulmonary artery.	

For Removal of the Catheter

1. Be sure that the balloon is not inflated.	
2. The catheter is removed without excessive force of traction; pressure dressing is applied over the site.	2. This site should be be checked periodically for bleeding.

order to maintain the digitalis effect without producing toxicity. The optimal dosage is the amount that relieves the patient's signs and symptoms of cardiac failure or slows the ventricular response therapeutically *without causing toxicity*. The patient is closely observed for relief of signs and symptoms: lessening dyspnea and orthopnea, decrease in crackles, and relief of peripheral edema.

Digitalis Toxicity. Anorexia, nausea, and vomiting are early effects of digitalis toxicity. There may be alterations in the heart rhythm, bradycardia, premature ventricular contractions, ventricular bigeminy (coupling of normal and premature beat), and paroxysmal atrial tachycardia.

- The apical heart rate is taken before digitalis is administered. If there is excessive slowing of the heart rate or change in rhythm, the drug is withheld and the physician is notified. Frequently the physician wants the digitalis preparation withheld if the rate is 60 or less.
- If prescribed, the serum digitalis level is checked prior to administration of the drug.

Diuretic Therapy. Diuretics are given to promote the excretion of sodium and water through the kidneys. These drugs may not be necessary if the patient responds to restricted activity, digitalis, and a low-sodium diet.

- When diuretics are given they should be administered early in the morning so that the resultant diuresis will not interfere with the patient's nighttime rest.
- An intake and output record is kept, because the patient may lose a large volume of fluid after a single dose of a given diuretic.
- As a basis for evaluating the effectiveness of therapy, a patient receiving diuretic drugs is weighed daily at the same time. In addition, skin turgor is examined for evidences of edema or dehydration. The pulse rate is also monitored.

The dosage schedule is determined by the patient's daily weight, physical findings, and symptoms. Table 26-1 summarizes the diuretics in common use. Furosemide (Lasix) is a particularly useful diuretic in the treatment of heart failure because it dilates the venules, thereby increasing venous capacitance, which in turn reduces preload (venous return to the heart).

Diuretic Side-Effects. Prolonged diuretic therapy may produce *hyponatremia* (deficiency of sodium in the blood), which results in apprehension, weakness, fatigue, malaise, muscle cramps and twitching, and rapid, thready pulse.

Profuse and repeated diuresis can also lead to *hypokalemia* (potassium depletion). Signs are weak pulse, faint heart sounds, hypotension, muscle flabbiness, diminished tendon reflexes, and generalized weakness. Hypokalemia poses new problems for the cardiac patient, because among the complications of hypokalemia are marked weakening of cardiac contractions and the precipitation of digitalis toxicity in persons receiving digitalis, both of which increase the likelihood of dangerous dysrhythmias.

- Periodic assessment of the electrolytes will alert to hypokalemia and hyponatremia.
- To lessen the risk of hypokalemia and its attendant complications, patients receiving diuretic drugs may be given a potassium supplement (potassium chloride). Bananas,

orange juice, dried prunes, raisins, apricots, dates, figs, peaches, and spinach are good dietary sources of potassium.

Other problems associated with diuretic administration are hyperuricemia, volume depletion, hyperglycemia, and diabetes mellitus.

The elderly male patient requires ongoing nursing surveillance because the incidence of urethral obstruction due to prostatic hypertrophy is high in this age group. Signs of bladder distention should be sought regularly by palpation over the bladder.

Vasodilator Therapy. Of particular significance in the management of cardiac failure are the vasoactive drugs.

Vasodilator drugs have been used to reduce impedance (resistance) to left ventricular ejection of blood. The drug action allows more complete ventricular emptying and increases venous capacity, so left ventricular filling pressure is reduced and a dramatic decrease in pulmonary congestion may be achieved rapidly.

Sodium nitroprusside may be given intravenously by means of carefully monitored infusions. The dosage is titrated to keep the arterial systolic pressure at the prescribed level, and the patient is monitored by measuring pulmonary artery pressures and cardiac output. Another commonly used vasodilator drug is nitroglycerin.

Providing Dietary Support

The rationale in dietary support is to provide the type of diet that will cause the heart the least possible work effort and muscular strain and to maintain good nutritional status, taking into consideration the patient's likes, dislikes, and cultural food habits.

Sodium Ion Manipulation. Restriction of the sodium ion is indicated for the prevention, control, or elimination of edema, as in hypertension or cardiac failure. Sodium should be specified in describing the regimen rather than "low-salt" or "salt-free," and the quantity should be indicated in milligrams. Very often mistakes are made in hospital units because of inconsistencies in the translation of salt to sodium. It is important to realize that salt is not 100% sodium. There are 393 mg, or approximately 400 mg, of sodium in 1 gram (1000 mg) of salt.

Although the major source of sodium in the average American diet is salt, many types of natural foods contain varying amounts of sodium. Therefore, even if no salt is added in cooking and if salty foods are avoided, the daily diet may still contain approximately 1000 mg to 2000 mg of sodium.

Other sources of sodium can be found in some processed foods. Added food substances—such as sodium alginate, which improves texture; sodium benzoate, which acts as a preservative; or disodium phosphate, which improves cooking quality in certain foods—increase the sodium intake when included in the daily diet. Therefore, patients on low-sodium diets should be advised not to buy processed foods and to check labels carefully for such words as "salt" or "sodium," especially on canned foods. For diets that call for less than 1000 mg of sodium, low-sodium milk and bread and salt-free butter should be considered.

Patients on sodium-restricted diets should also be cautioned against using nonprescription medications, such as alkalizers, cough syrups, laxatives, sedatives, or salt substitutes, because these products contain sodium or excessive amounts of potassium. Any over-the-counter medication of this type should not be purchased without first consulting the physician.

When diets are very restrictive of both fat and sodium, the patient may find the food unpalatable and may refuse to eat. A variety of flavorings such as lemon juice and herb seasonings may be used to improve the taste of the food and encourage the patient to accept the diet. Every effort should be made to take into account the patient's likes and dislikes.

► Nursing Process
The Patient With Cardiac Failure

▷ Assessment

The focus of the nursing assessment for the patient with cardiac failure is directed toward observing for signs and symptoms of pulmonary and systemic fluid overload. All untoward signs are recorded and reported to the physician.

Respiratory. The lungs are auscultated at frequent intervals to determine the presence or absence of crackles and wheezes. Crackles are produced by the movement of air through fluid, and therefore, if present, are evidence that pulmonary congestion is developing. The rate and depth of respirations are also noted.

Cardiac. The heart is auscultated for the presence of an S_3 or S_4 heart sound. The presence of these signs can mean that the pump is beginning to fail and that there is increased blood volume remaining in the ventricle with each beat. The rate and rhythm are also noted. Rapid rates indicate that the ventricle has had less time to fill and there is therefore some stagnation of blood in the atria and eventually the pulmonary bed.

Sensorium/Level of Consciousness. As the intravascular volume increases, the circulating blood becomes dilute and its oxygen transport capacity is compromised. The brain tolerates inadequate oxygenation poorly, and the patient becomes confused.

Periphery. The dependent parts of the patient's body are assessed for edema. If the patient is sitting upright, examine the feet and lower legs; if the patient is supine in bed, examine the sacrum and back for edema. Fingers and hands may also become edematous. In extreme cases of cardiac failure the patient may develop periorbital edema, in which the eyelids may be swollen shut.

The liver is examined for hepatojugular reflux (HJR). The patient is asked to breath normally while manual pressure is applied over the liver for 30 to 60 seconds. If neck vein distention increases more than one centimeter, the test is positive for increased venous pressure.

Jugular vein distention (JVD) is assessed. This is done by elevating the patient to a 45° angle. Estimate the distance between the angle of Louis and the level of jugular vein distension. (The *angle of Louis* is the junction between the body of the sternum and the manubrium.) A distance greater than 3 centimeters is said to be normal. Remember that this is an estimate and not an exact measurement.

Urinary Output. The patient may become oliguric or anuric. It is important to measure output frequently in order to develop a baseline to measure against in testing the efficacy of diuretic therapy. Intake and output records are rigorously maintained and the patient is weighed daily, at the same time and on the same scales.

▷ Nursing Diagnoses

Based on the assessment data, major nursing diagnoses for the patient may include the following:

- Activity intolerance related to fatigue and dyspnea secondary to decreased cardiac output
- Anxiety related to breathlessness and restlessness secondary to inadequate oxygenation
- Alteration in tissue perfusion—peripheral, related to venous stasis
- Potential deficit in knowledge of self-care program related to nonacceptance of necessary life-style changes

▷ Planning and Implementation

▷ ***Goals:*** The major goals of the patient may include (1) promotion of rest, (2) relief of anxiety, (3) attainment of normal tissue perfusion, and (4) knowledge of self-care program.

Nursing Interventions

Promotion of Rest. It is essential that the patient have both physical and emotional rest. Rest reduces the work of the heart, increases heart reserve, and reduces blood pressure. Periods of recumbency also promote diuresis by improving renal perfusion. Rest also decreases the work of the respiratory muscles and oxygen utilization. The heart rate is slowed, which prolongs the diastolic period of recovery and thus improves the efficiency of heart contraction. The patient will be impressed to hear that each day of complete rest spares the heart approximately 25,000 contractions.

Positioning. The head of the bed may be elevated on 20-cm to 30-cm (8-inch to 10-inch) blocks or the patient may be placed in a comfortable armchair. In this position the venous return to the heart (preload) and the lungs is reduced, pulmonary congestion is alleviated, and impingement of the liver on the diaphragm is minimized. The lower arms should be supported with pillows to eliminate the fatigue caused by the constant pull of their weight on the shoulder muscles. The orthopneic patient may sit on the side of the bed with feet supported on a chair, the head and arms resting on an over-the-bed table, and lumbosacral spine supported by a pillow. If pulmonary congestion is present, positioning the patient in an armchair is advantageous because this position favors the shift of fluid away from the lungs. Edema, which usually occurs in dependent parts of the body, shifts from the extremities to the sacral areas when the patient is confined to bed.

Relief of Anxiety. Because of their inability to maintain adequate oxygenation, patients in cardiac failure are apt to be restless and anxious. They feel overwhelmed by breathlessness. These symptoms tend to become exaggerated at night.

Raising the head of the bed and keeping a night light on are helpful. The presence of a member of the family provides necessary reassurance to some persons. The patient should be observed for possible respiratory irregularities such as Cheyne-Stokes respirations, a phenomenon that may occur in cardiac failure. If such a respiratory disturbance is present, it may be worthwhile to test the effect of oxygen inhalations administered (as prescribed) each night just before the hour of sleep. Oxygen may be given during the acute stage to diminish the work of breathing and to increase the comfort of the patient. Small doses of morphine may be prescribed for extreme dyspnea, and chloral hydrate may be given as needed for sleep.

- The patient with hepatic congestion is unable to detoxify drugs with normal rapidity and should be medicated with caution. As a result of cerebral hypoxia with superimposed nitrogen retention, the patient may react unfavorably to soporific drugs, becoming confused and increasingly anxious in response to medication. Such a patient should not be restrained; restraints are likely to be resisted, and resistance inevitably increases the cardiac load.

The patient who insists on getting out of bed at night should be seated comfortably in an armchair. As cerebral and systemic circulations improve, the quality of sleep will improve.

Avoiding Stress. Rest is not possible without relaxation. Emotional stress produces vasoconstriction, elevates arterial pressure, and speeds the heart. Promoting physical comfort and avoiding situations that tend to promote anxiety and agitation may help the patient to relax. The period of rest is continued for a few days to a few weeks until the cardiac failure is controlled.

Attainment of Normal Tissue Perfusion. The decreased tissue perfusion occurring in cardiac failure results from inadequate levels of circulating oxygen and stagnation of blood in the peripheral tissues. Moderate daily exercise will enhance the blood flow to peripheral tissues. Adequate oxygenation and appropriate diuresis will also serve to provide good tissue perfusion. Effective diuresis reduces hemodilution, thus providing more oxygen-carrying capacity to the vascular system.

Adequate rest is essential to the promotion of adequate tissue perfusion.

- There are dangers inherent in bed rest, such as pressure sores (especially in edematous patients), phlebothrombosis, and pulmonary embolism. Changes of position, deep breathing, elastic stockings, and leg exercises all help to improve muscle tone and at the same time aid venous return to the heart.

Knowledge About Self-Care. The self-care program is prepared in cooperation with the patient or significant other (Chart 26-5). Activities of daily living should be planned to minimize breathlessness and fatigue. The patient should remember that intolerable breathlessness and fatigue associated with normal activities are reasons to seek medical attention.

Patient Education. After cardiac failure is under control, the patient is encouraged to gradually resume the activities he was accustomed to prior to illness, particularly his job. The patient's earlier life-style should be retained if possible. However, some modifications in his habits, work, and interpersonal relationships usually have to be made. Any ac-

tivity that produces symptoms must be curtailed or other adaptations made. The patient should be helped to identify his emotional stresses and to explore ways in which these may be ventilated and discharged.

All too frequently patients keep returning to the clinic and hospital for recurring episodes of cardiac failure. Not only does this create psychological, sociological, and financial problems, but the physiological burden on the patient can be serious. Previously normal organs of the body may ultimately be damaged. Repeated attacks can lead to pulmonary fibrosis, liver cirrhosis, enlargement of the spleen and kidneys, and even brain damage due to insufficient oxygen during acute episodes.

To ensure that the patient will persevere in therapy requires patient education, involvement, and cooperation. Many of the recurrences of cardiac failure appear to be preventable. These include failure to follow the drug therapy properly, dietary indiscretions, inadequate medical follow-up, excessive physical activity, and failure to recognize recurring symptoms. A summary of what the patient should know is given in Chart 26-5.

It must be emphasized that many remedies such as cough medicines, alkalizers, and pain pills contain fairly large amounts of sodium. The patient must be warned against using these products and advised to rinse the mouth with clear water when using toothpaste and mouthwashes. In some areas the drinking water has a high sodium content. To find out what this content is, the patient should contact the local health department.

As an added precaution for older patients whose eyesight is dimming and whose fingers are less nimble as a result of arthritis, the printing on any drug bottle should be large and easily readable and the bottle should be equipped with an easy-open stopper.

Cardiac failure can be controlled. The patient must never become lax in following the prescribed therapeutic program. Careful follow-up, maintenance of correct weight, sodium restriction, prevention of infection, avoidance of noxious agents such as coffee and tobacco, and avoidance of unregulated or excessive exercise all aid in preventing the onset of cardiac failure. In patients with valvular heart disease, surgical correction of the defect at the appropriate time may spare the heart and prevent failure.

▷ *Evaluation*

▷ *Expected Outcomes*

1. Patient reduces fatigue and dyspnea.
   a. Obtains adequate physical and emotional rest
   b. Assumes positions that reduce fatigue and dyspnea
   c. Adheres to medication regimen
2. Experiences less anxiety
   a. Avoids situations that produce stress
   b. Sleeps comfortably at night
3. Attains normal tissue perfusion
   a. Obtains adequate rest
   b. Performs activities that promote venous return: moderate daily exercise; active range of motion of extremities if immobile or in bed for long periods of time; wearing support stockings
   c. Skin warm and dry; color is good.
   d. Exhibits no peripheral edema.

Chart 26-5
Patient Education: Cardiac Failure

A patient with heart disease should learn to regulate his activity according to his individual response.

Goal: To prevent progression of disease and the development of cardiac failure
The patient learns that to achieve these goals he will have to do the following:

I. Live within the limits of the cardiac reserve.
   A. Obtain adequate rest.
      1. Have a regular daily rest period.
      2. Shorten working hours if possible.
      3. Avoid emotional upsets.
   B. Accept the fact that taking digitalis and restricting sodium intake may be a permanent way of life.
      1. Take digitalis daily, exactly as prescribed.
         a. Avoid substituting another brand of digitalis for the one prescribed.
         b. Check own pulse rate daily.
         c. Have a check-off system to ensure that medicine(s) has been taken.
      2. Take diuretic as prescribed.
         a. Weigh at the same time daily to detect any tendency toward fluid accumulation.
         b. Report weight gain of more than 0.9 kg to 1.4 kg (2–3 pounds) in a few days.
         c. Know the signs and symptoms of potassium depletion; if taking oral potassium, keep a check-off system along with diuretic medication.
      3. Take vasodilator as prescribed.
         a. Learn to take own blood pressure at prescribed intervals.
         b. Know signs and symptoms of orthostatic hypotension and how to prevent it.
   C. Restrict sodium as directed.
      1. Consult the written diet plan and the list of permitted and restricted foods.
      2. Examine labels to ascertain sodium content (antacids, laxatives, cough remedies, and the like).
      3. Avoid using salt.
      4. Avoid excesses in eating and drinking.
   D. Review activity program.
      1. Increase walking and other activities gradually, provided that they do not cause fatigue and dyspnea.
      2. In general, continue at whatever activity level can be maintained without the appearance of symptoms.
      3. Avoid extremes of heat and cold, which increase the work of the heart. Air conditioning may be essential in a hot, humid environment.
      4. Keep regular appointments with physician or clinic.
II. Be alert for symptoms that may indicate recurring failure.
      1. Recall the symptoms experienced when illness began. Reappearance of previous symptoms may indicate a recurrence.
      2. Report immediately to the physician or clinic any of the following:
         a. Gain in weight
         b. Loss of appetite
         c. Shortness of breath on activity
         d. Swelling of ankles, feet, or abdomen
         e. Persistent cough
         f. Frequent urination at night

4. Adheres to self-care regimen. (See Chart 26-5, in which self-care activities are described.)

Cardiogenic Shock

Cardiogenic shock (power failure), the end stage of left ventricular dysfunction, occurs when the left ventricle is extensively damaged. The heart muscle loses its contractile power, and the result is a marked reduction in cardiac output with inadequate tissue perfusion to the vital organs (heart, brain, kidneys). The degree of shock is proportional to the level of left ventricular dysfunction. Although cardiogenic shock is seen most commonly as a complication of myocardial infarction, it can also occur with cardiac tamponade, pulmonary embolism, and epidural or general anesthesia.

Pathophysiology. The symptoms and signs of cardiogenic shock reflect the circular nature of the pathophysiology of cardiac failure. The damage to the myocardium results in a decrease in cardiac output, which in turn reduces arterial blood pressure in the vital organs. Flow to the coronary arteries is reduced. This results in a decrease in the oxygen supply to the myocardium, which in turn increases ischemia and further reduces the heart's ability to pump. Thus, a "vicious cycle" is set in motion.

- The classic signs of cardiogenic shock are low blood pressure, rapid and weak pulse, cerebral hypoxia manifested by confusion and agitation, and decreased urinary output.

Dysrhythmias are common and result from a decrease in oxygen to the myocardium. As in cardiac failure, the use of a pulmonary artery catheter to measure left ventricular pressure is important in assessing the severity of the problem and evaluating management. Continuing elevation of left ventricular end-diastolic pressure (LVEDP) accompanied by a fall in arterial blood pressure indicates the failure of the heart to function as an effective pump.

Medical Management. There are many approaches to the treatment of cardiogenic shock. Any major dysrhythmias are corrected because they may have caused or contributed to the shock. If low intravascular volume is suspected, or found through pressure readings (*i.e.*, hypovolemia), the patient is treated by infusion of volume expanders. If hypoxia is present, oxygen is given, often under positive pressure when regular flow is insufficient to meet tissue demands.

Drug therapy is selected and guided according to cardiac output and mean arterial blood pressure. One group of drugs used is the catecholamines, which raise blood pressure and increase cardiac output. However, they tend to increase the workload of the heart by increasing oxygen demand. Vasoactive drugs such as sodium nitroprusside and nitroglycerine are effective drugs that lower blood pressure and thus cardiac work. They cause arterial and venous dilatation, thereby shunting much of the intravascular volume to the periphery and causing a reduction in preload and afterload. These vasoactive drugs are usually given in tandem with dopamine, a vasopressor which assists in maintaining an adequate blood pressure.

Other therapeutic modalities employed in treating cardiogenic shock involve the use of circulatory assist devices. The most frequently used mechanical support system is the intra-aortic balloon pump (IABP). The IABP uses internal counterpulsation to augment the pumping action of the heart by the regular inflation and deflation of a balloon located in the descending thoracic aorta (Fig. 26-19). The device is connected to a control box that directs its activities by synchronization with the electrocardiogram. Hemodynamic monitoring is also essential to determine the patient's circulatory status during the use of the IABP. The balloon inflates during ventricular diastole and deflates during systole at a rate equal to the heart rate. The IABP augments diastole, which results in increased perfusion of the coronary arteries and myocardium and a decrease in left ventricular workload.

Nursing Implications. The patient with cardiogenic shock requires constant nursing care and observation. Careful patient assessment, measurement of hemodynamic parameters, and recording of fluid intake and urinary output are essential. The patient must be closely monitored for dysrhythmias, which must be corrected immediately.

Because of the technology required for effective medical management in such cases, this patient is always treated in a critical care environment. Critical care nurses with highly developed skills are responsible for the nursing management. Every nurse, however, needs to understand the concepts of treatment modalities.

Thromboembolic Episodes

The decreased mobility of the patient and the impaired circulation that accompanies cardiac diseases contribute to the development of intracardiac and intravascular thrombosis. As the patient increases activities, a thrombus may become detached (the detached thrombus is called an *embolus*) and may be carried to the brain, kidneys, intestines, or lungs.

The most common embolic episode is that of a pulmonary embolus. The symptoms of pulmonary embolism include chest pain, cyanosis, shortness of breath, rapid respirations, and hemoptysis. The pulmonary embolus may block the circulation to a part of the lung, producing an area of pulmonary infarction. The pain experienced is usually pleuritic—that is,

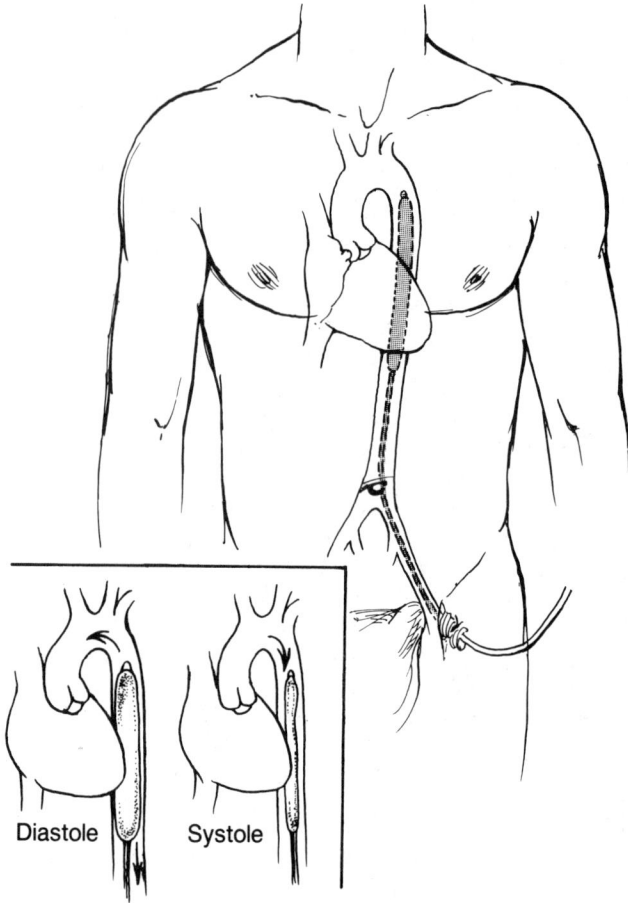

Figure 26-19
The intra-aortic balloon pump augments diastole, which results in increased perfusion of the coronary arteries and myocardium and a decrease in the left ventricular workload.

it increases with respiration and may disappear when the patient holds a breath. Cardiac pain is continuous, however, and usually does not vary with respirations. The treatment of pulmonary embolism is discussed in Chapter 23.

Systemic embolism may occur from the left ventricle, and the resulting vascular occlusion may present as stroke or renal infarct; it may compromise the blood supply to an extremity. The nurse must be aware of such possible complications and prepared to identify and report signs and symptoms.

Pericardial Effusion

Pathophysiology. *Pericardial effusion* refers to the escape of fluid into the pericardial sac. This may accompany pericarditis, advanced congestive heart failure, or cardiac surgery.

The characteristic sign of pericardial effusion is an extension of flatness to percussion across the anterior aspect of the chest wall. The patient may complain of a feeling of fullness within the chest or have substernal or ill-defined pain.

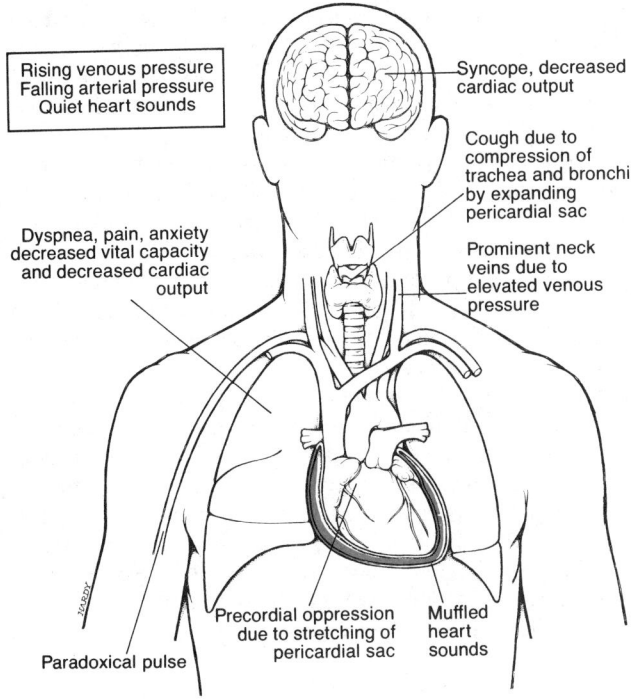

Rising venous pressure
Falling arterial pressure
Quiet heart sounds

Syncope, decreased cardiac output

Cough due to compression of trachea and bronchi by expanding pericardial sac

Dyspnea, pain, anxiety decreased vital capacity and decreased cardiac output

Prominent neck veins due to elevated venous pressure

Precordial oppression due to stretching of pericardial sac

Muffled heart sounds

Paradoxical pulse

Figure 26-20
Assessment for cardiac tamponade due to pericardial effusion.

Normally, the pericardial sac contains less than 50 ml of fluid. Pericardial fluid may accumulate slowly without causing noticeable symptoms. However, a *rapidly* developing effusion can stretch the pericardium to its maximum size and can cause decreased cardiac output and decreased venous return to the heart. The result is *cardiac tamponade* (compression of the heart). See Figure 26-20.

Clinical Manifestations. Symptoms include a feeling of precordial oppression due to the stretching of the pericardial sac; shortness of breath; and a drop and fluctuation in blood pressure. Blood pressure is lowest on inspiration (*pulsus paradoxus*), at which point the pulse may not be perceptible. The venous pressure tends to rise, as evidenced by the engorged neck veins.

The cardinal signs are falling arterial blood pressure, narrowing pulse pressure, rising venous pressure, and distant heart sounds. *This is a life-threatening situation, demanding immediate intervention.*

Diagnostic Evaluation. If the clinical manifestations are not immediately life-threatening, the physician may choose to confirm the diagnosis via echocardiogram. Bedside diagnosis based on clinical signs and symptoms is usually sufficient.

Management: Pericardial Aspiration (Pericardiocentesis). If the cardiac function becomes seriously impaired, a pericardial aspiration (puncture of the pericardial sac) is performed to remove fluid from the pericardial sac. The major goal for it is to prevent cardiac tamponade, which restricts normal heart action.

During the procedure the patient is monitored by ECG, and central venous pressure measurements are made. Emergency resuscitative equipment is readily available.

The head of the bed is elevated to a 45° to 60° angle so that the needle can be inserted into the pericardial sac more easily. If not already in place, a peripheral intravenous device is inserted and a slow intravenous drip of saline or glucose is started in case it becomes necessary to administer emergency drugs or blood.

The pericardial aspiration needle is attached to a 50-ml syringe by a three-way stopcock. The V lead (precordial lead wire) of the ECG may be attached to the hub of the aspirating needle with alligator clips, because the monitoring of ECG oscillation is useful in determining whether or not the needle has contacted the myocardium. Contact is evidenced by an elevation of the ST segment or stimulation of premature ventricular contractions.

There are several possible sites for pericardial aspiration. The needle may be inserted in the angle between the left costal margin and the xiphoid, near the cardiac apex, to the left of the fifth or sixth interspace at the sternal margin, or on the right side of the fourth intercostal space. The needle is advanced slowly until fluid is obtained.

A fall in central venous pressure associated with a rise in blood pressure indicates that relief of cardiac tamponade has occurred. The patient almost always feels immediate improvement. If there is a substantial amount of pericardial fluid, a small catheter may be left in place to drain recurrent bleeding or effusion.

During the procedure it is important to watch for the presence of bloody fluid. Pericardial blood does not clot readily, whereas blood obtained from inadvertent puncture of one of the heart chambers does clot.

Pericardial fluid is sent to the laboratory for examination for tumor cells, bacterial culture, chemical and serological analysis, and differential cell count. A hematocrit is done if the fluid is bloody.

- After pericardiocentesis, effective care involves careful monitoring of the blood pressure, venous pressure, and heart sounds to evaluate for the possible recurrence of cardiac tamponade. If it recurs, repeated aspiration is necessary. Sometimes cardiac tamponade is treated by open pericardial drainage. The patient is ideally in an intensive care unit.

Myocardial Rupture

When a myocardial infarction, infectious process, pericardial disease, or other myocardial dysfunction weakens the cardiac muscle, the heart may rupture, leading to immediate death in most cases. Cardiac rupture, although fairly rare, can occur.

Death is caused by cardiac tamponade (the heart is bleeding into its pericardial sac). Pericardiocentesis and repair of the myocardium can be life-saving measures.

Cardiac Arrest

Cardiac arrest is defined as the sudden, unexpected cessation of the heartbeat and effective circulation. All heart action may stop, or asynchronized muscular twitchings (ventricular fibrillation) may occur.

There is an immediate loss of consciousness and an absence of pulses and audible heart sounds. Dilation of the pupils of the eyes begins within 45 seconds. Convulsions may or may not be present.

- There is an interval of approximately 4 minutes between the cessation of circulation and the appearance of irreversible brain damage. The interval varies with the age of the patient. During this period, the diagnosis of arrest must be made and the circulation must be restored.
- *The most reliable sign of arrest is the absence of a carotid pulsation.* Valuable time should not be wasted taking the blood pressure or listening for the heartbeat.

Cardiopulmonary Resuscitation

Basic cardiopulmonary resuscitation (CPR) consists of the following sequence: Airway, Breathing, and Circulation (see Fig. 26-21). The resuscitation process consists of maintaining an open airway, providing artificial ventilation by means of rescue breathing, and providing artificial circulation by external cardiac compression.

The first step in CPR is to secure an airway. Remove any material from the airway and lift the jaw forward. Insert an oropharyngeal airway if available. Ventilate the patient with 12 breaths per minute using direct mouth-to-mouth breathing or using the bag and mask technique.

The next step after ventilation is external cardiac compression. This must be done with the patient on a firm surface. The heel of one hand is placed on the lower half of the sternum, 3.8 cm (1½ inches) from the tip of the xiphoid and toward the patient's head. Place the other hand on top of the first one. The fingers should not touch the chest wall. Using the body weight while keeping the elbows straight, apply quick, forceful compressions to the lower sternum, 3.8 cm to 5.0 cm (1½–2 inches) toward the spine. Regular compression and release are made 60 times per minute.

When two persons are available, the first person does the cardiac compressions and the second ventilates the patient after 5 compressions. If only one person is available, the rate is 2 ventilations to every 15 cardiac compressions.

The decision to terminate resuscitation is based on medical considerations and will take into account the cerebral and cardiac status of the patient.

TABLE 26-2
Drug Therapy in Cardiopulmonary Resuscitation

Drug	Indication	Side-Effects and Comments
Oxygen	To correct hypoxemia	No lung damage when used for less than 24 hours
Lidocaine	To suppress ventricular dysrhythmias. To raise the threshold for ventricular fibrillation (VF)	Myocardial and circulatory depression. CNS changes: drowsiness, disorientation, decreased hearing ability, paresthesias, muscle twitching, and agitation. Focal and grand mal seizures.
Procainamide Hydrochloride	To suppress ventricular dysrhythmias when lidocaine is ineffective	
Atropine	To accelerate cardiac rate by creating a positive chronotropic effect due to parasympatholytic action (reduces vagal tone) and by creating a positive dromotropic effect that accelerates AV conduction.	This increased heart rate may be deleterious in patients with acute MI. Atropine should be given to patients with acute MI only if the bradycardia results in hemodynamic changes.
Epinephrine	To increase perfusion pressure during cardiac compressions To improve the myocardial contractile state To stimulate spontaneous contractions (*e.g.,* in asystole) To increase the vigor of VF	Epinephrine should not be added directly to a bicarbonate infusion, because catecholamines may be inactivated by alkaline solution.
Sodium Bicarbonate (NaHCO₃)	To correct metabolic and respiratory acidosis	Because CO_2 production is increased, adequate ventilation is required. Excessive $NaHCO_3$ leads to metabolic alkalosis with displacement of oxyhemoglobin dissociation curve and consequent impairment of oxygen release to tissues. Hyperosmolality may also develop. Catecholamines and calcium salts should not be added to bicarbonate infusions because inactivation results. Because bicarbonate has a high *p*H, avoid mixing any drugs with it.

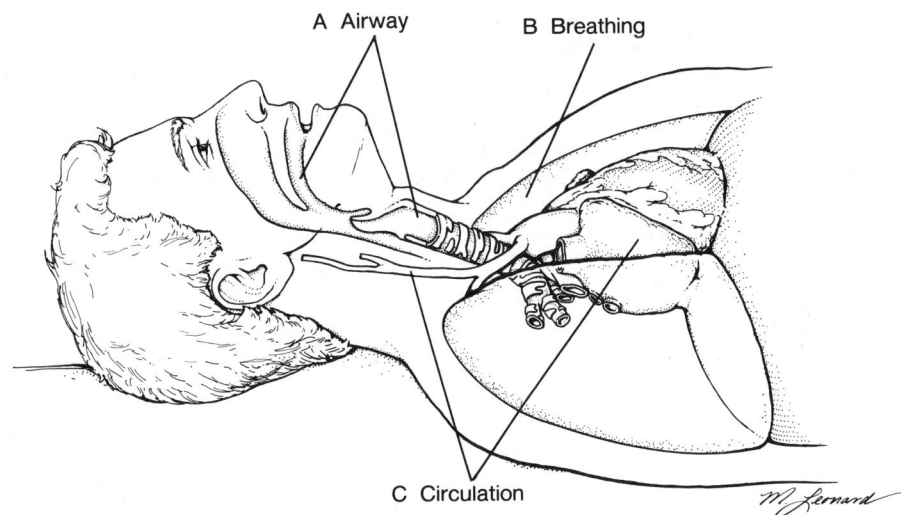

Figure 26-21
A, B, Cs of basic life support.

Following successful resuscitation after cardiac arrest, the nurse should carefully monitor the situation because the patient is at great risk for another cardiac arrest. Continuation of ECG monitoring is essential, and any abnormalities of rhythm must be corrected. Electrolyte and acid–base balances must be established and maintained. Hemodynamic monitoring should be initiated if it was not previously instituted. Selected drugs are used during and after resuscitation (Table 26-2), and should be immediately available.

Bibliography

Books

Abels L. Critical Care Nursing. St Louis, CV Mosby, 1986.

Andreoli K et al. Comprehensive Cardiac Care. St Louis, CV Mosby, 1984.

Basta L. Cardiovascular Disease: Essentials of Primary Care. New York, Medical Examination Publishing Co, 1983.

Bigger JT. A Primer on Calcium Ion Antagonists. Whippany, New Jersey, Knoll Pharmaceutical Co, 1981.

Braunwald E. Heart Disease: A Textbook of Cardiovascular Disease. Philadelphia, WB Saunders, 1984.

Bustin, D. Hemodynamic Monitoring for Critical Care. Norwalk, Appleton-Century-Crofts, 1986.

Chernow B. The Pharmacologic Approach to the Critically Ill Patient. Baltimore, Williams & Wilkins, 1983.

Chung EK. Artificial Cardiac Pacing. Baltimore, Williams & Wilkins, 1984.

Chung EK. Cardiac Emergency Care. Philadelphia, Lea & Febiger, 1985.

Conover MB. Understanding Electrocardiography. St Louis, CV Mosby, 1980.

Das Gupta DS. Principles and Practice of Acute Cardiac Care. Chicago, Year Book Medical Publishers, 1984.

Douglas MK and Shinn JA. Advances in Cardiovascular Nursing. Rockville, Maryland, Aspen Systems, 1985.

Guzetta CE and Dossey BM. Cardiovascular Nursing: Bodymind Tapestry. St Louis, CV Mosby, 1984.

Holloway N. Nursing the Critically Ill Adult. Menlo Park, California, Addison-Wesley, 1984.

Hurst JW. The Heart. New York, McGraw-Hill, 1982.

Josephson ME. Sudden Cardiac Death. Philadelphia, FA Davis, 1985.

Julian DG and Wenger NK. Management of Heart Failure. Boston, Butterworth, 1986.

Kloner R. The Guide to Cardiology. New York, John Wiley & Sons, 1984.

Marriott HL and Conover MR. Advanced Concepts in Arrhythmias. St Louis, CV Mosby, 1983.

Meltzer LE, Pinneo R, and Kitchell JR. Intensive Coronary Care: A Manual for Nurses. Bowie, Maryland, Prentice-Hall, 1983.

Metcalf K. Understanding Cardiac Pacing. Norwalk, Appleton-Century-Crofts, 1986.

Price S and Wilson L. Pathophysiology: Clinical Concepts of Disease Process. New York, McGraw-Hill, 1986.

Sadler D. Nursing for Cardiovascular Health. Norwalk, Appleton-Century-Crofts, 1984.

Sanderson RG and Kurth CL. The Cardiac Patient: A Comprehensive Approach. Philadelphia, WB Saunders, 1983.

Silver MD. Cardiovascular Pathology, Vol 1. New York, Churchill Livingstone, 1983.

Silver MD. Cardiovascular Pathology, Vol 2. New York, Churchill Livingstone, 1983.

Underhill SL et al. Cardiac Nursing. Philadelphia, JB Lippincott, 1982.

Warren JV and Lewis RP. Diagnostic Procedures in Cardiology. Chicago, Year Book Medical Publishers, 1985.

Wells SJ. Manual of Cardiovascular Assessment. Reston, Virginia, Reston Publishing Co, 1983.

Woods SL. Cardiovascular Critical Care Nursing. New York, Churchill Livingstone, 1983.

Yee BH and Zorb SL. Cardiac Critical Care Nursing. Boston, Little, Brown & Co, 1986.

Yurick AG et al. The Aged Person and the Nursing Process. Norwalk, Appleton-Century-Crofts, 1984.

Articles

Dysrhythmias

Berman N. Antiarrhythmic therapy in the elderly: Pacemakers and drugs. Geriatrics 1986 Feb; 41(2):61–72.

Burden LL et al. Bradycardia—The signals of a slowing heart. Nursing 84 1984 Sept; 14(9):50–55.

Catalano JT. Antiarrhythmic medications classified by their autonomic properties. Crit Care Nurse 1986 May/June; 6(3):44–48.

Cooke DH. Ventricular fibrillation: The state of the art. Emergency Med 1986 Mar 15: 116–138.

Geddes LE. Monitoring the patient with conduction disturbances and blocks. Nurs Clin North Am 1987 Mar; 22(1):33–47.

Glasser SP and Zoble RG. Management of cardiac arrhythmias. Hosp Practice 1985 Aug 15: 20(8):127–148.

Horowitz L. How do you manage the patient with VPCs? Cardiovasc Med 1986 April: 37–42.

Kupper NS et al. Tachycardia: Stay a step ahead of your patient's racing heart. Nursing 84 1984 Aug; 14(8):34–41.

Loeb JM. Cardiac electrophysiology: Basic concepts and arrhythmogenesis. Crit Care Quart 1984 Sept; 7(2):9–19.

Moser SA and Flake G. The new antiarrhythmics are coming. Nursing 85 1985 Sept; 15(9):56–58.

Ordonez RV. Monitoring the patient with supraventricular dysrhythmias. Nurs Clin North Am 1987 Mar; 22(1):49–59.

Reyes AV. Monitoring and treating life-threatening ventricular dysrhythmias. Nurs Clin North Am 1987 Mar; 22(1):61–76.

Schessl EC. Learning the basics of cardiac monitors. Nursing 84 1984 Oct; 14(10):42–43.

Sergeant LL. Tracking your outpatient's EKG with a Holter monitor. Nursing 86 1986 Oct; 16(10):47–49.

Sumner SM and Grau P. Guidelines for running a 12-lead EKG. Nursing 85 1985 Dec; 15(12):30–33.

Thielbar S. Antiarrhythmic drug therapy: An overview. Crit Care Quart 1984 Sept; 7(2):21–33.

Wessman JP. Preventing ventricular dysrhythmia following myocardial infarction. Dimens Crit Care Nurs 1985 Jan/Feb; 4(1):24–32.

Zhertlin T. Theory of patients with malignant ventricular arrhythmias. Crit Care Quart 1984 Sept; 7(2):35–48.

Pacemakers

Evans N. Clinical assessment of pacemaker functions: The ICHD code. DCCN 1985 May/June; 4(3):140–145.

Hawthorne JW. How to choose a cardiac pacing system. Cardiovasc Med 1986 Jan: 10–11.

Haywood D. Temporary A-V sequential pacing using an epicardial lead system. Crit Care Nurse 1985 May/June; 5(3):21–24.

Mickus D et al. Exciting external pacemakers. Am J Nurs 1986 April; 86(4):403–405.

Murdock D. Pacemaker malfunction: Fact or artifact? Heart Lung 1986 Mar; 15(2):150–154.

Owen PM. Defibrillating pacemaker patients. Am J Nurs 1984 Sept; 84(9):1129–1132.

Pietro DA. Recurrent dizziness and fatigue in a pacemaker patient. Cardiovasc Med 1985 Feb: 37–39.

Purcell JA and Burrows SG. A pacemaker primer. Am J Nurs 1985 May; 85(5):553–568.

Rosenthal M et al. When do you advise dual-chamber pacing? Cardiovasc Med 1986 Mar: 27–34.

Shirley D and Littrell K. Troubleshooting malfunctions of the dual-chambered pacemaker. DCCN 1985 May/June; 4(3):146–155.

Vacek JL and Cissik JH. Applications of physiologic pacemakers. Applied Cardiol 1986 May/June; 14(3):15–18.

Pulmonary Edema, Failure, Shock

Cardin S and Clark S. A nursing diagnosis approach to the patient awaiting cardiac transplantation. Heart Lung 1985 Sept; 14(5):499–504.

Gever LN. Anticoagulants. Nursing 84 1984 Nov; 14(11):64.

Glasbrenner K. Calcium channel antagonists. JAMA 1985 Apr 19; 253(15):2179–2180.

Goldberg L and Rajfer S. Cardiac failure: The role of adrenergic and dopamine receptors. Hosp Practice 1985 June 15; 20(6):67–80.

Goldsmith M. Recombinant plasminogen agent continues to show promise in trials. JAMA 1985 Mar 22; 253(12):1693–94.

Kleinhenz TJ. The inside story on preload and afterload. Nursing 85 1985 May; 15(5):50–56.

Koszuta LE. The ins and outs of measuring cardiac output. Nursing 86 1986 Mar; 16(3):55–56.

Lough ME. Introduction to hemodynamic monitoring. Nurs Clin North Am 1987 Mar; 22(1):89–110.

Murray JF. The lungs and heart failure. Hosp Practice 1985 Apr 15; 20(4):55–68.

Niemczura J. Rules to remember when caring for the patient with a Swan-Ganz catheter. Nursing 85 1985 Mar; 15(3):39–41.

Norsen LH and Fox GB. Understanding cardiac output and the drugs that affect it. Nursing 85 1985 Apr; 15(4):34–41.

Painvin GA et al. Cardiac transplantation: Indications, procurement, operation, and management. Heart Lung 1985 Sept; 14(5):484–489.

Parmley W. To rescue a failing heart. Emergency Med 1983 Mar 15; 15(3):178–189.

Rice V. Shock management. Crit Care Nurse 1985 Jan/Feb; 5(1):42–57.

Scordo C. Hemodynamic monitoring: Learning to read the waves. Nursing 85 1985 July; 15(7):40–42.

Urban N. Integrating hemodynamic parameters with clinical decision-making. Crit Care Nurse 1986 Mar/Apr; 6(2):48–61.

Thromboembolism

Beller LC and Neunaber KL. The 'simple' valsalva. Am J Nurs 1986 Apr; 86(4):398–399.

Fahey VA. Life-threatening pulmonary embolism. Crit Care Quart 1985 Sept; 8(2):81–88.

Hull RD. Suspected pulmonary embolism. Primary Cardiol 1985 May; 11(5):15–26.

Mok CK. Preventing thromboembolism in prosthetic heart valves. Cardiology Board Review 1986 July; 3(7):87–95.

Pericarditis/Rupture

Estes ME. Management of the cardiac tamponade patient: A nursing framework. Crit Care Nurse 1985 Sept/Oct; 5(5):17–26.

Feneley MP. Postinfarction myocardial rupture. Primary Cardiology 1986 Feb; 12(2):133–153.

Fowler NO. Constrictive pericarditis. Primary Cardiology 1985 Jan; 11(1):94–96.

Fowler NO. Cardiac tamponade. Primary Cardiol 1985 Feb; 11(2):81–87.

Miracle V. Anatomy of a murmur. Nursing 86 1986 July; 16(7):26–31.

Spodick DH. Acute pericardial disease. Heart Lung 1985 Nov; 14(6):599–604.

Spodick DH. Acute pericarditis: Clinical findings and ECG changes that confirm diagnosis. Consultant 1986 July; 26(7):145–156.

Arrest/Cardiopulmonary Resuscitation

Bauman EC. Code drugs. Nursing 85 1985 Dec; 15(12):50–55.

Buschiazzo L. What's new in CPR. Nursing 86 1986 Jan; 16(1):34–39.

Dennison R. Cardiopulmonary assessment. Nursing 86 1986 Apr; 16(4):34–39.

Hallstrom A et al. The potential use of automatic defibrillators in the home for management of cardiac arrest. Medical Care 1984 Dec 22; 12:1083–1087.

Jett GK and Isbell J. IV drugs for cardiac arrest. Hosp Therapy 1986 July: 41–53.

Porterfield JG et al. Sudden cardiac death. Focus Crit Care 1986 June; 13(3):23–31.

Sommer MS. Creating a therapeutic environment during cardiopulmonary resuscitation. Focus Crit Care 1985 June; 12(3):22–29.

Standards for CPR and ECC. JAMA 1986 June 6; 255(21):2915–2989.

Agencies

Governmental

National Heart, Lung, and Blood Institute; National Institues of Health, Building 31, Room 5A52, Bethesda, MD 20892.

Voluntary

American Heart Association, 7220 Greenville Avenue, Dallas, TX 75231.
Coronary Club, 3659 Green Road, Cleveland, OH 44122.
Heartlife, PO Box 54305, Atlanta, GA 30308.

Chapter 27

Management of the Cardiac Surgery Patient

Since the introduction of valvular heart surgery in the 1940s, continued advances in technology associated with cardiac diagnostics, anesthesia, and surgery have made it possible today to perform surgery to correct many congenital heart defects, to bypass obstructions in the coronary arteries, to resect foci of dysrhythmias, and to transplant hearts. Much progress has been made in the development of a totally artificial heart. The use of percutaneous laser angioplasty as a noninvasive measure to relieve atheromatous obstructions is becoming a reality.

In 1984, 202,000 coronary artery bypass graft (CABG) surgeries were performed in the United States. The high number of CABG surgeries can be attributed to improvements in cardiac cineangiography, cardiopulmonary bypass (extracorporeal circulation) techniques, and anesthesia procedures, and advances in hemodynamic pressure monitoring techniques that have refined postoperative assessment and enabled improved postoperative care and decreased mortality.

This chapter describes the surgical procedures and care required by adults with heart disease. Congenital heart defects are not covered but may be reviewed in a pediatric textbook.

Cardiac Surgery Procedures

Cardiopulmonary Bypass

Many of the cardiac surgical procedures are performed while the patient is placed on partial or complete cardiopulmonary bypass (extracorporeal circulation). All of the cardiac surgeries that require direct visualization by means of an incision into the heart (*e.g.*, valve replacements) or that require the heart to be arrested (*e.g.*, CABG) utilize cardiopulmonary bypass.

The bypass procedure provides a mechanical means of circulating and oxygenating the blood while diverting it from the heart and lungs. This allows for operative accessibility by affording the surgeon a quiet, bloodless field, yet preserves tissue and organ perfusion and viability.

The patient is placed on a machine that consists of a mechanical pump that simulates the pumping action of the left ventricle and an oxygenator that simulates the function of the lungs. The blood is removed from the systemic circulation by means of cannulas inserted into the right atrium or vena cavae. By means of a pump, the blood enters the venous reservoir and is then filtered and passed through the oxygenator and heat exchanger. The blood is usually returned by way of a cannula in the ascending aorta. However, the femoral artery is used for this purpose when the operative procedure involves the aortic arch or in patients where calcification of the aorta is extensive. The oxygenated blood is used by the tissues of the body and then returned to the pump or heart–lung machine, where the process is repeated (Fig. 27-1).

Because cardiopulmonary bypass is an artificial means of maintaining circulation, complications resulting from alterations in hemodynamics will occur if measures are not taken to provide for hemodilution, hypothermia, and anticoagulation.

The original practice of using whole blood to prime the pump has been replaced with the use of autologous blood (blood donated by the patient prior to the procedure) diluted with an isotonic crystalloid substance (*e.g.*, 5% dextrose and lactated Ringer's solution). This type of hemodilution has resulted in less extreme extravascular-to-interstitial fluid shifts, decreased blood viscosity and increased capillary perfusion, decreased formation of microthrombi, and reduced chances for blood incompatibilities and transmission of diseases such as hepatitis and acquired immunodeficiency syndrome (AIDS).

Hypothermia (and rewarming at the completion of the procedure) is accomplished by the heat exchange element in the pump. During the operative procedure, the patient is cooled to a temperature of 28° to 32°C (82.4° to 89.6°F), which decreases the tissue oxygen requirements by about 50% and protects the major organs from the ischemic injury that would result if it became necessary to slow perfusion during the surgery or if the pump should fail. Although hypothermia increases blood viscosity, this effect is compensated for by hemodilution.

Anticoagulation is necessary to decrease the risk of massive clotting in the mechanical parts of the bypass system. This is accomplished with heparin, the effects of which are closely monitored during the surgery. Immediately after discontinuation of the bypass, protamine sulfate is used to reverse the effects of heparin. The patient is observed closely during the first few postoperative hours for a heparin rebound effect, which results when heparin that has pooled in the peripheral circulation and has been trapped in fatty tissue gradually returns to the central circulation after the patient has been rewarmed. Additional protamine sulfate is usually needed to neutralize this heparin.

Although several types of machines have been used for cardiopulmonary bypass, at present the most commonly used are those with a bubble oxygenator or a membrane oxygenator. The bubble oxygenator bubbles oxygen through a long column of blood in a chamber. The blood is foamy when it reaches the top of the chamber and is defoamed when it passes over steel wool or a polypropylene mesh with a silicone antifoam compound on its surface. The membrane oxygenator uses a semipermeable membrane that separates blood from gas-containing oxygen and thus eliminates direct blood gas interface, which occurs in the bubble oxygenator. Oxygen

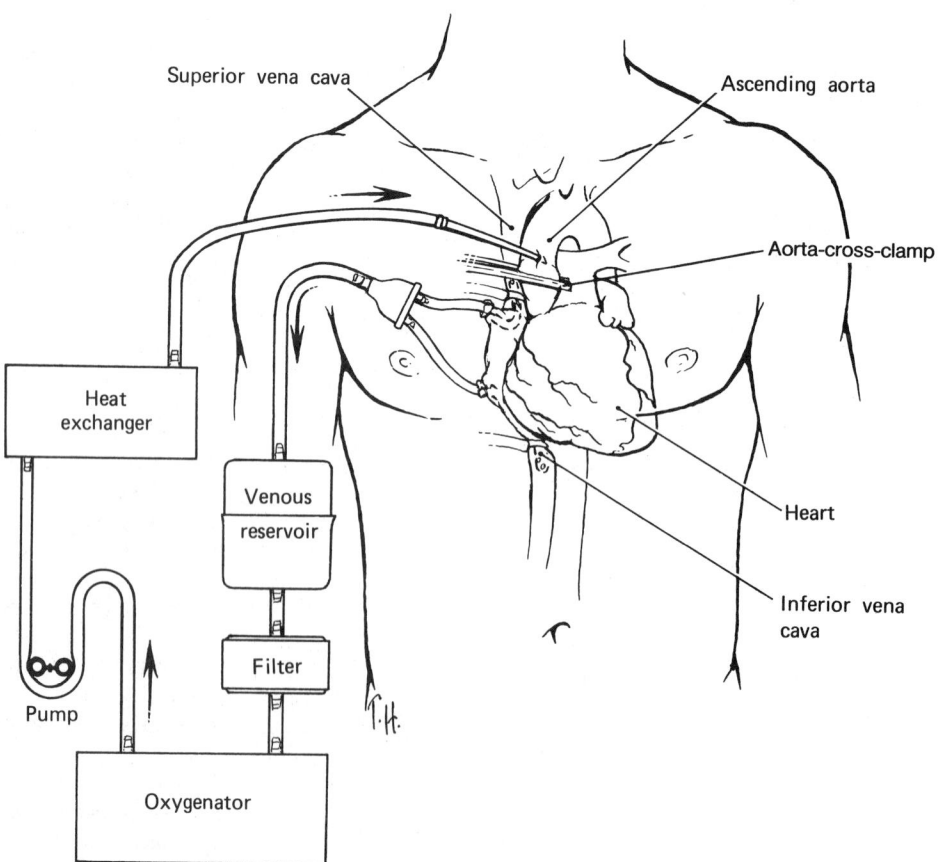

Figure 27-1
Schematic drawing of the cardiopulmonary bypass system.

diffuses across the membrane into the blood in a manner similar to the physiologic process that takes place between the alveoli and capillaries in the lungs.

While some physicians prefer the membrane oxygenator because it eliminates the direct blood gas interface, there seems to be little clinical difference between the bubble and the membrane oxygenators.

During surgery, the adequacy of tissue perfusion is determined by monitoring the electrocardiogram, arterial blood pressure, left atrial pressure, urine output, and arterial blood gases. Both the anesthesiologist and the pump perfusionist monitor these parameters.

Cardiopulmonary bypass is not without risk, and the risk increases when pump time exceeds 2 hours. When pump time exceeds 3 to 4 hours, the risk increases sharply. Excessive pump time increases the potential for development of hemolysis, increased capillary membrane permeability with resultant fluid and electrolyte shifts, tissue anoxia, embolism, and pulmonary complications. All these complications must be anticipated after surgery.

Mitral Valve Commissurotomy

Mitral valve stenosis is narrowing of the valve orifice secondary to thickening and loss of pliability of the valve leaflets and chordae tendineae. Progressive scarring with deformity and calcification causes fusion of the valve commissures and contraction of the chordae tendineae. The resultant narrowing of the valve orifice impedes the flow of blood through the valve. The left atrium dilates and hypertrophies, and in some cases pulmonary pressures increase, causing high pulmonary vascular resistance and variable degrees of right heart failure.

Mitral stenosis results almost exclusively from rheumatic endocarditis. Rarely, it results from congenital absence of one of the papillary muscles. Patients with mitral stenosis experience dyspnea associated with the increased pulmonary artery pressures. Some will experience hemoptysis and pulmonary edema. With more advanced disease, patients develop high pulmonary vascular pressure, right heart failure, and low cardiac output. In addition to dyspnea, fatigue, and weakness, these patients frequently have peripheral edema and hepatic engorgement. Most patients with longstanding mitral stenosis also develop atrial fibrillation secondary to dilatation of the left atrium. This irregular rhythm further reduces left ventricular filling and cardiac output because of the loss of atrial contraction in coordination with ventricular filling. Atrial fibrillation and atrial dilatation also allow blood to stagnate in the atrium, forming mural thrombi. Dislodgment of any of these thrombi can cause systemic or pulmonary embolization.

The patient with mitral stenosis can usually be managed initially with medical therapy. The goals of therapy are to reduce pulmonary edema and congestive heart failure, to prevent pulmonary and cardiac infections, to prevent embolization, and to maximize cardiac output by controlling heart rate (see Chap. 26). Patients with progressive symptoms are stabilized medically and then treated surgically. If the valve cusps are still pliable and if the chordae tendineae have not already shortened and thickened, mitral stenosis can be corrected with a mitral *commissurotomy* whereby the fused portion of the leaflets of the valve are opened. A pliable valve is indicated by the presence of an opening snap on auscultation and the absence of calcification on echocardiography or cinefluorography.

The *closed mitral commissurotomy* procedure is carried out without direct visualization of the mitral valve. The procedure is performed through a right anterolateral thoracotomy. A small incision is made in the left atrium, and the mitral valve is dilated by insertion of the surgeon's finger or a metal dilator through the valve. This procedure does not require cardiopulmonary bypass. However, the extracorporeal circulation equipment is prepared and available for use should the commissurotomy fail and valve replacement be required, or should complications occur that require direct visualization of and operation on the valve.

Open mitral commissurotomy is performed through a large incision in the left atrium, which provides direct visualization for the procedure. Open commissurotomy requires cardiopulmonary bypass. Some surgeons prefer this technique so they can observe any thrombi in the atrium or any calcium plaques on the valve leaflets. It may also be preferred when it is suspected that the commissurotomy may fail, necessitating valve replacement.

Mitral commissurotomy is associated with a low incidence of surgical complication and mortality.

Mitral Valve Replacement or Repair

Mitral insufficiency (regurgitation) results from incomplete closure of the mitral valve. The incomplete closure allows backward flow of blood (regurgitation) from the left ventricle to the atrium during ventricular systole. This regurgitated blood is returned to the left ventricle with the normal amount of circulating blood during atrial systole, thus increasing the volume of blood the left ventricle must handle. This increased volume results in dilatation and hypertrophy of both the left atrium and the left ventricle.

Mitral insufficiency is caused by rheumatic or bacterial endocarditis. These infectious processes cause fibrotic and calcific changes that thicken, shorten, and deform the valve cusps in such a way that they do not completely close. Other causes of mitral insufficiency include ischemia or infarction of the papillary muscles, ruptured chordae tendineae secondary to bacterial endocarditis, and congenital deformities.

Patients with mitral insufficiency have chronic pulmonary congestion and symptoms of fatigue, orthopnea, exertional dyspnea, and palpitations. They may develop atrial extrasystoles or atrial fibrillation secondary to dilatation of the left atrium (see Chap. 26). Some patients develop pulmonary edema and hemoptysis, especially if the mitral insufficiency develops suddenly, as from infarcted papillary muscle or ruptured chordae tendineae.

Mitral valve insufficiency is most often treated with drug therapy to increase cardiac contractility, to reduce the pressures the left ventricle must pump against, and to reduce congestive heart failure (see Chap. 26). Surgical treatment is indicated when the patient develops sudden dysfunction and severe failure from ruptured papillary muscle or when the patient with chronic insufficiency develops symptoms (fatigue, palpitations, and dyspnea) during minimal activity.

Whenever possible, the mitral valve is repaired rather than replaced in order to avoid the long-term risks associated with artificial valves. Repair, rather than replacement, can be performed confidently when the ruptured chordae tendineae affect a limited portion of the posterior leaflet of the valve and the anterior leaflet is normal. Repair of the mitral valve involves reconstruction of the valve leaflets and annulus. The procedure is called an *annuloplasty* and usually involves suturing of the valve tissue to a flexible ring (Carpentier's ring).

Should the mitral valve leaflets be calcified and immobile, a valve replacement is performed through a median sternotomy incision. The valve, chordae tendineae, and papillary muscles are excised and replaced with an appropriate mechanical prosthetic valve or a biological tissue valve. The mechanical valves have been used for several decades and have proven to be extremely durable. Two of the most common ones used for mitral valve replacement are the Starr-Edwards silastic ball-and-cage valve and the Bjork-Shiley tilting-disc valve (Fig. 27-2).

Patients who have one of these mechanical valve devices placed are usually maintained on anticoagulant therapy postoperatively to minimize the risk of embolization.

Biological tissue valves became popular in the early 1970s, but their use has been limited by their availability. They are obtained from animal heart tissue and human heart valves taken from cadaver donors. In addition to their limited availability, they present problems in sizing as well as the risk of rejection. They are commonly used for patients in whom anticoagulant therapy is contraindicated, such as children, young adult females, elderly persons, and patients with bleeding tendencies. The most commonly used biological valve is the Carpentier-Edwards porcine heterograft valve, which is preserved in a buffered glutaraldehyde solution to promote stability and reduce antigenicity and is mounted on a flexible stent (see Fig. 27-2).

Aortic Valve Replacement

Aortic valve replacement is done for patients with aortic stenosis or insufficiency. *Aortic stenosis* is narrowing of the valve orifice between the left ventricle and the aorta. Aortic stenosis can be congenital or it can result from rheumatic heart disease or calcification of unknown origin. Rheumatic changes include thickening and fibrosis of the cusps, fusion of the commissures, and valve calcification.

Aortic stenosis results in left ventricular hypertrophy and decreased ventricular function. The resulting decreased cardiac output reduces cardiac and cerebral perfusion and may cause syncope, angina, and dysrhythmias.

Severe aortic stenotic disease results in left ventricular

failure, decreased cardiac output, left atrial failure, pulmonary edema, and eventually right heart failure. Sudden death, probably due to ventricular fibrillation, occurs even in patients who are asymptomatic.

The goal of medical therapy is to reduce congestive failure and angina (see Chap. 26). If patients have heart failure, syncope, or angina, aortic valve replacement is indicated. Some physicians perform aortic valve replacement even on asymptomatic patients because of the risk of sudden death associated with aortic stenosis.

Aortic valve insufficiency is due to incomplete closure of the aortic valve cusps during ventricular diastole. This incomplete closure allows blood to flow backward (regurgitate) from the aorta into the left ventricle. With rheumatic heart disease and bacterial endocarditis, the valve leaflets become thickened and scarred, lose compliance, and eventually become calcified. This process causes deformity that prevents approximation of the valve cusps.

Other causes of aortic insufficiency include congenital bicuspid valves, traumatic tears, dissecting aortic aneurysms, and syphilitic aortitis. Syphilitic aortitis affects the ascending aorta, causing widening of the aorta and valve orifice. The resultant stress on the aortic valve causes fibrotic changes in the valve cusps, which worsens the insufficiency. The changes distort the aortic valve so that the cusps do not close completely, resulting in insufficiency (regurgitation).

The regurgitation of blood into the left ventricle results in dilation and hypertrophy of the ventricle. The ventricle pumps more forcefully to expel the blood, and as a result systolic blood pressure rises. The elevated systolic pressure triggers a reflex that dilates the peripheral arterioles and decreases peripheral vascular resistance and diastolic blood pressure. Patients with aortic insufficiency characteristically have an elevated systolic blood pressure, a low diastolic blood pressure, and thus a wide pulse pressure. These patients also develop symptoms associated with the increased force of ventricular systole, such as bounding pulse, palpitations, and awareness of pulsations in the neck. Other symptoms include dyspnea with exertion and dizziness with sudden postural change.

Patients who suddenly develop aortic insufficiency without compensatory changes develop heart failure and decreased cardiac output, which can result in death.

The treatment for patients who are symptomatic or for patients who have documented left ventricular hypertrophy and pressure changes is aortic valve replacement. The patient

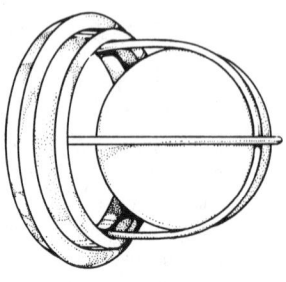 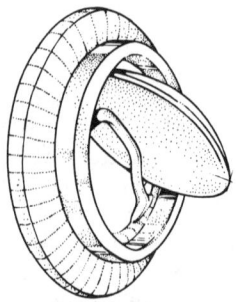 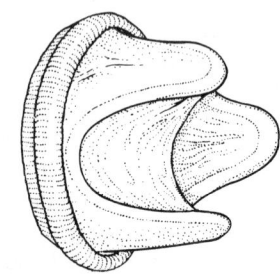

Figure 27-2
Common mechanical and biological valve replacements.

Caged ball valve
(Starr-Edwards/mechanical)

Tilting disc valve
(Bjork-Shiley/mechanical)

Porcine heterograft valve
(Carpentier-Edwards/biological)

who develops acute aortic insufficiency may require drug therapy to increase cardiac output and to reduce failure prior to emergency aortic valve replacement.

Aortic valve replacement is performed through a median sternotomy incision, using total cardiopulmonary bypass. The aortic valve tissue is removed through a transverse incision in the aorta, and a prosthetic valve is sutured in place. Aortic prosthetic devices that are used include the Bjork-Shiley tilting-disc valve and the Starr-Edwards silastic ball-and-cage valve (see Fig. 27-2). All mechanical valves necessitate prolonged anticoagulant therapy to prevent thromboembolism.

When anticoagulant therapy is contraindicated, a biological tissue valve (see Fig. 27-2) is used for replacement. These tissue valves are not thrombogenic and do not require anticoagulant therapy, but they may degenerate and necessitate replacement.

Tricuspid Valve Repair or Replacement

Tricuspid valve stenosis is characterized by the same fibrotic and calcific changes as stenosis of the other heart valves. These changes result in narrowing of the valve orifice, which impedes the flow of blood from the right atrium to the right ventricle. The right atrium dilates, and right-sided heart failure leads to venous congestion with cyanosis, hepatomegaly, peripheral edema, and ascites.

Tricuspid stenosis is caused by rheumatic heart disease, bacterial endocarditis, or congenital heart defects. With rheumatic heart disease, the tricuspid valve is frequently both stenotic and insufficient. Often the mitral valve, and sometimes the aortic valve, have rheumatic disease changes also.

If the stenotic tricuspid valve requires surgical repair, usually a commissurotomy is done. If the valve is both stenotic and insufficient, both a commissurotomy and an *annuloplasty* (reconstruction of the incompetent valve) may be performed. Replacement of the tricuspid valve is required infrequently. In such cases a mechanical valve or a biological tissue valve may be used, depending on suitability for the individual patient.

Tricuspid insufficiency is incomplete closure of the tricuspid valve during right ventricular systole (incompetence), resulting in backward flow of blood (regurgitation) from the right ventricle to the right atrium. Tricuspid insufficiency is most often a functional disorder caused by failure and dilation of the heart due to severe mitral valve insufficiency. The heart dilation distorts the orifice of the tricuspid valve. Insufficiency may also result from fibrotic and calcific changes caused by rheumatic or bacterial endocarditis.

The symptoms of tricuspid insufficiency are the same as those of tricuspid stenosis. In the symptomatic patient the treatment is annuloplasty and sometimes valve replacement. If the insufficiency is a functional disorder, the defects in the other heart valves are corrected first.

Tricuspid annuloplasty may be done using a Carpentier flexible ring that is modified to avoid the area of the septal leaflet associated with the atrioventricular node and the His bundle. If the leaflets of the valve are so distorted that function cannot be achieved with annuloplasty, then valve replacement is indicated. A stent-mounted human semilunar valve has been found to be an ideal replacement. When such a valve is not available, a large porcine valve can be used for patients over

the age of 50 and a mechanical valve can be used for younger patients.

Pulmonary Valve Disease

Diseases of the pulmonary valve are uncommon unless associated with congenital heart disease. Such defects are usually diagnosed and treated in the pediatric patient.

Repair of Traumatic Lesions of the Heart

Traumatic lesions of the heart are becoming more common as accidents due to high-speed transportation increase and crime rates rise. A wide variety of injuries is possible, such as laceration of a coronary artery or rupture of the chordae tendineae, papillary muscles, or valve cusps (blunt, nonpenetrating injuries). Survival from penetrating injuries, such as gunshot or stab wounds, depends largely on the location of the injury, the size of the wound, and the availability of emergency medical and surgical management of cardiac tamponade (acute compression of the heart due to rapid accumulation of blood in the pericardium) or shock. The particular lesion determines what therapy is required.

Removal of Cardiac Tumors

Cardiac tumors arising within the chambers or in the myocardium, especially primary tumors, are rare. Approximately 70% of all cardiac tumors are benign. The most common benign tumor is the *myxoma*, which is an intercavitary tumor that is formed on a stalk, or pedicle. It occurs most often in older adults and is 2 to 3 times more common in women than in men. It is often difficult to diagnose myxomas because of their similarity in appearance to thrombi. However, one distinguishing feature is that, unlike thrombi, they are covered with endothelium and have crevices and clefts that are lined with endothelium. Successful removal of these tumors has been achieved. The most common malignant primary tumor of the heart is sarcoma, which tends to metastasize widely and has a poor prognosis. Secondary malignant tumors of the heart are usually due to metastasis from a primary lesion elsewhere in the body.

Ascending Aorta Repair

Diseases of the ascending aorta, primarily aneurysms, are surgically repaired by cross-clamping the area above and below the aneurysm, removing the diseased or affected portion, and replacing it with a Teflon or Dacron graft. Cardiopulmonary bypass is used.

Pericardectomy

When inflammation or disease of the pericardium restricts the movement and filling of the heart, the pericardial sac may need to be surgically removed. Some of the causes of pericarditis include infection, connective tissue disorders, hypersensitivity states, neoplasms, and trauma (see Chap. 25).

Constrictive pericarditis restricts filling of the heart and thus reduces venous return and cardiac output. The patient suffers dyspnea and other adverse effects of reduced cardiac output.

Pericardectomy is removal of the pericardial sac. The surgical approach can be either through a left anterolateral thoracotomy or a median sternotomy, neither of which requires cardiopulmonary bypass. The pericardium is dissected and removed very gently and slowly. The left ventricle is freed first, so that the increased flow to the right side of the heart is prevented from overloading the lungs and causing pulmonary edema. This method also allows the left ventricle to adjust to the increased blood volume that it will receive as the constriction is removed.

The patient must be observed during and following the procedure for low cardiac output associated with the development of cardiac dilation during the pericardectomy. Patients most prone to developing low cardiac output are those who preoperatively had advanced disability, fluid retention, and ascites.

Left Ventricular Aneurysmectomy

An *aneurysm* is a ballooning enlargement of the ventricle due to weakening of the ventricular wall. Left ventricular aneurysms occur in 5% to 35% of patients who suffer myocardial infarction and are secondary to the injury and scarring caused by the infarction. In some patients the presence of an aneurysm may cause the heart to become ineffective as a pump, leading to congestive heart failure, peripheral emboli, and tachydysrhythmias, all of which can be difficult to treat. Surgical removal of the ballooned portion of the left ventricular wall (*aneurysmectomy*) may be indicated for the symptomatic patient. Patients often show a marked improvement in cardiac reserve following surgery, and the dysrhythmias usually disappear.

Surgical Removal of Dysrhythmia Foci and Pathways

Advances in direct electrophysiological study of the heart have made it possible to locate the origin or pathway of dysrhythmias. A catheter inserted into the chambers of the heart is used to incite dysrhythmias. The dysrhythmic activity is mapped and recorded, thus showing the pathway of the dysrhythmia throughout the heart. This direct cardiac mapping provides information that is valuable in determining medical and surgical therapies to be used. Direct cardiac mapping has been most successful in the localization of accessory pathways associated with Wolff-Parkinson-White (WPW) syndrome, a preexcitation syndrome in which one or more accessory pathways connect the atrial myocardium to the ventricular myocardium. Direct cardiac mapping can also be used to localize the site of origin of atrial or ventricular dysrhythmias and the site of myocardial ischemia and infarction.

Surgical resection of the dysrhythmia focus or pathway is indicated if the dysrhythmia is life-threatening and is refractory to medical therapy. Preoperatively, a complete electrophysiological study is performed to map and record the activity of the heart.

The surgical procedure is performed through a median sternotomy. Electrodes are placed directly on the heart and a recording is made. In the case of recurrent ventricular tachycardia following myocardial infarction, an aneurysmectomy and CABG procedure are often performed along with the endocardial resection. In WPW syndrome, direct cardiac mapping is performed to locate the accessory pathways. After the pathways are dissected, dysrhythmias are induced and further cardiac mapping is performed to exclude the presence of additional accessory pathways. These surgical procedures require the use of cardiopulmonary bypass. Perioperative care is the same as for other cardiac surgery procedures.

Surgical Intervention for Coronary Artery Disease

Coronary artery disease is a narrowing and distortion of the coronary arteries resulting in decreased blood flow to the myocardium. It is caused by atherosclerosis. The atherosclerotic process causes proliferation of smooth muscle cells and accumulation of lipids in the intima of the artery wall. The cause of this atherosclerosis is not known. Risk factors that have been identified include high blood pressure, hyperlipidemia, smoking, and obesity. Some of the symptoms associated with coronary artery disease are angina, myocardial infarction, and primary ventricular fibrillation.

The choice of medical or surgical intervention for the treatment of patients with coronary artery disease has been the subject of much controversy. Because surgical intervention cannot alter the atherosclerotic disease process, it may not prolong life or reduce the occurrence of myocardial infarction. However, because it reduces angina and increases activity tolerance, surgical intervention is used to improve the quality of life.

Generally, medical therapy (nitroglycerin, β-adrenergic blocking agents, calcium ion antagonists) is used initially to relieve the pain of angina, to improve the blood and oxygen supply to the myocardium, and to reduce the oxygen needs of the myocardium (see Chap. 25). A criterion generally accepted as rationale for surgical intervention is disabling angina pectoris unrelieved by medical therapy. Because the severity of angina that is disabling can only be determined by the patient, ultimately the decision of whether or not to have surgery must be made by the patient.

The location and amount of stenosis in the coronary arteries, the amount of myocardium served by a stenotic artery, and previous infarction related to an affected artery are all factors considered by the physician when recommending therapy. Patients with greater than 50% stenosis of the left main coronary artery have better prognostic results with surgical intervention. Stenosis of other coronary arteries exceeding 70% occlusion is considered significant disease and may be treated surgically. Generally, unstable angina, postinfarction angina, and myocardial infarction complicated by left ventricular failure or intractable ventricular dysrhythmias are treated surgically.

Coronary artery disease is treated surgically by myocardial revascularization (coronary artery bypass graft), by heart transplantation, and less invasively by percutaneous transluminal coronary angioplasty (dilation of diseased coronary arteries with a balloon-tipped catheter). Because the decision of when it is appropriate to use surgical therapy is somewhat controversial, it is imperative that the benefits and risks of the proposed therapy and alternative therapies be explained to the patient and family. The patient must ultimately define what limitations and risks are tolerable and what therapeutic approach is acceptable.

Myocardial Revascularization. *Coronary artery bypass graft (CABG) surgery* connects a segment of a vein or artery between the aortic root and the affected coronary artery at a point distal to the obstruction or stenosis caused by atherosclerosis. Usually a portion of the patient's saphenous vein is used for the graft(s).

The bypass graft surgery is done through a median sternotomy. The patient is supported on cardiopulmonary bypass so that the heart can be arrested and a *quiet field* provided for anastomosis of the saphenous veins to the coronary arteries.

The segments of saphenous vein are implanted in the aortic root with an end-to-side anastomosis. The veins are reversed from their normal direction so that their valves do not interfere with blood flow through the vein (Fig. 27-3).

Direct bypass of the occluded coronary arteries by attachment of a mammary artery distal to the obstruction has also been used (Fig. 27-4). Early in the development of coronary artery bypass surgery the internal mammary artery (IMA) was used for grafting. However, until recent years, many surgeons did not consider its use because the tedious dissection that is necessary to mobilize the IMA pedicle makes the procedure more time-consuming than the saphenous vein graft, and until recently the flow capabilities of the IMA as a graft were not known. Comparative studies now show that the IMA has a significantly higher patency rate than does the saphenous vein graft during both the immediate postoperative and long-term follow-up periods. The IMA has proven to be durable, and graft closure due to late atherosclerosis has rarely been seen. However, because the mammary artery is of limited length, it can only be used to revascularize the anterior surface of the heart supplied by the left anterior descending coronary artery.

Percutaneous Transluminal Coronary Angioplasty. Percutaneous transluminal coronary angioplasty (PTCA) can be performed instead of coronary artery bypass graft (CABG) surgery in some patients with single-vessel coronary artery disease. The procedure is usually performed on patients who have had angina for less than 1 year because these patients usually have atheromas that are soft, compressible, and easily dilated. Cardiac cineangiography is used to confirm that the patient has a single atherosclerotic lesion in the proximal portion of a single vessel, that it is not calcified, that there is no distal stenosis, and that the lesion is not at a bifurcation. Candidates for PTCA must also be candidates for CABG surgery, since complications of angioplasty would necessitate immediate bypass surgery.

Percutaneous transluminal coronary angioplasty is done by inserting a balloon-tipped catheter into the diseased coronary artery and reducing the stenosis by inflating the balloon with controlled pressure (Fig. 27-5). Local anesthesia is used. The procedure is performed in the cardiac catheterization facility. Preprocedure and postprocedure care is very similar to the care of the cardiac catheterization patient.

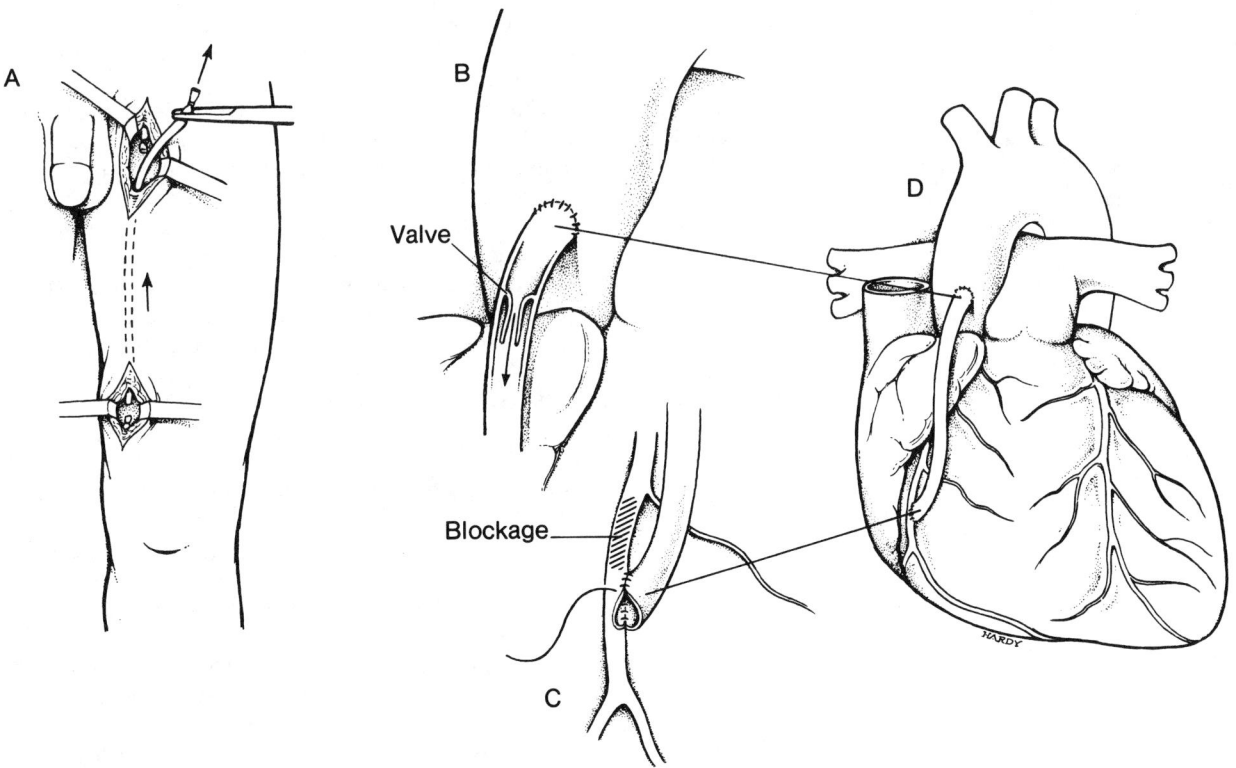

Figure 27-3
Saphenous vein revascularization procedure. (*A*) The saphenous vein is removed from the patient's leg. The vein is reversed so that the valves will not interfere with blood flow. (*B*) The distal end of the vein is sutured to the ascending aorta. (*C*) At a point distal to the blockage, the vein is sutured to the coronary artery by end-to-side anastomosis. (*D*) The completed bypass reestablishes the flow distal to the blockage.

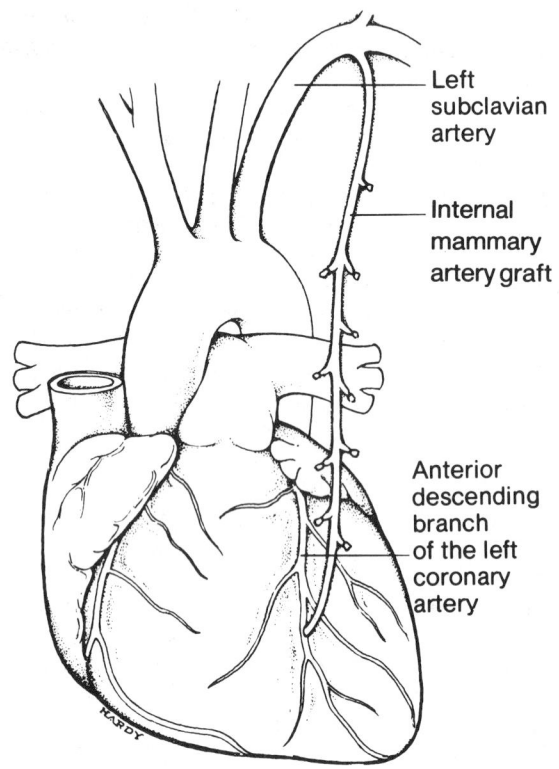

Left
subclavian
artery

Internal
mammary
artery graft

Anterior
descending
branch
of the left
coronary
artery

Figure 27-4
Mammary artery revascularization procedure, showing
mammary artery anastomosis to the anterior descending
branch of the left coronary artery.

Complications of PTCA are abrupt occlusion of the artery
through collapse, spasm, or clot; arterial dissection or rupture;
or myocardial infarction. The procedure is performed with
the cardiac surgery team and an operating room on standby.
Should a patient develop any of these complications, emergency CABG surgery is performed.

The patient who has PTCA is hospitalized for only 2 to
4 days and may immediately resume previous activity levels.
While the long-term effects of this procedure are not yet fully
documented, the advantages because the procedure is less
invasive make it preferable to CABG surgery for selected patients.

Heart Transplantation. Heart transplantation is performed for end-stage cardiac disease that has not been remedied by other surgical or medical therapies. It is currently
performed in only selected medical centers because of the
complex surgical and management techniques involved.

Selection criteria for transplant candidates are strict and
include (1) an upper age limit of 55 years, (2) less than a
10% chance of survival for 6 months, and (3) normal renal
and liver function, or dysfunction that is reversible. Transplantation is contraindicated in patients with active infection
or with donor-specific antibodies (*i.e.,* patients whose tissue
is not compatible with the donor tissue). It may be contraindicated for patients with other chronic diseases, cachexia,
severe pulmonary hypertension, a history of pulmonary infarction, insulin-dependent diabetes mellitus, peripheral vascular or cerebrovascular disease, or lymphocyte hyperactivity.
The patient's emotional acceptance of the transplantation

and family support systems are also important for the long
recovery period.

The principal factor that limits the number of transplants
performed is the limited number of suitable, available donors.
It is desirable that donors be between the ages of 15 and 35
if male and between the ages of 15 and 40 if female and have
no history of severe or chronic heart or liver disease. The
number of potential donors is slowly increasing because of
public information efforts of local and national organ banks.

Heart transplantation involves removal of the heart from
the donor by transecting the great vessels and the atria at a
point dorsal to the atrial appendages. In preparing the recipient, many surgeons retain portions of the recipient atria to
facilitate anastomosis of the donor heart. The atria of the
donor heart are sutured to the atria of the patient's heart, the
great vessels are connected, and then air is evacuated from
the heart chambers. Transplantation is performed through a
median sternotomy. The patient is supported by cardiopulmonary bypass during the procedure.

The primary focus of postoperative care is to prevent
infection and rejection. With the introduction of cyclosporine
immunosuppression, morbidity from serious infection and
cardiac rejection has been reduced. Endomyocardial biopsy
is used during and after hospitalization to assess the effectiveness of therapy and to detect early rejection. Other postoperative care is the same as that described later in the chapter
for other heart surgery procedures.

In rare cases, transplantation of both the heart and the
lungs is performed successfully. This procedure is advantageous for the patient whose heart disease has caused pulmonary disease. It is also done for the patient who needs
lung transplantation.

Artificial Heart. Because of the incidence of heart
disease, the complexities of donor heart transplantation, and
the limited supply of donor hearts, much research is being
done to perfect the totally artificial heart. For some time devices have been used to support the damaged heart until it
recovers and can completely take over its pumping function.
The intra-aortic balloon pump (IABP) (see Fig. 26-19) has
been used most successfully in supporting the damaged heart
before and after surgery. It has been less successful in reversing cardiogenic shock. The left heart assist device has
also been used to support the pumping function of the heart
until it recovers or until a donor heart is available for transplantation (Fig. 27-6).

Great strides have been made in the development of a
permanent device, a totally artificial heart. Advances in bio-
materials and pump and energy systems have led to the development of an artificial heart that has been implanted in
humans. The procedure remains investigational and much
experimentation is directed toward developing a drive system
that is smaller and more compact than the original one. It is
hoped that eventually current artificial heart devices will be
replaced by an electrohydraulic heart.

Laser Angioplasty. For several decades research efforts have been directed toward the use of laser radiation to
vaporize atherosclerotic plaques as a replacement for cardiac
surgery. Progress has been slow because of the risk of vessel
wall damage and perforation, which can only be minimized
by use of low energies and critical positioning of the laser
beam. The use of laser therapy as an adjunct to peripheral
vascular surgery has already been successful because the

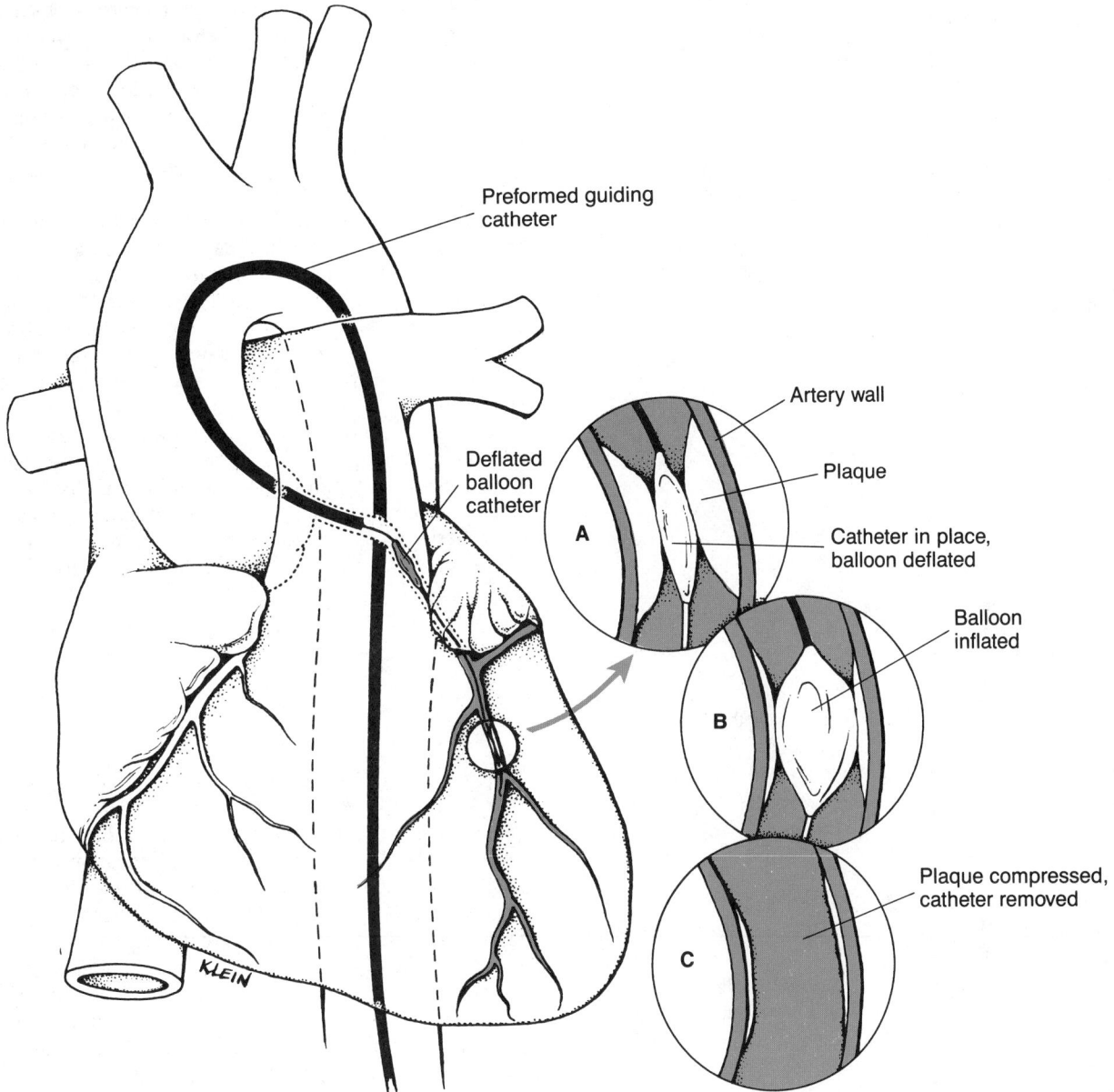

Figure 27-5
Percutaneous transluminal coronary angioplasty is a less invasive procedure than
coronary artery bypass surgery in selected patients. (*A*) A balloon-tipped catheter is
passed into the affected coronary artery and placed within the atherosclerotic lesion.
(*B*) The balloon is then rapidly inflated and deflated with controlled pressure. (*C*) After
the plaque is compressed, the catheter is removed, allowing improved blood flow of the
vessel. (Redrawn from Purcell JA and Giffin PA. Percutaneous transluminal coronary
angioplasty. Am J Nurs 1981 Sept; 81[9]:1621)

problem of vessel inaccessibility is not an issue. Percutaneous
use of lasers in peripheral arteries and eventually in coronary
arteries is the way the ultimate clinical benefit will be realized.
Some researchers believe that the greatest application of laser
angioplasty will be as an adjunct to PTCA—by use of lasers,
totally occluded arteries could be opened enough to allow
the advancement of the PTCA catheter and the dilation of
the remaining occlusion. It is believed that laser angioplasty
as a safe and effective therapy is on the horizon and will
become a reality within the decade.

Perioperative Nursing Management

The patient who is undergoing heart surgery has many of the
same needs and requires the perioperative care described
for other surgical patients in Chapters 17 to 19. In addition,
the patient and family are experiencing a major life crisis.
Their emotional and psychological responses to the surgery

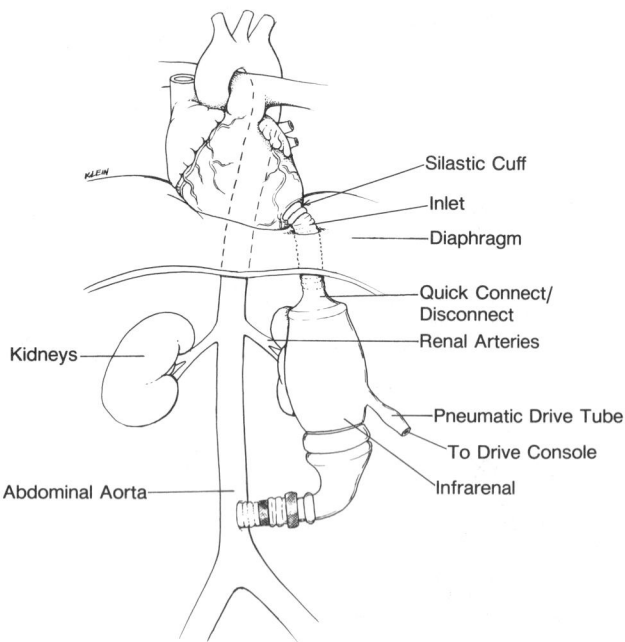

Figure 27-6
Left ventricular assist device.

are intense because of the association of the heart with life and death. Due to the intensified fears and anxieties that accompany heart surgery, the patient and family require extensive emotional support and teaching. The nature of the surgery and the incidence of postoperative problems also require that the patient receive intensive assessment, monitoring, and physical care.

While many of the fears of heart surgery patients are the same as those of other surgical patients, the fears are frequently intensified because of the special meaning attached to the heart, the realization of the risk of death associated with heart surgery, the infrequency with which the public encounters persons who have had heart surgery, and the extent to which the patient has been involved in the decision to have surgical or medical therapy for the cardiac condition. The nurse assists the patient in coping with fears. Emotional support should begin prior to hospitalization and continue through rehabilitation.

A major component of the physical care is timely assessment. Preoperatively, the patient is assessed to determine readiness for surgery and to establish baseline data for reference postoperatively. Immediately after surgery, the patient is managed in a postanesthesia recovery unit or an intensive care unit, where continuous assessment of cardiac function and prompt initiation of therapy are possible. Assessment continues in the rehabilitation phase, during which the patient is taught to do self-assessment in order to regulate activity and sometimes adjust medication.

Preoperative Nursing Management

The preoperative phase of patient preparation usually begins prior to hospitalization. This phase focuses on stabilizing any other disease conditions and optimizing cardiac function. The

patient with diabetes, high blood pressure, chronic obstructive pulmonary disease, or other respiratory, renal, or liver disease has these conditions assessed and medical therapy adjusted to stabilize them. Any sources of possible infection (*i.e.*, periodontal disease, skin lesions, stasis ulcer) are investigated and treated. Therapies are adjusted to control any heart failure, dysrhythmias, and fluid or electrolyte imbalances to optimize cardiac function.

Patients are instructed to avoid aspirin and any drugs containing aspirin for at least 9 days prior to surgery. Aspirin decreases platelet adhesion and may predispose the patient to surgical hemorrhage. Anticoagulant therapy is usually stopped 5 to 7 days before surgery. The patient is also encouraged to stop or reduce smoking a few weeks prior to surgery. If the patient is on digitalis, a short-acting preparation will be prescribed, and sometimes even this is discontinued 36 to 48 hours prior to surgery. Most antidysrhythmics, nitrates, and propranolol will be continued until the night before surgery. Special consideration is given to the anxiety associated with waiting for hospitalization and surgery, and a mild tranquilizer is prescribed as needed to help control increased heart rate, which may worsen the cardiac condition.

▶ *Nursing Process*

▷ *Assessment*

The patient with nonacute heart disease will usually be hospitalized only 1 or 2 days prior to surgery. Most of the preoperative medical evaluation is completed before the patient enters the hospital. A new history and physical examination, chest x-ray, electrocardiogram (ECG), serum electrolytes, coagulation screen, and typing and crossmatching of blood may be done at this time. These data provide information about other disease conditions and cardiac problems. Nursing assessment focuses primarily on obtaining baseline physiological data and assessing the patient's and family's emotional and teaching needs. The history includes a social assessment of family roles and support systems, and a description of the patient's usual functional level and typical activities. This information will assist with emotional care and rehabilitation planning.

Health Assessment. The preoperative history and health assessment should be thorough and well documented because they provide a basis for postoperative comparison. A systematic assessment of all systems is done, with emphasis on assessment of cardiovascular functioning. Functional status of the cardiovascular system is determined by reviewing the patient's symptomatology, including past and present experiences with chest pain, hypertension, palpitations, dyspnea, cyanosis, orthopnea, paroxysmal nocturnal dyspnea, peripheral edema, and intermittent claudication. Because alterations in cardiac output can effect renal, respiratory, gastrointestinal, and neurologic functioning, these systems are also assessed thoroughly. History of major illnesses, surgeries, and drug therapies, and use of alcohol and tobacco are also explored. A complete physical examination is performed, with special emphasis on the following parameters:

· General appearance and behavior
· Vital signs

- Nutritional and fluid status, weight, and height
- Inspection and palpation of the heart, noting the point of maximal impulse (PMI), abnormal pulsations, thrills
- Auscultation of the heart, noting pulse rate, rhythm, and quality, S_3, S_4, snaps, clicks, murmurs, friction rub
- Jugular venous pressure
- Peripheral pulses
- Peripheral edema

Psychosocial Assessment. The psychosocial assessment and the assessment of teaching–learning needs of the patient and family are as important as the physical examination. Anticipation of cardiac surgery is a source of great stress to the patient and family. They will be anxious and fearful and will have many unanswered questions. Their anxiety usually increases with the patient's admission to the hospital and the immediacy of surgery. An assessment of the level of anxiety is important. If it is low, this may indicate denial. If it is extremely high, it may interfere with the use of effective coping mechanisms and with preoperative teaching. Questions should be asked to obtain the following information about both the patient and the family:

- The meaning to the patient and family of the surgery
- Coping mechanisms that are being used
- Measures used in the past to deal with stress
- Anticipated changes in life-style
- Support systems in effect
- Fears regarding the present and the future
- Knowledge and understanding of the operative procedure, postoperative course, and long-term rehabilitation

Adequate time should be allowed for the patient and family to express their fears. The fears most often expressed are fear of the unknown, fear of pain, fear of body image change, and fear of dying.

- *Fear of the unknown.* This fear is difficult to express. Lack of past experience with heart surgery does not provide sufficient detail to attach fears to any specific aspects. Instead of specific fears which can be identified and for which coping mechanisms can be used, the patient and family often express a generalized dread.
- *Fear of pain.* The patient may openly express a fear of pain and the inability to tolerate it, or may indirectly express this fear by asking many questions about pain, pain medications, and the process of recovering from anesthesia. The family may fear that they will be unable to cope with watching the patient experience pain.
- *Fear of body image change.* Many patients have a fear of the scarring from surgery. This fear is frequently exaggerated due to lack of information. Patients may talk openly about this fear or express it indirectly through concern about continued love from others or excessive focus on postoperative pain.
- *Fear of dying.* Some patients share their fear of dying. Others only drop clues about their concern, such as questioning why they need to know about their surgery and postoperative course, asking for reassurance that someone will care for their family on the day of surgery, or becoming tearful around their family members or telling them to wait at home on the day of surgery. Likewise, family members who do not openly express this fear will often drop similar clues.

During the assessment, the nurse determines how much the patient and family know about the impending surgery and the expected postoperative events. They are encouraged to ask questions and to indicate how much information they wish to have. Some patients prefer not to have detailed information, while others want to know as much as possible. Patients should be approached as unique individuals with their own specific learning needs, learning styles, and levels of understanding.

Patients requiring emergency heart surgery may have both cineangiography and surgery within several hours of admission. The nurse will have little opportunity to assess and meet their emotional and teaching needs before surgery. As a result, they will need extra help postoperatively to adjust to the situation.

▷ Nursing Diagnoses

The nursing diagnoses for patients awaiting cardiac surgery will vary from patient to patient according to their cardiac disease process or abnormality and their symptomatology. The majority of patients will have a nursing diagnosis of decreased cardiac output (see Cardiac Failure, Chap. 26). In addition, preoperative nursing diagnoses for most patients will include the following:

- Fear related to the surgical procedure, its questionable outcome, and the threat to well-being
- Deficit in knowledge about the surgical procedure and the postoperative course

▷ Planning and Implementation

▷ *Goals.* The major goals of the patient may include reduction of fear and learning about the surgical procedure and postoperative course.

▷ Nursing Interventions

During the preoperative phase of cardiac surgery, the nurse develops a plan of care that includes emotional support and teaching for the patient and family. Establishing rapport, answering questions, listening to fears and concerns, clarifying misconceptions, and providing information about what to expect are all interventions the nurse uses to prepare the patient and family emotionally for the surgery and for the postoperative events.

Reduction of Fear. The patient and family are allowed adequate time and repeated opportunities to express their fears. If there is fear of the unknown, other surgical experiences that the patient has had can be compared to the impending surgery. Describe what the patient will feel. If the patient has already had a cardiac catheterization, compare the similarities and differences between that and the surgery. Also, encourage the patient to talk about any concerns related to previous bad experiences.

Encourage discussion of the patient's fears about pain. Make a comparison between the pain experienced with cardiac surgery and other pain experiences. Describe the preoperative sedation, the anesthetic, and the postoperative pain medication. Reassure the patient that the fear of pain is normal. Confirm that some pain will be experienced, but indicate that the patient will be closely observed and that the use of medication, positioning, and relaxation will make the pain more tolerable.

Patients who have a fear of the scarring from surgery are encouraged to discuss this. Misconceptions are corrected. Be sure to indicate that the health team members will keep the patient fully informed about the healing process.

Encourage the patient and family to talk about their fear about dying. Reassure them that this fear is normal. For those who only drop clues despite efforts to encourage them to talk about their fear, coach them to express it (*e.g.*, "Are you worrying about not making it through surgery? Most people who have heart surgery at least think about the possibility of dying."). Once the fear is expressed, the patient and family can be helped.

By alleviating undue anxiety and fear, emotional preparation of the patient for surgery lessens the chance of preoperative problems, aids in smooth anesthesia induction, and enhances the patient's involvement postoperatively in care and recovery. Likewise, preparation of the family for the events to come helps them to cope, to be supportive to the patient, and to participate in the postoperative and rehabilitative care.

Learning About the Surgical Procedure and Postoperative Course. Patient teaching is based on assessed learning needs. Teaching usually includes information about hospitalization, about the surgery (the preoperative care, the length of the surgery, what the patient will feel like, the visiting privileges in the intensive care unit), and about the recovery phase (length of hospitalization, when normal activities, such as housework, shopping, and work, can be resumed). Any changes made in medical therapy and preoperative preparations need to be explained and reinforced.

The patient is told that physical preparation usually involves several showers or scrubs with an antiseptic solution. Medication for sleep will be given the night before surgery and sedation just before surgery. With few exceptions, almost all cardiac surgical teams use prophylactic antibiotic therapy, and the antibiotics are started preoperatively.

If the preoperative hospitalization period is very short, teaching of the patient and family together may be most effective. The patient's anxiety increases with the admission process and the immediacy of surgery. Unless the nurse has met the patient before the day of hospitalization, the time may be too short to establish a relationship that contributes to patient learning. Teaching of the patient and family together capitalizes on their established support relationship. Teaching in this phase should be directed primarily by the patient's and family's questions. Too much detail may only increase anxiety. The patient may be offered a tour of the intensive care unit, the postanesthesia recovery room, or both. (In some hospitals, the patient will initially go to the postanesthesia unit.) The patient recovering from anesthesia is reassured by having already seen and heard the environment and having met someone from the unit. The patient and family should be informed about the tubes that will be present postoperatively and their purposes. They should know to expect several intravenous lines, chest tubes, and a urinary catheter. Explaining the purpose and the approximate time that these will be in place helps to reassure the patient. Most patients will remain intubated and on mechanical ventilation for 6 to 24 hours postoperatively. They need to be aware that this prevents them from talking, and should be reassured that the staff are skilled in other means of communication.

The patient's other questions about postoperative care and procedures should be answered. Deep breathing and coughing, using the incentive spirometer or intermittent positive pressure breathing (IPPB), and foot exercises should be explained and practiced by the patient preoperatively. The family's questions at this time will primarily focus on the length of the surgery, who will discuss the results of the procedure with them and when this may occur, where to wait during the surgery, the visiting privileges in the intensive care unit, and how they can support the patient preoperatively and in the intensive care unit.

▷ *Evaluation*

▷ *Expected Outcomes*

1. Patient experiences reduction of fear.
   a. Identifies fears
   b. Discusses fears with family
   c. Uses past experiences as a focus for comparison
   d. Expresses positive attitude about outcome of surgery
   e. Expresses confidence in measures to be used to relieve pain
2. Acquires knowledge about the surgical procedure and postoperative course
   a. Identifies the purposes of the preoperative preparation procedure
   b. Tours the intensive care unit, if appropriate
   c. Identifies limitations expected after surgery
   d. Discusses expected immediate postoperative environment, *e.g.*, tubes, machines, nursing surveillance
   e. Identifies expected activities after surgery, *e.g.*, deep breathing, coughing, foot exercises

Intraoperative Nursing Management

Most of the surgical procedures previously described are performed through a median sternotomy incision. Because of the possible problems associated with these surgeries, the patient is prepared for continuous monitoring. Electrodes and indwelling catheters and probes are placed prior to the procedure to facilitate assessment of the patient's status and the need for changes in therapy. In addition, the patient will be intubated and supported on mechanical ventilation. Intravenous lines will be placed as needed for administration of fluids, medications, and blood products.

Before the chest incision is closed, chest tubes are positioned to evacuate air and drainage from the mediastinum and the thorax. Epicardial pacemaker electrodes are implanted on the surface of the right atrium and sometimes the right ventricle. These epicardial electrodes can be used postoperatively to pace the heart or to monitor the heart for dysrhythmia differentiation via an atrial lead. Most of the indwelling catheters are retained for continuous monitoring and treatment of the patient in the immediate postoperative period.

In addition to assistance with the surgical, anesthetic, and extracorporeal procedures, the surgical nurses are responsible for the comfort and safety of the patient. Some of their areas of intervention include emotional support of the patient and family, positioning, skin care, and wound care.

Possible intraoperative complications include dysrhythmias, hemorrhage, myocardial infarction, cerebral vascular accident, embolization, and organ failure secondary to shock, embolus, or adverse drug reactions. Astute intraoperative patient assessment is critical in preventing these complications or in detecting symptoms and initiating prompt therapy.

Postoperative Nursing Management

The immediate postoperative period for the patient who has undergone cardiac surgery presents many challenges to the health team. All efforts are made to facilitate the transition from the operating room to the intensive care unit or post-anesthesia suite with a minimum of risk. Specific information about the operation and important factors about postoperative management are communicated by the surgical team and anesthesia personnel to the primary nurse, who then assumes responsibility for the patient's care (Fig. 27-7).

▶ Nursing Process

▷ Assessment

When the patient is admitted to the nursing unit, and frequently thereafter, a complete systematic assessment is performed to establish baseline information. Assessment of the following physiological parameters is imperative:

- *Neurologic status*—level of responsiveness, pupil size and reaction to light, movement of extremities, and hand grasp ability
- *Cardiac status*—blood pressure, heart rate and rhythm, heart sounds, arterial pressure, central venous pressure, pulmonary artery pressure, pulmonary capillary wedge pressure, cardiac output, jugular vein pressure
- *Respiratory status*—respiratory rate, chest movement, breath sounds, secretions, arterial blood gases, tidal volume, chest tube drainage
- *Peripheral vascular status*—peripheral pulses; color of skin, nail beds, lips, earlobes; skin temperature
- *Renal function*—urinary output, urine specific gravity and osmolarity
- *Fluid and electrolyte status*—intake; output from all drainage tubes; all cardiac output parameters, such as the following:
  - Hypokalemia: digitalis toxicity, dysrhythmias (U wave, AV block, flat or inverted T waves)
  - Hyperkalemia: mental confusion, restlessness, nausea, weakness, paresthesias of extremities, dysrhythmias (tall, peaked T waves; increased amplitude; widening QRS complex; prolonged QT interval)
  - Hyponatremia: weakness, fatigue, confusion, convulsions, coma
  - Hypocalcemia: paresthesias, carpal pedal spasm, muscle cramps, tetany
  - Hypercalcemia: digitalis toxicity, asystole
- *Pain*—nature, type, location, duration (incisional pain must be differentiated from anginal pain); apprehension; response to analgesics

Assessment also includes the observation of all machines and tubes to determine if they are functioning properly: endotracheal tube, ventilator, pulmonary artery catheter, central venous catheter, arterial catheters, cardiac monitor, pacemaker, chest tubes, indwelling catheter, intravenous fluid tubing, blood transfusion tubing.

As the patient regains consciousness and progresses through the postoperative period, the nurse expands the assessment to include parameters indicative of psychological and emotional status. The patient may exhibit behavior that reflects denial or depression, or may experience postcardiotomy psychosis. Characteristic signs of psychosis include (1) transient perceptual illusions, (2) visual and auditory hallucinations, and (3) disorientation and paranoid delusions.

The needs of the family should also be assessed. The nurse ascertains how they are coping with the situation; what their psychological, emotional, and spiritual needs are; and whether or not they are receiving adequate information about the patient's condition.

Assessing for Complications. The patient is continuously assessed for indications of impending complications. The nurse and the physician work as a team to recognize early signs and symptoms of complications and to institute measures to reverse their progress.

Decreased Cardiac Output. A decrease in cardiac output is always a threat to the patient who has had cardiac surgery. It can be due to a variety of causes:

- Hypovolemia resulting from blood loss during surgery
- Persistent bleeding after surgery
- Cardiac tamponade
- Cardiac failure
- Myocardial infarction after surgery
- Hypotension

Hypovolemia. Hypovolemia may result from blood loss during the surgical procedure, although the blood is usually replaced to within 10% of normal. The nurse observes for signs of hypovolemia: arterial hypotension and low venous pressure (CVP) with an increasing pulse rate, and low left atrial and pulmonary artery wedge pressures. These signs are reported to the physician. When indicated, the physician prescribes blood or blood components and additional solutions to replace any deficits in electrolytes and protein.

Persistent Bleeding. Persistent bleeding may be the result of tissue fragility, trauma to tissues, or some unexplained clotting defect. Therefore, accurate measurement of blood loss through dressings and drainage tubes is important. An accurate account of chest tube drainage is essential. Bloody drainage should not exceed 200 ml/hour for the first 4 to 6 hours. At the same time the patient is assessed for signs of hypovolemia. Medical management may include the administration of protamine sulfate to neutralize the heparin used during cardiopulmonary bypass, vitamin K, and blood products (fresh-frozen plasma, platelets, or specific blood factors). Preparations are made to return the patient to surgery should this be necessary.

Cardiac Tamponade. Cardiac tamponade results from bleeding into the pericardial sac or accumulation of fluids in the sac, which compresses the heart and prevents adequate filling of the ventricles. The nurse assesses for signs of tamponade: arterial hypotension accompanied by a rising left atrial pressure; muffled heart sounds; weak, thready pulse; neck vein distention; and decreased urinary output. A reduction in the amount of drainage in the chest-collection device

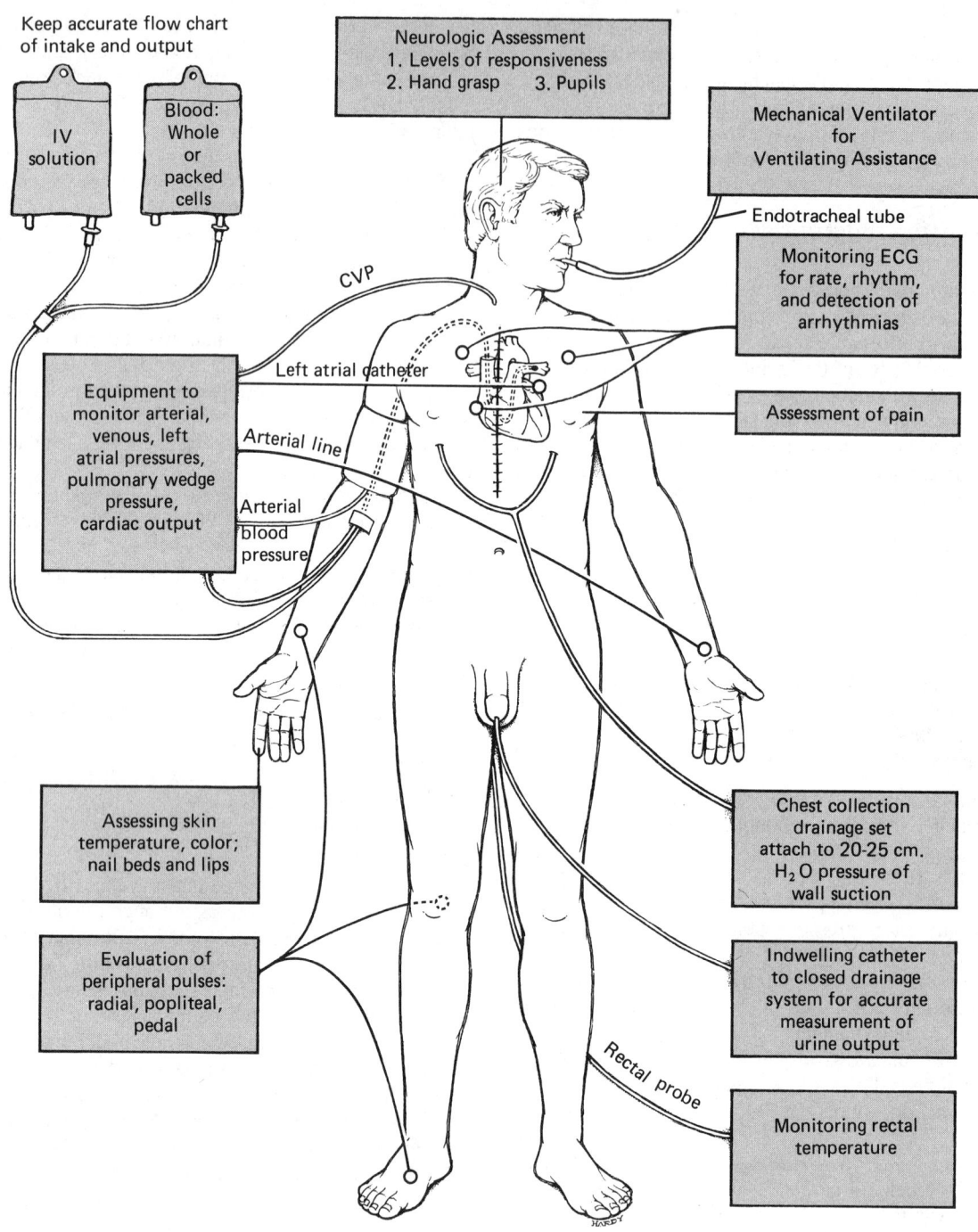

Figure 27-7
Postoperative care of the cardiac surgery patient.

dicates that the fluid may be accumulating elsewhere. The nurse assures the patency of the chest tubes by "milking" or "stripping" them and by making sure that they are free of kinks or obstructions. When tamponade is suspected, the physician obtains a chest x-ray which will indicate if fluid accumulation in the mediastinum is present. Medical management of tamponade includes pericardiocentesis (see Chap. 26).

Cardiac Failure. Cardiac failure results when the heart fails as a pump and the cardiac chambers are not adequately

emptied (see Chap. 26). The nurse observes for and reports the following signs and symptoms of cardiac failure: a falling mean arterial pressure, a rising venous pressure, an increasing tachycardia, restlessness and agitation, peripheral cyanosis, venous distention, labored respirations, tissue edema, and ascites. Medical management to avoid acute failure includes diuretic therapy and rapid digitalization.

Myocardial Infarction. Myocardial infarction may occur during the postoperative period. When assessing the patient, the nurse is aware that symptoms may be masked by the usual postoperative chest discomfort. A careful assessment of the pain is made in order to differentiate it from the incisional pain. The patient is suspected of having sustained an infarction if the mean arterial pressure falls in the presence of normal circulating volume and a normal venous pressure. The physician uses serial ECGs and cardiac enzymes to make a definitive diagnosis and to determine how serious the injury is. Analgesics are given with caution because they may cause peripheral vasodilatation and compound the hypotension. It may be necessary to reduce the rate at which the patient increases activity in order to allow the heart adequate time for healing.

Hypotension. Hypotension may be caused by inadequate cardiac contractility and blood volume and by mechanical ventilation, when the patient "fights" the ventilator or when positive end-expiratory pressure (PEEP) is used, causing a reduction in cardiac output. The development of inadequate circulating blood volume may occur after the patient has been removed from cardiopulmonary bypass. As the blood is rewarmed, vasodilatation occurs and increases vascular capacity. Normally, the fluid replacement that the physician prescribes is adequate to replenish blood volume.

Nursing assessment for hypotension includes the monitoring of left atrial pressure, CVP, pulmonary artery mean and wedge pressures, and arterial pressure. Chest tube drainage is monitored because hypotension may result from excessive drainage. When necessary, the physician prescribes blood and fluids to maintain left atrial pressure at a level that will promote good tissue perfusion. Vasopressors may be prescribed to maintain blood pressure at a desirable level. The rate and amount of vasopressor administered is carefully titrated to prevent excessive vasoconstriction.

Impaired Gas Exchange. Impaired gas exchange is another possible complication following cardiac surgery. All body tissues require an adequate supply of oxygen and nutrients for survival. To achieve this after surgery, endotracheal intubation with ventilator assistance may be left intact for 8 to 48 hours in the postoperative period, depending on the results of blood gas measurements. Studies have shown that patients who are stable following surgery may be extubated as early as 6 hours after surgery, which reduces their anxiety regarding their limited ability to communicate.

The patient is continuously assessed for indications of impaired gas exchange: restlessness, anxiety, cyanosis of mucous membranes and of peripheral tissues, tachycardia, and fighting the ventilator. Breath sounds are assessed frequently to detect fluid in the lungs, and arterial blood gas measurements are promptly reported to the physician.

Impaired Cerebral Circulation. The brain is dependent on a continuous supply of oxygenated blood. It does not have the capacity to store oxygen and must rely on adequate continuous perfusion by the heart. Thus it is important to observe the patient for any symptoms of hypoxia: restlessness, headache, confusion, dyspnea, hypotension, and cyanosis. An assessment of the patient's neurologic status is made hourly in terms of level of consciousness, response to verbal commands and painful stimuli, pupillary size and reaction to light, movement of extremities, hand grasp ability, presence of pedal and popliteal pulses, and temperature and color of extremities. Any indication of a changing status is documented and reported immediately to the surgeon, because it may signal the beginning of a complication in the postoperative period. Hypoperfusion or microemboli may produce CNS damage after cardiac surgery.

Altered Fluid and Electrolyte Balance. Alterations in fluid and electrolyte balance may occur after cardiac surgery. Nursing assessment for these complications includes monitoring of intake and output, weight, pulmonary wedge and left atrial pressure and CVP readings, hematocrit levels, distention of neck veins, tissue edema, liver size, breath sounds (*i.e.*, fine crackles, wheezing), and electrolyte levels.

Changes in serum electrolytes are reported promptly so that treatment can be instituted. Especially important are dangerously high or low levels of potassium, sodium, and calcium.

Hypokalemia. Hypokalemia (low potassium) may be caused by inadequate intake, diuretics, vomiting, diarrhea, excessive nasogastric drainage, and stress due to surgery (increased aldosterone secretion produces decreased potassium-ion (K^+) and increased sodium-ion (Na^+) retention). The patient must be observed carefully when serum potassium rises or falls outside the normal level (K^+ = 3.5–5.0 mEq/liter [3.5–5.0 mmol/L]). Some cardiac surgeons feel that it is important to maintain the K^+ level at 4.5 mEq/liter (4.5 mmol/L) or higher in order to avoid dysrhythmias in the postoperative period. The following effects of low K^+ may be noted: digitalis toxicity, dysrhythmias, metabolic alkalosis, a weakened myocardium, and cardiac arrest. One possible specific ECG change is the presence of a U wave that is more than 1 mm high. (A *U wave* is a positive deflection following the T wave). Additional signs are AV block, flat or inverted T waves, and low voltage. When necessary, the physician prescribes intravenous potassium replacement.

Hyperkalemia. Hyperkalemia (high potassium) may be caused by increased intake, red cell breakdown caused by the pump, acidosis, renal insufficiency, tissue necrosis, and adrenal cortical insufficiency. The following effects of high K^+ may be exhibited: mental confusion, restlessness, nausea, weakness, and paresthesias of the extremities. ECG changes specific for hyperkalemia are tall, peaked T waves; increased amplitude; a widening of the QRS complex; and a prolonged QT interval. When necessary, the physician prescribes an ion-exchange resin, sodium polystyrene sulfonate (Kayexalate), which binds the potassium. Alternative treatments are IV sodium bicarbonate or IV insulin and glucose to drive the potassium back into the cells from the extracellular fluid.

Hypernatremia and Hyponatremia. Both *hypernatremia* (high sodium) and *hyponatremia* (low sodium) may occur following cardiac surgery; however, the latter is more common. Hyponatremia may result from a reduction of total body sodium or from an increase in water intake which causes a dilution of body sodium. The patient must be observed for sodium values that vary from the normal ranges (*i.e.*, normal Na^+ = 135–145 mEq/liter [135–145 mmol/L]). The nurse observes for symptoms of hyponatremia: weakness, fatigue, confusion, convulsions, and coma. When there is a true loss of sodium from the body, the physician prescribes sodium replacement. Diuretics are prescribed when reduction in sodium is due to increased water intake.

Hypocalcemia. Hypocalcemia (low calcium) is caused by alkalosis, which reduces the amount of Ca^{++} in the extracellular fluid, and by multiple blood transfusions. When large amounts of citrated blood are given, the level of ionized Ca^{++} is reduced as some of the citrate binds calcium. The calcium

(Text continues on p. 616)

Postoperative Nursing Care of the Cardiac Surgery Patient

Nursing Interventions	*Rationale*	*Expected Outcomes*

Nursing Diagnosis: Decreased cardiac output related to blood loss and compromised myocardial function

Goal: Restoration of cardiac output

1. Monitor cardiovascular status. Serial readings of arterial pressure, heart rate, CVP, and left atrial or pulmonary artery pressure are observed, correlated with patient's condition, and recorded.
    a. Assess arterial pressure every 15 minutes until stable, and as directed thereafter.

    b. Auscultate for heart sounds and rhythm.

    c. Assess all peripheral pulses (pedal, tibial, popliteal, femoral, radial, brachial, carotid).

    d. Measure left atrial pressure or pulmonary artery wedge pressure to determine left ventricular end-diastolic volume and to assess cardiac output (see p. 584)
    e. Monitor central venous pressure to assess blood volume, vascular tone, and pumping effectiveness of the heart. *Remember: Changes in values are more important than isolated readings;* mechanical ventilator may elevate CVP.
    f. Monitor ECG pattern for cardiac dysrhythmias (see Chap. 26 for discussion of dysrhythmias).

    g. Check cardiac enzymes daily.

    h. Check urine output every ½ to 1 hour.

1. Effectiveness of cardiac output is determined by hemodynamic monitoring.

    a. Blood pressure is one of the most important physiological parameters to follow; vasoconstriction after cardiopulmonary bypass makes auscultatory blood pressure unobtainable.
    b. Auscultation provides evidence of cardiac tamponade (muffled distant heart sounds), pericarditis (precordial rub), dysrhythmias.
    c. Presence or absence and quality of pulses provide data about cardiac output as well as obstructive lesions.
    d. Rising pressures may indicate congestive heart failure or pulmonary edema.

    e. High CVP may result from hypervolemia, heart failure, cardiac tamponade; if blood pressure drop is due to low blood volume, CVP will show corresponding drop.

    f. Dysrhythmias are apt to occur with coronary ischemia, hypoxia, alterations in serum potassium, edema, bleeding, acid-base or electrolyte disturbances, digitalis toxicity, cardiac failure. PVCs occur most frequently following aortic valve replacement and coronary bypass surgery.
    g. Elevations may indicate myocardial infarction.
    h. Urine output less than 30 ml/hour indicates decreased cardiac output and decreased renal perfusion.

- The following parameters are within normal ranges:
    arterial pressure
    heart sounds
    peripheral pulses
    pulmonary artery wedge pressure
    central venous pressure
    cardiac rate and rhythm
    cardiac enzymes
    urine output
    skin and mucosal color
    skin temperature
    jugular vein pressure

(continued)

Nursing Interventions	*Rationale*	*Expected Outcomes*

Nursing Diagnosis: Decreased cardiac output related to blood loss and compromised myocardial function

Goal: Restoration of cardiac output

i. Observe buccal mucosa, nail beds, lips, ear lobes, and extremities.	i. Duskiness and cyanosis indicate decreased cardiac output.	
j. Assess skin; note temperature and color.	j. Cool moist skin indicates vasoconstriction and decreased cardiac output.	
k. Measure jugular vein pressure.	k. Increased JVP indicates diminishing cardiac capacity.	
2. Observe for persistent bleeding: steady, continuous drainage of blood; hypotension; low CVP; tachycardia. Prepare to administer blood, IV solutions.	2. Bleeding can result from cardiac incision, tissue fragility, trauma to tissues, clotting defects.	• Less than 300 ml/hour of drainage via chest tubes during first 4 to 6 hours • Vital signs stable
3. Observe for cardiac tamponade: hypotension; rising CVP; rising left atrial pressure; muffled heart sounds; weak, thready pulse; neck vein distention; decreasing urinary output. Check for diminished amount of blood in chest collection bottle. Prepare for pericardiocentesis (see p. 591)	3. Cardiac tamponade results from bleeding into the pericardial sac or accumulation of fluid in the sac, which compresses the heart and prevents adequate filling of the ventricles. Decrease may indicate fluid is accumulating in pericardial sac.	• Vital signs stable • Chest tube drainage expected amount • CVP and left atrial pressures within normal limits • Urinary output within normal limits
4. Observe for cardiac failure: hypotension, rising CVP and left atrial pressure, tachycardia, restlessness, agitation, cyanosis, venous distention, dyspnea, ascites. Prepare to administer diuretics and digitalis	4. Cardiac failure results from decreased pumping action of heart; can cause deficient blood perfusion to vital organs.	• Vital signs stable • CVP and left atrial pressures within normal limits • Skin color normal • Respirations unlabored
5. Observe for myocardial infarction: decreased cardiac output in presence of normal circulating volume and filling pressures. Obtain serial ECGs and isoenzymes. Differentiate myocardial pain from incisional pain.	5. Symptoms may be masked by incisional pain.	• Vital signs stable • Pain limited to incision • ECG and isoenzymes negative for ischemic changes

Nursing Diagnosis: Potential impaired gas exchange related to trauma and extensive chest surgery

Goal: Adequate gas exchange

Assess respiratory status and provide for adequate ventilation and tissue oxygenation.		
1. Maintain "assisted" or "controlled" ventilation (see p. 435).	1. Ventilatory support is used the first 8 to 24 hours to decrease work of the heart, to maintain effective ventilation, and to provide an airway in the event of cardiac arrest.	• Airway patent • ABGs within normal range • Endotracheal tube correctly placed, as evidenced by x-ray • Breath sounds clear

(continued)

Nursing Interventions	*Rationale*	*Expected Outcomes*

Nursing Diagnosis: Potential impaired gas exchange related to trauma and extensive chest surgery

Goal: Adequate gas exchange

2. Monitor arterial blood gas and tidal volume findings.	2. ABGs and tidal volume indicate effectiveness of ventilator and changes that need to be made to improve gas exchange.	• Respirations synchronous with ventilator
3. Ausculate chest for breath sounds.	3. Crackles indicate pulmonary congestion; decreased or absent breath sounds indicate pneumothorax.	• Tracheobronchial secretions adequately removed by suctioning
4. Sedate patient adequately, as prescribed, and monitor respiratory rate and depth if ventilations are not "controlled".	4. Sedation helps the patient to tolerate the endotracheal tube and to cope with ventilatory sensations; sedatives can depress respiratory rate and depth.	• Adequacy of color of skin and mucous membranes • Mental acuity consistent with amount of sedatives and analgesics received.
5. Provide chest physiotherapy as prescribed.	5. Aids in preventing retention of secretions and atelectasis	
6. Promote coughing, deep breathing, and turning.	6. Aids in keeping airway patent, preventing atelectasis, and facilitating lung expansion	
7. Suction tracheobronchial secretions as needed, using strict aseptic technique.	7. Retention of secretions leads to hypoxia and possible cardiac arrest; retained secretions promote infection.	
8. See page 441 for weaning process and endotracheal tube removal.		

Nursing Diagnosis: Potential alteration in fluid volume and electrolyte balance related to alternations in blood volume

Goal: Fluid and electrolyte balance

1. Maintain fluid and electrolyte balance.	1. Adequate circulating blood volume is necessary for optimum cellular activity; metabolic acidosis and electrolyte imbalance can occur after use of pump oxygenator.	• Fluid intake and output balanced • Hemodynamic assessment parameters negative for fluid overload and dehydration
a. Keep intake and output flow sheets; record urine volume every ½ to 1 hour.	a. Provides a method to determine positive or negative fluid balance and fluid requirements	
b. Assess the following parameters: blood pressure, CVP, pulmonary artery wedge pressure, weight, electrolyte levels, hematocrit, jugular vein pressure, tissue turgor, liver size, breath sounds.	b. Provides information about state of hydration	
c. Measure postoperative chest drainage (should not exceed 300 ml/hour for first 4 to 6 hours); cessation of drainage may indicate kinked or blocked chest tube.	c. Excessive blood loss from chest cavity can cause hypovolemia.	

(continued)

Nursing Interventions	*Rationale*	*Expected Outcomes*

Nursing Diagnosis: Potential alteration in fluid volume and electrolyte balance related to alternations in blood volume

Goal: Fluid and electrolyte balance

2. Be alert to changes in serum electrolyte levels.	2. A specific concentration of electrolytes is necessary in both extracellular and intracellular body fluids to sustain life.	• Blood *p*H 7.35 to 7.45 • Serum potassium 3.5–5.0 mEq/liter (3.5–5.0 mmol/L) • Serum sodium 135–145 mEq/liter (135–145 mmol/L) • Serum calcium 8.8–10.3 mg/100 ml (2.20–2.58 mmol/L)

a. Hypokalemia (low potassium)
   Effects: dysrhythmias, digitalis toxicity, metabolic acidosis, weakened myocardium, cardiac arrest
   Watch for specific ECG changes.
   Give IV potassium replacement as directed.
	a. *Causes:* inadequate intake, diuretics, vomiting, excessive nasogastric drainage, stress from surgery	

b. Hyperkalemia (high potassium)
   Effects: mental confusion, restlessness, nausea, weakness, paresthesias of extremities
   Be prepared to administer an ion-exchange resin (sodium polystyrene sulfonate [Kayexalate]), IV sodium bicarbonate or IV insulin and glucose.
	b. *Causes:* increased intake, hemolysis from pump, acidosis, renal insufficiency, tissue necrosis, adrenal cortical insufficiency.
	   The resin binds potassium and promotes intestinal excretion of it.
	   IV sodium bicarbonate drives potassium into the cells from extracellular fluid	

c. Hyponatremia (low sodium)
   Effects: weakness, fatigue, confusion, convulsions, coma
   Administer sodium or diuretics as directed.
	c. *Causes:* reduction of total body sodium, or increased water intake causing dilution of sodium	

d. Hypocalcemia (low calcium)
   Effects: numbness and tingling in fingertips, toes, ears, nose; carpopedal spasm; muscle cramps; tetany
   Administer replacement therapy as directed.
	d. *Causes:* alkalosis, multiple blood transfusions	

e. Hypercalcemia (high calcium)
   Effects: dysrhythmias, digitalis toxicity, asystole
   Institute treatment as directed.
	e. *Cause:* prolonged immobility	

Nursing Diagnosis: Potential sensory-perceptual alterations related to sensory overload

Goal: Reduction of symptoms of sensory overload; prevention of postcardiotomy syndrome

1. Observe for symptoms: perceptual distortions, hallucinations, disorientation, paranoid delusions.		

(continued)

Nursing Diagnosis: Potential sensory-perceptual alterations related to sensory overload

Goal: Reduction of symptoms of sensory overload; prevention of postcardiotomy syndrome

Nursing Interventions	Rationale	Expected Outcomes
2. Use measures to prevent postcardiotomy syndrome: a. Carefully explain all procedures and the need for patient cooperation. b. Plan nursing care to provide for periods of uninterrupted sleep with day–night pattern. c. Decrease sleep-preventing environmental stimuli as much as possible. d. Promote continuity of care from nurse to nurse. e. Orient to time and place frequently. Encourage family to visit at regular times.	2. Postcardiotomy syndrome may result from anxiety, sleep deprivation, increased sensory input, disorientation to night and day.	• Patient cooperates with procedures. • Sleeps for long intervals • Oriented to time, place, person • Experiences no perceptual distortions, hallucinations, disorientation, delusions

Nursing Diagnosis: Pain related to operative trauma and pleural irritation caused by chest tubes

Goal: Relief of pain

Nursing Interventions	Rationale	Expected Outcomes
1. Record nature, type, location, and duration of pain. 2. Differentiate between incisional pain and anginal pain. 3. Medicate as prescribed and observe for side-effects of lethargy, hypotension, tachycardia, respiratory depression.	1. Pain and anxiety increase pulse rate, oxygen consumption, and cardiac workload. 2. Anginal pain requires immediate treatment. 3. Analgesia promotes rest, decreases oxygen consumption caused by pain, and aids patient in performing deep breathing and coughing exercises.	• Complaints of pain decreased • Restlessness decreased • Vital signs stable • Patient participates in deep breathing and coughing exercises. • Verbalizes fewer complaints of pain each day

Nursing Diagnosis: Potential alteration in renal perfusion related to decreased cardiac output, hemolysis, or vasopressor drug therapy

Goal: Maintenance of adequate renal perfusion

Nursing Interventions	Rationale	Expected Outcomes
1. Assess renal function: a. Measure urine output every ½ to 1 hour. b. Measure urine specific gravity c. Report lab results: BUN, serum creatinine, urine and serum electrolytes.	1. Renal injury can be caused by deficient perfusion, hemolysis, low cardiac output, and use of vasopressor agents to increase blood pressure. a. Less than 20 ml/hour indicates decreased renal function. b. Indicates kidneys' ability to concentrate urine in renal tubules. c. Indicate kidneys' ability to excrete waste products	• Urine output consistent with fluid intake • Urine specific gravity 1.015–1.025 • BUN, creatinine, electrolytes within normal limits

(continued)

Nursing Interventions	*Rationale*	*Expected Outcomes*

Nursing Diagnosis: Potential alteration in renal perfusion related to decreased cardiac output, hemolysis, or vasopressor drug therapy

Goal: Maintenance of adequate renal perfusion

2. Prepare to administer rapid-acting diuretics or inotropic drugs (dopamine, dobutamine).	2. Promote renal function and increase cardiac output and renal blood flow	
3. Prepare patient for peritoneal dialysis or hemodialysis if indicated.		

Nursing Diagnosis: Potential hyperthermia related to infection or postpericardiotomy syndrome

Goal: Maintenance of normal body temperature

1. Assess temperature every hour.	1. Fever can indicate infectious process or postpericardiotomy syndrome.	• Normal body temperature • Incisions free of infection • Absence of symptoms of postpericardiotomy syndrome
2. Use sterile technique when changing dressings, suctioning endotracheal tube; maintain closed system for all intravenous and arterial lines and for Foley catheter.	2. Decreases chance of infection	
3. Observe for symptoms of postpericardiotomy syndrome: fever, malaise, pericardial effusion, pericardial friction rub, arthralgia.	3. Occurs in 10% to 40% of patients after cardiac surgery	
4. Administer salicylates and steroids as directed; promote bed rest.	4. Relieve symptoms	

Nursing Diagnosis: Deficit in knowledge about self-care activities

Goal: Ability to perform self-care activities

1. Develop teaching plan for patient and family. Provide specific instructions for the following:
  diet
  activity progression
  exercise
  coughing, deep breathing, lung expansion exercises
  temperature-monitoring
  medication regimen
	1. Each patient will have unique learning needs.	• Patient and family member explain all aspects of therapeutic regimen.
		• Patient and family member identify lifestyle changes necessitated by therapeutic regimen.
		• Patient has copy of discharge instructions.
		• Makes follow-up phone calls weekly
		• Keeps follow-up appointments with surgeon

2. Provide verbal and written instructions; provide several teaching sessions for reinforcement and answering questions.	2. Repetition promotes learning by allowing for clarification of misinformation.	
3. Involve family in all teaching sessions	3. Family member responsible for home care is usually anxious and requires adequate time for learning.	
4. Provide information regarding follow-up: weekly phone call to surgeon or cardiologist and assigned liaison nurse; follow-up visit with surgeon in 4 to 6 weeks.	4. Arrangements for phone contacts with health-care personnel help to allay anxieties.	
5. Make appropriate referrals: *e.g.,* Visiting Nurse service, community support groups, Mended Hearts Club.		

level is monitored to determine if it is within normal limits (Ca^{++} = 8.8–10.3 mg/100 ml [2.20–2.58 mmol/L]). The nurse assesses the patient for symptoms of reduced calcium: numbness and tingling in the fingertips, toes, ears, and nose; carpal pedal spasm; and muscle cramps and tetany. Any symptoms of hypocalcemia are reported promptly so that the physician can institute calcium replacement immediately.

Hypercalcemia. *Hypercalcemia* (high calcium) can cause dysrhythmias that imitate those caused by digitalis toxicity. Calcium is known to potentiate, or enhance, the action of digitalis. Therefore, the nurse assesses the patient for signs of digitalis toxicity and reports these immediately so that the physician can institute treatment to prevent asystole and death.

▷ Nursing Diagnoses

Based on the assessment data and the type of surgical procedure performed, major nursing diagnoses of the patient may include items such as the following:

- Decreased cardiac output related to blood loss and compromised myocardial function
- Potential impaired gas exchange related to trauma of extensive chest surgery
- Potential alteration in fluid volume and electrolyte balance related to alteration in circulating blood volume
- Potential sensory-perceptual alterations related to sensory overload (ICCU, surgical experience)
- Pain related to operative trauma and pleural irritation caused by chest tubes
- Potential alteration in tissue perfusion related to venous stasis, embolization, or coagulation problems
- Potential alteration in renal perfusion related to decreased cardiac output, hemolysis, or vasopressor drug therapy
- Potential hyperthermia related to infection or postpericardiotomy syndrome
- Deficit in knowledge about self-care activities

▷ Planning and Implementation

▷ *Goals.* The major goals of the patient include restoration of cardiac output, adequate gas exchange, maintenance of fluid and electrolyte balance, reduction of symptoms of sensory overload, relief of pain, promotion of rest, maintenance of adequate tissue perfusion, maintenance of adequate renal perfusion, maintenance of normal body temperature, and learning self-care activities.

Nursing Interventions

A typical postoperative nursing care plan for the cardiac surgery patient is presented in Nursing Care Plan 27-1, pp. 610–615.

Restoration of Cardiac Output. Nursing management of the patient involves continuous observation of the patient's cardiac status and immediate notification of the surgeon of any changes that indicate a decrease in cardiac output. The nurse and the surgeon then work as a team to correct the problem.

In evaluating the patient's cardiac status, the nurse primarily determines the effectiveness of cardiac output through clinical observations and routine measurements. Serial readings of blood pressure, heart rate, central venous pressure, arterial pressure, and left atrial or pulmonary artery pressure from monitors are observed and recorded.

Cardiac function is related to kidney function; therefore, urinary output is measured and recorded. If urine output falls below 30 ml/hour, this may indicate a decrease in cardiac output. Urine specific gravity is also assessed (normally 1.010–1.025), as is urine osmolality. Underhydration may be manifested by low urinary output and a high specific gravity, whereas overhydration is exhibited by high urinary output with low specific gravity.

The growth and function of body cells depend on adequate cardiac output to provide a continuous supply of oxygenated blood to meet the changing demands of the organs and body systems. Since the buccal mucosa, nail beds, lips, and earlobes are sites with rich capillary beds, they should be observed for cyanosis or duskiness as possible signs of reduced heart action. Moist or dry skin may indicate either vasodilation or vasoconstriction respectively. Venous distention of the neck veins or of the dorsal surface of the hand raised to heart level may signal a changing demand or diminishing capacity of the heart. If cardiac output has fallen, the skin becomes cool, moist, and cyanotic or mottled.

Irregularities of heart action, which may arise when poor perfusion of the heart exists, also serve as important indicators of heart function. The most common dysrhythmias encountered during the postoperative period are bradycardias, tachycardias, and ectopic beats. Continuous observation of the monitor for various dysrhythmias is an essential part of patient care and management.

Any indications of decreased cardiac output are reported promptly to the physician. These assessment data and further diagnostic tests are used by the physician to determine the cause of the problem. Once a diagnosis has been made, the physician and the nurse work together to restore cardiac output and prevent further complications. When indicated, the physician prescribes blood components, fluids, digitalis, diuretics, or vasopressors. When further surgery is necessary, the patient is prepared for the procedure.

Adequate Gas Exchange. To assure adequate gas exchange, the nurse assesses and maintains the patency of the endotracheal tube. The patient is suctioned frequently to minimize collection of secretions. 100% oxygen is delivered to the patient via a self-inflating bag (Ambu) prior to and following suctioning to prevent hypoxia that can result from the suctioning procedure. Arterial blood gas determinations are compared with baseline data and reported to the physician promptly.

Because an open airway enhances O_2 and CO_2 exchange, the endotracheal tube must be secured to prevent it from slipping into the right mainstem bronchus and occluding the airway. In addition, suctioning at frequent intervals is essential to remove secretions and mucus plugs. Frequent change of position also provides for optimum pulmonary ventilation and perfusion by allowing the lungs to expand more fully. When the patient's condition stabilizes, body position is changed every 1 to 2 hours and the nurse listens to breath sounds to detect the presence of wheezes and fluid in the lungs. Deep breathing and coughing are also encouraged to open the alveolar sacs and provide for increased perfusion. Physical support of the incision is provided when the patient coughs and breathes deeply at regular intervals.

When ready for extubation, the patient may gag or "fight" the ventilator. Other indications for extubation are an adequate tidal volume, toleration of O_2 with warmed humidification, and adequate blood gas determinations. Early extubation is considered when the patient's condition is stable. This means that the patient's hemodynamic pressures are not fluctuating and are within 20% of preoperative volumes—and hence are high enough to maintain peripheral perfusion as indicated by urinary output, provided that there are no dangerous dysrhythmias. With these parameters as guidelines, early extubation has been performed without any adverse effects on the patient's condition or prognosis. During this time the nurse assists with the weaning process and, eventually, the removal of the tube.

Maintenance of Fluid and Electrolyte Balance.

To promote fluid and electrolyte balance the nurse carefully assesses intake and output. Flow sheets are utilized to determine positive or negative fluid balance. All fluid intake is recorded, including intravenous fluids, flush solutions used in arterial and venous catheters and the nasogastric tube, and oral fluids. Likewise, all output is recorded including urine, nasogastric drainage, and chest drainage.

Hemodynamic parameters (blood pressure, pulmonary wedge and left atrial pressures, and CVP) are correlated with intake, output, and weight to determine the adequacy of hydration and cardiac output. Serum electrolytes are monitored and the patient is observed for signs of hypokalemia, hyperkalemia, hyponatremia, and hypocalcemia.

Any indications of dehydration, fluid overload, or electrolyte imbalance are reported promptly, and the physician and nurse work together to restore fluid and electrolyte balance. The patient's response to fluid and electrolyte replacements or restrictions is monitored closely.

Reduction of Symptoms of Sensory Overload.

Sensory overload is a common effect associated with the surgical experience and environmental factors in the ICCU. *Postcardiotomy psychosis* may occur after cardiac surgery. The term refers to a group of abnormal behaviors which occur in varying intensity and duration in a large number of patients. In the early years of cardiac surgery this phenomenon occurred more frequently than it does today. At that time it was attributed to inadequate cerebral perfusion during surgery, microemboli, and the length of time that the patient remained on the cardiopulmonary bypass machine. Advances in surgical techniques have significantly decreased these factors. Today, when it occurs, it is thought to be due to anxiety, sleep deprivation, increased sensory input, and disorientation to night and day when the patient loses track of time. An important finding is that patients who do not or cannot express anxiety before surgery are more prone to develop psychosis in the postoperative period. Psychosis may appear after a brief lucid interval.

The nurse should be watchful for signs of denial and should provide an opportunity for emotional expression during the preoperative period. Careful explanations of all procedures and of the need for cooperation help to keep the patient oriented throughout the postoperative course. Continuity of care, if at all possible, is desirable; a familiar face and a nursing staff with a consistent approach will prove to be assets in the delivery of nursing care. The use of a well-designed and individualized nursing care plan will provide guidelines to assist the nursing team in coordination of their efforts for the emotional well-being of the patient.

Relief of Pain.

Deep pain may not be reflected in the immediate area of injury but in a broader, more diffuse area. Patients who have had cardiac surgery experience pain caused by the severance of intercostal nerves along the incision route and irritation of the pleura by the chest catheters. It is essential to observe and listen to the patient for verbal and nonverbal clues about pain. The nurse should accurately record the nature, type, location, and duration of the pain. (Incisional pain must be differentiated from anginal pain.) The patient is medicated as often as prescribed to reduce the amount of pain and to improve the success of deep breathing and coughing exercises. If pain inhibits performance of these activities, progress will be jeopardized.

Pain produces tension, which may stimulate the central nervous system to release adrenalin and thus constrict the arterioles. This can cause increased afterload and decreased cardiac output. Morphine sulfate alleviates anxiety and pain and induces sleep, which reduces metabolic rate and oxygen demands. Following the administration of narcotics, any observations indicating relief of apprehension and pain are documented in the patient's record. The patient is observed for any respiratory depressant effects of the analgesic. If respiratory depression occurs, a narcotic antagonist (*e.g.*, Naloxone [Narcan]) is used to counteract the effect.

Promotion of Rest.

Basic comfort measures used in conjunction with prescribed analgesics will potentiate the effects of the analgesics and promote rest. The patient is assisted in changing positions every 1 to 2 hours and is positioned in such a way that strain on the incisional line and chest tubes is avoided. Physical support of the incision during coughing and deep breathing helps to minimize pain. Nursing activities are scheduled as much as possible to provide undisturbed periods of rest. As the condition stabilizes and the patient is disturbed less frequently for monitoring and therapeutic procedures, rest periods can become extended.

Maintenance of Adequate Tissue Perfusion.

Peripheral pulses (pedal, tibial, popliteal, femoral, radial, brachial) are routinely palpated to assess for arterial obstruction. If any pulse is absent, the cause may be recent catheterization of that extremity. The absence of any pulse is immediately reported to the physician.

Following surgery, measures are taken to prevent venous stasis that can cause thrombus formation and subsequent embolization: (1) applying antiembolic stockings, (2) discouraging leg crossing, (3) avoiding use of the knee gatch on the bed, (4) omitting pillows in the popliteal space, and (5) instituting passive exercises followed by active exercises to promote circulation and prevent loss of muscle tone.

Thrombus formation and resulting embolization can also result from injury to the intima of the blood vessels, dislodgment of a clot from a damaged valve, loosening of mural thrombi, and coagulation problems. Air embolism may occur as a result of cardiopulmonary bypass. The usual embolic sites are the lungs, coronary arteries, mesentery, extremities, kidneys, spleen, and brain.

Symptoms of embolization, which vary according to site, should be watched for: (1) midabdominal or midback pain; (2) pain, cessation of pulses, blanching, numbness, or coldness in an extremity; (3) chest pain and respiratory distress with pulmonary embolus or myocardial infarction; and (4) one-sided weakness and pupillary changes, such as occur in cerebral vascular accident. All such symptoms are promptly reported to the physician.

Maintenance of Adequate Renal Perfusion. Inadequate renal perfusion can occur as a complication of open heart surgery. One possible cause is low cardiac output. In addition, trauma to blood cells during cardiopulmonary bypass can cause hemolysis of red blood cells. This leads to a buildup of toxic substances because of the kidney's inability to excrete waste products. Use of vasopressor agents to increase blood pressure can also lead to reduction of the blood flow to the kidneys, when the vasopressors are ones that cause constriction of renal arteries (*e.g.,* levarterenol [Levophed]). Nursing management includes accurate measurement of urine output. An output of less than 20 ml/hour can indicate hypovolemia. Specific gravity tests should be carried out to determine the kidneys' ability to concentrate urine in the renal tubules. Rapid-acting diuretics or inotropic drugs (digitalis, isoproterenol) may be prescribed to increase cardiac output and renal blood flow. The nurse should be aware of the BUN and serum creatinine levels as well as urine and serum electrolytes. Abnormalities in these studies are reported promptly because it may be necessary to restrict fluids and limit the use of drugs that are normally excreted by the kidneys.

If efforts to maintain renal perfusion are not effective, the patient may require peritoneal dialysis or hemodialysis (see Chap. 39).

Maintenance of Normal Body Temperature. Following cardiac surgery the patient is at risk for developing raised body temperature caused by infection or postpericardiotomy syndrome. The resultant increase in metabolic rate increases tissue oxygen demands and thus increases cardiac workload. Measures are taken to prevent this sequence of events or to halt it as soon as it is recognized.

Sites of infection include the lungs, urinary tract, incisions, and intravascular catheters. Meticulous care is used in preventing contamination at the sites of catheter and tube insertions. Sterile technique is used when changing dressings and when providing endotracheal tube care and catheter care. Clearance of pulmonary secretions is accomplished by frequent repositioning of the patient, chest physical therapy, and suctioning. A closed system is used to maintain all intravenous and arterial lines.

Postpericardiotomy syndrome occurs in approximately 10% to 40% of patients who undergo cardiac surgery. Its precise etiology is unknown. A common factor appears to be trauma with residual blood in the pericardial sac following surgery. The syndrome is characterized by fever, pericardial pain, pleural pain, dyspnea, pleural effusion and pericardial friction, and arthralgia. There may be a combination of these signs and symptoms. Leukocytosis is present, along with elevation of the sedimentation rate. These symptoms frequently appear after the patient is discharged from the hospital.

The syndrome must be differentiated from other postoperative complications (incisional pain, myocardial infarction, pulmonary embolus, bacterial endocarditis, pneumonia, or atelectasis). The treatment is dependent on the severity of the symptoms. Bed rest and anti-inflammatory agents, such as salicylates and steroids, lead to a dramatic improvement in symptoms.

Patient Teaching/Home Health Care. Depending upon the type of surgery and postoperative progress, the patient may be discharged from the hospital as early as 7 to 10 days after surgery. Although the patient may be anxious to return home, usually both patient and family have apprehensions about this transition. The family often expresses the fear that they are not capable of caring for the patient at home. They are often concerned that complications will occur which they are unprepared to handle.

The nurse helps the patient and family to set realistic, achievable goals. A teaching plan that meets the patient's individual needs is developed with the patient and family. This is done several days prior to discharge to allow ample time for periodic review of the plan and answering of questions. Specific instructions are provided about diet; activity progression and exercise; coughing, deep breathing, and lung expansion exercises; weight and temperature monitoring; and the medication regimen.

The nurse may find that some patients will have difficulty learning and retaining information after cardiac surgery. Studies have shown that many patients experience difficulties in cognitive function after cardiac surgery which have not been shown to occur after other types of major surgery. The patient may experience recent memory loss, short attention span, difficulty with simple math, poor handwriting, and visual disturbances. Patients who experience these difficulties often become frustrated when they try to begin resuming normal activities and learning how to care for themselves at home. The patient and family are reassured that the difficulty is temporary and will subside in several weeks, 6 to 8 weeks at the most. In the meantime, instructions are given to the patient at a much slower pace than normal, and a family member assumes responsibility for making sure that the prescribed regimen is followed. If necessary, arrangements are made for community nurse services to provide home care such as dressing changes, monitoring of vital signs, diet counseling, and support for the patient and family.

Patient education postoperatively does not end at the time of discharge. The patient is encouraged to maintain telephone contact with the surgeon and cardiologist and with an assigned liaison nurse. This provides the patient and family with reassurance that questions can be answered and problems can be resolved when they arise. Many hospitals provide family support sessions that help family members to cope with their own stress related to the patient's home health care management. The patient is expected to have a follow-up visit with the surgeon 4 to 6 weeks after discharge.

Many patients and families benefit from supportive programs such as the postbypass rehabilitation programs offered by many medical centers. These programs provide exercise monitoring, instructions about diet and stress reduction, and support groups for patients and families. The American Heart Association sponsors the Mended Hearts Club, which provides information as well as an opportunity for families to share experiences.

▷ *Evaluation*

▷ *Expected Outcomes*
(See Nursing Care Plan 27-1 for specific outcomes.)

1. Patient achieves adequate cardiac output.
2. Maintains adequate gas exchange.
3. Maintains fluid and electrolyte balance.
4. Experiences decreased symptoms of sensory overload; is reoriented to person, time, and place.
5. Experiences relief of pain.

6. Maintains adequate tissue perfusion.
7. Gets adequate rest.
8. Maintains adequate renal perfusion.
9. Maintains normal body temperature.
10. Performs self-care activities.

Bibliography

Books

Baue AE & Glenn WWL. Thoracic and Cardiovascular Surgery. Norwalk, Appleton-Century-Crofts, 1983.

Behrendt DM & Austen WG. Patient Care in Cardiac Surgery. Boston, Little, Brown & Co, 1985.

Douglas MK & Shinn JA. Advances in Cardiovascular Nursing. Rockville, Maryland, Aspen Systems, 1985.

Hovath PT. Care of the Adult Cardiac Surgery Patient. New York: John Wiley & Sons, 1984.

Hudak CN, Lohr T, and Gallo BM. Critical Care Nursing. Philadelphia, JB Lippincott, 1986.

Hurst JW. The Heart, Arteries, and Veins. New York, McGraw-Hill, 1986.

Kirklin JW & Barratt-Boyes BG. Cardiac Surgery. New York, John Wiley & Sons, 1986.

McCauley KM, Brest AN, & McGoon DC. McGoon's Cardiac Surgery: An Interprofessional Approach to Patient Care. Philadelphia: FA Davis, 1985.

Roberts SL. Physiological Concepts and the Critically Ill Patient. Englewood Cliffs, New Jersey, Prentice-Hall, 1985.

Yee BH & Zorb SL. Cardiac Critical Care Nursing. Boston, Little, Brown & Co, 1986.

Articles

(Asterisks indicate nursing research articles.)

General

Dalsing MC, Dilley RS, and McCarthy M. Surgery of the aorta. Crit Care Quart 1985 Sept; 8(2):25–38.

*Dandalides PC, Rutala WA, and Sarubbi FA. Postoperative infections following cardiac surgery: Association with an environmental reservoir in a cardiothoracic intensive care unit. Infect Control 1984 Aug; 5(8):378–384.

Fogarty TJ et al. A new approach to transluminal angioplasty. CVP 1984 Feb/Mar; 12(2):14–24.

Forrester JS and Staniloff HM. Pericardial tamponade. Emerg Med 1984 Feb 29; 16(4):108–116.

*Grigas D et al. Cardiopulmonary function following post-cardiac surgical mediastinitis. Chest 1984 June; 85(6):729–732.

Gurevich I. Infectious complications after open heart surgery. Heart Lung 1984 Sept; 13(5):472–481.

Heyman S. Effects of cardiopulmonary bypass on coagulation. DCCN 1985 Mar/Apr; 4(2):70–80.

Kaiser AB. Risk factors for infection in cardiac surgery: Will the real culprit please stand up? Infect Control 1984 Aug; 5(8):369–370.

McClendon CE. Postpericardiotomy syndrome. Drug Intell Clin Pharm 1986 Jan; 20(1):20–23.

Ng L and Nuckols OJ. Nursing management of the postoperative cardiac surgical patient in the critical care unit. In Rackley CE. Advances in Critical Care Cardiology. Philadelphia, FA Davis, 1986.

Popovsky MA. Autologous transfusion. Present practice and future trends. NITA 1986 July/Aug; 9(4):292–295.

Rowe GG. Ventricular aneurysm: Current concepts. Hosp Med 1985 Sept; 21(9):21–34.

Seifert PC and Lefrak EA. Atrial septal defect: The adult patient. AORN J 1984 Mar; 39(4):617–630.

Smith EF. Acyanotic obstructive lesions: Coarctation of the aorta and congenital aortic stenosis. Nurs Clin North Am 1984 Sept; 19(3): 471–483.

Walsh M. The cardiac surgical patient: Guidelines for assessment. AORN J 1984 Nov; 40(5):739–743.

Weiland AP and Walker WE. Physiologic principles and clinical sequelae of cardiopulmonary bypass. Heart Lung 1986 Jan; 15(1):34–39.

Coronary Artery Bypass Surgery

Cave L et al. When families get together. Nursing 85 1985 Feb; 15(2): 58–61.

Clancey CA, Wey JM, and Guinn GA. The effect of patients' perceptions on return to work after coronary artery bypass surgery. Heart Lung 1984 Mar; 13(2):173–176.

*Eyherabide A and Yates BC. The effects of cardiac rehabilitation on compliance in the coronary artery bypass surgery patient. Cardiovasc Nurs 1985 Nov/Dec; 21(6):31–35.

*Gilliss CL. Reducing family stress during and after coronary artery bypass surgery. Nurs Clin North Am 1984 Mar; 19(1):103–112.

*Gortner SR et al. Expected and realized benefits from coronary bypass surgery in relation to severity of illness. Cardiovasc Nurs 1985 May/June; 21(3):13–18.

Horowitz BF, Fitzpatrick JJ, & Flaherty GG. Relaxation techniques for pain relief after open heart surgery. DCCN 1984 Nov/Dec; 3(6): 364–371.

Jansen KJ et al. Postoperative nursing management in patients undergoing myocardial revascularization with the internal mammary artery bypass. Heart Lung 1986 Jan; 15(1):48–54.

*King KB. Measurement of coping strategies, concerns, and emotional response in patients undergoing coronary artery bypass grafting. Heart Lung 1985 Nov; 14(6):579–586.

Loop FD. Progress in surgical treatment of coronary atherosclerosis, Part 1. Chest 1983 Nov; 84(5):611–624.

Loop FD. Progress in surgical treatment of coronary atherosclerosis, Part 2. Chest 1983 Dec; 84(6):740–755.

*Marshall J, Penckofer S, and Llewellyn J. Structured postoperative teaching and knowledge and compliance of patients who had coronary artery bypass surgery. Heart Lung 1986 Jan; 15(1):76–82.

Ng L. Coronary artery bypass surgery: Implications for occupational health nursing. Occup Health Nurs 1984 Feb; 32(2):78–117.

*Osborne D. Cardiovascular responses of patients ambulated 32 and 56 hours after coronary bypass surgery. West J Nurs Res 1984 Summer; 6(3):321–324.

*Penckofer S and Holm K. Early appraisal of coronary revascularization on quality of life. Nurs Res 1984 Mar/Apr; 33(2):60–63.

*Quinless F. The relationship between ego strength, field dependence–independence, and the development of postcardiotomy psychosis in adult male coronary artery revascularization patients. Cardiovasc Nurs 1984 July/Aug; 20(4):19–24.

Raymond M et al. Coping with transient intellectual dysfunction after coronary bypass surgery. Heart Lung 1984 Sept; 13(5):531–539.

Rodgers CD. Needs of relatives of cardiac surgery patients during the critical care phase. Focus Crit Care 1983 Oct; 10(5):50–55.

*Roviaro S, Holmes DS, and Holmsten RD. Influence of a cardiac rehabilitation program on the cardiovascular, psychological, and social functioning of cardiac patients. J Behav Med 1984 Mar; 7(1):61–81.

Slosky DA, Martinsen KS, and Doricette M. Post-bypass arrhythmia: Managing common postoperative rhythm disturbances. Consultant 1984 Oct; 24(10):115–128.

*Stanton BA et al. Perceived adequacy of patient education and fears and adjustments after cardiac surgery. Heart Lung 1984 Sept; 13(5): 525–531.

Valvular Surgery

Cohn LH. The long-term results of aortic valve replacement. Chest 1984 Mar; 85(3):387–396.

Georges JM and Stotts NA. Reducing cardiac cachexia before cardiac valve replacement. DCCN 1985 Nov/Dec; 4(6):349–353.

Gonzales JL and Rogers WJ. Follow-up of patients with prosthetic heart valves. Hosp Med 1984 June; 20(6):159–167.

Kostis, JB et al. Aortic valve replacement in patients with aortic stenosis. Chest 1984 Feb; 85(2):211–214.

Lamb LS and DiGiacomo BM. What to expect when your patient's scheduled for mitral valve replacement. Nursing 85 1985 Jan; 15(1):58–64.

O'Brien P. Surgical repair of cyanotic cardiac defects in young adults. Nurs Clin North Am 1984 Sept; 19(3):521–535.

Rahemtoola SH. Valvular heart disease: The decision to treat. Hosp Pract 1984 Nov; 19(11):63–78.

Santinga JT, Kirsh M, and Fekety R. Factors affecting survival in prosthetic valve endocarditis: Review of the effectiveness of prophylaxis. Chest 1984 Apr; 85(4):471–475.

Smith ND and Abrams J. Valvular heart disease of rheumatic origin. Hosp Med 1984 Oct; 20(1):77–92.

The problems with prosthetic valves. Emerg Med 1985 Feb 15; 17(3):133–134.

Tricuspid stenosis: Basic pathophysiology. Hosp Med 1985 Sept; 21(9):174.

Tricuspid stenosis: Checklist of clinical features. Hosp Med 1985 Sept; 21(9):171.

Heart Transplant/Artificial Heart

DeVries WC and Joyce LD. The artificial heart. Clin Symp 1983; 35(6):4–32.

Elzy PS and Marsh LC. Artificial heart implantation: Nursing protocol, preparation, participation. AORN J 1985 Aug; 42(2):171–178.

Humbecker RO et al. Heart and heart–lung transplantation. Heart Lung 1984 Jan; 13(1):1–4.

Mathias JM. Immunosuppression: Postoperative management of heart transplant recipients. AORN J 1985 Apr; 41(4):748–761.

Quaal SJ. The artificial heart. Heart Lung 1985 July; 14(4):317–327.

Schoer K and Hartin P. Cardiac transplants: The Stanford experience. AORN J 1984 Aug; 40(2):220–229.

Shinn JA. Heart and lung transplantation for end-stage pulmonary vascular hypertension. Nurs Clin North Am 1984 Sept; 19(3):547–558.

Vaughan-Cole B and Kee HK. A heart decision. Am J Nurs 1985 May; 85(5):535–536.

Agencies

International Society for Heart Transplantation, Thoracic and Cardiovascular Surgery, Newark Beth Israel Hospital, 201 Lyons Ave., Newark, NJ 07112.

Mended Hearts, 7320 Greenville Ave., Dallas, TX 75231.

Chapter 28

Assessment and Management of Patients With Vascular Disorders and Problems of Peripheral Circulation

Physiologic Overview

Adequate perfusion, which results in oxygenation and nutrition of body tissues, is dependent in part upon a functionally intact cardiovascular system. Efficient pumping action of the heart, patent and responsive blood vessels, and an adequate circulating blood volume are essential for adequate blood flow. Nervous system activity, blood viscosity, and the metabolic needs of tissues influence the rate of blood flow, and hence the adequacy of blood flow.

The peripheral vascular system consists of the systemic circulation and the pulmonary circulation serially connected in a closed system with the right and left heart. The blood vessels provide distensible channels for the transport of blood from the heart to the tissues and back to the heart. Cardiac ventricular contracton supplies the driving force for movement of blood through the vascular systems. *Arteries* distribute oxygenated blood from the left side of the heart to the tissues while the *veins* convey unoxygenated blood from the tissues to the right side of the heart. *Capillary vessels*, located within the tissues, connect the arterial and venous systems and constitute the site of exchange of nutrients and metabolic wastes between the circulatory system and the tissues. *Arterioles* and *venules* immediately adjacent to the capillaries, together with the capillaries, compose the *microcirculation*. A schematic representation of the circulation is shown in Figure 28-1.

The *lymphatic system* complements the function of the circulatory system. Lymphatic vessels transport *lymph* (a fluid similar to plasma) and tissue fluids (containing smaller proteins, cells, and cellular debris) from the interstitial space to systemic veins.

Anatomy of the Vascular System

Arteries and Arterioles. Arteries are thick-walled structures that carry blood from the heart to the tissues. The aorta, which has a diameter of approximately 25 mm (1 inch), gives rise to numerous branches, which in turn divide into smaller vessels that approach 4 mm (0.16 inch) in diameter

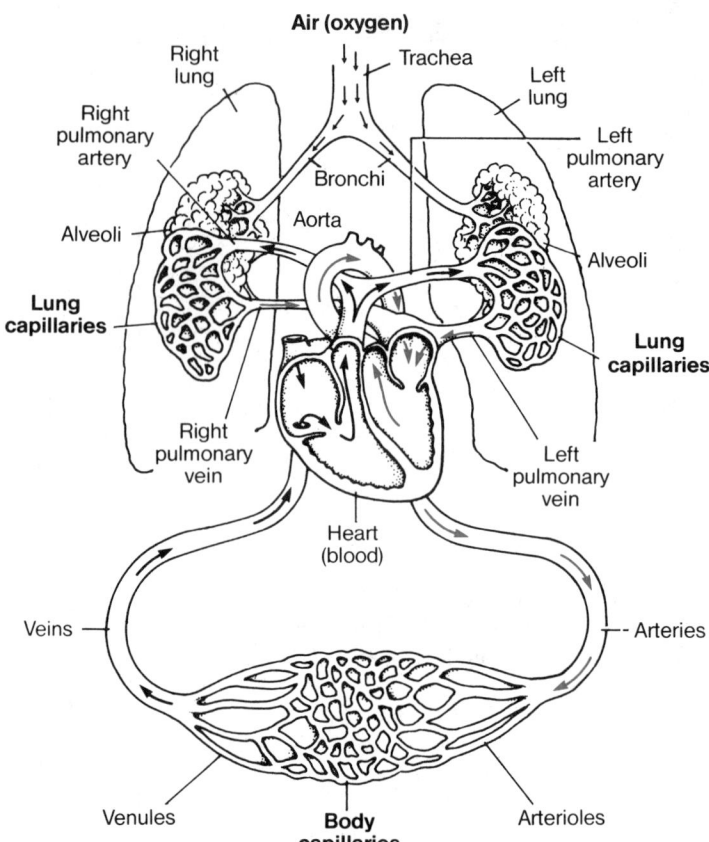

Figure 28-1
Schematic drawing of systemic circulation. (Start
at bottom of diagram.) Loaded with carbon
dioxide, blood from the body capillaries goes
through venules and veins into the right chamber
of the heart (*black arrows*). It is pumped into the
two lungs. Having dropped carbon dioxide and
picked up oxygen, it goes back to the left
chamber of the heart (*color arrows*). From there
it is pumped through the aorta into the body
circulation (arteries and arterioles) until it reaches
the body capillaries, where it gives up oxygen and
picks up carbon dioxide. (National Tuberculosis
and Respiratory Disease Association.)

by the time they reach the tissues. Within the tissues, the
vessels divide further, diminishing to approximately 30 microns in diameter; these vessels are called arterioles.

The walls of the arteries and arterioles are divided into
three layers: an inner endothelial cell layer called the *intima,*
which is in contact with the blood; a middle layer called the
media; and an outer layer called the *adventitia.* The intima
provides a smooth surface for contact with the flowing blood.
The adventitia is a layer of connective tissue that anchors the
vessel to its surrounding structures. The media makes up the
major portion of the vessel wall. In the aorta and other large
arteries of the body, this layer is composed chiefly of elastic
and connective tissue fibers that give the vessels considerable
strength and allow them to constrict and dilate for the purpose
of accommodating stroke volume and maintaining an even,
steady flow of blood. There is much less elastic tissue in the
smaller arteries and arterioles, and the media in these vessels
is composed primarily of smooth muscle.

Smooth muscle, by contraction and relaxation, controls
vessel diameter. Chemical, hormonal, and nervous system
factors influence the activity of smooth muscle. Because arterioles can alter their diameter, thereby offering resistance
to blood flow, they are often referred to as *resistance vessels.*
Arterioles regulate the volume and pressure in the arterial
system and blood flow to the capillaries.

Because of the large amount of muscle, the wall of the
arteries is relatively thick; it accounts for approximately 25%
of the total diameter of the artery and approximately 67% of
the total diameter of arterioles. The muscle and adventitia of
the arterial wall require their own blood supplies to meet

metabolic requirements. The blood vessels that supply the
wall are the *vasa vasorum.* The intima is thin and is in such
close contact with the blood within the vessel that it can
receive its nourishment directly from that source.

Capillaries.   Capillary walls lack muscle and adventitia
and are composed of a single layer of cells. This thin-walled
structure permits rapid and efficient transport of nutrients to
the cells and removal of metabolic wastes. The diameter of
capillaries ranges from 5 to 10 microns, so red blood cells
must alter their shape to pass through these vessels. Changes
in capillary diameter are passive and are influenced by
changes in the resistance of precapillary and postcapillary
vessels. A muscular sphincter, called the *precapillary sphincter,* is located at the arteriolar end of the capillary and is
responsible, along with the arteriole, for controlling capillary
blood flow.

Some capillary beds contain *arteriovenous anastomo-
ses,* through which blood passes directly from the arterial to
the venous system. These vessels are believed to regulate
heat exchange between the body and the external environment.

The distribution of capillaries throughout the tissues varies
with the type of tissue. For example, skeletal tissue, which is
metabolically active, has a more dense capillary network than
does less active tissue such as cartilage.

Veins and Venules.   Capillaries join together to form
larger vessels called venules, which in turn join to form the
veins. The venous system is therefore structurally analogous
to the arterial system. Venules correspond to arterioles, veins
to arteries, and the vena cavae to the aorta. Analogous types

of vessels in the arterial and venous systems have approximately the same diameters.

The walls of the veins, in contrast to those of the arteries, are thinner and considerably less muscular. The wall of the average vein amounts to only 10% of the vein diameter, in contrast to 25% in the artery. The wall of a vein, like that of an artery, is composed of three layers.

The thin, less muscular structure of the vein wall allows greater distensibility of these vessels. Greater distensibility permits the "storage" of large volumes of blood in the veins under low pressure. For this reason, veins are referred to as *capacitance vessels*. Approximately 75% of the total blood volume is contained in the veins. The sympathetic nervous system, which innervates the vein musculature, can stimulate venoconstriction, thereby reducing venous volume and increasing the general circulating blood volume.

Some veins, unlike arteries, are equipped with valves. In general, veins that transport blood against the force of gravity, as in the lower extremities, have one-way valves that prevent the distal reflux of blood as it is propelled toward the heart. Valves are composed of endothelial leaflets, the competency of which depends on the integrity of the vein wall.

Lymphatic Vessels. The lymphatic circulation begins in the tissues and is a one-way system that carries lymph from tissues back to the venous circulation. The lymphatics are thin-walled capillaries similar to the blood capillaries, except that lymphatic vessels are more permeable to large molecules because of wider spaces between endothelial cells and absence of a basement membrane. Peripheral lymphatics join larger lymph vessels and pass through regional lymph nodes before entering the venous system. The lymphatics converge into two main trunks, the thoracic duct and the right lymphatic duct. These ducts empty into the junction of the subclavian and the internal jugular veins. The thoracic duct drains most of the lymph vessels in the body. The right lymphatic duct conveys lymph primarily from the right side of the head, neck, thorax, and upper arms. Like veins, lymphatics contain one-way valves to prevent fluid reflux. Muscular contraction of the lymphatic walls and surrounding tissues aids in the propulsion of lymph toward venous drainage points.

Circulatory Needs of Tissues

The amount of blood flow needed by body tissues is constantly changing. The percentage of the cardiac output received by individual organs or tissues is determined by the metabolic needs of the cells and the function of the tissues (Table 28-1). When metabolic requirements increase, blood vessels dilate to increase the flow of oxygen and nutrients to the tissues. When metabolic needs decrease, vessels constrict and blood flow to the tissues decreases. Metabolic demands of tissues increase with physical activity or exercise, local heat application, fever, and infection. Reduced metabolic requirements of tissues accompany rest or decreased physical activity, local cold application, and cooling of the body. Failure of blood vessels to dilate in response to the need for increased blood flow will result in tissue *ischemia* (deficient blood supply).

As blood passes through tissue capillaries, oxygen is removed and carbon dioxide added. The amount of oxygen extracted by each tissue is different. For example, heart muscle tends to extract about half the oxygen from arterial blood in one passage through its capillary bed, whereas in the kidneys only about 7% of the oxygen is removed as blood passes through the organ. The average amount of oxygen removed collectively by all of the body tissues is about 25%. This means that the blood in the vena cavae contains about 25% less oxygen than aortic blood. This is known as the *systemic arteriovenous oxygen difference*. It increases when the amount of oxygen delivered to the tissues is decreased relative to their metabolic needs. More detailed information about the blood flow and oxygen extraction as blood passes through capillary beds in various tissues is summarized in Table 28-1.

TABLE 28-1
Typical Values for Blood Flow and Oxygen Consumption for Various Human Organs

| Organ | Organ Weight (kg) | Blood Flow During Rest | | | Oxygen Usage During Rest | | | |
		Organ Blood Flow (ml/min)	Blood Flow Unit Wt (ml/min/100 gm)	% Total Cardiac Output	AV O$_2$ Difference (ml/100 ml blood)	Organ O$_2$ Usage (ml/min)	O$_2$ Usage Unit Wt (ml/min/100 gm)	% Total O$_2$ Usage
Brain	1.4	750	55	14	6.0	45	3.00	18
Heart	0.3	250	80	5	10.0	25	8.00	10
Liver	1.5	1,300	85	23	6.0	75	2.00	30
GI tract	2.5	1,000	40					
Kidneys	0.3	1,200	400	22	1.3	15	5.00	6
Muscle	35.0	1,000	3	18	5.0	50	0.15	20
Skin	2.0	200	10	4	2.5	5	0.20	2
Remainder (*e.g.*, skeleton, bone marrow, fat, connective tissue)	27.0	800	3	14	5.0	35	0.15	14
TOTAL	70	6,500		100		250		100

(Folkow B and Neil E. Circulation. New York, Oxford University Press.)

Blood Flow

Blood flow through the cardiovascular system always proceeds in the same direction: left heart to aorta, arteries, arterioles, capillaries, venules, veins, vena cavae, and finally to the right heart. The reason for this unidirectional flow is that a pressure difference exists between the arterial and venous systems. Because arterial pressure (approximately 100 mm Hg) is greater than venous pressure (approximately 4 mm Hg), and fluid always flows from an area of high pressure to an area of low pressure, blood flows from the arterial to the venous system.

Although the pressure difference or gradient (ΔP) in the vascular system provides the impetus for propulsion of blood forward, a force opposing blood flow provided by the blood vessels also exists. This is termed *resistance* (R). Thus, the rate of blood flow is determined by dividing the change in pressure by the resistance.

(1) Flow = ΔP/R

From this equation it is clear that when resistance increases, a greater driving pressure is required in order to maintain the same degree of flow. Physiologically, an increase in driving pressure is accomplished by an increase in the force of contraction of the heart. If arterial resistance is chronically elevated, the heart muscle hypertrophies in order to sustain the greater contractile force.

In the majority of blood vessels, flow is *laminar* or streamlined, with blood in the center of the vessel moving slightly faster than the blood near the vessel walls. Laminar flow is silent. In some instances, particularly at vessel bifurcations, laminar flow becomes turbulent. Turbulent blood flow creates sounds that can be heard superficially with a stethoscope. The sound created by turbulent blood flow is called *bruit*. Turbulent blood flow may also occur when the velocity of blood flow is high, with decreased blood viscosity, with greater than normal vessel diameter, or when vessels have narrowed or constricted segments.

Blood Pressure. See page 520 for physiology and measurement.

Capillary Filtration and Reabsorption

Fluid exchange across the capillary wall is continuous. This fluid, which has the same composition as plasma without the proteins, forms the interstitial fluid. The equilibrium between hydrostatic and oncotic forces of the blood and interstitium, as well as capillary permeability, govern the amount and direction of fluid movement across the capillary. Normally, the blood pressure (*hydrostatic pressure*) at the arterial end of the capillary is relatively high, compared with that at the venous end. This high pressure at the arterial end of the capillaries tends to drive fluid out of the capillaries' blood and into the tissue. The plasma proteins in the capillaries exert an osmotic force (*osmotic pressure*) that tends to pull fluid back into the capillary from the tissue space, but this osmotic force cannot overcome the high hydrostatic pressure at the arterial end of the capillary. At the venous end of the capillary, however, the osmotic force predominates over the low hydrostatic pressure and there is a net reabsorption of fluid from the tissue space back into the capillary. Virtually all of the fluid that is filtered at the arterial end of the capillary bed

is reabsorbed at the venous end, except for a very small amount. This excess filtered fluid enters the lymphatic circulation. These processes of filtration, reabsorption, and lymph formation aid in the maintenance of tissue fluid volume and in the removal of tissue waste and debris. Capillary permeability, under normal conditions, remains constant.

Under certain abnormal conditions, the fluid filtered out of the capillaries may greatly exceed the amounts reabsorbed and carried away by the lymphatics. This can result from damage to capillary walls and resulting increased permeability, obstruction of lymphatic drainage, elevation of venous pressure, or decrease in plasma protein osmotic force. The accumulation of fluid that results from these processes is known as *edema*.

Hemodynamic Resistance

Peripheral vascular resistance is the opposition to blood provided by the blood vessels.

(2) $R = \dfrac{8\eta L}{\pi r^4}$ where

 r = radius of the vessel
 L = length of the vessel
 η = viscosity of the blood
 8/π = a constant

This equation shows that the resistance is proportional to the viscosity of the blood and the length of the vessel, but inversely proportional to the fourth power of the vessel radius.

The most important factor in the vascular system determining the resistance is the vessel radius. Small changes in vessel radius will lead to large changes in resistance. The predominant sites of change in caliber of blood vessels, and therefore in resistance, are the arterioles and the precapillary sphincter.

Blood viscosity and vessel length, under normal conditions, do not change significantly. Therefore, these factors do not usually play an important role in blood flow. However, a large increase in hematocrit may increase blood viscosity and reduce capillary blood flow.

Peripheral Vascular Regulating Mechanisms

Because the metabolic needs of body tissues, even at rest, are continuously changing, an integrated and coordinated system of regulation is necessary so that blood flow to individual areas is maintained in proportion to the needs of that area. As might be expected, this regulatory mechanism is complex and consists of central nervous system influences, circulating hormones and chemicals, and independent activity of the arterial wall itself.

Sympathetic (adrenergic) nervous system activity, mediated by the hypothalamus, is the most important factor in regulating the caliber, and thus the blood flow, of peripheral blood vessels. Arteries are relatively abundantly innervated by the sympathetic nervous system. Stimulation of the sympathetic nerves causes vasoconstriction. The neurotransmitter responsible for sympathetic vasoconstriction is norepinephrine. Sympathetic activation occurs in response to a number of physiological and psychological stressors. Removal of sympathetic activity, as by drugs or sympathectomy, will result in vasodilatation.

Other hormonal substances also affect peripheral vascular resistance. *Epinephrine*, released from the adrenal medulla, acts like norepinephrine in constricting peripheral blood vessels. However, in low concentrations epinephrine causes vasodilation in skeletal muscles, the heart, and the brain. *Angiotensin,* a substance formed from the interaction of renin (synthesized in the kidney) and a circulating serum protein, stimulates arterial constriction. Although the blood concentration of angiotensin is usually small, its vasoconstrictor effects become important in certain pathophysiologic states, such as congestive heart failure and hypovolemia.

Alterations in local blood flow are influenced by a number of circulating substances that have vasoactive properties. Potent vasodilator substances include histamine, bradykinin, and certain muscle metabolites. A reduction in available oxygen and nutrients and changes in local *p*H also affect local blood flow. Serotonin, a substance liberated from platelets that aggregate at the site of vessel wall damage, constricts arterioles. The application of heat to parts of the surface body will cause local vasodilatation, while the application of cold will cause vasoconstriction.

Pathophysiology of the Vascular System

Reduced blood flow through peripheral blood vessels characterizes all peripheral vascular diseases. The physiological effects of altered blood flow depend on the extent to which tissue demands for oxygen and nutrients exceed the flow of blood delivered to the tissues. If tissue needs are high, even modestly reduced blood flow may be inadequate to maintain tissue integrity, and tissues become *ischemic* (deficient in blood supply) and malnourished and will ultimately die if adequate blood flow is not restored.

Heart Failure. Inadequacy of peripheral blood flow occurs whenever the heart's pumping action becomes inefficient. Left-sided heart failure causes an accumulation of blood in the lungs and a reduction in forward flow or cardiac output, which results in inadequate arterial blood flow to the tissues. Right-sided heart failure causes systemic venous congestion and a reduction in forward flow.

Alterations in Blood and Lymphatic Vessels. Intact, patent, and responsive blood vessels are necessary for adequate delivery of oxygen to tissues and removal of metabolic wastes. Arteries can become obstructed by atherosclerotic plaque, thrombus, or embolus. Damage and subsequent obstruction of arteries follow chemical or mechanical trauma and infections or inflammatory processes. A complete arterial obstruction is associated with a greater incidence of tissue necrosis from deficient blood flow than is a partial obstruction. Likewise, a sudden arterial occlusion causes profound and frequently irreversible tissue ischemia and tissue death. When arterial occlusions develop gradually, the opportunity for the growth of new vessels to replace occluded ones (collateral circulation) is greater.

A reduction in venous blood flow can be caused by obstruction of the vein by a thrombus, incompetent venous valves, or a reduction in the effectiveness of the pumping action of surrounding muscles. Decrease in venous blood flow results in an increase in venous pressure, a subsequent rise in capillary hydrostatic pressure, a net filtration of fluid out of the capillaries, and thus edema. Edematous tissues cannot receive adequate nutrition from the blood and consequently are more susceptible to breakdown or injury and to infection.

Obstruction of lymphatic vessels also results in edema. Lymphatics can become obstructed by tumor or by damage resulting from mechanical trauma or inflammatory processes.

Gerontological Considerations. The aging process produces changes in the walls of the blood vessels that affect the transportation of oxygen and nutrients to the tissues. The intima thickens as a result of cellular proliferation and fibrosis. Elastin fibers of the media become calcified, thinned, and fragmented, and collagen accumulates in both the intima and the media. These changes cause stiffening of the vessels, which results in increased peripheral resistance, impairment of blood flow, and increased left ventricular workload.

Assessment of Circulatory Insufficiency of the Extremities

Despite the variety of specific peripheral vascular diseases, all patients with these disorders experience ischemia (deficiency of blood supply to a body part) and therefore will have some of the same symptoms. The type and severity of symptoms present depends, in part, on the type, stage, and extent of the disease process as well as the speed with which the disorder develops. The distinguishing features of arterial and venous insufficiency are presented in Table 28-2.

Pain. A severe cramp-type pain in the extremities following activity or exercise is experienced by patients with peripheral arterial insufficiency. This pain, referred to as *intermittent claudication,* is thought to be due to the inability of the arterial system to meet the oxygen demands of the muscles and to remove waste metabolites. Accumulation of metabolites in the ischemic tissues then produces muscle spasms. When the patient rests, and thereby decreases the metabolic needs of the muscles, the pain goes away. The progression of the vascular disease can be monitored by documenting the amount of exercise or the distance a patient can walk before pain occurs. Persistent pain in the extremities when the patient is resting can indicate a severe degree of arterial insufficiency or venous disease. This pain is often worse at night and may interfere with sleep.

The site of arterial disease can be deduced from the location of claudication. Calf pain may accompany reduced blood flow through the superficial femoral artery, while pain in the thigh may result from flow obstruction in the pelvic arteries.

Changes in Skin Appearance and Temperature. Adequate blood flow warms the extremities and gives them a rosy coloring. Inadequate blood flow results in cool and pale extremities. Further reduction of blood flow to these tissues, such as would occur with extremity elevation, results in an even whiter or more blanched appearance. A reddish blue discoloration of the extremities (*rubor*) may be observed and is indicative of severe peripheral arterial damage in which vessels are unable to constrict and remain dilated. *Cyanosis,* a bluish coloring of the skin, is manifested when the amount of oxygenated hemoglobin contained in the blood is reduced.

TABLE 28-2
Clinical Manifestations of Peripheral Vascular Disease

Arterial Insufficiency	Venous Insufficiency
Acute	
1. Asymmetrical symptoms (include only one leg)	1. Usually asymmetrical symptoms
2. Severe, unrelenting pain	2. Sharp, deep muscle pain; may be relieved by elevation of extremity
3. Cold, pale extremity	3. Skin warm, red or red blue; with severe edema, skin cool and cyanotic
4. Diminished sensation	
5. Inability to move the extremity	4. Pulses normal, or diminished
6. Absence of pulses below the occlusion	5. Superficial veins full
7. No edema, initially	6. Usually moderate to severe edema
Chronic	
1. Intermittent claudication, usually described as "cramps;" may progress to rest pain, usually described as "burning"	1. Discomfort described as aching, cramping, muscle fatigue; increased discomfort at end of day
2. Cool, pale extremity	2. Pigmentation, trophic changes, ulcers of lower legs and ankles
3. Diminished distal pulses	
4. Atrophy of skin, thickened nails, loss of hair	3. Superficial veins prominent
5. History of delayed wound healing	4. Edema moderate to severe
6. Reddish blue discoloration when extremity dependent	5. Paresthesias (burning, itching)
7. Presence of ulcers, superficial gangrene	6. Presence of ulcers around ankle

Additional adverse changes seen in the extremities as a result of chronically reduced nutrient supply include loss of hair, brittle nails, dry or scaling skin, atrophy, and ulcerations. Edema may be apparent either bilaterally or unilaterally. Gangrenous changes appear after prolonged severe ischemia and represent tissue death and decay.

Pulses. Determining the presence or absence, as well as the quality, of peripheral pulses is important in assessing the status of peripheral arterial circulation (Fig. 28-2). Occlusive arterial disease impairs blood flow and can reduce or obliterate palpable pulsations in the extremities. When pulses cannot be reliably palpated, it is sometimes helpful to use a Doppler ultrasound device to detect peripheral flow (Fig. 28-3).

Gerontological Considerations. In the elderly person the symptoms of peripheral vascular disease may be more pronounced than in the younger person because of the duration of the condition. Intermittent claudication may occur after walking only a few short blocks or after walking up a slight incline. Any prolonged pressure on the foot can cause pressure areas that become ulcerated, infected, and gangrenous. If chronic venous insufficiency is a problem, it can also lead to ulceration. The outcome of either arterial or venous insufficiency in the elderly person is increased impairment of mobility, activity, and independence.

Nursing Diagnoses

Based on assessment data, major nursing diagnoses for the patient may include the following:

Alteration in peripheral tissue perfusion related to compromised circulation

- Pain related to impaired ability of peripheral vessels to supply tissue with oxygen
- Potential impairment of skin integrity related to compromised circulation
- Deficit in knowledge about self-care activities

Planning and Nursing Implementation

Goals. The major goals of the patient may include increase in arterial blood supply to the extremities, decrease in venous congestion, promotion of vasodilatation, prevention of vascular compression, relief of pain, attainment or maintenance of tissue integrity, and adherence to the home health-care program.

Measures used by the patient and members of the health-care team to accomplish a single goal must be evaluated in terms of the positive as well as the negative effects they may have on the simultaneous achievement of other goals. A summary of the management of patients with peripheral vascular disease is presented in Nursing Care Plan 28-1 (pp. 629–630).

Increase in Arterial Blood Supply to the Extremities and Decrease in Venous Congestion

Arterial blood supply to a part can be enhanced when the part is placed below the level of the heart. For the lower

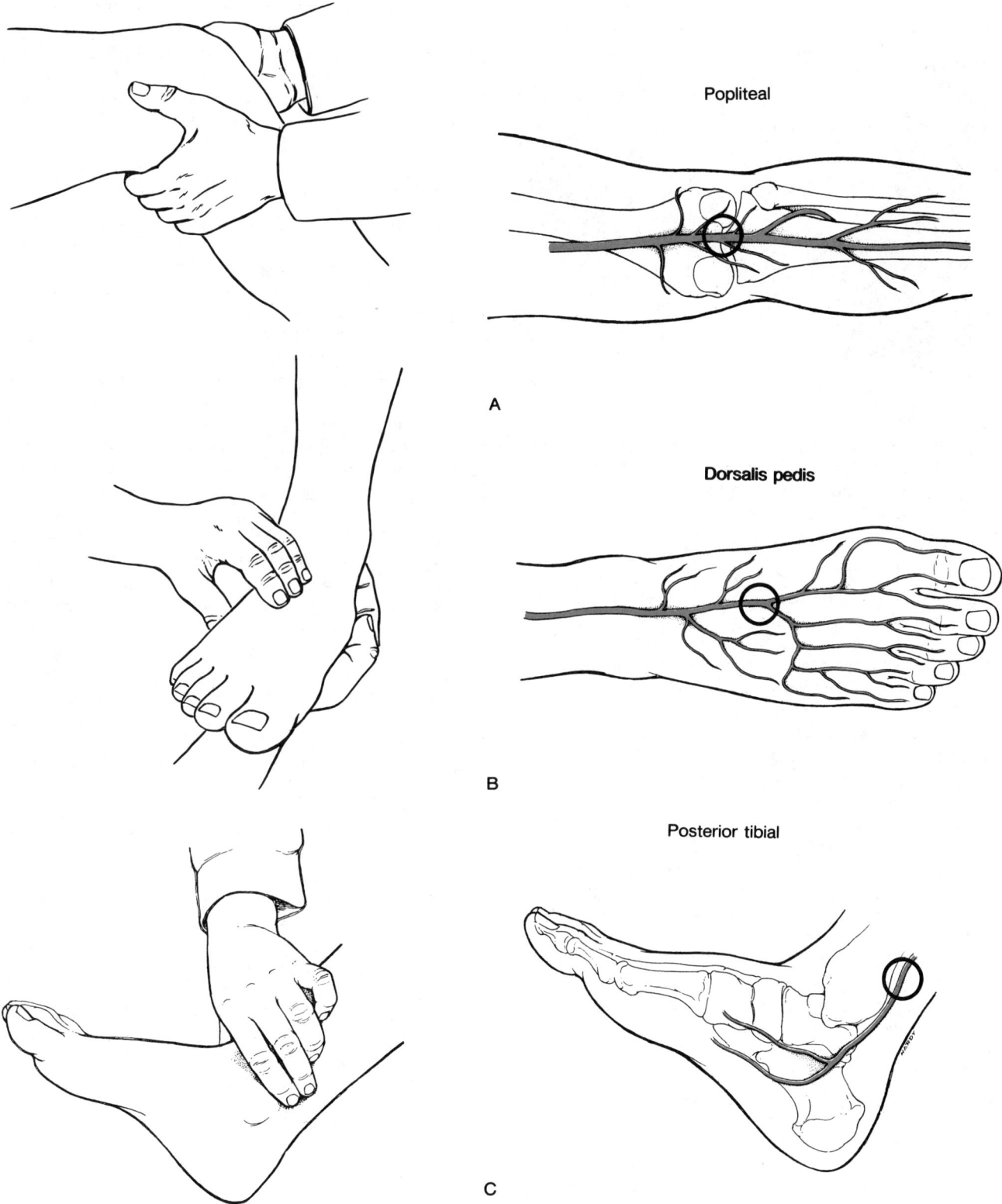

Figure 28-2
Assessing peripheral pulses. (*A*) Popliteal pulse. (*B*) Pedal pulse. (*C*) Posterior tibial pulse.

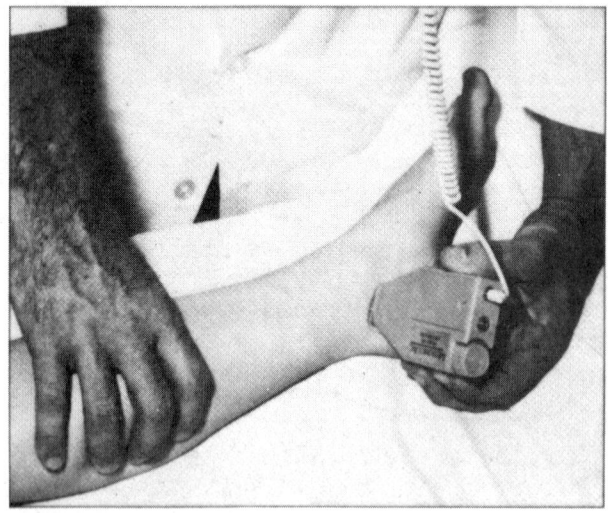

Figure 28-3
Doppler ultrasound transducer being used in screening for major deep-vein thrombosis. (Brunner LS and Suddarth DS. The Lippincott Manual of Nursing Practice, 4th ed. Philadelphia, JB Lippincott, 1986.)

extremities, this can be accomplished by elevating the head of the bed on 15-cm (6-inch) blocks or allowing the patient to assume a sitting position with feet resting on the floor. Walking or other moderate or graded exercises may be recommended to promote blood flow by muscular exercise and thus to encourage the development of collateral circulation. Pain can serve as a guide in determining the amount of exercise a person should engage in. The onset of pain indicates that tissues are not receiving adequate oxygen, so the patient should rest before continuing activity.

In patients with venous insufficiency, placing the lower extremities in a dependent position will only worsen the venous pooling associated with this condition. The pull of gravity impedes venous return to the heart and promotes venous stasis. Therefore, persons with venous insufficiency should elevate their legs above heart level as much as possible. When upright, these patients should avoid standing still or sitting for prolonged periods of time. Walking aids venous return by the activation of the "muscle pump." In bed, patients with venous insufficiency should have the foot of the bed elevated on blocks.

Active postural exercises, such as the *Buerger-Allen exercises,* may be prescribed for the patient with circulatory disorders of the lower extremities. The routine involves placing the extremities in three positions: elevation, dependency, and then at the horizontal position. The patient lies flat in bed with both legs elevated above the heart for 2 to 3 minutes. Then, sitting on the edge of the bed with the legs relaxed and dependent, the patient exercises the feet and toes (upward and downward, inward and outward) for about 3 minutes. Finally, the patient lies flat with the legs at the same level as the heart and covered for warmth for about 5 minutes. The times for each maneuver may vary. Pain and dramatic color changes indicate the need for termination of the maneuver and rest. This routine may be repeated several times a day (Fig. 28-4, p. 631).

Not all patients with peripheral vascular disease should exercise. Therefore, before recommending any program to patients, it is important to consult with the physician. Patients with leg ulcers, cellulitis, gangrene, or acute thrombotic occlusions require bed rest. These latter conditions can be made worse by activity.

Promotion of Vasodilatation and Prevention of Vascular Compression

Arterial dilation promotes increased blood flow to the extremities and is therefore a desirable goal in patients with peripheral arterial disease. However, in instances where the arteries are severely sclerosed, inelastic, or damaged, dilation is not possible. For this reason, measures to promote vasodilatation, such as drugs or surgery, may only be minimally effective.

Warmth promotes arterial flow by preventing chilling and thus the vasoconstriction associated with cold exposure. Adequate clothing and warm environmental temperatures protect the patient against chilling. If chilling occurs, a warm bath or drink is helpful. When heat is applied directly to ischemic extremities, the temperature of the heat source should not exceed body temperature. Burn injuries can occur at lower temperatures in ischemic extremities than in normal limbs. In addition, excess heat may increase the metabolic rate of the extremities, and thus increase the need for oxygen until it cannot be met by the reduced arterial flow through the diseased artery. Therefore, patients are instructed to test the temperature of bath water, hot water bottles, or heating pads before using them, or to avoid them altogether. Application of a heating pad to the abdomen can cause reflex vasodilatation in the extremities and is safer than direct application to affected extremities.

Nicotine causes vasospasm and can thereby dramatically reduce circulation to the extremities. Patients with arterial insufficiency who smoke must be fully informed of the circulatory consequences of this habit and be encouraged to stop completely. Emotional upsets stimulate the sympathetic nervous system, which results in peripheral vasoconstriction. Although emotional stress is unavoidable, it can be minimized to some degree by environmental manipulation and a consistent stress management program. Emotionally charged situations should be avoided. Counseling services or relaxation training may be indicated for persons unable to cope effectively with situational stressors.

Constricting clothing and accessories such as garters, belts, girdles, and shoe laces will impede circulation to the extremities and promote venous stasis, and therefore should be avoided. Likewise, leg crossing should be discouraged because it compresses vessels in the legs.

Relief of Pain

Frequently, the pain associated with peripheral vascular disease is chronic and continuous. It limits activities, affects work and responsibilities, disturbs sleep, and alters one's sense of well-being and optimism. Because of this, patients are often depressed, irritable, and unable to exert the energy necessary to execute prescribed therapies. As a result it can be more

Care of the Patient With Peripheral Vascular Problems

Nursing Interventions	Rationale	Expected Outcomes

Nursing Diagnosis: Alteration in peripheral tissue perfusion related to compromised circulation

Goal: Increase in arterial blood supply to extremities

1. Lower the extremities below the level of the heart.	1. Dependency of lower extremities enhances arterial blood supply.	• Extremities are warm to touch.
2. Encourage moderate amount of walking or graded extremity exercises.	2. Muscular exercise promotes blood flow and the development of collateral circulation.	• Patient has improved color of extremities
3. Encourage active postural exercise (Buerger-Allen exercises).	3. With postural exercises, gravity alternately fills and empties the blood vessels.	• Experiences decreased muscle pain with exercise • Performs Buerger-Allen exercise series 6 times, 4 times per day or as tolerated

Goal: Decrease in venous congestion

1. Elevate extremities above heart level.	1. Elevation of extremities counteracts gravitational pull, promotes venous return, and prevents venous stasis.	• Patient elevates lower extremities as prescribed
2. Discourage standing still or sitting for prolonged periods.	2. Prolonged standing still or sitting promotes venous stasis.	• Decreased edema of extremities • Patient avoids prolonged standing still or sitting.
3. Encourage walking.	3. Walking promotes venous return by activating the "muscle pump."	• Gradually increases walking time daily

Goal: Promotion of vasodilatation and prevention of vascular compression

1. Maintain warm temperature and avoid chilling.	1. Warmth promotes arterial flow by preventing the vasoconstriction effects of chilling.	• Patient protects extremities from exposure to cold.
2. Discourage smoking.	2. Nicotine causes vasospasm, which impedes peripheral circulation.	• Does not smoke
3. Counsel in ways to avoid emotional upsets; stress management.	3. Emotional stress causes peripheral vasoconstriction by stimulating the sympathetic nervous system.	• Uses stress management program to minimize emotional upset
4. Encourage to avoid constrictive clothing and accessories (*e.g.*, seat belts).	4. Constrictive clothing and accessories impede circulation and promote venous stasis.	• Avoids constricting clothing and appliances
5. Encourage to avoid leg crossing.	5. Leg crossing causes compression of vessels with subsequent impediment of circulation, resulting in venous stasis.	• Avoids leg crossing
6. Administer vasodilator drugs and adrenergic blocking agents as prescribed, with appropriate nursing considerations.	6. Vasodilators relax vascular smooth muscle; adrenergic blocking agents block the response to sympathetic nerve impulses or circulating catecholamines.	

(continued)

difficult to alleviate pain, because the best means to do so is through the institution of measures that augment circulation. Analgesics can be helpful in reducing pain to the point where the patient may be more able to participate in the therapies that will increase circulation and ultimately relieve pain more effectively.

Maintenance of Tissue Integrity

Poorly nourished tissues are more susceptible to damage and bacterial invasion. When lesions develop, healing may be delayed or inhibited due to the poor blood supply to the area.

Nursing Interventions	*Rationale*	*Expected Outcomes*

Nursing Diagnosis: Pain related to impaired ability of peripheral vessels to supply tissue with oxygen

Goal: Relief of pain

1. Promote increased circulation.	1. Enhancement of peripheral circulation increases the oxygen supplied to the muscle and decreases the accumulation of metabolites that cause muscle spasms.	• Patient utilizes measures to increase arterial blood supply to extremities. • Utilizes analgesics as prescribed.
2. Administer analgesics as prescribed, with appropriate nursing considerations.	2. Analgesics help to reduce pain and allow the patient to participate in activities and exercises that promote circulation.	

Nursing Diagnosis: Potential impairment of skin integrity related to compromised circulation

Goal: Attainment or maintenance of tissue integrity

1. Instruct in ways to avoid trauma to extremities.	1. Poorly nourished tissues are susceptible to trauma and bacterial invasion; healing of wounds is delayed or inhibited due to poor tissue perfusion.	• Patient inspects skin daily for evidence of traumatic injury. • Avoids trauma and irritation to skin • Wears protective shoes • Adheres to meticulous hygienic regimen • Eats well-balanced diet that contains adequate protein and vitamins B and C
2. Encourage to wear protective shoes and padding for pressure areas.	2. Protective shoes and padding prevent foot injuries and blisters.	
3. Encourage meticulous hygiene: bathing with neutral soaps, applying lotions, carefully trimming nails.	3. Neutral soaps and lotions prevent drying and cracking of skin.	
4. Caution to avoid scratching or vigorous rubbing.	4. Stratching and rubbing can cause skin abrasions and bacterial invasion.	
5. Promote good nutrition: adequate intake of Vitamins B and C and protein; control of obesity.	5. Good nutrition promotes healing and prevents tissue breakdown.	

Nursing Diagnosis: Knowledge deficit regarding the self-care program

Goal: Adherence to the self-care program

1. Include family/significant others in teaching program.	1–4. Adherence to the self-care program is enhanced when the patient receives support from family and from appropriate self-help groups and agencies.	• Patient practices frequent position changes as prescribed. • Practices postural exercises as prescribed. • Takes medications as prescribed. • Avoids vasoconstrictors • Utilizes measures to prevent trauma • Utilizes stress management program • Accepts condition as chronic but amenable to therapies that will decrease symptomatology
2. Provide written instructions about foot and leg care.		
3. Help to secure properly fitting clothing, shoes, stockings.		
4. Refer to self-help groups as indicated: *e.g.*, Smoke-Enders, stress management.		

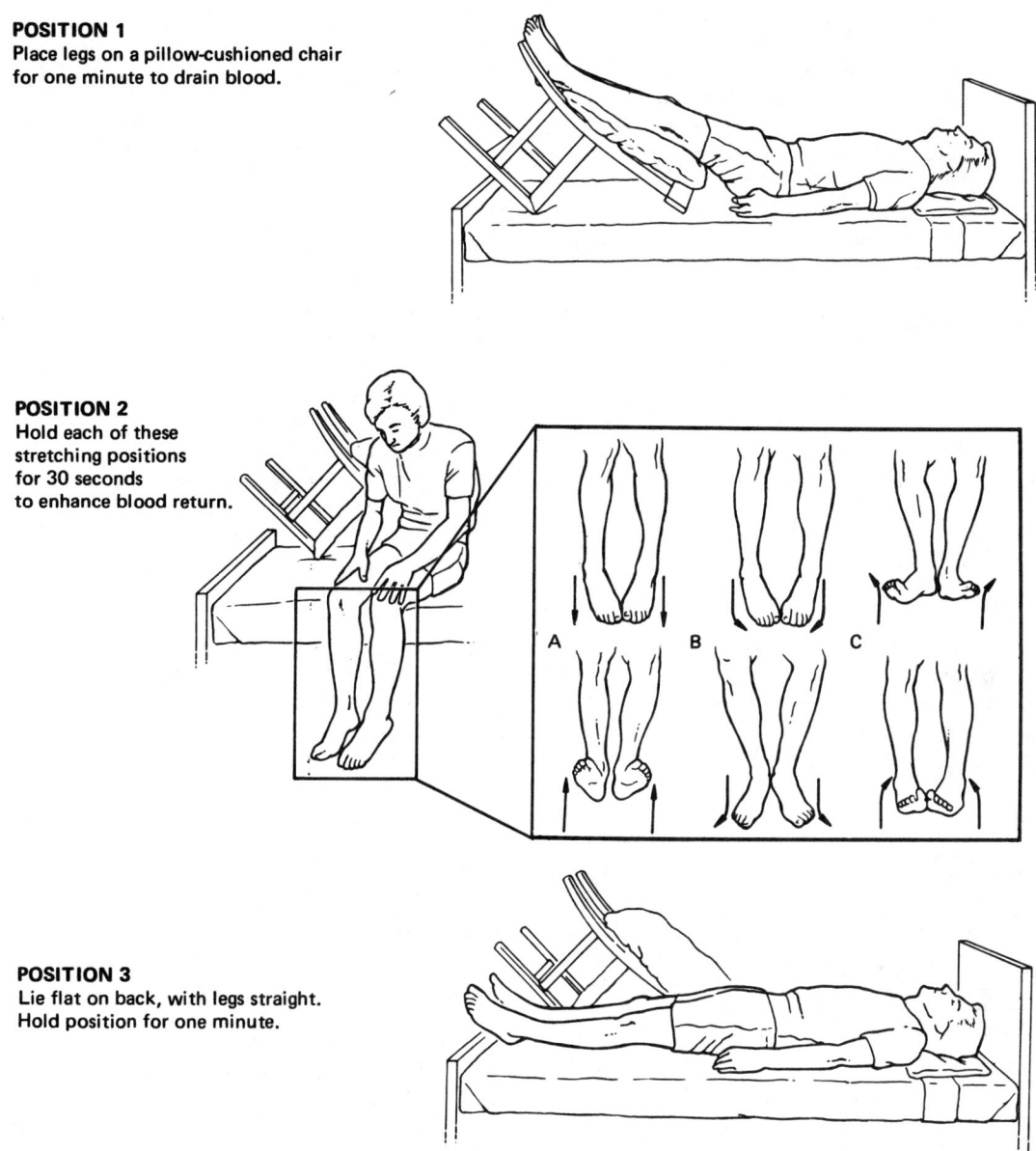

POSITION 1
Place legs on a pillow-cushioned chair for one minute to drain blood.

POSITION 2
Hold each of these stretching positions for 30 seconds to enhance blood return.

POSITION 3
Lie flat on back, with legs straight. Hold position for one minute.

Figure 28-4
Buerger-Allen exercises. Do exercise series 6 times, 4 times a day. (Forshee T and Minckley B. Lumbar sympathectomy. RN; 39[2].)

Infected, nonhealing ulcerations of the extremities can be very debilitating and can require prolonged, often expensive hospitalization and treatments. Amputation of the extremity may eventually be necessary. Thus, measures to prevent these complications should be of high priority and vigorously implemented.

Trauma to the extremities should be avoided. Sturdy, well-fitting shoes or slippers will prevent foot injuries and blisters. The use of neutral soaps and body lotions prevents drying and cracking of skin. Scratching and vigorous rubbing can abrade skin and create a site for bacterial invasion. Finger- and toenails should be carefully trimmed straight across. Protective padding over corns and callouses will prevent break-

down and alleviate pressure. All signs of blisters, ingrown toenails, infection, or other problems should be reported to health-care professionals for treatment and follow-up. Persons with diminished vision may require assistance in periodically examining the lower extremities for trauma.

Good nutrition will promote healing and prevent tissue breakdown, and is thus included in the overall preventive program for persons with peripheral vascular disease. Vitamins B and C and adequate protein are necessary. Obesity strains the heart, increases venous congestion, and reduces circulation. A diet low in lipids may be indicated for patients with atherosclerosis. The physician and dietitian should be consulted.

Patient Education

The self-care program should be designed to help the patient faithfully carry out those activities that will promote arterial and venous circulation, relieve pain, and promote tissue integrity. The patient and family should be helped to understand the reasons for each aspect of the program and the possible consequences of nonadherence. Care of the feet and legs is of prime importance in the prevention of trauma, ulceration, and gangrene. Detailed patient instruction in foot and leg care is provided in Chart 28-1.

Evaluation

Expected Outcomes

1. Patient increases arterial blood supply to extremities.
    a. Exhibits extremities warm to touch
    b. Has improved color of extremities (is free of rubor or cyanosis)
    c. Is free of or experiences decreased muscle pain with exercise
    d. Demonstrates palpable peripheral pulses
2. Decreases venous congestion
    a. Elevates lower extremities as prescribed
    b. Avoids prolonged standing still or sitting
    c. Has decreased edema in extremities
3. Promotes vasodilatation; prevents vascular compression
    a. Protects extremities from exposure to cold
    b. Does not smoke
    c. Uses stress management program to minimize emotional upset
    d. Avoids constricting clothing and appliances (*e.g.,* tight seat belts)
    e. Avoids leg crossing
4. Is free of pain
    a. Utilizes measures to increase arterial blood supply to extremities
    b. Utilizes analgesics as prescribed
5. Attains/maintains tissue integrity
    a. Inspects skin daily for evidence of traumatic injury
    b. Avoids trauma and irritation to skin
    c. Wears protective shoes
    d. Adheres to meticulous hygienic regimen
    e. Eats well-balanced diet that contains adequate protein and vitamins B and C
6. Performs self-care activities
    a. Practices frequent position changes as prescribed by physician
    b. Practices postural exercises as prescribed by physician

---

Chart 28-1
Patient Education: Care of the Feet and Legs for the Person With a Peripheral Vascular Problem

Cleanliness
1. Wash feet at least once daily.
2. Use warm water and bland soap.
3. Dry feet thoroughly, especially between the toes. Blot and pat with a towel, but do not rub.

Warmth
1. Wear cotton hose, because they are comfortable and absorb moisture.
2. Prevent feet from getting cold; this reduces blood supply.
3. Avoid applying heat to the feet or legs unless approved by a physician or nurse.
4. Avoid swimming in cold water.
5. Avoid sunburn.

Safety
1. Protect feet by performing exercises on level ground.
2. Avoid walking in crowds.
3. Use care in cutting toenails.
    a. First soak feet for 10 minutes in warm water to soften nails.
    b. Cut nails straight across; avoid cutting nails close to flesh.

Comfort Measures
1. Wear shoes that provide adequate toe room, have a good arch, and feel comfortable.
2. Apply powder if feet tend to become moist.
3. Apply a thin coating of lanolin if feet are dry and scaly.

Preventing Constriction of Blood Vessels
1. Avoid circular garters that cut off blood supply to legs and feet.
2. Do not cross legs at knees.
3. Place a pillow at foot end of bed under covers to prevent top bedding from exerting pressure on toes.
4. Apply lamb's wool between toes if they rub each other.

Exercise
Walking stimulates circulation and promotes tissue repair.

Medical Attention
1. Report redness, blistering, swelling, or pain.
2. Report athlete's foot, and peeling and itching between toes.
3. Do not use any medication on feet or legs unless prescribed by the physician.

Smoking
Avoid tobacco in any form because it aggravates peripheral vascular conditions.

stenosis- narrowing

c. Takes medications as prescribed
d. Avoids vasoconstrictors (*e.g.*, clothing, smoking, leg crossing)
e. Utilizes measures to prevent trauma
f. Utilizes stress management program
g. Accepts condition as chronic but amenable to therapies that will decrease symptomatology

Diseases of the Arteries

Arteriosclerosis and Atherosclerosis

Arteriosclerosis is the most common disease of the arteries; it literally means "hardening of the arteries." It is a diffuse process characterized by fibromuscular or endothelial thickening of the walls of small arteries and arterioles. Atherosclerosis refers to a generalized process characterized by focal changes in the intima of arteries. These changes consist of the accumulation of lipids, calcium, blood components, carbohydrates, and fibrous tissue (atheroma or plaque). Although the pathologic processes of arteriosclerosis and atherosclerosis differ, rarely does one occur without the other, and thus the terms are often used interchangeably. Because atherosclerosis is a generalized disease of the arteries, when it is present in the extremities it is usually present elsewhere in the body.

Pathophysiology and Etiology. The most common direct results of atherosclerosis in arteries include narrowing (stenosis) of the lumen, obstruction by thrombosis, aneurysm development (abnormal dilatation of a blood vessel), and rupture. Its indirect results are malnutrition and the subsequent fibrosis of the organs that the sclerotic arteries supply with blood. All actively functioning tissue cells require an abundant supply of nutrients and oxygen and are sensitive to any reduction in their supply. If such reductions are severe and permanent, these cells undergo ischemic necrosis (death of cells due to deficient blood flow) and are replaced by fibrous tissue, which requires much less nutrition.

Atherosclerosis primarily affects the main arteries throughout the entire arterial tree in varying degrees, usually in a patchy manner. Branch arteries are affected usually only at their bifurcation.

There have been many theories to explain why and how atherosclerosis develops. No single theory has been proven, but parts of several theories have been combined into the current response-to-injury theory. According to this theory, endothelial cell injury is perhaps due to prolonged hemodynamic factors, such as the shearing stresses and pressures that occur in hypertension because of the turbulence of blood flow through the arteries. Injury to the endothelium is thought to promote platelet aggregation and adherence and to alter the intima, with resultant permeation of lipids into the endothelium. However, it may be that there is not a single cause or mechanism for the development of atherosclerosis, but rather that multiple processes are involved.

Morphologically, atherosclerotic lesions are of three types: fatty streaks, fibrous plaque, and complicated lesions. *Fatty streaks* are yellow and smooth, protrude slightly into the lumen of the artery, and are composed of lipids, primarily cholesterol. These lesions have been found in the arteries of persons of all age groups, including infants. It is not clear whether fatty streaks predispose to the formation of fibrous plaques nor if they are reversible. They do not usually cause clinical symptoms.

The *fibrous plaque* characteristic of atherosclerosis is composed of smooth muscle cells, collagen fibers, plasma components, and lipids. It is yellowish gray and protrudes in varying degrees into the arterial lumen, at times completely obstructing it. This plaque is believed to be an irreversible lesion.

The *complicated* atherosclerotic lesion is almost always associated with complete occlusion of the artery with subsequent ischemia or infarction of the organ served by the involved vessel. In this lesion, fibrous plaque becomes calcified and ruptures. There is hemorrhage into the plaque or thrombus development (Fig. 28-5).

Gradual narrowing of the arterial lumen as the disease process progresses stimulates the development of collateral circulation (Fig. 28-6). While this vascular "bypass" allows continued perfusion to the tissues beyond the arterial obstruction, it is often inadequate to meet imposed metabolic demands, and ischemia results.

Risk Factors. Many factors are associated with the development of atherosclerosis. These factors have been determined from systematic observations of relationships between the development of atherosclerosis and certain characteristics. While it is not completely clear whether modification of these risk factors will prevent the development of cardiovascular disease, there is evidence that it may slow the disease process. Some risk factors, those that are genetically determined, are unavoidable. However, it is believed that genetic factors can be influenced by alteration of other risk factors and thereby can be modified indirectly.

A diet high in fat has been strongly implicated in the causation of atherosclerosis. Approximately 39% of the calories Americans ingest are derived from fats. Fats are classified according to their chemical structure as *saturated* or *unsaturated*. Saturated fats include fats of animal origin, such as those in meat, milk, butter, and eggs, and also solid vegetable oils. The intake of primarily saturated fats is positively correlated with the elevation of serum cholesterol and triglycerides and with the development of atherosclerotic cardiovascular disease. Serum triglycerides are also found to be elevated in diets high in refined carbohydrates (sugar). On the other hand, unsaturated fats, such as corn oil, cottonseed oil, safflower oil, and the fats in fish, may be capable of reducing blood cholesterol and triglyceride levels. Based on these findings, the American Heart Association recommends that, in order to reduce the risk of cardiovascular disease, persons should reduce the total amount of fat ingested in the diet, substitute unsaturated fats for saturated fats, and decrease the intake of cholesterol to no more than 300 mg per day.

Certain drugs are now being used to reduce blood lipid levels in conjunction with dietary modification. Among these are clofibrate, cholestyramine, colestipol, probucol, and niacin. Close supervision of patients on long-term therapy with these drugs is required.

Other risk factors include cigarette smoking, sedentary activity patterns, emotional stress, obesity, and hormones, particularly estrogen. The presence of hypertension or diabetes seems to accelerate the atherosclerotic process. In ad-

CONCEPT OF PATHOGENESIS OF ATHEROSCLEROTIC LESIONS

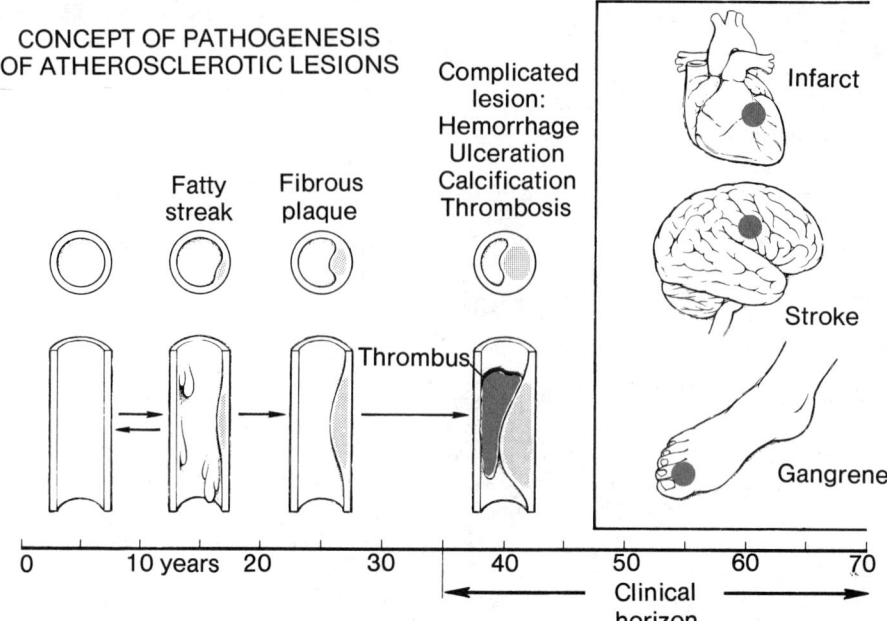

Figure 28-5
Schematic concept of the progression of atherosclerosis. Fatty streaks constitute one of the earliest lesions of atherosclerosis. Many fatty streaks regress, whereas others progress to fibrous plaques and eventually to atheromata. These may then become complicated by hemorrhage, ulceration, calcification, or thrombosis and may produce myocardial infarction. (Adapted from Hurst JW and Logue RB. The Heart. New York, McGraw–Hill.)

dition, many other factors, such as caffeine and alcohol, may contribute in a minor way to the development of the disease.

Although no single risk factor has been identified as the primary contributor to the development of atherosclerotic cardiovascular disease, it is clear that the greater the number of risk factors, the greater the likelihood of developing the disease. Therefore, the elimination of combined risk factors should be strongly emphasized.

Clinical Manifestations. The clinical symptoms and signs resulting from the atherosclerotic process depend on the organ or tissue affected. Coronary atherosclerosis (heart disease), angina pectoris, and acute myocardial infarction

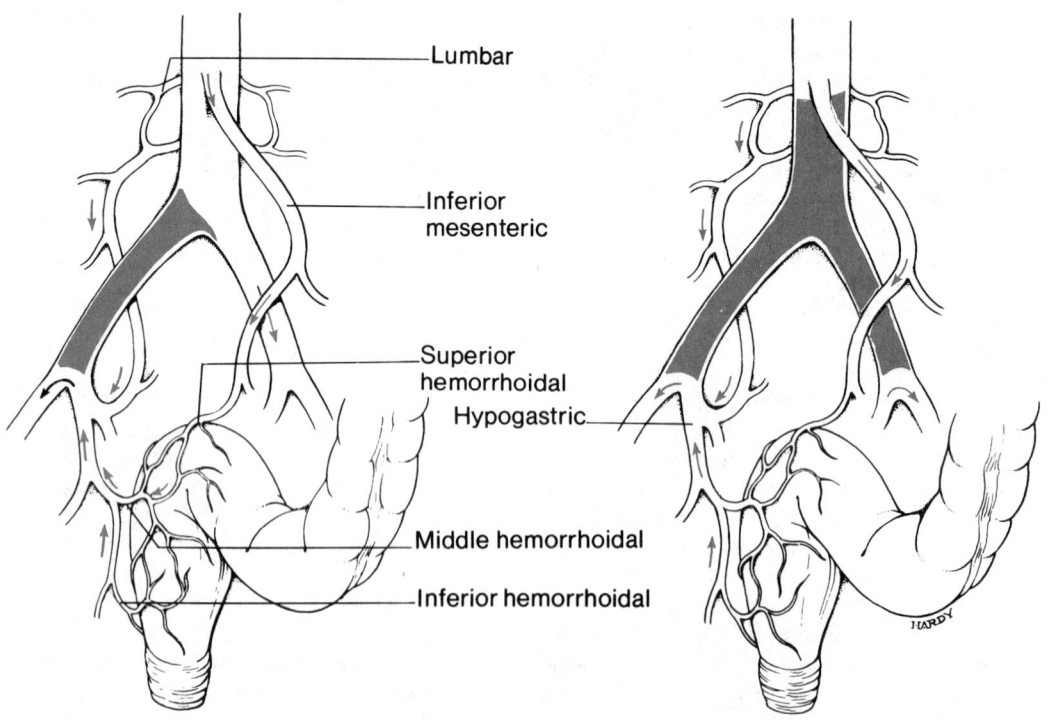

Figure 28-6
Development of collateral channels in response to occlusion of the right common iliac artery and the terminal aortic bifurcation.

are discussed in Chapter 25. Cerebrovascular disease, including transient cerebral ischemic attacks and stroke, is discussed in Chapter 53. Atherosclerosis of the aorta, including aneurysm, and atherosclerotic lesions of the extremities are discussed below.

Peripheral Arterial Occlusive Disease

Arterial insufficiency of the extremities is usually found in individuals over 50 years of age, most often in men, and predominantly in the lower extremities. The age of onset and severity are influenced by the type and number of atherosclerotic risk factors present. Obstructive lesions are predominantly confined to segments of the arterial system extending from the aorta, below the renal arteries, to the popliteal artery (Fig. 28-7).

Clinical Manifestations. The hallmark and only symptom of peripheral arterial insufficiency is *intermittent*

claudication, that is, pain or discomfort in the lower extremities (buttock, hip, thigh, calf, arch of the foot) occurring with exercise and terminating with rest. This pain is insidious in onset and is produced by muscle hypoxia and the accumulation of metabolites. The pain may be described as aching, cramping, tiredness, or weakness. One of the diagnostic features of intermittent claudication is that the amount of activity that produces claudication in a person on one occasion will produce it again on repeated occasions.

A feeling of coldness or numbness in the extremities may accompany intermittent claudication and is a result of the reduced arterial flow. Upon examination, the extremities may be cool and exhibit pallor on elevation or a ruddy, cyanotic color with dependency. Skin and nail changes, ulcerations, gangrene, and muscle atrophy may be evident. Bruits may be auscultated with a stethoscope (a *bruit* is the sound produced by turbulent flow of blood through an irregular, stenotic lumen or through a dilated [aneurysm] segment of the vessel). Peripheral pulses may be diminished or absent.

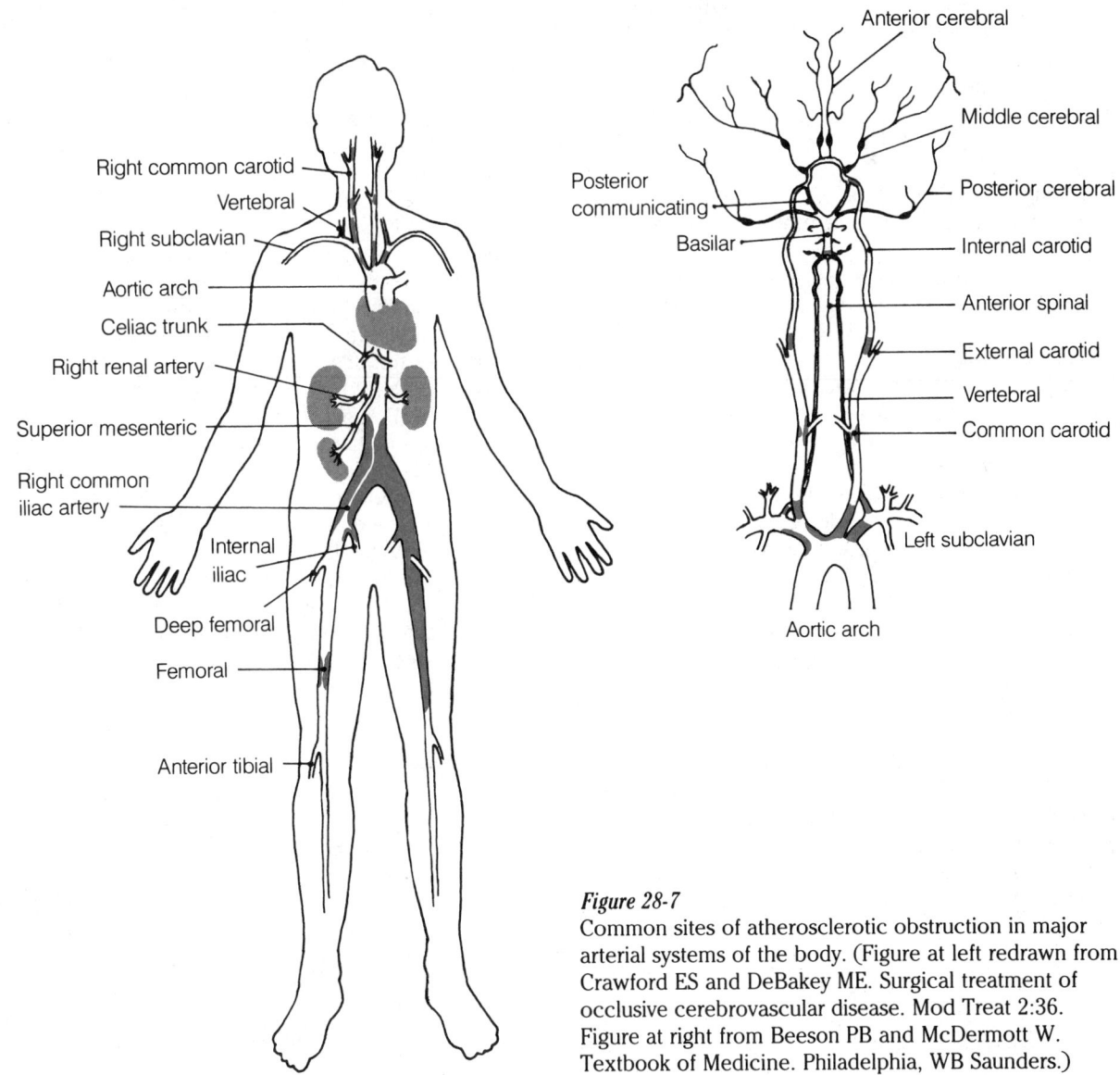

Figure 28-7

Common sites of atherosclerotic obstruction in major arterial systems of the body. (Figure at left redrawn from Crawford ES and DeBakey ME. Surgical treatment of occlusive cerebrovascular disease. Mod Treat 2:36. Figure at right from Beeson PB and McDermott W. Textbook of Medicine. Philadelphia, WB Saunders.)

The examination of the peripheral pulses is an important part of the examination for arterial occlusive disease and should include the femoral, popliteal, posterior tibial, and pedal pulses.

Inequality of pulses between extremities or the absence of a normally palpable pulse is a reliable sign of occlusion. The femoral pulse in the groin and the posterior tibial pulse behind the medial malleolus are most easily found. The popliteal pulse is sometimes difficult to palpate behind the knee in the obese patient, and the pedal artery varies in location on the dorsum of the foot and is normally absent in about 7% of the population (see Fig. 28-3).

Patients with peripheral arterial insufficiency may eventually develop *rest pain*, which is indicative of a severe obstruction of blood flow. The pain is persistent, aching, or boring and is usually present in the distal extremities. Elevation or horizontal placement of the extremity will aggravate the pain, while dependency of the extremity will reduce the pain. Some patients sleep with the affected leg hanging over the side of the bed in an attempt to relieve the pain.

Assessment. The presence, anatomical location, and physiological extent of arterial occlusive disease are determined by a careful history of the patient's symptoms and physical examination. Observations of extremity color and temperature are made and pulses palpated. The nails may be thickened and opaque, and the skin shiny, atrophic, and dry with sparse hair growth. A comparative assessment is made of the two extremities.

Diagnostic Evaluation. To determine the qualitative and quantitative aspects of the problem, Doppler ultrasonic flow studies can be done.

The Doppler is an electronic stethoscope through which blood flow can be heard, even at times when pulses are not palpable. In addition, lower extremity blood pressure measurements can be obtained by coupling the Doppler with a standard pneumatic cuff. When comparing leg blood pressures with arm pressures, the patient with arterial occlusive disease of the lower extremities may demonstrate pressure in the legs lower than that in the arms.

Additional diagnostic tests for evaluating peripheral arterial occlusive disease include *oscillometry* to measure alterations in pulse volume at different levels of the extremity; an *exercise test* to determine the amount of activity possible prior to the onset of intermittent claudication; *plethysmography*, which monitors changes in pulse and leg size with each heartbeat; and a *lumbar sympathetic block*. This last test, used to evaluate peripheral circulation, involves injection of a local anesthetic into the lumbar epidural space to block the sympathetic nerves that go to the legs. Because the sympathetic nerves control the tension in the muscles of the blood vessels, a block of these nerves should produce vasodilation and increased temperature in the legs if the vessels are normal. Atherosclerotic vessels are incapable of vasodilation; hence there is either no increase in temperature in the legs or only a slight one. This test is often used to determine whether or not *sympathectomy* (interruption of afferent pathways in the sympathetic division of the autonomic nervous system) would be of benefit to the patient with impaired circulation of the legs. This procedure eliminates vasospasm and improves peripheral blood supply.

Angiography may be used to confirm the diagnosis of occlusive arterial disease if surgery is contemplated. The procedure involves the injection of contrast medium directly into the vascular system and visualization of the vessels as the radiopaque material flows through them. In this manner, the location of vascular obstructions or aneurysms and the presence of collateral circulation can be demonstrated. Usually patients experience a temporary feeling of warmth as the contrast medium is injected. Local irritation at the injection site may occur. Infrequently, a patient may have an allergic reaction to the iodine contained in the contrast material. This reaction may appear immediately after the injection or may be delayed. Manifestations may include dyspnea, nausea and vomiting, sweating, tachycardia, and numbness of the extremities. Any such reaction is reported at once; treatment may include the administration of epinephrine (adrenalin), antihistamines, or steroids. In addition, there are risks of vessel injury and possibly stroke.

Digital subtraction angiography (DSA) is a radiologic visualization of arterial vessels utilizing computer technology. Usually, angiography requires hospital admission from the day before the test until 24 hours after the test, and there are risks of severe complications following the procedure. With DSA, no hospitalization is necessary and the risks are fewer because entry into the arterial system is not necessary.

The patient is asked not to eat for 2 hours prior to the test, to lie still in the supine position on the radiographic table, and to hold in a breath at the appropriate time.

Usually, the brachial vein is selected for lidocaine local injection; a small nick is made through which an angiocath is threaded toward the superior vena cava. Contrast medium is injected when the radiologist has positioned the patient under fluoroscopy for adequate exposure of the desired site. By the use of an image-intensifier video system, vessels are displayed on a TV monitor. By computer, those images not required are subtracted so that the final intense image of the desired area is heightened. The study takes about 30 to 40 minutes; upon completion, the catheter is removed. Pressure is applied to the nick site for several minutes, and thereafter the patient is instructed to increase fluid intake to about 2000 ml in the subsequent 24 hours in order to encourage excretion of the contrast medium. The rare side-effect is an allergic reaction to the iodine in the contrast medium.

Management. The general care measures for patients with peripheral arterial disorders were described earlier in this chapter and are summarized in Chart 28-1. Generally, patients feel better on some type of exercise program. If this program is combined with weight reduction and the cessation of smoking, patients can often improve their activity limitations. Patients should not be promised that their symptoms will be relieved if they stop smoking. If claudication persists they may lose their motivation not to smoke.

In some instances, *sympathectomy* may be beneficial to improve collateral circulation in patients with intermittent claudication. Excision of sympathetic ganglia will release arteriolar constriction and improve peripheral blood flow. In other patients, when intermittent claudication has become gravely disabling, vascular *grafting* or *endarterectomy* may be helpful. In the grafting procedure, either the diseased segment of artery is removed and a synthetic graft inserted in place of it, or the obstructed segment is left intact and instead "bypassed" by use of a graft. Material used for arterial bypass grafts may be synthetic (*e.g.*, Dacron, Teflon) or from autogenous veins (*e.g.*, saphenous vein). When an endarterectomy is performed, the atheromatous obstruction is "shelled out" through an incision into the artery. The artery is then sutured closed to restore vascular integrity.

Percutaneous transluminal angioplasty (PTA) of arteries of the lower extremities is gaining acceptance as an alternative to vascular surgery, especially for those patients who are considered at high risk for surgical complications. Under local anesthesia a balloon catheter is used to dilate mechanically the affected area of the artery and remodel the stenotic segment. Because surgery and general anesthesia are not required, the risks of morbidity are reduced, as are the length and cost of hospitalization. If reocclusion occurs, subsequent PTAs can be performed or, if that is not feasible, vascular surgery can be used to alleviate the obstruction.

Postoperative Nursing Management. The primary objective in postoperative management of patients who have had these vascular procedures is to maintain adequate circulation through the arterial repair. Extremity pulses should be checked and recorded frequently. Disappearance of a pulse may indicate thrombotic occlusion of the graft, so the surgeon is immediately notified. The color and temperature of the extremity are also monitored and any changes reported. An adequate circulating blood volume should be established and maintained. Continuous monitoring of urine output, central venous pressure, mental status, and pulse rate and volume will permit early recognition and treatment of fluid imbalances. Leg crossing and prolonged extremity dependency should be avoided in order to prevent thrombosis. Leg elevation will reduce edema.

Thromboangiitis Obliterans (Buerger's Disease)

Buerger's disease is characterized by recurring inflammation in the arteries and veins of the lower and upper extremities, and results in thrombus formation and occlusion of the vessels. It is differentiated from other vessel diseases by its microscopic appearance. In contrast with atherosclerosis, Buerger's disease has no lipid aggregates in the intimal coat, has more changes in the adventitia, results in a thrombosis that contains many more cells, and does not cause vessel wall necrosis. The disease begins in the small arteries and later progresses to the larger vessels. Although this condition is different from atherosclerosis, in older patients atherosclerosis of the larger vessels may occur following involvement of the smaller vessels.

Etiology and Clinical Manifestations. The cause of Buerger's disease is unknown. It occurs most often in men between the ages of 20 and 35, and it has been reported in all races in many areas of the world. There is considerable evidence that heavy smoking is either an etiologic or aggravating factor. Generally, the lower extremities are affected, but arteries in the upper extremities or viscera are also commonly involved. Superficial thrombophlebitis may be present. Arteriography confirms arterial occlusive disease.

Pain is the outstanding symptom of Buerger's disease. The patient complains of cramps in the feet or legs after exercise (intermittent claudication), which are relieved by inactivity; often there is considerable burning pain that is aggravated by emotional disturbances, smoking, or chilling. Rest pain in the digits, a feeling of coldness, or a sensitivity to cold may be early symptoms. Various types of paresthesias may develop, and pulses may be diminished or absent.

As the disease progresses, definite redness or cyanosis of the part appears when it is dependent. Color changes may affect only one extremity or only certain digits or certain parts of a digit. Ulceration with gangrene may occur.

Management and Nursing Interventions. The treatment of Buerger's disease is essentially the same as that for atherosclerotic peripheral vascular disease. The main objectives are to improve circulation to the extremities, prevent the spread of the disease, and protect the extremities from trauma and infection. The continuation of smoking is highly detrimental, and patients are advised to stop completely. Symptoms are often relieved by cessation of smoking.

Rest, adequate hydration, and scrupulous attention to cleanliness are essential. Daily washing of the feet with bland soap and warm water is desirable. Circumstances predisposing to extremity trauma and infection must be strictly avoided. Shoes and stockings must be fitted accurately, and the feet must be protected adequately from cold. Caustic antiseptics, such as iodine or phenol and its derivatives, should not be applied to the feet if the peripheral circulation is inadequate.

Vasodilators are rarely prescribed because these drugs only cause dilatation of healthy vessels; therefore, vasodilators may even divert blood away from the partially occluded vessels, which makes the situation worse. Regional sympathetic block or ganglionectomy may be useful in some instances to produce vasodilatation and thereby increase blood flow.

Prognosis. If gangrene of a toe develops as a result of arterial occlusive disease in the leg, it is unlikely that toe amputation or even a transmetatarsal amputation will succeed. Usually a below-knee amputation, or occasionally an above-knee amputation, is necessary. The indications for amputation are worsening gangrene, especially if moist; severe rest pain; or sepsis secondary to gangrene. If any of these are present in a situation where bypass surgery is not feasible, then amputation becomes necessary.

Aortic Diseases

The aorta is the main trunk of the arterial system and is divided into the ascending aorta (5 cm [2 inches] contained in the pericardium), the aortic arch (extending upward, backward, and downward), and the descending aorta. The entire aorta is designated as thoracic above the diaphragm and abdominal below the diaphragm.

Aortitis

Aortitis is inflammation of the aorta, particularly of the aortic arch. Two types are known to occur: Takayasu's disease and syphilitic aortitis. Takayasu's disease, or occlusive thromboaortopathy, is uncommon; syphilitic aortitis is almost never seen today.

Takayasu's Disease. Takayasu's disease is a chronic inflammatory disease of the aortic arch and its branches seen primarily in young or middle-aged females. It results in ischemic symptoms affecting the upper extremity, brain, and eyes. In the early stages, it may respond to corticosteroids.

Syphilitic Aortitis. Syphilitic aortitis, unlike the arteriosclerotic type, usually begins before the age of 50. It starts at the root of the aorta and spreads in the form of a few discrete patches scattered over an otherwise normal intima. In most cases, the inflammatory process produces moderate dilatation of the aorta, but it can produce more serious complications such as aortic insufficiency, aneurysm, or occlusion of the coronary ostia. Symptoms experienced by patients include sensations of substernal heaviness, vise-like feelings of constriction of the chest, or attacks of agonizing pain. Sudden, short attacks of dyspnea may also occur.

Aortic Aneurysms

Classification of Aneurysms. An aneurysm is a localized sac or dilatation of an artery formed at a weak point in the vessel wall (Fig. 28-8). Very small aneurysms due to local infection are designated *mycotic aneurysms*. An aneurysm that is somewhat larger but still limited in extent, projecting from one side of the vessel only, is called a *saccular aneurysm*. If an entire arterial segment becomes dilated, a *fusiform aneurysm* develops. Aneurysms are serious because rupture is always possible and can lead to hemorrhage and death.

The most common cause of aneurysm is atherosclerosis.

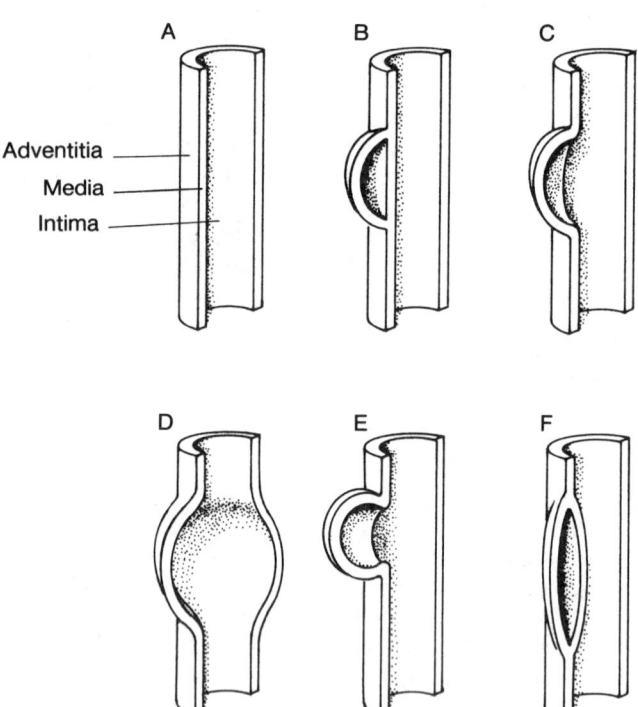

Figure 28-8
Characteristics of arterial aneurysm. (*A*) Normal artery. (*B*) False aneurysm—actually a pulsating hematoma. The clot and connective tissue are outside the arterial wall. (*C*) True aneurysm. One, two, or all three layers may be involved. (*D*) Fusiform aneurysm—symmetrical, spindle-shaped expansion of entire circumference of involved vessel. (*E*) Saccular aneurysm—a bulbous protrusion of one side of the arterial wall. (*F*) Dissecting aneurysm—this usually is a hematoma that splits the layers of the arterial wall.

However, wall trauma, infection (pyogenic or syphilitic), and congenital defects of the artery wall also give rise to aneurysms.

Aneurysm of the Thoracic Aorta

Approximately 85% of all cases of thoracic aortic aneurysm are caused by atherosclerosis. They occur most frequently in men between the ages of 40 and 70. The thoracic area is the most common site for the development of a dissecting aneurysm. About one third of patients with thoracic aneurysms die from rupture.

Clinical Manifestations. Symptoms are variable and depend on how rapidly the aneurysm dilates and how the pulsating mass affects surrounding intrathoracic structures. Most are asymptomatic. In most cases *pain* is the most prominent symptom. It is usually constant and boring in character and may only be perceived when the person is lying in a supine position. Other conspicuous symptoms are *dyspnea*, the result of the pressure of the sac against the trachea, a main bronchus, or the lung itself; *cough*, frequently paroxysmal and with a brassy quality ("goose cough"); *hoarseness*, stridor, weakness of the voice, or complete aphonia (manifestations of pressure against the left recurrent laryngeal nerve); and *dysphagia*, due to impingement on the esophagus.

Dilated superficial veins on the chest, the neck, or the arms; edematous areas on the chest wall; and cyanosis are often evident when large veins in the chest are compressed by the aneurysm. The pupils of the eyes may be unequal because of pressure against the cervical sympathetic chain. Diagnosis of a thoracic aortic aneurysm is principally by chest radiography and fluoroscopy.

Management. Whether medical or surgical treatment is selected for thoracic aortic aneurysms depends on the type of aneurysm present. The goal of surgery is to remove the aneurysm and restore vascular continuity using a vascular graft (Fig. 28-9). Intensive monitoring is usually required after this type of surgery, and the patient is placed in the critical care unit.

Medical management of the patient involves, in part, strict control of arterial blood pressure and a reduction in pulsatile aortic flow. Systolic pressure is maintained around 100 mm Hg to 120 mm Hg with antihypertensive drugs (*e.g.*, reserpine, guanethidine). Pulsatile flow is reduced by medications that reduce cardiac contractility (*e.g.*, propranolol).

Abdominal Aortic Aneurysm

The most common cause of abdominal aortic aneurysm is atherosclerosis; syphilis is present in less than 1% of patients. Men are affected four times more than women; the condition is most prevalent after age 60. Most of these aneurysms occur below the renal arteries. Untreated, the eventual outcome may be rupture and death.

Pathophysiology. The factor common to all aneurysms is a damaged media in the vessel. This may be caused by congenital weakness, trauma, or disease process. Once an aneurysm develops, the tendency is toward an increase in size.

Clinical Manifestations and Diagnosis. About two fifths of patients with abdominal aortic aneurysms have symptoms; the remainder are asymptomatic. Some patients complain that they can feel their "heart beating" in their ab-

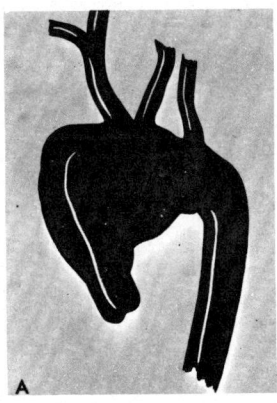 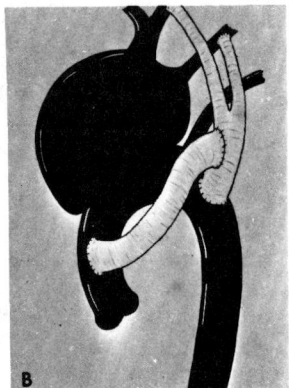 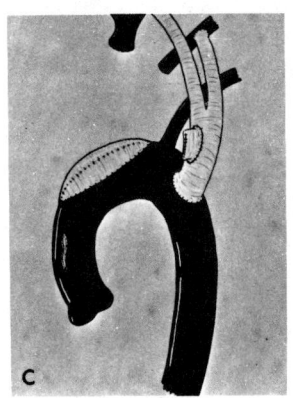 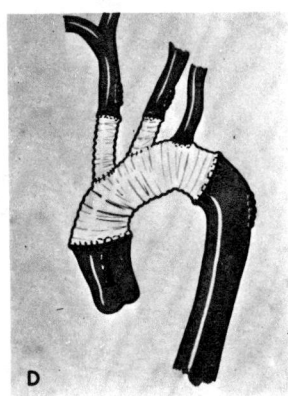

Figure 28-9
Surgical treatment of aortic aneurysm. (*A*) Location and extent of aortic aneurysm.
(*B*) Method of treatment utilizing temporary bypass graft to maintain normal aortic
circulation during excision of aneurysm. (*C*) Completed procedure with patch graft
angioplasty to repair excised segment of aortic arch and conversion of temporary bypass
graft to innominate and left common carotid arteries into the permanent graft.
(*D*) Temporary bypass grafts used to maintain normal aortic circulation during excision
and graft replacement of aneurysm have been completely removed, and aortic graft has
been inserted. (DeBakey ME. Changing concepts in vascular surgery. Figs 12B, 12E, 13C
and 13D. J Cardiovasc Surg; 1:3–44.)

domen when lying down. The most common symptom is
abdominal pain, which may be persistent or intermittent and
is often localized in the middle or lower abdomen to the left
of the midline. The next most common symptom is *low back
pain.* This is a serious symptom that usually signifies rapid
expansion or impending rupture of the aneurysm. Less frequently, the patient complains of *feeling an abdominal mass*
or *abdominal throbbing.* More than half of these patients
exhibit hypertension. An interesting finding is the comparison
of blood pressure readings of the thigh and arm. Ordinarily,
the systolic blood pressure of the thigh exceeds that of the
arm by 15 mm Hg or more. In about three quarters of patients
with abdominal aortic aneurysm, the systolic pressure in the
thigh is abnormally low in comparison with that in the arm.

A most important diagnostic indication of this type of
aneurysm is the presence of a pulsatile mass in the middle
and upper abdomen. A systolic bruit may be heard over the
mass. Confirmation of the aneurysm by abdominal x-ray is
possible if the aneurysm is calcified. An abdominal aortogram,
ultrasonography, or digital subtraction angiography (DSA)
may also be used to define and confirm the presence of the
aneurysm.

Management. The likelihood of rupture is significant
in patients with an expanding or enlarging abdominal aneurysm. Consequently, surgery is the treatment of choice for
abdominal aneurysms larger than 5 cm (2 inches) in diameter
or those that are enlarging. This involves resection of the
aneurysm and insertion of a bypass (synthetic) graft (Fig. 28-
10). Although this is a major operation, elective aneurysm
repair has been reported to have a mortality rate of 5%. The
prognosis for a patient with a ruptured aneurysm is poor, and
surgery is performed immediately.

Preoperatively, nursing assessment should be guided by
the fact that the aneurysm might rupture, and by the recognition that the patient may have cardiovascular, cerebral, and
pulmonary impairment secondary to atherosclerosis. There-

fore, the functional capacity of all organ systems should be
established. Medical therapies designed to stabilize physiological function should be promptly implemented. Postoperative care requires intense monitoring of pulmonary, cardiovascular, renal, and neurologic status. After the acute
recovery phase, an exercise schedule may be prescribed.
Prolonged sitting should be avoided.

Signs of a rupturing abdominal aortic aneurysm include
a constant intense back pain, falling blood pressure, decreasing red cell count and increasing white count, plus a soft
abdomen. Following a retroperitoneal rupture of an aneurysm,
hematomas have been noticed in the scrotum, perineum, or
penis. Signs of heart failure or loud bruit may suggest a rupture
into the vena cava. Rupture into the peritoneal cavity is rapidly
fatal. The overall surgical mortality rate for a ruptured aneurysm is 50% to 75%.

Dissecting Aneurysm of the Aorta

Pathophysiology. Occasionally, an aorta diseased by
arteriosclerosis develops an intimal tear due to a type of medial degeneration. This entity, which is often associated with
hypertension, is three times more common in men than in
women and occurs in the age group between 40 and 70.
Dissecting aneurysms are extremely dangerous, resulting in
death if untreated.

The intimal tear permits blood to dissect its way into the
substance of the aortic wall. The result is the formation of a
large hematoma in the arterial wall, which may extend for a
considerable distance and produces severe and persistent
pain. Death is usually caused by external rupture of the hematoma.

Clinical Manifestations and Assessment. The process
of dissection leads to shearing and occlusion of the arteries
branching from the aorta in the area involved by the process.
The tear occurs most commonly in the region of the aortic
arch. The dissection of the aorta may progress backward in

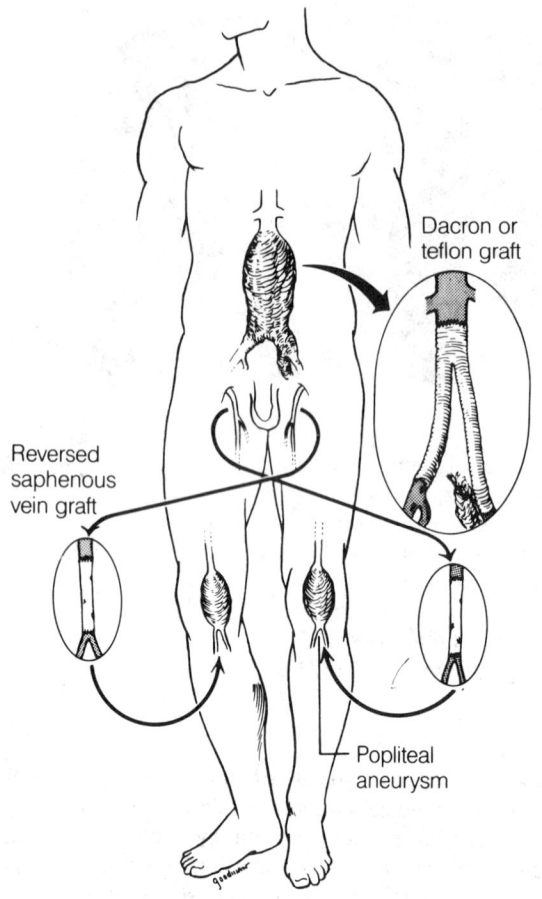

Reversed
saphenous
vein graft

Dacron or
teflon graft

Popliteal
aneurysm

Figure 28-10
Surgical treatment of a patient who had a large abdominal
aneurysm involving the iliac arteries plus bilateral
symptomatic popliteal aneurysms. These were resected and
the abdominal aneurysm was replaced with a Teflon graft.
The popliteal aneurysms were replaced by saphenous vein
grafts, which appear to function much better at the flexion
crease than the synthetic graft. (Hardy JD et al. Aneurysms
of the popliteal artery. Surg Gynecol Obstet 1975 Mar; 140:
402. By permission of Surgery, Gynecology & Obstetrics.)

the direction of the heart, obstructing the opening to the
coronary arteries or producing hemopericardium (effusion
of blood into the pericardial sac) or aortic insufficiency, or
it may extend in the opposite direction, causing occlusion of
the arteries supplying the gastrointestinal tract, the kidneys,
the spinal cord, and even the legs.

The onset of symptoms is usually sudden. Severe and
persistent pain, described as "tearing" or "ripping," may be
reported in the anterior chest or below the scapulae posteriorly. The patient may manifest pallor, sweating, and tachycardia. Blood pressure may be elevated, unobtainable, or
markedly different from one arm to the other. Other symptoms
are variable depending on the location and extensiveness of
the dissection. Because of the variable clinical picture associated with this condition, early diagnosis is often difficult.
Aortography and ultrasound aid in the diagnosis. Medical or
surgical treatment of a dissecting aneurysm again depends
on the type present and follows the general principles outlined
for treatment of thoracic aortic aneurysms (see p. 638).

Other Aneurysms

Aneurysms may also arise in the peripheral vessels, most often
as a result of atherosclerosis. These may involve such vessels
as the renal artery, the subclavian artery, or (most frequently)
the popliteal artery in the area of the knee. Such aneurysms
may be bilateral.

The aneurysm produces a pulsating mass and a disturbance of peripheral circulation distal to it. Pain and swelling
develop because of pressure on adjacent nerves and veins.
Surgical repair of such aneurysms is now carried out with
replacement grafts.

Arterial Embolism

Pathophysiology. Arterial emboli arise most commonly from thrombi that develop in the chambers of the
heart as a result of atrial fibrillation, myocardial infarction,
infective endocarditis, or chronic congestive heart failure.
These thrombi may become detached and be carried from
the left side of the heart into the arterial system, where they
can plug an artery that is too small to allow passage. Emboli
may also develop in advanced aortic atherosclerosis due to
roughening or ulceration of the atheromatous plaques. The
sequelae of arterial emboli depend primarily on the size of
the embolus, the organ involved, and the state of the collateral
vessels. The immediate effect is cessation of distal blood flow.
The clot can progress above and below the obstruction. Secondary vasospasm can contribute to the ischemia. Fragmentation of the embolus can occur, resulting in occlusion of
more distal vessels.

Emboli tend to lodge at arterial bifurcations and atherosclerotic narrowings. Cerebral, mesenteric, renal, and coronary arteries are often involved, in addition to the large arteries
of the extremities.

Clinical Manifestations. The symptoms of acute arterial embolism in extremities with poor collateral flow are
acute, severe pain and a gradual loss of sensory and motor
function. Pain may be aggravated by movement of the extremity. Distal pulses are lost, and the extremity becomes
pale, mottled, and numb. Superficial veins may be collapsed
because of decreased blood flow to the extremity. A sharp
line of color and temperature demarcation may occur distal
to the site of the occlusion as a result of ischemia.

Management. *Embolectomy* is the treatment of choice
when a major vessel has been occluded (Fig. 28-11). This
procedure involves incising the vessel and removing the clot.
The success of surgery in preserving extremity viability depends on the length of time the extremity has been ischemic.
After 6 to 10 hours, muscle necrosis develops and the extremity cannot be salvaged. Prior to surgery, the patient should
remain on bed rest with the extremity level or slightly (15
degrees) dependent. The affected part is kept at room temperature and protected from trauma. Padded side rails, pillows
between the legs, and bed cradles to keep the weight of linen
off the extremity are useful.

Medical management of an acute embolic occlusion includes intravenous anticoagulation with heparin, which will
prevent propagation of the clot and thus reduce muscle necrosis. Thrombolytic agents such as streptokinase and urokinase may be useful to hasten embolic lysis. The pain as-

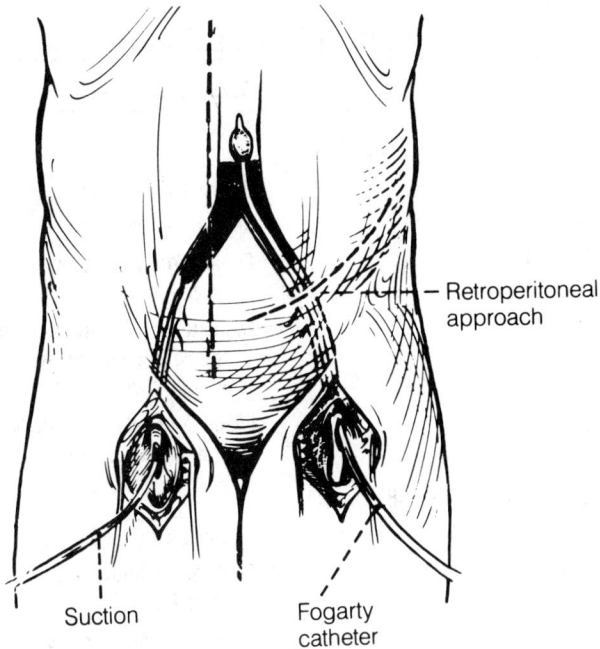

Figure 28-11
Aortic bifurcation embolectomy may be approached directly through the abdomen or in a retrograde fashion via the femoral arteries by suction or Fogarty catheter. (Rhoads et al. Surgery. Philadelphia, JB Lippincott)

sociated with vasospasm may be relieved by a small dose of the drug papaverine hydrochloride.

Postoperative Nursing Management. During the postoperative period, every effort is made to encourage movement of the leg in order to stimulate circulation and prevent stasis. Because each patient is different, the nurse collaborates with the surgeon about the appropriate level of activity needed. Anticoagulants may be continued for a period of time after surgery in order to prevent thrombosis of the affected artery and to diminish the development of thrombi at the initiating site. The nurse should frequently assess the surgical wound for evidence of hemorrhage, which can occur when anticoagulants are given.

Arterial Thrombosis

Arterial thrombosis can also acutely occlude an artery. This slowly developing clot usually occurs at the site of damage of the arterial wall, which is most commonly due to atherosclerosis. Thrombi may also develop in an arterial aneurysm. The manifestations of an acute thrombotic arterial occlusion are similar to those described for embolic occlusion. However, treatment is made more difficult with a thrombus because the arterial occlusion has occurred in a degenerated vessel. This requires more extensive reconstructive surgery to restore flow than is required with an embolic event.

Raynaud's Disease

Raynaud's disease is a form of intermittent arteriolar vasoconstriction that results in coldness, pain, pallor, and, oc-

casionally, ulceration of the fingertips. Involvement of the toes is seen occasionally. The etiology is unknown, although many patients with the disease seem to have immunologic disorders. Recent studies indicate that the symptoms may be the result of a defect in basal heat production that eventually decreases the ability of cutaneous vessels to dilate. Episodes may be triggered by emotional factors or by unusual sensitivity to cold. The disease is most common in females between the ages of 16 and 40 years and is seen much more frequently in cold climates and during the winter months. If the degree of vasoconstriction is moderate, there may still be some arterial flow. However, blood flow is relatively stagnant, which produces a cyanotic (blue) color in the fingers. If the spasm is severe, the fingers become a dead white color. After rewarming, the fingers develop a reactive hyperemia (increased blood flow) and appear red. Thus the characteristic color change of Raynaud's phenomenon is described as blue, white, and red. The aching, throbbing, burning pain occurs as the color changes from white to red and results from the mobilization of accumulated ischemic metabolic wastes. The involvement tends to be bilateral and symmetrical.

The term *Reynaud's phenomenon* is currently used to refer to localized, intermittent episodes of vasoconstriction of small arteries of the extremities, causing color and temperature changes. It is generally unilateral and affects only one or two digits. It is not usually indicative of the status of the entire peripheral vascular system. It may occur with scleroderma, systemic lupus erythematosus, rheumatoid arthritis, obstructive arterial disease, or trauma.

The prognosis for Raynaud's disease varies: some patients slowly improve, some grow slowly worse, and others show no change.

Nursing Management. Avoidance of the particular stimuli that provoke vasoconstriction is the prime objective in controlling Raynaud's disease. An effort should be made to avoid situations that may upset the patient. Because concern over serious complications such as gangrene and amputation are certainly upsetting, the patient should be reassured that serious sequelae are not usual with Raynaud's disease. Smoking should be avoided.

Exposure to cold must be minimized. In areas where the fall and winter months are cold, the patient should remain indoors as much as possible and wear protective clothing when outdoors. Sharp objects should be handled carefully to avoid injuring the digits. The physician may prescribe vasodilator and sympatholytic agents, such as reserpine or other rauwolfia derivatives, although their effectiveness is variable. The patient is cautioned about the postural hypotension that can result from these drugs and that this effect is increased by alcohol, exercise, and hot weather.

Interruption of the sympathetic nerves by removal of the sympathetic ganglia or division of their branches (*sympathectomy*) may afford some improvement in patients with Raynaud's disease.

Hypertension

Definition, Incidence, and Etiology

Hypertension can be defined arbitrarily as persistent levels of blood pressure in which the systolic pressure is above 140 mm Hg and the diastolic pressure is above 90 mm Hg. In the elderly population, hypertension is defined as systolic pressure above 160 mm Hg and diastolic pressure above 90 mm Hg. Hypertension is a major cause of heart failure, stroke, and kidney failure. It is called the "silent killer," because the person who has it is often symptom-free. The National Heart, Lung, and Blood Institute has estimated that 50% of persons with hypertension do not know they have it. Once it develops, a patient should have blood pressure checked frequently because hypertension is a lifetime condition.

About 20% of the adult population develop hypertension; more than 90% of these have *essential* (primary) hypertension, which has no identifiable medical cause. The remainder develop elevations in blood pressure with specific etiology, such as renovascular narrowing or parenchyma-renal disease, certain drugs, organ dysfunctions, tumors, and pregnancy.

Accompanying hypertension is the risk of premature morbidity and mortality, which increases as the systolic and diastolic pressures rise. The 1984 Report of the Joint National Committee on Detection, Evaluation, and Treatment of High Blood Pressure presented a recommended classification of blood pressure for persons aged 18 years and older (Table 28-3). This classification is helpful in diagnosing hypertension when it is used with the knowledge that a diagnosis cannot be based on a single elevated reading but that such a reading requires further evaluation (Table 28-4).

Essential hypertension usually begins as a labile (intermittent) process in a person's late 30s to early 50s and gradually becomes "fixed." On occasion it appears abruptly and severely and takes an accelerated or "malignant" course that causes rapid deterioration of the patient.

TABLE 28-4
Follow-Up Criteria for First-Occasion Measurement

Range, mm Hg	Recommended Follow-Up*
Diastolic	
<85	Recheck within 2 yr.
85–89	Recheck within 1 yr.
90–104	Confirm promptly (not to exceed 2 mo).
105–114	Evaluate or refer promptly to source of care (not to exceed 2 wk).
≥115	Evaluate or refer immediately to a source of care.
Systolic, when diastolic BP is <90	
<140	Recheck within 2 yr.
140–199	Confirm promptly (not to exceed 2 mo).
≥200	Evaluate or refer promptly to source of care (not to exceed 2 wk).

* If recommendations for follow-up of diastolic and systolic BPs are different for those aged 18 years or older, the shorter recommended time period supersedes and a referral supersedes a recheck recommendation.

(The 1984 Report of The Joint National Committee on Detection, Evaluation, and Treatment of High Blood Pressure [NIH Publication No. 84-1088]. Arch Intern Med 1984 May; 144[5]:1047.)

TABLE 28-3
Classification of BP

Range, mm Hg	Category*
Diastolic	
<85	Normal BP
85–89	High normal BP
90–104	Mild hypertension
105–114	Moderate hypertension
≥115	Severe hypertension
Systolic, when diastolic BP is <90	
<140	Normal BP
140–159	Borderline isolated systolic hypertension
≥160	Isolated systolic hypertension

* A classification of borderline isolated systolic hypertension (systolic BP 140 to 159 mm Hg) or isolated systolic hypertension (systolic BP > 160 mm Hg) takes precedence over a classification of high normal BP (diastolic BP, 85 to 89 mm Hg) when both occur in the same person. A classification of high normal BP (diastolic BP 85 to 89 mm Hg) takes precedence over a classification of normal BP (systolic BP < 140 mm Hg) when both occur in the same person.

(The 1984 Report of The Joint National Committee on Detection, Evaluation, and Treatment of High Blood Pressure [NIH Publication No. 84-1088]. Arch Intern Med 1984 May; 144[5]:1047.)

Emotional disturbances, obesity, excessive alcohol intake, and overstimulation with coffee, tobacco, and stimulatory drugs play a role, but the disease is strongly familial. It affects more women than men, but men, especially black men, are less able to tolerate the disease. The incidence increases with age in the U.S., and the incidence for black Americans far exceeds that for white Americans.

Prolonged elevation of blood pressure eventually damages blood vessels throughout the body, most notably in the eyes, heart, kidneys, and brain, so that failing vision, coronary occlusion, congestive heart failure, renal failure, and strokes are the usual consequences of prolonged, uncontrolled hypertension.

Increased peripheral resistance controlled at the arteriolar level is the basic cause for the elevated blood pressure, but the causes of increased resistance are poorly understood. Drug therapy is aimed at reducing peripheral resistance, in order to lower the blood pressure and lessen the stresses on the vascular system.

Pathophysiology of Essential Hypertension

The vasomotor center is situated in the medulla of the brain. Emanating from this vasomotor center are the sympathetic nervous system tracks, which go down the spinal cord and emerge from the spinal column at the sympathetic ganglia in the thorax and abdomen. Stimulation of the vasomotor center sets in motion impulses that travel down through the sympathetic nervous system to the sympathetic ganglia. At this point, the preganglionic neurons release acetylcholine, which stimulates the postganglionic nerve fibers in the blood vessel, where the release of norepinephrine results in constriction of the vessels. Numerous influences may affect the response of the blood vessel to these vasoconstrictor stimuli. Hypertensive persons are very sensitive to norepinephrine, although it is not known exactly why.

In the hypertensive patient, many factors moderate the vasomotor and vasoconstrictor responses, such as anxiety and fear.

Occurring concurrently with sympathetic nervous system stimulation of the blood vessels in response to emotional stimuli is stimulation of the adrenal gland. The adrenal medulla secretes epinephrine, which causes vasoconstriction. The adrenal cortex secretes cortisol and other steroids, which may enhance the vasoconstrictor response of the blood vessels. Vasoconstriction results in reduced blood flow to the kidney, causing the release of renin. Renin leads to the formation of angiotensin, a potent vasoconstrictor, which in turn stimulates secretion of aldosterone by the adrenal cortex. This hormone promotes sodium and water retention by the kidney tubules, causing an increase in intravascular volume. All of these factors tend to perpetuate the hypertensive state.

Gerontological Considerations. Changes in the peripheral vascular system are responsible for the changes in blood pressure that occur with age. As the age-related process of atherosclerosis evolves, the ability of the vessels to distend and recoil is reduced. Consequently, the aorta and large arteries are less able to accommodate the ejected stroke volume, and a decrease in cardiac output and increase in peripheral resistance result. Systolic blood pressure increases as a result of the increased peripheral resistance, and pulse pressure widens subsequent to the diastolic fall that accompanies reduced distensibility of the aorta.

The risk factors for high blood pressure that are present in the population in general continue into old age. These are approximately the same for elderly men and women.

Clinical Manifestations

Physical examination may reveal no abnormalities other than high blood pressure, but there may be changes in the retinae with hemorrhages, exudates (fluid accumulation), narrowed arterioles, and, in severe cases, papilledema (edema of the optic disc).

Persons with hypertension can be asymptomatic and remain so for many years. The appearance of symptoms usually indicates vascular damage, and specific manifestations are related to the organ systems served by the involved vessels. Coronary artery disease with angina is the most common sequela in hypertensive individuals. Left ventricular hypertrophy occurs in response to the increased work load placed on the ventricle as it contracts against higher systemic pressures. When the heart can no longer sustain the increased work load, left heart failure ensues. Pathologic changes in the kidneys may be manifested as nocturia and azotemia (increased BUN and creatinine). Cerebral vascular involvement may produce a stroke or transient ischemic attack manifested by temporary hemiplegia, blackouts, or alterations in vision. Cerebral infarcts account for 80% of the strokes and transient ischemic attacks in hypertensive persons.

Diagnostic Evaluation

A thorough history and physical examination are necessary. The retinas are examined, and laboratory studies are done to determine target organ damage. Left ventricular hypertrophy (LVH) can be assessed through the electrocardiogram; protein in the urine can be detected by urinalysis. Inability to concentrate the urine and an increase in the blood urea nitrogen may also be present. Special studies, such as renograms, intravenous pyelograms, renal arteriograms, split renal function studies, and the determination of renin levels, may also be done to identify patients with renovascular disease. The presence of additional risk factors is sought and evaluated.

Management

The type of treatment program selected for individual patients is determined by the degree of hypertension, the complications present, the number and extent of risk factors, and the personal, financial, and physical resources for adherence to the treatment program available to the patient. In cases of mild hypertension, conservative medical management may be the most beneficial approach. Patients are counseled and instructed in ways to change poor health habits. Dietary control of salt and cholesterol, weight reduction, a regular exercise program, abstinence from tobacco and alcohol, and stress management are addressed, and modifications are realistically planned with the patient.

When the conservative approach is ineffective, drug therapy is usually necessary. The selection of the appropriate drug or combination of drugs for the treatment of hypertension is highly individualized. In the "stepped care" approach, drugs are used that have the potential for the greatest effectiveness with the fewest side-effects and the best chance of acceptance by the patient (Table 28-5).

In an attempt to promote compliance, complicated drug therapy schedules should be avoided. Table 28-6 describes the various pharmacologic agents used in the treatment of hypertension.

▶ Nursing Process
The Patient With Hypertension

▷ Assessment

Assessment of the patient with hypertension involves careful monitoring of the blood pressure at frequent intervals. Blood pressure readings are taken in both arms to reveal any differences between them, and the readings are taken with the patient in the supine, sitting, and standing positions to reveal postural changes in pressure. Readings are also taken after activity and after anxiety-producing situations to indicate if such events have a significant effect on the pressure. When the patient is placed on an antihypertensive drug therapy regimen, blood pressure readings are imperative to demonstrate the effectiveness of the drugs and to reveal drops in pressure that would necessitate a change in the dosage of the drugs.

Physical examination also includes assessment of apical and peripheral pulses, their rate, rhythm, and character, to detect effects of the hypertension on the heart and the pe-

TABLE 28-5
Stepped-Care Approach to Drug Therapy

Step	Drug Regimens
1	Begin with less than a full dose of either a thiazide-type diuretic or a β-blocker*; proceed to full dose if necessary and desirable.
2	If BP control is not achieved, either add a small dose of an adrenergic-inhibiting agent† or a small dose of thiazide-type diuretic; proceed to full dose if necessary and desirable‡; additional substitutions may be made at this point§.
3	If BP control is not achieved add a vasodilator, hydralazine hydrochloride, or minoxidil for resistant cases.
4	If BP control is not achieved, add guanethidine monosulfate.

* β-Blockers include atenolol, metoprolol tartrate, nadolol, oxprenolol hydrochloride, pindolol, propranolol hydrochloride, and timolol maleate.

† These include centrally acting adrenergic inhibitors (clonidine hydrochloride, guanabenz acetate, and methyldopa), peripherally acting adrenergic inhibitors (guanadrel sulfate and reserpine), and an α_1-adrenergic blocker (prazosin hydrochloride).

‡ A high percentage (70% to 80%) of patients with mild hypertension will respond to the above regimen using steps 1 and 2.

§ An angiotensin-converting enzyme inhibitor (Table 5) may be substituted at steps 2 through 4 if side effects limit use of other agents or if other agents are ineffective. Slow channel calcium-entry blockers (diltiazem hydrochloride, nifedipine, and verapamil hydrochloride) have not been approved for therapy in hypertension but may be acceptable as drugs for steps 2 or 3.

(The 1984 Report of The Joint National Committee on Detection, Evaluation, and Treatment of High Blood Pressure [NIH Publication No. 84-1088]. Arch Intern Med 1984 May 144[5]:1048.)

ripheral vessels. The patient is questioned about symptoms that would be indicative of multisystem sequelae of hypertension, such as nosebleeds, anginal pain, shortness of breath, alterations in vision, vertigo, headaches, or nocturia. The patient who can sense when the blood pressure is elevated should be asked what symptoms create the awareness of such changes and what events or factors seem to precipitate the symptoms. A thorough assessment can yield valuable information about the extent of the effects of the hypertension throughout the body and any psychological factors related to the problem.

▷ *Nursing Diagnoses*

Based on the assessment data, nursing diagnoses for the patient may include items such as the following:

- Knowledge deficit regarding the relationship between the treatment regimen and control of the disease process
- Potential nonadherence to the self-care program related to negative side-effects of prescribed therapy and inability to believe that treatment is needed when symptoms are absent

▷ *Planning and Implementation*

▷ *Goals.* The major goals for the patient include understanding of the disease process and its treatment and adherence to the self-care program.

Nursing Interventions

Patient Education to Avoid Progression of Vascular Changes. The objective of treatment for hypertension is to lower the blood pressure to as close to normal levels as possible without introducing adverse effects. Adherence to therapy must be maximized in a cost-effective manner.

The treatment regimen consists of antihypertensive medications, dietary restrictions on sodium and fat, weight control, life-style changes, and follow-up health care at regular intervals. Because the therapeutic regimen becomes the responsibility of the patient, if able, or of a significant other, counseling and education are imperative on an ongoing basis. Many patients benefit from hypertensive clinics and support groups in which they can share their concerns with other patients with the same or similar problems. The family should be involved in the educational and counseling programs so that they can support the patient's efforts to control hypertension.

Regular follow-up care is imperative so that the disease process can be assessed in terms of control or progression and treated accordingly. Symptoms of progression of the disease with involvement of other body systems must be detected early so that appropriate changes in the treatment regimen can be made.

Adherence to the Self-Care Program. Nonadherence to the therapeutic program is a significant problem in people with hypertension. It is estimated that 50% discontinue their drug therapy within one year of its initiation, and that adequate blood pressure control is maintained in only 20%. Active participation of the patient in the program, including self-monitoring of blood pressure and diet, has been found to increase compliance.

A lot of energy is required of patients with hypertension to adhere to life-style, diet, and activity restrictions and to take regularly prescribed medications. The effort needed does not always seem reasonable, particularly when patients are symptom-free without medications but experience side-effects with the medications. Much supervision, education, and encouragement are often needed with hypertensive persons to arrive at an acceptable plan for living with their hypertension and the treatment regimen. Compromises may have to be made on some aspects of the therapy in order to achieve success in higher priority areas.

A thorough understanding of the disease process of hypertension as well as the impact of medication and health habits on this process is important. The concept of hypertension control rather than cure is important to explain. The temporary nature of medication side-effects shoud be emphasized. Consultation with a dietitian may be useful in exploring the number of possible ways to modify salt and fat intake. Lists of low-salt foods and beverages should be provided. Salt substitutes are readily available and inexpensive. Beverages containing caffeine should be avoided. Alcohol may have synergistic effects with the medications, so the patient should be fully informed of this and encouraged to abstain from the use of alcohol. Because nicotine causes vasoconstriction, the use of tobacco should be discouraged. Support groups for control of weight, smoking, and stress may be beneficial for some patients. Others may need more support from family and friends.

Written information about the expected effects and side-effects of medications is very useful in maintaining a safe self-

(Text continues on p. 648)

TABLE 28-6
Chemotherapy for Hypertension

Purpose: To maintain blood pressure within normal ranges by the simplest and safest means possible with the fewest side-effects for each individual patient

Medication	Major Action	Advantages	Contraindications	Effects and Nursing Considerations
Diuretics & Related Drugs				
Thiazide Diuretics				
Chlorthalidone (Hygroton) Quinethazone (Hydromox) Chlorothiazide (Diuril) Hydrochlorothiazide (Esidrix; HydroDiuril)	*At beginning of therapy:* Decrease of blood volume, renal blood flow, and cardiac output Depletion of extracellular fluid Negative sodium balance (from natriuresis), mild hypokalemia Directly affect vascular smooth muscle	Effective orally Effective during long-term administration Mild side-effects Enhance other antihypertensive drugs Counter sodium retention effect of other antihypertensive drugs	Gout Known sensitivity to sulfonamide-derived drugs Severely impaired kidney function	Dry mouth, thirst, weakness, drowsiness, lethargy, muscle aches, muscular fatigue, tachycardia, GI disturbance Postural hypotension may be potentiated by alcohol, barbiturates, or narcotics Because thiazides cause sodium loss, patient is instructed to watch for postural hypotension in the summer. (Eating salted pretzels in hot weather may avert this.) Administer supplementary potassium. *Gerontological Conditions:* Risk of postural hypotension is significant due to volume depletion; take blood pressure in three positions.
Loop Diuretics				
Furosemide (Lasix) Ethacrynic acid (Edecrin)	Volume depletion Block reabsorption of sodium and water in kidney Antagonize action of aldosterone	Action rapid Potent To be used only when thiazides fail	Same as for thiazides	Volume depletion is rapid— profound diuresis Electrolyte depletion— replacement is required. Thirst, nausea, vomiting, skin rash, postural hypotension Sweet taste noted; oral and gastric burning *Gerontological Conditions:* Same as Thiazides
Potassium-Sparing Diuretics				
Spironolactone (Aldactone) Triamterene (Dyrenium)	Competitive inhibitors of aldosterone Act on distal tubule independently of aldosterone	Spironolactone is effective in treating hypertension accompanying primary aldosteronism. Both spironolactone and triamterene retain potassium.	Renal disease Azotemia Severe hepatic disease	Drowsiness, lethargy, headache—decrease the dosage. Diarrhea and other GI symptoms—give drug after meals. Skin eruptions, urticaria

(continued)

TABLE 28-6 *(continued)*

Medication	Major Action	Advantages	Contraindications	Effects and Nursing Considerations
				Mental confusion, ataxia—perhaps dosage needs to be reduced.
				Gynecomastia (not for triamterene)
Adrenergic Inhibitors				
Reserpine (alkaloid of Rauwolfia serpentina)	Impairs synthesis and reuptake of norepinephrine	Slows pulse, which counteracts tachycardia of hydralazine	History of depression Psychosis Obesity Chronic sinusitis Peptic ulcer	May cause severe depression; report manifestations, since this may require that drug be omitted. Nasal stuffiness, which may require nasal vasoconstrictor Increases appetite—therefore, suggest stricter diet. Recurrence of peptic ulcer Administer with meals or milk. *Gerontological Conditions:* Depression and postural hypotension common in elderly
Methyldopa (Aldomet)	Dopa-decarboxylase inhibitor; displaces norepinephrine from storage sites	Effective in patients not controlled with thiazide-reserpine (with or without hydralazine) Useful in patients with renal failure Does not decrease cardiac output or renal blood flow Does not induce oliguria	Liver disease	Drowsiness, dizziness Dry mouth; nasal stuffiness (troublesome at first but then tends to disappear) Hemolytic anemia (a hypersensitization reaction)—positive Coombs's test; may not indicate drug discontinuance *Gerontological Conditions:* May produce mental and behavioral side-effects in the elderly
Propranolol (Inderal)	Blocks the sympathetic nervous system (β-adrenergic receptors), especially the sympathetics to the heart, producing a slower heart rate and lowered blood pressure	Reduces pulse rate in patients with tachycardia and blood pressure elevation and is useful as an adjunctive drug with drugs that act at the neuroeffector site of the blood vessel	Bronchial asthma Allergic rhinitis Right ventricular failure due to pulmonary hypertension Congestive heart failure	Mental depression manifested by insomnia, lassitude, weakness, and fatigue Lightheadedness and occasional nausea, vomiting, and epigastric distress

(continued)

TABLE 28-6 *(continued)*

Medication	Major Action	Advantages	Contraindications	Effects and Nursing Considerations
				Blood dyscrasias such as agranulocytosis and thrombocytopenic purpura do occur but are uncommon. *Gerontological Conditions:* Risk of toxicity is increased for elderly with decreased renal and liver function. Take blood pressure in three positions and observe for hypotension.
Prazosin hydrochloride (Minipress)	Peripheral vasodilator acting directly on the blood vessel; similar to hydralazine	Acts directly on the blood vessel and is an effective agent in patients with adverse reactions to hydralazine	Angina pectoris and coronary artery disease. Induces tachycardia if not preceded by administration of propranolol and a diuretic	Occasional vomiting and diarrhea, urinary frequency, and cardiovascular collapse, especially if given in addition to hydralazine without lowering the dose ot the latter. Patients occasionally experience drowsiness, lack of energy, and weakness.
Clonidine hydrochloride (Catapres)	Exact mode of action not understood, but acts through the central nervous system, apparently through centrally mediated α-adrenergic stimulation in the brain, producing blood pressure reduction	Little or no orthostatic effect. Moderately potent, and sometimes is effective when other drugs fail to lower blood pressure	Severe coronary artery disease, pregnancy, children	Most common side-effects are dry mouth, drowsiness, sedation, and occasional headaches and fatigue. Anorexia, malaise, and vomiting with mild disturbance of liver function have been reported. Skin rash, dreams and nightmares, insomnia, and anxiety have been reported but are not common.
Metoprolol (Lopressor)	Blocks access of norepinephrine to β_1-adrenergic receptors, especially in myocardium; decreases blood pressure by decreasing cardiac output and peripheral resistance	Rapid absorption	Cardiac failure Sinus bradycardia A-V conduction defects Diabetes mellitus	May cause bradycardia, congestive heart failure, intensification of heart block—take apical pulse before administration. May cause severe depression; report manifestations, since this may require that drug be omitted. Instruct patient to take radial pulse before each dose and report slow or irregular pulse to physician.

(continued)

TABLE 28-6 *(continued)*

Medication	Major Action	Advantages	Contraindications	Effects and Nursing Considerations
Nadolol (Corgard)	Blocks β-adrenergic receptors within the heart; reduces cardiac rate and output and decreases myocardial automaticity; exact mode of action for decreasing standing and supine blood pressures unknown	Can be used alone to treat hypertension, or in combination with a diuretic Long half-life; once daily administration	Cardiac failure Sinus bradycardia Bronchial asthma COPD	May cause bradycardia; instruct patient to take pulse before each dose and report slow pulse to physician. May cause dizziness, sedation, behavioral changes, depression; caution patient to avoid driving and other dangerous activities until response is known.
Guanethidine (Ismelin)	Prevents release of sympathetic transmitter, norepinephrine. Is a depressant of adrenergic activity Depletes tissue stores Causes venous pooling, decreased venous return, and decreased cardiac output Decreases pulse rate, cardiac output, and renal blood flow	Potency	Pheochromocytoma, because greatly enhances pressor effect of catecholamines	Severe postural hypotension accentuated by alcohol, exercise, hot weather Warn against suddenly standing or standing for a long time. Diarrhea and nausea, nocturia Failure of ejaculation; counsel about possible sexual dysfunction. Fatigue and giddiness; blackout
Vasodilators				
Hydralazine hydrochloride (Apresoline)	Decreases peripheral resistance but concurrently elevates cardiac output Acts directly on smooth muscle of blood vessels	Used as a third drug of choice when patient does not respond to thiazide-reserpine, thiazide-methyldopa, thiazide-guanethidine	Angina or coronary disease Congestive heart failure Hypersensitivity	Headache, tachycardia, flushing, and dyspnea may occur—can be prevented by pretreating with reserpine. Peripheral edema may require diuretics. May produce lupus erythematosus-like syndrome
Minoxidil	Direct vasodilating action on arteriolar vessels, causing decreased peripheral vascular resistance; reduces systolic and diastolic pressures	Hypotensive effect more pronounced than hydralazine No effect on vasomotor reflexes; thus does not cause postural hypotension	Pheochromocytoma	Tachycardia, angina pectoris, ECG changes, edema; take blood pressure and apical pulse before administration; monitor I&O and daily weights.

administration program. When side-effects do occur, patients need to know when and whom to contact. In addition, patients should be advised of the possibility of rebound hypertension with sudden discontinuation of antihypertensive medication, and of the possibility of sexual dysfunction related to the drugs.

Sometimes the patient is taught to measure blood pressure at home. Some authorities believe that this involves pa-tients in their own care and emphasizes the fact that failing to take the medication can lead to a rise in blood pressure. It is difficult to convince many patients that the blood pressure is normally variable and does not stay fixed at one number.

Gerontological Considerations. Adherence to the therapeutic program is even more difficult for the elderly person than for the general population. Drug therapy can be a significant problem because it must be continuous, it may require numerous doses daily, and it may be especially expensive for the person on a fixed income. Special care must be taken to make sure that the patient understands the drug regimen and is able to read the instructions, and that provisions are made for having prescriptions refilled as needed. The elderly patient's family should always be included in the teaching program so that they can understand the patient's needs, support adherence to the therapeutic program, and know when to seek guidance from health professionals.

The patient and family should be especially cautioned that the antihypertensive drug therapy may cause problems of hypotension, which should be reported immediately. Because of their impaired cardiovascular reflexes, the elderly are often more sensitive than are younger persons to the volume depletion caused by diuretic therapy and by the sympathetic inhibition effect of adrenergic antagonists. In an attempt to prevent the postural hypotension that may ensue, the patient should be very careful to change positions slowly and to use supportive aids if necessary to prevent falls that could result from dizziness and syncope.

▷ Evaluation

▷ Expected Outcomes

1. Patient exhibits no progression of vascular changes.
   a. Maintains blood pressure within acceptable range with medication or diet therapy
   b. Gives no evidence of symptoms of angina
   c. Reveals no ECG changes indicative of left ventricular hypertrophy
   d. Has normal BUN and serum creatinine levels
   e. Exhibits no progression of retinal pathology
   f. Gives no evidence of symptoms of cerebral infarction
2. Adheres to the self-care program
   a. Explains rationale for all aspects of therapeutic regimen
   b. Includes family in decisions regarding changes in life-style necessitated by therapeutic regimen
   c. Adheres to dietary regimen as prescribed: sodium, cholesterol, and calorie reduction
   d. Loses weight as prescribed
   e. Becomes involved in a regular program of exercise
   f. Takes own blood pressure daily (if appropriate)
   g. Takes medications as prescribed
   h. Reports side-effects of medications to physician prior to altering or discontinuing medications
   i. Abstains from tobacco, caffeine, and alcohol
   j. Uses available community resources for stress management and reduction
   k. Explains rationale for continuance of therapeutic regimen, even though symptom-free
   l. Keeps follow-up clinic or physician appointments

Hypertensive Emergencies

Occasionally, acute, life-threatening elevations in blood pressure occur that require prompt treatment. Hypertensive emergencies frequently occur in patients whose hypertension has been poorly controlled or in whom medications have been abruptly discontinued. The degree of organ failure present because of the hypertension will determine the rapidity with which the blood pressure must be lowered. The presence of acute left ventricular failure or cerebral dysfunction indicates the need for immediate reduction in blood pressure over the next 24 to 48 hours.

The drugs of choice in hypertensive emergencies are those that have immediate effect. Intravenous nitroprusside has an immediate vasodilating action that is short-lived, and is thus widely used as the initial treatment in crisis. Other drugs used for hypertensive emergencies include reserpine (Serpasil), methyldopa (Aldomet), phentolamine (Regitine), diazoxide (Hyperstat), and hydralazine (Apresoline). Most of these potent drugs are potentiated by diuretics. Extremely close monitoring of the patient's blood pressure and cardiovascular status is required during treatment with these medications. A precipitous drop in blood pressure can occur, and action must be taken immediately to prevent shock.

Vein Disorders

Venous Thrombosis, Thrombophlebitis, Phlebothrombosis, and Deep Vein Thrombosis (DVT)

Although the above terms do not necessarily represent an identical pathology, for clinical purposes they are often used interchangeably.

Pathophysiology and Etiology

Although the exact etiology of venous thrombosis remains unclear, three antecedent factors are believed to play a significant role in its development: stasis of blood, injury to the vessel wall, and altered blood coagulation. The presence of at least two factors appears to be necessary for thrombosis to occur.

Venous stasis occurs when blood flow is retarded, such as with heart failure or shock; when veins are dilated, such as following drug therapy; and when skeletal muscle contraction is reduced, such as with immobility, extremity paralysis, or anesthesia. Bed rest has been shown to reduce blood flow in the legs at least 50%.

Disruption of the lining of blood vessels creates a site for clot formation. Direct vessel trauma, such as after a fracture or dislocation; diseases of the veins; and chemical irritation of the vein from intravenous drugs or solutions can all damage veins.

Increased coagulability of blood occurs most commonly in patients who have been abruptly withdrawn from anticoagulant medications. Oral contraceptives and a number of blood dyscrasias can also lead to hypercoagulability.

Thrombophlebitis is inflammation of the walls of the veins with formation of a clot. When a clot develops initially in the veins without inflammation, the process is referred to as *phlebothrombosis*. Venous thrombosis can occur in any vein but is most frequent in the veins of the lower extremities. Both superficial and deep veins of the legs may be affected. Of the superficial veins, the saphenous vein is most frequently affected. Of the deep leg veins, the iliofemoral, popliteal, and small calf veins are most often involved.

Venous thrombi are composed of an aggregate of platelets attached to the vein wall and a taillike appendage containing fibrin, white blood cells, and many red blood cells. The "tail" can grow larger or propagate in the direction of blood flow as successive layering of the clot constituents occurs. The danger associated with a propagating venous thrombosis is that parts of a clot can become detached and produce an embolic occlusion of the pulmonary blood vessels. Fragmentation of the thrombus can occur spontaneously as the clot undergoes natural dissolution, or it can occur in association with elevation in venous pressure, such as occurs with sudden standing or muscular activity after prolonged inactivity. Other complications of venous thrombosis are described in Figure 28-12.

Clinical Manifestations

At least one third of all patients with venous thrombosis of the lower extremities have no symptoms. In others, symptoms are variable and not usually specific for thrombophlebitis. However, despite this uncertainty, the presence of clinical signs should always be investigated further.

Obstruction of the *deep* veins of the legs produces edema and swelling of the extremity because the outflow of venous blood is inhibited. The amount of swelling can be determined by measuring extremity circumference at various levels with a tape measure. One extremity is compared to the other at the same level for size differences. Bilateral swelling may be difficult to detect. The skin over the affected leg may become warmer, and superficial veins may become more prominent. Tenderness, which usually occurs later, is produced by inflammation of the vein wall and can be detected by gentle

palpation of the extremity. *Homans*'s sign, a pain in the calf following sharp dorsiflexion of the foot, is not specific for deep venous thrombosis because it can be elicited in any painful condition of the calf. In some cases, signs of a pulmonary embolus are the first indication of a deep venous thrombosis.

Thrombosis of *superficial* veins produces pain or tenderness, redness, and warmth of the involved area. The risk of dislodgment and embolization of superficial venous thrombi is very low because the majority of them undergo spontaneous lysis; thus, this condition can be treated at home with rest, extremity elevation, analgesics, and possibly anti-inflammatory agents.

Nursing Assessment

Careful nursing assessment is invaluable in detecting early signs of venous disorders of the lower extremities. Patients with a history of varicose veins, hypercoagulation, cardiovascular disease, or recent major surgery or injury, and the obese, the elderly, and women taking oral contraceptives are in the high-risk group (see Chart 28-2).

- Question the patient about the presence of leg pain, any functional impairment, or edema
- Inspect the legs from the groin to the feet, noting asymmetry and measuring and recording calf circumference. (One early indication of edema is engorgement of the concavity behind the medial malleolus.)
- Note any increase in temperature in the affected leg. (To determine temperature differences more effectively, cool hands in cold water, dry, and place them simultaneously on both of the patient's ankles and then on the calves.)
- To identify areas of tenderness and any thromboses (as evidenced by cordlike venous segments), palpate the leg carefully using three or four fingers, advancing the hands back and forth from the ankle to the knee and then to the groin.

Diagnostic Evaluation

Phlebography (venography) involves the injection of a radiographic contrast medium into the venous system through a dorsal foot vein. The diagnosis is based on the demonstration of an unfilled segment of vein in an otherwise completely filled vein with its connecting collaterals. Injection of the

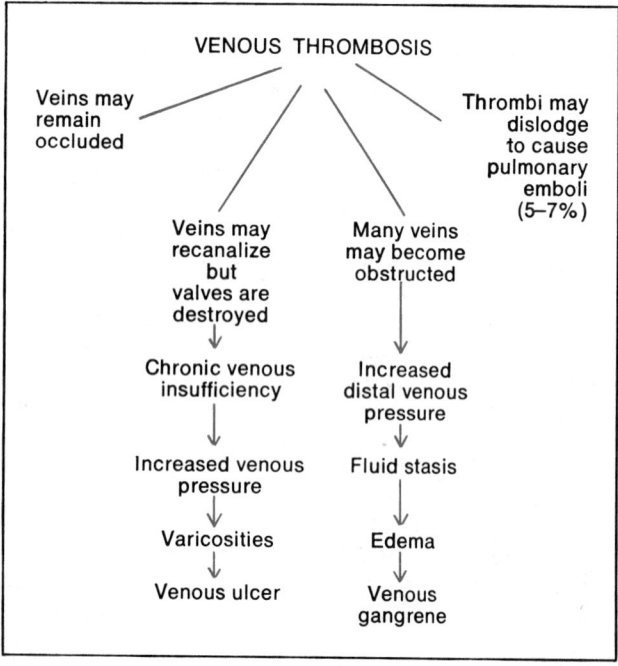

Figure 28-12
The seriousness of venous thrombosis is readily noted.

contrast medium can cause a brief but painful vein inflammation.

Another method used to measure alterations in the velocity of blood flow in leg veins is *Doppler ultrasonography*. When the Doppler probe is placed over veins that are obstructed, the Doppler flow reading will be diminished in comparison to that for the opposite extremity or absent. This method is relatively inexpensive, portable, simple, rapid, and noninvasive.

Impedance plethysmography is used to measure changes in venous volume. A blood pressure cuff is applied to the patient's thigh and is inflated enough to impede venous flow (about 50 to 60 mm Hg) but not enough to impede arterial flow. Calf electrodes are used to measure electrical resistance that results from venous volume changes. In the presence of deep vein thrombosis, the increase in venous volume that normally results from blood trapped below the level of the cuff will be less than expected. False positive results can be due to factors that cause vasoconstriction, increased venous pressure, decreased cardiac output, or external compression of the vein. False negative results can be due to the existence of an old thrombus with subsequent development of adequate collateral circulation or to superficial phlebitis. The use of both Doppler ultrasonography and impedance plethysmography can significantly increase the accuracy of diagnosis.

^{125}I-labeled fibrinogen scanning, a recently developed diagnostic procedure, has provided a sensitive method for early detection of venous thrombosis. The test relies on the fact that radioactive fibrinogen, when injected intravenously, will concentrate in the forming clot. The level of radioactivity can then be serially measured by an external counter, and the progression of the clot can be monitored. However, this test will not reveal thrombi that have already formed or thrombi in the groin or pelvic areas. A further drawback is the costliness of the test.

Preventive Measures

Venous thrombosis, thrombophlebitis, and deep vein thrombosis can often be prevented, especially if patients who are considered at high risk are identified and preventive measures are instituted without delay.

Elastic Stockings. One approach to prophylaxis is the use of elastic stockings, which are usually prescribed for patients on a regimen of restricted activity, particularly those who are confined to bed. These stockings, by exerting a sustained, evenly distributed pressure over the entire surface of the calves, reduce the caliber of the superficial veins of the lower extremities, resulting in increased flow in the deeper veins. It is important to note that any type of stocking, including the elastic type, can be converted into a tourniquet if applied incorrectly (*i.e.,* rolled tightly at the top). In such instances, the stockings will produce stasis instead of preventing it. Elastic stockings are removed for a brief interval at least twice daily. While they are off, the skin is inspected for signs of irritation and the calves are examined for possible tenderness. Any skin changes or signs of tenderness are reported.

Recent research studies have questioned the value of using elastic stockings and have indicated that the stockings may be ineffective or provide only modest benefit in some patients. It seems logical that, if elastic stockings are used as

the only preventive measure without adjunctive therapies, their efficacy would be substantially reduced.

Gerontological Considerations. Because of decreased strength and manual dexterity, elderly patients may be unable to apply elastic stockings properly. If such is the case, a family member should be taught how to assist the patient to apply the stockings so that they do not cause undue pressure on any part of the feet or legs.

Body Position and Exercise. When the patient is on bed rest, the feet and lower legs should be elevated periodically above heart level. The superficial and tibial veins empty rapidly in this position and remain collapsed. Active and passive leg exercises, particularly those involving calf muscles, should be performed preoperatively and postoperatively to increase venous flow. Early ambulation is most effective in preventing venous stasis. Deep-breathing exercises are beneficial because they produce increased negative pressure in the thorax, which assists in emptying the large veins.

Management

The objectives of medical treatment are to prevent propagation of the thrombus and the inherent risk of pulmonary embolism and to prevent recurrent thromboemboli.

Therapeutic anticoagulation can accomplish both of these goals. Heparin is administered by intermittent intravenous infusion or by continuous infusion. Drug dosage is regulated by the partial thromboplastin time (PTT).

Heparin is usually continued for 10 to 12 days until organization of the clot has taken place. The patient is then started on oral anticoagulants for long-term prevention.

Many centers use thrombolytic (fibrinolytic) therapy because lysis and dissolution of clots take place effectively. Such therapy is given within the first 3 days following acute arterial occlusion. Streptokinase and urokinase are both from biological sources and are about equal in thrombolytic activity. Urokinase is much more expensive than streptokinase.

The patient's partial thromboplastin time, prothrombin time, hemoglobin, and hematocrit are monitored frequently. If bleeding occurs and cannot be stopped, the drug is discontinued. During and 24 hours after infusion, parenteral injections are withheld because the likelihood of bleeding from puncture sites is great.

Occasionally, dextran has been used to decrease viscosity and aggregations of blood cells in patients with deep venous thrombosis. Use of this agent is associated with a relatively high incidence of allergic reaction and is therefore not widely practiced.

Surgical Management. Surgery for deep vein thrombosis is necessary when (1) the patient cannot be given anticoagulants; (2) the danger of pulmonary embolism is extreme; and (3) the venous drainage is so severely compromised that permanent extremity damage will probably result. A thrombectomy is the treatment of choice when surgery is necessary.

Nursing Management. Bed rest, elevation of the affected extremity, elastic stockings, and analgesics for pain are adjuncts to anticoagulant therapy. Usually, bed rest is required for 5 to 7 days following a deep venous thrombosis. This is approximately the length of time necessary for inflammatory symptoms to subside and organization of the thrombus to occur. When the patient begins to ambulate, elastic stockings are used. Walking is superior to standing or sitting for long periods. Bed exercises, such as dorsiflexion of the foot against a foot board, are also recommended.

Warm, moist packs to the affected extremity reduce discomfort associated with deep venous thrombosis. Mild analgesics for pain control, as prescribed, provide additional relief. A summary of the management of thrombophlebitis is presented in Table 28-7.

Anticoagulant Therapy for Thromboembolism

Anticoagulant therapy is the administration of a medication to delay the clotting time of blood, to prevent the formation of a thrombus in postoperative patients, and to forestall the extension of a thrombus once it has formed. Anticoagulants cannot dissolve a thrombus that has already formed.

Measures for the *prevention* or reduction of blood clotting within the vascular system are indicated in patients with thrombophlebitis, patients suspected of recurrent embolus formation, those with persistent leg edema secondary to heart failure, and the elderly person with a hip fracture who is likely to be immobilized for a considerable time. The usual treatment consists of the single or combined administration of heparin or coumarin derivatives, which reduce the normal activity of the clotting mechanism (Table 28-8).

Administration. *Continuous pump infusion* is the preferred method for administering heparin (provided there are appropriate facilities and adequate personnel for monitoring) because evidence suggests a lower incidence of hemorrhagic complications. Dosage is calculated on the basis of weight, and any possible bleeding tendencies are indicated by a pretreatment clotting profile. If renal insufficiency exists, lower doses are required. The nurse periodically checks for kinks or leaks in the tubing and inspects the entire system frequently to ensure that the exact dose is being administered. Periodic coagulation tests and hematocrit evaluations are obtained. The nurse watches for bleeding gums, ecchymotic areas, and signs of pain, which may be indicative of an overdose of anticoagulants.

Intermittent intravenous injection is another means of administering heparin, in this instance as a dilute aqueous solution given every 4 hours. Administration may be facilitated by the use of a "heparin lock"—a small, butterfly-type scalp vein needle with injection site at the end of tubing.

Oral anticoagulants, such as Coumadin, are monitored by the prothrombin time. Because Coumadin has a lag period of 3 to 5 days, it is usually administered in conjunction with heparin until desired anticoagulation has been achieved (*i.e.,* when the prothrombin time is kept at 1½ to 2 times the normal).

Precautions and Nursing Assessment. *The principal complication of anticoagulant therapy is the occurrence of*

TABLE 28-7
Comparison of Superficial and Deep Thrombophlebitis

Superficial	Deep
Clinical Manifestations	
Local swelling; bumpy and knotty	"Heaviness" on standing
Red, tender, local induration	Cramping leg pain
	Swelling:
	Calf vein thrombus—none
	Femoral vein thrombus—mild to moderate
	Ileofemoral vein thrombus—severe
	Positive Homans's sign
Diagnostic Evaluation	
Venography—to rule out deep vein thrombosis	Blood flow studies to show inflow, filling and emptying
	Venography—to determine presence of phlebitis, recanalization, extent of occlusion
Management	
Bed rest	Bed rest
Warm, moist compresses	Warm, moist compresses
Legs elevated; then elastic support after acute stage	Foot of bed elevated to 15 cm (6 inches)
Heparin, intermittent or continuous	Surgery, possibly, to prevent embolic development
Acetaminophen for pain	
Antibiotics if necessary	
If deep veins are patent, superficial phlebitic veins may be removed.	

TABLE 28-8
Comparison of Heparin and Coumarin Derivatives

Heparin Sodium	Coumarin Derivatives
Physiologic Action	
Interferes with clotting reaction at many points, but primarily acts as an antagonist to thrombin and prevents conversion of fibrinogen to fibrin	Blocks the formation of prothrombin from vitamin K, a conversion normally taking place in the liver
Therapeutic Action	
Advantages	
Used for short-term therapy primarily (may also be used for long-term therapy)	Used for long-term therapy
Action is prompt and predictable.	Is given orally and provides efficient absorption from gastrointestinal tract
It can be used outside the body as well as inside: it may be used in certain dialysis procedures and in place of sodium citrate in donor blood.	Uniform strength of medication because of synthetic production
	Less expensive than heparin sodium
	Control factor better than with heparin sodium
	Sodium warfarin more completely absorbed than bishydroxycoumarin
Disadvantages	
Must be given parenterally, intravenously, or into the fat subcutaneously.	Prolonged lag period (2–3 days) before the appearance of its effect
A few patients have developed allergic reactions, and transient hair loss or osteoporosis has been reported (after several months of therapy).	Unpredictable duration of anticoagulant action (at times persisting up to 3 weeks)
Administration	
Test clotting and partial thromboplastin time (PTT) first.	Test prothrombin time first (see below).
PTTs are obtained every 4 to 6 hours, at which time repeat doses of heparin are given.	Warfarin: Administer initial dose of 15 mg to 25 mg.
The object is to attain a PTT 1½ to 2½ times the normal control.	Give a second dose, somewhat smaller (10 mg), on following day.
Subcutaneous route—least recommended because of erratic absorption, possible puncture of vessels, and discomfort	Adjust subsequent doses on basis of daily prothrombin determinations.
The average therapeutic dose is 20,000 to 30,000 units daily either by *continuous infusion* with an infusion pump or in divided doses by *intermittent IV injection* every 4 to 6 hours.	Average dose is usually 5 mg/day.
Prolonged Therapy: May be given deep subcutaneously (into the fat) in lower abdomen. Use a fine, short, sharp needle (No. 25–27 gauge, 1.27 cm–1.60 cm [0.5–0.62 inches]).	Therapeutic level of hypoprothrombinemia may be reached in 3 to 5 days.
Grasp roll of fat gently, and in dartlike fashion insert needle at right angle to the skin surface.	
Following injection, do not rub site but firmly press site with an alcohol sponge.	
Each time use a new location on lower abdomen.	
Note: Intramuscular administration of heparin is avoided because of likelihood of local hematomas and tissue irritation.	
Action for Adverse Effects	
Discontinue heparin.	Administer vitamin K preparations:
Protamine sulfate (acts as a base to neutralize acidic heparin)	For mild bleeding control:
Blood transfusion when hemorrhage is present	Phytonadione tablets (oral use) (Mephyton) (vitamin K_1)
	For moderate to severe control:
	Phytonadione solution (Aqua-MEPHYTON) IV or IM. Transfusion may be required.

Prothrombin time is measured in seconds or percent of normal.
Normal: 12.5 seconds or 100%
Desired Therapeutic Range: 25 to 30 seconds when the control is 12 seconds (approximately 1½–2½ times the control in seconds). When the prothrombin time is measured in percent of normal, the desired therapeutic range is felt to be 20% to 30%.

spontaneous bleeding anywhere in the body. Bleeding from the kidneys will be manifested by microscopic hematuria and is often the first sign of anticoagulant overdose. Bruises, nosebleeds, and bleeding gums are also early signs of bleeding. To promptly reverse the effects of heparin, the physician may prescribe intravenous injections of protamine sulfate. The reversal of the effects of coumarin derivatives is more difficult, but effective measures that the physician may prescribe include administering phytonadione and possibly fresh whole blood or plasma.

A further possible complication of heparin therapy is that of heparin-induced *thrombocytopenia* (decrease in platelets), which generally occurs 7 to 10 days after the treatment has been started. When this occurs it is a serious complication that results in thromboembolic manifestations, and the prognosis is extremely guarded. The thrombocytopenia is thought to be the result of an immunologic mechanism that causes aggregation of platelets. Prevention of this syndrome is dependent upon regular monitoring of platelet counts and subsequent studies of platelet aggregation if thrombocytopenia becomes evident. The physician will discontinue heparin when this occurs and use protamine sulfate to reverse the heparin effects.

Oral anticoagulants interact with many other medications, and close monitoring of the patient's drug schedule is necessary. Drugs that potentiate oral anticoagulants include salicylates, anabolic steroids, chloral hydrate, glucagon, chloramphenicol, neomycin, quinidine, and phenylbutazone (Butazolidin). It is advisable to study drug interactions for patients taking specific oral anticoagulants.

Contraindications to anticoagulant therapy are summarized in Chart 28-3.

Patient Education About Oral Anticoagulants. The patient should be informed about the medication, its purpose, and the need to take the correct amount at the specific times prescribed, and should be aware that blood tests are scheduled periodically to determine how the blood is clotting and whether a change in medication dosage is required. If the patient is unable or unwilling to cooperate with the therapeutic program, continuation of the drug therapy should be questioned. Specific teaching directives should include the following points:

- Take the anticoagulant tablet at the same time each day, usually between 8:00 and 9:00 AM.
- Wear or carry identification indicating what anticoagulant is being taken.
- Keep all appointments for blood tests.
- Because other medications affect the way the anticoagulant normally acts, do not take any of the following medications without the physician's consent: vitamins, cold medicines, antibiotics, aspirin, mineral oil, and antiinflammatory drugs. The physician should be contacted prior to taking any over-the-counter drugs.
- Remember that alcohol may alter the body's response to an anticoagulant.
- Avoid food fads, crash diets, or marked changes in eating habits.
- Do not take Coumadin unless so directed by the physician.
- Do not stop taking Coumadin (when prescribed) unless so directed by the physician or nurse.

Chart 28-3
Contraindications to Anticoagulant Therapy (Risk Factors)

Lack of patient cooperation
Bleeding from the following tracts:
  Gastrointestinal
  Genitourinary
  Respiratory
Hemorrhagic blood dyscrasias
Aneurysms
Severe trauma
Alcoholism
Compulsive drug use
Recent or impending surgery of:
  Eye
  Spinal cord
  Brain
Severe hepatic or renal disease
Recent cerebrovascular hemorrhage
Infections
Open ulcerative wounds
Occupations that involve a significant hazard of injury

- When seeking treatment from another physician, a dentist, or a podiatrist, indicate that an anticoagulant is being taken.
- Contact one's personal physician prior to dental extraction or elective surgery.
- If any of the following signs appear, report them immediately to the physician:
  Faintness, dizziness, or increased weakness
  Severe headaches or stomach pain
  Red or brown urine
  Any bleeding, such as cuts that do not stop bleeding
  Bruises that increase in size, nosebleeds, or unusual bleeding from any part of the body
  Red or black bowel movements
  Skin rash
  Pregnancy
- Be extra careful to avoid injury that can cause bleeding.
- Women should notify their physicians if they suspect that they are pregnant.

Chronic Venous Insufficiency

Pathophysiology and Clinical Manifestations

Venous insufficiency is a disease state resulting from the incompetency of venous valves in the legs. Both superficial and deep leg veins can be involved. Valvular incompetence can occur whenever there has been a prolonged increase in venous pressure, such as occurs with deep venous thrombosis.

Because the walls of veins are thinner and more elastic than walls of arteries, they distend readily when venous pressure is consistently high. In this state, leaflets of the venous valves are stretched and prevented from closing completely, thereby allowing a backflow or reflux of blood in the veins. Venous stasis and edema result.

When the deep veins in the legs have incompetent valves following a thrombus, *postphlebitic syndrome* may develop. This disorder is characterized by chronic venous stasis resulting in edema, altered pigmentation, pain, stasis dermatitis, and stasis ulceration. Superficial veins may be dilated. The disorder is long-standing, difficult to treat, and often disabling.

Stasis ulcers develop as a result of the rupture of small skin veins and subsequent ulcerations. When these vessels rupture, red blood cells escape into surrounding tissues, and then degenerate and leave a brownish pigment that stains the tissues. The pigmentation and ulcerations usually occur in the lower part of the extremity in the area of the medial malleolus of the ankle. The skin becomes dry, cracks, and itches. Subcutaneous tissues fibrose and atrophy. The risk of injury and infection of the extremities is increased.

Leg ulcers can be associated with other conditions affecting the circulation of the lower extremities (see Fig. 28-14). The potential complications and the principles of care, however, will be similar for all types.

Management and Patient Education

Management of the patient with venous insufficiency is directed at reducing venous stasis and preventing ulcerations. Measures that increase venous blood flow are antigravity activities and compression of superficial veins with elastic stockings.

Elevation of the legs above the heart should be preformed frequently throughout the day (at least 30 minutes every 2 hours). At night, the patient should sleep with the foot of the bed elevated about 15 cm (6 inches). Prolonged sitting or standing still is detrimental, but walking should be encouraged. When sitting, the patient should avoid placing pressure on the popliteal spaces, such as occurs with leg crossing, or sitting with the legs dangling over the side of the bed. Constricting garments such as girdles or garters should be avoided.

Elastic compression of the legs reduces pooling of venous blood and enhances venous return to the heart. Thus, elastic hose are recommended for patients with venous insufficiency. The fit of the stocking is important. It should provide for a greater pressure at the foot and ankle, gradually declining to a lesser pressure at the knee or groin. If the top of the stocking is too tight or twisting has occurred, a tourniquet effect is created, which worsens venous pooling. Stockings should be applied following a period of leg elevation, when the venous blood volume is at its lowest. The technique for putting on elastic hose is depicted in Figure 28-13.

Extremities with venous insufficiency are conscientiously protected from trauma. The skin is kept clean, dry, and soft. Signs of ulceration are immediately reported to the healthcare professional for treatment and follow-up.

Leg Ulcers

Definition and Etiology

A *leg ulcer* is an excavation of the skin surface that is produced by the sloughing of inflammatory necrotic tissue. The most

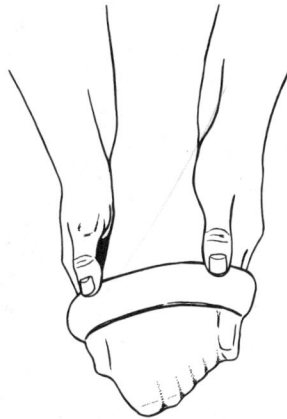

Figure 28-13
Method of applying a support stocking. A support stocking can be rolled, spread apart, and unrolled as the hands hold it in place—moving from foot to ankle and up the calf. Ideally, the stocking should be put on while the patient is in bed.

frequent cause is vascular insufficiency, either venous or arteriolar. It is estimated that, of all leg ulcers, postphlebitic and varicose ulcers account for about 70%; the remaining 30%, such as those caused by burns, sickle cell anemia, and neurogenic disorders, are of nonvenous origin.

Pathophysiology

Inadequate exchange of oxygen and other nutrients in the tissue is the metabolic abnormality underlying the development of leg ulcers. When the cellular metabolism cannot maintain energy balance, cell death (necrosis) results. Alterations in blood vessels at the arterial, capillary, and venous levels may affect cellular processes and lead to the formation of ulcers (see Fig. 28-14).

Clinical Manifestations

The patient with a leg ulcer usually complains of aching, fatigue, heaviness, and swelling of the leg. The symptoms will vary depending upon whether the problem is one that is arterial or venous in origin (see Table 28-2). The severity of the symptoms depends on the extent and duration of the vascular insufficiency. The ulcer itself appears as an open sore that is inflamed. Drainage may be present, or the area may be covered by a dark crust.

Diagnostic Evaluation

Because there are many causes of ulcers, it is important that an accurate causative diagnosis be made so that appropriate therapy can be prescribed. The history of the condition is important in determining the presence of venous or arterial insufficiency. The quality of all pulses of the lower extremities (femoral, popliteal, posterior tibial, and pedal) is carefully checked. More conclusive diagnostic aids are Doppler ultrasound studies, arteriography, and venography. Cultures of the ulcer drainage may be necessary to determine whether infection is the primary cause of the ulcer.

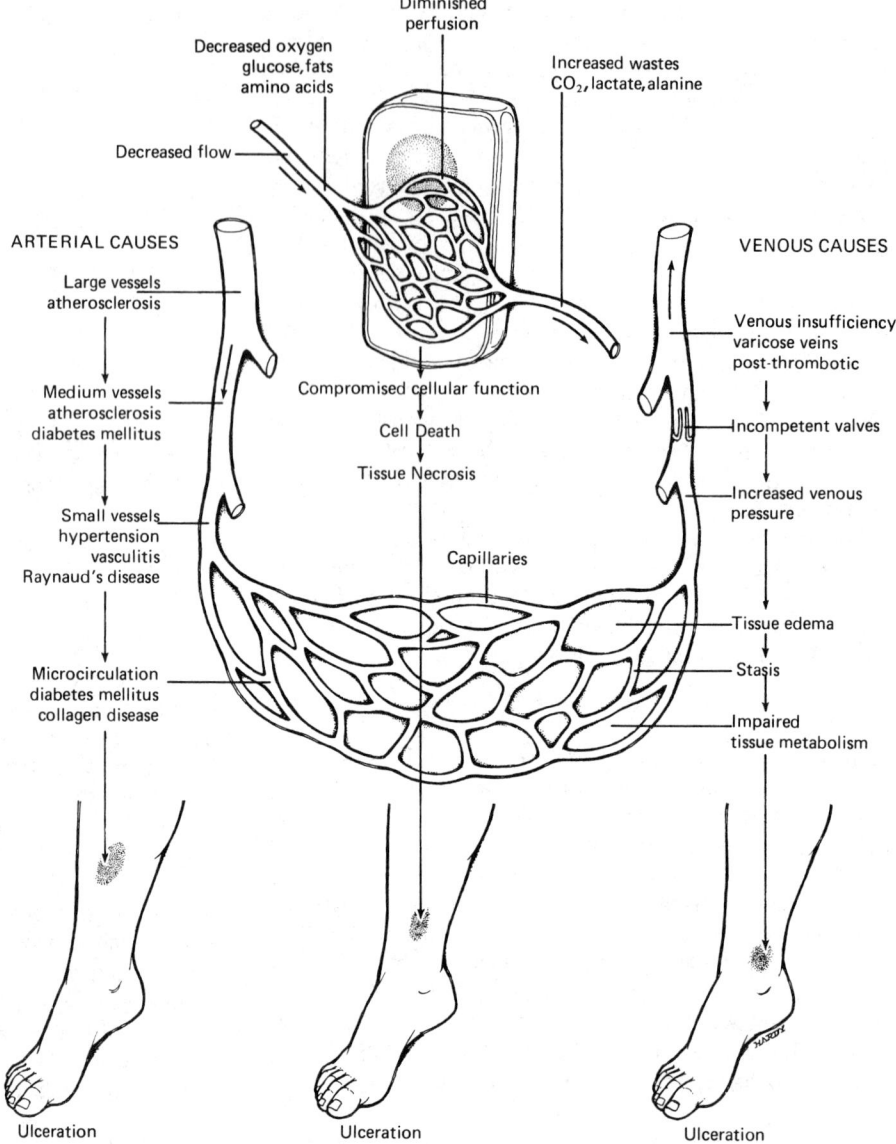

Figure 28-14
Pathophysiology of leg ulcers.
Some of the conditions that cause
diminished blood flow to
peripheral tissue are indicated on
the left. Oxygen and energy
sources are further aggravated by
capillary changes brought about
by diabetes mellitus and collagen
disease. Cellular function is
compromised when insufficient
oxygen and energy substrates are
supplied. Tissue necrosis takes
place and results in ulceration. A
somewhat similar situation occurs
when there is venous insufficiency
brought about by a different
hemodynamic pattern. Increased
venous pressure reduces capillary
flow. Edema and stasis result,
impairing cellular metabolism and
again leading to ulceration.

Management

Because most ulcers are infected and all ulcers have the potential for becoming infected, antibiotic therapy is prescribed when indicated by culture and sensitivity determinations. The route of administration prescribed is usually systemic because topical antibiotics have not proven to be effective for leg ulcers.

To promote healing, the wound is kept clean of drainage and necrotic tissue. This may be accomplished by flushing the area with normal saline; if that is unsuccessful, the physician may decide that debridement is necessary. Debridement can be performed using instruments to cut away devitalized tissue. It can also be done by applying isotonic saline dressings of fine mesh gauze to the ulcer bed. When dry, the dressing is removed along with the debris adhering to the gauze.

A variety of topical agents and soaps can be used in conjunction with washing and débridement therapies to promote healing of leg ulcers. The goals of treatment are to remove devitalized tissue and to keep the wound clean and moist while healing takes place.

Enzymatic débridement is preferred by some physicians, and enzyme ointments are used to treat the ulcer. The ointment is placed over the lesion but not over normal surrounding skin. The lesion and ointment are then covered with a saline-soaked sponge that has been thoroughly wrung out. A gauze dressing and a loose bandage are then applied. For the first 3 or 4 days applications are made every 4 hours, and then every 8 hours. When pink granulating tissue develops, saline wet dressings are used.

A newer method of treating ulcers involves the use of dextranomer (Debrisan) beads. These are small, highly porous, spherical beads (0.1 mm to 0.3 mm in diameter) that possess the ability to absorb wound secretions. Bacteria and products of tissue necrosis and protein degradation are actively suctioned into the bead layer, which changes color according to the infecting organism. When the beads are completely saturated they take on a greyish yellow color, at which point their cleansing action stops. When the beads become saturated, they are removed and a fresh layer is applied.

In patients where arterial insufficiency is the problem and the ulcer does not respond to antibiotics, cleansing, and débridement, more aggressive therapy may be necessary. Aortoiliac, aortofemoral, and femoropopliteal revascularization often are effective in correcting arterial insufficiency.

▶ Nursing Process
The Patient With Leg Ulcers

▷ Assessment

A careful nursing history and assessment of symptoms are important in determining venous or arterial insufficiency. The extent and type of pain are carefully assessed, as are the appearance and temperature of the skin of both lower extremities. The quality of all peripheral pulses is determined, and comparisons are made of the pulses bilaterally. The presence or absence of edema is determined. If the extremity is edematous, it is examined to see if pitting is present. Any limitation of mobility and activity that results from the vascular insufficiency is determined. In addition, the patient is questioned about nutritional status and about any chronic conditions that may exist, such as diabetes, collagen disease, or varicose veins, that could be associated with the leg ulcer.

▷ Nursing Diagnoses

Based on the assessment data, major nursing diagnoses for the patient may include the following:

- Impairment of skin integrity related to vascular insufficiency
- Impaired physical mobility related to the activity restrictions of the therapeutic regimen and the presence of pain
- Potential nutritional deficit related to increased need for nutrients that promote wound healing

▷ Planning and Implementation

▷ *Goals.* The major goals of the patient may include restoration of skin integrity, improvement of physical mobility, and attainment of adequate nutrition.

The nursing challenge in caring for these patients is great, whether the patient is in the hospital or at home. The physical problem is often a long-term one that casues a substantial drain on the patient's physical, emotional, and economic resources.

Nursing Interventions

Restoration of Skin Integrity. To promote wound healing, measures are used to keep the area clean. Cleansing requires very gentle handling; a mild soap, lukewarm water, and cotton balls may be used. Strict aseptic technique is used to prevent contamination. Ointments and dressings are applied as prescribed.

Positioning of the legs depends on whether the cause of the ulcer is arterial or venous in origin. If there is arterial insufficiency, blood flow can be improved by elevating the head of the bed on 7.5-cm to 15-cm (3-inch to 6-inch) blocks. This improved flow of blood increases oxygenation of the tissue and promotes healing. If there is venous insufficiency, resolution of dependent edema can be promoted by elevating the lower extremities. Decrease in the edema will allow for improved exchange of cellular nutrients and waste products in the area of the ulcer. Thus healing is promoted.

Avoidance of trauma to the lower extremities is imperative in promoting skin integrity. When the patient is ambulatory, all obstacles are moved from the path so that the patient's legs will not be bumped. When the patient is in bed, a bed cradle is used to relieve pressure from bed linens and to prevent anything from touching the legs. Heat in the form of heating pads, hot water bottles, or hot baths is avoided. Heat increases the oxygen demands and thus blood flow demands of the tissue, which in this case are already compromised.

Improvement of Physical Mobility. Generally, physical activity is restricted at first in order to promote healing. When infection has improved and healing has begun, ambulation will be resumed gradually and progressively. Activity aids arterial flow and venous return and is encouraged after the acute phase of the ulcer process.

Until full activity can be resumed, the patient is encouraged to move about when in bed, to turn from side to side frequently, and to exercise the upper extremities to maintain muscle tone and strength. Meanwhile, diversional activities that interest the patient are encouraged. Consultation with an occupational therapist may be helpful if the period of limited mobility and activity is prolonged.

If pain limits the patient's activity, analgesics are often prescribed by the physician. The pain of peripheral vascular disease is often chronic in nature, so nonnarcotic analgesics are more desirable than narcotics because the problem of drug dependency is less. It is often desirable to administer the analgesic prior to scheduled activity periods in order to help the patient participate more comfortably in the activity.

Attainment of Adequate Nutrition. Nutritional deficiencies are determined from the patient's account of usual dietary intake. Alterations in the diet are made to remedy these deficiencies. In addition, a diet that is high in protein, vitamin C, and iron is encouraged in an attempt to promote the healing process.

Many patients with peripheral vascular disease are elderly. The caloric intake of these patients may need to be adjusted because of their decreased metabolic rate and decreased level of activity. Particular consideration should also be given to their iron intake because many elderly people are anemic. Once a diet plan has been developed that meets the individual's nutritional needs, diet instruction is made available to the patient and family. The diet plan is designed to be compatible with the patient's and family's life-style and preferences.

▷ Evaluation
▷ Expected Outcomes

1. Skin integrity is restored.
   a. Absence of inflammation.

    b. Absence of drainage; negative culture report.
    c. Patient uses measures to avoid trauma to the legs.
    d. Patient uses prescribed position (head elevated or feet elevated) to promote circulation.
  2. Patient increases physical mobility.
    a. Progresses gradually to optimum level of activity.
    b. Relates that pain does not impede activity.
  3. Patient attains adequate nutrition.
    a. Select foods high in protein, vitamins, iron.
    b. Discusses with family member dietary modifications that need to be made at home.
    c. Plans, with family, a diet that is nutritionally sound.

Varicose Veins

Incidence

Varicose veins (varicosities) are abnormally dilated, tortuous, superficial veins caused by incompetent venous valves (Fig. 28-15). Most commonly, this condition occurs in the lower extremities, the saphenous veins, or the lower trunk; however, it can occur elsewhere in the body (*e.g.*, esophageal varices; see Chap. 35).

It is estimated that varicose veins of the lower extremities affect one out of five persons in the world. The condition is most common in women and in persons in occupations requiring prolonged standing, such as salespeople, barbers, beauticians, elevator operators, nurses, and dentists. A hereditary weakness of the vein wall may contribute to the development of varicosities, and it is not uncommon to see this condition occur in several members of the same family.

Pathophysiology and Manifestations

Varicose veins may be caused *primarily* (without involvement of deep veins) or *secondarily* (resulting from obstruction of deep veins). A reflux of venous blood in the veins results in venous stasis. If only the superficial veins are affected the person may have no symptoms, but cosmetically the ap-

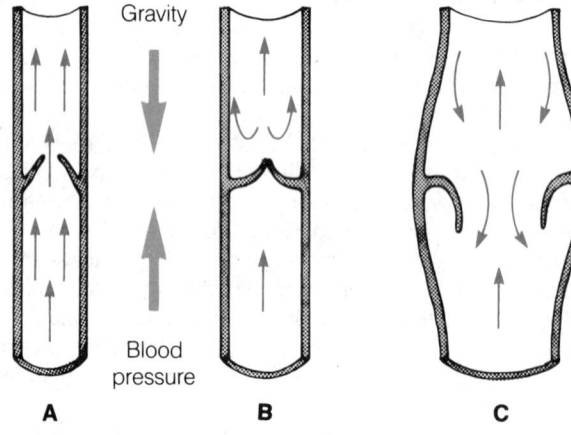

Gravity

Blood pressure

A   B   C

Figure 28-15
(*A, B*) *Competent valves* showing blood flow patterns when the valve is open (*A*) and closed (*B*), allowing blood to flow against gravity. (*C*) With faulty, or *incompetent*, valves, the blood is unable to move toward the heart.

pearance of the dilated veins may be unappealing. If symptoms are present, they may take the form of dull aches, muscle cramps, and increased fatigue of muscles in the lower legs. Ankle swelling and a feeling of heaviness of the legs may be manifested. Nocturnal cramps are a common symptom.

When deep venous obstruction results in varicose veins, patients may demonstrate the signs and symptoms of chronic venous insufficiency: edema, pain, pigmentation, and ulcerations. Susceptibility to injury and infection is greater.

Diagnostic Evaluation

A common diagnostic test for varicose veins is the *Brodie-Trendelenburg test*. This test will demonstrate backward flow of blood through incompetent valves of the superficial veins and of the branches that communicate with the deep veins of the leg. With the patient lying down, the affected leg is elevated to empty the veins. A soft, rubber tourniquet is then applied around the upper thigh to occlude the veins, and the patient is asked to stand. If the valves of the communicating veins are incompetent, blood flows into the superficial veins from the deep veins. If, upon release of the tourniquet, blood flows rapidly from above into the superficial veins, the inference is that the valves of the superficial veins are also incompetent. This test is used to determine the type of treatment to be recommended for the varicose veins.

The *Perthes' test* is a diagnostic procedure that easily indicates whether the deeper venous system and communicating veins are competent. A tourniquet is applied just below the knee and the patient is asked to walk. If the varicose veins disappear, the deep system and communicating vessels are competent. If the vessels do not empty and become even more distended on walking, incompetency or obstruction is inferred.

Additional diagnostic tests for the presence of varicose veins are the Doppler flow meter, phlebography, and plethysmography. The *Doppler flow meter* can detect the retrograde flow of blood in superficial veins with incompetent valves following compression of the leg proximally. *Phlebography* involves the injection of radiographic contrast into the leg veins so that vein anatomy can be visualized during various leg movements. *Plethysmography* allows measurement of changes in venous blood volume.

Prevention and Health Education

Activities that cause venous stasis should be avoided, such as wearing tight garters or a constricting panty girdle, crossing the legs at the thighs, and sitting or standing for long periods of time. Changing position frequently, elevating the legs when they are tired, and getting up to walk for several minutes of every hour promote circulation. The patient should be encouraged to walk 1 or 2 miles a day if there are no contraindications. Walking up the stairs rather than using the elevator or escalator is helpful in promoting circulation. Swimming is also good exercise for the legs.

Support hose or elastic stockings are useful. The overweight patient should be assisted in a weight-reduction plan.

Surgical Treatment

Surgery for varicose veins requires demonstrated patency of deep veins. Once this is established, *ligation* of the saphenous vein is accomplished under general anesthesia. The vein is ligated high in the groin where the saphenous vein meets the femoral vein. An incision is then made in the ankle, and a metal or plastic wire is passed the full length of the vein, "stripping" as it passes (Fig. 28-16). The branches of the saphenous vein break off at their junctions. Pressure and elevation keep bleeding at a minimum during surgery.

Postoperative Nursing Management. Elastic compression of the leg is maintained continuously for about 1 week after vein stripping. Exercise and movement of the legs and elevation of the foot of the bed are necessary. Walking may be started 24 to 48 hours after surgery. Standing still and sitting are contraindicated.

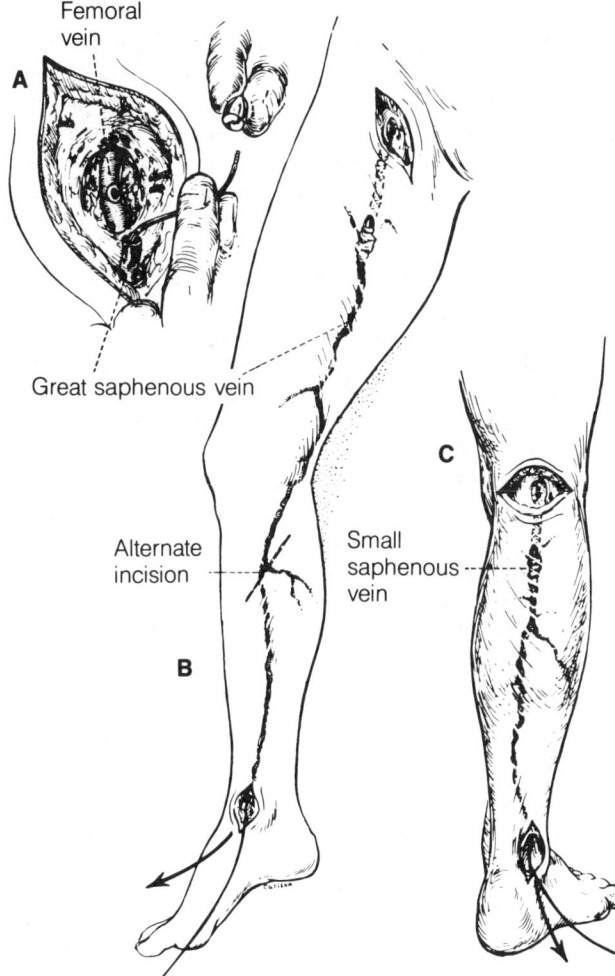

Figure 28-16
Ligation and stripping of the great and the small saphenous veins. (*A*) The tributaries of the saphenous vein have been ligated, and the saphenous vein has been ligated at the saphenofemoral junction. (*B*) Vein stripper has been inserted from the ankle superiorly to the groin. The vein is stripped from above downward. A number of alternate incisions may be needed to remove separate varicose masses. (*C*) The small saphenous vein is stripped from its junction with the popliteal vein to a point posterior to the lateral malleolus. (Rhoads et al. Surgery. Philadelphia, JB Lippincott.)

Analgesics may help patients move affected extremities more easily. The bandages are inspected for bleeding, particularly at the groin because the greatest risk of bleeding occurs there. Sensations of "pins and needles" or hypersensitivity to touch in the involved extremity may indicate a temporary or permanent nerve injury resulting from surgery. The saphenous vein and saphenous nerve are in close proximity to each other in the leg.

Patients will require long term elastic support of the leg after discharge from the hospital, and plans are made to provide adequate supplies. Exercises of the legs will also be necessary and the development of an individualized plan will require consultation with the patient and physician.

Sclerotherapy. In sclerotherapy an irritating chemical, such as 3% sodium tetradecyl sulfate (Sotradecal), is injected into the vein, which irritates the vein wall and produces localized phlebitis and fibrosis, thereby obliterating the vein lumen. This treatment may be done alone for small varicosities or may follow vein ligation or stripping. Sclerosing is a palliative, not curative, treatment. Following injection of the sclerosing agent, elastic compression bandages are applied to the leg. These are worn for approximately 6 weeks. Walking is important for maintenance of blood flow in the extremity and should be emphasized.

If the patient experiences a burning sensation in the injected leg for one or two nights, a mild sedative and walking will relieve the problem. The bandage should be removed for the first time under the direction of the physician. Because bathing may be a problem during this time, a plastic bag may be placed over the bandaged leg and secured above the bandage to allow the patient to shower.

Sclerotherapy has declined in popularity in recent years because of the possible complications of thrombosis, injection site necrosis, vasospasm, hemolysis, and allergic reactions.

The Lymphatic System

The lymphatic system consists of a set of vessels that spread throughout most of the body. These vessels start as lymph capillaries that drain tissue spaces of plasma that is not reabsorbed by the venular end of the capillaries. They unite to form the lymph vessels, which in turn pass through the lymph nodes and finally empty into the large thoracic duct that joins the jugular vein on the left side of the neck. *Lymph* is the fluid found in lymph vessels. *Tissue fluids* are found outside of vessels in the cellular interspaces. The lymphatic system of the abdominal cavity maintains a steady flow of digested fatty food (chyle) from the intestinal mucosa to the thoracic duct. In other parts of the body the lymphatic system's function is regional; the lymphatic vessels of the head, for example, empty into clusters of lymph nodes located in the neck, and those of the extremities into nodes in the axillae and the groin. The flow of lymph depends upon the intrinsic contractions of the lymph vessels, the contraction of muscles, respiratory movements, and gravity.

Diagnosis by Lymphangiography

Radiologic visualization of the lymphatic system is possible after the injection of contrast medium directly into lymphatic vessels in the hands and feet. This technique, *lymphangiography*, affords a means of detecting lymph node involvement by metastatic carcinoma, lymphoma, or infection in sites that are otherwise inaccessible to the examiner except by the direct surgical approach.

The first step in this procedure is the location of a lymphatic vessel in each foot (or hand) by injecting Evans blue contrast medium intradermally between the first and second digits. Approximately 15 to 20 minutes later, the skin proximal to the injection site is incised. A blue lymphatic segment is identified, isolated, cannulated with a 25- to 30-gauge needle, and infused very slowly with a contrast medium containing iodine and oil. Appropriate x-ray pictures are taken at the conclusion of the injection, 24 hours later, and periodically thereafter, as indicated.

Apart from its diagnostic value in cases of unsuspected lymph node disease, lymphangiography offers a means of evaluating the presence and the extent of metastases in patients who are known to have cancer. Moreover, because lymphomatous lymph nodes retain the contrast medium for up to 1 year after the injection, any change in their size that may occur in response to irradiation or chemotherapy can be measured and used as a criterion in determining therapeutic effect.

Lymphangitis and Lymphadenitis

Lymphangitis is an acute inflammation of the lymphatic channels. It arises most commonly from a focus of infection in an extremity. Usually, the infectious organism is the hemolytic streptococcus. The characteristic red streaks that extend up the arm or the leg from an infected wound outline the course of the lymphatics as they drain.

The lymph nodes located along the course of the lymphatic channels also become enlarged, red, and tender (*acute lymphadenitis*), and can become necrotic and form an abscess (*suppurative lymphadenitis*). The nodes involved most often are those in the groin, the axilla, or the cervical region.

Because these infections are nearly always caused by organisms that are sensitive to antibiotics, it is unusual to see abscess formation. Recurrent episodes of lymphangitis are often associated with progressive lymphedema.

After acute attacks, elastic support should be worn on the affected extremity for several months to prevent long-term edema.

Lymphedema and Elephantiasis

Lymphedema is a swelling of tissues in the extremities due to an increased quantity of lymph that results from an obstruction of lymphatics. It is especially marked when the extremity is in a dependent position. Initially the edema is soft, pitting, and relieved by treatment. As the condition progresses, the edema becomes firm, nonpitting, and unresponsive to treatment. The most common type is congenital lymphedema (lymphedema praecox), which is caused by hypoplasia of the lymphatic system of the lower extremity. This disorder is usually seen in females, and appears first between the ages of 15 and 25 years.

The obstruction may be in both the lymph nodes and the lymphatic vessels. At times it is seen in the arm, after a radical mastectomy for carcinoma, and in the leg in association with varicose veins or a chronic phlebitis. In the latter case the lymphatic obstruction usually is due to a chronic lymphangitis. Lymphatic obstruction caused by a parasite (*Filaria*) is seen frequently in the tropics. When chronic swelling is present, there may be frequent bouts of acute infection characterized by high fever and chills and increased residual edema after the inflammation has resolved. These lead to chronic fibrosis, thickening of the subcutaneous tissues, and hypertrophy of the skin. This condition, in which chronic swelling of the extremity recedes only slightly with elevation, is given the name *elephantiasis*.

Management

Lymphedema is currently managed by three modes of therapy: physical therapy, coumarin, and surgery. Lymphatic fluid can be compressed manually from the soft tissues by squeezing the extremity distally. In this manner, drainage of fluid proximally can be accomplished. Active and passive exercises assist in the movement of lymphatic fluid into the bloodstream. Mechanical pulsatile air pressure devices are also available.

Coumarin and similar types of drugs remove proteins from the interstitial spaces. Removal of protein reduces tissue colloid osmotic pressure and allows the interstitial fluid to move back into the capillaries, thereby reducing lymphedema.

Diuretics have been used palliatively for lymphedema in conjunction with elevation and elastic compression of the affected extremity. However, the use of diuretics is controversial because their action is not to remove protein.

Surgical treatment of lymphedema is performed in order to reduce the size of the extremity and improve its appearance, to reduce the incidence of inflammatory episodes, and to limit secondary skin changes associated with chronic lymphedema. One surgical approach involves the excision of affected subcutaneous tissue and fascia, with skin grafting to cover the defect. Another procedure involves the transfer of superficial lymphatics into the deep lymphatic system by a buried dermal flap to provide a conduit for lymphatic drainage.

Postoperatively, the management of skin grafts and of flaps is the same as when these therapies are used for other conditions. Prophylactic antibiotics may be prescribed for 5 to 7 days. Constant elevation of the affected extremity and observations for complications are essential. Complications can include flap necrosis, hematoma or abscess under the flap, and cellulitis.

Bibliography

Books

Bates B. A Guide to Physical Examination, 4th ed. Philadelphia, JB Lippincott, 1987.

Cardiovascular Disorders. Nursing 84 Books. Springhouse, Pennsylvania, Springhouse Corporation, 1984.

Guzzetta CE and Dossey BM. Cardiovascular Nursing. Bodymind Tapestry. St Louis, CV Mosby, 1984.

Haimovici H. Vascular Surgery, 2nd ed. Norwalk, Appleton-Century-Crofts, 1984.

Jarrett F and Hirsch SA. Vascular Surgery of the Lower Extremity. St Louis, CV Mosby, 1985.

McMahon FG. Management of Essential Hypertension: The New Low-Dose Era, 2nd ed. Mount Kisco, New York, Futura Publishing Co, 1984.

Page IH. Hypertensive Mechanisms. Orlando, Grune & Stratton, 1987.

Rakel RE (ed). Conn's Current Therapy. Philadelphia, WB Saunders, 1988.

Rutherford RB (ed). Vascular Surgery, 2nd ed. Philadelphia, WB Saunders, 1984.

Sadler D. Nursing for Cardiovascular Health. Norwalk, Appleton-Century-Crofts, 1984.

Strandness DE (ed). Vascular Diseases: Current Research and Clinical Applications. Orlando, Grune & Stratton, 1987.

Underhill SL et al. Cardiac Nursing. Philadelphia, JB Lippincott, 1982.

Articles

General

Beaver BM. Health education and the patient with peripheral vascular disease. Nurs Clin North Am 1986 June; 21(2): 265–272.

Dalsing MC et al. Surgery of the aorta. Crit Care Quart 1985 Sept; 8(2): 25–38.

Doyle JE. Treatment modalities in peripheral vascular disease. Nurs Clin North Am 1986 June; 21(2):241–253.

Ekins MA. Psychosocial considerations in peripheral vascular disease: Cause or effect? Nurs Clin North Am 1986 June; 21(2):255–263.

Gallino A et al. Percutaneous transluminal angioplasty of the arteries of the lower limbs: A 5-year follow-up. Circulation 1984 Oct; 70(4): 619–623.

Kotler MN, Goldman AP, and Parry WR. Geriatric cardiology: Managing the most common nonischemic disorders. Geriatr 1986 June; 41(6): 45–53.

Marinelli-Miller D. What your patient wants to know about angiography—but may not ask. RN 1983 Nov; 46(11):52–54.

McCarthy WJ and Williams LR. Femoral artery reconstruction. Crit Care Quart 1985 Sept; 9(2):39–50.

Pairitz D. Peripheral vascular surgery: Postoperative assessment. AORN J 1984 Nov; 40(5):712–713.

Sands D and Holman E. Does knowledge enhance patient compliance? J Gerontol Nurs 1985 Apr; 11(4):23, 26–29.

Turner JA. Nursing intervention in patients with peripheral vascular disease. Nurs Clin North Am 1986 June; 21(2):233–240.

Wagner MM. Pathophysiology related to peripheral vascular disease. Nurs Clin North Am 1986 June; 21(2):195–205.

Walker S. Sympathectomy in peripheral vascular disease. Nursing 83 1983 Apr; 2(12):349, 351.

Anticoagulant and Thrombolytic Therapy

Blakely WP et al. Standard care plan for systemic administration of streptokinase. Crit Care Nurs 1983 Jul/Aug; 3(4):86–89.

Böttiger LE. Heparin-induced thrombocytopenia. Acta Med Scand 1985; 218(3):257–259.

Gever LN. Streptokinase and urokinase: Minimizing the risks of these thrombolytics. Nursing 83 1983 Jan; 13(1):76.

Gever LN. Anticoagulants . . . and what to teach your patient about them. Nursing 84 1984 Nov; 14(11):64.

Gray D et al. Development of an anticoagulation clinic. QRB 1983 Jan; 9(1):6–10.

Hattersley PG et al. Adjusting heparin infusion rates from the initial response to activated coagulation time. Drug Intell Clin Pharm 1983 Sept; 17(9):632–634.

McConnell EA. APTT and PT: Two common-but-important coagulation studies. Nursing 86 1986 May; 16(5):47–48.

Statland BE and Ito RK. Thrombolytic therapy: Minimizing the risks. Diagn Med 1984 Jan; 7(1):24–29.

Walsh PN. Oral anticoagulant therapy. Hosp Pract 1983 Jan; 18(1):101–105.

Arterial Conditions

Coffman JD. Principles of conservative treatment of occlusive arterial disease. Cardiovasc Clin 1983; 13(2):1–13.

Conner CS. Nifedipine: Two new uses. Drug Intell Clin Pharm 1983 June; 17(6):457–458.

Czapinski N et al. Nursing plan for abdominal aortic aneurysms. AORN J 1983 Feb; 37(2):205–208, 210.

Dale WA. Differential management of acute peripheral arterial ischemia. J Vasc Surg 1984 Mar; 1(2):269–278.

Imparato AM. Abdominal aortic aneurysms. Hosp Med 1983 Oct; 19(10): 211–219.

Lee G et al. Current and potential uses of lasers in the treatment of atherosclerotic disease. Chest 1984 Mar; 85(3):429–434.

Lusby RJ and Wylie EJ. Acute lower limb ischemia: Pathogenesis and management. World J Surg 1983 May; 7(3):340–346.

Memon AS. Raynaud's vasospasm. Hosp Pract 1983 May; 19(5):141, 144, 149–150.

Pairolero PC. Lower limb ischemia in young adults: Prognostic implications. J Vasc Surg 1984 May; 1(3):459–464.

Quinless F. P.V.D.: Physiology, signs, and symptoms. Nursing 84 1984 Mar; 14(3):52–53.

Russell J et al. Abdominal aortic aneurysm: Standard post-operative care. Crit Care Nurse 1983 May/June; 3(3):124, 126.

Warbinek E and Wyness MA. Designing nursing care for patients with peripheral arterial occlusive disease. Cardiovasc Nurs 1986 Jan/Feb; 22(1):1–5.

Warbinek E and Wyness MA. Peripheral arterial occlusive disease (Part II): Nursing assessment and standard care plans. Cardiovasc Nurs 1986 Mar/Apr; 22(2):6–10.

Whittemore AD et al. Treatment of arterial occlusion disease of the lower extremities. Annu Rev Med 1985; 36:505–514.

Zimmerman TA et al. Thoracoabdominal aortic aneurysms: Treatment and nursing interventions. Crit Care Nurse 1983 Nov/Dec; 3(6):54–63.

Assessment and Diagnosis

Bastarache MM et al. Assessing peripheral vascular disease: Noninvasive testing. Am J Nurs 1983 Nov; 83(11):1552–1556.

Baum PL. Taking the PVD patient's history. Nursing 86 1986 May; 16(5): 30–33.

Baum PL. Heed the early warning signs of PVD. Nursing 85 1985 Mar; 15(3):50–58.

Cudworth-Bergin KL. Detecting arterial problems with a Doppler stethoscope. RN 1984 Jan; 47(1):38–41.

Durbin N. The application of Doppler techniques in critical care. Focus Crit Care 1983 June; 10(3):44–46.

Fogarty TJ and Kinney TB. A new approach to transluminal angioplasty. Appl Radiol 1984 May/June; 13(3):25, 28, 31.

Gilfillan RS et al. The prediction of healing in ischemic lesions of the foot: A comparison of Doppler ultrasound and elevation reactive hyperemia. J Cardiovasc Surg 1985 Jan/Feb; 26(1):15–20.

Herman JA. Nursing assessment and nursing diagnosis in patients with peripheral vascular disease. Nurs Clin North Am 1986 June; 21(2): 219–231.

Hudson B. Sharpen your vascular assessment skills with Doppler ultrasound stethoscope. Nursing 83 1983 May; 13(5):54–57.

Long RL et al. Physical assessment: Peripheral vascular and lymphatic systems. Drug Intell Clin Pharm 1985 Apr; 19(4):252.

Malott JC and Fodor J. Digital vascular imaging: Two years of clinical experience. Radiol Technol 1983 Nov/Dec; 55(2):633–637.

Massey JA. Diagnostic testing for peripheral vascular disease. Nurs Clin North Am 1986 June; 21(2):207–218.

Mathewson M. A Homans's sign is an effective method of diagnosing thrombophlebitis in bedridden patients. Crit Care Nurse 1983 Jul/Aug; 3(4):64–65.

Peterson FY. Assessing peripheral vascular disease at the bedside. Am J Nurs 1983 Nov; 83(11):1549–1551.

Rogers H. Digital subtraction angiography: First 900 cases. Radiography 1984 Mar/Apr; 50(590):67–70.

Smalling RW and Gould KL. Cardiovascular imaging: Ischemia and reperfusion. Hosp Pract 1984 Mar; 19(3):163–178.

Spittell JA. Occlusive arterial disease: Noninvasive diagnostic techniques to use in the office. Consultant 1984 July; 24(7):214–227.

Tobis JM et al. Digital subtraction angiography. Chest 1983 July; 84(1):68–75.

Hypertension

Barker WH et al. Community surveillance of stroke in persons under 70 years old: Contribution of uncontrolled hypertension. Am J Public Health 1983 Mar; 73(3):260–265.

Black HR. Hypertension Therapy: Prescribe for compliance, simplify the regimen. Consultant 1984 Feb; 24(2):333–340.

Border WA. Recent advances in β-blocker therapy for hypertension. Hosp Formul 1984 Dec; 19(12):1120–1126.

Bursztyn M et al. Nifedipine in antihypertensive therapy. Arch Inter Med 1985 May; 145(5):953–954.

Cressman MD et al. Geriatric hypertension controversies (Part I): Initial Rx. Geriatrics 1985 Sept; 40(9):45–57.

Dickson E et al. A hypertension follow-up program. Nurs Health Care 1983 Nov; 4(9):598–599.

Forsyth RA. Hypertension: Criteria for diagnosis and for initiating therapy. Consultant 1984 Oct; 24(10):306–318.

Fouad FM et al. Pathophysiology and treatment of hypertension. Appl Cardiol 1984 Nov/Dec; 12(6):17–21.

Gwen B and Given CW. Adherence to hypertensive therapy. Geriatr Nurs 1983 May/June; 4(3):172–175.

Hinds C. A hypertension survey: Respondents' knowledge of high blood pressure. Int Nurs Rev 1983 Jan/Feb; 30(1):12–14.

Hulley SB et al. Systolic Hypertension in the Elderly Program (SHEP): The first three months. J Amer Gerontol Soc 1986 Feb; 34(2):101–105.

Kerr JAC. Adherence and self-care. Heart Lung 1985 Jan; 14(1):24–31.

Lakatta EG. Geriatric hypertension: Aggressive therapy and its physiologic rationale. Geriatrics 1986 May; 41(5):44–53.

Lapierre G et al. Evaluation of hypertensive therapy in a skilled nursing facility. Drug Intell Clin Pharm 1983 Jan; 17(1):39–44.

Mathewson MA. Current vasodilator therapy. Focus Crit Care 1983 Feb; 10(1):49–53.

McMahon M and Palmer RM. Exercise and hypertension. Med Clin North Am 1985 Jan; 69(1):57–70.

McMillan E et al. Patient compliance with anti-hypertensive drug therapy. Nursing 84 1984 June; 2(26):761–764.

Moriskey DE et al. Five-year blood pressure control and mortality following health education for hypertensive patients. Am J Public Health 1983 Feb; 73(2):153–162.

Plunkett LW and Dustan HP. Mild hypertension: The continuing dilemma of treatment. Fam Community Health 1984 May; 7(1):38–46.

Rocella EJ. Progress of and lessons learned from the national high blood pressure education program. Patient Educ Couns 1984; 6(3):103–104.

Rush DR et al. Hypertensive crisis. Top Emerg Med 1983 July; 5(2):58–74.

Sackett DL et al. Hypertension: Attacking the problem of low compliance. Consultant 1983 Jan; 23(1):287–297.

The 1984 Report of The Joint National Committee on Detection, Evaluation, and Treatment of High Blood Pressure. Arch Intern Med 1984 May; 144(5):1045–1057.

Wyka-Fitzgerald C et al. Long-term evaluation of group education for high blood pressure control. Cardiovasc Nurs 1984 May/June; 20(3):13–18.

Leg Ulcers

Cornwall JV. Guidelines to leg ulcer care. Nursing 83 1983 Mar; 2(11):317–319.

Doyle JE. All leg ulcers are not alike: Managing and preventing arterial and venous ulcers. Nursing 83 1983 Jan; 13(1):58–63.

Ivancin LA. Healing those frustrating stasis ulcers. RN 1983 Aug; 46(8):38–40, 68.

Solid R. Give venous leg ulcers the boot . . . Unna's boot. Nursing 84 1984 Nov; 14(11):52–53.

Varicose Veins

Baron HC. Varicose veins: Definitive therapy and preventive measures both have a place. Consultant 1983 May; 23(5):108–118.

Gage AM et al. Varicose veins: To treat or not to treat. Hosp Med 1983 Sept; 19(9):97–108.

Green S et al. Varicose veins. Nursing 84 1984 June; 2(26):778–781.

Thompson NW. The diagnosis and treatment of varicose veins. NAPT J 1985 Jan/Feb; 17–23.

Venous Conditions

Brown SA. Venous Thrombosis: Another complication of cancer. Oncol Nurs Forum 1983 Spring; 10(2):41–47.

Fahey VA. An indepth look at deep vein thrombosis. Nursing 84 1984 Mar; 14(3):34–41.

Fahey VA et al. Venous reconstruction: Surgery for severe venous stasis. AORN J 1985 Feb; 41(2):423–429.

Moser KM and Fedullo PF. Venous thromboembolism: Three simple decisions (Part 1). Chest 1983 Jan; 83(1):117–121.

Moser KM and Fedullo PF. Venous thromboembolism: Three simple decisions (Part 2). Chest 1983 Feb; 83(2):256–260.

Taylor DL. Thrombophlebitis: Physiology, signs, and symptoms. Nursing 83 1983 July; 13(7):52–53.

Thomas DP. Venous thrombogenesis. Annu Rev Med 1985; 36:39–50.

Tikoff G. Axioms on venous thrombosis. Hosp Med 1984 Apr; 20(4):13–19.

Turpie AGG et al. Venous thromboembolism: Current concepts (Part 1). Hosp Med 1984 Oct; 20(10):151–159.

Turpie AGG et al. Venous thromboembolism: Current concepts (Part 2). Hosp Med 1984 Nov; 20(11):13–20.

Agencies

Joint National Commission on Detection, Evaluation and Treatment of High Blood Pressure; National Heart, Lung and Blood Institute; National Institutes of Health, Bldg 31, Rm 4A28, Bethesda, MD 20892.

National Heart, Lung and Blood Institute; National Institutes of Health, Bldg 31, Rm 5A52, Bethesda, MD 20205.

Chapter 29

Assessment and Management of Patients With Hematologic Disorders

Glossary

Agranulocytosis — acute disease in which the white blood cell count decreases to extremely low levels and neutropenia is pronounced

Aplasia — failure of an organ or tissue to develop normally

Band cell — immature granulocyte

Basophil — a granular leukocyte

Ecchymosis — a blue black macula that results from seepage of blood into skin or mucous membrane

Eosinophil — a granular leukocyte

Erythrocyte — red blood cell

Erythropoiesis — the formation of red blood cells

Erythropoietin — hormone that regulates red blood cell production

Glossitis — inflammation of the tongue

Granulocyte — granular leukocyte: polymorphonuclear leukocyte (neutrophil, basophil, or eosinophil)

Granulocytopenia — abnormal reduction of granulocytes in the blood

Hematocrit — fraction of the blood occupied by erythrocytes

Hematopoiesis — production and development of blood cells

Hematopoietic — blood-producing

Hemoglobin — iron-containing pigment of red blood cells

Hemolysis — destruction of red blood cells with liberation of hemoglobin into the surrounding fluid

Histiocyte — cell of loose connective tissue that shows phagocytic activity

Hyperplasia — excessive proliferation of normal cells in normal tissue

Hypochromia — blood possessing less than normal color and hemoglobin content

Leukocyte — white blood cell

Leukopenia — abnormal decrease of white blood cells

Lymphocyte — a mononuclear leukocyte

Lysis — disintegration or dissolution of cells

Macrocyte — a large-sized red blood cell

Macrophage — cells of the reticuloendothelial system that have the ability to phagocytose particulate matter

Megaloblast — abnormally large red blood cells

Microcyte — a small-sized red blood cell

Monocyte — a mononuclear leukocyte

Mononuclear leukocyte — agranulocyte (lymphocyte, monocyte)

Neutrophil — a granular leukocyte

Normochromic — normal color of cells

Normocytic — normal size of cells

Oxyhemoglobin — hemoglobin combined with oxygen

Pancytopenia — reduction in all cellular elements of the blood

Petechiae — small red or purple hemorrhagic spots on the skin

Phagocytosis — the process of ingestion and digestion of bacteria and particles

Plasma — liquid part of the blood

Platelet — thrombocyte; cell fragment found in the blood that plays an important role in coagulation, hemostasis, and thrombus formation

Reticulocyte — immature red blood cell

Reticuloendothelial system — cells scattered throughout the body that have the ability to phagocytose particulate matter (bacteria, colloidal particles)

Serum — the watery portion of the blood that remains after coagulation

Spherocyte — an erythrocyte that assumes a spheroid shape

Thrombocyte — platelet

Thrombocytopenia — abnormal decrease in number of platelets

Physiologic Overview

The hematologic system consists of the blood and the sites where blood is produced, including the bone marrow and lymph nodes. The blood is a specialized organ that differs from other organs in that it exists in a fluid state. The fluid consists of cellular components suspended in blood plasma. The blood cells are divided into *erythrocytes* (red blood cells, normally 5 million per mm³ of blood) and *leukocytes* (white blood cells, normally 5,000–10,000 per mm³ of blood). There are approximately 500–1000 erythrocytes for each leukocyte. Also suspended in the plasma are small, nonnucleated cell fragments called *platelets* (normally 150,000–450,000 platelets per mm³ of blood). These cellular components of blood normally make up 40% to 45% of the blood volume. The fraction of the blood occupied by erythrocytes is called the *hematocrit*. Blood appears as a thick, opaque, red fluid. Its color is imparted by the hemoglobin contained within the red blood cells.

The volume of blood in humans is approximately 7% to 10% of the normal body weight, which represents about 5 liters. The blood is recirculated through the vascular system and serves as a link between body organs, carrying oxygen absorbed from the lungs and nutrients absorbed from the gastrointestinal tract to the body cells for cellular metabolism.

The blood also carries waste products produced by cellular metabolism to the lungs, skin, liver, and kidneys for subsequent transformation and elimination from the body. It also carries hormones, antibodies, and other products of internal secretion to their sites of action or utilization.

In order to perform its functions, blood must remain in its normally fluid state. Because it is fluid, the danger always exists that trauma can lead to loss of blood from the vascular system. To prevent this, the blood has an intricate clotting mechanism that is activated when necessary to seal leaks in the blood vessels.

Excessive clotting is equally dangerous because it potentially obstructs blood flow to vital tissues. To prevent this complication, the body has a fibrinolytic mechanism that eventually dissolves the clots formed within blood vessels.

Bone Marrow

The bone marrow occupies the interior of spongy bones and the central cavity of the long bones of the skeleton. The marrow accounts for 4% to 5% of the total body weight and therefore is one of the larger organs of the body. The marrow can be either red or yellow. Red marrow is the site of active blood cell production and constitutes the major *hematopoietic* (blood-producing) organ. Yellow marrow, on the other hand, is composed mainly of fat and is not active in the production of blood elements. During childhood, the major portion of the marrow is red. As a person ages, a large portion of the marrow in the long bones is converted into yellow marrow, but it retains the potential for reversion to hematopoietic tissue if necessary. Red marrow in the adult is confined chiefly to the ribs, vertebral column, and other flat bones.

The marrow is a highly vascularized organ that consists of connective tissue containing free cells. The most primitive of this population of free cells are the stem cells, which are precursors of two different cell lines. The *myeloid line* includes erythrocytes, several types of leukocytes, and platelets. The *lymphoid line* differentiates into lymphocytes.

Erythrocytes

The normal red blood cell is a biconcave disc, its configuration resembling that of a soft ball compressed between two fingers. It has a diameter of about 8 microns but is a very flexible cell, so flexible that it is capable of passing easily through capillaries that may be as small as 4 microns in diameter. The volume of a red blood cell is about 90 cubic microns. The red blood cell membrane is so thin that gases such as oxygen and carbon dioxide can easily diffuse across it. Mature red blood cells consist primarily of hemoglobin, which makes up 95% of the cell mass. These cells have no nuclei and have many fewer metabolic enzymes than do most other cells. The presence of a large amount of hemoglobin enables the cell to perform its principal function, the transport of oxygen between lungs and tissues.

The oxygen-carrying pigment *hemoglobin* is a protein with a molecular weight of 64,000. The molecule is made up of four subunits, each containing a heme portion attached to a globin chain. Iron is present in the heme component of the molecule. An important property of the heme portion is its ability to bind to oxygen loosely and reversibly. When hemoglobin is combined with oxygen, it is called *oxyhemoglobin*. Oxyhemoglobin has a brighter red color than hemoglobin that does not contain oxygen (*reduced hemoglobin*), so arterial blood is a brighter red than venous blood. Whole blood normally contains about 15 gm of hemoglobin per 100 ml of blood (150 gm/L), or 30 μg of hemoglobin per million erythrocytes.

Production of Erythrocytes (Erythropoiesis). Erythroblasts arise from the primitive stem cells in bone marrow. The erythroblast is a nucleated cell that in the process of maturing within the bone marrow accumulates hemoglobin and gradually loses its nucleus. At this stage, the cell is known as a *reticulocyte*. Further maturation into an erythrocyte entails the loss of dark staining material and a slight shrinkage in size. The mature erythrocyte is then released into the circulation. Under conditions of rapid *erythropoiesis*, reticulocytes and other immature cells may be released prematurely into the circulation.

Differentiation of the primitive multipotential stem cell of the marrow into an erythroblast is stimulated by *erythropoietin*, a substance produced mostly by the kidney. Under conditions of prolonged hypoxia, as in the case of persons dwelling at high altitudes or after severe hemorrhage, erythropoietin levels are increased and red blood cell production is stimulated.

For normal erythrocyte production, the bone marrow requires iron, vitamin B_{12}, folic acid, pyridoxine (vitamin B_6), and other factors. If any of these factors is deficient during erythropoiesis, decreased red blood cell production and anemia result.

Iron Stores and Metabolism. Total body iron content in the average adult is approximately 3 gm, most of which is present in hemoglobin or one of its breakdown products. Normally, about 0.5 mg to 1 mg of iron is absorbed per day from the intestinal tract to replace losses of iron in the feces. Additonal amounts of iron, up to 2 mg per day, must be absorbed by the adult female to replace blood lost during menstruation. Iron deficiency in the adult (decreased total body iron content) generally indicates that blood has been lost from the body—for example, by hemorrhage or excessive menstruation.

The concentration of iron in blood is normally about 80–180 μg/dL (14–32 μmol/L) for men and 60–160 μg/dL (11–29 μmol/L) for women. With iron deficiency, bone marrow iron stores are rapidly depleted, hemoglobin synthesis is depressed, and the red blood cells produced by the marrow are small and low in hemoglobin.

Vitamin B_{12} and Folic Acid Metabolism. Vitamin B_{12} and folic acid are required for DNA synthesis in many tissues, but deficiencies of either of these vitamins has the greatest effect on erythropoiesis. Vitamin B_{12} or folic acid deficiency is characterized by the production of abnormally large red blood cells (called *megaloblasts*). Because these cells are abnormal, many are sequestered in the bone marrow and their rate of release is decreased. This condition results in megaloblastic anemia.

Both vitamin B_{12} and folic acid are derived from the diet. Vitamin B_{12} combines with intrinsic factor produced in the stomach. The vitamin B_{12}-intrinsic factor complex is absorbed in the distal ileum. Folic acid is absorbed in the proximal small intestine.

Red Blood Cell Destruction. The average lifespan of a circulating red blood cell is 120 days. Aged red blood cells are removed from the blood by the reticuloendothelial system, particularly in the liver and the spleen. The reticuloendothelial cells produce a pigment called bilirubin from the hemoglobin that is released from the destroyed red blood cells. *Bilirubin* is a waste product that is excreted in the bile. The iron, freed from the hemoglobin during bilirubin formation, is carried in plasma bound to the protein called *transferrin* to the bone marrow, where it is reclaimed for production of new hemoglobin.

Function of Erythrocytes. The major function of the red blood cells is to transport oxygen from the lungs to the tissues. Erythrocytes are uniquely capable of performing this function because of their high concentration of hemoglobin. If hemoglobin were not present, the oxygen-carrying capacity of blood would be decreased by 99% and would not be sufficient to meet the metabolic needs of the body. An important property of hemoglobin is that it binds oxygen loosely and reversibly. As a result, oxygen readily binds to hemoglobin in the lungs, is carried as oxyhemoglobin in arterial blood, and readily dissociates from hemoglobin in the tissues. In venous blood, hemoglobin combines with hydrogen ions produced by cellular metabolism and thus buffers excess acid.

Leukocytes

Leukocytes are divided into two general categories, granulocytes and mononuclear cells (agranulocytes). In normal blood, the total leukocyte count is 5,000 to 10,000 cells per cubic millimeter. Of these, approximately 60% are granulocytes and 40% are mononuclear cells. Leukocytes can be readily differentiated from erythrocytes by the presence of a nucleus, their larger size, and different staining properties.

Granulocytes. Granulocytes are defined by the presence of granules in their cytoplasm. The diameter of a granulocyte is generally two to three times that of an erythrocyte. Granulocytes are divided into three subgroups, which are characterized by their staining properties as seen on microscopic examination. *Eosinophils* have bright red granules in their cytoplasm, whereas the granules in *basophils* stain deep blue. The third, and by far the most numerous, cell in this series is the *neutrophil*, with granules that show a dull violet hue. The nucleus of the mature granulocyte generally has multiple lobes (usually two to four) connected by thin filaments of nuclear material. Because of their nuclear characteristics, these cells are called *polymorphonuclear* (PMN) leukocytes. The immature granulocyte has a single-lobed ovoid nucleus and is called a *band cell*. Ordinarily, band forms account for only a small percentage of circulating granulocytes, although their percentage can increase greatly under conditions in which the rate of production of polymorphonuclear leukocytes is increased. The number of circulating granulocytes found in the healthy person is maintained relatively constant, but in the presence of infection large numbers of these cells are rapidly released into the circulation. Granulocyte production from the stem cell pool is thought to be controlled in a manner similar to the regulation of erythrocyte production by erythropoietin.

Mononuclear Leukocytes (Agranulocytes). Mononuclear leukocytes (lymphocytes and monocytes) are white blood cells with a single-lobed nucleus and a granule-free cytoplasm. In normal adult blood, lymphocytes account for approximately 30% and monocytes approximately 5% of the total leukocytes. Mature *lymphocytes* are small cells with scanty cytoplasm. They are produced primarily in the lymph nodes and in the lymphoid tissue of the intestine, spleen, and thymus gland from precursor cells that originated as marrow stem cells. *Monocytes* are the largest of the blood leukocytes. They are produced by the bone marrow and give rise to tissue histiocytes, including Kupffer cells of the liver, peritoneal macrophages, alveolar macrophages, and other components of the reticuloendothelial system.

Function of the Leukocytes. The function of the leukocytes is to protect the body from invasion by bacteria and other foreign entities. The major function of neutrophilic polymorphonuclear leukocytes is to ingest foreign material (phagocytosis). Neutrophils arrive at the site within an hour of the onset of an inflammatory reaction and initiate phagocytosis, but are relatively short-lived. The influx of monocytes is later, but these cells continue their phagocytic activities for long periods.

The function of lymphocytes is primarily to produce substances that aid in the attack of foreign material. One group of lymphocytes (T-lymphocytes) kills foreign cells directly or releases a variety of *lymphokines*, substances that enhance the activity of phagocytic cells. The other group of lymphocytes (B-lymphocytes) produces antibodies, protein molecules that destroy foreign material by several mechanisms.

Eosinophils and basophils function as reservoirs of potent biological materials such as histamine, serotonin, and heparin. Release of these compounds alters the blood supply to tissues, such as occurs during inflammation, and helps to mobilize body defense mechanisms. The increase in the number of eosinophils in allergic states indicates that these cells are involved in the hypersensitivity reaction.

Platelets

Platelets are small particles, 2 to 4 microns in diameter, that are present in the circulating blood plasma. Because they disintegrate quickly and easily, their number varies normally between 150,000 and 450,000 per cubic millimeter of blood, depending on the numbers that are produced, how they are used, and how quickly they are destroyed. They are formed from the fragmentation (the pinching off of bits of membrane and cytoplasm) of giant cells of the bone marrow, called *megakaryocytes*. Platelet production is regulated by thrombopoietin.

Platelets play an essential role in the control of bleeding. When vascular injury occurs, platelets collect at the site. Substances released from platelet granules and other blood cells cause the platelets to adhere to each other and form a patch or plug, which temporarily stops bleeding. Additional substances released from platelets activate coagulation factors in the blood plasma.

Blood Coagulation

Blood coagulation is the process whereby the components of the liquid blood are transformed into a semisolid material called a *blood clot*. The blood clot is composed mainly of blood cells entrapped in a meshwork of fibrin. Fibrin is formed

TABLE 29-1
Clotting Factors

Official Number	Synonym	Contemporary Version	
I	Fibrinogen	I	(fibrinogen)
II	Prothrombin	II	(prothrombin)
III	Tissue thromboplastin	III	(tissue factor)
IV	Calcium	IV	(calcium)
V	Labile factor	V	(labile factor)
		VI	PF_3 (platelet coagulant activities)
		VI	PF_4
VII	Stable factor	VII	(stable factor)
VIII	Antihemophilic factor	VIII	AHF (antihemophilic factor)
		VIII	VWF (von Willebrand factor)
		VIII	RAg (related antigen)
IX	Christmas factor	IX	(Christmas factor)
X	Stuart-Power factor	X	(Stuart-Power factor)
XI	Plasma thromboplastin (antecedent)	XI	(plasma thromboplastin antecedent)
XII	Hageman factor	XII	HF (Hageman factor)
		XII	PK (Prekallikrein, Fletcher)
		XII	HMWK (high molecular weight kininogen)
XIII	Fibrin stabilizing factor	XIII	fibrin stabilizing factor

The Roman numerals and synonyms designating each clotting factor accepted by the International Committee on Blood Clotting Factors are located in the left-hand columns. Note the absence of factor VI. The version in the right-hand column incorporates more recently recognized clotting factors but is not officially recognized.

(Green D. General considerations of coagulation proteins. Ann Clin Lab Sci 8[2]:95–105.)

from proteins in the plasma as the result of a complex series of reactions.

Many factors are involved in the reaction cascade that forms fibrin. The clotting factors are listed in Table 29-1, and the extrinsic and intrinsic pathways for fibrin generation are shown diagrammatically in Figure 29-1. When tissue is injured, the extrinsic pathway is activated by the release from the tissue of a substance called thromboplastin. As the result of a series of reactions, prothrombin is converted to thrombin, which in turn catalyzes the conversion of fibrinogen to fibrin. Calcium (factor IV) is a necessary cofactor for many of these reactions. Clotting by the intrinsic pathway is activated when the collagen lining blood vessels is exposed. Clotting factors are then activated sequentially until, as with the extrinsic pathway, fibrin is ultimately formed. Although longer, this sequence is probably most often responsible for clotting *in vivo*. The intrinsic pathway is also responsible for initiating the clotting of blood that comes into contact with glass or other foreign surfaces, as when blood is withdrawn from the body into a test tube. It is for this reason that anticoagulants must often be used when drawing blood for chemical or other tests. The anticoagulants usually used are either citrate, which binds the plasma calcium, or heparin, which prevents the conversion of prothrombin to thrombin. Citrate cannot be used as an anticoagulant *in vivo* because binding of plasma

calcium would cause death. Heparin can be used clinically as an anticoagulant. Coumarins are also used clinically for their anticoagulant action of interfering with the production of several of the plasma coagulating factors.

Clots that form in the body are eventually dissolved by the action of the fibrinolytic system, which consists of plasmin and other proteolytic enzymes. Through the action of this system, clots are dissolved as tissue is repaired, and the vascular system is returned to its normal baseline state.

Blood Plasma

After cellular elements are removed from blood, the remaining liquid portion is called blood plasma. It contains ions, proteins, and other substances. If plasma is allowed to clot, the remaining fluid is called *serum*. Serum has essentially the same composition as plasma except that its fibrinogen and several of the clotting factors have been removed.

Plasma Proteins. Plasma proteins consist primarily of albumin and globulins. The globulins in turn consist of alpha, beta, and gamma fractions derived by a laboratory test called *serum protein electrophoresis*. Each of these groups is made up of distinct proteins. The gamma globulins, which consist mainly of antibodies, are called *immunoglobulins*. These proteins are produced by the lymphocytes and plasma cells. Im-

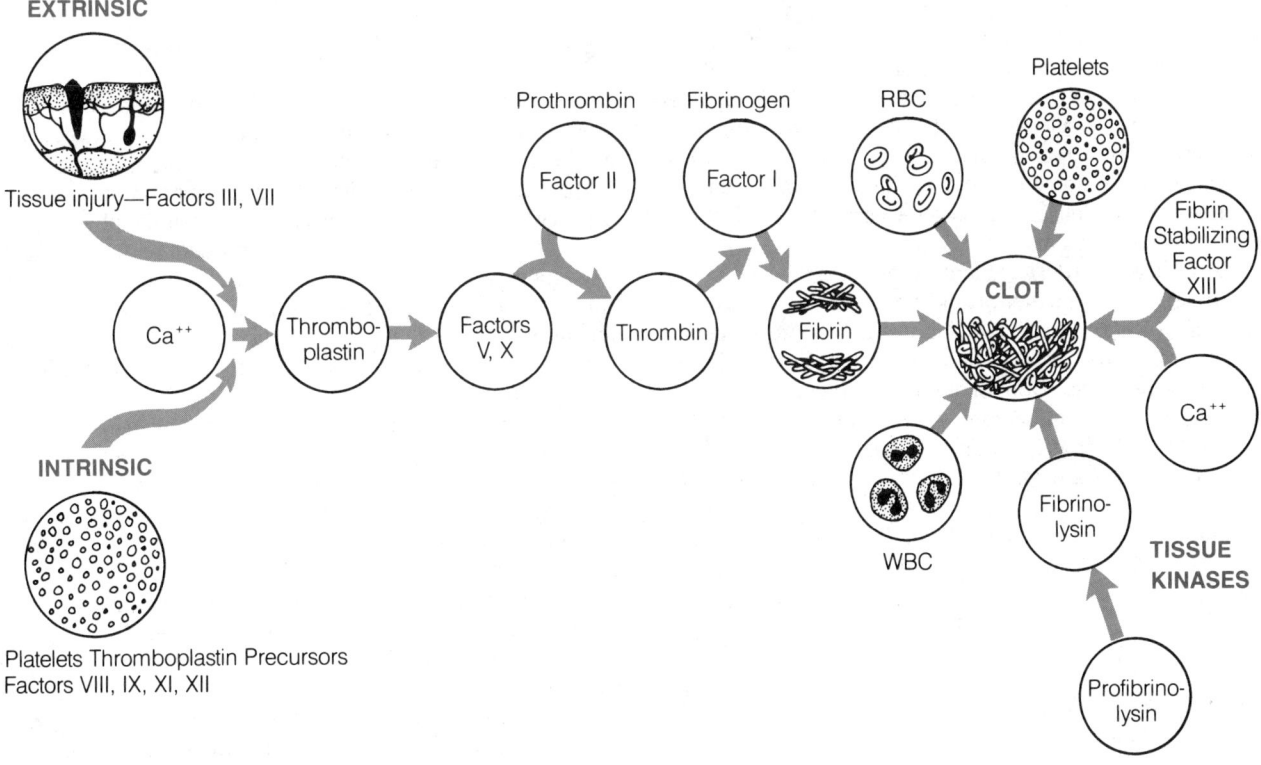

Figure 29-1

The blood-clotting mechanism. The schematic drawing represents the factors essential to change blood into a solid gel. The entire chain reaction in which fibrinogen (a plasma protein) is converted to fibrin (the clot) takes place at the site of vessel damage. (Adapted from Feller I and Archambeault C. Nursing the Burn Patient. Ann Arbor, Michigan, The Institute for Burn Medicine.)

portant proteins in the alpha and beta fractions are the transport globulins and the clotting factors, which are made in the liver. The transport globulins carry various substances in bound form around the circulation. For example, thyroid-binding globulin carries thyroxin, and transferrin carries iron. The clotting factors, including fibrinogen, remain in an inactive form in the blood plasma until activated by the clotting cascade.

Albumin is particularly important for the maintenance of fluid volume within the vascular system. Capillary walls are impermeable to albumin, so its presence in the plasma creates an osmotic force that keeps fluid within the vascular space. Albumin, which is produced in the liver, has the capacity to bind to a number of substances that are often present in plasma. In this way, it functions as a transport protein for metals, fatty acids, bilirubin, and drugs, among other substances.

Pathophysiology of the Hematologic System

Anemias. A frequent disorder of the hematologic system is a decrease in the number of circulating red blood cells. This condition, called *anemia,* can result from either underproduction of red blood cells by the bone marrow or increased destruction of circulating red blood cells. Underproduction of red blood cells can be due to a deficiency in cofactors for erythropoiesis, including folic acid, vitamin B_{12}, and iron. Red blood cell production may also be reduced if bone marrow is suppressed (by tumor or drugs) or is inadequately stimulated due to lack of erythropoietin, as occurs in chronic renal disease. Increased destruction of red blood cells may occur because of an overactive reticuloendothelial system (*e.g.,* hypersplenism) or because the bone marrow produces abnormal red blood cells (*e.g.,* sickle cell anemia). Because the red blood cell and its contained hemoglobin are important for the delivery of oxygen to tissues, anemias may result in tissue hypoxia.

Bleeding Disorders. Bleeding disorders can be attributed to deficiency in either platelets or clotting factors in the circulating blood. Platelet function in the blood plasma can be reduced as the result of bone marrow insufficiency, increased splenic destruction, or abnormal circulating platelets. Deficiencies of clotting factors are usually due to underproduction of these factors by the liver. Hemophilia is a hereditary disorder that results from deficiency of clotting factors VIII and IX.

Manifestations of Blood Disorders. Problems commonly seen in patients with blood disorders are outlined in Chart 29-1.

Blood Study Procedures

Methods of Obtaining Blood

Venipuncture. Most routine hematologic studies are performed on venous blood, which is usually obtained from an antecubital vein. Occasionally, in very obese persons or those whose veins have been thrombosed by chemotherapy, it may be necessary to puncture one of the veins on the dorsum of the hand.

After a tourniquet has been applied around the upper arm, the arm and hand veins become prominent. The vein chosen for venipuncture should be straight, not tortuous, and should be well fixed in the subcutaneous tissue so that it does not roll away. The skin below the vein is stretched with one hand while the opposite hand is used to push the needle through the skin and then slowly into the vein. Blood is immediately placed in the collection tube appropriate for the particular test required. The tubes are color coded to specify what, if any, additive they contain. For some tests the blood is allowed to coagulate; for others it is kept fluid by the presence of an anticoagulant in the collection tube.

Finger Puncture. The finger puncture method is used frequently for blood smears and counts. This method utilizes capillary blood, but for practical purposes the results are identical to those obtained with venous blood. Lances of various shapes are available. These make a puncture of 1 mm to 2 mm. Best results are obtained if the patient's hand is warm and if the pulp of the index or middle finger is punctured. The skin should be cleaned with alcohol first and then carefully wiped dry with a lint-free sponge. If any alcohol remains, it will alter red cell morphology. The drops of blood obtained by this method can be gently touched to glass slides or cover slips, for peripheral smears. Capillary blood can also be drawn into calibrated red cell and white cell pipettes and into microhematocrit tubes.

The most common hematologic tests are described in Chart 29-2.

Bone Marrow Aspiration

Bone marrow is usually aspirated from the sternum or iliac crest in adults. Most patients need no more preparation than a careful explanation of the procedure but, for some very anxious patients, meperidine (Demerol) or a minor tranquilizer may be useful. It is always important for the physician or nurse to describe and explain the procedure as it is being performed. First, the skin area is cleansed as for any minor surgery. Then a small area is anesthetized with lidocaine (Xylocaine), through the skin and subcutaneous tissue to the periosteum of the bone. The bone marrow needle is introduced with a stylet in place. When the needle is felt to go through the outer cortex of bone and enter the marrow cavity, the stylet is removed, a syringe is attached, and a small volume (0.5 ml) of blood and marrow is aspirated. The actual aspiration always causes brief pain, and the patient should be warned of this. Taking deep breaths or using relaxation techniques often helps.

If a bone marrow biopsy is necessary, it is best performed after the aspiration and with a special needle. Several types of needles are available, the procedure varying according to the type of needle used. Because these needles are large, the skin should be punctured first with a surgical blade (No. 9 or 11) to make a 3-mm or 4-mm incision. Only the iliac bone is used for this procedure (Fig. 29-2, p. 671), because the sternum is too thin.

The major hazard of these procedures is a slight risk of hemorrhage. This risk is increased if the patient's platelet count is low. Following bone marrow aspiration, pressure should be applied to the site for several minutes. After a biopsy, pressure is applied to the posterior iliac crest for 60 minutes by the combination of a pressure dressing and having

Chart 29-1
Common Problems of Patients With Blood Disorders

Problem	Nursing Interventions
Fatigue and weakness	Plan nursing care to conserve the patient's strength and emotional energy. Give frequent rest periods. Encourage ambulation activities as tolerated. Avoid disturbing activities, noise, and stress. Encourage optimal nutrition—high-protein and high-calorie foods and drinks.
Hemorrhagic tendencies	Keep the patient at rest during the bleeding episodes. Apply gentle pressure to the bleeding sites. Apply cold compresses to the bleeding sites when indicated. Do not disturb clots. Use small-gauge needles when administering medications by injection. Support the patient during transfusion therapy. Observe for symptoms of internal bleeding. Have a tracheostomy set available for the patient who is bleeding from the mouth or the throat.
Ulcerative lesions of the tongue, gums, or mucous membranes	Avoid irritating foods and beverages. Give frequent oral hygiene with mild, cool mouthwash solutions. Use applicators or soft-bristled toothbrush. Keep the lips lubricated. Give mouth care both before and after meals. Encourage regular visits to the dentist.
Dyspnea	Elevate the head of the bed. Use pillows to support the patient in the orthopneic position. Administer oxygen when indicated. Prevent unnecessary exertion. Avoid gas-forming foods.
Bone and joint pains	Relieve pressure of bedding by using a cradle. Administer either hot or cold compresses as prescribed. Administer analgesic as prescribed on a regular basis. Provide for joint immobilization when prescribed.
Fever	Administer cool sponges. Give antipyretic (acetaminophen) drugs as prescribed. Encourage fluid intake unless contraindicated. Maintain a cool environmental temperature.
Pruritus or skin eruptions	Keep the patient's fingernails short. Use soap sparingly. Apply emollient lotions in skin care.
Anxiety of the patient and family	Explain the nature, the discomforts, and the limitations of activity associated with the diagnostic procedures and treatments. Offer the patient the service of listening. Provide an atmosphere of acceptance and understanding. Promote the patient's relaxation and comfort. Remember the patient's individual preferences. Promote independence and self-care within the patient's limitations. Encourage the family to participate in the patient's care (as desired). Create a comfortable atmosphere for family visits with the patient.

Chart 29-2
Common Hematologic Laboratory Tests

Test	Definition
Complete blood count	Includes enumeration of number of white cells, red cells, and platelets per cubic millimeter of venous blood, as well as a differential count, percentage of each type of nucleated cell in the blood (*i.e.,* percent polymorphonuclears, percent lymphocytes, and so on).
Reticulocyte count	Percentage of young (1–2 days old), nonnucleated erythrocytes in peripheral blood; they are recognized in special stains of blood smears as cells with lacy inclusions, which consist of RNA.
Hemoglobin electrophoresis	A drop of blood placed on a solid medium (paper, starch block, gel, or cellulose acetate) is exposed to a current of electricity while being bathed by a buffer solution. The different hemoglobins (*e.g.,* A, A-2, F, S) travel at varying speeds, depending on their charge. At the end of the procedure, the paper or gel is stained, and the hemoglobins in each sample can be identified.
Sickling test	A drop of blood is mixed with a drop of a reducing agent (sodium metabisulfite). This substance deprives the red cells of oxygen and induces sickling if S hemoglobin is present. Sickling of red cells is observed under the microscope in 30 minutes if the blood was obtained from a person with either sickle trait or sickle cell anemia. Normal blood does not undergo any change.
Leukocyte alkaline phosphatase (LAP)	LAP is an enzyme present in high concentrations in granules of neutrophils. A special stain of peripheral blood smears is used to estimate the amount of LAP present per cell. The normal score is 20 to 130. Untreated chronic myelogenous leukemia patients have scores of less than 20, and the test is useful to help diagnose CML. High scores are seen in infection and steroid-induced leukocytosis.
Coombs's test	Determines the presence of immune globulin (hence, antibodies) on the surface of erythrocytes (direct Coombs's test) or in the plasma (indirect Coombs's test)
Bleeding time	A screening test for disorders of platelet function. It is the time taken for bleeding to cease after a standardized skin wound is produced, usually on the volar surface of the forearm. A prolonged time suggests an inherited or acquired platelet defect, *e.g.,* von Willebrand's disease or aspirin ingestion.
Platelet aggregation	A measure of the time and completeness of the formation of platelet aggregates in a sample of plasma, after the addition of an agent such as epinephrine or ADP.
Prothrombin time test	Measures the coagulant activity of the "extrinsic" system, including fibrinogen, prothrombin, and factors V, VII, and X. It is used to monitor therapy of coumarin derivatives, as well as for a screening test for liver disease.
Partial thromboplastin time test	A screening test for deficiencies of all plasma coagulation factors except VII and XIII. It is usually considered abnormally prolonged if levels of factors are less than 30% of normal. It is often used to monitor heparin therapy.

---

the patient lie recumbent in bed. Most patients have no discomfort after a bone marrow aspiration, but the site of a biopsy may ache for a day or two.

Anemia

Definition and Etiology

Anemia is a laboratory term that indicates a low red cell count and a below normal hemoglobin or hematocrit level. It is not a disease, but rather reflects a disease state or altered body function. Physiologically, anemia exists when there is an insufficient amount of hemoglobin to deliver oxygen to the tissues.

There are many different kinds of anemias. Some are due to inadequate production of red blood cells, while others are due to premature or excessive destruction of red blood cells. The most common cause is blood loss, but other etiologic factors include deficits in iron and other nutrients, hereditary factors, and chronic diseases.

Pathophysiology

The appearance of anemia reflects either marrow failure or excessive red cell loss, or both. Marrow failure (*i.e.,* reduced erythropoiesis) may occur as a result of a nutritional deficiency, toxic exposure, tumor invasion, or, as in many instances, from causes unknown. Red cells may be lost through hemorrhage or hyperhemolysis (increased destruction). In the latter case the problem may be rooted in some red cell defect that is incompatible with normal red cell survival or explainable on the basis of some factor extrinsic to the red cell that promotes red cell destruction.

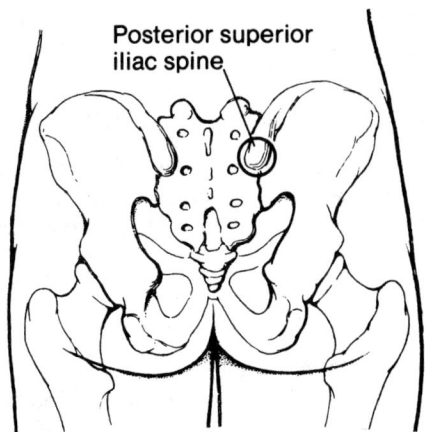

Posterior superior
iliac spine

Figure 29-2
Site of bone marrow biopsy.

Red cell lysis (dissolution) occurs mainly within the phagocytic cells of the reticuloendothelial system, notably in the liver and spleen. As a by-product of this process, bilirubin, formed within the phagocyte, enters the bloodstream, and any increase in hemolysis is promptly reflected by an increase in plasma bilirubin. (This concentration normally is 1 mg/dl or less; levels above 1.5 mg/dl produce visible jaundice of the sclerae.)

If, as happens in certain specific hemolytic disorders, red cells are destroyed within the circulating bloodstream, hemoglobin itself appears in the plasma (*hemoglobinemia*). If its concentration there exceeds the capacity of the plasma haptoglobin to bind it all (*i.e.,* if the amount is more than about 100 mg/dl), then this pigment is free to diffuse through the renal glomeruli and into the urine (*hemoglobinuria*). Thus, the presence or absence of hemoglobinemia and hemoglobinuria provides information about the location of abnormal blood destruction in a patient with hemolysis and can be a clue to the nature of the hemolytic process.

A conclusion as to whether the anemia in a particular patient is caused by hemolysis or by inadequate erythropoiesis usually can be reached on the basis of (1) the reticulocyte count in the circulating blood; (2) the degree to which young red cells are proliferating in the bone marrow and the manner in which they are maturing, as observed on biopsy, and (3) the presence or absence of hyperbilirubinemia and hemoglobinemia. Moreover, erythropoiesis can actually be quantitated by measuring the rate at which injected radioactive iron is incorporated into circulating erythrocytes. The life span of the patient's red cells (therefore, the hemolytic rate) can be measured by tagging a portion of these with radioactive chromium, reinjecting them, and following their disappearance from the circulating blood over the course of the ensuing days or weeks. Methods by which one particular type of marrow failure can be distinguished from another type, and one hemolytic disease from another, are specified in relation to each of the conditions discussed.

Gerontological Considerations. Anemia is common in older persons and is the most common hematologic condition that affects the elderly, but studies indicate that the aging process does not cause changes in hematopoiesis. The cause is usually unexplained. Anemia is generally considered to be part of a pathological process rather than a result of aging. Because the elderly person may be unable to respond adequately to the anemia with increased cardiac output or pulmonary ventilation, anemia in this population can have serious effects on cardiopulmonary function if not properly treated. Thus, it is particularly important to identify the cause of the anemia and not to attribute it to the aging process.

Clinical Manifestations

Aside from the severity of the anemia, several factors affect the anemic patient and tend to influence the severity and even the presence of symptoms: (1) the speed with which the anemia has developed, (2) its duration (*i.e.,* its chronicity), (3) the metabolic requirements of the particular patient, (4) any other disorders or disabilities with which the patient is currently afflicted, and (5) special complications or concomitant features of the condition that has produced this anemia.

The more rapidly an anemia develops, the more severe its symptoms. An otherwise normal person can tolerate as much as a 50% gradual reduction in hemoglobin, red count, or hematocrit without pronounced symptoms or significant incapacity, whereas the rapid loss of as little as 30% may precipitate profound vascular collapse in the same individual. A person who has been anemic for a very long period of time, with hemoglobin levels between 9 and 11 mg/dl (90 and 110 g/L), experiences few or no symptoms other than slight tachycardia on exertion. Exertional dyspnea is likely to occur below, but not above, 7.5 gm/dl (75 g/L); weakness, only below 6 gm/dl (60 g/L); dyspnea at rest, below 3 gm/dl (30 g/L); and cardiac failure, only at the profoundly low level of 2 to 2.5 g/dl (20 to 25 g/L).

Patients who customarily are very active are more likely to experience symptoms, and symptoms that are more pronounced, than a more sedentary person. A hypothyroid patient, who requires less than the usual amount of oxygen, may be perfectly asymptomatic, without tachycardia or increased cardiac output, at a hemoglobin level of 10 gm/dl (100 g/L). Contrary to this, at any given level of anemia patients with underlying heart disease are far more apt to experience angina or symptoms of congestive failure than someone without heart disease.

Finally, as will emerge in the discussions that follow, many anemic disorders are complicated by various other abnormalities that do not depend on the anemia but are inherently associated with these particular diseases. These abnormalities may give rise to symptoms that completely overshadow those of the anemia, as is exemplified by the painful crises of sickle cell anemia (see p. 677).

There are a number of hematologic disorders in which anemia is the presenting problem, or the problem of paramount concern, and that, as a group, exemplify all·of the etiologic factors that have been discussed and all of the pathogenic mechanisms that have been formulated to date with respect to anemia.

Diagnostic Evaluation

A variety of hematologic studies are done to determine the type and cause of the anemia. These include measurements of hemoglobin and hematocrit, red cell indices, white blood cell studies, serum iron level, measurement of total iron binding capacity, folate level, vitamin B_{12} level, platelet count, bleeding time, prothrombin time, and partial thromboplastin time. Bone marrow aspiration and biopsy may be included. In addition, diagnostic studies are done to determine the presence of acute or chronic illness and the source of any chronic blood loss.

Management

Management of anemia is directed toward reversing the cause and replacing any blood that has been lost. The discussion below of each specific type of anemia includes its management.

▶ Nursing Process
The Patient With Anemia

▷ Assessment

The nursing history and physical examination are important when caring for a patient with anemia. They will reveal clues that may hasten the diagnostic process and alert the nurse to problems and concerns that often can be alleviated. Weakness, fatigue, and general malaise are common, as are pallor of the skin and mucous membranes. Jaundice may be present in patients with pernicious anemia or anemia that is of a hemolytic nature. Dryness of the skin and hair and spooning (concave surface) of the nails are often seen in iron deficiency anemia.

Cardiac status is carefully assessed. When the hemoglobin is low, the heart will attempt to compensate by pumping faster and harder in an effort to deliver more blood to hypoxic tissue. This increased cardiac workload results in such symptoms as tachycardia, palpitations, dyspnea, dizziness, orthopnea, and exertional dyspnea. Congestive heart failure will eventually develop, as evidenced by cardiomegaly, hepatomegaly, and peripheral edema.

Neurologic examination is also important because of the effects of pernicious anemia on the central and peripheral nervous systems. The patient is assessed for peripheral numbness and paresthesias, ataxia, poor coordination, and confusion. Assessment of gastrointestinal function may reveal complaints of nausea, vomiting, diarrhea, anorexia, and glossitis (inflammation of the tongue).

The nursing history includes information about any drugs the patient may be taking that could depress bone marrow activity or interfere with folate metabolism. The patient is also questioned about any loss of blood, as evidenced by blood in the stools or, for women, excessive menstrual flow. Family history is important because certain anemias are inherited. A nutritional history may reveal deficiencies in essential nutrients such as iron, vitamin B_{12}, and folic acid.

▷ Nursing Diagnoses

Based on the assessment data, major nursing diagnoses for the patient may include the following:

- Activity intolerance related to weakness, fatigue, and general malaise
- Potential decreased cardiac output related to increased cardiac workload

- Alteration in nutrition related to inadequate intake of essential nutrients

▷ Planning and Implementation

▷ **Goals.**   The major goals of the patient may include tolerance of normal activity, attainment/maintenance of normal cardiac output, and attainment/maintenance of adequate nutrition.

Nursing Interventions

Tolerance of Normal Activity.   Nursing care is planned to conserve the patient's strength and physical and emotional energy. Frequent rest periods are encouraged, and family support is elicited to promote a restful environment. A regular schedule of rest and sleep is imperative for restoring strength and activity tolerance. Ambulation and activities of daily living are encouraged as tolerated. Conditioning exercises are used to increase endurance. As the anemia is treated and blood studies return to normal, the patient is encouraged to resume normal activities gradually. Activities that are found to cause undue fatigue are postponed until greater endurance becomes evident. Safety precautions are used to prevent falls resulting from poor coordination, paresthesias, and weakness.

Attainment/Maintenance of Normal Cardiac Output.   With longstanding reduction of oxyhemoglobin, the heart may begin to lose its ability to withstand the additional work of supplying blood to hypoxic tissue. It will begin to enlarge, and cardiac output will decrease. Nursing measures are directed toward decreasing activities and stimuli that cause an increase in heart rate and that necessitate increased cardiac output. The patient is encouraged to identify those situations that precipitate palpitations and dyspnea and to avoid them until the anemic condition improves. If dyspnea is a problem, measures such as elevation of the head of the bed and the use of pillows for support are used. Unnecessary exertion is avoided. Oxygen is administered when necessary. Vital signs are monitored frequently and the patient is observed for indications of fluid retention, *e.g.,* peripheral edema, decreased urinary output, and neck vein distention.

Attainment/Maintenance of Adequate Nutrition.   Inadequate intake of essential nutrients, such as iron and folic acid, can cause some anemias. The symptoms associated with anemias, such as fatigue and anorexia, can also lead to malnutrition. A well-balanced diet high in protein and high-calorie foods, fruits, and vegetables is encouraged. Spicy foods that can cause gastric irritation and foods that are gas-producing should be avoided. The patient's family is included in dietary teaching sessions because the diet plan should be acceptable to both patient and family.

▷ Evaluation

▷ *Expected Outcomes*

1. Patient tolerates normal activity.
   a. Follows a progressive plan of rest, activities, and exercises
   b. Paces activities according to energy level
2. Attains/maintains normal cardiac output
   a. Avoids activities that cause tachycardia, palpitations, dizziness, and dyspnea

b. Uses rest and comfort measures to alleviate dyspnea
c. Has normal vital signs
d. Experiences no signs of fluid retention, *e.g.*, peripheral edema, decreased urinary output, neck vein distention
3. Attains/maintains adequate nutrition
a. Eats foods high in protein, calories, and vitamins
b. Avoids foods that cause gastric irritation
c. Develops a meal plan that promotes optimal nutrition

Classification of Anemias

There are several ways to classify the anemias. The physiologic approach is to determine whether the deficiency in red cells is due to a defect in production of red cells (*hypoproliferative anemia*) or to destruction of the red cells (*hemolytic anemia*).

In the hypoproliferative anemias, red cells usually survive normally, but the marrow is unable to produce adequate numbers of cells; thus, the reticulocyte count is depressed. This situation may be a result of marrow damage by drugs or chemicals (*e.g.*, chloramphenicol, benzene) or may be due to lack of erythropoietin (as in renal disease) or to lack of iron, vitamin B_{12}, or folic acid.

When hemolysis (dissolution of red blood cells with liberation of hemoglobin into surrounding fluid) is the major cause of anemia, the abnormality is usually within the red cell itself (as in sickle cell anemia or G-6-PD [glucose-6-phosphate dehydrogenase] deficiency), in the plasma (as in the immune hemolytic anemias), or in the circulation (as in heart valve hemolysis). In all of these hemolytic anemias, the reticulocyte count is elevated and the indirect bilirubin is high, often enough to cause clinical jaundice.

Hypoproliferative Anemias

Aplastic Anemia

Pathophysiology. Aplastic anemia is anemia caused by a decrease in precursor cells in the bone marrow and replacement of the marrow with fat. It may be idiopathic, that is, without apparent cause; result from certain infections; or be caused by drugs, chemicals, or radiation damage. Agents that regularly produce marrow aplasia in sufficient dosage include benzene and benzene derivatives; antitumor agents such as nitrogen mustard; the antimetabolites, including methotrexate and 6-mercaptopurine; and certain toxic materials, such as inorganic arsenic. Other agents occasionally responsible for aplasia or hypoplasia include certain antimicrobials, anticonvulsants, antithyroid drugs, antidiabetic agents, antihistamines, analgesics, sedatives, phenothiazines, insecticides, and heavy metals. The most common offenders in this respect are the antimicrobials chloramphenicol and the organic arsenicals, the anticonvulsants mephenytoin (Mesantoin) and trimethadione (Tridione), the anti-inflammatory analgesic drug phenylbutazone, sulfonamides, and gold compounds.

In many situations, aplastic anemia occurs when a drug or chemical is ingested in toxic amounts. However, in a small minority of persons it develops after a drug has been taken in the recommended dosage. These latter cases may be considered a type of idiosyncratic drug reaction in persons who are hypersusceptible for reasons as yet unknown. Provided that their exposure is terminated early (*i.e.*, on the first appearance of reticulocytopenia, anemia, granulocytopenia, or thrombocytopenia), a prompt and complete recovery may be anticipated. (Unfortunately, one cannot be so optimistic in the case of chloramphenicol recipients. Reactions in persons hypersusceptible to this drug may be completely unrelated to dosage; they may develop without premonitory changes in the hemogram long after the drug has been discontinued and can progress to a complete and fatal aplasia despite all available therapy.)

Whatever the offending drug, if exposure is allowed to continue after signs of hypoplasia have appeared, bone marrow depression almost certainly progresses to the point of complete and irreversible failure—hence, the importance of frequent complete blood counts for every patient receiving a drug or exposed regularly to any chemical that has been implicated in the production of aplastic anemia.

Diagnostic Evaluation. Because the bone marrow is hypocellular, attempts at marrow aspiration frequently yield only a few drops of blood. A biopsy is usually necessary to demonstrate a severe decrease in normal marrow elements and replacement by fat. The abnormality is probably in the stem cell, the precursor for granulocytes, erythrocytes, and platelets. As a result, pancytopenia (deficiency in all of the cellular elements of the blood) occurs.

Clinical Manifestations. The onset of aplastic anemia characteristically is a gradual one, marked by weakness, pallor, breathlessness on exertion, and other manifestations of anemia. A presenting symptom in about a third of the patients is abnormal bleeding due to thrombocytopenia. When the granulocytic series is involved as well, the patient is likely to present with fever, acute pharyngitis, or some other form of sepsis, in addition to bleeding. Physical signs, except for pallor and skin hemorrhages, are unremarkable. The blood count is marked by variable degrees of pancytopenia. Red cells are normocytic and normochromic, that is, of normal size and color. Frequently, patients have no characteristic physical findings; adenopathy (enlargement of glands) and hepatosplenomegaly (liver and spleen enlargement) are lacking.

Management. As might be expected from a condition that affects all hematopoietic cells, aplastic anemia carries a very poor prognosis. Three methods of treatment are currently employed: (1) bone marrow transplantation, (2) administration of immunosuppressive therapy with antilymphocyte globulin (ALG), and (3) high-dose methylprednisolone therapy.

The goal of bone marrow transplantation is to provide the patient with an undamaged supply of functioning hematopoietic tissue. Successful transplantation requires the ability to match donor and recipient and to prevent complications during the recovery process. With the use of the immunosuppressant cyclosporine, incidence of graft rejection is less than 10%.

The goal of immunosuppressive therapy with ALG is to remove the immunologic functions that prolong the aplasia and thus allow the patient's bone marrow a chance to recover. ALG is given through a central venous catheter daily for 7 to 10 days. Patients who respond to the therapy usually do so within 6 weeks to 3 months, but response may be as late as

6 months after treatment. Patients who have nonsevere aplastic anemia and are treated early in the course of their disease have the best chance of responding to ALG.

The response rate to high-dose methylprednisolone is similar to that achieved with ALG. Currently, trials of moderately high doses of methylprednisolone with ALG are in progress to see if the response rate can be improved further.

Supportive therapy plays a major role in the management of aplastic anemia. Any offending drug is discontinued. The patient is supported with transfusions of red cells and platelets as necessary to prevent symptoms. Eventually, such patients may develop antibodies to minor red cell antigens and to platelet antigens, so that transfusions no longer raise the counts sufficiently Death is usually caused by hemorrhage or infection, although modern antibiotics, especially those active against gram-negative bacilli, have been a major advance for these patients. Patients with pronounced leukopenia are protected from contact with people who have infections. Antibiotics should not be used prophylactically in neutropenic patients, because this favors the emergence of resistant bacteria and fungi.

Preventive Management. An extremely important area is prevention of drug-induced aplastic anemia. Because it is not possible to predict which patients will react adversely to a particular drug, potentially toxic drugs should be used only when alternative therapies are not available. Blood cell counts must be carefully monitored in patients receiving potentially marrow-toxic drugs, such as chloramphenicol. Persons taking toxic drugs on a long-term basis should understand the need for periodic blood studies and know what symptoms to report.

Nursing Interventions. Patients with diagnosed aplastic anemia are vulnerable to the effects of leukocyte, erythrocyte, and platelet deficiencies. They should be assessed carefully for signs of infection, tissue hypoxia, and bleeding. Any wound, abrasion, or ulcer of mucous membrane or skin is a potential site of infection and should be guarded against. Oral hygiene also is very important. Depending on the degree of weakness and fatigue, care should be planned to preserve the patient's energy. When thrombocytopenia is present, minor trauma, including subcutaneous and intramuscular injections, must be avoided. Regular atraumatic bowel movements are important, because hemorrhoids can develop and become infected or bleed.

Red Cell Aplasia

Red cell aplasia is an isolated anemia caused by lack of red cell formation in the marrow. This is a rare disorder in which only the erythroid cells are affected. The marrow is cellular, but the erythroid element is almost absent. There is a severe anemia without granulocytopenia or thrombocytopenia. The condition is sometimes associated with tumors of the thymus or certain drugs, such as phenytoin (Dilantin), or it may arise during the course of a hemolytic anemia. Some patients can be shown to produce an antibody to immature red cells, and this may be the cause of the disease. Treatment measures include red cell replacement, thymectomy, and administration of immunosuppressive drugs, such as corticosteroids and cyclosporine.

Myelophthisic Anemias

Myelophthisic anemias are a varied group of anemias that differ as to cause but are similar in that all show partial re-

placement of normal marrow space by abnormal tissue. This tissue may be fibrous (in myelofibrosis) or it may consist of plasma cells (in multiple myeloma) or metastatic carcinoma cells. A marrow biopsy is often necessary for the diagnosis. Pancytopenia is present, although usually less severe than in aplastic anemia, but there are also young marrow cells circulating, apparently because there is abnormal release from the damaged marrow. Myeloblasts and nucleated red cells are seen in small numbers. The treatment is that for the primary disease. Androgens occasionally improve the patient's condition.

Anemias in Renal Disease

There is a great deal of variability in the degree of anemia seen in kidney disorders, but in general, patients with a blood urea nitrogen (BUN) greater than 10 mg/dl blood are anemic. The symptoms of anemia often constitute the patient's major problems. The hematocrit usually falls to between 20% and 30% and is lower for more severe uremia, although it rarely falls below 15%. The red cells appear normal on peripheral smear.

This anemia is due to both a mild shortening of red cell survival and a deficiency of erythropoietin. Some erythropoietin is evidently produced outside the kidney, because some erythropoiesis does continue, even in anephric patients (those whose kidneys have been removed), and developing red cells can be seen in the bone marrow.

- Patients undergoing chronic hemodialysis lose blood into the artificial kidney and may thus become iron deficient. Folic acid deficiency develops because this vitamin passes into the dialysate.
- Dialysis patients shold be treated with iron and folic acid and occasional transfusions.

Androgens have been shown to stimulate enough erythropoiesis to obviate the need for transfusions in some patients. Most patients with uremia can tolerate moderate anemia with few symptoms and should not be transfused unless symptoms are present.

Anemias in Chronic Diseases

Many chronic inflammatory diseases are associated with anemia of a normochromic, normocytic type (red cells are normal in color and size). These include rheumatoid arthritis, lung abscesses, osteomyelitis, tuberculosis, and many malignancies. The anemia is usually mild and nonprogressive. It develops gradually over a period of 6 to 8 weeks and then stabilizes at hematocrit levels that are seldom below 25%. The hemoglobin rarely falls below 9 gm/dl, and the bone marrow has normal cellularity with increased stores of iron. Erythropoietin levels are low, perhaps because of decreased production, and there is a block in the utilization of iron by erythroid cells. There is also a moderate shortening of red cell survival.

Most of these patients are comfortable and do not require treatment for the anemia. With amelioration of the underlying disorder, the marrow iron is used to make red cells, and the hemoglobin rises.

Iron Deficiency Anemia

Iron deficiency anemia is a condition in which the total body iron content is decreased below a normal level. (Iron is needed for the synthesis of hemoglobin.) It is the most common type of anemia in all age groups.

Etiology. The common cause of iron deficiency in men and postmenopausal women is bleeding (.*e.g.*, from ulcers, gastritis, ·or gastrointestinal tumors) or malabsorption, especially after gastric resection. The most common cause in premenopausal women is *menorrhagia* (excessive menstrual bleeding). Rarely, iron can be lost in the urine during intravascular hemolysis, as in paroxysmal nocturnal hemoglobinuria or heart valve hemolysis.

Clinical and Laboratory Manifestations. In persons who are iron deficient, the blood hemoglobin and the red blood cell count are reduced. The hemoglobin is reduced more than the red cell count, and for this reason the red cells tend to be small and relatively devoid of pigment, that is, *hypochromic.* Hypochromia is the hallmark of iron deficiency. The cause of this deficiency is the failure of the patient to ingest, or absorb, sufficient dietary iron to compensate for the iron requirements associated with body growth or for the loss of iron that attends bleeding, whether the bleeding is physiologic (*e.g.*, menstrual) or pathologic.

Patients with iron deficiency present primarily with the symptoms of anemia. If the deficiency is severe, they may also have a smooth, sore tongue; thin, spoon-shaped fingernails; and pica (a craving to eat unusual substances, such as clay, laundry starch, or ice). All of these symptoms subside after therapy.

The laboratory studies show a hemoglobin that is proportionately lower than the hematocrit and red count, because of the small, poorly hemoglobinized red cells (microcytosis and hypochromia). The serum iron concentration is low, the total iron-binding capacity is high, and the serum ferritin (a measure of the iron stores) is low. The white count is usually normal, and the platelet count is variable.

Management. It is always important to search for a cause of iron deficiency. It may be a sign of a curable gastrointestinal malignancy or of uterine fibroids or cancer. Except in pregnancy, when the cause is obvious, stool specimens should be tested for occult blood.

Several oral iron preparations are available for treatment: ferrous sulfate, gluconate, and fumarate. The cheapest and most effective preparation is ferrous sulfate. Tablets with enteric coating may be poorly absorbed and should be avoided. Usually, three or four doses a day are necessary. Although iron is absorbed best on an empty stomach, taking it with food is usually advised to minimize gastric distress. Patients may be better able to tolerate the therapy if the dose is started at one tablet daily and then raised. They should be warned that iron salts often change the stools to a darker color. Generally, the iron is continued for a year after the source of bleeding has been controlled. This allows for replenishing of the iron stores.

Nursing Interventions. Preventive education is important because iron deficiency anemia is so common in menstruating and pregnant women. Food sources high in iron include organ and other meats, cooked white beans, leafy vegetables, raisins, and molasses. Taking iron-rich foods with a source of vitamin C enhances absorption.

The selection of a well-balanced diet is encouraged. Nutritional counseling is provided for those whose normal diet is less than adequate. Patients who have a history of fad diets are counseled that such diets often contain limited amounts of absorbable iron.

Iron therapy usually has to be continued for many months to replenish iron stores. In some cases, intramuscular administration of iron may be prescribed; that is, when oral iron is not absorbed or is poorly tolerated or when iron is needed in large amounts. The injection causes some local pain and can stain the skin. A method for parenteral administration of iron preparations follows:

1. Discard needle used to draw medication into syringe; use new needle for injection to avoid tracking medication through subcutaneous tissue.
2. Allow a small amount of air into syringe.
3. Use a needle 5 cm (2 inches) long—medication is injected deep into upper outer quadrant of buttock.
4. Retract skin over muscle *laterally* before inserting needle, to prevent leakage and staining of skin.
5. Inject solution slowly followed by air in syringe; wait a few seconds before withdrawing needle.

Occasional febrile or allergic reactions are seen. Total iron replacement with a single intravenous injection is possible, but it can cause a severe anaphylactic reaction.

Patients with iron deficiency anemia are encouraged to continue their iron therapy as long as it is prescribed, even though they may no longer be fatigued. If the iron supplement causes gastric distress, the patient is told to take it with meals until the symptoms subside, and then to resume the between-meal schedule for maximum absorption. Because ferrous sulfate is apt to deposit on the teeth and gums, the patient is advised to use frequent oral hygiene measures.

Megaloblastic Anemias

The anemias caused by deficiencies of the vitamins B_{12} and folic acid show identical bone marrow and peripheral blood changes. This is because both vitamins are essential for normal DNA synthesis. In each case, *hyperplasia* (abnormal increase in the number of normal cells) of the marrow occurs, and the precursor erythroid and myeloid cells are large and bizarre; some are multinucleated. But many of these cells die within the marrow, so the mature cells, which leave the marrow, are decreased in number. Thus, a *pancytopenia* (deficiency of all cellular elements of the blood) develops. In a far advanced situation, the hemoglobin may be as low as 4 to 5 gm/dl, the white blood count 2,000 to 3,000 per cu mm, and the platelet count less than 50,000 per cu mm. The red cells are large and the polymorphonuclears are hypersegmented.

Vitamin B_{12} Deficiency

Etiology. A deficiency of vitamin B_{12} can occur in several ways. Inadequate dietary intake is very rare but can develop in strict vegetarians who consume no meat. Faulty absorption from the gastrointestinal tract is more common. An absence of intrinsic factor normally secreted by cells of the stomach is called *pernicious anemia.* This is primarily a disorder of elderly persons and has a familial tendency. The abnormality is in the gastric mucosa: the stomach wall becomes atrophic and fails to secrete intrinsic factor. This substance ordinarily binds with the dietary vitamin B_{12} and travels with it to the ileum, where the vitamin is absorbed. Without intrinsic factor, no orally administered B_{12} can enter the body.

Even if adequate vitamin B_{12} and intrinsic factor are present, a deficiency can occur if disease involving the ileum or pancreas impairs absorption. Gastrectomy can also cause vitamin B_{12} deficiency.

Clinical Manifestations. After the body stores of vitamin B_{12} are used up, patients begin to show signs of the anemia. They gradually become weak, listless, and pale. The hematologic effects of deficiency are accompanied by effects on other organ systems, particularly the gastrointestinal tract and nervous system. Patients with pernicious anemia develop a smooth, sore, red tongue and mild diarrhea. They may become confused, but more often have paresthesias in the extremities and difficulty keeping their balance because of damage to the spinal cord: they lose position sense. These symptoms are progressive, although the course may be marked by spontaneous partial remissions and exacerbations. Without treatment, patients die after several years, usually from congestive failure secondary to anemia.

Diagnostic Evaluation. One means of determining the cause of vitamin B_{12} deficiency is the *Schilling test*. After fasting for 12 hours, the patient is given a small dose of radioactive B_{12} in water to drink, followed by a large, nonradioactive intramuscular dose. When the oral vitamin is absorbed, it will be excreted in the urine; the IM dose helps to flush it into the urine. A 24-hour urine specimen is collected and measured for radioactivity. If very little has been excreted, the test is repeated several days later (the "second stage"), with a capsule of oral intrinsic factor added to the oral B_{12}. If the patient has pernicious anemia, this time much more radioactivity will be found in the 24-hour urine. If the problem is due to an ileal or pancreatic defect, administration of digestive enzymes will increase absorption and subsequently increase urine radioactivity.

Management. Vitamin B_{12} deficiency is treated by replacement. Strict vegetarians can prevent or treat deficiency with oral supplementation with vitamins or fortified soy milk. When, as is much more common, the deficiency is due to defective absorption or absence of intrinsic factor, replacement is by intramuscular injections of vitamin B_{12}.

At first, B_{12} is given daily, but eventually most patients are managed with 100 μg IM monthly. This can produce dramatic recoveries in desperately ill patients. The reticulocyte count rises within a week, and in several weeks the blood counts are all normal. The tongue improves in several days. The neurologic manifestations require more time for recovery; if there is severe neuropathy, paralysis, or incontinence, the patient may never recover fully.

- Vitamin B_{12} therapy must be continued for the life of the patient who has had pernicious anemia or noncorrectable malabsorption in order to prevent recurrence of the anemia.

Nursing Interventions. These patients may need support during the diagnostic tests and nursing care for several aspects of their disease: anemia, congestive failure, neuropathy. When they are incontinent or paralyzed, care must be taken to prevent pressure sores and contracture deformities. The Schilling test can be useful only if the urine collections are complete; here, the nurse's assistance is essential. Patients must be taught about the chronicity of their disorder and the necessity for monthly injections even when they are asymptomatic. The gastric atrophy associated with pernicious anemia increases the risk of gastric carcinoma, so these patients need to understand that ongoing medical follow-up is important.

Folic Acid Deficiency

Folic acid is another vitamin that is necessary for normal red blood cell production. It is stored as different compounds, referred to as *folates*. The folate stores in the body are much smaller than those of vitamin B_{12}, so it is much more common to see dietary folate deficiency. This occurs in patients who rarely eat uncooked vegetables or fruits (*i.e.*, primarily elderly people living alone or persons with alcoholism). Alcohol increases folic acid requirements, and at the same time persons suffering from alcoholism usually have a diet that is deficient in the vitamin. Folic acid requirements are increased in chronic hemolytic anemias and in pregnancy, so these patients may develop the anemia while ingesting an adequate diet.

- Patients on prolonged intravenous feeding or hyperalimentation may become folate deficient after several months, unless the vitamin is given intramuscularly. Some patients with small bowel diseases may not absorb it normally.

Clinical Manifestations and Laboratory Tests. All of these patients have the characteristic findings of megaloblastic anemia along with a sore tongue. Symptoms of folic acid and vitamin B_{12} deficiencies are quite similar, and the two anemias may coexist. However, the neurologic manifestations of vitamin B_{12} deficiency do not occur with folic acid deficiency, and persist if vitamin B_{12} is not replaced. Therefore, careful distinction between the two anemias must be made. Serum levels of both vitamins can be measured.

Management. Treatment is administration of a good diet and 1 mg of folic acid a day. This should be given intramuscularly only in patients with malabsorption. With the exception of the vitamins given during pregnancy, most proprietary vitamin preparations do not contain folic acid, so it must be given as a separate tablet. When the hemoglobin returns to normal, the folic acid replacement can be stopped. However, persons suffering from alcoholism should continue receiving folic acid as long as they continue drinking.

Hemolytic Anemias

In *hemolytic anemias*, the erythrocytes have a shortened life span. The bone marrow is usually able to compensate partially by producing new red cells at three or more times the normal rate. Consequently, all of these anemias have certain laboratory features in common: the reticulocyte count is elevated, the fraction of indirect bilirubin is increased, and the haptoglobin (a binding protein for free hemoglobin) is often low. The bone marrow is hypercellular, with erythroid proliferation. The only truly diagnostic test for hemolysis is the red cell survival study. This is usually necessary only for difficult diagnostic problems. About 20 ml to 30 ml of the patient's blood is removed, incubated with radioactive chromium-51, and then reinjected. The chromium-51 labels the red cells exclusively. After these cells have equilibrated with the circulating blood, small samples are taken at intervals over the next days and weeks, and the radioactivity is measured. A normal chromium-51 survival time is 28 to 35 days. Red cells of patients with severe hemolysis (such as sickle cell anemia) have survival times of 10 days or less.

Inherited Hemolytic Anemias

Hereditary Spherocytosis

Hereditary spherocytosis is a hemolytic anemia characterized by small, sphere-shaped red cells and splenomegaly (enlarged spleen). This is an uncommon disorder inherited in a dominant fashion.

Clinical Manifestations and Diagnostic Evaluation. An abnormality of the erythrocyte membrane causes cells to lose membrane as they pass through the spleen and to become spherical in shape. These spheres are relatively rigid and easily destroyed. The peripheral blood contains many of the characteristic small spherical cells, and the patient has an anemia that may be exacerbated during infections, even minor viral illnesses. In addition, the spleen is enlarged. The disorder is usually diagnosed in childhood, but may be missed until adult life because there are few symptoms.

Management. Surgical removal of the spleen (*splenectomy*) is the treatment. It does not change the erythrocyte defect but removes the site of membrane loss and hemolysis. After splenectomy (see p. 693), patients have normal hemoglobin levels, only slight shortening of red cell survival times, and few spherical cells in the peripheral smear. Patients have a normal life expectancy. The major complications are all prevented by splenectomy: (1) aplastic crises after infection, often with severe anemia; (2) nonhealing leg and ankle ulceration; and (3) gallstones.

Sickle Cell Anemia

Definition and Etiology. Sickle cell anemia is a severe hemolytic anemia resulting from a defective hemoglobin molecule and associated with attacks of pain. This disabling disease is found predominantly in Africans and in black Americans, but it also occurs in people from Mediterranean and Arab countries.

Pathophysiology. The defect is a single amino acid substitution in the β chain of hemoglobin. Because normal hemoglobin A contains two α and two β chains, there are two genes for synthesis of each chain. Persons with sickle cell trait have inherited only one abnormal gene, so their red cells can synthesize both normal β chains and β^s chains; thus, they have A and S hemoglobin. If two people with sickle trait marry, some of their children may inherit two abnormal genes and will then have only β^s chains and only S hemoglobin; these children have sickle cell anemia.

Clinical Manifestations. The sickle hemoglobin has the unfortunate property of acquiring a crystallike formation when exposed to low oxygen tension. The oxygen in venous blood is low enough to cause this change; consequently, the cell containing S hemoglobin becomes deformed, rigid, and

sickle-shaped when in the venous circulation (see Fig. 29-3). These long, rigid cells can become lodged in small vessels and, when they pile up against each other, blood flow to a region or an organ may be slowed. When ischemia or infarction results, the patient may experience pain, swelling, and fever. Such a chain of events is presumed to explain the painful crises of this disease, but what triggers the chain or how to prevent it is not understood.

Symptoms are secondary to hemolysis and thrombosis. Patients are always anemic, with hemoglobin values in the 7 to 10 g/dl (70 to 100 g/L) range. Jaundice is characteristic and is usually obvious in the sclerae. The bone marrow expands in childhood in a compensatory effort, sometimes leading to enlargement of the bones of the face and skull. As a result, patients may have prominent foreheads and high cheekbones. The chronic anemia is associated with tachycardia, flow murmurs, and often cardiomegaly. Dysrhythmias and heart failure may occur in older patients.

Like patients with spherocytosis, patients with sickle cell anemia may develop aplastic crises when infected and may have gallstones (due to increased hemolysis that leads to bilirubin stones) and leg ulcers. The latter may be chronic and painful and require skin grafting. These patients are unusually susceptible to infection, particularly pneumonias and osteomyelitis. Infection has been one of the most common causes of death.

All of the patient's tissues and organs are constantly vulnerable to microcirculatory interruptions by the sickling process, and therefore are susceptible to hypoxic damage or true ischemic necrosis at any time. Thrombotic episodes may result in minor pain in an extremity, in severe pain and swelling in a hand or knee, in chest pain due to pulmonary infarction, in pain simulating an acute abdominal crisis, or in the sudden appearance of a "stroke," with hemiplegia. These crises are completely unpredictable; they can occur monthly or very rarely and may last for hours, days, or weeks. Events that

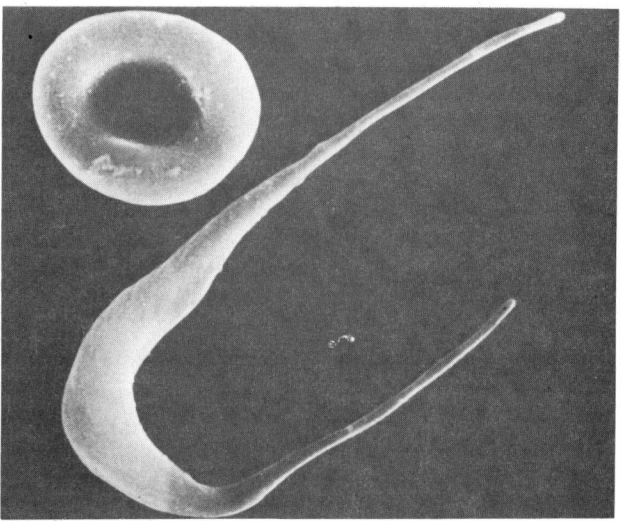

Figure 29-3
Unusual photo of a sickled cell and a normal red blood cell taken under the auspices of the Comprehensive Sickle Cell Center, University of Miami. (Photo by Dr. Bruce R. Cameron)

seem to precipitate crisis include dehydration, fatigue, menstruation, intake of alcohol, emotional stress, and acidosis. Certain effects of infarction are permanent, such as hemiplegia, aseptic necrosis of the femoral head, and renal concentrating defects.

Diagnostic Evaluation.   The diagnosis can be made by hemoglobin electrophoresis or by "sickle prep," in which a drop of blood is mixed with sodium metabisulfite and watched under the microscope for sickling. Sickling in this test occurs whether the patient has sickle trait or sickle cell anemia; only the electrophoresis can show the distinction. The patient with sickle trait has normal hemoglobin and hematocrit levels as well as a normal blood smear. In contrast, the patient with sickle cell anemia has a low hematocrit and sickled cells on smear.

Sickle Trait.   Patients with sickle trait are protected from crises because the hemoglobin A in their cells prevents the cells from sickling under ordinary circumstances. Such persons have no anemia and look and feel well. About 8% of black Americans have sickle trait.

Sickle Cell Anemia.   Patients with sickle cell anemia are usually diagnosed in childhood, because they are anemic in infancy and begin to have crises at 1 or 2 years of age. Many die in the first years of life, but antibiotics and patient and physician education about this disease have probably improved the outlook in the last 10 to 20 years, and some patients live into the sixth decade. All siblings of a patient with sickle cell anemia should be tested for the disease.

Management.   There is no specific treatment for the hemoglobin abnormality. The disease could be prevented only by intensive genetic counseling of the population at risk, a difficult and controversial task. Crises cannot now be prevented. Researchers are evaluating several chemicals with antisickling properties, but these are still in the investigational stage. Because infection seems to predispose to crises in children, all infections should be promptly treated or prevented when possible. Since dehydration and hypoxia promote sickling, patients are instructed to avoid high altitudes, anesthesia, or fluid loss. Because of the renal defect, these patients easily become dehydrated. Folic acid therapy is given continuously, because the marrow has an increased requirement.

When sickle crisis occurs, the mainstays of therapy are hydration and analgesia. Increased fluid intake helps to dilute the blood and reverse the agglutination of sickled cells within the small blood vessels. Patients and families can learn to handle minor crises at home but, if there is no relief after several hours, hospital admission may be necessary. The patients often have fever and leukocytosis with crisis, so infection or appendicitis or cholecystitis may be suspected and must be ruled out. Intravenous fluids (3–5 liters/day for adults) are essential. Narcotic analgesics are often necessary because of the severity of pain and should be given in adequate doses. They should never be used chronically, however, for some patients do become addicted. Relaxation techniques, breathing exercises, transcutaneous nerve stimulation, and whirlpool baths are helpful for some patients.

Transfusions are reserved for particular situations: (1) aplastic crisis, when the patient's hemoglobin falls rapidly; (2) severe painful crisis not responding to any other therapy after several days; (3) as a preoperative measure, to dilute the amount of sickled blood; and (4) sometimes during the latter half of pregnancy in an attempt to prevent crises.

▶ Nursing Process
The Patient With Sickle Cell Anemia

▷ Assessment

Because the sickling process can cause microcirculatory interruptions in any tissues and organs, with resultant hypoxia and ischemia, a careful assessment of all body systems is necessary. Particular emphasis is placed on assessing for pain, swelling, and fever. All joint areas are carefully examined for pain and swelling, as is the abdomen. A careful neurologic examination is important to elicit symptoms of cerebral hypoxia.

The patient is also questioned about symptoms indicative of gallstones, such as food intolerances, epigastric distress, and pain in the right upper abdominal quadrant.

Because these patients are so susceptible to infections, they are assessed for the presence of any infectious process. Particular attention is given to examination of the chest and long bones and femoral head, since pneumonia and osteomyelitis are especially common. Leg ulcers which may be infected are sometimes present. Chronic anemia, another common problem associated with sickle cell anemia, is also considered during the physical examination (see p. 672).

Patients in crisis are questioned about factors that could have precipitated the crisis. They are asked to recall whether they have recently had symptoms of infection or dehydration or have been experiencing situations that promote fatigue or emotional stress. History of alcohol intake is also discussed. In addition, patients are asked to recall factors that seemed to precipitate previous crises and measures that they use to prevent crises. This information will provide guidelines for identifying and meeting their learning needs.

▷ Nursing Diagnoses

Based on the assessment data, major nursing diagnoses for the patient may include the following:

- Pain related to agglutination of sickled cells within blood vessels
- Potential for infection related to increased susceptibility as a factor of the disease process
- Knowledge deficit regarding prevention of crisis

▷ Planning and Implementation

A care plan for the patient with sickle cell crisis is presented in Nursing Care Plan 29-1.

The nurse can help the patient and family adjust to this chronic disease and understand the importance of hydration and prevention of infection. When leg ulcers are present, they require careful dressing and protection from trauma and wound contamination. If they fail to heal, skin grafting may be necessary. Cardiac disease is managed in the same way as for any patient who does not have sickle cell anemia. During crisis, the patient is kept quiet and allowed to rest undisturbed. Swollen extremities should not be exercised and pain should be relieved. Male patients may develop sudden, painful episodes of priapism (persistent penile erection) and need to know that it is common and has no long-term deleterious effects.

Other Hemoglobinopathies

C Hemoglobin. C hemoglobin is less common among American blacks than S hemoglobin. The C trait is asymptomatic, and homozygous C disease is a mild hemolytic anemia with splenomegaly but no serious complications.

Thalassemia. Thalassemia is a group of hereditary disorders associated with defective hemoglobin-chain synthesis. These anemias occur worldwide, but the highest prevalence is found in persons of Mediterranean, African, and Southeast Asian ancestry. They are seen increasingly often in the United States with the influx of refugees from Southeast Asia. They are characterized by *hypochromia* (abnormal decrease in hemoglobin content of erythrocytes), *microcytosis* (smaller than normal erythrocytes), hemolysis, and variable degrees of anemia.

The thalassemias are classified into two major groups according to the affected globin chain of hemoglobin: α-thalassemias and β-thalassemias, which are associated with decreased or absent α-chain synthesis and β-chain synthesis respectively. The α-thalassemias occur mainly in people from southeast Asia and Africa, and the β-thalassemias are most prevalent in Mediterranean populations. The α-thalassemias are milder than the β-forms and are often without symptoms. Patients with severe β-thalassemia will die within the first few years of life if untreated; if treated with regular transfusion therapy they may survive into their 20s or 30s.

The β-thalassemias are classified according to their severity: minima, minor, intermedia, and major. Patients with *thalassemia minima* are asymptomatic; the majority of those with *thalassemia minor* are also wihout symptoms, although significant anemia that requires transfusion therapy may occur during pregnancy.

Thalassemia intermedia is more severe, with life expectancy of only about 3 or 4 decades. These patients often suffer from chronic fatigue, debilitating bone pain, cardiac disease, and hypersplenism. Because of an inadequate excretory pathway for iron, they often experience complications of iron overload (*e.g.*, hepatic fibrosis and cirrhosis) which is worsened by transfusion therapy.

Thalassemia major (Cooley's anemia) is characterized by severe anemia, marked hemolysis, and ineffective erythropoiesis. With early regular transfusion therapy, growth and development through childhood is facilitated. Organ dysfunction due to iron overload usually begins in adolescence, and death generally occurs in the second or third decade of life.

Glucose-6-Phosphate Dehydrogenase Deficiency

The abnormality in this disorder is in G-6-PD, an enzyme within the red cell that is essential for membrane stability. A few patients have inherited an enzyme so defective that they have a chronic hemolytic anemia, but the most common type of defect results in hemolysis only when the red cells are stressed by certain situations, such as fever or the presence of certain drugs. The disorder came to the attention of researchers during World War II, when some soldiers developed hemolysis while taking primaquine, an antimalarial drug. Drugs that are hemolytic for G-6-PD-deficient persons are antimalarial drugs, sulfonamides, nitrofurantoin, the common coal tar analgesics (including aspirin), the thiazide diuretics, the oral hypoglycemic agents, chloramphenicol, para-aminosalicylic acid (PAS), vitamin K, and, for certain individuals subject to "favism," the fava bean. Blacks and peoples of Greek or Italian origin are those primarily affected. The type of deficiency found in the Mediterranean group is more severe than that in the black group, resulting in greater hemolysis and sometimes in life-threatening anemias. All types are inherited as X-linked defects; thus, many more males are at risk than females. In the U.S., about 15% of black males are affected.

Clinical Manifestations. The patients are asymptomatic and have normal hemoglobin levels and reticulocyte counts most of the time. Several days after exposure to an offending drug, they may develop pallor, jaundice, and hemoglobinuria, and the reticulocyte count will rise. Special strains of the peripheral blood may then show *Heinz bodies* (degraded hemoglobin). Hemolysis continues for a week, and then spontaneously the counts begin to improve because the new young red cells are resistant to lysis. In the Mediterranean type, this recovery does not occur.

Diagnostic Evaluation and Management. The diagnosis is made by a screening test or a quantitative assay of G-6-PD. The treatment is removal of the drug. Transfusion is only necessary in the Mediterranean variety. The patient should be educated about the disease and given a list of drugs to avoid. These include sulfonamides, hypoglycemic agents, antimalarials, nitrofurantoin, phenacetin, aspirin (in high doses), and para-aminosalicylic acid.

Acquired Hemolytic Anemias

There are a variety of acquired hemolytic anemias, including paroxysmal nocturnal hemoglobinuria, immune hemolytic anemia, microangiopathic hemolytic anemia, heart valve hemolysis, and spur cell anemia, as well as those associated with infections and hypersplenism. Table 29-2 (p. 682) identifies the causes, manifestations, and treatment of these anemias. Immune hemolytic anemia is addressed in the text discussion.

Immune Hemolytic Anemia

When antibodies combine with red cells they can be either *isoantibodies*, reacting with foreign cells, as in transfusion reactions or erythroblastosis fetalis, or *autoantibodies*, which react with the cells of the host. The immune hemolysis that results may be very severe. Antibodies coat the red cells, producing a positive Coombs's test. These cells are then removed by the spleen and the rest of the reticuloendothelial system. Many cells are destroyed, and others return to the circulation as spherocytes with reduced membrane and a shortened survival rate.

In *idiopathic autoimmune hemolytic states*, what induces the immune system to produce the antibodies is not known. The disease usually begins suddenly, often in persons over 40 years of age. In some cases, the hemolysis is associated with systemic disease (especially systemic lupus erythematosus, chronic lymphatic leukemia, or lymphoma).

Nursing Care Plan 29-1

Care of the Patient With Sickle Cell Crisis

Nursing Interventions	*Rationale*	*Expected Outcomes*

Nursing Diagnosis: Pain related to agglutination of sickled cells within small blood vessels

Goal: Relief of pain

1. Assess severity and location of pain. Common sites of pain are— Joints and extremities Chest Abdomen	1. Tissues and organs are susceptible to microcirculatory thrombosis with resulting hypoxic damage; hypoxia causes pain.	• Patient verbalizes that pain is relieved after administration of analgesics • Moves body parts slowly and carefully to minimize pain • Increases fluid intake
2. Administer analgesics as prescribed.	2. Narcotic analgesics are necessary to relieve severe pain; avoid use of narcotics for chronic pain because of possibility of addiction.	• Gradually experiences longer pain-free periods • Expresses interest in diversional activities
3. Encourage oral intake of fluids and administer IV fluids as prescribed; monitor intake and output.	3. Fluids promote hemodilution and reverse agglutination of sickled cells within small blood vessels.	
4. Carefully position and support painful areas; encourage use of relaxation techniques and breathing exercises; apply moist heat to painful areas.	4. Joint pain can be minimized during a crisis by careful movement and with the use of moist heat; relaxation techniques and breathing exercises help the patient to focus attention away from the pain.	

Nursing Diagnosis: Potential for infection related to increased susceptibility as a factor of the disease process

Goal: Prevention of infection

1. Assess for signs and symptoms of infection. Common sites of infection are— Lungs Long bones; head of the femur Leg ulcers	1. The physiological stress that results from infection often precipitates crises; resolution of infection at its onset can prevent or limit the duration of a crisis episode.	• Temperature normal • Breath sounds clear • WBCs within normal range (5,000–10,000 cu mm) • Absence of pain of long bones • Cultures of wound drainage negative

(continued)

Other patients, with identical clinical pictures, can be shown to be producing antibodies to a drug (especially penicillin, cephalosporins, or quinidine). The antibodies or the drug–antibody complexes then attach to red cells, resulting in hemolysis. Patients taking large doses of methyldopa may develop antibodies to their own red cells; only a few of these patients have a significant hemolytic anemia.

Clinical Manifestations.   Presentation can be quite variable. A positive Coombs's test may be the only manifestation in mild cases. More often, signs of anemia are present, such as fatigue, dyspnea, palpitations, and jaundice. Occasionally, the anemia is so severe that the patient presents with overwhelming hemolysis and shock.

Management.   Any possibly offending drug should be discontinued. The treatment consists of high doses of corticosteroids until hemolysis decreases. When, usually after several weeks, the hemoglobin has returned toward normal, the steroid dose can be lowered; in some patients it can be discontinued entirely. In severe cases blood transfusions may be required. Because the antibody may react with all possible donor cells, transfusion requires careful typing and slow, cautious administration.

Splenectomy removes a major site of red cell destruction, so this operation is often performed if steroids do not produce a remission. If neither corticosteroids nor splenectomy is successful, immunosuppressive drugs may be administered.

Polycythemia

Polycythemia refers to an increased concentration of red cells; it is a term used when the red cell count is greater than 6 million/cu mm or the hemoglobin exceeds 18 gm/dl. True

Nursing Interventions	Rationale	Expected Outcomes

Nursing Diagnosis: Potential for infection related to increased susceptibility as a factor of the disease process

Goal: Prevention of infection

2. Encourage early ambulation and pulmonary hygiene.	2. Activity mobilizes pulmonary secretions; stagnant secretions are a prime medium for bacterial growth.	
3. Utilize aseptic technique when changing wound dressings.	3. Aseptic technique deters introduction of microorganisms into wound areas.	
4. Promote adequate nutrition and fluid intake.	4. Optimal nutrition and fluid balance promote tissue integrity.	

Nursing Diagnosis: Deficit in knowledge about prevention of crisis

Goal: Avoidance of situations that can precipitate crisis

1. Discuss factors that commonly precipitate crisis: 　Infection 　Dehydration 　Trauma 　Strenuous physical exertion 　Extreme fatigue 　Exposure to cold 　Hypoxia, *e.g.,* high altitudes 　Emotional stress	1. Avoidance of situations that precipitate crisis can often increase the intervals between crisis attacks.	• Patient identifies factors that can precipitate crisis • Identifies acceptable life-style changes necessary to prevent crisis • Elicits support of family in making changes in life-style • Maintains adequate fluid intake • Identifies sources of infection that can be avoided • Identifies the need to seek prompt medical attention when infection occurs
2. Discuss the chronic nature of the disease with patient and family; stress the importance of adequate hydration and avoidance of infection.	2. Understanding of the chronicity of the disorder and the ability to minimize crises promotes adherence to the therapeutic regimen.	

polycythemia is present when the total body red cell mass is increased. "Relative" polycythemia occurs when the red cell mass is normal but the plasma volume is reduced; this may be produced by diuretic therapy or by unknown factors. Red cell mass can be measured accurately by an isotopic technique.

Secondary Polycythemia

Secondary polycythemia is caused by excessive production of erythropoietin. This may occur in response to a hypoxic stimulus, as in chronic obstructive pulmonary disease or cyanotic heart disease, or in certain hemoglobinopathies in which the hemoglobin has an abnormally high affinity for oxygen (*e.g.,* hemoglobin$_{Chesapeake}$). In some cases of secondary polycythemia, the production of erythropoietin serves no purpose because there is no hypoxemia; this is the situation

in a few patients with renal carcinoma, renal cysts, cerebellar hemangioblastoma, hepatoma, or uterine fibroids.

Management of secondary polycythemia involves treatment of the primary problem. If the cause cannot be corrected, *phlebotomy* (withdrawal of blood) can be used to treat the symptoms of hypervolemia and hyperviscosity.

Polycythemia Vera

Polycythemia vera, or primary polycythemia, is a proliferative disorder in which all the marrow cells seem to have escaped from the normal control mechanisms. The bone marrow is intensely cellular, and in the peripheral blood the red count, white count, and platelets, are often all elevated. Patients typically have a ruddy complexion and *hepatosplenomegaly* (enlarged liver and spleen). The symptoms are referable to the increased blood volume (headache, dizziness, fatigue,

TABLE 29-2
Acquired Hemolytic Anemias

Name	Cause	Manifestations and Treatment
Paroxysmal nocturnal hemoglobinuria	Unknown—sometimes occurs after aplastic anemia	Dark urine (*hemoglobinuria*) especially in morning Sometimes pancytopenia Multiple venous thrombosis No treatment known
Immune hemolytic anemia	Antibodies produced, sometimes secondary to drug (methyldopa [Aldomet], penicillin)	Jaundice, spherocytes Responds to steroids
Microangiopathic hemolytic anemia	RBC damaged during flow through abnormal small blood vessels, as in malignant hypertension	Fragmented RBC seen on smears Treat primary disease.
Heart valve hemolysis	RBC damaged by regurgitant flow through incompetent valve prosthesis	Fragmented RBC Treatment: replace valve.
Spur cell anemia	Severe liver disease, usually hypertension Increased lipid in RBC membrane	Spur-shaped RBC No treatment
Infections	Malaria, *Clostridium welchii*, especially after septic abortion	Hemoglobinuria possible Treat the infection.
Hypersplenism	Large spleen from any cause: cirrhosis, lymphomas	Sometimes pancytopenia Treatment: splenectomy

and blurred vision) or to increased blood viscosity (angina, claudication, thrombophlebitis). Bleeding is also a complication, perhaps because of the engorged capillaries. Another common and unexplained problem is pruritus.

Management

The objective of management is to reduce the high blood viscosity. Phlebotomy is an important part of therapy and can be done repeatedly to keep the hemoglobin within normal range. Radioactive phosphorus or chemotherapeutic agents can be used to suppress marrow function but may increase the risk of leukemia. When the patient has an elevated uric acid level, allopurinol is used to prevent gouty attacks. Cyproheptadine may be administered to control pruritus.

Leukopenia and Agranulocytosis

Leukopenia is a condition in which the white cells number fewer than normal. Agranulocytosis is a potentially fatal condition in which there is almost complete absence of polymorphonuclear cells. A leukocyte count of fewer than 5000/cu mm or a granulocyte count of fewer than 2000/cu mm is abnormal and may be a signal of a generalized bone marrow disorder, such as megaloblastic anemia, aplasia, metastatic

tumor, myelofibrosis, or acute leukemia. Viral infections and overwhelming bacterial sepsis can also cause leukopenia. Most commonly, the etiology is drug toxicity: phenothiazines are implicated frequently, and antithyroid drugs, sulfonamides, phenylbutazone, and chloramphenicol are also contributing factors. The patient is not symptomatic unless infection develops, which usually occurs when the granulocytes are fewer than 1000/cu mm. Fever and severe sore throat with ulcerations are common complains. Bacteremia may follow soon after.

Management

Any possibly offending drugs are withdrawn. If the granulocyte count is very low, the patient is protected from any obvious sources of infection. Cultures of all orifices and blood are essential, and when fever occurs it is treated with broad spectrum antibiotics until the specific organism is known. Good oral hygiene is helpful.

Hot saline irrigations of the throat are employed to keep it clear of necrotic exudate. Comfort is provided by supplying an ice collar and whatever analgesic, antipyretic, and sedative drugs may be indicated. The essence of treatment, apart from eradicating the infection, is to eliminate, if possible, the factor responsible for the bone marrow depression. Spontaneous restoration of marrow function, except in the case of neoplastic diseases, often occurs in time, that is, within 2 or 3 weeks, if death from infection can be averted.

Hematopoietic Malignancies

Blood-forming tissues are characterized by rapid and continuous turnover of cells. Normally, production of specialized blood cells from stem cell precursors is carefully regulated according to the body's needs. If homeostatic control of production is disrupted, neoplastic proliferation may result. A wide variety of hematopoietic malignancies can develop and are often classified according to the cell line involved. *Leukemia,* literally white blood, is a neoplastic proliferation of white cells. The defect is believed to originate in the hematopoietic stem cell. The *lymphomas* are neoplasms of lymphoid tissue. Hodgkin's disease accounts for 40% of all lymphomas and is believed to result from defective T-lymphocytes. Many other lymphomas are derived from B-lymphocytes. Both Waldenström's macroglobulinemia and multiple myeloma are neoplasms affecting plasms cells produced by B-lymphocytes.

Leukemia

The common feature of the leukemias is an unregulated proliferation or accumulation of white cells in the bone marrow, replacing normal marrow elements. There is also proliferation in the liver, spleen, and lymph nodes, and invasion of non-hematologic organs, such as the meninges, gastrointestinal tract, kidney, and skin. The leukemias are often classified according to the cell line involved, as either lymphocytic or myelocytic, and according to the maturity of the malignant cells, as either acute (immature cells) or chronic (differentiated cells). The etiology is unknown, but there is some evidence that genetic influence and viral pathogenesis may be involved. Bone marrow damage with radiation (as in the atomic bomb survivors) or chemicals (benzene) can cause leukemia.

Acute Myelogenous Leukemia (AML)

Acute myelogenous leukemia (AML) affects the hematopoietic stem cell that differentiates into all myeloid cells: monocytes, granulocytes (basophils, neutrophils, eosinophils), erythrocytes, and platelets. All age groups are affected; incidence rises with age.

Clinical Manifestations. Most of the signs and symptoms evolve from insufficient production of normal blood cells. Vulnerability to infection results from granulocytopenia, weakness and fatigue occur due to anemia, and bleeding tendencies arise as a result of thrombocytopenia. The proliferation of leukemic cells within organs leads to a variety of additional symptoms: pain from enlarged liver or spleen; lymphadenopathy; headache or vomiting secondary to meningeal leukemia (most common in lymphocytic leukemia); and bone pain from expansion of marrow.

Onset is often insidious, with symptoms occurring over a period of 1 to 6 months. The peripheral blood will show a decrease in both erythrocyte and platelet counts. Although the total leukocyte count can be low, normal, or high, the percentage of normal cells is usually vastly decreased. A bone marrow specimen is diagnostic.

Management. Chemotherapy is the major form of therapy and in some instances results in remissions lasting a year or longer. Drugs commonly used include daunorubicin hydrochloride (Cerubidine), cytarabine (Cytosar-U), and mercaptopurine (Purinethol). Transfusions of red cells and platelets are administered to provide normal cells temporarily. When a tissue match with a close relative can be obtained, bone marrow transplantation is used to provide normal bone marrow after destruction of leukemic marrow by chemotherapy.

Prognosis. At the present time, survival of treated patients averages only 1 year, with death usually a result of infection. Untreated patients survive only about 2 months.

Chronic Myelogenous Leukemia (CML)

Chronic myelogenous leukemia (CML) is also believed to be a malignancy of myeloid stem cells. However, more normal cells are present than in the acute form, and therefore the disease is milder. Uncommon before age 20, the incidence of chronic myelogenous leukemia rises with age.

Manifestations. The clinical picture is similar to that of acute myelogenous leukemia, but signs and symptoms are less severe. Many patients are without symptoms for years. Onset is typically insidious. Leukocytosis is always present, sometimes at extraordinary levels.

Management and Prognosis. The drug of choice for chemotherapy is busulfan (Myleran). Survival has been significantly improved with bone marrow transplantation. The final event in most patients is a transformation into an acute myelogenous leukemia that is usually resistant to all therapy. Overall, patients live for 3 to 4 years. Death usually results from infection or hemorrhage. The nursing process is similar to that for acute leukemia (see p. 684).

Acute Lymphocytic Leukemia (ALL)

Acute lymphocytic leukemia (ALL) is believed to be a malignant proliferation of lymphoblasts. It is most common in young children, with a peak incidence at 4 years of age. After age

Manifestations. Lymphocytes proliferate in marrow and peripheral tissue and crowd the development of normal cells. As a result of marrow proliferation of malignant cells, normal hematopoiesis is inhibited and leukopenia, anemia, and thrombocytopenia develop. Erythrocyte and platelet counts are low, and leukocyte counts may be either low or high but always include immature cells. Manifestations of leukemic cell infiltration into other organs are more common with acute lymphocytic leukemia than with other forms.

Management and Prognosis. Therapy for this childhood leukemia has improved to the extent that approximately 50% of children survive at least 5 years. The major form of treatment is chemotherapy with combinations of vincristine, prednisone, daunorubicin, and asparaginase used for initial therapy and combinations of mercaptopurine, methotrexate, vincristine, and prednisone for maintenance. Irradiation of the craniospinal region and intrathecal injection of chemotherapeutic drugs help prevent central nervous system recurrence.

Chronic Lymphocytic Leukemia (CLL)

A disease of elderly people, chronic lymphocytic leukemia tends to be a mild disorder that primarily affects persons over age 35.

Clinical Manifestations. Many patients are asymptomatic and are diagnosed during physical examination or treatment for another disease. Possible manifestations are those of anemia, infection, or enlargement of lymph nodes and abdominal organs. The erythrocyte and platelet counts may be normal or decreased. Lymphocytosis is always present.

Management and Prognosis. If mild, chronic lymphocytic leukemia may require no treatment. When symptoms are severe, chemotherapy with steroids and chlorambucil (Leukeran) is often used. Highly variable in course, the average survival time is 7 years.

Patients who no longer respond to therapy may be hospitalized for supportive care. They have often experienced remissions and exacerbations of the disease, and have known hope and despair. They are very tired and ill and require knowledgeable nursing assessment, support, and expert physical care. (See also section on patients with advanced carcinoma, p. 294.)

▶ *Nursing Process*
The Patient With Leukemia

▷ *Assessment*

Although the clinical picture will vary with the type of leukemia involved, the nursing history may reveal a range of signs and symptoms reported by the patient and noted during the physical examination. Included in the clinical manifestations may be weakness and fatigue, bleeding tendencies, petechiae and ecchymoses, pain, headache, vomiting, fever, and infection. Blood studies may reveal alterations of the white blood cells, anemia, and thrombocytopenia. Specific manifestations are identified under the discussion of each of the types of leukemia.

▷ *Nursing Diagnoses*

Based on the assessment data, nursing diagnoses for the patient may include the following:

- Ineffective coping related to the diagnosis and prognosis
- Potential for bleeding related to thrombocytopenia
- Potential for infection related to neutropenia
- Activity intolerance related to anemia
- Alteration in comfort related to leukocytic infiltration of systemic tissues
- Inadequate nutrition related to gastrointestinal proliferative changes and toxic effects of chemotherapeutic agents
- Disturbance in body image related to alopecia

▷ *Planning and Implementation*

▷ *Goals.* The major goals of the patient may include ability to cope with the diagnosis and prognosis, absence of bleeding, absence of infection, tolerance of activity, attainment/maintenance of comfort, attainment/maintenance of adequate nutrition, and promotion of positive body image.

Nursing Interventions

Ability to Cope with the Diagnosis and Prognosis. Like other patients with malignant diseases, patients with leukemia are often depressed, frightened, and lonely. A well-informed and sympathetic nurse can contribute immeasurably to their comfort by explaining procedures, anticipating side-effects of drugs, and encouraging patients to participate in the therapeutic regimen. The therapy can become very complex, and too often patients feel that more is being done "to" them than "for" them. The nurse can be a sympathetic listener and help patients mobilize defenses to cope with the emotional and physical stresses.

Prevention of Bleeding. These patients should be approached in the same manner as those with aplastic anemia and should be assessed for thrombocytopenia, granulocytopenia, and anemia. The risk of bleeding correlates with the level of thrombocytopenia. In addition to having petechiae and ecchymoses, patients may develop major hemorrhages when their platelet counts drop below 20,000 per cubic millimeter of blood. For undetermined reasons, fever or infection also increases the likelihood of bleeding. Any increase in petechiae and any melena, hematuria, or nosebleeds should be reported. Undue trauma or intramuscular injections must be avoided, and acetaminophen, rather than aspirin, should be used for analgesia. Hemorrhage is treated by bed rest and transfusions of red cells and platelets.

Prevention of Infection. Because of the lack of mature and normal granulocytes, these patients are always threatened by infection, the major cause of death in leukemia. The likelihood of infection increases with the degree of neutropenia, so granulocyte counts under 100/milliliter of blood make the development of systemic infection highly probable. Immune dysfunction compounds the risk of infection. Patients must be systematically assessed for any evidence of infection.

Monitor for temperature elevation, flushed appearance, chills, tachycardia, appearance of white patches in mouth; redness, swelling, heat, or pain of eyes, ears, throat, skin, joints, abdomen, rectal and perineal areas; cough; changes in character and/or color of sputum, stool; skin rash.

- Remember that the usual manifestations of infection are altered in patients with leukemia. Prednisone may blunt the normal febrile response to infection.

Some typical signs of infection, such as the appearance of exudates, are often not apparent and make the need for careful observation even greater. Frequent oral hygiene may decrease the likelihood of infection originating from the oral cavity. Because of the high risk of infection arising from intravenous cannulas, gloves should be worn to start infusions, daily site care should be provided, and the cannula should be changed every 48 hours. Rectal abscesses are not unusual, so it is important to ensure normal elimination and avoid rectal thermometers, enemas, and rectal trauma. The urinary tract is another common site for infection. Avoidance of catheterization and, when catheterization is essential, scrupulous asepsis during catheter insertion and maintenance are important.

Improvement of Activity Tolerance. Anemia results from defective erythropoiesis, accelerated red cell destruction, and episodes of bleeding. If weak and easily fatigued, the patient may need assistance in choosing priorities and will need alternate rest and activity periods. Patients must also be assessed for dyspnea, tachycardia, and other evidence of inadequate oxygen supply to vital organs.

Attainment/Maintenance of Comfort. Infiltration of abnormal leukocytes into systemic tissues causes a variety of disabling symptoms. Pain is a common problem due to infiltration and enlargement of abdominal organs, lymph nodes, bones, and joints. Signs of central nervous system infiltration include headache, confusion, and other manifestations of meningeal irritation and increased intracranial pressure. Ongoing assessment of every body system will help to identify these widespread effects so that care can be planned to decrease symptoms as they occur.

Careful positioning is helpful in preventing undue pain in the abdomen, lymph node areas, bones, and joints. Sudden movements are avoided and soft supports, such as pillows, are used to promote comfort. When necessary, analgesics are administered as prescribed to relieve pain. To avoid bleeding at puncture sites, small-gauge needles are used when analgesics are given parenterally.

The massive cell destruction resulting from chemotherapy increases uric acid levels and makes patients vulnerable to renal stone formation and resulting renal colic. Therefore, patients need a high fluid intake to prevent crystallization of uric acid and subsequent stone formation.

Attainment/Maintenance of Adequate Nutrition. Gastrointestinal problems may result from the infiltration of abnormal leukocytes into the abdominal organs as well as from the toxicity of the chemotherapeutic agents. Anorexia, nausea, vomiting, diarrhea, and mucosal lesions in the mouth are common. Because good nutrition is so important for cancer patients, careful timing of chemotherapeutic drug administration, prophylactic use of prescribed antiemetics, and the encouragement of foods and fluids that are the least irritating are essential. Frequent oral hygiene helps to prevent oral lesions and to promote appetite. Small, frequent feedings of foods and fluids that are high in protein and vitamins and palatable to the patient are often helpful in maintaining nutrition.

Promotion of Positive Body Image. Because the hair is an important factor in a person's self-image, the development of alopecia is usually traumatic. Patients are prepared for the occurrence of this problem and helped to express and resolve their feelings about it. It is often helpful for them to obtain a wig that they find aesthetically appealing before the hair loss occurs. Family members are encouraged to assist in selecting the wig. Involvement and support of the family are often invaluable in helping patients adjust to the problem.

▷ *Evaluation*

▷ *Expected Outcomes*

1. Patient copes with diagnosis and prognosis.
   a. Verbalizes feelings about prognosis to family/support system
   b. Utilizes defense mechanisms appropriately
   c. Sets realistic goals
   d. Participates in the therapeutic regimen
2. Is free of bleeding
   a. Adheres to therapeutic regimen
   b. Avoids situations that predispose to physical trauma, *e.g.*, razor and other sharp objects, forceful nose blowing, straining with stool, contact sports
   c. Uses atraumatic measures of oral hygiene
   d. Monitors urine, stools, and vaginal discharge for evidences of bleeding
   e. Alerts health care personnel at first sign of bleeding
3. Is free of infection
   a. Attempts to maintain adequate nutritional intake
   b. Utilizes acceptable method and routine of oral hygiene
   c. Describes signs and symptoms of infection and preventive measures
   d. Avoids those with known infection
   e. Alerts health care personnel to first signs of infection
4. Experiences increased strength and endurance
   a. Explains causes for weakness and fatigue
   b. Spaces activities throughout the day
   c. Rests at specified intervals
   d. Makes appropriate alterations in life-style to accommodate decreased physical activity
   e. Shows progression in activity endurance from day to day
5. Attains/maintains comfort
   a. Identifies positions that promote comfort of abdomen and extremities
   b. Positions self to relieve abdominal and extremity pain
   c. Rests with head of bed elevated to decrease headache
   d. Uses analgesics as prescribed
   e. Drinks adequate fluids to prevent renal stone formation
6. Attains/maintains adequate nutrition
   a. Identifies factors that precipitate gastrointestinal discomfort
   b. Uses antiemetics as prescribed to prevent nausea and vomiting
   c. Chooses foods that have the least chance of causing gastric irritation
   d. Attempts to increase intake of foods high in protein and vitamins
   e. Performs frequent oral hygiene
   f. Maintains/gains weight
7. Maintains positive body image
   a. Discusses feelings about alopecia
   b. Accepts help from nursing personnel and family in preparing for and coping with alopecia
   c. Obtains a wig that patient finds appealing

Malignant Lymphomas

The lymphomas are neoplasms of the cells of the lymphoid system: the lymphocytes and histiocytes. They are often classified according to the degree of cell differentiation and the origin of the predominant malignant cell. These tumors usually start in lymph nodes, but can involve lymphoid tissue in the spleen, the gastrointestinal tract (for example, the tonsils or the wall of the stomach), the liver, or the bone marrow. They often spread to all of these areas and to extralymphatic tissues (lungs, kidneys, skin) by the time of death. The etiology of these tumors is unknown.

Hodgkin's Disease

Hodgkin's disease, like other lymphomas, is a malignant disease of unknown etiology that originates in the lymphatic system and involves predominantly the lymph nodes. It is somewhat more common in males and has two peaks of incidence: one in the early 20s and the other after age 50. Because many manifestations are similar to those occurring with infection, an infectious origin for the disease continues to be sought.

The malignant cell of Hodgkin's disease, its pathologic hallmark and its essential diagnostic criterion, is the "Reed-Sternberg cell," a gigantic atypical tumor cell, morphologically unique and of uncertain lineage, which many regard as an aberrant histiocyte.

Patients with Hodgkin's disease are customarily classified into subgroups based on pathologic criteria that reflect the grade of malignancy and suggest the prognosis. *Hodgkin's paragranuloma*, for example, with fewest Reed-Sternberg cells and least disturbance of nodal architecture, carries a much more favorable prognosis than *Hodgkin's sarcoma*, in which the lymph nodes are virtually replaced by tumor cells of the most primitive type. The majority of patients with so-called *Hodgkin's granuloma* (which includes two conditions currently designated "nodular sclerosis" and "mixed cellularity") are in an intermediate position with respect to the density and destructiveness of tumor cells, therapeutic responsiveness, and overall outlook.

Clinical Manifestations

Hodgkin's disease usually begins as a painless enlargement of the lymph nodes on one side of the neck, which becomes increasingly conspicuous. However, for months generalized pruritus may be the first and only symptom and later is often a most distressing one. The individual nodes remain firm and discrete (that is, they do not soften and do not fuse) and are seldom tender and painful. Soon the lymph nodes of other regions, usually the other side of the neck, also enlarge in the same manner. The mediastinal and retroperitoneal lymph nodes may also enlarge, causing severe pressure symptoms: pressure against the trachea results in dyspnea; pressure against the esophagus causes dysphagia; pressure on the nerves causes laryngeal paralysis and brachial, lumbar, or sacral neuralgias; pressure on the veins results in edema of one or both extremities and effusions into the pleura or peritoneum; and pressure on the bile duct causes obstructive jaundice. Later the spleen may become palpable, and the liver may enlarge. In some patients the first nodes to enlarge are those of one axilla or of one groin. Occasionally, the disease starts in mediastinal or peritoneal nodes and may remain limited to them. In still other cases the enlargement of the spleen is the only conspicuous lesion.

Sooner or later a progressive anemia develops. A leukocytosis often is observed with an abnormally high polymorphonuclear count and an elevated eosinophil count. About half of the patients have a slight fever, the temperature seldom rising above 38.3°C (101°F). However, patients with mediastinal and abdominal involvement present a remarkable intermittent fever. The temperature goes as high as 40.0°C (104°F) for periods of 3 to 14 days, returning to normal within a few weeks. Untreated, this disease is progressive in its course; the patient loses weight and becomes cachectic, the anemia becomes marked, *anasarca* (severe generalized edema) appears, the blood pressure falls, and death is likely to ensue in 1 to 3 years.

Diagnostic Evaluation

The diagnosis of Hodgkin's disease hinges on the identification of its characteristic histologic features in an excised lymph node. A diagnosis having been firmly established on the basis of the requisite criteria, it becomes necessary to assess as accurately as possible the total extent of tumor involvement and to define the manner in which it is distributed. In other words, one attempts to pinpoint the location of every tumor lesion inside and outside the lymphatic system and to exclude the presence of a tumor in organs and tissues that are not yet involved. This is a difficult, expensive, and uncertain undertaking but an extremely important one because these are the very considerations on which treatment is to be based.

Laboratory tests include a complete blood count, platelet count, sedimentation rate, and liver and renal function studies. A bone marrow biopsy and liver and spleen scans are done to determine if there is involvement in these ogans. Chest x-ray as well as bone scans of the pelvis, vertebrae, and long bones are done to identify any involvement in these areas.

Management

Current concepts of treatment stem from the following observations and premises:

1. Hodgkin's disease spreads from its original location (usually a single node) by way of the lymphatic channels to contiguous lymph nodes, which in turn become the sites of tumor growth; it rarely skips lymph nodes en route to more distant sites of metastasis.
2. Rarely does Hodgkin's disease spread beyond the lymphatic system to involve other organs and tissues until late in the disease.
3. Hodgkin's disease can be completely and permanently eradicated 95% of the time from any site that has received a radiation dose of 3500 to 4500 rads within the space of about 4 weeks. Megavoltage radiation techniques permit the delivery of such a dose to one or more entire lymph node chains.
4. Areas of the body in which the lymph node chains are located can tolerate doses of this magnitude without serious damage (as can the area of the spleen and the oronasopharynx, both of which may become involved in Hodgkin's disease), provided that vital structures such as the lungs, liver, gastrointestinal tract, kidneys, and bone marrow are protected by carefully shaped lead shields.

From the foregoing it is postulated that Hodgkin's disease is potentially curable by radiotherapy, provided it has not extended beyond the lymph node chains, spleen, and oro-nasopharynx. Failing signs of such extension, patients with this disease should have the benefit of "curative" radiotherapy in which doses large enough to destroy the tumors are delivered not only to obvious tumor nodes but to all adjacent nodes and lymph node chains as well. Conversely, any sign of spread beyond the treatable areas automatically disqualifies the Hodgkin's patient from such a program, in which case a combination of chemotherapy and palliative radiotherapy is indicated.

Staging of Hodgkin's Disease. For the sake of simplicity, uniformity, and convenience in categorizing patients with Hodgkin's disease with respect to the extent and activity of their disease and hence their eligibility for curative radiotherapy, the disease generally is classified, or "staged," as follows:

Stage I: Disease is limited to a single node and contiguous structures, or a single extralymphatic organ or site.

Stage II: Disease involves more than a single node or group of contiguous nodes, but is confined to one side of the diaphragm only.

Stage III: Disease is present both above and below the diaphragm and may include solitary involvement of the spleen, one extralymphatic site, or both.

Stage IV: Disease has disseminated diffusely to one or more extralymphatic sites with or without associated lymph node involvement.

Stages are further subdivided on the basis of the presence or absence of constitutional symptoms, *i.e.*, fever, night sweats, and unexplained weight loss. Patients without these symptoms are designated A and patients with them are designated B. Chemotherapy is often added for stage IIB and for stage IIIA. For stages IIIB and IV, combination chemotherapy is used, and radiation is generally reserved for the palliative treatment of local lesions that are especially damaging or painful. Currently, patients diagnosed at stage IA or IIA have a 5-year survival rate of 90% and can essentially be considered cured. Survival rates decrease progressively with more advanced stages.

Nursing Interventions

Radiation therapy often requires many weeks of daily trips to the hospital. The dose to the tumor and adjacent lymph node areas is generally 4500 rads.

Patients often develop esophagitis, anorexia, loss of taste, nausea and vomiting, diarrhea, skin reactions, and lethargy. Much ingenuity is needed to help patients cope with these unpleasant side-effects. They should be encouraged to make a concerted effort to eat. Bland soft foods that they normally like are usually most palatable and are tolerated best when served at mild temperatures. Aspirin in chewing gum form and anesthetic throat lozenges may be helpful in relieving the mouth and throat discomfort that often interfere with eating. The antiemetic that the physician prescribes should be given during the peak times of nausea.

Skin reactions that give the appearance of sunburned or tanned skin are common. Patients are alerted that these are expected and that rubbing of the area and application of heat, cold, or lotions should be avoided unless prescribed by the physician. If the reaction is severe and the skin is burned, the health care professional is to be notified.

The lethargy that accompanies radiation may cause patients to become discouraged about their progress. They are told that it is expected and that they must increase periods of rest and sleep in order to maintain a reasonable energy level. The family is encouraged to help patients in their attempts to rest. Diversional activities that require minimal energy expenditure may help to prevent boredom.

A commonly used chemotherapeutic regimen is a combination of nitrogen mustard, vincristine (Oncovin), prednisone, and procarbazine (MOPP). As for any patient receiving chemotherapy (see p. 272), support is necessary to help these patients tolerate the toxic effects, which include bone marrow depression, gastrointestinal disturbances, and alopecia. It often helps if patients are told that the therapy will end in a specific period of time. This, along with the knowledge that there is a high likelihood of cure, serves as an incentive for them to continue with the therapy. Helping patients to prepare for the alopecia by encouraging them to purchase a wig that is aesthetically acceptable to them before the problem occurs often averts some of the distress commonly associated with the loss of hair.

Patients with Hodgkin's disease are extremely vulnerable to infection, both as a result of radiation and chemotherapy and as a consequence of defective immune responses caused by the tumor. They are urged to report fever or any other signs of infection (skin redness, tenderness, lesions, cough) immediately so that treatment can be instituted. They are also apprised of the importance of avoiding contact with persons who are known to have infections.

Follow-up appointments with the physician are important for determining the effectiveness of the treatment. The patient and family are encouraged to keep all appointments.

Non-Hodgkin's Lymphomas

Lymphocytic lymphomas are more indolent and have a better prognosis than histiocytic lymphomas. Non-Hodgkin's lymphomas are a group of disorders that can be defined as malignancies of the lymphoid tissue other than Hodgkin's disease. They are relatively uncommon in the United States. The etiology is unknown. The prognosis is better than for Hodgkin's disease.

Manifestations are similar to those of Hodgkin's disease, but patients with these disorders are more likely to have generalized lymph node disease or extranodal disease when the disorder is first discovered. If the disease is localized, irradiation is the treatment of choice. If there is generalized involvement, chemotherapy is used. As with Hodgkin's disease, infection is a major problem. Central nervous system involvement is also common.

Mycosis Fungoides
(Cutaneous T-Cell Lymphoma)

Mycosis fungoides is a relatively rare lymphoma of the skin that is found equally among blacks and whites, and that is more common in men than women. It usually begins as a pruritic, red rash, and months or years later the skin becomes infiltrated with plaques and tumors of lymphoma. The specific lymphocyte involved is the T-cell lymphocyte. The body may be covered with mushroomlike growths varying in size from 1 cm to 5 cm (0.4–6 inches). Eventually, the malignant process reaches nodes, liver, spleen, and lungs. Patients are very uncomfortable with the itching and disfigurement of this disease. Treatment with nitrogen mustard (which may be used topically) or irradiation can achieve palliation.

The patient with painful ulcerative lesions will require skilled nursing. A bed cradle should be used to remove the weight of bedding from painful skin lesions. Bacteriostatic ointment may be prescribed as a preventive measure against secondary infection and to seal off air from open nerve endings. Other aspects of management are similar to those for the patient with Hodgkin's disease.

Multiple Myeloma

Multiple myeloma is a malignant disease of plasma cells that infiltrate bone, soft tissues, lymph nodes, liver, spleen, and kidneys. It is not classified as a lymphoma. The malignant cell is the plasma cell, the neoplastic proliferation taking place mainly in the bone marrow.

Patients generally present with a normochromic, normocytic anemia, back pain, and sometimes leukopenia or thrombocytopenia due to marrow infiltration by malignant plasma cells. The diagnosis of myeloma can be made by aspiration or biopsy of the bone marrow. X-rays showing destructive lesions of many bones are suggestive but not diagnostic for this disease. The malignant plasma cells produce large quantities of abnormal globulins, which appear in the serum electrophoresis as a paraprotein "spike." Fragments of these globulins are excreted in urine as Bence Jones proteins.

Patients may be incapacitated by constant bone pain. Plasma cell tumors can appear in many sites in these patients, including skin, mouth, and pleura; these are often painless. The osteolytic lesions are often associated with hypercalcemia, and bone fractures are common, especially in the vertebrae or ribs.

Management

Melphalan (Alkeran), cyclophosphamide, and steroids are the drugs used to decrease the tumor mass and relieve bone pain. They can prolong life from 1 year to 2 or 3 years. Radiation is very useful for palliation of bone pain and for reducing the size of extraskeletal plasma cell tumors. Good hydration is essential in order to prevent renal damage from precipitation of Bence Jones protein in the renal tubules, hypercalcemia, and hyperuricemia. Thus, it is important to assess these patients for signs and symptoms of renal insufficiency. Allopurinol is used to prevent uric acid crystallization. When patients have severe pain they need narcotic analgesics and local irradiation, and sometimes back braces to relieve pressure. Pathologic fractures are also possible. It is important to keep the patients as active as possible, because bed rest only increases the likelihood of hypercalcemia. Bacterial infections, especially pneumonia, are common in these patients, since they have impaired capacity for antibody production. Patients with multiple myeloma should not be put on fasting regimens for diagnostic tests because dehydrating procedures can precipitate acute renal failure.

Bleeding Disorders

Pathophysiology

The body is normally protected against excessive and lethal blood loss by numerous complicated and interrelated mechanisms. As indicated in Figure 29-1, hemostasis includes three phases. The first, the *vascular phase,* involves immediate vasoconstriction of injured vessels. This vessel spasm is sufficient to stop capillary bleeding. The second phase, or *platelet phase,* involves platelet aggregaton at the site. These tiny cells are rapidly attracted to the damaged endothelium and form loose plugs. More platelets gather, and eventually these fuse together and contract, forming stable plugs. The platelet plug effectively stops bleeding in small vessels such as venules, and provides temporary protection in larger injuries. Complete and permanent sealing of vascular wounds is accomplished through the clotting of the blood, which results in the production of an adherent gellike mass that effectively controls most types of hemorrhage. Initiated through either the intrinsic or the extrinsic pathway, a chain reaction occurs in which blood proteins are sequentially activated until factor Xa is formed. At this point, factor Xa interacts with favor V, calcium, and a platelet substance to convert prothrombin to thrombin. This is a very active enzyme that has several functions: one is to encourage further platelet aggregation; another is to convert fibrinogen to fibrin. Therefore, strands of fibrin begin to form in the vicinity of the platelet plug, reinforcing the plug and producing a larger clot. The fibrin clot is then further stabilized by the formation of bonds between the molecules, catalyzed by another plasma protein, factor XIII. The result is that the damaged vessel is sealed and blood flow in the area is slowed. Then, tissue repair of the vessel endothelium can proceed. Eventually, much of the fibrin clot will be lysed by another plasma protein system—the plasmin system, which produces fibrinolysis.

Several other homeostatic mechanisms contribute to hemostasis. Hemorrhage from a large, lacerated vessel is retarded as a result of an abrupt lowering of the arterial blood pressure (*i.e.,* "shock"), which reduces the rate of blood flow throughout the body and therefore reduces the rate of its escape. Further protection also may be furnished by compression of the leaking vessel by the swelling mass of blood (hematoma) surrounding the vessel. A final factor of great importance in the prevention of bleeding is the normal resistance of blood vessels to mechanical rupture, either by the pressure of blood exerted from within the vessel or by traumatic pressures exerted from the outside.

Abnormalities that predispose to hemorrhagic diseases can affect vessels, platelets, and any of the plasma coagulation factors, fibrin, or plasmin. Some patients can have defects at several sites simultaneously. Bleeding may be a manifestation of a primary coagulation defect (as in hemophilia), may occur secondary to another disease (as in cirrhosis, uremia, or leukemia), or may even be due to drugs (overdose of warfarin sodium).

Clinical Manifestations

The symptoms and signs of bleeding disorders vary, depending on the type of defect. A careful history can often give clues to the diagnosis. Abnormalities of the vascular system give rise to local bleeding, usually into the skin. Because platelets are primarily responsible for the cessation of bleeding from small vessels, patients with thrombocytopenia will have petechiae—small red or purple spots, often in clusters, seen on the skin and mucous membranes. Trauma results in excessive bruising but not large, uncontrolled hematomas. After cuts or skin puncture, bleeding stops promptly with local pressure and does not recur when pressure is released. In contrast, in hemophilia and abnormalities of other coagulation factors, the platelets function normally so that there are no petechial or superficial hemorrhages. Instead, deep bleeding occurs after minor trauma, such as intramuscular hematomas and hemorrhage into joint spaces. External bleeding recurs several hours after pressure is removed—as, for example, severe bleeding starting several hours after a tooth extraction.

Patients who have bleeding disorders or who have the potential for developing such disorders as a result of disease processes or therapeutic agents are observed carefully and frequently for bleeding. All drainage and excreta such as feces, urine, emesis, and gastric drainage are observed for occult as well as evident blood. The skin is observed for petechiae and ecchymoses, and the nose and gums are checked for bleeding. Abdominal, flank, or joint pain are promptly reported because they may be indicative of internal bleeding. In addition, the patient is closely observed for evidence of hypovolemia manifested by hypotension, tachycardia, pallor, cool clammy skin, altered responsiveness, and oliguria.

Vascular Disorders

Spontaneous rupture of small vessels that are defective or injured results in leakage of blood into the skin, mucous membranes, and serosal surfaces. The smallest hemorrhages, pinhead in size, are called *petechiae*. Hemorrhages up to 1 cm in diameter are referred to as *purpura*, and larger, blotchy lesions are *ecchymoses*.

Vascular dysfunction can be caused by a variety of mechanisms. Alterations in the connective tissue framework supporting blood vessels are believed to explain the bleeding associated with vitamin C deficiency and adrenocortical hormone excess. Vascular injury can also result from systemic diseases such as diabetes mellitus or the action of bacterial toxins. A particularly important cause of vascular injury is immunologically mediated. As a consequence of drug reactions, bacterial infections, allergic disorders, or collagen-vascular diseases, vascular damage occurs. Effects range from minor local injury to widespread thromboses or hemorrhage.

Platelet Defects

The sudden onset of petechiae, purpura, or excessive bruising or bleeding from the nose or gums should stimulate a search for a platelet defect. Deficiencies of platelet number, or thrombocytopenias, are most common, but there are also some rare disorders of platelet function in which the platelet count is normal but the clinical picture is identical to that in thrombocytopenia. The platelet function disorders can be diagnosed by special tests for platelet factor 3 and platelet adhesiveness and aggregation. The most important functional disorder to remember is that induced by aspirin; even small amounts of aspirin prevent normal platelet aggregation, and the bleeding time test is prolonged for several days after aspirin ingestion. Although this defect does not cause bleeding in most normal people, patients with another coagulation disorder (such as thrombocytopenia or hemophilia) can experience life-threatening hemorrhage after taking aspirin.

Thrombocytopenia

Thrombocytopenia is the most common cause of generalized bleeding. It can result either from decreased production of platelets by the marrow or from increased peripheral destruction. Some of the causes are listed in Table 29-3. If the platelet deficiency is secondary to an underlying disease, this can usually be diagnosed from the examination of the patient or the bone marrow. When peripheral destruction is the cause of thrombocytopenia, the marrow shows increased megakaryocytes and normal platelet production. Bleeding and petechiae usually do not occur with platelet counts above 50,000/cu mm, although excessive bleeding can follow surgery.

When the platelet count drops below 20,000/cu mm, petechiae appear and there are nose bleeds, excessive menstrual bleeding, and hemorrhage after surgery or dental extractions. When the platelet count is less than 5,000/cu mm, spontaneous fatal central nervous system hemorrhage or gastrointestinal hemorrhage can occur.

Management. The management for secondary thrombocytopenia is usually that for the underlying disease. If platelet production is impaired, platelet transfusions may help to raise platelet counts and stop bleeding or prevent intracranial hemorrhage. If excessive destruction is the problem, transfused platelets will also be destroyed and will not raise the count.

Idiopathic Thrombocytopenic Purpura (ITP)

Idiopathic thrombocytopenic purpura (ITP) is a disease of all ages but commonly affects children and young women. Although the precise etiology remains unknown, viral infections sometimes precede the disease in children. Antiplatelet antibodies are produced so platelet life span is markedly shortened. Occasionally, the antibodies can be demonstrated *in vitro*, but usually the diagnosis is made from the decreased platelet count and survival time and increased bleeding time. Other overt causes of thrombocytopenia must be ruled out. Symptoms may begin suddenly, with petechiae and mucosal bleeding. The platelet count is generally below 20,000/cu mm. Death may result from intracranial bleeding. There are no physical findings of note other than the hemorrhages.

Management. Corticosteroids are the treatment of choice; the bleeding ceases in 1 to 2 days, and platelet counts rise in a week or so. About three quarters of patients respond to steroids, but many have a relapse when the drug is withdrawn. These patients, as well as the nonresponders, are subjected to splenectomy. Splenectomy produces a lasting remission in 75% of patients, although transient recurrences of

TABLE 29-3
Thrombocytopenias

Cause	Treatment
I. Failure of Production	
Leukemia	Treat the leukemia.
Tumor invasion of marrow	
Aplastic anemia	Bone marrow transplant, androgens, antithrombocyte globulin
Megaloblastic anemia	B_{12} or folic acid
Toxins	Discontinue toxin.
Drugs: thiazides, heparin, chloramphenicol, cytotoxic drugs	Discontinue drug.
Infection, especially septicemia, viral infections, tuberculosis	Treat infection.
Alcohol	Discontinue alcohol.
II. Increased Destruction	
Due to antibodies	
ITP	Steroids, splenectomy
Lupus erythematosus	Steroids, immunosuppressive drugs
Malignant lymphoma	Steroids
Drugs: quinine, quinidine, digoxin, phenytoin, aspirin, sulfonamides, alcohol, gold	Discontinue drug.
Due to entrapment in large spleen	
Due to infections	Splenectomy
Bacteremia	
Postviral infections	Treat infection.
III. Increased Utilization	
Disseminated intravascular coagulation	Heparin

thrombocytopenia sometimes occur months or years later. The rare patients who do not respond to splenectomy are sometimes treated with the immunosuppressive drugs azathioprine or cyclophosphamide.

Clotting Factor Defects

Hemophilia

Definition and Etiology. There are two hereditary bleeding disorders that are indistinguishable clinically, but that can be separated by laboratory tests—hemophilia A and hemophilia B. Hemophilia A is due to a deficiency of factor VIII clotting activity, whereas hemophilia B stems from a deficiency of factor IX. Factor VIII deficiency is about five times more common. Both types of hemophilia are inherited as X-linked traits, so almost all affected persons are males; their mothers and some of their sisters are carriers but are asymptomatic.

Clinical Manifestations. The disease, which may be very severe, is manifested by large, spreading bruises and bleeding into muscles and joints after even minimal trauma. Patients often note pain in a joint before swelling and limitation of motion are apparent. Recurrent joint hemorrhages can result in damage so severe that chronic pain or ankylosis

(fixation) of the joint occurs. Many of the patients are crippled by the joint damage before they become adults. Spontaneous hematuria and gastrointestinal bleeding can occur. The disease is recognized in early childhood, usually in the toddler age group.

Prior to the availability of factor VIII concentrates, many patients died of the complications before reaching adulthood. Some patients with hemophilia have a milder deficiency, having between 5% and 25% of the normal level of factor VIII or IX. These patients do not experience the painful and disabling muscle and joint hemorrhages, but bleed only after dental extractions or surgery. Nevertheless, such hemorrhages can prove fatal if the cause is not recognized quickly.

Management. In the past, the only treatment was fresh frozen plasma, which had to be given in such large quantities that the patients became volume overloaded. Now factor VIII and IX concentrates are available to all blood banks. Patients are given concentrates when they are actively bleeding or as a prophylactic measure before dental extractions or surgery. Some families are taught how to administer the concentrate at home, at the first sign of bleeding.

A few patients eventually develop antibodies to the concentrates, so their factor levels cannot be elevated. Treatment of this problem is extremely difficult and often unsuccessful. Aminocaproic acid is an inhibitor of fibrinolytic enzymes. This drug can slow the dissolution of blood clots that do form, and is sometimes used after oral surgery in patients with hemophilia.

In terms of general care, patients with hemophilia should never be given aspirin or intramuscular injections. Dental hygiene is very important as a preventive measure, because dental extractions are so hazardous. Splints and other orthopedic devices may be very useful in patients who have suffered joint or muscle hemorrhages.

In recent years it has been found that patients with hemophilia are at high risk for developing AIDS (acquired immunodeficiency syndrome) as a result of the transfusions of blood and blood components that they receive. To prevent this problem, people with AIDS and those at high risk for developing AIDS are no longer considered for blood donation. In addition, all donated blood is now tested for the presence of antibodies to the AIDS virus.

▶ Nursing Process
The Patient With Hemophilia

▷ Assessment

Patients with hemophilia are carefully assessed for evidence of internal bleeding (abdominal, chest, or flank pain; hematuria; hematemesis; melena), muscle hematomas, and hemorrhage into joint spaces. Vital signs and hemodynamic pressure readings are assessed for indications of hypovolemia. All extremities and the torso are carefully examined for hematomas. All joints are assessed for swelling, limitation of mobility, and pain. Range of motion of the joints is done slowly and carefully to avoid further damage. At the first indication of pain, joint motion is stopped. Patients are questioned about any limitations of activities and movement experienced in the past and any need they have had for mobility aids such as splints, cane, or crutches.

If the patient has had recent surgery, the surgical site is assessed for bleeding frequently and carefully. Continuous monitoring of vital signs may be necessary until it is certain that excessive postoperative bleeding is not present.

All patients with hemophilia should be questioned about how they and their family cope with their condition, measures that they use to prevent bleeding episodes, and any limitations that the condition imposes on their life-style and daily activities. The patient who has frequent hospitalizations for bleeding episodes due to traumatic injury is carefully questioned about the factors that have led to these episodes. Such data are particularly helpful in determining the extent of the patient's acceptance of the condition and the need for patient and family education regarding measures to prevent unnecessary trauma.

▷ Nursing Diagnoses

Based on the assessment data, major nursing diagnoses for the patient may include the following:

- Pain related to joint hemorrhage and subsequent ankylosis
- Potential for decreased tissue perfusion related to bleeding

- Knowledge deficit regarding prevention of bleeding
- Ineffective coping related to the chronicity of the condition and its effects on life-style

▷ Planning and Implementation

▷ *Goals.* The major goals of the patient may include relief/minimization of pain, adequate tissue perfusion, utilization of measures to prevent bleeding, and coping with chronicity and altered life-style.

Nursing Interventions

Relief/Minimization of Pain. Generally, analgesics are required to alleviate the pain associated with large muscle hematomas and joint hemorrhage. The physician usually prescribes nonnarcotic analgesics when possible, because pain may be of long duration and dependency on narcotics becomes a problem with chronic pain. It is often helpful to administer the analgesic prior to activities that are known to precipitate pain. This not only helps the patient to accomplish the activity, but also tends to decrease the amount of analgesic that the patient requires.

All efforts possible are taken to prevent or minimize pain due to activity. The patient is encouraged to move slowly and to prevent undue stress on involved joints. Many patients report that warm baths promote relaxation, improve mobility, and lessen pain. Heat is avoided during bleeding episodes, however, because it potentiates further bleeding.

Since joint pain restricts mobility, patients with excessive pain during activity may benefit from orthopedic aids. Splints, canes, or crutches are helpful in some cases in shifting body weight off joints that are particularly painful. Splints must be properly applied and crutches must be properly fitted to prevent undue pressure on body surfaces that could cause tissue trauma and bleeding.

Attainment/Maintenance of Adequate Tissue Perfusion. The patient is assessed frequently for signs and symptoms of decreased tissue perfusion as evidenced by hypoxia to vital organs: restlessness, anxiety, confusion, pallor, cool clammy skin, chest pain, and decreased urinary output. Hypotension and tachycardia will occur as a result of volume depletion. The blood pressure, pulse, respirations, central venous pressure, and pulmonary artery pressure are monitored, as are the hemoglobin and hematocrit, coagulation and bleeding times, and platelet counts.

The patient is observed frequently for bleeding from the skin, mucous membranes, and wounds and for internal bleeding. During bleeding episodes the patient is kept at rest and gentle pressure is applied to any external bleeding sites. Cold compresses are applied to bleeding sites when indicated. Parenteral medications are administered with small-gauge needles to decrease trauma and the risk of bleeding. All possible efforts are made to protect the patient from trauma. The environment is kept free of obstacles that could cause falls, and the patient is turned and moved with care. Side rails are padded when necessary. Blood and blood components are administered as prescribed, and precautions are taken to avoid complications (see p. 696).

Use of Measures to Prevent Bleeding. The patient and family are informed of the risk of bleeding and the necessary safety precautions to be taken. They are encouraged to alter the home environment as necessary to prevent physical trauma. Obstacles that could cause falls are removed. An electric razor is used for shaving and a soft toothbrush is used for oral hygiene. Forceful nose blowing and coughing and straining at stool are avoided. A stool softener is used if necessary. Aspirin and aspirin-containing drugs are to be avoided.

Physical activity is encouraged, but with proper safety measures used. Noncontact sports such as swimming, hiking, and golf are acceptable activities, whereas contact sports are always to be avoided.

The necessity for regular check-ups and laboratory studies is explained. With knowledge of the reasons for continued medical evaluation, the patient will be more likely to keep appointments.

Coping with Chronicity and Altered Life-Style. Patients with hemophilia often require assistance in coping with the condition because it is chronic, it places restrictions on their lives, and it is an inherited disorder that can be passed to future generations. From childhood, patients are helped to accept themselves and the disease and to identify the positive aspects of their lives. They are encouraged to be self-sufficient and to maintain independence by preventing unnecessary trauma that can cause acute bleeding episodes and temporarily interfere with normal activities. As they work through feelings about the condition and progress to acceptance of it, they will accept more and more responsibility for maintaining optimal health. They will cooperate with health care providers, keep regular medical and dental appointments, and strive toward a healthy, productive family life. Many patients benefit from the services of hemophilia care centers and support groups. These provide coordinated, ongoing care and the opportunity to interact with others who are faced with the same situation.

▷ Evaluation

▷ Expected Outcomes

1. Experiences relief/minimization of pain.
   a. Reports decrease in pain after taking analgesic
   b. Exhibits increased ability to tolerate joint motion
   c. Uses orthopedic aids (when necessary) to decrease pain
2. Maintains adequate tissue perfusion
   a. Vital signs and hemodynamic pressure readings remain normal.
   b. Laboratory studies remain within normal ranges.
   c. Experiences no active bleeding.
3. Uses measures to prevent bleeding
   a. Avoids physical trauma
   b. Alters home environment to increase safety
   c. Keeps appointments with health-care professional
   d. Keeps appointments for laboratory studies
   e. Avoids contact sports
   f. Avoids aspirin and aspirin-containing drugs
   g. Wears Medic-Alert bracelet
4. Copes with chronicity and altered life-style
   a. Identifies the positive aspects of present life
   b. Involves family members in decisions about the future and changes to be made in life-style
   c. Strives toward independence
   d. Makes specific plans for continuation of health care

Von Willebrand's Disease

This is a common bleeding disorder, inherited as a dominant character and affecting males and females equally. It is due to a mild deficiency of factor VIII (15%–50% of normal) associated with an impairment of platelet function. The laboratory tests show normal platelet count, prolonged bleeding time, and slightly prolonged partial thromboplastin time. Patients commonly have nosebleeds, excessively heavy menses, bleeding from cuts, and postoperative bleeding. They do not suffer from massive soft tissue or joint hemorrhages. Both of the defects can be corrected by the administration of cryoprecipitate, which contains factor VIII, fibrinogen, and factor XIII.

Hypoprothrombinemia

Prothrombin, as was previously noted, is essential for the clotting process. This protein is produced in the liver by a vitamin K-dependent chemical process. Vitamin K enters the body from food sources as well as from synthesis by bacteria that reside in the intestine. Normal prothrombin activity in the blood depends on adequate absorption of this vitamin from the gastrointestinal tract and on adequate liver function. Therefore, prothrombin deficiency may arise as a result of diarrhea, from a lack of bile in the gastrointestinal tract (necessary for absorption of fat-soluble vitamin K) due to biliary tract obstruction, from surgical removal or mucosal damage of a large part of the small intestine, from prolonged antibiotic therapy, or as the result of liver disease.

The principal manifestation of prothrombin deficiency, as observed in patients with hemophilia, is prolonged hemorrhage from blood vessels that are damaged by trauma or disease, which explains the characteristic occurrence of ecchymoses, hematuria, gastrointestinal bleeding, and postoperative hemorrhages.

Coumarin Toxicity. The coumarins are drugs that are often employed for the express purpose of inducing a partial depression of prothrombin activity, because the drugs interfere with the action of vitamin K in the liver. Therapy is usually calculated to prolong the prothrombin time by 2 to 2½ times the normal time. In this range, thrombosis is inhibited and thrombophlebitis is prevented. However, if taken in excessive dosages, whether intentionally or mistakenly, or if certain other drugs are administered simultaneously that interfere with metabolism, the complete picture of prothrombin deficiency, with a severe hemorrhagic disorder, may be produced. Among drugs that enhance coumarin-induced anticoagulation are phenylbutazone, indomethacin, chloral hydrate, and salicylates. Other drugs, such as barbiturates, decrease coumarin effects.

Management. Hypoprothrombinemia, if due to vitamin K deficiency, responds to treatment with any of several preparations that are available for oral or parenteral administration. However, when corrective measures are urgently required, particularly in patients with liver disease or coumarin toxicity, the effective treatment requires the direct replacement of prothrombin by means of transfusion because purified preparations of prothrombin are not yet available.

Liver Disease. The liver cell makes all the plasma protein coagulation factors except factor VIII. Therefore, in severe hepatic disease of any sort, deficiencies in these factors may occur. The prothrombin time and partial thromboplastin time will both be prolonged. If the spleen is enlarged as well (as in cirrhosis), the platelet count may also be depressed. These patients frequently bruise easily and may have life-threatening hemorrhage from peptic ulcers or esophageal varices. Treatment includes fresh frozen plasma, fresh blood, and factor IX complex (Konyne). Vitamin K does not improve the disorder.

Disseminated Intravascular Coagulation (DIC)

Occasionally, widespread clotting in small vessels of the body occurs, causing clotting factors and platelets to be used up. Thus, paradoxically, the patient presents with a bleeding disorder characterized by low fibrinogen, prolonged prothrombin time and partial thromboplastin time, low factor VIII, and thrombocytopenia. Such patients may bleed from mucous membranes, venipuncture sites, and the gastrointestinal and urinary tracts. The bleeding can range from minimal occult internal bleeding to profuse hemorrhaging from all orifices. Patients may also develop renal failure due to fibrin deposition in small vessels of the kidney. Many serious illnesses may predispose to DIC, including septicemia, premature separation of the placenta in a pregnant woman, metastatic malignancies, hemolytic transfusion reactions, massive tissue trauma and shock. DIC should be suspected in any patient with a predisposing cause who develops purpura, a bleeding tendency, and signs of renal damage.

Serious hemorrhage requires replacement therapy: transfusions of red cells, platelet concentrates, and, if indicated by very low fibrinogen level, cryoprecipitate. The best treatment is correction of the underlying disease, but in the meantime intravenous heparin may retard the coagulation process and permit normalization of clotting tests and a decrease in the hemorrhagic manifestations.

Therapeutic Measures in Blood Disorders

Splenectomy

The surgical removal of the spleen is sometimes necessary following trauma to the abdomen. Because the spleen is very vascular, severe hemorrhage can result after splenic rupture. Under such circumstances splenectomy becomes an emergency procedure.

Splenectomy is also often performed as a treatment for a number of hematologic disorders. An enlarged spleen may be the site of excessive destruction of blood cells; when this destruction is life-threatening, the operation may prove palliative. This is the case in autoimmune hemolytic anemia or idiopathic thrombocytopenia purpura when these disorders do not respond to corticosteroids. Some patients with severe anemia due to inherited red cell defects (such as thalassemia or pyruvate kinase deficiency) may benefit from splenectomy. Patients with rheumatoid arthritis may develop splenomegaly

with destruction of granulocytes and granulocytopenia; removal of the spleen may improve the blood count and reduce the tendency toward infection.

Very large, bulky, and painful spleens (such as may occur in myelofibrosis or chronic myelogenous leukemia) usually do not need to be removed, but when the patient's symptoms and blood counts do not respond to drugs, splenectomy can be helpful. Most patients with hereditary *spherocytosis* (spheroid shape of erythrocytes) are essentially cured of their hemolytic process by splenectomy.

When the spleen is large, the operation can be difficult, but generally there is a very low mortality. Morbidity may result from postoperative atelectasis, pneumonia, abdominal distention, and subphrenic abscess formation. Young patients are at increased risk of pneumococcal infections for several years after splenectomy and should receive pneumococcal vaccine. All patients are instructed to seek prompt medical attention when even relatively minor symptoms of infection occur. Patients with high platelet counts (such as those with myelofibrosis) often are found to have even higher counts after splenectomy—greater than a million—and this can predispose the patient to serious thrombotic or hemorrhagic problems.

Blood Transfusion

Blood Donation

Because blood and blood components are used so frequently, nearly all hospitals now have blood banks, and most large hospitals also have facilities for removal of blood from donors. These donor clinics are often the responsibility of nurses, who must screen prospective donors, supervise the phlebotomies, and care for the health and safety of the donors.

Donor Interviewing

All prospective donors are examined and interviewed before the donation for their own protection and that of the recipients. The questioning must be tactful but complete, and an experienced interviewer will learn how to ask each question in several ways in order to obtain the most complete answers. Donors should appear to be in good health and should be free of any of the following disqualifying factors:

- A history of viral hepatitis, recently or at any time in the past, or a history of close contact with a hepatitis or dialysis patient within 6 months.
- A history of receiving a blood transfusion or injection of any fraction of blood other than serum albumin or immune globulin within 6 months.
- A history of untreated syphilis or malaria, because these can be transmitted by transfusion even years later. A person who has been free of symptoms and off therapy for 3 years after malaria may be a donor.
- A history of evidence of drug abuse in which drugs were self-injected, because addicts have a high hepatitis carrier rate, and because of the risk of AIDS.
- A history of possible exposure to the AIDS virus. A test for the presence of antibodies to AIDS virus in donated blood is now available. The population at risk includes

homosexual and bisexual men with multiple partners, intravenous drug abusers, persons with hemophilia, sexual partners of individuals at risk for AIDS, and persons with signs and symptoms suggestive of the appearance of the disease.

- A skin infection, because of the possibility of contamination of the phlebotomy needle.
- A history of recent asthma, urticaria, or allergy to drugs, because hypersensitivity can be passively transferred to the recipient.
- Pregnancy within 6 months, because of the nutritional demands of pregnancy on the mother.
- A history of tooth extraction or oral surgery within 72 hours, because such procedures are frequently associated with transient bacteremia.
- A history of recent tattoo, because of the higher risk of hepatitis.
- A history of exposure to infectious disease within the past 3 weeks, because of the risk of transmission to the recipient.
- Recent immunizations, because of the risk of transmitting live organisms (2-week waiting period for live, attenuated organisms; 2 months for rubella; 1 year for rabies).
- Presence of cancer, because of the lack of knowledge about transmission.
- A history of whole blood donation within the past 56 days.

Blood donors who pass this screen are then examined with regard to blood pressure, pulse, oral temperature, weight, and hemoglobin level. The last is often checked via a screening test that only estimates the hemoglobin. Persons under 17 and over 65 years of age are usually disqualified. Donors are expected to meet the following minimal requirements:

1. The body weight should exceed 50 kg (110 pounds) for a standard 450-ml donation. Donors weighing less than 50 kg (110 pounds) may be bled proportionately less.
2. The oral temperature should not exceed 37.5°C (99.6°F).
3. The pulse rate should be regular and between 50 and 100 beats per minute.
4. The systolic arterial pressure should be between 90 and 180 mm Hg, and the diastolic pressure between 50 and 100 mm Hg.
5. The hemoglobin level in the case of a woman should be at least 12.5 gm/dl (125 g/L), and in the case of a man, 13.5 gm/dl (135 g/L).

Phlebotomy

Phlebotomy consists of venipuncture and the withdrawal of blood. Donors are placed in a semirecumbent position, the skin over the antecubital fossa is carefully cleansed with an iodine preparation, a tourniquet is applied, and venipuncture is performed. Withdrawal of 450 ml of blood takes less than 15 minutes. Following removal of the needle, donors are asked to hold the involved arm straight up, and firm pressure is applied with sterile gauze for 2 or 3 minutes or until bleeding stops. A firm bandage is then applied. Donors are asked to remain recumbent until they feel able to sit up, usually 1 or 2 minutes. If weakness or faintness is experienced, they should

rest for a longer period. After getting up, they are given food and fluids in a reception area and asked to remain another 15 minutes. Donors should be instructed to leave the dressing on and avoid heavy lifting for several hours, to avoid smoking for 1 hour and alcoholic beverages for 3 hours, to increase fluid intake for 2 days, and to be sure to eat well-balanced meals for 2 weeks. The labels on the blood bag and tubes are checked carefully before and after donation to avoid any error that could prove fatal to a recipient.

Complications

Excessive bleeding at the site of venipuncture is sometimes due to a bleeding disorder in the donor, but more often is the result of a technical error: laceration of the vein, excessive tourniquet pressure, or failure to apply enough pressure following withdrawal of the needle.

Fainting is relatively common and may be related to emotional factors, vasovagal reaction, or prolonged fasting before donation. Sometimes, because of the loss of blood volume, hypotension and syncope occur when the donor assumes an erect position.

- A donor who appears pale or complains of faintness should immediately lie down or sit with head lowered below the knees. The nurse should observe the donor for another 30 minutes.

Anginal chest pain may be precipitated in patients with unsuspected coronary artery disease.

Convulsions may occur in patients with epilepsy. Both angina and convulsions require further medical evaluation.

Blood and Blood Components

A unit of blood that has been drawn from a donor consists of approximately 450 ml of whole blood and 60 to 70 ml of preservative-anticoagulant. The latter serves as the anticoagulant and also provides the red cells with a sugar for metabolism. This blood can be maintained at 1°C to 6°C in the blood bank for 21 to 35 days, depending on the type of preservative-anticoagulant used; after that it is discarded, because too many of the red cells are unable to survive *in vivo*. Whole blood stored more than 24 hours does not contain functional platelets or practical amounts of coagulation factors V and VIII.

Samples of the unit are always taken immediately after donation so that the blood can be typed and tested for the presence of syphilis, hepatitis, and antibodies. A test for the presence of AIDS antibodies in donated blood is now required. A label on the unit thereafter states the blood type and certifies that the unit is negative for syphilis serology, hepatitis B antigen, and AIDS antibodies.

Whole blood is a complex tissue with both cellular and many noncellular plasma components. Recently it has been recognized that whole blood is necessary only in certain clinical situations; many times, component therapy can replace the particular deficiency without subjecting the patient to unnecessary risks, such as circulatory overload. In addition, the use of components is more economical because it makes it possible to meet the needs of more than one patient from a single blood donation. Many blood banks are able to separate whole blood into these fractions, and all of the components are available from the American Red Cross.

Whole Blood. Whole blood may be used to treat acute, massive hemorrhage or hypovolemic shock due to hemorrhage. It is not indicated for the correction of anemia. Whenever possible, components should be used instead.

Packed Red Cells. Red cells are separated from whole blood by centrifugation or sedimentation; most of the plasma is removed, leaving a hematocrit of approximately 80%. Packed red cells are indicated for transfusions in all anemic patients, in surgical patients before and after operation, and in many cases of acute blood loss. The use of packed cells instead of whole blood reduces the volume load. Thus, this method is safer for patients with incipient congestive failure and reduces the incidence of transfusion reactions due to plasma factors.

Frozen Red Cells. The method of freezing red cells allows storage for long periods of time—even years—but is expensive. Hence, frozen cells are used only under unusual circumstances, such as for patients with very rare blood types or with antibodies to the common minor antigens.

Platelets. Patients with thrombocytopenia and hemorrhage often require transfusions of large numbers of platelets. Platelets taken from 4 to 8 units of blood are necessary to raise the count of a severely thrombocytopenic patient to a hemostatic level. Therefore, "platelet-rich plasma" with a small volume is used rather than whole blood. Several methods are available for harvesting fresh platelets: (1) Plasma can be removed after centrifugation of a unit of freshly collected whole blood; the plasma is then centrifuged again slowly to separate the platelets. Several such platelet "units" can then be pooled and given to the recipient, who thus receives platelets from several different donors. (2) A single donor can undergo *platelet apheresis,* in which blood is donated, the red cells are separated and returned to the donor immediately, and the plasma is spun down to obtain platelets in a volume of only 10 ml to 20 ml. In this way, multiple units can be donated.

Platelet concentrates are generally kept at room temperature with agitation and are administered within 48 hours of collection to ensure viability. Each unit of platelets will raise the recipient's platelet count by about 10,000/cu millimeter. For an adult with severe thrombocytopenia, 10 or more units of platelets may be needed daily. Even larger doses are needed for patients with fever or infection because these conditions decrease platelet effectiveness.

Single donor platelet transfusions are especially valuable for patients who have received many transfusions and have developed antibodies to all except HLA (transplantation antigen) matched blood products.

Granulocytes. Severely granulocytopenic patients with infection can sometimes benefit from transfusions of normal white cells. Large numbers of granulocytes less than 24 hours old must be administered. The donor's white cells are continuously removed as blood is drawn from one vein and constantly returned to another vein. The process requires about 4 hours of donor time, and the donor must be anticoagulated during the procedure.

Plasma. Whole plasma was originally used in the treatment of hypovolemic shock, but now, because plasma carries a risk of hepatitis equal to that of whole blood, other colloids (such as albumin) or electrolyte solutions (like Ringer's lac-

tate) are usually preferred. Plasma can be used to replace deficient coagulation factors in acquired or inherited bleeding disorders. Only fresh frozen plasma (which can be stored for 12 months) contains all the coagulation factors, including V and VIII. However, fractions of plasma have now been prepared that can replace all the factors except V, in small volume concentrates. Fresh frozen plasma may be administered to replace clotting factors in patients who are hemorrhaging and being massively transfused with whole blood or packed red cells. It is also used to treat patients with severe liver disease.

Albumin. Plasma albumin is a large protein molecule that usually stays within vessels and is a major contributor to plasma oncotic pressure. This material is used to expand the blood volume of patients in hypovolemic shock and to elevate the level of circulating albumin in patients with hypoalbuminemia. These preparations, in contrast to all other fractions of human blood, cellular or soluble, are subjected to heating at 60°C (140°F) for 10 hours, and therefore can be certified unequivocally as free of all viral contaminants, including hepatitis virus. Whereas the risk of hepatitis transmission is an important consideration in connection with every other type of transfusion therapy (except immune globulin), no such complication has ever been known to follow the use of albumin.

Cryoprecipitate. Cryoprecipitate is a plasma derivative that is rich in factor VIII, fibrinogen, factor XIII, and fibronectin. It is prepared by thawing one unit of fresh frozen plasma and removing all but 10 ml to 15 ml of plasma and the cold-insoluble globulins. The product is then refrozen and can be used for up to one year for the treatment of hemophilia A, Von Willebrand's disease, DIC, and uremic bleeding.

Factor IX Concentrate. A concentrated form of factor IX is prepared by pooling, fractionating, and freeze-drying large volumes of plasma. It is used primarily for treatment of patients with factor IX deficiency (also called hemophilia B, or Christmas disease). It carries a high risk of hepatitis because preparation requires plasma pooling from many donors and it is not processed to destroy infectious agents.

Prothrombin Complex. This fraction, commercially marketed as Konyne and Proplex, contains prothrombin and factors VII, IX, and X, and some factor XI. It is useful for the treatment of bleeding in congenital or acquired deficiencies in these factors. However, the hepatitis hazard is significant with this material.

Transfusion Technique

Administration of blood and blood components demands knowledge of correct techniques for administration and possible complications. After verifying the order and explaining the procedure to the patient, the nurse obtains the blood or blood component from the blood bank. Labels are carefully checked with another nurse. Vital signs should be recorded prior to initiating the transfusion.

Whole blood or packed red cells are generally administered through a 19-gauge or large needle into a large vein. Special tubing is used that contains a blood filter to screen out fibrin clots and other particulate matter. For the first 15 minutes, the transfusion is run very slowly, at about 2 ml per minute, and the patient is observed carefully for adverse effects. If no ill effects occur during this time, the flow rate is then increased unless the patient is at high risk for overload. The patient must continue to be observed frequently. A summary of major points to consider when administering blood components is listed in Table 29-4.

Assessment

Prior to initiating transfusion therapy it is important to check to see that the blood has been typed and cross-matched and that the ABO group and Rh type on the blood containers are in accordance with the compatability record. The blood should also be checked for the presence of gas bubbles and any abnormal color or cloudiness. Gas bubbles may indicate bacterial growth, and abnormal color or cloudiness may be a sign of hemolysis. The labels identifying the number and type of the donor blood and the recipient blood are noted. Patient identification is confirmed by asking for the patient's name and by checking the identification wrist band. At the same time, the patient's chart is checked for blood type and number. TPR and blood pressure are taken in order to provide a baseline for comparing vital signs at a later time.

After the blood transfusion is started, the patient should be watched closely for 15 to 30 minutes to assure that no signs of reaction or circulatory overload occur. Monitoring vital signs is carried out at regular intervals as indicated.

Complications and Nursing Management

Every patient who receives a blood transfusion is subject to the possible development of complications of transfusion therapy. Nursing management is directed toward the prevention of these complications and prompt initiation of measures

TABLE 29-4
Administration of Blood Components

Product	Administration Technique	Major Complications
Packed red cells	Use standard blood filter and make sure cells cover entire surface. Administer only with 0.9% NaCl. (Dextrose hemolyzes RBCs and Ringer's lactate causes coagulation.) Squeeze bag to mix cells every 20 to 30 minutes during administration. Administer 1 unit over 1 to 2 hours. If necessary to help cells infuse, add 50 ml to 100 ml 0.9% NaCl.	Transfusion reactions less frequent than with whole blood
Platelets	Use special nonwettable filter. (Do not use microaggregate filter.) Administer only with 0.9% NaCl. Administer as rapidly as tolerated, usually 4 units/hour, to prevent platelets from clumping and sticking to side of bag.	Febrile reactions common
Granulocytes	Use standard blood filter. (Do not use microaggregate filter.) Administer only with 0.9% NaCl. Administer over 2 to 4 hours to aid patient tolerance. (Do not use microaggregate filter.)	Febrile and allergic reactions common Leukoagglutinin reactions possible, leading to hypotension; anaphylaxis, and respiratory distress
Plasma	Use straight line set. (Do not use microaggregate filter.) Administer as rapidly as patient tolerates because coagulation factors become unstable after thawing.	Risk of circulatory overload Risk of hepatitis greater than with whole blood (if multiple donors)
Albumin	Undiluted 25% albumin should be administered at 1 ml/minute if patient is normovolemic. Use administration set supplied with it. Administer as rapidly as possible for patient in hypovolemic shock.	Risk of circulatory overload No risk of hepatitis
Factor VIII	Administer by syringe or component drip set.	Allergic and febrile reactions common Hepatitis risk same as with whole blood
Prothrombin	Administer through straight line set.	Allergic and febrile reactions possible Risk of hepatitis greater than with whole blood

to control any complications that occur. Transfusion complications include the following:

Circulatory overload
Febrile reaction
Allergic reaction
Septic reaction
Hemolytic reaction
Delayed hemolytic reaction
Diseases transmitted by the transfusion (*e.g.*, hepatitis, malaria, syphilis, AIDS)

Circulatory Overload. In patients with normal blood volume (as in chronic anemia) or increased blood volume (as in renal failure or heart failure), the addition of whole blood or packed cells can precipitate pulmonary edema. Packed red cells are safer to use and, if the rate of administration is sufficiently slow, circulatory overload may be prevented.

- The signs to look for are dyspnea, orthopnea, cyanosis, or sudden anxiety. If the transfusion is continued, severe dyspnea and coughing of pink, frothy sputum can occur. Neck vein distention, crackles at the base of the lungs, and rise in central venous pressure will occur.
- The patient is placed in an upright position with the feet in a dependent position, the blood is discontinued, and the physician is notified. The intravenous line is kept patent with a *very* slow infusion of normal saline to retain access to the vein in case intravenous medications are necessary. Phlebotomy or diuretics, oxygen, morphine, and aminophylline may be necessary if improvement does not occur rapidly.

Febrile Reaction. Patients may develop a fever during transfusion because of the presence of bacterial pyrogens, sensitivity to leukocytes or platelets, hemolytic episodes, or unknown factors. Due to the widespread use of disposable transfusion equipment, bacterial pyrogens are rarely a cause. Infrequently, blood can be grossly contaminated with large numbers of microorganisms that survive in the 4°C (39.2°F) storage. If such blood is infused, the patient develops fever and shaking chills within 30 minutes, and shock soon follows. Even when the cause of this reaction is recognized early (by gram stain of the donor blood), the mortality rate is high.

As soon as the reaction is recognized, the transfusion is discontinued and the intravenous line is kept open with normal saline. The physician and blood bank are notified and the blood bag is returned to the blood bank. The temperature is checked ½ hour after the chill and as indicated thereafter. Antipyretics are administered as prescribed.

Sensitivity to leukocyte or platelet antigens is much more common, especially in previously transfused patients or women who have borne children. The temperature rises during the administration of blood or shortly afterward and is rarely associated with chills, hypotension, or nausea. This type of reaction has a good prognosis; the treatment is aspirin. Subsequent transfusions should utilize leukocyte-poor blood.

Allergic Reaction. Some patients may develop urticaria (hives) or generalized itching or, rarely, wheezing or anaphylaxis. The cause of these reactions is thought to be sensitivity to a plasma protein in the transfused blood, or passive transfer of antibodies from the donor that react with some antigen (for example, in a drug or food) to which the recipient is exposed. To avoid this, allergic individuals are disqualified as donors. The reactions are usually mild and respond to antihistamines. If hives are the only symptom, the transfusion can sometimes be continued at a slower rate. If the reaction is severe, parenteral epinephrine is used.

Septic Reaction. *Septic reactions* are severe reactions that result from transfusion of blood or components contaminated with bacteria. Preventive measures include administering blood within 4 hours before warm room temperatures promote bacterial growth, and inspecting blood or components for gas bubbles, clotting, or abnormal color before administration. If the transfusion is contaminated, the patient will respond with rapid onset of chills, high fever, vomiting, diarrhea, and marked hypotension. In such a case the transfusion is discontinued immediately and the intravenous line kept patent with normal saline. The physician and blood bank are notified, and the blood bag is returned to the blood bank. Blood cultures are obtained, and the patient is treated for septicemia with antibiotics, IV fluids, vasopressors, and steroids.

Hemolytic Reaction. The most dangerous type of transfusion reaction occurs when the donor blood is incompatible with that of the recipient. Antibodies in the recipient's plasma rapidly combine with donor erythrocytes, and the cells are hemolyzed either in the circulation or in the reticuloendothelial system. The most rapid hemolysis occurs in ABO incompatibility (*e.g.*, if the donor is group A and the recipient is group O, and therefore has anti-A and anti-B antibodies). Rh incompatibility is often less severe.

- Symptoms consist of chills, low back pain, headache, nausea, or chest tightness, followed by fever and hypotension and vascular collapse. Severe reactions usually start within 10 minutes after the transfusion is begun. *Hemoglobinuria* (red urine) appears at the next voiding.
- The reaction must be recognized promptly and the transfusion discontinued immediately; the chances of a fatal episode are much reduced if less than 100 ml of incompatible blood are infused.

Treatment is directed toward correcting the hypotension and preventing the renal damage that can follow hemoglobinuria. The patient is supported with intravenous colloid and given mannitol as an osmotic diuretic to maintain a good urine flow, glomerular filtration, and renal blood flow. An indwelling catheter may be necessary for accurate measurement of output. If, after 24 hours, urine flow cannot be maintained, mannitol is contraindicated because it can be assumed that acute tubular necrosis has occurred. The management henceforth will be that for the renal disorder and will include fluid restriction and possibly dialysis until spontaneous healing takes place.

Delayed Hemolytic Reaction. Delayed hemolytic reactions occur at about 1 to 2 weeks and are recognized by fever, mild jaundice, a gradual fall in hemoglobin level, and a positive Coombs's test. There is no hemoglobinuria, and generally these reactions are not dangerous. However, recognition is important because subsequent transfusions may cause an acute hemolytic reaction.

Diseases Transmitted by Blood Transfusion. The following diseases are transmissible by blood transfusion.

Serum Hepatitis. Serum hepatitis is an important risk of transfusion therapy, both for whole blood and for most components (see above). Blood and blood products obtained from paid donors carry a higher risk than that from volunteer donors. Pooled blood products also constitute a significantly higher risk. Tests are currently used to detect hepatitis B virus, as well as non-A, non-B hepatitis. Hepatitis is further discussed in Chap. 35.

Malaria. Malaria is sometimes transmitted in blood donated by asymptomatic persons who have been exposed to the disease. Recipients develop high fever and headache several weeks after the transfusion.

Syphilis. Syphilis is rarely transmitted now because of the serologic tests required on all units of blood and because the organism does not survive refrigeration.

Acquired Immunodeficiency Syndrome (AIDS). AIDS has been associated with transfusion of blood products. For this reason persons in high-risk groups (*i.e.*, homosexual and bisexual men with multiple partners, intravenous drug abusers, persons with hemophilia, sexual partners of individuals at risk for AIDS, and persons with signs and symptoms suggestive of the appearance of the disease) should not donate blood. All donated blood is now tested for the presence of antibodies to the AIDS virus.

Summary of Nursing Interventions in Transfusion Reaction

If it is suspected that a transfusion reaction is occurring because of any of the conditions mentioned above, the nurse should stop the transfusion and call the physician immediately. The following steps are taken in order that a diagnosis may be made regarding the type and severity of the reaction:

- The transfusion set is disconnected, but the intravenous line is kept open with a saline solution in case intravenous medication should be needed rapidly.
- *The blood bag and tubing are saved, not thrown away.* They should be sent to the blood bank for repeat typing and culture.
- The patient's blood is drawn for plasma hemoglobin, culture, and retyping.
- A urine sample is collected as soon as possible and sent to the laboratory for a hemoglobin determination. Subsequent voidings of urine should be observed.
- The blood bank is notified that a suspected transfusion reaction has occurred.

Bone Marrow Transplantation

This is an exciting addition to the therapeutic possibilities for hematologic disease. Bone marrow can be aspirated by needle from multiple sites of an anesthetized normal donor and easily transfused intravenously into the recipient. The marrow cells immediately travel to the marrow spaces that have been emptied by disease (*i.e.*, aplastic anemia) or by chemotherapy. The donor cells proliferate in the marrow, releasing functional cells into the peripheral circulation. Complete marrow recovery may take 6 to 8 weeks.

The major barrier to the success of bone marrow transplantation is the antigenic difference between donor and recipient. Thus, transplants between identical twins are almost always successful, and sibling transplants are often successful. If the donor and the patient are not identical in HLA (transplantation antigen) types, pretreatment of the patient with

immunosuppression is necessary. Many recipients succumb to graft vs. host disease or severe infections while awaiting the recovery of the transplanted marrow. However, methods of immunosuppression and supportive care have improved greatly over the last few years, and this is currently the best treatment for severe aplastic anemia. Bone marrow transplantation is also used to treat some forms of leukemia and thalassemia.

Bibliography

Books

Boggs DR and Winkelstein A. White Cell Manual. Philadelphia, FA Davis, 1983.

Braunwald E et al. (ed). Harrison's Principles of Internal Medicine. New York, McGraw-Hill, 1987.

Corbett JV. Laboratory Tests in Nursing Practice. New York, Appleton-Century-Crofts, 1982.

DeVita VT, Hellman S, and Rosenberg SA. Cancer: Principles and Practice of Oncology. Philadelphia, JB Lippincott, 1985.

Gale RP. Leukemia Therapy. Boston, Blackwell Scientific Publications, 1986.

Griffin JP. Hematology and Immunology: Concepts for Nursing. Norwalk, Connecticut, Appleton-Century-Crofts, 1986.

Gunz F (ed). Leukemia. New York, Grune & Stratton, 1983.

Hillman RS and Finch CA. Red Cell Manual. Philadelphia, FA Davis, 1985.

Mollison P. Blood Transfusion in Clinical Medicine. St Louis, CV Mosby, 1982.

Price SA and Wilson LM. Pathophysiology: Clinical Concepts of Disease Processes. New York, McGraw-Hill, 1986.

Rifkind RA et al. Fundamentals of Hematology. Chicago, Year Book Medical Publishers, 1986.

Robbins SL and Cotran RS. Pathologic Basis of Disease. Philadelphia, WB Saunders, 1984.

Rutman R and Miller WV. Transfusion Therapy: Principles and Procedures. Rockville, Maryland, Aspen Systems, 1985.

Suitor CW and Hunter MF. Nutrition: Principles and Application in Health Promotion. Philadelphia, JB Lippincott, 1984.

Widmann FK. Clinical Interpretation of Laboratory Tests. Philadelphia, FA Davis, 1983.

Williams WJ et al. Hematology. New York, McGraw-Hill, 1983.

Articles

General

Baserger SJ and Benz EJ. Approach to blood disorders in elderly patients. Consultant 1984 Mar; 24(3):309–319.

Brandt B. A nursing protocol for the client with neutropenia. Oncol Nurs Forum 1984 Mar/Apr; 11(2):24–28.

Eddy JL, Selgan-Corden R, and Curran M. Cutaneous T-cell lymphoma. Am J Nurs 1984 Feb; 84(2):202–206.

Giardina PJV and Hilgartner MW. Thalassemia: Practical points. Hosp Med 1985 June; 21(6):162–182.

Hagemeister FB and Fuller LM. Lymphoma and Hodgkin's disease: New imaging techniques help guide diagnosis and referral. Consultant 1984 Feb; 24(2):128–148.

Kelly JO. Standards of clinical nursing practice for leukemia: Neutropenia and thrombocytopenia. Cancer Nurs 1983 Dec; 6(6):487–494.

Lamb C. Why is that hematocrit high? Patient Care 1986 Jan 15; 20(1): 46–75.

Lipschitz DA and Udupa KB. Age and the hematopoietic system. J Am Geriatr Soc 1986 June; 34(6):448–454.

McConnell EA. Leukocyte studies: What the counts can tell you. Nursing 86 1986 Mar; 16(3):42–43.

Neely SM. NonHodgkin's lymphomas: Classification and staging as guides to therapy. Consultant 1985 Nov 15; 25(26):67–85.

O'Rourke A. Bone marrow procedure guide. Oncol Nurs Forum 1986 Jan/Feb; 13(1):66–67.

Reheis CE. Neutropenia: Causes, complications, treatment, and resulting nursing care. Nurs Clin North Am 1985 Mar; 20(1):219–225.

Wheby MS. Polycythemia: Interpreting the "message" of an elevated hematocrit. Consultant 1984 Dec; 24(12):124–144.

Anemia

Brown EB. Anemia of chronic disease: Recognize it and exclude other red cell disorders. Consultant 1983 Nov; 23(11):235–243.

Conley CL. Anemia: Accurate diagnosis and appropriate therapy. Hosp Pract 1984 Sept; 19(9):57–66.

Freedman ML. Iron deficiency in the elderly. Hosp Pract 1986 Mar 30; 21(3):115–137.

Johnson CS. Microcytic anemia: When treatment is necessary, and when it isn't. Consultant 1985 Oct. 15; 25(14):75–78.

LaBounty LA. Iron metabolism and the identification of iron deficiency and anemia. J Med Technol 1986 Feb; 3(2):81–100.

Marchand A. Immune hemolytic anemia—Part 3: The role of drugs. Diag Med 1983 Nov/Dec; 6(8):24–36.

Merenstein A and Schenkman M. Pernicious anemia: The disease and physical management. Phys Ther 1984 July; 64(7):1076–1077,.

Nicolle LS. Anemia of chronic disorders. Nurse Pract 1984 Nov; 9(11): 19–20, 22.

Pale blood, thin blood. Emerg Med 1983 Dec 15; 15(21):26–47.

Patient compliance and relapsing anemia. Nurses Drug Alert 1983 Nov; 7(11):81–82.

Quick guide to common anemias. Nursing 83 1983 Dec; 13(12):24T–24U.

Smith ECG. Treatment of aplastic anemias. Hosp Pract 1985 May 15; 20(5):69–84.

Bleeding Disorders

Goodwin SA. Drug-induced coagulation alterations. Crit Care Quart 1985 Mar; 7(4):1–18.

Hamilton GC. Hemostasis out of order. Emerg Med 1985 Nov 15; 17(19): 82–116.

Harrington WJ. Generalized bleeding: Interpreting clinical findings. Hosp Pract 1985 Jan 30; 20(1):75–90.

King NH. Controlling bleeding when the platelet count drops. RN 1984 Aug; 47(8):25–27.

Koch PM. Thrombocytopenia: Don't let it make a big problem out of nothing. Nursing 84 1984 Oct; 14(10):54–57.

Luby CK and Wood PW. Thrombotic thrombocytopenia purpura. DCCN 1985 July/Aug; 4(4):209–214.

Lucas F. Lab tests plus clinical clues equals diagnosis of bleeding disorders. Diagn Med 1983 Nov/Dec; 6(8):65–77.

Schafer AI. Bleeding disorders: Finding the cause. Hosp Pract 1984 Nov; 19(11):88K–88HH.

Silinsky JJ. What you can learn from the platelet count. RN 1985 Jan; 48(1):87–88.

Statland BE and Ito RK. How cancer upsets hemostasis. Diagn Med 1983 May/June; 6(3):74–86.

Tabor PA. Antibiotic-related bleeding disorders. Focus Crit Care 1985 June; 12(3):31–35.

Bone Marrow Transplantation

Cogliano-Shutla NA et al. Bone marrow transplantation. Nurs Clin North Am 1985 Mar; 20(1):49–66.

McGlave PB. The status of bone marrow transplantation for leukemia. Hosp Pract 1985 Nov 15; 20(11):97–110.

Neischer R et al. Bone marrow transplantation. Am J Nurs 1984 June; 84(6):764–772.

Salinger JH. If your patient gets a bone marrow transplant. RN 1984 May; 47(5):62–68.

Stewart FM et al. Bone marrow transplantation: Three treatments for diseases. AORN J 1985 Aug; 42(2):196–211.

Disseminated Intravascular Coagulation

Caplin M. Disseminated intravascular coagulation: A multisystem problem. DCCN 1984 Mar/Apr; 3(2):76–83.

Detro CL. A review of disseminated intravascular coagulation. AANA J 1984 Feb; 52(1):68–71.

Greenberg HJ, Vogel JM, and Sanders M. Disseminated intravascular coagulopathy. Physician Assist 1985 Feb; 9(2):106–162.

Lamb C. When you suspect DIC. Patient Care 1985 Apr 15; 19(7):84–103.

Newland JR. Consumption coagulopathy: Coagulation and the tests for DIC. Consultant 1985 Feb 15; 25(3):112–120.

Rooney A and Hawley C. Nursing management of disseminated intravascular coagulation. Oncol Nurs Forum 1985 Jan/Feb; 12(1):15–22.

Sickle Cell Anemia

Alcorn R et al. Fluidotherapy and exercise in the management of sickle cell anemia. Phys Ther 1984 Oct; 64(10):1520–1522.

Lamb C. Managing sickle cell emergencies. Patient Care 1985 Jan 15; 19(1):92–141.

McLaurin SE. Sickle cell disease—a need for physical therapy intervention. Clin Manage Phys Ther 1986 Jan/Feb; 6(1):12–13, 28.

Nagel RL, Fabry ME, and Kaul DK. New insights on sickle cell anemia. Diagn Med 1984 May; 7(5):26–33.

To avoid a sickle cell CNS crisis. Emerg Med 1984 May 15; 16(9):130–134.

Transfusion Therapy

Berkman SA. The spectrum of transfusion reactions. Hosp Pract 1984 June; 19(6):205–219.

Brzica SM. Trouble with transfusions. Emerg Med 1983 Nov 30; 15(2):115–118.

Collins ML and Kafer ER. Lab rounds: Using blood components. Emerg Med 1985 June 15; 17(11):130–142.

Huestis DW. Platelet transfusion: Some general considerations. J Med Technol 1984 Sept; 1(9):703–707.

Krasnoff AR. Blood products: A review of uses and adverse reactions. Am J IV Ther Clin Nutr 1983 Nov/Dec; 10(10):17–22.

Leparc GF and Schmidt PJ. Stop! Transfusion reaction. Diagn Med 1984 Sept; 7(8):48–53.

Masoorli ST and Piercy S. A lifesaving guide to blood products. RN 1984 Sept; 47(9):32–37.

Pauley SY. Transfusion therapy for nurses (Part 1). NITA 1984 Nov/Dec; 7(6):501–511.

Pauley SY. Transfusion therapy for nurses (Part 2). NITA 1985 Jan/Feb; 8(1):51–60.

Querin JJ and Stahl LD. 12 simple sensible steps for successful blood transfusions. Nursing 83 1983 Nov; 13(11):34–44.

Silenieks A. Component therapy: Current concepts. J Med Technol 1984 June; 1(6):501–504.

Tannenbaum S. Blood—which component and why? Physician Assist 1983 Nov; 7(11):133–150.

Agencies

Governmental

National Heart, Lung and Blood Institute; National Institutes of Health Bldg 31, Rm 5A52, Bethesda, MD 20892.

Voluntary

American Cancer Society, 90 Park Ave., New York, NY 10016.

American Red Cross, 17th and D Sts., N.W., Washington, DC 20006.

Center for Sickle Cell Disease, Howard University, 2121 Georgia Avenue, N.W., Washington, DC 20059.

Leukemia Society of America, 733 Third Ave., New York, NY 10017.

National Association for Sickle Cell Disease, 3460 Wilshire Blvd., Suite 1012, Los Angeles, CA 90010.

National Hemophilia Foundation, 19 W. 34th St., Room 1204, New York, NY 10001.

Nursing Research Profile for Unit VII

Cardiovascular Nursing

Overview

In recent years a number of nursing research studies have focused on the needs of patients who have medical and surgical problems related to cardiovascular dysfunctions. Three groups of the patients studied are those who have experienced myocardial infarction, those with hypertension, and those who have had cardiac surgery. Many of the studies have investigated the educational needs of these patients, measures that have influenced their ability to cope with their condition, and strategies that have affected adherence to therapeutic regimens. The concerns and needs of the family and significant others have also been studied. Results of these studies have important nursing implications and indicate areas where further nursing research is needed.

The following studies are presented as examples of the research that has been conducted in this area. Although the subject populations are in many cases small and nonrandomized, and generalization of the findings is not always feasible, the nursing implications warrant consideration and further study.

Education and Support/Coping Needs

▷ *Mickus D. Activities of daily living in women after myocardial infarction. Heart Lung 1986 July; 15(4): 376–381.*

By means of a retrospective descriptive investigation (one based on description and documentation of experiences and phenomena that occurred in the past), Mickus studied 25 women who had sustained an uncomplicated myocardial infarction (MI) and compared their levels of physical activity during the postconvalescent period of recovery with their levels of activity before MI. Data were collected from chart review and from a questionnaire mailed to the subjects 5 to 11 months following the MI. The questionnaire provided subjective data about the subjects' perceived levels of activity pre-MI and post-MI. The activity levels studied were those related to activities of daily living, work, leisure, exercise, and sexual activity. The findings showed that 60% of the subjects spent less time, 24% spent the same amount of time, and 16% spent more time in activity post-MI than they did pre-MI. Shortness of breath on exertion was experienced by 92% and depression by 84%.

The decrease in activity experienced by 60% of the subjects may be related to dyspnea on exertion; this requires further study, especially in light of the fact that only 20% of the subjects participated in a structured cardiac rehabilitation program.

Nursing Implications. (1) Depression should be viewed as a possible sequela of MI, and appropriate psychological support should be provided during and after hospitalization. (2) Patient education should include the expected pace of activity resumption during the convalescent period. (3) Participation in cardiac rehabilitation and exercise programs after discharge should be encouraged.

▷ *Hentinen M. Need for instruction and support of the wives of patients with myocardial infarction. J Adv Nurs 1983 Nov; 8(6):519–529.*

Hentinen's study was based on the assumption that the illness of one family member affects the other members. The following questions were examined: Whether signs of stress are evidenced by wives of patients who have had myocardial infarction (MI), how much information about the hospital and home care of these patients the wives receive, who provides support for the wives during the patients' illness, and what wishes the wives had with respect to the instruction they received. The data were collected by means of a questionnaire completed by the wives of 59 patients eight weeks after the MI occurred.

Of the subjects who responded to the questionnaire, 83% indicated that they had suffered from insomnia in relation to their husbands' MI, and 69% had experienced fatigue. Other complaints included depression, anorexia, and sexual disinclination. Over half of the subjects reported that they had received no information about matters related to hospital or home care of their husbands. Those who had received information indicated that information on exercise, use of nitroglycerin, and smoking was provided most frequently. The majority reported that they wished that they had received instruction about home care, specifically about heart attack, diet, and support of the patient during the convalescent period. Sixty percent of the wives responded that they had received support from relatives, 37% from neighbors, 31% from registered nurses, and 24% from physicians.

Nursing Implications. (1) To cope with the stress associated with the MI of a spouse, wives need to receive information about the hospital and home care of the patient. (2) Wives need to receive support during the hospital and convalescent periods of their husbands' illness. Those who do not receive support from relatives and friends should be given particular attention by nurses and physicians to ensure that their emotional needs are met.

▷ *Hinds C. A hypertension survey: Respondents' knowledge of high blood pressure. In Nurs Rev 1983 Jan/Feb; 30(1):12–14.*

To assess knowledge about high blood pressure, a blood pressure screening survey was conducted on a college campus. Of the 347 persons who responded to the survey, 15% were less than 20 years of age, 78% were between 20 and 40 years, and 7% were 40 years of age or older. Ninety-three percent had never been treated for high blood pressure, and six percent had a history of high blood pressure treatment.

The survey results revealed that a large proportion of the subjects had inadequate knowledge and misinformation about high blood pressure despite the abundance of information available for laymen about hypertension. There was no significant difference in knowledge between those who had been treated for high blood pressure and those who had not.

Nursing Implications. (1) New and appropriate strategies for informing the public about high blood pressure need to be developed. (2) Persons with hypertension should be assessed to determine whether their knowledge about the condition is inadequate or incorrect and whether this contributes to the level of their compliance.

▷ *Stanton B, Savageau JA, and Aucoin R. Perceived adequacy of patient education and fears and adjustments about cardiac surgery. Heart Lung 1984 Sept; 13(5):525–531.*

Patients who were recovering from elective cardiac surgery were studied to determine their perceptions of the adequacy of the instruction they had received, whether or not they experienced common sources of fears and adjustments during the first 6 postoperative months, and whether a relationship exists between the perceived adequacy of instruction and the extent of fears and adjustments. A standardized home interview and a self-administered questionnaire were used to collect the data. Two hundred and forty-nine adult patients participated in the study.

In general, the subjects indicated that they had been most adequately instructed in the following areas: amount of exercise to resume, activities to avoid, and when to return to work. Almost 66% reported that they were either very well or adequately prepared for return to sexual functioning and for possible postoperative symptoms. Over 50% reported that they had not been prepared adequately with regard to emotional reactions that might be experienced and changes in the way other people might treat them (*e.g.,* overprotection).

The fears and worries reported most frequently were related to paying medical bills, not recovering completely, and having to rely too much on their spouses. However, each of these was rated by only 11% of the subjects. Over 25% responded that they had had to make moderate to extensive adjustments related to lack of energy, activity limitation, learning to slow down, being oversensitive, and having difficulty sleeping.

Nursing Implications. (1) Postoperative instructions for patients who have had cardiac surgery need to include emphasis on the areas of sexual functioning, possible postoperative physical and emotional symptoms, and changes in the ways that other people may respond to the patient. (2) Family members should be cautioned to avoid overprotecting the patient. (3) Postoperatively, patients need encouragement and assistance in coping with the recovery process. (4) Cardiac rehabilitation programs and self-help groups can offer assistance in coping and making adjustments after cardiac surgery.

▷ *Nicklin WM. Postdischarge concerns of cardiac patients as presented via a telephone callback system. Heart Lung 1986 May; 15(3):268–292.*

A telephone callback system was used to identify the types of problems encountered after discharge by patients and families of patients who had had cardiac surgery or who had medical cardiac problems. A sample of 217 telephone calls that related to concerns about 170 male and 47 female patients was used. Forty-nine percent of the calls were made by former patients, 35.5% by spouses, and the remaining 17.5% by community health nurses, other family members, or friends and colleagues. Patients who had had cardiac surgery composed 73% of the sample and medical patients made up the other 27%.

The most frequent concerns revealed were related to cardiopulmonary problems (31.3%); of these, 20% involved dysrhythmias or palpitations. Next in frequency were medication-related problems (14.7%), the majority of which were reported by the medical patients, and gastrointestinal problems (13.4%). Forty percent of the concerns occurred within the first week after discharge from the hospital, and 43.6% of the concerns were assessed as serious enough to warrant advice to seek treatment at an emergency department or to contact the physician.

Nursing Implications. (1) Since many of the concerns expressed arise during the first week after discharge, follow-up classes during this time may be helpful to allow patients and their families an opportunity to receive advice and share concerns. (2) Education about medications should be emphasized for medical patients before and after discharge. (3) Predischarge and postdischarge teaching programs should provide information that will allow decisions about seeking assistance from health professionals. (4) A telephone callback system is helpful in providing information, identifying learning needs, and reinforcing predischarge education.

▷ *Rodgers CD. Needs of relatives of cardiac surgery patients during the critical care phase. Focus Crit Care 1983 Oct; 10(5):50–55.*

Rodgers' study was designed to describe the needs of cardiac surgery patients' relatives during the critical postoperative period. Twenty relatives were studied, 10 of whom were spouses, 7 children, and 3 in-laws. A questionnaire was used to collect data during the first or second postoperative day. The results indicated that the relatives assigned highest priority to receiving reassurance and honest information about the patient's condition. The one need identified by all relatives as the most important was to know that they would be called at home should a change in the patient's condition occur.

Nursing Implications. (1) Nursing assessment of the needs of cardiac patients' relatives during the critical postoperative period is important. (2) Relatives should be assured that leaving the hospital is acceptable behavior and that they will be notified if the patient's condition changes.

Adherence to Therapeutic Regimens

▷ *Miller P, Wikoff RL, McMahon M, Garrett MJ and Ringel K. Indicators of medical regimen adherence for myocardial infarction patients. Nurs Res 1985 Sept/Oct; 34(5):268–272.*

The purpose of the Miller and co-workers study was to investigate the relationships between attitudes, intentions (self and perceived beliefs of others), and demographic variables and the performance of the prescribed medical regimen of the MI patient during hospitalization and adherence to the regimen 6 to 9 months posthospitalization. One hundred twelve first-time MI subjects whose ages ranged from 32 to 70 years (mean age of 56), were studied. Immediately prior to discharge from the hospital, attitude toward the medical regimen was assessed with the Miller Attitude Scale (MAS), intention to follow the medical regimen was measured with the Health Intention Scale (HIS), and demographic and medical data were obtained. A home visit was made 6 to 9 months later, at which time the MAS, the Health Behavior Scale (HBS), and a second demographic and medical data form were completed.

The findings revealed that attitudes both in the hospital and at home were favorable toward adherence. The scores for attitudes and intentions were highest for taking medications and performing activities and lowest for stopping smoking. Attitudes and perceived beliefs of others were indicators both of intentions toward adherence in the hospital and of actual adherence 6 to 9 months later. The findings suggest that patients are ready to receive information during hospitalization as well as postdischarge and that there is a need for the significant other to be included in this intervention.

Nursing Implications. (1) An individualized rehabilitation program for each MI patient should be developed for the hospital period and the home period of convalescence. (2) The significant other should be encouraged to offer continuing support to the patient and to assist him in identifying deterrents to adherence and in planning strategies for adaptation.

▷ *Kerr JAC. Adherence and self-care. Heart Lung 1985 Jan; 14(1):24–30.*

It is evident from many studies that adherence behaviors for patients with hypertension are a problem. This study was designed to investigate whether teaching patients about hypertension or self-monitoring of blood pressure, or a combination of both, without further supervision or support from health care personnel, would promote adherence to the antihypertensive regimen.

The subjects selected for the study were 116 volunteers from 3 occupational settings who were diagnosed as hypertensive and for whom antihypertensive medications had been prescribed. Their ages ranged from 29 to 64 years with a mean age of 50.3 years; 57% were men and 43% were women. Subjects were randomly assigned to one of four groups: (1) control group that received no intervention except the paper-and-pencil tests; (2) education and self-monitoring group; (3) self-monitoring only group; and (4) education only group. No significant differences existed in diastolic blood pressure at the beginning of the study among the four groups.

All subjects upon beginning the study had their blood pressure taken in the right arm by a nurse, were asked to complete a multiple-choice test that evaluated their general knowledge about hypertension, were given 3 medication tally sheets to record the number of antihypertensive pills taken each day for 3 months, and were asked to return once a month to have their blood pressure taken and to submit the tally sheet. In addition, the subjects who received education were given a 10- to 15-minute lecture on hypertension followed by discussion and a repeat of the multiple-choice test. The subjects who were to self-monitor their blood pressure were shown how to perform this procedure and how to record the results. They were given a self-monitoring blood pressure cuff to take home and tally sheets to use for recording the readings.

The results of the study showed that none of the intervention strategies yielded a significant increase in adherence when ongoing support was not provided. However, of the strategies used, self-monitoring of blood pressure seemed to be the most effective. All groups showed an improvement in blood pressure, with the total study population showing a significant improvement. This improvement can possibly be attributed to the use of the self-monitoring technique of keeping a tally of daily pill-taking behavior.

Nursing Implications. (1) Self-monitoring of blood pressure along with ongoing support or attention from health care personnel merits further study. (2) Research is needed on the long-term effects on adherence to the regimen produced by tallying the number of antihypertensive pills.

▷ *Marshall J, Penckofer S and Llewellyn J. Structured postoperative teaching and knowledge and compliance of patients who had coronary artery bypass surgery. Heart Lung 1986 Jan; 15(1):76–82.*

Determining the effects of a structured teaching program on knowledge and compliance of patients who had had coronary artery bypass surgery was the purpose of the Marshall and associates study. A convenience sample of two comparable groups of patients (N = 64) on a cardiovascular surgical step-down unit was studied. One group received education about normal postoperative recovery by means of an unstructured method. The other group received instruction with the use of a teaching guide developed by nurses experienced in the recovery of patients after cardiac surgery. Knowledge was measured before teaching, on discharge from the hospital, and 6 weeks after discharge.

The results showed that both groups had higher knowledge scores after surgery. The group that received the structured teaching walked more blocks after surgery than did the group that received unstructured teaching. The patients who received structured teaching had higher total compliance scores than did the patients of the other group.

Nursing Implications. (1) Structured teaching programs should be tested to determine whether they have a greater effect on knowledge and compliance than unstructured programs. (2) Nurses should critically evaluate the effectiveness of their role as educators and the effectiveness of the teaching strategies that they use.

Additional Studies

Burke LJ, Gabriel LM, Fischer LE and Zemke SL. Nursing diagnosis, indicators, and interventions in an outpatient cardiac rehabilitation program. Heart Lung 1986 Jan; 15(1):70–76.

Clancy CA, Wey JM, and Guinn GA. The effect of patients' perceptions on return to work after coronary artery bypass surgery. Heart Lung 1984 Mar; 13(2):173–176.

Dickson E, Robb JR, Hersman CJ, Ryan J and Dahl JC. A hypertension follow-up program. Nursing & Health Care 1983 Nov; 14(9):508–509.

Eyherabide A and Yates BC. The effects of cardiac rehabilitation on compliance in the coronary artery bypass surgery patient. Cardiovasc Nurs 1985 Nov/Dec; 21(6):31–35.

Gilliss CL. Reducing family stress during and after coronary artery bypass surgery. Nurs Clin North Am 1984 Mar; 19(1):103–112.

Hilbert GA. Spouse support and myocardial infarction patient compliance. Nurs Res 1985 July/Aug; 34(4):217–220.

Kerr JAC. Multidimensional health locus of control, adherence, and lowered diastolic blood pressure. Heart Lung 1986 Jan; 15(1):87–92.

King KB. Measurement of coping strategies, concerns, and emotional response in patients undergoing coronary artery bypass surgery. Heart Lung 1985 Nov; 14(6):579–586.

McMahon M, Wikoff R, and Ringel K. Life situations, health beliefs, and medical regimen adherence of patients with myocardial infarction. Heart Lung 1986 Jan; 15(1):82–86.

Mills G, Barnes R, Rodell DE and Terry L. An evaluation of an inpatient cardiac patient/family education program. Heart Lung 1985 July; 14(4):400–406.

Penckoffer SH and Holm K. Early appraisal of coronary revascularization on quality of life. Nurs Res 1984 Mar/Apr; 33(2):60–63.

Digestive and Gastrointestinal Problems

Unit VIII

Assessment and Management of Patients With Ingestive Problems and Upper Gastrointestinal Disorders

Since the process of ingestion begins with the mastication of food in the mouth, adequate nutrition is related to good dental health and the general condition of the mouth. The presence and condition of the teeth directly affect nutritional well-being by influencing the type of food ingested and the degree to which food particles are properly mixed with salivary enzymes. Any discomfort in the mouth, due to lip lesions, inflammation of the buccal mucosa, or other conditions, can have a deleterious effect on food intake. Esophageal problems related to the apparently simple act of swallowing can also adversely affect food and fluid intake, thereby jeopardizing general health and well-being.

Given the close interrelationship between adequate nutritional intake and all of the structures of the upper gastrointestinal tract (lips, mouth, teeth, esophagus), preventive health teaching should place heavy emphasis on helping people to avoid the discomfort caused by disorders associated with any of these structures.

Nursing Process Overview: Patients With Conditions of the Oral Cavity

▷ Assessment

The nursing history includes questions about the patient's normal routine for brushing and flossing his teeth, the frequency of his dental visits, and his awareness of any lesions or irritated areas in the mouth, tongue, or back of the throat that interfere with eating. Does he wear dentures? Does he have any capped teeth or a partial plate? Has he recently experienced sore throats (frequency, severity, duration, treatment used), difficulty with swallowing or chewing, gum problems (pain or bleeding), and voice changes? Does he avoid foods that are hard to chew? What constitutes his daily food intake?

Physical assessment includes inspection and palpation of both the internal and external structures of the mouth and throat. Removal of dentures and partial plates is necessary to ensure a thorough inspection of the gums. In general, the examination can be accomplished with the use of a bright light source (penlight) and a tongue depressor. If a suspicious lesion is observed, a finger cot or glove is worn to palpate the abnormality. The examination begins with inspection of the lips for moisture, hydration, color, and the presence of ulcerations or fissures. The patient is instructed to open his mouth wide; then a tongue blade is inserted to expose the buccal mucosa for an assessment of color and lesions (Fig. 30-1*A*). Stensen's duct of each parotid gland is visible as a small red dot in the buccal mucosa next to the upper molars.

The gums are inspected for inflammation, bleeding, retraction, and discoloration. The odor of the breath is also noted. The hard palate is examined for color and shape. The dorsum of the tongue is inspected for texture, color, and lesions. A thin, white coat and large, vallate papillae in a V formation on the distal portion of the dorsum of the tongue are normal findings (Fig. 30-1*B*). The patient is instructed to protrude his tongue and move it laterally. This provides the examiner with an opportunity to estimate the tongue's size as well as its symmetry and strength (the integrity of the 12th cranial nerve [hypoglossal] can be ascertained). Further inspection of the ventral surface of the tongue and the floor of the mouth is accomplished by asking the patient to touch the tip of his tongue to his palate. Any lesions of the mucosa or any abnormalities involving the frenulum or superficial veins are noted. This is a common area for oral cancer, which presents as a white or red plaque, an indurated ulcer, or a warty growth.

A tongue blade is used to depress the tongue for adequate visualization of the pharynx. It is pressed firmly beyond the midpoint of the tongue. Proper placement avoids a gagging response and minimizes the patient's aversion to future oral examinations. The patient is told to tip his head back, open his mouth wide, take a deep breath, and say "ah." Often this will flatten the posterior tongue and briefly expose a full view of the anterior and posterior pillars, the tonsils, uvula and posterior pharynx. These structures are inspected for color, symmetry, and evidence of exudate, ulceration, or enlargement. Normally, the uvula and soft palate rise with a deep inspiration or "ah," and indicate an intact vagus nerve (10th cranial nerve).

A complete assessment of the oral cavity is essential for diagnosing many disease conditions. Acquired immunodeficiency syndrome (AIDS) is associated with several oral manifestations: oral candidiasis, hairy leukoplakia, and oral herpes simplex. Lesions of Kaposi's sarcoma, which is reported to occur in 2% of the male homosexual population, may also be observed.

Gerontological Considerations. Assessment of the oral cavity of the elderly patient requires an understanding of age-related changes in the oral mucosa. Epithelial skin becomes drier and thinner and is more susceptible to injury. There is a decrease in salivation because of atrophy of the salivary glands. Sublingual varicosities are more common. The presence of caries increases with age, and many patients have lost all their teeth. There is also a decrease in oral motor functioning (swallowing, chewing) in the aged.

▷ Nursing Diagnoses

Based on all the assessment data, major nursing diagnoses may include the following:

- Alteration in the oral mucous membranes related to a pathologic condition, infection, or chemical/mechanical trauma (drugs, ill-fitting dentures)
- Alteration in nutrition, less than body requirements, related to inability to ingest adequate nutrients secondary to oral/dental disease conditions
- Disturbance in self-concept/body image, related to a physical change in appearance subsequent to a disease condition or surgical/medical treatment

▷ Planning and Implementation

▷ *Goals:* The major nursing goals for the patient may include improvement in the condition of the oral mucous membrane, improvement in nutritional intake, and attainment of a positive self-image.

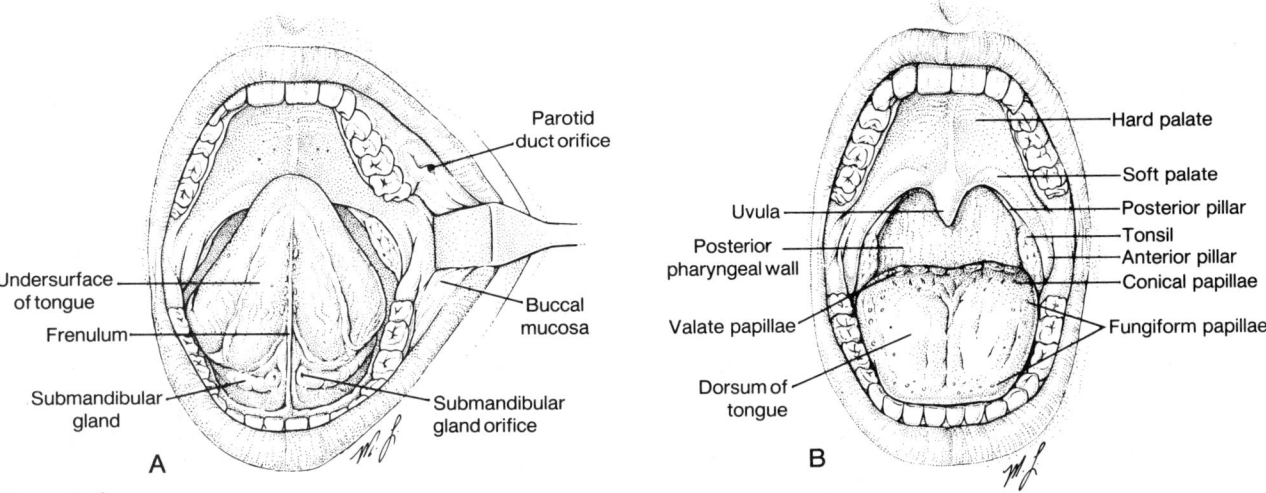

Figure 30-1
The mouth (*A*) and the pharynx (*B*). (Adapted from Bates B: A Guide to Physical Examination and History Taking, 4th ed. Philadelphia, JB Lippincott, 1987.)

Nursing Interventions

Mouth Care.   The cause of the oral mucous membrane disorder is identified so that it can be treated. The nurse monitors the intake of irritating substances (tobacco [including smokeless tobacco], alcohol, highly spiced foods) so that their influence as offensive agents can be evaluated. She recommends that the patient visit a dentist if a chipped tooth is irritating sensitive gums or a cavity is visible. A neglected cavity can lead to root canal damage. The need for frequent brushing and flossing of the teeth and visiting the dentist every 6 months is emphasized.

Nutritional Intake.   The patient's weight, age, and level of activity are recorded so an adequate daily calorie intake can be estimated. A daily calorie count is maintained to determine the exact quantity of food and fluid ingested. The frequency and pattern of eating is recorded to determine if there are psychosocial factors as well as physiologic factors influencing ingestion. The nurse suggests that the patient avoid eating any foods that interfere with digestion. She recommends changes in the consistency of foods and the frequency of eating based on the disease condition and the patient's preferences. The goal is to help the patient attain a desirable body weight.

Positive Self-image.   The patient is encouraged to verbalize his perceived change in body appearance and realistically discuss actual changes or losses. The nurse offers support while the patient verbalizes his fears and negative feelings. She encourages him to identify his reactions (withdrawal, depression, anger) and to describe himself and how he believes others see him so he has a better understanding of his emotions. The nurse listens attentively and determines if his needs are primarily psychosocial or cognitive-perceptual. This determination will help individualize a plan of care. The patient's strengths and achievements are praised and his positive attributes reinforced.

The nurse should determine the patient's major anxieties concerning interpersonal relations at home and at work. She can then recommend specific ways for him to interact with others and help him cope with his anxieties and fears. She emphasizes that his substance and worth is not diminished by a physical change in a body part.

The patient's progress in developing a positive self-esteem is recorded. The nurse should be alert to signs of grieving and should keep a record of emotional changes. Repeated opportunities are provided for listening, and the nurse should accept the patient's expressions of hostility. He is encouraged to relate his feelings in an atmosphere of acceptance.

▷ ## Evaluation

▷ ### Expected Outcomes

1. Patient shows evidence of an intact oral mucous membrane.
   a. Is free of pain/discomfort in the oral cavity.
   b. Avoids spicy foods.
   c. Is able to identify foods that are irritating to the gums (nuts, pretzels).
2. Attains a desirable body weight.
   a. Eats nutritionally balanced meals.
   b. Keeps a daily record of calories.

   c. Substitutes foods appropriately to maintain suggested caloric intake.
   d. Maintains a recommended body weight plus or minus 2 to 3 kg (4 to 6 pounds).
3. Attains a positive self-image.
   a. Freely discusses his body change.
   b. Verbalizes anxieties.
   c. Talks about self as an important person.
   d. Is able to accept change and modify his self-concept.
   e. Speaks positively about his appearance.
   f. Focuses energies away from self toward new identified goals.

Conditions of the Oral Cavity

Abnormalities of the Lips

Actinic Cheilitis.   Actinic cheilitis refers to irritation of the lips resulting from the cumulative effect of exposure to radiation from the sun. The inflammation is associated with scaling, crust formation, and fissuring and may lead to squamous cell carcinoma. It is manifested by whitish hyperkeratosis (an overgrowth of the horny layer of the epidermis), fissuring, and erythema. Treatment consists of protecting the lips with a good sunscreen ointment. In some instances, electrosurgery or cryosurgery is required to decrease the inflammatory reaction. Periodic checkups are mandatory to detect possible malignancy. Certain groups of people, such as farmers and fair-skinned people, who are sensitive to sun exposure, are especially susceptible.

Herpes Simplex.   A cold sore or fever blister is produced by the herpes simplex virus. Singular or clustered vesicles erupt on the lip. Vesicles rupture, forming ulcers that are covered with a gray membrane.

Chancre.   A chancre is a reddened, circumscribed lesion that ulcerates and becomes crusted. A hard papule is the primary lesion of syphilis.

Contact Dermatitis.   Lipsticks, cosmetics, ointments to prevent chapping, and even toothpaste and chewing gum may be the source of allergens that cause erythema, vesiculation, burning, and itching of the lips. These conditions are treated by eliminating the suspected contactant, applying topical corticosteroid ointment, and using hypoallergenic cosmetics.

Nursing Interventions.   An initial approach to the patient with lip lesions includes taking a nursing history concerning the length of time the lesions have existed, any known precipitating factors, methods of treatment used to date, known associates with similar problems, and a statement of the problem in the patient's words.

The nurse inspects the lesions, noting their appearance, location, size, and drainage, if any; and after identifying the abnormality, she recommends that the patient

- Avoid spicy/irritating foods.
- Use warm rinses to clean the mouth without irritating the lips.

- Apply cold soaks to the lips for 20 minutes, every 2 to 4 hours.
- Avoid emotional situations that increase stress and aggravate the condition.
- Eliminate causative factors (sun exposure, cosmetics).
- Refrain from direct contact with another through kissing.
- Seek health care if necessary.

Abnormalities of the Gums

Enlargement of the gingival tissue can occur in response to normal body changes (puberty, pregnancy).

Gingivitis. Gingivitis (inflammation of the gums) is the most common disease of oral tissues. At first there is inflammation and slight swelling of the superficial gingivae and interdental papillae. Bleeding in response to light contact may occur and prompt the patient to refrain from adequately cleaning his teeth. Such neglect compounds the problem, because food debris, bacterial plaque, and calculus (tartar) can result in chronic degenerative gingivitis, and, later, in periodontal disease.

Necrotizing gingivitis is a pseudomembranous ulceration affecting the edges of the gums, the mucosa of the mouth, the tonsils, and the pharynx. It is thought to be caused by a combination of two organisms, a spirochete and a fusiform bacillus. Smears made from the ulcerations are found to be teeming with the characteristic organisms and establish the diagnosis. However, the condition may also be due to poor oral hygiene, low tissue resistance, and infection produced by a complex of microorganisms.

The chief symptom is painful, bleeding gums. Swallowing and talking are also painful, especially when infection has spread to the tonsils and pharynx. There may be a mild fever and swelling of the lymph nodes in the neck.

Management. Conscientious mouth hygiene and periodic professional teeth cleaning can prevent plaque buildup and gum irritation. For necrotizing gingivitis the plan of care includes washing and irrigating the mouth hourly with prescribed solutions rich in free oxygen, such as sodium perborate in a 2% solution, to combat the anaerobic spirochete. Procaine penicillin, given intramuscularly, or potassium phenoxymethyl penicillin (penicillin V), given orally, is effective. Definitive measures such as dental prophylaxis and gingival massage are postponed until the acute inflammation has subsided.

Herpetic Gingivostomatitis. Herpes simplex infection may take the form of an acute herpetic gingivostomatitis. The patient frequently experiences a burning sensation 24 to 48 hours before blisters appear. Small vesicles, single or clustered, may erupt and rupture, forming sore, shallow ulcers that are covered with a gray membrane. Herpes infections appear often in association with other febrile infections, such as streptococcal pneumonia, meningococcal meningitis, and malaria.

Some patients may associate herpes simplex with hearsay stories relating this herpesvirus to cancer. Although herpesvirus type 2 has been associated with carcinoma of the cervix in women, there is no documented evidence to show the exact relationship between the two.

Management. Some relief is experienced with the application of topical analgesics. Other common therapies include (1) applying spirits of camphor twice a day; (2) applying a moistened styptic stick to the vesicles several times a day; and (3) rinsing with a topical anti-infective, chlorhexidine (Peridex solution).

Periodontitis. Periodontitis (periodontal disease, pyorrhea), which can result from untreated gingivitis, affects the gums and other supporting structure (bone, cementum, and periodontal membrane). At the onset, there is little discomfort and few other signs of the condition. Later there may be bleeding, infection, gum recession, and loosening of the teeth. As a result, the teeth may fall out or may need to be extracted. It is estimated that one in four people have the disease at some stage of its development, and up to 90% of all people in their 40s are affected. Dental authorities suggest that the principal reason why most people, after age 50, require dentures is the effect of this increasingly prevalent disease.

Malocclusion, poor fillings, and inadequate diet are suspected causes of periodontal disease; in addition, improper cleaning and poor mouth hygiene contribute to the problem. Tartar or calculus that cannot be brushed from the teeth tends to build up and requires professional removal twice a year. If this is not done, gums become swollen and tender, infection progresses, and pockets that collect pus and bacteria are formed between the gums and teeth. The protective layer that normally covers the gums is destroyed, exposing the blood vessels, which bleed easily. Bacteria thrive on the nutrients in the blood and tissues that fill and line the space. The bone supporting the teeth is destroyed, and the tooth becomes loose.

Some authorities believe that this condition is frequently associated with other systemic diseases, such as diabetes mellitus and certain skin and blood disorders; however, conclusive evidence is lacking.

Management. At present, the best advice is to brush the teeth and floss carefully, at least once a day, and to have the teeth cleaned professionally twice a year. Such a cleaning should include the area below the gum line. Poor occlusion should be corrected, crooked teeth straightened, and missing teeth replaced with bridgework or another form of splinting. Not too long ago, such work by an orthodontist was considered a luxury and done only for cosmetic reasons. Today the value of such treatment is seen in the prevention of periodontal disease and other mouth problems. However, because of cost, this type of therapeutic intervention is still generally available only to those with adequate dental health plans.

In the near future, perhaps, three-dimensional photography will assist periodontists in measuring the changes in the shape or elevation of the gum, signs that allow early detection of periodontal disease.

Nursing Interventions. The patient is advised to brush his teeth gently and prevent trauma to the gums. Foods that are soft in consistency are recommended; highly seasoned or strongly acidic foods are eliminated from the diet when the gums are swollen and painful. Use of tobacco products and alcohol causes irritation and is to be avoided, if possible, or restricted.

Adolescents are often afflicted with periodontitis because of poor eating habits, bowel irregularity, and insufficient rest. Patient education is directed toward correcting mouth problems and emphasizing proper oral hygiene to prevent a recurrence.

Abnormalities of the Teeth

Dental Plaque and Caries

At least 95% of Americans sooner or later experience tooth decay. This is an erosive process that results from the action of bacteria on fermentable carbohydrates in the mouth, which in turn produces acids that dissolve tooth enamel. The extent of damage to the teeth depends on several factors, the most significant of which are (1) the presence of dental plaque; (2) the strength of the acids and the ability of the saliva to neutralize them; (3) the length of time the acids are in contact with the teeth; and (4) susceptibility of the teeth to decay. Dental plaque is a gluey, gelatin-like substance that adheres to the teeth and affords protection for the bacteria. The initial action that causes damage to a tooth occurs under dental plaque.

Dental decay begins with a small hole, usually in a fissure or flaw of the enamel, or in an area that is hard to clean. Left unchecked, it penetrates the enamel into the dentin. Because the dentin is not as hard as the enamel, decay progresses somewhat more rapidly and in time reaches the pulp. When the blood, lymph vessels, and nerves are exposed, they become infected, and an abscess may form, either within the tooth or at the tip of the root. Soreness and pain usually accompany the abscess. As the infection increases, the face may become swollen, and there may be pulsating pain. The dentist can determine by x-ray films the extent of damage and the type of treatment needed. It may be necessary to extract the tooth.

Preventive Management. Measures used in the prevention and control of dental caries include reducing the intake of sugars (refined carbohydrates), practicing effective mouth care (as described below), applying fluoride to the teeth or drinking fluoridated water, and using resin sealants. According to recent research, dentists consider the use of pit and fissure sealants as the least effective measure for preventing caries, compared with diet counseling, plaque control, and topical fluoride applications.

Healthy teeth require conscientious and effective daily cleaning. The purpose of toothbrushing is to mechanically break up the bacterial plaque that collects around teeth. Proper brushing requires a toothbrush with soft bristles and rounded tips. The bristles of the brush are directed into the gingival sulcus in a horizontal scrubbing motion. Ten strokes are recommended for each surface. Dental floss should also be used every 24 hours to reach those areas between the teeth not accessible to the brush. The floss is inserted between the teeth and moved back and forth in a gentle sawing motion until it reaches under the gum line. Of course, the normal movement of the muscles of mastication and the normal flow of saliva also aid greatly in keeping the teeth clean. Even so, it is necessary to disorganize plaque once during each 24-hour period, preferably before bedtime. This practice prevents decay and periodontal disease.

Since many ill patients do not eat and salivate normally, the natural cleaning process of the teeth is reduced. If a patient is absolutely unable to brush his teeth, as in the case of patients with cerebrovascular disease or those disabled by trauma, then it becomes a nursing responsibility. In any case, merely swabbing the patient's mouth and teeth with glycerin and lemon juice is inadequate, since all it does is coat collections of bacteria without removing them. Again, the *most effective method is mechanical cleansing*. It is better to wipe the patient's teeth with a washcloth than to have him swish an antiseptic mouthwash several times and then emit it into the emesis basin. If a toothbrush is used, an electric brush is more effective in cleansing someone else's teeth than the conventional hand toothbrush. While the nondominant hand of the nurse retracts the lips and cheeks, the dominant hand can direct the electric brush to all surfaces of the patient's teeth. Even the tongue should receive a beneficial light brushing. Once any toothbrush is used, it should be cleansed thoroughly with soap and water and allowed to dry.

Fluoridation. Adjusting the fluoride level in the drinking water to an optimal healthful level of one part per million can help to prevent up to two thirds of tooth decay. Such a concentration of fluoride makes tooth enamel more resistant to the acids that are formed in the mouth. When ingested from birth to about 10 years of age, fluoridated water can give permanent protection. Some sections of the western United States have natural fluoridation; other areas of the country have enacted legislation for controlled fluoridation of public water supplies. In these areas, studies have demonstrated a reduction in dental decay. Fluoridation also lessens the possibility of malocclusion and gingival disease.

Most areas of this country, however, do not have fluoridated water, and people must find other ways of receiving the benefits of fluoride. Four other methods are possible:

- Vitamin preparations can include fluoride. Treatment must start early in life and continue until the age of 10.
- A concentrated fluoride solution can be applied directly to the teeth. This procedure is done by the dentist and has the advantage of providing professional control and encouraging regular checkups.
- Sodium fluoride can be added to the water in the home; however, home fluoridators that operate automatically are expensive and may do little good, since children drink most of their daily water supply in school.
- Sodium fluoride can be provided in tablet or liquid drops as a dietary additive; this, too, is expensive and often impractical.

Management. Treatment for dental caries includes fillings, extraction, and dental implants.

Fillings. A translucent tooth-filling material, made by mixing a special aluminosilicate glass powder with a solution of polyacrylic acid, has several advantages over conventional enamel fillings made with phosphoric acid. The polyacrylic acid is much milder than phosphoric acid (which can damage the tooth if the cavity is not lined before it is filled). Also, the new filling is adhesive, which eliminates the need for extensive drilling to secure the filling.

Technological advances in recent years have produced several new coatings that bond to the enamel of the tooth and protect it from decay. These composite dental resins consist of an epoxy resin product and a form of acrylic acid, plus reinforcing fillers, such as glass beads or quartz fillers. Dentists can use the new materials to seal pits and fissures when the teeth first grow in, thus preventing decay. The new materials can also be used to restore teeth eroded near the gum, a common site of periodontal disease.

Extraction. Sometimes dental extraction is necessary if a tooth is defective or severely damaged. Extraction of one or several teeth is usually done in the dental office. A local anesthetic is effective, and the procedure takes less than 30 minutes.

The patient will most likely be admitted to a hospital for same-day surgery when all four molars are to be extracted at one time. Using endotracheal general anesthesia, the oral surgeon inserts a mouth retractor to provide exposure. Incisions are made laterally in the mandible to approach the impacted tooth. The jaw eventually regenerates bone that has been removed. Closure of the mucous membrane is accomplished with black silk sutures.

It is likely that the patient who requires multiple tooth extraction for denture preparation is over 65 years of age. Therefore, hospitalization may be required.

Tooth extraction is a simple procedure that has few complications. However, there are several groups of people that require special considerations: the elderly, patients taking anticoagulants, and those diagnosed as having AIDS. The elderly may have a chronic illness that makes it difficult for them to sit or recline in a dental chair for periods greater than 15 minutes. The dentist can keep the dental chair in the upright position and perform the procedure in spaced intervals. Patients taking an oral anticoagulant are advised by the physician to withhold the medication and take oral vitamin K for 3 days prior to the dental procedure. The American Dental Association recommends that the infection control regimen that is used for patients with hepatitis be used when caring for a patient with AIDS. Salivary transmission of the virus seems unlikely but until more is known about the disease, special precautions are necessary.

Dental Implants. Sometimes dental implants or transplantations are suggested if a patient has had multiple tooth extractions. Successful research is being done involving the transplantation of teeth and the possible "storage" of teeth in a bank. Some researchers have restricted their transplants to undeveloped or "bud" teeth, whereas others are trying to transplant teeth at many stages of development. However, at present, homotransplants (transplanting teeth from one person to another) will have to await additional research to combat the rejection process. Successful autotransplants (using the patient's own teeth) have been reported. For example, a defective first molar has been replaced successfully by the patient's own third molar.

Implants are not to be considered as fully acceptable alternatives to other forms of dental treatment. Rather they are to be used only when other forms of treatment do not suffice to restore the mouth to its masticatory function. There is an element of unpredictability in the field of oral implants. Therefore, their use should be regarded as a last approach to sound dentistry.

Nursing Interventions. After tooth extraction, oozing of blood may be apparent the first day. The patient is advised to rest and not rinse his mouth for the first 24 hours to lessen the likelihood of bleeding. If heavy bleeding occurs, he is told to place a clean, folded gauze pad directly on the bleeding spot and close his teeth tightly over the pad and apply pressure for about 30 minutes. He is advised to notify the dentist if there is prolonged or severe pain, swelling, or bleeding.

If impacted molars have been removed, the patient is advised to use ice packs to both sides of his face for 20-minute periods every hour for 24 hours to relieve swelling and soreness. Liquids are recommended for the first 24 hours. Most patients enjoy ice cream or milk shakes because they are filling, and the cool liquid soothes swollen tissues. A spouted container can be used if sucking from a straw is painful. The patient is reminded that the sutures are removed after the fifth day. Mouthwashes can proceed from saline to sodium perborate monohydrate (Amosan). Brushing of the teeth is resumed when the gums have healed. Any pain or swelling after 1 week is reported; infection is common and can be easily treated with drainage, packing, and antibiotics.

Preventive patient education includes advising patients to brush and floss at least twice a day to prevent plaque formation, to decrease their intake of "sweets," to drink water with an adequate fluoride level or have routine topical fluoride applications, and to visit the dentist at least twice a year.

Gerontological Considerations. *Gerodontology* is the branch of dentistry that deals with the elderly. About 50% of adults in the United States over age 65 no longer have teeth (edentulous). However, tooth loss *is not* a normal result of aging; it results primarily from two preventable disease entities, caries and periodontitis. In periodontal disease, the gum tissue becomes inflamed and the tooth's supporting structures erode. Frequently the older person requires extensive dental work. Although the goal in dentistry today is to retain the permanent teeth, that goal is not always possible for an aged person who has neglected caring for his teeth. A partial or complete set of dentures may be necessary.

Dentures. It is common practice for people to postpone indefinitely the final decision to obtain dentures, even though there is no possibility of having the few remaining teeth repaired. Hesitant patients are encouraged to pursue this health need by pointing out to them the positive aspects of obtaining dentures: improved appearance, better nutrition, and reduced likelihood of infection. The nurse should stress that when dentures are obtained, patience is required in learning to use them effectively.

During the first 2 months of denture wear the patient is advised to

- Keep his dentures in place for 24 hours before the first adjustment so that any pressure areas or irritated tissue can be identified.
- Always put his dentures in place at least 6 hours before he sees his dentist for an adjustment.
- Be patient. It takes 6 to 8 weeks for gum tissue to adapt.
- Avoid large pieces of food, foods that irritate the gums (peanuts, celery, corn, seeds [as in fruits]), and foods that may get stuck between the gum tissue and the dentures because the tissues are still swollen.
- Keep dentures clean and maintain healthy gum tissue by brushing twice a day with a soft toothbrush.

Pressure or irritation caused by dentures is reported to the dentist, who can make the proper adjustment. Uncorrected pressure areas may cause lesions, which in turn may become malignant.

Dentures require careful scrubbing, using a firm denture brush, mild soap and water, salt, and sodium bicarbonate. The addition of a drop of household chlorine acts as a deodorant and gives a fresher taste. Most dentists recommend that dentures be removed at night, scrubbed, and allowed to soak in a proprietary cleaner.

Partial dentures should not be left in place for prolonged

periods without being removed for a good cleaning. They are held in place with metal clasps that encircle the teeth. These clasps can be spread: using gentle force with two index fingers, one side and then the other can be loosened. When reapplied, the cleaned partial dentures usually can be pressed into place.

Many people now prefer to have "immediate dentures." Usually, the back teeth are extracted first, which allows the tissues time to heal. Meanwhile, the artificial teeth are made and are ready for placement immediately after the front teeth have been extracted.

Dentoalveolar Abscess or Periapical Abscess

A dentoalveolar abscess results from a suppurative process involving the apical dental periosteum (fibrous membrane supporting the tooth structure) and the alveolar process in the periapical region (tissue surrounding the apex of the tooth where it is suspended in the tooth socket). It may appear in two forms. The acute form is usually secondary to a suppurative pulpitis that arises from an infection extending from dental caries. The infection of the dental pulp extends through the apical foramen of the tooth to form an abscess about the apex, its site of implantation in the alveolar bone. The abscess produces a dull, gnawing, continuous pain, often with a surrounding cellulitis and edema of the adjacent facial structures. The gum opposite the apex of the tooth is usually swollen on the cheek side, where the abscess is prone to point. Swelling and cellulitis of the facial structures may make it difficult to open the mouth. In well-developed abscesses there may be a systemic reaction, fever, and malaise.

Chronic dentoalveolar abscess is a slowly progressive infection with the same mode as the acute form. It differs from the acute form in that the process may progress to a fully formed abscess without the patient's knowing it. The infection eventually leads to a "blind dental abscess" that is really a periapical granuloma. It may enlarge to as much as 1 cm in diameter. It is often discovered in x-ray examination and is treated by extraction or root canal therapy, often with apicoectomy.

Management. In the early stages of an infection, a dental surgeon may drill an opening into the pulp chamber to relieve tension and pain and to provide drainage. Usually, the infection has progressed to a periapical abscess, and drainage is provided by an incision through the gingivae down to the jaw bone. Foul pus escapes under pressure. This procedure is usually done in the dental office. Occasionally the patient is admitted to the hospital for same-day surgery. After the inflammatory reacton has subsided, the tooth may have to be extracted or appropriate root canal therapy given.

Nursing Interventions. The patient is instructed to use warm saline mouthwashes every 2 hours while awake. External heat, in the form of a hot compress or heating pad, will relieve some of the soreness because heat hastens the subsidence of the inflammatory process. He is advised to expectorate any foul pus drainage into paper wipes and discard them into a plastic-lined receptacle. The plastic bag can be tied and thrown into a larger trash can. This keeps contaminated tissues in a contained area and prevents them from being handled by other family members.

Pain and swelling may interfere with an adequate fluid intake; therefore, the nurse recommends that fluids be taken with a straw for 24 to 48 hours. Soup is an excellent source

of fluid and nutrients during the first 2 days. A soft diet is introduced by the second day, and the patient progresses to a regular diet as tolerated.

Bed rest is suggested for several days. Analgesic drugs are taken every 3 to 6 hours as needed for pain. If the patient is taking an antibiotic, the nurse makes sure that he understands when to take the drug (usually every 6 hours around the clock to maintain therapeutic blood levels) and what foods to avoid that cause gastrointestinal upset or decreased drug effectiveness.

Malocclusion

Malocclusion is a faulty relationship between the teeth when the jaws are closed. Correction of malocclusion requires several factors: an orthodontist who has special training, a patient who is motivated and cooperative, and adequate time. Most treatments begin when the patient has shed his last primary tooth and the last permanent successor has erupted, usually around 12 or 13 years of age.

Currently "preventive orthodontics" is started at age 5 if malocclusion is diagnosed early. Studies have shown the reduced need for teeth-strengthening in adolescence if preventive orthodontics is started with the primary teeth.

Management. In order to realign the teeth, the orthodontist gradually forces the teeth into a new location by the use of wires or plastic bands. Although the patient may object to the effect of these devices on his appearance, this psychological burden must be overcome if good results are to be achieved in the future. In the final phase of treatment, a retaining device is worn for several hours each day to support the tissues as they adjust to the new location of the teeth.

Braces are also used as part of the means of correcting long or short jaw syndrome. These procedures, called *orthognathic surgery,* are done when the jaw is either too long or too short for proper mandibular alignment. When the jaw is too long, bony material is extracted; when the jaw is too short, a bone graft or inert material may be inserted. The postoperative care of these patients is similar to that needed by patients with a fractured mandible (see p. 721).

Nursing Interventions. During this time, it is essential that the patient keep his mouth meticulously clean. Encouragement is often necessary for the patient to persist in this most important part of the treatment. When an adolescent undergoing orthodontal correction is admitted to the hospital for some other problem, it may be necessary to remind him to continue wearing the retainer if it does not interfere with the problem requiring hospitalization.

Abnormalities of the Mouth

Leukoplakia. White patches that cannot be diagnosed as a specific disorder can be benign and hyperkeratotic (tissue overgrowth) or malignant. They occur most frequently between the ages of 50 and 70 years and are commonly found in the buccal and mandibular mucosa. The majority have no evidence of abnormal tissue development; however, a small percentage develop into squamous cell carcinoma so biopsy is recommended if the lesions persist for longer than 2 weeks.

Lichen Planus. Lichen planus is a mucocutaneous disease recognized as white papules at the intersection of a network of interlacing lesions. Often the lesions are ulcerated and painful. If asymptomatic, reassurance is all that is needed. For lichen planus, the diet is limited to soft, bland foods. If there is pain, small amounts of viscous lidocaine (Xylocaine viscous 2%) held in the mouth for 2 to 3 minutes may relieve soreness while eating. Direct application of triamcinolone acetonide (Kenalog in Orabase) after meals or at bedtime may promote healing. Corticosteroids given systemically or injected intralesionally have been effective. Periodic examinations of chronic lesions are necessary because of their potential for malignancy.

Candidiasis. Candidiasis (moniliasis, thrush) produces white, cheesy plaques that look like milk curds and can be rubbed off to leave an erythematous and, often, bleeding base. Diagnosis requires identifying the spores of *Candida albicans* from exfoliated cells (dead tissue cells scraped from the lesion). Predisposing factors may include diabetes mellitus, lymphoma, or other debilitating conditions; corticosteroids; and antibiotics. Treating the basic cause may improve the condition. In addition, nystatin (Mycostatin), taken orally or as an oral suspension, is effective. The suspension is a medicated fluid that should be swished about the mouth vigorously for at least 1 minute. If the condition becomes chronic, it is more difficult to treat and requires persistent attention to basic care.

Aphthous Stomatitis. Among the most common lesions of the mouth are recurrent aphthous ulcers (canker sores). Aphthous ulcers are shallow ulcers found in the mucous membrane of the mouth, most often on the inner side of the lips and cheeks, and in the sulcus between the lips and gums. However, they may appear anywhere in the mouth, including on the tongue. The lesions begin with a burning, tingling sensation and slight swelling of the mucous membrane, which soon becomes a shallow ulcer with a whitish center surrounded by a red border. These ulcers are especially painful when eating and are particularly aggravated by acid or spicy foods. Since these ulcers are tender to pressure, any abrasion or movement of the skin around the ulcer makes it painful to speak or move any of the facial muscles. The ulcers may be single or multiple, and they often tend to heal at one site and recur elsewhere. The sores may appear at any time in life; most often they begin in childhood or adolescence and may appear as frequently as once a month. In most cases, however, they do not occur more than once a year or so. These ulcers last only a short time (from 10 to 14 days) and eventually heal spontaneously, leaving no scar.

In spite of intense studies, no definite cause can be found for canker sores. An L-form of α-hemolytic *Streptococcus* has been proposed as the microbial cause. There seem to be definite predisposing factors, such as emotional or mental stress, related to their occurrence. In women, they seem to appear at the time of menstrual periods, and they occur much more frequently among women than men. Fatigue, change in a life situation, and anxiety are other predisposing factors.

Because no cause is known there is no specific treatment for canker sores. When anxiety is an obvious etiologic factor, tranquilizing drugs may be beneficial. A soft, bland diet may reduce pain. Various antibiotic and steroid preparations applied locally, or injected systemically, offer some relief. Fortunately, these ulcers eventually heal spontaneously in a relatively short time.

Leukoplakia Buccalis. Leukoplakia buccalis (also called "smoker's patch") and the related *keratosis labialis* are seen in middle-aged adults, more than 80% of whom are

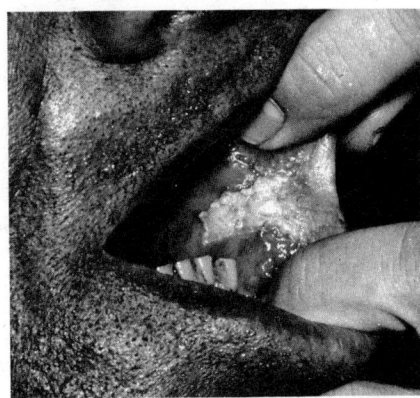

Figure 30-2
Leukoplakia. Note the white patches above and to the right of the teeth.

men. These conditions are characterized in the early stages by the appearance of one or two small, thin, often crinkled, pearly patches on the mucous membrane of the tongue, the mouth, or both, owing to keratinization of the mucosa and sclerosis of its underlying tissue (Fig. 30-2). In time, most of the tongue and the mouth may become covered by a creamy, white, thick, fissured or papillomatous mucous membrane that desquamates occasionally, leaving a beefy-red base. This condition results from chronic irritation by carious, infected, or poorly repaired teeth; by tobacco; and by highly spiced foods. It will disappear in time after cessaton of smoking. Occasionally, it is due to syphilis. Not infrequently, cancers start in the keratinized patches. Detection of these patches through a nursing history and examination is a prime nursing responsibility in this situation.

Erythroplakia. The lesions of erythroplakia are due to exudative or ulcerative processes that resemble a red patch on the oral mucous membrane. They are of short duration, are fairly easy to remove, and are nonspecific for an inflammatory disorder. Erythroplakia is more common than leukoplakia in the elderly and has a greater incidence of malignancy.

Kaposi's Sarcoma. Kaposi's sarcoma is a malignant mesenchymal skin tumor that occurs primarily on the legs of men between 50 and 70 years of age. Recently it has been seen with increased frequency as a nonsquamous tumor of the oral cavity in patients with AIDS. The lesions are purplish and nonulcerated and are composed of spindle-shaped cells. Irradiation is the treatment of choice.

Abnormalities of the Salivary Glands

The salivary glands consist of the parotid glands, one on each side of the face below the ear; the submaxillary and sublingual glands, both in the floor of the mouth; and the buccal gland, beneath the lips. About 1200 ml of saliva is produced daily. The glands' primary functions are lubrication, antibacterial protection, and digestion.

Parotitis. Parotitis (inflammation of the parotid gland) is the most common inflammatory condition of the salivary glands; however, infection can occur in the other glands as well. The essential lesion of mumps (epidemic parotitis) is an inflammation of the salivary gland (usually the parotid) and is primarily a pediatric communicable disease.

Elderly, acutely ill, and debilitated people whose salivary glands fail to secret sufficiently because of general dehydration often develop parotitis. The infecting organisms travel from the mouth through the salivary duct. Because older people tend to have parched mouths and do not chew solid foods adequately, they offer poor defense against invasion of the parotid ducts by pathogenic organisms.

The offending organism usually is *Staphylococcus aureus* (except in mumps). The onset of this complication is sudden, with an exacerbation of the fever and of the symptoms of the primary condition. The gland swells and becomes tense and tender. Pain is felt in the ear, and there is interference with swallowing. The swelling increases rapidly, and the overlying skin soon becomes red and shiny.

Nursing Interventions. In order to prevent postoperative parotitis, patients are advised to have necessary dental work done before surgery. In addition, optimal patient preparation includes maintaining an adequate nutritional and fluid intake along with good mouth hygiene.

After surgery, having the patient chew gum or suck hard candy may prevent obstruction of the salivary gland ducts. At the onset of the swelling, an icebag may be applied over the affected gland and chemotherapy may be instituted with penicillin or one of the sulfonamides. A suppurating gland may require incision and drainage.

Sialadenitis. *Sialadenitis* is caused by dehydration, stress, or improper oral hygiene and is associated with infection with *Staphylococcus aureus, Streptococcus viridans,* or pneumococcus. Characteristcs include pain, swelling, and a purulent discharge.

Management. Antibiotics are used to relieve acute symptoms. Massage, hydration, and steroids frequently cure the problem. Chronic sialadenitis, with uncontrolled pain, requires surgical excision of the gland and its duct.

Salivary Calculus (Sialolithiasis). More than 80% of all salivary stones are found in the submaxillary gland, following glandular infection or ductal stricture owing to trauma or inflammation. Sialograms (x-ray films taken with a radiopaque substance injected into the duct) may be required to show obstruction of the duct by stenosis. Salivary stones are formed mainly from calcium phosphate. If located within the gland, they are irregularly lobulated and vary in diameter from 3 to 30 mm. Stones in the duct are small and oval.

Calculi within the salivary gland cause no symptoms unless infection arises; but a calculus that obstructs the gland's duct causes sudden, local, and often colicky pain, which is suddenly relieved by a gush of saliva. This characteristic complaint can be elicited in a nursing history. Where this condition exists, the gland is swollen and quite tender, the stone itself often is palpable, and its shadow may be seen on x-ray films.

The calculus can be extracted fairly easily from the duct in the mouth; sometimes enlarging the orifice permits the stone to pass spontaneously. It may be necessary to remove the gland if there are repeated recurrences of symptoms and calculi in the gland itself.

Neoplasms. Neoplasms of almost any type develop in salivary glands; the majority are malignant. In 80% of these patients, tumors develop in one parotid gland. The tumors remain small and quiescent for years, then suddenly begin to increase in size. Diagnosis is based on the history and physical examination, frozen sections, and fine-needle aspiration biopsy. Biopsy has been demonstrated to be 90% as accurate as a frozen section, more convenient (can be done in a physician's office), and cost effective. Encouraging results in the detection of neoplasms have also been reported with radiosialography (scanning with Technetium 99m).

Minor salivary gland tumors are usually malignant and occur in patients around 70 years of age. *Pleomorphic adenoma* is the most common minor salivary gland tumor that is benign; *adenoid cystic carcinoma* is the most common malignant tumor. Biopsy determines tumor type, and surgical removal is recommended.

Management. The best treatment of a parotid tumor is the early and complete excision of the mass. Fortunately, most of these growths occur superficially, rather than in the deep retromandibular lobe. Partial excision of the gland, along with all of the tumor, combined with careful dissection to preserve the vulnerable facial (seventh) nerve, is the common procedure. For more involved tumors, it may be necessary to sacrifice the nerve when a parotidectomy is done. If the tumor is malignant or mixed, radiation therapy follows surgery. Local recurrences are common; the recurrent growth usually is more malignant than the original one.

Nursing Interventions. Preoperatively the patient is encouraged to ask questions about the procedure since there is the possibility that a radical neck dissection may be required. In the postoperative period, the nurse should be aware that the patient may have some facial paralysis (if the nerve was not excised) due to tissue trauma and edema. This paralysis will gradually subside. Dressings are removed after 24 hours, and the patient is allowed to shower and wash his hair.

Cancer of the Oral Cavity

Cancer of the oral cavity, which may occur in any part of the mouth, including the pharynx, is highly curable if discovered early. It accounts for less than 5% of all cancer deaths in the United States. Males are afflicted three times more often than females. The 5-year survival rate for cancer of the oral cavity and pharynx is 53% for whites and 34% for blacks. Of the 9400 annual deaths from oral cancer, the distribution by site is estimated as follows:

Lips	2% (175 cases)
Tongue	23% (2100 cases)
Mouth	30% (2825 cases)
Pharynx	46% (4300 cases)

Squamous cell (epidermoid) carcinoma constitutes over 90% of all mouth cancer. The next most common type, adenocarcinoma, arises frm the submucous glands. The third grouping includes malignancy of the jaw bone. The cure rate for these cancers is below 35%.

The tumor seen with *cancer of the lip* is usually called an epithelioma. It occurs most frequently as a chronic ulcer on the lower lip in men. Basal cell carcinoma usually occurs on the upper lip and squamous cell carcinoma on the lower lip. Predisposing factors may be chronic irritation of a warm pipe stem or prolonged exposure to the sun and wind. More significant, however, is the tendency for leukoplakia to progress to an epidermoid lip cancer. A typical lesion is a painless indurated ulcer with raised edges. Any wart or ulcer of the lip that does not heal in 3 weeks should be biopsied.

In *cancer of the tongue*, the constant expansion and contraction of the tongue can easily force small tumor cells into the lymphatic channels and eventually into the regional lymph nodes, where they become embedded. This cancer is most common in men in their later decades of life. Alcohol and tobacco are the two primary etiologic agents. Currently the male to female ratio is 2:1. The disease is not common before the age of 30; however, recent data show that the mortality rate for young males between the ages of 10 and 29 has doubled over the past 30 years owing to the use of smokeless tobacco (snuff).

Clinical Manifestations

Most oral cancers cause no symptoms in the early stages. Often the patient feels a roughened area with his tongue. The first complaints may be difficulty in chewing, swallowing, or speaking; swelling, numbness, or loss of feeling in any part of the mouth may also occur. A lump in the neck may indicate metastatic spread. Any patient with a white, patchy area, sore spot, or ulceration of lips, gums, or mouth that fails to heal in 3 weeks should be urged to see a physician.

Cancer of the lip is associated with discomfort and irritation due to the presence of a nonhealing sore that may be raised or ulcerated. Localized tenderness is characteristic; pain is usually absent.

With cancer of the tongue there is pain or soreness (when eating hot or highly seasoned foods) and limitation of motion. As the growth spreads to neighboring structures, other symptoms develop, such as excessive salivation, slurred speech, blood-tinged sputum, trismus (tonic contractions of the muscles of mastication), and pain on swallowing liquids. If the cancer is untreated, the patient is unable to swallow, and earache, faceache, and toothache become almost constant. Unable to eat or sleep, the patient finally dies of hemorrhage (lingual artery), cervical lymph node metastasis, or general debilitation.

Malignancy at the base of the tongue (posterior) produces less obvious symptoms: slight dysphagia, sore throat, salivation, and some blood-tinged sputum.

Diagnostic Evaluation

Oral exfoliative cytology is a means of screening intraoral lesions. As the first step in the screening process, the patient's mouth is examined carefully. Then the tongue is grasped with a 4×4-inch gauze pad and moved gently to expose the suspicious area. The lesion is then scraped with a moistened tongue blade. If a hyperkeratotic lesion is present, the surface keratin is scraped off so that the deeper epithelial cells are available for the specimen, since these cells are usually involved in early malignant change. The cells are smeared on a glass slide, immersed carefully in alcohol, and sent to the laboratory for cytologic examination.

The early stage of cancer of the anterior undersurface of the lateral aspects of the tongue is usually detected as a small ulcer that has not healed in 3 weeks or as an area of thickening. Confirmation by a biopsy is necessary.

Management

Management varies with the nature of the lesion and preference of the physician. Electrocoagulation, radiation therapy, resectional surgery, or combinations of therapy are effective.

In cancer of the lip, small lesions usually are excised liberally (Fig. 30-3); larger lesions involving more than one third of the lip may be treated best by radiation therapy because of superior cosmetic results. The choice depends on the extent of the lesion, the skill of the surgeon or radiologist, and what is necessary to cure the patient while preserving the best appearance. There is a 70% recurrence for tumors greater than 4 cm. Fortunately, only 10% to 15% of lip cancers metastasize. The survival rate is between 85% and 90%. When lymph nodes appear to be involved, a neck dissection is indicated.

For cancer of the tongue the two major treatments of choice are radiation therapy and surgery (Fig. 30-4). Laser excision and cryotherapy can be used along with local excision. Preoperative irradiation is often followed by surgery 4 to 6 weeks later. Enlargement of lymph nodes indicates metastasis, necessitating more extensive surgical neck dissection, combined with radium and x-ray therapy. When the tongue is involved, it is often necessary to perform a *hemi-*

Figure 30-3
The Estlander procedure for repair of carcinoma of the lower lip. (1) A V-shaped excision is made wide enough to remove tumor and allow for a small margin of tissue on either side of the tumor. (2) A flap of the same shape (*A–C*) is excised from the opposite lip. (3) The new flap is rotated downward to form a new buccal commissure. (Adapted with permission from del Regato JA, Spjut HJ, and Cox JD. Ackerman and del Regato's Cancer: Diagnosis, Treatment, and Prognosis. St Louis, CV Mosby, 1985.)

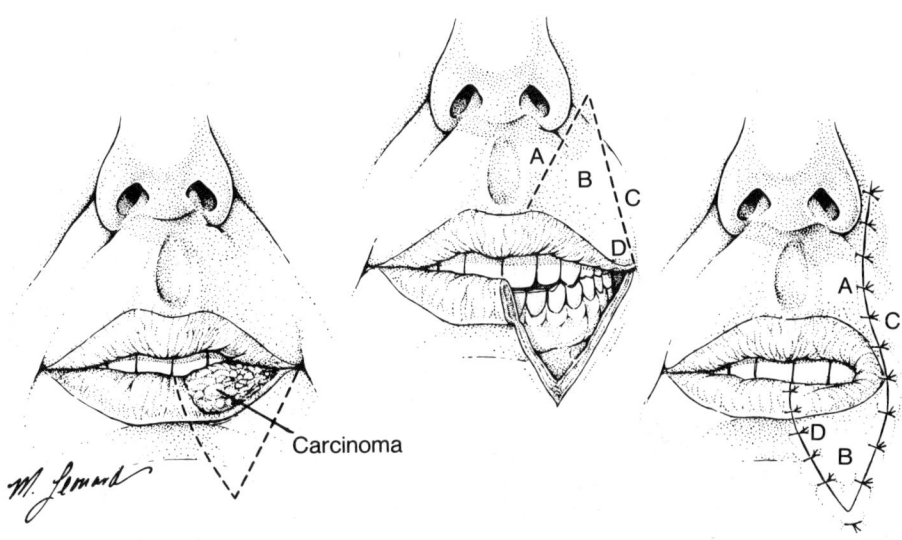

Carcinoma

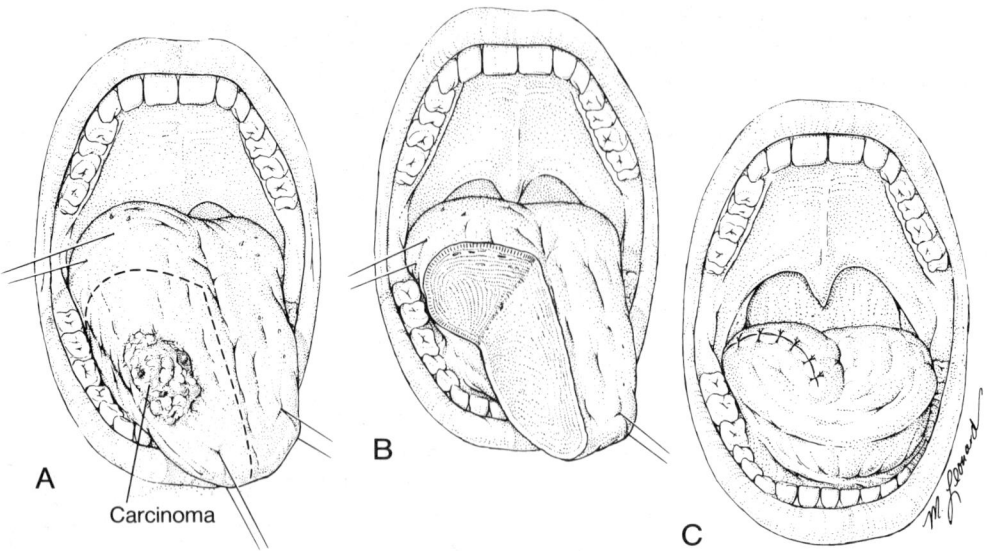

Figure 30-4
Surgery for cancer of the tongue. (*A*) Small invasive cancer of the tongue. Tongue is extended and incision margins are outlined. (*B*) A deep resection provides for removal of a generous portion of nonmalignant tissue. (*C*) Sutured area results in a shallow margin which is less defined when the tongue is extended. (Adapted with permission from McQuarrie DG, Adams GL, Shons AR et al. Head and Neck Cancer. Chicago, Year Book Medical Publishers, 1986.)

glossectomy (removal of a lateral segment of the tongue). The tongue is a difficult site for effective irradiation, and because of the mutilating effects of total glossectomy, and the likelihood of metastasis, the cure rate of posterior tongue cancer is very low. There is an 85% chance of a 5-year survival period with early detection and no lymph node spread. However, only 25% of cases are diagnosed early. In more extensive ablative procedures it may be necessary to graft tissue by flap or pedicle grafts (see Chap. 48). For even more advanced lesions involving the tongue, mandible, larynx, and neck, the trend is away from extremely radical surgery (which only ends in cosmetic and functional disaster) and toward combining chemotherapy and irradiation. If surgery is necessary, neck dissecton may be performed.

▶ *Nursing Process*
The Patient With Cancer of the Oral Cavity

▷ *Assessment*

The principal nursing activities in the assessment phase include a careful nursing history to detect symptoms requiring medical evaluation. Complaints of sores, lumps, pain in the mouth, stiffness in the neck, and difficulty with swallowing, chewing, or speaking require attention.

The nurse asks if the patient has an intolerance to hot, cold, or highly seasoned foods. Is there a history of heavy alcohol and tobacco use? Is the mucosa inflamed? Are there signs of dehydration?

To prepare the patient for examination of the oral cavity he is assisted into Fowler's position. Dentures are removed. Adequate examination of the oral cavity requires good lighting (penlight, flashlight, or head mirror). A wooden tongue blade is used to retract the cheek and hold back the tongue. A finger cot or rubber glove is used to palpate the area. White areas (leukoplakia), fissures, ulcers, red areas (erythroplakia), masses, or unusual pigmentation are searched for. Gingival tissue should be pink and the palate moist.

The lips are inspected for color (moist and pink), symmetry, texture (smooth, soft), and the absence of blisters, ulcerations, fissures, and lesions. The tongue is examined for cracks, fissures, lesions, and color (pink). Discoloration and keratinization may indicate the beginnings of cancer. Is there any pain? To assess the hypoglossal (12th cranial) nerve, the nurse asks the patient if he can touch his upper lip with the tip of his tongue.

▷ *Nursing Diagnoses*

Based on all the assessment data, the nursing diagnoses may include the following:

- Alteration of the oral mucous membrane related to irritation, inflammation, and dryness of the mouth secondary to the presence of a lesion
- Alteration in nutrition, less than body requirements, related to reduced intake of foods and fluids secondary to sensitive oral mucous membranes
- Disturbance in self-concept/body image, related to disfiguring appearance of an oral lesion or reconstructive surgery

- Fear of pain and social isolation and inability to cope related to the diagnosis and prognosis of the disease process
- Potential for injury or infection related to altered immunologic responses secondary to chemotherapy/irradiation
- Anticipatory grieving related to the diagnosis of cancer

▷ *Planning and Implementation*

▷ *Goals:* The patient's major goals may include maintenance of the integrity of the oral cavity, adequate intake of foods and fluids, attainment of a positive self-image and effective communication, acquisition of coping mechanisms, absence of infection, and acceptance of the diagnosis of cancer.

Nursing Interventions

Mouth Care. The nurse teaches the patient how to keep his mouth clean. Use of a soft toothbrush is recommended to minimize irritation of the gums. Flossing should be done at least once a day to prevent the accumulation of food debris, which can aggravate sensitive tissues. If the patient cannot tolerate brushing or flossing, an irrigating solution of 1 teaspoon of baking soda to 8 ounces of warm water is recommended. Gentle lavage with a catheter inserted between the cheek and teeth loosens mucus and is refreshing. A power spray has the advantage of getting the solution into inaccessible areas. Viscous lidocaine (Xylocaine Viscous 2%) may be prescribed as a mouth rinse. Commercial mouthwashes are not used because they contain alcohol, which can irritate the gums.

In the unconscious patient, the nurse is wholly responsible for maintaining good mouth hygiene. The use of a special mouth tray with all necessary applicator sticks, padded tongue depressors, mouthwashes, and lubricants encourages frequent mouth attention. Apply a lip moisturizer (petrolatum) as needed to soothe dry and cracking lips.

Dryness of the mouth is a frequent sequela of oral cancer, particularly when the salivary glands have been exposed to irradiation or major surgery. It is also noted in patients who are receiving psychopharmacologic agents or in those who are unable to close the mouth and therefore become mouth-breathers. To minimize this problem, the patient is advised to avoid dry, bulky, and irritating foods and fluids as well as alcohol and tobacco. He is also encouraged to increase his intake of fluids, if not contraindicated. Some degree of relief is obtained through the lubricating action of such substances as petrolatum, mineral oil, and cough drops with glycerin. Salivary flow can be stimulated with sugar-free lemon lozenges or sugar-free chewing gum. In a dry environment, the use of humidifiers may also help.

Adequate Food and Fluid Intake. Anorexia is a common problem in a patient with oral cancer because of the discomfort associated with eating. The nurse recommends the intake of soft, high-carbohydrate foods (pasta, potatoes) that are filling and have a protein-sparing action (*i.e.*, protein catabolism for energy needs is saved, or "spared," so that protein can be used for tissue regeneration). Creative approaches to food preparation are encouraged, such as the generous use of spices (cinnamon, mint, cloves) to enhance the taste of foods, marinating meats, stir-frying vegetables, and poaching fish. The nurse suggests three moderate meals a day, rather than frequent small servings, to limit the frequency of coping with the oral discomfort associated with eating. Supplementary feedings (Sustacal, Compleat-B) help maintain an adequate protein and calorie intake. Fluid requirements can be met by suggesting sweetened juices that are nonacidic (gelatin desserts in liquid form, colas, and milk shakes). Flexible straws or modified feeding utensils are helpful. Antiemetic agents are administered as prescribed.

The desires as well as the nutritional needs of the patient should be taken into consideration. If he is not able to take anything by mouth, it may be necessary to feed him parenterally to maintain fluid and electrolyte balance and to prevent starvation and negative nitrogen balance. Such feeding may be by way of parenteral hyperalimentation (see p. 766), a lateral pharyngostomy stab wound (to prevent nasal discomfort), or nasogastric intubation.

Coping Measures. The patient with a mouth or facial problem requires patience and understanding. Quite naturally, he tends to withdraw from people, is self-conscious about mouth odors, and is sensitive about his appearance. The nurse is challenged to communicate with him, encourage his expression of fears and concerns, and offer him support and explanations as necessary. The immediate family needs to be aware of their supporting role and, in turn, should be informed of the plan of therapy for the patient and urged to participate in the plan of care.

A particular area of concern that interferes with communication, feeding, and swallowing is excessive salivation or drooling. The measures taken to control drooling depend on the cause, severity, and relative permanence of the dysfunction. If the problem is moderate to severe but temporary, as may be the case following surgery, mechanical suction devices used with a soft catheter are effective. If drooling is mild, management may be obtained by training the patient to swallow more frequently, by providing emotional reassurance and support, and by using anticholinergic agents (antisialogogues), such as those containing atropine or belladonna (Banthine, Robinul). For more severe drooling, it may be necessary to resort to plastic reconstruction of the oral structures.

Mouth wipes, as well as a paper bag attached to the bed or the bedside stand to receive soiled tissues, always should be on hand. An effective way of holding dressings of the mouth or the lower jaw in place is by the use of a face mask. The strings can be tied at the top of the head.

The patient may express a strong desire for solitude and may be self-conscious about his appearance. (The need to remove, temporarily, any large mirrors in the room should be considered by the nurse.) The results of surgery or irradiation concern him, especially the fear of disfigurement; if the resection is extensive, the possibility of prosthetics (fitting an artificial part) may be explained.

The patient may have problems with speech. Providing him with a pad of paper and a pencil or "magic slate," so that he can express his needs and thoughts, may make a tremendous difference in his depressed condition. Often these patients are reluctant to associate with other patients and prefer to be alone. If there are two or more patients with a similar condition, they can help each other. It is easier for them, and for others, if they have their meals apart from other patients.

The patient's family and friends should be encouraged to visit so that he is aware that others care about him. He can be helped to care for his appearance. With speech training and adjustment to a prosthesis, he will become increasingly aware that the future holds promise for him.

Alleviation of Fear.   The nurse has the patient describe his fears related to pain, isolation, altered life-style, and loss of control. The description may provide a clue for managing the problem and developing a plan of care. She assesses his physical reactions to his fears. Common responses include muscle rigidity, fatigue, tachycardia, hypertension, dyspnea, and nausea.

The nurse can reduce fears in a number of ways. For example, the fear of pain can be managed by advising the patient that medication will be offered every 3 to 4 hours, and that if something more is needed the physician will be called to adjust the dosage or frequency. The nurse supports adaptive behaviors, encourages expressions of emotions, emphasizes the patient's abilities, and fosters positive self-esteem.

Distorted perceptions are corrected by providing accurate information. Control is encouraged by having the patient participate in the treatment process. Support groups are recommended, and the nurse can offer to contact a representative from a support group to visit the patient.

The nurse should be receptive to the patient's expressions of potential loss. Behaviors associated with defense mechanisms such as projection, displacement, and rationalization need to be recognized. Many patients withdraw, cry easily, and experience a sense of hopelessness. Some of them progress through certain behaviors in anticipating death: denial, anger, depression, bargaining, resolution, and acceptance. The nurse's role is one of offering support. She projects an optimistic attitude, especially if the lesion has a high incidence of cure (90% for cancer of the lip). Visits by an appropriate counselor, social worker, or member of the clergy can be suggested.

Infection Control.   Thrombocytopenia and leukopenia, side-effects of radiation and chemotherapy, weaken a patient's defense mechanisms, making him more susceptible to infections. Anemia, subsequent to malnutrition, is also common. Laboratory studies must be evaluated frequently, and the patient's temperature is checked every 6 to 8 hours for an elevation that may indicate an infection. Visitors who may transmit microorganisms are prohibited because the patient's immunologic system is depressed. Trauma to sensitive skin tissues is avoided to maintain skin integrity and prevent infection. Strict aseptic technique is necessary when changing dressings. Desquamation (shedding of the epidermis) is a reaction to radiation therapy that causes dryness and itching and can lead to a break in skin integrity and subsequent infection.

Viscous lidocaine, ice chips, and oral irrigations of saline may be prescribed for the patient who develops mouth ulcers, stomatitis, or xerostomia (dryness of the mouth caused by the arresting of salivary secretion) as a result of chemotherapy. The intake of a high-protein, high-carbohydrate diet with vitamin supplements is encouraged to promote tissue repair for the patient who is anorexic and anemic.

Patient Education.   The nurse has the responsibility to make sure that the patient receives accurate information about his disease process if he wants the information. Some patients want to know everything about their diagnosis, while others only want to know what is necessary for them to manage their daily activities. The participation of family members or significant others is encouraged in any discussions.

The nurse must determine what the patient already knows and what he wants to know about the type of treatment recommended (chemotherapy, radiation therapy, surgery), the process involved, and the implications for his care. Information is presented at his level of learning and when he is relaxed, pain free, and not distracted by visitors. A person must be physically and emotionally ready to learn for learning to occur. Pictures or diagrams can be used when appropriate, and family members are involved in the sessions whenever possible. The patient's active participation is encouraged, but it is important to remember that he must have the energy to attend the session. Important facts are emphasized and repeated by the patient as necessary.

Home Health Care.   The post-hospital objectives of patient care are similar to those in the hospital. The patient who is recovering from treatment of a mouth condition needs to breathe, to secure nourishment, to avoid infection, and to be alert for adverse signs. The patient, members of his family or the person responsible for his home care, the nurse, and whoever else may be involved, such as a speech therapist, dietitian, and psychologist, need to prepare an individualized plan. If suctioning the mouth or a tracheostomy tube is required, it is important to determine what equipment is needed and how to use it, as well as where it can be obtained. Consideration is given to the humidification and aeration of the room, as well as measures to control odors. How to prepare foods that are nutritious, properly seasoned, and of the right temperature can be explained. Perhaps it may be more feasible to use commercial baby food than to prepare liquid and soft diets in a blender. The use and care of prostheses must be understood. The importance of cleanliness with dressings and mouth care is reviewed. The person caring for the patient needs to know the signs of obstruction, hemorrhage, infection, depression, and withdrawal, as well as what to do about these problems. Follow-up visits to the clinic or physician are important to determine progression or regression and to receive any modifications in medication or general care.

Over 90% of recurrences will appear within the first 18 months; therefore, meticulous inspection by the physician every 4 to 6 weeks is essential. Early detection of local recurrences or metastasis, followed by aggressive treatment, can cure as many as 50% of these patients. Follow-up visits become less frequent after 2 years but must be continued for life, because of the frequency of other primary carcinomas. One important part of continuing care is the elimination of alcohol consumption and smoking. Because of further extension of a malignancy by metastasis and necrosis, it may not be possible medically to halt the spread of disease. All efforts are then directed toward the comfort measures—physical, psychological, and spiritual. With the family's help this may be continued in the hospital, a nursing home, a hospice setting, or the patient's own home.

▷ *Evaluation*

▷ *Expected Outcomes*

1. Patient practices oral hygiene measures.
   a. Brushes teeth and flosses daily; performs mouth care after each meal.

b. Inspects mouth routinely for the presence of lesions.

c. Avoids foods and fluids that irritate the gums or mouth.

d. Limits or avoids use of alcohol and tobacco (including smokeless tobacco).

e. Uses lubricating agents for the mouth (lozenges, chewing gum).

2. Maintains adequate intake of foods and fluids.

a. Eats soft, nonirritating foods several times a day.

b. Uses a modified eating utensil if necessary.

c. Maintains or gains weight.

d. Is hydrated.

e. Requests antiemetic agents as needed.

f. Adheres to parenteral feeding schedule.

3. Evidences a positive self-image.

a. Interacts appropriately with family members.

b. Is able to communicate effectively (verbally or by using a "magic slate").

c. Projects self-confidence.

d. Participates in social gatherings.

4. Expresses personal feelings about diagnosis.

a. Is aware of diagnosis and understands prognosis.

b. Discusses feelings with family members and significant others.

c. Verbally discusses emotional responses to the diagnosis.

5. Acquires information about disease process and course of treatment.

a. Is motivated to learn about treatment and its implications and participates in the teaching sessions.

b. Involves family members in teaching sessions as a means of support.

6. Reduces fears related to pain, isolation, and the inability to cope.

a. Accepts that pain will be managed if not eliminated.

b. Freely expresses fears and concerns.

c. Agrees to talk with a support group.

d. Communicates openly with family members and significant others.

e. Writes down one positive thing about self each day.

7. Is infection free.

a. Maintains normal laboratory values.

b. Is afebrile.

c. Maintains skin integrity.

d. Practices oral hygiene after every meal and at bedtime.

e. Avoids visitors with infectious conditions.

f. Eats a high-protein, high-carbodhydrate diet.

Radical Neck Dissection

Malignancies of the head and neck, including cancers of the lips, tongue, gums, palate, tonsils, and of the mucosa of the mouth, pharynx, and larynx, may be treated early by surgery, irradiation, or chemotherapy, with good results. These cancers (stages I and II) are in an area that can be easily seen, making early prognosis and treatment possible. Most observers agree that such patients do not die of recurrence at the site of the primary growth, but rather of metastasis to the cervical lymph nodes in the neck, which often takes place by way of the lymphatics before the primary lesion has been treated. Only the nodes on one side of the neck are involved, unless the tumor is located at or near the midline, in which case the nodes of both sides of the neck may contain metastatic tumors.

Because radiation does not by itself give good results in controlling the metastatic cancer in the lymph nodes in the neck, an operation called a *radical neck dissection* is performed. A radical neck dissection involves removal of all the tissue under the skin, from the ramus of the jaw down to the clavicle, and from the midline anteriorly back to the anterior border of the trapezius muscle posteriorly. This includes removing the sternocleidomastoid muscle and other smaller muscles, as well as the jugular vein in the neck, because the lymphatic nodes are found widely distributed throughout these tissues (Fig. 30-5).

A *functional or modified neck dissection* is similar to a radical neck dissection except that the sternocleidomastoid muscle, internal jugular vein, and the spinal accessory nerve are preserved. Obviously, this approach appears a reasonable alternative to radical radiation therapy and is a preferred alternative to traditional neck dissection in the control of regional metastasis when neck disease is either occult or still confined to mobile lymph nodes.

Nursing Interventions

The nursing interventions for patients requiring radical neck dissection include both physical and psychological preparation for major surgery. In addition to the impending physical rigors of this surgery, this patient is aware that his malignancy includes metastasis to his cervical nodes. This information is bound to cause concern and anxiety regarding the postsurgical outcome.

Before the operation, the patient should be informed about the impending surgery, what is to be done in the operating room (amplification of the surgeon's explanation), and what the postoperative period will be like. At the same time, the patient can be given an opportunity to express concerns about the upcoming surgery. During this exchange, the nurse has an opportunity to assess the patient's coping abilities, encourage questions, and develop a plan for offering assistance. A sense of mutual understanding and rapport will make the postoperative experience less troublesome for the patient. After the operation, any expressions of concern on the patient's part can guide the nurse in providing additional support. These intervention activities deliberately include supportive family members.

The general postoperative nursing intervention activities are similar to those described on pages 722 through 724 for the patient who has had extensive neck surgery and therefore may have problems with breathing and swallowing. The specific postoperative physical nursing interventions for this patient include maintenance of a patent airway and continuous assessment of respiratory status; wound care and attention to dressings, including careful observation for hemorrhage; and management of oral hygiene and nutritional needs.

Airway Management. After the endotracheal tube or airway has been removed and the effects of the anesthesia have worn off, the patient may be placed in Fowler's position to facilitate breathing and promote comfort. This position also increases lymphatic and venous drainage, facilitates swallowing, and decreases venous pressure on the skin flaps.

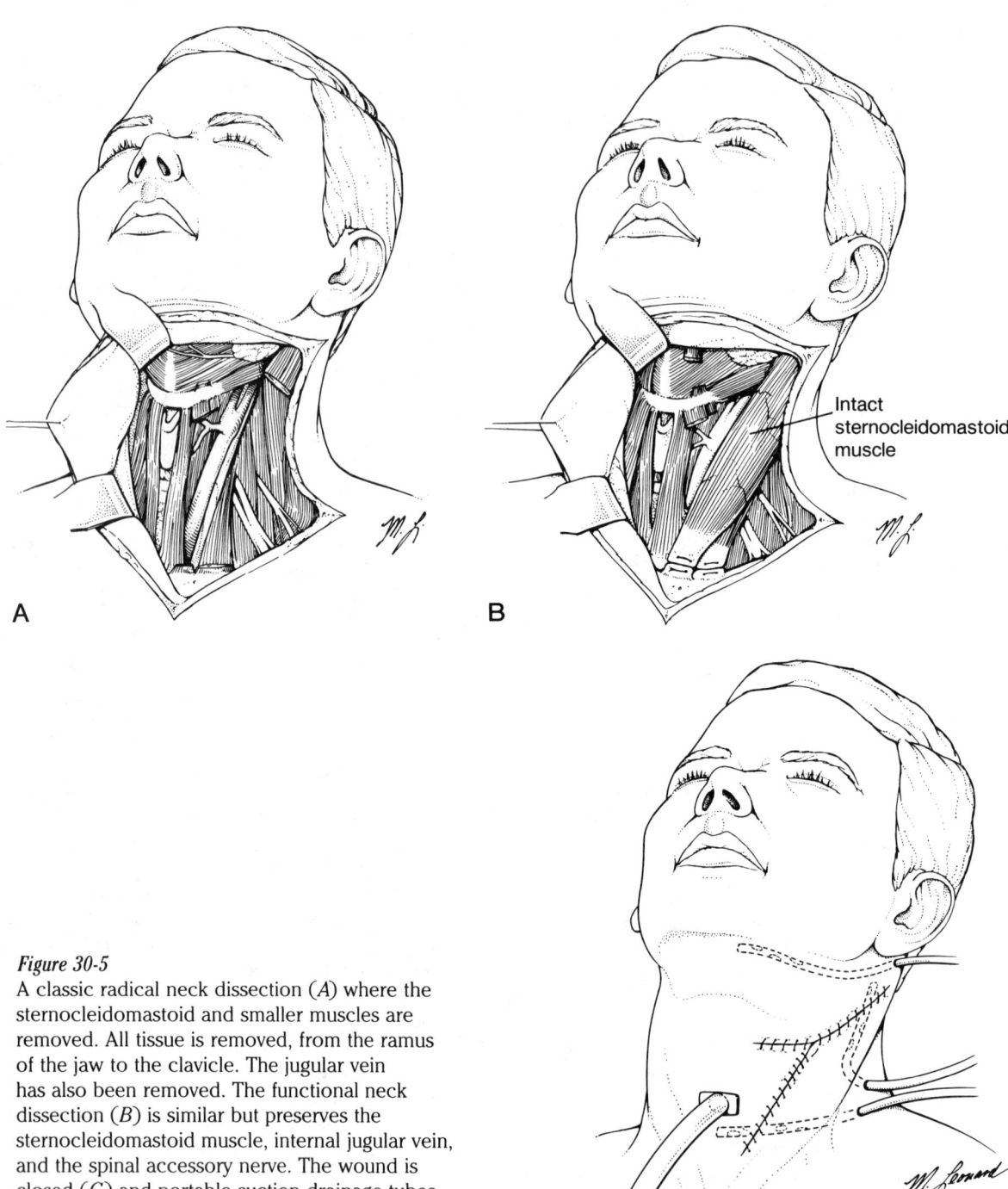

Figure 30-5
A classic radical neck dissection (*A*) where the
sternocleidomastoid and smaller muscles are
removed. All tissue is removed, from the ramus
of the jaw to the clavicle. The jugular vein
has also been removed. The functional neck
dissection (*B*) is similar but preserves the
sternocleidomastoid muscle, internal jugular vein,
and the spinal accessory nerve. The wound is
closed (*C*) and portable suction drainage tubes
are in place.

Signs of respiratory distress, such as dyspnea, cyanosis,
and changes in vital signs, are watched for, since they may
suggest edema, throat irritation from the endotracheal tube,
hemorrhage, or inadequate drainage. Temperature is usually
taken rectally.

In the immediate postoperative period, the nurse may
be able to detect the presence of stridor (coarse, high-pitched
sound on inspiration) by listening frequently at the trachea
with a stethoscope. In this situation, the physician should be
summoned.

Coughing is encouraged to aid in the removal of secretions. The patient should assume a sitting position, with the
nurse supporting his neck with her hands, so that he may be
able to bring up bothersome secretions. If this technique fails,
the patient's respiratory tract may have to be suctioned. Care
is exerted to protect the suture lines during suctioning. If a
tracheostomy tube is in place, suctioning is done through this
tube using sterile technique.

Wound Care.   With portable wound suction drainage,
there is no need for pressure dressings because the skin flaps
are drawn down tightly; 80 to 120 ml of serosanguineous
secretions is drawn off by a portable suction unit the first
day. This amount diminishes thereafter. If portable wound
suction is not used, drains may be placed in the wound and

pressure dressings applied to obliterate dead spaces and to provide immobilization. These pressure dressings may need to be reinforced from time to time. Dressings are observed for evidence of hemorrhage and constriction, which may affect respiration. Drains may be removed before the massive dressings are changed in about 5 days. Lighter dressings permit greater freedom of movement. Aeroplast or other antiseptic plastic sprays protect the wound. The patient usually is allowed out of bed the first postoperative day.

Possible Complications. Because of the extensiveness of the surgery, hemorrhage is a possible complication. Later, postoperative respiratory problems may cause pneumonia, unless the patient is turned and encouraged to breathe deeply. Wound infection has been reduced considerably, with the use of portable wound suction in place of pressure dressings. Neural complications can occur if the cervical plexus or spinal accessory nerves are severed.

Since lower facial paralysis may occur as a result of injury to the facial nerve during the dissection, this is watched for and reported if noted. Likewise, if the superior laryngeal nerve is damaged, the patient may have difficulty with swallowing liquids and food because of the partial lack of sensation of the glottis.

Prevention and Management of Hemorrhage. The following measures are indicated:

1. Assess vital signs. Tachycardia, tachypnea, and hypotension may indicate impending hypovolemic shock subsequent to hemorrhage.
2. Observe dressings and wound drainage for excessive bleeding. The expected postoperative drainage should be serosanguineous and less than 200 ml in the first 24 hours. Blood loss is excessive if there is ligature separation or rupture of a vessel.
3. If hemorrhage occurs, apply pressure over dressings and over the carotid and internal jugular vessels. Direct pressure over the wound will slow blood loss. Pressure on surrounding major vessels will decrease blood flow to the area, thus decreasing blood loss.
4. Stay with the patient and summon assistance. Hemorrhage requires the continuous application of pressure to the bleeding site and/or major associated vessel. A controlled, calm manner will allay patient anxiety. A physician is notified immediately because vessel or ligature tear will require surgical intervention.

Oral Hygiene and Nutrition. Mouth hygiene is necessary and welcomed by this patient. It is done frequently and helps to enhance the appetite. A nasogastric tube may be inserted for feeding purposes or to help decompress the stomach.

Coping Measures. The psychological postoperative nursing intervention is directed toward the support of a patient who has had a radical change in body image and who has major concerns regarding his prognosis. Such a patient also has difficulty in communication and is concerned about his continuing ability to breathe and swallow normally. Adjustment to the results of this surgery will take time, and the nurse enlists the support of family members in encouraging and reassuring the patient.

The person who has had extensive neck surgery often is sensitive about his appearance, either when the operative area is covered by bulky dressings or when an incision line is exposed, as with portable drainage. If the nurse conveys acceptance of the patient and his appearance and expresses a positive, optimistic attitude, the patient is more likely to be encouraged. In spite of the wide removal of tissue, the cosmetic and functional defects are less than might be expected. The patient also needs an opportunity to voice his concerns regarding the success of the surgery and his prognosis. Most of these patients are able to maintain and gain weight and are soon restored to economic independence.

Specific interventions for the care of the patient who has had radical neck surgery are presented in detail in Nursing Care Plan 30-1.

Rehabilitation Following Head and Neck Surgery

Many problems can be avoided with a conscientious exercise program. The purpose of the exercises depicted in Figure 30-6 (p. 725) is to regain maximum shoulder function and neck motion following neck surgery. These exercises are recommended by the physician when it is believed that the neck incision is sufficiently healed. Excision of muscle and nerves results in a weakness of the shoulder than can cause "shoulder drop," with some forward curvature of the shoulder. Exercises will assist the patient in returning to normal activity.

Exercises are done in the morning and evening. At first each exercise is done once; thereafter, it is gradually increased by one, every day, until each is done ten times. Sweeping, smooth motions are used, in a relaxed manner. After each exercise the patient is directed to go limp and relax. Between exercises and when not using the arm or hand, the patient is encouraged to rest the arm and hand on a padded support to keep the shoulder lifted slightly.

Fracture of the Mandible: Jaw Repositioning or Reconstruction

Fractures of the mandible may consist of simple fractures without displacement resulting from a blow on the chin. They may also be the result of planned surgical intervention, as in the correction of long or short jaw syndrome, or they may be very complicated, involving loss of tissue and bone from a severe accident. Mandibular fractures are usually closed fractures.

Management. In simple fractures, without loss of teeth, the lower jaw is immobilized by wiring it to the upper jaw. The wires are placed around the teeth in both the upper and lower jaw, on each side of the fracture line. The lower jaw is held tight against the upper jaw by cross-wires or rubber bands placed around the wires about the teeth. This simple form of fixation is used when there are teeth that can be used in the wire fixation. In other cases, in which teeth are missing or bone displacement has occurred, various other forms of fixation can be used. Some of these, such as metal arch bars, are applied in the mouth; other methods are more involved, requiring pins inserted into the bone, with fixation to a plaster head piece.

(Text continues on p. 724)

Care of the Patient Who Has Undergone a Neck Dissection

Nursing Interventions	*Rationale*	*Expected Outcomes*

Nursing Diagnosis: Ineffective airway clearance related to obstruction secondary to edema, hemorrhage, or inadequate wound drainage

Goal: Maintenance of normal respiratory function

1. Place the patient in high Fowler's position.	1. High Fowler's position facilitates expansion of the lungs because the diaphragm is pulled downward and the abdominal viscera are pulled away from the lungs. Breathing is promoted. This position also increases lymphatic and venous drainage, facilitates swallowing, and decreases venous pressure on the skin flaps. Regurgitation and aspiration of stomach contents is prevented postoperatively.	• Achieves a normal respiratory rate. • Breathes comfortably. • Avoids use of accessory muscles of respiration.
2. Monitor vital signs every 15 to 20 minutes initially then every 1 to 2 hours for the first 24 hours.	2. Edema, hemorrhage, or inadequate drainage will alter heart rate and respirations. Tachypnea and restlessness may indicate respiratory distress.	• Maintains vital signs within normal range.
3. Auscultate breath sounds as needed. Place the stethoscope over the trachea in the immediate postoperative period to assess for the presence of stridor.	3. Abnormal breath sounds may indicate ineffective ventilation, decreased perfusion, and fluid accumulation. Stridor, a harsh, high-pitched sound, primarily heard on inspiration, indicates airway obstruction.	• Shows evidence of normal breath sounds.
4. Encourage deep breathing and coughing. Place the patient in a sitting position and support the neck area with both hands.	4. Deep breathing prior to coughing promotes expansion of the airways and a more forceful cough. The coughing mechanism assists airway cilia with removal of secretions. Splinting the incision during coughing reduces strain and promotes the expulsion of secretions by allowing for deeper inspirations.	• Coughs effectively. • Maintains a patent airway.
5. Suction the airway as needed.	5. Suctioning mechanically clears the airway by removing secretions that the patient may be unable to bring up. Airway obstruction is prevented and coughing is stimulated. Atelectasis, caused by mucus blockage, is prevented.	• Breathes easier after suctioning.
6. Assess for hoarseness or dysphagia.	6. Edema, subsequent to surgical trauma, can cause pressure on the pharynx.	• Voice characteristics are unchanged. • Swallows without discomfort.

(continued)

Nursing Interventions	*Rationale*	*Expected Outcomes*

Nursing Diagnosis: Potential for injury: infection related to improper wound healing

Goal: Absence of infection

1. Monitor wound suction drainage.	1. Suction drainage negates the need for pressure dressings because the skin flaps are pulled down tightly. Drainage should approximate 80 to 120 ml of serosanguineous secretions for the first 24 hours. Then the secretions should decrease daily. Continuous bloody drainage indicates small vessel oozing.	• Wound drains less than 200 ml of sero-sanguineous drainage the first postoperative day.
2. Note drainage quantity and odor.	2. Purulent, malodorous drainage indicates an infection. Drainage greater than 300 ml in the first 24 hours is considered abnormal.	• Serosanguineous drainage is within normal limits.
3. Reinforce pressure dressings as needed.	3. If portable wound suction is not used, then pressure dressings are applied to obliterate dead spaces and provide immobilization. These are *reinforced,* not changed, as needed. Assess for any possible constrictions that would affect respirations.	
4. Use aseptic technique to cleanse skin around the drains and change the dressings after the fifth postoperative day.	4. Aseptic technique prevents wound contamination. Sterile saline effectively cleans the skin around the drains. A povidone-iodine solution, which is effective against a variety of microorganisms, can also be used.	• Wound and surrounding skin remain clean and free of infection.
5. Monitor vital signs. Assess for symptoms of infection: chills, diaphoresis, altered level of consciousness.	5. An elevated temperature, tachypnea, and tachycardia may indicate an infection.	• Is afebrile with normal respirations and a normal heart rate. • Is alert and aware of surroundings.

Nursing Diagnosis: Alteration in nutrition, less than body requirements related to anorexia and dysphagia

Goal: Attainment of an optimal level of nutrition

1. Provide oral hygiene before and after meals.	1. Mouth hygiene enhances the appetite.	• Expresses a desire for food.

2. Assist with oral intake:
  a. Offer easily chewed foods; mash or blenderize if necessary
  b. Suggest that the head be tilted to the unaffected side when swallowing.
	2. Soft textured foods facilitate swallowing.
	
	  b. Passage of food may be tolerated better when pressure occurs on the side opposite surgery.
		• Swallows food easily.

(continued)

Nursing Interventions	Rationale	Expected Outcomes

Nursing Diagnosis: Alteration in nutrition, less than body requirements related to anorexia and dysphagia

Goal: Attainment of an optimal level of nutrition

c. Add spices or sweeteners.	c. Taste sensation is enhanced to compensate for impaired taste or smell.	
d. Inquire if privacy is desired when eating.	d. Self-feeding difficulties may cause embarrassment and interfere with digestion.	• Is comfortable eating alone or with others.
3. Administer tube feedings as prescribed.	3. A nasogastric tube may be in place for several days.	• Tolerates tube feedings.

Nursing Diagnosis: Disturbance in self-concept and body image related to changes in appearance and alterations in communication

Goal: Attainment of a positive self-image

1. Help the patient to communicate effectively.	1. Temporary hoarseness is common after neck surgery.	• Recognizes that hoarseness is temporary.
a. Provide materials for writing messages.	a. A tracheostomy is usually performed and verbal communication may not be possible.	• Communicates nonverbally.
b. Make certain that the call bell is readily accessible.		
c. Develop nonverbal ways to communicate (*e.g.*, finger-tapping, sign language).	c. Communication with head movement may be impossible because of incisional pain.	
2. Encourage verbalizations of fears:		• Willingly talks about fears and concerns.
a. Provide time to listen		
b. Project a positive, optimistic attitude.	b. An optimistic approach conveys interest and hope.	
c. Reinforce reality.	c. Honesty will promote a trusting relationship. This includes confirming cosmetic and functional limitations.	• Accepts prognosis with realistic limitations.
d. Collaborate with family members to elicit their support and encouragement.	d. Family members or significant others can provide valuable support to the patient.	• Accepts support as offered.
3. Observe for facial paralysis.	3. Injury to the facial nerve will cause lower facial paralysis.	• Absence of facial paralysis.
4. Observe for excessive drooling.	4. Damage to the hypoglossal nerve will result in excessive drooling and decreased ability to swallow.	• Absence of drooling and dysphagia.
5. Check for normal shoulder position and function.	5. Damage to the spinal accessory nerve will result in drooping of the shoulder. Rehabilitation exercises are begun when the incision is healed.	• Maintains normal shoulder function.

Nursing Interventions. Preoperatively the nurse must assure the patient that he will be able to breathe comfortably and to swallow. Immediately following surgery, the patient is placed on his side, with his head slightly elevated. The nasogastric suction tube inserted during surgery is connected to low-pressure suction to remove stomach contents and lessen the danger of aspiration. Antiemetic drugs are administered to prevent vomiting. If the patient vomits and the wires are cut, surgery and rewiring have to be repeated later. A plier-type of wire cutter (or scissors, if rubber bands are used) must be taped to the head of the bed for emergency use.

Clearing of the nasopharyngeal area is done with a small catheter inserted through the nasal orifice. The oral cavity can be aspirated by first inserting a tongue blade to move

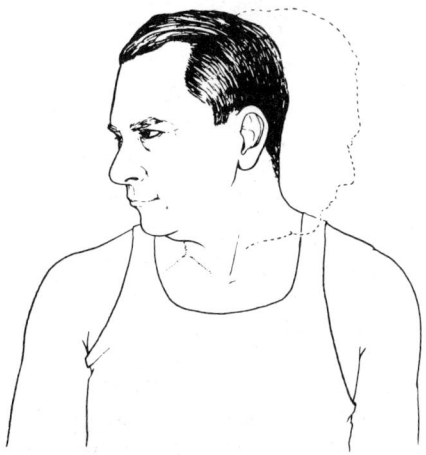

1a. Gently turn head to each side and look as far as possible.

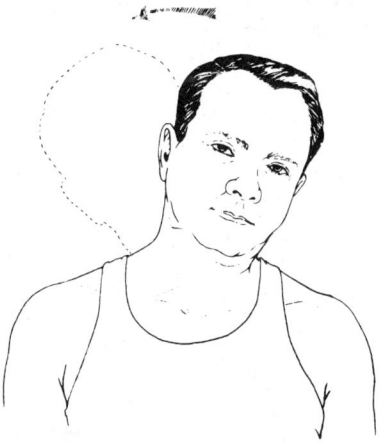

1b. Gently tip right ear toward right shoulder as far as possible. Repeat on left side.

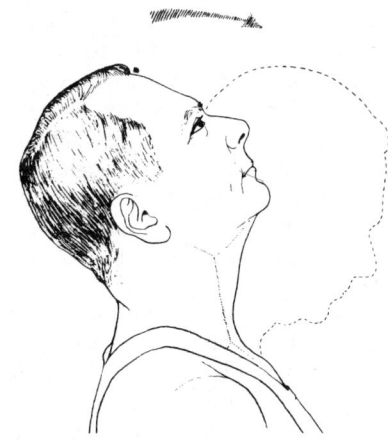

1c. Move chin to chest and then lift head up and back.

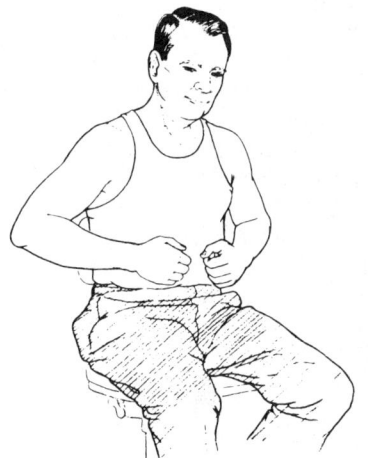

2a. Place hands in front with elbows at right angles away from body.

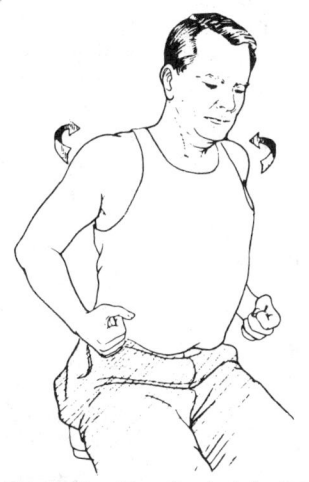

2b. Rotate shoulders back, bringing elbows to side.

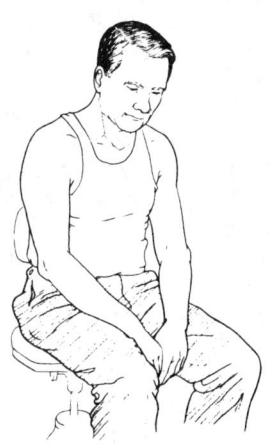

2c. Relax whole body.

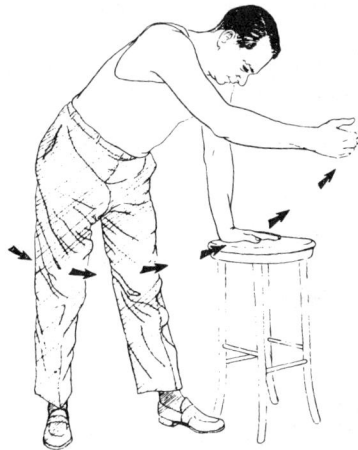

3a. Lean or hold onto low table or chair with hand on the unoperated side. Bend body slightly at waist and swing shoulder and arm from left to right.

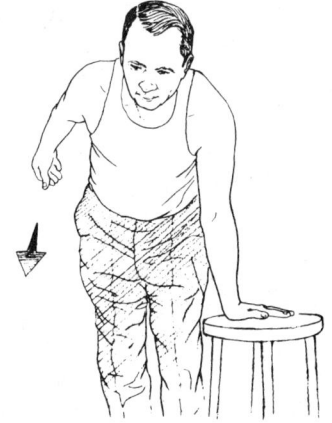

3b. Swing shoulder and arm from front to back.

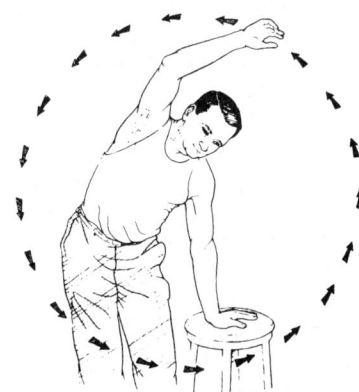

3c. Swing shoulder and arm in a wide circle, gradually bringing arm above head.

Figure 30-6
Three rehabilitation exercises following head and neck surgery. The objective is to regain maximum shoulder function and neck motion following neck surgery. (Exercise for Radical Neck Surgery Patients. Head and Neck Service, Department of Surgery, Memorial Hospital, New York, New York.)

the cheek away from the teeth; the catheter is inserted in an area where there is a space between teeth, where a tooth is missing, or in the space behind the third molar.

Constant attention by the nurse in the immediate postoperative period is necessary. As the patient regains consciousness, he needs to be reminded again that his jaw is wired but that he can breathe and swallow. As he emerges from anesthesia, his head is elevated. If an extraoral appliance is used to immobilize the mandible, the patient needs instruction on positioning himself so that he does not roll onto the device. To prevent dry and cracking lips, a lubricant is applied.

Careful attention to the hygiene of the mouth is insisted upon, using warm alkaline mouthwashes or oxygenating rinses at least every 2 hours, and after each feeding. In addition, the mouth is inspected at least once or twice daily to ensure thorough cleansing. A flashlight and a tongue blade to retract the cheeks are essential equipment. If permissible, a small, soft toothbrush can be used carefully.

The diet must necessarily be liquid, but sufficient caloric and fluid intake can be given easily to these patients. They can be fed through a straw without much difficulty, and soft foods are given with a spoon. Water is given after each liquid feeding, followed by a mouthwash.

Usually, the patient is out of bed the first postoperative day and discharged in 2 to 3 days in the absence of other trauma. The wiring is usually removed in 6 to 8 weeks.

Patient Education and Home Health Care. The patient needs very specific guidelines for mouth care and feeding. He is reminded to see his physician for scheduled visits and make sure the fixation appliance is functioning properly. Any irritated areas are to be reported. A wire cutter is readily available and the patient and a family member made aware how to cut the wires in an emergency.

Conditions of the Esophagus

The esophagus is a mucus-lined, muscular tube that allows food to enter the stomach. It begins at the base of the pharynx and ends about 4 cm below the diaphragm. Its ability to transport food and fluid is facilitated by two sphincters: the pharyngoesophageal at the junction of the pharynx and the esophagus, and the gastroesophageal at the junction of the esophagus and the stomach. An incompetent gastroesophageal sphincter allows reflux (backward flow) of gastric contents.

Difficulty in swallowing (dysphagia) is the most common symptom of esophageal disease. This symptom may range from an uncomfortable feeling that a bolus of food is "caught" in the upper esophagus (before it eventually passes into the stomach) to acute pain on swallowing (odynophagia). Obstruction to the passage of food (solid and soft) and even liquids may be felt anywhere along the esophagus. Often the patient can indicate if the problem is located in the upper, middle, or lower third of the esophagus.

There are many pathologic conditions of the esophagus, with the order of frequency beginning with achalasia and progressing to diffuse spasm, diverticula, perforation, foreign bodies, chemical burns, hiatal hernias, benign tumors, and carcinoma. A discussion of these conditions is preceded by an overview of nursing process for patients with esophageal disorders.

Nursing Process Overview: Patients With Conditions of the Esophagus

▷ *Assessment*

The nurse elicits a complete health history. If an esophageal disorder is suspected, she asks about the patient's appetite. Has it remained the same, increased, or decreased? Is there any discomfort with swallowing? If so, does it occur only with certain foods? Is it associated with pain? Does a change in position affect the discomfort? The patient is asked to describe the pain experience. Does anything aggravate it? Are there any other symptoms that occur regularly, such as regurgitation, nocturnal regurgitation, eructation (belching), heartburn, substernal pressure, a sensation that food is sticking in throat, a feeling of early satiety, nausea, vomiting, or weight loss? Are the symptoms aggravated by emotional upset? If the patient admits to any of these complaints, the nurse questions those factors that affect them, such as the time of their occurrence; their relationship to eating; factors that relieve or aggravate them, such as position change, belching, antacids, or vomiting. This history also includes questions about the existence of past or present causative factors, such as infections and chemical, mechanical, or physical irritants. A history of alcohol and tobacco use is elicited. The nurse determines if the patient looks emaciated and auscultates the patient's chest to determine if pulmonary complications exist.

▷ *Nursing Diagnoses*

Based on all the assessment data, the nursing diagnoses may include the following:

- Alteration in nutrition, less than body requirements, related to difficulty with swallowing
- Alteration in comfort, pain, related to ingestion of an abrasive agent, a tumor, or frequent episodes of gastric reflux
- Knowledge deficit about the esophageal disorder, diagnostic studies, medical management, surgical intervention, and rehabilitation

▷ *Planning and Implementation*

▷ *Goals:* The major goals for the patient may include attainment of an adequate nutritional intake, relief of pain, and improvement in knowledge level.

Nursing Interventions

Adequate Nutritional Intake. The patient is encouraged to eat slowly and chew his food thoroughly to facilitate its passage to the stomach. Small, frequent feedings of bland food are recommended to promote digestion and prevent tissue irritation. Sometimes liquid swallowed with food will facilitate passage. An atmosphere for eating that will help stimulate the appetite should be provided. The patient should avoid using irritants such as tobacco and alcohol. A baseline weight is obtained and daily weights are recorded. Calories are counted to estimate daily food intake.

Relief of Pain. Small, frequent feedings are recommended because large quantities of food overload the stomach and promote gastric reflux. The nurse suggests that the patient avoid very hot and cold beverages and spicy foods because they stimulate esophageal spasm and increase the secretion of hydrochloric acid. He is advised to avoid any activities that put strain on the thoracic area and increase pain. The patient should remain upright for 1 to 4 hours after each meal to prevent reflux by using gravity to decrease an elevated gastroesophageal pressure gradient. The head of the bed should be placed on 4- to 8-inch (10- to 20-cm) blocks. Eating is discouraged before bedtime.

The patient is advised not to abuse over-the-counter antacids because excessive use can cause rebound acidity. Antacid use should be directed by a physician who can recommend the daily, safe quantity needed to neutralize gastric juices and prevent esophageal irritation. Histamine antagonists (Pepcid, Tagamet, Zantac) are administered as prescribed to decrease gastric acid irritation.

Patient Education. The patient is prepared physically and psychologically for diagnostic tests, treatments, and possible surgical intervention. Reassurance and discussion about the purposes and procedures involved are the principal nursing interventions. Some disorders of the esophagus evolve over time, while others are the result of trauma (*e.g.*, chemical burns or perforation). The emotional and physical preparation for the latter groups is more difficult owing to the shortened time period and the circumstances of the injury. Evaluation of treatment interventions must be ongoing and directed to whether the patient has enough information to participate in care and diagnostic efforts. If surgery is involved, immediate and long-term evaluation is similar to that of a patient having chest surgery.

The goals of rehabilitation will reflect whether surgery or more conservative measures such as diet, positioning, and use of antacids were used in the treatment phase. If the condition is corrected, short-term evaluative measures may be sufficient. If an ongoing condition exists, the nurse must help the patient plan for needed physical and psychological adjustment and for follow-up care. Many elderly patients may be found in the group with ongoing conditions. These patients need support for realistic meal planning, use of medications, and participation in a full life. A multidisciplinary approach is helpful here, including the nutritionist, social worker, and family members.

Home Health Care. Chronic conditions (diffuse spasm, diverticula) require an individualized approach to home management. There may be a need for special food preparation (blenderized foods; bland, soft diets) and increased frequency of eating (four to six small servings per day). The medication schedule is adjusted to the patient's daily activities as much as possible. Analgesics and antacids can be taken as needed every 3 to 4 hours.

Emergency conditions (perforation, chemical burns) usually happen in the home or away from medical help and require emergency management. The patient is treated for shock and respiratory distress and transported as quickly as possible to a medical facility. Specific emergency measures for chemical burns can be found on page 730.

Foreign bodies in the esophagus do not pose an immediate threat to life unless pressure is exerted on the trachea resulting in dyspnea or the cessation of respirations. Educating the public to prevent accidental swallowing of foreign bodies or corrosive agents is a major health issue. (See page 882 for emergency resuscitation measures.)

Postoperative home health care focuses on nutritional support, management of pain, and respiratory function. Some patients are discharged from the hospital with parenteral hyperalimentation or a gastrostomy tube in place as a temporary measure. The patient and his family need specific instruction on the management of equipment and treatments. (See page 776 for caring for a patient receiving hyperalimentation and page 763 for the management of the patient with a gastrostomy. Postoperative nursing management for thoracic and/or abdominal surgery patients can be found on pages 343 and 447. Nursing management for a patient receiving irradiation or chemotherapy is discussed on pages 270 and 272.)

▷ *Evaluation*

▷ *Expected Outcomes*

1. Patient achieves an adequate nutritional intake.
   a. Eats small, frequent meals.
   b. Drinks water with small servings of food.
   c. Stops using irritants (alcohol, tobacco).
   d. Maintains a desired weight.
2. Is free of pain or able to control pain within an acceptable level.
   a. Avoids large meals and irritating foods.
   b. Takes antacids as prescribed.
   c. Maintains the upright position after meals for 1 to 4 hours.
   d. States that he has less eructation and chest pain.
3. Increases knowledge level of esophageal condition, treatment, and prognosis.
   a. Understands cause of condition.
   b. Expresses rationale for medical or surgical management and diet/medication regimen.
   c. Describes treatment program.
   d. Practices preventive measures so accidental injuries are avoided.

Achalasia

Achalasia is the term used to designate functional esophageal obstruction caused by neuromuscular changes that prevent relaxation of the inferior esophageal sphincter. Nerve degeneration, esophageal dilatation, and hypertrophy are parts of the clinical picture. Achalasia is usually associated with a lack of peristaltic activity in the esophagus itself and with a failure of the esophageal sphincter to relax in response to swallowing. Narrowing of the esophagus just above the stomach results in a gradually increasing dilatation of the esophagus in the upper chest.

Clinical Manifestations. The primary symptom of achalasia is that of difficulty in swallowing both liquids and solids. The patient has a sensation of food sticking in the lower portion of the esophagus. As the condition progresses, regurgitation of the food is common; this may occur spontaneously or may be brought about by the patient to relieve the discomfort that is produced by the prolonged distention of the esophagus by food that will not pass into the stomach. There may be secondary pulmonary complications due to spillover of esophageal contents (aspiration pneumonia).

Diagnostic Evaluation. Radiologic studies show esophageal dilatation above the narrowing at the cardioesophageal junction. The diagnosis is confirmed by manometry, which shows the absence of primary peristalsis. Esophagoscopy and cineradiography (motion images produced during fluoroscopy) help confirm the diagnosis.

Management. Two methods of management are recommended to treat the obstruction: forceful dilation (Fig. 30-7) and surgical separation of the muscle fibers (Fig. 30-8). Calcium channel blockers have been used to decrease esophageal pressure and improve swallowing.

The conservative approach to treating early achalasia involves stretching the narrowed area of the esophagus. This is done by passing a tube orally into the esophagus. A distensible bag (Mosher pneumatic) at the end of the tube is positioned and inflated. Vigorous dilatation has a 75% success rate and only a 3% incidence of perforation. The procedure can be painful; therefore, an analgesic or tranquilizer is administered before the treatment.

A cardiomyotomy is the preferred surgical approach. A longitudinal incision about 12 cm in length is made through the muscularis of the esophagus extending about 1 cm into the gastric area. All muscle fibers are separated to relieve the lower esophageal stricture. Esophagoscopy is recommended

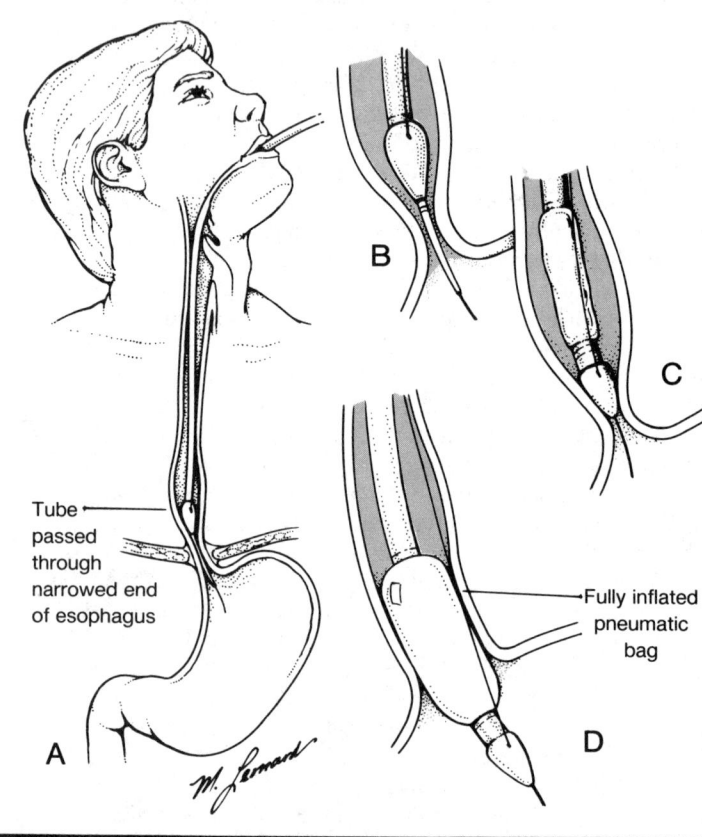

Figure 30-7
Treatment of achalasia: conservative approach. (*A*, *B*, *C*) The dilator is passed, guided by a previously swallowed thread, into the upper stomach. (*D*) When the balloon is in proper position, it is distended by pressure sufficient to dilate the narrowed area of the esophagus.

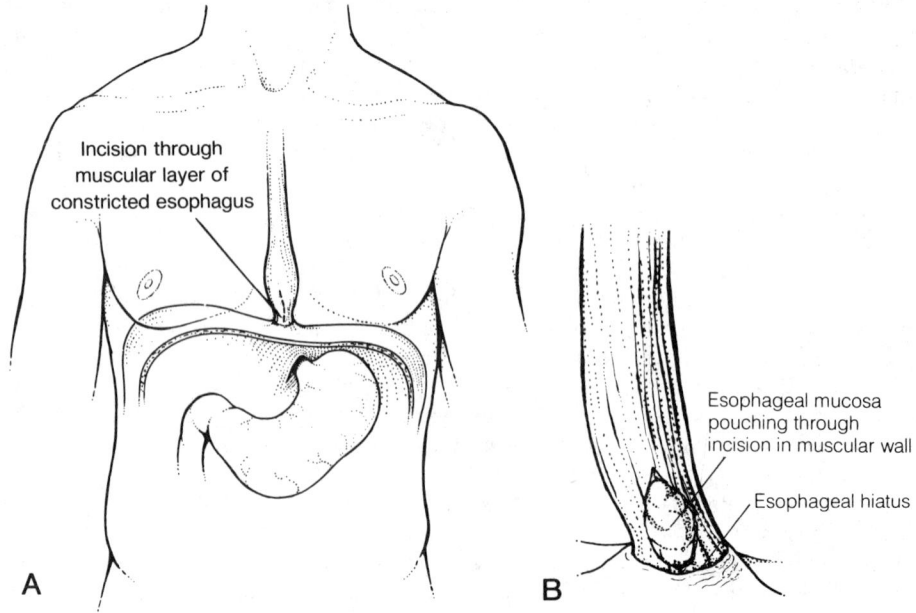

Figure 30-8
Treatment of achalasia: major surgical approach. (*A*) The esophagus is approached from the front, on the left side. An incision is made through the muscularis of the esophagus. (*B*) The incision is of sufficient size to allow a pouching of the esophageal mucosa. Separation of the muscular fibers relieves the narrowing at the lower end of the esophagus and permits the patient to swallow normally again.

every 3 to 5 years because esophageal carcinoma is associated with achalasia.

Diffuse Spasm

Diffuse spasm is a motor disorder of the esophagus characterized by dysphagia, odynophagia (painful swallowing), and chest pain similar to that of coronary artery spasm. Manometry indicates simultaneous contractions occurring irregularly. Radiographic studies show separated areas of spasm.

Conservative therapy includes administering sedatives and long-acting nitrates to relieve pain. Small, frequent feedings and a soft diet are usually recommended to decrease the esophageal pressure and irritation that leads to spasm. Pneumatic dilatation and esophageal myotomy may be necessary if pain becomes intolerable.

Diverticulum

A diverticulum is an outpouching of mucosa and submucosa that protrudes through a weak portion of the musculature (*pulsion* type). If there is a pulling outward of the esophageal wall from inflamed or scarred peribronchial lymph nodes, the term *traction diverticulum* is used (Fig. 30-9).

Pharyngoesophageal Diverticulum. The most common type of diverticulum, which is found three times more frequently in men than in women, is pharyngoesophageal pulsion diverticulum (Zenker's diverticulum), which occurs posteriorly through the cricopharyngeal muscle in the midline of the neck. It is usually seen in people over 60 years of age. The patient first notices difficulty in swallowing and a fullness

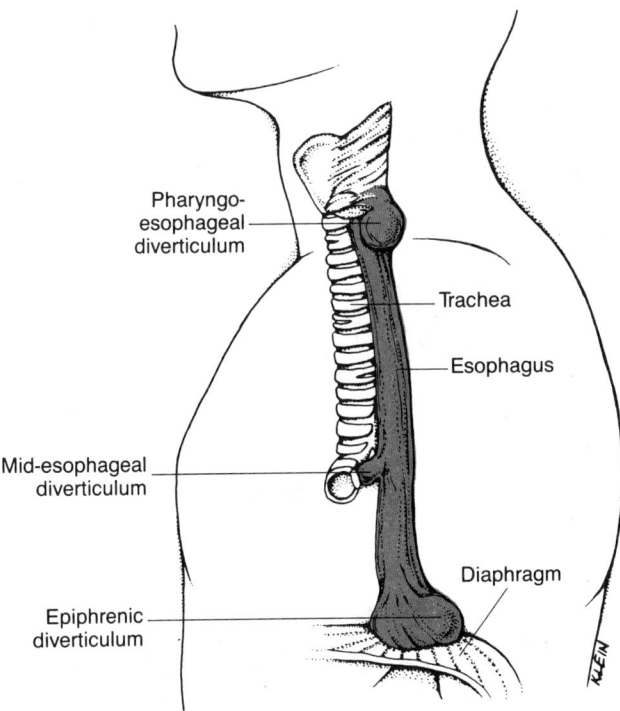

Figure 30-9
Possible sites for the occurrence of esophageal diverticula. The site will determine the location of the surgical incision to correct the problem.

in the neck. He may complain of belching, regurgitation of undigested food, and gurgling noises after eating. The diverticulum, or pouch, becomes filled with food or liquid. When the patient assumes a recumbent position, undigested food is regurgitated and may also cause coughing, owing to irritation of the trachea. Halitosis and a sour taste in the mouth are also common, because of the decomposition of food retained in the diverticulum.

Diagnostic Evaluation and Management. To determine the exact nature and location of a diverticulum, barium is ingested and x-ray films are taken. Esophagoscopy usually is contraindicated because of the danger of perforating the diverticulum, with resulting mediastinitis. The blind passing of a nasal tube should be avoided. The tube should be guided into the stomach under direct vision of a lighted scope. Because this patient is often a victim of unbalanced diet and fluid levels, an evaluation of his nutritional state is done to determine dietary needs.

Since the condition is progressive, the only means of cure is surgical removal of the diverticulum. Care is taken, surgically, to avoid undue trauma to the common carotid artery and internal jugular veins. The sac is dissected free and amputated flush with the esophageal wall. In addition to a diverticulectomy, a myotomy of the cricopharyngeal muscle is often done, in order to relieve spasticity of the musculature, which otherwise seems to contribute to a continuation of the previous symptoms.

Nursing Interventions. When a patient has difficulty in swallowing, the diet is limited to foods that pass more easily. Blenderized meals supplemented with vitamins are usually prescribed. The nurse arranges for the nutritionist to see the patient and his family to discuss plans for continuing this treatment at home.

Midesophageal and Epiphrenic Diverticula. The occurrence of diverticula in the midtubular esophagus is less common; symptoms are less acute, and usually the condition does not require surgery.

Traction diverticula are usually asymptomatic. They are found in the midesophageal area and occur when inflamed lymph nodes near the tracheal bifurcation create a tension sac by adhering to the esophagus as the tissue heals and contracts. No specific treatment is usually necessary.

Epiphrenic diverticula are usually larger pulsion diverticula occurring in the lower esophagus just above the diaphragm, and occasionally higher. They are thought to be related to the improper functioning of the lower esophageal sphincter.

Management. Surgery is indicated only if the symptoms are troublesome and growing progressively worse. A transthoracic (thoracotomy) approach is used, which means that preoperative and postoperative nursing management is similar to that for chest surgical patients (see p. 446).

Nursing Interventions. After surgery the patient is fed through a nasogastric tube that usually is inserted at the time of operation. The feedings may include any liquid, but a careful record of their kind, amount, and character must be kept. After each feeding, the tube is irrigated carefully with water. The wound also must be observed for evidence of leakage from the esophagus and a developing fistula.

If the operative risk is prohibitive, nursing management is similar to that advocated for the patient with a peptic ulcer: antacids, anticholinergics, and abstinence from coffee, alcohol, and smoking (see p. 780). In addition, reflux is avoided by (1) keeping the head elevated; (2) remaining upright for 2 hours in the postprandial period; (3) avoiding abdominal compression from garments and posture; (4) eating small meals; and (5) reducing, if overweight.

Perforation

The esophagus is not an uncommon site of injury. Perforation may result from stab or bullet wounds of the neck or chest, as well as from accidental puncture by a surgical instrument during examination or dilatation. Spontaneous perforation of the esophagus has been known to occur during vomiting.

The patient experiences spontaneous pain followed by dysphagia. Infection, fever, leukocytosis, and severe hypotension may be noted. Hyperpnea and cervical tenderness are early signs of injury and crepitation. In some instances, signs of pneumothorax are observed. Radiographic examination and fluoroscopy can localize the injury.

Management. Because of the high risk of infection, broad-spectrum antibiotic therapy is initiated. A nasogastric tube is passed, to provide suction and to reduce the amount of gastric juice that can reflux into the esophagus and mediastinum. Nothing is given by mouth, but nutritional needs are met by intravenous hyperalimentation. Surgery is performed to close the wound, and postoperative nutritional support then becomes a primary concern. Parenteral hyperalimentation is preferred to gastrostomy since the latter might cause reflux into the esophagus. Depending on the incisional site and nature of surgery, the postoperative nursing management will be similar to that for patients who have had thoracic or abdominal surgery.

Foreign Bodies

Swallowed foreign bodies (dentures, fishbones, pins) may injure the esophagus as well as obstruct its lumen. Pain and dysphagia may be present; dyspnea may occur as a result of pressure. Radiographic findings are useful in identifying the foreign body.

Usually, foreign bodies can be removed with the aid of the esophagoscope. When the foreign body is made of metal (bobby pins, safety pins, needles, jacks, nails, and tacks), it may not be safe to allow the object to make its way slowly through the stomach and intestinal tract. A bar magnet, fastened to a cable, may be maneuvered into place with the aid of fluoroscopy and the object withdrawn. A Foley catheter can be manipulated past the object, the balloon inflated, and the catheter and the foreign body removed. It is possible for a skilled esophagoscopist to remove open safety pins through the esophagoscope.

If an impacted bolus of meat is lodged in the esophagus, it can usually be dissolved with proteolytic enzymes. The injuries to the esophagus are the more serious part of the problem, because they may lead to deep cervical or mediastinal abscess or to stricture formation. Drainage of such abscesses requires thoracic surgery.

Chemical Burns

The patient who accidentally or intentionally swallows a strong acid or base (such as lye) is emotionally distraught as well as in acute physical pain. An acute chemical burn of the esophagus is accompanied by severe burns of the lips, mouth, and pharynx, with pain on swallowing and, sometimes, difficulty in respiration, due either to edema of the throat or to a collection of mucus in the pharynx. The patient may be profoundly toxic, febrile, and in shock. Emergency treatment consists of having the patient drink water for the purpose of dilution. Dilution is not carried out if the patient has acute airway obstruction or swelling or if there is evidence of esophageal, gastric, or intestinal perforation. The patient is treated immediately for shock, pain, and respiratory distress.

Management. Esophagoscopy is performed as soon as possible to determine the extent and severity of damage. If the patient is able to swallow, fluids are given in small quantities. Secretions are aspirated from the pharynx if respiration is affected. The necessity for high fluid intake may require administration by parenteral means.

Corticosteroid therapy is also administered to suppress inflammation and to minimize subsequent scar and stricture formation. Antibiotics are given to combat infection and to prevent mediastinitis. A nasogastric tube is passed for feeding purposes and to ensure patency of the esophageal lumen.

About a week after chemical ingestion, passage of a dilating bougie (cylindrical instrument) may be done daily, beginning with a No. 28 F. When the lumen is "stable," bougienage (use of bougie) can be terminated.

Occasionally a patient is admitted after the acute phase has subsided but multiple stricture levels have formed in the esophagus. These may be dilated by peroral use of bougies; if this is not successful, it may be necessary to try the retrograde bougienage method. A gastrostomy opening is made, and a braided silk string is swallowed. One end is brought out through the gastrostomy opening and the other end through the nose. The two ends are tied together and form a complete loop. Dilatation is obtained by pulling larger and larger bougies upward through the esophagus by means of the string. It is important that this string be left in place at all times. The gastrostomy is kept open by means of a gastrostomy tube, through which feedings may be given if necessary.

Hiatal Hernia

The esophagus enters the abdomen through an opening in the diaphragm, to empty, at its lower end, into the upper part of the stomach. The opening in the diaphragm normally encircles the esophagus tightly; therefore, the stomach lies completely within the abdomen. In a condition known as *hiatus* (or *hiatal*) *hernia*, the opening in the diaphragm through which the esophagus passes becomes enlarged and part of the upper stomach tends to come up into the lower portion of the thorax. There are two types of hernias, sliding hernias and paraesophageal hernias.

Sliding Hiatal Hernia. Sliding hiatal hernias occur when the upper stomach and the cardioesophageal junction are displaced upward and slide in and out of the thorax. About 90% of patients with esophageal hiatal hernias have sliding hernias. Diagnosis is confirmed by radiographic studies and fluoroscopy (see Fig. 30-10*A*).

Clinical Manifestations and Management. The patient may experience heartburn, regurgitation, and dysphagia. At least 50% of the patients are asymptomatic. Medical management includes frequent, small feedings that can pass easily

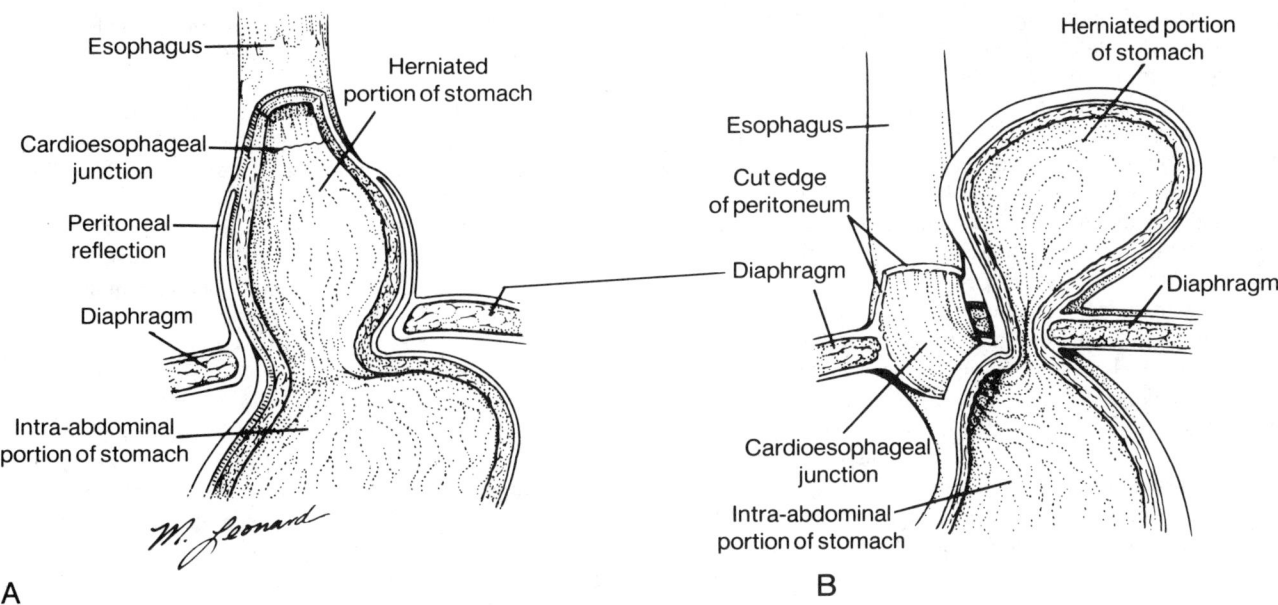

Figure 30-10
Sliding esophageal and paraesophageal hernias. (*A*) Sliding esophageal hernia. Upper stomach and cardioesophageal junction are moved upward and slide in and out of the thorax. (*B*) Paraesophageal hernia. All or part of the stomach pushes through the diaphragm next to the gastroesophageal junction.

through the esophagus. The patient is advised not to recline for 1 hour after eating to prevent reflux or movement of the hernia. The patient's bed should be elevated at the head on 10- to 20-cm (4- to 8-inch) blocks to prevent movement of the hernia by gravity. Surgery is indicated in about 15% of patients.

    Paraesophageal Hernia. Paraesophageal hernias occur when all or part of the stomach pushes through the diaphragm next to the gastroesophageal junction. Fewer than 10% of patients experience paraesophageal herniation and many are asymptomatic. Reflux does not usually occur because the gastroesophageal sphincter is intact (Fig. 30-10*B*).

    Clinical Manifestations and Management. The patient usually experiences a sense of fullness after eating. The complications of hemorrhage, obstruction, and strangulation can occur, so an anterior gastropexy (fixation of prolapsed stomach in its normal position by suturing to the abdominal wall) is the treatment of choice.

Esophageal Varices

Varices of the lower esophagus are really a secondary manifestation of cirrhosis of the liver. This subject is discussed on page 882.

Benign Tumors

Benign tumors may arise anywhere along the esophagus. The most common lesion is a leiomyoma, which can occlude the lumen of the esophagus. Most benign tumors are asymptomatic and are distinguished from cancerous growths by a biopsy. Small lesions are excised during esophagoscopy; thorocotomy may be necessary for intramural lesions.

Cancer of the Esophagus

Carcinoma of the esophagus occurs three times more frequently in men than in women in the United States and usually occurs during the fifth decade of life. There is a 1% incidence in the population.

    Pathophysiology and Clinical Manifestations. Unfortunately, the patient may have an advanced ulcerated lesion of the esophagus before symptoms present. Malignancy, usually of the squamous cell epidermoid type, may spread beneath the esophageal mucosa, or it may spread directly into, through, and beyond the muscle layers into the lymphatics. In the latter stages, obstruction of the esophagus is noted, with possible perforation into the mediastinum and erosion into the great vessels.

    Unfortunately, when symptoms exist that are related to esophageal cancer, the disease is generally advanced. Symptoms include dysphagia, initially with solid foods and eventually with liquids; a feeling of a lump in the throat; painful swallowing; substernal pain or fullness; and, later, regurgitation of undigested food with foul breath and hiccoughs. The patient is first aware of intermittent and increasing difficulty in swallowing. At first only solid food gives trouble, but as the growth progresses and the obstruction becomes more complete, even liquids cannot pass into the stomach. Regurgitation of food and saliva occurs, hemorrhage may take place, and there is a progressive loss of weight and strength owing to starvation. Later symptoms include substernal pain, hiccough, respiratory difficulty, and foul breath. *The delay between onset of early symptoms and the time when the patient seeks medical advice is often 12 to 18 months.* The nurse insists that anyone with swallowing difficulties be encouraged to see a physician immediately.

Diagnostic Evaluation. Diagnosis is confirmed in 95% of the cases by esophagoscopy with biopsy. Bronchoscopy usually is performed, especially in tumors of the middle and the upper third of the esophagus, to determine whether the trachea has been involved by the tumor and to help in determining whether the lesion can be removed. Mediastinoscopy is used to determine involvement of nodes and other mediastinal structures. Cancer of the lower end of the esophagus may be due to adenocarcinoma of the stomach extending upward into the esophagus.

Management. Treatment includes surgery, radiation, and chemotherapy. The patient may be treated by surgical excision of the lesion, radiation therapy, or a combination of both modalities. Usually, surgery is preferred for lower esophageal tumors, whereas irradiation is favored for upper esophageal lesions. With irradiation, the lesion may shrink, thereby expanding the lumen and permitting the patient to swallow. Relatively few patients are cured; hence palliative therapy may be required, including combinations of treatment such as gastrostomy, jejunostomy, cervical esophagostomy, dilatation of the stricture, insertion of the intraluminal prosthetic tube, and chemotherapy.

The surgical approach may be through the thorax, or through the abdomen and thorax, depending on the location of the tumor. A common approach for lesions of the lower esophagus is to remove the involved portion of the esophagus and re-form the continuity of the gastrointestinal tract by bringing the stomach into the chest and implanting the proximal end of the esophagus into it (esophagogastrostomy). The chest is closed after a drain is inserted into the pleural cavity and connected to closed suction.

Lesions in the middle and upper thirds of the esophagus, particularly, are often not suitable for surgical excision and, fortunately, occur less frequently. However, some success has been reported with a method in which a tunnel is created beneath the sternum and a resected segment of either jejunum or colon replaces the diseased esophagus. A palliative procedure in which a plastic tube is introduced through a cervical incision has been done with resultant symptomatic relief, improvement in nutrition, and amelioration of psychological symptoms.

Radiation therapy is used before surgery in some clinics; in others, it is used after surgery. The ideal method of treating this problem has not yet been found; each patient is approached in a way that appears best for him. If the growth is found to be inoperable, either before or at operation, a gastrostomy is performed as a palliative procedure to permit the administration of food and fluids (see p. 763).

Prognosis. If the malignancy is detected early, removal is simplified and the continuity of the digestive system is easily maintained. However, the mortality rate among patients with cancer of the esophagus is high, owing to three factors: (1) Usually, the patient is an older person, in whom the incidence of pulmonary and cardiovascular disorders is high. (2) Before significant symptoms occur, the tumor has already invaded surrounding structures. It is impossible to excise a liberal area of tissue because of the proximity of vital structures. (3) The malignancy tends to spread to nearby lymph nodes, and the unique relation of the esophagus to the heart and lungs makes these organs easily accessible to the extension of the tumor. In several series of operative cases, 45% to 80% showed evidence of metastasis when examined in the operating room.

Nursing Interventions. Intervention is directed toward improving the patient's nutritional and physical condition in preparation for surgery or radiation therapy. A weight-gaining program based on a high-caloric and high-protein diet, in liquid or soft form, is advocated, if it can be managed by mouth. If not, then intravenous or parenteral hyperalimentation is initiated.

The patient is educated about the nature of the postoperative equipment that will be used, including that required for closed chest drainage, nasogastric suction, parenteral fluid therapy, and perhaps gastric intubation. Immediate postoperative care is similar to that provided for patients undergoing thoracic surgery (see p. 450). Following emergence from anesthesia, the patient is placed in semi-Fowler's position, and later Fowler's position, to assist in preventing reflux of gastric secretions. He is observed carefully for regurgitation and dyspnea. A common postoperative complication is aspiration pneumonia. Temperature is monitored to detect any elevation that may indicate seepage of fluid through the operative site into the mediastinum.

If a prosthetic tube has been inserted or an anastomosis has been done, the patient will have a functioning continuum between the throat and the stomach. He will need encouragement and patience as he begins to swallow small sips of water and, later, pureed small feedings. When he is able to increase food intake to a significant amount, intravenous and parenteral findings are discontinued. If a prosthetic tube (such as a pliable latex tube held open with fine wire coils) is used, it may easily become obstructed if food is not chewed sufficiently. After each meal, he is to remain upright for at least 2 hours to assist in movement of food. The nurse is challenged to encourage this patient to eat, since his appetite is usually poor. Family involvement and home-cooked favorite foods may help the patient to eat. If he complains of gastric distress, antacids may help. When irradiation is part of the therapy, the patient's appetite is further depressed.

Often, in either the preoperative or postoperative period, an obstructed or nearly obstructed esophagus causes difficulty with excess saliva, so that drooling becomes a problem. This is also of concern in an esophagostomy. In this situation, the use of small plastic bags fastened to the stoma are helpful in collecting secretions, or a wick-type piece of gauze may be placed at the corner of the mouth to direct secretions to a dressing or emesis basin. Of more concern is the possibility of aspiration of saliva into the tracheobronchial tree, with the danger of pneumonia.

When the patient is ready to go home, the family is instructed in how to give nutritional care, what to observe, how to handle signs of complications, how to keep the patient comfortable, and how to obtain needed physical and emotional support.

Bibliography

Books

Ballenger JJ. Diseases of the Nose, Throat, Ear, Head and Neck. Philadelphia, Lea & Febiger, 1985.

Bates B. A Guide to Physical Examination and History Taking, 4th ed. Philadelphia, JB Lippincott Company, 1987.

Donovan M and Girton S. Cancer Care Nursing. Norwalk, Connecticut, Appleton-Century-Crofts, 1984.

Dychtwald K (ed). Wellness and Health Promotion for the Elderly. Rockville, Maryland, Aspen, 1986.

Frable WJ. Thin Needle Aspiration Biopsy. Philadelphia, WB Saunders, 1983.

Haskell CM (ed). Cancer Treatment. Philadelphia, WB Saunders, 1985.

Laskin DM. Oral and Maxillofacial Surgery. St Louis, CV Mosby, 1985.

Million RR and Cassisi NJ (ed). Management of Head and Neck Cancer, a Multidisciplinary Approach. Philadelphia, JB Lippincott, 1984.

Pilch YH. Surgical Oncology. New York, McGraw-Hill, 1984.

Regato JA, Spjut HJ, and Cox JD. Cancer: Diagnosis, Treatment and Prognosis. St Louis, CV Mosby, 1985.

Robbins SL, Cotran RS, and Kumar V. Pathologic Basis of Disease. Philadelphia, WB Saunders, 1984.

Sabiston DC (ed). Textbook of Surgery: The Biological Basis of Modern Surgical Practice. Philadelphia, WB Saunders, 1986.

Smith LH and Thier SO. Pathophysiology, The Biological Principles of Disease. Philadelphia, WB Saunders, 1985.

Way LW. Current Surgical Diagnosis and Treatment. Los Altos, California, Lange Medical, 1985.

Wilkins R and Levin KN (ed). Medicine: Essentials of Clinical Practice. Boston, Little, and Brown & Co, 1983.

Articles

Conditions and Cancer of the Oral Cavity

Alberico J. Breaking the chronic pain cycle. Am J Nurs 1984 Oct; 84(10): 1222–1225.

Anders J and Leach E. Sun versus skin. Am J Nurs 1983 July; 83(7): 1015–1020.

Anonsen C et al. Carcinosarcoma of the floor of the mouth. J Otolaryngol 1985 Aug; 14(4):215–220.

Arnet GF et al. Dentofacial reconstruction. Am J Nurs 1984 Dec; 84(12): 506–507.,

Ash CR. Cancer care for the elderly. Cancer Nurs 1986 Oct; 9(5):229.

Baranovsky A and Myers MH. Cancer incidence and survival in patients 65 years of age and older. CA 1986 Jan/Feb; 36(1):26–41.

Benoliel BDS et al. Dental treatment for the patient on anticoagulant therapy: Prothrombin time value—what difference does it make? Oral Surg 1986 Aug; 62(2):149–151.

Berktold RE. Carcinoma of the oral cavity: Selective management according to site and stage. Otolaryngol Clin North Am 1985 Aug; 18(3):445–450.

Bersani G and Williams C. Oral care for cancer patients. Am J Nurs 1983 Apr; 83(4):533–536.

Bogdasarian RS. Halitosis. Otolaryngol Clin North Am 1986 Feb; 19(1): 111–117.

Brady L. The changing role of radiation oncology in cancer management. CA 1983 Mar/Apr; 33(2):66–73.

Brugere J et al. Differential effects of tobacco and alcohol in cancer of the larynx, pharynx and mouth. Cancer 1986 Jan 15; 57(2):391–395.

Callery CD, Spiro RH, and Strong EW. Changing trends in the management of squamous carcinoma of the tongue. Am J Surg 1984 Oct; 148(10): 449–454.

Cohen MB, Ljung ME, and Boles R. Salivary gland tumors. Arch Otolaryngol Head Neck Surg 1986 Aug; 112(8):867–869.

Eversole LR et al. Oral Kaposi's sarcoma associated with acquired immunodeficiency syndrome among homosexual males. J Am Dent Assoc 1983 Aug; 107(2):248–253.

Fitzpatrick PJ. Cancer of the lip. Otolaryngology 1984 Jan; 13(1):32–36.

Gift HC and Frew RA. Sealants: Changing patterns. J Am Dent Assoc 1986 Mar; 112(3):391–392.

Glaser J. Geriatric dentistry: Its specialty and its literature. Med Ref Serv Q 1985/86 Winter; 4(4):29–46.

Gluckman JL and Barrord J. Nonsquamous cell tumors of the minor salivary glands. Otolaryngol Clin North Am 1986 Aug; 19(3):497–505.

Hauk L. Enabling clients to manage dentures. Geriatr Nurs 1986 Sept/Oct; 7(5):254–255.

Kahn R. Renewing the commitment to oral hygiene. Geriatr Nurs 1986 Sept/Oct; 7(5):244–247.

Khanna NN et al. Intensive combination chemotherapy for cancer of the oral cavity. Cancer 1983 Sept 1; 52:790–793.

La Camera DJ, Masur H, and Henderson DK. The acquired immunodeficiency syndrome. Nurs Clin North Am 1985 Mar; 20(1):241–254.

Levin LS and Johns ME. Lesions of the oral mucous membranes. Otolaryngol Clin North Am 1986 Feb; 19(1):87–102.

Longman AJ and Dewalt EM. A guide for oral assessment. Geriatr Nurs 1986 Sept/Oct; 7(5):252–253.

Luce EA. Carcinoma of the lower lip. Surg Clin North Am 1986 Feb; 66(1):3–11.

Markman M. Newer techniques in cancer chemotherapy. DM 1984 July; 30(10):6–45.

McQuaire DG. Cancer of the tongue: Selecting appropriate therapy. Curr Probl Surg 1986 Aug; 23(8):565–639.

Mettlin C. Dietary factors for cancer of specific sites. Surg Clin North Am 1986 Oct; 66(5):917–929.

Moore C, Flynn M, and Greenbery RA. Evaluation of size in prognosis of oral cancer. Cancer 1986 July 1; 58(1):158–162.

Morris CA. Self-concept as altered by the diagnosis of cancer. Nurs Clin North Am 1985 Dec; 20(4):611–630.

Ofstehage JC and Magilvy K. Oral health and aging. Geriatr Nurs 1986 Sept/Oct; 7(5):238–241.

Poulson TC, Lindermuth JE, and Greer RO. A comparison of the use of smokeless tobacco in rural and urban teenagers. CA 1984 Sept/Oct; 34(5):248–261.

Rabinov K, Kell T, and Gordon P. CT of the salivary glands. Radiol Clin North Am 1984 Mar; 22(1):145–159.

Ryan RJ. The accuracy of clinical parameters in detecting periodontal disease activity. J Am Dent Assoc 1985 Nov; 111(11):753–760.

Saunders JR Jr, Hirata R, and Jaques DA. Salivary glands. Surg Clin North Am 1986 Feb; 66(1):59–81.

Schuller DE et al. Preoperative reductive chemotherapy for locally advanced carcinoma of the oral cavity, oropharynx, and hypopharynx. Cancer 1983 Jan 1; 51(1):15–19.

Shack RB. Carcinoma of the tongue and tonsil (oropharynx). Surg Clin North Am 1986 Feb; 66(1):83–95.

Shaha AR et al. Squamous carcinoma of the floor of the mouth. Am J Surg 1984 Oct; 148(10):455–459.

Silverberg E and Lubera J. Cancer statistics, 1986. CA 1986 Jan/Feb; 36(1):9–25.

Silverman S, Gorsky M, and Lozada F. Oral leukoplakia and malignant transformation. Cancer 1984 Feb 1; 53(2):563–568.

Spiro RH. Squamous cancer of the tongue. CA 1985 July/Aug; 35(4): 252–256.

Squier CA. Smokeless tobacco and oral cancer: A cause for concern? CA 1984 Sept/Oct; 34(5):242–247.

Radical Neck Dissection and Conditions of the Esophagus

Ariyan S. Radical neck dissection. Surg Clin North Am 1986 Feb; 66(1): 133–147.

Bartelink H et al. The value of postoperative radiotherapy as an adjuvant to radical neck dissection. Cancer 1983 Sept 15; 52(6):1008–1013.

Cohn DJ et al. Surgery for reflux esophagitis: Experience with the antireflux prosthesis. AORN J 1986 Apr; 43(4):858–864.

Collin CF and Spiro RH. Carcinoma of the cervical esophagus: Changing therapeutic trends. Am J Surg 1984 Oct; 148(4):460–461.

Crozier RE et al. Esophageal spasm: A possible cause of atypical chest pain. Postgrad Med 1986 Nov; 80(6):73–78.

Dilawari JB et al. Corrosive acid ingestion in man: A clinical and endoscopic study. Gut 1984 Feb; 25(2):183–187.

Goldman LP and Weigert JM. Corrosive substance ingestion: A review. Am J Gastroenteral 1984 Feb; 79(2):85–89.

Henderson RD. Diffuse esophageal spasm. Surg Clin North Am 1983 Aug; 63(4):951–962.

Herang BS, Payne WS, and Cameron AJ. Surgical management for recurrent pharyngoesophageal (Zenker's) diverticulum. Ann Thorac Surg 1984 Mar; 37(3):189–191.

Jamieson WRE. Surgical management of primary motor disorders of the esophagus. Am J Surg 1984 July; 148(1):36–38.

Kelson DP. Esophageal carcinoma: How to spot it; what can be done about it. Consultant 1983 Nov; 23(11):247–256.

McCallum RW. Diagnosing motility disorders of the upper gastrointestinal tract. South Med J 1984 Aug; 77(8):947–955.

Pai GP et al. Two decades of experience with modified Heller's myotomy for achalasia. Ann Thorac Surg 1984 Sept; 38(3):201–206.

Payne WS and Knig RM. Treatment of achalasia of the esophagus. Surg Clin North Am 1983 Aug; 63(4):963–970.

Rapka ME. Corrosive esophagitis and stricture. Nursing '83 1983 Dec; 13(12):24x.

Reede DL, Whelan MA, and Bergeron RT. CT of the soft tissue structures of the neck. Radiol Clin North Am 1984 Mar; 22(1):239–250.

Richter JE and Castell DO. Diffuse esophageal spasm: A reappraisal. Ann Intern Med 1984 Feb; 100(2):242–245.

Robinson MG. Management of reflux esophageal disease. Am J Med 1984 Nov; 77(5B):106–110.

Skinner DB. Myotomy and achalasia. Ann Thorac Surg 1984 Mar; 37(3): 183–184.

Agencies

American Association of Public Health Dentists, New York University Dental Center, 421 First Avenue, New York, New York 10010.

American Dental Association, 211 E. Chicago Avenue, Chicago, Illinois 60611.

American Society of Geriatric Dentistry, 1121 West Michigan Street, Indianapolis, Indiana 46202.

American Cancer Society, 90 Park Avenue, New York, New York 10016.

Chapter 31

Assessment of Digestive and Gastrointestinal Function

Physiological Overview

Anatomy of the Gastrointestinal Tract

The gastrointestinal tract is a tube that is continuous with the external environment at both ends. The pathway extends from the mouth through the esophagus, stomach, and intestines to the anus. The esophagus is located in the mediastinum in the thoracic cavity, anterior to the spine and posterior to the trachea and heart. It is a collapsible tube about 25 cm (10 inches) in length that becomes distended when food passes through it.

The stomach is situated in the upper portion of the abdomen to the left of the midline, just under the left diaphragm. It is a distensible pouch with a capacity of approximately 1500 ml. The inlet to the stomach is called the esophagogastric junction. It is surrounded by a ring of smooth muscle, called the lower esophageal sphincter, which, on contraction, closes the stomach off from the esophagus. The outlet from the stomach is called the pylorus. Circular smooth muscle in the wall of the pylorus forms the pyloric sphincter and controls the size of the opening between the stomach and small intestine.

The small intestine is the longest segment of the gastrointestinal tract and accounts for about two thirds of the total length. It is folded back and forth on itself and occupies a major portion of the abdominal cavity. It is divided into three parts: an upper part, called the *duodenum;* the middle part, called the *jejunum;* and the lower part, called the *ileum.* The common bile duct, the conduit for both bile and pancreatic secretions, empties into the duodenum.

The junction between the small and large intestines usually lies in the right lower portion of the abdomen. It is in this area that the vermiform appendix is located. At the junction of the small and large intestines is the ileocecal valve, which functions in a similar fashion to the pyloric and esophageal sphincters. The large intestine consists of an ascending segment on the right side of the abdomen, a transverse segment that extends from right to left in the upper abdomen, and a descending segment on the left side of the abdomen. The terminal portion of the large intestine is the rectum, which is continuous with the anus. The anal outlet is surrounded by the external anal sphincter, which, unlike the other sphincters of the gastrointestinal tract, is composed of striated muscle and is under voluntary control.

Blood Supply to the Gastrointestinal Tract.   Since the gastrointestinal tract is so long, its blood supply is from arteries that originate along the entire length of the thoracic and abdominal aorta. Of particular importance are the vessels to the large and small intestines: the superior and inferior mesenteric arteries. These two arteries form small loops, or arcades, which encircle the intestine, supplying its wall with oxygen and nutrients. Blood in the veins that drain the intestine is enriched by nutrients absorbed from the lumen of the gastrointestinal tract. These veins merge with others in the abdomen to form a large vessel called the portal vein, which carries the nutrient-rich blood to the liver. The blood flow to the entire gastrointestinal tract is about 20% of the total cardiac output, and it is significantly increased after eating.

Innervation.   The gastrointestinal tract is innervated by both the sympathetic and parasympathetic parts of the autonomic nervous system. The parasympathetic fibers travel in the vagus nerve and in nerves that arise from the sacral segment of the spinal cord. In addition, the upper esophagus and the external anal sphincter are under voluntary control and are supplied by somatic nerves that arise from the cervical spinal cord and the sacral spinal cord, respectively.

The Digestive Process

In order to perform their functions, all cells of the body require nutrients, which must be derived from the intake of food that contains protein, fat, carbohydrates, vitamins, and minerals, as well as cellulose fibers and other vegetable matter without nutritional value. This diet provides the energy needs of the body and maintains body weight at approximately constant levels.

The intake of food is a voluntary act that is controlled by conscious sensations of hunger and satiety, modified by learned behavior. These sensations originate in the higher centers of the brain, probably in the hypothalamus. The hypothalamus itself is influenced by visual and olfactory sensations, nervous and hormonal signals originating in the digestive tract, and behavioral patterns.

The primary functions of the gastrointestinal tract are as follows:

- To break down food particles into their small constituent molecules for digestion
- To absorb the small molecules produced by digestion into the bloodstream
- To eliminate undigested and unabsorbed foodstuffs and other waste products from the body

The pathway that foodstuffs take in the digestive tract begins at the mouth, where they are chewed and swallowed. The bolus of food is then conveyed down through the esophagus into the stomach, where it remains for a variable length of time. It then enters the small intestine, where much of the digestion and absorption of nutrients takes place. The unabsorbed food passes from the small intestine into the colon (also called the large intestine) for further modification and storage prior to elimination (defecation). A schematic diagram of the structures of the gastrointestinal tract is shown in Figure 31-1. The total length of the gastrointestinal pathway, from mouth to anus, is approximately 7 to 8 meters (23–26 feet).

Large volumes of fluid containing hormones and enzymes are secreted into the gastrointestinal tract in order to aid in the process of digestion, absorption, and elimination. The total secretion into the lumen of the gastrointestinal tract is about 8 liters per day, but less than 200 ml per day of liquid is excreted in the feces. This illustrates the massive absorptive capacity of the gastrointestinal tract.

- Derangements of the absorption function of the digestive system can lead to serious alterations of body fluids.

Gastrointestinal Motility and Secretions

Motility refers to the coordinated contractions of the muscles in the walls of the gastrointestinal tract that propel food and secretions from the mouth toward the anus. These sequential rhythmic contractions are referred to as *peristalsis*. At the same time that the food is being propelled through the gastrointestinal tract, it comes into contact with a wide variety of secretions that aid in breaking down and digesting the food particles (Fig. 31-2).

Oral Digestion.   The process of digestion begins with the act of chewing, in which food is broken down into small particles that can be swallowed and mixed with digestive enzymes. The first secretion encountered is saliva, which is secreted in the mouth by the salivary glands at the rate of about 1.5 liters daily. Saliva contains an enzyme, *ptyalin*, or salivary amylase, that helps in the digestion of starches. It also serves as a solvent for the molecules in the food that stimulate the taste buds. Eating or even the sight, smell, or thought of food can cause reflex salivation. The major function of saliva is to lubricate the food as it is chewed, thereby facilitating swallowing.

Swallowing.   Swallowing, the initial act in the propulsion of food, is under voluntary control. It is regulated by a swallowing center in the medulla oblongata of the central nervous system. Voluntary efforts to initiate swallowing are ineffective unless there is something to swallow, such as air, saliva, or food. As the food is swallowed, the epiglottis moves to cover the tracheal opening and thus prevents aspiration of food into the lungs. Swallowing results in the propulsion of the bolus of food into the upper esophagus. The smooth muscle in the wall of the esophagus undergoes rhythmic contractions that move sequentially from above to below and help to propel the bolus of food from the upper esophagus toward the stomach. During this process of esophageal peristalsis, the lower esophageal sphincter, at the junction of the esophagus and the stomach relaxes and permits the bolus of food to enter the stomach. Subsequently, the lower esophageal sphincter closes tightly to prevent reflux of stomach contents into the esophagus.

- When there is reflux of the acid contents of the stomach into the esophagus, an uncomfortable sensation occurs beneath the sternum. This sensation is commonly called heartburn.

Gastric Action.   Within the stomach, food is exposed to gastric juice, the major characteristic of which is its very acid *p*H. The acidity (*p*H as low as 1) is due to the secretion of *hydrochloric acid* by the glands of the stomach. The volume

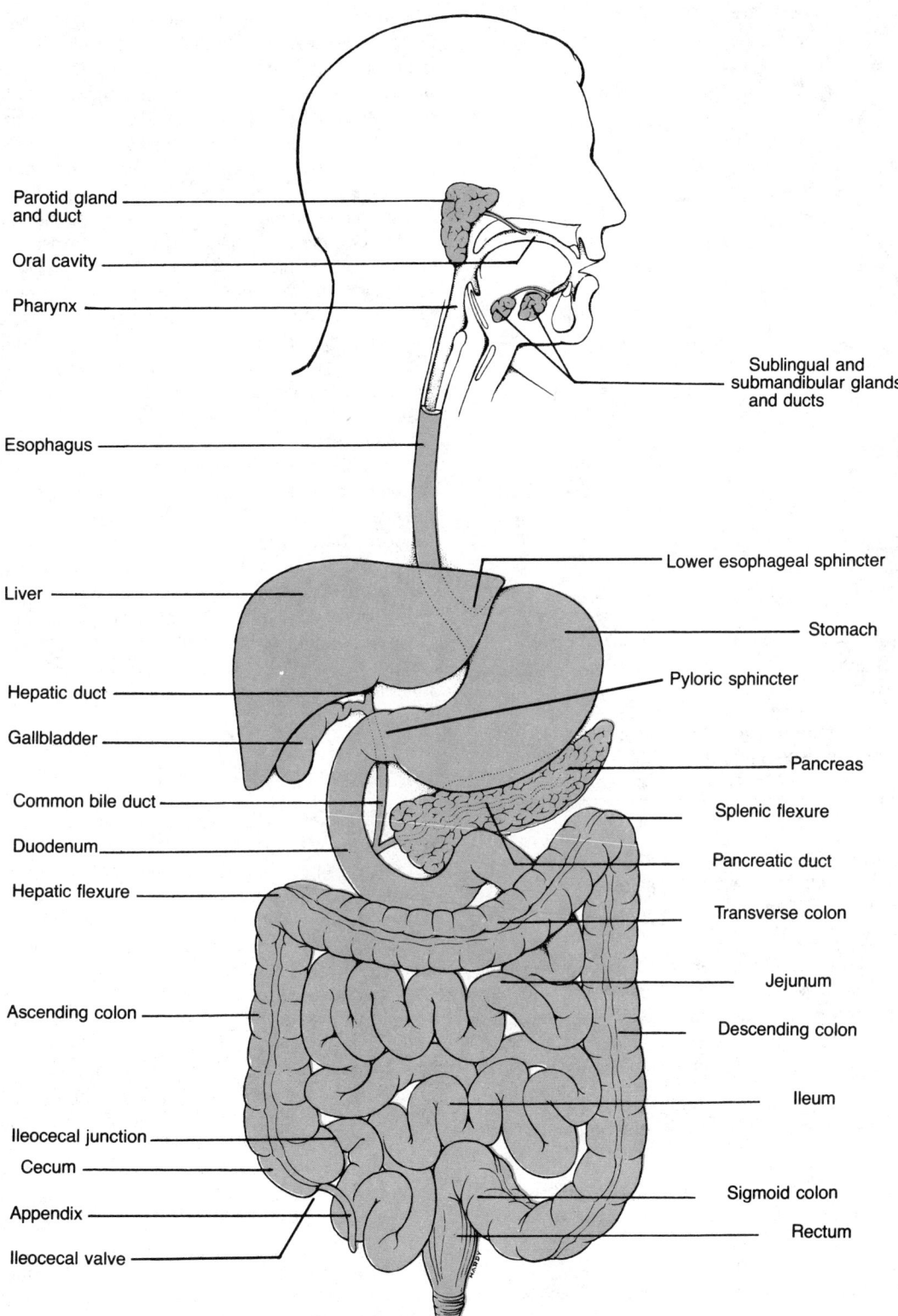

Figure 31-1
Diagram of the digestive system, showing the digestive or alimentary canal and sphincters. (Chaffee EE and Greisheimer EM. Basic Physiology and Anatomy, 3rd ed. Philadelphia, JB Lippincott.)

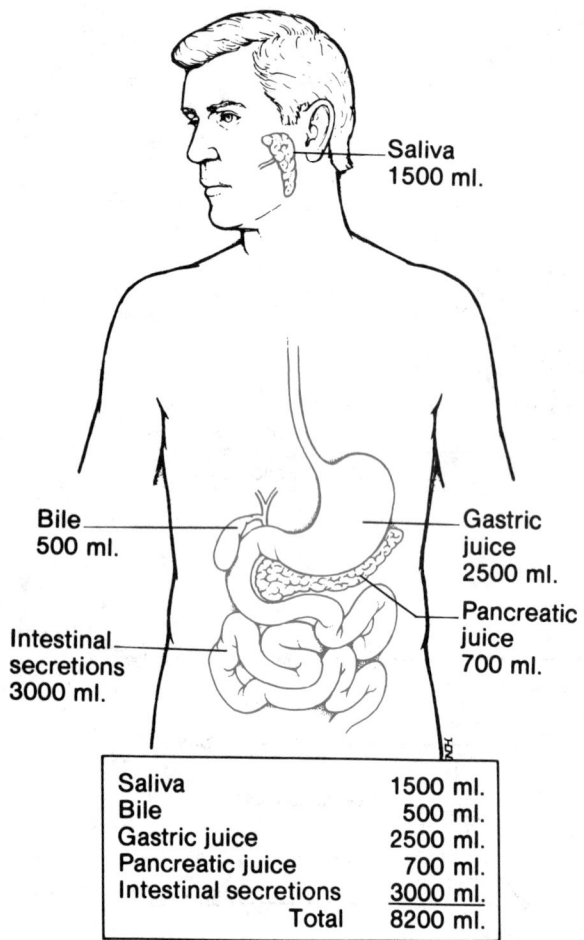

Saliva	1500 ml.
Bile	500 ml.
Gastric juice	2500 ml.
Pancreatic juice	700 ml.
Intestinal secretions	3000 ml.
Total	8200 ml.

Figure 31-2
Total volume of digestive secretions produced in 24 hours. (Adapted from Bowen A: Intravenous alimentation in surgical patients. Mod Med.)

of gastric secretion is 2.5 liters per day. The function of the highly acidic stomach secretion is to aid in digestion, breaking food down into more absorbable components. The secretion of hydrochloric acid occurs in response to a meal. Between meals, the rate of secretion of acid into the stomach is low.

- People who chronically secrete excessive amounts of gastric acid are susceptible to development of gastric and duodenal ulcers.

The gastric secretions also contain the enzyme *pepsin*, which is an important enzyme for the digestion of proteins (Table 31-1).

Another component of gastric secretions is *intrinsic factor*. This compound is synthesized by cells of the stomach and combines with vitamin B_{12} in the diet, so that the vitamin can be absorbed in the ileum.

- In the absence of intrinsic factor, vitamin B_{12} cannot be absorbed, resulting in pernicious anemia.

Peristaltic contractions in the stomach propel its contents toward the pylorus. Large food particles cannot pass through the pyloric sphincter and are churned back into the body of the stomach. In this way, food in the stomach is mechanically

agitated and broken down into smaller particles. Therefore, different types of meals remain in the stomach for times varying from a half hour to several hours, depending on the size of food particles, composition of the meal, and other factors.

Peristalsis in the stomach and contractions of the pyloric sphincter allow the partially digested food to enter the small intestine at a rate that permits efficient absorption of nutrients.

Intestinal Secretions. Secretions in the *duodenum* come from the pancreas, the liver, and the glands in the wall of the intestine itself. The major characteristic of these secretions is their high content of digestive enzymes.

Pancreatic secretion has an alkaline *p*H, owing to a high *bicarbonate* concentration. This serves to neutralize the acid entering the duodenum from the stomach. The pancreas also secretes digestive enzymes, including *trypsin*, which aids in the digestion of protein; *amylase*, which aids in the digestion of starch; and *lipase*, which aids in the digestion of fats.

Bile (secreted by the liver and stored in the gallbladder) contains bile salts, *cholesterol*, and *lecithin*, which emulsify the ingested fats and make them more accessible to digestion and absorption. The bile salts themselves are reabsorbed into the portal blood when they reach the ileum.

Secretions from the intestinal glands consist of mucus, which coats the cells and protects the duodenum from attack by hydrochloric acid; hormones; electrolytes; and enzymes. The total amount of intestinal secretions is approximately 1 liter per day of pancreatic juice, 0.5 liter per day of bile, and 3 liters per day from the glands of the small intestine.

Gastrointestinal Regulatory Substances and Bacteria

Hormones. Three major hormones and two neuroregulators have been found to control the rate of secretion of the gastrointestinal fluids and gastrointestinal motility (Table 31-2). Local regulators also play a role. Acetylcholine and histamine stimulate the gastric glands to increase the secretion of gastric acid. Norepinephrine and some prostaglandins inhibit gastric acid activity.

Gastrin is secreted by the cells of the stomach. It partially regulates the secretion of gastric acid and influences contraction of the lower esophageal and pyloric sphincters. The stimulus to gastrin release is distention of the stomach.

Secretin, secreted by the mucosa in the upper portion of the small intestine, stimulates the secretion of *bicarbonate* in pancreatic juice and inhibits the secretion of gastric acid. The stimulus to the release of secretin is acid entering the small intestine from the stomach.

Cholecystokinin-pancreozymin (CCK-PZ), also released from the cells in the upper small intestine, acts on both the gallbladder and the pancreas. It causes contraction of the gallbladder and release of digestive enzymes from the pancreas. The stimulus to the release of CCK-PZ is the presence of fatty acids and amino acids in the small intestine.

Bacteria. Bacteria are normal components of the contents of the gastrointestinal tract. Their presence is essential for normal gastrointestinal function. Few bacteria are present in the stomach or upper small intestine, probably because they are killed by the acid secretions in the stomach. However, the bacterial population increases in the ileum and becomes a major component of the contents of the large intestine.

TABLE 31-1
The Major Digestive Enzymes

Name of Enzyme	Substrate	Products of Reaction	Source of Enzyme	Site of Action
Action of Enzymes that Digest Carbohydrate				
Salivary amylase (ptyalin)	Starch (amylose) as in grains, potatoes, legumes	Dextrins, maltose, glucose	Secretions from parotid and submaxillary glands (saliva)	Mouth, if chewing is very thorough; some in fundus of stomach if mixing with acidic gastric juice is delayed
Pancreatic amylase (amylopsin)	Starch	α-limit dextrins, maltose, glucose	Secretions from pancreas	Small intestine
	Dextrins	Maltose, glucose		
Disaccharidases	Disaccharides	Monosaccharides	Mucosal cells of small intestine (brush border)	Brush border of intestinal wall
Maltase	Maltose (in corn syrup, beer)	Glucose		
Isomaltase	Isomaltose	Glucose		
Sucrase	Sucrose (in table sugar, fruits)	Glucose and fructose		
Lactase	Lactose (in milk)	Glucose and galactose		
Action of Enzymes that Digest Protein				
Pepsin (protease)	Protein	Large peptides	Chief cells of gastric mucosa (secreted as the inactive pro-enzyme pepsinogen*)	Stomach
Trypsin	Protein and polypeptides (Polypeptides are primarily from the partial digestion of protein.)	Polypeptides, dipeptides, amino acids	Pancreas (secreted as the inactive pro-enzymes trypsinogen, chymotrypsinogen, and procarboxypeptidase*)	Lumen of the small intestine
Chymotrypsin				
Carboxypeptidase				
Aminopeptidase	Polypeptides	Smaller peptides, amino acids	Mucosal cells of small intestine	Brush border of small intestine
Dipeptidase	Dipeptides	Amino acids		
Action of Enzymes that Digest Fat (Triglyceride)				
Pharyngeal lipase†	Triglycerides (in foods containing fat such as meat, butter, nuts, cheese)	Fatty acids, diglycerides, monoglycerides	Mucosa of pharynx	Fundus of stomach
Gastric lipase† (steapsin)	Short chain triglycerides (dairy fats)	Short chain fatty acids, diglycerides, monoglycerides	Gastric mucosa	Stomach
Pancreatic lipase	Triglycerides, diglycerides	Diglycerides, monoglycerides, fatty acids (short, long, and medium chain)	Pancreas	Lumen of small intestine

* Activation of proenzymes takes place in the lumen of the intestinal tract
† Not essential for adequate digestion of fat.
(Suitor CW and Hunter MF. Nutrition: Principles and Application in Health Promotion, p 219. Philadelphia, JB Lippincott, 1984.)

TABLE 31-2
Gastrointestinal Regulatory Substances

Substance	Stimulus for Production	Target Gland	Effect on Secretions	Effect on Motility
Neuroregulators				
Acetylcholine	Sight, smell, chewing food, stomach distention	Gastric glands, other secretory glands, gastrointestinal muscle	Increased gastric acid	Generally increased; decreased sphincter tone
Norepinephrine	Stress, other various stimuli	Secretory glands, gastrointestinal muscle	Generally inhibitory	Generally decreased; increased sphincter tone
Hormonal Regulators				
Gastrin	Myenteric reflexes caused by (1) distention of stomach with food; (2) secretagogues (partially digested protein; caffeine; other substances present in regular and decaffeinated coffee; alcohol; extractives)	Gastric glands	Increased secretion of gastric juice, which is rich in HCl	Increased motility of stomach, decreased time required for gastric-emptying. Relaxation of ileocecal sphincter. Excitation of colon. Constriction of gastroesophageal sphincter
Cholecystokinin	Fat in duodenum	Gallbladder	Release of bile into duodenum	
		Pancreas	Increased production of enzyme-rich pancreatic secretions	
		Stomach	May inhibit gastric secretion somewhat	
Secretin	pH of chyme in duodenum below 4–5	Stomach	May inhibit gastric secretion somewhat	Inhibits stomach contractions
		Pancreas	Increased production of bicarbonate-rich pancreatic juice	
*Vasoactive intestinal peptide	Unclear	Pancreas	Increased pancreatic secretions	
		Stomach	Decreased gastric acid and pepsin production	Relaxation of stomach muscles
*Gastric inhibitory peptide (GIP)	Peptides, amino acids, fats, and glucose	Gastric glands	Decreased gastric acid production. Increased insulin production	Decreased gastric motility
*Motilin	Alkaline pH in duodenum	Stomach, intestines		Increased stomach and intestinal activity
Local Regulators				
Histamine	Unclear; substances in food	Gastric glands	Increased gastric acid production	
*Prostaglandins (many types)	Possibly intestinal muscle contraction	Varied	Some (E_1, E_2, A) may inhibit gastric acid and pepsin secretion	PGE, PGF may cause contraction of longitudinal muscles

* Specific physiologic roles not clear

(Data from Grossman MI: Neural and hormonal regulation of gastrointestinal function: An overview. Ann Rev Physiol 1979; 41:27. Rattan S: Neural regulation of gastrointestinal motility: Nature of neurotransmission. Med Clin North Am 1981; 65:1129. Ouyang A, Cohen F: Effects of hormones on gastrointestinal motility Med Clin North Am 1981; 65:1111. Wilson D, Kaymakcalan H: Prostaglandins: Gastrointestinal effects and peptic ulcer disease. Med Clin North Am 1981; 65:773. Konturek SJ et al: Role of mucosal prostaglandins. Gut 1981; 11:927. Table from Suitor CW and Hunter MF. Nutrition: Principles and Application in Health Promotion, p 224. JB Lippincott, 1984.)

Bacteria function as an aid to digestion and also synthesize essential nutrients that otherwise might not be available for absorption. The bacterial mass comprises about 10% of the dry weight of the stool.

Digestion and Absorption of Nutrients

Food, ingested in the form of fats, protein, and carbohydrates, is broken down into its constituent nutrients by the process of digestion.

Carbohydrate digestion begins in the mouth with the breakdown of starches by the action of *salivary amylase*. It continues in the esophagus but is inhibited in the stomach by gastric acid. Continuation of carbohydrate digestion occurs in the duodenum by the action of *pancreatic amylase*. The end result of this process is the liberation of small sugar molecules known as *disaccharides* (*e.g.,* sucrose, maltose, galactose). Enzymes attached to the mucosal cells of the intestine convert the disaccharides into *monosaccharides,* such as glucose and fructose, which are then absorbed into the blood.

- Glucose is the major carbohydrate that the tissue cells use as fuel.

Proteins are long chains of amino acids linked together chemically. The hydrochloric acid in the stomach aids in breaking down proteins into smaller particles that are more easily attacked by the digestive enzymes. The process of protein digestion begins in the stomach by the action of pepsin and continues in the duodenum by the action of pancreatic enzymes, such as trypsin. When the proteins are broken down into their constituent amino acids, they are actively absorbed through the mucosal cells of the small intestine into the blood. The tissues use amino acids in synthesizing their constituent proteins.

Ingested fats must be dispersed into small droplets (emulsified) so that they can be attacked by digestive enzymes. Emulsification of fats takes place as the result of the churning action in the stomach and duodenum and contact with bile salts. Pancreatic lipase then breaks down the emulsified fats into monoglycerides and fatty acids. These are solubilized as *micelles,* which move to the mucosal surface of the intestine, where they are absorbed. Within the mucosal cells, the fatty acids are recombined into fats, which then enter the lacteals (part of the lymphatic system) and eventually enter the bloodstream. The tissues use fats as a fuel; excess fat is stored in the fat cells that are widely distributed throughout the body.

Vitamins in the diet are absorbed essentially unchanged from the gastrointestinal tract. The fat-soluble vitamins A, D, E, and K are absorbed by a mechanism similar to that described above for fats. Vitamin B_{12} is absorbed after combination with intrinsic factor, as previously described.

Minerals in the diet, such as calcium and iron, are absorbed in the small intestine. Calcium absorption requires the presence of vitamin D and is modified by the action of parathyroid hormone.

- Iron in the diet is needed to replace small amounts of iron normally lost by the body, but only a limited fraction of the ingested iron can be absorbed. Therefore, repletion of iron stores of the body by oral therapy, in a patient with iron deficiency, is a long-term process.

Little of the *water and electrolytes* in the diet, and in the 8 liters per day of gastrointestinal secretions, is excreted in the stool.

Intestinal Peristalsis

Peristalsis propels the contents of the small intestine toward the colon. Intense peristaltic waves may be responsible for the gurgling sounds emanating from the gastrointestinal tract at various times. Segmental contractions of the intestinal smooth muscle occur in addition to its peristaltic contractions. These segmental contractions do not propel contents toward the colon, but rather churn it back and forth, to permit more efficient digestion and absorption. Food leaving the small intestine must pass through the ileocecal valve to enter the colon. This valve is normally closed and helps prevent colonic contents from refluxing back into the small intestine. However, with each peristaltic wave of the small intestine, the valve opens briefly and permits some of the contents to pass through. The first part of a meal usually reaches the ileocecal valve in about 4 hours, and all of the unabsorbed food has entered the colon by 8 or 9 hours after eating.

Motility of the colon consists of relatively weak peristaltic activity that moves the colonic contents slowly, and strong peristaltic rushes that propel the contents for considerable distances. When the contents reach and distend the rectum, an urge to defecate is experienced. Eating stimulates the peristaltic rushes in the colon, resulting in desire to defecate shortly after a meal. This gastrocolic reflex is the reason that defecation after meals is the rule in children. However, in adults, habit and cultural factors are more important in determining the time for elimination of fecal contents. The first part of a meal reaches the rectum about 12 hours after eating. From the rectum to the anus, transport is much slower, and as much as one fourth of the meal may still be in the rectum 3 days after ingestion. This slow transport of colonic contents allows efficient reabsorption of water and electrolytes.

Defecation

Distention of the rectum reflexly initiates contractions of its musculature and relaxation of the internal anal sphincter, which is ordinarily closed. The internal sphincter is controlled by the autonomic nervous system; the external sphincter is under the conscious control of the cerebral cortex. When the desire to defecate is felt, the external anal sphincter voluntarily relaxes, permitting expulsion of colonic contents. Normally, the external anal sphincter is maintained in a state of tonic contraction. Thus, defecation is seen to be a spinal reflex that can be voluntarily inhibited by keeping the external anal sphincter closed. In this regard, it is similar to micturition. Contraction of abdominal muscles (straining) facilitates emptying of the colon.

- The presence of neurologic lesions that disrupt the innervation of the rectum lessens the effectiveness of reflex evacuation and can lead to abnormal retention of fecal material (fecal impaction).

The average frequency of defecation in humans is once daily, but the range is extremely variable. It is commonly observed that some people defecate several times daily, while others may defecate only a few times per week. More importantly, changes in bowel habits may signify colonic disease. An increase in frequency of defecation is called *diarrhea*, whereas decreased frequency is called *constipation*.

The elderly are prone to constipation because of limited mobility and a decreased intake of fiber and foods that are hard to chew. A detailed explanation of gastrointestinal problems in the aged population is presented in Chapter 35.

Feces and Flatus. Feces consist of undigested foodstuffs, inorganic materials, water, and bacteria. Their composition is relatively unaffected by alterations of diet, since a large fraction of the fecal mass is of nondietary origin, derived from the gastrointestinal tract. This is why appreciable amounts of feces continue to be passed despite prolonged starvation. The brown color of the feces is due to breakdown of bile by the intestinal bacteria. With obstruction of the bile ducts, bile is absent from the intestine and the stools become white (acholic stools). Formation of chemicals, especially indole and skatole, by the intestinal bacteria are responsible in large part for the fecal odor.

The gastrointestinal tract normally contains approximately 150 ml of gas. Gas expelled from the upper gastrointestinal tract (belching) has its origin as swallowed air. Gas expelled from the lower gastrointestinal tract (flatulence) consists of swallowed air, as well as gas produced by bacteria in the colon. The gas in the colon contains methane, hydrogen sulfide, ammonia, and other potentially harmful gases. These gases can be absorbed into the portal circulation and are detoxified by the liver.

- Patients with liver disease are frequently treated with antibiotics to reduce the number of colonic bacteria and thereby inhibit the production of toxic gases.

Pathophysiological Overview

Abnormalities of the gastrointestinal tract are numerous and exemplify every type of major pathology that can affect other organ systems. A composite view of the various types of gastrointestinal disorders that may occur is presented in Figure 31-3. Congenital, inflammatory, infectious, traumatic, and neoplastic lesions have been encountered in every portion, and at every site, along its length. In common with many other organ systems, it is subject to circulatory disturbances, faulty nervous control, and senescence.

Obstruction of the Gastrointestinal Tract. Various degrees of obstruction to the passage of intestinal contents

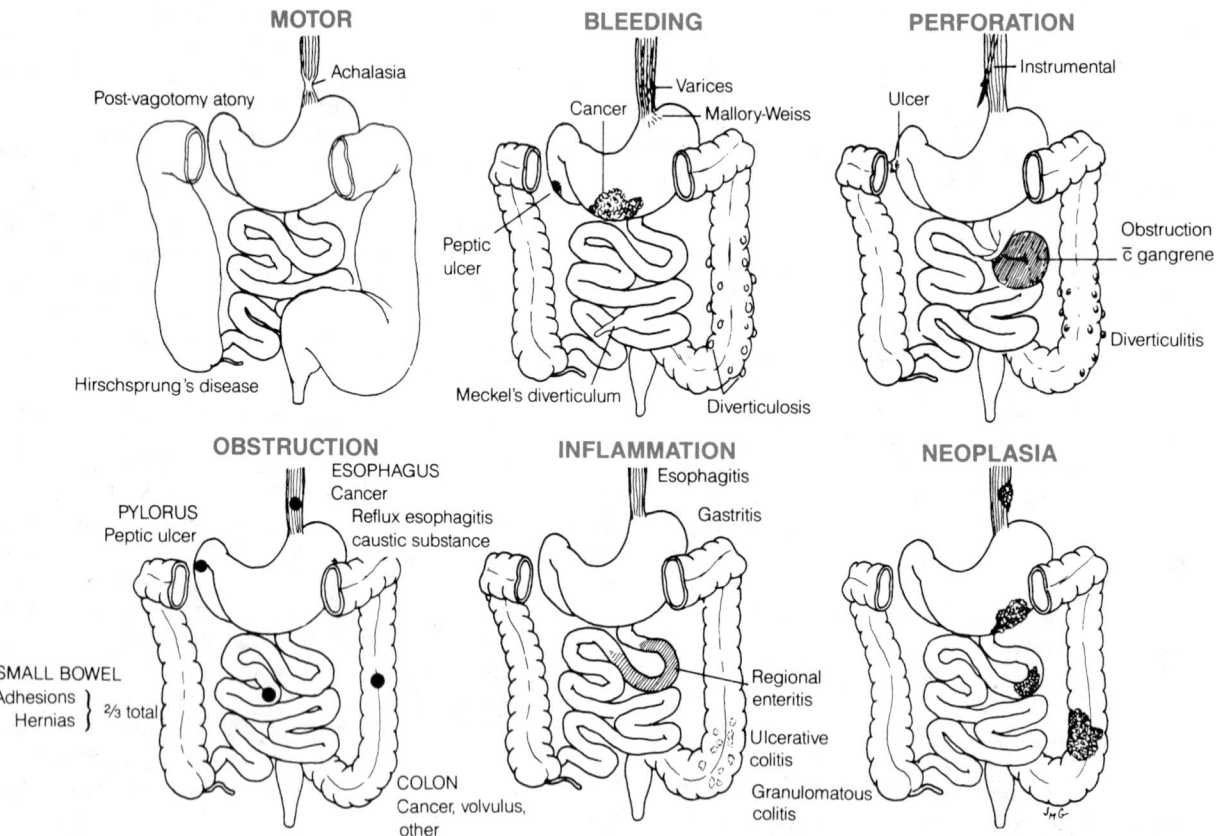

Figure 31-3
Pathophysiology of the gastrointestinal tract can be classified in many ways. The above illustration vividly shows the many conditions that can occur under the six classifications. (Hardy JD: Rhoads Textbook of Surgery, 5th ed. Philadelphia, JB Lippincott.)

in the gastrointestinal tract may result from tumors growing into the lumen, twisting or kinking of the intestine, infarction of tissue owing to interruption of the blood supply, aspirated foreign bodies, or other reasons. As a consequence of obstruction, the force of the intestinal contractions is increased, the intestine becomes distended above the point of obstruction, and abdominal pain and bloating result. The peristaltic waves may actually reverse their direction, leading to vomiting. Excessive vomiting may result in the loss of large volumes of fluid from the body, causing *dehydration,* and loss of large amounts of hydrochloric acid, causing *systemic alkalosis.* If the obstruction in the gastrointestinal tract occurs at, or below, the duodenum, biliary material will be in the vomitus, giving the characteristic green color. If the colon is obstructed, the ileocecal valve may become stretched and incompetent, colonic contents can reflux, and the patient may vomit fecal material.

Psychosocial Considerations in Gastrointestinal Disorders

Apart from the many organic diseases to which the gastrointestinal tract is susceptible, there are many extrinsic factors—some related to disease, others not—that can interfere with its normal function and produce symptoms. An anxiety state, for example, often finds its chief expression in indigestion, anorexia, or motor disturbances of the intestines, producing constipation or diarrhea. Students facing examinations or stressed executives facing major decisions can readily be susceptible to gastrointestinal disorders. Also, some psychological problems are thought to have a role in physical dysfunction. For example, personality factors are thought to have an influence in peptic ulcer disease.

In addition to the state of mental health, physical factors such as fatigue and an unbalanced or abruptly changed dietary intake can markedly affect the gastrointestinal tract. In both assessing the patient and instructing him, the nurse should realize that a combination of mental and physical factors affect the status of the gastrointestinal tract.

Surgical Considerations

Abdominal Topography

For purposes of convenience in description, the abdomen has been divided into nine regions by imaginary lines, as illustrated in Figure 31-4 (Chart 31-1).

The abdominal cavity normally contains a small amount of fluid that lubricates the peritoneal surfaces. This cavity is lined with a thin, glistening membrane called the *peritoneum,* which covers most of the abdominal organs, forming folds between which the coils of intestine are located. Some organs (such as the liver, pancreas, kidney, and urinary bladder) are not covered completely by peritoneum; hence inflammations of these structures may not always involve the general abdominal cavity but may develop into retroperitoneal extensions or abscesses.

Abdominal Incisions and Surgical Procedures

Laparotomy and *abdominal section* are terms used to describe any operation that involves opening the abdominal cavity. The gridiron, or McBurney, incision (see Fig. 31-4 in Chart 31-1) is the simplest. It opens the abdomen through a small wound made by spreading the fibers of the muscles through which it passes. This incision is especially suitable for operations on the appendix, and since it has the advantage of being closed without tension, it makes a firm wound in which hernias rarely form.

More widely useful, however, are the vertical incisions made in the midline or to either side of it. These are made to pass between or through the rectus muscles. Many other types of incisions may be made, depending on the preference of the surgeon.

Diagnostic Evaluation

Diagnostic assessment of the gastrointestinal tract includes the use of x-rays and ultrasound and the passage of various oral and anal tubes. In general, the nurse has a supportive and educative role. Patients requiring such tests are frequently anxious, elderly, or debilitated. The preparation for many of these studies includes fasting and the use of laxatives or enemas, measures that are poorly tolerated by weakened patients. In addition, many of these tests require seemingly endless waiting, either for the tests to begin or be completed or for the results to be known.

Roentgenography of the Upper Gastrointestinal Tract

The entire gastrointestinal tract can be delineated by x-rays, following the introduction of barium sulfate or a similar radiopaque liquid as the contrast medium. This material, a tasteless, odorless, nongranular, and completely insoluble (hence, not absorbable) powder, is ingested in the form of a thick or thin aqueous suspension for purposes of upper gastrointestinal tract study ("upper GI series") and is instilled rectally for visualization of the colon ("barium enema").

Patient Preparation. In preparation for a GI series, the patient is to receive nothing by mouth after midnight prior to the test. A laxative may be prescribed to clean out the intestinal tract. Since smoking can stimulate gastric motility, the patient is discouraged from smoking the morning before the examination.

Procedure. For purposes of examining the upper gastrointestinal tract, the patient is required to swallow barium under direct fluoroscopic examination.

As the contrast medium descends into the stomach, the position, patency, and caliber of the esophagus are visualized, enabling the examiner to detect or exclude any anatomical or functional derangement of that organ. An important observation can also be made in relation to the heart, namely, observing the presence or the absence of right atrial enlargement. An enlarged right atrium invariably impinges on the

Chart 31-1
Abdominal Incisions and Surgical Procedures

Before studying about patients with specific gastrointestinal problems and operations, the nurse should be familiar with the prefixes denoting abdominal organs and the suffixes used to denote the diseases of or operations on these organs. Suffixes used to denote the names of diseases and operations are listed below:

-itis—inflammation of, as *appendicitis,* an inflammation of the appendix
-otomy—to make a cut into, as *gastrotomy,* to make an opening into the stomach
-ostomy—to make a mouth or opening into, as *cystostomy,* to insert a tube into the urinary bladder
-ectomy—to cut or remove, as *salpingectomy,* to remove the uterine tube
-pexy—to sew up in position, as *nephropexy,* to sew the kidney up in position
-orrhaphy—to repair a defect, as *herniorrhaphy,* to repair a hernial defect
-plasty—to improve by changing the position of the tissue, as *pyloroplasty,* an operation to enlarge the pyloric opening of the stomach

Organ	Prefix	Example
Stomach	Gastr-	*Gastritis*—inflammation of stomach
Pylorus	Pylor-	*Pylorectomy*—removal of pyloric end of stomach
Liver	Hepa-	*Hepatitis*—inflammation of liver
Gallbladder	Cholecyst-	*Cholecystitis*—inflammation of gallbladder
Common bile duct	Choledoch-	*Choledochitis*—inflammation of common bile duct
Small intestine	Enter-	*Enteritis*—inflammation of intestine
Colon	Col-	*Colitis*—inflammation of large colon
Appendix	Appendic-	*Appendicitis*—inflammation of appendix
Loin or abdomen	Lapar-	*Laparotomy*—incision in the abdomen
Urinary bladder	Cyst-	*Cystitis*—inflammation of urinary bladder
Uterine tube	Salping-	*Salpingitis*—inflammation of uterine tube
Ovary	Oophor-	*Oophoritis*—inflammation of ovary
Pelvis of kidney	Pyel-	*Pyelitis*—inflammation of pelvis of kidney
Kidney	Nephr-	*Nephritis*—inflammation of kidney

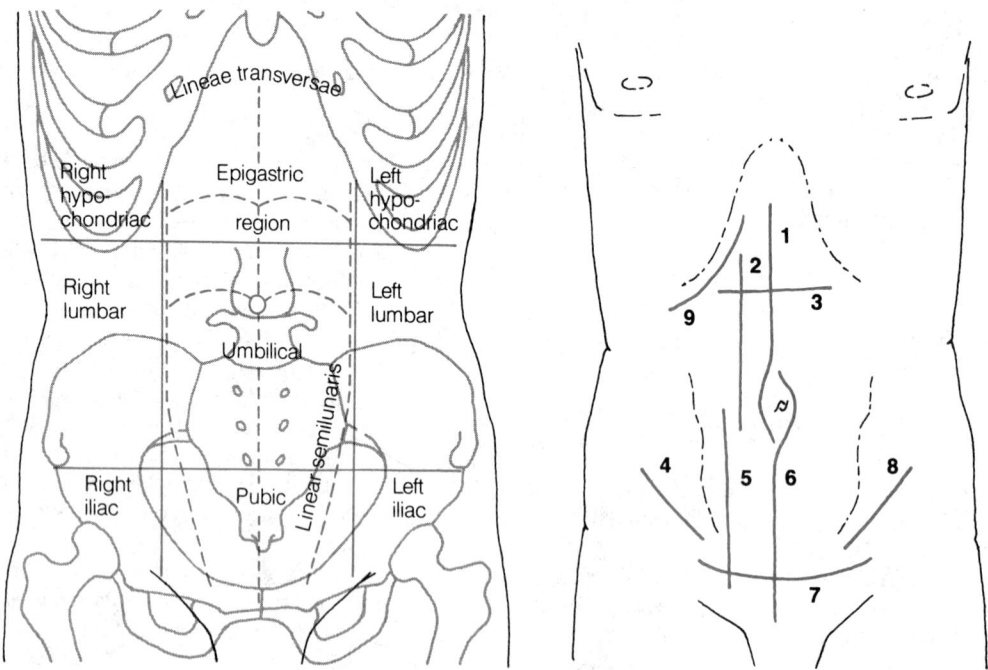

Figure 31-4
(*Left*) Regions of the abdomen. (*Right*) Diagram to show the various abdominal incisions that are used: (1) upper midline incision, (2) upper right rectus incision, (3) transverse incision in the upper abdomen, (4) gridiron incision on the right, (5) lower right rectus incision, (6) lower midline incision, (7) Pfannenstiel incision, (8) left gridiron incision, (9) subcostal incision.

esophagus and is revealed by the resulting pressure defect in the esophagus. The roentgenographic appearance of the lower esophagus after a swallow of thick barium suspension also allows for detection of esophageal varices, a manifestation of portal hypertension, as in cirrhosis of the liver.

Fluoroscopic examination next extends to the stomach, as its lumen fills with barium. The motility and the thickness of the gastric wall and the mucosal pattern are observed for evidence of spasms, ulcerations, malignant infiltrates, and other anatomical abnormalities, including pressure defects from without. The patency of the pyloric valve and the anatomy of the duodenum are also observed, with particular reference to possible ulceration of the mucosa, spasm of the wall, or displacement of the structure as a whole by a tumor in the adjacent area.

During the fluoroscopic examination, x-ray films are exposed in order to obtain a permanent record of the findings. Additional films are taken at intervals, for as long as 24 hours thereafter, as a means of estimating the rate of gastric emptying and the degree of small bowel motility.

Double Contrast Studies.   The double contrast method of examining the upper gastrointestinal tract involves administering a thick barium suspension medium to outline the stomach and esophageal wall. Next, tablets that release carbon dioxide in the presence of water are given. (To reduce these bubbles, simethicone is given.) The primary advantage of this technique is the finer detail that can be shown within the esophagus and stomach, permitting signs of early superficial neoplasms to be noted.

Continuous Infusion Method.   A truly detailed study of the small intestine involves the continuous infusion, through a duodenal tube, of 500 to 1000 ml of a thin barium sulfate suspension. This is carried out as a separate procedure. The barium column fills the intestinal loops and is observed continuously by fluoroscope and filmed at frequent intervals as it progresses through the jejunum and the ileum.

Roentgenography of the Colon (Barium Enema)

The purpose of a barium enema is to reveal the presence of polyps, tumors, and other lesions of the large intestine and to demonstrate any abnormal anatomy or malfunction of the bowel.

Patient Preparation.   The preparation of the patient includes those measures necessary to produce an empty and clean lower bowel. Usually, this includes clear liquids the day before, a laxative the evening before, taking nothing by mouth after midnight, and cleansing enemas until returns are clear.

- If the patient has active inflammatory disease of the colon, only gentle enemas should be used.

Procedure.   In the x-ray department, the radiopaque substance is instilled rectally; it is viewed in the fluoroscope and then filmed. If the patient has been prepared satisfactorily and the colonic contents have been evacuated completely by enemas, the contour of the entire colon, including cecum and appendix (if patent), is clearly visible and the motility of each portion readily observed. The procedure takes about 15 minutes and is followed by an evacuating enema or laxative to facilitate barium removal.

Gastric Analysis

Examination of the gastric juice offers a means of estimating the secretory activity of the gastric mucosa and of determining the presence, or the degree, of gastric retention in patients suspected of having pyloric or duodenal obstruction.

- A diagnosis of pernicious anemia is excluded by the finding of acid.
- A diagnosis of gastric carcinoma may be established by the discovery of cancer cells in the gastric juice.

The fasting patient is intubated through a nostril with a Levin duodenal tube, a small tube with catheter tip marked at various points from the distal end. (See p. 756 for nursing management during intubation.)

When the Levin tube is at a point slightly less than 50 cm (21 inches) distant, the tube should be within the stomach. Once in place, the tube is secured to the patient's cheek by means of a small strip of adhesive tape, and the patient is placed in a semireclining position. If he exhibits any tendency to gag, he is instructed to pant gently with his mouth wide open, the effect of which is to minimize contact between the tube and the soft palate. The entire stomach contents are aspirated by gentle suction into a syringe.

Histamine or betazole (Histalog) may be given to stimulate gastric secretions. The patient is told that he may experience a flushed feeling after the injection of this medication. Also, blood pressure and pulse are frequently monitored to detect hypotension. Emergency medications such as epinephrine and diphenhydramine (Benadryl) are to be kept nearby if required. Specimens are labeled to indicate time before and after histamine injections.

The acidity of the specimen is determined by means of an indicator, such as Töpfer's reagent, by indicator paper, or by a pH meter. Other examinations, in special instances, may include cytologic study by the Papanicolaou technique for the presence or absence of carcinoma cells. Enzyme analysis of the gastric juice is sometimes indicated.

One of the most important items of information to be gained from gastric analysis relates to the ability of the mucosa to secrete hydrochloric acid:

- Patients with pernicious anemia secrete no acid under basal conditions or after stimulation.
- Patients with severe chronic atrophic gastritis secrete little or no acid. Some patients with gastric cancer secrete little or no acid.
- Patients with peptic ulcer invariably secrete some acid; patients with duodenal ulcers usually secrete an excess amount.

Upper Gastrointestinal Fiberoscopy

Fiberoscopy of the upper gastrointestinal tract allows for direct visualization of the gastric mucosa through a lighted endoscope (gastroscope) and is especially valuable when gastric neoplasm is suspected (Fig. 31-5). Fiberscopes are flexible scopes equipped with fiberoptic lenses. Colored photographs or motion pictures can be taken through them. However, precautions must be taken to protect the scope, since the fiberoptic bundles may be broken if the scope is bent acutely. Mouth guards are essential to prevent the patient from biting the scope.

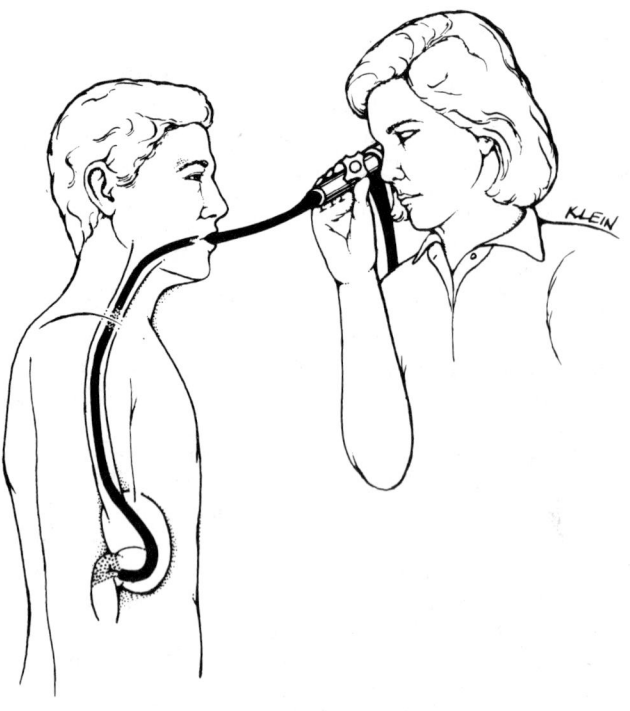

Figure 31-5
Patient undergoing gastroscopy. Note the extreme
flexibility of the tube with the patient in the sitting position.

An electronic video endoscope is available that is similar
to the conventional fiberscope except that there is no viewing
lens in the control section. The endoscope attaches directly
to the video processor, which converts electronic signals to
a television screen.

Currently a laser-compatible upper gastrointestinal endoscope is being developed. Endoscopic laser therapy for
gastrointestinal neoplasms is primarily palliative. It is used
mainly to relieve obstruction, reduce tumor size, enlarge an
obstructed lumen, and treat bleeding sites.

Patient Preparation.   The patient is placed in a fasting
state for 6 to 8 hours before the examination. One-half hour
before the procedure, he is given a narcotic analgesic. Usually,
gargling with a local anesthetic, along with the intravenous
administration of diazepam (Valium) just before the scope is
introduced, will suffice. Sometimes atropine may be helpful
in reducing secretions. Glucagon may be given to relax
smooth muscle.

Procedure.   The patient's lips, oral cavity, and pharynx
are sprayed with tetracaine (Pontocaine) or a liquid gargle
of ethyl aminobenzoate (Hurricane), after which the gastroscope is passed smoothly and slowly. The fiberoptic gastroscope is almost completely flexible and gives the physician
an opportunity to view a large part of the gastric wall. Experienced gastroscopists may recognize a cancer and remove
a piece of tissue for microscopic examination. Ulcers under
treatment can be monitored and degree of healing evaluated.

Follow-Up Care.   Following a gastroscopy the patient
is instructed not to eat or drink until the gag reflex returns in
3 to 4 hours; this is done to prevent aspiration into the lungs.
Postgastroscopy assessment by the nurse includes observation

for signs of perforation, such as pain, unusual discomfort,
and an elevated temperature. Minor throat discomfort can
be relieved with lozenges, cool saline gargle, and oral analgesic medications.

Anoscopy, Proctoscopy, Sigmoidoscopy, and Colonofiberoscopy

Procedures to view the lower bowel make use of tubular
instruments that incorporate small electric lights that allow
the lumen of the lower bowel to be viewed directly. The
anoscope is employed to examine the anal canal; procto-
scopes and sigmoidoscopes (Fig. 31-6) are used to inspect
the rectum and the sigmoid, respectively, for evidence of
ulceration, tumors, polyps, or some other pathologic process.

The flexible sigmoidoscope permits an examination of
up to 40 to 50 cm (16 to 20 inches) from the anus, more
than the 25 cm (10 inches) that can be seen with the rigid
sigmoidoscope. Although there is a more proximal distribution
of lesions of the colon, polyps and cancer are found more
commonly on the left side of the colon. Rectal bleeding and
anemia are indicators for a colonoscopy even if the patient
has a negative barium enema. A flexible sigmoidoscopy
should be performed at age 50, be repeated in 1 year, and
then performed every 3 years after that. Research has shown
that the majority of carcinoid tumors begin in the terminal
portion of the ileum.

Patient Preparation.   Such an examination requires
that the lower bowel be clean; therefore, a warm tap-water
enema or Fleet's enema is given until returns are clear. It
may be necessary for the patient to take clear liquids the day
before the examination. Generally, laxatives are not given.

Procedure.   The patient assumes the knee-chest position, resting on his knees, feet extending over the edge of
the bed or the examining table. With knees spread apart to
give steady support, the patient leans over and rests the side
of his face on the bed or the table, with his forearms on either
side of the head and his hands placed, one on top of the
other, above the head. His back is now inclined at about a
45-degree angle, and he is in proper position for the introduction of an anoscope, proctoscope, or sigmoidoscope.
Maximal convenience and comfort are afforded by a table
that has been especially designed for rectal endoscopy—the
so-called proctoscopic table, which tilts the patient into the
optimal position.

- The patient undergoing a proctosigmoidoscopic examination is kept informed about the progress of the examination and praised for his cooperation. Let him know
  that he will experience a feeling of pressure and will feel
  as though he is going to have a bowel movement. Explain
  that this is from the pressure of the instrument and will
  last only a brief period of time. It may be necessary to
  attach suction equipment through the scope to remove
  any secretion, exudate, blood, or excreta that might be
  obstructing the area of observation. After each use these
  tubes must be cleansed thoroughly and the collecting
  bottles emptied and cleansed likewise. Disposable sigmoidoscopes are now available. Although they eliminate
  the need for cleaning, they must be disposed of safely.

As part of the endoscopic examination, one or more
small pieces of tissue may be removed for histologic

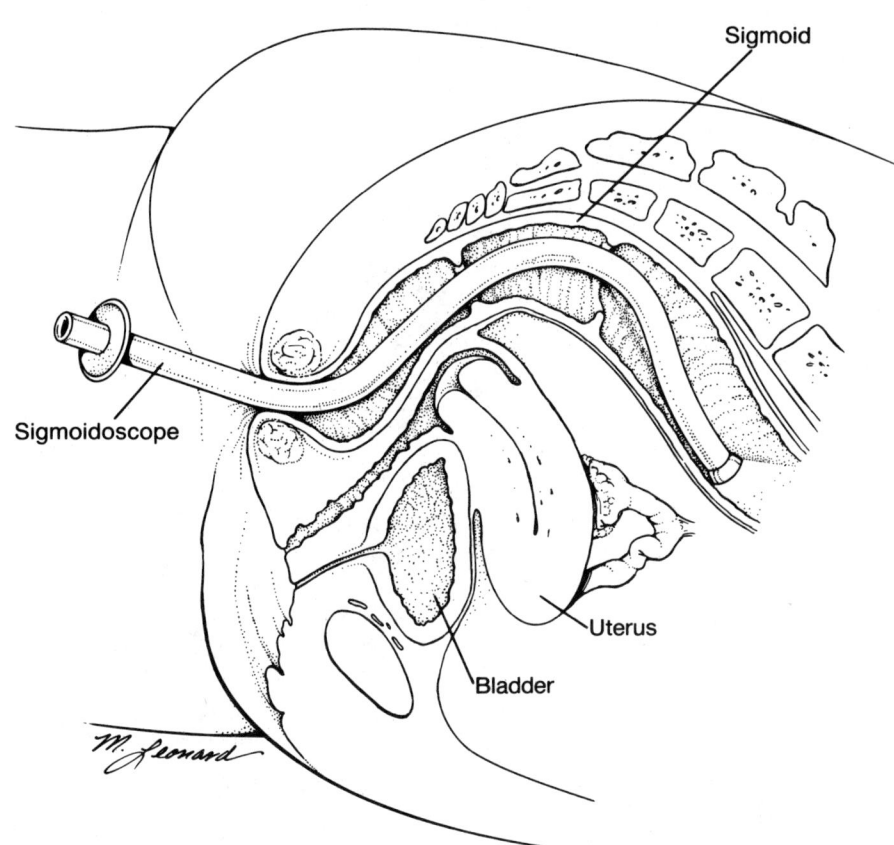

Figure 31-6
Sigmoidoscopy. Instrument is
advanced past proximal sigmoid
and then deflected into descending
colon. Patient is assisted to the
knee–chest position for the
procedure.

study, a procedure referred to as a *biopsy*. This is done with small biting forceps introduced through the instrument. Rectal and sigmoidal polyps, if present, may be removed by means of a wire snare, which is used to grasp the pedicle or stalk, and an electrocoagulating current, used to sever it and to prevent bleeding. It is extremely important that all tissue that is excised by the endoscopist be placed immediately in moist gauze or in an appropriate receptacle, labeled correctly and legibly, and then delivered without delay to the pathology laboratory.

Fiberoptic Colonoscopy

Direct visual inspection of the colon is possible by means of a flexible colonoscope. This procedure is used as a diagnostic aid, and the instrument may be used to remove foreign bodies, polyps, or tissue for biopsy (Fig. 31-7).

Patient Preparation. The patient is informed about the procedure and requested to cooperate and relax during the examination. In addition, the intestinal tract is emptied by limiting the patient's intake to liquids (perhaps for a 3-day period), cleansing the tract with a laxative for 2 nights, and giving a Fleet enema or saline enema until returns are clear the morning of the test. Currently, polyethylene glycol electrolyte lavage solutions (GoLYTELY, Colyte) are being used as effective intestinal lavages for cleansing the bowel. They are fast (rectal effluent is clear in about 4 hours) and tolerated well by elderly patients.

Before the examination, a narcotic analgesic, usually meperidine (Demerol), may be administered. During the ex-

amination, diazepam (Valium) may be useful in relieving anxiety.

Procedure. Colonoscopy is performed with the patient lying on his left side with his legs drawn up. Discomfort may result from instilling air to open the colon or from tugging the colon so that the scope can be maneuvered. Complications are rare following this procedure, although perforation or hemorrhage is possible.

Colonoscopic Polypectomy

Colonoscopic polypectomy involves resection of a colonic polyp and the use of cautery through a colonoscope. Many colon cancers begin with adenomatous polyps of the colon; therefore, the goal of colonoscopic polypectomy is prevention of colorectal cancer. Resection and biopsy are done to determine the cellular nature of the polyp, such as benign or malignant. All adenomatous colon polyps larger than 1.0 cm in diameter should be resected because malignancy is related to polyp size.

Stool Examination

The basic examination of the stool includes an inspection of the specimen for its amount, consistency, and color, and a screening test for occult blood. Special tests indicated in specific cases may include tests for fecal urobilinogen, fat, nitrogen, parasites, food residues, and other substances.

Stool Color. The color of stools varies from light to dark brown. (Milk-fed infants pass stools that are golden-yellow, owing to unchanged bilirubin.) Various foods and

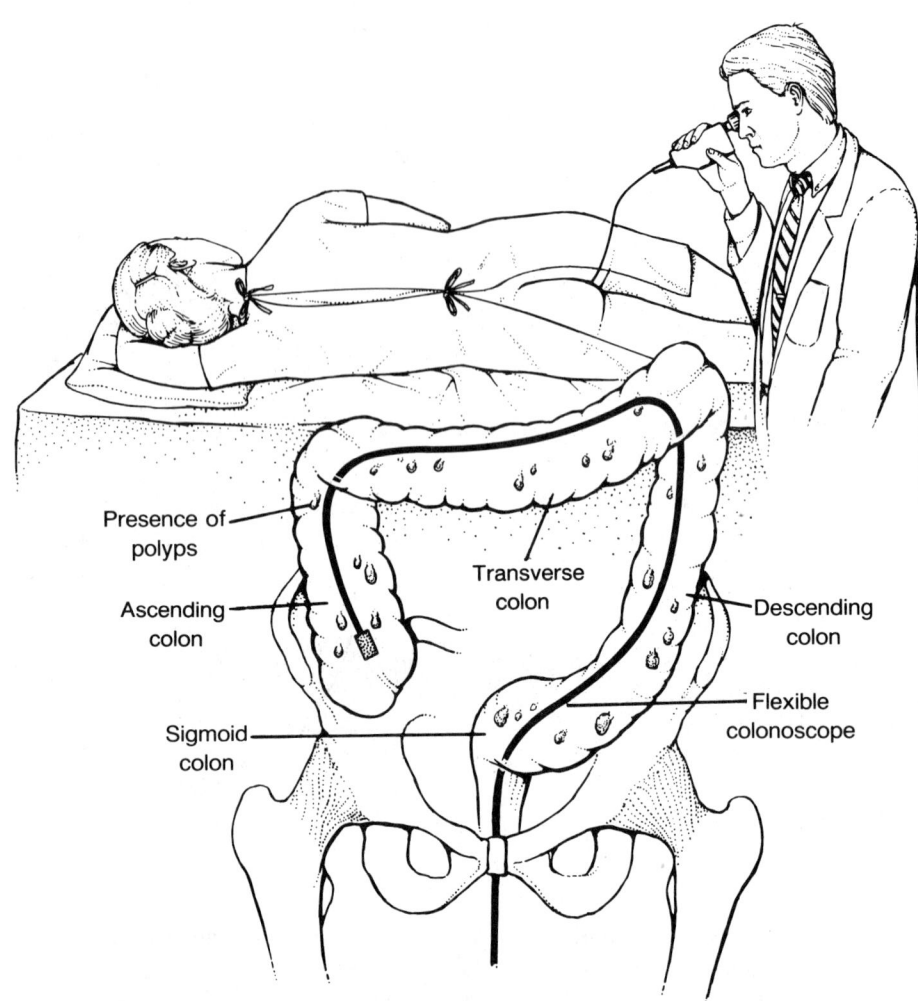

Figure 31-7
Colonoscopy. Flexible scope passes through rectum and sigmoid colon into the descending, transverse, and ascending colon.

medications affect stool color as follows: meat protein produces a dark brown coloration; spinach, a green hue; carrots and beets, red; cocoa, dark red or brown; senna and santonin, a yellowish hue; calomel, green; bismuth, iron, licorice, and charcoal, black; and barium, a milky white appearance.

- Blood in sufficient quantities, if shed into the upper gastrointestinal tract, produces a tarry black color (melena).
- Blood entering the lower portion of the gastrointestinal tract or passing rapidly through it will appear bright or dark red.
- Lower rectal or anal bleeding can be suspected if there is streaking of blood on the surface of the stool or if blood is noted on toilet tissue.

Even considerable quantities of hemoglobin may fail to produce a distinctive color, in which event it is termed *occult blood.*

Tests for Occult Blood or to Confirm Melena. The most common stool tests are based on the benzidine, gum guaiac, or the orthotolidin reaction. A form of the guaiac test is the Hemoccult test. A dry paper slide is used, on which the stool specimen is smeared. The slide comes in an envelope that can be mailed, if needed, and examined later.

The American Cancer Society recommends annual fecal guaiac screening beginning at age 50. The screening test re-quires a 3-day serial stool testing. It is easy, inexpensive, noninvasive, and easily done at home. It should not be done when there is hemorrhoidal bleeding.

Stool Consistency and Appearance. In various disorders the stool assumes a typical appearance:

In *steatorrhea*, the stools are generally bulky, greasy, foamy, and foul in odor; stool color is gray, with a silvery sheen.

With *biliary obstruction*, the stool becomes "acholic" and is light gray or "clay colored," owing to the absence of urobilin.

In *chronic ulcerative colitis*, mucus or pus may be visible on gross inspection of the stool.

Constipation, obstipation, or *fecal impaction* may result in the passage of small, dry, rocky-hard masses called *scybala.* This type of stool may traumatize the rectal mucosa sufficiently to cause hemorrhage, in which case the fecal masses are streaked with red blood.

Ultrasonography

Ultrasonography is a noninvasive diagnostic technique in which sound waves are passed into internal body structures; varying deflections of these sound waves are bounced back, much like a reflection. Reflections, in turn, are displayed on an oscilloscope. Vertical deflections from a horizontal baseline represent the depth of the reflected tissues. When scans are taken from several angles, and a computer is added to the system, a two-dimensional image of the abdominal organs can be produced. Usually, for abdominal examination, a transducer is placed on the abdomen after a coating of lubricant jelly has been applied to the skin.

The chief advantage of the ultrasonography is the spatial reproduction of masses in transverse and longitudinal directions. There is no ionizing radiation or any noticeable biological side-effects in the energy range used for diagnostic purposes. It is relatively inexpensive. This type of diagnostic procedure is useful in studying the liver, pancreas, spleen, gallbladder, and retroperitoneal tissues.

Disadvantages include the following:

- A high degree of skill is required of the operator.
- This technique cannot be used when a structure to be examined lies behind bony tissue, which prevents passage of sound waves to deeper structures.
- Gas in the abdomen or air in the lungs present a problem, since ultrasound is not well transmitted through gas or air.

Endoscopic ultrasonography provides a clearer image of lesions in the gastrointestinal tract than conventional abdominal ultrasonography because imaging is not distorted by gas in the intestines.

Computed Tomography

Computed tomography (CT scanning) is a diagnostic method in which a very narrow x-ray beam is used to detect the density differences from very small cubes of tissue. These data are computerized and then reconstructed so that transverse cross-sections of the body can be shown on a television monitor.

The indications for CT scanning are diseases of the liver, spleen, kidney, pancreas, and pelvic organs. However, good detail depends on the presence of fat, which means that this diagnostic tool is not useful for very thin, cachectic patients. Also, since a scanning time of 5 seconds is required, it is impossible to maintain complete stillness (*e.g.*, heartbeat) during the procedure. Therefore, motion artifacts are produced and the results are a less than clear picture. Finally, radiation doses are appreciable.

Magnetic Resonance Imaging (MRI)

Magnetic resonance imaging (MRI) for gastroenterology is currently used to supplement, not replace, ultrasonography and computed tomography. For MRI examination, the patient lies within a machine that is constructed around a cylindrical magnet that produces a static magnetic field. This magnetic field interacts with certain nuclei (*e.g.*, hydrogen and phosphorus) to produce a net magnetization. Detection of this magnetization is possible because atomic nuclei in cells absorb or emit radio frequency electromagnetic radiation. Radio frequency electromagnetic waves, applied using an antenna coil, interact with the nuclei to produce a net rotation of the magnetization. During a recovery period, the antenna coil receives the electromagnetic signal emitted by the nuclei as they reorient themselves to the original net magnetization. This signal contains the information necessary to reconstruct an image.

The entire procedure takes 30 to 90 minutes. There is no specific patient preparation except for abdominal or pelvic scans. Patients having magnetic resonance imaging of the abdomen or pelvis can have nothing by mouth for 6 hours before the procedure.

Nursing Assessment

The nurse performs a physical examination and takes a complete history. She focuses on symptoms common to gastrointestinal dysfunction. A sample assessment guide is found in Chart 31-2.

Pain.   Pain can be a major symptom of gastrointestinal disease. The character, duration, frequency, and time of the pain vary greatly, depending on the underlying cause, which affects the location and distribution of referred pain. Other factors, such as meals, rest, defecation, and vascular disorders, may directly affect pain.

Indigestion.   Indigestion can result from disturbed nervous control of the stomach or from a disorder in the stomach or elsewhere in the body. Fatty foods tend to cause the most discomfort because they remain in the stomach longer than proteins or carbohydrates. Coarse vegetables and highly seasoned foods can also cause considerable distress.

Upper abdominal pain associated with eating is the most common complaint of patients with gastrointestinal dysfunction. The basis for the abdominal distress may be the patient's own gastric peristaltic movements. Bowel movements may or may not relieve the pain.

Intestinal "Gas" (Belching and Flatulence).   The accumulation of gas in the gastrointestinal tract may result in *belching*, the expulsion of gas from the stomach through the mouth, or *flatulence*, the expulsion of gas from the rectum.

Air that reaches the stomach is quickly expelled, but not necessarily by belching. Periodically, stomach gas moves into the lower esophagus (simple reflux) and then returns to the stomach, owing to a peristaltic contraction of the distal esophagus. Belching occurs when simple reflux is accompanied by contraction of the anterior abdominal muscles. At the first urge to belch, simply swallowing may interrupt the belch.

Usually, gases in the intestine pass into the colon and are released as flatus. Patients often complain of bloating, distention, or being "full of gas."

So-called heartburn, acid eructation, and so forth, are due to reverse peristalsis, probably gastroesophageal reflux.

Vomiting.   The involuntary act of vomiting is preceded by closure of the glottis and pylorus, together with relaxation of the gastric wall and the cardiac orifice. With retching, the cardiac orifice remains closed so gastric contents are not expelled. Vomiting is usually preceded by nausea, an unpleasant sensation suggesting that vomiting is imminent.

Hematemesis.   Hematemesis is the vomiting of blood. When this happens soon after hemorrhage, the vomitus is bright red. If blood has been retained in the stomach, digestive processes change the hemoglobin to a brown pigment, which

Chart 31-2
Assessment of Gastrointestinal Functioning

General Nutritional Information

Patient name: _____

Current weight: _____ .   Ideal body weight: _____ .   Age: _____   Sex: _____ .

Height: _____ .

There has been a recent (weight gain, weight loss) _____ over _____ months of _____ pounds. At home, food is purchased by _____ and prepared by _____ .

Dietary record for past 72 hours: Food description and quantity

	Breakfast	Lunch	Dinner	Snack	Snack	Total Daily Calories
Day #1						
Day #2						
Day #3						

Symptoms of Gastrointestinal Dysfunction

Is (able, unable) to chew food. Description of any disorder _____ .

Has recently experienced _____ .

   Anorexia, the lack of appetite for food.

   Dysphagia, difficulty with swallowing.

   Polyphagia, a voracious appetite or excessive eating.

   Odynophagia, pain on swallowing.

The above symptom has existed for _____ (days, weeks, months). It is aggravated by _____ and relieved by _____ .

(Does, does not) experience indigestion. Foods that tend to cause the most discomfort are _____ .

Relief measures include _____ .

(Has, has not) experienced heartburn. Relief measures include _____ .

(Does, does not) experience pain. Pain can be described as _____ and of _____ duration. It occurs (frequency) _____ . It is aggravated by _____ and relieved by _____ . It seems to be localized in the _____ region.

It (does, does not) radiate to the _____ .

   Esophageal: Retrosternal; may radiate to back

   Gastric: Epigastric; may radiate to back, especially left subscapular

   Duodenal: Epigastric; may radiate to back, especially right subscapular

   Gallbladder: Right upper quadrant or epigastric; may radiate to back or right subscapular

   Pancreatic: Epigastric; may radiate to back or left lumbar

   Appendicular: Periumbilical, later to right lower quadrant

   Colonic: Hypogastrium, right or left lower quadrant

   Rectal: Pelvic area

Has recently experienced _____ .

   Vomiting, the forceful expulsion of gastric contents up through the esophagus.

   Retching, abdominal muscles contract in an attempt to expel contents.

   Hematemesis, the vomiting of blood that is bright red or "coffee ground" in appearance.

The above symptom has existed for _____ (days, weeks). It occurs _____ times per day.

It is aggravated by _____ and relieved by _____ . Description of vomitus:

   Quantity _____ Odor _____ Color _____ Taste _____

   Presence of _____ (food particles, blood, mucus).

Has recently experienced _____ (diarrhea, constipation).

The above symptom has existed for _____ (days, weeks, months). It is aggravated by _____ and relieved by _____ . Description of stool:

   Content _____ Color _____ Consistency _____ Odor _____ .

Associated factors: Daily fluid intake _____ Exercise pattern _____

Intake of high fiber foods _____ Activity pattern_____

Presence of (bleeding, hemorrhoids).

gives the vomitus a coffee-ground appearance. Occasionally, the patient has difficulty in differentiating between hematemesis and hemoptysis (expectoration of blood-tinged sputum), particularly if a coughing paroxysm has preceded it.

Diarrhea. Diarrhea, which is defined as the presence of more than the usual number of daily bowel movements or an increase in volume of stool, is a major abnormality of gastrointestinal function. A common mechanism for diarrhea is an increased rate of movement of the contents through the intestine and colon, so that inadequate time is available for absorption of the gastrointestinal secretions, resulting in an increased fluid content of the stool. Inflammation or other diseases of the colonic mucosa can also lead to diarrhea, as can infection from pathogens or parasites or overuse of cathartics. When these occur, water and electrolytes are not sufficiently reabsorbed and increased amounts of fluids or liquid reach the rectum, resulting in increased stool volume. *Steatorrhea,* defined as a large amount of fat in the stools, is commonly due to pancreatic disease. The decreased activity of pancreatic enzymes is responsible for decreased fat digestion. Disease of the biliary tract can also cause steatorrhea, owing to the absence of bile salts. The consequences of diarrhea are loss of potassium, causing electrolyte imbalance; loss of bicarbonate, leading to acidosis; and loss of nutrients, leading to malnutrition.

Constipation. Constipation is the retention of or a delay in expulsion of fecal content from the rectum. In this situation, water is absorbed from the fecal matter, producing stools that are hard and dry and of smaller volume than normal. A person is said to be constipated if he strains at stool more than 25% of the time or passes two or fewer stools per week.

A variety of factors can produce constipation, such as decreased food or fluid intake, or an intake of primarily low residue foods; decreased exercise or activity patterns; atony of the aged bowel; neuroses; colon or rectal lesions; and intestinal obstructions.

In the elderly, constipation and impaction can result from a decrease in the sensation to defecate due to the decreased response of tactile and stretch receptors in the rectum and the anal canal; decreased exercise; and decreased intake of high-fiber foods because of chewing difficulties secondary to ill-fitting dentures or lack of teeth.

Nursing Interventions

Nursing interventions for the patient requiring gastrointestinal diagnostic assessment include the following:

- Providing general information about a balanced diet and the nutritional factors that can cause gastrointestinal disturbances. Specific information cannot be provided until a diagnosis has been confirmed.
- Providing needed information about the test and the activities required of the patient; oral and written instructions should be given.
- Alleviating anxiety
- Assuring the patient that he will be helped to cope with his discomfort

- Encouraging family members, or others, to offer emotional support to the patient during the diagnostic testing

Bibliography

Books

Berk JE (ed). Bockus' Gastroenterology. Philadelphia, WB Saunders, 1985.

Drossman DA (ed). Manual of Gastroenterologic Procedures. New York, Raven Press, 1982.

Given BA. Gastroenterology in Clinical Nursing. St Louis, CV Mosby, 1984.

Kratzer GL and Demarest RJ. Office Management of Colon and Rectal Disease. Philadelphia, WB Saunders, 1985.

Porth CM. Pathophysiology: Concepts of Altered Health States, 2nd ed. Philadelphia, JB Lippincott, 1986.

Shinya H. Colonoscopy: Diagnosis and Treatment of Colonic Diseases. New York, Igaku-Shoin, 1982.

Williams SR. Nutrition and Diet Therapy. St Louis, Times Mirror/Mosby, 1985.

Articles

Al-Jurf AS. Upper abdominal pain: Identifying gastrointestinal causes. Consultant 1984 Dec; 24(12):67–82.

Bown SG et al. Endoscopic laser treatment of vascular anomalies of the upper gastrointestinal tract. Gut 1985 Dec; 26(12):1338–1348.

Christie JP. Malignant colon polyps: Cure by colonoscopy or colectomy? Am J Gastroenterol 1984 July; 79(7):543–547.

Cohen LB and Waye JD. Treatment of colonic polyps: Practical considerations. Clin Gastroenterol 1986 Apr; 15(2):359–376.

Cooper BT and Neumann CS. Upper gastrointestinal endoscopy in patients aged 80 years or more. Age Aging 1986 Nov; 15(6):343–349.

DiPalma JA, Brady CE, and Pierson WP. Colon cleansing: Acceptance by older patients. Am J Gastroenterol 1986 Aug; 81(8):652–655.

Engler MB and Engler MM. The hazards of magnetic resonance imaging. Am J Nurs 1986 June; 86(6):650.

Feczko PJ et al. Small colonic polyps: A reappraisal of their significance. Radiology 1984 Aug; 152(2):652–655.

Fleischer D. Lasers and gastroenterology. Am J Gastroenterol 1984 May; 79(5):406–410.

Fleischer D. Endoscopic palliative tumour therapy with laser irradiation. Clin Gastroenterol 1986 Apr; 15(2):273–278.

Freston JW. Chronic abdominal pain: Functional or organic? Hosp Pract 1985 Sept 30; 20(9):35–60.

Hoexter B et al. Common diseases of the anus and rectum. Hosp Med 1985 Sept; 21(9):110–137.

Ingegno AP and Dagradi AE. Historical note: The first total colonoscopy. Am J Gastroenterol 1985 Aug; 80(8):605–607.

Kleinman MS. Flexible fiberoptic sigmoidoscopy. Hosp Pract 1984 June; 19(6):106N–106O, 106S–106T.

Kreel L. Computed tomography in gastroenterology. Clin Gastroenterol 1984 June; 13(1):235–264.

Lamb C. Selecting a flexible signoidoscope. Patient Care. 1986 Mar 30; 20(16):26–29, 32, 34.

Lamy PP. Treating GI upset in older adults. J Gerontol Nurs 1985 July; 11(7):40, 42.

Lintott D and Herlinger H. Double-contrast examination. II: Small intestine. Clin Gastroenterol 1984 Jan; 13(1):73–98.

Macrae FA, Tan KG, and Williams CB. Towards safer colonoscopy: A report on the complications of 5000 diagnostic or therapeutic colonoscopies. Gut 1983 May; 24(5):376–383.

Meiri HB. Ultrasound in gastroenterology. Clin Gastroenterol 1984 Jan; 13(1):183–204.

Messner RL et al. Stop a killer with early detection . . . colorectal cancer. J Gerontol Nurs 1985 Nov; 11(11):8–10, 13–14.

Messner RL, Gardner SS, and Webb DD. Early detection: The priority in colorectal cancer. Cancer Nurs 1986 Feb; 9(1):8–14.

Newman FK, Ogburn-Russell L and Rutledge JN. Magnetic resonance imaging, the latest in diagnostic technology. Nursing '87 1987 Jan; 17(1):45–47.

Norfleet RG. Endoscopy: Lower GI tract. Hosp Med 1986 Mar; 22(3):93, 96, 98.

Palmer RC. Colorectal cancer: Current diagnostic screening of asymptomatic patients. Consultant 1986 Feb; 26(2):25–34.

Patras AZ and Brozenec SA. Gastrointestinal assessment. AORN J 1984 Nov; 40(5):726–731.

Salmon PR and Jong M. Endoscopic haemostasis of the upper gastrointestinal tract. Clin Gastroenterol 1986 Apr; 15(2):321–331.

Schuman BM. Endoscopy: Upper GI tract. Hosp Med 1986 Feb; 22(2): 111–120.

Simpkins KC. Double-contrast examination: Colon. Clin Gastroenterol 1984 Jan; 13(1):99–121.

Sivak MV. Video endoscopy. Clin Gastroenterol. 1986 Apr; 15(2):205–234.

Smith CE. Detecting acute abdominal distension: What to look for, what to do. Nursing '85 1985 Sept; 15(9):39–40.

Stone B et al. Hypercalcemia: A risk factor to patients undergoing gastrointestinal endoscopy. Am J Gastroenterol 1986 July; 81(7):516–518.

Sugarbaker PH. Endoscopy in cancer diagnosis and management. Hosp Pract 1984 Nov; 19(11):111–122.

Takemoto T et al. Endoscopic ultrasonography. Clin Gastroenterol 1986 Apr; 15(2):305–319.

Tytgat GNJ et al. Endoscopic palliative therapy of gastrointestinal and biliary tumors with prosthesis. Clin Gastroenterol 1986 Apr; 15(2): 249–271.

Trenkner SW and Larfer I. Double-contrast examination. I: Oesophagus, stomach and duodenum. Clin Gastroenterol 1984 Jan; 13(1):41–73.

Wilson C. The diagnostic work-up for the patient with inflammatory bowel disease. Nurs Clin North Am 1984 Mar; 19(1):51–59.

Zettel ER. Beaming in on the GI tract . . . laser treatment. Am J Nurs 1986 Mar; 86(3):280–282.

Chapter 32

Gastrointestinal Intubation and Special Nutritional Management

Gastrointestinal Intubation

Gastrointestinal intubation is the insertion of a short or a long flexible rubber or plastic tube into the stomach or intestine by way of the mouth or nose to (1) decompress the stomach and remove gas and fluid, (2) diagnose gastrointestinal motility, (3) administer medications and feedings, (4) treat an obstruction or bleeding site, and (5) obtain gastric contents for analysis. Any solution administered through a tube is either poured from a syringe or delivered by drip regulated by gravity or by an electric pump. Aspiration (suctioning) to remove gas and fluids is accomplished by using a syringe, an electric suction machine, or a built-in wall suction outlet.

A variety of tubes are used for decompression, aspiration, and irrigation (Miller-Abbott, Cantor, Harris, Ewald, Levin, Salem sump) and for administration of feedings and medications (Levin, Dobhoff, Keofeed, Flexiflo, Nutriflex, and Entriflex). The tubes differ in composition (rubber, polyurethane, silicone), length (90 cm to 3 m [36 inches to 10 feet]), size (No. 6 Fr to No. 18 Fr), purpose, and placement in the gastrointestinal tract (stomach, duodenum, jejunum).

Nasogastric Tubes

A nasogastric tube, or short tube, is introduced through the nose or the mouth into the stomach. Commonly used short tubes include the Levin tube, gastric sump tube, Nutriflex tube, and G. Moss tube, which are described below.

Levin Tube.   The Levin tube has a single lumen (No. 14 to 18 Fr) and is made of plastic or rubber with holes near its tip. The tube is used in adults to remove fluid and gas from the upper gastrointestinal tract, to obtain a specimen of gastric contents for laboratory studies, and to administer medications or feeding (gavage) directly into the gastrointestinal tract.

Circular markings at specific points on the tube serve as guides for insertion. A marking is made on the tube to indicate the midpoint (Fig. 32-1). The tube is advanced under close observation until this marking reaches the patient's nostril. When this occurs, the tube is in the stomach. Placement may be checked further by aspirating gastric contents with a syringe.

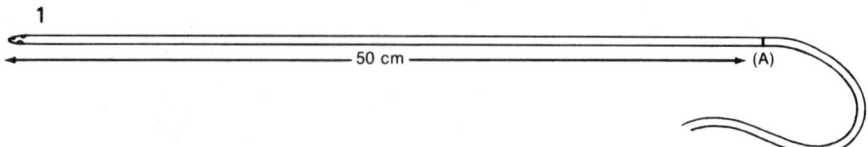

1. Mark the nasogastric tube at a point 50 cm. from the distal tip; call this point 'A'.

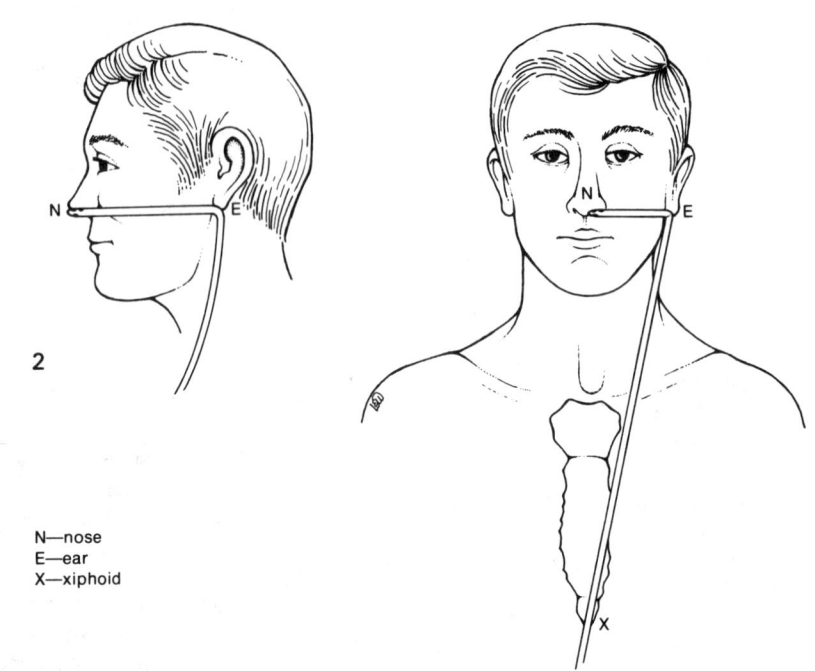

N—nose
E—ear
X—xiphoid

2. Have the patient sit in a neutral position with head facing forward. Place the distal tip of the tubing at the tip of the patient's nose (N); extend tube to the tragus (tip) of his ear (E), and then extend the tube straight down to the tip of his xiphoid (X). Mark this point 'B' on the tubing.

Figure 32-1
Nasogastric intubation using the Levin tube (short tube) or the Salem sump tube. (Based on research reported in Hanson RL. Predictive criteria for length of nasogastric tube insertion for tube feeding. J Parenteral Enteral Nutr 1979 May/June; 3[3]:160–163.)

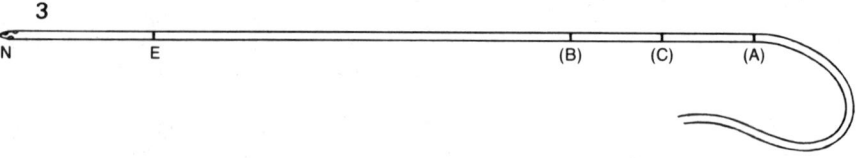

3. To locate point C on the tube, find the midpoint between points A and B. The nasogastric tube is passed to point C to ensure optimum placement in the stomach.

Gastric Sump Tube. The gastric sump tube (Salem, VENTROL) is a radiopaque, clear-plastic, double-lumen nasogastric tube (Fig. 32-2). It is used to decompress the stomach and keep it empty. The inner, smaller tube vents the larger suction-drainage tube to the atmosphere by means of an opening at the distal end of the tube. It is passed the same way as the Levin tube. It can protect gastric suture lines because, when used properly, the sump tube never allows the force of suction at the drainage "eyes," or outlets, to exceed 25 mm Hg, the level of capillary fragility. This action is controlled by a small vent tube (blue pigtail). Continuous suction is set at a low of 30 mm Hg with the pigtail (usually blue) outlet kept open. If available suction is intermittent, rather than continuous, it may be set at 80 to 120 mm Hg. Because of its cyclic setting, by the time suction reaches the gastric mucosa it will be reduced to about 25 mm Hg.

To prevent reflux of gastric contents through the vent lumen (blue pigtail), the vent lumen is kept above the patient's midline; otherwise it will act as a siphon. Irrigation may be done through either the main lumen or the vent lumen; if the vent lumen is used, irrigation is followed with 10 ml of air, to clear the lumen.

Nutriflex Tube. The Nutriflex nasogastric feeding tube is 76 cm (30 inches) long and has a mercury-weighted tip to facilitate insertion. It is coated with a Hydromer lubricant that is activated when moistened.

G. Moss Tube. The G. Moss nasoesophageal gastric decompression tube is 90 cm (35 inches) long and has a double lumen (see Fig. 32-5). It is anchored in the stomach by inflating the balloon. The decompression feeding catheter provides for esophageal and gastric aspiration as well as duodenal feeding.

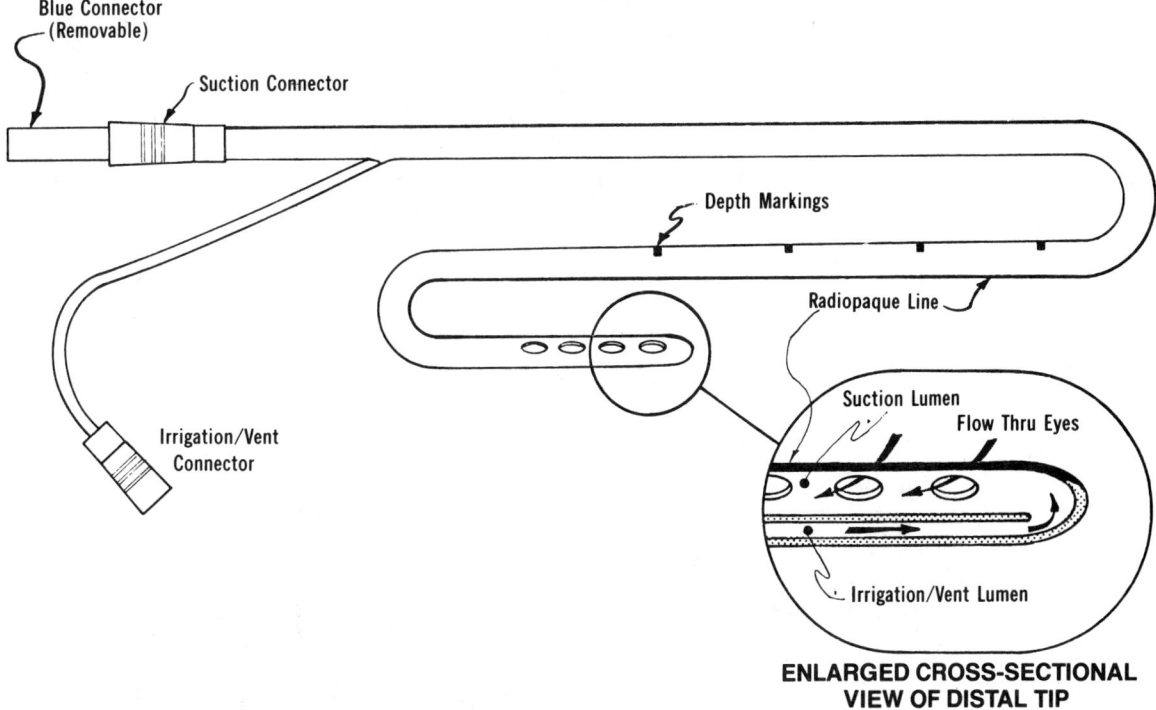

Figure 32-2
The VENTROL Levin (sump) tube. Note the blown-up version showing the direction of flow for suction and irrigation. (Courtesy of National Catheter Co, Argyle, New York.)

Nasoenteric Tubes

A nasoenteric tube, or long-tube, is introduced through the nose and passed through the esophagus and stomach into the intestinal tract. It is used to aspirate intestinal contents to prevent gas and fluid from distending the coils of intestine. This process is called *decompression*. Three major nasoenteric tubes that are used for aspiration and decompression are the Miller-Abbott tube, the Harris tube, and the Cantor tube. These tubes are used in the active treatment of intestinal obstruction of the small intestine. They are also used prophylactically, being inserted the night before an abdominal operation to prevent obstruction after the operation. The intestine is threaded on the tube and is thus shortened and held together compactly, making it relatively easier to pack off the intestine at the time of operation on the colon.

Because peristalsis either decreases or stops for 24 to 48 hours after an operation, owing to the effects of anesthesia and of visceral manipulation, nasogastric or nasoenteric suction are used for the following reasons:

- To evacuate fluids and flatus, so that vomiting is prevented and tension is reduced along the incision line
- To reduce edema, which can cause obstruction
- To enhance blood supply to the suture line, thereby providing nutrition to the site

Usually, the tubes are allowed to remain in place after operation until peristalsis is resumed, as determined by the presence of bowel sounds.

Miller-Abbott Tube. The Miller-Abbott tube is a double-lumen (No. 16 Fr) 3-meter (10-foot) tube, one lumen of which is used to introduce mercury or to inflate the balloon at the end of the tube; the other lumen, which is entirely independent, is used for aspiration. Before the tube is inserted, the balloon should be tested and its capacity measured; it is then deflated completely. The tube should be lubricated sparingly, and chilled well, before the tip is inserted through the patient's nose. Markings on the tube indicate the distance it has been passed.

Harris Tube. The Harris tube is a single-lumen (No. 14 F), mercury-weighted tube of about 1.8 meters (6 feet). This tube has a metal tip that is lubricated and introduced into the nostril. The mercury-weighted bag follows. The weight of the mercury carries the bag by gravity. Since this is a single-lumen tube that is used wholly for suction and irrigation, there is no difficulty in irrigating it. Usually, a Y tube is attached to the end of the tube, so that the suction apparatus is attached to one side and an outlet with a clamp is available on the other side for irrigating purposes.

Cantor Tube. The Cantor tube is 3 meters (10 feet) long with a No. 18 F lumen. Its distinguishing feature is that it is larger than the other long tubes and has 4 or 5 ml of mercury in the bag at the extreme end of the rubber tubing. Prior to insertion, the bag is wrapped about the tube. After the tube is lubricated, it is passed through the nostril and advanced to the esophagus (Fig. 32-3). The patient is in a sitting position and is offered sips of water to facilitate passage of the tube. Fluoroscopy is helpful in passing the tube into the duodenum.

Feeding Tubes. Several nasoenteric tubes that are commonly used for feeding include the Keofeed, Nyhus/Nelson, Moss, and Dobhoff tubes (Fig. 32-4). It usually takes

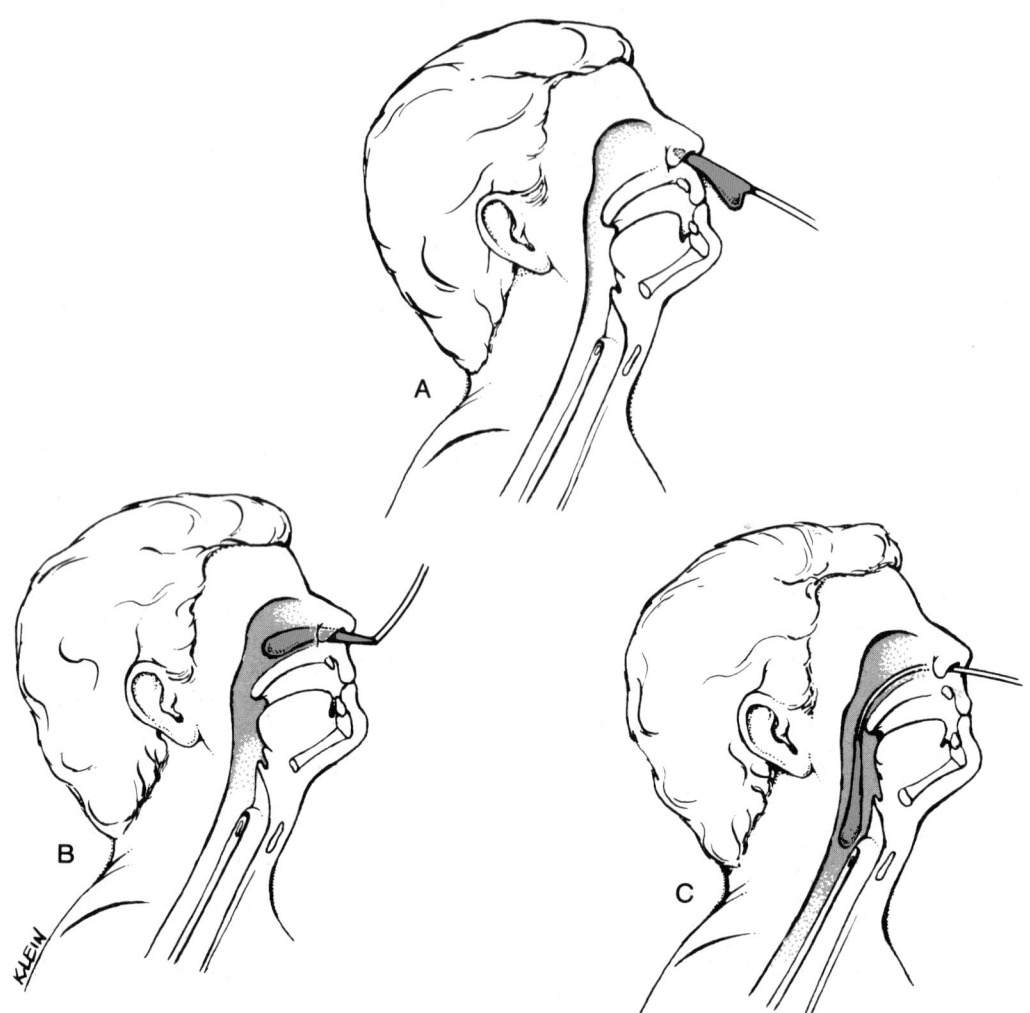

Figure 32-3
Passage of Cantor tube. (*A*) Tube with weighted mercury bag is introduced into the nostril. Note the natural tilt of the tubing. (*B*) After the mercury bag has entered the nostril, the catheter is tilted upward (head can also be tilted slightly upward) to facilitate gravity pull on the weighted bag. (*C*) The weight of the mercury pulls the bag downward. (Redrawn from Hardy JD. Rhoads Textbook of Surgery, 5th ed. Philadelphia, JB Lippincott.)

24 hours for the Dobhoff and the Keofeed tubes to pass through the stomach and into the intestines. Passage is facilitated by having the patient lie on his right side. The Nyhus/Nelson nasoenteral tube uses a twin balloon design to provide both gastric decompression and jejunal feeding. Both the Nyhus/Nelson and the Moss tubes are frequently used for postoperative enteral feeding to avoid negative nitrogen balance and to enhance wound healing (Fig. 32-5).

Nursing Interventions for Nasogastric and Nasoenteric Intubation

Nursing interventions are organized into the following areas:

- Instructing the patient about the purposes of the tube and the procedures required for insertion and advancement

- Inserting a nasogastric tube and assisting with the insertion of a nasoenteric tube
- Checking for placement of the nasogastric tube
- Advancing the nasoenteric tube
- Monitoring the patient
- Providing oral and nasal hygiene
- Removing the tube

Instruction. Before the patient is intubated, the nurse explains the purpose of the tube. This information may make the patient more cooperative and tolerant of an initially unpleasant procedure. The general activities related to the passage of the tube are then reviewed, including the fact that the patient may have to breathe through his mouth and that passage of the tube may cause him to gag until the tube has passed his gag reflex.

Insertion of the Tube. During insertion, the patient usually sits upright with a towel spread bib-fashion over his chest. Tissue wipes are made available. The patient is screened

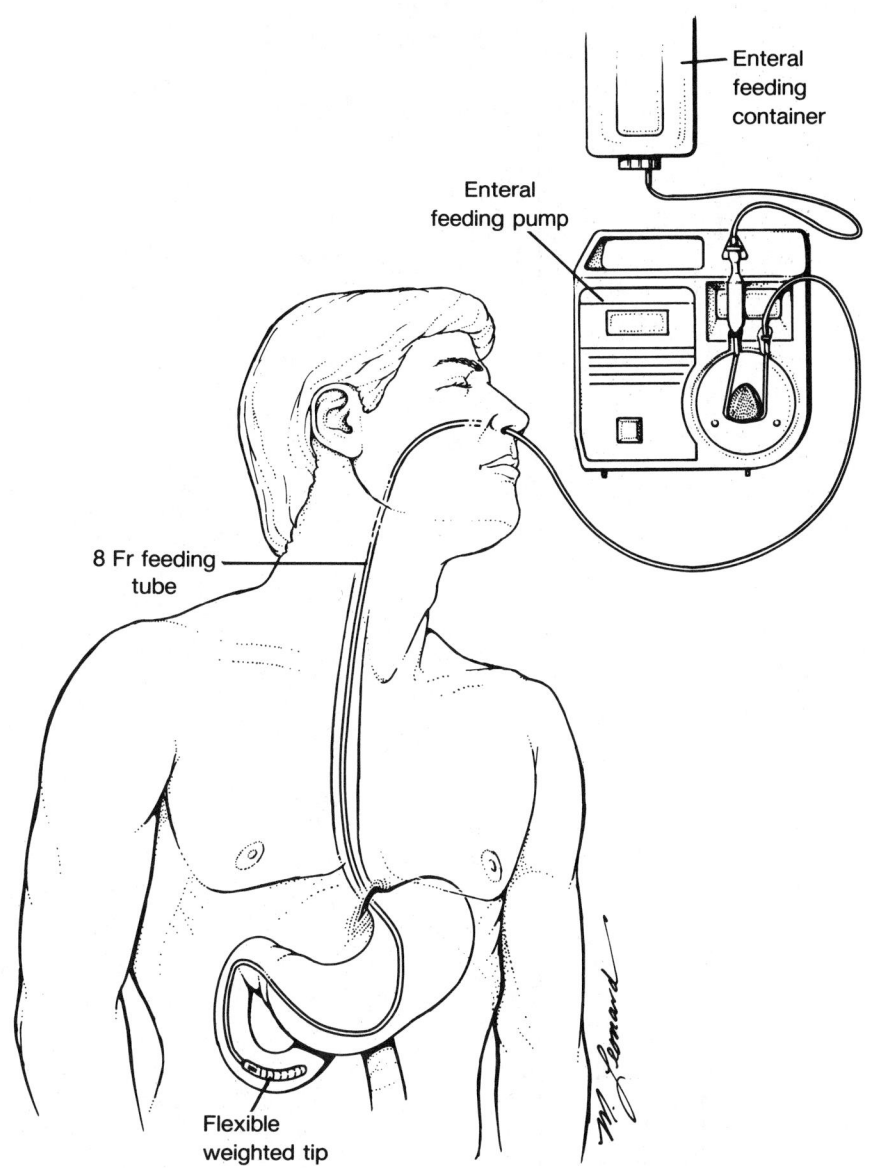

Enteral
feeding
container

Enteral
feeding pump

8 Fr feeding
tube

Figure 32-4
The enteral feeding tube (8 Fr) with a flexible weighted tip is readily passed into the stomach and through the pylorus into the duodenum or proximal jejunum.

Flexible
weighted tip

from other patients, and adequate light is provided. Occasionally, the physician will swab the nostril and spray the oropharynx with tetracaine (Pontocaine) to dull the nasal passage and the gag reflex and to make the procedure more tolerable. Gargling with a liquid anesthetic or holding ice chips in the mouth for a few minutes will have the same effect. Encouraging the patient to breathe through his mouth or pant often helps, as does swallowing water, if permitted.

A rubber nasogastric tube is sterilized and placed in a basin containing cracked ice for about 5 minutes before use to make the tubing firm. A polyurethane tube may need to be warmed to make it more pliable. The tube should be lubricated with a water-soluble substance (K-Y jelly) unless it has a dry coating called Hydromer, which, when moistened, provides lubrication for ease of insertion. After the tube is prepared, the patient is asked to tilt his head back so that the tube can be introduced through the nostril. When the tip is positioned in the stomach, the tube is secured to the nose or above the upper lip with tape. A recommended method is to apply tincture of benzoin to the skin where the nasogastric tube will be secured. The prepared area is covered

with a strip of hypoallergenic tape; then the tube is placed over the tape and secured with another piece of tape (Fig. 32-6). A nasoenteric tube can be secured with tape to the malar eminence (use a slight U-shaped loop) and then draped over the ear. This technique secures the tube during patient movement. Nasoenteric tubes are not taped immediately because it takes approximately 24 hours for these tubes to progress into the intestine.

Placement of the Nasogastric Tube. To check the placement of the nasogastric tube, a stethoscope is placed over the epigastrium and 5 ml of air is injected into the tube using a bulb syringe. A "whooshing" sound indicates that air is entering the stomach and not a bronchus. Another method is to aspirate stomach contents using a 10- to 20-ml syringe. Contents can be checked with pH paper. If the pH is above 7 (alkaline), the tube is in the intestine; if it is below 7 (acid), the tube is still in the stomach.

Advancement of the Nasoenteric Tube. After the tube has passed through the pyloric sphincter, it may be advanced 5 to 7.5 cm (2 to 3 inches) every hour, so that gravity and peristalsis will aid in the passage of the tube. The patient is

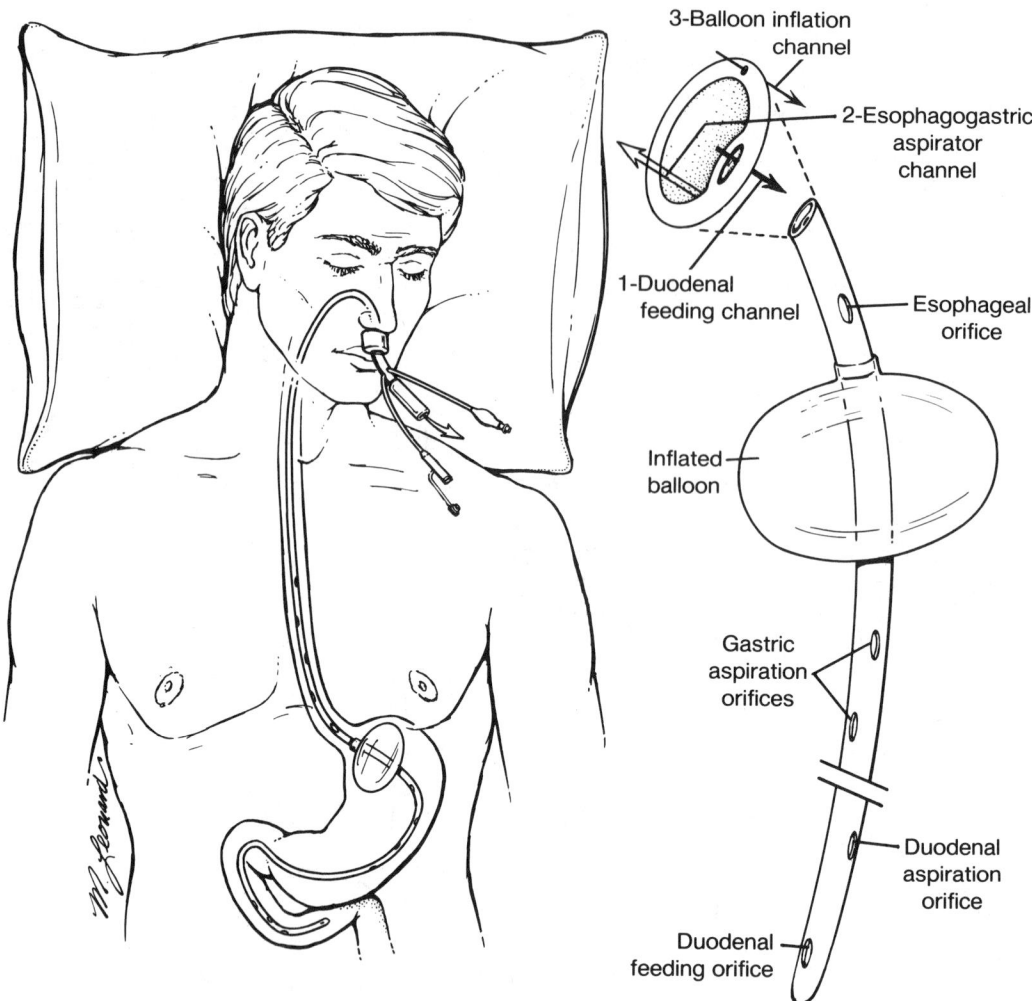

Figure 32-5
The G. Moss esophageal/duodenal decompression and feeding catheter. There are three channels: (1) the duodenal feeding channel; (2) the esophagogastric aspiration channel, which has additional openings into the proximal duodenum, as well as the stomach and the distal esophagus; and (3) the balloon inflation channel.

generally asked to lie on his right side for 2 hours, on his back for 2 hours, and then on his left side for 2 hours. Ambulation, if possible, also helps to advance the tube. If the tube is advanced too rapidly, it will curl and kink in the stomach.

Monitoring the Patient. The nasogastric tube is attached to straight drainage or intermittent low suction. If used for enteral nutrition, the end is wrapped in gauze and clamped closed between feedings. Confirmation of tube placement is essential before any fluids are instilled. Tube displacement is caused by tension on the tube (when the patient moves around in the bed or room), coughing, tracheal or nasotracheal suctioning, and airway intubation.

An accurate record is kept of all fluid intake, feedings, and irrigation. Normal saline is recommended for irrigations to avoid electrolyte loss through gastric drainage. The amount, color, and type of all drainage are recorded every 8 hours.

When double- or triple-lumen tubes are used, the individual tubes intended for aspiration, feeding, and balloon inflation are labeled. To avoid tension on the tube, the tube line from the nose to the drainage unit is fixed in position,

either with a safety pin or with adhesive-tape loops that are pinned to the patient's pajamas or gown. The tube must be looped loosely to prevent tension and dislodgment.

Oral and Nasal Hygiene. Regular and conscientious oral and nasal hygiene is a vital part of patient care, since the tube may be in place for several days. Applicator sticks dipped in water can be used to clean the nose. This can be followed by cleansing with water-soluble oil. Frequent mouth attention is comforting. If the nasal and pharyngeal mucosa is excessively dry, steam or cool vapor inhalations may be beneficial. Throat lozenges, an ice collar, chewing gum (if permitted), and frequent movement also assist in relieving discomfort. These activities will keep the mucous membranes moist and will help prevent infection of the parotid glands.

Removal of Tube. When it is desirable to remove the tube, it is necessary to deflate the balloon and withdraw it, gently and slowly, for 15 to 20 cm (6 to 8 inches), at intervals of 10 minutes, until the tip reaches the esophagus when the remainder is withdrawn rapidly from the nostril. If the tube does not come out easily, force should not be used—a physician is notified.

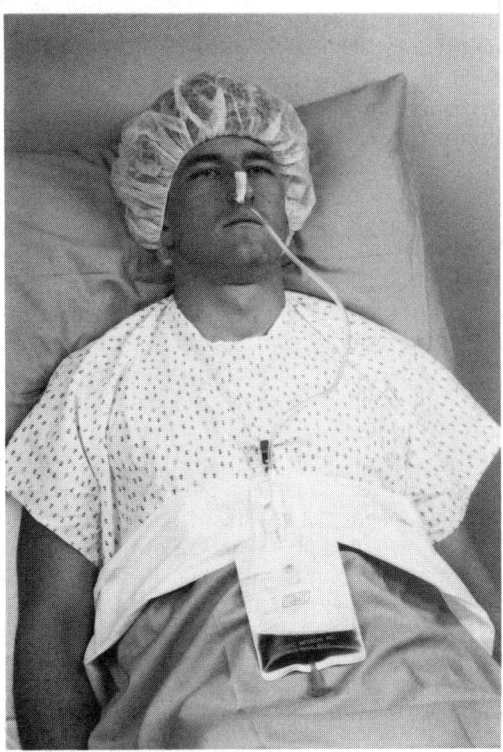

Figure 32-6
Nasogastric tube attachment and drainage bag. The tube is secured to the nose to prevent injury to the nasopharyngeal passages. The lightweight portable drainage bag is secured with a metal clip to the patient's gown or the bedclothes. (Photograph courtesy of Towic Medical, Inc., Park Ridge, Illinois).

As it is withdrawn, the tube is concealed in a towel, because the sight of it may cause the patient to vomit. After removal of the tube, the patient will be grateful for good mouth care.

Assessment for Possible Complications. Patients undergoing suction decompression are susceptible to a variety of problems, including fluid volume deficit. pulmonary complications, and parotitis, which require careful ongoing assessment, as follows:

Fluid Volume Deficit

1. Symptoms indicating a fluid volume deficit include

   - Dryness of skin and mucous membranes
   - Decreasing urinary output
   - Lethargy and exhaustion
   - Drop in body temperature

2. Assessment of fluid volume deficit involves maintaining an accurate record of the following:

   - Drainage—amount, color, and type, every 8 hours
   - Amount of fluid instilled by irrigation of the nasogastric catheter and the amount of water taken by mouth. An isotonic solution, such as normal saline, is used for irrigations in order to avoid electrolyte loss through gastric drainage.
   - Amount and character of vomitus, if any

- Duration of any period in which the suction apparatus did not appear to function
- Effects produced by the treatment

Pulmonary Complications

1. Nasogastric intubation produces a higher incidence of postoperative pulmonary complications by interfering with coughing and clearing of the pharynx.
2. The nurse examines the lung fields regularly, through auscultation, to determine the presence of congestion. In addition, the patient is encouraged to cough and to take deep breaths regularly. The nurse also carefully confirms the proper placement of the tube before instilling any fluids.

Parotitis

1. When administering oral hygiene, the nurse carefully inspects the mucous membranes for signs of irritation or excessive dryness. In addition, she palpates the area around the parotid glands to detect any soreness or lumps and any skin or mucous membrane irritation or necrosis.
2. The nostrils, oral mucosa, esophagus, and trachea are susceptible to irritation and necrosis. Visible areas are inspected frequently and the adequacy of hydration is assessed. In addition, the patient is assessed for the presence of esophagitis and tracheitis. Symptoms include sore throat and hoarseness.

Nasogastric and Nasoenteric Tube Feedings

Tube feedings are given to meet nutritional requirements when oral intake is inadequate or not possible. Tube feedings are delivered to the stomach (nasogastric) or the distal duodenum or proximal jejunum (nasoenteric) when it is necessary to bypass the esophagus and stomach. The numerous conditions requiring enteral nutrition are summarized in Table 32-1.

Liquid formulas are designed to improve nutritional intake by either oral or tube administration. Tube feedings have several advantages:

- Intraluminal delivery of nutrients preserves gastrointestinal integrity.
- Tube feedings preserve the normal sequence of intestinal and hepatic metabolism prior to nutrient delivery to the arterial circulation.
- The intestinal mucosa and liver are important in fat metabolism and are the only sites of lipoprotein synthesis.
- Normal insulin–glucagon ratios are maintained with the intestinal administration of carbohydrates.

Commercial formulas frequently present problems because the composition is "fixed." Some patients may not be able to tolerate certain ingredients, such as sodium, protein, or potassium. "Modular" diets can be prepared commercially, and the critical constituents of sodium, potassium, and fat can be added by the dietitian. Attention is given to including all essential minerals and vitamins. Total intake of calories

TABLE 32-1
Conditions Requiring Enteral Nutrition

Condition or Need	Cause
Preoperative preparation with elemental diet	
Gastrointestinal problems with elemental diet	Fistulas, short bowel syndrome, Crohn's disease, ulcerative colitis, nonspecific maldigestion or malabsorption
Cancer therapy	Radiation, chemotherapy
Convalescent care	Surgery, injury, severe illness
Coma, semiconsciousness*	Stroke, head injury
Hypermetabolic conditions	Burns, trauma, multiple fractures, sepsis
Alcoholism, chronic depression, anorexia nervosa*	Chronic illness, psychiatric or neurologic disorder
Debilitation*	Senility, disease
Maxillofacial or cervical surgery	Disease or injury
Oropharyngeal or esophageal paralysis*	Disease or injury
Mental retardation*	

* Some of these patients will be at risk for regurgitating or vomiting and aspirating administered formula. Accordingly, each case must be considered individually.

(Jensen T. Home enteral nutrition. Dietetic Currents, Ross Timesaver 1982 July/Aug; 9:15–20.)

and nutrients is assessed when there is a reduction in total intake, or excessive dilution, of feedings.

Many patients are highly resistant to tube feedings, particularly those feedings administered via nasogastric intubation. Often a medium- or fine-bore Silastic tube is tolerated better than a plastic or rubber tube. The finer-bore tube, however, requires a finely dispersed formula to prevent the tube from clogging.

A wide variety of containers, feeding tubes and catheters, delivery systems (Kangaroo 2, IMED-430, Dobhoff, Keofeed II, Flexiflo II), and pumps are available for use in tube or enteral feedings. The decision as to what to use is made after considering the most appropriate formula and delivery system for a given patient: nutrient sources, concentrations, osmolality, viscosity, and mineral content of a given formula, as well as the method and rate of administration, patient dexterity, available storage and refrigerator space, and cost of the formula and supportive equipment. Some commonly used commercial tube feedings include Ensure, Compleat-B, Isocal, Sustacal, and Vivonex. Pulmocare is a specialized formula for patients with pulmonary disorders that is high in fat and low in carbohydrates. Its high density (1.5 calories/ml) is ideal for patients who require fluid restriction, and it is also designed to reduce carbon dioxide production.

Some feedings are given as supplements, and others are provided to meet the patient's total nutritional needs. Nutritionists work closely with physicians and nurses in determining the best formula for the individual patient.

Osmosis and Osmolality. Solutions that are highly concentrated and foods that have certain characteristics can upset the normal water balance within the body. Fluid balance is maintained by the process of *osmosis*. It is accomplished within the body by moving water through membranes from a dilute solution of lower osmolality to a more concentrated one of higher osmolality until the solutions are nearly of equal osmolality. The osmolality of normal body fluids is approximately 300 mOsm/kg. The body attempts to keep the osmolality of the contents of the stomach and intestines at approximately this level.

The proteins are extremely large particles and therefore have little or no osmotic effect. However, individual amino acids and carbohydrates are smaller particles and therefore have greater osmotic effect. Fats are not water soluble and do not form a solution in water; thus, they have no osmotic effect. Since electrolytes such as sodium and potassium are comparatively small particles, they have a great effect on osmolality, and consequently on tolerance.

Osmolality is an important consideration for patients being fed past the pylorus. When a concentrated solution of high osmolality is taken in large amounts, water will move to the stomach and intestines from fluid surrounding the organs and the vascular compartment. The patient experiences a feeling of fullness, nausea, and diarrhea, which can bring about dehydration, resulting, in some cases, in hypotension and tachycardia. Collectively, these symptoms have been termed the *dumping syndrome*. This problem can generally be alleviated by starting the patient on a more dilute solution and by increasing the concentration over several days.

There is a wide range of tolerance among patients as to the effects of osmolality. Usually, debilitated patients are more sensitive to such disorders. Therefore, the nurse should be knowledgeable about the osmolality of formulas and should observe and prevent such disorders.

▶ Nursing Process
The Patient Receiving a Tube Feeding

▷ Assessment

The nurse participates in the assessment of patients with suspected nutritional problems. A preliminary assessment includes the family's need for information and should answer the following questions:

- What is the patient's nutritional status as judged by his current physical appearance; dietary history, including a history of food intolerance; and recent weight loss or gain?
- Are there any existing chronic illnesses or situations that will increase metabolic demands on the body?
- Is his fluid and electrolyte balance in order?
- Is his digestive tract functioning? Does it have good absorptive capacity?
- Are his kidneys and urinary system adequate?

- What medications is he on, and what other therapy is he receiving that may affect his digestive intake and digestive system?
- Does the dietary prescription fulfill his needs?

In addition, a more elaborate assessment is done on those patients who may require extensive nutritional therapy. This is done by a team that includes the nurse, physician, and nutritionist. In addition to the history and physical examination, nutritional assessment consists of recording any weight change, determining serum albumin and transferrin levels and total lymphocyte count, testing of delayed hypersensitivity reaction, and evaluating muscle function.

▷ *Nursing Diagnoses*

Based on all the assessment data, the major nursing diagnoses may include the following:

- Alteration in nutrition, less than body requirements, related to inadequate intake or nutrients
- Alteration in bowel elimination, diarrhea related to the dumping syndrome
- Potential ineffective airway clearance related to aspiration of tube feeding
- Potential ineffective individual coping related to the discomfort imposed by the presence of the nasogastric/nasoenteric tube

▷ *Planning and Implementation*

▷ *Goals:* The major goals of the patient may include attainment and maintenance of nutritional balance, maintenance of a normal bowel pattern, maintenance of a patent airway, and improvement in individual coping.

Nursing Interventions

Nutritional Balance. When preparing and administering a tube feeding, it is essential that all measures of cleanliness be observed. Temperature of the feeding, volume of the feeding, flow rate, and adequate fluid intake are critically important.

The schedule determining the quantity and frequency of tube feedings is maintained. The nurse must therefore carefully monitor the rate of drip and avoid too rapid administration of fluids. Commonly used electrical pumps to control the rate and pressure of the delivery of viscous fluids are relatively heavy and must be attached to an IV pole. However, several pumps that have been designed specifically for enteral tube feedings are lightweight and easy to handle, and require minimal instructions for use. Some examples are the Kangaroo Easy-Cap II (Chesebrough-Pond's, Inc); the Flexiflo II Portable Enteral Nutrition Pump (Ross Laboratories), which can be carried by using a nylon adjustable strap and can operate for 8 hours on a rechargeable battery; the Enteroport (Diatek, Inc), designed for continuous home feedings and available with a portable shoulder strap; the IMED 430 Enteral Delivery System (IMED); and the Flo Gard 2000 peristaltic pump (Travenol Laboratories).

The newer polyurethane or silicone rubber feeding tubes have small diameters (No. 6 to 8 Fr) and tungsten tips (rather than a weighted mercury-filled bag), and some have a water-activated lubricant that makes it easier to place the tube and insert and remove the stylet. The various tubes come with instructions for ease of passage. Since they are softer, more pliable, and much thinner than the conventional nasogastric tube, they provide greater patient comfort. However, kinking of tubing may present a problem. A guide or stylet is recommended for ease of passage. Essentially, such a tube is passed in the same way as a nasogastric tube, that is, with the patient in high Fowler's position. If this is not feasible, the patient is placed on his right side.

Residual gastric content is checked before each feeding. (This solution is returned to the patient.) If the amount of aspirated gastric content is greater than 150 ml, the feeding is delayed and the patient's condition reassessed in 2 hours. If this occurs twice, the physician is notified.

Before and after the administration of tube feedings, about 50 ml of water is administered to ensure tube patency and to decrease the chance of bacterial growth, tube crusting or occlusion.

Feedings are administered either by gravity (drip) or by continuous controlled pump that is either volumetric (ml/hour) or peristaltic (drops/hour). With jejunal feedings, continuous pump infusions are usually necessary.

Feedings are lactose free, with an osmolality of only 300 mOsm/kg; a feeding may be given undiluted and provides 1 calorie/ml. Feeding rates of about 100 to 150 ml/hr (2400 to 3600 calories/day) are effective in inducing positive nitrogen balance and progressive weight gain, without producing abdominal cramps and diarrhea. If the feeding is intermittent, 200 to 350 ml is given in 10 to 15 minutes. Additional water after feeding is important to prevent hypertonic dehydration. At the beginning of administration, the feeding is diluted to at least half the strength and not more than 50 to 100 ml given at a time, or 40 to 60 ml/hr in continuous drip administration. This gradual administration helps the patient to develop tolerance, especially for hyperosmolar solutions.

Continuous monitoring of the tube-feeding regimen is necessary to determine its effectiveness.

- Assess placement of tubing, position of patient, and flow rate.
- Observe patient's ability to tolerate the formula (assess for feeling of fullness, bloating, urticaria, nausea, vomiting, diarrhea, and constipation).
- Check clinical responses, as noted in laboratory findings: blood urea nitrogen, hemoglobin, serum protein, and hematocrit.
- Assess the patient's general condition by noting the appearance of the skin (turgor, dryness, color) and mucous membranes; urinary output; state of hydration; and weight gain or loss.
- Observe for signs of dehydration (dry mucous membranes, thirst, decreased urine output).
- Record the actual formula intake by the patient, including incidents of vomiting and diarrhea or distention.
- Note any signs of inability of the patient to communicate.
- Report a glucose concentration of +3 or +4, decreased urinary output, sudden weight gain, and periorbital or dependent puffiness.
- Assess for possible complications (Table 32-2).

Bowel Pattern. Patients on nasogastric or nasoenteric tube feedings frequently experience diarrhea (watery stools

TABLE 32-2
Complications of Enteral Therapy

Complication	Cause
Tube displacement	Excessive coughing
	Tension of the tube
	Tracheal suctioning
	Airway intubation
Nasopharyngeal irritation	Tube position
Diarrhea	Hyperosmolar feedings
	Rapid infusion
	Feeding administered at a temperature that is either too cold or too hot.
	Bacterial contamination
Dehydration and azotemia (excess of urea in the blood)	Hyperosmolar feedings with insufficient fluid intake
	Excessive urea from high-protein mixtures and formulas lacking fat
Atelectasis and possible pneumonia	Aspirated tube feeding

occurring three times in 24 hours). Pasty, unformed stool is expected with enteral therapy because most formulas (except Enrich and Compleat-B) have little or no residue. The dumping syndrome also leads to diarrhea. To confirm that the dumping syndrome is causing the diarrhea, other possible causes must be ruled out: zinc deficiency (15 mg of zinc every 24 hours is recommended via the feeding to maintain a normal serum level of 50 to 150 μg/dl [7.65 to 22.95 μmol/L]), contaminated formula, malnutrition (a decrease in the intestinal absorptive area resulting from malnutrition can cause diarrhea), and drug therapy. Antibiotics such as clindamycin (Cleocin) and lincomycin (Lincocin), antiarrhythmic drugs (quinidine, propranolol [Inderal]), aminophylline (Theophylline), and digitalis are known to increase the frequency of the dumping syndrome in certain patients.

The dumping syndrome (discussed in Chapter 33, p. 796) results from the rapid distention of the jejunum when hypertonic solutions are administered quickly (over 10 to 20 minutes). Foods high in carbohydrates and electrolytes draw extracellular fluid from the blood into the jejunum so that dilution and absorption can occur. The gastrointestinal symptoms (diarrhea, nausea) associated with the dumping syndrome can be managed by

- Decreasing the instillation rate to provide time for carbohydrates and electrolytes to be diluted
- Giving the feedings at room temperature, because temperature extremes stimulate peristalsis
- Administering the feeding by continuous drip rather than bolus (if permitted) to prevent sudden distention of the intestine

- Advising the patient to remain in semi-Fowler's position for 30 minutes after the feeding (this position prolongs transit time by decreasing the influence of gravity)
- Instilling the minimal amount of water needed to flush the tubing before and after a feeding because fluid given with a feeding increases transit time

Airway Management. Airway obstruction occurs when stomach contents or enteral feedings are regurgitated and aspirated or when a nasogastric tube is improperly placed and feedings are instilled into the pharynx or the trachea. Nasoenteric tubes, especially those that provide for gastric and esophageal/duodenal decompression (Nyhus/Nelson, Moss), have helped decrease the frequency of regurgitation and aspiration.

To maintain a patent airway, the nurse should always check tube placement before giving a feeding and always administer the feeding with the patient in the proper position to prevent regurgitation. The semi-Fowler's position is recommended for a nasogastric feeding; the patient's head should be elevated at least 30 degrees for a nasoenteric feeding.

If aspiration is suspected, the feeding is stopped, the nasogastric tube is removed, and the pharynx and trachea are suctioned if necessary. The nurse should notify a physician and maintain a calm affect. She must be supportive to the patient, who may feel that he is going to suffocate and die.

Promoting Coping Ability. The psychosocial goal of nursing care is to provide support, encouragement, and a warm acceptance of the patient, while conveying hope that daily progressive improvement is possible. If the patient is having difficulty adjusting to the treatment, the nurse intervenes by

- Praising him when he adheres to the medical plan of care
- Encouraging self-care within the parameters of his activity level (making his bed, recording his daily weight and intake and output)
- Reinforcing an optimistic approach by mentioning signs and symptoms that indicate progress (daily weight gain, electrolyte balance, absence of nausea and diarrhea)

Patient Education and Home Health Care. Preparation for home care management of enteral feedings begins when the patient is hospitalized. The nurse teaches while administering the feedings so that the mechanics of the procedure are observed and reinforced. Prior to discharge, information is provided about the equipment, formula purchase and storage, and administration of the feedings (frequency, quantity, rate of instillation). Family members who will participate in the patient's home care are invited to all teaching sessions. Available printed information about the delivery equipment and formula is distributed and reviewed. The patient is encouraged to handle the equipment under the supervision of a nurse.

When the patient is at home a visiting nurse will monitor his progress (weight, vital signs, activity level, electrolyte values) and assess for any complications (dumping syndrome, nausea/vomiting, weight loss, lethargy, confusion, excessive thirst). The patient is encouraged to keep a diary in which he records times and amounts of feedings and any symptoms that occur. The nurse can review the diary during home visits.

▷ *Evaluation*

▷ *Expected Outcomes*

1. Patient attains/maintains nutritional balance.
   a. Has positive nitrogen balance.
   b. Hematologic diagnostic studies within normal limits (*i.e.*, BUN, hemoglobin, hematocrit, serum protein).
   c. Attains or maintains desired body weight.
   d. Attains or maintains hydration of body tissue.
2. Is free from episodes of diarrhea.
   a. Has fewer than three watery stools a day.
   b. Does not have a bowel movement after a bolus feeding.
   c. States he has no intestinal cramping.
   d. Has normal bowel sounds.
3. Maintains an open airway.
   a. Has normal breath sounds.
   b. Evidences normal heart rate and respirations.
   c. Has a negative chest x-ray film.
4. Copes effectively with tube feeding regimen.
   a. Asks to help with administering the feedings.
   b. Projects a positive affect.
   c. Participates in self-care activities.
   d. Offers encouragement and support to others who are receiving tube feedings.

Gastrostomy

A gastrostomy is an operation performed to create an opening into the stomach for the purpose of administering food and fluids. In some instances, a gastrostomy is used for prolonged nutrition, as in the elderly or debilitated patient. Gastrostomy is preferred to nasogastric feedings in the comatose patient because the cardioesophageal sphincter remains intact. Also, regurgitation may occur in nasogastric feedings but is less likely in gastrostomy.

Several commonly employed feeding gastrostomies are the Stamm (temporary and permanent), Janeway (permanent), and percutaneous endoscopic gastrostomy (temporary). The Stamm and Janeway gastrostomies (Fig. 32-7) require either an upper abdominal midline incision or a left upper quadrant transverse incision. The Stamm procedure requires the use of concentric purse-string sutures to secure a tube to the anterior gastric wall. A stab wound exit is created in the left upper abdomen to provide for a gastrostomy. The Janeway procedure necessitates the creation of a tunnel (called a gastric tube) that is brought out through the abdomen to form a permanent stoma.

For the percutaneous endoscopic gastrostomy, a physician inserts a cannula into the stomach through a 1.0 cm abdominal incision using local anesthesia. He then threads a 150 cm (60 in.) silk suture through the cannula. A second physician, looking through an endoscope, uses the endoscopic snare to grasp the end of the suture and guide it up through the patient's mouth. The suture is knotted to the dilator tip at the end of the PEG tube. The endoscopist then advances the dilator tip through the patient's mouth while the other physician pulls the suture through the cannula site. The attached PEG tube is guided down the esophagus, into

the stomach and out through the abdominal incision. The mushroom catheter tip and internal crossbar secure the tube against the stomach wall. An external crossbar keeps the catheter in place. A tubing adaptor is in place between feedings and a clamp is used to close or open the tubing.

Patients with severe gastroesophageal reflux are at risk for aspiration pneumonia and therefore are not candidates for a gastrostomy. A jejunostomy is preferred, or jejunal feeding via a naso jejunal tube may be recommended.

▶ Nursing Process
The Patient Undergoing a Gastrostomy

▷ *Assessment*

Preoperative

The focus of the preoperative assessment is on determining the patient's ability to understand the surgical experience and the manner in which he is dealing with the impending surgery. The ability to adjust to a change in body image and to participate in self-care is evaluated, along with the patient's and the family's psychological states. Is the patient depressed, angry, withdrawn, or optimistic? Will the family be supportive?

The purpose of the operative procedure is explained to the patient so that he will have a better understanding of his postoperative course. He needs to know that the purpose of this surgery is to bypass his esophagus and that liquid feedings will be administered directly into the stomach by means of a rubber or plastic tube or a prosthesis. If the prosthesis is to be permanent, the patient should be aware of it. Psychologically, this is often difficult for the patient to accept. However, when the procedure is being done to relieve discomfort, prolonged vomiting, debilitation, and the inability to eat, it is more acceptable. Frequently a gastrostomy is performed on an elderly or a comatose patient who cannot tolerate nasogastric feedings.

The nurse evaluates the patient's skin condition and determines whether a delay in wound healing may be anticipated because of a systemic disorder (*e.g.*, diabetes mellitus, cancer).

Postoperative

In the postoperative period the patient's fluid and nutritional needs are assessed to ensure proper food and fluid intake. The nurse checks the status of the tube and the wound for proper maintenance and any signs of infection. At the same time, the patient's reaction to the change in body image and his understanding of the methods for carrying out the feeding procedure are evaluated to determine the interventions needed to help him cope with the presence of the tube and to learn self-care measures.

▷ *Nursing Diagnoses*

Based on all the assessment data, the major nursing diagnoses in the postoperative period may include the following:

- Alteration in nutrition, less than body requirements, related to enteral feeding problems

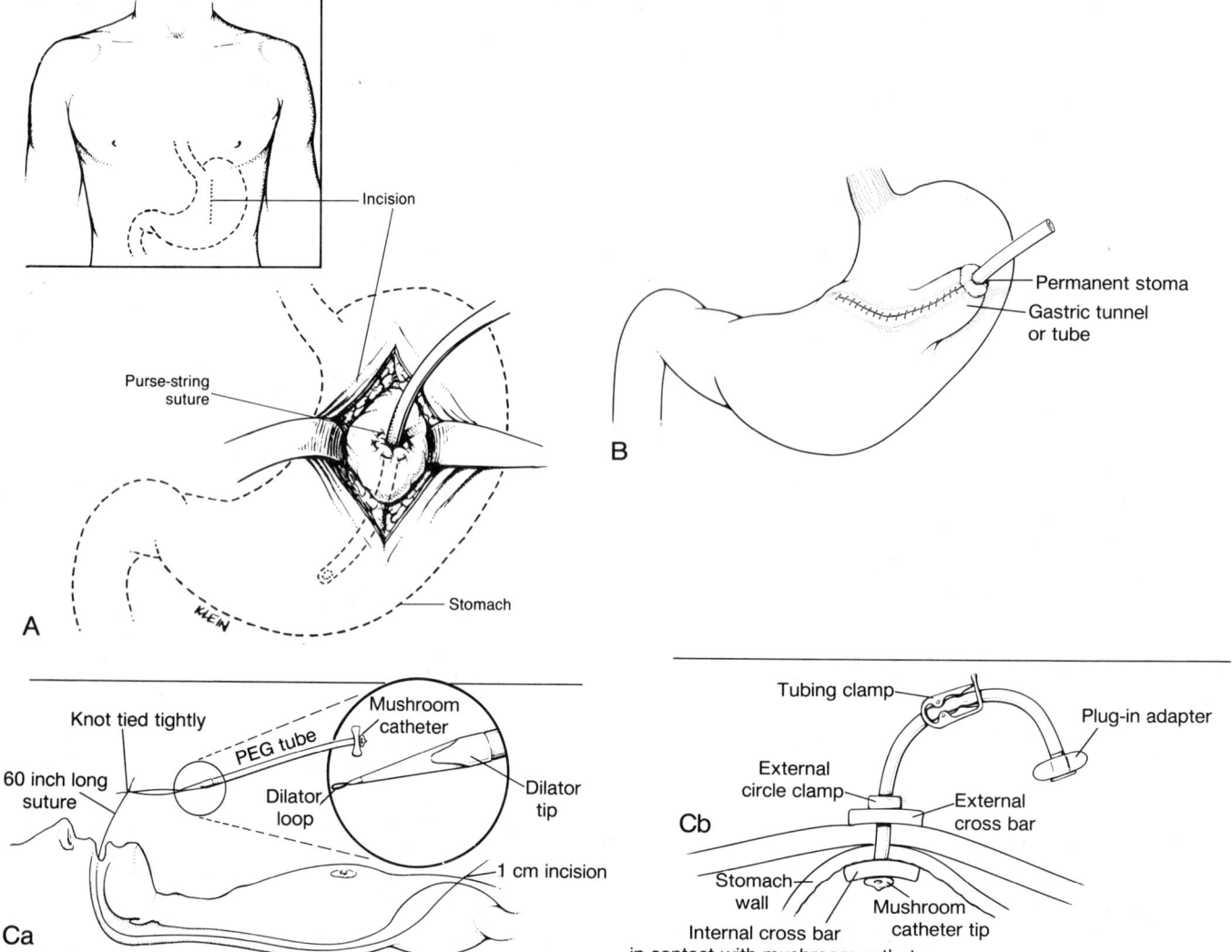

Figure 32-7
(*A*) Stamm gastrostomy, showing incision line and purse-string suture. (*B*) Janeway permanent gastrostomy. (*Ca*) Percutaneous endoscopic gastrostomy (PEG). (*Cb*) A close-up illustration of the abdomen showing catheter fixation.

- Potential for infection related to presence of wound and tube
- Potential impairment of skin integrity related to enteral feedings
- Ineffective coping related to the inability to eat normally
- Disturbance in self-concept/body image related to the presence of the tube
- Knowledge deficit about the feeding procedure

▷ *Planning and Implementation*

▷ *Goals:* The major goals for the patient may include attainment of the desired level of nutrition, maintenance of skin integrity, absence of infection, improvement in coping methods, adjustment to changes in body image, and acquisition of sufficient knowledge about the tube feeding regimen.

Nursing Interventions

Nutritional Needs. The first fluid nourishment is given by the surgeon soon after surgery. This is usually tap water and 10% glucose. At first only 30 to 60 ml (1 to 2 oz) is given at a time, but the amount is gradually increased. By the second day, from 180 to 240 ml (6 to 8 oz) may be given at one time, provided it is tolerated and there is no leakage of fluid around the tube. Water and milk can be instilled after 24 hours for a permanent gastrostomy. High-calorie liquids are added gradually. In some clinics, in the early postoperative period the nurse aspirates gastric secretions and reinstills them, after adding enough feeding to bring the volume to the desired total. By this method, gastric dilatation is avoided.

Blended foods are gradually added to clear liquids until a full diet is reached. Powdered feedings that are easily liquefied are commercially available. However, a food blender can be used to liquefy a normal diet, which can then be fed through the tube. Blenderized tube feedings allow the patient to follow his usual diet pattern, which proves to be psychologically more acceptable. In addition, good bowel function is promoted, since the fiber and residue are similar to that of a normal diet. Excessive intake of milk is to be avoided in patients with lactase deficiency.

Tube Care and Infection Precautions. The tube can be held in place by a thin strip of adhesive that is first twisted about the tube and then firmly attached to the abdomen. A catheter plug or rubber-tipped hemostat may close the outlet of the tube immediately following a feeding to prevent leakage. This can also be facilitated by having the patient relax for a short time after his feeding. A small dressing can be applied over the tube outlet; the tube can be coiled and held in place by Montgomery straps or a firm abdominal binder. This protects the skin surrounding the incision from the seepage of gastric acid contents and the spillage of feedings (Fig. 32-8). Thereafter, the tube is changed every 2 or 3 days and the patient taught how to do this for himself. Once the opening into the stomach has been established there is no need for sterile technique in changing and introducing a gastrostomy tube, which may be reinserted only when a feeding is given. However, items are to be thoroughly clean.

Skin Care. The skin surrounding a gastrostomy opening requires special care. It may become irritated owing to the enzymatic action of gastric juices that leak around the tube. If untreated, the skin becomes macerated, red, raw, and painful. Daily washing with soap and water around the tube, and the application of a bland ointment such as zinc oxide or petrolatum are protective measures.

Skin status is evaluated daily for signs of breakdown, irritation, or excoriation. The patient and family members should be encouraged to participate in this inspection and in hygiene activities.

Body Image Adjustment. The patient with a gastrostomy has experienced a major assault on his body image. A normal body function, eating, can no longer be taken for granted. The patient is also aware that gastrostomy as a therapeutic intervention is only done in the presence of a major, chronic, or perhaps terminal illness. Calm discussion of the purposes and routines of gastrostomy feeding can help keep gastrostomy from becoming an overwhelming situation. Talking with a person who has had a gastrostomy can also help the patient to accept the expected changes. Adjusting to a change in body image takes time and requires family support and acceptance. An evaluation of the existing family support system is necessary. One family member may emerge as the primary support person. If so that person will become the major communicator between the patient and health care personnel.

Patient Education and Home Health Care. The nurse assesses the patient's level of knowledge, interest in learning about the procedure, and ability to understand and apply the information. Detailed instructions about formula preparation and management of the tube feeding are provided. To facilitate self-care, the patient is instructed properly in post-hospital care and encouraged to establish as normal a routine as possible. These goals are achieved through teaching about tube feedings and tube and skin care and through ongoing evaluation by questioning and return-demonstrations. The patient (or caregiver in the home setting) must view himself as capable and responsible for care; know the method and frequency of administration of self-care activities; and have adequate supplies, including the physical, financial, and social resources to maintain care. In addition to individual teaching, the use of printed instruction is necessary as a reinforcement. Adequate provision of needed supervision and support must be arranged.

The demonstration begins by showing the patient how to check for residual gastric content before the feeding. The patient then learns how to determine the patency of the tube by administering water at room temperature before the feeding and after to clear the tube of food particles, which could decompose if allowed to remain in the tube. All feedings are given at room temperature or near body temperature.

For a bolus feeding, the patient is shown how to introduce the liquid into the catheter by using a funnel or the barrel of a syringe. The receptacle is tilted to allow air to escape while the liquid is initially being instilled. As the syringe or barrel fills with liquid, the feeding is allowed to flow into the stomach by gravity by holding the barrel or syringe perpendicular to the abdomen (Fig. 32-9). The rate of flow is regulated by raising or lowering the receptacle no higher than 45 cm (18 inches) above the abdominal wall.

With a bolus feeding, usually 300 to 500 ml is given for each meal and requires 10 or 15 minutes to complete. The amount is often determined by the patient's reaction. If he feels "full" it may be desirable to give smaller amounts more frequently. Keeping the head of the bed elevated for at least a half hour after feeding facilitates digestion. Any obstruction requires that the feeding be stopped and the physician notified.

Some patients smell, taste, and chew small amounts of food before taking their tube feedings. This procedure stimulates the flow of salivary and gastric secretions and may give some sensation of normal eating. The chewed food is then deposited by the patient into a funnel attached to his gastrostomy tube and not swallowed.

A tube feeding may also be given by intermittent or continuous pressure via a feeding pump. Instruction in the use of the particular pump is provided. Most enteral feeding systems have built-in alarms that signal when the bag is empty, when the battery is low, or if an occlusion is present.

▷ *Evaluation*

▷ *Expected Outcomes*

1. Patient achieves a balanced intake of nutrients.
   a. Tolerates quantity and frequency of tube feedings.
   b. Has 50 ml or less of residual gastric content prior to each feeding.
   c. States he has no diarrhea.

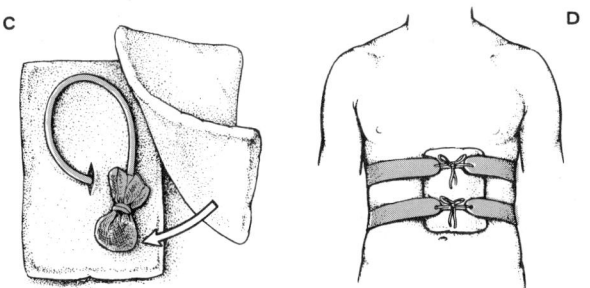

Figure 32-8
Tube care. After a feeding, the opening of the tube is covered with a sterile gauze square held by a rubber band. The tubing is coiled on a dressing, covered, and secured with Montgomery straps.

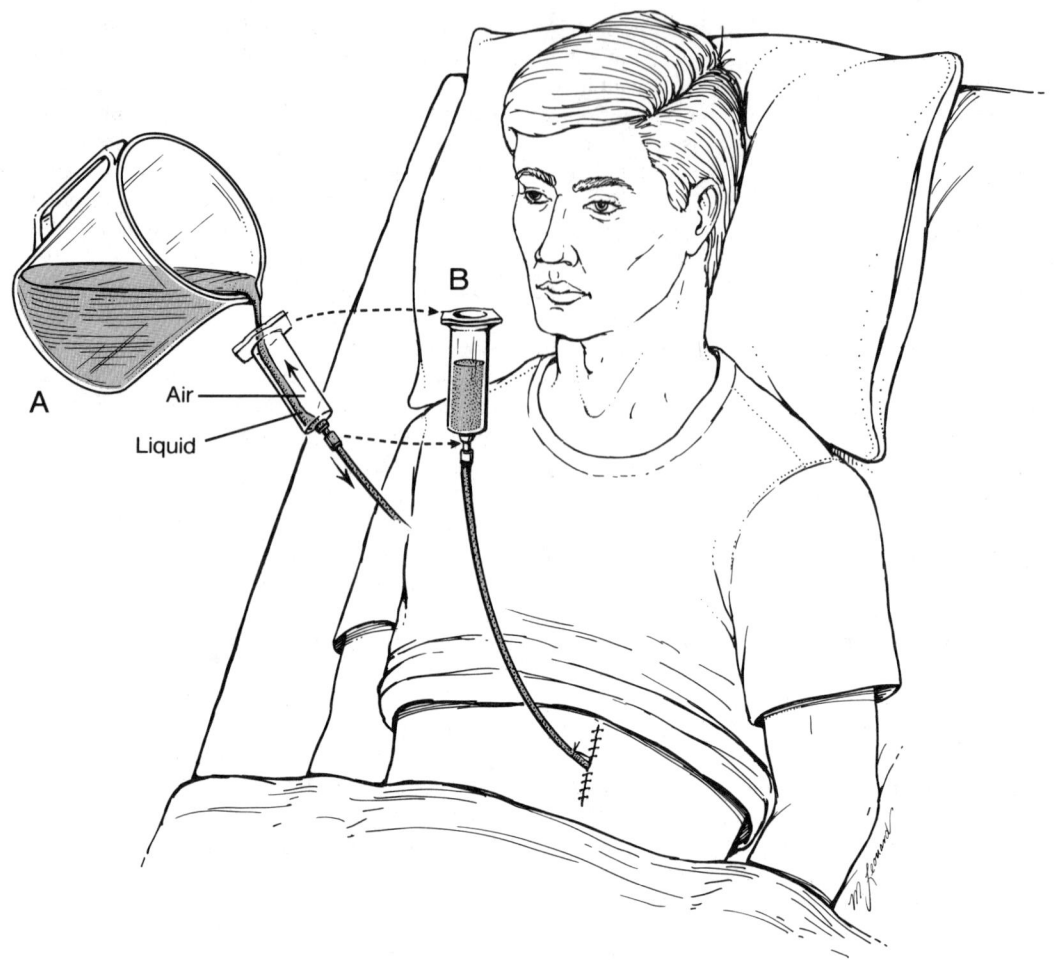

Figure 32-9
Gastrostomy feeding by gravity. (*A*) Feeding is instilled at an angle so that air does not enter the stomach. (*B*) Syringe is raised perpendicular to stomach so feeding can enter by gravity.

d. Maintains or gains weight.
e. Has normal electrolyte values.
2. Is free from infection and skin breakdown.
   a. Is afebrile.
   b. Has no drainage from the wound.
   c. Demonstrates pink skin surrounding the incision.
   d. Inspects incision twice a day.
3. Is adjusting to the idea of change in body image.
   a. Is able to discuss expected changes.
   b. Verbalizes concerns.
   c. Asks to speak with someone who has experienced this procedure.
4. Is knowledgeable about the tube feeding regimen.
   a. Helps prepare the prescribed formula or blenderized food.
   b. Handles equipment competently.
   c. Helps administer the feeding or does so independently.
   d. Demonstrates how to maintain the patency of the tube.
   e. Cleans the tubing as needed.

f. Keeps an accurate record of intake.
g. Is able to remove and reinsert the tube as needed for feedings.

Intravenous Hyperalimentation (Total Parenteral Nutrition)

When a patient's intake of nutrients is significantly less than that required by the body to meet energy expenditures, a state of *negative nitrogen balance* results. This means that protein use is greater than protein intake. Intravenous hyperalimentation is a method of supplying nutrients to the body. The goals of hyperalimentation are to attain improved nutritional status and weight gain and to improve healing ability.

Traditional intravenous feedings do not provide sufficient calories or nitrogen to meet the daily requirements of patients. In response, the body begins to convert protein to carbohydrates by the process of gluconeogenesis. However, intravenous hyperalimentation solutions contain water, amino acids, glucose, vitamins, and electrolytes in a concentration that provides enough calories and nitrogen to meet the patient's daily nutritional needs. In general, intravenous hyperalimentation provides 30 to 35 kcal and 1.0 to 1.5 gm of protein per kilogram of body weight.

The average adult postoperative patient requires approximately 1500 calories a day to spare body protein. If this patient has complications, such as fever, trauma, or hypermetabolic disease, he will require up to 10,000 additional calories daily. The amount of volume necessary to provide these calories would surpass fluid tolerance and lead to pulmonary edema or congestive heart failure. To provide the required calories in small volume, it is necessary to increase the concentration and use an avenue of administration that will rapidly dilute incoming nutrients to the proper levels of body tolerance.

When hypertonic glucose is administered, it satisfies caloric requirements and allows amino acids to be released for protein synthesis, rather than being used for energy. Additional potassium is added to provide proper electrolyte balance and to transport glucose and amino acids across the cell membranes. In order to prevent deficiencies and fulfill requirements for tissue synthesis, other elements, such as calcium, phosphorus, magnesium, and sodium chloride, are added.

Patients who need intravenous hyperalimentation and additional intravenous solutions (chemotherapy, blood products, antibiotics) may be candidates for cyclic parenteral nutrition. With cyclic parenteral nutrition there is a set time during a 24-hour period when parenteral therapy is infused and a set time when it is not. This assures the patient that his nutritional and pharmacologic needs will be met. Ideally, cyclic parenteral nutrition is infused over an 8 to 10-hour period during the night.

The pharmacy department prepares the prescribed nutritional intravenous solutions. These are mixed, using strict aseptic precautions, under a filtered-air laminar flow hood. Basically, the solution consists of 25% glucose and synthetic amino acids (FreAmine); this provides the patient with 1000 calories and 6 gm of nitrogen per liter. Electrolytes are added as determined by the serum electrolyte needs of the patient. Solutions delivered to the unit are refrigerated until needed and then allowed to warm to room temperature. Formulas for local hospital use can be made for individual patients. Commercial preparations (Amigen, Aminosol, FreAmine, Hyprotigen C, and others) are available and can be modified to meet individual needs.

Fat emulsions (Intralipid) can be administered simultaneously with intravenous hyperalimentation. Usually 500 ml of a 10% emulsion is administered over 6 hours, one to three times a week. Fat emulsions can provide up to 30% of the total daily calorie intake.

Clinical Indications

Intravenous hyperalimentation is indicated for the following patients:

- Patients whose intake is insufficient to maintain an anabolic state (*e.g.*, those with severe burns, malnutrition, short-bowel syndrome)
- Patients unable to ingest food orally or by tube (*e.g.*, those with paralytic ileus, Crohn's disease with obstruction, postirradiation enteritis)
- Patients who refuse to ingest adequate nutrients (*e.g.*, those with anorexia nervosa, geriatric postoperative patients)
- Patients who should not be fed orally or by tube (*e.g.*, those with acute pancreatitis or high enterocutaneous fistula)
- Patients who need preoperative and postoperative nutritional support (*e.g.*, following bowel surgery)

Certain criteria must be met before a patient receives total parenteral nutrition (*e.g.*, a 10% deficit in body weight; an inability to take oral food or fluids within 7 postoperative days; and hypercatabolic situations, such as major infection with fever).

Management

A nutritional support nurse or physician determines the patient's need for intravenous hyperalimentation by evaluating certain criteria: the degree of weight loss, the nitrogen balance, the amount of muscle loss and the total lean body mass, as well as the patient's inability to tolerate ingestion of food via the gastrointestinal tract. Ideally the nutritional support nurse, pharmacist, and physician collaborate to determine the specific formula needed.

Total intravenous alimentation is complicated and hazardous and is limited to carefully selected patients. Careful monitoring and conscientious care by experienced physicians and nurses can reduce the risk of many complications.

Partial parenteral nutrition is used to supplement oral intake when complete bowel rest is not indicated and nasogastric or nasoenteric suction is not required. Partial nutritional support is administered by peripheral vein because a less hypertonic solution is used. Dextrose concentrations above 10% should not be administered through peripheral veins. The usual length of therapy for partial, peripheral nutrition is less than 2 weeks.

Method of Administration

Because hyperalimentation solutions have five or six times the solute concentration of blood (and exert an osmotic pressure of about 2000 mOsm/liter) they are injurious to the intima of peripheral veins. Therefore, to prevent phlebitis and other venous complications, these solutions are administered into the circulatory system by means of a large-bore needle or catheter inserted into a high-flow large blood vessel (Fig. 32-10). Concentrated solutions are then diluted in this vessel, very rapidly, to isotonic levels.

Administering medications through the main catheter so that they may mix with the nutritional solution is not recommended because of the possibility of incompatibility (insulin is an exception). If incompatible drugs must be given, they should be infused through a peripheral IV line, not by piggyback. Transfusions of blood products also should not be given through the main catheter, since red cells may possibly coat the lumen of the catheter, thereby reducing the flow of solution.

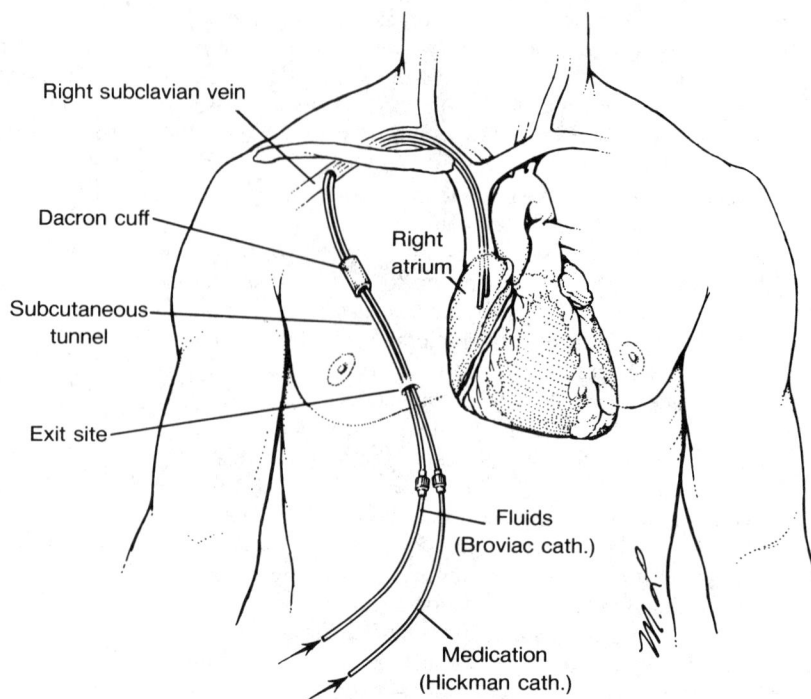

Figure 32-10
Double-lumen Hickman/Broviac
catheter used for intravenous
hyperalimentation.

Patient Preparation. The procedure is explained to
the patient so that he realizes the importance of not touching
the area where the catheter is inserted and is aware that he
will be able to be ambulatory during the extended time of
therapy. For the procedure, the patient is placed supine, in
head-low position (to produce dilatation of neck and shoulder
vessels, which makes entry easier and prevents air embolus).
A rolled sheet is placed vertically along the vertebral column,
from the neck to the end of the rib cage, in order to hyperextend the shoulders. The area is shaved, if necessary, and
the skin prepared with acetone or ether to remove surface
oils. Final skin preparation includes scrubbing with tincture
of iodine or povidone-iodine solution. The patient is instructed
to turn his head facing the side opposite from the site of
venipuncture; he is to remain motionless while the catheter
is inserted and the wound dressed, so as to afford maximum
accuracy in the placement of the tube.

Insertion of the Catheter. The preferred route is by
way of the subclavian vein, which leads into the superior vena
cava. An alternate route is the internal jugular to the superior
vena cava. With long-term use, an indwelling catheter is a
constant source of potential infection.

Sterile drapes are applied to the upper chest. Some physicians ask the patient to wear a face mask to prevent the
spread of microorganisms.

Procaine or lidocaine is injected for local anesthesia into
the skin and underlying tissues. The target area is the inferior
border at the midpoint of the clavicle (Fig. 32-11). A large-
bore needle on a syringe is inserted and moved parallel to
and beneath the clavicle until it enters the subclavian vein.
The syringe is then detached and a radiopaque catheter is
inserted through the needle into the vein. When the catheter
is positioned the needle is withdrawn and the catheter attached to the intravenous tubing. Until the syringe is detached
from the needle and the catheter inserted, the patient may
be asked to perform the Valsalva maneuver. (To do this, he

is instructed to take a deep breath, hold it, and bear down
with his mouth closed. Compression of the abdomen may
also accomplish the maneuver.) The Valsalva maneuver is

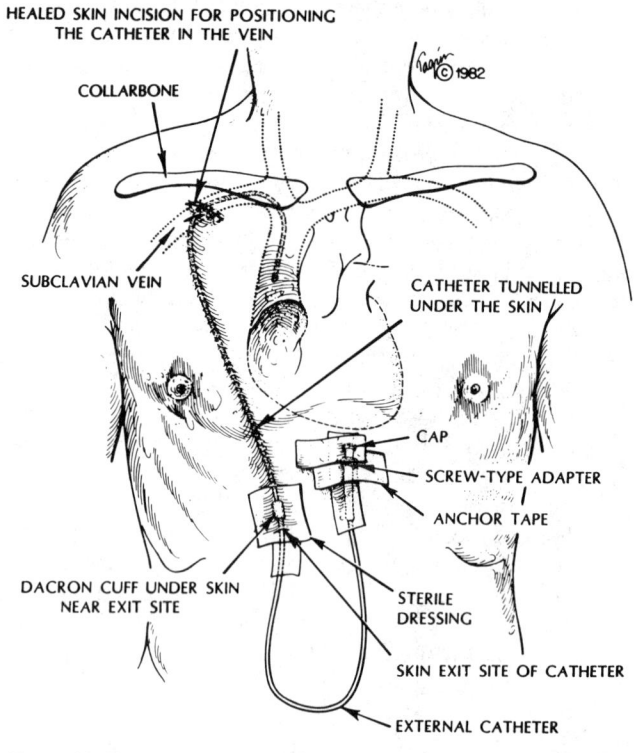

Figure 32-11
Right atrial catheter for parenteral hyperalimentation. The
Silastic catheter is threaded under the skin to the superior
vena cava and right atrium. (Wilson JM, et al. Silicone
catheters: Patient teaching pamphlet. NITA 1984 May/June;
7[3]:170.)

done to produce a positive phase in central venous pressure in order to lessen the possibility of air being drawn into the circulatory system.

The position of the tip of the catheter is checked at this point with an x-ray film to confirm its location before the hyperalimentation solution is administered. Following this, the area is again swabbed with germicide solution and antibiotic ointment is applied directly to the insertion site.

A gauze or transparent dressing is applied using strict aseptic technique. After the catheter position is confirmed, the prescribed hyperalimentation solution is started by connecting the catheter to the IV administration set.

Blood is not aspirated from hyperalimentation tubing for blood studies unless it is a life-saving measure. Because of the danger of emboli, a small amount of heparin is flushed into the central venous catheter. (Dosage ranges from 800 to 1000 units.)

Discontinuance of Intravenous Hyperalimentation

Parenteral hyperalimentation is discontinued gradually to allow for adjustment to decreased levels of glucose. Following hypertonic solution, isotonic glucose is administered for several hours to protect against rebound hypoglycemia. Oral carbohydrates will shorten tapering time. Specific symptoms include weakness, faintness, sweating, shakiness, feeling cold, confusion, and increased heart rate.

▶ Nursing Process
The Patient Receiving Intravenous Hyperalimentation

▷ Assessment

The nurse assists in identifying a patient who may be a candidate for intravenous hyperalimentation. Indicators to look for include any significant weight loss (10% or more of weight when healthy), a decrease in oral food intake for more than 1 week, any significant sign of protein loss (serum albumin levels below 3.2 gm/dl [32 g/L], muscle wasting, decreased tissue healing, or abnormal urea nitrogen excretion), and persistent vomiting and diarrhea. The nurse carefully monitors the patient's hydration, electrolyte status, and calorie intake.

During therapy the nurse evaluates daily body weight, intake and output record, fractional urine studies, blood glucose levels, serum electrolyte studies, and the complete blood cell count for any abnormalities. A number of major complications can occur with intravenous hyperalimentation. See Table 32-3 for a list of potential complications and associated nursing interventions.

▷ Nursing Diagnoses

Based on all the assessment data, the major nursing diagnoses may include the following:

- Alteration in nutrition, less than body requirements, related to inadequate intake of nutrients

- Potential for infection related to contamination of the catheter site
- Potential fluid volume deficit related to an altered infusion rate
- Potential for activity intolerance related to fear of dislodgement or occlusion of the catheter

▷ Planning and Implementation

▷ *Goals:* The major goals for the patient may include attainment of an optimal level of nutrition, absence of infection, maintenance of adequate fluid volume, and achievement of an optimal level of activity within individual limitations.

Nursing Interventions

Optimal Nutrition. A continuous, uniform infusion of hyperalimentation fluid over a 24-hour period is desired. Cyclic parenteral nutrition allows patients to receive optimal amounts of calories and electrolytes while receiving other needed intravenous agents through the same line. A set number of hours per day is provided for hyperalimentation.

An infusion pump is recommended for intravenous hyperalimentation. Rates are usually set at milliliters per hour. The rate is checked every ½ to 1 hour, and an alarm signals a problem. The infusion can usually be speeded up or slowed down by not more than 10% of the original rate (unless otherwise requested by the physician) to compensate for fluids that are infusing too quickly or too slowly.

- If the rate is too rapid, hyperosmolar diuresis occurs (excess sugar will be excreted) and if severe enough may cause intractable seizures, coma, and death. Symptoms of rapid fluid intake include headache, nausea, fever, chills, and increasing lassitude.
- If the flow goes too slowly, the patient does not get the maximum benefit of calories and nitrogen.

The patient is weighed daily at the same time, under the same conditions, for accurate comparison. Under this regimen, 0.11 to 0.45 kg (0.25 to 1 lb) per day weight gain of lean body tissue can be expected. Accurate intake and output records are kept, and if the patient also receives oral nutrients, this is recorded according to calorie count.

Absence of Infection. Dressings are changed aseptically on a regular basis and as needed. *Candida albicans* is the most common infectious organism. Others include *Staphylococcus aureus, S. epidermidis,* and *Klebsiella pneumoniae.*

The patient is placed in low Fowler's position for a dressing change. The nurse and patient may reduce the possibility of airborne contamination by wearing masks. Old dressings are removed very carefully, to prevent the catheter from becoming dislodged. The area is checked for leakage, kinked catheter, and skin reactions, such as inflammation, pain, or purulence. Using sterile gloves, the nurse cleanses the area with acetone, followed by tincture of iodine or thimerosal (Merthiolate), with the aid of a sponge holder and 3×3-inch gauze pledgets. Cleaning begins from the center and moves outward. Alcohol may be used in the same manner to remove iodine. Antibiotic ointment is applied to the insertion site if prescribed, and the site is covered with a small dressing, slit to fit around the catheter. The gauze pad or transparent

TABLE 32-3
Potential Complications of Intravenous Hyperalimentation

Complication	Cause	Nursing Action
Sepsis	Separation of dressings	Reinforce or change quickly using aseptic technique.
	Contaminated solution	Discard
	Infection at insertion site of catheter	Notify physician. Monitor vital signs every 4 hours.
Air embolism	Disconnected tubing	Replace tubing immediately and notify physician.
	Cap missing from unused lumen.	Replace cap and notify physician.
	Blocked segment of vascular system	Turn patient on his left side and place him in the head-low position. Notify physician.
Catheter displacement	Excessive movement possibly with a nonsecured catheter	Stop the infusion and notify physician.
Fluid overload	Fluid running rapidly.	Decrease infusion rate. Monitor vital signs. Notify physician. Treat respiratory distress by sitting patient upright and administering oxygen prn, if prescribed.
Pneumothorax	Improper catheter placement and inadvertent puncture of the pleura.	Place in the Fowler's position. Offer reassurance. Check vital signs. Be prepared for respiratory arrest. Initiate resuscitative measures. Prepare patient for thoracentesis or chest tube insertion.

dressing is centered over the area. The intravenous tubing, including piggyback lines, is replaced rapidly to prevent buildup of organisms along the lumen of the inner tubing. The union of the catheter and tubing is then covered and secured with adhesive tape to prevent separation and exposure to air.

If the patient has a draining wound, such as a tracheostomy, in the nearby area, additional precautions are taken to keep the wound dry by applying transparent plastic operating-room adhesive drape over the dressings, to ensure waterproofing. Hypoallergenic adhesive tape can be used if the patient complains of itching from conventional tape. The dressing change is recorded, and the condition of the local area as well as the patient's reaction are reported.

Maintenance of Adequate Fluid Volume. The flow rate is monitored every ½ to 1 hour and adjusted as needed. Intake and output are recorded every 8 hours so that fluid imbalance can be readily detected, and the patient is weighed daily; the patient should not show a weight loss. The nurse assesses for signs of dehydration (thirst, decreased skin turgor, lowered central venous pressure reading) and reports any findings to the physician immediately. It is essential to monitor blood glucose status because hyperglycemia can cause diuresis and excessive fluid loss.

Optimal Level of Activity. Activities and ambulation are encouraged when the patient is physically capable. With a plastic catheter in the subclavian vein, the patient has freedom to move his extremities and should be encouraged to maintain good muscle tone. The teaching and exercise program initiated in the occupational and physical therapy departments should be reinforced.

Patient Education and Home Health Care. Successful home parenteral nutrition requires teaching the patient and his family specialized skills by means of an intensive training program and follow-up supervision in the home. This must be done through a team effort. The financial costs of such programs are less than those incurred in a hospital. Initiation of a home program may be the only way the patient can be discharged. Ability to learn, availability of family interest and support, adequate finances, and the physical plan of the home are factors that must be assessed when the decision for home hyperalimentation is made. Institutions sponsoring home hyperalimentation programs have developed teaching brochures for every aspect of the treatment, including catheter and dressing care, use of an infusion pump for hyperalimentation, fat emulsions, and instillation of heparin flushes.

A home care teaching program prepares the patient to manage his specific form of intravenous hyperalimentation. He is taught how to store his solutions, set up his infusion, flush the line with heparin, change his dressings, and troubleshoot for complications. The most frequent complication is infection. The nurse emphasizes hand washing and strict asepsis in handling equipment, changing the dressing, and preparing the solution, if the patient is going to do so.

Mechanical problems usually arise from technical complications found within the infusion pump or catheter site. The patient is taught how to troubleshoot for catheter problems (leakage, loose cap, tear in the tubing, blood clot) and is given a list of directions explaining what to do for each problem. Malfunctioning pumps can usually be replaced in 24 hours. The patient is given a list of symptoms indicative of metabolic complications (neuropathies, mentation changes, diarrhea, nausea, skin changes) and directed to contact his home health care nurse or physician if he thinks he is experiencing a complication. He is asked to have weekly serum chemistry and hematology monitoring and to have the glucose level of his urine checked daily.

The nurse should be aware that the average patient will need about 2 weeks of instruction and reinforcement. Additional time will be needed from a nutritional support nurse or pharmacist for the patient who is going to mix his own solution at home instead of using a premixed solution supplied by an outside vendor. Compounding solutions at home requires an area that is free of traffic and clutter.

The psychosocial aspects of home parenteral nutrition are just as significant as the physiologic and technical concerns. These patients must cope with the loss of eating and the changes in life-style brought about by sleep disturbances (frequent urination during infusions, usually two to three times during the night). Major psychosocial reactions include depression, anger, withdrawal, anxiety, and altered self-image. A successful home parenteral nutrition program depends on motivation, emotional stability, and technical competence.

▷ *Evaluation*

▷ *Expected Outcomes*

1. Patient attains/maintains nutritional balance.
   a. Attains positive nitrogen balance.
   b. Has results of specific diagnostic studies within normal limits (blood urea nitrogen, serum protein, hemoglobin, hematocrit).
   c. Attains or maintains desired body weight.
   d. Attains or maintains hydration of body tissue.
2. Is infection free.
   a. Is afebrile.
   b. Has no purulent drainage from the catheter insertion site.
   c. States that the catheter site is not tender or painful.
3. Is hydrated.
   a. Has good skin turgor.
   b. Maintains a balanced daily intake and output.
   c. Maintains current weight or gains 1 to 2 pounds weekly until ideal body weight is achieved.

4. Achieves an optimal level of activity within self-limitations.
   a. Performs isometric and isotonic exercises as directed.
   b. Participates in exercise program recommended by physician and physiotherapists.
   c. Ambulates freely according to his abilities and the physician's direction.

Bibliography

Books

Alpers D et al. Manual of Nutritional Therapeutics. Boston, Little, Brown, & Co, 1983.

Bockus HL. Gastroenterology. Philadelphia, WB Saunders, 1985.

Cerra FB. Pocket Manual of Surgical Nutrition. St. Louis, CV Mosby, 1984.

Dietal M (ed). Nutrition in Clinical Surgery. Baltimore, Williams & Wilkins, 1985.

Dixon JA (ed). Surgical Application of Lasers. Chicago, Year Book Medical Publishers, 1984.

Eastwood GL. Core Textbook of Gastroenterology. Philadelphia, JB Lippincott, 1984.

Hudak CM, Gallo BM, and Lohr T. Critical Care Nursing, A Holistic Approach. Philadelphia, JB Lippincott, 1986.

Moghissi K and Boore JRP. Parenteral and Enteral Nutrition for Nurses. Rockville, Maryland, Aspen Systems Corporation, 1983.

Rombeau JL and Caldwell MD (eds). Clinical Nutrition, Vol I, Enteral and Tube Feeding. Philadelphia, WB Saunders, 1984.

Sabiston DC (ed). Textbook of Surgery: The Biological Basis of Modern Surgical Practice. Philadelphia, WB Saunders, 1986.

Shackelford RT and Zuidema GD. Surgery of the Alimentary Tract. Philadelphia, WB Saunders, 1983.

Sleisenger MH and Fordtran JS. Gastrointestinal Disease: Pathophysiology, Diagnosis and Management. Philadelphia, WB Saunders, 1983.

Spiro HM. Clinical Gastroenterology. New York, Macmillan, 1983.

Williams SR. Nutrition and Diet Therapy. St. Louis, Times Mirror/Mosby, 1985.

Wright RA and Heymsfield SB (eds). Nutritional Assessment. Boston, Blackwell Scientific Publications, 1984.

Zollinger RM and Zollinger RM Jr. Atlas of Surgical Operations. New York, Macmillan, 1983.

Articles

(Asterisks indicate nursing research articles.)

Nasogastric and Nasoenteric Intubation and Feedings

Anderson BJ. Tube feeding: Is diarrhea inevitable? Am J Nurs 1986 June; 86(6):704–706.

Brown JH. Endoscopic laboratory with laser: Organization, safety, and equipment. Am J Gastroenterol 1985 Sept; 80(9):713–714.

Carroll PF. Aspirated feeding solution. Nursing '86 1986 Jan; 16(1):33.

Flynn KT, Norton LC and Fisher RL. Enteral tube feeding: Indications, practices and outcomes. Image: J Nurs Scholarship 1987 Spring; 19(1):16–19.

Freedman J. Speaking out on nasogastric feeding. Geriatr Nurse 1987 Jan/Feb; 8(1):7.

Guiness R. How to use the new small-bore feeding tubes. Nursing '86 1986 Apr; 16(4):51–56.

Haynes-Johnson V. Tube feeding complications: Causes, prevention, and therapy. Nutr Supp Serv 1986 Mar; 6(3):17–18, 24.

Hearne BE et al. *In vitro* flow rates of enteral solutions through nasoenteric tubes. J Parenter Enteral Nutr 1984 July/Aug; 8(4):456–459.

*Heinz J. Validation of sublingual temperatures in patients with nasogastric tubes. Heart Lung 1985 Mar; 14(2):128–130.

Heitkemper M and Hansen BC. Gastric relaxation prior to enteral feedings. J Parenter Enteral Nutr 1984 Nov/Dec; 8(6):682–684.

Heymsfield SB et al. Enteral nutritional support: Metabolic, cardiovascular and pulmonary interrelations. Clin Chest Med 1986 Mar; 7(1):41–67.

McLean CK et al. Enteric alimentation: A radiologic approach. Radiology 1986 Aug; 160(2):555–556.

Metheny NM. 20 ways to prevent tube feeding complications. Nursing '85 1985 Jan; 15(1):47–50.

Metheny NA, Eisenberg P and Spies M. Aspiration pneumonia in patients fed through nasoenteral tubes. Heart Lung 1986 May; 15(3):256–261.

*Moore MC, Guenter PA, and Bender JH. Nutrition-related nursing research. Image 1986 Spring; 18(1):18–21.

Niemiec PW Jr et al. Gastrointestinal disorders caused by medication and electrolyte solution osmolality during enteral nutrition. J Parenter Enteral Nutr 1983 July/Aug; 7(4):387–389.

Olbrantz KR et al. Pneumothorax complicating enteral feeding tube placement. J Parenter Enteral Nutr 1985 Mar/Apr; 9(2):210–211.

Pagana KD. Preventing complications in jejunostomy tube feedings. Dimens Crit Care Nurs 1987 Jan/Feb; 6(1):28–38.

Patras AZ. Gastrointestinal assessment, identifying significant problems. AORN J 1984 Nov; 40(5):726–731.

Pipp TL. Nutritional product chart, #1: Enteral feeding pumps. Nutr Supp Serv 1986 Sept; 6(9):12–15.

Raizman DH and Braunschweig C. Fiber in enteral feedings. Nutr Supp Serv 1986 June; 6(6):29, 33.

Rajaratnam R. Method for anchoring nasogastric feeding tubes. Laryngoscope 1985 Feb; 95(2):219–220.

Randall HT. Enteral nutrition: Tube feeding in acute and chronic illness. J Parenter Enteral Nutr 1984 Mar/Apr; 8(2):113–136.

Shea M and McCreary M. Early postop feeding. Am J Nurs 1984 Oct; 84(10):1230–1231.

Thurlow PM. Bedside enteral feeding and tube placement into duodenum and jejunum. J Parenter Enteral Nutr 1986 Jan/Feb; 10(1):104–105.

Tiller HJ et al. Iatrogenic perforation of the esophagus by a nasogastric tube. Am J Surg 1984 Mar; 147(3):423–425.

Valentine RJ and Turner WW. Pleural complications of nasoenteric feeding tubes. J Parenter Enteral Nutr 1985 Sept/Oct; 9(5):605–607.

Wright B. Enteral feeding tubes as drug delivery systems. Nutr Supp Serv 1986 Feb; 6(2):33–37, 47–48.

Gastrostomies

Gauderer MWL and Stellato TA. Gastrostomies: Evolution, techniques, indications, and complications. Curr Probl Surg 1986 Sept; 23(9):661–710.

Kazarek RA, Ball TJ, and Ryan JA. When push comes to shove: A comparison between two methods of percutaneous endoscopic gastrostomy. Am J Gastoenterol 1986 Aug; 8(8):642–645.

Larson DE et al. Percutaneous endoscopic gastrostomy: Simplified access for enteral nutrition. Mayo Clin Proc 1983 Feb; 58(8):103–107.

Russell TR, Brotman M, and Norris F. Percutaneous gastrostomy: A new simplified and cost-effective technique. Am J Surg 1984 July; 148(1):132–135.

Shellito PC and Malt RA. Tube gastrostomy: Techniques and complications. Ann Surg 1985 Feb; 201(2):180–185.

Stein JS. Comparison of percutaneous endoscopic gastrostomy with surgical gastrostomy at a community hospital. Am J Gastoenterol 1986 Dec; 81(12):1171–1173.

Thatcher BS, Ferguson DR, and Paradis K. Percutaneous endoscopic gastrostomy: A preferred method of feeding tube gastrostomy. Am J Gastroenterol 1984 Oct; 79(10):748–750.

Wills JS and Oglesby JT. Percutaneous gastrostomy: Further experience. Radiology 1985 Jan; 154(1):71–74.

Wills JS and Oglesby JT. Percutaneous gastrostomy: A safe, cost-effective alternative to surgical gastrostomy and intravascular hyperalimentation. Nutr Supp Serv 1986 Feb; 6(2):10, 14, 19.

Intravenous Hyperalimentation

Baker DJ. 10 years of TPN at home. Am J Nurs 1984 Oct; 84(10):1248–1249.

Birdsall C. When is TPN safe? Am J Nurs 1985 Jan; 85(1):73.

Boblick P, Lundvick J, and Aramha GV. Detection of magnesium deficiency in the patient receiving parenteral nutrition. Nutr Supp Serv 1986 Feb; 6(2):51, 80.

Campbell SM. Delivery of cyclic parenteral nutrition via a single-lumen Hickman catheter. Nutr Supp Serv 1986 Feb; 6(2):27–28, 46.

Chwals WJ and Blackburn GL. Perioperative nutritional support in the cancer patient. Surg Clin North Am 1986 Dec; 66(6):1137–1165.

Dresser RS et al. Ethics, law and nutritional support. Arch Intern Med 1985 Jan; 145(1):122–124.

Fox B. Take precautions now. Nursing '85 1985 May; 15(5):48–49.

Hakki A et al: A simple formula for monitoring parenteral infusion. Crit Care Nurse 1986; 6(3):57–62.

Maillet JO. Calculating parenteral feedings: A programmed instruction. J Am Diet Assoc 1984 Nov; 84(11):1312–1320, 1323.

*Martyn PA, Hansen BC, and Jen KC. The effects of parenteral nutrition on food intake and gastric motility . . . rhesus monkeys. Nurs Res 1984 Nov/Dec; 33(6):336–342.

Meguid MM et al. Preoperative identification of the surgical cancer patient in need of postoperative supportive total parenteral nutrition. Cancer 1985 Jan 1; 55(suppl 1):258–262.

Olsen GB. Balanced parenteral nutrition. Nutr Supp Serv 1985 June; 5(16):16–17, 19–20.

Rodgers BL. Home parenteral nutrition. Nurse Pract 1984 Mar; 9(3):42, 47–48, 50.

Rudman D. Nutrient deficiencies during total parenteral nutrition. Nutr Rev 1985 Jan; 43(1):1–13.

Seltzer MH. Specialized nutrition support: Patterns of care. J Parenter Enteral Nutr 1984 Nov/Dec; 8(6):621.

Shatcky F and Kelts DG. Blood chemistry considerations for parenteral nutrition: I. Nutr Supp Serv 1986 June; 6(6):25–27.

Turner NC. Nutritional support at home: Parenteral and enteral hyperalimentation. Caring 1984 Nov; 3 (11):21–27.

Wilhelm L. Helping your patient "settle in" with TPN. Nursing '85 1985 Apr; 15(4):60–64.

Agencies

American Cancer Society, 90 Park Avenue, New York, New York 10016.

American Institute of Nutrition, 9650 Rockville Pike, Bethesda, Maryland 20014.

American Society for Gastrointestinal Endoscopy, 6 Beacon Street, Suite #620, Boston, Massachusetts 02108.

Nutrition Foundation, 489 Fifth Avenue, New York, New York 10017.

Nutrition Institute of America, 200 West 86th Street, New York, New York 10024.

Chapter 33

Management of Patients With Gastric and Duodenal Disorders

Gastritis

Acute Gastritis

Gastritis (inflammation of the stomach) is most often due to a dietary indiscretion. The person eats too much or too rapidly or eats food that is noxious because it is too highly seasoned or is infected. Other causes of acute gastritis include alcohol, aspirin, uremia, or radiation therapy. Gastritis may also be the first sign of an acute systemic infection.

Pathophysiology and Clinical Manifestations. The gastric mucous membrane becomes edematous and hyperemic and undergoes superficial erosion; it secretes a scanty amount of gastric juice, containing very little acid but much mucus. Superficial ulceration may occur and can lead to hemorrhage. The patient may have uncomfortable feelings in his abdomen, with headache, lassitude, nausea, and anorexia, often accompanied by vomiting and hiccuping. Some patients, however, are asymptomatic.

The gastric mucosa is capable of repairing itself after a bout of gastritis. Occasionally, hemorrhage may require surgical intervention. If the irritating food is not vomited but reaches the bowel, colic and diarrhea may result. As a rule, the patient is well in about a day, although he may not have much appetite for the next 2 or 3 days.

Chronic Gastritis

Inflammation of the stomach that exists for a prolonged period of time can be caused by either benign or malignant ulcers of the stomach, by cirrhosis of the liver complicated by portal hypertension, and by uremia (exact mechanism is unknown; the breakdown in the gastric mucosa is believed to be caused by the excess of urea in the blood).

Pathophysiology. Chronic gastritis may be classified as type A or type B. Type A disease results from parietal cell changes leading to atrophy and cellular infiltration. As time passes, both the lining and the walls become thinned and secretion lessens in quantity and in quality, eventually consisting almost entirely of mucus and water. The antrum of the stomach (lower end of the stomach near the duodenum) is not affected; however, in type B disease only the antrum is affected.

Clinical Manifestations.   Symptoms of chronic gastritis vary greatly. Iron deficiency anemia is seen in types A and B. Pernicious anemia is usually associated only with type A. The appetite may be poor (anorexia) or too good (bulimia); there is usually some distress ("heartburn") after eating, and often there are eructations of gas. The taste in the mouth is unpleasant; there is usually considerable nausea and perhaps some vomiting, especially early in the morning.

Diagnostic Evaluation.   In both types of gastritis, hydrochloric acid is absent from the gastric juices. Levels of serum gastrin will vary. In type A they are elevated; in type B they are normal. Distinguishing between types A and B is possible only about 70% of the time. A definitive diagnosis is determined by gastroscopy, upper gastrointestinal x-ray series, and histologic examination.

Corrosive Gastritis

A more severe form of acute gastritis is caused by the ingestion of strong acids or alkalies. The mucosa may become gangrenous or perforate. Scarring can occur, resulting in pyloric obstruction.

Management of Gastritis

For *acute gastritis,* management consists of permitting the patient to ingest nothing by mouth until symptoms subside. When the patient is able to take nourishment by mouth, a bland diet, perhaps supplemented by alkalies, is offered. If the symptoms persist, parenteral administration of fluids may become necessary. If bleeding is present, then management is similar to the procedures used for upper gastrointestinal tract hemorrhage (see p 775).

For *chronic gastritis,* management is directed toward diet modification, rest, stress reduction, and pharmacotherapy. Patients with diffuse atrophic gastritis usually evidence malabsorption of vitamin B_{12} due to the presence of intrinsic factor antibodies.

For *corrosive gastritis,* immediate treatment consists of diluting and neutralizing the offending substance.

- To neutralize acids, common antacids (*e.g.,* aluminum hydroxide) are used; to neutralize an alkali, diluted lemon juice or diluted vinegar is used.
- If corrosion is extensive or severe, emetics and lavage are avoided because of the danger of perforation.

Therapy thereafter is supportive, including nasogastric intubation, analgesics and sedatives, antacids, intravenous fluids, and electrolytes. It may be necessary to evaluate the situation by fiberoptic endoscopy. Emergency surgery may be required to remove gangrenous or perforated tissue. Gastrojejunostomy or gastric resection may be necessary to treat pyloric obstruction.

▶ Nursing Process
The Patient With Gastritis

▷ *Assessment*

During the history, the nurse asks questions about the patient's presenting signs and symptoms. Does the patient experience heartburn, indigestion, nausea, or vomiting? Do the symptoms occur at any specific time of the day, before or after meals, after ingesting spicy or irritating foods, or after the ingestion of certain drugs? Are the symptoms related to anxiety, stress, allergies, eating too much, or eating too quickly? How are the symptoms relieved? Is there any history of previous gastric disease or surgery? A diet history plus a 72-hour diet recall is helpful. A history is important to identify whether known dietary excesses or other indiscretions are associated with the current symptoms, whether others in the patient's environment have similar symptoms, whether the patient is vomiting blood, and whether any known caustic element has been swallowed.

The nurse performs a complete physical assessment. Signs to note include abdominal tenderness, dehydration (altered skin turgor, dry mucous membranes), and evidence of any systemic disorder that might be responsible for the symptoms of gastritis (chronic uremia, cirrhosis). The length of time that the current symptoms last and any interventions tried by the patient, and their effects, should also be identified.

▷ *Nursing Diagnoses*

Based on all the assessment data, the patient's major nursing diagnoses may include the following:

- Alteration in nutrition, less than body requirements, related to the intake of irritating food
- Potential for fluid volume deficit related to insufficient fluid intake and excessive fluid loss subsequent to vomiting
- Knowledge deficit related to dietary management

▷ *Planning and Implementation*

▷ *Goals:*   The major goals of the patient may include reduced intake of irritating foods, maintenance of fluid balance, and increased awareness of dietary management.

Nursing Interventions

Nutritional Measures.   For *acute gastritis,* physical and emotional support is provided and the patient is helped to deal with his symptoms, which may include nausea, vomiting, heartburn, and fatigue. Most patients are not allowed to ingest anything by mouth for hours or days until the acute symptoms subside. Intravenous therapy is monitored, and serum electrolyte values are evaluated daily. When the symptoms subside, ice chips followed by clear liquids are offered. Small, frequent, bland meals are introduced as soon as possible to provide oral nutrition, decrease the need for intravenous therapy, and minimize irritation to the gastric mucosa. As food is introduced, any symptoms suggesting a repeat episode of gastritis are evaluated and reported to the physician. The intake of caffeinated beverages is discouraged because caffeine is a central nervous system stimulant that increases gastric activity and pepsin secretion. Cigarette smoking is discouraged because nicotine reduces the secretion of pancreatic bicarbonate and thus inhibits the neutralization of gastric acid in the duodenum. Nicotine also increases parasympathetic stimulation, which increases muscular activity in the bowel and can lead to nausea and vomiting.

The nurse must always be alert for any indicators of hemorrhagic gastritis (hematemesis, tachycardia, hypotension).

If evident, the physician is alerted, vital signs are monitored every 5 to 15 minutes, and the guidelines for managing upper gastrointestinal tract bleeding are followed (see p. 783).

For *chronic gastritis*, the patient is asked to identify and eliminate any irritating foods that may stimulate inflammatory changes. Interventions are directed toward the symptoms. Chronic gastritis is nonspecific and flare-ups and remissions are not always consistent with the disease.

For *corrosive gastritis*, emergency measures are carried out as quickly as possible. Supportive therapy is offered to the patient and family during treatment and after the ingested acid or alkali has been neutralized or diluted. The patient may need to be prepared for additional diagnostic studies (endoscopy) or surgery. Anxiety about the pain and treatment modalities is usually present as well as fear of permanent damage to the esophagus. A calm manner is used, and questions are answered honestly. All procedures and treatments are explained according to the patient's interest and level of understanding.

Fluid Balance. Daily intake and output are monitored to detect early signs of dehydration (minimal output of 30 ml/hr; minimal intake of 1.5 liters/day). If food and fluids are withheld, 3 liters of intravenous fluids daily are prescribed. Fluid intake plus caloric value is measured (1 liter of 5% dextrose in water = 200 calories of carbohydrate). Electrolyte values (sodium, potassium, chloride) are assessed every 24 hours to detect early indicators of fluid imbalance.

Dietary Management. The patient's knowledge about gastritis is evaluated so that a teaching plan can be individualized. A bland diet is constructed that takes into account daily caloric needs, food preferences, and the desired frequency of eating. Smaller, more frequent meals are recommended to help control gastric secretions. This regimen may be difficult for the elderly patient, who may prefer to eat twice a day (a larger mid-morning brunch and an early evening meal).

The patient is given a list of irritating substances to avoid (*e.g.*, caffeine, nicotine, spicy foods, highly seasoned foods). Antacids, sedatives, and/or anticholinergics are administered as prescribed.

▷ *Evaluation*

▷ *Expected Outcomes*

1. Patient eats fewer irritating foods.
   a. Eliminates caffeinated beverages from diet.
   b. Avoids spicy foods and seasonings (pepper).
   c. Chooses nonirritating seasonings for foods (mint, parsley).
2. Maintains fluid balance.
   a. Drinks 6 to 8 glasses of water daily.
   b. Tolerates intravenous therapy of at least 3 liters daily.
   c. Has a urinary output of about 1.5 liters daily.
   d. Displays adequate skin turgor.
   e. Is not dehydrated.
   f. Increases oral intake of fluids and foods as symptoms wane.
3. Understands dietary management.
   a. Repeats dietary restrictions to the nurse.
   b. Identifies irritating foods and beverages.
   c. Modifies caloric intake to individual preferences.
   d. Eats smaller meals more frequently.
   e. Takes medications as prescribed.

Upper Gastrointestinal Tract Bleeding

Gastritis and hemorrhage from peptic ulcer are the two most common causes of upper gastrointestinal tract bleeding. *Hematemesis* refers to the vomiting of blood. The vomited blood can be bright red or have a "coffee-ground" appearance (hemoglobin changes to methemoglobin in the stomach). The passage of dark, tarry stools (melena) indicates upper gastrointestinal tract bleeding. Management depends on the amount of blood lost and the rate of bleeding.

Management. Management of upper gastrointestinal tract bleeding consists of (1) quickly determining the amount of blood lost and the rate of bleeding, (2) rapidly correcting the blood loss, (3) stopping the bleeding with ice water or iced saline lavage, (4) stabilizing the patient, and (5) diagnosing the cause. Specific medical and nursing interventions for upper gastrointestinal tract bleeding are discussed on pages 782–784 in the section Complications of Peptic Ulcers.

Once the patient has been stabilized, endoscopy is performed to possibly determine the cause. Endoscopy is about 80% effective. If the diagnosis is inconclusive, then upper gastrointestinal x-ray films can provide more information.

Rebleeding occurs in about 25% of patients and warrants surgical intervention. The patient is carefully monitored so that indicators of bleeding can be quickly detected. These signs include decreased central venous pressure, tachycardia, tachypnea, hypotension, mental confusion, thirst, and oliguria.

Peptic Ulcer

A peptic ulcer is an excavation formed in the mucosal wall of the stomach, the pylorus, the duodenum, or the esophagus (Fig. 33-1). A peptic ulcer is frequently referred to as a gastric, duodenal, or esophageal ulcer, depending on its location. It is caused by the erosion of a circumscribed area of mucous membrane. This erosion may extend as deeply as the muscle layers or through the muscle to the peritoneum. Peptic ulcers are more apt to be in the duodenum than in the stomach. As a rule, they occur singly, but there may be a number of them present at one time. Chronic gastric ulcers tend to occur in the lesser curvature of the stomach, near the pylorus. See Table 33-1 for a comparison of the features of gastric and duodenal ulcers.

Etiology and Incidence

The etiology of peptic ulcer is poorly understood. It is known that peptic ulcers occur only in the areas of the gastrointestinal tract that are exposed to hydrochloric acid and pepsin. The disease occurs with the greatest frequency between the ages of 40 and 60 but is relatively uncommon in women of childbearing age, although it has been observed in childhood and even in infancy. More men than women are affected (3:1),

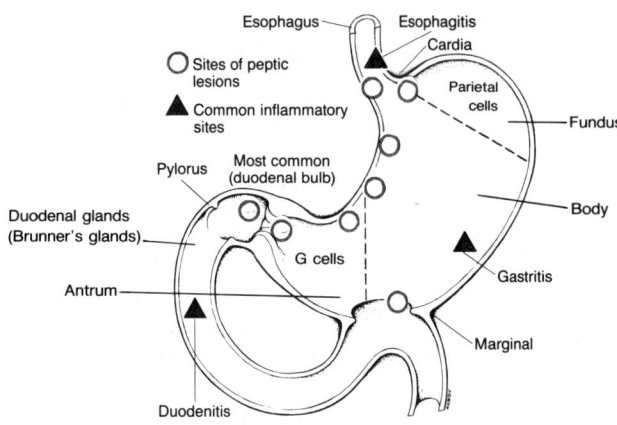

Figure 33-1
"Peptic" lesions may occur in the esophagus (esophagitis), stomach (gastritis), or duodenum (duodenitis). Note peptic ulcer sites and common inflammatory sites. Hydrochloric acid is formed by parietal cells in the fundus; gastrin is secreted by G cells in the antrum. The duodenal glands secrete an alkaline mucus solution.

although there is some evidence that the incidence in women is increasing. After menopause, the incidence of peptic ulcer in women is almost equal to that in men. Peptic ulcers in the body of the stomach can occur without excessive acid secretion; therefore, an attempt should be made to differentiate gastric from duodenal ulcers.

It is estimated that 5% to 15% of the population in the United States have ulcers, but only about half of these are recognized. Duodenal ulcer was first recognized around 1900, and the incidence increased until the 1950s. Duodenal ulcers are five to ten times more common than gastric ulcers. Since then there as been a steady decrease in the United States, but the reason is unclear. The incidence has declined by 50% over the past 20 years.

Predisposition

Attempts continue to be made to delineate the "ulcer personality." Psychoanalysts claim that an ulcer results from repression of strong dependency needs. Others claim that occupational stress, with no opportunity to express hostility, is another strong factor. It seems to develop in persons who are emotionally tense, but whether this is the cause or the effect of the condition is uncertain. Familial tendency also appears as a significant predisposing factor, revealing that three times as many ulcer patients have relatives with the same diagnosis. A further hereditary link is noted in the finding that persons in blood-group O are 35% more susceptible than persons with type A, B, or AB. Other predisposing factors associated with peptic ulcer include emotional stress, eating hurriedly and irregularly, and smoking excessively. Rarely, ulcers are due to excessive amounts of the hormone gastrin, produced by tumors (gastrinomas—Zollinger-Ellison syndrome).

Pathophysiology

Peptic ulcer occurs mainly in the gastroduodenal mucosa because this tissue is unable to withstand the digestive action of gastric acid and pepsin. The erosion is due to an increase in concentration or activity of acid-pepsin or to a decrease in the normal resistance of the mucosa. A damaged mucosa is unable to secrete enough mucus to act as a barrier against hydrochloric acid.

Gastric secretion occurs in three phases: (1) cephalic, (2) gastric, and (3) intestinal. Since these phases are interactive and not independent of one another, a disturbance in any one phase may be ulcerogenic.

Cephalic (Psychic) Phase. The first phase is initiated by stimuli such as the sight, smell, or taste of food, acting on cerebral cortical receptors that, in turn, stimulate the vagal

TABLE 33-1
Comparison of Duodenal and Gastric Ulcer

Chronic Duodenal Ulcer	Chronic Gastric Ulcer
Age	
Usually 50	Usually 45 and over
Sex	
Male–female: 4:1	Male–female: 2:1
Blood Group	
Most frequently—0	No differentiation
Social Class	
More frequently in those subjected to stress and responsibility: executives, leaders in competitive fields	More common among laboring persons
General Nourishment	
Usually well nourished	Often malnourished
Acid Production: Stomach	
Hypersecretion	Normal—hyposecretion
Pain	
2–3 hours after a meal; nighttime: often awakened between 1 AM and 2 AM	Occurs ½ to 1 hour after a meal; nighttime: rarely; relieved by vomiting
Ingestion of food relieves pain	Ingestion of food does not help; sometimes pain is increased
Vomiting	
Uncommon	Common
Hemorrhage	
Melena more common than hematemesis	Hematemesis more common than melena
Malignancy Possibility	
Never	Perhaps in less than 10%

nerves. Essentially, an unappetizing meal has little effect on gastric secretion, whereas a more tasty, appealing meal evokes a high secretion. This accounts for the traditional emphasis on serving a bland meal to the peptic ulcer patient. Today many gastroenterologists agree that the bland diet has no significant effect on gastric acidity or ulcer healing. However, excessive vagal activity during the night, when the stomach is empty, is a significant irritant.

Gastric Phase.   The gastric phase of gastric secretion is mediated by the hormone *gastrin*. Gastrin, which can be measured by a radioimmunoassay, enters the bloodstream from the antrum and is carried to glands in the fundus and body of the stomach; here it stimulates the production of gastric juice. Gastrin activity may be greater in patients with pyloric stenosis. The antrum of the patient with gastric ulcer contains less gastrin than that of the patient with a duodenal ulcer. Following partial gastrectomy or gastrojejunostomy, if part of the antrum is left in place but no longer is in contact with the acid-secreting portion of the stomach, the antrum continues to release gastrin, because acid no longer bathes the mucosa to inhibit gastrin release. Excess gastrin in the blood can lead to marginal ulcers. Excessive gastrin is also present in Zollinger-Ellison syndrome.

Intestinal Phase.   During the intestinal phase a hormone, secretin, is secreted when hydrochloric acid enters the duodenum. Secretin, in turn, stimulates bicarbonate secretion from the pancreas, which neutralizes the acid. Secretin also inhibits the gastric phase of gastric secretion.

Gastric Mucosal Barrier.   In humans, gastric secretion is a mixture of mucopolysaccharides and mucoproteins secreted continuously by the mucosal glands. This mucus adsorbs pepsin and protects it against acid. Hydrochloric acid is secreted continuously, but secretions increase owing to neurogenic and hormonal mechanisms that are initiated by gastric and intestinal stimuli. If hydrochloric acid were not buffered and neutralized, and if the outer layer of mucosa did not offer protection, hydrochloric acid, along with pepsin, would destroy the stomach. Hydrochloric acid comes into contact with only a small portion of the gastric mucosal surface: it diffuses into it with amazing slowness. This impenetrability of the mucosa is called the *gastric mucosal barrier*. It is the chief defense of the stomach against being digested by its secretions. Other factors that influence mucosal resistance are blood supply, acid–base balance, integrity of the mucosal cells, and epithelial regeneration.

Note then, that a person is likely to develop a peptic ulcer from one of two causes: (1) hypersecretion of acid-pepsin, and (2) a weakened gastric mucosal barrier. Anything that decreases the production of gastric mucus or damages gastric mucosa is ulcerogenic: salicylates, alcohol, and indomethacin fall into this category.

Clinical Manifestations

Symptoms of duodenal ulcer (the most common form of peptic ulcer) may last for a few days, weeks, or months and may even disappear only to reappear, often without an identifiable cause. Exacerbations seem to occur in the spring or fall, but even this pattern is inconsistent. Many persons have symptomless ulcers, and in 20% to 30% perforation or hemorrhage may occur without any preceding manifestations.

Pain.   As a rule, the patient with duodenal ulcer complains of pain or a burning, sharply localized sensation in the midepigastrium or in the back. It is believed that the pain occurs when the increased acid content of the stomach and duodenum erodes the lesion and stimulates the exposed nerve endings. Another theory suggests that contact of the lesion with acid stimulates a local reflex mechanism that initiates contraction of the adjacent smooth muscle.

Pain precedes meals from 1 to 3 hours and becomes progressively more severe toward the end of the day. It may also waken the person between midnight and 3 AM. However, there is no pain when the patient awakens in the morning because the flow of gastric acid is at its lowest at this time.

Pain typically is relieved quite promptly by food or alkalies, either of which neutralizes the free acid in contact with the ulcer. If the patient takes neither food nor alkali, the pain gradually wears off as the secretion of acid stops and empties into the intestine. The character of the pain may be described as a dull, burning sensation, a feeling of emptiness, or a gnawing so severe that the patient is in agony. When the ulcer has begun to affect the pancreas, pain in the back may become noticeable.

Sharply localized tenderness can be elicited by gentle pressure in the epigastrium at, or slightly to the right of, the midline. Some relief is obtained by local pressure on the epigastrium.

Pyrosis (Hypersialorrhea, Heartburn).   Some patients experience a burning sensation in the esophagus and stomach, which moves up to the mouth, occasionally with sour eructation. Eructation, or burping, is common when the patient's stomach is empty.

Vomiting.   Although rare in uncomplicated duodenal ulcer, vomiting may be a symptom of peptic ulcer. It is due to gastric outlet obstruction caused by either muscular spasm of the pylorus or mechanical obstruction. The latter may be due to scarring or to acute swelling of the inflamed mucous membrane adjacent to the acute ulcer. Vomiting may or may not be preceded by nausea; usually it follows a bout of severe pain, which is relieved by ejection of the acid gastric contents. The vomitus may contain food particles from the previous day.

Constipation and Bleeding.   Constipation may be apparent in the patient with duodenal ulcer, probably as a result of diet and medications.

- About 20% of patients who bleed from an acute duodenal ulcer have had no previous digestive complaints; however, they develop symptoms thereafter.

Diagnostic Evaluation

A physical examination may show pain, epigastric tenderness, and/or abdominal distention. Bowel sounds may be absent. A barium study of the upper gastrointestinal tract may reveal an ulcer. Upper gastrointestinal endoscopy is used to identify inflammatory changes, ulcers, and lesions. Endoscopy permits direct visualization of the duodenal mucosa and is used to augment radiographic studies. Endoscopy has been found to detect 20% of those lesions not evident in x-ray studies because of the size or location of the lesion. Stools should be collected daily until the laboratory reports are negative for occult blood. Gastric secretory studies are of value in diagnosing achlorhydria (the absence of hydrochloric acid in gastric juices) and Zollinger-Ellison syndrome. Pain that is relieved by ingesting food or antacids and the absence of pain on arising are also highly suggestive of duodenal ulcer.

A breath test has been developed that detects *Campylobacter pyloridis*, a bacterium linked to a variety of gastrointestinal disorders. This organism is present in patients with peptic ulcer disease and gastritis; however, no causative relationship has yet been established.

Management

From the beginning, once the diagnosis is established, the patient is informed that he can learn how to keep his problem under control, but he may expect both remissions and recurrences.

Control of Gastric Secretions. Gastric acidity can be managed with appropriate sedation and neutralization of the gastric juice at frequent and regular intervals with drugs, non-irritating foods, and antacids. Sometimes antispasmodics are given to reduce pylorospasm and intestinal motility. Anticholinergic agents may be prescribed to inhibit gastric secretion. Drugs that block the acid-secreting action of histamine (H_2 blockers), such as cimetidine, or that produce an acid-resistant barrier over the ulcer, such as sucralfate, have been shown to be effective in healing duodenal ulcers. Hospitalization, if required at all, can be limited to 2 or 3 days, unless bleeding, obstruction, perforation, or severe nocturnal pain are present.

Rest and Stress Reduction. Reducing environmental stress is a difficult task requiring physical and mental interventions on the patient's part and aid and cooperation of family members and significant others. The patient may need help in identifying situations that are stressful or exhausting. A rushed life-style and an irregular schedule may aggravate symptoms and interfere with regular meals taken in relaxed settings and with regular administration of medications. In addition to stress reduction suggestions, the patient may also benefit from suggestions about regular rest periods during the day, at least during the acute phase of the disease.

Smoking. Studies have been shown that smoking decreases the secretion of bicarbonate from the pancreas into the duodenum. Therefore the acidity to the duodenum is higher when one smokes.

Diet. Since there is little evidence to support the theory that bland diets are more beneficial than regular meals, patients have been encouraged to eat whatever agrees with them. However, there are a few precautions to consider in the early stages of healing. *The objective of the diet for peptic ulcers is to avoid oversecretion and hypermotility in the gastrointestinal tract.* These can be minimized by avoiding extremes of temperature and overstimulation by meat extracts, alcohol, seasonings (especially pepper and mustard), and coffee, (including decaffeinated coffee, which also stimulates acid secretion). In addition, an effort is made to neutralize acid by eating three regular meals a day. Small, frequent feedings are not necessary as long as antacids or a histamine blocker is taken.

Diet compatibility becomes an individual matter. If the patient tolerates a particular food, he may eat it. If it produces pain, he should avoid it. Milk and cream are no longer considered central to therapy. In fact, diets rich in milk and cream are potentially harmful over a long period because they increase serum lipids, a contributing factor in producing atherosclerosis. Skim milk stimulates acid secretion to some extent: the more effective the change in pH to neutral, the more

enhanced is the stimulus to new acid secretion. As alkalinity increases, gastrin release is stimulated and acid secretion is increased.

Antacids. Antacids continue to be a mainstay of peptic ulcer treatment even though they are not capable of maintaining a pH of 3.5 or above (necessary for pepsinogen inactivity) for longer than 45 minutes. The objective is to select the antacid that provides the safest and longest period of acid neutralization. Usually, antacids leave the stomach rapidly, so that frequent doses are required. Recommended dosages should not be exceeded because systemic alkalosis or rebound hyperacidity can occur.

Sodium bicarbonate is probably the best neutralizer of acid contents in the stomach but is not recommended because it is emptied from the stomach too rapidly and over a period of time can easily lead to alkalosis.

Antacids can be divided into those that contain magnesium or magnesium and aluminum and those that contain aluminum alone. Those that contain magnesium tend to cause diarrhea, and those that contain aluminum cause constipation. Antacids that contain calcium are not recommended because calcium produces an increase in serum gastrin and in acid secretion. Magaldrate (Riopan) is a low-sodium antacid that should be used for patients who are on sodium-restricted diets. All antacids have been found to be more effective if given in the liquid form.

Antacid intake is scheduled to correspond to the delay in gastric emptying. A recommended schedule is 1 to 2 tablespoons (15 to 30 ml), 1 to 3 hours after each meal and at bedtime (Chart 33-1). For convenience, most people use the tablet forms. Patients are advised to read the package directions and consult their physician for dosage and schedule. The effectiveness of antacid therapy can be prolonged if antacids are taken after a meal because gastric emptying is delayed by the presence of food. If the patient is awakened at night with epigastric pain, he notes the time, and thereafter sets his alarm clock for an hour earlier to take the antacid

---

Chart 33-1
Schedule for Prescribing Antacids in the Treatment of Peptic Disorders

This therapy concentrates antacid in the stomach and duodenum at those times when gastric secretion would be at its highest.

7:30–8:00 AM	Breakfast
9:00 AM	First dose of antacid
11:00 AM	Second dose of antacid
Noon–1:00 PM	Lunch
2:00 PM	Third dose of antacid
4:00 PM	Fourth dose of antacid
5:00–6:00 PM	Supper
7:00 PM	Fifth dose of antacid
9:00 PM	Sixth dose of antacid
Bedtime	Seventh dose of antacid

(Adapted from Eastwood GL. Core Textbook of Gastroenterology. Philadelphia, JB Lippincott, 1984.)

(see Duration of Treatment, this page, for continued pattern of antacid therapy).

Anticholinergics. Anticholinergics block acetylcholine, which is a major stimulant of acid secretion. Their effectiveness is limited because undesirable side-effects may occur at therapeutic doses. Therefore, they are only prescribed for those patients who suffer from severe, persistent nocturnal pain and are rarely recommended for long-term use. Anticholinergics decrease gastric motor activity and thus allow an antacid to remain in the stomach longer. They are occasionally used at nighttime with a double dose of antacid for persistent night pain.

Side-effects of anticholinergic drugs include dryness of the mouth and throat; excessive thirst; difficulty in swallowing; flushed, dry skin; rapid pulse and respiration; dilated pupils; and emotional excitement.

- Anticholinergic medications *should not be used* by patients with glaucoma, urinary retention, or pyloric obstruction because of drug side-effects (increased central nervous system stimulation, increased intraocular pressure, and urinary hesitation).

H₂ Receptor Antagonists. Histamine has two receptors for its action. H_1 receptor is located on bronchial and nasal mucosa, cardiac tissue, and blood vessels; H_2 receptor is found primarily in the parietal cells in the stomach, in uterine and bronchial muscle, and in T lymphocytes. Even though H_2 receptors are distributed in body tissue, only gastric receptors appear to be affected by this drug. Common antihistamines block the action of H_1 receptors but have no effect on H_2 receptors in the stomach. Cimetidine, a H_2 receptor antagonist, has a dramatic effect on lowering acid secretion in the stomach. A very high dose of the drug reduces acid secretion to an almost unmeasurable level.

Cimetidine is given orally with each meal and at bedtime. A 300-mg tablet can inhibit acid secretion by greater than 90% for about 5 hours. It also inhibits the body's secretory response to gastrin, acetylcholine, and histamine. Cimetidine relieves ulcer pain and thus decreases the need for antacids. Although research has shown that liquid antacids used appropriately are as effective as cimetidine, most patients prefer to take tablets rather than a liquid preparation throughout the day. Short-term treatment with cimetidine has resulted in complete ulcer healing, but low-dose maintenance therapy may be needed to prevent recurrence. Side-effects may include leukopenia, bone marrow depression, diarrhea, constipation, gynecomastia, and confusion in older patients. Cimetidine's effect on renal function is under investigation.

Ranitidine (Zantac) is another H_2 antagonist that is given in a tablet form twice a day. Studies have shown this drug to be as effective as cimetidine, and it causes fewer side-effects. Side-effects that have been noted include dizziness, constipation, gynecomastia, and depression. Depression usually begins in 6 to 8 weeks. It takes several weeks for the depression to lift after the drug has been stopped.

Famotidine (Pepcid) is an H_2 antagonist that is taken once a day, usually at bedtime. Trial clinical studies have shown rapid ulcer healing in 4 to 8 weeks for about 85% of those treated. Thereafter a reduced dosage is recommended for maintenance therapy. Famotidine's absorption rate is not significantly affected by antacids, which can be given at the same time. Studies on elderly patients have shown no significant changes in pharmacodynamics.

Other Drugs. Sucralfate (Carafate) is a locally acting drug that has also been shown to have antiulcer properties. Sucralfate forms complexes with proteinaceous exudates, such as albumin and fibrinogen, in the ulcer crater, producing an adherent barrier over the ulcer. This barrier is acid resistant, as opposed to acid reducing. The result is that acid is prevented from passing through to the ulcer, but the acid is not appreciably neutralized. Sucralfate is only minimally absorbed from the gastrointestinal tract and does not depend on systemic activity for its antiulcer effects.

Duration of Treatment. The patient should adhere to the drug program to ensure complete healing of the ulcer. Since most patients become free of symptoms in a week, it becomes a nursing goal to stress the imporance of following the prescribed regimen so that the breakdown of the healing process and the return of chronic ulcer symptoms are averted. Rest, sedatives, and tranquilizers add to the patient's comfort and are used as needed. Cimetidine therapy is generally continued for 4 to 6 weeks.

After the first week, the purpose of using antacids switches from that of relieving symptoms to preventing symptoms. The best plan appears to be to have the patient eat regular meals.

From the sixth or seventh week to 6 months, antacid is taken about an hour after meals and at bedtime. Thereafter, antacid therapy is usually dropped. If the person experiences a stressful situation or has been indiscreet in his diet and symptoms recur, he may resume antacid therapy until he is free of symptoms.

Prognosis

Recurrence of an ulcer is possible and may happen within 2 years in about one third of all patients, although this incidence may be affected with prophylactic use of such drugs as cimetidine, ranitidine, and famotidine. The likelihood of recurrence is lessened if the person avoids tea, coffee, and cola (including decaffeinated), alcohol, highly seasoned and fried foods, and ulcerogenic drugs, such as salicylates, corticosteroids, and phenylbutazone. If symptoms recur, he is to resume antacid medications hourly. Antacid tablets may be taken when required during a normal day's activities; however, it is necessary to chew them thoroughly and to recognize that three or four tablets are equal in potency to 1 tablespoon of liquid antacid. Medical treatment is sought if relief is not obtained.

▶ Nursing Process
The Patient With a Peptic Ulcer

▷ Assessment

The history serves as an important base for diagnosis. The patient is asked to describe the pain and methods that he uses to relieve it (food, certain antacids). Peptic ulcer pain is usually described as "burning" or "gnawing" and occurs about 2 hours after a meal. It frequently awakens the patient between midnight and 3 AM. The patient will usually state that the pain is relieved by taking antacids or foods or by vomiting. During the history the nurse asks the patient to list his usual food intake for a 72-hour period and to include his food habits (speed of eating, regularity of meals, preference for spicy foods, use of seasonings, use of caffeinated beverages). The patient's level of tension or nervousness is assessed. Does he smoke cigarettes? How does he manage the stressors of everyday life? How does he express anger? How does he describe his work and family life? Is there occupational stress or problems within his family? Is there a past family history of ulcer disease?

Vital signs are assessed for indicators of anemia (tachycardia, hypotension), and the stool is examined for occult blood. A physical examination is performed, and palpation of the abdomen for localized tenderness is emphasized.

▷ Nursing Diagnoses

Based on all the assessment data, the patient's nursing diagnoses may include the following:

- Alteration in comfort, pain, related to the effect of gastric acid secretion on damaged tissue
- Anxiety related to coping with an acute disease
- Nutritional impairment related to dietary intake, effect of acid on gastric mucosa, work habits, and methods of dealing with stress
- Activity intolerance related to lack of sleep
- Knowledge deficit related to prevention of symptoms and management of the condition

▷ Planning and Implementation

▷ *Goals:* The major goals of the patient may include relief of pain, reduction of anxiety, promotion of proper nutrition, attainment of adequate rest, and acquisition of knowledge about prevention and management.

Nursing Interventions

Relief of Pain. Pain relief can be attained by administering prescribed medications (antacids, anticholinergics, histamine antagonists). Aspirin and foods and beverages that contain caffeine (cola, tea, coffee, chocolate) and are spicy are avoided. The patient is told to eat regularly spaced meals slowly and in a relaxed atmosphere. He is encouraged to learn relaxation techniques to help him cope with stress and pain and to stop smoking. See Nursing Care Plan 33-1, Care of The Patient with Peptic Ulcer Disease.

Reduction of Anxiety. The nurse should assess what the patient knows and wants to know about his disease. His level of anxiety is evaluated. Peptic ulcer patients are usually anxious, but their anxiety is not always obvious. This attempt at coping frequently aggravates their disease process. Information is provided at the patient's level of learning, and his questions are answered. The patient is allowed to express his fears openly and without criticism. Diagnostic tests are explained, and medications are administered on schedule. Peptic ulcer patients are frequently time oriented, and any schedule deviation can cause anxiety and increase gastric secretion. The nurse emphasizes that nurses are nearby if there is a problem. She interacts with the patient in a relaxing manner and helps him identify his stressors and learn effective coping techniques and relaxation methods. She encourages the participation of his family in his care and emotional support if this is feasible.

Nutritional Considerations. The nurse should determine the patient's dietary habits and advise him to eliminate foods and beverages that stimulate hydrochloric acid and pepsin secretion. Regularly scheduled meals eaten in a relaxed manner are recommended so gastric acidity can be neutralized. The patient is advised that adherence to the medication regimen will help promote tissue healing and prevent additional irritation and inflammation. The patient is helped to identify stressful situations and to learn effective coping mechanisms and relaxation techniques.

Rest. The patient is helped to identify a realistic level of activity with scheduled rest periods that coincide with his treatment regimen. Energy-saving techniques (sit to cook, sit on a chair in the shower) are taught. He is encouraged to become aware of signs of overactivity (excessive fatigue, dizziness), and to take his medication on time so that he can sleep uninterrupted through the night.

Patient Education and Home Health Care. In order to deal successfully with ulcer disease, the patient must understand his situation and those factors that will help or aggravate his condition. Areas that need consideration and perhaps modification, along with evaluative questions, are the following:

1. *Medication:* Does the patient know what medications are to be taken at home, including name, dosage, frequency, and possible side-effects (*e.g.*, cimetidine, antacids, and anticholinergics)? Does the patient know what drugs to avoid (*e.g.*, aspirin, bicarbonate of soda)?
2. *Diet:* Does the patient know what particular foods tend to upset him? Does he know that coffee, tea, colas, alcohol, and spices have acid-producing potential? Does he know to take antacids if he overeats or overdrinks? Does he understand the importance of regular meals taken in a relaxed setting?
3. *Rest and stress reduction:* Is the patient aware of sources of stress in family and work environments? Has this illness or other situations produced symptoms of stress or poor coping in the family or work setting? Is the patient aware that smoking probably increases the irritation to his ulcer? Can the patient identify rest periods during the day? Can the patient plan for added periods of rest or relaxation after unavoidable periods of stress? Does the patient need extended psychological counseling?
4. *Awareness of complications:* Is the patient alert to signs and symptoms of complications that should be reported?

   - *Hemorrhage:* cool skin, confusion, increased heart rate, labored breathing, blood in the stool
   - *Perforation:* severe abdominal pain, rigid and tender abdomen, vomiting, elevated temperature, increased heart rate
   - *Pyloric obstruction:* nausea, vomiting, distended abdomen, abdominal pain
   - *Intractability:* persistent pain and discomfort related to stress, food intake, or drug regimen

5. *Follow-up care:* Does the patient realize that follow-up supervision is necessary for about 1 year? Does he realize that his ulcer could recur? Does he know to seek medical assistance if symptoms recur?

Care of the Patient With Peptic Ulcer Disease

Nursing Interventions	*Rationale*	*Expected Outcomes*

Nursing Diagnosis: Alteration in comfort, pain, related to irritated mucosa and muscle spasms

Goal: Relief of pain

1. Administer drug therapy as prescribed:
 	
  a. Antacids
  b. Histamine antagonists
  c. Anticholinergics
	1. Pharmacotherapy helps reduce pain as follows
	
	  a. Antacids neutralize acidity of gastric secretions
	  b. Histamine antagonists interfere with the secretion of gastric acid
	  c. Anticholinergics inhibit the release of gastric acid
		• Takes medications as prescribed.
		• Experiences less pain with drug therapy.

2. Recommend avoidance of ulcerogenic over-the-counter drugs.	2. Drugs that contain salicylates are irritable to the stomach mucosa.	• Substitutes acetaminophen (Tylenol) for aspirin. • Avoids over-the-counter drugs that contain acetylsalicylic acid (Contac, Alka-Seltzer) • Complies with recommended restrictions.
3. Advise patient to avoid foods/beverages that are irritating to the stomach lining: spicy, very hot or very cold, caffeinated foods/beverages.	3. Foods/beverages that contain caffeine or are very spicy stimulate the secretion of hydrochloric acid.	
4. Instruct patient to increase intake of water.	4. Water is considered a good antacid.	• Drinks 6 to 8 glasses of water daily.
5. Instruct patient to eat slowly and chew small pieces of food.	5. The greater the size of food particles, the greater the secretion of hydrochloric acid.	• Eats smaller amounts of food at one time and chews food slowly.
6. Advise patient to space meals and snacks at regular intervals.	6. Regularly scheduled meals help keep food particles in the stomach, which helps to neutralize the acidity of gastric secretions.	• Adheres to a schedule of regularly spaced meals and snacks.

Nursing Diagnosis: Alteration in nutrition, less than body requirements, related to pain associated with eating

Goal: Attainment of an optimal level of nutrition

1. Recommend nonirritating foods and beverages.	1. Nonirritating foods reduce epigastric pain.	• Avoids irritating foods and beverages.
2. Suggest that meals be eaten at regularly scheduled times.	2. Scheduled intervals between meals help neutralize gastric secretions.	• Eats meals and snacks at regularly scheduled intervals.
3. Encourage eating meals in a relaxed atmosphere.	3. A relaxed atmosphere is less anxiety producing. Decreasing anxiety helps decrease the secretion of hydrochloric acid.	• Chooses a relaxed atmosphere for meals.

(continued)

▷ *Evaluation*

▷ *Expected Outcomes*

1. Patient experiences less pain.
   a. Is free of pain between meals.
   b. Uses antacids to prevent pain.
   c. Avoids foods and fluids that cause pain.
   d. Eats meals at regular times.
   e. Experiences no side-effects of antacids (diarrhea, constipation, fluid retention).
   f. Uses anticholinergics as prescribed.
   g. Has no side-effects of anticholinergics.

Nursing Interventions	*Rationale*	*Expected Outcomes*

Nursing Diagnosis: Activity intolerance related to fatigue and difficulty with sleeping

Goal: Attainment of adequate rest

1. Recommend scheduled rest periods throughout the day.	1. Periods of rest alternating with periods of activity help maximize energy throughout the day.	• Verbalizes less fatigue. • Adheres to regularly scheduled rest periods throughout the day.
2. Suggest measures to conserve energy for activities of daily living (ADL): a. Sit on a stool while cooking b. Sit on a chair in the shower c. Allow 30 minutes to get dressed in the morning	2. Minimizing energy expenditure helps reduce fatigue and improve activity tolerance.	• Uses energy conserving measures for ADL.
3. Educate the patient to recognize signs of exhaustion: tachycardia, dizziness, and excessive weakness.	3. Fatigue stresses the body's normal compensatory mechanisms.	• Recalls symptoms associated with extreme fatigue. • Agrees to modify/stop activities if any signs of exhaustion occur. • Knows what symptoms indicate that a physician should be notified.

Nursing Diagnosis: Anxiety related to the fear of coping with an acute disease

Goal: Reduction of anxiety

1. Encourage the patient to express his concerns and fears and ask questions as needed.	1. Open communication fosters a trusting relationship, which helps reduce anxiety and stress.	• Expresses fears and concerns without fear of criticism.
2. Explain the reasons for adhering to a planned treatment schedule: a. Pharmacotherapy b. Diet restriction c. Modified activity levels d. Reduction or cessation of smoking	2. Knowledge reduces the anxiety found with "fear of the unknown." Knowledge can have a positive influence on behavior modification.	• Understands rationale for various treatments and restrictions. • Modifies behavior appropriately.
3. Help the patient identify anxiety-producing situations.	3. Stressors need to be identified before they can be managed.	• Identifies anxiety-producing situations.
4. Teach stress-reducing exercises: meditation, distraction, and imagery.	4. Decreased anxiety decreases hydrochloric acid secretion.	• Uses relaxation measures appropriately.

(continued)

2. Experiences less anxiety.
   a. Uses sedatives and tranquilizers as prescribed.
   b. Experiences no side-effects of sedatives and tranquilizers.
   c. Identifies situations that produce stress.
   d. Identifies life-style adjustments necessary to reduce stress.
   e. Alters life-style as appropriate.
   f. Involves family in decisions regarding life-style adjustments.
3. Maintains tissue integrity.
   a. Avoids irritating foods and beverages.
   b. Eats regularly scheduled meals.
   c. Eats slowly and in a relaxed atmosphere.
   d. Takes prescribed medications as scheduled.
   e. Uses coping mechanisms to deal with stress.
4. Attains adequate rest.
   a. Alternates activity with rest periods.
   b. Uses energy-saving techniques for activities of daily living.
   c. Recognizes signs of overactivity.

Complications of Peptic Ulcers

There are four major complications of peptic ulcer: hemorrhage, perforation, pyloric obstruction, and intractable ulcer.

Nursing Interventions	*Rationale*	*Expected Outcomes*

Potential Complications: Hemorrhage, perforation, pyloric obstruction

Goal: Prevention of complications

1. Encourage the patient to adhere to his planned treatment schedule.	1. Adherence to treatment schedule will minimize complications.	• Follows plan of care.
2. Make the patient aware of the signs/symptoms indicating one of the following complications:	2. Knowledge improves the patient's awareness of his disease condition. Knowledge can have a positive influence on behavior modification.	• Recognizes signs/symptoms of possible complications.
a. Hemorrhage		
1) Tachycardia		
2) Dyspnea		
3) Confusion		
b. Perforation		
1) Severe abdominal pain		
2) Rigid and tender abdomen		
3) Tachycardia		
c. Pyloric obstruction		
1) Nausea and vomiting		
2) Distended abdomen		
d. Intractability		
1) Pain related to stress		
2) Pain related to intake of irritating foods		

Nursing Diagnosis: Knowledge deficit regarding the prevention of symptoms and management of the condition

Goal: Acquisition of knowledge about prevention and management

1. Assess the patient's level of knowledge and "readiness to learn."	1. Attending to learning is dependent on a patient's physical condition, level of anxiety, and mental readiness.	• Expresses an interest in learning how to manage his disease.
2. Teach necessary information:		• Participates in teaching sessions.
a. Use words at the "level of learner."		• Asks questions.
b. Choose a time when the patient is rested and interested.		
c. Limit teaching sessions to 30 minutes or less.		
3. Reassure the patient that the disease can be managed.	3. Knowledge can have a positive influence on behavior modification.	• States a desire to be responsible for self-care.

Hemorrhage.   Manifested by hematemesis, melena, or both, hemorrhage is the *most common complication* of peptic ulcer. Hemorrhage occurs in 10% to 20% of patients with ulcers and has a mortality rate of 30% to 40%. The most frequent site is the distal portion of the duodenum. When the hemorrhage is of large proportions (2000 to 3000 ml), most of the blood is vomited. The patient may become almost exsanguinated, and rapid correction of blood loss will be required to save his life. When the hemorrhage is small, much or all of the blood may be passed in the stools, which will appear tarry black owing to the digested hemoglobin.

Assessment.   The nurse assesses the patient for early symptoms of faintness or giddiness; nausea may precede or accompany bleeding. Dyspepsia may not be present. Vital signs are evaluated for tachycardia, hypotension, and tachypnea. The hemoglobin and hematocrit are analyzed. The stool is tested for gross or occult blood, and 24-hour urinary output is recorded to detect anuria or oliguria.

Management.   Because bleeding can be fatal, the physician will identify the cause and severity of the hemorrhage and correct the blood loss to prevent hypovolemic shock.

• Preparations are made for a peripheral intravenous line for infusion of saline and blood and possibly a central line for infusion and measurement of central venous pressure. Whole blood or plasma transfusions are given

to keep the circulating blood volume at a safe level. The physician does not wait for a drop in blood pressure before starting transfusion therapy if there are signs of tachycardia, sweating, and coldness of the extremities.
- The hemoglobin and hematocrit are monitored to detect bleeding.
- An indwelling urinary catheter is inserted to monitor urinary output.
- Nasogastric intubation is used to distinguish fresh blood from "coffee-ground" material and administer iced saline for lavage (clot removal, vasoconstriction of superficial vessels). The normal saline solution may be taken by mouth and the fluid withdrawn through the tube by suction. Usually, the nasogastric tube is left in place during the cooling procedure. This removes acid, prevents nausea and vomiting, and provides a means of monitoring further bleeding. Antacids are administered after the bleeding has been controlled.
- Oxygen therapy may be instituted.
- The patient is placed in the recumbent position to prevent hypovolemic shock.
- Vital signs are monitored every 5 minutes initially and then every 15 to 30 minutes.
- Hypovolemic shock is treated as outlined on pages 365–367.

If bleeding cannot be managed by the measures just described, then the following may be done:

- *Intra-arterial vasopressin infusions via pump directly into a bleeding artery:* A repeat arteriogram is needed to evaluate the efficacy of treatment.
- *Selective embolization:* Emboli of autologous blood clots with or without Gelfoam (absorbable gelatin sponge), or a mixture of the patient's own blood. Amicar (ε-aminocaproic acid), and platelets are forced through a catheter to a point above the bleeding lesion.
- *Endoscopic laser photocoagulation:* Coagulation of the bleeding site is accomplished by a laser beam.

Surgical Treatment. If bleeding recurs in 48 hours after medical therapy has begun, or if more than 5 units of blood is required in 24 hours to maintain blood volume, the patient is likely to be scheduled for surgery. Some physicians recommend that if a patient with peptic ulcer hemorrhages three times, surgery is indicated.

Other determining factors for surgery are the patient's age (if he is over 60, massive hemorrhaging is three times more likely to be fatal), a history of chronic duodenal ulcer, and a coincidental gastric ulcer.

The ulcer-bearing area is removed, or the bleeding vessels are ligated. In many patients a procedure is included that is aimed at controlling the underlying causes of the ulcer (*e.g.*, vagotomy and pylorectomy, or gastrectomy).

Perforation. Perforation of a peptic ulcer may occur unexpectedly, without much evidence of preceding indigestion. Perforation into the free peritoneal cavity is an abdominal catastrophe and an indication that surgery is required.

Signs and symptoms to note during a nursing assessment include the following:

- Sudden, severe upper abdominal pain (persisting and increasing in intensity)

- Pain, which may be referred to the shoulders, especially the right shoulder, because of irritation of the phrenic nerve in the diaphragm
- Vomiting and collapse (fainting)
- Extremely tender and rigid (boardlike) abdomen
- Shock

Immediate surgical intervention is indicated, because chemical peritonitis develops within a few hours following perforation and is followed by a bacterial peritonitis. Therefore, the perforation must be closed as quickly as possible. In a few patients, it may be deemed safe and advisable that surgery be performed for the ulcer disease, in addition to the perforation being sutured.

Postoperatively, the stomach contents are drained by means of a nasogastric tube. The nurse monitors fluid and electrolyte balance and assesses the patient for peritonitis or localized infection (increased temperature, abdominal pain, paralytic ileus, increased or absent bowel sounds, abdominal distention). Antibiotic therapy is given parenterally as prescribed.

Pyloric Obstruction. Pyloric obstruction occurs when the area distal to the pyloric sphincter becomes scarred and stenosed from spasm or edema or from scar tissue that is formed when the ulcer alternately heals and breaks down. The patient has symptoms of nausea and vomiting, constipation, epigastric fullness, anorexia, and (later) weight loss.

In treating the patient, the first consideration is the relief of the obstruction by gastric decompression. At the same time, attempts are made to confirm that obstruction is the cause of discomfort. This is done by checking the amount of fluid aspirated from the nasogastric tube. A residual of over 200 ml is strongly suggestive of obstruction. Some physicians also use the load test, which involves infusing 750 ml of normal saline via the nasogastric tube into the mid-antrum of the stomach. The patient is rotated, to permit normal gastric emptying; 20 minutes later, aspiration is done, and if more than 400 ml is retrieved, obstruction is confirmed.

Before surgery is undertaken, decompression continues and extracellular fluid volume and electrolyte and metabolic derangements are corrected. Conscientious daily fluid monitoring is continued. With supportive measures, the patient's condition may improve. It may be feasible to repeat the load test; if negative, medical treatment continues. If positive, surgery, in the form of a vagotomy and antrectomy, may be required. If the patient is severely malnourished during this time, parenteral hyperalimentation may be used.

Intractability. An intractable ulcer is one that continues to give problems and is resistant to all forms of treatment. It is the most common, persistent problem seen with peptic ulcer disease and the most common reason given by patients for choosing surgery.

A careful patient history includes a thorough review of dietary and drug habits, which could reveal long-term use of caffeine-containing drinks or aspirin-containing medications. The entire gastrointestinal tract is carefully assessed to determine other possible problems, such as hiatus hernia, gallbladder disease, or diverticulitis.

The patient and family are informed of the fact that surgery is no guarantee that an ulcer is cured. Possible postoperative sequelae, such as intolerance to dairy products and sweet foods, are also discussed.

Surgical Approaches

Surgery for ulcer disease is done when medical therapy has not been successful or when complications arise, such as hemorrhage, perforation, or pyloric obstruction. Patients requiring ulcer surgery may have had a long illness, be discouraged, have interruptions in their work role, and experience pressures in their family life. Various types of surgical procedures may be used in treating peptic ulcer disease (Table 33-2).

- *Subtotal gastrectomy* is removal of one third to three fourths of the stomach. The remaining segment is anastomosed to the duodenum or the jejunum.
- *Antrectomy* involves removing the antral (lower) portion of the stomach (which contains the G cells that secrete gastrin) as well as a small portion of the duodenum and pylorus. The remaining segment is anastomosed to the duodenum (Billroth I) or the jejunum (Billroth II). See Figure 33-2. An antrectomy may also be performed in conjunction with a truncal vagotomy.
- *Vagotomy,* severing of the vagus nerves, may be done to reduce gastric acid secretion.

  Truncal vagotomy, severing of the right and left vagus nerves as they enter the stomach at the distal part of the esophagus, is the type of vagotomy most commonly used to decrease acid secretion and reduce gastric and intestinal motility.

  Selective vagotomy involves severing vagal innervation to the stomach but maintaining the innervation to the rest of the abdomen.

  Parietal cell vagotomy involves severing only those vagus nerves that innervate the parietal cell mass in the upper portion of the stomach. Antrum innervation remains intact, decreasing the need for a pyloroplasty.

- *Pyloroplasty* is a drainage operation in which a longitudinal incision is made into the pylorus and transversely sutured closed to enlarge the outlet and relax the muscle (see Fig. 33-2). A pyloroplasty usually accompanies truncal and selective vagotomies, which produce delayed gastric emptying.

Nursing Interventions. Preoperative nursing care for the patient undergoing surgery for peptic ulcer disease includes the following:

- *Preparing the patient for diagnostic tests:* The patient undergoes laboratory analyses, x-ray series, and a general physical examination before surgery. The nurse prepares

TABLE 33-2
Gastric Operations for Peptic Ulcers

Operation	Description	Mortality	Recurrence	Advantages	Sequelae
Vagotomy with drainage: pyloroplasty or gastroenterostomy	Vagotomy may be truncal or selective (preserving hepatic, celiac, and pancreatic branches)	Under 1%	5%–10%	Fairly simple Clinical results: 75%—excellent 10%—fair 10%—poor	Some patients experience problems of fullness after eating (33%), dumping syndrome (10%), diarrhea (10%), and gastritis (90%)
Vagotomy with antrectomy	Resection of vagus nerves and removal of antrum	3.9%	3.3%	Marginal ulceration rate lowest	In some patients, fullness after eating, dumping syndrome, diarrhea, anemia, malabsorption
Subtotal gastrectomy Billroth I (gastroduodenostomy; anastomosis after resection)	Removal of distal ⅓ to ½ of stomach; anastomosis with duodenum	2%	1%–3%	Restores normal continuity	Dumping syndrome, anemia, malabsorption, and weight loss. Billroth I has a 4% marginal ulceration rate.
Billroth II (gastrojejunostomy; anastomosis after resection)	Removal of distal segment of stomach and antrum: anastomosis with jejunum		1%–3%		Billroth II has a 2% marginal ulceration rate.
Proximal (parietal cell) gastric vagotomy without drainage	Denervation of acid-secreting parietal cells but preserving vagal innervation to gastric antrum and extragastric abdominal viscera	Under 1%	1%–9%	No dumping syndrome, reflex gastritis, or diarrhea No need for antibiotics, since gastrointestinal tract is not open	Appears to be a safe procedure; needs long-term assessment

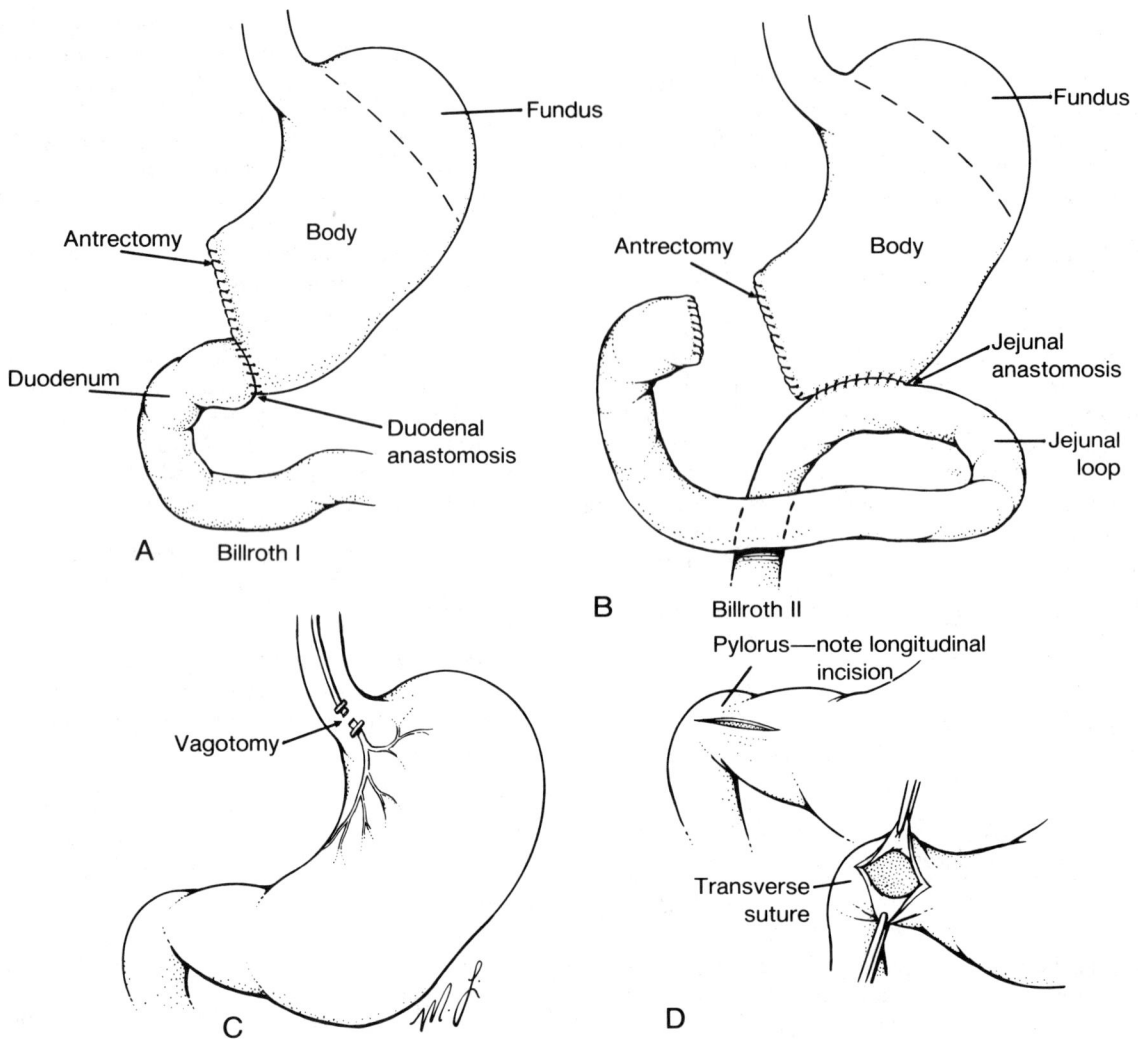

Figure 33-2
Surgical procedures for ulcer disease. (*A*) Antrectomy with anastomosis to the
duodenum (Billroth I). (*B*) Antrectomy with anastomosis to the jejunum (Billroth II).
(*C*) Severing of the vagus nerves (vagotomy). (*D*) A longitudinal incision into the pylorus
followed by a transverse suture to enlarge the opening (pyloroplasty).

the patient for each of these diagnostic measures by explaining their nature and significance.
- *Attending to the patient's fluid and nutritional needs:*
  The nutritional and fluid needs of the patient are of major
  importance. In those patients with pyloric obstruction,
  there usually is prolonged vomiting, with resultant weight
  and fluid loss. Every effort is made to restore an adequate
  nutritional level and to maintain an optimal fluid and
  electrolyte balance.
- *Clearing and emptying the gastrointestinal tract:* Nasogastric suction often is required to empty the stomach,
  especially in patients with pyloric obstruction. The tube
  is inserted before the operation and left in place for operative and postoperative use.

  It is important that the colon be empty when the
  patient comes to surgery; this is ensured by an enema

the day before surgery. If gastrointestinal films have been
made shortly before the day of surgery, it is most important that enemas be given to completely remove the
barium that may remain in the colon.
- *Limiting fluid intake:* The patient usually is limited to
  fluids during the 24-hour period preceding surgery.
- *Shaving and preparing the skin:* The abdomen should
  be prepared, from the nipple line to the symphysis, although the incision is usually made in the upper right
  quadrant or the midline.

Postoperative care is the same as that for gastric surgery.
(See pages 790–797, Nursing Management of the Patient Un-
dergoing Gastric Surgery, as well as pages 792–795, Nursing
Care Plan 33-2, Care of the Patient Experiencing a Gastric
Resection.)

Zollinger-Ellison Syndrome (Gastrinoma)

Zollinger-Ellison syndrome is considered a possibility when a patient presents with several peptic ulcers. It is identified by the following findings: hypersecretion of gastric juice, multiple duodenal ulcers (second and third portions), an increase in parietal cell mass, hypertrophied duodenal glands, and gastrinomas (islet cell tumors) in the pancreas. The gastrinomas may also be found in the duodenum and stomach. The incidence of malignancy is approximately 65%. The huge amounts of secreted hydrochloric acid almost have the effect of the stomach's trying to digest itself. The serum gastrin level is increased. In Zollinger-Ellison syndrome, secretin stimulates gastrin secretion rather than inhibits it. Steatorrhea (unabsorbed fat in the stool) may be evident, because excessive gastric acid inactivates lipase in the intestine, thereby precipitating bile salts and decreasing fat digestion. The result is steatorrhea and diarrhea. Gastrin also decreases water and salt absorption, which in turn leads to diarrhea.

Management. Hypersecretion of acid can be controlled with cimetidine (Tagamet) in doses up to 1200 mg, four to six times a day. However, there is a high failure rate with prolonged drug therapy. The recommended surgical procedure is antrectomy with a truncal or parietal cell vagotomy (see p. 785). Total gastrectomy is the most successful treatment for those who cannot be managed with H_2 receptor blockers. Preoperatively, the patient's weight needs to be monitored and fluid and electrolyte balance must be brought under control. In the postoperative period, dietary instruction is necessary. Lifelong parenteral vitamin B_{12} therapy will be necessary if a total gastrectomy is done because intrinsic factor, secreted by the gastric mucosal cells and necessary for vitamin B_{12} absorption, can no longer be produced. Careful follow-up monitoring is done to detect possible metastasis.

Nursing Assessment. Diarrhea and hypercalcemia are common problems. A nursing assessment frequently reveals that the patient's symptoms are often refractory (unyielding) to large amounts of antacids. He may disclose taking several pints of milk a day with no apparent relief from pain.

Stress Ulcer

Stress ulcer is the term given to a group of duodenal or gastric ulcers that occur following physiologically disturbing conditions.

Pathophysiology and Etiology. Stressful conditions such as burns, shock, severe sepsis, and multiple organ trauma can initiate the development of such ulcers. Fiberoptic endoscopy within 24 hours of injury reveals shallow erosions of the stomach wall; by 72 hours, multiple gastric erosions are observed. As the stressful condition continues, the ulcers spread. When the patient recovers, the lesions are reversed. This is typical of stress ulceration.

Differences of opinion exist as to the actual causation of mucosal ulceration. Usually, it is preceded by shock; this leads to a decrease in gastric mucosal blood flow and a reflux of duodenal content into the stomach. In addition, large quantities of pepsin are released. The combination of ischemia, acid, and pepsin creates an ideal climate to produce ulceration. When acute stress ulceration is combined with central nervous system trauma, stress ulcers (Cushing's ulcers) are often deeper and more penetrating. Gastric erosions are frequently observed about 72 hours after extensive burns (Curling's ulcers).

Management. Antacids are the basis of treatment. If the patient is acutely ill, antacids may be given through the nasogastric tube. Frequent gastric aspiration is done to check pH, in an attempt to get it to, or above, 3.5. Antacid therapy can also inhibit the activity of the proteolytic enzyme, pepsin. Stress ulcers are treated aggressively with antacid therapy and cimetidine therapy. Other methods of management of upper gastrointestinal tract hemorrhage are discussed on page 775.

Morbid Obesity

Morbid obesity is a term applied to people who are twice their ideal body weight. Management consists of placing the person on a reducing diet, implementing behavioral modification, and encouraging enrollment in a weight loss clinic. Some physicians recommend acupuncture and hypnosis. When conservative measures have been tried for more than 5 years and have failed, a surgical procedure is recommended.

Surgical Management

Maxillomandibular Fixation. In maxillomandibular fixation the person's jaws are wired to prevent the mouth from opening more than a fraction. The object is to restrict the patient's oral intake to fluids. Weight loss with this method is slow, and most patients regain their weight.

Intragastric Balloon. The intragastric balloon is a soft polyurethane sac that is inserted into the stomach, where its presence reduces the space available for food. The patient is sedated for the procedure, and the balloon, which is about the size of a small juice can, is inserted into the stomach by means of an endoscope. Although the exact mechanism of action is not known, it is believed that the balloon stimulates gastric nerve fibers that induce satiety. Patients feel full and eat smaller meals. The balloon is meant to supplement diet management and behavior modification. It must be removed after 4 months and is reinserted if needed. A major concern with this method of treatment is the danger that the balloon may break, necessitating removal via endoscope to prevent it from passing through the duodenum.

Jejunoileal Bypass. Jejunoileal bypass is the anastomosis of the proximal jejunum to the terminal ileum. It is preferred only for those patients weighing more than 500 pounds and only as a temporary measure. It is usually followed by gastric bypass or gastroplasty when the patient has lost sufficient weight to be considered a good surgical candidate. Jejunoileal bypass is associated with an unacceptable amount of metabolic complications (hepatic cirrhosis, renal stones, hypoproteinemia) and is therefore not recommended for long-term management of morbid obesity.

Gastric Bypass and Vertical Banded Gastroplasty. Gastric bypass and vertical banded gastroplasty are the current gastric restrictive operations of choice for gastric morbidity. In gastric bypass surgery, the proximal segment of the stomach is transected to form a small pouch with a small gastroenterostomy stoma. The Roux-en-Y gastric bypass is the recommended procedure for long-term weight loss. In the Roux-en-Y bypass, a horizontal row of staples creates a stomach pouch with a 1-cm stoma that is anastomosed with a portion of distal jejunum creating a gastroenterostomy. The transected proximal portion of the jejunum is anastomosed to the distal jejunum (Fig. 33-3).

In vertical banded gastroplasty a double row of staples is applied vertically along the lesser curvature of the stomach beginning at the angle of His. A small stoma is created at the end of the staples by adding a circle of staples or a band of polypropylene mesh or silicone tubing (Fig. 33-4).

Nursing Interventions. General postoperative nursing care is similar to that for any patient experiencing gastric resection (see Nursing Care Plan 33-2). Patients are usually discharged in 1 week with detailed dietary instruction. Usually a 600- to 800-calorie diet is recommended, and fluid intake is encouraged to prevent dehydration. Patients are instructed to report any excessive thirst or concentrated urine to their physician. Outpatient visits are scheduled monthly.

Psychosocial considerations are essential for these patients. All efforts are directed toward helping them modify

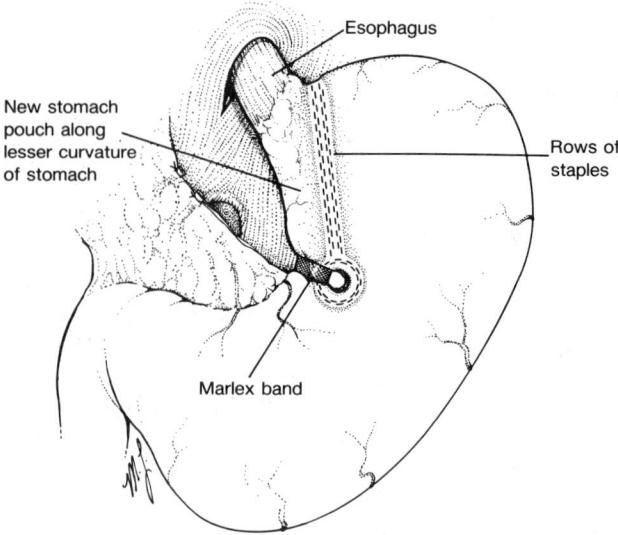

Figure 33-4
Vertical banded gastroplasty. A vertical row of staples along the lesser curvature of the stomach creates a new, smaller stomach pouch.

their eating behaviors and cope with their body image change. Noncompliance usually results in patients eating too much or too fast. If this happens, vomiting and painful esophageal distention may occur.

Postoperative complications usually occur in the immediate postoperative period and include peritonitis, stomal obstruction, stomal ulcers, atelectasis and pneumonia, thromboembolism, and metabolic sequelae resulting from prolonged vomiting and diarrhea.

Gastric Cancer

Cancer of the stomach continues to decrease in the United States, for some unexplained reason (a 60% decline in the United States in the past 30 years). However, it is still a serious problem, accounting for 14,200 deaths annually, mostly in people over 40, and occasionally in younger people. More than 90% of cases arise from the mucosa but less than 5% appear as gastric ulcers. The incidence of gastric cancer is four times greater in Japan, which has led to mass surveys for earlier diagnosis in that country. Heredity appears to be a factor, as do chronic inflammation of the stomach, pernicious anemia, and achlorhydria (25%). The prognosis is poor. About 60% of patients have clinical findings at the time of diagnosis, resulting in a low cure rate.

Clinical Manifestations

The early symptoms of gastric cancer are often indefinite, since most of these tumors start on the lesser curvature, where they cause little disturbance to gastric functions. Later, after

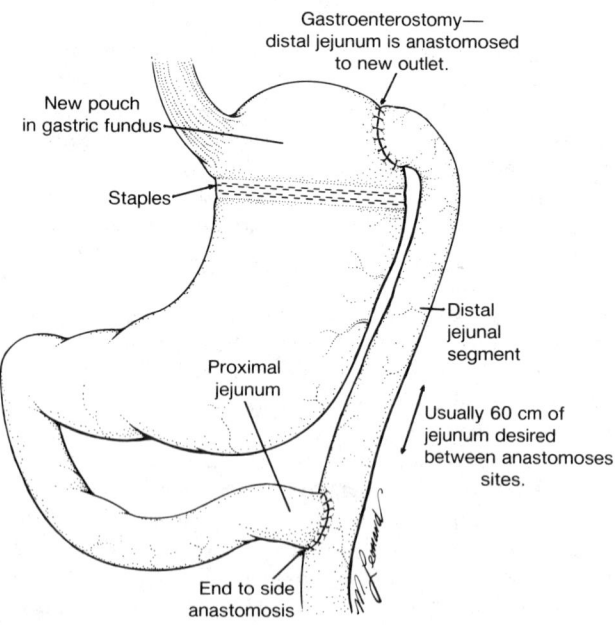

Figure 33-3
Gastric bypass with Roux-en-Y. A horizontal row of staples creates a pouch with a capacity of 50 ml or less. The proximal jejunum is transected and the distal end anastomosed to the new pouch. The proximal segment is anastomosed to the jejunum.

they have spread to the cardiac orifice, or especially to the pylorus, the suffering may be distressing; this is due not as much to the cancer as to the disturbance in gastric motility. Weight loss, weakness, anemia, and sometimes icterus appear late in the disease. Pain, in gastric cancer, as in cancer in almost all other parts of the body, is a late symptom. Whereas pain is a sensitive indicator of disturbed physiology or disease, it is ironic that pain rarely warns the person who has cancer while there is still an opportunity of curing it. The most important early symptoms of gastric cancer are

- A progressive loss of appetite and weight
- The appearance of, or change in, gastrointestinal symptoms that have been increasingly apparent for only a matter of weeks or months
- The appearance of blood in the stools
- Vomiting (If the tumor causes obstruction at the cardiac orifice, vomiting or a feeling of fullness will immediately follow a meal. If the tumor is near the pylorus, it eventually obstructs this channel, and vomiting becomes a prominent sign.)
- Occasional vomiting of "coffee-ground" vomitus or signs of blood in the stool

The blood that leaks slowly from the cancer (large hemorrhages are rare in patients with gastric cancer) is altered chemically and forms small clots or precipitates. The patient may not vomit, but traces of blood may be found in the stools when examined in the laboratory.

Diagnostic Evaluation

When gastric juice, obtained by aspiration, reveals no free hydrochloric acid, gastric neoplasm is suspected. Biopsies through the gastroscope are most helpful. Cytologic studies verify the diagnosis. Occasionally, the tumor is palpable, especially if it is located near the pylorus. Since metastasis frequently occurs before warning signs are experienced, x-ray films, fluoroscopy, and gastroscopy are most valuable in determining the extent of the problem. Occult blood may be found in stools. Serum protein levels would be low. Dyspepsia of more than 4 weeks' duration in any person over age 40 calls for complete x-ray examination of the gastrointestinal tract.

Management

There is no successful treatment of gastric carcinoma except removal of the tumor. If the tumor can be removed while it is still localized to the stomach, the patient can be cured. If the tumor has spread beyond the area that can be excised surgically, cure cannot be effected. However, in many of these patients, effective palliation may be obtained by resection of the tumor (see pp. 790–797, Nursing Management of Patients Undergoing Gastric Surgery). If a *radical subtotal gastrectomy* has been performed, the stump of the stomach is anastomosed to the jejunum, as in the gastrectomy for ulcer. When *total gastrectomy* is performed, gastrointestinal continuity is restored by an anastomosis between the ends of the esophagus and jejunum. Palliative, rather than radical, surgery is done if there is metastasis to other vital organs, such as the liver.

▶ ## Nursing Process
The Patient With Gastric Cancer

▷ ### Assessment

The nurse asks the patient if there is a family history of cancer. If so, are immediate members or close or distant relatives afflicted? This information is helpful when determining possible support systems. What is the patient's marital status? Is there someone who is going to provide emotional and financial support?

The patient's occupation is recorded. Has he been exposed to an environmental carcinogen? Is he currently employed? Is he happy in his job? Is he experiencing job-related stress? If so, for how long? Stress increases the incidence of gastric mucosal irritation.

Does he smoke cigarettes? If so, how many a day? How long has he been smoking? Does he notice any stomach discomfort during or after smoking?

He is asked to describe his eating pattern, including frequency and size of meals, number of snacks per day, food preferences, and intake of fats, fiber, and starches. Has he lost weight? If so, how much and over what period of time? His ideal body weight is recorded, and a 24-hour diet recall is elicited to aid in nutritional counseling. Is he having nausea, vomiting, hematemesis, or anorexia?

During the physical examination it may be possible to palpate a mass. Other organs are examined for tenderness or a tumor. Pain is usually a late symptom.

▷ ### Nursing Diagnoses

Based on all the assessment data, the patient's major nursing diagnoses may include the following:

- Anxiety related to anticipating the surgical procedure
- Alteration in nutrition, less than body requirements related to anorexia
- Alteration in comfort, pain, related to the presence of abnormal epithelial cells
- Anticipatory grieving related to the diagnosis of cancer
- Knowledge deficit regarding self-care activities

▷ ### Planning and Implementation

▷ *Goals:* The major goals of the patient may include reduction of anxiety, attainment of optimum nutrition, relief of pain, and adjustment to the diagnosis and to anticipated lifestyle changes.

Nursing Interventions

Reducing Anxiety. A relaxed, nonthreatening atmosphere is provided so that the patient can express his fears, concerns, and possibly anger with the diagnosis and prognosis. The nurse encourages the family to listen or ventilate as appropriate. She offers assurance and supports positive coping measures. She advises the patient about any procedures and treatments so that he knows what to expect and suggests that he discuss his feelings with a member of the clergy if he so desires.

Promoting Optimum Nutrition. Small frequent feedings of nonirritating foods are encouraged to decrease gastric irritation. Food supplements should be high in vitamins A and C and iron so that tissue repair is facilitated. If a total gastrectomy is to be done, then parenteral vitamin B_{12} will need to be given indefinitely. The nurse monitors the rate and frequency of intravenous therapy. She records intake, output, and daily weights to make sure the patient is maintaining or gaining weight. Signs of dehydration (thirst, dry mucous membranes, poor skin turgor, tachycardia) are assessed and results of daily laboratory studies are reviewed to note any metabolic abnormalities (sodium, potassium, glucose, blood urea nitrogen). Antiemetics are administered as prescribed.

Relief of Pain. Analgesics are administered as prescribed. A continuous drip infusion may be necessary for severe pain. The frequency, intensity, and duration of the pain is assessed to determine the effectiveness of the analgesic being administered. The nurse works with the patient to help him manage his pain (*e.g.,* position changes, decreased environmental stimuli, restricted visiting). Nonpharmacologic methods for pain relief such as imagery, distraction, relaxation tapes, backrubs, and massage are suggested, and periods of rest and relaxation are encouraged.

Psychosocial Support. The nurse helps the patient express his fears and concerns about his diagnosis. He is allowed the freedom to grieve in his own way. His questions are answered honestly, and he is encouraged to participate in his treatment decisions. Some patients mourn the loss of a body part and perceive their surgery as a type of mutilation. Some express disbelief and need reality reinforcement. Privacy should be provided during periods of crying if the patient wants to be alone.

The nurse offers emotional support and involves family members and significant others whenever possible. She must be aware of mood swings and defense mechanisms (denial, rationalization, displacement, regression) and reassure the patient and family members that emotional responses are normal and expected. Professional services are provided if necessary, including those of clergy, psychiatric nurse clinical specialists, psychologists, social workers, and psychiatrists. The nurse projects an empathetic approach and spends time with the patient. Most patients will begin to participate in self-care activities when they have acknowledged their loss.

Patient Education and Home Health Care. The patient is advised that it may take 6 months before regular meals can be eaten after a partial resection. Small, frequent feedings are given initially, or he will be fed via a tube; intravenous hyperalimentaion may be necessary. With any enteral feeding the possibility of the dumping syndrome exists, so it must be explained and ways to manage it reviewed.

The patient is told that it may take 3 months before normal activities can be resumed. Daily periods of rest are necessary, and he will have to visit his physician frequently after he is discharged. Changes in life-style will be affected by irradiation or chemotherapy. The patient needs to know what to expect: length of treatments, expected reactions (nausea, vomiting, anorexia, fatigue), need for transportation to and from the treatments, and need for a support person for the first 24 hours after the treatment because of generalized weakness. Psychological counseling may be necessary for some.

Nutritional counseling is started in the hospital and reinforced at home. Any tube feeding procedure is supervised by a visiting nurse who teaches the patient and family members how to use the equipment and formulas and how to detect complications. (See p. 759 to review management of tube feedings.) The patient learns to record his daily intake, output, and weight and is taught how to cope with pain, nausea, vomiting, and bloating. He is made aware of those complications that require medical attention, such as bleeding (overt or covert hematemesis, melena), obstruction, perforation, or any symptoms that become consistently worse.

The nurse teaches the patient how to care for his incision and how to examine the wound for signs of infection (malodorous drainage, pain, heat, inflammation, swelling). Any irradiation or chemotherapy regimen is explained. The patient as well as his family need to know what kind of care will be needed during and after treatments. Patients who live alone or who are responsible for the care of children need to make arrangements for help for about 24 hours after a treatment.

▷ *Evaluation*

▷ *Expected Outcomes*

1. Patient experiences less anxiety.
   a. Understands the surgical procedure.
   b. Expresses his fears and concerns about surgery.
   c. Seeks emotional support.
   d. Discusses feelings about surgery with family.
   e. Discusses the surgical procedure and postoperative course.
2. Attains optimum nutrition.
   a. Eats small, frequent meals.
   b. Eats foods high in iron and vitamins A and C.
   c. Maintains a reasonable weight.
3. Experiences less pain.
   a. Takes prescribed medications as scheduled.
   b. Rests periodically during the day.
   c. Uses relaxation techniques.
4. Adjusts to diagnosis.
   a. Freely expresses his fears and concerns.
   b. Seeks emotional support from family members.
   c. Discusses his prognosis.
5. Performs self-care activities and adjusts to life-style changes.
   a. Resumes normal activities within 3 months.
   b. Alternates periods of rest and activity.
   c. Tolerates three regular meals daily within 6 months after surgery.
   d. Manages tube feedings.
   e. Adjusts to intravenous hyperalimentation.
   f. Adheres to irradiation/chemotherapy regimen.
   g. Keeps follow-up clinic or physician appointments.

Nursing Management of Patients Undergoing Gastric Surgery

The major considerations in the nursing care of patients undergoing gastric surgery include providing physical and psychological support in the preoperative period, assessing and monitoring for complications in the postoperative period, and preparing the patient to deal with the post-hospitalization regimen and required self-care activities.

Preoperative Nursing Interventions. An important part of preoperative nursing care involves allaying the patient's fears and anxieties about the impending surgery and its implications. The nurse encourages the patient to express his feelings and answers his questions. It is also necessary to explain the surgical procedure to the patient and prepare him for what to expect after the operation, such as nasogastric intubation and intravenous fluid therapy. However, if the operation is an emergency, because of hemorrhage, perforation, or acute obstruction, adequate psychological preparation may not be possible. In this event, the nurse caring for the patient in the postoperative period should anticipate his concerns, fears, and questions and be available for support and explanation.

Gastric Resection (Partial Gastrectomy)

Postoperative nursing strategies following gastric resection include the following:

1. *Positioning the patient:* When recovery from anesthesia is complete, the patient is placed in a modified Fowler's position, for comfort and for easy drainage of the stomach.

2. *Avoiding pulmonary complications:* Pain medications are administered as prescribed, so that deep breathing and productive coughing may be effective in preventing pulmonary complications. This will overcome the patient's tendency to take shallow breaths for fear of incisional pain. The patient will be asked to take deep breaths and to cough hourly in the immediate postoperative period. The nurse should listen with a stethoscope for lung congestion.

3. *Checking nasogastric tube drainage:* Drainage from the nasogastric tube may contain some blood for the first 12 hours, but excessive bleeding should be reported. Since a nasogastric tube is in place and peristalsis has not yet returned, fluids by mouth are withheld. The nurse should evaluate the patient for the return of peristalsis by listening to the lower abdomen with a stethoscope. It is also important to observe for signs of distention (increased girth) and to contact the surgeon for any needed readjustment of the nasogastric tube.

4. *Giving nose and mouth care:* The nostrils can be cleaned with an applicator stick moistened with water, followed by swabbing with another applicator stick dipped in mineral oil. To relieve dryness of the mouth, mouthwashes may be given frequently. Cool water sponges to the lips are preferred to cracked ice chips, since ice often intensifies thirst.

5. *Attending to fluid needs:* Parenteral fluids are given to meet fluid and nutritional needs, as well as to compensate for fluid lost in drainage and vomitus. Fluid intake as well as output is recorded.

   Following the return of peristalsis and the removal of the nasogastric tube, fluids by mouth may be restricted for several hours, then begun sparingly. Small amounts of water are used at first, after which the amount is gradually increased as tolerated. Cold fluids usually cause distress. Therefore, warm, weak tea with sugar and lemon is preferred.

6. *Providing dietary intake:* Bland foods are gradually added until the patient is able to eat six small meals a day and drink 120 ml of fluid between meals. The key to increasing the dietary content is to offer increments gradually as tolerated and to recognize that each person is different. If regurgitation occurs, the patient may be eating too fast or too much. It also may indicate that edema along the suture line is preventing fluids and food from moving into the intestinal tract. If gastric retention does occur, it may be necessary to reinstitute nasogastric suction.

7. *Encouraging ambulation:* Usually on the first postoperative day, the patient is encouraged to get out of bed. Ambulation is then increased daily.

8. *Providing wound care:* Wound dressings may have serosanguineous drainage because of drainage tubes left in the wound. Dressings are reinforced if necessary; however, undue drainage saturation is reported.

Total Gastrectomy

Nursing interventions for the patient having a total gastrectomy include the care described on pages 792–795 (under Nursing Process: Caring for the Postoperative Patient) and pages 446–458 (The Patient Undergoing Thoracic Surgery), since the chest cavity may be entered. Because of the location of the incision, respiration is painful and limited. The importance of breathing exercises is emphasized (practice is encouraged before the operation), and the patient is assisted with breathing after surgery. The nutritional status of the patient with gastric cancer or another long-standing gastric condition often needs to be improved before surgery, usually by total parenteral nutrition for several days.

Postoperatively, nasogastric suction will not involve as much drainage, since the stomach is no longer present to produce secretions or to act as a receptacle. The nasogastric tube is removed as soon as normal bowel sounds are heard. Clear fluids are given hourly and small feedings offered after 2 or 3 days, providing there is no evidence of anastomosis leakage (temperature elevation), edema, or obstruction (regurgitation). If there is regurgitation or an increase in temperature, it must be reported immediately.

Additional interventions are described in Nursing Care Plan 33-2, Care of the Patient Experiencing a Gastric Resection.

Nutritional Management After Gastric Surgery

Often a patient who has had gastric surgery has been undernourished before the operation because of food intolerance or preoperative diagnostic testing. There may be significant protein deficiency, which may require parenteral nutritional support (see p. 766) for the first 5 or 6 postoperative days. Mouth feeding is resumed as soon as the patient feels hungry and bowel sounds are elicited.

Dysphagia may be noticed in those patients who have had truncal vagotomy, which causes trauma to the lower

(Text continues on p. 795)

Care of the Patient Experiencing a Gastric Resection

Nursing Interventions	*Rationale*	*Expected Outcomes*

Preoperative

Nursing Diagnosis: Knowledge deficit regarding the surgical procedure and postoperative course

Goal: Attainment of information about the procedure and postoperative course

1. Make certain the patient understands what type of surgery he is to have.	1. Preoperative knowledge helps the patient understand the reasons for postoperative procedures.	• Improves adherence to treatment regimen.
2. Advise the patient that he will be placed in a modified Fowler's position after recovery from anesthesia.	2. Modified Fowler's position promotes comfort and drainage of the stomach.	
3. Advise the patient that he will be asked to breathe deeply and cough, postoperatively.	3. Coughing and deep breathing will prevent pulmonary complications.	• Avoids shallow breathing associated with incisional pain.
4. Advise the patient that he will have a nasogastric tube in place postoperatively and fluids will be withheld until peristalsis returns.	4. The nasogastric tube provides for gastric drainage that may contain some blood for the first 12 hours.	• Tolerates discomfort of nasogastric tube.
5. Inform the patient that he will be receiving parenteral fluids. Oral fluids will be withheld until the nasogastric tube is removed and peristalsis returns.	5. Parenteral fluids meet fluid and nutritional needs and compensate for fluids lost in drainage and vomitus.	• Accepts fluid restriction by mouth.
6. Let the patient know that bland foods are added gradually.	6. Small increments of food and fluid (120 ml between meals) are initiated to determine the patient's tolerance.	• Adheres to dietary regimen.
7. Inform the patient that ambulation will usually be encouraged on the first postoperative day.	7. Early ambulation prevents venous stasis and phlebothrombosis.	• Is anxious to get up out of bed as soon as possible.
8. Tell the patient that wound dressings may have drainage. Excessive drainage or bright red blood will be reported immediately.	8. Serosanguineous drainage is expected postoperatively especially if tubes are left in the wound.	• Understands that dressings will have drainage and will be reinforced.

Postoperative

Potential Complications: Shock, hemorrhage, pulmonary problems, thrombosis and embolism, wound evisceration, dumping syndrome, leakage from duodenal stump, pancreatitis

Goal: Avoidance of complications

1. Assess patient for signs of shock:
  a. Evaluate drainage from dressing and drainage bottle.
  b. Evaluate blood pressure, pulse, and respiratory rates.
  c. Give blood and fluid replacement at time prescribed.
	1. Decreased circulating blood volume can lead to hypovolemic shock.	• Alerts nurse to any dizziness, increased heart rate, confusion, excessive fatigue, or clammy skin.

(continued)

Nursing Interventions	*Rationale*	*Expected Outcomes*

Postoperative

Potential Complications: Shock, hemorrhage, pulmonary problems, thrombosis and emoblism, wound evisceration, dumping syndrome, leakage from duodenal stump, pancreatitis

Goal: Avoidance of complications

2. Be alert to signs of hemorrhage:
  a. Watch gastric aspirate in drainage bottle for evidence of blood.
  b. Observe the suture line for bleeding.
  c. Evaluate blood pressure, pulse, and respiratory rates.
  d. Prepare patient for blood transfusion, and start replacement if indicated.
  e. If bleeding continues, prepare patient for surgical intervention.
	2. Hemorrhage can lead to hypovolemic shock and death.	• Alerts nurse to any signs of bleeding.

3. Assess for pulmonary complications:
  a. Auscultate for clear lung sounds.
  b. Encourage deep breathing and coughing to counteract voluntary diaphragm splinting.
  c. Promote frequent turning and moving to mobilize bronchial secretions.
  d. Ambulate, when prescribed, to increase respiratory exchange.
	3. Inactivity encourages the pooling of pulmonary secretions.	• Cooperates with pulmonary routine.
		• Ambulates early as prescribed.

4. Examine for thrombosis and embolism:
  a. Encourage participation in self-care activities to increase circulation.
  b. Encourage early ambulation to minimize stasis of venous blood.
  c. Use elastic stockings as indicated to prevent venous stasis.
  d. Check dressing and binders for tightness that impairs circulation.
	4. Inactivity results in venous stasis, which can lead to the formation of a phlebothrombosis and possible embolism.	• Ambulates early as prescribed.

5. Be aware of possible wound evisceration:
  a. Use abdominal binders if prescribed for support.
  b. Prevent distention and wound infection.
  c. Support incision when coughing.
  d. Promote good nutrition.
  e. Inspect dressing frequently.
	5. Unnecessary strain on a suture line may result in evisceration.	• Supports incision as directed.

6. Teach the patient how to avoid the dumping syndrome:
  a. Eat small meals.
  b. Avoid salty, or highly concentrated carbohydrate foods.
  c. Take fluids between meals.
	6. Hypertonic intestinal contents draw fluid, by osmosis, from the extracellular fluid into the jejunum increasing the density of the intestinal mass and rapidly distending the jejunum.	• Eats meals in a semirecumbent position. Lies down for 20 to 30 minutes after the meal.
		• Takes fluids 1 hour after meals.
		• Eats low carbohydrate diet.
		• Takes anticholinergics as prescribed.

(continued)

Nursing Interventions	Rationale	Expected Outcomes

Postoperative

Potential Complications: Shock, hemorrhage, pulmonary problems, thrombosis and emoblism, wound evisceration, dumping syndrome, leakage from duodenal stump, pancreatitis

Goal: Avoidance of complications

Nursing Interventions	Rationale	Expected Outcomes

d. Avoid liquids with meals.
 e. Eliminate sweets from the diet.
 f. Eat regularly, slowly, and in a relaxed environment.
 g. Lie down after meals.
 h. Take anticholinergic drugs before meals (as directed) to lessen gastrointestinal activity.
 7. Check for leakage from the duodenal stump:
   a. Evaluate for pain, elevation of temperature, accelerated pulse rate, abdominal rigidity, and deteriorating clinical course.
   b. Observe for appearance of bile-stained drainage.
   c. Prepare for surgical drainage:
     1) Obtain drainage equipment.
     2) Prepare for intravenous infusions and blood transfusions.
     3) Institute nasogastric suction.
     4) Protect skin from irritating drainage.
 8. Assess for signs of pancreatitis: abdominal pain, rapid pulse, and temperature elevation.
   a. Establish continuous gastric suction.
   b. Maintain fluid and blood volume and electrolyte balance.
   c. Control pain.
   d. Give medications and antibiotics as prescribed.
	7. Decreased circulating blood volume can lead to hypovolemic shock.
	
	 8. Pain, tenderness and elevated temperature are abjective indicators of inflammation.
		• Alerts nurse to any abdominal tenderness, rigidity, or pain.

Nursing Diagnosis: Alteration in comfort, pain, related to the surgical incision

Goal: Relief of pain

Nursing Interventions	Rationale	Expected Outcomes
1. Promote frequent turning for comfort and for the prevention of pulmonary and vascular complications.	1. Inactivity encourages the pooling of pulmonary secretions.	• Cooperates with pulmonary routine.
2. Give analgesics or narcotics as prescribed.	2. Pain control results from selective depression of the central nervous system.	• Requests pain medication as needed.
3. Withhold oral fluids until prescribed.	3. Sealing of the suture line is enhanced if patient is NPO.	• Remains NPO.
4. Use gastric suction to remove liquids, blood, and gas from stomach.	4. Promotes healing of suture line. Prevents unnecessary distention and pain.	

(continued)

Nursing Interventions	*Rationale*	*Expected Outcomes*

Nursing Diagnosis: Alteration in nutrition, less than body requirements, related to the surgical procedure

Goal: Attainment of optimum nutrition

1. Give intravenous fluids as prescribed.	1. Intravenous fluids help prevent shock and maintain fluid and electrolyte balance.	• Cooperated with intravenous therapy.
2. Give oral fluids when audible bowel sounds are present.	2. Positive bowel sounds indicate peristalsis is present.	
3. Increase fluids according to patient's tolerance.	3. Maintain fluid balance.	• Accepts fluids as tolerated.
4. Keep patient on bland diet with vitamin suppliments as indicated by his condition.	4. Bland foods are less irritating to stomach mucosa.	• Adheres to diet therapy.
5. Maintain supplementary iron–vitamin therapy.	5. Iron–vitamin therapy is necessary to supplement postoperative diet to promote tissue repair and prevent anemia.	• Takes iron–vitamin supplement as prescribed.
6. Avoid foods that may initiate development of dumping syndrome: moderate amount of fat, low carbohydrate.	6. Decreased hypertonicity of intestinal contents prevents the osmotic pull of extracellular fluid into the intestinal area.	• Adheres to diet therapy.

Nursing Diagnosis: Potential nonadherence to the therapeutic regimen related to denial

Goal: Adherence to therapeutic regimen

1. Help patient to modify his environmental stresses.	1. Stress increases the secretion hydrochloric acid, which irritates a compromised/damaged stomach mucosa.	• Employs stress reduction methods (biofeedback, imagery, distraction).
2. Encourage him to remain under medical supervision.	2. Periodic hematologic studies are necessary to monitor for anemia. A complete physical examination may yield data about possible metatasis.	• Sees physician every 6 to 12 months as scheduled.
3. Arrange for some person or agency to help the patient cope: home health worker, clergyman, psychologist, nurse practitioner.	3. Long-term coping requires a support system.	• Seeks help when needed.

esophagus. This patient may be more comfortable on a soft diet for the first 10 days to 2 weeks. To encourage the patient to eat, attractive and appetizing food should be served in a pleasant atmosphere. With regard to long-term management of this patient, weight loss is a common problem because the patient experiences early fullness that curbs his appetite. Anorexia may also be due to the dumping syndrome, which occurs in about one fifth of patients following partial gastrectomy (see p. 796).

Appropriate nursing intervention is to suggest the following patient teaching points:

- Fluids should be taken before or between meals, rather than with meals.
- Smaller but more frequent meals should be eaten.
- Meal composition should be more dry than fluid-filled.
- Diets with small-molecule carbohydrates, such as sucrose and glucose, should be avoided, but fat may be consumed to tolerable levels.
- It may be advisable to supplement the diet with vitamins and medium-chain triglycerides.

Other dietary deficiencies of which the nurse should be aware include (1) malabsorption of organic iron, which may require supplementation with oral or parenteral iron, and (2) low serum level of vitamin B_{12}, which may require supplementation by the intramuscular route.

Postoperative Complications

For an overall outline of the complications following gastric resection and related nursing management, see Nursing Care Plan 33-2.

Shock.   Shock has been mentioned as a complication, especially in very ill patients. The restoration of normal temperature and the administration of fluids are the prophylactic measures necessary. For symptoms and treatment of shock, see pages 363–367.

Hemorrhage.   Hemorrhage is occasionally a complication after gastric operations. The patient exhibits the usual signs (see p. 367) and may vomit bright red blood in considerable amounts. Since this experience can prove upsetting to the patient, diazepam (Valium) or phenobarbital is effective in lessening the patient's apprehension. Nasogastric drainage or lavage may be physician-initiated. Epinephrine may be given to produce vasoconstriction.

- When hemorrhage occurs, it is important to initiate antishock measures and notify the physician. Blood, blood substitutes, and intravenous equipment are made available.
- Nursing support of the patient is given concurrently with emergency therapy.

Pulmonary Complications.   Pulmonary complications frequently follow upper abdominal incisions because of the tendency for shallow respirations. Therefore, the nurse uses foresight and initiates appropriate preventive measures to promote optimum oxygen–carbon dioxide exchange and adequate circulation.

Steatorrhea.   Steatorrhea (unabsorbed fat in the stool) is partially the result of rapid gastric emptying, which prevents adequate mixing with pancreatic and biliary secretions. In mild cases, steatorrhea can be controlled by reducing the intake of fat and taking an antimotility drug.

Dumping Syndrome.   The term dumping syndrome designates an unpleasant set of vasomotor and gastrointestinal symptoms that occur after meals in 10% to 50% of patients who have had gastrointestinal surgery or a form of vagotomy.

Clinical Manifestations.   Early symptoms may include a sensation of fullness, weakness, faintness, dizziness, palpitations, diaphoresis, cramping pains, and diarrhea. Later, there is a rapid elevation of blood glucose followed by a compensatory reaction of insulin secretion. This results in a reactive hypoglycemia, which is also unpleasant for the patient. Symptoms that may occur 10 to 90 minutes after eating are vasomotor and are manifested by pallor, perspiration, palpitations, headache, and feelings of warmth, dizziness, and even drowsiness.

Pathophysiology.   The pathophysiology underlying this syndrome is not completely understood, but there may be several causes for its occurrence. One is the mechanical result of surgery in which a small gastric remnant connects into the jejunum through a large opening. Foods that are high in carbohydrates and electrolytes have to be diluted in the jejunum before absorption can take place; yet the passage of food from the stomach remnant into the jejunum is too rapid. The ingestion of fluid at mealtime is another factor that causes the stomach contents to empty rapidly into the jejunum. The symptoms that occur are probably brought about by rapid distention of the jejunal loop anastomosed to the stomach. The hypertonic intestinal contents draw extracellular fluid from the circulating blood volume into the jejunum to dilute the high concentration of electrolytes and sugars.

Nursing Strategies.   In anticipation of the possibility of the patient's experiencing the dumping syndrome, nursing intervention is directed toward proper dietary instruction.

- The patient should be positioned in a semirecumbent position during mealtime. Following the meal, he should lie down for 20 to 30 minutes to delay stomach emptying.
- Fluids are discouraged with meals but may be given up to an hour before mealtime or 1 hour following mealtime.
- Fat may be given to tolerance, but carbohydrate intake should be kept low (sucrose and glucose are avoided).
- Antispasmodics, as prescribed, also may aid in delaying the emptying of the stomach.

Surgery is resorted to only if absolutely necessary (less than 1% of patients).

Gastritis and Esophagitis.   With the removal of the pylorus, which acts as a barrier to the reflux of duodenal contents, a bile reflux gastritis and esophagitis may occur. This is manifested by burning epigastric pain and the vomiting of bilious material. Eating or vomiting does not relieve the situation. Binding agents such as cholestyramine, aluminum hydroxide gel, or metoclopramide hydrochloride (Reglan, Maxeran) have been used with some success.

Bezoars (Phytobezoar).   Bezoars are gastrointestinal concretions (hardened particles) of digested plant material (such as skins, seeds, and fibers of fruit and vegetables). The patient complains of a feeling of upper abdominal fullness and a "dragging" sensation. The undigested fibers congeal to form a mass that becomes coated by mucous secretions; this produces a *bezoar.* Bezoars may erode the gastrointestinal mucosa and cause ulceration, hemorrhage, perforation, or obstruction. On x-ray or endoscopy, a freely movable mass is observed. The endoscope can be used to break up the concretion. Restricting cellulose-containing foods (especially citrus fruits, such as oranges) is a good prophylactic measure, as is proper mastication of food.

Vitamin B_{12} Deficiency.   Total gastrectomy brings to an abrupt, complete, and final halt the production of "intrinsic factor," the gastric secretion that is required for the absorption of vitamin B_{12} from the gastrointestinal tract (see p. 738). Therefore, unless this vitamin is supplied by parenteral injection throughout life, the patient inevitably suffers from vitamin B_{12} deficiency, which leads in time to a condition identical to that of a patient with pernicious anemia in relapse. All of the manifestations of pernicious anemia, including macrocytic anemia and combined system disease, may be expected to develop within a period of 5 years or less, to progress in severity therafter, and, in the absence of therapy, to prove fatal. This complication is avoided by the regular monthly intramuscular injection of 100 to 200 μg of vitamin B_{12}, a regimen that should be started without delay after gastrectomy.

Evaluation

Nursing evaluation of the patient who has had gastric surgery involves confirming that the patient is free of physical complications and is coping effectively with the surgical experience and his postoperative concerns. Points to be noted include the following:

- *Stable respiratory status:* Respiratory rate between 14 and 20 per minute; clear breath sounds
- *Lack of infection or excessive drainage or hemorrhage:* Vital signs stable; minimal blood in gastric drainage after 12 hours
- *Stable hydration and nutrition:* Adequate intake and output; adequate urinary drainage; gradually tolerating

fluids and bland foods; maintaining or possibly gaining weight; absence of dumping syndrome
- *Daily increases in activity and ambulation*
- *Effective coping behavior:* Patient understands the purposes of the surgical procedure and the postoperative course; verbalizes his concerns about the surgical outcome; uses support of family or significant others appropriately

Patient Education and Home Health Care

Patient teaching is based on an assessment of the patient's physical and psychological readiness to return to his home and the community. (If the patient has gastric cancer, goals are for maintenance and palliation.) The patient and family will benefit from a team approach to discharge care. The team members include the community nurse, physician, nutritionist, and perhaps the social worker. Written instructions about meals, activities, medications, and follow-up care are helpful. The postdischarge plan has to be individualized, and the patient's physical status, resources, and prognosis taken into account. The plan should include the following areas:

- *Nutrition and hydration:* The patient may be on small, frequent feedings or may have progressed to regular meals. Resumption of regular meals may require a period of 6 months. If a major portion of the stomach was removed, the patient may require enteral tube feedings or perhaps parenteral hyperalimentation therapy (see Chap. 32).
- *Activity and rest:* Gradual resumption of activities is encouraged according to the patient's abilities. This could require a period of at least 3 months but is dependent on the patient's previous activity schedule. Daily rest periods are encouraged.
- *Analgesics:* If the patient requires medication for pain, instructions regarding usage and administration are given.
- *Follow-up supervision:* The patient should understand that follow-up care is necessary. Travel arrangements for clinic and office visits may be necessary.
- *Long-term coping:* The need for assistance for the patient and family in coping with the situation should be anticipated. Appropriate community agencies (*e.g.,* church, hospice, home health worker) are identified and referrals made as needed.

Bibliography

Books

Bockus HL (ed). Gastroenterology. Philadelphia, WB Saunders, 1984.

Brandt LJ. Gastrointestinal Disorders of the Elderly. New York, Raven Press, 1984.

Eastwood GL. Core Textbook of Gastroenterology. Philadelphia, JB Lippincott, 1984.

Gilman AG et al (eds). The Pharmacological Basis of Therapeutics. New York, Macmillan, 1985.

Given BA and Simmons SJ. Gastroenterology in Clinical Nursing. St. Louis, CV Mosby, 1984.

Griffin J. Critical Care of the Cancer Patient. Chicago, Year Book Medical Publishers, 1985.

Griffin J. Hematology and Immunology, Concepts for Nursing. New York, Appleton-Century-Crofts, 1986.

Hamilton H. Gastrointestinal Disorders. Springhouse, Pennsylvania, Springhouse Corporation, 1985.

Howland M. Critical Care of the Cancer Patient. Chicago, Year Book Medical Publishers, 1985.

Sleisenger MH and Fordtran JS. Gastrointestinal Disease: Pathophysiology, Diagnosis, Management. Philadelphia, WB Saunders, 1983.

Articles

(Asterisks indicate nursing research articles.)

Peptic Ulcer and Gastritis

Bankhead CD. *Campylobacter* and GI diagnosis. Med World News 1986 Nov; 2(21):30–31.

Bardhan KD. Refractory duodenal ulcer. Gut 1984 July; 25(7):711–717.

Blum AL. Therapeutic approach to ulcer healing. Am J Med 1985 Aug 30; 79(2C):8–14.

Bruckstein AH. Peptic ulcer disease: New concepts, new and current therapeutics. Consultant 1986 Apr; 26(4):157–168.

Crawshaw JP. Managing acid reflux: A stepped approach. Patient Care 1986 Apr 15; 20(7):72–90.

Ferrara JJ et al. Preoperative serum creatinine as a predictor of survival in perforated gastroduodenal ulcer. Ann Surg 1985 Oct; 51(10): 551–555.

Fisher RS. Modern concepts of peptic ulcer disease: Advances in treatment. Med Times 1983 Jan; 111(1):111–121.

Goldberg MA. Medical treatment of peptic ulcer disease: Is it truly efficacious? Am J Med 1984 Oct; 77(4):589–591.

Holt KM and Isenberg JI. Peptic ulcer disease: Physiology and pathophysiology. Hosp Pract 1985 Jan; 20(1):89–106.

Johnston IDA. The adverse effects of gastric surgery for peptic ulceration. Med Times 1984 May; 112(5):63–69.

Johnston JH et al. Comparison of heater probe and YAG laser in endoscopic treatment of major bleeding from peptic ulcers. Gastrointest Endosc 1985 June; 31(3):175–180.

Kaushik SP, Ralphs DNL, and Hobsley M. Influences on the occurrence of dumping syndrome. Am J Gastroenterol 1983 Mar; 78(3):155–158.

Kleinman MS. Gastroesophageal reflux disease. Hosp Pract 1985 May 15; 20(5):40I, 40L, 40N.

Lamy PP. Treating GI upset in older adults. J Gerontol Nurs 1985 July; 11(7):40, 42.

*Mathewson M et al. Milk therapy in ulcer disease: Yes or no? . . . Milk is no longer the ideal. Crit Care Nurs 1984 May/June; 4(3):75.

McCarthy DM. Smoking and ulcers, time to quit. N Engl J Med 1984 Sept 13; 311(11):726–728.

Medley ES. Peptic ulcer disease. J Fam Pract 1984 Mar; 18(3):443–451.

Meeroff JC. Ulcer disease of the upper gastrointestinal tract. Hosp Pract 1984 Oct; 19(10):177–192.

Moody FG. Answers to questions on stress ulcer. Hosp Med 1983 Nov; 19(11):84–85.

Negre J. Seasonal periodicity of peptic ulcer: A myth. Lancet 1985 June 29; 1(8444):1504–1505.

Peters MN and Richardson CT. Stressful life events, acid hypersecretion and ulcer disease. Gastroenterology 1983 Jan; 84(1):114–119.

Pounder RE. Duodenal ulcers that will not heal. Gut 1984 July; 25(7): 697–702.

Rubin M et al. Dysphagia: A clinical guide. Hosp Med 1984 Sept; 20(9): 231–246.

Shorvon PJ et al. Preliminary clinical experience with the heat probe at endoscopy in acute upper gastrointestinal bleeding. Gastrointest Endosc 1985 Dec; 31(6):364–366.

Sontag SJ. Prostaglandins and acid peptic disease. Am J Gastroenterol 1986 Nov; 81(11):1021–1028.

Steer ML and Silen W. Diagnostic procedures in gastrointestinal hemorrhage. N Engl J Med 1983 309(11):646–649.

Strickland RG. Acute and chronic gastritis. Hosp Med 1983 June; 19(6): 148–176.

Swain CP et al. Which electrode? A comparison of four endoscopic methods of electrocoagulation in experimental bleeding ulcers. Gut 1984 Dec; 25(12):1424–1431.

Zimmerman TW. Problems associated with medical treatment of peptic ulcer disease. Am J Med 1984 Nov 19; 77(5B):51–56.

Gastrointestinal Bleeding

Brearley S et al. Endoscopic prediction of major rebleeding. Gastroenterology 1985 Feb; 90(2):507–508.

Briones T. Nursing care plan for the patient with acute gastrointestinal bleeding. Crit Care Nurs 1984 Mar/Apr; 4(2):22–24.

Bullas JB et al. Upper gastrointestinal hemorrhage. Crit Care Nurs 1984 May/June; 4(3):72–74.

*Dusek JL. Iced gastric lavage slows bleeding in gastric hemorrhage. Crit Care Nurs 1984 July/Aug; 4(4):8.

Fleischer D. Etiology and prevalence of severe persistent upper gastrointestinal bleeding. Gastroenterology 1983 Mar; 84(3):538–543.

Fuller E. Finding the site of upper GI bleeding. Patient Care Feb 29; 18(4):80–92.

Gever LN. Controlling upper GI tract bleeding with vasopressin. Nursing '85 1985 Nov; 15(11):81.

Greenburg AG et al. Changing patterns of gastrointestinal bleeding. Arch surg 1985 Mar; 120(3):341–344.

Griffin JP. Be prepared for the bleeding patient. Nursing '86 1986 June; 16(6):34–42.

Langman MJS. Upper gastrointestinal bleeding: The trials of trials. Gut 1985 Mar; 26(3):217–220.

Meeroff JC. Management of massive gastrointestinal bleeding: I. Hosp Pract 1986 May 15; 21(5):154 A-C, 154 G-H, 154 J-L.

Meeroff JC. Management of massive gastrointestinal bleeding: II. Hosp Pract 1986 May 30; 21(5):93–106.

Patras AZ, Paice JA, and Lanigan K. Managing GI bleeding: It takes a two-tract mind. Nursing '84 1984 July; 14(7):26–33.

Rottenberg R. GI bleeding . . . emergency handbook. Patient Care 1986 Sept 15; 20(14):72–87.

Morbid Obesity

Besson A. The Roux-Y loop in modern digestive tract surgery. Am J Surg 1985 May; 149(5):656–664.

Carey LC, Martin EW Jr, and Mojzisik C. The surgical treatment of morbid obesity. Curr Probl Surg 1984 Oct; 21(10):8–78.

Earlam R. Bile reflux and the Roux-en-Y anastomosis. Br J Surg 1983 July; 70(7):393–397.

Freeman JB and Burchett HJ. Failure rate with gastric partitioning for morbid obesity. Am J Surg 1983 Jan; 145(1):113–119.

Freeman JB, Deitel M, and MacLean LD. Morbid obesity. Contemp Surg 1985 Jan; 26(1):71–118.

Griffin WO. Stapling in gastroesophageal surgery. Surg Clin North Am 1984 June; 64(3):529–542.

*Orr J. Obesity. J Adv Nurs 1985 Jan; 10(1):71–78.

Payne WS. Prevention and treatment of biliary-pancreatic reflux esophagitis: The role of long-limb Roux-Y. Surg Clin North Am 1983 Aug; 63(4):851–858.

*Torrington KG at al. Postoperative chest percussion with postural drainage in obese patients following gastric stapling. Chest 1984 Dec; 86(6):891–895.

Gastric Cancer

Classification of early gastric carcinoma. Hosp Med 1984 July; 20(7):132B.

Hagin GD and Jain A. Gastric cancer: Complete chemotherapy response in an elderly woman: Current status of treatment. Am J Gastroenterol 1985 Nov; 80(11):835–837.

Hattori T. Development of adenocarcinomas in the stomach. Cancer 1986 Apr 15; 57(8):1529–1534.

Lawrence W. Gastric cancer. CA 1986 July/Aug; 36(4):216–236.

Leichman L et al. Cisplatin: An active drug in the treatment of disseminated gastric cancer. Cancer 1984 Mar 15; 53(1):18–22.

Perez D et al. Gastric carcinoma after peptic ulcer surgery. Am Surg 1984 Oct; 50(10):538–540.

Rhoads JE. Nutrition and cancer: An introduction. Surg Clin North Am 1986 Oct; 66(5):869–872.

Shiratori Y et al. Significance of a gastric mass screening survey. Am J Gastroenterol 1985 Nov; 80(11):831–834.

Shiu MH et al. Recent results of multimodal therapy of gastric lymphoma. Cancer 1986 Oct 1; 58(7):1389–1399.

Stockbrugger RW et al. Gastroscopic screening in 80 patients with pernicious anaemia. Gut 1983 Dec; 24(12):1141–1147.

Zollinger-Ellison Syndrome

Andersen BN et al. Development of cimetidine resistance in the Zollinger-Ellison syndrome. Gut 1985 Nov; 26(11):1263–1265.

Haught JM. Zollinger-Ellison syndrome: An overview. SGA J 1983 Winter; 6(3):14–17.

Jin GL et al. Surgical management of gastrinoma. Surg Clin North Am 1985 Apr; 65(2):285–290.

Thompson JC et al. The role of surgery in the Zollinger-Ellison syndrome. Ann Surg 1983 May; 197(5):594–607.

Therapy

Collen MJ et al. Comparison of ranitidine and cimetidine in the treatment of gastric hypersecretion. Ann Intern Med 1984 Jan; 100(1):52–57.

Deveney CW, Stein S, and Way LW. Cimetidine in the treatment of Zollinger-Ellison syndrome. Am J Surg 1983 July; 146(1):116–128.

Gever LN. Ranitidine: New relief for peptic ulcers. Nursing '84 1984 June; 14(6):22.

Griffin JW Jr. H$_2$ blocker update . . . success of H$_2$ receptor antagonists in ulcer disease. Hosp Formul 1984 Nov; 19(11):1032–1038.

Heading RC. Antacids and duodenal ulcer. Gut 1984 Nov; 25(11):1195–1198.

Howard JM et al. Famotidine, a new potent long-acting histamine H$_2$ receptor antagonist: Comparison with cimetidine and ranitidine in the treatment of Zollinger-Ellison syndrome. Gastroenterology 1985 Apr; 88(4):1026–1033.

Isenberg JI et al. Healing of benign gastric ulcer with low-dose antacid or cimetidine. N Engl J Med 1983 June 2; 308(22):1319–1324.

*Pearson BD. Pain control: An experiment with imagery. Geriatr Nurs 1987 Jan/Feb; 8(1):28–30.

Rawls DE et al. Peptic ulcer: Previewing new drugs, reviewing current therapy. Consultant 1984 Feb; 24(2):85–98.

Rottenberg R. Planning drug therapy for peptic ulcer. Patient Care 1986 Apr 30; 20(8):27–36.

Shorvon PJ et al. Preliminary clinical experience with the heat probe at endoscopy in acute upper gastrointestinal bleeding. Gastrointest Endosc 1985 Dec; 31(6):364–366.

Weintraub M et al. Pirenzepine: A new anticholinergic agent for the treatment of peptic ulcer disease. Hosp Form 1985 Oct; 20(10):1057–1059.

Wicklund S (ed) et al. Ranitidine-induced depression. Am J Nurs 1986 Oct; 86(10):1151.

Agencies

American Cancer Society, 90 Park Avenue, New York, New York 10016.

American Digestive Disease Society, 420 Lexington Avenue, New York, New York 10017.

American Gastroenterological Association, 6900 Grove Road, Thorofare, New Jersey 08086.

National Interagency Council on Smoking and Health, 419 Park Avenue, South, New York, New York 10016.

Chapter 34

Management of Patients With Intestinal Disorders

Digestive diseases constitute a major health problem afflicting more than 34 million Americans. About 20 million of them have a chronic disorder and about 2 million are permanently disabled. Long-term disability drains the economy. Digestive diseases account for 200,000 absences from work daily and for males are the leading cause of time lost from work. About $100 million is paid annually in benefits to veterans who receive payments for service-connected disabilities due to digestive conditions. The greatest cost, however, is in the number of lives lost annually (200,000).

Two of the major intestinal problems afflicting many people, especially the elderly, are constipation and diarrhea. In all age groups, a fast-paced life-style, high levels of stress, irregular eating habits, insufficient intake of fiber and water, and lack of daily exercise contribute to these problems. Laxatives are among the most popular over-the-counter medications purchased in the United States today, and laxative abuse is becoming a serious problem in the aged population. Nurses can have an impact on the chronicity of these problems by identifying behavior patterns that put patients at risk, by educating the public about prevention and management, and by helping those afflicted improve their condition and prevent complications.

Constipation

Constipation refers to an abnormal infrequency of defecation, and also to abnormal hardening of stools that makes their passage difficult and sometimes painful.

Chronic Constipation

Most individuals have one bowel movement a day. However, the range of normal extends from three movements per day to three or fewer per week. In persons who are constipated, defecation is irregular and is complicated by hardened stools. Some constipated persons occasionally have a diarrhea of liquid stools as a result of the irritation caused by the presence in the colon of hard, dry fecal masses. Such stools contain a good deal of mucus, secreted by glands in the colon in response to these irritating masses. In severe constipation, the rectum may become impacted, that is, filled with masses of hard feces that must be removed by the fingers or first softened by instillations of oil before they can be washed out by an enema.

Constipation can be caused by certain medications (tranquilizers, anticholinergics, narcotics, antacids with aluminum), rectal/anal disorders (hemorrhoids, fissures), obstruction (cancer of the bowel), metabolic and neurologic conditions (diabetes mellitus, multiple sclerosis), lead poisoning, and connective tissue disorders (scleroderma, lupus erythematosus). Other etiologic factors include weakness, debility, fatigue, and inability to increase intra-abdominal pressure to facilitate the passage of stools, such as occurs with emphysema. One of the most common types of constipation in the United States is irritable bowel syndrome, which occurs when colon spasms delay the propulsion of feces. Many people develop constipation because they are busy and cannot or will not take the time to defecate. In the U.S. constipation is also seen as a result of dietary habits (low consumption of fiber), lack of regular exercise, and a stress-filled life.

Constipation can also result from the chronic use of laxatives, which eventually override the bowel's sensitivity to the need to eliminate. Chronic laxative use is a major health concern in the U.S., where it has been estimated that $250 million is spent annually for laxatives.

Acute Constipation

Acute constipation, in contrast to chronic constipation, always indicates an acute and frequently a serious disorder.

It must be remembered that acute constipation may be an early symptom of acute appendicitis, and that a laxative given in this instance may produce perforation of the inflamed appendix. In general, a cathartic should not be given while the patient has fever, nausea, or pain merely because the bowels fail to move. A cathartic should never be prescribed in the presence of inflammatory bowel disease.

Pathophysiology

The pathophysiology of constipation is poorly understood. However, it is believed to be related to interference with one of three major functions of the colon: mucosal transport (mucosal secretions facilitate movement of colon contents), myoelectric activity (mixing of the rectal mass and propulsive

actions), or the processes involved in defecation. The urge to defecate is normally stimulated by rectal distention, which initiates a series of four actions: stimulation of the inhibitory rectoanal reflex, relaxation of the internal sphincter muscle, relaxation of the external sphincter muscle and muscles in the pelvic region, and increased intra-abdominal pressure. Interference in any of these four processes can thus lead to nonorganic or idiopathic constipation.

When the urge to defecate is ignored, the rectal mucous membrane and musculature become insensitive to the presence of fecal masses, and consequently a stronger stimulus is required to produce the necessary peristaltic rush for defecation. The initial effect of this fecal retention, or hoarding, is to produce irritability of the colon, which, at this stage, frequently goes into spasm, especially after meals, giving rise to colicky midabdominal or low abdominal pains. After several years of this process the colon loses muscular tone; it is essentially unresponsive to normal stimuli. At this point, the patient may be said to have *atonic constipation*, whereas in the earlier stage the condition is sometimes referred to as *spastic constipation*, although neither type should be regarded as a separate entity. Atony of the bowel also occurs with aging, and this can be complicated with constant use of laxatives.

Clinical Manifestations

Clinical manifestations include abdominal distention, *borborygmus* (intestinal rumbling), pain and pressure, decreased appetite, headache, fatigue, indigestion, a sensation of incomplete emptying, straining at stool, and the elimination of small-volume, hard, dry stool.

Diagnostic Evaluation

Diagnosis is based on a complete physical examination, a sigmoidoscopy, a radiographic examination, and stool testing for occult blood. Idiopathic constipation is diagnosed after an organic cause is eliminated.

Gerontological Considerations. Elderly persons report problems with constipation five times more frequently than younger people. A number of factors contribute to this increased frequency. Persons who have loose-fitting dentures or have lost their teeth have difficulty chewing and frequently choose soft, processed foods that are low in fiber. Convenience foods, also low in fiber, are popular for those who have lost interest in eating. Some older people reduce their fluid intake if they are not eating regular meals; decreased

TABLE 34-1
Correlations Between Diet, Fecal Characteristics, and Intestinal Elimination

Diet	Movement	Bulk	Consistency	Intralumen Pressure	Susceptibility to Disease
High-residue Bulky Unrefined	Rapid	Large	Soft	Low	Low
Low-residue Concentrated Refined	Slow	Small	Hard	High	High

fluid intake decreases bulk and makes passage of stool more difficult. Lack of exercise and prolonged bed rest also contribute to constipation by decreasing abdominal muscle tone.

Sometimes older persons imagine that they are constipated because they do not have a daily bowel movement and have misconceptions about what is and is not normal. This self-diagnosis frequently leads to laxative abuse or the habitual use of enemas.

Management

Management includes discontinuing abusive laxative use, recommending the inclusion of fiber in the diet, prescribing an exercise routine to strengthen abdominal muscles, and patterning behaviors related to establishing a normal bowel movement (responding to reflexes, "heeding the call," setting a daily defecation time, drinking warm water with a meal). The daily addition to the diet of 6 to 12 teaspoonfuls of unprocessed bran is recommended, especially for the treatment of constipation in the elderly. See Table 34-1 for relationships between diet, fecal characteristics, and intestinal elimination.

If laxative use is necessary, one of the following may be prescribed: bulk-forming agents, saline/osmotic agents, lubricants, stimulants, or fecal softeners. The physiologic action and patient teaching related to these laxatives is described in Table 34-2. Enemas and rectal suppositories are not recommended for constipation and should be reserved for the treatment of impaction or for bowel preparation for surgery or diagnostic procedures. If long-term laxative use is absolutely necessary, the physician will prescribe a bulk-forming agent in combination with an osmotic laxative.

▶ Nursing Process
The Patient With Constipation

▷ Assessment

When talking with patients about their bowel habits, it is helpful to keep in mind that some may be embarrassed to discuss such a personal body function. Tact and respect for the reserved patient are generally appreciated. Questions of a more personal matter may be placed later in the history after rapport has been established.

TABLE 34-2
Laxatives: Classification, Agent, Action, and Patient Education

Classification	Sample Agent	Action	Patient Education
Bulk-Forming	Psyllium hydrophilic muciloid (Metamucil)	Polysaccharides and cellulose derivatives mix with intestinal fluids, swell, and stimulate peristalsis.	Take with 8 ounces of water and follow with 8 ounces of water. Do not take dry. Report abdominal distention or unusual amount of flatulence.
Saline/Osmotic Agent	Magnesium hydroxide (Milk of Magnesia)	Nonabsorbable magnesium ions alter stool consistency by drawing water into the intestines by osmosis; peristalsis is stimulated. Action occurs within 2 hours.	The liquid preparation is more effective than the tablet form. Only short-term use is recommended because of toxicity (CNS or neuromuscular depression, electrolyte imbalance). Magnesium laxatives should not be taken by patients with renal insufficiency.
Lubricant	Mineral oil	Nonabsorbable hydrocarbons soften fecal matter by lubricating the intestinal mucosa. The passage of stool is facilitated. Action occurs within 6–8 hours.	Do not take with meals because mineral oils may impair the absorption of fat-soluble vitamins and delay gastric emptying. Swallow carefully because drops of oil that gain access to the pharynx may produce a lipid pneumonia.
Stimulant	Bisacodyl (Ducolax)	Irritates the colon epithelium by stimulating sensory nerve endings and increasing mucosal secretions. Action occurs within 6–8 hours.	Catharsis may cause fluid and electrolyte imbalance, especially in the elderly. Tablets should be swallowed, not crushed or chewed. Avoid milk or antacids within 1 hour of taking the drug because the enteric coating may dissolve prematurely.
Fecal Softener	Dioctyl sodium sulfosuccinate (Colace)	Hydrates the stool by its surfactant action on the colonic epithelium (increases the wetting efficiency of intestinal water). Aqueous and fatty substances are mixed. The drug does not exert a laxative action.	Can be used safely by patients who should avoid straining (cardiac patients, patients with anorectal disorders)

(Adapted from Malseed RT. Pharmacology: Drug Therapy and Nursing Considerations. Philadelphia, JB Lippincott, 1985.)

A complete nursing history includes onset and duration of constipation, life-style (exercise, nutrition, stress), occupation, past elimination pattern, current elimination pattern, laxative/enema use, current drug therapy, and past medical-surgical history. The patient is asked to describe the color, odor, and consistency of the stool as well as any associated intestinal symptoms (rectal pressure/fullness, abdominal pain, pain and straining at defecation, watery diarrhea, flatulence). Does the patient have bleeding when trying to defecate?

The nurse auscultates the abdomen for bowel sounds and notes if they are infrequent or absent and high-pitched or gurgling. The abdomen is also palpated for distention (absent, slight, moderate, severe). The perianal area is inspected for hemorrhoids, fissures, and signs of irritation. A physician's request is required in some health care agencies for digital examination for impaction in cardiac patients because pressure in the rectum may stimulate the vagal nerve to slow down the heart rate.

▷ *Nursing Diagnoses*

Based on all the assessment data, the patient's major nursing diagnoses may include the following:

- Alteration in bowel elimination, constipation, or fecal impaction related to health habits
- Alteration in comfort related to abdominal pressure
- Fluid volume deficit related to inadequate fluid intake
- Anxiety related to concern about irregular elimination pattern
- Knowledge deficit about health maintenance practices to prevent constipation

▷ *Planning and Implementation*

▷ *Goals:* The major goals of the patient may include restoration/maintenance of a regular pattern of normal bowel function, relief of pain, adequate intake of fluids and roughage foods, relief of anxiety, and understanding of methods for avoiding constipation.

Nursing Interventions

Patient Education and Home Health Care. Most of the patient's goals can be achieved through a thorough teaching program that presents information about the causes of constipation and the dietary practices and exercise activity that can promote healthy bowel habits.

In functional constipation, the role of the nurse is to assist with the reeducation of the patient. The physiology of defecation should be explained carefully, with particular emphasis on the importance of heeding promptly the urge to defecate. Instruct the patient to have a regular time for defecation, preferably after a meal. Thinking about the act of defecation, that is, "autosuggestion," may be an aid in initiating the reflex. A small footstool to promote flexion of the hips ensures an optimal posture during defecation.

The patient must know what constitutes a normal diet and should be aware of the similarities and differences between the prescribed diet and the normal diet. In general, a high-residue, high-fiber diet is prescribed for atonic constipation; a bland or low-residue diet is indicated for the patient

with an irritable colon (Table 34-1). For the elderly, the addition of 2 grams of bran to cereal daily can markedly increase the number of spontaneous bowel movements and decrease the use of cathartics, stool softeners, and enemas.

The nurse recommends frequent ambulation and abdominal muscle toning exercises to promote defecation. Abdominal toning exercises consist of contracting abdominal muscles 4 times daily, doing sit-ups with knees flexed and heels on the floor, and doing straight leg lifts while in a lying position. A patient confined to bed is encouraged to perform range-of-motion exercises, turn frequently from side to side and lie prone (if not contraindicated) for 30 minutes every 4 hours. These exercises increase abdominal muscle tone, which helps propel colon contents.

Patients who worry about having a *daily* bowel movement need reassurance. Carefully explain that some healthy persons have a bowel movement three times daily while others do so only two or three times a week. Knowing that some of the food eaten may normally remain in the intestinal tract 48 hours after ingestion will help the patient to understand and accept the fact that a daily bowel evacuation is not always necessary. The use of laxatives should be discontinued. If the feces remain in the rectum too long and become dehydrated and hardened, the patients may be instructed to instill 60 ml to 90 ml (2-3 oz) of warm oil into the rectum at bedtime. A small enema of physiologic saline the next morning should help to alleviate this condition.

If a laxative regimen has been prescribed, explain the consequences of laxative dependency and possible fecal impaction. Preventive measures include the gradual tapering off of laxative use; sufficient fluid and fiber intake; an adequate exercise program; and modification of contributory life-style factors (*e.g.*, ignoring the urge to defecate, stress).

▷ *Evaluation*

▷ *Expected Outcomes*

1. Patient establishes a regular pattern of bowel function
   a. Includes a time for defecation as part of daily routine
   b. Participates in a regular exercise program
   c. Avoids laxative abuse
   d. Drinks 2-3 liters of water daily
   e. Includes foods high in bulk in the diet (fresh fruits, bran, nuts, whole grain breads and cereals, cooked fruits and vegetables)
   f. Reports soft, formed stool every day or every 2-3 days
2. Experiences less abdominal discomfort
   a. Performs abdominal muscle toning exercises
   b. Is as physically active as possible

Complications of Constipation

The maintenance of elimination is basic to the care of every patient. The effort entailed in defecation is considerable. With the use of a bedpan the muscular strain is inevitably greater; when constipation is imposed in addition, the performance of this function can be extremely fatiguing if not altogether exhausting. This is a serious consideration in the management of patients with congestive heart failure, those who have suffered a recent myocardial infarction and are susceptible to cardiac rupture, and those with arterial hypertension.

To facilitate elimination, the patient should assume the normal position for defecation. The semi-squatting position maximizes the use of the abdominal muscles and the force of gravity. Hospitalized patients who cannot use the bathroom experience less strain if assisted to a bedside commode, or seated on a bedpan at the side of the bed with feet supported on a chair. If the patient cannot sit up, a small support should be placed under the lumbosacral curve to minimize strain and increase comfort while using the bedpan.

Valsalva Maneuver. Straining at stool has a striking effect on the arterial blood pressure (*Valsalva maneuver*). During the period of active straining, the flow of venous blood in the chest is temporarily impeded due to an increase in intrathoracic pressure that tends to collapse the large veins in the chest. The atria and the ventricles receive less blood, and consequently less is delivered by the systolic contractions of the left ventricle; the cardiac output is decreased, and there is a transient drop in arterial pressure. Almost immediately after this period of hypotension, a rise in arterial pressure occurs; the pressure is elevated momentarily to a point far exceeding the original level (the "rebound" phenomenon). In patients with arterial hypertension, this compensatory reaction may be exaggerated greatly, and the peaks of pressure attained may be dangerously high—sufficient, indeed, to rupture a major artery in the brain or elsewhere.

It is not possible to make more than a rough estimate of the frequency with which straining at stool is the event that brings on vascular accidents that result in death. The danger is not sufficiently appreciated, however, particularly in patients with vascular diseases of the type described. Because straining is promoted by constipation, it must be concluded that the regularity and the consistency of the stools, as well as the mechanical aspects of defecation, are matters or primary concern.

Fecal Impaction. Fecal impaction refers to an accumulated mass of dry feces that cannot be expelled. The mass may be palpable on digital examination, may cause pressure on the colon mucosa that results in ulcer formation, and may cause the frequent seepage of liquid stools. Treatment consists of mineral oil and saline enemas and the digital extraction of the stool.

Megacolon. Megacolon refers to a dilated and atonic colon caused by a fecal mass that obstructs the passage of colon contents. Symptoms include constipation, liquid fecal incontinence, and abdominal distention. The obstruction, which is diagnosed on radiographic examination, can lead to perforation and an emergency colectomy.

Cathartic Colon. Cathartic colon refers to mucosal atrophy of the colon with muscle thickening and fibrosis subsequent to the chronic use of laxatives. Symptoms include hypokalemia, metabolic alkalosis, malabsorption, and liquid fecal seepage. Treatment is directed at relieving the symptoms.

Diarrhea

Diarrhea is a condition in which there is an unusual frequency of bowel movements, as well as changes in the amount, the character, and the consistency of the stools. It is best described, quantitatively, as more than 200 grams of stool per day. Three factors determine its severity: intestinal secretions, altered mucosal absorption, and increased motility.

Diarrhea can be classified as large-volume, small-volume, or infectious. It can also be described as mild, moderate, or severe depending on the quantity of daily unformed stools. See Table 34-3 for classification of diarrhea based on the number of unformed stools in 24 hours and the recommended medical treatment.

Acute or large-volume diarrhea is caused by an increased secretion of water and electrolytes by the intestinal mucosa. This occurs because water is pulled into the intestines by the osmotic pressure of nonabsorbed particles or because intestinal secretions are increased. *Small-volume diarrhea* is caused by increased peristaltic action of the intestines and is usually due to inflammatory bowel disease (ulcerative colitis, Crohn's disease). *Infectious diarrhea*, which is caused by an infectious agent, results in an acute increase in the water content of feces due to increased mucosal cell secretion of water. Peristaltic action is also increased. Common infectious agents are *Shigella, Escherichia coli,* and *Campylobacter jejuni.*

TABLE 34-3
Diarrhea Classification and Recommended Medical Management

Classification	Number of Unformed Stools in 24 Hours	Recommended Medical Treatment
Mild	1 to 3	Fluids only
Moderate	3 to 6	Nonspecific drugs Diphenoxylate (Lomotil)
Severe	More than 6, with associated symptoms (fever, blood in the stools)	Antimicrobial agents Ampicillin (Amcill)

(Based on DuPont HL. Nonfluid therapy and selected chemoprophylaxis of acute diarrhea. Am J Med 1985 June 28;78[6B]:81–90.)

Pathophysiology.   The most common intestinal irritants are the products of certain bacteria grown either in the intestine or in the food before it was eaten. In the case of the enteric pathogens, the organisms causing bacillary dysentery, bacterial growth with release of the irritating toxins takes place in the intestine. On the other hand, many cases of food poisoning are due to the ingestion of food that is contaminated and already contains the toxin. *Staphylococcus aureus,* for example, if given an opportunity to grow in food, produces an exotoxin that is extremely irritating to the intestinal tract.

The inflammatory response to mild irritants is slight; little or no mucous membrane lining is destroyed on exposure to them unless their concentration in the intestinal fluid is excessive. Their chief effect is to produce hyperemia (vascular dilatation, with local increase in blood flow) of the intestinal mucosa and an increase in mucous secretion. A motor response of hyperperistalsis also occurs, persisting until the irritant is excreted, which explains the symptoms of crampy diarrhea.

Clinical Manifestations.   In acute cases the stools are grayish brown, foul smelling, and filled with undigested particles of food and mucus. The patient complains of abdominal cramps, distention, intestinal rumbling (borborygmus), anorexia, and thirst. Painful straining (tenesmus) of the anus may attend each defecation.

The diarrhea in food poisoning is explosive in onset, develops within a very few hours following the toxic meal, and, except in severe cases, subsides within 1 or 2 days—as soon as the toxin is excreted and the inflammatory response lessens. There is little or no fever, and usually the only associated symptoms are those directly attributable to the diarrhea, namely, dehydration and weakness.

Dysentery resulting from the growth of gastrointestinal pathogens within the gastrointestinal tract, on the other hand, develops with a more gradual onset and persists for several days or weeks, with striking constitutional symptoms in addition to the diarrhea.

Gerontological Considerations.   Older persons can quickly become dehydrated and hypokalemic from episodes of diarrhea. Exact intake and output records are kept to determine fluid loss. All output is measured, including liquid stools. Urinary output of less then 30 ml/hour for 2 to 3 consecutive hours is reported to the physician. Hypokalemia is manifested by muscle weakness, paresthesia, hypotension, anorexia, and drowsiness. A potassium level below 3.0 mEq/L is reported to the physician because decreased potassium causes cardiac arrhythmias that can lead to death (atrial and ventricular tachycardia, ventricular fibrillation, and premature ventricular contractions). The older person taking digitalis must be aware of the signs of hypokalemia because low levels of potassium potentiate the action of digitalis, which can lead to digitalis toxicity.

Older persons need to have ready access to a bathroom because they may not be able to control elimination fully. They may need help with ambulation if a mobility problem exists.

The older person's skin is very sensitive because of decreased turgor and reduced subcutaneous fat layers. Enzymes from diarrheal stool are irritating and can cause excoriation. Teach the patient to keep the anal area dry and clean. Washing with a mild soap is recommended. The area is patted dry, and petrolatum can be applied after stool passage to serve as a protective barrier.

Preventive Health Measures.   Precautions include ensuring that proper storage and refrigeration facilities are available and are used for the handling of all fresh fruits and meats. Meat products should be cooked thoroughly and either consumed promptly or refrigerated immediately. Milk and milk products should be refrigerated and protected against exposure. Food items that are particularly apt to cause infection, because they provide the best environment for bacterial growth, include custards and cream fillings such as those prepared for use in éclairs, cream pies, layer cakes, and cream puffs. Such materials should be cooked thoroughly and then brought to refrigerator temperature immediately.

Proper housekeeping, especially in the kitchen, is obviously very important in the prevention of epidemic diarrhea. All materials used in the preparation and the serving of food must be cleaned rigorously and kept in immaculate condition. All food handlers should receive detailed instructions in hygienic principles and practices and, upon the development of any illness that is potentially infectious, should be relieved of their duties immediately.

Diagnostic Evaluation.   The diagnosis of an acute diarrhea is based on the course of the disease: the type of onset and progression, the presence or absence of fever, and a study of the stools, which are examined for bacteria as well as for blood and pus. The majority of cases (60%) are diagnosed by microbiologic, serologic, or tissue culture techniques; undiagnosed cases are usually of an infectious nature.

Management.   Oral fluids are immediately increased and an oral glucose and electrolyte solution may be prescribed to rehydrate the patient. Nonspecific drugs such as diphenoxylate (Lomotil) and loperamide (Imodium) are prescribed to decrease motility for diarrhea of a noninfectious source. Antimicrobial agents are prescribed when an infectious agent has been identified. Intravenous therapy may be necessary for rapid hydration, especially for the very young or the elderly.

▶ *Nursing Process*
The Patient With Diarrhea

▷ *Assessment*

Diarrhea and its associated symptoms occur in a variety of disorders. The nurse will facilitate the diagnosis in each case by recording discerning observations, including the patient's symptoms, behavior, and remarks. Ask the patient to describe the onset and pattern of the diarrhea. Is it associated with abdominal pain, cramping or urgency? Does it occur at any specific time of the day? Assess stool frequency, consistency, color and odor. Watery stools are characteristic of small-bowel disease, whereas loose, semisolid stools are associated more often with disorders of the colon. Voluminous, greasy stools suggest intestinal malabsorption, and the presence of mucus and pus in the stools denotes inflammatory enteritis or colitis. Oil droplets in the toilet water are almost always diagnostic of pancreatic insufficiency. Nocturnal diarrhea may be a manifestation of diabetic neuropathy.

Inspect the abdomen for distention and auscultate bowel sounds for frequency (hyperactivity) and sound characteristics (borborygmus). Review the patient's usual daily dietary intake and drug therapy to identify any possible causative agents. Ask if the patient is suffering from any chronic disease, has any known allergies, or has recently been exposed to an acute illness or an infected person. Note whether the patient has traveled recently and, if so, to what geographic area.

Assess for dehydration by checking for postural hypotension, tachycardia, a weak, thready pulse, decreased skin turgor, dry mucous membranes, and inadequate urinary output. Laboratory results are analyzed for abnormalities such as increased serum osmolality, increased hematocrit, increased specific gravity of urine, and decreased serum potassium. Because dehydration exists when weight loss exceeds 6.0% of body weight, the patient is weighed daily and an accurate intake and output record is kept.

▷ Nursing Diagnoses

Based on all the assessment data, the patient's major nursing diagnoses may include the following:

- Alteration in bowel elimination, diarrhea, related to the infection and ingestion of irritating foods
- Potential for fluid volume deficit related to frequent passage of stools and insufficient fluid intake
- Anxiety related to frequent, uncontrolled elimination
- Potential impairment of skin integrity related to the passage of frequent, loose stools
- Potential for transmission of infection related to fecal contamination

▷ Planning and Implementation

▷ *Goals:* The major goals of the patient may include cessation of diarrhea, avoidance of fluid volume deficit, reduction of anxiety, maintenance of skin integrity, and prevention of spread of infection.

Nursing Interventions

Measures to Control Diarrhea. During an episode of acute diarrhea, the patient is encouraged to rest in bed and take liquids and foods that are low in bulk until the acute period subsides. When food intake is tolerated the nurse recommends a bland diet. Caffeine intake is limited because caffeine stimulates intestinal motility. Milk may be restricted for several days because transient lactase deficiency may be seen in some forms of acute diarrhea. Antidiarrheal drugs such as diphenoxylate (Lomotil) are administered as prescribed.

Maintaining Fluid Balance. Fluid balance is difficult to maintain during an acute episode of diarrhea because the rapid propulsion of feces through the intestines decreases water absorption; output exceeds intake. The nurse assesses for dehydration (decreased skin turgor, tachycardia, decreased pulse volume, decreased serum sodium) and keeps an accurate record of intake and output. The patient is weighed daily. The nurse encourages oral fluid replacement in the form of water, juices, bouillon, and commercial preparations such as Gatorade. Parenteral fluids are mentioned.

Reducing Anxiety. Provide an opportunity for the patient to express fears/worry about being embarrassed by lack of control over bowel elimination. This fear of embarrassment is a major concern.

Suggest that the patient identify irritating foods and stressors that precipitate an attack of diarrhea. Elimination or reduction of these factors helps control defecation. Encourage the patient to be sensitive to body clues that warn of impending urgency (abdominal cramping, hyperactive bowel sounds). Recommend special absorbant underwear, similar to a plastic diaper, that will protect clothes if there is accidental fecal discharge.

Project an understanding, tolerant, and relaxed demeanor. Support the patient's efforts to use coping mechanisms. Give antianxiety medications as prescribed.

Skin Care. The perianal area becomes excoriated because diarrheal stool contains digestive enzymes that cause local irritation. The nurse instructs the patient to follow a perianal care routine such as the following: wipe or pat the area dry after defecation, cleanse with a mild soap and warm water, pat dry immediately with cotton balls, and apply lotion/ointment as a skin barrier. If necessary, the patient can expose the perianal area to a heat lamp for 30 minutes, 4 times a day.

Precautionary Infection Measures. All patients with diarrhea should be treated as potentially infectious until they are proven otherwise. If the diarrhea is of an infectious origin, the nurse should determine whether there is any diarrhea among the family and neighbors. Proper precautions must be taken to prevent the spread of the disease through contamination of hands, clothing, bed linens, and other objects with feces or vomitus.

The nurse tries to determine if there is a causal relationship between episodes of diarrhea and food intake. If a food contaminant is suspected, food is tested by bacteriologic cultures. Food that is not contaminated can still act as an irritant to the patient's gastrointestinal tract.

▷ Evaluation

▷ *Expected Outcomes*

1. Patient avoids irritating foods
   a. Identifies foods that act as an irritant
   b. Eliminates irritating foods from diet
   c. Reports a decrease in number and frequency of daily stools
   d. Reports formed stools
2. Maintains fluid and electrolyte balance
   a. Takes sufficient fluids orally
   b. Tolerates parenteral fluid/electrolyte replacement
   c. States absence of fatigue and muscle weakness
   d. Is alert and oriented
   e. Displays moist mucous membranes and normal tissue turgor
   f. Has a balanced intake and output
   g. Has normal urine specific gravity
3. Experiences less anxiety
   a. Verbalizes concerns and fears
   b. Recognizes symptoms that signal an impending attack

TABLE 34-4
Pathophysiologic and Clinical Aspects of Diseases of Malabsorption and Maldigestion

Diseases/Disorders	Physiologic Pathology	Clinical Features
Gastric resection with gastrojejunostomy	Decreased pancreatic stimulation because of duodenal bypass; poor mixing of food, bile, pancreatic enzymes; decreased intrinsic factor; bacterial stasis in afferent loop	Weight loss, moderate steatorrhea, anemia (combination of iron, vitamin B_{12} malabsorption, folate deficiency)
Pancreatic insufficiency (chronic pancreatitis, pancreatic carcinoma, pancreatic resection, cystic fibrosis)	Reduced intraluminal pancreatic enzyme activity, with maldigestion of lipid and protein	History of abdominal pain followed by weight loss; marked steatorrhea, azotorrhea; also frequent glucose intolerance (70% in pancreatic insufficiency)
Ileal dysfunction (resection or disease)	Loss of ileal absorbing surface leads to reduced bile-salt pool size and reduced vitamin B_{12} absorption; bile in colon inhibits fluid absorption.	Diarrhea, weight loss with steatorrhea, especially when greater than 100 cm resection, decreased vitamin B_{12} absorption
Stasis syndromes (surgical strictures, blind loops, enteric fistulas, multiple jejunal diverticula, scleroderma)	Overgrowth of intraluminal intestinal bacteria, especially anaerobic organisms, to greater than 10^6 per ml, results in deconjugation of bile salts, leading to decreased effective bile-salt pool size, also bacterial utilization of vitamin B_{12}.	Weight loss, steatorrhea; low vitamin B_{12} absorption; may have low D-xylose absorption
Zollinger-Ellison syndrome	Hyperacidity in duodenum inactivates pancreatic enzymes.	Ulcer diathesis, steatorrhea
Lactose intolerance	Deficiency of intestinal lactase results in high concentration of intraluminal lactose with osmotic diarrhea.	Affects 80% of U.S. black persons and probably all other nonCaucasian races; varied degrees of diarrhea and cramps after ingestion of lactose-containing foods; positive lactose tolerance test, decreased intestinal lactase
Celiac disease (gluten enteropathy)	Toxic response to a gluten fraction by surface epithelium results in destruction of absorbing surface.	Weight loss, diarrhea, bloating, anemia (low iron, folate), osteomalacia, steatorrhea, azotorrhea, low D-xylose absorption; folate and iron malabsorption; diagnostic biopsy change
Tropical sprue	Unknown toxic factor results in mucosal inflammation, partial villous atrophy.	Weight loss, diarrhea, anemia (low folate, vitamin B_{12}); steatorrhea; low D-xylose absorption, low vitamin B_{12} absorption; typical but nonspecific biopsy change
Whipple's disease	Bacterial invasion of intestinal mucosa	Arthritis, hyperpigmentation, lymphadenopathy, serous effusions, fever, weight loss; steatorrhea, azotorrhea, diagnostic biopsy change
Certain parasitic diseases (giardiasis, stronglyoidiasis, coccidiosis, capillariasis)	Damage to, or invasion of, surface mucosa	Diarrhea, weight loss; steatorrhea; organism may be seen on jejunal biopsy or recovered in stool
Immunoglobulinopathy	Decreased local gut defenses, lymphoid hyperplasia, lymphopenia	Frequent association with *Giardia;* hypogammaglobulinemia or isolated IgA deficiency; diagnostic or typical biopsy changes

(Halsted JA. The Laboratory In Clinical Medicine. Philadelphia, WB Saunders.)

c. Uses coping mechanisms effectively
d. Wears special absorbant underwear that protects clothing from soiling if needed
4. Maintains skin integrity
   a. Keeps area clean after defecation
   b. Uses lotion/ointment as a skin barrier
   c. Uses a heat lamp to the perianal area, 4 times a day, if needed

Diseases of Malabsorption

Digestion is the process whereby nutrients are reduced to appropriate form for intestinal absorption. Intestinal absorption transports nutrients across the mucosa to the portal blood system.

Along with nutrients, the intestinal tract is the recipient of a large volume of fluid and electrolytes. Of about 1500 ml of ingested liquid, plus about 7000 ml from the gastrointestinal tract (salivary, gastric, biliary, pancreatic, and intestinal sources), all but 500 ml are absorbed proximal to the ileocecal valve. Thus, the intestine continually shifts the volume and composition of its contents to fulfill its major function of absorption.

Interruptions in the complex digestive process may occur anywhere to cause malabsorption, the inability of the digestive system to absorb one or more of the major nutrients—carbohydrates, fats, and proteins. Malabsorption occurs when the digestive process has been altered by:

- The inability of nutrients to be readily catabolized and transported (gastric resection, Zollinger-Ellison Syndrome, pancreatic insufficiency)
- The decreased absorption of nutrients by the intestinal mucosa (jejunal diverticula, ileal dysfunction)
- A combination of causes (parasitic diseases, Whipple's disease, celiac disease)

In addition to these causes, certain inflammatory bowel disorders, such as ulcerative colitis and regional enteritis (Crohn's disease), cause increased protein breakdown (catabolism) in the small intestine, with resulting loss of protein into the lumen of the intestine (protein-losing enteropathy).

Pathophysiology and Clinical Manifestations. Three primary malabsorption diseases are (1) tropical sprue, (2) adult celiac disease (nontropical sprue, gluten-induced celiac disease), and (3) lactose intolerance. Tropical sprue and adult celiac disease are similar in clinical manifestations and pathologic changes, but differ in their geographic incidence and causes, and also respond to different treatments. In adult celiac disease, protein malabsorption is frequently seen as an allergic reaction to gluten, which is found in wheat, rye, oats, and barley. Gluten causes the mucosal villi to atrophy, thus restricting their absorptive abilities. Lactose intolerance occurs when there is a deficiency of lactase, a digestive enzyme that breaks down milk sugar (the disaccharide lactose). The resulting high concentration of lactose in the intestines causes an osmotic retention of water, which results in abdominal cramping, nausea, and possibly diarrhea.

The hallmarks of the *malabsorption syndrome*, of whatever cause, are diarrhea or frequent loose, bulky, foul stools that have increased fat content and are often greyish in color;

associated weakness, weight loss, and lack of well-being are often present. The chief result of malabsorption is malnutrition, manifested by weight loss.

Patients with the malabsorption syndrome, if untreated, become weak and emaciated due to starvation. Failure to absorb the fat-soluble vitamins A, D, and K causes these patients to develop a corresponding avitaminoses. Manifestations of abnormal bleeding are likely to appear as a result of vitamin K deficiency and hypoprothrombinemia (see p. 692). Anemia develops, which is of the macrocytic type characteristic of folic acid deficiency (see p. 676). Impaired absorption of calcium may be responsible for gradual demineralization of the skeleton. Moreover, calcium deficiency may lead to extreme neuromuscular hyperirritability, including attacks of hypocalcemic tetany.

See Table 34-4 for the clinical and pathophysiological aspects of malabsorption and maldigestion diseases.

Management. Diagnostic studies are helpful in determing the disorder responsible for the malabsorption syndrome (Table 34-5). Dietary considerations are preeminent

TABLE 34-5

Suggested Diagnostic Studies for Disorders Resulting in Malabsorption

Diagnostic Study	Test Result With Malabsorption Syndrome
Hemoglobin and hematocrit	Decreased if anemia is present
Mean corpuscular volume (MCV)	Decreased values are found with malabsorption of vitamin B_{12}.
Serum carotene level	Decreased values are associated with steatorrhea and fat malabsorption syndrome.
Upper G.I. series	Abnormal findings with malabsorption syndrome may include thickening of the intestinal mucosa, a change in fecal transit time, or narrowed mucosa of the terminal ileum.
Sudan stain for fecal fat	Abnormally large numbers of fat droplets can help to distinguish malabsorption from maldigestion.
A 72-hour stool collection for fat	A diet containing 80 grams of fat must be ingested for 2 days before and during the test. Stool fat greater than 5 grams/24 hours indicates a fat digestion disorder.
D-Xylose absorption test	Urine excretion over 5 hours after the ingestion of 5 grams of D-xylose should be 5 grams of xylose. Decreased excretion is indicative of malabsorption or enterogenous steatorrhea (fatty stools caused by a disease of the small intestines).

(Adapted from Eastwood GL. Core Textbook of Gastroenterology. Philadelphia, JB Lippincott, 1984.)

in the treatment of adult celiac disease and lactose intolerance. In celiac disease, the elimination of gluten from the patient's diet is followed by striking clinical improvement. The diarrhea ceases and nutritional status is restored to normal. This gratifying remission may be expected to last as long as the patient remains on a gluten-free diet, and no longer. Unfortunately, the total exclusion of gluten is difficult to accomplish because this substance is incorporated into many foods as a binder and filler. It is contained in almost every bakery product, "wheat-free" or otherwise, and is an ingredient of other foodstuffs as well, including some brands of ice cream.

The treatment for lactose intolerance consists of removing lactose-containing foods from the diet *e.g.,* milk, ice cream. Soy milk products can be substituted. Most adults can digest fermented milk products such as cheese and yogurt. These products supply a vital need for calcium, and their use is encouraged.

The factors primarily reponsible for the onset and the progression of tropical sprue have not as yet been clarified. Its clinical course appears to be unaffected by the presence or the absence of gliadin in the diet; hence gliadin intolerance seemingly plays no role in its pathogenesis. Of greatest benefit in this condition is the administration of folic acid, which usually is prescribed for a period of 4 to 6 months after remission has occurred. Broad-spectrum antibiotics are equally important. The beneficial effects of folic acid in patients with tropical sprue appear with such regularity and on occasion are so striking as to suggest that this particular malabsorption syndrome may be attributable to, as well as productive of, folic acid deficiency.

Acute Inflammatory Intestinal Disorders: Appendicitis and Peritonitis

Acute inflammatory intestinal disorders such as appendicitis and peritonitis may at first have similar clinical manifestations: abdominal pain and tenderness, nausea and vomiting, anorexia, a low-grade temperature, tachycardia, and leukocytosis. Diagnosis is based on a complete history and physical examination. Surgery is the treatment of choice. Common nursing goals are relief of pain, prevention of fluid volume deficit, reduction in anxiety, elimination of infection due to the potential/actual disruption of the gastrointestinal tract, maintenance of skin integrity, and attainment of optimum nutrition.

Appendicitis

The appendix is a small, fingerlike appendage about 10 cm (4 inches) long, attached to the cecum just below the ileocecal valve. No definite function can be assigned to it in humans. The appendix fills with food and empties as regularly as does the cecum, of which it is a part. It empties inefficiently, however, and its lumen is very small, so that it is prone to become

obstructed and is particularly vulnerable to infection (appendicitis).

Appendicitis is the most common cause of acute inflammation in the right lower quadrant of the abdominal cavity. About 7% of the population will have appendicitis at some time in their lives; males are affected more than females, and teenagers more than adults. It occurs most frequently between the ages of 10 and 30.

The disease is more prevalent in countries in which people consume a diet low in fiber and high in refined carbohydrates. In the United States about 200,000 appendectomies are performed annually for acute appendicitis.

Pathophysiology and Clinical Manifestations

The appendix becomes inflamed and edematous due to either kinking or an occlusion, possibly caused by a fecalith (hardened mass of stool), tumor, or foreign body. The inflammatory process increases intraluminal pressure, initiating a progressively severe generalized or upper abdominal pain which, within a few hours, becomes localized in the right lower quadrant of the abdomen. This pain is usually accompanied by a low-grade fever, nausea, and often vomiting. At *McBurney's point* (Figure 34-1), located halfway between the umbilicus and the anterior spine of the ilium, local tenderness is noted when pressure is applied and there is some rigidity of the lower portion of the right rectus muscle. A moderate leukocytosis is often present. Loss of appetite is common.

Just how much tenderness there will be, how much muscle spasm, and whether or not there is constipation or diarrhea depend not so much on the severity of the appendiceal infecton as on the location of the appendix. If the appendix curls around behind the cecum (*retrocecal* appendix), pain and tenderness may be felt in the lumbar region; if its tip is in the pelvis, these signs may be elicited only on rectal examination. Pain on defecation suggests that its tip is against the rectum; pain on micturition suggests that it is near the bladder or impinges on the ureter. Eventually, the inflamed appendix fills with pus and then is apt to perforate. Once it has ruptured, the pain becomes more diffuse; abdominal distention develops as a result of paralytic ileus, and the patient's condition worsens.

Diagnostic Evaluation

The patient has a low-grade temperature and a leukocyte count greater than 10,000/cu mm. The neutrophil count is frequently elevated above 75%. However, in about 10% of those with acute appendicitis, leukocyte and differential cell counts are normal.

Upon physical examination, common findings include slight muscular rigidity, normal bowel sounds, and local and *rebound tenderness* (production or intensification of pain when pressure is released). Early palpation of the abdomen reveals diffuse tenderness around the umbilicus and mid-epigastrium. As the condition progresses, pain shifts to the lower right quadrant. If the patient coughs or the anterior abdominal wall is percussed, pain is enhanced. An interesting *Rovsing's sign* may be elicited by palpating the left lower quadrant (Fig. 34-1), which, paradoxically, causes pain to be felt by the patient in the right lower quadrant.

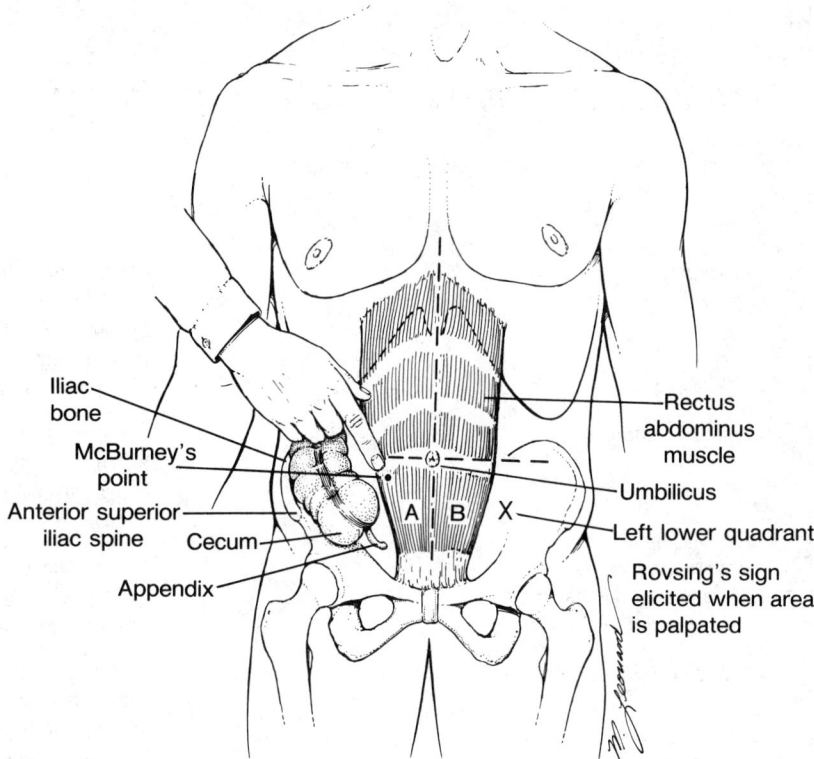

Figure 34-1
McBurney's point. When the appendix is inflamed, tenderness can be noted in the right lower quadrant at McBurney's point (*A*), which is between the umbilicus and the anterior superior iliac spine. Rovsing's sign occurs when pain is felt in the right lower quadrant after the left lower quadrant has been palpated (*B*).

The more severe the pain, the more the patient will guard and protect the abdomen and the greater will be muscular rigidity.

A posture of right hip flexion is a protective maneuver used by the patient, suggesting irritation of the psoas muscle (*positive psoas sign*) by the inflamed appendix. Radiologic signs in about 50% of the patients show right lower quadrant density or localized air-flow levels.

Complications

The major complications of acute appendicitis are perforation, peritonitis, appendiceal abscess formation, and pyelophlebitis. With perforation, the pain is severe and the temperature is elevated to about 37.7°C (100°F). The physician is immediately notified. Patients over 50 years of age are considered high risk because they have the highest mortality rate. Perforation can lead to an appendiceal abscess (a mass that is walled off from the peritoneal cavity by the omentum, or small bowel) or peritonitis. An abscess is managed with parenteral antibiotics that help localize the infection until surgical drainage can be performed; an appendectomy is done in about 6 weeks. The management of peritonitis is described on pages 811–812. See Chart 34-1 for a summary of nursing management for postoperative complications.

Management

Surgery is always indicated if acute appendicitis is suspected, unless there is good evidence that perforation has occurred recently and that a generalized peritonitis has developed. The patient treated conservatively is given parenteral elec-

trolyte and amino acid solutions, gastric suction, and antibiotics, in the expectation that the infection will localize and then be susceptible to surgical drainage. As long as the question of operation is undecided, a narcotic analgesic is withheld, even in the face of moderate pain, because it may mask the patient's symptoms. After the decision has been made, the patient may be given medication for pain.

Surgical Management

When an operation is necessary, the patient is carefully prepared. An intravenous infusion is used to establish adequate urinary output and replace existing fluid loss. Aspirin may be prescribed to lower the elevated temperature. Antibiotic therapy is often instituted as a preventive measure against infection. If there is evidence or likelihood of paralytic ileus, a nasogastric tube may be passed. The patient is asked to void, the abdomen is prepared, and the prescribed preoperative medications are given. Usually, an enema is not given, but if one is requested it is given slowly.

The patient who has been suffering from acute abdominal pain may view the operation as a means of relief. This acceptance of surgery makes the anesthetic and postanesthetic course a relatively easy one. The operation may be performed under general or spinal anesthesia. The usual incisions are the McBurney, the muscle-splitting or the grid-iron, and the Rockey-Davis (transverse).

Appendectomy Without Drainage. Immediately upon recovery from the anesthesia, the patient is placed in Fowler's position. A narcotic analgesic, usually morphine sulfate, is given at intervals of 3 or 4 hours. Fluids are usually given when they can be tolerated unless the patient has been de-

Chart 34-1
Potential Complications Following Appendectomy

Prompt recognition by the nurse and effective management of treatment can prevent prolonged disability for the patient.

Complication	Nursing Assessment and Interventions
Peritonitis	Observe for abdominal tenderness, fever, vomiting, abdominal rigidity, and tachycardia. Employ constant nasogastric suction. Correct dehydration. Give antibiotic agents as prescribed.
Pelvic or lumbar abscess	Evaluate for anorexia, chills, fever, and diaphoresis. Watch for "diarrhea," which may indicate pelvic abscess. Prepare patient for rectal examination. Prepare patient for operative drainage procedure.
Subphrenic abscess (abscess under the diaphragm)	Assess patient for chills, fever, and diaphoresis. Prepare for x-ray examination. Prepare for surgical drainage of abscess.
Ileus (paralytic and mechanical)	Assess for bowel sounds. Employ nasogastric intubation and suction. Replace fluids and electrolytes by intravenous route. Prepare for operation, if diagnosis of mechanical ileus is established.

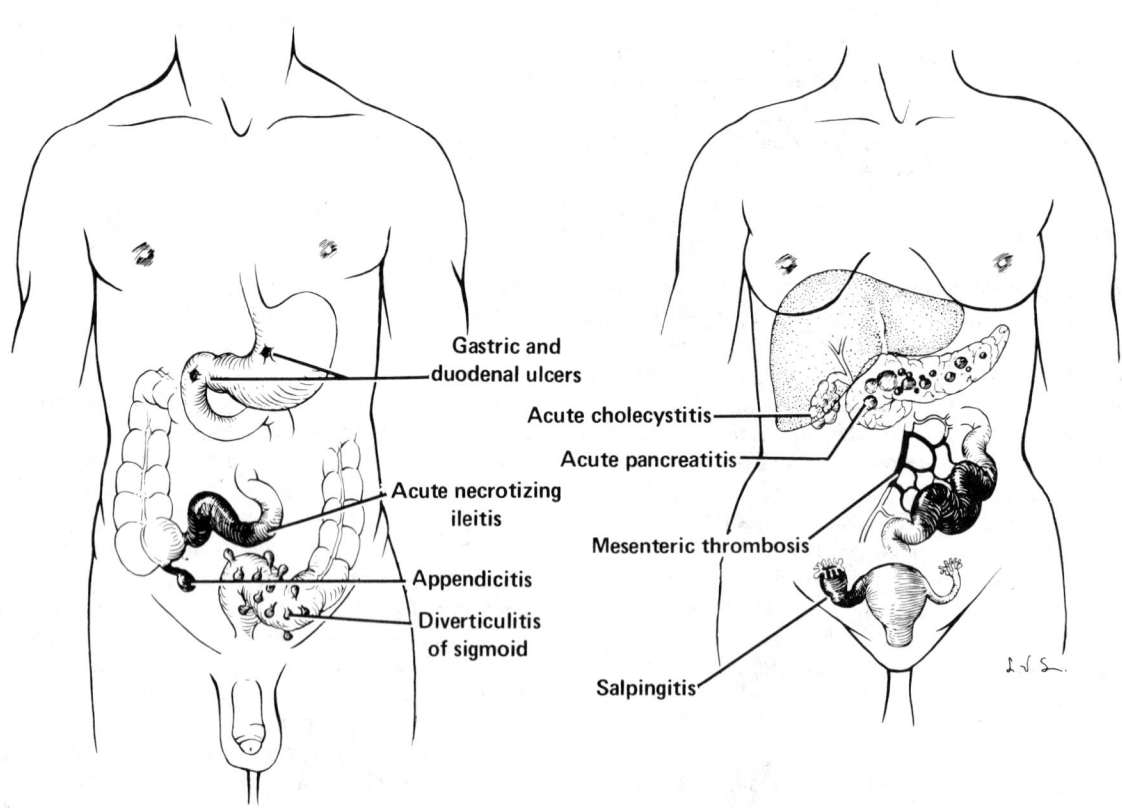

Figure 34-2
Common primary causes of peritonitis. (Dunphy JE and Way LW. Current Surgical Diagnosis and Treatment. Los Altos, California, Lange Medical Publishers.)

hydrated, in which case they are given intravenously. Food may be given as desired on the day of operation, if the patient's condition permits.

For the uncomplicated appendectomy, the patient can be discharged on the day of surgery if the temperature is within normal limits and there is no undue discomfort in the operative area. The sutures are removed from the incision between the fifth and seventh days, in the physician's office. However, an appendectomy is usually an emergency procedure, and frequently complications such as perforation are present. Hospitalization for 5 to 7 days may be necessary, depending on the complication.

Appendectomy With Drainage. If drainage is required following the appendectomy, there is a possible complication of local or general peritonitis. These patients are placed in Fowler's position as soon as they recover from the anesthetic, and treatment for peritonitis is instituted (as described below). Patients are monitored carefully for many days for signs of intestinal obstruction and secondary hemorrhage. Secondary abscesses may form in the pelvis, under the diaphragm, or in the liver. These cause an elevation of temperature and pulse rate, with an increase in the leukocyte count. A fecal fistula, with discharge of feces through the drainage tract, sometimes develops. This complication may occur after the drainage of an appendiceal abscess. Any sign of feces on the dressing is brought to the attention of the surgeon.

Peritonitis

Peritonitis is inflammation of a part or all of the parietal and visceral surfaces of the abdominal cavity. Usually it is a result of bacterial infection, the organisms coming from disease of the gastrointestinal tract or, in women, the internal reproductive organs (Fig. 34-2). Secondary peritonitis comes from external sources by injury, or by extension of inflammation from an extraperitoneal organ, such as the kidney. The most common bacteria found are *Escherichia coli*, *Klebsiella*, *Proteus*, and *Pseudomonas*. *Inflammation* and *ileus* are the direct effects of the infection. Common causes of peritonitis are presented in Table 34-6. In addition to these causes, peritonitis may be associated with continuous ambulatory peritoneal dialysis (see p. 1020).

Pathophysiology. Peritonitis is caused by leakage of contents from abdominal organs into the abdominal cavity, usually as a result of inflammation, infection, ischemia, trauma, or tumor perforation, or, in the case of peritoneal dialysis, through the inadvertent introduction of contaminated material. Initially, the material that spills into the abdominal cavity is sterile (except in the case of peritoneal dialysis), but within 6 to 12 hours bacterial contamination occurs. Edema of tissues results, and in a short while exudation develops. Fluid in the peritoneal cavity becomes turbid with increasing amounts of protein, white cells, cellular debris, and blood. The immediate response of the intestinal tract is hypermotility, but this is soon followed by paralytic ileus, with an accumulation of air and fluid in the bowel.

Clinical Manifestations. Symptoms depend on the location and extent of the inflammaiton, which are determined by the infection causing the peritonitis. At first a diffuse type of pain is felt. This tends to become constant, localized, and more intense near the site of the process. It is usually aggravated by movement. The affected area of the abdomen becomes extremely tender, and the muscles become rigid. Rebound tenderness and ileus may be present. Usually, nausea and vomiting occur and peristalsis is diminished. The temperature and pulse rate increase, and there is almost always an elevation of the leukocyte count. Shock may result from hypovolemia or septicemia. These early clinical manifestations of peritonitis frequently are the symptoms of the disorder causing the condition.

TABLE 34-6
Common Causes of Peritonitis

Severity	Cause	Mortality Rate
Mild	Appendicitis Perforated gastroduodenal ulcers Acute salpingitis	<10%
Moderate	Diverticulitis (localized perforations) Nonvascular small bowel perforation Gangrenous cholecystitis Multiple trauma	<20%
Severe	Large bowel perforations Ischemic small bowel injuries Acute necrotizing pancreatitis Postoperative complications	20–80%

(Reproduced with permission from Way LW [ed]. Current Surgical Diagnosis and Treatment, 7th ed. Los Altos, California, Lange Medical Publishers, 1985.)

Management

Fluid, colloid, and electrolyte replacement is the major focus of medical management. Hypovolemia occurs because massive amounts of fluids and electrolytes move from the intestinal lumen into the peritoneal cavity and deplete the vascular space. This in turn decreases renal perfusion. In addition, the fluid in the abdominal cavity can impair ventilation by causing pressure on the diaphragm. Several liters of an isotonic solution are prescribed.

Intestinal intubation and suction assist in relieving abdominal distention and in promoting intestinal function. Oxygen therapy by nasal cannula or mask will promote ventilatory function, but occasionally a tracheostomy and ventilatory assistance may be required.

If the cause of the peritonitis is removed at an early stage, the inflammation subsides and the patient recovers. Frequently, however, the inflammation is not localized and the whole abdominal cavity becomes involved, in which case the patient is acutely ill, has severe pain, and must be treated compassionately.

Because sepsis is the major cause of death from peritonitis, massive antibiotic therapy is usually initiated early in the treatment. Cultures of peritoneal fluid are taken but, until the laboratory reports are available, large doses of a broad-spectrum antibiotic are given intravenously. When laboratory results are completed, the usual regimen of antibiotic therapy consists of an aminoglycoside with clindamycin.

Eventually, unless the cause of peritonitis is eliminated, the patient may succumb to intestinal obstruction. This is brought about by small bowel adhesions and even local abscess formation. If these can be localized, surgical drainage is effective.

Surgical objectives include removing the infected material and correcting the cause. Surgical treatment is directed toward excision (appendix), resection with or without anastomosis (intestine), repair (perforation), and drainage (abscess). With extensive sepsis, the creation of an ostomy is preferred to intestinal anastomosis because the colon could be damaged as a result of ischemia.

Nursing Interventions

Accurate assessment of pain is important. A description of the nature of the pain, its location in the abdomen, and any shifts in location may help ascertain the source of difficulty.

Accurate recording of input and output, including vomitus, assists in calculating fluid replacement. In addition, determination of central venous pressure (see p. 534) may be helpful. A rise in pressure levels to 15 cm H_2O or higher may indicate circulatory overload.

Drains are frequently inserted during the operation, and it is essential that the nurse observe and record the character of the drainage. Care must be taken in moving and turning the patient to prevent the drains from being dislodged accidentally.

Signs that the peritonitis is subsiding include a fall in temperature and pulse rate, softening of the abdomen, return of peristaltic sounds, passing of flatus, and bowel movements. Foods and fluids (taken by mouth) will be gradually increased and parenteral fluids reduced.

Two of the most common complications that must be watched for are wound evisceration and abscess formation. Any suggestion from the patient that an area of the abdomen is tender or painful or "feels as if something just gave way" should be reported. The sudden occurrence of serosanguineous wound drainage strongly suggests wound dehiscence (see p. 361).

Diverticular Disorders

A *diverticulum* is an outpouching or herniation of the mucous membrane lining of the bowel through a defect in the muscle layer. Diverticula, in fact, may occur anywhere along the course of the gastrointestinal tract, from the esophagus to the rectum.

Diverticulosis exists when multiple diverticula are present without inflammation or symptoms. *Diverticulitis* results when food and bacteria retained in a diverticulum produce infection and inflammation that can impede drainage and lead to perforation or abscess formation. Diverticulitis is found in approximately 10% of the United States population, but is more common in those over 60 years. Its incidence is approximately 60% in those over 80 years of age. A congenital predisposition is likely when the disorder is present in those under 40 years of age. A low intake of dietary fiber is considered a major cause of the disease.

It has been estimated that approximately 20% of patients with diverticulosis experience diverticulitis at some point. Di-

verticulitis is most common in the sigmoid colon (95%). It may occur in acute attacks or may persist as a long-continued, smoldering infection.

Pathophysiology

A diverticulum forms when the mucosa and submucosal layers of the colon herniate through the muscular wall because of high intraluminal pressure (thickened muscle layers occlude the lumen), low volume in the colon (fiber-deficient contents), and decreased muscle strength in the colon wall (muscular hypertrophy from hardened fecal masses). A diverticulum can become obstructed and then inflamed if the obstruction continues. The inflammation tends to spread to the surrounding bowel wall, giving rise to irritability and spasticity of the colon. An abscess may develop, leading to peritonitis, and erosion of the blood vessels (arterial) may produce bleeding.

Clinical Manifestations

Constipation from spastic colon syndrome often precedes the development of diverticulosis by many years. Other signs of diverticulosis are bowel irregularity and diarrhea. A moderately severe acute diverticulitis has as its most common symptom crampy pain in the *left lower quadrant* of the abdomen, and a low-grade fever. Following local inflammation of the diverticula, there may be a narrowing of the large bowel with fibrotic stricture, leading to cramps, narrow stools, and increased constipation. With the development of granulation tissue, occult bleeding may occur, producing iron-deficiency anemia. In addition, weakness and fatigue are evident. If an abscess develops, there is tenderness, a palpable mass, fever, and leukocytosis. If an inflamed diverticulum perforates, abdominal pain results that is localized over the involved segment—usually the sigmoid; local abscess or peritonitis results. With the development of peritonitis, the symptoms of rigidity, abdominal pain, loss of bowel sounds, and shock develop. Uninflamed or slightly inflamed diverticula may erode areas adjacent to arterial branches, thus causing massive rectal bleeding.

Gerontological Considerations

The incidence of diverticular disease increases with age. There are structural changes in the circular muscle layers of the colon as well as cellular hypertrophy. The elderly may not notice abdominal pain until infection occurs. They may delay reporting symptoms because they fear surgery or may be afraid that they may have cancer.

Although blood in the stool is a common sign of diverticular disease in the elderly, it is frequently overlooked because a person fails to examine the stool or cannot see slight changes because of diminished vision.

Diagnostic Evaluation

Diverticulosis may be diagnosed from radiographic studies that show narrowing of the colon and thickened muscle layers.

A history generally elicits the two main presenting symptoms of diverticulitis: pain in the lower left quadrant, along with a marked change in bowel habits (diarrhea or constipation). Diagnosis is made on the basis of sigmoidoscopy (direct visualization), colonoscopy, and x-ray findings with a barium enema (after inflammation has subsided). An obstruction may show with localized inflammation. A CT scan can reveal abscesses.

Management

In diverticulosis, a high-fiber diet is prescribed to prevent constipation. In diverticulitis, the bowel is rested by withholding oral fluids, administering intravenous fluids, and instituting nasogastric suctioning. Broad-spectrum antibiotics and analgesics are prescribed. Oral intake is increased as symptoms subside. A low-fiber diet may be necessary until signs of infection decrease.

If mastication is a problem, foods should be puréed. For spastic pain, antispasmodics such as propantheline bromide (Pro-Banthine) and oxyphencyclimine (Daricon) are taken before meals and at bedtime. Sedatives and tranquilizers, as well as bowel antimicrobials, may also be required. Stool normalization can be achieved by the use of one or more of the following: bulk preparations, such as Metamucil; stool softeners, such as dioctyl sodium sulfosuccinate (Colace); instillation of warm oil into the rectum; and an evacuant suppository, such as bisacodyl (Dulcolax). Such a prophylactic plan will reduce the bacterial flora of the bowel, diminish the bulk of the stool, and soften the fecal mass, so that it traverses more easily the area of inflammatory obstruction.

Surgery for diverticulosis is usually necessary only if severe hemorrhage occurs, and even then is controversial because studies show that in 50% of cases, surgery is followed by a recurrence of diverticula. If surgery is decided upon, a total colectomy with an ileorectal/ileoanal anastomosis is recommended. In this surgery, the entire colon is removed

and the end of the small intestine is joined to the rectum or the anus.

Although acute diverticulitis usually subsides with medical management, about 25% of the cases require surgical intervention for perforation, peritonitis, abscess formation, hemorrhage, and obstruction. There are two types of surgery: (1) one-stage resection of the involved sigmoid section, for recurrent attacks, and (2) multiple-staged procedures for complications, such as obstruction, perforation, and fistulae (Fig. 34-3). Surgery is preceded by barium studies. In preparing the patient for surgery, it is important to avoid irritating the colon, which is already sensitive and susceptible to perforation. A mild saline laxative and carefully administered cleansing enemas may be sufficient.

The surgery performed varies with the operative findings. When possible, the area of diverticulitis is resected and the remaining bowel joined end to end (primary resection and end-to-end anastomosis). A two-stage resection is sometimes done, in which the diseased colon is resected, as in a one-stage operation, but no anastomosis is performed and both ends of the bowel are brought out onto the abdomen as stomas. The "double-barrel" colostomy is then anastomosed in a later procedure. In some patients such an operation may appear impossible or inadvisable, in which case a colostomy is performed in the right transverse colon. Diverting the fecal flow from the area of diverticulitis allows the inflammatory process to subside, and a later operation removing the colon containing the diverticulitis is done, followed by an anastomosis. When this method of treatment is chosen, the colostomy is only temporary; after the area of diverticulitis has been removed and the intestinal continuity established by the anastomosis, the colostomy is closed. This is thus a three-stage procedure, requiring care for a colostomy during only a part of the treatment (see p. 835). A colostomy on the right

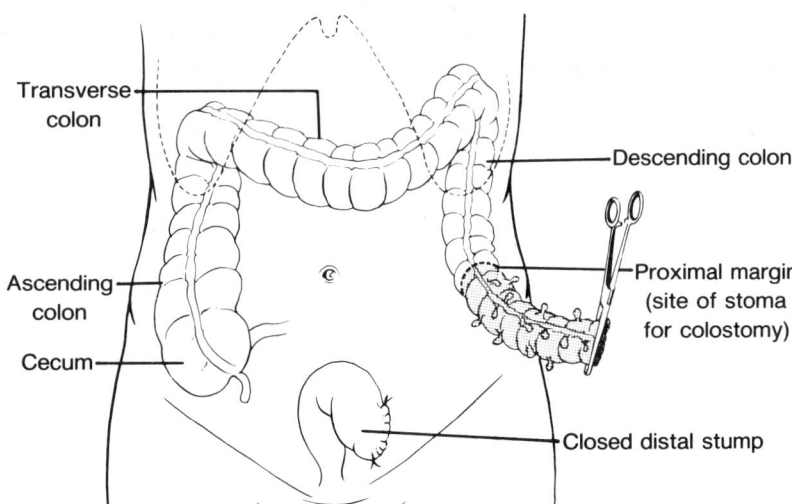

Figure 34-3
The Hartmann procedure for diverticulitis. Primary resection for diverticulitis of the colon. The affected segment (shaded) has been divided at its distal end. If primary anastomosis is to be done, the proximal margin (dotted line) is transected, and the bowel is anastomosed end-to-end. If a 2-stage procedure will be used, a colostomy is formed at the proximal margin, and the distal stump is oversewn (Hartmann procedure, as shown), or exteriorized as a mucous fistula. The second stage consists of colostomy takedown and anastomosis. (Way LW [ed]. Current Surgical Diagnosis and Treatment. Los Altos, California, Lange Medical Publishers, 1985.)

side of the transverse colon drains liquid or mushy feces and requires that a bag be worn constantly. Irrigations are rarely of value in this type of colostomy, but ordinary cleanliness is obtained by baths or showers, using soap and water to cleanse the skin around the colostomy stoma.

▶ *Nursing Process*
The Patient With Diverticulitis

▷ *Assessment*

The main symptoms of diverticulitis are left lower quadrant pain and abdominal tenderness. The sigmoid may be palpated as a firm mass. The patient reports intermittent rectal bleeding and constipation, although episodes of diarrhea may occur. The following questions should be asked: Does the patient strain at stool? Is tenesmus experienced? Is the abdomen distended?

A review of dietary habits usually indicates a history of low fiber intake. The stool is examined for pus, mucus, and blood. Elevations in temperature and pulse rates are signs of inflammation, as are elevations in the white blood cell count and the sedimentation rate.

▷ *Nursing Diagnoses*

Based on all the assessment data, the patient's major nursing diagnoses may include the following:

- Alteration in bowel elimination, constipation, related to narrowing of the colon secondary to thickened muscular segments and strictures
- Alteration in comfort, pain, related to inflammation and infection
- Alteration in gastrointestinal tissue perfusion related to infection secondary to abscess formation, perforation, and peritonitis

▷ *Planning and Implementation*

▷ *Goals:* The major goals of the patient may include attainment of normal elimination, reduction in pain, and improvement in gastrointestinal tissue perfusion.

Nursing Interventions

Elimination. Recommend a fluid intake of 2–3 liters/ day (within limits of the patient's cardiac reserve), and suggest foods that are soft but have increased fiber, such as peas and prunes, to promote defecation. For uncomplicated diverticular disease, suggest the addition of unprocessed bran to soups, salads, and cereals. Develop an individualized exercise program to improve abdominal muscle tone. Review the patient's daily routine and help to establish a schedule for meals and a set time for defecation. Help the patient identify undesirable habits that may have been used to suppress the urge to defecate. Recommend the daily intake of bulk laxatives such as Metamucil, which helps to propel feces through the colon. Administer stool softeners as prescribed to decrease straining at stool which, in turn, decreases intestinal pressure. Oil-re-

tention enemas may be prescribed to soften the stool and decrease inflammation.

Pain Relief. Administer analgesics and antispasmodic drugs as prescribed. A low-fiber diet is recommended until the inflammation subsides. Record the intensity, duration, and location of pain to determine severity and progression/ remission of the inflammatory process. Pain is felt in the left lower quadrant and can be referred to the back. Immediately report any abdominal rigidity, which may indicate perforation and peritonitis.

Preventing Complications. The major nursing focus is prevention through identification of persons at risk and management of those suffering from diverticular disease. The nurse encourages fluid intake to promote hydration in order to maintain normal stool consistency and prevent straining. During acute inflammation, however, oral foods and fluids may be restricted, in which case intravenous fluids are prescribed to prevent dehydration.

If food is tolerated while infection is present, a low-fiber diet is prescribed and the nurse advises the patient about dietary management. The nurse assesses for indicators of perforation: a tender, rigid abdomen; an elevated white blood cell count; an elevated sedimentation rate; the presence or absence of pain; increased temperature; tachycardia, and hypotension. Perforation constitutes a surgical emergency.

The patient should understand the nature of the problem and recognize that the objective is to rest the intestinal tract. Heretofore, diverticulosis of the colon was considered relatively harmless, but, because of the potential for developing complex problems, prevention is now given major emphasis.

▷ *Evaluation*

▷ *Expected Outcomes*

1. Patient attains a normal pattern of elimination
   a. Reports less abdominal cramping and pain
   b. Reports the passage, without pain, of soft, formed stool
   c. Adds unprocessed bran to foods
   d. Drinks at least 10 glasses of fluid a day (if fluid intake is tolerated)
   e. Exercises daily
2. Experiences less pain
   a. Requests analgesics as needed
   b. Adheres to a low-fiber diet
3. Achieves normal gastrointestinal tissue perfusion
   a. Complies with food restrictions
   b. Remains on bed rest
   c. Is afebrile
   d. Has a soft, nontender abdomen with normal bowel sounds

Meckel's Diverticulum

Meckel's diverticulum is a congenital abnormality consisting of a blind tube, comparable to the appendix, that usually opens into the distal ileum near the ileocecal valve. A portion of this duct persists as a diverticulum in approximately 2% of the population. It is more common in men than in women.

The importance of Meckel's diverticulum lies in the fact that its mucosal lining not infrequently may become inflamed and may lead to intestinal obstruction, or it may perforate, causing peritonitis.

The most common symptoms of a diseased Meckel's diverticulum are abdominal pain, typically umbilical in location, or the passage of stools containing blood. The blood is a dark crimson color. (A slowly bleeding gastric or upper intestinal lesion is tarry black; a colonic hemorrhage usually produces bright red bleeding). The treatment is surgical excision of the diverticulum.

Chronic Inflammatory Bowel Disease: Regional Enteritis (Crohn's Disease) and Ulcerative Colitis

The term *inflammatory bowel disease* is used to designate two chronic inflammatory gastrointestinal disorders: regional enteritis (Crohn's disease, granulomatous colitis) and ulcerative colitis. The incidence of inflammatory bowel disease in the United States is estimated to be between 4% and 10%, with 25,000 new cases occurring annually. The disease is seen more frequently in whites and most frequently in the Jewish population. A familial history is found in 20% to 40% of patients.

The current belief is that regional enteritis and ulcerative colitis are separate entities with similar etiologies. Both are characterized by exacerbations and remissions. Both diseases are associated with ankylosing spondylitis and the HLA antigen B27. A specific chromosomal abnormality has not been identified. Each disease may be triggered by environmental agents such as pesticides, food additives, tobacco, and radiation. An immunologic influence has been suggested because of studies that show abnormalities in humoral and cell-mediated immunity in people with these disorders. Lymphocytotoxic antibodies have been found in patients with inflammatory bowel disease, but more definitive research is needed to link immunologic and environmental factors.

A psychological factor has also been suggested. Many individuals with ulcerative colitis are found to be dependent, passive, immature, perfectionist, and anxious to please. Coping behaviors are often inappropriate and can include withdrawal, denial, and repression. Some people have a decreased level of tolerance for the pain and discomfort associated with intestinal cramping and diarrhea. They may react by being depressed or violent. Some clinicians suggest that the personality traits are the cause—not the result—of the disease symptoms, but more clinical research is needed to establish a causal relationship.

Pathophysiology

Although both diseases share certain similarities, they differ in many ways. Regional enteritis is an inflammatory disorder that erodes the wall of the intestine. It may involve any part of the intestine, although the ileum is most commonly affected. Ulcerative colitis is a recurrent ulcerative and inflammatory disease of the colon and rectum, with rare involvement

of the distal ileum. It is a serious disease, accompanied by systemic complications and a high mortality rate. Eventually 10% to 15% of the patients develop carcinoma of the colon. See Table 34-7 for a comparison of regional enteritis and ulcerative colitis.

Regional Enteritis. Regional enteritis (Crohn's disease) is a subacute and chronic inflammation that extends through the intestinal mucosa. This transmural involvement accounts for the formation of fistulas, fissures, and abscesses. The lesions are characteristically discontinuous or separated by normal tissue. Granulomas occur in 50% of the cases. Advanced cases present with a "cobblestone" appearance. As the disease advances, the intestinal lumen narrows, causing obstruction.

Ulcerative Colitis. Ulcerative colitis affects the superficial mucosa of the colon and is characterized by multiple ulcerations, diffuse inflammations, and desquamation of the colonic epithelium, with alternating periods of exacerbation and remission. The lesions are continuous and ultimately spread throughout the large intestine. Eventually the bowel narrows, shortens, and thickens due to muscular hypertrophy and the deposition of fat.

Clinical Manifestations

Regional enteritis. With regional enteritis, the onset of symptoms is usually insidious, but abdominal pain, diarrhea, and weight loss are prominent, and are unrelieved by defecation. Diarrhea is present in 90% of patients. Scar tissue and formation of granulomas interfere with the ability of the intestine to transport products of the upper intestinal digestion through the constricted lumen, resulting in crampy abdominal pains. Because intestinal peristalsis is stimulated by the eating of food, the crampy pains occur after meals. To avoid these bouts of crampy pain, the patient avoids food or takes it only in amounts and types inadequate for normal nutritional requirements, so that weight loss, malnutrition, and secondary or macrocytic anemia occur. In addition, ulcers form in the lining membrane of the intestine and other inflammatory changes take place, resulting in a constant irritating discharge that is emptied into the colon from the weeping, swollen intestine. This causes a chronic diarrhea. The end result is a very uncomfortable person who is thin and emaciated from inadequate food intake and constant fluid loss. In some patients, the inflamed intestine may perforate and form intraabdominal and anal abscesses. Melena may occur, along with malabsorption syndrome. Fever and leukocytosis occur. Abscesses, fistulas and fissures are common.

Ulcerative Colitis. The predominant symptoms of ulcerative colitis are diarrhea, abdominal pain, intermittent tenesmus, and rectal bleeding. In addition, anorexia, weight loss, fever, vomiting, and dehydration may be evident, as well as cramping and the feeling of an urgent need to defecate. The patient may report passing 10 to 20 liquid stools daily. Hypocalcemia and anemia frequently develop. Rebound tenderness may occur in the right lower quadrant.

Diagnostic Evaluation

Regional enteritis. For regional enteritis, the most conclusive diagnostic aid is a barium study of the upper gastrointestinal tract that reveals the classic "string sign" on x-ray of

TABLE 34-7
Comparison of Regional Enteritis (Crohn's Disease) and Ulcerative Colitis

	Regional Enteritis, Granulomatous Colitis (Transmural)	Ulcerative Colitis (Mucosal)
History	Crippling: indolent	Exacerbations, remissions; may be lethal
		Toxic megacolon
Pathology		
Early	Transmural thickening	Mucosal ulceration
Late	Deep, penetrating granulomas	Mucosal minute ulceration
Clinical Manifestations		
Location	Ileum, right colon (usually)	Rectum, left colon
Bleeding	Usually not, but may occur	Common—severe
Perianal involvement	Common	Rare—mild
Fistulas	Common	Rare
Rectal involvement	About 20%	Almost 100%
Diarrhea	Less severe	Severe
Diagnostic Studies:	Skip areas	Diffuse involvement
X-ray films	Shortening of colon	No shortening of colon
	Mucosal edema	No mucosal edema
	Stenosis, fistulas	Stenosis, rare; no fistulas
Therapeutic Management	Steroids, Sulfonamides (Sulfasalazine [Azulfidine])	Steroids, sulfonamides; Azulfidine is useful in preventing recurrence
	Intravenous alimentation	
	Partial or complete colectomy, with ileostomy or anastomosis	Proctocolectomy, with ileostomy
	Rectum can be preserved in some patients.	Rectum can be preserved in only a few patients "cured" by colectomy.
	Recurrence common	
Complications	Right-sided hydronephrosis	Pyelonephritis
	Nephrolithiasis	
	Cholelithiasis	Cholangiocarcinoma
		Pericholangitis
	Retinitis, iritis	Same
	Finger clubbing	Same
	Erythema nodosum	Same

the terminal ileum, indicating the constriction of a segment of intestine.

A proctosigmoidoscopic examination is usually done initially to establish whether there is an inflammatory process in the rectosigmoid area. If this area is normal, the diagnosis of ulcerative colitis is ruled out.

A stool examination may be positive for occult blood and steatorrhea. Leukocytosis and an elevated sedimentation rate may be present. Bowel sounds are hyperactive over the right lower quadrant.

Ulcerative Colitis. In the diagnosis of chronic ulcerative colitis, careful stool examination is done to rule out dysentery caused by the common intestinal organisms, especially *Entamoeba histolytica* infection. The stool is positive for blood. Leukocytosis, anemia, and bone marrow depression are common. Other indicators include a loss of plasma proteins due to liver dysfunction, electrolyte imbalance, thrombocytosis due to the inflammatory process, and decreased serum iron levels secondary to blood loss. Sigmoidoscopy and barium enema x-ray examination are of value in distinguishing this condition from other diseases of the colon with similar symptoms.

- In acute ulcerative colitis, cathartics are contraindicated when the patient is being prepared for barium enema because they may cause severe exacerbation of the condition, which may lead to megacolon (excessive dilatation of the colon), perforation, and death. If the patient is required to have this diagnostic test, pehaps a liquid diet for a few days before the x-ray and a gentle tap water enema on the day of examination are sufficient preparation.

Management

Medical treatment for both regional enteritis and ulcerative colitis is aimed at reducing inflammation, suppressing inappropriate immune responses, and providing rest for a diseased bowel, so that healing may take place.

Well-balanded, low-residue, high-protein diets with supplemental vitamin therapy and iron replacement are effective in meeting nutritional needs. Fluid and electrolyte imbalance due to dehydration caused by diarrhea is corrected by intravenous therapy. Any foods that exacerbate diarrhea should be avoided. Milk may contribute to diarrhea if lactose intolerance is present. In addition, cold foods are to be avoided, along with smoking, because both increase intestinal motility.

Sedation and antidiarrheal/antiperistaltic medications are given to reduce to a minimum the colonic peristalsis, in order to rest the inflamed bowel. They are continued until the patient's stools approach normal frequency and consistency. Sulfonamides such as sulfasalazine (Azulfidine) or sulfisoxazole (Gantrisin) are often effective for mild or moderate inflammation. Antibiotics are used for secondary infections, particularly for purulent complications such as abscesses, perforation, and peritonitis. Azulfidine is helpful in preventing recurrences.

ACTH and corticosteroids are most effective early in the course of the acute inflammatory phase rather than in the chronic phase. When steroids are reduced or stopped, the symptoms of disease are likely to return. If steriods are continued, adverse sequelae such as hypertension, fluid retention, subcapsular cataracts, and hirsutism may develop.

Psychotherapy is aimed at determining what factors distress the patient, dealing with these factors, and attempting to resolve conflicts so that they no longer aggravate the patient.

Surgical Intervention for Inflammatory Bowel Disorders

When conservative measures fail to relieve the severe symptoms of inflammatory bowel disease, surgery may be recommended by the physician.

Regional enteritis. If a lesion can be delineated in regional enteritis (obstruction, abscess, fistula, stricture), it is resected (excised, removed), and the remaining portions of the bowel are anastomosed (joined together). Loss of 50%

of the small bowel can usually be tolerated. The surgical procedures of choice are the following:

- Total colectomy (excision of the entire colon) with ileostomy (surgical creation of an opening into the ileum, usually by means of an ileal stoma on the abdominal wall)
- Segmental colectomy (removal of a segment of the colon) with colocolonic anastomosis (joining of the remaining portions of the colon)
- Subtotal colectomy (removal of nearly all of the colon) with ileorectal anastomosis (joining of the ileum and rectum)

The rate of recurrence following surgery is 20% to 40% for the first 5 years. Patients under 25 years of age have the highest recurrence rate.

Ulcerative Colitis. Approximately 15% to 20% of the patients with ulcerative colitis require surgical intervention. Indications for surgery include lack of improvement and continued deterioration, profuse bleeding, perforation, stricture formation, and indications that carcinoma has developed. The operation of choice is a total colectomy and ileostomy; any procedure more limited will prove to be of only temporary benefit in most patients. A proctocolectomy (complete excision of colon, rectum, and anus) is recommended when the rectum is severely involved.

In the 1970s a surgical procedure was introduced that combined protocolectomy with a continent ileal reservoir (*Kock's pouch*). This procedure eliminates the need for an external fecal collection bag. Approximately 30 cm of the distal ileum is reconstructed to form a reservoir with a nipple valve that is created by intussusception of a portion of the terminal ileal loop. See Figure 34-4*A*. Gastrointestinal effluent can be stored in the pouch for several hours and is then removed by means of a catheter inserted through the nipple valve. The major problem with the Kock pouch is malfunction of the nipple valve, which is seen in 20% to 40% of the patients.

A new surgical procedure is being performed for chronic ulcerative colitis and familial polyposis that eliminates the permanent ileostomy, establishes an ileal reservoir, and retains anal sphincter control of elimination. The procedure involves an ileoanal anastomosis done in conjunction with a total abdominal colectomy and a mucosal proctectomy. A temporary diverting-loop ileostomy is constructed at the time of surgery and closed about 3 months later (Fig. 34-4*B*). With ileoanal anastomosis, the diseased colon and rectum are removed, voluntary defecation is maintained, and anal continence is preserved. The ileal reservoir decreases the number of bowel movements by 50%, from approximately 14–20 per day to 7–10 per day. Nighttime elimination is gradually reduced to 1 bowel movement. Complications of the ileoanal anastomosis include perianal skin excoriation from leakage of fecal contents, stricture formation at the anastomosis site, and small bowel obstruction. See Table 34-8 for an description of common intestinal ostomies.

Preoperative Nursing Interventions

A period of preparation, with intensive fluid, blood, and protein replacement, is necessary before surgery is attempted. Antibiotics may be prescribed. If the patient has been taking

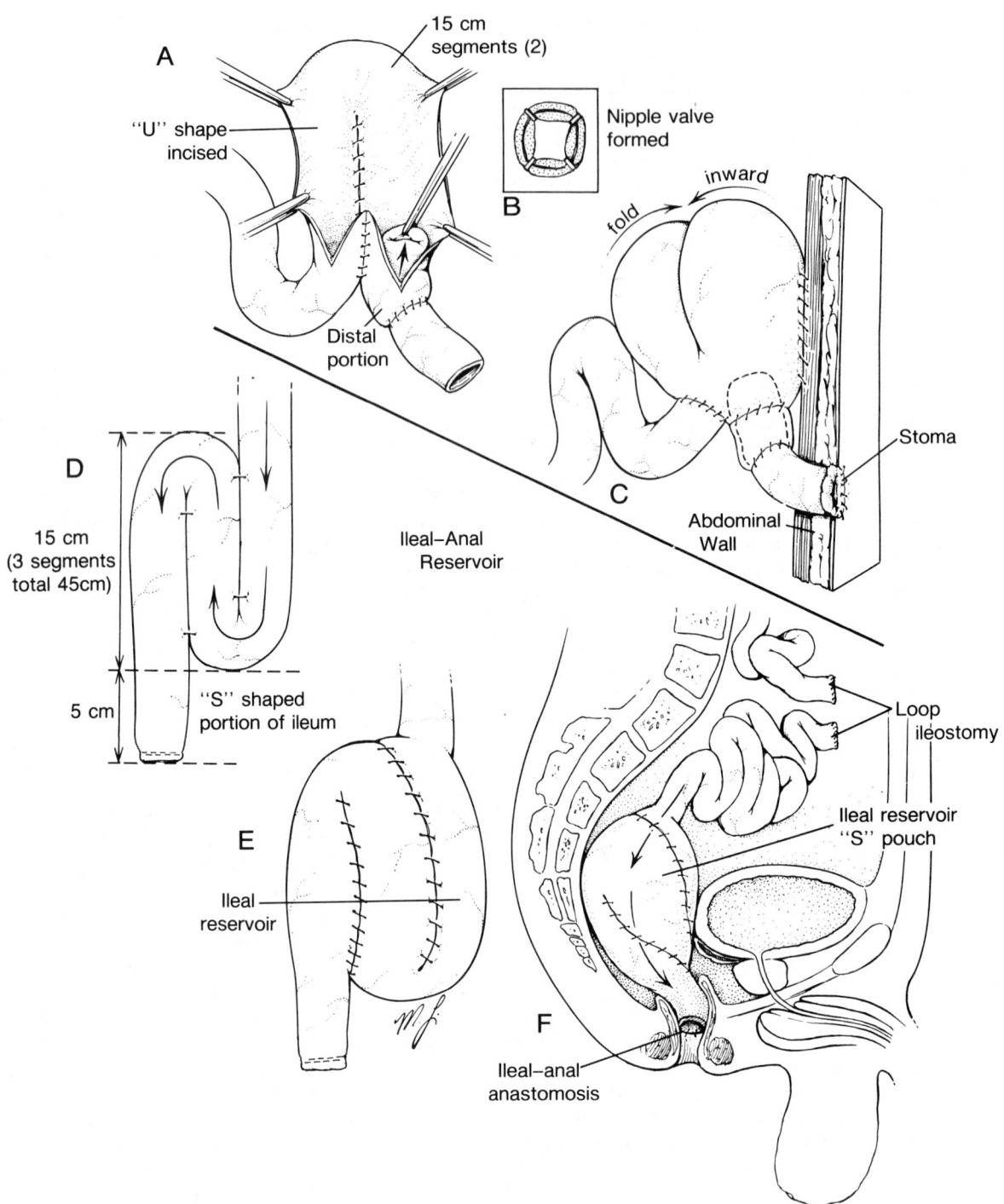

Figure 34-4
An ileal reservoir for the Kock pouch and for an ileoanal anastomosis.
   For the Kock pouch: (*A*) A 30-cm portion of the ileum is sutured together to form a "U" shape. It is then excised open and the distal portion is pulled back into the ileum (similar to an intussusception). (*B*) A nipple valve is formed by suturing the pulled-back portion of the intestine to itself. (*C*) The top of the ileum is folded onto itself and a stoma is formed from the distal portion.
   For the ileoanal anastomosis: (*D*) A 50-cm portion of the distal ileum is aligned in an "S" shape. (*E*) The bowel is opened along the antimesenteric surface and then adjacent walls are anastomosed to create a reservoir. (*F*) A mucosal proctectomy precedes anastomosis of the ileal reservoir. A temporary loop ileostomy diverts effluent discharge for several months.

TABLE 34-8
Common Intestinal Ostomies

Ileostomy	Ileal Loop (Urinary Conduit)	Transverse Colostomy	Descending or Sigmoid Colostomy
Intestinal Segment Involved			
End of ileum	Loop of ileum is made into a pouch into which transplanted ureters drain urine.	Transverse colon	Descending or sigmoid colon
Effluent			
Liquid, semi-liquid, soft	Urine only	Soft and, at occasional intervals, fairly firm; softer toward ileum	Descending—fairly firm stool; sigmoid—even more solid
Odor			
Slightly odorous	Nonodorous	Very malodorous	Usually malodorous
Skin Effect			
Enzymes highly irritating	Urine is irritating to unprotected skin.	Irritating, with continuous discharge	Fairly irritating
Types of Appliances			
Open-ended pouch worn at all times; if Kock pouch, no appliance is worn	Open-ended pouch worn at all times	Pouch worn at all times. (Either a large stoma with two openings, or two separate stomas; fecal discharge from one and mucus from the other)	Depends on patient's level of control. Some wear no appliance and irrigate regularly. Others wear closed pouch, if effluent is firm; open-ended, if discharge is more liquid continuously.
Indications			
Use meticulous skin care. Avoid irritating foods. Wear nonconstricting garments.	Use meticulous skin care. Protect clothes from seepage. Drink sufficient fluids to maintain recommended daily output.	Avoid irritating and gas-producing foods. Modify clothing to protect pouch. Protect skin.	Avoid irritating foods. Protect skin.

steroids for a long period of time, steroids will probably be continued during the surgical phase, and then gradually tapered off. Meanwhile the patient should be assessed for adrenal insufficiency by observing and recording pulse, blood pressure, urinary output, general appearance, and reactions.

Usually, the patient is given a low-residue diet offered frequently in small feedings. All other preoperative measures are similar to those for general abdominal surgery. The abdomen is marked for the proper placement of the stoma by the surgeon or the ostomy nurse. Care is taken to see that the ostomy or stoma is conveniently placed. Information about an ileostomy is presented to the patient by means of literature, models, and discussion. The patient should have a fairly good idea of what the surgery is all about and what to expect postoperatively, and may even be encouraged to wear an ileostomy appliance for a day or two before surgery to facilitate adjustment to it after the operation.

Preoperative preparation for a continent ileostomy is similar to that for the patient having a traditional ileostomy. Teaching before surgery will relate to managing the drains from the outlet, the nature of drainage, and the need for nasogastric intubation, parenteral fluids, and perineal packing and care.

Postoperative Nursing Interventions

General abdominal surgery wound care is required. As soon as the operation is completed, a temporary plastic bag with an adhesive facing is placed over the ileostomy and firmly pressed onto surrounding skin. The opening of the small intestine on the abdomen continuously discharges the liquid contents of the small intestine, because the stoma does not have a controlling sphincter. The contents draining from the ileostomy drain into the plastic bag and are thus kept from coming into contact with skin. They are collected and measured as the bag becomes full. After the ileostomy has had a chance to heal, a permanent appliance is obtained and held in place on the skin with a special cement. The stomal size should be rechecked in 3 weeks, when the edema has subsided. The final size and type may be selected in 3 months, after the patient's weight has stabilized and the stoma shrinks to a stable shape.

Because these patients lose much fluid and food in the early postoperative period, an accurate record of fluid intake, urinary output, and fecal discharges is necessary to help gauge the fluid needs of the patient. Fluids and a low-residue, high-calorie diet are given until the patient becomes accustomed to the new digestive arrangement.

Nasogastric suction is also a part of immediate postoperative care, with the tube requiring frequent irrigation, as requested. The purpose of nasogastric suction is to facilitate healing and to relieve pressure on the suture line by preventing a buildup of gastric contents. The patient receives parenteral fluids for 4 to 5 days. Thereafter, sips of clear liquids are offered, and the diet progresses gradually. Nausea and abdominal distention are observed as signs of an obstruction. Should they occur, the physician is notified.

As with other patients undergoing abdominal surgery, early ambulation is encouraged. Prescribed pain medications are given if required.

By the end of the first week, rectal packing is removed. Because this procedure may be uncomfortable, the patient may be given a sedative an hour before it is done. Changing the perineal dressings may also be facilitated by moistening the dressings a day before they are removed. After the packing is removed, the perineum is irrigated 2 to 3 times daily until full healing takes place.

Psychosocial Considerations

The patient understandably may think that everyone is aware of the ileostomy, and may view the stoma as mutilative in comparison with other abdominal incisions that heal and are hidden. Because there is loss of a body part and a major change in anatomy, the ileostomy patient often goes through the various phases of grieving. The nurse can expect the patient to experience shock, disbelief, denial, rejection, anger, and restitution. Nursing support through these phases is important, and understanding of the patient's emotional outlook in each instance should determine the nurse's approach. For example, any form of teaching is of no avail until the patient has reached the stage of restitution.

Concern over body image may lead to questions related to family relationships, sexual function, and the ability to become pregnant and to deliver normally.

Finally, such patients need to know that someone understands and cares about them. Sincere friendliness and a nonjudgmental attitude exhibited by the nurse will aid in gaining the patient's confidence, so important to therapy and preoperative preparation. It is important to recognize the dependency needs of these patients.

Such patients probably are the most challenging of all to the nurse. Their prolonged illness can make them irritable, anxious, and depressed. The nurse can coordinate patient care through nursing conferences attending by consultants such as the physician, psychologist, psychiatrist, social worker, and dietitian. The team approach lends support in approaching a complex nursing problem.

On the other hand, an operation establishing an ileostomy can produce dramatic changes in patients who have suffered from colitis for several years. Once the misery of the disease has lifted and patients learn how to take care of an ileostomy, they can become normal, affable people. But until they progress to this phase, an empathetic and tolerant approach by the nurse will play an important part in recovery.

The support of other ostomates is also a help. A nonprofit health service agency that is dedicated to the rehabilitation of ostomates is the United Ostomy Association.* This organization gives patients useful information on living with an ostomy through an educational program of literature, lectures, and exhibits. Local associations provide visiting services by qualified members who give hope, as well as rehabilitation services, to new ostomy patients. Local hospitals may have an enterostomal therapist on the staff; this is a valuable resource person for the ileostomy patient.

Rehabilitation and Patient Education Following an Ileostomy

There are certain rehabilitation problems unique to the ileostomy patient, one of which is irregularity of bowel evacuation. The patient with an ileostomy cannot establish regular bowel habits because the contents of the ileum are fluid and are discharging continuously. Therefore, the patient must wear an appliance (a vinyl or plastic bag) day and night. The appliance is regarded, then, as an intestinal prosthesis.

Several days after the operation, the ileostomy diameter is carefully measured with a stoma-measuring card (various apertures indicate different sizes) so that a suitable opening in the mounting ring will be available in the permanent appliance. The ring is sealed to the skin with an adhesive disc that permits the patient to carry on normal activities without fear of leakage or odor.

The location and length of the stoma are significant in the management of the ileostomy by the patient. The surgeon places the stoma as close to the midline as possible and in a position where even an obese patient with a protruding abdomen can care for it readily. Usually, the ileostomy stoma is about 2.5 (1 inch) long, which makes it convenient for the attachment of an appliance.

The ileostomy may be noisy at first, due to edema caused by slight obstruction of tissues. Eventually it will become quieter. A low-fiber diet is followed at first, with strained fruits and vegetables. These foods are important for vitamins A and C. Later there are few dietary restrictions, except for avoiding foods that are high in fiber or hard-to-digest kernels, such as celery, popcorn, corn-on-the-cob, poppy seeds or caraway seeds, and coconut. Fluids may be a problem during the summer, when they are lost during perspiration as well as through the ileostomy. Drinks such as Gatorade are helpful in maintaining electrolyte balance. If the effluent (fecal discharge) is too water, fibrous foods (such as whole grain cereals, fresh fruit skins, beans, corn, and nuts) are restricted.

* 2001 W. Beverly Blvd., Los Angeles, California 90057

If the effluent is excessively dry, salt intake is increased. An increased intake of water or fluid will not increase the effluent because excess water is excreted in the urine.

Another possible problem is skin excoriation around the stoma. Not only does the ileostomy drainage contain enzymes that rapidly excoriate the skin but, if cement is used in putting the appliance on, the skin may be irritated when the appliance is removed. To prevent irritation and yeast growth, nystatin powder (Mycostatin) is dusted lightly on the peristomal skin.

A regular schedule for changing the appliance before leakage occurs is established. In teaching the patient to use and care for his appliance, stress the following essential points:

To Remove the Appliance

1. Sit or stand in a comfortable position.
2. Fill a container with the prescribed solvent. Apply a few drops of solvent with a medicine dropper between the disc of the appliance and the skin. *Do not pull off the appliance.* As the solvent works, the pouch loosens and pulling is unnecessary.

To Cleanse the Skin

1. Use a cotton ball soaked in solvent. Wet the skin around the stoma. During the time the skin is being cleansed, a gauze dressing may cover the stoma or a vaginal tampon can be inserted gently to absorb excess drainage. Avoid rubbing, because solvents are irritating.
2. Wash the skin with a soft cloth moistened with *tepid* water and mild soap, or shower or bathe either before putting on the clean appliance or before removing the bag. Micropore tape applied to the sides of the disc will keep it secure during bathing.

To Put on the Appliance

1. When there is no irritation, a disposable plastic bag can be applied directly to the skin after the cover has been removed from the adherent surface of the bag. Press firmly in place for 30 seconds.
2. When there is a skin irritation, after skin cleansing apply Kenalog spray (antibiotic); blot excess moisture with a cotton pledget and dust lightly with nystatin (Mycostatin) powder.
3. Moisten a Karaya gum washer and apply when it is tacky or "sticky."
4. Press the adhesive disc on the faceplate of the pouch against the washer. This will allow skin to heal while the appliance is in place.

The amount of time that a person can keep the appliance sealed to the body depends on the location of the stoma and on body structure. Usually, the normal wearing time is 2 to 4 days. The appliance is emptied every 4 to 6 hours, or at the same time the patient empties his bladder. An emptying spout at the bottom of the appliance is closed with a rubber band or special clip made for this purpose.

The appliance is cleaned and aired according to the manufacturer's directions. Usually, thorough washing with soap and water using a soft nylon brush is effective. There are many deodorizers and cleaning aids available that the patient can use. Full-strength distilled vinegar, rather than strong bleaches, is effective for soaking the bag. Commercial liquid deodorizers are also available, and are preferred by some patients. Other inexpensive deodorants are pieces of charcoal, or two aspirin tablets crushed and dropped into the bag. Foods such as spinach and parsley act as deodorizers in the intestinal tract; foods that cause odors are cabbage, onions, and fish. Most patients alternate bags and allow the cleaned bag to be exposed to moving fresh air, out of direct sunlight. Bismuth subcarbonate tablets taken by mouth 3 or 4 times a day are effective in reducing odor. Some physicians prescribe a stool thickener, such as diphenoxylate (Lomotil) (by mouth), to assist in odor control.

Continent Ileostomy. The following considerations apply specifically to the patient with a continent ileostomy.

Irrigation. A continent ileostomy is irrigated to stimulate the discharge of fecal contents. After the operation, a catheter extends from the stoma and is attached to a closed suction system. Drainage is maintained for approximately 2 weeks. The catheter is irrigated, usually every 3 hours, to assure its patency. About 10 to 20 ml of normal saline are introduced gently into the pouch by means of a syringe. Return flow is not aspirated, but permitted to drain by gravity.

After 2 weeks, when the healing process has progressed to the point at which the catheter is removed from the stoma, it is time for the patient to learn to manage draining the pouch.

The equipment required includes a catheter, tissues, water-soluble lubricant, gauze squares, a syringe, irrigating solution in a bowl, and an emesis or receiving basin.

1. Lubricate the catheter and gently insert about 5 cm (2 inches), at which point some resistance may be felt at the valve or "nipple." When gentle pressure is used, the catheter usually will enter the pouch.
2. If there is much resistance, fill a syringe with 20 ml of air or water and inject it through the catheter, while still exerting some pressure on the catheter. This will permit the catheter to enter into the pouch (Fig. 34-4*A*).
3. Place the other end of the catheter in a drainage basin held below the level of the stoma so that gravity will facilitate drainage. Later, of course, this process can be carried out at the toilet, with drainage delivered into the toilet bowl. Drainage may include flatus as well as effluent.
4. Following drainage, the catheter is removed and the area around the stoma is gently washed with warm water. Pat dry and apply an absorbent pad over the stoma. Fasten the pad with hypoallergenic tape.

The whole procedure should not require more than 5 to 10 minutes. At first, irrigation is done every 3 hours. The time between irrigations is gradually lengthened so that it is done about 3 times daily.

When discharge is thick, water can be injected via the catheter to loosen and soften it. Effluent consistency is affected by food intake. At first drainage is only 60 to 80 ml, but as time goes on it will increase significantly. The pouch will stretch, eventually accommodating 500 to 1000 ml. The gauge to determine frequency of drainage is the sensation of pressure in the pouch.

Patient Education and Home Health Care. The spouse and family should be familiar with the adjustment that will be necessary when the patient returns home. They need to know why it is necessary for the ileostomate to occupy the bathroom for 10 minutes at certain times of the day, and why certain equipment is needed. Their understanding is necessary to reduce tension—a relaxed patient tends to have fewer problems.

Psychosocial needs of the patient are stressed. Knowledge that it will not be necessary to wear an ileostomy bag is often sufficient encouragement for the patient to master control over the pouch.

A successful cover for the stoma for home use consists of a dressing that is absorbent on one side and plasticized on the other. (High-quality disposable diapers can be cut into 7.5 cm × 7.5 [3″ × 3″] squares; this makes an ideal dressing.) The dressing is held in place with tape. To reduce skin excoriation, the tape is placed differently with each application so that it does not contact the same area of skin each time.

A water-soluble lubricant, rather than petrolatum, should be used. The latter has a tendendy to clog the catheter and is difficult to wash from it.

The position to assume in the bathroom is one of individual preference and convenience. The patient may sit on the toilet seat, stand in front of the toilet, or sit on a chair in front of the toilet. It is suggested that an adapter and a length of tubing be available to attach to the catheter, so that effluent does not splatter but drains easily into the toilet bowl.

Encourage experimentation when there are problems with drainage. If the catheter meets resistance when attempts are made to insert it, the patient is encouraged to relax before draining the pouch and to be sure to lubricate the catheter well. It may be easier for the patient to lie down when the catheter is inserted and then stand up for drainage purposes.

Injection of air or water may help in passing the catheter through the stoma into the pouch. (Skin care, odor reduction, diet, and activities are similar to those recommended for other ostomy patients; see p. 824.)

Complications

Minor complications occur in about 40% of patients who have an ileostomy; less than 20% of the complications require surgical intervention. *Peristomal skin irritation,* the most common complication of an ileostomy, is due to leakage of effluent. An ill-fitting pouch is frequently the cause. The pouch is adjusted by the nurse or an enterostomal therapist and skin barriers are applied. *Diarrhea,* manifested by very irritating effluent that rapidly fills the pouch (every hour or sooner), can quickly lead to dehydration and electrolyte losses. Supplemental water, salt, and potassium are given to prevent hypovolemia and hypokalemia. Antidiarrheal agents are administered. *Stenosis* is caused by circular scar tissue formation at the stoma site. The scar tissue is surgically released. *Urinary calculi* occur in about 10% of ileostomy patients because of dehydration secondary to decreased fluid intake. Intense lower abdominal pain that radiates to the legs, hematuria, and signs of dehydration alert the nurse to strain all urine. Sometimes small stones are passed during urination; otherwise an invasive procedure is necessary to crush or remove the calculi. *Cholelithiasis* (formation of gallstones) due to cholesterol is seen three times more frequently than in the general population because of changes in the absorption of bile acids that occurs preoperatively. Spasm of the gallbladder causes severe upper right abdominal pain that can radiate to the back and right shoulder. *Ileitis* is usually seen with a recurrence of inflammatory bowel disease.

▶ Nursing Process
The Patient With a Chronic Inflammatory Bowel Disease

▷ Assessment

The nurse obtains a complete history, which includes patient concerns about diarrhea, abdominal cramping, tenesmus, nausea, anorexia, and weight loss. Exacerbations related to stress or dietary indiscretions and remissions are reported. Job-related stress factors are identified. A family history of inflammatory bowel disease is explored, because 15% of those diagnosed have a family member with the disease. Any known allergies are recorded, especially an allergy to milk, because lactose intolerance is common with regional enteritis. The amounts of alcohol, caffeine, and nicotine used daily/weekly are noted, because these agents stimulate the bowel and can initiate diarrhea and abdominal cramping.

Nutritional status needs to be assessed. Malabsorption is not uncommon, and some patients can lose 10 to 20 pounds in 2 months. Because patients with inflammatory bowel disease may have 20 diarrheal stools per day, they isolate themselves from family and friends and become anxious, dependent, and depressed. Sleep disturbances are common. Assessment includes psychosocial evaluation of the individual's coping mechanisms and emotional status.

Regional enteritis. With regional enteritis, pain is usually localized in the right lower quadrant where hyperactive bowel sounds can be heard due to borborygmus and increased peristalsis. Abdominal tenderness is noted on palpation. The most prominent symptom is intermittent pain associated with diarrhea that does not decrease with defecation. Pain in the periumbilical region usually indicates involvement of the terminal ileum.

Ulcerative Colitis. With ulcerative colitis, the abdomen may be distended and rebound tenderness present. Rectal bleeding is a dominant sign.

▷ Nursing Diagnoses

Based on all the assessment data, the patient's major nursing diagnoses may include the following:

- Alteration in bowel elimination, diarrhea, related to the inflammatory process
- Alteration in comfort, abdominal pain and cramping, related to increased peristalsis
- Fluid volume and electrolyte deficits related to anorexia, nausea, and diarrhea
- Alteration in nutrition, less than body requirements related to anorexia secondary to diarrhea
- Activity intolerance related to fatigue
- Anxiety related to impending surgery
- Ineffective individual coping related to repeated episodes of diarrhea
- Knowledge deficit concerning the process and management of the disease

▷ Planning and Implementation

▷ **Goals:** The major goals of the patient may include attainment of normal bowel elimination, reduction in abdominal pain and cramping, prevention of fluid volume deficit, maintenance of optimum nutrition, avoidance of fatigue, reduction of anxiety, attainment of emotional balance, and acquisition of knowledge and understanding of the disease process.

Nursing Interventions

Bowel Elimination. The nurse ascertains if there is a relationship between diarrhea and certain foods, activity, or emotional stress. Any precipitating factors are reported, as well as stool frequency, consistency, and amount. Ready access to a bathroom or bedpan is provided, and the environment is kept clean and odor-free. Anti-diarrheal agents are administered as prescribed, and the frequency and consistency of stools are recorded after therapy has started. Bed rest is encouraged to decrease peristalsis.

Pain Relief. The character of the pain is documented as dull, burning, or cramplike. Its onset is relevant: Does it occur before or after meals, during the night, or before elimination? Is the pattern constant or intermittent? Is it relieved with medications?

Anticholinergic medications are given as prescribed, 30 minutes before a meal to decrease intestinal motility, and analgesics are given as needed for pain. Pain can also be reduced by position changes, the local application of heat (as prescribed), diversional activities, and the prevention of fatigue.

Fluid Intake. To detect fluid volume deficit, an accurate record of oral and intravenous fluids is kept as well as a record of output (urine, liquid stool, vomitus, wound or fistula drainage). Daily weights are taken because they indicate rapid fluid gains or losses. The nurse assesses for signs of fluid volume deficit: dry skin and mucous membranes, decreased skin turgor, oliguria, exhaustion, temperature decrease, increased hematocrit, elevated urine specific gravity, and hypotension. Oral intake of fluids is encouraged, and intravenous flow rate is monitored. Measures to decrease diarrhea are initiated: dietary restrictions, stress reduction, and administration of antidiarrheal agents.

Nutritional Measures. Total parenteral nutrition (TPN) is used when the symptoms of inflammatory bowel disease are severe. With TPN the nurse maintains an accurate record of fluid intake and output as well as the patient's daily weight. The patient should gain 0.5 kg daily during therapy. The urine is tested for sugar, acetone, and specific gravity daily when TPN is being used. Elemental feedings that are high in protein and low in fat and residue are instituted after TPN therapy because they are digested primarily in the jejunum, do not stimulate intestinal secretions, and allow the bowel to rest. Intolerance is noted if the patient exhibits nausea, vomiting, diarrhea, or abdominal distention.

If oral foods are tolerated, small, frequent feedings are given to avoid overdistending the stomach and stimulating peristalsis. Activities are restricted to conserve energy, reduce peristalsis, and limit calorie depletion.

Rest. Intermittent rest periods during the day are recommended and activities are restricted in order to conserve energy and reduce the metabolic rate. Activity within the limit of the patient's capacity is desirable, so that he will not regard himself as an invalid. Bed rest is suggested for a patient who is febrile, has frequent diarrheal stools, or is bleeding. Active and passive exercises are encouraged for anyone on bed rest to maintain muscle tone and prevent thromboembolic complications. Activity restrictions are evaluated and modified on a day-to-day basis.

Reducing Anxiety. Establish rapport by being attentive and displaying a calm, confident manner. Provide time for the patient to ask questions and express feelings. Listen carefully and be sensitive to nonverbal indicators of anxiety (restlessness, tense facial expressions). The patient may be emotionally labile because of the conditions of the disease, so information about impending surgery should be tailored to the patient's level of understanding and desire for detail. Some persons need to know everything to lessen their anxiety, while others want to know very little. If necessary, use pictures and illustrations to explain the surgical procedure and help the patient visualize what a stoma looks like.

Coping Measures. Because the patient feels isolated, helpless, and out of control, offer understanding and emotional support. The patient may be demanding and angry, and may exhibit inappropriate responses to stress: infantile behavior, perfectionism, denial, and social self-isolation.

The nurse needs to recognize that the patient's behavior may be affected by innumerable factors unrelated to inherent emotional characteristic. Any patient who is suffering from the discomforts of frequent bowel movements and rectal soreness is anxious, discouraged, and depressed. Thus, it is important to develop a relationship with the patient that gives him a feeling that he is receiving support in his attempts to deal with the stresses that have plagued him. Let him know that his complaints are understood, encourage him to talk and ventilate his feelings, and listen to matters that are disturbing to him, even if they seem trivial. Try to direct his attention to himself rather than his intestinal tract. Recommend stress reduction measures: relaxation techniques, breathing exercises, and biofeedback.

Patient Education and Home Health Care. Assess the patient's understanding of the disease process and need for additional information about medical management (medications, diet) and surgical interventions. Mention that control is possible when the cause of exacerbations is determined.

Provide information about nutritional management. A bland, low-residue, high-protein, high-calorie, and high-vitamin diet relieves symptoms and decreases diarrhea. Explain the rationale for the use of steroids, anti-inflammatory agents, antibacterial and antidiarrheal drugs, and antispasmodics. Emphasize that medications are to be taken as prescribed and not abruptly discontinued (especially the steroid agents, which can cause serious medical problems if suddenly stopped).

If surgery is required the nurse explains the procedure and the pre- and postoperative care. Ileostomy care is reviewed if necessary. See Nursing Care Plan 34-1 for the patient with an intestinal ostomy, on pages 824–827.

Patients who are being medically managed at home need to understand that their disease can be controlled and they can lead a healthy life between exacerbations. Control implies management based on an understanding of inflammatory bowel disease and its treatment.

(Text continues on p. 826)

Care of the Patient With an Intestinal Ostomy

Nursing Interventions	*Rationale*	*Expected Outcomes*

Nursing Diagnosis:　Disturbance in self-concept related to altered body image

Goal:　Attainment of a positive self-concept

1. Encourage the patient to verbalize feelings about the stoma.	1. Free expression of feelings allows the patient the opportunity to verbalize and identify concerns. Expressed concerns can be therapeutically addressed by health care team members.	• Freely expresses concerns • Accepts support • Seeks help as needed • States is willing to talk with an ostomate
2. Offer to be present when the stoma is first viewed and touched.	2. Anxiety can be reduced if questions are immediately answered.	
3. Suggest that the spouse or significant other view the stoma.		
4. Offer counseling, if desired.		
5. Arrange for a visit with an ostomate.	5. Ostomates provide an empathetic approach because they can share mutual feelings, and offer support	

Nursing Diagnosis:　Anxiety related to the loss of bowel control

Goal:　Reduction of anxiety

1. Provide information about expected bowel function: 　a. Characteristics of effluent 　b. Frequency of discharge	1. Emotional adjustment is facilitated if adequate information is provided at the level of the learner.	• Expresses interest in learning about expected bowel function • Handles equipment correctly. • Changes the pouch unassisted • Irrigates colostomy successfully • Progresses toward a regular schedule of elimination
2. Teach the patient how to prepare the pouch for an adequate fit. 　a. Choose the drainage pouch that will provide a secure fit around the stoma. Measure the stoma size with a measuring guide provided by the ostomy manufacturer and compare to the opening on the pouch. About 3 mm (1/8-inch) clearance should be provided around the stoma.		
	a. The pouch opening should be larger than the stoma for an adequate fit. Available brands come in different sizes to fit the stoma. Adjustments can be made if necessary.	
b. Remove any plastic covering that protects the pouch adhesive. 　*Note:* The pouch is applied by pressing the adhesive for 30 seconds to the skin or skin barrier.	b. The pouch is ready to apply directly to the skin or skin protector.	
3. Demonstrate how to change the pouch before leakage occurs. Be aware that the elderly person may have diminished vision and difficulty handling equipment.	3. Manipulation of the appliance is a learned motor skill that requires practice and positive encouragement.	
4. Demonstrate how to irrigate the colostomy (usually on the 4th-5th day.) Recommend that irrigating be done on a regular time depending on the type of colostomy.		

(continued)

Nursing Interventions	*Rationale*	*Expected Outcomes*

Nursing Diagnosis: Potential impairment of skin integrity related to irritation of the peristomal skin by the effluent

Goal: Attainment of skin integrity

1. Provide information about signs/symptoms of irritated or inflamed skin. Use pictures if possible. 2. Teach patient how to cleanse gently the peristomal skin.	1. Peristomal skin should be slightly pink without abrasions and similar to that of the entire abdomen. 2. Mild friction with warm water and a gentle soap cleanses the skin and minimizes irritation and possible abrasions. Patting the skin dry prevents tissue trauma.	• Describes appearance of healthy skin • Correctly cleanses the skin • Successfully applies a skin barrier • Gently removes the drainage pouch without skin damage • Demonstrates intact skin around the colostomy stoma
3. Demonstrate how to apply a skin barrier (powder, gel, paste, wafer). 4. Demonstrate how to remove the pouch.	3. Skin barriers protect the peristomal skin from enzymes and bacteria. 4. Gently separate adhesive from the skin to avoid irritation. Never pull!	

Nursing Diagnosis: Potential alteration in nutrition, inadequacy of nutrients related to avoidance of foods secondary to a fear of gastrointestinal discomfort

Goal: Achievement of an optimum nutritional intake

1. Do a complete nutritional assessment to identify any foods that may increase peristalsis by irritating the bowel. 2. Advise the patient to avoid food products with a cellulose or hemi-cellulose base (nuts, seeds).	1. Patients react differently to certain foods because of individual sensitivity. 2. Cellulose food products are the nondigestable residue of plant foods. They hold water, provide bulk, and stimulate elimination.	• Modifies diet to avoid offensive foods yet maintains a balanced nutritional intake • Avoids foods such as peanuts • Modifies intake of certain fruits
3. Recommend moderacy in intake of certain irritating fruits such as prunes, grapes, and bananas.	3. These fruits tend to increase the quantity of effluent.	

Nursing Diagnosis: Sexual dysfunction related to altered body image

Goal: Attainment of satisfactory sexual performance

1. Encourage the patient to verbalize his fears. The sexual partner is welcomed to participate in the discussion. 2. Recommend alternative sexual positions.	1. Expressed needs help the therapist develop a plan of care. 2. Avoid patient embarrassment with the visual appearance of the stoma. Avoid peristomal skin irritation secondary to friction.	• Expresses fears and concerns • Discusses alternative sexual positions • Accepts services of a professional counselor
3. Seek assistance from a sexual therapist or psychiatric clinical specialist.	3. Some patients need professional sexual counseling.	

(continued)

Nursing Interventions	*Rationale*	*Expected Outcomes*

Nursing Diagnosis: Deficit in knowledge concerning the surgical procedure and preoperative preparation

Goal: Understands the surgical process and the necessary preoperative preparations

1. Ascertain if the patient has had a previous surgical experience and ask for recollections of positive and negative impressions.	1. Fear of a repeated negative experience increases anxiety. Talking about the experience with a nurse helps clarify misconceptions and helps the patient ventilate any repressed emotions. Positive experiences are reinforced.	• Expresses anxieties and fears about the surgical process • Projects a positive attitude toward the surgical procedure • Repeats in own words information supplied by the surgeon • Understands normal anatomy and physiology of gastrointestinal tract and how it will be altered. Can point to expected location of abdominal wound and stoma. Describes stoma appearance and size
2. Determine what information the surgeon provided and whether it was understood. Clarify and elaborate as necessary. Know whether the stoma is permanent or temporary. Be aware of the patient's prognosis if carcinoma exists.	2. Clarification prevents misunderstandings and alleviates anxiety. A positive affect may be more difficult to project if the ostomy is permanent and/or the prognosis poor.	
3. Use pictures or drawings to illustrate the location and appearance of the wounds (abdominal, perineal) and the stoma if the patient is interested and receptive.	3. Knowledge, for some, alleviates anxiety because they have decreased their fear of the unknown. Others choose not to know because it makes them more anxious.	• Adheres to "bowel prep" regimen of antimicrobials and/or mechanical cleansing • Tolerates the presence of nasogastric/nasoenteric tube
4. Explain that oral/parenteral antimicrobials will be administered to cleanse the bowel preoperatively. Mechanical cleansing may also be required.	4. Antimicrobials and mechanical cleansing will reduce intestinal bacterial flora.	
5. Assist the patient during nasogastric/nasoenteric intubation. Measure drainage from the tube.	5. Nasoenteral intubation is used for decompression and drainage of gastrointestinal contents prior to surgery.	

(continued)

During a flare-up, patients are encouraged to rest as needed and modify activities according to energy levels. If possible they should limit activities to one floor in the house. Patients are advised to limit their housecleaning tasks and to avoid running the vacuum cleaner because this activity imposes strain on the lower abdominal muscles. Patients should sleep in a bedroom with an adjacent or nearby bathroom because of frequent diarrheal stools (10–20/day). Quick access to a toilet helps alleviate the worry of embarrassment if an accident occurs. Room deodorizers help control odors.

Patients in the home setting need information about their medications (drug name, dosage, side-effects, frequency of administration) and need to take them on schedule. Medication reminders are helpful (containers that separate pills according to day and time, daily checklists, programmed phone messages).

Dietary modifications can control but not cure the disease. A low-residue, high-protein, high-calorie diet is recommended, especially during an acute phase. Patients are encouraged to keep a record of those foods that irritate the bowel and eliminate them from the diet.

The prolonged nature of the disease causes a strain on family life and financial resources. Family support is vital; however, some family members experience resentment, guilt, fatigue, and an inability to continue coping with the emotional demands of the illness as well as with the physical demands of caring for another.

Some persons will not socialize for fear of being embarrassed. Many prefer to eat alone. Because they have lost control over elimination they feel that they have lost control over other aspects of their life. They need time to ventilate their fears and frustrations.

Nursing Interventions	*Rationale*	*Expected Outcomes*

Nursing Diagnosis: Potential for fluid volume deficit related to anorexia and vomiting

Goal: Attainment of fluid balance

1. Estimate fluid intake and output: a. Strict intake and output	a. An early indicator of fluid imbalance is a daily, significant difference between intake and output. The average person ingests (food, fluids) and loses (urine, feces, lungs) about 3.0 liters of fluid every 24 hours.	• Maintains fluid balance • Maintains normal serum and urinary values for sodium and potassium • Normal skin turgor • Surface of tongue is pink with a moist mucous membrane.
b. Daily weights	b. A gain/loss of 1.0 liter of fluid is reflected in a body weight change of 2.2 pounds.	
2. Assess serum and urinary values of sodium and potassium.	2. Sodium is the major electrolyte regulating water balance. Vomiting results in decreased urinary and serum sodium levels. Urinary sodium values, in contrast to serum values, reflect early, sensitive changes in sodium balance. Sodium works in conjunction with potassium, which is also decreased with vomiting. A significant deficiency in potassium is associated with a decrease in intracellular potassium bicarbonate, which leads to acidosis and compensatory hyperventilation.	
3. Observe and record skin turgor and the appearance of the tongue.	3. Adequate hydration is reflected by the skin's ability to return to its normal shape after being grasped between the fingers. *Note:* In the older person, it is normal for the return to be delayed. Changes in the mucous membrane covering of the tongue are an accurate and early indicator of hydration status.	

▷ *Evaluation*

▷ *Expected Outcomes*

1. Patient reports a decrease in the frequency of diarrheal stools.
   a. Recognizes a causal relationship between certain foods, activity or stress, and elimination
   b. Complies with activity restrictions; maintains bed rest
   c. Takes medications as prescribed
2. Experiences less pain
   a. Uses diversional activities to decrease anxiety and pain
   b. Takes anticholinergics before meals
   c. Takes analgesics as needed

3. Maintains fluid volume balance
   a. Takes 1 to 2 liters of oral fluids daily
   b. Has a normal body temperature
   c. Displays adequate skin turgor and moist mucous membranes
4. Attains optimum nutrition
   a. Tolerates small, frequent feedings without diarrhea
   b. Complies with total parenteral nutrition therapy
   c. Accepts elemental feedings if necessary
5. Avoids episodes of fatigue
   a. Rests periodically during the day
   b. Adheres to bed rest restrictions
   c. Performs exercises as needed
6. Feels less anxious
   a. Discusses fears and worries
   b. Describes the surgical procedure in own words

c. Handles equipment with ease
d. Asks to speak with an ostomate
7. Copes successfully with diagnosis
   a. Ventilates feelings freely
   b. Socializes with family members and friends
   c. Uses appropriate stress reduction behaviors
8. Acquires an understanding of the disease process
   a. Modifies diet appropriately to decrease diarrhea
   b. Adheres to medication regimen
   c. Describes possible surgical interventions

Intestinal Obstruction

The normal flow of the intestinal contents through the intestinal tract can be impeded by two types of intestinal obstruction:

1. *Mechanical* (dynamic ileus, organic ileus, spastic ileus), in which there is an intraluminal obstruction or a mural obstruction from pressure on the intestinal walls, and
2. *Paralytic* (adynamic ileus), in which the intestinal musculature is unable to propel the contents along the bowel. (Stimuli that may inhibit intestinal peristalsis are laparotomy, trauma, infection, mesenteric ischemia, and metabolic disorders.)

An obstruction is partial or complete. Its seriousness depends on the region of bowel that is affected, the degree to which the lumen is occluded, and, especially, the degree to which the blood circulation in the bowel wall is disturbed.

Small Bowel Obstruction

Adhesions are the most common cause of small bowel obstruction (60% incidence), followed by hernias and neoplasms. Other causes include intussusception, volvulus, paralytic ileus, inflammatory bowel disease, strictures, and foreign bodies.

Pathophysiology

Proximal to the intestinal obstruction there is an accumulation of intestinal contents, fluid, and gas. In the small intestine, distention reduces the absorption of fluids and stimulates gastric secretion. As a result, fluids and electrolytes are lost. With increasing distention, pressure within the intestinal lumen causes a decrease in venous and arteriolar capillary pressure. This, in turn, causes edema, congestion, necrosis, and eventual rupture or perforation of the intestinal wall.

With vomiting, there is a loss of hydrogen ions and potassium from the stomach, producing hypochloremia, hypokalemia, and metabolic alkalosis. Then dehydration and acidosis develop because of water loss and sodium loss. When there are acute fluid losses, hypovolemic shock may occur.

Clinical Manifestations and Diagnostic Evaluation

The initial symptom is usually pain that is wavelike in character. The patient may pass blood and mucus, but no fecal matter and no flatus. Vomiting occurs. This pattern is often characteristic. If the obstruction is complete, the peristaltic waves become extremely vigorous and assume a reverse direction, the intestinal contents being propelled toward the mouth instead of toward the rectum. If the obstruction is in the ileum, fecal vomiting takes place. First, the patient vomits the stomach contents, then the bile-stained contents of the duodenum and the jejunum, and finally, with each paroxysm of pain, the darker, fecal-like contents of the ileum. Soon, due to the loss of water, sodium, and chlorides in the vomitus, the unmistakable signs of dehydration become evident. The patient complains of intense thirst, drowsiness, generalized malaise, and aching. The tongue and the mucous membranes become parched; the face acquires a pinched appearance. The abdomen becomes distended, the lower the obstruction in the gastrointestinal tract, the more marked is the distention. If the situation is allowed to continue uncorrected, shock appears, due to dehydration and loss of plasma volume. The patient is prostrated; the pulse becomes increasingly weak and rapid; the temperature and the blood pressure are lowered; the skin is pale, cold, and clammy. At this point, death may supervene rapidly.

Radiographic studies indicate dilated bowel loops. With strangulation, the patient experiences severe abdominal pain and tenderness, high fever with leukocytosis, and symptoms of shock.

Management

Decompression of the bowel via a nasoenteral tube is successful in the majority of cases. When the bowel is completely obstructed, the possibility of strangulation warrants surgical intervention.

The surgical treatment of intestinal obstruction depends largely on the cause of the obstruction. In the most common causes of obstruction, such as stangulated hernia and obstruction by adhesions, the operation consists of repair of the hernia or division of the adhesion to which the intestine is attached. In some hernias, the strangulated portion of bowel may be removed and an anastomosis performed. Operation for intestinal obstruction may be simple or complicated, depending on the duration of the obstruction and the condition of the intestine found at operation.

Preoperatively, the patient's vital signs are stabilized, parenteral electrolyte solutions are administered for hydration, and a nasogastric tube is inserted to prevent vomiting.

Postoperative Adhesions

After abdominal operations, there are many areas within the abdomen that may not be completely healed, and loops of intestine may become adherent to these areas. Such inflammatory adhesions usually are only temporary and of no particular importance. However, occasionally these adhesions may produce a kinking of an intestinal loop, which causes obstruction of the intestinal flow. This obstruction usually appears on the third or fourth day after operation, when peristalsis is normally resumed and when food and fluids are being given to the patient for the first time. The symptoms are typical of any intestinal obstruction—crampy abdominal pain, distention, vomiting, etc.

The difficulty is usually relieved by nasoenteric suction. Decompressing the bowel above the site of the obstruction allows the inflammation to subside and relieves the obstruction. When the obstruction cannot be relieved by this conservative means, an operation may be necessary to free the adherent intestine and to permit the intestinal flow to be resumed.

Intussusception

Intussusception is a condition in which one part of the intestine slips into another part located below it, much as a telescope is shortened by pushing one section into the next. This occurs through peristalsis. The point at which intussusception develops most commonly is at or near the ileocecal valve. The telescoping, or *invagination,* also may start at the point of attachment of a tumor in the colon—particularly a pedunculated tumor—as a result of its becoming engaged by a peristaltic wave and propelled along the colon, dragging into the lumen that portion of the wall to which its pedicle is attached. (See Fig. 34-5*A*)

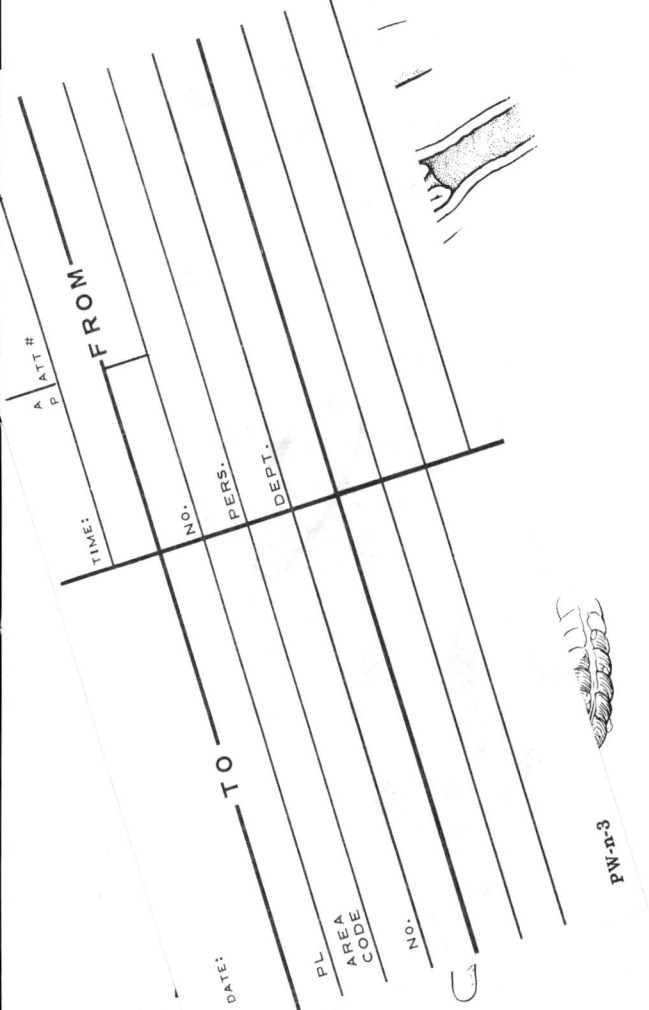

Figure 34-5
Two courses of intestinal obstruction. (*A*) Intussusception. Note invagination or shortening of colon by the movement of one segment of bowel into another. (*B*) Volvulus of the sigmoid colon. The twist is counterclockwise in most cases of sigmoid volvulus. Note the edematous bowel. (*B*: Way LW [ed]. Current Surgical Diagnosis and Treatment. Los Altos, California, Lange Medical Publishers, 1985.)

Volvulus

A volvulus (Fig. 34-5*B*) is a life-threatening obstruction in which the bowel is twisted upon itself and the intestinal lumen is obstructed both proximally and distally. The accumulation of gas and fluid in the trapped bowel leads to necrosis, perforation, and peritonitis.

Paralytic Ileus (Adynamic Ileus)

A paralytic ileus is a paralysis of peristaltic movement due to the effect of trauma or toxins on the nerves that regulate intestinal movement. Functional paralytic ileus following abdominal surgery may last 12 to 36 hours. Because of this, food and fluids are withheld until normal peristalsis returns, as indicated by bowel sounds (heard with the stethoscope) or the passing of flatus. Paralytic ileus may also happen after back injuries, after operation on the kidney, and frequently with peritonitis.

The lack of peristalsis results in a distention of the intestine with gas produced by decomposition of the intestinal contents or by swallowing of air. Few or no peristaltic sounds can be heard, and the patient may be extremely uncomfortable, if not in marked pain. Relief of the distention associated with paralytic ileus is often obtained by intestinal intubation (see p. 755).

Abdominal Hernias

A hernia ("rupture") is a protrusion of an organ, tissue, or structure through the wall of the cavity in which it is naturally contained. This definition may apply to any part of the body; for instance, the protrusion of the brain after a subtemporal decompression is called *cerebral hernia.* However, in general the term is applied to the protrusion of an abdominal viscus through an opening in the abdominal wall.

Inguinal hernia is a major reason for surgery, especially among men, in whom it occurs three times more frequently than in women. Most hernias result from congenital or acquired weakness of the abdominal wall, coupled with sustained increased intra-abdominal pressure from coughing or straining, or from an enlarging lesion within the abdomen. Once the hernia occurs, it has a tendency to increase in size.

The hernial sac is formed by an outpouching of the peritoneum and may contain the large or small intestine, the omentum, and occasionally the bladder. When the hernia is initially formed, the sac is filled only when the patient is standing up; the contents return to the abdominal cavity as soon as the patient lies down.

Indirect inguinal hernia is the most common type of hernia (see Table 34-9). It is due to a weakness of the abdominal wall at the point through which the spermatic cord emerges in the male, and the round ligament in the female. Through this opening the hernia extends down the inguinal canal and often into the scrotum or the labia (Fig. 34-6). It is common in the male, and it may appear at any age.

Direct inguinal hernia passes through the posterior inguinal wall. It also is more common in males. It is more difficult to repair than indirect inguinal hernia, and often recurs after surgery. It is believed to be hereditary or related to a defect in the synthesis of collagen.

Umbilical hernia results from failure of the umbilical orifice to close. It is most common in obese women and in children, as a protrusion at the umbilicus. This hernia is also

TABLE 34-9
Incidence of Hernia

Type	Frequency (Approximate %)
Inguinal, indirect	70
Inguinal, direct	15
Umbilical	3–5
Incisional	10
Femoral	6 or less
Others	3

seen with increased intra-abdominal pressure in cirrhosis and ascites.

Ventral or incisional hernias occur because of a weakness in the abdominal wall. They are due most frequently to previous operations in which drainage was necessary, complete closure of the tissues being impossible. Weakened byinfection, only a slight bulge results at first, but this increases gradually in size until a definite hernial sac is produced.

Femoral hernia appears below the inguinal (Poupart's) ligament (*i.e.,* below the groin) as a round bulge. It is more frequent in women because of changes during pregnancy.

A hernia is referred to as *reducible* when the protruding mass can be placed back into the abdominal cavity. This can occur naturally when the patient lies down, or it may require manual reduction (the mass is pushed back into the cavity). As time goes on, adhesions form between the sac and its contents, so that the hernia becomes *irreducible* or *incarcerated*. Such a hernia is one that cannot be reduced and in which the intestinal flow may be obstructed completely.

In a *strangulated hernia,* not only are the contents irreducible, but the blood and intestinal flow through the intestine in the hernia is stopped completely. This condition develops when the loop of intestine in the sac becomes twisted or swollen and a constriction is produced at the neck of the sac. The result then is an acute intestinal obstruction, with the added danger of gangrene of the bowel. The symptoms are pain at the site of strangulation, followed by colicky abdominal pain, vomiting, and swelling of the hernial sac.

Mechanical Reduction. Very often patients can reduce their own hernias. In order to keep the mass from protruding when a standing position is assumed, a *truss* (a pad made of firm material that is placed externally over the hernia and held in place with a belt) may be worn. Most authorities agree that a truss creates more problems than it can solve. Skin irritation and lesions may result from constant rubbing. When improperly fitted, it may cause strangulation of the hernia. However, a truss may be recommended (1) for infants, when there is need to wait for a weight gain before surgery or for remission of another problem, such as bronchitis or diaper rash; (2) for adults who have an underlying problem that needs to be resolved first; or (3) when a patient has worn a truss for years, is terrified of the hospital, and will not part with the truss. In this last instance, the proper fitting of the truss must be done by a qualified person. The Valsalva maneuver can also be used to check for the effectiveness of the truss. Daily bathing and the use of corn starch powder can lessen the possibility of skin irritation. Usually the truss is worn directly over the hernia and not over clothing, which could cause slipping. It must be emphasized that *a truss does not cure a hernia;* it simply prevents the abdominal contents from entering the hernial sac.

The hernia should always be repaired by surgery; otherwise, it is in continual danger of strangulation. When strangulation occurs, an operation becomes imperative and is attended invariably by considerable risk.

The operation involves removal of the hernial sac after it has been dissected free from surrounding structures, the contents have been replaced in the abdominal cavity, and the neck has been ligated. The muscle and the fascial layers then are sewn together firmly over the hernial orifice to prevent a recurrence. The incidence of recurrence is 5–25%. When the tissues are not sufficiently strong, reinforcement can be obtained by overlaying the suture line with synthetic sutures or mesh, which is also sutured in place (*hernioplasty*). The presence of the mesh stimulates more than the usual amount of fibroblastic activity and thereby enhances the strength of the repair. When strangulation has occurred, the operation is complicated by intestinal obstruction and injury to the bowel.

Preoperative Nursing Interventions. Most patients undergoing a *herniorrhaphy* (surgical repair of a hernia) are in good physical condition and have elected to have the surgery. They may be prompted by the knowledge that an unrepaired hernia can become a serious emergency, or that the condition can cause difficulty in securing employment. The patient may come into the hospital the morning of surgery or the night before, or the procedure can be done in a surgical clinic/center. In emergency conditions of strangulated or incarcerated hernia, the nurse prepares the patient as in any other acute surgical problem.

An important nursing checkpoint is to determine whether the patient has an upper respiratory infection, chronic cough from excessive smoking, or sneezing due to an allergy. It may be necessary to postpone the operation, because coughing or sneezing could weaken the postoperative wound, thereby negating the purpose of surgery.

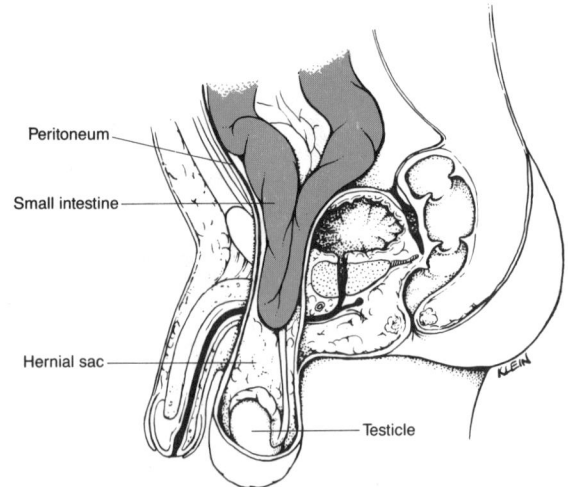

Figure 34-6
Inguinal hernia. Note that the sac of the hernia is a continuation of the peritoneum of the abdomen and that the hernial contents are intestine, omentum, or other abdominal contents that pass through the herinal opening into the hernial sac.

Postoperative Nursing Interventions. The patient is allowed out of bed several hours after surgery. Young, healthy patients without other diseases are often discharged on the day of surgery. Following local or spinal anesthesia, diet is determined by the desires of the patient. When general anesthesia is used, fluid and food are restricted until peristalsis returns.

Urinary retention is common in the postoperative period. However, if the patient gets out of bed to void within several hours after surgery, there usually is no difficulty. In any case, it is necessary to prevent bladder distention; this may require catheterization if other nursing measures fail.

The patient who coughs or sneezes after the operation is instructed to splint the incision site with one hand, both to lessen the pain and to protect the incision site from the increased intra-abdominal pressure caused by the coughing and sneezing.

Following repair of an inguinal hernia, swelling of the scrotum may occur. Because this is extremely painful, the patient is reluctant to move. Elevating the scrotum on a rolled towel and applying small ice bags intermittently are helpful. A narcotic may be prescribed for pain, and antibiotics to prevent epididymitis. A suspensory bandage or a jock strap may be applied for support and comfort.

Infection that interferes with healing occurs occasionally. Soreness in the operative region and temperature elevation may suggest such a problem. Systemic antibiotics or local wound treatment with heat application, followed by incision and drainage, may be required.

For more extensive hernia repair, such as may be required following umbilical or large incisional hernia, nasogastric suction may be used to prevent distention, vomiting, and straining. Stool softeners are prescribed to prevent straining during defecation.

Patient Education and Home Health Care Considerations. Hospitalized patients may go home the day following herniorrhaphy or may stay 3 to 5 days or longer, depending on their age and medical condition. Many patients have same-day surgery with local anesthesia. The patient at home needs to know that pain and scrotal swelling will be present after surgery for 24 to 48 hours. Local applications of ice, elevation of the scrotum, use of a scrotal support, and pain medication should relieve the pain. The patient is instructed to report severe pain to the physician.

Some surgeons permit patients to do whatever they wish if they agree not to engage in painful activity, thereby preventing injury to the incision. Most, however, recommend limited activities for 5 to 7 days, and restriction of heavy lifting for 4 to 6 weeks. The use of correct body mechanics at all times is encouraged.

The patient is advised to report any drainage from the incision to the physician. Straining during defecation is avoided by diet modification, bulk cathartics, or stool softeners, and a daily fluid intake of 2000 ml. Pain or difficulty with urination is reported to the physician.

Evaluation. Short-term evaluation of nursing interventions can be carried out through an assessment of the return of peristalsis, adequate urinary output, decrease in scrotal swelling, absence of infection, relief of pain, and avoidance of straining at stool. Long-term evaluation can be carried out through an assessment of the patient's understanding of the restrictions established.

Large Bowel Obstruction

About 15% of intestinal obstructions occur in the large bowel, and most are found in the sigmoid. The most common causes are carcinoma, diverticulitis, inflammatory bowel disorders, and benign tumors.

Pathophysiology

Obstruction at the ileocecal valve produces changes similar to those in small bowel obstruction. Obstruction in the colon can lead to severe distention and perforation unless some gas and fluid can flow back through the ileum (incompetent valve). Large bowel obstruction, even if complete, is also comparatively undramatic if the blood supply to the colon is not disturbed. However, if the blood supply is cut off, intestinal strangulation and necrosis (tissue death) occur, and the patient's life is in jeopardy. In the large intestine, dehydration occurs more slowly than in the small intestine because the colon is able to absorb its fluid contents and can distend to a size considerably beyond its normal full capacity.

Clinical Manifestations and Diagnostic Evaluation

Large bowel obstruction differs clinically from the small bowel type in that the symptoms develop and progress relatively slowly. In patients with obstruction in the sigmoid or the rectum, constipation may be the only symptom for days. Eventually, the abdomen becomes markedly distended, loops of large bowel become visibly outlined through the abdominal wall, and the patient suffers from crampy lower abdominal pain. Finally, fecal vomiting develops. The terminal features are essentially those of ileum obstruction.

Radiographic studies show a distended colon. Barium studies are contraindicated.

Management

The usual treatment is surgical resection, with the formation of a colostomy or ileostomy in right colon obstruction and perforation. Sometimes an ileoanal anastomosis is performed. A *cecostomy* (insertion of a tube into the lumen of the cecum) may be done for those patients who are poor surgical risks and need relief from the obstruction. The procedure provides a vent for releasing gas and a small amount of drainage.

Cancer of the Large Intestine: Colon and Rectum

Tumors of the small intestine are rare; on the other hand, tumors of the colon are relatively common, In fact, second only to lung cancer, cancer of the colon and rectum is now the most common type of internal cancer in men in the United States. In women, colorectal cancer ranks third as a cause of death, following cancer of the lung and cancer of the breast. More than 95% of the cancer tumors are adenocarcinomas. The incidence increases with age (most patients are over age 50), and is higher in persons with a family history of colon cancer and those with ulcerative colitis. The distribution of cancer sites throughout the colon can be seen in Figure 34-7. Changes in the percentage distribution have been recorded recently. The incidence of cancer in the sigmoid and rectal areas has decreased, whereas the incidence in the ascending and descending colon has increased.

More than 130,000 North Americans are afflicted annually; about half that number die of it annually—although almost 3 out of 4 patients might be saved by early diagnosis and prompt treatment. The low 5-year survival rate of 40% to 50% is due primarily to late diagnosis. Most people are asymptomatic for long periods of time and only seek medical help when they notice a change in bowel habits or rectal bleeding. Risk factors are listed in Chart 34-2.

Pathophysiology and Clinical Manifestations

Cancer of the colon and rectum always arises from the epithelium lining the intestine. The effects produced depend largely on the location of the cancer.

The chief symptoms are changes in bowel habits (the most common presenting symptom), the passage of blood in the stools (second most common symptom), mucus, rectal/abdominal pain, anemia, weight loss, obstruction, and perforation. A suddenly developing obstruction may be the first symptom of cancer involving the colon anywhere between the cecum and the sigmoid, for in this region, where the bowel contents are liquid, a slowly developing obstruction will not become evident until the lumen is practically closed. Cancer of the sigmoid and the rectum causes earlier symptoms of partial obstruction, with constipation alternating with diarrhea, lower abdominal crampy pains, and distention.

- Any patient with a history of unexplained change in bowel habit, with changes in the shape of the stool, or with

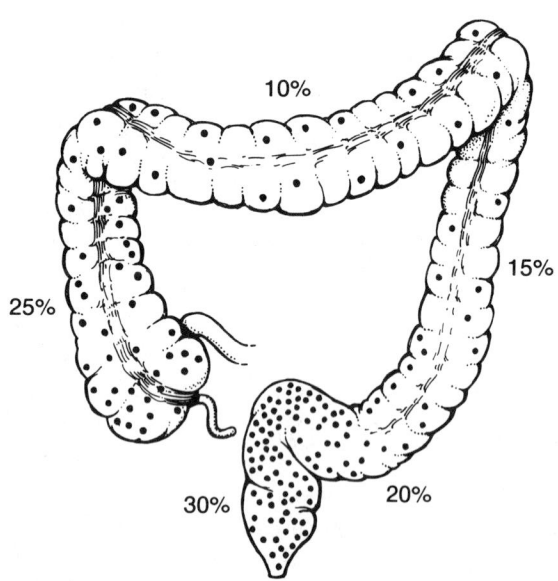

Figure 34-7
Distribution of cancer of the colon and rectum. (After Way LW [ed]. Current Surgical Diagnosis and Treatment. Los Altos, California, Lange Medical Publishers, 1985.)

Chart 34-2
Risk Factors for Cancer of the Colon

Age—over 40
Blood in stool
History of rectal polyps
Presence of adenomatous polyps or villous adenomas.
Family history of colon cancer or familial polyposis
History of chronic inflammatory bowel disease

---

passage of blood in the stools should be studied carefully to rule out cancer of the large bowel.

The possibility that a rectal carcinoma exists—detectable, but still asymptomatic and still operable—is one important reason for the inclusion of a rectal examination as part of every routine physical examination (see p. 842). A digital examination can reveal about 20% of colorectal cancers. Additional symptoms, often present, are those of progressive weakness, anorexia, weight loss, anemia, and lower abdominal pain.

Gerontological Considerations. The incidence of carcinoma of the colon and rectum increases with age. These cancers are considered the most common malignancies in old age except for prostatic cancer in males. The presentation of symptoms is often insidious. Fatigue is almost always present, due primarily to iron deficiency anemia. The symptoms most commonly reported by the elderly are abdominal pain, obstruction, tenesmus, and rectal bleeding.

Colonic carcinoma in the elderly has been closely associated with dietary carcinogens. Lack of fiber is a major causative agent because fecal transit time is prolonged, which in turn prolongs exposure to possible carcinogens. Excess fat is believed to alter bacterial flora and convert steroids into compounds that have carcinogenic properties.

Diagnostic Evaluation

Along with the abdominal and rectal examination, the most important diagnostic procedures for cancer of the colon are fecal occult blood testing, barium enema, proctosigmoidoscopy, and colonoscopy. As many as 60% of colorectal cancers can be identified by sigmoidoscopy.

The level of carcinoembryonic antigen (CEA) found in colon cancer tissue was previously believed to be a highly reliable indicator in diagnosing colon cancer. However, recent studies show that CEA levels are only 30% to 40% accurate as a basis for diagnosis, although they are reliable in predicting prognosis. With complete tumor excision, the elevated levels of CEA should return to normal within 48 hours. Elevations of CEA at a later date suggest recurrence.

Guaiac-based tests for fecal occult blood are being replaced by a quantitative assay known as the *Hemo Quant test*, which detects *heme* (the iron-containing nonprotein portion of the hemoglobin molecule) that is altered during fecal transit. Results are reported as milligrams of hemoglobin per gram of stool.

Surgical Management

The operative treatment will depend on the location and the extent of the cancer. When the tumor can be removed, the involved colon is excised for some distance on each side of the growth to remove the tumor and the area of its lymphatic spread (Fig. 34-8). If distant (liver) metastasis has occurred, the tumor may be excised for palliation (relief of symptoms without cure). The intestine is reunited by an end-to-end anastomosis of the colon. When the growth is situated low in the sigmoid or the rectum, the colon is cut above the growth and brought out through the abdominal wall, forming an abdominal anus called a *colostomy*. The growth then is removed from below by a perineal incision (*abdominoperineal resection*, Fig. 34-9).

In the event that the tumor has spread and involves surrounding vital structures, it is considered to be inoperable.

When the growth in the rectum or the sigmoid is inoperable, and especially when symptoms of partial or complete obstruction are present, a colostomy is performed. A loop of the colon, near the junction of the descending colon and the sigmoid, is brought out of the abdomen through a lower left rectus incision and maintained in place by a plastic rod or rubber tube inserted underneath the loop. If the obstruction is complete, the loop may be drained by the insertion of a rubber tube or by the use of a right-angled tube, held in the intestine by a purse-string suture. When the obstruction is incomplete, the colostomy loop is allowed to remain unopened for several days to permit the peritoneal cavity to become thoroughly sealed off. During this time, the patient is given a liquid diet. The intestine is opened by electrocautery, because hemorrhage is slight after its use.

In some instances, when a tumor cannot be resected, a bypass procedure is performed; *colocolostomy* is the pre-

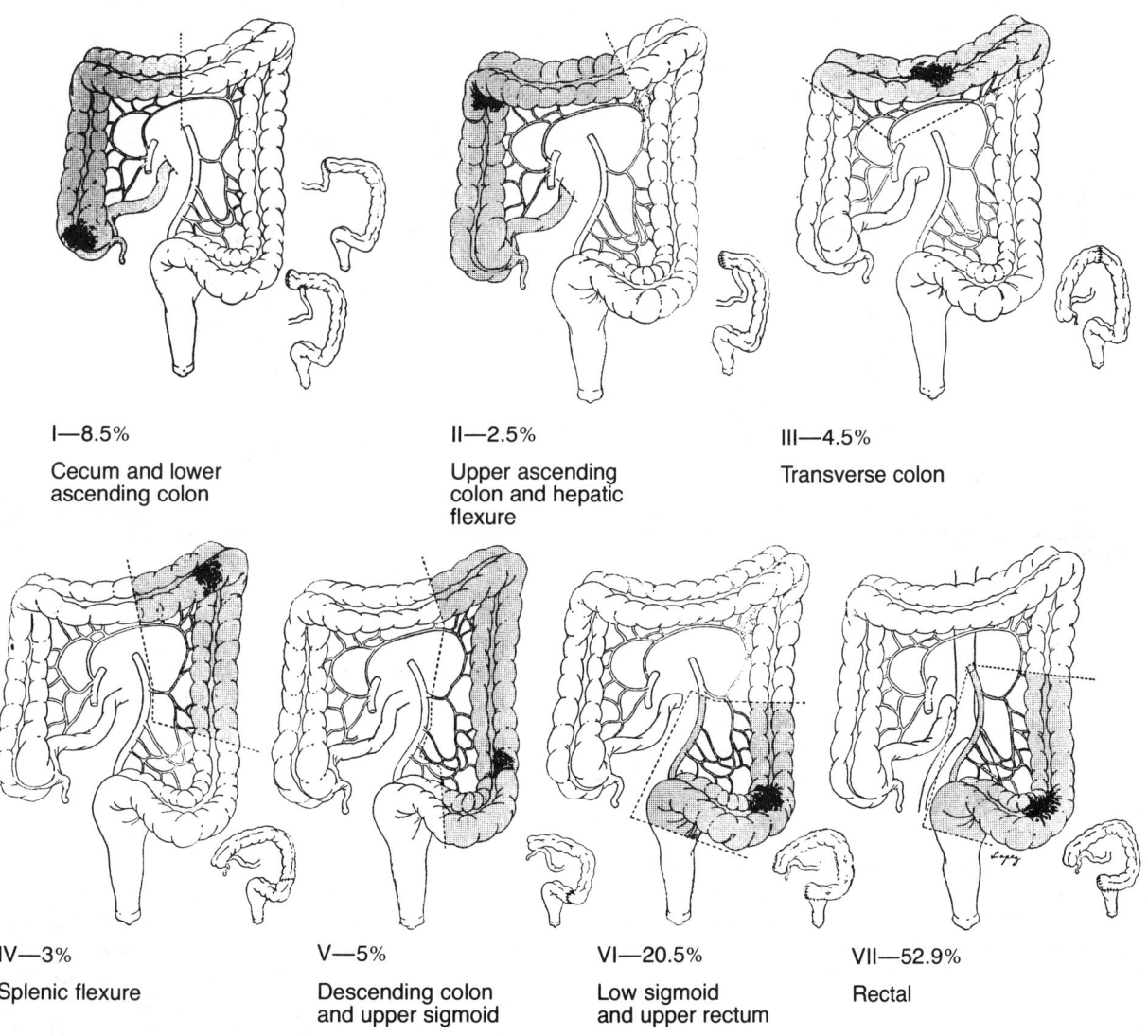

I—8.5%

Cecum and lower
ascending colon

II—2.5%

Upper ascending
colon and hepatic
flexure

III—4.5%

Transverse colon

IV—3%

Splenic flexure

V—5%

Descending colon
and upper sigmoid

VI—20.5%

Low sigmoid
and upper rectum

VII—52.9%

Rectal

Figure 34-8
Cancer of the colon. Diagrams show areas where cancer can occur, what area is removed, and (in the very small diagrams) how the anastomosis is done. For rectal cancer, an abdominoperineal resection is done with colostomy. (Adapted from American Cancer Society.)

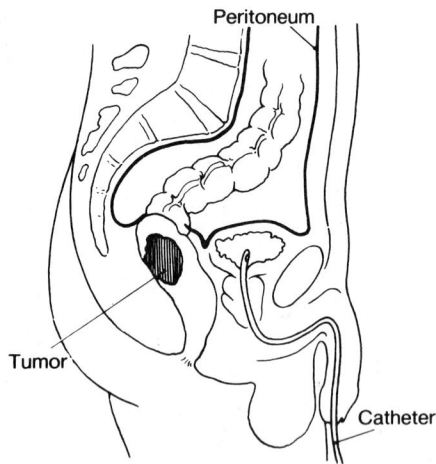

1. Presurgical patient. Note tumor in rectum.

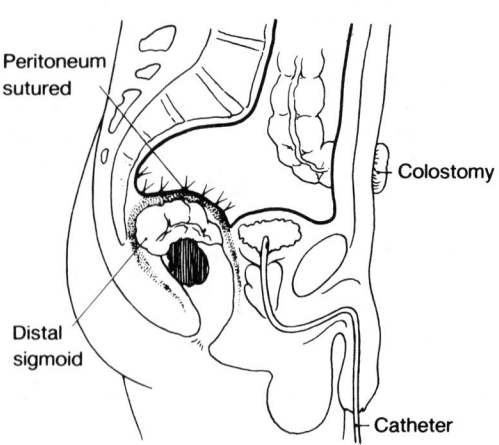

2. At operation, sigmoid is removed and colostomy established. The distal bowel has been dissected free to a point below pelvic peritoneum, which is sutured over the closed end of the distal sigmoid and rectum.

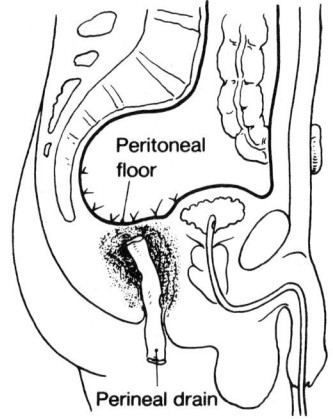

3. Perineal resection includes removal of the rectum and free portion of the sigmoid from below. A drain is inserted in this void.

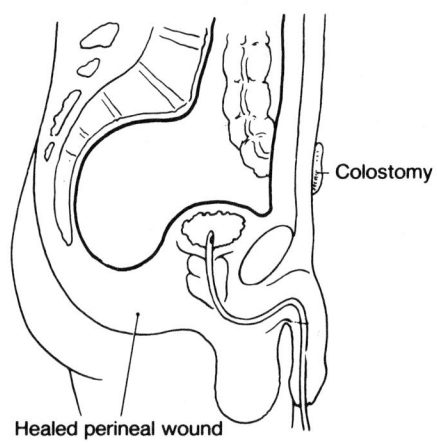

4. The final result after healing. Note healed perineal wound and the permanent colostomy.

Figure 34-9
Abdominoperineal resection for carcinoma of rectum.

ferred method. In this procedure the ends of the remaining colon are joined, eliminating the need for a stoma. When the rectum is involved, a major concern is to save the sphincter, which controls defecation. A low anterior resection of the rectum is done through an abdominal incision. However, the lesion must be located in the upper two thirds of the rectum, and there must be sufficient normal bowel tissue (2.5 cm [1 inch]) below the lesion to be resected and 10 cm (4 inches) of normal bowel proximal to the lesion to be removed. The sigmoid is anastomosed to the rectum, and no colostomy is needed.

Medical Management

Radiation is recommended for lesions that may not be resectable. Intracavitary and implantable devices are becoming more popular as a mode of treatment. Little benefit is obtained when chemotherapy and immunotherapy are used alone. However, radiation plus chemotherapy has been shown to result in longer survival rates.

Complications

The incidence of complications for colostomies is about half that seen with ileostomies. Some common complications are *prolapse of the stoma* (usually due to obesity), *perforation* (due to improper stoma irrigation), *stoma retraction, fecal impaction,* and *skin irritation. Leakage from an anastomotic site* can occur if remaining bowel segments are diseased or weakened. Leakage from an intestinal anastomosis causes abdominal distention and rigidity, temperature elevation, and signs of shock. Surgical repair is necessary.

Pulmonary complications are also always a concern with abdominal surgery. Patients over 50 years of age are considered to be at high risk, especially if they are hospitalized, are or have been receiving antibiotics or sedatives, or are being maintained on bed rest for a prolonged period of time. Two primary pulmonary complications are pneumonia and atelectasis. *Pneumonia* can be prevented by frequent movement (turning the patient from side to side every 2 hours), deep abdominal breathing, coughing, and early ambulation. Pneumonia is manifested by a high fever (39.5°C–40.5°C [101°F–105°F]), severe chest pain, tachypnea, and tachycardia. These symptoms, although just as severe, are less evident in the elderly, who frequently have compromised pulmonary functions. For treatment, the nurse administers prescribed antipyretics and antibiotics such as penicillin G or erythromycin. Bed rest is maintained when the symptoms are severe. *Atelectasis*, a collapse of a lobule or lung unit, is manifested by dyspnea, cyanosis, and tachycardia. Preventive measures are similar to those used for pneumonia. Treatment consists of aspiration or bronchoscopy.

Care of the Patient With a Colostomy

When the possibility of a colostomy exists, the patient is informed by the surgeon. This is a lifesaving arrangement that is compatible with active participation in social and business life. The nurse is in a position to help the patient accept a colostomy; with courage, optimism, and determination, the patient can adjust to a new life-style, improving daily until an individual pattern of management has been established. Members of the health team, the enterostomal therapist, the family, and other ostomates are available for assistance and support.

To give adequate support, care, and instruction to these patients, the nurse must know not only basic information about their physical condition, nutritional status, and proposed surgery, but also the patients themselves. What do they think, feel, express, suppress, desire, fear, *etc.?* In daily contacts with patients who have a colostomy, valuable rapport can be established to facilitate their adjustment. The nurse must understand and practice psychology and the principles of learning as they apply to each particular individual. In addition to the shock of the colostomy, these patients are perhaps also dealing with a diagnosis of cancer. These two issues together can tax their coping ability and that of their families.

Gerontological Considerations.
Elderly patients usually have some degree of decreased vision and impaired hearing, as well as difficulty with skills that require fine motor coordination. Have the patient handle the ostomy equipment preoperatively and simulate cleaning the peristomal skin and irrigating the stoma. Note those skills that require assistance.

Accidents resulting from falls occur frequently among the elderly. Determine whether the patient can walk unassisted to the bathroom. Is the bathroom nearby?

Skin care is a major concern for the elderly ostomate because of skin changes that occur with aging. The epithelial and subcutaneous fatty layers thin out; the skin is less hydratedand easily irritated. To prevent breakdown, special attention is paid to skin cleansing and the proper fit of an appliance. Arteriosclerosis causes decreased blood flow to the wound and stoma site. As a result, transport of nutrients is delayed, and healing takes longer.

Some patients experience delayed elimination after ir

rigation because of decreased peristalsis and reduced mucus production. Most require 6 months before they feel comfortable with their ostomy care.

For additional interventions, see Nursing Care Plan 34-1 for a patient with an intestinal ostomy, on pages 824–827.

Preoperative Nursing Interventions

Psychosocial Support.
A patient diagnosed with cancer of the colon/rectum may require a permanent colostomy and may grieve about the diagnosis and the impending surgery. Assess emotional reactions and evaluate the family's ability to offer support and encourage coping behaviors. Those undergoing surgery for a temporary colostomy may express fears and concerns similar to those of a person with a permanent stoma. A temporary colostomy can become permanent for a patient whose condition deteriorates and who cannot tolerate additional surgery. Encourage emotional expressions and observe for adaptive behaviors.

Identify the level of anxiety (mild, moderate, severe) and any measures the patient uses to cope with the diagnosis and impending surgery. Does he know what the stoma will look like, where it will be located, and how it will function? Is he aware of the type and frequency of drainage that is expected? Has he seen the available drainage pouches? Has he spoken to an enterostomal therapist? Does he know anyone who has a stoma? Does he wish to speak with an ostomate (a person with an ostomy)?

Speaking with a person who is successfully managing a colostomy is often helpful. The United Ostomy Association is a nonprofit agency that gives patients useful information on living with an ostomy, through an educational program of literature, lectures, and exhibits. Visiting services by qualified members and rehabilitation services for new ostomy patients are provided by national organizations. (See p. 848.)

Anticipated changes in body image and lifestyle are profoundly disturbing, and patients will need empathetic support in trying to adjust to them. Because the excretory orifice is located on the abdomen, the patient may think that everyone will be aware of the ostomy. The nurse can help reduce this apprehension by presenting factual information about the surgical procedure and the creation and management of the ostomy. If the patient is receptive, diagrams, photographs, and appliances may be used to explain and clarify. Because the patient is experiencing emotional stress, the nurse may need to repeat some of the information. Time should be provided for the patient to ask questions. The nurse's acceptance and understanding of the patient's concerns and feelings convey a caring, competent attitude that promotes confidence and cooperation.

Preparation for Operation.
Usually, a high-calorie, low-residue diet is given for several days before operation, if time and the patient's condition permit. If an emergency does not exist, prescribed intestinal anti-infectives, such as kanamycin, erythromycin, and neomycin, are given by mouth for several days to reduce the bacterial content of the colon and to soften and decrease the bulk of the contents of the colon. In addition, mechanical cleansing of the bowel may be done by laxatives, enemas, or colonic irrigations.

Careful attention is given to complaints of pain, which are assessed and described as to their nature, location, and duration. The nurse records fluid losses such as occur with vomiting and diarrhea. This will aid in regulating the fluid intake and maintaining adequate balance. If the hemoglobin is below 12 gm, a blood transfusion may be prescribed because anemia is common. Preoperative nasogastric intubation facilitates the performance of intestinal surgery and minimizes postoperative distention. An indwelling catheter is inserted as prescribed to ensure that the bladder is empty during surgery. This will aid in keeping postoperative perineal dressings dry. The abdomen and perineum are prepared for surgery.

Postoperative Nursing Interventions

Postoperative nursing care for patients undergoing a colectomy is similar to nursing care for any abdominal surgery patient (see p. 343). The patient is monitored for signs of the complications discussed earlier in this section (page 834). These include leakage from an anastomotic site, prolapse of the stoma, perforation, stoma retraction, fecal impaction, and skin irritation, as well as pulmonary complica-tions associated with abdominal surgery. Patients experiencing a colostomy are helped out of bed on the first postoperative day and encouraged to care for the colostomy from the very first irrigation. The return to normal diet is rapid, and every effort is made to encourage them to live as they did before the operation. Psychologically, this appears to deemphasize the abnormality of the situation.

The colostomy is opened by the surgeon on the second or third postoperative day, at which time there is often an evacuation of loose stools. In anticipation of this procedure, the nurse protects the bedding with a plastic sheet covered with a towel and places an emesis basin at the patient's side.

Regulating the Colostomy

It is valuable to observe a usual time for doing certain activities (*e.g.*, mealtime, irrigation time, bedtime, and so forth). A reg-ular schedule for meals, irrigation, exercise, and sleep will be helpful in achieving colostomy regularity.

Irrigating Equipment

Irrigation can be accomplished by using a catheter or a bulb syringe. Catheter irrigation requires equipment that is used to administer an enema (2-liter bag, tubing, adapter, clamp, catheter, and irrigating solution). Commercial irrigation sets (Fig. 34-10) are available and all contain similar equipment: an irrigation sleeve or plastic irrigation bag that fits over the stoma, a belt to secure the sleeve/bag in place, an irrigating bag with tubing and flow regulator, and a soft catheter or irrigation cone tip that fits over the catheter.

Colostomy Irrigations

The stoma on the abdomen does not have voluntary muscular control and may empty at irregular intervals. Regulation is achieved either by irrigation or by training the bowel to evacuate naturally without irrigations. The choice often depends on the individual and the nature of the colostomy. The type and frequency of effluent vary according to the type of colostomy:

- Ascending colostomy—fluid feces
- Colostomy near hepatic flexure—semifluid feces
- Transverse colostomy—mushy feces
- Splenic flexure colostomy—semimushy feces
- Descending colostomy—solid feces

The purpose of irrigating a colostomy is to empty the colon of gas, mucus, and feces so that the patient can go about social and business activities without fear of fecal drainage. By irrigating the stoma at a *regular* time, there is less gas and retention of irrigating fluids.

The time of irrigation should be selected with regard to the schedule the person will pursue after leaving the hospital.

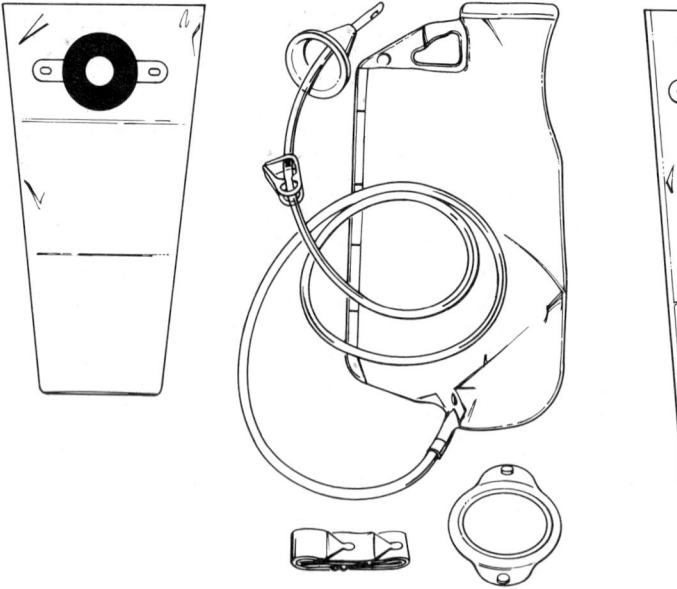

Figure 34-10
Colostomy irrigating kit. (Courtesy of John F. Greer Co.)

It is best to irrigate after a meal, because ingestion of food stimulates peristalsis and defecation. An ascending colostomy is difficult to control and usually requires daily irrigation. Sigmoidostomy may require irrigation only every 2 or 3 days, if at all.

The initial irrigation is usually done on the fourth or fifth postoperative day. There are two methods of irrigating a colostomy: the conventional way, using an enema irrigation-procedure, and a second method utilizing a bulb syringe. (See Fig. 34-11.)

Irrigation by Catheter

- Have the patient sit on the toilet (or on a chair facing the toilet).
- Remove the drainage pouch or the stoma dressing.
- Clean the stoma and the surrounding skin with gauze pads to remove mucus or fecal material.
- Fill the bag with irrigating solution and hang it at shoulder height. Remove air from the tubing.
- Attach the irrigating sleeve and secure with a belt.
- Insert a lubricated catheter 5.0–7.0 cm (2–3 inches) or a cone tip 1.2 cm (½ inch) into the stoma. The lubricated catheter can be advanced 10–15 cm (4–6 inches). *Force is contraindicated because it is possible to perforate the bowel.*

- Allow the irrigating solution (plain water, saline, or soapy solution) to run in for 5–10 minutes. At first, only about 500 ml of solution is given, after which the amount may be increased gradually every day up to 1500 ml. The temperature of the solution is about 40.5°C (105°F). Because distention of the colon is an effective stimulus for bowel evacuation, the irrigating solution should be introduced in such amount, and with such pressure, as to distend the bowel and give the patient a feeling of fullness. If the patient complains of cramps, the level of the can may be lowered to lessen the force of flow. The patient should be taught that the rate of flow of solution varies with the pressure and the caliber of the tube. Pressure depends on height; therefore, when increased pressure is desired the container of solution may be raised, and vice versa. The irrigation may be given daily, every other day, or every 3 days, according to the need and preference of the patient.
- Remove the catheter or cone tip when the urge to expel stool occurs.
- Direct the drainage through the irrigating sleeve/bag and into the toilet.
- Remove sleeve/bag and belt.
- Wipe stomal area dry.
- Apply a drainage pouch or clean dressing.

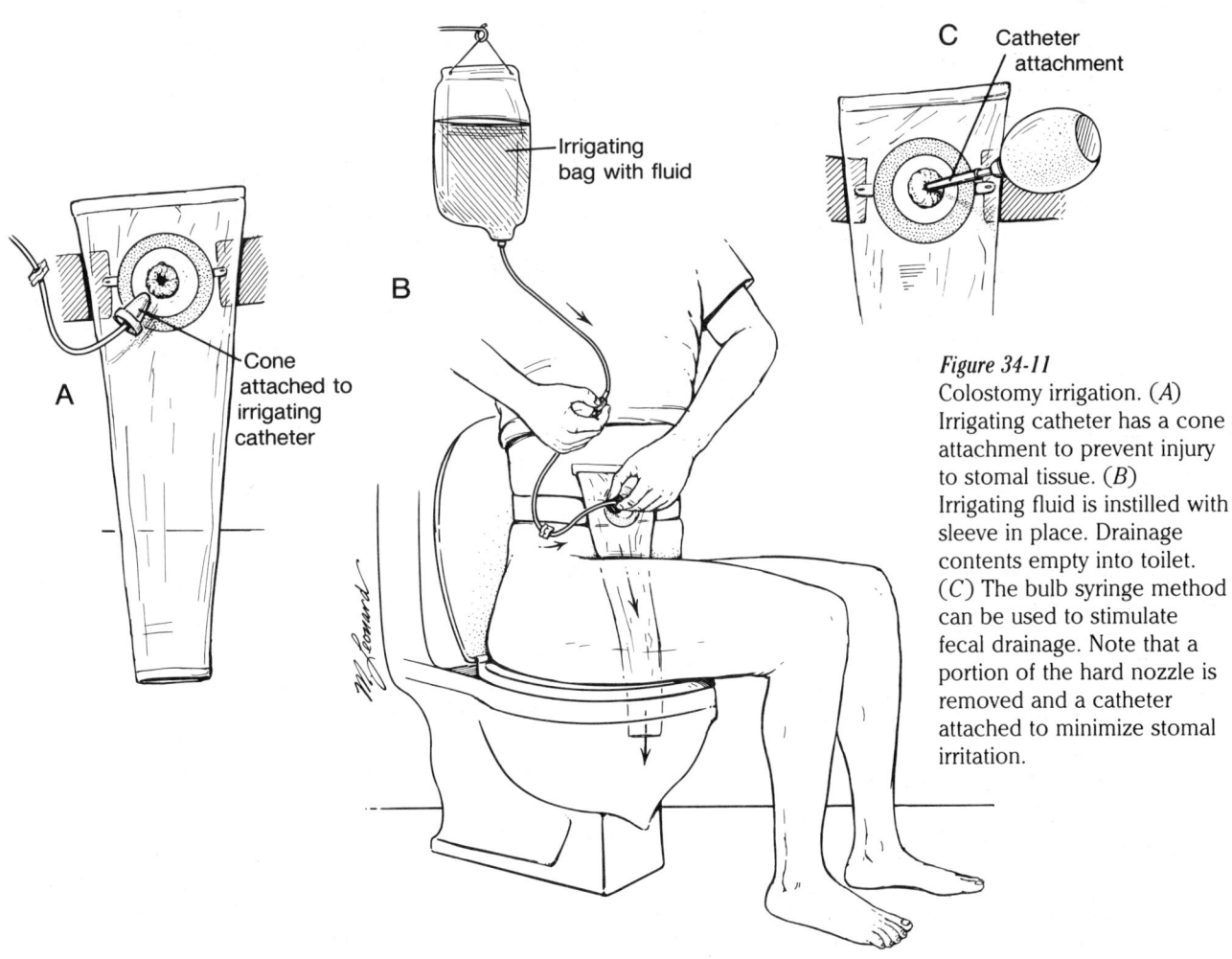

C Catheter attachment

—Irrigating bag with fluid

B

—Cone attached to irrigating catheter

A

Figure 34-11
Colostomy irrigation. (*A*) Irrigating catheter has a cone attachment to prevent injury to stomal tissue. (*B*) Irrigating fluid is instilled with sleeve in place. Drainage contents empty into toilet. (*C*) The bulb syringe method can be used to stimulate fecal drainage. Note that a portion of the hard nozzle is removed and a catheter attached to minimize stomal irritation.

Irrigation by Bulb Syringe

The second method of colostomy irrigation is the *bulb syringe* method, which stimulates fecal return rather than washing the feces out. There is no prolonged trapping of water in the colon and no spillage or accidents during the day.

The patient is seated on the toilet. A 250-ml (8-oz) soft rubber bulb syringe is used. The hard nozzle is cut off, and a No. 24 French catheter is attached to the end of the bulb syringe. *No more than 750 ml (24 oz) of water is used.* The bulb syringe method is shown in Figure 34-11.

The patient may massage the lower part of the abdomen to ensure adequate return. The bag is left in place for 15 minutes and then removed, after which the stoma is covered with a piece of gauze and held in place by a girdle, elasticized shorts, or an elastic belt. The patient completes the procedure by washing the pitcher and bulb syringe with soapy water.

Colostomies That Are Not Irrigated

"Wet" colostomies are colostomies through which both urine and feces are excreted, because of transplantation of ureters into the colon. These colostomies are never irrigated, because of the danger that contaminated material will be forced into the ureters and produce infection.

Skin Care

The effluent discharge will vary with the type of ostomy. The stool is soft and mushy but irritating with a transverse colostomy, and fairly solid and slightly irritating with a descending or sigmoid colostomy. Advise the patient to protect the peristomal skin by frequently washing the area with a mild soap, applying a protective skin barrier around the stoma, and securely attaching the drainage pouch. Nystatin powder (Mycostatin) can be dusted lightly on the peristomal skin to prevent irritation and yeast growth.

Cleanse the skin gently with a moist, soft cloth and a mild soap or solvent. Gently remove any excess Karaya. Soap acts as a mild abrasive agent to remove enzyme residue from fecal spillage. During the time the skin is being cleansed, a gauze dressing may cover the stoma or a vaginal tampon can be inserted gently to absorb excess drainage. The patient may be permitted to bathe or shower before putting on the clean appliance. Micropore tape applied to the sides of the disc will keep it secure during bathing. Pat the skin completely dry with a gauze pad and avoid rubbing the area. Patting the skin prevents irritation because solvents can be damaging. Use a skin barrier (wafer, paste, powder) around the stoma to protect the skin from fecal drainage.

Application of the Drainage Pouch

Measure the stoma to determine the correct size for the pouch. The pouch opening should be about 0.6 cm (¼ inch) larger than the stoma. Cleanse the skin according to the above procedure. Apply a peristomal skin barrier. Remove the backing from the adherent surface of the pouch and press the drainage bag down over the stoma for 30 seconds. Mild skin irritation may require dusting the skin with Karaya powder before attaching the pouch.

Management of the Drainage Pouch

Colostomy bags may be worn immediately after irrigation; then a change to a simple dressing may be effective. Patients are instructed in the care and the cleaning of equipment to prolong its life and keep it free of odors. Cleaning by soap or a detergent and water and exposure to fresh air usually are sufficient; however, it may still be necessary to deodorize the appliance. Liquid deodorizers are available to use in washing and soaking equipment. The other aspect of the problem is the control of odors arising from the body excreta as they collect in the appliance. Inserting readily soluble deodorizing tablets in the appliance or putting a few drops of chlorophyll solution into the bag will help in the control of odors. Powdered charcoal, two crushed aspirin tablets, or a teaspoon of baking soda may be sprinkled into the bag to absorb odors. Also effective are commercially available colostomy deodorants.

As a rule, colostomy bags are not necessary. As soon as the patient has learned a routine for evacuation, bags may be dispensed with and a simple dressing of disposable tissue (often covered with plastic wrap) is used, held in place by an elastic belt or girdle. Except for the escape of gas and a slight amount of mucus, nothing comes from the colostomy opening between irrigations; therefore, the inconvenience of a colostomy bag is unnecessary.

Removal of the Appliance

The drainage appliance is changed when it is ¼ to ⅓ full so that the weight of its contents does not cause the pouch to separate from the adhesive disc and spill the contents. Have the patient assume a comfortable sitting or standing position and *gently* push the skin down from the adhesive disc while pulling the pouch up and away from the stoma. Gentle pressure prevents traumatizing the skin as well as preventing the spillage of any liquid fecal contents.

Care of Perineal Wound

If the malignancy has been removed by the perineal route, the wound is observed carefully for signs of hemorrhage. This wound usually contains a drain or packing that is removed gradually, so that about the seventh day all drains are out. There usually are sloughing bits of tissue that will come away for the following week or 10 days. This process is hastened by the mechanical irrigation of the wound.

It is appreciated by the patient if the prescribed medication for pain is administered before the procedure is begun. An irrigating container with normal saline is effective. Enzymes (streptokinase or streptodornase) are also effective in liquefying necrotic tissue. This may be done 2 or 3 times a day, and then gradually less frequently. Observe and record the condition of the perineal wound; note any bleeding, infection, or necrosis. During the procedure it is important to protect the bed with an extra waterproof sheet and absorbentpads, and it may be well to plan the irrigation so that it can be performed before the patient receives morning care.

Changing the patient's position from one side to the other every 2 to 4 hours is desirable, because not only is it uncomfortable to lie in a dorsal recumbent position, but such a position may also interfere with healing by causing wound separation. By the beginning of the second postoperative week, sitz baths may be prescribed, to improve circulation and promote healing and cleanliness. A half-inflated rubber ring is comfortable to sit on.

An indwelling catheter remains in place for several days to prevent urinary retention and pressure on the perineal area.

Continuing assessment of the patient's urinary status is maintained to control infection and maintain hydration.

Patient Education and Home Health Care

The spouse and family should be familiar with the adjustment that will be necessary when the patient returns home. They need to be encouraged to verbalize their concerns. Their understanding is necessary to reduce tension; a relaxed patient tends to have fewer problems.

Prior to discharge from the hospital an individualized routine for stoma care and irrigation is reviewed with the patient and family. Supplemental literature is helpful, because those involved may have questions when the patient is back in the home setting. Someone in the family should assume responsibility for purchasing the equipment and supplies that will be needed at home.

Nutritional Status

In general, the patient needs to be reminded that good health practices will materially aid feelings of well-being and positiveadjustment to the colostomy. Diet is individualized as long as it is well-balanced and does not cause diarrhea or constipation.

Do a complete nutritional assessment and recommend the avoidance of certain foods that cause excessive odor and gas: foods in the cabbage family, eggs, fish, beans, and cellulose products such as peanuts. Is the elimination of food causing any nutritional deficiencies? If so, confer with the physician/dietition about nonirritating foods to substitute for those that are restricted so that deficiencies are corrected. Advise the patient to experiment with an irritating food several times before restricting it, because the reaction may be an initial sensitivity that will decrease with use.

Assess hydration status (skin turgor, mucous membranes, intake and output, weight) and report signs of dehydration. If the patient has problems with diarrhea, note the frequency of diarrheal stools plus the occurrence of abdominal cramping, urgency, and hyperactive bowel sounds. The use of paregoric, bismuth subgallate, bismuth subcarbonate, or diphenoxylate with atropine (Lomotil) will control the diarrhea. For constipation, prune or apple juice or a mild laxative is effective. Help the patient identify any specific foods that may precipitate elimination: milk, fruits, sodas, coffee, tea, carbonated beverages, and high-fiber foods. For dietary support of complications, see Table 34-10.

Sexual Activity

The patient is encouraged to discuss plans to return to usual sexual activity. Some patients may initiate questions about sexual activity directly or give indirect clues about their fears. Some may view the surgery as mutilative and a threat to their sexuality; some fear impotence. Others may express worry about odor/leakage from the pouch during sexual activity. Alternative sexual positions are recommended as well as alternative methods of stimulation to satisfy sexual drives. The nurse assesses the patient's needs and attempts to identify specific concerns. If the nurse is uncomfortable with this, or if the patient's concerns seem complex, the nurse should seek assistance from an appropriate source, such as the "ostomy nurse," sex educator, or psychiatric clinical specialist.

▶ Nursing Process
The Patient With Cancer of the Colon or Rectum

▷ Assessment

Interview the patient and ask for a description of the symptoms that led him to seek medical care. Is there any abdominal pain? If so, ask for a description of it (where it occurs and

---

TABLE 34-10
Dietary Support in Common Complications of Surgical Treatment for Cancer

Procedure	Complications	Dietary Support
Small bowel resection	Poor absorption Weight loss Absorptive capacity improves with time.	Immediate support after surgery: long-term enteral or parenteral nutrition Later: Oral intake of high-protein, high-calorie, low-fat diet Medium-chain triglycerides
Ileostomy Colostomy	Initial loss of water and electrolytes	Daily replacement of electrolytes; full liquid diet, high in protein
Bypass surgery	For relief of pain and obstruction Malabsorption syndrome Maldigestion, diarrhea	Feedings by natural route High-protein, high-vitamin C diet Adequate vitamins and minerals

(Adapted from Valassi K. Nutritional management of cancer patients in a variety of therapeutic regimens. Arch Phys Med Rehabil 58: Sept 1977.)

how often, how long it lasts, and whether it is associated with food intake or activities). Has there been a change in bowel habits? If so, what were the exact changes? Have blood or mucous been noticed in the stools? Has he lost weight? How many pounds and over what period of time? How much does the patient eat every day (amount and variety of foods)? Has there been unusual fatigue? Is a nap required during the day? Is the patient able to sleep well during the night?

Elicit a history of habits (smoking, alcohol intake, exercise) and dietary preferences. Are fruits and vegetables eaten daily? How often does the patient eat fatty meats, dairy products (butter, ice cream, cheese) and "junk foods" (potato chips, chocolate candy)? How does he cope with stress? Has the patient ever had ulcerative colitis?

The physical examination includes abdominal palpation for areas of tenderness and auscultation for bowel sounds. Any stool is examined for appearance and the presence of blood.

▷ Nursing Diagnoses

Based on all the assessment data, the patient's major nursing diagnoses may include the following:

Preoperative
- Anxiety related to impending surgery and the diagnosis of cancer
- Alteration in comfort, pain, related to tissue compression secondary to obstruction
- Alteration in nutrition, less than body requirements, related to nausea and anorexia
- Potential for fluid volume deficit related to vomiting and dehydration

Postoperative
- Potential for infection related to possible contamination of the abdominal cavity during the surgical procedure
- Knowledge deficit concerning the diagnosis, the surgical procedure, and self-care after discharge
- Actual impairment of skin integrity related to the surgical incisions (abdominal and perianal) and the formation of a stoma

▷ Planning and Implementation

▷ **Goals:** The major goals of the patient may include reduction in anxiety, reduction/alleviation of pain, attainment of an optimal level of nutrition, maintenance of fluid and electrolyte balance, prevention of infection, acquisition of information about the diagnosis, surgical procedure, and self-care after discharge, and maintenance of optimal tissue healing.

Nursing Interventions

Reducing Anxiety. Identify the patient's level of anxiety (mild, moderate, severe). Are any coping mechanisms being used to deal with stress? Provide supportive efforts: arrange for periods of privacy if desired for meditation, relaxation exercises, biofeedback; set time aside to sit with the patient who wishes to ventilate, cry, or ask questions. Offer to contact a member of the clergy if desired; arrange a time for the family to meet with the physicians and nurses if the patient wishes to discuss the treatment/prognosis with them; arrange a meeting with an enterostomal therapist if that seems useful; and suggest that an ostomate be asked to visit.

Project a relaxed and empathetic attitude. Always be honest when answering questions. Explain all tests and treatment procedures at the level of the patient's understanding. Clarify any information the physician has provided, if necessary. Sometimes anxiety is relieved if the patient knows what physical preparation is necessary preoperatively and what to expect postoperatively. Some patients appreciate seeing pictures or drawings, while others would prefer not to know details. Assess what the patient needs and wants to know.

Pain Reduction/Alleviation. Administer analgesics as prescribed. Make the environment conducive to relaxation by dimming the lights, turning off the television or radio, and restricting visitors and telephone calls. Offer additional comfort measures: position changes, a back rub, distraction, and relaxation techniques.

Nutritional Measures. If the patient's condition permits, a diet high in calories, protein, and carbohydrates and low in residue is given preoperatively for several days to provide adequate nutrition and decrease excessive peristalsis, in order to minimize cramping. A full-liquid diet may be prescribed 24 hours before surgery to decrease bulk. Total parenteral nutrition is required for some patients to supply depleted nutrients, vitamins, and minerals. Record daily weights and notify the physician if the patient continues to lose weight while receiving parenteral nutrition.

Anemia is common. If the hemoglobin falls below 12 grams (1.86 mmol/L), a blood transfusion may be prescribed by the physician. When administering a blood transfusion, carefully follow normal safety guidelines and agency policy regarding safety. Be alert for indicators of an allergic reaction (rash, flushing, hives, chills, dyspnea, vomiting, tachycardia) and stop the transfusion if a reaction appears.

Maintenance of Fluid and Electrolyte Balance. Measure intake and output, including vomitus, to have an accurate record of fluid balance. The patient's intake of oral food and fluids is restricted to prevent vomiting. If vomiting is expected, administer antiemetics as prescribed. Full or clear liquids may be tolerated, or the patient may be allowed nothing by mouth. A nasogastric tube will be inserted preoperatively to drain accumulated fluids and prevent abdominal distention. An indwelling catheter may be inserted to allow monitoring of hourly output. An output of less than 30 ml/hr is reported to the physician.

Monitor intravenous administration of fluids and electrolytes. Check serum electrolytes to detect hypokalemia and hyponatremia, which occur with gastrointestinal fluid loss. Monitor vital signs to detect hypovolemia: tachycardia, hypotension, and decreased pulse volume. Assess hydration status and report decreased skin turgor, dry mucous membranes, concentrated urine, and increased urine specific gravity.

Prevention of Infection. Administer prescribed intestinal anti-infectives such as kanamycin sulfate (Kant Rex) erythromycin (Erythrocin), and neomycin sulfate (Mycigvent) to reduce intestinal bacteria in preparation for bowel surgery. These are given by mouth to reduce the bacterial content of the colon and to soften and decrease the bulk of the contents of the colon. In addition, the bowel can be cleansed by laxatives, enemas, or colonic irrigations.

Preoperative Patient Education. Determine the patient's present knowledge about the diagnosis, prognosis, surgical procedure, and expected level of functioning postoperatively. Assess learning ability and interest. Decide what information is needed, how it should be presented, when the patient would be most receptive, and who should be present during the instruction. Encourage the patient to participate in the learning process. Choose a time and location conducive to learning. Use repetition and praise to reinforce learning.

Review information the patient needs about the physical preparation for surgery, the expected appearance and care of the wound postoperatively, the technique of ostomy care, dietary restrictions, pain control, and medication management. (See Nursing Care Plan 34-1 for the patient with an intestinal ostomy, pp. 824–827.)

Wound Care. Examine the abdominal wound frequently during the first 24 hours to make sure that it is healing without complications (infection, dehiscence, hemorrhage, excessive edema). Change dressings as needed to prevent infection. Show the patient how to splint the abdominal incision during coughing and deep breathing to lessen tension on the edges of the incision. Monitor temperature, pulse rate, and respirations for elevations that may indicate an infectious process. A temperature higher than 38.3°C (101°F) is reported to the physician.

Examine the stoma for swelling (slight edema due to surgical manipulation is normal), color (a healthy stoma should be pink), discharge (a small amount of oozing is normal), and bleeding (an abnormal sign). Cleanse the peristomal skin gently and pat it dry to prevent irritation. Carry out perineal wound care as described on page 838.

Patient Education and Home Health Care. Discharge planning requires the combined efforts of the physician, nurse, enterostomal therapist, social worker, and dietitian. Patients being discharged are given specific information, individualized to their needs, about ostomy care and complications to observe for: obstruction, infection, stoma stenosis, retraction or prolapse, and peristomal skin irritation. Dietary instructions are essential to help patients identify and eliminate irritating foods that can cause diarrhea or constipation. Patients are given a list of the medications prescribed for them, with information on the action, purpose, and possible side-effects of each. A system for remembering when to take the medication is developed with the patient.

Treatments (irrigations, wound cleansing) and dressing changes are reviewed, and the family is encouraged to participate. Patients need very specific directions about when to call the physician. They need to know exactly what complications require prompt attention (bleeding, abdominal distention and rigidity, diarrhea, and the "dumping syndrome"— see p. 796). Patients are directed to weigh weekly and notify a physician if they experience continued or abrupt weight loss of 1 to 2 pounds per week. If radiation therapy is necessary, the possible side-effects of anorexia, vomiting, diarrhea, and exhaustion are reviewed.

▷ *Evaluation*

▷ *Expected Outcomes*

1. Patient experiences less anxiety.
   a. Verbalizes concerns and fears freely
   b. Uses coping measures to deal with stress
   c. Shares feelings/concerns with family members
   d. Meets with support persons (clergy, social worker, ostomate)
2. Experiences less pain
   a. Requests analgesics as needed
   b. Uses diversional activities successfully
   c. Reports a decrease in pain
3. Achieves an optimal level of nutrition
   a. Eats a low-residue, high-protein, high-calorie diet
   b. Reports less abdominal cramping
   c. Tolerates parenteral nutrition therapy
4. Achieves fluid balance
   a. Restricts oral intake of foods and fluids when nauseated
   b. Urinates about 1.5 L/24 hrs
   c. Denies paresthesia, dizziness, unusual fatigue (signs of hypokalemia), excessive thirst
   d. Denies dry, itchy, or scaly skin
   e. Maintains desired weight
5. Avoids infection
   a. Takes oral intestinal anti-infectives
   b. Cooperates with bowel cleansing
   c. Is afebrile
6. Acquires information about the diagnosis, surgical procedure, and self-care after discharge
   a. Discusses the diagnosis, surgical procedure, and postoperative self-care
   b. Asks specific questions
   c. Relates concerns and fears
   d. Participates actively in the learning process (listens attentively, clarifies procedures, restates important concepts, answers questions correctly)
   e. Communicates individual needs for self-care after discharge
   f. Understands technique of ostomy care
7. Maintains clean incision, stoma, and perineal wound
   a. Describes the appearance of incision site accurately
   b. States that there is some pain in the incisional area, but that it is relieved by analgesics
   c. Discusses the appearance of the stoma as raised and pink, with minimal edema
   d. Describes peristomal skin as pink in color and without irritation
   e. Assists the nurse with dressing changes
   f. Begins to clean the stoma and peristomal skin whenever necessary
   g. Cooperates with perineal wound irrigations
   h. Splints incisional area with hand when coughing and taking deep breaths
   i. Is afebrile

Polyps of the Colon and Rectum

Benign polyps are much more common in the large intestine than in the small intestine. If there are numerous growths, the condition is referred to as *polyposis*, often a congenital abnormality. Polyps occur in 10% to 60% of the population; occurrence is most frequent in the fifth decade of life, with the majority of polyps found in the sigmoid and rectum.

Clinical manifestations depend on the size of the polyp and the amount of pressure it exerts on intestinal tissue. The most common symptom is rectal bleeding. Diagnosis can be made by digital rectal examination, barium enema studies, proctosigmoidoscopy, and colonoscopy, depending on the lesion's location and size. Once they are identified, polyps are excised because of the possibility that malignancy is already present or may develop.

Familial polyposis coli refers to a condition in which there are hundreds of polyps in the large intestines. Surgery is always recommended because untreated cases invariably turn malignant, usually by age 40. A total colectomy with ileoanal anastomosis is the preferred surgical procedure.

Diseases of the Anorectum

Patients with anorectal disorders seek medical care primarily because of pain and rectal bleeding. Other frequent complaints are protrusion of hemorrhoids, anal discharge, itching, swelling, anal tenderness, stenosis, and ulceration. Constipation occurs because defecation is delayed due to pain.

Rectal Examination and Patient Preparation

Visual inspection and digital examination of the anus and the rectum are indispensable for detecting and identifying lesions involving these structures. Moreover, rectal examination is extremely useful in diagnosing or excluding many intra-abdominal and pelvic conditions, including appendicitis; diverticulitis; salpingitis; tumors of the ovary, uterus, and colon; and prostatic lesions of various types.

Rectal examinations may be done with the patient in the knee–chest, Sims's lateral, or inverted position or on a special proctoscopic table. Whatever position is used, the patient is informed of the procedure and how it is to be done, and is draped so that only the rectal area is exposed.

Anorectal Abscess

Anorectal abscess is located in the pararectal spaces. Usually, it is caused by infection of pathogenic microorganisms. Incidence is higher in men than women.

Clinical Manifestations and Management. An abscess may occur in a variety of spaces in and around the rectum. Often it contains a quantity of foul-smelling pus and is painful. If the abscess is superficial, swelling, redness, and tenderness are observed. A deeper abscess may result in toxic symptoms and even lower abdominal pain, as well as fever. More than half of rectal abscesses will result in fistulas.

Palliative therapy consists of sitz baths and analgesics. Surgical treatment consists of incision and drainage; this may be all that is necessary. When deeper infection exists, with the possibility of a fistula, it is necessary to remove the fistulous tract. This may be done initially, or it may require a second operation. Often no packing is used; if it is used, usually the wound is lined with petrolatum gauze. Later, when it is necessary to remove the packing, soaking it first with saline solution is helpful.

These wounds are allowed to heal by granulation. Bowel movements should be formed, rather than liquid or soft. Cathartics or mineral oil are not usually used.

Fistula in Ano

Fistula in ano is a tiny tubular tract that extends into the anal canal from an opening located beside the anus (Fig. 34-12*A*). Fistulas usually result from an infection. Pus or stool leak constantly from the cutaneous opening, making it necessary for the patient to wear a protective pad. This condition may be an early sign of regional enteritis.

Management. A *fistulectomy* (excision of the fistulous tract) is the recommended surgical procedure. Three or four hours before the operation, the perineum is shaved and the lower bowel evacuated thoroughly with several prescribed enemas. The last enema should return clear and should be evacuated entirely.

The patient usually is placed in the lithotomy position, and the sinus tract is identified by inserting a probe into it or by injecting the tract with methylene blue solution. The fistula is dissected out or laid open by an incision from its rectal opening to its outlet. The wound is packed with gauze.

Fissure in Ano

Fissure in ano is a longitudinal ulcer in the anal canal (see Fig. 34-12*B*). Fissures are usually caused by diarrheal stools and persistent tightening of the anal canal secondary to stress and anxiety (leading to constipation). Other causes include childbirth, trauma, and cathartic abuse. The most pronounced symptom is extreme pain during defecation.

Clinical Manifestations and Management. Fissures are characterized by painful defecation and bleeding. The pain may be excruciating. More than half of these fissures will heal if treated by conservative measures, and the remainder will require minor surgery. Stool softeners and an increase in water intake are helpful; a bland laxative will prevent constipation. A suppository combining an anesthetic with

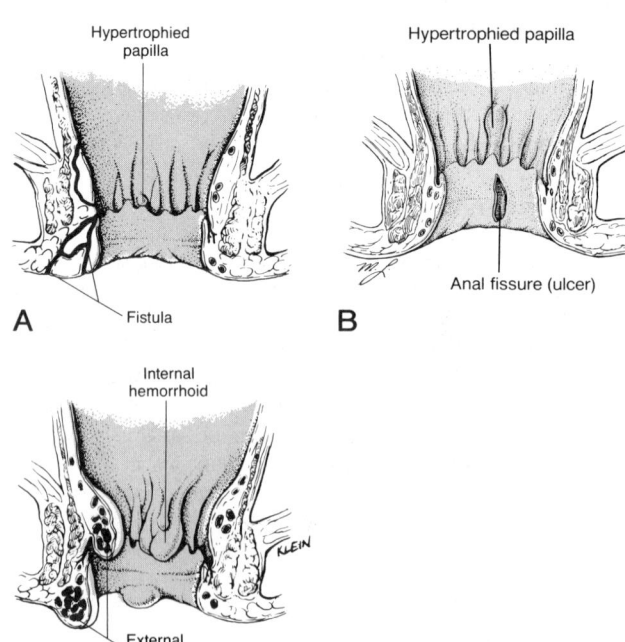

Figure 34-12
Various types of anal lesions. (*A*) Fistula. (*B*) Fissure. (*C*) External and internal hemorrhoids.

a steroid is comforting. Anal dilatation under anesthesia may be required.

In surgical management, the same preoperative preparation as for fistula in ano is indicated. Several types of operations may be performed: in some cases, the anal sphincter is dilated and the fissure is excised; in others, a part of the external sphincter is divided. This establishes a paralysis of the external sphincter, with consequent relief of spasm, and permits the ulcer to heal. When there is a large, overhanging sentinel hemorrhoid, excision of the ulcer and of the hemorrhoid is performed.

Hemorrhoids

Hemorrhoids are simply varicose veins in the anal canal. They may come and go, and almost everyone has them at some time. They are very common in pregnancy. When they fadeaway, they may leave a telltale skin tag. They occur in two locations. Those occurring above the internal sphincter are called *internal hemorrhoids,* and those appearing outside the external sphincter are called *external hemorrhoids* (see Fig. 34-12C). They cause itching, bleeding during bowel movements, and pain. Internal hemorrhoids prolapse frequently through the sphincter and cause considerable discomfort. If the blood within them clots and becomes infected, they grow painful and are said to be *thrombosed.*

Clinical Manifestations and Management. External hemorrhoids are associated with severe pain due to inflammation and edema caused by thrombosis. Internal hemorrhoids are not usually painful until they bleed or prolapse with enlargement. Hemorrhoid symptoms and discomfort can be relieved by good personal hygiene and by avoiding excessive straining during defecation. A diet that contains fruit and bran may be all the treatment that is necessary; failing this, perhaps a hydrophilic laxative will help. Sitz baths, astringents (witch hazel), and bed rest are only palliative measures. Surgery is required when prolapsed hemorrhoids can no longer be reduced spontaneously or manually.

Many physicians have one or another preferred medications that, when injected above the sensitive squamous mucosa through an anoscope, has no direct effect on thrombosed veins, *per se,* but induces a fibrous reaction. This reaction in submucosal tissues of the upper anal canal and lower rectum tends to draw tissue upward toward its normal site. This method has little effect on advanced hemorrhoids.

A conservative measure is the rubber-band ligation treatment. As the hemorrhoid is visualized through the anoscope, its proximal portion above the mucocutaneous lines is grasped with an instrument, and a small rubber band is slipped over it. Tissue distal to the rubber band becomes necrotic after several days and is removed. Because of fibrosis, lower anal mucosa is drawn up and adheres to the underlying muscle. While this treatment has been satisfactory in some patients, it has proved painful in others and may cause some secondary hemorrhage.

Cryosurgical hemorrhoidectomy involves freezing the tissues of the hemorrhoid for a sufficient time to cause necrosis. Although it is painless, it is not popular because the discharge is very foul-smelling and wound healing is prolonged.

Excision of an external hemorrhoidal tag can be done with laser therapy. The treatment is usually performed in the physician's office, and is quick and relatively painless.

The methods of treating hemorrhoids just described are not effective for advanced thrombosed veins, which are usually treated by surgical hemorrhoidectomy.

The operation usually involves digital dilatation of the rectal sphincter and removal of the hemorrhoids by the use of a clamp and cautery or by ligation and excision. After completion of the operative procedures, a small tube, often covered with petrolatum gauze, may be inserted through the sphincter to permit the escape of flatus and also of blood, if there should be any bleeding. Instead of the tube, some surgeons place pieces of Gelfoam or Oxycel gauze over the anal wounds. Dressings, in such cases, are held in place by a T-binder.

Patient Education and Home Health Care. Stool softeners are usually prescribed for several days to prevent pain and discomfort during elimination. Local cooling astringents such as witch hazel help reduce discomfort. The physician usually recommends aspirin or acetaminophen for pain. Normal bowel elimination without pain should occur within a week. (See Nursing Process, p. 844.)

Pilonidal Sinus (Cyst)

A pilonidal sinus or cyst is found in the intergluteal cleft on the posterior surface of the lower sacrum (Fig. 34-13). It is

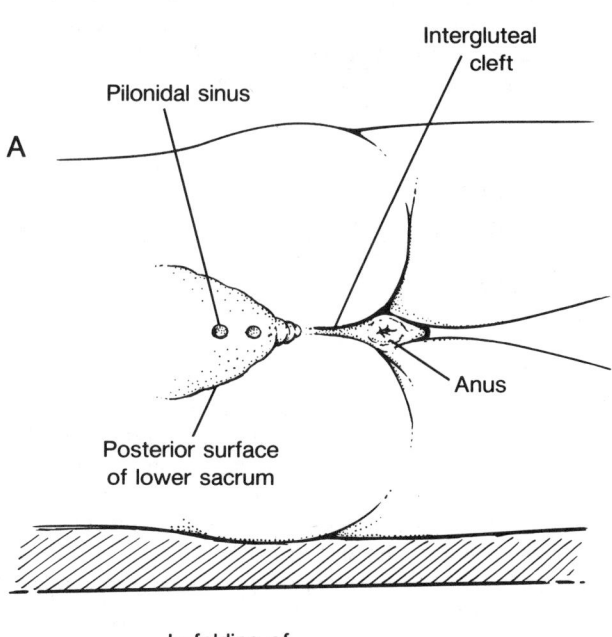

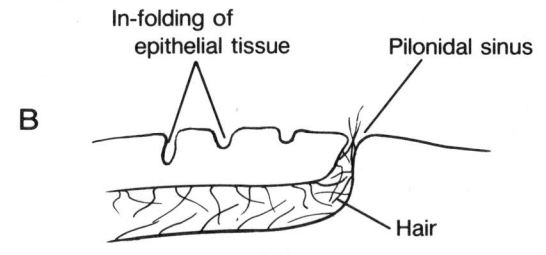

Figure 34-13

(*A*) Pilonidal sinus on lower sacrum about 5 cm (2 inches) above the anus in the intergluteal cleft. (*B*) Note hair particles emerging from sinus tract. Localized indentations of the skin (pits) can occur near the sinus openings.

thought by some to be formed by an infolding of epithelial tissue beneath the skin, which may communicate with the skin surface through one or several small sinus openings. Hair frequently is seen protruding from these openings, and this gives the cyst its name—*pilonidal*—a nest of hair. The cysts rarely give symptoms until adolescence or early adult life, when infection produces an irritating drainage or an abscess. This area is easily irritated by perspiration and friction.

Management. In the early stages of the inflammation, the infection may be controlled by antibiotic therapy. Once an abscess has formed, as in cases of a hair-containing sinus, surgery is indicated. When an abscess is present, incision and drainage are performed. In patients with hair-containing sinuses without marked inflammatory reaction, surgery is also necessary to remove hair and debris, a potential source of irritation and infection. The entire cyst and the secondary sinus tracts are excised. In many patients the resulting defect may be sutured, but in some the defect may be so large that it cannot be closed entirely, and it is allowed to heal by granulation. Extensive excisions are no longer considered necessary.

Nursing Interventions. The nursing care of these patients is relatively simple. In those with abscess, hot, moist applications are used frequently. After excision of the cyst, the care is that of any superficial wound. Shaving of hair around the wound is recommended to avoid recurrence. For the first few days, the patient often is more comfortable lying on his abdomen or side with a pillow between the legs. Most patients are allowed out of bed soon after surgery, and their postoperative care is managed at home.

▶ Nursing Process
The Patient With an Anorectal Condition

▷ Assessment

Bleeding is frequently seen in anorectal disease. (The most common cause of rectal bleeding is hemorrhoids.) Ask the patient to describe the bleeding. It may be bright red, but occasionally it is a darker color, due to its remaining in the rectal ampulla before expulsion and also its admixture with feces. Bleeding from the anal canal usually has a bright red appearance. Examine the stool to see if blood is mixed with the feces or just coating the stool.

Ask the patient to describe the pain. Does it occur during evacuation? Is there associated abdominal pain? How long does the pain last after evacuation? Is there a discharge? Can it be described as mucoid, purulent, or bloody?

Take a dietary history to note if there is an absence of fiber intake. Is there a history of constipation? How has it been handled before? Does the patient abuse laxatives? Is there straining at stool? Has any protrusion from the anus after defecation ever been noticed? If so, did it spontaneously resolve?

Does the patient have a job that requires prolonged standing or sitting? Is there a pregnancy history? Was the childbirth experience normal?

▷ Nursing Diagnoses

Based on all the assessment data, the patient's major nursing diagnoses may include the following:

- Alteration in bowel elimination, constipation, related to ignoring the urge to defecate because of pain during elimination
- Anxiety related to impending surgery and embarrassment
- Alteration in comfort, pain, related to irritation, pressure, and sensitivity in the rectal/anal area secondary to anorectal disease and sphincter spasms postoperatively
- Alteration in urinary elimination pattern related to postoperative fear of pain
- Potential for injury, hemorrhage, related to the surgical incision
- Potential nonadherence to the therapeutic regimen

▷ Planning and Implementation

▷ *Goals:* The major goals of the patient may include attainment of adequate elimination, reduction in anxiety, relief of pain, promotion of urinary elimination, prevention of hemorrhage, and adherence to the therapeutic regimen.

Nursing Interventions

Measures for Relief of Constipation. Encourage the intake of at least 2000 ml of water daily to provide adequate hydration. Recommend high-fiber foods to promote bulk in the stool and facilitate easy passage through the rectum. Recommend bulk laxatives such as Metamucil. Administer stool softeners as prescribed. Advise the patient to set aside a time for defecation and to heed the urge. Relaxation exercises might be helpful before defecation to relax the abdominal perineal muscles that may be constricted or in spasm due to anticipated pain with elimination.

Reducing Anxiety. Patients facing rectal surgery are usually upset and irritable because of discomfort, pain, and embarrassment. Identify specific psychosocial needs and individualize a plan of care. Promote privacy by limiting visitors, if agreeable to patient. Always maintain the patient's privacy when giving care. Remove soiled dressings from the room to prevent unpleasant odors. Room deodorizers may be needed if dressings are foul-smelling.

Relieving Pain. During the first 24 hours after rectal surgery, there may be painful spasms of the sphincter and perineal muscles. Therefore, control of pain is a prime consideration. Encourage the patient to assume positions of comfort (bed rest with prolapsed internal hemorrhoids, avoidance of walking with an abscess). Apply ice and analgesic ointments to decrease pain, warm compresses to promote circulation and soothe irritated tissues. Sitz baths, 3 or 4 times a day, will relieve soreness and pain by relaxing sphincter spasm. After 24 hours have elapsed, topical anesthetic agents may be beneficial for relief of local irritation and soreness.

Wet dressings saturated with equal parts of cold water and witch hazel help relieve edema. When wet compresses are being used continuously, petrolatum should be applied around the anal area to prevent skin maceration. Instruct the patient to assume a prone position at intervals, since this position promotes dependent drainage of edema fluid.

Chart 34-3
Summary of Potential Complications Following Surgery
of Small and Large Intestines

Anticipation of and vigilance for complications have first priority in caring for postoperative patients. Prompt recognition and management of these complications can prevent prolonged disability and, in some instances, death.

Complication	*Nursing Assessment and Interventions*
Paralytic Ileus	Initiate or continue nasogastric intubation. Prepare patient for x-ray study. Ensure adequate fluid and electrolyte replacement. Give prescribed antibiotics if patient has symptoms of peritonitis.
Mechanical Obstruction	Evaluate patient for intermittent colicky pain, nausea, and vomiting.
Intraperitoneal Infection and Abdominal Wound Infection	Assess for evidence of constant or generalized abdominal pain, rapid pulse, and elevation of temperature. Prepare for tube decompression of bowel. Restore fluid and electrolytes by IV route. Give antibiotics as directed.
Intra-abdominal Septic Conditions: Peritonitis	Evaluate patient for nausea, hiccups, chills, spiking fever, tachycardia. Give antibiotics as prescribed. Prepare patient for drainage procedure. Institute intravenous fluid and electrolyte therapy. Prepare patient for reoperation if condition deteriorates.
Abscess Formation	Administer antibiotics as directed. Apply warm compresses as prescribed. Prepare for surgical drainage.
Wound Complications	
Infection	Watch temperature graph for evidences of spiking fever. Observe for redness, tenderness, and pain around wound. Assist in establishing local drainage. Obtain specimen of drainage material for culture and sensitivity studies.
Wound disruption	Watch for sudden appearance of profuse serous drainage from wound. Cover wound area with sterile towels held in place with binder. Prepare patient immediately for surgery.
Anastomotic Complications	
Dehiscence of anastomosis	Prepare patient for surgery.
Fistulas	Assist in bowel decompression. Give parenteral fluids as prescribed to correct fluid and electrolyte defects.

Medications may include *suppositories* that contain anesthetics, astringents, antiseptics, tranquilizers, antinauseants, and even bronchodilators. Patients will be more compliant, and less apprehensive and uncomfortable, if the suppository is inserted properly. The most effective position for the patient to assume while the suppository is being inserted is side-lying, with the uppermost leg flexed. The suppository is unwrapped; the buttocks are spread apart with one hand and the suppository is inserted with the other. If the suppository was stored in the refrigerator (to prevent melting), it may be warmed to room temperature to lessen irritation of rectal mucosa. Water-soluble suppositories may be lubricated with water or lubricating jelly; however, cocoa butter suppositories are self-lubricating.

Promoting Urinary Elimination. Voiding may be a problem, due to a reflex spasm of the sphincter at the outlet of the bladder and a certain amount of muscle-guarding from apprehension and pain. All methods to encourage voluntary micturition (increasing fluid intake, listening to running water, dripping water over the urinary meatus) should be tried before resorting to catheterization. After rectal operations, patients are usually allowed out of bed to void.

Preventing Hemorrhage. Examine operative site for rectal bleeding. Assess for systemic indicators of excessive bleeding (tachycardia, hypotension, restlessness, thirst). Report any unusual signs to the physician. After hemorrhoidectomy, hemorrhage may occur from the veins that were cut. If a tube has been inserted through the sphincter after operation, evidence of bleeding should be apparent on the dressings. If bleeding is obvious, apply direct pressure to the area, make sure the patient remains in bed, and elevate the buttocks on a pillow. Seek medical help.

Patient Education and Home Health Care. The patient should keep the perianal area as clean as possible. This is accomplished by gentle cleansing with warm water and *drying* with absorbent cotton wipes. The patient is instructed to avoid rubbing the area with toilet tissue.

The patient prevents constipation by responding quickly to the urge to defecate. Over-the-counter laxatives should be avoided. Diet is modified to increase fluids and fiber. The patient is encouraged to ambulate as soon as possible.

See Chart 34-3 (p. 845) for a list of possible complications to watch for following small and large bowel surgery.

When it is time for discharge from the hospital, the patient should know how to take sitz baths and how to test the temperature of the water. Sitz baths may be given in a bathtub 3 or 4 times a day, or a plastic sitz bath unit (usually sold in a drugstore) can be used.

The patient is informed about the prescribed diet, made aware of the significance of proper eating habits, and told what laxatives can be taken safely and why exercise is important. The surgeon usually outlines a schedule in detail to cover the daily routine. This can be reviewed with the patient by the nurse.

▷ *Evaluation*

▷ *Expected Outcomes*

1. Patient attains a normal pattern of elimination.
   a. Sets aside a time for defecation, usually after a meal or at bedtime
   b. "Heeds the call" and takes the time to sit on the toilet and try to eliminate
   c. Uses relaxation exercises as needed
   d. Increases fluid intake to 2.0 L/24 hours
   e. Adds high-fiber foods to diet
   f. Reports passage of soft, formed stools
   g. Reports less abdominal discomfort
2. Projects less anxiety
   a. Discusses fears and concerns
   b. Understands surgical procedure
   c. Describes postoperative recovery procedures
   d. Communicates privacy needs

3. Experiences less pain
   a. Modifies body position and activities to minimize pain and discomfort
   b. Applies heat/cold to rectal/anal area
   c. Takes sitz baths 4 times a day
   d. Changes dressing frequently; requests assistance if needed
   e. Reports less pain
4. Achieves voluntary micturition
   a. Voids without difficulty
   b. Is free of urinary pain/discomfort
5. Is free of any bleeding problems
   a. Has a clean incision
   b. Exhibits normal vital signs
   c. Is free of hemorrhage
6. Adheres to a therapeutic regimen
   a. Keeps perianal area dry
   b. Eats bulk-forming foods
   c. Has soft, formed stools on a regular basis
   d. Ambulates as soon as possible

Bibliography

Books

Allan RN et al (eds). Inflammatory Bowel Diseases. New York, Churchill Livingstone, 1983.

Bockus HL. Bockus Gastroenterology Intestine (Parts I and II). Philadelphia, WB Saunders, 1985.

Bolt RJ et al. The Digestive System. New York, John Wiley & Sons, 1983.

Chernecky CC and Ramsey PW. Critical Nursing Care of the Client with Cancer. Connecticut, Appleton-Century-Crofts, 1984.

Cohen S (ed). Clinical Gastroenterology: A Problem-Oriented Approach. New York, John Wiley & Sons, 1983.

Corman ML. Colon and Rectal Surgery. Philadelphia, JB Lippincott, 1984.

Donovan MI and Girton SE. Cancer Care Nursing. Connecticut, Appleton-Century-Crofts, 1984.

Ferrari BT, Ray JE, and Gathright JB. Complications of Colon and Rectal Surgery. Philadelphia, WB Saunders, 1985.

Given B and Simmons S. Gastroenterology in Clinical Nursing. St Louis, CV Mosby, 1983.

Goldner FC and Draft SC. Idiopathic Inflammatory Bowel Disease: Internal Medicine. Boston, Little, Brown & Co, 1983.

Goligher J. Surgery of the Anus, Rectum, and Colon. London, Bailliere Tioudall, 1984.

Jagelman DG (ed). Mucosal Ulcerative Colitis. New York, Futura Publishing Co, 1986.

Magrina E de Los Rios. Color Atlas of Anorectal Diseases. Philadelphia, WB Saunders, 1980.

Price AL. Ileostomy Care: Stoma Care and Management Techniques. Springfield, Illinois, Charles C Thomas, 1984.

Shackelford RT and Zuidema GD. Surgery of the Alimentary Tract. Philadelphia, WB Saunders, 1986.

Sleisenger MH and Fordtran JS. Gastrointestinal Disease: Pathophysiology, Diagnosis, Management. Philadelphia, WB Saunders, 1983.

Spiro HM. Clinical Gastroenterology. New York, Macmillan Publishing Company, 1983.

Spratt JS. Neoplasms of the Colon, Rectum, and Anus. Philadelphia, WB Saunders Company, 1984.

Truelove SC and Kennedy HJ (Ed). Topics in Gastroenterology. London, Blackwell Scientific Publications, 1980.

Way LW. Current Surgical Diagnosis and Treatment. Los Altos, California, Lange Medical Publishers, 1985.

Welch CE, Ottinger LW, and Welch JP. Manual of Lower Gastrointestinal Surgery. New York: Springer-Verlag, 1986.

Articles

(Asterisks indicate nursing research articles.)

Constipation and Diarrhea

Behm RM. A special recipe to banish constipation. Geriatr Nurs 1985 July/Aug; 6(4):216–217.

Binder HJ. The pathophysiology of diarrhea. Hosp Pract 1984 Oct; 19(10): 107–113.

Cantey JR. Infectious diarrhea: Pathogenesis and risk factors. Am J Med 1985 June 28; 78(6B):65–67.

Coralli CH. Promoting health in international travel. Nurse Pract 1985 Oct; 10(10):28–32.

Donald IP et al. A study of constipation in the elderly living at home. Gerontology 1985 Feb; 31(2):112–118.

DuPont HL. Diarrheal diseases: An overview. Am J Med 1985 June 28; 28(6B):63–64.

DuPont HL. Nonfluid therapy and selected chemoprophylaxis of acute diarrhea. Am J Med 1985 June 28; 78(6B):81–90.

Elliot DL et al. Constipation: Mechanisms and management of a common clinical problem. Postgrad Med 1983 Aug; 74(2):143–149.

Iseminger M and Hardy P. Bran works! Geriatr Nurs 1982 June; 1(6): 402–404.

Karmali MA. Bacterial diarrhea: An update. Diagnostic Med 1985 May; 8(5):12–19.

Kasanof DM. Constipation: Is it functional or? Patient Care 1984 Feb 29; 18(4):128–130, 133, 137.

Lewis B. Streamlining the process of elimination. Am J Nurs 1985 July; 85(7):774.

Mager-O'Conner E. How to identify and remove fecal impactions. Geriatr Nur 1984 May/June; 5(3):158–161.

McShane RE et al. Constipation: Consensual and empirical validation . . . nursing diagnosis. Nurs Clin North Am 1985 Dec; 20(4):801–808.

Meeroff JC. Approach to the patient with constipation. Hosp Pract 1985 Jan 15; 20(1):148, 152–153.

Poisson J et al. Severe chronic constipation as a surgical problem. Surg Clin North Am 1983 Feb; 63(1):193–217.

Quinn TC, Bender BS, and Bartlett JG. New developments in infectious diarrhea. DM 1986 Apr; 32(4):174–240.

Resnick B. Constipation: Common but preventable. Geriatr Nurs 1985 July/Aug; 6(4):213–215.

Rogers A. Answers to questions on diarrhea. Hosp Med 1983 Feb; 19(2): 267–275.

Shefts DL et al. Bowel management protocol. Home Health Care Nurse 1984 Sept/Oct; 2(5):17–20.

Diseases of Malabsorption

Cerda JJ et al. Nutritional aspects of malabsorption syndromes. Compr Ther 1983 Nov; 9(11):35–46.

Cosnes J et al. Compensatory enteral hyperalimentation for management of patients with severe short bowel syndrome. Am J Clin Nutr 1985 May; 41(5):1002–1009.

Fuller E. Differentiating malabsorption causes. Patient Care 1983 Jan 30; 17(2):96–108.

Gillian JS et al. Malabsorption and mucosal abnormalities of the small intestine in the acquired immunodeficiency syndrome. Ann Intern Med 1985 May; 102(5):619–622.

Iles M. Effective use of total parenteral nutrition in an ileostomy patient. J Am Diet Assoc 1984 Nov; 84(11):1324–1328.

Jett MF et al. Functional loss of the ileum: Consequences and management. Nurse Pract 1984 Nov; 9(11):24, 29–30, 32–34.

Meerpff JC. Etiologic evaluation and treatment of malabsorption syndrome. Hosp Pract 1984 Apr; 19(4):88.

Appendicitis

Arnbjornsson E. Acute appendicitis: A familial disease? Curr Surg 1982 Jan/Feb; 39(1):18–20.

Ballantine TV. Appendicitis. Surg Clin North Am 1981 Oct; 61(5):1117–1124.

Cooperman M. Complications of appendectomy. Surg Clin North Am 1983 Dec; 63(6):1233–1247.

Feicher I et al. Scoring system to aid in diagnosis of appendicitis. Ann Surg 1983 Dec; 198(6):753–759.

Rottenbery R. RLQ pain: Is it what you think? Patient Care 1985 Jan 30; 19(2):70–74, 76, 78.

Strom PR et al. Safety of incidental appendectomy. Am J Surg 1983 June; 145(6):819–822.

Peritonitis

Dougherty SH. Role of amikacin in the management of intra-abdominal sepsis. Am J Med 1985 July 15; 79(1A):28–36.

Hau T. Management of peritonitis. Curr Surg 1984 May/June; 41(3):165–167.

Jones LM. Bacterial peritonitis: Protecting the high-risk patients. Am Surg 1984 July; 50(7):358–361.

Lobato V et al. Peritoneal lavage as an aid to diagnosis of peritonitis in debilitated and elderly patients. Am Surg 1985 Sept; 51(9):508–510.

Stone HH et al. Reliability of criteria for predicting persistent or recurrent sepsis. Arch Surg 1985 Jan; 120(1):17–20.

Hernias

Stoppa RE et al. The use of dacron in the repair of hernias of the groin. Surg Clin North Am 1984 Apr; 64(2):269–285.

Wantz GE. Complications of inguinal hernial repair. Surg Clin North Am 1984 Apr; 64(2):287–298.

Regional Enteritis

Ashley N et al. Inflammatory bowel disease. Practitioner 1984 Sept; 228(139):803–810.

Butler C et al. Supporting the patient with Crohn's disease. Nursing '83 1983 Nov; 13(11):46–51.

Cantor DS. Crohn's disease and psychiatric illness. Gastroenterology 1984 Aug; 87(2):478–479.

Fazio VW. Regional enteritis (Crohn's disease): Indications for surgery and operative strategy. Surg Clin North Am 1983 Feb; 63(1):27–45.

Fazio VW. Crohn's disease: Surgical procedures, sequelae, and management of recurrence. Consultant 1983 Jan; 23(1):49–68.

Greenstein AJ. The surgery for Crohn's disease. Surg Clin North Am 1987 June; 67(3):573–596.

Heimann TM et al. Early complications following surgical treatment for Crohn's disease. Ann Surg 1985 Apr; 201(4):494–498.

Jones VA et al. Crohn's disease; Maintenance of remission by diet. Lancet 1985 July 27; 2(8448):177–180.

Lessman M. Painful chronicle. Am J Nurs 1985 May; 85(5):551–552.

Lewicki LJ and Leeson MJ. The multisystem impact on physiological processes of inflammatory bowel disease. Nurs Clin North Am 1984 Mar; 19(1):71–80.

Myer SA. Overview of inflammatory bowel disease. Nurs Clin North Am 1984 Mar; 19(1):3–9.

Peppercorn MA. Current status of drug therapy for inflammatory bowel disease. Compr Ther 1985 Dec; 11(12):14–19.

Peppercorn MA et al. Inflammatory bowel disease: Medication for ulcerative colitis and Crohn's disease. Consultant 1985 Nov 30; 25(17): 37–39, 43–45.

Simmons MA. Using the nursing process in treating inflammatory bowel disease. Nurs Clin North Am 1984 Mar; 19(1):11–25.

Sparacino LL. Psychosocial considerations for the adolescent and young adult with inflammatory bowel disease. Nurs Clin North Am 1984 Mar; 19(1):41–49.

Steinberg SE. Zinc deficiency in Crohn's disease. Compr Ther 1985 Dec; 11(12):34–38.

Wright R. Crohn's disease: Diagnosis and management. Compr Ther 1985 Apr; 11(4):38–44.

Ulcerative Colitis

Baille J et al. Systemic complications of inflammatory bowel disease. Geriatrics 1985 Feb; 40(2):53–60.

Buls J and Goldberg S. Surgical options in ulcerative colitis. Postgrad Med 1983 Dec; 74(6):175–188.

Das KM. Pharmacotherapy of inflammatory bowel disease. Part I: Sulfasalazine. Postgrad Med 1983 Dec; 74(6):141–151.

Datta PK. Inflammatory bowel disease and carcinoma. Practitioner 1985 May; 229(1403):465–469.

Farmer RG. Extended management of chronic ulcerative colitis and the problem of carcinoma. Primary Care 1981 June; 8(2):321–323.

Hively-Petillo M. Psychologic factors and inflammatory bowel disease: A review of the literature. J Enterostom Ther 1985 Nov/Dec; 12(6): 214–216.

Horowitz I et al. Diagnosis: Inflammatory bowel disease. Hosp Med 1985 Feb; 21(2):99–109.

Lamont JT and Kandel GP. Toxic megacolon in ulcerative colitis: Early diagnosis and management. Hosp Pract 1986 Sept; 21(9):102A–102Z.

Mayberry JF. Some aspects of the epidemiology of ulcerative colitis. Gut 1985 Mar; 26(9):968–974.

Metz G. Medical management of inflammatory bowel disease. J Enterostom Ther 1984 May/Jun; 11(3):114–115.

Oakley JR et al. Complications and quality of life after ileorectal anastomosis for ulcerative colitis. Am J Surg 1985 Jan; 149(1):23–30.

Rubin DM. New hope for colitis patients . . . a successful colectomy and ileoanal anastomosis. AORN J 1983 Nov; 38(5):783–794.

Simmons MA. Using the nursing process in treating inflammatory bowel disease. Nurs Clin North Am 1984 Mar; 19(1):11–25.

Sparberg M. Ulcerative colitis. Compr Ther 1984 Oct; 10(10):26–35.

Ileostomy, Kock Pouch

Alterescu KB. The ostomy: What about special procedures? Am J Nurs 1985 Dec; 85(12):1363–1367.

Barnett WO. Modified techniques for improving the continent ileostomy. Am J Surg 1984 Feb; 50(2):66–69.

Bush AMH. Conventional ileostomy converted to a Kock continent ileostomy: Social and psychological significance as perceived by two individuals with conversions. J Enterostom Ther 1985 Mar/Apr; 12(2):55–60.

Gouge TH et al. Stoma management: Caring for the colostomy and the ileostomy. Consultant 1983 Feb; 23(2):45–58.

Knobler H et al. Pouch ileitis—recurrence of the inflammatory bowel disease in the ileal reservoir. Am J Gastroenterol 1986 Mar; 81(6): 199–201.

Melzl MT et al. The rodless stoma: An alternative to the conventional loop. J Enterostom Ther 1985 May/June; 12(3):93–98.

Pearl RK. Early local complications from intestinal stomas. Arch Surg 1985 Oct; 120(10):1145–1147.

Rothenberger, DA. Restorative proctocolectomy with ileal reservoir and ileoanastomosis. Am J Surg 1983 Jan; 145(1):82–85.

Schoetz DJ, Coller JA, and Veidenheimer MC. Ileoanal reservoir for ulcerative colitis and familial polyposis. Arch Surg 1986 Apr; 121(4): 404–408.

Taylor BM et al. The endorectal ileal pouch-anal anastomosis. Dis Colon Rectum 1984 June; 27(6):347–350.

Watt RC. The ostomy: Why is it created? Am J Nurs 1985 Nov; 85(11): 1242–1245.

Williams NS and Johnston D. The current status of mucosal proctectomy and ileo-anal anastomosis in the surgical treatment of ulcerative colitis and adenomatous polyposis. Br J Surg 1985 Mar; 72(3):159–168.

Diverticulosis

Gramse CA. Diverticular disease. Nursing '83 1983 June; 13(6):56–57.

Hackford AW and Veidenheimer MC. Diverticular disease of the colon: Current concepts and management. Surg Clin North Am 1985 Apr; 65(2):347–363.

Johnson HC and Block MA. Diverticular disease: Current trends in therapy. Postgrad Med 1985 Sept 1; 78(3):75–79, 82.

Rodkey GV and Welch MD. Changing patterns in the surgical treatment of diverticular disease. Ann Surg 1984 Oct; 200(4):466–478.

Thayer WR et al. Diagnosis and management of irritable bowel syndrome. Compr Ther 1984 Oct; 10(10):20–25.

Colon Cancer

Bristol JB et al. Sugar, fat, and the risk of colorectal cancer. Br Med J 1985 Nov 23; 291(6507):1467–1470.

Burkett DP. Etiology and prevention of colorectal cancer. Hosp Pract 1984 Feb; 19(2):67–77.

Fink DJ. Facts about colorectal cancer detection. CA 1983 Oct; 44(10): 4633–4637.

Garland C et al. Dietary vitamin D and calcium and risk of colorectal cancer: A 19-year prospective study in men. Lancet 1985 Feb 9; 1(8424):307–309.

Gnauck R. Occult-blood screening. Lancet 1986 Feb 22; 1(8478):444.

Khan AH. Colorectal carcinoma: Risk factors, screening, early detection. Geriatrics 1984 Jan; 39(1):42–47.

Kleinman, MS et al. Inflammatory bowel disease and cancer. Hosp Pract 1984 Oct; 19(10):56.

Messner RL. Colorectal cancer screening in the workplace. Occup Health Nurs 1985 Nov; 33(11):561–565.

Messner RL, Gardner SS, and Webb DD. Early detection, the priority in colorectal cancer. Cancer Nurs 1986 Feb; 9(1):8–14.

Messner RL et al. Stop a killer with early detection . . . colorectal cancer. J Gerontol Nurs 1985 Nov; 11(11):8–10, 13–14.

Minton JP. Colon cancer: Special surgical considerations. Cancer 1982 Dec 1: 50(11 suppl):2624–2626.

Moore JR and LaMont JT. Colorectal cancer: Risk factors and screening strategies. Arch Intern Med 1984 Sept; 144(9):1819–1823.

Norflact RG. Stool blood testing for colorectal cancer. Arch Intern Med 1985 May; 145(5):954.

Raina S et al. Changing attitudes toward management of cancer of the colon and rectum. Am Surg 1985 Jan; 51(1):26–30.

Swedberg J et al. Screening for colorectal cancer: The role of the primary physician in improving survival. Postgrad Med 1986 Feb 15; 79(3): 67–71, 74.

Colostomy

Conklin WT et al. A simple technique for securing a loop colostomy. Am Surg 1984 Sept; 50(9):502.

*Frainor MA. Acceptance of ostomy and the visitor role in a self-help group for ostomy patients. Nurs Res 1982 Mar/Apr; 31(2):102–106.

Gebhart EM. Perioperative care of the ostomy patient. AORN J 1982 Aug; 36(2):296–310.

Harocopos CJ. Stoma management: The nursing perspective. Practitioner 1984 Sept; 228(1395):822–823.

McDowell DE. The special needs of the older colostomy patient. J Gerontol Nurs 1983 May; 9(5):294–296.

Penny CJ. There's more to stoma care than the care of stomas. Practitioner 1984 Sept; 228(1395):820–821.

Weakley FL. Cancer of the rectum: A review of surgical options. Surg Clin North Am 1983 Feb; 63(1):129–136.

Agencies

American Cancer Society, 90 Park Avenue, New York, New York 10016.

International Association for Enterostomal Therapy, 505 North Tustin, Suite 219, Santa Ana, California 92705.

National Foundation for Ileitis and Colitis, Inc., Dept N-80, 295 Madison Avenue, New York, New York 10017.

United Ostomy Association, 2001 W. Beverly Blvd., Los Angeles, California 90057.

Nursing Research Profile for Unit VIII

Gastrointestinal Nursing

Overview

Over the last few years nursing research on the gastrointestinal system has been concentrated in the areas of enteral nutrition and ostomy management. Current nursing practice research is concerned with the complications of displacement and pulmonary aspiration encountered with the use of small-bore feeding tubes. Researchers are attemting to define high-risk populations and suggest nursing interventions to prevent these complications. The effectiveness of various methods of oral hygiene, especially for the dependent patient, is also being explored. In addition, several groups of nurse researchers are conducting studies on the psychosocial aspects of patient management for ostomy care. Body image, sexuality, and independence in self-care activities are being studied.

The following studies are representative of some of the significant current nursing research. Although some of the patient populations studied were limited in number, the implications of the studies are significant and can be used as a stimulus for additional research.

Oral Hygiene

▷ Roth PT and Creason NS. Nurse administered oral hygiene: Is there a scientific basis? J Adv Nurs 1986 May; 11(3):323–331.

Roth and Creason identified practices in oral hygiene where nursing intervention is needed. They also critically reviewed relevant nursing research and discussed tools, chemicals, and the frequency of nurse-administered oral hygiene in relation to dental theory.

Nursing researchers studied the significance of frequent brushing and flossing for plaque removal. Firm bristles and horizontal strokes were found to cause gum inflammation and laceration, especially in older people. Studies showed that foamsticks were ineffective in plaque removal, and in one group of 22 subjects, only 20% preferred the foamstick.

Antimicrobial mouthwashes have been accepted as adjuncts to brushing and flossing. However, in one nursing study, the alkaline mouthwash was found to be less effective than hydrogen peroxide. Since recent research indicates that adult dental enamel does incorporate topical fluoride, fluoride-containing toothpastes, classified as dentifrices, are recommended for use.

Studies of lemon and glycerol solutions have failed to show a significant correlation between their use and effective cleansing and moisturizing. Additionally, local dehydrating effects are well documented in the nursing literature.

Studies indicated that the frequency of oral hygiene should be increased when the patient is exposed to dehydrating stressors such as nasal oxygen, mouth-breathing, continuous suctioning, and restricted oral intake of food and fluid. Some research indicates that mouth care given at 4-hour intervals is insufficient to maintain comfort; 2-hour intervals are recommended.

Nursing Implications. Oral hygiene is an effective measure to prevent dental caries and periodontal disease. Patients should be reminded to brush twice daily with a soft-bristled toothbrush and floss after each brushing. This should be done for the patient who is unable to provide his own care. Avoid foamsticks and the use of lemon and glycerol solutions because neither have been shown to be effective. Encourage more frequent brushing for patients who have dehydrating stressors.

Parenteral Nutrition

▷ *Martyn PA, Hansen BC and Kai-Len CJ. The effects of parenteral nutrition on food intake and gastric motility. Nurs Res 1984 Nov/Dec; 33(6):336–342.*

Martyn and co-workers addressed postparenteral nutrition satiety, a condition that frequently causes significant weight loss before the patient can tolerate normal calorie intake. The condition follows a course of parenteral therapy during which most patients report frequent episodes of hunger even when receiving 4000 to 5000 calories a day.

The study was conducted on four healthy rhesus monkeys. Animal subjects were chosen because the researchers could not justify altering levels of parenteral nutrition in patients. The monkeys were fed Ensure through a silastic cannula inserted through the jugular vein into the superior vena cava. Additional oral food was available between 8 AM and 4 PM if the monkeys felt hungry.

Gastric motility was determined by reading pressure recordings on a Beckman dynograph. Readings were recorded for 24 hours on the last day of each parenteral nutrition level, and comparisons were made with feeding patterns and intake. Periodic blood tests (CBC, electrolytes, glucose) were taken to determine parenteral nutrition tolerance.

Two protocols, incremental and cyclic, were followed. The incremental protocol involved progressively increasing calories over 16 days, during which three monkeys received continuous intravenous feedings until 100% of the total needed calories were given. Twenty-five percent of the total calorie intake was administered on days 1 to 4, 50% on days 5 to 8, 75% on days 9 to 12, and 100% on days 13 to 16. These feedings were suddenly stopped on day 17. The cyclic protocol involved three 7-day cycles during which three monkeys were given 100% of their total calories for 7 days, saline for the next 7 days, and then 100% for the last 7 days. For both protocols, the monkeys were allowed to feed freely from a feeder available for 8 hours a day.

During parenteral nutrition, appetite suppression was directly proportional to the amount of calories infused. At 100% parenteral nutrition levels, oral intake was reduced, but the monkeys showed a 3% to 9% gain in body weight, indicating that hunger was present. Research findings also suggested a delay in the beginning of satiety when the nutrition route was changed from oral to intravenous.

After parenteral nutrition, the appetite was suppressed for 8 to 14 days and body weight decreased. Gastric motility patterns indicated that the amplitude of the gastric contractions correlated with the amount of calories delivered. Large-amplitude contractions were minimal during 100% infusions yet present during decreased calorie intake.

Nursing Implications. Patients receiving parenteral nutrition may experience hunger even when 100% of the required calories are being infused. They need to be informed that the feeling of hunger is a normal occurrence with parenteral nutrition and counseled not to take additional calories by mouth. Patients also need to be advised that appetite

suppression can occur following parenteral nutrition and may last for 2 weeks. During this time, methods to improve the appetite should be incorporated into the nursing plan of care. The nursing goal is optimal nutritional balance and desired weight maintenance.

Intubation

▷ *Kacan MJ and Jickisch SM. A comparison of continuous and intermittent enteral nutrition in NICU patients. J Neurosurg Nurs 1986 Dec; 18(6):333–337.*

Kacan and Jickisch's study compared continuous with intermittent tube feedings in neurologically impaired patients to determine whether one method had advantages over the other. The object was to see whether the two methods produced different results in the following areas: stool frequency and consistency, occurrence of aspiration, average gastric residuals, and amount of nursing care time required for skin care and bed changing because of fecal incontinence. The study also investigated whether the patient's level of consciousness (determined by the Glasgow Coma Scale) affected the occurrence of aspiration, and if there was a difference in time required to achieve 100% of caloric needs.

A convenience sample of patients (N = 34) in the neurological intensive care unit (NICU) was studied over a 20-month period. Only those patients who had no previous gastrointestinal pathology and who were receiving tube feedings could be chosen as subjects. Subjects were randomly assigned to group A (9 men, 8 women) or group B (10 men, 7 women). All received Magnacal, an enteral formula that supplies 2 calories/ml, by way of an infusion pump. Continuous feedings (group A) ran over 24 hours at a maximum flow rate of 120 ml/hr and were only interrupted for patient care activities that demanded it. Intermittent feedings (group B) were administered every 4 hours and over a 1-hour period at a maximum rate of 370 ml/hr.

Results indicated no significant differences in the frequency or consistency of stools. There was no significant difference in the incidence of aspiration as determined by the presence of a blue indicator contrast medium in pulmonary secretions. The difference in the incidence of intubation was nonsignificant. The average gastric residual for each group was similar. The amount of nursing time required by each group was similar: 12.6 minutes for group A and 9.3 minutes for group B. There were no correlations between level of consciousness and occurrence of aspiration. There was also no significant correlation in time required to achieve 100% calorie intake; group A required 4.18 days, and group B needed 5.20 days. Calorie requirements were similar. Patients in group A needed a mean of 1882 calories and those in group B needed 2046.

Nursing Implications. Gastrointestinal functioning and nutritional balance are similar whether continuous or intermittent enteral feedings are given. Therefore, physician preference and patient tolerance may be significant criteria in selecting a delivery mode.

▷ *Metheny NA, Spies M and Eisenberg P. Frequency of nasoenteral tube displacement and associated risk factors. Res Nurs Health 1986 Sept; 9(3):241–247.*

Metheny and associates studied risk factors believed to be associated with tube displacement and pulmonary aspiration in 105 patients with nasogastric or nasointestinal feeding tubes. They also studied the frequency of tube displacement.

A descriptive, longitudinal study was conducted on 105 patients over a 6-month period. Of 98 nasogastric tubes studied, the majority were weighted No. 8 French polyurethane (N = 82), and the remainder were No. 12–18 French polyvinyl (N = 16). Of the 115 nasointestinal tubes studied, the majority were unweighted. Weighted tubes had a bolus of mercury or tungsten at the distal tip, whereas unweighted tubes did not have the bolus.

Small-bore feeding tubes became popular during the 1970s because they decreased the incidence of mechanical irritation to the nares, stomach, and duodenum that was seen with large-bore tubes. However, nursing research studies conducted in the early 1980s reported easy dislocation of small-bore feeding tubes, even those with mercury or tungsten weights. The results of this study are noteworthy because 92% of the patients studied had small-bore feeding tubes in place.

Two instruments were developed by the nurse researchers to record the presence of risk factors seen with tube displacement and pulmonary aspiration. Since one third of the tubes were monitored by radiographs, the actual frequency of tube displacement was not known. When spontaneous tube displacement was documented, a comparison of risk factors was determined using chi-square statistics. Risk factors included coughing, retching, vomiting, upper airway intubation, nasotracheal or tracheal suctioning, round-the-clock use of narcotics, failure to maintain elevation of the head of the bed at all times, restlessness, and decreased levels of consciousness.

Data analysis yielded several significant results. For weighted small-bore nasogastric tubes, coughing was a significant risk factor. For unweighted nasointestinal tubes, three risk factors were significant: coughing, upper airway intubation, and the use of tracheal or nasotracheal suctioning. There were no significant risk factors for patients with weighted nasointestinal tubes.

Nursing Implications. Small-bore nasoenteric feeding tubes are used more frequently, and in some cases, to the exclusion of large-bore feeding tubes. Small-bore pliable feeding tubes also dislodge more easily than firm tubes because they do not offer enough resistance to upward movement when risk factors such as coughing, nasotracheal/tracheal suctioning, upper airway intubation, and decreased levels of consciousness are present. Patients with these risk factors need careful monitoring for tube displacement. Radiographic studies should be used to confirm tube placement prior to instilling any feeding.

▷ *Treloar DM and Stechmiller J. Pulmonary aspiration in tube-fed patients with artificial airways. Heart Lung 1984 Nov; 13(6):667–671.*

The purpose of Treloar and Stechmiller's study was to determine whether a significant number of critically ill patients with artificial airways, who were receiving enteral feedings continuously, were aspirating any of the tube feedings. The sample (N = 30) consisted of 20 men and 10 women ranging from 18 to 76 years of age. All had a tracheostomy or endotracheal tube in place and were receiving continuous enteral tube feedings by way of an IMED infusion using a Dobbhoff feeding tube.

Methylene blue dye (1%), one milliliter per 500 ml of tube feeding, was used as an indicator, and the mixture was administered through the IMED volumetric pump. Tracheal suctioning was done at least every 2 hours, which was the standard nursing protocol for the institution where the study was conducted. Aspiration of blue-stained, suctioned, tracheobronchial secretions was considered a positive indicator of pulmonary aspiration.

None of the 30 patients studied evidenced any blue stained secretions. The researchers concluded that the use of the small-bore Dobbhoff enteral feeding tube in critically ill patients with artificial airways is a safe procedure. They felt that the weighted Dobbhoff tube kept its position in the upper small bowel, thus helping to prevent aspiration.

Nursing Implications. Critically ill patients with artificial airways who are receiving continuous enteral feedings are at risk for pulmonary aspiration. Occurrence of aspiration can be decreased or prevented by using small-bore feeding tubes, by verifying proper tube placement with radiographic studies prior to initiating the feeding, and by keeping the patient's head and chest elevated at a 30- to 45-degree angle. Keeping the patient's head and chest elevated during the feeding eliminates gravitational forces that can elevate intragastric pressure and promote regurgitation.

▷ *Gloeckner MR. Perceptions of sexual attractiveness following ostomy surgery. Res Nurs Health 1984 Jun; 7(2):87–92.*

Gloeckner's study was conducted to determine changes in body image perception by exploring a subject's feelings of sexual attractiveness after ostomy surgery. An interview schedule was developed that consisted of 21 questions about information the patient received on sexuality, changes in sexual attractiveness and sexual functioning, and reactions of the sexual partner. The study report was limited to analyzed data on sexual attractiveness.

The interview questions used a Likert-type rating scale from 1 to 5, with 1 indicating the lowest range and 5 the highest. Subjects were asked to indicate periods of time during which certain feelings occurred: (1) 1 year before ostomy surgery, (2) during the year of ostomy surgery, and (3) at the time of interview. All interviews were 60 minutes in length and took place in the subject's home. Attractiveness scores were tabulated for feelings before surgery, 1 year postoperatively, and at the time of interview.

Results indicated that 60% of the subjects (N = 24) experienced a decline in their feelings of sexual attractiveness during the year after surgery. Many subjects used the terms "ugly" or "disfigured" to describe self-perceptions of body image. In comparison to feelings during the first postoperative year, 67.5% (N = 27) experienced an increased sense of sexual attractiveness at the time of interview (mean of 4.6 postoperative years). Only one subject felt less attractive.

The only variable related to feeling and time was gender. Women's feelings of sexual attractiveness tended to increase from the first postoperative year to the time of interview. The type of ostomy surgery had some effect on self-perception of attractiveness, but the difference was not statistically significant. Generally, the subjects who had the highest attractiveness scores were those who had undergone an ileostomy, followed by colostomy patients and those with urinary diversion. Subjects who successfully managed their ostomies felt significantly more attractive than those with management problems. Those subjects who were ill for more than 10 years before surgery evidenced higher attractiveness scores after surgery than those who were not ill preoperatively.

Nursing Implications. The effect of an ostomy on sexuality should be discussed with the patient and his sexual partner if both desire the information. Nurses need to examine their own feelings about sexuality and should attempt not to convey personal values or biases. The patient is encouraged to express his concerns, and counseling is offered if necessary.

▷ *Trainor MA. Acceptance of ostomy and the visitor role in a self-help group for ostomy patients. Nurs Res 1982 Mar/Apr; 31(2):102–106.*

Trainer's study examined whether an ostomate who belonged to the United Ostomy Association (UOA) and served as a visitor demonstrated a greater acceptance of his ostomy than a UOA member who did not serve as a visitor. Extraneous variables that were analyzed were sex, age, type of ostomy, length of time that had elapsed since surgery, education, amount of time the subject served in the visitor role, and the usual number of patients seen by the subject each year.

The instrument used was "The Acceptance of Disability Scale," and the term *ostomy* was substituted for the term *disability*. There were 50 statements that required a response within a 6-point Likert scale that ranged from "I disagree very much" to "I agree very much." Data were collected in three phases over a 9-month period. Volunteers from 25 UOA chapters in the Middle Atlantic region made up the total respondents (N = 318). Fifty-four percent of the subjects (N = 171) were visitors, and 46% (N = 147) were nonvisitors. The majority of subjects had a colostomy (55.2%); 31.8 % had an ileostomy and 11.5% a urinary diversion.

Chi-square analysis showed no significant relationship between ostomy type and visitor/nonvisitor classification. Chi-square analysis also indicated that visitors had more education (p < .05) than nonvisitors and had their ostomy for a longer period of time (p < .001). Seventy-nine percent of the subjects had been working as visitors for 4 years or less.

Analysis of variance indicated that visitors had a significantly higher level of ostomy acceptance than nonvisitors (p < .001). There was a significant correlation between the visitor's ADM score and the amount of time he had been in the visitor role (r = .27, p < .006). The number of years a subject had the ostomy was significant (p < .003) in predicting his participation in a visitor role.

Nursing Implications. Visits from a member of a self-help group (*e.g.*, the United Ostomy Association) can provide support for the patient and also help the visitor cope with accepting his own condition. Social recognition, an improved sense of self-worth, and positive feedback are behavioral reactions experienced by visitors. Nurses should recommend that patients participate in self-help groups whenever possible.

Additional Studies

Cataldi-Betcher E et al. Complications occurring during enteral nutrition support: A prospective study. J Parenter Enter Nutr 1983 Nov/Dec; 7(6):546–552.

Heinz J. Validation of sublingual temperatures in patients with nasogastric tubes. Heart Lung 1985 Mar; 14(2):128–130.

Meguid M, Gray G and Debonis D. The use of enteral nutrition in the patient with cancer. In Rombeau J and Caldwell M (eds). Clinical Nutrition: Enteral and Tube Feeding. Philadelphia, WB Saunders, 1984.

Metheny N, Eisenberg P and Spies M. Monitoring patients with nasally placed feeding tubes (abstract). Heart Lung 1985 May; 14(3):285–286.

Metheny N, Spies M and Eisenberg P. Aspiration pneumonia in patients fed through nasoenteral tubes. Heart Lung 1986 May; 15(3):256–261.

Mims FH and Swenson M. A model to promote sexual health care. Nurs Outlook 1978 Feb; 26(2):121–125.

Moore MC et al. Nutrition-related nursing research. Image 1986 Spring; 18(1):18–21.

Ricci JA. Alcohol-induced upper GI hemorrhage: Case studies and management. Crit Care Nurs 1987 Jan/Feb; 7(1):56–63.

Speedie G. Nursology of mouth care: Preventing, comforting and seeking activities related to mouth care. J Adv Nurs 1983 Jan; 8(1):33–40.

Taylor TT. A comparison of two methods of nasogastric tube feedings. J Neurosurg Nurs 1982 Feb; 14(1):49–54.

Metabolic and Endocrine Problems

Unit IX

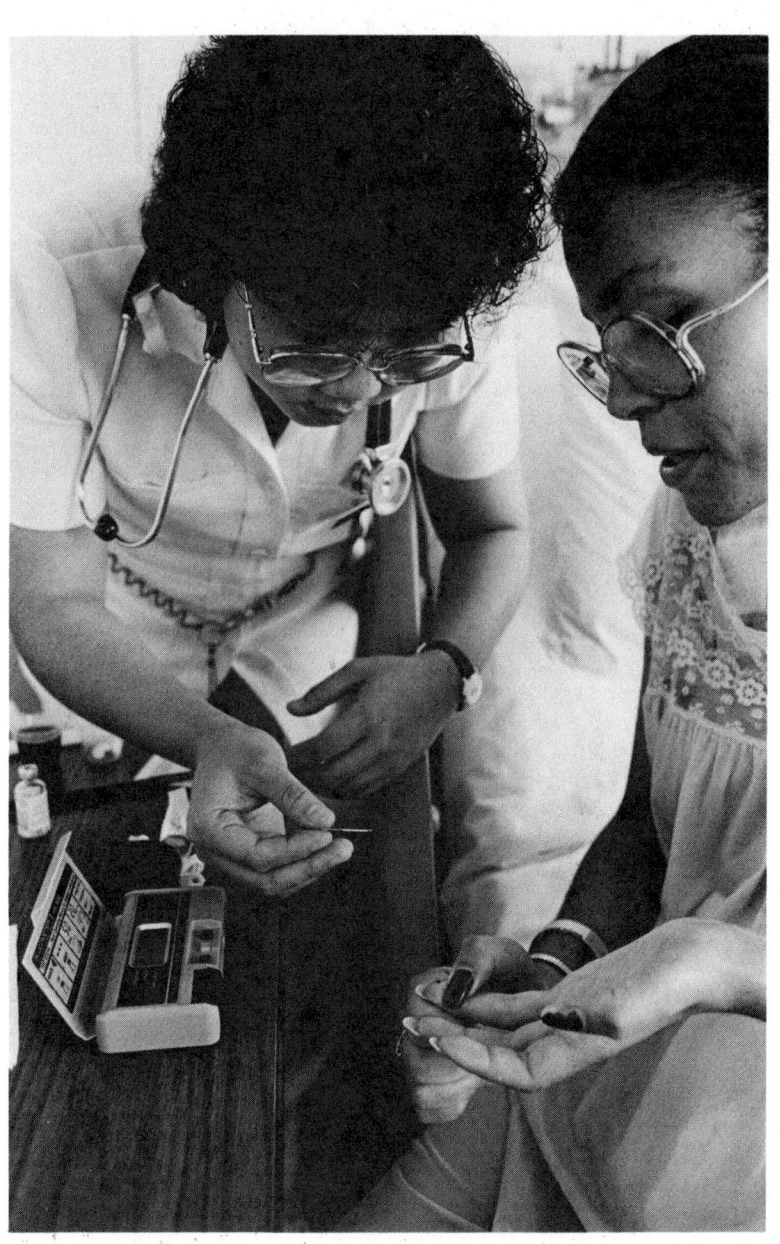

Chapter 35

Assessment and Management of Patients With Hepatic and Biliary Disorders

Physiologic Overview

The liver, the largest gland of the body, can be considered a chemical factory whose job is to manufacture, accumulate, alter, and excrete a large number of substances involved in metabolism. The location of the liver is essential in this function, since it receives nutrient-rich blood directly from the gastrointestinal tract and then either stores or transforms these nutrients into chemicals that are used elsewhere in the body for metabolic needs. The liver's role is especially important in the regulation of glucose and protein metabolism. The liver manufactures and secretes bile, which has a major role in the digestion and absorption of fats in the gastrointestinal tract. It functions as an organ of excretion by removing waste products from the bloodstream and secreting them into the bile. The bile produced by the liver is stored temporarily in the gallbladder until it is needed for the process of digestion, at which time the gallbladder empties and bile enters the intestine.

Anatomy

The liver is located behind the ribs in the upper right portion of the abdominal cavity. It weighs about 1500 gm and is divided into four lobes. Each lobe is surrounded by a thin layer of connective tissue, which extends into the lobe itself and divides the liver mass into small units, called *lobules*. A schematic diagram of the liver and its anatomical relationships is shown in Figure 35-1.

The circulation of the blood into and out of the liver is of major importance in its function. The blood that perfuses the liver is derived from two sources. Approximately 75% of the blood supply comes from the portal vein, which drains the gastrointestinal tract and is rich in nutrients. The remainder of the blood supply enters by way of the hepatic artery and is rich in oxygen. Terminal branches of these two blood supplies join to form common capillary beds, which constitute the sinusoids of the liver. Liver cells (hepatocytes) are thus bathed by a mixture of venous and arterial blood. The sinusoids empty into a venule that occupies the center of each liver lobule and is called the *central vein*. The central veins

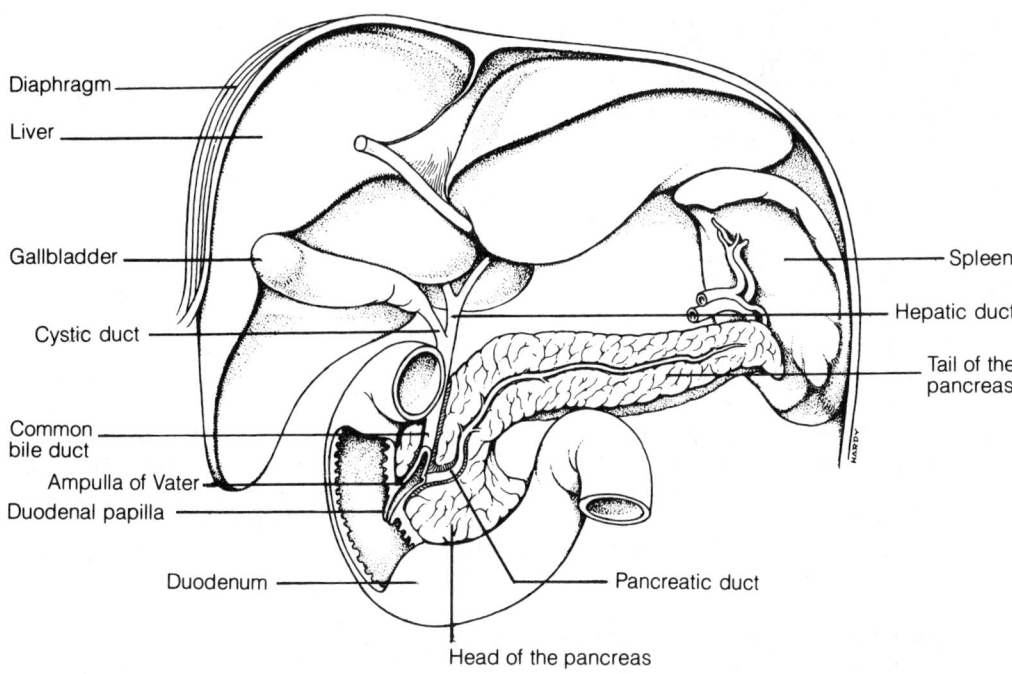

Figure 35-1
Liver and biliary system. (Chaffee EE and Greisheimer EM. Basic Physiology and
Anatomy, 4th ed. Philadelphia, JB Lippincott.)

join to form the hepatic vein, which constitutes the venous drainage from the liver and empties into the inferior vena cava, close to the diaphragm. Thus, there are two sources of blood flowing into the liver but there is only one exit pathway.

In addition to hepatocytes, phagocytic cells belonging to the reticuloendothelial system are present in the liver. Other organs that contain reticuloendothelial cells are the spleen, bone marrow, lymph nodes, and lungs. In the liver, these cells are called *Kupffer cells*. Their main function is to engulf particulate matter such as bacteria that enters the liver through the portal blood.

The smallest bile ducts, called *canaliculi*, are located between the lobules of the liver. These canaliculi receive secretions from the hepatocytes and carry them to larger bile ducts, which eventually form the *hepatic duct*. The hepatic duct from the liver and the cystic duct from the gallbladder join to form the *common bile duct*, which empties into the small intestine. The flow of bile into the intestine is controlled by the sphincter of Oddi, located at the junction where the common bile duct enters the duodenum.

The gallbladder, a pear-shaped, hollow, saclike organ, 7.5 to 10 cm (3 to 4 inches) long, lies in a shallow depression on the inferior surface of the liver, to which it is attached by loose connective tissue. The capacity of the gallbladder is 30 to 50 ml of bile. Its wall is composed largely of smooth muscle. The gallbladder is connected to the common bile duct by the cystic duct.

Metabolic Functions of the Liver

The liver plays a major role in the regulation of blood glucose concentration. After a meal, glucose is taken up from the portal venous blood by the liver and converted into glycogen, which is stored within the hepatocytes. Subsequently, the gly-

cogen is converted back to glucose and released as needed into the bloodstream, in order to maintain normal levels of blood sugar. Additional glucose can be synthesized by the liver through a process called *gluconeogenesis*. For this process, the liver can use amino acids from protein breakdown or lactate produced by exercising muscles.

Use of amino acids for gluconeogenesis results in the formation of ammonia as a by-product. The liver converts this metabolically generated ammonia into urea. Ammonia produced by bacteria in the intestines is also removed from portal blood for urea synthesis. In this way, the liver converts ammonia, a potential toxin, into urea, a harmless compound that can be excreted in the urine.

The liver also plays an important role in protein metabolism. It synthesizes almost all of the plasma proteins (except γ-globulin), including albumin, α-and β-globulins, blood-clotting factors, specific transport proteins, and most of the plasma lipoproteins. Vitamin K is required by the liver for synthesis of prothrombin and some of the other clotting factors. Amino acids serve as the building blocks for protein synthesis.

The liver is also active in fat metabolism. Fatty acids can be broken down for the production of energy and production of ketone bodies (acetoacetic acid, β-hydroxybutyric acid, and acetone). Ketone bodies are small compounds that can enter the bloodstream and provide a source of energy for muscles and other tissues. Breakdown of fatty acids into ketone bodies occurs predominantly when the availability of glucose for metabolism is limited, as during starvation or in diabetic patients. Fatty acids and their metabolic products are also used for the synthesis of cholesterol, lecithin, lipoproteins, and other complex lipids. Under some conditions, lipids may accumulate in the hepatocytes and result in the abnormal condition called fatty liver.

Vitamins A, B_{12}, D, and several of the B complex vitamins are stored in large amounts in the liver. Certain metals, such as iron and copper, are also stored within the liver. Because the liver is rich in these substances, liver extracts have been used for therapy of a wide range of nutritional disorders.

Drug Metabolism

Many drugs, such as barbiturates and amphetamines, are metabolized by the liver. Metabolism generally results in loss of activity of the drug, although in some cases activation may occur. One of the important pathways for drug metabolism involves alteration of the drug by the cytochrome P-450 system. Another pathway of importance involves conjugation (binding) of the drug with a variety of compounds, such as glucuronic or acetic acid, to form more soluble substances. The conjugated products may be excreted in the feces or urine, similar to bilirubin excretion.

Bile

Bile is continuously formed by the hepatocytes and collected in the canaliculi and bile ducts. It is composed mainly of water and electrolytes, such as sodium, potassium, calcium, chloride, and bicarbonate, and also contains significant amounts of lecithin, fatty acids, cholesterol, bilirubin, and bile salts. Bile is collected and stored in the gallbladder and is emptied into the intestine when needed for digestion. The functions of bile are excretory, as in the excretion of bilirubin, and as an aid to digestion through the emulsification of fats by bile salts.

Bile Salts. Bile salts are made by the hepatocytes from cholesterol. After conjugation with amino acids (taurine and glycine), they are excreted into the bile. The bile salts, together with cholesterol and lecithin, are required for emulsification of fats in the intestine. This process is necessary for efficient digestion and absorption. Bile salts are then reabsorbed, primarily in the distal ileum, into portal blood for return to the liver and are again excreted into the bile. This pathway from hepatocytes to bile to intestine and back to the hepatocytes is called the *enterohepatic circulation*. Because of the enterohepatic circulation, only a small fraction of the bile salts that enter the intestine is excreted in the feces. This decreases the demand for active synthesis of bile salts by the liver cells.

Bilirubin Excretion

Bilirubin is a pigment derived from the breakdown of hemoglobin by cells of the reticuloendothelial system, including the Kupffer cells of the liver. Hepatocytes remove bilirubin from the blood and chemically modify it through conjugation to glucuronic acid, which makes the bilirubin more soluble in aqueous solutions. The conjugated bilirubin is secreted by the hepatocytes into the adjacent bile canaliculi and is eventually carried in the bile into the duodenum. In the small intestine, bilirubin is converted into urobilinogen, which is in part excreted in the feces and in part absorbed through the intestinal mucosa into the portal blood. Much of this reabsorbed urobilinogen is removed by the hepatocytes and is secreted into the bile once again (enterohepatic circulation). Some of the urobilinogen enters the systemic circulation and is excreted by the kidneys in the urine. Elimination of bilirubin in the bile represents the major route of excretion for this compound. The bilirubin concentration in the blood may be increased either in the presence of liver disease or when the flow of bile is impeded (*e.g.*, with gallstones in the bile ducts). With bile duct obstruction, bilirubin does not enter the intestine and, as a consequence, urobilinogen will be absent from the urine.

Gallbladder

The gallbladder functions as a storage depot for bile. Between meals, when the sphincter of Oddi is closed, bile produced by the hepatocytes enters the gallbladder. During storage, a large portion of the water in bile is absorbed through the walls of the gallbladder, so that gallbladder bile is five to ten times more concentrated than that originally secreted by the liver. When food enters the duodenum, the gallbladder contracts, and the sphincter of Oddi relaxes, allowing the bile to enter the intestine. This response is mediated by secretion of the hormone cholecystokinin-pancreozymin (CCK-PZ) from the intestinal wall.

Pathophysiology

Liver dysfunction results from damage to the liver parenchymal cells, either directly, from primary liver diseases, or indirectly, due to obstruction to bile flow or to derangements of hepatic circulation.

Disease processes that lead to hepatocellular dysfunction may be caused by infectious agents, such as bacteria and viruses, and by anoxia, metabolic disorders, toxins and drugs, nutritional deficiencies, and states of hypersensitivity. Probably the most common cause of parenchymal damage is malnutrition, especially in alcoholism. The response of the parenchymal cells is much the same for most noxious agents: replacement of glycogen by lipids, producing fatty infiltration, with or without cell death or necrosis. This is commonly associated with inflammatory cell infiltration and growth of fibrous tissue. Cell regeneration can occur if the disease process is not too toxic to the cells. The end result of chronic parenchymal disease is the shrunken, fibrotic liver seen in cirrhosis.

Hepatocellular dysfunction is manifested by alteration of the metabolic and excretory functions of the liver. Serum bilirubin concentration rises, leading to jaundice or yellowing of the skin; this results from intrahepatic obstruction of bile channels. Abnormalities of carbohydrate, fat, and protein metabolism occur with liver dysfunction. Abnormal protein metabolism results in decreased serum albumin concentration and edema. Ammonia, a by-product of metabolism, is absorbed from the gastrointestinal tract but is not converted to urea by the damaged liver cells. An increased serum ammonia level may produce signs of central nervous system impairment.

The vascular architecture of the liver may be disturbed, causing increased portal vein blood pressure, which results in leakage of fluid into the peritoneal cavity, or ascites, and esophageal varices. The lack of normal production of various blood-clotting factors can lead to bleeding from any site, but the patient is particularly prone to gastrointestinal bleeding.

Many endocrine abnormalities also occur with liver dysfunction as a result of the inability of the liver to metabolize hormones normally, including androgens or sex hormones. Although the exact mechanisms for their appearance are not well established, gynecomastia, amenorrhea, testicular atrophy, and other disturbances of sexual function and sex characteristics are thought to result from failure of the damaged liver to normally inactivate estrogens.

Acute liver damage may cause acute liver failure, may be completely reversible, or may progress to chronic disease. The end result of chronic liver damage is cirrhosis, characterized by replacement of parenchymal cells with fibrotic tissue. Liver failure is present when the ability of the liver to carry out its excretory and metabolic functions falls below the needs of the body. Hepatic coma results when liver dysfunction is so severe that the liver is unable to remove end products of metabolism from the bloodstream.

Gerontological Considerations

The most frequently observed change in the liver in the elderly is a decrease in the size and weight of the liver accompanied by a decrease in total hepatic blood flow. In general, however, these decreases are in proportion to the decreases in body size and weight seen in normal aging. Results of liver function tests do not normally change in the elderly; abnormal results in an elderly patient indicate abnormal liver function and are not the result of the aging process itself.

The immune system is altered in the aged, and a less responsive immune system may be responsible for the increased incidence and severity of hepatitis B in the elderly and the increased incidence of liver abscesses secondary to decreased phagocytosis by the Kupffer cells.

Drug metabolism by the liver appears to be decreased in the elderly, but such changes are usually also accompanied by changes in intestinal absorption, renal excretion, and altered body distribution of some drugs secondary to changes in fat deposition. These alterations necessitate careful administration of all medications with reduction of dosage to prevent drug toxicity.

Diagnostic Evaluation of Hepatic Function

Liver Function Tests. Over 70% of the parenchyma of the liver may be damaged before liver function tests become abnormal. Function is generally measured in terms of serum enzyme activity (*e.g.,* alkaline phosphatase, transaminases, lactic dehydrogenase), clearance of indocyanine green (ICG) or sulfobromophthalein (Bromsulphalein or BSP), and serum concentrations of proteins, bilirubin, ammonia, clotting factors, and lipids. Several of these tests may be helpful for assessment of patients with liver disease; however, the nature and extent of hepatic dysfunction cannot be determined by these tests alone. Many other disorders can influence their results; therefore, the tests are not sensitive indicators of liver dysfunction. A list of the commonly used liver function tests is shown in Table 35-1.

Examination of the Liver. The liver may be palpable in the right upper quadrant. A palpable liver presents as a firm, sharp ridge with a smooth surface (Fig 35-2, p. 860). The size of the liver is estimated by percussion of the liver's upper and lower borders. When the liver is not palpable, but tenderness is suspected, tapping the lower right thorax briskly may elicit tenderness. The patient's response is then compared by performing a similar maneuver on the left lower thorax.

If the liver is palpable, the examiner notes and records its size, consistency, whether it is tender, and whether its outline is regular or irregular. If the liver is enlarged, the degree to which it descends below the right costal margin is recorded to provide some indication of its size. The liver of a patient with cirrhosis is small and hard, while the liver of a patient with acute hepatitis is quite soft and the edge is easily moved by the hand. Tenderness of the liver implies recent acute enlargement with consequent stretching of the liver capsule. The absence of tenderness may imply that the enlargement is of long standing. The liver of a patient with viral hepatitis is tender, while that of a patient with alcoholic hepatitis is not. The examiner determines if the liver edge is sharp and smooth or blunt and if the enlarged liver is nodular or smooth. Enlargement of the liver is an abnormal finding requiring further evaluation.

Liver Biopsy. A procedure that greatly facilitates the diagnosis of most hepatic disorders is the liver biopsy (*i.e.,* the sampling of liver tissue by needle aspiration for the purpose of histologic study). Nursing responsibilities in relation to liver biopsy and the rationale of the nurse's participation in this procedure are summarized in Chart 35-1 (p. 860). A graphic presentation is found in Figure 35-3 (p. 861).

Clinical Manifestations of Hepatic Dysfunction

The complications of liver disease are numerous and varied. In many instances their ultimate effects are incapacitating or lethal; their presence is ominous, and their treatment is notoriously difficult.

Among the most frequent and important of these complications are the following:

- Jaundice, resulting from increased bilirubin concentration in the blood
- Portal hypertension and ascites, resulting from circulatory changes within the diseased liver and producing severe gastrointestinal hemorrhages and excessive sodium and water retention
- Nutritional deficiencies, attributable to the inability of the malfunctioning liver cells to metabolize certain vitamins, and responsible for impaired central and peripheral nervous systems and abnormal bleeding tendencies
- Hepatic coma, reflecting the incomplete metabolism of protein by the diseased liver

Nursing care of the patient with impaired liver function is summarized in Nursing Care Plan 35-1, pages 862–863.

Jaundice

When, for any reason, the bilirubin concentration in the blood becomes abnormally increased, all the body tissue, including the sclerae and the skin, becomes tinged yellow or greenish yellow. This condition is called *jaundice*. There are several types of jaundice: (1) hemolytic, (2) hepatocellular, (3) obstructive, and (4) jaundice due to hereditary hyperbilirubinemia. Hepatocellular and obstructive jaundice are the two types commonly associated with liver disease.

TABLE 35-1
Liver Function Studies

Test	Normal	Clinical Functions
Pigment Studies		
Serum bilirubin, direct	0–0.3 mg/dl (0–5.1 μmol/L)	These studies measure the ability of liver to conjugate and excrete bilirubin. Results are abnormal in liver and biliary tract disease and are associated with jaundice clinically.
Serum bilirubin, total	0–0.9 mg/dl (1.7–20.5 μmol/L)	
Urine bilirubin	0 (0)	
Urine urobilinogen	0.05–2.5 mg/24 hr (0.09–4.23 μmol/24 hr)	
Fecal urobilinogen (infrequently used)	40–200 mg/24 hr (0.068–0.34 mmol/24 hr)	
Dye Clearances		
Indocyanine green	500–800 ml/M^2/min	Dye is extracted from blood and excreted by liver; its clearance depends on hepatic blood flow, functioning liver cells, and lack of obstruction. It is replacing the BSP test because of its fewer side-effects.
Bromsulphalein excretion (BSP test)	<5% Retention 45 minutes after dye injection fraction retention: <0.05 at 45 minutes after dye injection)	BSP binds to albumin in blood. Liver cells unbind BSP, conjugate it, and excrete it in bile. Normal clearance depends on hepatic blood flow, functioning liver cell mass, and lack of obstruction. Retention is increased in liver cell damage or decreased liver blood flow.
Protein Studies		
Total serum protein	7.0–7.5 gm/dl (70–75 g/L)	Proteins are manufactured by the liver. Their levels may be affected in a variety of liver impairments.
Serum albumin	3.5–5.5 (35–55 g/L)	
Serum globulin	1.5–3.0 gm/dl (15–30 g/L)	Albumin (cirrhosis, chronic hepatitis, edema, ascites)
Serum protein electrophoresis	3.2–5.6 m/dl (32–56 g/L)	
Albumin		Globulin (Cirrhosis, liver disease, chronic obstructive jaundice, viral hepatitis)
α_1-Globulin	0.1–0.4 gm/dl (1–4 g/L)	
α_2-Globulin	0.4–1.2 gm/dl (4–12 g/L)	
β-Globulin	0.5–1.1 gm/dl (5–11 g/L)	
γ-Globulin	0.5–1.6 gm/dl (5–16 g/L)	
Albumin/globulin (A/G) ratio	A > G or 1.5:1–2.5:1	A/G ratio is reversed in chronic liver disease (decreased albumin and increased globulin)
Prothrombin Time		
Response of prothrombin time to vitamin K	100% return to normal	Prothrombin time may be prolonged in liver disease. It will not return to normal with vitamin K in severe liver cell damage.
Serum Alkaline Phosphatase	Varies with method: 2–5 Bodansky units 20–90 IU/liter at 30° (20–90 U/L at 30°)	Serum alkaline phosphatase is manufactured in bones, liver, kidneys, and intestine and excreted through biliary tract. In absence of bone disease, it is a sensitive measure of biliary tract obstruction.

(continued)

TABLE 35-1 (continued)

Test	Normal	Clinical Functions
Serum Transaminase Studies		
SGOT or AST	10–40 units (4.8–19 U/L)	The studies are based on release of enzymes from damaged liver cells. These enzymes are elevated in liver cell damage.
SGPT or ALT	5–35 units (2.4–17 U/L)	
LDH	165–400 units (80–192 U/L)	
Blood Ammonia	20–120 μg/dl (11.1–67.0 μmol/L)	Liver converts ammonia to urea. Ammonia level rises in liver failure.
Cholesterol		
Ester	150–250 mg/dl (3.90–6.50 mmol/L)	Cholesterol levels are elevated in biliary obstruction and decreased in parenchymal liver disease.
	60% of total (fraction of total cholesterol: 0.60)	

Additional Studies	Clinical Functions
Radiologic Studies	
Barium study of esophagus	For varices, which indicate increased portal pressure
Plain film of abdomen	To determine gross liver size
Liver scan with radio-tagged iodinated rose bengal, gold, or technetium	To show size and shape of liver; to show replacement of liver tissue with scars, cysts, or tumor
Cholecystogram and cholangiogram	For gallbladder and bile duct visualization
Celiac axis arteriography	For liver and pancreas visualization
Splenoportogram (splenic portal venography)	To determine adequacy of portal blood flow
Peritoneoscopy or Laparoscopy	Direct visualization of anterior surface of liver, gallbladder, and mesentery through a trocar
Liver Biopsy	To determine anatomical changes in liver tissue
Measurement of Portal Pressure	Elevated in cirrhosis of the liver
Esophagoscopy/Endoscopy	To search for esophageal varices and abnormalities
Electroencephalogram	Abnormal in hepatic coma and impending hepatic coma
Ultrasonography	To show size of abdominal organs and presence of masses
Computed Tomography (CT scan)	To detect hepatic neoplasms; diagnose cysts, abscesses, and hematomas; and distinguish between obstructive and nonobstructive jaundice
Angiography	Visualizes hepatic circulation and detects presence and nature of hepatic masses

Hemolytic Jaundice. Hemolytic jaundice is the result of an increased destruction of the red blood cells, the effect of which is to flood the plasma with bilirubin so rapidly that the liver, although functioning normally, cannot excrete the bilirubin as quickly as it is formed. This type of jaundice is encountered in patients with hemolytic transfusion reactions and other hemolytic disorders. The bilirubin in the blood of these patients is predominantly of the unconjugated, or "free," type. Fecal and urine urobilinogen are increased; on the other hand, the urine is free of bilirubin. Patients with this type of jaundice, unless their hyperbilirubinemia is extreme, do not experience symptoms or complications as a result of the jaundice *per se*. However, very prolonged jaundice, even if mild, predisposes to the formation of "pigment stones" in the gallbladder, and extremely severe jaundice (*e.g.*, in patients with levels of free bilirubin above 20 to 25 mg/dl) is attended by a definite risk of possible brain stem damage.

Hepatocellular Jaundice. Hepatocellular jaundice is caused by the inability of diseased liver cells to clear normal amounts of bilirubin from the blood. The cellular damage

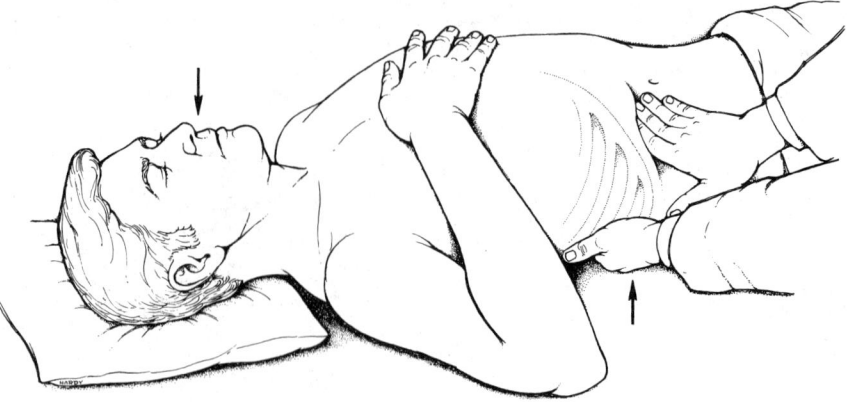

Figure 35-2
Technique for palpation of the liver. As the patient inhales, a palpable liver edge will descend to meet the index finger of the right hand. At the height of inspiration, the examiner releases the pressure of the right hand slightly and tries to feel the liver edge "slip" under the fingertips.

Chart 35-1
Liver Biopsy and the Role of the Nurse

Nursing Activities	*Rationale*
1. Ascertain in advance that hemostasis tests have been requisitioned, completed, and reported and that compatible donor blood is available.	Many patients with liver disease have clotting defects and are prone to bleed abnormally.
2. Measure and record the patient's pulse, respirations, and arterial pressure immediately prior to biopsy.	Prebiopsy values provide a basis on which to compare the patient's vital signs and evaluate his status following the procedure.
3. Describe to the patient in advance: • Steps of the procedure • Sensations expected • Aftereffects anticipated • Restrictions of activity to be imposed afterward	Explanations serve to allay his fears and ensure his cooperation.
4. Give support to the patient during the procedure.	The presence of an understanding nurse enhances comfort and promotes a sense of security.
5. Expose the right side of the patient's upper abdomen (right hypochondriac).	The skin at the site of penetration will be cleansed and infiltrated with local anesthetic.
6. Instruct the patient to inhale and exhale deeply several times, finally to exhale, and to hold his breath at the end of expiration (see Fig. 39-2). • The physician promptly introduces the biopsy needle by way of the transthoracic (intercostal) or transabdominal (subcostal) route, penetrates the liver, aspirates and withdraws. The entire procedure is completed within 5 to 10 seconds.	Holding the breath immobilizes the chest wall and the diaphragm; penetration of the diaphragm thereby is avoided, and the risk of lacerating the liver is minimized.
7. Instruct the patient to resume breathing.	
8. Immediately following the biopsy, assist the patient to turn on his right side; place a pillow under his costal margin, and caution him to remain in this position, recumbent and immobile, for several hours.	In this position, the liver capsule at the site of penetration is compressed against the chest wall, and the escape of blood or bile through the perforation is impeded.
9. Measure and record the patient's pulse and respiratory rates and his arterial pressure at 10- to 20-minute intervals for the prescribed period of time, or until his status proves to be stable, and his condition is satisfactory. Be alert to and report promptly any increase in pulse rate or any decrease in arterial pressure, any complaint of pain or manifestations of apprehension.	These signs may indicate the presence and the progress of hepatic bleeding, severe hemorrhage, or bile peritonitis, the most frequent complications of liver biopsy.

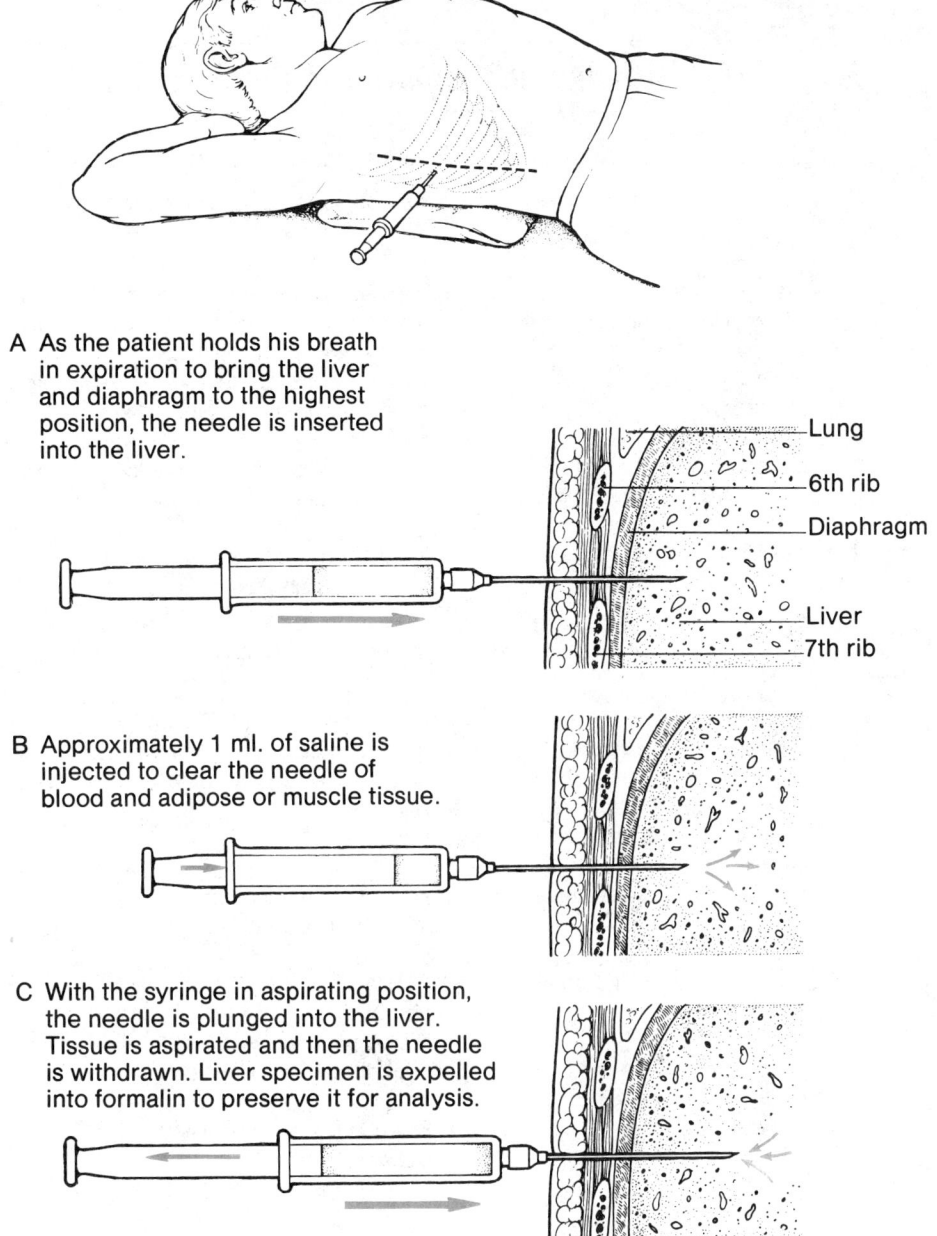

A As the patient holds his breath
in expiration to bring the liver
and diaphragm to the highest
position, the needle is inserted
into the liver.

Lung
6th rib
Diaphragm
Liver
7th rib

B Approximately 1 ml. of saline is
injected to clear the needle of
blood and adipose or muscle tissue.

C With the syringe in aspirating position,
the needle is plunged into the liver.
Tissue is aspirated and then the needle
is withdrawn. Liver specimen is expelled
into formalin to preserve it for analysis.

Figure 35-3
Technique of liver biopsy.

may be from infection, such as in hepatitis A, hepatitis B, non-A, non-B hepatitis (from virus-infected blood transfusion), or yellow fever virus, or from drug or chemical toxicity (*e.g.*, carbon tetrachloride, chloroform, phosphorus, arsenicals, certain psychotherapeutic drugs, or ethanol).

Cirrhosis of the liver is a form of hepatocellular disease that may produce jaundice; it is usually associated with excessive alcoholic intake. It may be a late result of liver cell necrosis caused by viral infection. In prolonged obstructive jaundice, cell damage eventually develops, so that both types appear together.

Clinical Manifestations. Patients with hepatocellular jaundice may be mildly or severely ill, with lack of appetite, nausea, loss of vigor and strength, and possible weight loss. In some instances of hepatocellular disease there may be no jaundice clinically. However, the serum bilirubin concentration and urine urobilinogen level may be elevated. In addition, levels of serum glutamic oxaloacetic transaminase (SGOT)

and serum glutamic pyruvic transaminase (SGPT)* may be increased, indicating cellular necrosis. At onset there may be complaints of headache, chills, and fever, if the cause is infectious. Depending on the cause and extent of the liver cell damage, hepatocellular jaundice may or may not be completely reversible.

Obstructive Jaundice. Obstructive jaundice of the extrahepatic type may be caused by the bile duct's being plugged by a gallstone, by an inflammatory process, by a tumor, or by pressure from an enlarged gland. The obstruction may also involve the small bile ducts within the liver substance (*i.e.*, intrahepatic obstruction), caused, for example, by pressure on these channels from inflammatory swelling of the liver substance or by an inflammatory exudate within the ducts themselves. Intrahepatic obstruction due to stasis and inspis-

(Text continues on p. 864)

---

* Aspartate aminotransferase (AST) and alanine aminotransferase (ALT)

Care of the Patient With Impaired Liver Function

Nursing Interventions	Rationale	Expected Outcomes

Nursing Diagnosis: Activity intolerance related to fatigue, lethargy, and malaise

Goal: Increased activity tolerance

1. Assess level of activity tolerance and degree of fatigue, lethargy, and malaise.	1. Provides baseline for further assessment and criteria for assessment of effectiveness of interventions.	• Exhibits increased interest in activities and events.
2. Assist with activities and hygiene when fatigued.	2. Promotes some exercise and hygiene within patient's level of tolerance.	• Participates in activities and gradually increasing exercise within physical limits.
3. Encourage rest when fatigued or when abdominal pain or discomfort occurs.	3. Conserves energy and protects the liver.	• Reports increased strength and well-being.
4. Assist with selection of desired activities and exercise.	4. Stimulates patient's interest in activities of interest to him.	• Reports absence of abdominal pain and discomfort.

Nursing Diagnosis: Alterations in nutrition related to abdominal distention and discomfort and anorexia

Goal: Improved nutritional status

1. Assess dietary intake and nutritional status through diet history and diary, daily weight measurements, laboratory data, and anthropometric assessment.	1. Identifies deficits in nutritional intake and adequacy of nutritional state.	• Exhibits improved nutritional status by increased weight (without fluid retention), improved laboratory data and anthropometric measurements.
2. Provide diet high in carbohydrates with protein intake consistent with liver function.	2. Provides calories for energy, "sparing" protein for healing.	• States rationale for dietary modifications.
3. Elevate the head of the bed during patient's meals.	3. Reduces discomfort from abdominal distention and decreases sense of fullness produced by pressure of abdominal contents and ascites on the stomach.	• Identifies foods high in carbohydrates and within protein requirements (high in cirrhosis and hepatitis, low in hepatic failure).
4. Provide oral hygiene before meals and pleasant environment for meals at meal time.	4. Promotes positive environment and increased appetite.	• Reports improved appetite.

Nursing Diagnosis: Potential impaired skin integrity related to jaundice and edema

Goal: Improved skin integrity

1. Assess degree of discomfort related to pruritus and edema experienced by patient.	1. Assists in determining appropriate strategies.	• Exhibits intact skin without redness, excoriation, or breakdown.
2. Note and record degree of jaundice and extent of edema.	2. Provides baseline for detecting changes and evaluating effectiveness of interventions.	• Reports relief of pruritis. • Exhibits no skin excoriation from scratching.
3. Keep patient's fingernails short and smooth.	3. Prevents skin excoriation and infection from scratching.	• Uses nondrying soaps and lotions. States rationale for use of nondrying soaps and lotions.
4. Provide frequent skin care avoiding use of soaps and alcohol-based lotions.	4. Removes waste products deposited in skin while preventing dryness of skin.	• Turns self periodically. Exhibits reduced edema of dependent parts of the body.
5. Massage bony prominences and turn frequently.	5. Minimizes prolonged pressure on bony prominences susceptible to breakdown and promotes mobilization of edema.	

(continued)

Nursing Interventions	*Rationale*	*Expected Outcomes*

Nursing Diagnosis: Potential injury related to altered clotting mechanisms and altered level of consciousness

Goal: Reduced risk of injury

1. Assess level of consciousness and cognitive level.	1. Assists in predicting patient's ability to protect self and comply with required self-protective actions; may detect deterioration of hepatic function.	• Is oriented to time, place, and person. • Exhibits no ecchymoses (bruises), cuts, or hematoma. • Exhibits no hallucinations, and demonstrates no efforts to get up unassisted or to leave hospital.
2. Provide safe environment (pad side rails, remove obstacles in room, prevent falls).	2. Minimizes falls and accidents and damage if falls occur.	
3. Provide frequent surveillance to orient patient and minimize use of restraints.	3. Protects patient from harm while stimulating and orienting patient; minimizes use of restraints, which may disturb patient further.	

Nursing Diagnosis: Altered body image related to changes in appearance, sexual dysfunction, and role function

Goal: Improvement of body image and self-esteem

1. Assess changes in appearance and the meaning these changes have for patient and family.	1. Provides information for assessing impact of changes in appearance, sexual function, and role on the patient and his significant other.	• Verbalizes concerns related to changes in appearance, life, and life-style. • Shares concerns with significant others. • Identifies past coping strategies that have been effective. • Uses past effective coping strategies to deal with changes in appearance, life, and life-style. • Maintains good grooming and hygiene. • Identifies short-term goals and strategies to achieve them. • Exercises an active role in decision making about self and care. • Identifies resources that are not harmful. • Verbalizes that some of previous life-style practices have been harmful. • Uses healthy expressions of frustration, anger, etc.
2. Encourage patient to verbalize his reactions and feelings about these changes.	2. Enables patient to identify and express concerns; encourages patient and significant others to share these concerns.	
3. Assess patient's and significant other's previous coping strategies.	3. Permits encouragement of those coping strategies that are familiar to patient and have been effective in the past.	
4. Assist and encourage patient to maximize appearance and explore alternatives to previous sexual and role functions.	4. Encourages patient not to abandon those roles and functions that may return with appropriate treatment while encouraging exploration of alternatives.	
5. Assist patient in identifying short-term goals.	5. Accomplishing these goals serves as positive reinforcement and increases self-esteem.	
6. Encourage and assist patient in decision making about care.	6. Promotes patient's taking control of life and improves sense of well-being and self-esteem.	
7. Identify with patient resources to provide additional support (counselor, clergy).	7. Assists patient in identifying resources and accepting assistance from others when indicated.	
8. Assist patient in identifying previous practices that may have been harmful to self (alcohol and drug abuse).	8. Recognition and admission of the harmful effects of these practices is necessary for identifying a more healthy life-style.	

sation of bile within the canaliculi is an occasional occurrence, following the ingestion of certain drugs, which accordingly are referred to as "cholestatic" agents. These include phenothiazines, antithyroid medications, sulfonylureas, tricyclic antidepressants, and nitrofurantoin.

Clinical Manifestations. Whether the obstruction is intrahepatic or extrahepatic, and whatever its cause may be, if bile cannot flow normally into the intestine, but is dammed back in the liver substance, it is reabsorbed into the blood and carried throughout the entire body, staining the skin, the mucous membranes, and the sclerae. It is excreted in the urine, which becomes deep orange and foamy. Because of the decreased amount of bile in the intestinal tract, the stools become light or clay-colored. The skin may itch intensely, requiring repeated starch or oil baths. Dyspepsia, and especially an intolerance to fatty foods, may develop temporarily, owing to impairment of fat digestion in the absence of intestinal bile. Here the SGOT and SGPT levels rise only moderately, but the bilirubin and alkaline phosphatase levels are elevated.

Hereditary Hyperbilirubinemia. Increased serum bilirubin levels (hyperbilirubinemia) due to several inherited disorders can also produce jaundice. *Gilbert's syndrome* is a familial disorder that is due to a diminution of glucuronyl transferase and an increased unconjugated bilirubin level that causes jaundice. Although serum bilirubin levels are increased, liver histology and liver function test results are normal, and there is no hemolysis. Other conditions that are probably caused by inborn errors of biliary metabolism include *Dubin-Johnson syndrome* (chronic idiopathic jaundice, with pigment in the liver) and *Rotor's syndrome* (chronic familial conjugated hyperbilirubinemia without pigment in the liver); "benign" cholestatic jaundice of pregnancy, with retention of conjugated bilirubin, probably secondary to unusual sensitivity to the hormones of pregnancy; and probably also benign recurrent intrahepatic cholestasis.

Portal Hypertension and Ascites

One set of problems associated with hepatic cirrhosis arises as a result of obstruction to the flow of portal venous blood through the liver, the effect of which is to elevate the blood pressure throughout the entire portal venous system. Although portal hypertension is commonly associated with hepatic cirrhosis, it can also occur with noncirrhotic liver disease.

There are two major sequelae of portal hypertension:

1. The formation of esophageal, gastric, and hemorrhoidal varicosities occurs because of the elevated pressures transmitted to all of the veins that drain into the portal system. These varicosities are prone to rupture and often are the source of massive hemorrhages from the upper gastrointestinal tract and the rectum (see p. 882). The likelihood of bleeding is increased by the blood clotting abnormalities frequently present in patients with cirrhosis.
2. The second important manifestation of portal hypertension is accumulation of fluid (ascites) in the abdominal cavity. As ascites develops, intravascular volume tends to fall and renin is released by the kidneys. This results in secretion of increased quantities of the hormone aldosterone by the adrenal glands, which, in turn, causes the kidneys to retain sodium and water in

an attempt to return intravascular volume to normal. Unfortunately, if portal hypertension continues, fluid retention will contribute to the formation of even more ascites.

Assessment

The presence and extent of ascites can be determined by percussing the abdomen. When fluid has accumulated in the peritoneal cavity, the flanks will bulge when the patient assumes a supine position. The presence of fluid accumulation can be confirmed either by percussing for shifting dullness (Fig. 35-4*A, B*) or by detecting a fluid wave (Fig. 35-4*C*). A fluid wave is likely to be found only when there is a large amount of fluid present. Daily measurement and recording of abdominal girth and body weight are indicated to assess the progression of ascites and its response to treatment. The role of dietary modification, drug therapy, paracentesis, and shunting in controlling ascites is discussed below.

Controlling Fluid Retention and Ascites

Nutritional Control. The goal of treatment for the patient with ascites is a negative sodium balance to reduce fluid retention. Table salt, salty foods, salted butter and margarine, and all the ordinary canned and frozen foods should be avoided. The taste of unsalted foods can be improved by using salt substitutes, such as lemon juice, oregano, and thyme. Commercial substitutes need to be cleared with the physician; for example, those containing ammonia could precipitate hepatic coma. Liberal use should be made of powdered, low-sodium milk and milk products. If fluid accumulation is not controlled on this regimen, the salt restriction must be more stringent, with the daily sodium allowance reduced to 200 mg, and diuretics administered.

Diuretics. Another method of reducing edema and ascites is to induce diuresis. This involves the reduction of sodium intake to 9 to 22 mEq (200–500 mg) daily; restriction of fluids, if the serum sodium is low; and administration of an oral diuretic drug such as chlorothiazide (Diuril). Spironolactone (Aldactone), an aldosterone-blocking agent, also may be administered to supplement the action of these diuretics and to help prevent undue potassium loss. If these medications fail, it may be necessary to use a more potent diuretic, such as furosemide (Lasix). Beyond this, ethacrynic acid (Edecrin) may be prescribed. These latter diuretic medications are used cautiously, since with long-term use they may induce severe sodium depletion (hyponatremia). Ammonium chloride and acetazolamide (Diamox) are contraindicated because of the possibility of precipitating hepatic coma. Daily weight loss should not exceed 0.227 kg (or less than ½ lb) daily.

Diuretic therapy is carefully monitored by the nurse to detect possible complications: fluid and electrolyte disturbances and encephalopathy. Possible fluid and electrolyte problems include hypovolemia, hypokalemia, hyponatremia, and hypochloremic alkalosis. Encephalopathy may be precipitated by dehydration and hypovolemia. Additionally, when potassium stores are depleted, the amount of ammonia in the systemic circulation increases, which may cause impaired cerebral functioning and encephalopathy. Careful intake and output documentation, daily assessment of abdominal girth, and daily weighing of the patient are required.

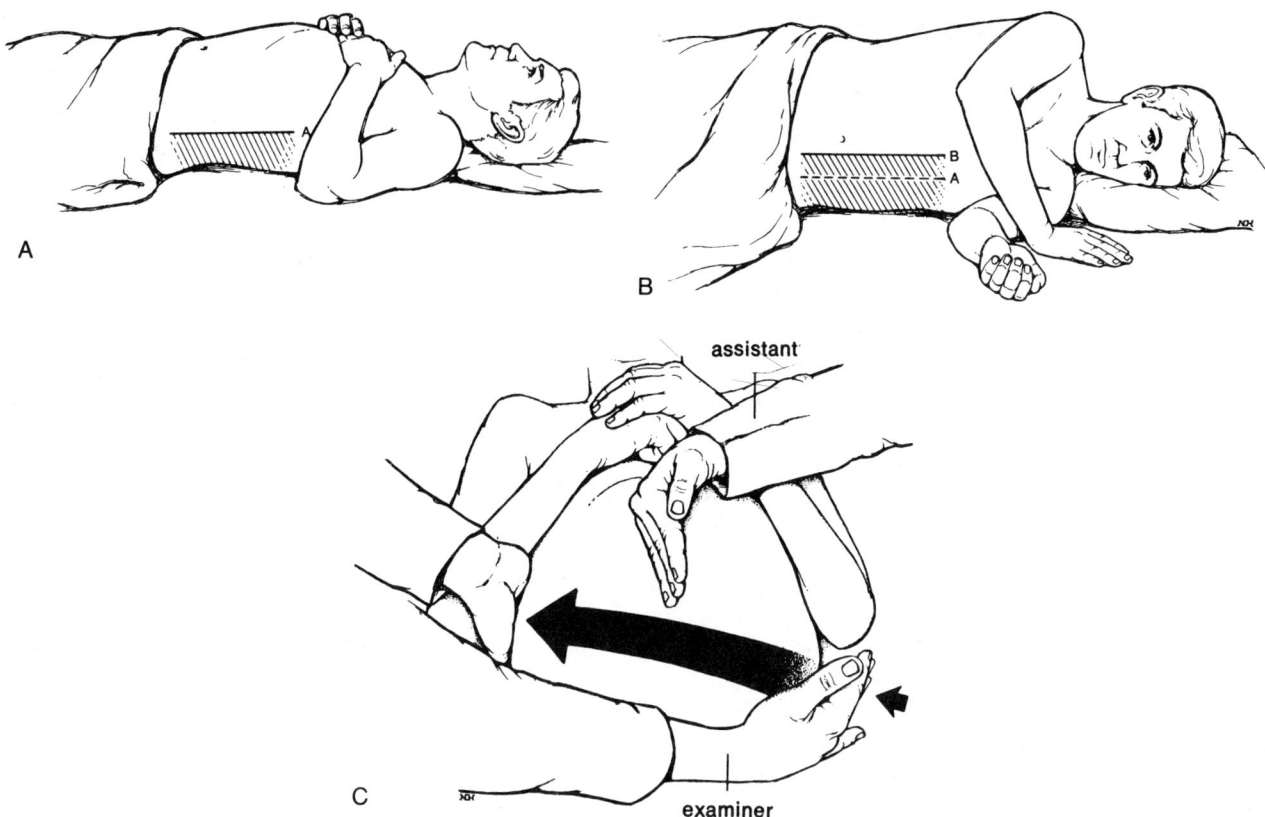

Figure 35-4
Assessing for ascites. (*A*) To percuss for shifting dullness, each flank is percussed with
the patient in a supine position. If fluid is present, dullness will be noted at each flank.
The most medial limits of the dullness should be marked as indicated in *A*. The patient
should then be shifted to his side. (*B*) Note what happens to the area of dullness if fluid
is present. (*C*) To detect the presence of a fluid wave, the examiner places one hand
alongside each flank. A second person then places a hand, ulnar side down, along the
patient's midline, and applies light pressure. The examiner then strikes one flank sharply
with one hand, while the other hand remains in place to detect any signs of a fluid
impulse. The assistant's hand dampens any wave impulses traveling through the
abdominal wall. (Copyright © 1974, American Journal of Nursing Company. Reproduced
with permission from American Journal of Nursing, 74, No. 9, Sept. 1974.)

Skin integrity will be affected if meticulous care is not
carried out. Pressure over bony prominences and edematous
tissue must be relieved by frequently changing body position,
or possibly by using an alternating pressure mattress. Lower
extremities may have to be elevated and support hose applied.
Salt-poor albumin may be given intravenously to temporarily
elevate the serum albumin level, which increases serum osmotic pressure. This helps reduce edema by causing the ascitic
fluid to be drawn back into the bloodstream and ultimately
eliminated by the kidneys.

Paracentesis

Paracentesis is the removal of fluid (ascites) from the peritoneal cavity through a small surgical incision or puncture
made through the abdominal wall. Once considered an acceptable form of treatment for ascites, paracentesis is now
primarily for diagnostic examination of ascitic fluid, for treatment of massive ascites resistant to other therapy and causing
severe problems to the patient, and as prelude to other pro-

cedures, including radiography, peritoneal dialysis, ascites
reinfusion, or surgery.

If paracentesis is warranted (Fig. 35-5), the aspiration is
limited to the slow removal of 2 to 3 liters, to relieve acute
symptoms. Removing large amounts of fluid may cause hypotension, oliguria, and hyponatremia. If fluid in excess of
this amounts is removed, ascitic fluid tends to form again,
drawing fluid from extracellular tissue throughout the body.

Nursing Interventions. The nurse prepares the patient
for paracentesis by providing the necessary information, instructions, and reassurance.

▷ *Have the patient void as completely as possible just
prior to paracentesis, to lessen the danger of inadvertently piercing the bladder.*

Sterile equipment and appropriate collection receptacles
are made ready. Preparatory to the procedure, the patient is
placed in the upright position on the edge of the bed or in a
chair, fully supported, with his feet resting on a stool and one
arm fitted with a sphygmomanometer cuff. The trocar is in-

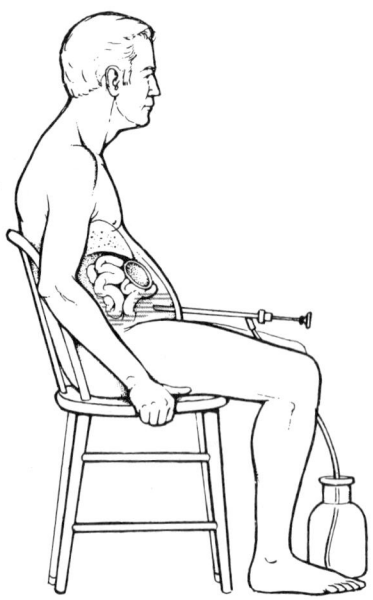

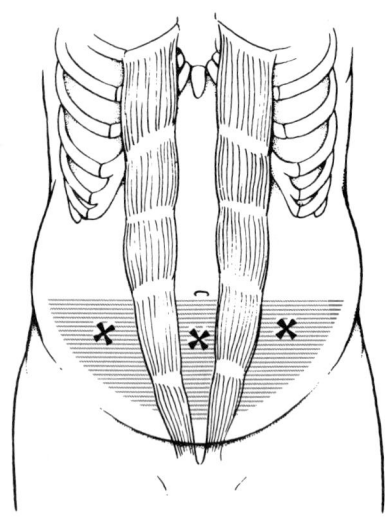

Figure 35-5
The patient undergoing paracentesis.

Sitting position is preferred since the intestines will float away from the site of paracentesis

The indicated sites for performing the procedure avoid injury to the deep inferior epigastric vessels

troduced with aseptic technique through a stab wound in the midline below the umbilicus, and the fluid is drained through an effluent tube into a container.

During the procedure the nurse helps the patient to maintain the proper posture.

▷ *Observe the patient closely for evidence of vascular collapse, such as the appearance of pallor, increase in pulse rate, or decline in blood pressure. Blood pressure readings are recorded at frequent intervals from the beginning of the procedure.*

When the procedure is concluded, the patient is placed in a comfortable position. The amount of fluid collected is measured, described, and recorded; and samples of the fluid, properly labeled, are sent to appropriate laboratories for examination of the cellular sediment, its specific gravity, protein concentration, and bacterial content.

Shunts

Although surgical bypass procedures or shunts performed to treat esophageal varices may also decrease ascites formation, the high operative mortality in patients with severe liver dysfunction limits surgical shunting as an effective treatment for ascites.

Attempts have been made to treat ascites through reinfusion of ascitic fluid into the general circulation; however, there is risk of infection from such treatment. In addition, this treatment is temporary, and reaccumulation of ascites occurs within 2 months in more than 70% of patients.

The insertion of a LeVeen or peritoneojugular shunt has been successful in reducing ascites and maintaining intravasular protein and fluid volume by "shunting" or redirecting the ascitic fluid from the peritoneal cavity into the systemic circulation (Fig. 35-6). In this method, a perforated silicon tube is directed through a small transverse abdominal incision into the peritoneal cavity. The proximal end of the tube is attached to a valve; from the valve another tube emerges and

is threaded subcutaneously to the superior vena cava. The valve is normally closed but opens when the pressure in the peritoneal cavity rises 3 cm H_2O above the pressure of the intrathoracic vena cava, which is located in the thorax. When

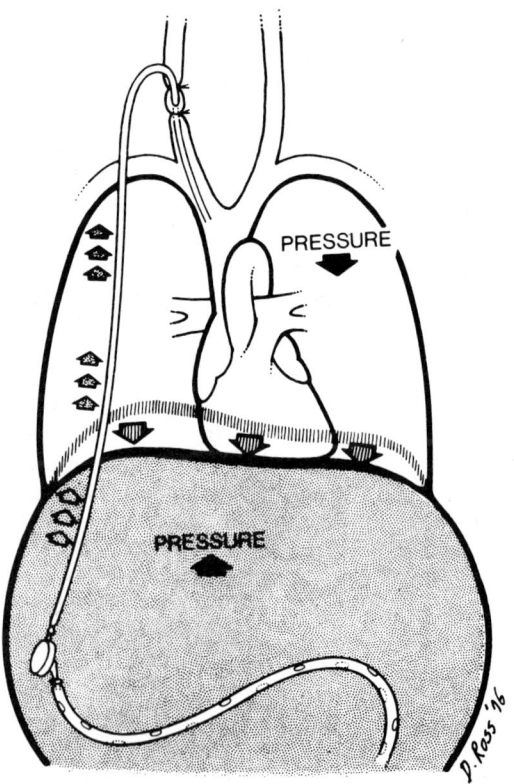

Figure 35-6
Peritoneojugular shunt for reducing ascites. The valve lies in the lower right side extraperitoneally, and a perforated collecting tube extends into the peritoneal cavity. (Schiff L [ed]. Diseases of the Liver, 6th ed. Philadelphia, JB Lippincott, 1987.)

the valve opens, the ascitic fluid is transported to the superior vena cava. When pressure falls, the valve closes.

In the postoperative period, the patient is observed closely and the hematocrit is measured every 4 hours to monitor vascular volume expansion and hemodilution which may result from the inflow of ascitic fluid. Excessive hemodilution may be interrupted by placing the patient in a sitting position, which reduces the difference between the pressures of the peritoneal cavity and intrathoracic pressure, closing the valve and temporarily stopping the drainage of ascitic fluid to the vena cava. A diuretic such as furosemide may be prescribed to avoid the possibility of pulmonary edema. Blood studies include careful monitoring of the coagulation profile, because reabsorption of substances in the ascitic fluid may inhibit clotting and lead to bleeding. Body weight, abdominal girth, and urinary output are recorded every 2 hours. Ordinarily, the hematocrit falls, abdominal girth decreases, weight drops, and urinary output rises. Reversal of these changes may indicate that the shunt is no longer patent and that the ascitic fluid is reaccumulating.

Following the relief of ascites, fluid and sodium intake will depend on the cardiac status and presence of peripheral edema. These patients require continued care and monitoring, for even though the ascites may be cleared, the liver problem is not improved by the insertion of a peritoneojugular shunt.

Nutritional Deficiencies

Another group of complications that is common to patients with severe chronic liver disease of all types is caused by inadequate intake of proper vitamins. Among the specific deficiency states that occur on this basis are (1) vitamin A deficiency, beriberi, polyneuritis, and Wernicke-Korsakoff psychosis, all attributable to a deficiency of thiamine; (2) skin and mucous membrane lesions characteristic of riboflavin deficiency; (3) pyridoxine deficiency, once referred to as "rum fits"; hypoprothrombinemia (see p. 688), characterized by spontaneous bleeding and ecchymoses, due to vitamin K deficiency; (5) the hemorrhagic lesions of scurvy (*i.e.*, vitamin C deficiency); and (6) the macrocytic anemia of folic acid deficiency.

- The threat of these avitaminoses provides the rationale for supplementing the diet of every patient with chronic liver disease (especially when alcoholism is involved) with ample quantities of vitamins A, B complex, C, K, and folic acid.

Hepatic Coma

Hepatic coma, one of the dreaded complications of liver disease, occurs with profound liver failure and results from the accumulation of ammonia and other identified toxic metabolites in the blood. Ammonia accumulates because damaged liver cells fail to detoxify and convert to urea the ammonia that is constantly entering the bloodstream as a result of its absorption from the gastrointestinal tract and its liberation from kidney and muscle cells. The increased ammonia concentration in the blood causes brain dysfunction and damage, resulting in hepatic encephalopathy and hepatic coma.

Assessment and Clinical Manifestations. The earliest symptoms of hepatic coma include minor mental aberrations and motor disturbances. The patient appears to be slightly confused and experiences alterations in mood. He becomes untidy and experiences altered sleep patterns. He tends to sleep during the day and to experience restlessness and insomnia at night. As hepatic coma progresses, he may be difficult to awaken. He may exhibit asterixis or flapping tremor of the hands. Simple tasks, such as handwriting, become difficult. A sample of handwriting, taken daily, may provide graphic evidence of progression of hepatic coma. In the early stages of hepatic coma, the patient's reflexes are hyperactive; with deepening of coma these reflexes disappear and the extremities may become flaccid.

The electroencephalogram (EEG) shows generalized slowing and an increase in amplitude of brain waves. Except for the triphasic waves, all of the other manifestations noted are also observable in other conditions. Occasionally, fetor hepaticus, a characteristic breath odor like freshly mowed grass, acetone, or old wine, may be noticed. In a more advanced stage there are gross disturbances of consciousness and the patient is completely disoriented with respect to time and place. With further progression of the disorder, he lapses into frank coma and may have convulsions. Approximately 35% of all patients with cirrhosis of the liver die in hepatic coma.

Aggravating and Precipitating Factors. Circumstances that increase blood ammonia content tend to aggravate or precipitate hepatic coma. The largest source of blood ammonia is the enzymatic and bacterial digestion of dietary and blood proteins in the gastrointestinal tract. Ammonia from these sources is increased as a result of gastrointestinal bleeding, a high-protein diet, bacterial growth in the small and large intestines, and uremia. The ingestion of ammonium salts will also increase the blood ammonia level. In the presence of alkalosis or hypokalemia, increased amounts of ammonia are absorbed from the gastrointestinal tract and from the renal tubular fluid. On the other hand, serum ammonia is *decreased* by elimination of protein from the diet and by the administration of antibiotics, such as neomycin sulfate, that reduce the number of intestinal bacteria capable of converting urea to ammonia.

Other factors unrelated to increased blood ammonia that may induce hepatic coma in susceptible patients include overdiuresis, dehydration, infections, surgery, fever, and consciousness-altering drugs, such as sedatives, tranquilizers, and narcotics.

Management

Principles of management of hepatic coma include the following:

- The patient with impending hepatic coma is observed frequently to assess neurologic status. A daily record is kept of handwriting and performance in arithmetic.
- Fluid intake and output and body weight are recorded each day.
- Vital signs are measured and recorded every 4 hours.
- Evidence suggesting pulmonary or other infection is sought frequently and reported promptly if observed.
- Serum ammonia level is monitored daily.
- If it becomes apparent that hepatic coma is impending, the patient's protein intake is reduced sharply or eliminated altogether, for the time being.

- To reduce ammonia absorption from the gastrointestinal tract, a high cleansing enema may be prescribed.
- In addition, an antibiotic drug such as neomycin is given as an intestinal antiseptic.
- Electrolyte status is carefully monitored and corrected if abnormal.
- Sedative and analgesic drugs, if prescribed at all, are administered to this patient in very conservative doses and under very close observation.

Lactulose (Cephulac) is given to reduce blood ammonia, which probably acts by a combination of mechanisms that promote the excretion of ammonia in the stool: (1) ammonia is kept in the ionized state, resulting in a fall in colon *pH*—this reverses the normal passage of ammonia from the colon to the blood; (2) catharsis takes place, which decreases the ammonia absorbed from the colon; and (3) the fecal flora is changed to organisms that do not produce ammonia from urea.

Two or three soft stools per day are hoped for; this means lactulose is performing as intended. However, watery diarrheal stools indicate drug overdose. Possible side-effects include intestinal bloating and cramps, which usually disappear in a week. To overcome the sweet taste to which some patients object, lactulose can be diluted with fruit juice. The patient is closely monitored for hypokalemia and dehydration. Other laxatives are not given during lactulose administration because their effects would disturb dosage regulation. Lactulose enemas have also been used effectively in acute hepatic encephalopathy for patients who are comatose or in whom oral administration is contraindicated or impossible.

Other Manifestations of Liver Dysfunction

Many patients with liver dysfunction develop generalized edema due to hypoalbuminemia that results from decreased hepatic production of serum albumin. The production of blood clotting factors by the liver is also reduced, leading to an increased incidence of bruising, nosebleeds, bleeding from wounds, and, as described above, gastrointestinal bleeding. Decreased production of several clotting factors may be due, in part, to deficient absorption of vitamin K from the gastrointestinal tract. This probably is caused by the inability of liver cells to use vitamin K to make prothrombin. Absorption of the other fat-soluble vitamins (vitamins A, D, and E) as well as dietary fats may also be impaired, owing to decreased secretion of bile salts into the intestine.

Abnormalities of glucose metabolism also occur; the blood sugar may be abnormally high shortly after a meal (*i.e.*, a diabetic-type glucose tolerance test), but hypoglycemia may occur during fasting because of decreased hepatic glycogen reserves and decreased gluconeogenesis.

- Because of decreased ability to metabolize drugs, usual drug dosages must be reduced for the patient with liver failure.

Decreased metabolism of estrogens by the damaged liver can lead to gynecomastia, testicular atrophy, loss of pubic hair in the male, and menstrual irregularities in the female, as well as spider angiomata and reddened palms ("liver palms"). Splenomegaly (enlarged spleen) with possible hypersplenism occurs commonly as a manifestation of portal hypertension. Patients with liver dysfunction due to biliary obstruction commonly develop severe itching (pruritus) due to retention of bile salts.

Hepatic Disorders

Viral Hepatitis

The increasing incidence of viral hepatitis is a growing public health concern. Although the mortality rate is low, the disease is important because of its ease of transmission, morbidity, and the prolonged loss of time from school or employment that it can cause.

Breakthroughs in better understanding of viral hepatitis in the past have been due to recognition in 1968, by Blumberg, that Australian (Au) antigen was a specific immunologic marker for hepatitis B infection. This led to a series of new designations, and Australian antigen now is referred to as hepatitis B surface antigen: HB_sAg. More recently, a specific antigen for hepatitis A has been identified (HA Ag). Also, tests have been developed to detect anti-HAV, anti-HB_s, and anti-HB_c antibodies, as well as the e-antigen and anti-e-antibody associated with hepatitis B. This means that diagnostic tests, including complement fixation, immune adherence, and radioimmunoassay, are available for recognizing hepatitis A and hepatitis B. The existence of one or more agents capable of producing non-A, non-B hepatitis has also been recognized.

A guide to the terminology associated with viral hepatitis is provided in Chart 35-2.

Nursing Implications. The nurse is especially concerned with four major problem areas of viral hepatitis: (1) the care of the patient with hepatitis; (2) the increased risks in hemodialysis units and in users of illicit injectable drugs; (3) the fact that many people who have the disease are asymptomatic, which may present serious epidemiologic problems; and (4) the apparent health needs of the community required for its elimination. The last category includes the following considerations:

- Proper community and home sanitation
- Conscientious individual hygiene at all times
- Safe practices for preparing and dispensing food
- Effective health supervision in schools, dormitories, extended care facilities, barracks, and camps
- Continuous health education programs
- Reporting of every case of viral hepatitis to the local health department

For a comparison of the many aspects of the major forms of viral hepatitis, see Table 35-2.

Hepatitis A Virus

Hepatitis A, formerly designated infectious hepatitis, is probably an RNA virus of the enterovirus family. The mode of transmission of this disease is the fecal–oral route, primarily through the ingestion of food or liquids infected by the virus. The virus has been found in the stool of infected patients prior to the onset of symptoms and during the first few days of illness. Typically, a young adult acquires the infection at school and brings it home, where haphazard sanitary habits

Chart 35-2
Hepatitis Glossary

Hepatitis A

HAV	Hepatitis A virus
Anti-HAV	Antibody to hepatitis A virus; appears in serum soon after onset of symptoms

Hepatitis B

HBV	Hepatitis B virus
HB$_s$AG	Hepatitis B surface antigen (Australian antigen); indicates acute or chronic hepatitis B or carrier state; indicates infectious state
Anti-HB$_s$	Antibody to hepatitis B surface antigen; indicates prior exposure and immunity to hepatitis B; may persist for prolonged time
HB$_e$Ag	Hepatitis B e-antigen; present in serum early in course; indicates highly infectious stage of hepatitis B; persistence in serum indicates progression to chronic hepatitis
Anti-HB$_e$	Antibody to hepatitis B e-antigen
HB$_c$Ag	Hepatitis B core antigen; found in liver cell; not easily detected in serum
Anti-HB$_c$	Antibody to hepatitis B core antigen; most sensitive indicator of hepatitis B; appears late in the acute phase of the disease

Non-A, Non-B Hepatitis

NANBH	Hepatitis non-A, non-B virus

TABLE 35-2
Hepatitis

	Hepatitis A Virus (HAV)	Hepatitis B Virus (HBV)	Non-A, Non-B Hepatitis Virus (NANBH)
Other Names	Type A hepatitis, infectious or epidemic hepatitis; IH virus	Type B hepatitis, serum hepatitis, SH virus, Dane particle	Hepatitis "C", "D"; Type C
Epidemiology			
Cause	Hepatitis A virus	Hepatitis B virus	Another virus
Method of transmission	Fecal-oral route; poor sanitation Person to person Waterborne, foodborne—shellfish Rarely, if at all, by blood transfusion	Parenterally, or by intimate contact with carriers or those with acute disease; male homosexuals. Vertical transmission from mothers to infants Contaminated instruments, syringes, needles; renal dialysis*	Transfusion of blood and blood products Personnel in renal transplant and dialysis units Parenteral drug abusers Institutions with long-term residents*
Source of virus/antigen	Blood, feces, saliva	Blood, saliva, semen, vaginal secretions	Appears to be blood-borne
Distribution by age	Young adults (15–29) and middle-aged who have escaped childhood infection	Affects all ages, but mostly young adults	Same as HBV
Incubation period	3–5 weeks; average: 30 days	2–5 months; average: 90 days	Variable: 14–115 days; average: 50 days

(continued)

TABLE 35-2 (continued)

	Hepatitis A Virus (HAV)	*Hepatitis B Virus (HBV)*	*Non-A, Non-B Hepatitis Virus (NANBH)*
Epidemiology			
Occurrence	Worldwide	Worldwide	Worldwide Accounts for 20% of sporadic cases
Antibody	Anti-HAV Present in convalescent sera and immune serum globulin (ISG)	Anti-HB$_c$ (core antigen) Anti-HB$_s$ (surface antigen)	
Immunity	Homologous	Homologous	
Severity	Most anicteric and asymptomatic	More severe than HAV	Wide spectrum of severity, resembling HAV or HBV; often prolonged illness—months May progress to chronic hepatitis.*
Nature of Illness			
Signs and symptoms	May occur with or without symptoms: flulike illness Preicteric phase: Headache, malaise, fatigue, anorexia, lassitude, fever Icteric phase: Dark urine, scleral icterus, jaundice, liver tenderness, and perhaps enlargement	May occur without symptoms 1000 IU/liter-serum transaminase level May develop antibodies to virus Similar to HAV, but more severe Fever and respiratory symptoms rare, but may have arthralgias, rash	Similar to HBV Less severe and anicteric
Diagnosis and method	Elevated serum transaminase Complement fixation rate Radioimmunoassay	Check serum for HB$_s$Ag, HB$_e$Ag, anti-HB$_c$, in absence of anti-HB$_s$ (obtainable as a panel) Elevated serum transaminase Radioimmunoassay—hemagglutination	
Severity	Usually mild Fatality rate 0%–1%	Variable, may be severe Fatality rate varies: 1%–10%	
Specific treatment	Adequate fluids, rest, nutrition	Same as HAV In research: vaccine antiviral chemotherapy to eliminate chronic HBV carrier state (being tested)	
Prevention	Good sanitation Proper personal hygiene Effective sterilization procedures Careful screening of food handlers Immune globulin given within a few days of exposure	Specific hepatitis B immune globulin (HBIG) probably useful after exposure by ingestion, inoculation, or splash involving hepatitis B surface antigen (HB$_s$Ag) Hepatitis B vaccine recommended for preexposure immunization of those at high risk	Mandatory screening of blood donors: For HB$_s$Ag, 20% For non-A, non-B, 80%

* Recent intensive research suggests probably the same for HBV and NANBH.

spread it through the family. It is more prevalent in underdeveloped countries or in instances of overcrowding and poor sanitation. An infected food handler can spread the disease, and people can contract it by consuming water or shellfish from sewage-contaminated waters. Animal handlers can contract it by consuming water or shellfish from sewage-contaminated waters. Animal handlers can contract hepatitis A from infected primates. It is rarely, if ever, transmitted by blood transfusions.

The incubation period is estimated to be from 1 to 7 weeks, with an average of 30 days. The course of the illness may be prolonged, lasting from 4 to 8 weeks. It generally lasts longer and is more severe in those over age 40.

Assessment and Clinical Manifestations. Most patients are anicteric (without jaundice) and symptomless. When symptoms appear, they are of a mild, flulike upper respiratory tract infection, with low-grade fever. Anorexia is an early symptom and is often severe. It is thought to result from release of a toxin by the damaged liver or by failure of the damaged liver cells to detoxify an abnormal product. Later, jaundice and dark urine may become apparent. Indigestion is present, in varying degrees, marked by vague epigastric distress, nausea, heartburn, and flatulence. The patient may also develop a strong aversion to the taste of cigarettes or the presence of cigarette smoke and other strong odors. These symptoms tend to clear as soon as the jaundice reaches its peak—perhaps 10 days after its initial appearance. The liver and the spleen are often moderately enlarged for a few days after onset; otherwise, apart from jaundice, there are few physical signs to be elicited.

Management. Bed rest during the acute stage and the provision of a diet that is both acceptable and nutritious are part of the treatment and nursing care. During the period of anorexia, the patient should receive frequent small feedings, supplemented, if necessary, by intravenous infusions of glucose. Since this patient would rather not look at food, or eat, it requires gentle persistence and ingenuity to whet his appetite. Optimal food and fluid levels need to be maintained to counteract probable weight loss and prolonged recovery. Even before the icteric phase, however, many patients recover their appetites and thereafter need no reminders to maintain a good diet.

The patient's sense of well-being as well as laboratory test results are generally appropriate guides to bed rest and restriction of physical activity. Gradual but progressive ambulation seems to hasten recovery, provided the patient rests after activity and does not ambulate or participate in activities to the point of fatigue.

Patient Education and Home Health Care. The patient is usually managed at home unless symptoms are particularly severe. Therefore, the patient and family need to be assisted to cope with the incapacitation and fatigue that are common problems in hepatitis and to be aware of the indications to seek additional health care if the patient's condition persists or worsens. Additionally, the patient and family need specific guidelines about diet, rest, follow-up blood work, as well as sanitation and hygiene measures, particularly handwashing, to prevent spread of the disease to other family members.

Prognosis. Recovery from hepatitis type A is the rule; a rare case progresses to acute liver necrosis or fulminant hepatitis, terminating in cirrhosis of the liver, or death. Hepatitis A confers immunity against itself; however, the person may contract other forms of hepatitis. The mortality rate of hepatitis A is approximately 0.5%. No carrier state exists, and no chronic hepatitis is associated with hepatitis A.

Control and Prevention. Ways to reduce the risk of contracting hepatitis A are

- Good personal hygiene, stressing careful handwashing (after bowel movement and before eating)
- Environmental sanitation—safe food and water supply, as well as effective sewage disposal
- Administration of immune globulin: Type A hepatitis can be prevented by the administration of globulin intramuscularly during the period of incubation, if this treatment is instituted within 2 to 7 days following exposure. This bolsters the person's own antibody production and provides 6 to 8 weeks of passive immunity. Immune globulin may suppress overt symptoms of the disease; the resulting subclinical case of hepatitis A would produce active immunity to subsequent attacks of the virus. Although rare, systemic reactions to immune globulin may occur.

Caution is required when anyone who has previously had angioedema, hives, or other allergic reactions is treated with any human immune globulin. Epinephrine should be available for use during systemic or anaphylactic reactions.

Hepatitis B Virus

Hepatitis B virus is a double-shelled particle containing DNA. This particle is composed of the following:

HB_cAg—hepatitis B core antigen (antigenic material in an inner core)
HB_sAg—hepatitis B surface antigen (antigenic material in an outer coat)
HB_eAg—an independent protein circulating in the blood
Each antigen elicits its specific antibody:
anti-HB_c—persists during the acute phase of illness; may indicate continuing hepatitis B virus in the liver
anti-HB_s—detected during late convalescence; usually indicates recovery and development of immunity
anti-HB_e—usually signifies reduced infectivity

HB_sAg can be detected transiently circulating in the blood in 80% to 90% of infected patients. HB_cAg cannot be detected in blood. HB_sAg may be noted in the blood for months and years, which suggests that these patients may be asymptomatic carriers, if HB_eAg is absent. If it is present, these patients may have chronic hepatitis and may be more infectious.

From the community health point of view, about 15% of American adults are positive for anti-HB_s, which indicates that they have had hepatitis B. Anti-HB_s may be positive in as many as two thirds of users of illicit injectable drugs.

Unlike hepatitis A, which is transmitted primarily by the fecal–oral route, hepatitis B is transmitted primarily through blood (percutaneous and permucosal routes). The virus has been found in blood, saliva, semen, and vaginal secretions and can be transmitted through mucous membranes and breaks in the skin. Therefore, those at risk of developing hepatitis B include the general surgeon, clinical laboratory worker, dentist, nurse, and respiratory therapist. Staff and patients in hemodialysis and oncology units and homosexually active males are also at increased risk. Mandatory screening of blood donors for HB$_s$Ag has greatly reduced the occurrence of hepatitis B following blood transfusion.

Assessment and Clinical Manifestations.   Clinically, the disease closely resembles hepatitis A. However, the incubation period is relatively much longer (between 2 and 5 months). The mortality is appreciable, ranging from 1% to 10%, depending on the infective dose and the condition of the patient. Symptoms and signs of hepatitis B may be insidious and variable. Fever and respiratory symptoms are rare: some patients have arthralgias and rashes. The patient may lose his appetite and experience dyspepsia, abdominal pain, generalized aching, malaise, and weakness. Jaundice may or may not be evident. If jaundice occurs, it is accompanied by light-colored stools and dark urine. The patient's liver may be tender and enlarged to 12 to 14 cm vertically. The spleen is enlarged and palpable·in a small number of patients; the posterior cervical nodes may also be enlarged.

Gerontological Considerations.   The elderly patient who contracts hepatitis B has a serious risk of severe liver cell necrosis or fulminant hepatic failure, particularly if other illnesses are present. The patient is seriously ill and the prognosis is poor.

Management.   It is important that bed rest be continued until the hepatitis has definitely subsided. Subsequently, the patient's activities should be restricted until the hepatic enlargement and the elevation of the level of serum bilirubin have disappeared. Adequate nutrition should be maintained; proteins are restricted when the liver has a decreased ability to metabolize protein by-products, as demonstrated by symptoms. Other therapeutic measures employed to control the dyspeptic symptoms and general malaise include the use of alkalies, belladonna, and antiemetics. However, all medications should be avoided if emesis is a problem. This patient should be hospitalized and treated with fluid therapy.

Convalescence may be prolonged, with complete symptomatic recovery sometimes requiring 3 to 4 months or longer. During this stage, gradual restoration of physical activity is permitted and encouraged, following complete clearing of the jaundice.

Psychosocial considerations are identified by the nurse, particularly the effects of isolation and separation from family and friends during the acute and infective stages. Special planning is required to minimize alterations in sensory perception. The family is included in planning to decrease the fears and anxieties of the patient and family about the spread of the disease.

Patient Education and Home Health Care.   Because of the prolonged period of convalescence, the patient and family must be prepared for home care. Provision for adequate rest and nutrition must be ensured prior to the patient's discharge. Those family members and friends who have had intimate contact with the patient should be informed about the risks of contracting hepatitis B, and arrangements should be made for them to receive hepatitis B vaccine or hepatitis B immune globulin. Those at risk must be aware of early signs of hepatitis B and of ways to reduce risk to themselves. Follow-up home visits by a community health nurse are indicated to assess the patient's progress and answer family members' questions about transmission of the disease. A home visit also permits evaluation of the understanding of the patient and family about the importance of adequate rest and nutrition.

Prognosis.   Mortality of hepatitis B has been reported to be as high as 10%. Another 10% of patients who have hepatitis B progress to a carrier state or develop chronic hepatitis.

Control and Prevention.   The goals are (1) to interrupt the chain of transmission, (2) to protect those people at high risk through the use of hepatitis B vaccine, and (3) to use passive immunization for unprotected people exposed to hepatitis B virus.

Continued screening of potential blood donors for the presence of HB$_s$Ag will further decrease the risk of transmission by blood transfusion. A reduction in the number of people acquiring hepatitis B could occur if paid blood donors could be replaced by an all-volunteer donor population. Washed red blood cells appear to reduce the risk of hepatitis transmission. The use of disposable syringes, needles, and lancets reduce the risk of spreading this infection from one patient to another in the process of collecting blood samples or administering parenteral therapy. Good personal hygiene practices are fundamental to infection control. In the laboratory, work areas should be disinfected daily. Gloves are to be worn when handling HB$_s$Ag-positive specimens. Eating is prohibited in the laboratory.

Administering medication by individual-dose ampules is essential. Where users of illicit injectable drugs share the same needle, serious outbreaks of hepatitis have occurred.

Hepatitis B Vaccine.   Hepatitis B vaccine is available for prevention of hepatitis B. Its use is recommended for those at high risk of developing hepatitis B, including health care workers exposed to blood, hemodialysis and oncology patients and staff, homosexually active males, and users of illicit injectable drugs. Studies have shown that hepatitis B vaccine produces active immunity to hepatitis B virus in 90% of healthy persons. It provides no protection against other types of hepatitis and does not provide protection to those already exposed to the virus. Side-effects are infrequent. The most common postinjection complaint is soreness and redness at the injection site.

Hepatitis B Immune Globulin.   Hepatitis B immune globulin (HBIG) is recommended for unprotected people exposed to hepatitis B virus through accidental contamination of mucous membranes or breaks in the skin. HBIG is prepared from pooled venous plasma of donors with a high titer of anti-HB$_s$ antibodies and provides passive immunity. The United States Public Health Service Advisory Committee on Immunization Practices recommends HBIG for a single exposure to blood containing hepatitis B virus, either by accidental inoculation via needle stick or by splashing contaminated material on mucous membranes, such as might occur while pipetting blood or fluid. HBIG is given intramuscularly as soon as possible, but no later than 7 days after exposure. A second dose is given 25 to 30 days after the first.

Non-A, Non-B Hepatitis

Those varieties of hepatitis that are not identified as hepatitis A or B are classified as non-A, non-B hepatitis. Repeated episodes of non-A, non-B hepatitis and variations in incubation periods of this form of hepatitis suggest the existence of multiple causative agents. Non-A, non-B hepatitis is blood borne, and the possibility of a carrier state is likely. This form of hepatitis is now the major cause of transfusion-related viral hepatitis and is often observed in parenteral drug abusers.

Non-A, non-B hepatitis occurs not only in patients (following blood transfusion) and among drug users but also in personnel associated with renal transplantation units and in residents in homes for the mentally retarded. Another community health-related implication is that whereas only 10% to 20% of post-transfusion hepatitis is type B, 80% to 90% is non-A, non-B hepatitis. Transmission of hepatitis virus is more likely from commercial or paid blood donors than from volunteer donors.

Incubation time is variable, and severity covers a wide spectrum that most resembles hepatitis B. Most manifestations are anicteric (without jaundice). Illness may be prolonged, lasting several months and resulting in chronic hepatitis. It is possible that immune globulin may offer limited protection against non-A, non-B hepatitis.

Toxic Hepatitis and Drug-Induced Hepatitis

Certain chemicals have poisonous effects on the liver and when taken by mouth or injected parenterally produce acute liver cell necrosis, or *toxic hepatitis*. The chemicals most commonly implicated in this disease are carbon tetrachloride, phosphorus, chloroform, and gold compounds. These are true hepatotoxins.

Many drugs may induce hepatitis but are sensitizing rather than toxic. The result, *drug-induced hepatitis,* is similar to acute viral hepatitis; however, parenchymal destruction tends to be more extensive. Some examples of drugs that can lead to hepatitis are cinchophen, isoniazid, halothane, acetaminophen, and certain antibiotics and antimetabolites.

Clinical Manifestations and Management. Toxic hepatitis resembles viral hepatitis in onset. Obtaining a history of exposure to hepatotoxic chemicals, drugs, or other agents assists in earlier initiation of treatment and removal of the offending agent. Anorexia, nausea, and vomiting are the usual symptoms; jaundice and hepatomegaly are noted on physical assessment. Symptoms are more intense for the more severely poisoned patient.

Recovery from acute toxic hepatitis is rapid if the hepatotoxin is identified early and removed or if exposure to the agent has been limited. Recovery, however, is unlikely if there is a prolonged period between exposure and onset of symptoms. There are no effective antidotes. The fever rises; the patient becomes deeply toxic and prostrated. Vomiting may be persistent, with the vomitus containing blood. Clotting abnormalities may be severe, and hemorrhages may appear under the skin. The severe gastrointestinal symptoms may lead to vascular collapse. Delirium, coma, and convulsions develop, and within a few days the patient usually dies.

There is little to be done by way of treatment, except to provide comfort measures, blood, fluids, and electrolytes. A few patients recover from an acute toxic hepatitis only to develop chronic liver disease.

Drug-induced hepatitis may progress to hepatic failure. In the event that the liver heals, there may be scarring, followed by postnecrotic cirrhosis. Manifestations of sensitivity to a drug may occur on the first day of its use or not until several months later, depending on the drug. Usually, the onset is abrupt, with chills, fever, rash, pruritus, arthralgia, anorexia, and nausea. Later, there may be jaundice and dark urine and an enlarged and tender liver. When the offending drug is withdrawn, symptoms may gradually subside. However, once provoked, reactions may be severe and even fatal, even though the drug is stopped. If fever, rash, or pruritus occur from any medication, its use should be stopped immediately.

Concern has been expressed regarding the effect on the liver of halothane (Fluothane) a commonly used nonexplosive inhalation anesthetic. Since halothane may cause serious, and sometimes fatal, liver damage, precautions should preclude its use in (1) patients with known liver disease; (2) repeated instances, particularly in patients who have had a fever of unknown cause after the first administration of halothane; and (3) patients with evidence of prior sensitization. Such sensitization would have been in evidence during the second postoperative week, with such manifestations as fever, rash, eosinophilia, arthralgia, or jaundice.

Hepatic Cirrhosis

Cirrhosis of the liver refers to scarring of the liver. Three kinds are generally considered:

1. *Laennec's portal cirrhosis* (alcoholic, nutritional), in which the scar tissue characteristically surrounds the portal areas. This is most frequently due to chronic alcoholism and is the most common type of cirrhosis.
2. *Postnecrotic cirrhosis,* in which there are broad bands of scar tissue, as a late result of a previous acute viral hepatitis.
3. *Biliary cirrhosis,* in which there is pericholangitic, perilobular scarring. This type usually is the result of chronic biliary obstruction and infection (cholangitis) and is much more rare than Laennec's and postnecrotic cirrhosis.

The portion of the liver chiefly involved consists of the portal and the periportal spaces, where the bile canaliculi of each lobule communicate to form the liver bile ducts. These areas become the site of inflammation, and the bile ducts become occluded with inspissated bile and pus. An attempt is made by the liver to form new bile channels; hence, there is an overgrowth of tissue made up largely of disconnected, newly formed bile ducts and surrounded by scar tissue.

Clinical manifestations of this disease include intermittent jaundice and fever and the finding of an enlarged, hard, irregular liver, which eventually becomes atrophic. The treatment is the same as that described for portal cirrhosis, that is, the treatment of any form of chronic liver insufficiency and, when indicated, surgical drainage to eradicate the biliary tract infection.

Pathophysiology

Although several factors have been implicated in the etiology of cirrhosis, alcohol consumption is considered the major causative factor. Cirrhosis occurs with greatest frequency among alcoholics. However, many explain cirrhosis on the basis of nutritional deficiency with reduced protein intake, rather than on alcohol toxicity, and certainly some cases of cirrhosis are observed among people who do not drink alcoholic beverages. Nonetheless, several investigators have shown that although nutritional factors are undoubtedly involved, alcohol itself has to be incriminated in the pathogenesis of the alcoholic fatty liver and the associated effects, because cirrhosis has been observed in those with a high alcohol intake despite a normal diet.

Some people appear to be more susceptible than others to this disease, whether they are alcoholics or malnourished or not. Other factors may play a role, such as exposure to certain chemicals (carbon tetrachloride, chlorinated naphthalene, arsenic, or phosphorus) or infectious schistosomiasis. Twice as many men as women are affected, and the majority of patients are between 40 and 60 years of age.

Laennec's cirrhosis is a disease characterized by episodes of necrosis involving the liver cells, sometimes occurring repeatedly throughout the course of the disease. The destroyed liver cells are replaced by scar tissue, the amount of which, in time, may exceed that of the functioning liver tissue. Islands of residual normal tissue and regenerating liver tissue may project from the constricted areas giving the cirrhotic liver its characteristic hobnail appearance. The disease usually has a particularly insidious onset and a very protracted course, occasionally proceeding over a period of 30 or more years.

Clinical Manifestations

Early in the course of cirrhosis, the liver tends to be large and its cells loaded with fat (Fig. 35-7). The liver is firm and has a sharp edge noticeable on palpation. Abdominal pain may be present due to recent, rapid enlargement of the liver, producing tension on Glisson's capsule (the fibrous covering of the liver). Later in the course of the disease, the liver decreases in size as scar tissue contracts the liver tissue. The liver edge, if palpable, is nodular.

The late manifestations are due partly to chronic failure of liver function and partly to obstruction of the portal circulation. Practically all the blood from the digestive organs is collected in the portal veins and carried to the liver. Since a cirrhotic liver does not allow the blood free passage, it is dammed back into the spleen and the gastrointestinal tract,

with the result that these organs become the seat of chronic passive congestion; that is, they are stagnant with blood and thus cannot function properly. Such patients are apt to have chronic dyspepsia and changes in bowel habit, with constipation or diarrhea. There is gradual weight loss. Fluid may accumulate in the peritoneal cavity, producing ascites. This can be demonstrated through percussion for shifting dullness or a fluid wave (see Fig 35-4). Splenomegaly may also be present. Spider telangiectases, or dilated superficial arterioles resembling bluish red spiders, are frequently observed on inspection of the face and trunk.

The obstruction to blood flow through the liver resulting from the fibrotic changes also results in the formation of collateral blood vessels in the gastrointestinal system and shunting of blood from the portal vessels into blood vessels with lower pressures. As a result, the cirrhotic patient will often have prominent, distended abdominal blood vessels, which are visible on abdominal inspection (caput medusae), and distended blood vessels throughout the gastrointestinal tract. The esophagus, stomach, and lower rectum are common sites of collateral blood vessels. These distended blood vessels form varices or hemorrhoids, depending on their location. Because these vessels were not intended to carry the high pressure and volume of blood imposed by cirrhosis, they may rupture and bleed. Therefore, assessment must include observation for occult and frank bleeding from the gastrointestinal tract. Approximately 25% of patients develop small hematemesis; others have profuse hemorrhage from the stomach and esophageal varices.

Other late symptoms of cirrhosis are attributable to chronic failure of liver function. The concentration of plasma albumin is lowered, predisposing to the formation of edema. Overproduction of aldosterone occurs in cirrhosis, causing sodium and water retention and potassium excretion. Because of inadequate formation, use, and storage of certain vitamins (notably vitamins A, C, and K), signs of their deficiency fre-

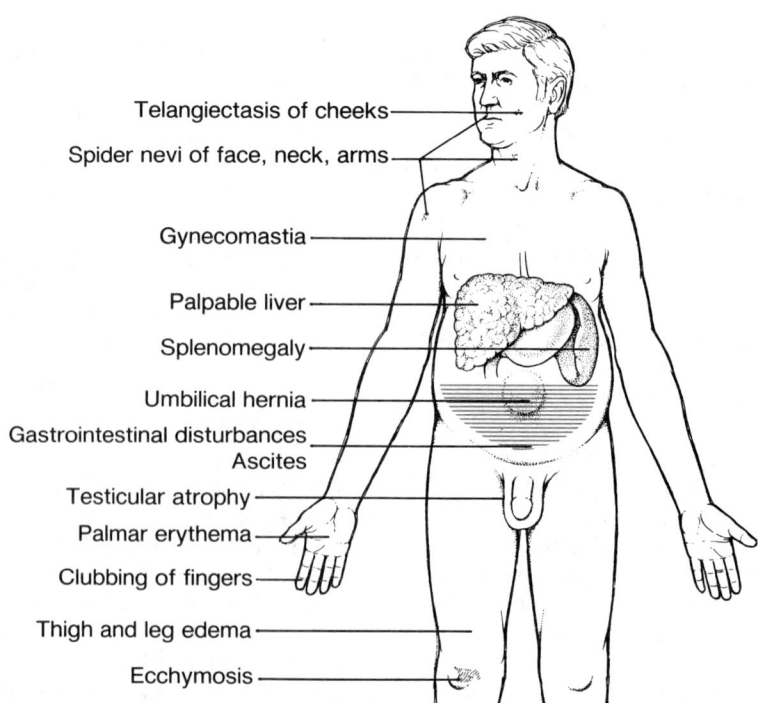

Figure 35-7
Common clinical findings in assessment of the patient with cirrhosis.

quently are encountered, particularly hemorrhagic phenomena associated with vitamin-K deficiency. Chronic gastritis and poor gastrointestinal function, together with the factors of poor diet and impaired liver function, account for the anemia often associated with this disease. The anemia and the patient's poor nutritional status and poor state of health result in severe fatigue, which interferes with the ability to carry out routine daily activities.

Additional clinical manifestations include deterioration of mental function with impending hepatic encephalopathy and hepatic coma. Therefore, neurologic assessment is in order and should include the patient's general behavior, cognitive abilities, orientation to time and place, and speech patterns.

In addition to noting the occurrence of clinical manifestations, the nurse should obtain accurate information about the patient's dietary and alcohol intake. It is also important to note exposure to toxic agents encountered during work or recreation. Any medications or drugs taken by the patient are recorded and checked for hepatotoxicity. Exposure to general anesthetics that may be hepatotoxic is also noted.

Diagnostic Evaluation

The extent of liver disease and the kind of treatment are determined after studying the laboratory findings. Because the liver is a complex, functioning organ, the tests are many (see Table 35-1). The patient needs to know why these tests are being done, why they are important, and how he can cooperate. In severe parenchymal liver dysfunction, the serum albumin level tends to decrease, and the serum globulin level rises. Enzyme tests indicate liver cell damage: serum alkaline phosphatase, SGOT, and SGPT levels increase, and the serum cholinesterase level may decrease. Excretory function is tested by the liver's ability to eliminate sulfobromophthalein (Bromsulphalein) and indocyanine green dye. In cirrhosis, the sulfobromophthalein and indocyanine green dye are retained. Bilirubin tests are done to measure bile excretion or bile retention. Photolaparoscopy, in conjunction with biopsy, permits direct visualization of the liver.

Ultrasound scanning will measure the difference in density of parenchymal cells and scar tissue. Computed tomography (CT scan) and radioisotopic liver scans give information about liver size and hepatic blood flow and obstruction.

Management

The management of the patient with cirrhosis is usually based on the patient's presenting symptoms. For example, antacids are prescribed to decrease gastric distress and minimize the possibility of gastrointestinal bleeding. Vitamins and nutritional supplements promote healing of damaged liver cells and improve the patient's general nutritional status. Potassium-sparing diuretics (*e.g.,* spironolactone) may be indicated to decrease ascites, if present, and minimize fluid and electrolyte changes common with other diuretic agents. The physician also strongly encourages the patient to avoid further alcohol use, a recommendation that should be encouraged and reinforced in a nonjudgmental way by the nurse. The fibrosis of the cirrhotic liver cannot be cured, but its progression may be halted or slowed by such measures.

▶ Nursing Process
The Patient With Hepatic Cirrhosis

▷ Assessment

Nursing assessment focuses on history of precipitating factors, particularly long-term alcohol abuse, as well as changes in the patient's physical and mental status. The amount and duration of the patient's alcohol use are obtained and noted. Mental status is assessed through interview and other interaction with the patient; orientation to person, place, and time is noted. The patient's ability to carry on a job or household activities provides some information about physical and mental status. Additionally, the patient's relationship with family, friends, and co-workers may give some indication about incapacitation secondary to alcohol abuse and cirrhosis. Abdominal distention and bloating, bruising, gastrointestinal bleeding, and weight changes are noted.

▷ Nursing Diagnoses

Based on all the assessment data, the patient's major nursing diagnoses may include the following:

- Activity intolerance related to fatigue, general debility, muscle wasting, and discomfort
- Alterations in nutrition related to chronic gastritis, decreased gastrointestinal motility, and anorexia
- Impairment of skin integrity related to edema, jaundice, and compromised immunologic status
- Potential for injury related to altered clotting mechanisms and portal hypertension
- Alteration in thought processes related to deterioration of liver function and increased serum ammonia level

The patient is also at risk for bleeding, owing to altered clotting mechanisms, and for portal hypertension.

▷ Planning and Implementation

▷ *Goals:* The goals of the patient may include independence in activities, improvement of nutritional status, improvement of skin integrity, decreased potential for injury, and improvement of mental status.

Nursing Interventions

To assist in accomplishing these goals, the major objectives of therapy are (1) to promote rest to reduce the demands on the dysfunctional liver, (2) to meet the patient's nutritional needs, (3) to prevent further threats to skin integrity, (4) to minimize risk of bleeding, and (5) to minimize metabolic derangements and limit those factors causing further deterioration of mental function.

Rest. The patient with active liver disease requires rest and other supportive measures to permit the liver to reestablish its functional ability. The patient's weight and the volume of his fluid intake and output are measured and recorded daily. His position in bed is adjusted for maximal respiratory efficiency, which is especially important if ascites is marked.

Oxygen therapy may be required in liver failure to oxygenate the weakened cells, lest more die.

Rest permits the liver to restore itself by limiting the demands of the body and increasing the liver's blood supply. Since the patient is more susceptible to infection, efforts to prevent respiratory, circulatory, and vascular disturbances need to be initiated. These measures may help prevent such problems as pneumonia, thrombophlebitis, and pressure sores. When the patient's nutritional status improves and the patient gains strength, he is encouraged to increase his activity gradually. Activity and mild exercise, as well as rest, are planned.

Improved Nutritional Status. The cirrhotic patient who has no ascites or edema and exhibits no signs of impending coma should receive a nutritious, high-protein diet supplemented by vitamins of the B complex and others as indicated (including vitamins A, C, and K and folic acid). Since proper nutrition is so important, every effort must be made to encourage the patient to eat. This is as important as any medication. Often small, frequent meals are tolerated better than three large meals because of the abdominal pressure exerted by ascites.

Patient preferences are considered. Patients with prolonged or severe anorexia, or those who are vomiting or eating poorly for any reason, can be fed by nasogastric tube or parenteral hyperalimentation.

Patients with fatty stools (steatorrhea) should receive water-soluble forms of fat-soluble vitamins—A, D, and E (Aquasol A, D, and E). Folic acid and iron are prescribed to prevent anemia. If the patient shows signs of impending or advancing coma, a low-protein diet should be given temporarily; too much high-protein food such as meats may produce portal-systemic encephalopathy (PSE), and too little may cause negative nitrogen balance and wasting. Suggested protein foods are dairy products (eggs, skim milk), cereal (wheat germ, white rice), and fish (shellfish, salmon sardines). A high-caloric intake should be maintained, and supplementary vitamins and minerals should be supplied (*e.g.*, oral potassium, if the serum potassium is normal or low and if renal function is normal). As soon as the patient's condition permits, the protein intake should be restored to normal, or above. Diet therapy is determined on an individualized basis.

Skin Care. Skin care is observed meticulously, because of the presence of subcutaneous edema, the immobility of the patient, jaundice, and increased susceptibility to skin breakdown and infection. Frequent position changes are necessary to prevent pressure sores. Irritating soaps and use of adhesive tape are avoided to prevent trauma to the skin. Lotion may be soothing to irritated skin; measures are taken to minimize the patient's scratching of the skin.

Prevention of Bleeding. Because of decreased production of prothrombin and the diseased liver's decreased synthesis of substances used in blood coagulation, hemorrhage is possible. Precautionary measures include protecting the patient with padded side rails, applying pressure to an injection site, and avoiding injury from sharp objects. The nurse should observe for melena and check stools for blood as signs of possible internal bleeding.

Improved Mental Function. Portal-systemic encephalopathy (PSE) is a possible neurologic syndrome that includes deteriorating mental status and dementia as well as physical signs such as abnormal voluntary and involuntary movements. It has occurred in postshunt patients and in those with advanced cirrhosis. PSE is mainly caused by ammonia and its effect on cerebral metabolism. Many factors predispose the patient with cirrhosis to PSE; some are unforeseeable, but many are avoidable. The nurse is in a position to observe early evidence of this condition and promote early treatment. The nurse also uses strategies to orient the patient to reality.

Patient Education and Home Health Care. During hospitalization, the patient is prepared for discharge by the nurse and other health care providers through dietary instruction. Of greatest importance is the exclusion of alcohol from the diet. The patient may need referral to Alcoholics Anonymous, psychiatric care, or support from a trusted clergyman.

Sodium restriction will continue for a considerable period of time, if not permanently. If this diet is to be followed correctly, the patient will require written instructions, teaching, reinforcement, and support from the staff as well as the family members.

The success of treatment depends on convincing the patient of the need to adhere completely to the therapeutic plan. This includes rest; probably a change in life-style; an adequate, well-balanced diet; and the elimination of alcohol. The patient and family are also instructed about the symptoms of impending encephalopathy and the possibility of bleeding tendencies and easy susceptibility to infection. Recovery is neither rapid nor easy; there are frequent setbacks and apparent lack of improvement. Many patients find it difficult to refrain from using alcohol for comfort or escape. The understanding nurse can play a significant role in offering support and encouragement to this patient. Referral of the patient to a community health nurse who visits the patient in the home following discharge may assist the patient in dealing with the transition from hospital to home, where use of alcohol may have been an important part of the patient's normal home life. The community health nurse is able to observe the patient's progress at home and the manner in which he and his family cope with the elimination of alcohol and restrictions on diet. Additionally, the nurse is able to reinforce previous teaching and answer questions that may not have occurred to the patient or family until the patient was back home and trying to reestablish new patterns of eating, drinking, and lifestyle.

Summary. For an overall view of the nursing management of the patient with cirrhosis, refer to Nursing Care Plan 35-2.

▷ *Evaluation*

▷ *Expected Outcomes*

1. Patient demonstrates ability to participate in activities.
   a. Plans activities and exercises to allow alternating periods of rest and activity.
   b. Reports increased strength and well-being.
   c. Displays increased weight gain without increased edema and ascites formation.
   d. Participates in hygienic care.
2. Increases nutritional intake.
   a. Demonstrates intake of appropriate nutrients and avoidance of alcohol as reflected in diet log.
   b. Gains weight without increased edema and ascites formation.

(Text continues on p. 882)

Care of the Patient With Cirrhosis

Nursing Interventions	Rationale	Expected Outcomes

Nursing Diagnosis: Activity intolerance related to fatigue and weight loss

Goal: Increased energy and increased participation in activities

Nursing Interventions	Rationale	Expected Outcomes
1. Offer high-protein, high-caloric diet.	1. Provides calories for energy and protein for healing.	Increases participation in activities: • Reports increased strength and well-being.
2. Give supplementary vitamins (A, B-complex, C, and K).	2. Provides additional nutrients.	• Plans activities to allow ample periods of rest.
3. Encourage alternating periods of rest and exercise.	3. Conserves patient's energy while encouraging exercise within patient's tolerance.	• Increases activity and exercise as strength increases.
4. Encourage and assist with gradually increasing periods of exercise.	4. Improves general well-being and self-esteem.	• Gains weight without increased edema or ascites formation. • Demonstrates adequate intake of nutrients and excludes alcohol from diet.

Nursing Diagnosis: Hyperthermia related to inflammatory process of cirrhosis

Goal: Maintenance of normal body temperature

Nursing Interventions	Rationale	Expected Outcomes
1. Record temperature regularly.	1. Provides baseline to detect fever and to evaluate interventions.	• Reports normal temperature and absence of chills or sweating.
2. Encourage fluid intake.	2. Corrects fluid loss from perspiration and fever and increases patient's level of comfort.	• Demonstrates adequate intake of fluids.
3. Apply cool sponges and/or icebag for elevated temperature.	3. Promotes reduction of fever by conduction and evaporation and increases patient's comfort.	
4. Administer antibiotics as prescribed.	4. Promotes appropriate serum concentration of antibiotics to treat infection.	
5. Avoid exposure to infections.	5. Minimizes risk of further infection and further increases in body temperature and metabolic rate.	
6. Keep patient at rest while temperature is elevated.	6. Reduces metabolic rate.	

Nursing Diagnosis: Altered skin integrity related to edema formation

Goal: Improved skin integrity and protection of edematous tissue

Nursing Interventions	Rationale	Expected Outcomes
1. Restrict sodium as prescribed.	1. Minimizes edema formation.	• Exhibits normal turgor of skin of extremities and trunk.
2. Give careful attention and care to the skin.	2. Edematous skin and tissue has compromised nutrient supply and is very vulnerable to pressure and trauma.	• Exhibits absence of skin breakdown. • Exhibits normal tissue without evidence of redness, discoloration, or increased warmth over bony prominences.
3. Turn and change position of patient frequently.	3. Minimizes prolonged pressure and promotes mobilization of edema.	• Changes position frequently.

(continued)

Nursing Care Plan 35-2 *(continued)*

Nursing Interventions	Rationale	Expected Outcomes

Nursing Diagnosis: Altered skin integrity related to edema formation

Goal: Improved skin integrity and protection of edematous tissue

4. Weigh patient daily and record intake and output.	4. Permits best estimate of fluid status and monitoring of fluid retention and loss from tissues.
5. Carry out passive range of motion exercises; elevate edematous extremities.	5. Promotes mobilization of edema.
6. Provide small foam-rubber supports under heels, malleoli, and other bony prominences.	6. Protects bony prominences and minimizes trauma *if used correctly*.

Nursing Diagnosis: Impairment of skin integrity related to jaundice and compromised immunologic status

Goal: Improved skin integrity and minimization of skin irritation

1. Note and record degree of jaundice of skin and sclerae.	1. Provides baseline for detecting changes and evaluating interventions.	Demonstrates improved skin integrity: • Exhibits intact skin without evidence of breakdown or infection.
2. Provide frequent skin care, bathing without soap, and massage with emollient lotions.	2. Prevents dryness of skin and minimizes pruritus.	• Reports absence of pruritus. • Demonstrates decreasing jaundice of skin and sclerae.
3. Keep patient's fingernails short.	3. Prevents skin excoriation from scratching.	• Uses emollients and avoids soaps in daily hygiene.

Nursing Diagnosis: Alterations in nutrition related to anorexia and gastrointestinal disturbances

Goal: Improved nutritional status

1. Encourage patient to eat meals and supplementary feedings.	1. Encouragement is essential for the patient with anorexia and gastrointestinal discomfort.	Increased intake of nutritious diet: • Demonstrates intake of sufficient high-protein, high-caloric meals.
2. Offer frequent, small feedings.	2. Small meals are frequently easier for the anorexic patient to tolerate.	• Identifies foods and fluid that are nutritious and permitted on diet.
3. Provide attractive meals and an aesthetically pleasing setting at meal time.	3. Promotes appetite and sense of well-being.	• Gains weight without increased edema or ascites formation.
4. Eliminate alcohol.	4. Eliminates "empty calories" and avoids the gastric irritation produced by alcohol.	• Identifies the rationale for small, frequent meals.
5. Provide oral hygiene before meals.	5. Reduces unpleasant taste and stimulates appetite.	• Reports increased appetite and well-being. • Excludes alcohol from diet.
6. Apply an ice collar for nausea.	6. May reduce incidence of nausea.	• Participates in oral hygiene measures before meals and to counteract nausea.
7. Administer medications prescribed for nausea, vomiting, diarrhea, or constipation.	7. Reduces gastrointestinal symptoms and discomforts that decrease the appetite and interest in food.	• Takes medications for gastrointestinal disorders as prescribed.
8. Encourage increased fluid intake and exercise if the patient reports constipation.	8. Promotes normal bowel pattern and reduces abdominal discomfort and distention.	• Reports normal gastrointestinal function with regular bowel function.
9. Observe for evidence of gastrointestinal bleeding.	9. Detects serious gastrointestinal complications.	• Identifies reportable symptoms of abnormal gastrointestinal function: melena, gross bleeding.

(continued)

Nursing Care Plan 35-2 *(continued)*

Nursing Interventions	Rationale	Expected Outcomes

Nursing Diagnosis: Potential for injury related to portal hypertension, altered clotting mechanisms, and impaired detoxification of drugs.

Goal: Decreased risk of injury

Nursing Interventions	Rationale	Expected Outcomes
1. Observe each stool for color, consistency, and amount.	1. Permits detection of bleeding in gastrointestinal tract.	• Exhibits absence of frank bleeding from gastrointestinal tract.
2. Be alert for symptoms of anxiety, epigastric fullness, weakness, and restlessness.	2. May indicate early signs of bleeding and shock.	• Exhibits absence of restlessness, epigastric fullness, and other indicators of hemorrhage and shock.
3. Test each stool and emesis for occult blood.	3. Detects early evidence of bleeding.	• Exhibits negative results of test for occult gastrointestinal bleeding.
4. Observe for hemorrhagic manifestations: ecchymosis, epistaxis, petechiae, and bleeding gums.	4. Indicates altered clotting mechanisms.	• Is free of ecchymotic areas or hematoma formation.
5. Record vital signs at frequent intervals.	5. Provides baseline and evidence of hypovolemia, shock.	• Exhibits normal vital signs.
6. Keep patient quiet and limit activity.	6. Minimizes risk of bleeding and straining.	• Maintains rest and remains quiet if active bleeding occurs.
7. Assist physician in passage of tube for esophageal balloon tamponade.	7. Promotes nontraumatic insertion of tube in anxious and combative patient for immediate treatment of bleeding.	• Identifies rationale for blood transfusions and measures to treat bleeding.
8. Observe during blood transfusions.	8. Permits detection of transfusion reactions (risk is increased with multiple blood transfusions needed for active bleeding from esophageal varices).	• Uses measures to prevent trauma (*e.g.,* uses soft toothbrush, blows nose gently, avoids bumps and falls, avoids straining during defecation).
9. Measure and record nature, time, and amount of vomitus.	9. Assists in evaluating extent of bleeding and blood loss.	• Experiences no side-effects of medications.
10. Maintain patient in fasting state, if indicated.	10. Reduces risk of aspiration of gastric contents and minimizes risk of further trauma to esophagus and stomach by preventing vomiting.	• Takes all medications as prescribed.
11. Administer vitamin K as prescribed.	11. Promotes clotting by providing fat-soluble vitamin necessary for clotting mechanism.	• Identifies rationale for precautions with use of all medications.
12. Stay in constant attendance during episodes of bleeding.	12. Reassures anxious patient and permits monitoring and detection of further needs of the patient.	
13. Offer cold liquids by mouth when bleeding stops (if prescribed).	13. Minimizes risk of further bleeding by promoting vasoconstriction of esophageal and gastric blood vessels.	
14. Institute measures to prevent trauma: a. Maintain safe environment.	a. Minimizes risk of trauma and bleeding by avoiding falls and cuts, etc.	
b. Encourage *gentle* blowing of nose	b. Reduces risk of nosebleed (epistaxis) secondary to trauma and decreased clotting.	
c. Provide soft toothbrush and avoid use of toothpicks.	c. Prevents trauma to oral mucosa while promoting good oral hygiene.	

(continued)

Nursing Interventions	*Rationale*	*Expected Outcomes*

Nursing Diagnosis: Potential for injury related to portal hypertension, altered clotting mechanisms, and impaired detoxification of drugs.

Goal: Decreased risk of injury

d. Encourage intake of foods with high content of vitamin C.	d. Promotes healing.	
e. Apply cold compresses where indicated.	e. Minimizes bleeding into tissues by promoting local vasoconstriction.	
f. Record location of bleeding sites.	f. Permits detection of new bleeding sites and monitoring of previous sites of bleeding.	
g. Use small-gauge needles for injections.	g. Minimizes oozing and blood loss from repeated injections.	
15. Administer medications carefully; watch for side-effects.	15. Reduces risk of side-effects secondary to damaged liver's inability to detoxify (metabolize) drugs and medications normally.	

Nursing Diagnosis: Alteration in comfort related to enlarged tender liver and ascites

Goal: Increased level of comfort

1. Maintain bed rest when patient experiences abdominal discomfort.	1. Reduces metabolic demands and protects the liver.	• Maintains bed rest and decreases activity in presence of pain.
2. Administer antispasmodics and sedatives as prescribed.	2. Reduces irritability of the gastrointestinal tract and decreases abdominal pain and discomfort.	• Takes antispasmodics and sedatives as indicated and as prescribed.
3. Observe, record, and report presence and character of pain and discomfort.	3. Provides baseline to detect further deterioration of status and to evaluate interventions.	• Reports decreased pain and abdominal discomfort. • Reports pain and discomfort if present.
4. Reduce sodium and fluid intake if prescribed.	4. Minimizes further formation of ascites.	• Reduces sodium and fluid intake to prescribed levels if indicated to treat ascites. • Obtains pain relief. • Exhibits decreased abdominal girth and appropriate weight changes.

Nursing Diagnosis: Fluid volume excess related to ascites and edema formation

Goal: Restoration of normal fluid volume

1. Restrict sodium and fluid intake if prescribed.	1. Minimizes formation of ascites and edema.	• Consumes diet low in sodium and within prescribed fluid restriction.
2. Administer diuretics, potassium, and protein supplements as prescribed.	2. Promotes excretion of fluid through the kidneys and maintenance of normal fluid and electrolyte balance.	• Takes diuretics, potassium, and protein supplements as indicated without experiencing side-effects.
3. Record intake and output.	3. Assesses effectiveness of treatment and adequacy of fluid intake.	• Exhibits increased urine output.
4. Measure and record abdominal girth daily.	4. Monitors changes in ascites formation and accumulation.	• Exhibits decreasing abdominal girth.
5. Explain rationale for sodium and fluid restriction.	5. Promotes patient's understanding of restriction and cooperation with it.	• Identifies rationale for sodium and fluid restriction.

(continued)

Nursing Interventions	*Rationale*	*Expected Outcomes*

Nursing Diagnosis: Impaired thought processes related to deterioration of liver function and increased serum ammonia level

Goal: Improved mental status

1. Restrict dietary protein as prescribed.	1. Reduces source of ammonia (protein foods).	Demonstrates improved mental status:
2. Give frequent small feeding of carbohydrates.	2. Promotes adequate carbohydrate for energy requirements and "spares" protein from breakdown for energy.	• Exhibits serum ammonia level within normal limits. • Is oriented to time, place, and person. • Reports normal sleep patterns.
3. Protect from infection.	3. Minimizes risk of further increase in metabolic requirements.	• Demonstrates an interest in events and activities around him.
4. Keep environment warm and draft-free.	4. Minimizes shivering, which would increase metabolic requirements.	• Demonstrates normal attention span. • Follows and participates in conversations appropriately.
5. Pad the side-rails of the bed.	5. Provides protection for the patient in the event that hepatic coma and seizure activity occur.	• Reports urinary and fecal continence. • Experiences no seizures.
6. Limit visitors.	6. Minimizes patient's activity and metabolic requirements.	
7. Provide careful nursing surveillance to ensure patient's safety.	7. Provides close monitoring of new symptoms and minimizes trauma to the confused patient.	
8. Avoid narcotics and barbiturates.	8. Prevents masking of symptoms of hepatic coma and prevents drug overdose secondary to reduced ability of the damaged liver to metabolize narcotics and barbiturates.	
9. Arouse at intervals.	9. Provides stimulation to the patient and opportunity for observing the patient's level of consciousness.	

Nursing Diagnosis: Alteration in respiratory function related to ascites and restriction of thoracic excursion secondary to ascites, abdominal distention, and fluid in the thoracic cavity

Goal: Improved respiratory status

1. Elevate head of bed.	1. Reduces abdominal pressure on the diaphragm and permits fuller thoracic excursion and lung expansion.	Experiences improved respiratory status: • Reports decreased shortness of breath.
2. Conserve patient's strength.	2. Reduces patient metabolic and oxygen requirements.	• Reports increased strength and sense of well-being.
3. Change position at intervals.	3. Promotes expansion and oxygenation of all areas of the lungs.	• Exhibits respiratory rate (12–18/min) with no adventitious sounds.
4. Assist patient during thoracentesis.	4. Thoracentesis (performed to remove fluid from the thoracic cavity) may be frightening to the patient. Helps obtain patient's cooperation with the procedure, minimizing discomfort and risks.	• Exhibits full thoracic excursion without shallow respirations. • Exhibits normal blood gases. • Experiences absence of confusion or cyanosis.
a. Support and maintain position during procedure.		
b. Record both the amount and the character of fluid aspirated.	b. Provides record of fluid removed and indication of severity of limitation of lung expansion by fluid.	
c. Observe for evidence of coughing, increasing dyspnea, or pulse rate.	c. Indicates irritation of the pleural space and evidence of ventilatory function compromised by pneumothorax or hemothorax (air or blood accumulating in pleural space).	

c. Reports decrease in gastrointestinal disturbances and anorexia.

d. Identifies foods and fluids that are nutritious and allowed on diet.

e. Identifies foods restricted from diet.

f. Adheres to vitamin therapy regimen.

g. Describes the rationale for small, frequent meals.

h. Excludes alcohol from diet.

3. Demonstrates improved skin integrity.

a. Shows intact skin without evidence of breakdown or infection.

b. Achieves decreased edema in extremities and trunk.

c. Demonstrates normal turgor of skin of extremities and trunk.

d. Changes position frequently.

e. Inspects bony prominences daily.

f. Avoids trauma to skin.

g. Reports decreased or absent pruritus.

h. Uses lotions to decrease pruritus.

4. Experiences decreased risk of bleeding.

a. Is free of ecchymotic areas or hematoma formation.

b. Reports absence of frank bleeding from gastrointestinal tract (*e.g.*, absence of melena and hematemesis).

c. Reports negative results of test for occult gastrointestinal bleeding.

d. Uses measures to prevent trauma (*e.g.*, uses soft toothbrush, blows nose gently, arranges furniture to prevent bumps and falls, avoids straining during defecation).

5. Demonstrates improved mental function.

a. Has serum ammonia level within normal limits.

b. Is oriented to time, place, and person.

c. Demonstrates normal attention span (*e.g.*, is able to complete reading of desired articles, books; able to watch television with interest).

d. Converses with family and health care team members appropriately.

e. Reports urinary and fecal continence.

f. Identifies early, reportable signs of impaired thought processes.

Bleeding Esophageal Varices

Signs of jaundice, ascites, and portal hypertension are manifestations of advanced liver disease. Usually, the patient has impaired clotting and requires careful monitoring of laboratory blood studies, hematemesis, and melena.

Pathophysiology and Clinical Manifestations

Esophageal varices are dilated tortuous veins usually found in the submucosa of the lower esophagus; however, they may develop higher in the esophagus or extend into the stomach. Such a condition nearly always is caused by portal hypertension, which, in turn, is due to obstruction of the portal venous circulation within the substance of a cirrhotic liver (see p. 873). Hemorrhage from ruptured esophageal varices is the most common single cause of death in patients with cirrhosis.

Because of increased obstruction of the portal vein, venous blood from the intestinal tract and spleen seeks an outlet through collateral circulation (new avenues of return to the right atrium). The pathophysiologic effect is increased strain, particularly on the vessels in the submucosal layer of the lower esophagus and upper part of the stomach. These collateral vessels are not very elastic but rather are tortuous and fragile and bleed easily. Other less common causes of varices are abnormalities of the circulation in the splenic vein or superior vena cava and hepatic venothrombosis.

Bleeding esophageal varices are life threatening and can result in hemorrhagic shock, producing decreased cerebral, hepatic, and renal perfusion. In turn, there will be an increased nitrogen load from bleeding into the gastrointestinal tract and an increased serum ammonia level which increase the risk of encephalopathy. Bleeding esophageal varices should be suspected in the presence of hematemesis and melena, especially in the patient who has been addicted to alcohol. Usually, the dilated veins cause no symptoms unless the mucosa over them becomes ulcerated. Then massive hemorrhage takes place. Factors that contribute to rupture and hemorrhage are muscular strain from lifting heavy objects, straining at stool, sneezing, coughing or vomiting, esophagitis, or irritation of vessels by poorly chewed foods or irritating fluids. Salicylates and any drug that erodes esophageal mucosa or interferes with cell replication may also cause bleeding.

Assessment

The patient's history and physical examination serve as a basis for identifying the problem. Neurologic assessment will assist in identifying possible hepatic encephalopathy resulting from the breakdown of blood in the gastrointestinal tract and a rising serum ammonia level. Manifestations range from drowsiness to coma. Portal hypertension may be suspected if dilated abdominal veins and rectal hemorrhoids are detected. Also apparent may be a palpable enlarged spleen (splenomegaly) and ascites. Laboratory tests that may be required are various liver function tests, such as BSP retention, serum transaminase, bilirubin, alkaline phosphatase, and serum proteins. Esophagoscopy or endoscopy most clearly confirms the diagnosis because even the site of hemorrhage may be seen. The site of bleeding must be identified, since one third or more patients bleed from other sources. Gastritis and duodenal ulcer frequently coexist with cirrhosis. Nursing support before and during examination by esophagoscopy or endoscopy can be effective in relieving a stressful experience. Careful monitoring can detect early signs of cardiac arrhythmias, perforation, and hemorrhage. After the examination, fluids are not given until the gag reflex returns. Lozenges and gargles may be used to relieve throat discomfort if the patient's condition permits and he is able to participate in his care.

Portal vein pressure can be measured in the operating room by introducing a needle into the spleen; a manometer reading above 20 ml saline is abnormal. Combined umbilical-portal and hepatic vein catheterization is the most practical method for measuring portal pressure and at the same time permits radiologic study of the hepatic vascular bed. Blood flow studies may also be done, which assists in determining cardiac output.

Splenoportography is studied in serial or segmental x-ray films to detect extensive collateral circulation in esophageal vessels, which would be indicative of varices. Other tests are hepatoportography and celiac angiography. These are usually done in the operating room or radiology department.

Overall nursing assessment includes an evaluation of the emotional concerns of the patient and any physical problems. Vital signs are taken, and the nutritional needs are assessed. Bleeding from esophageal varices can quickly lead to hemorrhagic shock and should be considered an emergency.

Management

The patient with bleeding varices is critically ill, requiring aggressive medical care and expert nursing care (Chart 35-3). Assessment requires that the extent of bleeding be evaluated and vital signs monitored continuously when hematemesis and melena are present. Signs of potential hypovolemia are to be noted, such as cold, clammy skin, tachycardia, a drop in blood pressure, decreased urine output, restlessness, and increased or shallow peripheral pulse. Blood volume is monitored by means of a central venous pressure or arterial

---

Chart 35-3
Management Modalities and Nursing Care for the Patient With Bleeding Esophageal Varices

Treatment Modality*	Action	Nursing Priorities
Nonsurgical Modalities		
Pharmacologic agents		
Vasopressin (Pitressin)	Reduces portal pressure by constricting splanchnic arteries	Observe response to therapy.
Propranolol (Inderol)	Reduces portal pressure by β-adrenergic blocking action.	Monitor for side-effects (*Vasopressin*: angina. *Propranolol*: decreased pulse and blood pressure, impaired cardiovascular response to hemorrhage).
		Administer medication as prescribed.
		Support patient during treatment.
Balloon tamponade	Exerts pressure directly to bleeding sites in esophagus and stomach	Monitor closely to prevent accidental removal or displacement of tube and subsequent airway obstruction.
		Explain procedure to patient briefly to obtain cooperation with insertion and maintenance of esophageal-tamponade tube and reduce patient's fear of the procedure.
		Provide frequent oral hygiene.
Iced saline lavage	Produces vasoconstriction of the esophageal and gastric blood vessels	Ensure patency of the nasogastric tube to prevent aspiration.
		Observe gastric aspirate for evidence of bleeding and its cessation.
		Protect the patient from chilling.
Injection sclerotherapy	Promotes thrombosis and sclerosis of bleeding sites by injection of sclerosing agent into the esophageal varices	Observe for aspiration, perforation of the esophagus, and recurrence of bleeding following treatment.
Surgical Modalities		
Portal-systemic shunts	Reduces portal hypertension by diverting blood flow away from obstructed portal system.	Observe for development of portal systemic encephalopathy (altered mental status, neurologic dysfunction), hepatic failure, and rebleeding.
		Requires intensive, expert nursing care for prolonged period.
Surgical ligation of varices	Ties off blood vessels at the site of bleeding	Provide post-thoracotomy care.
		Observe for rebleeding.

* Several modalities may be used concurrently or in sequence.

catheter. Oxygen is required to prevent hypoxia and to maintain adequate blood oxygenation. Blood transfusion also may be needed.

Since patients with bleeding esophageal varices are subject to electrolyte imbalance, intravenous fluids are provided to restore fluid volume and replace deficient electrolytes. Urinary output is carefully monitored; an indwelling catheter may be indicated.

Nonsurgical Management.   Nonoperative treatment is the treatment of choice because of the high mortality of emergency surgery for control of bleeding esophageal varices and because of the poor physical condition of the patient with severe liver dysfunction.

Pharmacologic Therapy.   Vasopressin (Pitressin) may be the initial mode of therapy because of its constriction of the splanchnic arterial bed and resulting decrease in portal pressure. It may be given intravenously or by intra-arterial infusion. Either method requires monitoring by the nurse. Gastric as-

piration and vital signs offer indices of the effectiveness of vasopressin.

- Coronary artery disease in this patient would be a contraindication to the use of vasopressin, since coronary vasoconstriction is a side-effect that may precipitate myocardial infarction.

Electrolyte evaluation and monitoring of fluid intake and output are necessary, since hyponatremia may occur and vasopressin may have an antidiuretic effect.

Balloon Tamponade.   To control the hemorrhage in certain patients, pressure is exerted on the cardia (upper orifice of the stomach) and against the bleeding varices by a double-balloon tamponade (Sengstaken-Blakemore tube) (Fig. 35-8). The three openings in the tube are for specific purposes: gastric aspiration, inflation of the gastric balloon, and inflation of the esophageal balloon.

The balloon in the stomach is inflated, and the tube is

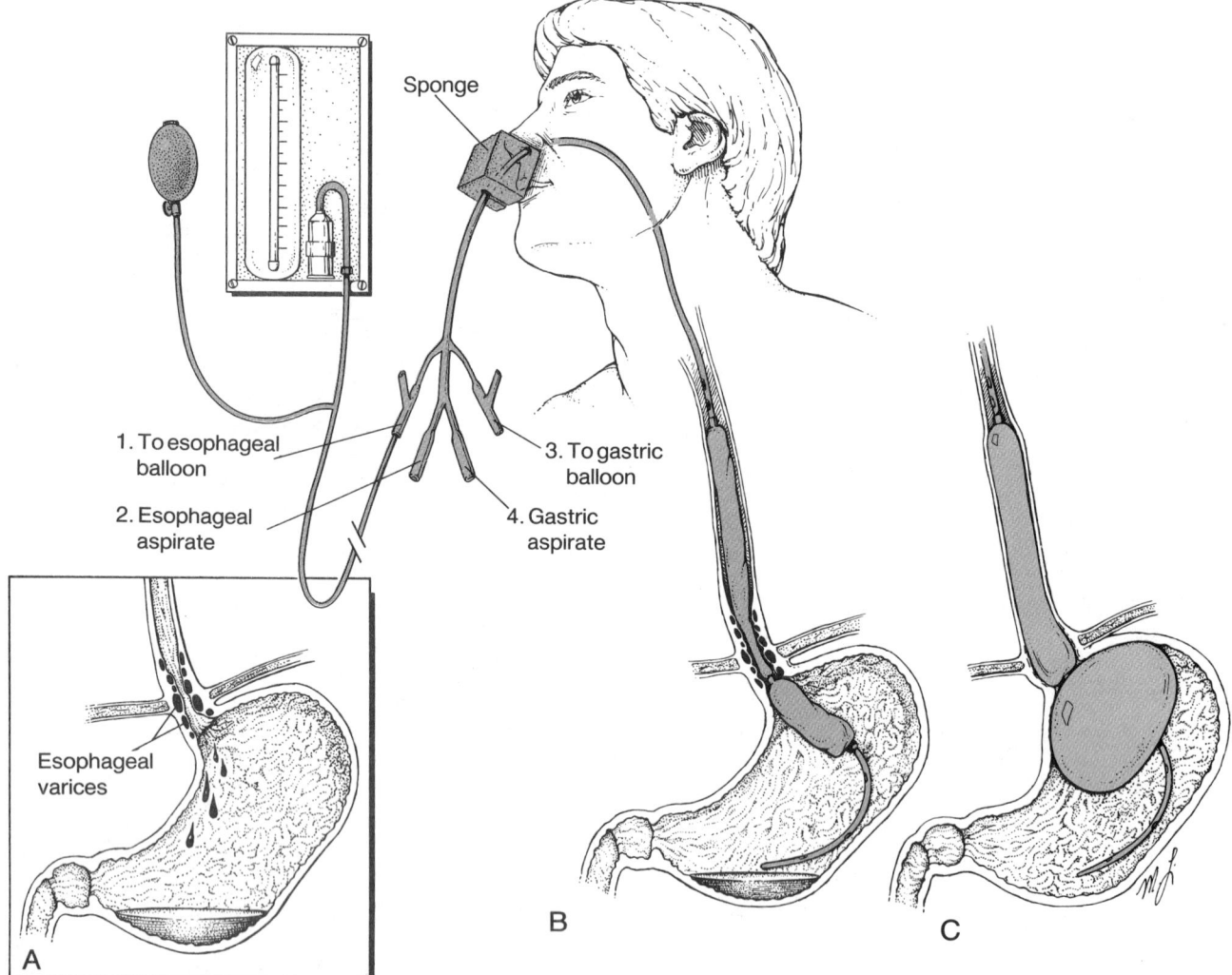

Figure 35-8
Esophageal balloon tamponade to treat bleeding esophageal varices. (*A*) Dilated, bleeding esophageal veins (varices) of the lower esophagus. (*B*) A four-lumen esophageal tamponade tube with balloons (uninflated) in place. (*C*) Compression of bleeding esophageal varices by inflated esophageal and gastric balloons. The gastric and esophageal outlets permit aspiration of secretions.

pulled gently to exert a force against the cardia. Irrigation of the tubing is performed to detect bleeding; if returns are clear, the esophageal balloon is not inflated. If bleeding continues, the esophageal balloon is inflated. The desired pressure in both balloons is 25 to 30 mm Hg, as measured by the manometer. After the balloon is inflated, there is a possibility of injury or rupture of the esophagus. Constant nursing surveillance is necessary at this time. Traction is placed on the tube at the site of insertion. A nasogastric tube may be inserted through the other nares to aspirate esophagopharyngeal secretions if a three-lumen tube is used. This is not necessary with the four-lumen tube (Fig. 35-8*C*), because a fourth lumen provides a direct route for esophageal aspiration.

Usually, a cathartic such as magnesium sulfate is introduced through the tube to eliminate blood in the gastrointestinal tract; otherwise, ammonia absorption could occur, which may lead to hepatic coma and death. Thereafter, neomycin is administered to reduce intestinal bacterial flora, which are a source of ammonia-forming enzymes.

Gastric suction is provided by connecting the proper catheter outlet to suction. The tubing is irrigated hourly, and drainage will indicate whether bleeding has been controlled. Iced saline lavage or irrigation may be used in the stomach balloon in order to constrict the gastric vessels. In such instances, the nurse will anticipate possible chilling of the patient and provide comfort measures. The pressures on the tubes and traction are released periodically, as prescribed. Balloon tamponade is continued for several days and then cautiously released, followed by removal of the tube if no bleeding recurs.

Although this method has been fairly successful, it is important to note some inherent dangers. If the tube is left in place or inflated too long or at too high a pressure, ulceration and necrosis can develop in the stomach or esophagus. If the tube suddenly ruptures, the result is disastrous—airway obstruction and aspiration of gastric contents into the lungs. Using a new, tested tube may prevent this calamity. Asphyxiation is another problem, caused by the counterweight pulling the tube into the oropharynx. These potential dangers suggest the need for intensive and expert care. The balloon may be deflated for 5 minutes at 8- to 12-hour intervals if prescribed, to prevent erosion and necrosis of the stomach and esophagus.

Nursing comfort measures include frequent mouth and nasal care. For secretions that accumulate in the mouth, tissues should be within easy reach of the patient. The patient who has experienced esophageal hemorrhage is usually anxious and frightened. The patient is less anxious if he knows that the nurse is nearby and will respond immediately to his call.

Injection Sclerotherapy. In injection sclerotherapy (Fig. 35-9), a sclerosing agent is injected through a fiberoptic endoscope into the bleeding esophageal varices to promote thrombosis and eventual sclerosis. Although controlled studies have not yet demonstrated that injection sclerotherapy is superior to other treatments or improves long-term survival, the procedure has been used successfully to treat gastrointestinal hemorrhage. In addition, it has been used as a prophylactic measure to treat esophageal varices before bleeding has occurred. Following treatment, the patient must be observed for bleeding, perforation of the esophagus, aspiration pneumonia, and esophageal stricture. Antacids may be given

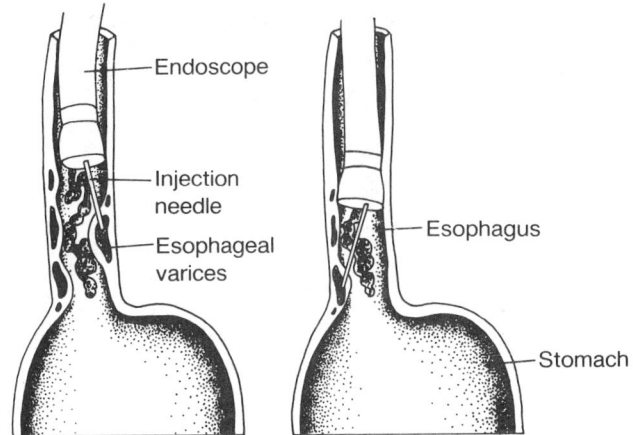

Figure 35-9
Injection sclerotherapy. Injection of sclerosing agent into esophageal varices through an endoscope.

following the procedure to counteract the effects of peptic reflux.

Repeated courses of sclerotherapy may be needed to obliterate all the varices. The patient and family need to be aware of the importance of these additional treatments even though the patient may not be actively bleeding.

Other Measures. Bleeding is also treated by sedation and complete rest of the esophagus (parenteral feedings). Straining and vomiting must be prevented. Gastric suction usually is employed to keep the stomach as empty as possible. The patient complains of severe thirst, which may be relieved by frequent oral hygiene and moist sponges to the lips. The nurse keeps close surveillance on the patient's blood pressure. Vitamin K therapy and multiple blood transfusions often are indicated. A quiet environment and calm reassurance will help to relieve the patient's anxiety.

Surgical Management. Surgical procedures that may be employed for esophageal varices are direct surgical ligation of varices and portacaval and splenorenal venous shunt operations.

Surgical Bypass Procedures. The most common procedure is to create an anastomosis between the portal vein and the inferior vena cava, which is spoken of as a *porta caval anastomosis* (Fig. 35-10). When portal blood is shunted into the vena cava, the pressure in the portal system is decreased, and consequently the danger of hemorrhage from esophageal and gastric varices is reduced. When the portal vein cannot be used because of thrombosis, or for other reasons, a shunt may be made between the splenic vein and the left renal vein (*splenorenal shunt*) following splenectomy. Some surgeons prefer this shunt to the portacaval shunt, even when the portal vein can be used.

A *mesocaval* shunt is a third type of bypass procedure, to which the inferior vena cava is severed and the proximal end of the vena cava is anastomosed to the side of the superior mesenteric vein.

These operations are extensive procedures and are not always successful, because of secondary clotting in the veins used for the shunt. Nevertheless, a shunt is the only method by which a lowering of pressure in the portal system may be brought about, and since hemorrhages from the esophageal

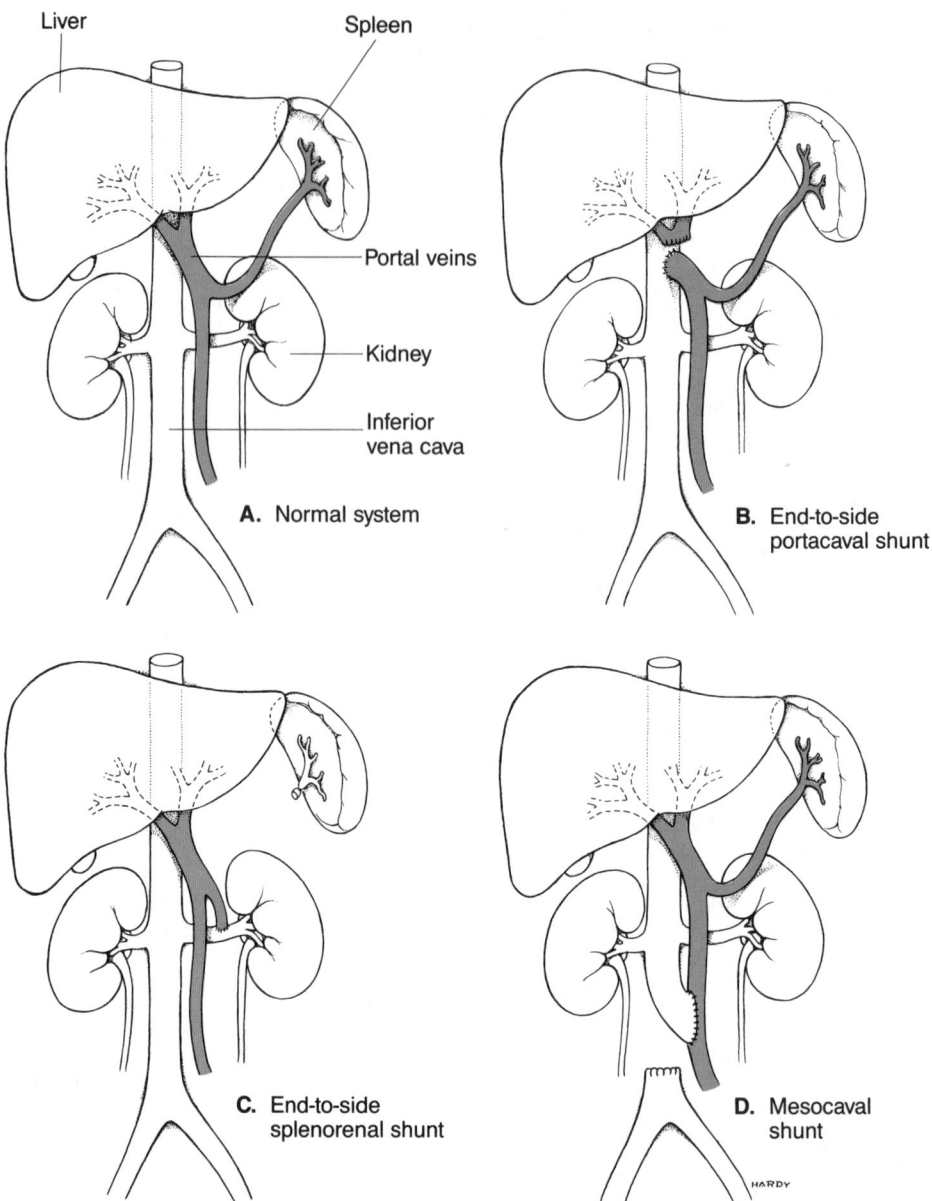

Figure 35-10
Normal portal system and examples of portal-systemic shunts.

varices are often fatal, many of these relatively poor-risk patients must be subjected to these attempts to save their lives.

Postoperative Nursing Interventions. Bleeding anywhere in the body is anxiety provoking, resulting in a crisis situation for the patient and his family. If the patient is an alcoholic, behavioral problems secondary to alcohol withdrawal can further complicate the situation. The nurse provides support and pertinent explanations regarding medical and nursing interventions. Monitoring the patient closely will help in detecting and managing complications.

Postoperative care is similar to that for any abdominal operation, but complications may arise, including hemodynamic shock, hepatic encephalopathy, electrolyte imbalance, metabolic and respiratory alkalosis, delirium tremens, and seizures. These procedures do not alter the course of the progressive liver disease, and bleeding may recur as new collateral vessels develop.

Management modalities and nursing care of the patient with bleeding esophageal varices are summarized in Chart 35-3 (p. 883).

Cancer of the Liver

Hepatic tumors generally are cancerous. It has only been in recent years that benign liver tumors have gained any significance, since their incidence has increased with the use of oral contraceptives.

As for cancerous tumors, few cancers originate in the liver. Those that are primary tumors ordinarily occur in patients with cirrhosis, especially of the postnecrotic type. Such a *hepatoma* is generally inoperable because of rapid extension and metastasis elsewhere. *Cholangiocarcinoma* is a primary malignant tumor, usually arising in normal liver. If found early, there may be cure; however, the likelihood of early detection is small.

Metastases are found in the liver in about one half of all late cancer cases. The primary growth may be almost anywhere, and since the bloodstream and the lymphatics from the body cavities nearly all reach the liver, malignant tumors anywhere in the trunk are likely to reach this organ eventually.

Moreover, the liver apparently is an ideal place for these malignant cells to thrive. Often the first evidence of a cancer in an abdominal organ is the appearance of liver metastases, and, unless exploratory operation or autopsy is performed, the primary growth may never be discovered.

Diagnosis of malignant disease of the liver is made, regardless of the location of the primary tumor, when there is a recent loss of weight, loss of strength, and anemia, which are the most common early manifestations of any cancer that interferes with nutrition. Abdominal pain may be present and accompanied by rapid enlargement of the liver, which on palpation presents an irregular surface. Jaundice is present only if the larger bile ducts are occluded by the pressure of malignant nodules in the hilum of the liver. Ascites occurs if such nodules obstruct the portal veins or if tumor tissue is seeded in the peritoneal cavity.

Nonsurgical Management

Radiation Therapy and Chemotherapy. Radiation therapy and chemotherapy have been used in the treatment of malignant disease of the liver with varying degrees of success. Although these therapies may prolong survival of some patients, the major effect is palliative.

An implantable pump has been used to deliver a high concentration of chemotherapy to the liver through the hepatic artery. This method provides a reliable, controlled, and continuous infusion of drug that can be done in the patient's home.

Patient Education and Home Health Care. The patient and family are instructed to assess and report complications and side-effects of the drug. Therefore, they need to be well informed about its actions and desired and undesirable effects. They are instructed by the nurse about the importance of follow-up visits to permit frequent checks on the response of the patient and the tumor to chemotherapy, the condition of the site of the pump insertion, and the occurrence of toxic effects. The patient is encouraged to resume routine activities as soon as possible but warned to avoid contact sports, which may damage the pump.

Percutaneous Biliary Drainage. Percutaneous biliary or transhepatic drainage is used to bypass biliary ducts obstructed by liver, pancreatic, or bile duct tumors in patients with inoperable tumors or in those considered poor surgical risks. Under fluoroscopy, a catheter is inserted through the abdominal wall, past the obstruction into the duodenum. Such procedures are used to reestablish biliary drainage, relieve pressure and pain from buildup of bile behind the obstruction, and decrease pruritus and jaundice. As a result, the patient's survival is increased and he is more comfortable. For several days after its insertion, the catheter is opened to external drainage. The bile is observed closely for amount, color, and the presence of blood and debris.

Complications of percutaneous biliary drainage include sepsis, leakage of bile, hemorrhage, and reobstruction of the biliary system by debris in the catheter or from encroaching tumor. Therefore, the patient is observed for fever and chills, bile drainage around the catheter, changes in vital signs, and evidence of biliary obstruction, including increased pain or pressure, pruritus, and recurrence of jaundice.

Patient Education and Home Health Care. The patient and his family often fear that the catheter will be dislodged and need reassurance and instruction to reduce their fear that the catheter will fall out easily. Additionally, the patient and family require verbal and written instruction as well as demonstration of catheter care. They are instructed in techniques to keep the catheter site clean and dry and to assess the catheter and its insertion site. Irrigation of the catheter with sterile normal saline or water may be indicated to keep the catheter patent and free of debris. The patient and his caregivers are taught proper technique to avoid introducing bacteria into the biliary system or catheter during irrigation. They are instructed not to aspirate or draw back on the syringe during irrigation to prevent entry of irritating duodenal contents into the biliary tree or catheter. The patient and his caregivers also learn the signs of complications and are encouraged to notify the nurse or physician if problems or questions occur.

Surgical Management

Successful hepatic lobectomy for cancer can be done when the primary hepatic tumor is localized or when, in the case of metastasis, the primary site can be completely excised and the metastasis is limited. Metastases to the liver, however, are rarely limited or solitary. Capitalizing on the regenerative capacity of the liver cells, some surgeons have successfully removed 90% of the liver.

Preoperative Evaluation and Preparation. As the patient is being prepared for surgery, his nutritional, fluid, emotional, and physical needs are evaluated and met. Meanwhile, he may be undergoing extensive and exhausting diagnostic studies. The support, explanation, and encouragement by the nurse will help him to achieve the most desirable level for surgery. It may be necessary to prepare the intestinal tract by way of cathartic, colonic irrigation, and intestinal antibiotics to minimize the possibility of ammonium accumulation and to anticipate the possibility of incision into the intestines at surgery. Specific studies may include liver scanning, liver biopsy, cholangiography, selective hepatic angiography, percutaneous needle biopsy, peritoneoscopy, laparoscopy, ultrasound and CT scans, and blood tests, particularly determinations of serum alkaline phosphatase and serum glutamic oxaloacetic acid levels.

Surgical Intervention. If it is necessary to restrict blood flow from the hepatic artery and portal vein beyond 15 minutes (under normothermic conditions, 15-minute occlusion is permissible), it is likely that hypothermia will be used. The nurse needs to be aware of the extent of surgical resection carried out in order to anticipate the patient's care. The usual true (functional) division of the liver is into two lobes, the larger (by six times) right lobe and the left lobe, with two smaller segments sandwiched between, the caudate and the quadrate. Most surgeons prefer the anatomical (surgical) division of the lobes. Here the liver is divided into a right and a left lobe by a lobar fissure that is almost in line with the gallbladder bed and the inferior vena cava on the visceral surface. According to this division, the branching of hepatic vessels and the portal vein lend themselves to a more even segmentation. A right-liver lobectomy according to the surgical division is less extensive than it would be in the functional division.

For a right-liver lobectomy or an extended right lobectomy (including medial left lobe), a thoracoabdominal incision is used. An extensive abdominal incision is made for a left lobectomy.

Postoperative Nursing Interventions. There are potential problems related to cardiopulmonary involvement, portal and general circulation, and respiratory and liver dysfunction. Metabolic abnormalities require careful attention. A constant infusion of 10% glucose may be required in the first 48 hours to prevent a precipitous fall in blood sugar, resulting from decreased gluconeogenesis. Protein synthesis and lipid metabolism are also altered, necessitating infusions of albumin. Extensive blood loss may occur, and, as a result, the patient will receive infusions of blood and intravenous fluids. The patient requires constant attention for the first 2 or 3 days, as described for abdominal and thoracic post-surgical nursing care (see pp. 343, 447). Early ambulation is encouraged. Liver regeneration is rapid; in one patient who had a 90% resection of the liver, a normal liver mass was restored in 6 months.

Liver Abscesses

Whenever an infection develops anywhere along the gastrointestinal tract, there is danger that the infecting organisms may reach the liver through the biliary system, portal venous system, or hepatic arterial or lymphatic systems. Most bacteria are promptly destroyed, but occasionally some gain a foothold. The bacterial toxins destroy the neighboring liver cells, and the necrotic tissue produced serves as a protective wall for the organisms. Meanwhile, leukocytes migrate into the infected area. The result is an abscess cavity full of a liquid containing living and dead leukocytes, liquified liver cells, and bacteria. Pyogenic abscesses of this type may be either single or multiple and small. The result is a life-threatening disease. In the past the mortality rate was 100% due to vague clinical symptoms, inadequate diagnostic tools, and inadequate surgical drainage of the abscess.

The clinical picture is one of sepsis with few or no localizing signs. The temperature is increased and may be accompanied by chills. The patient may complain of dull abdominal pain and tenderness in the right upper quadrant of the abdomen. Hepatomegaly, jaundice, and anemia may develop. With the aid of a CT scan and a liver scan for early diagnosis, and surgical drainage of the abscess, mortality has been greatly reduced.

Treatment includes intravenous antibiotic therapy; the specific antibiotic used in treatment depends on the organism identified. Although a protozoan, *Entamoeba histolytica* is the most common cause of liver abscess. In certain geographic areas, gram-negative bacilli have been implicated with increased frequency. Continuous supportive care is indicated because of the serious condition of the patient.

Liver Transplantation

Human liver transplantation has in most instances been done for life-threatening liver disease for which no other form of treatment was available. This includes biliary atresia, liver cirrhosis, chronic aggressive hepatitis, and primary liver malignancies. Orthotopic liver transplantation is the preferred surgical procedure because it is technically the easiest to perform and has been successful. This procedure involves total replacement of the liver, with anatomical reconstruction of the vasculature, or replacement of the liver with a transplant in the same area of the right upper quadrant.

The main difficulties in hepatic transplantation are technical problems causing obstruction, drug toxicity, immunochemical rejection, hepatic arterial thrombosis, or hepatic abscess. Because hepatic transplantation is performed only for severe liver disease, the patient is a poor surgical risk and frequently has many systemic problems that influence preoperative and postoperative care.

Cyclosporin, an immunosuppressive agent, used in combination with corticosteroids has considerably improved the success rate of liver transplantation. However, the patient must be monitored closely because of the regimen's toxic effects on the liver and kidneys.

Postoperative Nursing Interventions

The patient is maintained in as germ free an environment as possible, because immunosuppressive drugs reduce the body's natural defense. The patient is monitored constantly for all cardiovascular parameters, as well as arterial pressures, blood gases, and *p*H. Respiratory assistance is provided via a mechanical ventilator. Suctioning is performed as required, and sterile humidification is provided. Rejection signs are monitored through such liver function tests as SGOT, liver scans, bilirubin level, and cholangiography. Coagulation studies indicate the functioning of the transplanted liver. Cultures of urine and blood and throat swabs are taken frequently.

Hourly progress determines when the patient is ready to be weaned from the ventilator, when he may take oral fluids, and when physical activity may gradually be resumed.

The family members must be informed about the patient's condition at frequent intervals, since extensive care required in the immediate postoperative period minimizes their contact with the patient. Constant emotional support is provided to assist the patient and family through the difficult and uncertain postoperative period.

The patient and family members will require teaching about immunosuppressive drugs, signs and symptoms of rejection, and the importance of follow-up care. Long-term survival after liver transplantation is uncertain. However, advances in donor organ transplantation techniques and immunosuppressive therapy are expected to improve survival rates.

Biliary Conditions

Several disorders affect the biliary system and interfere with normal drainage of bile into the duodenum. These disorders include carcinoma that obstructs the biliary tree and infection of the biliary system. However, gallbladder disease with gallstones is the most common disorder of the biliary system. Estimates indicate that approximately 500,000 people a year in the United States are hospitalized for gallbladder disease and that about two thirds of these are treated surgically. Although not all occurrences of gallbladder infection (*cholecystitis*) are related to gallstones (*cholelithiasis*), 95% of patients with acute cholecystitis have gallstones. However, a majority of the 15 million Americans with gallstones have no pain and are unaware of the presence of stones. For a guide to the terminology associated with biliary disorders and procedures see Chart 35-4.

Cholecystitis

At times the gallbladder may be the site of an acute infection (cholecystitis) that causes acute pain, tenderness, and rigidity of the upper right abdomen, associated with nausea and vomiting and the usual signs of an acute inflammation. This condition is referred to as *acute cholecystitis*. If the gallbladder is found to be filled with pus, there is an *empyema* of the gallbladder.

Cholelithiasis

Cholelithiasis (calculi, or gallstones) usually form in the gallbladder from the solid constituents of bile and vary greatly in size, shape, and composition (Fig. 35-11).

Gallstones are uncommon in children and young adults but become increasingly prevalent after age 40. The incidence of cholelithiasis increases thereafter to such an extent that it has been estimated that by the age of 75, one of every three people will have gallstones.

Pathophysiology

There are two major types of gallstones: those composed predominantly of pigment and those composed primarily of cholesterol. Pigment stones probably form when unconjugated pigments in the bile precipitate to form stones. The risk of developing such stones is increased in patients with cirrhosis, hemolysis, and infections of the biliary tree. These stones cannot be dissolved and must be removed surgically.

Cholesterol stones account for most gallbladder disease in the United States. Cholesterol, a normal constituent of bile, is insoluble in water. Its solubility depends on bile acids and lecithin (phospholipids) in bile. In gallstone-prone patients, there is decreased bile acid synthesis and increased cholesterol synthesis in the liver, resulting in a bile supersaturated

---

> ## Chart 35-4
> ## Terminology—Biliary Disorders and Procedures
>
> Cholecystitis—inflammation of the gallbladder
> Cholelithiasis—calculi in the gallbladder
> Cholecystectomy—removal of the gallbladder
> Cholecystostomy—opening and drainage of the gallbladder
> Choledochotomy—opening into the common duct
> Choledocholithiasis—stones in the common duct
> Choledocholithotomy—incision of common bile duct for removal of stones
> Choledochoduodenostomy—anastomosis of common duct to duodenum
> Choledochojejunostomy—anastomosis of common duct to jejunum

---

with cholesterol, which precipitates out of the bile to form stones. The cholesterol-saturated bile predisposes to the formation of gallstones and acts as an irritant, producing inflammatory changes in the gallbladder.

Four times more women than men develop cholesterol stones and gallbladder disease; they are usually over 40 years of age, multiparous, and obese. There is increased incidence of stone formation in users of oral contraceptives, estrogens, and clofibrate, which are known to increase biliary cholesterol saturation. The incidence of stone formation increases with age as a result of increased hepatic secretion of cholesterol and decreased bile acid synthesis. In addition, there is increased risk because of malabsorption of bile salts in patients with gastrointestinal disease or T-tube fistula or in those who have had ileal resection or bypass.

Clinical Manifestations

Gallstones may be silent, producing no pain and only mild gastrointestinal symptoms. Such stones may be detected in-

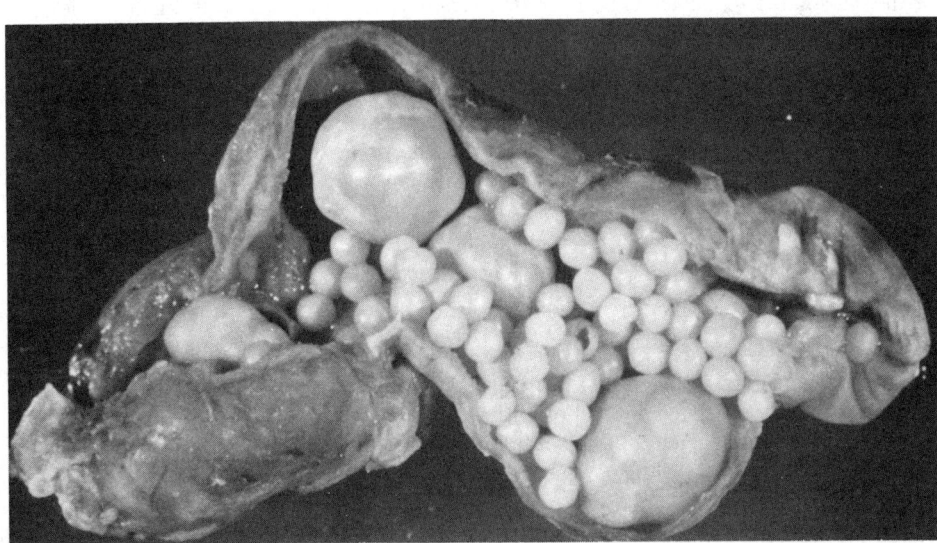

Figure 35-11
Multiple gallstones in a gallbladder. (Courtesy of National Institute of Diabetes and Digestive and Kidney Diseases.)

cidentally during surgery or evaluation for nonrelated problems.

The patient with gallbladder disease due to gallstones may develop two types of symptoms: those due to disease of the gallbladder itself and those due to obstruction of the bile passages by a gallstone. The symptoms may be acute or chronic. Epigastric distress, such as fullness, abdominal distention, and vague pain in the right upper quadrant of the abdomen, may occur following a meal high in fried or fatty foods.

If a gallstone obstructs the cystic duct, the gallbladder becomes infected and distended. The patient develops a fever and may have a palpable abdominal mass. The patient experiences biliary colic with excruciating upper right abdominal pain that radiates to the back or right shoulder, is usually associated with nausea and vomiting, and is noticeable several hours after a heavy meal. The patient moves about restlessly, unable to find a comfortable position.

Such a bout of biliary colic is caused by contraction of the gallbladder, which has been stimulated by fat and cannot release bile because of obstruction by the stone. When distended, the fundus of the gallbladder comes in contact with the abdominal wall in the region of the right ninth and tenth costal cartilages. This produces marked tenderness in the right upper quadrant on deep inspiration and prevents full inspiratory excursion. The pain of acute cholecystitis may be so severe that analgesics such as meperidine are required; nitroglycerin has also been used effectively. Morphine is thought to increase spasm of the sphincter of Oddi and its use is therefore avoided.

Jaundice occurs in a small percentage of patients with gallbladder disease and usually occurs with obstruction of the common bile duct. Obstruction of the flow of bile into the duodenum results in the following characteristic symptoms: the bile, no longer carried to the duodenum, is absorbed by the blood, giving the skin and mucous membrane a yellow color. This is frequently accompanied by marked itching of the skin.

The excretion of the bile pigments by the kidneys gives the urine a very dark color. The feces, no longer colored with bile pigments, are grayish, like putty, and usually described as "clay-colored."

Obstruction of bile flow also interferes with absorption of the fat-soluble vitamins A, D, E, and K. Therefore, the patient may exhibit deficiencies of these vitamins if biliary obstruction has been prolonged. Vitamin K deficiency will interfere with normal blood clotting.

If the gallstone is dislodged and no longer obstructs the cystic duct, the gallbladder drains and the inflammatory process subsides after a relatively short time. If the gallstone continues to obstruct the duct, abscess, necrosis, and perforation with generalized peritonitis may result.

Diagnostic Evaluation

Abdominal X-ray Films. An abdominal x-ray film may be obtained if gallbladder disease is suspected and to exclude other causes of symptoms. However only 15% to 20% of gallstones are sufficiently calcified to be visible on such films.

Ultrasonography. Ultrasonography has replaced oral cholecystography as the diagnostic procedure of choice because it is rapid and accurate and can be used in patients with liver dysfunction and jaundice. Additionally, it does not expose patients to ionizing radiation. The procedure is most accurate if the patient fasts overnight so that the gallbladder is distended. The use of ultrasound is based on reflected sound waves. Ultrasonography can detect calculi in the gallbladder or a dilated common bile duct. It is reported to detect gallstones with 95% accuracy.

Radionuclide Imaging. Cholescintigraphy is another test that has been used successfully in diagnosis of acute cholecystitis. In this procedure a radioactive agent is administered intravenously. It is then taken up by the hepatocytes and rapidly excreted through the biliary system. The biliary tract is then scanned, and images of the gallbladder and biliary tree are obtained. This test is more expensive than ultrasonography, takes longer to perform, exposes the patient to radiation, and cannot detect gallstones. Its use may be limited to those cases in which ultrasonography is not conclusive.

Cholecystography. Although it has been replaced by ultrasonography as the test of choice, cholecystography is still used if ultrasound equipment is not available or if the ultrasound results are questionable in a patient with chronic symptoms. Oral or intravenous cholangiography may be performed to detect gallstones and to assess the ability of the gallbladder to fill, concentrate its contents, contract, and empty. An iodide-containing contrast medium that is excreted by the liver and concentrated in the gallbladder is administered to the patient. The normal gallbladder fills with this radiopaque substance. If gallstones are present, they appear as negative shadows on the x-ray film.

Drugs given as contrast media include iopanoic acid (Telepaque), iodipamide meglumine (Cholografin), and sodium ipodate (Oragrafin). These preparations are given in oral doses, 10 to 12 hours before x-ray study. Intravenous cholecystography involves the injection of an iodide approximately 10 minutes prior to roentgenography. During the interval between the administration of the iodide and the x-ray study, the patient is permitted nothing by mouth to prevent contraction and emptying of the gallbladder.

Nursing Interventions. Before administering the contrast medium to the patient, it is important to question him about allergies to iodine or seafood. The use of iodine in such patients may produce a severe allergic reaction.

Instructions to patients who are scheduled for x-ray studies of the gallbladder (cholecystogram, gallbladder series) include the following:

1. One hour or more after the evening meal, and approximately 10 hours before roentgenography, the patient receives tablets or capsules of contrast medium by mouth. These are to be taken with at least 8 ounces of water. (If the patient vomits after ingestion of the tablets, the test may be postponed or the physician may request that the medication be given again after the nausea subsides.)
2. The patient then is to receive nothing by mouth, except water, until bedtime. Until the test is completed, the patient is not permitted anything by mouth, including water, laxatives, or breakfast.
3. A saline enema may be administered early in the morning of the test.

Procedure. An x-ray film of the right upper abdominal quadrant is made. If the gallbladder is found to fill and empty normally and to contain no stones, it is concluded that no gallbladder disease is present. If gallbladder disease is present, the gallbladder may not be visualized because of obstruction by gallstones. If the gallbladder is visualized, shadows of gallstones may be present. A repeat of the oral cholecystogram with a second dose of the contrast medium may be necessary if the gallbladder is not visualized on the first attempt.

Note: Oral or intravenous cholecystography in the obviously jaundiced patient is not useful since the liver cannot excrete the radiopaque dye into the gallbladder in a jaundiced patient. If jaundice develops in a patient scheduled for cholecystography, the nurse should notify the physician so that the test can be cancelled.

Endoscopic Retrograde Cholangiopancreatography.
Endoscopic retrograde cholangiopancreatography (ERCP) permits direct visualization of structures once available only during laparotomy. It involves insertion of a flexible fiberoptic endoscope into the esophagus to the descending duodenum (Fig. 35-12). The common bile duct and pancreatic duct are cannulated, and contrast material is injected into the ducts, permitting visualization and evaluation of the biliary tree. ERCP also permits direct visualization of these structures and access to the distal common bile duct to retrieve a retained gallstone.

Nursing Interventions. The procedure requires a cooperative patient to permit insertion of the endoscope without damage to the gastrointestinal tract. Prior to the procedure, the patient needs an adequate explanation of the procedure and his role in it. He receives sedation immediately prior to the procedure. During ERCP, the nurse may be called on to monitor intravenous fluids, administer medications, and position the patient. Following the procedure, the nurse monitors

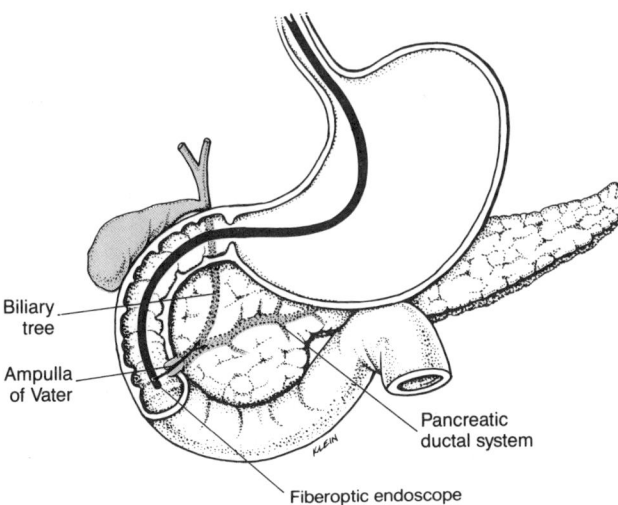

Figure 35-12
Endoscopic retrograde cholangiopancreatography (ERCP). By means of a side-viewing fiberoptic duodenoscope, the ampulla of Vater is catheterized and the biliary tree injected with contrast material. The pancreatic ductal system is also assessed, if indicated. This procedure is of special value in ampullary or periampullary neoplasms, which may be simultaneously visualized and biopsied. Acute pancreatitis is a contraindication. (Redrawn from Misra PS and Bank S. Gallbladder disease: Guide to diagnosis. Hosp Med 1982 Feb; p 136.)

the patient's condition, observing vital signs and checking for signs of perforation or infection. The nurse also monitors the patient for side-effects of any medications received during the procedure and return of the patient's gag reflex following the use of local anesthetics.

Percutaneous Transhepatic Cholangiography.
Percutaneous transhepatic cholangiography (PTC) involves the injection of dye directly into the biliary tree. Because of the relatively large concentration of dye that is introduced into the biliary system, all components of the system, including the hepatic ducts within the liver, the entire length of the common bile duct, the cystic duct, and the gallbladder, are clearly outlined.

This procedure can be carried out even in the presence of liver dysfunction and jaundice. It is useful in distinguishing jaundice caused by liver disease (hepatocellular jaundice) from that due to biliary obstruction; for investigating the gastrointestinal symptoms of patients whose gallbladders have been removed; for locating stones within the bile ducts; and in diagnosing cancer involving the biliary system.

Procedure. The patient, who is fasting and well sedated, lies supine on the x-ray table. The injection site, which is usually in the midclavicular line immediately beneath the right costal margin, is disinfected and anesthetized with lidocaine (Xylocaine). A small incision is made at this point and a thin, flexible needle ("skinny" needle) with stylet is inserted cephalad, posteriorly at a 45-degree angle and parallel to the midline. When the needle has penetrated to a depth of approximately 10 cm (4 inches), the stylet is removed and replaced by a plastic connector tube with 50-ml syringe attached. Gentle suction is applied while the needle is slowly withdrawn, until bile appears in the syringe. As much bile as possible is withdrawn, a radiopaque dye is injected, and an x-ray film obtained.

Before the needle is removed as much dye and bile as possible are aspirated in order to forestall subsequent leakage into the needle tract and eventually into the peritoneal cavity, to minimize the risk of bile peritonitis.

Nursing Interventions. Although the complication rate following this procedure is low, the patient must be observed closely for symptoms of bleeding, peritonitis, and septicemia. Pain and indicators of these complications should be reported immediately. Antibiotics should be administered as prescribed to minimize the risk of sepsis and septic shock.

Nonsurgical Management

The major objectives of medical therapy are to reduce the incidence of acute attacks of gallbladder pain and cholecystitis by supportive and dietary management, and, if possible, to remove the cause of cholecystitis by pharmacotherapy, endoscopic procedures, or surgical intervention.

Supportive and Dietary Management. Approximately 80% of the patients with acute gallbladder inflammation achieve a remission with rest, intravenous fluids, nasogastric suction, analgesia, and antibiotics. Unless the patient's condition deteriorates, surgical intervention is delayed until the patient's acute symptoms subside and complete evaluation can be carried out.

The diet, immediately after an attack, is usually limited to low-fat liquids. Powdered supplements high in protein and carbohydrate can be stirred into skim milk. The following may then be added as tolerated: cooked fruits, rice or tapioca, lean meats, mashed potatoes, non-gas-forming vegetables, bread, coffee, or tea. Eggs, cream, pork, fried foods, cheese and rich dressings, gas-forming vegetables, and alcohol are avoided. The patient needs to be reminded that fatty foods may bring on an attack.

Dietary management may be the major mode of therapy in those patients who have experienced only dietary intolerance to fatty foods and vague gastrointestinal symptoms.

Pharmacotherapy. Chenodeoxycholic acid (chenodiol or CDCA) has been effective in dissolving about 60% of radiolucent gallstones composed primarily of cholesterol. The mechanism of action is the inhibition of liver synthesis and secretion of cholesterol, thereby desaturating bile. Existing stones can be decreased in size, small ones dissolved, and new stones prevented from forming. The therapy is most effective if the stones are small. The effective dose of chenodiol depends on body weight. Chenodiol is generally indicated for those patients who refuse surgery or for whom it is considered too risky.

Certain other medications, such as estrogens, oral contraceptives, clofibrate, and dietery cholesterol, may adversely affect the results of treatment with chenodeoxycholic acid. If the patient is taking these drugs, the physician should be made aware of this.

Cholesterol stones may recur in a small percentage of patients after chenodeoxycholic acid is terminated; therefore, a low dose of this drug may be continued to prevent recurrence. Patients' adherence to this mode of therapy requires further study and follow-up.

If acute symptoms of cholecystitis continue or recur, pharmacotherapy is inappropriate as a substitute for surgery, and surgical intervention is indicated.

Long-term follow-up and monitoring of the patient's liver enzymes are indicated. The patient is instructed to report adverse side-effects and the recurrence of symptoms of cholecystitis.

Ursodeoxycholic acid (UDCA), another drug with similar effects, is also used to dissolve gallstones. UDCA has fewer side-effects than chenodiol and can be given in smaller doses to achieve the same effect.

Nonsurgical Removal of Gallstones. Methods of treating gallstones by infusion of solvents into the gallbladder are under investigation. One method involves infusion of a solvent through a tube or catheter inserted percutaneously directly into the gallbladder. Other procedures may involve infusion of the solvent via tube or drain inserted through a T-tube tract to dissolve stones not removed at the time of surgery, through an ERCP endoscope, or through a transnasal biliary catheter. In this last procedure, the catheter is introduced through the mouth and inserted into the common bile duct. The tube is then rerouted from the mouth to the nose and left in place. This enables the patient to eat and drink normally while passage of stones is monitored or chemical solvents are infused to dissolve the stones.

Several nonsurgical methods are used to remove stones that were not removed at the time of cholecystectomy or have become dislodged in the common bile duct. The procedures, however, cannot be used to remove stones from the gallbladder itself. A catheter and instrument with a basket attached are threaded through the T-tube tract or fistula formed at the time of T-tube insertion; the basket is used to retrieve and remove the stone lodged in the common bile duct. A second procedure is use of the ERCP endoscope. After the endoscope is inserted, a cutting instrument is passed through the endoscope into the ampulla of Vater of the common bile duct. It may be used to cut the submucosal fibers, or papilla, of the sphincter of Oddi, enlarging the opening, which may allow the lodged stone to pass spontaneously into the duodenum. Another instrument with a small basket or balloon at its tip may be inserted through the endoscope to retrieve the stone (Fig. 35-13). Although complications following this procedure are rare, the patient must be observed closely for bleeding, perforation, and the development of

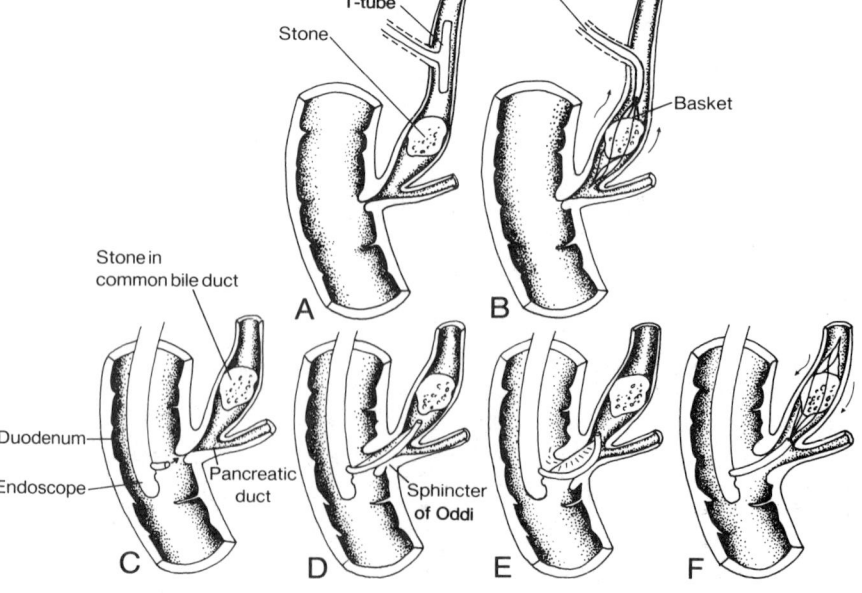

Figure 35-13
Removal of gallstone. (*A*) Use of T-tube tract for removal of retained stone. (*B*) Removal of stone with basket attached to catheter threaded through T-tube tract. (*C*) ERCP endoscope inserted into duodenum. (*D*) Papillotome inserted into common bile duct. (*E*) Enlarging opening of sphincter of Oddi. (*F*) Retrieval and removal of stone with basket inserted through endoscope.

pancreatitis. This procedure is particularly useful in the diagnosis and treatment of patients presenting with symptoms after biliary tract surgery, for those patients with intact gallbladders, and for patients in whom surgery is particularly hazardous.

Extracorporeal shock wave therapy (lithotripsy) has also been successfully used for nonsurgical fragmentation of gallstones in selected patients. This method (see Chap. 40) uses repeated shock waves directed at the gallstone located in the gallbladder or common bile duct to break up the stones. The fragments then pass the gallbladder or common bile duct spontaneously, are removed by endoscopy, or are dissolved with previously described solvents. It is expected that this mode of treatment will continue to be used only for select patients whose gallstones are not amenable to other forms of treatment.

These nonsurgical methods of removing stones are expected to decrease the need for surgery, reduce the length of hospital stay, and enable patients to return to their normal activities more quickly than they could if they had undergone surgical removal of the stones.

Surgical Management

Surgical treatment of gallbladder disease and gallstones is necessary for the relief of long-continued symptoms, for the removal of the cause of biliary colic, and for treatment of acute cholecystitis. Surgery may be elective when the patients's symptoms have subsided or may be performed as an emergency procedure if the patient's condition necessitates it.

Preoperative Management. In addition to x-ray studies of the gallbladder, chest x-rays, electrocardiogram, and liver function tests (see Table 35-1) may be performed. Vitamin K may be administered if the patient's prothrombin level is low. If this level is unusually low, a fresh blood transfusion may be given before surgery is done to ensure adequate blood clotting.

Nutritional requirements are considered; if the patient is not eating properly, it may be necessary to provide intravenous glucose with protein hydrolysate supplements to aid wound healing and help prevent liver damage.

Preparation for a gallbladder operation is similar to that for any upper abdominal laparotomy. Instruction and explanation are given prior to surgery with regard to turning and deep breathing. Because the abdominal incision is high on the abdomen (subcostal), the patient is often reluctant to move and turn; pneumonia and atelectasis are possible postoperative complications that are to be avoided by breathing deeply and by turning. Since drainage tubes are usually required after operation, the patient should be informed of this, so that he knows what to expect. The patient should also be informed about the likelihood of nasogastric suction during the immediate postoperative period.

Surgical Intervention and Drainage Systems. Patients usually are placed on the operating table with the upper abdomen raised somewhat by an air pillow or sandbag to make the biliary area more accessible.

Cholecystectomy. In this operation, the gallbladder is removed after ligation of the cystic duct and artery. The operation is performed in most cases of acute and chronic cho-

lecystitis. A drain (Penrose) is placed in the gallbladder and brought out through a stab wound for drainage of blood, serosanguineous fluids, and bile into absorbent dressings.

Choledochostomy. In choledochostomy, an incision is made into the common duct for removal of stones. After the stones have been evacuated, a tube usually is inserted into the duct for drainage of bile until edema subsides. This tube is connected to gravity drainage tubing. The gallbladder also contains stones and, as a rule, a cholecystectomy is performed at the same time.

Cholecystostomy. Cholecystostomy is performed when the patient's condition prevents more extensive surgery or when an acute inflammatory reaction obscures the biliary system. The gallbladder is opened, the stones and the bile or the pus are removed, and a tube is secured with a purse-string suture. As soon as the patient is returned to bed, the nurse should connect this tube to a drainage bottle placed at the side of the bed. Failure to do this may result in the leakage of bile around the tube and in its escape into the peritoneal cavity. Following recovery from the acute episode, the patient may return for cholecystectomy.

Gerontological Considerations. Surgical intervention for disease of the biliary tract is the most common operative procedure performed in the elderly. Although the incidence of gallstones increases with age, the symptoms experienced by the elderly patient may not be the typical fever, pain, chills, and jaundice. Biliary tract disease in the elderly may be accompanied or preceded by symptoms of septic shock: oliguria, hypotension, mental changes, tachycardia, and tachypnea.

Although surgery in the elderly presents risk because of preexisting associated diseases, the mortality from serious complications from biliary tract disease itself is also high. The risk of mortality and morbidity is increased in the elderly patient who undergoes emergency surgery for life-threatening disease of the biliary tract. Despite associated or preoperative medical illness in the elderly, elective cholecystectomy is usually well tolerated and can be carried out with low risk if expert assessment and care are provided before, during, and after the surgical procedure.

▶ Nursing Process
The Patient Undergoing Surgery for Gallbladder Disease

▷ Assessment

The nursing history and examination focus on the occurrence of abdominal pain and discomfort as well as those factors that tend to precipitate discomfort. The presence of abdominal pain several hours after eating a meal high in fats is noted. The history and examination also include information about respiratory status since the high abdominal incision required during surgery may interfere with full respiratory excursion. A history of smoking or previous respiratory problems is obtained. Shallow respirations, a persistent or ineffective cough, and the presence of adventitious breath sounds are noted. Nutritional status is obtained through dietary history and general examination.

▷ *Nursing Diagnoses*

Based on all the assessment data, the major nursing diagnoses of the patient with gallbladder disease and undergoing surgery may include the following:

- Pain and discomfort related to obstruction of the biliary system and inflammation and distention of the gallbladder
- Potential respiratory impairment related to the high abdominal surgical incision
- Potential alterations in skin integrity related to altered biliary drainage following surgical intervention
- Alterations in nutrition related to inadequate bile secretion.
- Knowledge deficit about self-care activities following discharge.

▷ *Planning and Implementation*

▷ *Goals:*   The patient's goals include relief of pain, absence of respiratory complications, absence of complications of altered biliary drainage related to surgical intervention, improved nutritional intake, and understanding of self-care routines.

Nursing Interventions

Postoperative Nursing Interventions.   As soon as the patient has recovered from anesthesia, he is placed in low Fowler's position. Fluids may be given intravenously, and nasogastric suction (tube probably inserted immediately prior to surgery) may be instituted to relieve distention. Water and other fluids may be given in about 24 hours, and a soft diet started later, after bowel sounds return.

Relief of Pain.   The location of the subcostal incision is likely to cause the patient to avoid turning and moving and to splint the operative site by taking shallow breaths to prevent pain. Since full aeration of the lungs and gradually increased activity are necessary to prevent postoperative complications, analgesics should be given as prescribed and the patient assisted to turn, cough, breathe deeply, and ambulate as indicated. Use of a pillow or binder over the incision may reduce the amount of pain during these maneuvers.

Improvement of Respiratory Status.   These patients are especially prone to pulmonary complications, as are all patients with upper abdominal incisions. Thus, they should be taught to take deep breaths every hour to aerate the lungs fully. Other complications, such as thrombophlebitis and pulmonary atelectasis, may be avoided by promoting early ambulation as soon as permissible. Such complications are more likely to occur in the more obese patient.

Biliary Drainage and Skin Care.   As was mentioned before, in patients who have undergone a cholecystostomy or choledochostomy, the drainage tubes must be connected immediately to a drainage receptacle. In addition, tubing should be fastened to the dressings or to the bottom sheet, with enough leeway for the patient to move without dislodging it. The patient must know why he cannot roll onto the tube and that it must remain patent at all times. Since a drainage receptacle remains attached when the patient is ambulating,

the collecting bag may be placed in a bathrobe pocket or fastened so that it is below the waist or common duct level. If a Penrose drain is used, as it is for cholecystectomy, the dressings are changed as required. Montgomery straps are helpful in maintaining a comfortable dressing.

Following these surgical procedures, the patient is observed for indications of infection, leakage of bile into the peritoneal cavity, and obstruction of bile drainage. If bile is not draining properly, an obstruction is probably causing bile to be forced back into the liver and bloodstream. Since jaundice may result, the nurse should be particularly observant of the color of the sclerae. The nurse should also note and report right upper quadrant abdominal pain, nausea and vomiting, bile drainage around the T tube, clay-colored stools, and a change in vital signs.

Bile may continue to drain from the drainage tract in considerable quantities for a time, necessitating frequent changes of the outer dressings and protection of the skin from irritation. Skin pastes of zinc oxide, aluminum, or petrolatum prevent the bile from literally digesting the skin.

In order to prevent total loss of bile, the drainage tube or collecting receptacle may be elevated above the level of the abdomen, so that the bile drains through the apparatus only if pressure develops in the duct system. The bile collected should be measured and recorded every 24 hours, and its color and character are also documented. After several days of drainage, the tubes may be clamped for an hour before and after each meal, with the purpose being to deliver bile to the duodenum to aid in digestion. Within 7 to 14 days, the drainage tubes are removed from the gallbladder or common bile duct.

In all patients with biliary drainage, the stools should be observed daily and their color recorded. Specimens of both urine and feces may be sent to the laboratory for examination for bile pigments. In this way, it is possible to determine that the bile pigment is disappearing from the blood and is draining again into the duodenum. A careful record of fluid intake and output is kept and totaled for each 24 hours.

Improvement of Nutritional Status.   The diet of these patients may be low in fats and high in carbohydrates and proteins immediately after surgery. At the time of hospital discharge, there are usually no special dietary instructions, other than to maintain a nutritious diet and avoid excessive fats. Fat restriction usually is lifted in 4 to 6 weeks when biliary ducts dilate to accommodate the volume of bile once held by the gallbladder, and when the ampulla of Vater again functions effectively. After this, when one eats fat, adequate bile will be released into the digestive tract to emulsify the fats and allow their digestion. Prior to this, fats would not be completely or adequately digested in some persons, and flatulence might occur. However, one purpose of gallbladder surgery is ultimately to allow for a normal diet.

Patient Education and Home Health Care.   Because the patient may be discharged from the hospital while the drainage system is still in place, the patient and family will need instructions about its management. They must be instructed in proper care of the drainage tube and should know to report changes in the amount or characteristics of drainage to the physician promptly. Assistance in securing the appropriate dressings will reduce the patient's anxiety about going home with the drain or tube still in place.

The patient should be instructed about which medications are required (vitamins, anticholinergics, and antispasmodics) and why they are given. He also should be aware of symptoms that are reportable to his physician—jaundice, dark urine, pale-colored stools, pruritus, or signs of inflammation, such as pain or fever.

Some patients note "looseness of the bowels," consisting of one to three bowel movements a day—the reason being a continual trickle of bile through the choledochoduodenal junction following cholecystectomy. Usually, such frequency diminishes over a period of a few weeks to several months. Follow-up visits are essential for this patient.

▷ *Evaluation*

▷ *Expected Outcomes*

1. Patient achieves relief of pain.
   a. Reports decrease in pain of cholecystitis and cholelithiasis, and absence of postoperative incisional pain.
   b. Splints abdominal incision to decrease pain.
   c. Avoids foods that cause pain.
   d. Uses postoperative analgesia as prescribed.
   e. Uses appropriate preventive activities when painfree postoperatively (*e.g.*, turns, coughs, breathes deeply, ambulates).
2. Is free of respiratory complications.
   a. Is free of temperature elevation, cough, and increased respiratory rate.
   b. Demonstrates full respiratory excursion with deep inspiration and expiration.
   c. Coughs effectively, using pillow to splint abdominal incision.
   d. Uses postoperative analgesia as prescribed.
   e. Exercises as prescribed (*e.g.*, turns, ambulates).
3. Exhibits normal skin integrity around biliary drainage site.
   a. Is free of temperature elevation, abdominal pain, change in vital signs, or drainage around drainage tube.
   b. Exhibits or reports gradual decrease in bile drainage.
   c. Reports skin, mucous membranes, stool, and urine to be of normal color.
   d. Demonstrates proper management of catheter; identifies reportable complications (*e.g.*, redness or purulent drainage at site).
   e. Demonstrates that skin around T-tube or drainage tube is intact and free of excoriation.
   f. Identifies signs and symptoms of biliary obstruction to be noted and reported.
   g. Has serum bilirubin level within normal range.
4. Obtains relief of dietary intolerance.
   a. Maintains adequate dietary intake.
   b. Avoids foods that cause gastrointestinal symptoms.
   c. Reports decreased incidence or absence of nausea, vomiting, diarrhea, flatulence, and abdominal discomfort.

Bibliography

Books

Berk JE. (ed). Gastroenterology, vol 7. Philadelphia, WB Saunders, 1985.

Csomos G and Thaler H. Clinical Hepatology. New York, Springer-Verlag, 1983.

Gitman G. Controversies in Gastroenterology. New York, Churchill Livingstone, 1984.

Given BA and Simmons SJ. Gastroenterology in Clinical Nursing. St Louis, CV Mosby, 1984.

Guyton AC. Textbook of Medical Physiology. Philadelphia, WB Saunders, 1986.

Hall P. Alcoholic Liver Disease. New York, John Wiley & Sons, 1985.

Moody FG et al. Surgical Treatment of Digestive Disease. Chicago, Year Book Medical Publishers, 1986.

Ravenscroft MM and Swan CHJ. Gastrointestinal Endoscopy and Related Procedures: A Handbook for Nurses and Assistants. Baltimore, Williams & Wilkins, 1984.

Schiff L and Schiff ER. Diseases of the Liver, 6th ed. Philadelphia, JB Lippincott, 1987.

Seitz HK and Kommerell B. Alcohol-related Diseases in Gastroenterology. New York, Springer-Verlag, 1985.

Articles

General

Chopra S and Griffin PH. Laboratory tests and diagnostic procedures in evaluation of liver disease. Am J Med 1985 Aug; 79(2):221–230.

DeVore NE, Jackson YM, and Piening SL. TORCH infections. Am J Nurs 1983 Dec; 83(12):1600–1665.

Dice JF. Cellular theories of aging as related to the liver. Hepatology 1985 May/June; 5(3):508–513.

Dodd RP. Ascites: When the liver can't cope. RN 1984 Oct; 47(10):26–30.

Friedman LS and Maddrey WC. Surgery in the patient with liver disease. Med Clin North Am 1987 May; 71(3):453–476.

Gannon RB and Pickett K. Jaundice. Am J Nurs 1983 Mar; 83(3):404–407.

James OFW. Gastrointestinal and liver function in old age. Clin Gastroenterol 1983 Sept; 12(3):671–691.

Klopp A. Shunting malignant ascites. Am J Nurs 1984 Feb; 84(2):212–213.

Lacy JH, Wieman TJ, and Shively EH. Management of malignant ascites. Surg Gynecol Obstet 1984 Oct; 159(4):397–412.

Popper MJ. Relations between liver and aging. Semin Liver Dis 1985 Aug; 5(3):221–227.

Rodman MJ. An update on the new drugs you're dispensing now. RN 1984 Apr; 47(4):68–82.

Schumann K. Correction of ascites with peritoneovenous shunting: A study of clinical management. Heart Lung 1983 May; 12(3):248–255.

Stassen WN and McCullough AJ. Management of ascites. Semin Liver Dis 1985 Aug; 5(3):291–307.

Liver Dysfunction

Anderson FD. The cirrhotic process in the alcoholic. Crit Care Q 1986 Mar; 8(4):74–78.

Baker CH and Brenna JM. Keeping health-care workers healthy: Legal aspects of hepatitis B immunization programs. N Engl J Med 1984 Sept 6; 311(10):684–688.

Bizer LC. Theoretical and practical considerations in the treatment of portal hypertension secondary to hepatic cirrhosis. Am Surg 1984 Oct; 50(10):524–529.

Bluett MK, Woltering E, and Adkins RB. Management of penetrating hepatic injury. Am Surg 1984 Mar; 50(3):132–142.

Brechot C et al. Hepatitis B virus DNA in patients with chronic liver disease and negative tests for hepatitis B surface antigen. N Engl J Med 1985 Jan 31; 312(5):270–276.

Burbige EJ. Hepatorenal syndrome. Hosp Med 1984 Dec; 20(12):32, 34–36.

Cozzi E et al. Nursing management of patients receiving hepatic arterial chemotherapy through an implanted infusion pump. Cancer Nurs 1984 June; 7(3):229–234.

Del Guercio LRM, Kinkhabwalla MN, and Berman HL. Current concepts in portal hypertension. Bull NY Acad Med 1985 Oct; 61(8):753–762.

Dong B, Barton EC, and Mancini BA. Viral hepatitis. Nurs Pract 1984 Mar; 9(3):27–32, 79.

Epstein M. Renal complications of liver disease. Clin Symp 1985; 37(5):3–37.

Foster JH. Treatment of metastatic disease of the liver: A skeptic's view. Semin Liver Dis 1984 May; 4(2):170–179.

Fredette SL. When the liver fails. Am J Nurs 1984 Jan; 84(1):64–67.

Friedman LS and Dienstag JL. Recent developments in viral hepatitis. DM 1986 June; 32(6):320–385.

Galambos JT. Portal hypertension. Semin Liver Dis 1986 Aug; 5(3):277–290.

Gullatte MM and Foltz AT. Hepatic chemotherapy via implantable pump. Am J Nurs 1983 Dec; 83(12):1674–1676.

Gurevich I. Viral hepatitis. Am J Nurs 1983 Apr; 83(4):571–585.

Hornbaker AE. Hematologic disorders in the critically ill alcoholic. Crit Care Q 1986 Mar; 8(4):29–39.

Jensen DM. Portal-systemic encephalopathy and hepatic coma. Med Clin North Am 1986 Sept; 70(5):1081–1092.

Johnson D. Fluid and electrolyte dysfunction in alcoholism. Crit Care Q 1986 Mar; 8(4):53–62.

Keith JS. Hepatic failure: Etiologies, manifestations, and management. Crit Care Nurs 1985 Jan./Feb; 5(1):60–86.

Kirkman-Liff B and Dandoy S. Hepatitis B: What price exposure? Am J Nurs 1984 Aug; 84(8):988–990.

Kolts BE and Spindel E. Chronic active hepatitis. Am Fam Physician 1984 June; 29(6):228–243.

MacSween HM, MacLeod JE, and Aterman K. Viral hepatitis: Practical aspects of "in-hospital" infection control. Can J Public Health 1984 Sept/Oct; 75(5):379–383.

Maletic-Staschak S. Orthotopic liver transplantation. AORN J 1984 Jan; 39(1):35–39.

Malt RA. Current concepts: Surgery for hepatic neoplasms. N Engl J Med 1985 Dec 19; 313(25):1591–1596.

Miller B and Gavant ML. Biliary catheter care. Am J Nurs 1985 Oct; 85(10):1115–1117.

Murray BJ. The hepatitis B carrier state. Am Fam Physician 1986 Apr; 33(4):127–133.

Newell J. Portal systemic encepthalopathy. Nurs Pract 1984 July; 9(7):26–37.

Pagana TJ. A new technique for hepatic infusional chemotherapy. Semin Surg Oncol 1986; 2(2):99–102.

Payne JA. Fulminant liver failure. Med Clin North Am 1986 Sept; 70(5):1067–1079.

Pimstone NR and French SW. Alcoholic liver disease. Med Clin North Am 1984 Jan; 68(1):39–56.

Rikkers LF, Soper NJ, and Cormier RA. Selective operative approach for variceal hemorrhage. Am J Surg 1984 Jan; 147(1):89–96.

Rocco VK and Ware AJ. Cirrhotic ascites: Pathophysiology, diagnosis, and management. Ann Intern Med 1986 Oct; 105(4):573–585.

Rossi RL, Jenkins RL, and Nielsen-Whitcomb FF. Management of complications of portal hypertension. Surg Clin North Am 1985 Apr; 65(2):231–262.

Schaffner F. The management of chronic liver disease. Semin Liver Dis 1985 Aug; 5(3):209–307.

Smith SL. Liver transplantation: Implications for critical care nursing. Heart Lung 1985 Nov; 14(6):617–627.

Starzl TE et al. Immunosuppression and other nonsurgical factors in the improved results of liver transplantation. Semin Liver Dis 1985 Nov; 5(4):334–343.

Traiger GL and Bohachick P. Liver transplantation: Care of the patient in the acute postoperative period. Crit Care Nurs 1983 Sept/Oct; 3(5):96–103.

Valenti WM. Hepatitis B prevention: I. A review of ACIP's newest guidelines. Infect Control 1986 Feb; 7(2):74–77.

Vargo J. Viral hepatitis: How to protect patients and yourself. RN 1984 July; 47(7):22–29.

Vitale G, Heuser LS, and Polk HC. Malignant tumors of the liver. Surg Clin North Am 1986 Aug; 66(4):723–741.

Warnes TW. Treatment of primary biliary cirrhosis. Semin Liver Dis 1985 Aug; 5(3):228–240.

Bleeding Esophageal Varices

Bell RH, Miyai K, and Orloff MJ. Outcome in cirrhotic patients with acute alcoholic hepatitis after emergency portacaval shunt for bleeding esophageal varices. Am J Surg 1984 Jan; 147(1):78–84.

Berger M, Mattioli CA, Dobbs SM, and Jackson D. Bleeding esophageal varices in an adolescent. Heart Lung 1983 Nov; 12(6):661–665.

Bernuau J and Rueff B. Treatment of acute variceal bleeding. Clin Gastroenterol 1985 Jan; 14(1):185–207.

Burroughs AK et al. Controlled trial of propranolol for the prevention of recurrent variceal hemorrhage in patients with cirrhosis. N Engl J Med 1983 Dec 22; 309(25):1539–1542.

Cello JP et al. Endoscopic sclerotherapy versus portacaval shunt in patients with severe cirrhosis and acute variceal hemorrhage. N Engl J Med 1987 Jan 1; 316(1):11–15.

Eckstein MR and Athanasoulis CA. Gastrointestinal bleeding: An angiographic perspective. Surg Clin North Am 1984 Feb; 64(1):37–51.

Galambos JT. Portal hypertension. Semin Liver Dis 1985 Aug; 5(3):277–290.

Gibb SP, Laney JS, and Tarshis AM. Use of fiberoptic endoscopy in diagnosis and therapy of upper gastrointestinal disorders. Med Clin North Am 1986 Nov; 70(6):1307–1324.

Gruber M. Endoscopic injection sclerotherapy: Nursing responsibilities. Crit Care Q 1985 Mar; 7(4):73–80.

Health and Public Policy Committee, American College of Physicians. Endoscopic sclerotherapy for esophageal varices (position paper). Ann Intern Med 1984 Apr; 100(4):608–610.

Maloney JP. Surgical intervention in the alcoholic patient with portal hypertension. Crit Care Q 1986 Mar; 8(4):63–73.

Rikkers LF, Soper NJ, and Cormier RA. Selective operative approach for variceal hemorrhage. Am J Surg 1984 Jan; 147(1):89–96.

Wexler MJ. Esophageal procedures to control bleeding from varices. Surg Clin of North Am 1983 Feb; 63(4):905–914.

Gallbladder Disease

Allen MJ et al. Rapid dissolution of gallstones by methyl *tert*-butyl ether. N Engl J Med 1985 Jan 24; 312(4):217–220.

Einarsson K et al. Influence of age on secretion of cholesterol and synthesis of bile acids by the liver. N Engl J Med 1985 Aug 1; 313(5):277–282.

Fisher MM et al. The Sunnybrook gallstone study: A double-blind controlled trial of chenodeoxycholic acid for gallstone dissolution. Hepatology 1985 Jan/Feb; 5(1):102–107.

Huber DF, Martin EW, and Cooperman M. Cholecystectomy in elderly patients. Am J Surg 1983 Dec; 146(6):719–722.

Jakimowicz JJ et al. Postoperative choledochoscopy. Arch Surg 1983 July; 118(7):810–812.

Kozarek RA. Transnasal pancreaticobiliary drains. Am J Surg 1983 Aug; 146(2):250–253.

Laing FC. Diagnostic evaluation of patients with suspected cholecystitis. Surg Clin North Am 1984 Feb; 64(1):3–22.

Lauschner U. Endoscopic therapy of biliary calculi. Clin Gastroenterol 1986 Apr; 15(2):333–356.

Lygidakis NJ. Operative risk factors of cholecystectomy-choledochotomy in the elderly. Surg Gynecol Obstet 1983 July; 157(1):15–19.

Mack E. Chemical dissolution of biliary stones. Contemp Surg 1986 June; 28(6):20–23.

Mogadam M et al. Gallbladder dynamics in response to various meals: Is dietary fat restriction necessary in the management of gallstones? Am J Gastroenterol 1984 Oct; 79(10):745–747.

Morran CG, Finley IG, and Mathieson M et al. Randomized controlled trial of physiotherapy for postoperative pulmonary complications. Br J Anaesth 1983 Nov; 55(11):1113–1117.

Mulley, AG. Shock-wave lithotripsy (editorial). N Engl J Med 1986 Mar 27; 314(13):845–847.

Munro R and Sorrell TC. Biliary sepsis. Drugs 1986; 31(5):449–454.

Peternel E. A high-tech approach to a GI problem. RN 1985 June; 44–47.

Ransohoff DF et al. Prophylactic cholecystectomy or expectant management for silent gallstones: A decision analysis to assess survival. Ann Intern Med 1983 Aug; 99(2):199–204.

Roberts JW. Carcinoma of the extrahepatic bile ducts. Surg Clin North Am 1986 Aug; 66(4):751–756.

Roberts JW and Daugherty SF. Primary carcinoma of the gallbladder. Surg Clin North Am 1986 Aug; 66(4):743–749.

Safrany L and Cotton PB. Endoscopic management of choledocholithiasis. Surg Clin North Am 1982 Oct; 62(5):825–836.

Sauerbruch T et al. Fragmentation of gallstones by extracorporeal shock waves. N Engl J Med 1986 Mar 27; 314(13):818–822.

Scharschmidt BF, Goldgerg HI, and Schmid R. Current concepts in diagnosis: Approach to the patient with cholestatic jaundice. N Engl J Med 1983 June 23; 308(25):1515–1519.

Thistle JL et al. The natural history of cholelithiasis: The national cooperative gallstone study. Ann Int Med 1984 Aug; 101(2):171–175.

Tytgat GNJ et al. Endoscopic palliative therapy of gastrointestinal and biliary tumours with prostheses. Clin Gastroenterol 1986 Apr; 15(2):249–271.

van Rensburg LCJ. The management of acute cholecystitis in the elderly. Br J Surg 1984 Sept; 71(9):692–693.

Ward A et al. Ursodeoxycholic acid: A review of its pharmacological properties and therapeutic efficiency. Drugs 1984 Feb; 27(2):95–131.

Welch CE and Malt RA. Surgery of the stomach, duodenum, gallbladder, and bile ducts. N Engl J Med 1987 April 16; 316(16):999–1008.

Zimmon DS and Clemett AR. Endoscopic stents and drains in the management of pancreatic and bile duct obstruction. Surg Clin North Am 1982 Oct; 62(5):837–843.

Agencies

National Institute on Alcohol Abuse and Alcoholism, Rockville, Maryland 20857.

Alcoholics Anonymous World Services (AA), P.O. Box 459, Grand Central Station, New York, New York 10163.

National Council on Alcoholism, Inc., 12 W. 21st Street, New York, New York 10010.

Chapter 36

Assessment and Management of Patients With Diabetes Mellitus

Definition

Diabetes mellitus is a disease resulting from a breakdown in the body's ability to produce or utilize insulin. *Insulin* is a powerful hormone secreted by the beta cells in the islets of Langerhans of the pancreas. It plays a major role in the metabolic processes of the body by controlling the storage and metabolism of ingested metabolic fuels. Following a meal, the secretion of insulin facilitates the uptake, utilization, and storage of glucose, amino acids, and fat. It promotes the storage of glycogen in the liver, the utilization of glucose in the muscles, and the storage of fat in adipose tissues by enhancing the transport of glucose across the cell membrane. Insulin regulates the level of blood glucose, which is formed from ingested carbohydrates or from the conversion of amino acids and fatty acids to glucose by the liver (*gluconeogenesis*).

   Diabetes mellitus is defined as a genetically heterogenous group of disorders that are characterized by glucose intolerance. Previously it was defined as chronic multisystem disorder characterized by hyperglycemia caused by insulin insufficiency or inadequate insulin action. The current definition reflects the latest research findings in epidemiology, genetics, virology, immunology, and biochemistry. This new knowledge has not negated the old definition. Rather, it has pointed out how little we knew about this complex disease. Diabetes is characterized by disorders in the metabolism of carbohydrate, protein, fat, and insulin, as well as the structure and function of blood vessels. These abnormalities account for both the acute and the chronic complications of the disease.

Epidemiology

Diabetes mellitus is a chronic disease of major importance in the United States today. It is the third leading cause of death by disease, and currently affects an estimated 11 million people. According to the National Diabetes Data Group of the National Institutes of Health, 5.8 million cases have been diagnosed; the remainder are undiagnosed. About 500,000 new cases of diabetes are diagnosed yearly.

Diabetes reduces life expectancy by one third, and the frequency of disability in diabetic persons is 2 to 3 times that in the general population. Diabetes is especially prevalent in the elderly. Among people over 65 years old, 8.6% have non-insulin-dependent diabetes. This figure includes 15% of the nursing home population. Blacks, Hispanics, and Asian Americans have higher rates of diabetes than do whites. Some American Indian tribes have the highest known rates of diabetes in the world—20% to 50% of the adults have diabetes.

The economic cost of diabetes continues to rise because of increasing medical costs and an aging population. Costs directly related to diabetes are conservatively estimated at $13.8 billion annually ($7.4 billion for direct medical care expenses, mostly for hospitalizations and nursing home care, and $6.4 billion in indirect costs due to disability and premature death). The actual costs for all medical care related to diabetes and its complications are estimated to be twice these figures.

Hospitalization rates are 2.4 times greater for adults and 5.3 times greater for children with diabetes than for the general population. The rate of hospitalization increases for the elderly with diabetes. Half of all persons with diabetes who are over 65 are hospitalized each year. Severe and life-threatening complications often contribute to increased rates of hospitalization with diabetes.

Types of Diabetes

Research has revealed more than one cause of diabetes and much diversity in definition, pattern, and course of disease. In 1978, conditions formerly called diabetes were reclassified for the following reasons:

- To eliminate the confusion of terminology and diagnosis
- To remove the psychological and socioeconomic labels
- To standardize research reporting
- To assist in more accurate diagnosis

The new classification system was adopted by the American, British, Australian, and European diabetes associations in 1979. The major groups are labelled as follows:

Type I—Insulin-dependent diabetes mellitus (IDDM)
Type II—Noninsulin-dependent diabetes mellitus (NIDDM)
Impaired glucose tolerance (IGT)
Gestational diabetes mellitus (GDM)
Diabetes mellitus associated with other conditions or syndromes

About 5% to 10% of people with diabetes have Type I, insulin-dependent diabetes (IDDM). In this form of diabetes, inadequate amounts of insulin are produced by the pancreas, resulting in the need for injection of insulin (exogenous insulin).

About 90% to 95% of people with diabetes have Type II, noninsulin-dependent diabetes (NIDDM). Type II diabetes may result from a decrease in the amount of insulin produced or an insensitivity of the cells to insulin. In the latter situation, excessive amounts of circulating insulin may be present.

Table 36-1 summarizes the major categories of diabetes, current terminology, old labels, and major clinical characteristics. It is important to recognize that this classification system is dynamic rather than static in two ways. First, as research findings become available, it appears that there are many differences among individuals within each category. Second, with time, patients may move from one category to another. For example, a woman with gestational diabetes may, after delivery, move into the noninsulin-dependent (type II) category. These types also differ in their etiology, pathology, clinical course, management, and long-term complications.

Etiology

The etiology of the disease is not completely understood. There are probably several causative factors within each type, varying from patient to patient. It remains to be proven whether the etiology is related to an inherited defect, an environmental factor (*e.g.*, viruses, obesity), or the interaction of both inheritance and environmental factors. In Type I (insulin-dependent) diabetes, it is felt that genetics or viruses or an autoimmune response, alone or in combination, are involved. In type II (noninsulin-dependent) diabetes, genetics and obesity play a more significant role.

Genetic Factors. Diabetes has always been thought of as a genetic or inherited disease. To date, no single mode of inheritance can explain all the types of diabetes adequately. In fact, many modes of inheritance have been proposed. Different types of diabetes may be inherited in different ways in different families—"genetic heterogeneity."

Both type I and type II diabetes have a genetic component, although the exact roles of genetics and environmental factors differ in each type.

Type I diabetes results from the destruction of the beta cells in the islets of Langerhans in the pancreas. This destruction usually results from an immunological defect that produces antibodies against the beta cells. These antibodies may be present months or years before clinical symptoms of diabetes develop. Type II diabetes results from inadequate insulin production or insensitivity to the insulin that is produced. The exact role that heredity and obesity play is not yet completely understood.

The search for a genetic marker for diabetes has important implications for the understanding of the inheritance of diabetes. Research with the human leukocyte antigen (HLA) system that is used in tissue typing has demonstrated a relationship with some HLA antigens and diabetes. Certain of these antigens are consistently found in insulin-dependent diabetes.

However, not all persons with these antigens develop diabetes. Therefore, environmental factors such as viruses may act to trigger the autoimmune response. Some researchers have observed a relationship between various HLA antigens and those diabetic persons with long-term complications. Although much of this work is still inconclusive, it appears that having certain HLA patterns increases a person's risk for developing diabetes. It may be possible in the future to identify potential diabetes by these markers and then attempt to offset the disease itself.

TABLE 36-1
Classification of Diabetes Mellitus and Related Glucose Intolerances

Current Classification	Previous Classifications	Clinical Characteristics	Nursing Implications
Type I: Insulin-dependent diabetes mellitus (IDDM) (5–10% of all diabetes)	Juvenile diabetes Juvenile-onset diabetes (JOD) Ketosis-prone diabetes Brittle diabetes	Any age, but usually young Mostly thin at diagnosis Causes may be genetic or viral but probably involve abnormal immune responses. Often have islet cell antibodies Little or no endogenous insulin Need insulin to preserve life Ketosis-prone	Critical to maintain normal range of blood glucose Potential future vaccine for immunization of susceptible persons Essential to monitor status of blood glucose for good control Knowledge emphasis on: • Relationship between food, exercise, and insulin in controlling blood glucose • Adjusting insulin • Interpreting glucose test results Skills emphasis on: • Insulin administration • Testing for glucose and ketones • Pump care • Foot care • Life-threatening situation, crucial for patient to detect and treat or prevent Peer pressure during adolescence and adulthood regarding compliance with diet, insulin, and testing
Type II: Noninsulin-dependent diabetes mellitus (NIDDM) (90–95% of all diabetes: nonobese—20% of type II; obese—80% of type II)	Adult-onset diabetes Maturity-onset diabetes Ketosis-resistant diabetes Stable diabetes Maturity-onset diabetes of youth (MODY)	Any age, usually over 40 but occasionally under 21 Causes may be related to genetic, obesity, or environmental factors. Mostly obese at diagnosis No islet cell antibodies Varying amounts of endogenous insulin present, often higher than normal levels May need insulin to avoid hyperglycemia Rare ketosis, except in stress or infection Nonketotic hyperosmolar coma	Very important to maintain near normal range of blood sugars Weight reduction crucial, but problems with motivation and compliance Insulin often overused as treatment; inappropriate use increases obesity Less life-threatening than Type I, but majority of diabetics in this class Life-threatening and often fatal
Impaired glucose tolerance (IGT)	Asymptomatic diabetes Chemical diabetes Subclinical diabetes Borderline diabetes Latent diabetes	Blood glucose levels between normal and that of diabetes Above normal susceptibility to atherosclerotic disease Renal and retinal complications usually not significant	Both obese and nonobese should be screened periodically for diabetes, but obese should reduce weight.

(continued)

Recent research has begun to assess the potential benefits of immunosuppressive therapy in the treatment of newly-diagnosed diabetes patients. To date, there appears to be a high incidence of remission (no need for endogenous insulin) as long as therapy is continued. However, there are disadvantages as well as hazards and ethical considerations in using long-term immunosuppressive therapy.

Viral Factors. Although viruses have been *indirectly* associated with diabetes for more than 100 years, it was not until 1965 that viral research on this association increased

TABLE 36-1 (continued)

Current Classification	Previous Classifications	Clinical Characteristics	Nursing Implications
Gestational diabetes (GDM)	Gestational diabetes	Begins or is recognized during or after pregnancy	
		Above normal risk of perinatal complications	Usually highly motivated to maintain normal blood glucose because of baby
		Glucose intolerance transitory, but frequently recurs:	Nursing challenge—maintain or reduce weight to ideal; may delay onset
		• 50% go on to develop overt diabetes within 15 years	
		• 80% go on to develop overt diabetes after 20 years, particularly postmenopausally	
Diabetes mellitus associated with other conditions or syndromes	Secondary diabetes	Accompanied by conditions known or suspected to cause the disease: pancreatic or hormonal conditions, drug or chemical toxicity, certain genetic syndromes	See above for type I or II
Previous abnormality of glucose tolerance (PrevAGT)	Latent diabetes Prediabetes	Previous history of hyperglycemia Current normal glucose metabolism	With a family history of diabetes, periodic screening of blood glucose, probably yearly after age 40 or if symptoms develop
Potential abnormality of glucose tolerance (PotAGT)	Potential diabetes Prediabetes	No history of glucose intolerance Likely to become diabetic: • Positive family history • Evidence of islet cell antibodies • Mothers of babies over 9 lb at birth • Pima Indians • Obesity	Maintain or reduce to ideal weight (same as above—PrevAGT)

significantly. The genetic makeup of cells in an individual probably determines whether the virus can attach itself to the cell surface, enter the cell, and change its metabolism.

The characteristically abrupt appearance of insulin-dependent diabetes could be the result of an infection with a diabetogenic virus in a person already genetically predisposed. The infection might cause an autoimmune (antigen–antibody) reaction. Other diseases of self-destruction have been known for some time. For instance, thyroiditis is a disease in which an infection of the thyroid gland causes the body to produce antibodies against its own thyroid gland. Antibodies that attack pancreatic islet cells have been found in at least 50% of all insulin-dependent diabetics.

The evidence for a viral cause of diabetes comes *indirectly* from epidemiologic studies, and more *directly* and recently from clinical cases. Insulin-dependent diabetes occurs abruptly and at a time of year when viral infections are frequent, so it is possible that its cause is a diabetogenic virus. It is now felt that this type of diabetes is related to an environmental cause (*e.g.*, viruses that perhaps cause an autoimmune destruction of a person's own beta cells).

Some viral strains cause the death of beta cells in genetically susceptible animals. In order for insulin-dependent diabetes to develop, at least 90% of the individual's beta cells must stop producing insulin. This could result from one very potent viral attack, or it could be the result of a series of viral infections that eventually destroy the beta cells.

There is apparently no relationship between viruses and the etiology of noninsulin-dependent diabetes. Antibodies against one of the suspected viruses, Coxsackie B4, have been found in the blood of newly diagnosed insulin-dependent diabetics and not in noninsulin-dependent diabetics.

Evidence that suggests a viral cause for insulin-dependent diabetes includes the following:

1. It usually occurs in young people, whose systems are more prone to viral infections.
2. It occurs suddenly, like viral infections.
3. It occurs when viral infections are prevalent.
4. Beta cells are inflamed early in the viral infection.
5. A viral infection develops before the diabetes develops.
6. It often develops in a child with no family history of diabetes.

Because less than 0.2% of the population has insulin-dependent diabetes and it is not known what percentage of these cases are caused by a virus, much research needs to be done. At least 20 other viruses in addition to Coxsackie B4 have been associated with the development of insulin-dependent diabetes—a fact that hampers development of a vaccine. These viral infections that lead to diabetes might be prevented if the type of virus causing beta cell damage can be isolated and if it can be proven that viruses are more than a minor cause of diabetes.

Combined Factors.   Viruses, heredity (including an immunological defect) and an autoimmune response may contribute to the development of insulin-dependent diabetes. Heredity by itself appears to be the least important contributor. Heredity and obesity significantly contribute to the development of non-insulin-dependent diabetes.

Although the exact mechanism of inheritance has not yet been explained, blood relatives of known patients with diabetes should maintain life-long vigilance for this condition. Obese persons and mothers who have delivered large babies are also susceptible. These and other high-risk individuals (Chart 36-1) should be examined regularly for signs of diabetes.

Pathophysiology

As was indicated previously, diabetes results from the inability of the body to produce and use insulin.

In the nondiabetic person, insulin is released from the pancreas in proportion to the amount of glucose in the blood. Normally, the beta cells in the pancreas stimulate or inhibit insulin secretion minute by minute, according to changing blood glucose levels. In diabetes, insulin is not secreted in proportion to blood glucose levels because of several possible factors: deficiency in the production of insulin by the beta cells; insensitivity of the insulin secretory mechanism of the beta cells; delayed or insufficient release of insulin; or excessive inactivation by chemical inhibitors or "binders" in the circulation.

In some noninsulin-dependent persons with diabetes, however, insulin secretion is increased, resulting in higher circulating insulin levels. Although excess insulin is present, it is not utilized because of an inadequate number of insulin receptors present on cells. This mechanism has been observed in obese noninsulin-dependent patients. With weight loss, the number of insulin receptors on the cells increases, thereby allowing glucose to enter the cell. This may result in return of a normal glucose tolerance.

An elevated fasting blood glucose level in diabetes reflects decreased uptake of glucose by the tissues or increased gluconeogenesis. If the concentration of glucose in the blood is sufficiently high, the kidney may not reabsorb all of the filtered glucose; the glucose then appears in the urine (*glucosuria*).

With increased gluconeogenesis (which is in part under the control of the adrenocortical hormones), protein and fats are mobilized, rather than stored or deposited in the cells. When there is deficiency of insulin, muscles cannot utilize glucose. Free fatty acids are then mobilized from adipose tissue cells and broken down by the liver into ketone bodies for energy. *Ketoacidosis* is characterized by excessive amounts of ketone bodies in the blood. Patients with ketoacidosis exhibit hyperventilation and loss of sodium, potassium, chloride, and water from the body. The net metabolic result of acute, uncontrolled diabetes mellitus is loss of fat stores, liver glycogen, cellular protein, electrolytes, and water. Over a period of years, blood glucose levels that are consistently above normal appear to hasten the complications that affect the large vessels in the brain, heart, kidneys, and extremities, and the small vessels in the eyes, kidneys, and nerves. The mechanisms have not yet been precisely determined, but several hypotheses have been proposed and will be discussed below with long-term complications. Chart 36-2 presents an overview of the complications of diabetes.

Clinical Manifestations

Type I Diabetes

Insulin-dependent diabetes mellitus (IDDM) usually begins in childhood, but may occur at any age and is not uncommon in adults. Measurable circulating insulin may still be present early in the course of the disease, but it soon disappears. In most instances the onset is abrupt, with weight loss, weakness, *polyuria* (excessive excretion of urine), *polydipsia* (excessive thirst), and *polyphagia* (excessive ingestion of food). As insulin production decreases, hyperglycemia develops as a result of the body's inability to use glucose. Hyperglycemia exceeds the renal threshold of glucose due to inability of the kidneys to absorb the extra glucose. Fluid loss through the kidneys results as the kidneys work to excrete the increased load of glucose, producing losses of water, sodium, magne-

---

Chart 36-1
Persons at Risk for Diabetes Mellitus

1. Persons with a family history of diabetes
2. Obese persons
3. Mothers delivered of large babies (over 9 lb) or those who have had an abnormal obstetrical history
4. Persons with early onset of arteriosclerosis
   a. Premenopausal women with myocardial infarction
   b. Men having myocardial infarctions before the age of 40
5. Persons with frequent or chronic infections (*e.g.,* gallbladder disease, pyelonephritis, pancreatitis)
6. Patients exhibiting temporary reduction of glucose tolerance during stress (myocardial infarction, infection, trauma, surgery)
7. Patients developing glucose intolerance during drug therapy (thiazides, glucocorticoids, ovulatory suppressants)
8. Persons with retinopathy, nephropathy, neuropathy, or other vascular manifestations

Chart 36-2
Complications of Diabetes

Eye Complications

- Diabetes is a leading cause of new cases of blindness in adults between 20 and 74 years of age.
- People with diabetes experience higher rates of cataracts and glaucoma.
- The cost of blindness from diabetes amounts to $75 million annually in lost income and public welfare expenses.
- About 40,000 people with diabetes are blind, and there are about 6,000 new cases of blindness from diabetes yearly.

Kidney Complications

- 25% of all new cases of end-stage renal disease are related to diabetes.
- Total cost to Medicare for end-stage renal disease related to diabetes is estimated to be $330 million a year.
- After 15 years of diabetes:
  $\frac{1}{3}$ of insulin-dependent cases of diabetes develop kidney disease.
  $\frac{1}{5}$ of noninsulin-dependent cases of diabetes develop kidney disease.
- People who develop diabetes during childhood die of renal disease at 500 times the expected rate.
- Renal disease causes 50% of all deaths among adults with insulin-dependent diabetes.

Peripheral Vascular Complications

- After 20 years of diabetes, 45% have peripheral vascular disease (4–7 times higher than the general population).
- 40–45% of all nontraumatic amputations each year are a result of diabetes.
- Hospitalization costs for lower-extremity amputations were $300 million in 1980 (not including costs of rehabilitation, premature death, or disability).

Cardiovascular Complications

- People with diabetes are twice as likely to die of heart disease as is the general population.
- Ischemic heart disease is implicated in:
  60% of deaths of adults with diabetes
  15% of deaths in young people with diabetes
- The incidence of strokes for people with diabetes is 2–6 times higher than that for the general population.
- After a stroke people with diabetes have a survival rate of 20%, while the rate for the general population is 40%.
- Hypertension is twice as common in persons with diabetes.
- More than 2.5 million Americans have both diabetes and hypertension.
- Diabetes and hypertension occur more frequently in black persons (twice the incidence in whites)
- Both diabetes and hypertension are more common among the lower socioeconomic groups.

Perinatal Complications

- The death rate in infants of mothers with diabetes is 2–4 times that for the general population.
- Congenital malformations are 2–3 times higher in infants of mothers with insulin-dependent diabetes.
- $\frac{1}{3}$ of all congenital anomalies are fatal.

Ketoacidosis

- Ketoacidosis contributes to 10% of diabetes-related deaths per year.

---

sium, calcium, potassium chloride, and phosphate. Because the body is not able to utilize ingested calories, body tissues are broken down to supply carbohydrate. An increased appetite is seen at first, but the hearty appetite may soon disappear as the metabolism becomes more unbalanced. Breakdown of protein and lipid (*catabolism*) produces loss of weight and muscular wasting. The patient is prone to develop *ketosis* (elevated level of ketone bodies in body tissues and fluids). Often the diagnosis is first made when the patient is brought to the hospital in a coma due to ketoacidosis. Insulin is always required.

Management includes subcutaneous injection of insulin, which is necessary for life. Diet and exercise are other essential components of therapy. Mortality and morbidity result from the acute or chronic complications of the disease. Hypoglycemia and hyperglycemia are for the most part preventable. It is thought that the onset of retinopathy, neuropathy, nephropathy, and cardiovascular effects may be delayed,

if not prevented, by maintaining blood glucose levels within the normal range.

Type II Diabetes

Noninsulin-dependent diabetes mellitus (NIDDM) usually occurs after the age of 40. It can also occur in younger persons who do not require insulin and who are not prone to developing ketosis. This type of diabetes is referred to as *maturity onset diabetes of the young (MODY)*. In general, these patients may never require insulin and are usually managed adequately by diet alone.

The majority (about 80%) of noninsulin-dependent diabetes mellitus patients are overweight when the condition is first diagnosed. The symptoms may be so minor that the diabetes is undetected for many years, and the diagnosis may be suspected as the result of a routine urinalysis. Frequently, the diabetes is discovered when the patient seeks health care for treatment of complications such as deteriorating vision, pain in the legs, or impotence. Often blood glucose tests are normal, with hyperglycemia being seen only postprandially (following a meal) or as a result of a glucose tolerance test.

The onset is insidious and may take years to develop. Fatigue, tendency to drowse after a meal, irritability, nocturia, itching of the skin (especially of the vulva in the female), skin wounds that heal poorly, blurring of vision, and cramps in the muscles are all warning symptoms of noninsulin-dependent diabetes.

Management includes diet and exercise; medications (insulin and/or oral agents) may be added if diet and exercise are unsuccessful after a reasonable trial period. Management goals are to achieve normal glucose levels and to prevent vascular complications. The vascular problems present in patients with type II diabetes account for most of the morbidity and mortality. Most of the vascular complications that develop in this category are macrovascular—that is, they involve the larger blood vessels, as in myocardial infarction or cerebral vascular accident. Microvascular problems, which involve the small blood vessels, are found in type I insulin-dependent diabetes.

Diagnostic Evaluation

Blood Glucose Tests

The presence of abnormally high blood glucose levels is the criterion on which the diagnosis of diabetes should be based. Blood glucose levels elevated above 120 mg/dl (SI: 6.6 mmol/L) on more than one occasion suggest a diagnosis of diabetes. If fasting glucose levels are normal or nearly normal, the diagnosis must be based on a glucose tolerance test.

Glucose Tolerance Test. Currently, the oral glucose tolerance test or OGTT is more sensitive than the intravenous glucose tolerance test (IVGTT), which is only used in special circumstances, *.e.g.*, for the patient who has had gastric surgery. The OGTT is now carried out through administration of a simple carbohydrate solution rather than a test meal.

The patient ingests high-carbohydrate (150–300 gm) meals for 3 days preceding the test. After an overnight fast, a blood sample is drawn. Then a 75-gm carbohydrate load, usually in the form of a carbonated sugar beverage (Glucola), is given to the patient. The patient is instructed to sit quietly during the test and to avoid exercise, smoking, coffee, and any other oral intake except water.

Blood samples are drawn ½ hour, 1 hour, and 2 hours after glucose ingestion. See Chart 36-3 for specific diagnostic criteria for diabetes mellitus.

Several factors affect the OGTT, including the method of analysis, source of the specimen (whole blood, plasma, or serum; capillary or venous blood), diet, activity level, amount of bed rest, presence of chronic disease, medication, and amount of the glucose load. In the elderly, diet, activity level, and medications present particular problems in interpreting the test results.

Dietary preparation for the test is very important because it may affect test results. It may be necessary to give written instructions to the patient to ensure the required intake of carbohydrate. If the diet is normal and the person's weight is stable, 150 gm per day are usually sufficient.

Medications that affect glucose tolerance should be discontinued, if possible, for about 3 days before the test. Four commonly prescribed drugs affect the OGTT: diuretics (usually thiazides), glucocorticoids, synthetic estrogens, and phenytoin (Dilantin). Other interfering agents include high doses of nicotinic acid, ethanol, and chronic ingestion of salicylates and monoamine oxidase inhibitors (especially hydrazine derivatives).

Special circumstances that affect the OGTT are pregnancy, gastric surgery, and advanced age. There is a special modification of the diagnostic criteria for the pregnant patient. In patients who have had gastric surgery, the IVGTT is necessary because an oral glucose load passes quickly into the small intestine, leading to a rapid absorption of glucose and therefore to glucose levels that are abnormal.

Gerontological Considerations. Elevated blood glucose levels appear to be age-related and occur in both men and women throughout the world. Elevation of blood glucose

---

Chart 36-3
Diagnostic Criteria for Diabetes Mellitus in Nonpregnant Adults

1. Classic symptoms of diabetes (polyuria, polydipsia, polyphagia, ketonuria, rapid weight loss)

   or

2. Elevated *fasting* glucose on more than one occasion:
   Venous whole blood greater than 120 mg/dl (6.6 mmol/L)
   Capillary whole blood greater than 120 mg/dl (6.6 mmol/L)

   or

3. Fasting glucose less than 120 mg/dl (6.6 mmol/L) but sustained elevated glucose during OGTT on more than one occasion. Both the 2-hour sample and some other sample taken between administration of the 75-gm glucose dose and 2 hours later must meet the following criteria:
   Venous whole blood greater than 180 mg/dl (9.9 mmol/L)
   Capillary whole blood greater than 200 mg/dl (11 mmol/L)

appears in the fifth decade of life and increases in frequency with advancing age. When elderly people with overt diabetes are excluded from the statistics, about 10% to 30% of elderly people have age-related hyperglycemia.

The question then arises as to whether age-related hyperglycemia is part of the normal aging process and benign, or whether it is pathological and requires therapeutic intervention. Several studies have suggested that the hyperglycemia is pathological because it leads to macrovascular complications.

The cause of age-related changes in carbohydrate metabolism is still not resolved. Apparently, delayed absorption from the gastrointestinal tract is not a factor. Other possibilities include poor diet, physical inactivity, a decrease in the lean body mass in which ingested carbohydrate may be stored, altered insulin secretion, and insulin resistance.

Screening Tests for Diabetes. Mass screening tests for diabetes in general use are 2-hour post-prandial blood glucose tests based on a capillary blood sample. However, there are many drawbacks in doing mass or community screening programs. The value of these programs has been questioned because they are nonspecific and because treatment may possibly be given to persons who may not have diabetes.

Urine Tests

Urine tests should not be used for diagnosis because both false-negative and false-positive results occur. Renal glucosuria occurs when the renal threshold for glucose is decreased. In this instance, glucose appears in the urine despite normal blood glucose values. In the elderly, renal threshold levels are higher than normal, so no glucose is found in the urine despite elevated blood glucose values.

Management

The basic problem of diabetes is impaired insulin secretion with a resulting abnormal carbohydrate metabolism. Over a period of years, this carbohydrate abnormality often leads to the vascular complications associated with diabetes. The main goal of treatment is to try to normalize insulin activity and blood glucose levels in an attempt to reduce the development of the vascular complications. The therapeutic goal within each type of diabetes is to lower blood glucose levels as much as possible without seriously disrupting the patient's usual activity patterns.

Treatment is variable throughout the course of the disease because of changes in life-style and physical and emotional status and improvements in therapy resulting from research. Therefore, treatment involves constant assessment and modification by health professionals as well as daily adjustments in therapy by the patients themselves. Although the health care team directs the treatment, it is the patient who is faced with the daily charge of managing the intricacies of a complex therapeutic regimen. The nurse is then the most accessible person qualified to teach the patient the range of skills needed for this daily management.

There are two essential components of management for *all* types of diabetes—*diet* and *exercise*. The use of medication, either insulin or oral hypoglycemic agents, depends

on the type of diabetes and/or the levels of glucose intolerance.

Dietary Management

Diet and weight control constitute the foundation of diabetes management. Nutritional management of the patient with diabetes can reasonably be expected to accomplish the following:

1. Provide all the essential food constituents (vitamins, minerals, etc.)
2. Achieve and maintain ideal weight
3. Meet energy needs
4. Achieve more normal blood glucose levels
5. Lower blood lipid levels, if elevated

The meals should be measured, and spaced at regular intervals. The menu is varied, with emphasis placed on what the patient is allowed rather than on what is forbidden, taking into consideration the patient's food likes and dislikes, lifestyle, and ethnic and cultural background in the daily selection of food.

Obesity

Obesity is corrected as soon as possible, since obese people are more resistant to both endogenous and exogenous insulin because of a decreased number of insulin receptors. Many patients who are overweight may achieve normal levels of blood glucose by losing weight because weight loss restores the number of insulin receptors on the cells. Success with diet for the patient with diabetes can be achieved more readily if the diet is fitted to the person instead of fitting the person to the diet.

A 1986 consensus panel convened by the National Institutes of Health considered the role of diet and exercise in non-insulin-dependent diabetes. The panel concluded that weight loss is the only proven treatment for type II diabetes.

Diet remains the basis of therapy. Overweight persons should lose weight, and those with a family history of diabetes should avoid becoming overweight. However, because approximately half of persons with type II diabetes remain undiagnosed, some researchers advise all overweight adults to consider themselves at risk and to have their blood glucose levels tested.

A subgroup of the obese particularly at risk to develop type II diabetes are the "apple-shaped" individuals with large amounts of abdominal fat.

The consensus statement acknowledged the poor prognosis for long-term weight maintenance. It recommended that obese type II patients be maintained on diets only moderately restricted in calories, and also suggested behavioral therapy, group support, and nutrition counseling to assist patients in weight loss and maintenance.

Calorie Intake

Calorie Requirements. The first step in preparing the meal plan is to determine the patient's basic calorie requirements, taking into consideration age, sex, body weight, and degree of activity. There are several methods of assessing calorie needs. A simple method, for instance, in most weight-maintenance diets is to multiply ideal weight by 30 to 35 cal/kg. For weight reduction a 15- to 20-cal/kg ideal weight is suitable. For most people, long-term reduction diets can be achieved with caloric levels between 1000 and 1200 calories. The calorie requirement can be raised to a maintenance level when the patient achieves the desired weight.

The most important objective in the dietary treatment of diabetes is control of total calorie intake to attain or maintain ideal weight. Success of this measure alone is often associated with reversal of the glucose intolerance. In the instance of a young, underweight patient with insulin-dependent diabetes, priority should be given to providing a diet with enough calories to maintain normal growth and development.

Calorie Distribution. While sources of calories are also to be taken into consideration, there is less emphasis now on restricted carbohydrate levels than in past years. This provides greater flexibility in diet and improves the ability of patients to adhere to an effective program of calorie restriction. Special attention is also given to lowering the fat content of diabetic diets. The Nutrition Committee of the American Diabetes Association issued a statement in 1971 pointing to the disadvantages of standard diets for diabetes that are high in fat. Epidemiologic evidence has been cited suggesting the favorable effects of high-starch, low-fat diets on both serum triglyceride levels and vascular disease in diabetes.

The caloric distribution preferred at present, as recommended by the American Diabetes and the American Dietetic Associations (1979), is as follows: for all levels of caloric intake, 55% to 60% of calories to be derived from complex carbohydrates, 20% to 30% from fat, and the remaining 12% to 20% from protein.

Carbohydrates. Within the established calorie distribution, carbohydrates should be taken in the form of polysaccharides (complex sugars). Approximately 15% to 20% of the carbohydrate should also be derived from disaccharides and monosaccharides in the form of lactose and fructose, from foods such as milk and fruits, respectively. It has been found that increasing the amount of carbohydrate without increasing the total daily number of calories does not increase the insulin needed. Patients can tolerate more carbohydrate than was formerly supposed.

Fat. The increase of carbohydrate has been made at the expense of fat, which is presently set at a level of 20% to 30% of caloric intake. The lowering of the proportion of dietary fat may reduce factors predisposing to the development of coronary heart disease, the most important cause of death and debility in diabetes.

Protein. The protein level of 12% to 20% of calories is considered appropriate.

Fiber

The use of fiber in diabetes has received increasing attention in the past 10 years as researchers study the effects in diabetes of a high-carbohydrate, high-fiber diet. This type of diet significantly reduces fasting blood glucose levels more than do the older traditional diets; both improvements in blood glucose levels and a decreased need for exogenous insulin have been seen.

Fiber, the indigestible part of certain foods, is important in the diet as roughage or bulk. Soluble fiber has high water-retaining capability and gels during digestion. This type of fiber, unlike the insoluble fiber, plays an important role in glucose absorption.

The mechanism of action remains unclear, although soluble fiber slows the emptying of the stomach and the movement of food through the upper digestive tract, and therefore the rate of glucose absorption.

Other benefits of fiber include relief of constipation, possibly prevention of diverticulitis and hemorrhoids, and possibly reduction of cholesterol and fat levels in the blood.

One risk involved in suddenly increasing fiber intake is that it may require adjusting the dosage of insulin or oral agents. Other problems include abdominal fullness, nausea and vomiting, increased flatulence, increased bowel movements, and vitamin/mineral deficiencies.

If fiber is added to or increased in the meal plan, it should be done gradually and in consultation with a dietitian. The 1986 *Exchange Lists for Meal Planning* is an excellent guide for increasing fiber intake. Food choices within the vegetable, fruit, and starch/bread exchanges are highlighted in the lists.

The manner in which food is prepared can also have an effect on blood glucose. Raw, whole, or solid foods cause less of a rise in blood glucose than do cooked, ground, or liquid forms.

More research is needed to determine how fiber works, which fibers are best, and the amount of fiber that is optimal for blood glucose control. However, it does appear that adding more fiber to the meal plan is beneficial.

Dietary Adaptation

Adapting dietary therapy to specific needs of individual patients on the basis of diagnostic tests is essential. If, for instance, a patient with diabetes is found to have type IV hyperlipoproteinemia, a lower carbohydrate intake would be beneficial in controlling this type of lipid abnormality. Patients with high levels of triglycerides, however, will benefit from a lowered fat intake (less than 30% of the diet). High cholesterol levels may require even greater reductions of dietary cholesterol and saturated fat. Guidelines for the treatment of hyperlipoproteinemias in diabetes are available.

Exchange Lists

The 1986 revision of the *Exchange Lists for Meal Planning* by the American Diabetes Association and the American Dietetic Association reflects the current thinking in the area of nutrition for the patient with diabetes.

The exchange lists are groups of foods that are approximately equal in calories and in carbohydrate, protein, and fat content. Foods may be selected or "exchanged" within a list but not between lists. These exchange lists allow for variety and flexibility in meal planning.

The 1986 exchange list emphasizes a high-carbohydrate, high-fiber diet and reflects the order in which foods are usually considered in meal planning. Some of the exchange list names have been modified in an attempt to incorporate into practice the most recent research findings. High-fiber foods and those with a high sodium content are identified to aid in diet planning for patients on special diabetic diets that are high in fiber and low in sodium.

The following foods should not be included in the meal plan: sugar, candy, honey, jam, jelly, cookies, syrup, condensed milk, chewing gum, pies, cakes, and soft drinks with sugar.

The patient should be taught to read labels. Foods that are advertised and labeled as "dietetic," "sugar-free," and "fat-free" often contain high proportions of carbohydrate and should be avoided. In addition, they are very expensive and often not as tasty as the items they are imitating.

The use of alcoholic beverages and sugar substitutes should be discussed with the physician or dietitian for possible inclusion in the meal plan.

Exchange Lists for Meal Planning (1986) includes a list of combination foods (*e.g.*, pizza, chili, chow mein), foods for use only occasionally (*e.g.*, ice cream, granola bars, cookies) because of their high fat or sugar content, and "free" foods (*e.g.*, seasonings, club soda, unsweetened pickles) that contain less than 20 calories per serving. A glossary, management tips, and nutritional goals are also included.

Sweeteners

It is probably unrealistic to ask patients to eliminate all food sweeteners from their diets. Adherence may even be improved if the patient is instructed in the use of sweeteners. Each has advantages and disadvantages. A summary of available sweeteners that may be used by the person with diabetes is listed below.

1. *Nutritive Sweeteners*—provide about 4 calories per gram of nutrient; use sparingly.

Aspartame

- Amino acid derivative
- Loses sweetness over time
- Heat stability—not stable
- Carcinogenicity unknown
- Anticariogenicity—none
- Contains phenylalanine; persons with phenylketonuria (PKU) advised against its use

Fructose

- Not useful in weight reduction (1 tbsp = 1 fruit exchange)
- Expensive
- Large amounts may have laxative effect

Sorbitol, xylitol, mannitol

- Found only in commercial products; not available for home use
- Half as sweet as sucrose
- Large amounts may have laxative effect
- Used in sugarless gums; do not promote tooth decay

2. *Nonnutritive Sweeteners*—no caloric or other nutrient value and no effect on blood glucose levels

Cyclamates

- 30 times sweeter than sucrose
- Removed from U.S. market (1969)
- May be carcinogenic

Saccharin

- 300 times sweeter than sucrose
- Use in meal plan as a free item
- May have cumulative carcinogenic effect; limit use

- May leave aftertaste
- Cannot be used in baked products

The Glycemic Index

It had long been thought that simple carbohydrates cause the greatest rise in blood glucose and that complex carbohydrates cause a lower rise. However, it appears that some complex carbohydrates act more like the simple carbohydrates. It has also been found that certain foods with equal carbohydrate content have different effects on the blood glucose level.

The Glycemic Index was created by Jenkins of the University of Toronto. It is a measure of how much a given food raises the blood glucose level. Glucose is assigned a value of 100%. Other foods are then assigned percentages based on glucose. See Table 36-2.

New studies point to a more complex response than that originally proposed. At the present time, not enough is known about the glycemic response to be able to predict consistently and accurately a person's response to a certain food. The glycemic response is further complicated by the patient's digestive, absorptive, and metabolic processes. Other factors that affect the response include the following:

- Dietary fiber content
  Alone or with other foods
  Percentage of carbohydrates in diet
  Type of fiber
  Level of blood glucose
  Amount of fat in meal
  Rate of digestion
- Food form
- Digestibility

TABLE 36-2
The Glycemic Index of Selected Foods*

Foods	%
Glucose	100
Carrots	92
Cornflakes	80
Potato (instant)	80
Rice (white)	72
Potato (new)	70
Bread (white)	69
Rice (brown)	66
Raisins	64
Banana	62
Corn	59
Peas (frozen)	51
All-Bran	51
Sponge cake	46
Spaghetti (whole-meal)	42
Apple (golden delicious)	39
Ice cream	36
Peas (chick)	36
Lentils	29
Peanuts	13

* Equal amounts of carbohydrates were compared.

- Cooking process
- Content and time of previous meals
- Rate of meal intake
- Glucose tolerance effect
- Liquids ingested at the meal

Despite the varied effects of all these factors, the concept of a glycemic index holds the potential for improving the ability to control blood glucose levels through dietary means. Patients can create their own glycemic index by monitoring their blood glucose level after ingesting a particular food. Many patients who practice frequent monitoring of blood glucose levels use this information to adjust their insulin doses.

The consensus panel of the National Institutes of Health (NIH) has carefully scrutinized the current ADA diet, which is high in complex carbohydrates and fiber. More research is needed to establish its safety and efficacy. The Glycemic Index was also examined. Much more work needs to be done in delineating the many variables that affect the Glycemic Index in any particular individual as well as its practical application.

The importance of exercise, advocated as an aid to weight loss and as a way to normalize blood glucose levels, was also debated. If exercise is to benefit persons with diabetes, they must exercise regularly.

In summary, the NIH consensus panel stressed weight control as the one beneficial treatment for type II diabetes, and the avoidance of obesity as the method for its prevention.

Health Teaching About Diet

To be practical and effective, a dietary program must be based on the patient's life-style and motivation, coupled with careful dietary instruction and follow-up.

Several cookbooks for diabetes are available and contain recipes that yield food portions with defined amounts of carbohydrate, fat, and protein, translated into food exchanges per portion. The patient should be cautioned to avoid recipes that contain excessive amounts of sugar.

A number of sources of information show popular food exchanges. The H. J. Heinz Company and the Campbell Soup Company have published lists showing the composition of their soups in terms of food exchanges. The local affiliates of the American Diabetes Association also have lists for ethnic and regional foods.

The nurse plays an important role in reinforcing the patient's understanding of the importance of diet in diabetes and the effective use of the exchange lists. The effect of this counseling is to reinforce the patient's motivation to follow the prescribed dietary regimen.

Exercise

Exercise is extremely important in the management of diabetes because of its effects on blood glucose and free fatty acids. Exercise lowers blood glucose by increasing the uptake of glucose by body muscles. It also improves circulation and muscle tone. These effects are useful in diabetes in relation to losing weight, easing stress or tension, and maintaining a feeling of well-being. Exercise also raises the levels of high-density lipoproteins (HDL), thereby lowering cholesterol and triglyceride levels. This is especially important to the person

with diabetes because of an increased risk of cardiovascular disease.

However, patients with blood glucose levels over 300 mg/dl (16.5 mmol/L) or who have ketones in their urine should not begin exercising until their blood glucose levels are in the normal range. Exercising with elevated blood glucose levels will cause increased secretions of glucagon, growth hormone, and catecholamines. The liver will then release more glucose, resulting in an increase in blood glucose. Therefore, exercise should not be performed until blood glucose levels are normalized.

The insulin-dependent patient should be taught to eat a 15-gm carbohydrate snack (a fruit exchange) before engaging in moderate exercise, in order to prevent unexpected hypoglycemia. Extra food is required for extra activity and need not be deducted from the regular meal plan. The exact amount of food needed can be determined only through trial and error.

Avoiding hypoglycemia during and after strenuous exercise may be accomplished by ingesting extra food as well as adjusting insulin. In addition, blood glucose testing should be performed before, during, and after the extended exercise period. A source of carbohydrate should be available during and after exercise. Other participants or observers should be aware that the person exercising has diabetes and should know what assistance to give if severe hypoglycemia occurs.

In obese persons with noninsulin-dependent diabetes, exercise in addition to dietary management not only improves glucose metabolism but also enhances loss of body fat and protects against the loss of lean body mass, the majority of which is muscle. The noninsulin-dependent patient who is not taking insulin or an oral agent does not require extra food before exercise. Exercise increases the number of insulin receptors in these patients and, if coupled with weight loss, increases still further the numbers of these receptors. Eventually, the patient's glucose tolerance may return to normal.

Persons with diabetes should be taught to exercise at the same time (preferably when blood sugar levels are at their peak) and in the same amount each day. Regular daily exercise, rather than sporadic exercise, should be encouraged.

Complications of diabetes may change the physiologic response to exercise because of microvascular problems, which affect the ability of blood vessels to dilate, and thus impair exercise tolerance. In addition, capillary permeability to fluids and proteins is increased. Exercise also decreases blood flow to the kidneys. Proteinuria is increased, and these factors may aggravate diabetic nephropathy. Exercise may also aggravate diabetic retinopathy by increasing blood pressure, thereby increasing the risk of a hemorrhage into the vitreous or retina. In patients with ischemic heart disease, there is a risk of triggering angina or a myocardial infarction.

If the patient is over 30 years of age and has two or more of the risk factors for heart disease, an exercise stress test is recommended. Risk factors include hypertension, obesity, high cholesterol levels, abnormal resting electrocardiogram, sedentary life-style, smoking, and a family history of heart disease. In general, persons with diabetes should discuss an exercise program with their physician.

Most research on exercise in diabetes has examined the effects of acute exercise. Fewer studies are available regarding the long-term effects of exercise training in diabetes. It has recently been shown that extremely intense exercise can raise blood glucose levels from normal levels. If the patient is in training, endurance should be built up gradually.

Gerontological Considerations. Physical activity that is consistent and realistic is beneficial for the elderly person with diabetes. Advantages include an improvement in glucose tolerance, a decreased need for oral antidiabetic agents or insulin, a general sense of well-being, and the utilization of ingested calories, resulting in weight reduction. Because there is an increased incidence of cardiovascular problems in the elderly, a pattern of slow, consistent exercise should be planned that does not exceed the patient's physical capacity. Both physical impairment from other chronic diseases and psychological capacity must be kept in mind.

Oral Antidiabetic Agents

Oral antidiabetic agents (previously referred to as oral hypoglycemic agents) may be effective for selected stable, non-insulin-dependent, nonketotic patients who cannot be treated by diet alone or who are unable or unwilling to take insulin. (See Table 36-3 for a list of these agents.) These drugs may be useful for the aged; those with poor vision, crippling arthritis of the fingers, and tremor of the hands; and those who for some reason refuse to take insulin. (Insulin is preferable to oral antidiabetic agents in some cases if dietary treatment fails to control diabetes.)

In the United States, the oral antidiabetic agents available are the sulfonylureas. They are thought to exert their primary action by directly stimulating the pancreas to secrete insulin. Therefore, a functioning pancreas is necessary for these drugs to be effective, and they cannot be used in the treatment of patients who are insulin-dependent and prone to ketoacidosis.

The sulfonylureas can be divided into short-, intermediate-, and long-acting agents with varying duration of action. Side-effects of these drugs are relatively rare, but include hematologic, hepatic, and dermatologic reactions. Hypoglycemia may occur when an excessive dose of a sulfonylurea is used or when meals are omitted or food intake is decreased. Hypoglycemia should be treated as usual, but special emphasis should be given to patients taking chlorpropamide (Diabinese) because of the possibility of prolonged hypogly-

cemia due to its long-time action. The sulfonylureas also interact with various drugs: *e.g.,* sulfonamides, salicylates, phenylbutazones, barbiturates, thiazides, alcohol, and catecholamines.

For successful treatment with oral antidiabetic agents, the diet must be restricted in total calories and carbohydrates, and the patient's blood glucose values monitored.

- Oral antidiabetic drugs must be abandoned temporarily in favor of insulin if the patient develops an infection with fever, suffers trauma, or undergoes major surgery.

If, as time goes on, the patient's blood glucose values are no longer responsive to oral antidiabetic therapy, the patient is then treated with insulin. This is referred to as a *secondary failure*. A *primary failure* occurs when the blood glucose level remains high a month after drug use.

A study by the National Institutes of Health, called the University Group Diabetes Program, has given rise to many questions concerning the safety and effectiveness of long-term oral antidiabetic agents. This study group found a higher death rate from heart disease in their tolbutamide-treated patients than in those treated with a placebo. However, since the tolbutamide-treated patients were older and had more baseline cardiac disease than did the control patients, the conclusions may not be justified.

At this time, the use of oral antidiabetic agents with insulin is again being proposed. This is an option for some patients who are not able to achieve near-normal blood glucose levels despite large doses of insulin. This combination must be accompanied by blood glucose monitoring. Weight gain is often a problem, but it can be minimized if insulin dosage is decreased.

Insulin Therapy

As was stated earlier, insulin is secreted by the beta cells of the islets of Langerhans. It works to lower the blood glucose by facilitating the uptake and utilization of glucose by muscle and fat cells and by decreasing the release of glucose from the liver.

TABLE 36-3
Oral Antidiabetic Agents in the United States

Trade Name	Generic Name	Major Manufacturer	Duration of Action
First Generation			
Orinase	Tolbutamide	Upjohn	6–12 hours
Dymelor	Acetohexamide	Lilly	12–24 hours
Tolinase	Tolazamide	Upjohn	12–24 hours
Diabinese	Chlorpropamide	Pfizer	1–2 days
Second Generation			
Glucotrol	Glipizide	Pfizer	12–24 hours
Diabeta	Glyburide	Hoechst-Roussel	Approximately 24 hours
Micronase	Glyburide	Upjohn	Approximately 24 hours

When the patient's body fails to produce enough insulin, and when diet alone cannot control the diabetes, then insulin must be administered. One or more insulin injections each day are usually taken by persons with insulin-dependent diabetes as well as by those with noninsulin-dependent diabetes that cannot be adequately controlled by diet alone or by diet and oral agents.

Since the insulin dose required by the individual patient is determined by the level of glucose in the blood, accurate monitoring of blood glucose levels is essential. Self-monitoring of blood glucose levels has become the cornerstone of insulin therapy because of its effectiveness in determining appropriate insulin dosage and promoting better control of blood glucose levels. This method is described in detail later in this section.

Obese noninsulin-dependent patients who have no complications, few symptoms, and no ketonuria can usually control their diabetes by means of calorie restriction. However, these same patients, whose diabetes is usually controlled by diet alone or by diet and an oral antidiabetic agent, may require insulin temporarily during illness, infection, pregnancy, surgery, or some other stressful event.

Sources of Insulin.   Insulin traditionally has been extracted from either beef or pork pancreases obtained from animals going to slaughter. Because of potential shortages of beef and pork sources, research into ways to produce insulin has received increased emphasis.

Insulin has been produced semi-synthetically. This method replaces an amino acid in pork insulin to produce human insulin (available from Squibb-Novo).

Biosynthetic human insulin has also been produced by using genetically-altered bacteria (*Escherichia coli*). It has been tested in humans and is now available in the United States. One of the proposed advantages of human insulins over those from animal sources is the lower levels of antibodies produced by the patient's body against the human insulin. It is thought that the production of this low level of antibodies is caused by the route of administration (subcutaneous), which is not physiologic, as well as the kind of insulin that is used. Whether these insulin antibodies are in any way harmful is still undetermined. Human insulins are often given to patients with newly diagnosed insulin-dependent diabetes or those who have an allergy to insulin obtained from animal sources.

Insulin Preparations

A number of insulin preparations are available, which vary in onset of action, time of peak or maximum effect, and duration or length of action (Table 36-4). These preparations are classified into three groups: (1) short-acting insulin, (2) intermediate-acting insulin, and (3) long-acting insulin. In many patients, combinations of short- and intermediate-action insulins are given to maintain metabolic control. Other combinations are also used with less frequency.

Insulin (which is prescribed in units) is available in two concentrations (strengths) that correspond to the number of units of insulin per milliliter of solution: U-40 (40 units per ml) and U-100 (100 units per ml). In the United States, the aim is to have only one strength, U-100, available in all varieties of insulin. The insulin syringe must correlate with the strength of insulin used. For example, U-100 insulin is given with a U-100 syringe.

Insulin Mixtures.   When insulins are mixed, the stability of the mixture depends on the ratio of the insulins as well as the time between mixing and injecting. These considerations are especially important in planning for home care and for elderly or visually impaired patients who depend on others (*e.g.*, neighbors) to prepare their insulin. Mixtures of regular/NPH insulin or regular/Lente should be administered within 5 minutes after being mixed or after a period of 24 hours. Consistency in the method of preparation is essential, because different ratios of insulin will be delivered depending on whether the mixture is injected within 5 minutes of mixing or whether 24 hours or more have elapsed. Community health nurses who prepare a week's supply of insulin syringes need to be aware of the stability of the insulin mixture.

Buffered regular insulin should not be used in combination with other insulin because of the incompatibility resulting from the buffering agent.

Regulation of Dosage

The dosage of insulin is adjusted according to the levels of blood glucose, the degree to which glucose is present, and the time when high glucose levels appear in relation to insulin administration and meals. Meals are planned at certain times to conform to insulin peaks and the exercise patterns of the patient receiving one or more insulin injections per day. Insulin curves vary from patient to patient, and the response of individual patients may be highly variable.

In the absence of complications, treatment may be started with 10 to 20 units of intermediate-acting insulin combined with a shorter-acting insulin, given subcutaneously before breakfast. This dosage is increased gradually, as indicated by the patient's response to the previous dose, until the urine is free of glucose and the blood glucose level before each meal is near normal. Larger doses may be necessary at the onset, depending on the degree of insulin insufficiency. The meals must coincide with the action of the insulin. During initial regulation, and when insulin requirements are changing rapidly (during an acute illness), it is common practice to give supplemental injections of regular insulin before each meal, depending on the results of a recent test for glucose and the previous response of the patient. Constant monitoring of blood glucose levels and close attention to insulin dose and food intake are crucial during an acute illness.

There is a narrow margin between the therapeutic and the hypoglycemic effects of insulin. It is important that the patient and the nurse know when hypoglycemia is most likely to occur with each type of insulin. While insulin is being regulated or during periods of illness, the patient is instructed to test for blood glucose and urine ketones before each meal and at bedtime. Patients who are unable to adjust insulin dosage themselves should keep a record of the test results and take it to the physician or clinic with each visit, so that insulin adjustments can be made.

Other factors that affect the dosage of insulin include the age of the patient, diet, the amount of insulin secretion, the level of insulin antibodies, exercise/activity levels, obesity, hormones (pregnancy, menstruation), oral contraceptives, other drugs and diseases, anxiety, stress, and smoking.

The Honeymoon Period.   Soon after initiation of insulin therapy, some type I patients begin to secrete some insulin, resulting in a decreased need for exogenous insulin. This

TABLE 36-4
Insulin Preparations Available in the U.S.

Manufacturer	Product	Species Source	Type
Rapid-Acting			
Lilly	Iletin I	Beef/pork	Regular
Lilly	Iletin II	Beef or pork	Regular
Squibb/Novo	Actrapid	Human or pork	Regular
Nordisk	Velosulin	Pork	Regular
Squibb/Novo	Insulin Injection	Pork	Regular
Squibb/Novo	Purified Insulin Injection	Pork	Regular
Lilly	Humulin R	Human	Regular
Squibb/Novo	Novolin R	Human	Regular
Lilly	Semilente Iletin I	Beef/pork	Semilente
Squibb/Novo	Semitard	Pork	Semilente
Squibb/Novo	Semilente Insulin	Beef	Semilente
Intermediate-Acting			
Lilly	NPH Iletin I	Beef/pork	NPH
Lilly	NPH Iletin II	Beef or pork	NPH
Squibb/Novo	NPH Protaphane	Pork	NPH
Nordisk	NPH Insulatard	Pork	NPH
Squibb/Novo	Purified Isophane Insulin	Beef	NPH
Lilly	Humulin	Human	NPH
Squibb/Novo	Novolin N	Human	NPH
Lilly	Lente Iletin I	Beef/pork	Lente
Lilly	Lente Iletin II	Beef or pork	Lente
Squibb/Novo	Monotard	Human or pork	Lente
Squibb/Novo	Lentard	Beef/pork	Lente
Squibb/Novo	Insulin Zn Susp.	Beef	Lente
Squibb/Novo	Purified Insulin Zn Susp.	Beef	Lente
Squibb/Novo	Novolin L	Human	Lente
Long-Acting			
Lilly	Protamine, Zn Iletin I	Beef/pork	PZI
Lilly	Protamine, Zn Iletin II	Beef or pork	PZI
Squibb/Novo	Protamine, Zn Insulin	Beef	PZI
Lilly	Ultralente Iletin I	Beef/pork	Ultralente
Squibb/Novo	Ultratard	Beef	Ultralente
Squibb/Novo	Ultralente Insulin	Beef	Ultralente
Mixed			
Nordisk	Mixtard	Pork	70% NPH 30% Regular
Squibb/Novo	Novolin 70/30	Human	70% NPH 30% Regular

transient period, or period of remission, is often referred to as the "honeymoon" period. It can last for a few weeks to a few months. It can be extremely frustrating to both patient and family because they may feel that a cure has occurred and thus find it difficult to understand the need to inject a small amount of insulin (only a few units). Eventually, self-secreted insulin production decreases and there is a need for more exogenous insulin. As insulin therapy is initiated, the patient and family should be warned that such a process may occur and about the eventual consequences. In the past, some researchers have tried without success to extend this honeymoon period with the use of oral agents.

Insulin Absorption. Individual variations in insulin absorption can affect the degree to which blood glucose levels can be controlled. Some of the factors involved can be controlled if they are recognized. For example, exercising the site of the insulin injection, injecting the insulin deep into the tissues, massaging the site, and taking an injection after a warm bath or shower all increase absorption.

Health Teaching: Self-Injection of Insulin

As soon as the need for insulin has been established, the patient is instructed in the technique of self-injection, and is

---

Chart 36-4
Teaching Insulin Administration

Choosing and Buying the Right Equipment

1. Know the manufacturer, type, and concentration of prescribed insulin.
2. U-80 insulins are no longer available. U-40 insulins will soon be phased out.
3. Any change in insulin should be made cautiously and only under medical supervision. Changes in purity, strength (U-40, U-100), brand (manufacturer), type (*e.g.*, Lente, NPH), or source (beef, pork, beef/pork, human) may result in the need for a change in dosage. When you change to a "purified insulin," a dosage decrease may be necessary. Adjustment may be needed with the first dose or over a period of several weeks. A small number of patients may require a significant change in dosage.
4. Insulin prices may vary greatly depending on preparation/purity, species source, and concentration.
5. Check insulin expiration dates when purchasing.
6. Store insulin in a cool place. Avoid temperature extremes.
7. Select insulin syringes based on comfort, convenience, and cost.
   - Disposable syringes are usually 1.25-cm (½-inch), 27-gauge, with a lubricated needle.
   - If taking less than 50 units, disposable syringes also available in a ½-ml size that measures up to 50 units.
   - Glass syringes are cheaper but are harder to find and involve time and dexterity in daily cleansing (*e.g.*, arthritic patients).

Before Injection

1. Match the syringe to the insulin concentration to avoid serious problems with either hypoglycemia or hyperglycemia. Use U-100 insulin with a U-100 syringe.
2. Know when insulin works—its onset, peak, and duration—and time snacks, meals, and exercise accordingly.
3. Understand that many patients take more than one type of insulin and inject more than once daily in order to achieve near-normal blood glucose levels.
4. Store insulin being used at a cool room temperature. Extra insulin may be kept in the refrigerator. The most important fact regarding storage is to avoid extremes in temperature.

Injection

1. Choose the right site. Choices include arms, thighs, abdomen, and buttocks.
2. Rotate sites to prevent *lipodystrophy*—lumps or indentations that can be caused by repeated injections in one area.
3. Rotate injection sites to help absorption. Injecting in the same site repeatedly often results in a less painful injection *but* poorer absorption. This may account for delayed insulin action, which can cause serious problems.
4. Avoid injecting into areas you plan to exercise that day (*e.g.*, avoid right arm if you are a right-handed tennis player). Exercise can cause a more rapid absorption of insulin and unexpected hypoglycemia can result.

After Injection

1. Always be prepared for hypoglycemia; carry hard candy or sugar. Chocolate candy takes longer to absorb because of its fat content.
2. If in doubt about whether person is experiencing hypoglycemia or hyperglycemia, *always* treat for hypoglycemia.
3. Quick-acting, commercially-prepared sugar products are available:
   - Glutose (Paddock laboratories)
   - Monojel (Monject)

   These are to be used if the hypoglycemic person can still swallow.
4. Glucagon (Eli Lilly Company) is a pancreatic hormone that raises blood sugar. It is available only by prescription and is injected subcutaneously, using an insulin syringe. The patient may need to self-administer it if vomiting. If the patient is unconscious, it should be administered by someone who knows how to give an injection (*e.g.*, a family member, neighbor, friend).
5. The patient should always wear medical identification stating that the person has diabetes and is on insulin. Carrying a card in a wallet is inadequate, because emergency personnel may not find it.

encouraged to begin self-injection as soon as possible. An optimistic but firm approach will offer the patient encouragement. Another family member or friend should also be taught. Charts 36-4 and 36-5 summarize the important factors to include in teaching insulin administration.

Rotation of Sites. Systematic rotation of injection sites (Fig. 36-1) is necessary to prevent localized changes in fatty tissue (lipodystrophy or lipohypertrophy) and to allow for uniform absorption of insulin. To ensure a definite rotation schedule, the patient is encouraged to keep a record of each injection site.

The rate of insulin absorption varies with the site used. Regular insulin is absorbed faster when injected into certain areas. Speed of absorption is greatest in the abdomen and decreases progressively in the arm (deltoid area), the thigh, and the buttock. In general, although site rotation is still im-

---

Chart 36-5
Self-Injection of Insulin

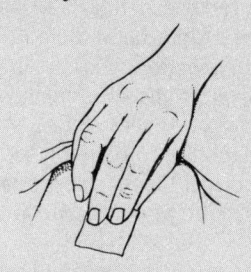

- The technique of filling the syringe is demonstrated, and the skin is disinfected with alcohol.

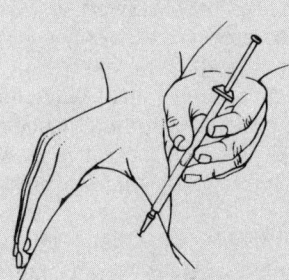

- The person is instructed to pull the skin taut on the anterior surface of the thigh or to form a skin fold by picking up subcutaneous tissue between the thumb and forefinger. Either of these techniques ensures that the needle tip is inserted into subcutaneous tissue and outside the muscle. The skin should not be pressed tightly together between the fingers, since this is a cause of local induration.
- The person is instructed to insert the needle with a quick thrust into deep subcutaneous tissue.
- When the arm is used as the site of injection, another person may need to assist, or the arm can be stabilized by leaning against a wall or door.
- The angle of injection should be between 45 and 90 degrees depending on the amount of adipose tissue present.

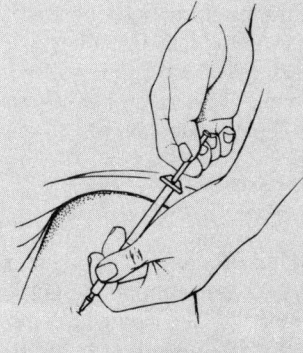

- The person then pulls back slightly on the plunger of the syringe to assure that the needle is not in a blood vessel before the insulin is injected. (If blood appears, the needle should be removed and a new site and a new syringe used.)

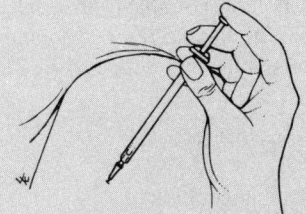

- The insulin is then injected. After injecting the insulin, the person holds the alcohol sponge against the needle, while gently withdrawing it, to prevent painful pulling of the skin while the needle is withdrawn.

- Massaging the site of injection will increase the absorption rate of the insulin.

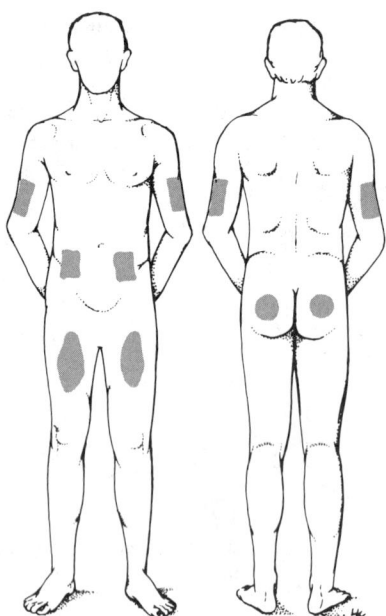

Figure 36-1
Suggested sites for insulin injections.

portant, it is better to rotate within a site and then move on to another site instead of rotating daily from arm to thigh to abdomen and onward around the circuit again.

Some patients do not rotate sites because repeated injections into the same site become less painful. However, lipohypertrophy may occur; insulin will then not be absorbed as well, and episodes of hypoglycemia or hyperglycemia may occur. Each injection should be separated from the previous injection by approximately 2.5 cm (1 inch), and each site should be used no more often than every 3 weeks.

Areas that are about to be exercised (*e.g.*, right arm for playing tennis) should be avoided that day, because injection in an exercising site can result in a more rapid absorption of insulin. Areas with loose skin and a sufficient amount of subcutaneous fat are sites suitable for insulin injection; that is, lateral surface of the arms, anterior aspect of the thighs, anterior and lateral aspects of the abdominal wall, and lateral areas of the back, just above the buttock.

Problems With Insulin

Local Allergic Reactions.   A local allergic reaction in the form of redness, swelling, tenderness, and induration, or a wheal may appear at the site of injection. These reactions usually occur during the beginning stages of therapy and disappear with continued use of insulin. These allergic reactions are becoming less frequent because of the increased purity of insulins. The physician may prescribe an antihistamine to be taken 1 hour before the injection if such a local reaction occurs.

Occasionally, if alcohol is not allowed to dry on the skin before injection, it is carried into the tissues. This results in a localized reddened area.

Systemic Allergic Reactions.   Systemic allergic reactions to insulin range from hives to general edema and anaphylaxis. The treatment is desensitization, with small volumes of insulin given as desensitizing doses.

Insulin Lipodystrophy.   *Lipodystrophy* refers to a localized disturbance of fat metabolism, in the form of either lipoatrophy or lipohypertrophy. These reactions occur at the site of injection and may appear separately, in combination, or in succession, in the same patient. *Insulin-induced atrophy* is loss of subcutaneous fat and appears as slight dimpling or more serious pitting of subcutaneous fat. It occurs most commonly in women and children. The use of U-100 insulin, which is 99% pure, has almost eliminated this disfiguring complication. Lipoatrophy is treated by injection of purified insulin into the periphery of the lipoatrophic area.

Lipohypertrophy is the development of fibrofatty masses at the injection site; it occurs more often in children and adult men and is caused by the repeated use of an injection site. If insulin is injected into scarred areas, the absorption is irregular and the action of the insulin unpredictable. This is one reason why the rotation of injection sites is so important. The patient should avoid injecting insulin into these areas until the hypertrophy disappears.

Insulin Edema.   A generalized retention of fluid is sometimes seen after near-normal blood glucose levels are suddenly established in a patient who has had prolonged hyperglycemia.

Insulin Resistance.   Most patients at one time or another have some degree of insulin resistance. This may occur for various reasons, the most common being obesity, which can be overcome by weight loss.

True insulin resistance has been defined as a daily requirement of 200 units or more. Some patients need as many as 500 to 2000 units daily for a certain period of time.

In most insulin-dependent patients with diabetes, immune antibodies develop and bind the insulin, thereby decreasing the insulin available for use. All animal insulins as well as human insulins to a lesser degree cause antibody production in humans.

Some patients develop high levels of antibodies. Many of these patients give a history of insulin therapy interrupted for several months or more. Treatment consists of administering a purer insulin preparation, and occasionally prednisone may be needed. This is usually followed by a dramatic reduction in insulin requirement.

During treatment, U-500 insulin may be needed and is available on special order from the Lilly Company.

In rare instances, insulin may be degraded when given subcutaneously and may need to be given intravenously or intranasally. The latter is still experimental.

Monitoring for Glucose and Ketones

Self-Monitoring of Blood Glucose.   Self-monitoring of blood glucose (SMBG) has become important during the past 10 years in managing diabetes and calculating insulin dosage because it provides a direct measurement of blood glucose levels. Approximately one million patients with insulin-dependent diabetes now use SMBG, at an estimated annual cost of $750 per patient. Persons with diabetes must be taught the following key elements:

· To understand the purpose of self-monitoring of blood glucose
· To perform the technique accurately
· To record the results
· To utilize the test results properly

Because the use of SMBG has become so widespread, a national consensus conference was convened in November, 1986, to examine current issues. Panel members recommended SMBG for insulin-treated patients. They *emphasized* its importance in the following circumstances:

- Pregnancy complicated by diabetes
- Unstable diabetes
- A tendency to severe ketosis or hypoglycemia
- Hypoglycemia in patients without warning symptoms
- Practice of intensive insulin regimens, *e.g.*, insulin pumps, multiple daily injections
- Presence of abnormal renal glucose thresholds

SMBG may also be useful in patients not treated with insulin. However, it should not be used to diagnose diabetes, and its usefulness in screening programs still remains uncertain. Additional recommendations include the following:

- Development of monitors that are easier to use and less dependent on the skill of the user
- Development of a monitor for the visually-impaired
- Implementation of quality control programs
- Development of monitors that are accurate in both high and low blood glucose ranges and not influenced by hematocrit

The proper use of SMBG is as an aid in making day-to-day decisions about insulin dosage, exercise, and meal planning, and in recognizing and responding to emergency situations (*e.g.*, hypoglycemia, influenza).

Procedure. A drop of blood is obtained from either the fingertip or the earlobe with one of a variety of lancetlike devices. The drop of blood is placed on one of the testing strips for a specific amount of time, determined by the manufacturer. The blood is then *wiped* off the strip. The results can be read either visually or with an electronic meter. If the visual method is used, the color block on the strip is compared to the color chart on the package (after an appropriate waiting period). If the meter is used, the strip is inserted into the meter for an exact reading (Fig. 36-2).

While approximating blood glucose visually is accurate enough for many insulin-dependent diabetics, a meter is either preferred or necessary for others. Costs for these methods of monitoring blood glucose must be considered by the patient, as well as the time and commitment they each require.

Hemoglobin A₁c (Glycosylated Hemoglobin A₁c). At the present time, the hemoglobin A_{1c} test is done only in a laboratory and not at home. It is a blood test that shows the *pattern* of blood glucose levels over a period of approximately 3 months. When blood glucose levels are elevated, a glucose molecule attaches itself to hemoglobin in a red blood cell. The longer the glucose in the blood remains above normal, the more glycosylated hemoglobins form. This complex (the hemoglobin attached to the glucose) is permanent and lasts for the life of the red blood cell, approximately 120 days. If near-normal blood glucose levels are maintained, with only occasional rises in blood glucose, the overall value will not be greatly elevated. However, if the *pattern* of blood glucose values is consistently high, then the test result will also be elevated. The normal values vary from laboratory to laboratory, but a value of 6 to 8 is considered within the "normal" range. Values within the normal range indicate consistently near-normal blood glucose levels, a goal easier to attain for insulin-dependent patients who monitor blood glucose levels themselves, particularly if they use multiple insulin injections or insulin pump (continuous subcutaneous insulin injection) therapy.

Urine Testing for Glucose. Urine testing for glucose may be adequate for noninsulin-dependent diabetics, because their diabetes is fairly stable. However, many clinicians now feel that blood glucose monitoring in these patients is indicated. It has been found to be especially useful in the obese type II patient because of increased motivation to lose weight after seeing the daily blood glucose levels drop in response to diet therapy. Urine tests do not provide enough accuracy for the insulin-dependent patient, who must adjust insulin doses based on accurate test results in order to maintain near-normal blood glucose levels. Urine testing for glucose should be performed by insulin-dependent patients who cannot, for some reason, use blood glucose testing, because it can approximate levels of blood glucose.

As was indicated earlier, urine testing for glucose is also affected by the aging process. Aging raises the renal threshold, so that negative tests for urinary glucose may occur when the blood glucose is elevated.

There are several methods of testing urine for glucose: Clinitest, Tes-tape and Diastix. False tests may be obtained if deteriorated reagent tablets or strips are used or if the directions are not followed accurately. Certain drugs taken by the

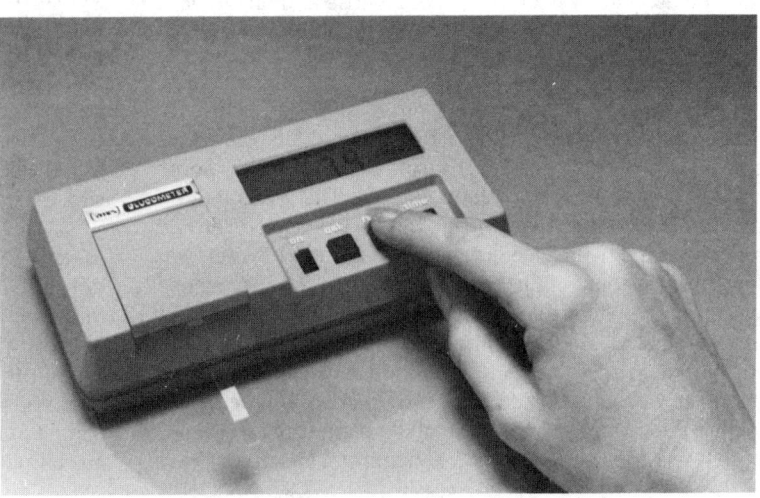

Figure 36-2
An example of a commercially available meter which measures electronically the amount of glucose in the blood. (Courtesy Ames Division, Miles Laboratory, Inc.)

patient can also produce false test results. Blood glucose testing on a *routine* basis by the patient has replaced urine testing as a tool the patient can use to keep blood glucose in the near-normal range. Blood glucose testing shows the *exact* amount of glucose in the blood at the time of testing, while urine testing shows only the *percentage* of glucose present in the urine when the sample is taken.

Urine Testing for Ketones. Ketones in the urine signal that control of diabetes is deteriorating and that the body has started to break down stored fat for energy. Mobilization of fat results in acetonemia and acetonuria, and can be detected by testing the urine for acetone. Tests for ketone bodies are done when there is persistent glucosuria or elevated blood glucose levels, or when the patient is not feeling well.

Tests can be done by the patient to determine the presence of acetone (ketone bodies) in the urine. The *Acetest* uses a chemical reagent that reacts with ketone bodies in the urine to yield a colored product; the depth of color is roughly correlated with the ketone-body concentration.

The *Ketostix* or *Chemstrip uK* is a reagent strip that is dipped in the urine. After the time specified on the product information sheet, a lavender color appears if the urine contains ketones. The depth of color is compared with the color chart.

Keto-Diastix or *Chemstrip uGK* is a combined reagent strip designed for the determination of ketones and glucose in urine. Large amounts of ketones may depress the color development of the glucose test area.

Testing urine for ketones is still very important in insulin-dependent patients who test their blood for glucose, because ketones signal a dangerous condition—ketosis.

Insulin Delivery Systems

It was not until the early 1960s that plasma insulin levels could be measured, which allowed researchers to see how inadequate conventional insulin therapy was.

In a person with a properly functioning pancreas, the beta cells produce smooth, rapid bursts of insulin secretion with each meal. This secretion of insulin is regulated through

1. The nervous system (vagus, catecholamines)
2. Gastrointestinal hormones (*e.g.*, gastric-inhibitory peptide)
3. Islet hormonal factors (somatostatin, glucagon) as well as substrate concentrations of glucose and amino acids, which affect the amount and duration of insulin secretion by the pancreas

Insulin-dependent persons with diabetes lack this type of secretion. Insulin injections, at best, can produce only peaks and valleys of insulin levels that are irregular and usually poorly coordinated with rises in blood glucose. The levels that are produced by one or more injections a day can prevent ketoacidosis and hypoglycemia in many patients. However, very few insulin-dependent patients can avoid swings of glucose, glucagon, free fatty acids, growth hormone, and the like that are not physiologic. With more and more evidence pointing to "tight control" (near-normal blood glucose levels) as a factor in preventing or delaying the dreaded long-term vascular complications, and the fact that near-normal blood glucose levels impart a feeling of well-being and an improvement

of growth and development in children with diabetes, it seemed logical to search for a better insulin delivery system.

Insulin Pump Development

Research on developing means to duplicate mechanically the work of the beta cell began around 1972. If a device could be made small enough to be implanted in the patient and still function as an insulin delivery system, then the patient would, in effect, be the recipient of an artificial beta cell. The ultimate goals of this approach, therefore, were to develop an artificial beta cell that would be implantable, functional, and convenient. However, development of this insulin delivery system has produced two similar, yet dissimilar, products, the "closed"-loop and the "open"-loop systems.

Closed-Loop System. In 1973, Albisser developed the first insulin delivery system (closed-loop system) at the Hospital for Sick Children in Toronto, Canada. In this system, the patient is connected to the machine via a venous catheter. The closed-loop system (feedback) devices are capable of monitoring glucose concentrations in the blood. "Closed loop" refers to the closed loop formed by the pancreas that delivers insulin in response to the body's glucose levels. The main components of such a device include a glucose sensor, an insulin pump, and a computer. Intravenous blood glucose levels are continuously monitored by a sensor in the device. The computer determines the insulin rate by means of algorithms, and the insulin pump adjusts itself without any participation on the part of the patient in order to control blood glucose concentrations. It also adjusts the rate of either glucagon or glucose delivery. This is the type of system that could be the answer to the beta cell problem in diabetes. However, two criteria must be met: miniaturization and implantability. The first has been solved, but the second has not. One of the current research problems is the immune response to the implanted cell.

These closed-loop systems have been developed and are in use clinically. The first one available commercially, the Biostator, a bedside device, was developed by Life Science Instruments (a division of Miles Laboratories). It is large, must be connected to the patient intravenously, and is used only in large medical centers and in special circumstances, usually during labor and delivery or lengthy surgical procedures, and for treating complicated cases of ketoacidosis.

Open-Loop Systems. The open-loop systems lack a built-in feedback component for blood glucose regulation. In other words, the patient acts as the glucose sensor via self-monitoring of blood glucose. These pump systems (continuous subcutaneous insulin infusion [CSII]) require strict dietary compliance and are dependent on the patient for delivery of the appropriate premeal insulin dose, based on the results of blood glucose self-monitoring, which is critical to the system's success.

Insulin Pumps in Use. Basically, insulin pumps in use today in persons with diabetes outside the hospital are battery-driven syringes that deliver a basal rate of insulin continuously throughout a 24-hour period (Fig. 36-3). In addition, they can deliver a premeal (bolus) dose. The amount of insulin delivered in the 24-hour period is determined by the results of numerous (4 to 8) blood glucose measurements done by the patient to maintain blood glucose levels in the normal range. Insulin physiologically follows a pattern of a low rate of se-

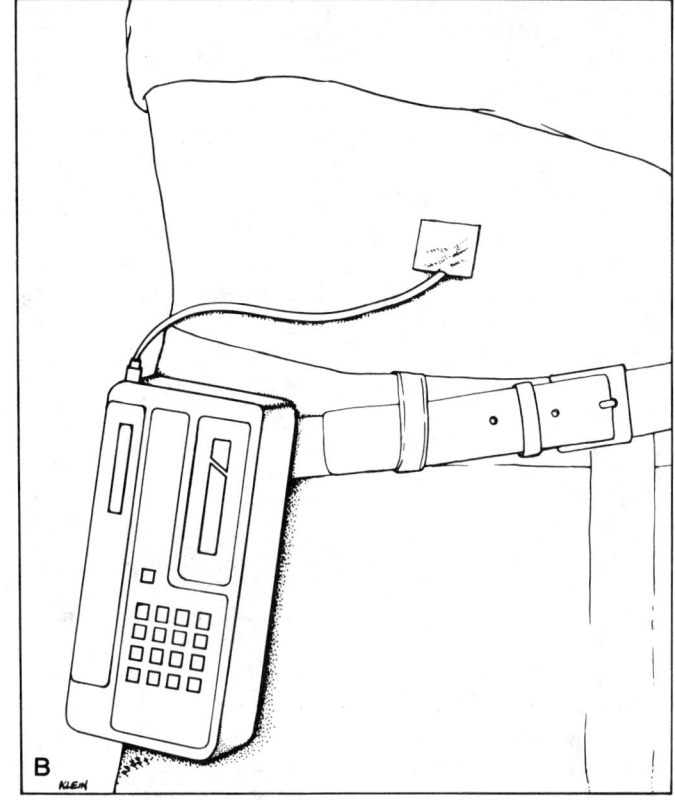

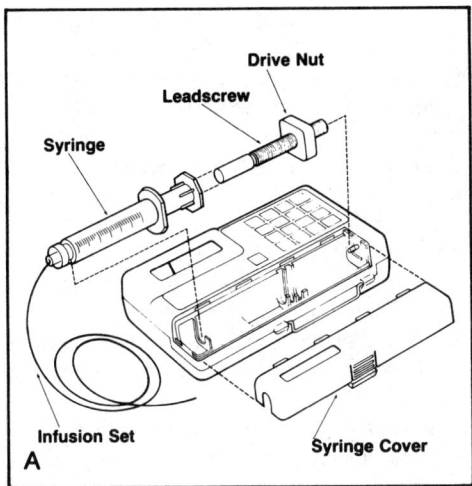

Figure 36-3
Infusion insulin pump. (*A*) Schematic drawing of infusion pump. (*B*) Insulin pump in
place. (*A:* Courtesy of Cardiac Pacemakers, Inc., St. Paul, Minnesota.)

cretion during fasting and a high output after meals. Algorithms have been developed to allow the pump to deliver
small quantities of insulin between meals and through the
night with bolus doses at mealtimes, taking into consideration
individual variations in daily living, food intake, and exercise.

At the present time, the insulin pump, which must be
used in conjunction with blood glucose monitoring by the
patient, attempts to mimic the normal insulin function of the
pancreas. It must be used only under a physician's direct
supervision.

The pump (Fig 36-3) consists of a case containing a battery (disposable or rechargeable), electronic circuit, motor
and gear box, and syringe mover or pump. This is attached
to a plastic tubing of varying length, which is then connected
to a 27-gauge needle inserted in subcutaneous tissue. Usual
sites are either the abdomen or the thigh. Pump users keep
a needle in place 1 to 3 days before replacing it.

The battery supplies power to the electronic circuit that
drives the motor. The motor causes the syringe to empty.

Supplies needed to use the pump include syringes, batteries, infusion sets (catheters), diluent, dilution chart, short-
acting (regular) insulin, tape, a carrying case, and blood glucose monitoring equipment. These cost $10–$20 weekly.
Third-party reimbursement varies from full coverage of the
pump and weekly supplies to partial coverage to none.

At the present time, there are many types of pumps being
used by more than 9000 insulin-dependent diabetics. They
vary in size, manner of operation, and price. The price range
for the pump alone is $1500 to $3000.

Candidates for Pump Therapy. Not all insulin-dependent patients are pump candidates. The American Diabetes
Association has issued the following guidelines for selection
of pump therapy candidates.

*Closed-Loop System (Intravenous Delivery in a Hospitalized
Setting)*
Use of an insulin pump in the hospital setting is recom-
mended in the following circumstances:

1. Initial treatment of ketoacidosis
2. Maintenance of blood glucose control during surgery
   and the immediate postoperative period
3. Maintenance of blood glucose control during pregnancy, especially during labor and delivery and periods of ketoacidosis
4. Maintenance of blood glucose control during severe
   and complicated medical illnesses when conventional
   insulin treatment is unsatisfactory. Examples of these
   illnesses would be a myocardial infarction or severe infection. Continuous intravenous delivery could also be
   advantageous for insulin-dependent patients receiving
   hyperalimentation or who are under restricted oral intake, such as during treatment of a bleeding peptic ulcer.
5. Treatment of the rare patient with excessive subcutaneous degradation of injected insulin, when other
   measures fail. This situation may necessitate continuous intravenous delivery with a central line at home.

Open-Loop System (Subcutaneous Delivery With a Portable Pump as a Long-Term Outpatient Procedure)

The following are candidates for portable insulin pump use in type I diabetes:

1. Pregnant patients with early long-term complications
2. Patients who are candidates for a renal transplant or who have had a renal transplant

Additional requirements are that the patient be motivated to accomplish the extra tasks needed for pump therapy; willing to be educated regarding all aspects of pump care; and responsible, willing, and able to perform at least 4 to 6 blood glucose determinations daily.

Chart 36-6 provides guidelines for health teaching.

Other Types of Insulin Delivery

Button Infuser. The button infuser allows the patient to inject insulin through a buttonlike device attached to a subcutaneous needle in the skin. Although the device must be changed every few days, like the needle used in the insulin pump, the patient is spared multiple daily skin punctures when intensive insulin therapy is required.

NovoPen. NovoPen, a portable insulin delivery system first introduced in Denmark by Novo, is a penlike device that measures insulin delivered from a small disposable insulin cartridge through a disposable needle. Depressing the device once will deliver two units of insulin. It is also possible to deliver an odd number of units. The cartridge contains 750 units of regular (human) insulin, and a package of 4 cartridges costs the same as a bottle of regular human insulin. The advantages of the NovoPen over the insulin pump are lower cost, greater convenience, and avoidance of pump malfunction and infections. It can be used with only one hand, an important consideration in patients recovering from a stroke. It can also be useful for a visually-impaired patient as long as someone checks the insulin supply remaining. It is currently available in the United States, Europe, Canada, and New Zealand.

Jet Insulin Injectors. Jet insulin injectors have been available as an alternative to needle injections for a number of years. The jet pressure delivers insulin through the skin in an extremely fine stream that some patients seem to prefer to a needle injection. Some injectors deliver up to 50 units of insulin, and others deliver up to 100 units in either single or mixed doses. Cost to the patient is often a concern, although some insurance plans cover a significant part of the cost. The device, which is about 6 inches long, is larger than a syringe–needle combination. It can be used by more than one person in a family, since no part of the system penetrates the skin; only the insulin does. Insulin may be absorbed faster than with the conventional injection method.

Patients should be cautioned that absorption rates, peak insulin activity, and insulin levels may be different when switching to a jet injector.

Multiple Insulin Injections. Although there are approximately 9000 insulin pumps in use in the United States today, many research studies have questioned the benefits of pump therapy for all type I diabetes patients. Within the past 5 years, many patients who might have been candidates

---

Chart 36-6
Health Teaching for Patients Using Insulin Pumps

1. The goal of insulin pump therapy is to achieve normoglycemia, not to provide an easier means of giving insulin.
2. The pump restores to normal circulating lipids and amino acids as well as the concentrations of anti-insulin hormones.
3. A basal infusion rate of insulin coupled with premeal boluses attempts to mimic the way a healthy pancreas works.
4. The daily insulin dose via the pump is usually reduced.
5. Only fast-acting (regular) insulin is used in insulin pumps.
6. Use only the proper syringe for the pump to give the correct flow rate.
7. The life of a disposable battery in the pump varies with the freshness of the battery and the storage conditions. For longest life, batteries should be stored in the refrigerator, but not in the freezer.
8. Use usual techniques of asepsis when inserting the needle. It should be inserted at a 45-degree angle. The needle is then taped as one would tape an intravenous needle. An application of Betadine may be applied to the site.
9. Implantable pumps are now being tested in humans.
10. The patient does not simply put on the pump and achieve good control. It serves as a "constant" reminder that the rules of living with diabetes must be followed.
11. Emotions about the pump range from utter devotion to tolerance to downright contempt. A patient may experience all or only one. The attitudes about the pump are the result of having a device that improves blood sugars and, therefore, how well one feels, but that in addition requires enormous amounts of motivation, time, energy, and money.
12. Patients complain that the pumps are "too bulky" and are a constant reminder that they "have diabetes." Wearing a pump may possibly alter body image or make a patient feel dependent on a mechanical device. The pump is cosmetically unacceptable to many patients. Initially, patients have difficulty sleeping with a pump. This can usually be resolved by the patient within a few days. Care must be taken when toileting and showering, since the pump is not waterproof. Some patients find wearing a pump bothersome during some types of activity (*e.g.*, sexual activity).
13. Few research studies have yet been conducted about the effects of using the pump.
14. Insurance companies may pay for all or part of the cost for meters used in monitoring blood glucose.

for pump therapy have been started on intensified insulin therapy (multiple injections using insulin mixtures). Current studies suggest that multiple injections can produce normoglycemia in most patients without the added risks of pump therapy (*e.g.*, mechanical breakdown, clogged tubing, pump deaths due to hypoglycemia or ketoacidosis) or the added inconveniences (*e.g.*, disconnecting the pump during swimming, showering, sexual activities, sleep).

The objectives of intensified insulin therapy include the following:

- To achieve normal blood glucose levels (70–150 mg/dl, or 3.85–8.25 mmol/L)
- To prevent hypoglycemia <70 mg/dl (3.85 mmol/L) hyperglycemia >150 mg/dl (8.25 mmol/L)
- To prevent, minimize, or reverse long-term complications
- To promote performance of ADL with a positive attitude
- To increase life-style flexibility
- To maintain normal weight
- To prevent infections
- To promote a sense of well-being

To achieve these objectives, the patient must monitor blood glucose levels at least 4 times daily, and pay close attention to dietary intake and the timing of meals as well as the amount and timing of daily exercise.

Disadvantages of multiple insulin injections include the cost of supplies and equipment; the possibility of hypoglycemia; and a change in self-image, either positive or negative, as a result of being mindful of some aspect of self-care daily.

Advantages of multiple daily injections of insulin include a physiologically closer approximation of blood glucose levels, increased life-style flexibility, lower cost than pump therapy, more predictable response to exercise, and an increased sense of well-being. In general, the advantages far outweigh the disadvantages, and this method of blood glucose control is advocated for all insulin-dependent patients with diabetes unless major physical or psychological problems exist (*e.g.*, a mentally-retarded person with diabetes who has little or no assistance).

Pen Pump. The pen pump may be used to facilitate multiple insulin injections. This device, which looks like a pen, contains an insulin syringe that is attached to plastic tubing and a subcutaneous needle. The needle of the pen pump remains in place, somewhat like an insulin pump; in contrast, the NovoPen, previously described, involves repeated injections. However, the pen pump is not a "pump" because it cannot deliver a basal dose of insulin. The patient clicks the device corresponding to the number of units of insulin desired. The device eliminates the need for several daily injections, while still providing multiple insulin doses. Some patients find this device helpful, although others do not.

Implantable Insulin Pumps. Implantable pumps are much more experimental at this time than the external pumps. Some of these hockey puck-sized pumps have been implanted experimentally in humans (Minnesota, 1980). Problems related to these pumps involve the insulin reservoir and the membrane of the pump through which the insulin must pass. This pump cannot hold a lifetime supply of insulin, and so it must be filled by means of an injection from the outside. Another problem is that it cannot deliver an extra dose of insulin at mealtimes, an important factor in controlling blood glucose levels. The ideal pump would be one that adds more insulin automatically as the blood glucose level rises, just as the normal pancreas does. The implantable pump currently in use, with special permission from the U.S. Food and Drug Administration, is limited to persons with some residual insulin function. An improved version of the pump with a magnetically activated valve is now being tested. This type allows the delivery of an extra mealtime dose by holding a magnet over the pump in the chest for a minute or two.

The implantable pump is similar to implantable pumps that have been used for the last few years to deliver constant doses of either blood-thinning or cancer therapy drugs.

The pump consists of two chambers, one of which holds the insulin while the other holds a compressible fluorocarbon gas. Once every 2 weeks, the drug reservoir is filled with about 1⅓ ounces of insulin solution, using a syringe with a needle inserted through the skin. The injection of the liquid compresses the fluorocarbon into a liquid, and its gradual expansion over the next 12 to 14 days drives the insulin through a narrow nozzle into a tube.

Research in Pancreatic Transplantation

Whole Organ. Most studies of pancreatic transplantation have focused on using pancreatic tissues that consist of both endocrine and exocrine parts. Although with this approach one can avoid isolating human islets from the pancreas, it creates other problems. For example, the drainage of pancreatic enzymes must be provided for, as well as an adequate supply of blood to the newly-transplanted organ. Additional problems include the requirement for immunosuppressive therapy and the accompanying increase in serious infection. The whole pancreas or segments of the pancreas are currently being transplanted, but usually only in conjunction with a kidney transplant (because of nephropathy).

Islet Cells. Advantages in using isolated islets include easy manipulation of the cells (which, because of their small size, can be injected through a small-gauge needle), easy provision of oxygen and food supply, avoidance of problems with enzymes, and lower incidence of immunogenic problems.

Acute Complications of Diabetes

There are three major conditions that can produce coma in the diabetic: hypoglycemia, diabetic ketoacidosis, and hyperosmolar coma. Other acute complications include lactic acidosis and the dawn phenomenon.

Hypoglycemia ("Insulin Reactions")

Hypoglycemia (abnormally low blood glucose level) occurs when the blood glucose falls below 50 mg/dl (2.75 mmol/L). It can be caused by too much insulin, too little food, or excessive physical activity. Hypoglycemia may occur 1 to 3 hours after regular insulin, 4 to 18 hours after NPH or Lente insulin, and 18 to 30 hours after protamine zinc or ultralente insulin. Most episodes occur before meals, but they may occur at any time of the day or night.

When the blood glucose falls rapidly, the sympathetic nervous system is stimulated to produce adrenalin, causing sweating, tremor, tachycardia, palpitation, and nervousness. When the blood glucose falls slowly, there is depression of the central nervous system, resulting in headache, lightheadedness, confusion, emotional changes, memory lapses, numbness of the lips and tongue, slurred speech, incoordination, staggering gait, double vision, drowsiness, convulsions, and eventually coma. Because the brain depends on glucose for its energy supply, as hypoglycemia progresses, brain function deteriorates. Permanent central nervous system damage may result from prolonged hypoglycemia.

The combination of symptoms varies considerably in different patients and in the same patient at different times.

- Every patient taking insulin should be familiar with the warning symptoms so that sugar can be taken promptly.
- Any abnormal behavior in a patient taking insulin should be considered to be due to hypoglycemia and treated as such until proven otherwise.
- Hypoglycemia must be treated promptly, because sustained hypoglycemia can lead to convulsions or coma and death. When the first warning symptoms appear, the patient should take some form of simple, fast-acting sugar orally: orange juice, sugar, hard candy (Lifesavers), or a soft drink containing sugar. If the symptoms persist for 10 to 15 minutes, the snack should be repeated. If it is more than an hour until the next meal, the patient should also eat a complex carbohydrate and protein.
- Every patient taking insulin should always carry candy, a few lumps of sugar, or Glutose or Monojel for the prompt relief of hypoglycemia.

Somogyi Phenomenon. The Somogyi phenomenon is a paradoxical situation in which sudden falls in blood glucose are followed by rebound hyperglycemia. This situation is usually caused by gradual excessive administration of insulin. The underlying mechanism is that the hormonal responses to hypoglycemia counteract the effect of insulin. The patient's condition becomes uncontrollable, because the effect of the administered insulin is antagonized. The situation remains out of control when more insulin is given, and the patient has periods of hyperglycemia interspersed with hypoglycemia. One is alerted to this possibility when there are symptoms of hypoglycemia (*e.g.*, irritability, confusion), with morning hyperglycemia. The treatment consists of gradually lowering the amount of insulin until the appropriate dosage is reached. See section on ketoacidosis for differential diagnosis of morning hyperglycemia.

Defective Glucose Counterregulation and Hypoglycemia in Type I Diabetes. Hypoglycemia is an uncommon clinical occurrence except in people who use insulin or oral agents to lower blood glucose. A deficient amount of insulin has been recognized as the pathology underlying type I diabetes. However, recent studies also demonstrate that a deficient secretion of *glucose-raising* (counterregulatory) *hormones*, which include glucagon and epinephrine in the insulin-dependent patient, is also a factor. Therefore, the risk of hypoglycemia in type I diabetes is determined by the imperfect methods of insulin replacement and an altered response of the counterregulatory system.

Many type I patients, within a few years after diagnosis, develop a glucagon deficiency. They are then partially dependent on epinephrine to prevent or correct hypoglycemia, and are not at any additional risk for hypoglycemia. However, as the duration of diabetes increases, some patients demonstrate an epinephrine deficiency. This aspect appears to be part of autonomic neuropathy. The precise mechanism for this event is unknown. There are no warning symptoms of hypoglycemia, and the patient is literally defenseless against severe hypoglycemia, especially if attempting to maintain blood glucose levels in near-normal ranges.

This phenomenon can also be induced by other medications, *e.g.*, β-adrenergic antagonists such as propranolol.

Because all insulin replacement therapy is imperfect at the present time, hypoglycemia will occur in patients with type I diabetes. If the glucose counterregulatory system is intact, hypoglycemia may still occur, but will not be as severe as it would be in the patient with many defects in the system.

In general, the integrity of the glucose counterregulatory system may determine whether or not hypoglycemia will occur and, if it does, to what degree.

In patients with altered hormonal responses to hypoglycemia, self-monitoring of blood glucose is crucial to prevent severe episodes of hypoglycemia and death from undetected, symptomless hypoglycemia that remains untreated.

Prevention and Patient Education. Hypoglycemia is prevented by following a regular pattern and timetable for eating, administering insulin, and engaging in daily exercise. Between-meal and bedtime snacks are often needed to counteract the maximum insulin effect. In general, the patient should cover the time of peak activity of insulin by eating a snack and by taking additional food when engaging in an increased level of physical activity. Routine glucose tests are performed so that changing insulin requirements may be anticipated and adjusted.

Because unexpected hypoglycemia may occur, all patients treated with insulin should wear an identification bracelet or tag indicating that they have diabetes.

Some diabetes patients with autonomic neuropathy or those taking propranolol may not experience symptoms of hypoglycemia. It is very important for these patients to perform blood glucose tests to determine blood glucose levels.

If the patient is unconscious and unable to swallow, glucagon hydrochloride is administered subcutaneously. This hormone, which is made in the alpha cells of the pancreas, causes glycogenolysis in the liver (if hepatic glycogen stores are not depleted). Glucagon raises the blood glucose level high enough for most patients to wake up after the first dose and take orange juice or ginger ale by mouth. This additional "sugar" intake is important, because the elevation of blood glucose following glucagon administration is only temporary, and a hypoglycemic relapse is a real and constant danger. Glucagon is packaged as a powder in 1-mg vials and given in the same manner as insulin. It comes with a vial of diluent and, once mixed, must be used. It should not be used after the expiration date. It is sold by prescription only, and should be part of the emergency supplies kept available by insulin-dependent persons with diabetes. It is useful for patients who receive little or no warning of their attacks and go into hypoglycemia.

If the patient cannot swallow and is unconscious, the intravenous administration of 50 ml of 50% glucose in water is the most effective treatment for hypoglycemia in a hospital. It is used when it is available or when a second dose of glucagon is ineffective.

Diabetic Ketoacidosis and Coma

Diabetic ketoacidosis is caused by an absence or inadequate amount of insulin, which results in hyperglycemia and leads to a series of biochemical disorders. The pathophysiology is the result of insulin deficiency affecting many aspects of the metabolism of carbohydrate, protein, and fat. As a result, the amount of glucose entering the cells is reduced, and fat is metabolized instead of carbohydrate. Free fatty acids are mobilized from adipose tissue. Liver oxidases act upon these fatty acids to produce ketone bodies. The ketone bodies escape into the blood, and metabolic acidosis results, with lowering of serum bicarbonate, PCO_2, and pH. The overall clinical picture is one of hyperglycemia, water and electrolyte loss, acidemia, and coma.

Causes. Ketoacidosis may be precipitated by failure to take insulin, by insufficient insulin intake, or by resistance to insulin. It may be caused by infection (of the respiratory tract, urinary tract, gastrointestinal tract, or the skin), by physiological stresses such as acute illness, surgery, trauma, pregnancy, and/or by emotional stresses that reduce the effectiveness of the available insulin. (Chart 36-7 presents guidelines for persons with diabetes to follow during periods of illness.) Anti-insulin factors (growth hormone, glucagon, cortisol) are released during stress and may play a part in the development of ketoacidosis. Ketoacidosis occurs more commonly in insulin-dependent diabetes. It is a serious complication, with a mortality rate ranging from 5% to 10%.

Clinical Manifestations. The clinical manifestations occur as a result of changes in body fluid, electrolytes, and acid–base status. Early manifestations are *polyuria* (excessive urination), *polyphagia* (excessive appetite), and *polydipsia* (excessive thirst). Osmotic diuresis causes water loss (*dehydration*) and electrolyte depletion. As the patient becomes more dehydrated, *oliguria* (diminished urination) develops. Malaise and visual changes may be noted by the patient. Headache, muscle aches, and abdominal pain are frequent complaints, as are nausea, vomiting, and gastric stasis and ileus. If infection has precipitated the ketoacidosis, fever may be present. The patient's respiratory rate increases to compensate for acidosis. Coma and severe acidosis are ushered in with *Kussmaul breathing* (very deep, but not labored, respirations) and a sweetish odor of the breath, due to acidemia.

The patient is drowsy and soon becomes comatose. The blood glucose is elevated, the serum bicarbonate and the blood pH are decreased, the blood urea is increased, and the plasma ketone is strongly positive. The urine is strongly positive for acetone. The patient's condition is serious at this stage, but recovery can be anticipated after prompt and vigorous treatment with insulin and intravenous fluids.

Management. The immediate goals in the management of ketoacidosis are (1) to restore normal carbohydrate, protein, and fat metabolism; (2) to reverse hypovolemia; and (3) to correct electrolyte imbalance. A flow sheet is kept of vital signs and ketone measurements, as well as of blood glucose and electrolytes, arterial blood gases, and the medications and treatment given. A rapid physical examination is carried out to detect evidence of infection, myocardial infarction, stroke, and other disease.

- An infusion of isotonic or hypotonic saline is started immediately to rehydrate the patient and improve tissue perfusion. The fluid deficit may range between 6 and 10 liters, and the rate of replacement depends on the patient's condition.
- Insulin is given to reduce blood glucose by promoting glucose utilization and to inhibit lipolysis (splitting up of fat), thereby preventing accumulation of ketones in the blood. The insulin regimens in current use are variable in both amounts and routes of administration.

Until recently, high doses of insulin were given by intravenous boluses or by the intramuscular or subcutaneous routes, and repeated every 4 hours. It was difficult to maintain steady plasma levels by this protocol.

Low-dose insulin regimens are being used with increasing frequency. Continuous low-dose intravenous therapy with insulin may be given to obtain immediate insulin action and to maintain steady blood levels of insulin. Low-dose insulin is controllable and gives a more predictable response. A constant infusion pump or pediatric drip (with insulin placed in 250 ml of half normal saline) may be used. Albumin or some other colloid may be added to the intravenous solution to prevent adherence of insulin to the infusion bottle and tubing. There are variations in the low-dose insulin regimens, including administration of insulin by intermittent subcutaneous injection.

As the blood glucose level declines, glucose is added to the infusion, and the insulin concentration is decreased to reduce the risk of hypoglycemia.

- Close monitoring of the patient is essential, since metabolic parameters change and call for continuing assessment of the patient and of fluid and electrolyte status. Frequent laboratory determinations of blood glucose, serum ketones, serum bicarbonate, and serum potassium are needed.

At first the patient's serum potassium may be normal or raised, but when the blood glucose level begins to approach normal, hypokalemia threatens the patient. Hypokalemia occurs when serum potassium levels are reduced as a result of potassium "migrating" into the cells along with glucose, under the influence of insulin. Hypokalemia also results when extracellular potassium ions are exchanged for intracellular hydrogen ions, in the correction of acidosis.

Chart 36-7
Guidelines to Follow During Periods of Illness

- Take insulin or oral antidiabetic agents as usual.
- Insulin-dependent patients may need even more insulin to compensate for increased blood glucose levels as a result of the illness.
- Report nausea, vomiting, and diarrhea to your physician, since extreme fluid loss may be dangerous.
- Test blood frequently for glucose. If only blood tests are being done for glucose, test urine for ketones.
- Follow your meal plan. Soft foods and liquids may be substituted for regular food to supply needed calories.
- Keep in touch with your physician.

- Frequent estimates of serum potassium and ECG monitoring are essential for early recognition of hypokalemia. Potassium replacement is usually started early; adequacy of renal function is essential before potassium is administered. Tingling, paresthesia, decreased tendon reflexes, and respiratory depression are clinical manifestations of hypokalemia.

Hypotension that does not respond to intravenous fluids is treated with albumin, plasma, and vasopressors. Monitoring of central venous pressure is important to achieve safe fluid balance, especially in elderly patients or those with myocardial disease. Nasogastric intubation and suctioning relieve vomiting and acute dilatation of the stomach and reduce the possibility of aspiration.

Consciousness should be restored and metabolic disturbances corrected within 12 to 24 hours. After the acute problem is corrected, the patient is regulated as described earlier. The precipitating cause of the coma should be determined to prevent a recurrence.

Hyperosmolar Nonketotic Coma

Hyperosmolar hyperglycemic coma is a syndrome in which hyperglycemia and hyperosmolarity predominate, with possible alterations of the sensorium (sense of awareness). At the same time, ketosis is minimal or absent. This condition occurs most frequently in older people (50 to 70 years) who have had no previous history of diabetes, or only mild non-insulin-dependent diabetes. The acute development of the condition can be traced to some precipitating event, such as an acute illness (pneumonia, myocardial infarction, stroke), ingestion of drugs known to provoke insulin insufficiency (thiazide diuretics, propranolol), or therapeutic procedures (peritoneal dialysis/hemodialysis, hyperalimentation). In the more chronic picture, there is a history of days to weeks of polyuria, with inadequate fluid intake. Upon admission to the hospital, the patient is found to have severe hyperglycemia ("syrupy blood"), profound dehydration, and variable neurologic signs ranging from sleepy confusion to coma.

The basic biochemical effect is lack of effective insulin. The patient's persistent hyperglycemia causes osmotic diuresis, resulting in losses of water and electrolytes. To maintain osmotic equilibrium, water shifts from the intracellular fluid space to the extracellular fluid space. With glucosuria and dehydration, hypernatremia and increasing hyperosmolality occur. The reasons why these patients show minimal ketosis is not clear.

The clinical picture is one of hypotension, dehydration (dry mucous membranes, poor skin turgor), fever, tachycardia, and variable neurologic signs (*e.g.*, alteration of sensorium, seizures, hemiparesis). This is a serious condition, with a mortality rate ranging from 5% to 50%.

Management. The objective of management is to correct the volume depletion and hyperosmolar state. A search is then made for the precipitating cause. Fluid therapy is started with hypotonic saline that is titrated by CVP or arterial pressure monitoring. Insulin may be given by either a high-dose or low-dose regimen. Potassium chloride is added when the urinary output is adequate, and is guided by ECG monitoring. Other therapeutic modalities are determined by the condition of the patient and the results of continuing clinical and laboratory evaluation.

Lactic Acidosis

Lactic acidosis occurs in diabetes, but the etiology remains unknown. Lactate levels in the blood reflect a delicate balance between lactate production and utilization. If even a small change in the balance occurs (as little as 1–2%), lactic acidosis may ensue over a very short period of time; it is associated with a high mortality rate. Any factor that interferes with oxidative phosphorylation may cause lactic acidosis. The diagnosis in diabetes is established when lactate levels in the plasma are over 7 mM per liter. Ethanol and phenformin (a first-generation oral antidiabetic agent) are often reported as the precipitating causes of lactic acidosis. However, phenformin no longer poses a problem in the United States because it has been removed from the market.

Management. The foundation of treatment is alkali infusion, usually in amounts greater than that indicated for ketoacidosis. Sodium bicarbonate is the alkali of choice. In addition, fluids, insulin, and electrolytes are indicated. Along with the general supportive measures that may be employed, there should be an attempt to discover and correct the underlying cause of the lactate imbalance.

The Dawn Phenomenon

The dawn phenomenon is characterized by a relatively normal blood glucose level until approximately 3 AM, when blood glucose levels begin to rise. The phenomenon is thought to result from nocturnal surges in growth hormone secretion that create a greater need for insulin in the early morning hours in patients with type I diabetes. It must be distinguished from insulin waning or the Somogyi effect (rebound hyperglycemia).

It is often difficult to tell from the patient's history which of these causes is responsible for morning hyperglycemia. In order to determine the cause, the patient needs to be awakened once or twice during a night to test blood glucose levels. Testing the blood glucose level at bedtime, at 3 AM, and upon awakening will provide information that can be used in making an insulin adjustment to avoid morning hyperglycemia caused by the dawn phenomenon. Table 36-5 summarizes the differences between insulin waning, the dawn phenomenon, and the Somogyi effect.

Long-Term Complications of Diabetes

There has been a steady decline in deaths of diabetic patients due to ketoacidosis and infection, but an alarming rise in deaths due to cardiovascular and renal complications. Long-term complications are becoming more common as more patients live longer with their diabetes.

Atherosclerotic complications, with myocardial infarction, cerebrovascular accidents, uremia, and gangrene cause 70% of deaths among persons with diabetes. There is no effective means of preventing or postponing the development of atherosclerosis in anyone. However, there is more and more evidence demonstrating that maintenance of blood

TABLE 36-5
Causes of Morning Hyperglycemia

Characteristic	Treatment
Insulin Waning	
Progressive rise in blood glucose from bedtime to morning	Increase the insulin dose at bedtime or institute a dose of insulin before the evening meal if one is not already in use.
Dawn Phenomenon	
Relatively normal blood glucose until about 3 AM, when the level begins to rise	Increase the amount of insulin before the evening meal, or alter the usual insulin mixture if this is being used.
Somogyi Effect	
Elevated blood glucose at bedtime, a decrease at 2–3 AM to hypoglycemic levels, and a subsequent increase caused by the production of counterregulatory hormones	Adjust the bedtime insulin dose to prevent nocturnal hypoglycemia, and/or adjust the bedtime snack.

glucose levels in the normal or near-normal range may delay the long-term complications. Even though much has been written on this subject, we still do not know why atherosclerosis occurs earlier and progresses more rapidly in diabetes.

Vascular Complications

Diabetes mellitus is accompanied by changes in the entire vascular system. During the course of diabetes, changes develop in the blood vessels that lead to the long-term complications of the disease. These changes in blood vessels involve either the large or the small vessels. Complications of the larger vessels (*macrovascular disease* or *macroangiopathy*) are cardiovascular in nature and involve the heart and the peripheral circulation, especially the legs. Complications of the smaller vessels (*microvascular disease* or *microangiopathy*) involve the eyes (*retinopathy*), kidneys (*nephropathy*), and nervous sytem (*neuropathy*).

The specific pathologic lesion of long-standing diabetes is characterized by thickening of the capillary basement membrane in the affected organ.

The incidence of retinopathy, neuropathy, and nephropathy increases with increasing duration of the diabetes. A common pathological "microvascular process" is probably not present, because a patient may be affected by only one or two complications. All of these complications are related to a prolonged hyperglycemia and are histologically similar in the late clinical stages.

The basement membrane of the capillary, which lies next to the cytoplasmic membrane, consists of a glycoprotein layer. This layer can incorporate sugars into its structure without depending on insulin. When blood glucose levels remain high

for long periods of time, excessive amounts are incorporated into the glycoproteins. Pathological swelling of the basement membrane results, with an increased permeability to plasma proteins and other substances. This pathology is common in the long-term complications.

Involvement of the capillaries of the retina may lead to blindness, due to diabetic retinopathy (see below).

Intracapillary glomerulosclerosis (Kimmelstiel-Wilson syndrome) is the specific renal disease of diabetes and is related to thickening of the capillary basement membrane in the glomerulus. It appears that blood glucose levels above normal are responsible for the pathologic changes in the kidney. Renal failure is common in type 1 diabetes that develops at an early age. (The pathophysiology and treatment of renal failure are discussed in Chap. 40.)

Microangiopathy of the vessels supplying the skin, peripheral nerves, and walls of the large arteries may be a factor in skin diseases and neuropathy. In addition, when excess glucose is present, it begins to be metabolized by a pathway (polyol) that produces excessive amounts of sorbitol. Sorbitol can be absorbed by nerve tissue. Water accompanies the sorbitol into these tissues, causing the nerve cell to expand. The result is decreased nerve conduction speed and eventual irreversible nerve damage.

The enzyme aldose reductase is required for the process of metabolizing glucose to sorbitol. Drugs that inhibit aldose reductase are currently undergoing clinical trials and may prove useful in decreasing the complications that result from increased production of sorbitol.

The changes in the larger arteries appear to be the same atherosclerotic changes that occur in nondiabetic persons as a result of the aging process. However, in diabetes the changes tend to occur at an earlier age. Occlusion of major vessels due to atherosclerosis causes strokes, myocardial infarction, intermittent claudication, and gangrene. Advanced vascular disease in the large and small arteries of the legs is common in diabetes and is often severe enough to lead to gangrene of the affected extremity. Such changes may be extensive enough to result in ossification of the wall of the artery. These changes in the smaller arteries present a serious problem, since a subsequent occlusion of one of the large arteries cannot be followed by the formation of adequate collateral circulation.

High blood glucose levels can also cause defects in the blood clotting process by increasing the clotting capability of the red blood cell. During hyperglycemia, there is an increase in the adhesiveness of platelets (blood components active in coagulation). In addition, red blood cells lose their flexibility and are unable to change shape and travel through narrow capillaries.

In general, the pathogenesis of the long-term complications of diabetes is just beginning to be understood. However, prolonged periods of hyperglycemia are known to contribute to the pathology of these complications (Chart 36-8).

Eye Disorders and Diabetes

The vision in diabetes can be affected in many ways. Each part of the eye and the visual system is susceptible to the complications of diabetes. The severity of the problem can range from a change in eyeglass prescription to total blindness. These changes are extremely important because even

---

Chart 36-8
Effects of Prolonged Hyperglycemia

• Increased thickening of capillary basement membrane
• Increased platelet adhesiveness
• Decreased erythrocyte flexibility
• Increased levels of hemoglobin A_{1c}
• Impairment of phagocytosis
• Increased sorbitol levels, resulting in glucose metabolism via polyol pathway

---

the smallest change can affect life-style (*e.g.*, insulin measurement, testing for glucose in blood, ability to drive or read).

Types of visual problems in diabetes may include:

• Refractive changes
• Extraocular muscle palsy
• Corneal problems
• Glaucoma
• Cataracts
• Retinopathy

Vision may be affected by some of these problems but, in general, if the pathology includes the macula and its function, then vision will be decreased.

Refractive changes in diabetes accompanied by prolonged periods of hyperglycemia are caused by a change in the shape of the lens brought about by fluid retention. This blurring of vision, if caused by hyperglycemia, will gradually subside as the blood glucose levels approach and are maintained in the near-normal range. Therefore, it is advisable not to purchase new eyeglasses during this period. Glaucoma, cataracts, and retinopathy are strongly influenced by long periods of hyperglycemia.

Extraocular muscle palsy is a neuropathic change and is explained in the section on neuropathy.

Diabetic Retinopathy

The eye pathology referred to as *diabetic retinopathy* is caused by changes in the small blood vessels in the retina of the eye. The retina is the area of the eye that receives images and sends information about the images to the brain. It is richly supplied with blood vessels of all kinds—small arteries and veins, arterioles, venules, and capillaries. The pathology involves the walls of the blood vessels, particularly the capillaries in the retina.

Diagnostic Evaluation. Retinopathy is frequently seen years after the diagnosis of diabetes, and is rarely totally absent in a patient with diabetes who has had the disease for years. Occasionally, it may be the first clinical sign of diabetes—the sign that brings the patient to the physician and eventually leads to the diagnosis of diabetes. It is often associated with the presence of hypertension in the patient with diabetes.

Diagnosis is by direct visualization with an ophthalmoscope or with a technique known as fluorescein angiography. Fluorescein angiography can document the type and activity of the retinopathy. It is a technique in which a dye is injected into an arm vein. The dye is carried to various parts of the

body through the blood, but especially through the vessels of the retina of the eye. This technique allows the ophthalmologist, using special instruments, to see the retinal vessels in bright detail and gives useful information that cannot be obtained with just an ophthalmoscope. Photographs of the fundus of the eye are taken through a series of filters that excite and record the fluorescence of the dye. The dye is bound to the blood proteins and first appears in the choroid and then in the arterial branches of the retina. Areas of leakage from the vessels and areas of neovascularization (new vessel formation) are stained with fluorescein.

Side-effects of this diagnostic procedure performed in an outpatient setting may include:

• Nausea during the dye injection
• A yellowish, fluorescent discoloration of the skin and urine that may last 12 to 24 hours
• An occasional allergic reaction, usually hives or itching

However, it is generally a safe diagnostic procedure.

Patient preparation includes explaining the following:

• The sequence of the procedure
• The fact that the procedure is painless
• The potential side-effects
• The type of information the technique can provide
• That the flash of the camera may be slightly uncomfortable for a short period of time

Problems in the blood-retinal barrier are possible before they become clinically visible in the fundus. The pathology increases with the duration of the diabetes and hyperglycemia.

Pathology. The pathologic changes in the vessels begin as bulges in the walls of the capillaries (*microaneurysms*). Eventually fluids leak into the surrounding areas of the retina (Fig. 36-4). If the changes are limited to the retina, the problem is referred to as *background retinopathy*. This does not generally interfere with vision, and occurs in 50% of all patients with diabetes after 10 to 15 years with diabetes. In some patients, this condition progresses to *proliferative retinopathy*, the stage of new vessel formation (neovascularization) in and around the retina. These vessels branch out and grow into other areas of the eye. These vessels have thin, leaky walls and can cause damage by hemorrhage and scar formation. Unless the macula of the eye is involved, considerable retinopathy can be present before interfering with vision.

Electron microscopy has shown an increased production of basement membrane material as the microaneurysms form. As this material ages, thickening of the basement membrane continues. The wall fragments and the debris leak from the capillary to the surrounding areas. Since the integrity of the basement membrane is impaired, the capillary loses its selective permeability. The capillaries continue to change, losing cells from their walls, and gradually the lumina of the capillaries are obliterated. This leads to a loss of adequate blood flow in this important area of the eye, and to the formation of "shunt" vessels (neovascularization). These defective vessels are grown in an attempt to supply areas of the retina deprived of blood (*retinal hypoxia*) because of the disease process. If no treatment is instituted at this time, the condition will progress to proliferative retinopathy in which vessels grow into the vitreous humor. These vessels hemorrhage into the vitreous, causing major problems that can lead to severe visual impairment, glaucoma, retinal detachment, and finally blindness.

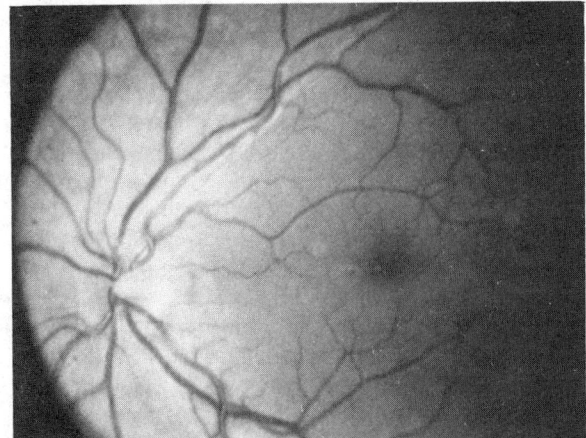

A

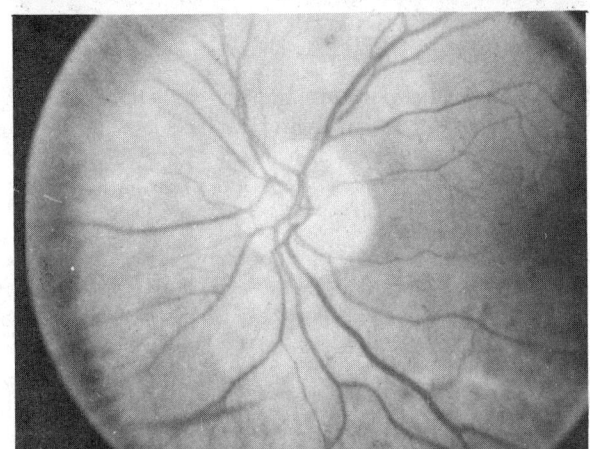

B

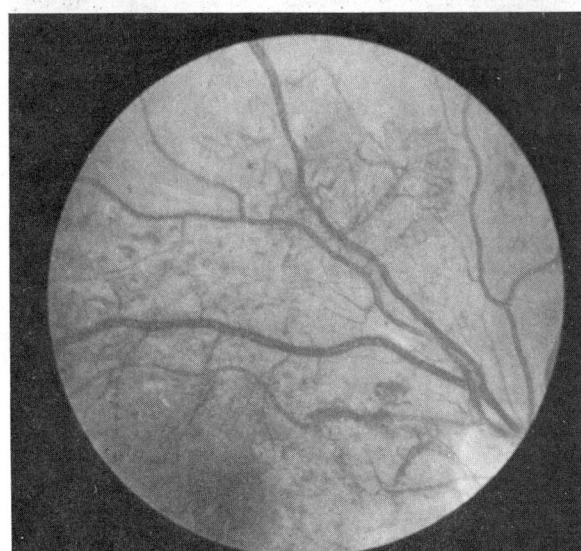

C

Nonproliferative (Background) Retinopathy. Classifying retinopathy into nonproliferative and proliferative types is useful in diagnosis, treatment, and counseling. Eighty percent of all cases of retinopathy fall in this group. It is more common in type II diabetes. This aspect of retinopathy waxes and wanes with time. An increase in the number of microaneurysms usually means an increase in the activity of the retinopathy or changes that may lead to reduced vision. The pathology seen in the nonproliferative stage includes:

- Microaneurysm formation (appearing as red spots on the fundus)
- Intraretinal hemorrhages
- Venous changes: dilation, beading, or sausaging, and occasionally venous loops
- Exudate deposition*
     Hard: glistening yellow fatty deposits in the retina
     Soft: "cotton-wool spots"—fluffy, white opacities in the nerve fiber layer of the retina; actually, infarcts—areas of ischemia
- Macular edema*

Preproliferative Retinopathy. The preproliferative stage will soon progress to proliferative retinopathy in 3% to 10% of all diabetic patients. The pathology seen in this stage includes:

- Increased venous abnormalities
- "Cotton-wool spots"
- Areas of nonperfusion or capillary closure in the retina
- Large clusters of microaneurysms
- Dot/blot hemorrhages
- Diffuse macular edema

This stage progresses to the next if new vessels increase. The best way to keep track of the activity is to have photographs taken of the fundus. These can be compared with previous photos to determine if the retinopathy is stable or progressing.

Proliferative Retinopathy. The proliferative stage is the most serious. It begins with the appearance of new blood vessels on the optic disc or on the surface of the retina, and is associated with generalized retinal ischemia. These vessels are fragile and prone to hemorrhage. These can cause preretinal or vitreous hemorrhages and traction retinal detachments.

Macular Edema. It has recently been realized that a significant loss of vision can occur as a result of macular edema. In this aspect of the disease, there is a breakdown of the blood-retinal barrier with an accumulation of fluid within the retina. Retinal structures become distorted; damage occurs in the neural part of the retina. At first, this damage is reversible; later it is not. The process occurs slowly, often

* May cause reduced vision.

Figure 36-4
Diabetic retinopathy. (*A*) In the fundus photograph of a normal eye, the light circular area to the left, over which a number of blood vessels converge, is the optic disc, where the optic nerve meets the back of the eye. To the right of the optic disc is a smaller, dark spot on the photograph, the macula. The macula is the part of the retina on which images in the center of a person's visual field are focused. This part of the retina has a high concentration of light-sensitive cells, called *cones*, which provide sharp, clear color vision in bright light. (*B*) The fundus photograph of a patient with diabetic retinopathy shows neovascularization—growth of a fine network of abnormal new vessels—directly on the optic disc. Small dots on the photograph are microaneurysms, while larger blotches are hemorrhages. One example of a hemorrhage in this photo is an almost horizontal streak on the lower left. (*C*) This fundus photograph showing severe diabetic retinopathy reveals widespread neovascularization, microaneurysms, and hemorrhaging. (Photo courtesy of National Eye Institute.)

with no ophthalmologically visible hemorrhages or exudates. The first symptom the patient notices is a distortion of vision, which, if left untreated, progresses to visual impairment.

Neovascularization. This growth of new blood vessels impairs the normal functioning of the eye. Part of the eye, especially the vitreous, which should remain clear if it is to transmit light, becomes clouded with a network of new blood vessels. In addition, the new vessels leak badly and further cloud the vitreous. Fibrous tissue replaces the free blood and, as the vitreous contracts, it pulls the retina from its normal attachment, resulting in retinal detachment.

Management

Photocoagulation. The principle of photocoagulation is that strong light energy can be converted into heat energy when it is absorbed by the two pigments in the retina—melanin (a natural retinal pigment) and hemoglobin (in the red blood cell of the retinal blood vessels; Fig. 36-5). The heat energy burns the area being treated and creates a controlled scar.

If the laser treatment is performed early enough, it will usually cause the abnormal vessels to shrink and disappear. The procedure is usually done in a retinal specialists's office with highly specialized equipment. Patients do not experience intense pain; discomfort varies with the patient.

Vitrectomy. When a major hemorrhage into the vitreous occurs, the vitreous fluid becomes mixed with blood and prevents light from passing through the eye, which can cause blindness. Until 1971 little could be done in such cases, even with a laser. To use a laser, it is necessary to see the retina.

A vitrectomy is a surgical procedure that uses an instrument containing a drill and a suction. It is inserted into the eyeball and is used to remove the hemorrhage, replacing it with saline or another liquid. The instrument is then removed and the hole sealed. It can then be determined if laser therapy is needed. The use of vitrectomy is still limited; the procedure is undergoing evaluation in a double-blind study being conducted at the National Institutes of Health.

The instrument can also be used to cut the fibrous bands that cause traction on the retina that might cause retinal detachment.

Only eyes in which hemorrhage is not resolving spontaneously are appropriate candidates for the procedure.

Side-effects of the procedure include vitreal and retinal hemorrhages, rubeosis iridis, and neovascularization.

Health Teaching

In all forms of therapy for retinopathy, something is destroyed in the process of saving vision. The facts must be presented to the patient and family as honestly as possible. The course of the retinopathy will be long and stressful. In counseling the patient, it is important to stress:

- That the appearance of retinopathy can be expected after many years of diabetes, and its appearance does not necessarily mean that the diabetes is on a downhill course
- That the odds for maintaining vision are in the patient's favor
- That frequent eye examinations are the best way to preserve vision, because they allow for the detection of any retinopathy

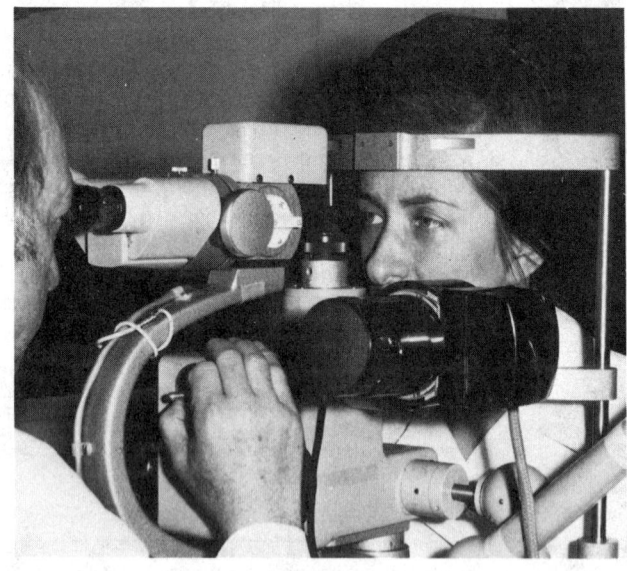
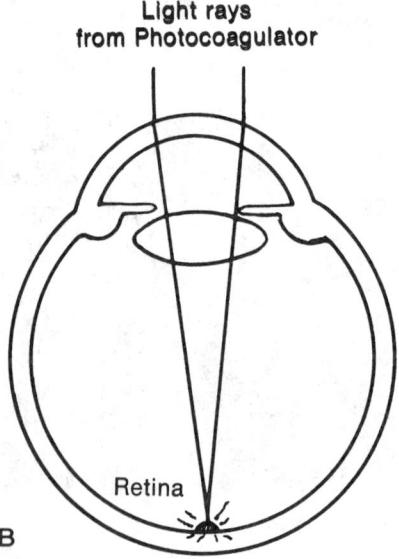

A   B

Figure 36-5
Photocoagulation. (*A*) The photograph shows a model receiving treatment with the argon laser, which generates a fine but intense blue-green beam of light. In this therapy the intense beam of light is directed into the eye and focused on a tiny spot in the retina. (*B*) Principle underlying photocoagulation. The intense beam of light acts in much the same way as the sun's rays focused through a magnifying glass produce a small burn on a leaf. (*A:* Courtesy of Dr. Arnall Patz, Wilmer Eye Institute, Johns Hopkins Hospital, Baltimore, Maryland. *B:* Reproduced with permission from American Association of Workers for the Blind, Inc., Blindness Annual.)

Some additional points to keep in mind when the patient with diabetes has some type of visual impairment are the following:

- Visual impairment can be a shock to anyone. A person's response to vision loss depends on personality, self-concept, and coping mechanisms.
- As in any loss, blindness and its acceptance by the patient will occur in stages; some patients may learn to accept blindness in a rather short period of time, while others may never accept it.
- Although retinopathy occurs bilaterally, the severity may differ in the two eyes.
- Many of the chronic complications of diabetes happen simultaneously. For example, a blind diabetic patient may also have peripheral neuropathy and may experience impairment of manual dexterity and tactile sensation.

Nephropathy

People with diabetes account for about 25% of cases of newly diagnosed kidney disease (renal failure) in the United States each year. Renal disease occurs more frequently in patients who develop diabetes before the age of 20 than in those who develop it later. Patients who develop diabetes before age 20 have a 50% chance of developing renal disease 20 years after diagnosis. Those who develop diabetes after age 20 have about a 2% chance. It appears that those who develop diabetes during periods of rapid growth are more likely to have kidney disease. However, the exact cause remains unclear.

Patients with type I diabetes frequently show initial signs of kidney disease after 15 to 20 years, while patients with type II develop kidney disease less frequently but more rapidly—usually within 10 years after diagnosis of diabetes. It has been theorized that this occurs because people with type II diabetes are older and already have cardiovascular problems worsened by diabetes. Many of these patients may have had diabetes for many years before it was diagnosed and treated.

To date, there is no reliable method to predict whether a person will develop kidney disease. Maintaining blood glucose levels at the near-normal range may prevent or delay its onset.

Pathology. New evidence suggests that, soon after the onset of diabetes, increased filtering by the kidneys occurs. The molecular makeup of the basement membrane of the kidney capillaries (*glomeruli*) is structured to serve as a selective filter. Over a period of years, the basement membrane thickens as a result of chronic high blood glucose levels. Not only is the amount of basement membrane increased, but the proportion of the various glycoproteins is altered so that the molecular architecture of the membrane is changed. The membrane is thicker as well as more permeable, and blood proteins are lost in the urine.

Soon after development of diabetes, and especially if the blood glucose levels are elevated, the kidney's filtration mechanism is stressed. As a result, the pressure in the blood vessels of the kidney increases. It is thought that the elevated pressure serves as the stimulus for the development of nephropathy. Various medications and diets are being tested to prevent these complications.

Diagnostic Evaluation. Early in the diagnostic process, it is important to differentiate between renal disease unrelated to diabetes and that induced by or directly related to diabetes. While a renal problem not related to diabetes may be more difficult to manage because of the accompanying diabetes, the prognosis is generally more favorable than in kidney disease induced by diabetes.

One of the most important blood proteins that begins leaking in the urine is albumin. Small amounts may leak for years undetected. Early microalbuminuria may be discovered in a 24-hour urine sample. Some people with small amounts of albumin loss may never develop a greater degree of kidney dysfunction. In others with diabetes, albumin loss increases as renal damage increases. Carefully designed low-protein diets appear to reverse early leakage of small amounts of protein from the kidney.

When a urine dipstick test reads consistently positive for significant amounts of albumin, the patient will need to be tested for creatinine and blood urea nitrogen.

At this point in the development of renal disease, the patient may also require diagnostic testing for cardiac or renal problems. Some of the tests involve injection into the body of special dyes that are not easily cleared by the damaged kidney. Therefore, the value of the diagnostic test must be weighed against the potential risks.

Patients with diabetes who are in the early stages of kidney disease also frequently develop hypertension. Several different forms of hypertension may develop. One is *essential hypertension*, like that experienced by people who do not have diabetes. This form is probably unrelated to the kidney disease. Hypertension in a person with diabetes does not necessarily indicate kidney disease. Another form of hypertension is *renal hypertension* or *hypertension in diabetes*.

Clinical Manifestations. Most of the signs and symptoms of renal dysfunction in the person with diabetes are similar to those seen in patients without diabetes. (See Chap. 39 on the management of patients with renal disorders.) Additionally, as renal failure progresses, the catabolism (breakdown) of both exogenous and endogenous insulin decreases, and frequent hypoglycemic episodes result. Not only do insulin needs change, but the dietary requirements change as well. Male patients are also faced with impotence. The stress of kidney disease affects self-esteem, family relationships, marital relations, and virtually all aspects of daily life. As renal function decreases, the patient frequently experiences multiple system failure—*e.g.*, declining visual acuity, impotence, foot ulcerations, congestive heart failure, and nocturnal diarrhea. Frequently, health professionals begin to avoid this patient at a time when the person is most in need of support systems.

Prevention and Management. In addition to achieving and maintaining near-normal blood glucose levels, management in all patients with diabetes should include careful attention to the following:

- Control of hypertension
- Prevention and/or vigorous treatment of urinary tract infections
- Avoidance of nephrotoxic substances
- Adjustment of medications during changing of renal function
- A diet low in sodium and protein

In renal failure, two types of treatment are available: dialysis (hemodialysis or peritoneal dialysis) and transplantation from a relative or a cadaver.

Hemodialysis for the patient with diabetes is similar to that for patients without the disease (see Chap. 39). Because hemodialysis creates additional stress on patients with cardiovascular disease, it may not be indicated in certain patients. In addition, it is extremely intrusive into a patient's life.

Both *continuous ambulatory peritoneal dialysis (CAPD)* and *intermittent peritoneal dialysis* are being used by an increasing number of patients with diabetes, mainly because of the independence they allow to patients. In addition, insulin can be mixed into the dialysate, which may result in better blood glucose control and end the need for insulin injections. However, these patients may require more insulin because the dialysate contains sugar. A major risk of peritoneal dialysis is a higher incidence of infection.

Renal disease is frequently accompanied by advancing retinopathy that may require laser treatments and surgery. Severe hypertension also worsens eye disease because of the additional stress it places on the blood vessels. Patients being treated by hemodialysis who require eye surgery may be switched to peritoneal dialysis and have their hypertension aggressively controlled for several weeks before surgery. The rationale for this change is that hemodialysis requires anticoagulants that can increase the risk of bleeding after the operation, and peritoneal dialysis minimizes pressure changes in the eyes.

In recent years, the success rate for kidney transplantation in patients with diabetes has improved. In medical centers performing large numbers of transplants, the chances are 75% to 80% that the transplanted kidney will continue to function in the patient with diabetes for at least 5 years. Like the original kidneys, transplanted kidneys in patients with diabetes can eventually be damaged if blood glucose levels are consistently high following the transplantation. Therefore, monitoring blood glucose levels frequently and adjusting insulin levels in diabetic patients with transplanted kidneys are essential for long-term success.

The mortality rate for patients undergoing dialysis or transplantation is closely related to the severity of cardiovascular problems.

The Neuropathies of Diabetes

Neuropathy in diabetes refers to a group of diseases that affect the peripheral nerves. These disorders affect all three types of peripheral nerves: motor, sensory, and autonomic. They involve either the entire neuron or selected levels. The disorders appear to be clinically diverse, and depend on the following:

- Severity of the disease process
- Rate of progression
- The structures of affected cells and their location
- The type of cells
- The underlying pathological process

The prevalence increases with the age of the patient and the duration of the disease. Higher blood glucose levels over a period of years have also been implicated in the etiology.

The exact causes are diverse, complex, and not completely understood. The pathogenesis may be due to either a vascular or a metabolic mechanism or both, but their relative contributions have not yet been determined.

The metabolic aberrations of neurons or their myelin sheaths may be responsible for the nerve damage seen in diabetes. In patients with prolonged high levels of blood glucose, an enzyme system (the sorbitol pathway) may become overactive during periods of insulin insufficiency. Overproduction of fructose in the myelin sheath may result, causing rupture of the sheath and disruption of nerve conduction. Another possibility is the formation of complexes (protein joined to glucose-glycoproteins) when abnormally high blood glucose levels are present. It appears unlikely that glucose damages the nerve cells directly.

Clinical Manifestations. The neuropathies of diabetes can produce symptoms of wide variety and differing intensity. There is some evidence that the first few years after neuropathy develops are critical in determining its progress. It appears that, if severe neuropathy is to develop, it will do so during this early period. If it does not develop then, there is a decreased likelihood that the neuropathy will become disabling in the future.

There are several types of neuropathy. Each has specific symptoms, and medical management is directed toward alleviation of these symptoms. Regardless of type or symptom, maintaining near-normal levels of blood glucose is the chief priority.

Management. There is no evidence that treatment will reverse neuropathy, but some clinicians feel that careful attention to maintaining near-normal blood glucose levels may halt or delay its progress. Additional treatment is symptomatic, palliative, and supportive. Pain and other symptoms usually disappear within months. Various medications that are often used include analgesics, phenytoin, and antidepressants. Nonnarcotic analgesics are preferred.

Inhibitors of aldose reductase constitute a new group of drugs that block the sorbitol pathway, which is involved in the pathology of the long-term complications of diabetes. They are currently being evaluated in a multi-center study in the United States.

Autonomic Neuropathy

Involvement of the autonomic nervous system covers a broad range of dysfunctions, including orthostatic hypotension, pupillary changes, abnormal sweating, bladder paralysis, and nocturnal diarrhea. A common example of autonomic neuropathy involves sexual dysfunction.

Sexual Problems and Diabetes. Sexual dysfunction occurs with the same frequency in females and males. However, most of the research involving sexual problems secondary to diabetes has focused on the male. This may be due in part to the lack of any objective measurement of female sexual performance and the need for researchers to rely on the patient's reports. Studies have not yet determined whether diabetes affects female sexual performance as well as that of the male. It is known, however, that some women with diabetes have inadequate vaginal lubrication, which may lead to reduced enjoyment of intercourse and subsequent problems in a woman's relationship with her partner.

Although impotence in the male with diabetes has been recognized for a number of years, it is only recently that the frequency, pathology, and clinical implications have been established. In addition to impotence, retrograde ejaculation has been noted in the male with diabetes. These changes are affected by different mechanisms and may appear singly or in combination.

Retrograde Ejaculation. Retrograde ejaculation refers to the propulsion of seminal fluid through the posterior urethra backwards into the urinary bladder through a muscle that is relaxed due to diabetic neuropathy. These patients are not impotent, despite the presence of diabetic neuropathy. The patient experiences an orgasm but has no accompanying ejaculation. Examination of the urine confirms the diagnosis because of the large number of active sperm present.

Impotence. Impotence, the difficulty or inability of the penis to become rigid and sustain sexual intercourse, occurs in 50% to 60% of all males with diabetes. This incidence is 4 to 5 times that found in the general population. It is usually present in diabetic patients with other symptoms of diabetic autonomic neuropathy. In most cases, the patient does not mention impotence unless specifically asked about it.

It must also be remembered that males with diabetes are subject to the same tensions and occasional lack of sexual performance as are other males. It cannot be assumed that the impotence of a patient is caused by diabetes. Typical causes of sexual impotence in the male who has diabetes follow:

- Psychological factors
- Organic factors

    Congenital abnormality
    Trauma
    Systemic disease
    Vascular disease
    Endocrine deficiency (rarely)

- Neurologic factors

    Central factors
    Spinal factors
    Peripheral neuropathy

- Drug-induced effects (by some of the drugs used to treat hypertension)

These factors are not more prevalent in diabetes. In many men, impotence is the first sign of diabetes. If a middle-aged man who has previously been potent develops impotence, the presence of diabetes must be suspected and investigated.

Another factor that may lead to impotence is diminished penile blood flow due to atherosclerosis, which is common in diabetes.

The mechanism of erection may be the only sexual function affected by the neuropathy, and the patient may continue to experience desire, orgasm, and ejaculation because these functions are controlled by different nerves.

When poorly-controlled diabetes causes impotence, it is generally due to associated malnutrition and weakness. A man with sustained hyperglycemia is probably unable to perform other activities, including sustaining an erection. After normoglycemia is attained, which restores normal health and vigor, potency if often restored. If the impotence is psychological, then the approach must be psychological evaluation followed by the appropriate therapy. If medications are involved, especially those being used for the treatment of hypertension, a switch to another antihypertensive agent may be indicated.

In most cases, the cause of impotence in diabetes is neurogenic. Unfortunately, there is no preventive therapy or systemic treatment available. Attempts to revascularize the penis have been unsuccessful for the most part. However, mechanical devices or prostheses, have been developed and may be used in some instances.

Foot and Leg Problems in Diabetes

Diabetic neuropathy most commonly manifests itself in the lower extremities. Pain and paresthesia are the outstanding manifestations. The pain has been described as dull or aching, cramping, burning, lancinating, or crushing. The pain is usually intensified at night and may be relieved by pacing the floor, which distinguishes this pain from the pain due to peripheral vascular insufficiency, which is intensified by walking.

The paresthesias have been described as sensations of tingling or burning, or of coldness and numbness. Because of these varied discomforts, it is quite common for the patient to be depressed and irritable and to suffer from anorexia.

Loss of sensation can lead to infection, gangrene, and amputation. The patient may be unaware of a blister, a protruding nail in a shoe, a burn from an electric blanket, or other injury. Instruction and reinforcement of previous learning about foot care are vital.

The feet in diabetes are subject to sepsis and ischemia from deficient nerve function and poor circulation. Diabetic neuropathy may cause pain and paresthesia, but the greatest problem is loss of the sensation of pain and temperature in the feet.

Without pain perception, repeated trauma to the feet is tolerated until calluses and ulcers form, and the joints become damaged. Because of numbness of the feet, the patient may fail to notice injury to the foot. Burns may occur when the patient is unable to recognize that a heating pad or a footbath is too hot. External heat is the most common single cause of gangrene. In view of these dangers, heat should not be applied below the knee of any patient with diabetes.

Vascular involvement of the feet may lead to occlusion of large, medium, and small arteries and cause atrophic changes in the skin. The swelling that results from cellulitis may cause decreased circulation at a time when it needs to be increased. (Occlusive vascular disease can coexist with neuropathy.) If there is no response to antibiotics and débridement, the ischemia may cause gangrene to start in the tips of the toes and then spread slowly up the leg.

Large-vessel insufficiency causes intermittent claudication (pain on walking, relieved by rest), blanching of the feet upon elevation, dusky redness of the feet when dependent, atrophic skin changes, cold feet, and finally pain at rest. Involvement of the autonomic nervous system may lead to an absence of sweating, which causes dry, cracked skin that permits bacterial invasion.

Thus, the triad of neuropathy, vascular disease, and infection leads to gangrene and amputation in older patients with diabetes. In the presence of gangrene, amputation is done at the lowest level that has an adequate blood supply and is free of infection. The care of the patient undergoing amputation of an extremity is discussed on pages 1604–1610.

Management. Patients who have neuropathy and vascular problems should be under the supervision of a podiatrist. However, often the nurse is the only member of the health care team who is available to provide direct care and guidance. The patient must be taught to wash and examine both feet every day. Unless the nails are thick, the vision is poor, or the neuropathy is severe, patients should learn to trim their own nails.

Pentoxifylline (Trental) is indicated in the treatment of intermittent claudication because of its beneficial effects on red blood cell flexibility, blood viscosity, and platelet adhesiveness. Because pentoxifylline produces few side-effects and is able to improve blood flow in ischemic areas, it is a drug of choice in peripheral vascular disease.

Special Problems in Diabetes

Stress

Stress in the life of patients with diabetes has an important effect on the management of their condition. Stressors vary widely and may include taking a vacation, the divorce of parents, an infection, moving, surgery, a change in schools, loss of a close friend or a pet, or the development of one of the chronic complications of diabetes. Whether its origin is physiological or psychological, stress activates an increased production of epinephrine. This in turn stimulates glycogenolysis, which results in increased levels of blood glucose. At the same time or shortly thereafter, ACTH is released from the pituitary gland and stimulates the adrenal cortex to release large quantities of cortisol. Cortisol increases lipid, protein, and carbohydrate metabolism, resulting in an increase of blood glucose and liver glycogen. The hepatic store of glycogen is converted into glucose, which is released into the blood stream. The elevated blood glucose requires increased amounts of insulin, which the pancreas is unable to provide. Stress also impairs utilization of insulin by the peripheral circulation, creating a demand for increased release of hepatic glucose, which in turn increases blood glucose levels.

Psychological (emotional) stress must be dealt with not only because of its effect on blood glucose levels but also because it may alter normal eating and exercise habits. For example, the patient may respond to emotional stress by overeating, not eating, or eating abnormal amounts of carbohydrates, and may decrease or omit normal physical exercise. The patient may also purposely omit insulin or report blood glucose results incorrectly.

The Patient With Diabetes Undergoing Surgery

Because of the possibility of generalized vascular disease, decreased resistance to infection, and changing insulin requirements due to stress, the patient must be followed very closely at the time of surgery. Surgical stress aggravates hyperglycemia because of an increased secretion of epinephrine and glucocorticoids. The metabolic stress of anesthesia also accentuates problems of hyperglycemia and ketosis. In addition, the patient's normal schedule of food intake, which is the foundation of diabetic treatment, is interrupted.

Preoperative Management. In the preoperative period, the aim is to have the diabetes well controlled and to correct any problems of hydration and electrolyte imbalance. The greatest danger is hypoglycemia, since the central nervous system is very sensitive to glucose deprivation and the clinical signs of hypoglycemia are difficult to interpret when the patient is unconscious from anesthesia.

If the patient has been on an oral antidiabetic agent or long-acting insulin, then regular insulin is substituted a day or two before surgery. The preoperative medication is kept to a minimum, since these patients are susceptible to sedatives and narcotics.

There is a wide variety of protocols for the management of the patient's nutrient and insulin requirements before, during, and after surgery, depending on the degree of diabetes, the nature of the surgery, the degree and persistence of glucosuria, and whether or not ketonuria is present. The key to control is careful monitoring for potentially rapid changes that will affect the patient's metabolic state.

On the morning of surgery, a fasting blood glucose is drawn 1 hour before the operation. Usually, the patient is given an intravenous infusion of 5% or 10% dextrose in water to provide necessary calories and carbohydrates, accompanied by the subcutaneous injection of insulin in a somewhat smaller dose than was required before surgery.

Postoperative Management. During the postoperative period, nutrition is maintained with intravenous dextrose until the patient is able to tolerate food by mouth. The insulin is adjusted on a sliding scale according to the results of the blood tests for glucose. Supplemental doses of regular insulin may be given as required. It is desirable to give insulin subcutaneously, since insulin added to an intravenous solution may adhere to the walls of the bottle and tubing, and IV fluids may be given at different rates, making insulin dosages difficult to adjust.

Following surgery, the diabetes may intensify and become difficult to control. Healing may be delayed due to vascular disease, poor circulation, and altered metabolism. A higher incidence of vascular complications (myocardial infarction, stroke) may occur due to the increased incidence of atherosclerosis.

Infections

There appears to be a correlation between diabetes and susceptibility to infection, perhaps because of depleted host defenses and higher than normal glucose concentration in the tissues. High blood glucose may impair the ability of granulocytes to carry out a number of vital functions. Hyperglycemia also depresses leukocyte phagocytosis.

Infections are more serious in diabetes because resistance to infection is decreased by hyperglycemia, and because diabetes becomes temporarily more severe in the presence of infection. Infections in diabetes are exacerbated by dehydration, insulin antagonism, impaired phagocytosis, and neuropathy. Infection is a common precipitating cause of acute complications, such as ketoacidosis.

The extremities may be vulnerable to infection because of diminished arterial circulation, which lowers resistance to bacterial invasion and local injury. Cellulitis may spread rapidly. Fungal infections between the toes may produce fissures that provide further portals of entry for bacteria. Infections of the foot can lead to gangrene, with loss of toes or foot and lower leg. A patient with an infected foot generally requires hospitalization. (The prevention of foot problems is discussed on pp. 937–938.)

Dermatologic problems are common in diabetes with hyperglycemia. Fungal infections, particularly candidiasis of the skin and vagina, are frequently found during prolonged periods of hyperglycemia. The presence of boils or carbuncles and severe pruritus should raise the suspicion of possible diabetes.

The increased prevalence of urinary tract infections in diabetes is related to incomplete emptying of the bladder due to poor bladder tone, a neurologic complication that may result from diabetic neuropathy, and possibly to an increased frequency of catheterization. Bladder infection produces ascending infections of the urinary tract. Serious complications from renal infection are more frequent in the person with diabetes.

Management. When the blood glucose level is elevated, the leukocytes are unable to destroy bacteria effectively. All infections, and especially those associated with leukocytosis and a spreading infection, cause an increased need for insulin. Ketoacidosis may result if the insulin dose is not increased adequately. Frequent blood glucose determinations are necessary to ascertain and compensate for rapidly changing insulin requirements. The cause of the infection should be determined by culture, so that the appropriate antibiotic may be given.

Influenza Vaccine. The Centers for Disease Control recommend that persons with diseases like diabetes and elderly persons receive the influenza vaccine yearly, because they are at the highest risk for the serious complications of influenza. Individuals with diabetes whose blood glucose levels are consistently above normal are more susceptible to infections like influenza, and are therefore candidates for the vaccine.

Periodontal Disease

Periodontal disease is an infection of gum tissue and supporting bone structures of the teeth. It is the leading cause of tooth loss in adults, and tends to be more severe in people with diabetes. Periodontal disease can be both a cause and a result of abnormal blood glucose levels. Continued infection can interfere with normal glucose maintenance. Poor dentition may lead to chewing problems, which may interfere with proper nutrition, a cornerstone of diabetes therapy.

More than half of the population over 18 years of age have periodontal disease, and in people with diabetes it can develop as early as 11 years of age. Age, more than duration of diabetes, appears to be a significant factor in its development.

The major cause is *dental plaque*, a collection of bacteria that grow on food particles, on tissue cells, and in saliva on the surface of teeth. These bacteria produce toxins that irritate and damage teeth and surrounding tissues. If the process continues, the bone around the tooth deteriorates, causing tooth loss and/or infection.

If plaque is not removed regularly, it combines with minerals in saliva to form *calculus* (tartar), a hard cementlike material. Calculus irritates gum tissues and creates pockets that may deepen and cause the loss of bone surrounding the teeth.

Plaque accumulates more readily in people with diabetes. As a result, periodontal disease begins at a younger age and usually progresses more rapidly in these patients.

There is also a loss of collagen in the gum tissue in diabetes, as well as an increase in collagenase activity. Collagenase is a naturally-occurring enzyme that destroys collagen, which is necessary for adequate support of the teeth.

Also present in the oral cavity of persons with diabetes are elevated salivary glucose levels, elevated calcium concentrations, higher oral *Candida albicans* counts, and alterations in the oral microbial flora. Elevated counts of *C. albicans*, associated with high salivary glucose levels, may result in thrush, which is more prevalent in diabetes.

Although the exact cause of periodontal disease in diabetes is not known, it is suggested that diabetes accelerates microangiopathy of the blood vessels in the gum tissue and decreases the capacity for collagen synthesis.

Treatment consists of normalizing blood glucose, and controlling plaque by mechanical and chemical means. The nurse outlines an adequate home care program and demonstrates the necessary skills, *e.g.*, brushing and flossing.

A medium-soft-bristle toothbrush can be used to remove plaque, and regular daily flossing can help to prevent periodontal disease and decay. A diet rich in vitamins and minerals, such as that prescribed in diabetes, will also help to keep teeth healthy. Achieving and maintaining near-normal blood glucose levels will delay or prevent dental caries and periodontal disease. The dental care performed daily by the patient should be supplemented with regularly-scheduled dental appointments to clean hidden deposits of calculus that the patient is unable to reach.

Premenstrual Syndrome (PMS)

The exact cause of premenstrual syndrome (PMS), is unknown, but changing hormone levels (estrogen and progesterone) may trigger symptoms in patients. In women with diabetes, blood glucose levels begin to rise approximately 5 days before menstruation. The higher the blood glucose level rises, the more severe the symptoms of PMS become. Symptoms include bloating, headache, food cravings, anxiety, mood swings, irritability, and depression. Additionally, anxiety and depression cause increases in blood glucose. Foods that are high in simple sugars, salt, and caffeine should be avoided during this time, and the frequency of blood glucose monitoring should be increased.

Use of Recreational Drugs

An increasing proportion of people in the U.S. are using recreational drugs (drugs used for reasons other than to treat an illness) today. Although there are harmful effects of the use of these drugs for the general population, there are specific effects on blood glucose levels and the general health of persons with diabetes. The information that exists about alcohol and diabetes is adequate, but there are conflicting reports about the use of nicotine, caffeine, marijuana, cocaine, and psychedelic (hallucinogenic) drugs. Persons with diabetes need to be aware of how these drugs affect blood glucose.

Alcohol. Alcohol and its effect on diabetes have been studied rather extensively. Alcohol interferes with the synthesis, storage, and release of glycogen, and may cause hypoglycemia if the person drinking alcohol has not eaten recently. It can also cause facial flushing in patients taking chlorpropramide. Alcohol can increase blood lipids, increase blood glucose levels, and make weight control more difficult.

Nicotine. Nicotine constricts blood vessels. As a result, smoking is not recommended for persons with diabetes because it is an additional risk factor for vascular disease. Research findings have implicated nicotine in decreased insulin absorption, in the development of nephropathy in insulin-dependent diabetes, and in the need for changes in insulin dosage.

Caffeine. In general, caffeine has a mild effect on blood glucose levels. However, the symptoms of too much caffeine (irritability, shakiness, and anxiety) may be confused with those of hypoglycemia. It is important for the patient to be aware that caffeine is found in tea, cola-type softs drinks, and many over-the-counter medications.

Marijuana. The specific effect of marijuana on blood glucose levels is not known. However, its use causes the following problems that may then affect blood glucose: impaired lung function, decreased sperm counts, effects on ovulation and pregnancy, lowered resistance to infection, increased heart rate, orthostatic hypotension, increased appetite, diarrhea, and drowsiness. Some of these effects may mimic the symptoms of hypoglycemia, while others may interfere with daily management of the patient's disease.

Sedatives-Hypnotics. Some sedatives or hypnotics may result in the rapid metabolism of other medications that the patient is taking.

Stimulants. Many stimulants are similar to epinephrine, which specifically causes an increase in blood glucose levels.

Hallucinogens and Inhalants. Most hallucinogenic and inhalant drugs act as stimulants and also depress appetite, which may cause a decrease in blood glucose levels. Because they also alter perception, a patient may forget to eat or take medication. Peripheral nerve damage and toxicity to the liver, kidneys, and bone marrow have also been reported.

Opiates. The effect of opiates on blood glucose levels is uncertain. There are some reports of impaired glucose tolerance.

Summary. Although the direct effects of recreational drugs vary, most create perceptual changes that could disrupt the routine of self-care. Motivation to carry out the prescribed regimen may also be affected.

Gerontological Considerations

Many elderly patients with diabetes have three or four chronic illnesses. These diseases may interact with diabetes and affect its management. Age-related changes may cause problems with medications, and *polypharmacy* (use of a large number of prescription and nonprescription drugs) is common. The incidence of noninsulin-dependent diabetes increases with age, affecting 10% of the population at age 60, and 20% at age 80. Hypertension and vascular disease are particularly common in the elderly with diabetes. Diabetes after age 50 is associated with increased levels of very-low-density lipoprotein (VLDL) cholesterol, decreased levels of high-density lipoprotein (HDLP) cholesterol, obesity, the use of diuretics, and the existence of vascular disease.

The pathology of noninsulin-dependent diabetes in the elderly involves diminished insulin secretion related to the patient's need and insulin resistance. The ability of older patients to secrete insulin is inversely related to the degree of hyperglycemia. Although insulin is released in response to glucose, the timing, pattern, and amount of insulin secretion are altered. Insulin resistance in the type II patient is a combination of altered sensitivity because of decreased numbers of insulin receptors and decreased responsiveness to insulin.

Blood glucose levels should be maintained in the near-normal range in order to prevent both short-term and long-term complications.

Acute complications in the elderly are common. In the elderly person with a diminished sense of thirst, osmotic diuresis secondary to hyperglycemia may lead to sodium depletion and dehydration, resulting in hypotension. High glucose levels place the older patient with diabetes at risk for hypotension (with the possibility of falls and fractures) and for hypokalemia (especially if the patient takes diuretics), and at increased risk for cardiac irregulatiries, dehydration, thrombotic events, and the development of hyperosmolarity.

Chronic complications include those that result from the macrovascular complications (such as accelerated atherosclerosis and its sequelae) and the microvascular complications (such as retinopathy, nephropathy, and neuropathy). Hypertension is prevalent, and, if untreated, worsens the course of retinopathy and nephropathy.

Severe hypoglycemia, especially in patients with possible vascular compromise, can lead to increased morbidity and mortality in the elderly.

Changes with aging should be kept in mind when planning care for the older patient with diabetes. Chart 36-9 summarizes changes in the elderly that may affect the outcome of the treatment plan.

▶ Nursing Process
The Patient With Diabetes

▷ Assessment

Nursing assessment of the patient with diabetes focuses on the presence and duration of the classical symptoms of hyperglycemia. The history identifies the existence of factors that affect blood glucose:

1. Changes in dietary habits with increased intake
2. Reduction or omission of required insulin or oral antidiabetic agents
3. Drugs or other therapies
4. Symptoms of infection—influenza, dental, urinary, respiratory, and skin infection
5. Symptoms of stress—psychological stress, acute illness, pregnancy, trauma, surgery

A complete physical assessment is essential because diabetes can affect every system in the body. Assessment includes the following:

Chart 36-9
Changes in the Elderly That May Affect Diabetes

Sensory Changes

- Decreased vision
- Decreased smell
- Taste changes
- Decreased proprioception

Gastrointestinal Changes

- Dental problems
- Appetite changes
- Delayed gastric emptying
- Decreased bowel motility

Activity/Exercise Pattern Changes

Renal Function Changes

- Decreased function
- Decreased drug clearance

Hepatic Function Changes

- Decreased function
- Insulin degradation decreased

Affective/Cognitive Disorders

- Medications/meals omitted or erratic

Socioeconomic Factors

- Fad diets
- Loneliness/living alone
- Lack of money

Chronic Diseases

- Hypertension
- Arthritis
- Neoplasms
- Acute/chronic infections

Drug Interactions

- Variable compliance
- Use of another's medications
- Consulting multiple physicians for different illnesses
- Alcohol

Skin

- Check groin, axillae, and inframammary areas in women (especially obese patients). High moisture and high glucose levels support the growth of *Candida albicans.*
- Assess pretibial area for *"shin spots"* (diabetic dermopathy) and *necrobiosis* (raised, reddened lesions with sharply-defined borders; may indicate undiagnosed diabetes).
- Check elbows, knees for *xanthomas* (yellow deposits of fat-laden cells on the skin).
- Check insulin injection sites for atrophy, hypertrophy.

Mouth

- Check teeth for periodontal disease and dental caries.
- Check mouth and tongue for the presence of thrush.

Eyes

- Check visual acuity.
- Use an ophthalmoscope to assess for the following:

  Cataracts
  Retinopathy (Other than hemorrhages that are fairly large needing referral, most of the early changes are not detectable by the inexperienced examiner without the benefit of a dilated pupil.)

Cardiovascular System

- Check weight, blood pressure, and pulses.
- Assess for signs and symptoms of cardiac disease (*e.g.,* dyspnea, chest pain, irregular heart beat).

Peripheral Vascular System

- Check legs and feet for compromised circulatory status:

  Cool, thin, shiny skin
  Thick, ridged nails
  Hair loss over dorsum of foot

  Pulse strength
  Ulcerations

Kidneys

- Assess for edema (swelling) of ankles, face (may indicate renal involvement and fluid retention).
- Assess for evidence of hypoglycemia, urinary tract infections.
- Note nonspecific signs and symptoms: fatigue, muscle weakness, exhaustion, pallor.

Neuromuscular System (Neuropathies)

- Check hands for atrophy of small muscles and burns (which may occur with decreased sensation).
- Check for extraocular muscle dysfunction.
- Note gastrointestinal disturbances—which may be due to delayed gastric emptying, diarrhea (particularly at night).
- Check for bladder dysfunction—frequent urinary infections because of neurogenic bladder.
- Check for reproductive dysfunction—male impotence, retrograde ejaculation; female sexuality problems (?), menstrual irregularities, vaginal infections (especially yeast).
- Check for peripheral neuropathy—*paresthesias* (tingling sensation, numbness, decreased ability to detect vibration).

Psychosocial assessment focuses on the impact of living with diabetes as a chronic disease. For newly-diagnosed patients, denial or depression may be present. As patients move through the initial stages of the disease and are faced with the complexity of the regimen, they may feel overwhelmed and powerless, deny the need for some or all aspects of the treatment plan, or have difficulty in coping or adapting to certain expected behaviors. A careful assessment of patients' attitudes about the disease, understanding of the treatment plan, and participation in their own care is critical for future self-care activities. Current life-style, including employment, living arrangements, hobbies, and family/friend relationships, may be affected by this disease, both at the time of diagnosis and as the disease progresses.

For patients who have lived with diabetes for a number of years, life-style and physical/emotional status need to be reassessed. Life experiences present new challenges and problems to be surmounted. This is especially true for the elderly patient, who may be faced with multiple chronic illnesses.

In addition, the patient's understanding of diabetes and ability to carry out the treatment are carefully assessed, both at the time of diagnosis and periodically throughout the course of the disease. Changes in meal planning, medication dosage or type, and exercise levels need to be examined in light of life-style changes as well as degree of interest, ability, and motivation for self-care.

▷ *Nursing Diagnoses*

Based on the assessment data, the major nursing diagnoses for the patient with diabetes may include the following:

- Deficit in knowledge concerning methods for maintaining near-normal blood glucose levels
- Alterations in nutrition related to dietary regulations to combat abnormal metabolism of carbohydrates, proteins, and fats
- Feelings of powerlessness related to the uncertainties of the disease and the development of complications
- Potential nonadherence to the prescribed therapeutic regimen related to its complexity
- Potential impairment of skin integrity secondary to hyperglycemia and vascular problems
- Potential for injury related to decreased tactile sensation and diminished visual activity
- Potential sexual dysfunction in the male related to erectile problems secondary to neuropathy

Potential Complications

- Potential for development of hypoglycemia related to imbalance between insulin need and insulin dose
- Potential for development of ketosis/ketoacidosis related to insulin deficiency and faulty fat metabolism
- Potential development of long-term complications related to persistent hyperglycemia and accelerated vascular disease

▷ *Planning and Nursing Implementation*

▷ *Goals:* The major goals for the patient may include maintenance of normoglycemia with few episodes of hypoglycemia or hyperglycemia; improved metabolism of carbohydrates, proteins, and fats; ability to control the day-to-day management of the disease and its potential complications; adherence to the therapeutic regimen; decreased incidence of hypoglycemia; absence of ketosis/ketoacidosis; prevention, delay, or control of the long-term complications of diabetes; maintenance of skin integrity; prevention of injury; and maintenance or improvement of sexual function.

Although specific treatment depends on the type of diabetes, the American Diabetes Association has established as a general goal for all diabetics the achievement of levels of blood glucose as close to those in the nondiabetic as feasible.

Management focuses on dietary control, exercise, and antidiabetic medications. Chart 36-10 summarizes the differences in the management of patients with insulin-dependent diabetes and those with noninsulin-dependent diabetes. Patient education about self-care is the foundation for the patient's successful attainment of goals.

▷ *Nursing Interventions*

Health Education for Diabetes. Since the responsibility for the management of diabetes rests with the individual, each patient is taught to perform duties usually done by the physician, nurse, dietitian, and laboratory technician. The educational program is started at the time of diagnosis and must be continued throughout the life of the patient. Continuing education reinforces learning and is necessary for better control of the disease and for greater self-reliance of the patient or significant other. A responsible member of the patient's family should be included in the educational program. The community health nurse also has a role. Group instruction may be an effective method of education in diabetic clinics, hospitals, and community health departments.

Realistic educational outcomes for the newly diagnosed patient include understanding of (1) the pathophysiology of diabetes; (2) basic concepts of dietary management; (3) administration of insulin; (4) exercise regimen; (5) urine or blood testing; (6) recall of signs and symptoms of hypoglycemia and hyperglycemia; and (7) basic principles of foot care.

A summary of detailed information necessary for the education of diabetic patients is found in Chart 36-11, p. 937.

Maintaining Normoglycemia. Maintenance of normoglycemia involves close daily attention to meal planning, exercise, medications, prevention of acute episodes of illness, and self-monitoring of blood glucose. Self-monitoring of blood glucose is probably the most important factor in daily management by the patient, because the exact level of blood glucose can serve as an indicator for adjustments in meal planning, exercise, and medications.

The nurse outlines goals with the patient about diet, exercise, medications, and method of monitoring blood glucose.

The *meal plan* needs to be realistic and to take into consideration the patient's food preferences, culture, socio-economic status, and support systems. Weight loss and gain are special situations often confronted by the patient. In general, the patient who needs to lose weight needs not only adequate information about food choices and meal timing but also counselling and social support during this period. Proper spacing of meals, and types and amounts of food, are important for all patients, but even more so for the patient with type I diabetes if normoglycemia is to be maintained. A more flexible life-style is now possible for this type of patient through use of such tools as insulin pumps, multiple injections, and direct coordination of meals with insulin delivery.

Exercise should be done daily and in the same amounts if at all possible. If the patient is hospitalized for diagnosis, stabilization of blood glucose levels, and patient teaching, exercise or some form of physical activity should be structured into the daily hospital routine. Some hospitals use the physical therapy department to assist patients in attempting to mimic

Chart 36-10
Summary: Differences In Nursing Management of Insulin-Dependent Diabetes Mellitus (Type I) and Noninsulin-Dependent Diabetes Mellitus (Type II)

Type I

Insulin-Dependent Diabetes Mellitus (IDDM)

1. Nursing assessment, diagnosis, and treatment should be focused on the state of insulin dependency. There is a greater need for "normalizing" blood glucose because of higher risk of serious long-term complications.
2. Etiology is thought to be less genetic and more viral/autoimmune; therefore, the future role of the nurse might be to encourage susceptible persons to be immunized.
3. Short-term problems involve balancing (avoiding hypoglycemia and hyperglycemia) and "normalizing" blood glucose, on a daily basis.

4. Obesity is usually not a problem. Diet, exercise, and insulin are the management tools available to the patient. These tools need to be thoroughly understood and used by a motivated patient. Patient gains from following the treatment plan, in an attempt to normalize blood glucose, are not always immediate. In addition, current techniques for attaining normal blood glucose values (*e.g.,* multiple injections, insulin pumps) are still far from perfect. Lifetime motivation for this patient is a nursing challenge.
5. There are long-term problems with serious, expensive, and often fatal complications: that is, retinal, renal, neuropathic, and arterial disease (microvascular and macrovascular complications).
6. Because this type is more life-threatening, nursing tends to focus on the acute problems and neglect the potential long-term patient problems. In addition, dealing effectively with a patient who has long-term complications is time-consuming and at times difficult because of the presence at one time of many complications with a poor prognosis.
7. Since this group is such a small percentage of the diabetic population, it is often regarded as "interesting" by nurses. If these patients pay close attention daily to normalizing blood glucose levels and manage to keep blood glucose levels fairly normal, they can avoid hospitalization. Based on nursing research, these patients need a reemphasis on knowledge and skills throughout life. This can have tremendous implications for long-term nursing care, health care costs, patient well-being, and the delay or prevention of long-term complications.

Type II

Noninsulin-Dependent Diabetes Mellitus (NIDDM)

1. Nursing assessment, diagnosis, and treatment should be focused on maintaining effective insulin levels.

2. Familial patterns of more frequent inheritance suggest a strong genetic basis that is greatly influenced by obesity.

3. Short-term problems are related to hyperglycemia and weight control/maintenance. Hyperglycemia related to infection, stress, and surgery may temporarily need to be treated with insulin.
4. Because 80% to 90% of these patients are obese, hyperglycemia and glucose intolerance are usually improved and occasionally reversed with weight reduction.

5. Long-term problems are related to obesity/weight reduction and to an increase in arterial disease (macrovascular). Renal and retinal complications (microvascular) are infrequent but can occur in this type.
6. Noninsulin-dependent diabetes is not especially life-threatening in the short term, but the majority of diabetic patients fall in this class.

their activity at home. This is extremely important, because insulin doses are calculated during hospitalization.

The relationship between diet, exercise, and specific antidiabetic medication must be understood by the patient, regardless of type of diabetes. Hypoglycemia, if experienced in the hospital, should be used as an opportunity to teach the patient about prevention and/or treatment.

Medications for treatment of diabetes should not be omitted by patients because they feel well or ill. In the event

of acute illness, more insulin may be needed by the type I patient because of insulin resistance that occurs temporarily. Many patients who have influenza, for example, feel that insulin should be omitted because of either vomiting or diarrhea. This rationale can easily lead to ketoacidosis.

Careful instruction is given, and special skills are demonstrated and practiced.

The results of the hemoglobin A_{1c} test should be shared with the patient. Positive results (normal values) serve to underscore good self-care practices, while negative results serve as a guide for improvement in some or all aspects of self-care.

Maintaining appropriate blood glucose levels involves close attention to situations that may disrupt normal metabolic processes, such as acute illnesses, menstruation, puberty, menopause, or pregnancy. Frequent blood glucose monitoring and attention by the patient to bodily symptoms warn the patient that some adjustment in diet, exercise, or medication needs to be made. Planning and preventive measures by patient and family need to be emphasized in the initial patient teaching sessions and reemphasized later on in the disease process as the need arises. Problem-solving techniques for the patient and significant others are an important tool for successful self-care management.

Creativity and use of a wide variety of community resources may be necessary for diabetic patients who have limited resources, live alone, or are unable to prepare their own food. Meals On Wheels or other community resources are utilized when appropriate to assure adequate dietary management. The community health nurse works with the patient and family to identify these needs and resources. Follow-up and planning are necessary to assist the patient to manage dietary requirements and to plan for emergencies and other unexpected situations (*e.g.*, failure of community resources to deliver meals during bad weather).

Adherence to the Therapeutic Regimen. Teaching of the knowledge and skills needed by the patient with diabetes will enhance adherence to the prescribed regimen. In addition, motivation must be assessed by the nurse and reinforced, not only during the initial contact with the patient but throughout the course of the disease. This is especially important during periods of stress and crisis, such as adolescence, marriage, attendance at college, or travel. Simplification and flexibility of the treatment regimen will increase adherence. The nurse can assist the patient in identifying barriers to adherence and planning alternatives.

Avoiding Hypoglycemia. Careful daily attention to all aspects of meal planning, exercise, medications, acute illness, and blood glucose monitoring can help in decreasing the incidence of hypoglycemia. In addition, the nurse emphasizes the need for insulin-dependent patients to carry with them at all times some form of simple carbohydrate for use if the need arises. The patient and family members need to be aware of the symptoms and signs of hypoglycemia, ways to differentiate them from those of hyperglycemia, and actions to take. Additionally, patients are urged to carry with them at all times medical identification information to alert others that they have diabetes and are dependent on insulin in case they are unable to convey this information in an emergency.

Avoiding Ketosis/Ketoacidosis. The nurse emphasizes repeatedly the warning signs of hyperglycemia and the need for frequent blood glucose monitoring, especially by the type I patient. The nurse periodically reviews the adjustments the patient should make with respect to diet, exercise, and medication. Most patients need to be reassessed throughout the course of their diabetes, since life events may interfere with self-care management. Information and instructions are provided about actions to take during acute illness to prevent hyperglycemia and ketoacidosis.

Avoiding Long-Term Complications. The nurse reinforces the importance of normoglycemia and its relationship to the prevention or delay of long-term complications. In addition, special attention is focused on the positive approaches the patient may employ. For example, the nurse discourages smoking or helps the patient to "kick the habit." Smoking is known to aggravate peripheral vascular problems. These measures are often difficult to incorporate into daily life with diabetes because of an uncertain future or denial of the possibility of development of the complications. Positive feedback and a system of rewards for the patient who does take the time and effort are important and often neglected components of care.

Maintaining Skin Integrity. The nurse needs to constantly remind *all* patients with diabetes about the importance of checking the skin, particularly the feet. Paying close attention to dry skin, cuts, bruises, and infections by detection and prompt treatment can help to prevent serious problems in the future. Preventive care is best accomplished by the patient on a daily basis. If the patient is obese or has diminished vision, family, friends, or neighbors can often help to perform skin assessments and should be encouraged to do so by the nurse. During hospitalization and clinic, office, or home visits, the nurse also carefully inspects the patient's feet and skin. While performing this assessment, the nurse demonstrates and reinforces the thorough examination that is necessary to detect cuts, calluses, and signs of impaired circulation. The patient's management and care of the skin and feet can also be assessed. The importance of seeking professional care of the feet and care to prevent ingrown nails is emphasized.

Preventing Injury. The presence of retinopathy or other eye diseases that compromise vision can lead to injury. The nurse needs to remind the patient to be mindful of possible sources of injury. It is also important to suggest aids to assist the patient in mobility and prevent injury.

Neuropathy, either alone or with retinopathy, poses special threats as the patient's decreased sensation prevents awareness of injuries.

During home visits, the community health nurse assesses the patient's home environment to identify potential sources of injury. Small rugs, slippery floors, hazardous electrical cords, and other objects in the home that may pose risks to the patient and others are identified. Alterations are made to promote a safe environment. Careful attention is given to the kitchen and bathroom, sites of many home accidents.

Enhancing Coping Strategies. Denial in the early stages of the disease is common and indeed may persist and interfere with self-care. Denial may serve initially to alleviate anxiety, but if it persists may be pathological. It is important for the nurse to discuss the issues openly with the patient and perhaps family members. The patient may need time to accept the diagnosis before treatment can be discussed. Often this period of time extends beyond the period of hospitalization. It is therefore important to plan for adequate home follow-up. Referral to classes for people with diabetes, to be attended after discharge, can be useful. Equally important is referral to support groups conducted by health care agencies in the community. Because diabetes is a chronic disease and demands long-term cooperation and responsibility on the part of patients, it is imperative that the nurse help patients to incorporate diabetes care into their life-styles rather than change life-styles because of the diabetes care regimen.

In addition to problems with daily aspects of living with diabetes, the development of one or many of the long-term complications also offers opportunities for denial. Again, these

Chart 36-11
Patient Education for Diabetes Mellitus (Expected Outcomes)

The person with diabetes mellitus must accept a major role in the management of the disease. Education must be amplified, reinforced, and updated continuously, because diabetes is a life-long disease.

Objective: To maintain the best possible control of diabetes

Patient's Expected Outcomes

A. Patient describes diabetes and how it affects the body.
   1. Visits the physician on a regular basis
   2. Studies and reviews available literature from reputable sources
   3. Secures booklets and pamphlets from the American Diabetes Association (see bibliography for address)
   4. Attends available classes
B. Maintains health at an optimal level
   1. Maintains a consistent daily routine
   2. Gets adequate rest and sleep
   3. Exercises regularly and consistently
      a. Avoids "spurts" of arduous exercise before meals
      b. Exercises after meals
      c. Keeps some form of carbohydrate (sugar, candy, orange juice) available during exercise periods
      d. Takes extra food for extra physical activity
   4. Seeks employment with regular hours when possible; adjusts diet and medication to work schedule
   5. Has teeth and gums checked regularly for periodontal disease
C. Follows the prescribed dietary regimen
   1. Eats 3 or more regularly spaced meals each day, timed to coincide with the action of insulin
   2. Becomes thoroughly familiar with the food exchange lists
   3. Learns how to follow a calculated diet
   4. Uses household measures or a gram scale until serving sizes can be judged accurately
   5. Avoids concentrated carbohydrates
   6. Avoids periods of fasting and feasting
   7. Keeps weight at optimal level; normalizes body weight
      a. Weighs weekly
      b. Keeps a weight record
   8. If taking insulin, eats extra calories when unusual physical activity is anticipated
   9. Eats a bedtime snack when taking insulin, if prescribed
   10. Avoids foods high in cholesterol
D. Utilizes measures to determine the degree of diabetic control
   1. Tests blood for glucose at specified intervals
   2. Tests urine for ketones when blood sugar evaluations are high or during periods of illness
   3. Knows that acetone in the urine indicates need for *more insulin*
   4. Protects all urine testing equipment from light, moisture, and heat (to prevent false interpretation due to deterioration of test materials)

E. Utilizes proper practices of insulin therapy
   1. Knows when the prescribed insulin is having its peak action
   2. Adjusts insulin dosage according to blood sugar test, as prescribed
   3. Rotates the sites of insulin injections in a systematic manner
   4. Keeps a reserve supply of insulin in the refrigerator; is aware of expiration date on bottle
      a. Keeps bottle in current use at *room temperature*
      b. Avoids injecting cold insulin, because it may contribute to tissue reaction
   5. Has extra syringes available
   6. Avoids conditions that produce insulin reactions
      a. Omission or delay of a meal
      b. Unaccustomed or strenuous exercise
      c. Too much insulin
   7. Recognizes symptoms of an insulin reaction
      a. Any unfamiliar or peculiar sensation
      b. Hunger, perspiration, weakness, tremor, pallor, palpitation, tachycardia
   8. Takes precautions to prevent an insulin reaction
      a. Eats carbohydrates (orange juice, sugar, candy) when symptoms first occur
      b. Tests blood
      c. Carries extra carbohydrate at all times (sugar lumps, candy)
      d. Eats extra carbohydrates before strenuous exercise and during periods of prolonged exercise, or reduces insulin dosage
      e. Eats a snack at bedtime if prescribed.
   9. Keeps a check-off system, to ensure taking insulin
   10. Wears identification bracelet or necklace
   11. When traveling, carries diabetic supplies in hand luggage
      a. Has letter from physician confirming diagnosis of diabetes and prescription for extra syringes
      b. Keeps watch from the time-of-departure point until arrival at destination; does not change diabetic regimen en route
F. Takes prescribed oral hypoglycemic medication
   1. Adheres faithfully to the prescribed diet
   2. Tests urine daily
   3. Takes the medication exactly as directed
G. Practices proper foot care to prevent infection
   1. Inspects feet carefully and routinely for calluses, corns, blisters, cracks, abrasions, redness, and nail abnormalities
      a. Uses a small mirror to check bottom of each foot (if unable to see foot)

(continued)

Chart 36-11 *(continued)*

Patient's Expected Outcomes

  b. Uses a magnifying glass under good light if eyesight is poor, or has someone else check feet
2. Bathes feet daily in warm (never hot) water
   a. Does not soak feet for prolonged periods
   b. Dries feet carefully, especially between toes
3. Massages feet with a lubricating lotion, except between toes
4. Prevents moisture between toes, to avert maceration of skin
   a. Inserts lamb's wool between overlapping toes
   b. Uses powder in the web spaces, especially if feet perspire
5. Wears well-fitting, noncompressive shoes and socks—long enough, wide enough, soft, supple, and low-heeled
   a. Buys shoes in the afternoon—feet are larger in the afternoon than in the morning
   b. Has each foot measured before buying shoes—feet enlarge with age
   c. Has the measurement taken while standing, since foot is larger in the standing position
   d. Does not "break in" shoes all at one time
   e. Checks shoes repeatedly for protruding nails
   f. Avoids rubber- or plastic-soled shoes, which cause feet to perspire and may lead to fungal infections
   g. Avoids working in bedroom slippers or other casual foot attire
6. Goes to a podiatrist on a regular basis if corns, calluses, and ingrown toenails are present
   a. Cuts toenails straight across, to prevent ingrown toenails
7. Avoids heat, chemicals, and injuries to the feet—does not go barefoot or expose feet to hot water bottles, heating pads, caustic solutions, etc.
   a. Switches off electric blanket before going to bed; wears socks at night to keep feet warm, if necessary
   b. Avoids overheated baths and sitting too close to the fire
8. If an injury occurs to the foot:
   a. Washes the area with mild soap and water

  b. Covers with a dry, sterile dressing, *without* adhesive
  c. Wears white socks—dye in colored socks and wool serves as an irritant when skin is already irritated
  d. Consults physician
H. Maintains diabetic control during periods of illness
   1. Calls physician immediately when any unusual symptoms become evident; does not allow diabetes to get out of control
   2. Makes dietary adjustments during illness according to physician's directions
   3. Continues taking insulin; physician may increase dosage during illness
   4. Monitors blood glucose
   5. Tests urine for acetone more frequently; keeps records
   6. Describes the conditions that bring about diabetic acidosis
      a. Nausea and vomiting
      b. Failure to increase insulin when blood sugar is increasing
      c. Failure to take insulin
      d. Dietary excesses
      e. Infections
      f. Stress
   7. Takes precautions to prevent impending diabetic acidosis
      a. Examines urine for acetone, and reports results to physician
      b. Takes additional insulin as advised by physician
      c. Goes to bed and keeps warm
      d. Alerts someone to be in attendance
      e. Drinks a glass of liquid hourly, if possible
      f. Ensures oral intake of enough calories to prevent sudden drop in blood sugar
I. Follows other health directives
   1. Avoids tobacco—nicotine constricts blood vessels, causing reduction in blood flow to feet
   2. Reports excessive itching—may indicate elevated blood sugar
   3. Takes only medications prescribed by physician—many drugs enhance effect of insulin and oral antidiabetic agents

need to be resolved by the patient with the assistance of other professionals as coordinated by the nurse.

Some of the other responses seen in patients attempting to cope with the diagnosis include anxiety, questioning, ambivalence, suspicion, hostility, regression, loneliness, and rejection. The nurse's role is to identify the existence of any of these behaviors, assist patient and family in dealing with them, and help to incorporate the illness into a wellness role for the person with diabetes. The success of this process depends on the coping strategies already developed by the patient in other areas of life.

Improving Sexual Function.   Asking about details of sexual practice and functioning is an important part of the nurse's assessment and subsequent patient teaching of both

men and women with diabetes. It is probably best to begin with general questions. If the answers to the general sex questions do not elicit enough information, the nurse should ask if there are any problems.

If the patient or partner indicates that sexual function or the level of sexuality has changed and is unsatisfactory, further evaluation is indicated. Diabetes and diabetic neuropathy are not the only causes of altered sexual function in diabetic patients; further evaluation may detect other causes that require or would benefit from treatment unrelated to diabetes. Sexual counselling may be indicated to encourage the couple to discuss their concerns openly with each other, to identify additional or alternative means of sexual expression, or to explore some of the definitive modes of therapy for sexual dysfunction such as penile implants. The importance of sexual function and sexuality to the patient and spouse should be respected regardless of the age of the patient.

▷ *Evaluation*

▷ *Expected Outcomes*
(Refer to outcomes in Chart 36-11.)

Bibliography

Books

American Diabetes Association. Diabetes in the Family. Bowie, Maryland, Robert J Brady, 1982.

American Diabetes Association and The American Dietetic Association. A Guide for Professionals: The Effective Application of "Exchange Lists for Meal Planning." New York, 1977.

American Diabetes Association and The American Dietetic Association. Family Cookbook, Vol II. Englewood Cliffs, New Jersey, Prentice-Hall, 1984.

American Diabetes Association and The American Dietetic Association. Exchange List for Meal Planning. Alexandria, Virginia, 1986.

Bernstein R. Diabetes: The Glucograf Method for Normalizing Blood Sugar. New York, Crown Publishers, 1981.

Bierman J and Toohey B. The Diabetic's Sport and Exercise Book: How to Play Your Way to Better Health. Philadelphia, JB Lippincott, 1977.

Bierman J and Toohey B, The Diabetic's Book: All Your Questions Answered. Los Angeles, JP Tarcher, 1981.

Bradoff B and Bleicher S (eds). Diabetes Mellitus and Obesity. Baltimore, Williams & Wilkins, 1982.

Bressler R and Johnson D (eds). Management of Diabetes Mellitus. Boston, John Wright–PSG, 1982.

Christy A and Germann J. Diabetes: Recipes for Health. Bowie, Maryland, Robert J Brady,1983.

Davidson M. Diabetes Mellitus: Diagnosis and Treatment, 2nd ed. New York, John Wiley & Sons, 1986.

Ellenberg M and Rifkin H. Diabetes Mellitus, 3rd ed. New Hyde Park, Medical Examination, 1983.

Feste C. The physician within: Taking charge of your well-being. Wayzata, Minnesota, Diabetes Center, Inc., 1987.

Guthrie D and Guthrie R (eds). Nursing Management of Diabetes Mellitus, 2nd ed. St Louis, CV Mosby, 1982.

Hamburg B et al (eds). Behavioral and Psychosocial Issues in Diabetes: Proceedings of the National Conference. U.S. Department of Health and Human Services, NIH Publication No. 80-1993, 1979.

Kahn AP. Diabetes Control and the Kosher Diet. Skokie, Illinois, Word-scope Associates, 1985.

Kivelowitz T. Diabetes: A Guide to Self-Management for Patients and Their Families. Englewood Cliffs, New Jersey, Prentice-Hall, 1981.

Kozak GP. Clinical Diabetes Mellitus. Philadelphia, WB Saunders, 1982.

Peterson C and Jovanovic L. The Diabetes Self-Care Method. New York, Simon & Schuster, 1984.

Podolsky S (ed). Clinical Diabetes: Modern Management. New York, Appleton-Century-Crofts, 1980.

Rifkin H and Raskin P (eds). Diabetes Mellitus, Vol V. Bowie, Maryland, Robert J Brady, 1981.

Steiner G and Lawrence P (eds). Educating Diabetic Patients. New York, Springer-Verlag, 1981.

Strauss A and Corbin J. Chronic Illness and the Quality of Life, 2nd ed. St Louis, CV Mosby, 1984.

Tupling H et al. You've Got to Get Through the Outside Layer: A Handbook for Health Educators, Using Diabetes as a Model. Sydney, New South Wales, Royal North Shore Hospital, 1981.

Van Son A (ed). Diabetes and Patient Education: A Daily Nursing Challenge. New York, Appleton-Century-Crofts, 1982.

Articles

Agner E et al. Impaired glucose tolerance and diabetes in elderly subjects. Diabetes Care 1982 Nov/Dec; 5(6):600–604.

Alogna M. Perceptions of severity of disease and health locus of control in compliant and noncompliant diabetic patient. Diabetes Care 1980 July/Aug; 3(4):523–524.

American Diabetes Association. The UGDP controversy: Policy statement. Diabetes Care 1979 Jan/Feb; 2(1):1–3.

American Diabetes Association. Indications for use of continuous insulin delivery systems and self-measurement of blood glucose: Policy statement. Diabetes Care 1982 Mar/Apr; 5(2):140–141.

American Diabetes Association. Glycemic effects of carbohydrates: Policy statement. Diabetes Care 1984; 7(6):607.

American Diabetes Association. Continuous subcutaneous insulin infusion: Policy statement. Diabetes Care 1985; 8:516.

Anderson JW and Ward K. Long-term effects of high-carbohydrate, high-fiber diets on glucose and lipid metabolism: A preliminary report on patients with diabetes. Diabetes Care, 1978 Mar/Apr; 1(2):77–82.

Barbosa J et al. Long-term, ambulatory, subcutaneous insulin infusion versus multiple daily injections in brittle diabetic patients. Diabetes Care 1981 Mar/Apr; 4(2):269–274.

Blankenship GW and Skyler JS. Diabetic retinopathy: A general survey. Diabetes Care 1978 Mar/Apr; 1(2):127–137.

Bodansky HJ et al. Risk factors associated with severe proliferative retinopathy in insulin-dependent diabetes mellitus. Diabetes Care 1982 Mar/Apr; 5(2):97–100.

Boyles V. Injection aids for blind diabetic patients. Am J Nurs 1977 Sept; 77(9):1456–1458.

Cianciola LJ et al. Prevalence of periodontal disease in insulin-dependent diabetes mellitus (juvenile diabetes). J Am Dent Assoc 1982 May; 104(5):653–660.

Clements R and Vourganti B. Fatal diabetic ketoacidosis: Major causes and approaches to their prevention. Diabetes Care 1978 Sept/Oct; 1(5):314–325.

Colwell J et al. Pathogenesis of atherosclerosis in diabetes mellitus. Diabetes Care 1981 Jan/Feb; 4(1):121–133.

Coughlin WR et al. Diabetes retinopathy. Diabetes Forecast 1978 Nov/Dec; 31(6):26–28.

Crapo, PA. Theory vs. fact: The glycemic response to foods. Nutrition Today 1984 Mar/April; 19(2):6–11.

Crapo PA and Olefsky JM. Food fallacies and blood sugar. N Engl J Med 1983 July 7; 309(1):44–45.

Cryer PE and Gerich JE. Glucose counterregulation, hypoglycemia, and intensive therapy of diabetes mellitus. N Engl J Med 1985 July 25; 313(4):232–241.

Danowski T et al. Diabetic complications and their prevention or reversal. Diabetes Care 1980 Jan/Feb; 3(1):94–99.

Davis W et al. Factors affecting the educational diagnosis of diabetes patients. Diabetes Care Mar/Apr; 4(2):275–278.

DeFronzo R. Glucose intolerance and aging. Diabetes Care 1981 July/Aug; 4(4):493–501.

Doody R and Grose N. The family medical history: Assessing patient understanding of diabetes mellitus. Diabetes Care 1981 Mar/Apr; 4(2):285–288.

Dyck PJ. The causes, classification, and treatment of peripheral neuropathy. N Engl J Med 1982 July 29; 307(5):283–286.

Eisenbarth GS. Type I diabetes mellitus: A chronic autoimmune disease. N Engl J Med 1986 May 22; 314(21):1360–1368.

Ellenberg M. Sex and diabetes: A comparison between men and women. Diabetes Care 1979 Jan/Feb; 2(1):4–8.

Ewing DJ and Clarke BF. Diabetic autonomic neuropathy: Present insights and future prospects. Diabetes Care 1986 Nov/Dec; 9(6):648–665.

Funnell MM and McNitt P. Autonomic neuropathy: Diabetics' hidden foe. Am J Nurs 1986 Mar; 86(3):266–270.

Graber A et al. Planning for sex, marriage, contraception, and pregnancy. Diabetes Care 1978 May/June; 1(3):202–203.

Hauser S and Pollets D. Psychological aspects of diabetes: A critical review. Diabetes Care 1979 Mar/Apr; 2(2):227–232.

Jackson C. Diabetes: How your patient looks at it. Nursing '81 1981 May; 11(5):82–83.

Jenkins DJA et al. The glycemic index of foods tested in diabetic patients: A new basis for carbohydrate exchange favouring the use of legumes. Diabetologia 1983 Apr; 24(4):257–264.

Jensen SB. Diabetic sexual dysfunction: A comparative study of 160 insulin-treated diabetic men and women and an age-matched control group. Arch Sex Behav 1981 Dec; 10(6):493–504.

Kahn CR. Insulin resistance: A common feature of diabetes mellitus. N Engl J Med 1986 July 24; 315(4):252–254.

Keon H and Hanna A. Self-administration of insulin by a hemiplegic individual. Diabetes Care 1980 Nov/Dec; 3(6):705.

Kolata G. Diabetics should lose weight, avoid diet fads. Science 1987 Jan 9; 235(4785):163–164.

Korvisto VA and Felig P. Effects of leg exercise on insulin absorption in diabetic patients. N Engl J Med 1987 Jan 12; 298(2):279–283.

LaCroix A et al. Coffee consumption and the incidence of coronary heart disease. N Engl J Med 1986 Oct 16; 315(6):977–982.

Leichter S et al. Readability of self-care instructional pamphlets for diabetic patients. Diabetes Care 1981 Nov/Dec; 4(6):627–630.

Levine E. Nutritional care of patients with renal failure and diabetes. J Am Diet Assn 1982 Sep; 81(3):261–267.

Liang JC and Goldberg MF. Review: Treatment of diabetic retinopathy. Diabetes 1980 Oct; 29(10):841–851.

Lipson L. Diabetes and hypertension. Diabetes Forecast 1985 May/June; 53–54:74.

Madsbad S et al. Influence of smoking on insulin requirement and metabolic status in diabetes mellitus. Diabetes Care 1980 Jan/Feb; 3(1):41–43.

McCarthy J. Diabetic nephropathy. Am J Nurs 1981 Nov; 81(11):2030–2034.

Mecklenburg RS et al. Long-term metabolic control with insulin pump therapy: Report of experience with 127 patients. N Engl J Med 1985 Aug 22; 313(8):465–468.

Medalie J. Risk factors other than hyperglycemia in diabetic macrovascular disease. Diabetes Care 1979 Mar/Apr; 2(2):77–84.

Nadig PW et al. Noninvasive device to produce and maintain an erectionlike state. Urology 1986 Feb; 27(2):126–131.

National Diabetes Data Group: Classification of diabetes mellitus and other categories of glucose intolerance. Diabetes 1979 Dec; 28(7):1039–1051.

Nemchik R. Diabetes today: A startling new body of knowledge. RN 1982 Oct; 45(10):31–37.

Nemchik R. Diabetes today: A very different diet: a new generation of oral drugs. RN 1982 Nov; 45(11):41–45, 97–99.

Nemchik R. Diabetes today: The news about insulin. RN 1982 Dec; 45(12):49–54.

Nemchik R. Diabetes today: The new insulin pumps: Tight control—at a price. RN 1983 May; 46(5):52–59.

Nemchik R. Diabetes today: Diabetic retinopathy: The current status of therapy. RN 1983 June; 46(6):34–63.

Nemchik R. Diabetes today: Facing up to the long-term complications. RN 1983 July: 46(7):38–45.

Nemchik R. Educating the older diabetic. The Diabetes Educator 1983; 9(Special Issue):41–44.

Nuttal FQ and Brunzell JD. Principles of nutrition and dietary recommendations for individuals with diabetes. Diabetes 1979 Nov; 28(11):1027–1030.

Page P et al. Patient recall of self-care recommendations in diabetes. Diabetes Care 1981 Jan/Feb; 4(1):96–98.

Pietri A and Raskin P . Cutaneous complications of chronic continuous subcutaneous insulin infusion therapy. Diabetes Care 1981 Nov/Dec; 4(6):624–626.

Plasse N. Monitoring blood glucose at home: A comparison of three products. Am J Nurs 1981 Nov; 81(11):2028–2029.

Prater B. Education guidelines for self-care living with diabetes. J Am Diet Assoc 1983 Mar; 82(3):283–286.

Robertson C. How to teach patients to monitor blood glucose. RN 1985 Dec; 48(12):24–25.

Resler MM and Bovington MM. Symposium on diabetes mellitus. Nurs Clin North Am 1983 Dec; 18(4):615–825.

Rosenberg C. Insulin pump therapy for older adults: Case report. Diabetes Educator 1986 Spring; 12(2):110–112.

Rotter J et al. Diabetes mellitus: The search for genetic markers. Diabetes Care 1979 Mar/Apr; 2(2):215–226.

Sanborn C et al. Shift work: How to adjust patterns of diabetes care. Occup Health Nurs 1982 Dec; 30(12):25–28.

Schade D and Eaton RP. Pathogenesis of diabetic ketoacidosis: A reappraisal. Diabetes Care 1979 May/June; 2(3):296–306.

Schade D et al. Future therapy of the insulin-dependent diabetic patient—the implantable insulin delivery system. Diabetes Care 1981 Mar/Apr; 4(2):319–327.

Schiffrin A and Belmonte MM. Comparison between continuous subcutaneous insulin infusion and multiple injections of insulin: A one-year prospective study. Diabetes 1982 Mar; 31(3):255–264.

Schlenk EA and Hart LK. Relationship between health locus of control, health value, and social support and compliance of persons with diabetes mellitus. Diabetes Care 1984 Nov/Dec; 7(6):566–574.

Sheppard M and Wright AD. The effect on mortality of low-dose insulin therapy for diabetic ketoacidosis. Diabetes Care 1982 Mar/Apr; 5(2):111–113.

Skyler J. The spectrum of insulin resistance. Diabetes Care 1979 May/June; 2(3):319–322.

Skyler JS. Diabetes and exercise: Clinical implications. Diabetes Care 1979 May/June; 2(3):307–311.

Skyler JS. Complications of diabetes mellitus: Relationship to metabolic dysfunction. Diabetes Care 1979 Nov/Dec; 2(6):499–509.

Skyler J et al. Algorithms for adjustment of insulin dosage by patients who monitor blood glucose. Diabetes Care 1981 Mar/Apr; 4(2):311–318.

Stiller CR et al. Effects of cyclosporine immunosuppression in insulin-dependent diabetes of recent onset. Science 1984 Mar 30; 223(4643):1362–1367.

Streja D et al. Nutritional therapy in noninsulin-dependent diabetes mellitus. Diabetes Care 1981 Jan/Feb; 4(1):81–84.

Sutherland D et al. Pancreas transplantation—an historical overview and its current status. Diabetes Educator 1982 Spring; 8(1):11–13.

Taub S et al. Gastrointestinal manifestations of diabetes mellitus. Diabetes Care 1979 Sept/Oct; 2(5):437–447.

Taylor A and Cox D. Job stress: Its impact on the diabetic worker. Occup Health Nurs 1982 Dec; 30(12):29–32.

Tyrer G et al. Sexual responsiveness in diabetic women. Diabetologia 1983 Mar; 24(3):166–171.

Unger R. Meticulous control of diabetes: Benefits, risks, and precautions. Diabetes 1982 June; 31(6):479–483.

U.S. Department of Health and Human Services. Diabetic neuropathies. NIH Publication No. 79-1641, 1979.

Villeneuve ME et al. Dental care for the person with diabetes mellitus. Diabetes Educator 1986 Fall; 11(3):44–47.

Weinrauch S and Tomky D. Commonly-asked questions about pump therapy. Diabetes Educator 1983 Spring; 9(1):30–31.

White NH et al. Identification of Type I diabetic patients at increased risk for hypoglycemia during intensive therapy. N Engl J Med 1983 Mar 3; 308(9):485–491.

Winegrad AS et al. Has one diabetic complication been explained? N Engl J Med 1983 Jan 20; 308(3):152–154.

Manuals

American Diabetes Association, Clinical Education Program. The Physician's Guide to Type II Diabetes (NIDDM): Diagnosis and Treatment. New York, American Diabetes Association, 1984.

Diabetes in America: Diabetes data compiled in 1984. National Diabetes Data Group, U.S. Department of Health and Human Services, National Institutes of Health, National Institute of Arthritis, Diabetes, and Digestive and Kidney Diseases. NIH Publication No. 85-1468, August 1985.

Emergency Personnel Program. New York, Amerian Diabetes Association, 1985.

Feet First: A Booklet About Foot Care for Older People and People Who Have Diabetes. U.S. Department of Health, Education and Welfare, 1970.

National Diabetes Advisory Board. The Prevention and Treatment of Five Complications of Diabetes: A Guide for the Primary Care Practitioner. Bethesda, Maryland, National Diabetes Advisory Board, 1983.

National Diabetes Advisory Board. Diabetes 1986 Annual Report. U.S. Department of Health and Human Services, Public Health Service, National Institutes of Health, NIH Publication No. 86-1587, April 1986.

Patient and Professional Education Guidelines. Atlanta, Centers for Disease Control, Center for Prevention Services, Division of Diabetes Control, 1983.

Reeves-Ellington D (ed). Blood Glucose Monitoring: For the Phases of Your Life. New York, Health Education Technologies, 1986.

Agencies

Voluntary

American Association of Diabetes Educators, 500 North Michigan Avenue, Suite 1400, Chicago, IL 60611.

American Diabetes Association, Diabetes Information Service Center, 1660 Duke Street, Alexandria, VA 22314.

American Dietetic Association, 430 North Michigan Avenue, Chicago, IL 60611.

American Foundation for the Blind, 15 West 16th Street, New York, NY 10011.

Independent Living Aids, 1500 New Horizons Boulevard, Amityville, NY 11701.

Joslin Diabetes Foundation, One Joslin Place, Boston, MA 02215.

Juvenile Diabetes Foundation International, 23 East 26th Street, New York, NY 10010.

Government

National Diabetes Data Group, National Institutes of Health, Bethesda, MD 20892.

National Diabetes Information Clearinghouse, Box NDIC, Bethesda, MD 20892.

Selected Resources for the Person With Diabetes With Visual Impairment

American Foundation for the Blind, 15 West 16th Street, New York, NY 10011. (Catalog of devices, vision aids, insulin syringes.)

Braille Volunteers of Huntington, P.O. Box 9422, Huntington, WV 25704. (Exchange Lists in braille and basic information about diabetes.)

Iowa Commission for the Blind, 4th and Ecoway, Des Moines, IA 60309. (Exchange lists in large print.)

Library of Congress, Division for the Blind and Physically Handicapped, 1291 Taylor Street, N.W., Washington, DC 20542.

Meditec, 9485 East Orchard Drive, Englewood, CO 80110. (Insulin gauges for visually handicapped.)

Office of Vocational Rehabilitation. (Check your own state office.)

Seeing Eye Dog, Washington Valley Road, Morristown, NJ 07960.

Social Security Administration. (Check your local office.)

Chapter 37

Assessment and Management of Patients With Endocrine Disorders

Physiologic Overview

Endocrine glands, which secrete their products directly into the bloodstream, are clearly differentiated from exocrine glands, such as sweat glands, which secrete through ducts onto epithelial surfaces. The chemical substances secreted by the endocrine glands are called *hormones*. Hormones help to regulate organ function in concert with the nervous system. This dual regulatory system, in which rapid action by the nervous system is balanced by slower hormonal action, permits precise control of body function in response to varied changes within and outside the body.

There are steroid hormones, such as hydrocortisone; peptide or protein hormones, such as insulin; and amine hormones, such as epinephrine. These different classes of hormones act on the target tissues by different mechanisms, as discussed below. A schematic diagram of the important endocrine glands is shown in Figure 37-1. Table 37-1 lists the important hormones, their target tissue, and some of their properties.

Certain anatomical features are common to the endocrine glands. The glands are composed of secretory cells arranged in minute clusters (acini). No ducts are present, but the glands have a rich blood supply, so that the chemicals they produce can rapidly enter the bloodstream.

The concentration in the bloodstream of most hormones is maintained at a relatively constant level. If the hormone concentration rises, further production of that hormone is inhibited. When the hormone concentration falls, the rate of production of that hormone increases. This mechanism for regulation of hormone concentration in the bloodstream is called *feedback control*. The principle of feedback control is important in the regulation of many biologic processes.

Mechanism of Hormone Action.   Hormones can alter the function of the target tissue by interacting with chemical receptors located either on the cell membrane or in the interior of the cell. Peptide and protein hormones interact with receptor sites on the cell surface, which results in the stimulation of the intracellular enzyme adenyl cyclase. This in turn results in increased production of cyclic 3',5'-adenosine monophosphate (cyclic AMP). The cyclic AMP inside the cell

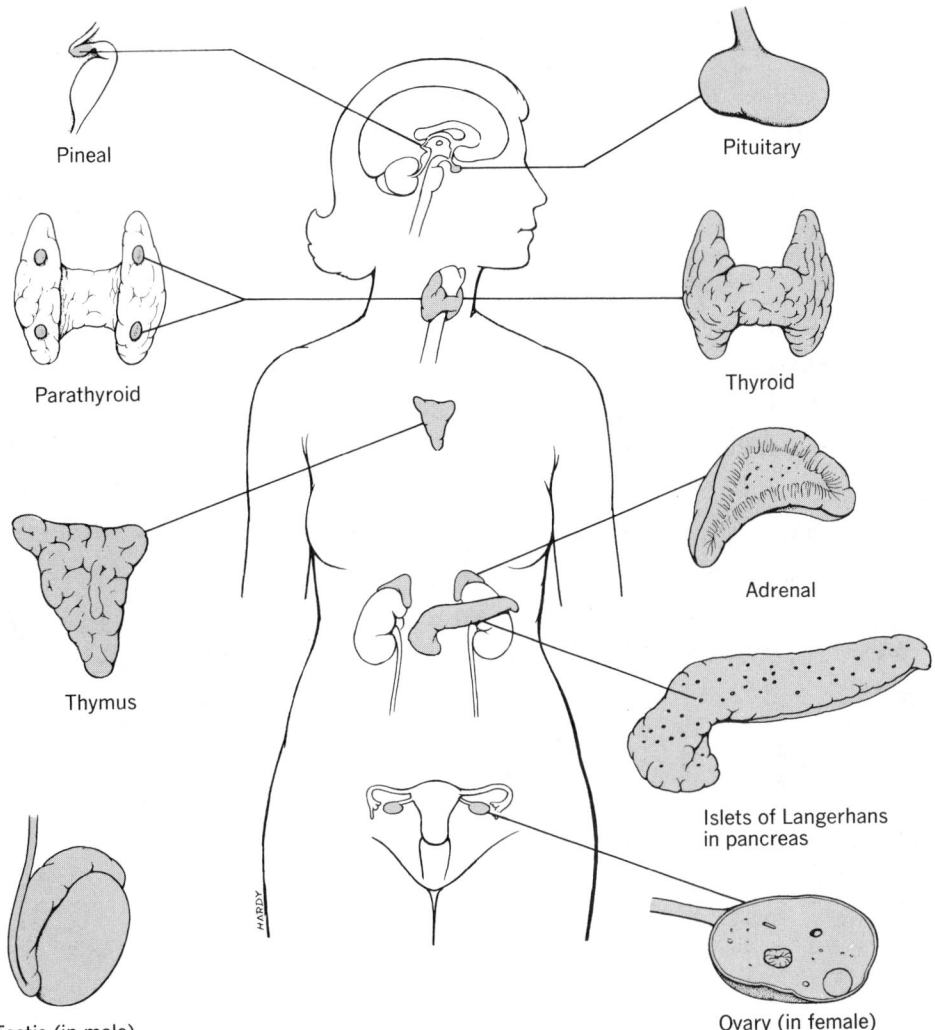

Figure 37-1
General location of the major endocrine glands. (Chaffee EE and Greisheimer EM. Basic Physiology and Anatomy, 4th ed. Philadelphia, JB Lippincott.)

alters enzyme activity. Thus, cyclic AMP is the "second messenger" that links the peptide hormone at the cell surface to a change in the intracellular environment. Some of the protein and peptide hormones may also act by changing membrane permeability. These hormones act relatively rapidly, within seconds or minutes. The mechanism of action for amine hormones is similar to that for peptide hormones.

Because of their smaller size and higher lipid solubility, steroid hormones penetrate the cell membranes and interact with intracellular receptors. This steroid-receptor complex modifies cell metabolism and formation of messenger ribonucleic acid (RNA) from deoxyribonucleic acid (DNA). The messenger RNA then stimulates protein synthesis within the cell. Steroid hormones, because they exert their action by the modification of protein synthesis, require several hours in order to exert their effects.

The Pituitary Gland

The pituitary gland, or the hypophysis, has been referred to as the "master gland" of the endocrine system. It secretes hormones that, in turn, control the secretion of hormones by other endocrine glands. The pituitary itself is controlled in large part by the hypothalamus, an adjacent area of the brain.

The pituitary gland is a round structure about 1.27 cm ($\frac{1}{2}$ inch) in diameter located on the inferior aspect of the brain and connected to the hypothalamus by the pituitary stalk. The pituitary gland is divided into anterior, intermediate, and posterior lobes.

The important hormones secreted by the posterior lobe of the pituitary gland are *vasopressin* (antidiuretic hormone [ADH]) and *oxytocin*. These hormones are synthesized in the hypothalamus and travel down the nerve cells that connect the hypothalamus to the posterior pituitary gland, where they are stored. Vasopressin secretion is stimulated by an increase in the osmolality of the blood or by a decrease in blood pressure. The primary function of vasopressin is to control the excretion of water by the kidney. Oxytocin secretion is stimulated during pregnancy and at the time of childbirth. The primary functions of oxytocin are to facilitate milk ejection during lactation and to increase the force of uterine contractions during labor and delivery. Exogenous oxytocin can be used therapeutically to initiate labor.

The important hormones of the anterior pituitary gland are follicle-stimulating hormone (FSH), luteinizing hormone (LH), prolactin, adrenocorticotropic hormone (ACTH), thyroid-stimulating hormone (TSH), and growth hormone. The secretion of each of these major hormones is controlled by

TABLE 37-1
Endocrine System in Summary

Endocrine Gland and Hormone	Principal Site of Action	Principal Processes Affected
Pituitary Gland		
Anterior Lobe		
Growth hormone (somatotropin)	General	Growth of bones, muscles, and other organs
Thyrotropin	Thyroid	Growth and secretory activity of thyroid gland
Adrenocorticotropin	Adrenal cortex	Growth and secretory activity of adrenal cortex
Follicle-stimulating	Ovaries	Development of follicles and secretion of estrogen
	Testes	Development of seminiferous tubules, spermatogenesis
Luteinizing or interstitial cell stimulating	Ovaries	Ovulation, formation of corpus luteum, secretion of progesterone
	Testes	Secretion of testosterone
Prolactin or lactogenic (luteotropin)	Mammary glands and ovaries	Secretion of milk; maintenance of corpus luteum
Melanocyte-stimulating	Skin	Pigmentation (?)
Posterior Lobe	Kidney	Reabsorption of water; water balance
Antiduiretic (vasopressin)	Arterioles	Blood pressure (?)
Oxytocin	Uterus	Contraction
	Breast	Expression of milk
Pineal Gland		
Melatonin	Gonads (?)	Sexual maturation (?)
Thyroid Gland		
Thyroxine and triiodothyronine	General	Metabolic rate; growth and development; intermediate metabolism
Thyrocalcitonin	Bone	Inhibits bone resorption; lowers blood level of calcium
Parathyroid Glands		
Parathormone	Bone, kidney, intestine	Promotes bone resorption; increases absorption of calcium; raises blood calcium level
Adrenal Glands		
Cortex		
Mineralocorticoids (*e.g.,* aldosterone)	Kidney	Reabsorption of sodium; elimination of potassium
Glucocorticoids (*e.g.,* cortisol)	General	Metabolism of carbohydrate, protein, and fat; response to stress; anti-inflammatory
Sex hormones	General (?)	Preadolescent growth spurt (?)
Medulla		
Epinephrine	Cardiac muscle, smooth muscle, glands	Emergency functions: same as stimulation of sympathetic system
Norepinephrine	Organs innervated by sympathetic system	Chemical transmitter substance; increases peripheral resistance
Islet Cells of Pancreas		
Insulin	General	Lowers blood sugar; utilization and storage of carbohydrate; decreased gluconeogenesis
Glucagon	Liver	Raises blood sugar; glycogenolysis

(continued)

TABLE 37-1 (continued)

Endocrine Gland and Hormone	Principal Site of Action	Principal Processes Affected
Islet Cells of Pancreas		
Somatostatin	General	Lowers blood sugar by interfering with release of growth hormone and glucagon
Testes		
Testosterone	General	Development of secondary sex characteristics
	Reproductive organs	Development and maintenance; normal function
Ovaries		
Estrogens	General	Development of secondary sex characteristics
	Mammary glands	Development of duct system
	Reproductive organs	Maturation and normal cyclic function
Progesterone	Mammary glands	Development of secretory tissue
	Uterus	Preparation for implantation; maintenance of pregnancy
Gastrointestinal Tract		
Gastrin	Stomach	Production of gastric juice
Enterogastrone	Stomach	Inhibits secretion and motility
Secretin	Liver and pancreas	Production of bile; production of watery pancreatic juice (rich in $NaHCO_3$)
Pancreozymin	Pancreas	Production of pancreatic juice rich in enzymes
Cholecystokinin	Gallbladder	Contraction and emptying

(Chaffee EE and Greisheimer EM. Basic Physiology and Anatomy, 4th ed. Philadelphia, JB Lippincott.)

releasing factors (RF) that are secreted by the hypothalamus. These releasing factors reach the anterior pituitary by way of the bloodstream in a special circulation called the pituitary portal blood system.

The hormones released by the anterior pituitary enter the general circulation and are transported to their target organs. TSH, ACTH, FSH, and LH have as their main function the release of hormones from other endocrine glands. Prolactin acts on the breast to stimulate milk production. Growth hormone has widespread effects on many target tissues and is discussed below. The other trophic hormones will be discussed in conjunction with their target organs.

Growth Hormone. Growth hormone, also referred to as somatotropin, is a protein hormone that increases protein synthesis in many tissues, increases the breakdown of fatty acids in adipose tissue, and increases the glucose levels in the blood. These actions of somatotropin are essential for normal growth, although other hormones, such as thyroid hormone and insulin, are required as well. The secretion of growth hormone is increased by stress, exercise, and low blood sugar. The half-time of growth hormone activity in the bood is 20 to 30 minutes. It is largely inactivated in the liver. If secretion of growth hormone is insufficient during childhood, generalized limited growth and dwarfism result. Conversely, oversecretion during childhood results in gigantism,

with a person reaching 7 or even 8 feet in height. Excess growth hormone in adults results in deformities of bone and soft tissue and enlargement of viscera (acromegaly) but no increase in height.

Abnormal Pituitary Function. Abnormalities of pituitary function are caused by oversecretion or undersecretion of any of the hormones produced or released by the gland. Abnormalities of the posterior and anterior portions of the gland may occur independently. Oversecretion (hypersecretion) most commonly involves ACTH or growth hormone, resulting in the conditions known as Cushing's disease or acromegaly, respectively. Undersecretion (hyposecretion) commonly involves all of the anterior pituitary hormones and is termed *panhypopituitarism*. In this condition, the thyroid gland, the adrenal cortex, and the gonads atrophy owing to loss of the trophic hormones. The most common disorder related to posterior lobe dysfunction is diabetes insipidus, a condition in which abnormally large volumes of dilute urine are excreted as a result of deficient production of vasopressin.

The Thyroid Gland

The thyroid gland is a butterfly-shaped organ located in the lower neck anterior to the trachea. It consists of two lateral lobes connected by an isthmus. The gland is approximately

5 cm long and 3 cm wide and weighs about 30 gm. The blood flow to the thyroid, per gram of gland tissue, is very high (about 5 ml/min/gm of thyroid), approximately five times the blood flow to the liver. This reflects the high metabolic activity of the thyroid gland. The thyroid gland produces three different hormones: *thyroxine (T$_4$)* and *triiodothyronine (T$_3$)*, which are referred to collectively as thyroid hormone, and *calcitonin.*

Thyroid Hormone. Thyroid hormone is composed of two separate hormones made in the thyroid gland, thyroxine and triiodothyronine. These hormones are amino acids that have the unique property of containing iodine molecules bound to the amino acid structure. T$_4$ contains four iodine atoms in each molecule, while T$_3$ contains only three. These hormones are synthesized and stored bound to a glycoprotein called thyroglobulin in the cells of the thyroid gland until needed for release into the bloodstream.

Iodine Uptake and Metabolism. Iodine is essential to the thyroid gland for synthesis of its hormones. In fact, the major use of iodine in the body is by the thyroid and the major derangement in iodine deficiency is alteration of thyroid function. Iodide is ingested in the diet and absorbed into the blood in the gastrointestinal tract. The thyroid gland is extremely efficient in taking up iodide from the blood and concentrating it within the cells. There, iodide ions are converted to iodine molecules, which react with tyrosine (one of the common amino acids) to form the thyroid hormones.

Regulation of Thyroid Function. The secretion of thyrotropin, or thyroid-stimulating hormone (TSH), by the pituitary gland controls the rate of thyroid hormone release. In turn, the release of TSH is determined by the level of thyroid hormones in the blood. If thyroid hormone concentration in the blood decreases, release of TSH increases, which causes increased output of T$_3$ and T$_4$. This is an example of feedback control. Thyrotropin-releasing hormone (TRH), secreted by the hypothalamus, exerts a modulating influence on the release of TSH from the pituitary. Environmental factors, such as a fall in temperature, may lead to increased secretion of TRH and, thereby, result in elevated secretion of thyroid hormones.

Function of Thyroid Hormones. The primary function of the thyroid hormones T$_3$ and T$_4$ is to control the cellular metabolic activity. These hormones serve as a general pacemaker by accelerating metabolic processes. The effects on the metabolic rate are frequently produced by increasing the level of specific enzymes that contribute to oxygen consumption and altering the responsiveness of tissues to other hormones. The thyroid hormones influence cell replication and are important in brain development. The presence of adequate thyroid hormone is also necessary for normal growth. The thyroid hormones, through their widespread effects on cellular metabolism, influence every major organ system.

Calcitonin. Calcitonin, or thyrocalcitonin, is another important hormone secreted by the thyroid gland. Its secretion is not controlled by TSH. It is secreted by the thyroid gland in response to high plasma levels of calcium, and it reduces the plasma level by increasing calcium deposition in bone.

Abnormalities of Thyroid Function. Inadequate secretion of thyroid hormone during fetal and neonatal development will result in stunted physical and mental growth (cretinism), owing to general depression of body metabolic

activity. In the adult, hypothyroidism (myxedema) is manifested by lethargy, slow mentation, and generalized slowing of body functions. Oversecretion of thyroid hormones (hyperthyroidism) is manifested by greatly increased metabolic rate. Many of the other characteristics of hyperthyroid patients result from the increased response to circulating catecholamines (epinephrine and norepinephrine). Hypothyroidism and hyperthyroidism are discussed in detail in a later section of this chapter. Oversecretion of thyroid hormones is usually associated with an enlarged thyroid gland (goiter). Goiter also commonly occurs in the presence of iodide deficiency. In this latter condition, lack of iodide results in low levels of circulating thyroid hormones, which causes increased release of TSH; the elevated TSH causes overproduction of thyroglobulin and hypertrophy of the thyroid gland. *Euthyroid* refers to thyroid hormone production that is within normal limits.

The Adrenal Glands

There are two adrenal glands in the human, each attached to the upper portion of a kidney. Each adrenal gland is, in reality, two endocrine glands. The adrenal medulla at the center of the gland secretes catecholamines, while the outer portion of the gland, the adrenal cortex, secretes corticosteroids.

Adrenal Medulla. The adrenal medulla functions as part of the autonomic nervous system. Stimulation of preganglionic sympathetic nerve fibers, which travel directly to the cells of the medulla, causes release of the catecholamine hormones epinephrine and norepinephrine. About 90% of the secretion of the human adrenal medulla is epinephrine (also called adrenalin). Catecholamines regulate metabolic pathways to promote catabolism of stored fuels to meet caloric needs from endogenous sources. The major effects of epinephrine release are involved in preparation to meet a challenge (fight-or-flight response). Secretion of epinephrine causes decreased blood flow to tissues that are not needed in emergency situations, such as the gastrointestinal tract, and causes increased blood flow to those tissues that are important for effective fight or flight, such as cardiac and skeletal muscle. Catecholamines also induce release of free fatty acids, increase the basal metabolic rate, and elevate the level of blood sugar.

Adrenal Cortex. The three kinds of steroid hormones produced by the adrenal cortex are glucocorticoids, the prototype of which is hydrocortisone; mineralocorticoids, mainly aldosterone; and sex hormones, mainly androgens (male sex hormones).

Glucocorticoids. The glucocorticoids are given their name because they have an important influence on glucose metabolism; increased hydrocortisone secretion results in elevated blood sugar levels. However, the glucocorticoids have major effects on the metabolism of almost all organs of the body. Glucocorticoids are secreted from the adrenal cortex in response to the release of ACTH from the anterior lobe of the pituitary gland. This system represents an example of negative feedback. The presence of glucocorticoids in the blood inhibits the release of corticotropin-releasing factor (CRF) from the hypothalamus and also inhibits ACTH secretion from the pituitary. The resultant decrease in ACTH secretion causes diminished release of glucocorticoids from the adrenal cortex. A functioning adrenal cortex is necessary for life, although survival is possible by appropriate replacement with exogenous adrenocortical hormones.

The glucocorticoids are frequently administered to inhibit the inflammatory response to tissue injury and suppress allergic manifestations. Toxic effects of glucocorticoids include possible development of diabetes, osteoporosis, peptic ulcer, increased protein breakdown resulting in muscle wasting and poor wound healing, and redistribution of body fat. The presence of large amounts of exogenously administered glucocorticoids in the blood inhibits release of ACTH and endogenous glucocorticoids. Because of this, the adrenal cortex can atrophy. If exogenous glucocorticoid administration is suddenly discontinued, adrenal insufficiency results, owing to the inability of the atrophied cortex to respond adequately.

Mineralocorticoids. Mineralocorticoids exert their major effects on electrolyte metabolism. They act principally on renal tubular and gastrointestinal epithelium to cause increased sodium ion absorption in exchange for excretion of potassium or hydrogen ions. Aldosterone secretion is only minimally influenced by ACTH. It is primarily secreted in reponse to the presence of angiotensin II in the bloodstream. Angiotensin II is a substance that elevates the blood pressure by constricting arterioles. Its concentration is increased when renin is released from the kidney in response to decreased perfusion pressure. The resultant increased aldosterone levels promote sodium reabsorption by the kidney and the gastrointestinal tract, which tends to restore blood pressure to normal. The release of aldosterone is also increased by hyperkalemia. Aldosterone is the primary hormone for the long-term regulation of salt balance.

Adrenal Sex Hormones (Androgens). Androgens, the third major type of steroid hormones produced by the adrenal cortex, exert effects similar to male sex hormones. The adrenal gland may also secrete small amounts of some estrogens, or female sex hormones. Secretion of adrenal androgens is controlled by ACTH. When secreted in normal amounts, the adrenal androgens probably have little effect, but when secreted excessively, in certain inborn enzyme deficiencies, masculinization may result. This is termed the *adrenogenital syndrome.*

The Parathyroid Gland

The parathyroid glands, normally four in number, are situated in the neck, embedded in the posterior aspect of the thyroid gland. These small glands are easily overlooked and can be removed accidentally at the time of thyroid surgery. Inadvertent surgical removal is the most common cause of hypoparathyroidism.

Parathormone, the protein hormone from the parathyroid glands, regulates calcium and phosphorus metabolism. Increased secretion of parathormone results in increased calcium absorption from the kidney, the intestine, and bones, thereby raising the blood calcium level. Some actions of this hormone are increased by the presence of vitamin D. Parathormone also tends to lower the blood phosphorus level. Excess parathormone can result in markedly elevated levels of serum calcium, a potentially life-threatening situation. When the product of serum calcium and serum phosphorus becomes high, calcium phosphate may precipitate in various organs of the body and cause tissue calcification.

The output of parathormone is regulated by the serum level of ionized calcium. Increased serum calcium results in decreased parathormone secretion, forming a feedback system.

The Pancreas

The pancreas, located in the upper abdomen, has both exocrine (digestive enzymes) and endocrine gland function. In contrast to endocrine glands, an exocrine gland is one whose secretions travel through a duct to their site of utilization and are not secreted into the bloodstream.

Exocrine Pancreas. The secretions of the exocrine portion of the pancreas are collected in the pancreatic duct, which joins the common bile duct and enters the duodenum at the ampulla of Vater. Surrounding the ampulla is the sphincter of Oddi, which partially controls the rate at which the secretions from both the pancreas and the gallbladder enter the duodenum.

The secretions of the exocrine pancreas are digestive enzymes high in protein content and an electrolyte-rich fluid. The secretions are very alkaline because of their high concentration of sodium bicarbonate and are capable of neutralizing the highly acid gastric juice that enters the duodenum. The enzyme secretions include *amylase*, which aids in the digestion of carbohydrates; *trypsin*, which aids in the digestion of proteins; and *lipase*, which aids in the digestion of fats. Other enzymes that aid in the breakdown of more complex foodstuffs are also secreted.

The stimulus for secretion of these exocrine pancreatic juices are hormones originating in the gastrointestinal tract. *Secretin* is the major stimulus for increased bicarbonate secretion from the pancreas, while the major stimulus for digestive enzyme secretion is the hormone *cholecystokinin-pancreozymin* (CCK-PZ). The vagus nerve also influences exocrine pancreatic secretion.

Endocrine Pancreas. The islets of Langerhans, the endocrine part of the pancreas, are collections of cells embedded in the pancreatic tissue. They are composed of alpha, beta, and delta cells. The hormone produced by the beta cells is called *insulin;* the alpha cells secrete *glucagon,* and the delta cells secrete *somatostatin.* A major action of insulin is to lower blood sugar by permitting entry of the sugar (glucose) into the cells of the liver, muscle, and other tissues where the glucose can be either stored as glycogen or burned for energy. Insulin also promotes the storage of fat in adipose tissue and the synthesis of proteins in various body tissues. In the absence of insulin, glucose is not able to enter the cells and is excreted in the urine. This condition, called diabetes mellitus, can be diagnosed by high levels of glucose in the blood and urine. In diabetes mellitus, stored fats and protein are used for energy instead of glucose, with consequent loss of body mass. The rate of insulin secretion from the pancreas is normally regulated by the level of sugar in the blood. The effects of glucagon are chiefly to raise the blood sugar (opposite to those of insulin) by converting glycogen to glucose in the liver. Glucagon is secreted by the pancreas in response to a fall in the level of blood glucose. Somatostatin exerts a hypoglycemic effect by interfering with release of growth hormone from the pituitary and glucagon from the pancreas, both of which tend to raise blood sugar levels.

Endocrine Control of Carbohydrate Metabolism.
Glucose for body energy needs is derived by metabolism of ingested carbohydrates and also from proteins by the process of gluconeogenesis. Glucose can be stored temporarily in the liver, muscles, and other tissues in the form of glycogen. The endocrine system controls the level of blood glucose by regulating the rate at which glucose is synthesized, stored, and moved to and from the bloodstream. Through the action of hormones, blood glucose is normally maintained at approximately 100 mg/dl (5.5 mmol/L) of blood. Insulin is the primary hormone that leads to a lowering of the blood glucose level. Hormones that act to raise the blood sugar level are glucagon, epinephrine, adrenocorticosteroids, growth hormone, and thyroid hormone.

The Thyroid Gland

Assessment: Tests of Thyroid Function

Several tests are available and may be necessary to give a complete and accurate picture of thyroid function. In addition, clinical signs and symptoms are evaluated and provide useful information about the function of the thyroid gland.

The stimulating effect of the thyroid gland is exerted through the production and distribution of two hormones: thyroxine (T_4), which maintains body metabolism in a steady state, and triiodothyronine (T_3), which is approximately five times as potent as T_4 and has a more rapid metabolic action. In testing, reliance is placed on the measurement of the levels of thyroid hormones in the blood.

Serum T_4.   The test most commonly used is the determination of serum T_4 by radioimmunoassay or competitive binding techniques. The range of T_4 in serum is normally between 4.5 and 11.5 µg/dl (58.5 to 149.5 nmol/L); T_4 is bound mainly to thyroxine-binding globulin (TBG) and prealbumin; T_3 is bound less firmly. T_4 is normally bound to proteins. Any factor that alters these binding proteins also changes the T_4 levels. Serious nonthyroidal illnesses, drugs (*i.e.*, oral contraceptives, steroids, phenytoin, salicylates), and protein-wasting as a result of nephrosis and use of androgens interfere with accurate test results.

Serum T_3.   The serum T_3 test measures free and bound, or total, serum content of T_3. Its secretion occurs in response to TSH secretion, as does T_4. Although T_3 and T_4 serum levels generally increase or decrease together, T_3 levels appear to be more accurate indicators of hyperthyroidism, which causes a greater rise in T_3 than T_4 levels. The normal range for serum T_3 is 70 to 220 ng/dl (1.15 to 3.10 nmol/L).

Resin T_3 Uptake.   The resin T_3 uptake test uses a reagent of radioactive T_3 to measure thyroid hormone levels in the serum by determining the amount of hormone bound to TBG and the number of available binding sites. Normally, TBG is not fully saturated with thyroid hormone, and additional binding sites are available to combine with radioiodine-labeled T_3 added to the patient's blood specimen. Measurement of the number of free binding sites, therefore, provides an index to the amount of thyroid hormone already present in the patient's circulation. The normal T_3 uptake value is 25% to 35% (relative uptake fraction: 0.25 to 0.35), which indicates that approximately one third of the available sites of TBG are occupied by thyroid hormone. If the number of free or unoccupied binding sites is low, as in hyperthyroidism, the T_3 uptake is greater than 35% (0.35). If the number of available sites is high, as occurs in hypothyroidism, the test results are less than 25% (0.25).

T_3 uptake is useful in evaluation of thyroid hormone levels in patients who have received diagnostic or therapeutic doses of iodine. The test results may be altered by the use of estrogens, androgens, salicylates, phenytoin, anticoagulants, or steroids.

Tests of Thyroid-Stimulating Hormone.   The secretion of T_3 and T_4 by the thyroid gland is under the control of TSH (thyrotropin) from the anterior pituitary gland. Measurement of serum TSH concentration is valuable in diagnosis and management of thyroid disorders and in differentiation between disorders due to disease of the thyroid gland itself and disorders due to disease of the pituitary or hypothalamus.

TSH Radioimmunoassay.   The level of TSH in the serum can be measured by radioimmunoassay. It is increased in patients with primary hypothyroidism.

Thyrotropin-Releasing Hormone Test.   The TRH stimulation test provides a direct means of testing pituitary reserve for TSH and is useful when T_3 and T_4 test results are inconclusive. The patient fasts overnight. Just before and 30 minutes after intravenous administration of TRH, blood samples are drawn for TSH levels. In hypothyroidism due to primary disease of the thyroid gland there is an increased serum TSH level; in hypothyroidism due to disease of the pituitary or hypothalamus there is an absent or delayed response to TRH. Prior to the test, the patient is warned that the intravenous administration of TRH may cause temporary facial flushing, nausea, or a desire to urinate.

Thyroglobulin.   Thyroglobulin, a precursor for T_3 and T_4, can be measured reliably in the serum by radioimmunoassay. Those factors that increase or decrease thyroid gland activity and the secretion of T_3 and T_4 have a similar effect on thyroglobulin synthesis and secretion. Thyroglobulin levels are increased in thyroid carcinoma, hyperthyroidism, and subacute thyroiditis. They may be high in normal physiologic conditions such as pregnancy. They may be increased or decreased by medications or by diagnostic and therapeutic procedures that temporarily increase the serum levels of thyroglobulin. Measuring the thyroglobulin level is useful in follow up and management of patients with thyroid carcinoma and metastatic thyroid disease.

Radioactive Iodine Uptake.   The radioactive iodine uptake test measures the rate of iodine uptake by the thyroid gland. The patient is given a tracer dose of ^{131}I, and a count is made over the thyroid, using a scintillation counter, which detects and counts the gamma rays released from the breakdown of ^{131}I in the thyroid. Thyroid activity divided by the amount of administered activity (expressed as a percentage) is the uptake value. It is a simple test and provides reliable results. It is affected by the patient's intake of iodide or thyroid hormone; therefore, a careful preliminary clinical history is essential in evaluating results. Normal values vary from one geographic region to another and with the intake of iodine. Patients with hyperthyroidism accumulate a high proportion of the [131]I (in some patients up to 90%), whereas patients with hypothyroidism exhibit a very low uptake. This test is also used to determine what dose of ^{131}I should be given to treat a hyperthyroid patient.

Thyroid Scan, Radioscan, or Scintiscan. Similar to the radioactive iodine uptake test, in a thyroid scan a highly focused scintillation detector moves back and forth across the area to be studied in a series of parallel tracks that move progressively downward. At the same time, a printing device records a mark whenever a predetermined number of counts has been received. This produces a visual representation of the localization of radioactivity in the area being scanned. Although ^{131}I has been the most commonly used isotope, ^{125}I, and especially ^{99m}Tc (sodium pertechnetate), are being used because of their physical and biochemical properties, which allow a lower radiation dose to be given to the patient.

Scanning is helpful in determining location, size, shape, and anatomical function of the thyroid gland, particularly when thyroid tissue is substernal or large. Identification of areas of increased function ("hot" areas) or decreased function ("cold" areas) can assist in diagnosis. Although most areas of decreased function are not malignancies, lack of function increases the likelihood of malignancy, particularly if only one nonfunctioning area is present. Scanning of the entire body, to obtain the total body profile, may be carried out in a search for a functioning thyroid metastasis.

Protein-Bound Iodine. Protein-bound iodine is a conjugated molecule formed when T_4 becomes attached to certain plasma protein components. Thyroid function may be assessed in relation to the concentration of protein-bound iodine in the blood. In this test, serum proteins are precipitated, washed, and then measured for iodine content. Normal values range from 4 to 8 μg/dl (0.32–0.63 μmol/L) of plasma. Values above 8 μg/dl indicate thyroid overactivity; conversely, concentrations below 4 μg/dl are considered evidence of hypothyroidism. Unreliable results that may occur if the patient has taken medications containing iodine have decreased the use of this test.

Nursing Implications of Thyroid Tests. When a patient is scheduled for thyroid tests, it is necessary to determine if he has taken medications or drugs that contain iodine because these will alter the results of some of the scheduled tests. Iodide-containing medications include contrast media and those used in treatment of thyroid disorders (Table 37-2). Other less obvious sources of iodine are topical antiseptics, multivitamin preparations and food supplements frequently found in health food stores, cough syrups, and amiodarone, an antidysrhythmic agent. Other medications that may affect thyroid function test values are estrogens, salicylates,

TABLE 37-2
Inorganic and Organic Iodides

Examples of Inorganic Iodides	*Examples of Organic Iodides*
Lugol's solution	X-ray contrast media: time
Diiodohydroxyquin (Diodoquin)	required for elimination of
Potassium iodide (Quadrinal)	contrast media from body:
Iodochlorhydroxyquin (Entero-Vioform)	Cholangiographic ...... months
Sodium iodothiouracil (Itrumil)	Bronchographic .... years
	Myelographic .... life
	Pyelographic .... rapidly

amphetamines, chemotherapeutic agents, antibiotics, steroids, and mercurial diuretics. The patient should be questioned about the use of these medications, and their use should be noted on the laboratory requisition for thyroid function tests.

Examination of the Thyroid Gland

Inspection and palpation of the thyroid gland are done routinely on all patients. The identification of specific anatomical landmarks is required to ensure an accurate assessment. The lower neck region between the sternocleidomastoid muscles is inspected for anterior swelling or asymmetry. The patient is instructed to extend his neck slightly and swallow. Thyroid tissue rises normally with swallowing. The thyroid is then palpated for size, shape, consistency, symmetry, and the presence of tenderness.

The examiner may perform this portion of the examination from an anterior or a posterior position. For the beginning examiner, the thyroid is most effectively palpated from the rear, with both hands encircling the patient's neck (Fig. 37-2). The thumbs are rested on the nape of the patient's neck, while the index and middle fingers palpate for the thyroid isthmus and the anterior surfaces of the lateral lobes. When felt, the isthmus is perceived as firm and of a rubber-band consistency. The left lobe is examined by positioning the patient with his neck flexed slightly forward and to the left. The thyroid cartilage is then displaced to the left with the fingers of the right hand. This maneuver displaces the left lobe deep into the sternocleidomastoid muscle, where it can

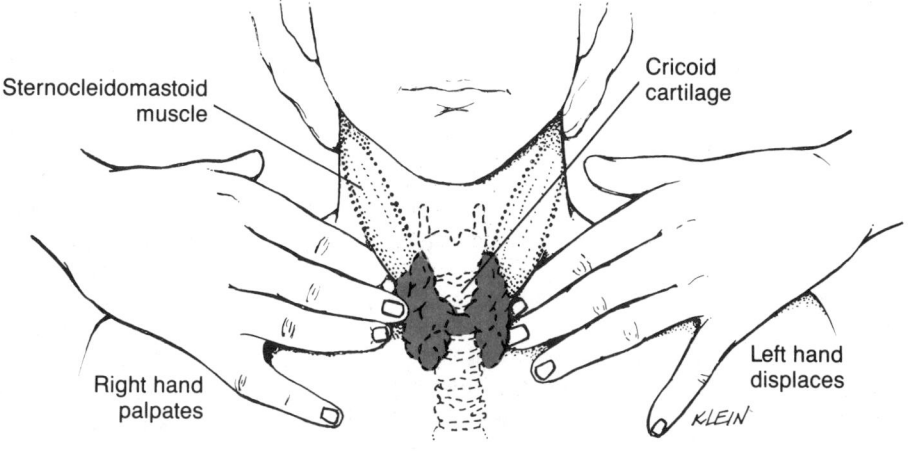

Figure 37-2
Technique of palpation of the thyroid gland. The isthmus of the thyroid may be felt in the midline, approximately 1 cm below the cricoid cartilage. The gland is felt laterally beneath the tendinous insertion of the sternocleidomastoid muscle.

be more easily palpated. The left lobe is then palpated by placing the left thumb deep into the posterior area of the sternocleidomastoid muscle, while the index and middle fingers exert opposite pressure in the anterior portion of the muscle. Having the patient swallow during the maneuver may assist the examiner to locate the thyroid as it ascends in the neck. The procedure is reversed for an examination of the right lobe. The isthmus is the only portion of the thyroid that is normally felt. If a patient has a very thin neck, occasionally two thin, smooth, nontender lobes may also be appreciated.

If the thyroid gland is enlarged on palpation, auscultation over both lobes with the diaphragm of the stethoscope is necessary. Auscultation will identify the localized audible vibration of a bruit. This is an abnormal finding and necessitates referral to a physician. The presence of tenderness, enlargement, or nodularity within the thyroid also requires additional evaluation by a physician.

Hypothyroidism and Myxedema

Hypothyroidism is a condition in which there is a slow progression of thyroid hypofunction, followed by symptoms indicating thyroid failure. More than 95% of patients with hypothyroidism have primary dysfunction of the thyroid gland itself. When the thyroid dysfunction is due to failure of the pituitary gland, it is known as *secondary hypothyroidism;* when failure of the hypothalamus is the underlying cause, the term *tertiary hypothyroidism* is used. When thyroid deficiency is present at birth, the condition is known as *cretinism.* In such instances, the mother may also suffer from thyroid deficiency.

The most common cause of hypothyroidism in adults is autoimmune thyroiditis. (Hashimoto's thyroiditis), in which the immune system attacks the thyroid gland. Symptoms of hyperthyroidism (see p. 952) may later be followed by those of hypothyroidism and myxedema. Hypothyroidism also commonly occurs in patients with previous hyperthyroidism who have been treated with radioiodine, surgery, or antithyroid drugs. It occurs most frequently in older women.

Clinical Manifestations

Early symptoms of hypothyroidism are nonspecific, but extreme fatigue makes it difficult for the person to complete a full day's work or activities. Complaints of hair loss, brittle nails, and dry skin are common, and numbness and tingling of the fingers may occur. On occasion, the voice may become husky, and the patient may complain of hoarseness. Menstrual disturbances such as menorrhagia or amenorrhea occur, in addition to loss of libido.

With more severe hypothyroidism, the temperature and pulse rate become subnormal. The patient usually begins to gain weight even without an increase in food intake. (Severely hypothyroid patients, however, may be cachectic.) The skin becomes thickened because of an accumulation of mucopolysaccharides in the subcutaneous tissues (the origin of the term *myxedema*). The hair thins and falls out; the face becomes expressionless and masklike.

At first the patient may be irritable and may complain of fatigue, but as the condition progresses, the emotional responses are subdued. The mental process becomes dulled, and the patient appears apathetic. Speech is slow, the tongue enlarges, and hands and feet increase in size. The patient frequently complains of constipation and intolerance to cold. Deafness also may occur. The advanced myxedematous state may produce personality changes.

Myxedema affects women five times more frequently than men and occurs most often between 30 and 60 years of age. It is not without its complications, because there is an associated tendency to the rapid development of atherosclerosis, with all the undesirable features of that disease. The patient with advanced myxedema is hypothermic and abnormally sensitive to sedatives, opiates, and anesthetic agents. Therefore, these drugs are given with extreme caution.

Management

The prime objective is to restore a normal metabolic state by replacing the missing hormone. Synthetic levothyroxine (Synthroid) is the preferred preparation for treating hypothyroidism and suppressing nontoxic goiters. The dosage for hormone replacement is based on the patient's normal or suppressed serum TSH concentration. Desiccated thyroid is used less frequently since it often results in transient elevated serum concentrations of T_3, with occasional symptoms of hyperthyroidism. If replacement therapy is adequate, the symptoms of myxedema disappear and normal metabolic activity is resumed.

The treatment consists of maintaining vital functions. Arterial blood gases may be measured to determine carbon dioxide retention and to guide the use of assisted ventilation to combat hypoventilation. Fluids are administered cautiously because of the danger of water intoxication. External heat application is discouraged, since it will increase oxygen requirements and may lead to vascular collapse. If hypoglycemia is evident, concentrated glucose may be given, to prevent fluid overload. Thyroid hormone (usually Synthroid) is given intravenously until consciousness is restored. Then the patient is continued on oral thyroid hormone therapy. Because of an associated adrenocortical insufficiency, steroid therapy may be initiated.

Precautionary Concerns

Myocardial ischemia or infarction may occur in response to therapy in patients with myxedema. Any patient who has been myxedematous for a long period of time is almost certain to have elevated serum cholesterol levels, atherosclerosis, and coronary artery disease. As long as metabolism is subnormal and the tissues, including the myocardium, require relatively little oxygen, a reduction in blood supply is tolerated very well. However, when thyroid hormone is given, the oxygen demand increases but oxygen delivery cannot be increased unless, or until, the atherosclerosis improves. This will occur very slowly, if at all. The signal that the oxygen needs of the myocardium exceed its blood supply is angina pectoris. Angina or dysrhythmias may also occur when thyroid replacement is initiated, because thyroid hormones enhance the cardiovascular effects of catecholamines.

The nurse must be alert for signs of angina, especially during the early phase of treatment, and if detected, it must be heeded at once in order to avoid a fatal myocardial infarction. Obviously, the administration of thyroid hormone must be discontinued immediately, and later, when it can be resumed safely, substitution therapy should be given cautiously at a lower level of dosage and under the close observation of the physician and the nurse.

Elderly arteriosclerotic patients may also become confused and agitated if their metabolic rates are raised too quickly in myxedema.

Marked clinical improvement follows the administration of hormone replacement; such medication must be continued for life, even though signs of myxedema disappear over a 3- to 12-week period.

Precautions must be taken during the course of therapy because of interaction of thyroid hormones with other drugs. Thyroid hormones may increase blood glucose levels, which may necessitate adjustment in doses of insulin or oral hypoglycemic agents. The effects of thyroid hormone may be increased by phenytoin and tricyclic antidepressants. Thyroid hormones may also increase the pharmacologic effects of digitalis glycosides, anticoagulants, and indomethacin, requiring careful observation and assessment by the nurse for side-effects of these drugs.

Severe untreated hypothyroidism is attended by an increased susceptibility to all hypnotic and sedative drugs. These agents, even in small doses, may induce profound somnolence, lasting far longer than anticipated. Moreover they are prone to cause respiratory depression, which could easily prove fatal.

With this in mind, the dosage of any such drug is most conservative (*e.g.*, no more than a half or one third the dosage ordinarily employed in patients of similar age and weight who are not myxedematous). Sedative and hypnotic agents are not used unless the indications are very specific, and if they are given, the nurse must be unusually alert for signs of impending narcosis or respiratory failure.

Nursing Management

The patient with hypothyroidism experiences decreased energy and moderate to severe lethargy. As a result, he is at risk of the complications of immobility. His ability to exercise and participate in activities is further limited by the changes in cardiovascular and pulmonary status resulting from the myxedematous state. A major role of the nurse is to support the patient by assisting with care and hygiene while encouraging him to participate in activities within his tolerance to prevent complications of immobility. The patient's vital signs and cognitive level are monitored closely during diagnostic workup and initiation of treatment to detect 1) deterioration of his physical and mental status, 2) symptoms indicating that an increased metabolic rate resulting from treatment is outstripping his cardiovascular and pulmonary status, and 3) continued limitations or complications of myxedema.

▷ *Medications are administered to the patient with hypothyroidism very cautiously because of his altered metabolism and excretion and the patient's already depressed metabolic rate and respiratory status.*

The patient often experiences chilling and extreme intolerance to cold even if the room temperature feels comfortable or hot to others. Extra clothing and blankets are provided, and the patient is protected from drafts. Although he may ask for a heating pad or electric blanket to decrease chilling and discomfort, these measures are avoided because of the risk of causing peripheral vasodilation, further loss of body heat, and vascular collapse. Additionally, the patient could be burned by using these items without being aware of it because of delayed responses and decreased mental status.

The patient and his family are often very concerned about the changes they have observed as a result of the hypothyroid state. It is often reassuring to be informed that many of the symptoms will disappear as treatment becomes effective. The patient is instructed to continue to use medications as prescribed even after he experiences symptomatic improvement. Dietary instruction is provided to promote weight loss once medication has been initiated and to promote return of normal bowel patterns. Because of the decreased mentation that occurs with hypothyroidism, it is important that a family member also be informed and instructed about treatment goals, medication schedules, and side-effects that are to be reported to the physician. Additionally, these instructions and guidelines are provided in writing for the patient, family, and community health nurse to refer to once the patient returns home.

The patient with moderate to severe hypothyroidism may experience severe emotional reactions to his altered physical state. Changes in appearance and body image and the frequent delay in diagnosis of the disorder because of the nonspecific, early symptoms often produce negative reactions by family members and friends. The patient may have been labeled by family and friends as mentally unstable, uncooperative, or unwilling to take proper care of himself. As hypothyroidism is treated successfully and symptoms subside, he may experience depression and guilt as a result of the progression and severity of symptoms that occurred. The patient and family are informed that the symptoms and inability to recognize them are common occurrences and part of the disorder itself. The patient and family may require assistance and counseling to deal with the emotional concerns and reactions that occurred.

Patient Education and Home Health Care. The patient with hypothyroidism and myxedema, who usually is an older woman, is in need of considerable follow-up teaching and health care. Prior to hospital discharge, arrangements are made to ensure that the patient is returning to an environment that will promote adherence to the prescribed treatment plan. The patient will require encouragement and assistance in daily administration of medications. The nurse assists the patient in devising a schedule or record to ensure accurate and complete administration of medications. The importance of thyroid hormone replacement is reinforced, and the patient and family members are instructed about the signs of over- and undermedication. A weekly visit from the community health nurse is arranged to assess the patient's physical and cognitive status and ability to cope with the recent changes.

Gerontological Considerations. The majority of patients with primary hypothyroidism are 40 to 70 years of age and present with long-standing mild-to-moderate hypothyroidism. The higher prevalence of hypothyroidism in the elderly may be related to alterations in immune function with age. The signs and symptoms of hypothyroidism are often atypical in the elderly; the elderly patient may have few or no symptoms until the dysfunction is severe. In all patients with hypothyroidism, the effects of analgesics, sedatives, and anesthetic agents are prolonged; particular caution is necessary in administration of these agents to the elderly because of concurrent changes in liver and renal function.

In the elderly patient with mild-to-moderate hypothyroidism, thyroid hormone replacement must be started with low doses and increased gradually to prevent serious cardiovascular and neurologic side-effects. Angina, for example, may occur because of rapid thyroid replacement in the presence of coronary disease secondary to the hypothyroid state. Congestive heart failure and tachydysrhythmias may worsen during the transition from the hypothyroid to normal metabolic state. Dementia may become more apparent during early thyroid hormone replacement in the elderly patient.

Myxedema and myxedema coma generally occur exclusively in patients over 50 years in age. The high mortality of myxedema mandates immediate intravenous administration of high doses of thyroid hormone as well as supportive care.

Nursing care of the patient with hypothyroidism/myxedema is summarized in Nursing Care Plan 37-1 (pp. 954–955).

Hyperthyroidism (Graves' Disease)

Hyperthyroidism constitutes a well-defined disease entity, commonly designated as *Graves' disease* or *exophthalmic goiter*. Its etiology is unknown, but the excessive output of thyroid hormones is thought to be due to abnormal stimulation of the thyroid gland by circulating immunoglobulins. Long-acting thyroid stimulator (LATS) is found in significant concentration in the serum of many of these patients and may be related to a defect in the patient's immune surveillance system. The disorder, which affects women five times more frequently than men and peaks in incidence in the third and fourth decades, may appear after an emotional shock, stress, or an infection, but the exact significance of these relationships is not understood.

Clinical Manifestations

Patients with well-developed hyperthyroidism exhibit a characteristic group of symptoms and signs. Their presenting symptom is often nervousness. They are often emotionally hyperexcitable, irritable, and apprehensive; they cannot sit quietly; they suffer from palpitations; and their pulse is abnormally rapid at rest as well as on exertion. They tolerate heat poorly and perspire unusually freely; the skin is flushed continuously, with a characteristic salmon color, and is likely to be warm, soft, and moist. A fine tremor of the hands may be observed. Many patients exhibit bulging eyes (exophthalmos), which produce a startled facial expression.

Other important symptoms include an increased appetite and dietary intake (unless gastrointestinal symptoms develop), progressive loss of weight, abnormal muscular fatigability and weakness, amenorrhea, and changes in bowel function, with constipation or diarrhea. The pulse rate of these patients ranges constantly between 90 and 160 beats/min; the systolic, but characteristically not diastolic, blood pressure is elevated; atrial fibrillation may occur, and cardiac decompensation in the form of congestive heart failure is common, especially in elderly patients.

The thyroid gland invariably is enlarged to some extent. It is soft and may pulsate; a thrill often can be felt and a bruit heard over the thyroid arteries, which are signs of greatly increased blood flow through the organ.

In the more advanced cases, the diagnosis is made on the basis of the symptoms and the tests described previously: an increase in serum T_4 and an increased ^{131}I uptake by the thyroid, in excess of 50%.

The course of the disease may be mild, characterized by remissions and exacerbations and terminating with spontaneous recovery in the course of a few months or years. On the other hand, it may progress relentlessly, with the untreated person becoming emaciated, intensely nervous, delirious, even disoriented, and the heart eventually fails.

Symptoms of hyperthyroidism may occur with release of excessive amounts of thyroid hormone as a result of inflammation following irradiation of the thyroid or destruction of thyroid tissue by tumor. Such symptoms may also occur with excessive administration of thyroid hormone for treatment of hypothyroidism.

Management

As yet, no treatment for hyperthyroidism has been discovered that combats its basic cause. However, reduction of thyroid hyperactivity provides effective symptomatic relief and removes the principal source of its most important complications.

Three forms of treatment are available for treating hyperthyroidism and controlling excessive thyroid activity: (1) pharmacotherapy, employing antithyroid drugs that interfere with the synthesis of thyroid hormones and other agents that control manifestations of hyperthyroidism; (2) irradiation, involving the administration of the radioisotope ^{131}I or ^{125}I for destructive effects on the thyroid gland; and (3) surgery, whereby most of the thyroid gland is removed.

Pharmacotherapy.   The objective of pharmacotherapy is to inhibit one or more stages in hormone synthesis or hormone release; another goal may be to reduce the amount of thyroid tissue, thereby reducing hormone production.

Antithyroid drugs (thiocarbamides, thioamides) effectively block the utilization of iodine by interfering with the iodination of thyrosine and the coupling of iodothyrosines in the synthesis of thyroid hormones. Since this prevents the synthesis of thyroid hormone, the patient with hyperthyroidism is greatly benefitted. The most commonly used medications are propylthiouracil (Propacil, PTU) or methimazole (Tapazole), until the patient is euthyroid (*i.e.*, neither hyperthyroid nor hypothyroid). These drugs block extrathyroidal conversion of T_4 to T_3. Since antithyroid drugs do not interfere with release or activity of previously formed thyroid hormones, it may take several weeks to stabilize the patient, at which time the maintenance dose is established, followed by a gradual withdrawal of the medication over the next several months.

Therapy is controlled on the basis of clinical criteria, including changes in pulse rate, pulse pressure, body weight, size of the goiter, and basal metabolic rate. Perhaps up to half of the patients experience prolonged remission of hyperthyroidism after thiocarbamide therapy is withdrawn. Toxic complications of thiocarbamides are relatively uncommon; nevertheless, periodic examinations cannot be neglected, in view of the possibility that drug sensitization, followed by fever, rash, urticaria, or even agranulocytosis and thrombocytopenia, may develop. With any sign of infection, especially pharyngitis and fever, the patient is advised to stop the medication, call the physician, and have hematologic studies performed. Rash, arthralgias, and fever occur in 5% of patients.

Agranulocytosis is the most feared toxic side-effect and occurs in 1 in every 200 patients. Its incidence is higher in those patients over 40 years of age who are treated with high doses of methimazole. It generally occurs within the first 3 months of therapy.

Patients on antithyroid drugs are instructed not to use decongestants for nasal stuffiness because they are poorly tolerated. These drugs are contraindicated in late pregnancy since they may produce goiter and cretinism in the fetus.

Thyroid hormone may occasionally be given with antithyroid drugs to put the thyroid gland at rest. In this approach, hypothyroidism from excess antithyroid drug is avoided, as is stimulation of the thyroid gland by TSH. Thyroid hormone is available as desiccated thyroid, thyroglobulin (Proloid), and levothyroxine sodium (Synthroid). These are slow-acting preparations that take about 10 days to achieve their full effect. Liothyronine sodium (Cytomel) has a more rapid onset and lasts a short time.

Adjunctive Therapy. Iodine or iodide compounds, once the only therapy available for patients with hyperthyroidism, are no longer used as the sole method of treatment. Such compounds decrease the release of thyroid hormones from the thyroid gland and reduce the vascularity and size of the thyroid. Compounds such as potassium iodide, Lugol's solution, and saturated solution of potassium iodide (SSKI) are used in combination with antithyroid agents or β-adrenergic blockers to prepare the patient with hyperthyroidism for surgery. These drugs reduce the acvitity of the thyroid hormone and the vascularity of the thyroid gland, making the surgical procedure safer.

Solutions of iodine and iodide compounds are more palatable in milk or fruit juice and are administered through a straw to prevent staining of the teeth. These compounds reduce the metabolic rate more rapidly than antithyroid drugs, but their action does not last as long.

- Patients receiving these drugs should be observed for the development of goiter and should be cautioned against use of over-the-counter medications that contain iodides and can increase the response to iodide therapy. Cough medications, expectorants, bronchodilators, and salt substitutes may contain iodide and should be avoided by the patient receiving iodide therapy.

Adrenergic blocking agents may also be used to control the sympathetic nervous system effects that occur in hyperthyroidism. Examples are reserpine, propranolol, and guanethidine, which are useful in controlling nervousness, tachycardia, tremor, anxiety, and heat intolerance.

Radioactive Iodine. The goal of treatment with radioactive iodine (^{131}I) is to destroy the overactive thyroid cells. Almost all the iodine that enters and is retained in the body becomes concentrated in the thyroid gland. Therefore, radioactive isotope of iodine will be concentrated in the thyroid gland, where it will destroy thyroid cells without jeopardizing other radiosensitive tissues. Over a period of weeks or months, those thyroid cells exposed to the radioactive iodine will be destroyed, resulting in reduction of the hyperthyroid state and eventually hypothyroidism.

Prior to treatment with radioactive iodine, the patient receives antithyroid drugs for 6 to 18 months. When drugs are given as temporary therapy for the purpose of reducing the production of hormones to normal, radiation or surgical therapy can then be undertaken safely.

The patient is instructed as to what to expect of this tasteless, colorless radioiodine, which is administered by the physician. If the patient is hospitalized during administration of ^{131}I, radiation safety precautions identified by the hospital's radiation safety committee should be followed. Following treatment with ^{131}I, the patient is discharged and usually followed closely until the euthyroid state is reached.

A single dose of the drug is given by mouth, based on 80 to 160 μCi/gm of estimated thyroid weight. The patient is observed for signs of thyroid storm (see p. 957). Seventy to 85% of patients are cured by one dose of ^{131}I. An additional 10% to 20% require two doses, and rarely is a third dose necessary.

In 3 to 4 weeks, symptoms of hyperthyroidism subside. Close supervision is required by periodic visits to the physician to evaluate thyroid function. If hypothyroidism results from gland destruction, thyroid hormones will have to be taken by the patient.

Radioactive iodine has been used in toxic adenomas or multinodular goiter and in most varieties of thyrotoxicosis (rarely permanently successful) and is preferred for the treatment of patients beyond the childbearing years with diffuse toxic goiter. It is contraindicated in pregnancy and in nursing mothers because radioiodine crosses the placenta and is secreted in breast milk.

Those caring for the patient need to give reassurance, since patients often fear such medications as radioactive drugs, which require special supervision.

Surgical Invervention. The surgical removal of about five sixths of the thyroid tissue (subtotal thyroidectomy) practically assures a prolonged remission in most patients with exophthalmic goiter. Before surgery, the patient is given propylthiouracil until signs of hyperthyroidism have disappeared. Iodine is prescribed to reduce the size and the vascularity of the goiter. It may be given in the form of Lugol's solution, potassium iodide, or hydriodic acid.

- Patients receiving iodine medication must be watched for evidence of iodine toxicity (iodism), the appearance of which is the signal for immediate withdrawal of the drug. Symptoms of iodism include swelling of the buccal mucosa, excessive salivation, coryza, and skin eruptions.

Thyroidectomy for treatment of hyperthyroidism usually is scheduled within a few days after the patient's basal metabolic rate has been reduced to normal.

In appraising the value of surgery, it is considered a less than ideal form of treatment, because there is a possibility of permanent postoperative hypothyroidism, of hypoparathyroidism, and of damage to the recurrent laryngeal nerve. (See p. 959 for pre- and postoperative management of the patient undergoing thyroidectomy.)

Gerontological Considerations

Patients over age 60 account for 10% to 20% of the cases of thyrotoxicosis. Although some older patients develop typical signs and symptoms of thyrotoxicosis, in most a less typical picture is present. The major symptoms of the elderly patient with hyperthyroidism may be depression and apathy, often accompanied by significant weight loss. In addition, the patient may report cardiovascular symptoms and difficulty climbing stairs or rising from a chair because of muscle weakness. Weight loss occurs but is often accompanied by anorexia

(Text continues on p. 956)

Care of the Patient With Hypothyroidism/Myxedema

Nursing Interventions	*Rationale*	*Expected Outcomes*

Mild to Moderate Myxedema

Nursing Diagnosis: Activity intolerance related to fatigue and depressed cognitive processes

Goal: Increased participation in activities and increased independence

1. Promote independence in self-care activities.
   a. Space activities to promote rest and exercise as tolerated.
   b. Assist with self-care activities when fatigued.

   c. Provide stimulation through conversation and nonstressful activities.
   d. Monitor patient's response to increasing activities.

a. Encourages activities while allowing time for adequate rest.
b. Permits patient to participate to the extent possible in self-care activities.
c. Promotes interest without overly stressing the patient.

d. Guards against over- and underexertion by the patient.

- Participates in self-care activities.
- Reports decreased level of fatigue.
- Displays interest and awareness in environment.
- Participates in activities and events in environment.
- Participates in family events and activities
- Reports no chest pain, increased fatigue, or breathlessness with increased level of activity.

Nursing Diagnosis: Discomfort related to intolerance to cold

Goal: Relief of discomfort of cold intolerance

1. Provide extra layer of clothing or extra blanket.
2. Avoid and discourage use of external heat source (*e.g.*, heating pads, electric or warming blankets)
3. Monitor patient's body temperature and report decreases from patient's baseline value.
4. Protect from exposure to cold and drafts.

1. Minimizes heat loss.
2. Reduces risk of peripheral vasodilatation and vascular collapse.
3. Detects decreased body temperature and onset of myxedema coma.
4. Increases patient's level of comfort and decreases further heat loss.

- Experiences relief of discomfort and cold intolerance.
- Maintains baseline body temperature.
- Reports adequate feeling of warmth and lack of chilling.
- Uses extra layer of clothing or extra blanket.
- Explains rationale for avoiding external heat source.

Nursing Diagnosis: Alteration in bowel function (constipation) related to depressed gastrointestinal function

Goal: Return of normal bowel function

1. Encourage increased fluid intake within limits of fluid restriction.
2. Provide foods high in fiber.

3. Instruct patient about foods high in fluid.
4. Monitor bowel function.

5. Encourage increased mobility within patient's exercise tolerance.
6. Encourage patient to use laxatives and enemas sparingly.

1. Promotes passage of soft stools.
2. Increases bulk of stools and more frequent bowel movements.
3. Provides rationale for patient to increase fluid intake.
4. Permits detection of constipation and return to normal bowel pattern.
5. Promotes evacuation of the bowel.
6. Minimizes patient's dependence on laxatives and enemas and encourages normal pattern of bowel evacuation.

- Attains return of normal bowel function.
- Reports normal bowel function.
- Identifies and consumes foods high in fiber.
- Drinks recommended amount of fluid each day.
- Participates in gradually increasing exercises.
- Uses laxatives as prescribed and avoids excessive dependence on laxatives and enemas.

(continued)

Nursing Interventions	*Rationale*	*Expected Outcomes*

Mild to Moderate Myxedema (continued)

Nursing Diagnosis: Knowledge deficit about the therapeutic regimen for life-long thyroid replacement therapy

Goal: Knowledge and acceptance of the prescribed therapeutic regimen

1. Explain rationale for thyroid hormone replacement	1. Provides rationale for patient to use thyroid hormone replacement as prescribed.	• Understands therapeutic regimen. • Explains rationale for thyroid hormone replacement.
2. Describe effects of medication to patient.	2. Provides encouragement to patient by identifying improved physical status and well-being that will occur with thyroid hormone therapy.	• Identifies positive outcomes of thyroid hormone replacement. • Administers medication to self as prescribed.
3. Assist patient to develop schedule and checklist to ensure self-administration of thyroid replacement.	3. Increases assurance that medication will be taken as prescribed.	• Identifies adverse side-effects that should be reported promptly to physician: recurrence of symptoms of hypothyroidism and occurrence of symptoms of hyperthyroidism.
4. Describe signs and symptoms of over and underdose of medication.	4. Serves as check for patient to determine if therapeutic goals are met.	

Severe Myxedema

Nursing Diagnosis: Alteration in breathing pattern related to depressed ventilation

Goal: Improved respiratory status and maintenance of normal breathing pattern

1. Monitor respiratory rate, depth, and pattern.	1. Identifies patient's baseline to monitor further changes and evaluate effectiveness of interventions.	• Shows improved respiratory status and maintenance of normal breathing pattern.
2. Encourage deep breathing and coughing.	2. Prevents atelectasis and promotes adequate ventilation.	• Demonstrates normal respiratory rate, depth, and pattern.
3. Administer medications (hypnotics and sedatives) with caution.	3. Myxedema patients are *very* susceptible to respiratory depression because of use of hypnotics and sedatives.	• Takes deep breaths and coughs when encouraged. • Demonstrates normal breath sounds without adventitious sounds on auscultation.
4. Maintain patent airway through suction and ventilatory support if indicated (see Chap. 22 for care of patients with ventilator).	4. Use of an artificial airway and ventilatory support may be necessary with respiratory depression.	• Explains rationale for cautious use of medications. • Cooperates with suction procedure and ventilator when necessary.

Nursing Diagnosis: Alteration in cognitive function related to depressed metabolism and altered cardiovascular and respiratory status

Goal: Improved cognitive functioning

1. Orient patient to time, place, date, and events around him.	1. Provides reality orientation to patient.	• Shows improved cognitive functioning. • Identifies time, place, date, and events correctly.
2. Provide stimulation through conversation and nonthreatening activities.	2. Provides stimulation within patient's level of tolerance for stress.	• Responds when stimulated. • Responds spontaneously as treatment becomes effective.
3. Explain to patient and family that change in cognitive and mental functioning is a result of disease process.	3. Reassures patient and family about the cause of the cognitive changes and that a positive outcome is possible with appropriate treatment.	• Interacts spontaneously with family and environment.
4. Monitor cognitive and mental processes and response of these to medication and other therapy.	4. Permits evaluation of the effectiveness of treatment	• Explains that change in mental and cognitive processes is a result of disease process. • Takes medications as prescribed to prevent decrease in cognitive processes.

in the elderly patient with thyrotoxicosis. These general symptoms may mask the underlying thyroid disease. Spontaneous remission of hyperthyroidism is rare in the elderly.

The use of ^{131}I is generally recommended for treatment of thyrotoxicosis in the elderly rather than surgery unless an enlarged thyroid gland is pressing on the airway. However, the hypermetabolic state of thyrotoxicosis must be controlled by antithyroid drugs before ^{131}I is used since radiation may precipitate thyroid storm by increasing the release of hormone from the thyroid gland. Thyroid storm, if it occurs, has a mortality rate of 10% in the elderly.

Use of β-blockers may be indicated to decrease the cardiovascular and neurologic signs and symptoms of thyrotoxicosis. However, these agents must be used with extreme caution to minimize adverse effects on cardiac function that may produce congestive heart failure. If antithyroid agents are used, the patient must be monitored closely since the elderly patient is more likely to develop granulocytopenia.

Use of other medications to treat other chronic illnesses in the elderly patient may need modification because of the altered rate of metabolism in hyperthyroidism.

► Nursing Process
The Patient With Hyperthyroidism

▷ Assessment

The nursing history and examination focus on the occurrence of symptoms related to accelerated or exaggerated metabolism. These include the patient's and family's report of irritability and increased emotional reaction. It is also important to determine the impact that these changes have had on the patient's interaction with family, friends, and co-workers. The history includes other stressful situations encountered and the patient's ability to cope with these stresses. Nutritional status and the presence of symptoms are assessed. The occurrence of symptoms related to excessive output of the nervous system and changes in vision and the appearance of the eyes are noted.

▷ Nursing Diagnoses

Based on all the assessment data, the major nursing diagnoses of the patient with hyperthyroidism include the following:

- Ineffective coping related to irritability, hyperexcitability, apprehension, and emotional instability
- Disturbance in self-esteem related to changes in appearance, excessive appetite, weight loss
- Discomfort related to heat intolerance
- Alteration in nutrition related to exaggerated metabolic rate, excessive appetite, and increased gastrointestinal activity

▷ Planning and Implementation

▷ *Goals:* The patient's goals may be improved coping ability, improved self-esteem, relief of discomfort, and improved nutritional status.

Nursing Interventions

Coping Measures. The patient with hyperthyroidism needs assurance that the emotional reactions that he is experiencing are a result of the disorder and that with effective treatment those symptoms will be controlled. Because of the negative effect that these symptoms have on interaction and communication of the patient with family and friends, they too need reassurance that these symptoms are expected to disappear with treatment. It is important to use a calm, unhurried approach with the patient. Additionally, the patient needs to be isolated from stressful experiences; therefore, the patient is not placed in a hospital room with very ill or talkative patients. The environment is kept quiet and uncluttered. Noises, such as loud music, conversation, and equipment alarms, are minimized. Relaxing activities are encouraged if they do not overstimulate the patient.

If thyroidectomy is planned, the patient is likely to be apprehensive and anxious about the surgery. The patient is informed that while surgery is planned, a period of nonsurgical treatment is necessary to prepare the patient and the thyroid gland for surgical treatment. The patient is assisted by the nurse to take the medications as prescribed by the physician and to develop a plan to encourage adherence to the therapeutic regimen. The patient's hyperexcitability and shortened attention span may necessitate repetition of this information and instruction.

Improved Self-Esteem. The hyperthyroid patient is likely to experience changes in appearance, appetite, and weight that are beyond his control. These factors along with the patient's recognition that he is not coping well with his family, environment, and illness may result in loss of self-esteem. The nurse conveys to the patient an understanding of his concern about these problems and expresses willingness to assist him to deal with them. The patient needs to know that these changes are a result of the dysfunction of the thyroid gland and are in fact out of his control. If changes in appearance are very disturbing to the patient, the nurse suggests that mirrors be removed from the room so that the patient is not constantly reminded of his changed appearance. In addition, family members and personnel are reminded to avoid bringing these changes to the patient's attention. The nurse explains to the patient that most of these changes are expected to disappear after effective treatment. If the patient experiences eye changes secondary to hyperthyroidism, eye care and protection may become necessary. The patient may need instructions in how to instill eyedrops or ointment prescribed to soothe the eyes and protect the exposed cornea.

The patient may be embarrassed by the very large meals that he consumes as a result of his greatly increased metabolic rate. Therefore, the nurse arranges the setting so that the patient eats alone if desired and avoids commenting on the large dietary intake of the patient, while at the same time making sure that the patient does receive sufficient food.

Relief of Discomfort. The patient with hyperthyroidism frequently finds a normal room temperature too warm or often unbearably uncomfortable because of his exaggerated metabolic rate and heat production. The nurse provides a cool, comfortable environment for the patient and provides fresh bedding and gown as needed. Giving cool baths, providing cool or cold fluids, and monitoring body temperature are important in providing relief. The reason for the patient's discomfort and the importance of providing a cool environment are explained to the family and staff.

Improvement of Nutritional Status. Hyperthyroidism affects the gastrointestinal system. The patient's appetite is increased but may be satisfied by several well-balanced meals of small size, even up to 6 meals a day. Foods and fluids are selected to replace fluid lost through diarrhea and diaphoresis and to control diarrhea that results from increased peristalsis. Rapid movement of food through the gastrointestinal tract may result in nutritional imbalance and further weight loss. In order to reduce diarrhea, highly seasoned foods and stimulants such as coffee, tea, cola, and alcohol are discouraged. High-calorie, high-protein foods are encouraged. A quiet atmosphere during mealtime may aid digestion. The patient's weight and dietary intake may be recorded to monitor nutritional status.

Patient Education and Home Health Care. The patient with hyperthyroidism is instructed how and when to take prescribed medication. Additionally, he needs to know how the medication regimen fits in with the broader therapeutic plan. Because of the patient's hyperexcitability and decreased attention span, the nurse provides the patient with a written plan to use at home. The type and amount of information given to the patient are individualized because of the resulting stress and possible emotional reactions by the patient. The patient and family members receive verbal and written information about the desired effects as well as possible side-effects of the medications. The patient is instructed by the nurse about which adverse effects should be reported to the physician. The importance of long-term follow-up is stressed because of the possibility of hypothyroidism following thyroidectomy or treatment with antithyroid drugs or [131]I.

If the patient is expected to have a total or subtotal thyroidectomy, he is informed about what to expect. This information, however, will be repeated to the patient as the time of surgery approaches. The patient is also instructed to avoid those situations that have the potential to stimulate the life-threatening occurrence of thyroid storm.

▷ *Evaluation*

▷ *Expected Outcomes*

1. Patient demonstrates effective coping methods in dealing with family, friends, and co-workers.
   a. Reports more effective conversation and interaction with family, friends, and co-workers.
   b. Explains reasons for irritability and emotional instability.
   c. Identifies situations, events, and people that are stress producing.
   d. Avoids stressful situations, events, and people.
   e. Participates in relaxing, nonstressful activities.
   f. Explains to family and friends reasons for irritability and expectation that behavior will change when treatment takes effect.
   g. Identifies expected goals/outcomes of surgery or other treatment.
   h. Explains reason for delay in surgery and identifies own role during waiting period.
   i. Takes medications as prescribed in preparation for surgery or other treatment.

2. Achieves increased self-esteem.
   a. Verbalizes feelings about self and illness.
   b. Describes feelings of frustration and loss of control to others.
   c. Describes reasons for increased appetite.
   d. Discusses events in environment rather than concentrating on changes in own appearance.
   e. Dresses in attractive clothes that do not emphasize changes in physical appearance.

3. Experiences relief of discomfort.
   a. Reports relief of discomfort and a more comfortable environment.
   b. Uses clothing or bedding that is cool and comfortable.
   c. Notifies staff when fresh clothing or bedding is needed.
   d. Reports normal body temperature.
   e. Drinks cool fluids within fluid allowance.
   f. Uses air conditioner or fan if indicated.
   g. Avoids hot, uncomfortable environments.

4. Improves nutritional status
   a. Reports adequate dietary intake and decreased feelings of hunger.
   b. Reports stabilization of weight.
   c. Identifies high-calorie, high-protein foods.
   d. Explains reasons for increased appetite.
   e. Identifies foods to be avoided on diet.
   f. Avoids use of alcohol and other stimulants.
   g. Reports decreased episodes of diarrhea.
   h. Demonstrates normal skin turgor and normal fluid balance.

Thyroid Storm (Thyrotoxic Crisis)

Thyroid storm (thyrotoxicosis, thyrotoxic crisis) is a form of severe hyperthyroidism, usually of abrupt onset and characterized by high fever (hyperpyrexia), extreme tachycardia, and altered mental state, which frequently appears as delirium. Thyroid storm is a life-threatening condition and is usually precipitated by stress such as injury, infection, nonthyroid surgery, thyroidectomy, tooth extraction, insulin reaction, diabetic acidosis, pregnancy, digitalis intoxication, abrupt withdrawal of antithyroid drugs, or vigorous palpation of the thyroid. These factors will precipitate thyroid storm in the partially controlled or completely untreated hyperthyroid patient. Patients who are maintained in a euthyroid state through the proper adjustment of an antithyroid drug may go through many of these episodes without a crisis being precipitated.

Although thyroid crisis may be difficult to identify, the following signs are suggestive: (1) tachycardia (over 130 beats/min), (2) temperature above 37.7°C (100°F), (3) exaggerated symptoms of hyperthyroidism, and (4) disturbances of a major system, for example, gastrointestinal (weight loss, diarrhea, abdominal pain), neurologic (psychosis, somnolence, coma), or cardiovascular (edema, chest pain, dyspnea, palpitations).

Untreated thyroid storm is almost always fatal, but with proper treatment, the mortality rate can be reduced substantially.

Management. The immediate objective is to reduce body temperature and heart rate. Measures to reduce the temperature include a hypothermia mattress or blanket, ice packs, a cool environment, and hydrocortisone. Salicylates are not used since they displace thyroid hormone from binding proteins and worsen the hypermetabolism. Humidified oxygen is administered to improve tissue oxygenation and meet the high metabolic demand. Dextrose-containing intravenous fluids are administered to replace liver glycogen stores that have been decreased in the hyperthyroid patient. Propylthiouracil (PTU) or methimazole is given to impede formation of thyroid hormone and block conversion of T_4 to T_3, the more active form of thyroid hormone. Hydrocortisone is prescribed to treat shock or adrenal insufficiency. Iodine is administered to decrease output of T_4 from the thyroid gland. For cardiac problems such as atrial fibrillation, dysrhythmias, and congestive heart failure, sympatholytic agents may be given. Propranolol in combination with digitalis has been effective in reducing severe cardiac symptoms.

- The patient with thyroid storm or crisis is critically ill and requires astute observation and aggressive and supportive nursing care during and after the acute stage of illness. Care of the patient with hyperthyroidism is the basis of nursing management of the critically ill patient with thyroid storm or crisis.

Thyroiditis

Subacute or granulomatous thyroiditis (deQuervain's thyroiditis), an inflammatory disorder of the thyroid gland that predominantly affects women in their 50s, presents as a painful swelling in the anterior neck that lasts 1 or 2 months and then disappears without residual effect. Evidence indicates that this disorder may be due to a viral infection. The thyroid enlarges symmetrically and occasionally is painful. The overlying skin is often reddened and warm. Swallowing may be difficult and uncomfortable. Irritability, nervousness, insomnia, and weight loss—manifestations of hyperthyroidism—are common, and many patients experience chills and fever as well.

Another form of thyroiditis occurs in the postpartum period and is thought to be an autoimmune reaction.

The purpose of treatment is to control the inflammation. In general, acetylsalicylic acid (aspirin) controls the symptoms of inflammation in mild cases but should be avoided if symptoms of hyperthyroidism occur, because it displaces thyroid hormone from its binding sites and increases the amount of circulating thyroid hormone. In more severe cases, glucocorticoids are effective but do not usually affect the underlying cause.

Chronic Thyroiditis (Hashimoto's Thyroiditis). Chronic thyroiditis, which occurs most frequently in women 30 to 50 years of age, has been termed *Hashimoto's disease*, depending on the histologic appearance of the inflamed gland. In contrast to acute thyroiditis, the chronic varieties are usually not accompanied by pain, pressure symptoms, or fever, and thyroid activity is apt to be normal or low, rather than increased.

There is evidence that cell-mediated immunity plays a significant role in the pathogenesis of thyroiditis. A genetic predisposition also seems to be significant in etiology. If un-

treated, the disease runs a slow, progressive course, leading eventually to myxedema.

The objective of treatment is to reduce the size of the thyroid gland and prevent myxedema. Thyroid hormone therapy is prescribed to reduce thyroid activity and the production of thyroglobulin. If hypothyroid symptoms are present, thyroid hormone is given. Antithyroid drugs may be given if an associated thyrotoxicosis exists. Surgery may be required if pressure symptoms persist.

Thyroid Tumors

Tumors of the thyroid gland are classified on the basis of being benign or malignant, as well as on the presence or absence of associated thyrotoxicosis and the diffuse or irregular quality of the glandular enlargement. If the enlargement is sufficient to cause a visible swelling in the neck, the tumor is referred to as a "goiter."

All grades of goiter are encountered, from those that are barely visible to those producing an unsightly disfigurement. Some are symmetrical and diffuse, others nodular. Some are accompanied by hyperthyrodism, in which case they are described as "toxic"; others are associated with a euthyroid state and are called "nontoxic" goiters.

Endemic (Iodine-Deficient) Goiter. The most common type of goiter, encountered chiefly in geographic regions where the natural supply of iodine is deficient (*e.g.*, the Great Lakes areas of the United States), is the so-called *simple* or *colloid goiter*. Aside from being caused by an iodine deficiency, simple goiter may also be caused by an intake of large quantities of goitrogenic substances in patients with unusually susceptible glands. These substances include excessive amounts of iodine or of lithium, which is currently used in the treatment of manic-depressive states.

Simple goiter represents a compensatory hypertrophy of the thyroid gland, presumably due to stimulation by the pituitary gland. The pituitary gland produces a hormone controlling thyroid growth, and this production is excessive if there is subnormal thyroid activity, as when insufficient iodine is available for production of the thyroid hormone. Such goiters usually cause no symptoms except for the swelling in the neck, which may result in tracheal compression, when excessive.

Management. Many goiters of this type recede after iodine imbalance is corrected. Supplementary iodine such as saturated solution of potassium iodide (SSKI) is prescribed in order to depress the pituitary's thyroid-stimulating activity.

When surgery is recommended, postoperative complications can be minimized when certain criteria exist: (1) a relatively young person without the complications of concurrent medical illnesses, such as diabetes, heart disease, drug allergies; (2) a preoperative euthyroid state resulting from treatment with antithyroid drugs; (3) proper preoperative iodide administration to reduce the size and vascularity of the goiter; and (4) a surgeon experienced in thyroid surgery.

Patient Education. Simple or endemic goiter can be prevented by providing children in iodine-poor districts with iodine compounds. If the mean iodine intake is less than 40 μg/day, the thyroid hypertrophies. The World Health Organization recommends that salt be iodized to a concentration of one part in 100,000, which is adequate for the prevention of endemic goiter. In the Uinted States, salt is iodized to one part in 10,000. The introduction of iodized salt has been the single most effective means of preventing goiter in susceptible populations.

Nodular Goiter. Certain thyroid glands are nodular because of the presence of one or several areas of *hyperplasia* (overgrowth) that appear to develop under conditions similar to those responsible for the colloid or simple goiter. No symptoms may arise as a result of this condition, but, not uncommonly, these nodules slowly increase in size, with some descending into the thorax, where they cause local pressure symptoms. Some nodules become malignant and some become associated with a hyperthyroid state. Thus, many nodular thyroids eventually require surgical intervention.

Thyroid Cancer

Cancer of the thyroid is much less prevalent than other forms of cancer. According to the American Cancer Society, approximately 1000 patients die annually of this malignancy. The most comon type is papillary adenocarcinoma, which accounts for over half of thyroid malignancies. This neoplasm starts in childhood or early adult life, remains localized, and eventually metastasizes along the lymphatics and lymph nodes if untreated. It appears as an asymptomatic nodule in a normal gland. If papillary adenocarcinoma occurs in the elderly, it is generally more aggressive as are other types of thyroid cancer when they occur in the elderly.

An association exists between external radiation of the head and neck in infancy and childhood and subsequent development of thyroid carcinoma. Between 1940 and 1960 radiation therapy was occasionally used to shrink enlarged tonsillar and adenoid tissue, to treat acne, or to reduce an enlarged thymus.

For people exposed in childhood, there appears to be a continuing increase in thyroid cancer 5 to 40 years after irradiation. Consequently, people who underwent such treatment should consult a physician, request an isotope thyroid scan as part of the evaluation, either submit to surgical thyroidectomy or take thyroid hormones if prescribed for abnormalities of the gland, and continue with annual checkups if all is normal.

Follicular adenocarcinoma appears in later life, usually over age 40, and accounts for 20% to 25% of thyroid neoplasms. It is encapsulated and feels elastic or rubbery on palpation. This tumor eventually spreads by hematogenous routes to bone, liver, and lung. The prognosis is not as favorable as for papillary adenocarcinoma.

Other types of cancer are medullary (5%), which present as solid, hard nodular tumors, and anaplastic (5%), which are hard, irregular masses that grow quickly and may be painful and tender. Almost 50% of anaplastic thyroid carcinomas are found in patients over 60 years of age. These tumors have an exceedingly poor prognosis.

Diagnostic Evaluation. The tests of thyroid function may be helpful in evaluation of thyroid nodules and masses. However, their results are rarely conclusive.

Needle biopsy of the thyroid gland is used as an outpatient procedure to make a diagnosis of thyroid cancer and to differentiate cancerous thyroid nodules from noncancerous ones. The procedure is safe and usually painless for the patient. However, patients who undergo the procedure are followed closely because cancerous tissues may be missed during the procedure.

Management. The treatment of choice of thyroid carcinoma is surgical removal. Total or near-total thyroidectomy is performed when possible.

Modified neck dissection is done if there is lymph node involvement. Following surgery, ablation procedures are carried out with ^{131}I to eradicate residual thyroid tissue if the tumor is radiosensitive. Radioactive iodine also maximizes the chance of discovering thyroid metastasis at a later state if total body scans are carried out.

Following surgery, thyroid hormone is administered in suppressive doses to lower the levels of TSH to a euthyroid state.

Patient Education. Postoperatively, the patient will require instructions about the need to take exogenous thyroid hormone to prevent the occurrence of hypothyroidism. Later follow-up includes clinical assessment for recurrence of nodules or masses in the neck and signs of hoarseness, dysphagia, or dyspnea. Chest x-ray films are done as recommended. Total body scans are advised annually for the first 3 postoperative years and less frequently thereafter. Prior to planned total body scans, thyroid hormones are stopped for about a month preceding the tests.

T_4, TSH, serum calcium, and phosphorus levels are assessed to determine if the thyroid hormone supplementation is adequate and to note whether calcium balance is maintained.

Although local and systemic reactions to radiation may occur and may include neutropenia or thrombocytopenia (see p. 689), these complications are rare when ^{131}I is used. Surgery combined with radioiodine produces a higher survival rate than does surgery alone.

Thyroidectomy

Partial or complete thyroidectomy may be carried out as primary treatment of thyroid carcinoma or hyperparathyroidism. The type and extent of the surgery depends on the diagnosis, goal of surgery, and prognosis.

Preoperative Management. Before undergoing surgery for treatment of hyperthyroidism (see p. 952), the patient will be treated with appropriate drug therapy to return his thyroid hormone levels and metabolic rate to normal and to reduce the risk of thyroid storm and hemorrhage during the postoperative period. One important approach in the preoperative period is to gain the confidence of the patient and lessen his anxiety. Some forms of occupational therapy are recommended because they are quieting and relaxing.

The patient with hyperthyroidism often comes from a home made tense and unhappy by his restlessness and nervousness. It it necessary to protect the patient from such unpleasantness and unhappiness in order to avoid precipitating thyroid storm. If there is evidence of nervous upsets when family or friends visit, it may be advisable to limit visiting privileges during the preoperative period.

Nutritional intake is regulated to include adequate carbohydrate and protein foods. A high daily caloric intake is necessary because of the increased metabolic activity and rapid depletion of glycogen reserves. Supplementary vitamins, particularly thiamine and ascorbic acid, are to be provided. Tea, coffee, cola, and other stimulants are to be avoided.

If the patient is to undergo diagnostic testing prior to surgery, he is informed of the purpose of the test and the preoperative preparations in order to reduce anxiety. In addition, a special effort is made to ensure a good night's rest preceding surgery.

Preoperative teaching includes demonstrating to the patient how to support his neck with his hands to prevent stress on the incision; that is, raising his elbows and placing his hands behind his neck will provide support and put much less strain and tension on the neck muscles and the surgical incision.

Postoperative Management. The patient is moved and turned carefully so as to support the head and avoid tension on the sutures. The most comfortable position is the semi-Fowler's position with the head elevated and supported by pillows. Narcotics are given as prescribed for pain. Occasionally, the patient is given humidified oxygen to facilitate breathing. The nurse should anticipate apprehension in the patient and inform him that oxygen will assist his breathing and help him to feel less tired. Intravenous fluids will be administered during the immediate postoperative period, but water may be given by mouth as soon as nausea ceases. Usually, there is a little difficulty in swallowing; initially, cold fluids and ice may be taken better than other fluids. Often patients prefer a soft diet to a liquid diet.

The surgical dressings should be checked periodically and reinforced when necessary. It is important to remember that when the patient is in the dorsal position, evidence of bleeding should be looked for at the sides and the back of the neck as well as anteriorly. In addition to checking the pulse and the blood pressure for any indication of internal bleeding, it is also important to be on the alert for complaints from the patient of sensation of pressure or fullness at the incision site. Such signs may indicate hemorrhage subcutaneously and should be reported.

Occasionally, difficulty in respiration occurs, with the development of cyanosis and noisy breathing, as a result of edema of the glottis or an injury to the recurrent laryngeal nerve. This complication requires that an airway be inserted. Therefore, a tracheostomy set is kept at the patient's bedside at all times, and the surgeon is summoned at the first indication of distress.

The patient is advised to talk as little as possible, but when he does speak, the nurse should note any voice changes that might indicate injury to the recurrent laryngeal nerve that lies just behind the thyroid next to the trachea.

When the nurse is not in attendance, an overbed table may be used to afford easy access to those materials and items that are needed frequently, such as paper wipes, water pitcher and glass, and a small emesis basin. These are kept within easy reach so that the patient will not need to turn his head in search of them. It is also convenient to use this table when vapor-mist inhalations are given for the relief of excessive mucous secretions.

The patient usually is permitted out of bed as soon as he feels able, and is provided his choice of diet. A well-balanced, high-calorie diet is prescribed to regain any weight lost. Sutures or skin clips usually are removed on the second day. The patient is usually ready for discharge from the hos-pital the day of surgery or soon afterward if the postoperative course is uncomplicated.

Complications. Hemorrhage, edema of the glottis, and injury to the recurrent laryngeal nerve are complications that have been reviewed previously. Occasionally, in thyroid operations, the parathyroid glands may be injured or removed, producing a disturbance of the calcium metabolism of the body. As the blood calcium level falls, hyperirritability of the nerves, with spasms of the hands and feet and muscular twitchings occurs. This group of symptoms is termed *tetany*, and its appearance should be reported at once since laryngospasm, although rare, may occur, blocking off the patient's airway. Tetany of this type is usually treated by the administration of calcium gluconate. This calcium abnormality may be temporary following thyroidectomy.

Patient Education and Home Health Care. The necessity for rest, relaxation, and nutrition is explained to both the patient and his family. Specific instructions are issued regarding follow-up visits to the physician or the clinic, which are inevitably necessary and invariably important. The patient should be permitted to resume his former activities and responsibilities completely once thyrotoxicosis has been eliminated.

Responsibilities and factors relating to the home environment that engender emotional tension often have been implicated as precipitating causes of thyrotoxicosis. The patient's hospitalization affords an opportunity to evaluate these factors and possibly alter the environmental situation.

Prevention of Radiation-Induced Thyroid Damage and Cancer. The thyroid gland has a very efficient mechanism to remove iodine from the bloodstream and concentrate or "trap" it for subsequent synthesis of thyroid hormone. The effectiveness of this mechanism to concentrate iodide is reflected in a concentration of iodide 20 to 40 times the concentration of iodide in the plasma. If milk and other food sources become contaminated with radioactivity as a result of a nuclear detonation or a nuclear power plant accident, the radioactive iodide would become concentrated in the thyroid gland at this very high concentration, irradiate the thyroid gland, and increase the risk of thyroid gland cancer. Therefore, in communities exposed to increased radioactivity, attempts have been made to block the uptake of radioactive iodide by flooding or saturating the thyroid gland with non-radioactive iodide. Saturated solutions of potassium iodide (SSKI) or other iodide preparations administered as soon as possible after exposure occurs almost completely inhibit thyroid absorption of the radioactive iodide and promote rapid excretion of any that is absorbed.

The Parathyroid Glands

Hyperparathyroidism

Hyperparathyroidism, which is due to overproduction of parathyroid hormone by the parathyroid glands, is characterized by bone calcification and the development of renal stones containing calcium in the kidneys. Primary hyperparathyroidism occurs two to four times more often in women than in men and is most frequently seen in patients over 70 years of age. Secondary hyperparathyroidism with similar manifestations occurs in patients with chronic renal failure and so-called renal rickets, as a result of phosphorus retention, increased stimulation of the parathyroid glands, and increased parathyroid hormone secretion.

Clinical Manifestations and Diagnosis. The patient may have no symptoms or may experience signs and symptoms resulting from involvement of several body systsms. He may have signs and symptoms of apathy, fatigue, muscular weakness, nausea, vomiting, constipation, and cardiac dysrhythmias, all attributable to an increased concentration of calcium in the blood. Psychological manifestations may vary from emotional irritability and neurosis to psychoses due to the direct effect of calcium on the brain and nervous system. An increase in calcium produces an increase in the excitation potential of nerve and muscle tissue. Occasionally, the patient may be misdiagnosed as "psychoneurotic."

The formation of stones in one or both kidneys, related to the increased urinary excretion of calcium and phosphorus, is one of the important complications of hyperparathyroidism and occurs in 55% of patients with primary hyperparathyroidism. Renal damage results from the precipitation of calcium phosphate in the renal pelvis and parenchyma, resulting in nephrocalcinosis, obstruction, pyelonephritis, and uremia.

Musculoskeletal symptoms accompanying hyperparathyroidism may result from demineralization of the bones or bone tumors, composed of benign giant cells resulting from overgrowth of osteoclasts. The patient may develop skeletal pain and tenderness, especially of the back and joints; pain on weight-bearing; pathologic fractures; deformities; and shortening of body structure.

The incidence of peptic ulcer and pancreatitis is increased with hyperparathyroidism and may be responsible for many of the gastrointestinal symptoms that occur.

The diagnosis of primary hyperparathyroidism is established on the basis of increased serum calcium levels and an elevated level of parathormone. Radioimmunoassays for parathormone are very sensitive and differentiate primary hyperparathyroidism from other causes of hypercalcemia in more than 90% of patients with elevated serum calcium levels. An elevated serum calcium level is a nonspecific finding since serum levels may be altered by diet, medications, and renal and bone changes. Bone changes may be detected on x-ray films in advanced cases of the disease.

Management. The insidious onset and chronic nature of hyperparathyroidism, and its diverse and often vague symptoms, may result in depression and frustration of the patient. The family may have considered the patient's illness to be psychosomatic. An awareness of the course of the disorder and an understanding approach by the nurse may help the patient and family to deal with their reactions and feelings.

The treatment of primary hyperparathyroidism is the surgical removal of abnormal parathyroid tissue. In the preoperative period it must be recognized that kidney involvement is possible, since these patients are subject to renal calculi. A fluid intake of 2000 ml or more is encouraged to help prevent calculi formation. Cranberry juice is suggested because it is effective in lowering urinary *p*H. It can be added to juices and ginger ale for variety. Because of the possibility of stone formation, urine is strained and any evidence of calculi is saved for laboratory analysis. The patient is observed for other manifestations of renal calculi, such as abdominal pain and hematuria. Thiazide diuretics should not be used in the patient with hyperparathyroidism since they decrease the renal excretion of calcium, thereby causing further elevations in serum calcium levels.

Mobility of the patient, with walking or use of a rocking chair, is encouraged as much as possible because bones subjected to normal stress give up less calcium. Bed rest, on the other hand, increases calcium excretion and predisposes the patient to renal calculi formation.

Oral phosphate lowers the serum calcium level in some patients. Long-term use is not recommended because of ectopic calcium–phosphate deposits in soft tissues.

Nutritional needs are met, but foods high in calcium and phosphorus, such as milk and milk products, are limited. If the patient has a coexisting peptic ulcer, specifically prescribed antacids and protein feedings will be necessary. Since anorexia is common, efforts are made to encourage the patient's appetite. Prune juice, stool softeners, and physical activity, along with increased fluid intake, should offset constipation, which is a common postoperative problem for this patient.

The nursing management of the patient undergoing parathyroidectomy is essentially the same as that for a thyroidectomy patient (see p. 959). Although not all parathyroid tissue will be removed during surgery in an effort to maintain control of calcium-phosphorus balance, the patient must be watched closely to detect symptoms of tetany, which may be an early postoperative complication. Most patients quickly regain function of the remaining parathyroid tissue and experience only mild, transient postoperative hypocalcemia. In patients with significant bone disease or bone changes, a more prolonged period of hypocalcemia should be anticipated.

Although it is rare, acute hypercalcemic crisis can occur in hyperparathyroidism. This occurs with extreme elevation of serum calcium levels. Serum calcium levels higher than 15 mg/dl (3.7 mmol/L) result in neurologic, cardiovascular, and renal symptoms that can be life threatening. Treatment includes rehydration with large volumes of intravenous fluids, diuretic agents to promote renal excretion of excess calcium, and phosphate therapy to correct hypophosphatemia and decrease serum calcium levels by promoting calcium deposit in bone and decreasing gastrointestinal absorption of calcium. Cytotoxic agents, calcitonin, and dialysis may be used in emergency situations to decrease serum calcium levels quickly. The patient in acute hypercalcemic crisis requires close monitoring for complications, deterioration of condition, or reversal of serum calcium levels.

A combination of calcitonin and glucocorticoids has been administered in emergencies to reduce the serum calcium level by increasing calcium deposition in bone.

The patient requires expert assessment and care to minimize complications and reverse the life-threatening hypercalcemia. Medications are administered with care and attention is given to fluid balance to promote return of normal fluid and electrolyte balance in this patent. Supportive measures are necessary for the patient and family.

Hypoparathyroidism

The most common cause of hypoparathyroidism is inadequate secretion of parathyroid hormone following interruption of the blood supply or surgical removal of parathyroid gland tissue during thyroidectomy, parathyroidectomy, or radical neck dissection. Atrophy of the parathyroid glands of unknown etiology is a less common cause of hypoparathyroidism.

Pathophysiology.   Symptoms of hypoparathyroidism are due to a deficiency of parathormone that results in an elevation of blood phosphate, hyperphosphatemia, and a decrease in the concentration of blood calcium—hypocalcemia. Hypocalcemia results because in the absence of parathormone there is decreased intestinal absorption of dietary calcium and decreased resorption of calcium from bone and through the renal tubules. Decreased renal excretion of phosphate causes hypophosphaturia, and low serum calcium levels result in hypocalciuria.

Clinical Manifestations.   Hypocalcemia causes irritability of the neuromuscular system and contributes to the chief symptom of hypoparathyroidism, *tetany*—a general muscular hypertonia, with tremor and spasmodic or uncoordinated contractions occurring with or without efforts to make voluntary movements. In latent tetany there is numbness, tingling, and cramps in the extremities, with the patient complaining of stiffness in the hands and feet. In overt tetany the signs include bronchospasm, laryngeal spasm, carpopedal spasm (flexion of the elbows and wrists and extension of the carpophalangeal joints—Fig. 37-3), dysphagia, photophobia, cardiac dysrhythmias, and convulsions. Other symptoms include anxiety, irritability, depression, and even delirium.

Diagnostic Evaluation.   Latent tetany is suggested by a positive Trousseau's sign or a positive Chvostek's sign. *Trousseau's sign* is positive when carpopedal spasm is induced by occluding the blood flow to the arm for 3 minutes using a blood pressure cuff. *Chvostek's sign* is positive when a sharp tapping over the facial nerve just in front of the parotid gland and anterior to the ear causes the mouth, nose, and eye to twitch.

The diagnosis is often difficult because of vague symptoms of aches and pains. Therefore, laboratory studies are especially helpful. Tetany develops at serum calcium levels of 5 to 6 mg/dl (1.2 to 1.5 mmol/L) or below. Serum phosphate levels are increased, and x-ray studies of bone show increased density. Calcification is noticed on x-ray films of subcutaneous or paraspinal basal ganglia of the brain.

Management.   The objective of therapy is to raise the serum calcium level to 9 to 10 mg/dl (2.2 to 2.5 mmol/L) and to eliminate the symptoms of hypoparathyroidism and hypocalcemia. When hypocalcemia and tetany occur following a thyroidectomy, the immediate treatment is to administer calcium gluconate intravenously. If this does not control convulsive tendencies immediately, it may be necessary to administer sedatives such as chloral hydrate or pentobarbital.

Parenteral parathormone can be administered to treat acute hypoparathyroidism with tetany. The high incidence of allergic reactions to injections of parathormone limits its use to acute episodes of hypocalcemia. The patient receiving parathormone is monitored closely for changes in serum calcium levels and allergic reactions.

Because of neuromuscular irritability, the patient with hypocalcemia and tetany requires an environment that is free of noise, sudden drafts, bright lights, or sudden movement.

Tracheostomy or mechanical ventilation may become necessary, along with bronchodilating medications, if the patient develops respiratory distress.

Nursing management of the patient with possible acute hypoparathyroidism includes the following actions:

- The attention of the nurse in the care of postoperative patients having thyroidectomy, parathyroidectomy, and radical neck dissection is directed toward anticipating signs of tetany, convulsions, and respiratory difficulties.
- Calcium gluconate is kept at the bedside with equipment necessary for intravenous administration. If the patient has cardiac problems, is subject to dysrhythmias, or is receiving digitalis, then calcium gluconate is administered by slow infusion.
- Calcium and digitalis increase systolic contraction, and, furthermore, they potentiate each other. This may produce potentially fatal dysrhythmias. Consequently, the cardiac patient requires constant vigilance and undoubtedly should be on continuous cardiac monitoring.

Therapy for the patient with chronic hypoparathyroidism is determined after serum calcium levels are obtained. The prescribed diet is high in calcium and low in phosphorus. Although milk, milk products, and egg yolk are high in calcium, they are restricted because they also contain high levels of phosphorus. Spinach is also avoided because it contains oxalate, which would form insoluble calcium substances. Oral tablets of calcium salts, such as calcium gluconate, may supplement the diet. Aluminum hydroxide gel or aluminum carbonate (Gelusil, Amphojel) is also given after meals to bind phosphate and promote its excretion through the gastrointestinal tract.

Variable dosages of a vitamin D preparation—dihydrotachysterol (AT 10 or Hytakerol) or ergocalciferol (vitamin D_2) or cholecalciferol (vitamin D_3)—are usually required and enhance calcium absorption from the gastrointestinal tract.

The convalescent phase of patient care is the time to instruct the patient in drug and diet therapy. He needs to know the reason for a high calcium and low phosphate intake and the symptoms of hypocalcemia and hypercalcemia so that he may immediately contact his physician should these symptoms occur.

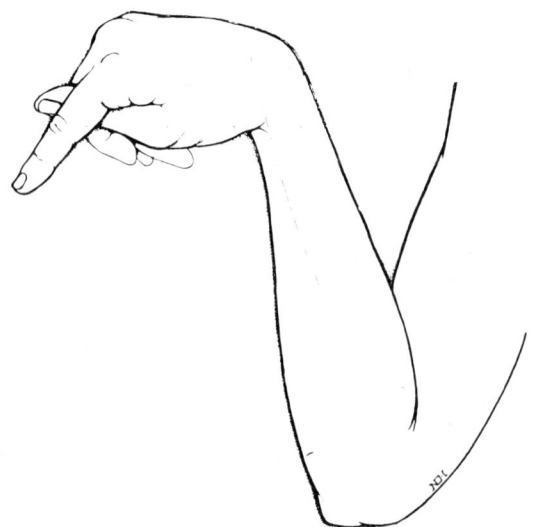

Figure 37-3
Carpopedal spasm.

The Adrenal Gland

Pheochromocytoma

A pheochromocytoma is a tumor that usually is benign and originates from the chromaffin cells of the adrenal medulla. In 80% to 90% of patients, the tumor arises in the medulla, and in the remaining patients it occurs in the extra-adrenal chromaffin tissue located in or near the aorta, ovaries, spleen, or other organs. Pheochromocytoma occurs at any age, but the peak incidence is between ages 25 and 50. It affects men and women equally. The patient's family should also be screened for this tumor because of the high incidence of pheochromocytoma in family members. Fewer than 10% of pheochromocytomas are malignant.

Although uncommon, pheochromocytoma is the cause of high blood pressure in 0.1% to 0.5% of patients with hypertension. It is one form of hypertension that is usually treated successfully by surgery.

Clinical Manifestations. Functioning tumors of the adrenal medulla cause arterial hypertension and other cardiovascular disturbances. The nature and severity depend on the relative proportions of epinephrine and norepinephrine secretion.

The hypertension may be intermittent or persistent. However, only 50% of patients with pheochromocytoma have sustained or persistent hypertension. If the hypertension is of the sustained type, it may be difficult to distinguish from so-called essential hypertension. In addition to hypertension, the symptoms are essentially the same as those encountered after the administration of epinephrine in large doses, namely, tachycardia or palpitations, excessive perspiration, tremor, headache, flushing, and nervousness. Hyperglycemia may result from conversion of liver and muscle glycogen to glucose by epinephrine secretion, occasionally requiring insulin to maintain normal blood glucose levels.

The clinical picture in the paroxysmal form of pheochromocytoma usually is characterized by acute, unpredictable attacks, lasting seconds or several hours, during which the patient feels excessively anxious, tremulous, and weak and suffers from headache, vertigo, blurring of vision, tinnitus, air hunger, and dyspnea. Other symptoms include polyuria, nausea, vomiting, diarrhea, abdominal pain, and fear. Palpitations and tachycardia are common. Postural hypotension occurs in 70% of untreated cases of pheochromocytoma.

Blood pressures as high as 350/200 mm Hg have been recorded. Such blood pressure elevations are dangerous and may precipitate life-threatening complications, including cardiac dysrhythmias, dissecting aneurysm, stroke, and acute renal failure.

Diagnostic Evaluation. The diagnosis of pheochromocytoma is suspected if signs of sympathetic nervous system overactivity occur in association with marked elevation of blood pressure. However, determination of the catecholamines in urine and blood offers the most direct and conclusive test for overactivity of the adrenal medulla. Determination of levels of vanillylmandelic acid (VMA), an end product of catecholamine catabolism, is particularly useful (normal urinary values: 2 to 6 mg/24 hr [10.1 to 30.3 micronmol/24 hr]). In addition, urine collected over a 2- to 3-hour period after a spontaneous or induced attack of hypertension should be assayed for catecholamine content. Coffee, vanilla, chocolate, and certain fruits, vegetables, and drugs are eliminated from the diet before assessment for VMA, since these substances may alter the test results.

With the introduction of reliable means of measuring catecholamines or their end products in urine and plasma, provocative and adrenolytic pharmacologic tests are rarely necessary unless clinical symptoms strongly suggest pheochromocytoma and the results of testing of urinary catecholamines are negative. Pharmacologic tests depend on the reaction of the blood pressure to *provocative* drugs and to *adrenergic blocking* drugs. Provocative agents are those that stimulate a sharp rise in arterial pressure, while adrenergic blocking drugs precipitate a definite fall in arterial pressure in patients with this disease. Both tests produce false-negative and false-positive results and have been associated with vascular complications. Almost 90% of cases of pheochromocytoma can be diagnosed by a single test for urinary norepinephrine and epinephrine or VMA levels. Pharmacologic tests are generally used in diagnosing only the small percentage of patients with atypical symptoms or inconclusive urine and serum test results because of the dangerous side-effects of these tests.

Diagnostic tests may also be carried out to localize the pheochromocytoma and to determine if more than one tumor is present. Computed tomography, ultrasonography, intravenous pyelography, and aortography or arteriography may be performed. However, these procedures are carried out only after the patient is prepared with blocking agents to prevent hypertensive attacks.

Management. During an episode or attack of hypertension, tachycardia, anxiety, and the other symptoms of pheochromocytoma, the patient is placed on bed rest with the head of the bed elevated to promote an orthostatic decrease in blood pressure. The patient is moved to the intensive care unit to permit close monitoring of electrocardiographic changes and careful administration of α-adrenergic blocking agents such as phentolamine (Regitine) or smooth muscle relaxants (sodium nitroprusside [Nipride]) to quickly lower the blood pressure. Phenoxybenzamine (Dibenzyline) is a long-acting α-blocker that may be used after the patient's blood pressure is stable to begin preparation of the patient for surgery.

The treatment of pheochromocytoma is surgical removal of the tumor, usually with adrenalectomy, which occasionally is bilateral. Preliminary patient preparation includes effective control of blood pressure and blood volumes. Usually, this is carried out over 10 days to 2 weeks. Phentolamine or phenoxybenzamine (Dibenzyline) may be used safely without causing undue hypotension. These agents inhibit the effects of catecholamines but do not alter their synthesis or degradation. β-Adrenergic blocking agents may be used in patients with cardiac dysrhythmias or in those not responsive to α-adrenergic blocking drugs. α-Adrenergic and β-adrenergic blocking agents must be used with caution, because patients with pheochromocytoma may have increased sensitivity to them. Still another group of drugs that may be used preoperatively are catecholamine synthesis inhibitors such as α-methyl-*p*-tyrosine (metyrosine). These are occasionally used when the effects of catecholamines are not reduced by adrenergic blocking agents.

Manipulation of the tumor during surgical excision causes release of stored epinephrine and norepinephrine with marked increases in blood pressure and changes in heart rate. Therefore, use of sodium nitroprusside and α-adrenergic blocking agents may be required during and after surgery. Exploration of other possible sites of tumor is frequently undertaken to ensure removal of all tumor. As a result, the patient is subject to the stress and effects of a long surgical procedure, which may increase the risk of hypertension postoperatively.

Corticosteroid replacement is required if bilateral adrenalectomy has been necessary. Intravenous administration of corticosteroids (methylprednisolone sodium succinate [Solu-Medrol]) may begin the evening before surgery and continue during the early postoperative period to prevent adrenal insufficiency. Oral preparations of corticosteroids (prednisone) will be prescribed after the acute stress of surgery diminishes.

The patient will be monitored for several days in the intensive care unit with special attention given to electrocardiographic changes, arterial pressures, fluid and electrolyte balance, and blood glucose levels. Several intravenous lines will be inserted for administration of fluids and medications. Hypotension and hypoglycemia may occur in the postoperative period owing to the sudden withdrawal of excessive amounts of catecholamines. Therefore, careful attention is directed to monitoring these changes.

Hypertension usually disappears with treatment. However, it can persist or recur if the blood vessels have been damaged by severe and prolonged hypertension or if all pheochromocytoma tissue has not been removed.

Several days after surgery, 24-hour urine excretion of catecholamines and their metabolites is measured to determine whether surgery has been successful. When levels have returned to normal, the patient may be discharged. Thereafter, periodic checkups are required, especially in young patients or in patients whose families have a history of pheochromocytoma. Pre- and postoperative nursing care is summarized in Nursing Care Plan 37-2 (pp. 966–967).

Patient Education and Home Health Care. The patient who has undergone surgery to treat pheochromocytoma has experienced a stressful preoperative and postoperative course and may remain fearful of repeated attacks. Although it is usually expected that all pheochromocytoma tissue has been removed, there is a possibility that other sites were undetected and that attacks may recur. The patient is scheduled for periodic follow-up appointments to observe for return of normal blood pressure and serum and urine levels of catecholamines. He may be required to collect urine specimens for 24 hours before follow-up visits to the clinic or physician's office and is given verbal and written instructions about the procedure. If long-term steroid replacement is necessary, the patient is given instructions on the correct schedule to follow (see p. 973 for care of patients on long-term steroid therapy). A visit from a community health nurse may be arranged to assure the patient that he is adhering to the medication schedule correctly and to assist him in dealing with problems that may result from long-term steroid use.

Disorders of the Adrenal Cortex

The adrenal cortex is necessary for life. Adrenocortical secretions make it possible for the body to adapt to stress of all kinds. How well one adapts to stress varies from person to person. Without the adrenal cortex, severe stress will cause peripheral circulatory failure, shock, and prostration. Life would be maintained only with nutritional and electrolyte replacement and replacement of adrenocortical hormones.

Adrenocortical hormones are classified into three groups: mineralocorticoids, glucocorticoids, and sex hormones. *Mineralocorticoids* are concerned with sodium and water retention and potassium excretion. Examples are aldosterone and desoxycorticosterone, a natural precursor of aldosterone. *Glucocorticoids* are concerned with metabolic effects, including carbohydrate metabolism. Examples are cortisol and corticosterone. Glucocorticoids enhance the metabolic breakdown of body proteins and fat to provide fuel during periods of fasting. They antagonize the action of insulin, enhance protein catabolism, and inhibit protein synthesis. They affect defense mechanisms of the body and influence emotional functioning either directly or indirectly. In high concentrations, they suppress inflammation and inhibit scar tissue formation. In adrenal insufficiency, patients may be depressed and upset, whereas with excessive replacement they tend to become euphoric. The *sex hormones* secreted by the adrenal cortex are androgens and estrogens.

Disorders of the adrenal cortex develop as a result of hyposecretion or hypersecretion of the adrenocortical hormones. Adrenal insufficiency may result from disease, atrophy, hemorrhage, or surgical removal of the adrenal gland or glands.

Chronic Primary Adrenocortical Insufficiency (Addison's Disease)

Pathophysiology. Addison's disease, caused by a deficiency of cortical hormones, results when the adrenal cortex is surgically removed with bilateral adrenalectomy or is destroyed, often as a result of idiopathic atrophy or infections such as tuberculosis or histoplasmosis. Inadequate secretion of ACTH from the pituitary gland results in adrenal insufficiency because of decreased stimulation of the adrenal cortex. The symptoms of adrenocortical insufficiency may also result from sudden cessation of exogenous adrenocortical hormonal therapy, which suppresses the body's normal response to stress and interferes with normal feedback mechanisms.

Clinical Manifestations. Addison's disease has a characteristic clinical picture. The chief clinical manifestations include muscular weakness, anorexia, gastrointestinal symptoms, fatigue, emaciation, generalized dark pigmentation of the skin, hypotension, low blood sugar, low serum sodium, and high serum potassium. In severe cases the disturbance of sodium and potassium metabolism may be marked with depletion of the sodium and water and severe chronic dehydration.

As the disease progresses, with acute hypotension developing due to hypocorticism, the patient moves into addisonian crisis, which is a medical emergency marked by cyanosis, fever, and the classic signs of shock: pallor, apprehension, rapid and weak pulse, rapid respirations, and low blood pressure. In addition, the patient may complain of headache, nausea, abdominal pain, and diarrhea and show signs of confusion and restlessness. Even slight overexertion, exposure to cold, acute infections, or a decrease in salt intake may lead to circulatory collapse. The stress of surgery or dehydration resulting from preparation for diagnostic tests or surgery may precipitate an addisonian or hypotensive crisis.

Diagnostic Evaluation. Although the clinical manifestations presented appear specific, the onset of Addison's disease usually occurs with nonspecific symptoms. The diagnosis of Addison's disease is confirmed by laboratory test results. Suggestive laboratory findings include a decrease in the concentrations of blood sugar and sodium (hypoglycemia and hyponatremia), an increased concentration of serum potassium (hyperkalemia), and an increased white blood cell count (leukocytosis).

The definitive diagnosis is confirmed by low levels of adrenocorticol hormones in the blood or urine. Serum cortisol levels are decreased in adrenal insufficiency. If the adrenal cortex is destroyed, baseline values are low and ACTH injection fails to cause the normal rise in plasma cortisol and urinary 17-hydroxycorticosteroids. If the adrenal gland is normal but not stimulated properly by the pituitary, a normal response to repeated dosages of exogenous ACTH is seen but no response follows the administration of metyrapone, which stimulates endogenous ACTH.

Management. Immediate treatment is directed toward combating shock: restoring blood circulation, administering fluids, monitoring vital signs, and positioning the patient in a recumbent position with legs elevated. Hydrocortisone (Solu-Cortef) is given intravenously and followed with 5% dextrose in normal saline. Vasopressor amines may be required if hypotension persists.

Antibiotics may be prescribed if infection has precipitated adrenal crisis in a patient with chronic adrenal insufficiency. Additionally, the patient will be examined closely to determine other factors or illnesses that led to the acute episode.

Oral intake may be initiated as soon as tolerated by the patient. Fruit juice and salted broth are given to provide sodium and correct electrolyte imbalance. Gradually, intravenous fluids are decreased as oral fluids are accepted.

If the adrenal gland does not regain function, the patient will require life-long replacement of corticosteroids and mineralocorticoids to prevent recurrence of adrenal insufficiency and to prevent addisonian crisis in times of stress and illness. Additionally, the patient will probably be required to supplement his dietary intake with added salt during times of gastrointestinal losses of fluids through vomiting and diarrhea.

► Nursing Process
The Patient With Adrenal Insufficiency

▷ Assessment

The nursing history and examination focus on the presence of symptoms of fluid imbalance and on the patient's level of stress. The blood pressure and pulse rate are observed as the patient moves from a lying to a standing position to detect inadequate fluid volume. Additionally, the patient's skin color and turgor are assessed for changes related to chronic adrenal insufficiency and decreased blood volume. A history of weight changes, presence of muscle weakness, and level of fatigue are obtained. The patient and family members are asked about

the onset of illness or increased stress that may have precipitated the acute crisis.

▷ Nursing Diagnoses

Based on all the assessment data, the major nursing diagnoses of the patient with adrenal insufficiency include the following:

- Fluid volume deficit related to inadequate fluid intake and to fluid loss secondary to inadequate adrenal hormone secretion
- Inadequate response to stress related to inadequate production of adrenal hormones
- Knowledge deficit related to the need for hormone replacement and dietary modification

▷ Planning and Implementation

▷ **Goals:** The patient's goals may include improved fluid balance, improved response to stress and decreased stress in life, and increased knowledge about the need for hormone replacement and dietary modifications.

Nursing Interventions

Fluid Balance Measures. Weight changes are recorded daily since they provide very useful information about the adequacy of the patient's fluid and hormone replacement. Additionally, the patient's skin turgor and mucous membranes are assessed to provide information about fluid balance. The patient is instructed to report increased thirst, which may indicate impending fluid imbalance. Frequent monitoring of lying, sitting, and standing blood pressure also provides a useful indicator of fluid balance.

The patient is encouraged to consume foods and fluids that will assist in restoring and maintaining fluid and electrolyte balance. With the assistance of the dietitian, the nurse can provide guidance to the patient to select foods high in sodium during gastrointestinal disturbances and very hot weather.

In collaboration with the physician, the nurse assists the patient in learning to administer hormone replacement as prescribed and to modify the dosage during illness and other stressful occasions. The patient is provided written and verbal instructions about the administration of mineralocorticoid (Florinef) and/or glucocorticoid (prednisone) as prescribed (see p. 973 for care of patient on corticosteroid therapy).

Stress Reduction. When the patient's condition is stabilized, precautions are taken to avoid stressful conditions, since stress could precipitate another hypotensive episode. Attempts are made to detect signs of infection or other stress that may have triggered the crisis in the first place. The nurse assists the patient to assess his level of stress and to determine if alternative approaches to dealing with stress are indicated.

During the acute crisis, a quiet, nonstressful environment is maintained. All procedures are explained to the patient in order to reduce fear and anxiety. The nurse explains to family members the rationale for minimizing stress during the acute crisis and the measures for helping the patient reduce or avoid stress.

Patient Education. Because of the need for life-long replacement of adrenal cortex hormones to prevent adrenal

Care of the Patient With Pheochromocytoma

Nursing Interventions	*Rationale*	*Expected Outcomes*

Preoperatively and During Acute Attacks

Nursing Diagnosis: Anxiety and fear related to excessive amount of circulating catecholamines and resulting symptoms

Goal: Relief of fear and anxiety

1. Remain with patient during acute episode/attack. Be calm in approach.	1. Remaining with patient will help decrease his fear and level of panic.	• Reports decreased level of fear and anxiety.
2. Reassure patient that attack will end and that assistance to treat problem will be provided.	2. Fear and anxiety may further stimulate production of adrenal medulla hormones and increase blood pressure.	• Expresses hope and expectation that problem will be handled effectively by health care team.
3. Decrease external stimulation.	3. Quiet environment will stimulate patient less than a hurried one.	• Rests comfortably and quietly in intensive care unit.
4. Explain all procedures and events but in a factual, brief way.	4. Procedures and events will be less frightening if the patient understands their purpose and the expected outcomes.	• Explains rationale for procedures and events. • Exhibits no further increase in blood pressure, heart rate, or other symptoms.

Potential Complication: Recurrence of attacks due to excessive circulating catecholamines

Goal: Reduction of factors that have the potential to precipitate attacks

1. Explain to patient activities that may precipitate attacks:
  a. Palpation of tumor
  b. Anxiety
  c. Vigorous exercise
  d. Trauma
  e. Exerting pressure on tumor
  f. Lying in certain positions (differs with each patient)
	1. Certain activities may cause stimulation of the tumor and produce release of excess catecholamines.	• Identifies events and activities to be avoided to reduce the risk of further attacks.
		• Explains rationale for avoiding events and activities that increase risk of further attacks.
		• Does not permit palpation of tumor by all health care team members.
		• Identifies foods that increase risk of attacks.

(continued)

insufficiency and acute adrenal crises with vascular collapse, the patient and family members receive explicit instructions about the rationale for replacement therapy and proper dosage. Additionally, they receive instructions from the nurse and physician about how to balance the drug dosage and increase salt intake in times of illness and other stressful situations. The patient and family are frequently provided with a syringe and a vial of injectable steroid, such as Solu-Cortef, for use in emergencies and they need careful guidance and instructions from the nurse and physician about how and when to use it. The patient is advised to inform other health care providers, such as dentists, that he is receiving steroids and to wear a Medic Alert bracelet and to have information about his need for steroids with him at all times.

The patient and family need to know the signs of excessive or insufficient hormone replacement. The development of edema may signify too high a dose of hormone, and postural hypotension (lightheadedness and dizziness on standing) frequently signifies too low a dose.

The patient is also instructed about modifications in diet that are helpful in maintaining fluid and electrolyte balance. During illness and very hot weather the patient should increase foods high in sodium to counteract increased sodium loss. Adequate fluids are also encouraged to maintain normal fluid balance. The patient is encouraged to weigh himself daily to detect any significant changes in weight that may indicate too much or too little hormone or a recurrence of adrenal insufficiency with changes in stress level.

Home Health Care.   Although many patients are able to return to job and family responsibilities soon after hospital discharge, others are unable to do so because of concurrent illnesses or incomplete recovery from the episode of adrenal insufficiency. In these circumstances, it is useful for the nurse to make a referral to the community health nurse who will

Nursing Interventions	*Rationale*	*Expected Outcomes*

Preoperatively and During Acute Attacks (continued)

Potential Complication: Recurrence of attacks due to excessive circulating catecholamines

Goal: Reduction of factors that have the potential to precipitate attacks

2. Caution patient to avoid certain foods (beer, red wines, aged cheese, yogurt) and drugs (*i.e.,* antitussive agents [cough syrup], MAO inhibitors, isoproterenol, amphetamines, *etc.*)	2. Certain foods and drugs may precipitate an attack by direct effects on the tumor, causing release of catecholamines.	• Consumes no foods that increase the risk of attacks. • Explains rationale for avoiding foods that may precipitate attacks. • Experiences no attacks.

Postoperatively

See Chapter 19 for care of the postoperative patient.

Potential Complications: Rapid changes in blood pressure, fluid and electrolyte imbalances, pain, surgical stress

Goal: Reduction of risk of postoperative complications

1. Monitor blood pressure and fluid and electrolyte status.	1. Manipulation of the tumor during surgery and sudden withdrawal of catecholamines postoperatively make the patient susceptible to rapid changes in blood pressure and fluid and electrolyte balance.	• Exhibits normal blood pressure and fluid and electrolyte status. • Reports pain relief and comfort. • Exhibits normal response to stress. • Maintains normal blood pressure and pulse rate.
2. Administer pain medication to assure patient of adequate pain relief.	2. Postoperative pain and surgical stress increase the risk of postoperative complications (changes in blood pressure, fluid imbalance).	• Exhibits appropriate psychological response to stressful events. • Explains rationale for steroid replacement.
3. Monitor patient's response to stressful events.	3. Surgical removal of one or both adrenal glands makes the patient more susceptible to stress and less able to respond to stressors.	• Takes medication as prescribed. • Identifies side-effects of corticosteroids and ways to minimize side-effects and complications.
4. Instruct patient how and when to administer own corticosteroids, if indicated (see p. 973 for care of patient on long-term steroid therapy).	4. Lifetime replacement of corticosteroids will be necessary if a bilateral adrenalectomy was performed.	

visit the patient at home, assess recovery, monitor hormone replacement, and assess stress in the home. Additionally, the nurse will have the opportunity to assess the knowledge the patient and family have about drug therapy and dietary modifications. A home visit also provides the opportunity to assess the patient's plans for follow-up visits to the clinic or physician's office.

▷ *Evaluation*

▷ *Expected Outcomes*

1. Patient achieves improved fluid balance.
   a. Exhibits normal skin turgor and moist mucous membranes.
   b. Reports stable weight and no excessive thirst.
   c. Reports absence of symptoms of postural hypotension (lightheadedness, dizziness, fainting on rising).
   d. Explains rationale for increasing salt and fluid intake in times of illness, increased stress, and very hot weather.
   e. Identifies foods high in sodium.
   f. Consumes high-sodium foods during illness, in very hot weather, and in times of increased stress.
   g. Seeks health care when illness or stress level exceeds the ability of patient to manage.
2. Improved response to stress and decreased stress level.
   a. Reports normal daily stresses without development of symptoms of adrenal crisis.
   b. Identifies sources of excessive stress and ways to avoid them.
3. Increases knowledge about the need for hormone replacement and dietary modifications.
   a. Explains rationale for hormone replacement.

b. Identifies consequences of inadequate hormone replacement.

c. Demonstrates proper technique of administering injectable hormone for use in emergencies.

d. Explains how to modify hormone dosage and diet to meet changing needs during illness, stress, and hot weather.

e. Wears Medic Alert bracelet and carries medical information with him at all times.

f. Designs schedule to ensure adherence to required medication therapy.

g. Takes medication as prescribed.

h. Identifies signs and symptoms of overdosage and underdosage of hormone.

i. Exhibits absence of signs and symptoms of overdosage and underdosage of hormone.

Cushing's Syndrome

Cushing's syndrome is the opposite of Addison's disease, with its clinical characteristics reflecting excessive, rather than deficient, adrenocortical activity. The syndrome may result from excessive administration of cortisone or ACTH or from hyperplasia of the adrenal cortex.

Pathophysiology. The basic lesion responsible for Cushing's syndrome may be a tumor arising in the cortex of one of the adrenal glands or a basophilic adenoma of the pituitary glands (see p. 973) involving an overgrowth of pituitary cells, producing ACTH, which stimulates the adrenal cortex despite adequate amounts of circulating adrenocortical hormones. The normal feedback mechanisms that control the function of the adrenal cortex become ineffective, and the usual diurnal pattern of cortisol is lost. The signs and symptoms of Cushing's syndrome are primarily a result of unregulated secretion of glucocorticoids and androgens or sex hormones, although there may also be altered mineralocorticoid secretion.

Clinical Manifestations. When overproduction of the adrenal cortical hormone occurs, growth arrest, obesity, and musculoskeletal changes occur.

The classic picture of Cushing's syndrome in the adult shows a characteristic central type obesity, with a fatty "buffalo hump" in the neck and supraclavicular areas, a heavy trunk, and relatively thin extremities (Fig. 37-4). The skin is thinned, fragile, and easily traumatized; ecchymoses and striae develop. The patient complains of weakness and lassitude. Sleep is disturbed because of altered diurnal secretion of cortisol. Excessive protein catabolism occurs, producing muscle wasting and osteoporosis. Kyphosis, backache, and compression fractures of the vertebrae may result. Retention of sodium and water occurs as a result of increased mineralocorticoid activity, contributing to the hypertension and congestive heart failure commonly seen in Cushing's syndrome.

The patient takes on a "moon-faced" appearance and may experience increased oiliness of the skin and acne. There is increased susceptibility to infection. Hyperglycemia or overt diabetes may develop.

In females of all ages, virilization may occur as a result of excess androgens. Virilization is characterized by the appearance of masculine traits and the recession of feminine traits. There is an excessive growth of hair on the face (hir-

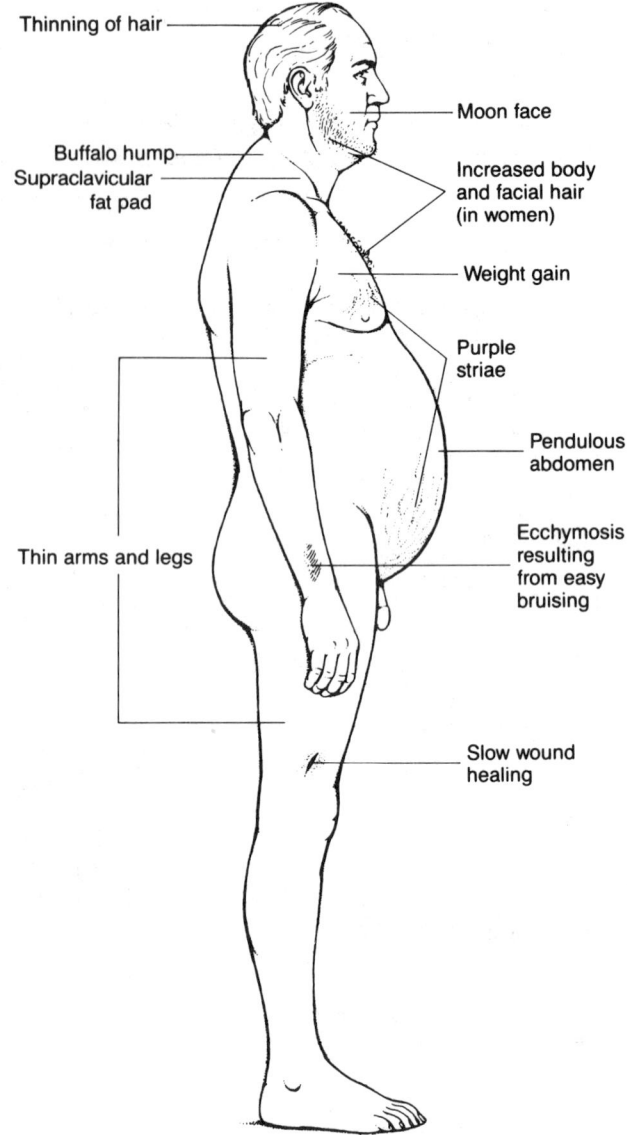

Figure 37-4
Features of Cushing's syndrome invariably include truncal obesity, thin extremities, moon face, buffalo hump, and supraclavicular fullness. Broad purple striae appear at stretch points, such as the abdomen, hips, and shoulders. Body and facial hair is increased, and thinning of scalp hair may be noted only if androgens are increased.

sutism), the breasts atrophy, menses cease, the clitoris enlarges, and the patient's voice deepens. Libido is lost in males and females.

Changes occur in mood and mental activity; a psychosis may develop on occasion. Distress and depression are common and are increased by the magnitude of the physical changes that occur with this syndrome. If the Cushing's syndrome is a consequence of pituitary tumor, visual disturbances may occur.

The patient may also report weight changes, and slow healing of minor cuts and bruises.

Diagnostic Evaluation. Diagnosis of this syndrome includes an increase in serum sodium and blood glucose levels and a decreased serum concentration of potassium, a reduction in the number of blood eosinophils, and a disappearance of lymphoid tissue. Measurements of plasma and urinary cortisol levels are obtained. Several blood samples may be collected to determine if the normal diurnal variation in plasma levels is present. This variation is frequently abolished in adrenal dysfunction. If several blood samples are required, it is essential that they be collected at the times specified and the time of collection be noted on the requisition slip. Diagnostic studies frequently also include 24-hour urine collection for levels of 17-hydroxycorticosteroids and 17-ketosteroids, the urinary metabolites of cortisol and androgens. In Cushing's syndrome, these levels and plasma cortisol levels are elevated.

A low-dose dexamethasone suppression test may be conducted in which a low dose of dexamethasone, a potent synthetic glucocorticoid, is administered and plasma cortisol and urine 17-hydroxycorticosteroid levels are obtained. In patients with normal adrenal function, even low doses of the glucocorticoid will produce decreased cortisol and 17-hydroxycorticosteroid levels. In patients with bilateral adrenal hyperplasia or adrenal tumors, there will be no decrease in these levels.

A CT scan may be performed to localize adrenal tissue and detect tumors of the adrenal gland.

Management. If possible, the cause of Cushing's syndrome is removed. For pituitary disorders, hypophysectomy or pituitary irradiation may be required. Adrenalectomy (see p. 970) remains the treatment of choice in cases of adrenal hyperplasia. Rare hyperplasia cases may benefit from a primary therapy directed against the pituitary, for example, patients with large pituitary adenomas or those with mild adrenal hyperfunction. In the latter, slow but successful responses to radiation therapy may be anticipated.

Postoperatively, symptoms of adrenal insufficiency may begin to appear 12 to 48 hours after surgery because of removal of the source of high levels of adrenal hormones. Temporary replacement therapy with hydrocortisone may be necessary for several months until the remaining adrenal gland regains its ability to respond normally to the body's needs. If both adrenal glands have been removed (bilateral adrenalectomy), life-time replacement of adrenal cortex hormones will be necessary.

If the Cushing's syndrome is a result of externally administered (exogenous) corticosteroids, an attempt will be made to reduce or taper the drug dose to the minimum level adequate to treat the underlying disease process (*e.g.*, autoimmune and allergic diseases and rejection of transplanted organs). Frequently, alternate-day therapy decreases the symptoms of Cushing's syndrome and allows recovery of the adrenal glands' responsiveness to ACTH.

▶ *Nursing Process*
The Patient With Cushing's Syndrome

▷ *Assessment*

The nursing history and examination focus on the effects on the body of high concentrations of adrenal cortex hormones and on the inability of the adrenal cortex to respond to changes in cortisol and aldosterone levels. The history includes information about the patient's level of activity and ability to carry out routine and self-care activities. The patient's skin is observed and assessed for trauma, infection, breakdown, bruising, and edema. Changes in physical appearance are noted, and the patient's responses to these changes are elicited. Throughout the interview and examination, the nurse assesses the patient's mental function, including mood, responses to questions, awareness of his environment, and level of depression.

▷ *Nursing Diagnoses*

Based on all the assessment data the major nursing diagnoses of the patient with Cushing's syndrome include the following:

- Impaired ability to carry out self-care activities related to weakness, fatigue, muscle wasting, and altered sleep patterns
- Impaired skin integrity related to edema, impaired healing, and thin and fragile skin
- Increased susceptibility to injury and infection related to altered protein metabolism and inflammatory response
- Altered body image related to altered physical appearance, impaired sexual functioning, and decrease in activity level
- Altered mental function related to mood swings, irritability, and depression

▷ *Planning and Implementation*

▷ *Goals:* The patient's major goals include increased ability to carry out self-care activities, improved skin integrity, decreased risk of injury and infection, improved body image, and improved mental function.

Nursing Interventions

Rest and Activity. Weakness, fatigue, and muscle wasting make it difficult for the patient with Cushing's syndrome to carry out normal activities. Yet moderate activity should be encouraged to prevent complications of immobility and promote increased self-esteem. Insomnia often contributes to the patient's fatigue. Rest periods are planned and spaced throughout the day. Efforts are made to promote a relaxing, quiet environment for rest and sleep.

Skin Care. Meticulous skin care is necessary to avoid traumatizing the patient's fragile skin. Use of adhesive tape is avoided because it can irritate the skin and tear the fragile skin when the tape is removed. The skin and bony prominences are assessed frequently, and the patient is encouraged to change position frequently to prevent skin breakdown.

Decreased Risk of Injury and Infection. A protective environment must be established to prevent falls, fractures, and other injuries to bones and soft tissues. The patient who is very weak may require assistance in ambulating to prevent falls or bumping into sharp corners of furniture. Unnecessary exposure to visitors, staff, or patients with infections is avoided. The patient is assessed frequently for subtle signs of infection since the anti-inflammatory effects of glucocorticoids may mask the common signs of inflammation and infection. Foods high in protein, calcium, and vitamin D are recommended to minimize muscle wasting and osteoporosis.

Improved Body Image. If removal of the cause of Cushing's syndrome is possible and is carried out, the major physical changes will disappear in time. However, the patient may benefit from discussion of the impact the changes have had on self-concept and relationships with others. The weight gain and edema seen with Cushing's syndrome may be modified by a low-carbohydrate, low sodium diet. A high-protein intake may reduce some of the other bothersome symptoms.

Improved Mental Function. Explanations to the patient and family members about the cause of emotional instability are important in helping them cope with the mood swings, irritability, and depression that may occur. Psychotic behavior may occur in a few patients and should be reported. The patient and family members are encouraged to verbalize their feelings.

Additionally, the patient is prepared for adrenalectomy if indicated, and postoperative care (see below). Peptic ulcer and diabetes mellitus are common in the patient with Cushing's syndrome; therefore, management includes assessment of stools for blood and urine for glucosuria and appropriate intervention if indicated.

▷ *Evaluation*

▷ *Expected Outcomes*

1. Patient increases participation in self-care activities.
   a. Plans activities and exercises to allow alternating periods of rest and activity.
   b. Participates in hygienic care.
   c. Reports improved well-being.
   d. Sleeps soundly at night and during planned rest periods.
   e. Is free of complications of immobility.
2. Attains/maintains skin integrity.
   a. Has intact skin, without evidence of breakdown or infection.
   b. Shows evidence of decreased edema in extremities and trunk.
   c. Avoids trauma to skin.
   d. Changes position frequently.
   e. Inspects bony prominences daily.
3. Decreases risk of injury and infection.
   a. Is free of fractures or soft tissue injuries.
   b. Is free of ecchymotic areas.
   c. Uses measures to prevent trauma (*e.g.*, seeks assistance when necessary, arranges rugs and furniture to prevent falls and bumps).
   d. Avoids people with cold or flu symptoms.
   e. Experiences no temperature elevation, redness, pain, and other signs of infection and inflammation.
   f. Explains rationale for foods high in protein, calcium, and vitamin D.
   g. Selects and eats foods high in protein, calcium, and vitamin D.
4. Achieves improved body image.
   a. Uses makeup appropriately and selects clothes that enhance appearance.
   b. Socializes with others.
   c. Uses good grooming (*e.g.*, skin care, hair care).
   d. Is not gaining weight.
   e. Adheres to diet (*e.g.*, consumes high-protein, low-carbohydrate, low-sodium diet).
   f. Verbalizes feelings about changes in appearance, sexual function, and activity level.
   g. States that physical changes are a result of excessive corticosteroids.
5. Exhibits improved mental functioning.
   a. Identifies reason for mood changes as excessive corticosteroid level.
   b. Verbalizes feelings to nurse and to family.
   c. Participates in family activities.
   d. Notifies nurse, physician, and family if feelings become overwhelming.

Primary Aldosteronism

The principal action of aldosterone is to conserve body sodium. Under the influence of this hormone, the kidneys excrete less sodium and more potassium and hydrogen.

Excessive production of aldosterone, which occurs in some patients with functioning tumors of the adrenal gland, causes a distinctive pattern of biochemical changes and a corresponding set of clinical manifestations that are diagnostic of this condition. Such patients exhibit a profound decline in the blood levels of potassium (hypokalemia) and hydrogen ions (alkalosis), as demonstrated by an increase in *p*H and carbon-dioxide combining power. The serum sodium level is normal or elevated depending on the amount of water reabsorbed with the sodium. Hypertension is usually present, although aldosteronism is the primary cause of only 3% of cases of hypertension.

Hypokalemia is responsible for the variable muscle weakness in patients with aldosteronism, as well as an inability on the part of the kidneys to acidify or concentrate the urine. Accordingly, the urine volume is excessive, leading to complaints of polyuria. Serum, by contrast, becomes abnormally concentrated, contributing to excessive thirst (polydipsia) and arterial hypertension. A secondary increase in blood volume and possible direct effects of aldosterone on nerve receptors such as the carotid sinus are other factors producing the hypertension. Hypokalemic alkalosis may decrease the plasma-ionized calcium level and predispose the patient to tetany and paresthesias. Trousseau's and Chvostek's signs can be used to assess neuromuscular irritability before overt paresthesia and tetany occur (see p. 962).

Diagnostic studies reveal, in addition to a high or normal serum sodium level and low serum potassium level, high serum aldosterone levels and low serum renin levels.

Treatment of primary aldosteronism usually involves surgical removal of the adrenal tumor through adrenalectomy.

Adrenalectomy

Adrenalectomy is the treatment of choice in primary Cushing's syndrome and aldosteronism. In addition, it is also used in the treatment of adrenal tumors and for malignancy of the breast and prostate gland.

For Adrenal Tumors. All of the endocrine disturbances associated with a functioning tumor of the adrenal cortex or medulla can be relieved completely, and the patient improved dramatically, by surgical removal of the involved gland. Adrenalectomy is performed through an incision in the loin or the abdomen. In general, the postoperative care resembles that given for any abdominal operation. Following surgery for adrenal cortical tumors, the patient is susceptible to fluctuations in adrenocortical hormones and may require administration of corticosteroids, fluids, and other agents to maintain blood pressure and prevent acute complications. Attention is also directed toward maintenance of a normal serum glucose level with insulin and appropriate intravenous fluids and dietary modifications.

Nursing management in the postoperative period includes frequent assessment of vital signs so that early indications of hemorrhage and possible adrenal crisis may be detected and treated. Stressful situations can be avoided by explaining the treatment, promoting comfort measures, establishing priorities of care, and providing rest periods.

For Malignancy of Breasts or Prostate. Certain malignancies, notably those of the breast and the prostate, are affected by the hormones produced by endocrine glands. Thus, ovarian hormones are known to have an effect on carcinoma of the breast, and hormones of the testes on carcinoma of the prostate. In some patients, even after suppression of endocrine stimulation, the hormones are still present, and they have been found to arise from adrenal glands. For this reason, bilateral adrenalectomy may be performed in an effort to control recurrent carcinoma of the breast or the prostate. The adrenals are approached either transabdominally or through the posterior bed of the 12th rib.

Postoperatively, adrenocortical hormone must be administered in appropriate dosage to overcome the sudden deprivation of those hormones by the operation. The dosage of adrenocortical hormone may be reduced gradually as the body adjusts itself to its new level of hormone production.

Corticosteroid Therapy

Corticosteroids are used extensively for adrenal insufficiency and are also widely used in suppressing inflammation, controlling allergic reactions, and reducing the rejection process in transplantation. Commonly used steroid preparations are listed in Table 37-3. Their *anti-inflammatory* and *antiallergy* actions make corticosteroids effective in treating rheumatic or connective tissue diseases such as rheumatoid arthritis and systemic lupus erythematosus. High doses seem to permit patients to tolerate high degrees of stress. Such *antistress* action may be due to the ability of corticosteroids to aid circulating vasopressor substances in keeping the blood pressure elevated, or it may be due to other effects, such as the maintenance of the plasma glucose level.

Although the synthetic steroids are safer for some patients because of relative freedom from mineralocorticoid activity, most natural and synthetic corticosteroids produce similar kinds of chronic toxicity. The size of the dose required to bring about desired anti-inflammatory and antiallergy effects also causes metabolic effects, pituitary gland suppression, and changes in the function of the central nervous system. Such changes may be disabling and even dangerous.

In view of these possible effects, it is obvious that while adrenocorticosteroids are highly effective therapeutically, they may also be very dangerous. Dosages of these medications are frequently altered to allow high concentrations when absolutely necessary and then tapered in an attempt to avoid undesirable effects. This requires that patients be closely observed for side-effects and the dose reduced when high doses are no longer required. Suppression of the adrenal cortex

TABLE 37-3
Commonly Used Steroid Preparations

Commonly Used Names	Other Names
Glucocorticoids	
Hydrocortisone*	Cortisol, Hydrocortone, Cortef, Compound F
Cortisone*	Cortone, Cortogen, Compound E
Dexamethasone	Decadron, Hexadrol, 9α-fluoro-16α-methylprednisolone
Prednisone*	Meticorten, Deltasone, 1,2-dehydrocortisone
Prednisolone*	Meticortelone, 1,2-dehydrocortisol
Methylprednisolone	Medrol
Triamcinolone	Aristocort, Kenacort
Mineralocorticoids	
DOC or DOCA†	Percorten, Cortate
Fludrocortisone	Florinef, F-Cortef, 9α-fluorohydrocortisone
Aldosterone	Electrocortin, Aldocorten

* Glucocorticoids that also have mineralcorticoid actions
† Desoxycorticosterone and desoxycorticosterone acetate.

may persist up to a year after a course of corticosteroids of only 2 weeks' duration.

Therapeutic Effects and Complications of Corticosteroid Therapy

The dosage of corticosteroids is determined by the nature and chronicity of the illness as well as by any other medical problem the patient has. Rheumatoid arthritis and bronchial asthma are chronic disorders that corticosteroids do not cure; however, these drugs may be useful when other measures no longer provide adequate control of symptoms. In such a situation, the adverse effects of steroids are weighed against the current problems of the patient. These drugs may be used for a period of time but then should be gradually reduced as the patient's symptoms subside. The nurse plays an important role in providing encouragement and understanding during the times the patient may feel less comfortable while taking smaller doses.

Acute flare-ups and crises are treated with large doses of corticosteroids, as in emergency treatment for bronchial obstruction in status asthmaticus and shock from septicemia caused by gram-negative bacteria. Of course other measures are used as required, such as anti-infective agents or drugs and measures to treat shock.

At times corticosteroids are continued past the acute flare-up stage for the purpose of combating possible complications that are deemed worse than the side-effects of steroids. Systemic lupus erythematosus is an example of such a condition.

A different problem exists when glucocorticosteroids are used in treating eye infections. Outer eye infection can be treated by topical application of eye drops, since these do not cause systemic toxicity. However, long-term application may cause an increase in intraocular pressure, which may lead to glaucoma in some patients. In other patients, prolonged use of steroids may lead to cataract formation.

Topical administration of steroids in the form of creams, ointments, lotions, and aerosols is especially effective in many dermatologic disorders. It may be more effective in some conditions to use occlusive dressings around the affected part so that maximum absorption of the drug is achieved. Steroid penetration and absorption are also increased if the drug is applied when the skin is hydrated or moist (*e.g.*, immediately after bathing). Absorption of topical steroids varies with body location. For example, absorption is greater through the layers of skin on the scalp, face, and genital area than on the forearm, and as a result these sites are more susceptible to the side-effects of the drug than other sites. The recent availability of over-the-counter topical steroids increases the risk of side-effects of steroids in patients who are unaware of the potential risks of these drugs or use them indiscriminately. Excessive use of these agents, especially to large surface areas of inflamed skin, can lead to decreased therapeutic effects and increased side-effects.

Major Side-Effects of Corticosteroid Therapy

Adverse effects are more likely to occur when steroid therapy is used for long periods of time. In general, such effects are classified as follows:

Metabolic Effects. Changes in the metabolism may occur following large doses of glucocorticoids or mineralocorticoids. Excessive glucocorticoid activity (hypercorticism) causes clinical manifestations of Cushing's syndrome (see p. 968), including the characteristic rounding of the face and an abnormal distribution of body fat.

Because of changes in the metabolism of carbohydrate, protein, and fat, certain other complications may occur. For example, some patients may develop peptic ulcer, diabetes mellitus, or osteoporosis. This does not mean that steroid therapy is to be avoided. It does mean that supportive therapy is required to minimize the threat of these other conditions. For example, it is necessary for the patient with a history of peptic ulcer to continue with antacids and perhaps antispasmodic medications, at the same time recognizing that peptic ulcer pain may not be present as a warning sign during the administration of corticosteroids. For the patient with diabetes, oral hypoglycemic agents should be continued or insulin dosages adjusted as needed. For the patient with osteoporosis, it is helpful to adhere to a high-protein diet and to take calcium salt and vitamin D supplement, looking out for possible hypercalciuria. Special efforts are made to prevent an injury that may result in a fracture.

Infection may spread with minimal symptoms, because the patient's defense against invading organisms is lowered by the metabolic effects of the steroid. Viral and fungal infections create further problems because of the difficulty in treating these conditions.

Endocrine Effects. Prolonged steroid therapy has a tendency to suppress certain functions of the anterior portion of the pituitary gland. Hence, growth in children may be halted following long-term treatment with steroids owing to adrenal atrophy and suppression of the pituitary's capacity to release ACTH. Although this effect may not be apparent under ordinary circumstances, it is obvious during times of unusual stress. During these periods of acute adrenal insufficiency, massive doses of corticosteroids are required to prevent adrenal collapse.

Central Nervous System Effects. Euphoria results from the action of corticosteroids on the central nervous system. Since such a reaction often creates psychological dependency on steroids, the patient may resist being removed from these drugs. With prolonged use of corticosteroids, the patient may experience mood swings that include excitement, restlessness, depression, and sleeplessness. Nursing support and understanding are required as the patient moves through these experiences. Any tendency to emotional, psychological, or psychotic difficulties needs to be brought to the attention of the physician before steroids are prescribed.

Chart 37-1 provides an overview of the management of the patient on steroid therapy.

Dosage Schedule

Attempts have been made to determine the best time to administer pharmacologic doses of steroids. Once the patient's symptoms have been controlled on a 6-hour or 8-hour program, a switch is made to a once-daily or every-other-day schedule. In keeping with the natural secretion of cortisol, the best time of the day for the total steroid dose is in the early morning from 7 to 8 AM. Large-dose therapy at 8 AM, when the gland is most active, produces maximal suppression of the gland. A large 8 AM dosage is more physiologic, since it allows the body to escape effects of the steroids from 4 PM to 6 AM, when serum levels are normally low, hence minimizing cushingoid effects. If symptoms of the disease being treated are successfully suppressed, alternative-day therapy is helpful in reducing pituitary-adrenal suppression in patients requiring chronic therapy. Taking the total steroid dose every other day presents some problems in that patients complain of discomfort on the second day. It may be necessary for the nurse to explain to the patient that this regimen may be necessary to prevent toxic reactions.

Tapering of Steroids. Corticosteroid dosages are reduced gradually to allow normal adrenal function to return and to prevent steroid-induced adrenal insufficiency. Up to 1 year or more after use of corticosteroids, the patient is at risk of adrenal insufficiency in times of stress. For example, if surgery for any reason is necessary, the patient is likely to receive intravenous steroids during and after surgery to prevent the occurrence of acute adrenal crisis.

The Pituitary Gland

Hypopituitarism

Hypopituitarism is pituitary insufficiency resulting from destruction of the anterior lobe of the pituitary gland. *Panhypopituitarism* (Simmonds' disease) is total absence of all pituitary secretions and is rare.

Chart 37-1
The Patient on Steroid Therapy

Side-Effects	Nursing Management	Possible Medical Management
Cardiovascular system effects: Hypertension Thromboembolic complications Arteritis	Report to physician. Continue assessment of patient.	Reduce dosage of steroids.
Infection	Assess for atypical indicators of infection. Report to physician. Limit visitors and prevent exposure to infection if possible. Promote cleanliness.	Prescribe antimicrobial agents.
Eye complications: Glaucoma Corneal lesions	Report to physician.	Refer to ophthalmologist.
Adrenal insufficiency as manifested by peripheral circulatory collapse (orthostatic hypotension)	Report to physician. Remain with patient. Decrease sources of stress. Assist with administration of fluids and steroids.	Prescribe hydrocortisone and intravenous normal saline; prescribe oral corticosteroid when patient's condition is stable.
Musculoskeletal effects	Encourage diet high in calcium and vitamin D. Use caution in moving and ambulating patient. Avoid trauma and falls.	Prescribe synthetic estrogens or androgens. Prescribe calcium supplement and oral preparations of vitamin D.
Moon face (Cushing's syndrome)	Suggest caloric restriction.	Consider switching steroid medication.
Weight gain, and edema	Suggest sodium restriction.	Prescribe diuretics.
Potassium loss	Report symptoms to physician. Suggest foods high in potassium.	Prescribe potassium supplement.
Acne	Suggest frequent washing.	Prescribe topical medications.
Increased urinary frequency and nocturia	Assess for urinary tract infection and glycosuria.	Evaluate for diabetes mellitus and order urinalysis.

Counseling of Patients on Long-Term Steroids

1. Recognize that steroids are valuable and useful medications but if taken longer than 2 weeks, certain side-effects may be noticed.
2. Side-effects that are to be reported to the physician include dizziness when rising from chair or bed (postural hypotension indicative of adrenal insufficiency), nausea, vomiting, thirst, abdominal pain, pain of any type, feelings of depression or nervousness, and development of an infection.
3. Other side-effects may include weight gain (perhaps due to water retention), acne, headaches, fatigue, and increased urinary frequency.
4. If the patient has a fall or is in an accident, his condition may precipitate adrenal failure. He requires an immediate injection of hydrocortisone phosphate. (Patients on long-term steroid therapy should wear a Medic Alert tag and have a kit with hydrocortisone.)

The total destruction of the pituitary gland by trauma, tumor, or vascular lesion removes every stimulus that is normally received by the thyroid, the gonads, and the adrenal glands. The resulting endocrinopathy is characterized by extreme weight loss, emaciation, atrophy of all endocrine glands and organs, hair loss, impotence, amenorrhea, hypometabolism, and hypoglycemia. Coma and death will ensue without replacement of the missing hormones.

Tumors of the pituitary gland are three principal types, representing an overgrowth of (1) eosinophilic cells, (2) basophilic cells, or (3) chromophobic cells (*i.e.*, cells with no affinity for either eosinophilic or basophilic stains).

Eosinophilic tumors, if they develop early enough in life, result in gigantism. The person thus affected may be over 7 feet tall and large in all proportions, yet so weak and lethargic that he can hardly stand. If the disorder begins during adult life, the excessive skeletal growth occurs only in the feet, the hands, the superciliary ridges, the molar eminences, the nose, and the chin, giving rise to the clinical picture called *acromegaly*. Enlargement, moreover, is not confined to the skeleton but involves every tissue and organ of the body. Many of these patients suffer from severe headaches and visual disturbances because the tumors exert pressure on the optic nerves. Assessment of central vision and visual fields may reveal loss of color discrimination, diplopia (double vision), or blindness of a portion of a field of vision. Decalcification of the skeleton, muscular weakness, and endocrine disturbances, similar to those occurring in patients with hyperthyroidism, also are associated with tumors of this type.

Basophilic tumors give rise to the so-called *Cushing's syndrome* (see p. 968) with features largely attributable to hyperadrenalism, including masculinization and amenorrhea in females, truncal obesity, hypertension, osteoporosis, and polycythemia.

Chromophobic tumors, which comprise 90% of pituitary tumors, produce no hormones but destroy the rest of the pituitary gland, causing hypopituitarism. Patients with this disease are inclined to be obese and somnolent, exhibiting fine, scanty hair; dry, soft skin; pasty complexion; and small bones. They also experience headaches, loss of libido, and visual defects progressing to blindness. Other symptoms include polyuria, polyphagia, a lowering of the basal metabolic rate, and a subnormal body temperature.

Hypophysectomy

Hypophysectomy, or removal of the pituitary gland, may be done for several reasons, including treatment of primary tumors of the pituitary gland. In diabetic retinopathy (see p. 924) it is used to halt the progress of hemorrhagic retinopathy and avoid blindness. Hypophysectomy is also done as a palliative measure to relieve bone pain secondary to metastasis of malignant lesions of the breast and prostate. Pituitary hormones influence the growth of the normal breast and stimulate the function of the ovaries and the adrenal glands. Hypophysectomy removes the hormonal influences of these glands and reduces stimuli to the continued growth of the neoplasm.

There are several methods of pituitary ablation (removal). It can be done surgically through the transfrontal, subcranial, or oronasal-transsphenoidal approaches. The pituitary can also be destroyed by irradiation or cryosurgery. (See Chap. 53 for the transsphenoidal approach to the removal of a pituitary tumor and for the nursing management of a patient undergoing cranial surgery.)

The absence of the pituitary gland alters the function of many parts of the body. Menstruation ceases and infertility occurs after total or nearly total ablation of the pituitary gland. Substitution therapy with adrenal steroids (hydrocortisone) and thyroid hormone may be necessary.

Diabetes Insipidus

Diabetes insipidus is a disorder of the posterior lobe of the pituitary gland due to a deficiency of vasopressin, the antidiuretic hormone (ADH). It is characterized by great thirst (polydipsia) and large volumes of dilute urine. The cause is unknown, although it may be secondary to head trauma, brain tumor, or surgical ablation or irradiation of the pituitary gland. Without the action of vasopressin on the distal nephron of the kidney, an enormous daily output of very dilute, water-like urine with a specific gravity of 1.001 to 1.005 occurs. The urine contains no abnormal substances, such as sugar and albumin. Because of the intense thirst, the patient tends to drink 4 to 40 liters of fluid daily, with a special craving for cold water.

In the hereditary form of diabetes insipidus, the primary symptoms may begin at birth. When it occurs in adults, the polyuria may have an insidious onset, although sometimes it occurs suddenly and may be related to an injury.

The disease cannot be controlled by limiting the intake of fluids since urine loss of high volumes of urine continues even without fluid replacement. Attempts to do this cause the patient to suffer extremely from an insatiable craving for fluid and to develop severe dehydration and hypernatremia.

Diagnostic Evaluation. The fluid deprivation test is carried out, in which fluids are withheld for 8 to 12 hours or until 3% of the body weight is lost. The patient is weighed frequently during the time fluid is withheld. Plasma and urine osmolality studies are done at the beginning and end of the test. Inability to increase specific gravity and osmolality of the urine are characteristic of diabetes insipidus. The patient with diabetes insipidus will continue to excrete large volumes of urine with low specific gravity and will experience weight loss, rising serum osmolality, and elevated serum sodium levels. The patient's condition needs to be assessed frequently during the test, and the test is terminated if the patient develops problems such as tachycardia, excessive weight loss, or hypotension.

Management. The objectives of therapy are (1) to assure adequate fluid replacement, (2) to replace vasopressin (which is usually a life-long therapeutic program), and (3) to search for and correct the underlying intracranial pathology.

Desmopressin (DDAVP), synthetic vasopression without the vascular effects of natural ADH, is particularly valuable because its action lasts longer and it has fewer adverse effects than other preparations previously used to treat the disease. It is administered intranasally with the patient sniffing the solution into his nose through a flexible plastic tube. Two administrations daily appear to control the symptoms.

Another form of therapy is the intramuscular administration of ADH, vasopressin tannate in oil, which is given at intervals of 36 to 48 hours or longer. The effect is a reduction in urinary volume for 24 to 48 hours. The vial of medication should be warmed or shaken vigorously prior to administration. The injection is given in the evening so that maximum results are obtained during sleep. Abdominal cramps are a side-effect of this drug.

The drug lypressin (Diapid) is absorbed through the nasal mucosa into the blood and is another method of administering vasopressin. Its duration may be too short for patients with severe disease. The patient should be observed for chronic rhinopharyngitis if this modality of treatment is used.

Clofibrate, a hypolipidemic agent, has been found to have an antidiuretic effect on patients with diabetes insipidus who have some residual hypothalamic vasopressin. Chlorpropamide (Diabinese) and thiazide diuretics are also used in mild forms of the disease, since they potentiate the action of vasopressin. The patient receiving chlorpropamide should be warned of the possibility of hypoglycemic reactions.

The patient will require encouragement and support if he is undergoing studies of a possible cranial lesion. The patient and family members are instructed about follow-up care and emergency measures. The patient is also advised to wear a Medic Alert bracelet and to carry information about this disorder and his medications with him at all times.

Syndrome of Inappropriate Antidiuretic Hormone Secretion

The syndrome of inappropriate antidiuretic hormone secretion (SIADH) refers to excessive ADH secretion from the pituitary gland even in the face of subnormal serum osmolarity. Patients with this disorder cannot excrete a dilute urine. They retain fluids and develop a sodium deficiency (dilutional hyponatremia). SIADH is often of nonendocrine origin. That is, the syndrome may occur in patients with bronchogenic carcinoma in which malignant lung cells synthesize and release ADH. SIADH has also occurred with severe pneumonia, pneumothorax, and other disorders of the lungs in addition to malignant tumors that affect other organs.

Disorders of the central nervous system, such as head injury, brain surgery or tumor, or meningitis are thought to produce SIADH by direct stimulation of the pituitary gland. Some drugs (vincristine, phenothiazines, tricyclic antidepressants, and others) have been implicated in SIADH; they either directly stimulate the pituitary gland or increase the sensitivity of renal tubules to circulating ADH.

This syndrome is generally managed by eliminating the underlying cause if possible and restricting the patient's fluid intake. Since retained water is slowly excreted through the kidneys, the extracellular fluid volume contracts and the serum sodium concentration gradually increases toward normal. Diuretics may be used along with fluid restriction if severe hyponatremia is present.

The Pancreas

The pancreas has both endocrine and exocrine functions, and these functions are interrelated. The major exocrine function is to facilitate digestion through secretion of enzymes into the proximal duodenum. Secretin and cholecystokinin-pancreozymin (CCK-PZ) are hormones from the gastrointestinal tract that aid in digestion of food substances by control of secretions of the pancreas. Additionally, neural factors also influence pancreatic enzyme secretion. Considerable dysfunction of the pancreas must occur before enzyme secretion decreases and protein and fat digestion becomes impaired. Pancreatic enzyme secretion is normally 1000 to 4000 ml per day, with the amount depending on the quantity and type of food intake.

Gerontological Considerations. There is little change in the size of the pancreas with age. There is, however, an increase in fibrous material and some fatty deposition in the normal pancreas in patients over age 70. Additionally, there may be some slight focal changes of arteriosclerosis with age. Studies have suggested a decreased pancreatic secretion

rate and bicarbonate output in older patients (decreased lipase, amylase, and trypsin). There may be some impairment of normal fat absorption with increasing age, possibly owing to delayed gastric emptying and pancreatic insufficiency. Decreased calcium absorption may also occur. These changes require care in interpreting diagnostic tests in the normal elderly person and in providing dietary counseling.

Pancreatitis

Pancreatitis (inflammation of the pancreas) is a serious disorder of the pancreas that can assume several forms. *Acute pancreatitis,* in which the structure and function of the pancreas usually return to normal after the acute attack, occurs most frequently as a result of gallstones. *Chronic pancreatitis* is characterized by permanent abnormalities of pancreatic function and is usually a result of long-term alcohol use. Patients with long-standing, undiagnosed chronic pancreatitis may develop acute episodes of pancreatitis, making the clinical picture less clear.

Several classification systems have been used to categorize the various stages and forms of pancreatitis. One classification system describes acute pancreatitis on the basis of findings on laparotomy or autopsy. These include interstitial (edematous) and hemorrhagic (acute necrotizing) pancreatitis. The 1984 International Symposium on Classification of Pancreatitis categorizes the disease as acute or chronic pancreatitis, with obstructive chronic pancreatitis added as a type of chronic pancreatitis.

Several theories exist about the cause and mechanism of pancreatitis, which is generally described as the autodigestion of the pancreas. Generally, these theories state that obstruction of the pancreatic duct is present and is accompanied by hypersecretion of the exocrine enzymes of the pancreas. These enzymes enter the bile duct where they are activated and, together with bile, back up (reflux) into the pancreatic duct, causing pancreatitis.

Acute Pancreatitis

Pathophysiology and Etiology. Acute pancreatitis or inflammation of the pancreas is brought about by the digestion of this organ by the very enzymes it produces, principally trypsin. Biliary tract disease occurs in up to 80% of patients with acute pancreatitis; however, only 5% of patients with gallstones develop pancreatitis. Gallstones enter the common bile duct and lodge at the ampulla of Vater, obstructing the flow of pancreatic juice or causing a reflux of bile from the common bile duct into the pancreatic duct, thus activating the powerful pancreatic enzymes within the gland. Normally, these remain in an inactive form until the pancreatic juice reaches the lumen of the duodenum. Spasm and edema of the ampulla of Vater, resulting from duodenitis, can probably produce pancreatitis.

Long-term alcohol use is a common cause of acute episodes of pancreatitis, but the patient usually has had undiagnosed chronic pancreatitis before the first episode of acute pancreatitis occurs. Other less common causes of pancreatitis include bacterial or viral infection, with pancreatitis a complication of mumps virus. Blunt abdominal trauma, ischemic vascular disease, hyperlipidemia, hyperparathyroidism, and the use of corticosteroids, thiazide diuretics, and oral contraceptives have been associated with an increased incidence of pancreatitis. In addition, there is a small incidence of hereditary pancreatitis.

Mortality of acute pancreatitis remains high (10%) owing to toxemia, shock, anoxia, hypotension, or fluid and electrolyte imbalances. Attacks of acute pancreatitis may result in complete recovery, may recur without permanent damage, or may progress to chronic pancreatitis. The patient admitted to the hospital with a diagnosis of pancreatitis is acutely ill and requires skilled nursing and medical care.

Classification. Pancreatitis ranges in severity from a relatively mild, self-limiting disorder to a rapidly fatal disease that does not respond to any treatment. Edema and inflammation usually confined to the pancreas itself are the major events in the more mild form of pancreatitis, which is termed *interstitial* or *edematous pancreatitis*. Although this is considered the more mild form of pancreatitis, the patient is acutely ill and at risk of developing shock, fluid and electrolyte disturbances, and sepsis.

Acute hemorrhagic pancreatitis represents a more advanced form of acute interstitial pancreatitis. Enzymatic digestion of the gland is more widespread and complete. The tissue becomes necrotic, and the damage extends to its vascular radicles, so that blood escapes into the substance of the pancreas and beyond into the retroperitoneal tissues. Late complications consist of pancreatic cysts or abscesses. The mortality rate of acute hemorrhagic pancreatitis is 30%.

Clinical Manifestations. Severe abdominal pain is the major symptom of pancreatitis that brings the patient to medical care. Abdominal pain and tenderness, along with back pain, result from irritation and edema of the inflamed pancreas that stimulate the nerve endings. An increase in tension on the pancreatic capsule and obstruction of the pancreatic ducts also contribute to the pain. Typically, the pain occurs in the midepigastrium but can be supraumbilical. It is frequently acute in onset, occurring 24 to 48 hours after a very heavy meal or alcohol ingestion, and it may be diffuse and difficult to locate. It is generally more severe after meals and is unrelieved by antacids. Pain may be accompanied by abdominal distention and a poorly defined palpable abdominal mass.

The patient appears acutely ill. Abdominal guarding is present. A rigid or boardlike abdomen may occur and is generally a grave sign. Ecchymosis (bruising) in the flank or around the umbilicus may indicate severe, hemorrhagic pancreatitis.

Nausea and vomiting are common in acute pancreatitis. The vomitus is usually gastric in origin but may also be bile stained. Fever, jaundice, mental confusion, and agitation may also occur.

Although hypertension is not rare in acute pancreatitis, hypotension is more typical and may reflect hypovolemia and shock in acute hemorrhagic pancreatitis. Hypovolemia is due to loss of large amounts of protein-rich fluid into the tissues and peritoneal cavity. The patient may develop tachycardia, cyanosis, and cold, clammy skin in addition to hypotension.

Respiratory distress is common, and the patient may develop diffuse pulmonary infiltrates, dyspnea, tachypnea, and arterial hypoxemia.

The diagnosis of acute pancreatitis is based on a history of abdominal pain, the presence of known risk factors, physical examination findings, and selected diagnostic findings.

Diagnostic Evaluation. *Blood Studies.* Serum amylase and lipase are the most important aids in diagnosing acute pancreatitis. Peak levels are reached in 24 hours, with a rapid fall to normal levels within 48 to 72 hours. Serum lipase and amylase levels in the urine also become elevated and remain elevated longer than serum amylase. The white blood cell count is usually elevated; hypocalcemia is present in many patients and appears to be correlated with the severity of pancreatitis.

Transient hyperglycemia and glucosuria and elevated serum bilirubin levels occur in some patients with acute pancreatitis.

X-Ray Studies. X-ray films of the abdomen and chest are obtained to differentiate pancreatitis from other disorders that may cause similar symptoms and to detect the development of pleural effusions.

Ultrasonography and Computed Tomography. Sonograms and tomograms are used to identify an increase in the diameter of the pancreas and to detect pancreatic cysts or pseudocysts.

Stools. Usually the stools of patients suffering with pancreatic disease are bulky, pale, and foul smelling. Fat content varies between 50% and 90% in pancreatic disease; normally, the fat content is 20%.

Management. Management of the patient with acute pancreatitis is symptomatic and is directed toward preventing or treating complications. All oral intake is withheld to inhibit pancreatic stimulation and secretion of pancreatic enzymes. Although there is some controversy about the use of parenteral hyperalimentation in acute pancreatitis because of the possibility that it may stimulate pancreatic secretion, it is usually an important part of therapy, particularly in debilitated patients. Nasogastric suction is frequently used to decrease painful abdominal distention and paralytic ileus and to remove hydrochloric acid so that it does not enter the duodenum and stimulate the pancreas. Cimetidine (Tagamet) is also used to decrease hydrochloric acid secretion.

Systemic treatment is necessary if vascular collapse and shock occur. Adequate correction of fluid and blood loss is necessary to maintain fluid volume and prevent renal failure. The patient is usually acutely ill and is monitored in the intensive care unit. Antibiotics are frequently administered to control infection; insulin may be required if hyperglycemia occurs. Peritoneal lavage has been effective in severe pancreatitis or if ascites is significant.

Intense respiratory care is indicated because of the increased likelihood of elevation of the diaphragm, pulmonary infiltrates and effusion, and atelectasis. Hypoxemia occurs in a significant number of patients with acute pancreatitis even without abnormalities present on x-ray films. Respiratory care may range from close monitoring of arterial blood gases to use of humidified oxygen to intubation and use of a ventilator. Adequate pain relief is essential during the course of acute pancreatitis.

Antacids may be used when the acute episode of pancreatitis begins to resolve. Oral feedings that are low in fat and protein content are initiated very gradually. Caffeine and alcohol are eliminated from the diet. If the episode of pancreatitis occurred during treatment with thiazide diuretics, glucocorticoids, or oral contraceptives, these medications are discontinued. Follow-up of the patient may include ultrasound, x-ray studies, or endoscopic retrograde cholangiopancreatography (ERCP) to determine if the pancreatitis is resolving and to assess for abscesses and pseudocysts. ERCP may also be used to identify the cause of acute pancreatitis if it is in question.

► Nursing Process
The Patient With Acute Pancreatitis

▷ Assessment

The nursing history focuses on the presence and character of the patient's abdominal pain and discomfort. The presence of pain, its location, its relationship to eating and to alcohol consumption, and the effect of the patient's efforts to bring about relief of pain are noted. The patient's nutritional status and history of gallbladder attacks and alcohol use are assessed. A history of gastrointestinal problems including nausea, vomiting, diarrhea, and passage of stools containing fat is elicited. Respiratory status, respiratory rate and pattern, as well as the breath sounds are assessed. Normal and adventitious breath sounds and abnormal findings on chest percussion, including dullness at the bases of the lungs and abnormal fremitus, are documented.

▷ Nursing Diagnoses

Based on all the assessment data, the major nursing diagnoses of the patient with acute pancreatitis include the following:

- Severe pain and discomfort related to inflammation, edema, distention of the pancreas, and peritoneal irritation
- Altered fluid and nutritional status related to vomiting, inadequate fluid intake, fever and diaphoresis, and fluid shifts
- Alterations in respiratory function related to severe pain, pulmonary infiltrates, pleural effusion, and atelectasis

▷ Planning and Implementation

▷ *Goals:* The major goals for the patient include relief of pain and discomfort, improved fluid and nutritional status, and improved respiratory function.

Nursing Interventions

Relief of Pain and Discomfort. Since the pathologic process responsible for pain is autodigestion of the pancreas, the objectives of therapy are to relieve pain and to decrease secretion of the enzymes of the pancreas. The pain of acute pancreatitis is often very severe, necessitating the liberal use of analgesics. Meperidine (Demerol) is the drug of choice; morphine sulfate is to be avoided because it causes spasm of the sphincter of Oddi. Oral feedings are withheld to decrease the formation and secretion of secretin. The patient is maintained on parenteral fluids and electrolytes to restore fluid balance. Nasogastric suction is used to remove gastric secretions and to relieve abdominal distention. The patient will require frequent explanations by the nurse about the necessity of withholding fluid intake and maintaining gastric suction. Additionally, the nurse provides frequent oral hygiene

and care to decrease discomfort from the nasogastric tube and relieve dryness of the mouth, which will be even more of a problem for the patient if he is receiving anticholinergic drugs to decrease pancreatic secretions.

The acutely ill patient will be maintained on bed rest to decrease the metabolic rate and reduce the secretion of pancreatic and gastric enzymes. If the patient experiences increasing severity of pain, this is reported to the physician because the patient may be experiencing hemorrhage of the pancreas or the dose of analgesic may be inadequate.

Fluid Balance and Nutritional Status. Nausea, vomiting, gastric suction, movement of fluid from the vascular compartment to the peritoneal cavity, and diaphoresis and fever increase the patient's need for fluid and electrolyte replacement. Intravenous fluids will be administered and may be accompanied by transfusion of blood and albumin to maintain the patient's blood volume. The nurse assesses the patient's fluid and electrolyte status by noting skin turgor and moistness of mucous membranes. The patient is weighed daily, and fluid intake and output are carefully measured, including urine output, nasogastric secretions, and diarrhea. The nurse observes the patient for the presence of ascites and measures abdominal girth if ascites is suspected.

During the attack of acute pancreatitis, the patient will not be permitted food and oral fluid intake; however, it is important for the nurse to assess the patient's nutritional status and to note any events that alter the patient's fluid and nutritional needs. These signs include increased body temperature, restlessness and increased physical activity, and fluid and nutrient loss through diarrhea. Circulatory collapse and shock are possible complications; therefore, frequent assessment of the patient is indicated and emergency medications are kept readily available.

As the patient's acute symptoms subside, oral feedings are reintroduced gradually. Between acute attacks, the patient receives a diet high in carbohydrates and low in fat and proteins. Heavy meals are to be avoided, as are alcoholic beverages.

Improvement of Respiratory Function. The patient is maintained in semi-Fowler's position to decrease pressure on the diaphragm by a distended abdomen and to increase respiratory expansion. Frequent changes of position are necessary to prevent atelectasis and pooling of respiratory secretions. Anticholinergic medications, if given to decrease gastric and pancreatic secretions, also dry the secretions of the respiratory tract, predisposing the patient to obstruction and infection. Pulmonary assessment is essential to observe for any changes in respiratory status. The patient is instructed in techniques of coughing and deep breathing to improve respiratory function.

Patient Education and Home Health Care. The patient who has experienced and survived an episode of acute pancreatitis has usually been acutely ill. He will require a prolonged period of time to regain strength and return to his previous level of activity. Because of the severity of the acute illness, the patient may not recall many of the facts and explanations that have been given to him during hospitalization. As a result, this patient often requires repetition and reinforcement of information and instructions. If acute pancreatitis is a result of biliary tract disease such as gallstones and gallbladder disease, the patient requires reinforcement about the need for a low fat diet and avoidance of heavy meals. If the pancreatitis is a result of alcohol abuse, the patient needs to be reminded of the importance of eliminating *all* alcohol. When the acute attack has subsided and he returns to his previous environment, he may be inclined to return to his previous habits. This patient needs to be given specific information about resources and support groups that may be of assistance in avoiding alcohol in the future. Referral to Alcoholics Anonymous or other support groups is essential.

A referral to the community health nurse is often indicated to permit the nurse to assess the patient's home situation, reinforce instructions about fluid and nutrition intake and avoidance of alcohol, and permit the patient and family members to discuss their questions and concerns.

A summary of nursing management of the patient with acute pancreatitis is provided in Nursing Care Plan 37-3.

▷ *Evaluation*

▷ *Expected Outcomes*

1. Patient experiences relief of pain and discomfort.
   a. Reports relief of pain and discomfort.
   b. Explains rationale for nasogastric tube and suction.
   c. Uses analgesics as prescribed, without overuse.
   d. Participates in oral hygiene measures.
   e. Maintains bed rest as prescribed.
   f. Uses anticholinergics appropriately if prescribed.
   g. Avoids alcohol to decrease abdominal pain.
2. Achieves improved fluid and nutritional balance.
   a. Demonstrates normal skin turgor and moist mucous membranes.
   b. Reports stabilization of weight.
   c. Demonstrates no increase in abdominal girth.
   d. Reports decrease in number of episodes of diarrhea.
   e. Identifies and consumes high-carbohydrate, low-protein foods.
   f. Explains rationale for eliminating alcohol intake.
   g. Maintains adequate fluid intake within prescribed guidelines.
3. Experiences improved respiratory function.
   a. Maintains semi-Fowler's position when in bed.
   b. Changes position in bed frequently.
   c. Coughs and takes deep breaths at least every hour.
   d. Demonstrates normal respiratory rate and pattern and full lung expansion.
   e. Demonstrates normal breath sounds and absence of adventitious breath sounds.
   f. Drinks at least 8 glasses of nonalcoholic fluids per day (if within fluid allowance) to liquefy pulmonary secretions.
   g. Demonstrates normal body temperature and absence of indications of respiratory infection.

Chronic Pancreatitis

Chronic pancreatitis is an inflammatory disease characterized by progressive anatomical and functional destruction of the pancreas. As cells are replaced by fibrous tissue with repeated attacks of pancreatitis, pressure within the pancreas increases. The end result is mechanical obstruction of the pancreatic and common bile ducts and the duodenum. Additionally,

there is atrophy of the epithelium of the ducts, inflammation, and destruction of the secreting cells of the pancreas.

Alcohol consumption in Western societies and malnutrition worldwide are the major causes of chronic pancreatitis. In alcoholism, the incidence of pancreatitis is 50 times the rate in the nondrinking population. Chronic consumption of alcohol produces a hypersecretion of protein in pancreatic secretions. The result is protein plugs and calculi within the pancreatic ducts. There is also evidence that alcohol has a direct toxic effect on the cells of the pancreas. Damage to these cells is more likely to occur and to be more severe in patients whose diets are poor in protein content and either very high or very low in fat. The incidence of chronic pancreatitis is increased in adult men and is characterized by recurring attacks of severe upper abdominal and back pain, accompanied by vomiting. Attacks often are so painful that narcotics, even in large doses, do not provide relief. As the disease progresses, recurring attacks of pain will be more severe, more frequent, and of longer duration. Some patients complain of continuous severe pain; others have a dull, nagging constant pain. The risk of addiction to opiates is increased in pancreatitis because of the nature of the pain.

Weight loss is a major problem in chronic pancreatitis; over 75% of patients experience significant weight loss usually due to decreased dietary intake secondary to anorexia or fear that eating will precipitate another attack. Malabsorption occurs late in the disease when as little as 10% of function remains. As a result, the digestion of foodstuffs, especially proteins and fats, is disrupted. The stools become frequent, frothy, and foul smelling, owing to the impairment of fat digestion, which results in a stool with a high fat content. This condition is referred to as *steatorrhea*. As the disease progresses, calcification of the gland may occur and calcium stones may form within the ducts.

Diagnostic Evaluation. Endoscopic retrograde cholangiopancreatography (ERCP) is the most helpful study in the diagnosis of chronic pancreatitis. It provides detail about the anatomy of the pancreas and of the pancreatic and biliary ducts. It is also helpful in obtaining tissue for analysis and in differentiating pancreatitis from other conditions such as carcinoma. A CT scan or ultrasonography is helpful to detect the presence of pancreatic cyst formation. A glucose tolerance test evaluates pancreatic islet cell function, information necessary for making decisions about surgical resection of the pancreas. An abnormal glucose tolerance test indicative of diabetes may be present. In contrast to the patient with acute pancreatitis, serum amylase levels and the white blood cell count are unremarkable.

Management. The management of chronic pancreatitis depends on its probable cause in each patient. Nonsurgical approaches may be indicated for the patient who refuses surgery, is a poor candidate for surgery, or whose disease and symptoms do not warrant surgical intervention. Treatment includes prevention and management of acute attacks, the relief of pain and discomfort, and management of exocrine and endocrine insufficiency of pancreatitis. Treatment and prevention of abdominal pain and discomfort are similar to those used in acute pancreatitis; however, the focus is usually on use of nonopiate methods to prevent or treat pain. The physician as well as nurse and dietitian emphasize to the patient and family the importance of avoiding alcohol and other foods that the patient has found tend to produce ab-

(Text continues on p. 982)

Care of the Patient With Acute Pancreatitis

Nursing Interventions	Rationale	Expected Outcomes

Nursing Diagnosis: Severe pain and discomfort related to edema, distention of the pancreas, and peritoneal irritation

Goal: Relief of pain and discomfort

Nursing Interventions	Rationale	Expected Outcomes
1. Administer meperidine (Demerol) frequently, as prescribed, based on patient's level of pain and discomfort.	1. Meperidine acts by depressing the central nervous system and thereby increasing the patient's pain threshold. Morphine is not usually given because it has a tendency to produce spasm of the sphincter of Oddi.	• Reports relief of pain. • Moves and turns without increasing pain and discomfort. • Rests comfortably and sleeps for increasing periods of time. • Reports less frequent episodes of pain, discomfort, and cramping.
2. Assess pain level before and after administration of analgesic.	2. Assessment and control of pain are important because restlessness increases body metabolism, which stimulates the secretion of pancreatic and gastric enzymes.	
3. Report unrelieved pain or increasing intensity of pain.	3. Pain may increase pancreatic enzymes and may also indicate pancreatic hemorrhage.	
4. Assist the patient to assume positions of comfort.	4. Frequent turning relieves pressure and aids in preventing pulmonary and vascular complications.	

Goal: Reduction of stimulation of the pancreas

Nursing Interventions	Rationale	Expected Outcomes
1. Give anticholinergic drugs as prescribed.	1. Anticholinergic drugs reduce gastric and pancreatic secretion.	• Reports relief of pain, discomfort, and abdominal cramping. • Takes no fluid and food during acute phase. • Maintains bed rest. • Explains rationale for fluid and dietary restrictions and use of nasogastric drainage.
2. Withhold oral intake.	2. Pancreatic secretion is increased by food and fluid intake.	
3. Keep the patient on bed rest.	3. Bed rest decreases body metabolism and thus reduces pancreatic and gastric secretions.	

4. Use continuous nasogastric suction.
  a. Measure gastric secretions at specified intervals.
  b. Observe and chart color and viscosity of gastric secretions.
  c. Ensure that the nasogastric tube is patent, to permit free drainage.
	4. Nasogastric suction removes gastric contents and prevents gastric secretions from entering the duodenum and stimulating the secretin mechanism. Decompression of the intestines (if intestinal intubation is used) also assists in relieving respiratory distress.	

Goal: Relief of discomfort associated with nasogastric drainage

Nursing Interventions	Rationale	Expected Outcomes
1. Use water-soluble lubricant around external nares.	1. Prevents irritation.	• Exhibits intact skin and tissue of nares at site of nasogastric tube insertion. • Reports no pain or irritation of nares or oropharynx. • Exhibits moist, clean mucous membranes of mouth and nasopharynx. • States that thirst is relieved by oral hygiene. • Restates rationale for nasogastric tube and suction.
2. Turn patient at intervals.	2. Relieves pressure of tube on esophageal and gastric mucosa.	
3. Give oral hygiene and gargling solutions.	3. Relieves dryness and irritation of oropharynx.	
4. Explain rationale for use of nasogastric drainage.	4. Assists patient to cope with the drainage nasogastric tube and suction.	

(continued)

Nursing Interventions	Rationale	Expected Outcomes

Nursing Diagnosis: Fluid volume deficit related to vomiting, decreased fluid intake, fever and diaphoresis, and fluid shifts

Goal: Improvement in fluid and electrolyte status

1. Assess fluid and electrolyte status (skin turgor, mucous membranes, urine output, vital signs).	1. The amount and type of fluid and electrolyte replacement are determined by the status of the blood pressure, the laboratory evaluations of serum electrolyte and blood urea nitrogen levels, the urinary volume, and the assessment of the patient's condition.	• Exhibits moist mucous membranes and normal skin turgor. • Exhibits normal blood pressure without evidence of postural (orthostatic) hypotension. • Excretes adequate urine output. • Exhibits normal, not excessive, thirst.
2. Assess sources of fluid and electrolyte loss (vomiting, diarrhea, nasogastric drainage, excessive diaphoresis).	2. Electrolyte losses occur from nasogastric suctioning, severe diaphoresis, emesis, and as a result of the patient's being in a fasting state.	• Maintains normal blood pressure, pulse, and respiratory rate. • Remains alert and responsive. • Exhibits normal arterial pressures and arterial blood gases.

3. Combat shock if present.
  a. Administer corticosteroids as prescribed to those who do not respond to conventional treatment.
  b. Evaluate the amount of urinary output. Attempt to maintain this at 50 ml/hr.
	3. Extensive acute pancreatitis may cause peripheral vascular collapse and shock. Blood and plasma may be lost into the abdominal cavity, and therefore there is a decreased blood and plasma volume. The toxins from the bacteria of a necrotic pancreas may cause shock.	• Exhibits normal electrolyte levels.
		• Exhibits no signs or symptoms of calcium deficit (*e.g.,* tetany, carpopedal spasm).
		• Exhibits no additional losses of fluids and electrolytes through vomiting, diarrhea, or diaphoresis.

4. Give intravenous electrolytes (sodium, potassium, chlorides) as prescribed.	4. Patients with hemorrhagic pancreatitis lose large amounts of blood and plasma, which decreases effective circulation and blood volume.	• Reports stabilization of weight. • Demonstrates no increase in abdominal girth. • Demonstrates no fluid wave on palpation of the abdomen.
5. Give plasma, albumin, and blood as prescribed.	5. Replacement with blood, plasma or albumin, assists in ensuring effective circulating blood volume.	
6. Keep a supply of intravenous calcium gluconate readily available.	6. May be prescribed to prevent or treat tetany.	

7. Assess abdomen for ascites formation:
  a. Measure abdominal girth daily.
  b. Weigh patient daily.
  c. Palpate abdomen for fluid wave (p. 865).
	7. During acute pancreatitis, plasma may be lost into the abdominal cavity, which diminishes the blood volume.	

Nursing Diagnosis: Alteration in nutrition: Less than body requirements related to inadequate dietary intake, impaired pancreatic secretions, increased nutritional needs secondary to acute illness, and increased body temperature

Goal: Improvement in nutritional status

1. Assess current nutritional status and increased metabolic requirements.	1. Alteration in pancreatic secretions interferes with normal digestive processes. Acute illness, infection, and fever increase metabolic needs.	• Maintains normal body weight. • Demonstrates no increase in weight loss. • Maintains normal serum glucose levels.
2. Montor serum glucose levels and give insulin as prescribed.	2. Impairment of endocrine function of the pancreas leads to increased serum glucose levels.	• Reports decreasing episodes of vomiting and diarrhea. • Reports return of normal stool characteristics and bowel pattern.

(continued)

Nursing Interventions	*Rationale*	*Expected Outcomes*

Nursing Diagnosis: Alteration in nutrition: Less than body requirements related to inadequate dietary intake, impaired pancreatic secretions, increased nutritional needs secondary to acute illness, and increased body temperature

Goal: Improvement in nutritional status

3. Administer intravenous fluid and electrolytes and parenteral nutrition as prescribed.	3. Parenteral administration of fluids, electrolytes, and nutrients is essential to provide fluids, calories, electrolytes, and nutrients when oral intake is prohibited.	• Consumes foods high in carbohydrate, low in fat and protein. • Explains rationale for high-carbohydrate, low-fat, low-protein diet. • Eliminates alcohol from diet.
4. Provide high-carbohydrate, low-protein, low-fat diet when tolerated.	4. These foods increase caloric intake without stimulating pancreatic secretions beyond the ability of the pancreas to respond.	• Explains rationale for limiting coffee intake and avoiding spicy foods.
5. Instruct patient to eliminate alcohol.	5. Alcohol intake produces further damage to pancreas and precipitates attacks of acute pancreatitis.	
6. Counsel patient to avoid excessive use of coffee and spicy foods.	6. Coffee and spicy foods increase pancreatic and gastric secretions.	

Nursing Diagnosis: Alterations in respiratory function related to splinting from severe pain, pulmonary infiltrates, pleural effusion, and atelectasis

Goal: Improvement in respiratory function

1. Assess respiratory status (rate, pattern, breath sounds).	1. Acute pancreatitis produces retroperitoneal edema, elevation of the diaphragm, pleural effusion, and inadequate lung ventilation. Intra-abdominal infection and labored breathing increase the body's metabolic demand, which further decreases pulmonary reserve and leads to respiratory failure.	• Demonstrates normal respiratory rate and pattern and full lung expansion. • Demonstrates normal breath sounds and absence of adventitious breath sounds. • Demonstrates normal arterial blood gases.
2. Maintain semi-Fowler's position	2. To decrease pressure on diaphragm and allow greater lung expansion.	• Maintains semi-Fowler's position when in bed. • Changes position in bed frequently.
3. Instruct and encourage patient to take deep breaths and to cough every hour.	3. Taking deep breaths and coughing will clear the airways and reduce atelectasis.	• Coughs and takes deep breaths at least every hour. • Demonstrates normal body temperature.
4. Assist patient to turn and change position every 2 hours.	4. Changing position frequently assists aeration and drainage of all lobes of the lungs.	• Exhibits no signs or symptoms of respiratory infection or impairment. • Is alert and responsive to environment.

5. Reduce the excessive metabolism of the body.
  a. Give antibiotics as prescribed.
  b. Place patient in an air-conditioned room.
  c. Administer nasal oxygen as required for hypoxia.
  d. Use a hypothermia blanket if necessary.
	5. Pancreatitis produces a severe peritoneal and retroperitoneal reaction that causes fever, tachycardia, and accelerated respirations. Placing the patient in an air-conditioned room and supporting him with oxygen therapy decreases the work load of the respiratory system and the tissue utilization of oxygen. Reduction of fever and pulse rate decreases the metabolic demands on the body.	

dominal pain and discomfort. The fact that no other treatment will be successful in relieving pain if the patient continues to consume alcohol is stressed to the patient.

Diabetes mellitus resulting from dysfunction of the pancreas islet cells is treated with diet, insulin, or oral hypoglycemic agents. The hazard of severe hypoglycemia if alcohol use continues is stressed to the patient and family members. Pancreatic enzyme replacement is indicated in the patient with malabsorption and steatorrhea.

Surgery is generally carried out to relieve abdominal pain and discomfort, to restore drainage of pancreatic secretions, and to reduce the frequency of acute attacks of pancreatitis. The surgical procedure to be performed depends on the anatomical and functional abnormalities of the pancreas, including the location of disease within the pancreas, the presence of diabetes, exocrine insufficiency, biliary stenosis, and pseudocysts of the pancreas. Other factors taken into consideration in determining if surgery is to be performed and what procedure is to be carried out include the presence of alcoholism and the ability of the patient to manage the endocrine or exocrine changes that are expected from surgical alterations.

Pancreaticojejunostomy with a side-to-side anastomosis or joining of the pancreatic duct to the jejunum allows drainage of the pancreatic secretions into the jejunum. Pain relief occurs by 6 months in over 80% of the patients who undergo this procedure, but pain returns in a substantial number of these patients as the disease itself progresses. A variety of other surgical procedures are performed for different degrees and types of disease, ranging from revision of the sphincter of the ampulla of Vater, internal drainage of a pancreatic cyst into the stomach, to wide resection or removal of the pancreas. Attempts have been made to preserve the endocrine function of the pancreas by autotransplantation or implantation of the patient's pancreas islet cells. Testing and refinement of this procedure continue in an effort to improve the results. Morbidity and mortality following these surgical procedures are high because of the poor physical condition of the patient prior to surgery and the concomitant occurrence of cirrhosis.

Despite these operative procedures the patient is likely to continue having pain and digestive difficulties from the pancreatitis unless he abstains completely from the use of alcohol. This point should be emphasized by the nurse in the course of instructing the patient and the family.

Pancreatic Cysts

As a result of the local necrosis that occurs at the time of acute pancreatitis, collections of fluid may form in the vicinity of the pancreas. These become walled off by fibrous tissue and are called pancreatic cysts. They are the most common type of pancreatic cyst; other types develop as a result of congenital anomalies or secondary to chronic pancreatitis or trauma to the pancreas.

Diagnosis of pancreatic cysts is made by ultrasound, CT scan, and ERCP. ERCP may be used to define the anatomy of the pancreas and to evaluate the patency of pancreatic drainage. Pancreatic cysts may attain considerable size. Because of their location behind the posterior peritoneum, when they enlarge, they impinge on and displace the stomach or

the colon, which are adjacent. Eventually, through pressure or secondary infection, they produce symptoms, requiring that they be drained.

Management. Drainage into the gastrointestinal tract or through the skin surface of the abdominal wall may be established. In the latter instance, the drainage is likely to be profuse and destructive to tissue because of the enzyme contents. Hence, steps must be taken to protect the skin in areas adjacent to the drainage site to prevent excoriation. Ointments protect the skin, provided that they are applied before excoriation takes place. Another method involves the constant aspiration of digestive juice from the drainage tract by means of a suction apparatus, so that contact with the digestive enzymes is avoided. This method demands expert nursing attention to be sure that the suction tube does not become dislodged from the drainage tract and that the entire apparatus functions properly without interruption.

When chronic pancreatitis develops in association with gallbladder disease, efforts are made to relieve the difficulty by surgically exploring the common duct and removing the stones; usually, the gallbladder is removed at the same time. In addition, an attempt is made to improve the drainage of the common bile duct and the pancreatic duct by dividing the sphincter of Oddi, a muscle that is located at the ampulla of Vater (this operation is known as a *sphincterotomy*). Nursing management after such an operation is the same as that indicated for all patients undergoing biliary tract surgery. A T tube usually is placed in the common bile duct, requiring a drainage system to collect the bile after the operation.

Pancreatic Tumors

Carcinoma of the Pancreas

The incidence of pancreatic cancer has been steadily increasing for the past 20 to 30 years, especially in nonwhite males. It is the fourth leading cause of cancer deaths in the United States and occurs most frequently in the sixth and seventh decades of life. Exposure to chemicals, a high-fat diet, and cigarette smoking are associated with an increased incidence of pancreatic cancer, although their role in the etiology is unclear.

Cancer may arise in any portion of the pancreas (in the head, the body, or the tail), producing clinical manifestations that vary, depending on the location of the lesion and whether or not functioning, insulin-secreting pancreatic islet cells are involved. Tumors that originate in the head of the pancreas, the most common location, give rise to a distinctive clinical picture (see p. 983). Functioning islet cell tumors, whether benign (adenoma) or malignant (carcinoma) are responsible for the syndrome of hyperinsulinism (see p. 987). With these exceptions, the symptoms are nonspecific and patients usually do not seek medical attention until late in the course of their illness; eighty to 85% of patients have advanced, unresectable disease when the tumor is first detected.

Clinical Manifestations. Anorexia, weight loss, abdominal pain, or jaundice may be the initial symptom and may develop only when the disease is far advanced. Other signs include rapid, profound, and progressive weight loss, as well as vague, upper or midabdominal pain or discomfort that is unrelated to any gastrointestinal function and difficult to describe. Such discomfort radiates as a boring pain in the midback and is unrelated to posture or activity. Patients with pancreatic carcinoma often find that they get some relief from pain by sitting hunched forward; pain is often accentuated by lying supine. A full-length foam-rubber pad placed under the patient has proven beneficial and protects the bony prominences from pressure. Pain is often progressive and severe, requiring the use of narcotic analgesics. The formation of ascites is common.

A very important sign, when present, is the onset of symptoms of insulin deficiency: glucosuria, hyperglycemia, and abnormal glucose tolerance. Diabetes may be an early sign of carcinoma of the pancreas. Meals often aggravate epigastric pain, which usually occurs weeks before the appearance of jaundice and pruritus. A gastrointestinal x-ray series may demonstrate deformities in adjacent viscera caused by the impinging pancreatic mass. Ultrasonography, CT scanning, and ERCP are useful in establishing the diagnosis.

Percutaneous fine needle aspiration biopsy of the pancreas is used to diagnose pancreatic tumors and to confirm the diagnosis in patients whose tumors are not resectable, eliminating the stress and postoperative pain of ineffective surgery. In candidates for surgery, a preoperative diagnosis of the tumor is helpful in planning the surgical procedure. In this procedure, a needle is inserted through the anterior abdominal wall into the pancreatic mass under the guidance of CT scan, ultrasound, ERCP, or other imaging techniques. The aspirated material is examined for malignant cells.

Management.   Therapy usually is limited to palliative measures. Definitive surgical treatment (*i.e.*, total excision of the lesion) often is not feasible because of the extensive growth when the lesion is finally diagnosed and the probable widespread metastases—especially to the liver, lungs, and bones.

The surgical procedure is usually extensive if carried out to remove resectable localized tumors. Although pancreatic tumors may be resistant to standard radiation therapy, the patient may be treated with radiation and chemotherapy. Pain management and attention to nutritional requirements are important measures to improve the patient's level of comfort.

Tumors of the Head of the Pancreas

Assessment.   Tumors in this region of the pancreas cause obstruction of the common bile duct where it passes through the head of the pancreas to join the pancreatic duct and empty at the ampulla of Vater into the duodenum. Obstruction to the flow of bile produces jaundice, clay-colored stools, and dark urine.

Malabsorption of nutrients and fat-soluble vitamins may result from the obstruction and from the absence of bile from the gastrointestinal tract. Some degree of abdominal discomfort or pain and of pruritus may be noted. Nonspecific symptoms such as anorexia, weight loss, and malaise may be present. If present, suspicion of visceral cancer is heightened.

This disease must be differentiated from the jaundice due to a biliary obstruction caused by a gallstone in the common duct, which usually is intermittent and appears typically in obese patients, most often women, who have had previous symptoms of gallbladder disease. The tumors producing the obstruction may arise from the pancreas, from the common bile duct, or from the ampulla of Vater.

Management.   When these patients come to the hospital, they are in such a poor nutritional and physical state that a fairly long period of preparation is necessary before operation can be attempted. Various liver and pancreatic function studies are carried out, vitamin K is given to restore the blood prothrombin activity, and diets high in protein often are given with pancreatic enzymes. Blood transfusions frequently are used as well.

Following conventional blood and x-ray studies, more sophisticated diagnostic aids may be used, including duodenography, angiography by hepatic or celiac artery catheterization, pancreatic scanning, percutaneous transhepatic cholangiography, ERCP, and percutaneous needle biopsy of the pancreas. Laparotomy with biopsy of the pancreas is a valuable diagnostic aid.

Surgical Management.   A biliary-enteric shunt may be performed to relieve the jaundice and, perhaps, provide time for a suspicious lesion to be proven nonmalignant. Pancreatoduodenectomy (Whipple's procedure), which involves the

(Text continues on p. 986)

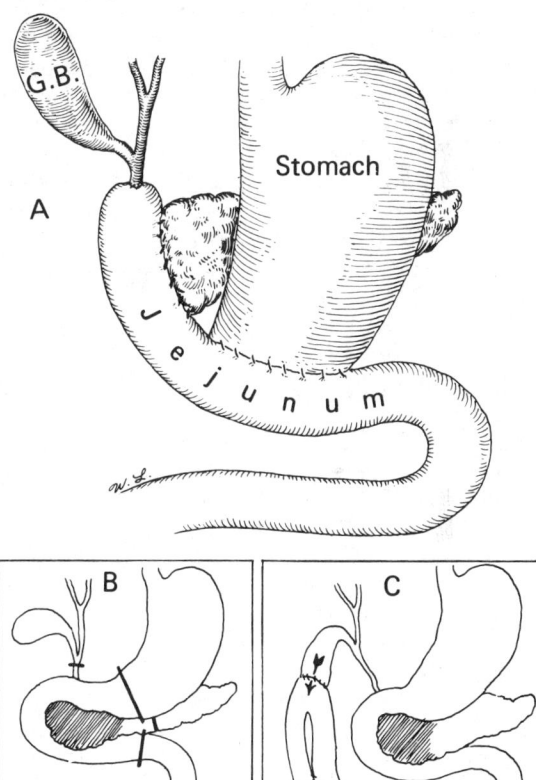

Figure 37-5
Pancreatoduodenectomy (after Whipple). (*A*) End result of resection of the carcinoma of the head of the pancreas or the ampulla of Vater. The common duct is sutured to the end of the jejunum, and the remaining portion of the pancreas and the end of the stomach are sutured to the side of the jejunum. (*B*) Lines indicate removal of head of pancreas, duodenum, adjacent stomach, and distal segment of common bile duct. (*C*) Cholecystojejunostomy is an alternative operation if tumor of the head of the pancreas is inoperable. Bile flows into the intestine through the anastomosis of the jejunum and gallbladder.

Care of the Patient Following Pancreatoduodenectomy (Whipple's Procedure)

Nursing Interventions	*Rationale*	*Expected Outcomes*

Nursing Diagnosis: Pain and discomfort related to extensive surgical incision and presence of nasogastric tube

Goal: Relief of pain and discomfort

1. Assess pain frequently before and after administration of analgesics.	1. Increasing pain may indicate occurrence of complications (pancreatitis, peritonitis, perforation of organ or leakage of anastomosis).	• Reports decreasing pain and discomfort. • Experiences no increase in severity or frequency of pain.
2. Administer pain medication frequently, as prescribed.	2. Previous use of pain medications for past persistent pain may alter patient's response to pain medications and necessitate larger doses.	• Takes pain medication as prescribed. • Turns frequently with assistance to positions of comfort.
3. Assist patient to assume position of comfort.	3. Position changes relieve pressure areas and decrease pressure and stress on suture lines.	• Rests comfortably without pain and discomfort. • Exhibits intact, nonirritated skin and tissue of nares at site of nasogastric tube insertion.
4. Use water-soluble lubricant around external nares.	4. Lubricates the tissues and decreases friction at site of nasogastric tube insertion.	• Reports no pain or irritation of nasopharynx, oropharynx, or nares.
5. Give oral hygiene and gargling solutions.	5. Relieves dryness and irritation of oropharynx.	• Exhibits moist, clean mucous membranes of mouth and nasopharynx. • Reports no excessive thirst.
6. Explain reasons for nasogastric tube and drainage.	6. Information increases the patient's ability to cope with nasogastric tube and drainage.	• States rationale for nasogastric tube and suction.

Nursing Diagnosis: Alterations in respiratory function related to extensive surgical incisions, immobility, prolonged anesthesia.

Goal: Improvement of respiratory function

1. Assess patient's respiratory status: a. Dependence on mechanical ventilator b. Respiratory rate and pattern c. Thoracic excursion d. Breath sounds and adventitious sounds	1. Splinting from extensive surgical excisions, prolonged immobility, and anesthesia frequently produce ineffective respiratory patterns and retained pulmonary secretions.	• Exhibits respiratory rate of 12 to 18/min with adequate thoracic excursion. • Breathes effectively without the mechanical ventilator. • Exhibits normal breath sounds without adventitious sounds.
2. Aspirate pulmonary secretions from the endotracheal tube or tracheostomy tube, as indicated.	2. Retained secretions interfere with adequate oxygen–carbon dioxide exchange.	• Takes deep breaths and coughs hourly while splinting abdominal incisions. • Coughs productively clear or white sputum.
3. Encourage and assist patient to cough and take deep breaths every hour.	3. Coughing and deep breathing aid in removal of pulmonary secretions and prevent atelectasis.	• Changes position frequently. • Exhibits normal body temperature and absence of respiratory infection.
4. Assist patient to change positions every hour.	4. Frequent changes of position will assist drainage of all lobes of the lungs.	

(continued)

Nursing Interventions	*Rationale*	*Expected Outcomes*

Nursing Diagnosis: Alteration in nutrition: Less than body requirements related to inadequate nutrition prior to surgery, increased metabolic demands secondary to extensive surgery, tissue repair, and altered gastrointestinal function

Goal: Improved nutritional state

1. Assess and report changes in factors affecting nutritional needs and status:
  a. Increased body temperature
  b. Increased gastrointestinal drainage and fluid loss
  c. Signs of infection
  d. Stress level
	1. Fever, increased gastrointestinal drainage, infection, and increased level of stress increase metabolic and nutritional needs.	• Maintains or increases body weight without edema formation.
		• Demonstrates no increase in metabolic rate and nutritional requirements:
		  Exhibits normal body temperature.
		  Experiences no excessive gastrointestinal losses of fluid or nutrients.
		  Demonstrates absence of signs of infection and inflammation.
		  Exhibits decreasing levels of stress.

2. Administer parenteral fluids, electrolytes, and nutrients as prescribed.	2. Parenteral administration of fluid, electrolytes, and nutrients is essential for healing when oral intake is prohibited.	• Exhibits rapid healing of incisions and no fistula formation.
3. Examine skin and tissue for breakdown and fistula formation.	3. The likelihood of breakdown of tissue increases with malnutrition and in turn increases need for nutrients.	• Exhibits intact skin without evidence of breakdown. • Exhibits normal serum glucose levels.
4. Monitor serum glucose level and observe for symptoms of hyperglycemia and hypoglycemia.	4. The insulin-secreting islets of Langerhans of the pancreas may be impaired or may be removed during surgery, increasing the risk of hypoglycemia or hyperglycemia.	• Consumes foods high in carbohydrates, proteins, and vitamins. • Reports enhanced appetite. • Explains rationale for foods high in carbohydrates, proteins, and vitamins.
5. Provide a high-carbohydrate, high-protein, high-vitamin diet as prescribed when oral intake is tolerated.	5. A high-carbohydrate, high-protein, high-vitamin diet is necessary to meet increased nutritional needs, prevent loss of muscle mass, promote healing of surgical incisions, and maintain weight.	• Identifies foods high in carbohydrates, proteins, and vitamins. • Takes pancreatic enzymes with meals as prescribed. • Reports decreasing episodes of diarrhea and steatorrhea.
6. Administer pancreatic enzymes (Pancrease or Viokase) with meals if prescribed.	6. Surgical resection of the pancreas may result in inadequate pancreatic enzymes, leading to malabsorption and further malnutrition.	• Explains rationale for use of pancreatic enzymes with meals.

Nursing Diagnosis: Potential impairment of skin and tissue integrity

Goal: Improvement of skin and tissue integrity

1. Avoid pressure on anastomoses and sutures:
  a. Irrigate nasogastric tube and other drainage tubes *gently* and *only* if prescribed.
 	
  b. Assess for adequate drainage from T tube, nasogastric tube, and any other drainage systems.
  c. Prevent kinking of tubing.
	a. Ensures patency of drainage tubes but avoids increased intraluminal pressure and disruption of anastomosis and suture lines.
	b. Ensures patency of drainage tubes and assesses type and amount of drainage.
	c. Prevents buildup of intraluminal pressure and pressure on anastomosis.
		• Exhibits expected type and amount of drainage from T tube, nasogastric tube, and other drainage tubes.
		• Exhibits no untoward effects after irrigation of drainage tubes, if irrigation is needed.
		• Demonstrates return of normal bowel sounds.
		• Exhibits no abdominal distention.
		• Passes flatus.

(continued)

Nursing Care Plan 37-4 (continued)

Nursing Interventions	Rationale	Expected Outcomes

Nursing Diagnosis: Potential impairment of skin and tissue integrity

Goal: Improvement of skin and tissue integrity

2. Withhold oral intake until gastrointestinal function returns and diet and fluids are prescribed.	2. Too early intake of foods and fluid may cause abdominal distention and vomiting, increasing the risk of disrupting surgical anastomoses.	• Reports no nausea or vomiting. • Exhibits clean surgical incision without signs of inflammation, infection, or abscess formation.
3. Assess bowel sounds and abdomen for distention.	3. Provides data about gastrointestinal function and early intestinal obstruction.	• Exhibits normal body temperature. • Exhibits pink, intact skin without signs of breakdown, irritation, or excoriation.
4. Inspect surgical incisions for inflammation, infection, and abscess formation.	4. Poor nutritional state and extensive surgery increase susceptibility to poor wound healing and increased skin and tissue breakdown.	• Demonstrates no purulent drainage or leakage of gastrointestinal secretions to skin surface.
5. Inspect skin for breakdown, irritation, and excoriation.	5. Leakage of gastrointestinal drainage may cause digestion and excoriation of skin.	• Reports no increased pressure or pain at surgical incisions or sites of drainage tubes.
6. Maintain aseptic technique in handling wound dressings and drainage and all secretions.	6. Minimizes the risk of infection in susceptible patient.	
7. Apply paste or salve to skin at sites of drainage.	7. Protects skin from further excoriation and damage.	

removal of the gallbladder, distal portion of the stomach, duodenum, and head of the pancreas and anastomosis of the remaining pancreas, stomach, and common duct to the jejunum, is the operation of choice for potentially curable cancer of the head of the pancreas (Fig. 37-5*A, B,* p. 983). The result is removal of the tumor, allowing flow of bile into the jejunum. When excision of the tumor cannot be performed, the jaundice may be relieved by diverting the bile flow into the jejunum by anastomosing the jejunum to the gallbladder, a procedure known as cholecystojejunostomy (Fig. 37-5*C,* p. 983).

Nursing Management. Extensive preoperative preparation is indicated and includes adequate hydration and nutrition, correction of prothrombin deficiency with vitamin K, and treatment of anemia to minimize postoperative complications.

The postoperative management of patients who have undergone a pancreatoduodenectomy or Whipple procedure is similar to the management of patients following extensive gastrointestinal and biliary surgery. The psychosocial considerations, however, are more specific and must be properly approached by the nurse. In view of the fact that the patient has undergone major and risky surgery and is severely ill, he most likely will experience anxiety and depression that will affect his response to therapy.

The mortality rate following this procedure has decreased recently because of advances in methods of nutritional support and improved techniques of surgical anastomosis. Preoperatively and postoperatively, the challenge for the nurse is to promote patient comfort, prevent complications, and assist the patient in returning to and maintaining as normal and comfortable a life as possible.

Hemorrhage, vascular collapse, and hepatorenal failure remain the major complications of this extensive surgical procedure. The patient will be monitored closely in the intensive care unit following surgery, have multiple intravenous and arterial lines in place for fluid and blood replacement as well as monitoring arterial pressures, and be on a mechanical ventilator in the immediate postoperative period. Careful attention is given to changes in the patient's vital signs, arterial blood gases and pressures, laboratory values, and urine output. Although the patient's physiologic status is the focus of the physician and nurse, his psychological and emotional state must be considered along with that of his family. The immediate and long-term outcome of this extensive surgical resection is uncertain, and the patient and family require emotional support and understanding in the critical and stressful preoperative and postoperative periods.

See Nursing Care Plan 37-4 (pp. 984–986) for care of the patient following pancreatoduodenectomy (Whipple's procedure).

Pancreatic Islet Tumors

The pancreas contains the islet (islands) of Langerhans—small nests of cells that secrete directly into the bloodstream and, therefore, are part of the endocrine system. The secretion, insulin, is essential for metabolism of glucose. Diabetes mellitus (Chap. 36) is the result of deficient secretion of insulin.

At least two types of tumors of the pancreatic islet cells are known: those that secrete insulin and those in which insulin secretion is not increased, known as "nonfunctioning" islet cell cancer.

Tumors of the islet cells frequently produce hypersecretion of insulin and an excessive rate of metabolism of glucose. Hypoglycemia, the resulting fall in serum glucose level, produces symptoms of weakness, mental confusion, and even convulsions. These may be relieved almost immediately by taking sugar by mouth or by intravenous administration of glucose. The 5-hour glucose tolerance test is helpful in diagnosing insulinoma, the tumor of the pancreatic islet cells that produces excessive insulin, and in distinguishing it from the more common functional hypoglycemia.

Once the diagnosis of a tumor of the islet cells has been made, surgical treatment with removal of the tumor usually is recommended. The tumors may be benign adenomas or they may be malignant. Complete removal usually results in a dramatic cure. In some patients, such symptoms may not be produced by an actual tumor of the islet cells but by a simple hypertrophy of this tissue. In such cases a partial *pancreatectomy*—removal of the tail and part of the body of the pancreas—is performed.

Management. In preparing these patients for operation, the nurse must be alert for symptoms of hypoglycemia and be ready to give sugar, usually with orange juice, should they appear. After operation, the nursing management is the same as that following any upper abdominal operation with special emphasis on observation of serum glucose levels.

Hyperinsulinism

Hyperinsulinism results from the overproduction of insulin by the pancreatic islets. Symptoms resemble those of excessive doses of insulin and are attributable to the same mechanism—an abnormal reduction in the concentration of blood sugar. Clinically, it is characterized by episodes during which the patient experiences unusual hunger, nervousness, sweating, headache, and faintness; in severe cases, convulsive seizures and episodes of unconsciousness may occur. The findings at operation or postmortem examination may indicate hyperplasia (overgrowth) of the islets of Langerhans or a benign or malignant tumor involving the islets and capable of producing large amounts of insulin (see preceding discussion). Occasionally, tumors of nonpancreatic origin produce an insulin-like material that can cause hypoglycemia. This condition occasionally is responsible for convulsions coinciding with decreases in the blood glucose to levels that are inadequate to sustain normal brain function (*i.e.*, below 30 mg/dl [1.6 mmol/L]).

All of the symptoms that accompany spontaneous hypoglycemia are relieved by the oral or parenteral administration of glucose. Surgical removal of the hyperplastic or neoplastic tissue from the pancreas offers the only successful method of treatment. About 15% of patients with spontaneous or functional hypoglycemia eventually develop diabetes mellitus.

Ulcerogenic (Zollinger-Ellison) Tumors

Some tumors of the islets of Langerhans are associated with a hypersecretion of gastric acid that produces ulcers in the stomach, the duodenum, and even the jejunum. The hypersecretion is so great that even after partial gastric resection enough acid to produce further ulceration may remain. When a marked tendency to develop gastric and duodenal ulcers is noted, an ulcerogenic tumor of the islets of Langerhans is suspected.

These tumors, which may be benign or malignant, are treated, when possible, by excision. Frequently, however, because of extension beyond the pancreas, removal is not possible. In many patients, a total gastrectomy may be necessary to reduce the secretion of gastric acid sufficiently to prevent further ulceration.

Bibliography

Books

Gyr KE, Singer MV, and Sarles H. Pancreatitis: Concepts and Classification. Amsterdam, Excerpta Medica, 1984.

Hennemann G (ed). Thyroid Hormone Metabolism. New York, Marcel Dekker, 1986.

Ingbar SH and Braverman LE. The Thyroid. Philadelphia, JB Lippincott, 1986.

Jubiz W. Endocrinology: A Logical Approach for Clinicians. New York. McGraw-Hill, 1985.

Kohler PO (ed). Clinical Endocrinology. New York, John Wiley, & Sons, 1986.

Ravenscroft MM and Swan CHJ. Gastrointestinal Endoscopy and Related Procedures: A Handbook for Nurses and Assistants. Baltimore, Williams & Wilkins, 1984.

Toledo-Pereyra LH. The Pancreas: Principles of Medical and Surgical Practice. New York, John Wiley & Sons, 1985.

Vestal RE. Drug Treatment in the Elderly. Boston, ADIS Health Science Press, 1984.

Williams RH, Wilson JD, and Foster DW. Williams Textbook of Endocrinology. Philadelphia, WB Saunders, 1985.

Articles

General

Bagdale JD. Endocrine emergencies. Med Clin North Am 1986 Sept; 70(5):1111–1128.

Didonato K. Highdose, short-term steroid therapy (40 days). Cancer Nurs 1984 June; 7(3):251–255.

Donham J. The weakness of steroids. Am J Nurs 1986 Aug; 86(8):917–919.

Eil C. Hormone receptor physiology in clinical medicine. Crit Care Q 1983 Dec; 6(3):86–95.

Goldman DR. Surgery in patients with endocrine dysfunction. Med Clin North Am 1987 May; 71(3):499–509.

Jordan RM. Endocrine emergencies. Med Clin North Am 1983 Nov; 67(6): 1193–1213.

Mooradian AD and Morley JE. Endocrine dysfunction in chronic renal failure. Arch Intern Med 1984 Feb; 144(2):351–353.

Nasr H. Endocrine disorders in the elderly. Med Clin North Am 1983 Mar; 67(2):481–495.

Noth RH and Walter RM. The effects of alcohol on the endocrine system. Med Clin North Am 1984 Jan; 68(1):133–143.

O'Toole K, Fenoglio-Preiser C, and Pushparaj N. Endocrine changes associated with the human aging process: III. Effect of age on the number of calcitonin immunoreactive cells in the thyroid gland. Hum Pathol 1985 Oct; 16(10):991–1000.

Savin JA. Some guidelines to the use of topical corticosteroids. Br Med J 1985 June 1; 290(6482):1607–1608.

Sheehy SB. Metabolic and endocrine emergencies. J Emerg Nurs 1985 Jan/Feb; 11(1):49–52.

Solomon B. Endocrinology: A future challenge for critical care nurses. Dimens Crit Care Nurs 1984 Mar/Apr; 3(2):68–69.

Vernoski B and Chernow B. Steroids: Use and abuse. Crit Care Q 1983 Dec; 6(3):28–38.

Zaloga GP and Chernow B. Hormones as therapeutic agents in the intensive care unit. Crit Care Q 1983 Dec; 6(3):75–83.

Zaritsky A and Chernow B. Catecholamines in critical care medicine. Crit Care Q 1983 Dec; 6(3):39–47.

Thyroid Disorders

Burman KD. Interpretation of thyroid function tests in systemically ill patients. Crit Care Q 1983 Dec; 6(3):1–11.

Cooper DS and Ridgway EC. Clinical management of patients with hyperthyroidism. Med Clin North Am 1985 Sept; 69(5):953–971.

Dillmann WH. Mechanism of action of thyroid hormones. Med Clin North Am 1985 Sept; 69(5):849–861.

Emerson CH. Central hypothyroidism and hyperthyroidism. Med Clin North Am 1985 Sept; 69(5):1019–1034.

Evangelisti JT and Thorpe CJ. Thyroid storm—A nursing crisis. Heart Lung 1983 Mar; 12(2):184–193.

Flaherty RJ. Postpartum thyroiditis. Am Fam Physician 1984 Feb; 29(2):195–197.

Gambert S and Brensinger JF. Assessing thyroid function in the elderly. Nurse Pract 1983 July/Aug; 8(7):38–43.

Gharib H, Goellner JR, Zinsmeister AR, Grant CS, and Van Heerden JA. Fine-needle aspiration biopsy of the thyroid: The problem of suspicious cytologic findings. Ann Intern Med 1984 July; 101(1):25–28.

Hilyard N. Solitary thyroid nodules in adults. Nurse Pract 1983 Feb; 8(2):14–15.

Hollingsworth DR. Graves' disease. Clin Obstet Gynecol 1983 Sept; 26(3):615–634.

Hurley JR. Thyroid disease in the elderly. Med Clin North Am 1983 Mar; 67(2):497–516.

Jacobson DH and Gorman CA. Diagnosis and management of endocrine ophthalmopathy. Med Clin North Am 1985 Sept; 69(5):973–988.

Kabadi UM. Laboratory evaluation of anatomic disorders of the thyroid. Am Fam Physician 1983 Nov; 28(5):195–203.

Kaplan MM. Clinical and laboratory assessment of thyroid abnormalities. Med Clin North Am 1985 Sept; 69(5):863–880.

Klein IL and Levey GS. Thyroid emergencies: Thyroid storm and myxedema. Top Emerg Med 1984 Jan; 5(4):33–39.

Leeper RD. Thyroid cancer. Med Clin North Am 1985 Sept; 69(5):1079–1096.

Levine SN. Current concepts of thyroiditis. Arch Intern Med 1983 Oct; 143(10):1952–1956.

Maxon HR. Radiation-induced thyroid disease. Med Clin North Am 1985 Sept; 69(5):1049–1061.

Mazzaferri EL. Thyrotoxicosis: Clinical syndromes and laboratory diagnosis. Postgrad Med 1983 Apr 73(4):85–98.

Miller JM. Evaluation of thyroid nodules: Accent on needle biopsy. Med Clin North Am 1985 Sept; 69(5):1063–1077.

Nicoloff JT. Thyroid storm and myxedema coma. Med Clin North Am 1985 Sept; 69(5):1005–1017.

Refetoff S and Lever EG. The value of serum thyroglobulin measurement in clinical practice. JAMA 1983 Nov 4; 250(17):2352–2357.

Rossi RL, Nieroda C, Cady B, and Wool MS. Malignancies of the thyroid gland: The Lahey Clinic experience. Surg Clin North Am 1985 Apr; 65(2):211–230.

Sawin CT. Hypothyroidism. Med Clin North Am 1985 Sept; 69(5):989–1004.

Schneider AB et al. Radiation-induced thyroid carcinoma. Ann Intern Med 1986 Sept; 105(3):405–412.

Silva JE. Effects of iodine and iodine-containing compounds on thyroid function. Med Clin North Am 1985 Sept; 69(5):881–889.

Spaulding SW and Lippes H. Hyperthyroidism: Causes, clinical features, and diagnosis. Med Clin North Am 1985 Sept; 69(5):937–951.

Tajiri J et al. Successful treatment of thyrotoxic crisis with plasma exchange. Crit Care Med 1984 June; 12(6):536–537.

Tibaldi JM and Surks MI. Effects of nonthyroidal illness on thyroid function. Med Clin North Am 1985 Sept; 69(5):899–911.

Tibaldi JM et al. Thyrotoxicosis in the very old. Am J Med 1986 Oct; 81(4):619–622.

Torres J et al. Thyroid cancer: Survival in 148 cases followed for 10 years or more. Cancer 1985 Nov 1; 56(9):2298–2304.

Volpé R. Immunoregulation in autoimmune thyroid disease. N Eng J Med 1987 Jan 1; 316(1):44–46.

Wall JR and Kuroki T. Immunologic factors in thyroid disease. Med Clin North Am 1985 Sept; 69(5):913–936.

Weber CA and Clark OH. Surgery for thyroid disease. Med Clin North Am 1985 Sept; 69(5):1097–1115.

Werk EE, Vernon BM, Gonzalez JJ, Ungaro PC, and McCoy RC. Cancer in thyroid nodules: A community hospital survey. Arch Intern Med 1984 Mar; 144(3):474–476.

Woolf PD. Thyroiditis. Med Clin North Am 1985 Sept; 69(5):1035–1048.

Zaloga GP and O'Brian JT. Euthyroid sick syndrome. Am Fam Physician 1985 Feb; 31(2)236–250.

Parathyroid Disorders

DeRubertis FR. Hypercalcemia and hypocalcemia. Top Emerg Med 1984 Jan; 5(4):64–73.

Evans RA. Hypercalcaemia: What does it signify? Drugs 1986; 31(1):64–74.

Forster J et al. Hypercalcemia in critically ill surgical patients. Ann Surg 1985 Oct; 202(4):512–518.

Gaz RD and Wang C. Management of asymptomatic hyperparathyroidism. Am J Surg 1984 Apr; 147(4):498–502.

McFadden EA, Zaloga GP, and Chernow B. Hypocalcemia: A medical emergency. Am J Nurs 1983 Feb; 83(2):225–230.

Okerlund MD et al. A new method with high sensitivity and specificity for localization of abnormal parathyroid hormones. Ann Surg 1984 Sept; 200(3):381–388.

Patten BM and Pages M. Severe neurological disease associated with hyperparathyroidism. Ann Neurol 1984 May; 15(5):453–456.

Rossi RL, ReMine SG, and Clerkin EP. Hyperparathyroidism. Surg Clin North Am 1985 Apr; 65(2):187–209.

Sneid D. Hypercalcemia. Top Emerg Med. 1983 July; 5(2):8–17.

Disorders of the Adrenal Medulla

Camunas C. Pheochromocytoma. Am J Nurs 1983 June; 83(6):887–891.

Harris RB and DelaRoca RR. Pheochromocytoma: A medical review. Heart Lung. 1984 Jan; 13(1):73–80.

Harris RB and Heany G. Comprehensive nursing care of the patient with pheochromocytoma. Heart Lung 1984 Jan; 13(1):82–87.

Levine SN and McDonald JC. The evaluation and management of pheochromocytomas. Adv Surg 1984; 17:281–313.

Rock RC. Finding the needle in the haystack: Pheochromocytoma. Diagn Med 1985 May; 8(5):21–27.

Disorders of the Adrenal Cortex

Bullas JB and Pfister S. Adrenal insufficiency. Crit Care Nurs 1985 Jan/Feb; 5(1):8, 10, 11.

Glascow BJ, Steinsapir KD Anders K, and Layfield LJ. Adrenal pathology in the acquired immune deficiency syndrome. Am J Clin Pathol 1985 Nov; 84(5)594–597.

Graham B and Tucker WS. Opportunistic infections in endogenous Cushing's syndrome. Ann Intern Med 1984 Sept; 101(3):334–338.

Guerin CK, Wahner HW, Gorman CA, Carpenter PC, and Sheedy PF. Computed tomographic scanning versus radioisotope imaging in adrenocortical diagnosis. Am J Med 1983 Oct; 75(4):653–657.

Hamburger S and Rush DR. Adrenal crisis. Top Emerg Med 1983 July; 5(2):75–78.

Meuleman J and Katz P. The immunologic effects, kinetics, and use of glucocorticosteroids. Med Clin North Am 1985 July; 69(4):805–816.

Miller PH. Primary aldosteronism: A challenging case. Dimens Crit Care Nurs 1984 Mar/Apr; 3(2):84–90.

Robinson AG. Acute adrenal insufficiency: Addisonian crisis. Top Emerg Med 1984 Jan; 5(4):40–44.

Sheahan SL. Weakness and fatigue. Nurse Pract 1985 Aug; 10(8):48–49.

Sheretz EF and Flowers FP. Rational use of topical corticosteroids. Am Fam Physician 1984 Jan; 29(1):262–266.

Vernoski B and Chernow B. Steroids: Use and abuse. Crit Care Q 1983 Dec; 6(3):28–38.

Pituitary Gland Disorders

Hagen TC. Early clues that suggest acromegaly. Diagnosis 1985 Nov; 7(11):63–64, 69.

Kruger LB. Complications of transsphenoidal surgery. J Neurosurg Nurs 1985 June; 17(3):179–183.

Propst CL. Nursing care of a patient undergoing transsphenoidal hypophysectomy. J Neurosurg Nurs 1983 Dec; 15(6):332–338.

Randall RV. Pituitary failure? Answer three questions. Diagnosis 1986 Apr; 8(4):57–59, 63–64.

Reid RL, Quigley ME, and Yen SSC. Pituitary apoplexy: A review. Arch Neurol 1985 July; 42(7):712–719.

Resio MJ. Nursing diagnosis: Alteration in oral/nasal mucous membranes related to trauma of transsphenoidal surgery. J Neurosurg Nurs 1986 June; 18(3):112–115.

Sheeler LR. Profiles of pituitary disease. Diagnosis 1985 Apr; 7(4):59–62, 64, 68.

Verbalis JG and Robinson AG. Hypopituitarism. Top Emerg Med 1984 Jan; 5(4):74–78.

Volner JS. Endocrine dysfunction associated with pituitary adenomas and pituitary surgery. J Neurosurg Nurs 1983 Dec; 15(6):325–331.

Zucker AR and Chernow B. Diabetes insipidus and the syndrome of inappropriate antidiuretic hormone release. Crit Care Q 1983 Dec; 6(3):63–74.

Disorders of the Pancreas

Axon ATR. Endoscopy in the diagnosis and therapy of pancreatic disorders. Clin Gastroenterol 1986 Apr; 15(2):279–303.

Braasch JW and Rossi RL. Pyloric preservation with the Whipple procedure. Surg Clin North Am 1985 Apr; 65(2):263–271.

Feller ER. Endoscopic retrograde cholangiopancreatography in the diagnosis of unexplained pancreatitis. Arch Intern Med 1984 Sept; 144(9):1797–1799.

Frey CF and Bodai BI. Surgery in chronic pancreatitis. Clin Gastroenterol 1984 Sept; 123(3):913–940.

Geokas MC. Ethanol and the pancreas. Med Clin North Am 1984 Jan; 68(1):57–75.

James OFW. Gastrointestinal and liver function in old age. Clin Gastroenterol 1983 Sept; 12(3):671–691.

Lankisch PG. Acute and chronic pancreatitis: An update on management. Drugs 1984 Dec; 28(6):554–564.

Lankisch PG and Creutzfeldt W. Therapy of exocrine and endocrine pancreatic insufficiency. Clin Gastroenterol 1984 Sept; 13(3):985–999.

Levine CD. Preventing complications in the pancreatoduodenectomy patient. Dimens Crit Care Nurs 1983 Mar/Apr; 2(2):90–97.

Managing the patient with concurrent life-threatening conditions. Nurs '84 1984 June; 14(6):60–64.

Neff CC and Ferrucci JT. Pancreatitis. Surg Clin North Am 1984 Feb; 64(1):23–35.

Prinz RA, Aranha GV, and Greenlee HB. Combined pancreatic duct and upper gastrointestinal and biliary tract drainage in chronic pancreatitis. Arch Surg 1985 Mar; 120(3):361–366.

Prinz RA et al. "Nonfunctioning" islet cell carcinoma of the pancreas. Am Surg 1983 July; 49(7):345–349.

Rossi RL, Heiss FW, and Braasch JW. Surgical management of chronic pancreatitis. Surg Clin North Am 1985 Feb; 65(1):79–101.

Teplick SK et al. Interventional radiology of the biliary system and pancreas. Surg Clin North Am 1984 Feb; 64(1):87–119.

Warshaw AL and Richter JM. A practical guide to pancreatitis. Curr Probl Surg 1984 Dec; 11(12):7–79.

Renal and Urinary Problems

Unit X

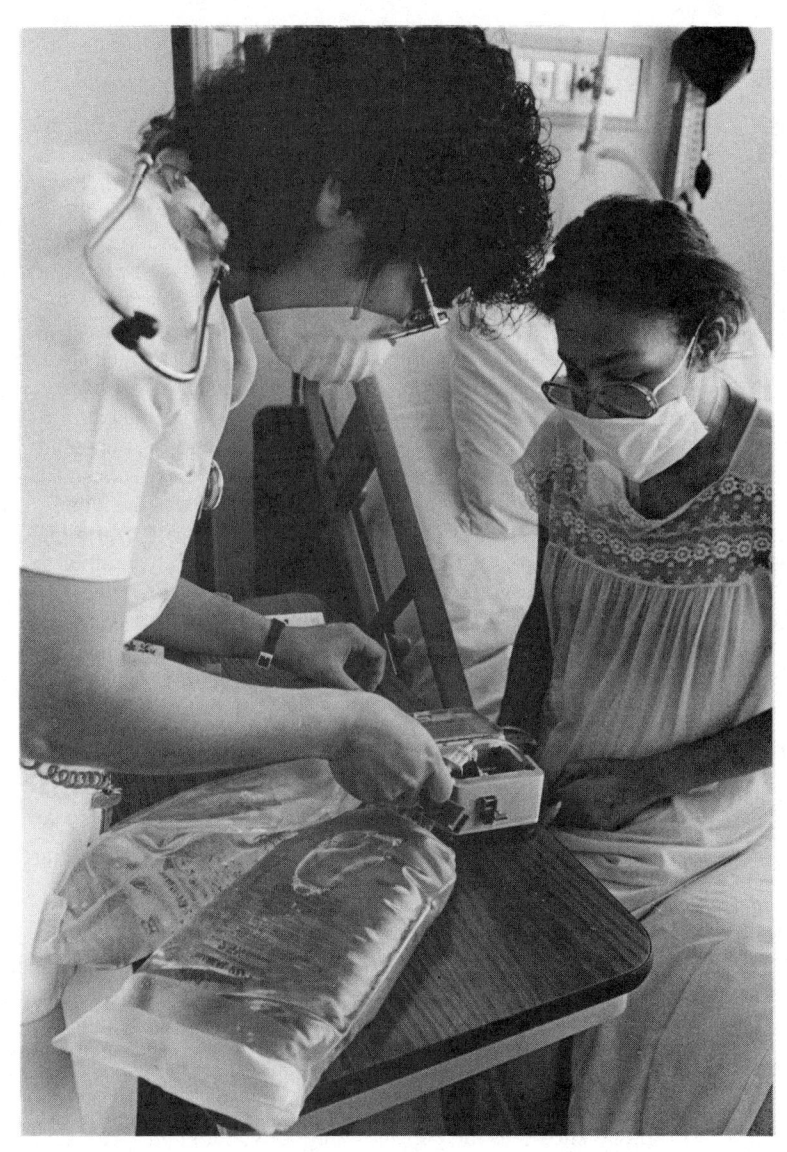

Chapter 38

Assessment of Renal and Urinary Function

Physiologic Overview

The kidneys, ureters, bladder, and urethra compose the urinary system. The kidneys' main function is to remove unwanted substances, including water, from the blood. These materials form the urine which is transported through the ureters for temporary storage in the urinary bladder. During the act of *micturition* (urination), the bladder contracts and the urine is excreted from the body through the urethra. Urine formation regulates the water content and electrolyte composition of the body fluids. Although fluid and electrolytes can be lost by other routes, such as in perspiration or feces, it is the kidneys that precisely regulate the internal environment of the body. The renal excretory function is necessary for maintenance of life. However, unlike the cardiovascular and respiratory systems, complete malfunction of the kidneys may not cause death for several days. Use of the artificial kidney and other treatment modalities make it possible to substitute for certain functions of the kidneys.

An important feature of the urinary system is its ability to adapt to wide variations in fluid load based on individual habits and patterns. Basically, the kidneys must be able to excrete that which is ingested in the diet and not eliminated by other organs. This usually amounts to 1 to 2 liters of water per day, 6 to 8 gm of salt (sodium chloride) per day, 6 to 8 gm of potassium chloride per day, and 70 mg of acid equivalents per day. In addition, protein is ingested and metabolized by the body into urea and other waste products that must also be excreted in the urine.

Anatomy of the Urinary System

The kidneys are paired organs, each weighing approximately 125 gm, located in a position lateral to the bodies of the lower thoracic vertebrae, a few centimeters to the right and left of the midline. They are surrounded by a thin, fibrous tissue known as the capsule. Anteriorly, the kidneys are separated from the abdominal cavity and its contents by layers of peritoneum. Posteriorly, they are shielded by the lower thoracic wall. Blood is supplied to each kidney through the renal artery and is drained through the renal vein. The renal arteries arise from the abdominal aorta, and the renal veins carry blood back into the inferior vena cava. The kidneys can efficiently clear the blood of waste materials, in part because their total blood flow is great and represents 25% of cardiac output.

Urine is formed within the functional units of the kidneys, known as nephrons. The urine formed within these nephrons passes into collecting ducts that join to form the pelvis of each kidney. Each kidney pelvis gives rise to a ureter. The ureter is a long tube (25 cm) with a wall composed largely of smooth muscle. It connects each kidney to the bladder and functions as a conduit for urine.

The urinary bladder is a hollow organ that is situated anteriorly just behind the pubic bone. It acts as a temporary storage reservoir for the urine. The walls of the bladder consist largely of smooth muscle called the detrusor muscle. Contraction of this muscle is mainly responsible for emptying the bladder during urination. The urethra arises from the bladder; it runs through the penis in the male and opens just anterior to the vagina in the female. A short distance from its origin, the urethra is encircled by a small bundle of muscle fibers that is called the external urinary sphincter. This sphincter is the major site for control of the initiation of urination.

The Nephron.   The kidney is divided into an outer portion called the cortex and an inner portion known as the medulla (Fig. 38-1). In the human, each kidney is composed of approximately 1 million nephrons, the functional unit of the kidney. Each nephron consists of a glomerulus and a tubule (Fig. 38-2); the glomerulus is about 0.2 mm in diameter and the tubule approximately 25 to 45 mm in length. The glomerulus, the beginning of the nephron, is composed of tufts of capillaries that are supplied with blood by an afferent arteriole and drained by an efferent arteriole. The latter is a thick-walled muscular vessel that helps to maintain a high pressure in the glomerular capillaries. Like capillaries in general, the walls of the glomerular capillaries are composed of

a layer of endothelial cells and a basement membrane. On the other side of the basement membrane are the epithelial cells that form the beginning of the tubule. The tubule itself is divided into three parts: a proximal tubule, the loop of Henle, and a distal tubule. The distal tubules coalesce to form collecting ducts that are about 20 mm long. The ducts pass through the renal cortex and the medulla to empty into the pelvis of the kidney. The total length of a typical nephron, including the collecting duct, ranges from 45 mm to 65 mm.

Function of the Nephron.   The process of urine formation begins as blood flows through the glomerulus. Fluid is filtered through the walls of the glomerular capillary tufts into the proximal tubule. Under normal conditions, approximately 20% of the plasma passing through the glomerulus is filtered into the nephron, amounting to about 180 liters of filtrate per day. The filtrate, very similar to blood plasma without its proteins, consists essentially of water, electrolytes, and other small molecules. Within the tubule and collecting ducts, some of these substances are selectively reabsorbed into the blood. Other substances are secreted into the filtrate as it travels down the tubule. The urine is the remaining fluid (along with its contents) that reaches the pelvis of the kidney. Some substances, such as glucose, are usually completely reabsorbed in the tubule and do not appear in the urine. The processes of reabsorption and secretion in the tubule frequently involve active transport and require the utilization of metabolic energy. The amount of various substances normally filtered by the glomerulus, reabsorbed by the tubules, and excreted in the urine is shown in Table 38-1.

Urine Composition

The kidney functions as the main excretory organ of the body. It disposes of unwanted materials that are ingested as well as the byproducts of the body's metabolism. In the normal person, the amounts of these materials excreted per day are

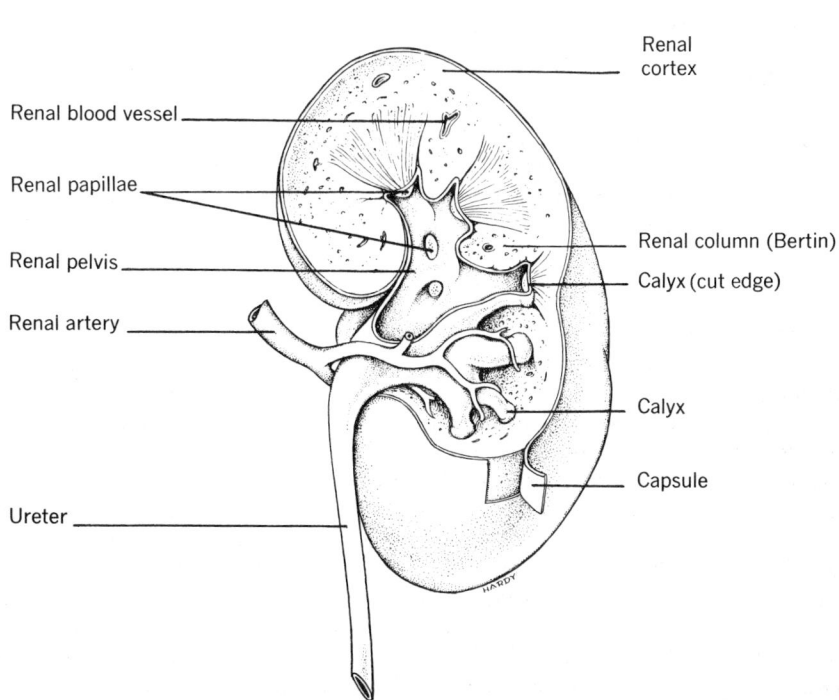

Figure 38-1
Diagram of internal structure of kidney, showing relations of renal pelvis and calyces to pyramids in medullary region. (Chaffee EE and Greisheimer EM. Basic Physiology and Anatomy, 4th ed. Philadelphia, JB Lippincott.)

Renal blood vessel

Renal papillae

Renal pelvis

Renal artery

Ureter

Renal cortex

Renal column (Bertin)

Calyx (cut edge)

Calyx

Capsule

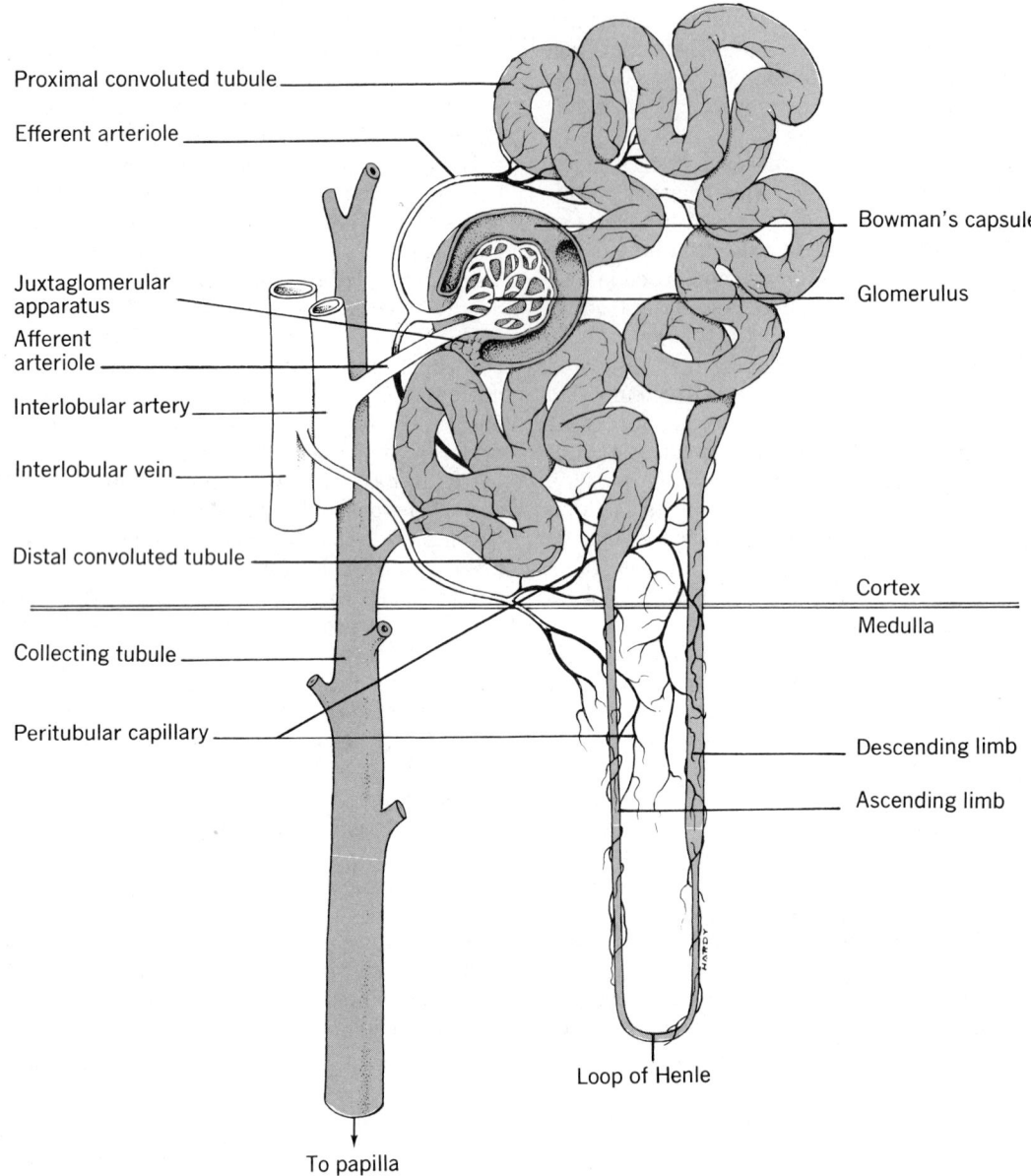

Figure 38-2
A nephron and its blood supply. The collecting tubule receives urine from neighboring nephron units. Note that the loop of Henle dips into the medullary layer of the kidney. (Chaffee EE and Greisheimer EM. Basic Physiology and Anatomy, 4th ed. Philadelphia, JB Lippincott.)

exactly equal to the amounts ingested and formed, so that over a period of time there is no net change in the total body composition.

Urine is composed primarily of water. A normal person ingests approximately 1 to 2 liters of water per day, and normally all but 400 to 500 ml of this fluid intake is excreted in the urine. The remainder is lost from the skin, from the lungs during breathing, and in the feces. The second major class of substances excreted in the urine is the electrolytes, including sodium, potassium, chloride, bicarbonate, and other less abundant ions. The average American diet contains about 6 to 8 gm each of sodium chloride (salt) and potassium chloride per day, and nearly all of this is excreted in the urine.

The third group of substances appearing in the urine is made up of the breakdown products of protein metabolism. The major breakdown product is urea, of which about 25 gm are produced and excreted per day. Other products of protein metabolism that must be excreted are creatinine, phosphates, and sulphates. Uric acid, formed as a breakdown product of nucleic acid metabolism, is also eliminated in the urine.

It is important to recognize that some substances that are present in high concentrations in the blood are ordinarily completely reabsorbed by active transport in the renal tubule. Amino acids and glucose, for example, are usually filtered at the glomerulus and reabsorbed so that none of either is excreted in the urine. Glucose, however, will appear in the urine

TABLE 38-1

Filtration, Reabsorption, and Excretion of Certain Normal Constituents of Plasma

	Filtered 24 Hr		Reabsorbed 24 Hr		Excreted 24 Hr*
Sodium	540	gm	537	gm	3.3 gm
Chloride	630	gm	625	gm	5.3 gm
Bicarbonate	300	gm	300	gm	0.3 gm
Potassium	28	gm	24	gm	3.9 gm
Glucose	140	gm	140	gm	0.0 gm
Urea	53	gm	28	gm	25.0 gm
Creatinine	1.4	gm	0	gm	1.4 gm
Uric acid	8.5	gm	7.7	gm	0.8 gm

* These are typical normal values. Wide variation is found, depending on diet.

if its blood level is so high that its concentration in the glomerular filtrate exceeds the capacity of the tubules to reabsorb it. Normally, the glucose is completely reabsorbed when its concentration in the blood is less than 200 mg/dl (11 mmol/L). In diabetes, in which the blood glucose levels exceed the kidney's reabsorption capacity, glucose will appear in the urine. Protein is also not normally found in the urine. These molecules are not filtered at the glomerulus because of their large size. The appearance of protein in the urine usually signifies damage to the glomeruli that causes them to become "leaky."

Regulation of Acid Excretion

The breakdown of proteins involves the generation of acid compounds, in particular phosphoric and sulfuric acids. In addition, a certain amount of acid material is ingested daily. Unlike CO_2, these are nonvolatile acids and cannot be eliminated by the lung. Because accumulation of these acids in the blood would lower its *p*H, (more acidic) and inhibit cell function, they must be excreted in the urine. A normal person excretes approximately 70 mEq of acid each day. The kidney is able to excrete some of this acid directly into the urine to the extent of lowering its *p*H to 4.5, 1000 times more acidic than blood.

More acid usually needs to be eliminated from the body than can be excreted directly as free acid in the urine. This is accomplished by the renal excretion of acid that is bound to chemical buffers. The acid (H^+) is secreted by the renal tubular cells into the filtrate, where it is buffered chiefly by phosphate ions and ammonia (NH_3). Phosphate is present in the glomerular filtrate, and ammonia is produced by the kidney cells and secreted into the tubular fluid. Through the buffering process, the kidney is able to excrete large quantities of acid in a bound form without further lowering the *p*H of the urine.

Regulation of Electrolyte Excretion

The amount of electrolytes and water that must be excreted by the kidney each day varies greatly, depending on the amounts ingested. The 180 liters of filtrate formed by the glomeruli each day contain about 1100 gm of sodium chlo-

ride. Approximately 2 liters of water and 6 to 8 gm of sodium chloride are normally excreted per day in the urine. The small amounts excreted relative to the amount filtered reflect reabsorption of sodium from the filtrate into the blood as it travels down the tubules. Water from the filtrate follows the reabsorbed sodium in order to maintain osmotic balance. Thus, more than 99% of the water and sodium filtered at the glomerulus is reabsorbed into the blood by the time the urine leaves the body. By regulating the amount of sodium (and therefore water) reabsorbed, the kidney can regulate the volume of body fluids.

- If sodium is excreted in excess of the amount ingested, the patient will become dehydrated.
- If less sodium is excreted than is ingested, the patient will retain fluid.

The regulation of the amount of sodium excreted depends on aldosterone, a hormone synthesized and released from the adrenal gland. In the presence of increased aldosterone in the blood, less sodium is excreted in the urine.

Release of aldosterone from the adrenal gland is largely under the control of angiotensin, a peptide hormone manufactured in the liver and activated in the lung. Angiotensin levels are in turn controlled by the hormone renin, which is released from cells in the kidneys. This complex system is activated when pressure in the renal arterioles falls below normal levels, as occurs with shock and dehydration. The effect of activation of this system is to increase the retention of water and expansion of intravascular fluid volume.

Another electrolyte whose concentration in the body fluids is regulated by the kidney is potassium, the most abundant intracellular ion. The excretion of potassium by the kidney is increased by elevated aldosterone levels, in contrast to the effects of aldosterone on sodium excretion.

- Retention of potassium is the most life-threatening effect of renal failure.

Regulation of Water Excretion

Regulation of the amount of water excreted is also an important function of the kidney. With a large water intake, a large volume of dilute urine must be excreted. Conversely, with a low water intake, the urine that is excreted must be concentrated. The relative degree of dilution or concentration of the urine can be measured in terms of its *osmolality*. This term refers to the amount of solid material (electrolytes and other molecules) dissolved in the urine. The filtrate in the glomerular capillary normally has the same osmolality as the blood, with a value of approximately 300 mOsm/liter (300 mmol/L). As the filtrate passes through the tubules and collecting ducts, the osmolality may vary from 50 to 1200 mOsm/liter, reflecting the maximal diluting and concentrating abilities of the kidney.

The osmolality of the urine specimen can be measured. *Osmolality* reflects the number of particles of solute in a unit of solution, unlike *specific gravity*, which is less precise and reflects both the quantity and the nature of particles. Therefore, protein, glucose, and intravenous contrast medium affect specific gravity more than osmolality. Osmolality is measured when a precise assessment of the concentrating and diluting abilities of the kidney is needed. Normal urine osmolality is

500 to 800 mOsm/liter. Normal specific gravity is 1.003 to 1.030.

Regulation of water excretion and urine concentraton is carried out in the tubule by varying the amount of water that is reabsorbed in relation to electrolyte reabsorption. The glomerular filtrate has essentially the same electrolyte composition as the blood plasma without the proteins. The amount of water that is reabsorbed is under the control of antidiuretic hormones (ADH, vasopressin). ADH is a hormone that is secreted by the posterior part of the pituitary gland in response to changes in osmolality of the blood. With decreased water intake, blood osmolality tends to rise and stimulate ADH release. ADH then acts on the kidney in order to cause increased reabsorption of water, thereby returning the osmolality of the blood toward normal. With excess water intake, the secretion of ADH by the pituitary is suppressed and, therefore, less water is reabsorbed by the kidney tubule. This latter situation leads to increased urine volume (*diuresis*).

- Loss of the ability to concentrate and dilute the urine is the most common early manifestation of kidney disease. A dilute urine of fixed specific gravity (approximately 1.010) or fixed osmolality (approximately 300 mOsm/liter) is excreted.

Renal Clearance

The test most commonly used to evaluate how well the kidney performs its excretory function is termed *clearance*. Clearance of a substance A is shown by the following equation: clearance equals (the urine concentration of A) times (the urine volume in a given time) divided by the plasma concentration of A.

Clearance =

$$\frac{(\text{urine concentration of A}) \times (\text{urine volume in a given time})}{\text{plasma concentration of A}}$$

For example, if the arterial plasma concentration of a substance is 0.1 mg/ml, the urine concentration of the same substance is 50 mg/ml, and the urine volume is 1.0 ml/min, the clearance of that substance according to the above equation is 500 ml/min. This means that 500 ml of blood are completely cleared of that substance in one minute. In the body, few substances are actually completely cleared from the blood during a single pass through the kidney. In the example given above, if the blood is cleared of only 50% of the substance, urine concentration of the substance would be 25 mg/ml and the calculated renal clearance would be 250 ml/min. It is possible to measure the renal clearance of any substance, but the one that has proven particularly useful is the creatinine clearance. *Creatinine* is an endogenous waste product of skeletal muscle that is excreted by glomerular filtration and is not appreciably reabsorbed or secreted by the renal tubules. Therefore, creatinine clearance is a good measure of the glomerular filtration rate (GFR). The normal adult GFR is about 100 to 120 ml/min (1.67–2.00 ml/sec).

Storage of Urine and Micturition

Urine formed by the kidney is transported from the renal pelvis through the ureters and into the bladder. This movement is facilitated by peristaltic waves occurring about 1 to 5 times per minute and generated by the smooth muscle in the ureter wall. Urine flows into the bladder sporadically, propelled by peristaltic contractions. There are no sphincters between the bladder and the ureters, although reflux of urine from the bladder in normal subjects is prevented by the unidirectional nature of the peristaltic waves and because each ureter enters the bladder at an oblique angle. However,

- with overdistention of the bladder due to disease, the elevated pressure in the bladder can be transmitted back through the ureters, leading to ureteral distention and possible reflux or back-up of urine. This can lead to kidney infection (pyelonephritis) and damage from the elevated pressure (hydronephrosis).

The pressure in the bladder is normally very low, even as the urine accumulates, because the bladder's smooth muscle adapts to the increased stretch as the bladder is slowly filled. The first sensations of bladder filling ordinarily occur when about 100 to 150 ml of urine are present in the bladder. In most cases, there is a desire to void when the bladder contains approximately 200 to 300 ml. With 400 ml a marked feeling of fullness is usually present.

Voiding of urine is controlled by contraction of the *external urethral sphincter*. This muscle is under voluntary control and is innervated by nerves from the sacral area of the spinal cord. Voluntary control is a learned behavior that is not present at birth. When there is a desire to urinate, the external urethral sphincter is relaxed, and the *detrusor muscle* (bladder smooth muscle) contracts and expels the urine from the bladder through the urethra. The pressure generated in the bladder during micturition (urination) is approximately 50 to 150 cm of water. Residual urine in the urethra drains by gravity in the female and is expelled by voluntary muscle contractions in the male.

The contraction of the detrusor muscle is regulated by a reflex involving the parasympathetic nervous system. The reflex is integrated in the sacral portion of the spinal tract. The sympathetic nervous system plays no essential part in micturition, but does prevent semen from entering the bladder during ejaculation.

- If the pelvic nerves to the bladder and sphincter are destroyed, voluntary control and reflex urination are abolished and the bladder becomes overdistended with urine. If the spinal pathways from the brain to the urinary system are destroyed (for example, after a spinal cord transection), reflex contraction of the bladder is maintained but voluntary control over the process is lost. In both of these types of loss of innervation, the muscle of the bladder can contract and expel urine, but the contractions are generally insufficient to empty the bladder completely, and residual urine is left behind.

Catheterization—passage of a catheter through the urethra into the bladder—can be used to assess bladder function by permitting measurement of the amount of urine left in the bladder after voiding (*residual urine*). Normally this is no more than 50 ml. However, catheterization is avoided whenever possible, because it increases the risk of infection. Another test for bladder dysfunction is to measure the pressure in the bladder after instillation of various volumes of saline. This latter procedure is called a *cystometrogram* (see p. 1005).

Renal Pathophysiology

Diseases of the kidney can be classified according to the segment of the nephron that is primarily affected. Glomerulonephritis and the various forms of the nephrotic syndrome primarily affect the renal glomerulus. Vascular diseases, infections, and toxins primarily affect the renal tubule, although some degree of glomerular dysfunction may coexist. Obstruction to the outflow of urine due to calculi (stones), protein, or other material in the collecting ducts or ureters may eventually lead to damage throughout the nephron. When the degree of kidney damage is severe, renal failure occurs and may result in the condition called *uremia*.

Glomerular Diseases

Nephritic Syndrome. The nephritic syndrome occurs in response to a group of diseases in which inflammation of the glomerulus (glomerulonephritis) is predominant. The major manifestations are hematuria, proteinuria, sodium and fluid retention, hypertension, and occasionally oliguria. These abnormalities are due to damage to the glomerular capillaries that permits leakage of red blood cells into the tubular lumen. Glomerulonephritis most commonly results from immune reactions. Common causes are the reaction to some streptococcal infections, predominantly in children, and the autoimmune diseases such as Goodpasture's syndrome and lupus erythematosus. Glomerulonephritis may resolve completely, although in some patients renal failure may result.

Nephrotic Syndrome. The nephrotic syndrome results from a group of glomerular diseases associated with increased permeability to proteins of the glomerulus. Frequently there are no alterations of kidney structure observable by light microscopy. The primary manifestation of the disease is the loss of plasma proteins, particularly albumin, in the urine. Although the liver is capable of increasing its production of albumin, it is unable to keep up with the daily loss of albumin through the kidney; thus, hypoalbuminemia results. The resultant decreased oncotic pressure leads to generalized edema as fluid moves from the vascular system into the extracellular fluid spaces. A decreased circulating blood volume activates the renin-angiotensin system, leading to retention of sodium and further edema. Patients with nephrotic syndrome also exhibit an elevated lipid concentration in their blood (*lipemia*), the cause of which is not known. The nephrotic syndrome can occur with almost any intrinsic renal disease or systemic disease that affects the glomerulus. See page 1047 for further discussion.

Renal Failure

Renal failure is present when the excretion of water, electrolytes, and metabolic waste products is insufficient because of kidney damage that prevents the kidneys from maintaining the normal internal environment of the body. Acute renal failure has a sudden onset and is frequently reversible. Chronic renal failure usually develops gradually, but can also occur as a consequence of an acute episode. One normal kidney is generally sufficient for normal urinary function, so renal failure requires bilateral kidney damage. The signs and symptoms of renal failure are in large part a result of altered fluid and electrolyte balance of the body. The diagnosis is generally made by the finding of *azotemia*, defined as elevation of nitrogenous waste products in the blood. *Uremia*, characterized by the signs and symptoms resulting from accumulation of these waste products, occurs when the condition is severe.

Pathogenesis of Renal Failure. Decreased excretion of metabolic waste products can occur as a result of decreased blood flow to the kidney (pre-renal), acute obstruction to the flow of urine from the kidney (post-renal), or damage to the kidney itself (intra-renal).

- Decreased renal blood flow can occur with hypotension, congestive heart failure, dehydration, or thrombosis of renal arteries. Acute decrease in renal blood flow may lead to secondary renal damage and renal failure. Decreased excretion of waste products due to decreased renal blood flow in the absence of kidney damage is called *pre-renal azotemia*.
- Decreased urine output due to complete urinary obstruction can occur in patients who have an enlarged prostate, stones (calculi) in the ureters or urethra, or infiltrating tumors. Secondary damage to the kidneys and renal failure will result if the obstruction is not relieved promptly. This is termed *obstructive* or *post-renal* failure.
- Acute renal failure due to direct injury to the kidney results from acute vasculitis, acute glomerulonephritis, severe ("malignant") hypertension, or, more commonly, acute damage to the renal tubules (acute tubular necrosis, ATN). The clinical conditions that may result in acute tubular necrosis include hypotension (shock), exposure to nephrotoxic chemicals, disintegration of blood components (intravascular hemolysis) leading to a buildup of hemoglobin in the urine (due to transfusion reactions, extensive burns, or infusion of water intravenously), or crush injury of an extremity that damages muscle tissue. These injuries cause a release of myoglobin which is carried to the kidneys and excreted in the urine (myoglobinuria).

Chronic renal failure may result from the same causes as acute renal failure, in addition to chronic infection (pyelonephritis), nephrosclerosis, diabetic nephropathy, collagen diseases, and other chronic, progressive kidney diseases. See page 1036 for further discussion.

Uremia/Uremic Syndrome

Uremia is a term used to designate the manifestations of chronic renal dysfunction that leads to an accumulation in the blood of substances normally excreted in the urine. Uremia is a generalized condition that affects all organ systems of the body.

Fluids and Electrolytes. The fluid and electrolyte abnormalities that occur in renal failure are the result of a decreased number of functional nephrons. The basic pathophysiologic alteration in kidney function is a decreased glomerular filtration rate (GFR) due to a reduced number of filtering glomeruli, leading to decreased clearance of substances that depend on filtration for their excretion. Decreased GFR can be diagnosed by a decreased inulin, urea, or creatinine clearance. As creatinine clearance decreases, serum creatinine increases. Because of creatinine's constant production, it is the most specific and sensitive indicator of kidney disease. The blood urea nitrogen (BUN) also rises with kidney damage, but its level is also affected by protein intake and tissue breakdown. Uric acid also rises.

In addition to decreased GFR, a decrease in the number of functioning nephrons results in decreased ability of the tubules to modify the glomerular filtrate prior to its excretion as urine. As a result, the urine resembles plasma, having a fixed specific gravity or osmolality. This inability to concentrate or dilute the urine prevents appropriate responses by the kidneys to changes in daily intake of water and electrolytes. Decreased intake of fluid or salt can lead to dehydration or sodium depletion; excess salt or water intake may cause water intoxication or sodium overload. Decreased tubular function also results in inability to excrete increased loads of potassium (K^+) and acid (H^+). With advanced renal disease, the normal production of H^+ by body metabolism or release of K^+ from damaged cells of the body can result in acidosis or hyperkalemia. Decreased excretion of acid results primarily from the inability of the tubules to secrete ammonia (NH_3) and to reabsorb sodium bicarbonate ($NaHCO_3$). There may also be decreased excretion of phosphates and organic acids. Decreased excretion of potassium results from inability of the tubules to secrete this ion into the urine. In addition, the excretion of drugs may be markedly altered, necessitating adjustment of their usual dosages.

Calcium Metabolism and Bone Changes. Disorders of calcium metabolism with secondary bone changes are among the major manifestations of uremia. The primary finding is usually a decreased serum calcium concentration. Several mechanisms have a role in the development of hypocalcemia. Calcium levels are dependent on the amount of phosphorus present. Thus, a decreased excretion of phosphorus in the urine and an elevation of the serum phosphorus level cause a decrease in the amount of free calcium in the body. An additional mechanism for hypocalcemia is decreased conversion of vitamin D to its active form by the damaged kidneys, leading to diminished absorption of calcium from the gastrointestinal tract.

Decreased serum calcium secondarily stimulates the parathyroid glands to produce increased parathormone, resulting in the condition called secondary *hyperparathyroidism*. This condition is characterized by demineralization of bone and formation of bone cysts. The bone changes are worsened by decreased deposition of calcium due to decreased active vitamin D and increased resorption of calcium due to chronic acidosis. The demineralization of bone leads to frequent fractures and bone pain. The term *renal osteodystrophy* is frequently used to designate the complex bone changes that occur with uremia.

Anemia. Anemia, another common manifestation of uremia, is generally caused by a decreased rate of production of red blood cells by the bone marrow and increased rates of red blood cell destruction. Decreased erythropoiesis (the formation of erythrocytes or red blood cells) is related to a decreased rate of production of erythropoietin by the kidneys. In this form of anemia, the red cells in the peripheral blood generally appear to be of normal size and of normal hemoglobin concentration (normocytic, normochromic anemia). Blood loss due to bleeding from the gastrointestinal tract or other sites may contribute to the anemia.

Cardiovascular Manifestations. Hypertension, frequently associated with chronic renal failure, may be either the cause or the result of renal damage. Primary hypertension leads to kidney damage as a result of atherosclerosis of the renal vasculature manifested by nephrosclerosis. Secondary hypertension occurs due to increased renin production by the diseased kidney, leading to generalized vasoconstriction as well as salt retention, which leads to fluid retention and an expansion of the vascular volume.

- Patients with impaired renal function are more prone than normal persons to volume overload because they are less able to compensate for acute increases in water and salt intake.
- Chronic congestive heart failure with pulmonary and peripheral edema frequently occurs as a consequence of hypertensive cardiac disease complicated by the effects of fluid overload and anemia.
- Congestive heart failure results in decreased renal blood flow with elevation of blood urea nitrogen (BUN) out of proportion to the degree of kidney damage.

Other Manifestations of Uremia. Among the diverse manifestations of uremia are gastrointestinal symptoms, including anorexia, nausea, vomiting, and hiccups; neuromuscular symptoms, including mental clouding, inability to concentrate, drowsiness, lethargy, twitching, convulsions, and tetany which is related to the low serum calcium. Dermatologic symptoms, including severe itching (pruritus) are common. Uremic frost, the deposit of urea on the skin by perspiration, is less common today because of early treatment of uremia. Patients with uremia also have altered cellular immunity, with decreased delayed hypersensitivity and increased susceptibility to infection probably related to a decreased ability of leukocytes to kill bacteria.

The precise mechanisms for many of these diverse conditions have not been identified. However, retention of products normally excreted in the urine, such as ammonia, phenols, and other organic and inorganic compounds, is the probable cause.

Course of Renal Failure

The basic mechanisms underlying the pathophysiologic changes of acute and chronic renal failure are similar. However, their clinical presentations are markedly different. There are two phases of acute renal failure: the oliguric phase and the polyuric or diuretic phase.

Oliguric Phase. Acute renal failure occurs due to sudden insults to the kidney that result in a decreased rate of urine formation. This is called the *oliguric phase* of acute renal failure.

- During the oliguric phase, the potential life-threatening complications are related to fluid and electrolyte retention (in particular, hyperkalemia and acidosis).

Polyuric Phase (Diuretic). If the original insult is removed, the recovery process begins with a gradually increasing glomerular filtration rate. At this stage, the renal tubular cells may still be unable to reabsorb the water and electrolytes in the increasing volume of glomerular filtrate. As a result, the volume of urine rises above normal, resulting in the *polyuric* phase of acute renal failure.

- The potential life-threatening complications of the polyuric phase are dehydration and electrolyte depletion.

Complete recovery from acute renal failure, if it occurs, may require several months or up to a year. Some patients with acute renal failure, despite the removal of the initial insult, will not recover normal renal function and will develop chronic renal failure. More commonly, however, chronic renal failure develops gradually and insidiously. The disease is frequently not discovered until the patient develops symptoms related to fluid and electrolyte abnormalities. At this stage, kidney function has generally decreased by more than 50% and the creatinine concentration in the blood has risen above normal. The nursing care of patients with renal failure is discussed on page 1036.

Assessment of Urinary Function

Clinical Manifestations of Urinary Dysfunction

The following symptoms and signs are suggestive of urinary tract disease: pain, changes in micturition, and gastrointestinal symptoms.

Pain

Genitourinary pain is not always present in renal disease, but is generally seen in the more acute conditions. Pain of renal disease is caused by sudden distention of the renal capsule. Its severity is related to how quickly the distention develops.

Kidney pain may be felt as a dull ache in the costovertebral angle (the area formed by the rib cage and vertebral column) and may spread to the umbilicus. Ureteral pain produces pain in the back that radiates to the abdomen, upper thigh, testis, or labium. Pain in the flank (the side between the ribs and ilium), radiating to the lower abdomen or epigastrium and often associated with nausea, vomiting, and paralytic ileus, may indicate renal colic. Bladder pain (low abdominal pain or pain over the suprapubic area) can be due to an overdistended bladder or bladder infection. Urgency, tenesmus (painful straining), and terminal dysuria (pain at the end of voiding) are usually present. Pain at the urethral meatus occurs with irritation of the bladder neck or urethra due to infection (urethritis), trauma, or a foreign body in the lower urinary tract.

Severe pain in the scrotal region results from inflammation and edema of the epididymis or testicle or from torsion of the testicle, while perineal and rectal fullness and pain signal acute prostatitis or prostatic abscess. Back and leg pain may be due to metastasis of cancer of the prostate to the pelvic bones. Pain in the penile shaft may originate from urethral problems, while pain in the glans penis is usually due to prostatitis.

Changes in Micturition (Voiding)

Normal micturition is a painless function occurring 5 to 6 times daily and occasionally once at night. The average person voids 1200 to 1500 ml of urine in 24 hours. This amount, of course, is modified by fluid intake, sweating, outside temperature, vomiting, or diarrhea.

Urinary frequency is voiding that occurs more often than usual when compared to the patient's usual pattern or the generally accepted norm of once every 3 to 6 hours. It may result from a variety of conditions: infection, diseases of the urinary tract, metabolic disease, hypertension, and certain medications (diuretics).

Urgency (strong desire to void) may be due to inflammatory lesions in the bladder, prostate, or urethra; acute bacterial infections or chronic prostatitis in men; and chronic posterior urethrotrigonitis (inflammation of the urethra and trigone of the bladder) in women.

Burning on urination is seen in patients with urethral irritation or bladder infection. Urethritis frequently causes burning during the act of voiding, whereas cystitis may produce burning both during and after urination.

Dysuria (painful or difficult voiding) stems from a wide variety of pathologic conditions.

Hesitancy (undue delay and difficulty in initiating voiding) may indicate compression of the urethra or neurogenic bladders, or outlet obstruction.

Nocturia (excessive urination at night) suggests decreased renal concentrating ability, heart failure, diabetes mellitus, or poor bladder emptyings.

Urinary incontinence (involuntary loss of urine) may result from injury of the external urinary sphincter, acquired neurogenic disease, or severe urgency from infection.

Stress incontinence (intermittent leakage of urine due to sudden strain) results from weakness of the sphincteric mechanism.

Enuresis (involuntary voiding during sleep) is physiologic to the age of 3 years. After this it may be functional or symptomatic of obstructive disease of the lower urinary tract.

Polyuria (a large volume of urine voided in a given time) may be due to diabetes mellitus, diabetes insipidus, chronic renal disease, diuretics, or excessive fluid intake.

Oliguria (a small volume of urine; output between 100–500 ml/24 hours) and *anuria* (absence of urine in the bladder; output less than 50 ml/24 hours) indicate a serious renal dysfunction requiring immediate medical intervention. These conditions may result from such causes as from shock, trauma, incompatible blood transfusion, and drug toxicity. Complete absence of urine (absolute anuria) is usually indicative of complete obstruction of the urinary tract.

Hematuria (red blood cells in the urine) is considered a serious sign because it may indicate cancer of the genitourinary tract, acute glomerulonephritis, or renal tuberculosis. The color of bloody urine is dependent upon the *p*H of the urine and the amount of blood present; acid urine is a dark, smoky color, while alkaline urine is red. Hematuria may also be due to systemic causes such as blood dyscrasias (abnormalities of clotting), anticoagulant therapy, neoplasms, trauma, and extreme exercise.

Proteinuria (*albuminuria*) (abnormal amounts of protein in the urine) is characteristically seen in all forms of acute and chronic renal disease. Normal urine does not contain persistent protein in significant quantities.

Gastrointestinal Symptoms

Gastrointestinal symptoms may occur with urologic conditions because the gastrointestinal and urinary tracts have common autonomic and sensory innervation and because of renointestinal reflexes. The anatomical relation of the right kidney to the colon, duodenum, head of the pancreas, common bile duct, liver, and gallbladder may cause gastrointestinal disturbances. The proximity of the left kidney to the colon (splenic flexure), stomach, pancreas, and spleen may also result in intestinal symptoms. These may include nausea, vomiting, diarrhea, abdominal discomfort, paralytic ileus, and gastrointestinal hemorrhage.

Appendicitis also may be accompanied by urinary symptoms.

Health History and Nursing Assessment

When obtaining a health history, it is essential that the nurse use language and terms understandable to the patient and be aware of the patient's embarrassment or discomfort in discussing genitourinary functions and symptoms. The patient may "forget" or deny symptoms because of anxiety or embarrassment. The following information related to urinary function is sought:

- What is the patient's chief concern, reason for seeking help?
- What is the patient's present and past occupation(s)? (Look for occupational hazards relevant to the urinary tract, including contact with chemicals, plastics, pitch, tar, or rubber.)
- Has the patient been exposed to any environmental toxins?
- What is the patient's smoking history?
- What is the past history in relation to urinary problems?
- Is there a family history of renal disease?
- What childhood diseases did the patient have?
- Is there a history of urinary infections?
- Did enuresis extend beyond the usual age (past 3 years old)?
- Is nocturia present or absent? Date of onset?
- Are there any disorders of voiding?
    Dysuria? When does it occur? Where is it felt? Initial or terminal dysuria?
    Hesitancy? Straining? Pain during or after urination?
    Changes in color of urine? Diminished urine output?
    Incontinence? Stress incontinence? Urgency incontinence?
    Any history of hematuria?
- Is pain present?
    Location? Character? Radiation? Duration? Related to voiding? What brings it on? What relieves it?
- Has the patient had fever? Chills? Passage of stones?
- Any history of genital lesions or sexually transmitted diseases?
- For the female patient:
    Number of children? Their ages? Forceps deliveries?
    Catheterized? When? Why?
    Any signs of vaginal discharge? Vaginal/vulvar itch or irritation?
- Does the patient have diabetes mellitus? Hypertension? Allergies?
- Has the patient ever been hospitalized with urinary tract infection?
    Before the age of 12?
    Cystoscopy? Indwelling catheter? Kidney x-ray procedures?

- Is the patient receiving any prescription or over-the-counter drugs that may affect urinary or renal function? Have any drugs been prescribed for treatment of renal or urinary problems?
- Is the patient at risk for urinary tract infection?

The nurse not only elicits information about the patient's physical complaints, but also assesses psychosocial status and educational needs. The nurse evaluates the patient's anxiety, perceived threats to body image, support systems, and sociocultural patterns. By putting together the information gathered during the initial and subsequent nursing assessments, the nurse finds valuable clues regarding misunderstandings, lack of knowledge, and needs for patient teaching.

Physical Assessment

Because renal dysfunction affects all body systems, a general assessment is indicated (see specific discussions in following sections). Additionally, the assessment focuses on the urinary tract specifically.

By direct palpation it is sometimes possible to determine the size and mobility of the kidneys.

- With the patient in a supine position, place one hand under the patient's back so that the fingers are clear of the lower ribs. The other hand (palm down) is located anterior to the kidney, with the fingers just above the level of umbilicus.
- Ask the patient to inhale deeply, and then push the anterior hand forward.

It may be possible to feel the smooth, rounded lower pole of the kidney between your hands; the right is more easily felt than the left because it is somewhat lower than the left.

Renal disease may produce tenderness over the costovertebral angle, which lies where the twelfth or bottom rib joins the spine.

In a rectal examination in the male, the prostate gland may be palpated digitally as a part of the study of urinary difficulty that occurs when there is hyperplasia of the prostate in older men (see p. 1154).

The inguinal area is examined for enlarged nodes, an inguinal or femoral hernia, and a varicocele. In women the vulva, urethra, and vagina are examined.

Diagnostic Evaluation

Urinalysis

Although its value is often underestimated, urinalysis provides a wealth of important clinical information and is regarded as an indispensable part of every clinical study. Urine examination of every patient includes evaluation of the following:

1. Urine color and clarity
2. Urine odor
3. Measurement of urine acidity and specific gravity
4. Tests for the presence of protein, glucose, and ketone bodies in the urine (proteinuria, glucosuria, and ketonuria, respectively)

5. Microscopic examination of the urine sediment after centrifuging for the detection of red blood cells (hematuria), white blood cells, casts (cylindruria), crystals (crystalluria), pus (pyuria), and bacteria (bacteriuria)

Numerous additional tests are applicable in special situations.

Collection of Urine Samples

All urine tests are ideally performed on fresh specimens, preferably of the first voiding of the day because this specimen is most concentrated and more likely to reveal abnormalities. Random specimens are satisfactory for most analyses, provided that they have been collected in clean containers and have been adequately protected against bacterial contamination and chemical deterioration. All specimens should be refrigerated as soon as possible after they are obtained. If left standing at room temperature, the urine becomes alkaline due to contamination of urea-splitting bacteria from the environment. Microscopic examination should be done within a half hour after collection; delay allows dissolution of cellular elements and bacterial overgrowth in nonsterile specimens. Urine cultures should be processed immediately. If this is not possible, they should be stored at 4°C (39°F).

Urine specimens should be collected from the patient by means of the clean-catch midstream technique, using a wide-mouthed container (see Fig. 38-3).

24-Hour Urine Collection

Many quantitative analytic tests are carried out on specimens of urine collected over a 24-hour period. The procedure is as follows:

The patient is instructed to empty the bladder at a specified time (such as 8:00 AM). This urine is discarded. All urine voided during the next 24 hours is collected. The last specimen is collected and saved 24 hours after the collection began (*i.e.*, 8:00 AM).

The patient's bladder should be empty when the test starts and empty when it ends. The urine is collected in a clean container. Depending on the test to be performed, a preservative may be added or the urine may need to be refrigerated. Discarding even one specimen voided during the test period invalidates the test. A successful collection requires the complete understanding and cooperation on the part of the patient and of all unit personnel concerned with the patient's care.

Clean-Catch Midstream Urine Specimens

Urine specimens voided in the usual manner are practically useless for bacteriologic study because of inevitable contamination by organisms residing in the vicinity of the urethral meatus. Such contamination can be avoided by catheterizing the urinary bladder. However, catheterization is no longer recommended except for specific indications because of the risk of infection. Reliable bacteriologic studies are possible without catheterization, utilizing the clean-catch midstream technique.

Instructions to the Male Patient

- Expose the glans and cleanse the area around the meatus with soap. Remove all soap with water-soaked pledgets.
- Do not collect the first portion of the voiding; discard it.
- Collect the next portion by voiding into a sterile wide-mouthed bottle or large-caliber tube that is protected by a sterile closure.
- Do not collect the last few drops of urine because prostatic secretions may be introduced into the urine at the end of the urinary stream.

Instructions to Female Patient

- Separate the labia to expose the urethral orifice (see Fig. 38-3).
- Cleanse around the urinary meatus with sponges soaked in liquid soap.
- Wipe the perineum from the front to the back.
- Remove all soap with water-soaked pledgets, wiping from front to back.
- Keep the labia separated and void forcibly, but do not collect the first portion of the voiding. (The distal portion of the urethral orifice is colonized by bacteria; the initial voiding washes away the urethral contaminants.)

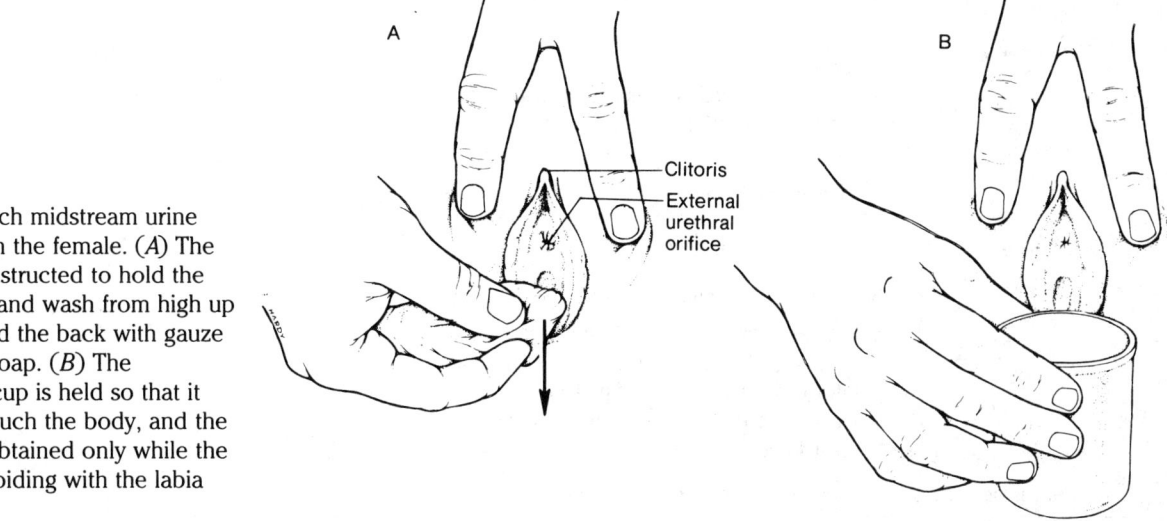

Figure 38-3
A clean-catch midstream urine specimen in the female. (*A*) The patient is instructed to hold the labia apart and wash from high up front toward the back with gauze soaked in soap. (*B*) The collection cup is held so that it does not touch the body, and the sample is obtained only while the patient is voiding with the labia held apart.

· Collect the midstream portion of the urinary flow, making sure that the container does not come in contact with the genitalia.

Renal Function Tests

Renal function tests are used to evaluate the severity of kidney disease and to follow the patient's clinical progress. These tests also give information concerning the kidneys' effectiveness in carrying out their excretory function. Results of function tests may be within normal limits until about 50% of renal function has been lost. Best results are obtained by combining a number of clinical tests. Table 38-2 lists the more common tests of renal function. Because of the important role of the kidneys in maintaining fluid and electrolyte balance, serum electrolyte levels also are assessed.

X-Ray Films

The examination usually begins with a plain film of the abdomen or KUB (kidney, ureters, and bladder) to delineate the size, shape, and position of the kidneys, and to reveal

TABLE 38-2
Tests of Renal Function

Test	Purpose/Rationale	Test Protocol
Renal Concentration Test		
Specific gravity Osmolality of urine	Tests the ability to concentrate solutes in the urine. Concentration ability is lost early in kidney disease; hence, this test shows early defects in renal function.	Fluids may be withheld for 12 to 24 hours to assess the concentrating ability of the tubules under controlled conditions. Specific gravity measurements of urine are taken at specific times to determine urine concentration.
Phenolsulfonphthalein Excretion Test (PSP)		
	A diagnostic agent (phenolsulfonphthalein) is given to determine the functional capacity of the kidney. (PSP test can also be used as a measure to assess residual urine.) Delayed excretion is seen in renal disease, cardiac failure, primary vascular disease.	Encourage fluids 1 to 1½ hours before the test. Phenolsulfonphthalein is given IV. 1. Record exact time dye is administered. 2. Collect urine in 15 minutes, 30 minutes, and 1 hour.
Creatinine Clearance* (Endogenous Creatinine Clearance) Test		
	Provides an approximation of rate of glomerular filtration Measures volume of blood cleared of creatinine in 1 minute Most sensitive indication of early renal disease Useful to follow progress of patient's renal status	Collect all urine over 24-hour period. Draw one sample of blood within the period.
Serum Creatinine Test		
	A test of renal function reflecting the balance between production and filtration by renal glomerulus Most sensitive measure of renal function	Do test on blood serum.
Serum Urea Nitrogen (Blood Urea Nitrogen—BUN) Test		
	Serves as index of renal excretory capacity Serum urea nitrogen is dependent on the body's urea production and on urine flow. (Urea is the nitrogenous end product of protein metabolism.) Affected by protein intake, tissue breakdown	Do test on blood serum.

* Clearance is the amount of blood cleansed of a constituent per unit of time.

any deviations, such as calcifications (stones) in the kidneys or urinary tract, hydronephrosis, cysts, tumors, or kidney displacement by abnormalities in the surrounding tissues.

Computed Tomography. Computed tomography (*CT* or *CAT scan*) is a noninvasive technique that provides an excellent cross-sectional view of the kidney and urinary tract. It provides information on the extension of invasive lesions of the kidney. No special patient preparation is needed.

Infusion Drip Pyelography. Infusion drip pyelography is an intravenous infusion of a large volume of dilute solution of contrast material to produce opacification of the renal parenchyma and complete filling of the urinary tract. This method of examination is useful when regular urographic techniques fail to show the drainage structures satisfactorily (*e.g.*, in a patient with an elevated blood urea nitrogen) or when prolonged opacification of the drainage structures is desired so that *tomograms* (body section radiography) can be made. Films are obtained at specified intervals after the start of the infusion to demonstrate the filled and distended collecting system. The patient preparation is the same as for excretory urography (see below), except that fluids are not restricted.

Excretory Urography (Intravenous Urogram or Intravenous Pyelogram). An excretory urogram or intravenous pyelogram (IVP) permits visualization of the kidneys, ureter, and bladder. A radiopaque contrast medium is administered intravenously, and is cleared from the bloodstream and concentrated by the kidneys. A *nephrotomogram* may be carried out as part of the study to visualize different layers of the kidney and the diffuse structures within each layer and to differentiate solid masses or lesions from cysts in the kidneys or urinary tract.

Excretory urography is conducted as part of the initial assessment of any suspected urologic problem, especially in the diagnosis of lesions in the kidneys and ureters. It also provides a rough estimate of renal function. After the contrast material (sodium diatrizoate or meglumine diatrizoate) is given intravenously, multiple films are taken serially to visualize drainage structures.

Patient Preparation. The patient may be prepared for the procedure as follows:

1. The patient's history should be checked for any indications of allergies that might cause an adverse reaction to the contrast material. The physician and the radiologist are notified of allergy (especially to iodine or shellfish) or suspicion of allergy so that appropriate measures are taken to prevent serious allergic reactions. The suspected allergy is also noted prominently in the patient's record.
2. A laxative may be given the night before the scheduled examination to eliminate feces and gas in the intestinal tract.
3. Liquids may be restricted 8 to 10 hours before the test to promote a concentrated urine. However, elderly patients with marginal renal reserve or function, patients with multiple myeloma, and those with uncontrolled diabetes mellitus may not tolerate dehydration. With the approval of the physician, the nurse may give such patients water to drink during the hours before the test. The patient should not be overhydrated, which may dilute the contrast material and thus cause inadequate visualization.

4. The procedure itself and the sensations produced by injection of the contrast medium and during the procedure (*e.g.*, a temporary feeling of warmth and flushing of the face) are described to the patient.

If the patient has a positive allergic history, a test dose of the contrast material may be injected intradermally. If no skin reaction occurs in 15 minutes, the regular intravenous test dose of contrast material is given. Although rare, as with the administration of any intravenous drug, an anaphylactoid reaction may occur. (This reaction may occur even if the skin sensitivity test has been negative.)

- All IV urogram rooms should have emergency drugs (epinephrine, corticosteroids, vasopressors), as well as oxygen, tracheostomy, and other equipment, ready for immediate therapy in case an anaphylactoid reaction occurs.

Retrograde Pyelography. In retrograde pyelography, ureteral catheters are passed up through the ureters into the renal pelvis by means of cystoscopic manipulation. A contrast material is then introduced into the catheters by gravity or syringe. Retrograde pyelography is usually done if intravenous urography provides inadequate visualization of the collecting systems. It is being used less frequently because of improved techniques in excretory urography.

Cystogram. A catheter is inserted into the bladder and contrast material instilled to outline the bladder wall and to aid in evaluation of *vesicoureteral reflux* (backflow of urine from the bladder into one or both ureters). Cystograms are also taken in conjunction with simultaneous pressure recordings inside the bladder.

Cystourethrogram. A cystourethrogram provides visualization of the urethra and bladder either by retrograde injection of the contrast material into the urethra and bladder or by x-ray films taken while the patient excretes the contrast material. See page 1005 for a description of a *voiding cystourethrogram*.

Renal Angiography. The purpose of this procedure is to visualize the renal arterial supply. A special needle is used to pierce the femoral (or axillary) artery, and a catheter is threaded up through the femoral and iliac arteries into the aorta or renal artery. Contrast material is injected to opacify the renal arterial supply. Angiography enables evaluation of blood flow dynamics, demonstrates abnormal vasculature, and helps to differentiate renal cysts from renal tumors.

Nursing Interventions. Before the procedure, a cathartic may be prescribed to eliminate fecal material and gas from the colon so that unobstructed x-rays will be visualized. The proposed injection sites (groin for femoral approach or axilla for axillary approach) are shaved. The peripheral pulse sites (radial, femoral, dorsalis pedis) are marked for easy access in postprocedural assessment. The patient is informed that a transient feeling of heat may be sensed along the course of the vessel when the contrast material is injected.

Following the procedure, the vital signs are taken until stable. If the axillary artery was punctured, the blood pressure is taken on the opposite arm. The puncture site is examined for swelling and hematoma development. The peripheral pulses are palpated. The color and temperature of the involved extremity are noted and compared with those of the uninvolved extremity. Cold compresses may be applied to the puncture site to decrease edema and pain.

Ultrasound

Ultrasound (ultrasonic scan) uses sound waves that are passed into the body. Organs in the urinary system create characteristic ultrasonic images. Abnormalities such as masses, malformations, or obstructions can be identified. Ultrasound is a noninvasive technique, and no special patient preparation is required.

Endourology (Urologic Endoscopic Procedures)

The Cystoscopic Examination

The cystoscopic exam (*cystoscopy* or "*cysto*") is a method of direct visualization of the urethra and bladder. The cystoscope, which is inserted through the urethra into the bladder, has a self-contained optical lens system that provides a magnified, illuminated view of the bladder. The cystoscope can be manipulated to allow complete visualization of the urethra and bladder as well as the ureteral orifices and prostatic urethra. Small ureteral catheters can be passed through the cystoscope, allowing assessment of the ureter and the pelvis of the kidney. The cystoscope also permits the urologist to obtain a urine specimen from each kidney to evaluate renal function. Cup forceps can be inserted through the cystoscope for biopsy. Calculi may be removed from the urethra, bladder, and ureter via cystoscopy.

The endoscope is passed under direct vision. After inspection of the urethra, the bladder is inspected. Sterile irrigating solution is instilled to distend the bladder and wash away blood clots, thereby allowing better visualization (Fig.

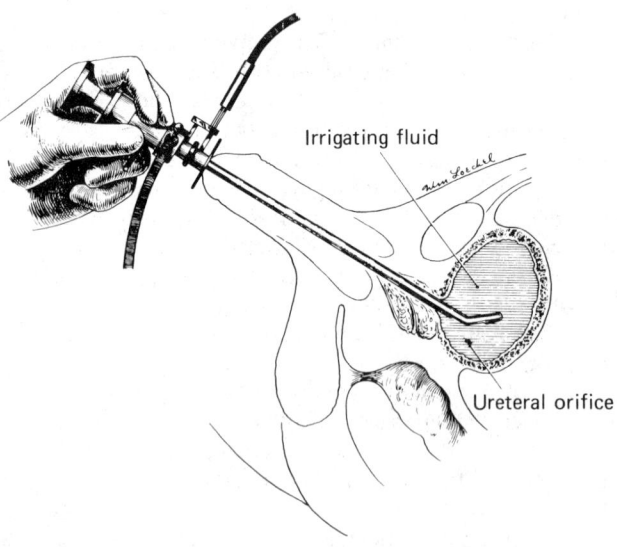

Figure 38-4
Cystoscopic examination. A cystoscope is introduced into the bladder of the male. The upper cord is an electric line for the light at the distal end of the cystoscope. The lower tubing leads from a reservoir of sterile irrigating fluid that is used to inflate the bladder.

38-4). The use of a high-intensity light and interchangeable lenses allows excellent visualization and permits still and motion pictures to be taken of these structures.

Prior to the procedure, a sedative may be given. A local topical anesthetic is instilled into the urethra by the urologist before the cystoscope is inserted. Intravenous diazepam (Valium) in combination with topical urethral anesthesia may be administered. Occasionally, it may be necessary to use spinal or general anesthesia.

Nursing Interventions. As with any diagnostic procedure, the nurse describes the examination and procedure in order to inform the patient and allay fears. Additional preprocedure preparation may include having the patient drink 1 or 2 glasses of water before going to the radiology department.

Postprocedure management is directed at relieving any possible discomfort resulting from the examination. Some burning upon voiding, blood-tinged urine, and urinary frequency from trauma to the mucous membrane may be expected after cystoscopic examination. Moist heat to the lower abdomen or warm sitz baths are helpful in relieving pain and promoting muscle relaxation. Occasionally, following cystoscopic examination the patient with obstructive pathology may experience urinary retention as a result of edema caused by the instrumentation. The patient with prostatic hyperplasia is carefully monitored for urinary retention. Warm sitz baths and relaxant medications are helpful for relieving retention, but an indwelling catheter may have to be inserted.

Renal and Ureteral Brush Biopsy

Brush biopsy techniques provide specific information when abnormal x-ray findings for the ureter or renal pelvis raise uncertainty as to whether the defect is a tumor, a stone, a blood clot, or an artifact. First, a cystoscopic examination is conducted. Then a ureteral catheter is introduced, followed by a biopsy brush that is passed through the catheter. The suspected lesion is brushed back and forth in order to obtain cells and surface tissue fragments for histologic analysis.

Following the procedure, the patient may be given an intravenous infusion to help clear the kidneys and prevent clot formation. Urine may show blood (usually clearing in 24 to 48 hours) from oozing at the brushing site. Postoperative renal colic occasionally occurs, and responds to analgesics.

Renal Endoscopy (Nephroscopy)

Renal endoscopy (nephroscopy) is the introduction of a fiberscope into the pelvis of the kidney, through an incision (pyelotomy) or percutaneously, to view the interior of the renal pelvis, remove calculi, biopsy small lesions, and aid diagnosis of renal hematuria and selected renal tumors.

Needle Biopsy of the Kidney

Needle biopsy of the kidney is performed by percutaneous needle biopsy through renal tissue or by open biopsy through a small flank incision. It is useful in evaluating the course of renal disease and in securing specimens for electron and immunofluorescent microscopy, particularly for glomerular disease. Before the biopsy is carried out, coagulation studies are conducted to identify any patient at risk for postbiopsy bleeding.

The patient may be placed on a fasting regimen 6 to 8 hours before the test. An intravenous line is established. A urine specimen is obtained and saved for comparison with the postbiopsy specimen. The patient is informed that it will be necessary to hold his breath in (to stop movement of the kidney) during insertion of the renal biopsy needle.

The sedated patient is placed in a prone position with a sandbag under the abdomen. A local anesthetic agent is infiltrated into the skin at the biopsy site. The biopsy needle is introduced just inside the renal capsule of the outer quadrant of the kidney. The location of the needle may be identified by fluoroscopy or by ultrasound, in which a special probe is used. Open biopsy may also be carried out, through a small flank incision.

Postbiopsy Nursing Management. After the specimen is obtained, pressure is applied to the biopsy site. The patient may be kept in a prone position immediately following biopsy and on bed rest for 24 hours to minimize risk of bleeding.

The nurse observes for hematuria, which may appear soon after biopsy. The kidney is a highly vascular organ, and approximately one fourth of the entire cardiac output passes through it in about 1 minute. The passage of the biopsy needle punctures the kidney capsule, and bleeding can occur in the perirenal space. Usually, the bleeding subsides on its own, but a large amount of blood can accumulate in this space in a short period of time without noticeable signs until cardiovascular collapse is evident.

- To detect early signs of bleeding, it is important that the vital signs be taken every 5 to 15 minutes for the first hour and then with decreasing frequency as indicated.
- Signs suggestive of bleeding include a rise or fall in blood pressure, anorexia, vomiting, and the development of a dull, aching discomfort in the abdomen.
- Any signs of backache, shoulder pain, or dysuria are reported to the physician.

Flank pain may occur, but usually represents bleeding into the muscle rather than around the kidney. Colicky pain similar to that of ureteral colic may develop when a clot is present in the ureter and may cause excruciating, sharp flank pain that radiates to the groin.

All urine voided by the patient is scrutinized for evidence of bleeding and compared with the prebiopsy specimen and subsequent voiding samples. If bleeding persists, as indicated by an enlarging hematoma, avoid palpating or manipulating the abdomen. A hematocrit and hemoglobin study is done within 8 hours to assess for anemia. Usually, the fluid level is kept at 3000 ml daily unless the patient has renal insufficiency. If bleeding occurs, the patient is prepared for blood transfusion and surgical intervention for control of hemorrhage, which may necessitate surgical drainage or nephrectomy (removal of kidney).

Patient Education. The nurse should keep in mind that a delayed hemorrhage can occur a number of days after biopsy. The patient is cautioned to avoid strenuous activity, strenuous sports, and heavy lifting for at least 2 weeks. The physician or clinic is to be notified if any of the following occurs: flank pain, hematuria, lightheadedness and fainting, rapid pulse, or any other signs and symptoms of bleeding.

Radioisotope Studies

Radioisotope studies are noninvasive procedures that do not interfere with normal physiological processes and require no specific patient preparation. Radiopharmaceuticals (^{99}Tc-labeled compound or ^{131}I-hippurate) are injected intravenously. Studies are obtained with a scintillation camera placed posterior to the kidney, with the patient in a supine, prone, or sitting position. The resultant image (called a *scan*) indicates the distribution of the radiopharmaceutical within the kidney.

The *Tc scan* provides information about kidney perfusion and is useful when renal function is poor. The *hippurate scan* provides information about kidney function.

Urodynamic Measurements

Urodynamic measurements provide physiologic and structural tests to evaluate bladder and urethral function by measuring the (1) rate of urine flow, (2) bladder pressures during voiding and at rest, (3) internal urethral resistance, and (4) bladder contraction and relaxation. Abdominal, bladder, and detrusor pressures, sphincter activity, bladder innervation, muscle tone, and sacral reflex are assessed.

The following are the urodynamic measurements most frequently performed.

Uroflowmetry (flow rate) is the record of the volume of urine passing through the urethra per time unit (ml/second).

A *cystometrogram* is a graphic recording of the pressures in the bladder (intravesical) at various phases of filling and emptying of the urinary bladder to assess its function. During the procedure, the amount of fluid instilled into the bladder and voided, as well as the patient's sensations of bladder fullness and urge to void, are recorded. These are then compared to the pressures measured in the bladder during bladder filling and voiding. The patient is first asked to void, and the physician observes the time it takes to initiate voiding; the size, force, and continuity of the urinary stream; and the degree of straining and hesitancy. A retention catheter is passed through the urethra and into the bladder. The residual volume is measured and the catheter left in place. The urethral catheter is connected to a water manometer, and sterile fluid or water is allowed to flow into the bladder, usually at the rate of 1 ml/second. The patient informs the examiner when the first desire to void is felt, and again when the bladder feels full. The degree of bladder filling at these points is recorded. The pressures above the zero level at the symphysis pubis are measured, and the pressures and volumes within the bladder are plotted and recorded.

The *urethral pressure profile* measures urethral resistance along the length of the urethra. Gas and fluid are instilled through a catheter that is withdrawn while the pressures along the urethral wall are obtained.

A *cystourethrogram* is visualization of the urethra and bladder either by retrograde injection or by voiding of contrast material.

In a *voiding cystourethrogram*, the bladder is filled with contrast medium, and the patient voids while rapid spot films are taken. The presence or absence of vesicoureteral reflux or congenital abnormalities in the lower urinary tract can be demonstrated. The voiding cystourethrogram is also used to investigate difficulty in bladder emptying and incontinence.

Nursing Care Plan 38-1

Care of the Patient Undergoing Assessment for Renal/Urinary Dysfunction

Nursing Interventions	*Rationale*	*Expected Outcomes*

Nursing Diagnosis: Deficit in knowledge about procedures and diagnostic tests

Goal: Patient acquires knowledge and understanding of the procedure and tests and expected behaviors

1. Assess patient's current level of understanding of planned tests and procedures.	1. Provides basis for further explanations and teaching and gives indication of patient's perception of procedures.	• Patient states rationale for planned diagnostic procedures and tasks and behaviors expected during the procedures.
2. Provide factual description of tests in language and terms the patient understands.	2. Understanding what is expected enhances patient's compliance and cooperation.	• Complies with urine collection, fluid modifications, or other procedures required for diagnostic evaluation.
3. Assess patient's understanding of test results following their completion.	3. Apprehension may interfere with patient's ability to understand information and results provided by physician and other health care providers.	• Restates in own terminology results of diagnostic assessment.
		• Asks for clarification of terms and procedures.
4. Reinforce information provided to patient about test results and implications for follow-up care.	4. Provides opportunity for patient to clarify points and anticipate follow-up care.	• Explains rationale for follow-up care.
		• Participates in follow-up care.

Nursing Diagnosis: Alteration in comfort—pain and discomfort related to infection, edema, obstruction, or bleeding along urinary tract

Goal: Relief of discomfort and pain

1. Assess level of pain and discomfort.
  a. dysuria
  b. burning on urination
  c. abdominal pain and discomfort
  d. flank pain
  e. bladder spasm
	1. Provides baseline for evaluating success of interventions and/or progression of dysfunction.	• Patient reports decreasing levels of pain and discomfort.
		• Uses sitz bath as indicated.
		• Consumes increased fluid intake.
		• Reports absence of local symptoms (urgency, frequency, dysuria, and burning on urination).

2. Encourage fluid intake (unless contraindicated).	2. Promotes dilute urine and flushing of lower urinary tract.	• States is able to start and stop urinary stream without discomfort.
3. Encourage warm sitz baths.	3. Relieves local discomfort and promotes relaxation.	• Identifies symptoms and signs to be reported to health care provider.

(continued)

Electromyography uses the placement of electrodes in the pelvic floor/musculature or anal sphincter to evaluate neuromuscular function of the lower tract.

Nursing Care of Patients Undergoing Assessment of the Renal/Urinary System

All patients, regardless of the extent or type of urinary tract dysfunction, undergo tests to assess the function of the urinary tract. Even those who have had these tests repeatedly in the past experience fear and apprehension about the procedures and the results. Additionally, they frequently feel discomfort and embarrassment about a previously private and personal function: voiding. Although this is a function that health care providers deal with frequently in the course of providing care, it is important to remember that it is not so routine to patients.

Nursing Diagnoses

Potential nursing diagnoses for these patients include the following:

- Deficit in knowledge about the procedures and their meaning
- Alteration in comfort; pain and discomfort related to renal dysfunction
- Fear related to possible diagnoses of serious illness
- Anxiety and embarrassment related to invasive techniques associated with private parts of the anatomy

Nursing Interventions	*Rationale*	*Expected Outcomes*

Nursing Diagnosis: Alteration in comfort—pain and discomfort related to infection, edema, obstruction, or bleeding along urinary tract

Goal: Relief of discomfort and pain

4. Report increased pain to physician.	4. May indicate progression or dysfunction, recurrence of dysfunction, or untoward signs (*e.g.*, bleeding, calculi).	• Takes medications as prescribed
		• Does not delay in emptying bladder
		• Uses appropriate hygienic practices:
		   Avoids use of bubble bath
		   Uses appropriate hygiene after bowel movements

5. Administer analgesics and antispasmodics for pain and spasm as prescribed.	5. May be prescribed for pain and spasm.	
6. Assess voiding patterns and practices of hygiene and provide instructions about recommended voiding patterns and hygienic practices.	6. Delayed emptying of the bladder and some poor practices of hygiene contribute to discomfort and pain secondary to renal or urinary tract dysfunction.	

Nursing Diagnosis: Fear related to (1) potential alteration in renal function and body part, and (2) embarrassment secondary to invasion of urinary tract

Goal: Reduces fear

1. Assess patient's level of fear and apprehension.	1. A high level of fear or apprehension can interfere with learning and cooperation.	• Patient appears relaxed with low level of fear and apprehension. • States rationale for tests and procedures in a calm, relaxed manner • Maintains usual privacy and modesty • Discusses own urinary tract dysfunction in correct terminology without overt indications of embarrassment or discomfort • Is able to relate fears and concerns • Shows correct understanding of procedures and possible outcomes
2. Explain all procedures and tests to patients.	2. Knowledge about what is expected helps to reduce fear and apprehension.	
3. Provide privacy and maintain patient's modesty by closing doors, keeping patient covered and clothed. Keep urinal and bedpan covered and out of sight.	3. Communicates that you are aware of and accept patient's need for privacy and modesty.	
4. Use correct terminology in factual manner when questioning patient about urinary tract dysfunction.	4. Conveys that nurse is comfortable discussing patient's urinary dysfunction and symptoms with patient.	
5. Assess patient's fears about perceived changes associated with tests and other procedures.	5. May reveal unfounded fears and misperceptions that can be alleviated by correct understanding.	

Planning, Implementation, and Evaluation

The goals, nursing interventions, rationales for interventions, and expected outcomes are discussed in more detail in Nursing Care Plan 38-1, Care of the Patient Undergoing Assessment for Renal/Urinary Dysfunction.

Bibliography

Books

Brenner B et al. Principles of Renal Medicine. Philadelphia, WB Saunders, 1986.

Bricker N and Kirchenbaum MA. The Kidney: Diagnosis and Management. New York, John Wiley & Sons, 1984.

Fischbach F. A Manual of Laboratory Diagnostic Tests. Philadelphia, JB Lippincott, 1984.

Hanno PM and Wein AJ. A Clinical Manual of Urology. East Norwalk, Connecticut, Appleton-Century-Crofts, 1986.

Hepinstall RH. Pathology of the Kidney. Boston, Little Brown & Co, 1983.

McConnell EA and Zimmerman MF. Care of Patients with Urologic Problems. Philadelphia, JB Lippincott, 1983.

Articles

Abraham PA and Smith CL. Medical evaluation and management of calcium nephrolithiasis. Med Clin North Am 1984 Mar; 68(2):281–299.

Arger PH. Computed tomography of the lower urinary tract. Urol Clin N Am 1985 Nov; 12(4):677–686.

Chait A. Current status of renal angiography. Urol Clin North Am 1985 Nov; 12(4):687–698.

Checchio LM and Como AJ. Electrolytes, BUN, creatinine: Who's at risk? Ann Emerg Med 1986 Mar; 15(3):363–366.

Coleman BG. Ultrasonography of the upper genitourinary tract. Urol Clin North Am 1985 Nov; 12(4):633–644.

Diokno AC et al. Urologic evaluation of urinary tract infection in pregnancy. J Reprod Med 1986 Jan 31; (1):23–26.

Engram BW. Do's and don'ts of urologic nursing. Nursing '83 1983 Oct; 13(10):49.

Free AH and Free HM. Urinalysis: Its proper role in the physician's office. Clin Lab Med 1986 June; 6(2):253–266.

Haber ME and Lindner LE. New life for microscopic urinalysis. Diagnostic Med 1985 Apr; 8(4):14–20.

Haggar AM and Kressel HY. Magnetic resonance imaging of the genitourinary tract. Urol Clin North Am 1985 Nov; 12(4):725–736.

Hillman BJ. Renal digital subtraction angiography. Urol Clin North Am 1985 Nov; 12(4):699–713.

Jenkins RD, Fenn JP, and Matsen JM. Review of urine microscopy for bacteriuria. JAMA 1986 June 27; 255(24):3397–3403.

Kulberg A. Urinalysis and urine culture. Top Emerg Med 1983 Apr; 5(1): 47–61.

Lantz EJ and Hattery RR. Diagnostic imaging of urothelial cancer. Urol Clin North Am 1984 Nov; 11(4):567–583.

Latham RH et al. Laboratory diagnosis of urinary tract infection in ambulatory women. JAMA 1985 Dec 20; 254(23):3333–3336.

McGuire EJ. Clinical evaluation of the female lower urinary tract. Urol Clin North Am 1985 May; 12(2):225–229.

Morgan DB. Plasma urea and electrolytes: The clinical need. Clin Endocrinol Metab 1984 July; 13(2):399–412.

Needham CA. Rapid methods in microbiology for in-office testing. Clin Lab Med 1986 June; 6(2):291–304.

Pollack HM and Banner MP. Current status of excretory urography. Urol Clin North Am 1985 Nov; 12(4):585–601.

Reid G. The office microbiology laboratory. Urol Clin North Am 1986 Nov; 13(4):569–576.

Rifkin MD. Ultrasonography of the lower genitourinary tract. Urol Clin North Am 1985 Nov; 12(4):645–656.

Sandler CM, Raval B, and David CL. Computed tomography of the kidney. Urol Clin North Am 1985 Nov; 12(4):657–675.

Sewell DL. Urine cultures. Diagnosis 1985 Apr; 7(4):15,16, 25.

Shannon GW. Urinalysis: High yield, low cost. Diagnosis 1983 June; 5(6): 89–93, 97, 101.

Sheldon CA and Gonzalez R. Differentiation of upper and lower urinary tract infections: How and when? Urol Clin North Am 1984 May; 11(2):321–333.

Stamm WE. When should we use urine cultures? Infect Control 1986 Aug; 7(8):431–433.

Uehara DT. Indications for intravenous pyelography in trauma. Ann Emerg Med 1986 Mar; 15(3):266–269.

Uehara DT and Eisner RF. Indications for retrograde cystograde cystourethrography in trauma. Ann Emerg Med 1986 Mar; 15(3):270–272.

Valeri AM and Appel GB. Determining the type of interstitial nephritis. Diagnosis 1986 Apr; 8(4):38–44.

Velchik MG. Radionuclide imaging of the urinary tract. Urol Clin North Am 1985 Nov; 12(4):603–631.

Voith AM. Conceptual framework for nursing diagnoses: Alteration in urinary elimination. Rehabil Nurs 1986 Jan/Feb; 11(1):18–21.

Werman HA and Brown CG. Utility of urine cultures in the emergency department. Ann Emerg Med 1986 Mar; 15(3):302–307.

Agencies

Governmental

National Institute of Diabetes and Digestive and Kidney Diseases, National Institutes of Health, Bethesda, Maryland 20892.

Voluntary

American Society for Artificial Internal Organs, P.O. Box 777, Boca Raton, Florida 33432.

National Association of Patients on Hemodialysis and Transplantation, 150 Nassau Street, New York, New York 10038.

National Kidney Foundation, 116 East 27th Street, New York, New York 10016.

United Ostomy Association, 2001 W. Beverly Boulevard, Los Angeles, California 90057.

Chapter 39

Management of
Patients With
Renal and
Urinary Dysfunction

Psychosocial Considerations

Conditions of the genitourinary tract may generate emotional stresses and feelings of guilt and embarrassment when the external genitalia are examined and treated or urinary function is discussed. Problems of incontinence may cause disgust and feelings of helplessness. Some patients are constantly uneasy over the possibility of an "accident," although others appear indifferent.

Surgical procedures affecting the male reproductive organs can pose a threat to the masculinity of the patient, no matter what his age. Although many men may hide their fears of impotency by blaming "prostate trouble," many sexual problems of males (such as difficulty in achieving erection and premature ejaculation) are psychological in origin and related to a variety of causes—fear, guilt, aversion to partner, and fatigue. Because of such fears and feelings, a male patient may react with anger and hostility to those caring for him, or he may turn his anger inward, resulting in more than the usual amount of pain. Patients with urinary infections may become depressed when they undergo prolonged periods of treatment. Anxiety in any stressful situation can produce urinary frequency and urgency.

Urologic patients, like any other patients, need to be respected as individuals and understood. They want their questions answered, fears allayed, and discomfort relieved. Additionally, their modesty and privacy need to be maintained. These patients may require reassurance, support, and acceptance from the nurse.

Fluid and Electrolyte Imbalance

A major problem for patients with renal disorders is fluid and electrolyte imbalance. The nurse must be skilled in observing and documenting the clinical condition of the patient. Every patient with a urologic disorder has a fluid intake–output chart on which is recorded all fluid intake, whether by ingestion or by parenteral administration. The volume of urine excreted and of other output is recorded. In addition, other sources of fluid loss and the patient's weight are monitored and recorded. These records are essential in determining the patient's fluid allowance.

The nurse is alert to manifestations of body fluid disturbances (see Chap. 9 and also pp. 1034 and 1037). For example, the following signs and symptoms may occur in patients with renal disease:

1. Acute weight loss (in excess of 5%), a drop in body temperature, dryness of skin and mucous membranes, longitudinal wrinkles or furrows of tongue, and oliguria or anuria—could indicate fluid volume deficit.
2. Acute weight gain (in excess of 5%), edema, moist crackles in lungs, puffy eyelids, and shortness of breath—could indicate fluid volume excess.
3. Abdominal cramps, apprehension, convulsions, fingerprinting on sternum, and oliguria or anuria—could indicate sodium deficit.
4. Dry, sticky mucous membranes, flushed skin, oliguria or anuria, thirst, and rough and dry tongue—could indicate sodium excess.
5. Anorexia, gaseous distention of intestines, silent intestinal ileus, weakness, and soft, flabby muscles—could indicate potassium deficit.
6. Diarrhea, intestinal colic, irritability, and nausea—could indicate potassium excess.
7. Abdominal cramps, carpopedal spasm, muscle cramps, tetany, and tingling of ends of fingers—could indicate calcium deficit.
8. Deep bone pain, flank pain, and muscle hypotonicity—could indicate calcium excess.
9. Deep, rapid breathing (Kussmaul), shortness of breath on exertion, stupor, and weakness—could indicate primary base bicarbonate deficit.
10. Depressed respiration, muscle hypertonicity, and tetany—could indicate primary base bicarbonate excess.
11. Chronic weight loss, emotional depression, pallor, fatigue, and soft, flabby muscles—could indicate protein deficit.
12. Positive Chvostek's sign, convulsions, disorientation, hyperactive deep reflexes, and tremor—could indicate magnesium deficit.

The nurse needs a thorough understanding of the patient's gains and losses of body fluids, and shares this information with other members of the health care team. When supervising intravenous therapy, the nurse adjusts the flow rate in accordance with the physician's prescription, which is based on collaborative assessment of the patient's fluid requirements.

Repeated blood samples are obtained for surveillance of electrolyte balance. The nurse explains the purpose of the studies and prepares the patient for venipuncture.

Maintaining Adequate Urinary Drainage

For the patient with urologic disease, as for any other person, urinary excretion of waste materials is necessary for life. The composition of the body fluids is determined not so much by what the patient ingests as by what the kidneys retain. In health, the kidneys are very efficient, excreting the substances that are not needed and retaining those that are. But in the patient with damaged kidneys, therapeutic efforts are necessary to ensure that the limited function of the kidneys is not exceeded.

When artificial drainage of the urinary system becomes necessary, catheters may be inserted directly into the bladder, the ureters, or the kidney pelves. Catheters are available in various sizes, shapes, and lengths, and may have one or more openings placed in various positions near the tip. A catheter may be constructed of hard or soft rubber, woven fabric, silicone, metal, glass, or plastic. The tip may be open or closed and may have a mushroom shape, such as the Pezzer catheter; have a winged shape, such as the Malecot catheter; or simply be round and blunt. The type of catheter chosen depends on its purpose.

Catheterization

Principles of Management

There are times when the catheter is a lifesaving instrument, as is the case when the patient is unable to void. At other times, catheterization may be necessary in determining the amount of residual urine in the bladder after the patient has voided, to bypass an obstruction that blocks the flow of urine, to provide postoperative drainage following bladder, vaginal, or prostate surgery, or in monitoring of hourly urinary output in critically ill patients.

- A patient should be catheterized only if absolutely necessary because catheterization commonly leads to urinary tract infection.

Urinary tract infections are responsible for 35% of all hospital-acquired infections. Most of these follow instrumentation of the urinary tract, usually catheterization. The pathogens responsible for catheter-associated urinary tract infections include *Escherichia coli, Klebsiella, Proteus, Pseudomonas, Enterobacter, Serratia,* and *Candida.* Many of these are part of the patient's endogenous bowel flora or are acquired through cross-contamination by patients or hospital personnel or through exposure to nonsterile equipment.

When catheters are used, microorganisms may gain access to the urinary tract by three main pathways: (1) by introduction from the urethra into the bladder at the time of catheterization; (2) from the thin film of urethral fluid outside of the catheter at the catheter–mucosa interface; and (3) by migration to the bladder along the internal lumen of the catheter after contamination (most common).

To safeguard the patient, the following points of care are essential in urethral catheter management:

- Strict surgical asepsis is employed.
- The urethra is adequately cleansed.
- The catheter should be smaller than the external urinary meatus to minimize trauma and allow secretions to drain out alongside the catheter.
- The catheter is well lubricated with an appropriate antimicrobial lubricant.
- The catheter is passed gently and skillfully.
- The catheter is removed as soon as possible.

Nursing Care of the Patient With an Indwelling Catheter and a Closed Urinary Drainage System.   When an indwelling catheter is necessary, a closed drainage system— one designed to minimize or prevent disconnection and risk of contamination—is essential. Such a system may consist of an indwelling catheter, a connecting tube, and a collecting bag emptied by a drainage valve; it may consist of a triple-lumen indwelling urethral catheter attached to a closed sterile drainage system. The three-way catheter allows urinary drainage through one channel, inflation of the bag with water or air through the second channel, and continuous irrigation of the bladder with antibacterial solution through the third channel.

▶ *Nursing Process*
The Patient With an Indwelling Catheter and a Closed Urinary Drainage System

▷ *Assessment*

The patient with an indwelling catheter is observed for signs and symptoms of urinary tract infection: cloudy urine, hematuria, fever, chills, anorexia, and malaise. The area around the urethral orifice is observed for drainage and excoriation. Urine cultures provide the most accurate means for assessment of infection. The color, odor, and volume of urine are also monitored.

Nursing assessment includes observation of the drainage system to ensure that the system provides adequate drainage of urine. The catheter itself is observed to make sure that it is properly anchored, to prevent pressure on the urethra at the penoscrotal junction in the male patient, and tension and traction of the bladder in both male and female patients. An accurate record of the patient's fluid intake and urine output provides additional information about the adequacy of urine elimination.

Additionally, patients at risk for urinary tract infection from catheterization are identified; these include persons who are elderly, debilitated, chronically ill, immunosuppressed, or diabetic. The patient's understanding of the purpose of catheterization is also assessed. Because of the increased risk of infection and subsequent septicemia, assessment for signs and symptoms of bacteriuria, infection, and sepsis is essential.

▷ *Nursing Diagnoses*

Based on the assessment data, the patient's major nursing diagnoses for the patient may include the following:

- Potential for infection of the urinary tract related to contamination of the urinary tract
- Potential impairment of the tissue integrity (urethra and bladder) related to catheterization

▷   *Goals:*   The major goals for the patient may include absence of urinary tract infection and absence of trauma to the urethra and bladder.

Nursing Interventions

Infection Control.   Certain principles of care are essential when managing a closed urinary drainage system.

- Strict asepsis is necessary during insertion of the catheter.
- A preassembled and sterile closed urinary drainage system is necessary and should not be disconnected before, during, or after insertion of the catheter.
- To prevent contamination of a closed system, the tubing is never disconnected. No part of the collection bag or drainage tube should ever be contaminated.
- The bag is never raised above the level of the patient's bladder because this will cause flow of contaminated urine into the patient's bladder from the bag. Urine flows by gravity.
- Urine should not be allowed to collect in the tubing because a free flow of urine must be maintained to prevent infection. Improper drainage occurs when the tubing is kinked or twisted, allowing pools of urine to collect in the loops of the tubing.
- The drainage bag is not allowed to touch the floor. The bag and collecting tubing are changed if contamination occurs, if the urine flow becomes obstructed, or if the tubing junctions start to leak at the connections.
- The bag is emptied at least every 8 hours through the drainage valve, and more frequently if there is a large volume of urine, to lessen the risk of bacterial proliferation.
- Care is taken to see that the drainage tube (valve/spout) is not contaminated. Each patient should have a urine receptacle in which to empty the bag.
- Irrigation of the catheter is *not* carried out routinely.
- The catheter is not disconnected from the tubing to obtain urine samples, irrigate the catheter, or ambulate or transport the patient.
- Inadvertent handling or manipulation of the catheter by the patient or staff is avoided.
- Hand washing is necessary before and after handling of the catheter, tubing, and drainage bag.

The catheter is a foreign body in the urethra, and produces a reaction in the urethral mucosa with some urethral discharge. However, meatal care during catheterization is discouraged, as catheter manipulation during cleansing may result in increased rates of infection. Gentle washing with soap during the daily bath is warranted to cleanse and to remove obvious encrustations from the external catheter surface. The catheter is anchored as securely as possible to prevent to-and-fro movement in the urethra. Drainage and encrustation occur at the exit of any tube. Encrustation arising from urinary salts may enter the bladder when the catheter is removed and may serve as a nucleus for stone formation. There appears to be significantly less crust formation when silicone catheters are used.

A liberal fluid intake and an increased urine output must be assured to mechanically flush the catheter and to dilute urinary elements that might form encrustations. (The intake must be within limits of the patient's cardiac reserve.) Keeping the urine acid helps to prevent tube obstruction and encrustation of urinary sand and calculus deposits. An acid ash diet helps to acidify urine, as does oral intake of ascorbic acid and potassium acid phosphate.

Urine cultures are obtained as prescribed or indicated in monitoring for infection. Many catheters have an aspiration (puncture) port from which a specimen can be obtained.

Measures must be taken to prevent cross-contamination because many urinary tract infections are due to extrinsically acquired organisms transmitted by cross-contamination. Patients at risk are women, elderly debilitated patients, and those who are critically ill.

- There must be renewed emphasis on *hand washing* between patients and before and after handling any part of the catheter or drainage system.
- Catheterized patients with bacteria in the urine should not be in the same room with noninfected catheterized patients. It is best to assign only one patient with an indwelling catheter to a room to minimize risk of cross-contamination.

Minimizing Trauma. The catheter selected is of an appropriate size to minimize trauma to the urethra during its insertion. The catheter is lubricated adequately so that it can be inserted easily and gently. It is inserted far enough into the bladder to prevent trauma to the urethral tissues when the retention balloon of the catheter is inflated. The catheter is secured properly to prevent it from moving, causing traction on the urethra, or being accidentally removed. Care is taken to ensure that any patient who is confused does not accidentally remove the catheter with the retention balloon still inflated, because such an action would cause considerable trauma to the urethra and bleeding.

In the male patient, the catheter is taped laterally to the thigh or to the abdomen (Fig. 39-1) to prevent pressure on the urethra at the penoscrotal junction, which can eventually lead to the formation of a urethrocutaneous fistula.

In the female patient, the drainage tubing attached to the catheter is taped to the thigh to prevent tension and traction on the bladder.

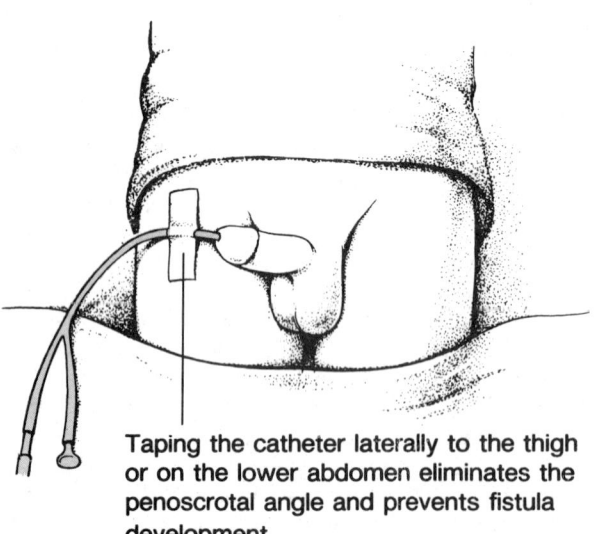

Taping the catheter laterally to the thigh or on the lower abdomen eliminates the penoscrotal angle and prevents fistula development.

Figure 39-1
For the male patient, the catheter is taped to the thigh or to the abdomen.

▷ *Evaluation*

▷ *Expected Outcomes*

1. Patient is free of urinary tract infection.
   a. Excretes urine that is clear and yellow or amber, with a specific gravity of 1.005 to 1.025
   b. Has a urine culture negative for microorganisms
   c. Has a normal temperature
   d. Demonstrates adequate fluid intake and urine output
   e. Does not have excessive drainage or excoriation around the urethral orifice
   f. Avoids kinking or twisting of the catheter or drainage tubing
   g. Maintains position of the drainage bag below the level of the bladder when in bed, sitting, or ambulating
   h. Maintains proper anchoring of the catheter to prevent movement and accidental removal of the catheter
2. Is free of trauma to urethra and bladder
   a. Reports absence of pain or discomfort in urethra or bladder
   b. Demonstrates no blood in urine or irritation of urethra
   c. Is free of pain or discomfort on voiding following catheter removal
   d. Eliminates 200 to 400 ml of urine with each voiding following catheter removal
   e. Shows no signs of urinary incontinence

Intermittent Self-Catheterization

Intermittent self-catheterization provides periodic drainage of urine from the bladder. It is the treatment of choice following spinal cord injury and other neurological disorders in which bladder emptying is impaired. Aseptic techniques are required during the in-hospital training period because of the risk of cross-contamination. The patient may use a "clean" (nonsterile) technique at home, where the risk is reduced. Self-catheterization promotes independence, results in fewer complications, and permits more normal sexual relations. The objectives are to decrease the morbidity associated with the long-term use of an indwelling catheter and to achieve catheter-free status if possible.

Teaching emphasizes the importance of frequent catheterization and the emptying of the bladder at the prescribed time irrespective of the circumstances. (If the bladder becomes overdistended, blood flow through the bladder wall is decreased and the risk of infection is increased.)

The female patient requires a mirror to help locate the urinary meatus. She is taught to catheterize herself by inserting a catheter 7.5 cm (3 inches) into the urethra in a downward and backward direction. The male patient is taught to lubricate the catheter and retract the foreskin of the penis with one hand while grasping the penis and holding it at a right angle to the body. (This maneuver straightens the urethra and makes it easier to insert the catheter.) The catheter is inserted 15 to 25 cm (6–10 inches) until the urine begins to flow. After the catheter is removed, it is washed in soapy water, rinsed, and wrapped in a paper towel, plastic bag, or case. A patient following this routine should be seen by a urologist at regular intervals for assessment of the patient's urinary function and the occurrence of complications.

If the patient is unable to perform intermittent self-catheterization, frequently a family member is taught to carry out the procedure at regular intervals during the day.

Suprapubic Bladder Drainage

Suprapubic bladder aspiration is a method of establishing drainage from the bladder by inserting a catheter or tube into the bladder through a suprapubic ("above the pubis") incision or puncture. It is used as a temporary measure to divert the flow of urine from the urethra when the urethral route is impassable (due to injuries, strictures, prostatic obstruction), after gyneocologic operations when bladder dysfunction is likely to occur (vaginal hysterectomy, vaginal repair surgery), and after pelvic fractures.

To facilitate insertion of the suprapubic catheter, the patient is placed in a supine position and the bladder is distended by administration of oral or intravenous fluids or by instillation of sterile saline into the bladder via a urethral catheter. These measures make it easier to locate the bladder.

The suprapubic area is surgically prepared and the puncture site located approximately 5 cm above the symphysis pubis. The bladder may be entered through an incision in the bladder or through a puncture made by a small trocar. The catheter or suprapubic drainage tube is threaded into the bladder and secured with sutures or tape (Fig. 39-2). The area around the catheter is covered with a sterile dressing. The catheter is connected to a sterile closed drainage system, and the tubing is secured to prevent tension on the catheter.

Suprapubic bladder drainage may be maintained continuously for several weeks. If the patient's ability to void is to be tested, the catheter is clamped for 4 hours, during which time the patient attempts to void. After the patient voids, the catheter is unclamped and the residual urine measured. Usually, if the amount of residual urine is less than 100 ml on two separate occasions (morning and evening), the catheter is removed. However, if the patient complains of pain or discomfort, the suprapubic catheter is usually left in place until the patient is able to void successfully.

Patients with suprapubic drainage are usually able to void sooner after surgery than those with urethral catheters. Suprapubic drainage may be more comfortable than an indwelling catheter. It also provides greater patient mobility, allows measurement of residual volume without urethral instrumentation, and presents less of a risk for bladder infection. The suprapubic catheter is removed when it is no longer necessary, and a sterile dressing is placed over the site.

Alterations in Voiding Patterns

Urinary Retention

Urinary retention (both acute and chronic) refers to the inability to urinate despite the patient's urge or desire to do so.

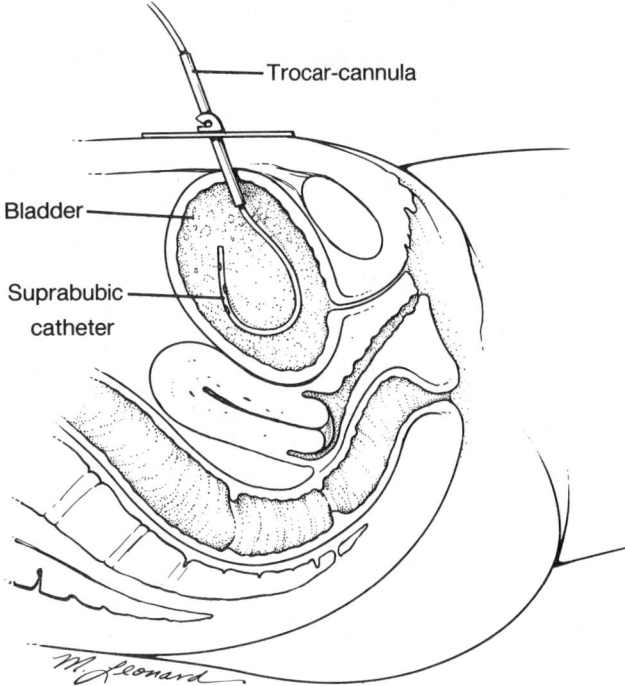

Figure 39-2
Suprapubic bladder drainage. A trocar-cannula is used to puncture the abdominal and bladder walls. The catheter is threaded through the trocar-cannula, which is then removed, leaving the catheter in place. The catheter is secured by tape or sutures to prevent accidental removal.

Chronic retention will often lead to overflow incontinence (due to pressure of retained urine in the bladder) or residual urine. *Residual urine* refers to urine that remains in the bladder after voiding.

Retention may occur in any postoperative patient, particularly in those who have undergone surgery on the perineal or anal regions that resulted in reflex spasm of the sphincters. It may also occur in the acutely ill, the elderly, or the bedridden. Urinary retention may be due to anxiety, prostatic enlargement, urethral pathology (infection, tumor, calculus), trauma, neurogenic bladder dysfunction, and other conditions. Some medications cause urinary retention, including anticholinergics–antispasmodics, such as atropine; antidepressant–antipsychotic agents, such as phenothiazine; antihistamine preparations, such as pseudoephedrine hydrochloride (Sudafed); β-adrenergic blockers, such as propranolol; and antihypertensive agents, such as hydralazine.

Urinary retention may lead to infection, which may develop as a result of overdistention of the bladder, compromised blood supply to the bladder wall, and proliferation of bacteria. Impaired renal function may also occur, particularly if obstruction of the urinary tract is present.

Management. Measures are instituted to prevent overdistention of the bladder and to treat infection or obstruction. Many problems, however, can be prevented by careful nursing assessment and appropriate nursing interventions.

▶ *Nursing Process*
The Patient With Urinary Retention

▷ *Assessment*

The signs and symptoms of urinary retention may easily be overlooked unless the nurse consciously assesses for them.

- Determine the time and volume of the last voiding.
- Is the patient passing small amounts of urine frequently?
- Is the patient dribbling?
- Is the patient complaining of pain or discomfort in the lower abdomen? (Note, however, that discomfort may be relatively mild if the bladder distends slowly.)
- Check for signs of a rounded swelling arising out of the pelvis, which could indicate retention.
- Palpate the suprapubic area for an oval-shaped mass, and percuss for dullness of a full bladder.
- Assess the patient for other indicators of urinary retention, such as restlessness and agitation.

▷ *Nursing Diagnoses*

Based on the assessment data, nursing diagnoses for the patient may include the following:

- Urinary retention related to pain, tension, lack of privacy, or unfamiliar surroundings and position for voiding
- Discomfort related to bladder distention

▷ *Goals:* The patient's major goals may be return of normal voiding patterns and relief of discomfort.

Nursing Interventions

Promoting Urinary Elimination. Nursing measures to encourage voiding include providing privacy, helping the patient to the bathroom or commode in order to provide a more natural setting for voiding, or allowing the male patient to stand beside the bed while using the urinal (because most men find this position more comfortable and natural for urination). Additional measures include providing warmth to relax the sphincters (*i.e.*, sitz baths, warm compresses to the perineum, showers), giving the patient hot tea to drink, and offering psychological reassurance and support.

Following surgical procedures, the prescribed analgesic should be administered because pain in the incisional area can make voiding difficult. When the patient cannot void, careful catheterization is used to prevent overdistention of the bladder. In the case of prostatic obstruction, attempts at catheterization (by the urologist) may not be successful, requiring that a suprapubic catheter be inserted.

Relief of Discomfort. Relief of urinary retention generally brings relief of abdominal distention and discomfort. Treatment of the cause (*i.e.*, obstruction) usually relieves the patient's fear that the problem will recur.

▷ *Evaluation*

▷ *Expected Outcomes*

1. Patient demonstrates normal voiding patterns.
   a. Voids 300–400 ml of urine every 3 hours

   b. Exhibits no abdominal distention
   c. Is free of sensation of bladder fullness
2. Experiences relief of discomfort
   a. Reports no abdominal or bladder pain and discomfort
   b. Uses appropriate measures to prevent recurrence of urinary retention and bladder discomfort

Urinary Incontinence

Urinary incontinence is the involuntary or uncontrolled loss of urine from the bladder. If urinary incontinence results from an inflammatory condition (cystitis), it will probably be temporary in nature. However, if it results from a serious neurologic condition (paraplegia), it could easily be a permanent problem.

Stress incontinence is the involuntary loss of urine through an intact urethra as a result of a sudden increase in intra-abdominal pressure. It is seen mostly in women, and is due to congenital conditions (exstrophy of the bladder, ectopic ureter) or to obstetrical injury, lesions of the bladder neck, extrinsic pelvic disease, fistulae, detrusor dysfunction, and a variety of other conditions.

The therapy for this type of incontinence is usually surgical correction. There is a wide range of surgical procedures: vaginal repair, abdominal suspension of the bladder, and elevation of the bladder neck. A modified artificial sphincter that uses a silicone-rubber balloon as a self-regulating pressure mechanism is being used to close the urethra. Another method of controlling stress incontinence is through the application of electronic stimulation to the pelvic floor by means of a miniature pulse generator with electrodes mounted on an intra-anal plug.

Nursing Interventions. Most patients with urinary incontinence can be conditioned to gain urinary control through systematic habit training or the establishment of an automatic bladder. Such a program helps a patient lose fear of embarrassment as progress is made in rehabilitation. The rehabilitation of the patient with urinary incontinence is discussed on pages 237–238.

Neurogenic Bladder

Neurogenic bladder refers to a bladder disturbance that results from a lesion of the nervous system. It may be caused by spinal cord injury or tumor, certain neurologic diseases (multiple sclerosis), congenital anomalies (spina bifida, myelomeningocele), and infection. There are two types of neurogenic bladders: (1) *spastic* or *hypertonic* bladder, characterized by automatic, reflex, or uncontrolled expulsion of urine from the bladder with incomplete emptying, and (2) *flaccid* bladder, with loss of sensation of bladder fullness and thus overfilling and distention of the bladder.

The major complication of neurogenic bladder is infection that results from stasis of urine and subsequent catheterization. Hypertrophy of the bladder walls also results, ultimately leading to *vesicoureteral reflux* (backing up of urine from the bladder to the ureters) and *hydronephrosis* (dilation of the internal structures of the kidney by increased pressure of the backed-up urine). *Urolithiasis* (stones in the urinary tract) may develop from urinary stasis and infection and from demineralization of bone due to the patient's prolonged bed rest. Renal failure is the major cause of death of patients with neurologic impairment of the bladder.

Nursing Interventions

The care of the patient with neurogenic bladder is a major challenge to the health care team. There are several long-term objectives appropriate for all types of neurogenic bladders: (1) to prevent overdistention of the bladder, (2) to empty the bladder regularly and completely, (3) to maintain urine sterility with no stone formation, and (4) to maintain adequate bladder capacity without vesicoureteral reflux.

The immediate management of the patient with a neurogenic bladder consists of catheterizing the patient intermittently or inserting a three-way catheter with closed drainage to avoid overdistention. In intermittent catheterization, the bladder is catheterized at designated intervals (4, 6, or 8 hours) with a small catheter. This intermittent emptying approximates physiologic bladder function and circumvents complications usually encountered with an indwelling catheter; however, strict asepsis is necessary. An hourly fluid intake and output record is kept to assess individual output patterns.

If continuous catheterization and drainage are used in a male patient, the catheter is taped laterally to the thigh or to the abdomen to avoid the sharp angulation of the catheter and prevent pressure at the penoscrotal angle.

With the use of either intermittent or continuous catherization, a liberal fluid intake is encouraged to reduce the urinary bacterial count, reduce stasis, decrease the concentration of calcium in the urine, and minimize the precipitation of urinary crystals and subsequent stone formation. The patient is kept as mobile as possible, through early ambulation if feasible, or through use of a wheelchair or tilt table. The diet is low in calcium to prevent calculi.

The problems of patients with neurogenic bladder disease vary considerably from patient to patient. It is difficult to assess initially what the long-term rehabilitation potential and eventual urologic disability may be.

Diagnostic Evaluation

As soon as the patient's condition permits, evaluation studies are performed to assess for bladder and bladder neck problems. The initial studies provide a baseline against which later changes can be measured. Serial studies of BUN, creatinine clearance, and serum creatinine are done to determine the status of renal function. A cystogram determines the presence of vesicoureteral reflux. A urethrogram may be done to detect the presence of urethral complications. Pressure and flow studies and an IV urogram are also carried out. A cystoscopic examination may be requested to assess loss of muscle fibers and elastic tissues and to provide an opportunity for biopsy if necessary.

Spastic Bladder

The spastic (reflex, automatic, or hypertonic) bladder disorder is caused by any lesion of the cord above the voiding reflex arc (upper motor neuron lesion). The result is a loss of conscious sensation and cerebral motor control. There is reduced bladder capacity and marked hypertrophy of the bladder wall.

As a result, the bladder empties on reflex, with minimal or no controlling influence to regulate its activity.

The objective of the bladder program is to develop effective spontaneous reflex voiding, which is accomplished in the following manner:

- Ask the patient to drink a measured amount of fluid from 8 AM to 10 PM; no fluids (except sips) are taken after 10 PM to avoid bladder overdistention.
- At a specific time(s), the patient attempts to void by applying pressure over the bladder, by tapping the abdomen, or by stretching the anal sphincter with a finger to trigger the bladder.
- Immediately following the voiding attempt, the patient is catheterized to determine the amount of residual urine.
- The volumes of urine voided and catheterized are measured.
- The bladder is palpated at repeated intervals to determine whether it is being emptied.
- The patient is cautioned to be alert for any signs that indicate a full bladder, such as perspiration, coldness of hands or feet, feelings of anxiety.
- The intervals between catheterizations are lengthened and the patient's program progresses as residual urine decreases. Catheterization is usually discontinued when the volume of residual urine is at an acceptable level compatible with urine sterility and radiologic normalcy of the upper urinary tract.

Flaccid Bladder

The flaccid (atonic, nonreflex, or autonomous) neurogenic bladder is caused by a lower motor neuron lesion, most commonly due to trauma. The bladder continues to fill and becomes greatly distended. The bladder muscle does not contract forcefully at any time. Sensory loss may accompany a flaccid bladder, so the patient feels no discomfort. Overdistention causes damage to the bladder musculature, infection due to stagnant urine, and damage to the kidneys as a result of pressure from the urine.

A patient with a flaccid bladder may be placed on the type of bladder routine outlined above under Spastic Bladder. A 2-hour voiding schedule is established to prevent overdistention. Parasympathomimetic drugs (bethanechol [Urecholine]) may help to increase the contraction of the detrusor muscle. This approach may be very effective, especially for a hypotonic bladder in which there is no significant obstruction of the bladder outlet.

Patients can also be taught to perform self-catheterization at intervals until spontaneous complete emptying of the bladder is achieved. Although intermittent catheterization may have to be carried out for a prolonged period of time, it is a safe and successful method of managing patients who have neurogenic bladders.

Sometimes it is not possible for the patient to achieve reflex bladder control or self-catheterization. The male patient then may use an external (condom catheter) collecting device if the bladder empties well and no residual urine remains. The female patient may need to wear pads or waterproof pants. Surgical intervention may be carried out to correct bladder neck contractures or vesicoureteral reflux or to perform some type of urinary diversion procedure (see Chap. 40).

Dialysis

Dialysis is a process used to remove unwanted fluid and waste products from the body when the kidneys are unable to do so because of impaired function or when toxins or poisons must be removed immediately to prevent permanent or life-threatening damage. In dialysis, solute molecules diffuse through a semipermeable membrane, passing from the side of higher concentration to that of lower concentration. Fluids pass through the semipermeable membrane by means of osmosis or ultrafiltration (application of external pressure to the membrane).

The purposes of dialysis are to maintain the life and well-being of the patient until kidney function is restored and to remove unwanted substances from the blood. Methods of therapy include *hemodialysis, hemofiltration,* and *peritoneal dialysis.*

Dialysis is used in renal failure to remove toxic substances and body wastes normally excreted by healthy kidneys, and in the management of patients with intractable (not responsive to treatment) edema, hepatic coma, hyperkalemia, hypertension, and uremia. The main indications for *acute dialysis* are a high and rising level of serum potassium, fluid overload (or impending pulmonary edema), pronounced acidosis, pericarditis, and severe mental confusion. It may also be used to remove certain drugs or other toxins taken in accidental or intentional poisonings or drug overdose.

The reasons for initiating *chronic dialysis* in renal failure are nausea and vomiting with anorexia, mental confusion, chronic high potassium, fluid overload (in the presence of diuretics and fluid restriction), and a general lack of well-being.

Hemodialysis

Hemodialysis is a process used for patients who are acutely ill and require short-term dialysis (days to weeks) or for patients with end-stage renal disease (ESRD) who require long-term therapy. A synthetic, semipermeable membrane replaces the renal glomeruli and tubules and acts as the filter for the impaired kidneys.

For patients with chronic renal failure, hemodialysis provides reasonable rehabilitation and life expectancy. However, hemodialysis does not cure renal disease and is not able to compensate for losses of the kidneys' endocrine or metabolic activities. These patients must undergo dialysis treatment for the rest of their lives (usually 3 times a week for 4 hours per treatment) or until they receive a successful kidney transplant. Patients are placed on chronic dialysis when they require dialysis therapy for survival.

The requirements for hemodialysis for a patient with end-stage renal failure are (1) access to the patient's circulation, (2) a dialyzer with a semipermeable membrane (the artificial kidney), and (3) an appropriate dialysate bath.

Access to the Patient's Circulation

Access to the patient's circulaton is achieved through an arteriovenus (A–V) *shunt* (external silastic tubing placed in an adjacent artery and vein), a *fistula* (internal access using the patient's own vessels), or a *graft* (internal access using a foreign material).

A–V Shunt. The A–V shunt can be placed wherever an artery and vein are close together. Usually, the silastic tubing is placed in the radial artery and the adjacent vein, but the ankle can also be used. The shunt was the first type of vascular access used for chronic dialysis, but now it is used only temporarily (while the patient awaits maturation of a newly-created fistula or graft) or as an immediate access to treat acute renal failure. (The use of femoral and subclavian catheters has greatly reduced the use of the A–V shunt.)

With the shunt, the tubing from the artery and vein exits the skin and joins with a connecting piece to form a closed arc, through which the blood flows between dialyses. When dialysis is performed, the connector is removed and the tubing coming from the artery is inserted into tubing *going to* the artificial kidney. Tubing *from* the artificial kidney is inserted into the venous segment of the shunt. The blood then can pass from the patient's vascular system through the artificial kidney filtering system, and back again into the patient's blood vessel (vein). The blood is traveling via a blood pump from 200 to 300 ml/min, depending on the patient's size, the condition of the blood vessels being used, and the overall condition of the patient's vascular system.

The shunt is cleaned before each dialysis with antiseptic solution, after which a dry sterile dressing is applied and secured with a stretchable gauze bandage. The patient is instructed to observe the shunt several times a day for evidence of clotting and to avoid wearing a watch or jewelry or carrying a handbag over the shunt arm. Use of a tourniquet on the arm with the shunt for venipuncture and application of a blood pressure cuff are avoided. While the shunt provides ready access to the patient's circulation, it has a limited life span due to infection or clotting. It can separate at the connection site, producing hemorrhage and death. It is also a visible reminder to patients of their disability.

Fistula. The fistula is created surgically by connecting or joining (anastomosis) an artery to a vein, either side to side or end to side. The fistula takes 4 to 6 weeks to be ready for use. This gives time for healing to take place and for the venous segment of the fistula to dilate in order to accommodate two large-bore (14-gauge or 16-gauge) needles. The needles are inserted into the vessel to obtain blood flow adequate to pass through the dialyzer. The arterial segment of the fistula is used for arterial flow and the venous segment for retransfusion of the dialyzed blood. The fistula has greatly reduced the problems of infection and clotting.

Graft. A graft is created by suturing a piece of bovine carotid artery, Gore Tex material (heterograft), or umbilical cord graft into the patient's own vessel (Fig. 39-3). This is done to provide an available segment in which to place the needles for dialysis. Usually, the graft is created when the patient's own vessels are not suitable to be used for a fistula. Grafts are usually placed in the forearm, upper arm, or upper thigh. Patients with compromised vascular systems, such as those with diabetes, often need to have a graft in order to have hemodialysis.

Underlying Principles of Hemodialysis

The objectives of hemodialysis are to extract toxic nitrogenous substances from the blood and to remove excess water. Hep-

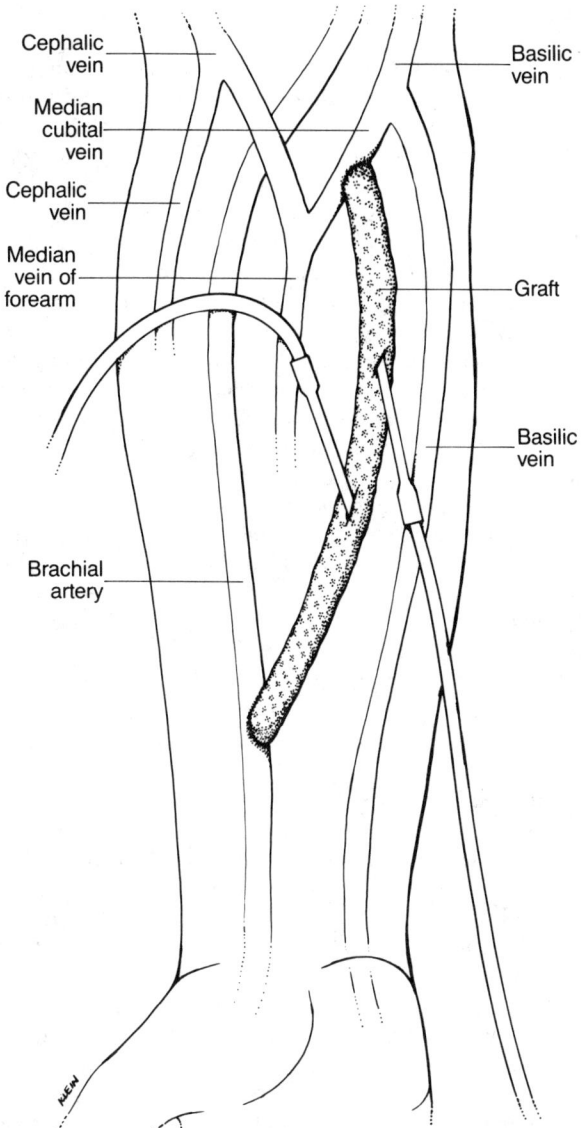

Figure 39-3
A graft (vascular access) in midarm used for hemodialysis.

Labels on figure:
Cephalic vein
Median cubital vein
Cephalic vein
Median vein of forearm
Brachial artery
Basilic vein
Graft
Basilic vein

arin is added to the blood to prevent clotting. The blood passes, by means of a pump, through the artificial kidney machine to the semipermeable membrane or artificial kidney, and the dialysate bath flows on the other side of the membrane. The toxins and wastes in the blood are removed by diffusion, moving from an area of greater concentration in the blood to an area of lesser concentration in the dialysate. The blood and dialysate do not mix. The dialysate is composed of all the important electrolytes in their ideal extracellular concentrations. The electrolytes in the blood can be brought under control by proper adjustment of the dialysate bath. (Small pores in the semipermeable membrane do not allow the loss of red blood cells and proteins.)

Excess water is removed from the blood by osmosis. The removal of water can be controlled by creating a desired pressure gradient (*ultrafiltration*). The body's buffer system is maintained by the addition of acetate, which is diffused from the dialysate into the patient and metabolizes to form

bicarbonate. Purified blood is returned to the body through the patient's vein. At the end of the dialysis treatment, the majority of poisonous wastes have been removed, electrolyte and water balance has been restored, and the buffer system has been replenished.

During dialysis, the patient, the dialyzer, and the dialysate bath require constant monitoring to detect the numerous complications that can arise—(*e.g.*, air embolism, inadequate or excessive ultrafiltration, blood leaks, contamination, and shunt or fistula complications). The nurse in the dialysis unit has an important role in monitoring and supporting the patient and in carrying out a continuing program of patient assessment and education.

Dialyzers and Dialysate Bath. There have been unprecedented developments in dialyzers and technology for treatment of end-stage renal disease, but most dialyzers conform to one of the following types: the coil dialyzer, the flat plate dialyzer, and the hollow fiber artificial kidney.

Management of the Patient on Long-Term Hemodialysis

An optimum dietary program is important for patients on hemodialysis because of the effects of uremia (wasting, poor dietary intake, the reduced palatability of the restricted diet, the loss of nutrients during dialysis, and any concurrent illnesses).

- With the effective use of hemodialysis, the patient's dietary intake can be improved. However, the diet usually involves some adjustment or restriction of protein, sodium, potassium, or fluid intake. Protein intake must be of high biological quality and of complete amino acid composition (eggs, meat, milk, fish) to prevent poor protein utilization and to maintain positive nitrogen balance and replace amino acids lost during dialysis. If many water-soluble nutrients and metabolites have been removed from the tissues as a result of the effects of dialysis, the patient may require additional vitamins and minerals. After dialysis procedures are initiated, the patient's clinical condition usually improves, and there is usually a diminished need for stringent dietary restrictions.

Many drugs are excreted wholly or in part by the kidneys. Patients requiring drug therapy (cardiac glycosides, antibiotics, antiarrhythmic agents, antihypertensive agents) are monitored closely to ensure that blood and tissue levels of these drugs are maintained without toxic accumulation. This type of information is kept in mind when the patient asks, "Is it all right to take this medicine for a headache?" It is also important to keep in mind that some medications are removed from the blood during dialysis, requiring the physician to modify the dosage.

Complications

Although hemodialysis can prolong life indefinitely, it does not halt the natural course of the underlying kidney disease, nor does it completely control uremia. The patient is subjected to a number of problems and complications. The leading cause of death among patients undergoing chronic hemodialysis is arteriosclerotic cardiovascular disease. Disturbances of lipid metabolism (*hypertriglyceridemia*) appear to be accentuated by hemodialysis. Congestive heart failure, coronary heart disease and anginal pain, stroke, and peripheral vascular insufficiency may incapacitate the patient. Anemia and fatigue contribute to diminished physical and emotional well-being, lack of energy and drive, and loss of interest. Gastric ulcers and other gastrointestinal problems occur from the physiologic stress of chronic illness, medication, and related problems. Disturbed calcium metabolism leads to renal osteodystrophy that produces bone pain and fractures. Other problems include fluid overload associated with congestive heart failure, malnutrition, and disequilibrium syndrome from rapid fluid and electrolyte changes. Patients with virtually no renal function have been maintained for a number of years by intermittent hemodialysis. For some, a successful kidney transplant would eliminate the need for chronic, long-term hemodialysis treatment.

Long-term therapy presents a problem for the patient (and for society) as to cost and reimbursement. With improved techniques and a greater number of patients on treatment, the cost of chronic dialysis is of great concern.

Psychosocial Considerations

Persons undergoing long-term hemodialysis are concerned with very real problems. Generally, their medical status is unpredictable and their lives are disrupted; they often have financial problems, difficulty in holding a job, waning sexual desires and impotence, depression from living the life of a chronically ill person, and fear of dying. Younger persons worry about marriage, having children, and the burden that they bring to their families. A regimented life-style necessitated by the need for frequent dialysis treatments and restrictions in food and fluid intake is often demoralizing to the patient and family.

Dialysis imposes an altered life-style on the family. The amount of time required for dialysis decreases social activities and can create conflict, frustration, guilt, and depression in the family. Frequently, family and friends regard the patient as a "marginal person" with a limited life expectancy. It may be difficult for the patient, spouse, and family to express anger and negative feelings.

The nurse can support the family by letting them know that feelings of anger and dismay are normal emotional reactions in this situation. It also helps to provide verbal and written instructions and to inform them of resources that are available for help. The family should be involved in treatment and decision making.

The patient should be given a chance to express any feelings of anger and concern over the limitations imposed by the disease and treatment, as well as possible financial problems, job insecurity, pain, and discomfort. If anger is not expressed, it may be directed inward and lead to depression. This may lead to despair and attempts at suicide, the incidence of which is increased in dialysis patients. If the anger is projected outward to other people, it may destroy an already threatened family relationship. The patient needs a close relationship with someone to turn to in times of stress and discouragement. Some patients will use the mechanism of denial to deal with the overwhelming array of medical problems (*e.g.*, infections, hypertension, anemia, neuropathy). The nurse can help by supporting the patient in coping with these ever present problems and fears.

Dialysis Settings

For selected patients, hemodialysis is carried out in the home. However, not all people are candidates because this procedure requires a highly motivated patient who is willing to take responsibility for the dialysis procedure and able to adjust each treatment to meet the body's changing needs.

The patient with kidney failure and the family member who will serve as helper must undergo a training program to learn how to prepare, operate, and disassemble the dialysis machine; maintain and clean the equipment; administer drugs (heparin) into the machine lines; and handle emergency problems (hemodialysis coil rupture, shock, convulsions). The home is surveyed to see if electrical outlets and plumbing facilities are adequate. The emphasis is on the patient's assuming primary responsibility for the treatment and a more normal life-style.

When financial assistance became available for long-term dialysis, most patients elected to have their dialysis performed in outpatient centers (satellite or limited-care dialysis centers) rather than in the home. Research continues in the area of "the wearable kidney," shortened dialysis times, and computerized dialysis, in the hope of greatly minimizing the patient's treatment and minimizing the dangers to the patient undergoing treatment for kidney failure.

Hemofiltration

Hemofiltration or *continuous arteriovenous hemofiltration (CAVH)* is another system for temporarily replacing kidney function. It is used for patients with fluid overload secondary to oliguric (low urinary output) renal failure or those patients whose kidneys are unable to handle their acute high metabolic or nutritional needs. The blood is circulated through a small-volume, low-resistance filter by the pressure of the patient's own arterial pressure rather than that of the blood pump used in hemodialysis (Fig. 39-4). Blood flows from an artery (via arteriovenous shunt or arterial catheter, as described in the section on hemodialysis) to a hemofilter. Here excess fluids, electrolytes, and nitrogenous waste products are removed by ultrafiltration. The blood then returns to the patient's circulation via the venous arm of the arteriovenous shunt or a venous catheter. The ultrafiltrate resulting from filtration of the blood contains unwanted solutes and fluid. The ultrafiltrate is discarded. Intravenous fluids may be administered to replace fluid removed by the procedure. The process of hemofiltration is continuous and slow, making it particularly suitable for patients with unstable cardiovascular systems.

Although hemofiltration shares many of the limitations and problems of hemodialysis, its advantage is that it does not require dialysis machines or dialysis personnel, and it can be initiated quickly in hospitals without dialysis facilities.

Peritoneal Dialysis

In peritoneal dialysis, the surface of the peritoneum, which amounts to approximately 22,000 sq cm, acts as the diffusing surface. An appropriate sterile dialyzing fluid (dialysate) is introduced into the peritoneal cavity at intervals. Urea and creatinine, both metabolic end-products normally excreted by the kidneys, are removed (cleared) from the blood during

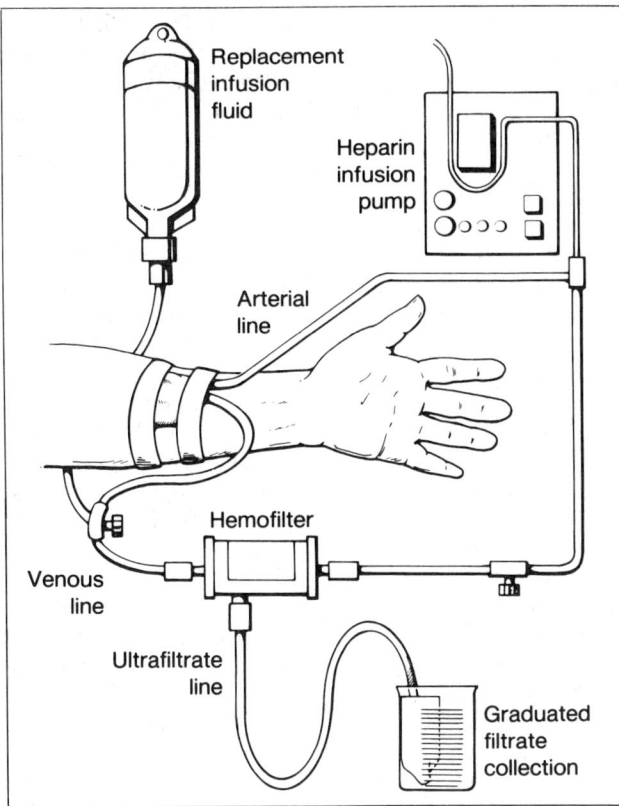

Figure 39-4
Continuous arteriovenous hemofiltration system. Blood
flows from the arterial shunt into the arterial hemofilter
tubing, where it is heparinized. Replacement intravenous
solution is infused into the venous infusion port. A sterile,
metered drainage bag is connected to the ultrafiltration
line to collect fluid removed from the patient. (Whittaker
AA et al. Preventing complications in continuous
arteriovenous hemofiltration. Dimens Crit Care Nurs, Mar/
Apr 1986; 5[2]:72–79.)

peritoneal dialysis. Urea is cleared at a rate of 15 to 20 ml/
min, while creatinine is removed more slowly.

With the development of nonirritating silicone catheters
and improvements in commercial dialyzing solution, peritoneal dialysis has become easier to perform. In addition to
the indications previously mentioned, peritoneal dialysis has
been used to treat peritonitis (inflammation of the peritoneum) by adding antibiotics to the dialysate, which comes
in direct contact with the infected site during dialysis. It is
also occasionally used as a means of lavage in abdominal
trauma and acute pancreatitis. Peritoneal dialysis can be carried out a few days after abdominal surgery.

It usually takes 36 to 48 hours to achieve with peritoneal
dialysis what hemodialysis accomplishes in 6 to 8 hours. Peritoneal dialysis can be intermittent (several times per week,
each 6 to 48 hours) or continuous.

Because of the development of a surgically implantable
silastic catheter for permanent access to the peritoneal cavity,
automated closed-cycle peritoneal dialysis machines, and
plastic bags to hold the dialysate, this procedure is being
done in the home for long-term therapy of patients with
chronic renal failure.

Although there are variations in the scheduling of dialysis
treatments with the different forms of peritoneal dialysis, the
underlying principles are the same.

Principles of Peritoneal Dialysis. Approximately 2
liters of sterile dialyzing solution (dialysate) are infused
through an abdominal catheter into the peritoneal cavity. The
solution flows into the cavity by gravity. The fluid comes in
close contact with the blood vessels of the peritoneal cavity,
which serves as the dialyzing membrane. Toxic wastes and
excess fluid move from the patient's circulation by diffusion
and osmosis into the peritoneal cavity during the *dwell time,*
the period in which the fluid remains in the abdominal cavity
before it is drained. At the end of the dwell time, the solution
is allowed to drain from the abdominal cavity and is discarded.
A new container of fluid is added and infused. An exchange
(infusion, dwell time, and drainage) may range from less than
an hour (as may be indicated in acutely ill patients) to many
hours (overnight or throughout the day as in continuous ambulatory peritoneal dialysis or continuous cycling peritoneal
dialysis).

Goals and Indications for Peritoneal Dialysis. The
goals of this method of treatment are to assist in the removal
of toxic substances and metabolic wastes, to reestablish normal fluid balance by removing excessive fluid, and to restore
electrolyte balance. Peritoneal dialysis may be the treatment
of choice for patients with renal failure who are unable or
unwilling to undergo hemodialysis or renal transplantation.
It may be more effective than hemodialysis in patients who
are susceptible to the rapid fluid, electrolyte, and metabolic
changes that occur during hemodialysis. Therefore, patients
with diabetes or cardiovascular disease and those who may
be at risk of side-effects of systemic use of heparin would be
likely candidates for peritoneal dialysis to treat their renal
failure. Additionally, severe hypertension, congestive heart
failure, and pulmonary edema not responsive to usual treatment regimens have been successfully treated with peritoneal
dialysis.

Preparation of the Patient for Peritoneal Dialysis.
The patient about to undergo peritoneal dialysis may be
acutely ill, thus requiring the treatment to correct extreme
changes in fluid and electrolyte status, or may be undergoing
one of many peritoneal dialysis treatments. Therefore, the
nurse's preparation of the patient and family for peritoneal
dialysis is dependent on the patient's physical and psychological status, level of alertness, previous experience with
dialysis, and understanding of and familiarity with the procedure.

The procedure is explained to the patient and a signed
consent is obtained. Baseline vital signs, weight, and serum
electrolyte levels are obtained and recorded. Emptying of the
bladder and bowel may be indicated to minimize the risk of
puncture of internal organs and structures. The nurse also
has an opportunity to assess the patient's anxiety about the
procedure and to provide support and instruction.

***Preparation of the Equipment for Peritoneal Dial-
ysis.*** In addition to assembling the equipment for peritoneal
dialysis, the nurse consults with the physician to determine
the concentration of dialyzing solution to be used and the
medications to be added to the dialysate. Heparin may be
added to prevent fibrin clot formation and occlusion of the
peritoneal catheter. Potassium chloride may be prescribed
to treat hyperkalemia without inducing hypokalemia. Antibiotics may be added to treat peritonitis. Prior to the adding

of these medications, the dialysate is warmed to body temperature to prevent patient discomfort and abdominal pain and to increase urea clearance by dilation of the vessels of the peritoneum. Immediately prior to initiation of dialysis, the administration set and tubing are assembled. The tubing is filled with the prepared dialysate fluid in order to reduce the amount of air entering the catheter and peritoneal cavity, which could increase abdominal discomfort and impede fluid instillation and drainage.

Insertion of the Catheter for Peritoneal Dialysis. The catheter may be inserted at the patient's bedside under strict asepsis by the physician. Prior to the procedure, the skin is prepared with a local antiseptic to reduce skin bacteria and reduce the risk of contamination and infection of the catheter site. The physician infiltrates the patient's skin and subcutaneous tissues with a local anesthetic prior to the procedure. A small incision or stab wound is made in the lower abdomen, 3 to 5 cm below the umbilicus; this area is relatively free of large blood vessels and little bleeding should occur. A *trocar* (sharp pointed instrument) is used to puncture the peritoneum as the patient tightens the abdominal muscles by raising the head. The catheter is threaded through the trocar and positioned. Dialysis fluid that has been previously prepared is infused into the peritoneal cavity, pushing the *omentum* (peritoneal lining extending from the abdominal organs) away from the catheter. A purse-string suture may be used to secure the catheter in place.

The dialyzing solution is allowed to flow freely into the peritoneal cavity. Five to ten minutes are usually required for infusion of 2 liters of fluid. The fluid is allowed to remain in the peritoneal cavity for the prescribed period of time (dwell or equilibration time) to allow diffusion and osmosis to occur. Diffusion of small molecules such as urea and creatinine takes place maximally in the first 5 to 10 minutes of the dwell time. At the end of the dwell time, the drainage tube is unclamped and the peritoneal cavity is drained by siphon and gravity through a closed system. Drainage is normally completed in 10 to 30 minutes, and the drained fluid is normally colorless or straw-colored. It should not be cloudy; bloody drainage should not appear after the first few exchanges. Guidelines for care of the patient during peritoneal dialysis are included in Chart 39-1.

Continuous Ambulatory Peritoneal Dialysis (CAPD)

Continuous ambulatory peritoneal dialysis (CAPD) is a form of dialysis for patients with end-stage renal disease who want to take an active part in their treatment. However, it is not appropriate for all patients requiring chronic dialysis. It is performed at home by the patient. Sometimes a family member is trained to perform the exchanges for the patient. The technique is adjusted to the patient's physiological requirements for dialysis and ability to learn the procedure.

Traditional peritoneal dialysis requires skilled nurses and technicians to perform the procedure. Treatments are intermittent, necessitating repeated sessions usually lasting from 6 to 48 hours, during which the patient is immobile. In contrast, CAPD is continuous and usually self-administered.

The dialysate is delivered from flexible plastic containers through a permanent peritoneal catheter (Fig. 39-5, p. 1023). After the dialysate is infused into the peritoneal cavity, the bag is folded and tucked underneath the clothing during the dwell or equilibration time. This provides the patient with some freedom and reduces the number of connections and disconnections necessary at the catheter end of the tubing, thereby reducing the accompanying risk of contamination and peritonitis.

The use of the titanium connector to connect the catheter to the tubing of the fluid administration set eliminated the possibility of the catheter and tubing becoming accidentally disconnected and eliminated the greatest source of contamination, infection, and peritonitis.

The success of CAPD also depends upon the maintenance of the permanent catheter placed in the peritoneal cavity. Catheter problems that can arise include one-way obstruction, dislodgment from the pelvis, omental wrapping, dialysate leak, exit-site infection, fibrin-clot formation, and bacterial/fungal contamination.

Patients who want control over their lives and are willing to be compliant in their care do well on CAPD. Almost half of all new end-stage renal disease patients are choosing CAPD for their form of therapy. The number of patients receiving CAPD is expected to continue to increase.

Principles. CAPD works on the same principles as do other forms of peritoneal dialysis: diffusion and osmosis. However, because CAPD is a continuous treatment, a steady state of blood values of the nitrogenous waste products results. The precise blood levels depend on the residual kidney function, on the daily dialysate volume, and, of course, on the rate of production of the waste products. There are less extreme fluctuations in the serum chemistries on CAPD, as the dialysis is constantly in progress. The serum electrolytes usually stay in the normal range.

The longer length of time that the dialysate stays in the peritoneal cavity has a positive effect on clearance of middle-sized molecules. It is thought that these middle molecules may be significant uremic toxins. Their clearance is greatly enhanced by CAPD. Low-molecular-weight substances, such as urea, diffuse more rapidly than middle-sized molecules in dialysis, but they are removed more slowly during CAPD than during hemodialysis.

The removal of excess water during peritoneal dialysis is achieved by the addition of hypertonic glucose to the dialysate, creating an osmotic gradient. Glucose solutions of 1.5%, 2.5%, and 4.25% are available in several sizes, from 500 ml to 3000 ml, thus allowing the dialysate selection to fit the patient's tolerance, size, and physiological needs. Usually, the patient is assisted in choosing appropriate solutions in the home setting.

An exchange is performed usually 4 times a day and the fluid is changed 4 times a day. This technique is continuous, 24 hours a day, 7 days a week. The patient performs the exchanges at intervals spread throughout the day (*e.g.,* at 8 AM, noon, 5 PM, and 10 PM) and sleeps during the night. No exchange is performed at night. Each exchange usually takes from 30 to 40 minutes to perform. This consists of a 20-minute drain period, a 5- or 10-minute exchange period, and a 5- or 10-minute period of infusion.

Indications. CAPD is the treatment of choice for most patients who want to perform their own dialysis at home. CAPD is indicated for those patients on maintenance or

Chart 39-1
Guidelines for Nursing Care of the Patient During Peritoneal Dialysis

Nursing Action	Rationale
I. Promote patient comfort during procedure.	
A. Provide physical comfort measures.	The dialysis period is lengthy, and the patient becomes fatigued.
1. Provide frequent back care and massage of pressure areas.	
2. Rotate from side to side.	
3. Elevate head of bed at intervals.	
4. Allow patient to sit in chair for brief periods if condition permits. (Only with surgically implanted catheter. With trocar, patient is on strict bed rest.)	
B. Keep patient informed of progress and results.	Being informed helps the patient to cope and cooperate with the lengthy procedure.
1. Reinforce teaching about the procedure and its goals.	
2. Give patient information about progress (*e.g.*, fluid loss, weight loss, return of electrolyte balance).	
C. Provide care of the whole patient.	Focus on the dialysis procedure, rather than on the patient, threatens the patient's psychological well-being and may result in failure to detect physiological and emotional problems.
1. Provide physiological and psychological care throughout procedure, remembering patient's pre-dialysis needs, reactions, concerns, and health problems.	
2. Keep family informed about the patient's status and progress.	
II. Maintain peritoneal dialysis fluid infusion and drainage.	
A. If the fluid is not draining properly, move the patient from side to side to facilitate the removal of peritoneal drainage. The head of the bed may also be elevated. *Never push in the catheter.* Ascertain if the catheter is patent. Check for closed clamp, kinked tubing, or air lock.	If the drainage stops, or starts to drip before the dialyzing fluid has been adequately drained, this may indicate that the catheter tip is buried in the omentum. Turning the patient may be helpful (or it may be necessary for the physician to reposition the catheter). Pushing in the catheter is avoided as it introduces bacteria into the peritoneal cavity.
B. Use strict aseptic technique when adding exchanges or emptying drainage containers.	
C. Take blood pressure and pulse every 15 minutes during the first exchange, and every hour thereafter. Monitor the heart rate for signs of dysrhythmia.	A drop in blood pressure may indicate excessive fluid loss due to the glucose concentrations of the dialyzing solutions. Changes in vital signs may indicate impending shock or over-hydration.
D. Take the patient's temperature every 4 hours (especially after catheter removal).	An infection may become evident after dialysis has been discontinued.
E. The procedure is repeated until the blood chemistry levels improve. The usual time is 36 to 48 hours; the patient will receive 24 to 48 exchanges (the number dependent on patient's condition). In acute conditions, catheters are usually removed within 48 to 72 hours. A new trocar is inserted for the next treatment.	The duration of the dialysis depends on the severity of the condition and on the size and weight of the patient.
III. Monitor changes in fluid and electrolyte status, weight changes, vital signs, and intake and output records.	
A. Keep an exact record of the patient's fluid balance during the treatment.	Complications (dehydration, circulatory collapse, hypotension, shock, and death) may occur if the patient loses too much fluid through peritoneal drainage. Large fluid losses around the catheter may be missed unless the dressings are checked carefully.
1. Know the status of the patient's loss or gain of fluid at the end of each exchange; check dressing for leakage, and weigh on gram scale if significant.	
2. The fluid balance should be about even or should show slight fluid loss or gain, depending on the patient's fluid status.	

(continued)

Chart 39-1 (continued)

Nursing Action	*Rationale*

Nursing Action

3. Make sure that the record includes the following:
   a. Exact time of beginning and end of each exchange; starting and finishing time of drainage
   b. Amount and type of solution infused and drained
   c. Fluid balance (cumulative)
   d. Number of exchanges
   e. Medications added to dialyzing solution
   f. Pre- and post-dialysis weight, plus daily weight
   g. Level of responsiveness at beginning, throughout, and at end of treatment
   h. Assessment of vital signs and patient's condition
IV. Monitor for complications.
   A. Peritonitis
      1. Watch for nausea and vomiting, anorexia, abdominal pain, tenderness, rigidity, and cloudy dialysate drainage.
      2. Send specimen of dialysate for WBC and full set of cultures.
   B. Bleeding
      1. Observe catheter site and drainage for bleeding.
      2. Monitor vital signs.
      3. Monitor serum hemoglobin and hematocrit.

   C. Respiratory difficulty
      1. Slow the inflow rate.
      2. Make sure tubing is not kinked.
      3. Prevent air from entering the peritoneal cavity by keeping the drip chamber of the tubing three fourths full of fluid.
      4. Elevate head of bed; encourage coughing and breathing exercises.
      5. Turn patient from side to side.
   D. Abdominal pain
      Encourage patient to move about.

   E. Leakage
      1. Change the dressings frequently around the trocar, being careful not to dislodge the catheter.
      2. Use sterile, plastic drapes to prevent contamination.
   F. Constipation
      1. Assist patient to move about.
      2. Provide high-fiber foods and fluid within dietary restrictions.
   G. Low serum albumin
      1. Monitor serum protein levels.
      2. Assess for edema, hypotension, weight changes.

Rationale

Peritonitis is the most common complication. Antibiotics may be added to the dialysate and also are given systemically.

A small amount of bleeding around a new catheter is not significant if it does not persist. During the first few exchanges, blood-tinged fluid from subcutaneous bleeding is not uncommon. Small amounts of heparin may be added to inflow solution to prevent the catheter from becoming clogged. A hematocrit of the drainage fluid may be taken to help determine the amount of bleeding.

Respiratory difficulty is caused by pressure from the fluid in the peritoneal cavity and the upward displacement of the diaphragm, producing shallow respirations.

In severe respiratory difficulty, the fluid from the peritoneal cavity should be drained immediately and the physician notified.

Pain may be caused by the dialyzing solution's not being at body temperature, incomplete drainage of the solution, chemical irritation, irritation by the catheter, peritonitis, or air pressing on the diaphragm and causing referred shoulder pain.

Leakage around the catheter predisposes to peritonitis.

Inactivity, decreased nutrition, phosphate binders, and the presence of fluid in the abdomen tend to cause constipation.

Small amounts of albumin are lost with each exchange, resulting in a lowered serum albumin. Edema may occur with possible hypotension.

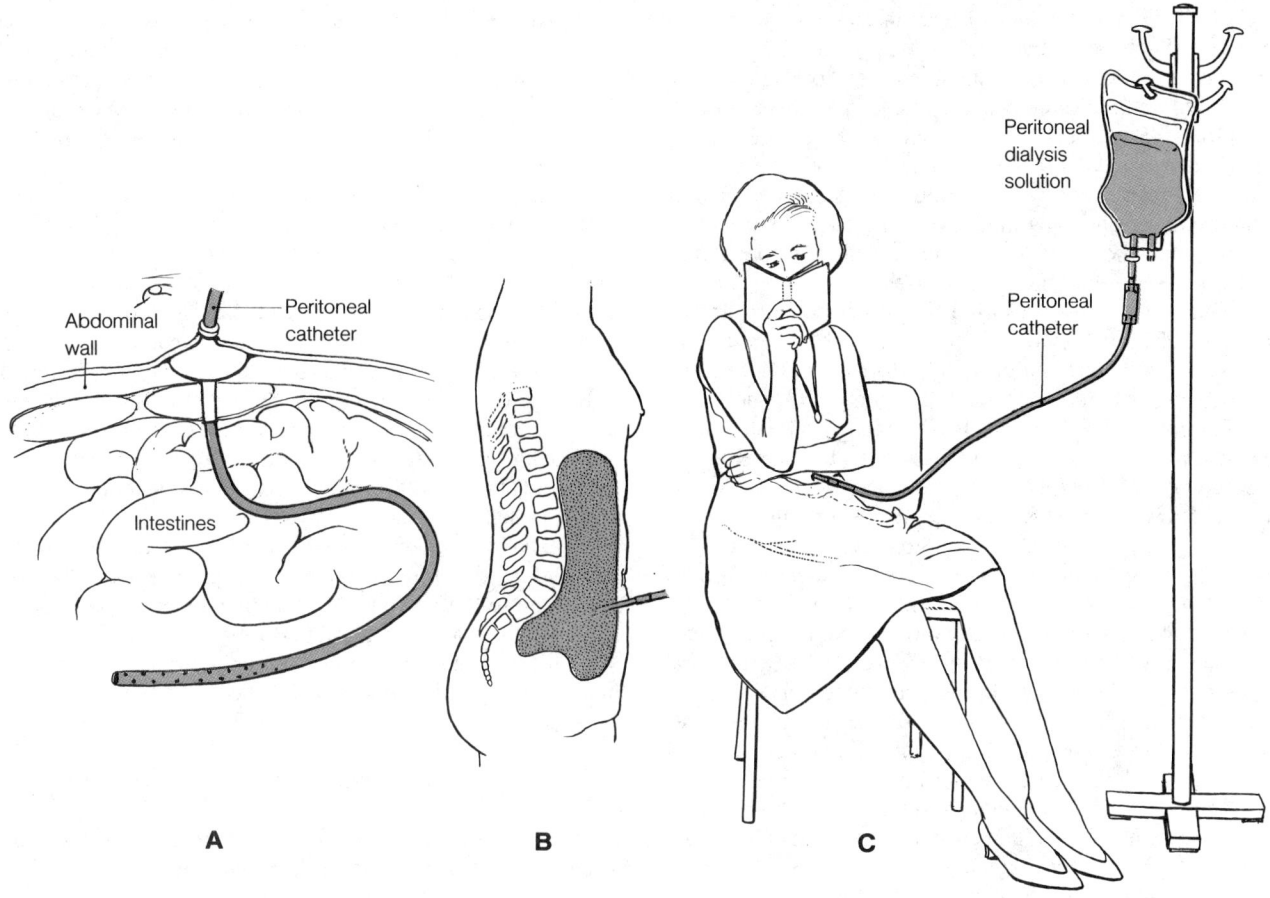

Figure 39-5
Continuous ambulatory peritoneal dialysis. (*A*) The peritoneal catheter is implanted
through the abdominal wall. (*B*) Fluid infusing into the peritoneal cavity. (*C*) The patient
allows for the prescribed dwell time and then drains the peritoneal cavity by gravity.
(Brunner LS and Suddarth DS. The Lippincott Manual of Nursing Practice, 4th ed.
Philadelphia, JB Lippincott, 1986.)

chronic hemodialysis who have problems with their present
treatment modality, such as vascular access, excessive thirst,
severe hypertension, postdialysis headaches, and severe anemia requiring frequent transfusion.

Patients awaiting a kidney transplant can be safely maintained on CAPD. Diabetic persons with end-stage renal disease may be a group for whom CAPD is an *absolute* indication. The excellent control of hypertension, the control of
uremia, and the satisfactory control of glycemia by intraperitoneal administration of insulin may arrest the diabetic
complications.

Older patients generally do well on CAPD if family or
community supports are adequate. Patients who want to take
an active part in their treatment, want more freedom, and
are motivated and willing to carry out the required treatment
also do well on CAPD. When deciding on the treatment modality, it is important to consider the patient's family support
system, as well as ability to perform self-dialysis.

Patients choose CAPD to gain freedom from a machine,
to have control over their daily activities, to avoid dietary
restrictions, to have greater fluid intake, to elevate the serum
hematocrit, to have blood pressure under greater control, to
have freedom from venipuncture, and, hopefully, to gain a
general overall feeling of well-being.

Contraindications. Contraindications for CAPD include poor clearance of solutes, due to adhesions from previous operations or to systemic inflammatory disease. Another
contraindication is recurrent chronic backache with preexisting disc disease (which could be aggravated by the continuous pressure of dialysis fluid in the abdomen). The presence of a colostomy, ileostomy, nephrostomy, or ileal conduit
may increase the risk of peritonitis. Patients receiving immunosuppressive treatment have increased complications due
to poor healing of the catheter exit site(s).

Patients with arthritis or poor hand strength may have
difficulty performing the exchange. Blind or partially blind
patients have been instructed successfully to perform CAPD.

Complications

CAPD is not without complications. Most complications are
minor in nature, but several, if left unattended, can have serious consequences for the patient.

Peritonitis.   Peritonitis is the most common complication and also the most serious. Most peritonitis episodes are due to accidental contamination caused by *Staphylococcus epidermidis.* Fortunately, these episodes result in mild symptoms and have a good prognosis. Peritonitis due to *Staphylococcus aureus* produces a higher morbidity rate, has a more serious prognosis, and runs a longer course. Gram-negative organisms may originate in the bowel, particularly when there is more than one organism in the peritoneal fluid and when the organisms are anaerobic.

Peritonitis is treated in the hospital if patients are not well enough to do their own exchanges. The patient is usually put on intermittent peritoneal dialysis for 48 hours or more while receiving parenteral antibiotic therapy. If the symptoms are minor, the patient who feels well enough is treated as an outpatient. Antibiotics are usually added to the dialysate and are also taken orally for 10 days. The infection usually clears in 2 to 4 days. Careful culture techniques are important for the treatment of the organism by the correct antibiotic.

With a persistent catheter exit-site infection (usually *Staphylococcus aureus*), removal of the permanent catheter may be necessary to prevent the development of peritonitis.

Patients with fungal peritonitis need to have the peritoneal catheter removed in order to clear the infection. Peritonitis with three positive peritoneal fluid cultures also necessitates catheter removal. The patient is maintained on hemodialysis for about 1 month before a new catheter is inserted.

Leakage.   Leakage of dialysate through the incision/insertion site may be noted immediately after catheter insertion. Usually, the leak stops spontaneously if dialysis is withheld for several days to give the incision and exit site enough time to heal. During this period, it is important to reduce factors that might delay healing, such as undue abdominal muscle activity and straining during bowel movement.

Late leaks can occur spontaneously months or years after catheter placement. They may be leaks through the exit site or into the abdominal wall.

Bleeding.   A bloody effluent (drainage) may be observed occasionally, especially in young, menstruating females. In most cases, no cause can be found for the bleeding. Catheter displacement from the pelvis has occasionally been associated with the bleeding. Some patients have had bloody effluent following an enema or from minor trauma. Invariably, bleeding stops after a day or two and requires no specific intervention. More frequent exchanges during this time may be necessary to prevent plugging of the catheter by blood clots.

Other complications include abdominal hernias, probably resulting from the continuously increased intra-abdominal pressure, and hypertriglyceridemia. The types of hernias that have developed include incisional, inguinal, diaphragmatic, and umbilical. The persistently raised intra-abdominal pressure also aggravates symptoms of hiatal hernia and hemorrhoids.

Hypertriglyceridemia, frequently found in patients on CAPD, raises the possibility that this therapy may accelerate atherogenesis. However, in some patients, concentration of HDL cholesterol has increased, providing a beneficial effect.

Low back pain and anorexia due to the presence of fluid in the abdomen and the constant sweet taste related to absorption of glucose may also occur in CAPD patients.

Altered Body Image and Sexuality.   Although CAPD has given end-stage renal disease patients more freedom and control over their treatment, it is not without its problems. The patients often experience an altered body image due to the abdominal catheter and the presence of the bag and tubing. Waist size increases from 1 to 2 inches (or more) with the presence of fluid in the abdomen, and this affects patients' clothing selection as well as their feeling of "being fat." Body image may be so altered that the patient does not want to look at or care for the catheter for days or weeks. Talking with other patients who have a positive attitude may help. Some patients seem to have no psychological problems with the catheter; they think of it as their lifeline and are quite glad to have it as a life-sustaining device. Patients sometimes feel they are doing exchanges all day long and have no free time, particularly in the beginning. They may experience depression over going home, as they feel overwhelmed with the responsibility of self-care.

Sexuality and sexual activity can be altered; the patient and partner may be reluctant to engage in sexual activities, partly due to the presence of the catheter being psychologically "in the way" of natural performance. The presence of the 2 liters of dialysate, peritoneal catheter, and empty bag may interfere with the sexual function and body image of these patients.

Patient Education and Home Health Care

Patients are taught to carry out CAPD when they are medically stable. They may be taught as inpatients or outpatients. The training usually takes 5 days to 2 weeks.

During the training period patients are taught basic anatomy and physiology about the kidney, the disease process, the exchange procedure, possible complications and the appropriate way to respond to these problems, the measurement of vital signs, catheter care, proper hand washing techniques, and, most importantly, when and whom to call with a problem. The dietitian and social worker meet with the patient and the family during the training period and at intervals afterward.

Additionally, information about diet is provided. Although the diet of CAPD patients can be liberal, some recommendations are necessary. Because of protein loss with continuous peritoneal dialysis, patients are instructed to eat a high-protein, well-balanced diet. They are also encouraged to eat bran daily to help prevent constipation. Often patients gain from 3 to 5 pounds within a month after being on CAPD, so they are asked to keep carbohydrate ingestion to a minimum in order not to gain an excessive amount of weight. Potassium, sodium, and fluid restrictions are not usually needed.

Patients usually lose about 2 liters of fluid over and above the 8 liters of dialysate infused into the abdomen during a 24-hour period, allowing a normal fluid intake even in an anephric patient (a patient without kidneys).

Patients are taught according to their own learning ability and learning level, and only as much at one time as they can handle without feeling uncomfortable or highly stressed. Follow-up care during phone calls and visits to the outpatient department as well as continuing home care assist patients in the transition to the home and to the role of active participants in their own health care. Patients depend on being able to check with the nurses to see if they are making the right choices as to dialysate or control of blood pressure, or simply to discuss a problem. They are seen by the CAPD team as outpatients once a month or more if needed. The patient's exchange procedure is checked at that time to see that good aseptic technique is being used. The patient's administration tubing is changed by the CAPD nurses every 4 to 8 weeks. Infrequent tubing changes decrease the chance of possible contamination. Blood chemistries are followed closely to make certain the therapy is adequate treatment for the patient.

CAPD is not for everyone with end-stage renal disease, but it is a viable form of therapy for those patients who not only want to do self-care, but experience a feeling of independence from a machine and its accompanying rigid schedule. If patients are willing to do the exchange as taught, and able to fit the therapy into their own routines, they can live relatively normal lives and feel a measure of accomplishment and success with CAPD. Often patients relate that they "feel better" on CAPD, have more energy, and feel more like they did before they had renal failure.

It would be wrong to encourage all patients to seek CAPD. Instead, patients should be helped to find the therapy most suitable for their particular life-style and with which they can best reach an optimal state of well-being.

Continuous Cycler Peritoneal Dialysis

Continuous cycler peritoneal dialysis (CCPD) is a combination of overnight intermittent peritoneal dialysis with a prolonged dwell during the day.

The patient is connected to a cycler machine every evening and receives three to five 2-liter exchanges during the night; in the morning the patient caps off the catheter after infusing 1 to 2 liters of fresh dialysate. This dialysate stays in the abdominal cavity until the patient's reattachment to the cycler machine at bedtime. The patient is able to sleep because the machine is very quiet, and extra long tubing from the machine allows the patient to move normally during sleep.

This technique decreases the infection rate and permits the patient to be free of exchanges throughout the day, making it possible to work more freely and carry out activities of daily living.

The Patient Undergoing Kidney Surgery

Preoperative Considerations

All operations on the kidney should be attempted only after a period of study and preparation. *Every effort is made to ensure that renal function is as good as possible.* This is the major preoperative goal. Fluids are encouraged to promote increased excretion of waste products before surgery, unless contraindicated because of preexisting renal dysfunction. If kidney infection is present preoperatively, a wide-spectrum antimicrobial agent may be given to avoid the hazards of bacteremia. Coagulation studies (prothrombin time, partial thromboplastin time, platelet count) may be done if the patient

has a history of bruising and bleeding. The general preoperative preparation is similar to that described on pages 306 to 318.

Patients facing kidney surgery are apprehensive. They may enter the hospital with pain, fever, and hematuria. Thus, the nurse encourages the patient to recognize and express any feelings of anxiety. Confidence is reinforced by establishing a relationship of trust and by providing expert and considerate care. Patients faced with the prospect of losing a kidney may think that they will be dependent on dialysis for the rest of their lives. However, normal function may be maintained by a single kidney.

Perioperative Management

Trends in Renal Surgery *Extracorporeal renal surgery* (bench surgery, ex vivo surgery) may be carried out for certain renal disorders. Certain operations on the kidney and ureter are done with considerable risk because of bleeding, difficult exposure, and poor illumination. Tumor resections and complicated renal reconstructive procedures temporarily interrupt renal circulation for variable lengths of time. Permanent damage to renal function can occur after 30 minutes of ischemia at normal body temperature.

It has become possible to correct several pathologic conditions of the renal artery and kidney and to perform reconstructive surgery on the kidney by removing the kidney, placing it on the "bench" (surgical table), repairing the lesion, and reimplanting the kidney. Damage to renal function is prevented by hypothermia of the kidney, which allows renal preservation by depressing renal metabolic activity and preventing ischemic damage. Kidney preservation is achieved during extracorporeal renal surgery by cooling (immersing kidney in a cold salt solution and flushing with a cold perfusate) or by continuous perfusion with a kidney preservation machine. This technique is useful in the repair of certain vascular lesions (renal artery stenosis/thrombosis, renal artery aneurysm) and for the removal of renal neoplasms.

Surgery on the kidney may be performed—

1. To remove obstructions (tumors, calculi)
2. To insert a tube for drainage of the kidney
3. To remove the kidney itself (may be removed to treat unilateral kidney disease, in preparation for transplantation, or to treat renal carcinoma)

Perioperative Concerns

The operative incisions for renal surgery include flank, intercostal, lumbodorsal, and transverse abdominal or thoracoabdominal incisions (Fig. 39-6). The difficulties in renal surgery are related to difficulty in access to the kidney. Additionally, plans are made for managing altered urinary drainage and drainage systems.

Postoperative Management

Because the kidney is such a vascular organ, hemorrhage and shock are the chief complications following renal surgery. Fluid and blood replacement is frequently indicated in the

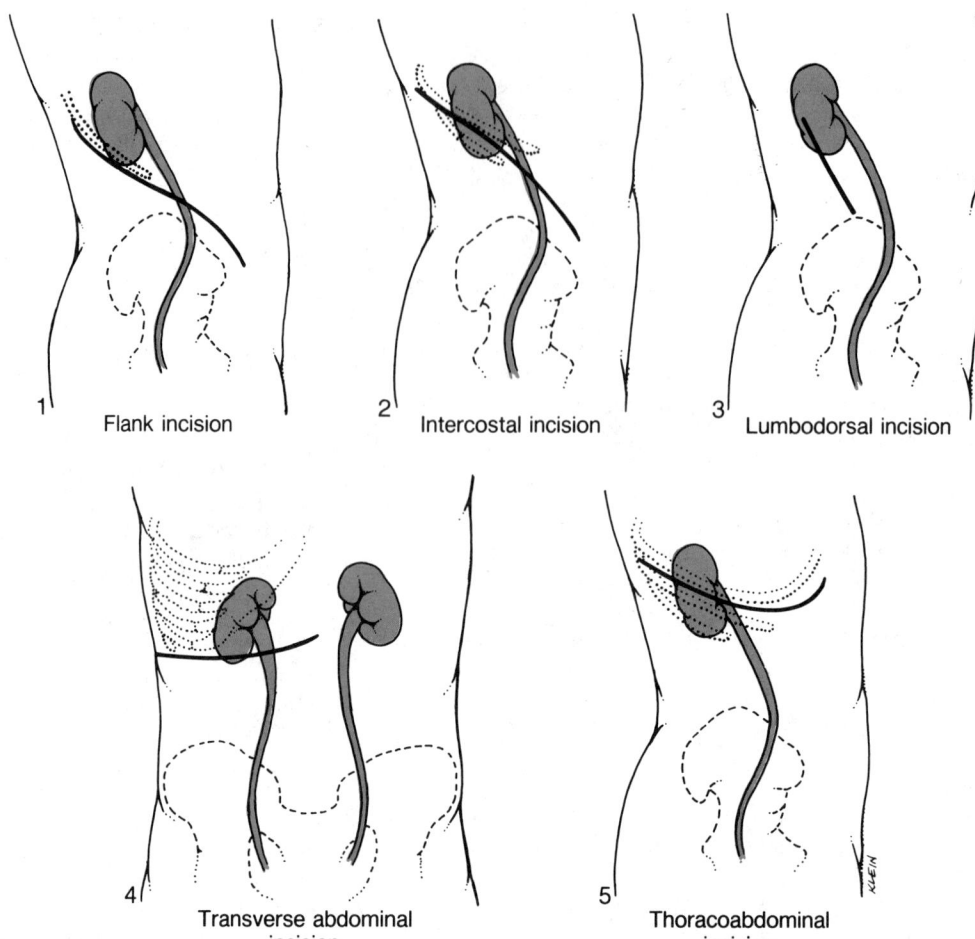

1 Flank incision

2 Intercostal incision

3 Lumbodorsal incision

4 Transverse abdominal incision

5 Thoracoabdominal incision

Figure 39-6
Standard incisions for urologic surgical procedures.

immediate postoperative period to prevent or treat intraoperative blood loss.

Abdominal distention and paralytic ileus are fairly common following operations on the kidney and ureter, and are thought to be due to a reflex paralysis of intestinal peristalsis and to manipulation of the colon or duodenum in gaining access to the kidney during surgery. Oral fluids are avoided until auscultation reveals active bowel sounds or until the passage of flatus is noted. Abdominal distention is relieved by decompression via a nasogastric tube. (See p. 350 for treatment of paralytic ileus.)

Antibiotics are given as necessary on the basis of culture identification of the causative organism. The toxic manifestations of these agents must be kept in mind when assessing the patient. Therapy with low doses of heparin subcutaneously has been shown to prevent thromboembolism in urologic patients.

Management may also include insertion of a nephrostomy or other drainage tube, and the use of ureteral stents. See page 1027 for a description of these devices and nursing implications.

Management of Drainage Tubes

Almost all postoperative kidney and urologic patients, and many other patients with kidney and urologic disturbances, have drains, tubes, or catheters in place. Following operations such as nephrostomy, pyelotomy, and ureterotomy, drainage tubes may be placed directly in the kidney, pelvis, or ureter in order to divert the urine and keep the wound dry. All catheters and tubes must remain functioning (*e.g.*, draining) to prevent obstruction by blood clots which can cause infection. Pain similar to renal colic is caused by the passage of clotted blood down the ureter.

Nephrostomy Drainage. A nephrostomy tube is inserted directly into the kidney for temporary or permanent urinary diversion either by open operation or percutaneously. This may be accomplished by a single tube or by a self-retaining U-loop or circular nephrostomy tube. (See p. 1061.) The purposes of nephrostomy drainage are to provide drainage from the kidney after surgery, conserve and permit physiologic restoration of renal tissue traumatized by obstruction, and provide drainage when the ureter is no longer draining. The nephrostomy tube is attached to closed gravity drainage or to a urostomy appliance.

Percutaneous nephrostomy is the insertion of a tube through the skin into the renal collecting system. It is done to provide external drainage of urine from an obstructed ureter, to provide a route for insertion of an ureteral stent (see following discussion), to dissolve renal calculi, to dilate strictures, to close fistulas, to administer drugs, to allow insertion of a brush biopsy instrument and nephroscope, and to perform selected surgical procedures.

The skin site is prepared and anesthetized, and the patient

is asked to hold a breath in while a spinal needle is advanced into the renal pelvis. Urine is aspirated for culture, and contrast material may be injected into the pyelocalyceal system. An angiographic catheter guidewire is introduced through the needle to the kidney. The needle is withdrawn and the tract dilated by the passage of tubes or guidewires. Then the nephrostomy tube is introduced and positioned within the kidney or ureter, fixed by skin sutures, and connected to a closed drainage system.

The patient and tubing are observed for signs of bleeding (immediate or delayed), urinary debris and stones, fistulae formation, and infection.

- Assess for bleeding at the nephrostomy site (main complication).
- Assure unobstructed drainage of the nephrostomy tube/catheter. Obstruction of the tube produces pain, trauma, pressure and stress on the suture lines, and infection. If the tube is dislodged inadvertently, it must be immediately replaced by the surgeon because the nephrostomy opening will contract, making it difficult to reinsert the tube.
- A *nephrostomy tube is never clamped,* as such an action will precipitate acute pyelonephritis.
- The nephrostomy tube is rarely irrigated. If necessary, irrigation may be carried out by the surgeon.

If irrigation is necessary, only 10 ml of warm, sterile saline are used for irrigation because of the small size of the renal pelvis and the risk of mechanical damage to the kidney or infection from pyelorenal backflow. Fluid intake is encouraged, to produce good mechanical flushing and to dilute urinary particles that cause calculus formation. The urine is kept acidic to prevent tube encrustation by urinary sediments. If the patient has a nephrostomy tube in each kidney, separate output records for each catheter are kept. The catheters are attached to leg collection bags when the patient becomes ambulatory.

Ureteral Stents

A ureteral stent is a tubular device designed for placement within the ureter to maintain ureteral flow in patients with ureteral obstruction (from edema, stricture, fibrosis, advanced malignancy), to restore kidney function, to divert urine, to promote healing, and to maintain the caliber/patency of the ureter after surgery (Fig. 39-7).

The stent, usually of soft, flexible silicone, may be temporary or permanent. It may be inserted through a cystoscope or nephrostomy tube or by open operation. Complications include infection from a foreign body in the genitourinary tract, tube encrustation, bleeding or clot obstruction within the stent, and dislodgment of the stent.

Newer stent designs avoid some of these problems. The double-J ureteral stent has a J-shaped curve molded into each end, which prevents upward or downward migration. This stent can be used in place of a nephrostomy or pyelostomy for short- or long-term urinary drainage. The double-pigtail ureteral stent has a pigtail coil at each end of the stent, which permits placement of the upper coil (pigtail) in the renal pelvis, with the lower coil at the ureteral orifice. The coils prevent the stent from moving and allow free body movement.

The nursing interventions are to monitor for bleeding;

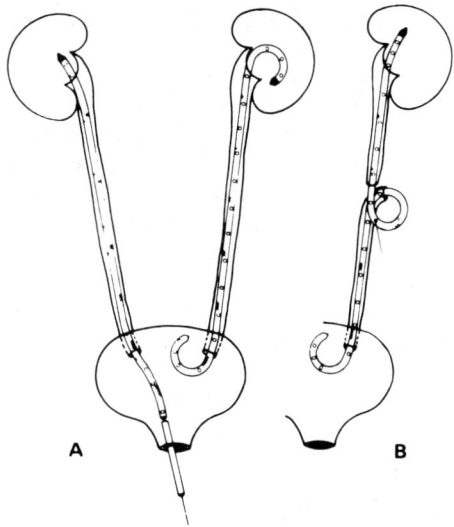

Figure 39-7
Ureteral stents. (*A*) Retrograde passage of ureteral stent. The Double-J ureteral stent is shaped to resist migration. The proximal J hooks into the lower calix or renal pelvis, and the distal J curves into the bladder. (*B*) Open surgical placement of Double-J stent prior to an ureteral anastomosis. (Courtesy of Medical Engineering Corporation, Racine, Wisconsin.)

observe and measure output; evaluate for purulent drainage at the insertion site or in the drainage bag; and monitor for stent dislodgment, which is denoted by colicky pain and a decrease in urine output.

An indwelling stent usually induces local ureteral reaction, including mucosal edema, which can cause temporary obstruction of the ureter.

▶ Nursing Process
The Patient Undergoing Kidney Surgery

▷ Assessment

Immediate concerns of the nurse caring for the postoperative patient who has undergone surgery of the kidney include assessment of respiratory and circulatory status, pain level, and patency and adequacy of urinary drainage.

The patient's respiratory status is assessed by monitoring the rate, depth, and pattern of respirations. The location of the surgical incision frequently causes pain on inspiration and coughing. Therefore, the patient tends to splint the chest wall and respirations tend to be shallow. Auscultation for normal and adventitious breath sounds is carried out. The location of the surgical incision provides a guide for anticipating respiratory problems and pain.

The vital signs and arterial or central venous pressure are monitored. Skin color and temperature and urine output will also provide information about the adequacy of circulatory status. The surgical incision and drainage tubes are observed frequently to aid in detection of unexpected blood loss and hemorrhage.

Pain is a major problem for the patient postoperatively because of the site of the surgical incision and the position assumed on the operating table to permit adequate access to the kidney. The location and severity of pain are assessed before and after administration of analgesics. Abdominal distention, which increases the patient's level of discomfort, is also noted.

The patient's urinary output and drainage from tubes inserted during surgery are monitored for amount, color, and type of output and drainage. Decreased or absent drainage is reported promptly to the physician, as it may indicate obstruction that may cause pain, infection, and disruption of the suture lines.

▷ Nursing Diagnoses

Based on the history and assessment data and the type of surgical procedure carried out, major nursing diagnoses for the patient include the following:

- Potential impaired gas exchange related to the location of the surgical incision
- Potential decreased cardiac output related to blood loss
- Pain and discomfort related to the location of the surgical incision, the position assumed on the operating table during surgery, and abdominal distention
- Alteration in urinary elimination related to urinary drainage

▷ Planning and Implementation

▷ *Goals:* The major goals for the patient may include adequate gas exchange, maintenance of cardiac output, relief of pain and discomfort, and maintenance of urinary elimination.

Nursing Interventions

Assuring Gas Exchange. The surgical approaches to the kidney predispose the patient to respiratory complications and paralytic ileus. Also, with a subcostal or posterior incision, the patient may have severe pain on breathing and coughing. If the pleura has been opened, pneumothorax may be a problem. The incision is generally close to the diaphragm and, with a substernal incision, the nerves may be stretched and bruised.

Adequate use of analgesic medications is necessary to relieve pain so that the patient is able to take deep breaths and cough. If the narcotic is given at proper intervals, the patient will be able to perform deep-breathing and coughing exercises more effectively. The incentive spirometer may be used to help maximize lung inflation. The patient is encouraged to cough after each deep breath to loosen secretions. Relief of abdominal distention will promote fuller respiratory effort and thoracic excursion.

Assessing for Complications. Bleeding, hemorrhage, hypovolemia, and shock are the major complications of kidney surgery. The nurse's role is to observe for these complications, to report their signs and symptoms, and to administer prescribed parenteral fluids and blood if complications occur. Continuing to monitor the patient's vital signs, skin condition, urinary drainage system, and surgical incision is necessary to detect evidence of decreased circulating blood and fluid volume and cardiac output.

Relieving Pain. In addition to the incisional pain, the patient may experience discomfort from distention of the renal capsule (tumor, blood clot), ischemia (from occlusion of blood vessels), and stretching of the intrarenal blood vessels. Adequate pain relief is necessary to permit the patient to take deep breaths, cough, turn, and move about. This patient also frequently experiences muscular aches and pains resulting from the position assumed on the operating table, which places anatomical and physiological stresses on the body. Massage, moist heat, and analgesic medications provide relief.

Promoting Urinary Elimination. Attention to the patient's urinary output and drainage is essential to preserve and protect the patient's remaining kidney function. Therefore, adequate drainage is critical to prevent obstruction and infection. The output from each urinary drainage tube is recorded separately; very accurate output measurements are essential in monitoring renal function and the patency of the urinary drainage system. Strict asepsis is used during manipulation of the drainage catheter and tube. Hand washing is indicated before and after touching any parts of the system. Use of closed drainage systems is essential to reduce contamination of the system and infection. The patient's urinary drainage is monitored closely for changes in volume, color, odor, and constituents. Urinalysis and urine cultures are important in following the patient's progress. Care is taken to be sure that the collection bag is suspended below the patient's bladder to prevent reflux of urine back into the urinary tract. (However, the bag is kept off the floor to prevent contamination.) Most urinary drainage systems do not require routine irrigation. If irrigation is necessary and prescribed, however, it should be performed carefully, using sterile solution, with minimal pressure, consistent with the physician's instructions, and with strict asepsis without interruption of the closed drainage system.

Patient Education and Home Care. If the patient is to be discharged from the hospital with the drainage system in place, measures are taken to be sure that both patient and family understand the importance of maintaining the system correctly and preventing infection. Written instructions and guidelines are provided to the patient prior to discharge.

Arrangements are made to have the patient visited at home by the community health nurse. The specific instructions and guidelines given to the patient are shared with the visiting nurse prior to the home visit. The visiting nurse will assess the patient's ability to carry out the instructions and guidelines in the home and answer questions the patient or family may have about the procedure. Additionally, the nurse assesses the patient for infection and obstruction of the urinary tract, encourages an adequate fluid intake, and assesses the patient's compliance with recommendations. She reviews with the patient and family those signs, symptoms, problems, and questions that should be referred to the physician or other primary health care provider.

Specific nursing interventions for the patient undergoing kidney surgery are presented in Nursing Care Plan 39-1.

Care for the Patient Undergoing Surgery of the Kidney

Nursing Interventions	Rationale	Expected Outcomes

Nursing Diagnosis: Altered gas exchange related to pain of high abdominal or flank incision, abdominal discomfort, and immobility

Goal: Improved gas exchange

1. Administer analgesics as prescribed.	1. Pain relief enables patient to take deep breaths and cough.	• Patient takes deep breaths and coughs adequately when encouraged and assisted.
2. Use hands or pillow to assist patient in coughing.	2. Splints incision and promotes adequate cough and prevention of atelectasis	• Exhibits respiratory rate of 12–18/minute
3. Assist patient to change positions frequently	3. Promotes drainage and inflation of all lobes of the lungs	• Exhibits normal breath sounds without adventitious sounds
4. Encourage use of incentive spirometer or blow bottles if indicated or prescribed.	4. Encourages adequate deep breaths	• Exhibits full thoracic excursion without shallow respirations
5. Assist with and encourage early ambulation.	5. Mobilizes pulmonary secretions	• Uses incentive spirometer or blow bottles with encouragement
		• Splints own incision while taking deep breaths and coughing
		• Reports progressively less pain and discomfort with coughing and deep breaths
		• Exhibits normal blood gases and x-ray
		• Exhibits normal body temperature with no signs of atelectasis or pneumonia on assessment

Nursing Diagnosis: Pain and discomfort related to surgical incision, positioning, and stretching of muscles during kidney surgery

Goal: Relief of pain and discomfort

1. Administer analgesics as prescribed.	1. Promotes pain relief	• Patient reports relief of severe pain and discomfort.
2. Apply moist heat and massage to areas with muscular aches and discomfort.	2. Promotes relaxation and relief of muscle pain and discomfort	• Takes analgesia as prescribed
		• States rationale for use of moist heat and massage
3. Use hands or pillow to splint incision during movement or deep breathing and coughing exercises.	3. Minimizes sensation of pulling or tension on incision and provides sense of support to the patient	• Exercises aching muscles within recommendations
4. Assist and encourage early ambulation	4. Promotes resumption of muscle activity exercise	• Gradually increases physical activity and exercise
		• Uses distraction, relaxation exercises, and imagery for pain relief
		• Exhibits absence of behavioral manifestations of pain and discomfort (*e.g.*, restlessness, perspiration, verbal expressions of pain)
		• Participates in deep-breathing and coughing exercises

(continued)

Nursing Interventions	*Rationale*	*Expected Outcomes*

Nursing Diagnosis: Fear and anxiety related to diagnosis, outcome of surgery, and alteration in urinary function

Goal: Reduction of fear and anxiety

1. Assess patient's anxiety and fear levels prior to surgery if possible.	1. Provides a baseline for postoperative assessment	• Verbalizes reactions and feelings to staff
2. Assess patient's knowledge about procedure and expected surgical outcome preoperatively.	2. Provides a basis for further teaching	• Shares reactions and feelings with spouse or significant other
3. Evaluate the meaning alterations have for patient and spouse or significant other.	3. Enables understanding of patient's reactions/responses to expected and unexpected results of surgery	• Grieves appropriately for self and for changes in role and function
4. Encourage patient to verbalize reactions, feelings, and fears.	4. Verbalization of responses is often necessary for patient's understanding of them and ultimate resolution.	• Identifies information needed to promote own adaptation and coping
5. Encourage patient to share feelings with spouse or significant other.	5. Enables patient and spouse to receive mutual support and reduces sense of isolation from each other	• Participates in activities and events going on around immediate environment
6. Offer and arrange for visit from member of support group (*e.g.*, ostomy group, if indicated).	6. Provides support from another person who has encountered the same or a similar surgical procedure and an example of how others have coped with the alteration	• Accepts visit from support person or support group
		• Identifies support person from own experience and peer group

Nursing Diagnosis: Alteration in urinary elimination related to urinary drainage

Goal: Maintenance of urinary elimination

1. Assess urinary drainage system immediately.	1. Provides basis for further assessment and action	• Exhibits adequate urinary output and patent drainage system
2. Assess adequacy of urinary output and patency of drainage system.	2. Provides baseline	• Exhibits urine output consistent with fluid intake
3. Use asepsis and hand washing when providing care and manipulating drainage system.	3. Prevents or reduces risk of contamination of urinary drainage system	• Demonstrates normal laboratory values: BUN, creatinine, and urine specific gravity
4. Maintain closed urinary drainage system.	4. Reduces risk of bacterial contamination and infection	• Exhibits sterile urine on urine culture
5. If irrigation of the drainage system is necessary, use gloves and sterile irrigating solution, and a closed drainage and irrigation system.	5. Permits irrigation when necessary while maintaining closed drainage system, minimizing risk of infection	• Exhibits clear, dilute urine without debris or encrustation in the drainage system
		• States rationale for avoiding manipulation of catheter, drainage or irrigation system

(continued)

▷ *Evaluation*

▷ *Expected Outcomes*

1. Patient achieves adequate gas exchange
   a. Exhibits clear and normal breath sounds
   b. Demonstrates normal respiratory rate and unrestricted thoracic excursion
   c. Performs deep-breathing exercises and coughs every 2 hours
   d. Uses the incentive spirometer as directed

   e. Demonstrates normal temperature and vital signs
2. Maintains cardiac output
   a. Demonstrates normal vital signs and arterial and central venous pressures
   b. Exhibits normal skin turgor, temperature, and color
   c. Demonstrates no additional losses of blood or fluid
   d. Exhibits absence of signs and symptoms of shock and hypovolemia (*e.g.*, decreased urine output, restlessness, rapid pulse)
3. Experiences reduced pain and discomfort
   a. Reports progressive decrease in pain

Nursing Interventions	*Rationale*	*Expected Outcomes*

Nursing Diagnosis: Alteration in urinary elimination related to urinary drainage

Goal: Maintenance of urinary elimination

6. If irrigation is necessary and prescribed, it is carried out gently, using sterile saline and the prescribed amount of irrigating fluid.	6. Maintains patency of the catheter or drainage system and prevents sudden increases in pressure in the urinary tract that may cause trauma, pressure on sutures or urinary tract structures, and pain	• Exhibits normal placement of urinary stent or ureteral catheters until removed by physician
7. Assist patient in turning and moving in bed and when ambulating to prevent displacement or accidental removal of urinary stent or ureteral catheters if in place.	7. Prevents trauma from accidental displacement of urinary stent or ureteral catheter, necessitating repeated instrumentation of the urinary tract (*e.g.,* cystoscopy) to replace them	• Maintains closed urinary drainage system
• Exhibits normal body temperature without signs or symptoms of urinary tract infection
• Cleans urinary meatus and catheter with soap and water.
8. Observe urine color, volume, odor, and constituents.	8. Provides information about adequacy of urine output, condition and patency of drainage system, and debris in urine	• Consumes adequate fluid intake (6–8 glasses of water or more per day unless contraindicated)
9. Minimize trauma and manipulation of catheter, drainage system, and urethra.	9. Reduces risk of contamination of drainage system and eliminates site of bacterial invasion	• Urinary drainage system remains in place until removed or discontinued by physician
10. Clean meatus gently with soap during bath.	10. Removes debris and encrustations without causing trauma or contamination of urethra	• Maintains urinary drainage system without infection or obstruction
11. Anchor drainage tube.	11. Prevents movement or slipping of drainage tube, minimizing trauma and contamination of urethra or catheter	• Maintains urinary drainage system without infection or obstruction
• Maintains urinary diversion as instructed
12. Maintain adequate fluid intake.	12. Promotes adequate urinary output and prevents urinary stasis	• Maintains self-care so that environment is odor-free
13. Assist with and encourage early ambulation while assuring placement of urinary drainage system.	13. Minimizes cardiovascular and pulmonary complications while preventing loss, dislodging, or disruption of drainage system	• States rationale for close follow-up and maintains recommended schedule of appointments with health care providers
14. If patient is to be discharged with urinary drainage system (catheter) in place or a urinary diversion, instruct patient and family member in care.	14. Knowledge and understanding of the drainage system or urinary diversion are essential to prevent infection and other complications.	

b. Requires analgesics at less frequent intervals
c. Turns, coughs, and takes deep breaths as suggested
d. Ambulates progressively
e. Uses moist heat and massage to reduce muscular aches
4. Maintains urinary elimination
  a. Demonstrates unobstructed urine flow from drainage tubes
  b. Exhibits normal fluid and electrolyte balance (normal skin turgor, serum electrolytes within normal, absence of symptoms of imbalances)

c. Reports no increase in pain, tenderness, or pressure at drainage site
d. Exhibits cautious handling of own drainage system
e. Washes hands before and after handling drainage system and handles it only when necessary
f. States rationale for use and maintenance of a closed drainage system
g. Identifies signs and symptoms that should be reported to the health care provider
h. Exhibits absence of signs of infection (such as fever and pain)

Bibliography

Books

Blandy J. Operative Urology. Boston, Blackwell, 1986.

Brenner B et al. Principles of Renal Medicine. Philadelphia, WB Saunders, 1986.

Bricker N and Kirchenbaum MA. The Kidney: Diagnosis and Management. New York, John Wiley & Sons, 1984.

Fischbach F. A Manual of Laboratory Diagnostic Tests. Philadelphia, JB Lippincott, 1984.

Gonick HC. Current Nephrology, Vol. 8. Chicago, Year Book Medical Publishers, 1985.

Hanno PM and Wein AJ. A Clinical Manual of Urology. East Norwalk, Connecticut, Appleton-Century-Crofts, 1986.

Harrison LH and Kandel LB. Techniques in Urologic Stone Surgery. Mt Kisco, New York, Futura Publishing Co, 1986.

Hepinstall RH. Pathology of the Kidney. Boston, Little Brown & Co, 1983.

McConnell EA and Zimmerman MF. Care of Patients with Urologic Problems. Philadelphia, JB Lippincott, 1983.

Resnick MI, Caldamone AA, and Sprinak JP. Decision Making in Urology. Toronto, Decker, 1985.

Schoengrund L and Balzer P. Renal Problems in Critical Care. New York, John Wiley & Sons, 1985.

Vestal RE. Drug Treatment in the Elderly. Boston, ADIS Health Science Press, 1984.

Articles

(Asterisks indicate nursing research articles.)

General

Corwin HL and Bonventre JV. Acute renal failure. Med Clin North Am Sept 1986; 70(5):1037–1054.

Ethical controversies in nephrology. Dial Transplant 1986 June; 15(5): 300–302, 305, 348–351.

Ouslander JG. Urinary incontinence: Geriatric challenge. Diagnosis 1986 July; 8(7):42–50, 52.

Voith AM. A conceptual framework for nursing diagnoses: Alterations in elimination. Rehabil Nurse 1986 Jan; 11(1):18–21.

*Voith AM and Smith DA. Validation of the nursing diagnosis of urinary retention. Nurs Clin North Am 1985 Dec; 20(4):723–729.

Catheterization

Anderson RU. Urinary tract infections in compromised hosts. Urol Clin North Am 1986 Nov; 13(4):727–734.

Andriole VT. Genitourinary infections in the patient at risk: An overview. Am J Med 1984 May 15; 76(5A):155–157.

Beaman E. I'll never take bladder catheters for granted again. RN 1985 Dec; 48(12):30–32.

Burke JP, Larsen RA, and Stevens LE. Nosocomial bacteriuria: Estimating the potential for prevention by closed sterile urinary drainage. Infect Control 1986 Feb; 7(2 Suppl):96–99.

Gurevich I. Selection of closed urinary drainage systems—An update. Infect Control 1985 July; 6(7):289–290.

*Hart JA. The urethral catheter—A review of its implication in urinary-tract infection. Int J Nurs Stud 1985; 22(1):57–70.

Kniefe-Hardy MJ, Votava K, and Stubbings MJ. Managing indwelling catheters in the home. Ger Nurs 1985 Sept/Oct; 6(5):280–285.

Kunin CM. The drainage bag additive saga (editorial). Infect Control 1985 July; 6(7):261–262.

Kunin CM. Genitourinary infections in the patient at risk: Extrinsic risk factors. Am J Med 1984 May 15; 76(5A):131–139.

Larson RA and Burke JP. The epidemiology and risk factors for nosocomial catheter-associated bacteriuria caused by coagulase-negative staphylococci. Infect Control 1986 Apr; 7(4):212–215.

MacFarlane DE. Prevention and treatment of catheter-associated urinary tract infections. J Infection 1985 Mar; 10(2):96–106.

*Roe B. Catheter care: An overview. Int J Nurs Stud 1985; 22(1):45–56.

Schaeffer AJ. Catheter-associated bacteriuria. Urol Clin North Am 1986 Nov; 13(4):735–747.

Simpson RA. Systemic and topical antimicrobial agents in the prevention of catheter-associated bacteriuria and its consequences. Infect Control 1986 Feb; 7(2):100–103.

Stamm WE. Prevention of urinary tract infections. Am J Med 1984 May 15; 76(5A):148–154.

Sweet DE et al. Evaluation of H_2O_2 prophylaxis of bacteriuria in patients with long-term indwelling Foley catheters: A randomized controlled study. Infect Control 1985 June; 6(7):263–266.

*Wilde MH. Living with a Foley. Am J Nurs 1986 Oct; 86(10):1121–1123.

Yoshikawa TT. Unique aspects of urinary tract infection in the geriatric population. Gerontol 1984 Sept/Oct; 30(5):339–344.

Dialysis (General)

Bonomi V et al. Benefits of early initiation of dialysis. Kidney Int 1985; 28(Suppl 17):S57–S59.

Comty CM and Collins AJ. Dialytic therapy in the management of chronic renal failure. Med Clin North Am 1984 Mar; 68(2):399–425.

McKevitt PM, Jones JF, and Marion RR. The elderly on dialysis: Physical and psychosocial functioning. Dial Transplant 1986 Mar; 15(3):133–137.

Paganini EP and Vidt DG. Renal replacement therapy utilizing hemodialysis and peritoneal dialysis. Urol Clin North Am 1983 May; 10(2):347–367.

Hemodialysis and Hemofiltration

Avram MM et al. Predialysis BUN and creatinine do not predict adequate dialysis, clinical rehabilitation, or longevity. Kidney Int 1985 Dec; 28(Suppl 17):S-100–S-104.

Birdsall C. Hemofiltration: When? why? how? Am J Nurs 1985 June; 85(6):646.

Carbone V and Bonato J. Nursing implications in the care of the chronic hemodialysis patient in the critical care setting. Heart Lung 1985 Nov; 14(6):570–578.

Chambers JK. Bowel management in dialysis patients. Am J Nurs 1983 July; 83(7):1051–1052.

*Ferrans CE and Powers MJ. The employment potential of hemodialysis patients. Nurs Res 1985 Sept/Oct; 34(5):273–277.

Whittaker AA et al. Preventing complications in continuous arteriovenous hemofiltration. Dimens Crit Care Nurs 1986 Mar/Apr; 5(2):72–79.

Peritoneal Dialysis

Binkley LS. Keeping up with peritoneal dialysis. Am J Nurs 1984 June; 84(6):729–733.

Golper TA and Hartstein AI. Analysis of the causative pathogens in uncomplicated CAPD-associated peritonitis: Duration of therapy, relapse, and prognosis. Am J Kidney Dis 1986 Feb; 7(2):141–145.

*Luker KA and Box D. The response of nurses towards the management and teaching of patients on continuous ambulatory peritoneal dialysis (CAPD). Int J Nurs Stud 1986; 23(1):51–59.

Agencies

Governmental

National Institute of Diabetes and Digestive and Kidney Diseases, National Institutes of Health, Bethesda, Maryland 20892.

Voluntary

American Society for Artificial Internal Organs, P.O. Box 777, Boca Raton, Florida 33432.

National Association of Patients on Hemodialysis and Transplantation, 150 Nassau Street, New York, New York 10038.

National Kidney Foundation, 116 East 27th Street, New York, New York 10016.

United Ostomy Association, 2001 Beverly Boulevard, Los Angeles, California 90057.

Chapter 40

Management of Patients With Renal and Urinary Disorders

Renal Failure

Renal failure results when the kidneys are unable to remove the body's metabolic wastes or perform their regulatory functions. The substances normally eliminated in the urine accumulate in the body fluids as a result of impaired renal excretion and lead to a disruption in endocrine and metabolic functions as well as fluid, electrolyte, and acid–base disturbances. Renal failure is a systemic disease and is a final common pathway of many different kidney and urinary tract diseases. Each year an estimated 42,000 Americans die of irreversible kidney failure.

Acute Renal Failure

Pathophysiology

Acute renal failure is a sudden and almost complete loss of kidney function caused by failure of the renal circulation or by glomerular or tubular dysfunction. It is manifested by sudden oliguria (less than 500 ml of urine per day), high urinary output, or anuria (less than 50 ml of urine per day). Regardless of the volume of urine excreted, the patient with acute renal failure experiences rising serum creatinine and blood urea nitrogen (BUN) levels and retention of other metabolic waste products normally excreted by the kidneys. Any condition that causes reduction in renal blood flow, such as volume depletion, hypotension, or shock, leads to a reduction in glomerular filtration, renal ischemia, and tubular damage. Renal failure may also result from the adverse effects of burns, crushing injuries, and infection as well as from nephrotoxic agents that cause acute tubular necrosis and temporary cessation of renal function. With burns and crush injuries, myoglobin (a protein released from muscle when injury occurs) and hemoglobin are liberated, causing renal toxicity, ischemia, or both. Severe transfusion reactions may also cause renal failure as the hemoglobin, released through hemolysis, filters through the kidney glomeruli and becomes concentrated in the kidney tubules to such a degree that precipitation occurs, halting the excretion of urine. Following these events,

Chart 40-1
Causes of Acute Renal Failure

1. Ischemia (severe hemorrhagic shock, open heart surgery, cross clamping of the aorta, surgery of the aorta or renal vessels or of the biliary tree, and extensive surgery in the elderly)
2. Septic shock
3. Pigment
   a. Hemoglobin (transfusion reaction, hemolytic anemia due to G-6-PD deficiency)
   b. Myoglobin (crush injury, exercise, electrical shock, seizures, diabetes)
4. Nephrotoxins
   a. Aminoglycoside antibiotics (*e.g.,* streptomycin, gentamicin)
   b. Other antibiotics
   c. Arsenic
   d. Mercury and other heavy metals
   e. Nonsteroidal anti-inflammatory drugs

the kidneys become swollen and edematous, and the epithelial cells in the tubules may undergo necrosis (Chart 40-1).

Although the exact pathogenesis of acute renal failure and oliguria is not always known, various possible mechanisms have been suggested. In many instances, there is a clear-cut underlying disease, mechanical obstruction of the urinary tract by calculi or tumor, or renal artery obstruction. A new causative factor in acute renal failure is the use of nonsteroidal anti-inflammatory agents, especially in the elderly. These agents interfere with prostaglandins that normally protect renal blood flow, and their use impairs this protective mechanism, leading to hypoperfusion of the kidneys.

It is important to know that some of the factors that lead to acute renal failure may be reversible if identified and treated promptly, before kidney function is impaired. This is true of the following conditions that reduce blood flow to the kidney and impair kidney function: (1) hypovolemia; (2) hypotension; (3) reduced cardiac output and congestive heart failure; (4) obstruction of the kidney or lower urinary tract by tumor, blood clot, or kidney stone; and (5) bilateral obstruction of the renal arteries or veins. If treated and corrected before the kidneys are permanently damaged, the increased BUN, oliguria, and other signs associated with these conditions may be reversed.

There are three clinical phases of acute renal failure: the period of oliguria, a period of diuresis, and a period of recovery. The *period of oliguria* (urinary volume less than 400 to 600 ml/24 hr) is accompanied by a rise in the serum concentration of the elements usually excreted by the kidneys (urea, creatinine, uric acid, organic acids, and the intracellular cations—potassium and magnesium). The oliguric phase lasts approximately 10 days.

In some patients, there can be a decrease in renal function with increasing nitrogen retention, yet the patient is actually excreting 2 or more liters of urine daily. This is the so-called high-output failure or nonoliguric form of renal failure

and occurs predominantly after nephrotoxic antibiotics are administered to the patient; it may occur with burns, traumatic injury, and halogenated anesthesia.

In the second phase, the *period of diuresis*, the patient experiences a gradually increasing urinary output, which signals that glomerular filtration has started to recover. Although the volume of urinary output may reach normal or elevated levels, renal function may be markedly abnormal in the diuretic phase. Therefore, expert medical and nursing management is still required.

The *period of recovery* signals the improvement of renal function and may take from 3 to 12 months. Usually, there is a permanent partial reduction in the glomerular filtration rate and the ability to concentrate urine.

Clinical Manifestations

Almost every system of the body is affected when there is failure of the normal renal regulatory mechanisms. The patient appears critically ill and is lethargic with persistent nausea, vomiting, and diarrhea. The skin and mucous membranes are dry from dehydration, and the breath may have the odor of urine. Central nervous system manifestations include drowsiness, headache, muscle twitching, and convulsions. The urinary output is scanty, may be bloody, and has a low specific gravity (1.010 compared with 1.025 normally). There is a steady daily rise in the serum creatinine value with the rate of rise dependent on the degree of catabolism (breakdown of protein).

A patient with renal disease in which the glomerular filtration rate is reduced has a decreased ability to excrete potassium. Protein catabolism results in the release of cellular potassium into the body fluids, causing serious potassium intoxication. High serum potassium levels are dangerous and lead to cardiac dysrhythmias and arrest. Sources of potassium are tissue breakdown; dietary intake; blood anywhere outside the vascular system, such as in the gastrointestinal tract; or blood transfusion and other sources (intravenous infusions, potassium penicillin, and extracellular shift in response to metabolic acidosis).

Additionally, there may be large losses of sodium from the gastrointestinal tract from diarrhea and vomiting. Patients with acute oliguria cannot eliminate the daily metabolic load produced by the normal metabolic processes. This is reflected by a fall in the blood carbon dioxide combining power and blood pH. Thus, progressive acidosis accompanies renal failure. There may be an increase in serum phosphate concentrations, and serum calcium levels may be low in response to decreased absorption of calcium from the intestine and in association with an elevation of serum phosphate levels.

Anemia inevitably accompanies acute renal failure from blood loss due to uremic gastrointestinal lesions, reduced red cell life span, and reduced erythropoietin production.

Prevention and Health Maintenance

A careful history is indicated to determine if the patient has been taking potentially nephrotoxic antimicrobial agents. The kidneys are especially susceptible to the adverse effects of drugs because they receive such a large blood flow (25% of the cardiac output at rest) and are a major excretory pathway for antimicrobial drugs. The nephrons are exposed to high concentrations of antimicrobials as a result of glomerular filtration and tubular secretion and reabsorption and thus are more likely to suffer toxic effects of drugs. Therefore, in patients taking potentially nephrotoxic drugs (aminoglycosides, gentamicin, tobramycin, colistimethate, polymyxin B, amphotericin B, vancomycin, amikacin, capreomycin) renal function should be monitored by evaluating BUN and serum creatinine levels within 24 hours of initiation of drug therapy and at least twice a week while the patient is receiving therapy. Any agent that reduces renal blood flow (*i.e.*, chronic analgesic abuse) may cause renal deterioration. Chronic analgesic abuse causes interstitial nephritis and papillary necrosis as the result of a complicated metabolic insult.

Other precautionary measures taken to avoid renal complications include the following:

- Adequate hydration procedures are initiated before, during, and after operative measures.
- Shock, in any clinical situation, is prevented or treated promptly with blood and fluid replacement.
- Critically ill patients are monitored by measuring central venous pressure and hourly urinary output to detect the onset of renal failure as early as possible.
- Hypertension is treated promptly.
- Patients undergoing intensive diagnostic studies requiring fluid restriction (*e.g.*, barium enema, intravenous pyelogram) should have "rest days," especially elderly patients who may not have adequate renal reserve. Dehydration is avoided.
- All precautions are taken to ensure that the correct person receives the appropriate blood in order to avoid severe transfusion reactions, which can precipitate renal complications.
- Infections, which may produce progressive renal damage, are controlled and avoided.
- Special attention is paid to draining wounds, burns, and other causes of sepsis and to septicemia.
- Meticulous care is given to patients with indwelling catheters to prevent ascending infections. Catheters are removed as soon as possible.

Management

The kidney has a remarkable ability to recover from insult. Therefore, the objective of treatment of acute renal failure is to restore normal chemical balance and prevent complications so that repair of renal tissue and restoration of renal function can take place. A search is made to treat and eliminate any possible cause.

Early dialysis is indicated to prevent serious complications of uremia, such as hyperkalemia (potassium intoxication), pericarditis, and seizures. Dialysis produces a more sustained correction of biochemical abnormalities; allows for liberalization of fluid, protein, and sodium intake; diminishes bleeding tendencies; and may help wound healing. Hemodialysis, hemofiltration, or peritoneal dialysis may be carried out. These forms of dialysis are discussed in Chapter 39, which covers treatment modalities for patients with renal dysfunction.

Fluid and electrolyte imbalances are a major problem in acute renal failure; hyperkalemia is the most life-threatening of these disturbances. Thus monitoring for hyperkalemia includes evaluating serum electrolyte levels (potassium value above 6.0 mEq/liter—SI: 6.0 mmol/L), electrocardiographic

assessment (peaked T waves), and patient evaluation. The elevated potassium levels may be reduced by giving ion exchange resins (sodium polystyrene sulfonate [Kayexalate]) orally or by retention enema. The drug's action depends on the ability to move resin through the intestinal tract. Sorbitol induces water loss in the gastrointestinal tract and may be given orally or as an enema with Kayexalate. The patient should be watched for the development of fecal impaction. If a retention enema is given (the colon is the major site for potassium exchange), a rectal catheter with a balloon may be prescribed to facilitate retention if necessary. The patient should retain the resin 30 to 45 minutes to remove potassium.

- A patient with a high and rising level of serum potassium requires immediate peritoneal dialysis, hemodialysis, or hemofiltration.
- Intravenous glucose and insulin or calcium gluconate is sometimes used as an emergency and temporary measure for potassium intoxication.
- Sodium bicarbonate may be given to promote an elevation of plasma *p*H. Sodium bicarbonate increases the *p*H, which causes potassium to move into the cell, and the result is lowering of potassium in the plasma. This is short-term therapy and is used with other long-term measures.
- All external sources of potassium are eliminated or reduced.

Guides to establishing fluid balance include daily body weight, serial measurements of central venous pressure, serum and urine concentrations, fluid losses, blood pressure, and the clinical status of the patient. This information should be kept on a flow chart to indicate the degree to which the patient's condition is improving or deteriorating. The parenteral and oral input and output of urine, gastric drainage, stools, wound drainage, and perspiration are calculated and are used as the basis for fluid replacement. The fluid lost through the skin and lungs and produced through the normal metabolic processes is also considered in fluid management.

The patient is weighed daily and can be expected to lose 0.2 to 0.5 kg (½-1 lb) daily. This occurs if the patient is in negative nitrogen balance (*i.e.*, receiving inadequate caloric support). This weight loss represents tissue breakdown. If the patient fails to lose weight or develops hypertension, fluid retention should be suspected. Fluid excesses can be evaluated by the clinical findings of dyspnea, tachycardia, and distended neck veins. The lungs are auscultated for signs of moist crackles (rales). Since pulmonary edema may be caused by excessive administration of parenteral fluids, the development of generalized edema is assessed by examining the presacral and pretibial areas several times daily.

Sodium losses are measured (by evaluating serum and urine sodium levels) and corrected.

Adequate blood flow to the kidneys in some patients may be restored by intravenous fluids and medications. Mannitol, furosemide, or ethacrynic acid may be prescribed to initiate a diuresis and prevent or minimize subsequent renal failure. If acute renal failure is caused by hypovolemia secondary to hypoproteinemia, an infusion of albumin may be given. Shock, if present, is controlled, and any infection is treated.

When severe acidosis is present, the arterial blood gases must be monitored and appropriate ventilatory measures instituted if respiratory problems develop. The patient may require sodium bicarbonate therapy or dialysis.

The patient's elevated serum phosphate concentration may be controlled with phosphate-binding agents (aluminum hydroxide) to keep phosphate from being absorbed into the bloodstream and to help prevent a continuing rise in serum phosphate levels.

Dietary proteins are limited to approximately 1 gm/kg during the oliguric phase to minimize protein breakdown and to prevent accumulation of toxic end products. Caloric requirements are met with high carbohydrate feedings, since carbohydrates have a protein-sparing effect (in a high-carbohydrate diet, protein is not used for meeting energy requirements but is "spared" for growth and tissue healing). Foods and fluids containing potassium and phosphorus (bananas, citrus fruits and juices, coffee) are restricted. Potassium intake is usually restricted to 40 to 60 mEq/day, and sodium is usually restricted to 2 gm/day. The patient may require hyperalimentation (see p. 766).

The oliguric phase of acute renal failure may last from 10 to 20 days and is followed by the diuretic phase, at which time urinary output begins to increase, signaling that glomerular filtration is taking place. Blood chemistry evaluations are made to determine the amounts of sodium, potassium, and water needed for replacement along with assessment for overhydration or underhydration.

After the diuretic phase, the patient is placed on a high-protein, high-caloric diet and is encouraged to resume activities gradually since muscle weakness will be present from excessive catabolism.

Nursing Interventions

The nurse has an important role in management of the patient with acute renal failure. In addition to directing attention to the patient's primary disorder, which may be a factor in the development of acute renal failure, the nurse monitors the patient for complications, participates in emergency treatment of fluid and electrolyte imbalances, assesses the patient's progress and response to treatment, and provides physical and emotional support. Additionally, the nurse keeps the patient's family informed about the patient's condition, assists them in understanding the treatments, and provides psychological support. Although the development of acute renal failure may be the most life-threatening problem, the nurse must continue to include in the plan of care those nursing measures indicated for the patient's primary disorder (*e.g.*, burns, shock, trauma, obstruction of the urinary tract).

The serious fluid and electrolyte imbalances that can occur with acute renal failure require the nurse to closely monitor the patient's serum electrolyte levels and physical indicators of these complications during all phases of the disorder. Additionally, parenteral fluids, all oral intake, and all medications are screened carefully to ensure that hidden sources of potassium are not inadvertently administered or consumed. The patient's cardiac function and musculoskeletal status are monitored closely for changes suggestive of hyperkalemia. The patient's fluid status is monitored by careful attention to fluid intake, urine output, changes in body weight, the presence of edema, distention of the jugular veins, alterations in heart sounds and breath sounds, and increasing

difficulty in breathing. Indicators of deterioration of fluid and electrolyte status are reported immediately to the physician and preparation is made for emergency treatment, including use of glucose and insulin, calcium gluconate, or cation-exchange resins (Kayexalate) to treat hyperkalemia and initiation of hemodialysis, peritoneal dialysis, or hemofiltration to correct fluid and electrolyte disturbances.

The nurse also directs attention to reducing the patient's metabolic rate during the acute stage of renal failure to reduce catabolism and the subsequent release of potassium and accumulation of endogenous waste products (urea and creatinine). Bed rest may be indicated to reduce exertion and the metabolic rate during the most acute stage of the disorder. Fever and infection, both of which increase metabolic rate and catabolism, are prevented or treated promptly. Attention is given to pulmonary function, and the patient is assisted to turn, cough, and take deep breaths frequently to prevent atelectasis and respiratory infection. Drowsiness and lethargy may prevent the patient from moving and turning without encouragement and assistance. Asepsis is essential with invasive lines and catheters to minimize the risk of infection and increased metabolism. An indwelling catheter is avoided if possible because of the high risk of urinary tract infection.

Skin care is an important part of nursing intervention because the patient's skin may be dry or susceptible to breakdown because of edema. Additionally, excoriation and itching of the skin may result from the deposit of irritating toxins in the patient's tissues. Massaging bony prominences, turning the patient frequently, and bathing with cool water are frequently comforting and prevent skin breakdown.

The patient with acute renal failure will require treatment with hemodialysis, peritoneal dialysis, or hemofiltration to prevent serious complications; the length of time that these treatments will be necessary varies with the cause and extent of damage to the kidneys. The patient and family will need assistance, explanation, and support during this time. The purpose and rationale of the treatments will be explained to the patient and family by the physician. However, their high levels of anxiety and fear may necessitate repeated explanation and clarification by the nurse. The family members may initially be afraid to touch and talk to the patient during the procedure but should be encouraged and assisted to do so. Although many of the nurse's functions will be devoted to the technical aspects of the procedure, the feelings of the patient and family cannot be ignored. Continued assessment of the patient for complications of acute renal failure and of its precipitating cause is essential.

Chronic Renal Failure (Uremia)

Chronic renal failure or end-stage renal disease is a progressive, irreversible deterioration in renal function in which the body's ability to maintain metabolic and fluid and electrolyte balance fails, resulting fatally in uremia (an excess of urea and other nitrogenous wastes in the blood). It may be caused by chronic glomerulonephritis; pyelonephritis; uncontrolled hypertenison; hereditary lesions, such as in polycystic kidney disease; vascular disorders; obstruction of the urinary tract; renal disease secondary to systemic disease; drugs; toxic agents; or infections. Dialysis or kidney transplantation eventually becomes necessary to maintain life.

Pathophysiology. As renal function declines, the end products of protein metabolism, which are normally excreted in urine, accumulate in the blood. There are imbalances in the body chemistry and in the cardiovascular, hematologic, gastrointestinal, neurologic, and skeletal systems. Skin and reproductive changes are also seen.

The patient tends to retain sodium and water. This is one factor that leads to edema formation, congestive heart failure, and hypertension. Hypertension may also result from activation of the renin–angiotensin axis and concomitant increased aldosterone secretion.

Other patients have a tendency to lose salt and run the risk of hypotension and hypovolemia. Episodes of vomiting and diarrhea may produce sodium and water depletion, which worsens the uremic state. Metabolic acidosis occurs as a result of the reduced ability of the kidney to excrete hydrogen ions, produce ammonia, and conserve bicarbonate.

The body's serum calcium and phosphate levels are reciprocal: as one rises, the other decreases. With decreased filtration through the kidney's glomerulus, there is an increase in the serum phosphate level and a reciprocal or corresponding decrease in the serum calcium level. Secretion of parathormone increases in response to this decreased calcium level. However, in renal failure the body does not respond normally to the increased secretion of parathormone and, as a result, calcium leaves the bone often producing bone changes and bone disease. Uremic bone disease (renal osteodystrophy) develops from changes in calcium, phosphate, and parathormone balance. Also, the active metabolite of vitamin D (1,25-dihydroxycholecalciferol) normally manufactured by the kidney, decreases with the progression of renal disease. In other patients, the calcification process in the bone may fail, resulting in osteomalacia. The serum magnesium level may rise from the inability of the kidney to excrete magnesium.

Anemia develops owing to inadequate erythropoietin production, the shortened life span of red cells, and the uremic patient's tendency to bleed, particularly from the gastrointestinal tract. Erythropoietin, a substance normally produced by the kidney, stimulates bone marrow to produce red blood cells. In renal failure, erthyropoietin production decreases and anemia results.

Neurologic complications of renal failure may occur from renal failure itself, severe hypertension, electrolyte imbalance, water intoxication, and drug effects. Such manifestations include altered mental function, changes in personality and behavior, convulsions, and coma.

A decrease in libido, impotence, and amenorrhea are sexual and menstrual changes that occur. Skin changes include pruritus (in part from calcium/phosphate imbalance), which adds to the patient's distress.

Clinical Manifestations

Although at times the onset of chronic renal failure is sudden, in the majority of patients it begins with one or more symptoms—fatigue and lethargy, headache, general weakness, gastrointestinal symptoms (anorexia, nausea, vomiting, diarrhea), bleeding tendencies, and mental confusion. There is decreased salivary flow, thirst, a metallic taste in the mouth, loss of smell and taste, and parotitis or stomatitis. If active treatment is begun early, the symptoms may disappear. Otherwise, these symptoms become more marked, and others appear as the metabolic abnormalities of uremia affect virtually every body system.

The patient gradually becomes more and more drowsy; the respiration becomes Kussmaul in character; and a deep coma develops, often with convulsions, which may occur as muscle twitchings or severe spasms (myoclonic jerks) quite similar to those of epilepsy. A white, powdery substance, "uremic frost," composed chiefly of urates, appears on the skin. Unless treatment is initiated, death soon follows.

Management

The aim of management is to help the diseased kidneys to maintain homeostasis for as long as possible. All factors that contribute to the problem and those that are reversible (*e.g.*, obstruction) are identified and treated.

With the deterioration of renal function, dietery intervention is necessary with careful regulation of protein intake, fluid intake to balance fluid losses, sodium intake to balance sodium losses, and some restriction of potassium. At the same time, adequate calorie intake and vitamin supplementation must be ensured. There is some restriction of protein since urea, creatinine, uric acid and organic acids—the breakdown products of dietary and tissue proteins—will accumulate rapidly in the blood when there is impaired renal clearance (the ability to remove or "clear" these substances from the blood). The allowed protein must be of high biologic value: dairy products, eggs, meats. High biologic value proteins are those that are complete proteins and supply the essential amino acids that are necessary for growth and cell repair. Usually, the fluid allowance is 500 to 600 ml of fluid more than the 24-hour urine output.

Sodium and potassium allowance is determined by concentrations of these electrolytes in the serum and urine. If a patient has a tendency to lose sodium, appropriate supplementation is given. Aluminum hydroxide antacids are given because they bind phosphorus in the intestinal tract, resulting in a lowering of serum phosphorus. (These antacids should be given when food is in the intestinal tract.) Calories are supplied by carbohydrates and fat to prevent wasting. Vitamin supplementation is necessary, since a protein-restricted diet does not give the necessary complement of vitamins. (Also, the patient on dialysis may lose water-soluble vitamins from the blood during the dialysis treatment.)

Hypertension is managed by intravascular volume control and a variety of antihypertensive medications. The metabolic acidosis of chronic renal failure usually produces no symptoms and requires no treatment; however, sodium bicarbonate supplements or dialysis may be needed to correct the acidosis.

The patient is observed for early evidence of cerebral abnormalities. These may vary from slight twitching, headache, or delirium. The patient is protected from injury during involuntary movements; thus, it is advisable to pad the side rails of the bed. The onset of seizures is recorded as well as their type, duration, and general effect on the patient. The physician is notified immediately. Intravenous diazepam (Valium) or phenytoin (Dilantin) is usually given to control seizures. (The nursing management of the patient having seizures is discussed on p. 1489.) Heart failure, infection, and volume depletion may also require treatment.

The patient is referred to a dialysis and transplantation center early in the course of progressive renal disease. Dialysis is usually begun when the patient cannot maintain a reasonable life-style with conservative treatment. The details of dialysis treatment can be found on pages 1016–1025.

Nursing Interventions

The patient with chronic renal failure requires astute nursing care to avoid the complications of reduced renal function and the stresses and anxieties of dealing with a life-threatening illness.

Potential nursing diagnoses for these patients include the following:

- Alterations in fluid and electrolyte balance related to decreased urine output and dietary and fluid restrictions
- Alteration in nutrition, less than body requirements, related to anorexia, gastrointestinal discomfort, and dietary restrictions
- Knowledge deficit about the condition and the treatment regimen
- Activity intolerance related to fatigue
- Altered self-concept related to dependency and role changes

Nursing care is directed at assessing fluid and electrolyte status and identifying potential sources of imbalance, implementing a dietary program to ensure proper nutritional intake within the limits of the treatment regimen, providing explanations and information to the patient and family concerning the ramifications of reduced renal function and the need to follow the protocols prescribed by the physician, and promoting positive feelings by encouraging increased self-care and greater independence. Specific interventions, along with rationale and evaluation criteria, are presented in more detail in Nursing Care Plan 40-1 for a patient with chronic renal failure.

Gerontological Considerations

Changes in kidney function with normal aging increase the susceptibility of the elderly to kidney dysfunction and renal failure. Alterations in renal blood flow, glomerular filtration, and renal clearance increase the risk of drug-associated changes in renal function. Precautions are indicated with administration of all medications because of the frequent use of multiple prescription and over-the-counter drugs and the risk of side-effects. The incidence of systemic diseases such as atherosclerosis, hypertension, cardiac failure, diabetes, and malignancy increases with advancing age, predisposing the elderly to renal disease associated with these disorders. Fluid and electrolyte balance in the elderly is usually maintained in normal circumstances. However, with age, the kidney is less able to respond to acute fluid and electrolyte changes. Therefore, acute problems need to be prevented if possible or recognized and treated quickly. Precautions are warranted when the elderly patient must undergo extensive diagnostic tests or when new medications (*e.g.*, diuretics) are added, to prevent dehydration which can compromise marginal renal function and lead to acute renal failure. The elderly patient may develop nonspecific and atypical signs of disturbed renal function and fluid and electrolyte imbalances. Recognition of these problems is further hampered by their association with previously existing disorders and the mistaken belief that they are normal changes of the aging.

Kidney Transplantation

Kidney transplantation involves transplanting a kidney from a living donor or human cadaver to a recipient who has end-stage renal disease. Most patients have been on dialysis for months or years prior to transplantation. Transplantation provides the patient with a more normal life-style and is less expensive than dialysis. Selected patients with irreversible end-stage renal disease are considered for kidney transplantation. Kidney transplants from well-matched living donors who are related to the patient (those with compatible ABO and HLA antigens) are more successful than those from cadaver donors.

The patient's kidneys, which are nonfunctioning, may or may not be removed, and dialysis is instituted until a kidney from a suitable donor is obtained. The transplanted kidney is placed in the patient's iliac fossa anterior to the crest of the ilium. The ureter of the newly transplanted kidney is transplanted into the bladder or anastomosed to the ureter of the recipient (Fig. 40-1, p. 1044).

Preoperative Management

The preoperative goal of management is to bring the patient's metabolic state to a level as close to normal as possible. Tissue typing is done to determine compatibility of the tissues and cells of the donor and recipient. Antibody screening is also carried out. Immunosuppressive drugs (azathioprine [Imuran] and prednisone) are given to suppress the body's immunologic defense mechanism and prevent later rejection of the transplanted kidney. Hemodialysis is usually performed the day before the scheduled transplant. The patient must be free of infection at the time of renal transplantation because of immunosuppression and the risk of spread of infection. The mouth must be treated for gingival disease and dental caries. The lower urinary tract is studied to assess bladder neck function and to detect ureteral reflux.

Nursing Interventions. The nursing aspects of preoperative management are essentially the same as those for patients undergoing renal and vascular surgery. The patient may have experienced considerable discouragement, depression, and anxiety while on dialysis awaiting a cadaver kidney. Dealing with these concerns is part of the nurse's role in preoperative management.

Postoperative Management

The goal of care is to maintain homeostasis until the transplanted kidney is functioning well. The major limiting factor of this procedure is the body's immunologic response, which may lead to rejection and destruction of the transplanted kidney. The survival of a transplanted kidney depends on the success of techniques that suppress this immunologic reac-

(Text continues on p. 1042)

Care of the Patient With Chronic Renal Failure

Nursing Interventions	Rationale	Evaluation

Nursing Diagnosis: Altered fluid and electrolyte balance related to decreased urine output and dietary and fluid restrictions

Goal: Maintenance of fluid and electrolyte balance

Nursing Interventions	Rationale	Evaluation
1. Assess fluid and electrolyte status: a. Serum electrolyte levels b. Daily weight changes c. Intake and output balance d. Skin turgor and presence of edema e. Distention of neck veins f. Blood pressure and pulse rate and rhythm g. Signs of calcium imbalance (Chvostek's and Trousseau's signs) h. Respiratory rate and effort	1. Assessment provides baseline and continuing data base for monitoring changes and evaluating interventions for disturbances in fluid balance, sodium balance, and potassium and calcium balance.	• Exhibits normal or acceptable serum electrolyte levels. • Demonstrates no rapid weight increases or decreases. • Maintains dietary and fluid intake within restrictions. • Exhibits normal skin turgor without evidence of edema. • Exhibits normal blood pressure. • Exhibits regular pulse rhythm. • Exhibits no distention of neck veins. • Reports no difficulty breathing or shortness of breath. • Demonstrates absence of Chvostek's and Trousseau's signs.
2. Identify potential sources of fluids or electrolytes that are to be reduced or eliminated: a. Medications b. Foods c. Intravenous fluids used to administer antibiotics d. Oral fluids used to ingest oral medications	2. Unrecognized sources of excessive fluid, sodium, potassium, phosphate, etc., may be uncovered.	• States rationale for dietary restrictions and limited fluid intake. • Reads labels of prepared foods and correctly identifies foods to be avoided. • Takes antacids as prescribed avoiding those antacids that contain magnesium. • States rationale for avoiding magnesium-containing antacids. • States rationale for use of antacids as prescribed. • Consumes foods and fluids within dietary restrictions. • Uses oral hygiene frequently. • Reports decreased dryness of oral mucous membranes. • Reports decreased thirst. • Exhibits interest in activities not related to food or fluid.
3. Explain to patient and family rationale for restrictions of certain foods and fluids.	3. Patient and family can cooperate with necessary food and fluid restrictions.	
4. Assist family in identifying hidden sources of restricted electrolytes.	4. Independence and involvement of patient and family in maintaining fluid and dietary restrictions are encouraged.	
5. Administer antacids as prescribed.	5. Antacids promote binding of phosphate in intestinal tract and normal calcium and phosphorus levels.	
6. Avoid use of antacids and other medications containing magnesium.	6. Magnesium toxicity is avoided.	
7. Provide foods and fluids within dietary restrictions.	7. Adequate dietary intake and fluid and electrolyte balance are promoted.	
8. Assist patient to cope with the discomforts resulting from restrictions. a. Provide or encourage frequent oral hygiene. b. Encourage use of distraction.	8. Increasing patient comfort promotes compliance with dietary restrictions. a. Oral hygiene minimizes dry oral mucous membranes. b. Focus on food and fluid restrictions is reduced.	

(continued)

Nursing Interventions	*Rationale*	*Evaluation*

Nursing Diagnosis: Altered nutrition: less than body requirements related to anorexia, gastrointestinal discomfort, and dietary restrictions

Goal: Maintenance of adequate nutritional intake

1. Assess nutritional status: a. Weight changes b. Anthropometric measures c. Laboratory values	1. Baseline data are provided for monitoring changes and evaluating interventions.	• Identifies foods within dietary restrictions that are appealing. • Consumes high biologic value proteins. • Consumes foods high in calories within other dietary allowances. • Reports increased appetite at meal time. • Takes antacids on a schedule that does not produce a feeling of fullness before meals. • Explains in own words the rationale for dietary restrictions and the relationship of dietary restrictions to urea and creatinine levels. • Consults written lists of acceptable foods when selecting foods. • Identifies ways of increasing food's palatability without using sodium or potassium. • Identifies foods that are prohibited on diet and rationale for their exclusion. • States rationale for dietary changes when dialysis is initiated. • Uses oral hygiene before each meal. • Reports increased appetite in more pleasant surroundings. • Reports no rapid increases or decreases in weight. • Demonstrates normal skin turgor without edema; healing; and acceptable plasma protein and albumin levels.
2. Assess patient's nutritional dietary patterns: a. Diet history b. Food preferences c. Calorie counts	2. Past and present dietary patterns can be considered in planning meals.	
3. Assess for factors contributing to altered nutritional intake: a. Anorexia b. Nausea and vomiting c. Unpalatable diet d. Depression e. Lack of understanding of dietary restrictions f. Stomatitis	3. Information about other factors that may be altered or eliminated to promote adequate dietary intake is provided.	
4. Provide patient's food preferences within dietary restrictions.	4. Increased dietary intake is encouraged.	
5. Promote intake of high biologic value protein foods: eggs, dairy products, meat.	5. Complete proteins are provided for positive nitrogen balance necessary for growth and tissue healing within protein restriction.	
6. Encourage high-calorie, low-protein, low-sodium, and low-potassium snacks between meals.	6. This diet eliminates/reduces sources of restricted foods and provides calories for energy while sparing protein for growth and tissue healing.	
7. Alter schedule of medications so that they are not administered right before meals.	7. Ingestion of medications right before meals may produce anorexia or a feeling of fullness that may interfere with dietary intake. (Antacids given to bind phosphate in the intestinal tract and reduce serum phosphate level frequently produce a feeling of fullness.)	
8. Explain rationale for dietary restrictions and their relationship to kidney dysfunction and increased urea and creatinine levels.	8. Patient can relate concrete relationships between diet and urea and creatinine levels to disturbed kidney function.	
9. Provide written lists of foods allowed and suggestions for improving their taste without the use of sodium or potassium.	9. Lists provide a positive approach to dietary restrictions and a reference for the patient and his family to use when at home.	
10. Provide written lists of foods that are to be used in limited amounts or avoided entirely.	10. Lists emphasize those foods that must be avoided to prevent serious electrolyte and nutritional problems.	

(continued)

Nursing Interventions	*Rationale*	*Evaluation*

Nursing Diagnosis: Altered nutrition: less than body requirements related to anorexia, gastrointestinal discomfort, and dietary restrictions.

Goal: Maintenance of adequate nutritional intake

11. Explain changes in diet and more liberal dietary intake if dialysis is initiated.	11. Frequent dialysis removes end products (*e.g.,* urea, creatinine); protein is removed by peritoneal dialysis and hemodialysis.	
12. Provide oral hygiene before meals.	12. Oral hygiene temporarily improves the patient's sense of taste by eliminating waste products and moistens mucous membranes.	
13. Provide pleasant surroundings at meal time.	13. Unpleasant factors that contribute to patient's anorexia are eliminated.	
14. Weigh patient daily.	14. Nutritional status can be monitored.	
15. Assess for evidence of inadequate protein intake: a. Edema formation b. Delayed healing c. Decreased serum albumin levels	15. Inadequate protein intake can lead to decreased albumin and other plasma proteins, edema formation, and delay in healing.	

Nursing Diagnosis: Knowledge deficit concerning condition and treatment regimen

Goal: Increased knowledge about condition and related treatment

1. Assess knowledge and understanding of cause of renal failure, consequences of renal failure, and its treatment: a. Cause of patients's renal failure b. Meaning of renal failure c. Understanding of renal function d. Relationship of fluid and dietary restrictions to renal failure e. Rationale for substitute for kidney function (hemodialysis, peritoneal dialysis, kidney transplantation)	1. Baseline information is provided for further explanations and teaching.	• Verbalizes relationship of cause of renal failure and consequences. • States relationship of renal failure and need of substitute for renal function in own words. • Explains fluid and dietary restrictions as they relate to failure of kidneys' regulatory functions. • Asks questions about treatment options indicating readiness to learn. • Verbalizes plans to continue as normal a life as possible. • Uses written information and instructions to clarify questions and seek additional information.
2. Provide explanations of renal function and consequences of renal failure at patient's level of understanding in language understood by patient guided by patient's level of readiness.	2. Patient can learn about renal failure and its treatment as he becomes ready to understand and accept the diagnosis and its consequences.	
3. Assist patient to identify ways to incorporate changes and treatment into life.	3. Patient can see that his life does not have to change completely or revolve around his disease and its treatment.	

(continued)

Nursing Interventions	*Rationale*	*Evaluation*

Nursing Diagnosis: Knowledge deficit concerning condition and treatment regimen

Goal: Increased knowledge about condition and related treatment

4. Provide verbal and written information and instructions as appropriate about
  a. Renal function and failure
  b. Fluid and electrolyte restrictions
  c. Dietary restrictions
  d. Medication schedule
  e. Reportable problems, signs and symptoms
  f. Follow-up schedule
  g. Community resources
  h. Treatment options
	4. Patient has information that he can refer to for further clarification during hospital stay and at home.	

Nursing Diagnosis: Activity intolerance related to fatigue

Goal: Participation in activity within tolerance

1. Assess factors contributing to fatigue:
  a. Anemia
  b. Fluid and electrolyte imbalances
  c. Accumulation of end products of metabolism (*e.g.,* urea and creatinine)
  d. Depression
	1. Indications of severity of fatigue are provided.	• Participates in increasing levels of exercise and activity.
		• Reports increased energy and sense of well-being.
		• Alternates rest and activity.
		• Participates in selected self-care activities.
		• Identifies activities and events of importance to him.

2. Promote independence in self-care activities within patient's activity tolerance.	2. Mild/moderate activity and improved self-esteem are promoted.	
3. Encourage alternating activity with rest.	3. Activity and exercise within limits are promoted and adequate rest encouraged.	
4. Assist with self-care activities when fatigued.	4. Adequate hygiene and opportunity for rest are promoted.	
5. Assist patient to determine which activities are of most value to him.	5. Patient can use energy to participate in those activities and events of most importance to him.	

(continued)

tion. In order to overcome or minimize the body's defense mechanism, immunosuppressive drugs such as azathioprine (Imuran) and corticosteroids (prednisone) are given. Plasmaleukapheresis (PLP), lymph drainage, antilymphocytic globulin (ALG), cyclophosphamide, and cyclosporine are other immunosuppressive agents that may be used. The doses are gradually tapered over a period of several weeks, depending on the patient's immunologic response to the transplant. This therapy is continued indefinitely.

Renal graft rejection and failure may occur early (24 to 72 hours), within a few days (3 to 14 days), or later (after 3 weeks). Ultrasound may be used to detect enlargement of the kidney, while renal biopsy and radiographic techniques are used to evaluate a failing renal transplant. When severe rejection occurs or when excessive immunosuppression is required to maintain the kidney, the transplanted kidney is removed (graft nephrectomy) and the patient is returned to dialysis.

Postoperative Nursing Interventions

Assessing for Rejection and Infection. Following a kidney transplant, the patient is assessed for signs and symptoms of threatened graft rejection: oliguria, edema, fever, in-

Nursing Interventions	*Rationale*	*Evaluation*

Nursing Diagnosis: Altered self-concept related to dependency and role changes

Goal: Improved self-concept

1. Assess patient's (and family's) responses and reactions to illness and its treatment.	1. Data are provided about problems encountered by patient and family in coping with changes in life and life-style.	• Identifies previously used coping styles that have been effective
2. Assess relationship of patient and significant family members.	2. Strengths and supports of patient and family are identified.	• Identifies previously used coping styles that are no longer possible because of renal failure and its treatment (alcohol and drug use; extreme physical exertion, etc.)
3. Assess usual coping patterns of patient and family members.	3. Coping patterns that may have been effective may be potentially destructive in view of restrictions imposed by renal failure and its treatment.	• Patient and family identify and verbalize their responses and feelings in reaction to renal failure and the necessary changes in their life and life-style.
4. Encourage patient and family to express concerns and reactions to changes produced by renal failure and its treatment: a. Role changes b. Changes in life-style c. Changes in occupation d. Sexual changes e. Dependence on health care team f. Altered food and fluid patterns g. Lack of energy	4. Patient can identify concerns and steps necessary to deal with them.	• Seeks professional counseling, if necessary, to cope with changes resulting from renal failure and its treatment. • Seeks information from nurse and other health care providers about treatment options. • Identifies own strengths and those of supportive family members when considering treatment options. • Takes active role in decision making about treatment options.
5. Assist patient and family in seeking professional counseling to deal with severe reactions if necessary.	5. Additional source of support and strength to deal with complex reactions and feelings is provided.	
6. Provide realistic descriptions of treatment options (hemodialysis, peritoneal dialysis, transplantation) to patient and family.	6. The patient and family have the data to assist in making decisions about treatment options in a positive, future-oriented manner.	

creasing blood pressure, apprehension, weight gain, and swelling or tenderness over the graft. Results of blood chemistry tests and leukocyte and platelet counts are monitored closely, since immunosuppression depresses the formation of leukocytes and platelets.

The patient is constantly monitored for infection since the kidney recipient is susceptible to faulty healing and infection owing to immunosuppressive therapy and complications of renal failure.

• A distinction must be made between infection and rejection since impaired renal function and fever are evi-

dence of both infection and rejection, and treatment differs.

Immunosuppressive drugs make the transplant patient more vulnerable to opportunistic infections (candidiasis, cytomegalic viral disease, *Pneumocystis carinii* pneumonia) and infection with other relatively nonpathogenic viruses, fungi, and protozoa, which can be a major hazard. The patient is protected from exposure to hospital staff, visitors, and other patients who have active infections. Careful hand washing is imperative, and face masks may be worn by hospital staff and visitors to reduce the risk of transmitting infectious agents

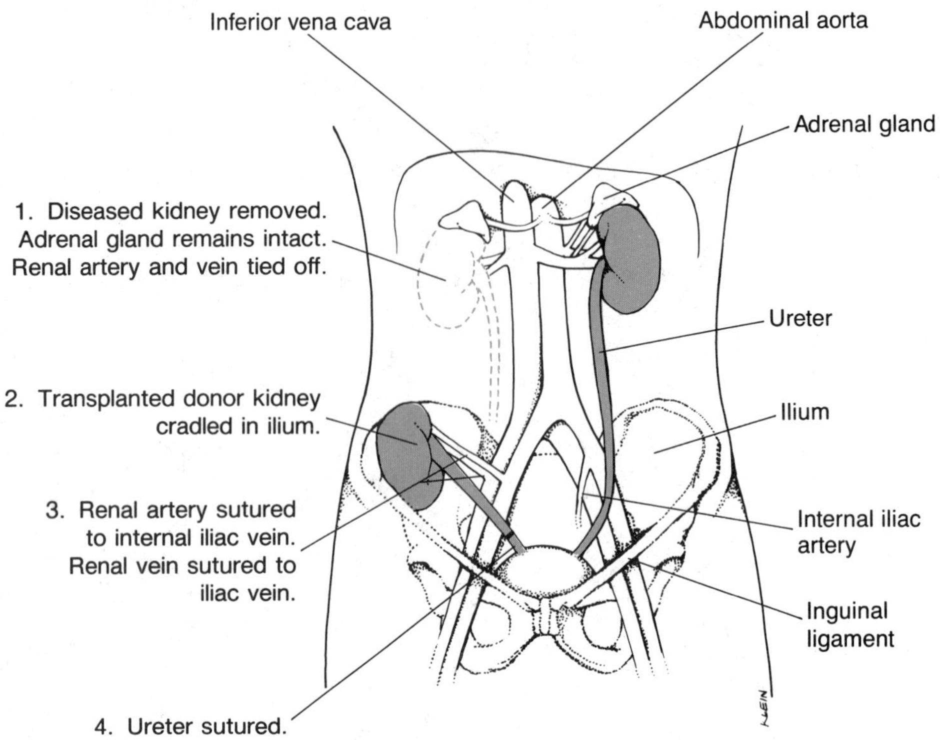

Inferior vena cava

Abdominal aorta

Adrenal gland

1. Diseased kidney removed.
   Adrenal gland remains intact.
   Renal artery and vein tied off.

Ureter

Figure 40-1
Renal transplantations (*1*) The diseased kidneys may be removed and the renal artery and vein are tied off. (*2*) The transplanted kidney is placed in the iliac fossa. (*3*) The renal artery of the donated kidney is sutured to the internal iliac vein, and the renal vein is sutured to the iliac vein. (*4*) The donated kidney's ureter is sutured to the bladder or to the patient's ureter.

2. Transplanted donor kidney cradled in ilium.

Ilium

3. Renal artery sutured to internal iliac vein. Renal vein sutured to iliac vein.

Internal iliac artery

Inguinal ligament

4. Ureter sutured.

while the patient is receiving high doses of immunosuppressive drugs. Septicemia (bacteremia or fungemia) in renal transplant patients is responsible for a significant number of the deaths.

- Clinical manifestations of septicemia include shaking chills, fever, rapid heartbeat and respirations (tachycardia and tachypnea), and either an increase or a decrease in white blood cells (leukocytosis or leukopenia).

The portal of entry for infection may be the urinary tract, the lung, the operative site, and other sources. Urine cultures are done frequently in view of the high incidence of bacteriuria during both the early and the late stages of transplant. Any type of wound drainage should be viewed as a potential source of infection since drainage is an excellent culture medium for bacteria. Catheter and drain tips are cultured on removal by cutting off the tip of the catheter or drain (using aseptic technique) and placing it in a sterile container for laboratory culture.

Monitoring Urinary Function. The vascular access (shunt or fistula) for hemodialysis is monitored to ensure patency and to evaluate for evidence of infection. Following a successful renal transplant the vascular access usually clots. This may result from improved coagulation with the return of renal function. Hemodialysis may be necessary postoperatively to maintain homeostasis until the transplanted kidney is functioning well.

Donor kidneys function immediately after grafting and may produce large quantities of dilute urine. A cadaver kidney may or may not undergo tubular necrosis and may not function for 2 or 3 weeks. The kidney may produce amounts of urine varying from extremes of no urine to large volumes of urine. During this stage, the patient may experience significant changes in fluid and electrolyte status; therefore, careful assessment is indicated. The output from the urinary catheter

(connected to a closed drainage system) is measured every 30 minutes to an hour. After the catheter is removed, the patient is instructed to void frequently to avoid stressing the bladder suture line. Intravenous fluids are given in accordance with urine volume and serum electrolyte levels and as prescribed by the physician.

Other Possible Complications. Gastrointestinal ulceration and steroid-induced bleeding may occur. Fungal colonization of the gastrointestinal tract (especially the mouth) and urinary bladder may occur secondary to steroid and antibiotic administration.

Psychological Considerations. The rejection of a transplanted kidney remains a matter of concern to the patient, the patient's family, and the supporting health care team for many months. The fears of kidney rejection and the complications of immunosuppressive therapy (cushingoid facies, diabetes, capillary fragility, osteoporosis, glaucoma, cataracts, acne) place tremendous psychological stresses on the patient. An additional problem is possible tumor growth, since patients on long-term immunosuppressive therapy have been found to develop malignancies more frequently than the general population. This requires understanding and the expert management of emotional crises by all concerned with the person's care.

Patient Education and Home Health Care. The patient is advised that follow-up care after transplantation is a lifelong necessity. He receives individual and written instructions concerning diet, medication, fluids, daily weight, daily measurement of urine, management of intake and output, prevention of infection, and resumption of activity and avoidance of contact sports in which the transplanted kidney may be injured.

The nurse works closely with the patient and family to ensure their understanding of the need for continuing the immunosuppressive drug as prescribed. Additionally, the patient and family are instructed to assess for and report signs of rejection of the transplanted kidney, signs of infection, or significant side-effects of the immunosuppressive drugs. These include decrease in urinary output; weight gain; malaise; fever; respiratory distress; tenderness over graft; anxiety; depression; changes in eating, drinking, or other habit patterns; and changes in blood pressure readings. The National Association of Patients on Hemodialysis and Transplantation, Inc.* is a nonprofit organization that serves the needs of kidney patients. Its quarterly publication, *NAPHT News,* has many helpful suggestions for patients and family members learning to cope with dialysis and transplantation.

Organ Donation. For those interested in donating a kidney, the National Kidney Foundation* will provide written information describing the organ donation program and a card specifying the organ to be donated in the event of death. The card is signed by the donor and two witnesses and is to be carried by the donor at all times. Procurement of an adequate number of kidneys for potential recipients is still a major problem; however, many states have recently passed legislation requiring physicians to ask relatives of deceased patients with potential cadaver kidneys if they would consider donation. Nurses are often called on by family members to explain or clarify donation and the possible outcomes.

Acute Glomerulonephritis

Acute glomerulonephritis refers to a group of kidney diseases in which there is an inflammatory reaction in the glomeruli. It is not an infection of the kidney *per se* but rather the result of untoward side-effects of the defense mechanism of the body. In most types of glomerulonephritis, IgG the major immunoglobulin (antibody) found in the serum of humans can be detected in the glomerular capillary walls. As a result of an antigen–antibody reaction, aggregates of molecules (complexes) are formed and circulate throughout the body. Some of these complexes lodge in the glomeruli, the filtering bed of the kidney, and induce an inflammatory response.

In most cases, the stimulus of the reaction is group A streptococcal infection of the throat, which ordinarily precedes the onset of glomerulonephritis by an interval of 2 to 3 weeks. The streptococcal product, acting as an antigen, generates circulating antibodies and results in deposit of the complexes in the glomeruli and injury to the kidney. Glomerulonephritis may also follow scarlet fever and impetigo (infection of the skin). The many forms of glomerulonephritis include proliferative, membranous, membranoproliferative, focal proliferative, and rapidly progressive. The pathology of these various types of glomerulonephritis has yet to be defined satisfactorily.

Pathophysiology. Cellular proliferation (increased production of endothelial cells lining the glomerulus), infiltration of the glomerulus by leukocytes, and thickening of the glomerular filtration membrane or basement membrane result in scarring and loss of filtering surface. In acute glomerulonephritis, the kidneys become large, swollen, and congested. All the renal tissues—glomeruli, tubules, and

* See bibliography at end of chapter for address.

blood vessels—are affected in all forms of glomerulonephritis, but in each form, the tissues are involved in varying degrees. In some patients, antigens outside the body (bacteria, viruses) initiate the process, resulting in the complexes being deposited in the glomerulus. In other patients, the membrane tissue of the kidney becomes altered by disease and serves as the inciting antigen. With electron-microscopy and immunofluorescent identification of the immune mechanism, the nature of the lesion can be studied.

Clinical Manifestations. The disease may be so mild that it is discovered accidentally through a routine urinalysis, or the history may reveal a preceding episode of pharyngitis or tonsillitis with fever. In the more severe form of the disease, the patient presents with headache, malaise, facial edema, and flank pain. Mild to severe hypertension is seen, and tenderness over the costovertebral angle is common. (The costovertebral angles, used as landmarks, are the angles formed on each side of the body by the bottom rib of the rib cage and the vertebral column.)

Acute glomerulonephritis is predominantly a disease of youth. Some cases that develop later are acute exacerbations of a glomerulonephritis that is already present but undetected.

Diagnostic Evaluation. The urine is scanty and bloody; there may even be *no* urine (anuria) for 1 or more days, although this is rare. Usually, early in the disease, the patient voids 50 to 200 ml daily of a cola-colored urine, with a specific gravity between 1.020 and 1.025 and a thick sediment of red blood cells, leukocytes, and all kinds of casts. (RBC casts mean glomerular injury.) The urine contains large amounts of protein. A large percentage of patients have an increased antistreptolysin titer as a result of a reaction to the streptococcal organism. Usually, there are rising values of BUN and serum creatinine. The patient may be anemic because of loss of the red blood cells in the urine and changes in the hematopoietic mechanism of the body.

As the patient improves, the amount of urine increases, while the urinary protein and urinary sediment diminish. Usually, more than 90% of children recover. The percentage of recovery for adults is not well established but is probably about 70%. Some patients become severely uremic within weeks and require dialysis for survival. Others, after a period of apparent recovery, insidiously develop chronic glomerulonephritis.

Management. The goals of management are to protect the patient's poorly functioning kidneys and to treat complications promptly. If residual streptococcal infection is suspected, penicillin is given. Bed rest is encouraged during the acute phase until the urine clears and the BUN, creatinine, and blood pressure return to normal. Rest also facilitates diuresis. The urine of the patient may serve as a guide to the duration of bed rest, since excessive activity may increase proteinuria and hematuria.

Dietary protein is restricted when renal insufficiency and nitrogen retention (elevated BUN) develop. Sodium is restricted when hypertension, edema, and congestive heart failure are present. Carbohydrates are given liberally to provide energy and reduce the catabolism of protein.

Fluids are given according to the patient's fluid losses and daily body weight. Insensible fluid loss through respiration and feces is estimated at 500 to 1000 ml. The intake and output are measured and recorded. Usually, diuresis starts 1 to 2 weeks after the onset of symptoms. Edema decreases and hypertension lessens. However, proteinuria and microscopic hematuria may persist for many months. In some patients, the disease may progress to chronic glomerulonephritis. Complications include hypertensive encephalopathy, congestive heart failure, and pulmonary edema. Hypertensive encephalopathy is considered a medical emergency, and therapy is directed toward reducing the blood pressure without impairing renal function.

Patient Education and Home Health Care. Instructions to the patient include explanations and scheduling for follow-up evaluations of (1) blood pressure, (2) urinalysis for protein, and (3) blood for BUN and creatinine studies to determine if there is exacerbation of disease activity. The patient is instructed to call the physician if symptoms of renal failure occur (*e.g.,* fatigue, nausea, vomiting, diminishing urinary output). Any infection must be treated promptly. A referral to the community health nurse may be indicated for those patients who live alone to provide an opportunity for careful assessment of the patient's progress and to detect the onset of early symptoms of renal insufficiency. Blood pressure is monitored, and serum and urine specimens may be collected to detect changes in renal function.

Chronic Glomerulonephritis

Pathophysiology. Chronic glomerulonephritis may have its onset as acute glomerulonephritis or may represent a milder type of antigen–antibody reaction, one so mild that it is overlooked. After repeated occurrences of these reactions, the kidneys are reduced to as little as one fifth their normal size, consisting largely of fibrous tissue. The cortex shrinks to a layer of 1 to 2 mm in thickness or less. Bands of scar tissue distort the remaining cortex, making the surface of the kidney rough and irregular. Many glomeruli and their tubules become scarred and the branches of the renal artery are thickened. The result is severe glomerular damage which results in chronic glomerulonephritis, a common cause of chronic renal failure.

Clinical Manifestations. The symptoms of chronic glomerulonephritis are variable. Some patients with severe disease have no symptoms at all for a long time. They may discover their condition as the result of a blood test or when their blood pressure is found to be elevated. The diagnosis may be suggested during a routine eye examination when vascular changes or hemorrhages are found. The first indication of disease may be a sudden, severe nosebleed, a stroke, or a convulsion. Many patients merely notice that their feet are slightly swollen at night. The majority of all patients also have such general symptoms as loss of weight and strength, increasing irritability, and nocturia. Headaches, dizziness, and digestive disturbances are common.

Physical examination may reveal a poorly nourished patient with a yellow-gray pigmentation of the skin and periorbital and peripheral (dependent) edema. Blood pressure may be normal or severely elevated. Retinal findings include hemorrhage, exudate, narrowed tortuous arterioles, and papilledema. Mucous membranes are pale owing to anemia.

As chronic glomerulonephritis progresses, the patient develops the following signs and symptoms of renal insufficiency and chronic renal failure: The neck veins may be distended as a result of fluid overload. Cardiomegaly, a gallop rhythm, and other signs of congestive heart failure may be present. Crackles can be heard in the lungs. Peripheral neuropathy with depressed deep tendon reflexes and neurosensory changes occurs late in the illness. When frank uremia occurs, the patient becomes confused and his attention span will be limited. An additional late finding includes evidence of pericarditis with a cardiac friction rub and pulsus paradoxus (an exaggerated drop in blood pressure or weakening of pulse amplitude with inspiration secondary to impaired cardiac flow during inspiration).

A number of laboratory abnormalities occur. Urinalysis reveals a fixed specific gravity of 1.010, variable proteinuria, and urine sediment changes. As glomerular filtration becomes depressed, hyperkalemia and decreased serum bicarbonate (metabolic acidosis) develop. Fatal hypermagnesemia may develop if magnesium-containing antacids are given to patients with renal failure. Anemia secondary to decreased erythropoiesis (production of red blood cells) and shortened red cell survival time, hypoalbuminemia with edema secondary to protein loss through the damaged renal glomeruli, and depressed serum calcium and increased serum phosphorus values occur as renal failure progresses. Impaired nerve conduction velocity develops in about 50% of patients once the glomerular filtration rate decreases below 50 ml/min as a result of rising levels of waste products in the tissues and nervous system and electrolyte abnormalities. Chest films may show cardiac enlargement and pulmonary edema. The electrocardiogram may be normal but may also reflect hypertension with left ventricular hypertrophy and electrolyte disturbances, such as hyperkalemia and spiked T waves.

Management. The treatment of the ambulatory patient is guided by the patient's symptoms. Therefore, if hypertension is present, treatment is directed toward readjusting the diet and fluid intake in an effort to maintain as normal a metabolic state as possible. Protein intake (of high biologic value) is adjusted according to the response of the patient with adequate calories to prevent protein from being used for energy. If there is a urinary tract infection, a possible factor in producing further renal damage, steps are taken to diagnose it and to treat it.

If severe edema develops, the patient is placed on bed rest and the head of the bed is elevated to promote comfort and diuresis. Weight is monitored daily, and diuretics are used to reduce fluid overload. Sodium and fluid intake is adjusted according to the ability of the patient's kidneys to excrete water and sodium.

Initiation of dialysis, which was previously used only in extreme cases of chronic glomerulonephritis, is considered early in the course of the disease to keep the patient in optimal physical condition, prevent fluid and electrolyte imbalances, and minimize the risk of complications of renal failure. The course of dialysis is smoother if treatment is initiated before the patient develops significant complications.

Nursing Interventions. The nurse has a major role in explaining to the patient and family what is occurring. Additionally, the nurse provides emotional support throughout the course of the disease and treatment by providing opportunities for the patient and family to verbalize their concerns and have their questions answered and their options discussed.

The nurse observes the patient for changes in fluid and electrolyte status and for signs of deterioration of renal function. Changes in fluid and electrolyte status and in cardiac and neurologic status are reported promptly to the physician. If dialysis is initiated, the patient and family will require considerable assistance and support in dealing with the need for this therapy and its long-term implications.

Nephrotic Syndrome

The nephrotic syndrome is a clinical disorder characterized by (1) marked increase in protein in the urine (proteinuria), (2) decrease in albumin in the blood (hypoalbuminemia), (3) edema, and (4) excess cholesterol in the blood (hypercholesterolemia). It is seen in any condition that seriously damages the glomerular capillary membrane. Causes include chronic glomerulonephritis, diabetes mellitus with intercapillary glomerulosclerosis, amyloidosis of the kidney, systemic lupus erythematosus, and renal vein thrombosis. The pathophysiology of nephrotic syndrome is discussed on page 997.

Clinical Manifestations. There is slow onset of fluid retention that progresses to pitting edema. The patient loses protein in the urine, leading to depletion of body proteins. In addition, the blood cholesterol level is high. The diagnosis is made on assessment of the patient's signs and symptoms, physical examination, renal function tests, measurements of 24-hour urine protein, and serum electrolyte evaluations. Urinalysis shows microscopic hematuria, urinary casts, and other abnormalities. Needle biopsy of the kidney is done for histologic examination of renal tissue to confirm the diagnosis.

Management. The objective of management is to preserve renal function. It may be necessary to keep the patient on bed rest a few days to promote diuresis to reduce the edema. A high-protein diet is given to replenish wasted tissues and restore body proteins. If the edema is severe, the patient is placed on a low-sodium diet. Diuretics are given in severe edema, and adrenocorticosteroids (prednisone) may be used to reduce proteinuria.

Nursing Interventions. In the early stages, the nursing management is similar to that of the patient with acute glomerulonephritis, but as the disease worsens, management is similar to the care of the patient with chronic renal failure (see pp. 1039–1043).

Nephrosclerosis

Nephrosclerosis is hardening, or sclerosis, of the arteries of the kidney and is usually seen in association with hypertension. It is the renal manifestation of generalized arteriosclerosis. There are two forms: malignant and benign. Malignant nephrosclerosis is thought to be a generalized vascular disease that starts in the kidney and finally involves the entire vascular tree. Patients with the malignant type progress rapidly through the stages of proteinuria, increasing hypertension, failing renal function, and retinal vessel changes. They usually die within several months. The factor responsible for death may be uremia, congestive heart failure due to hypertensive heart disease, or a cerebrovascular accident. It occurs most commonly from the third to the fifth decade of life.

Patients who develop benign nephrosclerosis are found in older age-groups. These patients rarely complain of renal symptoms, although for years the urine has a low and fixed specific gravity and contains a small amount of protein and an occasional hyaline or granular cast. Only late in the disease does renal insufficiency appear.

Hydronephrosis

Hydronephrosis due to obstruction of urinary flow is dilatation of the pelvis and calyces of one or both kidneys with resulting thinning of the renal parenchyma. Obstruction to the normal flow of urine causes the urine to back up, resulting in increased pressure in the kidney. If the obstruction is in the urethra or the bladder, the back-pressure affects both kidneys, but if the obstruction is in one of the ureters due to a stone or kink, only one kidney is damaged.

Partial or intermittent obstruction may be caused by a renal stone that has formed in the renal pelvis but has dropped into the ureter and blocked it. Or the obstruction may be due to a tumor of some other abdominal or pelvic organ pressing on the ureter or to bands of scar tissue resulting from an abscess or inflammation near the ureter that pinches it. The disorder may be due to an odd angle of the ureter as it leaves the renal pelvis or to an unusual position of the kidney, favoring a ureteral twist or kink. In elderly males, the most common cause is urethral obstruction at the bladder outlet by an enlarged prostate.

Whatever the cause, as the fluid accumulates in the renal pelvis it distends the pelvis and its calyces. In time, atrophy of the kidney results. As one kidney undergoes gradual destruction, the contralateral kidney gradually enlarges (compensatory hypertrophy). Ultimately, there is impairment of renal function.

Clinical Manifestations. The patient may be asymptomatic if the onset is gradual. Acute obstruction may produce aching in the flank and back. If infection is present, there are symptoms of bladder irritability (dysuria) and chills, fever, tenderness, and pyuria. The hydronephritic kidney may bleed from congestion, causing hematuria. Signs and symptoms of chronic renal failure develop as the condition progresses.

Management. The goals of management are to identify and correct the cause of the obstruction, to treat infection, and to restore and conserve renal function.

To relieve the obstruction, the urine may have to be diverted by nephrostomy (see p. 1026) or other types of diversion. The infection is treated with antimicrobials since residual urine in the calyces produces infection and pyelonephritis. The patient is prepared for surgical removal of obstructive lesions (calculus, tumor, obstruction of the ureter). If one kidney is severely damaged and its function is destroyed, nephrectomy (removal of the kidney) is performed. (See Management of the Patient Undergoing Renal Surgery, pp. 1025 and 1029–1031.)

Infections of the Urinary Tract

Urinary tract infections (UTIs) are caused by the presence of pathogenic microorganisms in the urinary tract, with or without signs and symptoms. Infection may occur at any site within the urinary tract and may affect the bladder (cystitis), urethra (urethritis), prostate (prostatitis), or kidney (pyelonephritis).

The normal urinary tract is sterile except near the urethral orifice.

Bacteriuria refers to the presence of bacteria in the urine. A colony count of at least 100,000 colonies per milliliter of urine on a clean-catch midstream or catheterized specimen usually indicates infection. However, urinary tract infection and subsequent sepsis have been reported with lower bacterial colony counts. Infections in any part of the urinary tract may persist for months or even years without symptoms.

The bacteria most commonly responsible for urinary tract infections are *Escherichia coli* (80%–90%); *Proteus mirabilis;* one or more species of *Klebsiella, Enterobacter, Proteus,* and *Pseudomonas;* and the various enterococci. All these are normally found in the fecal flora.

Factors Contributing to Urinary Tract Infections

The majority of urinary tract infections result from bowel organisms that ascend from the perineum to the urethra and the bladder, adhering to the mucosal surfaces. A higher rate of bacteria adhering to the urethral epithelium has been associated with a higher rate of urinary tract infection. Defense mechanisms of the bladder, including an "antiadherence" defense or fluid on the surface of the bladder wall and a "washout factor" (flushing bacteria away with voiding), normally protect the urinary tract from infection. Interference with these mechanisms by inflammation, abrasion of the urethral mucosa, or incomplete emptying of the bladder increases susceptibility to urinary tract infection.

Women are more prone to develop bladder infections because of the short female urethra and its anatomical proximity to the vagina, periurethral glands, and rectum. In the male, the length of the urethra and the antibacterial properties of the prostatic secretions tend to ward off ascending urethral infections. Adult males who develop urinary tract infections should be examined for urinary obstruction, prostatic infection, renal stones, or systemic disease.

Urethrovesical reflux refers to the reflux (flowing back) of urine from the bladder into the urethra. It is caused by an increase in intrabladder pressure (coughing, sneezing), which may squeeze the urine out of the bladder into the urethra. When the pressure returns to normal, the urine flows back into the urethra, bringing back into the bladder the bacteria from the anterior portions of the urethra. Urethrovesical reflux is also caused by dysfunction of the bladder neck or urethra.

Ureterovesical or *vesicoureteral reflux* refers to the flowing back of urine from the bladder into one or both ureters. In the normal person, the ureterovesical junction prevents urine from traveling back into the ureter, particularly at the time of voiding. When the ureterovesical valve is incompetent (congenital causes, ureteral abnormalities), the bacteria may reach the kidneys and there may be subsequent dilatation of the ureter, renal pelvis, and calyces with ultimate kidney destruction.

Fecal contamination of the urethral meatus is a common way in which bacteria are introduced into the urinary tract. *Sexual intercourse* plays a role in the ascent of organisms from the perineum to the bladder in women. *Instrumentation* (from catheterization, cytoscopic examinations) is also implicated in producing infections. *Stasis of urine in the bladder* may lead to infection, which may ultimately spread through the entire urinary system. Any *obstruction* to urinary flow renders the kidney more susceptible to infection. Common causes of urinary tract obstruction are congenital anomalies, urethral strictures, contracture of the bladder neck, bladder tumors, ureteral stones, compression of the ureters, and neurologic abnormalities. Infections may spread to the urinary tract by way of the blood (hematogenous spread) or the lymphatic system (lymphogenous spread). Diabetes mellitus also predisposes to urinary tract infections. Common causes of urinary tract infection are summarized in Fig. 40-2.

Clinical Manifestations

Signs and symptoms of urinary tract infections cover a broad range. Frequently, the patient is asymptomatic and is found to have bacteria in the urine (bacteriuria) while undergoing a periodic health checkup. Signs and symptoms of lower urinary tract infection (cystitis) include frequent painful and burning urination, sometimes accompanied by bearing-down sensations and spasms in the region of the bladder and suprapubic area. Hematuria and back pain may also be present. Signs and symptoms of upper urinary tract infection (pyelonephritis) include fever, chills, flank pain, and painful urination. Upon examination there is pain and tenderness in the area of the costovertebral angle (CVA). If extensive destruction of the kidneys has resulted, features of renal failure may be present, including nausea, vomiting, pruritus, weight loss, edema, and shortness of breath. Acute flareups or episodes of reinfection may be asymptomatic.

Diagnostic Evaluation

Urinary tract infection is diagnosed by bacteria in the urine specimen collected by a midstream clean-catch technique. A bacterial count of 100,000 organisms (colonies) per milliliter of urine indicates a urinary infection. Urine cultures are also obtained to identify the bacterial species present. In men, a culture is made of prostatic fluid or urine voided after prostatic massage. In persons at high risk of complicated or recurring infection, diagnostic studies such as intravenous pyelography (IVP) and cystography may be carried out to determine if the infection is secondary to abnormalities of the urinary tract.

Cystitis (Lower Urinary Tract Infection)

Cystitis is an inflammation of the urinary bladder that is most often caused by an ascending infection from the urethra. It may be caused by urine flowing back from the urethra into the bladder (urethrovesical reflux), fecal contamination, or the use of various instruments such as a catheter or cystoscope.

Cystitis is seen more commonly in women. The distal portion of the urethra is frequently colonized with bacterial flora following colonization of the vaginal vestibule. A defect of the mucosa of the urethra, vagina, or external genitalia of these patients may allow enteric organisms to adhere and colonize at periurethral sites and to invade the bladder. Acute cystitis in women is usually caused by *Escherichia coli* and often follows sexual intercourse, which implicates the ascending urethral pathway in its pathogenesis.

About half of the women who present with symptoms

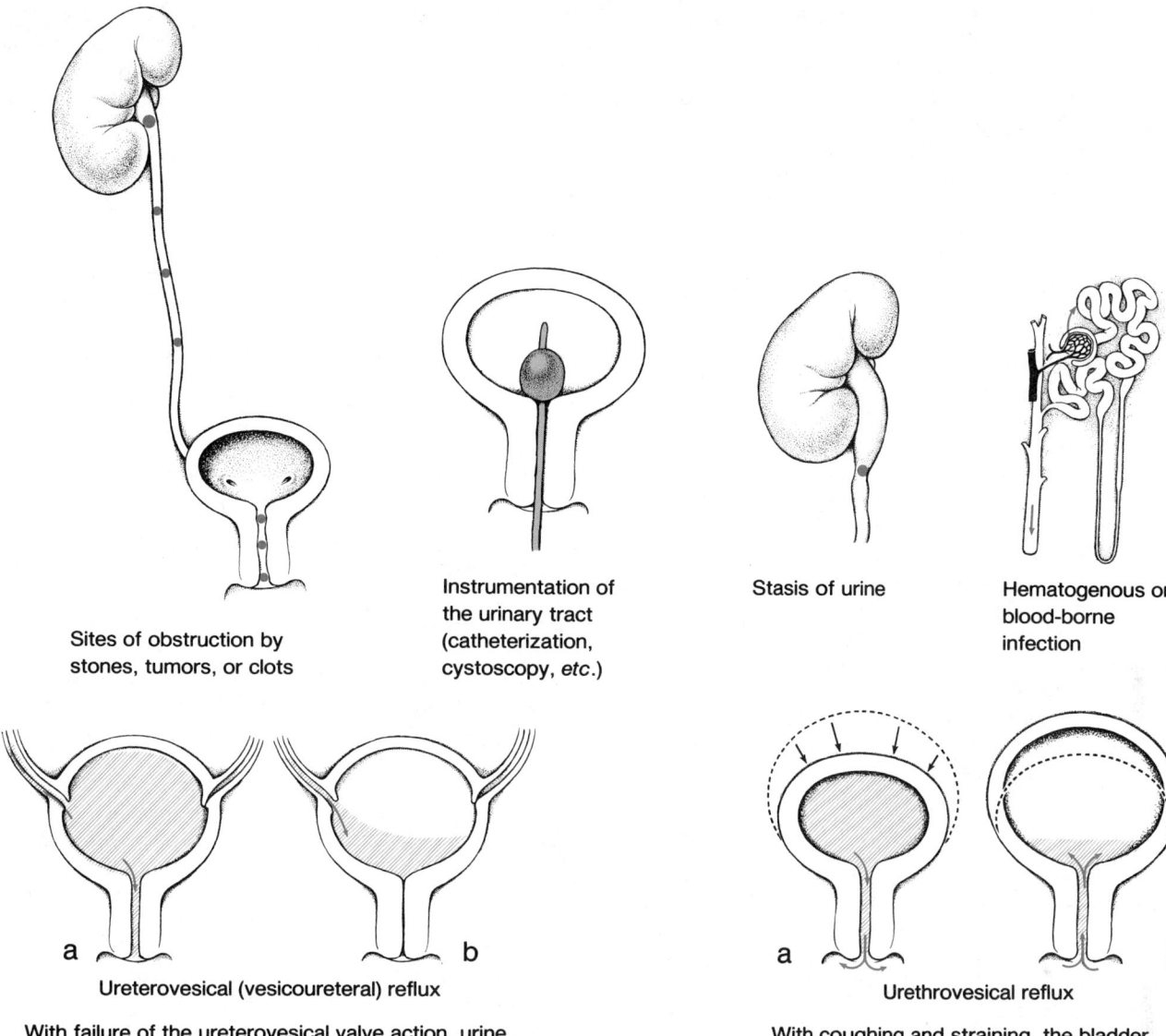

Sites of obstruction by stones, tumors, or clots

Instrumentation of the urinary tract (catheterization, cystoscopy, *etc.*)

Stasis of urine

Hematogenous or blood-borne infection

a   b

Ureterovesical (vesicoureteral) reflux

With failure of the ureterovesical valve action, urine moves up the ureters during voiding (*a*) and flows into the bladder when voiding has stopped (*b*). This prevents complete emptying of the bladder, stasis, and contamination of the ureters with bacteria-laden urine.

a   b

Urethrovesical reflux

With coughing and straining, the bladder pressure rises, which may force urine from the bladder into the urethera (*a*). When bladder pressure returns to normal, the urine flows back to the bladder (*b*), which introduces bacteria from the urethra to the bladder.

Figure 40-2
Causes of urinary tract and kidney infections.

of acute cystitis (frequency, dysuria) without bacteriuria have *acute urethral syndrome* (symptoms suggesting urinary tract infection but occurring in the presence of urine with fewer than 100,000 organisms). Cystitis in men is secondary to some other factor, such as infected prostate; epididymitis by reflux of urine along the vas or perivesical lymphatics, as from an infected prostate; or bladder stones. Therefore, men undergo diagnostic testing usually after the first episode of cystitis to identify and treat the cause.

The patient with cystitis complains of urgency, frequency, burning and pain on urination, nocturia, and a bearing-down sensation in the region of the bladder and suprapubic area. There is pus, bacteria, and often red cells in the urine.

Management

The goals of medical management are to eradicate the causative pathogens, to decrease morbidity, and to prevent recurrences. The specific treatment depends on the cause and location of the infection. A urine specimen is usually obtained for smears and culture so that the appropriate drug may be selected.

For an uncomplicated, nonobstructed lower urinary tract infection, the female patient may be treated with single-dose or short-term therapy with an antimicrobial agent to which the organisms are susceptible. These infections usually respond favorably to antimicrobials that result in high urinary drug levels. Amoxicillin, sulfonamide, nitrofurantoin, trimethoprim-sulfamethoxazole, and tetracycline derivatives have been used successfully. A potentially effective drug should *rapidly* eradicate the organism and relieve the patient's symptoms. The urine is reexamined 24 hours to 3 days after initiation of treatment to determine if the urine is free of bacteria. In the male patient, prostatitis may require prolonged antimicrobial therapy.

There is a tendency for these infections to recur. Recurrences are of two types: (1) reinfection, the occurrence of sequential infections caused by different organisms, and (2) persistent infection, the occurrence of repeated infections caused by the same organism. Repeated or persistent infection due to the same organism usually results from a persistent source of infection in the urinary tract, such as infected urinary tract stones or structural anomalies of the urinary tract. Although the incidence of such infections is relatively small, the potential for irreversible kidney damage and its prevention, if the source of persistent infection is treated, make differentiation of the type of recurrent infection important.

Patients with spaced recurrent infections may require long-term, low-dose antimicrobial prophylaxis. It is usually given at bedtime. The rationale is that the antibacterial agent is maintained in the bladder urine/periurethral zone, thus blocking reinfection. Periodic urine cultures are done to be certain that prophylaxis is effective.

Further diagnostic studies are carried out in patients with persistent infections, suspected complicated infections (obstruction, calculi), or infections secondary to repeated lack of response to antimicrobial therapy.

The effectiveness of certain antimicrobial drugs is affected by the reaction (*p*H) of the urine. Aminoglycoside antibiotics (streptomycin, kanamycin, neomycin, and gentamicin) are more active when the urine is alkaline. Sodium bicarbonate may be given to alkalinize the urine. The tetracyclines, methenamine mandelate, and nitrofurantoin are more active when the urinary *p*H is acidic, and ascorbic acid may be given to acidify the urine.

Since there is a marked tendency for infection to recur, follow-up urine studies are recommended for at least 2 years to determine if asymptomatic infection is present. It is especially important to have follow-up studies if urinary tract infections occur during pregnancy.

▶ *Nursing Process*
The Patient With Lower Urinary Tract Infection

▷ *Assessment*

A history of urinary signs and symptoms is obtained from the patient with a possible urinary tract infection. The presence of pain, frequency, urgency, and hesitancy and changes in urine are assessed, documented, and reported. The patient's usual pattern of voiding is assessed to detect factors that may predispose the patient to urinary tract infection. Infrequent emptying of the bladder, the association of symptoms of urinary tract infection with sexual intercourse, and personal hygiene are assessed. The patient's knowledge about prescribed

antimicrobial medications and preventive health care measures is also assessed. Additionally, the patient's urine is checked for volume, color, concentration, cloudiness, and odor, all of which are altered by bacteria in the urinary tract.

▷ *Nursing Diagnoses*

Based on the assessment data, the nursing diagnoses may include the following:

- Alteration in comfort related to inflammation and infection of the urethra, bladder, and other urinary tract structures
- Knowledge deficit of factors predisposing to recurrence, detection and prevention of recurrence, and pharmacologic therapy

▷ *Planning and Implementation*

▷ *Goals:* The patient's major goals may include relief of pain and discomfort and increased knowledge of preventive measures and treatment modalities.

Nursing Interventions

Relieving Pain and Discomfort. Dysuria, frequency, hesitancy, urgency, and other types of discomfort associated with urinary tract infection are frequently relieved quickly once antimicrobial therapy is initiated. Antispasmodic drugs may be useful in relieving bladder irritability and pain. Aspirin, heat to the perineum, and hot tub baths help relieve urgency, discomfort, and spasm. The patient is encouraged to drink liberal amounts of fluids to promote renal blood flow and to flush the bacteria from the urinary tract. However, fluids that may be irritating to the bladder (*e.g.*, coffee, tea, colas) are avoided. Frequent voiding (every 2 to 3 hours) is encouraged to empty the bladder completely since this can significantly lower urine bacterial counts, reduce urinary stasis, and prevent reinfection.

Patient Education and Home Health Care. Women who have repeated urinary tract infections should receive detailed instructions on the following points:

1. Reduce concentrations of pathogens at the vaginal introitus by hygienic measures:
   a. Shower rather than bathe in a tub, since bacteria in the bath water may enter the urethra.
   b. Cleanse around the perineum and urethral meatus (cleansing from the front to the back) after each bowel movement.
2. Drink liberal amounts of fluid during the day to flush out bacteria.
3. Void every 2 to 3 hours during the day and completely empty the bladder. This prevents overdistention of the bladder and compromised blood supply to the bladder wall, which predisposes the patient to urinary tract infection.
4. If sexual intercourse is the initiating event for development of bacteriuria:
   a. Void immediately after sexual intercourse.
   b. Take the prescribed single dose of an oral antimicrobial agent following sexual intercourse.
5. If bacteria continue to appear in the urine, long-term

antimicrobial therapy may be required to prevent colonization of the periurethral area and recurrence of infection. The drug should be taken after emptying the bladder just before going to bed to ensure adequate concentration of the drug during the overnight period.

6. If prescribed, monitor and test the urine for bacteria with dipslides (Microstix) as follows:
   a. Wash around the urethral meatus several times, using different washcloths.
   b. Collect a midstream specimen.
   c. Remove a slide from its container, dip it into the urine sample, and return it to the container.
   d. Incubate the slide at room temperature according to product directions.
   e. Read the results by comparing the slide with the colony density chart that comes with the product.
7. See health care provider regularly for follow-up, recurrence of symptoms, infections nonresponsive to treatment, or further involvement of the urinary tract.

▷ *Evaluation*

▷ *Expected Outcomes*

1. Patient experiences relief of pain, urgency, dysuria, and fever.
   a. Reports absence of pain, urgency, dysuria, hesitancy on voiding.
   b. Takes antimicrobial agent as prescribed.
   c. Takes analgesics and hot tub baths for discomfort.
   d. Drinks 8 to 10 glasses of fluids daily.
   e. Voids every 2 to 3 hours.
   f. Voids urine that is clear and free from odor.
2. Increases knowledge of preventive measures and prescribed treatment modalities.
   a. States rationale for using shower rather than tub for daily hygiene.
   b. Uses appropriate cleansing action (front to back) following each bowel movement.
   c. States rationale for appropriate cleansing method following each bowel movement.
   d. Consumes 7 to 8 glasses of fluid per day.
   e. Voids frequently during day and at bedtime to prevent overdistention of bladder.
   f. Voids immediately after sexual intercourse.
   g. Takes oral antimicrobial agents as prescribed following sexual intercourse.
   h. Takes entire course of antimicrobial agent as prescribed.
   i. Demonstrates correct use of dipslides to monitor for urinary tract infection.
   j. Reports recurrence of symptoms to health care provider.
   k. Adheres to follow-up schedule as recommended by health care provider.
   l. Reports symptoms of further involvement of the urinary tract.

Gerontological Considerations

Urinary tract infection is the most common cause of sepsis in the elderly. Gram-negative sepsis resulting from urinary tract infection in the elderly is associated with a mortality rate exceeding 50%. Obstruction from an enlarged prostate is the most frequent cause of urinary tract infection in elderly men; elderly women often have incomplete emptying of the bladder and urinary stasis. Postmenopausal women also are susceptible to colonization and increased adherence of bacteria to the vagina and urethra in the absence of estrogen. The recognition of urinary tract infection and sepsis in the elderly is made more difficult by the frequent lack of typical symptoms. Although frequency, urgency, and dysuria may occur, nonspecific symptoms such as altered sensorium, lethargy, anorexia, hyperventilation, and a low-grade fever may be the only clues to the presence of a urinary tract infection. The probability of frequent reinfection appears with advancing age.

Age-related changes in intestinal absorption of drugs and reduced renal function and hepatic flow may necessitate alterations in the antimicrobial treatment of urinary tract infection in the elderly. Treatment is usually initiated as soon as the infection and bacteremia are suspected because of the high mortality associated with sepsis.

Pyelonephritis (Upper Urinary Tract Infection)

Pyelonephritis is a bacterial infection of the renal pelvis, tubules, and interstitial tissue of one or both kidneys. Bacteria may gain access to the bladder via the urethra and ascend to the kidney or may reach the kidney through the bloodstream. Pyelonephritis is frequently secondary to ureterovesical reflux in which an incompetent ureterovesical valve allows the urine to back up (reflux) into the ureters, usually at the time of voiding (see Fig. 40-2). Urinary tract obstruction (which renders the kidneys more susceptible to infection) and renal diseases are among other causes. Pyelonephritis may be acute or chronic.

Acute pyelonephritis is an active infection that presents with chills and fever, flank pain, costovertebral angle tenderness, leukocytosis, bacteria and pus in the urine, and frequently symptoms of lower urinary tract involvement, such as dysuria and frequency. Upper urinary tract infection is associated with antibody coating of the bacteria in the urine. (Antibodies coat the bacteria in the renal medulla; when the bacteria are excreted in the urine, the immunofluorescent test can detect the antibody coating.)

There are areas of inflammation in the kidney with interstitial infiltrations of inflammatory cells which in time may produce tubular destruction and abscess formation. Low-grade interstitial inflammation may result in atrophy and destruction of tubules and the glomeruli. Eventually, when pyelonephritis becomes chronic, the kidneys become scarred, contracted, and nonfunctioning.

Diagnostic Evaluation and Management. An intravenous urogram and other diagnostic tests are carried out to locate any obstruction in the urinary tract. The relief of obstruction is essential to save the kidney from destruction. The treatment is essentially the same as that of cystitis. Culture and sensitivity tests are done on the urine since the choice of antimicrobial is determined by the causative organism. Medication should produce sustained antibacterial concentration of the drugs within the renal parenchyma. The antimicrobial drug must be given for a long enough period to prevent reseeding of residual foci of infection.

A possible problem in treatment is a chronic or recurring infection persisting for months or years without symptoms. After the initial antimicrobial regimen, the patient is kept on continuous antimicrobial treatment until there is no evidence of infection, all causative factors have been treated or controlled, and kidney function is stabilized. The patient is monitored with serum creatinine determinations and blood counts for the duration of the long-term therapy.

Chronic Pyelonephritis

Repeated bouts of acute pyelonephritis may lead to chronic pyelonephritis (chronic interstitial nephritis).

The patient with chronic pyelonephritis usually has no symptoms of infection unless an acute exacerbation occurs. Noticeable signs may include fatigue, headache, poor appetite, polyuria, excessive thirst, and weight loss. Persistent and recurring infection may produce progressive scarring of the kidney with ultimate kidney failure.

Complications of chronic pyelonephritis include uremia (from progressive loss of nephrons secondary to chronic inflammation and scarring), hypertension, and formation of kidney stones (from chronic infection with urea-splitting organisms, resulting in stone formation).

Diagnostic Evaluation and Management. The extent of the disease is assessed by intravenous urogram and measurements of BUN, creatinine levels, and creatinine clearance. Eradication of bacteria from the urine is undertaken if present. The choice of an antimicrobial is based on culture identification of the pathogen. If the urine cannot be made bacteria free, nitrofurantoin or a combination of sulfamethoxazole and trimethoprim may be used to suppress bacterial growth. Hypertension and chronic renal failure are the major complications of chronic pyelonephritis.

Perinephric Abscess

Perinephric abscess is an abscess in the fatty tissue of the kidney that may arise secondary to an infection of the kidney or as a hematogenous (spread through the bloodstream) infection originating elsewhere in the body. It may be secondary to a staphylococcal infection of the kidney or to the spread of infection from adjacent areas, such as from diverticulitis or appendicitis. The symptoms often are acute in onset, with chills, fever, leukocytosis, and other signs of suppuration. Locally, there is flank or abdominal tenderness or pain. The patient usually appears seriously ill.

Management. The treatment consists of administration of the appropriate antimicrobial agent and incision and drainage of the abscess. Drains are usually inserted and left in the perinephric space until all significant drainage has ceased. Because the drainage often is profuse, frequent changes of the outer dressings may be necessary. As in the treatment of an abscess in any site, the patient is monitored for sepsis, fluid intake and output, and general response to treatment.

Carbuncle of the Kidney

Carbuncle of the kidney is an infection of hematogenous origin that is caused usually by *Staphylococcus*. It usually follows a cutaneous boil or carbuncle and is characterized by fever, malaise, and dull pain in the region of the kidney. This type of infection, if recognized, usually subsides with chemotherapy and penicillin. Recently, carbuncles of the kidney from gram-negative bacteria have increased in incidence.

Tuberculosis of the Kidney and Genitourinary Tract

Pathophysiology and Clinical Manifestations. Tuberculosis of the kidney and urinary tract is caused by the organism *Mycobacterium tuberculosis* and usually spreads from the lungs by way of the bloodstream to the kidneys and to other organs of the genitourinary tract. At first the symptoms are mild; there is usually a slight afternoon fever and a loss of weight and appetite. The process of tuberculosis generally starts in one of the renal pyramids; ulceration into the kidney pelvis follows. The organisms are carried down with the urine into the bladder so that the bladder is likely to become infected.

Tuberculosis of the lower genitourinary tract is always secondary to renal tuberculosis, with the infection having disseminated downward. In the male, the prostate and epididymis may become infected.

Tuberculosis of the urinary bladder is an extension of tuberculosis of a kidney. This disease gives rise to several small ulcers, the majority of them near the trigone of the bladder. The symptoms of bladder tuberculosis are those of cystitis in general but with an unusual degree of bladder irritability because of the location of the lesions. Suggestive early symptoms of this disease are an increased urinary output that contains considerable pus and yet is acid in reaction (in nearly all other pyurias the urine is alkaline) and hematuria (either microscopic or gross). The features of pain, dysuria, and urinary frequency, when they occur, are due to bladder infection. Signs of bladder irritability (frequency, nocturia) are a later manifestation of the disease.

Management. A search for tuberculosis elsewhere in the body is conducted when tuberculosis of the kidney or urinary tract is found. Inquiry is made to determine if the patient has had known exposure to tuberculosis. Three or more clean-voided first morning urine specimens are obtained for culture for *M. tuberculosis*.

The objective of treatment is to eradicate the offending organism. Combinations of ethambutol, isoniazid, and rifampin are used to delay the emergence of resistant organisms. Shorter-course chemotherapy (4 months) has been proven effective in eradicating the organism and in penetrating renal tissue. Since renal tuberculosis is a manifestation of a systemic disease, all measures to promote the general health of the person are used. Surgical intervention may be necessary to prevent obstructive problems and to remove an extensively diseased kidney. The patient is counseled about the need for follow-up examinations (urine cultures, excretory urograms) usually for a period of a year.

Treatment will need to be reinstituted if a relapse occurs

and the tubercle bacilli again invade the genitourinary tract. Ureteral stenosis or bladder contractures are complications that may develop during the healing process.

Urolithiasis

Urolithiasis refers to the presence of stones (calculi) in the urinary system. Stones are found in the urinary tract by the deposit of crystalline substances (calcium oxalate, calcium phosphate, uric acid) excreted in the urine. They may be found anywhere from the kidney to the bladder and vary in size from minute granular deposits, called sand or gravel, to bladder stones the size of an orange. The different sites of calculus formation in the urinary tract are shown in Figure 40-3.

Certain factors favor the formation of stones, including infection, urinary stasis, and periods of immobility (produces slowing of renal drainage and altered calcium metabolism). Hypercalcemia (abnormally high concentration of blood calcium compounds) and hypercalciuria (abnormally large amounts of calcium in the urine) may be caused by hyperparathyroidism, renal tubular acidosis, excessive intake of vitamin D, excessive intake of milk and alkali, and certain myeloproliferative diseases (leukemia, polycythemia vera, multiple myeloma), which produce an unusual proliferation of blood cells derived from bone marrow. These factors promote increased calcium concentrations in blood and urine, causing precipitation of calcium and formation of stones. Some stones are caused by an excessive excretion of uric acid, the end product of purine metabolism. Urinary stone formation may also occur with inflammatory bowel disease and in those with an ileostomy or bowel resection, particularly of the small bowel since these persons absorb more oxalate. Vitamin A deficiency may be another cause. In many patients, however, no cause may be found.

The problem occurs predominantly in the third to fifth decades and affects men more than women. Persons who have had two stones tend to have recurrences. The majority of stones contain calcium or magnesium in combination with phosphorus or oxalate. Most stones are radiopaque and can be detected by roentgenography.

Clinical Manifestations

The clinical manifestations of stones in the urinary tract depend on the presence of obstruction, infection, and edema. When the stones block the flow of urine, obstruction develops, and the constant irritation of the stone may be followed by a secondary infection that causes pyelonephritis and cystitis with chills, fever, and dysuria. Some stones cause few if any symptoms while slowly destroying the functional units of the kidney (nephrons); others cause excruciating pain and discomfort. Stones in the renal pelvis may be associated with intense, deep ache in the loin (part of the back between the thorax and pelvis) and with voiding of increased amounts of urine containing blood and white blood cells (pus). The stone produces an increase in hydrostatic pressure and distends the renal pelvis and proximal ureter. Thus, painful afferent sensations are initiated. Pain originating in the renal area radiates anteriorly and downward toward the bladder in the female and toward the testis in the male. If the pain suddenly becomes acute, the loin exquisitely tender, and nausea and vomiting appear, the patient is having an attack of *renal colic*. Diarrhea and abdominal discomfort may accompany the attack. These gastrointestinal symptoms are due to renointestinal reflexes and the anatomical proximity of the kidneys to the stomach, pancreas, and large intestines.

When stones lodge in the ureter, acute, excruciating, colicky pain is experienced, radiating down the thigh and to the genitalia. The pain usually occurs in waves. There is usually a frequent desire to void, but very little urine is passed, and it usually contains blood because of the abrasive action of the stone. This group of symptoms is called *ureteral colic*. In general, the patient will spontaneously pass stones 0.5 to 1 cm in diameter. Those over 1 cm in diameter usually must be removed or broken up so that they can be removed or passed spontaneously. When stones lodge in the bladder, they usually produce symptoms of irritation and may be associated with urinary tract infection and hematuria. If the stone obstructs the bladder neck, there will be urinary retention.

Diagnostic Evaluation

The diagnosis is confirmed by intravenous urography or retrograde pyelography. Blood chemistries and a 24-hour urine test for measurement of calcium, uric acid, creatinine, sodium,

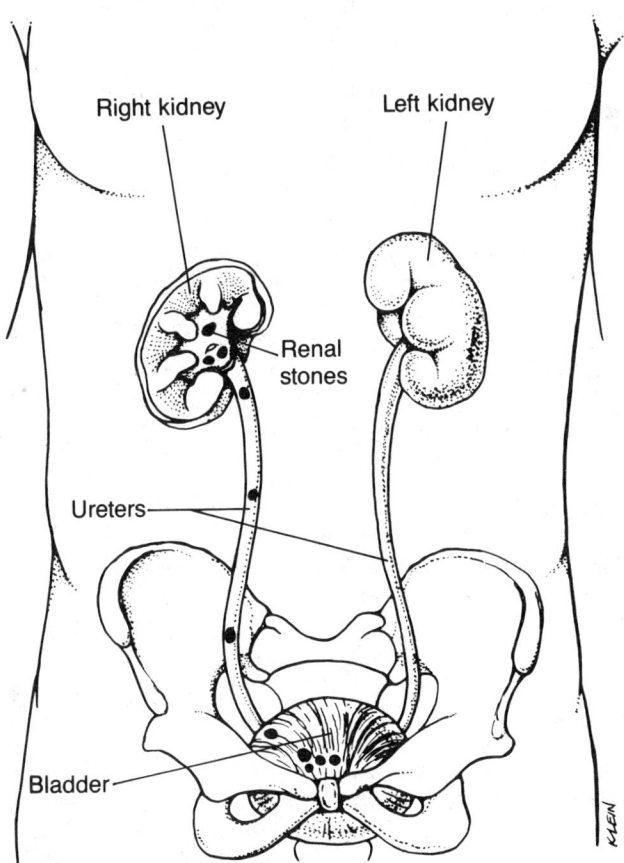

Figure 40-3
Various sites of calculous disease of the urinary tract (urolithiasis).

*p*H, and total volume are part of the diagnostic workup. A dietary and drug history and family history of renal stones are obtained to identify factors predisposing the patient to the formation of stones.

Management

The basic goals underlying the management of the patient's disease are to eradicate the stone, to determine the stone type, to prevent nephron destruction, to control infection, and to relieve any obstruction that may be present. Infection and back-pressure of obstructed urine can destroy the renal parenchyma.

The immediate objective of treatment for renal or ureteral colic is to relieve the pain until its cause can be eliminated; morphine or meperidine is administered to prevent shock and syncope that may result from the excruciating pain. Hot baths or moist heat to the flank areas is also useful. Unless the patient is vomiting, fluids are encouraged, since this treatment tends to increase the hydrostatic pressure behind the stone and thus assists it in its downward passage. A high round-the-clock fluid intake reduces the concentration of urinary crystalloids and ensures a high urinary output. Encouraging fluid intake also lowers the specific gravity of the urine.

Cystoscopic examination and passage of a small ureteral catheter to dislodge the obstructive stone (when possible) immediately relieves back-pressure on the kidney and alleviates the intense pain.

When stones are recovered, chemical analysis is carried out to determine their composition. For example, calcium oxalate or calcium phosphate stones usually indicate disorders of oxalate or calcium metabolism, while urate stones suggest a disturbance in uric acid metabolism. Struvite stones (infection stones) account for 15% to 20% of urinary calculi. Specific antibacterial agents are administered if infection is present.

Diet and Drug Therapy. Diet therapy is most effective when stones are caused by metabolic abnormalities resulting in increased excretion of stone constituents (hypercalciuria) or altered physiochemical properties of the urine (urine acidity). Most stones contain calcium combined with phosphate or other substances. For these patients, the diet selected is moderately reduced in calcium and phosphorus content (Chart 40-2). The urine is acidified. Sometimes stones will cease enlarging simply by ensuring an adequate fluid intake and limiting certain foods in the diet that make up the main ingredient of the stone (*e.g.,* calcium).

Sodium cellulose phosphate has been reported to be effective in preventing calcium stones. It binds calcium from food in the intestinal tract, reducing the amount of calcium absorbed into the circulation. If increased parathormone production (resulting in increased serum calcium levels in blood and urine) is a factor in formation of stones, thiazide therapy may be beneficial in reducing the calcium loss in the urine and lowering the elevated parathormone levels.

Patients who develop phosphatic calculi may have a diet low in phosphorus prescribed (see Chart 40-2). To offset excess phosphorus, aluminum hydroxide gel often is prescribed, since it combines with the excess phosphorus, causing it to be excreted through the intestinal tract rather than in the urinary system.

Chart 40-2
Moderately Calcium- and Phosphorus-Restricted Diet Plan*

Foods Used

Milk: Limited to 1 cup (½ pint) a day. Cream may be substituted for part of the milk.
Cheese: Pot or cottage cheese only; limited to 2 oz.
Fats: As desired.
Eggs: Limited to 1 a day; egg whites as desired.
Meat, fish, fowl: Limited to 4 oz daily of beef, lamb, pork, veal, chicken, turkey, fish. See those to be avoided.
Soups and broths: All; cream soups made with milk allowance only.
Vegetables: At least 3 servings besides potato. One or 2 servings of deep green or deep yellow vegetables to be included daily. See list of those to be avoided.
Fruits: All except rhubarb. Include citrus fruit daily.
Breads, cereals, Italian pastas: White, enriched bread, rolls, and crackers except those made from self-rising white flour; farina (not enriched); cornflakes; corn meal; hominy grits; rice; Rice Krispies; Puffed Rice; macaroni; spaghetti; noodles.

Desserts: Fruit pies, fruit cobblers, fruit ices, gelatin, puddings made with allowed milk and egg, angel food cake. (Do not use packaged mixes.)
Beverages: Coffee, Postum, Sanka, tea, gingerale.
Condiments: Sugar, jellies, honey, salt, pepper, spices.

Foods to Be Avoided

Cheese: All except pot or cottage cheese.
Meats, fish, fowl: Brains, heart, liver, kidney, sweetbreads, game (pheasant, rabbit, deer, grouse), sardines, fish roe.
Vegetables: Beet greens, chard, collards, mustard greens, spinach, turnip greens, dried beans, peas, lentils, soybeans.
Fruits: Rhubarb.
Breads, cereals, Italian pastas: Whole-grain breads, cereals, and crackers, rye bread; all breads made with self-rising flour; oatmeal; brown and wild rice; bran; Bran Flakes; wheat germ; all dry cereals except those allowed.
Desserts: All except those allowed.
Beverages: Carbonated "soft" drinks, cocoa.
Miscellaneous: Nuts, peanut butter, chocolate, cocoa, condiments having a calcium or a phosphate base (read labels).

* This diet will contain from 500 to 700 mg of calcium and from 1000 to 1200 mg of phosphorus.
(Anderson L et al. Nutrition in Health and Disease, 17th ed. Philadelphia, JB Lippincott Co.)

For uric acid stones, the patient is placed on a low-purine diet to reduce the output of uric acid in the urine. Foods high in purine (shellfish and organ meats) are avoided, and other proteins may be limited. Allopurinol (Zyloprim) may be given to reduce serum and urinary uric acid excretion. The urine is alkalinized. For cystine stones, a low-protein diet is given, the urine is alkalinized, and penicillamine is given to reduce the amount of cystine in the urine.

For oxalate stones, a dilute urine is maintained and the intake of oxalate is limited. This means avoiding green, leafy vegetables, beans, celery, beets, rhubarb, chocolate, tea, coffee, and peanuts.

If the stone cannot be passed spontaneously or complications occur, the stone must be removed surgically or through a percutaneous nephrostomy. It may also be fragmented through extracorporeal shock wave lithotripsy (ESWL) or dissolved.

Surgical Removal. Surgical intervention is indicated if the stone is causing obstruction, unremitting pain, infection that does not respond to treatment, or progressive renal damage. Surgery is also done to correct any anatomical abnormalities within the kidney to improve urinary drainage.

If the stone is in the kidney, the operation performed may be a *nephrolithotomy* (incision into the kidney with removal of the stone) or a *nephrectomy*, if the kidney is non-functional secondary to infection or hydronephrosis. Stones in the kidney pelvis are removed by a *pyelolithotomy*, those in the ureter by *ureterolithotomy*, and those in the bladder by *cystotomy*. Sometimes an instrument is inserted through the urethra into the bladder, and the stone is crushed in the jaws of this instrument. Such an operation is called a *cystolitholapaxy*.

In prolonged operations for the removal of branched or multiple renal calculi, extracorporeal surgery allows better visualization and provides access for irrigation to remove stone fragments (see p. 1025). The postoperative nursing management following kidney surgery is discussed on page 1029.

Endourologic Methods of Stone Removal. The field of endourology integrates the skills of the radiologist and urologist to extract renal calculi without major surgery. A percutaneous nephrostomy is performed (see p. 1026), and a nephroscope is introduced through the dilated percutaneous tract into the renal parenchyma. Depending on its size, the stone may be extracted with forceps or by a stone basket or an ultrasound probe is introduced through the nephrostomy tube and ultrasonic waves are used to pulverize the stone. Small stone fragments and stone dust are irrigated and suctioned out of the collecting system. Larger stones may be further reduced by ultrasonic disintegration and then removed with forceps or stone basket. Using a similar method, an electrical discharge is used to create a hydraulic shock wave to crack the stone (electrohydraulic lithotripsy). A probe is passed through the cystoscope, and the tip of the lithotriptor is placed near the stone. The strength of the discharge and pulse frequency can be varied. This procedure is performed under topical anesthesia.

After stone extraction, the percutaneous nephrostomy tube is left in place for a time to ensure that the ureter is not obstructed from edema or blood clots. The most common complications are hemorrhage, infection, and urinary extravasation. Only a very small skin incision is required to remove the stone, a shorter hospital stay is required, and postoperative morbidity is minimal. After tube removal, the nephrostomy tract closes spontaneously.

Extracorporeal Shock Wave Lithotripsy. Extracorporeal shock wave lithotripsy (ESWL; Fig. 40-4) is a new, nonsurgical procedure used to break up stones in the calyx of the kidney. After the stones are reduced to small fragments the size of grains of sand, the remnants of the stones are passed in the urine through the lower urinary tract and voided.

Lithotripsy is carried out after the patient is given anesthesia (epidural or general anesthesia) and is lowered into a water bath. Shock waves are generated by the lithotriptor, transmitted through the water bath, and directed precisely at the stone identified in the renal pelvis by fluoroscopy. The shock waves are timed with the patient's electrocardiogram to prevent cardiac dysrhythmias. Multiple shocks are necessary, with their number depending on the size of the kidney stone to be fragmented. Although the shock waves usually do not damage other tissue, discomfort from the multiple shocks may occur. Additionally, the patient is observed for damage to lung tissue as well as obstruction and infection resulting from blockage of the urinary tract by stone fragments. All urine is strained following the procedure; voided gravel or sand is sent to the laboratory for chemical analysis. The patient is encouraged to increase his fluid intake to assist in passage of stone fragments, which may occur for 6 weeks to several months after the procedure.

Although lithotripsy is a costly treatment, it is expected to decrease hospital stay and expenses by reducing the amount of time required by the patient to recover, since an invasive surgical procedure to remove the kidney stone is avoided.

Stone Dissolution. Infusions of chemolytic solutions (*e.g.*, alkylating agents, acidifying agents) for the purpose of stone dissolution may be done as an alternative to surgery in patients who are poor risks or have easily dissolved (struvite) stones. Usually, a percutaneous nephrostomy is performed (see p. 1026) and the warm irrigating solution is allowed to flow continuously onto the stone. The irrigating solution leaves the renal collecting system via the ureter or the nephrostomy tube. The pressure inside the renal pelvis is monitored during the procedure.

▶ *Nursing Process* *The Patient With Renal Stones*

▷ *Assessment*

The patient with suspected renal stones is assessed for pain and discomfort. The severity and location of pain are assessed along with the area of radiation of the pain. The patient is also assessed for the presence of associated symptoms such as nausea, vomiting, diarrhea, and abdominal distention. Additionally, the nursing assessment includes observations for signs of urinary tract infection (chills, fever, dysuria, frequency, and hesitancy) and obstruction (frequent urination of small amounts, oliguria, or anuria). The urine is observed for the presence of blood and strained for stones or gravel.

The history focuses on factors that predispose the patient to urinary tract stones or that may have precipitated the current episode of renal or ureteral colic. Factors that predispose

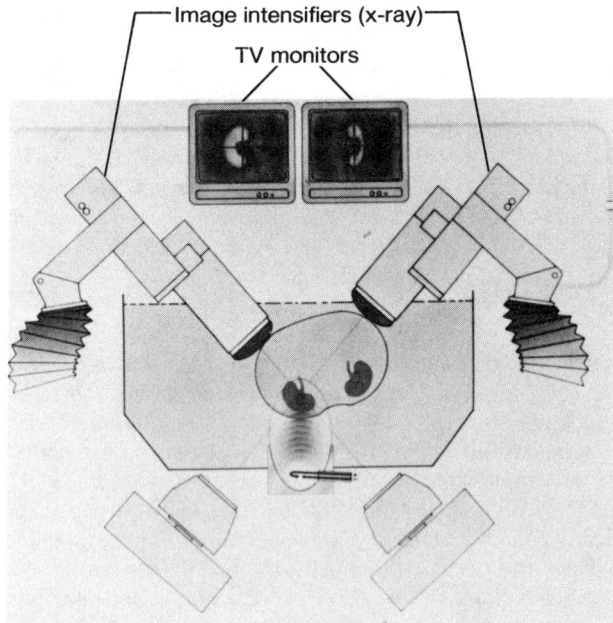

A

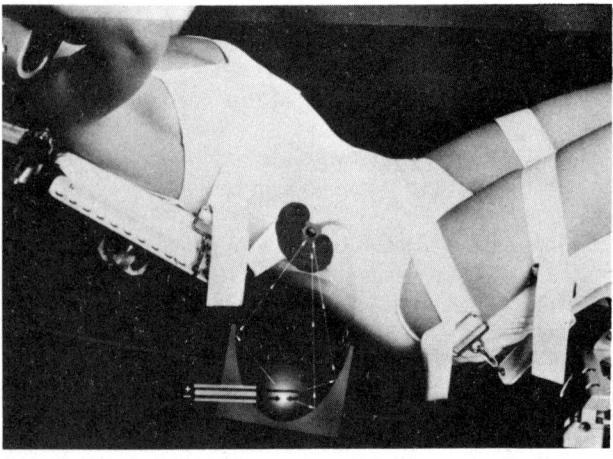

C

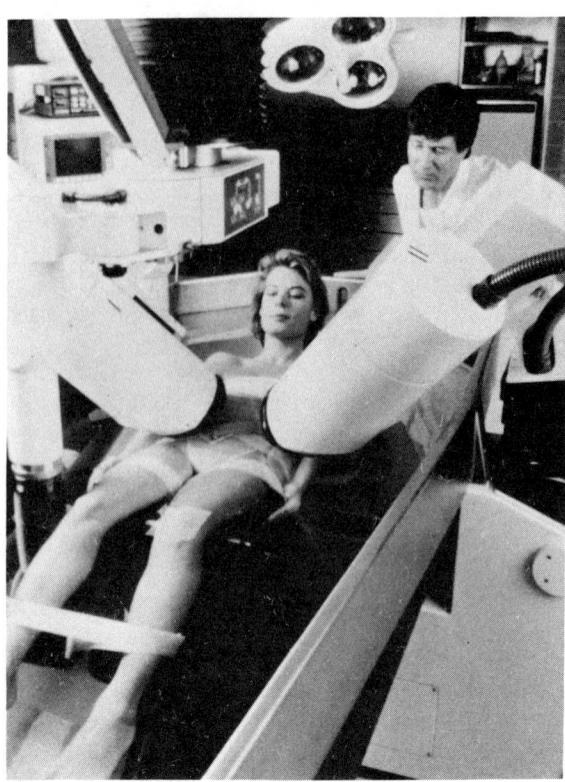

B

Figure 40-4
Extracorporeal shock wave lithotripsy (ESWL).
(*A*) Schematic diagram of the lithotripter directed
toward a stone located in a patient's kidney (seen
in cross-section). The patient is positioned to
ensure precise three-dimensional localization of the
kidney stone using fluoroscopy to visualize the
stone on the TV monitors. (*B*) Patient positioned in
the water bath for treatment, (*C*) Shock waves are
directed at the kidney stone. (Courtesy of Dornier
Medical Systems, Inc.)

the patient to stone formation may include family history of
stones, the presence of cancer or bone marrow disorders or
use of chemotherapeutic agents, inflammatory bowel disease,
or a diet high in calcium or purines. Factors that may precipitate stone formation in the patient predisposed to renal calculi
include episodes of dehydration, prolonged immobilization,
and infection. The patient's knowledge about renal stones
and measures to prevent their occurrence or recurrence is
also assessed.

▷ Nursing Diagnoses

Based on the assessment data, the nursing diagnoses of the
patient with renal stones may include the following:

- Alterations in pain and discomfort related to inflammation, obstruction, and abrasion of the urinary tract
- Potential for infection and obstruction related to blockage of the urinary tract by a stone or edema
- Knowledge deficit regarding prevention of recurrence
  of renal stones

▷ Planning and Implementation

▷ *Goals:*   The patient's major goals may include relief of
pain and discomfort, prevention of infection and obstruction,
and prevention of recurrence of renal stones.

Nursing Interventions

Relieving Pain.   Immediate relief of severe pain from
renal or ureteral colic is promoted through use of narcotic
analgesics as prescribed. Intravenous or intramuscular administration may be prescribed to provide rapid relief and
prevent shock from developing as a result of the excruciating
pain. Moist heat to the flank may also be prescribed and may
provide some relief. The patient is encouraged and assisted
to assume a position of comfort. If the patient obtains some
pain relief by ambulating, he is assisted to do so. The patient's
pain is monitored closely, and increases in severity are reported promptly to the physician so that relief can be provided
and additional treatment initiated. The patient is prepared

for other treatment (*e.g.*, surgery, lithotripsy) if severe pain is unrelieved and the stone is not passed spontaneously.

Preventing Infection and Obstruction. The patient with suspected renal stones is at risk of infection and obstruction of the urinary tract. He is instructed to report decreased urine volume and bloody or cloudy urine. The total urine output as well as patterns of voiding are monitored. Increased fluid intake will be encouraged to prevent dehydration and increase hydrostatic pressure within the urinary tract to promote passage of the stone. If the patient is unable to take adequate fluids orally, intravenous fluids will be prescribed. The patient is assisted with walking since ambulation may help to move the stone through the urinary tract.

The nursing care of patients with calculi requires constant observation to detect the spontaneous passage of a stone. All urine should be strained through gauze, since uric acid stones may crumble. Any blood clots passed in the urine should be crushed and the sides of the urinal and bedpan inspected for clinging stones.

Patient Education and Home Health Care. Because it is known that urinary calculi may recur after the first stone is found, the patient is encouraged to follow a regimen to avoid further stone formation. One facet of prevention is to *maintain a high fluid intake* since stones form more readily in a concentrated urine. A patient who has shown a tendency to form stones should drink enough to excrete 3000 to 4000 ml of urine every 24 hours, should adhere to the prescribed diet, and should avoid sudden increases in environmental temperatures, which may cause a fall in urinary volume. Occupations and sports that produce excessive sweating can lead to severe temporary dehydration; therefore, fluid intake should be increased. Sufficient fluids should be taken in the evening to prevent urine from becoming too concentrated at night. Urine cultures are done every 1 to 2 months the first year and periodically thereafter. Recurrent urinary infection must be treated vigorously.

Since prolonged immobilization slows renal drainage and alters calcium metabolism, increased mobility is to be encouraged whenever possible. In addition, excessive ingestion of vitamins (especially vitamin D) and minerals should be discouraged.

If medications are prescribed for prevention of stone formation, the actions and importance of the medications are explained to the patient. Additionally, detailed information about foods to be included and excluded are provided verbally and in writing. The patient may be instructed to monitor his urinary *p*H; he will be instructed by the nurse about the procedures of determining the *p*H and interpreting the results. Because of the high risk of recurrence, the patient with renal stones is taught the signs and symptoms of stone formation, obstruction, and infection. He is directed to report these to the physician promptly.

▷ *Evaluation*

▷ *Expected Outcomes*

1. Patient experiences relief of pain.
   a. Reports decreased pain and discomfort.
   b. Assumes a position of comfort.
   c. Ambulates progressively with assistance.
   d. Requests analgesia as prescribed.
   e. Uses moist heat to flank area and hot baths to relieve discomfort.
   f. Exhibits no signs of pain-induced shock or syncope.
2. Exhibits no indications of urinary tract infection or obstruction.
   a. Voids clear urine without red blood cells.
   b. Voids 200 to 400 ml of urine/voiding.
   c. Reports absence of dysuria, frequency, hesitancy.
   d. Exhibits normal body temperature.
   e. Reports no chills.
3. Exhibits increased knowledge of health behaviors to prevent recurrence.
   a. Consumes high fluid intake (10 to 12 glasses of fluid/day).
   b. Voids dilute urine that is clear in color and free of blood.
   c. Identifies actions to take to avoid dehydration.
   d. Avoids prolonged periods of immobilization and activity if possible.
   e. Consumes diet prescribed to reduce dietary factors predisposing to stone formation (high calcium, phosphorus, oxalate, or purine foods).
   f. Identifies symptoms to be reported to health care provider (fever, chills, flank pain, hematuria).
   g. Monitors urinary *p*H as directed.
   h. Takes prescribed medication as directed to reduce stone formation.

Renal Tumors

Renal tumors may arise from the renal capsule, parenchyma (renal cell carcinomas), connective tissue (sarcomas), or fatty tissue, or they may be neurogenic or vascular. Almost 90% of all tumors are adenocarcinomas. These tumors occur more frequently in males and may metastasize early to the lungs, bone, liver, brain, and contralateral kidney. One fourth to one half of patients will have metastatic disease at the time of diagnosis.

Clinical Manifestations

Many renal tumors produce no symptoms and are discovered on a routine physical examination as a palpable abdominal mass. The classic triad, occurring late in the course of the disease, is blood in the urine (hematuria), pain, and a mass in the flank. *The usual sign that first calls attention to the tumor is painless hematuria,* which may be either intermittent and microscopic or gross. There may be a dull pain in the back from back-pressure produced by compression of the ureter, extension of the tumor into the perirenal area, or hemorrhage into the substance of the kidney. Colicky pains occur if a clot or mass of tumor cells passes down the ureter. Symptoms from metastasis may be the first manifestation of renal tumor and include unexplained weight loss, increasing weakness, and anemia.

The diagnosis of renal tumor may require intravenous urography, cystoscopic examination, nephrotomograms, renal angiograms, ultrasonography, or computed tomography (CT scan). These tests may be exhausting for a patient already debilitated by the systemic effects of a tumor, for the elderly patient, and for one anxious about the diagnosis and outcome. The nurse assists the patient physically and psychologically in preparation for these procedures and monitors him carefully for signs of dehydration and exhaustion.

Management

The goal of management is to eradicate the tumor before metastasis occurs. A radical nephrectomy is the preferred treatment if the tumor can be removed. This includes removal of the kidney (and tumor), adrenal gland, surrounding perinephric fat and Gerota's fascia, and lymph nodes. In patients with a solitary kidney or with bilateral renal tumors, extracorporeal renal surgery in which the kidney is removed, surgically treated, and then reinserted (as described on p. 1025), allows a meticulous dissection and separation of the tumor from surrounding normal renal tissue. (See pp. 1029–1031 for nursing management following renal surgery.) Radiation therapy may be used adjunctively with surgery. Chemotherapy or hormonal therapy may be tried. Immunotherapy may be helpful.

Renal Artery Embolization.   In patients with metastatic renal carcinoma, embolization of the renal artery is performed to cut off the blood supply to the tumor and thus cause the death of tumor cells. In other words, an infarct (area of dead cells) is created. Several days after completion of angiographic studies, a catheter is advanced into the renal artery, and embolizing materials (Gelfoam, autologous blood clot, steel coils) are injected into the artery and carried with the arterial blood flow to mechanically occlude the tumor vessels. This decreases the local blood supply, making removal of the kidney (nephrectomy) easier, and theoretically stimulates an immune response. This is based on the concept that infarction of the renal cell carcinoma will release tumor-associated antigens that will enhance the patient's response to metastatic lesions. The procedure may also reduce the number of tumor cells entering the venous circulation during surgical manipulation.

Following renal artery embolization and tumor infarction, a characteristic symptom-complex labeled ''postinfarction syndrome'' occurs, lasting 2 to 3 days. The patient has pain localized to the flank and abdomen, an elevated temperature, and gastrointestinal complaints. Pain is treated with parenteral analgesics, while aspirin controls the fever; antiemetics, restriction of oral intake, and maintenance with intravenous fluids are used to treat the gastrointestinal complaints.

Nursing Interventions

The patient with a renal tumor may undergo extensive diagnostic and therapeutic procedures, including surgery, radiation therapy, and chemotherapy. Following surgery, the patient usually has catheters and drains in place to ensure a patent urinary tract, to remove drainage, and to permit very accurate measurement of urine output. Because of the location of the surgical incision and the position of the patient during the surgical procedure, pain and muscle soreness are common. The patient requires frequent analgesia during the postoperative period and assistance with turning. He needs to be encouraged to turn, cough, and take deep breaths to prevent atelectasis and other pulmonary complications. The patient and his family require assistance and support to cope

with the diagnosis and uncertainties about outcome. (See Chapter 39 for postoperative care of the patient undergoing renal surgery and Chapter 16 for care of the oncology patient).

Follow-up care is essential to detect signs of metastases as well as to reassure the patient and family about the patient's continued well-being. The patient who has had surgery for renal carcinoma should undergo a yearly physical and roentgen examination of the chest throughout life, since late metastases are not uncommon. All subsequent symptoms should be evaluated with possible metastases in mind.

Renal Cysts

Cysts of the kidney may be multiple (polycystic) or single. Polycystic disease of the adult is inherited as an autosomal dominant trait and usually involves both kidneys. The patient presents with abdominal or lumbar pain, hematuria, hypertension, palpable renal masses, and recurrent urinary tract infections. Renal insufficiency and failure usually develop in the terminal stages. Polycystic renal disease is also associated with cystic diseases of other organs (liver, pancreas, spleen) and aneurysms of the cerebral arteries. It is characteristically seen in midlife.

Management.   Since there is no specific treatment for polycystic renal disease, care of the patient is directed toward relief of pain, symptoms, and complications. Hypertension and urinary tract infections are treated aggressively. Dialysis is indicated when signs of renal insufficiency and failure occur. Genetic counseling is part of patient education, since polycystic kidney disease is a hereditary disease. The patient is advised to avoid sports and occupations that present a risk of trauma to the kidney.

Simple cysts of the kidney usually occur unilaterally and differ clinically and pathophysiologically from polycystic kidney disease. The cyst may be drained percutaneously.

Congenital Anomalies

Congenital anomalies of the kidney are not uncommon. Occasionally, there is fusion of the two kidneys, forming what is called a *horseshoe kidney*. One kidney may be small and deformed and often is nonfunctioning. Not infrequently there may be a double ureter or congenital stricture of the ureter. The treatment of these anomalies is necessary only if they cause symptoms, but it is important to determine that the other kidney is present and functioning before surgery is undertaken.

Renal Trauma

Various types of injuries of the flank, back, or upper abdomen may result in bruising, lacerations, or rupture of the kidney or pedicle injury. The kidneys are protected by the musculature of the back posteriorly and by a cushion of abdominal wall and viscera anteriorly. They are highly mobile and are ''fixed'' only at the renal pedicle. With traumatic injury, the kidney can be thrust against the lower ribs, resulting in contusion and rupture. Rib fractures occurring with renal displacement or a fracture of the transverse process of the upper lumbar vertebrae may be associated with renal contusion or laceration. Injuries may be blunt (auto and motorcycle accidents, falls, athletic injuries) or penetrating (gunshot wounds, stabbings). Renal trauma is frequently associated with other injuries.

The most common renal injuries are contusions, laceration, rupture, and renal pedicle injuries or small internal laceration of the kidney. The kidneys receive half of the blood flow from the abdominal aorta; therefore, a fairly small renal laceration can produce massive bleeding.

Clinical Manifestations. The clinical manifestations include pain, renal colic (due to clots/fragments obstructing the collecting system), hematuria, flank mass, ecchymoses, and lacerations or wounds of the lateral abdomen and flank.

Management. The goals of management are to control hemorrhage, pain, and infection; to preserve and restore renal function; and to maintain urinary drainage.

Hematuria is the most common manifestation of renal trauma; therefore, the appearance of blood in the urine following an injury to the loin indicates the possibility of renal injury. There is no correlation between the degree of hematuria and the degree of injury. Hematuria may be absent or detectable only on microscopic examination. Therefore, all urine is saved and sent to the laboratory for analysis to detect the presence of red cells and to follow the course of bleeding. The time the urine is voided and the volume should be recorded. Decreased hematocrit and hemoglobin levels indicate hemorrhage.

The patient is monitored for oliguria and signs of hemorrhagic shock since a pedicle injury or shattered kidney can lead to rapid exsanguination (lethal blood loss). An expanding hematoma may cause rupture of the kidney capsule. To detect the presence of hematoma, the area around the lower ribs, upper lumbar vertebrae, flank, and abdomen is palpated for tenderness. A palpable flank or abdominal mass with local tenderness, swelling, and ecchymosis suggests renal hemorrhage or extravasation. The area of the original mass can be outlined with a marking pencil so that the observer can evaluate the area for change. Skin abrasions, lacerations, and entry and exit wounds in the muscles of the upper abdomen, flank, and lower thoracic regions are important signs to check. Severe flank or costovertebral pain may signal a pedicle injury, which can cause ischemic necrosis of the kidney. It is important to remember that renal trauma is often associated with other injuries to the abdominal organs (liver, colon, small intestines).

In minor injuries to the kidney, healing may take place with conservative measures. The patient is kept on bed rest until hematuria clears. Intravenous infusions may be necessary, because retroperitoneal bleeding may produce a reflex paralytic ileus.

Antimicrobial drugs may be given to prevent infection from perirenal hematoma or urinoma (a cyst containing urine). Patients with retroperitoneal hematomas may develop a low-grade fever as absorption of the clot takes place.

The patient should be evaluated frequently during the first few days following injury in order to detect flank and abdominal pain, muscle spasm, and swelling over the flank.

- Any *sudden* change in the patient's condition may indicate hemorrhage and require surgical intervention. The

vital signs are monitored to detect evidence of bleeding. Narcotic analgesia is avoided since this may mask accompanying abdominal symptoms.
- The patient is prepared for surgical exploration if increasing pulse rate, hypotension, and impending shock occur.

Most penetrating injuries require surgical exploration because of the high incidence of involvement of other organ systems and serious complications if untreated. The damaged kidney may have to be removed (nephrectomy), although on occasion it is possible to repair it.

The postoperative management is discussed on pages 1029–1031. Early complications (within 6 months) include rebleeding, abscess, sepsis, urine extravasation, and fistula formation.

Patient Education and Home Health Care. Follow-up care includes monitoring the blood pressure to detect hypertension that may occur on a renovascular basis. Other complications include stone formation, infection, cysts, vascular aneurysms, and loss of renal function. Activity is usually restricted for 1 month following trauma to minimize the incidence of delayed or secondary bleeding. The patient is instructed about what changes should be reported to the physician. Guidelines for increasing activity gradually are also provided.

Bladder Injuries

Injury to the bladder may occur with pelvic fractures and multiple trauma or from a blow to the lower abdomen when the bladder is full. Blunt trauma may result in contusion (an ecchymosis or large discolored bruise resulting from escape of blood into the tissues and involving a segment of the bladder wall) or in rupture of the bladder, extraperitoneally, intraperitoneally, or a combination of both. Complications from these injuries (hemorrhage, shock, sepsis, and extravasation of blood into the tissues) must be treated promptly.

A retrograde urethrogram is done first to evaluate for urethral injury. The patient is catheterized after the urethrogram is done.

Management. Treatment for traumatic rupture of the bladder involves immediate surgical exploration and repair of the laceration, with suprapubic drainage of the bladder and the perivesical space (around the bladder) along with insertion of an urethral indwelling catheter.

In addition to the usual postoperative care following urologic surgery (see pp. 1029–1031), the drainage systems (suprapubic, indwelling urethral catheter, and perivesical drains) are observed to ensure adequate drainage until healing takes place. The patient with a ruptured bladder may have gross bleeding for several days after repair. Complications of urethral injuries include stricture, incontinence, and impotence.

Cancer of the Bladder

Cancer of the urinary bladder is seen more frequently in persons from age 50 onward and affects men more than women (3:1). Statistics indicate that these tumors make up approximately 2% of all cancers in the body and are on the increase. The most common type is transitional cell cancer.

Risk factors for cancer of the bladder include cigarette smoking and carcinogens in the work environment, such as dyes, rubber, leather, ink, or paint. There may be a relationship between coffee drinking and bladder cancer. Chronic schistosomiasis (parasitic infection that irritates the bladder) is also a risk factor. Cancers arising from the prostate, colon, and rectum in males and from the lower gynecologic tract in females may metastasize to the bladder.

Clinical Manifestations. These tumors usually arise at the base of the bladder and involve the ureteral orifices and bladder neck. *Gross, painless hematuria* is the most common symptom of cancer of the bladder. Infection of the urinary tract is a common complication, producing frequency, urgency, and dysuria. However, any disturbance of micturition or change in the urine may indicate cancer of the bladder. Pelvic or back pain may be due to metastasis.

The diagnostic evaluation may include excretory urography, computed tomography (CT scan), ultrasonography, cystoscopy, and bimanual examination under anesthesia. Biopsies of the tumor and mucosa adjacent to the tumor are the definitive diagnostic procedures.

Transitional cell carcinomas and carcinomas *in situ* shed recognizable cancer cells. Cytologic examination of fresh urine and saline bladder washings provide information about the patient's prognosis, especially for those at high risk for recurrence of primary bladder tumors.

Management. Treatment of bladder cancer depends on the grade of the tumor (based on the degree of cellular differentiation), the stage of growth (the degree of local invasion and the presence or absence of metastasis), and the multicentricity (having many centers) of the tumor. The patient's age and physical, mental, and emotional status are considered in determining treatment modalities.

Transurethral resection or fulguration may be done for simple papillomas (benign epithelial tumors), although aggressive malignancies may develop from these tumors. These procedures eradicate the tumors through surgical incision or electrical current using instruments inserted through the urethra. One of the greatest challenges is the management of superficial bladder cancers, as it is now known that there are widespread abnormalities in the bladder mucosa of these patients. The entire lining of the urinary tract, or urothelium, is at risk, since carcinomatous changes are not only found in the mucosa of the bladder but also in that of the renal pelvis, ureter, and urethra. Recurrences are a serious problem, and approximately 60% of superficial bladder tumors recur after transurethral resection or fulguration. Persons with benign papillomas should be followed with cytology and cystoscopy periodically for the rest of their lives.

Topical chemotherapy (intravesical chemotherapy or instillation of antineoplastic agents into the bladder so that they come in contact with the bladder wall) is considered when there is high risk of recurrence, when cancer *in situ* is present, or when tumor resection has been incomplete. Topical chemotherapy delivers a high concentration of drug (thiotepa, doxorubicin, 5-fluorouracil) to the tumor to promote tumor destruction. Fluid intake may be limited during instillation of the drug to prevent the need to void during the procedure, which takes approximately 2 hours. At the conclusion, the patient is encouraged to void and drink liberal amounts of fluid to flush the drug from the bladder.

The tumor may be irradiated preoperatively to reduce microextension of the neoplasm and viability of tumor cells, thus reducing the chances that the cancer may recur in the immediate area or spread by way of the circulatory or lymphatic systems. Radiation therapy is also used in combination with surgery or to control the disease in the inoperable patient.

A simple cystectomy (removal of the bladder) or a radical cystectomy is done for invasive or multifocal bladder cancer. Radical cystectomy in the male involves removal of the bladder, prostate, and seminal vesicles and immediate adjacent perivesical tissues. In the female, radical cystectomy involves removal of the bladder, lower ureter, uterus, tubes, ovaries, anterior vagina, and urethra. It may or may not include a pelvic lymphadenectomy (removal of lymph nodes). Removal of the bladder requires a urinary diversion procedure (see below).

The transitional cell variety of bladder cancer responds poorly to chemotherapy. Cisplatin, doxorubicin, and cyclophosphamide have been administered in various doses and schedules and appear most effective.

Bladder cancer may also be treated by direct infusion of the cytotoxic agent through the arterial supply of the involved organ. Thus, a higher concentration of the chemotherapeutic agent can be achieved with lessened toxicity to the system. For more advanced bladder cancer or for patients with intractable hematuria (especially following radiation therapy), a large water-filled balloon placed within the bladder produces tumor necrosis by reducing the blood supply of the bladder wall (hydrostatic therapy). The instillation of formalin, phenol, or silver nitrate has achieved relief of hematuria and strangury (slow and painful discharge of urine) in some patients.

Urinary Diversion

Urinary diversion refers to a means of diverting the urinary stream from the bladder so that it exits via a new route and opening in the skin (stoma). This is done primarily when a large or invasive bladder tumor requires that the entire bladder be removed. Other conditions requiring urinary diversion include pelvic malignancy, birth defects, strictures and trauma to ureters and urethra, neurogenic bladder, and chronic infection causing severe ureteral and renal damage.

There is controversy concerning the best means of establishing permanent diversion of the urinary tract. The age of the patient, condition of the bladder, body build, degree of obesity, degree of ureteral dilation, state of renal function, and the patient's acceptance of the results of the procedure and his learning ability are all taken into consideration.

The most common methods of urinary diversion are listed below:

1. *Ileal conduit:* transplanting the ureters to an isolated section of the terminal ileum and bringing one end to the abdominal wall (Fig. 40-5A). The ureter may also be transplanted into the transverse colon (colon conduit) or proximal jejunum (jejunal conduit).

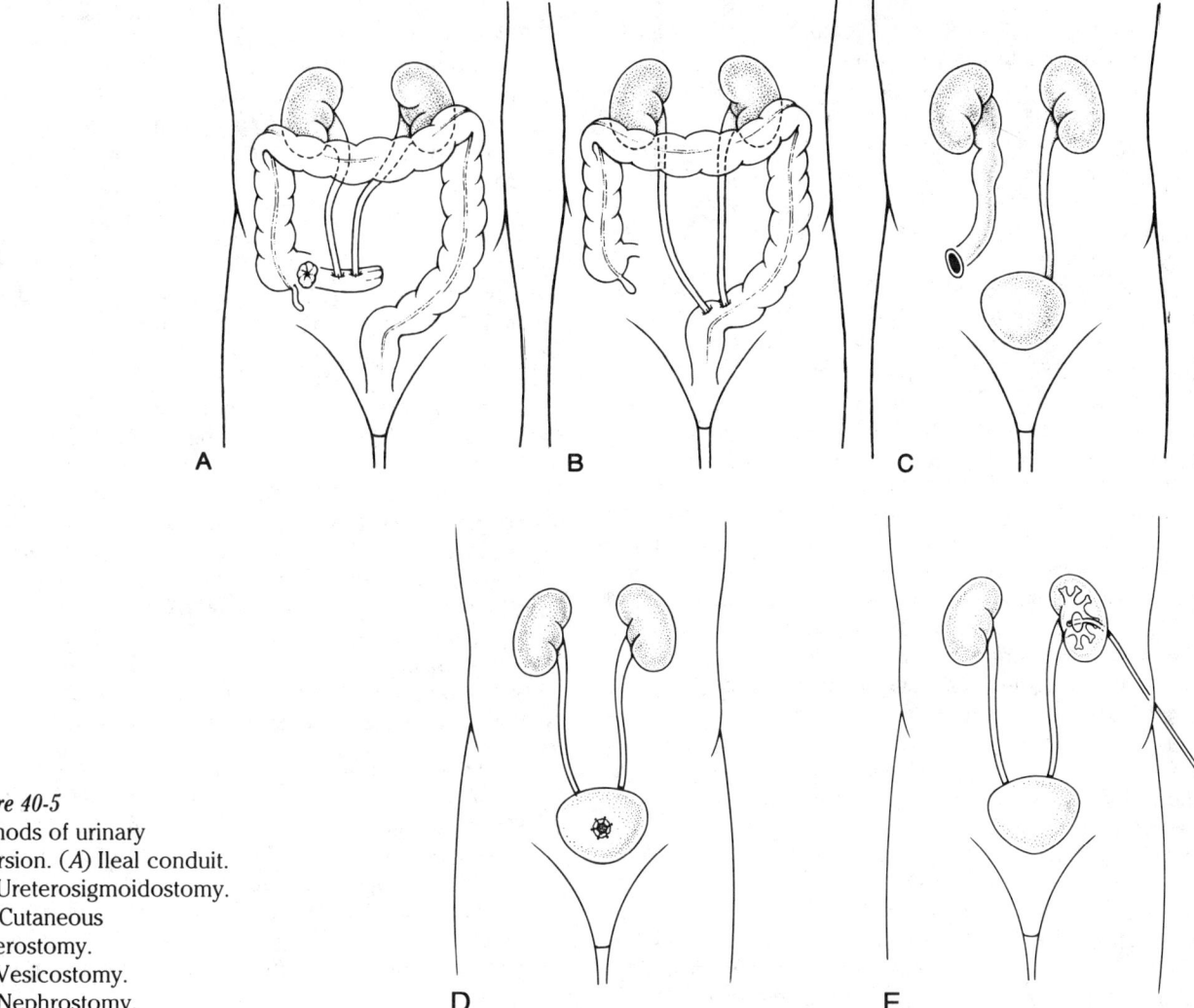

Figure 40-5
Methods of urinary
diversion. (*A*) Ileal conduit.
(*B*) Ureterosigmoidostomy.
(*C*) Cutaneous
ureterostomy.
(*D*) Vesicostomy.
(*E*) Nephrostomy.

2. *Ureterosigmoidostomy:* introducing the ureters into the sigmoid, thereby allowing urine to flow through the colon and out of the rectum (Fig. 40-5*B*).
3. *Cutaneous ureterostomy:* bringing the detached ureter through the abdominal wall and attaching it to an opening in the skin (Fig. 40-5*C*).
4. *Vesicostomy:* suturing the bladder to the abdominal wall and creating an opening (stoma) through the abdominal and bladder walls for urinary drainage (Fig. 40-5*D*).
5. *Nephrostomy:* inserting a catheter into the renal pelvis via an incision into the flank or by percutaneous catheter placement into the kidney (Fig. 40-5*E*).
6. *Continent ileal urinary reservoir (Kock pouch):* transplanting the ureters to an isolated segment of ileum (pouch) with a nipple-like one-way valve; urine is drained by catheter (Fig. 40-7, p. 1064.)

Ileal Conduit Urinary Diversion (Ileal Loop)

In an ileal conduit, the urine is diverted by implanting the ureter into a loop of ileum that is led out through the abdominal wall. This loop of ileum is a simple conduit (passageway)

for urine from the ureters to the surface. A loop of the sigmoid colon may also be used. An ileostomy bag is used to collect the urine. The resected (cut) ends of the remaining intestine are anastomosed (connected) to provide an intact bowel.

After surgery, a skin barrier and a transparent, disposable urinary drainage bag are applied around the conduit and connected to drainage. A temporary appliance is used until the edema subsides and the stoma shrinks to normal size. The clear bag allows the stoma to be visualized and the patency of the stent and the urinary output to be better monitored. The ileal bag drains urine constantly but not feces. The appliance (bag) usually remains in place as long as it is watertight. Then it is changed.

Nursing Interventions. Urine volumes are checked hourly, since an output below 30 ml/hr may indicate an obstruction in the ileal conduit with possible backflow or leakage from the ureteroileal anastomosis. A catheter may be inserted through the urinary conduit to check for possible stasis or residual urine from a tight stoma.

The stoma is inspected frequently for bleeding. Minimal bleeding may be seen and implies good blood supply. A change in color of the stoma from a normal pink to red color to a dark purplish color suggests that the vascular supply may be compromised. If cyanosis and compromised blood supply persist, surgical intervention may be required.

The stoma is insensitive to touch, but the skin around the stoma is exquisitely sensitive if it becomes irritated by urine or the appliance. The skin is inspected for (1) signs of irritation and bleeding of the stomal mucosa; (2) alkaline encrustation with skin irritation around the stoma (from alkaline urine coming in contact with exposed skin); and (3) wound infections.

The odor of urine around the patient should alert the nursing personnel to the possibility of leakage from the appliance, the presence of an infection, or a problem in hygienic management. Since severe alkaline encrustation can accumulate rapidly around the stoma, the urine *p*H is kept below 6.5. Urine *p*H can be determined by testing the urine draining from the stoma, not from the collecting appliance. A properly fitted appliance is essential to prevent the peristomal skin (skin around the stoma) from being exposed to urine. If the urine is foul smelling, the stoma may be catheterized if prescribed in order to obtain a specimen for culture and sensitivity or to determine if the stoma is patent and draining properly and to detect the presence of residual urine. Scarring of the stoma can interfere with urine drainage.

A high-fluid diet is encouraged, in order to flush the ileal conduit and prevent mucus from congealing. The patient may excrete a fairly large amount of mucus with the urine as a result of the urine's irritating the intestine. To relieve anxiety, the patient is reassured that this is a normal occurrence following an ileal conduit.

Complications. Complications following this method of urinary diversion include wound infection or wound dehiscence, urinary leakage, ureteral obstruction, small bowel obstruction, and stomal gangrene. Delayed complications include ureteral obstruction, contraction or narrowing of the stoma (stomal stenosis), pyelonephritis, and renal calculi.

Patient Education and Home Care

Appliance Selection. The urinary appliance may consist of one or two pieces and may be temporary/disposable (applied once and discarded) or semidisposable (reusable). The choice of appliance is determined by the location of the stoma and the patient's normal activity, body build, and economic status. A reusable appliance has a faceplate that is attached to the body with cement or adhesive. A semidisposable appliance has a reusable faceplate to which disposable pouches are attached. Disposable appliances are discarded after each use. They have the advantage of having a surface that is already prepared and of being lightweight and easy to conceal. See Fig. 40-6 for examples of appliances.

Determining the Stoma Size. As the postoperative edema subsides, the stoma opening is recalibrated every 3 to 6 weeks for the first few months postoperatively. The correct appliance size is determined by measuring the widest part of the stoma with a ruler. The permanent appliance should not be more than 1.6 mm ($^1/_{16}$ inch) larger than the diameter of the stoma to prevent skin reaction to the urine.

Changing the Appliance; Skin Care. The appliance is changed at a time that will be most convenient to the patient. Early in the morning, before drinking fluids, when urinary output is lower, is the most preferred time. Ideally, the collecting appliance is changed every 5 to 7 days.

- Prepare the new appliance according to the manufacturer's directions. (The center opening is tailored to the individual stomal opening.)
- Moisten the edge of the faceplate with water or adhesive solvent, or soap and water, and gently remove it. Adhesive solvent is not used if skin barriers are used.
- Instruct the patient to bend over quickly and remain in that position a minute to allow the conduit to empty before the skin is washed and dried.

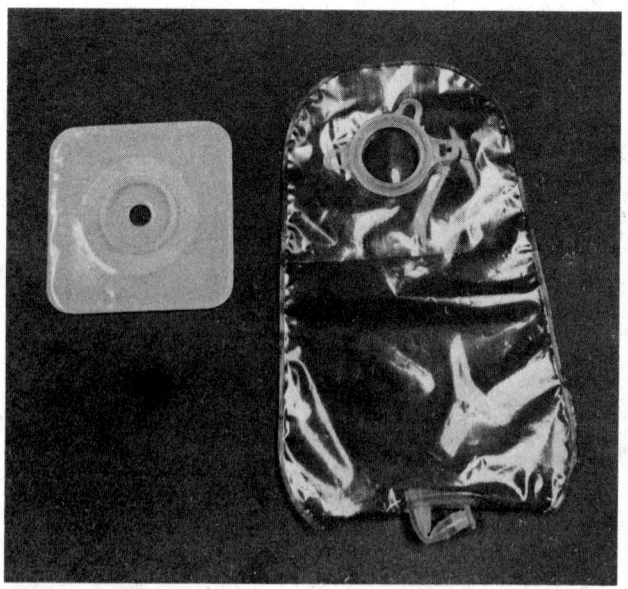
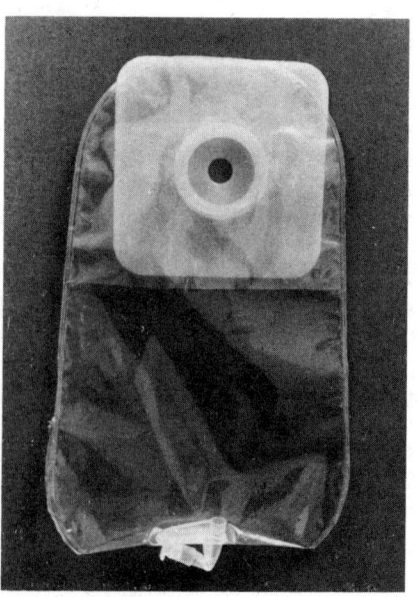

A   B

Figure 40-6
Skin-protective barrier used with urostomy pouch. (*A*) Squibb Stomahesive wafer (*left*) and Sur-Fit urostomy pouch (*right*). (*B*) Stomahesive wafer with pouch attached.

- Clean all adhesive cement from the skin with warm water or adhesive solvent, using a soft cloth. Wash the skin with a noncream-based soap and water. Rinse well, since a soap film will prevent the appliance from adhering to the skin. Pat dry. *The skin must be dry or the appliance will not adhere.*

  1. Insert a tampon or gauze or tissue wick at the stoma opening to absorb the urine and keep the skin dry while the appliance is being changed.
  2. Inspect the skin for signs of irritation. Keep the skin free from direct contact with urine.
  3. Apply a skin protector or barrier if required (Fig. 40-7). Center the appliance directly over the stoma and apply it carefully. Apply gentle pressure around the appliance to remove air bubbles and creases so that it will adhere securely.

- Apply hypoallergenic tape in a picture-frame effect around the pouch. The skin under the appliance may be dusted with pure talcum powder. An appliance cover may be used to absorb perspiration and eliminate warmth from the appliance.

Since the degree to which the stoma protrudes is not the same in all patients, there are various accessories and custom-made appliances to solve individual problems.

Odor Control. The patient should be advised to avoid foods and medications that give the urine a strong odor. A few drops of liquid deodorizer or diluted white vinegar may be introduced through the drain spout into the bottom of the pouch with a syringe or eyedropper. Taking ascorbic acid by mouth helps acidify the urine and suppresses urine odor problems. Also, the patient should be reminded that the pouch will develop an odor if it is worn too long and not cared for properly.

Managing the Ostomy Appliance. The pouch is emptied by a drain valve when it is one third to one half full, since the weight of the urine may cause it to separate from the skin. Some patients prefer wearing a leg bag attached with an adaptor to the drainage apparatus. To ensure uninterrupted sleep, the collecting bottle and tubing (one unit) are snapped onto an adaptor that screws into the ileal appliance. A small amount of urine is left in the bag when the adaptor is screwed on to prevent the bag from collapsing against itself. The tubing may be threaded down the pajama leg to prevent kinking.

Cleaning and Deodorizing the Appliance. Usually, the reusable appliance is rinsed in warm water and soaked in a solution of water and white vinegar or a commercial deodorizing solution for 30 minutes. It is rinsed and airdried away from direct sunlight. After drying, the appliance may be powdered with cornstarch and stored. Two appliances are necessary—one to be worn while the other is air drying.

The patient is encouraged to contact the local ostomy association for visits, reassurance, and practical information.*

Ureterosigmoidostomy

Ureterosigmoidostomy is an implantation of the ureters into the sigmoid colon. It is usually done for the patient who has had extensive pelvic irradiation, previous small bowel resection, or coexisting small bowel disease. In addition to the usual preoperative regimen, the patient may be placed on a

---

* See bibliography at end of chapter for address.

liquid diet for several days preoperatively to reduce residue in the colon. Antimicrobial agents (neomycin, kanamycin) are administered for bowel disinfection. Ureterosigmoidostomy requires a competent anal sphincter, adequate renal function, and active renal peristalsis. The degree of anal sphincter control may be determined by assessing the patient's ability to retain enemas.

The patient will be informed that, following surgery, voiding will occur from the rectum for the rest of his life and that an adjustment in life-style will be necessary because of urinary frequency (as often as every 2 hours), which will have a consistency equivalent to a watery diarrhea. There will be some degree of nocturia. Activities will have to be planned around the frequent need to urinate, which in turn may restrict the patient's social life. However, the patient has the advantage of urinary control without having to wear an external appliance.

Postoperatively, a catheter is placed in the rectum to drain the urine and prevent reflux of urine into the ureters and kidneys. The tube is taped to the buttocks and special skin care given around the anus to prevent excoriation. Irrigations of the rectal tube may be prescribed, but force should not be used because of the danger of introducing bacteria into the newly implanted ureters.

In this operation, larger areas of the bowel mucosa are exposed to urine and electrolyte reabsorption; as a result, electrolyte imbalance and acidosis may occur. Potassium and magnesium imbalances may occur from the presence of urine in the bowel, which simulates diarrhea. Fluid and electrolyte balance is maintained in the immediate postoperative period by serum chemical determinations and appropriate intravenous infusions. Acidosis may be prevented by placing the patient on a low-chloride diet supplemented with sodium potassium citrate. The patient should be instructed never to wait longer than 3 hours before emptying urine from the intestine in order to keep rectal pressure low and to minimize absorption of urinary constituents from the colon.

After the rectal catheter is removed, the patient learns to control the anal sphincter through special sphincteric exercises. At first urination is frequent. With reassurance and encouragement and the passage of time, the patient will gain greater control and will learn to differentiate between the need to void and the need to defecate.

Pyelonephritis (upper urinary tract infection due to reflux of bacteria from the colon) is fairly common in some patients who may have to take prophylactic antimicrobial therapy for the rest of their lives.

Specific diet instructions include avoidance of gas-forming foods, since flatus can cause stress incontinence and offensive odors. Other ways to avoid gas are to avoid chewing gum, smoking, and any other activity that involves swallowing air. Salt intake may be restricted to prevent hyperchloremic acidosis. Potassium intake is increased through foods and medication since potassium may be lost in acidosis. A late complication is adenocarcinoma of the sigmoid colon, possibly due to the exposure of colonic mucosa to urine, leading to cellular changes.

Cutaneous Ureterostomy

A cutaneous ureterostomy is accomplished by bringing the detached ureters through the abdominal wall and attaching them to an opening in the skin. This procedure is used in selected patients with ureteral obstruction (advanced pelvic cancer); for poor-risk patients, since it requires less extensive surgery than other urinary diversion procedures; and for patients who have had previous abdominal irradiation.

A urinary appliance is fitted immediately following surgery. The management of the patient with a cutaneous ureterostomy is very similar to the care of the patient with an ileal conduit (see p. 1061).

Cystostomy

An infrequently used method of urinary diversion is the suprapubic cystostomy, which is accomplished by inserting a special catheter through the abdomen into the bladder either through an incision in the lower abdominal wall or by a trochar punch technique. It is usually done under local anesthesia. Generally, a cystostomy is done on the patient with an obstruction below the bladder (prostatic obstruction) when it is not possible to insert a urethral catheter. A cystostomy may be temporary (until corrective surgery can be done) or permanent.

The patient with a cystostomy requires liberal amounts of fluid to prevent encrustation around the catheter. Other problems encountered include the formation of bladder stones, acute and chronic infections, and problems in collecting urine. The advice and assistance of an enterostomal therapist is needed in choosing the most suitable urine collection bag and to instruct the patient in its use.

Continent Ileal Urinary Reservoir (Kock Pouch)

The continent ileal urinary reservoir is another type of urinary diversion created for patients whose bladder is removed or can no longer function (neurogenic bladder). In this procedure, a segment of the small intestine is surgically isolated from the intestine and serves for storage of urine (Fig. 40-7). The ureters are implanted in the isolated segment and an opening is created connecting the new "bladder" to the abdominal wall. A nipple-like valve is created by intussuscepting (telescoping) the intestine to prevent leakage of urine. To drain the stored urine, a catheter is inserted through the nipple valve and urine is drained. The advantage of this urinary diversion is that the valve prevents leakage of urine and the drainage of urine is under the control of the patient. The pouch must be drained at regular intervals to prevent absorption of metabolic waste products from the urine and reflux of urine to the ureters.

General Management of Patients Undergoing Urinary Diversion Procedures

Preoperative Management

A careful preoperative assessment of cardiopulmonary function is done since patients undergoing cystectomy (excision of the urinary bladder) are usually older people who may not fare well in a lengthy complex procedure. As part of preoperative management, the bowel is cleansed (to minimize fecal stasis, to decompress the bowel, and to minimize postoper-

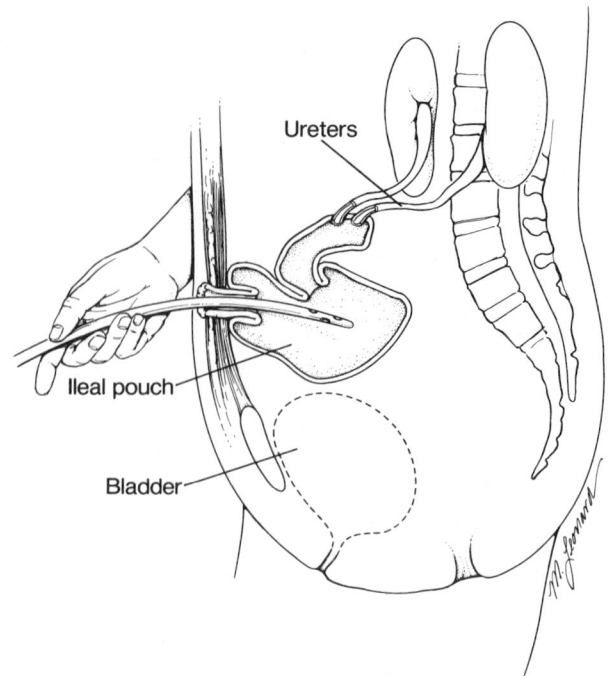

Figure 40-7
Continent ileal urinary reservoir (Kock pouch). Insertion of a catheter through the valve to drain stored urine.

ative ileus), a low-residue diet is prescribed, and antimicrobial drugs are administered for bowel disinfection to reduce pathogenic flora and to lessen potential complications of wound infection and sepsis. Adequate preoperative hydration is imperative to ensure urine flow during surgery and to prevent hypovolemia during the prolonged operative procedure. The patient with urogenital tract cancer may have severe problems with malnutrition because of increased tumor mass and decreased food intake. Enteral or intravenous hyperalimentation can be used to support the patient, minimize toxicity, promote healing, and improve response to treatment.

Postoperative Management

Postoperative management focuses on maintaining urinary function, preventing postoperative complications (respiratory complications, fluid and electrolyte imbalances), and promoting patient comfort. Catheters or drainage systems are observed and urine output monitored carefully. A nasogastric tube is inserted during surgery to allow for decompression and to relieve pressure on the intestinal anastomosis. It is usually kept in place for several days following surgery. As soon as bowel function resumes, as manifested by bowel sounds, the passage of flatus, and a soft abdomen, the patient is given fluids by mouth. Until that time, fluids and electrolytes are given intravenously. The patient is ambulated as soon as possible.

Nursing Interventions

The role of the nurse in the immediate postoperative phase is to assess the patient for complications and prevent their occurrence. The catheters and urinary collection receptacle inserted during surgery are monitored closely. Urine volume, patency of the drainage system, and color of drainage are noted. A sudden decrease in urine volume or increase in drainage is reported promptly to the physician since this may indicate obstruction of the urinary tract, inadequate blood volume, or bleeding. Analgesia is administered as prescribed to promote patient comfort and permit the patient to turn, cough, and take deep breaths without excessive pain and discomfort. The nursing care indicated for this patient includes measures for the patient undergoing intestinal surgery (see Chap. 34) and surgery of the urinary tract (pp. 1025 and 1029–1031). The remainder of the postoperative management and the nursing care related to the physical needs of the patient are covered under the previous discussions of the specific urinary diversion procedures.

▶ *Nursing Process*
The Patient Undergoing a Urinary Diversion Surgical Procedure

▷ *Assessment*

The patient admitted to the hospital for a urinary diversion surgical procedure is assessed thoroughly. The nursing history focuses on the patient's and the family's understanding of the procedure and the changes in physical structure and function that will result from the surgery. The patient's self-concept and self-esteem are also assessed in addition to his usual way of coping with stress and loss. The patient's mental status, hand dexterity, and preferred method of learning are noted since these will influence his ability to participate in self-care postoperatively.

▷ *Nursing Diagnoses*

Based on the assessment data, the nursing diagnoses for the patient undergoing urinary diverson surgery may include the following:

Preoperative Diagnoses

- Anxiety related to anticipated losses associated with the surgical procedure
- Knowledge deficit related to outcomes of the surgical procedure

Postoperative Diagnoses

- Knowledge deficit concerning management of urinary function
- Potential alterations in self-concept related to altered body image
- Ineffective individual coping related to fear of the diagnosis and the impact of surgery
- Self-care deficit related to ostomy maintenance
- Altered sexuality patterns related to aftereffects of surgery and self-consciousness about stoma

▷ *Planning and Implementation*

▷ *Preoperative Goals:* The patient's major goals may include relief of anxiety and increased knowledge about expected outcomes of the surgery.

▷ *Postoperative Goals:* The patient's major goals may include increased knowledge about management of urinary function, improved self-concept, and appropriate coping mechanisms to accept and deal with altered urinary function.

Preoperative Nursing Interventions

Relieving Anxiety. The threat of bladder removal and cancer creates fear related to losses—loss of love, body image, and security. In addition to problems in adapting to an external appliance, a stoma, and a scar, the patient must also adapt to alterations in toileting habits, and the male patient must also adapt to sexual impotency. (A penile implant is considered if the patient is a candidate for the procedure.) Women face the fear of loss of appearance because of changed body image. A supportive approach is needed that includes physical, psychological, and psychosocial support. It involves taking a personal interest in the patient, assessing the patient's concept and perception of self and the manner in which he responds to stress and loss, and helping him to maintain his usual life-style and independence with as few modifications as possible. The patient is encouraged to express his fears and anxiety. A visitor from the "Ostomy Visitation Program" of the American Cancer Society can give emotional support and make adaptation easier both before and after surgery.

Patient Education. An enterostomal therapist is invaluable for preoperative teaching. Explanations of the surgical procedure and the reasons for wearing a collection device postoperatively are given to the patient and the family. The stoma site is planned preoperatively with the patient standing, sitting, and lying in order to locate the stoma away from bony prominences, skin creases, and fat folds. *The patient should be able to see the site for ease of self-care.* The optimum site is marked with indelible ink for intraoperative location. It is desirable to have the patient practice wearing the appliance partially filled with water before surgery.

Postoperative Nursing Interventions

Patient Education. A major postoperative objective is to assist the patient to achieve the highest level of independence and self-care possible. The nurse, or enterostomal therapist, if available, works closely with the patient and family to instruct and assist them in all phases of management of the ostomy. The patient is encouraged to participate in decisions regarding type of collecting appliance and time of day to change the appliance. The patient is assisted and encouraged to look at and touch the stoma early so that he overcomes his fears.

The patient and family are instructed about the signs and symptoms to be reported to the physician and about problems that they can handle themselves. Information and increased responsibility for self-care are provided according to the patient's physical recovery from surgery and his ability to accept and acquire knowledge and skill needed for independence. Verbal and written instructions are provided, and the patient is given the opportunity to practice and demonstrate his skill in management of his urinary drainage.

Improving Self-Concept. In addition to alterations in urinary drainage, the patient with a urinary diversion also experiences loss or fear of loss of relationships with others, altered sexuality and sexual function, dependence, and changes in life-style. The patient's ability to cope with these potential changes depends to some degree on his body image and self-esteem before the surgery and the support and reaction of others around him. The nurse can assist the patient to improve his self-concept by providing him with the skills and confidence to be independent in management of his altered urinary drainage. Additionally, acceptance of his feelings and reactions as he adjusts to alteration of the previously private and routine act of urinary drainage or voiding may assist him in accepting these changes. The patient who experiences altered sexual function as a result of the surgical procedure may mourn this loss and its meaning to him and his partner. Encouraging the patient and partner to share their feelings about this loss with each other and acknowledging the importance of sexual function and expression may assist the patient and spouse to seek sexual counseling if necessary and to explore alternative ways of expressing sexuality. A visit from another "ostomate" who is functioning fully in society and family life may also assist the patient and family in recognizing that full recovery is possible.

▷ *Evaluation*

▷ *Expected Outcomes*

Preoperative

1. Patient experiences reduced anxiety.
   a. Verbalizes fears and anxieties about surgery and its outcomes.
   b. Grieves about alterations openly as appropriate.
   c. Shares fears, anxieties, and concerns with partner.
   d. Accepts visit from "Ostomy Visitation Program."
   e. Reports reduction in level of anxiety.
   f. Exhibits interest in other activities and events.
2. Increases knowledge about expected outcomes of surgery.
   a. States purpose and expected outcomes of surgical procedure.
   b. Describes anticipated alterations in urinary drainage in own words.
   c. Asks nurse or enterostomal therapist relevant questions related to postoperative course.
   d. Exhibits cooperation with nurse, enterostomal therapist, or surgeon in identifying stoma site.

Postoperative

1. Increases knowledge about management of urinary function.
   a. Participates in management of urinary drainage system.
   b. Verbalizes own preferences and opinions in making decisions about care and management.
   c. Describes anatomical alteration due to surgery.
   d. Describes and uses recommended skin care measures.
   e. Revises daily routine to accommodate urostomy (urinary drainage) management.
   f. Identifies potential problems and measures to handle them.
   g. Identifies reportable signs and symptoms.
   h. Asks questions relevant to care at home.

2. Exhibits improved self-concept.
   a. Verbalizes acceptance of urinary diversion, stoma, and appliance.
   b. Demonstrates increasing independence in self-care.
   c. Verbalizes plans to resume normal activities of daily living and return to usual life-style.
   d. Identifies alternative ways of sexual expression (if impotent).
   e. Verbalizes acceptance of support and assistance from family members and health care providers.
   f. Exhibits proper hygiene and grooming.
   g. Accepts visit from "ostomate."
   h. Volunteers to visit other patients about to undergo urinary diversion.

Urethral Conditions

Caruncle

A caruncle is a small, red, extremely vascular polyp-like growth situated just within, and protruding from, the external urethral meatus of women. On rare occasions, it causes no subjective symptoms. However, it may be acutely sensitive, causing a local burning pain exaggerated by exertion and frequency of urination, which is exquisitely painful. Local excision of the caruncle will relieve the symptoms.

Urethritis

Urethritis, inflammation of the urethra, is usually an ascending infection and may be classified as gonorrheal (see Chap. 59) or nongonorrheal. However, both conditions may be present in the same patient.

Gonorrheal Urethritis. Gonorrheal urethritis is caused by *Neisseria gonorrhoeae* and is transmitted by sexual contact. In the male, inflammation of the meatal orifice occurs with burning on urination. A purulent urethral discharge appears 3 to 14 days (or longer) after sexual exposure. However, the disease may be asymptomatic. In the female, a urethral discharge is not always present and the disease also is often essentially asymptomatic. Therefore, gonorrhea in the female is frequently not reported and diagnosed. In the male, the infection involves the tissues around the urethra, causing periurethritis, prostatitis, epididymitis, and urethral stricture. Sterility may occur as a result of vasoepididymal obstruction. Treatment of gonorrhea is discussed and patient education information is provided in Chapter 59.

Nongonorrheal Urethritis. Urethritis not associated with *Neisseria gonorrhoeae* is usually caused by *Chlamydia trachomatis* or *Ureaplasma urealyticum*. If the male patient is symptomatic, he will complain of mild to severe dysuria and a scanty to moderate urethral discharge. Nongonorrheal urethritis requires prompt antimicrobial treatment with tetracycline or doxycycline, or in those patients who do not respond or are allergic to the tetracyclines, erythromycin may be substituted. Follow-up care is necessary to make certain that a cure is achieved. All persons who are sexual partners of patients with nongonorrheal urethritis must be examined for sexually transmitted disease and treated.

Urethral Strictures

A urethral stricture is a narrowing of the lumen of the urethra due to scar tissue and contraction. Strictures result from urethral injury (caused by insertion of surgical instruments during transurethral surgery, indwelling catheters, or cystoscopic procedures), straddle injuries and automobile accidents, untreated gonorrheal urethritis, and congenital abnormalities.

The force and size of the urinary stream is diminished and symptoms of urinary infection and retention occur. Stricture causes urine to back up, resulting in cystitis, prostatitis, and pyelonephritis. An important element of prevention is to treat all urethral infections promptly. Prolonged urethral catheter drainage is to be avoided and utmost care taken in any type of instrumentation involving the urethra, including catheterization.

Management. The treatment may be palliative (gradual dilatation of the narrowed area with metal sounds or bougies) or operation under direct vision (internal urethrotomy). If the stricture has become so small as to prevent the passage of a catheter, the urologist uses several small filiform bougies in search of the opening. When one bougie passes beyond the stricture into the bladder, it is fixed in place, and urine will drain from the bladder. The stricture then can be dilated to larger size by the passage of a larger sound (a dilating instrument) following behind the filiform as a guide. Following dilatation, hot sitz baths and nonnarcotic analgesics are given to control the pain. Antimicrobials are given for several days after dilatation to minimize the infectious reaction, thus lessening discomfort.

Surgical excision or urethroplasty may be necessary for severe cases. Sometimes a suprapubic cystostomy must be performed. The postoperative treatment for cystostomy is described on page 1064.

Bibliography

Books

Blandy J. Operative Urology. Boston, Blackwell, 1986.

Brenner B et al. Principles of Renal Medicine. Philadelphia, WB Saunders, 1986.

Bricker N and Kirchenbaum MA. The Kidney: Diagnosis and Management. New York, John Wiley & Sons, 1984.

Fischbach F. A Manual of Laboratory Diagnostic Tests. Philadelphia, JB Lippincott, 1984.

Gonick HC. Current Nephrology, vol. 8. Chicago, Year Book Medical Publishers, 1985.

Hanno PM and Wein AJ. A Clinical Manual of Urology. East Norwalk, Connecticut, Appleton-Century-Crofts, 1986.

Harrison LH and Kandel LB. Techniques in Urologic Stone Surgery. Mt. Kisco, New York, Futura, 1986.

Hepinstall RH. Pathology of the Kidney, Boston, Little, Brown & Co, 1983.

McConnell EA and Zimmerman MF. Care of Patients with Urologic Problems. Philadelphia, JB Lippincott, 1983.

Schoengrund L and Balzer P. Renal Problems in Critical Care. New York, John Wiley & Sons, 1985.

Vestal RE. Drug Treatment in the Elderly. Boston, ADIS Health Science Press, 1984.

Articles

(Asterisks indicate nursing research articles.)

General Articles

Checcio LM and Como AJ. Electrolytes, BUN, creatinine: Who's at risk? Ann Emerg Med 1986 Mar; 15(3):363–366.

Ethical controversies in nephrology. Dial Transplant 1986 June; 15(6): 300–305, 348–351.

Glassrock RJ. Nephrology. JAMA 1985 Oct 25; 254(16):2274–2276.

Peterson PK. Host defense abnormalities predisposing the patient to infection. Am J Med 1984 May 15; 76(5A):2–10.

Reid G. The office microbiology laboratory. Urol Clin North Am 1986 Nov; 13(4):569–576.

Werman HA and Brown CG. Utility of urine cultures in the emergency department. Ann Emerg Med 1986 Mar; 15(3):302–307.

Acute Renal Failure

Baer CL. Acute renal failure: Mortality or magic? Dimens Crit Care Nurs 1983 Nov/Dec; 2(6):324–326.

Burke JF and Francos GC. Surgery in the patient with acute or chronic renal failure. Med Clin North Am 1987 May; 71(3):489–497.

Cameron JS. Acute renal failure in the intensive care unit today. Intensive Care Med 1986; 12(2):64–70.

Coleman EA. When the kidneys fail. RN 1986 July; 28–34.

Goldstein MB. Acute renal failure. Med Clin North Am 1983 Nov; 67(6): 1325–1341.

Lazarus JM. Editorial. Acute renal failure. Intensive Care Med 1986; 12(2): 61–63.

The patient in acute renal failure. RN 1986 July; 35–37.

Whittaker AA. Acute renal dysfunction: Assessment of patients at risk. Focus Crit Care 1985 June; 12(3):12–17.

Chronic Renal Failure

Chubon RA. Quality of life and persons with end-stage renal disease. Dial Transplant 1986 Aug; 15(8):450–459.

Comty CM and Collins AJ. Dialytic therapy in the management of chronic renal failure. Med Clin North Am 1984 Mar; 68(2):399–425.

Eschbach JW and Adamson JW. Anemia of end-stage renal disease (ESRD). Kidney Int 1985 July; 28(1):1–5.

Evans RW et al. The quality of life of patients with end-stage renal disease. N Engl J Med 1985 Feb 28; 312(9):553–559.

Freeman RB. Treatment of chronic renal failure: An update. N Engl J Med 1985 Feb 28; 312(9):577–579.

Friedman EA and Lundin AP. Forces determining selection of uremia therapy. Adv Nephrol 1984;13:151–162.

Gibson TP. Renal disease and drug metabolism: An overview. Am J Kidney Dis 1986 July; 8(1):7–17.

Holliday MA. Nutrition therapy in renal disease. Kidney Int 1986 July; 30(suppl 19):S-3–S-6.

Norris MK. Management of acute conditions in chronic renal failure. Dimens Crit Care Nurs 1983 Nov/Dec; 2(6):328–337.

Trompeter RS et al. Neurologic complications of renal failure. Am J Kidney Dis 1986 Apr; 7(4):318–323.

Kidney Transplantation

Banowsky LHW. Current results and future expectations in renal transplantation. Urol Clin North Am 1983 May; 10(2):337–346.

Calne RY. The current state of renal transplantation. Kidney Int 1986 July; 29(suppl 19):S-23–S-24.

Gulledge AD, Buszta C, and Montague DK. Psychosocial aspects of renal transplantation. Urol Clin North Am 1983 May; 10(2):327–335.

Harwood CH and Cook CY. Cyclosporine in transplantation. Heart Lung 1985 Nov; 14(6):529–540.

McEnery PT et al. Renal transplant immunity and immunosuppression. Am J Kidney Dis 1986 Apr; 7(4):312–317.

Rao KY. Status of renal transplantation: A clinical perspective. Med Clin North Am 1984 Mar; 68(2):427–453.

Steinmuller DR. Evaluation and selection of candidates for renal transplantation. Urol Clin North Am 1983 May; 10(2):217–229.

Transplanting islet cells along with kidneys. Am J Nurs 1985 July; 85(7): 773.

Urinary Tract Infections

Anderson RU. Urinary tract infections in compromised hosts. Urol Clin North Am 1986 Nov; 13(4):727–734.

Andriole VT. Genitourinary infections in the patient at risk: An overview. Am J Med 1984 May 15; 76(5A):155–157.

Bahnson RR. Urosepsis. Urol Clin North Am 1986 Nov; 13(4):627–635.

Burke JP, Larsen RA, and Stevens LE. Nosocomial bacteriuria: Estimating the potential for prevention by closed sterile urinary drainage. Infect Control 1986 Feb; 7(suppl 2):96–99.

Carlson KJ and Mulley AG. Management of acute dysuria. Ann Intern Med 1985 Feb; 102(2):244–249.

Diokno AC et al. Urologic evaluation of urinary tract infection in pregnancy. J Reprod Med 1986 Jan; 31(1):23–26.

Farrar WF. Infections of the urinary tract. Med Clin North Am 1983 Jan; 67(1):187–201.

Fowler JE. Urinary tract infections in women. Urol Clin North Am 1986 Nov; 13(4):673–683.

Foxman B and Frerichs RR. Epidemiology of urinary tract infection: I. Diaphragm use and sexual intercourse. Am J Pub Health 1985 Nov; 75(11):1308–1313.

Foxman B and Frerichs RR. Epidemiology of urinary tract infection: II. Diet, clothing, and urination habits. Am J Pub Health 1985 Nov; 75(11):1314–1317.

Hanno P. Therapeutic principles of antimicrobial therapy and new antimicrobial agents. Urol Clin North Am 1986 Nov; 13(4):577–590.

*Hart JA. The urethral catheter—a review of its implication in urinary tract infection. Int J Nurs Stud 1985; 22(1):57–70.

Kunin CM. Genitourinary infections in the patient at risk: Extrinsic risk factors. Am J Med 1984 May 15; 76(5A):131–139.

Kunin CM. Use of antimicrobial agents in treating urinary tract infection. Adv Nephrol 1985;14:39–65.

Latham RH et al. Laboratory diagnosis of urinary tract infection in ambulatory women. JAMA 1985 Dec 20; 254(23):3333–3336.

Macfarlane DE. Prevention and treatment of catheter-associated urinary tract infections. J Infect 1985 Mar; 10(2);96–106.

Mulholland SG. Female urinary tract infection. Prim Care 1985 Dec; 12(4): 661–673.

Naeye RL. Urinary tract infections and the outcome of pregnancy. Adv Nephrol 1986; 15:95–102.

Parsons CL. Pathogenesis of urinary tract infections: Bacterial adherence, bladder defense mechanisms. Urol Clin North Am 1986 Nov; 13(4): 563–568.

Roberts JA. Pyelonephritis, cortical abscess, and perinephric abscess. Urol Clin North Am 1986 Nov; 13(4):637–645.

*Roe B. Catheter care: An overview. Int J Nurs Stud 1985; 22(1):45–56.

Ronald AR. Current concepts in the management of urinary tract infections in adults. Med Clin North Am 1984 Mar; 68(2):335–349.

Schaeffer AJ. Catheter-associated bacteriuria. Urol Clin North Am 1986 Nov; 13(4):735–747.

Sheehan G, Harding GKM, and Ronald AR. Advances in the treatment of urinary tract infection. Am J Med 1984 May 15; 76(5A):141–147.

Sheldon CA and Gonzalez R. Differentiation of upper and lower urinary tract infections: How and when? Med Clin North Am 1984 Mar; 68(2):321–333.

Simpson RA. Systemic and topical antimicrobial agents in the prevention of catheter-associated bacteriuria and its consequences. Infect Control 1986 Feb; 7(2):100–103.

Smith CI. Urinary tract infection: Pathogenesis and management. Female Patient 1986 May; 11(5):70–88.

Sobel JD and Kaye D. Host factors in the pathogenesis of urinary tract infections. Am J Med 1984 May 15; 76(5A):122–130.

Stamm WE. Prevention of urinary tract infections. AM J Med 1984 May 15; 76(5A):148–154.

Uehling DT. Future approaches to the management of urinary tract infections. Urol Clin North Am 1986 Nov; 13(4):749–758.

Urinary tract infection in women (Test yourself). Am J Nurs 1986 Jan; 86(1):71, 94.

Yoshikawa TT. Unique aspects of urinary tract infection in the geriatric population. Gerontology 1984 Sept/Oct; 30(5):339–344.

Glomerulonephritis

Glassock RJ. Natural history and treatment of primary proliferative glomerulonephritis: A review. Kidney Int 1985 Dec; 28(suppl 17):S-136–S-142.

Joyce KM, Austin HA, and Balow JE. The patient with lupus nephritis: A nursing perspective. Heart Lung 1985 Jan; 14(1):75–79.

Mann R and Neilson EG. Pathogenesis and treatment of immune-mediated renal disease. Med Clin North Am 1985 July; 69(4):715–750.

What is interstitial cystitis—and what can be done about it? Am J Nurs 1986 Jan; 86(1):13–14.

Whitley K, Keane WF, and Vernier RL. Acute glomerulonephritis: A clinical overview. Med Clin North Am 1984 Mar; 68(2):259–279.

Kidney Stones

Abraham PA and Smith CL. Medical evaluation and management of calcium nephrolithiasis. Med Clin North Am 1984 Mar; 68(2):281–299.

Boyce WH. Surgery of urinary calculi in perspective. Urol Clin North Am 1983 Nov; 10(4):585–594.

Chaussy C and Schmiedt E. Shock wave treatment for stones in the upper urinary tract. Urol Clin North Am 1983 Nov; 10(4):743–750.

Coe FL and Parks JH. Recurrent renal calculi: Causes and prevention. Hosp Prac 1986 Mar 30; 21(3A):49–57.

Cubler AJ and Whalen-Myers MA. Ureteroscopy. AORN J 1985 Dec; 42(6):853–858.

Harwood CT. Pulverizing kidney stones: What you should know about lithotripsy. RN 1985 July; 32–37.

Marshall S. Coagulum pyelolithotomy. Urol Clin North Am 1983 Nov; 10(4):659–664.

Menon M and Krishnan CS. Evaluation and medical management of the patient with calcium stone disease. Urol Clin North Am 1983 Nov; 10(4):595–615.

Percutaneous lithotripsy for urinary calculi. Am J Nurs 1985 July; 85(7): 772–773.

Ruge CA. Shock (wave) treatment for kidney stones. Am J Nurs 1986 Apr; 86(4):400–401.

Shortliffe LMD and Spigelman SS. Infection stones: Evaluation and management. Urol Clin North Am 1986 Nov; 13(4):717–726.

Smith AD and Lee WJ. Percutaneous stone removal procedures including irrigation. Urol Clin North Am 1983 Nov; 10(4):719–727.

Spirnak JP and Resnick MI. Urinary stones. Prim Care Dec 1985; 12(4): 735–759.

Stafford SA and Deluca SA. Urinary tract stones. Am Fam Physician 1985 Feb; 31(2):219–221.

Webb DR, Payne SR, and Wickham JEA. Extracorporeal shockwave lithotripsy and percutaneous renal surgery. Br J Urol 1986 Feb; 58(1): 1–5.

Urinary Diversion

Brogna L and Lakaszawski ML. The continuent urostomy. Am J Nurs 615t Feb; 86(2):160–163.

Kosko JW, Kursh ED, and Resnick MI. Metabolic complications of urologic intestinal substitutes. Urol Clin North Am 1986 May; 13(2):193–200.

Montie JE et al. Continent ileal urinary reservoir (Kock pouch). Urol Clin North Am 1986 May; 13(2):251–260.

Penninger JI, Moore SB, and Frager SR. After the ostomy: Helping the patient reclaim his sexuality. RN 1985 Apr; 46–50.

Resnick MI and Caldamone AA (eds). The use of large and small bowel in urologic surgery. Urol Clin North Am 1986 May; 13(2):177–359.

Skinner DG, Lieskovsky G, and Boyd SD. Technique of creation of a continent internal ileal reservoir (Kock pouch) for urinary diversion. Urol Clin North Am 1984 Nov; 11(4):741–749.

Thorne ID and Resnick MI. The use of bowel in urologic surgery: An historical perspective, Urol Clin North Am 1986 May; 13(2):179–191.

Toth JM. When your patient faces a urostomy. RN 1985 Nov; 50–55.

Urothelial Cancer

Flanigan RC, Rapp RP, and McRoberts JW. Nutritional assessment and therapy in advanced urothelial cancer. Urol Clin North Am 1984 Nov; 11(4):623–635.

Gittes RF. Carcinogenesis in ureterosigmoidostomy. Urol Clin North Am 1986 May; 13(2):201–205.

Loening S. Chemotherapy as an adjuvant for cystectomy and for advanced urothelial cancer. Urol Clin North Am 1984 Nov; 11(4):699–708.

Martinez A and Gunderson LL. Intraoperative radiation therapy for bladder cancer. Urol Clin North Am 1984 Nov; 11(4):693–698.

Morrison AS. Advances in the etiology of urothelial cancer. Urol Clin North Am 1984 Nov; 11(4):557–566.

Soloway MS. Intravesical and systemic chemotherapy in the management of superficial bladder cancer. Urol Clin North Am 1984 Nov; 11(4):623–635.

van der Werf-Messing BHP. Carcinoma of the urinary bladder treated by interstitial radiotherapy. Urol Clin North Am 1984 Nov; 11(4):659–699.

Whitemore WF and Betata M. Status of integrated irradiation and cystectomy for bladder cancer. Urol Clin North Am 1984 Nov; 11(4):681–691.

Agencies

Governmental

National Institute of Diabetes and Digestive and Kidney Disease, National Institutes of Health, Bethesda, Maryland 20892.

National Cancer Institute, Office of Cancer Communications, Bethesda, Maryland 20205.

Voluntary

American Cancer Society, 90 Park Avenue, New York, New York 10016.

American Society for Artificial Internal Organs, PO Box 777, Boca Raton, Florida 33432.

National Association of Patients on Hemodialysis and Transplantation, 150 Nassau Street, New York, New York 10038.

National Kidney Foundation, 116 E. 27th Street, New York, New York 10016.

United Ostomy Association, 2001 W. Beverly Blvd., Los Angeles, California 90057.

Nursing Research Profile for Unit X

Renal and Urologic Nursing

Overview

Two major areas that have been the focus of recent nursing research in renal and urologic nursing have been the patient undergoing dialysis for treatment of end-stage renal disease (ESRD) and aspects of management of indwelling catheters.

The psychological reactions of hemodialysis patients have been an area of concern to nurses as well as to other health care providers. Since hemodialysis requires the patient's co-operation and understanding, a greater knowledge of patient reactions to treatment is important in planning teaching strategies and nursing care.

Further research in the area of hemodialysis and urologic nursing management is necessary to increase our understanding of the experiences of patients experiencing renal dysfunction, treatment modalities such as hemodialysis, peritoneal dialysis, and transplantation, and alteration in urinary drainage.

Hemodialysis

▷ *Laborde JM and Powers MK. Satisfaction with life for patients undergoing hemodialysis and patients suffering from osteoarthritis. Res Nurs Health 1980 Mar; 3(1):19–24.*

The Laborde and Powers study focused on the effects of two different chronic illnesses on the quality of life. The quality of life of 20 hemodialysis patients was compared to that of 20 patients with osteoarthritis. Cantril's Self-Anchoring Life Satisfaction Scale, a measure of general sense of well-being, was modified for this study and used by the subjects to rate their past, present, and future life satisfaction. The hemodialysis patients viewed their present life as significantly better than did patients with osteoarthritis. The hemodialysis patients also viewed their present life as better than their past life, while the patients with osteoarthritis viewed the quality of their past life as better than that of their present life.

The authors speculated that the chronic pain of osteoarthritis may explain the reduced satisfaction with quality of life experienced by this group. The hemodialysis patients' view of their present life as better than their past life may be related to improved physiological well-being despite the restrictions accompanying lifesaving dialysis treatments. The supportive group and environment provided during dialysis by staff and other dialysis patients may also promote more positive perceptions. One of the implications of this study is that the impact of different chronic illnesses on perception of well-being and quality of life may differ considerably and that hemodialysis patients do have the capacity to live a satisfying life.

▷ *Ferrans CE and Powers MJ. The employment potential of hemodialysis patients. Nurs Res 1985 Sept/Oct; 34(5):273–277.*

The Ferrans and Powers study compared two groups of hemodialysis patients, some currently employed and some unemployed, in an effort to identify variables that might affect their employment status. All subjects in both groups had been employed before beginning hemodialysis and were assessed by their physicians as physically able to work. Illness-related variables, occupation-related variables, and psychosocial variables were assessed. Data collected for analysis included laboratory data (*i.e.*, predialysis serum potassium, BUN, phosphorus, creatinine levels and hematocrit, mean arterial blood pressure, and interdialytic weight gain). The subjects' level of dependency and their self-rating of health status and life satisfaction, as well as their assessment of impediments to job performance or return to work, were also included in data analysis.

No significant differences were found in the biophysiological and subjective health status of the two groups. However, the impact of illness was different for the two groups. Those unemployed after starting dialysis had previously held jobs requiring heavier physical labor than was required by the jobs of those currently employed. Additionally, they reported more job discrimination than those who were employed. Subjects in the unemployed group also experienced a greater decrease in life goals since beginning dialysis than those employed. The authors note that although there are significant differences in job-related variables, the subjects in this study were assessed by their physicians as able to return to work. Therefore, employment status and problems in returning to work among dialysis patients may be underrepresented in this sample.

Nursing Implications. The authors suggest that in view of the findings of this study, special attention be given to those patients who previously held jobs requiring moderate-to-heavy physical labor and that job retraining be initiated during initial hospitalization for renal failure.

▷ *Goddard HA and Powers MJ. Educational needs of patients undergoing hemodialysis: A comparison of patient and nurse perceptions. Dialysis and Transplantation 1982 Jul; 11(7):578–579, 582–583.*

Goddard and Powers studied the perceptions of patients and nurses about the importance of several categories of educational information. Twenty-four hemodialysis patients and nine hemodialysis nurses were surveyed about their perceptions of the importance of specific information related to kidney disease and its treatment. A 31-item rating scale developed by the authors for this study was used to assess the perceived importance of nine categories of information. These categories included information about medications, blood pressure, diet and fluids, prevention of infection, care of the fistula, mechanisms of dialysis, adherence to medical orders, disease process, and activities. A 5-point Likert scale was used by patients and nurses to rate each item's importance. The ratings of patients and nurses were compared.

The nurses rated the information needs of hemodialysis patients as significantly more important than did patients. Additionally, nurses and patients differed about those areas of information that they considered more and less important.

Nursing Implications. The implications of this study are that patients' perceptions about what is important to know may be different from the perceptions of nurses. Patients' perceptions about what they consider important need to be identified and taken into account when planning and carrying out formal and informal education programs if those teaching efforts are to be successful.

Catheter Management

Another major area of interest to nurse researchers is indwelling or long-term catheter management. Although use of indwelling catheters has decreased because of the high incidence of urinary tract infection associated with them, they continue to be used in some instances. Research has focused on efforts to prevent premature or accidental removal requiring replacement and strategies to return the patient to the previous level of urinary function as rapidly as possible.

▷ *Barnes KE and Malone-Lee J. Long-term catheter management: Minimizing the problem of premature replacement due to balloon deflation. J Adv Nurs 1986 May; 11(3):303–307.*

Barnes and Malone-Lee speculated that improper catheter and balloon size may be associated with inadvertent removal of catheters and needed replacement. They investigated several types of long-term urinary catheters in a laboratory and clinical setting to determine the extent of fluid loss from the catheter balloon over time. Additionally, they studied the degree of deflation of the balloon and the effective diameter of the catheter balloon after the fluid was withdrawn.

Various types of catheters were studied in the laboratory: 20 silicone-coated latex catheters and 40 100% silicone catheters (20 from each of two manufacturers). These catheters were inflated with 10 ml of sterile water and immersed in artificial urine at 37°C. Fluid loss from the catheter balloons was measured twice a week, and deflated catheters were measured to determine whether there was a change in effective diameter of the catheter shaft resulting from incomplete balloon deflation despite fluid removal.

Patients who were expected to have an indwelling catheter in place for at least 10 days were sequentially assigned to have either 100% silicone catheters or silicone-coated latex catheters inserted. The volume of water in the balloon was measured by withdrawal at weekly intervals and upon removal of the catheter.

The findings in the laboratory study revealed that silicone-coated latex catheter balloons retained their fluid to a greater degree than did 100% silicone catheters. By the third week, the 100% silicone catheters had lost 50% of their volume of fluid. All catheters showed a significant increase in effective shaft diameter after deflation as a result of incomplete collapse of the balloon after fluid removal.

Although it was anticipated that the patients in the clinical setting would have the catheter in place for at least 10 days, permitting comparison of the laboratory and clinical findings of the study, early removal of many catheters because of blockage prevented comparison of the laboratory and clinical findings. However, all catheters except one silicone-coated latex catheter showed some deflation of the balloon.

Nursing Implications. The laboratory findings of this study suggested that silicone-coated latex catheters be reserved for those patients who are expected to have the catheter in place for a prolonged period of time, to prevent its accidental removal because of progressive fluid loss from the balloon. They further suggest careful removal of the catheter because complete collapse of the balloon may not occur even with removal of all the fluid from the balloon.

▷ *Oberst MT et al. Catheter management programs and postoperative urinary dysfunction. Res Nurs Health 1981 Mar; 4(1):175–181.*

The effectiveness of two approaches to urinary catheter management in promoting normal urinary dysfunction or reducing postoperative urinary dysfunction was investigated by Oberst and co-workers. Patients who had either an abdominal perineal resection (APR) or a low anterior bowel resection (LAR) for cancer of the bowel were stratified by sex and surgical procedure and randomly assigned to one of two groups. Beginning on the fourth postoperative day, the first group of patients had their urinary catheters clamped for increasingly longer periods of time, beginning at 1 hour and progressing to a maximum 4-hour interval by the sixth postoperative day. The catheter was drained after each clamping period for a period of 5 minutes. The second group had their catheters connected to straight drainage throughout the period the catheter was in place. The presence of urinary dysfunction following catheter removal was defined as failure to void or residual urine volume of more than 150 ml 20 to 24 hours after catheter removal.

No differences in urinary dysfunction occurred in men in the two groups following either APR or LAR; no urinary dysfunction occurred in women with LAR. However, significant differences in incidence of urinary dysfunction did occur in women in the catheter clamping group (27%) and straight drainage group (67%).

Nursing Implications. These findings suggest that systematic bladder training has the potential to reduce some types of urinary dysfunction associated with low abdominal surgery and has the greatest effect in women who have APR.

Sexual and Reproductive Problems

Unit XI

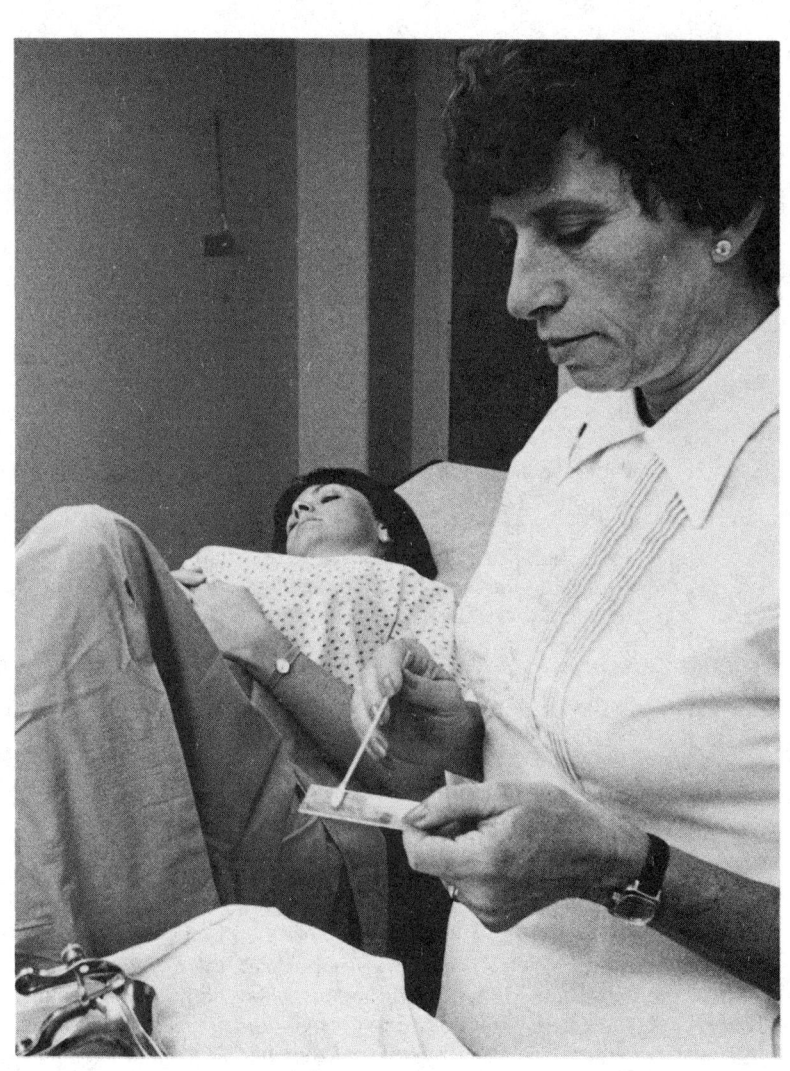

Chapter 41

Management During the Reproductive Cycle

Physiologic Overview

The female reproductive system consists of two ovaries, two uterine tubes, a uterus, and a vagina. The *vulva* is the region of the external genitalia; it includes two thick folds of tissue called the *labia majora* and two smaller lips of delicate tissue called the *labia minora,* which lie within the labia majora. The upper portions of the labia minora unite to form a partial covering for the *clitoris,* a highly sensitive organ made of erectile tissue. Between the labia minora, below and posterior to the clitoris, is the urinary meatus, the external opening of the female urethra, which measures a little more than 3 cm (1½ inches). Below this orifice is a larger opening, the vaginal orifice (Fig. 41-1). On each side of the vaginal orifice is a *vestibular (Bartholin's) gland,* which is a small bean-sized structure that empties its mucous secretion by way of a small duct. The orifice of the duct is found within the labia minora, external to the hymen. The tissue between the external genitalia and the anus is called the *perineum.*

The *vagina* is the canal lined with mucous membrane that is 7.5 to 10 cm (3 or 4 inches) long and extends downward and forward from the uterus to the vulva. Anterior to it are the bladder and the urethra, and below it lies the rectum. The anterior and posterior walls of the vagina normally lie in contact with one another. The upper part of the vagina, the *fornix,* surrounds the *cervix* (the neck of the uterus).

The *uterus* is a pear-shaped muscular organ that is about 7.5 cm (3 inches) long and about 5.0 cm (2 inches) wide at its upper part. Its walls are about 1.25 cm (½ inch) thick. The uterus is divided into a narrow neck, or cervix, that projects into the vagina and a larger upper part, the *fundus* or body, that is covered posteriorly and partly anteriorly by peritoneum. The uterus lies posterior to the bladder and is held in position in the pelvic cavity by several ligaments. The *round ligaments* extend anteriorly and laterally to the internal inguinal ring and down the inguinal canal, where they blend with the tissues of the labia majora. The *broad ligaments* are folds of peritoneum extending from the lateral pelvic walls and enveloping the uterine tubes. The uterosacral ligaments extend posteriorly to the sacrum, and the uterovesical ligaments pass anteriorly. The inner portion of the fundus is triangular. It narrows to a

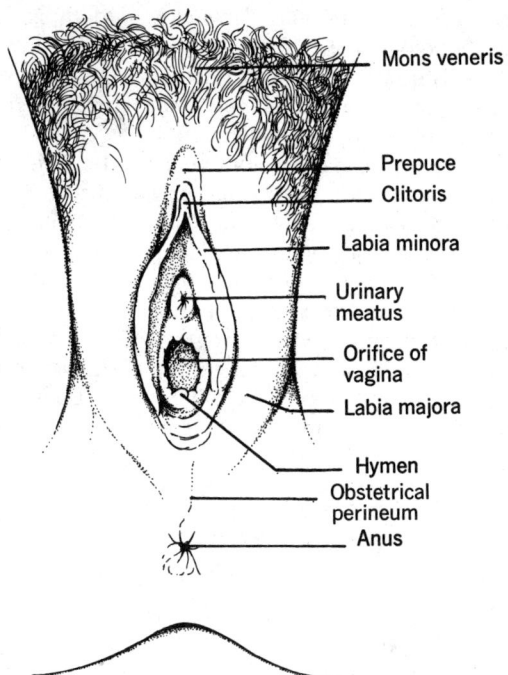

Figure 41-1
External female genitalia. (Chaffee EE and Greisheimer EM. Basic Physiology and Anatomy. Philadelphia, JB Lippincott.)

small canal in the cervix that has a constriction at each end, referred to as the external and internal ossa. The upper lateral parts of the uterus are called the *cornua*. From here the oviducts or uterine tubes extend outward, with their lumen continuous internally with the uterine cavity.

The *ovaries* lie behind the broad ligaments, behind and below the tubes. They are oval bodies, 2.5 to 5.0 cm (1 to 2 inches) long, that contain thousands of tiny egg cells or ova. The ovaries and the uterine tubes are called the *adnexae* (Fig. 41-2).

The ovary, which normally contains from 30,000 to 40,000 ova, remains quiescent in early life, but at the time of puberty (usually between the 12th and 14th years) the ova begin to ripen or mature, enlarging as a type of cyst known as a *graafian follicle*. The cyst enlarges until it reaches the surface of the ovary, where rupture occurs, and the ovum is discharged into the peritoneal cavity. This periodic discharge of matured ova is referred to as *ovulation*. The ovum usually finds its way into the uterine tube, where it is carried to the uterus. If it meets a spermatozoon, the male reproductive cell, a union occurs and *conception* takes place. Following the discharge of the ovum, the cells of the graafian follicle undergo a rapid change. Gradually they become yellow (*corpus luteum*) and produce a secretion that has the function of preparing the uterus for the reception of the fertilized ovum.

If conception does not occur, the ovum dies and the mucous membrane lining the uterus (*endometrium*), which has become thickened and congested, becomes hemorrhagic. The upper layer of lining cells and the blood that appears in the uterine cavity are discharged through the cervix and the vagina. This flow of blood (*menstruation*) mixes with mucus and cells and occurs approximately every 28 days during the sexual life of females. The period of flow usually lasts from 4 to 5 days, during which time 50 to 60 ml of blood is lost. After the cessation of the menstrual flow the endometrium returns to an inactive state until stimulated again by ovulation. Ovulation usually occurs midway between menstrual periods.

Between the ages of 45 and 55 years, the menstrual flow ceases in most women. This period, called the *menopause* (change of life, climacteric), is associated with atrophy of the

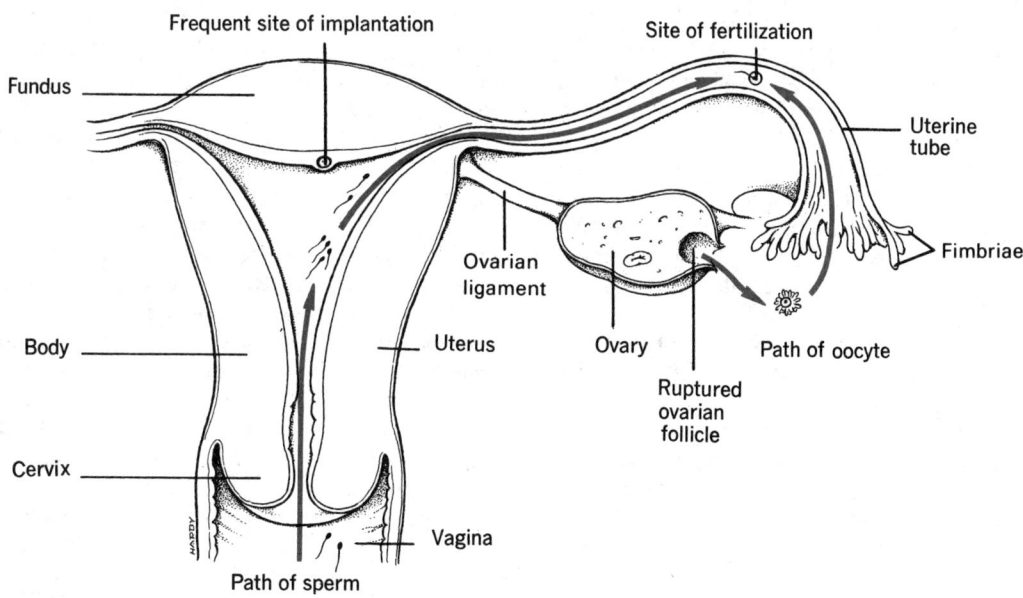

Figure 41-2
Schematic drawing of female reproductive organs, showing path of oocyte from ovary into uterine tube, path of spermatozoa, and the usual site of fertilization. (Chaffee EE and Greisheimer EM. Basic Physiology and Anatomy. Philadelphia, JB Lippincott.)

breasts and genital organs and sometimes with psychic and vascular disturbances.

Health Maintenance

Over the past 2 decades increased interest has been focused on women's health problems and health maintenance. Biological as well as psychosocial changes that have a direct bearing on the health of women continue to be studied from conception to death.

As women have moved into the labor market, they have faced changes in life-style, such as new family patterns; competition; exposure to environmental hazards; and greater participation in damaging health practices, such was smoking and drinking. Greater responsiblity for one's personal health (self-care) is being assessed. Delaying the time of having children until well after a career is established is a common practice. The use of oral contraceptives and intrauterine devices (IUDs) has become more popular than the use of the diaphragm and other contraceptive methods, although recent problems traced to certain IUDs have dampened the enthusiasm for this form of contraception. Physical exercise and competitive sports that once were considered nonfeminine are now popular. Stress-related illnesses have increased, and programs to control stress are common in women's circles.

Nurses are becoming more knowledgeable about preventive care for women, particularly with regard to their unique needs. The nurse encourages female clients to determine their own goals and behaviors. This can be facilitated by assessing health and illness manifestations; offering intervention strategies; and providing support, counseling, and ongoing monitoring as women move toward their health goals.

Hygienic Features: Client/Patient Education

The nurse is in a key position to teach and to advise girls and women about the principles of good health and personal hygiene, especially principles dealing with feminine hygiene related to those parts of the female body concerned with reproduction. The reproductive system, like any other part of the anatomy, will function well if nutrition, exercise, rest, and elimination are adequate. Aside from teaching female patients about these general aspects of care, the nurse should provide instruction about sexually transmitted diseases and prenatal and postnatal care.

It is important to recognize that concepts of feminine hygiene vary greatly with different cultures. What may be considered appropriate care for a European woman may be viewed very differently by an American or Japanese woman. In some societies, an emphasis on cleanliness and neatness may be considered unnecessary, while in others, climate and local customs may affect the habits practiced. Even members of the same family may have different opinions about personal tidiness.

Nurses need to understand the variations in attitudes and practices of hygiene and their relation to sexual function. Because many methods of feminine hygiene are empirical, it is necessary to apply common sense. Douching of the vagina has come down from certain old cultures as a traditional practice of feminine hygiene. However, modern studies of vaginal physiology make clear that it has no health virtue; indeed, many douches that were once considered to be necessary may irritate the vaginal mucosa or reduce the normal mechanisms of resistance to infection.

Contrary to popular opinion, genital odor rarely arises from the vagina but is of external origin, arising from the interaction of oil secreted by the vulvar skin with surface bacteria. Occasionally, old menstrual blood or seminal fluid ejaculated in coitus will give some vaginal odor. A simple, low-pressure, warm water irrigation or, at most, a douche of a solution of 30 ml of white vinegar to a liter of water is appropriate. Significant malodor from the vagina can result from a retained tampon or some other foreign body or from a pathologic condition, indicating the need for examination.

Assessment

Nursing History

Complications of gynecologic disturbances can be prevented if proper medical attention and supervision are available. The nurse is in a unique position to teach the normal physiologic processes of menstruation and menopause. Many difficulties encountered by the young girl or the middle-aged woman usually can be corrected quite easily; if allowed to go untreated, they may cause irreparable damage.

▷ *Danger signals that every woman should report to a health care professional are spotting, irregular or excessive bleeding, or any bleeding after menopause.*

Persistent painful menstruation, leukorrhea, and urinary disturbances also should be investigated. Many of these early signs can be corrected simply and permanently. An annual pelvic examination is especially important for women who are past 30 years of age or for those who are sexually active, regardless of age.

The gynecologic patient often requires more understanding than other patients because of the emotional as well as physical considerations that govern the situation. A woman may resent any reference to her genitourinary system, feeling that she is suspected of questionable social or sexual habits. Or she may have a real fear of disturbance of the reproductive process. Perhaps an explanation of the anatomy involved and the proposed treatment will clarify the stiuation. Any intention of sterilization must be explained carefully to the patient and her partner by the physician. Perhaps religious belief is more important to a patient than physical treatment. The decision rests with the patient, and, when it is made, must be respected and supported.

Psychic factors may present during the menopausal period. The loss of the reproductive capacity may cause disappointment if the woman has had no children. For a woman with a grown family, it may mean that she feels that she is no longer useful. Circumstances affect the problems of each patient and must be considered on an individual basis.

Because gynecologic conditions often are of such a personal and private nature, the nurse is expected to respect the confidentiality of the patient's problems. This information is shared only with those directly involved in professional patient care.

Physical/Pelvic Examination

The pelvic examination is a facet of physical assessment that may be accomplished by the nurse. Competency can be attained in an environment that fosters practice and clinical supervision.

Although several positions may be used for performing the pelvic examination, the supine lithotomy position is used most frequently. A newer technique employs the lithotomy position in which the woman assumes a semi-sitting stance. This position offers several advantages: (1) it is more comfortable, (2) it allows better eye contact between patient and examiner, (3) it provides an easier means for the examiner to carry out the bimanual examination, and (4) it enables the woman to use a mirror to see her anatomy, note the presence of any lesions, and learn methods for certain types of contraceptive techniques (Swartz, 1984).

If the examiner is required to perform the pelvic assessment in the hospital on a patient who is too ill to be placed on a table equipped with stirrups, the Sims' position may be used. In the Sim's position, the patient lies on her left side, with her left arm behind her and her right leg bent at a 90-degree angle. The right labia may be retracted for adequate access to the vagina.

The patient is instructed to void prior to the pelvic examination. The urine is retained if a urine specimen is part of the total assessment procedure. The patient is then placed on the table with her legs in stirrups; she is encouraged to relax so that her buttocks are presented at the edge of the examination table and her thighs are spread as widely apart as possible. The patient is appropriately draped to avoid embarrassment. The following equipment is necessary: good light source, vaginal speculum, unsterile gloves, lubricant, spatula, cotton-tipped applicators, glass slides, fixative solution or spray, and appropriate material for occult blood screening.

When the patient is prepared, the labia majora and minora are examined. The epidermal tissue of the labia majora, with its hair follicles characteristic of skin, fades to the pink mucous membrane of the vaginal introitus. In the nulliparous woman the labia minora should come together at the opening of the vagina. In women who have borne children, the labia minora may gape, and vaginal tissue may protrude. The patient is asked to "bear down." Birth damage to the anterior vaginal wall may have resulted in incompetency of musculature, so that a bulge representing bladder intrusion into the submucosa of the anterior vaginal wall may be seen. This is called a *cystocele*. Birth trauma may also have affected the posterior vaginal wall, so that a bulge representing the cavity of the rectum may protrude, presenting as a *rectocele*. The cervix or the uterus itself may descend under pressure through the vaginal canal and present itself at the introitus. This is termed *prolapse* of the uterus.

The introitus should be free of hair follicles and of superficial mucosal lesions. The labia minora may be separated by the fingers of the gloved hand and the lower part of the vagina palpated. In virginal women, a *hymen* of variable thickness may be felt circumferentially within 1 or 2 cm of the vaginal opening. The hymenal ring will usually permit the admission of two fingers but occasionally is sufficiently restricting so that only one finger may enter the vagina. Rarely, the hymen totally occludes the vaginal entrance. In nonvirginal women, a rim of scar tissue representing the remnants of the hymenal ring may be felt circumferentially around the vagina near its opening. The greater vestibular glands (Bartholin's glands) lie between the labia minora and the remnants of the hymenal ring. These glands frequently become infected in gonococcal disease. Patients may occasionally present with an abscess of one of these glands.

Speculum Examination

Assorted sizes of the bivalved speculum are available in metal or plastic. A metal speculum is warmed with running tap water to make it less uncomfortable when it is inserted. The speculum is not lubricated, since lubrication with commercial jellies may interfere with the examination of the cervical cytology. Two setscrews may be seen on the speculum. One is along the handle and holds the two valves of the speculum together; this one is tightened. The setscrew that holds the thumbrest in place is loosened. The speculum is grasped in the right hand, with the thumb against the back of the thumbrest in order to keep the tips of the valves closed.

The speculum is rotated slightly counterclockwise, and the vaginal orifice is held open by the thumb and the forefinger of the gloved left hand. The speculum is gently inserted into the posterior portion of the introitus and slowly advanced to the top of the vagina (Fig. 41-3). The tip of the speculum may then be elevated and the speculum rotated to a transverse position. The speculum is then slowly opened to reveal the cervix of the uterus. The cervix having been brought into view, the setscrew of the thumbrest may be tightened to hold the speculum open.

If any purulent material appears at the cervical os, it is cultured with a sterile cotton-tipped applicator and immediately placed in an appropriate medium for transfer to a laboratory. Some authorities now advocate routine culture for gonococcus in light of the high incidence of the disease in the general population.

The cervix is inspected. In nulliparous women, the cervical os is 2 to 3 mm in diameter and smooth. Women who have borne children may have a laceration, usually transverse, frequently giving the cervical os a "fishmouth" appearance. Moreover, epithelium from the endocervical canal may have grown out onto the surface of the cervix, appearing as beefy red surface epithelium circumferentially arranged around the os. This is commonly called a *cervical erosion*. Although not always differentiable from a cervical carcinoma, the cervical erosion is, in general, less sharply outlined than malignant tissue. Indeed, malignant change may not be obviously differentiated from the remainder of the cervical mucosa. The presence of endocervical epithelium around the cervical os can lead to chronic infection and discharge from the orifice. Small cysts may appear on the surface of the cervix under these circumstances. These are usually bluish and are termed *nabothian cysts*. A polyp of endocervical mucosa may protrude through the os and appears dark red. A carcinoma may appear as a cauliflower-like growth. It is friable and will bleed easily when traumatized. A bluish color of the cervix is a sign of early pregnancy (Chadwick's sign).

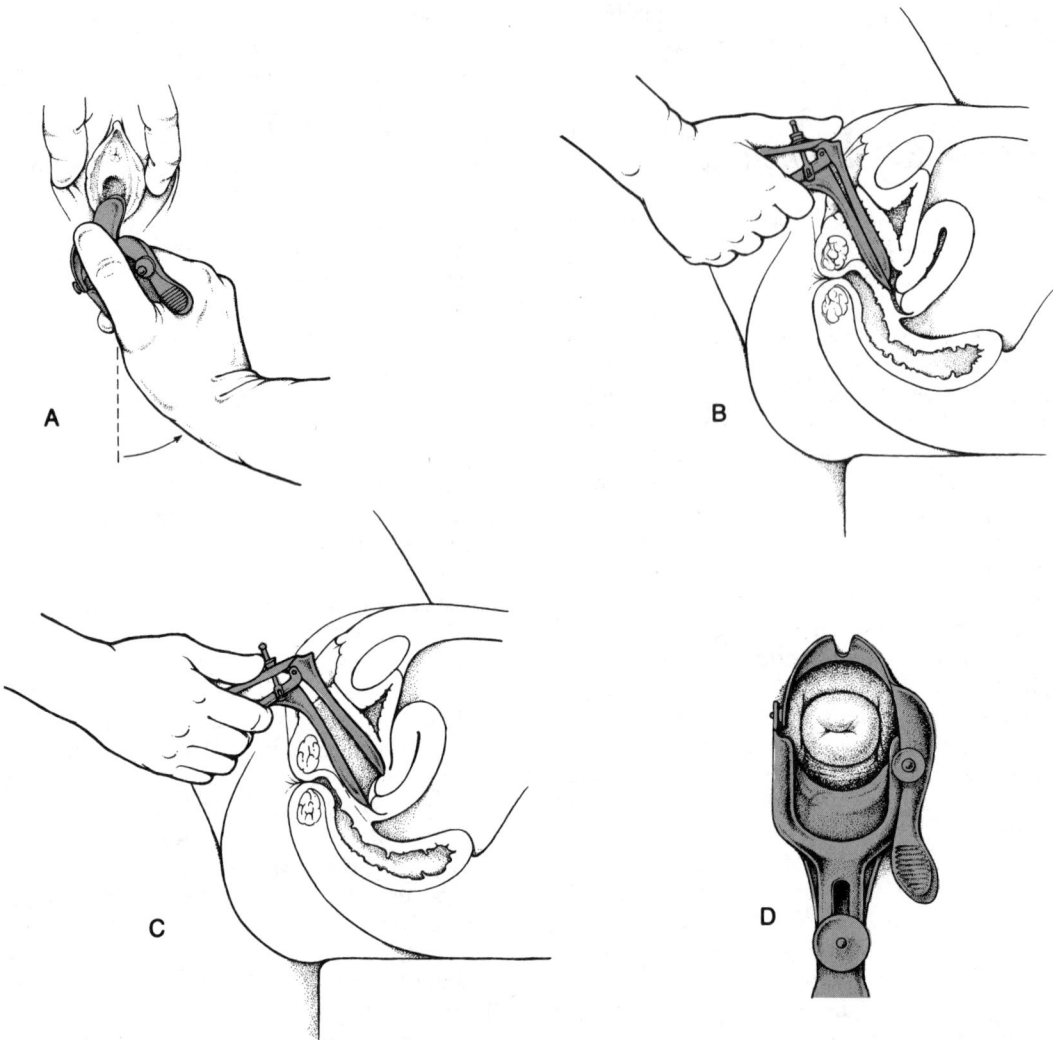

Figure 41-3
Technique for speculum examination of the vagina and cervix. (*A*) The labia are spread
apart with a gloved left hand, while the speculum is grasped in the right hand and turned
counterclockwise before being inserted into the vagina. (*B*) The closed speculum is
inserted into the vagina. (*C*) The blades of the speculum are then spread apart to reveal
the cervical os, as shown in *D*.

The vagina is examined as the speculum is withdrawn.
It is smooth in young girls and becomes more thickened after
puberty, with many rugae and much redundancy in the epithelium. Vaginal discharge may be present. Discharge due to
bacteria is yellow and has a purulent appearance. Discharge
due to *Trichomonas* is thin and watery, often yellow, and
occasionally frothy and malodorous. Discharge due to *Candida* is thick and white and may have a cheesy appearance.

Bimanual Examination

The examiner assumes a standing position for the bimanual
examination. This examination is performed with the forefinger and middle finger of the gloved and lubricated hand (Fig.
41-4). These fingers are placed in the vaginal orifice, while
the other fingers are held tightly out of the way, with the
thumb completely adducted. The fingers are advanced vertically along the vaginal canal, and the vaginal wall is palpated.
Firmness of any part of the vaginal wall may represent old

scar tissue from birth trauma. Such tissue may be tender.
Anterior tenderness or burning may represent urethritis associated with a urinary tract infection.

The cervix is palpated and noted for its consistency, mobility, size, and position. The normal cervix is uniformly firm
but not hard. Softening of the cervix and elongation of the
cervical canal are seen in early pregnancy. Hardness may
reflect invasion by neoplasia. The cervix and uterus are normally freely movable. Fixation in the pelvis may reflect extension of malignancy. The body of the uterus is normally
twice the diameter and twice the length of the cervix. The
body may be felt on either side of the cervix, curving anteriorly
toward the abdominal wall. One of five women will, however,
have a *retroflexed uterus,* which curves posteriorly toward
the sacrum.

The opposite hand is now placed halfway between the
umbilicus and the pubis and pressed firmly toward the opening of the pelvis. If the uterus is in an appropriate position,
movement of the abdominal wall will cause the body of the

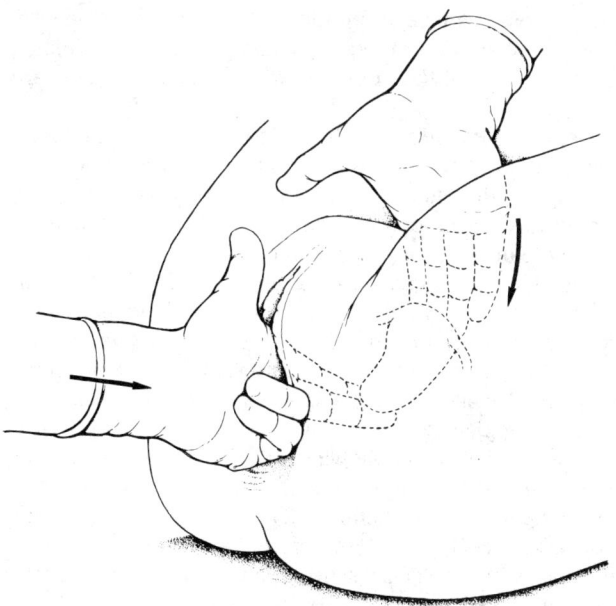

Figure 41-4
Technique for the bimanual examination of the pelvis in the female.

uterus to descend and the pear-shaped organ will be freely movable between the abdominal hand and the examining fingers of the pelvic hand. A reasonably accurate impression can be gained of the size, mobility, and regularity of the contour of the uterus.

The right and left parametria are now palpated. The tube and ovary are contained within these structures. The fingers of the pelvic hand are moved first to one side, then to the other, while the abdominal hand is moved correspondingly to either side of the abdomen. The adnexae are trapped between the two examining hands and are palpated for an obvious mass, tenderness of adnexal tissue, and mobility of the parametrial contents.

It is common for the ovaries to be slightly tender. Bimanual palpation of the vagina and cul-de-sac is accomplished by placing the index finger in the vagina and the middle finger in the rectum. A gentle movement of these fingers toward each other compresses the posterior vaginal wall and the anterior rectal wall and assists the examiner in identifying the integrity of these structures. This procedure may give the patient the sensation of having a bowel movement. The examiner reassures the patient that although she has the urge to defecate, she is not in fact doing so.

To prevent cross-contamination between the vaginal and rectal orifices, the examiner changes gloves between these examinations.

Diagnostic Evaluation

Tests Performed During the Gynecologic Examination

Cytologic Test for Cancer (Papanicolaou Test). The cytologic test is done to detect cervical cancer. Vaginal secretions are aspirated or scraped from the posterior fornix,

and a smear is transferred to a glass slide (Fig. 41-5). The secretion usually is "fixed" immediately by immersing the slide in a fixative. The patient should be instructed not to douche before this examination, since such cleansing will wash away cellular deposits.

The pathologist examines and interprets the cytologic smear. The classification for cytologic findings as suggested by Papanicolaou is as follows:

Class 1: Absence of atypical or abnormal cells
Class 2: Atypical cytology, but no evidence of malignancy
Class 3: Cytology suggestive of, but not conclusive for, malignancy
Class 4: Cytology strongly suggestive of malignancy
Class 5: Cytology conclusive for malignancy

The finding of an abnormal smear (with the exception of Class 5) does not necessarily mean that the patient has cancer but points out that additional procedures, such as

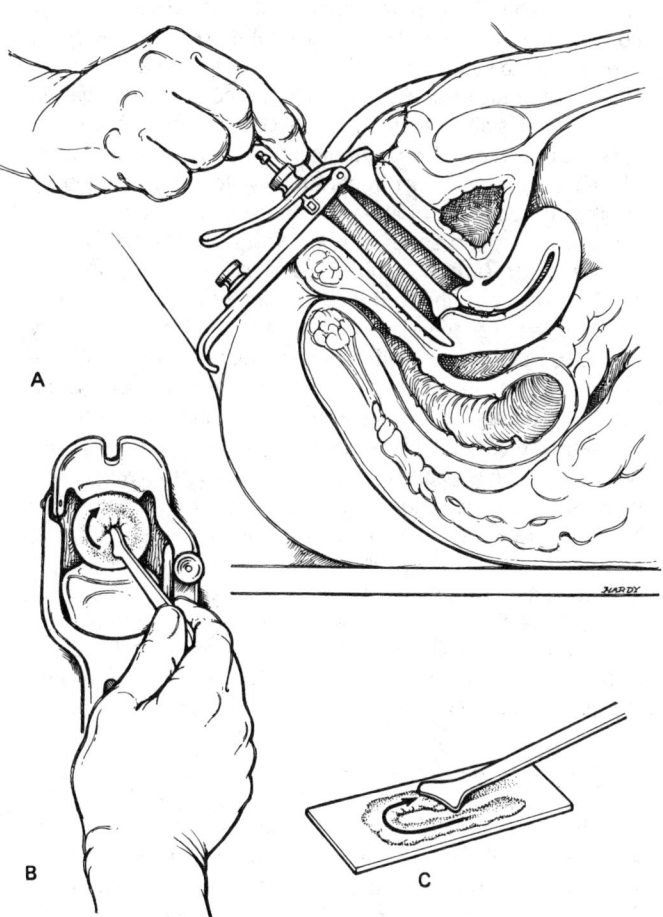

Figure 41-5
Method of using a wooden Ayre spatula to obtain cervical secretions for cytology. (*A*) Speculum in place and the Ayre spatula in position at the cervical os. (*B*) The tip of the spatula is placed in the cervical os and the spatula rotated 360 degrees, firmly but nontraumatically.
(*C*) Cellular material clinging to the spatula is then smeared smoothly on a glass slide, which is promptly placed in a fixative solution.

biopsies or a dilatation and curettage, are indicated. The patient will be grateful for this explanation.

Endometrial (Aspiration) Smears and Biopsy. A smear obtained directly from the endometrium provides an even more accurate method of cytologic diagnosis. There are many ways of obtaining endometrial tissue for cytologic analysis. Evaluation can be made of endometrial secretions, cells, or lavage solutions introduced into the endometrial cavity. These procedures are quite effective in diagnosing cancer but are not suitable for diagnosing hyperplasia and polyps.

Endometrial biopsy is done as an outpatient procedure during the gynecologic pelvic examination. It can usually be done without anesthesia; however, a paracervical block is effective if required. A sound is inserted into the uterus followed by a thin, hollow currette. Suction (Vabra aspirator) may also be used for retrieving endometrial tissue for laboratory analysis. This procedure is probably the most accurate outpatient method for evaluating endometrial cancer.

Schiller Test. With the patient in the lithotomy position (cervix exposed by speculum), a long cotton-tipped applicator is used to paint the cervix with aqueous iodine solution. The appearance of a mahogany-brown color covering the entire surface indicates a reaction between the iodine and the glycogen of normal cells. Such a reaction is considered negative. If the cervix is abnormal, immature cells are present and tissues are not stained brown, indicating that the test is positive. The absence of staining directs attention to the sites requiring additional study (*i.e.*, biopsy), such as those related to cancer, scars, erosion, and zones of nonmalignant leukoplakia.

Cervical Biopsy. The type and extent of biopsy of the cervix vary according to the abnormality or to the results of an abnormal Papanicolaou smear. When a lesion is clearly visible or can be seen with a magnifying instrument called a *colposcope,* one or more punch biopsies may be done as an office procedure without anesthesia because the cervix is less sensitive to cutting procedures than the vagina. However, when no lesion is visible, but the Papanicolaou smear is "suspicious," biopsy excision of an inverted cone of tissue (cone biopsy) is usually needed. This procedure requires anesthesia and probably operating room facilities.

The patient is advised to rest for 24 hours after a biopsy and to leave the packing or tampon in place for the recommended time—usually 8 to 24 hours. Any excess bleeding is to be reported. Sexual intercourse is delayed until the physician indicates that it is permissible.

Dilatation and Curettage

In a dilatation and curettage (D&C) the cervical canal is widened with a dilator and the uterine endometrium is scraped with a curette. This procedure is done to secure endometrial or endocervical tissue for cytologic examination, to control abnormal uterine bleeding, and as a therapeutic measure for incomplete abortion.

Since this procedure usually is carried out under anesthesia and requires surgical asepsis, it is performed in the operating room. Many gynecologists perform D&Cs under local anesthesia, supplemented with diazepam (Valium) or meperidine (Demerol). Explanations as well as psychological and physical preparations are done by the nurse. The patient has a right to know what the procedure will involve (usually explained by her gynecologist) and what to expect in the

way of postoperative discomfort, drainage, or incapacity. Many physicians do not require perineal shaving, but voiding and evacuation of the intestinal tract by a small enema are usually desired.

In the operating room, the patient is placed in the lithotomy position, the cervix is dilated with an instrument, and scrapings of the endometrium are obtained by means of a curette. Tissue for biopsy also may be obtained with an electric needle or a punch biopsy forceps. A cone of tissue may be obtained with a cautery or scalpel. Packing is placed in the cervical and vaginal canal, and a sterile perineal pad is placed over the perineum. A sanitary belt is used to hold the pad in place, or a "stick-on" pad is used. When the pad must be changed while the packing is still in place (usually 24 hours), it is replaced with a sterile pad. Evidence of excessive bleeding is reported. Following the operation, the patient remains in bed for the remainder of the day, although she may get up to go to the bathroom. No restrictions are placed on dietary intake. If pelvic discomfort or low back pain occurs, mild analgesics will usually suffice. The physician will indicate when sexual intercourse may be resumed.

Endoscopic Examinations

Pelvic Endoscopy: Culdoscopy. In this procedure, an incision is made in the posterior vaginal cul-de-sac to admit the *culdoscope* (a tubular, lighted instrument similar to a cystoscope or laparoscope). The patient is prepared as for a vaginal operation, and anesthesia may be local, regional, or general. This procedure makes it possible to visualize directly the uterus, uterine tubes, broad ligaments, uterosacral ligaments, rectal wall, sigmoid colon, and small intestine. The procedure is done in the operating room with the patient in a knee–chest positon.

Culdoscopy is usually used to investigate infertility and is indicated in suspected ectopic pregnancy, in unexplained pelvic pain, and in the presence of undetermined pelvic masses. Following this examination, the scope is withdrawn and the patient is returned to her room. The incision through the posterior vaginal septum heals readily without sutures. Until healing takes place, the patient is directed not to douche or have intercourse until so instructed.

Laparoscopy (Pelvic Peritoneoscopy). A laparoscopy is the insertion of a scope (diameter about 10 mm) into the peritoneal cavity through a 2-cm (¾-inch) subumbilical incision (Fig. 41-6), to allow visualization of the pelvic structures. Indications for laparoscopy are similar to those for culdoscopy. It is also possible to perform minor operative procedures, such as tubal sterilization, ovarian biopsy, and lysis of peritubal adhesions, by means of laparoscopy. A D&C precedes this procedure, not only because it affords additional information but also because a surgical instrument (intrauterine sound or cannula) may be positioned to permit manipulation of the uterus during laparoscopy, affording better visualization.

A better view of the pelvis, lower abdomen, and visceral contents is also facilitated by the injection of a prescribed amount of carbon dioxide intraperitoneally into the cavity (insufflation). This separates the intestines from the pelvic organs. The tubes may be electrocoagulated, and a segment removed for histologic verification. After the purpose of the laparoscopy has been accomplished, the scope is withdrawn and carbon dioxide is allowed to escape through the outer

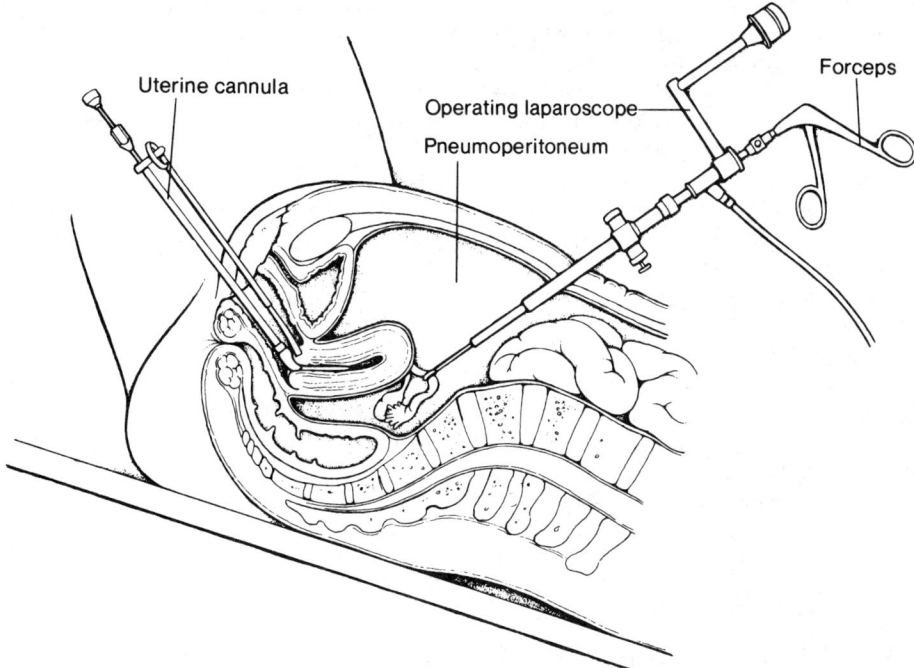

Figure 41-6
Laparoscopy. The laparoscope (*on the right*) is inserted through a small incision in the abdomen. A forceps is inserted through the scope to grasp the uterine tube. To improve the view, a uterine cannula (*on the left*) is inserted into the vagina to push the uterus upward. Insufflation of gas creates an air pocket (pneumoperitoneum), and the pelvis is elevated (note the angle), which forces the intestines higher in the abdomen.

cannula. The skin incision is closed with stitches and covered with a bandage.

The patient is carefully observed for several hours to detect any untoward signs indicating bleeding, injury, or burns from the coagulator. However, these complications rarely occur. Laparoscopy is a cost-effective outpatient procedure.

Hysteroscopy. Hysteroscopy allows direct visualization of all parts of the uterine cavity by means of a lighted optical instrument. The procedure is best performed about 5 days after completion of menstruation (estrogenic phase of the menstrual cycle). The vagina and vulva are cleansed, and a pericervical anesthetic block is done. The instrument used for the procedure, a *hysteroscope*, is passed into the cervical canal and advanced under direct vision 1 or 2 cm; uterine-distending fluid (saline or 5% dextrose) is passed through the instrument to dilate the uterine cavity and provide better visualization.

Hysteroscopy is most commonly indicated as a diagnostic procedure in complex situations: infertility, unexplained bleeding, and retained IUD. Hysteroscopy is contraindicated in patients with cervical or endometrial carcinoma.

Colposcopy and Colpomicroscopy. The *colposcope* (magnification, 10 to 25 times) and *colpomicroscope* (magnification to 400 times) are optical instruments designed to permit three-dimensional views of stained or unstained cervical epithelium *in situ*. These instruments are an additional tool to provide visual access to areas of suspicion, but biopsy of the tissue and other diagnostic methods are required for accurate diagnosis in many instances.

Radiographic Diagnostic Procedures

Many radiologic procedures are helpful in diagnosing pelvic conditions. Ordinary x-ray films, barium enemas, gastrointestinal x-ray series, intravenous urography and cystography are just a few examples.

Hysterosalpingogram (Uterotubogram). A uterotubogram is an x-ray study of the uterus and the uterine (fal-lopian) tubes after the injection of a contrast medium. The diagnostic procedure is done to study sterility problems, to evaluate tubal patency, and to determine the presence of a pathologic condition in the uterine cavity.

The patient is placed in the lithotomy position, and the cervix is exposed with a bivalved speculum. A cannula is inserted into the cervix, and contrast medium is injected into the uterine cavity and the tubes. X-ray films are taken to show the path and the distribution of the contrast materials.

In preparation for a salpingogram, the intestinal tract is prepared by a cathartic and an enema so that gas shadows do not distort the x-ray films. An analgesic is prescribed for comfort, since some patients experience nausea, vomiting, cramps, and faintness. Following the test, it may be advisable for the patient to apply a perineal pad for several hours, because the radiopaque medium may stain clothing.

Computed Tomography. Computed tomography (CT scanning) has several advantages over ultrasound (described below), even though it involves radiation exposure and is more costly. It is more effective with obese patients or a patient with a distended bowel or stomach. A CT scan also can reveal the presence of cancer and its extension into retroperitoneal lymph nodes and skeletal involvement although it is of limited value in diagnosing other gynecologic abnormalities.

Angiography and Radioisotope Scanning. The procedures of angiography and radioisotope scanning are also used as required. Since the uterus and adnexa are in close proximity to the kidneys, ureter, and bladder, urologic diagnostic aids, such as the KUB (kidney, ureter, and bladder) and pyelogram, are frequently used.

Other Diagnostic Aids

Ultrasonography. Ultrasonography employs a simple procedure based on transmission of sound waves similar to the sonar detection used in submarines. Diagnostic ultrasonic scanning equipment uses pulsed ultrasound waves of a frequency exceeding 20,000 cycles per second; the pelvis and abdomen are scanned in linear fashion. The transducer, which is placed in contact with the abdomen, converts mechanical energy into electrical impulses, which in turn are amplified and recorded on an oscilloscope screen. (A photograph is taken of the pattern.) The entire procedure takes about 10 minutes. The findings of this test, in combination with other diagnostic tools, provide useful adjuncts, particularly in the obstetric patient and the obese patient in whom pelvic examination and x-ray studies may hve been unsatisfactory. A definite advantage of ultrasound scanning is that exposure to ionizing radiation is avoided. Patients will appreciate knowing this fact.

Magnetic Resonance Imaging. Magnetic resonance imaging produces patterns that are more delicate and definitive than other radiographic processes. Its chief advantage is absence of radiation. However, it is more costly and less generally available.

Nursing Interventions for Patients With Gynecologic Conditions

Douches are common therapeutic measures in the treatment of patients with gynecologic diseases. They are used both before and after operation and are of two types: vulvar and vaginal.

Vaginal irrigations are used therapeutically to cleanse or disinfect the vagina and adjacent parts, both before and after operation. They also serve to soothe inflamed tissues and to stimulate relaxed tissues. Occasionally, warm or cold douches are indicated in the treatment of oozing.

The patient is placed on the bedpan in the dorsal position with the knees apart and the labia separated. Undue exposure of the patient is prevented, and the bed is protected by placing a plastic sheet under the bedpan. Commonly used solutions include sterile water, normal saline, and antiseptic solutions.

Douches should be given at a temperature of 43.3°C (110°F) or as prescribed. The douch bag is hung not more than 60 cm (2 feet) above the level of the patient's hips. The nurse then puts on sterile gloves, and, separating the labia with the thumb and the forefinger of the left hand, cleans the vaginal orifice and inserts the douche nozzle gently into the vagina for a distance of 5 cm (2 inches), with the tip directed toward the hollow of the sacrum. The clamp then is removed from the tube, and the solution is allowed to flow. Pressure should be avoided to prevent the douche fluid from refluxing through the uterus and the tubes. The solution can be allowed to flow intermittently until at least 1 liter of solution has been used.

The treatment should not be done hastily if therapeutic benefits are to be achieved; it should take from 20 to 30 minutes. After the solution has been instilled, the nozzle may be removed and the patient should be asked to strain as if trying to move the bowels. This act tends to expel the fluid remaining in the vagina. Then, the bedpan is removed, and the perineum is dried with cotton. The patient is instructed to remain recumbent for at least an hour following a warm douche.

After the douche has been completed, the apparatus is cleansed and sterilized again (if not disposable), including

the bedpan. When douching is done at home, the patient usually lies in the bathtub and follows the same principles just described.

Vulvar irrigations are indicated chiefly after operations on the perineum. They should be given after each urination or bowel movement in an effort to keep the incision free from infection. The patient is prepared for a vulvar irrigation in the same manner as for a vaginal douche. Warm, sterile water then is poured gently over the vulva from a sterile container. The area is dried with sterile gauze or cotton, and a sterile dressing or pad is applied and held in place with a T-binder, or stick-on pad is used.

Vaginal antiseptic jellies are another form of medication that the patient can apply herself by means of an applicator. Creams or jellies can be used before and after operation, and in many instances they are substituted for the therapeutic and cleansing douche. It may be necessary for the patient to wear a perineal pad following application of medication.

Menstruation

Physiologic Overview

The *gonads* are the organs that produce either the egg cells (ova) or the sperm cells of an organism. In the female, the gonads are called *ovaries* and are located in the abdomen. In the male, the gonads are the *testes* and are contained within the scrotum. In addition to their reproductive function, the gonads are important endocrine glands.

Ovarian Hormones. The ovaries produce steroid hormones, predominantly *estrogens* and *progesterone*. Several different estrogens are produced by the ovarian follicle, which consists of the developing ovum and its surrounding cells. The most important of the ovarian estrogens is *estradiol*. Estrogens are responsible for the development and maintenance of the female reproductive organs and the secondary sexual characteristics associated with the adult female. Estrogens have an important role in breast development and in the cyclic changes of the uterus that occur monthly.

Progesterone is also important in regulating the changes that occur in the uterus during the menstrual cycle. It is secreted by the *corpus luteum,* which consists of the ovarian follicle after the ovum has been released. Progesterone is the most important hormone for conditioning the lining of the uterus (endometrium) in preparation for implantation of the fertilized ovum. If pregnancy occurs, the secretion of progesterone becomes largely a function of the placenta. This secretion is important for the maintenance of normal pregnancy. In addition, progesterone, working in concert with estrogen, prepares the breast for production and secretion of milk.

Androgens are also produced by the ovaries, but only in very small amounts. Very little is known about the function of androgens in the female.

Regulation of Ovarian Hormone Secretion. *Follicle-stimulating hormone (FSH)* secreted by the pituitary is primarily responsible for stimulating estrogen secretion. *Luteinizing hormone (LH)* is primarily responsible for stimulating the production of progesterone. Feedback mechanisms in part regulate FSH and LH secretion. Increased estrogen levels in the blood inhibit FSH secretion but promote LH secretion.

Elevated progesterone levels inhibit LH secretion. In addition, stimuli from the hypothalamus (releasing factors) affect the rate of gonadotropin (FSH and LH) release.

Menstrual Cycle. In the female, secretion of ovarian hormones follows a cyclic pattern that results in changes of the uterine endometrium (the inner lining of the uterus) and in menstruation (Fig. 41-7). At the begining of the cycle (just after menstruation), FSH output is increased and estrogen secretion is stimulated. This causes the endometrium to thicken and become more vascular. Near the middle portion of the cycle, LH output increases and progesterone secretion is stimulated. It is at this time that ovulation occurs. Under the combined stimulus of estrogen and progesterone, the endometrium reaches its peak of thickening and vascularization. If the ovum has been fertilized, estrogen and progesterone levels remain high and the complex hormonal changes of pregnancy follow. If fertilization has not occurred, the output of FSH and LH diminishes; secretion of estrogen and progesterone falls rapidly; and the vascularized, thickened endometrium is sloughed, with resultant vaginal bleeding (menstruation). The cycle then begins again.

Psychosocial Considerations

The girl between the ages of 11 and 14 who is approaching the *menarche*, or onset of menstruation, should be instructed about this normal process. Psychologically, it is more healthy to refer to this event as "my period" rather than as "being sick" or "having the curse." With adequate nutrition, rest, exercise, and good posture, there will be little discomfort. Some girls do experience breast tenderness and a feeling of fullness a day or two before the onset of menstruation. There may be a greater tendency to fatigue and some discomfort of the lower back, legs, and pelvis on the first day; temperament and mood changes may be apparent. Slight deviations from the usual healthy pattern of daily living is considered normal, but signs of excessive deviations may require investigation. The perineal pad is a widely used method of disposing of menstural discharge; deodorant pads are available. Tampons are also used extensively; usually, there is no significant evidence of untoward effects from their use, providing there is not difficulty in inserting them.* Should the "tail" string break and difficulty be encountered in removing the tampon, the woman's physician should be consulted. A third type of protection is the internal rubber cup, but this is used less frequently.

As was mentioned earlier, menstruation may be handled differently in different cultures. Some women believe that it is detrimental to change a pad or tampon too frequently; they believe that by allowing this discharge to accumulate, an increased flow is stimulated, which is considered desirable. For the nurse to insist that a pad be changed before the time the patient believes proper may cause conflict. These differences must be carefully reconciled so that proper understanding develops.

Other psychosocial aspects may need to be considered, such as belief in the vulnerability of women to illness during menstruation. Many believe it is detrimental to swim, take a cold shower, receive a "permanent wave," get teeth filled, or eat certain foods during one's period. Such myths need to be recognized and corrected. Many other examples of

---

* See toxic shock syndrome, p. 1108.

---

misunderstanding could be listed; however, the objective is to alert the nurse to these unexpressed, deep-rooted beliefs. Aspects of gynecologic problems cannot always be expressed easily. The nurse needs to convey confidence and trust, as well as offer sound advice, in order to set up a communication exchange.

Premenstrual Syndrome

Premenstrual syndrome (PMS) is a combination of symptoms experienced by some women prior to the onset of each menstrual cycle. The etiology is unknown, but several theories suggest estrogen–progesterone imbalance, vitamin deficiencies, excessive prostaglandins, and/or abnormal magnesium metabolism. Major symptoms include headache, fatigue, low back pain, engorged or painful breasts, and a feeling of abdominal fullness. General irritability may even include mood swings, fear of losing control, binge eating, and crying spells. Symptoms vary widely from one woman to another and from one cycle to the next in the same person. A generally stressful life appears related to the intensity of physical symptoms. Women report moderate to severe life disruption, even affecting interpersonal exchanges among family members. PMS can be a factor in reduced productivity, work-related accidents, and absenteeism.

The *timing* of the above symptoms is what helps in determining the diagnosis. Symptoms recur regularly at the same phase of each menstrual cycle and, in the same cycle, are followed by a symptom-free phase.

Management. There is no single treatment for PMS and no specific medication. Women are encouraged to chart their own symptoms, which can help in learning to anticipate what symptoms to record and when they occur. Such a chart is helpful in ruling out other problems such as anemia, diabetes, and thyroid disorders. Some physicians prescribe pain relievers, diuretics, and natural progesterone.

▶ Nursing Process
The Patient With Premenstrual Syndrome (PMS)

▷ Assessment

The nurse should establish a comfortable rapport with the patient while taking a nursing history, which should note when symptoms began and their intensity. She determines whether the onset is related to a major hormonal change, such as following oral contraceptives, a pregnancy, tubal ligation, or after a period of amenorrhea. In addition to obtaining a record of symptoms and times of occurrence, the nurse can offer guidance in drawing up a chart showing the timing and intensity of symptoms as shown in Figure 41-8. Such a record, to be meaningful, is done over a minimum of three cycles. A nutritional history is also elicited to determine dietary excesses or deficiencies of salt, alcohol, and caffeine.

▷ Nursing Diagnoses

Based on the nursing and nutritional history as well as other assessment data, the patient's major nursing diagnoses may include the following:

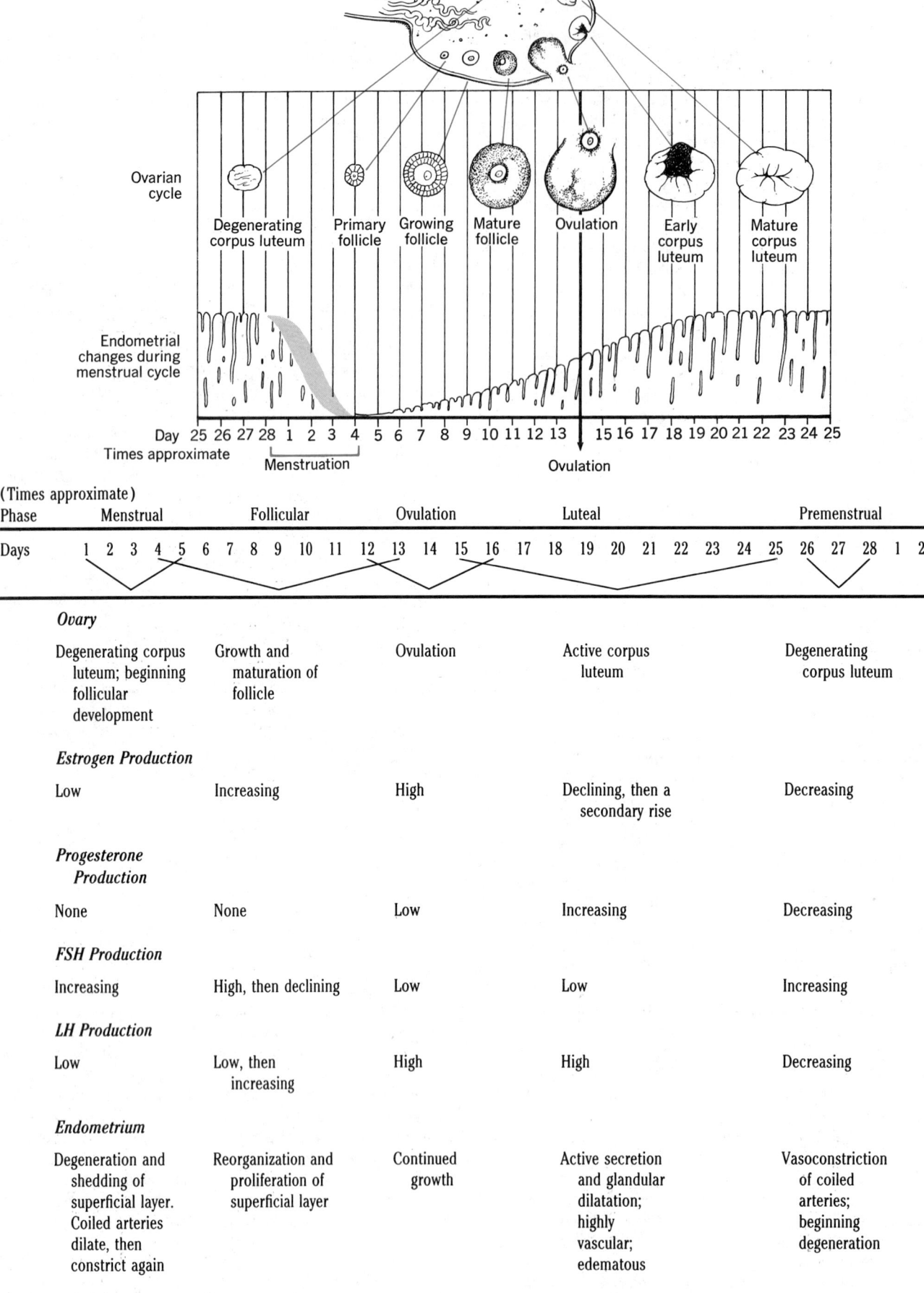

Figure 41-7
Correlation of hormonal activities with ovarian and uterine changes. (Adapted from Chaffee EE and
Greisheimer EM. Basic Physiology and Anatomy, 3rd ed. Philadelphia, JB Lippincott.)

	Jan	Feb	Mar	Apr
1				
2				
3				
4				
5				
6		h		
7				
8				
9				
10				
11				
12				
13			Hd	
14			HD	
15			HD	
16		D	HD	
17		Hd	Md	
18	d	HD	M	
19	Hd	HD	M	
20	D	M	M	
21	HD	M	M	
22	HD	M		
23	Mh	M		
24	M			
25	M			
26	M			
27	M			
28				
29				
30				
31				

Figure 41-8
Chart for recording timing pattern of premenstrual symptoms as an aid to diagnosis of premenstrual syndrome. Capital letters signify intense symptoms; lowercase letters, mild symptoms. M, menstruation; H, h, headache; D, d, depressive symptoms. (Lindemann JC. Premenstrual syndrome—a practical approach. Wisc Med J 1984; 83[11]:32.)

- Anxiety related to the effects of PMS
- Ineffective coping of both patient and family related to effects of PMS
- Potential for violence directed at family members related to symptoms of PMS
- Inadequate knowledge of the causes and treatment of PMS

▷ *Planning and Implementation*

▷ *Goals:* The major goals of the patient may include reduction of anxiety (mood swings, crying, binge eating, fear of losing control), ability to cope with usual interpersonal relations with family and at work, absence of violent reactions, improved knowledge regarding PMS and use of control measures.

Nursing Interventions

Reducing Anxiety. General support and counseling are provided. The patient is asked to participate in her care by keeping a chart of her symptoms (see Fig. 41-8) and daily temperature; she is encouraged to plan activities around the troublesome times. Her partner and children are included in discussing her problem, since sharing this information leads to mutual understanding and lessened tension for the patient. Taking analgesics/tranquilizers as prescribed is encouraged.

Coping Measures. Positive coping measures are facilitated, such as recommending to the partner how he can help his mate. This may include offering support, increased involvement with child care, and seeking marital counseling if problems get out of control. The patient can try to plan her working time to accommodate the days she will be less productive owing to PMS.

Reducing Stress. The nurse intervenes at times of increased stress by removing those activities, conversations, or disruptions that appear to worsen the patient's problem. The nurse is attentive and understanding since it provides relief to the patient; it is helpful to the patient to know that others recognize and understand what she is experiencing.

Patient Education. The nurse can suggest that the patient keep a 3-month record of daily temperature and symptoms and consult with a health care professional in determining the specific diagnosis. She is encouraged to follow the recommendations for additional testing to rule out other possible causes of the annoying symptoms.

The patient should assume responsibility for following a dietary plan of eating small meals and eliminating or restricting sugar, alcohol, caffeine and nicotine. Supplements of vitamin B_6, calcium, and magnesium may be prescribed. Exercise and relaxation each day are encouraged, and the importance of participating in various health promotion strategies such as weight reduction if applicable is emphasized. Perhaps flexible work schedules can be arranged to accommodate the troublesome period each month. Enrolling in a PMS group that meets to discuss mutual problems can also be helpful. Such groups provide support and have a tendency to make problems more bearable when others have the same or worse symptoms.

Much research is being done on PMS, and new clues for its treatment are likely to appear.

▷ *Evaluation*

▷ *Expected Outcomes*

1. Patient experiences less anxiety.
   a. Verbalizes awareness of the nature of the problem.
   b. Relates that her new support system (health care personnel) has reduced her concerns.
2. Demonstrates adequate coping mechanisms.
   a. Keeps a monthly calendar of her symptoms and temperature.
   b. Schedules activities around her "problem times."
   c. Reports greater comfort and reduced stress.

3. Follows dietary practices that improve behavior.
   a. Increases intake of protein and reduces intake of refined sugar and salt.
   b. Increases intake of magnesium-rich foods (whole grains, nuts, green vegetables).
   c. Avoids caffeine and cigarettes.
   d. Takes vitamin B$_6$ (pyridoxine) as prescribed.

Dysmenorrhea

Primary dysmenorrhea is painful menstruation with no identifiable pelvic pathology. It usually occurs within a few years after the menarche and appears to be related to the establishment of ovulatory cycles. It is a common condition occurring in approximately 35% of all older adolescent girls, 25% of female college students, and 60% to 70% of single women in their 30s. Painful cramps are the result of excessive production of prostaglandins, which causes increased uterine hypercontractility and arteriolar vasospasm. Psychological factors, such as anxiety, tension, and dependency, may also contribute to dysmenorrhea. As the woman grows older, pain tends to decrease and often completely resolves after childbirth.

In *secondary dysmenorrhea* a pelvic pathologic process is confirmed, such as endometriosis, tumor, and pelvic inflammatory disease. These conditions are discussed in Chapter 42.

Assessment and Clinical Manifestations. In primary dysmenorrhea, the symptoms are mild cramps that may begin 12 to 24 hours preceding the onset of flow and become more acute with the flow, lasting an additional 12 to 24 hours. The pain is crampy, is located in the lower midabdomen and may radiate to lower back and upper thighs, and may be associated with chills, nausea, vomiting, headache, and irritability. In secondary dysmenorrhea, patients are usually older and pain is not always limited to the time of menses and first day of flow.

A complete physical examination is done to rule out possible abnormalities, such as strictures of the cervix or vagina or an imperforate hymen, as well as other conditions, such as endometriosis, pelvic inflammatory disease, and fibroid uterus. For organic causes, a hysterosalpingogram or ultrasound examination may be required.

Management and Nursing Interventions. In primary dysmenorrhea, the reason for the discomfort is explained, and the patient is assured that menstruation is a normal function of the reproductive tract. If the patient is a young girl and is accompanied by her mother, then the mother too can be reassured. Many daughters are conditioned to expect dysmenorrhea because their mothers experienced it. The pain, which is real, can be treated once worry and concern over its possible significance are dispelled through accurate understanding. Symptoms subside in a few years or with normal sexual function and childbearing.

More specific methods of affording relief are as follows. The patient is encouraged to carry on her usual activities, since mind-occupying functions and physical exercise provide a neurophysiologic basis for relief. Taking analgesics before cramps start, in anticipation of discomfort, is advised. Aspirin or acetaminophen may be taken at recommended doses every 4 hours. If necessary, antiemetics, antispasmodics, and mild tranquilizers may be prescribed by the physician. Prostaglan-

dins have been cited as causing dysmenorrhea, so prostaglandin antagonists appear helpful (Ibuprofen [Motrin], naproxen [Naprosyn], mefenamic acid [Ponstel], naproxin [Anaprox]). If one inhibitor does not provide relief, the patient is advised to try another. Usually these medications are well tolerated, but some women experience gastrointestinal side-effects. Contraindications may include allergy, peptic ulcer history, or sensitivity to aspirin-like medications. Low-dose oral contraceptives often provide relief in over 90% of patients.

Management of secondary dysmenorrhea is directed to treating the underlying cause (*e.g.*, endometriosis, pelvic inflammatory disease).

Amenorrhea (Absence of Menstrual Flow)

Primary amenorrhea (delayed menarche) refers to those instances when a young woman over age 17 has not yet begun to menstruate but otherwise shows evidence of sexual maturation. This may be of considerable concern to the person as well as to her mother but is more than likely due to minor variations in body build, heredity, and environment, as well as in physical, mental, and emotional development.

The understanding nurse will provide an opportunity for the girl to express her concerns and anxiety about this problem, since she may feel that she is not like her peers and that she may not be able to fulfill her role as a woman. A complete physical examination, careful history, and simple laboratory studies will assist in excluding physiological disorders, metabolic or endocrine difficulties, and other systemic diseases. Treatment is directed toward correction of any anomalies.

Secondary amenorrhea (at least 6 to 12 months in duration) occurs after a normal menarche and during pregnancy and lactation. In the adolescent, the most common cause is a minor emotional upset related to being away from home, attending college, tension from school work, or interpersonal problems. Since the second most common cause is pregnancy, this possibility should always be investigated.

Secondary nutritional disturbances may also be apparent, such as weight loss or weight gain. This psychogenic or hypothalamic amenorrhea may last for a few years. On occasion there may be a pituitary or thyroid dysfunction that may be helped by appropriate measures. At any rate, consultation with a physician is necessary.

Abnormal Uterine Bleeding

Menorrhagia. Menorrhagia is excessive bleeding at the time of the regular menstrual flow. In early life, it may be due to endocrine disturbances, but with increase in duration of the menstrual periods in later life, it is usually due to inflammatory disturbances or tumors of the uterus. Emotional disturbance may also affect bleeding.

A woman with menorrhagia is encouraged to see her gynecologist and relate the nature of the excessive bleeding. Although difficult to measure, an estimate might be given in terms of numbers of pads or tampons used in excess of those used for the regular flow.

Metrorrhagia. Metrorrhagia is the appearance of blood from the uterus between the regular menstrual periods or after menopause. It is always the symptom of some disease, often cancer or benign tumors of the uterus; therefore, it merits early diagnosis and treatment. Metrorrhagia is probably the most significant form of menstrual dysfunction; the fact that it occurs warrants further investigation.

Perimenopause

Perimenopause is the period extending from the first signs of menopause, usually hot flashes, to beyond the complete cessation of menses (1 year beyond). *Menopause* is described as the physiologic cessation of menses associated with failing ovarian function. It is often diagnosed in retrospect when a year has passed with no menses. The *climacteric* period is the transition period in the life of a woman during which the reproductive function gradually diminishes and is lost. *Post-menopause* is the period about 1 year past the cessation of menses and beyond.

Physiologic Overview

The menopausal period of a woman's life marks the end of her active reproductive life. It usually occurs between the ages of 49 and 52, but it may occur in some women as early as 42 or as late as 55. Menstruation then ceases, and as a result of the complete cessation of activity on the part of the ovaries, the reproductive organs and the mammary glands atrophy. No more ova mature; therefore, no ovarian hormones are produced. A similar situation prevails earlier if the ovaries are removed or destroyed by irradiation, producing an artificial menopause.

Menopause is not a pathologic phenomenon; in addition to estrogen deficiency, there are multifaceted psychological and physiologic changes, including neuroendocrinologic, biochemical, and metabolic changes related to the aging process.

Clinical Manifestations

Usually, symptoms of menopause can be classified according to cause, as arising from (1) endocrine changes due to a lack of estrogen or (2) psychological changes. The process starts gradually and is recognized by the change in menstruation. The monthly flow becomes smaller in amount, then irregular, and finally ceases. Often, the time between periods gets longer—there may be a lapse of several months between them. Any prolonged menstrual flow or bleeding between periods should be reported promptly to the physician.

Hot or warm flashes and night sweats are reported by most women and are directly attributable to hormonal changes. The hot flash is a symptom denoting vasomotor instability. Flashes may be mild, moderate, and severe, varying from a warm feeling, often fleeting, that is barely noticed to an extremely hot feeling accompanied by profuse sweating that is quite uncomfortable. The latter may require the woman to seek relief by fanning, showering, and lying down. She may have associated feelings of dizziness, chills, chest pains, and inability to concentrate.

The middle-aged woman will note beginning changes in her physical appearance and a lower level of physical energy. Additional physical manifestations may include atrophic changes, suggestion of stress incontinence, sagging structures, senile vaginitis, skin dryness, weight gain, and signs of calcium deficiency (shrinking in stature—osteoporosis). Although the entire genitourinary system is affected by lessened estrogens, the vulvovagina area is most apparent. There is a thinning of hair (mons veneris) and a gradual shrinkage of the labia. Vaginal secretions diminish, and dispareunia (painful intercourse) may be experienced. The vaginal *p*H rises, predisposing to bacterial infections (vaginitis). Itching and burning of vulvar tissues may be noted.

Psychological Manifestations

Symptoms of a more psychological type may occur before or during these changes in the monthly periods (*e.g.,* dizziness, weakness, nervousness, insomnia, headaches, and inability to concentrate). This often is the time in a woman's life when the children have grown up and left home; thus, she may no longer feel needed. This realization, added to an acute awareness of the aging process, can have an effect on symptoms expressed. Fear of growing old may trigger feelings of depression. These feelings may be more of a problem for women who have not worked outside the home. For those who are involved with interesting and meaningful work, such reactions are infrequent. Many woman have very mild symptoms, and some have none.

Management

The majority of patients will respond to a program of education, reassurance, modification of their living habits, and an improved regimen of health. In some patients, mild sedatives and tranquilizers are necessary to control nervousness and to counteract depression, which is not at all unusual at this time. Sometimes even simple, everyday problems are too much to handle.

Persistent and severe hot flashes require treatment by estrogen therapy given on a cyclic basis. The dosage is regulated by the physician according to a desired schedule, such as taking the medication for the first 25 days of each month. A progestational agent is usually added for the last 10 days of estrogen administration.

Continued use of estrogen therapy to prevent widespread degenerative changes, including physical aging, is still controversial. Most authorities are conservative and prescribe estrogen replacement on an individual basis for acute estrogen deprivation or annoying signs of estrogen deficiency, such as atrophic vaginitis or osteoporosis. Restraint in prescribing estrogens for all menopausal women arises from concern that protracted treatment will induce neoplastic changes in estrogen-sensitive aging tissue.

Nursing Interventions

Measures should be taken to promote the woman's general health. The nurse can explain to the patient that the cessation of the menses is a physiologic function that is not inevitably accompanied by extreme nervous symptoms and illness. Women whose children have left home are *not* at increased risk for depression.

The current expected life span after menopause for the average woman is 30 to 35 years. This is an optimistic thought, since it encompasses as many years as the childbearing phase of her life.

The menopause is not a complete change of life. The normal sexual urges remain, and women retain their usual reaction to sex long after menopause. There is nothing abnormal about the change of life, and nothing unusual about the continuation of happy marital relations afterward. Many women enjoy better health after the menopause than they have had for years. This is especially true with persons who have always suffered pain during their menstrual periods.

Patient Education. The following factors are stressed in patient teaching:

- The climacteric period is normal and self-limiting.
- Overfatigue and environmental problems exaggerate the symptoms.
- A nutritious diet and weight control will improve the physical condition.
- An exercise program in keeping with the patient's needs promotes vitality.
- Interest and participation in outside activities help to absorb anxiety and to lessen tension.
- Changes are expected in former support networks: departure of children, aging and dependent parents, death of loved ones.
- Old friendships should be revived, new friendships sought, and self-fulfillment provided.
- This is an excellent time for intellectual growth and the stimulation of new ideas and experiences.
- Menopause does not mean a termination of the patient's sex life.
- An annual physical examination is essential to the maintenance of continuing good health.

For the handling/prevention of physical annoyances, the following may be helpful:

- For itching or burning vulvar areas, obtain prescription for a recommended cortisone cream (*e.g.,* Mycolog).
- To prevent dyspareunia, use a water-soluble lubricant, such as K-Y jelly.
- Improve perineal muscle tone and bladder control by practicing Kegel's exercises daily:
  When lying on the back with a pillow under the knees, contract the perineal muscles as though stopping urination; hold for 5 seconds and release. Repeat 10 times for 3 or 4 times a day. It can be done while sitting or standing.
- Use bland skin cream and lotions to prevent drying, itching, and cracking skin.
- Avoid bubble baths since most ingredients are drying to the skin.
- Pay increased attention to good grooming, including attractive color coordination of clothes, make-up, and hairstyling to give a needed lift when it is most needed.
- Join a weight-reduction support group such as *Weight Watchers* or a similar support group if being overweight is a problem. There is a tendency to gain weight particularly around the hips, thighs, and abdomen.
- Observe a proper level of calcium intake since calcium requirements increase after menopause. Milk and calcium supplements are necessary to offset osteoporosis (see Chap. 58 for discussion of this condition).

The individual woman's evaluation of herself and her worth, now and in the future, certainly affects her emotional reaction to this change in her life.

Gerontological Considerations

Frequent examinations can help in preventing problems of the reproductive tract in the aging female. Often older women do not have regular gynecologic examinations; many who have been delivered of their children at home have never had a pelvic examination. Some regard it as an embarrassing and unpleasant procedure. The role of the nurse in emphasizing an annual pelvic examination for all women is of major health teaching significance.

With aging, the vulva loses hair and subcutaneous fat, accompanied by general tissue atrophy. As a result, the woman is easily susceptible to irritation and infection. Pruritus is a common symptom. Physiologic changes include diminished vaginal lubrication and elasticity.

The primary change is the absence of responsive follicles in the ovary. This results in the reduction of estrogen secretion and concomitant changes in androgen production. Estrogen deficiency directly affects the ovaries, endometrium, vaginal epithelium, and skin, which is known to possess estrogen receptors. Clinical effects are dyspareunia and increased susceptibility to vaginal trauma and infection.

With relaxing pelvic musculature, prolapse of the uterus is common; sagging structures produce low back pain, stress urinary incontinence, and later difficulty in voiding and defecation. This usually causes the patient to become more sedentary, which leads to osteoporosis, vertebral collapse, pain, unstable gait, falls, and fractures. Appropriate evaluation and proper vaginal surgery could provide more years of an active and happy life. When surgery is indicated in the aging woman, it must be recognized that more time is needed for the healing and repair of tissues. In addition, concern needs to be given to the psychosocial aspects of relating to family, friends, and partners. Support resources are essential in achieving the desired outcomes of self-sufficiency in the woman.

The incidence of cancer is more apparent in the aging person. Gerontological implications are presented in Chapter 16. Sexual changes are discussed in Chapter 13.

Conception Control

Control of human reproduction has been practiced for various reasons since ancient times. Many methods exist and their acceptance has fluctuated. An ideal method has not been developed; all have advantages and disadvantages. Most methods apply to women.

Family planning refers to limiting or spacing the number of children born. In preventing unwanted or unplanned births, the means described below are available:

> *Natural planning*—using any natural means of pregnancy prevention to the exclusion of chemical or mechanical means
> *Contraception*—a means of temporarily avoiding pregnancy
> *Sterilization*—a means of permanently preventing pregnancy
> *Induced abortion*—the voluntary evacuation of the fetus before it becomes viable

In the United States, sterilization has become the most popular method of contraception. The second most popular method is the birth control pill.

Patient Education. Much has been written about family planning and the availability and use of contraceptive devices. The nurse is in a strong position to help patients understand the options available. Religious groups have made clear their teaching and dogma regarding birth control, and these beliefs need to be respected and understood as couples make their decision. Research is changing the methods used in fertility control, and more acceptable and longer-lasting types are sought.

Natural Methods

The advantages of natural methods of contraception include the following: (1) they are not hazardous to a person's health, (2) they are inexpensive, and (3) they are preferred by some religions. The disadvantages are that they require discipline by the couple and periods of abstinence. Also, they are less effective than other methods. *Abstinence* or *celibacy* is the only completely effective means of preventing pregnancy. *Coitus interruptus* is the withdrawal of the penis from the vagina before ejaculation, which requires strong willpower. The uncertainty in this method is due to the presence of sperm in the pre-ejaculatory fluid.

Rhythm Method. The rhythm method of contraception can be difficult to use because it is based on the woman's ability to determine her time of ovulation and on the avoidance of intercourse during the fertile period. The fertile phase (which requires sexual continence) is estimated to occur about 14 days before menstruation, although it may occur between the 10th and 17th days. It is assumed that spermatozoa can fertilize an ovum up to 72 hours after intercourse and that the ovum can be fertilized for about 24 hours after it leaves the ovary. Studies reveal that of 100 women practicing the rhythm method, up to 40 will conceive during a year.

According to some researchers, if a woman carefully determines her "safe period," based on precise recording of her menstrual dates for at least 1 year, and follows a carefully worked out formula, she may achieve 80% protection. However, it requires a long period of abstinence during each cycle. New methods of detecting ovulation (*e.g.*, ovulimeter) have improved statistics.

For ensuring best success, the woman is encouraged to

- Keep a daily chart recording the nature of cervical mucus; this changes as the menstrual cycle progresses
- Check her temperature at waking (temperature rises for a few days after ovulation)
- Estimate when ovulation will occur based on past experience

It is encouraging to note that a group of researchers are working on how to predict ovulation. They have discovered that the presence of the enzyme *guaiacol peroxidase* in cervical mucus signals ovulation 6 days beforehand and controls viscosity. Sperm can get through the cervical canal *only* when mucus is watery (ovulation time) and an egg is present. When research in this area is developed further, the woman will be able to sample her cervical mucus using a color-coded device from a test kit.

Oral Steroids—"The Pill"

Physiologic Basis. Oral synthetic steroid preparations of estrogen and progesterone tend to block the stimulation of the ovary by the central nervous system by preventing the release of the follicle-stimulating hormone (FSH) from the anterior pituitary. In the absence of FSH, a follicle does not ripen and ovulation does not take place. This is the mechanism of action of oral contraceptives. Progestin suppresses the luteinizing hormone (LH) surge, preventing ovulation. It also renders cervical mucus impenetrable to sperm.

Synthetic estrogens and progestins vary in potency as well as in androgenic and anabolic activity. Usually, a single pill is taken on the fifth day of menstruation and each day thereafter for 20 or 21 days; this is repeated on the fifth day of each ensuing menstrual period. Some companies provide 28 pills in a convenient case; 7 to 8 are placebos. This means the woman takes a pill each day.

There are two kinds of therapy: "combined" and "gestagen only." The difference lies in the dosage of progestogens. In the *combined therapy*, estrogen and progestogen are present in every pill. The majority of women taking oral contraceptives take this type. Progestogen interferes with cervical mucus production and prevents uterine endometrium from fully developing to receive the fertilized ovum, resulting in a lighter-than-normal menstrual flow. Progestogen (*gestagen only*) in a smaller dose given daily is the other major kind of oral contraceptive. A small percentage of women take this type.

Side-Effects. In a small percentage of patients, side-effects may be noted, such as nausea, pelvic discomfort, backache, irritability, depression, headache, weight gain, leg cramps, breast soreness, hirsutism, and acne. Usually, these disappear after 3 or 4 months. Because such symptoms are related to sodium and water retention caused by estrogen, a smaller dose of the hormone and salt reduction in the diet may alleviate the problem.

Other problems encountered are the occurrence of thromboembolic disorders, more rapid growth of uterine fibroids, and jaundice. Therefore, these drugs should not be used by women who have had thromboembolic disorders, uterine fibroids, diabetes, or liver or gallbladder disease. Noted also is an increased incidence of heart attacks in smokers over the age of 35 who are on the pill. Occasionally, neuro-ocular complications arise, but a cause-and-effect relationship is unknown at present. Should visual disturbances occur, the drug should be terminated. An increased incidence of candidal vulvovaginitis has also been reported.

Women with scanty or irregular periods are strongly advised to use another method of contraception. If they use oral contraceptives, they may have difficulty becoming pregnant or may fail to have menstrual periods after discontinuing the pill. With respect to how soon fertility returns after taking oral contraceptives, resumption of fertility is delayed 2 to 3 months in approximately 20% of users. For some women it is longer; since ovulation may be delayed for varying periods, it is probably helpful (for calculating expected delivery date) for the woman desiring to become pregnant to use a mechanical contraceptive barrier for the first month.

Regarding a possible link with breast cancer, a recent study indicates that regardless of the age when a woman starts using the pill or how long she uses it, she is at no greater risk of breast cancer than those women who have never used birth control pills.

It is generally accepted that no definite long-term undesirable effects following prolonged use of oral contraceptives have been observed. Fetal anomalies do not appear to be a concern, and normal reproductive tract function and fertility are restored (although somewhat delayed, as was indicated above) following discontinuance of the oral contraceptive. Meanwhile, research and experimentation continue toward the development of a single monthly pill or injection that would be safe as well as effective. The risk factors of oral contraceptives are listed in Chart 41-1.

Mechanical Barriers

Diaphragm. The diaphragm is an effective contraceptive device. It is a round flexible spring (50 to 90 mm in diameter) that is covered with a domelike latex rubber cup. A spermicidal jelly or cream is used to coat the concavity of the diaphragm before it is inserted deep into the vagina. The combination of a diaphragm and spermicide prevents spermatozoa from entering the cervical canal. The diaphragm presents no discomfort, since it is lodged against the back wall of the vagina and anteriorly against the edge of the pubic bone. Since women vary in size, diaphragms are designed to fit the client; therefore, it is necessary for the woman to be fitted for the proper size by a physician or a nurse practioner. At this time the woman is instructed in its use and care. A return-demonstration will ensure that the diaphragm is inserted correctly to cover the cervix and upper vagina.

Each time the diaphragm is used, it must be examined carefully by holding it up to a bright light and making sure it has no pinpoint holes, cracks, or tears. Contraceptive jelly or cream is applied in a prescribed manner to the dome of the diaphragm. If it is applied more than 2 hours before intercourse, it must be reapplied. The diaphragm is then positioned to cover the cervix completely. The diaphragm is left in place at least 6 hours after coitus. Upon removal it is cleansed thoroughly with mild soap and water, rinsed, and dried before it is stored in its original container.

Cervical Cap. The cervical cap is much smaller (22 to 35 mm) than the diaphragm and covers only the cervix; it is used with a spermicide. If the woman knows how to insert a diaphragm, it is easy to apply a cervical cap. The chief advantage is that the cap may be left in place for several days.

Sponge and Spermicide. A more recent contraceptive is a sponge made of urethane and a spermicide (nonoxynol-9) that is marketed under the trade name of *Today*. It is inserted into the vaginal tract, fits loosely over the cervix, and may be left in place up to 24 hours. A polyester loop attached to the sponge permits its retrieval. It is available without prescription and appears according to some tests to be as effective as the diaphragm.

Condom. The condom is an impermeable snug-fitting rubber or plastic cover applied to the erect penis before it enters the vaginal canal. The penis with condom in place is to be removed from the vagina while still erect to prevent leakage of ejaculate.

Intrauterine Device

An intrauterine device (IUD) is a plastic or metal piece (frequently copper) of varying shapes, usually 2.5 × 2 cm (1 × ¾ inches), that is inserted by a gynecologist through the cervix into the endometrial cavity to prevent pregnancy. The method by which an IUD prevents contraception is thought to be due to a local inflammatory reaction caused by the presence of a foreign body in the uterus. The inflammatory reaction appears to be toxic to spermatozoa and blastocytes. One type of IUD, the Progestasert-T, releases progestin and is replaced each year. Other types are replaced every 2 to 3 years unless there is a problem.

The advantages of this method are that it is effective over

Chart 41-1
Conception Control: Risk Factors and Patient Monitoring

Absolute Contraindications to the Use of Oral Contraceptives (FDA)

1. Known or suspected estrogen-dependent neoplasia
2. Known or suspected cancer of the breast
3. Thrombophlebitis or thromboembolic disease
4. A history of thrombophlebitis, thromboembolism, or thrombotic disease
5. Cerebrovascular and coronary artery disease
6. Abnormal uterine bleeding from an unknown cause
7. Known or suspected pregnancy

Other Contraindications

Hypertension, congenital hyperlipidemia, diabetes mellitus, liver disease, cholestatic jaundice, amenorrhea, migraine headache, leiomyoma of the uterus, heavy cigarette smoking
Oral contraceptives are mainly recommended for young women; systemic disease and the mortality risk in using the pill both increase with age.

a long period of time, appears to have no systemic effects, and reduces the factor of patient error. The disadvantages are that such a device may cause excessive bleeding, become displaced, perforate the cervix and uterus, and may cause infection. There is also the risk of pregnancy-related complications, such as congenital anomalies, spontaneous or septic abortion, and ectopic pregnancy.

Because several commonly used IUDs have caused problems, many have been taken off the market. The popularity of this method has consequently decreased.

Interception (Postcoital Conception Control)

A properly timed administration of an adequate dosage of estrogen following intercourse will prevent pregnancy. Such a ''morning after'' pill is not applicable for use in long-term contraception, but is of real value in emergency situations such as rape, defective or torn condom or diaphragm, or other ''accidental'' intercourse. Such medication given immediately after fertilization and before the occurrence of implantation is effective. Usually, the therapy is continued over 5 days using diethylstilbestrol or ethinyl estradiol. Nausea can be minimized by taking the medication with meals and with an antiemetic drug. Other side-effects may be experienced, such as breast soreness and irregular menses, but these are transient.

''Permanent'' Conception Control

Sterilization is becoming increasingly popular, and in fact is the preferred method of contraception for couples who no longer desire to have children. Sterilization may be achieved by hysterectomy, oophorectomy, or tubal ligation in the female and by vasectomy in the male. With increasing research, ligations may be reversible; however, they are still considered a permanent means of sterilization.

Tubal Sterilization. Tubal sterilization (ligation or electrocoagulation of uterine tubes) terminates a woman's ability to have children without affecting her ovulatory or menstrual function. Various surgical techniques have been developed using the abdominal or vaginal approach.

Laparoscopy is the most common method of tubal ligation in the United States. The small incision is either sub-umbilical or at the pubic hairline (see p. 744).

The surgeon performs a *laparotomy* (an abdominal incision) and locates the uterine (fallopian) tubes. The tubes are then occluded using clips or sutures to prevent ova entering from the ovaries. Another possible technique is to resect a segment of the tube. This operation may be done during other abdominal surgery or a cesarean section, provided an informed consent has been obtained.

Tubal ligation may also be done through a *mini-laparotomy* (small abdominal incision). The surgeon places an instrument into the vagina and moves the uterus and tubes up against the abdominal wall where he has access through the small incision to ligate the tube.

Sterilization can also be done through a *colpotomy* (incision of the vagina). A culdoscope is inserted into the vagina and through a colpotomy incision. The fimbriated uterine tube is then ligated and excised or occluded by tantalum clips. With the clips, however, there is the possibility that sterilization will be reversed at some point in the future. The advantage of this method is the absence of an abdominal scar and less intraperitoneal insufflation (injection of gas, as is done with an abdominal laparoscope).

Patient Education. Usually before a sterilization is done, an IUD, if present, is removed. If the patient is on the ''pill,'' it is usually stopped for a month before the procedure. Postoperatively there is some abdominal soreness for a few days. The patient is to report any of the following: bleeding, pain that continues or increases, and elevated temperature. For one week she is to avoid intercourse and strenuous excercises or lifting. A comparison of female sterilization with vasectomy is shown in Chart 41-2.

Vasectomy. A vasectomy is the ligation and transection of a section of the vas deferens in the male, with or without removal of a segment of the vas. The severed ends are occluded with ligatures or clips, or the lumen of each vas is coagulated. A bilateral vasectomy may be done as a sterilization procedure, since it interrupts the transportation of the sperm. (The spermatozoa, which are manufactured in the testis, are unable to travel up the vas deferens because of surgical interruption.)

Seminal fluid is mostly manufactured in the seminal vesicles and prostate gland, which are unaffected by vasectomy. Thus, there will be no noticable decrease in the amount of ejaculated fluid, except that it contains no spermatozoa. Because the sperm cells have no exit, they are reabsorbed into the body. The procedure has no effect on sexual potency, erection, ejaculation, or production of male hormones.

Two behavioral responses seem to be common after vasectomy. Persons who were anxious about intercourse because of fear of pregnancy due to contraceptive failure often report a decrease in anxiety and an increase in spontaneous sexual arousal. Some men adopt stereotyped masculine behavior, supposedly to allay concerns that the surgery has decreased their masculinity. Concise and factual preoperative discussion may minimize or prevent the latter behavior. Some studies purport that vasectomy can lead to autoimmune disorders, in that antibodies that agglutinate the patient's own spermatozoa may form and persist for many years after the procedure. However, an increased incidence of autoimmune disorders following vasectomy has not yet been clinically proven, and the implications are not clear.

The patient is advised that he will be sterile but that potency will not be altered following a bilateral vasectomy. The procedure does not prevent sexually transmitted disease. On rare occasions, a spontaneous reanastomosis of the vas deferens occurs, which may result in pregnancy of the partner. A legal consent form (usually signed by both the man and his partner) must be obtained before the procedure is carried out.

Complications of vasectomy include scrotal ecchymoses and swelling, superficial wound infection, vasitis (inflammation of the vas deferens), epididymitis or epididymo-orchitis, hematomas, and sperm granuloma. A *sperm granuloma* is an inflammatory response to the collection of sperm in the scrotum due to leakage from the severed end of the proximal vas. This can initiate recanalization of the vas, possibly resulting in pregnancy of the partner.

For a comparison of vasectomy and female sterilization, see Chart 41-2.

Chart 41-2
Comparison of Vasectomy and Female Sterilization

Vasectomy	Female Sterilization
Effectiveness	
Very effective, but slightly higher rate of spontaneous recanalization and pregnancy	Very effective; slightly lower failure rate
Effective 6 to 10 weeks after surgery	Effective immediately
Complications	
Procedure involves almost no risk of internal injury or other life-threatening complications	Procedure involves slight risk of serious internal injuries and other life-threatening complications
Very slight possibility of serious infection	Slight possibility of serious infection
No anesthesia-related deaths	Few anesthesia-related deaths
Acceptability	
Minute scar	Scar can be small but still visible
Slightly more reversible	Slightly less reversible
Less expensive	More acceptable in many cultures
Personnel	
Can be performed by one trained person with or without an assistant	Team needed, including one doctor, one trained anesthetist, and at least two assistants with more training than needed for vasectomy assistant
Can usually be performed in half the time of most female sterilizations	Usually only physicians with training in gynecology can perform laparoscopy and laparotomy; minilaparotomy is simpler
Equipment	
Requires no specialized equipment; equipment readily available	Laparoscopy requires expensive complex equipment that needs to be carefully maintained; minilaparotomy requires only simple standard surgical instruments
Can usually be performed under local anesthesia	Systemic sedation necessary as well as local anesthesia
Back-Up Facilities	
No back-up facilities needed for immediate complications	Back-up facilities needed in case of damage to abdominal organs and blood vessels or other complications that require laparotomy
Possible Long-Term Side-Effects	
None demonstrated	Slight risk of ectopic pregnancy

(Adapted from Liskin L, Pile JM, and Quillin WF. Population Reports Series D, No. 4, Nov/Dec 1983, published by Johns Hopkins University, Population Information Program.)

Patient Education. Ice bags are applied intermittently to the scrotum for several hours after surgery to reduce swelling and relieve discomfort. The patient is advised to wear cotton jockey-type briefs for added comfort and support. He may become greatly concerned about the discoloration of the scrotal skin and superficial swelling. This occurs frequently after vasectomy and responds to sitz baths.

Sexual intercourse may be resumed as desired by the patient, although he should be informed that he will still be fertile for a varying length of time after vasectomy until the spermatozoa that are stored distal to the point of interruption of the vas have been evacuated.

Contraceptives should be used until the patient is de-

clared infertile. This declaration is made on examination of ejaculate. Some physicians examine a specimen 4 weeks after the vasectomy to determine sterility; others use two consecutive specimens 1 month apart, and still others consider a patient sterile after 36 ejaculations.

Vasovasostomy (Sterilization Reversal). Microsurgical techniqes are being used for vasectomy reversal (vasovasostomy), which restores patency to the vas deferens. However, the success rate of this procedure is still under investigation.

Sperm Banking. Storage of fertile semen in a sperm bank *before* a vasectomy is a possibility should unforeseen life events cause a desire in the patient to father a child. The success rate in achieving pregnancy with frozen sperm is uncertain.

Investigational Conception Control

Researchers recognize that the perfect method of conception control (barring abstention or sterilization) does not exist; every device has some risk. Research and testing of types of contraception control have decreased considerably because of the cost of testing and the risk of liability. The following are considered investigational:

- Ovulation-inhibiting hormone, progestin, is released from a Silastic synthetic rubber implant, inserted under local anesthesia beneath the skin in the arm (Norplant). By steadily and slowly releasing low-dose progestin from 3 to 5 years, it is claimed to be almost as effective as sterilization.
- A special "vaginal ring" also releases progestin. It is placed around the cervix for 3 weeks each month and removed for menstruation. This method requires careful vaginal hygiene.
- "Once-a-month pill" (RU-486) is a hormone that blocks progesterone; this in effect induces an abortion.
- Male "pill." To date a satisfactory male contraceptive is still being sought. A steroid comparable to the "pill" for the female has been associated with undesirable side-effects in the male.

Pregnancy Termination

Interruption of pregnancy or expulsion of the contents of the pregnant uterus before the fetus is viable (up to 20 weeks) is called *abortion;* interruption between 20 to 28 weeks is commonly referred to as *miscarriage.* The viability of the fetus is usually considered to be any time after the sixth month of gestation; however, legal periods of viability vary in different states in the United States.

The aborted fetus weighs less than 1000 gm; beyond this weight, the fetus is usually viable, and the term *premature labor* is used, instead of abortion, to describe the situation. It is estimated that one of every five or ten conceptions results in abortion. Most of these occur because of an abnormality in the fetus, so that abortion is nature's method of rejecting a defective conception. Other causes may be due to systemic diseases, hormonal imbalance, or anatomical abnormalities.

Spontaneous Abortion

Spontaneous abortion occurs most commonly in the second or third month of gestation, probably owing to a defective ovum and subsequent developmental defects of the fetus and placenta.

There are various kinds of spontaneous abortion, depending on the nature of the process (threatened, inevitable, incomplete, and complete). Uterine bleeding and pain (uterine contractions) are suggestive of an abortion in a woman of childbearing age. In such a *threatened abortion,* the cervix does not dilate; with bed rest and conservative treatment, it may be prevented. If it cannot be prevented, an *inevitable*

abortion is imminent. If some of the tissue, but not all, is passed, the abortion is referred to as *incomplete;* however, if the fetus and all related tissue are expressed (removed), the abortion is *complete.*

Habitual Abortion

Habitual abortion is successive (three), repeated abortions of unknown cause; immunologic rejection is suspected. Ultraconservative measures are employed in an attempt to save the pregnancy, such as complete bed rest, administration of progesterone to prevent sloughing of the endometrium, thyroid extract therapy, and psychotherapy.

In the condition known as "incompetent cervical os," the cervix dilates painlessly in the second trimester of pregnancy, resulting in spontaneous abortion. A surgical procedure called the Shirodkar operation (cervical cerclage) is designed to prevent the cervix from dilating prematurely. A purse-string suture of fascia, polyethylene, or dermal graft strip obtained from the patient's lower abdominal skin is tied snugly around the cervix at the level of the internal os. It is most important that the patient and the nurses attending her, including those in community health agencies and industry, be informed that such a suture is in place. As soon as labor occurs, the physician should be notified immediately so that the suture can be cut and labor allowed to proceed; otherwise, the uterus may possibly rupture. Usually, delivery is by cesarean section.

Therapeutic Abortion

Under certain circumstances, the physician may consider terminating a pregnancy; such a termination is called a therapeutic abortion and is performed by skilled medical personnel. On January 22, 1973, the United States Supreme Court handed down its ruling on abortions, which in effect states the following:

1. In the first trimester of pregnancy, the abortion decision is to be left to the woman and her physician.
2. During the second trimester, the state may not prohibit abortion but may regulate its practice in the interest of protecting the woman's health. (Permissible regulations could determine who are qualified to do abortions and where they might be done.)
3. During the final weeks of pregnancy, the state may choose to protect the potential life of the fetus by prohibiting abortion, except when necessary to preserve the life or health of the woman.

Even though the liberalization of abortion laws makes many abortions legally permissible, the religious beliefs of the woman involved must be respected. Baptism of all stillborn and aborted fetuses is required in the Roman Catholic faith.

Management. Usually, the opinions of two or more physicians are documented to identify the reasons for performing a therapeutic abortion. Appropriate informed permission is obtained from the patient.

Vacuum aspiration of uterine contents within 14 days of a missed menstrual period may be performed in a physician's office; this is called *menstrual regulation* or *menstrual extraction.*

Therapeutic abortions may be carried out in the following ways, usually in the operating room:

Dilatation and Evacuation (Suction Curettage). The cervix is dilated, and a uterine aspirator is introduced. Suction from a pump is applied, and fetal tissue is removed from the uterus. This method is not used if the pregnancy has advanced beyond 12 weeks, since the fetus at this stage is supposedly too firm. More recently, some clinics have extended the period to 16 weeks and even beyond.

Intra-amniotic Injection of Oxytocic Agent. This procedure is used beyond the 14th week of pregnancy. Under local anesthesia, a needle is inserted in the mid-abdomen, and an amniocentesis is performed. Over 200 ml of fluid is withdrawn and replaced by hypertonic saline. In some clinics, after 6 hours, oxytocin is administered intravenously, with lactated Ringer's solution, to initiate labor. If no oxytocics are administered, labor will usually begin spontaneously within 8 to 20 hours, but may be delayed for several days. Subsequent curettage may be necessary to completely remove any remaining placental and residual tissue. The dangers of this procedure, such as accidental intravenous injection of saline, cerebral convulsion, and acute renal failure, need to be realized.

Prostaglandins. Intra-amniotic instillation of natural or synthetic prostaglandins produces strong uterine contractions, causing cervical dilatation and expulsion of the fetus and placenta within 24 hours. This method appears safer than using hypertonic saline, because it avoids the complication of disseminated intravascular coagulation (DIC) and hypernatremia.

Prostaglandins continue to be studied; side-effects such as nausea, vomiting, diarrhea, tachycardia, substernal "pressure," and paralytic ileus may occur, although the incidence and frequency of such problems vary according to the medication, dosage, and technique of administration. Transvaginal extra-amniotic administration is used to initiate uterine contractions, as are vaginal suppositories and intramuscular prostaglandins. The latter methods are noninvasive with decreased morbidity and ease of administration.

Laminaria. An age-old method of cervical dilatation is being revived in medical practice. *Laminaria* tents are made from a species of seaweed that grows in cold ocean waters; the stem is dried and cut into lengths of 6 to 8 cm (2.4 to 3.1 inches) and shaped into cylindrical (tampon-shaped) forms for sizing, from 2 to 4 mm, 4 to 6 mm, 6 to 8 mm, and 8 to 10 mm in diameter. A string is looped through one end. When placed in a moist environment, the tent, which is highly hygroscopic, swells to three or five times its original diameter. The tent may be placed in the cervix in order to dilate it. The greatest amount of swelling occurs in 4 to 5 hours; however, additional dilatation may be expected over the next few hours.

Advantages of *Laminaria* tents over metal-instrument dilators are many: tents cause limited cervical trauma, hold little risk of other serious complications, and are readily accepted and tolerated by patients. Disadvantages include the following: there is some discomfort and slight uterine cramping immediately after insertion, and mild-to-severe intermittent cramps may be experienced in some women for several hours. There is also risk of low-grade endometritis. Removal of the tent is difficult at times and, on occasion, has resulted in the tent's slipping into the uterus. Tents are sterilized in gamma radiation or ethylene oxide gas.

An alternative to *Laminaria* is a synthetic, Lamicel, which consists of a polyethylene sponge impregnated with magnesium sulfate and compressed into a rod. It works more rapidly than *Laminaria* tents.

Hysterotomy. A hysterotomy is a "miniature" cesarean section; usually, this method is reserved for pregnant women who also want to be sterilized at the same time. The patient remains in the hospital for 3 to 6 days; care is essentially the same as for a patient having an abdominal operation.

Septic Abortion

When unskilled attempts to end a pregnancy are made, the methods usually include administering large amounts of drugs (effects are toxic and never really evacuate the uterus) or performing a curettage, with an associated high risk of rupture of the uterus, hemorrhage, or infection.

Although this has been a major problem in the past, with the widespread dissemination of birth control information and the liberalization of abortion laws, a decline in septic abortion is anticipated.

If a woman who has had a simple, uncomplicated septic abortion receives proper medical attention early enough, the prognosis is excellent with treatment using broad-spectrum antibiotics. Fluid and blood replacement is required before very careful attempts are made to evacuate the uterus.

For the treatment of septic abortion complicated by impending shock, see the discussions of shock (p. 362) and pelvic inflammatory disease (p. 1110).

Management of Abortion Patients

Signs of a threatening abortion are vaginal discharge or bleeding and abdominal cramps. The woman is encouraged to see a physician, who will probably recommend bed rest, light diet, and no straining on defecation. According to some estimates, when first seen, fewer than 30% of patients who are actually threatening to abort have viable fetuses, and 80% or more will proceed to abortion regardless of management. Sedation or tranquilizers may be prescribed, and if infection is suspected, antibiotics may be given.

Nursing Interventions. All tissue passed vaginally is saved for examination by the physician. In the hospital, all personnel caring for the patient are alerted to save the contents of the bedpan for possible placenta tissue or fetus. If there is much bleeding, the patient may require transfusions and fluid replacement. An estimate of the amount of bleeding can be determined by recording the number of perineal pads and the nature of saturation per 24 hours. For an incomplete abortion, oxytocin may be prescribed to contract the fundus prior to the woman's having a dilatation and evacuation (D&E) or undergoing suctioning of the uterus. A patient with such an evacuation of retained secretions requires the same nursing care as a person having a D&C (see p. 1080).

Since this person often experiences a severe emotional reaction, the component of "caring" for her is an important aspect of nursing. The cause of the abortion colors the problem and the patient's reaction. The response of the woman who desperately wants the baby is quite different from that of the woman who does not want to be pregnant but may be frightened of the possible consequences of an abortion. The nurse must not overlook the fact that in many instances, particularly for the woman having a spontaneous abortion, there is a grieving period that must be handled. Such grieving may be delayed or unresolved, resulting in other problems until the grief reaction has been worked out. There are many reasons for delayed grief reaction: friends may not have known the woman was pregnant; the woman may not have seen the lost fetus and can only imagine the sex, size, and so forth of the person who never developed; there is no burial service; those who know about the abortion (family, friends, caregivers) encourage denial and rarely encourage crying and talking about the loss.

In any event, providing opportunities for the patient to talk and vent her emotions will not only help her but will also provide clues for the nurse in planning more specific care. Those persons closest to the woman are encouraged to hug her and allow her to talk and cry. If grief is unresolved, it may manifest itself by persistent vivid memories of the events surrounding the time of loss, persistent sadness or anger, and frequent flooding of emotion when recalling the loss. Signs of pathologic grief may require the assistance of a therapist skilled in grief work.

It is well to remember that the incidence of complications and death is higher for abortion than for other methods of contraception. Because of this, contraception and sterilization are preferred to prevent unwanted pregnancy. Therapeutic abortion should be considered only when these measures fail. See Chart 41-3 for points on patient education after a therapeutic abortion.

Infertility

Infertility usually refers to a couple's failure to achieve a pregnancy in 1 or 2 years of unprotected intercourse. *Primary* infertility refers to a couple who have never had a child. *Secondary* infertility means that at least one conception has occurred but currently the couple is unable to achieve a pregnancy. In the United States, infertility is a major medical and social problem. Both partners are urged to seek health care for complete examinations and evaluation.

Etiology. Possible causative factors of infertility include uterine displacement, tumors, congenital anomalies, and inflammation. For an ovum to become fertilized, the vagina, cervix, and uterus must be patent and the mucosal secretions must be receptive to the sperm. Semen is alkaline, as is cervical secretion; normal vaginal secretion is acid. Often more than one factor may be responsible for the problem. Such tests may require the services of a gynecologist, urologist, endocrinologist, and internist.

Diagnostic Evaluation

Careful evaluation includes not only anatomical and endocrinologic investigation but also consideration of psychosocial factors. A complete history, physical examination, and laboratory studies are done on both partners to rule out such causative factors as previous sexually transmitted disease, anomalies, injuries, tuberculosis, mumps, orchitis, abortions, and psychosocial disorders.

Five types of factors are considered basic to the infertility: for the female, (1) ovarian, (2) tubal, (3) cervical, or (4) uterine conditions; and for the male, (5) seminal conditions. A composite estimate of the relative frequency of these factors as the major cause of the infertility is usually ovarian, 20%; tubal, 30%; cervical, 18%; seminal, 30%.

Ovarian Factor. Tests are done to determine whether there is regular ovulation and a progestational endometrium adequate for implantation. This includes keeping a basal body temperature chart for at least four cycles, taking an endometrial biopsy, and performing other tests for ovulation and progesterone production.

Tubal Factor (Tubal Insufflation or Rubin's Test). To determine tubal patency, carbon dioxide is introduced through

---

Chart 41-3
Post-therapeutic Abortion: Patient Education

1. Note that bleeding similar to menstruation will continue for 7 days or less. Report:
   a. If bleeding is heavier than usual menstrual flow
   b. If bleeding is followed by severe cramps, backache, nausea
2. During bleeding:
   a. Do not take tub baths; showers or sponge baths are permitted.
   b. Do not douche or go swimming.
   c. Do not use tampons—use sanitary pads. (Tampons may be used during your next period.)
   d. Do not have intercourse; preferably, wait until you have one normal period.
   e. Avoid strenuous exercise for at least 1 week, since it may cause further bleeding.
3. Medication for bleeding: If medication has been prescribed to prevent bleeding, expect a few cramps or clots.
4. Take your temperature for 5 to 7 days. Report:
   a. If it is elevated for 24 to 48 hours
   b. If it is elevated and accompanied by symptoms mentioned in 1.
5. Normal expected signs due to hormonal changes (these will pass):
   a. Some women experience depression.
   b. Breasts may be sore and perhaps leak. To combat this, wear a supportive brassiere and restrict fluids.
6. Follow-up: In about a month (or when requested), report to your physician or clinic for a checkup.

(Adapted from Easterbrook B and Rust B. Abortion counseling. Can Nurse 1977 Jan; 73:30.)

a sterile cannula into the uterus and the uterine tubes, and then into the peritoneal cavity. By listening with a stethoscope on the abdomen, the physician may hear gas swishing into the abdomen, indicating that the tubes are open. Another positive indication of tubal patency is the feeling by the patient of referred pain under the scapula or shoulder on the side of the patent tube. This suggests that the gas is under the diaphragm, exerting pressure on the phrenic nerve. If normal patency is present, there is a rise in pressure of 80 to 120 mm, with a sudden drop to 50 to 70 mm as gas passes into the peritoneal cavity. If the gas pressure gauge reaches 200 mm, the test is considered negative, indicating an occlusion.

Hysterosalpinogography (see p. 1081) is an x-ray study that is useful when tubal occlusion is apparent since other abnormalities may be found.

Culdoscopy or *laparoscopy* (see p. 1080) permits direct visualization of tubes and adnexa, including the status of ovarian function.

Cervical Factor. Cervical mucus can be examined to determine whether proper changes occur at ovulation that are favorable to sperm penetration, survival, and growth.

A postcoital cervical mucus test (Sims-Huhner or P-K test) is done between 6 and 12 hours after intercourse. The physician aspirates cervical secretions, using a medicine dropper or special cannula. The woman has been instructed not to void, bathe, or douche between coitus and the examination; a perineal pad is worn until she is placed in a lithotomy position in the examination room. Aspirated material is placed on a slide and examined under the microscope for presence and viability of sperm cells.

Uterine Factor. Fibroids, polyps, and congenital malformations are possible problems in this category. Their presence may be determined by pelvic examination or by hysterosalpingography.

Seminal Factor. After 4 or 5 days of sexual abstinence, the sperm specimen is collected in a clean, dry glass container; kept at or below room temperature; and examined within 2 to 4 hours for volume, sperm motility, morphology, and cell count. Three to 5 ml of viscid alkaline semen is normal; a normal count is 60 to 100 million per milliliter.

Miscellaneous Factors. Miscellaneous factors, including immunologic factors, are currently being investigated.

Management

Sterility may be difficult to treat, since it is often due to a combination of several factors. Statistics show that many couples undergoing study conceive without the cause of infertility coming to light; likewise, although some couples undergo all tests, the cause of the problem may remain undiscovered. Between these extremes, many problems, simple as well as complex, can be discovered and corrected, to the happy benefit of the couple. Between 25% and 50% of all infertile couples can be cured.

Therapy may require correction of faulty coital technique, surgery to correct a malfunction or anomaly, hormonal supplements, attention to proper timing, and recognition and correction of psychological or emotional factors.

Reproductive Technologies

Numerous technologies have been developed to help in the reproduction process and to assist in the basic right of pro-

creativity. Mechanisms already exist under U.S. law to foster safe medical procedures while safeguarding the integrity of the participants. Institutional review boards and procedures for informed consent are two such mechanisms.

Artificial Insemination. Artificial insemination is the deposition or introduction of semen into the female genital tract by artificial means. If the sperm cannot penetrate the cervical canal normally, consideration may be given to *artificial insemination,* using the husband's semen (AIH). In the event of azospermia (lack of sperm in the semen), semen from carefully selected donors may be used (AID).

Indications for using artificial insemination are (1) inability of the male to deposit semen in the vagina, which may be due to premature ejaculation, pronounced hypospadias, or dyspareunia (painful intercourse experienced by the female), and (2) inability of semen to be transported from the vagina to the uterine cavity; this is usually due to faulty chemical conditions, such as may be produced with an abnormal cervical discharge. The latter may be corrected with chemotherapeutic agents. Another indication for artificial insemination is the desire of a single woman to have a child.

Husband's Semen. Certain conditions need to be established before semen is transferred to the vagina. The wife must have no abnormalities of the genital system, the tubes must be patent, and ova must be available. In the husband, sperm need to be normal in shape, amount, motility, and endurance. The time of ovulation in the wife should be determined as accurately as possible, so that the 2 or 3 days during which fertilization is possible each month can be utilized. Fertilization seldom occurs from a single insemination. Usually, insemination is attempted between the 10th and 17th days of the cycle; three different attempts are made. Semen is collected in a wide-mouth, 2-ounce jar following masturbation or withdrawal.

Donor's Semen. A donor may be used when the husband's sperm is defective or absent, or when, for hereditary reasons, it is feared that an undesirable disease may be transmitted. Safeguards need to be set up to prevent legal, ethical, emotional, and religious problems. Written consent may protect the wife, donor, donor's wife, and legal status of the child.

The donor is selected on the basis of close resemblance to the husband, both physically and intellectually; there should be no family history of epilepsy, diabetes, or known genetic defects, and a negative test result for syphilis should be obtained.[*] Preferably, precautions should be taken so that the donor is not known to the recipient, and vice versa.

Insemination Procedure. The recipient is placed in the lithotomy position on the examining table, a speculum is inserted, and the vagina and cervix are swabbed clean with a cotton-tipped applicator. Semen is drawn into a sterile syringe, and a cannula is attached. The semen is then directed to the external os. If this is contraindicated, the semen may be inserted directly into the cervical canal. Following the careful withdrawal of the syringe, the patient is to lie flat on the examining table for a half hour. Thereafter, there are no restrictions on the activities of the woman.

The success rate for artificial insemination is about 50%. About three to six inseminations are required over a 2- to 4-month period. Since this procedure is opposed by the Roman

---

[*] There are commercial firms that bank sperm in Chicago, New York City, Los Angeles, and St. Paul.

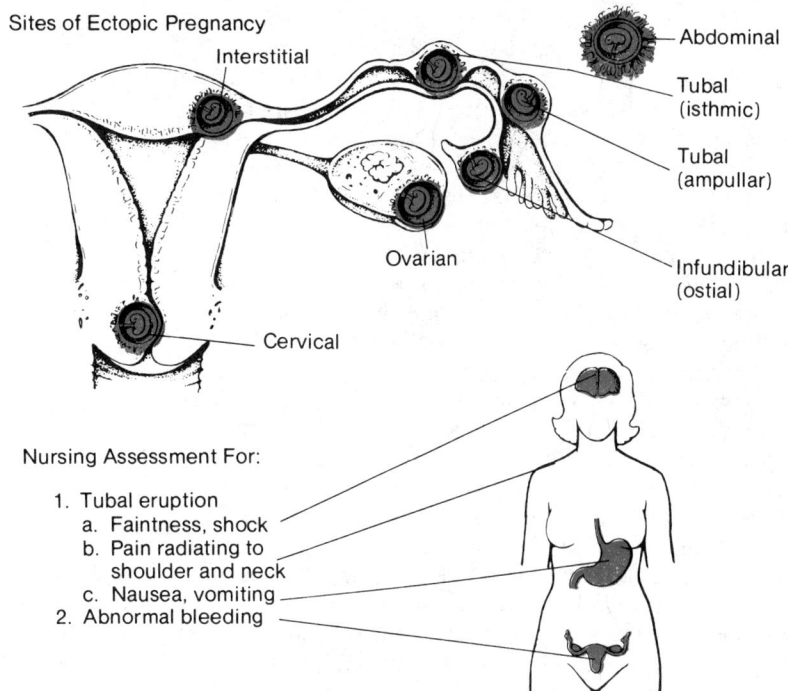

Sites of Ectopic Pregnancy

Nursing Assessment For:

1. Tubal eruption
   a. Faintness, shock
   b. Pain radiating to shoulder and neck
   c. Nausea, vomiting
2. Abnormal bleeding

Figure 41-9
Ectopic pregnancy. The various possible sites for ectopic pregnancy are shown in the upper diagram of the uterus and uterine tube.

Catholic Church, this method should not be suggested to members of this faith.

In Vitro *Fertilization.* *In vitro* fertilization (IVF) is accomplished by first stimulating the ovary to produce multiple eggs because pregnancy success rates are greater with more than one preembryo.* At the appropriate time, the egg is recovered either by laparoscopy and follicle aspiration or by ultrasound. Sperm and eggs are coincubated for 12 to 18 hours so that fertilization can occur. Following an additional 48 to 72 hours, the resulting preembryo is transferred to the uterine cavity via a catheter positioned transcervically. Within 2 to 3 days, implantation takes place. Success rates vary.

The most common indications for IVF are tubal damage or destruction, endometriosis that has not responded to therapy, and anomalies of the uterus and reproductive tract. IVF may also be considered if the male has oligospermia (very low sperm concentration).

Many reservations have been expressed about IVF: procreation is separated from sexual union, the procedure may lead to other types of questionable procedures, and much in the way of expertise and resources are being used. However, on the whole IVF is considered an acceptable method for treating intractable infertility.

Tubal Ectopic Pregnancy

Ectopic pregnancy occurs when the fertilized ovum does not reach the cavity of the uterus but becomes caught and implanted on any tissue other than the lining of the uterine cavity, such as the uterine tube or, occasionally, in the ovary or the abdomen, or even the cervix of the uterus (Fig. 41-9).

---

* *Preembryo* is the term applied during the first 14 days of gestastion. The term *embryo* is used after the second week following fertilization.

As the fertilized ovum increases in size, the tube becomes more and more distended, until finally, 4 to 6 weeks after conception, rupture takes place, and the ovum is discharged into the abdominal cavity.

Etiology and Incidence. The highest incidence of ectopic pregnancy occurs in women ages 35 to 44. Precipitating causes may be salpingitis, endometriosis, pelvic inflammatory disease, chemotherapy for pelvic tuberculosis, congenital anomalies of the tubes, or spasm of the tubes with muscular insufficiency. Factors inherent in the embryo (embryonic abnormalities) may also predispose to ectopic gestation. The Centers for Disease Control report that increasing use of fertility-control measures such as tubal ligation and abortion has been directly associated with ectopic pregnancy. Studies have shown the incidence to vary from 0.5% to 2.5% (1 in 50 to 1 in 250 pregnancies).

Clinical Manifestations. Delay in menstruation from 1 to 2 weeks followed by slight bleeding (spotting) may suggest the problem of an ectopic pregnancy. Or amenorrhea may continue several weeks. Symptoms may start with vague soreness on the affected side, probably due to uterine contractions and distention of the tube; frequently the patient experiences sharp, colicky pain at times.

When tubal rupture occurs, there is agonizing pain, dizziness, faintness, and some nausea and vomiting (see Fig. 41-9 for nursing assessment). These symptoms are related to peritoneal reaction to blood escaping from the tube. Air hunger and symptoms of shock indicate that the patient is desperately ill; all the signs of hemorrhage—rapid, thready pulse; subnormal temperature; restlessness; pallor; sweating—are in evidence. Later the pain becomes generalized in the abdomen and radiates to the shoulder and neck because of intraperitoneal accumulation of blood that causes an irritation to the diaphragm. By vaginal examination, the surgeon is able to feel a large mass of clotted blood that has collected in the pelvis behind the uterus.

Diagnostic Evaluation. Usually, the clinical picture makes the diagnosis relatively simple; however, when it is questionable, other aids are of value. Pelvic aspiration from the cul-de-sac of Douglas (culdocentesis) may be useful. Laparoscopy is especially helpful because the physician can visually note an unruptured ectopic pregnancy, thereby circumventing the risks to the patient of a tubal rupture. Ultrasonography may be effective in differentiating an intrauterine pregnancy from an unruptured tubal gestation.

Management. The goal of treatment is the surgical removal of the ectopic pregnancy, since it is a life-threatening problem; the woman is then relieved of pain and discomfort.

When the operation is performed early, practically all patients recover with remarkable rapidity, but without operation the mortality is 60% to 70%. The type of surgery is determined by the size and extent of local tubal damage; surgery ranges from conservative to more extensive. Very conservative surgery would include "milking" an ectopic pregnancy from the tube. Perhaps a resection of the involved tube with end-to-end anastomosis may be effective. Some surgeons today perform a salpingostomy, which involves opening and evacuating the tube, controlling bleeding, and resuturing the tube to preserve it. More radical surgery includes salpingectomy or salpingo-oophorectomy. Depending on the amount of blood lost, blood transfusions and treatment for shock may be necessary preoperatively and operatively.

Prognosis. The pregnancy rate following treatment is enhanced; the expectancy of another ectopic pregnancy or miscarriage is five to six times greater than for a woman who has not had an ectopic gestation.

▶ *Nursing Process*
The Patient With a Tubal Ectopic Pregnancy

▷ *Assessment*

The nursing history will include the menstrual pattern and any (even slight) bleeding since conception. The patient's description of pains and their location are elicited. Did she experience any sharp, colicky pains? The nurse notes whether pain eventually radiates to the shoulder and neck, which may be due to pressure on the diaphragm. Signs and symptoms of rupture are more prominent and suggest hemorrhage and shock.

The meaning of a tubal pregnancy to the patient should be assessed, if possible, noting its psychological impact, how she is coping with the problem, and evidence of grief. Vital signs, level of consciousness, and nature and amount of vaginal bleeding are monitored.

▷ *Nursing Diagnoses*

Based on the assessment data, the patient's major nursing diagnoses may include the following:

- Alteration in comfort—pain, related to the progression of the tubal pregnancy
- Grieving related to the loss of pregnancy and effect on future pregnancies

- Knowledge deficit of treatment and impact on future pregnancies

A potential complication of ectopic pregnancy is hemorrhage and shock. Careful assessment is essential to detect the development of this serious problem.

▷ *Planning and Implementation*

▷ *Goals:* The major goals of the patient may include relief of pain, correction of fluid volume deficit (shock and hemorrhage), acceptance and resolution of grief and pregnancy loss, and achievement of understanding of the unnatural pregnancy, its treatment, and its outcome.

Nursing Interventions

Potential Hemorrhage. Continuous monitoring of vital signs, level of consciousness, amount of bleeding, and intake and output will provide information regarding the possiblity of hemorrhage and the need to prepare for intravenous therapy. Bed rest, of course, is indicated. Laboratory results relative to hematocrit and hemoglobin, as well as blood gases, are noted. Significant deviations in these laboratory values are reported to the physician, and the patient is prepared for the possibility of surgery.

Relief of Pain. After determining location of pain, the nurse uses measures to relieve discomfort by position changes, distraction, and relaxation techniques. She provides emotional support by listening and correcting misconceptions. Prescribed analgesics are administered if other interventions are ineffective. If the patient is to have surgery, preanesthetic medications will also provide pain relief.

Grief Support. The loss of early pregnancy may or may not be expressed verbally. The impact may not be fully realized or even accepted until much later. The nurse should be available to listen and provide support. The patient's partner should share in this obvious loss and sad time. Other professionals such as a psychotherapist or clergyman can be consulted if required.

Patient Education. With rapid changes, confusion may occur in the early hospital experience of the patient. Life-threatening symptoms resulting from possible hemorrhage and shock must be addressed and treated first. At this time the patient's attention is focused on a crisis and not on learning. Therefore, it may be later that the patient is in a position to learn and ask questions about what has happened and why certain diagnostic measures and interventions were carried out. Treatments are explained as they are presented and understood by the patient. The patient's partner is included when possible. On recovering from the postoperative discomforts, the time may be more appropriate to address any questions and deep-seated problems, such as the effect of this aborted pregnancy on future pregnancies.

▷ *Evaluation*

▷ *Expected Outcomes*

1. Patient experiences a lessening of pain and discomfort.

2. Shows no signs of hemorrhage and shock.
   a. Has lessened amounts of discharge (vaginal pad).
   b. Has normal skin color and turgor.
   c. Has stable vital signs.
3. Begins to accept pregnancy loss/expresses grief.
   a. Expresses sorrow over loss.
   b. Expresses the future hope for another child.
4. Acquires knowledge about tubal pregnancy and its resolution.
   a. Demonstrates an understanding of the causes of tubal pregnancy.
   b. Describes the need for careful health assessment during any future pregnancy.

Bibliography

Books

Benson RC (ed). Current Obstetric and Gynecologic Diagnosis and Treatment, 5th ed. Los Altos, California, Lange Medical Publications, 1984.

Corson SL, Sedlacek TV, and Hoffman JJ. Greenhill's Surgical Gynecology, 5th ed. Chicago, Yearbook Medical Publishers, 1986.

Dalton K. The Premenstrual Syndrome and Progesterone Therapy, 2nd ed. Chicago, Year Book Medical Publishers, 1984.

DiSara PJ and Creasman WT. Clinical Gynecologic Oncology, 2nd ed. St. Louis, CV Mosby, 1984.

Harrison M. Self Help for Premenstrual Syndrome. New York, Random House, 1982.

Jensen MD and Bobak IM. Maternity and Gynecologic Care: The Nurse and the Family, 3rd ed. St. Louis, CV Mosby, 1985.

Kistner RW. Gynecology, 4th ed. Chicago, Year Book Medical Publishers, 1986.

Lark SM. Premenstrual Syndrome Self Help Book. Los Angeles, Forman, 1984.

Laursen NH and Stukane E. Premenstrual Syndrome and You. New York, Simon and Schuster, 1983.

Nichols DH and Evrard JR. Ambulatory Gynecology. Philadelphia, Harper & Row, 1985.

Norris RV and Sullivan C. PMS: Premenstrual Syndrome. New York, Rawson Associates, 1983.

Salzer LP. Infertility: How Couples Can Cope. Boston, GK Hall & Co, 1986.

Storch M and Carmichael C. How to Relieve Cramps and Other Menstrual Problems. New York, Workman, 1982.

Articles

(Asterisks indicate nursing research articles.)

General Articles

Abrums M. Health care for women. JOGNN 1986 May/June; 15(3):250–255.

Bernhard LA and Dan AJ. Redefining sexuality from women's own experiences. Nurs Clin North Am 1986 Mar; 21(1):125–136.

Leslie LA and Swider SM. Changing factors and changing needs in women's health care. Nurs Clin North Am 1986 Mar; 21(1):111–123.

Nolan JW. Developmental concerns and the health of midlife women. Nurs Clin North Am 1986 Mar; 21(1):151–159.

Webb C. Gynaecological nursing: A compromising situation. J Adv Nurs 1985 July; 10(1):47–54.

Gerontological Considerations

Labby DH. Aging's effects on sexual function. Postgrad Med 1985 Nov 15; 78(7):32–43.

McElmurry BJ and LiBrizzi SJ. The health of older women. Nurs Clin North Am 1986; Mar; 21(1):161–171.

Masters WH. Sex and aging—expectation and reality. Hosp Pract 1986 Aug 15; 21(8):175–198.

Walbroehl GS. Sexuality and aging. Am Fam Physician 1984 Feb; 29(2):239–242.

Diagnostic Evaluation

*Dougherty MC, Abrams R, and McKey PL. An instrument to assess the dynamic characteristics of the circumvaginal musculature. Nurs Res 1986 July/Aug; 35(4):202–206.

Edelin KC and Hamid MA. Abnormal Pap smears. Hosp Pract 1985 May 30; 20(5A):23–30.

Pelvic sonography: When to order it. Patient Care 1984 Mar 15; 18(5):65–97.

Stenkvist B et al. Papanicolaou smear screening and cervical cancer. JAMA 1984 Sept 21; 252(11):1423–1426.

Swartz WH. The semi-sitting position for pelvic examination. JAMA 1984 Mar 2; 251(9):1163.

Tupa B and De Coux M. Preparing for diagnostic and operative laparoscopy. Today's OR Nurse 1985 July; 7(7):8–16.

*Willard MD, Heaberg GL, and Bettmann J. The educational pelvic examination. JOGNN 1986 Mar/Apr; 125(2):135–140.

Zbella EA, Nemec LA, and Vermesh M. Vaginal douching. Postgrad Med 1984 Dec; 76(8):93–97.

Zima RE. The Pap smear revisited. Postgrad Med 1984 Nov 1; 76(6):36–46.

Premenstrual Syndrome

Brecher DB and Birrer RB. Premenstrual syndrome update. Med Times 1985 Apr; 113(4):13FM–16FM.

*Brown MA and Zimmer PA. Personal and family impact of premenstrual symptoms. JOGNN 1986 Jan/Feb; 15(1):31–38.

Frank EP. What are nurses doing to help PMS patients? Am J Nurs 1986 Feb; 86(2):137–140.

Goldman L. Premenstrual syndrome: Is it oversold or underdiagnosed? Mod Med 1985 June; 53(6):11.

Havens C. Premenstrual syndrome. Postgrad Med 1985 May 15; 77(7):32–37.

Laversen NH. Recognitition and treatment of premenstrual syndrome. Nurs Pract 1985 Mar; 10(3):11–22.

Lindemann JC. Diagnosis of premenstrual syndrome. Postgrad Med J 1985 Feb 15; 77(3):119, 160.

Lindeman JC. Premenstrual syndrome—a practical approach. Wisc Med J 1984 Nov; 83(11):30–32.

Muse KN et al. The premenstrual syndrome: Effects of "medical ovariectomy." N Engl J Med 1984 Nov 22; 311(21):1345–1349.

Price WA and Giannini AJ. Premenstrual tension syndrome. Res Staff Physician 1985 May; 31(5):34–37.

Progesterone for premenstrual syndrome. Med Lett Drug Ther 1984 Nov 9; 26(674):101–102.

Walton J and Youngkin E. The effect of a support group on self-esteem of women with premenstrual syndrome. JOGNN 1987 May/June; 16(3):174–178.

Wilhelm-Hase E. Premenstrual syndrome: Its nature, evaluation and management. JOGN Nurs 1984 July/Aug; 13(4):223–229.

Menstruation

*Brown MA and Woods NF. Correlates of dysmenorrhea. JOGN Nurs 1984 July/Aug; 13(4):259–266.

DeBrovner CH. Initial work-up of dysmenorrhea. Hosp Med 1985 Mar; 21(3):63–80.

*Cooper KH and Abrams RM. Attributes of the oral cavity as a site for basal body temperature measurements. JOGN Nurs 1984 Mar/Apr; 13(2):125–129.

*Estok PJ and Rudy EB. Intensity of jogging relationships with menstrual/reproductive variables. JOGN Nurs 1984 Nov/Dec; 13(6):390–395.

Friedman AJ and Schiff I. Dysmenorrhea. In Conn's Current Therapy, p 870. Philadelphia, WB Saunders 1986.

Gibbons WE. Diagnosis: Amenorrhea. Hosp Med 1983 Dec; 19(12):57-69.

Hansen AM, Immordino KF, and Farber M. The diagnostic evaluation and therapy of secondary amenorrhea. JOGN Nurs 1984 May/June; 13(3):180-184.

*Havens B and Swenson I. Menstrual perceptions and preparation among female adolescents. JOGN Nurs 1986 Sept/Oct; 15(50):406-411.

*McKeever P and Galloway SC. Effects of nongynecologic surgery on the menstrual cycle. Nurs Res 1984 Jan/Feb; 33(1):42-46.

Olive DL and Hammond CB. Evaluation of the anovulatory patient. Postgrad Med 1985 Apr; 77(5):205-216.

*O'Rourke M. Self-reports of menstrual and nonmenstrual symptomatology in university-employed women. JOGN Nurs 1983 Sept/Oct; 12(5):317-324.

*O'Rourke M. Subjective appraisal of psychological well-being and self-reports of menstrual and nonmenstrual symptomatology in employed women. Nurs Res 1983 Sept/Oct; 32(5):288-293.

*Patterson ET and Hale ES. Making sure: Integrating menstrual care practices into activities of daily living. Adv Nurs Sci 1985 Apr; 7(3):18-31.

*Samples JT and Abrams RM. Reliability of urine temperature as a measurement of basal body temperature. JOGN Nurs 1984 Sept/Oct; 13(5):319-323.

*Shelley S and Anderson C. The influence of selected variables on the experience of menstrual distress in alcoholic and nonalcoholic women. JOGN Nurs 1986 Nov/Dec; 15(6):484-491.

Wilson MA. Menstrual disorders. JOGN Nurs 1984 Mar/Apr; 13(suppl 2):11s-19s.

*Woods NF. Relationship of socialization and stress to perimenstrual symptoms, disability, and menstrual attitudes. Nurs Res 1985 May/June; 34(3):145-149.

Woods NF, Most A, and Dery G. Prevalence of perimenstrual symptoms. Am J Pub Health 1982 Nov; 72(11):1257-1264.

*Woods NF, Most A, and Longenecker. Major life events, daily stressors, and perimenstrual symptoms. Nurs Res 1985 Sept/Oct; 34(5):263-267.

Menopause

Aloia JF et al. Risk factors for postmenopausal osteoporosis. Am J Med 1985 Jan; 78(1):95-100.

Beauchamp PJ and Held B. Estrogen replacement therapy. Postgrad Med 1984 May 15; 75(7):42-49.

*Bowles C. Measure of attitude toward menopause using the semantic differential model. Nurs Res 1986 Mar/Apr; 35(2):81-85.

Braunstein GD. The benefits of estrogen to the menopausal woman outweigh the risks of developing endometrial cancer. CA 1984 July/Aug; 34(4):210-219.

Estradiol skin patch may relieve hot flashes. Am J Nurs 1986 Nov; 86(11):1215.

Gambrell RD Jr. The menopause: Benefits and risks of estrogen-progestogen replacement therapy. Indust Med 1985 Oct; 6(10):135-163.

*Havens B and Swenson I. Menstrual perceptions and preparation among female adolescents. JOGNN 1986 Sept/Oct; 15(5):406-411.

Huppert LC. Hormonal replacement therapy: Benefits, risks, doses. Med Clin North Am 1987 Jan; 71(1):23-37.

Iddenden DA. Sexuality during the menopause. Med Clin North Am 1987 Jan; 71(1):87-93.

Kreisberg RA. Pathophysiology and treatment of menopause. Med Times 1985 May; 113(5):65-72.

Kreisberg RA. Pathophysiology and treatment of menopause. Res Staff Physician 1985 Apr; 31(4):25-30.

*MacPherson KI. Osteoporosis and menopause: A feminist analysis of the social construction of a syndrome. Adv Nurs Sci 1985 July; 7(4):11-22.

Morrow CP. The benefits of estrogen to the menopausal women outweigh the risks of developing endometrial cancer (Opinion): Con. CA 1984 July/Aug; 34(4):220-231.

*Muhlenkamp AF, Waller MM, and Borune AE. Attitudes toward women in menopause: A vignette approach. Nurs Res 1983 Jan/Feb; 32(1):20-23.

Nolan JW. Developmental concerns and the health of midlife women. Nurs Clin North Am 1986 Mar; 21(1):151-159.

Notelovitz M. The symptomatic menopausal patient. Hosp Med 1985 Jan; 21(1):21-30.

Riis B, Thomsen K and Christiansen C. Does calcium supplementation prevent postmenopausal bone loss? N Engl J Med 1987 Jan 22; 316(4):173-177.

Silver SJ and Lindsay R. Postmenopausal osteoporosis. Med Clin North Am 1987 Jan; 71(1):41-55.

Waxman J and Zatzkis SM. Fibromyalgia and menopause. Postgrad Med 1986 Sept 15; 80(4):165-171.

Conception Control

Block M and Rubin MC. Managing patients on oral contraceptives. Am Fam Physician 1985 Aug; 32(2):154-168.

Cupit LG. Contraception. JOGN Nurs 1984 Mar/Apr; 13(suppl 2):23s-29s.

D'Arcy PF. Drug interactions with oral contraceptives. Drug Intell Clin Pharm 1986 May; 20(5):353-360.

Goldzieher JW. Hormonal contraceptives. Postgrad Med 1984 Apr; 75(5):75-86.

Goldzieher JW and Poindexter AN. Medical aspects of contraception. Hosp Pract 1987 March 30; 22(3A):93-108.

Johnson MA. The cervical cap as a contraceptive alternative. Nurs Pract 1985 Jan; 10(1):37-45.

*Klein PM. Contraceptive use and perceptions of change and ability of conceiving in women electing abortion. JOGN Nurs 1983 May/June; 12(3):167-171.

*Kugel C and Vercon H. Relationship between weight change and diaphragm size change. JOGNN 1986 Mar/Apr; 15(2):123-129.

*Orne R and Hawkins JW. Reexamining the oral contraceptive issues. JOGNN 1985 Jan/Feb; 14(1):30-33.

*Sachs B. Contraceptive decision-making in urban, black female adolescents: Its relationship to cognitive development. Int J Nurs Stud 1985; 22(2):117-126.

Stoehr GP and White J. Managing drug interactions with oral contraceptives. JOGN Nurs 1983 Sept/Oct; 12(5):327-331.

Wilbur AE. The contraceptive crisis. Sci Digest 1986 Sept; 94(9):54-85.

Sterilization

Female sterilization. Population Rep 1985 May; 13(2):C125-C168.

Pool F and Kohn I. What to tell patients about sterilization. RN 1986 May; 55-61.

Risks associated with tubal sterilization. AORN 1983 Sept; 38(3):415.

Infertility

*Christianson CAT. Support groups for infertile patients. JOGNN 1986 July/Aug; 15(4):293-296.

*D'Andrea KG. The role of the nurse practitioner in artifical insemination. JOGN Nurs 1984 Mar/Apr; 13(2):75-78.

Daling JR et al. Primary tubal infertility. Intrauterine devices. N Engl J Med 1985 April; 312(15):937-941.

*Darland NW. Infertility associated with luteal phase defect. JOGNN 1986 May/June; 14(3):212-217.

Davis DC. A conceptual framework for infertility. JOGNN 1987 Jan; 16(1):30-35.

Kredentser JV and Schiff I. Infertility: An overview. Med Times 1985 July: 113(7):85-93.

Larsen JL and Odell WD. An approach to the men with infertility. Med Times 1985 Sept; 113(9):31-39.

Robertson BJ and Blake RE. Tuboplasty: Uses, resources, and nursing implications. Periop Nurs Q 1985 June; 1(2):49–56.

*Sandelowski M and Pollock C. Women's experiences of infertility. IMAGE: J Nurs Scholarship 1986 Winter; 18(4):140–144.

Abortion

*Beeman PB. Peers, parents, and partners. Determining the needs of the support person in an abortion clinic. JOGNN 1985 Jan/Feb; 14(1): 54–57.

Brown MA. Adolescents and abortion. JOGN Nurs 1983 July/Aug; 12(4): 241–247.

Hassett MR. Abortion by hysterotomy—an ethical dilemma. Periop Nurs Q 1986 Sept; 2(3):64–70.

Neidhardt A. Why me? Second trimester abortion. Am J Nurs 1986 Oct; 86(10):1133–1135.

*Well-Haas CL. Women's perceptions of first trimester spontaneous abortion. JOGNN 1985 Jan/Feb; 14(1):50–53.

Agencies

American College of Obstetrics and Gynecology, 600 Maryland Avenue SW, Suite 300, Washington DC 20024.

American Fertility Society, 2131 Magnolia Avenue, Suite 201, Birmingham, Albama 35256.

Association for Voluntary Sterilization, 708 Third Avenue, New York, New York 10017.

Chapter 42

Management of Patients With Gynecologic Disorders

Infections of the Female Reproductive System

Vulvovaginal Infections

Overview and Prevention

The vagina is protected against infection by its normally low pH (3.5 to 4.5), which is maintained by the actions of Döderlein's bacilli (a part of the normal vaginal flora) and the hormone estrogen. The risk of infection is greater if the woman's resistance is lowered, the pH is altered, and the number of invading organisms is increased.

Vulvovaginal disorders are common female problems. The nurse has a key role in providing information that will assist in preventing and treating many of these conditions. Young girls and many women need to understand female anatomy, proper personal hygiene, and the wearing of proper clothing.

The epithelium of the vagina is highly responsive to estrogen, which induces the formation of glycogen. The breakdown of glycogen into lactic acid produces a low vaginal pH. When estrogen decreases, such as during lactation and menopause, there is a decrease in glycogen. In adolescents or young women who take oral contraceptives, the normal vaginal flora and glycogen formation are reduced. Compounding the problem, many in this age-group develop acne for which tetracycline is prescribed; this drug further destroys the normal vaginal flora, which are needed to maintain the lower pH that inhibits the growth of most organisms. With reduction in glycogen formation, infections are common and require careful diagnosis for proper treatment to be prescribed.

As the vaginal epithelium matures during the reproductive years, other causative factors initiate infections, such as sexual intercourse with an infected partner, poor feminine hygiene, and the wearing of tight, nonabsorbent, and heat-retaining clothing.

During the perimenopausal period when estrogen production ceases, the vaginal labia and tissue become atrophied and fragile, making the area more susceptible to injury and infection.

Risk factors for vulvovaginal infections are summarized in Chart 42-1.

Vulvitis, Leukorrhea, and Nonspecific Vaginitis

Vulvitis, an inflammation of the vulva, usually occurs in conjunction with other local or systemic disorders, such as a dermatologic problem, poor local hygiene, or sexually transmitted disease, or it may be secondary to a specific vaginitis.

Vaginitis, an inflammation of the vagina, occurs when organisms such as *Escherichia coli*, staphylococci, and streptococci invade the vagina. The normal whitish vaginal discharge (known as *leukorrhea*), which occurs in slight amounts during ovulation or just prior to menarche or the onset of menstruation, becomes more profuse and yellowish when vaginitis occurs. Often vaginitis is accompanied by urethritis because of the proximity of the urethra to the vagina. The discharge may cause itching, redness, burning, and edema, which may be aggravated by voiding and defecation.

Treatment for vaginitis may be directed toward enhancing the natural flora of the vagina. This can be accomplished by a weak acid douche, 15 ml of vinegar to 1 liter of warm water (1 tablespoon of white vinegar to 1 quart of warm water). In addition, β-lactose, a sugar, can be administered as a vaginal suppository. On insertion into the vagina, the suppository dissolves with body heat; the sugar then stimulates the growth of Döderlein's bacilli. An additional objective is to initiate chemotherapy. Local intravaginal applications may be dispensed from a tube with an applicator. The applicator is inserted into the vagina, and medication is expressed in the desired amount. Hydrocortisone vulvar ointment or cream may be applied locally after douching or sitz baths, as prescribed for symptomatic relief of itching. Cleanliness after voiding and defecation is stressed. During menstrual periods, tampons are preferred, since pads often cause chafing.

Gerontological Considerations. Older postmenopausal women are prone to infection by pyogenic bacteria as a result of atrophy of the vaginal mucosa (atrophic vaginitis). An annoying leukorrhea (vaginal discharge) causes itching and burning. Management is similar to that for nonspecific vaginitis. In addition, estrogenic hormones taken orally or applied locally as an ointment are effective in restoring epithelium.

Specific Vaginal Infections

Specific vaginal infections include candidiasis, *Gardnerella*-associated vaginitis, trichomoniasis, and chlamydial infections (Table 42-1).

Candidiasis. Candidiasis is a fungal infection caused by *Candida albicans*. This organism is frequently a normal inhabitant of the mouth, throat, large intestine, and vagina; it propagates where it is moist and warm, such as in mucous membranes and folds of tissue. *C. albicans* is also found in patients who have been on penicillin, cephalosporin, or tetracycline therapy, since these medications probably reduce the number of natural protective organisms usually present in the vaginal tract. Clinical infection may occur during pregnancy, when there is a systemic condition such as diabetes mellitus, or when the patient is taking steroids or oral contraceptives.

Clinical manifestations are a vaginal discharge that causes intense pruritus; is irritating, watery, and tenacious; and may contain white, cheesy particles. A burning sensation may follow urination especially if there is excoriation from scratching. Symptoms are often more severe just before menstruation but are more refractory (less yielding to treatment) during pregnancy. Diagnosis is made by identifying the spores on a wet potassium hydroxide slide. In most cases, this organism can also be cultured from the intestinal tract.

Management. The goal is to eliminate this infection. Assessment of the patient includes identifying any underlying factors that may contribute to the overgrowth of candidal organisms, such as pregnancy, diabetes, or estrogenic or oral contraceptive medications.

Preferred medications are antifungal agents such as clotrimazole, miconazole, and nystatin (Mycostatin). Clotrimazole cream is applied topically by vaginal applicator, usually at bedtime for 7 nights or longer if the problem is chronic. The cream may be applied to the vulvar area for pruritus. Treatment is continued even through a menstrual cycle. For sensitivity to this medication, boric acid powder may be prescribed.

Gardnerella-Associated Vaginitis. *Gardnerella vaginalis* acting with a vaginal anaerobic causes a nonspecific vaginitis that is characterized by excessive discharge and odor (fishy odor, especially after intercourse). This condition occurs throughout the menstrual cycle and does not produce local discomfort. The discharge is creamy grayish white to yellowish white. The odor can be detected readily ("whiff test") by using a dropper to deposit 10% potassium hydroxide solution onto a sample of the discharge that clings to the removed vaginal speculum.

Management. Metronidazole given twice or three times a day for a week is effective. If this medication is contraindicated, ampicillin is administered. If the infection recurs, the male partner is also treated.

Trichomoniasis. *Trichomonas vaginalis* is a flagellated protozoan that causes a common sexually transmitted disease (see also Chap. 59). If trichomoniasis is transferred sexually, the male may be an asymptomatic carrier who harbors the organisms in his urogenital tract.

Clinical manifestations are a vaginal discharge that is thin,

---

Chart 42-1
Risk Factors for Vulvovaginal Infections

Premenarche	Allergies
Pregnancy	Oral contraceptives
Perimenopause	Broad-spectrum antibiotics
Poor personal hygiene	Diabetes mellitus
Tight undergarments	Low estrogen levels
Synthetic clothing	Intercourse with infected partner
Frequent douching	

TABLE 42-1
Vaginal Infections

Condition	Cause	Clinical Manifestations	Management Goals
Candidiasis	*Candida albicans*	Inflammation of vaginal epithelium producing itching, reddish irritation White, cheeselike discharge clinging to epithelium	Eradicate the fungus: Administer clotrimazole. Review other causative factors: stop antibiotic therapy: determine if diabetes or other systemic disease is present.
Gardnerella-associated	*Gardnerella vaginalis* and vaginal anaerobes.	Usually no edema or erythema of vulva or vagina. Grayish white to yellow-white discharge clinging to external vulva and vaginal walls	Administer metronidazole. If infection is recurrent, treat partner. Apply intravaginal acidifying agents.
Trichomonas vaginalis vaginitis (STD)	*Trichomonas vaginalis*	Inflammation of vaginal epithelium, producing burning and itching Frothy yellowish white or yellowish brown vaginal discharge	Remove exudate, relieve inflammation, restore acidity, and reestablish normal bacterial flora: oral metronidazole. For stubborn infections: oral plus vaginal metronidazole. For recurrence: repeat treatment and include sexual partner.
Bartholinitis (infection of greater vestibular gland)	*Escherichia coli* *Trichomonas vaginalis* *Staphylococcus* *Streptococcus* Gonococcus	Erythema around vestibular gland Swelling and edema Development of vestibular gland abscess	Drain the abscess; provide antibiotic therapy; excise gland of patients with chronic bartholinitis.
Cervicitis: acute and chronic	Gonorrhea *Streptococcus* Many pathogenic bacteria	Profuse purulent vaginal discharge Backache Urinary frequency and urgency	Determine the cause: perform cytologic examination of cervical smear. Eradicate the gonococcus, if present: penicillin (as directed) or spectinomycin or tetracycline, if patient is allergic to penicillin. Eradicate other causes: cervical cauterization.
Atrophic vaginitis	Lack of estrogen; glycogen deficient	Discharge and irritation with alkaline *p*H	Provide estrogen therapy for vaginal epithelialization; provide topical vaginal estrogen therapy; improve nutrition.

(sometimes frothy), yellow to yellow-brown, malodorous, and very irritating. An accompanying vulvitis may result, with intense vulvovaginal burning and itching. In some women, the problem tends to become chronic. It is diagnosed by microscopic detection of the pear-shaped, mobile, flagellate organisms. On inspection with a speculum, tissue may reveal generalized vaginal erythema with multiple small petechiae ("strawberry spots").

Management. The most effective treatment appears to be metronidazole (Flagyl), given as a tablet orally one or two times a day with meals for 7 days. Both partners should be treated because of inaccessible trichomonads in the urinary system. Some clinics suggest treating the patient and her sexual partner in 1 day by giving them one or two concentrated doses of metronidazole under physician supervision. Some patients complain of an unpleasant but temporary metallic taste when taking metronidazole. Some also note nausea and vomiting, as well as a hot and flushed feeling when this medication is taken in combination with an alcoholic beverage. In view of these possible side-effects, the patient should be advised not to take alcohol while on the drug.

In addition, intercourse is avoided unless a condom is used. For those who have uncomfortable side-effects from metronidazole, antitrichomonal suppositories are available (*e.g.*, Vagisec Plus). Relief may be experienced but not a complete cure. Metronidazole therapy is contraindicated in patients with some blood dyscrasias or central nervous system diseases or those who are pregnant or breast-feeding their infants.

Chlamydial Infections. Sexually transmitted infection with *Chlamydia trachomatis,* a bacterium, is on the increase (see Chap. 59). Clinical manifestations in women resemble those of gonorrhea (cervicitis and mucopurulent discharge). In males, urethritis and epididymitis are noted. Chlamydia attack the genitourinary tract and can cause dysuria. The condition also may be asymptomatic. Diagnosis can be confirmed by cytologic and serologic studies. Direct smear packets are commercially available but are expensive.

The Centers for Disease Control recommends treatment with tetracycline, doxycycline, or erythromycin usually for 1 week at prescribed doses. Pregnant women are cautioned not to take tetracycline because of potential adverse effects on the fetus.

Results of treatment are usually good if it is begun early enough. Possible complications from delayed treatment are tubal disease, pelvic inflammatory disease, and infertility.

Gerontological Considerations. A common postmenopausal occurrence is atrophy of the vaginal mucosa, which then becomes more prone to infection by pyogenic bacteria—*atrophic vaginitis.* An annoying leukorrhea (vaginal discharge) causes itching and burning. Management is similar to that for nonspecific vaginitis (see p. 1103). In addition, estrogenic hormones, either taken orally or applied locally as an ointment, are effective in restoring epithelium.

Management

For more painful vulvovaginal infections such as an abscess, the patient may require an incision to drain the affected area. This procedure is performed by the physician when the patient first seeks medical attention. Relief is almost immediate, but soreness may continue for 1 or 2 days.

▶ Nursing Process
The Patient With a Vulvovaginal Infection

▷ *Assessment*

The woman with a vulvovaginal problem should be examined soon after the onset of symptoms. As part of the preparation she is instructed not to douche, since this practice would alter the appearance of the perineal area. A nursing history and physical examination include inspection of vaginal mucosa and vulvar surfaces. The area is observed for erythema, edema, excoriation, and discharge. Each of the organisms producing infections appears to have its own characteristic discharge and effect (Table 42-1). The patient is asked if there has been an increase in the amount of secretions and how she would describe any sensations, such as itching or burning. Dysuria often occurs as a result of local irritation of the urinary meatus. Abdominal cramps and fullness may indicate spread of infection of the pelvic area.

Factors that may be involved should be assessed: (1) physical and chemical factors, such as increased perspiration plus decreased evaporation (from tight or synthetic clothing), antiperspirants, perfumes and powders, soaps, bubble bath, a soiled perineal area, contraceptive jellies, feminine hygiene products, and vaginal discharges; (2) psychogenic factors; and (3) medical conditions or endocrine factors such as a predisposition for vulvar involvement in the diabetic, geriatric, or chronically ill patient. The medications the patient has been taking are noted, since hormones and antibiotics, for example, may have altered the vaginal flora, resulting in an overgrowth of *C. albicans.*

The nurse may prepare a vaginal smear (wet mount) to assist in diagnosing the nature of the infection. A common method is for the examiner to collect vaginal secretions with a cotton-tipped applicator and place the secretions at opposite ends of a glass slide. Then a drop of physiologic saline is added to one end and a drop of potassium hydroxide 10% to 20% is added to the other end. Examining the slide under the microscope reveals *C. albicans* at the potassium hydroxide side and white cells, epithelial cells, trichomonads, and bacteria at the other side.

▷ *Nursing Diagnoses*

Based on the nursing assessment and other data, the patient's major nursing diagnoses may include the following:

- Alteration in comfort—pain and discomfort related to burning or itching from the infectious process
- Potential for reinfection or spread of infection
- Knowledge deficit of proper hygiene and preventive measures

▷ *Planning and Implementation*

▷ *Goals:* The major goals of the patient may include relief of pain and discomfort; prevention of reinfection, complications, and infection of sexual partner; and acquisition of knowledge about methods for preventing vulvovaginal infections and managing self-care.

Nursing Interventions

Relief of Discomfort and Pain. Vulvovaginal conditions are usually treated on an outpatient basis, unless the patient has other medical problems. Tact and gentleness in all contacts is important in providing comfort. Psychosocial comfort is also significant since many women express embarrassment and even guilt that the infection may have been acquired from a sex partner. In some instances, treatment plans may include the partner.

The nurse's role is to reinforce instructions for warm perineal irrigations that can provide comfort and also cleanse the infected area. Irrigations are also recommended after each voiding and defecation. A sitz bath may be taken in a bathtub or with the use of a small disposable unit that fits over the toilet seat. If chafing of the upper thighs is present, a dusting of cornstarch powder may alleviate the discomfort.

Generally, sexual intercourse is discouraged until a cure is achieved. Use of a condom is suggested to prevent reinfection and irritation of sensitive tissues. If dyspareunia is experienced, the woman is counseled about other ways of showing affection.

Prevention of Reinfection or Spread of Infection. One of the basic goals of preventing reinfection is to reduce tissue irritation, such as may be caused by scratching or wearing tight clothing. The area is to be kept clean by daily bathing and adequate cleansing after voiding and defecation.

In postmenopausal patients, the level of naturally secreted estrogen decreases. Vaginal mucosal cells and vulvar skin lose glycogen. Vaginal acidity declines, and the atrophic tissues become more fragile and susceptible to trauma and infection. Therefore, gentleness and proper lubricating ointments are essential.

In teaching the patient how to use medications such as suppositories and applicators to dispense cream or ointment, the nurse may demonstrate by using a model of the pelvis. The importance of hand washing is stressed before and after administration of each medication. To prevent loss of medication from the vagina, the patient should lie down for 30 minutes following insertion. If there is some medication seepage, a perineal pad is worn to prevent soilage of clothing. When certain drugs are prescribed, the nurse can instruct the patient about certain precautions. For example, tetracycline, if prescribed for infection with *Gardnerella*, is taken 1 to 2 hours after meals and not with dairy products, iron, or other mineral-containing substances. In addition, sunlight exposure should be avoided when this medication is taken. In general, long-term use of antibiotics should be avoided to prevent candidiasis, which can result when normal flora is destroyed by the antibiotics.

If boric acid powder is prescribed, it is usually in a size 0 gelatin capsule inserted vaginally at night for 10 to 14 days. (This treatment is usually not prescribed if the patient is pregnant because of possible toxic effects.) Vaginal suppositories are stored in the refrigerator to prevent softening.

The patient is advised that her sex partner should be treated if infection recurs.

Patient Education and Self-Care. In addition to reviewing ways of preventing reinfection, the nurse assesses the individual learning needs of the patient relative to the immediate problem. The patient needs to know the characteristics of a normal vs abnormal discharge. Questions often arise about douching. Normally douching is unnecessary, since daily bathing and proper cleaning after voiding and defecation keep the perineal area clean. Many patients are misinformed about the presumed necessity for douching or using feminine hygiene products. Douching has a tendency to eliminate normal flora that nature provides; this tends to reduce the woman's ability to ward off infection. Repeated douching may result in vaginal epithelial breakdown and chemical irritation. However, douching may be recommended and prescribed to reduce malodors, to remove excessive discharge, to change the *p*H (such as vinegar douches), and to serve as an antiseptic irrigating solution. The procedure is reviewed, as is the care and cleaning of equipment so that it is properly disinfected.

Following douching, and whenever necessary, the woman should keep the perineum dry; a hair dryer turned on low is an effective aid. She is advised to wear loose-fitting cotton underwear, not tight-fitting synthetic, nonabsorbent, heat-retaining garments (pantyhose, tight pants and slacks). It is suggested that the woman also avoid wearing damp swimsuits for long periods of time.

Sexual intercourse should be avoided until cure is achieved. If pain during intercourse (dyspareunia) is no longer a problem, a condom may be used and efforts made not to injure the vaginal tissue. The use of water-soluble lubricant (K-Y jelly) will decrease excoriation. If infection recurs, it may be necessary to repeat the treatment regimen and include the partner.

▷ Evaluation

▷ Expected Outcomes

1. Patient experiences reduced pain and discomfort.
   a. Irrigates the perineum as prescribed.
   b. Reports that itching is relieved.
2. Is free from infection.
   a. Has no signs of inflammation, pruritus, or dysuria.
   b. Notes vaginal discharge appears normal (thin, clear, nonfrothy).
   c. Reports that her partner is free from infection.
3. Acquires helpful information related to self-care.

Herpesvirus Type 2 Infection (Herpes Genitalis, Herpes Simplex Virus)

Herpes genitalis is a viral infection that causes herpetic (blisters) lesions on the cervix, vagina, and external genitalia; it is a sexually transmitted disease.

This form of herpes is of major concern to health care providers and consumers because of the increasing prevalence of the disease (400,000 to 500,000 new cases each year). Not only is the infection painful, but it also can recur and affect future well-being. There is no cure at present. The condition requires accurate diagnosis, effective care, and specific measures to prevent possible complications.

Etiology and Pathophysiology

Of the known herpesviruses, six affect humans: (1) herpes simplex type 1 (HSV-1), usually causing "cold sores" of lips; (2) herpes simplex type 2 (HSV-2); (3) varicella zoster; (4) Epstein-Barr virus; (5) cytomegalovirus; and (6) HBLV (human B-lymphotropic virus). Herpes simplex type 2 appears to be the causative virus in over 80% of genital and perineal lesions; about 20% are HSV-1.

There is considerable overlap between the two forms, which are clinically indistinguishable. Close human contact via mouth, oropharynx, mucosal surface, vagina, and cervix seems necessary to acquire the infection. Other susceptible sites are skin lacerations and conjunctivae. Usually the virus is killed at room temperature by drying. When virus replication diminishes, the virus ascends the peripheral sensory nerves and remains inactive in the nerve ganglia. Another outbreak occurs when the host is subjected to stressors, such as fatigue or illness.

It is significant to note that cervical cancer is higher in women who have had cervical herpes. In pregnant women with cervical herpes, babies delivered vaginally may become infected with the virus; there is significant fetal morbidity and mortality.

Clinical Manifestations

Itching and pain accompany the process as the area becomes red and edematous. The vesicular state may appear as a pimple, which later coalesces, ulcerates, and encrusts. In the female, the cervix is the usual primary site, and then possibly the labia, vulva, vagina, and perianal skin. The male is affected on the glans penis, foreskin, and penile shaft. Flulike symptoms occur 3 to 4 days after the appearance of lesions. Inguinal lymphadenopathy, temperature elevation, malaise, headache, myalgia, and dysuria are noted. In the female, a purulent discharge may develop from a secondary bacterial infection. Pain is evident during the first week and then lessens. The lesions disappear in about 3 weeks unless they become secondarily infected.

Complications arise from extragenital spread, such as to the buttocks or upper thighs and even to the eyes as a result of touching them with unclean hands. Other potential problems are hepatitis, aseptic meningitis, autonomic nervous system dysfunction, and psychological stress.

Management

There is no cure for herpesvirus type 2 infection, but treatment is aimed at relieving the symptoms. The goals are to prevent the spread of infection, to make the patient comfortable, to decrease potential health risks, and to be supportive and initiate a counseling and education program. Acyclovir (Zovirax), an antiviral agent that can alter the course of the infection, is available for topical, oral, and intravenous use. In general, acyclovir may reduce the duration of the infection but is only marginally effective in preventing recurrences. Of concern is the potential for drug resistance and long-term side-effects. The most effective management at present remains the care of local lesions and supportive care of systemic illness. Antibacterial agents assist in combating secondary infections.

▶ Nursing Process
The Patient With a Genital Herpesvirus Infection

▷ Assessment

The nursing history, physical and pelvic examination plus collaboration with other health care personnel taking care of this patient will establish the nature of the infectious condition.

▷ Nursing Diagnoses

Based on all the assessment data, the patient's major nursing diagnoses may include the following:

- Alteration in comfort—pain related to the presence of genital lesions
- Potential for reinfection or spread of infection
- Anxiety and distress related to embarrassment over the presence of the disease
- Knowledge deficit of the disease process and methods for avoiding spread or reinfection

▷ Planning and Implementation

▷ *Goals:* The major goals of the patient may include relief of pain and discomfort, control of infection and its spread, relief of anxiety, and knowledge of and adherence to treatment regimen and self-care.

Nursing Interventions

Relief of Pain. The local lesions are to be kept clean, and proper hygienic practices are advocated. Small ice packs may be applied intermittently to painful areas to bring relief. Clothing should be clean, loose, soft, and absorbent. Tepid sitz baths are comforting and cleansing. Aspirin and other analgesics are effective to control pain. A topical anesthetic such as lidocaine cream is effective. Occlusive ointments and powders are to be avoided since they will prevent the lesions from drying, which in turn helps to kill the virus.

If there is considerable pain and malaise, bed rest may be required. It is necessary to assess the fluid intake of the patient, the presence of bladder distention, and the frequency of voiding. Adequate fluid intake is encouraged; voiding is assisted by pouring warm water over the vulva. Such measures will help in preventing urinary retention and infection. Acyclovir is taken as prescribed, and side-effects such as rash, headache, insomnia, acne, sore throat, muscle cramps, and lymphadenopathy, are monitored. Rest and an appropriate diet are recommended. An indwelling urinary catheter may be necessary in severe cases of urethritis.

Control of Infection. Since herpesvirus can spread from the discharge of lesions, efforts are made to keep these areas dry. Using a hair dryer turned on low and cool is comforting and drying. Acyclovir as prescribed may be applied locally to the lesions four to five times daily to control the spread of infection. Other forms of administration may be recommended by the physician. For general methods of preventing the spread of the infection, see the recommendations mentioned in the next section on self-care instruction.

Patient Education. The problems of genital herpes are both physical and psychological. Usually, the patient experiences a great deal of stress on learning the diagnosis, and this in itself aggravates the problem. Therefore, when counseling the patient, the nurse should review the causes of the condition and the manner in which it progresses. The client's questions are encouraged since such questions indicate a receptive time to learn. The highly individual nature of the disease, its widespread incidence, the prevention of complications, and promising research are discussed. The nurse can reassure the patient that in time she will be able to function normally both socially and sexually. Self-care measures for the person with genital herpes are listed in Chart 42-2.

▷ Evaluation

▷ *Expected Outcomes*

1. Patient experiences minimal pain and discomfort.
   a. Takes aspirin/analgesic/acyclovir as prescribed.
   b. Rests and conserves energy.
   c. Uses warm sitz baths.
   d. Wears clean, loose, cotton clothing.

Chart 42-2
Patient Education and Self-Care for Genital Herpes

- Herpes is transmitted essentially only by direct contact; abstinence is required for a brief period.
- Control of the condition will not require a major life-style change. Intercourse is avoided during treatment, but hand-holding and kissing are permissible.
- Women can be reassured that they can have children; their obstetrician needs to know that they have the condition so they can be monitored appropriately.
- Conscientious hygienic practices of cleanliness (handwashing, perineal cleanliness) must be practiced.
- The patient should wear proper clothing, eat nutritionally good foods, get rest and relaxation.
- Lesions should be washed gently with mild soap and running water and lightly dried
- Prolonged exposure to the sun should be avoided.
- Occlusive ointments, strong perfumed soaps, or bubble bath should be avoided.
- Medications must be taken as prescribed; follow-up appointments with health care personnel should be kept and recurrences, which are not as severe as the initial episode, reported.
- The patient is encouraged to join a group to share solutions and experiences and hear about newer treatments. Information can be obtained from HELP (Herpetics Engaged in Living Productively), 260 Sheridan Avenue, Palo Alto, California 94306.
- Usually precautions are unnecessary in the absence of active lesions.
- Lesions away from the mouth or perineum can be covered with a dressing and an impermeable cover during intercourse.
- For a partner with no history of genital herpes, a condom should be used.

e. Abstains from sexual activity while infected.
f. Develops a plan of relaxation/stress reduction.
2. Keeps infection under control.
a. Practices proper hygienic techniques.
b. Washes hands after going to the bathroom/cleansing perineum.
c. Avoids use of occlusive ointments.
3. Acquires knowledge and keeps updated.
a. Defines the limitations of social and sexual practices as the condition permits.
b. Describes intent to follow proper health habits and to control stress.
c. Indicates a willingness to arrange for follow-up care.

Toxic Shock Syndrome

Toxic shock syndrome (TSS), a condition first identified in the late 1970s, is caused by the bacterium *Staphylococcus aureus* and usually occurs in women under age 30 who are menstruating and using tampons (particularly highly absorbent tampons). Research studies suggest that magnesium-absorbing fibers in the tampons may lead to lower levels of magnesium in the body. Such low levels contribute to providing an ideal condition for toxins to be produced by the bacteria. TSS has also occurred in nonmenstruating women and in men and has been associated with such conditions as cellulitis, surgical wound infections, and subcutaneous abscesses.

Clinical Manifestations. In an otherwise healthy person the onset of TSS occurs with a sudden fever (up to 38.9°C [102°F]), vomiting, diarrhea, myalgia, hypotension, and signs suggesting the onset of septic shock. At times sore throat, headache, and myalgia are noted. A red, macular rash often develops. In some patients, this rash makes its first appearance

on the torso, and in others, it first appears on the hands (palms and fingers) and feet (soles and toes); it may then desquamate in 7 to 10 days.

Urine output is decreased and the urea nitrogen level becomes elevated; such urinary dysfunction may initiate disorientation due to fluid deficit and toxins. Respiratory distress or signs of "shock lung" have been reported as a result of pulmonary edema. Inflammation of mucous membranes may also occur. Blood studies indicate leukocytosis and elevated bilirubin, urea nitrogen, and creatine phosphokinase values.

Diagnostic Evaluation. Blood and urine cultures are taken, along with throat cultures when appropriate. Vaginal and possibly cervical specimens are also evaluated.

Management. The patient is placed on bed rest, and the treatment plan is directed primarily at controlling the infection with chemotherapeutic agents. General assessment may reveal shock and fluid imbalance, which is corrected. If there is respiratory distress, oxygen therapy is instituted; if signs of acidosis appear, sodium bicarbonate is given. Calcium is prescribed for hypocalcemia.

The entire treatment plan is adjusted according to the individual patient's condition, which may vary from mild to very acute. Certainly not overlooked are the patient's emotional and psychological concerns.

▶ Nursing Process
The Patient With Toxic
Shock Syndrome

▷ Assessment

The nursing history is directed toward determining if the patient has used tampons recently, what kind she used, how long she retained a single tampon before changing it, and whether she noted any problems when inserting the tampon, which may have injured the vaginal tissue. Sometimes, rough edges on the cardboard applicator can scratch or injure the mucosa when the tampon is inserted. The injured or broken tissue becomes an open avenue through which organisms invade the bloodstream.

▷ Nursing Diagnoses

Based on the nursing assessment and other data, the patient's major nursing diagnoses may include the following:

- Anxiety related to the severity and suddenness of the symptoms
- Fluid volume deficit related to vomiting and diarrhea
- Alteration in comfort—generalized "sick feeling" due to systemic toxicity
- Knowledge deficit regarding use of tampons and personal hygiene

▷ Planning and Implementation

▷ *Goals:* The major goals of the patient may include reduction of anxiety and emotional stress, absence of vomiting and diarrhea, absence of discomfort, absence of complications, and acquisition of relevant knowledge.

Nursing Interventions

The nursing interventions will follow the goals according to priority of needs. The patient will be reassured that any and all treatment modalities that are necessary will be available and that members of the health care team will do everything to keep her comfortable and improve her condition. Such reassurance will relieve anxiety and apprehension. Close monitoring and documentation of vital signs and blood gases provide valuable indices regarding the patient's physical status. The nurse notes skin changes as well as fluid intake and loss inasmuch as these data will assist in evaluating hydration and kidney function.

Cultures of all body excretions and of the nose, throat, vagina, and cervix are taken. The results of these studies will assist the physician in prescribing appropriate antibiotic therapy.

Since disseminated intravascular coagulation (DIC) has been observed in patients with TSS, it is essential for the nurse to be observant for hematomas; petechiae; oozing from needle puncture sites; cyanosis; and coolness of the nose, fingertips, and toes.

Patient Education and Home Health Care. Since the use of tampons during menstruation has been linked with TSS, it is recommended that superabsorbent tampons not be used. If tampons are preferred, women should be advised to alternate their use with pads. Other instructions should advocate that tampons be changed frequently (every 4 hours) and not left in place longer than 8 hours. Tampons should be inserted carefully to avoid abrasions (applicators with rough edges should not be used). If a diaphragm is used, it should not be left in place longer than 6 hours. Use of tampons is discouraged if the patient has had TSS.

▷ Evaluation

▷ Expected Outcomes

1. Patient exhibits reduced anxiety and emotional stress.
2. Is free of fluid loss and imbalance.
   a. Notes absence of vomiting and diarrhea.
   b. Takes fluids and food well.
3. Is comfortable and oriented.
   a. Reports absence of pain, and of feeling "sick."
   b. Has normal vital signs.
   c. Is free of purulent discharge.
   d. Has normal laboratory values.
   e. Is free of infection.
4. Demonstrates awareness of self-care measures.

Endocervicitis

Endocervicitis is an inflammation of the mucosa and the glands of the cervix. It is a fairly common problem that may occur when organisms gain access to the cervical glands after abortion, intrauterine manipulation, or delivery. It is an infection that, if untreated, may extend into the uterus, uterine tubes, and pelvic cavity. In the majority of patients, the inflammation is caused by the ordinary pyogenic organisms, but gonorrheal infection of the glands can occur.

Inflammation can cause erosion of the cervical tissue, resulting in spotting or bleeding. The chief symptom is leukorrheal discharge, at times associated with sacral backache, low abdominal pain, and urinary and menstrual disturbances.

Management. Treatment should be preventive as well as curative. Prevention of gonorrhea will reduce the incidence of endocervicitis. Proper obstetric care can also prevent the occurrence of this condition. Delivery ought not to be attempted until the cervix completely dilates spontaneously; cervical lacerations should be repaired immediately.

Palliative treatment consists of antibiotics, douches, and the application of antiseptics to the cervix, but often a cure is effected only after the cervical glands are destroyed with a cautery or after the diseased tissue is excised. Anesthesia may or may not be required, since cauterization in the cervical area is a painless procedure.

For more severe chronic cervicitis, conization may be done. Anesthesia is optional. In the operating room, the tip of an electric instrument is inserted into the external os of the cervix and rotated to cut and coagulate a cone of tissue. Aftercare may require packing, but otherwise it is similar to that following electric cauterization.

Patient Education and Home Health Care. Following cauterization, the patient should rest more than usual for the next few days. The nature of vaginal discharge is explained to the patient so that she can expect a grayish green, malodorous discharge for up to 3 weeks, because of sloughing cervical tissue. A follow-up visit is recommended by the gynecologist in 2 to 3 weeks, when the cervix is checked for possible stenosis, which may require dilatation. Usually, 6 to 8 weeks are required for healing. Sexual relations are resumed on recommendation of the physician. The patient should note any excess bleeding and report it to her physician.

Pelvic Infection
(Pelvic Inflammatory Disease)

Pelvic infection is an inflammatory condition of the pelvic cavity that may involve the uterine tubes (salpingitis), ovaries (oophoritis), pelvic peritoneum, or pelvic vascular system. Infection may be acute, subacute, recurrent, or chronic and may be localized or widespread. It is usually bacterial but may also be caused by a virus, fungus, or parasite.

Etiology. Pathogenic organisms usually enter the body through the vagina, pass through the cervical canal and into the uterus, and under various conditions may proceed to one or both uterine tubes and ovaries and into the pelvis. In bacterial infections that occur after childbirth or abortion, and in some IUD-related infections, pathogens are disseminated directly through the tissues that support the uterus by way of the lymphatics and blood vessels (Fig. 42-1A). The increased blood supply required by the placenta provides more pathways for infection. These postpartal and postabortion infections tend to be unilateral. In gonorrheal infections, the gonococci pass through the cervical canal and into the uterus, where the environment, especially during menstruation, allows them to multiply rapidly and spread to the uterine tubes and into the pelvis (Fig. 42-1B). The infection is usually bilateral. In rare instances some diseases (*e.g.*, tuberculosis) gain access to the reproductive organs by way of the bloodstream from the lungs (Fig. 42-1C).

Clinical Manifestations. The onset of pelvic infection is usually manifested by vaginal discharge and lower abdominal and pelvic pain and tenderness that occurs following the menses. The type of discharge varies with the infecting organism. It is usually heavy and purulent for gonorrhea or staphylococcal infection; for streptococcal infection, the discharge tends to be more mucoid and thinner. Systemic symptoms include fever, general malaise, anorexia, nausea, headache, and possibly vomiting. On pelvic examination, intense tenderness may be noted.

Management. The goal of therapy is to control and eradicate the infection by preventing the infection from spreading to other systems in the patient or to other persons. Even before the specific infective organism is determined,

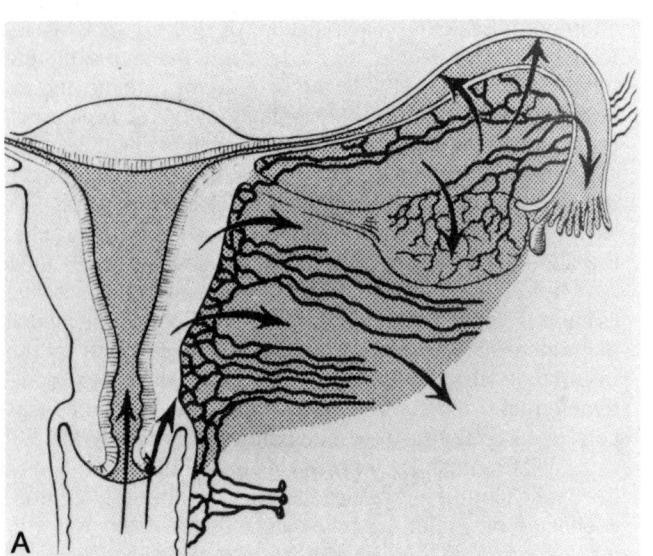
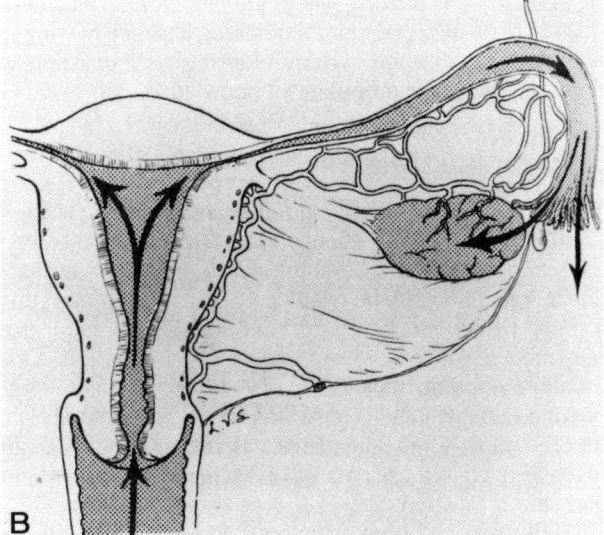
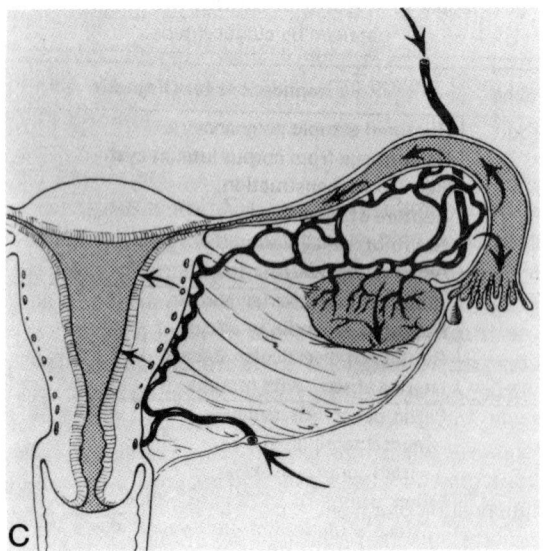

Figure 42-1
Pelvic infections: Avenues of invasion of the female reproductive system by various infectious organisms. (*A*) Spread of nongonorrheal bacterial infection from the vagina through the uterus and uterine tube to the ovary and pelvis. Dissemination is accomplished by way of lymphatics and blood vessels of the parametrium (loose connective tissue within the broad ligament that supports the uterus). (*B*) Spread of gonorrheal infection from the vagina through the uterus and uterine tubes to the peritoneal region. (*C*) Top and bottom arrows depict circulatory pathways carrying such organisms as tubercle bacilli from the lungs to the vascular structures of the reproductive system. (Benson RC [ed]: Current Obstetrics and Gynecologic Diagnosis and Treatment, 5th ed. Los Altos, California, Lange Medical Publications, 1984.)

the patient is placed on broad-spectrum antibiotic therapy. Women with mild to moderately severe infections are usually treated as outpatients. However, patients who are acutely ill may be hospitalized.

In the hospital, intensive therapy includes bed rest and intravenous fluids to correct dehydration and acidosis. If abdominal distention or ileus is present, nasogastric intubation and suction will be initiated. Careful monitoring of vital signs and symptoms will assist in evaluating the movement of the infection.

Complications. Pelvic or generalized peritonitis may develop, as may abscess formation, strictures, and obstruction in the uterine tubes. Obstruction may result in an ectopic pregnancy at some future time if a fertilized egg is unable to pass the stricture. Or, scar tissue may close the uterine tubes, resulting in sterility. Adhesions are a common development that eventually may require removal of the uterus, tubes, and ovaries. Other complications include bacteremia with septic shock and thrombophlebitis with possible embolization.

Nursing Interventions

The "caring" for the patient with pelvic infections is just as important as the "curing." This infection may be very distressing, both physically and emotionally. The patient may feel well one day and develop vague symptoms and discomfort the next. She often suffers from constipation and menstrual difficulties.

The hospitalized patient is maintained on bed rest and usually placed in semi-Fowler's position to facilitate dependent drainage. For comfort, heat (heating pad) can be applied to the abdomen externally and warm douches may be prescribed to improve local circulation. In addition, the patient is supported nutritionally and with selective antibiotic therapy as prescribed. Catheterization and the use of tampons are avoided to prevent the spread of the infection.

Proper recording of vital signs and the nature and amount of vaginal discharge are necessary as a guide in future therapy.

The dissemination of infection to others can be controlled in many ways:

- Perineal pads are handled carefully with an instrument or gloves, and the soiled pad is deposited in a paper bag for proper disposal.
- Hands are washed carefully with a germicidal soap.
- All items that come in contact with the patient (utensils, bedpans, toilet seats, and linens) are properly disinfected by the correct procedure for controlling the specific organisms responsible for the infection.

The patient must be informed of the need for these precautions and encouraged to take part in plans to prevent contamination of others as well as to protect herself from reinfection.

If reinfection or spread of infection occurs, symptoms may include abdominal pain, nausea and vomiting, elevation of temperature, malaise, malodorous purulent vaginal discharge, and leukocytosis.

Patient Education and Home Health Care. Patient teaching consists of explaining how pelvic infections occur and how they can be controlled.

- Be aware that organisms can gain entrance to the reproductive area during sexual intercourse or following pelvic surgery, abortion, and childbirth.
- Realize that users of intrauterine devices are more susceptible to infections.
- Follow proper perineal care, especially wiping from front to back.
- Do not douche frequently since this practice will reduce natural flora that can combat infecting organisms.
- Wear clean, cotton, loose-fitting undergarments.
- Avoid strong soaps, bubble bath, sprays, powders, and deodorants in the perineal area.
- Consult with a health care provider if unusual vaginal discharge or odor is noted.
- Avoid tampons if they have caused problems.
- Do not wear pads or tampons longer than 6 hours; preferably change them every 4 hours.
- Remember to remove a diaphragm after using it for 6 hours.
- Maintain optimum health practices with proper nutrition, exercise, weight control, and relaxation.
- Visit a gynecologist at least once a year.
- Insist on a partner's wearing a condom if there is any question of infection prior to intercourse.

Structural Disorders

Fistulas of the Vagina

A fistula is an abnormal, winding opening between two internal hollow organs or between an internal hollow organ and the exterior of the body. The name of the fistula indicates the two areas that are connected abnormally; a *ureterovaginal fistula* is an opening between the ureter and vagina; a *vesicovaginal fistula*, an opening between the bladder and the vagina; and a *rectovaginal fistula*, an opening between the rectum and the vagina (Fig. 42-2).

Etiology. Fistulas may occur congenitally, but in the adult, breakdown often occurs because of tissue damage resulting from injury sustained during surgery, delivery, radiation therapy, or disease processes such as carcinoma.

Clinical Manifestations. The immediate problem becomes one of infection and resulting excoriation. For example, the patient who has a vesicovaginal fistula has a continuous trickling of urine into the vagina. With a rectovaginal fistula, there is fecal incontinence, and flatus is discharged through the vagina. When such a discharge combines with a leukorrhea, a malodorous condition develops that is difficult to control.

Methylene blue dye can be used to delineate the course of the fistula. In vesicovaginal fistula, the dye is instilled into the bladder and appears in the vagina. Following a negative methylene blue test, indigo carmine is injected intravenously; if the dye appears in the vagina, a ureterovaginal fistula is indicated.

Management. The goal is to eliminate the fistula, thereby also controlling infection and excoriation. Frequently, a fistula will heal without surgical intervention. Otherwise sur-

Figure 42-2
Common sites for fistulas:
Uterocolic
—uterus and colon
Vesicocolic
—bladder and colon
Vesicovaginal
—bladder and vagina
Urethrovaginal
—urethra and vagina
Vaginoperineal
—vagina and perineal area
Vesicouterine
—bladder and uterus
Ureterovaginal
—ureter and vagina
Rectovaginal
—rectum and vagina

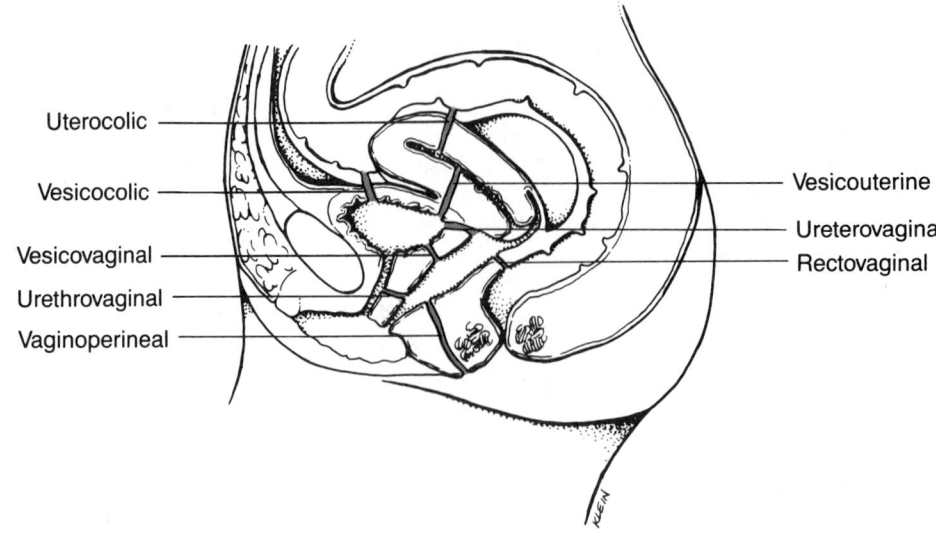

Figure 42-3
Diagrammatic representation of the four most common types of pelvic floor relaxation: cystocele, urethrocele, rectocele, and enterocele. Arrows depict sites of maximum protrusion. (Kistner RW. Gynecology: Principles and Practice, 4th ed. Chicago, Year Book Medical Publishers, 1986.)

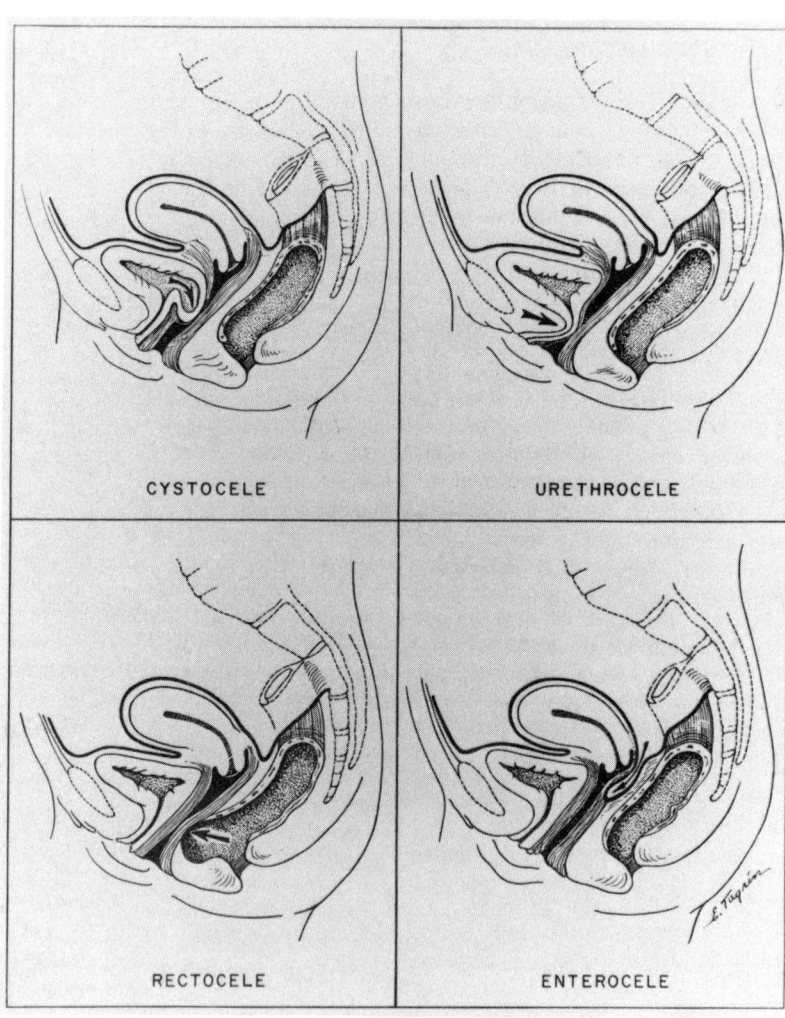

gery is indicated. Usually the vaginal approach is used for vesicovaginal and urethrovaginal fistulas. The abdominal approach is used for fistulas higher in the abdomen. Fistulas that are difficult to repair or very large may require urinary or fecal diversion.

Nursing Interventions. Nursing measures are planned to relieve discomfort, prevent infection, and improve the patient's self-perception, and self-care abilities.

Healing of the tissues is promoted by proper nutrition with an increase in intake of vitamin C and protein, by local cleanliness through douching and enemas, by rest, and by taking prescribed intestinal antibiotics. A rectovaginal fistula will heal faster if the patient is placed on a low-residue diet and if proper drainage of affected tissues is initiated.

If the person is older, more rest is required than in most postoperative patients because of a higher incidence of debilitation and the delicate as well as sensitive nature of the tissues. Warm perineal irrigations and controlled heat-lamp treatments are effective in stimulating the healing process.

For the patient who has had repair of a vesicovaginal fistula, an indwelling catheter is usually inserted. Drainage from the catheter is observed carefully, and care is taken to ensure that the catheter is functioning properly. If the catheter becomes clogged, urine may collect in the bladder, causing pressure that may damage the repaired tissue. Bladder irrigation and vaginal irrigations are done gently, with minimal pressure.

Effective measures to assist the woman whose fistula cannot be repaired must be planned on an individual basis. Cleanliness, frequent sitz baths, and deodorizing douches are required, as well as the use of perineal pads and protective undergarments. Particular attention to skin care is necessary to prevent excoriation. Bland creams or a light dusting of cornstarch may be soothing. Morale boosters and attention to the social and psychological needs of this patient are essential components of effective care.

Cystocele, Rectocele, Enterocele, and Lacerations of the Perineum

Cystocele is a downward displacement of the bladder toward the vaginal orifice (Fig. 42-3). Occasionally, it is caused by tissue weakness, but most often it is a result of injuries received during childbirth. The condition appears some years later when genital atrophy associated with aging takes place.

Rectocele and lacerations of the perineum may occur as injuries to the muscles and the tissues of the pelvic floor and may happen at the time of childbirth. Because of tears in muscles below the vagina, the rectum may pouch upward, pushing the posterior wall of the vagina in front of it. This condition is termed a rectocele. At times, the lacerations may extend to such a degree as to sever completely the fibers of the anal sphincter (complete tear). An enterocele is a protrusion of intestinal wall into the vagina.

Clinical Manifestations. A cystocele occurs as a bulging downward of the interior vaginal wall that causes a sense of pelvic pressure, fatigue, and often such urinary symptoms as incontinence, frequency, and urgency. Back pain (dragging and strain type) and pelvic pain are experienced.

The symptoms of rectocele are similar to those of cystocele with one exception—instead of urinary symptoms, the patient experiences constipation and incontinence of gas and liquid feces when complete tears have occurred.

Management. Perineal exercises are sometimes prescribed and help to strengthen the weakened muscles. These are more effective in the early stages of a cystocele. If surgery is contraindicated, or refused, a pessary may be used. Such a device may be prescribed for mild problems.

A *pessary* is a device inserted in the upper vagina and positioned to assist in keeping an organ, such as the bladder, uterus, or intestine, in proper alignment. It is usually shaped as a ring or doughnut and is made of a variety of materials, such as rubber or plastic. The size and type of pessary are selected and fitted by the gynecologist. The patient can be taught to remove the pessary at bedtime and to reinsert it in the morning. If it remains in place and is not removed by the patient, she should have it removed, checked, and cleaned by the physician or nurse practitioner periodically. At this time, tissues need to be inspected for pressure points or signs of irritation. Normally, there is no pain, discomfort, or discharge with its use. Douching may be recommended if there is a discharge.

Surgical Management. The treatment of cystocele is surgical, the operation for the repair of the anterior vaginal wall being termed *anterior colporrhaphy*. The operation for the repair of rectocele and lacerations of the perineum is called a *perineorrhaphy* or a *posterior colporrhaphy*.

Displacements of the Uterus

The uterus lies normally with the cervix at right angles to the long axis of the vagina and with the body of the uterus inclined slightly forward. However, it is freely movable, owing to the requirements of pregnancy. The strain of this physiologic function, the formation of adhesions, or a weakening of its natural supports may produce changes in the normal position of the uterus that usually cause no severe problems to the patient but may give rise to many troublesome symptoms.

Backward Displacements. Backward displacements (*retroversion* and *retroflexion*) of the uterus (Fig. 42-4) may give rise to such symptoms as bachache, a sense of pelvic pressure, easy fatigue, and leukorrheal discharge. Most retrograde displacements are asymptomatic.

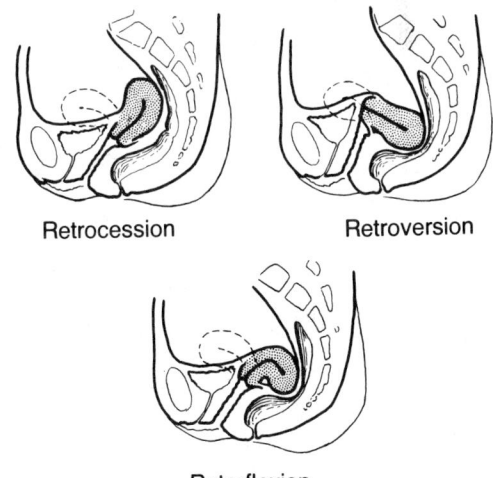

Retrocession

Retroversion

Retroflexion

Figure 42-4
Retrodisplacements of the uterus. The dotted line indicates the normal position of the uterus. In *retrocession,* the uterus tilts posteriorly. In *retroversion,* the uterus turns posteriorly as a whole unit. In *retroflexion,* the fundus bends posteriorly above the cervical end. (Hardy JD. Hardy's Textbook of Surgery, 2nd ed. Philadelphia, JB Lippincott, 1988.)

Surgery for backward displacements of the uterus is carried out only if the condition is incapacitating. An abdominal incision allows access to the uterus, which is brought forward into its normal position and is then maintained there by shortening its ligaments. Some patients with retroversion may be treated by the use of *pessaries*. These are instruments of hard rubber or crystal-clear Plexiglas that maintain the uterus in a forward position by exerting pressure on ligaments attached to the posterior wall of the cervix. They are of great value as a test of the patient's symptoms and often effect a cure. Pessaries must be removed and cleaned at frequent intervals.

Prolapse and Procidentia. Because of the weakening of the supports of the uterus, most often brought about by childbirth, the uterus may work its way down the vaginal canal (prolapse) and even appear outside the vaginal orifice (procidentia) (Fig. 42-5).

In its descent, the uterus pulls with it the vaginal walls and even the bladder and the rectum. The symptoms caused

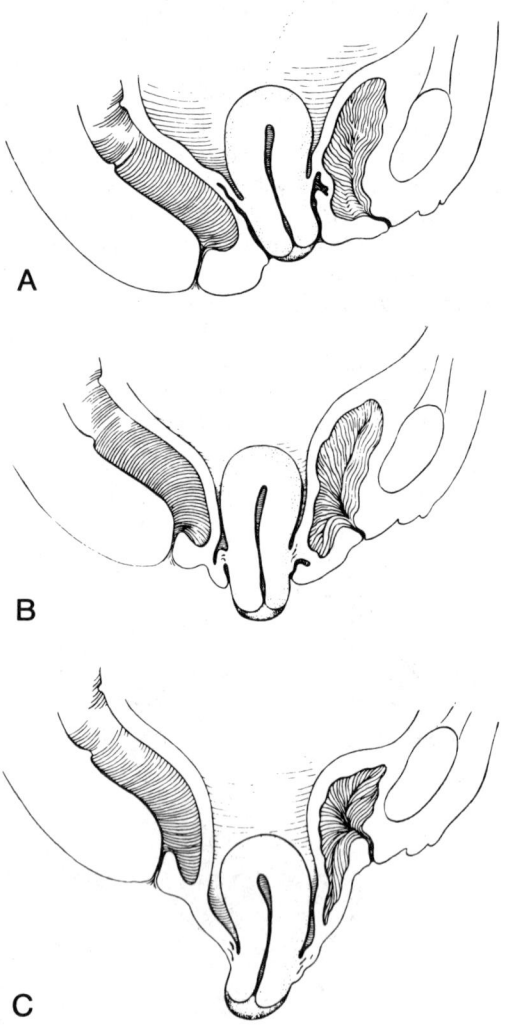

Figure 42-5
Prolapse of the uterus and the vagina. (*A*) First-degree prolapse—cervix comes down to introitus. (*B*) Second-degree prolapse—cervix protrudes through introitus. (*C*) Third-degree prolapse—total procidentia: uterus protrudes through introitus. (Adapted from Gray LA. Postgrad Med 30:209.)

are similar to those mentioned for backward displacements, plus urinary symptoms (incontinence and retention) from displacement of the bladder. These symptoms are aggravated when the woman coughs, lifts a heavy object, or stands for a long while. Normal activities are troublesome tasks; even walking up the steps may aggravate the problem. The nurse can encourage women who have such difficulties to seek medical attention, because time is not likely to correct the problem.

The best treatment is surgical. The uterus is sutured back into place, and repair work is done to strengthen and tighten muscle bands. In postmenopausal women, the uterus may be removed (hysterectomy). For elderly women or those who are too ill to stand the strain of surgery, pessaries may be the treatment of choice.

Nursing Interventions

Patient Education and Home Health Care. Many of the problems related to relaxation of the pelvic muscles (cystocele, rectocele, uterine prolapse) might have been prevented. During obstetrical care, early visits to the nurse midwife or obstetrician permit early detection of potential problems. During the postpartum period, perineal exercises can be taught so that the woman develops the ability to tighten and relax gluteal and perineal floor muscles. Learning to start and stop the urinary stream also enhances perineal muscle tone.

It is incorrect to assume that these problems are the direct result of aging or of having had children. Such misconceptions have a tendency to prevent the woman from seeking professional evaluation and treatment. Delays may result in further complications such as infection, cervical ulceration, cystitis, and hemorrhoids.

If the patient is to have a pessary, she needs to know how to insert it, how long it may remain in place and how to clean it, as well as reinsert it.

Preoperative Nursing Management. Before surgery, the patient needs to know the extent of the proposed surgery, the expectations for the postoperative period, and the effect of surgery on future sexual functions. Often, a midstream clean-catch urine specimen is required. The specimen is sent to the laboratory immediately. For a rectocele repair, a cathartic and a cleansing enema may be prescribed. Some surgeons require a perineal shave.

In the operating room, special attention is given to placing both of the patient's legs in and out of stirrups simultaneously in order to prevent muscular strain and excess pressure on the legs and thighs. Other preoperative details are similar to that described on page 306.

Postoperative Nursing Management and Rehabilitation. In the postoperative period, the immediate goals are to prevent infection and pressure on the suture line. This will require perineal care and may preclude the use of dressings. The patient is always urged to void within a few hours after operations for cystocele and complete tear. If the patient does not void within this period, feels uncomfortable, or has pain in the region of the bladder after 6 hours, catheterization is performed. Some physicians prefer to have an indwelling catheter in place for 2 to 4 days. There are various other methods of bladder care, as described in Chapter 39.

After each urination or bowel movement, the perineum

is irrigated with warm sterile saline (see vulvar douche, p. 1082) and the area blotted dry with sterile cotton.

There are several methods used in caring for the sutures. In one method, the sutures are left alone until healing occurs (*i.e.*, for 5 to 10 days). Thereafter, daily vaginal douches of sterile saline are given during the period of convalescence. In another method—the wet method—small douches of sterile saline are given twice daily, beginning on the day after operation and continuing throughout convalescence.

A heat lamp or hair dryer may be used to help dry the area and enhance the healing process. Commercially available sprays containing a combination of antiseptic and anesthetic solutions are soothing and effective. An ice pack applied locally may relieve discomfort. For effective relief of this type, a plastic bag can be filled with ice chips. However, the weight of the bag must rest on the bed and not on the patient.

The routine postoperative care is much like that for an abdominal operation. The patient is placed in bed, with the head and the knees elevated slightly. A liquid diet (many surgeons omit milk) is given on the first day, and then a full diet is begun as soon as desired.

After an operation for a complete perineal laceration (through the rectal sphincter), special care and attention are required. The bladder is emptied by catheterization to prevent strain on sutures.

Throughout the convalescence of all patients who have had plastic surgery, liquid petrolatum or another stool-softening agent is given each night after the patient is permitted a soft diet.

Patient Education and Home Health Care. Predischarge instructions include information pertaining to douching, the use of mild laxatives, the amount of exercise recommended, and the need to avoid lifting heavy objects or standing for prolonged periods. The patient is reminded to return to the gynecologist for a follow-up visit and to check with the physician regarding the resumption of sexual intercourse.

In particular, the patient is instructed to report any pelvic pain, observation of unusual discharge, inability to care for personal hygiene, and bleeding from the vagina. She is advised to continue with perineal exercises, which are recommended to assist in strengthening muscles. The patient is instructed as follows: tense the perineal muscles by pressing the buttocks together; hold this position; relax. This exercise, done 10 to 20 times each hour, can be performed while the person is sitting or standing.

Benign Tumors and Conditions

Vulvar Cysts

A cyst of the greater vestibular gland is a cystic dilation of the duct of the Bartholin's gland resulting from obstruction. This is the most common of vulvar tumors and is located in the posterior third of the vulva, near the vestibule. A simple cyst may be asymptomatic. Infection may be due to the gonococcus organism, *Escherichia coli*, or *Staphylococcus aureus* and can cause an abscess with or without inguinal adenopathy. The best treatment is incision and drainage, plus antibiotics.

Lichen Sclerosus

Lichen sclerosus et atrophicus, often mistaken for leukoplakia, is noted as very slightly raised whitish papules or macules of the vulvar dermis. Symptoms are usually mild or absent, in contrast to the intense pruritus of leukoplakia. It is believed that at least 10% of patients with cancer of the vulva have an associated lichen sclerosus, with or without leukoplakia. Biopsy and a careful follow-up program are definitely recommended. If cancer cells are detected on biopsy, a simple vulvectomy is performed, with continued follow-up.

Ovarian Cysts

Pathophysiology. The ovary is a frequent site for the development of cysts. These may be simply pathologic enlargements of normal ovarian constituents, the graafian follicle or corpus luteum, or they may arise from abnormal growth of the ovarian epithelium. They are considered benign tumors with a possibility of becoming malignant.

Dermoid cysts are tumors that are believed to arise from parts of the ovum that disappear normally as ripening (maturation) takes place. Since their origin is undefined, all that can be said is that they are tumors made up of undifferentiated embryonal cells. They grow slowly and at operation are found to contain a thick, yellow, sebaceous material arising from a skin lining. Hair, teeth, bone, brain, eyes, and many other tissues often are found in a rudimentary state within these cysts.

Clinically, cysts are manifested by their obvious presence as an ovarian mass. There may be lower abdominal pain that may be acute or chronic. Rupture may occur and simulate a variety of acute abdominal emergencies, such as appendicitis or ectopic pregnancy. Larger cysts may produce abdominal swelling and pressure on adjacent abdominal organs.

Management. The treatment of ovarian cysts is surgical removal. However, if malignant degeneration has taken place, with invasion of the abdomen and general emaciation (general carcinomatosis), operation is of little benefit. The patient may be given roentgen therapy and testosterone. The abdomen may be tapped to relieve distention from ascites. The postoperative nursing care after cystectomy is similar to that for abdominal surgery, with one exception. The marked decrease in intra-abdominal pressure incidental to the removal of a large cyst often leads to considerable abdominal distention. This complication may be prevented to some extent by the application of a snug-fitting abdominal binder.

Benign Tumors of the Uterus: Leiomyomas ("Fibroids," Myomas, or Fibromyomas)

Myomatous or fibroid tumors of the uterus are benign tumors arising from the muscle tissue of the uterus. They are common, occurring in about 20% of white women and 40% to 50% of black women. They develop slowly between the ages of 25 and 40 and often become large in size after this period. There are instances in which such a tumor causes no symptoms. The most common symptom is abnormal endometrial bleeding. Other symptoms are due to pressure on the surrounding organs—pain, backache, constipation, and urinary symptoms. In addition, such tumors often cause metrorrhagia and even sterility.

Management. The treatment of uterine fibroids depends to a large extent on their size and location. The patient with minor symptoms is watched closely. If she wishes to have children, treatment is as conservative as possible. As a rule, large tumors that produce pressure symptoms should be removed. Usually, the uterus is removed (hysterectomy), while the ovaries are preserved, if possible. If the tumor is small, it may be removed (myomectomy); the wound in the uterus is then closed. This is the procedure of choice in young women. If the tumor is producing excessive bleeding, the uterus and the tumor are removed (hysteromyomectomy).

The nursing process for a patient having a hysterectomy is on pages 1119–1120.

Endometriosis

Endometriosis is a benign lesion in which cells similar to those lining the uterus are found growing aberrantly in the pelvic cavity outside the uterus. It is a very puzzling disease because symptoms vary and may be misleading. Extensive endometriosis may cause few symptoms, whereas an isolated lesion may produce considerable symptomatology.

Pathophysiology. In order of frequency, pelvic endometriosis attacks the ovary, ureterosacral ligaments, culde-sac, rectovaginal septum, uterovesical peritoneum, cervix, umbilicus, laparotomy scars, hernial sacs, and appendix. The misplaced endometrium responds to ovarian hormonal stimulation and is indeed dependent on this stimulation. When the uterus goes through the process of menstruation, this ectopic tissue bleeds—mostly into areas having no outlet—which then causes pain and adhesions. At surgery, these lesions are typically small, puckered, and brown or blue-black, indicating concealed bleeding. If the endometrial tissue is within an ovarian cyst, there is no outlet for the bleeding and the formation is referred to as a *pseudocyst* (chocolate cyst).

Incidence. Endometriosis has been on the increase in the past several decades. There is a high incidence among patients who marry later, bear children later, and have fewer children. In countries such as India, where tradition favors early marriage and early childbearing, endometriosis is rare.

It is characteristically found in the young, nulliparous female, aged 25 to 35. A similar condition affecting the uterine lining in older, multiparous patients is referred to as adenomyosis. At present, these two conditions, which at one time were thought to be related, are now considered separate entities. There appears to be a predisposition to endometriosis; it is about seven times more common in women whose close female relatives have this condition.

Etiology. The more popular theories regarding the origin of endometrial lesions are the transplantation theory and the metaplasia theory. The transplantation theory suggests that a backflow of menses (retrograde menstruation) causes endometrial tissue to be transported to ectopic sites through the uterine tubes. Transplantation can also occur during surgery if endometrial tissue is transferred inadvertently by way of instruments. Endometrial tissue can also be spread by lymphatic or venous channels. The metaplasia theory relates to retained remnants of embryonic epithelial tissue, which during

the growth process may be transformed into endometrial tissue by means of outside stimuli. The real cause of endometriosis may be a combination of factors.

Clinical Manifestations and Diagnostic Evaluation. Symptoms vary with the location of endometrial tissue. Usually the chief symptom is a type of dysmenorrhea, unlike typical uterine cramps. The patient complains of a deep-seated aching in the lower abdomen, vagina, posterior pelvis, and back that occurs 1 or 2 days before the menstrual cycle and lasts 2 or 3 days. Some patients, however, have no pain. Abnormal uterine bleeding and dyspareunia (painful intercourse) may also be evident in sexually active women. Infertility is another possible effect.

A health history including the menstrual pattern is necessary to elicit specific symptoms. On bimanual pelvic examination, fixed tender nodules may be detected and the uterus may be restricted in motility, indicating the presence of adhesions. Laparoscopy confirms the diagnosis.

Management. Treatment depends on the nature of the symptoms, desire for pregnancy, and the extent of the disease. If the woman is asymptomatic, observation every 6 months may be all that is required. Other therapy for varying degrees of symptoms may be palliation, hormone administration, or surgery. Palliative efforts include analgesics, prostaglandin inhibitors, and pregnancy; the latter will alleviate symptoms because of the residual reaction in the various endometrial sites.

Hormonal therapy, in which estrogen-progestogene is given for 6 to 9 months, will suppress menstruation (pseudopregnancy) and relieve menstrual pain (dysmenorrhea). However, there may be side-effects such as fluid retention (diuretics may be recommended), nausea, weight gain, some vaginal discharge, and possibly thromboembolism. If these side-effects are troublesome, this form of therapy is stopped. Another type of hormonal therapy involves the use of a synthetic androgen, danazol (Danocrine), which causes atrophy of the endometrium and subsequent amenorrhea. The drug inhibits the release of gonadotropin with minimal overt sex hormone stimulation. This medication is expensive and may cause troublesome side-effects such as fatigue, depression, weight gain, oily skin, decreased breast size, mild acne, hot flashes, and atrophy of the vagina.

If conservative measures are not helpful, surgery may be necessary. The procedure selected will depend on the individual patient's needs. A laparoscopy may be performed during which it may be feasible to fulgurate (cut with high-frequency current) endometrial implants and to lyse (cut) adhesions. Laser surgery is another option made possible by laparoscopy. Lasers are used to vaporize the endometrial implants or to coagulate the implant, thereby destroying it.

Depending on circumstances, other surgical procedures may be used, including laparotomy, uterine suspension, abdominal hysterectomy, bilateral salpingo-oophorectomy, and appendectomy.

Prognosis. In mild to moderate endometriosis, the use of hormonal or surgical treatment relieves pain and enhances the chance of pregnancy. For women over age 35 or those willing to sacrifice reproductive capability, definitive surgery (total hysterectomy) provides good results.

Nursing Interventions. A nursing history and physical examination concentrate on identifying the specific symptoms and determining when and how long they have been bothersome and on what the woman's reproductive desires are. This information is most helpful in contributing to the treatment plan.

Patient goals include relief of pain, relief of dysmenorrhea and dyspareunia, and avoidance of infertility. Nursing interventions will include assessment of pain and evaluation of the techniques and prescribed medications that provide relief. Explanations of the various diagnostic procedures will afford assurance that therapy can be recommended specifically for this problem.

Emotional support is provided to the woman and her partner who are desirous of having a child. As the treatment plan progresses, it may become apparent that pregnancy is not possible. The psychosocial impact of this realization on the couple must

The nurse's
such as a causa
and endometr
upward statis
encouraged
menstrual
gated.

Aden
the uterin
to 50 year
and prolo
norrhea (
staining. (
enlarged, t
of bleedin
more cons

Malig

ance. Whatever measures are followed, an increase in the number of women having this simple, painless test will save lives that otherwise would be claimed by cancer.

There are two main types of primary uterine cancer—carcinoma of the cervix, which is predominantly epidermoid cancer, and carcinoma of the endometrium (corpus and body of the uterus).

Cancer of the Cervix

Cancer of the cervix is the most common cancer of the reproductive system in women. Although it rarely occurs before the age of 20, it is most common between the ages of 30 and
te that sexual activity has some relationship
f cancer of the cervix; before age 25, it is
those who have had many sex partners
ancies. Studies made on the incidence of
ong prostitutes also tend toward this con-

valuation. A valuable tool for the phy-
al staging of a disease. By estimating the
ase, treatment can be planned more spe-
osis reasonably predicted. The International
ted by the International Federation of Gy-
tetrics (Table 42-2) is most widely used;
ion is also used in describing malignancies
269). In this system T refers to extent of
lymph node involvement, and M to extent

ptoms are evaluated, and x-ray and labo-
special examinations such as punch biopsy
re done. Depending on the stage, other
including dilatation and curettage (D&C),
raphy, lymphangiography, and possibly
e imaging.

festations. Early cancer of the cervix is
tic. The two chief symptoms of early car-
ix are leukorrhea (vaginal discharge) and
leeding or spotting. For a long time, leu-
e only abnormal symptom. The discharge
in amount and becomes watery and, fi-
smelling because of necrosis and infection
The bleeding occurs at irregular intervals,
metrorrhagia) or after menopause. It may
enough to spot the undergarments, and it
fter some form of trauma (intercourse,
cation). As the disease continues, the
me constant and may increase in amount.
ions and erosions of the cervix seem to
art in the development of cervical cancer.
comes evident as a large reddish growth
ng crater before any symptoms appear.
advances, the tissues outside the cervix
cluding the lymph glands anterior to the
d of patients with invasive cervical cancer,
es the fundus. The nerves in this region
producing excruciating pain in the back
relieved only by large doses of narcotics.
hen untreated, is one of extreme emacia-
ften with irregular fever due to secondary
esses in the ulcerating mass.

To Do List...

TABLE 42-2
International Classification of Carcinoma of the Uterine Cervix

Stage of Lesion	Area	Description
Stage 0	Carcinoma *in situ*	Cancer limited to epithelial layer; no evidence of invasion
Stage I	Carcinoma strictly confined to cervix	Size is not a criterion
Stage IA		Microinvasive
Stage IB		Clinically obvious stage I
Stage II	Vaginal cancer	Lesion has spread beyond cervix to involve vagina (not lower third) or paracervical region on one or both sides
Stage IIA		Vaginal extension only
Stage IIB		Paracervical extension with or without vaginal involvement
Stage III	Cancer involves lower third of vagina or has extended to one or both pelvic walls	Unequivocal palpable lymph node disease on the pelvic wall IV pyelogram shows one or both ureters obstructed by the tumor
Stage IIIA		Extends to lower third of vagina only
Stage IIIB		Isolated carcinomatous metastases are palpable on the pelvic wall
Stage IV	Bladder extension	Evidence that carcinoma involves the bladder seen in cystoscopic examination or by presence of vesicovaginal fistula
	Rectal extension Distant spread	Carcinoma spreads outside true pelvis to other organs

Management. When precursor lesions are found by colposcopy, punch biopsy, or endocervical curettage, conservative nonsurgical removal is possible. Cryotherapy (freezing with nitrous oxide refrigerant) or CO_2 laser therapy are effective. Conization (removing a cone-shaped section of cervix) is done when the lesion is small. This is preferable for young women concerned about a future pregnancy. Frequent subsequent periodic examinations are done to check for recurrence. For invasive cervical cancer, radiation is the most frequent form of treatment. However, radical pelvic surgical procedures may be required for the more advanced lesions. The method selected depends on the stage of the lesion (Table 42-2) and on the judgment and skill of the physician. Radical surgery is advocated by some authorities, especially when a patient is unable to withstand the effects of radiation or has a radiation-resistant cancer. Surgical procedures commonly carried out include the following:

Hysterectomy—surgical removal of the uterus.
Total hysterectomy—removal of the uterus, including cervix.
Subtotal (partial) hysterectomy—removal of the uterus, leaving the cervix in place.
Radical hysterectomy (Wertheim)—an abdominal incision is made, and the uterus, adnexa, proximal vagina, and bilateral lymph nodes are removed en masse.
Radical vaginal hysterectomy (Schauta)—a vaginal approach is used to remove the uterus, adnexa, and proximal vagina.
(Note: "Radical" used before each of the above procedures means that an extensive area of the paravaginal, paracervical, parametrial, and uterosacral tissues is removed with the uterus.)
Bilateral pelvic lymphadenectomy—Removal of the common iliac, external iliac, hypogastric, and obturator lymphatics and nodes.
Pelvic exenteration—removal of the pelvic organs.
Salpingo-oophorectomy—removal of uterine tube and ovary.

Cancer of the Endometrium

Cancer of the endometrium (fundus or corpus) of the uterus has increased in incidence partly because people are living longer and there is more accurate reporting. The major emphasis for the nurse is to encourage all women over the age of 18 to have annual checkups, including a gynecologic examination.

ersome and on what the woman's reproductive desires are. This information is most helpful in contributing to the treatment plan.

Patient goals include relief of pain, relief of dysmenorrhea and dyspareunia, and avoidance of infertility. Nursing interventions will include assessment of pain and evaluation of the techniques and prescribed medications that provide relief. Explanations of the various diagnostic procedures will afford assurance that therapy can be recommended specifically for this problem.

Emotional support is provided to the woman and her partner who are desirous of having a child. As the treatment plan progresses, it may become apparent that pregnancy is not possible. The psychosocial impact of this realization on the couple must be respected and addressed.

The nurse's role in patient education is to dispel myths, such as a causative relationship between the use of tampons and endometriosis, which is not true. In order to combat the upward statistical trend of endometriosis, women should be encouraged to have regular physical examinations. Unusual menstrual bleeding patterns should be reported and investigated.

Adenomyosis. In this condition, endometriosis involves the uterine wall; the incidence is highest in women from 40 to 50 years of age. Symptoms are hypermenorrhea (excessive and prolonged bleeding), acquired dysmenorrhea, polymenorrhea (abnormally frequent bleeding), and premenstrual staining. On physical examination, the uterus is felt to be enlarged, firm, and tender. Treatment depends on the severity of bleeding and pain; hysterectomy offers greater relief than more conservative forms of therapy.

Malignant Conditions

Cancer of the Uterus

Malignant tumors of the female reproductive system (excluding the breast) rank as the second cause of death in the United States, accounting for approximately 10,000 deaths yearly (uterine corpus and endometrium, 3,000; cervix, 7,000). The death rate for uterine cancer has shown a steady decline in recent years because more women are being educated to seek annual checkups that include the Papanicolaou test. However, when it is realized that a significant number of women in the United States over the age of 20 have never had a Papanicolaou test, it is obvious that much remains to be done.

Why a woman who knows about the Papanicolaou test does not have it done is a question to be explored by all those concerned with community health. Are women who feel and look healthy afraid to "look for trouble?" Is getting to the clinic or physician inconvenient because of hours, transportation, or babysitting difficulties? Not only is the continued dissemination of information necessary, but it may be necessary for health personnel to "go more than halfway" in order to ensure the broadest possible application of this test. Perhaps a routine Papanicolaou test could be a required part of preemployment examinations, applications for marriage license, admissions to a hospital, and applications for insur-

ance. Whatever measures are followed, an increase in the number of women having this simple, painless test will save lives that otherwise would be claimed by cancer.

There are two main types of primary uterine cancer—carcinoma of the cervix, which is predominantly epidermoid cancer, and carcinoma of the endometrium (corpus and body of the uterus).

Cancer of the Cervix

Cancer of the cervix is the most common cancer of the reproductive system in women. Although it rarely occurs before the age of 20, it is most common between the ages of 30 and 50. Statistics indicate that sexual activity has some relationship to the incidence of cancer of the cervix; before age 25, it is more prevalent in those who have had many sex partners and several pregnancies. Studies made on the incidence of cervical cancer among prostitutes also tend toward this conclusion.

Diagnostic Evaluation. A valuable tool for the physician is the clinical staging of a disease. By estimating the extent of the disease, treatment can be planned more specifically and prognosis reasonably predicted. The International Classification adopted by the International Federation of Gynecology and Obstetrics (Table 42-2) is most widely used; the TNM classification is also used in describing malignancies (see Chart 16-2, p. 269). In this system T refers to extent of primary tumor, N to lymph node involvement, and M to extent of metastasis.

Signs and symptoms are evaluated, and x-ray and laboratory studies plus special examinations such as punch biopsy and colposcopy are done. Depending on the stage, other tests may be used, including dilatation and curettage (D&C), computed tomography, lymphangiography, and possibly magnetic resonance imaging.

Clinical Manifestations. Early cancer of the cervix is usually asymptomatic. The two chief symptoms of early carcinoma of the cervix are leukorrhea (vaginal discharge) and irregular vaginal bleeding or spotting. For a long time, leukorrhea may be the only abnormal symptom. The discharge increases gradually in amount and becomes watery and, finally, dark and foul smelling because of necrosis and infection of the tumor mass. The bleeding occurs at irregular intervals, between periods (metrorrhagia) or after menopause. It may be very slight, just enough to spot the undergarments, and it is noted usually after some form of trauma (intercourse, douching, or defecation). As the disease continues, the bleeding may become constant and may increase in amount.

Chronic infections and erosions of the cervix seem to play a significant part in the development of cervical cancer. Such pathology becomes evident as a large reddish growth or a deep, ulcerating crater before any symptoms appear.

As the cancer advances, the tissues outside the cervix may be invaded, including the lymph glands anterior to the sacrum. In one third of patients with invasive cervical cancer, the disease involves the fundus. The nerves in this region become involved, producing excruciating pain in the back and the legs that is relieved only by large doses of narcotics. The final picture, when untreated, is one of extreme emaciation and anemia, often with irregular fever due to secondary infection and abscesses in the ulcerating mass.

TABLE 42-2
International Classification of Carcinoma of the Uterine Cervix

Stage of Lesion	Area	Description
Stage 0	Carcinoma *in situ*	Cancer limited to epithelial layer; no evidence of invasion
Stage I	Carcinoma strictly confined to cervix	Size is not a criterion
Stage IA		Microinvasive
Stage IB		Clinically obvious stage I
Stage II	Vaginal cancer	Lesion has spread beyond cervix to involve vagina (not lower third) or paracervical region on one or both sides
Stage IIA		Vaginal extension only
Stage IIB		Paracervical extension with or without vaginal involvement
Stage III	Cancer involves lower third of vagina or has extended to one or both pelvic walls	Unequivocal palpable lymph node disease on the pelvic wall
		IV pyelogram shows one or both ureters obstructed by the tumor
Stage IIIA		Extends to lower third of vagina only
Stage IIIB		Isolated carcinomatous metastases are palpable on the pelvic wall
Stage IV	Bladder extension	Evidence that carcinoma involves the bladder seen in cystoscopic examination or by presence of vesicovaginal fistula
	Rectal extension	Carcinoma spreads outside true pelvis to other organs
	Distant spread	

Management. When precursor lesions are found by colposcopy, punch biopsy, or endocervical curettage, conservative nonsurgical removal is possible. Cryotherapy (freezing with nitrous oxide refrigerant) or CO_2 laser therapy are effective. Conization (removing a cone-shaped section of cervix) is done when the lesion is small. This is preferable for young women concerned about a future pregnancy. Frequent subsequent periodic examinations are done to check for recurrence. For invasive cervical cancer, radiation is the most frequent form of treatment. However, radical pelvic surgical procedures may be required for the more advanced lesions. The method selected depends on the stage of the lesion (Table 42-2) and on the judgment and skill of the physician. Radical surgery is advocated by some authorities, especially when a patient is unable to withstand the effects of radiation or has a radiation-resistant cancer. Surgical procedures commonly carried out include the following:

Hysterectomy—surgical removal of the uterus.
Total hysterectomy—removal of the uterus, including cervix.
Subtotal (partial) hysterectomy—removal of the uterus, leaving the cervix in place.
Radical hysterectomy (Wertheim)—an abdominal incision is made, and the uterus, adnexa, proximal va-

gina, and bilateral lymph nodes are removed en masse.
Radical vaginal hysterectomy (Schauta)—a vaginal approach is used to remove the uterus, adnexa, and proximal vagina.
(*Note:* "Radical" used before each of the above procedures means that an extensive area of the paravaginal, paracervical, parametrial, and uterosacral tissues is removed with the uterus.)
Bilateral pelvic lymphadenectomy—Removal of the common iliac, external iliac, hypogastric, and obturator lymphatics and nodes.
Pelvic exenteration—removal of the pelvic organs.
Salpingo-oophorectomy—removal of uterine tube and ovary.

Cancer of the Endometrium

Cancer of the endometrium (fundus or corpus) of the uterus has increased in incidence partly because people are living longer and there is more accurate reporting. The major emphasis for the nurse is to encourage all women over the age of 18 to have annual checkups, including a gynecologic examination.

Menopausal and postmenopausal women who take estrogens have an increased risk of acquiring endometrial cancer. The Federal Drug Administration strongly supports warnings that advise health professionals and female patients that the risk is much lower if estrogens are taken in the lowest possible doses.

For older women, the increased risk of endometrial cancer from estrogen use is proportional to the length of time during which the estrogens are taken (particularly 5 years or longer). Estrogens are effective for the vasomotor symptoms of menopause if doses are kept low and treatment is limited to less than a year.

Clinical Manifestations. About 50% of all patients with postmenopausal bleeding have cancer of the fundus. Its progress is slow, metastasis occurs later, and the symptom of irregular vaginal bleeding often appears early enough in the disease to allow cure by removal of the uterus. In late metastasis, radium and roentgen rays are the usual therapeutic measures.

Diagnostic Evaluation. Heretofore, dilatation and curettage was the only means of early diagnosis. The Papanicolaou smear is inadequate because it alerts the physician only to about 25% of endometrial lesions; consequently, diagnosis is made only after the development of overt symptoms. Endometrial smears (p. 1080) are more accurate and relatively inexpensive.

Hysterectomy

A total hysterectomy involves the removal of the uterus, including the cervix. This procedure is done for many conditions, including dysfunctional uterine bleeding; endometriosis; malignant and nonmalignant growths on uterus, cervix, and adnexa; problems of pelvic relaxation and prolapse; and irreparable injury to the uterus.

▶ *Nursing Process* *The Patient Undergoing a Hysterectomy*

▷ *Assessment*

The nursing history and physical and pelvic examination plus a review of the laboratory studies enable the nurse to establish a broad picture of the patient's problems. Additional questions will include psychosocial implications since a hysterectomy in most instances affects very personal and deep-seated experiences and relationships.

▷ *Nursing Diagnoses*

Based on all the assessment data, the patients major nursing diagnoses may include the following:

- Anxiety related to the diagnosis of cancer, fear of pain, loss of femininity and disfigurement
- Disturbance in self-concept related to altered body image, sexuality, fertility, and relationships with family and partner

- Alteration in comfort—pain related to surgery and other adjuvant therapy
- Grieving related to loss of significant reproductive organs
- Knowledge deficit of the perioperative aspects of hysterectomy as well as adjustment to postoperative recovery and convalescence

▷ *Planning and Implementation*

▷ *Goals:* The major goals of the patient may include relief of anxiety, acceptance of self as altered, absence of pain/discomfort, reduction of grief, and acquisition of knowledge and understanding of what a hysterectomy means.

Nursing Interventions

Relief of Anxiety. Anxiety in the woman undergoing a hysterectomy stems from a number of variables: unfamiliar environment, effects of surgery on body image and reproductive ability, fear of pain and other discomforts, and sensitivity and possibly feelings of embarrassment about exposure of the genital area in the perioperative period. She may fear that a sexually transmitted disease may be discovered or that she may no longer fulfill her role as a woman. Conflicts between medical treatment and religious beliefs may trouble her. It is necessary for the nurse to determine the meaning of this experience to the patient, and it is also necessary for the patient to verbalize her feelings to someone who understands and can help.

The nurse identifies the patient's strengths that will produce a positive effect. Through the preoperative period, explanations are given relative to the phases of physical preparation.

Preoperative Preparation. The physical preparation differs little from the details described for the preparation of a patient undergoing a laparotomy. The lower half of the abdomen and the pubic and perineal regions usually are carefully shaved and cleansed with soap and water (some clinics do not require shaving). The intestinal tract and the bladder are empty before the patient is sent to the operating room. This is most important to prevent contamination and accidental injury to the bladder or intestinal tract. An enema and antiseptic douche are probably required the evening before surgery to be followed by sedation for a restful night. Preoperative medications the morning of surgery will help the patient relax.

Self-Concept. The nursing history will reveal how the woman feels about having a hysterectomy. It is a personal experience that is affected by the nature of the diagnosis, significant others who may be involved (family, partner, occupational associates), religious beliefs, and prognosis. Concerns may surface such as the inability to have children, loss of femininity, and questions about the impact on sexual relationships. The patient needs to be reassured that she will still have a vagina and that sexual intercourse can be experienced following a temporary period of abstinence postoperatively while the tissues heal.

Moreover, when hormonal balances are upset, as often occurs in disturbances of the reproductive system, the patient may exhibit depression and heightened emotional sensitivity to people and situations. Each patient must be understood in the light of such factors and be approached and evaluated individually. This understanding must be shared by the family as well as the health care providers. The nurse who exhibits interest, concern, and willingness to listen to the patient's fears will add immeasurably to the patient's progress throughout the surgical experience, however temporary or prolonged that may be. Since the decision to have a hysterectomy rests with the patient, this must be respected and supported.

Postoperative Care. Postoperatively, with careful monitoring and nursing attention, the patient will have minimal discomfort. The principles of general postoperative care for abdominal surgery apply. Particular attention is given to peripheral circulation, such as noting presence of varicosities and promoting circulation with leg exercises and antiembolic stockings.

In addition, because of the proximity of the surgical intervention to the bladder, problems of voiding may be expected; edema or nerve trauma may cause temporary atony, and an indwelling catheter may be used. If no catheter is in place, catheterization may be necessary if the patient has not voided after 8 hours. If the catheter is in place, it is usually removed shortly after ambulation. During surgery, the handling of the bowel may cause ileus and interfere with bowel functioning.

To combat the discomfort of abdominal distention, a nasogastric tube may be inserted before the patient leaves the operating room, especially if excessive handling of viscera has taken place. If a large tumor was present, its excision could cause edema because of the sudden release of pressure. In the postoperative period, fluids and food may be restricted for 1 or 2 days. If there is abdominal flatus, a rectal tube may be prescribed, as well as heat to the abdomen. When peristalsis begins, as determined by abdominal auscultation, the patient is served additional fluids and a soft diet. Ambulation facilitates the return to normal peristalsis.

Patient Education and Home Health Care. Information is provided to the patient according to her needs and desires. It is important for her to know what kind of an operation she has had and what limitations or restrictions (if any) may be expected. Menstruation will no longer occur; symptoms of menopause will not result if ovaries are intact, but if they have been removed, hormonal replacement may be considered. Although a hysterectomy is often thought of as "simply a bit more than an appendectomy" it does cause some reduced strength and a "tired feeling" for a few weeks. This is to be expected and should gradually improve.

The patient should assume activities gradually; however, this does not mean sitting for long periods of time since this may cause pooling of the blood in the pelvis and the potential for thromboembolism. Showers are preferable to tub bathing in order to reduce the possibility of vaginal irritation and infection and to avoid the dangers of injury from stepping in and out of the tub. The patient is advised to avoid straining, lifting, sexual intercourse, or driving until these activities are permitted by the physician. Vaginal discharge, foul odor, excessive amount of bleeding, and an elevated temperature are reported to a health care professional.

The nurse will reinforce information given to the patient by the physician regarding the resumption of sexual intercourse. Perhaps other methods of sexual experiences are in order or other less strenuous coital positions might be suggested.

▷ *Evaluation*

▷ *Expected Outcomes*

1. Patient is free of anxiety.
   a. Asks specific questions regarding the effects of surgery on menstruation, procreation, sexual relations, and cancer.
   b. Discusses the surgical procedure and postoperative course.
2. Accepts herself as she now is.
   a. Includes her partner in planning her convalescence.
   b. Verbalizes understanding of her problem and projected solution.
   c. Takes time and care with her appearance.
   d. Shares her plans with the nurse regarding her first 2 weeks at home.
   e. Displays no depression or sadness.
3. Experiences minimal pain and discomfort.
   a. Is afebrile for 24 hours prior to discharge.
   b. Has stable vital signs.
   c. Ambulates early.
   d. Notes absence of calf pain, redness, tenderness, or swelling in extremities.
   e. Reports no urinary problems or abdominal distention.
4. Confirms her acquisition of knowledge and understanding of self-care.
   a. Practices deep breathing, turning, and leg exercises as taught.
   b. Increases activity and ambulation daily.
   c. Reports adequate fluid intake and adequate urinary output.
   d. Alternates periods of rest with activity.
   e. Tells what symptoms to report.
   f. Relates what hormonal replacement she is prescribed and its purpose.
   g. Keeps follow-up clinic appointments.

Cancer of the Vulva

Primary cancer of the vulva represents 3% to 4% of all gynecologic malignancies and is seen mostly in postmenopausal women. More whites than nonwhites are afflicted. Epidermoid cancer is the most common type. Intraepithelial cancer includes squamous cell carcinoma *in situ* and extramammary Paget's disease. Less common are Bartholin's gland cancer, basal cell carcinoma, and malignant melanoma. Little is known of the etiology of this condition.

Clinical Manifestations and Diagnostic Evaluation. Long-standing pruritus is the most common symptom of vulvar cancer. Bleeding, foul-smelling discharge, and pain may also be present. Early lesions appear as a chronic dermatitis; later a lump may be noted that continues to grow and becomes a hard ulcerated, cauliflower-like growth. Biopsy is the chief means of diagnosing vulvar cancer. *Any vulvar lesion that is persistent and/or ulcerated or does not heal quickly with proper therapy should be biopsied.*

The nurse is in a unique position to encourage a woman with this disease to seek help, since this is one of the most curable of all malignant conditions: it is visible and accessible and grows relatively slowly. Although it begins on the skin surface and is easily noticed as a small ulcer that becomes infected and causes pain, women so affected seem reluctant to seek medical attention. Procrastination causes more extensive involvement, jeopardizing cure.

Management. Vulvectomy is preferred to radiation therapy. The extensiveness of the vulvectomy depends on the extent of the malignancy. For example, leukoplakic changes call for simple vulvectomy; carcinoma *in situ* requires a total vulvectomy; and invasive carcinoma necessitates a wide radical vulvectomy with pelvic and groin lymph node dissection. Occasionally, even a part of the urethra, vagina, and rectum may have to be removed. With such extensive surgery (pelvic exenteration) there have been encouraging recovery rates. Chemotherapy, radiation therapy, and immunotherapy have been used as adjunctive measures.

▶ Nursing Process
The Patient Undergoing a Vulvectomy

▷ Assessment

In addition to the findings on physical and pelvic examination, the nursing history is a valuable tool since it is at this relaxed talking time that rapport on a one-to-one basis can be developed between nurse and patient. Why the patient has sought health counsel is apparent. What needs to be determined is the reason for the delay—was it modesty, economics, denial, or simply neglect? How will this affect her future care and needs? Health habits are ascertained, and receptability for learning is evaluated. An appraisal of the psychosocial factors is also determined. Preoperative preparation and psychological encouragement is also begun at this time.

▷ Nursing Diagnoses

Based on all the assessment and other data, the patient's major nursing diagnoses may include the following:

- Anxiety related to the diagnosis and aftermath of surgery
- Alteration in skin integrity related to wound drainage
- Potential for infection related to proximity of excretory function
- Alteration in comfort related to surgical incision and subsequent wound care
- Sexual dysfunction related to change in body part and functioning—vulvectomy
- Self-care deficit related to lack of understanding of perineal care and general health status

▷ Planning and Implementation

▷ *Goals:* The major goals of the patient may include acceptance of and preparation for surgical intervention, avoidance of infection and postsurgical complications, recovery of the best possible sexual function, and ability to perform adequate and appropriate self-care.

Preoperative Nursing Interventions

Relieving Anxiety. The patient must be allowed time to talk and ask questions. Fear of mutilation and loss of function is lessened when a woman of childbearing age learns that the possibility of having sexual relations is good and that

pregnancy is possible following a simple vulvectomy. Of course, the nurse must know what the physician has told the patient in this regard.

Physical Preparation. In addition to the nursing care described in Chapter 17 regarding physical and psychological preparation, wide preparation of the skin may include cleansing the lower abdomen, inguinal areas, upper thighs, and vulva with a detergent germicide for several days prior to the operation. The extent of surgery is dependent on the extent of the spread; more extensive lesions require deep pelvic node dissection. Antibiotic and heparin prophylaxis may be prescribed preoperatively and continued postoperatively.

Postoperative Nursing Interventions

Wound Care. When the patient returns from the operating room, perineal dressings are more likely to remain in place and be comfortable if a T-binder is used. Groin wounds may be exposed or covered with simple dressings. Pressure dressings may be placed over the wounds to aid in preventing the accumulation of lymph and serum. Many surgeons insert plastic tubes through stab wounds in each inguinal area with attachment to portable suction. This arrangement facilitates apposition of tissue flaps and prevents accumulation of serum.

The wound is cleansed daily with warm normal saline irrigations or other antiseptic solutions as prescribed. After a *gentle* cleansing, a warm-water spray is pleasant and nontraumatizing and enhances circulation. The wound should be exposed to the air at frequent intervals to decrease moisture and maceration of the incision site. While stitches are in, some physicians prefer dry heat from a heating lamp or hair dryer, and later, perineal packs or soaks.

Comfort Measures. Since stitches may be taut because of the surgeon's attempt to approximate tissues, comfortable positioning is required. Perhaps a low Fowler's position, or occasionally a pillow placed under the knees, will relieve tension on the incision. When placed on her side, it is more comfortable for the patient and reduces tension on the wound to have a pillow placed between her legs and against the lumbar region.

An air mattress or "egg crate" pad or mattress can assist in distributing weight and relieving pressure points. Moving from one position to another requires time and patience on the part of both patient and nurse. An overbed trapeze bar helps the patient to move herself. Ambulation may be attempted on the second day.

Analgesics are given as required for comfort. Since primary healing rarely occurs, debridement is usually performed to provide satisfactory conditions for healing by secondary intention. Because the healing process is slow and the nature of the surgery is often disquieting to a female patient, she is apt to be discouraged. The nurse must be aware of the patient's uneasiness about being "caught" unduly exposed when visitors arrive or someone enters the room. She will tend to be sensitive and apologetic about odors. Thus, cleanliness, deodorant sprays, immediate removal of soiled dressings, and adequate ventilation contribute to a more pleasant environment.

Prevention of Infection. A low-residue diet will prevent straining on defecation and wound contamination. Of particular concern is urethral and catheter care, inasmuch as an indwelling catheter is usually in place. The incidence of infection is high, which emphasizes the need for the best in nursing intervention. Many nursing researchers frown on the use of sitz baths for vulvectomy patients because of the likelihood of reinfecting the wound.

Patient Education and Home Health Care. The patient is encouraged to share her concerns as she convalesces and begins to assume increasing responsibility for her care. As she participates in changing her dressings and cleansing herself, she can use a mirror to see the perineal area involved. By commenting on how well the tissues are healing, and that they are looking more and more normal, the nurse will be able to lift the patient's spirits.

The nurse explains the need for the patient to share her concerns with her partner. She can relay her daily progress to him. Activities are gradually increased and words of encouragement mean a great deal.

Post-hospital care requires giving complete instructions to a family member who will assist in caring for this patient at home or to the community nurse who will be visiting her. Graduate resumption of physical and social activities is to be encouraged. The cure rate of properly treated vulvar carcinoma is 50% to 60%. In the absence of lymph node metastasis, the cure rate is around 85% to 90%.

A radical vulvectomy is often extensive and may require a second admission and operation for skin grafting. This is determined on an individual basis, but the possibility is cleared with the physician.

▷ *Evaluation*

▷ *Expected Outcomes*

1. Patient adjusts to the surgical experience.
   a. Uses available resources in coping with and alleviating emotional stress.
   b. Asks questions relating to postoperative expectations.
   c. Demonstrates willingness to discuss alternate methods for expressing love.
2. Avoids infection and postoperative complications.
   a. Is free of any signs and symptoms of infection: normal vital signs
   b. Demonstrates the procedure of taking a sitz bath (as prescribed).
   c. Begins to move with a minimum of discomfort.
   d. Maintains cleanliness of the site following micturition or defecation.
3. Assumes appropriate self-care.
   a. Participates more each day in caring for her dressing changes.
   b. Uses the mirror to check progress in wound healing.
   c. Irrigates the wound for comfort and to stimulate healing.

Cancer of the Vagina

Cancer of the vagina usually occurs as a result of metastasis from choriocarcinoma or from cancer of the cervix or adjacent organs, such as from the uterus, vulva, bladder, or rectum. Primary cancer of the vagina is rare. Prior to 1970, cancer of the vagina was considered to be a condition that occurred predominantly in the postmenopausal woman. In the 1970s it was revealed that maternal ingestion of diethylstilbestrol

(DES) affected female offspring who were exposed *in utero*. Benign genital tract abnormalities have occurred in a majority of these young women. Adenosis of the vagina is a common finding.

Kistner (1986) indicates that in view of studies establishing a relationship between DES exposure *in utero* and clear cell adenocarcinoma of the vagina and the increased likelihood for the development of adenosis, there is justification for examining all women exposed to this drug. If adenosis or a significant cervical lesion is found, follow-up two or three times a year appears reasonable. Prophylactic resection of vaginal adenosis does not appear justified at present.

Nursing Interventions. Encouraging close cooperation with health care personnel is the prime target of nursing intervention with daughters who have been exposed to DES *in utero*. They are at an age when sexuality in all its ramifications including pregnancy is of significance. Emotional support for mothers and daughters undoubtedly needs constant bolstering. For young women who have had vaginal reconstructive surgery, specific vaginal dilating procedures may be initiated. Water-soluble lubricants are helpful in reducing dyspareunia. If a possible malignancy develops, requiring treatment, all aspects and effects of radiation therapy, chemotherapy, or surgery need to be explored on an individual basis.

Cancer of the Ovary

Ovarian cancer is a particularly frustrating cancer for several reasons: it is difficult to diagnose and is unique in that it may give rise to many primary cancers and may be the recipient of metastases from other cancers. It carries an annual mortality rate of over 11,700 and is the sixth most prevalent cancer in women. The peak incidence is in the sixth to eighth decades of life, and it is slightly more common in blacks than whites.

Of the many studies attempting to relate some causative link to ovarian cancer, the most significant study by the Centers for Disease Control indicated that a protective effect was identified in those women who used oral contraceptives during their reproductive years. Hereditary factors are being studied for additional clues.

Clinical Manifestations. Because early signs and symptoms are similar to those of functional ovarian cysts or endometriosis, other means of differentiating benign from potentially malignant growths must be used. Manifestations include irregular menses, increasing premenstrual tension, menorrhagia with breast tenderness, and an early menopause. Before puberty and after menopause there may be precocious breast development and uterine bleeding. Virilization may be noted. Ovarian malignancy may be observed more frequently in women who are infertile, nulliparous, anovulatory, or habitual aborters. In addition to a long history of ovarian dysfunction or malfunction, persistent gastrointestinal symptoms in a woman aged 40 or over that cannot be definitely diagnosed should raise a suspicion of ovarian malignancy. Early and insidious symptoms include vague abdominal discomfort, dyspepsia, flatulence, eructations, and a feeling of fullness after a light meal.

Diagnostic Evaluation. Because these tumors are located deep in the abdomen and are often painless, it is difficult to obtain an early diagnosis. Pelvic examination is not likely to detect early ovarian cancer. Pelvic imaging techniques also are not helpful in screening when the patient is relatively asymptomatic. Tumor antigens are being studied for their potential as tumor markers.

Management. For ovarian cancer, surgical removal is the goal. Because of high morbidity and mortality, every effort is made to stage the tumor as accurately as possible and to direct treatment accordingly. A total abdominal hysterectomy with bilateral salpingo-oophorectomy may be done. Radiation therapy and chemotherapy using cisplatin in combination with other agents such as doxorubicin (Adriamycin) may be used. It is not uncommon to do an exploratory laparotomy ("second look") following adjunct therapies in order to determine whether any malignancy persists. Further irradiation may be required.

Several investigational therapies are promising. Intraperitoneal administration of chemotherapeutic agents provides an opportunity to deliver high concentrations of agents directly to the tumor. Biological modifiers such as interferon are being considered. Radiation therapy in fractionated amounts is also being studied.

Nursing Management. The combination of two major clues—(1) a long history of ovarian dysfunction and (2) vague, undiagnosed, persistent gastrointestinal symptoms in the woman over 40—should alert the nurse to the possibility of early malignancy. Usually ovarian malignancy is extensive at the time of diagnosis. Following assessment and evaluation of other data, nursing measures will include those related to the various treatment modalities of surgery, irradiation, chemotherapy, and palliation. Emotional support and comfort measures plus attentiveness and caring are meaningful aids to this patient and her family.

Radiation Therapy

Radiation therapy plays a pivotal role in the treatment of gynecologic malignancy (see also Chap. 16, p. 270). In the treatment of squamous cell carcinoma of the cervix, it is frequently the procedure of choice. In the management of uterine and ovarian cancers, it is usually employed as an adjunct to surgery. In the definitive treatment of cervical disease by irradiation, a combination of external pelvic irradiation and internal intracavitary irradiation is used. Only in the earliest microinvasive carcinomas of the cervix is internal (intracavitary) irradiation used alone. Cure rates of 85% or greater can be expected with cervical cancer that is limited to the cervix alone. As the disease extends into the parametrium, the cure rate drops to approximately 65%. However, once the disease extends to the pelvic sidewalls, perhaps only one third of the patients will be cured, although many more will benefit from the palliative effects of irradiation as a result of the reduction in tumor bulk and the control of infection, pain, and bleeding.

External pelvic irradiation delivered by supervoltage equipment usually extends over 4 to 6 weeks. Thereafter, intracavitary radiation is performed. This sequence may be reversed, depending on anatomical considerations. The cervix and uterus lend themselves naturally to internal irradiation since they act as a receptacle for radioactive sources. Radium and cesium are two isotopes that are the mainstays of intracavitary irradiation.

External Beam Therapy. Betatrons, linear accelerators, and cobalt 60 units are capable of delivering high doses of well-collimated irradiation deep within the pelvis to the site of the tumor. Radiation side-effects are cumulative and tend to express themselves as the total dose exceeds the body's natural capacity to repair the radiation effect. Radiation enteritis, expressed by diarrhea and abdominal cramping, and radiation cystitis, manifested by frequency, urgency, and dysuria, may ensue. This clearly does not indicate an overdosage. It is a natural manifestation of the normal tissues' response to the radiation therapy program. The radiation therapist and nurse inform the patient in advance of these possible side-effects and employ a variety of measures to modify their impact when they occur. These measures include dietary control (by restricting the amount of fiber and roughage), the maintenance of fluid intake, and the use of antispasmodic drugs. On occasion, severe reactions will require that treatment be suspended briefly until the normal tissues repair themselves.

Internal (Intracavitary) Irradiation. In the operating room, an examination is performed under anesthesia, after which specially prepared applicators are inserted into the endometrial cavity and vagina. These devices are not loaded with radioactive material until the patient has returned to her room. X-ray films are obtained to determine the precise relationship of the applicator to the normal pelvic anatomy and to the tumor. Only when this study is completed does the radiation therapist load the applicators with predetermined amounts of radioactive material. This is called *after loading* and allows for precise control of the radiation exposure received by the patient, with minimal exposure of the physician and the nursing and health care team. A patient undergoing internal radiation treatment is placed in a private unit until the application is completed (Chart 42-3).

Various applicators have been developed for intracavitary treatment. Some are inserted into the endometrial cavity and endocervical canal as multiple small irradiators (*e.g.*, Heyman's capsules). Others consist of a central tube (tandem or intrauterine "stem") placed through the dilated endocervical canal into the uterine cavity, which remains in fixed relationship with irradiators placed in the upper vagina on each side of the cervix (vaginal ovoids) (Fig. 42-6).

At the time of insertion of the applicator, an indwelling bladder catheter is inserted. The applicator is secured in place with vaginal packing. The objective of the internal treatment is to maintain the distribution of internal radiation at a fixed dosage throughout the application. Such applications usually last 24 to 72 hours, depending on dose calculations made by the radiation therapist and the radiation physicist.

Nursing Management During Cesium Treatment

During the application, diligent nursing care must be given. The patient is carefully observed and attended, although the nursing staff must try to reduce as much as possible the radiation exposure to themselves. Nurses should stay in the immediate vicinity of the patient no longer than is necessary to give proper care and attention, and no nurse should attend the patient more than a half hour per day (see Chart 42-3). Of course, a pregnant nurse should not be involved in the immediate care of such patients. Visits to the patient should not be aimless; nurse-patient contacts provide a good opportunity for the patient to talk about her anxiety and fear. To minimize radiation exposure, the nurse may stay at the foot of the bed or at the entrance to the room.

Chart 42-3
Nursing Care of Patients Undergoing Treatment With Encapsulated Radioactive Sources

_____ is being treated with _____ mg Ra Eq
(name)

of radioactive _____   _____ at
(cesium, iridium seeds, etc.)   (date)

_____ m. The type of application or implantation is _____
(time)

Precautions for hospital personnel to observe when handling patients who are undergoing treatment with encapsulated radioactive materials:

1. The PATIENT must be placed in a single room.
2. PREGNANT NURSES SHOULD NOT CARE FOR THESE PATIENTS.
3. NURSES should not stay in the immediate vicinity of the patient longer than is necessary (less than ½ hour per day) to give proper care and attention.
4. VISITORS should stay at least six (6) feet from the bed and limit the visit to less than 1 hour per day. Children under age 18 and pregnant women may not visit.
5. If a radioactive source or applicator becomes dislodged from the patient, pick up the source with the long forceps provided and place it in the lead container located in the patient's room. NOTIFY THE RADIOTHERAPIST IMMEDIATELY. NEVER PICK UP A RADIOACTIVE SOURCE WITH YOUR HANDS.
6. Save all dressings, bed linens, etc. Do not vacuum the floor. Save floor sweepings in the room. Dishes, trays, and eating utensils can leave the room. Do not save any of the patient's excreta or body fluids unless requested to do so by the radiotherapist.
7. Before the patient is discharged, a radiation survey will be made to ensure that no radiation hazard remains. The Radiation Therapy Department will then NOTIFY THE HEAD NURSE THAT USED LINENS AND DRESSINGS CAN BE REMOVED.

Notify the Radiotherapy Department Immediately:
1. In case of any doubt as to safe procedure
2. In case of any emergency
3. If any unexpected complications arise
4. In case of death:
   Before postmortem care is given
   Before an autopsy is performed
   Before the body is released
During the day, call the Radiation Therapy Department
During the night, call the Page Operator and request the physician on call be contacted either by telephone or beeper.

(A form similar to that used at American Oncologic Hospital, Fox Chase Cancer Center, Philadelphia, Pennsylvania)

During the application, the patient will be on absolute bed rest. She may move from side to side with her back supported by a pillow, and the head of the bed may be raised to 45 degrees. The patient should be encouraged to practice deep-breathing and cough exercises and to flex and extend the feet to stretch the calf muscles in order to promote venous return. Back care is much appreciated by the patient, but adequate care is given within the minimum amount of time at the bedside.

Usually, the patient is on a low-residue diet to prevent frequent bowel movements. One is less concerned here with dislodging the radium applicator than with the social and physical discomforts that the patient may experience. The nurse should inspect the catheter frequently to make sure that it is draining properly. The chief hazard of improper drainage is that the bladder may become distended. Although perineal care is omitted at this time, any profuse discharge should be reported immediately to the radiation therapist or gynecologic surgeon.

The patient is observed for evidence of temperature elevation, nausea, and vomiting. These symptoms should be reported, since they may indicate infection or perforation. Finally, the radiation therapist takes steps to secure the internal applicator in place. Nursing personnel need not be preoccupied with the fear that the applicator will be prematurely extruded. However, one should check from time to time to see that the applicator or the radioactive sources have not been dislodged. Should this happen, the radioactive source is grasped with a long forceps and held at arm's length and returned to the lead container located in the patient's room. Radioactive sources should never be grasped with the bare hand. The radiation therapist should be notified immediately.

Cesium Removal. The radiation therapist calculates precisely the radiation dose delivered. At the end of the prescribed period, the nurse may be requested to assist the physician in removing the applicator. Since the sources are "afterloaded," they can be removed by the physician in the same manner as they were inserted. This does not require local or

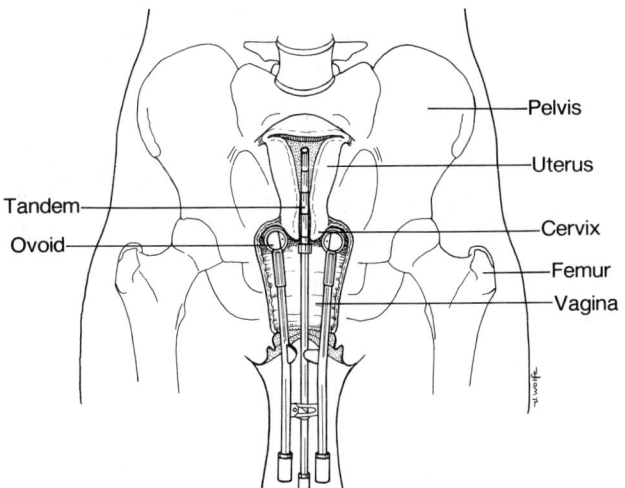

Figure 42-6
Placement of tandem and ovoids for internal radiation therapy. (© 1987 J. Wolfe)

general anesthesia and is done in the patient's room. Medication with a mild sedative may be required before the applicator is removed.

Postinsertion Care. Progressive ambulation is recommended after the period of enforced bed rest. The patient may shower as soon as she wishes; a vinegar or dilute saline douche may be prescribed. The diet may be offered as tolerated.

Bibliography

Books

Cavanagh D, Ruffolo EH, and Marsden DE. Gynecologic Cancer. Norwalk, Connecticut, Appleton-Century-Crofts, 1985.

Corson S. Greenhill's Surgical Gynecology, 12th ed. Chicago, Year Book Medical Publishers, 1986.

DiSara PJ and Creasman WT. Clinical Gynecologic Oncology, 2nd ed. St. Louis, CV Mosby, 1984.

Griffith NW, McEvers J, and Becker R. Instructions for Obstetric and Gynecologic Patients. Philadelphia, WB Saunders, 1984.

Hacker N. Essentials of Obstetrics and Gynecology. Philadelphia, WB Saunders, 1986.

Holmes KK et al. Sexually Transmitted Diseases. New York, McGraw-Hill, 1984.

Kistner RW. Gynecology, 4th ed. Chicago, Year Book Medical Publishers, 1986.

Nichols DH and Evrard JR. Ambulatory Gynecology. Philadelphia, Harper & Row, 1985.

Articles

(Asterisks indicate nursing research articles.)

General Articles

Gelfant BB. Preoperative teaching of gynecological patients. Point of View (Ethicon) 1984 Jan; 21(1):4–7.

Hill EC. Obstetrics and gynecology. JAMA 1985 Oct 25; 254(16):2308–2309.

Huppert LC. Hormonal replacement therapy: Benefits, risks, doses. Med Clin North Am 1987 Jan; 71(1):23–39.

King LA. Pelvic inflammatory disease. Postgrad Med 1987 Mar; 81(4):105–114.

Manzagol KA. Gynecologic surgery using the CO_2 laser. Point of View (Ethicon) 1984 Jan; 21(1):14–16.

Gerontological Considerations

Hooyman N and Cohen HJ. Medical problems associated with aging. Clin Obstet Gynecol 1986 June; 29(2):353–373.

Parker RT and Piscitelli J. Gynecologic surgery in the elderly patient. Clin Obstet Gynecol 1986 June; 29(2):453–461.

Soper JT and Creasman WT. Vulvar dystrophies. Clin Obstet Gynecol 1986 June; 29(2):431–439.

Steege JF. Sexual function in the aging woman. Clin Obstet Gynecol 1986 June; 29(2):462–469.

Steinke EE and Berge MB. Sexuality and aging. J Gerontol Nurs 1986 June; 12(6):6–10.

Vulvovaginal Infections

Bertholf ME and Stafford MJ. An office laboratory panel to assess vaginal problems. Am Fam Physician. 1985 Sept; 32(3)113–125.

Bourcier KM and Seidler AJ. Chlamydia and condylomata acuminata: An update for the nurse practitioner JOGNN 1987 Jan; 16(1):17–22.

*Burnhill MS. Taking a serious approach to vulvovaginitis. Contemp OB/GYN 1986 Sept; 28(3):69–79.

Chlamydia: The silent epidemic. Time 1985 Feb 4; 125(5):67.

Friedrich EG Jr. Vaginitis. Am Fam Physician 1983 Nov; 28(5):238–242.

Gilly PA. Vaginal discharge. Postgrad Med 1986 Dec; 80(8):231–237.

Kaufman CA and Jones PG. Candidiasis. Postgrad Med 1986 July; 80(1):129–134.

Kaufman RH. Common causes of vaginitis. Hosp Med 1986 Nov; 22(11):23–44.

King J. Vaginitis. JOGN 1984 Mar/Apr; 13(2):41s–48s.

King LA. Pelvic inflammatory disease. Postgrad Med 1987 Mar; 81(4):105–114.

Ladogana L. Pelvic inflammatory disease: Diagnosis and management. Med Times 1985 Nov; 113(11):25–31.

Lossick JG. Sexually transmitted vaginitis. Urol Clin North Am 1984 Feb; 11(1):141–153.

McKay M. Vulvodynia versus pruritus vulvae. Clin Obstet Gynecol 1985 Mar; 28(1):123–133.

Paavonen J. Mucopurulent cervicitis: An often ignored STD. Med Aspects Human Sexuality 1985 June; 19(6):132–140.

Pruessner HT, Hansel MK, and Griffiths M. Diagnosis and treatment of chlamydial infections. Am Fam Physician 1986 July; 34(1):81–91.

Rein MF. How to treat the three most common vaginal infections. Mod Med 1985 Mar; 53(3):126–137.

Salvio K and Aprezzio JJ. New antibiotics in the treatment of pelvic infections. JOGN 1984 Sept/Oct; 13(5):308–311.

Schmid GP and Larsen SA. Finding the elusive *T. vaginalis*. Diagn Med 1984 Dec; 7(10):38–40.

Smith LS and Lauver D. Assessment and management of vaginitis and cervicitis. Nurs Pract 1984 June; 9(6):34, 39–47, 67.

Van Slyke KK et al. Treatment of vulvovaginal candidiasis with boric acid and powder. Am J Obstet Gynecol 1981 Sept 15; 141(2):145–148.

Washington D. Helping the patient with vaginitis. RN 1984 Sept; 47(9):63–71.

Herpes Genitalis

Bryson YG et al. Treatment of first episodes of genital herpes simplex virus infection with oral acyclovir. N Engl J Med 1983 Apr 21; 308(16):916–921.

Corey L et al. Intravenous acyclovir for the treatment of primary genital herpes. Ann Intern Med 1983 Jan; 98(6):914–921.

Fife KH, Raab B, and Strauss SE. New options for genital herpes: Diagnosis/treatment. Patient Care 1986 Apr 15; 20(7):20–46.

Goldberg CB. Controlled trial of "Intervir-A" (IVA) in herpes simplex virus infections. Lancet 1986 Mar 29; 1(8483):703–706.

Mertz G and Corey L. Genital herpes simplex infections in adults. Urol Clin North Am 1984 Feb; 11(1):103–119.

Oral acyclovir for genital herpes simplex infection. Med Lett Drugs Ther 1985 May 10; 27(687):41–43.

Reichman RC et al. Treatment of recurrent genital herpes simplex infections with oral acyclovir. JAMA 1984 Apr 27; 251(16):2103–2107.

Warmbrodt L. Herpes: The shock, the stigma, the ways you can ease the emotional pain. RN 1983 May; 46(5):47–49.

Toxic Shock Syndrome

Cibulka NJ. Toxic shock syndrome and other tampon-related risks. JOGN 1983 Mar/Apr; 12(2):94–99.

Greenman RL and Immerman RP. Toxic shock syndrome. Postgrad Med 1987 Mar; 81(4):147–160.

MacDonald KL et al. Toxic shock syndrome. JAMA 1987 Feb 27; 257(8):1053–1059.

Morrison VA and Olafield EC. Postoperative toxic shock syndrome. Arch Surg 1983 July; 118(7):791–794.

Smirniotopoulos TT. Update on toxic shock syndrome. Postgrad Med 1983 Oct; 74(4):369–372.

Tofte RW and Williams DN. Toxic shock syndrome. Postgrad Med 1983 Jan; 73(1):275–288.

Toxic shock syndrome. Nurs '85 1985 Oct; 15(10):74.

Wheltam J. Update on toxic shock: How to spot it and treat it. RN 1984 Feb; 47(2):55–60.

Wiesenthal AM. Toxic shock syndrome: An update. Drug Ther 1983 Mar; 83(3):33–39.

Endometriosis

Buttram VC Jr, Meldrum DR, and Ward AB. When you suspect endometriosis. Patient Care 1986 Mar 15; 20(5):69–84.

Davis GD. Management of endometriosis and its associated adhesions with the CO_2 laser laparoscope. Obstet Gynecol 1986 Sept; 68(3):422–425.

Parmley TH. Diagnosis: Endometriosis. Hosp Med 1983 Oct; 19(10):152–167.

Radwanska E and Dmowski WP. Dyspareunia due to endometriosis. Med Aspects Human Sexuality 1985 June; 19(6):256–258.

Prolapse

Rogers SF. Variations in vaginal surgery: Severe uterine prolapse and vaginal wall defects. Point of View (Ethicon) 1984 Jan; 21(1):8–10.

Reproductive Malignancy

Adams-Greenley MA, Beldoch N, and Moynihan R. Helping adolescents whose parents have cancer. Semin Oncol Nurs 1986 May; 2(2):133–138.

Benedict JL and Murphy KJ. Cervical cancer screening. Postgrad Med 1985 Dec; 78(8):69–79.

Ferenczy A. Cryosurgery and CO_2 laser therapy in the prevention of cervical cancer. Infect Surg 1985 Oct; 4(10):753–758.

Hartz A et al. Obesity and endometrial cancer. Intern Med 1985 Sept; 6(9):61–66.

Jones PG and Alvarez ME. Gyn cancers: Common infections and how to treat them. Your Patient and Cancer 1984 June; 4(6):50–59.

Kaplan A. Carcinoma of the uterine corpus. Hosp Med 1984 Sept; 20(8):93–122.

Mansey FM. Vulvovaginal reconstruction following radical resections. Clin Obstet Gynecol 1986 Sept; 29(3):617–627.

*Nelson JH Jr, Averette HE, and Richart RM. Dysplasia, carcinoma *in situ* and early invasive cervical carcinoma. CA 1984 Nov/Dec; 34(6):306–327.

Richardson GS and MacLaughlin DT. The status of receptors in the management of endometrial cancer. Clin Obstet Gynecol 1986 Sept; 29(3):628–637.

Robertson BJ. Tuboplasty: Use, resources, and nursing implications. Periop Nurs Q 1985 June; 1(2):49–56.

Rubin D. Gynecologic cancer: Cervical, vulvar, and vaginal malignancies. RN 1987 May; 56–63.

Wabrek AJ and Gunn JL. Sexual and psychological implications of gynecologic malignancy. JOGN 1984 Nov/Dec; 13(6):371–376.

Hysterectomy

Hemsell DL, Hemsell PG, and Nobles BJ. Doxycycline and cefamandole prophylaxis for premenopausal women undergoing vaginal hysterectomy. Surg Gynecol Obstet 1985 Nov; 161(5):462–463.

O'Laughlin KM. Changes in bladder function in the woman undergoing radical hysterectomy for cervical cancer. JOGNN 1986 Sept/Oct; 15(5):380–385.

*Webb C and Wilson-Barnett J. Self-concept, social support and hysterectomy. Int J Nurs Stud 1983; 20(2):97–107.

Wells MP and Villano K. Total abdominal hysterectomy. AORN J 1985 Sept; 42(3):368–373.

Ovarian Cancer

Barber HRK. Ovarian cancer. CA 1986 May/June; 36(3):149–183.

Copeland LJ. Second-look laparotomy for ovarian carcinoma. Clin Obstet Gynecol 1985 Dec; 28(4):816–823.

Freedman RS. Recent immunologic advances affecting the management of ovarian cancer. Clin Obstet Gynecol 1985 Dec; 28(4):853–871.

Hanauske AR and VonHoff DD. The value of the human tumor cloning assay in ovarian cancer. Clin Obstet Gynecol 1986 Sept; 29(3):638–646.

*Jenkins JF, Hubbard SM, and Howser DM. Managing intraperitoneal chemotherapy: A new assault on ovarian cancer. Nurs '82 1982 May; 12(5):76–83.

Jolles CJ. Ovarian cancer: Histogenetic classification, histologic grading, diagnosis, staging, and epidemiology. Clin Obstet Gynecol 1985 Dec; 28(4)787–799.

Kavanagh JJ. Investigational therapies for epithelial ovarian cancer. Clin Obstet Gynecol 1985 Dec; 28(4):846–852.

Malfetano JH. Current approaches to treatment of advanced ovarian cancer. Curr Concepts Oncol 1985 Fall; 7(3):3–9.

Weiss GR. Second-line chemotherapy for ovarian cancer. Clin Obstet Gynecol 1986 Sept; 29(3):665–677.

Wharton JT et al. Chemotherapy and radiation therapy in the treatment of ovarian carcinoma of common epithelial origin. Clin Obstet Gynecol 1985 Dec; 28(4):806–815.

Vaginal and Vulvar Cancer

DiSaia P. Management of superficially invasive vulvar carcinoma. Clin Obstet Gynecol 1985 Mar; 28(1):196–203.

Hurley M, Meyer-Ruppel A, and Evans E. Emma needed more than standard teaching (radical vulvectomy). Nurs '83 1983 Mar; 13(3):63–64.

Iverson T. New approaches to treatment of squamous cell carcinoma of the vulva. Clin Obstet Gynecol 1985 Mar; 28(1):204–210.

Kaplan AL. Vulvar reconstruction. Clin Obstet Gynecol 1985 Mar; 28(1):211–219.

Peters WA, Kumar NB, and Morley GW. Carcinoma of the vagina: Factors influencing treatment outcomes. Cancer 1985 Feb 15; 55(4):892–897.

Piver MS. Early diagnosis and treatment of vulvar cancer. Hosp Med 1984 Feb; 20(2):163–177.

Smerz LR et al. Second-look laparotomy after chemotherapy in the management of ovarian malignancy. Am Obstet Gynecol 1985 July 15; 152(6):661–668.

Wilkinson EJ. Superficial invasive carcinoma of the vulva. Clin Obstet Gynecol 1985 Mar; 28(1):188–175.

Woodruff JD. Carcinoma *in situ* of the vulva. Clin Obstet Gynecol 1985 Mar; 28(1):230–239.

Radiation Therapy

Jankowski CB. Preventing radiation exposure in critical care. DCCN 1986 Sept/Oct; 5(5):270–276.

Vigliotti APG et al. Radiotherapy research in gynecologic cancer. Clin Obstet Gynecol 1986 Sept; 28(3):647–664.

Chapter 43

Assessment and Management of Patients With Breast Disorders

Physiology of Breast Development

Up to the time of puberty, no microscopic difference can be found in the breasts of the two sexes. At puberty, some slight swelling appears in the male breast. At the same time, a pronounced increase in size occurs in the female organ. This begins around age 10 and increases rapidly up to ages 14 to 16. The development of the mammary gland is a result of hormonal action that begins with puberty in the female. At this time, the nipple takes on its natural protruding form. In the male, contrary to some statements, breast tissue always exists and may grow.

The breast is a glandular organ with many lobules; its secretion passes through collecting ducts to the nipple. In some women, there is a cyclic engorgement of the breasts, associated with tingling and tenderness; this is hormonal in origin. The symptoms begin usually in the latter part of the menstrual cycle and disappear when menstruation occurs. During pregnancy, about 8 weeks after a woman conceives, her breasts enlarge greatly, the nipples become more prominent and sensitive, and the breasts are prepared to nourish the infant. When pregnancy is over and lactation has ceased, the breasts shrink, lose their excessive fat, and often become flabby and flattened.

Psychosocial Implications

In Western cultures, the breast is considered a significant component of feminine beauty. Shapeliness is a quality much desired and is emphasized in a woman's choice of clothing. Particularly in the United States, the social value placed on looking young has led to consumer demands for brassieres that further contribute to a trim, fit look. Thus, a woman's reaction to any actual or suspected disease or injury affecting her breast tends to reflect the prevailing societal view of the female breast. Not only do social values play a significant role in the rehabilitation of a patient who has undergone radical breast surgery, but the fear of disfigurement may also prevent a woman from seeking immediate medical attention after she has detected suspicious signs or changes in her breast.

A major goal of the health professions is to spread sound advice about the prevention of illness and the detection of disease in its early stages. Every woman should be alerted to the early signs of breast disease and should be well informed on what to do about suspicious changes. The nurse has a major responsibility in the area of prevention and early detection of breast diseases and in handling the concomitant psychosocial concerns of the patient. The nurse's association with industry, diagnostic clinics, and community health agencies offers opportunities to teach and disseminate information, particularly about the value of breast self-examination.

Incidence of Breast Disease

Although most of the disorders of the female breast are benign, the breast is one of the two female organs (the other is the uterus) that are most frequently the primary site of cancer. The breast normally changes during menstruation, pregnancy, lactation, and menopause, and these variations must be differentiated from pathologic changes. Although the breast is fairly accessible to examination, the detection and accurate diagnosis of breast disease can be difficult.

About one fourth of all women have irregular areas in their breasts at some time. Just before menstruation, irregularities produced by hyperplasia and involution occur. These irregularities, which feel granular or finely nodular, usually occur in the upper outer quadrants. Some women have persistently irregular breast tissue that feels shotlike or plaquelike between periods. Such masses are not considered true masses because they usually are bilateral and neither increase in size nor consolidate. On the other hand, true masses do not fluctuate in size and are usually unilateral.

In both women and men, benign lesions of the breast occur more frequently than malignant lesions (70% benign vs. 30% malignant). Of the malignant tumors, 99% occur in females. Benign lesions occur frequently in premenopausal women.

The benign lesions, presented according to order of frequency and the common ages at which they occur, are fibrocystic disease (20 to 45 years), fibroadenoma (20 to 39 years), and intraductal papilloma (35 to 45 years). By way of contrast, cancer of the breast is manifested chiefly in the menopausal and postmenopausal years, with the incidence increasing progressively as the woman gets older. Approximately 75% of breast cancers occur in patients over the age of 40; less than 2% occur before the age of 30.

According to 1987 annual statistics of the American Cancer Society, approximately 130,900 new cases of malignant breast tumors were discovered, and approximately 41,300 women died of the disease.

Assessment

Breast Examination

Examination of the female breast is conducted during any general physical or gynecologic examination, or whenever the patient presents with suspicion, complaint, or fear of breast disease. A professional breast examination is recommended every 3 years for women 20 to 40 years of age, and every year for those over age 40.

Inspection. The patient is disrobed to the waist and initially is seated in a comfortable position facing the examiner with her hands in her lap. The breasts are inspected for size and symmetry. A slight difference in the sizes of the two breasts is common and is generally a normal finding. The skin is inspected for color, thickening or edema, and venous pattern. Erythema may indicate local inflammation or superficial lymphatic invasion by a neoplasm. Likewise, an increased venous pattern may signal the accessory blood supply of a growing neoplasm. Lymphatic blockage by tumor cells may create edema and pitting of the skin and give the skin surface an orange peel (peau d'orange) appearance.

The nipples, although variable from patient to patient, are normally similar in size and shape. A slight inversion of one or both nipples is not uncommon and is only a significant finding when of recent origin. The position of the nipples is observed for symmetry. The presence of ulceration, rashes, or nipple discharge is an abnormal finding that requires the attention of a physician. In order to elicit a dimpling or retraction that may otherwise go undetected, the examiner instructs the patient to raise both arms overhead. This maneuver normally elevates both breasts equally. Next, the patient is instructed to place the palms of both hands together, pushing forcibly. This facilitates contraction of the pectoral muscles and normally does not alter the breast contour or nipple direction. Any dimpling or retraction of the breast during these movements is highly suggestive of an underlying malignancy. Lastly, the clavicular and axillary regions are inspected for signs of discoloration, swelling, or lesions.

Palpation. Palpation of the axillae and clavicular areas is easily performed with the patient in a sitting position. To examine axillary lymph nodes, the patient's arm is gently abducted from the thorax by the examiner's hand. The patient's left forearm is grasped and supported with the examiner's left hand (Fig. 43-1). The right hand is then free to palpate the axilla, noting the presence or absence of nodes that may be lying against the thoracic wall. The fingertips are used to gently palpate the areas of the central, lateral, subscapular and pectoral nodes. Normally these lymph nodes are not palpable. If enlarged, their size, location, mobility, consistency, and tenderness are noted. The arm is put through a full range of motion in order to uncover any nodes or masses that may be hidden under the pectoralis muscle or under subcutaneous fat. The procedure is reversed to examine the right axilla. In a similar fashion, the supraclavicular and infraclavicular areas are palpated.

The patient is now assisted to a supine position on the examining table. Prior to palpation of the breast, the shoulder is elevated on a small pillow in order to balance the breast on the chest wall (Fig. 43-1*B*). Otherwise, a mass may be missed in the thick tissue if the breast is allowed to fall to the side.

Light palpation in an orderly fashion includes the entire surface of the breast, including the breast tail. The examiner may choose to proceed in a clockwise direction following imaginary concentric circles from the outer limits of the breast toward the nipple. Another acceptable method is to palpate from each "number" on the face of the clock toward the nipple in a clockwise fashion (Fig. 43-1*C*).

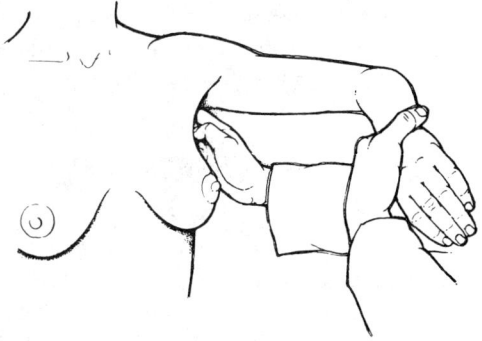

A. Palpation of axillae. Positioning of patient.

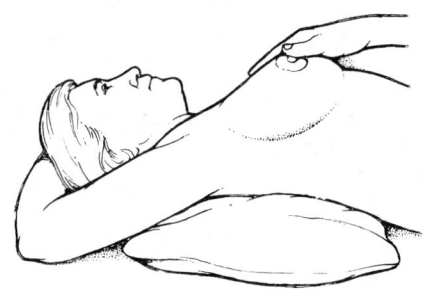

B. Palpation of breast. The patient's shoulder is elevated on a small pillow.

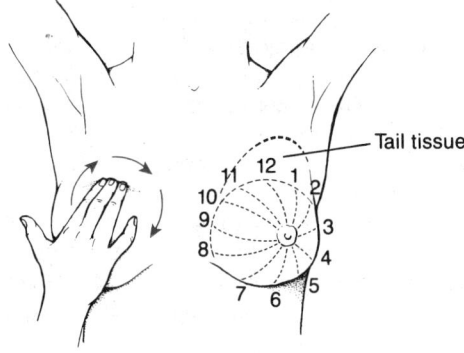

Tail tissue

C. The entire surface of the breast, including the tail, is palpated in a clockwise fashion.

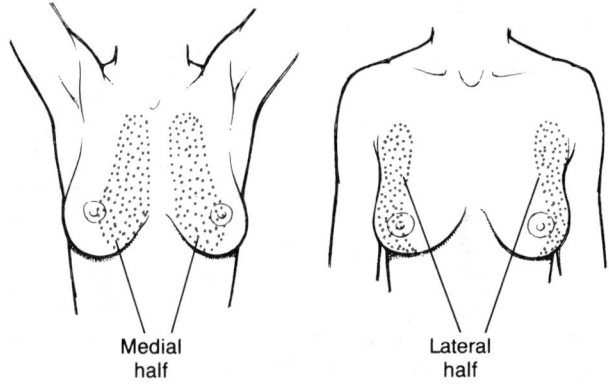

Medial half   Lateral half

D. The medial half of the breast is examined with the patient's arm overhead, the lateral half with the arm at the side.

Figure 43-1
Breast examination: Palpation of the axilla and the breast.

When the medial half of the breast is palpated, the arm may be actively or passively moved above the head in order to tense the pectoralis muscles and provide a flatter surface. When the lateral half of the breast is palpated, the arm is brought back to the patient's side (Fig. 43-1*D*). The examiner may do this by simple manipulation of a relaxed elbow. A prolongation or "tail" of breast tissue may extend toward the axilla along the pectoralis tendon toward its insertion. This breast tissue also requires palpation and is not to be mistaken for disease.

During palpation, the consistency of the tissue and the presence of tenderness or masses are noted. If a mass is felt, it is described by its location (*e.g.*, left breast, 2 cm from nipple at 2 o'clock), size, shape, consistency, delimitation, mobility, and presence of tenderness.

Lastly, the areola around the nipple is gently compressed to determine the presence or absence of abnormal secretion.

The breast tissue of the adolescent is firm and lobular, while the postmenopausal women often has breast tissue that feels stringy and granular. During pregnancy and lactation, the breasts are larger and firmer, and the lobules are more distinct. Cysts are a common finding in menstruating women and are usually well defined and freely movable. Premenstrually, they may be larger and more tender. Malignancies, on the other hand, tend to be hard, poorly defined, fixed to the skin or underlying tissues, and often nontender. Any abnormalities detected during inspection and palpation require additional evaluation by the physician.

The Male Breast. Examination of the male breast and axillae is not to be overlooked. The nipple and areola are inspected for masses, lesions, or discharge. The areola is palpated for masses. Gynecomastia (overdeveloped mammary glands in the male) is differentiated from the soft, fatty enlargement of obesity by the firm enlargement of glandular tissue beneath and immediately surrounding the areola. The same procedure for inspection and palpation of the female axillae is employed during an assessment of the male axillae.

Self-Examination of the Breast. Because 95% of breast cancers and 65% of early minimal breast cancers are detected by women themselves, top priority must be given to teaching all women how and when to examine their breasts. It is estimated that only a minority (25% to 30%) perform breast self-examination (BSE) on a monthly basis. Even among women who perform BSE there often are delays in seeking medical attention. The reasons for this must continue to be explored; among them are economic factors, lack of education, reluctance to do anything if there is no pain, psychological factors, fear (a predominant deterrent), false modesty, and depression. Whatever the reason, the nurse is in a unique position in all contacts with women to inform and educate.

The nurse can offer advice and arrange for showings of the film *Breast Self-Examination,* available from local chapters of the American Cancer Society. The method of BSE, which should be performed monthly, is shown in Figure 43-2.

The importance of this examination should be stressed, especially in the light of recent findings related to the occurrence of "interval cancers" (cancer that may develop after a negative screening visit and prior to the subsequent examination in the physician's office). Breast self-examination is essential in detected these "interval cancers."

Some cancers grow very rapidly, whereas others grow very slowly. It has been reported that the course of a cancer from its inception to the death of the patient can be as short as 120 days; conversely, a chronic breast cancer has been known to last for 23 years without treatment.

Mammography

Mammography is a breast-imaging modality that does not require the injection of a contrast medium but can detect hidden nonpalpable lesions. The procedure takes about 20 minutes, can be done at most health centers, and is painless. Usually, two views are taken of each breast: a craniocaudal view, taken from above while the patient is seated, and a mediolateral view.

With mammography, breast cancer may be diagnosed before the appearance of any clinical manifestations, permitting recognition of abnormal breast masses smaller than 1 cm, the minimal size detectable by BSE. However, a skilled roentgenologist is required to interpret the findings. At the same time, it should be noted that this form of diagnostic examination has limitations, since some carcinomas noted on clinical examination are not detectable by mammography. In addition, mammography is not as effective in studying very small breasts as it is for "fatty" breasts. More recently, certain architectural patterns of the breast have been distinguished, making it possible to identify patients who are at high risk for developing breast cancer.

Concern about the possibility of inducing breast cancer by exposing the breast to the low-dose radiation of mammography is invalid. Advocates of mammography indicate that today's radiographic techniques are much safer and better at detecting early cancers in women of all ages. Various organizations such as the American Cancer Society, American College of Obstetricians and Gynecologists, American College of Radiology, and National Institute of Health publish guidelines for mammography. A baseline mammography is often done with a physical examination for women between 35 and 50. Following this baseline evaluation and other examinations, the physician determines the frequency of mammography for each individual patient.

Indications for immediate mammography include the following:

· A mass or other abnormality is noted on physical examination.
· The patient falls into a high-risk classification (Chart 43-1).
· Physical examination is difficult because of scarring, implants, large breasts.
· Cancer is present in the other breast.

Nurses as health teachers should inform patients and women with whom they come in contact of the advantages and risks of mammography and the recent decisions about its use.

Thermography and Xeroradiography

Thermography is a diagnostic procedure that provides a picture of the surface temperature of the skin area of the breast. Abnormal circulatory signs may be detected by infrared photography. Signals are electronically converted to an oscilloscopic display. Following patient preparation and instruction similar to those for mammography, the patient is placed in a room under basal conditions (*i.e.,* the room has been cooled to 21°C [70°F]) for 20 to 30 minutes. By means of a sophisticated heat-sensing apparatus, it is possible to detect minute amounts of heat generated in and around areas of increased blood supply, indicating the existence of disease. The method requires a well-trained radiologist to interpret abnormal patterns. Thermography is recommended only as an adjunct to, and not instead of, physical examination and mammography.

Xeroradiography provides an x-ray film of the soft tissue of the breast using a very limited amount of radiation. In this procedure, a selenium-coated plate is subjected to an electrical charge, the x-ray exposure is made, and the plate is then developed by a special process under careful monitoring. The result is a xeroradiograph in which all tissues of the breast, including the skin, are protrayed in a bas-relief effect.

Other Diagnostic Methods

Ultrasound (*sonography*) is the use of a transducer to focus a beam of high-frequency sound waves through the skin and into the breast. These sound waves reflect back to the transducer like an echo that varies with the density of the underlying tissues. The waves are then processed by computer for display on a screen to be interpreted.

Diaphanography uses a fiberoptic light (transillumination of the breast) and synchronizes mapping of the breast to show areas through which the light does not pass.

The above two diagnostic methods are used much less frequently than mammography but have potential for greater use in the future. It is believed that *magnetic resonance imaging* (*MRI*), introduced as a diagnostic tool for other body systems, will eventually replace all other diagnostic modalites for breast conditions.

Biopsy: Aspiration Cytology

Biopsy of the breast, which involves obtaining tissue specimens for examination, can be done on an outpatient basis or in the physician's office. Following the injection of a local anesthetic, a No. 22 (fine) needle is directed into the site to be sampled. Suction is applied to a syringe, and tissue is drawn into the needle. This material is spread on an albuminized glass slide and stained before being sent to the laboratory. Over 90% of lesions can be accurately diagnosed by this technique.

Incisional vs. Excisional Biopsy. Biopsies may be done in the operating room under general anesthesia or as an outpatient procedure under local anesthesia. A biopsy may

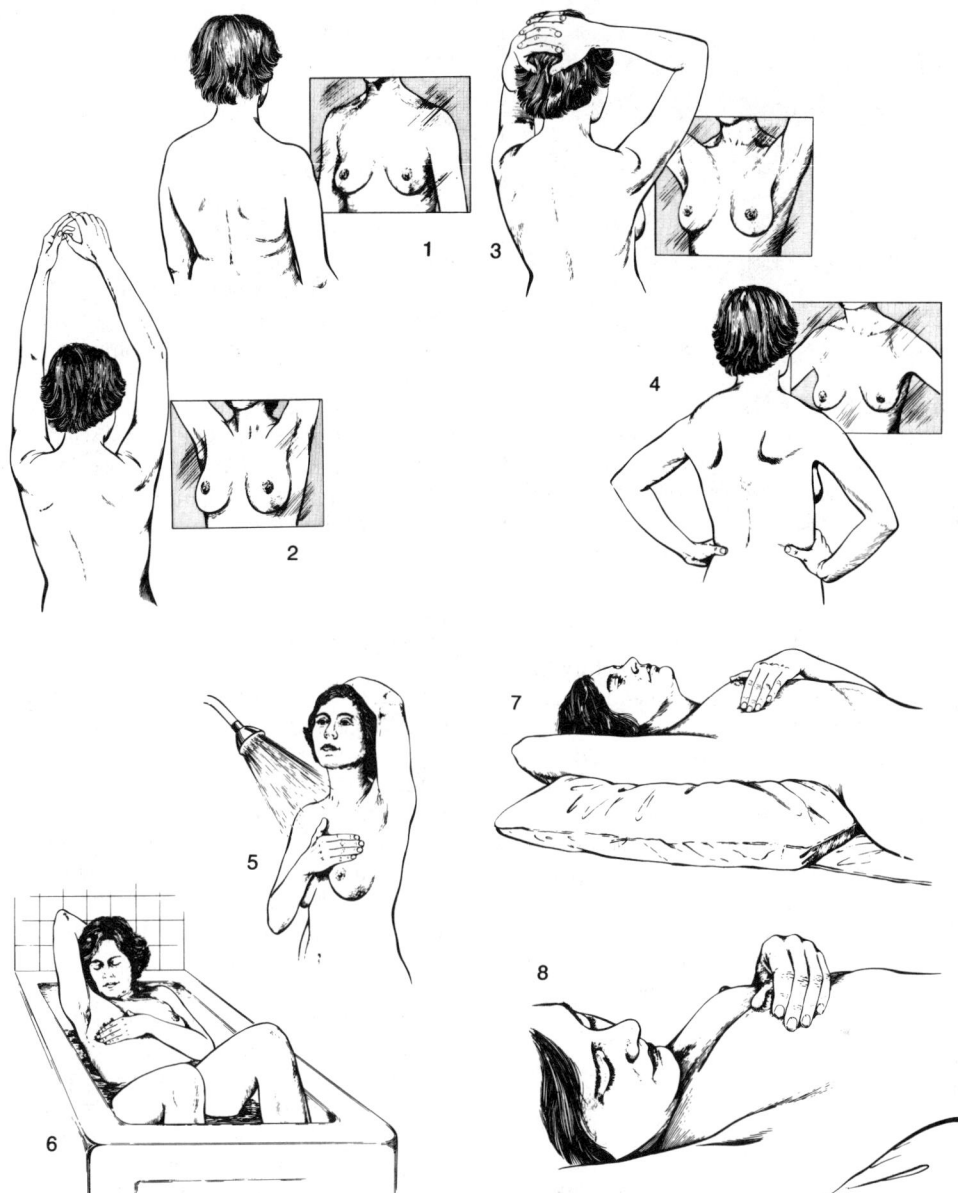

Figure 43-2

(*1*) Breast self-examination is begun with inspection using a mirror. Attention is given to contours of breast and to skin. (*2*) Arms are extended high above the head in a search for abnormal motion or skin retraction. (*3*) Pressure is placed on back of head to tense the pectoralis major muscles that underlie mammary tissues. (*4*) Inward pressure on hips serves to tense pectoralis major muscles. Retraction of skin is a sign of abnormality.
(*5*) Wet soapy skin facilitates manual examination of breast for lumps. (*6*) Tub bathing provides an optimal time for discovering lumps. Wet skin permits easy motion of the examining hand, and a reclining position flattens breast tissues on the chest wall.
(*7*) Palpatory examination is best performed in a supine position with the side to be examined elevated on a pillow or blanket. Lumps are most evident when the breast is flattened and evenly distributed on the chest wall. As a woman gains familiarity with the appearance and feel of her breast through repeated examinations, she becomes more capable of appreciating changes. (*8*) Self-examination is completed with a squeeze of the nipple to detect abnormal discharge. (Danforth DN and Scott JR (eds). Obstetrics and Gynecology 5th ed. Philadelphia, JB Lippincott, 1986.)

Chart 43-1
Women at High Risk for Breast Cancer (High Risk Factors)

Women over age 40 (North American, Western European)
Familial history of breast cancer (especially a sister or mother)
Early menarche
Nulliparous women or those whose first parity occurred after age 34
Natural menopause occurring after age 50
Exposure to carcinogens; ionizing radiation
Chronic psychological stress
Presence of other cancer, such as endometrial, colon-rectum, salivary gland, ovarian

comprise the entire lesion (excisional) or a piece of the specimen (incisional). Tissue may be sent to the laboratory to be frozen for subsequent study, or it may be examined as quickly as possible if a 24-hour report is requested. Very thin slices containing a good cross-section of tissue are stained with a dye to facilitate microscopic observation.

If cancer is diagnosed, a frozen tissue specimen should undergo estrogen receptor assay to determine the presence or absence of estrogen receptors. More than half of patients with metastatic breast cancer will respond to hormonal manipulation if their tumors contain estrogen receptors. When tumors do not contain estrogen receptors (estrogen-receptor negative) fewer than 10% can be successfully treated with hormonal manipulation.

Conditions Affecting the Nipple

Fissure of the Nipple. A fissure of the nipple is a longitudinal ulcer that tends to develop in any woman who is nursing a baby. The ulcer is irritated constantly by the baby's sucking and causes the mother considerable pain, often associated with bleeding of the nipple. Prophylactic treatment, cleanliness, and washing and drying of the nipple after each nursing usually prevent the occurrence of this condition. In the prenatal period, the woman can wash, dry, and lubricate the nipples in preparation for nursing, in order to help prevent fissure development. If a fissure develops, it should be washed at frequent intervals with sterile solution, and nursing should continue only with the use of an artificial nipple. If healing does not occur promptly, or if the case is severe and painful, nursing should be stopped and a breast pump used instead. Persistent ulceration suggests carcinoma or a primary syphilitic lesion.

Bleeding or Bloody Discharge From the Nipple (Intraductal Papilloma). At times, a bloody discharge may seep from the nipple and stain the clothes. Often, pressure at one area of the edge of the areola produces the discharge. Although a bloody nipple discharge may be caused by malignancy, it is most commonly due to a wartlike benign epithelial tumor (papilloma) growing in one of the larger collecting ducts just at the edge of the areola, or in an area of cystic disease. This bleeds on trauma, and the blood collects in the duct until it is pressed out at the nipple. The duct can be identified in the nipple and traced down, so that the duct and the papilloma can be excised.

Paget's Disease of the Breast. Paget's disease of the breast is seen most frequently in women over age 45; usually, it is unilateral. Most often, it begins as a mild eczematoid condition of the nipple that may spread over the areola and even part of the breast; later, it may become ulcerated or eroded. In the more advanced stages, retraction of the nipple may occur. This is a true carcinoma of the ducts of the breast that converge at the nipple.

When any lesion of the nipple has not healed after a few weeks of treatment by simple cleansing and protective measures, a suspicion of Paget's disease should be confirmed by biopsy examination. This disease demands early and total removal of the breast.

Breast Infection

Lactational Mastitis. Lactational mastitis may occur at the beginning or the end of lactation. Mastitis may result from the transfer of microorganisms to the breast by the hands of the patient or those of the personnel caring for her. The baby with an oral, eye, or skin infection may be a source of infection. Mastitis may be caused by blood-borne organisms. An infection of the ducts results, causing stagnation of milk in one or more lobules. The breast becomes tough or doughy, and the patient complains of dull pain in the region affected. A nipple that is discharging pus, serum, or blood demands investigation.

Treatment consists of taking the baby off the breast temporarily. A broad-spectrum antibiotic may be given to the mother for 7 to 10 days. Progesterone has been found to reduce breast congestion, which in turn relieves the pain. The patient should wear a firm breast support and follow good habits of personal hygiene.

Lactational Mammary Abscess. A breast abscess usually develops as a sequela of an acute mastitis, although it may occur independently of lactation. The area affected becomes very tender and dusky red, and pus may be expressed from the nipple. Nursing is stopped and adequate support is provided for the breasts. Chemotherapy and antibiotic therapy are prescribed; however, incision and drainage may be performed when fluctuation indicates the presence of pus. Warm, wet dressings increase the drainage and hasten resolution.

Benign Cysts and Tumors of the Breast

Every growth within the breast should be viewed with suspicion and should be removed unless there is a contraindication.

Cystic Disease of the Breast. In cystic disease of the breast, many small cysts are produced owing to an overgrowth of fibrous tissue in the area of the ducts. The disease occurs most commonly between the ages of 30 and 50. These cysts are labile, that is, they may develop quickly to a considerable size in a few days and also decrease in size just as rapidly. They may be noted as lumps, which may be either painless or tender when palpated or pressed, particularly before menstruation. Occasionally, shooting pains may be felt. For tenderness, a supporting brassiere worn day and night may be helpful. The cyst itself rarely has any malignant potential, although breasts containing cysts may be more prone to developing cancer than normal breasts. Most cysts can be treated by simple aspiration of the fluid under local anesthesia. Usually, the fluid will not reaccumulate. If the fluid is uncharacteristic on aspiration, biopsy may be recommended.

When pain and tenderness are more severe (enough to warrant suppression of ovarian function), danazol (Danocrine) may be prescribed. By inhibiting secretion of FSH and LH, ovarian production of estrogen is suppressed. This hypoestrogenic effect may be the reason for a decrease in breast pain and nodularity. Possible side-effects are fluid retention and hepatic disturbance.

Fibroadenoma (Adenofibroma). Fibroadenomas are firm, round, movable, benign tumors of the breast, usually appearing in the breasts of girls in their late teens and early 20s. They cause no pain and are not tender. They can be removed through a small incision and have no malignant potential.

Patient Education. The psychological and physical needs of the woman with benign breast problems determine the kind of teaching and assistance that is required. These needs are ascertained on an individual basis. Obviously, there is greater risk of additional breast problems, including precancerous manifestations. The nurse can emphasize the need for monthly BSE. Comfort measures that can be suggested are as follows:

- Wear a well supporting bra 24 hours a day.
- Make a determination as to whether warm or cool appliances are effective (warm compresses, heating pad, cool compresses, ice bag).
- Use mild analgesics, such as aspirin or acetaminophen.
- Reduce or eliminate use of methylxanthines (coffee, tea, cola, theophylline) since this appears to reduce fibrocystic masses.
- Adhere to a low-salt diet, especially the 2 weeks before menstruation (diuretics may be helpful).

The nurse can reduce the patient's fear and anxiety through education, reassurance, and follow-up support.

Breast Cancer

"The concept of breast cancer as a systemic disease in which micrometastases have disseminated long before the primary tumor is detected has now firmly taken hold."* This statement implies that *early detection* of breast cancer can be accomplished only by sophisticated diagnostic measures such as mammography or ultrasound. At present the main means of

* Hermann RE and Cooperman A. Foreword: Symposium on Breast Cancer. Surg Clin North Am 1984 Dec; 64(6):1029.

detection of over 90% of breast cancers is by women doing BSE. When cancer is discovered by this method, the average size of the tumor is 2.5 cm. About 50% already have lymph node spread, and the majority will die of their cancer.

Incidence. Worldwide, breast cancer is diagnosed in approximately 1 million women annually. According to the latest statistics of the American Cancer Society, 130,900 new cases were discovered, and approximately 41,300 women will die of the disease. The incidence of breast cancer has continued to rise over the past 35 to 40 years, whereas the mortality rate has changed very little. This appears to be a hopeful sign in the battle against this disease and undoubtedly means that a higher proportion of women are being treated earlier and that the methods of treatment have improved. Mortality continues to increase with age except during the menopause, at which time there is a slight decrease in incidence (the reason is unknown). The highest incidence is found in the unmarried female, and the lowest incidence occurs among those who have had multiple pregnancies or those who gave birth to their first child before the age of 34. Low incidence is also noted in women who have had an early artificial menopause brought on by a hysterectomy. Racial differences have been noted, but no explanation is offered as to why, for example, the women of Japan have the lowest incidence. However, among Japanese women who immigrate to the United States and adopt our culture, mortality rate from breast cancer increases (see Chart 43-1).

Pathophysiology. Basically, breast cancer is a disease of breast tissue but can progress to systemic involvement. It begins as an atypical area, progresses to a carcinoma *in situ* (either ductal or lobular), and then enters a minimally invasive stage (up to 5 mm [$^3/_{16}$ inch]). Once the carcinoma passes this stage, there is a higher likelihood of its invading the lymph nodes and the systemic circulation. Because the same factors affect both breasts, the opposite breast must be carefully watched for the development of a second carcinoma.

The tumor is located most frequently in the upper outer quadrant of the breast. As it grows, it becomes attached to the chest wall or the overlying skin. If no treatment is given, the tumor invades the surrounding tissues and extends to the lymph glands of the adjacent axilla. When the tumor arises in the medial half of the breast, its extension may involve the lymph nodes within the chest along the internal mammary artery (Fig. 43-3). Metastases occur most commonly in the lungs, bone, mediastinal lymph nodes, or liver. In untreated cases, death usually results in 2 or 3 years.

Etiology. The cause of breast carcinoma is not known; however, several factors appear to influence its occurrence. The strongest factor is genetic; women of succeeding generations are not only predisposed to develop breast cancer, but they develop it 10 to 12 years earlier than women without a family history of breast cancer. Women who have more menstrual periods are more prone to have breast cancer, whereas women with more children have a lower incidence. Obviously, bearing children reduces the number of menstrual periods. Breast feeding also appears to protect against breast cancer.

The question continues regarding the effect of estrogens in promoting breast cancer. This uncertainty has a bearing on the use of the "pill" for contraceptive purposes. Although the long-range effects of using the pill are incomplete, there is reason to suggest that other means of contraception should be used by women who have a family history of breast cancer

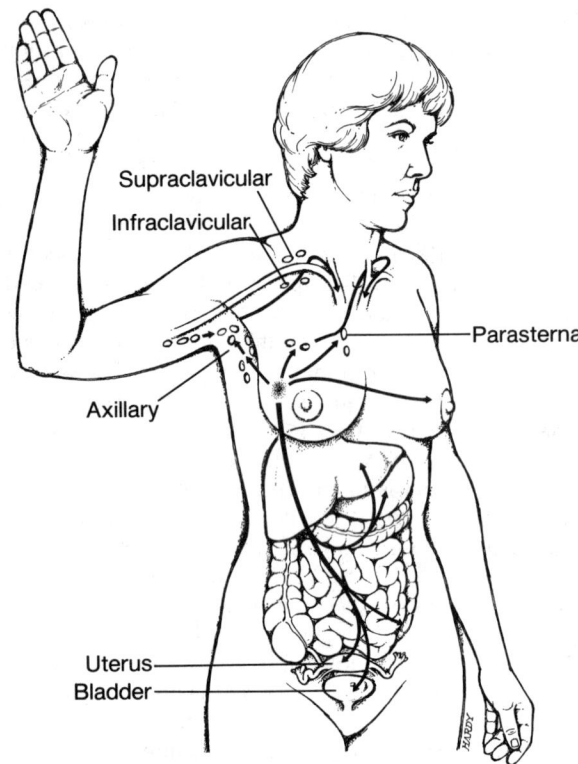

Figure 43-3
Lymphatic drainage of the mammary gland. Metastases from cancer of the mammary gland may follow several lymphatic pathways: (*1*) Upper outer quadrant to axillary, infraclavicular, and supraclavicular nodes, *etc.* (*2*) Upper inner quadrant directly to intercostal and parasternal nodes. (*3*) Upper inner quadrant directly to parasternal nodes. (*4*) Directly across midline to opposite breast. (*5*) Lower quadrants, particularly inner aspect, through pectoralis major, external oblique, and linea alba to subperitoneal lymphatic plexus, followed by abdominal and pelvic spread.

or by those who have gross cystic disease, multiple breast papillomas, or cancer in one breast.

Dietary patterns are also significant; there is a positive correlation between fat consumption and rates of breast cancer.

Clinical Manifestations. The symptoms of the disease, unfortunately, are insidious. A nontender lump, which may be movable, appears in the breast, usually in the upper outer quadrant. Pain is usually absent, except in the very late stages. Some women are first made aware of a problem by a well-localized discomfort that may be described as burning, stinging, or aching. Eventually, dimpling or "orange peel" appearance of the skin may be observed. On examination in the mirror, the patient may note asymmetry and an elevation of the affected breast. Nipple retraction may be evident. Later, the breast becomes more or less fixed on the chest wall, and nodules appear in the axilla. Finally, ulceration occurs and malnutrition and general ill health become prominent.

Inflammatory carcinoma is a rare type of breast cancer (1%–2%) that produces symptoms different from those of other breast cancers. The localized tumor is tender and painful; the breast is abnormally firm and enlarged. The skin over

it is red and dusky. Often edema and nipple retraction occur. These symptoms rapidly increase in severity and usually prompt the woman to seek medical help sooner than the ordinary breast cancer patient.

Prognosis. Breast cancer is more unpredictable than most other cancers because of hormone dependence, immune response, host resistance, and other variable factors. If the lymph nodes have not been involved, the prognosis is better than in those instances when cancer cells are found in the nodes. In clinical assessment, the absence of palpable nodes does not necessarily mean absence of malignancy (the growth may be microscopic). However, the presence of a palpable node, even a large node, may reflect an inflammation rather than a tumor. Tumor spread at the time of treatment appears to be more significant in prognosis than the type of treatment.

Diagnostic Evaluation. The key to better cure rates is to diagnose the disease as early as possible before the stage of microscopic metastasis has been reached. When the mass is less than 1 cm in size (stage 0), the likelihood of recovery (for at least 10 years) is 85%.

Staging is done to assess the local extent of the disease, regional lymph node involvement, status of opposite breast, and possibility of systemic metastasis (see Chart 43-2 and Fig. 43-4).

Management

The approach to treating breast cancer has altered during the past few decades, reflecting the basic premise that *this disease is not local but systemic*. Because of this assumption, not only is the local cancer treated, but the micrometastatic cancer, which may have disseminated throughout the body or may be present within the surrounding breast tissue, is also treated. More specifically, surgery combined with adjuvant chemotherapy is more effective than surgery alone for certain groups of patients. The use of postoperative radiation therapy (following simple or modified radical mastectomy) decreases local recurrence but does not improve survival. Studies are being conducted to determine the best strategy, the correct combination of chemotherapeutic agents, and the optimum timing in the multidisciplinary approach.

Surgical Management. The usual treatment of carcinoma of the breast is removal or destruction of the whole tumor. It is evident that complete removal of the tumor can be accomplished most surely when the cancer is still confined to the breast. This is borne out by clinical experience, which shows a rate of cure better than 80% if the tumor is confined to the breast. When cancer cells have spread to the nodes of the axilla, the cure rate falls to 40%.

Types of surgical intervention include the following:

1. Simple excision (*lumpectomy* or *tumorectomy*) followed by irradiation of unremoved breast tissue and axillary nodes.
2. *Quadrantectomy:* resection of the involved breast quadrant (usually upper outer quadrant), dissection of axillary lymph nodes, and irradiation to the residual breast tissue.
3. *Simple (total) mastectomy:* resection extends from the clavicle to the costal margin and from the midline to the latissimus dorsi. The entire axillary tail and the pectoral fascia are removed. Usually this is followed by ir-

Chart 43-2
Clinical Stages: Carcinoma of the Breast

Stage	Size Primary Tumor	Regional Lymph Node Involvement	Metastasis
I	Small (<2 cm)	Negative	Not detectable
II	>2 cm but <5 cm	Negative or Positive	No distant metastasis detectable
III	Large (>5 cm) or Any size with invasion of skin or chest wall	Positive lymph nodes in clavicular area	No distant metastasis detectable
IV	Tumor of any size	Positive or negative nodes	Distant metastasis

radiation of unremoved axillary nodes plus radiation boost to the scar area.

4. *Modified radical mastectomy:* entire breast and axillary lymph nodes are removed along with the pectoralis major but not pectoralis minor.
5. *Radical mastectomy:* removal of entire breast, axillary lymph nodes, and both pectoral muscles.

Following the removal of the tumor mass, bleeding points are ligated and the skin is closed as well as possible over the chest wall. Skin grafting is done if the skin flaps are not of sufficient size to close the wound. Nonadhering dressing (Adaptic) permits serum and blood to escape between the strips. Pressure dressings may then be applied. Two drainage tubes may be placed in the axilla and beneath the superior skin flap; portable suction may be preferred by some surgeons. Final dressings may be held in place by wide elastic bandages.

Functional Considerations. The objective is to restore normal function to the hand, arm, and shoulder girdle on the affected side. Before surgery is performed, the surgeon plans an incision that will provide maximum opportunity to excise

Figure 43-4
Clinical staging of patients with carcinoma of the breast. Staging is determined by the extent of the spread. (*A*) Stage I. Carcinoma is confined to the mammary lobules; no evidence in the regional nodes. (*B*) Stage II. Extension evident outside the lobules with tethering to the skin; axillary nodes may contain metastases. (*C*) Stage III. Tumor has infiltrated the skin and may have caused ulceration, or it has invaded the lymphatics and produced peau d'orange over the tumor site. Penetration extends to the deep fascia and perhaps the pectoralis major. Metastases over axillary nodes have extended beyond the capsules (*D*) Skin is grossly ulcerated, peau d'orange appears over the whole breast, and deep fixation has occurred to the ribs. There is distant metastasis.

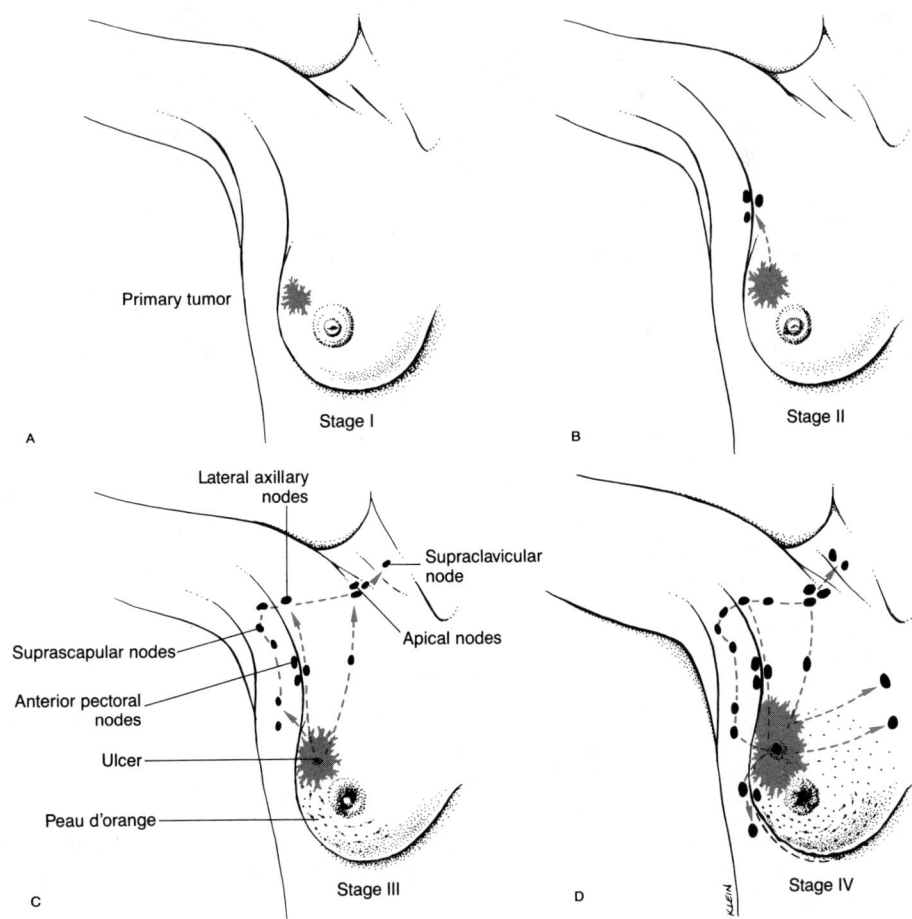

Primary tumor

Stage I

A

Stage II

B

Lateral axillary nodes

Supraclavicular node

Apical nodes

Suprascapular nodes

Anterior pectoral nodes

Ulcer

Peau d'orange

Stage III

C

Stage IV

D

the tumor and the affected nodes. At the same time, the patient's life-style should be considered, and efforts should be made to avoid a scar that will be visible and restrictive. Skin flaps and tissue are handled meticulously to ensure proper viability, hemostasis, and drainage. A valuable technique involves injecting fluorescein contrast medium into the peripheral vein at the time of surgical closure and actually inspecting the blood supply to the flaps with a Wood's lamp. When the light is turned off, the manner in which the blood has been distributed to the flaps can be assessed.

Variations in Approach.   There has been a gradual but marked departure from the radical mastectomy to more conservative surgery for primary breast tumors. Often a biopsy of the breast is not followed by an immediate mastectomy on the pathologist's report that the tissue is malignant. A two-stage approach spares the patient from awakening after a biopsy to discover that she has had a mastectomy. Instead, time is taken to confirm the biopsy report and discuss alternative methods of treatment with the patient. These modalities vary with the stages of the malignancy. In most instances, therapy includes combinations of chemotherapy, immunotherapy, antiestrogens, or oophorectomy and adrenalectomy for estrogen receptor–positive patients. Another trend followed in some clinics is to do a breast reconstruction immediately following mastectomy or subsequently (*e.g.*, 6 months later).

Hormonal Therapy.   Hormonal therapy for breast cancer is greatly influenced by the index of estrogen receptor protein (ERP), an assay done on tumor tissue taken at the original biopsy. Normal breast tissue contains receptor sites for estrogen. However, only about one third of breast malignant tumors are estrogen dependent, or ERP positive. An ERP-positive assay indicates that tumor growth depends on estrogen supply and that surgical measures to cut down on hormone production (oophorectomy, adrenalectomy, or hypophysectomy) would be appropriate. These procedures are effective for palliative treatment. If ERP is negative, surgery of this type is ineffective. Hormones may also be manipulated by antiestrogen drugs (tamoxifen and nafoxadine).

Adjuvant Chemotherapy of Breast Cancer.   Cytotoxic drugs may be given as adjuvant chemotherapy (combined with or to supplement some other treatment modality—in this case, surgery) following primary excisional therapy; the purpose is to eliminate hidden or micrometastatic spread of the disease. It is important that this type of therapy be initiated before drug resistance develops. Therefore, the drugs must be started almost immediately following definitive treatment of the primary neoplasm. The other strategy is to use combined chemotherapy (combining two or three chemotherapeutic agents). When assessing the value of any form of therapy, it is important to weigh its efficacy against its toxic effects.

Common chemotherapeutic regimens include

CMF: cyclophosphamide, methotrexate, 5-fluorouracil
CMF-VP: cyclophosphamide, methotrexate, 5-fluorouracil, plus vincristine and prednisone
CAF: cyclophosphamide, doxorubicin (Adriamycin), fluorouracil
L-PAM: melphalan or phenylalanine mustard

Radiation Therapy.   Radiation therapy, when used, is usually instituted following excision of the tumor mass. An external beam irradiates the area including nearby lymph nodes and is repeated at specified intervals for several weeks. Another method of irradiation is to surgically place hollow needles in the desired breast area into which radioactive seeds or needles are later inserted for a prescribed time (see pp. 270–272). The purpose of both methods is to destroy migrant or remaining cancer cells after surgical removal of the tumor mass.

▶ Nursing Process
The Patient With Breast Cancer

▷ Assessment

The nursing history can be significant in revealing the reaction of the patient to her diagnosis and her ability to cope. Some pertinent questions are

- How does the patient feel about the fact that she has breast cancer?
- What coping measures is she planning to use? What inner resources or strengths can she draw upon?
- Can she identify support persons who can assist her at this time?
- If appropriate, is there a close partner who can help her in making decisions about the treatment choices?
- Can problem areas such as misinformation about the therapeutic plan or unwarranted self-incrimination related to the subsequent development of cancer be identified?
- Is she experiencing any discomfort?

Family members and/or persons significant to her can be helpful in eliciting data that can be used in developing a nursing care plan.

A breast examination is performed as described on pp. 1128–1130. Results of other diagnostic modalities such as mammography, breast biopsy, thermography, and transillumination are reviewed.

▷ Nursing Diagnoses

Based on the nursing and other assessment data, the patient's major nursing diagnoses may include the following:

- Fear and ineffective coping related to the diagnosis of cancer, its treatment, and prognosis
- Disturbance in self-concept related to extensiveness of surgery and side-effects of radiation and/or chemotherapy
- Alterations in comfort—pain, related to tissue trauma from incision(s)
- Self-care deficit related to partial immobility of upper extremity on side of breast surgery
- Possible sexual dysfunction related to loss of body part and fear of partner's reaction to this loss

Potential Complications: Infection, injury, edema formation, neurovascular deficits in upper extremity on affected side

▷ Planning and Implementation

▷   *Goals:*   The major goals of the patient may include reduction of emotional stress, fear, and anxiety and improvement in ability to cope with the problem; realistic adaptation to changes that will occur relative to treatment modalities; absence of pain/discomfort; avoidance of impaired mobility and achievement of self-care to the fullest possible level; and identification of alternative satisfying/acceptable sexual experiences.

Preoperative Nursing Interventions

Psychosocial Preparation. Emotional preparation of the patient begins at the moment she is told that hospitalization and treatment may be required. When informed of possible breast disorders, she is encouraged to avoid delay in following through on suspicious findings. It must be recognized that on admission to a hospital for a questionable breast tumor, most women have a real fear of cancer. Unfortunately, many times this fear has made them delay seeking treatment until the tumor has metastasized. Fear also stems from the emotional trauma of knowing that the breast may be removed or that she may sustain disfigurement. This may be perceived as affecting her sexual attractiveness and loss of femininity.

Opportunity is provided to discuss her concerns and correct her misapprehensions. When the specific treatment plan has been developed, the patient is assisted in understanding what is involved. She and her partner may need to know that a variety of resources and options may be available, such as prosthetic implants, reconstructive surgery, organizations such as "Reach to Recovery," and other services. She also will be followed closely and be informed of the next step. When appropriate, the details of additional diagnostic measures, treatments, and preoperative preparation are described. Should skin grafting or transplantation of tissue (muscle or fat) be required, the nature of the incision is described as well as consideration for the cosmetic result. This may be of particular concern for one who enjoys swimming (swim suit wear), participating in sports, and wearing certain styles of clothing.

Preoperative Preparation. Once the treatment plan has been established, it is initiated with due consideration to preparing the patient to be in the best physical, psychological, and nutritional condition. She is to be aware of the treatment plan after adequate discussion with the health care team in which she is a participant. Possibilities and deviations in the plans are explained by the physician, as determined by her progress. Details of surgery include the location and extent of the incision(s). If blood loss is expected, provision is made for replacement. Radiation includes extent and potential side-effects as well as their treatment; chemotherapy includes the nature of the medication, frequency and method of administration, side-effects that may be encountered, and the expected goal to be achieved.

Whatever physical changes in appearance are anticipated, methods to compensate for these deviations are explained, such as prosthesis, alternatives in garments and dress, and plastic surgery.

Radiation therapy may be prescribed after the operation or as adjunct therapy as a means of destroying any cancer cells that may have escaped removal at operation. Wound healing may be delayed during concomitant irradiation. Anorexia, nausea, and vomiting can occur after irradiation; abstinence from eating and drinking for 3 hours before and after these treatments often helps.

Postoperative Nursing Interventions

Postoperative care is given with special attention to pulse and blood pressure, since they are valuable indices in detecting shock and hemorrhage. Blood pressure readings are not taken on the arm of the affected side in order to avoid further constriction of blood vessels.

Dressings are inspected for bleeding, especially under the axilla and in the area on which the patient is lying. At the same time, tube drainage is monitored for proper functioning. The patient is encouraged to turn and take deep breaths to avert pulmonary complications. The dressing usually is fairly snug; however, it should not be so tight that lung expansion is restricted. Most surgeons eliminate pressure dressings early in the postoperative period and use portable suction to promote adherence of the skin flap to the chest wall, which reduces the potential for infection and promotes wound healing.

All graft areas (skin, muscle, fatty tissue) are assessed for unusual redness, pain, swelling, or drainage. Such monitoring will enhance healing and alert the health care team to early signs of infection.

Positioning. Positioning of the patient depends on the dressing; a semi-Fowler position is usually desirable. If free, the arm should be elevated with each joint positioned higher than the more proximal joint. Thus, gravity helps to remove the fluid via the lymphatic and venous pathways. Whether the arm is flexed or extended depends on the preference of the physician. Elevation of the arm helps to prevent lymphedema, which may occur after surgery because of interference with the circulatory and lymphatic systems (especially following radical mastectomy). Whether there will be satisfactory postmastectomy lymph drainage depends on how many collateral lymphatic avenues were not destroyed during surgery.

Pain Relief. After the patient has recovered from the anesthesia, analgesics are given for the relief of pain. The nurse will frequently assess for manifestations of discomfort and initiate comfort measures by keeping the involved upper extremity elevated on pillows (about 30 degrees when the patient is in bed or sitting in a chair). This is done to reduce tension on the arm and to decrease the amount of fluid accumulation.

When dressings are changed and the wound site is cleansed, gentleness is required to avoid injury and discomfort. The area is blotted rather than scrubbed. Exercises are introduced gradually and only increased in keeping with the ability of the healing tissues to withstand added stresses and strains.

Lymphedema. Although the cause of lymphedema is not known, it will result if the number of properly functioning lymphatic channels is insufficient to ensure a return flow of lymph into the general circulation. Although edema may affect only the upper arm, often the entire arm on the operated side is involved. Such swelling can occur immediately following operation (postoperative surgical edema) or may occur many months or years after surgery (secondary surgical edema).

When axillary nodes and the lymphatic system have been removed, a collateral system for lymphatic drainage from the hand and arm must be developed (Fig. 43-5). This is done within a month and is facilitated by exercise. Although most postmastectomy patients escape massive lymphedema, this complication would occur even less frequently if the nurse

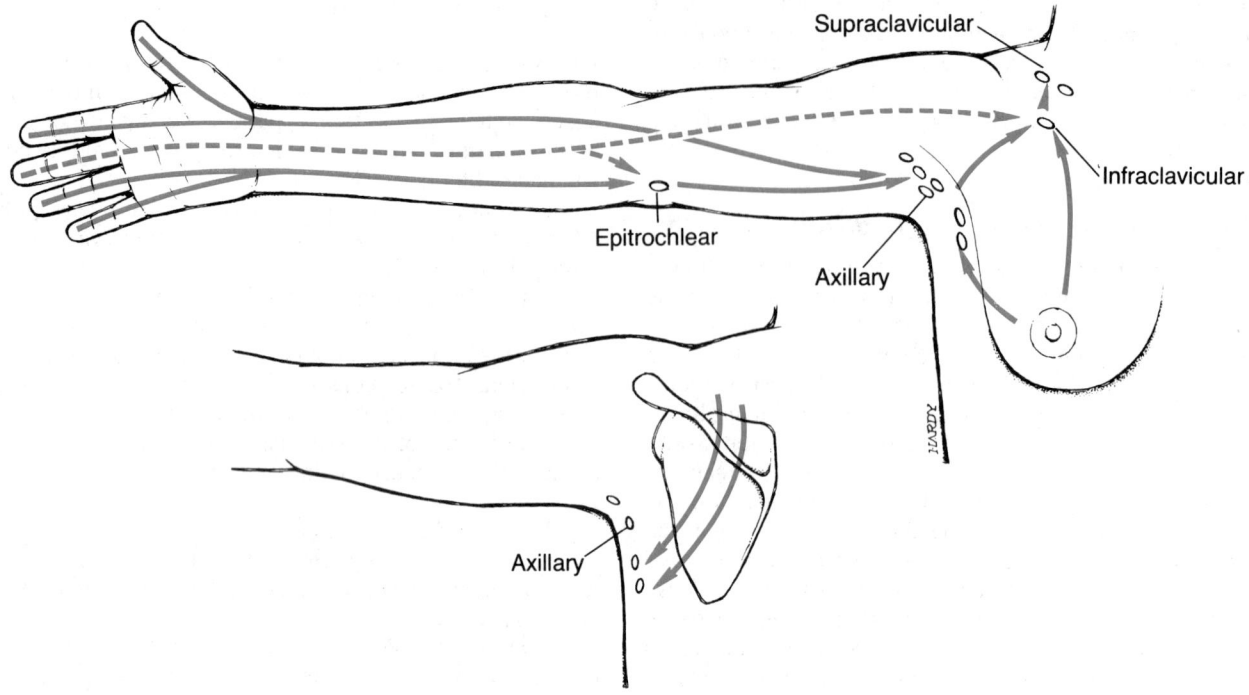

Figure 43-5
Lymphatic drainage of the upper extremity. The lymphatic vessels draining the fingers
and the hand converge on the dorsum of the hand. From here the lymphatic drainage
pursues three courses. The lymph vessels draining the ulnar aspect (little finger and ring
finger) accompany the basilic vein and drain into the epitrochlear nodes and thence into
the axillary nodes. The lymph vessels draining the thumb and the index fingers bypass
the epitrochlear nodes and go directly to the axillary nodes. The lymph vessels draining
the middle fingers may drain into the epitrochlear or the axillary, or they may bypass
both of these groups of nodes to drain directly into the intraclavicular, and thence into
the supraclavicular, and finally into the bloodstream. The axillary nodes also receive
lymph from the posterior scapular region (*insert*).

impressed on patients the importance of elevating, massaging,
and exercising the affected arm for 3 or 4 months following
the operation.

For marked lymphedema, the arm should be elevated,
but not in adduction since this position is uncomfortable and
constricts the axilla. The elbow is elevated on a pillow so
that the elbow is higher than the shoulder. The hand is further
elevated on another pillow so that the hand is higher than
the elbow. Elastic bandages are not recommended at this
time since they may interfere with the formation of collateral
lymphatic pathways.

When acute infection has subsided, some physicians
recommend the use of intermittent pneumatic compression
of the arm, but many doubt its value. For the chronic stage,
the patient may wear an elastic sleeve (custom-made) from
the wrist to the shoulder during the day when she is up and
about.

Patient Education. Since secondary surgical edema may
occur much later, one of the most important teaching points
to emphasize with the patient is that for months and years
she must take extra precautions to avoid cuts, bruises, and
infection of the hand and arm on the side of her operation.
She should also avoid undue stress on the suture line during
shoulder range of motion exercises and gravity-dependent
positions for prolonged periods of time. Carrying hand bags

for extended periods should also be avoided. Other precautions are listed in Chart 43-3.

Care of Incision Site. When dressings are changed,
the nature of the incision, the way it looks and feels, and how
it will gradually change are explained. The patient needs to
know that sensation in the newly healed area may have decreased because nerves have been severed; however, the
area should be bathed gently and blotted dry to avoid injury.
Signs of irritation and possible infection are described, so
that if they occur, the patient will recognize them and report
them to her physician. When talking about the incision, the
nurse should use the term *incision* rather than *scar*, since
scarring connotes defect, deformity, and ugliness in the minds
of many persons. The arm on the affected side may be supported in a sling for a time to prevent tension on the wound.
Gentle massage of the healed incision with cocoa butter or
other lotions helps to increase the elasticity of the skin and
encourages circulation.

Psychosocial Considerations. A real problem may
arise if the patient is reluctant to look at the incision site.
Although the presence of the scar must eventually be faced,
the patient should not be forced at this time to look at her
chest area. Her psychological defenses may require that she
be spared this added shock at this time. It is sometimes helpful
to direct the patient to acceptance by first drawing a picture

Chart 43-3
Patient Education: Hand and Arm Care Following Mastectomy

Suggested Activities:	*Avoid:*
• Protect the hand and arm on the operated side. • Apply lanolin hand cream several times daily. • Use a thimble when sewing. • Stay out of strong sun. • Wear a Medic Alert tag engraved as follows: *Caution—recent mastectomy—no tests—no needle injections* • Call a health care person if the arm gets red or swollen or becomes unusually hard.	• Cuts, bruises, insect bites, burns • Injury to cuticles or hangnails • Strong detergents • Working near thorny bushes • Digging in the garden • Holding a cigarette • Reaching into a hot oven • Having blood drawn; injections • Having a blood pressure cuff applied • Wearing jewelry or a wrist watch • Carrying heavy bags or purse

of the incision line on a piece of paper. Then at a later time, when the dressings are being changed, the patient may show signs of being willing to look at her chest. However, the nurse must explore this area in a very gentle manner. Any resistance on the part of the patient must be sensed and respected. Each woman must work her way to acceptance on the basis of her own individual psychological needs.

Ambulation and Exercise. Ambulation is encouraged on the first day following surgery when the effects of the anesthetic have worn off and the patient is free from nausea and has been able to take fluids and nutrients. Assistance is given when needed; the nurse supports the patient from the unoperated side. After the physician's assessment postoperatively and the removal of drainage tubes, passive range of motion of the affected arm is initiated to increase circulation and muscle strength and to prevent stiffness of the shoulder. Hand exercises are also begun. These activities can be increased as the patient is encouraged to do more for herself by brushing her teeth, washing her face, and combing her hair with the hand on the affected side. Failure to encourage such exercises as "climbing the wall with the fingers" may prolong the disuse of the arm and promote the development of a contracture. Exercise should not be accompanied by pain; if the patient has had a skin graft or if the incision was closed with considerable tension, such exercises are greatly limited and must be done very gradually. At the bedside, pulley-type ropes from the over-bed or curtain frame can be used for one kind of exercise. Turning a jump rope that is attached to the doorknob can be arranged easily (see muscle-training exercises, Fig. 43-6). In all exercises, it is important to emphasize bilateral activity. Likewise, the value of proper posture must be emphasized; if the patient hunches over and favors the affected side as she combs her hair, the purpose of the exercise will be defeated.

Naturally, difficulty with arm movement is much greater in the patient who has undergone radical mastectomy. Limitation of motion after simple and modified radical mastectomy is unusual, and the patient is encouraged to use the arm to the point of complete mobility almost immediately.

The exercises done in the hospital and illustrated in Figure 43-6 can be related to household activities. Putting dishes on a shelf, dusting window sashes, typing, and piano playing are activities that promote and maintain muscle tone. Other suggestions are to swing the arm while walking; wear loose or nonconstricting clothing; keep the mastectomy site, underarm, and arm scrupulously clean; and avoid injury to the hand and arm.

Follow-up visits are very important for the evaluation of incision healing, mental outlook, general physical condition, and any evidence of recurrence. If there is a need for consultation with a community nurse, the availability of such a service is pointed out to the patient.

▷ *Evaluation*

▷ *Expected Outcomes*

1. Patient demonstrates willingness to deal with the anxiety of the diagnosis and the impact of surgery on sexual functioning and self-image.
   a. Talks about her concerns related to possible future course of disease.
   b. Expresses an understanding that mastectomy need not have a negative effect on sexuality.
2. Experiences little or no discomfort.
   a. Is afebrile 48 hours prior to discharge.
   b. Experiences minimal pain in operative area.
   c. Demonstrates a drainage-free incision site.
   d. Has satisfactory wound healing; knows to report signs of redness, heat, and pain.
3. Participates actively in self-care activities.
   a. Carries out exercises as prescribed.
   b. Performs additional activities that will enhance the exercise plan.
4. Uses means that will help in preventing complications.
   a. Relates what signs and symptoms are reportable and suggestive of complications.
   b. Describes side-effects of chemotherapeutic agents; understands what measures to take in minimizing these effects.
   c. Avoids cuts, bruises, infection, and excessive stress on hand and arm on operative side.

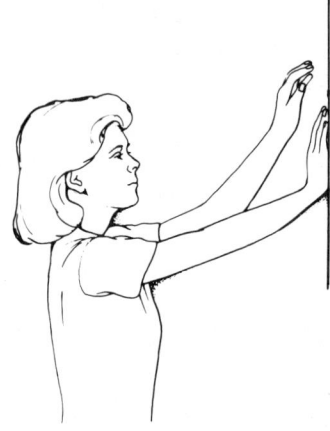

A. *Wall handclimbing.* Stand facing the wall, with the toes as close to the wall as possible—feet apart. With elbows somewhat bent, place the palms on the wall at shoulder level. By flexing the fingers, work hands up the wall until arms are fully extended. Work hands down to starting point.

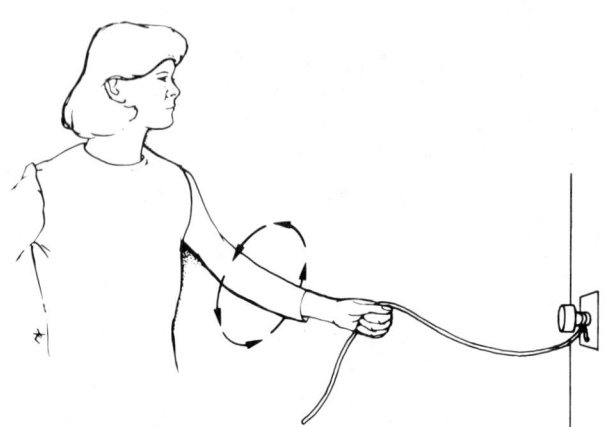

B. *Rope turning.* Stand facing the door. Take free end of light rope in hand of the operated side. Place other hand on hip. With arm extended and held away from the body—nearly parallel with the floor—turn rope, making as wide swings as possible. Slow at first—speed up later.

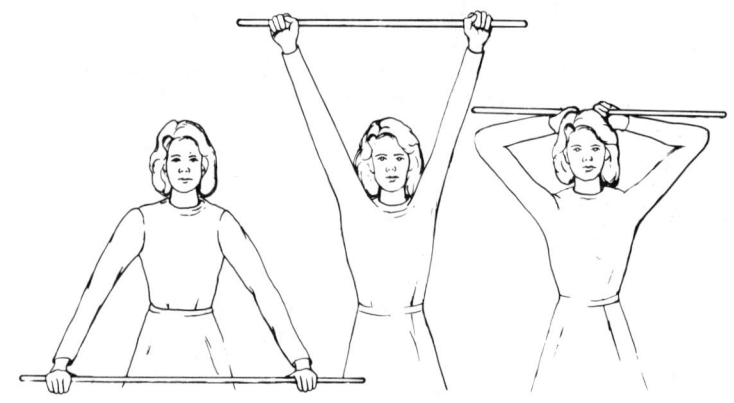

C. *Rod or Broom.* Grasp rod with both hands, held about 2 feet apart. With arms straight, raise rod over the head. Bend elbows lowering rod behind the head. Reverse maneuver, raising rod above the head, then to starting position.

D. *Pulley.* Toss rope over shower curtain rod or doorway curtain rod. Stand as nearly under rope as possible. Grasp an end in each hand. Extend arms straight and away from body. Pull left arm up by tugging down with right arm, then right arm up and left down—like a seesaw.

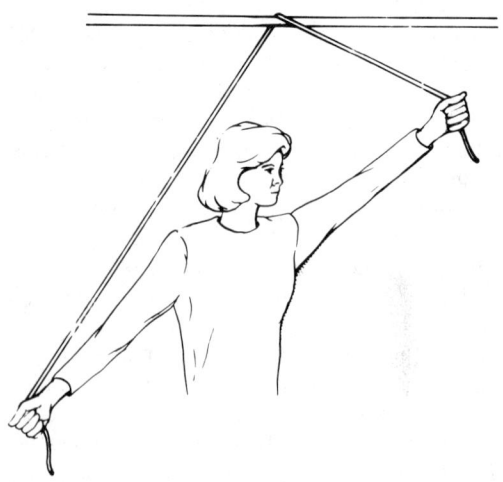

Figure 43-6
Exercises after mastectomy. The purpose of the exercise program is to secure a complete range of motion of the affected shoulder joint. (Adapted from Radler. A Handbook for Your Recovery. New York, The Society of Memorial Center.)

d. Relates that she will see her physician for follow-up visits.

e. Notes the phone number of health care personnel to call should untoward signs arise.

Care of the patient with breast cancer is summarized in Nursing Care Plan 43-1, pages 1142 to 1144.

Care of the Patient With Advanced Breast Cancer

Following a radical mastectomy, the woman is asked to adhere to a schedule of follow-up visits to her physician. Usually, visits take place every 3 months for 2 or 3 years, every 6 months for 5 years, and then annually. The hope is that the patient will be free from disease as long as possible. Unfortunately, many women have recurrences of the tumor or metastatic spread. Likewise, many women who seek medical assistance have a primary cancer that is so far advanced as to be inoperable. Advanced breast cancer may indicate extensive spread within the breast or to adjacent tissues, or even metastasis to other parts of the body. The status of dissemination can be determined by a metastatic x-ray series (chest, skull, long bones, and pelvis); liver chemistries; a mammogram of the other breast; and available imaging procedures of the bone, liver, and brain.

Of the patients who have recurrences, almost half show evidence of recurrence locally and in regional lymph nodes; over a fourth have visceral involvement; and a similar percentage have bone involvement of the spine, ribs, hips, or pelvis.

Nursing Interventions. Regression or abatement of symptoms for as long as possible is the goal for nursing intervention. However, individual differences make its attainment unpredictable. The emphasis is on improving the quality of survival.

The nurse is challenged to use many skills in assessing the physical as well as the psychosocial condition of the patient. Information about changes in behavioral patterns can be elicited from the patient's family. The nurse can also assist the physician in determining the specific kind of palliation suitable for the individual patient. Such therapy is designed to keep the woman as comfortable as possible, although it may not arrest the disease.

A wide range of treatment is available, depending on the specifics of the patient's condition. For a detailed outline of the various treatment modalities that are frequently used, see Table 43-1 (pp. 1145–1147), and also refer to Chapter 16, Oncology: Nursing the Patient With Cancer.

Reconstructive and Plastic Surgery of the Breast

Hypertrophy of the Breast

The breasts are such an important part of the female figure that abnormalities often lead to requests for surgical management. The variations most often encountered are in size: breasts are too large or too small. Those that are too large are said to be hypertrophied; when the condition occurs in early life, it is called *virginal breast hypertrophy*. The condition is usually bilateral but may occur on only one side. The hypertrophied breasts that occur in later life are always bilateral.

Symptoms of Breast Hypertrophy. Patients with breast hypertrophy complain of tender breasts, diffuse pains, and fatigue. The tenderness and pain is particularly marked at the time of the menstrual period. The weight of the breasts causes a dragging sensation on the shoulders, and efforts to support these tremendous breasts with brassieres are futile. Most patients with virginal hypertrophy have deep grooves in the shoulder tissue caused by pressure from brassiere straps.

Not only are physical symptoms present, but psychological difficulties develop, especially in girls and younger women. They become too embarrassed to wear swim suits, sweaters, or evening gowns. Their social life is restricted, and they become introverts, avoiding social contacts and even marriage. Because they think that they are unattractive, married women with this condition develop a sense of insecurity, fearing the loss of their husband's affection and, possibly, divorce. These are very real difficulties, which cause emotional repercussions that may be very serious.

Mammoplasty. The operation performed to reduce the size of the breasts is termed a *reduction mammoplasty*. In this operation, the surgeon makes one incision beneath the breast and a similar curved incision in the skin of the anterior breast. The nipple is transplanted to a new location after the redundant tissue is cut away. The remaining skin edges are approximated with sutures, and the nipple is sutured to its new location. Drains are placed in the incision and remain for only 1 or 2 days. Simple gauze dressings are used without pressure.

Postoperative Nursing Intervention. Following mammoplasty, nursing intervention is relatively basic. These patients sit up in bed the same day or day after operation and may be out of bed and eating a normal diet thereafter. The results of these plastic operations are good for both relief of symptoms and appearance. There is no recurrence of the hypertrophy, and the operation is not a serious one. The new transplanted nipple may turn black and be covered by a dry scab. This is to be expected, but the scab will come away after a week or two as the nipple regains a blood supply in its new location. It must be accepted that the breast cannot function for lactation after such an operation.

Usually, these patients are euphoric about the results, but it is not uncommon for some patients to experience negative psychological reactions related to the loss of a part of the body. The patient may feel anxious about this reaction, but it helps to let her know that these feelings occur frequently.

Operations to Enlarge or Uplift the Breasts

Operations to enlarge or uplift the breasts are requested fairly frequently. Although padded brassieres and other devices are available, they do not always give the desired result. The operations are performed through an incision along the undermargin of the breast (circumareolar). The breast is elevated, and a pocket is formed between the breast and the chest wall, into which are inserted various types of plastic and synthetic materials intended to enlarge and uplift the breast. This procedure is called an *augmentation mammoplasty* and may be done on an outpatient basis with local anesthesia by an experienced plastic surgeon. These operations are not serious, but complications do occur occasionally,

(Text continues on p. 1144)

Care of the Patient With Cancer of the Breast

Nursing Interventions	*Rationale*	*Expected Outcomes*

Nursing Diagnosis: Fear and ineffective coping related to the diagnosis of breast cancer, its treatment and prognosis

Goal: Reduction of emotional stress, fear, and anxiety

1. Begin emotional preparation of the patient (and partner) as soon as she is told that hospitalization and treatment are required.	1. The earlier the patient accepts the reality of the situation, the more readily will coping mechanisms be effective.	• Displays a reduction of emotional stress and anxiety and exhibits an ability to cope with the problem.
2. Inform the patient of recent research and newer treatment modalities for breast cancer.	2. Increasing options and improved results both statistically and cosmetically greatly reduce the fear and promote acceptance of the treatment plan.	• Participates in the treatment plan and asks questions relating to the best choice for her particular needs.
3. Describe the experiences the patient will face and encourage her questions.	3. Fear of the unknown is eliminated.	• Responds positively to the information she is accumulating.
4. Acquaint her with the increasing number of team-related resources to facilitate her recovery.	4. The information about new prosthetics, reconstruction specialists, and other resources confirm that a great deal of attention is being given to newer treatment methods for breast cancer.	• Describes her appreciation of social support of family, friends, and women who have had breast surgery as a significant aid in coping with a stressful experience.
		• Is aware that husband or "significant other" has been advised and prepared with regard to this role in providing support.

Nursing Diagnosis: Disturbance in self-concept related to nature of surgery and side-effects of radiation and/or chemotherapy

Goal: Realistic adaptation to changes that will occur relative to treatment modalities

1. Establish with the physician the nature of the treatment anticipated.	1. This sets the basis for a cooperative therapeutic plan that will prevent conflicting information from reaching the patient.	• Appears to be accepting the treatment plan.
2. Explain that it is normal to experience grief at the loss of a body part.	2. When this fact is established the patient can then be free to move to the next level of coping.	• Verbalizes that grief must run its course.
3. Encourage visits by loved ones and understanding friends.	3. Support systems that are meaningful to the patient are more endurable than from relative strangers.	• Uses her support personnel effectively; plans future activities with them.
4. Tell her that it is normal not to want herself/partner to view the incision (do not refer to this as a 'scar'); further reinforce the fact that each day the site will look better.	4. This reduces the feeling that she will never be able to accept her altered body.	• Eventually looks at her incision site and participates in dressing changes.
		• Conveys an understanding of the many options; collects brochures and data; asks questions.
5. Discuss the use of prosthesis, reconstruction possibilities, and clothing adjustment as realistic and attainable expectations.	5. The emphasis on the positive and the availability of adaptations will enhance her self-concept and promote positive acceptance of the treatment plan.	• Expresses an understanding of the long-term benefits of chemotherapy/radiation (if prescribed) even though there may be uncomfortable side-effects.

(continued)

Nursing Interventions	*Rationale*	*Expected Outcomes*

Nursing Diagnosis: Alterations in comfort related to tissue trauma from incision(s)

Goal: Absence of pain/discomfort

1. Explain that nerves are severed or damaged but that analgesics and narcotics are available.	1. Analgesics and narcotics can intercept nerve pathways to the brain and spinal cord.	• Reports when pain is worsening and accepts prescribed pain medication.
2. Proper body positioning will promote comfort, such as semi-Fowler's position postanesthetically and elevation of the arm on the affected side.	2. Stress on the incision site is reduced; gravity reduces fluid accumulation in the arm.	• Adjusts her position to relieve discomfort; uses small pillows effectively.
3. Promote passive and then active exercises of the hand, arm, and shoulder on the affected side.	3. This will stimulate circulation, promote neurovascular competence, and prevent stasis with subsequent stiffening of the shoulder girdle.	• Exercises frequently; moves affected arm gently and shows progress in moving from passive to active exercises.
4. Encourage protection and the avoidance of anything that can break through the skin barrier or impose stress on the arm and shoulder (cuts, burns, strong detergents, infections, carrying a heavy bag or purse).	4. Impaired circulation and weakened nerves are vulnerable to sudden or prolonged stress.	• Describes home-related activities that will provide the required range of motion of the affected arm. • Lists various activities that must be avoided because of potential for injury to the breast site and affected arm.
5. Suggest application of an effective cream several times a day.	5. Such practice will keep the skin healthy, intact, pliable, and resistant to breakdown.	• Relates procedures to follow if accidental injury is sustained.
6. Instruct patient to contact a health care person if the arm or incision site becomes painful, swollen, or red.	6. Early treatment of possible infection or injury will avoid further discomfort and complications.	• Orders Medic Alert bracelet when arm lymphedema is diagnosed.
7. Suggest the wearing of a Medic Alert tag if there is a potential for edema.	7. A recognized alert tag will serve as a precaution against injections, taking of blood pressure, and other forms of injury.	

Nursing Diagnosis: Self-care deficit related to partial immobility of upper extremity on side of breast surgery

Goal: Avoidance of impaired mobility and achievement of self-care to the fullest possible level

1. Invite patient's active participation in postoperative care.	1. Patient involvement enhances and facilitates the recovery process.	• Participates in dressing change; expresses interest in working with rehabilitative team including physical therapist.
2. Encourage patient's socialization, particularly with patients who have successfully recovered in similar circumstances.	2. Humans thrive more effectively and happily when they are socially able to relate to others.	• Shows concern about her appearance and accepts suggestions from rehabilitation support groups.
3. Make progressive modifications in the patient's exercise program as dictated by comfort and tolerance levels.	3. There is lessened strain on tissues; improvement is steadily consistent.	• Shows her relatives how she can raise her arm and fix her own hair.
4. Commend the patient when ingenuity and creativity are in evidence, such as an attractive hair style or make-up application.	4. Psychological well-being compounds the effects of optimum physical good health.	• Anticipates eagerly and displays happiness when partner visits; relates the compliments she receives about her good progress.

(continued)

Nursing Interventions	*Rationale*	*Expected Outcomes*

Potential for Complications: Infection, injury, lymphedema, neurovascular deficits

Goal: Avoidance of complications

1. Encourage the elevation of the arm if not contraindicated, with each joint positioned higher than the more proximal joint.	1. Swelling is reduced and there is less pressure on the nerves and blood vessels; pain and discomfort are lessened.	• Demonstrates how to place pillows so that proper elevation of arm is maintained.
2. Inform patient to avoid injury, strenuous activity, or infection.	2. These can stimulate fluid accumulation and compromise the neurovasculature of the arm.	• Lists activities that are to be avoided, including injections and having blood pressure taken on the affected side.
3. Describe and demonstrate exercises in a step-up fashion from simple to more involved.	3. A graduated exercise program will improve muscle tone and hasten full range of activities with avoidance of impairment such as a frozen shoulder.	• Gradually moves the arm freely so that hair combing and 'climbing the wall' can be achieved with no discomfort. Avoids the discomfort of a frozen shoulder.
4. Recommend physical therapy and a weight reduction program if indicated.	4. Properly prescribed activities and exercise plus diet modification are general health measures that enhance well-being and thwart complications.	• Acquires good health habits and avoids complications at the same time.

Nursing Diagnosis: Possible sexual dysfunction related to loss of body part and fear of partner's reaction to this loss

Goal: Identification of alternative satisfying/acceptable sexual experiences

1. Be comfortable in discussing this topic; display a caring, nonjudgmental supportive attitude.	1. The patient will easily sense insincerity, insecurity, lack of knowledge, and inexperience in the health care person.	• Responds by conveying trust and a desire to obtain assistance; asks appropriate questions.
2. Encourage, at the appropriate time, both partners to discuss their concerns; this can be done before and after major treatment.	2. The patient will not feel that she is alone in facing problems that may concern both partners.	• Includes partner in aspects of the medical problem that concern both.
3. Arrange for privacy when discussing personal problems with the patient.	3. Sensitive personal problems are not revealed when people not close to the patient are present.	• Expresses appreciation for promoting confidentiality regarding very personal matters.
4. Describe the incision site and its appearance with the partner before he actually sees it.	4. Partner will know what to expect and not likely register shock in front of the patient.	• Accepts the incision site as evidenced by assisting with dressings and using an appropriate prescribed emollient such as cocoa butter.
5. Emphasize that behavioral changes take time and should not be interpreted as rejection.	5. The very nature of undergoing any surgery takes time in acceptance, recuperation, and perhaps altered life-style.	• Expresses awareness that any adjustments take time but that with patience and understanding the desired goals can be approached and possibly reached.

in some instances requiring the removal of the inserted substance.

Breast Reconstruction Following Mastectomy

Restoration of the female breast following mastectomy in patients who have an early stage cancer and favorable prognosis is becoming increasingly popular. The skin and subcutaneous tissue have been found to be far looser and more supple than was previously thought, and the blood supply to the area has been shown to be sufficient.

Opinions differ about whether postmastectomy breast reconstruction should be done immediately after surgery or delayed. The concern about immediate reconstruction stems from the fear that any recurrence of a local tumor will not

TABLE 43-1
Treatment Modalities for the Patient With Advanced Cancer of the Breast

Palliative Therapy	Objectives of Therapy	Concomitant Effects	Essential Nursing Intervention
Hypophysectomy			
Method:	Removes source of adrenocorticotropic hormone as well as hormones that seem to stimulate the breast directly	May cause salt wastage ⟶	Replace adrenal salt-regulating hormone fludrocortisone acetate (Florinef). Many patients do not require this.
1. Major craniotomy		Following hypophysectomy, diabetes insipidus may occur (inability to conserve body water because of absence of posterior pituitary and its secretion, antidiuretic hormone).	Recognize need for additional steroid replacement during stress periods, such as minor illness, infection, injury, serious vomiting, surgery.
2. Transnasal implantation of radioactive Yttrium (^{90}Y)			
3. Transsphenoidal excision of pituitary			
4. Stereotactic cryohypophysectomy		In 4–6 weeks, hypothalamus takes over function of antidiuretic hormone.	Otherwise, adrenal insufficiency results (symptoms similar to crises described above).
5. Stereotactic radiofrequency to destroy pituitary			For transsphenoidal hypophysectomy: Frequent oral care is required. Observe for hemorrhage, especially after nasal packing is removed. Clear nasal drip and patient swallowing constantly may indicate cerebrospinal leak. Keep patient in Fowler's position to facilitate cerebrospinal fluid drainage.
			Advise patient to wear Medic Alert bracelet with operation and the name of replacement medication.

Note: Medical adrenalectomy: When it is impossible to do an adrenalectomy or hypophysectomy (because of age, patient refusal, poor condition), administer high doses of cortisone to achieve adrenal suppression. This is combined with 5-fluorouracil (5-FU).

Chemotherapy

1. Antimetabolites: 5-fluorouracil (5-FU) combined with adrenalectomy (see p. 970, chemotherapy)	Permits a satisfactory mode of palliation and allows return to normal activity	Toxic effects: stomatitis, nausea and vomiting, diarrhea, alopecia, burning sensation in mouth from acid foods	Provide frequent mouth care. Use topical anesthesia for mouth before meals. Administer antiemetics. Change narcotics as tolerance for each develops.
2. Alkylating agents	When above are no longer effective, switch to other chemotherapeutic agents: cyclophosphamide (Cytoxan); (Thiotepa).	Bone marrow depression, cystitis, alopecia, jaundice	

(continued)

TABLE 43-1 (*continued*)

Palliative Therapy	Objectives of Therapy	Concomitant Effects	Essential Nursing Intervention
Chemotherapy			
3. Corticosteroids (prednisone)	Suppresses estrogen production by the adrenals and decreases urinary estrogenic metabolites	Does not bring about hypercalcemia as does androgen or estrogen therapy It is a good hormonal treatment for brain metastasis. Induces some degree of Cushing's syndrome: fullness of face, gain in body weight, and edema of lower extremities	(See p. 971, steroid therapy)
4. Antiestrogen tamoxifen citrate (Nolvadex)	Effective in palliative treatment in postmenopausal women with positive assays for estrogen receptors May permit delay or avoidance of adrenalectomy of hypophysectomy	Adverse effects usually transient: thrombocytopenia, leukopenia Appears less toxic than other agents	Expect nausea, vomiting, hot flashes. May cause weight gain, vaginal bleeding and discharge, rashes, thrombophlebitis, hypercalcemia.
5. Enzyme antagonist (aminogluthemide)	Inhibition of estrogen synthesis with enzyme antagonists	Adrenal inhibitor	
Radiation (see p. 270)	Effective in relieving pain More effective in skeletal metastasis; less effective in visceral metastasis	Depends on area affected: Chest: esophagitis, pneumonitis, shortness of breath, slight cough Abdomen: affects digestion Body: general lethargy	Administer pain-relieving medication as required until effects of radiation lessen the need for such drugs. Recognize that fatigue and weakness often result from radiation. When pain is controlled, instruct patient to take extra precautions in order to avoid pathologic fractures: avoid lifting heavy packages and children and strenuous arm movements, such as those used in sweeping.
Oophorectomy	Castration removes cyclic hormone stimulation of the tumor. Preferred for premenopausal women: 1. Surgical ⟶ Immediate estrogen withdrawal 2. Radiation ⟶ Estrogen withdrawal takes 4–6 weeks If breast cancer is localized to breast, oophorectomy may or may not be advised.		(See p. 343 for surgical care.)

(*continued*)

TABLE 43-1 *(continued)*

Palliative Therapy	Objectives of Therapy	Concomitant Effects	Essential Nursing Intervention
Hormonal Therapy	Androgens, fluoxymesterone (Halotestin) for premenopausal women Estrogens (diethylstilbestrol) for postmenopausal patients	Masculinization ⟶ Fluid retention Cholestatic jaundice Hypercalcemia ⟶	Watch for signs of increased libido, deepening voice, facial hirsutism. Note serum calcium levels. Observe for signs of: lethargy, insomnia, thirst, nausea, vomiting, thickened speech, fluid retention, collapse, coma. Assist with treatment: Moderately high doses of corticosteroids, vigorous hydration, low-calcium diet
Adrenalectomy Bilateral posterior (flank), or anterior with oophorectomy	Removes another source of endogenous estrogens Effective for metastasis to viscera or bone	Removes a hormone essential to life ⟶	Replace cortisone daily for rest of patient's life. Otherwise, adrenal crisis results. Symptoms: hypotension, diarrhea, nausea and vomiting, elevated temperature, weakness, abdominal pain

be recognized early enough because of the musculocutaneous flap used in reconstruction or the presence of the implanted prosthesis. Proponents for immediate reconstruction argue that such a delay in diagnosis would be minimal, especially in view of the psychological benefits to be gained from the procedure. Meanwhile, the criteria used for selecting patients for breast reconstruction following mastectomy are being developed to reduce the risk of potential recurrence of malignancy. Varying opinions for delay suggest waiting 2 to 5 years after completion of chemotherapy or radiation therapy or 6 months after mastectomy.

Procedures. The choice of the method used for reconstruction is based on the condition of the overlying skin and the status of the underlying muscle. The latissimus dorsi and the abdominis myocutaneous flap are two of the more popular sources of tissue. The surgical procedures are described in Figures 43-7 and 43-8.

Postoperative Nursing Management. Suction tubes attached to closed drainage are placed in the breast and the donor area. Measures are used to reduce tension on the incisions. Elevating the head of the bed 30 degrees and flexing the knees will relieve tension on the abdominal incision. Antiemetics may be prescribed to control nausea and vomiting. Analgesics may help to relieve discomfort. The color and temperature of the newly reconstructed breast area should

be observed frequently to assess circulation. Mottling or an obvious temperature drop should be reported immediately as possible signs that circulation is impaired. Drainage of more than 50 ml/hr must also be reported. Dietary and other measures (described on p. 348) are taken to prevent flatus and abdominal distention.

When ambulating the first postoperative day, the patient may assume positions that favor incision-line protection; gradually a more upright positon is encouraged and will be achieved. A brassiere is not worn for several weeks, and the breast is not massaged until the physician indicates that no injury will result. As expected, the woman should not elevate her arms above the shoulder level or lift more than 5 pounds for at least a month.

Diseases of the Male Breast

In the male, *gynecomastia* (overdeveloped breast tissue) is the most frequently encountered breast condition. It affects about 40% of adolescent males, probably in relation to hormones being secreted by the testes, and disappears within 1 or 2 years. It may occur in prepubertal boys as well as adult males. Gynecomastia is usually unilateral and presents as a

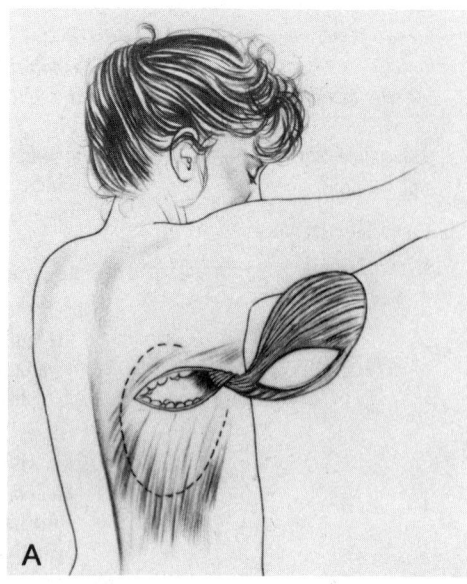

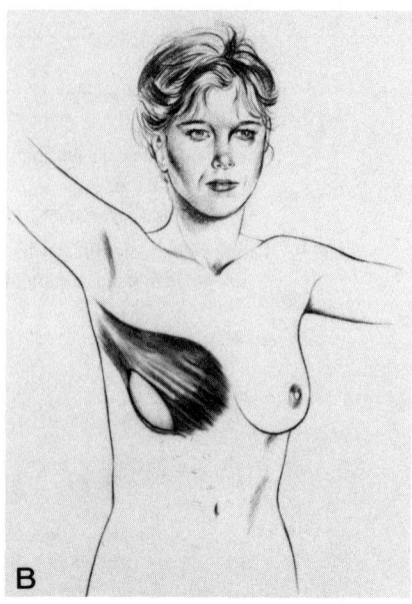

An elliptical incision identifies the skin tissue (island) that will be attached to dissected latissimus dorsi muscle (dissected underneath skin in area of dotted line). When freed but with one end attached, this muscle and skin flap (note arrow) is then threaded through a tunnel under the skin (subaxillary) and brought out at the breast site.

Flap in place after being tunneled from back to front of the chest.

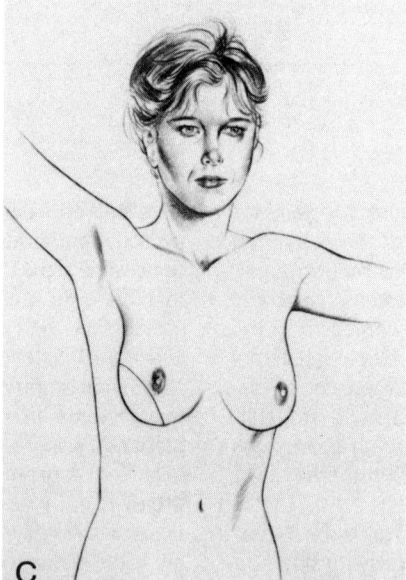

Flap is in place re-creating breast contour with reconstructed nipple and areola.

Figure 43-7
Breast reconstruction: Myocutaneous flap procedure using latissimus dorsi muscle. (Adapted from The Breast Cancer Digest, 2nd ed. Bethesda, Maryland, US Department of Health and Human Services, Public Health Service.)

firm, circular, tender mass beneath the areola. In the adult male, diffuse gynecomastia may occur and may be related to certain drugs the patient is taking, such as digitalis, reserpine, ergotamine, and phenytoin. Pain and tenderness are initial symptoms. One percent of malignant breast lesions occur in the male. Usually, the man discovers the malignancy as a painless lump beneath the areola. Other symptoms are nipple discharge (occasionally bloody), possible nipple retraction, and skin ulceration. Diagnostic and treatment modalities are similar to those used for women. Since the average age of the male breast cancer patient is 5 years older than women, the death rate appears higher. When the age difference is taken into account, the mortality rate is about the same.

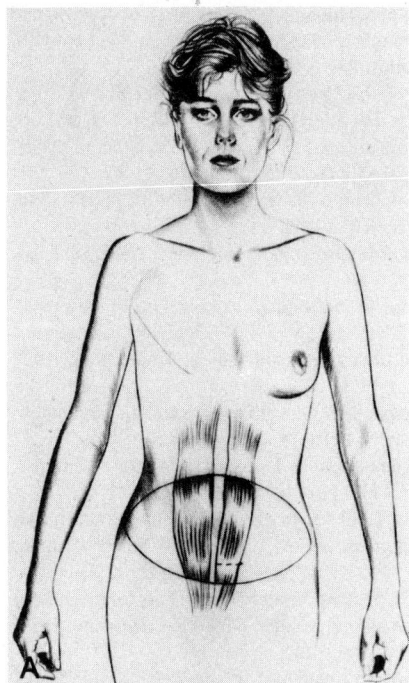

An elliptical lower abdominal incision is made, and one of two vertical abdominal muscles is cut.

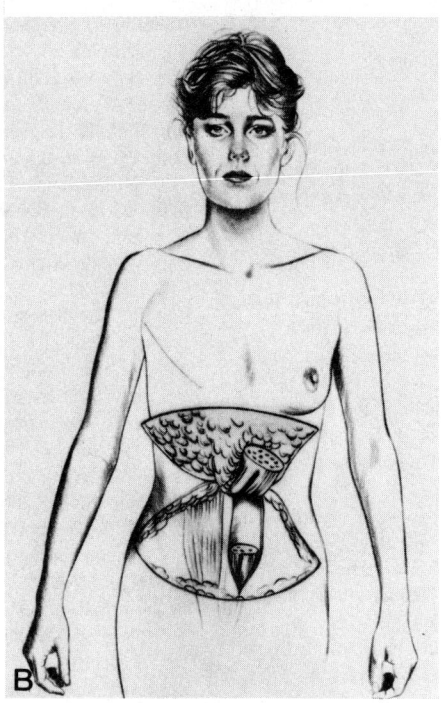

The skin flap including muscle and fat is then tunneled under the skin of upper abdominal and lower chest to the breast site.

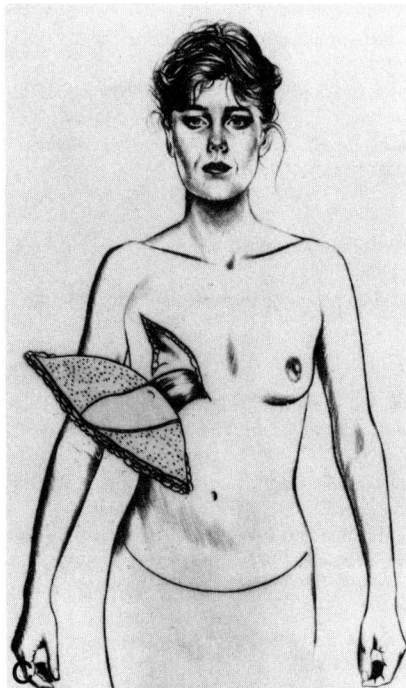

The flap will be positioned and molded to the contour of the breast. Blood supply continues with flap.

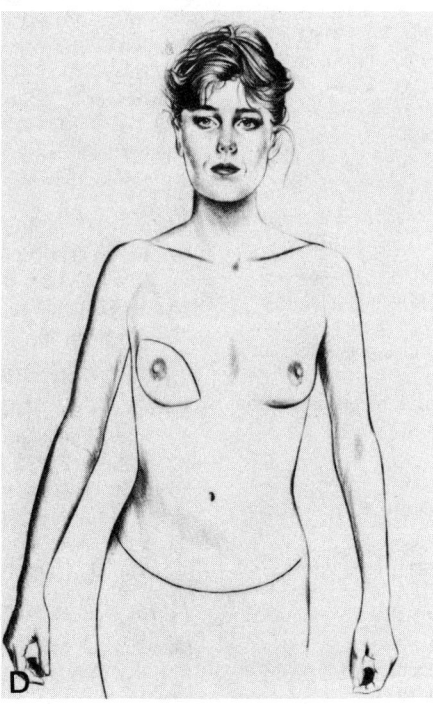

Flap in place re-creating breast contour with reconstructed nipple and areola.

Figure 43-8
Breast reconstruction: Myocutaneous flap procedure using abdominis rectus muscle. (Adapted from The Breast Cancer Digest, 2nd ed. Bethesda, Maryland, US Department of Health and Human Services, Public Health Service.)

Bibliography

Books

Ariel IM and Cleary JB. Breast Cancer. New York, McGraw-Hill, 1987.

Breast Cancer Digest, 2nd ed, publication No. 84-1691. Bethesda, Maryland, U.S. Department of Health and Human Services, National Cancer Institute, 1984.

Graham J. In the Company of Others. New York, Harcourt Brace Jovanovich, 1982.

Haagensen C. Diseases of the Breast. Philadelphia, WB Saunders, 1986.

Harris JR et al. Breast Diseases. Philadelphia, JB Lippincott, 1987.

Harris J et al. Conservative Management of Breast Cancer. Philadelphia, JB Lippincott, 1983.

Ichinoe K. Functional Preservation of Gynecologic Reproductive Organs. Sapporo, Japan, Hokkaido University School of Medicine, 1986.

Kisner C and Colby LA. Therapeutic Exercises: Foundations and Techniques. Philadelphia, FA Davis, 1985.

Kushner R. If You've Thought about Breast Cancer (booklet). Kensington, Maryland, Women's Breast Cancer Advisory Center, 1985.

Nealon TF (ed). Problems in General Surgery: Controversies in Cancer of the Breast and Colon, vol 2, No. 2. Philadelphia, JB Lippincott, 1985.

Pfeiffer CH and Mulliken JB (eds). Caring for the Patient with Breast Cancer. Reston, Virginia, Reston Publishing Co, 1984.

Articles

(Asterisks indicate nursing research articles.)

General Articles

Holleb AI: Interview: Progress against breast cancer. Cancer Nurs 1984 Spring/Summer; 38(2):7-9.

LaCroix AZ and Hukla BS. Are OCS (oral contraceptives) dangerous for women with benign breast disease or a family history of breast cancer? Your Patient and Cancer 1984 May; 9(6):27-32.

*Rutledge DN. Factors related to women's practice of breast self-examination. Nurs Res 1987 Mar/Apr; 36(2):117-121.

Etiology

Hildreth NG et al. Risk of breast cancer among women receiving radiation treatment in infancy for thymic enlargement. Lancet 1983 July 30; 2(8344):273.

*Larson E. Epidemiological correlates of breast, endometrial, and ovarian cancers. CA Nurs 1983 Aug; 6(4):295-301.

Rosenberg L et al. Breast cancer and cigarette smoking. N Engl J Med 1984 Jan 12; 310(2):92-94.

Senie RT, Rosen PP, and Kinne DW. Epidemiologic factors associated with breast cancer. CA Nurs 1983 Oct; 6(5):367-371.

Assessment and Detection

Arter AM. Now—a better way for patients to learn BSE. Your Patient and Cancer 1984 Feb; 4(2):23, 27.

Baines CJ. Breast self-examination: The doctor's role. Hosp Pract 1984 Mar; 19(3):120-127.

Bennett SE et al. Profile of women practicing breast self-examination. JAMA 1983 Jan 28; 249(4):488-491.

Bolsen B. Ultrasound breast scanning: (only) a complement to mammography? JAMA 1982 Sept 3; 248(9):1025-1027.

*Brailey LJ. Effects of health teaching in the workplace on women's knowledge, beliefs, and practices regarding breast self-examination. Res Nurs Health 1986 Sep; 9(3):223-231.

*Champion VL. Use of the health belief model in determining frequency of breast self-examination. Res Nurs Health 1985 Dec; 8(4):373-379.

Cohen MI et al. Mammography in women less than 40 years of age. Surg Gynecol Obstet 1985 Mar; 160(3):220-222.

*Edgar L, Shamian J, and Patterson D. Factors affecting the nurse as a teacher and practicer of breast self-examination. Int J Nurs Stud 1984; 2(4):255-265.

Hallal JC. The relationship of health beliefs, health locus of control, and self-concept to the practice of breast self-exam in adult women. Nurs Res 1983 May/June; 31(3):137-142.

Harper AP. Mammography. Hosp Med 1985 Apr; 21(4):189-208.

Kegels SS. Breast self-exam. Pat Educ Lett 1984 Apr; 7(2):1-2, 8.

Keith LG et al. Breast examination: I. The physician's dilemma "What am I feeling?" Prim Care Cancer 1984 Sept; 4(8):41-47.

Keith LG et al. Breast examination: II. Narrowing the diagnosis. Prim Care Cancer 1984 Oct; 4(9):37-42.

King M. Mammography: Good news, bad news. Cancer News 1985 Autumn; 2-5.

King RC. Detailed guidelines for a thorough examination of the breast. RN 1982 July; 45(7):57-63.

*Lashley ME. Predictors of breast self-examination. Adv Nurs Sci 1987 July; 9(4):16-24.

*Lauver D. Theoretical perspectives relevant to breast self-examination. Adv Nurs Sci 1987 July; 9(4):16-24.

Lee Y-TM. Limitation of mammography in detecting breast carcinoma. Med Times 1986 Apr; 114(4):31-39.

Marty PJ, McDermott RJ, and Gold RS. An assessment of three alternative formats for promoting breast self-examination. CA Nurs 1983 June; 6(3):207-211.

McDermott RJ and Marty PJ. Seeking an effective strategy for promoting breast self-examination among women. Pat Educ Counselling 1984; 6(3):116-124.

Moskowitz M. Benefit/risk ratio for mammography screening. Med Times 1985 Oct; 113(10):48-52.

Newsome JF and McLelland R. A word of caution concerning mammography. JAMA 1986 Jan 3; 255(1):528.

Oberst MT. Testing approaches to teaching breast self-examination. CA Nurs 1981 June; 4(3):246.

Rudolph A and McDermott RJ. The breast physical examination. Cancer Nurs 1987 Apr; 10(2):100-106.

Scanlon EF. How we do a breast palpation. Primary Care Cancer 1984 July; 4(6):35-43.

Schydlower M. Breast masses in adolescents. Am Fam Physician 1982 Feb; 25(2):141-145.

Wertheimer MD et al. Increasing the effort toward breast cancer detection. JAMA 1986 Mar 14; 255(10):1311-1315.

Risks

Webster LA et al. Alcohol consumption and risk of breast cancer. Lancet 1983 Sept 24; 2(8352):724-726.

Wynder EL and Rose DP. Diet and breast cancer. Hosp Pract 1984 Apr; 19(4):73-88.

Psychosocial Implications

Meyerowtiz BE, Watkins IK, and Sparks FC. Quality of life for breast cancer patients receiving adjuvant chemotherapy. Am J Nurs 1983 Feb; 83(2):232-235.

Scott DW. Quality of life following the diagnosis of breast cancer. Topics Clin Nurs 1983 Jan; 4(4):20-37.

*Scott DW. Anxiety, critical thinking and information processing during and after breast biopsy. Nurs Res 1983 Jan/Feb; 32(1):24-28.

Fibrocystic Breast Disease

Humphrey LJ. Relieving the symptoms of fibrocystic disease. Your Patient and Cancer. 1984 Apr; 4(4):49-52.

Lesnick GJ. How best to proceed when the diagnosis is fibrocystic breast disease. Your Patient and Cancer 1983 Feb; 3(2):39-48, 53.

Love SM, Gelman RS, and Silen W. Fibrocystic "disease" of the breast a non-disease? N Engl J Med 1982 Oct 14; 16(307):1010-1014.

Breast Cancer

Ashikari RH. Modified radical mastectomy. Surg Clin North Am 1984 Dec; 64(6):1095-1102.

Baker RR. Preoperative assessment of the patient with breast cancer. Surg Clin North Am 1984 Dec; 64(6):1039-1050.

Breast cancer: The challenge of early detection. Harvard Med School Lett 1983 Feb; 8(4):2-3, 5.

Bullough B. Nurses as teachers and support persons for breast cancer patients. CA Nurs 1981 June; 4(3):221–225.

Charlson ME. Delay in the treatment of carcinoma of the breast. Surg Gynecol Obstet 1985 May; 160(5):393–398.

Cohen RJ. Diagnosis: Breast cancer. Hosp Med 1984 July; 20(7):81–102.

Cooperman AM and Hermann RE. Breast cancer: An overview. Surg Clin North Am 1984 Dec; 64(6):1031–1038.

Fisher B and Wickerham L. Answers to questions about breast cancer. Am Fam Physician 1986 Apr; 33(4):214–222.

Foster RS. Breast cancer: Detection, diagnosis, staging, and adjuvant systemic therapy. Curr Concepts Oncol 1984 Summer; 6(2):2–9.

Goldie JH. Breast cancer: Why some women respond to chemotherapy while others don't. Your Patient and Cancer 1984 Jan; 4(1):59–68.

Glick JH. Breast cancer: Endorsing two therapies. Almanac (University of Pennsylvania) 1985 Sept 17; 32(4):1.

Greifzu S. Breast cancer: The risks and the options. RN 1986 Oct; 26–31.

Greiner L and Weiler C. Early-stage breast cancer. What do women know about treatment choices? Am J Nurs 1983 Nov; 83(11):1570.

Gump FE. Premalignant diseases of the breast. Surg Clin North Am 1984 Dec; 64(6):1051–1059.

Harris JR. Management of localized breast cancer. Hosp Pract 1986 Oct 15; 21(10):61–72.

Hermann RE et al. Partial mastectomy without radiation therapy. Surg Clin North Am 1984 Dec; 64(6):1103–1113.

Holmes P. 'Why me?' Nurs Times 1986 Jan 8; 82(2):16–17.

*Kramer MA Sr, Albrecht S, and Miller RA. Handedness and the laterality of breast cancer in women. Nurs Res 1985 Nov/Dec; 34(6):333–337.

Leis HP, Cammarota A, and LaRaja RD. Update in primary potentially curable breast cancer therapy. Contemp Surg 1985 Feb; 26(2):13–43.

*Lierman LM. Support for mastectomy: A clinical nursing research study. AORN J 1984 June; 39(7):1150–1157.

Lipnick RJ et al. Oral contraceptives and breast cancer. JAMA 1986 Jan 3; 255(1):58–61.

Lippman ME. Management of breast cancer with hormones and drugs. Hosp Pract 1986 May 15; 21(5):119–131.

*Massey V. Perceived susceptibility to breast cancer and practice of breast self-examination. Nurs Res 1986 May/June; 35(3):183–185.

*Ray C et al. Nurses' perceptions of early breast cancer and mastectomy, and their psychological implications, and of the role of health professionals in providing support. Int J Nurs Stud 1984; 21(2):101–111.

Wertheimer MD et al. Increasing the effort toward breast cancer detection. JAMA 1986 Mar 14; 255(10):1311–1315.

Wolberg WH. Convention and controversies in the surgical approach to benign and malignant breast disease. Surg Ann 1985; 17:271–286.

Male Breast Cancer

Male breast cancer. In the Breast Cancer Digest, 2nd ed, Chap 12, publication No. 84-1691. Bethesda, Maryland, U.S. Department of Health and Human Services, National Cancer Institute, 1984.

Roses DF and Harris MN. Male Breast Cancer. Hosp Med 1985 Oct; 21(10):23–40.

Management

Surgery

Aitken DR and Minto JP. Complications associated with mastectomy. Surg Clin North Am 1983 Dec; 63(6):1331–1352.

Gilliland MD et al. The implications of local recurrence of breast cancer as the first site of therapeutic failure. Ann Surg 1983 Mar; 197(3):284–290.

O'Brien RL. Breast cancer treatment—current status. Postgrad Med 1983 Sept; 74(3):124–125.

Pilch YH. Breast cancer treatment: I. Mastectomy, standard surgical approach. Postgrad Med 1983 Sept; 74(3):126–134.

Pilch YH. Breast cancer treatment: II. Segmental mastectomy, alternative to total breast excision? Postgrad Med 1983 Sept; 74(3):139–146.

Science and the citizen: More or less? (Lumpectomy vs mastectomy). Sci Am 1985 Aug; 253(2):59.

Radiation

Carrier R and Martel G. Working with radiation: Reducing the risks. Can Nurse 1985 Oct; 81(9):18–20.

Gilman CJ. Primary radiotherapy in early breast cancer. Am Fam Physician 1982 Apr; 25(4):113–117.

Hassey KM, Bloom LS, and Burgess SL. Radiation—alternative to mastectomy. Am J Nurs 1983 Nov; 83(11):1567–1569.

Rosenal L. Radiotherapy nurse: Developing a new role. Can Nurse 1985 Oct; 81(9):21–23.

Wilson JF. Breast cancer treatment: III. Simple excision with irradiation. Postgrad Med 1983 Sept; 74(3):151–158.

Chemotherapy

Derby CE. Alternate methods of chemotherapy administration. Can Nurse 1985 Oct; 81(9):44–45.

Hopkins MB. Information-seeking and adaptational outcomes in women receiving chemotherapy for breast cancer. Cancer Nurs 1986 Oct; 9(5):256–262.

Kiang DT et al. A randomized trial of chemotherapy and hormonal therapy in advanced breast cancer. N Engl J Med 1985 Nov 14; 313(20):1283–1284.

Ludwig Breast Cancer Study Group. Toxic effects of early adjuvant chemotherapy for breast cancer. Lancet 1983 Sept 3; 2(8439):542–544.

Mitchell MS. Breast cancer treatment. Postgrad Med 1983 Sept; 74(3):161–175.

Breast Augmentation/Reconstruction

Dinner MI. Postmastectomy reconstruction. Surg Clin North Am 1984 Dec; 64(6):1193–1207.

DiNobile C. Reduction mammoplasty. Today's OR Nurse 1985 Nov; 7(11):18–21.

Frazier TG and Noone RB. An objective analysis of immediate simultaneous reconstruction in the treatment of primary carcinoma of the breast. Cancer 1985 Mar 15; 55(6):1202–1205.

Hoffman LA et al. Avoiding complications in postmastectomy breast reconstruction. Infect Surgery 1983 Sept; 2(9):651–661.

Hutcheson HA. TAIF: New option for breast reconstruction. Nurs '86 1986 Feb; 16(2):52–53.

McGrath MH. The argument for immediate post-mastectomy breast reconstruction. In Nealon TF Jr. Problems in General Surgery: Controversies in Cancer of the Breast and Colon, vol 2, No. 2, pp. 185–195. Philadelphia, JB Lippincott, 1985.

Noone RB et al. A 6-year experience with immediate reconstruction after mastectomy for cancer. Plast Reconstr Surg 1985 Aug; 76(2):258–269.

Snyderson RK. Delayed reconstruction of the breast after mastectomy. In Nealon TF Jr. Problems in General Surgery: Controversies in Cancer of the Breast and Colon, vol 2, No. 2, pp. 196–199. Philadelphia, JB Lippincott, 1985.

Solomon J. The good news about breast reconstruction. RN 1986 Nov; 47–54.

Walsh KC. Breast augmentation: Your patient's adjustment to a new body image. Today's OR Nurse 1986 Sept; 8(9):20–26.

Wellisch DK et al. Psychosocial correlates of immediate versus delayed reconstruction of the breast. Plast Reconstr Surg 1985 Nov; 76(5):713–718.

Advanced Breast Cancer

Cristina AG et al. Intraosseous metastatic breast cancer treatment with internal fixation and study of survival. Ann Surg 1983 Feb; 197(2):128–134.

Agencies

American Cancer Society, 90 Park Avenue, New York, New York 10016.

American Society of Plastic and Reconstructive Surgeons, Inc., 233 North Michigan Avenue, Suite 1900, Chicago, Illinois 60601.

Chapter 44

Management of the Male Patient With Disorders Related to the Reproductive System

In the male, several organs serve as parts of both the urinary tract and the reproductive system. Disease of these organs may produce functional abnormalities of either or both systems. For this reason, diseases of the entire reproductive system in the male usually are treated by the urologist.

Physiologic Overview

The structures included in the male reproductive system are the testes, the vas deferens and the seminal vesicles, the penis, and certain accessory glands, such as the prostate gland and Cowper's gland (Fig. 44-1). The testes are formed in embryonal life within the abdominal cavity near the kidney. During the last month of fetal life, they descend posterior to the peritoneum, to pierce the abdominal wall in the groin. Later they progress along the inguinal canal into the scrotum. In this descent they are accompanied by blood vessels, lymphatics, nerves, and ducts, which, along with supporting tissue, make up the spermatic cord. This cord extends from the internal inguinal ring through the abdominal wall and the inguinal canal to the scrotum. As the testes descend into the scrotum, a tubular process of peritoneum accompanies them. This normally is obliterated, the only remaining portion being that which covers the testes, the *tunica vaginalis*. (When this peritoneal process is not obliterated but remains open into the abdominal cavity, a potential sac remains, into which abdominal contents may enter to form an indirect inguinal hernia.)

The testes proper consist of numerous seminiferous tubules in which are formed the male reproductive elements, the spermatozoa. These are transmitted by a system of collecting tubules into the epididymis, which is a hoodlike structure lying on the testes and containing tortuous ducts that lead into the vas deferens. This firm tubular structure passes upward through the inguinal canal to enter the abdominal cavity behind the peritoneum and then extends downward toward the base of the bladder. An outpouching from this structure is the seminal vesicle, which acts as a reservoir for the secretion of the testes. The tract is continued as the ejaculatory duct, which then passes through the prostate gland

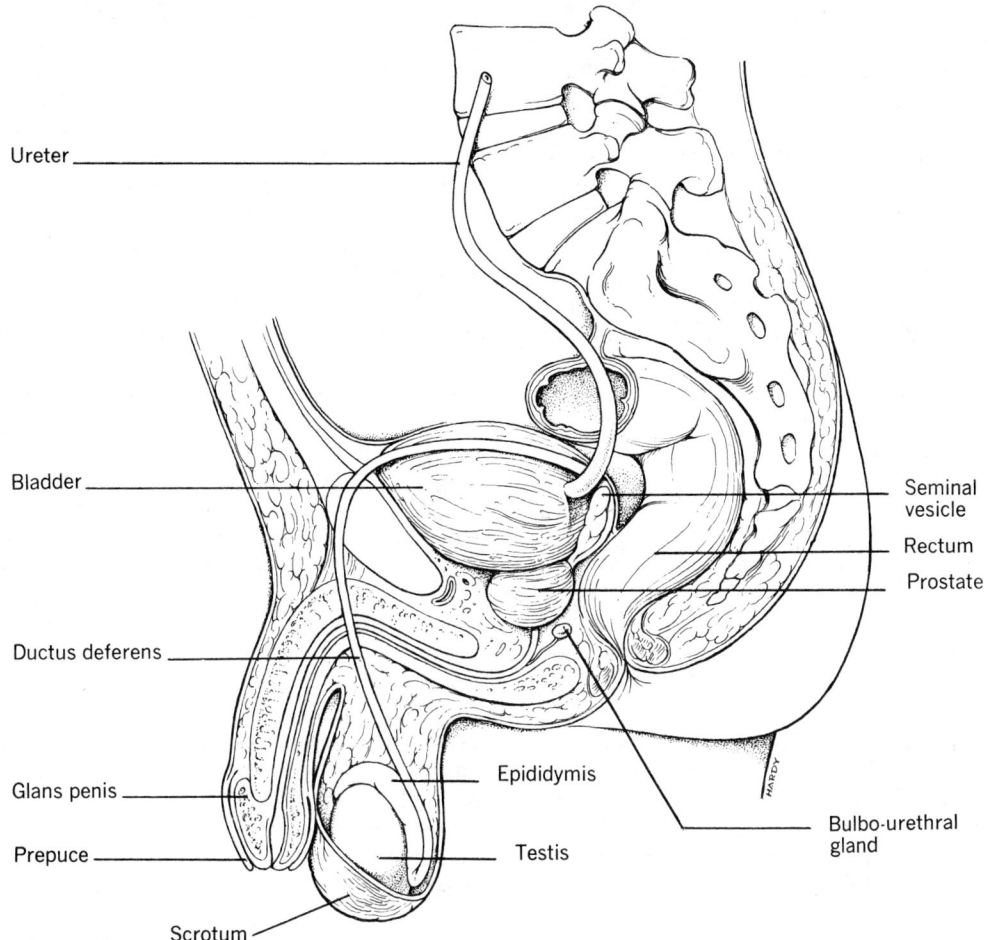

Figure 44-1
Organs of the male reproductive system. (Chaffee EE and Greisheimer EM. Basic
Physiology and Anatomy, 3rd ed. Philadelphia, JB Lippincott.)

to enter the urethra. The secretion of the testes is carried by
this pathway to the end of the penis in the reproductive act.

The testes have a dual function. The primary function is
reproduction—the formation of spermatozoa from the germinal cells of the seminiferous tubules. However, the testes
are also important glands of internal secretion. This secretion
is produced by the so-called interstitial cells and is called the
male sex hormone, or testosterone,which induces and preserves the male sex qualities.

The prostate gland lies just below the neck of the bladder.
It surrounds the urethra posteriorly and laterally and is tra-
versed by the ejaculatory duct, the continuation of the vas
deferens. This gland produces a secretion that is chemically
and physiologically suitable to the needs of the spermatozoa
in their passage from the genital glands.

The penis has a dual function of being the organ of co-
pulation and of urination. Anatomically, it consists of a glans
penis, a body, and a root. The glans penis is the soft, rounded
portion at the end that retains its soft structure even when
erect. The urethra opens at the extremity of the glans. The
glans normally is covered or protected by an elongation of
the skin of the penis—the foreskin—which may be retracted
to expose the glans. The body of the penis is composed of
erectile tissues that contain numerous blood vessels that may

become distended during sexual excitement. Through it
passes the urethra, which extends from the bladder through
the prostate to the end of the penis.

Congenital Malformations.   Of the many disturbances
of normal growth that may occur, the most common is a
failure of the testes to descend into the scrotum. This condition is called *cryptorchidism*.

Failure of the urethra to form normally in the penis can
result in hypospadias or epispadias. *Hypospadias* occurs
when the urethral opening is a groove on the underside of
the penis; when the urethral opening is on the dorsum of the
penis the condition is called *epispadias*. These anatomical
abnormalities may be repaired by various types of plastic
surgery.

Gerontological Considerations

As the male ages, the prostate gland hypertrophies (enlarges),
prostate secretion decreases, the scrotum hangs lower, the
testes become smaller and more firm, and pubic hair becomes
sparser and stiffer.

Changes in gonad function include a decline in the concentration of plasma testosterone and a reduction in the
amount of progesterone produced.

Male reproductive capability is maintained with advancing age. Although degenerative changes occur in the seminiferous tubules, spermatogenesis (production of sperm) remains. However, sexual function, involving libido (desire) and potency, lessens. This decline is more evident in men over age 70 but is also noted in males in their 60s. The lessening of sexual function is affected by a number of factors such as psychological problems, illnesses, and medications. In general, the sexual act takes longer. Sexual activity is closely correlated with the man's sexual activity of his earlier years; if he was more active than the average male as a young man, he will most likely continue to be more active than average in his later years.

Impotence is usually due to either organic or psychogenic factors. Organic causes include vascular insufficiency, diabetes mellitus, and neuropathy that cause erectile dysfunction. Drugs may also affect sexual performance.

Conditions of the Prostate

Prostatitis

Prostatitis is an inflammation of the prostate gland caused by infectious agents (bacteria, fungi, mycoplasma) or by a variety of other problems (*e.g.*, urethral stricture, prostatic hyperplasia). Microorganisms usually are carried to the prostate from the urethra. Prostatitis may be classified as bacterial or abacterial depending on the presence or absence of microorganisms in the prostatic fluid.

The symptoms of prostatitis are many and include perineal discomfort, burning, urgency, and frequency. *Prostatodynia* (pain in the prostate) is manifested by pain on voiding or perineal pain symptoms, but there is no evidence of inflammation or bacterial growth in the prostatic fluid.

Acute bacterial prostatitis may produce a sudden onset of fever and chills and perineal, rectal, or low back pain. Urinary symptoms of burning, frequency, urgency, nocturia, and dysuria may be evident. Some patients, however, are asymptomatic.

Diagnosis requires a careful history, culture of prostatic fluid or tissue, and, occasionally, a histologic examination of tissue. In order to locate the source of the lower genitourinary infection (bladder neck, urethra, prostate), it is necessary to collect a divided urinary specimen for segmental urine culture. After the patient cleanses the glans penis and retracts the foreskin (if present), he voids 10 to 15 ml of urine into the first container. This represents urethral urine. A second voiding of 50 to 75 ml of urine is then collected in a second container without interruption; this represents bladder urine. If the patient does not have acute prostatitis, the physician immediately performs a prostatic massage and any prostatic fluid that is expressed is collected by gravity drainage into a third container. If it is not possible to collect prostatic fluid, the patient voids a small quantity of urine. This specimen may contain the bacteria present in the prostatic fluid.

Management. The goal of management is to avoid the complications of abscess formation and septicemia. A broad-spectrum antimicrobial (to which the organism causing the infection is susceptible) is given for a period of 10 to 14 days.

Intravenous administration of the drug may be necessary to achieve high serum and tissue levels. The patient is encouraged to remain on bed rest since this will alleviate symptoms rapidly. Comfort is promoted with analgesics (pain relief), antispasmodics and bladder sedatives (relieves bladder irritability), sitz baths (relieves pain and spasm), and stool softeners (prevent straining at stool, which increases pain).

Swelling of the gland may produce urinary retention. Other complications include epididymitis, bacteremia or septicemia, and pyelonephritis.

Chronic bacterial prostatitis is a major source of relapsing urinary tract infection in men. The treatment of chronic prostatitis is difficult, because of poor diffusion of most antimicrobials from the plasma into the prostatic fluid. Antimicrobials (trimethoprim-sulfamethoxazole, tetracycline, minocycline, doxycycline) may be given. Continuous suppressive treatment with low-dose antimicrobial drugs may be indicated. The patient is advised of the possibility of relapsing infection. Comfort is promoted with antispasmodics (to relieve bladder irritability), sitz baths, and stool softeners.

The treatment of *nonbacterial prostatitis* is directed toward symptomatic relief: sitz baths, analgesics, etc. The sexual partner should be investigated because of the possibility of cross-infection.

Patient Education. The patient is instructed to take the prescribed antibiotic for the full time period. Hot sitz baths (10–20 minutes) may be taken several times daily. Fluids are encouraged to satisfy thirst, but fluids are not "forced" because an effective drug level must be maintained in the urine. Foods and drink that have diuretic action or increase prostatic secretions should be avoided: alcohol, coffee, tea, chocolate, cola, and spices. During periods of acute inflammation, sexual arousal and intercourse should be avoided. However, sexual intercourse may be beneficial in the treatment of chronic prostatitis. The patient should avoid sitting for long periods of time. Medical follow-up is necessary for at least 6 months to 1 year since recurrence of prostatitis due to the same or different organisms can occur.

Benign Prostatic Hyperplasia

In many patients over 50 years of age, the prostate gland enlarges, extending upward into the bladder and obstructing the outflow of urine by encroaching on the vesical orifice. This condition is known as benign prostatic hyperplasia (enlargement, or hypertrophy, of the prostate). The etiology is uncertain, but evidence suggests a hormonal cause as initiating hyperplasia of the supporting stromal tissue and of glandular elements in the prostate.

Since enlargement of the prostate gland produces an obstruction to flow of urine, a gradual dilatation of the ureters (hydroureter) and kidneys (hydronephrosis) results. The hypertrophied lobes may obstruct the vesical neck or prostatic urethra and thus cause incomplete emptying and urinary retention. Urinary tract infection may result from urinary stasis.

Clinical Manifestations and Diagnostic Evaluation. The symptom complex (referred to as *prostatism*) includes increasing frequency of urination, nocturia, hesitancy in starting urination, a decrease in size and force of urinary stream; interruption of urinary stream; terminal dribbling, in which urine dribbles out after urination; a sensation of incomplete emptying of the bladder; and acute urinary retention. Other generalized symptoms may be noted, including fatigue secondary to nocturia, anorexia, nausea and vomiting due to impaired renal function, and perhaps epigastric discomfort from a distended bladder.

A battery of diagnostic examinations may be performed to determine the degree of prostatic enlargement, the presence of any bladder wall changes, and the efficiency of renal function. Renal function studies may be carried out to determine if there is renal impairment from prostatic back-pressure and to evaluate renal reserve. A complete hematologic investigation is done. Since hemorrhage is a major postoperative complication, all clotting defects must be corrected. A high percentage of these patients have cardiac or respiratory complications, or both.

Management.　The plan of treatment depends on the cause, the severity of the obstruction, and the condition of the patient. If a patient is admitted as an emergency because he is unable to void, he is immediatedly catheterized. The ordinary catheter frequently will be too soft and pliable to pass through the urethra into the bladder. A thin wire, called a stylet, is introduced (by a urologist) into the catheter in order to prevent the catheter from collapsing when it encounters resistance. In severe cases, metal catheters with a pronounced prostatic curve may be used. Sometimes an incision is made into the bladder (a suprapubic cystostomy) to give adequate drainage. Surgery to remove the hyperplastic prostatic tissue is frequently necessary to provide permanent relief of the obstruction. The procedure is referred to as a prostatectomy.

The Patient Undergoing Prostatectomy

The preoperative objectives prior to prostatectomy (removal of the prostate) are to assess the patient's general health status and to establish optimum kidney function. The operation should be done before the development of acute urinary retention and infection and certainly before the upper urinary tract and collecting system are damaged.

Four different approaches are possible in removing the hypertrophied fibroadenomatous portion of the prostate gland (Table 44-1). In all four techniques, all hyperplastic tissue is removed, leaving behind the surgical capsule of the prostate. The transurethral approach is a closed procedure, while the other three are open surgical procedures.

A *transurethral resection* of the prostate is the most common procedure and can be carried out by means of an endoscopic instrument that has ocular and operating systems. The instrument is introduced directly through the urethra to the prostate, which can be viewed directly. The gland is then removed in small chips with an electrical cutting loop (Fig. 44-2*A*). The real advantage of this method is the absence of an incision. It may be used for glands of varying size (urologists differ on how large the prostate must be before considering an open procedure), and it is ideal for most poor-risk patients with small glands. This approach means a shorter hospital stay; however, strictures are more frequent, and repeat operations may be necessary.

Suprapubic prostatectomy is one method of removing the gland through an abdominal wound. An opening is made into the bladder, and the gland is removed from above (Fig. 44-2*B*). Such an approach can be used for a gland of any

size, and few complications occur, although blood loss may be greater than with other methods. Another disadvantage is the need for an abdominal incision with the concomitant hazards of any major surgical procedure.

Perineal prostatectomy involves the removal of the gland through an incision in the perineum (Fig. 44-2*C*). This approach is practical when other approaches are blocked. It is a useful procedure when open biopsy is needed. In the postoperative period, the wound may become contaminated rather easily because of the location of the incision. Incontinence, impotence, or rectal injury are more likely sequelae when this approach is used.

Retropubic prostatectomy is another technique that is more popular than the suprapubic approach. A low abdominal incision is made, and the prostate gland is approached between the pubic arch and the bladder (without entering the bladder) (Fig. 44-2*D*). This procedure is suitable for large glands located high in the pelvis. Blood loss is controlled more easily, and there is better visualization. However, infections can readily start in the retropubic space.

▶ *Nursing Process*
The Patient Undergoing Prostatectomy

▷ *Assessment*

The nurse asks the patient how benign hypertrophy of the prostate has affected his life-style during the past few months. Has he been reasonably active for his age? What is the presenting urinary problem (as described in the patient's words): decreased force of urinary flow, decreased ability to initiate voiding, urgency, frequency, nocturia, dysuria, urinary retention, hematuria? Are there associated aches or pains with the above problems, such as back pain, flank pain, and lower abdominal or suprapubic discomfort? If such discomfort is present, possible causes might be infection, retention, and possibly renal colic.

The nurse determines the patient's family history of cancer and heart or kidney disease, including hypertension. Has he lost weight? Does he appear "colorless" (pallor)? Can he raise himself out of bed and return to bed without assistance? This may help in determining how soon he will be returned to normal activities following prostatectomy.

▷ *Nursing Diagnoses*

Based on the nursing history and all other assessment data, the patient's major nursing diagnoses may include the following:

Preoperative

- Anxiety related to the inability to void
- Knowledge deficit of factors related to his problem and the treatment protocol

Postoperative

- Fluid volume deficit related to fluid loss and possible bleeding
- Alteration in comfort: pain related to the surgical incision, catheter placement, and bladder spasms

TABLE 44-1
Comparison of Surgical Approaches for Prostatectomy

The operation of choice depends on (1) the size of the gland, (2) the severity of the obstruction, (3) the age of the patient, (4) the condition of patient, and (5) the presence of associated diseases.

Surgical Approach	Advantages	Disadvantages	Nursing Implications
Transurethral Resection (removal of prostatic tissue by instrument introduced through urethra)	Avoids abdominal incision Safer for surgical-risk patient Shorter period of hospitalization and convalescence Lower morbidity rate Causes less pain	Requires highly skilled operator Recurrent obstruction, urethral trauma, and stricture may develop. Delayed bleeding may occur.	Watch for evidence of hemorrhage (drainage in bag). Observe for symptoms of urethral stricture (dysuria, straining, small urinary stream).
Open Surgical Removal			
Suprapubic	Technically simple Offers wider area of exploration Permits exploration for cancerous lymph nodes Allows more complete removal of obstructing gland Permits treatment of associated lesions in bladder	Requires surgical approach through the bladder Control of hemorrhage difficult Urinary leakage around suprapubic tube Convalescence more prolonged and uncomfortable	Watch for indications of hemorrhage and shock. Give meticulous aseptic attention to area around suprapubic tube.
Perineal	Offers direct anatomical approach Permits gravity drainage Particularly efficacious for radical cancer therapy Allows hemostasis under direct vision Low mortality rate Less incidence of shock Ideal for very old, feeble, and poor-risk patient with large prostate	Higher postoperative incidence of impotence and urinary incontinency Problem of damage to rectum and external sphincter Restricted operative field Greater potential for infection	Avoid use of rectal tubes, rectal thermometers, and enemas after perineal surgery. Use drainage pads to absorb excess urinary drainage. Provide foam rubber ring for patient comfort in sitting. Urinary leakage may occur around wound for several days after catheter removal.
Retropubic	Avoids incision into the bladder Permits easier visualization and control of bleeders Shorter period of convalescence Less bladder sphincter damage	Cannot treat associated bladder disease Increased incidence of hemorrhage from prostatic venous plexus; osteitis pubis	Watch for evidences of hemorrhage. Posturinary leakage may occur for several days after catheter is removed.

- Potential for infection related to bacterial invasion of the incision
- Knowledge deficit related to postoperative and convalescent management

▷ *Planning and Implementation*

▷ *Goals:* The patient's major *preoperative* goals may include reduction of anxiety and learning about the prostate problem and the perioperative experience. His major *postoperative* goals may include correction of fluid volume dis-

turbances, relief of pain and discomfort, prevention of infection, and ability to perform self-care activities.

Preoperative Nursing Interventions

Reduction of Anxiety. The nurse familiarizes the patient with his hospital environment and initiates measures to reduce his anxiety. Communication is established regarding his understanding of his problem and what the physician has already told him. He may be sensitive and embarrassed to discuss problems related to the genital area. Privacy is pro-

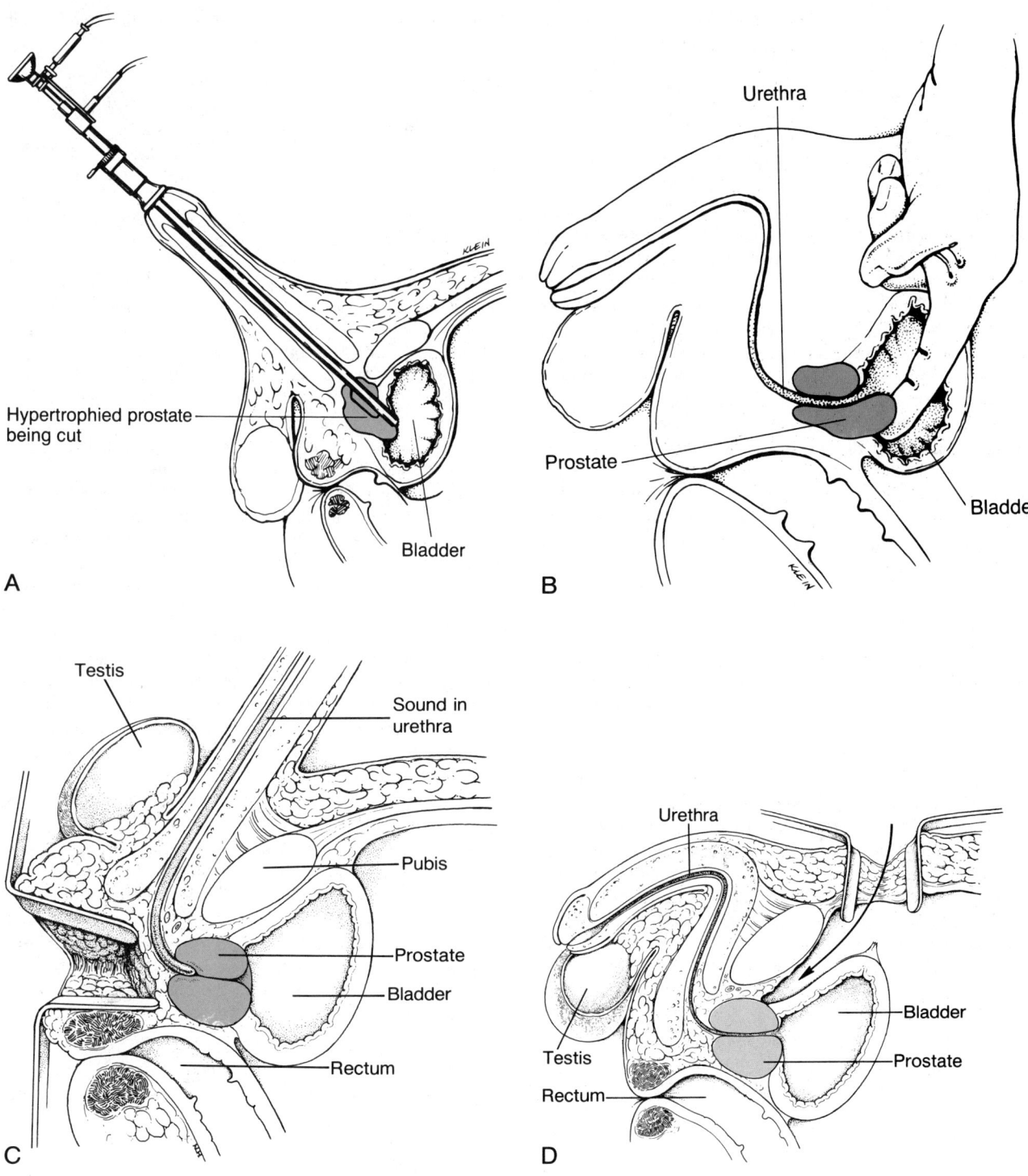

Figure 44-2

Prostatectomy procedures. (*A*) Transurethral resection (TUR). A loop of wire connected with a cutting current is rotated in the cystoscope to remove shavings of prostate at the bladder orifice. (*B*) Suprapubic prostatectomy. Using an abdominal approach, the prostate is shelled out of its bed by the surgeon's fingers. (*C*) Perineal prostatectomy. Two retractors on the left spread the perineal incision in providing a view of the prostate. (*D*) Retropubic prostatectomy is done through a low abdominal incision. Note two abdominal retractors and arrow approaching the prostate gland.

vided, and a trusting and professional relationship is developed with the patient since he often has related sexual concerns that may need to be discussed. Guilt feelings often surface as he falsely assumes a cause-and-effect relation between early sexual practices and his current problems. In short, his verbalization of concerns is encouraged.

Patient Education.   A convenient time is established for the patient (ensuring his privacy) to review the anatomy of the affected parts and how they function in relation to the urinary and reproductive systems. Diagrams may be effective in the teaching process. The nurse reinforces what will take place as the patient is prepared for diagnostic tests and then for surgery. (The protocol is differentiated as it relates to the specific type of prostatectomy planned for the particular patient). The nurse describes the nature of the incision because this varies—it could be directly over the bladder, low on the abdomen, in the perineal area, or performed through a resectoscope, in which case there is no external incision. The patient is informed of drainage expectations, the type of anesthesia, and the recovery room procedure. The amount of information is limited to the point of meeting the patient's needs and relieving his concerns. All procedures about the immediate perioperative period are explained, questions are answered, and support is provided.

Comfort Measures.   If the patient presents with signs and symptoms of discomfort, he is placed on bed rest and comfort measures such as reducing his anxiety and administering the prescribed sedation are initiated. The nurse monitors the patient's voiding patterns, observes for bladder distention, and assists with catheterization for retention. An indwelling catheter is introduced if the patient has continuing urinary retention or if there is evidence of azotemia (accumulation of nitrogenous waste products in the blood). It may be desirable to decompress the bladder gradually over a period of several days, especially if the patient is elderly and hypertensive and has diminished renal function or an excessive amount of urinary retention that has existed for many weeks. *The blood pressure may fluctuate and renal function declines the first few days after bladder drainage is instituted.* If the patient cannot tolerate a urethral catheter, he is prepared for a cystostomy (see pp. 1013 and 1064).

Preoperative Preparation.   When the patient is scheduled for a prostatectomy, the preparation described in Chapter 17 is followed. Antiembolism stockings are applied before the operation and are particularly important if the patient is placed in a lithotomy position during surgery. The preoperative enema may prevent postoperative straining, which can induce postoperative bleeding.

Postoperative Nursing Interventions

Assessing for Potential Complications.   Following prostatectomy, it is important to be on the alert for major complications such as hemorrhage, infection, thrombosis, and catheter obstruction.

Hemorrhage.   Since a hyperplastic prostate gland is very vascular, the immediate dangers following a prostatectomy are bleeding and shock. Bleeding may occur from the bed of the prostate. Bleeding may also result in the formation of clots, which then obstruct the flow of urine. The drainage

begins as reddish pink and then clears to a light pink within 24 hours after operation.

- Bright red bleeding with increased viscosity and numerous clots usually indicates arterial bleeding. Venous bleeding appears darker and less viscous.
- Arterial hemorrhage usually requires surgical intervention (*e.g.,* suturing of bleeders or transurethral coagulation of bleeders), while venous bleeding may be controlled by applying traction to the catheter so that the balloon applies pressure to the prostatic fossa.

Infection and Thrombosis.   Following perineal prostatectomy, the urologist changes the dressing on the first postoperative day; after that it may become the nurse's responsibility. Careful aseptic technique is practiced, since the possibility of infection is great. Dressings can be held in place by a double-tailed T-binder bandage or a padded athletic supporter. The tails cross over the incision to give double thickness, and then each tail is drawn up on either side of the scrotum to the waistline and is fastened.

Rectal temperatures, rectal tubes, and enemas are to be avoided because of the danger of causing trauma and bleeding in the prostatic fossa. After the perineal sutures are removed, the perineum is cleansed as requested. A heat lamp may be directed to the perineal area to promote healing. The scrotum is protected with a towel while the heat lamp is in use. Sitz baths are also used to encourage healing.

In addition to hemorrhage, urinary tract infections and epididymitis are possible complications following prostatectomy. A vasectomy may be performed during surgery to prevent retrograde spread of infection from the prostatic urethra through the vas and into the epididymis. If epididymitis occurs, it is managed as discussed on page 1161.

Patients undergoing prostatectomy (with the exception of transurethral resection) have a high incidence of deep-vein thrombosis and pulmonary embolism. Low-dose heparin therapy may be required prophylactically.

Catheter Obstruction.   Following a transurethral prostatic resection, *the catheter must drain well;* an obstructed catheter will produce distention of the prostatic capsule with resultant hemorrhage. Sometimes furosemide is prescribed to initiate postoperative diuresis, thereby helping to keep the catheter patent.

- Watch and palpate the lower abdomen to see that no blockage of the catheter is occurring. An overdistended bladder presents a distinct rounded swelling above the pubis.
- Check the drainage bag, dressings, and incision site for evidence of bleeding. Note color of urine; change in color from pink to amber indicates lessened bleeding.
- Monitor the blood pressure, pulse, and respirations and compare with the preoperative vital signs to assess for hypotension. Observe the patient for restlessness; cold, sweating skin; pallor; fall in blood pressure; and an increasing pulse rate.

Drainage of the bladder may be accomplished by gravity through a closed sterile system of drainage. A three-way system is useful in cleansing the bladder and preventing clot formation. Some urologists prefer to leave an indwelling catheter attached to dependent drainage. The catheter can be gently irrigated with a plunger syringe to remove any obstructing clots.

- If the patient complains of pain, check the tubing and irrigate the system, thereby correcting any obstruction, before administering an analgesic. Usually, the catheter is irrigated with 50 ml of irrigating fluid at a time, making sure that the same amount is recovered in the drainage bag.
- Avoid overdistending the bladder, which can produce secondary hemorrhage by stretching the coagulated vessels in the prostatic capsule.
- Maintain an input and output record, including the amount of fluid used for irrigation.

The drainage tube (not the catheter) is taped to the shaved inner thigh to prevent traction on the bladder. If a cystostomy catheter is in place, it is taped to the abdomen. The nurse reexplains to the patient the purpose of the catheter and assures him that the urge to void is from the presence of the catheter and bladder spasms. He is cautioned not to pull on the catheter, since this causes bleeding, subsequent plugging of the tubing, and urinary retention.

Catheter Removal. After the catheter is removed (usually when the urine clears), urinary leakage may occur around the wound for several days in patients who have undergone perineal, suprapubic, and retropubic surgery. The cystostomy tube may be removed before or after the urethral catheter is removed. Some urinary incontinence may occur after the catheter is removed. The patient is told that this will probably disappear in time.

Pain Relief. Usually following a prostatectomy, the patient is kept on bed rest for the first 24 hours. If pain occurs, the cause and location must be determined. It may be related to the incision; it may be due to excoriation of the skin at the catheter site; it may be in the flank area, indicating a kidney problem; or it may be due to bladder spasms. Bladder irritability can initiate bleeding and result in clot retention.

Before administering the prescribed medication for pain relief, the patient's vital signs, including blood pressure are checked; then the drainage tubing is checked and the system is irrigated as prescribed, thus correcting any obstruction that may cause discomfort. Usually, the catheter is irrigated with 50 ml of irrigating fluid at a time, making sure that the same amount is recovered in the drainage receptacle.

Discomfort may be caused by dressings that are too snug or have become saturated with drainage or are not properly placed.

Patient Education and Home Health Care. When the patient is ambulatory, he is encouraged to walk but not to sit for prolonged periods, since this increases intra-abdominal pressure and increases the possibility of discomfort and bleeding. The bowel movements are kept soft (prune juice, stool softeners) to prevent excessive straining. If an enema is prescribed, it is administered with caution to avoid possible rectal perforation.

As the days pass and drainage tubes are removed, the patient often shows signs of discouragement and depression because he is not able to regain bladder control immediately. Urinary frequency and burning may occur after the catheter is removed. The following exercises are helpful for regaining urinary control:

- Tense the perineal muscles by pressing the buttocks together; hold this position; relax. This exercise, done 10 to 20 times each hour, can be performed while sitting or standing.
- Try to shut off the urinary stream after starting to void; wait a few seconds and then continue to void.

Perineal exercises are continued until full urinary control is gained. The patient should be instructed to urinate as soon as the *first* desire to do so is felt. It is important for the patient to know that regaining urinary control is a gradual process, and that even though he may continue to "dribble" after being discharged from the hospital, the dribbling should gradually diminish (up to 1 year). The urine may be cloudy for several weeks but should clear as the prostate area heals.

While the prostatic fossa is healing (6 to 8 weeks), the patient should not engage in any Valsalva efforts (straining at stool, heavy lifting), since this increases venous pressure and may produce hematuria. He should avoid long automobile rides and strenuous exercise, which increase the tendency to bleed. He will also benefit from knowing that certain foods (spicy), alcohol, and coffee may cause discomfort. The patient is cautioned to drink enough fluids to avoid dehydration, which increases the tendency for a clot to form and obstruct the flow of urine. Any bleeding or decrease in the size of the urinary stream is to be reported to the physician.

Sexual Function. A prostatectomy does not usually cause impotence. (Perineal prostatectomy may cause impotence due to unavoidable damage of the pudendal nerves.) In most instances, sexual activity may be resumed in 6 to 8 weeks, the time required for the prostatic fossa to heal. Following ejaculation, the seminal fluid will go into the bladder and is excreted with the urine. (The anatomical changes in the posterior urethra lead to retrograde ejaculation).

After total prostatectomy (usually for cancer), impotence is almost always expected. For the patient who does not desire to give up sexual activity, a plastic insert may be used to make the penis rigid for sexual intercourse. Incidentally, if it is known that there is no evidence of sexually transmitted disease present, this information is often reassuring to the patient.

▷ *Evaluation*

▷ *Expected Outcomes*

Preoperative

1. Patient is free of anxiety.
   a. Verbalizes his concerns and accepts solutions offered.
   b. Expresses relief that the bladder problem can be treated and that the condition is not a malignant tumor.
2. Relates his understanding of the surgical procedure and postoperative course.
   a. Discusses the surgical procedure and expected postoperative course.
   b. Practices perineal muscle exercises and other techniques useful in facilitating control of bladder function.
   c. Participates in all preoperative preparations for surgery.

Postoperative

1. Maintains acceptable level of urinary elimination.
   a. Maintains optimum drainage of catheter/drainage tubes.
   b. Verbalizes his understanding that urinary incontinence will gradually disappear.
2. Is free of pain.
   a. Relates relief of discomfort.
   b. Relates signs/symptoms of problems that are to be reported.
3. Is free of infection and hemorrhage.
   a. Maintains vital signs within normal limits.
   b. Exhibits good wound healing; no signs of inflammation.
   c. Relates what signs are to be reported if an infection is developing.
4. Responds positively to self-care measures.
   a. Increases activity and ambulation daily.
   b. Keeps urinary output within normal ranges and consistent with intake.
   c. Uses perineal exercises and interruption of urinary stream to promote bladder control.
   d. Drinks adequate amounts of fluids daily.
   e. Avoids straining and lifting of heavy objects.
   f. Says he is looking forward to resuming sexual activity when permitted.

Cancer of the Prostate

Cancer of the prostate is the second most common cause of cancer, the second most common cause of cancer deaths in American males (over age 55), and the most prevalent cancer overall in black men. With increasing numbers of men in the older age-group, greater attention will be focused on this condition.

Clinical Manifestations. Early cancer of the prostate does not usually produce symptoms. The obstructive symptoms occur late in the disease. This cancer tends to be variable in its course. If the neoplasm is large enough to encroach on the bladder neck and cause obstruction of urine, there are symptoms and signs of obstruction, namely, difficulty and frequency of urination, urinary retention, and decreased size and force of the urinary stream. Prostatic cancer commonly metastasizes to bone, lymph nodes, brain, and lungs. Symptoms due to metastases are backache, hip pain, perineal and rectal discomfort, anemia, weight loss, weakness, nausea, and oliguria. Hematuria may be present from urethral or bladder invasion, or both.

Early Detection. Every male over age 40 should have a digital rectal examination as part of his health checkup. Earlier detection is the clue to a higher cure rate. Routine repeated rectal palpation of the gland (preferably by the same examiner) is important because early cancer may be felt as a nodule within the substance of the gland or as a diffuse induration in the posterior lobe. A digital rectal examination in addition to being more accurate, readily available, and less costly than other screening tests for prostatic cancer provides useful clinical information regarding the rectum, anal sphincter, and quality of stool.

Diagnostic Evaluation. On rectal examination, an area of increased firmness within the prostate is noted. The more advanced lesion is "stony hard" and fixed. The diagnosis is made on histologic examination of tissue removed surgically by transurethral resection, open prostatectomy, or needle biopsy (perineal or transrectal). Fine needle aspiration is a quick painless method of obtaining prostate cells for cytologic examination. It is a helpful method for determining staging of the tumor if cancer is present. The serum acid phosphatase level is frequently increased when cancer extends outside the prostatic capsule. (Acid phosphatase is seen in most body tissues, but is 1000 times more concentrated in the prostate gland.) Smaller amounts of acid phosphatase can be detected with radioimmunoassay.

Other tests include bone scans to detect metastatic bone disease, skeletal x-rays to reveal osteoblastic metastases, excretory urograms to demonstrate changes from ureteral obstruction, and renal-function tests and lymphangiography to seek evidence of metastases to the pelvic nodes.

Management

Treatment selection is based on the stage of the disease and on the patient's age and symptoms. A radical prostatectomy (removal of the prostate and seminal vesicles) still remains the standard operative procedure for patients who have potentially curable disease and a life expectancy of 10 years or more. This procedure may be followed by bilateral orchiectomy. Sexual impotency follows radical prostatectomy, and 5% to 10% of the patients have various degrees of urinary incontinence. (See p. 1158 for care of the patient following a prostatectomy.)

If the cancer is found in the early stage, the treatment may be curative radiation therapy, either using teletherapy with a linear accelerator or interstitial irradiation (implantation of radioactive iodine or gold combined with pelvic lymphadenectomy). Radiation therapy is also used for palliation in patients with late stage disease. Side-effects, which usually are transitory, include proctitis (inflammation of the rectum) and cystitis due to the radiation doses and the proximity of the bladder and rectum. There is better preservation of sexual potency with radiation therapy; therefore, younger patients may prefer this treatment modality.

Since approximately half of the patients have locally advanced tumors or evidence of metastatic disease at the time they present for treatment, palliative measures are indicated. Hormonal therapy may be selected to suppress all androgenic stimuli to the prostate. This is accomplished by either orchiectomy (removal of the testes) or administration of estrogens (see below). Hormonal therapy is a method of control rather than cure, since adenocarcinoma of the prostate is hormone dependent. The rationale underlying hormone treatment is that prostatic epithelium becomes atrophied or inactivated when androgen hormones are greatly reduced or inactivated.

Orchiectomy lowers plasma testosterone levels, since 93% of circulating testosterone is of testicular origin. This results in completely removing the testicular stimulus required for continued prostatic growth. Prostatic atrophy occurs after this procedure. Orchiectomy is preferred over hormonal therapy by many urologists because it does not result in the potential side-effects of estrogen therapy. However, castration in the male carries a significant emotional impact. The administration of *estrogen* is thought to inhibit the gonadotropins that are responsible for testicular androgenic activity, thus removing the androgenic hormone, on which the growth of the malignancy depends. Diethylstilbestrol is the most widely used estrogen at this time.

Diethylstilbestrol gives symptomatic control, lessens tumor size, lessens pain from metastatic nodules, and imparts an improved sense of well-being. However, there is evidence that giving higher doses of diethylstilbestrol carries a significant risk of death from cardiovascular disease, especially from thromboembolic phenomena. A lower dose apparently is as effective and does not contribute to cardiovascular death.

Gynecomastia (enlargement of breasts in the male) is an annoying complication of estrogen therapy that may be lessened by pretreatment radiation of breast tissue. Impotence almost always occurs following estrogen therapy.

Cryosurgery of the prostate gland has been advocated by some for the poor-risk patient. Chemotherapy may also be tried. Doxorubicin, cisplatin, and cyclophosphamide are under investigation.

For patients failing to respond to conventional therapy, estramustine phosphate (Emcyt), a conjugate of estradiol and nitrogen mustard, has shown to be promising in giving rapid pain relief. It is based on the premise that a hormone can be used as a carrier to bring a chemotherapeutic agent (nitrogen mustard) to hormone-sensitive tissues (prostate). The drug is available in capsule form. Side-effects include nausea, vomiting, and occasionally diarrhea.

To maintain patency of the urethral passage, repeated transurethral resections may have to be performed. When this is impractical, catheter drainage is instituted by way of the suprapubic or transurethral route.

Patients with recurring symptoms are treated symptomatically. Corticosteroids may give relief but do not affect the tumor.

Blood transfusions are given to maintain adequate hemoglobin levels when bone marrow is replaced by tumor. Radiation therapy to skeletal lesions can relieve bone pain. Pain may be controlled by estrogens and narcotics and, if necessary, by severing spinal cord pain fibers via neurosurgery.

See also p. 249, Nursing Management of the Patient With Pain; p. 294, The Care of the Patient With Advanced Cancer; and p. 1155, The Care of the Patient with a Prostatectomy. Care of the patient with cancer of the prostate is summarized in Nursing Care Plan 44-1 (pp. 1162–1166).

Conditions Affecting the Testes and Adjacent Structures

Undescended Testis (Cryptorchidism)

Cryptorchidism is the absence of one or both testes from the scrotum. The testes may be located in the abdominal cavity or inguinal canal. If the testis does not descend, hormone therapy or surgery (orchiopexy) is employed to secure proper positioning.

In orchiopexy, an incision is made over the inguinal canal, and the testis is brought down and placed in the scrotum. To maintain proper position of the testis, traction may be applied to the thigh by means of a suture drawn from the lower end of the scrotum.

Orchitis

Orchitis is an inflammation of the testes (testicular congestion). The etiology is usually pyogenic, viral, spirochetal, parasitic, traumatic, chemical, or idiopathic.

When mumps is contracted in the postpubertal male 4 to 7 days after swelling of the jaw and neck, approximately one in five men will develop some form of orchitis. The testis may show some atrophy. In past years, sterility and impotence often resulted. Current practice is for the man who has not previously had mumps and is now exposed to the disease to receive γ-globulin immediately. The disease is likely to be less severe, with reduced or no complications.

Management. If the causes are bacterial, viral, or fungal, therapy is specific. Rest, elevation, ice packs, antibiotics, analgesics, and anti-inflammatory medications are recommended.

Epididymitis

Epididymitis is an infection of the epididymis that usually descends from an infected prostate or urinary tract. It may also develop as a complication of gonorrhea. In men under 35 years of age, the major cause of epididymitis is *Chlamydia trachomatis*. The infection passes upward through the urethra and the ejaculatory duct, and thence along the vas deferens to the epididymis.

The patient complains of pain and soreness in the inguinal canal along the course of the vas deferens, and then develops pain and swelling in the scrotum and the groin. The epididymis becomes swollen and extremely painful; the temperature is elevated. The urine may contain pus (pyuria) and bacteria (bacteriuria), and the patient may experience resulting chills and fever.

Management. If the patient is seen within the first 24 hours after onset, the spermatic cord may be infiltrated with a local anesthetic agent to relieve pain. If the epididymitis is chlamydial in origin, the patient and the patient's sexual partners must also be treated with antibiotics. The patient is observed for abscess formation. If no improvement occurs within 2 weeks, an underlying testicular tumor should be considered. An epididymectomy (excision of the epididymis from the testis) may be performed for patients with recurrent, incapacitating episodes or for those with chronic, painful conditions.

Nursing Considerations. The patient is placed on bed rest with the scrotum elevated with a scrotal bridge or folded towel to prevent traction on the spermatic cord and to improve venous drainage and relieve pain. Antimicrobials are given as prescribed until all evidence of the acute inflammatory reaction has subsided.

Intermittent cold compresses to the scrotum may help ease the pain. Local heat or sitz baths later in the infection may hasten resolution of the inflammatory process. Analgesics are given for pain relief as prescribed.

Patient Education and Home Health Care. The patient should avoid straining (lifting) and sexual excitement until the infection is under control. He should be instructed to continue with analgesics for pain and antibiotics as prescribed

(Text continues on p. 1166)

Care of the Patient With Cancer of the Prostate

Nursing Interventions	Rationale	Expected Outcomes

Nursing Diagnosis: Anxiety related to concern and lack of knowledge about the diagnosis, treatment plan, and prognosis

Goal: Reduced stress and improved ability to cope

Nursing Interventions	Rationale	Expected Outcomes
1. Take a nursing history to determine the following: a. Patient's reasons for concerns b. His level of understanding of his health problem c. His past experience with cancer d. Whether he knows his diagnosis of malignancy/prognosis e. His support systems and coping potential	1. Nurse and patient become partners in resolving myths and developing understanding.	• Appears more relaxed. • Responds verbally in a positive manner. • States that he understands the problem now. • Admits that for the time being his immediate problems can be relieved. • Relates positively to his family. • Says he is prepared to undergo surgery if this is required.
2. Explain in simple terms what diagnostic measures he will have, how long they will take, and what will happen to him during each test.	2. With his understanding, the patient will be more relaxed and cooperative during each test.	
3. Assess his mental reaction to his diagnosis and how he hopes to accept it.	3. This will provide clues in determining pertinent measures to assist him in coping.	

Nursing Diagnosis: Alteration in fluid and electrolyte balance related to urinary dysfunction because of prostate tumor

Goal: Maintain adequate fluids, electrolytes, and acid–base balance

Nursing Interventions	Rationale	Expected Outcomes
1. Monitor output hourly if indicated.	1. If output is excessive, the patient's fluid volume may become depleted.	• Maintains desirable fluid and electrolyte levels. • Maintains blood pressure within normal range. • Is free of symptoms of shock.
2. Check blood pressure and pulse hourly.	2. Falling blood pressure and rising pulse rate may suggest hypovolemia.	
3. Note skin characteristics: dry, clammy, warm, cool. Note also patient's mental level of concern that may suggest physiologic changes	3. These assessments are for manifestations of shock.	
4. Suggest the patient remain quiet and rest.	4. Reduces cardiac workload.	
5. Administer intravenous fluids as prescribed and monitor patient for their effect.	5. Fluid replacement properly prescribed and given at optimal rate should control and normalize the imbalance.	

(continued)

Nursing Interventions	*Rationale*	*Expected Outcomes*

Nursing Diagnosis: Alteration in nutrition related to decreased oral intake because of anorexia, nausea, and dysphagia brought on by cancer and/or its treatment

Goal: Improved nutritional states

1. Assess the extent of food intake at each mealtime.	1. A concrete assessment of food eaten aids in determining level of intake.	• Responds positively to his favorite foods.
2. Listen to patient's explanation of why he is unable to eat more.	2. His explanation may present easily corrected practices.	• Assumes responsibility for his oral hygiene since the "bad taste" in his mouth inhibited his interest in food.
3. Cater to his individual food requests (*e.g.,* food too spicy or too cold).	3. He will be more likely to consume larger servings if food is palatable to him.	• Notes increase in weight following improved appetite.
4. Recognize effect of medication on his appetite.	4. Some chemotherapeutic agents promote anorexia.	
5. Tell patient that aging and the disease process can reduce taste sensitivity.	5. By the body's absorbing by-products of cellular destruction (brought on by malignancy), smell and taste are altered.	
6. Use measures to control vomiting since this can affect one's appetite.	6. Vomiting can depress interest in food.	
7. Ensure oral hygiene following episodes of vomiting. Use antiemetic prescribed drugs.	7. These measures will enhance the desire for food.	
8. Provide frequent small meals and a compatible pleasant environment.		

Nursing Diagnosis: Alteration in comfort: pain related to treatment modalities and progression of disease

Goal: Relief of pain

1. Evaluate nature of patient's pain and its location.	1. Determining nature and causes of pain helps to select proper relief modality and provide baseline for later comparison.	• Reports control of pain.
2. Avoid activities that aggravate or worsen pain.	2. Bumping the bed is an example of an action that can intensify the patient's pain.	• Expects exacerbations, reports their quality or intensity, and obtains relief.
3. Since pain usually is related to bone (metastasis), ensure that patient's bed has a bed board on a firm mattress and protect from falls/injuries.	3. This will provide added support and is more comfortable.	
4. Provide support for affected extremities.	4. The more support coupled with reduced movement of the part helps in pain control.	
5. Prepare patient for radiation therapy if so prescribed.	5. Radiation therapy may be effective in controlling pain.	
6. Administer analgesic or narcotic as prescribed.	6. These medications alter perception of pain and provide comfort.	

(continued)

Nursing Interventions	*Rationale*	*Expected Outcomes*

Nursing Diagnosis: Impaired physical mobility/activity intolerance related to tissue hypoxia, malnutrition, and exhaustion and to spinal cord or nerve compression from metastatic spread

Goal: Improved physical mobility

1. Assess for reasons causing limited mobility (*e.g.,* pain, hypercalcemia, limited exercise tolerance).	1. This information offers clues to the cause; if possible, this is treated.	• Achieves improved physical mobility. • Relates that short-term goals are encouraging him because they are attainable.
2. Provide pain relief by administering prescribed medications.	2. Analgesics/narcotics allow the patient to increase his activity more comfortably.	
3. Encourage use of assistive devices: cane, walker	3. Support may offer the security needed to become mobile.	
4. Involve significant others in helping patient with range of motion exercises, positioning, and walking.	4. Assistance from partner or others encourages patient to repeat activities and achieve goals.	
5. Praise the patient for achieving small gains.	5. Encouragement stimulates improvement of performance.	

Nursing Diagnosis: Alteration in urinary elimination patterns related to urethral obstruction secondary to prostatic enlargement/ tumor and loss of bladder tone due to prolonged distention/retention

Goal: Improved pattern of urinary elimination

1. Determine patient's usual pattern of bladder elimination.	1. Provides a baseline for comparison and goal to work toward.	• Voids at normal intervals. • Reports absence of frequency, urgency, or bladder fullness. • Displays no suprapubic palpable distention after voiding. • Maintains balanced intake and output.
2. Assess for signs/symptoms of urinary retention: amount and frequency of urination, suprapubic distention, complaints of urgency and discomfort.	2. Suspect retention if he voids 20 to 30 ml frequently and if output is less than intake.	
3. Catheterize patient to determine amount of residual urine.	3. This is done after voluntary urination is completed in order to determine amount remaining.	
4. Initiate measures to treat retention: a. Encourage assuming normal position for voiding.	a. Usual position provides relaxed conditions conducive for voiding.	
b. Recommend using Valsalva maneuver.	b. By exerting pressure, this has a tendency to force urine out of bladder.	
c. Administer prescribed cholinergic drug.	c. Stimulates bladder contraction.	
d. Monitor effects of medication.	d. If unsuccessful, another measure may be required.	
5. Consult with physician regarding intermittent or indwelling catheterization; assist with procedure as required.	5. Catheterization will relieve urinary retention until the specific cause is determined; it may be an obstruction that only can be corrected surgically.	
6. Monitor catheter function; maintain sterility of closed system; irrigate as required.	6. Adequate functioning of catheter is to be ensured to achieve purpose and to prevent infection.	
7. Prepare patient for surgery if indicated.	7. Surgical removal of obstruction may be the only solution.	

(continued)

Nursing Interventions	*Rationale*	*Expected Outcomes*

Nursing Diagnosis: Sexual dysfunction related to effects of therapy: chemotherapy—hormonal—radiation—surgery

Goal: Ability to assume/enjoy modified sexual functioning

1. Determine from nursing history what effect patient's medical condition is having on his personal life. (Full assessment will follow guidelines in Chapter 13, Human Sexuality, p. 202.)	1. Usually decreased libido and, later, impotence may be experienced.	• Describes the reasons for changes in sexual functioning. • Discusses what practices have been substituted and appreciated with appropriate health care personnel.
2. Inform patient of the effects of chemotherapy, irradiation, hormonal therapy, prostate surgery, and orchiectomy (when applicable) on patient's sexual function.	2. Treatment modalities may alter sexual function, but each is evaluated separately with regard to its effect on a particular patient.	
3. Include his partner in developing understandings and in discovering alternative satisfying close relations with each other.	3. Often the bonds between a couple are strengthened with new appreciation and support that had not been thought about prior to the current illness.	

Nursing Diagnosis: Knowledge deficit related to a new health problem: cancer, urinary difficulties, and treatment modalities

Goal: Understanding of health problem and ability to care for self

1. Encourage communication with the patient.	1. This is designed to establish rapport and trust	• Discusses his concerns and problems freely. • Asks questions and shows interest in his condition. • Describes activities that help or harm his recovery. • Identifies ways of attaining/maintaining bladder control. • Demonstrates satisfactory technique and understanding of catheter use. • Lists signs and symptoms that must be reported should they occur.
2. Review the anatomy of the involved area.	2. Orientation to one's anatomy is basic to understanding its function.	
3. Be specific in selecting information that is relevant to the patient's particular treatment plan.	3. This is based on the treatment plan since it varies with each patient; individualization is desirable.	

4. Suggest ways in which pressure on the operative area can be reduced or avoided.
  a. Avoid prolonged sitting (in a chair, long automobile rides), standing, walking.
  b. Avoid straining, such as during exercises, bowel movement, lifting, and even sexual intercourse.
	4. This is to prevent bleeding; such precautions are in order for 6 to 8 weeks postoperatively.	

5. Familiarize patient with ways of attaining/maintaining bladder control.	5. These measures will help him to control frequency, dribbling and aid in preventing retention.	
a. Encourage urination when he feels the need—usually every 2 to 3 hours; discourage his voiding when supine.	a. By sitting or standing, he is more likely to empty his bladder.	
b. Avoid drinking cola and caffeine beverages; urge a cut-off time in the evening for drinking fluids to minimize getting out of bed frequently at night.	b. Spacing the kind and amount of liquid intake will help to prevent frequency.	

(continued)

Nursing Interventions	*Rationale*	*Expected Outcomes*

Nursing Diagnosis: Knowledge deficit related to a new health problem: cancer, urinary difficulties, and treatment modalities

Goal: Understanding of health problem and ability to care for self

c. Describe perineal exercises to be performed every hour.	c. Exercises will assist him in starting and stopping the urinary stream.
d. Develop a schedule with patient so that it will fit into his routine.	d. A schedule will assist in developing a workable pattern of normal activities.
6. Demonstrate catheter care: encourage his questions; stress the importance of position of urinary receptable.	6. By requiring return-demonstration of care, collection, and emptying of his device, he will become more independent and also can prevent backflow of urine, which can lead to infection.
7. Alert the patient to those changes that may occur (after he leaves the hospital) that need to be reported: a. Continued bloody urine; passing of blood clots b. Pain; burning around the catheter c. Frequency of urination d. Diminishing output e. Increasing loss of bladder control	7. These are signs and symptoms of complications (hemorrhage, infection, obstruction) and are to be reported to health care personnel.

and to use ice packs if necessary for discomfort. It may take 4 weeks or longer for the epididymis to return to normal.

Tumors of the Testes

Testicular cancer accounts for only 1% of all malignant tumors, but it ranks first in cancer deaths among males in the 20- to 35-year age-group. Such cancers are classified as *germinal* or *nongerminal*. Germinal tumors arise from the germinal cells of the testes (seminomas, teratocarcinomas, and embryonal carcinomas); nongerminal tumors are from epithelium. Most neoplasms are germinal, with about 40% of these being seminoma. The etiology of testicular tumors is unknown, but cryptorchidism, infections, and genetic and endocrine factors appear to play a part in their development. These tumors are usually malignant and tend to metastasize early.

Clinical Manifestations. The symptoms appear very gradually with a mass in the scrotum and generally painless enlargement of the testis. The patient may complain of heaviness in the scrotum. Backache (from retroperitoneal node extension), pain in the abdomen, loss of weight, and general weakness may be from metastatic disease. The metastatic growth may be more marked than the local testicular one. *The enlargement of the testis without pain is a significant diagnostic finding.*

One method of early detection of testicular cancer is self-examination. Part of health promotion practices for men should include testicular self-examination. Teaching men to perform self-examination as depicted in Figure 44-3 is an important intervention for early detection of this disease.

Diagnostic Evaluation. α-Fetoprotein and human chorionic gonadotropin are tumor markers that may be elevated in patients with testicular cancer. (Tumor markers are substances synthesized by the tumor cells and released into the circulation in abnormal amounts.) Newer immunocytochemical techniques have made possible the identification of the cells that apparently produce these markers. Other diagnostic tests include an intravenous urogram to detect ureteral deviation secondary to tumor mass, lymphangiography to assess extent of lymphatic spread of the tumor, computed tomography to identify lesions in the retroperitoneum, or abdominal ultrasound.

Management. The goals of management are to eradicate the disease and achieve a cure. Treatment selection is based on the cell type and the anatomical extent of the disease. The testis is removed (orchiectomy) through an inguinal incision with a high ligation of the spermatic cord. Retroperitoneal lymph node dissection (RPLND) to prevent lymphatic spread may be employed after orchiectomy although controversy exists over this approach. Some believe that the after effects of the surgical procedure (including ejaculatory dysfunction with resultant infertility) are not justified when more than 50% of patients have negative lymph nodes. The proponents of RPLND are quick to claim that it may be a curative procedure and as such spares the patient the greater discomforts of chemotherapy should relapse occur. Following

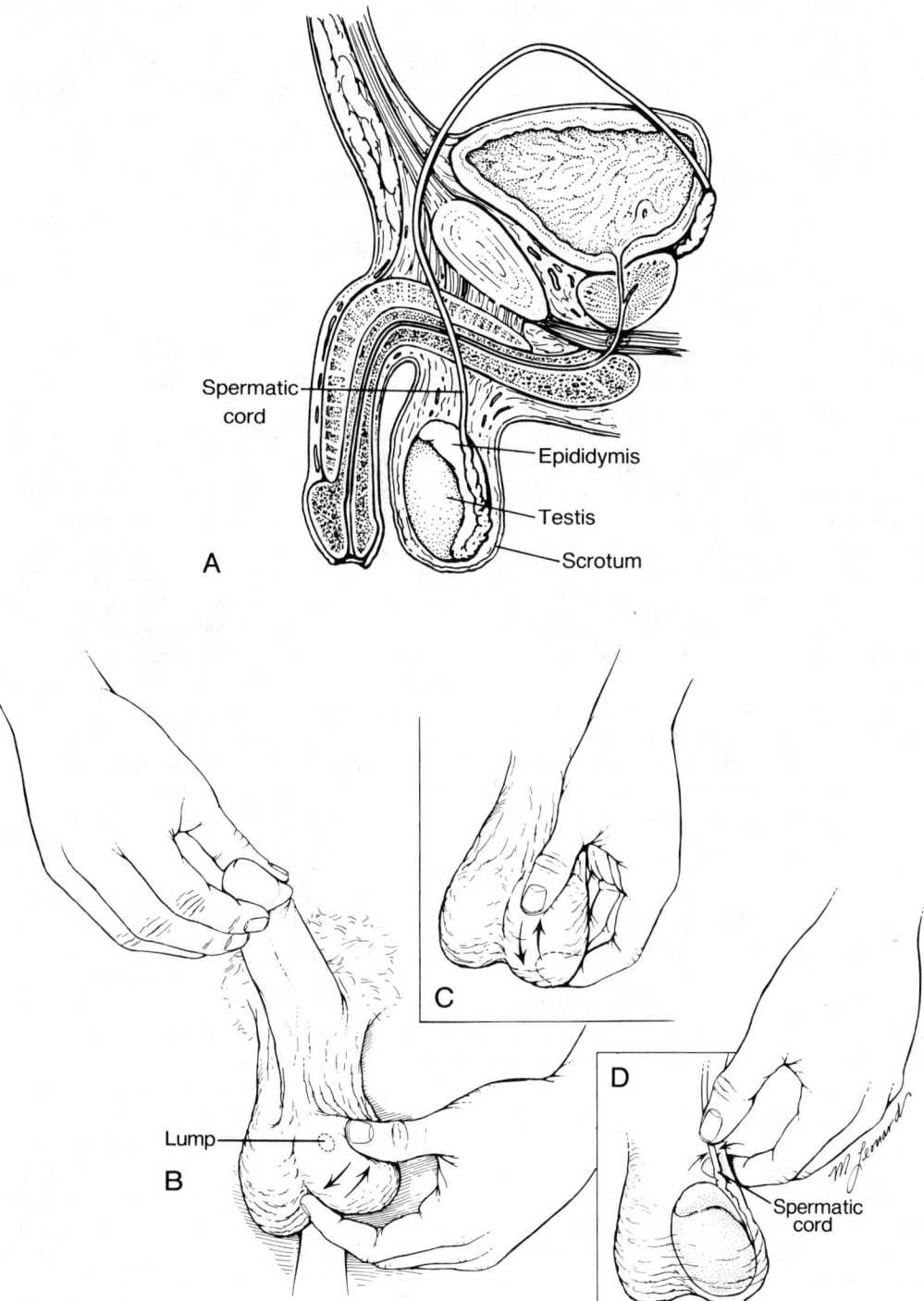

Figure 44-3
Testicular self-examination (TSE) is to be performed once a month; it is neither difficult nor time-consuming. A convenient time is often after a warm bath or shower when the scrotum is more relaxed. Both hands are used to palpate the testis; the normal testicle is smooth and uniform in consistency. (*A*) Normal anatomy. (*B*) With the index and middle finger under the testis and the thumb on top, roll the testis gently in a horizontal plane between the thumb and fingers, feeling for any evidence of a small lump or abnormality. (*C*) Follow the same procedure for palpation in the "vertical" plane. (*D*) Locate the epididymis (cordlike structure on the top and back of the testicle that stores and transports sperm). Repeat the examination for the other testis; it is normal to find one testis larger than the other. Any evidence of a small, pea-size lump should be checked by a physician. It may be due to an infection or a tumor growth.

RPLND, normal libido and orgasm are usually unimpaired but the patient will not be fertile. Postoperative irradiation to the lymphatic drainage pathways may be done and is the treatment of choice when the tumors are identified as seminomas. Such radiation is limited to the side of the tumor. The other testis is shielded from radiation to preserve fertility.

Sperm banking before surgery may be considered for the young man as a "hedge" against sterility after surgery. A gel-filled prosthesis can be implanted to offset the absence of one testis.

Testicular carcinomas are highly responsive to drug therapy. Multiple chemotherapy using cisplatin with other agents (vinblastine, bleomycin, dactinomycin, cyclophosphamide) gives a high percentage of complete remission. The program of therapy is probably best prescribed by those trained in oncology, since these regimens are toxic and require intensive therapeutic support. Good results may be obtained by combining different types of treatment, including surgery, radiation therapy, and chemotherapy. Disseminated testicular cancer is regarded as a treatable and probably curable disease.

Patient Education. The patient may have difficulty in accepting his condition. He needs encouragement to maintain a positive attitude during what may be a long course of therapy. Radiation therapy does not necessarily prevent the patient from fathering children, nor will unilateral excision of a tumor necessarily lessen virility.

A patient with a history of one tumor of the testes has a greater chance of developing another. Follow-up evaluation includes chest films, excretory urography, radioimmunoassay of human chorionic gonadotropins and α-fetoprotein, and examination of lymph nodes to detect recurrence of malignancy.

Hydrocele

A hydrocele is a collection of fluid generally in the tunica vaginalis of the testis, although it may also occur within the spermatic cord. The tunica vaginalis becomes widely distended with fluid. Hydrocele may be acute or chronic and is differentiated from a hernia by the fact that a hydrocele transmits light when transilluminated.

Acute hydrocele occurs in association with acute infectious diseases of the epididymis or as a result of local trauma or systemic infectious diseases, such as mumps. The cause of chronic hydrocele is unknown.

Usually, therapy is not required. Treatment is necessary only if the hydrocele becomes tense and compromises testicular circulation or if the scrotal mass becomes large, uncomfortable, or embarrassing.

In the surgical treatment of hydrocele, an incision is made through the wall of the scrotum down to the distended tunica vaginalis. The sac is resected or, after being opened, is sutured together to collapse the wall. Postoperatively, an athletic supporter is worn for comfort and support. The major complication is the formation of a hematoma in the loose tissues of the scrotum. The nursing management is the same as for a varicocele.

Varicocele

A varicocele is an abnormal dilation of the veins of the pampiniform venous plexus in the scrotum (network of veins from the testis and the epididymis, constituting part of the spermatic cord). Varicoceles occur most frequently in the veins on the left side in adults. In some men, a varicocele has been associated with infertility. Very few, if any, subjective symptoms may be produced by the enlargement of the spermatic vein, and as a rule, no treatment is required unless fertility is a matter of concern. Symptomatic varicocele (pain, tenderness, and discomfort in the inguinal region) is corrected surgically by ligating the external spermatic vein at the inguinal area. An ice bag may be applied to the scrotum for the first few hours after operation to relieve edema. The patient then wears a scrotal support.

Impotence

Impotence is the alteration of a man's sexual capability to either achieve or maintain an erection sufficient to accomplish intercourse. Impotence can be either erectile or ejaculatory. Erectile impotence has both psychogenic and organic causes. Causes of psychogenic impotence include anxiety, fatigue, depression, and cultural pressure to perform sexually. Research suggests, however, that organic impotence may account for a larger percentage of cases of impotence than previously realized. Organic causes include occlusive vascular disease, endocrine disease (diabetes, pituitary tumors, hypogonadism), genitourinary conditions (radical pelvic cancer surgery), hematologic conditions (Hodgkin's disease, leukemia), neurologic disorders (neuropathies, parkinsonism), trauma to the pelvic or genital area, and drugs (alcohol, psychoactive drugs, anticholinergics) and drug abuse.

Diagnosis of impotence includes a sexual and medical history, an analysis of presenting symptoms, physical examination, and various laboratory studies. The advent of sleep laboratories has made the nocturnal penile tumescence test (NPT) possible. Research revealed that normal males have nocturnal penile erections closely paralleling rapid eye movement (REM) sleep in their occurrence and duration. Organically impotent men show inadequate sleep-related erections that correspond to their waking performance. Changes in penile circumference are monitored (using a mercury strain gauge placed around the penis) and recorded. The NPT test is a means of determining whether erectile impotence has organic or psychogenic etiology.

Arterial blood flow to the penis is measured with the Doppler probe. Nerve conduction tests and psychological evaluation of the patient are part of the diagnostic workup.

Management. Treatment, which depends to some extent on the cause, can be medical, surgical, or a combination of both. A patient's response to nonsurgical therapy, such as treatment of alcoholism and readjustment of hypertensive agents or other medications, is examined. Impotence secondary to hypothalamic-pituitary-gonadal dysfunction may be reversible with endocrine therapy. Insufficient penile blood flow may be treated with recently developed vascular surgery. Patients with impotence from psychogenic causes are directed to a professional specializing in sex therapy. Patients with impotence secondary to organic causes are considered candidates for penile implants.

Two basic types of penile implants are available: the semirigid rod and the inflatable prosthesis. The semirigid rod, such as the Small-Carrion prosthesis, has no moving parts, unlike the inflatable prosthesis, which stimulates natural erections and natural flaccidity. Complications following implant procedures include infection, erosion of the prosthesis through the skin, and persistent pain, which may require removal of the implant.

Impotence, regardless of its cause, has vast psychological and psychosocial implications for most men. Therefore, the nurse must listen and be supportive to both the patient and his partner.

Conditions Affecting the Penis

Phimosis

Phimosis is a condition in which the foreskin is constricted so that it cannot be retracted over the glans. There has been a trend away from routine circumcision of newborns. Therefore, the child and adult will require early instruction in cleansing of the prepuce. In the adult, when the cleansing of the preputial area is neglected or no longer possible, the accumulation of normal secretions and subsequent inflammation (*balanitis*) occur. This causes adhesions and scarring. The thickened secretions become encrusted with urinary salts and calcify, forming preputial concretions. In the aged, penile carcinoma may develop. Phimosis is corrected by circumcision (see below). The patient is instructed in proper hygienic care of the foreskin.

Paraphimosis is a condition in which the foreskin is retracted behind the glans and, because of narrowness and subsequent edema, cannot be reduced back to its usual position (covering the glans). It is treated by manual reduction (compressing the glans firmly, to reduce its size, and then pushing the glans back as the prepuce is moved forward). Circumcision is usually indicated once the inflammation and edema subside.

Circumcision

Circumcision is the excision of the foreskin (prepuce) of the glans penis. It is usually done in infancy for hygienic purposes. In adults, it is indicated for phimosis, paraphimosis, recurrent infections of the glans and foreskin, and personal desire of the patient.

Postoperatively, the patient is watched for bleeding. The petrolatum (Vaseline) gauze dressing is changed as indicated. Since the adult male may experience a considerable amount of pain following circumcision, analgesics are given when needed.

Cancer of the Penis

Cancer of the penis occurs in the skin of the penis and rarely in circumcised individuals. It appears as a painless, wartlike growth or ulcer on the glans or coronal sulcus under the prepuce and represents about 0.5% of malignancies in men in the United States. In some countries, however, the incidence is up to 10%. Often diagnosis is delayed for more than a year, probably because of guilt, embarrassment, or ignorance. Smaller lesions involving only the skin may be controlled by excisional biopsy. Topical chemotherapy with 5-fluorouracil cream may be one option in selected patients. Radiation therapy or radioactive needle implant produces varying results. Partial penectomy (removal of the penis) is preferred to total penectomy if possible; approximately 40% of patients are then able to participate in sexual intercourse and to stand for voiding. Total penectomy is indicated when the tumor is not amenable to conservative treatment. Radiation therapy may be used as treatment for small squamous cell carcinomas of the penis or for palliation in advanced tumors or lymph node metastasis.

Patient Education. Circumcision in infancy almost eliminates the possibility of penile cancer, since chronic irritation and inflammation of the glans penis predisposes to penile tumors. Personal hygiene is an important preventive measure in uncircumcised males.

Priapism

Priapism is an uncontrolled, persistent erection of the penis that causes the penis to become very large, hard, and often painful. It occurs from either neural or vascular causes, including sickle cell thrombosis, spinal cord tumors, and tumor invasion of the penis or its vessels. This condition may result in gangrene and often results in impotence, whether treated or not.

Priapism is considered a urologic emergency. The goal of therapy is to improve venous drainage of the corpora cavernosa to prevent ischemia, fibrosis, and impotence. Initially, treatment is directed at relieving the erection and includes bed rest and sedation. The corpora may be irrigated with an anticoagulant, which allows aspiration of stagnant blood. Shunting procedures to divert the blood from the turgid corpora cavernosa to the venous system (corpora cavernosa-saphenous vein shunt) or into the corpus spongiosum-glans penis compartment may be tried.

Bibliography

Books

Brenner B et al. Principles of Renal Medicine. Philadelphia, WB Saunders, 1986.

Corriere JN Jr. Essentials of Urology. New York, Churchill Livingstone, 1986.

Hanno PM and Wein AJ. A Clinical Manual of Urology. Norwalk, Connecticut, Appleton-Century-Crofts, 1986.

Kaufman JJ. Current Urologic Therapy, 2nd ed. Philadelphia, WB Saunders, 1986.

Kaye JW. Outpatient Urologic Surgery. Philadelphia, Lea & Febiger, 1986.

Resnick MI, Caldamone AA, and Sprinak JP. Decision Making in Urology. Toronto, BC Decker, 1985.

Smith DR. General Urology, 11th ed. Los Altos, California, Lange Medical Publications, 1984.

Spagna VA and Prior RB. Sexually Transmitted Diseases. New York, Marcel Dekker, 1985.

Swanson JM and Forrest KA. Men's Reproductive Health. New York, Springer, 1984.

Articles

(Asterisks indicate nursing research articles.)

General Articles

Baum N. Treatment of impotence. Part 1. Non surgical methods. Part 2. Surgical methods. Postgrad Med 1987 May 15; 81(7):133–140.

Cowling WR III and Campbell VG. Health concerns of aging men. Nurs Clin North Am 1986 Mar; 21(1):75–83.

Cozad J. Penile implants: The surgical treatment for impotence. Ethicon (Point of View) 1984; 21(1):20–21.

Forrester DA. Myths of masculinity: Impact upon men's health. Nurs Clin North Am 1986 Mar; 21(1):15–23.

Kniefe-Hardy MJ, Votava K, and Stubbings MJ. Managing indwelling catheters in the home. Geriatr Nurs 1985 Sept/Oct; 6(5):280–285.

Masters WH. Sex and aging: Expectations and reality. Hosp Pract 1986 Aug 15; 21(8):175–198.

Murphy NJ and Weiss BD. Hematospermia. Am Fam Physician 1985 Oct; 32(4):167–171.

Parker C. Ambulatory surgery for a penile prosthesis. AORN J 1982 Sept; 36(3):487–494.

Rowan RL. Maintaining sexual function regardless of age or infirmity. Mod Med 1985 Aug; 53(8):11–16.

Schover LR et al. Sexual rehabilitation of urologic cancer patients: A practical approach. CA 1984 Mar/Apr; 34(2):66–73.

Srinevas V and Ali Khan S. Penile carcinoma. Hosp Pract 1985 Jan 15; 20(1):154–159.

Assessment

Gault PL. Testicular cancer. Nurs '81 1981 May; 11(5):47–50.

Ramsey FB. Testicular self-examination. Postgrad Med 1986 Sept 15; 80(4):172.

Prostatic Conditions

Ashmann FR. Dilemmas in managing prostate carcinoma: II. Metastatic disease. Geriatrics 1985 Sept; 40(9):61–70.

Crawford ED. Diagnosis and treatment of prostatitis. Hosp Pract 1985 Sept 30; 20(9A):77–88.

Creaven PJ et al. New potential treatment modalities for disseminated prostatic cancer. Urol Clin North Am 1984 May; 11(2):343–356.

Drago JR. Diagnostic techniques in prostatic cancer. Postgrad Med 1986 July; 80(1):214–224.

Elder JS and Catalona WJ. Management of newly diagnosed metastatic carcinoma of the prostate. Urol Clin North Am 1984 May; 11(2):283–295.

Fuselier HA Jr et al. Practical clues to managing impotence. Patient Care 1985 Sept 15; 19(15):61–75.

Fuselier HA et al. Diagnosing and managing chronic prostatitis. Patient Care 1985 Aug 15; 19(14):97–105.

George FW. Prostate cancer: Newer radiation therapy causes fewer side-effects. Your Patient and Cancer 1984 Apr; 4(4):96–109.

Greene LF. Rational management of prostatitis. Hosp Med 1984 Mar; 20(3):13–31.

Kadmon D and Fair WR. Prostate cancer: Managing its complications and the side-effects of treatment. Primary Care Cancer 1984 Sept; 4(89):78–90.

LaFollette SS. Radical retropubic prostatectomy. AORN J 1987 Jan; 45(1):57–71.

Lange PH. Management of localized prostatic cancer. Postgrad Med 1986 July; 80(1):235–245.

Lawler PE. Benign prostatic hyperplasia. AORN J 1984 Nov; 40(5):745–750.

Potency-sparing radical prostatectomy. Med Lett Drug Ther 1986 Jan 17; 28(705):8.

Schmidt JD. Treatment of localized prostatic carcinoma. Urol Clin North Am 1984 May; 11(2):305–309.

Slack NH et al. Criteria for evaluating patient response to treatment modalities for prostatic cancer. Urol Clin North Am 1984 May; 11(2):378–342.

Soloway MS. Treatment of prostatic cancer. Postgrad Med 1986 July; 80(1):249–258.

Walsh PC. How the new prostatectomy can preserve sexual function. Your Patient and Cancer 1984 June; 4(6):78–79.

Testicular Conditions

Belis JA. Testicular tumors. Hosp Med 1982 Apr; 18(4):37–52.

Clinical features of testicular tumors. Hosp Med 1986 Mar; 22(3):77–81.

Flickinger CJ. The effects of vasectomy on the testis. N Engl J Med 1985 Nov 14; 313(20):1283–1284.

*Hubbard S and Jenkins J. An overview of current concepts in the management of patients with testicular tumors of germ cell origin: I. Pathophysiology, diagnosis and staging. Cancer Nurs 1983 Feb; 6(1):39–47.

*Hubbard S and Jenkins J. An overview of current concepts in the management of patients with testicular tumors of germ cell origin: II. Treatment strategies by histology and stage. Cancer Nurs 1983 Apr; 6(2):125–139.

LaFollette SS. Effective treatment: Testicular cancer. AORN J 1983 Oct; 38(4):622–636.

Nursing Grand Rounds. Managing the patient with testicular cancer. Nurs '86 1986 Aug; 16(8):42–45.

Roth BJ and Lochrer PJ. Testicular cancer: New directions in therapy. Curr Concepts Oncol 1985 Spring; 7(1):7–16.

Thomas GM. Current controversies in the management of seminoma. Cancer Ther Update 1985 July/Aug; 5(4):3–5.

Wheatley JK. Evaluating male infertility. Hosp Med 1983 Aug; 19(8):157–179.

Cancer

Leuprolide (Lupron). New drug for prostatic cancer. Am J Nurs 1985 Sept; 85(9):951.

Schover LR et al. Sexual rehabilitation of urologic cancer patients: A practical approach. CA 1984 Mar/Apr; 34(2):66–74.

Srinivas V and Khan SA. Penile carcinoma. Hosp Pract 1985 Jan 15; 20(1):154–159.

Nursing Research Profile for Unit XI

Gynecologic Nursing

Overview

A number of factors have influenced nurse investigators to pursue research studies in this area. The nursing profession is more than 95% female, hence an inherent interest in the concerns and health of women. In addition, many assumptions and old wives' tales (unquestioned traditional beliefs) that have persisted with little or no scientific backing need to be investigated. Treatments for female disorders have been recommended for the most part by male physicians and, again, may not have been based on research findings.

Current investigation has concentrated on life change events (menstruation, menopause), gynecologic surgery (including breast surgery), and the significance of social supports. Nursing implications are many and significant, and have been included in the following summaries.

Potential areas for additional research are rich, and include the effects of contraceptives and abortion, the impact of infection, (toxic shock syndrome, AIDS), the increasing aging population, hormonal therapy, strenuous exercise, and changing work habits.

There is a noticeable lack of nursing research on conditions of the male reproductive system. Prostatic, testicular, and hormonal disorders, as well as malignancy, are general areas that need to be investigated.

Menstruation and Menopause

▷ *Jordan J and Meckler JR. The relationship between life change events, social supports, and dysmenorrhea. Res Nurs Health 1982 June; 5(2):73–79.*

The Jordan and Meckler study proposed to determine the relationship between life change events and dysmenorrhea, and the significance of social supports in this relationship. The survey included 156 female undergraduate nursing students. Support systems were viewed in four broad ways: (1) actual number of support persons—friends, family, counsellors/teachers; (2) quantitative aspects of meeting these persons (how often); (3) qualitative evaluation of their value; and (4) whether the subject had one particular person in whom to confide. Several questionnaires were used in one junior and one senior nursing class. The use of oral and other forms of contraceptives was also determined.

The results were surprising in that the degree of social support (high or low) did little to modify the relationship between life change events and dysmenorrhea. The only support dimension that seemed to make a difference was the confidant. Even the pain symptom was lower with a confidant than without one. The one problem with this study was that only 8% reported not having a confidant. This would indicate the desirability of doing a study with more evenly balanced groups: those having and those not having a confidant.

Nursing Implications. (1) As a result of the discussion of this research, it was noted that in a separate study of elderly subjects, maintaining a stable, intimate relationship was more closely associated with mental health than any other social factor—a point to consider in understanding and caring for elderly persons. (2) It may be worthwhile when taking a nursing history to determine whether the patient has a confidant.

(3) An interesting study would be to determine whether high use of health services correlates positively with lack of social supports such as confidants.

▷ *McKeever P and Galloway SC. Effects of nongynecological surgery on the menstrual cycle. Nurs Res 1984 Jan/Feb; 33(1):42–46.*

The purpose of McKeever and Galloway's study was to determine the nature and frequency of alterations in the menstrual cycle following nongynecological surgery in women.

All subjects studied had surgery under general anesthesia, and none were pregnant. There were 46 women age 19 to 25, and 31 women age 12 to 18. They were carefully screened to exclude any with menopausal symptoms or grossly irregular menstrual cycles, those taking medications known to alter the menstrual cycle, and those undergoing neurologic and gynecologic surgery. They were interviewed in the hospital 72 or more hours following surgery and again about 6 weeks later by telephone. Preoperatively, no adult subject had been advised of the possibility of an alteration in the length of the menstrual cycle after surgery. Most subjects (71%) who experienced an early menses after surgery were distressed by its occurrence; some expressed concern and others experienced pain that increased their general postoperative discomfort.

Nursing Implications. (1) Information on the likelihood of a change in the menstrual cycle length could be included in preoperative teaching of female surgical patients. (2) Menstrual distress may account for some of the physical discomfort and depression experienced by women in the early postoperative period. (3) Nurses need to be aware that many women find it embarrassing to be dependent on others for menstrual hygiene care.

▷ *Woods NF, Most A and Dery GK. Estimating perimenstrual distress: A comparison of two methods. Res Nurs Health 1982 Jun; 5(2):81–91.*

Two methods of measuring menstrual distress were presented to 73 women, ages 18 to 35, selected from lower middle to upper middle income neighborhoods. First, the women were asked to keep a daily diary for 2 months to record all symptoms. After 2 months, they were asked to respond to a questionnaire called Menstrual Distress Questionnaire (MDQ), which asked about symptoms experienced 1 week before the last menstruation, during menstruation, and during the remainder of the cycle. The collected diaries were compared with the questionnaires, using the data in the diaries for the comparable menstrual period only. Symptoms reported on the MDQ exceeded those documented in the diaries. It was interpreted that the MDQ probably indicated the effect of menstrual stereotypes and bias recall. That is, there appears to be a tendency to recall the discomforts and minimize the reporting of the more comfortable times.

Nursing Implications. Diaries are an effective means of recording symptoms and problems; however, to produce a meaningful data base, it is important to document symptom-free periods as well. In other words, stressing the positive is an effective tool in minimizing the negative. This would apply to any recording of symptoms by patients.

▷ *Feldman BM, Voda A and Gronseth E. The prevalence of hot flash and associated variables among perimenopausal women. Res Nurs Health 1985 Sep; 8(3): 261–268.*

The intent of Feldman and co-workers' study is to make an accurate assessment of the prevalence of hot flash in perimenopausal women. Common definitions of hot flash and menopause are presented, as well as a general review of pertinent studies.

A telephone survey of 594 women between ages 35 and 60 was done in a large midwestern metropolitan area. Questions used related to the subject's perception of menopause, experience of hot flash, use of estrogen, surgical procedures on the reproductive system, age hot flashes were first experienced, and their frequency.

The prevalence of hot flash was between 86% and 88%, indicating that most women experience this phenomenon. How long hot flash is experienced is highly variable, but frequency is greatest when the menstrual period first terminates; frequency continues to diminish through the postmenopausal years.

Nursing Implications. (1) The variability in occurrence of hot flash needs to be recognized by the nurse; hot flash may be experienced from a period of 1 to 11 years. (2) Frequency of hot flash also varies, from 72 in a day to too infrequent to count. (3) There is a greater prevalence of hot flash in the surgical menopause group and in those using estrogen; this information should be included in patient teaching of this group. (4) Encourage patients to keep careful records of their symptoms, including date and length of discomfort. Such a record assists health care personnel in their evaluation of the patient.

Hysterectomy

▷ *Webb C and Wilson-Barnett J. Self-concept, social support and hysterectomy. Int J Nurs Stud 1983; 20(2):97–107.*

Webb and Wilson-Barnett's study was designed to examine the effect of a simple hysterectomy on a woman's self-concept and the possible role of social support in the recovery process.

A review of more than 60 articles in medical journals suggested that a woman recovering from hysterectomy may find her image of herself radically changed even though her body shows no visible change. It was extrapolated that this operation may pose a profound threat to a woman's self-concept as a feminine person and an attractive sexual being, when childbearing is a highly valued social role.

Women having bilateral ovariectomy or surgery for malignant disease were excluded from the study. Structured interviews were done 5 to 6 days postoperatively, and follow-up interviews were done 4 months postsurgery, when recovery was well advanced but recollections still accurate. The study included over 100 subjects and was conducted in two hospitals.

Contrary to many literature reports, self-concept did not appear to be damaged. There was improvement in the categories of Negative and Helplessness scores. Women did not feel devalued or defeminized. With improved health and decreased levels of depression, an increase in Positive Self-

Concept scores was expected but did not occur (may be due to insensitivity of the scale). Results may reflect disappointment regarding the quality and quantity of partner support.

Nursing Implications. (1) There is a need to counsel women before hysterectomy and recovery; concerns should be elicited and misinformation corrected at this time. (2) It should be recognized that depression has not been proven to occur postoperatively. (3) Anxiety that femininity and sex life will be adversely affected has no basis in fact. (4) Health should be restored and even improved with recovery. (5) Support, guidance, and counseling should be given to the woman and her partner jointly.

Breast Conditions

▷ Lewis FM, Ellison ES and Woods NF. The impact of breast cancer on the family. Semin Oncol Nurs 1985 Aug; 1(3):206–213.

The unique and excellent article by Lewis and co-workers sought to focus attention in a direction other than that of the patient: to review selected concepts that characterize the impact on the family of the partner/mother who had nonmetastatic breast disease. In addition, the study highlighted selected research results and sought implications for nursing clinical practice. Information was obtained on initial at-home interviews with the mother, her partner, and their school-age children.

Family's adaptation to breast cancer may be characterized by conceptual themes that characterize all phases of illness: powerlessness, ambivalence (higher in families in which conflict was perceived as a dominant characteristic of the family's interaction), interdependence, uncertainty, restructuring, and resiliency.

The paper further briefly reviewed another area, that of the impact of divorce on a child, and attempted to relate psychosocial research to this study and the impact on the child. The child's perception is well presented in three age groupings: 7 to 10 years, 10 to 13 years, and 14 to 19 years. In addition, the demands of the illness on both mother and partner were analyzed.

Nursing Implications. (1) The entire article is well worth reading by the nurse caring for a woman with breast cancer. (2) Young children experience concern and fear for their safety when their mother has been diagnosed as having breast cancer. Strong assurances need to be made that, under all circumstances, the integrity of the family and the care of the children will be maintained. (3) Children age 10 to 13 need to have their competence, self-sufficiency, and self-control promoted and supported. (4) Adolescents' conflicts must be recognized: they are at an age when they want to "do their own thing" and yet are expected to spend time with and assist their mother. (5) Nearly 50 demands were identified as affecting the partners; for example, change in self-image, alopecia, weakness, and vulnerability to recurrence. A clear delineation of the demands of such an illness needs to be made (including the different ways in which women and men are affected by them). (6) Additional research is needed on including services to the isolated patient. On the whole, a number of avenues need to be explored and are identified in the last section of this study on future directions for service and research.

▷ Lierman L. Psychological preparation and supportive care for mastectomy patients. West J Nurs Res 1982 Summer; 4(3):13–19.

The intent of Lierman's study was to test the effectiveness of a systematic program of psychological preparation and supportive care for women diagnosed as having breast cancer and treated by mastectomy.

Of the 108 subjects, 23 control and 19 experimental subjects had mastectomies; 30 other control and 36 experimental subjects had biopsies. The latter grouping served as an additional control for the mastectomy groups.

The protocol consisted of the following: (1) Preoperative nursing history and needs assessment followed by preoperative teaching; (2) postoperative visits (twice daily) focusing on physical appearance, breast prosthesis, exercises, and anticipation of posthospital experiences (including coping mechanisms and support systems as well as community resources); and (3) consistent supportive relationship including empathy, reassurance, encouragement, trust, and confidence.

On the whole, the experimental group did slightly better postoperatively than the control group. Posthospital assessments at 1 month and 3 months indicated that the experimental group was slightly less depressed. Upon retrospective evaluation, it was noted that some women did not desire advance information about expected stress events. In addition, their high anxiety levels suggested that they were unable to process and comprehend this information.

Nursing Implications. (1) Psychological preparation and supportive care during the acute hospital phase may be effective in reducing the stress of a patient having a mastectomy. (2) More importantly, it appears that therapeutic interventions need to extend to the posthospital phase of recovery. The reason for this is that the multiple and complex stress situations extend over a prolonged period of time.

▷ Morra ME. Breast self-examination today: An overview of its use and its value. Seminars in Oncol Nurs 1985 Aug; 1(3):170–175.

The purpose of Morra's overview was to review the primary studies on awareness and use of breast self-examination (BSE), the value of BSE, and the latest research.

Some recent studies extol the values of the examination and state that it affects survival; others do not corroborate these findings. Some indicate no significant reduction in the average size of breast cancers in large unselected populations. Additional studies were done of various methods used to promote BSE. These include presenting demonstrations on how to do BSE using silicone models, training on the person's own breast, or combining the silicone model and the person's own breast; sending reminders by mail; and giving stickers or calendars in some instances. Rewards such as lottery tickets or Susan B. Anthony dollars were offered for those who reported more frequent BSEs and returned more records than other women. The need for additional research was advocated.

Nursing Implications. (1) Most women do not perform BSE monthly and they do not do all the steps; rewards do not have a lasting effect. (2) Questions that need to be addressed: Since about 50% of breast cancers occur in the upper outer breast quadrant, should this area be emphasized?

Are all the steps necessary? (3) Is there a way in which women could find lumps smaller than 2 cm? (Physicians seem to find them.) (4) The study proved that BSE teaching can be integrated into nursing service schedules without imposing a major burden.

Additional Studies

Bailey LJ. Effects of health teaching in the workplace on women's knowledge, beliefs, and practices regarding breast self-examination. Res Nurs Health 1986 Sept; 9(3):223–231.

Champion VL. Use of the health belief model in determining frequency of breast self-examination. Res Nurs Health 1985 Aug; 2(8):373–379.

Edgar L, Shamian J and Patterson D. Factors affecting the nurse as a teacher and practicer of breast self-examination. Int J Nurs Stud 1984; 2(4):255–265.

Hallal JC. The relationship of health beliefs, health locus of control, and self-concept to the practice of breast self-exam in adult women. Nurs Res 1982 May/Jun 31(3):137–142.

Kramer Sr MA, Albrecht S and Miller RA. Handedness and the laterality of breast self-examination. Nurs Res 1986 May/June; 35(3):183–185.

Massey V. Perceived susceptibility to breast cancer and practice of breast self-examination. Nurs Res 1986 May/Jun; 35(3):183–185.

Olshansky EF. Infertility of self as infertile: An example of theory-generating research. Adv Nurs Science 1987 Jan; 9(2):54–63.

Ray C et al. Nurses' perceptions of early breast cancer and mastectomy, and their psychological implications, and of the role of health professionals in providing support. Int J Nurs Stud 1984; 21(2):101–111.

Riddle LB. Expansion exercises: Modifying contracture of the augmented breast. Res Nurs Health 1986 Dec; 9(4):341–345.

Rutledge DN. Factors related to women's practice of breast self-examination. Nurs Res 1987 Mar/Apr; 36(2):117–121.

Scott DW. Anxiety, critical thinking and information processing during and after breast biopsy. Nurs Res 1983 Jan/Feb; 32(1):24–38.

Shaver JF and Woods NF. Concordance of perimenstrual symptoms across two cycles. Res Nurs Health 1985 Dec; 8(4):313–320.

Uphold CR and Susman EJ. Child-rearing, marital, recreational and work role integration and climacteric symptoms in midlife women. Res Nurs Health 1985 Mar; 8(1):73–82.

Webb C. Gynaecological nursing: A compromising situation. J Adv Nurs 1985 Jan; 10(1):47–54.

Immunology-Related Problems

Unit XII

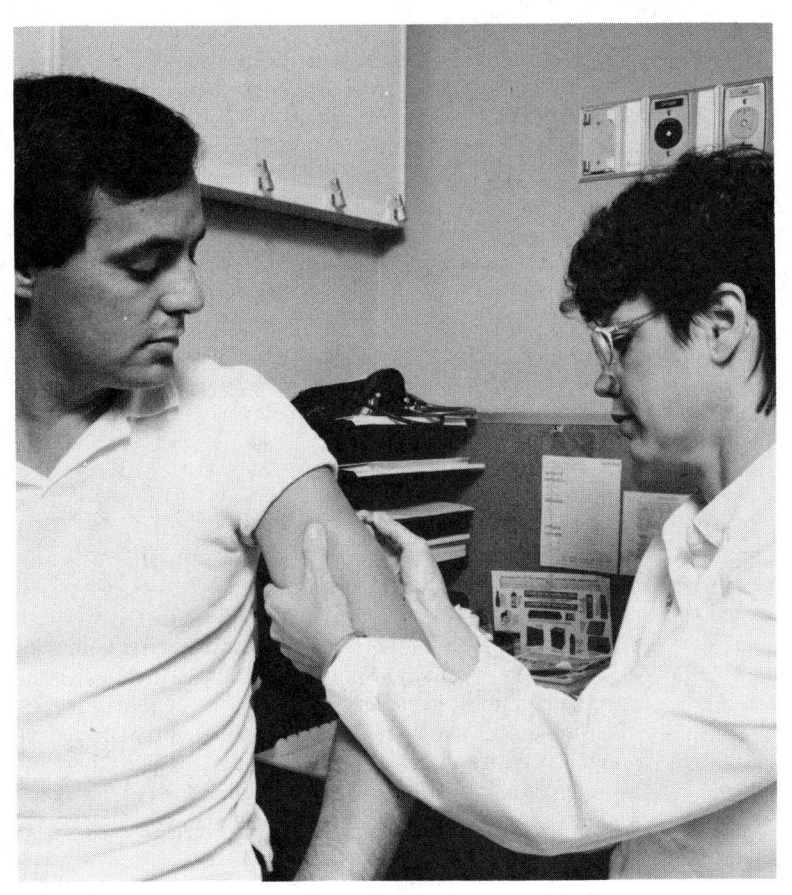

Chapter 45

The Immune System, Immunopathology, and Immunodeficiency

The term *immunity* refers to the body's specific protective response to an invading foreign agent or organism. However, pathological developments within the immune system lead to certain disease manifestations. Therefore, the term *immunopathology* is used to describe the study of diseases caused by the *immune reaction*—the protective response that the body initiates but which paradoxically turns against the body and causes tissue damage and disease. *Immunodeficiencies*, on the other hand, are disorders characterized by a defect in the immune system that leads to suppression of the immune response. To understand immunopathology and immunodeficiency, one must first understand how the body's immune system functions normally.

Types of Immunity: Natural and Acquired

There are two general types of immunity: natural immunity and acquired immunity. Natural immunity, which is a nonspecific immunity, is present at birth, while acquired or specific immunity develops after birth. Although each type of immunity plays a distinct role in the defense against harmful invaders, it is important to remember that the various components often act in an interdependent manner.

Natural Immunity

Natural immunity provides a nonspecific response to any foreign invader, regardless of the composition of the invader. The basis of natural defense mechanisms is merely the ability to distinguish between "self" and "nonself." Such natural mechanisms include physical and chemical barriers, the action of white blood cells, and inflammatory responses.

Physical barriers consist of intact skin and mucous membranes, which prevent pathogens from gaining access to the body, and the cilia of the respiratory tract along with coughing and sneezing responses, which act to clear pathogens from the upper respiratory tract before they can invade the body further. *Chemical barriers* such as acid gastric juices, enzymes in tears and saliva, and substances in sebaceous and sweat secretions act in a nonspecific way to destroy invading bacteria and fungi. Viruses are countered by other means, such as interferon (one of the *biologic response modifiers* currently being investigated), which is a nonspecific viricidal substance naturally produced by the body and capable of stimulating the activity of other components of the immune system.

White blood cells, or *leukocytes*, participate in both the natural and the acquired immune responses. Granular leukocytes, or *granulocytes* (so called because of granules in their cytoplasm), include neutrophils, eosinophils, and basophils. *Neutrophils* (also called polymorphonuclear leukocytes or PMNs because their nucleus has multiple lobes) are the first cells to arrive at the site of inflammation. *Eosinophils* and *basophils*, other type of granulocytes, increase in number during allergic reactions and stress responses. Granulocytes assist in fighting invasion by foreign bodies or toxins by releasing cell mediators, such as histamine, bradykinin, and prostaglandins, and engulfing the foreign bodies or toxins. *Nongranular leukocytes* include *monocytes* or *macrophages* (referred to as *histiocytes* when they enter tissue spaces) and lymphocytes. Monocytes also function as phagocytic cells and are able to engulf greater numbers and quantities of foreign bodies or toxins than granulocytes. *Lymphocytes*, consisting of B and T cells or lymphocytes, play major roles in humoral and cell-mediated immunity, as will be discussed later.

The *inflammatory response* is a major component of the nonspecific or natural immune system elicited in response to tissue injury or invading organisms. Chemical mediators assist in the inflammatory response to minimize blood loss, wall off the invading organism, activate phagocytes, and promote fibrous scar formation and regeneration of injured tissue. (The inflammatory response is discussed in detail on p. 83.)

Acquired Immunity

Acquired immunity consists of immunological responses that are not present at birth but acquired during life. Most acquired immunity develops as a result of contracting a disease or generating a protective immune response through immunization. Weeks or months after exposure to the disease or immunization, an immune response develops sufficiently to prevent contraction of the disease on re-exposure to it. This type of acquired immunity is referred to as *active acquired immunity* because the immunological defenses are developed by the body of the person being defended. Active acquired immunity generally lasts many years or even the person's lifetime. (Acquired immunity is discussed further in Chap. 46.)

Passive acquired immunity is temporary immunity transmitted from another source that has developed immunity through previous disease or immunization. Gamma globulin and antiserum, obtained from blood plasma of persons with acquired immunity, are used in emergencies to provide passive immunity to diseases when risk of contracting a specific disease is great and there is not time for a person to develop adequate active immunity.

Both types of acquired immunity involve humoral and cell-mediated (cellular) immunological responses, described below.

The Immune System

General Immune Responses

When the body is invaded or attacked by bacteria or viruses, it has three means of defending itself—the phagocytic immune response, the humoral or antibody immune response, and the cellular immune response.

The first line of defense, the *phagocytic immune response*, involves the white blood cells (granulocytes and macrophages), which have the ability to ingest foreign particles. These cells can move to the point of attack to engulf and destroy the foreign agents.

The second protective response, the *humoral or antibody response*, begins with the lymphocyte cells, which can transform themselves into plasma cells that manufacture antibodies. It is the antibodies, which are highly specific proteins, that are transported in the bloodstream and have the ability to disable the invaders.

A third mechanism of defense, the *cellular immune response*, also involves the lymphocytes, which, in addition to transforming themselves into plasma cells, can also turn into special killer T cells that can attack the microbes themselves.

Antigens and Antibodies

The part of the invading or attacking organism that is responsible for stimulating the production of an antibody is called an *antigen* or an *immunogen*.* An antigen is a small patch of proteins on the outer surface of the microorganism. A single bacterium, even a single large molecule such as a toxin (diphtheria or tetanus toxin), may have several such antigens or "markers" on its surface and can therefore induce the body to produce a number of different antibodies. Once an antibody is produced, it is released into the bloodstream and carried to the attacking organism, where it combines with the antigen on its surface, binding with it like a complementary piece of a jigsaw puzzle (Fig. 45-1).

Stages of the Immune System Response

There are four well-defined stages in an immune response: recognition, proliferation, response, and the effector stage. An overview of these stages is presented here, followed by descriptions of humoral immunity, cell-mediated or cellular immunity, and the complement system.

Recognition

The basis of any immune reaction is, first and foremost, recognition. It is our immune system's ability to recognize antigens on materials as "foreign," or "nonself," that is the initiating event in any immune reaction. The body must first recognize invaders as "foreign" before it can react to them.

Surveillance by Lymph Nodes and Lymphocytes. The body accomplishes its surveillance in two ways. First, the immune system is widely dispersed—distributed close to all

---

* The newer term *immunogen* is currently being used widely as an alternative to *antigen*.

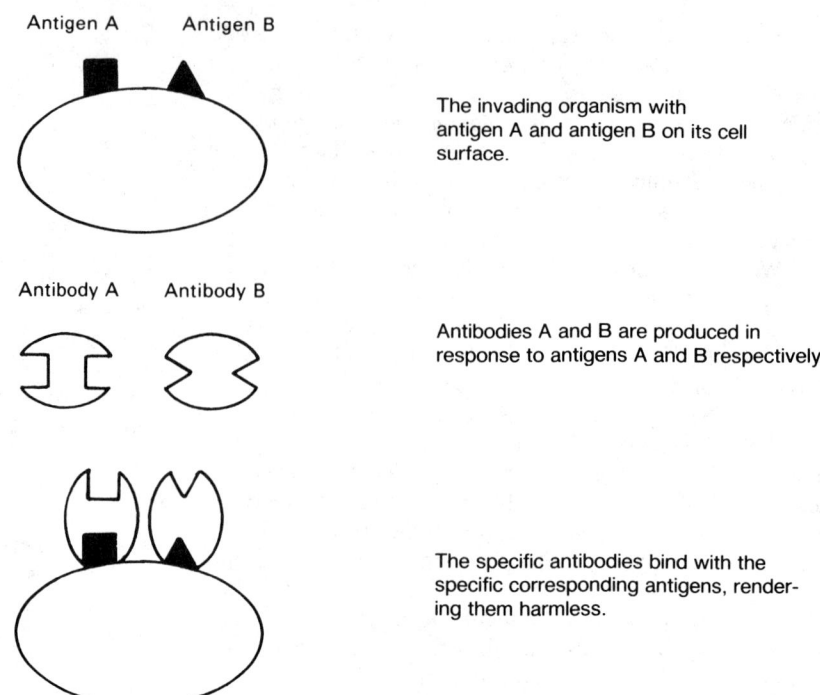

Antigen A   Antigen B

The invading organism with antigen A and antigen B on its cell surface.

Antibody A   Antibody B

Antibodies A and B are produced in response to antigens A and B respectively.

The specific antibodies bind with the specific corresponding antigens, rendering them harmless.

Figure 45-1
Antibody specificity. Antibodies are produced by B-cell lymphocytes to bind with specific antigens.

of the body's surfaces, internal as well as external, in the form of tiny organs called lymph nodes. Second, small lymphocytes are continuously being discharged from each lymph node into the bloodstream, where they patrol the tissues and vessels that drain the areas served by that node. Basically, it is the lymph nodes and lymphocytes that make up our immune system.

Circulating Lymphocytes.   There are lymphocytes in the lymph nodes themselves and those that circulate. Taken in aggregate, the total number of lymphocytes in the body adds up to a mass of cells of impressive size. Radioactive labeling of circulating lymphocytes has shown that these cells recirculate from the blood to lymph nodes and from their lymph nodes back into the bloodstream again, in a never-ending series of patrols. Some circulating lymphocytes can survive for decades. Some of these small, hardy cells maintain their solitary circuits for the lifetime of the person.

The exact way in which circulating lymphocytes recognize antigens on foreign surfaces is not known. At present, the accepted theory is that recognition depends on specific receptor sites on the surface of the lymphocytes. It appears that *macrophages*, a type of nongranular leukocyte found in the tissues of the body, play an important role in helping these circulating lymphocytes to process the antigens. Foreign materials enter the body, and a circulating lymphocyte comes into physical contact with the surfaces of these materials. Upon contact, the lymphocyte, with the help of macrophages, either removes the antigen from the surface or in some way picks up an imprint of its structure. For example, during a streptococcal throat infection, the streptococcal organism gains access to the mucous membranes of the throat, and a circulating lymphocyte moving through the tissues of the neck comes in contact with the organism. The lymphocyte, familiar with the surface markers on the cells of its own body, recognizes the antigens on the microbe as being different (nonself) and the streptococcus as being antigenic (foreign). This

triggers the second phase, the immune response—proliferation.

The Proliferation Stage

The circulating lymphocyte containing the antigenic message returns to the nearest lymph node. Once in the node, these "sensitized" lymphocytes stimulate certain of the dormant lymphocytes residing there to enlarge, divide, proliferate, and differentiate into either T lymphocytes or B lymphocytes. Enlargement of the lymph nodes in the neck in conjunction with a sore throat is one example of the immune response.

The Response Stage

In the response stage, the changed lymphocytes will function in either a humoral or a cellular fashion.

Humoral.   The production of antibodies to a specific antigen is called a humoral response, *humoral* referring to the fact that the antibodies are released into the bloodstream and so reside in the plasma or fluid fraction of the blood, one of the classical four "humors" of the body. (An explanation of humoral immunity and antibody function can be found on p. 1179.)

Cellular.   The returning sensitized lymphocytes migrate to areas of the lymph node (other than those areas containing lymphocytes programmed to become plasma cells), where they stimulate the residing lymphocytes to become cells that will attack microbes directly rather than through the action of antibodies. These transformed lymphocytes have been given the descriptive name *killer T cells*. The *T* stands for the fact that during the embryologic development of the immune system these lymphocytes spent some time in the thymus of the developing fetus, at which time they were genetically programmed to become T cells rather than the antibody-producing B lymphocytes. Viral rather than bacterial antigens induce a cellular response. This response is manifested by the increasing number of lymphocytes seen in the blood smears of people with viral illnesses—for instance, in the lymphocytosis occurring in infectious mononucleosis. (Cellular or cell-mediated immunity is discussed in detail on p. 1182.)

Most immune reactions to antigens involve both humoral and cellular responses, though usually one predominates. During transplantation rejections the cellular reaction predominates, whereas in the bacterial pneumonias and sepsis it is the humoral response that plays the dominant protective role (Chart 45-1).

The Effector Stage

In the effector stage, the antibody of the humoral response or the killer T cell of the cellular response reaches and couples with the antigen on the surface of the foreign object. The coupling initiates a series of events that in the majority of instances results in the total destruction of the invading microbes or the complete neutralization of the toxin. The events involve an interplay of antibodies (humoral immunity), complement, and action by the killer T cells (cellular immunity).

Figure 45-2 summarizes the phases of the immune response.

Humoral Immune Response

The humoral response is characterized by production of antibodies by the B-cell lymphocytes in response to a specific antigen. Although the B lymphocyte is ultimately responsible for the production of antibodies, both the macrophages of natural immunity and the special T-cell lymphocytes of cellular immunity are involved in recognition of the foreign substance and in antibody production.

Antigen Recognition

Several theories exist about the mechanisms by which the B cells recognize the invading antigen and produce appropriate antibodies in response. The existence of several theories probably results from the fact that there are several different methods of recognition of antigens by the B lymphocyte or cell. These different means of antigen recognition may also be responsible for different types of antibody response. Some antigens seem to have the ability to trigger antibody formation by the B lymphocytes directly, while others require the assistance of T cells.

T cells, or T lymphocytes, are part of a surveillance system dispersed throughout the body. These lymphocytes recycle through the general circulation, tissues, and lymphatic system. It is suggested that, with the assistance of macrophages, the T lymphocyte recognizes the antigen of a foreign invader. The T lymphocyte picks up the antigenic message or "blueprint" of the antigen and returns to the nearest lymph node with that message.

Antibody Production

B lymphocytes, which are stored in the lymph nodes, are subdivided into thousands of clones, each responsive to a single group of antigens having almost identical characteristics. The T lymphocyte carries the antigenic message back to the lymph node and stimulates specific clones of the B lymphocyte to enlarge, divide, proliferate, and differentiate into plasma cells capable of producing specific antibodies to the antigen. Other B lymphocytes differentiate into B-cell clones with a memory for the antigen. These "memory cells" are responsible for the more exaggerated and rapid immune response in a person who is repeatedly exposed to the same antigen.

Antibody Structure

Antibodies are large proteins that are referred to as *immunoglobulins* because they are found in the globulin fraction of the plasma proteins. Each antibody molecule consists of two subunits, each of which contains a light and a heavy peptide chain (Fig. 45-3). The subunits are held together by a chemical link composed of disulphide bonds. Each subunit has a portion that serves as a binding site for a specific antigen. This site, referred to as the *Fab* fragment, provides the "lock" portion that is highly specific for an antigen. An additional portion, known as the *Fc* fragment, allows the antibody molecule to take part in the complement system (to be discussed later).

The body is able to produce five different types of antibodies or immunoglobulins. Immunoglobulins in general are designated by the symbol *Ig*, and each of the five types, or classes, is identified by a specific letter of the alphabet (IgA, IgD, IgE, IgG, and IgM). Classification is based on the chemical

---

Chart 45-1
Comparison of Cellular and Humoral Immunologic Responses

Cell-Mediated Immune Responses	Humoral-Mediated Immune Responses
Transplant rejection	Bacterial phagocytosis and lysis
Delayed hypersensitivity—tuberculin reaction	Anaphylaxis
Contact dermatitis	Allergic hay fever and asthma
Graft-vs.-host reactions	Immune complex disease
Tumor surveillance or destruction	Defense against bacterial and some viral infections
Intracellular infections	
Defense against viral, fungal and parasitic infection	

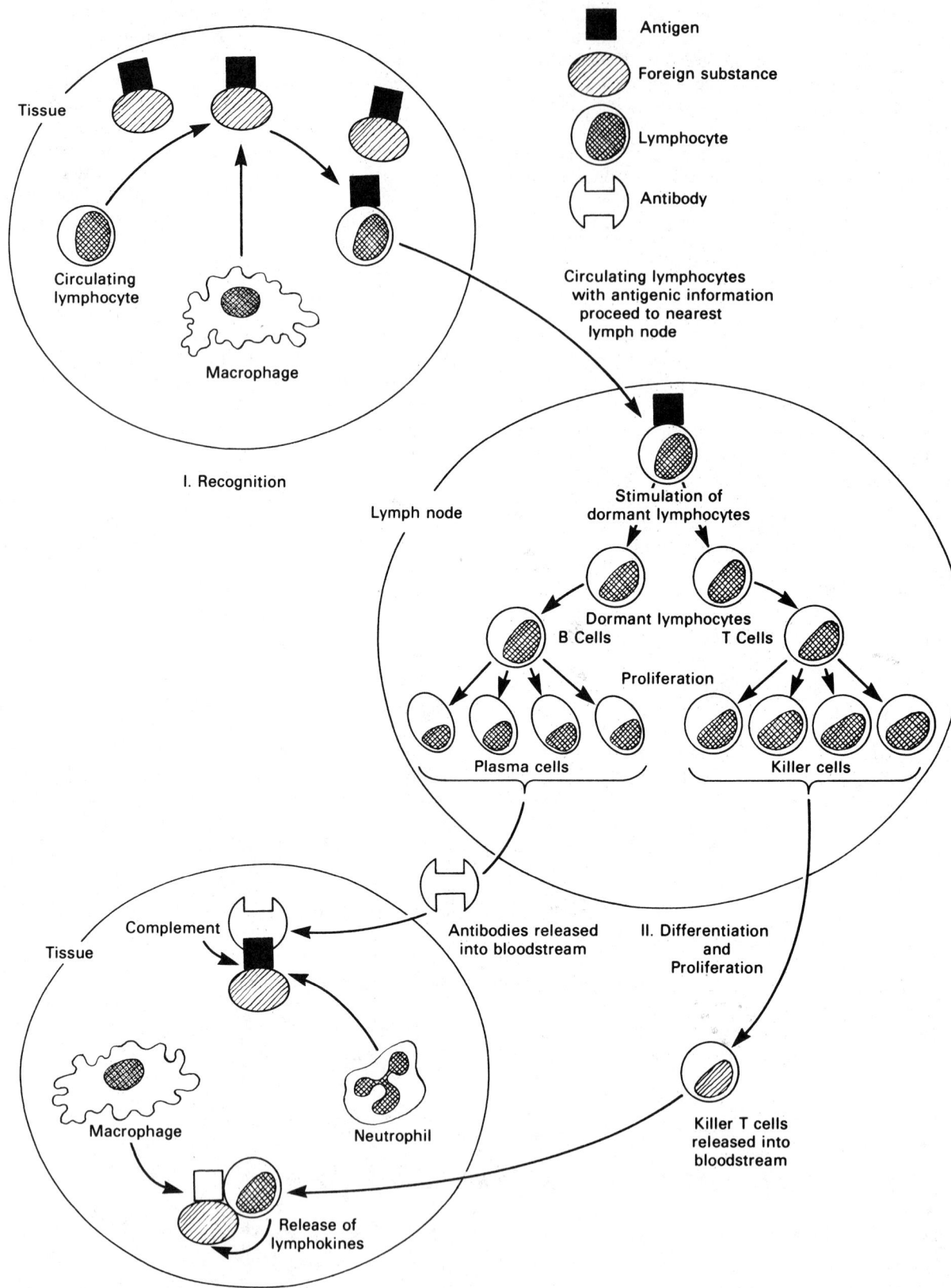

Figure 45-2

The phases of the immune response. I. Recognition of the antigen by circulating lymphocytes and macrophages. II. Stimulation of dormant lymphocytes, and differentiation and proliferation of T cells and B cells with formation and release of antibodies. III. Destruction or neutralization of antigens through the action of antibodies, complement, macrophages, and killer T cells.

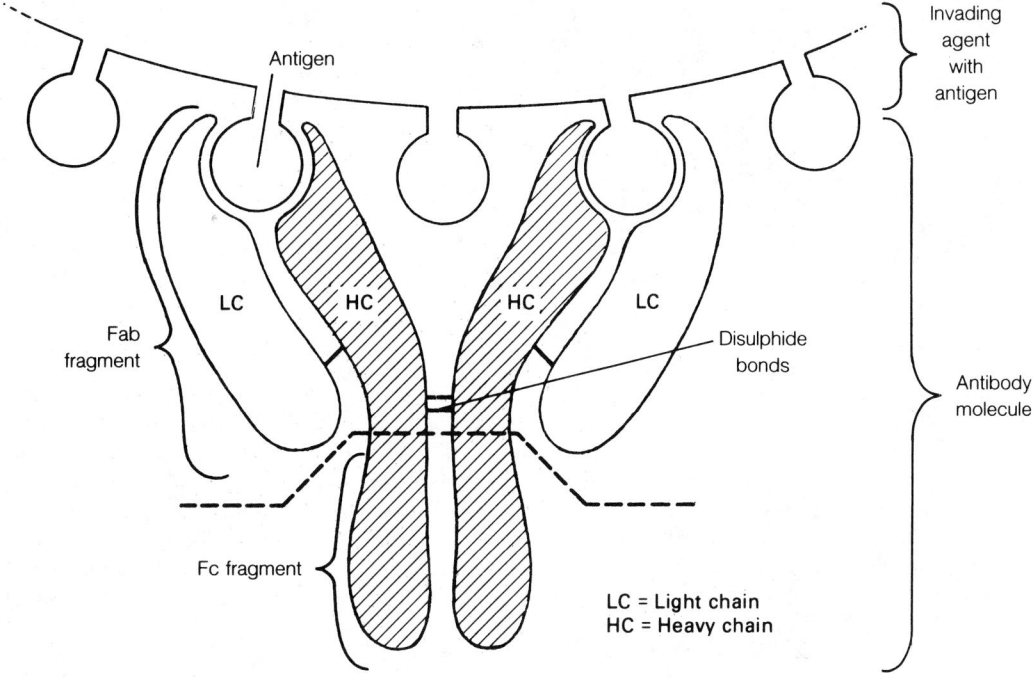

Figure 45-3
An antibody molecule. The Fab fragment serves as the binding site for a specific antigen.
The Fc fragment allows the antibody molecule to take part in the complement system.

structure and biologic role of the individual immunoglobulin.
Some of the outstanding characteristics of the immunoglobulins may be summarized as follows:

1. *IgG* (75% of total)

   · Present in serum and tissues (interstitial fluid)
   · Major role in bloodborne and tissue infections
   · Activates complement system
   · Enhances phagocytosis
   · Crosses placenta

2. *IgA* (15% of total)

   · Present in body fluids (blood; saliva; tears; breast
     milk; and pulmonary, gastrointestinal, prostatic, and
     vaginal secretions)
   · Protects against respiratory, gastrointestinal, and
     genitourinary infections
   · Prevents absorption of antigens from food
   · Passed in breast milk to protect neonate

3. *IgM* (10% of total)

   · Mostly limited to intravascular serum
   · First immunoglobulin produced in response to bac-
     terial and viral infections
   · Activates complement system

4. *IgD* (0.2% of total)

   · Present in small amounts in serum
   · Role unclear; may influence B-lymphocyte differ-
     entiation

5. *IgE* (0.004% of total)

   · Present in serum
   · Involved in allergic and hypersensitivity reactions
   · May help in defense against parasites

Antibody Function

Antibodies defend against foreign invaders in several ways.
The type of defense employed depends on the structure and
composition of both the antigen and the immunoglobulin. As
discussed above, the antibody molecule has at least two
combining sites known as the Fab fragments. One antibody
can act as a cross-link between two antigens, causing them
to bind or clump together. This clumping effect, referred to
as *agglutination,* helps in clearing the body of the invading
organism by facilitating phagocytosis. Some antibodies have
the ability to assist in the removal of offending organisms
through the process of *opsonization*. In this process, the
antigen–antibody molecule is coated with a sticky substance
that also facilitates phagocytosis.

Antibodies also promote the release of vasoactive substances, such as histamine and slow-reacting-substance (SRS),
two of the chemical mediators of the inflammatory response.
In addition, antibodies are involved in the activation of the
complement system.

Antigen–Antibody Binding

The portion of the antigen involved in binding with the antibody is referred to as the *antigenic determinant.* The binding
of the Fab fragment (antibody binding site) to the antigenic
determinant can be likened to a "lock and key" situation
(Fig. 45-4). The most efficient immunological responses occur
when the antibody and antigen fit exactly. Poor fit can occur
with an antibody that was produced in response to a different
antigen (Fig. 45-4). This phenomenon is known as *cross-
reactivity.* For example, in acute rheumatic fever, the antibody
produced against *Streptococcus pyogenes* in the upper respiratory tract may cross-react with the patient's heart tissue,
leading to damage to valves of the heart.

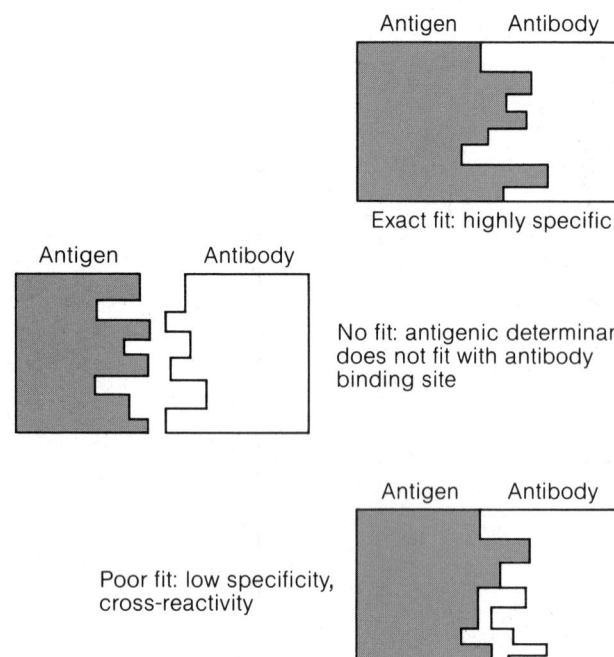

Antigen Antibody

Exact fit: highly specific

Antigen Antibody

No fit: antigenic determinant does not fit with antibody binding site

Antigen Antibody

Poor fit: low specificity, cross-reactivity

Figure 45-4
Antigen–antibody binding. (*Top*) A highly specific antigen–antibody complex. (*Middle*) No match and therefore no immune response occurs. (*Bottom*) Poor fit or match with low specificity; antibody reacts to antigen with *similar* characteristics, producing cross-reactivity. (Adapted from Kirkwood EM and Lewis CJ: Understanding Medical Immunology. Chichester, Sussex PO19 1UD, England, John Wiley & Sons, Ltd., © 1983, page 24. Used by permission of John Wiley & Sons, Ltd.)

Cell-Mediated (Cellular) Immune Response

While the B lymphocytes are the soldiers of humoral immunity, the T lymphocytes, also referred to as T cells, are primarily responsible for cellular immunity. These lymphocytes spend time in the thymus, where they are programmed to become T cells rather than antibody-producing B lymphocytes. There are several types of T cells, each with designated roles in the defense against bacteria, viruses, fungi, parasites, and malignant cells. T cells attack foreign invaders directly rather than through the production of antibodies.

Cell-mediated reactions are initiated by the binding of an antigen with an antigen receptor located on the surface of a T cell. This may occur with or without the assistance of macrophages. The T cells then carry the antigenic message or blueprint to the lymph nodes, where the production of other T cells is stimulated. Some T cells remain in the lymph nodes and retain a memory for the antigen. Other T cells, known as killer T cells, migrate from the lymph nodes into the general circulatory system and ultimately to the tissues, where they remain until they either come in contact with their respective antigens or die.

Upon contact with foreign cells (or antigens), some killer T cells release chemical mediators known as *lymphokines*.

These lymphokines are low-molecular-weight proteins with the ability to influence the inflammatory and immune responses to facilitate destruction and removal of the foreign cells or toxins. Lymphokines can recruit, hold, and activate other lymphocytes and macrophages to assist in removing the invading antigen. The actions of specific lymphokines are described in Table 45-1. One killer lymphocyte can, by releasing lymphokines, quickly recruit a large number of other cells into the area of antigenically foreign cells, amassing in a short time a large number of effector cells to protect the body. Unfortunately, such cellular activation can cause tissue injury and disease if the supposedly "foreign" cell under attack is in reality part of the person.

Other types of T-cell lymphocytes also contribute to the destruction and removal of antigens. Other T-cell lymphocytes include cytotoxic T cells, K cells, and helper and suppressor T cells. *Cytotoxic T cells* attack the antigen directly by altering its cell membrane and ultimately causing cell lysis (destruction). *K cells*, a subpopulation of lymphocytes that lack the usual characteristics of T cells, defend against antigens already coated with antibody. These cells have special Fc receptor sites on their surfaces that allow them to couple to the Fc end of antibodies.

The discovery of T-lymphocytes known as helper and suppressor cells has contributed to the understanding that humoral and cellular immune responses are not separate,

TABLE 45-1
Lymphokines and Their Biological Effects

Lymphokine	Effect
Permeability factor	Increases vascular permeability, allowing white cells into area
Interferon	Interferes with viral growth, stopping the spread of viral infection
Migration inhibitory factor	Suppresses movement of macrophages, keeping macrophage in area of foreign cells
Skin reactive factor	Induces inflammatory response
Cytotoxic factor (Lymphotoxin)	Kills certain antigenic cells
Macrophage chemotatic factor	Attracts macrophages into the area
Lymphocyte blastogenic factor	Stimulates more lymphocytes, recruiting additional lymphocytes into the area
Macrophage aggregation factor	Causes clumping of macrophages and lymphocytes
Macrophage activation factor	Causes macrophages to adhere to surfaces more readily
Proliferation inhibitor factor	Inhibits growth of certain antigenic cells
Cytophilic antibody	A factor that binds to an Fc receptor on macrophages that permits them to bind to antigens

unrelated processes, but branches of the immune response that can and do affect each other. Upon contact with the antigen, *helper T cells* (T_h or T_4 cells) release substances that enhance B-lymphocyte function and the production of antibodies. In addition, helper T cells contribute to differentiation of K cells and killer T cells. *Suppressor T cells* have the ability to decrease B-cell production, thereby keeping the immune response at a level that is compatible with health, (*e.g.,* sufficient to fight infection adequately without attacking the body's healthy tissues).

Complement

The term *complement* refers to circulating plasma proteins made in the liver that can be activated when an antibody couples with its antigen. Once activated, these proteins interact sequentially with one another in a cascade or "falling domino" effect. This causes alterations of the cell membranes on which antigen and antibody complex form, permitting fluid to enter the cell and leading eventually to cell lysis and death. In addition, activated complement molecules attract macrophages and granulocytes to areas of antigen–antibody reactions. These cells continue the body's defense by devouring the antibody-coated microbes and by releasing bacterial agents.

Complement plays a very important role in the immune response. Destruction of an invading or attacking organism or toxin is not achieved merely by the binding of the antibody and antigens, but also requires activation of complement, the arrival of killer T cells, or the attraction of macrophages.

Classical Complement Activation. There are two ways to activate the complement system. One, termed the classical pathway because it was the first method discovered, involves the reaction of the first of the circulating complement proteins (C_1), with the receptor site of the Fc portion of an antibody molecule following formation of an antigen–antibody complex. The activation of the first complement component then activates all the other components in the sequence in which the other components were discovered, namely C_1, C_4, C_2, C_3, C_5, C_6, C_7, C_8, and C_9.

Alternate Pathway of Complement Activation. The alternative method of complement activation occurs without the formation of antigen–antibody complexes. This alternate pathway can be initiated by the release of bacterial products such as endotoxins. When complement is activated through this pathway, the process bypasses the first three components (C_1, C_4, and C_2) and begins with C_3. Whatever the method of activation, however, once activated, the complement can and does destroy cells by altering or damaging the cell membrane of the antigen, by chemically attracting phagocytes to the antigen (*chemotaxis*), and by rendering the antigen more vulnerable to phagocytosis (*opsonization*). The complement system enhances the inflammatory response by the release of vasoactive substances.

This response is usually therapeutic and can be lifesaving if the cell attacked by the complement system is a true foreign invader, such as a streptococcus or staphylococcus. However, if that cell is in reality part of the person—a cell of the brain or liver, the tissue lining the blood vessels, or the cells of a transplanted organ or skin graft—the result can be devastating disease and even death. The result of the immune response—

the vigorous attack on any material read as foreign, the deadliness of the struggle—is obvious in the pus (the remains of microbes, granulocytes, and macrophages, T-cell lymphocytes, plasma proteins, complement, and antibodies) that accumulates in wound infections and abscesses.

Interferons

Biologic response modifiers are currently under investigation to determine their roles in the immune system and their potential therapeutic effects in disorders characterized by disturbed immune responses. *Interferons,* one example of the compounds known as *biologic response modifiers,* have antiviral and antitumor properties. In addition to responding to viral infection, they are produced by T cells, B cells, and macrophages in response to antigens. They are thought to have a role in modifying the immune response by suppressing antibody production and cellular immunity. They also facilitate the cytolytic role of macrophages and natural killer cells. Interferons are undergoing extensive study to determine their effectiveness in treatment of tumors and acquired immunodeficiency syndrome (AIDS).

Factors Affecting Immune System Functioning

Age. Persons at the extremes of the life span are more likely to develop problems related to immune system functioning than those in their middle years. There is an increased frequency and severity of infections in the elderly, which may be a result of a decreased ability to respond adequately to invading organisms. Both the production and the function of T- and B-cell lymphocytes may be impaired. The incidence of autoimmune diseases also increases with aging; this may be related to a decreased ability of antibodies to differentiate between "self" and "nonself." Failure of the surveillance system to recognize mutant, or abnormal, cells may be responsible for the high incidence of cancer associated with increasing age.

Declining function of various organ systems associated with increasing age also contributes to impaired immunity. Decreased gastric secretions and motility allow normal intestinal flora to proliferate and produce infection, causing gastroenteritis and diarrhea. Decreased renal circulation, filtration, absorption, and excretion contribute to urinary tract infections. Prostatic enlargement and neurogenic bladder can hinder the passage of urine and subsequently bacterial clearance through the urinary system. Urinary stasis, common in the elderly, permits the growth of organisms.

Exposure to tobacco and environmental toxins will impair pulmonary function. Prolonged exposure to these agents causes decreased elasticity of lung tissue, decreased effectiveness of cilia, and a decreased ability to cough effectively. These impairments hinder the removal of infectious organisms and toxins, increasing the elderly person's susceptibility to pulmonary infections and malignancies.

Finally, with age the skin becomes thinner and less elastic. Peripheral neuropathy and the accompanying decreased sensation and circulation may facilitate stasis ulcers, pressure sores, abrasions, and burns. Impaired skin integrity predisposes the aging person to infection from organisms that are part of normal skin flora.

Nutrition.   Adequate nutrition is essential for function of the immune system. Depletion of protein reserves results in atrophy of lymphoid tissues, depression of antibody response, reduction in the number of circulating T cells, and impairment of phagocytic function. As a result, susceptibility to infection is greatly increased. During periods of infection and serious illness, nutritional requirements may be exaggerated further, potentially contributing to protein depletion and an even greater risk of impaired immune response and sepsis.

Existence of Other Organ Diseases.   Conditions such as burns or other forms of trauma, infection, and cancer may contribute to altered immune system function. Major burns or other factors cause impaired skin integrity and compromise the body's first line of defense. Loss of large amounts of serum with burn injuries depletes the body of essential proteins, including immunoglobulins. The physiological and psychological stressors induced during surgical disruption of tissue integrity stimulate cortisol release from the adrenal cortex; increased serum cortisol also contributes to suppression of normal immune responses.

Cancer.   Immunosuppression contributes to the development of malignancies. However, cancer itself is immunosuppressive. Large tumors are able to release antigens into the blood that combine with circulating antibodies and prevent them from attacking the tumor cells. Furthermore, tumor cells may possess special blocking factors that coat tumor cells and prevent destruction by killer T lymphocytes. During the early development of tumors, the body may fail to recognize the tumor antigens as foreign and subsequently fail to initiate destruction of malignant cells.

Medications.   Certain drug therapies are capable of causing both desirable and undesirable alterations in immune system functioning. Four major classifications of medications have the potential for causing immunosuppression: antibiotics, corticosteroids, nonsteroidal anti-inflammatory drugs (NSAIDS), and cytotoxic drugs (Table 45-2). Therapeutic use of these agents requires striking a delicate balance between therapeutic benefit and dangerous suppression of host defense mechanisms.

Radiation.   Radiation therapy may be used in the treatment of cancer or in the prevention of allograft rejection. Radiation destroys lymphocytes and decreases the population of cells required to replace them. The size or extent of the irradiated area determines the extent of immunosuppression. Whole-body radiation renders the individual totally immunoincompetent.

Disorders of the Immune System

Disorders of the immune system can be divided into two general categories, one related to immunopathology and the other to immunodeficiencies. Disorders related to *immunopathology* are those diseases in which the normally protective immune response paradoxically turns against or attacks the body, leading to tissue damage. Disorders related to *immu-*

nodeficiencies are those diseases in which there is either an unexplained (primary) or explained (secondary) defect in one or more components of the immune response.

Immunopathology

When the body fails to differentiate between self and nonself, *immunopathology* may develop. This is a determining factor that allows the disease-producing potential of the immune response to take precedence over its protective nature. If the antigen is truly foreign, we are protected; if not, autoimmune disease and associated tissue damage result. The underlying problems of immunopathology may involve any component of the immune system in a variety of adverse interactions referred to as *hypersensitivity reactions*.

Allergic/Anaphylactoid Reaction (Hypersensitivity Type I)

An *allergic reaction* is a result of antigen–antibody reactions (specifically IgE) that attract and destroy mast cells. *Mast cells* are found in most tissues of the body, but are particularly abundant in connective tissue found in the lungs, intestinal mucosa, skin, and blood vessels. These cells serve as storage sites for histamine. As a result of mast cell destruction, histamine is released, causing sneezing, rhinitis, and watery eyes. Anaphylaxis, the most extreme reaction, involves laryngobronchospasm, shock, hypotension, and potentially death.

Cytotoxicity Reaction (Hypersensitivity Type II)

A cytotoxicity reaction occurs when the system mistakenly identifies a normal constituent of the body as foreign. Such reactions may be a result of a cross-reacting antibody and eventually lead to cell and tissue damage. An example of this is seen in myasthenia gravis, in which the body mistakenly generates antibodies against normal receptors of nerve endings. Another example is seen in Goodpasture's syndrome, in which antibodies against lung and renal tissue are generated, producing lung damage and renal failure.

Immune-Complex-Mediated Reaction (Hypersensitivity Type III)

Immune complexes (antigen–antibody molecules) normally circulate in the blood stream during the course of infectious diseases. Usually, these complexes cause no symptoms and eventually disappear from the circulation. However, in some persons these large complexes are deposited in the lining of blood vessels or on tissue surfaces. As a result, the complement system is activated and vasculitis (inflammation of blood vessels) and other tissue damage may occur. The vessels of the joints and kidneys are particularly susceptible to this type of injury. Examples of this process include glomerulonephritis and systemic lupus erythematosus (SLE). Antigen–antibody complexes involving streptococcus are often responsible for glomerulonephritis. In SLE, abnormal suppressor T-cell function may contribute to the development of antibodies gen-

TABLE 45-2
Drugs That Can Compromise the Inflammatory–Immune Response

Classification and Examples of Drugs	Effects on Inflammatory–Immune Response
Antibiotics (in large doses)	
Dactinomycin (Cosmagen)	Decreased antibody production
Chloramphenicol (Chloromycetin)	Hypoplasia of bone marrow
Mitomycin (Mutamycin)	Destruction of normal bacteria flora of gastrointestinal and respiratory tracts, allowing overgrowth of fungi or resistant strains of bacteria
Corticosteroids (in large doses)	Decreased antibody production
	Decreased fibroplasia
	Decreased polymorphonuclear (PMN) leukocyte responses
	Decreased prostaglandin synthesis
Cytotoxic Drugs	
Purine antagonists	Decreased antibody production in presence of antigen
Mercaptopurine (6-MP) (Purinethol)	
Azathioprine (Imuran)	
Folic acid antagonists	Blocked conversion of folic acid to tetrahydrofolic acid, which is
Methotrexate	necessary for DNA and RNA synthesis, particularly in leukocytes
Alkylating agents	Decreased antibody production
Mechlorethamine (Mustargen)	Destruction of circulating lymphocytes
Cyclophosphamide (Cytoxan)	Suppression of bone marrow production of leukocytes
Alcohol (in large amounts)	Depressed bone marrow production of leukocytes
	Decreased Kupffer cell activity
Heroin Addiction	Unknown action
Aspirin (in large doses)	Inhibition of prostaglandin synthesis and release
Indomethacin (Indocin) (in large doses)	Inhibition of prostaglandin synthesis and release

(Jett MF and Lancaster LE. The inflammatory immune response: The body's defense against invasion. Crit Care Nurs 1983 Sep/Oct; 3[5]:64–86. Used with permission.)

erated against the body's own DNA. DNA/antiDNA complexes may lead to arthritis and a form of glomerulonephritis associated with SLE.

Delayed Hypersensitivity (Hypersensitivity Type IV)

A delayed hypersensitivity reaction may occur as a result of exposure to microbial infections or to skin irritants, such as chemicals found in cosmetics or poison ivy. This type of hypersensitivity is dependent on lymphokines released from T-cell lymphocytes. As a result of the release of the lymphokines, inflammatory reactions can occur, leading to such problems as contact dermatitis, graft rejection, and the formation of granulomas.

In an attempt to isolate, contain, and block an invading microbe, the body may recruit a large mass of cells. This mass of cells surrounds and "walls off" the organism from the rest of the body in order to prevent dissemination and further infection. As a result, a granuloma is formed. An example of this type of response is the body's response to the tubercle bacillus. Unfortunately, as in tuberculosis, large caseating lung abscesses may be formed, compromising organ function.

Management

Treatment of immunopathology falls into two categories: (1) removal of the offending antigens, and (2) suppression of the immune response through immunosuppression. Unfortunately, the vast majority of antigens that cause immune disease have not yet been identified or, if known, cannot be removed from the body because they constitute normal cellular elements. Use of immunosuppression has become the most common method for dealing with immune reactions.

Immunosuppressive drugs may be classified according to their chemical structure and/or mechanism of action. Regardless of classification, most immunosuppressive drugs work by interfering with normal cell growth and metabolism. Some of these drugs were first used by cancer specialists in the treatment of malignancies because of their detrimental effects on cancer cells. We now know that immunosuppressive drugs also impede the growth and metabolism of T- and B-cell lymphocytes. For this reason, they are used in the treatment of immunopathology.

Immunosuppressive therapy, however, is not without potential adverse effects. The use of antimetabolites, for example, may increase the risk of infections and malignances such as leukemia and non-Hodgkin's lymphoma. Steroid therapy may increase the risk of infections or mask the signs and symptoms of infection. In addition, steroids may contribute to the development of hypertension, diabetes, gastrointestinal bleeding, cataracts, changes in appearance, and psychosis.

In view of the potential adverse effects of immunosuppressive therapy, the nurse has a key role in patient education and continuing assessment for potential complications. This role has special importance for nurses involved in the care of the older adult, who is already at risk for immune dysfunction.

Immunodeficiency

The second type of disorder of the immune system is immunodeficiency. Regardless of the underlying cause of immunodeficiency, the cardinal symptoms include recurrent, severe infections often involving unusual organisms. Immunodeficiencies may be classified as either primary or secondary, and also according to which components of the immune system are affected.

Primary Immunodeficiencies

Immunodeficiencies for which there are no known causes or underlying medical conditions are referred to as primary im-

TABLE 45-3
Primary Immunodeficiencies

Immune Component	Underlying Abnormality
Nonspecific immunity	Phagocytic dysfunction: chemotaxis, opsonization, ingestion, and digestion
Humoral immunity	Immunoglobulin production: decrease in or absence of one or all of the immunoglobulins (hypogammaglobulinemia)
Cellular immunity	Abnormal or absent T-lymphocyte production
Combined deficiencies	Abnormalities of more than one component of the immune system

TABLE 45-4
Factors Contributing to Secondary Immunodeficiencies

Immune Deficit	Examples
Alteration in skin integrity	Venipunctures, burns, trauma
Alteration in nutrition (deficit)	Anorexia, malabsorption, and impaired ingestion, digestion, and assimilation; severe protein losses in urine
Alteration in urinary elimination	Urinary stasis, bladder catheterization
Immunosuppressive therapy	Chemotherapy, antibiotics
Malignancy	Leukemia, lymphoma
Infectious processes	Septicemia, HIV (AIDS)

munodeficiencies. They may involve one or a combination of components of the immune system (Table 45-3).

Secondary Immunodeficiencies

Secondary immunodeficiencies, which are more common than primary deficiencies, often occur in the course of underlying disease or health care problems as a result of the treatment or of the conditions themselves. Persons with secondary immunodeficiencies are immunosuppressed and are often referred to as *immunocompromised hosts*. A variety of factors contribute to the development of secondary immunodeficiency (Table 45-4). The goals of treatment include elimination of the contributing factors and use of sound principles of infection control. Acquired immunodeficiency syndrome (AIDS) is an example of a devastating secondary immunodeficiency that results in increased susceptibility of the patient to a variety of infections and rare malignancies. This syndrome will be discussed in detail in the section that follows.

Acquired Immunodeficiency Syndrome (AIDS)

Acquired immunodeficiency syndrome (AIDS) is defined as the most severe form of a continuum of illness associated with *human immunodeficiency virus (HIV) infection*. HIV has previously been referred to as human T-cell lymphotropic virus type III (HTLVIII) and lymphadenopathy-associated virus (LAV). Manifestations of HIV infection range from mild abnormalities in the immune response without overt signs and symptoms to profound immunosuppression associated with a variety of life-threatening infections and rare malignancies.

Pathology

HIV belongs to a group of viruses known as *retroviruses*. The designation of retrovirus indicates that these viruses carry their genetic material in RNA rather than DNA. HIV is known to selectively infect helper T-cell lymphocytes. Through the use of an enzyme known as *reverse transcriptase,* HIV is able to reprogram the genetic materials of the infected T_4 cell. As a result, HIV can use the T_4 cell to reproduce the virus instead of itself. Consequently, whenever the infected T_4 cell is stimulated to reproduce by invading organisms, HIV is reproduced instead of the T_4-lymphocyte. The newly produced virus can then infect other T_4-lymphocytes.

As was discussed earlier in this chapter, the T_4-lymphocyte plays several important roles in the immune response, including recognition of foreign antigens, activation of antibody-producing B-cell lymphocytes, stimulation of cytotoxic T lymphocytes, production of lymphokines, and defense against parasitic infections. When T_4-lymphocyte function is impaired, organisms that do not usually cause disease are given the opportunity to invade and cause serious illness. Infections and malignancies that develop as a result of immune system impairment are referred to as *opportunistic diseases.*

Incidence

The Surgeon General of the U.S. has estimated that by the end of 1991, 270,000 cases of AIDS will have occurred in the U.S. and 5 to 10 million Americans will have been infected with HIV. An estimated 179,000 deaths from AIDS will have occurred by 1991, only 10 years after AIDS was first recognized.

Approximately 70% of AIDS victims in this country are male homosexuals and bisexuals. Users of intravenous drugs make up 25% of AIDS victims. Other risk groups include sexual partners of those infected with HIV, persons who have received blood products and transfusions infected with HIV (before screening of blood and blood products was possible), and children born to mothers infected with HIV. However, in large urban areas such as New York, San Francisco, Los Angeles, and Newark, proportionately greater numbers of AIDS cases are related to male homosexuality and intravenous drug use than to other risk factors.) AIDS is largely a disease of young people, the majority of cases affecting men between the ages of 20 and 49. This is expected to change, however, as heterosexual transmission and the number of AIDS victims increase in the next few years. AIDS has reached epidemic proportions in other parts of the world.

Transmission

The routes of transmission of HIV are very similar to those of hepatitis type B. In male homosexuals, anal intercourse or manipulation increases chances of trauma to the rectal mucosa and subsequently increases chances of exposure to the virus through body secretions. Increased frequency of this practice and multiple sexual partners have contributed to the spread of this disease. Heterosexual intercourse with individuals who have been directly exposed to HIV is also a means of transmission.

Transmission among intravenous drug users occurs through direct blood exposure to contaminated needles and syringes. Blood products, including those used by hemophiliacs, are capable of transmitting HIV to the recipients. The virus may also be transmitted *in utero* from mother to child. Transmission through breast milk has been suggested but not clearly documented.

In an attempt to screen blood products for evidence of HIV, the Food and Drug Administration (FDA) licensed an HIV antibody assay for all blood and plasma donations. The *ELISA (enzyme-linked-immunosorbent assay) test* determines the presence of antibodies directed specifically against HIV. The ELISA test does not establish a diagnosis of AIDS, but rather indicates that the individual has been exposed to or infected with HIV. Persons whose blood contains antibodies for HIV are said to be *seropositive.* The *Western blot assay* is another test that can identify the presence of HIV antibodies, and is used to confirm seropositivity as identified by the ELISA procedure. These tests are also used by physicians to assist in identifying patients with AIDS. It is expected that, in the future, HIV infections related to blood products will be largely eliminated as a result of screening efforts.

Diagnostic Evaluation

The manifestations of HIV infections vary. Diagnosis is based on clinical history, identification of risk factors, physical examination, laboratory evidence of immune dysfunction, presence of opportunistic disease based on biopsy or culture (Chart 45-2), and identification of HIV antibodies.

In the earliest stages of HIV infection, persons who are seropositive may be without signs or symptoms or laboratory evidence of immune dysfunction. Others may have laboratory evidence of immune dysfunction (Chart 45-3) without signs or symptoms of illness. Some persons in the early stages of HIV infection do develop a mononucleosis-type syndrome that is characterized by fevers, chills, muscle and joint aching, maculopapular rash, abdominal cramps, and diarrhea, and some may also develop enlarged lymph nodes and an enlarged spleen.

Persistent generalized lymphadenopathy (*PGL*) is another syndrome associated with HIV infection. PGL refers to the presence of at least two or more enlarged noninguinal lymph nodes that remain enlarged for 3 months or longer. Occasionally, PGL is accompanied by fevers. The term *AIDS-related complex* (*ARC*) is used to describe persons with HIV infection who have at least two symptoms indicative of immunodeficiency (Chart 45-3) as well as two or more laboratory abnormalities. It is currently estimated that approximately 10% to 20% of individuals with PGL or ARC go on to develop AIDS. Only the passing of time will reveal the true incidence of developing AIDS in those with PGL or ARC. The diagnosis of AIDS is reserved for those persons who develop life-threatening opportunistic infections and/or malignancies.

Clinical Manifestations

The clinical manifestations of AIDS are widespread and may involve the pulmonary, gastrointestinal, and neurologic systems as well as several types of malignancy and chronic illness due to opportunistic pathogens.

Pulmonary. Shortness of breath, dyspnea, cough, chest pain, and fever are associated with a variety of opportunistic infections such as those caused by *Mycobacterium avium intracellulare,* cytomegaloviruses, and *Legionella.* However, the most common infection in persons with AIDS is *Pneumocystis carinii pneumonia* (*PCP*), which has a mortality

Chart 45-2
Opportunistic Diseases

Protozoan Infections

Pneumocystis carinii pneumonia
Toxoplasma gondii encephalitis or disseminated infection
(excluding congenital infection)
Chronic *Cryptosporidium enteritis* (longer than 1 month)

Fungal Infections

Candidiasis (esophageal, bronchial, or pulmonary)
Chronic cryptosporidiosis (meningitis or disseminated)

Bacterial Infections

Disseminated *Myobacterium avium intracellulare*
Mycobacterium kansasii

Viral Infections

Cytomegalovirus
Chronic mucocutaneous or disseminated herpes simplex
Multidermatomal herpes zoster
Progressive multifocal leukoencephalopathy

Malignancies

Kaposi's sarcoma
Primary brain lymphoma
NonHodgkins lymphoma

Helminthic Infections

Strongyloidiasis
Isosporiasis

(Adapted from Opportunistic Infections and Diseases Indicative of Immunodeficiency [slide presentation]. U.S. Department of Health and Human Services, Centers for Disease Control)

rate of approximately 60%. *Pneumocystis carinii*, a protozoan, causes disease only in immunocompromised hosts. It invades and proliferates within the pulmonary alveoli, resulting in consolidation of the pulmonary parenchyma.

The clinical presentation of PCP in the AIDS patient is generally less acute than in persons who are immunosuppressed as a result of other conditions. The period of time between the onset of symptoms and the actual documentation of disease may be weeks to months. Patients with AIDS initially develop nonspecific signs and symptoms such as fevers, chills,

nonproductive cough, shortness of breath, dyspnea, and occasionally chest pain. PCP may be present despite the absence of crackles or rhonchi. Room air arterial oxygen concentrations may be mildly decreased, indicating minimal hypoxemia. Untreated, PCP will eventually progress to cause significant pulmonary impairment and ultimately respiratory failure. A small number of patients have a dramatic onset and fulminant course, involving severe hypoxemia, cyanosis, tachypnea, and altered mental status. Respiratory failure can develop within 2 to 3 days of initial onset of symptoms.

Chart 45-3
Signs and Symptoms and Laboratory Studies Indicating Immune Dysfunction

Clinical Signs/Symptoms
Chronic condition present for 3 months or longer, *unexplained.*
Lymphadenopathy $\geq$ 2 noninguinal sites
Fever $\geq$ 38°C, intermittent or continuous
Unexplained diarrhea
Unexplained fatigue/malaise
Unexplained night sweating

Laboratory Studies
Decreased number of T-helper cells
Decreased ratio of T-helper: T-suppressor lymphocytes
Anemia *or* leukopenia *or* thrombocytopenia *or* lymphopenia
Increased serum globulin levels
Decreased blastogenic response of lymphocytes to mitogens
Cutaneous anergy to multiple skin-test antigens
Increased levels of circulating immune complexes

(Gottlieb MS and Groopman JE [eds]. AIDS, p. 70. New York, Alan R Liss, 1984. Reprinted with permission.)

PCP can only be diagnosed definitively by identification of the PCP protozoan in bronchial secretions or lung tissue. The most common means of isolating the organism is transbronchial biopsy obtained by using a fiberoptic bronchoscope.

Gastrointestinal. The gastrointestinal manifestations of AIDS include loss of appetite, nausea, vomiting, oral and esophageal candidiasis, and chronic diarrhea. *Diarrhea* is a problem for 50% to 90% of all AIDS patients. Some of the enteric pathogens that occur most frequently, which are identified by stool cultures or intestinal biopsy, include *Cryptosporidium muris*, *Salmonella*, cytomegalovirus (CMV), *Clostridium difficile*, and *Mycobacterium avium intracellulare*. For patients with AIDS, the effects of diarrhea can be devastating in terms of profound weight loss (more than 10% of body weight), fluid and electrolyte imbalances, perianal skin excoriation, weakness, and inability to carry out usual activities of daily living. Although many forms of infectious diarrhea respond to treatment, it is not unusual for the infections to recur and become a chronic problem.

Oral candidiasis, a fungal infection, is nearly universal in all patients with AIDS and AIDS-related conditions. The development of oral candidiasis often precedes other life-threatening infections. It is characterized by the presence of creamy white patches in the oral cavity. When untreated, oral candidiasis will progress to involve the esophagus. Associated signs and symptoms include difficult and painful swallowing and retrosternal pain. Some patients also develop ulcerating oral lesions, and are particularly susceptible to dissemination of candidiasis to other body systems.

Neurologic. Approximately 30% to 40% of all patients with AIDS experience some form of neurologic involvement during the course of HIV infection. Neurologic complications may involve both the central and the peripheral nervous systems. Signs and symptoms may be subtle and difficult to distinguish from fatigue, depression, or the adverse effects of treatment for infections and malignancies.

Subacute encephalitis accounts for approximately 25% of the neurologic dysfunctions in AIDS. This syndrome is characterized by memory deficits, headache, fever, progressive confusion, and visual disturbances. As the syndrome progresses, patients develop seizures and coma followed by death. Extensive neurologic evaluation, including radiologic procedures, lumbar puncture, and brain biopsy, may fail to identify the underlying etiology. Although the exact cause of subacute encephalitis is unclear, some investigators believe that it may result from CMV infection of the central nervous system.

Progressive multifocal leukoencephalopathy (*PML*) is a central nervous system demyelinating disorder that is associated with AIDS. This disorder, which is caused by a virus, may begin with mental confusion and rapidly progress to include blindness, aphasias, paresis, and ultimately death. Other common infections involving the nervous system include *Toxoplasma gondii* and *Cryptococcus neoformans*. Computed tomography and brain biopsy are often useful in identifying the source of neurologic impairments.

Malignancy. Kaposi's sarcoma (KS), some forms of non-Hodgkin's lymphoma, and primary brain lymphoma are associated with AIDS. *Kaposi's sarcoma*, the complication that occurs most commonly, is a disease involving the endothelial layer of blood and lymphatic vessels. When first noted in 1872, KS characteristically presented as lower extremity skin lesions in elderly men of Eastern European ancestry. In that population, the disease was slow to progress and easily treated. However, in the AIDS population KS is far more aggressive and often widely disseminated at the time of diagnosis. KS can effect any organ system, including skin, lymphatic, pulmonary, gastrointestinal, and central nervous systems. Skin involvement may range from purple lesions found on the trunk, face, oral mucosa, or extremities to fungating wounds that increase the patient's susceptibility to infection (Fig. 45-5). Involvement of internal organs may eventually lead to organ failure, hemorrhage, and death. Diagnosis of KS is confirmed through biopsy of suspected lesions.

Chronic Illness. Almost all AIDS patients develop at least one opportunistic infection during the course of their disease. Although many infections are successfully treated, some persons never fully recover and are at increased risk for developing a second infection or malignancy. Treatment is often complicated by the debilitating signs and symptoms of HIV infection that include unexplained fatigue, headache, profuse night sweats, unexplained weight loss, dry cough, shortness of breath, extreme weakness, diarrhea, and persistent lymphadenopathy. Chronic illness develops when opportunistic diseases and the symptoms of HIV do not resolve.

The effects of chronic illness—repeated and prolonged hospitalizations—can be devastating. Persons who progress to the terminal phases of HIV infection are usually severely immunocompromised. Multiple local and disseminated infections involving several organ systems are common. Many persons become profoundly malnourished as a result of impaired oral intake, gastrointestinal malabsorption, and the effects of opportunistic diseases. Pulmonary, renal, and hepatic failure may develop as a result of infection or malignancy. Skin breakdown related to immobility, profuse diarrhea, and progression of KS is common. Neurologic impairments may progress to coma and eventually death.

Patients in the advanced stages of AIDS are often no longer able to work, maintain current roles or relationships, or care for themselves independently. Although the length of survival varies from months to years, approximately half of all the cases that have occurred since 1981 have resulted in death. Death occurs because either there is no known effective treatment for the opportunistic diseases or the patient no longer responds to standard therapy.

Management

At this time, no effective treatment exists for the underlying viral infection and subsequent immunodeficiency seen in AIDS. Medical management is aimed at treating opportunistic infections and malignancies, and includes supportive care for the debilitating effects of chronic illness such as malnutrition, skin breakdown, weakness, immobility, and altered mental status.

Trimethoprim-sulfamethoxazole (TMP/SMZ) is an antibacterial drug that is used to treat a variety of organisms causing infection. It has long been the treatment of choice for *Pneumocystis* pneumonia (PCP) in nonAIDS patients. Unfortunately, AIDS patients with PCP who are treated with TMP/SMZ have experienced an increased incidence of adverse effects such as rashes, decreased white blood cell counts, and drug-related fevers. These adverse effects have been re-

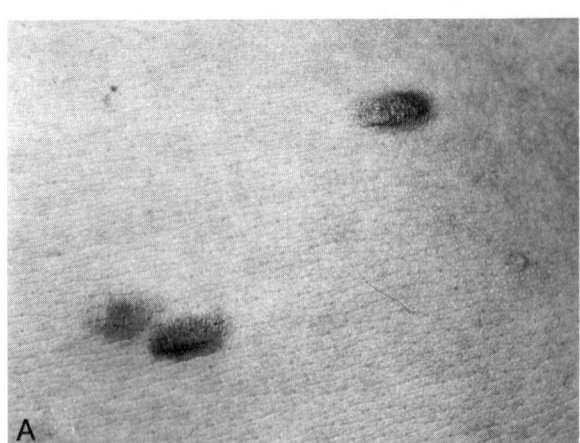
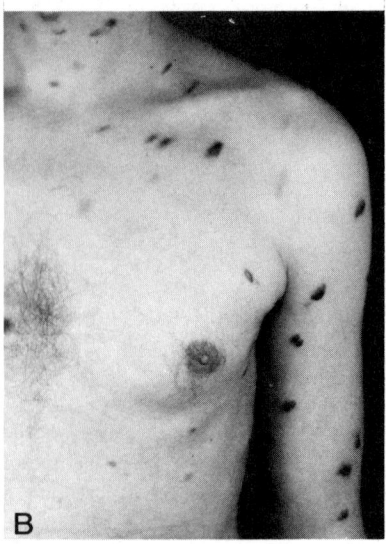

Figure 45-5
Epidemic Kaposi's sarcoma. (*A*) The ovoid shape of the lesions is a common feature of
AIDS-associated Kaposi's sarcoma. (*B*) With time, an increasing number of patch,
plaque, and eventually nodular lesions may appear throughout the course of the disease.
The symmetrical distribution of lesions along the lines of skin cleavage (Langer's lines) is
typical of AIDS-associated Kaposi's sarcoma. (DeVita VT Jr, Hellman S, and Rosenberg
SA. AIDS Etiology, Diagnosis, Treatment, and Prevention. Philadelphia, JB Lippincott,
1985.)

ported in as many as 65% of all AIDS patients treated with
TMP/SMZ. Pentamidine, an antiprotozoal drug, is a second
option for combatting PCP. Many physicians initiate treatment
with TMP/SMZ and change to pentamidine if adverse effects
develop or patients do not show evidence of clinical improvement when treated with TMP/SMZ. The adverse effects
of pentamidine include the formation of sterile abscesses at
the site of intramuscular injection, impaired glucose metabolism, renal damage, and bone marrow suppression.

The treatment of Kaposi's sarcoma remains experimental
and has had limited success. Radiation therapy has been used
to eradicate localized lesions that are disfiguring and anatomically inconvenient. Unfortunately, recurrence of irradiated lesions is not uncommon. Various single-agent and
combination chemotherapy regimens have been tried with
limited effectiveness. Chemotherapeutic drugs attempt to stop
the growth of malignant tumors by interfering with cell metabolism and reproduction. Some of the chemotherapeutic
agents that have been used in treating Kaposi's sarcoma are
vinblastine, etoposide, adriamycin, and bleomycin. Unfortunately, chemotherapy may induce bone marrow suppression
and opportunistic infections in an already immunocompromised patient.

Persons who become weak and debilitated as a result
of chronic illness associated with HIV infection often require
many forms of supportive care. Nutritional support may be
as simple as providing assistance for obtaining or preparing
meals. For persons with more advanced nutritional impairment that results from decreased intake or gastrointestinal
malabsorption associated with diarrhea, parenteral feedings
such as intravenous hyperalimentation may be required. Fluid
and electrolyte imbalances that result from nausea, vomiting,
and profuse diarrhea often necessitate intravenous replace-

ment. Skin breakdown associated with Kaposi's sarcoma,
perianal skin excoriation, and immobility is managed with
thorough and meticulous skin care involving turning schedules, cleansing, and application of ointments and dressings
as prescribed by the physician. Pulmonary symptoms such
as dyspnea and shortness of breath may be related to infection, Kaposi's sarcoma, or fatigue. For these patients oxygen
therapy, relaxation training, and energy conservation techniques may be helpful. Patients with severe respiratory dysfunction may require mechanical ventilation in order to sustain
life. Pain associated with skin breakdown, abdominal cramping, or Kaposi's sarcoma is managed by analgesics given at
regular intervals around the clock. Relaxation and guided
imagery can be helpful in reducing pain and anxiety.

Future Treatment Options

Throughout the world, researchers are searching for ways to
halt the human immunodeficiency virus. A variety of antiviral
drugs are being investigated—for example, Suramin, HPA-
23, ansamycin, phosphonoformate, ribavirin, and azido-
thymidine (AZT). These drugs act by inhibiting the activity
of reverse transcriptase. It is believed that these agents, in
doing so, can stop virus replication by preventing the virus
from reprogramming the genetic material of helper T lymphocytes. Considerable attention has been focused on AZT,
which has demonstrated promising results in patients with
AIDS-related complex and in patients with *Pneumocystis*
pneumonia. In clinical trials, orally-administered AZT has been
shown to halt reproduction of HIV, allowing the infected T
cells to recover, multiply, and regain their immunologic functions. Although preliminary results of AZT have been quite
positive, the long-term effects of AZT and other antiviral

agents remain unknown. In addition, these drugs are associated with potentially serious side-effects such as hemolytic anemia and bone marrow suppression.

In addition to identifying ways to halt HIV replication, investigators are also studying a variety of approaches that will reconstitute and enhance immune system functions. Interferons and interleukin-2 (IL2) are examples of substances occurring naturally in the body that enhance immune system functions. Their success in clinical trials has been mixed. Although interferon has shown positive results in the treatment of Kaposi's sarcoma, its effectiveness in the treatment of patients with opportunistic infections has been disappointing. Other attempts to restore the immune system include bone marrow transplantation and lymphocyte transfusions. Patient improvement and survival depend not only on eliminating the HIV but also on restoring the damaged immune system.

▶ Nursing Process
The Patient With Acquired Immunodeficiency Syndrome (AIDS)

The nursing care of persons with AIDS is quite challenging because of the potential for any organ system to be the target of infections or malignancies. In addition, this disease is complicated by several controversial emotional and ethical issues. The plan of care for the patient with AIDS is individualized to meet the needs of the patient.

▷ Assessment

Nursing assessment includes identification of potential risk factors, including sexual history and history of intravenous drug use. The patient's physical status and psychological status are assessed. All factors reflecting immune system functioning are thoroughly explored.

Nutritional status is assessed by obtaining a dietary history and identifying factors that may interfere with oral intake, such as anorexia, nausea, vomiting, oral pain, or difficulty swallowing. In addition, the patient's ability to purchase and prepare food is investigated. Weight, triceps skin fold measurements, and blood urea nitrogen, serum protein, albumin, and transferrin levels provide objective measurements of nutritional status.

The *skin and mucous membranes* are inspected daily for evidence of breakdown, ulceration, and infection. The oral cavity is monitored for redness, ulcerations, and the presence of white creamy patches indicative of candidiasis. It is especially important to assess the perianal area for excoriation and infection in those patients with profuse diarrhea. Wound cultures are obtained in order to identify infectious organisms.

Respiratory status is assessed by monitoring the patient for cough, sputum production, shortness of breath, orthopnea, tachypnea, and chest pain. The presence and quality of breath sounds are also assessed. Other objective parameters of pulmonary function include chest x-rays, arterial blood gas concentrations, and pulmonary function tests.

Neurologic status is determined by assessing the patient's level of consciousness and orientation to person, place, and time, and the occurrence of memory lapses. The patient is also observed for sensory impairments such as visual changes, headache or numbness, and tingling in the extremities. Motor impairments such as altered gait and paresis may also occur. Finally, the patient is observed for evidence of seizure activity.

Fluid and electrolyte status is assessed by examining the skin and mucous membranes for turgor and dryness. Increased thirst, decreased urine output, low blood pressure or a decline in systolic blood pressure of 15 mm Hg with concurrent rise in pulse when the patient sits up, weak rapid pulse, and specific gravity of 1.025 or more may indicate dehydration. Electrolyte imbalances such as decreased serum sodium, potassium, calcium, magnesium, and chloride often result from profuse diarrhea. The patient is assessed for signs and symptoms of electrolyte depletion. These may include decreased mental status, muscle twitching, muscle cramps, irregular pulse, nausea and vomiting, and shallow respirations.

The patient's *level of knowledge* about the disease and means of transmission is evaluated. In addition, the level of knowledge of family and friends is investigated. The patient's psychological reaction to the diagnosis of AIDS is important to explore. Reactions vary among individuals and may include denial, anger, fear, shame, withdrawal from any social interactions, and depression. It is often helpful to gain an understanding of how the patient has dealt with illness and major life stressors in the past. The patient's resources for support are also important to identify.

▷ Nursing Diagnoses

The list of potential nursing diagnoses is quite extensive because of the complex nature of this disease. However, based on assessment data, major nursing diagnoses for the patient may include the following:

- Alteration in perianal skin integrity related to excoriation and diarrhea
- Alteration in bowel elimination: diarrhea related to enteric pathogens and/or HIV infection
- Potential for infection related to immunodeficiency
- Activity intolerance related to weakness, fatigue, malnutrition, impaired fluid and electrolyte balance, and hypoxia associated with pulmonary infections
- Alteration in thought processes related to shortened attention span, impaired memory, confusion, and disorientation associated with AIDS encephalitis
- Alteration in fluids and electrolyte balance related to losses associated with persistent diarrhea
- Ineffective airway clearance related to *Pneumocystis* pneumonia, increased bronchial secretions, and decreased ability to cough related to weakness and fatigue
- Alteration in comfort: pain related to diarrhea and impaired perianal skin integrity
- Inadequate nutritional status related to decreased oral intake
- Deficit in knowledge concerning means of preventing transmission of HIV
- Social isolation related to stigma of the disease, withdrawal of support systems, isolation procedures, and fear of infecting others
- Grieving related to changes in life-style and roles and to unfavorable prognosis

▷ Planning and Implementation

▷ **Goals:** Goals for the patient may include achievement and maintenance of perianal skin integrity, resumption of usual bowel habits, absence of infection, improved activity tolerance, improved thought processes, maintenance of fluid and electrolyte status, improved airway clearance, increased comfort, improvement of nutritional status, increased knowledge concerning means of preventing disease transmission, decreased sense of social isolation, and expression of grief.

Nursing Interventions

Perianal Skin Care. The patient's perianal region is assessed frequently for impairment of skin integrity and infection. The patient is instructed to keep the area as clean as possible. The perianal area is cleaned after each bowel movement with nonabrasive soap and water to prevent further excoriation and breakdown of the skin and infection. If the area is very painful, soft cloths or cotton sponges may prove to be less irritating than washcloths. In addition, sitzbaths or gentle irrigation may facilitate cleansing and promote comfort. The area is dried thoroughly after cleansing. The physician is consulted concerning topical lotions or ointments to promote healing. Wounds are cultured if infection is suspected so that the appropriate antimicrobial treatment can be initiated. Debilitated patients may require assistance in maintaining hygienic practices.

Resumption of Usual Bowel Habits. The patient's bowel patterns are assessed for signs and symptoms of diarrhea, including frequency and consistency of stools and the presence of abdominal pain or cramping associated with bowel movements. Factors that exacerbate the frequency of diarrhea are also assessed. The quantity and volume of liquid stools are measured in order to document fluid volume losses. Stool cultures are obtained in order to identify pathogenic organisms.

The patient is counseled about ways to decrease diarrhea. Restriction of oral intake may be indicated and recommended by the physician in order to rest the bowel during periods of acute bowel inflammation associated with severe enteric infections. As the patient's dietary intake is advanced, the patient is advised to avoid foods that act as bowel irritants such as raw fruits and vegetables, popcorn, carbonated beverages, spicy foods, and foods of extreme temperatures. Small, frequent meals will also help to prevent abdominal distention. The physician may prescribe medications such as anticholinergic antispasmodics or opiates, which decrease diarrhea by decreasing intestinal spasms and motility. Antibiotics and antifungal agents may also be prescribed in order to combat offending pathogens that are identified by stool cultures.

Preventing Infection. The patient and caregivers are instructed to monitor for signs and symptoms of infection: fever, chills, night sweats, cough with or without sputum production, shortness of breath, difficulty breathing, oral pain or difficulty swallowing, creamy white patches in the oral cavity, unexplained weight loss, swollen lymph nodes, nausea, vomiting, persistent diarrhea, or frequency, urgency, or pain of urination; headache, visual changes or memory lapses; redness, swelling, or drainage from skin wounds, and vesicular lesions on the face, lips, or perianal area. The nurse also monitors laboratory values that indicate the presence of infection such as the white blood cell count and differential blood cell count. The physician may request culture specimens of wound drainage, skin lesions, urine, stool, sputum, mouth, and blood in order to identify pathogenic organisms and the most appropriate antimicrobial therapy.

The patient will require education about ways of preventing infection. The importance of personal hygiene is emphasized. Kitchen and bathroom surfaces should be cleansed regularly with disinfectants in order to prevent fungal and bacterial growth. Patients with pets are instructed to use gloves when cleaning areas soiled by animals such as bird cages and litter boxes. Patients are advised to avoid exposure to others who are sick or who have been recently vaccinated. Patients with AIDS and their sexual partners are strongly urged to avoid exposure to body fluids during sexual activities and to use condoms for any form of sexual intercourse. Intravenous drug use is strongly discouraged because of risk to the patient of other infections and transmission of HIV infection to others. The importance of avoiding smoking and maintaining a balance between diet, rest, and exercise is also addressed. All health professionals must remember to maintain strict aseptic technique when performing invasive procedures such as venipunctures and bladder catheterizations.

Improving Activity Tolerance. Activity tolerance is assessed by monitoring the patient's ability to ambulate and perform activities of daily living. Patients may be unable to maintain usual levels of activity because of weakness, fatigue, shortness of breath, dizziness, and neurological involvement. Assistance in planning daily routines that maintain a balance between activity and rest may be necessary. In addition, patients benefit from instructions about the use of energy conservation techniques, such as sitting while washing or while preparing meals. Personal items that are frequently used should be kept within the patient's reach so that they can be obtained without walking any distance. Measures such as relaxation and guided imagery may be beneficial in decreasing anxiety that contributes to weakness and fatigue.

Promoting Improvement of Thought Processes. Thought processes are assessed by monitoring the patient for decreased attention span, memory lapses, confusion, disorientation, agitation, and decreased levels of consciousness which may range from somnolence to coma. The nurse consults with the family and the physician in order to identify factors that might contribute to altered thought processes, such as use of illegal drugs, prescribed medications, hypoxia, fluid and electrolyte disturbances, and severe depression.

The patient and family are helped to understand and cope with changes in thought processes. The patient is reoriented to person, place, and time whenever necessary. It is often helpful to have a clock and calendar within the patient's view to facilitate sustained orientation. The patient's family and friends are encouraged to bring favorite objects from home in order to provide a familiar and less threatening environment while the patient is hospitalized. All instructions given to the patient are delivered in a slow, simple, and clear manner. Measures to protect the patient from injury are instituted. These may include placing the call bell within easy reach, keeping side rails up and the bed in a low position, instructing the patient to wear shoes and slippers with nonskid soles, and monitoring the patient who is smoking or shaving.

Maintaining Fluid and Electrolyte Balance. Fluid and electrolyte status is monitored on an ongoing basis. The skin is assessed for dryness and turgor. Fluid intake and output and specific gravity of urine are measured daily. The patient is also monitored for decreases in systolic blood pressure or increases in pulse associated with sitting or standing. Signs and symptoms of electrolyte disturbances such as muscle cramping, weakness, irregular pulse, decreased mental status, nausea, and vomiting are documented and reported to the physician. Serum electrolyte values are monitored and abnormalities reported to the physician when indicated. The nurse assists the patient in selecting foods that will replenish electrolytes, such as oranges and bananas (potassium) and cheese and soups (sodium). A fluid intake of 2500 ml or more, unless contraindicated, is encouraged in order to regain fluid lost from diarrhea. In addition, measures to control diarrhea are initiated. If fluid and electrolyte imbalances persist, the nurse may administer intravenous fluid and electrolytes as prescribed by the physician. It then becomes important for the nurse to monitor the therapeutic or potentially adverse effects of parenteral therapy.

Improving Nutritional Status. Nutritional status is assessed by monitoring weight, dietary intake, anthropometric measurements, and serum albumin, BUN, protein, and transferrin levels. The patient is also assessed for factors that interfere with oral intake, such as anorexia, nausea, pain, weakness, and fatigue. Based on the results of assessment, the nurse can implement specific measures to facilitate oral intake.

When fatigue and weakness interfere with intake, the patient is encouraged to rest prior to meals. In addition, meals should be planned so that they do not occur immediately after painful or unpleasant procedures. The patient with diarrhea and abdominal cramping is encouraged to avoid foods that stimulate intestinal motility and distention, such as foods high in fiber or of extreme temperatures. The dietitian is consulted to determine the patient's nutritional requirements. The patient is instructed about ways in which to supplement nutritional value of meals. The addition of eggs, butter, margarine, and fortified milk to gravies, soups, or milkshakes can provide additional calories and protein. Use of commercial supplements such as puddings, powders, and milkshakes may be advised. Patients who are unable to maintain nutritional status through oral intake often require enteral or parenteral feedings. Instruction is provided to patients and families about how to administer such feedings when patients are able to return home. Community health nurses provide additional teaching and support for these patients after discharge from the hospital. The nurse often consults with social workers in order to identify sources of financial support for patients who are unable to purchase or prepare meals. Referral to the AIDS Task Force or other community resources may be indicated if the patient is unable to shop for or prepare meals. These resources are often able to provide volunteers who can assist patients after discharge from the hospital.

Patient Education. Patients, families, and friends are instructed about the routes of transmission of AIDS. All fears and misconceptions are thoroughly discussed. In addition, the nurse discusses precautions necessary to prevent transmission of HIV, including use of condoms during vaginal or

(Text continues on p. 1198)

Chart 45-4
Precautions to Prevent Transmission of HIV

- Sharp items (*e.g.,* needles, scalpel blades) should be considered potentially infective and be handled with extraordinary care to prevent accidental injuries.
- Disposable syringes and needles, scalpel blades, and other sharp items should be placed in puncture-resistant containers located as near as is practical to the area in which they were used. Needles should not be recapped, purposely bent, broken, removed from disposable syringes, or otherwise manipulated by hand.
- When the possibility of exposure to blood or other body fluids exists, routinely recommended precautions should be followed. The anticipated exposure may require gloves alone, as in handling items soiled with blood or equipment contaminated with blood or other body fluids, or may require gowns, masks, and eye-coverings when performing procedures involving more extensive contact with blood or potentially infective body fluids, as in some dental or endoscopic procedures or post mortem examinations. Hands should be washed thoroughly and immediately if they accidentally become contaminated with blood.
- To minimize the need for emergency mouth-to-mouth resuscitation, mouth pieces, resuscitation bags, or other ventilation devices should be located strategically and available for use in areas where the need for resuscitation is predictable.
- Health care workers who are pregnant are not known to be at greater risk of contracting HIV infection than those who are not pregnant; however, if a health care worker develops HIV infection during pregnancy, the infant is at increased risk of infection resulting from perinatal transmission. Because of this risk, pregnant health care workers should be especially careful and maintain proper precautions.
- In the home setting, blood and body fluids may be flushed down the toilet.
- Contaminated items that cannot be flushed down the toilet should be wrapped securely in a plastic bag and placed in a second bag before being discarded in a manner consistent with local regulations for solid waste disposal.
- Spills of blood or other body fluids should be cleaned with soap and water or a household detergent. Freshly prepared solutions of sodium hypochlorite (household bleach) in concentrations of 1:10 dilution are effective disinfections. Persons cleaning spills should wear gloves.

(U.S. Department of Health and Human Services. Recommendations for prevention of transmission of HTLV-III/LAV among health care workers in the workplace. MMWR 1985 Nov; 34(45):684–685.)

Care of the Patient With Acquired Immunodeficiency Syndrome (AIDS)

Nursing Interventions	*Rationale*	*Expected Outcomes*

Nursing Diagnosis: Alteration in bowel elimination: diarrhea related to enteric pathogens and/or HIV infection

Goal: Resumption of usual bowel habits

1. Assess patient's normal bowel habits.	1. Provides baseline for evaluating effectiveness of measures	• Bowel habits return to normal.
2. Assess for signs and symptoms of diarrhea: frequent, loose stools; abdominal pain or cramping.		• Patient reports decreasing episodes of diarrhea and abdominal cramping.
a. Measure amount of liquid stools.	a. Quantifies loss of fluids	• Identifies and avoids foods that irritate the gastrointestinal tract.
b. Identify exacerbating and alleviating factors.	b. Provides basis for nursing measures	• Appropriate therapy is initiated as prescribed.
3. Obtain stool cultures as prescribed by physician. Administer antimicrobial therapy as prescribed.	3. Identifies pathogenic organism.	• Exhibits normal stool cultures.
4. Initiate measures to reduce hyperactivity of bowel:	4. Bowel rest may decrease acute episodes.	• Maintains adequate fluid intake
a. Maintain food and fluid restrictions as prescribed by physician.	a. Reduces stimulation of bowel	• Maintains body weight and reports no additional weight loss
b. Discourage smoking.	b. Nicotine acts as bowel stimulant.	• States rationale for avoiding smoking
c. Avoid bowel irritants such as foods high in fat, fried foods, raw vegetables and fruits, nuts, onions, popcorn, carbonated beverages, spicy foods, and foods of extreme temperatures.	c. Prevents stimulation of bowel and abdominal distention	• Enrolls in program to stop smoking
d. Offer small, frequent meals.		• Patient uses medication as prescribed
5. Administer anticholinergic antispasmodics as prescribed (propantheline bromide, dicyclomine hydrochloride).	5. Decreases intestinal spasms and motility	• Patient maintains adequate fluid status
6. Administer opiates or opiate-like medications as prescribed by physician (tincture of opium, loperamide, or diphenoxylate hydrochloride).		• Exhibits normal skin turgor, moist mucous membranes, adequate urine output, and no excessive thirst
7. Maintain fluid intake of at least 2500 ml unless contraindicated.	7. Prevents hypovolemia	

Nursing Diagnosis: Potential for infection related to immunodeficiency

Goal: Absence of infection

1. Monitor for signs and symptoms of infection: Fever, chills, and diaphoresis; cough; shortness of breath; oral pain or painful swallowing; creamy white patches in oral cavity; urinary frequency, urgency, or dysuria; redness, swelling, or drainage from skin wounds; vesicular lesions on face, lips, or perianal area.	1. Early detection of infection is essential for prompt initiation of treatment. Repeated and prolonged infections contribute to patient's debilitation.	• Patient identifies reportable signs and symptoms of infection.
		• Reports signs and symptoms of infection if infection does occur
		• Exhibits and reports absence of fever, chills, and diaphoresis
		• Exhibits normal (clear) breath sounds without adventitious breath sounds
		• Maintains weight

(continued)

Nursing Interventions	*Rationale*	*Expected Outcomes*

Nursing Diagnosis: Potential for infection related to immunodeficiency

Goal: Absence of infection

2. Teach patient or caregiver about need to report above signs and symptoms of infection.	2. Allows early detection of infection	• Reports adequate energy level without excessive fatigue
3. Monitor white blood cell count and differential	3. Elevated WBC is associated with infection.	• Reports absence of shortness of breath and cough
4. Obtain cultures of wound drainage, skin lesions, urine, stool, sputum, mouth, and blood as prescribed by physician. Administer antimicrobial therapy as prescribed by physician.	4. Offending organism must be identified in order to initiate appropriate treatment.	• Exhibits pink, moist oral mucous membranes without fissures or lesions • Appropriate therapy is administered. • Infection is prevented. • States rationale for strategies to avoid infection.

5. Instruct patient in ways in which to prevent infection:
  a. Cleanse kitchen and bathroom surfaces with disinfectants.
  b. Cleanse hands thoroughly after exposure to body fluids.
  c. Avoid exposure to others' body fluids or sharing eating utensils.
  d. Turn, cough, and deep breathe, especially when activity is decreased.
  e. Maintain cleanliness of perianal area.
	5. Minimizes exposure of patient to infection and transmission of HIV infection to others	• Modifies activities to reduce exposure to infection or infectious persons
		• Practices "safe sex"
		• Avoids sharing eating utensils and tooth brush
		• Exhibits normal body temperature
		• Uses recommended techniques to maintain cleanliness of skin, skin lesions, and perianal area

6. Maintain aseptic technique when performing invasive procedures such as venipunctures, bladder catheterizations, and injections.	6. Prevents hospital-acquired infections	

Nursing Diagnosis: Alteration in thought processes related to shortened attention span, impaired memory, confusion, restlessness, and disorientation associated with AIDS encephalitis

Goal: Improved thought processes

1. Assess patient for evidence of impaired thought processes such as decreased attention span, impaired memory, confusion, disorientation, agitation, and decreased level of consciousness.	1. HIV is able to invade the CNS, resulting in subacute encephalitis; this is believed to account for approximately 25% of all neurologic symptoms seen in patients with AIDS.	• Patient demonstrates intact orientation to time and place. • Responds appropriately to interactions and conversation of others • Exhibits interest in events and surroundings
2. Reorient patient to person, place, and time as necessary; keep calender and clock within patient's view; leave soft light on at night.	2. Facilitates patient's orientation to environment	• Experiences no falls or other consequences of trauma • Explains treatments and other instructions in own words
3. Encourage family and friends to bring patient's favorite objects from home to place in hospital room.	3. Provides familiar and less threatening environment	• Follows recommendations to reduce safety hazards and to protect self and others from injury
4. Repeat instructions slowly as necessary, using simple, clear language.	4. Prevents overwhelming and frustrating patient	• Calls for assistance from others when appropriate
5. Implement measures to protect patient from injury	5. Prevents injuries from falling, cuts, burns, and other accidents	

(continued)

Nursing Interventions	Rationale	Expected Outcomes

Nursing Diagnosis: Ineffective airway clearance related to pneumocystis pneumonia, increased bronchial secretions, decreased ability to cough related to weakness and fatigue

Goal: Improved airway clearance

Nursing Interventions	Rationale	Expected Outcomes
1. Assess and report signs and symptoms of altered respiratory status: tachypnea, use of accessory muscles, cough, color and amount of sputum, abnormal breath sounds, dusky or cyanotic skin color, restlessness, confusion, or somnolence.	1. Indicates abnormal respiratory function	• Patient maintains normal airway clearance: —Respiratory rate <20/minute —Unlabored breathing without use of accessory muscles and flaring of nares (nostrils) —Skin color pink (without cyanosis) —Patient alert and aware of surroundings —Arterial blood gases normal —Normal breath sounds without adventitious breath sounds
2. Obtain sputum sample for culture prescribed by physician. Administer antimicrobial therapy as prescribed.	2. Aids in identification of pathogenic organisms	• Appropriate therapy is initiated • Takes medication as prescribed. • Reports improved breathing
3. Provide pulmonary care (cough, deep breathing, postural drainage, and vibration) every 2 to 4 hours.	3. Prevents stasis of secretions and promotes airway clearance	• Airway clearance is maintained • Coughs and takes deep breaths every 2–4 hours as recommended.
4. Assist patient in attaining semi- or high Fowler's position.	4. Facilitates breathing and airway clearance	• Demonstrates appropriate positions for postural drainage
5. Encourage adequate rest periods.	5. Maximizes energy expenditure and prevents excessive fatigue	• Practices postural drainage every 2–4 hours
6. Initiate measures to decrease viscosity of secretions: a. Maintain fluid intake of at least 2500 ml per day unless contraindicated. b. Humidify inspired air as prescribed by physician. c. Consult with physician concerning use of mucolytic agents delivered through nebulizer or IPPB treatment.	6. Facilitates expectoration of secretions; prevents stasis secretions	• Reports reduced breathing difficulty when in semi- or high Fowler's position • Practices energy-conserving strategies • Plans schedule to allow alternating periods of rest and activity • Demonstrates reduction in thickness (viscosity) of pulmonary secretions • Reports increased ease in coughing up sputum • Uses humidified air or oxygen as prescribed and indicated
7. Perform tracheal suctioning as needed.		• Indicates need for assistance with removal of pulmonary secretions
8. Administer oxygen therapy as prescribed.		• States rationale for endotracheal intubation and use of a mechanical ventilator
9. Assist with endotracheal intubation; maintain ventilator settings as prescribed.	9. Maintains ventilation	• Cooperates with intubation procedure and use of mechanical ventilator • Verbalizes fears and anxieties about increased respiratory difficulty and need for intubation and mechanical ventilation

(continued)

Nursing Interventions	*Rationale*	*Expected Outcomes*

Nursing Diagnosis: Inadequate nutritional status related to decreased oral intake

Goal: Improvement of nutritional status

1. Assess patient for evidence of malnutrition through the following: height, weight, age, BUN, serum protein, albumin, transferrin levels, hemoglobin, hematocrit, cutaneous anergy, and anthropometric measurements.	1. Provides objective measurement of nutritional status	• Deficient values will return to normal. • Patient identifies factors limiting oral intake. • Identifies and uses resources to assist in adequate dietary intake • Reports increased appetite • States understanding of nutritional needs
2. Obtain dietary history, including likes and dislikes and food intolerances.	2. Helps to identify need for nutritional education; assists in planning individualized interventions	• Identifies ways to minimize factors limiting oral intake • Rests before meals
3. Assess factors that interfere with oral intake.	3. Provides basis and direction for interventions	• Eats in pleasant, odor-free environment • Arranges meals to coincide with visitors' visits
4. Consult with dietitian to determine patient's nutritional needs.	4. Facilitates meal planning	• Reports increased dietary intake • Uses oral hygiene prior to meals
5. Reduce factors limiting oral intake:		• Takes pain medication prior to meals as prescribed
a. Encourage patient to rest prior to meals.	a. Minimizes fatigue, which can decrease appetite	• Patient states ways to increase protein and caloric intake
b. Plan meals so that they do not occur immediately after painful or unpleasant procedures.	b. Decreases noxious stimuli	• Identifies foods high in protein and calories
c. Encourage patient to eat meals with visitors or others in the home when possible.	c. Limits social isolation	• Consumes foods high in protein and calories • Reports decreased rate of weight loss
d. Encourage patient to prepare simple meals or to obtain assistance with meal preparation if possible.	d. Limits energy expenditure	• Maintains adequate intake • Patient states rationale for enteral or parenteral nutrition if needed
e. Serve small, frequent meals: 6 per day.	e. Prevents overwhelming patient and reduces satiety	• Demonstrates skill in preparing alternate sources of nutrition
f. Limit fluids 1 hour prior to meals and with meals. —Provide mouth care prior to eating.		
6. Instruct patient in ways to supplement nutritional value of meals: consume foods high in protein (meat, poultry, fish, legumes, dairy products) and carbohydrates (pasta, fruit, breads).	6. Provides additional proteins and calories	
7. Consult with physician about alternate means of providing nutrition, such as enteral feedings or parenteral nutrition.	7. Provides nutritional support if patient unable to take sufficient amounts by mouth	
8. Consult with social worker or AIDS Task Force to identify means of obtaining financial assistance if patient unable financially to obtain food.		

(continued)

Nursing Interventions	*Rationale*	*Expected Outcomes*

Nursing Diagnosis: Knowledge deficit related to means of preventing transmission of HIV

Goal: Increased knowledge concerning means of preventing disease transmission

1. Instruct patient, family, and friends about routes of transmission of HIV.
2. Instruct patient, family, and friends about means of preventing transmission of HIV:
  a. Avoid sexual contact with multiple partners.
	1. Knowledge about disease transmission can help prevent spread of disease; may also alleviate fears.
	
	  a. The risk of infection increases with the number of sexual partners, male or female, and sexual contact with members of high-risk groups.
		• Patient, family, and friends state means of transmission.
		• Reports and demonstrates practices to reduce exposure of others to HIV.
		• Avoids intravenous drug use
		• Demonstrates safe sexual practices
		• Identifies means of preventing disease transmission
		• States that sexual partners are informed about positive HIV antibodies in blood

b. Use precautions when it is not absolutely certain that the sexual partner has not been exposed to HIV through intravenous drug abuse, sexual contact with members of high-risk groups, or receiving blood or blood products before screening efforts were instituted.		

c. Use condoms during sexual intercourse (vaginal or anal).
  d. Avoid mouth contact with the penis, vagina, or rectum.
  e. Avoid sexual practices that can cause cuts or tears in the lining of the rectum, vagina, or penis.
	c. Reduces risk of transmission of HIV	

f. Avoid sex with prostitutes and others in high-risk groups.	f. Many prostitutes are infected with HIV through sexual contact with multiple partners or intravenous drug abuse.	
g. Do not abuse intravenous drugs; if addicted and unable or unwilling to change behavior, use clean needles and syringes.	g. Clean needles and syringes are the only way to prevent HIV transmission for those who continue to abuse drugs. Taking precautions is especially important for those who are antibody-positive to transmit HIV to others.	

(continued)

anal intercourse, avoiding oral contact with the penis, vagina, or rectum, avoiding sexual practices that might cause cuts or tears in the lining of the rectum, vagina, or penis, and avoiding sexual contact with multiple partners or members of high-risk groups. The dangers of intravenous drug use and sharing of needles and syringes are also discussed. Patients with AIDS or members of high-risk groups are instructed not to donate blood.

Improving Airway Clearance.   Respiratory status including rate, rhythm, use of accessory muscles, breath sounds, mental status, and skin color must be assessed at least daily. The presence of cough and the quantity and characteristics of sputum are documented. Sputum specimens are tested for the possible presence of infectious organisms. Pulmonary measures (coughing, deep breathing, postural drainage, percussion, and vibration) are provided as often as every 2 hours to prevent stasis of secretions and promote clearance of airways. Because of weakness and fatigue, many patients may require assistance in attaining a position (such as a high or semi-Fowler's) that will facilitate breathing and airway clear-

Nursing Interventions	*Rationale*	*Expected Outcomes*

Nursing Diagnosis: Knowledge deficit related to means of preventing transmission of HIV

Goal: Increased knowledge concerning means of preventing disease transmission

h. Women who may have been exposed to AIDS through sexual or drug practices should consult with a physician prior to becoming pregnant.	h. AIDS can be passed from mother to child in utero.	

Nursing Diagnosis: Social isolation related to stigma of the disease, withdrawal of support systems, isolation procedures, and fear of infecting others

Goal: Decreased sense of social isolation

1. Assess patient's usual patterns of social interaction.	1. Establishes basis for individualized interventions.	• Patient shares with others the need for valued social interaction.
2. Observe for behaviors indicative of social isolation, such as decreased interaction with staff or friends and family, hostility, noncompliance, sad affect, and verbalization of feelings of rejection or loneliness.	2. Social isolation may be manifested in several ways.	• Demonstrates interest in events, activities, and communication
		• Verbalizes feelings and reactions to diagnosis, prognosis, and resulting changes in life
3. Provide instruction concerning means of transmission of HIV.	3. Provision of accurate information corrects misconceptions and alleviates anxiety.	• Identifies means of transmission of AIDS.
		• States ways of preventing transmission of AIDS virus to others while maintaining contact with valued friends and relatives
4. Assist patient to identify and explore resources for support and positive mechanisms for coping (*e.g.,* contact with family, friends, AIDS task force).		• Reveals AIDS diagnosis to others when appropriate
		• Identifies resources (*i.e.,* supportive family, friends, and support groups)
5. Allow time to be with patient other than for medications or procedures.	5. Promotes feelings of self-worth and provides social interaction	• Uses resources when appropriate
		• Accepts offers of assistance and support from others
6. Encourage participation in diversional activities such as reading, television, or hand crafts.	6. Provides distraction	• Reports decreased sense of social isolation
		• Maintains contacts with those of importance to self
		• Develops or continues hobbies that effectively serve as diversion or distraction

ance. The provision of adequate rest periods is essential to maximize the patient's energy expenditure and prevent excessive fatigue. The patient's fluid volume status is evaluated so that adequate hydration can be maintained. Unless contraindicated by renal or cardiac disease, intake of 3 to 4 liters of fluid daily is encouraged. Humidified oxygen may be prescribed and nasopharyngeal or tracheal suctioning may be indicated to maintain adequate ventilation. Mechanical ventilation may be necessary for patients who are unable to maintain adequate ventilation as a result of pulmonary infection, fluid and electrolyte imbalance, or respiratory muscle paresis.

Increasing Comfort. The patient is assessed for the quality and quantity of pain associated with diarrhea and impaired perianal skin integrity. In addition, the effects of pain on elimination, nutrition, sleep, affect, and communication are explored, along with exacerbating and relieving factors. Cleansing the perianal area as previously described can promote comfort. Topical anesthetics or ointments may be prescribed. Soft cushions or foam pads may be used to increase comfort while sitting. The patient is instructed to avoid foods that act as bowel irritants, such as milk products, caffeine, prunes, cabbage, spicy foods, carbonated beverages, and extremely hot or cold foods. Antispasmodics and antidiarrheal preparations may be prescribed to reduce discomfort and frequency of bowel movements. If necessary, systemic analgesics may also be prescribed.

Decreasing Sense of Social Isolation. AIDS patients are at risk for "double stigmatization." They have what society often refers to as "a dread disease," and they may have a life-style (homosexuality or drug abuse) that differs from what is considered acceptable. The majority of persons with AIDS are young adults at a developmental stage in which they should be establishing intimate relationships and personal and career goals. Their focus changes as they are faced with a disease that has no cure and a limited life expectancy. In addition, they may be forced to reveal hidden life-styles to family, friends, co-workers, and health care providers. As a result, AIDS patients are often flooded with emotions such as anxiety, guilt, shame, and fear. Patients may be faced with multiple losses, such as rejection by family and friends and loss of financial security, normal roles and functions, self-esteem, privacy, ability to control bodily functions, ability to interact meaningfully with the environment, and sexual functioning. Some patients may harbor feelings of guilt because of chosen life-style or because of the possibility of having infected others in current or previous relationships. Other patients may feel anger towards sexual partners who may have been responsible for transmission of the virus. Infection control measures used in the hospital or at home may further contribute to the patient's emotional isolation. Any or all of these stressors may cause the AIDS patient to withdraw both physically and emotionally from social contact.

Nurses are in a key position to provide an atmosphere of acceptance and understanding of AIDS patients and their families and partners. A patient's usual level of social interaction is assessed as early as possible, to provide a baseline for monitoring changes in behavior indicative of social isolation (*e.g.*, decreased interaction with staff or family, hostility, noncompliance). Patients are encouraged to express feelings of isolation and aloneness, and assured that these feelings are not unique or abnormal.

Providing information about how to protect themselves and others can help to prevent patients from avoiding social contact. Patients, family, and friends must be assured that AIDS is not spread through casual contact. Educating ancillary personnel, nurses, and physicians will help to reduce factors that might contribute to feelings of isolation. Patient care conferences concerning the psychosocial considerations regarding AIDS patients may help sensitize nurses to patients' needs.

The nurse can help patients explore and identify resources for support and mechanisms of coping. Patients are encouraged to telephone family and friends as well as local or national AIDS support groups and hotlines. If at all possible, barriers to social contact are identified and eliminated. For patients who are able to participate, social interaction with family, friends, or co-workers is encouraged. Patients are also encouraged to engage in their usual diversional activities whenever possible.

Home Health Care Considerations. Many persons with AIDS are able to return to the community and resume their usual daily activities. Others who return home are unable to continue employment or maintain their preexisting level of independence. Families or caregivers need assistance in providing supportive care. They must receive instructions about how to prevent disease transmission, including hand washing and methods of safely handling items soiled with body fluids. Caregivers in the home are taught how to administer medications, including intravenous preparations. Guidelines about infection, follow-up care, diet, rest, and activities are also necessary. Both the patient and caregivers will require support and guidance in coping with this debilitating and usually fatal disease.

Community health nurses and hospice nurses are in an excellent position to help provide the support and guidance so often needed in the home setting. As hospital costs continue to rise and insurance coverage continues to undergo major changes, the complexity of home care continues to increase. Community nurses are frequently able to assist in administration of parenteral antibiotics, chemotherapy, and nutrition. In addition, complicated wound care or respiratory care is often required in the home. Both patients and families are often unable to meet these skilled care needs without the assistance of nurses. Hospice nurses are increasingly called upon to provide emotional support to patients and families as AIDS patients enter the terminal stages of disease. This support takes on special meaning when AIDS patients lose the support of friends and families who have turned away from them because of fear of the disease or anger concerning life-styles adopted by patients.

Prevention of HIV Transmission. As discussed earlier in this chapter, AIDS is not transmitted by casual contact. Epidemiological evidence has indicated that HIV is transmitted only through intimate sexual contact, parenteral exposure to infected blood or blood products, and perinatal transmission from mother to neonate. Studies of nonsexual household contacts of AIDS patients as well as nonsexual person-to-person contact that generally occurs in the work place have not demonstrated any increased risk for transmission of AIDS through such contact.

HIV has been isolated from blood, semen, saliva, tears, breast milk, urine, and other body fluids, secretions, and excretions. In the interest of public health, the Centers for Disease Control and the Surgeon General of the U.S. have issued recommendations for preventing transmission of HIV. These guidelines apply to health care workers in the hospital setting as well as in the home. The guidelines are also applicable to family or friends providing care for patients in the home (Chart 45-4, p. 1193).

▷ *Evaluation*

▷ *Expected Outcomes*

The outcomes expected for the patient with AIDS are as follows:

1. Patient resumes usual bowel habits
2. Experiences no infections
3. Maintains usual level of thought processes
4. Maintains fluid and electrolyte balance
5. Maintains effective airway clearance
6. Experiences increased sense of comfort
7. Maintains perianal skin integrity

8. Maintains adequate nutritional status
9. Understands means of preventing disease transmission
10. Experiences decreased sense of social isolation
11. Maintains adequate level of activity tolerance
12. Progresses through grieving process

Specific outcomes are discussed in Nursing Care Plan 45-1, pages 1194 to 1199.

Bibliography

Books

Amos WMG. Basic Immunology. London, Pergamon Press, 1981.

Armstrong D and Ma P (eds). The Acquired Immune Deficiency Syndrome and Infections of Homosexual Men. New York, York Medical Books, 1984.

Barrett JT. Textbook of Immunology: An Introduction to Immunochemistry and Immunobiology, 4th ed. St Louis, CV Mosby, 1983.

Biggar RJ et al (eds). AIDS: A Basic Guide for Clinicians. Copenhagen, Sanders, 1984.

Brostoff RJ, Roitt IM, and Male DK. Immunology. London, Gower Medical Publishing, 1985.

Cooper EL. General Immunology. Oxford, Pergamon Press, 1982.

Coping With AIDS: Psychological and Social Considerations in Helping People with HTLV-III Infection. U.S. Department of Health and Human Services, National Institute of Mental Health, 1986.

DeVita V, Hellman S, and Rosenberg S. AIDS: Etiology, Diagnosis, Treatment, and Prevention. Philadelphia, JB Lippincott, 1985.

Gottlieb MS and Groopman JE (eds). AIDS. New York, Alan R Liss, 1984.

Griffin JP. Hematology and Immunology: Concepts for Nursing. Norwalk, Connecticut, Appleton-Century Crofts, 1986.

Articles

Immunology (General)

Barber JS. Immunologic responses to trauma. Crit Care Quart 1986 June; 9(1):57–67.

Corman LC and Katz P. Symposium on Clinical Immunology II. Med Clin North Am 1985 July; 69(4):621–840.

Esperson S. Nursing support of host defenses. Crit Care Quart 1986 June; 9(1):51–56.

Griffin JP. Nursing care of the critically ill immunocompromised patient. Crit Care Quart 1986 June; 9(1):25–34.

Groenwald SL. Physiology of the immune system. Heart Lung 1980 July/Aug; 9(4):645–650.

Gurevich I. The competent internal immune system. Nurs Clin North Am 1985 Mar; 20(1):151–162.

Gurevich I and Tafuro P. Nursing measures for the prevention of infection in the compromised host. Nurs Clin North Am 1985 Mar; 20(1):257–260.

Kemp D. Development of the immune system. Crit Care Quart 1986 June; 9(1):1–6.

MacClamrock EA and Suppers VJ. Biologicals in cancer treatment: Future effects on nursing practice. Oncol Nurs Forum 1985 May/June; 12(3):27–32.

Murasko DM et al. Immunologic response in an elderly population with a mean age of 85. Am J Med 1986 Oct; 81(4):612–618.

The new immunology: Helping the body heal itself. Am J Nurs 1987 Apr; 87(4):455–473.

Nossal GJV. Current concepts: Immunology—the basic components of the immune system. N Engl J Med 1987 May 21; 316(21):1320–1325.

Smith SL. Immunosuppressive drugs used in clinical practice. Crit Care Quart 1986 June; 9(1):19–24.

Smith SL. Physiology of the immune system. Crit Care Quart 1986 June; 9(1):7–13.

AIDS

Anderson D. AIDS: An update on what we know now. RN 1986 Mar; 49(3):49–56.

Banks RA, Lindley KJ, and Pozniak AL. AIDS: A problem for intensive care (Editorial). Intensive Care Med 1985; 11(4):169–171.

Bennett JA. AIDS: Epidemiology update. Am J Nurs 1985 Sept; 85(9):968–972.

Bennett JA. HTLV-III/AIDS link. Am J Nurs 1985 Oct; 85(10):1089–1090.

Bennett JA. What we know about AIDS. Am J Nurs 1986 Sept; 86(9):1016–1021.

Brock RB. On a nursing AIDS task force: The battle for confident care. Nurs Man 1986 Mar; 41(2):4–6.

Brosnan S. Our first home care A.I.D.S. patient: Maria. Nursing '86 1986, Sept; 16(9):37–39.

Calliari D. Administrative perspectives on care of patients with AIDS. Top Clin Nurs 1984 July; 6(2):72–75.

Carr GS and Gee G. AIDS and AIDS-related conditions: Screening for populations at risk. Nurse Pract 1986 Oct; 11(10):25–48.

Cassen BJ. AIDS update: HTLV-III/LAV infection. Penn Med 1986 Jan; 89(1):324–326.

Cecchi R. Living with AIDS: When the system fails. Am J Nurs 1986 Jan; 86(1):45–47.

Coleman DA. How to care for an AIDS patient. RN 1986 July:16–21.

Cooney TG and Ward TT (ed). AIDS and other medical problems in the male homosexual. Med Clin North Am 1986 May; 70(3):499–719.

Crovella AC. The person behind the disease . . . AIDS. Nursing '85 1985 Sept; 15(9):42–43.

Curtain LL. AIDS: A balance of sorrows. Nurs Man 1986 Mar; 17(3):7–8.

Donehower MG. Malignant complications of AIDS. Oncol Nurs Forum 1987 Jan/Feb; 14(1):57–64.

Durham JD and Hatcher B. Reducing psychological complications for the critically ill AIDS patient. Dimens Crit Care Nurs 1984 Sept/Oct; 3(5):300–306.

Farthing CF, Shanson DC, and Gazzard BG. The acquired immune deficiency syndrome: Problems associated with the management of *Pneumocystis carinii* pneumonia. J Infect 1985 Sept; 11(2):103–106.

Fauci AS and Lane HC. Overview of clinical syndromes and immunology of AIDS. Top Clin Nurs 1984 July; 6(2):12–18.

Faulstich ME. Psychiatric aspects of AIDS. Am J Psychiatry 1987 May; 144(5):551–556.

Gall RC. The AIDS virus. Sci Am 1987 Jan; 256(1):46–56.

Gold JW. Clinical spectrum of infections in patients with HTLV-III associated diseases. Cancer Res 1985 Sept; 45(s):4652s–4654s.

Graf TM. Unmasking AIDS. Home Healthcare Nurse 1984; 2(1):44–47.

Groopman JE. Clinical spectrum of HTLV-III in humans. Cancer Res 1985 Sept; 45(s):4649s–4651s.

Henderson DK. AIDS: Epidemiology and potential for nosocomial transmission. Top Clin Nurs 1984 July; 6(2):1–11.

Howes AC. Nursing diagnoses and care plans for ambulatory care patients with AIDS. Top Clin Nurs 1984 July; 6(2):61–66.

Irich AC. Straight talk about gay patients. Am J Nurs 1983 Aug; 83(8):1169.

Klein CA. AIDS and employment issues. Nurse Pract 1986 May; 11(5):87, 88, 90.

LaCamera DJ. AIDS: Precautions for health care personnel. Top Clin Nurs 1984 July; 6(2):45–52.

LaCamera DJ, Masur H, and Henderson DK. The acquired immunodeficiency syndrome. Nurs Clin North Am 1985 Mar; 20(1):241–256.

Layon J, Warzynski M, and Idris A. Acquired immunodeficiency syndrome in the United States: A selective review. Crit Care Med 1986 Sept; 14(9):819–827.

Lotze MT. Surgical considerations in the diagnosis and management of AIDS. AIDS Research 1986 Spring; 2(2):141–148.

Luce JM and Hopewell PC. The acquired immunodeficiency syndrome: A San Francisco perspective. Intens Care Med 1985; 11(4):172–173.

Masur H. Immunotherapy and therapy of complications of AIDS. Top Clin Nurs 1984 July; 6(2):53–60.

Mitchell C and Smith L. If it's AIDS, please don't tell. Am J Nurs 1987 July; 87(7):911–914.

Neurberger J. Fear and loathing . . . lack of compassion in dealing with AIDS victims. Nurs Times 1986 Feb; 82(6):22.

Newmark DA. Review of a support group for patients with AIDS. Top Clin Nurs 1984 July; 6(2):38–44.

Peabody B. Living with AIDS: A mother's perspective. Am J Nurs 1986 Jan; 86(1):45–46.

Perry SW et al. Psychiatric problems of AIDS inpatients at New York Hospital: Preliminary report. Public Health Ref 1984 Mar/Apr; 99(2):200–205.

Popkin B. Caring for AIDS patients fearlessly. Nursing '83 1983 Sept; 13(9):50–55.

Price DM and Scimeca AM. The epidemic of the 80s: AIDS. Cancer Nurs 1984 Aug; 7(4):283–289.

Robinson L. Acquired immunodeficiency syndrome: An update. Crit Care Nurs 1984 Sept/Oct; 4(5):75–83.

Rubinow DR. The psychological impact of AIDS. Top Clin Nurs 1984 July; 6(2):26–37.

Schietinger H. A home care plan for AIDS. Am J Nurs 1986 Sept; 86(9):1021–1028.

Selwyn PA. AIDS: What is now known. I. History and immunovirology. Hosp Prac 1986 May 15; 21(5):67–76, 81–82.

Selwyn PA. AIDS: What is now known. II. Epidemiology. Hosp Prac 1986 June 15; 21(6):127–164.

Selwyn PA. AIDS: What is now known. III. Clinical aspects. Hosp Prac 1986 Sept 15; 21(9):119–153.

Selwyn PA. AIDS: What is now known. IV. Psychosocial aspects, treatment prospects. Hosp Prac 1986 Oct; 21(10):125–164.

Sherertz RJ. Acquired immune deficiency syndrome. Med Clin North Am 1985 July; 69(4):637–655.

Siegal FP. Immune function and dysfunction in AIDS. Semin Oncol 1984 Mar; 11(1):29–37.

Sunder JA. AIDS: A neurological nursing challenge. Top Clin Nurs 1984 July; 6(2):67–71.

Thornton JE and Vinogradov S. If I have AIDS, then let me die now. Hastings Cent Rep 1984 Feb; 14(1):24–25.

U.S. Department of Health and Human Services. AIDS: Meeting of WHO collaborating centers on AIDS. MMWR 1985 Nov; 34(44):678–679.

U.S. Department of Health and Human Services. Additional recommendations to reduce sexual and drug abuse related transmission of HTLV-III/LAV. MMWR 1986 Mar; 35(10):152–155.

U.S. Department of Health and Human Services. HTLV-III/LAV antibody testing at alternative sites. MMWR 1986 May; 35(17):285–287.

Valenti WM. AIDS update: HTLV-III testing, immune globulins, and employees with AIDS. Infect Control 1986 Aug; 7(8):427–430.

Viele CS et al. Caring for acquired immunodeficiency syndrome patients . . . experiences of one AIDS nursing unit. Oncol Nurs Forum 1984 May/June; 11(3):56–60.

Williams AB. Public health implications of HIV infection. Nurse Pract 1986 Oct; 11(10):8–10, 19–20.

Wolff PH and Colletti MA. AIDS: Getting past the diagnosis and on to discharge planning. Crit Care Nurs 1986 July/Aug; 6(4):76–81.

Resources for Support and Information

Telephone Hotlines (Toll Free)

National Gay Task Force AIDS Information Hotline: (800) 221-7044; (212) 807-6016 (NY State)

National Sexually Transmitted Disease Hotline/American Social Health Association: (800) 227-8922

PHS AIDS Hotline: (800) 342-AIDS; (800) 342-2437

Information Sources

AIDS Action Council 729 Eighth Street, S.E., Suite 200, Washington, DC 20003. *Phone:* (202) 547-3101.

American Red Cross AIDS Education Office, 1730 D Street, N.W., Washington, DC 20006. *Phone:* (202) 737-8300 (or local Red Cross).

Gay Men's Health Crisis Network, P.O. Box 274, 132 West 24th Street, New York, NY 10011. *Phone:* (212) 807-6655.

Hispanic AIDS Forum, c/o APRED, 853 Broadway, Suite 2007, New York, NY 10003. *Phone:* (212) 870-1902 or 870-1864.

Minority Task Force on AIDS, c/o New York City Council of Churches, 475 Riverside Drive, Room 456, New York, NY 10115. *Phone:* (212) 749-1214.

Mothers of AIDS Patients (MAP), c/o Barbara Peabody, 3403 E Street, San Diego, CA 92102. *Phone:* (619) 234-3432.

National AIDS Network, 729 Eighth Street, S.E., Suite 300, Washington, DC 20003. *Phone:* (202) 546-2424.

National Association of People with AIDS, P.O. Box 65472, Washington, DC 20035. *Phone:* (202) 483-7979.

National Coalition of Gay Sexually Transmitted Disease Services, c/o Mark Behar, P.O. Box 239, Milwaukee, WI 53201. *Phone:* (414) 277-7671.

National Council of Churches/AIDS Task Force, 475 Riverside Drive, Room 572, New York, NY 10115. *Phone:* (212) 870-2421.

U.S. Public Health Service Public Affairs Office, Hubert H. Humphrey Building, Room 725-H, 200 Independence Avenue, SW, Washington, DC 20201. *Phone:* (202) 245-6867.

Chapter 46

Assessment and Management of Patients With Allergic Disorders

The human body is menaced by a host of potential invaders—for the most part, microbial organisms—that are constantly threatening its surface defenses. Having penetrated those defenses, these agents compete with the body for its nutrients and, if allowed to flourish unimpeded, disrupt its enzyme systems and destroy its vital tissues. Against these agents, the body is equipped with an elaborate blockade system. The first line of defense consists of the epithelial cells that coat the skin and make up the lining of the respiratory, gastrointestinal, and genitourinary tracts. The structure and continuity of these surfaces and the resistance to penetration are initial deterrents to invaders.

One of the most effective of the body's defense mechanisms is its capacity to equip itself rapidly with weapons (antibodies) individually designed to meet each new invader, namely, specific protein *antigens*. Antibodies react with antigens in a variety of ways: (1) by coating their surface if they are particular substances, (2) by neutralizing them if they are toxic, or (3) by precipitating them out of solution if they are dissolved. In any event, the antibodies prepare the antigen for handling by the phagocytic cells of the blood and the tissues.

Allergic Reaction: Physiologic Overview

Immunity

Some people are born with the ability to resist invasion by certain types of foreign agents. Most persons, however, acquire resistance by actually fighting off the invader. It is also possible to acquire resistance by two other methods.

1. By *actively acquired immunization*, whereby an antigenic substance (one that has lost its ability to produce illness, but is able to stimulate antibody formation) is injected into the body (*e.g.*, virus vaccine and tetanus toxoid)
2. By *passively acquired immunization*, whereby resistance is brought about by the transfer of antibody-con-

taining serum from a sensitized donor to a normal recipient (*e.g.*, human gamma globulin)

Allergic Reaction

The term *allergy* has historically been defined as "altered reactivity," meaning that the body's response to a substance is different from its original response when initially exposed to that substance. Although such a definition proved to be fairly workable during the first half of this century, concepts and definitions have changed somewhat as a result of a better understanding of the events that take place when the body recognizes "foreignness." Thus, the definition of allergy has changed.

We have come to think of an *allergic reaction* as a manifestation of tissue injury resulting from an immunologic process (an interaction between an antigen and an antibody). When the host is invaded by the antigen, usually a protein that is recognized as foreign, a series of events takes place designed to render the invader harmless and to expel it. If white blood corpuscles of the lymphocyte series respond to such an invasion, antibodies may be produced by these cells.

An *antigen*, then, is any substance that, in the course of repeated contacts with the body, stimulates the body to produce another substance called an *antibody*, capable of combining with it in a very specific manner. This antibody may circulate freely in the blood as globulins or may be "fixed" in the tissues. Ordinarily, the net effect is protection of the host, in which case immunity results and the stimulus is then defined as an *immunogen* (Fig. 46-1*A*). If, on the other hand, tissue injury results from the body's attempt to become immune, the stimulus is then defined as an *allergen* (Fig. 46-1*B*).

Exposure to the specific allergen causes the release of *mediators* (active chemical substances; Fig. 46-2). These act directly or indirectly on the muscles and glands of the tracheobronchial tree to produce bronchial constriction, excess mucus, and edema. Such chemical mediators include histamine and kinins: serotonin, bradykinin, SRS-A (slow-reacting substance of anaphylaxis), and acetylcholine.

Immunogens and allergens are usually protein in nature, but occasionally large-molecular-weight carbohydrates may also stimulate the initiation of an immune response. Many small-molecular-weight molecules may unite firmly with a tissue protein, the resultant combination then being recognized

as foreign. These small molecules, which form a union with proteins, are called *haptens*. The metal nickel and many drugs, such as penicillin, are examples of haptens.

Immunoglobulins

Antibodies that are formed by lymphocytes and plasma cells in response to an immunogenic stimulus constitute a group of serum proteins called *immunoglobulins*. These can be found in the lymph nodes, tonsils, appendix, and Peyer's patches of the intestinal tract, or circulating in the blood and lymph. These antibodies combine with antigens in a very special way, which has been likened to keys fitting into a lock. Antigens (keys) only fit certain antibodies (locks); hence, the term *specificity* has been coined in relation to the specific reaction of an antibody to an antigen. There are many variations and complexities in these patterns.

Antibody molecules are *bivalent*, which means that they have two combining sites. Because of this, the antibody easily becomes a cross-link between two antigen groups, causing them to clump together (*agglutination*). By this action, invaders in the bloodstream are cleared. Agglutination is the means of determining blood group in laboratory tests.

There are five classes of immunoglobulins, designated as follows: IgG, IgA, IgM, IgD, and IgE. Antibodies of the IgM, IgG, and IgA classes have definite and well-established protective functions. These include neutralization of toxins and viruses, and precipitation, agglutination, or lysis of bacteria and other foreign cellular material.

IgM ("gamma-M") is the largest molecule, which tends to stay in the bloodstream and is thus primarily engaged in defense in the intravascular compartment, such as in bloodstream infections. If it occurs in a pregnant woman, it will not cross the placenta from the mother to the fetus. Thus, the finding of a high concentration of IgM in the newborn's circulation is suggestive of an intrauterine infection.

IgG ("gamma-G"), the most abundant of the immunoglobulins, is one of the smallest immunoglobulins and thus can diffuse readily into the tissue spaces to assist in combating tissue toxins or infections. IgG has the property of crossing the placenta, so that antibodies of this family provide the baby with temporary immunity to many common diseases.

IgA ("gamma-A") circulates in the blood, but its role in that compartment of the body is uncertain. It is distinct in that it is produced in the external secretion, where it provides

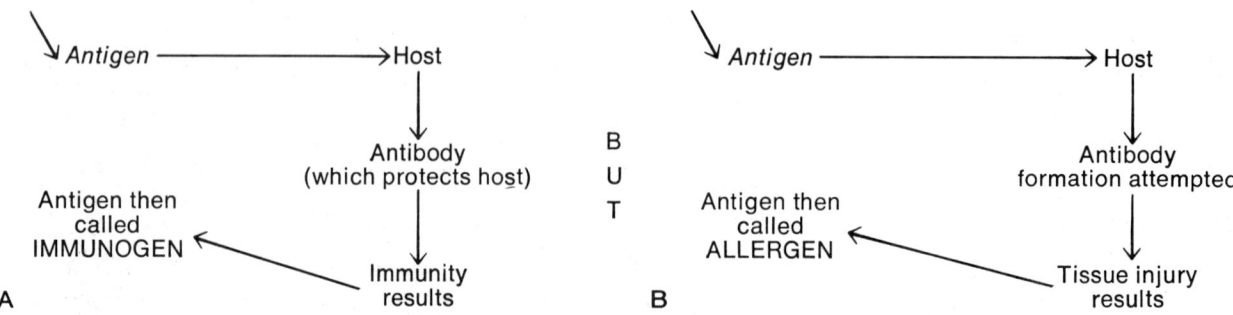

Figure 46-1
(*A*) Diagram describes the effect of an immunogen. (*B*) Diagram describes the effect of an allergen.

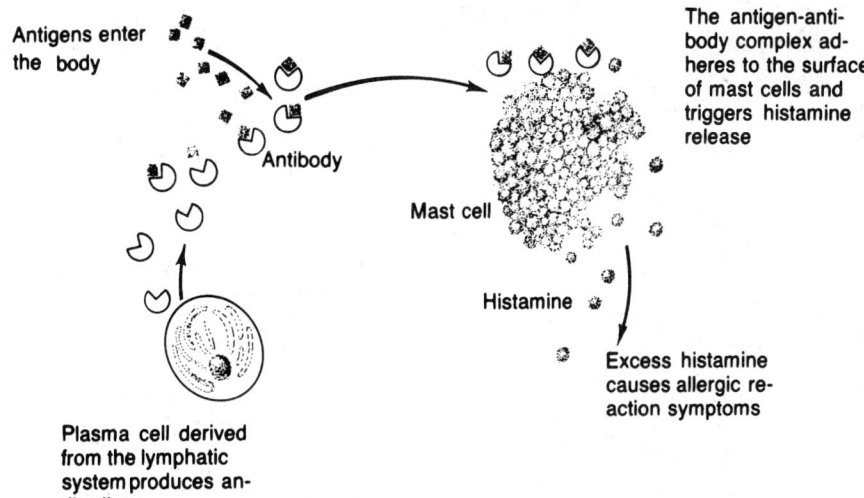

Antigens enter the body

Antibody

The antigen-antibody complex adheres to the surface of mast cells and triggers histamine release

Mast cell

Histamine

Excess histamine causes allergic reaction symptoms

Plasma cell derived from the lymphatic system produces antibodies

Figure 46-2
How allergic reactions begin.
(Patient Care, Sept 15, 1973.
Copyright © 1973. Patient Care
Corp. Darien, Conn. All rights
reserved.)

a primary defense mechanism. IgA is found in saliva, tears, and the respiratory, genitourinary, and gastrointestinal tracts.

The function of *IgD* ("gamma-D") has not yet been determined. It is small, like IgG, and has a molecular pattern distinct from the other known immunoglobulins.

IgE ("gamma-E"), the most recently described immunoglobulin, is responsible for most of the immediate types of allergic reactions, which will be discussed later. It is present only in minute amounts in the blood serum. (In the normal person, 1 of 5000 immunoglobulin molecules are of this class.) The unique feature of IgE is its great affinity for attaching to human epithelium.

A protective role for IgE has not yet been established, but it has been postulated that antibodies in this class may play a role in ridding the host of certain parasites. Deficiency of IgE has been associated with increased susceptibility to infection. The most important aspect regarding IgE is its association with immediate allergic reactions of the anaphylactic type. These reactions appear within minutes of an injection of antigen into a person having anaphylactic antibodies (or after 2 hours, if precipitin antibodies are present). Anaphylactic reactions are discussed more fully at the end of the chapter.

Delayed Hypersensitivity

Delayed hypersensitivity occurs when an antigen is brought into contact with the skin surface of a sensitized person, with the inflammatory reaction reaching its peak within 24 to 48 hours. The reaction consists of erythema (redness) and induration (hardness).

Delayed hypersensitivity is mediated not by circulating immunoglobulins (described above), but rather by sensitized "T" (thymus-dependent) lymphocytes. Such lymphocytes, when stimulated on a second or subsequent occasion, elaborate a variety of factors that enhance the host's defense mechanism. The tuberculin skin test is an example of a delayed hypersensitivity reaction, and advantage is taken of this action for diagnostic purposes. Also, contact dermatitis (dermatitis venenata), such as poison ivy, detergent allergy, and skin reactions to a variety of chemicals, including medications,

is an example of tissue injury resulting from reexposure of a sensitized person.

Atopic Disorders

Atopic disorders (allergic rhinitis, bronchial asthma, allergic dermatoses) are allergic manifestations that occur in persons who are genetically predisposed to forming *reagin*, a special antibody of the IgE class, when exposed to a variety of environmental allergens. Such allergens include various plant pollens, mold spores, domestic animal danders, and foods. An estimated 7% to 10% of the population are subject to atopic disorders. A family history of related allergies can usually be elicited, but this is not always the case. There is recent evidence to show that the immune response gene resides near the HLA (tissue-type) locus on the chromosome. (HLA stands for histocompatibility locus antigen and pertains to compatibility of tissue, that is, whether the recipient can tolerate a particular graft.)

If sensitized persons are reexposed to an allergen to which they have become sensitive, histamine and other mediators are released, producing prompt and profound effects on the tissues of the organ involved. These include (1) dilatation of the walls of small blood vessels with loss of fluid from the blood into the tissue, causing swelling, and (2) constriction of the smooth muscles surrounding the bronchi and the gastrointestinal tract. While clinical manifestations of *atopy* (genetically induced hypersensitivity) are most frequently caused by antigen–antibody interactions, some are initiated by other mechanisms. Nonspecific factors such as autonomic nervous system imbalance, hormonal disturbances, psychic factors, exertion, and changes in barometric pressure may result in tissue changes that mimic allergic reactions.

Assessment

The chief problem for the nurse is to get the patient to avoid medications or attitudes that can aggravate the condition.

Chart 46-1
Allergy Assessment Sheet

Name _____ Age _____ Sex _____ Date _____

  I.   Chief complaint: _____

 II.   Present illness: _____

III.   Collateral allergic symptoms: _____

      Eyes: Pruritus _____ Burning _____ Lacrimation _____
                         Swelling _____ Injection _____ Discharge _____

      Ears: Pruritus _____ Fullness _____ Popping _____
                         Frequent infections _____

      Nose: Sneezing _____ Rhinorrhea _____ Obstruction _____
                         Pruritus _____ Mouth-breathing _____
                         Purulent discharge _____

      Throat: Soreness _____ Postnasal discharge _____
                         Palatal pruritus _____ Mucus in the morning _____

      Chest: Cough _____   Pain _____   Wheezing _____
                         Sputum _____   Dyspnea _____
                         Color _____   Rest _____
                         Amount _____   Exertion _____

      Skin: Dermatitis _____   Eczema _____   Urticaria _____

 IV.   Family allergies

  V.   Previous allergic treatment or testing: _____
      Prior skin testing: _____

      Drugs: Antihistamines   Improved _____   Unimproved _____
                Bronchodilators   Improved _____   Unimproved _____
                Nose drops   Improved _____   Unimproved _____
                Hyposensitization   Improved _____   Unimproved _____
                      Duration _____
                      Antigens _____
                      Reactions _____
                Antibiotics   Improved _____   Unimproved _____
                Steroids   Improved _____   Unimproved _____

 VI.   Physical agents and habits: _____

Bothered by:

      Tobacco for _____ years   Alcohol _____   Air cond. _____
      Cigarettes _____ packs/day   Heat _____   Muggy weath. _____
      Cigars _____ per day   Cold _____   Weath. chngs. _____
      Pipes _____ per day   Perfumes _____   Chemicals _____
      Never smoked _____   Paints _____   Hair spray _____
      Bothered by smoke _____   Insecticides _____ Newspapers _____
                                  Cosmetics _____

VII.   When symptoms occur: _____
      Time and circumstances of 1st episode: _____
      Prior health: _____

(continued)

The nurse must understand the patient with an allergy, offering necessary services and lending an interested, friendly ear, as well as showing empathy for problems. In the many contacts with the patient, the nurse gathers enough data and impressions to characterize the patient fairly accurately from the psychological standpoint, to discern with clarity the environment in which the patient habitually dwells, and to discover what factors are most important from the standpoint of "triggering" attacks. An assessment sheet such as is presented in Chart 46-1 is effective in obtaining and organizing this information.

The nurse must be prepared to meet the dangerous emergency that allergy creates on occasion in the form of anaphylactic shock or fulminating asthma, when swift and effective countermeasures may spell the difference between life and death (see Anaphylaxis, p. 1214).

Chart 46-1 (continued)

Course of illness over decades: progressing _____ regressing _____
Time of year: _____ Exact dates: _____
    Perennial _____
    Seasonal _____
    Seasonally exacerbated _____
Monthly variations (menses, occupation): _____
Time of week (weekends vs. weekdays): _____
Time of day or night: _____
After insect stings: _____
VIII. Where symptoms occur: _____
Living where at onset: _____
Living where since onset: _____
Effect of vacation or major geographic change: _____
Symptoms better indoors or outdoors: _____
Effect of school or work: _____
Effect of staying elsewhere nearby: _____
Effect of hospitalization: _____
Effect of specific environments: _____
Do symptoms occur around: _____
    old leaves _____ hay _____ lakeside _____ barns _____
    summer homes _____ damp basement _____ dry attic _____
    lawnmowing _____ animals _____ other _____
Do symptoms occur after eating:
    cheese _____ mushrooms _____ beer _____ melons _____
    bananas _____ fish _____ nuts _____ citrus fruits _____
    other foods (list) _____
Home: city _____ rural _____
          house _____ age _____
          apartment _____ basement _____ damp _____ dry _____
          heating system _____
          pets (how long) _____ dog _____ cat _____ other _____

Bedroom:	Type	Age	*Living room:*	Type	Age
Pillow	_____	_____	Rug	_____	_____
Mattress	_____	_____	Matting	_____	_____
Blankets	_____	_____	Furniture	_____	_____
Quilts	_____	_____			
Furniture	_____	_____			

Anywhere in home symptoms are worse: _____
IX. What does patient think makes symptoms worse? _____
X. Under what circumstances is patient free of symptoms? _____
XI. Summary and additional comments: _____

(Patterson R. Allergic Diseases. Philadelphia, JB Lippincott)

Allergic Rhinitis ("Hay Fever," Chronic Allergic Rhinitis, Pollinosis)

Allergic rhinitis is the most common form of respiratory allergy presumed to be mediated by an immunologic reaction. It affects approximately 8% to 10% of the U.S. population (20–30% of adolescents). When untreated, many complications may result, such as allergic asthma, chronic nasal obstruction, chronic otitis media with hearing loss, anosmia (absence of the sense of smell), and, in children, orofacial dental deformities. Consequently, early diagnosis and adequate treatment are strongly recommended.

Because allergic rhinitis is induced by airborne pollens or molds, it is characterized by seasonal occurrences.

Time	Source	Example
Early spring	Tree pollen	Oak, elm, poplar
Early summer, ("rose fever")	Grass pollen	Timothy, red-top
Early fall	Weed pollen	Ragweed

Each year the attacks begin and end approximately on the same dates. Airborne mold spores require warm, damp weather. Although there is no rigid seasonal pattern, these spores appear in early spring, are rampant during the summer, and taper off and disappear by the first frost. Regional patterns for the appearance of pollens and molds are shown in Table 46-1.

Pathophysiology. Antibodies of IgE that coat the mucosa of the nose and conjunctiva and are specific for a given pollen (antigen) combine with the pollen. As a result, cell injury occurs (causing copious secretions, edema, sneezing, local itching). When the offending pollen is blown away, the allergic condition ceases.

Clinical Manifestations. Sneezing is the most characteristic symptom of allergic rhinitis. Sneezing episodes consisting of 10–20 sneezes in rapid succession are common. Usually the rhinitis starts in the mucous membrane of the nose, which may become so edematous and swollen that the nostrils are closed completely. The nasal mucous membrane burns and secretes a thin, irritating discharge. The eyes are usually involved, and become red, with burning and tearing. Pruritus affects the eyes, nose, ears, and throat. If nasal obstruction is severe, headache and earache may be apparent. Some patients exhibit systemic symptoms: weakness, malaise, fatigue, irritability, and anorexia. During the "off seasons," a nasal examination reveals normal findings.

Diagnostic Evaluation. The patient's hypersensitivity to the pollens that induce the attacks can usually be confirmed by appropriate skin, conjunctival, or intradermal tests. These reactions are not necessarily specific, because a positive skin test does not necessarily mean that symptoms are due to that antigen. When properly performed and interpreted, these tests are quite specific in demonstrating reagin to the antigen in question. Accurate identification of the offending antigen, of course, depends on close examination of the patient's history.

Management

The goal of therapy is to provide relief from the annoying symptoms just described. Therapy usually takes one or all of the following tracks:

1. *Avoidance Therapy.* Removal of the offending pollen or antigen (stripping the environment of irritants, using air conditioning, or moving to another locale as dictated by climate)
2. *Pharmacotherapy*
   a. Administration of antihistamines (substances that protect cells against the effects of histamine)
   b. Suppression of the immune response by means of corticosteroids—(used for more advanced allergic reactions, such as asthma)
   c. Cromolyn sodium—usually reserved for asthma
3. *Immunotherapy.* Hyposensitization by repeated injections of the offending pollens in low concentration

Avoidance Therapy

In avoidance therapy, every attempt is made to remove those allergens that act as precipitating factors. For example, allergy due to animal dander would require removing the pet from the home environment and replacing a feather pillow with a hypoallergenic Dacron pillow.

Aeroallergens are most difficult to avoid because they are so widely distributed; however, the immediate surroundings may be altered. For example, irritating pollens, dusts, and molds can be avoided by remaining in a building that has central air conditioning with an electrostatic precipitating filter. The limitation here is that one cannot remain indoors all the time. When the controlled environment provided by central air conditioning with filtered air is not available, the rooms where the person spends most time can be modified. Room air conditioners can be used. Mattress and box springs are encased in elastic fabric casings; upholstered furniture, stuffed toys, chenille bedspreads, and the like are removed from the bedroom.

Another method is to travel to areas where the offending allergen is absent during certain times of the year. This method is becoming less effective (as well as more expensive) because the atmosphere is becoming increasingly permeated with allergens.

Pharmacotherapy

Histamine is found in all body tissue and fluid and is concentrated in skin, lung, and gastrointestinal tissues. An enzyme, histidine decarboxylase, acts as a catalyst in the biosynthesis of histamine from histidine (a precursor amino acid). Histamine is concentrated in mast cells and basophils. Certain agents can cause the histamine in these cells to be discharged, resulting in an anaphylacticlike reaction. Hence, the mast cell is considered the major target cell in acute allergic reactions.

Nasal Decongestants. Nasal decongestants are used for relief of nasal congestion when applied topically (by spray or nasal drops) to the nasal mucosa. They activate the α-adrenergic receptor sites on the smooth muscle of the nasal mucosal blood vessels. This reduces local blood flow, fluid exudation, and mucosal edema. Examples are:

- Oxymetazoline (Afrin, Duration)
- Pseudoephedrine (Afrinol, Novafed, Sudafed)

Antihistamines. Antihistamines are classified as H_1 or H_2 receptor antagonists, and are associated synonymously with H_1 antagonists. Examples are as follows:

- Alkylamine (most widely used): Chlorpheniramine (Chlor-Trimeton, Teldrin, Dimetane)
- Tripelennamine (Pyribenzamine, PBZ)
- Diphenhydramine (Benadryl)
- Terfenadine (Seldane)

Antihistamines given orally are readily absorbed. They are most effective when given at the first sign of symptoms, because they prevent the development of new symptoms by preventing further histamine release. In actual practice, the effectiveness of these drugs is limited to certain patients with hay fever, vasomotor rhinitis, urticaria (hives), and mild asthma; they are rarely effective in other conditions or in

TABLE 46-1
Approximate Time of Appearance of Major Pollens and Molds in Various Regions of the U.S.*

	Jan	Feb	Mar	Apr	May	June	July	Aug	Sept	Oct	Nov	Dec
Northeast				Elm Maple	Oak	Grass	Alternaria †Hormod.	Ragweed Alternaria Hormod.	Ragweed Alternaria Hormod.	Alternaria Hormod.		
Southeast		Elm	Ash Maple	Oak Sycamore	Pecan Oak Bermuda grass	Bermuda grass Hormod.	Alternaria Hormod.	Ragweed Alternaria Hormod.	Ragweed Alternaria Hormod.	Ragweed Alternaria Hormod.	Hormod.	
North Central				Elm Maple	Oak	Grass Hormod.	Alternaria Hormod.	Ragweed Alternaria Hormod.	Ragweed Alternaria Hormod.	Alternaria Hormod.		
South Central		Elm	Oak Maple Sycamore	Pecan Alternaria	Bermuda grass Alternaria Hormod.	Bermuda grass Alternaria Hormod.	Alternaria Hormod.	Ragweed Alternaria Hormod.	Ragweed Alternaria			
Plains			Maple	Cottonwood		Grass Hormod.	Russian thistle Kochia Hormod.	Ragweed Russian thistle Kochia Hormod. Alternaria	Ragweed Sagebrush			
Southwest	Alternaria	Alternaria Cottonwood	Alternaria Ash Mountain cedar	Alternaria Bermuda grass False ragweed	Bermuda grass	Bermuda grass Hormod.		Alternaria Russian thistle Kochia	Alternaria Russian thistle Kochia	Alternaria		
Intermountain Basin			Elm	Cottonwood	Sycamore	Grass		Russian thistle Kochia	Sagebrush			
Pacific Coast North			Alder	Maple Oak	Grass	Grass Plantain	Grass					
Pacific Coast South	Alternaria		Oak Walnut	Oak Walnut Olive	Bermuda grass	Bermuda grass	Bermuda grass	Various ‡Compos.	Elms Compos.	Elm Compos. Alternaria	Alternaria	Alternaria

*There is some variation from year to year. Locations in the northern parts of the region usually lag behind locations in the southern parts. Small amounts of the various pollens and molds often are presented before and after the season indicated in the table. Bermuda grass, which flourishes in the South, contains different antigens from those of the northern grasses, but the two regions overlap somewhat. There are many aero-allergens which are not listed that occur in small amounts or in restricted locations.

† Hormod.: Hormodendrum

‡ Compos.: Compositae

(Asthma, A Practical Guide for Physicians. American Lung Association in cooperation with the Allergy Foundation of America)

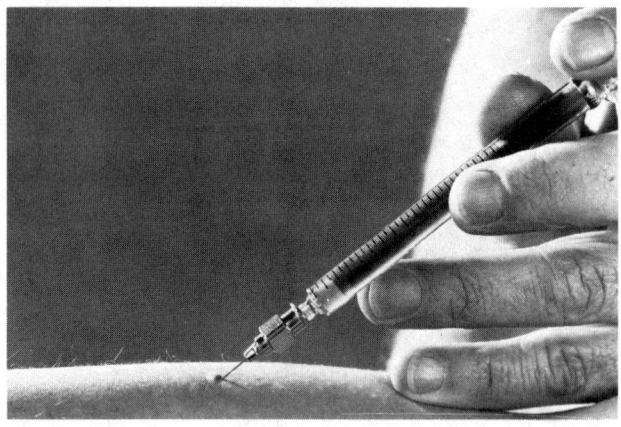

Figure 46-3
Intradermal testing. Cleanse the testing site with alcohol or ether. Tests are made on the volar surface of the lower arm and the outer surface of the upper arm, omitting the antecubital space. Intradermal tests are limited to 10 or 20 at most. (Courtesy, Hollister-Stier Laboratories.)

severe conditions of any sort. Side-effects vary with the individual; therefore, individualization of dosage is required. The most common side-effects are dryness of mouth, dizziness, irritability, drowsiness, and gastrointestinal upset. These are often mild and temporary. Steroid hormones frequently are helpful in ameliorating manifestations of allergy.

Sensitivity Tests and Immunotherapy (Hyposensitization)

A knowledge of the general concepts regarding assessment and therapy in allergic diseases is important, since the nurse is very apt to be an active participant in the treatment of these disorders and will almost certainly be in the position to advise patients who are potential candidates for one or another of these procedures.

Skin Tests. The most common method of treatment is the serial injection of one or more antigens that are selected in each particular case on the basis of skin tests. Skin testing (Fig. 46-3) entails the simultaneous intradermal inoculation (or superficial application), at separate sites, of several solutions containing individual antigens representing an assortment of allergens deemed most likely to be implicated in the patient's disease. A positive reaction, evidenced by the appearance of an urticarial wheal (Fig. 46-4) or by localized erythema (redness) in the area of inoculation or contact, is regarded as evidence of sensitivity to the corresponding antigen.

Skin tests lend important weight to other evidence obtained from the patient's history, indicating which of several antigens are most likely to provoke symptoms and providing some clue to the intensity of the patient's sensitization.

The dosage of the pollen injected is important also. The majority of patients are hypersensitive not to one but to several pollens, and under testing conditions they may not react to the specific pollens that induce their attacks, but they usually do. Ragweed seems to be the most potent of all.

If there is any doubt about the validity of the skin tests,

a RAST (see below) or a provocative challenge test may be done. In the provocative challenge test, the suspected antigen is applied to the sensitive tissue (such as the conjunctiva, nasal or bronchial mucosa, or gastrointestinal tract) and the response is observed.

Immunotherapy. Correlation of a positive skin test with a positive history is an indication for immunotherapy *if* the allergen cannot be avoided. The value of such injections has been fairly well established in instances of allergic rhinitis and bronchial asthma that are clearly due to sensitivity to one of the common pollens or molds or to house dust. Although referred to as a "hyposensitization" procedure, the effects are most likely attributable to the opposite process (*i.e.*, immunization), for it appears to stimulate the production of a new antibody with the capacity of neutralizing the allergy-provoking properties of the responsible allergen.

Immunotherapy, while helpful in a majority of patients, does not cure the condition. Before such a program is launched, the physician discusses with the patient what may be expected from immunotherapy and why it is important to continue the therapy for several years. When skin tests are done, they are to be correlated with clinical manifestations; the treatment is based on the patient's needs rather than on the skin tests.

Specific treatment consists of injecting extracts of the pollens or mold spores that cause symptoms in a particular patient. Injections begin with very small amounts and are gradually increased, usually at weekly intervals, until a maximum tolerated dose is attained. Maintenance "booster" injections are then given at 2- to 4-week intervals, frequently for a period of several years, before maximum benefit is achieved.

There are three methods of injection therapy: coseasonal, preseasonal, and perennial. When treatment is given on a *coseasonal basis,* it is initiated during the season in which the patient experiences symptoms. This method has been used less widely in recent years; it is not an effective form of therapy, and there is increased risk of systemic reactions. *Preseasonal therapy* injections are given 2 to 3 months before symptoms appear, allowing time for hyposensitization to take place. This treatment is discontinued after the season. *Perennial therapy* is administered all year round, usually on a monthly basis, and is the preferred method because of more effective, longer-lasting results.

Precautions. Since there is a possibility that the injection of an allergen may induce systemic reactions, it is only given in a physician's office where epinephrine is immediately available. Because of the dangers involved, injections ought not to be given by a lay person or by the patient. The patient remains in the physician's office for a minimum of 20 to 30 minutes and is observed for the possible development of systemic symptoms. If a large, local swelling develops, the next dose should not be increased because this may be a warning of a possible systemic reaction.

Complications. A systemic reaction is a serious complication that ranges from mild hives to an acute asthmatic attack, hypotension, or even anaphylactic shock. Emergency treatment is described on page 1215.

RAST. The radioallergosorbent test (RAST) is a laboratory technique for determining the presence of IgE antibodies in serum. The sensitivity of this procedure correlates very well with carefully conducted skin tests in the detection

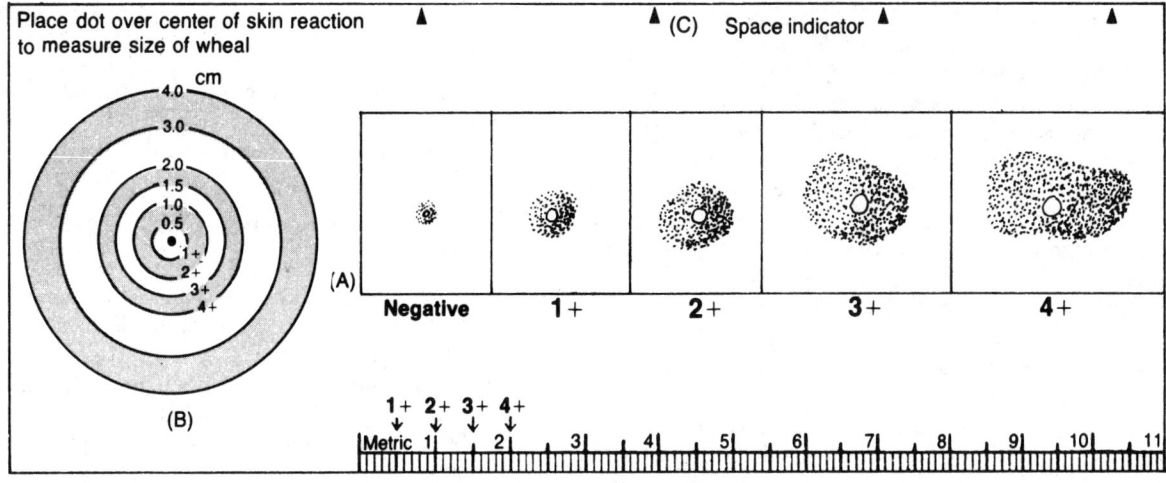

Place dot over center of skin reaction to measure size of wheal

cm
4.0
3.0
2.0
1.5
1.0
0.5
1+
2+
3+
4+

(B)

(A)

Negative   1+   2+   3+   4+

(C)   Space indicator

1+ 2+ 3+ 4+

Metric 1 2 3 4 5 6 7 8 9 10 11

Figure 46-4

Method for evaluating wheals. (*A*) This series of reactions indicates the sizes of wheals as they are referred to by the allergist (1+, 2+, *etc.*). A negative reaction is shown at the left. (*B*) The target wheal guide can be traced on a transparent sheet (acetate or x-ray film) and then placed over the wheal to measure the size in centimeters or according to plus-size. The relationship between the two is indicated on the lower metric scale. (*C*) Showing placement of test sites spaced uniformly. (Patient Care, Sept. 15, 1973. Copyright © 1973, Patient Care Corp., Darien, Conn. All rights reserved.)

of immediate-type hypersensitivity. The RAST is probably no more specific than direct skin testing, but may be used to corroborate skin-test findings, especially in questionable cases. The RAST may also substitute for skin testing when the latter is considered hazardous or when a generalized dermatitis may preclude direct skin testing.

▶ Nursing Process
The Patient With Allergic Rhinitis

▷ *Assessment*

The examination and history of the patient reveal sneezing, often in paroxysms, thin and watery nasal discharge, itching eyes and nose, lacrimation, and occasionally headache. The nursing history includes a personal or family history of allergy. The pertinent parts of the Allergy Assessment Form on p. 1206 will determine the nature of antigens, seasonal upswings, and medication history. The nurse also obtains subjective data about how the patient feels just before symptoms become obvious, such as feelings of pruritus, breathing problems, and tingling sensations. In addition to the symptoms described, note signs of hoarseness, wheezing, hives, rash, erythema, or edema. Elicit any relation between emotional problems/stress and the triggering of allergy symptoms.

▷ *Nursing Diagnoses*

Based on the assessment data, major nursing diagnoses for the patient may include the following:

- Alteration in comfort related to an allergic response of the nasal mucosa to a prevalent antigen

- Ineffective individual coping related to symptoms produced by an allergic condition
- Knowledge deficit concerning specific environmental modification, avoidance procedures, and self-care information

▷ *Planning and Implementation*

▷ *Goals:* The major goals of the patient may include relief of discomfort through control of allergic manifestations insofar as possible, ability to cope with the signs and symptoms of the particular allergy, and knowledge about the causes and control of allergic symptoms.

Nursing Interventions

Relieving Discomfort. The best way to prevent allergic reactions is to remove whatever produces sensitizing antigens. To some extent it is possible to prevent discomfort by reducing, eliminating, or avoiding the particular allergens. If the problem is instigated by seeds, trees, and plants, perhaps moving to an area where such vegetation is not present is the best and most effective treatment. If the person is allergic to pet fur or dander, it may be best to give the pet away. Should symptoms occur as a result of dust and mold, the environment in which the patient spends most time may have to be modified.

Enhancing Coping Abilities. Allergy is a common condition; other persons with similar problems have learned how to circumvent the discomforts, and this patient can do so also. Hearing about what allergens cause their reactions give allergy patients better insight into their particular needs and problems.

If the patient is to undergo desensitization, the nurse can reinforce the physician's explanation regarding the purpose and procedure as described on p. 1210. It is necessary to follow instructions thereafter regarding the subsequent series of inoculations, usually given every 2 weeks or monthly. These include (1) remaining in the physician's office at least 20 minutes after the injection so that emergency treatment may be given if the patient sustains a reaction, (2) avoiding rubbing or scratching the site of the injection, and (3) continuing with the series for the period of time required.

Patient Education and Home Health Care. In addition to avoiding situations that bring on the allergic symptoms, the patient needs to understand any medications prescribed to control the allergy problem.

Because antihistamines often produce drowsiness, the patient is cautioned about this and other side-effects of the particular medication. Operating machinery, driving a car, and activities requiring intense concentration should be postponed. The patient is also informed about the dangers in drinking alcohol when taking these drugs because they tend to potentiate the effects of alcohol.

The patient must be aware of the effects caused by *overuse* of sympathomimetic agents in nose drops or sprays. A condition referred to as *rhinitis medicamentosa* may result. After topical application of the drug, a rebound period may occur in which the nasal mucous membranes become more edematous and congested than they were before the medication was used. Such a reaction encourages the use of more drug. A circular pattern of activity results, much like a "cat chasing its tail." The topical agent must be discontinued immediately and completely in order to correct this problem.

Rhinitis Medicamentosa

Nasal congestion → Topical application of sympathomimetic drugs → Relief → Rebound reaction → Nasal congestion

The instruction program is geared to the individual needs of the patient, as determined by the results of tests, the medication prescribed, and the degree to which patient and family are motivated to deal with the condition. Some general suggestions for those sensitive to dust and mold in the home include the following:

1. Try to maintain a dust-free environment, particularly in the bedroom:

    - Reduce contents to barest minimum; remove drapes, curtains, and venetian blinds and replace with pull shades.
    - Remove carpets; wash woodwork and floor and thereafter dust and vacuum daily. Waxed flooring is preferable to rugs.
    - Replace stuffed furniture with wooden pieces that can be dusted easily.
    - Avoid tufted bedspreads, stuffed toys, feather pillows; replace them with easily washable cotton material.
    - Cover the mattress with a hypoallergenic cover that can be zippered to fit snugly.
    - Avoid wearing fabrics that cause itching.

2. Within the house as a whole, reduce dust by the following practices:

    - Use steam or hot water for heating rather than hot air.
    - Utilize filters/air conditioning.
    - Wear a mask if cleaning is being done.

3. For patients sensitive to pollen/mold, reduce exposure to them:

    - Determine times of the year when pollen count is highest; reduce exposure at these times.
    - Avoid barns, weeds, dry leaves, and freshly cut grass.
    - Wear a mask at times of increased exposure (*e.g.,* windy days, when grass is being cut).
    - Seek air-conditioned areas at the height of the season.
    - Take antihistamines as prescribed.
    - Avoid sprays and perfumes; use hypoallergenic cosmetics.

4. For insect stings, see emergency section in Chapter 60.
5. Determine specific foods that may be a problem:

    - Pursue a plan of avoiding what appears to be a troublesome food for a period of time. By trial, one can develop a list of foods that are to be avoided. Examples may be fish, nuts, eggs, or chocolate.

▷ *Evaluation*
Expected Outcomes

1. Patient obtains relief from allergenic reactions by following specific directives:
    a. Removes items that retain dust from the bedroom environment
    b. Wears a dampened mask if dust/mold may be a problem
    c. Avoids smoke-filled rooms, dust-filled or freshly sprayed areas
    d. Uses air-conditioned areas for a major part of the day
    e. Takes antihistamines as prescribed; participates in hyposensitization program
2. Is able to cope with the inconveniences of the allergy
    a. Demonstrates understanding of the problem and ways of keeping symptoms under control
    b. Shows ability to distinguish symptoms for which professional health consultation may be needed
    c. States understanding that there is often an association between general physical condition and severity of allergy manifestations
3. Describes knowledge gained about the allergy problem and how to control symptoms
    a. Names the particular antigens that cause the symptoms
    b. Relates how contact with these antigens is minimized
    c. Describes the type of medication taken and how it functions
    d. Tells what activities are feasible to participate in and how his involvement in them can be maximized without activating the allergies

Allergic Dermatoses

Contact Dermatitis

Contact dermatitis (dermatitis venenata) is an inflammatory, often eczematous, condition caused by a skin reaction to a variety of irritating or allergenic materials. Almost any substance can produce contact dermatitis. Poison ivy is probably the most common example; cosmetics, soaps, detergents, and industrial chemicals are frequent offenders. The skin sensitivity may develop after brief or prolonged periods of exposure, and the clinical picture may appear hours or weeks after the sensitized skin has been exposed.

The symptoms include itching, burning, erythema, skin lesions (vesicles), and edema, followed by weeping, crusting, and finally drying-up and peeling of the skin. In very severe responses, hemorrhagic bullae may develop. Repeated reactions may be accompanied by the development of thickening of the skin and pigmentary changes.

Secondary invasion by bacteria may develop in skin abraded by rubbing or scratching. Usually, there are no systemic symptoms unless the eruption is widespread.

Diagnosis may sometimes be made easily on the basis of the location of the eruption and history of exposure. However, in cases of obscure irritants or an unobservant patient, diagnosis may be extremely difficult and many trial-and-error procedures may be involved before the etiology is correctly determined. Patch tests on the skin with suspected offending agents may clarify the picture.

The most important aspect of treatment is to remove the patient from further contact with the irritant or allergen. Burow's solution soaks (aluminum acetate) soothe the blistered erythematous skin and may be followed by application of corticosteroid ointments or creams. Antimicrobials are given if secondary invasion is present.

Atopic Dermatitis. Atopic dermatitis is chronic, pruritic, and familial in nature. It involves principally the skin of the neck, the face, and the flexural creases (Fig 46-5), and will wax and wane in activity. It has a more prolonged course than simple contact dermatitis. It is frequently associated with allergic respiratory disorders, but the true cause remains unknown. Family history is usually positive for allergies such as allergic rhinitis, asthma, or eczema. Drying of the skin is an aggravating factor; wool and lanolin commonly compound the skin irritation of these patients. Allergy to foods has probably been overstressed but is, nonetheless, a factor. Emotional stress and nervousness aggravate the condition. The principles of treatment are the same as those for contact dermatitis.

Drug Reactions (Dermatitis Medicamentosa)

Dermatitis medicamentosa is the term applied to skin rashes induced by the internal administration of certain drugs. While as a rule certain drugs tend to induce eruptions of similar types, individuals react differently to each drug.

In general, it may be said that drug rashes appear suddenly, have a particularly vivid color, present characteristics that are more spectacular than the somewhat similar eruptions of infectious origin, and, with the exception of the bromide and the iodide rashes, disappear rapidly after the drug is withdrawn. Some drug rashes are accompanied by constitutional symptoms. Upon discovery of a drug allergy, such patients

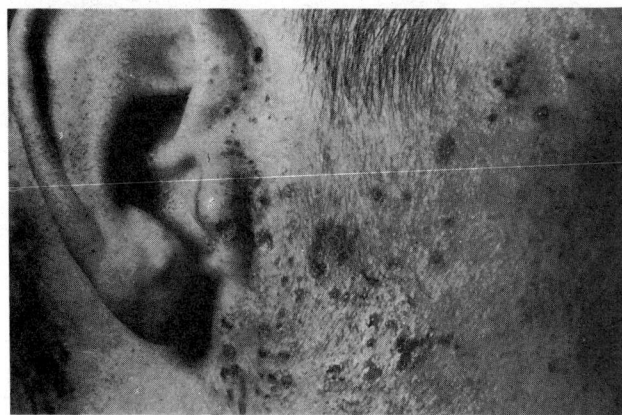

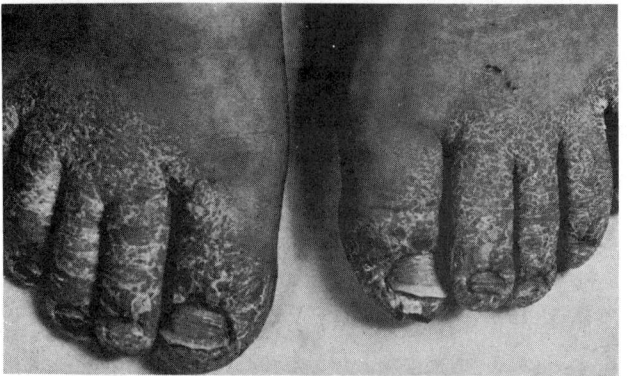

Figure 46-5
Atopic eczema. (Sauer GC. Manual of Skin Diseases. Philadelphia, JB Lippincott.)

are warned that they have an idiosyncracy to a particular drug and are advised not to take it again.

The nurse has an important responsibility in relation to drug eruptions, for these lesions suggest more serious idiosyncrasies. By being in a primary position of initial contact with the patient, the nurse is able to report the appearance of the eruption so that early treatment is initiated.

Urticaria and Angioneurotic Edema

Urticaria (hives) is an allergic affection of the skin characterized by the sudden appearance of pinkish edematous elevations, which vary in size and shape, and itch and smart. They may involve any part of the body, including the mucous membranes, especially those of the mouth, the larynx (occasionally with serious respiratory complications), and the gastrointestinal tract. Each hive remains for a period varying from a few minutes to several hours, and then disappears. For hours or days, crops of these lesions may come, go, and return, in a most capricious manner. If this sequence continues indefinitely, the condition is called *chronic urticaria*.

The swellings of *angioneurotic edema* involve the deeper layers of the skin, resulting in more diffuse swelling, rather than the discrete lesions characteristic of hives. Occasionally one may be seen that covers the entire back. The skin over it may appear normal, but often has a reddish hue. It does not pit on pressure, as ordinary edema does. The regions most often involved are lips, eyelids, cheeks, hands, feet, genitalia, and tongue; the mucous membranes of the larynx, the bronchi, and the gastrointestinal canal may also be affected, particularly in cases of the hereditary type. An eye may be completely closed; one lip may become so large that eating is impossible; one hand may become so huge that the fingers cannot be flexed. These swellings may appear suddenly, in a few seconds or minutes, or slowly, in 1 or 2 hours. In the latter case, their appearance often is preceded by itching or burning sensations. Seldom does more than a single swelling appear at one time, although one may develop while another is disappearing. Only infrequently do they recur in the same region. The individual lesions usually last from 24 to 36 hours. On rare occasions, they recur with a remarkable periodicity at intervals of 3 or 4 weeks.

Hereditary Angioedema

Hereditary angioedema, although not an immunologic disorder in the usual sense, is included in this section because of its resemblance to allergic angioedema and because of the seriousness of this condition. Symptoms are due to edema of the skin, the respiratory tract, or the digestive tract. Attacks may be precipitated by trauma or may seem to occur spontaneously.

When the skin is involved, the swelling is usually rather diffuse, does not itch, and is usually not accompanied by urticaria. Gastrointestinal edema may cause abdominal pain severe enough to suggest the need for surgery. Edema of the upper respiratory tract may cause marked swelling of the uvula and of the larynx, resulting in suffocation. Acute laryngeal edema is the most serious manifestation of this disorder and has resulted in death due to asphyxiation in nearly 20% of these patients. Attacks usually subside within 3 to 4 days, but during this time the patient should be observed carefully for signs of laryngeal obstruction, which may necessitate tracheostomy as a lifesaving measure. Epinephrine, antihistamines, and corticosteroids are usually employed in treatment, but the success of these agents is limited.

Food Allergy

Immune reactions to food are more complex than reactions to inhalants. Inhalant allergy usually involves an abnormal increase in IgE, whereas ingestant reactions involve all known immune mechanisms. This complicates the understanding, diagnosis, and treatment of food allergies.

Symptoms of food allergies may include itching, wheezing, sneezing, cough, throat clearing, nausea, vomiting, abdominal cramps, and urinary frequency. Several types of tests are available to detect the specific food or foods to which the patient is allergic, but they take time. One method is to place the patient in an environmentally controlled unit to fast for several days while avoiding the use of drugs, tobacco, cosmetics, and water additives and contaminants. After ridding the body of irritative food and chemical residues, the patient then ingests organically grown foods in specified proportions. As foods are added, reactions to certain foods become apparent. This method is time-consuming and expensive.

Other methods are based on avoiding or eliminating suspect foods. The foods that most commonly present problems are cereal grains, dairy products, and processed foods containing additives, refined sugars and preservatives.

Treatment must be individualized. If a certain food has been identified as the cause of an allergic reaction, that food as well as any related foods (*i.e.*, foods in the same "food family," such as the parsley family, mint family, maple family) should be avoided.

Whether the food allergy is fixed or cyclic is also determined. *Fixed food allergy* is one that occurs each time the food is consumed. *Cyclic food allergy* is related to whether the food is eaten frequently or in great quantities.

Researchers continue to explore the complex problem of food allergies. There is much that has been learned in the past several years, but much remains to be done.

Serum Sickness

The illness known as serum sickness traditionally has resulted from the administration of therapeutic antisera of animal sources for the treatment or prevention of infectious diseases such as tetanus, pneumonia, rabies, diphtheria, and botulism and for bites of venomous snakes and black-widow spiders. With the advent of human antitetanus serum and antibiotics, true serum sickness is much less common now than in previous years. However, various drugs, chief of which is penicillin, are now the main cause of a syndrome identical to that caused by foreign sera.

Clinical Manifestations.   The symptoms are due to a reaction and immunologic attack upon the serum or the drug. Antibodies appear chiefly to be of the IgE and IgM classes. Early manifestations, beginning 6 to 10 days after the administration of the drug, include an inflammatory reaction at the site of injection of the drug, followed by regional and generalized lymphadenopathy. There is nearly always a skin rash, which may be urticarial or purpuric, and joints are frequently tender and swollen. Vasculitis may occur in any organ but is most commonly observed in the kidney, resulting in proteinuria and, occasionally, casts. Cardiac involvement, mild to severe in nature, may occur. Peripheral neuritis may cause temporary paralysis of the upper extremities or may be widespread, causing the Guillain-Barré syndrome.

The usual untreated course lasts for several days to a few weeks, but ordinarily the patient responds promptly and completely if treated with antihistamines and corticosteroids.

Anaphylaxis

Anaphylaxis is an immediate, shocklike (life-threatening) allergic reaction following exposure to a substance to which the person is exquisitely sensitive. Drugs, such as foreign sera and penicillin; insect stings; and allergenic extracts used in immunotherapy for extrinsic allergic conditions are the most common causes of anaphylaxis. Iodinated contrast media occasionally present the same clinical picture and are similarly treated. Commonly implicated foods to which some persons are sensitive are eggs, cow's milk, nuts, shellfish, legumes, and chocolate. Food additives such as metabisulfite tartrazine ("sulfites") and monosodium glutamate can produce severe reactions in persons with asthma.

Clinical Manifestations.   Initial symptoms may include a generalized feeling of warmth, apprehension, uneasiness,

TABLE 46-2
Manifestations of Anaphylactic Reaction

System Site	Mild	Moderate	Severe
Cutaneous			
Skin	Warm, tingling	Urticaria	Urticaria
Mucosa	Nasal congestion	Angioedema	Angioedema
	Pruritus		Pallor
	Lacrimation		Cyanosis
	Periorbital edema		
Respiratory			
Upper	Sneezing	Laryngeal edema	Stridor
	Rhinorrhea	Edema of epiglottis, tongue, pharynx, trachea	Hoarseness
Lower	None	Wheezing, cough	Bronchospasm
		Dyspnea	
		Bronchospasm	
Central nervous	None	Apprehension	Seizures
		Anxiety	Coma
		Worry	
Gastrointestinal	None	Nausea	Abdominal Cramps
		Vomiting	Diarrhea
Circulatory	None	None	Tachycardia
			Hypotension
			Shock

weakness, itching of the palms and soles, itching around the eyes, itching in the ears, hoarseness, dysphagia, a sense of constriction in the throat, and a feeling of impending doom. The patient may experience tightness in the chest, with an audible expiratory wheeze. Fright may be evident, and pruritus severe. Hives may be localized and progress to massive facial angioedema, suggestive of upper respiratory edema. Death may occur within minutes to several hours, due to respiratory failure brought on by laryngeal edema or bronchospasm, but if recovery occurs, it is usually complete and without sequelae. Manifestations of an anaphylactic reaction are summarized in Table 46-2.

Prevention. A careful history is taken before the administration of any drug, to be certain that there is no known hypersensitivity to it. Any person who is known to be susceptible to anaphylaxis should carry an identification tag.*

Anyone who is endangered by the sting of Hymenoptera (bees, wasps, hornets, yellow jackets) should carry an emergency kit (during spring and summer) containing parenteral epinephrine. An ANA-Kit (Hollister-Stier), which is available commercially, contains a prefilled syringe with epinephrine and the equipment required for self-administration.

* Medic Alert Foundation, 1000 North Palm, Turlock, California 05380.

If animal serum is to be given, it is mandatory that careful skin testing be carried out prior to injection of therapeutic doses. (Horse serum, for example, is still used for patients needing snake antivenom and antilymphocyte serum.)

The injection of any drug should, whenever possible, be given sufficiently distal on an extremity so that a tourniquet may be applied proximally in order to retard the absorption of the drug into the circulation.

In the presence of a positive skin test for a drug that must be given, a procedure of "desensitization" may be carried out. This is done by giving a minute amount of diluted drug or serum, followed by gradually increasing doses every 10 to 15 minutes until a full therapeutic dose has been achieved. When carefully done, this is a fairly safe procedure but does not obviate the later development of a serum-sicknesslike reaction (described above).

Management and Nursing Intervention. Help should be summoned immediately, but the person suffering the attack should not be left unattended. Immediate assessment of vital functions is done to determine the status of respiration and heart beat. If these have stopped, cardiopulmonary resuscitation is initiated.

Epinephrine (Adrenalin) is the most effective treatment of an acute allergic reaction. An intramuscular injection of epinephrine 1:1000 is given immediately into the upper arm, and the area is massaged. A tourniquet is then applied, if possible, proximal to the site of injection of the allergen. An additional 0.01 ml/kg up to 0.2 ml of epinephrine is injected into the site of the allergen injection to assist in the reduction of antigen into the system. Routine measures for shock, including assuring an adequate airway, assuming the shock position, providing supplementary oxygen, and giving intravenous fluids, are also indicated. It is not necessary to wait for blood gas determinations to administer oxygen, because it directly relieves hypoxemia and alveolar hypoxia.

Later, on the basis of individual clinical assessment, the following may be required:

For *anaphylaxis:* diphenhydramine
For *bronchospasm:* intravenous aminophylline; intravenous fluids; intravenous corticosteroids
For *hypotension:* volume expanders, vasopressors, isoproterenol
For *laryngeal obstruction:* tracheostomy and oxygen therapy.
For *respiratory arrest:* intubation, oxygen therapy
For *cardiac arrest:* cardiopulmonary resuscitation, sodium bicarbonate

Bibliography

Books

Altman LC. Clinical Allergy and Immunology. Boston, GK Hall, 1984.
Klaustermeyer WD. Practical Allergy and Immunology. New York, John Wiley & Sons, 1983.
Lockey RF and Bukantz SC. Fundamentals of Immunology and Allergy. Philadelphia, WB Saunders, 1986.
Lockey RF and Bukantz SC. Principles of Immunology and Allergy. Philadelphia, WB Saunders, 1986.
Middleton E Jr et al. Allergy: Principles and Practice. St Louis, CV Mosby, 1983.
Patterson R. Allergic Diseases: Diagnosis and Management, 3rd ed. Philadelphia, JB Lippincott, 1985.
Speer F. Handbook of Clinical Allergy. Littleton, Massachusetts, Wright PSG, 1982.

Articles

General

Adkinson NF Jr. Keeping current on allergy treatment. Patient Care 1984 Feb 15; 18(3):137–173.
Boyles JH Jr. Chemical sensitivity. Otolaryngol Clin North Am 1985 Nov; 18(4):787–795.

Chandler MJ and Patterson R. Immunotherapy update. Ear, Nose, and Throat J 1986 May; 65(5):226–229.
Chandler MJ and Patterson R. Psychosomatic nasal disorder. Allergy and Clin Immunol 1986 Aug; 78(2):329–331.
Cohen SH and Fink JN. The allergic patient: Office evaluation. Hosp Med 1983 Feb; 19(2):105–125.
de Shazo RD and Salvaggio JE. Allergy and immunology. JAMA 1985 Oct 25; 254(16):2257–2259.
Eckmann SF. New office assay for theophylline. Patient Care 1986 July 15; 20(12):21, 182.
Girsh LS. Avoidance of allergens. Postgrad Med 1982 Oct; 72(4):54–56.
King HC. Endpoint titration and immunotherapy. Otolaryngol Clin North Am 1985 Nov; 18(4):703–717.
Lapp L. Taming of the vernal sneeze. Vital Signs (University of Pennsylvania) 1986 Spring:23–25.
Mangi RJ. Allergy skin tests: An overview. Otolaryngol Clin North Am 1985 Nov; 18(4):719–723.
Mennies JH et al. An overview of adult allergic disorders. Nurs Pract 1985 June; 10(6):16–27.
Minimizing risks of penicillin allergy. Patient Care 1984 Apr 30; 18(8): 21–47.
Nalebuff DJ. PRIST, RAST, and beyond. Otolaryngol Clin North Am 1985 Nov; 18(4):725–744.
Terfenadine—a nonsedating antihistamine. Med Letter Drug Ther 1985 Aug 2; 27(693):65–66.
Trofatter KF. Immune responses and aging. Clin Obstet Gynecol 1986 June; 29(2):384–396.

Food Allergy

Boyles JH Jr. Food allergy: Diagnosis and treatment. Otolaryngol Clin North Am 1985 Nov; 18(4):775–785.
Corman LC. The relationship between nutrition, infection, and immunity. Med Clin North Am 1985 May; 69(3):519–529.
Panush RS and Webster EM. Food allergies and other adverse reactions to food. Med Clin North Am 1985 May; 69(3):533–542.
Podell RN. Is migraine a manifestation of food allergy? Postgrad Med 1984 Mar; 75(4):221–225.
Schultz CM. Sulfite sensitivity. Am J Nurs 1986 Aug; 86(8):914.

Anaphylactic Reaction

Cohen GA and Hamburger RN. Anaphylaxis: When time is of the essence. Mod Med 1985 Mar; 53(3):117.
Horrow JC. Systemic anaphylactic reactions. Med Times 1984 Mar; 112(3): 29–35.

Agencies

American Academy of Allergy and Immunology (AAAI), 611 East Wells, Milwaukee, WI 53202.
Asthma and Allergy Foundation of America, 9604 Wisconsin Avenue, Bethesda, MD 20814.
National Institutes of Allergy and Infectious Diseases (NAID), National Institute of Health, Bethesda, MD 20892.

Chapter 47

Management of Patients With Rheumatic Disorders

The Arthritis Foundation classifies more than 100 different types of rheumatic disorders. Simply stated, a *rheumatic disease* is a widespread disorder, primarily affecting skeletal muscles, bones, and joints. Many rheumatic diseases are subclassified as diffuse connective tissue diseases (rheumatoid arthritis, systemic lupus erythematosus, progressive systemic sclerosis) because they share a common pathology, involving disruption of the protein components and collagen portion of the connective tissue. Most rheumatic diseases are chronic in nature and are characterized by joint inflammation (arthritis) or degenerative joint changes. The disease onset may be acute or insidious, and the course is usually marked by remissions and exacerbations. Common abbreviations for rheumatic diseases can be found in Chart 47-1.

Physiologic Overview

Because the rheumatic disorders presented here are primarily connective tissue diseases, the physiologic overview will be specific to connective tissue. Connective tissue is distributed throughout the body in three forms: loose connective tissue, hematopoietic tissue, and strong supporting connective tissue. *Loose connective tissue* is divided into three major types: *collagen,* the most abundant type, consists of proteins clustered in bundles to increase strength; *elastin,* fibers whose elastic properties allow tissues to stretch; and *reticulin,* delicate networks of fibers that support capillaries, nerve fibers, and the smallest units of organs. *Hematopoietic tissue* includes the bone marrow, blood cells, and lymphatic tissue. *Strong supporting connective tissue* is the main component of cartilage, bone, tendons, ligaments, and serous organ coverings. The function of connective tissue is to provide mechanical support, warmth, structure, and movement.

Assessment

Management of rheumatic diseases begins with a complete and accurate assessment of the patient's signs and symptoms.

Chart 47-1
Common Abbreviations for
Rheumatic Diseases

Rheumatic Disease	Abbreviation
Connective tissue disease	CTD
Rheumatoid arthritis	RA
Systemic lupus erythematosus	SLE
Degenerative joint disease	DJD
Progressive systemic sclerosis	PSS

The patient history is the most valuable diagnostic aid to the physical assessment. In instances of suspected connective tissue disease, it is particularly important to elicit information about the patient's pain. Pain is the symptom that most commonly causes a person to seek medical attention. Other common symptoms include joint swelling, limited movement, stiffness, weakness, and fatigue.

Inspection of the patient's general appearance occurs during initial contact. Gait, posture, and general musculoskeletal size and structure are observed. Gross deformities and abnormalities in movement are noted. Deviations away from the body midline are called *varus* deformities (*e.g.*, bow legs); deviations toward the midline are called *valgus* deformities (*e.g.*, knock knees). The symmetry, size, and contour of other connective tissues, such as the skin and adipose tissue, are also noted and recorded.

Because connective tissue is found in nearly all body systems, a complete physical assessment is performed. Special attention is given to the examination of each joint and its adjacent structures. The procedure for musculoskeletal assessment is found in the discussion of rheumatoid arthritis (see p. 1220).

Diagnostic Evaluation

In addition to the history and physical assessment, a battery of diagnostic studies is used to confirm or support a tentative diagnosis.

X-rays are important in evaluating patients with musculoskeletal conditions. Bone films determine bone density, texture, erosion, and changes in bone relationships. X-rays of the bone cortex detect widening, narrowing, and signs of irregularity. Joint x-rays reveal the presence of fluid excess, irregularity, bony overgrowth, narrowing, and changes in the joint structure.

Arthrography is another diagnostic tool used to detect connective tissue disorders. A radiopaque substance or air is injected into the joint cavity, especially of the knee or shoulder, in order to outline the contour of the joint. This procedure usually takes 30 to 45 minutes. The joint is put through passive range of motion while a series of x-rays is taken. After the test, the patient is reassured that the radiopaque substance will be absorbed systemically and joint swelling will consequently subside. No special post-test precautions are neces-

sary, but the patient is observed for signs of infection and hemarthrosis (bleeding into the joint).

An *arthrocentesis* is performed to obtain a sample of synovial fluid, especially from the knee or shoulder. The joint is anesthetized locally, and a large-bore needle is inserted into the joint space to aspirate a fluid specimen. Since this procedure has the potential for introducing bacteria into the joint, aseptic technique must be followed. Following aspiration, no special precautions are necesary, but the patient is observed for signs of infection and hemarthrosis.

Normally, synovial fluid is clear, viscous, straw-colored, and scanty in volume with few cells. The fluid is examined for volume, viscosity, glucose value, white blood cells, and its ability to form a mucin clot. It is examined microscopically for cell count, cell identification, Gram's stain, and formed elements. In inflammatory joint disease, the fluid often becomes cloudy, milky, or dark yellow and contains numerous inflammatory cells, such as leukocytes (white blood cells) and complement, a plasma protein associated with immunologic reactions. The viscosity is reduced in inflammatory disease, and copious amounts of fluid may be present. Blood in the fluid specimen suggests trauma or a tendency to bleed.

Arthroscopy is an endoscopic procedure that allows direct visualization of a joint, especially the knee (see Chap. 55). Although it is performed primarily to detect trauma or lesions, it may be used to obtain a biopsy of synovial tissue for microscopic examination. A synovial biopsy may also be obtained by needle or surgical incision.

Myelography is performed to confirm a diagnosis of degenerative joint disease of the spinal column. A radiopaque substance, air, or metrizamide (Amipaque), a new water-soluble material, is injected into the subarachnoid space of the lumbar or cervical spine.

A *bone scan* reflects the degree to which the crystal lattice of bone "takes up" a bone-seeking radioactive isotope that is injected into the system, such as technetium-99. The degree of uptake of isotope is evaluated. An area of increased uptake is considered abnormal and possibly related to connective tissue disease.

A *joint scan* procedure is similar to that of the bone scan and allows determination of joint damage throughout the body. It is the most sensitive study for the detection of early disease.

Electromyography and muscle biopsy may be performed when skeletal muscle is directly affected by connective tissue disease, to determine the presence of muscle inflammation or degeneration. In *electromyography,* an electrode is placed into a muscle and electrical activity is measured. A *muscle biopsy* is carried out for microscopic examination of skeletal muscle. The procedure may be performed in the operating room under local or general anesthesia. A surgical incision is made, and the desired specimen is obtained. A pressure dressing is applied, and the affected extremity is immobilized for 12 to 24 hours. A less invasive type of biopsy, the needle biopsy, may be chosen as an alternative to the incisional procedure.

Arterial biopsy is carried out to examine a specimen of an arterial vessel wall. Most frequently, the temporal artery is selected, but other arteries may be biopsied as indicated. The procedure is similar to that for the incisional muscle biopsy, but is generally performed under local anesthesia in the operating room. Arterial biopsy most often confirms inflammation of the vessel wall, or *arteritis*, a type of vasculitis.

A *skin biopsy* may be performed to confirm inflammatory connective tissue diseases, such as lupus erythematosus or progressive systemic sclerosis (scleroderma). A specimen may be lightly scraped from the patient's skin without discomfort. Deeper skin biopsies may need to be carried out when scraping is not sufficient.

Thermography measures the degree of heat radiating from the skin surface. It is used to investigate the pathophysiology of inflamed joints and to assess the patient's response to anti-inflammatory drug therapy.

In general, *serum laboratory studies* in rheumatology rely on the theory that most connective tissue diseases are autoimmune. While many of the tests are highly complex and technical, no one test *sufficiently* supports a diagnosis of CTD. In Table 47-1, some of the most common serum studies are listed with corresponding normal value ranges and primary indications. Because many of the tests are relatively new and rather costly, they may not be used in every health care facility.

TABLE 47-1
Common Serum Laboratory Diagnostic Studies for Rheumatic Diseases

Description	Normal Value	Nursing Significance
Antinuclear Antibody (ANA)		
Measures the presence of antibodies that react with a variety of nuclear antigens	Negative	Positive test (titer 1:10–1:30) is associated with SLE, RA, PSS, Raynaud's disease, Sjögren's syndrome, necrotizing arteritis.
If antibodies are present, further testing determines the type of ANA circulating in the blood (anti-DNA, anti-DNP).	A small number of healthy adults have a positive ANA.	The higher the titer, the greater the degree of inflammation.
C₄ Complement Component		
Complement is a protein substance that binds with antigen–antibody complexes for the purpose of lysis. When the number of complexes increases markedly, complement is used for lysis, thus depleting the amount available in the blood.	*Men* 12–72 mg/dl *Women* 13–75 mg/dl	Decrease may be seen in RA and SLE. Decrease indicates autoimmune and inflammatory activity.
C-Reactive Protein Test (CRP)		
Shows presence of abnormal glycoprotein due to inflammatory process	Trace 6 μg/ml	A positive reading indicates active inflammation. Positive for RA, disseminated lupus erythematosus
Erythrocyte Sedimentation Rate (ESR)		
Measures the rate at which RBCs settle out of unclotted blood in 1 hour	Westergren = *Men* 0–15 mm/hr, *Women* 0–20 mm/hr. Wintrobe = *Men* 0–9 mm/hr, *Women* 0–15 mm/hr	Increase often seen in any inflammatory CTD. An increase indicates increased inflammation, resulting in clustering of RBCs which make them heavier than normal. The higher the sedimentation rate, the greater the inflammatory activity.
HLA-B27 Antigen		
Measures presence of HLA antigens, which are used for tissue recognition	Negative	Found in 80–90% of those with ankylosing spondylitis and Reiter's syndrome
Immunoglobulin Electrophoresis		
Measures the values of immunoglobulins	IgA 85–385 mg/dl IgG 565–1700 mg/dl IgM 55–370 mg/dl	Increased levels are found in people who have autoimmune disorders.

(continued)

TABLE 47-1 (continued)

Description	Normal Value	Nursing Significance
LE prep (LE test)		
Essentially, a type of ANA (anti-DNP)	Negative	Positive in 75–80% of patients with SLE
Should be repeated on 3 consecutive days		Positive results may also be associated with RA and PSS.
Red Blood Cell Count (RBC)		
Measures the number of circulating erythrocytes	*Men:* Average 4.8 million/cu mm.	Decreased in RA, LE
	Women: Average 4.3 million/cu mm.	
Rheumatoid Factor (RF)		
Determines the presence of abnormal antibodies seen in CTD	Negative	Positive titer > 1:80
		Present in 80% of those with rheumatoid arthritis
		Positive RF may also suggest SLE, Sjögren's syndrome, or mixed CTD. The higher the titer (number at right of colon), the greater the degree of inflammation.

Rheumatoid Arthritis

Rheumatoid arthritis (RA) is a chronic, systemic, progressively deteriorating connective tissue disease characterized by inflammation of the synovial membrane of the joints, immobility, and pain, as well as a generalized feeling of fatigue. Exacerbations of this disease are frequently associated with periods of increased physical or emotional stress. Rheumatoid arthritis is commonly referred to as an "immune complex disease." It is estimated that 1 in every 100 persons throughout the world has the disease, which indicates a 1% incidence rate. According to the National Center for Health Statistics, women have 2 to 3 times the incidence rate of men, with no significant racial difference noted between whites and blacks in the United States. With increasing age, the incidence rate for women and men tends to equalize. Research data continue to support the manifestation of symptoms in the second to third decade of life, with peak incidence occurring in the fourth and fifth decades.

The etiology still remains a mystery. Rheumatoid arthritis is believed to be an immune response to an unknown antigen of internal or external origin. It occurs in people with a genetic predisposition to the disease. The stimulus for the immune response may be viral (Epstein-Barr) or bacterial, or related to an alteration in the normal production and function of collagen or immunoglobulin. Immunoglobulin is an antibody that generally neutralizes toxic antigens, which are then destroyed and removed by phagocytosis. The altered immune response leads to an inflammatory response localized in the joints that is characteristic of rheumatoid arthritis. Recent research has identified two possible risk factors: a deficiency of α-1-antitrypsin or the presence of human leukocyte-associated histocompatibility antigen (HLA-DwR).

Pathophysiology

To understand the pathophysiology of rheumatoid arthritis, the normal anatomy and physiology of joints are reviewed. A *joint,* an area where two or more bones meet, is primarily comprised of connective tissue. Joints are of three main types: (1) synarthrodial, or immovable (*e.g.,* the joints between the cranial bones); (2) amphiarthrodial, or slightly movable (*e.g.,* the joints between the vertebrae); and (3) diarthrodial, or freely movable (*e.g.,* the knee joint). The *diarthrodial* or *synovial* joint is most commonly affected by inflammation and degeneration as seen in rheumatoid arthritis.

Synovial joints are classified further according to the shapes of the bone surfaces that meet. The *ball and socket* type, or spheroidal joint, best exemplified by the hip and shoulder, permits full freedom of movement. *Hinge* joints, such as the elbow, permit motion in one plane, flexion, and extension. A *condylar* joint, such as the knee, is similar to the hinge but additionally allows a small degree of rotation. The carpal (wrist) joints are examples of the *plane,* or biaxial joints, and permit only gliding movement. The *pivot* joint is characterized by the articulation between the radius and ulna in the forearm; it permits rotation only.

Articular cartilage covers the bone end of a joint and provides a smooth, resilient surface for movement. Because the cartilage has no vascular supply, it cannot regenerate. Once the cartilage is damaged, it cannot be repaired.

The space between the bone ends is maintained by a

sheath of fibrous tissue, the *joint capsule*. The joint capsule is strengthened by bands of connective tissue, or *ligaments*, which help to keep the bones in proper relationship to each other. Ligaments are located both along the outside of the joint capsule and also within the capsule, where they bridge the gap between the bones. *Synovial membrane* lines the inner surface of the fibrous capsule and secretes fluid into the space between the bones. This *synovial fluid* functions as a shock absorber and a lubricant, to allow the joint to move freely in the appropriate direction.

The pathologic changes of rheumatoid arthritis are first seen in the synovial tissue, where the immune response tends to localize. The antigen stimulus activates monocytes and T-lymphocytes. The immunoglobulin antibodies form immune complexes with other antibodies or antigens. Phagocytosis of the immune complexes is initiated, which generates an inflammatory reaction (joint swelling, pain, and edema). Phagocytic cells produce enzymes that create more destruction, hyperemia, edema, swelling, and thickening of the synovial lining. Granulation tissue covers the articular cartilage, causing the formation of collagen and the change to fibrous scar tissue (*pannus*). As the process spreads, the joint is destroyed as the articular cartilage becomes eroded, exposing

the bone in the joint (Fig. 47-1). Destruction of the joint produces *ankylosis* (immobility and consolidation of the joint) and deformity. The muscles are affected as the muscle fibers undergo degenerative changes with loss of muscle elasticity and contractile power.

Clinical Manifestations

The clinical picture of rheumatoid arthritis is variable, but may generally be determined by the stage and severity of the disease process. Joint swelling that is soft or spongy to the touch is a *classic clinical feature* of rheumatoid arthritis. Joint swelling may be due to fluid accumulation or hypertrophied synovium; swelling due to bony overgrowth tends to be associated with osteoarthritis. A severely swollen joint, particularly in the hand, appears taut and shiny, causing the normal ''wrinkles'' of the skin to disappear. Swelling may occur in areas around the joint in the form of generalized edema or nodules.

Redness, a sign of joint inflammation, often begins in the fingers, particularly involving the proximal interphalangeal joints (PIPs) and the metacarpophalangeal joints (MCPs), bilaterally and symmetrically (Fig. 47-2). Additional joints such

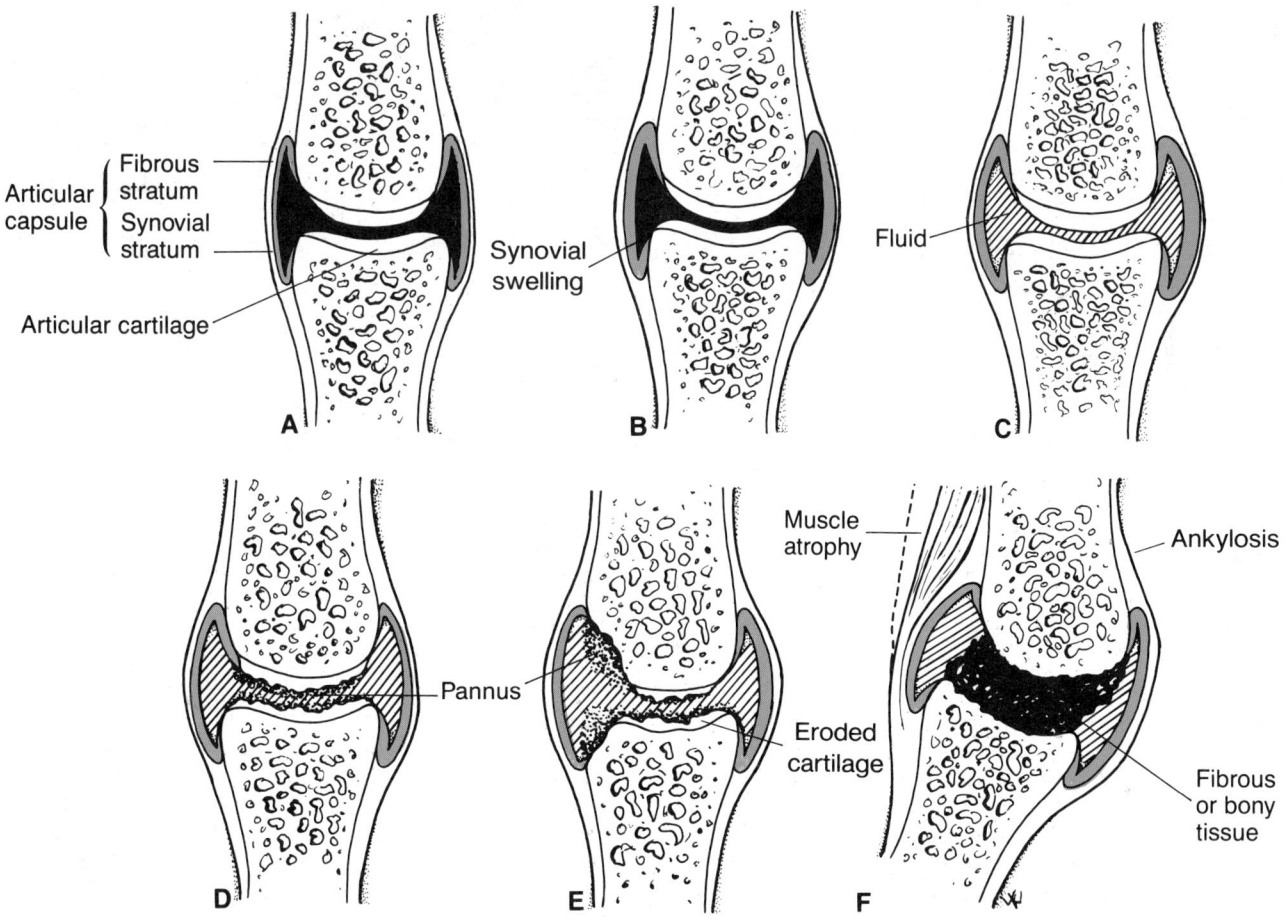

Figure 47-1
Pathophysiology of rheumatoid arthritis. (*A*) Normal. (*B*) Synovial swelling. (*C*) Fluid collects in joint. (*D*) Pannus. (*E*) Eroded articular cartilage. (*F*) Ankylosis and muscle atrophy.

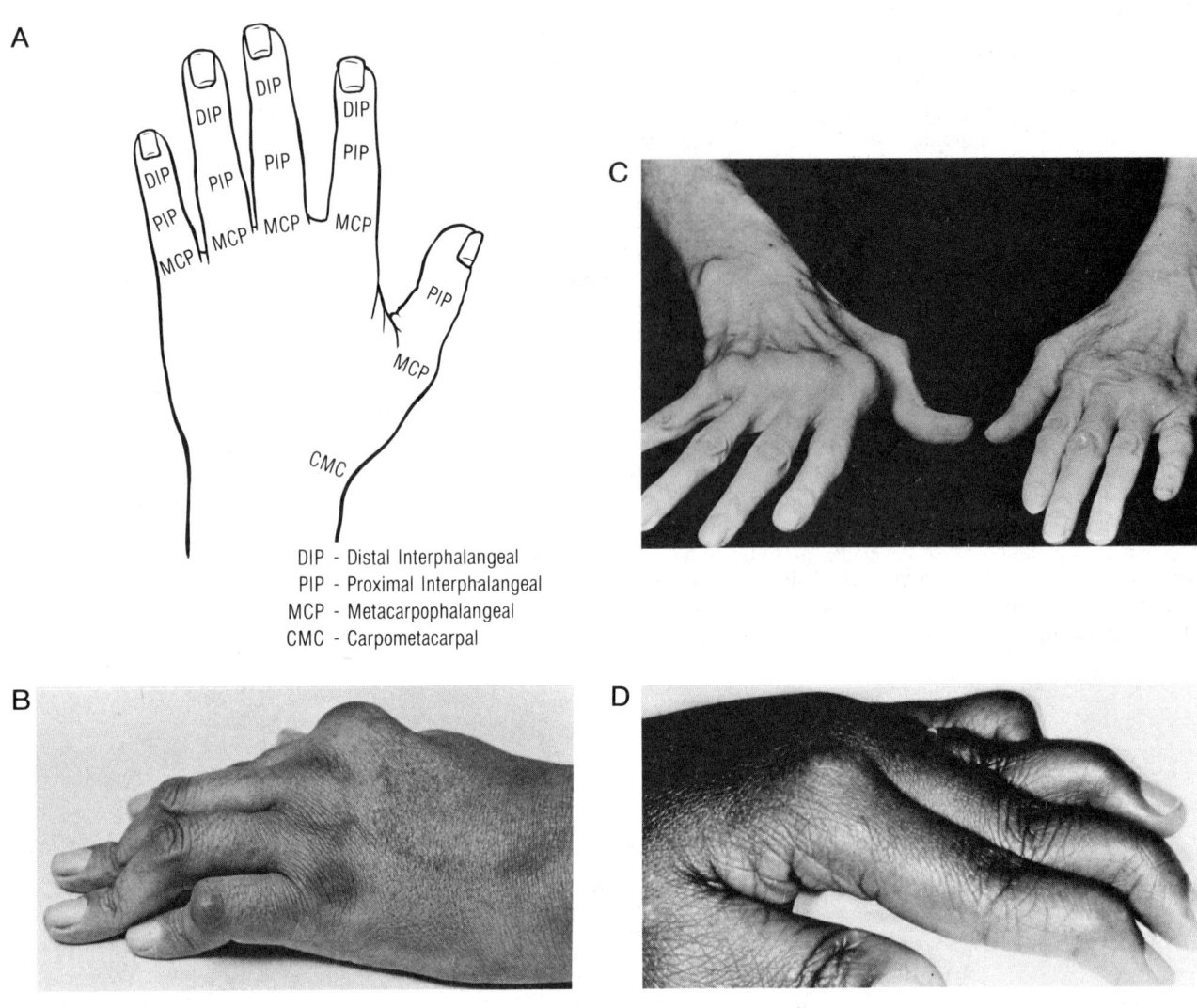

Figure 47-2
Rheumatoid arthritis of the hand. (*A*) Common reference points. (*B*) Boutonnière deformity, characterized by flexion of the proximal interphalangeal joint, hyperextension of the distal interphalangeal joint, and inability to straighten the joint. (*C*) Swelling and atrophy of the metacarpophalangeal joints in both hands. Ulnar deviation and subluxation of the metacarpophalangeal joints occur (as seen in right hand). (*D*) Swan neck deformity, in which the proximal interphalangeal (middle) joint is hyperextended and the distal interphalangeal joint is in flexion. (Reprinted from the Arthritis Teaching Slide Collection, © 1980. Used by permission of the Arthritis Foundation.)

as the wrists, elbows, shoulders, knees, and hips soon become involved, and mobility is impaired.

Fixed deformities of the hands and feet are common in rheumatoid arthritis (Fig. 47-2). In severe cases, the temporomandibular joints (jaws) and spinal column may also be involved. *Ulnar drift* occurs when the fingers point to the ulna (inner bone of the forearm, on the side opposite that of the thumb). *Swan-neck deformity* occurs when the PIP joints hyperextend, and *Boutonnière's deformity* occurs when the PIP joints develop flexion deformities. In approximately 25% of patients, rheumatoid nodules are present. When occurring in the subcutaneous tissue adjacent to joints, these nodules are movable and "spongy." They may also occur in major organs, particularly the heart and lungs.

Because rheumatoid arthritis is a systemic disease, patients frequently show evidence of fatigue, morning stiffness, weight loss related to anorexia, and a low-grade fever. A decreased red blood cell count occurs with anemia, and an elevated white blood cell count is seen with inflammation. In the later stages of rheumatoid arthritis, patients may develop Sjögren's syndrome, which is characterized by *leukopenia* (low white cell count), neuropathy, and decreased salivary and lacrimal gland secretions.

Gerontological Considerations

In the elderly, males and females have the same incidence of rheumatoid arthritis. About 25% of the elderly will experience a sudden onset of the severe form, but it is usually managed conservatively. Interpretation of a positive rheumatoid factor is viewed cautiously because the elderly tend to have an increased number of positive tests even in the absence of the disease.

Symptoms suggestive of the rheumatoid disease process are carefully evaluated in the elderly. A false positive diagnosis may be made if the normal musculoskeletal degenerative processes associated with aging are incorrectly viewed as indicators of rheumatoid arthritis. For example, diminished muscle strength may result from disuse; structural joint changes may result from bone demineralization (*osteoporosis*) or osteoarthritis, and/or overall restricted joint mobility may be related to compromised range of motion subsequent to aging rather than to actual joint pathology. There is evidence that the prognosis for rheumatoid arthritis is the same in the elderly as in the younger population.

Diagnostic Evaluation

Physical examination reveals information about the size, symmetry, and movement of involved joints. The presence of Bouchard's nodes (p. 1232) can be noted. Joint inflammation is detected on palpation.

Radiographic examination of involved joints shows atrophic, frayed, or degraded cartilage. Joint debris may also be present.

An arthroscopic examination is a popular diagnostic tool that allows for visualization of the synovium, cartilage, menisci, and ligaments. Rheumatoid arthritis is associated with synovial villi (slender projections of the synovial membrane) that appear swollen, thick, and pale. Cartilage destruction with fibrous scar formation (pannus) can also be seen.

An arthrocentesis shows synovial fluid that is cloudy, milky, or dark yellow and contains numerous inflammatory cells, such as leukocytes and complement.

Certain serum laboratory studies are significant. Rheumatoid factor (RF) is present in more than 80% of patients with rheumatoid arthritis. The erythrocyte sedimentation rate (ESR) is significantly elevated with rheumatoid arthritis. The red blood count and C_4 complement component are decreased. The C-reactive protein (CRP) and antinuclear antibody (ANA) tests are positive.

Management

The major goal for medical management is suppression of the autoimmune inflammatory process. For *early, mild* rheumatoid arthritis, most physicians prescribe application of heat or cold and recommend therapuetic exercises spaced with periods of rest.

The salicylates (aspirin) are used initially in full therapeutic dosages for their analgesic, anti-inflammatory, and antipyretic action. Salicylates reach their peak level in the blood approximately 2 hours after oral ingestion and then gradually decline. For the drug to be most effective, the patient takes aspirin every 3 to 4 hours, first on awakening and then regularly throughout the day. The serum salicylate level is kept at 20 to 30 mg/dl, which usually requires 12 to 20 tablets daily.

If aspirin is not successful in relieving pain and inflammation, other anti-inflammatory drugs are used with salicylate therapy. Nonsteroidal anti-inflammatory drugs (NSAIDs) include a large variety of drugs that both decrease inflammation and have an analgesic action. Examples are ibuprofen (Motrin, Advil), naproxen (Naprosyn), indomethacin (Indocin), and meclofenamate (Meclomen). NSAIDs and aspirin have similar toxic effects.

Additional analgesia may be prescribed for periods of extreme pain. Care should be taken to avoid narcotic analgesics, as the patient may become drug dependent due to the chronic need for pain relief.

Reconstructive surgery is indicated when pain cannot be relieved by conservative measures. Surgical procedures include *synovectomy* (excision of the synovial membrane), *tenorrhaphy* (suturing of a tendon), *arthrodesis* (surgical fusion of the joint), and *arthroplasty* (surgical repair of the joint). *Plasmapheresis, lymphopheresis,* and total *lymphoid irradiation* are new, controversial procedures that are limited to extreme cases where conventional therapy has failed.

Table 47-2 summarizes the drugs used in the treatment of rheumatoid arthritis. By decreasing inflammation and pain, these drugs can help relieve discomfort. It is important that the nurse, in either a hospital or a home care setting, be familiar with the side-effects and potential toxicity of these drugs. Patients who take three or more anti-inflammatory drugs concurrently should receive additional monitoring. All patients on drug therapy should be thoroughly instructed regarding drug type, purpose, dosage, side-effects, and toxic effects.

For *moderate, erosive* rheumatoid arthritis, supportive (orthotic) devices are usually prescribed along with a program of occupational and physical therapy. Acupuncture and hypnosis are also effective for some patients. Hydroxychloroquine sulfate (Plaquenil) is usually prescribed in doses of 200 mg daily. The therapeutic effectiveness of Plaquenil is determined 6 to 12 months after beginning therapy. When Plaquenil is used, retinal examinations are scheduled every 6 months because irreversible retinal damage has been seen with prolonged therapy. If therapy with Plaquenil is ineffective, then intramuscular gold therapy is usually initiated. The patient should be advised of possible dermatologic, hematologic, and renal complications resulting from gold therapy.

Penicillamine (Cuprimine), an oral chelating agent, may be used as an alternative to gold therapy. Its anti-inflammatory action is not understood, but it has been useful in suppressing the progress of rheumatoid arthritis in some patients. Its adverse effects are similar to those of gold.

For *active, erosive* rheumatoid arthritis, glucocorticoids and reconstructive surgery are usually prescribed.

Systemic therapy with one of the corticosteroids (such as prednisone [Orasone]) does not alter the course of rheumatoid arthritis, but reduces inflammation and pain and suppresses the production of lymphocytes (part of the immune system). Corticosteroids are used when the patient has a rapid downhill course or when extra-articular (outside the joints) manifestations occur. As a systemic disease, rheumatoid arthritis can affect not only the joints but also other body tissues as in Sjögren's syndrome and vasculitis. Corticosteroid therapy has undesirable side-effects, including sodium and water retention, potassium depletion, hypertension, hyperglycemia, menstrual irregularities, and other features of the Cushing syndrome, as well as cataracts, osteoporosis, psychosis, and psychological dependency.

(Text continues on p. 1227)

TABLE 47-2
Drugs Used in Rheumatic Diseases

Drug	Action, Use, and Indications	Nursing Implications and Assessment for Drug Intolerance
Salicylates		
Aspirin (may be buffered or enteric-coated)	Has anti-inflammatory, antipyretic, and analgesic effects. Long-term therapy requires 10–16 tablets/day to achieve optimum anti-inflammatory effects. Aspirin is the cornerstone of treatment, especially in early phase of diseases such as rheumatoid arthritis. Optimum dosage (4–6 grams/day) will produce blood salicylate levels of 20–30 mg/dl. Can be used in combination with other analgesics and anti-inflammatory agents.	Take salicylates with antacid or milk to protect against gastric irritation. Watch for complaints of tinnitus, gastric intolerance, or GI bleeding and purpuric tendencies.
Nonsteroidal Anti-inflammatory Agents		
Ibuprofen (Motrin, Advil)	Anti-inflammatory action, particularly in joints Effective for rheumatoid and osteoarthritis	Gastrointestinal irritation and hemorrhagic erosions, but less frequently than aspirin Used in patients who cannot tolerate or who do not respond to aspirin Administer with milk or food.
Fenoprofen (Nalfon)	Mechanism of action may be related to inhibition of prostaglandin synthetase (prostaglandins have role in inflammatory process, pain, and fever). It reduces platelet aggregation and increases bleeding time.	Variation among patients in response to drug. Side-effects include dizziness, tachycardia, blurred vision, hematuria, and leukopenia.
Salsalate (Disalcid)	Has an anti-inflammatory effect by selectively inhibiting prostaglandin synthesis	Low potential for serious gastric side-effects. Can be safely given to aspirin-sensitive persons.
Mefanamic acid (Ponstel)	Anti-inflammatory, analgesic, and antipyretic that inhibits prostaglandin synthesis	Give with milk or food. Be alert to drowsiness, bowel inflammation, leukopenia. Stop drug and alert physician if they develop.
Naproxen (Naprosyn)	Longer half-life, which permits less frequent administration	Dosage individualized for each patient
Tolmetin (Tolectin)	Anti-inflammatory, analgesic, and antipyretic properties. It lowers plasma levels of prostaglandin E.	Therapeutic response can usually be seen within a week. Used for acute flare-ups and long-term management
Sulindac (Clinoril)	Anti-inflammatory, analgesic, antipyretic properties	Peptic ulceration and gastrointestinal bleeding are common side-effects. Retinal damage can occur with long-term use.
Meclofenamate sodium (Meclomen)	Anti-inflammatory and analgesic action	Not recommended as initial drug because of gastrointestinal side-effects. Administer with meals or milk. Diarrhea can be severe.
Other Anti-inflammatory Agents		
Indomethacin (Indocin)	Used for short-term treatment of active synovitis	Can produce significant side-effects: gastrointestinal effects, CNS effects
Phenylbutazone (Butazolidin)	Nonsteroidal antirheumatic agents for adjunctive treatment of rheumatoid arthritis	Observe for untoward effects.

(continued)

TABLE 47-2 (continued)

Drug	Action, Use, and Indications	Nursing Implications and Assessment for Drug Intolerance
Other Anti-inflammatory Agents		
Oxyphenbutazone (Tandearil)	Exerts analgesic, antipyretic, anti-inflammatory action Sometimes remarkably effective in control of articular symptoms Patient should be under close medical supervision. Can cause salt and water retention Usually used only for short periods	Gastrointestinal: Nausea, vomiting, epigastric distress, precipitation and reactivation of peptic ulcer *Hematologic:* Bone marrow depression, anemia, leukopenia, agranulocytosis, thrombocytopenia purpura *Irreversible blood element depression may occur rapidly despite careful supervision and frequent testing.*
Antimalarial Compounds		
Hydroxychlorquine sulfate (Plaquenil)	No rational basis for the comparative success of this drug has been established at this time. Used primarily in discoid lupus and rheumatoid arthritis Takes 3–6 months to achieve therapeutic blood levels.	Useful for severe and destructive forms of arthritis Stress that patient should have regular ophthalmologic examination every 4–6 months; *drug has potential adverse retinal effects.* Toxic effects: Headache, dizziness, GI complaints, ocular toxicity, retinopathy, and hepatotoxicity
Chloroquine phosphate (Aralen)	Believed to suppress antigen formation required for hypersensitivity reactions	Response usually takes 2 months.
Antirheumatic Agents		
Gold sodium thiomalate (Myochrysine) (water-based)	Gold salts may be used when rheumatoid activity is not controlled by nonsteroidal therapy. Primarily a remission-inducing drug that is used before penicillamine and after the antimalarial agents	Administered along with nonsteroidal anti-inflammatory agents until benefits from gold therapy are achieved The most common side-effects are dermatitis and stomatitis.
Aurothioglucose (Solganal) (oil-based)	Gold therapy is cumulative with slow onset of beneficial effects	Question patient at each visit concerning pruritus, rash, sores in mouth, metallic taste.
Auranofin (Ridaura)	Mechanism of action unknown; exerts an inflammatory-suppressive effect, *given orally* Can produce a long-sustained remission when treatment continued indefinitely Induces remission; 8–14 weeks may pass before benefit is noted Gradual decrease in administration intervals from weekly through monthly	Diarrhea is the major toxic side-effect. Be alert for hematologic reactions and proteinuria.
Penicillamine	Mechanism unknown	Benefits are not seen for 2 months. Be alert for serious complications of nephrotic syndrome and glomerulonephritis. Bone marrow suppression may occur. Patient should have monthly CBC, platelet count, and urinalysis. Patient should report any sore throat or fever.

(continued)

TABLE 47-2 (continued)

Drug	Action, Use, and Indications	Nursing Implications and Assessment for Drug Intolerance
Corticosteroids		
Prednisone (Deltasone) Prednisolone (Delta-Cortef) Hydrocortisone (Cortef)	Corticosteroids used in treatment of incapacitating active rheumatoid arthritis, systemic lupus erythematosus, progressive systemic sclerosis, necrotizing arteritis Use of corticosteroids for long periods has wide range of adverse effects. Steroids are used with caution and are tapered to minimal maintenance dose if possible.	Toxic effects: Osteoporosis, fractures, avascular necrosis Gastric ulcers, psychiatric problems, infection susceptibility Hirsutism, acne, moon facies, abnormal fat deposition, edema, emotional disorders, menstrual disorders Hyperglycemia, hypokalemia Hypertension Cataracts and glaucoma
Corticosteroids Intra-articular Injections	Given when arthritic reaction has been suppressed and one or two joints are not responding to treatment Given when only one or two joints are affected Given to patient with extremely painful joints so he can undergo physical therapy Relieves pain. Benefit may last from weeks to months.	An inflamed joint may respond to local injection when it has failed to come under control through other general systemic measures. Joints most amenable to corticosteroid injections are ankles, knees, hips, shoulders, and hands.
Immunosuppressive Agents		
Azathioprine (Imuran)	Used in advanced rheumatoid arthritis or systemic lupus erythematosus that is unresponsive to conventional therapy These drugs have teratogenic potential. Action is believed to result from drug's cytotoxic effects of inhibiting lymphocytes or macrophages and thus interfering with joint inflammation.	Highly toxic: Bone marrow depression, GI ulcerations Skin rashes, alopecia Bladder toxicity *Reduces patient's resistance to infections* Patient must be monitored with weekly blood evaluation and urinalysis. Advise patient of contraceptive measures.
Uricosuric Agents		
Probenecid (Benemid)	Inhibits renal reabsorption of urates and increases the urinary excretion of uric acid. Prevents tophi formation	Be alert for nausea, rash, and constipation.
Agents Used in Gout		
Allopurinol (Zyloprim)	Interrupts the breakdown of purines before uric acid is formed. Inhibits xanthinoxidase because it blocks uric acid formation.	Side-effects include bone marrow depression, vomiting, and abdominal pain.
Colchicine	Action is unknown. It does not alter serum or urine levels of uric acid. It lowers the deposition of uric acid and interferes with leukocytes and kinin formation, thus reducing inflammation.	Prolonged use may decrease vitamin B_{12} absorption. Causes gastrointestinal upset in the majority of patients Must be given when attack first begins. Dosage is increased until pain is relieved or diarrhea develops.

When the disease does not respond sufficiently to daily administration of oral steroids, high doses of intravenous steroids may be administered as "pulse therapy." This consists of a single dose or a series of daily doses for a specified length of time or until inflammation decreases.

Joints that are severely inflamed and fail to respond promptly to the measures outlined above may be treated by the local injection of a corticosteroid. This maneuver suppresses local inflammation and provides temporary relief from pain and disability.

For *advanced, severe* rheumatoid arthritis, immunosuppressive drugs are prescribed because of their ability to affect the production of antibodies at the cellular level. These include methotrexate (Mexate), cyclophosphamide (Cytoxan), and azathioprine (Imuran). However, these drugs are highly toxic and can produce bone marrow depression, anemia, gastrointestinal disturbances, and skin rashes.

▶ *Nursing Process*
The Patient With Rheumatoid Arthritis

▷ *Assessment*

Data collection begins with an interview and physical examination. During the interview process the nurse assesses the patient's self-image related to musculoskeletal changes and determines if the patient is experiencing unusual fatigue, generalized weakness, morning stiffness, fever, or anorexia. Fatigue and morning stiffness are the *two classic clinical symptoms* seen with rheumatoid arthritis. Morning stiffness lasting longer than 30 minutes after rising and subsiding as activity increases is characteristic of rheumatoid arthritis.

The Arthritis Impact Measurement Scales (AIMS; Chart 47-2) is an outcome assessment instrument that uses a questionnaire format to assess health status. It can be used to help direct questions during data collection.

Physical examination for a patient with rheumatoid arthritis includes assessment of the cardiovascular, pulmonary, and renal systems as well as the musculoskeletal system, because the disease has an inflammatory effect on many body systems. Musculoskeletal assessment is presented here in detail because alterations in this system are an early indicator of rheumatoid disease.

The nurse begins the assessment with the joints of the upper extremities and proceeds to the joints of the trunk and lower extremities. The patient should be comfortable and relaxed during the physical assessment. The nurse initially observes for symmetry of paired joints (shoulders, hands, hips, and knees) and then observes each joint for size, shape, color, and appearance.

After the joint is inspected, it is palpated anteriorly, posteriorly, and laterally for skin temperature, joint swelling, tenderness, and irregularity. A warm, swollen, and tender joint indicates inflammation; a cool joint suggests a decrease in blood supply. Tenderness is associated with joint swelling as nerve endings are compressed by excess fluid, synovium, or bone. Irregularities of the bony surfaces within a joint may produce an audible, grating sound known as *crepitus*. Percussion over the joint may also elicit tenderness or indicate the presence of fluid.

During the palpation process, the nurse checks peripheral pulses, particularly when vascular supply deficits are. suspected. When edema is present, the amount and location are recorded.

Following inspection and palpation, joints are evaluated for their passive range of motion. Range of motion is recorded in approximate degrees of deviation from a defined neutral zero point and from a normal range of motion for each joint.

During the range-of-motion process, the nurse supports each joint. If a joint is severely inflamed or painful, range of motion testing is not done because inflammation and pain will increase.

Skeletal muscle is inspected for contour and size. A bilateral inspection allows comparison of symmetry in size and shape; hypertrophy or atrophy is noted. Disuse atrophy is seen frequently in patients who have joint pain and limited joint movement due to a disease such as rheumatoid arthritis.

Muscle strength is also tested. The patient is asked to perform a number of voluntary tasks—for example, picking up a book. Actual strength measurement may be ascertained by devices such as the grip or pinch manometer. Otherwise, muscle strength may be graded on a 0-to-5 scale, on which 0 represents no muscle strength (paralysis) and 5 indicates normal strength. Other types of grading scales may be used, but the parameters of each are similar.

If impairments of joint and muscle functions are present, an assessment of the patient's mobility is determined. The desired mobility level is one that allows the patient to be independent in activities of daily living (ADLs). The patient is questioned about his ability to feed, dress, bathe, and ambulate. Precise tools are available to provide a numerical index of the patient's ability to perform these tasks.

Some patients may be asked to perform certain tasks while the examiner observes ability level. One such task is the ability to walk 15.24 meters (50 feet) as quickly as possible. The time it takes to walk the prescribed distance is recorded and used as a measure of mobility. This test may be performed at intervals to assess patient progress.

▷ *Nursing Diagnoses*

Based on all the nursing assessment data, major nursing diagnoses for the patient may include the following:

- Alterations in comfort, pain, related to movement of inflamed joints
- Impaired physical mobility related to restricted joint movement
- Self-care deficits (feeding, bathing, dressing, toileting) related to fatigue and joint stiffness
- Disturbance in self-concept related to the physical and psychological dependency seen with chronic illness and a loss of independence
- Alteration in nutrition related to inadequate food intake

▷ *Planning and Implementation*

▷ *Goals:* The major goals of the patient may include relief of pain and discomfort, increased mobility, activity, and exercise tolerance, achievement of an optimal, individual level of independence in activities of daily living, attainment/maintenance of a positive self-concept, and attainment/maintenance of optimal nutrition.

Chart 47-2
Arthritis Impact Measurement Scales (AIMS)*

Mobility

4* Are you in bed or in a chair for most or all of the day because of your health?
3 Are you able to use public transportation?
2 When you travel around your community, does someone have to assist you because of your health?
1 Do you have to stay indoors most or all of the day because of your health?

Physical Activity

5 Are you unable to walk unless you are assisted by another person or by a cane, crutches, artificial limbs, or braces?
4 Do you have any trouble either walking several blocks or climbing a few flights of stairs because of your health?
3 Do you have any trouble either walking several blocks or climbing a few flights of stairs because of your health?
2 Do you have trouble bending, lifting, or stooping because of your health?
1 Does your health limit the kinds of vigorous activities you can do, such as running, lifting heavy objects, or participating in strenuous sports?

Dexterity

5 Can you easily write with a pen or pencil?
4 Can you easily turn a key in a lock?
3 Can you easily button articles of clothing?
2 Can you easily tie a pair of shoes?
1 Can you easily open a jar of food?

Social Role

7 If you had to take medicine, could you take all your own medicine?
6 If you had a telephone, would you be able to use it?
5 Do you handle your own money?
4 If you had a kitchen, could you prepare your own meals?
3 If you had laundry facilities (washer, dryer), could you do your own laundry?
2 If you had the necessary transportation, could you go shopping for groceries or clothes?
1 If you had household tools and appliances (e.g., vacuum, mops), could you do your own housework?

Social Activity

5 About how often have you been on the telephone with close friends or relatives during the past month?
4 Has there been a change in the frequency or quality of your sexual relationships during the past month?
3 During the past month, about how often have you had friends or relatives to your home?
2 During the past month, about how often have you gotten together socially with friends or relatives?
1 During the past month, how often have you visited with friends or relatives at their homes?

Activities of Daily Living

4 How much help do you need to use the toilet?
3 How well are you able to move around?
2 How much help do you need in getting dressed?
1 When you bathe, by sponge bath, tub, or shower, how much help do you need?

Pain

4 During the past month, how often have you had severe pain from your arthritis?
3 During the past month, how would you describe the arthritis pain you usually have?
2 During the past month, how long has your morning stiffness usually lasted from the time you wake up?
1 During the past month, how often have you had pain in two or more joints at the same time?

Depression

6 During the past month, how often have you felt that others would be better off if you were dead?
5 How often during the past month have you felt so down in the dumps that nothing could cheer you up?
4 How much of the time during the past month have you felt downhearted and blue?
3 How often during the past month have you felt that nothing has turned out for you the way you wanted it to?
2 During the past month, how much of the time have you been in low or very low spirits?
1 During the past month, how much of the time have you enjoyed the things you do?

Anxiety

6 During the past month, how much of the time have you felt tense or "high-strung"?
5 How much have you been bothered by nervousness and your "nerves" during the past month?
4 How often during the past month have you found yourself having difficulty trying to calm down?
3 How much of the time during the past month have you been able to relax without difficulty?
2 How much of the time during the past month have you felt calm and peaceful?
1 How much of the time during the past month have you felt relaxed and free of tension?

* Higher scores reflect more limitation.
(Meenan RF, Gertman PM and Mason JH. Measuring health status in arthritis: The arthritis impact measurement scales. Arthritis Rheum 1980 23[2]:146–152. Used by permission of the American Rheumatism Association.)

Nursing Interventions

Relieving Pain and Discomfort. Nursing measures to relieve pain include warm and cold applications, promotion of rest, proper positioning, and the use of supportive devices.

Warm and Cold Applications. Heat applications are often helpful in relieving pain, stiffness, inflammation, and muscle spasm. Superficial heat may be supplied in the form of warm tub baths and warm, moist compresses. Paraffin baths (dips) offer concentrated heat and are helpful to patients with wrist and small joint involvement. Therapeutic exercises can be carried out more comfortably and effectively after heat has been applied. However, in some patients, heat may actually increase pain, muscle spasm, and synovial fluid volume. If the inflammatory process is acute, cold applications may be tried in the form of moist packs or an ice bag. Both heat and cold are analgesic to nerve pain receptors and relax muscle spasms.

Rest. Rest also helps to allay pain. Since rheumatoid arthritis is a systemic disease, the whole patient—not merely the joints—must be treated. The amount of rest required is indicated by the amount of inflammatory involvement and the feelings of the patient. When in bed, the patient should lie flat on a firm mattress with only one pillow under the head because of the risk of dorsal kyphosis. (At no time should a pillow be placed under the knees, as this promotes flexion contractures of those joints.)

Frequent periods of bed rest during the day take the weight off the joints and relieve fatigue. If joint inflammation is severe, the patient may be placed on complete bed rest for a brief period. (Range-of-motion exercises should still be carried out.) During bed rest, the patient should lie flat with feet propped against a footboard. All joints should be supported in a position of optimum function.

Positioning and Posture. For the patient in pain, proper body posture is essential to minimize stress on those joints that are inflamed. Proper body posture includes walking erect and sitting in chairs that have straight backs so that the feet can rest flat on the floor and the shoulders and hips can rest against the back of the chair. When in bed, extreme joint flexion is avoided and the knees are not flexed on pillows. The patient lies on the abdomen several times daily to prevent flexion deformities. Passive range-of-motion exercises are encouraged because they prevent joint stiffness.

Assistive and Supportive Devices. If neck pain exists, cervical collars may be used to support the weight of the head and limit cervical motion. For joint pain in the hands, stretch gloves provide a splinting action that presumably reduces joint swelling. A metatarsal bar or special pads may be put into standard shoes if foot pain or deformity is present. Braces and splints can be used to support and immobilize a joint.

If acutely inflamed, the affected joints are rested by applying splints, bivalved casts, or other mechanical devices that will maintain the joints in functional positions. Simple splints provide rest, support the joint in optimal position to relieve pain and spasm, and help prevent deformity. Above all, the joints should not be permitted to "freeze" in positions of flexion, which is their natural tendency because of the predominant strength of flexor muscles. The knee is splinted at full extension, and the wrist at slight dorsiflexion. Splints may need to be modified when changes occur in joint structure.

Holistic Methods. Muscle relaxation techniques decrease inflammatory pain by reducing muscle tension and anxiety. These techniques involve a sequence of muscle contraction and relaxation exercises in association with controlled breathing exercises. Imagery is used to encourage the patient to concentrate on a pleasant scene or experience so that attention is drawn away from the pain experience. Self-hypnosis is a process whereby the state of consciousness is altered so the patient is able to relax and focus on pleasant images to the exclusion of unpleasant events or painful stimuli. Distraction is an easy method of pain control, in which a patient is encouraged to pay attention to events other than the pain experience. Biofeedback is used to help patients develop their ability to control their autonomic nervous system, heart rate, and skin temperature.

Pharmacotherapy. Drug therapy is used to relieve inflammation and pain and arrest the progress of the disease. Nursing responsibilities include assessing the patient's need for medication, preparing and administering the medication, and observing for side-effects (Table 47-2, p. 1244).

Increasing Mobility, Activity, and Exercise Tolerance. Inflammation, scarring, or other structural damage to joint structures results in pain and disability. The patient, in an effort to avoid pain, tends to immobilize the affected joints, and muscular spasm further limits their motion. Muscle atrophy and deformity may occur. This loss can be prevented to a large extent by systematic range-of-motion and specific muscle-strengthening exercises. If activity is painful, the nurse may help the patient perform the required motions. Emphasis is placed on the need to carry out a regular exercise routine on a daily basis in order to increase muscle strength. Exercises are essential in restoring joint mobility and strengthening the muscles that support the joints (Table 47-3).

Improving Self-Care Activities. In order to become independent, the patient must be instructed and supervised by the nurse and others of the rehabilitation team in ADLs. It is important that the nurse work with the patient to achieve the goals of self-care and independence.

The patient with rheumatoid arthritis is allowed to perform as many ADLs as possible, even though additional time might be needed to complete them. Manual assistance from the nurse is given only when absolutely necessary. Often the patient has the greatest difficulty with fine, delicate movements, such as those required for fastening items of clothing

---

TABLE 47-3

Exercise Tolerance Related to Inflammatory Process: Suggested Exercises

Inflammatory Process/Pain	Recommended Exercise	Patient Performance Level
Acute exacerbation	Passive range-of-motion	Unable to perform exercises alone
Subacute; minimal pain	Assistive	Can perform with help from another person or an assistive mechanical device
Inactive; remission; absence of pain	Active	Can do alone

and opening small packages. The nurse should work with occupational or physical therapists to teach the patient how to perform difficult tasks. There are many self-help devices available to assist with dressing, bathing, grooming, and eating when the patient cannot perform these activities alone (Fig. 47-3).

When there is difficulty in ambulation, canes or walkers are prescribed as assistive devices to reduce the amount of weight bearing on the joints of the lower extremities. Well-fitted, supportive shoes should be worn when walking to protect joints and prevent falls. Custom-made corrective shoes are used to prevent further foot deformity and provide support.

When physical mobility is severely impaired and relief of pain by conventional drug therapy fails, reconstructive joint surgery may restore some function and reduce pain. Many patients receive total joint replacements to achieve pain control and increase mobility (see p. 1561).

Promoting a Positive Self-Concept.
Patients with arthritis show the same fundamental psychological responses to their disease as persons with other chronic diseases: fear, anxiety, depression, anger, and loss. The unpredictability and uncertainty of the course of the disease frequently cause the patient to react in an angry, bitter, and hostile manner.

All aspects of the patient's life, including work role, social life, sexual function, and financial status, may be altered. Body image changes may cause social isolation and depression. The resulting strain on the patient and family contributes to the often negative attitude of the patient. Such behavior should not be reciprocated with an equally negative response by the nurse. It is better for the patient to express hostility or depression than to suppress it and to ultimately stop trying to communicate with the health care team. Failure of communication also leads to deterioration of interfamily relationships.

The nurse and the family should try to understand the patient's personality and emotional reactions to the disease. Presenting a realistic but optimistic view by pointing out that only a small percentage of patients become totally disabled can help reassure the patient. At the same time, the favorable outcome must be linked to a faithful adherence to the rehabilitation program that is designed to improve functioning. Social workers, psychiatric liaison nurses, sex counselors, and clergy may serve as valuable resources for reassurance and promotion of a patient's positive self-concept.

Promoting Optimal Nutrition.
Patients with rheumatoid arthritis frequently experience anorexia, weight loss, and anemia. A dietary history is taken on each patient to determine usual eating habits and food preferences. The patient is taught how to select foods to include the daily requirements from the basic four food groups, with emphasis on foods high in vitamins, protein, and iron for tissue building and repair. For the extremely anorexic patient, small, frequent feedings with increased protein supplements may be prescribed.

Care must be taken to prevent obesity. Excess weight causes increased stress on weight-bearing joints, creating further joint damage. If obesity is already present, a weight-reduction diet is prescribed.

Patient Education and Home Health Care.
Patients are usually unfamiliar with their disease process and treatment regimen and need to be able to verbalize their concerns and ask questions. The nurse begins by assessing the patient's knowledge base, interest level, ability to learn, and degree of physical comfort. Information is provided in a quiet and private area at a time when the patient is comfortable and well rested. Teaching sessions should not exceed 30 minutes at one sitting. A family member or support person should be present when home care instructions are given for treatments (compresses, baths), positioning, exercises, and the use of assistive devices. Allow the patient sufficient time to ask questions, handle equipment, and practice as necessary. Provide reinforcement and encouragement as needed.

After the patient's discharge from the hospital, a com-

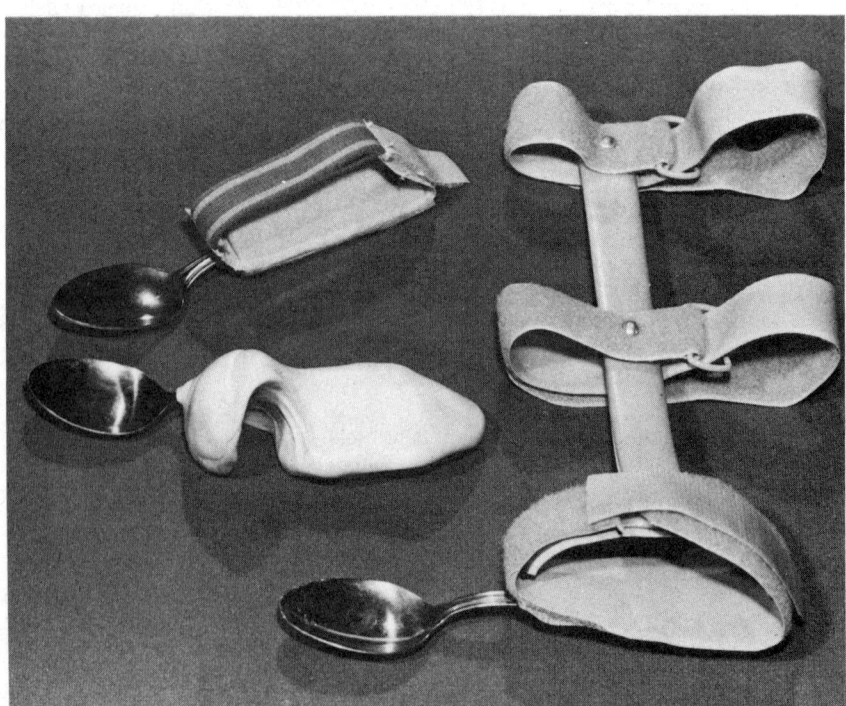

Figure 47-3
Assistive devices to aid in holding eating utensils. (Hopkins HL and Smith HD. Willard and Spackman's Occupational Therapy, 7th ed. Philadelphia, JB Lippincott, 1988.)

munity nurse can visit the home to make sure the patient is able to function as independently as possible with mobility problems and to safely manage treatments and pharmacotherapy. Alert the patient/family to local support services. For example, some regional chapters of the Arthritis Foundation sponsor exercise and swimming programs and will provide an annual allowance toward the purchase of equipment.

▷ *Evaluation*

▷ *Expected Outcomes*

1. Patient experiences relief of pain and discomfort
   a. Identifies measures that decrease the pain experience
   b. Demonstrates improved joint mobility
   c. Uses pharmacotherapy/holistic methods of pain management successfully
2. Demonstrates increased mobility and tolerance of activity and exercise
   a. Demonstrates measures to increase mobility with or without assistive devices
   b. Maintains or increases muscle strength and endurance
   c. Adheres to an individualized program of exercise
3. Achieves an optimal level of independence in activities of daily living
   a. Performs daily tasks of dressing, bathing, grooming, and eating at an optimal level of functioning
   b. Uses safety measures to prevent injury
   c. Uses adaptive devices successfully
4. Attains/maintains a positive self-concept
   a. Expresses feelings freely to family and members of the health team
   b. Socializes appropriately with family members, peers, and friends
   c. Participates in a hobby or diversional activities
   d. Accepts limitations and accomplishments
5. Attains/maintains optimal nutrition
   a. Adheres to a nutrition program that maintains body weight by limiting weight gain or loss to 10% of ideal body weight
   b. Prepares meals on a regular schedule with or without assistance
   c. Seeks assistance for the purchase of food if necessary

Osteoarthritis (Degenerative Joint Disease)

Osteoarthritis, also known as degenerative joint disease (DJD), is the most common type of connective tissue disease in the U.S. and, among Caucasians, affects between 16 and 40 million people. Osteoarthritis refers to a "wear and tear" process in which there is degeneration of articular cartilage with resultant formation of *osteophytes* (irregular bony overgrowths).

Etiology is related to age and joint degeneration. Osteoarthritis begins as early as the second decade of life and peaks between the fifth and sixth decades. By age 70, more than 80% of people have some form of bone degeneration. Osteoarthritis affects women twice as often as men over age 55, whereas the distribution between the sexes appears equal between 40 and 50 years. It is less prevalent in whites than in blacks. Although seen most often in the elderly, the disease may be associated with athletics, obesity, previous trauma, or strenuous physical labor in any age group in which repeated wear and tear can cause joint damage. The degenerative process is associated with mechanical injury or derangement, anatomic damage, or prolonged use of a joint.

Pathophysiology

Cartilage destruction and new bone formation at the edges of the joints are the most common pathologies seen with osteoarthritis. These pathologies are associated with inflammatory and biochemical changes that occur in response to joint insult. The process initiates the degeneration of the matrix of the cartilage. As a joint undergoes repeated mechanical stress, the elasticity of the joint capsule, articular cartilage, and ligaments is reduced. The articular plate is thinned, and its function as a shock absorber is decreased. There is narrowing of the joint space and loss of stability. When the articular plate disappears, bony spurs form at the edges of the joint surfaces and the capsule and synovial membranes thicken. The joint cartilage degenerates and atrophies, the bones harden and hypertrophy at their articular surfaces, and the ligaments calcify. As a result, sterile joint effusions and secondary synovitis may be present, particularly in the knees (Fig. 47-4).

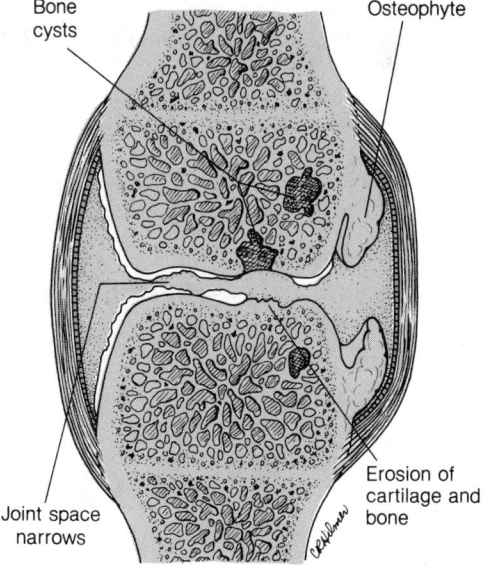

Figure 47-4
Joint changes in osteoarthritis. The left side denotes early changes, joint space narrowing with cartilage breakdown. The right side shows more severe disease progression with lost cartilage and osteophyte formation. (Porth CM. Pathophysiology: Concepts of Altered Health States, 2nd ed. Philadelphia, JB Lippincott, 1986.)

Clinical Manifestations

The primary clinical manifestations are pain, stiffness, and functional impairment. Stiffness, which is most commonly experienced in the morning after awakening, usually lasts less than 30 minutes. Functional impairment is due to limited joint motion, which occurs when structural changes develop in the joints. Joint *crepitus* (crackling sound produced by grating of joint parts) and altered alignment are two other prominent clinical manifestations.

Although osteoarthritis occurs most often in weight-bearing joints (hips and knees), finger joints are frequently involved. Osteoarthritis is seen in the uppermost and middle joints of the fingers (distal interphalangeal joints and the proximal interphalangeals). Characteristic bony nodules may be present which, on inspection, may be painful and inflamed. When present on the distal interphalangeal joints, the nodules are called *Heberden's nodes*. Nodes on the proximal interphalangeals are called *Bouchard's nodes*. Both are bony enlargements that appear in a bilateral and symmetrical pattern (Fig. 47-5).

Gerontological Considerations

Osteoarthritis ranks as the most frequent articular disorder in the elderly; as many as 80% are believed to have some form of osteoarthritis, but 20% of the 80% may be asymptomatic. With the elderly population, emphasis is placed on encouraging those afflicted to maximize their abilities to perform activities of daily living. Inactivity, frequently seen with osteoarthritis, can result in falls and fractures because bone resorption is accentuated with inactivity. The presence of osteoporosis should be determined, because it is a disorder seen with aging that can compound the problems found with osteoarthritis. Because osteoarthritis is so common in the elderly, the symptoms are carefully assessed and evaluated to confirm a wear-and-tear process and rule out other pathology.

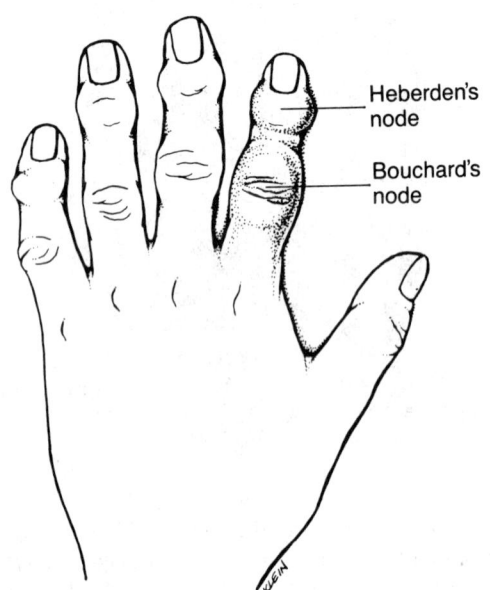

Figure 47-5
Hand deformities commonly seen in osteoarthritis.

Diagnostic Evaluation

A physical examination of the musculoskeletal system will show tenderness and enlargement of the joints. Radiographic examination of degenerating joints demonstrates bony hypertrophy, spur formation, cartilage destruction, and gross irregularities of the joint structures. Serum laboratory diagnostic studies are not useful in the diagnosis of this disorder. Occasionally, local synovitis may cause a slight elevation in the sedimentation rate.

Management

Medical management focuses on treating the symptoms because there is no treatment available that slows the degenerative joint disease process. Therapeutic modalities consist of pharmacotherapy, supportive measures, and surgical intervention when pain is intractable.

The pharmacological regimen centers on analgesics and anti-inflammatory agents. The use of acetaminophen is prescribed in preference to the use of salicylates because effective analgesia can be provided without subjecting the patient to the potential side-effects of aspirin. Nonsteroidal anti-inflammatory agents are usually recommended during inflammatory flare-ups because research has shown NSAIDs to be as effective as aspirin. Intra-articular injections of corticosteroids are used cautiously for an immediate, short-term effect when a joint is acutely inflamed.

Conservative measures include the use of heat, weight reduction, joint rest and avoidance of joint overuse, orthotic devices to support inflamed joints (splints, braces), and isometric and postural exercises. Occupational and physical therapy is encouraged in the elderly. Recently, transcutaneous electrical nerve stimulation has been used, especially for osteoarthritis of the spinal cord. Surgery is recommended when conservative measures are ineffective. Popular surgical modalities include *osteotomy* (transection of the bone), *joint débridement*, *arthrodesis* (fusion), and *arthroplasty* (replacement).

▶ Nursing Process
The Patient With Osteoarthritis

▷ *Assessment*

The nursing history is structured to obtain information about mobility, social activities, and the emotional response to the disorder. The patient's ability to perform activities of daily living adequately is assessed. Because osteoarthritis is specific to the musculoskeletal system, the nurse uses the techniques of inspection, palpation, and joint movement to assess function or impairment. The patient's gait and mobility and any difficulties with ambulation are observed, and muscle spasm and crepitus are noted if present. Joints are palpated for swelling, effusion, enlargement, and the presence of bony nodules. Palpation may elicit tenderness in early degeneration or severe pain in advanced degeneration. Pain which tends to worsen with activity and improve with rest is the most common symptom of osteoarthritis.

Once the joints are inspected and palpated, they are evaluated for range of motion. In severe disease, joint movement is markedly compromised. The vertebral column is assessed because the spine is frequently involved in patients with degenerative disease. Limitations in movement of the cervical and lumbar areas, with an accompanying increase in pain, are indicative of spinal involvement. A detailed discussion of the technique for joint assessment is found in the discussion of rheumatoid arthritis.

▷ Nursing Diagnoses

Based on all the assessment data, major nursing diagnoses for the patient may include the following:

- Alteration in comfort, pain, related to joint degeneration and muscle spasm
- Impaired physical mobility related to limited joint movement
- Self-care deficits related to limited joint movement

▷ Planning and Implementation

▷ *Goals:*   The major goals of the patient may include relief of pain and discomfort, increased physical mobility and endurance, and attainment of an optimal level of independence in activities of daily living.

Nursing Interventions

Relief of Pain and Discomfort.   Measures for relief of pain, stiffness, and muscle spasm are generally the same as those used in rheumatoid arthritis: rest with alternating periods of activity, an exercise program, heat application, splinting, and joint protection. A weight-reduction diet may be required to reduce stress on weight-bearing joints. The nurse explains the purpose for the prescribed regimen and works with the patient in planning the implementation of rest, exercise, diet, and heat therapy. The purpose, action, side-effects, and schedule for taking the prescribed drugs are also part of the teaching program.

Increased Physical Mobility and Endurance, and Independence in Activities of Daily Living.   Nursing interventions for promoting mobility and independence are the same as those employed for patients with rheumatoid arthritis. Although gross deformity is not usually present in DJD, joint pain and muscle spasm decrease joint movement and the ability of patients to care for themselves.

▷ Evaluation

▷ *Expected Outcomes*

1. Patient experiences relief of pain and discomfort
   a. Reduces factors or avoids situations that cause pain
   b. Uses pain management measures successfully
2. Increases mobility and endurance
   a. Reports improved use of affected joints
   b. Performs measures to increase mobility and endurance
3. Achieves an optimal individual level of independence in activities of daily living
   a. Performs daily activities of living at an optimal level of functioning
   b. Uses assistive devices successfully

Lupus Erythematosus

Lupus erythematosus is a chronic, autoimmune collagen vascular disease that may involve multiple body systems (*systemic*) or affect only the skin (*discoid*). About 500,000 people in the U.S. are afflicted with this disease. Women tend to be affected 9:1 over men; the average age at onset is 30 years, with predominance in nonwhites.

The etiology of lupus is unknown. Although a genetic link has not been found, there is a familial association which suggests that a genetic predisposition may be related to environmental factors or susceptibility to certain viruses. Certain drugs, such as hydralazine hydrochloride (Apresoline), procainamide hydrochloride (Pronestyl), and some anticonvulsants, have been thought to trigger the onset of symptoms or aggravate an existing disease. A hormonal abnormality is a possible risk factor because an increased incidence has been noted during the childbearing years. Ultraviolet radiation is also considered a possible risk factor.

Pathophysiology

The pathophysiology is believed to be related to one or several immune system defects that produce inflammation and local tissue damage subsequent to the clustering of antigens and antibodies (immune complexes). A reduction in the number of T-lymphocytes causes the body to synthesize immunoglobulins and autoantibodies, which then form immune complexes that cause tissue damage. Inflammation stimulates antigens, which in turn stimulate additional antibodies, and the cycle continues.

Clinical Manifestations

The onset of systemic lupus erythematosus (SLE) may be insidious or acute. If insidious, as in most cases, the symptoms may be mild and vague. For this reason, the patient with SLE may be undiagnosed for many years. Initially, the patient may experience extreme fatigue, generalized weakness, and anorexia. *Fatigue* has been reported to be the most frustrating symptom.

Weight loss, fever, rash, and signs of joint inflammation alert the physician to the suspected diagnosis of SLE. More than 80% of patients experience fever, fatigue, and weight loss. A characteristic "butterfly" rash appears around the eyes in fewer than half of these patients (Fig. 47-6), but other cutaneous lesions may be present on the trunk or extremities. Typically, the rash either has a diffuse, flat pattern or is a raised, scaly patch.

Other common manifestations include *polymyositis* (skeletal muscle inflammation); *alopecia* (hair loss), which occurs in less than 40% of patients; and *photosensitivity* (sensitivity to sunlight), which is present in one third of the patients. Life-threatening *vasculitis* (vessel wall inflammation) decreases the blood supply to major organs, causing necrosis and dysfunction. Patients experience hepatomegaly, splenomegaly, pericarditis, and pleurisy. Gastrointestinal problems, such as nausea and vomiting, esophagitis, and abdominal pain are common. Pneumonitis, chronic obstructive lung disease, and interstitial fibrosis are typical when lung involvement occurs. Hypertension and peripheral vascular disease result

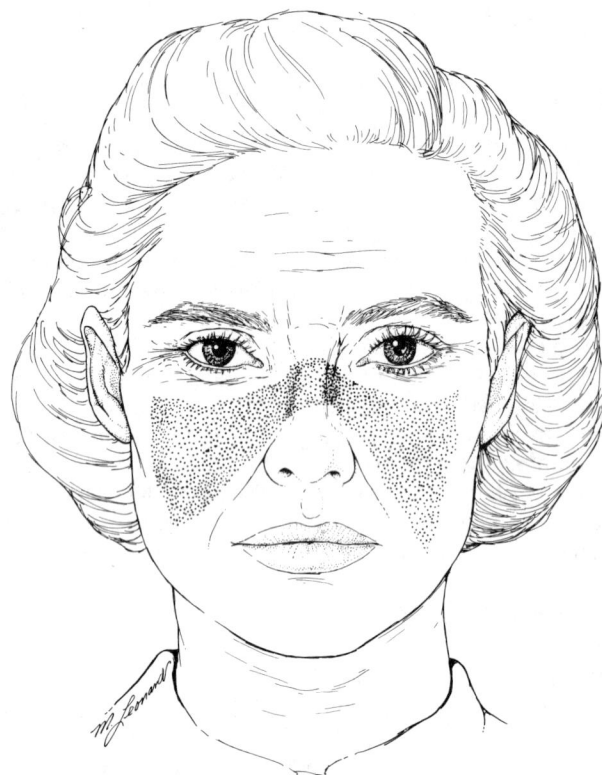

Figure 47-6
Butterfly rash of systemic lupus erythematosus.

from peripheral vasculitis. About 5% of patients experience psychiatric disorders (seizures or organic psychoses). Acute glomerular nephritis occurs early in the disease in 50% of patients, with renal failure the major cause of death in patients with renal involvement.

Raynaud's phenomenon is common in systemic lupus erythematosus and results from vasospasm of smaller vessels in the hands and feet. On exposure to cold, the vessels constrict, resulting in the characteristic white to blue to red color changes. These "attacks" of vasoconstriction are painful and may lead to necrosis with eventual distal digit autoamputation.

Diagnostic Evaluation

Diagnosis is based on a complete history and analysis of blood work. The physician is looking for the classic symptoms of fever, fatigue, and weight loss, and assessing for arthritis, pleurisy, and pericarditis. There is no single definitive laboratory test in the diagnosis of SLE. Serum testing reveals moderate to severe anemia, thrombocytopenia, and leukocytosis or leukopenia. Other diagnostic immunologic tests support but often do not confirm the diagnosis.

Management

Management is directed toward quick treatment of the clinical symptoms. The patient is advised to avoid extreme stress and fatigue and overexposure to sunlight. Counseling and individual education for both the patient and the family are emphasized. A program of moderate exercise combined with rest periods is established, and some people participate in a

physical therapy program. The mainstay of treatment is pharmacotherapy. The major classes of drugs used are nonsteroidal anti-inflammatory drugs, antimalarials, corticosteroids, and immunosuppressive and cytotoxic agents. Antibiotics and certain other drugs are used with caution because of the possibility of hypersensitivity reactions. Because of their reduced resistance to infection, persons with SLE are advised to avoid exposure to people with infections, particularly of the respiratory and urinary tracts. Some physicians are experimenting with the use of *plasmapheresis*, in which 3 to 4 liters of plasma are exchanged weekly for normal plasma from a donor.

▶ Nursing Process
The Patient With Lupus Erythematosus

▷ Assessment

The nurse performs a thorough, systematic physical assessment of the patient, beginning with the major body organs. The *skin* is inspected for any rashes, which are examined for appearance, size, and sensitivity to sunlight. The typical "butterfly" rash over the bridge of the nose is characteristic of systemic lupus erythematosus (Fig. 47-6). Skin bruises (ecchymosis) or ulcerations due to vasculitis may be present. If alopecia is present, the patient is advised that the hair loss is usually temporary. A *neurological* assessment is performed to determine any central nervous system involvement. Any behavioral changes, neuroses, or psychoses are noted. The *heart* is assessed for size, rate, and rhythm, because valvular damage can occur when scar tissue forms as a result of tissue inflammation. Pericarditis and myocarditis may be present along with friction rubs, tamponade, and heart murmurs. Peripheral pulses are palpated for rate and volume. The *lungs* are assessed for any signs of respiratory insufficiency (pleural effusion, infiltrations).

The *kidneys* are involved in 50% of patients with SLE. Acute glomerular nephritis is one of the most common complications. The nurse assesses for edema, hematuria, and proteinuria. A 24-hour urinary output record is kept, and serum creatinine levels are monitored. Any behavioral changes indicating confusion or extreme lethargy are immediately reported to the physician. The *spleen* is palpated for size and tenderness, because splenomegaly (enlarged spleen) exists in 10% to 20% of SLE patients. Laboratory values should be examined for thrombocytopenia.

The *joints* usually exhibit inflammation associated with swelling and pain; paralysis and paresthesia may be present. A complete joint assessment, similar to that presented under rheumatoid arthritis, should be conducted. Patients with SLE usually have a low-grade fever, fatigue, and a diminished sense of self-worth related to coping with the dependency of a chronic illness.

▷ Nursing Diagnoses

Based on all the assessment data, major nursing diagnoses for the patient may include the following:

- Impairment of skin integrity related to photosensitivity and vasculitis

- Activity intolerance related to fatigue
- Disturbance in self-concept related to body-image changes
- Alteration in comfort, pain, related to restricted joint movement
- Anticipatory grieving related to the unpredictability of a chronic, potentially fatal disease.
- Self-care deficits related to musculoskeletal impairment
- Alteration in nutrition related to inadequate food intake

▷ *Planning and Implementation*

▷ *Goals:* The major goals of the patient may include maintenance of skin integrity, decreased fatigue and weakness, attainment of a positive self concept, relief of pain and discomfort, appropriate use of the grieving process, attainment of independence in activities of daily living, and attainment or maintenance of optimal nutrition.

Nursing Interventions

Maintenance of Skin Integrity. The skin rash of DLE or SLE is often scaly and itchy. Cool baths may decrease discomfort and scaliness. The skin should be kept clean and void of powders or other irritants. Topical corticosteroid creams or ointments may be applied, as prescribed, to decrease inflammation. In some cases, an antimalarial drug, such as hydroxychloroquine sulfate (Plaquenil), is given to reduce the inflammatory response of the skin. The main side-effects and toxic effects to be on the alert for include nausea and vomiting, rash, and diminished visual acuity (from retinal damage).

The nurse reinforces the physician's explanations concerning the need to avoid sunlight and ultraviolet lights (such as fluorescent lighting). Long-sleeved clothing, wide-brim hats, and long pants are worn to protect the skin. A sunscreen with the maximum solar protection factor rating should be applied to uncovered skin areas, and sunglasses should be worn to decrease photosensitivity.

The nurse checks for the presence or spread of superficial vasculitic lesions. Appropriate skin hygiene measures, such as keeping the skin clean and dry but moisturized, help to prevent skin breakdown.

Meticulous mouth care is given to prevent and manage oral lesions. Care is taken when brushing the teeth to prevent gum irritation with subsequent bleeding. Antifungal mouth rinses or tablets may be prescribed for secondary oral yeast infections.

Decreased Fatigue and Weakness. The patient with SLE often experiences severe fatigue and generalized weakness. The nurse develops a teaching program to guide the patient in conserving energy. Frequent rest periods combined with a 10- to 12-hours of sleep each night are usually helpful in decreasing fatigue. Principles of energy conservation must be followed to avoid severe fatigue. The patient is advised to participate in a moderate exercise program, which can increase endurance, strengthen some muscle groups, and improve activity tolerance.

Promoting a Positive Self-Concept. One of the major changes in body image is the presence of the erythematous rash on the face and other parts of the body. Even when the

disease is in remission, the rash may not disappear. Lupus patients, particularly young women, are usually very concerned about the disfigurement caused by the rash. The patient may be advised to consult a cosmetologist who specializes in skin disorders to help select appropriate cosmetics to cover the rash and make it less noticeable.

In addition to the skin abnormalities, joint deformity, severe fatigue and weakness, and the unpredictability of the disease contribute to a poor self-concept. The nurse and the family should try to understand this reaction and approach the patient in a realistic but optimistic manner. Further discussion of this goal is found in the section on rheumatoid arthritis.

Relief of Pain and Discomfort. In addition to administering anti-inflammatory or other prescribed drugs for the relief of joint and muscle pain, the nurse helps the patient achieve maximum comfort by establishing a therapeutic lifestyle. Because fatigue, a major symptom of SLE, increases vulnerability to pain, the nurse reinforces adherence to the physician's recommendations for adequate sleep and daily rest periods balanced with moderate exercise. Because stress also exacerbates pain, the patient is encouraged to express feelings about the problems associated with SLE. The patient and family are involved in planning daily activities to prevent the build-up of pressure and in promoting a supportive environment that helps reduce emotional stress. Pain relief measures previously described in this chapter are employed. They include muscle relaxation techniques, guided imagery and other forms of distraction, and self-hypnosis.

Promotion of the Grieving Process. The patient with a diagnosis of SLE may be overwhelmed by the effects and implications of the condition. Grief is a common reaction to the discomforts and restrictions imposed by the disease and to the possibility of severe, life-threatening complications. The nurse accepts and validates these feelings and encourages the expression of fear and concern. The patient and family are helped to identify their individual and collective strengths and to support one another. Support groups may be available, or a network of understanding friends may gradually encourage the patient to resume some activities that were enjoyed previously. The nurse and other members of the health care team are supportive throughout the grief process.

Independence in Activities of Daily Living. Joint involvement combined with fatigue, weakness, and muscle inflammation may alter a patient's ability to perform ADLs independently. The nurse assesses the coping ability of patients and helps them to identify coping mechanisms that have worked in the past. They are encouraged to resume activity gradually and to increase efforts as they gain skill in managing their lives. Activity is alternated with rest periods, to avoid overfatigue and stress. A program of moderate exercise builds confidence and skill. Additional interventions for achieving independence are discussed in the section on rheumatoid arthritis.

Promotion of Nutrition. Anorexia may be compounded by dysphagia from esophagitis. Food selection for the dysphagic patient includes foods of soft, bolus-type consistency, such as mashed potatoes and gelatin. Liquids and hard, brittle foods are the most difficult for a dysphagic patient to swallow. Foods high in protein, vitamins, and iron are encouraged, with supplemental feedings added as necessary to maintain weight.

▷ *Evaluation*

▷ *Expected Outcomes*

1. Patient maintains skin integrity
   a. Applies topical creams or ointments as prescribed
   b. Identifies factors that contribute to skin alterations
   c. Describes measures to decrease erythema of skin rash and skin ulceration
   d. Participates in a treatment program to maintain skin integrity
2. Decreases fatigue and weakness
   a. Identifies activities that cause fatigue
   b. Follows energy conservation principles
   c. Uses proper body mechanics to improve endurance
3. Attains positive self-concept
   a. Expresses feelings freely to family and members of the health team
   b. Accepts physical appearance
   c. Socializes appropriately with family members, peers, and friends
   d. Participates in social activities, such as parties and clubs
   e. Demonstrates active interest and participation in a hobby or diversional activity
4. Experiences relief of pain and discomfort
   a. Uses pharmacotherapy methods of pain management successfully
   b. Experiences optimal joint movement
5. Uses the grieving process appropriately
   a. Expresses feelings to family, significant others, and health team members
6. Achieves independence in ADLs
   a. Performs ADLs at an individual level of optimal functioning
   b. Uses assistive devices safely
7. Attains/maintains optimum nutrition
   a. Prepares food independently or seeks assistance as needed
   b. Eats foods high in protein, iron, and vitamins daily
   c. Keeps body weight at ideal or no less than 10% below ideal weight

Systemic Sclerosis

Systemic sclerosis is a progressive disease of connective tissue characterized by inflammatory, fibrotic, and degenerative changes associated with immunologic abnormalities. Systemic sclerosis is divided into three subgroups: *diffuse scleroderma* which is manifested by widespread skin involvement; *CREST syndrome,* characterized by limited skin involvement (see further description under Clinical Manifestations); and *overlap* the occurrence of systemic sclerosis along with additional connective tissue disorders.

It is important to distinguish systemic sclerosis from localized scleroderma because organ involvement is different with each. *Scleroderma* means hardening of the skin, and is an inflammatory disease in which there is chronic hardening and thickening of connective tissue throughout the body.

Systemic sclerosis is thought to be an autoimmune disease that affects women of all races 3 to 4 times more often than men. The first symptoms usually appear between the ages of 30 and 50. Some studies indicate that white women are at a lower risk than black women.

The exact cause is unknown and believed to be related to many factors. Collagen overproduction and fibrous thickening seem to be triggered by environmental factors (plastics, working with coal) and alcohol abuse. A genetic or familial association has not been determined.

Pathophysiology

Like lupus erythematosus, systemic sclerosis has a variable course with remissions and exacerbations; its prognosis, however, is not as optimistic as that of lupus.

The disease often begins with skin involvement. Mononuclear cells cluster on the skin, and stimulate lymphokines to stimulate procollagen. Insoluble collagen is formed and accumulates excessively in the tissues. Initially, the inflammatory response causes edema formation, with a resulting taut, smooth, and shiny skin appearance. The skin then undergoes fibrotic changes leading to loss of elasticity and movement. Eventually the tissue degenerates and becomes nonfunctional. This chain of events, from inflammation to degeneration, also occurs in blood vessels, major organs, and body systems, often resulting in death.

Clinical Manifestations

The disease starts insidiously on the face and hands, where the skin acquires a tense, wrinkle-free, bound-down appearance. The skin and the subcutaneous tissues become increasingly hard and rigid and cannot be pinched up from the underlying structures (hidebound). Wrinkles and lines are obliterated. The skin is dry, because sweat secretion over the involved region is suppressed.

The face appears masklike, immobile, and expressionless, and the mouth becomes rigid. The buccal mucous membrane likewise may be affected. For years these changes may remain localized in the hands and the feet; the condition spreads slowly. The extremities become stiff and immobile; the fingers semiflexed, immobile, and useless; the hands, clawlike.

The changes within the body, while not visible directly, are vastly more important than the visible changes. The heart muscle becomes fibrotic, causing dyspnea; the esophagus is hardened, interfering with swallowing; the lungs are scarred, impeding respiration; digestive disturbances occur due to hardening of the intestine; progressive renal failure may occur.

The patient may manifest a variety of symptoms referred to as the *CREST syndrome.* The letters CREST stand for: *c*alcinosis (calcium deposits in the tissues); *R*aynaud's phenomenon; *e*sophageal hardening and dysfunctioning; *s*clerodactyly (scleroderma of the digits), and *t*elangiectasis (capillary dilatation that forms a vascular lesion).

Diagnostic Evaluation

There is no one conclusive test to diagnose progressive systemic sclerosis. A complete history and physical examination are performed to note any fibrotic changes in the skin, lungs, heart, or esophagus. The skin is biopsied to identify cellular changes specific to scleroderma. Lung tests will show ventilation–perfusion abnormalities; pericardial effusion will be present with heart involvement. Hypermotility will be present in 50% of those with involvement of the esophagus. The presence of antinuclear antibodies indicates a connective tissue disorder.

Management

Treatment is dependent on the clinical manifestations associated with the sub-group classification. All patients require personal counseling in which individual realistic goals are determined. There is currently no pharmacological drug regimen that has proved effective; however, several agents are used to treat the symptomatology: anti-inflammatory drugs, d-penicillamine (Depen), colchicine, and immunosuppressive and vasoactive agents. Supportive measures include decreasing pain and limiting disability. A moderate exercise program is encouraged to promote joint involvement. Patients are advised to avoid extremes in temperature and to use lotions to minimize excessive skin dryness.

▶ Nursing Process
The Patient With Systemic Sclerosis

▷ Assessment

Because of the inflammatory processes seen with progressive systemic sclerosis, the nurse assesses for joint pain, stiffness, tenderness, and localized edema; polyarthritis may also be present. The fingers and hands are inspected for any color changes or skin disruption indicative of Raynaud's disease. The patient is asked if stiffness or blanching occurs in the fingers after exposure to cold or stress, because either can trigger vasospasm. A complete musculoskeletal examination is performed, as described in the assessment section of Rheumatoid Arthritis (p. 1227).

Because progressive systemic sclerosis is a systemic disorder, the nurse also inspects and palpates the skin (calcinosis, sclerodactyly, and telangiectasis); evaluates gastrointestinal functioning (dysphagia, constipation, diarrhea); and assesses the pulmonary and renal systems (tachypnea, fibrosis, oliguria, hematuria). Any assessment is incomplete without an estimate of the impact of body changes on the patient's self-image.

▷ Nursing Diagnoses

Based on all the assessment data, major nursing diagnoses for the patient may include the following:

- Impairment of skin integrity related to disruption of the skin surface and tissue layers
- Activity intolerance related to fatigue
- Self-care deficits related to musculoskeletal impairment
- Disturbance in self-concept related to body image changes
- Alteration in nutrition related to inadequate food intake
- Alteration in comfort, pain, related to restricted joint movement

▷ Planning and Implementation

▷ *Goals:* The major goals of the patient may include attainment or maintenance of optimum skin integrity, activity tolerance without fatigue, attainment of optimal independence in activities of daily living, attainment of a positive self-con-

cept, attainment or maintenance of optimal nutrition, and management of pain and discomfort.

▷ Nursing Interventions and Evaluation

Nursing care for a patient with systemic sclerosis includes maintaining joint mobility by encouraging range-of-motion exercises and keeping the hands and fingers warm if Raynaud's disease is present. For patients with gastrointestinal involvement, the nurse administers prescribed medications (antacids, antibiotics) and helps patients cope with the discomforts of constipation or diarrhea. The patient with dysphagia needs frequent, small feedings and encouragement to chew food thoroughly. If there is pulmonary involvement, the patient needs encouragement to take periodic deep breaths and to rest at prescribed intervals throughout the day. Vital signs, breath sounds, and fluid intake are evaluated. Oxygen therapy, at a low flow-rate, is administered along with bronchodilators, steroids, and antimicrobials as prescribed. For those who show evidence of renal failure, the nurse assesses daily weight and keeps hourly urinary output records, monitors the urine specific gravity and serum sodium levels, and inspects the skin for signs of excess fluid volume. The patient is also encouraged to verbalize feelings about self-esteem and the socioeconomic impact of living with a chronic illness.

Evaluation outcomes are similar to those presented in the sections on rheumatoid arthritis and lupus erythematosus.

Gout

Primary gout is a disease manifested by joint inflammation, caused by the deposit of uric acid crystals in the joints and connective tissues. Uric acid is the end product of purine metabolism. *Hyperuricemia,* the persistent elevation of urates in the blood, is usually found in gout and is caused by overproduction or undersecretion of uric acid.

Between 1.5 and 2.0 million people in the United States are afflicted with gout. The disorder occurs most frequently in males, usually in the fourth to sixth decades of life. Etiology seems to be related to a genetic defect of purine metabolism or a renal defect resulting in decreased excretion of uric acid. This disorder is also associated with an overindulgence in foods that are high in purines (such as shellfish and organ meats) and alcohol. There seems to be a genetic predisposition to an elevated serum uric acid level.

In *secondary gout* (an acquired disease), hyperuricemia occurs in conditions in which there is an increase in cell turnover (leukemia, multiple myeloma, psoriasis) and an increase in cell breakdown, or it may occur because renal excretion of uric acid is somehow blocked. Other causes of hyperuricemia and gout include prolonged ingestion of certain diuretic agents (thiazides) and aspirin, trauma, or the treatment of myeloproliferative disease.

Pathophysiology

Because of its low solubility, uric acid tends to precipitate and form deposits at various sites where blood flow is least active, including cartilaginous tissue. These masses of sodium urate crystals, called *tophi,* are deposited in the vicinity of the joints, particularly the great toe, on the knuckles (Fig. 47-7), and in the ears. An inflammatory cycle is triggered and tophi cause pressure symptoms, deformity, and ulceration of overlying tissues. These are generally considered to be late signs.

In some patients, renal urate lithiasis (*kidney stones*) may be the earliest manifestation of gout. Chronic renal disease secondary to urate deposition may develop.

Clinical Manifestations

An acute attack of gout usually begins with sudden onset of severe pain in one or more of the peripheral joints, which may be accompanied by intense inflammation, swelling, and tenderness. The first joint of the great toe is most often affected; large joints may also be affected. Sometimes fever is present. An untreated attack of gout subsides in about 1 week. Gouty attacks may be precipitated by starvation, alcohol, fad diets, stress, and certain medications such as aspirin and thiazide diuretics.

The attacks usually recur at irregular intervals. After repeated acute attacks, gout may become chronic, leaving certain joints (particular those of the hands) permanently disabled, deformed, and painful.

Diagnostic Evaluation

Diagnosis is based on the presence of urate crystals in fluid aspirated from a joint cavity. Subcutaneous deposits of urates

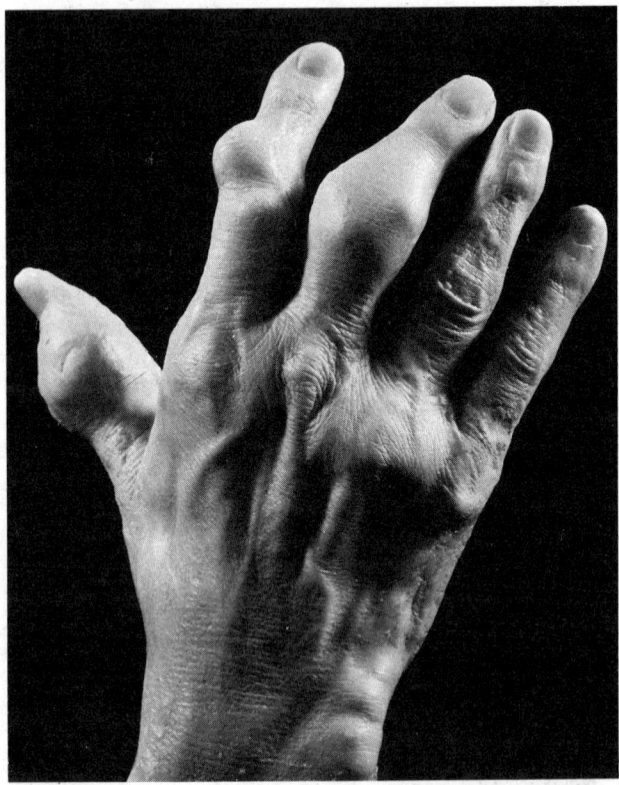

Figure 47-7
Accumulation of uric acid crystals on the knuckles of a patient with gout. (Photo courtesy of National Institute of Arthritis, Metabolism, and Digestive Diseases.)

(tophi) are considered to be positive signs of gout. Roentgenograms of the joints reveal tophi and urate deposits.

Almost one half of chronic gout patients have renal involvement secondary to the development of urate kidney stones. Renal function tests are conducted to determine the extent of kidney involvement (see p. 1002).

Management

The treatment of the acute attack is directed toward relieving pain and inflammation. The pharmacological regimen includes a potent uricosuric agent (colchicine, probenecid [Benemid], NSAIDs and a xanthinoxidase inhibitor (allopurinol [Zyloprim]). Colchicine, given early in the attack, often provides dramatic relief although it has no effect on uric acid metabolism. A response to colchicine is regarded as diagnostic evidence of the disorder. An initial dose of colchicine is given, followed by doses every 1 to 2 hours until the pain is relieved or the patient develops symptoms of gastrointestinal irritability: diarrhea, nausea, and vomiting. (The drug is then stopped temporarily.) Joint pain and swelling start to subside 6 to 12 hours after therapy is started.

For patients in whom there is an overproduction of uric acid or those who have nephrolithiasis or renal impairment, allopurinol (Zyloprim) may be given. Allopurinol is a xanthinoxidase inhibitor that interferes with the conversion of the products of purine metabolism to uric acid and thus inhibits uric acid synthesis. The administration of allopurinol generally produces a prompt fall in both serum and urinary uric acid. It is also used prophylactically during chemotherapy for myeloproliferative disorders.

Many persons with chronic gout have been relieved of their joint pain and have experienced increased joint mobility. Tophaceous deposits cease to form and draining urate sinuses tend to heal on this regimen. The dosage is based on serum urate determinations.

Agents that lower uric acid are used for long-term management to prevent complications (destructive joint disease, nephropathy) and to reduce the occurrence of acute attacks. Such drugs inhibit the reabsorption of uric acid by the renal tubules, resulting in increased excretion of uric acid and thereby lowering the serum urate level. In time, the size of tophi is reduced, and the formation of new tophi is prevented.

Medical treatment includes management of associated conditions, such as cardiovascular complications and nephrolithiasis.

▶ Nursing Process
The Patient With Gout

▷ Assessment

The findings from the joint assessment of a patient with gout will depend on the phase of the disease process. During an acute "gouty attack," the patient displays *severe* joint inflammation, particularly in the great toe (podagra), ankle, and knee, causing extreme pain. The patient with acute gout cannot tolerate light touch on an inflamed joint.

During the intercurrent, or intercritical, phase, the patient is usually asymptomatic and no abnormalities are noted on physical assessment. In late-stage or chronic gout, the patient presents with tophi, which may be palpable near joints and in the ears or may be internal. Joint deformity may also be present.

▷ *Nursing Diagnoses*

Based on all the assessment data, major nursing diagnoses for the patient may include the following:

- Alteration in comfort, pain, related to restricted joint movement
- Impairment of skin integrity related to changes in joint structure due to presence of tophi
- Potential alteration in nutrition related to intake of foods high in purines

▷ *Planning and Implementation*

▷ *Goals:* The major goals of the patient may include relief of joint pain, maintenance of skin integrity, and attainment of optimum nutrition.

Nursing Interventions

Relief of Joint Pain. The patient is encouraged to rest in bed or in a chair, with the affected extremity protected by a bed cradle. The limb should be elevated. Weight-bearing is avoided until the attack subsides, because early ambulation may precipitate a recurrence. If joints in the hand, wrist, or elbow are involved, a splint may be worn to immobilize the hot and tender joint. Cold applications to an affected joint may be helpful.

Maintenance of Skin Integrity. Tophi may become ulcerated and infected due to irritation by clothing and subsequent draining. Care is taken to provide meticulous skin hygiene measures and to prevent injury to tophaceous areas. Draining tophi are covered and topical antibiotic ointment is applied.

Nutrition. Foods high in purines are avoided in the diet; sardines, anchovies, shellfish, and organ meats are particularly high in purine content. The physician may prescribe a protein-restricted diet in an attempt to decrease purine intake.

It is more difficult for uric acid to precipitate as urate crystals in the presence of alkaline urine. Therefore, the patient is instructed to eat alkaline-ash foods, such as milk, potatoes, and citrus fruits. Sodium bicarbonate or citrate solution may be given to maintain a high urine *p*H.

The patient's life-style may need to be modified to include a balanced diet, a low intake of purine-containing foods, a low level of "social" alcohol consumption, and a clear fluid intake of at least 3 liters/day.

▷ *Evaluation*

▷ *Expected Outcomes*

1. Patient achieves management of joint pain
   a. Adheres to medication regimen
   b. Limits weight-bearing on affected joints
   c. Applies ice appropriately to reduce inflammation and pain
2. Maintains skin integrity
   a. Experiences a decrease in or elimination of tophi
   b. Applies medications/dressings to existing tophi to prevent ulceration and infection
3. Attains optimum nutrition
   a. Manages to eat a well-balanced diet
   b. Eats foods low in purines
   c. Maintains a daily fluid intake of at least 2000 ml
   d. Limits alcohol consumption

Other Connective Tissue Disorders

Seronegative Spondyloarthropathies

The spondyloarthropathies are inflammatory disorders of the skeleton that include ankylosing spondylitis, Reiter's syndrome, and psoriatic arthritis.

Ankylosing Spondylitis. Ankylosing spondylitis is a systemic inflammatory disease of unknown etiology that affects the cartilaginous joints of the spine and surrounding tissues. It ranks third in the list of rheumatic diseases commonly occurring in the U.S. Its most characteristic clinical feature is back pain. Diagnosis is based on a comprehensive history, physical examination, and radiologic studies. Sacroiliac joint changes are considered an early sign. An elevated sedimentation rate and a negative rheumatoid factor are relevant laboratory clues.

As the disease progresses, the entire spine may become ankylosed, causing respiratory compromise and complications. Other manifestations such as iritis (inflammation of the iris) and cardiac conduction disturbances may also occur. The disease affects between 1% and 2% of the population and is believed to be slightly more prevalent in males. It is usually diagnosed around the third decade of life, and is believed to be associated with inherited histocompatability antigen HLA-B27. Medical management focuses on treating the pain and maintaining mobility. The drugs of choice are salicylates and NSAIDs. Surgical management may include spinal fusion.

Reiter's Syndrome. Reiter's syndrome affects young adult males and is characterized primarily by urethritis, arthritis, and conjunctivitis. Symptoms occur after a sexually transmitted or enteric infection. Dermatitis and ulcerations of the mouth and penis may also be present. A genetic association with the antigen HLA-B27 has been theorized over the last decade. Management involves treatment of the symptoms, because no cure is available. Salicylates, nonsteroidal anti-inflammatory agents, corticosteroids, and supportive measures for arthritis are recommended.

Psoriatic Arthritis. Psoriatic arthritis occurs in fewer than 10% of patients who have psoriasis, and is characterized by synovitis, polyarthritis, and spondylitis depending on its clinical classification (Group I, II, or III). The symptoms seen with Group III psoriatic arthritis are similar to those seen with ankylosing spondylitis. Salicylates, NSAIDs, and corticosteroids often produce marked improvement in skin and joint symptoms.

Necrotizing Arteritis

Arteritis is a term referring to a group of disorders in which vasculitis (particularly of the arteries) is the major manifestation. Vital organs and body systems are deprived of blood supply because of arterial wall inflammation. Examples of these disorders are periarteritis nodosa (polyarteritis), giant cell arteritis (such as temporal arteritis), and Takayasu's (aortic) arteritis. In most cases, corticosteroid therapy is the treatment of choice, but immunosuppressants may also be given.

Bibliography

Books

Black CM and Myers AR. Systemic Sclerosis (Scleroderma). New York, Gower Medical, 1985.

Blau SP (ed). Emergencies in Rheumatoid Arthritis. New York, Futura Publishing Company, 1986.

Brena SF and Chapman SL. Management of Patients with Chronic Pain. New York, SP Medical and Scientific Books, 1983.

Calin A. Diagnosis and Management of Rheumatoid Arthritis. California, Addison-Wesley, 1983.

Carty DJ. Arthritis and Allied Conditions: A Textbook of Rheumatology. Philadelphia, Lea & Febiger, 1985.

Eliopoulos C (ed). Health Assessment of the Older Adult. California, Addison-Wesley, 1984.

Eschleman MM. Introductory Nutrition and Diet Therapy. Philadelphia, JB Lippincott, 1984.

Fischbach F. A Manual of Laboratory Diagnostic Tests. Philadelphia, JB Lippincott, 1984.

Gupta S and Talal N. Immunology of Rheumatic Diseases. New York, Plenum, 1985.

Hadler NM. Medical Management of the Regional Musculoskeletal Diseases. Orlando, Grune & Stratton, 1984.

Kelley WN et al (eds). Textbook of Rheumatology. Philadelphia, WB Saunders, 1985.

Kuettner KE, Schleyerbach R, and Hascall VC (eds). Articular Cartilage Biochemistry. New York, Raven Press, 1986.

Maskowitz RW et al (eds). Osteoarthritis: Diagnosis and Management. Philadelphia, WB Saunders, 1984.

Maskowitz RW and Haug MR. Arthritis and the Elderly. New York, Springer Publishing, 1986.

McCarthy D (ed). Arthritis and Allied Conditions. Philadelphia, Lea & Febiger, 1984.

Moll J. Management of Rheumatic Disorders. New York, Raven Press, 1983.

Pigg JS, Driscoll PW, and Caniff R. Rheumatology Nursing: A Problem-Oriented Approach. New York, John Wiley & Sons, 1985.

Riggs GK and Gall EP. Rheumatic Diseases: Rehabilitation and Management. Boston, Butterworth, 1984.

Rodman GP and Schumacher HR. Primer of Rheumatic Diseases. Atlanta, Arthritis Foundation, 1983.

Roth SH. Rheumatic Therapeutics. New York, McGraw-Hill, 1985.

Utsinger PD, Avaifler NJ, and Ehrlich GE. Rheumatoid Arthritis: Etiology, Diagnosis, Management. Philadelphia, JB Lippincott, 1985.

Articles

(Asterisks indicate nursing research articles.)

Bentley G and Dowd GSE. Surgical treatment of arthritis in the elderly. Clin Rheum Dis 1986 Apr; 12(1):291-327.

Blechman W. Managing the older arthritic: Can the family help? Geriatrics 1984 Sept; 39(9):131-132.

*Burckhardt CS. The impact of arthritis on quality of life. Nurs Res 1985 Jan/Feb; 34(1):11-15.

Calin A (ed). Factors affecting arthritis health care. Am J Med 1986 June 23; 80(6A):1-20.

Drutzen P. Living with and adjusting to arthritis. Nurs Clin North Am 1984 Dec; 19(4):629-636.

Fox RI et al. Ocular and oral problems in arthritis. Postgrad Med 1985 Sept 1; 78(3):87-97.

Johnson JA and Repp EC. Nonpharmacologic pain management in arthritis. Nurs Clin North Am 1984 Dec; 19(4):583-591.

Koerner ME and Dickinson GR. Adult arthritis: A look at some of its forms. Am J Nurs 1983 Feb; 83(2):255-262.

Liang MH et al. Evaluation of comprehensive rehabilitation services for elderly homebound patients with arthritis and orthopedic disability. Arthritis Rheum 1984 Mar; 27(3):258-266.

Meenan RF. New approaches to outcome assessment: The AIMS questionnaire for arthritis. Adv Intern Med 1986; 31:167-185.

Price JH et al. The public's perceptions and misperceptions of arthritis. Arthritis Rheum 1983 Aug; 26(8):1023-1028.

Sakalys J et al. Outcomes evaluation: Continuing education in rheumatology for nurses. J Contin Educ Nurs 1986 Sept/Oct; 17(5):170-175.

Simpson CF and Dickinson GR. Adult arthritis: Exercise. Am J Nurs 1983 Feb; 83(2):273-274.

Soric R, Tepperman PS, and Devlin HTM. Arthritis rehabilitation: A multifaceted process. Postgrad Med 1986 Dec; 80(8):175-182.

Stevens MB. Connective tissue disease in the elderly. Clin Rheum Dis 1986 Apr; 12(1):11-32.

Wolfe F. Arthritis and musculoskeletal pain. Nurs Clin North Am 1984 Dec; 19(4):565-574.

Yelin EH, Henke CJ, and Epstein WV. Work disability among persons with musculoskeletal conditions. Arthritis Rheum 1986 Nov; 29(11): 1322-1333.

Ziminski CM. Treating joint inflammation in the elderly: An update. Rheumatol 1985 Jan; 40(1):73-85.

Rheumatoid Arthritis

Aho K. When does rheumatoid disease start? Arthritis Rheum 1985 May; 28(5):485-489.

Bach JF and Jacob L. Prospects in the immunological treatment of rheumatoid arthritis. Clin Rheum Dis 1984 Aug; 10(2):219-227.

Cooke TD. Rheumatoid arthritic pannus: True or false? Arthritis Rheum 1985 Oct; 28(10):1195-1198.

Feinberg JR. Allied health team management of rheumatoid arthritis patients. Am J Occup Ther 1984 Sept; 38(9):613-620.

Healey LA. Rheumatoid arthritis in the elderly. Clin Rheum Dis 1986 Apr; 12(1):173-179.

Krane SM and Simon LS. Rheumatoid arthritis: Clinical features and pathogenetic mechanisms. Med Clin North Am 1986 Mar; 70(2): 263-284.

Mitrovic D. The mechanism of cartilage destruction in rheumatoid arthritis. Arthritis Rheum 1985 Oct; 28(10):1192-1195.

Shern MA and Fireman BH. Stress management and mutual support groups in rheumatoid arthritis. Am J Med 1985 May; 78(5):771-775.

St Clair EW and Polisson RP. Therapeutic approaches to the treatment of rheumatoid disease. Med Clin North Am 1986 Mar; 70(2):285-301.

Wolfe F. Remission in rheumatoid arthritis. J Rheumatol 1985 Apr; 12(2):245-252.

Osteoarthritis

Altman R. Development of criteria for the classification and reporting of osteoarthritis. Arthritis Rheum 1986 Aug; 29(8):1039-1049.

Bellamy N. The clinical evaluation of osteoarthritis in the elderly. Clin Rheum Dis 1986 Apr; 12(1):131-151.

Brandt KD and Fife RS. Aging in relation to the pathogenesis of osteoarthritis. Clin Rheum Dis 1986 Apr; 12(1):117-130.

Cooke TDV and Dwash IL. Clinical features of osteoarthritis in the elderly. Clin Rheum Dis 1986 Apr; 12(1):155-172.

Hadler NM. Osteoarthritis as a public health problem. Clin Rheum Dis 1985 Aug; 11(2):175-185.

Hochberg MC. Osteoarthritis: Pathophysiology, clinical features, management. Hosp Pract 1984 Dec; 19(12):41-50, 53.

Jacobs RP. Osteoarthritis: Current concepts in pathogenesis and medical management. Consultant 1984 Nov; 24(11):29-43.

*Laborde JM et al. Life satisfaction, health control orientation, and illness-related factors in persons with osteoarthritis. Res Nurs Health 1985 June; 8(2):183–190.

Ling MH et al. Cost-effectiveness of total joint arthroplasty in osteoarthritis. Arthritis Rheum 1986 Aug; 29(8):937–943.

Ryer J, Treadwell BV, and Mankin HJ. Biochemical and metabolic abnormalities in normal and osteoarthritic human cartilage. Arthritis Rheum 1984 Jan; 27(1):49–57.

Swanson AB and Swanson G. Osteoarthritis in the hand. Clin Rheum Dis 1985 Aug; 11(2):393–420.

Systemic Lupus Erythematosus and Systemic Sclerosis

Blau SP. Systemic lupus erythematosus: In management, less is often more. Consultant 1986 Oct; 26(10):95–108.

Joyce KM et al. The patient with lupus nephritis: A nursing perspective. Heart Lung 1985 Jan; 14(1):75–79.

Liang MH et al. The psychosocial impact of systemic lupus erythematosus and rheumatoid arthritis. Arthritis Rheum 1984 Jan; 27(1):13–19.

Searle L et al. Honoring the personal side of chronic illness . . . systemic lupus erythematosus. Nuring '85 1985 Nov; 15(11):52–57.

Steen VD et al. Factors predicting the development of renal involvement of PSS. Am J Med 1984 May; 76(5):779–786.

Wallace DJ. Systemic lupus erythematosus, rheumatology, and medical literature: Current trends. J Rheumatol 1985; 12(5):913–915.

Ziegler GC. Systemic lupus erythematosus and systemic sclerosis. Nurs Clin North Am 1984; 19(4):673–695.

Diagnosis and Pharmacotherapy

Adams ME et al. Magnetic resonance imaging in rheumatology. J. Rheumatol 1985 Dec; 12(6):1038–1040.

Doyle DV and Lanham JG. Routine drug treatment of osteoarthritis. Clin Rheum Dis 1984 Aug; 10(2):277–291.

Gibson T. Use of simple analgesics in rheumatoid arthritis. Ann Rheum Dis 1985 Jan; 44(1):27–29.

Harris ED. Synovial inflammation in rheumatoid arthritis. Hosp Pract 1986 Sept; 21(9):71–82.

Lipsky PE. Remission-inducing therapy in rheumatoid arthritis. Am J Med 1983 Oct 31; 75(4B):40–49.

Myles A. Corticosteroid treatment in rheumatoid arthritis. Br J Rheumatol 1985 May; 24(2):125–127.

Sims RE and Genant HK. Magnetic resonance imaging of joint disease. Radiol Clin North Am 1986 June; 24(2):179–188.

Strand CV and Clark SR. Drugs and remedies. Am J Nurs 1983 Feb; 83(2):266–269.

Miscellaneous

Borgatti RS. Management decisions in hyperuricemia. Patient Care 1986 Sept 30; 20(15):93–104.

Calin A. Ankylosing spondylitis. Clin Rheum Dis 1985 Apr; 11(1):41–60.

German DC and Holmes EW. Hyperuricemia and gout. Med Clin North Am 1986 Mar; 70(2):419–436.

Laurent MR. Psoriatic arthritis. Clin Rheum Dis 1985 Apr; 11(1):61–85.

Meyers OL. Gout in females. Clin Exp Rheumatol 1985 Apr/June; 3(2):105–109.

Nakayama DA et al. Tophaceous gout: A clinical and radiographic assessment. Arthritis Rheum 1984 Apr; 279(40):468–471.

Agencies

American Coalition of Citizens with Disabilities, 1346 Connecticut Avenue, N.W., Room 817, Washington, DC 20036.

American Lupus Society, 23751 Madison Street, Torrance, CA 90505.

Lupus Foundation of America, Inc., 11921A Olive Drive, St Louis, MO 63141.

The National Arthritis Foundation, 1314 Spring Street, Atlanta, GA 30309.

National Council on the Aging, 1828 L Street N.W., Washington, DC 20036.

National Institute of Arthritis and Musculoskeletal and Skin Diseases, National Institutes of Health, Bethesda, MD 20892.*

Integumentary Problems

Unit XIII

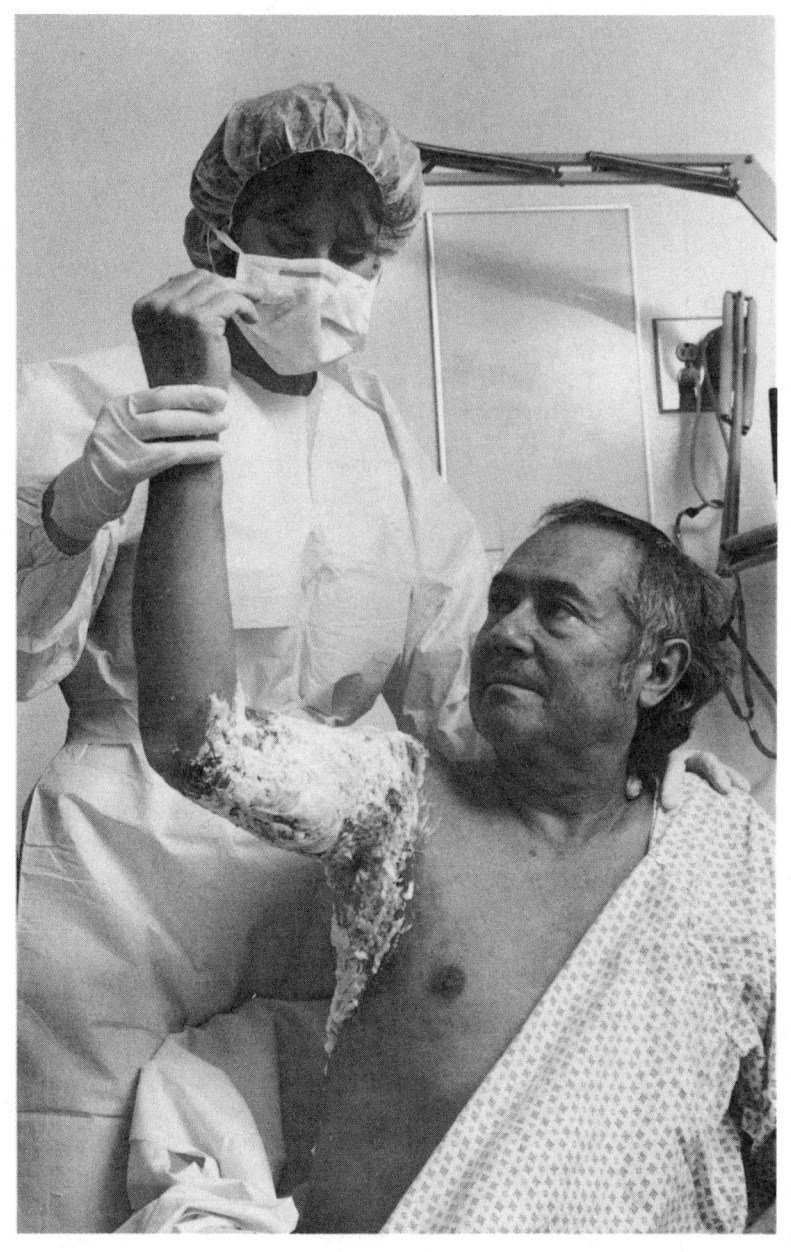

Chapter 48

Management of Patients With Dermatologic Problems

Skin problems are encountered frequently in nursing practice. Skin-related complaints account for 5% to 10% of all ambulatory patient visits in this country. Because the skin mirrors the general condition of the patient, many systemic conditions may be accompanied by dermatologic manifestations. Any patient hospitalized with a medical or a surgical problem may suddenly develop itching and a rash. In certain systemic conditions, such as hepatitis and cancer, dermatologic manifestations may be the first sign that these disorders are present.

Physiologic Overview

The skin is a structure that is indispensable for human life. It forms a barrier between the internal organs and the external environment and participates in many vital functions of the body. The skin is continuous with the mucous membrane at the external openings of the organs of the digestive, respiratory, and urogenital systems. Because disorders of the skin are readily visible, dermatologic complaints are frequently the primary reason for patient visits.

Anatomy of the Skin

The skin is composed of two layers of tissue, the *epidermis,* an outer layer in contact with the environment, and a deeper layer called the *dermis.* The epidermis consists of live, continuously dividing epithelial cells covered on the surface by dead cells that were originally deeper in the dermis but were pushed upward by newly developing cells underneath. The dead cells are constantly flaking off from the skin, frequently in irregular patches. These dead cells contain large amounts of *keratin,* an insoluble, fibrous protein that forms the outer barrier of the skin. The epidermis is devoid of blood vessels and has few nerve endings. The superficial layers of the epidermis can be shaved from the body without pain or blood loss. The epidermis is modified in different areas of the body. Over the palms of the hands and the soles of the feet it is thickened and contains increased amounts of keratin, in contrast to the thin epidermis over most of the rest of the body. The thickness of the epidermis can increase with use, as is the case, for example, with the hands of a laborer.

The dermis is a broad layer of connective tissue that underlies the epidermal layer. It is composed of collagen and elastic fibers and contains blood and lymph vessels, nerves, sweat and sebaceous glands, and hair roots. Interdigitation (interlocking) between dermis and epidermis produces ripples on the surface of the skin. On the fingertips, these ripples are called *fingerprints.* They are perhaps a person's most individualistic characteristic, and they almost never change. With aging, the number of elastic fibers in the dermis progressively decreases, and the skin becomes wrinkled.

The color of the skin is determined by the pigment called *melanin,* which is produced by the cells in the epidermis called *melanocytes.* The skin of black persons and the darker areas of the skin on white persons (for example, the nipple) contain large amounts of this pigment. Production of melanin by melanocytes is largely under the control of a hormone secreted from the hypothalamus of the brain, called melanocyte-stimulating hormone (MSH). Increased production of melanin occurs on exposure to ultraviolet light, such as occurs with suntanning.

The skin is anchored to the muscles and bones underneath by subcutaneous tissue composed of connective tissue interlaced with fat. Fat is deposited and distributed according to the person's sex, and in part accounts for the difference in body shape between men and women. Overeating results in increased deposition of fat beneath the skin.

Hair. Hair is present over the entire body except for the palms of the hands and soles of the feet. The hair consists of a root formed in the dermis and a hair shaft that projects beyond the skin. It grows in a cavity called a *hair follicle.* The proliferation of cells in the bulb of the hair causes the hair to form. Hairs in different parts of the body serve different functions. The hairs of the eyes (eyebrows and lashes), nose, and ears screen dust, bugs, and airborne debris. Hair of the skin serves as thermal insulation in lower animals. This function in enhanced during cold or fright by the piloerection (hairs "standing on end"), caused by contraction of the tiny arrector muscles attached to the hair follicle. The piloerector response that occurs in humans is probably vestigial. The color of hair is due to the presence of varying amounts of melanin within the hair shaft. Gray or white hair is the result of loss of pigment. Growth of hair in certain locations on the body is under the control of sex hormones. The best examples are the hair on the face (beard and mustache) and on the body trunk that are controlled by the presence of the male hormones (androgens).

Nails. On the dorsal surface of the fingers and toes, a hard, transparent plate of keratin, called the *nail,* overlies the skin. The nail grows from its root, which lies under a thin fold of skin called the *cuticle.* The nail helps to protect the fingers and toes, in order to preserve their highly developed sensory function, and aids in the performance of certain fine functions of the fingers, such as picking up small objects.

Glands of the Skin. *Sebaceous glands* are associated with hair follicles. The ducts of the sebaceous glands empty an oily secretion onto the space between the hair follicle and the hair shaft. For each hair there is a sebaceous gland, whose secretions oil the hair and render the skin soft and pliable.

Sweat glands are found in the skin over most of the body surface. They are heavily concentrated on the palms of the hands and soles of the feet. Only the glans penis, the margins of the lips, the external ear, and the nail bed are devoid of sweat glands. Sweat glands are subclassified into two categories: *eccrine* and *apocrine.* The eccrine sweat glands are found in all areas of the skin. Their ducts open directly onto the skin surface. The apocrine sweat glands are larger and, in contrast to that of the eccrine glands, their secretion contains parts of the secretory cells. They are located in the axillae, anal region, scrotum, and labia majora. Their ducts generally open onto hair follicles. The apocrine glands become active at the time of puberty. In the female, they enlarge and recede with each menstrual cycle.

Apocrine glands produce a milky sweat that is broken down by bacteria to produce the characteristic underarm odor. Specialized apocrine glands called *cerumenous glands* are found in the external ear, where they produce wax (*cerumen*).

The thin, watery secretion called *sweat* is produced in the basal coiled portion of the eccrine gland and is released into its narrow duct. Sweat is composed predominantly of water and contains about half of the salt content of the blood plasma. Sweat is released from eccrine glands in response to elevated ambient temperature. The rate of sweat secretion is under the control of the sympathetic nervous system. Excessive sweating of the palms and soles, axillae, forehead, and other areas may occur in response to pain and stress.

Functions of the Skin

Protective Function. The skin protects the body against invasion by bacteria and foreign matter. The thickened skin of the palms and soles provides the tough covering necessary for the constant trauma occurring in these areas.

The epidermis is relatively impermeable to most chemical substances. It is this property of skin that allows it to be an effective barrier for protection. Some substances go through the skin more readily than others. A variety of different lipids (fatty substances) may be absorbed through the skin. Fat-soluble vitamins (A and D) and steroid hormones are examples. Substances may enter the skin through the epidermis—the transepidermal route—or via the orifices of the follicles (follicular "holes").

Sensory Function. Stimulation of the receptor endings of nerves in the skin allows us to monitor constantly the conditions of our immediate environment. The primary functions of the receptors in the skin are to sense temperature, pain, light touch, and pressure (or heavy touch). Different nerve endings are responsible for responding to each of the different stimuli. Although the nerve endings are distributed over the entire body, they are more concentrated in some areas than in others. For example, the fingertips are much more densely innervated than the skin of the back.

Water Balance. Skin forms a barrier that prevents loss of water and electrolytes from the internal environment and also prevents the subcutaneous tissues from drying out. When skin is damaged, as occurs with a severe burn, for example, large quantities of fluids and electrolytes can be lost rapidly, possibly leading to circulatory collapse, shock, and death. On the other hand, the skin is not completely impermeable to water. Small amounts of water continuously evaporate from the skin surface. This evaporation, called *insensible perspiration*, amounts to approximately 500 ml per day for a normal adult. Insensible water loss may vary with the body temperature, and in the presence of fever these losses can increase. During immersion in water, the skin can accumulate water up to approximately 3 or 4 times its normal weight. A common example of this is the swelling of the skin after prolonged bathing.

Temperature Regulation. The body continuously produces heat as a result of the metabolism of foodstuffs to produce energy. This heat is dissipated primarily through the skin. Three major physical processes are involved in loss of heat from the body to the environment. The first process, *radiation*, is the ability of a body to give off its heat to another object of lower temperature situated at a distance. The second process, *conduction*, is the transfer of heat from the body to a cooler object in contact with it. Heat transferred by conduction to the air surrounding the body is removed by the third process, *convection*, which consists of bulk movement of warm air molecules away from the body. Evaporation from the skin aids the process of heat loss by conduction. Heat is conducted through the skin into water molecules on its surface, causing the water to evaporate. The source of the water on the skin surface may be insensible perspiration, sweat, or water from the environment. Normally, all of these mechanisms for heat loss are utilized. However, when the ambient temperature is very high, radiation and convection are not effective, and evaporation from the skin constitutes the only means for heat loss.

Under normal conditions, metabolic heat production is exactly balanced by heat loss, and the internal temperature of the body is maintained constant at approximately 37°C (98.6F). The rate of heat loss depends primarily on the surface temperature of the skin, which is in turn a function of the skin blood flow. Skin is richly supplied with blood vessels that carry heat to the skin from the core of the body. Blood flow through these vessels is controlled primarily by the sympathetic nervous system. Increased blood flow to the skin results in delivery of more heat to the skin and a greater rate of heat loss from the body. On the other hand, decreased skin blood flow decreases the skin temperature and helps conserve heat for the body. When the temperature of the body begins to fall, as occurs on a cold day, the blood vessels of the skin constrict and reduce heat loss from the body.

Sweating is another process by which the body can regulate the rate of heat loss. Sweating is increased when body temperature starts to rise. In extremely hot environments, the rate of sweat production may be as high as 1 liter per hour. Under some circumstances, for example, with emotional stress, sweating may occur on a reflex basis unrelated to the necessity to lose heat from the body.

Wheal and Flare Reaction. Stroking the skin with sufficient firmness to cause local injury results in local reddening. This is followed within a few minutes by localized swelling and more diffuse redness around the injury site. The combination of the swelling (called a *wheal*) and the diffuse redness (called a *flare*) constitutes a normal reaction of the skin to injury.

The flare reaction is due to an increased temperature in the area (from the stimulus) and to dilation of the arterioles and venules. It is also dependent upon local nervous mechanisms. The wheal is caused by increased capillary permeability induced by trauma. Fluid-containing protein leaks out of the capillaries locally and produces edema at the site of injury.

These responses have also been attributed to the release of some diffusible substance (histamine; bradykinin) by the injured cells.

Assessment

Physical Assessment

Assessment of the skin includes all body surfaces, mucous membranes, and the nails. The skin is a reflection of a person's overall health, and alterations often correspond to disease in other organ systems. Inspection and palpation constitute the chief techniques of the skin assessment.

A thorough examination of the skin includes an assessment of color, lesions, vascularity, temperature, texture, mobility, and the presence of edema. Skin color varies from person to person and ranges from ivory to deep brown. The skin of exposed portions of the body, especially in sunny, warm climates, tends to be more pigmented than that of the rest of the body. The vasodilative effects of fever, sunburn, and inflammation produce a pink or reddish hue in the skin. Pallor is an absence of or decrease in normal skin tones and vascularity, and is best observed in the conjunctivae. The bluish hue of cyanosis indicates cellular hypoxia and is easily observed in the nail beds, lips, and mucous membranes. Jaundice, a yellowing of the skin, is directly related to elevations in serum bilirubin and is often noted in the sclerae and mucous membranes.

Assessing color changes in the dark-skinned or black person may be difficult. Additional lighting may be helpful during inspection. The overall surface of dark skin normally has a reddish base or undertone; the buccal mucosa, tongue, lips, and nails have a pink color. Erythema is often visible as a purplish grey cast to the skin. Dark-skinned persons normally have yellow conjunctivae; thus, it may be necessary to inspect the hard palate for the yellowing hue of jaundice. Rashes are more easily identified by palpation. Differences in skin texture are detected and borders of the rash defined.

The presence of any eruptions or lesions on the skin is noted. Careful observation of the eruption or lesion helps to identify the type of dermatosis (abnormal skin condition) and indicates whether the lesion is primary or secondary. At the same time, the anatomical distribution of the eruption is noted, because certain diseases affect certain sites of the body and are distributed in characteristic patterns and shapes. To determine the extent of the distribution, the left and right sides of the body are compared while the color and shape of the lesion are noted. Following observation, the lesions are palpated to determine their texture and to see if they are hard or soft or filled with fluid. A metric ruler is used to measure the size of the lesions so that any further extension can be compared with this initial baseline measurement. The dermatosis is then documented clearly and in detail.

It is essential for the examiner to use precise and accurate terminology in any verbal or written communication about the status of the skin. This facilitates the ultimate identification and diagnosis of local and systemic diseases, and requires memorization and the reinforcement of clinical experience.

Once the color of the skin has been inspected and lesions have been noted, an assessment of vascular changes in the skin is carried out. A description of vascular changes includes location, distribution, color, size, and the presence of pulsations. Common vascular changes include petechiae, ecchymosis, telangiectasia, angiomas, and venous stars.

Skin moisture, temperature, and texture are assessed primarily by palpation. The elasticity (*turgor*) of the skin, which lessens in normal aging, may be a factor in assessing the hydration status of a patient.

A brief inspection of the nails includes observation of configuration, color, and consistency. Many of the alterations seen in the nail or nail bed reflect local or systemic abnormalities in progress, or are the result of past events. Transverse depressions (*Beau's lines*) in the nails may reflect retarded growth of the nail matrix secondary to severe illness or, more commonly, are the result of local trauma. Ridging, hypertrophy, and other changes may also be visible with local trauma. Inflammation of the skin around the nail (*paronychia*) is usually accompanied by tenderness and erythema. The angle between the normal nail and its base is 160 degress. When palpated, the base of the nail is usually firm. *Clubbing* is manifested by a straightening of the normal angle (180 degrees or greater) and a softening of the nail base. This softening is perceived as spongelike when palpated.

Gerontological Considerations

The major changes in the skin of older people include dryness, wrinkling, laxity, uneven pigmentation, and a variety of proliferative lesions. The histologic features of skin associated with aging include a thinning at the junction of the dermis and epidermis, loss of dermal and subcutaneous tissue, reduction of the vascular bed (especially of the capillary loops), marked reduction of the vascular network surrounding hair bulbs and the eccrine, apocrine, and sebaceous glands, and reduced numbers of melanocytes, specialized epidermal cells, and mast cells (Fig. 48-1).

Loss of dermal thickness approaches 20% in elderly persons, accounting for the thin, sometimes nearly transparent quality of their skin. The aging skin, like all other aging organ systems, has a loss of functional capacity. Functions affected include cell replacement, the barrier function, sensory perception, thermoregulation, and sweat and sebum production.

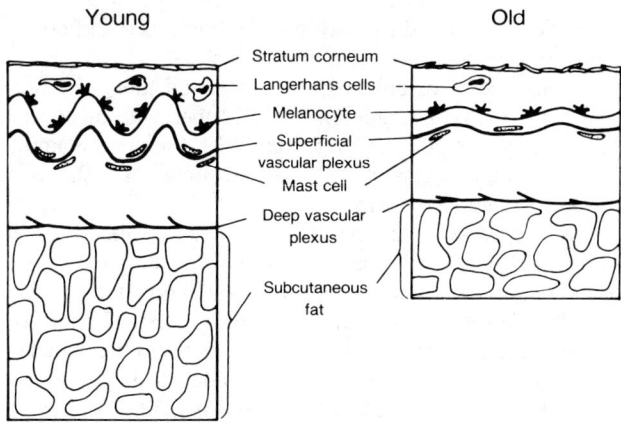

Figure 48-1
Histologic changes in aging normal skin. Schematic drawings emphasize the age-associated flattening of the dermo-epithelial junction; loss of dermal and subcutaneous mass; shortened capillary loops; and reduced numbers of melanocytes, Langerhans cells, and mast cells. (Reprinted with permission from the American Geriatrics Society, "Age-associated changes in the skin," by Barbara A. Gilchrest, M.D. Journal of the American Geriatrics Society, Vol. 30, No. 2, pg. 140, 1982.)

The result is an increasing vulnerability to injury and to certain disease. Skin problems are common among older people.

Diagnostic Evaluation

Dermatology is a visually-oriented speciality. In addition to listening to the patient's history, the examiner inspects the appearance of the primary and secondary lesions and their configuration and distribution. Certain diagnostic procedures may also be used to help in identifying skin conditions.

A *skin biopsy* is performed to obtain tissue for microscopic examination. It may be obtained by scalpel excision or by a skin punch that removes a small core of tissue. Biopsies are performed on skin nodules of uncertain etiology to rule out malignancy, on plaques of unusual shapes and colors, and to secure an exact diagnosis in blistering and other disorders.

Immunofluorescence (IF) testing is a technique in which antigen or antibody is combined with a fluorochrome dye and used to localize the site of an immune reaction. (Antibodies can be made fluorescent by attaching them to a dye). Immunofluorescence tests on skin (*direct IF test*) are techniques to detect autoantibodies directed against portions of the skin. The *indirect IF test* detects specific antibodies in the patient's serum.

Patch testing is done to identify substances to which the patient has developed an allergy. The suspected allergens are applied to normal skin under occlusive patches. After about 48 hours, the patches are removed and the underlying skin is inspected. If dermatitis develops, the presence of redness, fine bumps, or itching is considered a *weak* positive reaction; fine blisters, papules, and severe itching may show a *moderate* positive reaction; and the presence of blisters, pain, and ulceration indicates a *strong* positive reaction. During testing the patient is advised to leave the patch in place and not to bathe or scratch under the patch site.

Skin scrapings are taken of suspected fungal lesions. This is done with a scalpel blade moistened with oil so that the scraped skin adheres to the blade. The scraped material is transferred to a glass slide, covered with a cover slip, and examined microscopically.

A *Tzanck smear* is used to examine cells from blistering skin conditions. The suspected lesion is opened and its contents are applied to a glass slide and examined after staining.

The *Wood's light examination* uses a special lamp for producing long-wave ultraviolet rays that gives a characteristic fluorescence in the presence of some microbial agents. The color of this fluorescent light, seen best in a darkened room, is characteristic of a disease or condition. The patient is reassured that the light is not harmful to skin or eyes.

Clinical photographs are taken to show the nature and extent of the skin condition and to reveal progress or improvement resulting from treatment.

Skin Lesions

Skin lesions represent the most prominent characteristic of dermatologic conditions. They vary in size, shape, and cause, and are classified according to their appearance and origin.

Skin lesions can be described as primary or secondary. *Primary* lesions are the initial lesions and are characteristic of the disease itself. *Secondary* lesions result from external causes, such as scratching, trauma, infections, or changes caused by wound healing. Depending on the stage of development, skin lesions are further divided according to type and appearance, as indicated in the following definitions and illustrated in Figure 48-2.

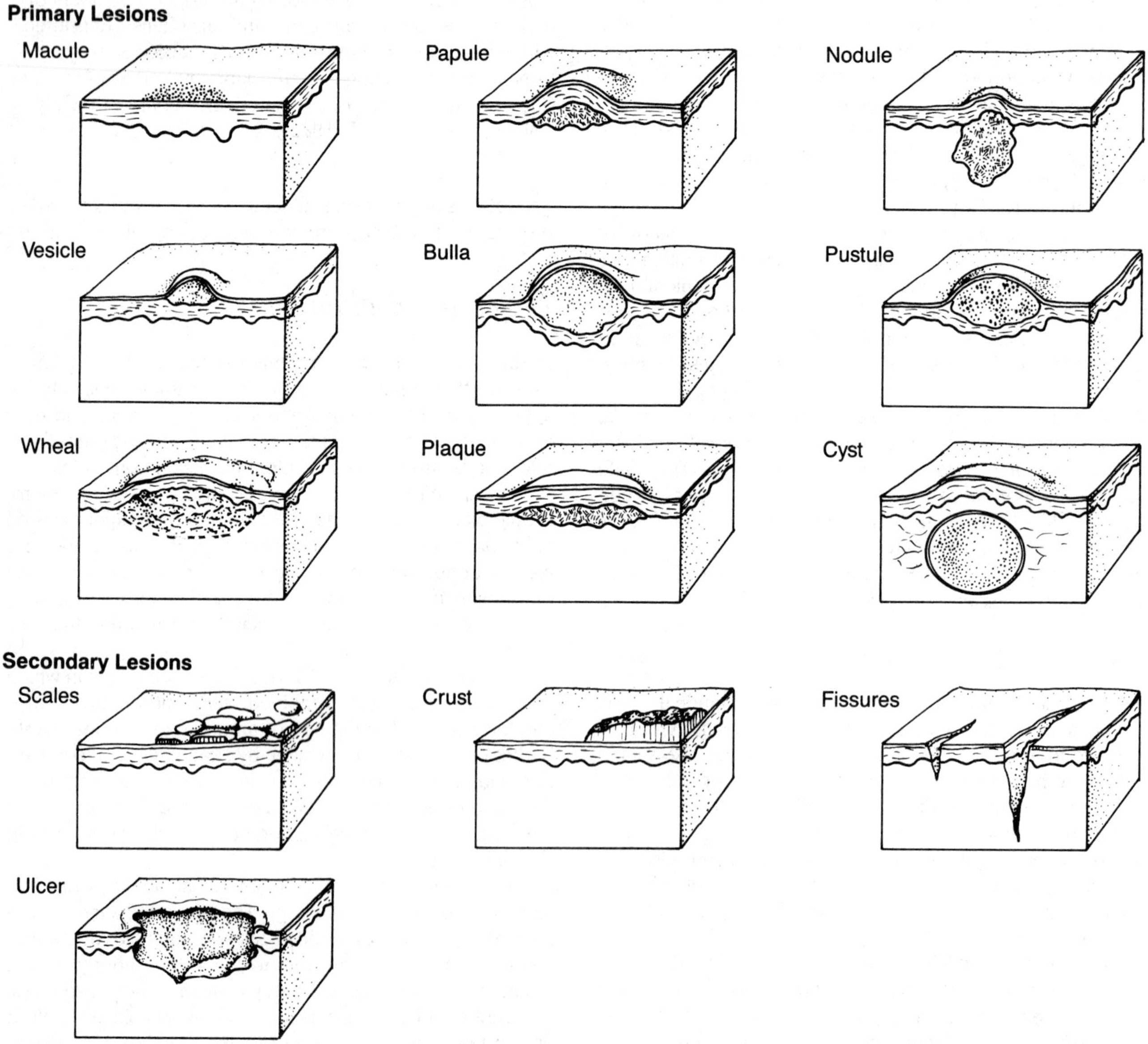

Primary Lesions

Macule Papule Nodule

Vesicle Bulla Pustule

Wheal Plaque Cyst

Secondary Lesions

Scales Crust Fissures

Ulcer

Figure 48-2
Types of skin lesions.

Primary Lesions (Initial Lesions)

Macule—a flat, circumscribed discoloration of the skin

Papule—a solid, elevated, palpable lesion smaller than 1 cm (0.4 inch) in diameter; lesions may vary in color

Nodule—a raised, solid lesion larger than 1 cm in diameter

Vesicle—a small elevation of the skin that is filled with clear fluid

Bulla—a large vesicle or blister larger than 1 cm (0.4 inch) in diameter

Pustule—a lesion that contains pus; may form as a result of purulent changes in a vesicle

Wheal—transient elevation of the skin caused by edema of the dermis and surrounding capillary dilatation

Plaque—a solid, elevated lesion on the skin or mucous membrane, larger than 1 cm (0.4 inch) in its largest diameter

Cyst—a tumor that contains semisolid or liquid material

Secondary Lesions

As the term implies, secondary lesions are the changes that take place in primary lesions and possibly modify them. Secondary lesions include the following:

Scales—heaped-up, horny layers of dead epidermis; may develop as a result of inflammatory changes

Crusts—a covering formed from serum, blood, or pus drying on the skin

Excoriations—linear scratch marks or traumatized area of skin

Fissures—cracks in the skin, usually from marked drying and longstanding inflammation

Ulcers—lesions formed by local destruction of the epidermis and part or all of the underlying dermis

Lichenification—thickening of skin accompanied by accentuation of skin markings

Scar—a fibrotic change in the skin following a destructive process

Atrophy—loss of one or more of the skin components

Shape and Configuration

Once the type of lesion is identified, the shape of the lesion and the configuration (arrangement) of the lesions relative to each other are noted. "Shape" may refer to a single lesion or to the appearance of multiple lesions. The following are descriptions frequently employed:

Annular—ring-shaped

Circinate—circular

Confluent—lesions run together or join

Discoid—disc-shaped

Discrete—lesions remain separate

Generalized—widespread eruption

Grouped—clustering of lesions

Guttate—droplike

Herpetiform—grouped vesicles

Iris—a ring or a series of concentric rings

Keratosis—horny thickening

Linear—in lines

Multiform—more than one kind of skin lesions

Nummular—coin-shaped

Polymorphous—more than one kind of skin lesion

Reticulated—lacelike network

Serpiginous—snakelike or creeping eruption

Telangiectasia—tiny, superficial, dilated cutaneous vessel; can be seen as a red thread or line

Zosteriform or dermatomal—bandlike distribution limited to one or more dermatomes of skin

Management of Skin Disorders

Therapeutic modalities used in the treatment of patients with dermatologic problems include topical and systemic medications, wet dressings, other special dressings, and therapeutic baths.

The major objectives of therapy are (1) prevent damage to the healthy skin, (2) prevent secondary infection, (3) reverse the inflammatory process, and (4) relieve the symptoms.

Preventing Damage to Healthy Skin. Some skin problems are markedly aggravated by soap and water. Therefore, bathing routines are modified according to the condition being treated.

Denuded skin, whether the area of desquamation is large or small, is excessively prone to damage by chemicals and trauma. The friction of a towel, if applied with vigor, is sufficient to excite a brisk inflammatory response that causes any existing lesion to flare up and increase in extent. Thus, the essence of skin care and protection in bathing a patient with abnormal skin is to use a mild, superfatted soap or soap substitute and to ensure the complete removal of the soap when rinsing, before blotting the area dry with a soft cloth. Deodorant soaps should be avoided in these patients.

Pledgets saturated with oil will aid in loosening crusts, removing exudates, or freeing an adherent dry dressing. The dressing also may be saturated with sterile saline or another prescribed solution, which softens it and permits it to be pulled away gently.

Preventing Secondary Infection. Potentially infectious skin lesions should be regarded strictly as such, and proper precautions should be observed until the diagnosis is established. Some lesions with pus contain infectious material. Although some genital lesions are suspect, most are minor irritations.

- If the condition is infectious, disposable gloves are worn by the nurse and the physician. Dressings removed from infected skin should be wrapped in paper and burned as soon as possible.

Reversing the Inflammatory Process. The type of skin lesion (oozing, infected, or dry) usually suggests the local medication or treatment that is prescribed. As a rule, if the skin is acutely inflamed (hot, red, and swollen) and is oozing, it is best to apply wet dressings and soothing lotions. In chronic conditions in which the skin surface is dry and scaly, water-soluble emulsions, creams, ointments, and pastes are used. The therapy must be changed as the response indicates. Explain that the patient must contact the physician or clinic if the medication or compresses seem to irritate the dermatosis. Success or failure of skin therapy rests upon adequate instruction and motivation of the patient and the interest and support of the health personnel.

Wet Dressings

Wet dressings (wet compresses applied to areas of the skin) are usually used for acute, weeping, inflammatory lesions. They may be either sterile or unsterile, depending on the condition being treated. The purposes of wet dressings are (1) to reduce inflammation by producing constriction of blood vessels (thus decreasing vasodilatation and the local blood flow in inflammation); (2) to cleanse the skin of exudates, crusts, and scales; and (3) to maintain drainage of infected areas. Before these dressings are applied, the hands should be washed thoroughly.

Wet dressings are used for vesicular, bullous, pustular, and ulcerative disorders, as well as for acute inflammatory disorders, erosions, and exudative, crusted surfaces.

The solutions generally consist of room-temperature tap water or saline. Other agents may be used to precipitate protein, thus acting as mild astringents and antibacterials. Medication may be applied after wet dressings are removed.

Although some dressings must be covered to prevent evaporation, most are allowed to remain open. The *open dressing* requires frequent changes because evaporation is rapid. The *closed dressing* is changed less frequently. However, there is always a danger that it will cause not only softening but actual maceration of the underlying skin.

Areas of normal skin that may be exposed to moisture for any extended period should first be coated with petrolatum jelly, a silicone oil, or zinc oxide paste to avoid skin maceration.

Smooth muslin or cotton materials can be cut and folded to make dressings that are 2 to 4 layers thick. The dressing is saturated with the prescribed solution before it is applied. Usually wet dressings are kept cool or at room temperature. Compresses are removed, wrung out of the solution, and reapplied every 5 minutes to ensure their wetness. Wet dressings are usually applied for 15-minute periods, 3 to 4 times daily during the acute phase unless otherwise prescribed. Medications applied to moist skin immediately after treatment with compresses are absorbed better than when applied to dry skin. If extensive areas are to be treated with wet compresses, the patient must be kept warm and not more than one third of the body treated at one time.

If warm compresses are prescribed, the area must be watched carefully because the skin may be burned. If a closed dressing is used, it may be covered with sterile towels to hold the dressing in place and further protected with a plastic film. In this way, the temperature can be maintained for a longer period.

Dressing materials should be laundered or discarded every 24 hours. Usually, the acute stage of dermatitis subsides after 48 to 72 hours of treatment. Wet dressings continued beyond this point can lead to dryness of skin.

Therapeutic Baths (Balneotherapy)

Baths or soaks are useful when large areas are involved, to remove crusts, scales, and old medications, and to relieve the inflammation and itching that accompany acute dermatoses. The temperature of the water should be comfortable, and the bath should not exceed 20 to 30 minutes because of the tendency of baths/soaks to produce maceration. For the different types of therapeutic baths and their uses, see Table 48-1.

Pharmacotherapy: Topical Medications

Medications in the form of lotions, creams, ointments, and powders are frequently used to treat skin lesions. In general, wet dressings, with or without medication, are used in the acute stage; lotions and creams are reserved for the subacute

TABLE 48-1
Types of Therapeutic Baths

Bath Solution and Medication	Desired Effect	Nursing Interventions
Water	Same effects as wet dressings	• Fill the tub half full.
Saline	Used for widely disseminated lesions	• Keep the water at a comfortable temperature.
Colloidal—Oatmeal or Aveeno	Antipruritic; soothing	• Do not allow the water to cool excessively.
Sodium bicarbonate	Cooling	• Use a bath mat—*medications may cause tub to be slippery.*
Starch	Soothing	• Apply a lubricating agent to wet skin after bath if emollient action is desired—increases hydration. Since tars are volatile, the bath area should be well ventilated.
Medicated tars—Alma-Tar, Balnetar (follow package directions)	Tar baths are used for psoriasis and chronic eczematous conditions.	
Bath oils—Alpha-Keri, Lubath, Domol	Bath oils are used for antipruritic and emollient actions.	• Dry by blotting with a towel.
	Used for acute and subacute eczematous eruptions	• Keep room warm to minimize temperature fluctuations.
		• Encourage patient to wear light, loose clothing after the bath.

stage; ointments are used when inflammation has become chronic and the skin is dry with scaling and *lichenification* (leathery thickening of the skin).

Lotions exert a cooling action through water evaporation; they also have a protective effect, relieve itching, and promote drying. They may also act as sunscreens. Lotions are applied easily with a soft paintbrush or cotton gauze, or by hand, and are not usually washed off between applications.

Powders usually have a talc, zinc oxide, bentonite, or cornstarch base and are dusted on the skin with a shaker or with cotton sponges. Although their medical action is brief, powders act as hygroscopic agents, absorbing moisture and reducing friction between skin surfaces and between the skin and bedding.

Creams are suspensions of oil and water, are easily applied, and usually are the most cosmetically acceptable to the patient. Creams are generally rubbed into the skin by hand. They are used for their moisturizing and emollient effects.

Gels are semisolid emulsions that become liquid when applied to the skin. They are cosmetically acceptable to the patient, as they vanish after application, and are greaseless and nonstaining. Most topical steroids are prescribed in gel form because the gel appears to penetrate more effectively than other skin preparations.

Pastes are mixtures of powders and ointments and are used in inflammatory conditions. They adhere best to the skin and may need to be removed with mineral or olive oil.

Ointments retard water loss, lubricate and protect the skin, and are preferred in the more chronic or localized skin conditions. Both pastes and ointments are applied with a wooden tongue depressor or by hand, with gloves if necessary.

Sprays and *aerosols* may be used on extensive lesions. These evaporate on contact and are used infrequently.

In all types of topical medication, the patient should be taught to apply the medication gently but thoroughly and, when necessary, to cover these medications with a dressing to prevent soiling of clothing.

Corticosteroids are being widely used in the treatment of many dermatologic conditions. Topical steroids frequently are used to suppress inflammation, thus relieving pain and itching. The patient is taught to apply this medication sparingly on hydrated skin and to rub it in thoroughly. Topical corticosteroids may be covered with occlusive dressings to enhance skin penetration. (See below.) However, this can cause obstruction of sweat glands and overgrowth of skin bacteria.

Wet dressings may be used with topical steroids to enhance steroid absorption by softening and hydrating the skin. Other techniques to enhance skin penetration include the application of hot wet dressings before applying the medication or using a heating pad over a wet dressing on treated skin areas.

When steroids are applied around the eyes, a great deal of caution is required, as chronic use around the eyes may cause glaucoma, cataracts, and viral and fungal infections. Also, when strong (fluorinated) steroids are put on the face, precautions must be taken because they may produce an acnelike dermatitis (*perioral dermatitis*), steroid-induced *rosacea* (characterized by lesions around the nose and cheeks), and *hypertrichosis* (excessive hair growth).

Intralesional therapy consists of the injection of a sterile suspension of medication (usually a corticosteroid) into or just below a lesion. Although this treatment may have an anti-inflammatory effect, local atrophy may result if the injection is made into subcutaneous fat. Skin lesions treated with intralesional therapy include psoriasis, keloids, and cystic acne. Occasionally, immunotherapeutic and antifungal agents are given by intralesional therapy.

Systemic medications are also given for skin conditions. These include the corticosteroids, antibiotics, antifungals, antihistamines, sedatives and tranquilizers, analgesics, and cytotoxic drugs.

Dressings for Skin Conditions

Skin dressings are used to keep topical medication in place and to allay itching and pain. One very effective type of dressing is the *occlusive dressing*, which increases the local skin temperature and hydration and enhances the absorption of topically applied medications. Occlusive dressings also promote the retention of moisture, which keeps the medication from evaporating and reduces the expense of topical corticosteroid treatment. An airtight plastic film, such as Saran Wrap, is applied to cover the medicated skin. Plastic film is advantageous because it is thin and adapts itself readily to anatomical structures of all sizes and shapes. Plastic surgical tape containing corticosteriod in the adhesive layer can be cut to size and applied to individual lesions. Plastic wrap should generally be used no more than 10 to 12 hours a day. The patient is given the following instructions: (1) wash the area, then pat dry; (2) rub the medication into the lesion while the skin is moist; (3) cover with plastic wrap (*e.g.*, Saran Wrap, vinyl gloves, plastic bags); and (4) cover with an ace bandage, stocking, dressing, or paper tape to seal the edges.

It is important to remember that prolonged use of occlusive dressings may cause local skin atrophy, *striae* (band-like streaks), *telangiectasia* (small red lesions caused by dilation of blood vessels), inflammation of hair follicles, nonhealing ulceration or erythema, and systemic absorption of corticosteroids. Dressings should be removed for 12 out of 24 hours to prevent some of these complications.

There are other forms of dressing that can be used to cover topical medications. The best material is soft cotton cloth. Stretchable cotton dressings (Surgitube, Tubegauze) can be used for fingers, toes, and extremities. The hands can be covered with disposable polyethylene or vinyl gloves, sealed at the wrists, while the feet can be wrapped in plastic bags covered by cotton socks. When large areas of the body need to be covered, cotton cloth covered with tubular material can be used. Disposable diapers or cloths folded diaper-fashion are also useful as dressings for the groin and the perineal areas. Sanitary napkins manufactured with an adhesive strip may be used for draining lesions in hairy areas, where tape can cause difficulty. Axillary dressings can be made of cotton cloth taped in place or held by dress shields. A turban or plastic shower cap is useful for holding dressings on the scalp. A face mask may be made from gauze with holes cut out for the eyes, nose, and mouth and held in place with gauze ties looped through holes cut in the four corners of the mask.

If the patient is troubled with itching at nighttime that interferes with sleep, the nurse can advise that wearing cotton clothes next to the skin may be helpful. Excessive warmth is avoided, and the room is kept cool and humidified. The fingernails can be trimmed to prevent injury from scratching while asleep.

▶ *Nursing Process*
The Patient With an Abnormal Skin Condition

▷ *Assessment*

Nursing History

The data base that constitutes the basis of the nursing history may be obtained by asking the following questions:

- When did you first notice this skin problem? (onset, duration, intensity)
- Has it occurred previously?
- Are there any other symptoms?
- What site was first affected?
- What did the rash/lesion look like when it first appeared?
- Where and how fast did it spread?
- Are there itching, burning, tingling, or crawling sensations? loss of sensation?
- Is it worse at a particular time? season?
- Do you have any idea how it started?
- Do you have a history of hay fever, asthma, hives, eczema, allergies?
- Does anyone in your family have skin problems or rashes?
- Did the eruptions appear after certain foods were eaten?
- Had there been recent intake of alcohol?
- Was there a relationship between a specific event and the outbreak of the rash/lesion?
- What medications are you taking?
- What medication (ointment, cream, salve) have you put on the lesion? (Include over-the-counter medications.)
- What skin products do you use?
- What is your occupation?
- What in your immediate environment (plants, animals, chemicals, infections) might be precipitating this problem? Anything new or any changes in the environment?
- Does anything touching your skin cause a rash?
- Is there anything else you wish to talk about in regard to this problem?

Physical Assessment

Assessment of the skin involves the entire skin area, including the mucous membranes, scalp, and nails. *Inspection* and *palpation*, constitute the chief procedures used in examining the skin, and require that the room be well-lighted and warm. The patient should completely disrobe and should be adequately draped.

Examine the general appearance of the skin, observing color, temperature, moisture, dryness, skin texture (rough or smooth), and the condition of the hair and nails. Skin turgor and elasticity are also determined by palpation.

A preliminary look at the eruption or lesion should help to identify the type of dermatosis (abnormal skin condition) and indicate whether the lesion is primary or secondary. At the same time, the anatomical distribution of the eruption should be noted because certain diseases tend to affect certain sites of the body and are distributed in characteristic patterns and shapes. To determine the extent of the regional distribution, the left and right sides of the body should be compared while the color and shape of the lesion(s) are noted. Following observation, the lesions are palpated to determine their texture, shape, and border and to see if they are soft or filled with fluid, or hard and fixed to the surrounding tissue.

A metric ruler is used to measure the size of the lesions so that any further extension can be compared with this initial baseline measurement. The dermatosis is then documented on the patient's record; it should be described clearly and in detail, using precise terminology.

After the characteristic distribution of the lesions has been determined, the following information should be obtained and described clearly and in detail:

- What is (are) the color(s) of the lesion(s)?
- Is there redness, heat, pain, or swelling?
- How large an area is involved? Where is it?
- Is the eruption macular, papular, scaling, oozing, discrete, confluent?
- What is the distribution of the lesion(s)—symmetrical, linear, circular?

Assessing Patients With Dark or Black Skin

The gradations of color that occur in dark-skinned persons are largely determined by genetic transmission; they may be described as light, medium, or dark. In dark-skinned persons, melanin is produced at a faster rate and in larger quantities than in lighter-skinned persons. Healthy, dark skin has a reddish base or undertone. The buccal mucosa, tongue, lips, and nails normally appear pink.

In examining the dark-skinned or black patient, it is important to have good lighting and to look at the skin and the nail beds as well as in the mouth. All suspicious areas should be palpated.

The degree of pigmentation of the black patient's skin may affect the appearance of the lesion. Lesions may be black, purple, or gray instead of the tan or red color seen in white patients.

Erythema.   Because there is a tendency for black skin to assume a purplish grayish cast when an inflammatory process is present, it may be difficult to detect *erythema* (redness of skin due to congestion of the capillaries). To determine possible inflammation, the skin should be palpated for increased warmth or for signs of smoothness (edema) or hardness. The adjacent lymph nodes are also palpated.

Rash.   In instances of itching, the patient should be asked to indicate what areas of the body are involved. The skin is then stretched gently to decrease the reddish tone and make the rash stand out. The differences in skin texture are then palpated by running the tips of the fingers lightly over the skin. Usually, the borders of the rash can be felt. Included in the examination are the patient's mouth and ears. (Sometimes rubeola will cause a red cast to appear on the tip of the ears.) Finally, the patient's temperature is checked and the lymph nodes are palpated.

Cyanosis.   When a person with black skin goes into shock, the skin usually assumes a grayish cast. To determine signs of cyanosis, the areas around the mouth and lips and over the cheekbones and earlobes should be checked. Other indicative signs to check for include a cold, clammy skin; a rapid, thready pulse; and rapid, shallow respirations. When the conjunctivae of the eyelid are checked for *petechiae* (small red spots due to escape of blood), it is important to realize that deposits of melanin may normally appear in this area and should not be misinterpreted as petechiae.

Changes in Skin Color. Changes in skin color that occur in black persons are noticeable and often cause distress to the patient. For example, *hypopigmentation* (loss of or decrease in skin color), which may be due to *vitiligo* (a condition characterized by destruction of melanocytes in limited or extensive skin areas), may cause more concern in the dark-skinned person because it is so readily visible. *Hyperpigmentation* (increase in color) may occur after disease or injury to the skin. A pigmented nasal crease below the eye may be an external sign of allergy. However, pigmented streaks in the nails are considered to be normal.

In general, persons with black skin suffer from the same skin conditions as those with white skin, although they are less apt to have skin cancer and scabies. On the other hand, black and other dark-skinned persons have a greater propensity for keloid or scar formation and for disorders resulting from occlusion or blockage of hair follicles.

Psychosocial Assessment

Because patients with skin conditions (1 in 20 persons) can see and feel their problems, they are more apt to be disturbed by their ailments than are patients with other conditions. Skin conditions can lead to cosmetic disfigurement, social isolation, and economic hardship. Some conditions are often erroneously associated with immorality and contagion. Some conditions can cost the patient a job, with devastating effects on the person's life. Others may subject the patient to a protracted course of illness, leading to feelings of depression, frustration, self-consciousness, and rejection. Itching and skin irritation may also be a constant annoyance and are common features of most skin diseases. The result of these discomforts may be loss of sleep, anxiety, and depression, all of which reinforce the general distress and fatigue that so frequently accompany skin disorders. The meanings attached to skin diseases are often concerns of self-image and interpersonal relationships.

Patients suffering from such physical and psychological discomforts require understanding, explanations of the problem and its treatment, nursing support, unending patience, and continual encouragement. It takes time to help patients gain insight into their problems and work out their difficulties. It becomes imperative, therefore, to overcome any aversion that might be felt when caring for patients with unattractive skin disorders. There must be no sign of hesitancy when approaching these patients. Such behavior would only reinforce the psychological trauma of the disorder. Since very few conditions are contagious, there is no need to fear touching the patient. In fact, touching reduces the patient's sense of isolation, and conveys human warmth and compassion.

▷ Nursing Diagnoses

The nursing diagnoses for patients with dermatoses (abnormal skin conditions) may include the following:

- Potential alteration in skin integrity related to change in barrier function of the skin
- Disturbance in self-image related to unsightly appearance of the skin
- Alteration in comfort (itching) related to skin lesions
- Knowledge deficit of skin care and methods of treating the skin ailment, and about sleep pattern disturbance related to pruritus
- Knowledge deficit of the treatment regimen related to length of treatment or the life-style adjustment required
- Potential fluid volume deficit related to loss of tissue fluids and serum from denuded skin
- Potential sexual dysfunction related to feelings of self-rejection and loss of self-esteem
- Ineffective individual coping related to emotional drain of dealing with an unsightly and often uncomfortable skin condition

▷ Planning and Implementation

▷ *Goals:* The major goals of the patient may include maintenance of skin integrity, relief of discomfort, achieving restful sleep, development of self-acceptance, and acquiring knowledge of skin care.

Nursing Interventions

Maintaining Skin Integrity. Many persons have dry and sensitive skin that is easily irritated. This is especially true of the elderly. Too much washing and scrubbing can increase the problem. Soaps are also irritating. Persons with sensitive skin should be bathed in tepid water with minimal soaping, taking care to rinse well and dry by gently patting the skin with a towel. An emollient can be applied to moist skin to trap moisture. Dry air is irritating because it reduces skin moisture, so keeping the environment humidified is also helpful.

Skin problems of the hands are a common complaint. The skin of the back of the hand is thin, accounting for its sensitivity and dryness and its poor resistance to soaps and detergents. Persons with this problem should protect the hands from contact with soaps, solvents, detergents, and other chemicals by wearing cotton-lined heavy-duty vinyl gloves when handling these agents. Persons with hand irritations can be advised to wear white cotton gloves (cosmetic gloves) for dry housework. The hands should be kept out of water.

In patients with diagnosed skin conditions, the skin should be protected from maceration (excessive hydration of stratum corneum) when applying wet dressings. Thermal injuries should be carefully guarded against.

The patient with a compromised immune system is at increased risk for cutaneous infection. Nursing Care Plan 48-1 (p. 1256) summarizes nursing interventions for persons with dry skin changes related to trauma and infection.

Relieving Discomfort. A rash that seems trivial to the observer may be causing extreme discomfort to the patient. Cystic lesions may be tender and painful. Many skin disorders produce itching, making the patient irritable and unable to sleep. Itching is a significant symptom which scratching does not relieve. The patient is advised to keep cool, especially at night, and to avoid taking hot baths and wearing woolen clothing. If itching persists, the sufferer is advised to see the physician, who may prescribe a topical agent.

In providing care for a patient with itching skin lesions, the nurse attempts to discover the cause of discomfort. A *sudden* onset of generalized rash may indicate a drug allery. Other causes are discussed under "Pruritus" (below).

Nursing interventions appropriate for the relief of itching include humidifying the environment with a room humidifier, maintaining a cool temperature, removing excess bedding and clothing, and limiting the use of soap to one made for sensitive skin. The nails are trimmed to decrease skin damage from scratching. Every effort should be made to keep the skin hydrated and moistened to avoid skin breakdown. The patient is advised to refrain from using over-the-counter preparations to relieve itching because the skin problem may be caused by irritation or sensitization from self-medication.

Gradual evaporation of water from dressings cools the skin and relieves pruritus. The nurse reinforces this teaching, making sure that the patient understands that normal skin should be protected during the application of wet dressings. In removing an adherent dressing, the patient is taught to moisten it before removal to relieve discomfort. When taking therapeutic baths (a form of wet dressing), the patient is advised to limit bathing time to no longer than 30 minutes to prevent skin maceration. Generally, therapeutic baths may be taken twice daily.

Achieving Restful Sleep. Irritation and itching interfere with normal sleep. The nurse may advise the patient of the following measures to promote sleep:

- Keep a regular schedule for sleeping; go to bed at the same time and get up at the same time.
- Avoid caffeinated drinks late in the evening.
- Use a bedtime routine or ritual to ease the transition from wakefulness to sleep.
- Exercise regularly.

In addition, the bedroom should be well-ventilated and humidified. Other measures to promote skin comfort so that the patient may feel more relaxed are found in Nursing Care Plan 48-1 (p. 1256).

Increasing Self-Acceptance. Physical appearance exerts a profound influence in the social world and in the way people are treated. Preferential treatment is often bestowed on someone who is perceived as being attractive. A clean and healthy skin is intimately correlated with one's self-regard.

Skin diseases can be unattractive, causing emotional suffering and affecting social relationships and business and recreational opportunities. Persons with eczema often have difficulty convincing others that their disease is not contagious. Those with flaking and scaling conditions are usually wary of meeting new people. Comments from strangers may be difficult to deal with. A lowering of self-confidence, excessive fixation on skin defects, and worry about scarring are frequently found in persons with acne. All of these factors can generate negative emotions in the patient.

The nurse understands that body image is a complex psychological concept that is related to the mental concept of self and self-esteem. Allowing patients to express their feelings freely gives them a sense of support and acceptance from which strength can be gained. Mutual trust and respect between patient and nurse are necessary to clear the lines of communication. Explore with the patient the strategies that may be used to cope with body image changes.

Informed patients are usually less anxious and more cooperative. Thus, teaching them about their condition and its treatment may make them more hopeful, which may reinforce their ability to use their resources effectively.

Self-care, particularly hair and skin care, can make a difference in the perceptions of others. Appropriate cosmetics can bring substantial benefits to a person with a chronic skin condition or disfigurement. A referal to an expert cosmetitian to camouflage birthmarks, mottled skin, scars, and chronic dermatitis can work wonders. Persons who remain depressed over their condition may benefit from psychological counseling.

Patient Education. A healthy skin reflects one's general health. Principles of good nutrition, exercise, rest, and sleep are emphasized in any teaching program dealing with skin care. Each person can learn that sunlight can permanently damage skin, leading to roughening, freckling, and wrinkling. It is not possible to tan safely without incurring some skin damage.

A patient who is under treatment for a skin condition is usually told by the physician what the skin condition is, its etiology, and what to expect from treatment. The nurse reinforces this teaching. It may be advisable to have a relative or friend of the patient nearby for emotional support and also to listen to the instructions. Some patients do not listen, do not hear, or hear only part of what is being said.

The patient is taught how to apply topical medication, particularly the amount to be used, the size of area to be treated, and the frequency of application. The topical medication is massaged gently onto the affected areas, never rubbed vigorously. In general, the medication is not used on normal skin. Potential side-effects of the medication are discussed. Printed instruction sheets serve to reinforce what has been told.

▷ *Evaluation*

▷ *Expected Outcomes*

1. Patient maintains skin integrity
   a. Indicates absence of skin cracking
   b. Protects skin from contact with irritating substances
   c. Applies emollient to skin as prescribed
2. Achieves relief of discomfort
   a. Uses topical medication and treatments as taught
   b. Reports relief of itching
3. Achieves more restful sleep
   a. States he is "sleeping better"
   b. Reports an increased feeling of well-being
4. Demonstrates increasing self-acceptance
   a. Voices fewer self-depreciating remarks
   b. Pays attention to appearance
5. Acquires understanding of skin care
   a. Verbalizes rationale of prescribed treatment
   b. Demonstrates ability to perform treatments

Nursing management is discussed further in Nursing Care Plan 48-1.

Pruritus

Pruritus (itching) is one of the most common complaints in dermatologic disorders, causing alteration in comfort and changes in the integrity of the skin. Although pruritus is most frequently due to primary skin disease, it may also reflect systemic disease. Thus, it may be the first indication of an internal disease such as diabetes mellitus, blood disorders, or cancer. Itching may also accompany renal, hepatic, and thyroid diseases. Pruritus may be caused by certain oral medications; by the external application of certain drugs, soaps, and chemicals; by prickly heat (*miliaria*); and by contact with woolen garments. Patients may also experience pruritus as a side-effect of radiation therapy or reaction to chemotherapy, analgesics, or antibiotic therapy or as a symptom of infection. Prurutis may occur in the elderly as a result of dry skin. Itching may also be caused by psychological factors.

Because pruritus usually leads to scratching, the secondary effects include excoriations, redness, raised areas on the skin (*wheals*), infections of the skin, and changes in pigmentation. Severe itching is debilitating.

Management

The cause of pruritus, if known, should be removed. The presence of signs of infection and environmental clues such as warm, dry air or irritating bed linens should be checked. In general, washing with soap and hot water is avoided. The application of a cold agent to the skin to help constrict the blood vessels may be helpful. Bath oils (Lubath, Alpha-Keri bath oil) containing a surfactant that makes the oil mix with water in the bath may be sufficient for cleansing. (However, an elderly patient should not add oil to the bath because of the danger of slipping in the bathtub.) Soothing baths containing starch or water-soluble tar derivatives may be prescribed.

Topical steroids may prove useful, not only for their emollient effect but also for their anti-inflammatory effect, which may decrease itching.

Nursing Interventions: Patient Education. The nurse reinforces the reasons for the prescribed medical regimen and guides the patient on specific points of care. If baths have been prescribed, the patient is reminded to use tepid, not hot, water, and to shake off the excess water and blot between intertriginous areas with a towel. Rubbing vigorously with the towel is avoided because this overstimulates the skin, causing more itching. It also removes water from the stratum corneum. Immediately after bathing, the skin should be lubricated with an emollient that traps moisture.

Perianal Itching

Pruritus of the anal and genital regions may be caused by small particles of fecal material lodged in the perianal crevices or attached to anal hairs, or by perianal skin damage caused by scratching, moisture, and decreased skin resistance due to steroids or antibiotics. Other possible causes of perianal itching include local irritants such as scabies and lice, local lesions such as hemorrhoids, fungal or yeast infections, and pinworm infestation. Conditions such as diabetes mellitus, the anemias, hyperthyroidism, and pregnancy may also result in perianal pruritus.

Patient Education and Home Health Care. The patient is instructed to follow proper hygienic measures and to discontinue home and over-the-counter remedies. The perianal area should be rinsed with lukewarm water and the area blot-ted dry with cotton balls. If cleansing after defecation is not possible, premoistened tissues may be used.

As part of health teaching, the patient is instructed to avoid bathing in water that is too hot and to avoid using bubble baths, sodium bicarbonate, or detergent soaps, all of which aggravate dryness. To keep the perianal skin as dry as possible, patients should avoid wearing underwear made of synthetic fabrics. Local anesthetic agents should not be used because of possible allergenic effects. The patient should avoid vasodilating agents or stimulants that increase emotional tension (alcohol, coffee), and mechanical irritants such as rough or woolen clothing. Increasing the humidity with a room humidifier may be useful.

Secretory Disorders

The main secretory function of the skin is performed by the sweat glands, which help to regulate body temperature. These glands excrete a fluid, perspiration, which evaporates and thus cools the body. The sweat glands are located in various parts of the body and respond to different stimuli; those on the trunk generally repond to thermal stimulation; those on the palms and soles respond to nervous stimulation; and those in the axillae and forehead respond to both kinds of stimulation.

As a rule, moist skin is warm, and dry skin is apt to be cool. However, this is not a hard and fast rule. It is not unusual to observe cold sweats; warm, dry skin in a dehydrated patient; and very hot, dry skin peculiar to some febrile states.

Seborrheic Dermatoses

Seborrhea is excessive production of sebum (secretion of sebaceous glands) in those areas where glands are normally found in large numbers (face, scalp, eyebrows, eyelids, at the sides of the nose and upper lip, malar or cheek regions, ears, axillae, under the breasts, groin, gluteal crease of the buttocks).

Seborrheic dermatitis is a chronic inflammatory disease of the skin with a predilection for areas that are well supplied with sebaceous glands or lie between folds of the skin, where the bacterial count is high.

The characteristic lesions are remarkably variable, but this is a dermatitis of the seborrheic areas. It may start in childhood with fine scaling of the scalp or other areas, and may continue throughout life. The scales may be dry, moist, or greasy. There may be patches of sallow, greasy-appearing skin, with or without scaling, and slight erythema, predominantly on the forehead, nasolabial fold, and scalp, and between adjacent skin surfaces in the regions of the axillae, groin, and breasts.

The dry, flaky desquamation of the scalp with a profuse amount of fine, powdery scales is commonly called *dandruff*. The mild forms of the disease are asymptomatic. When scaling is present, it is often accompanied by pruritus, which may lead to scratching and result in secondary complications, such as infections and excoriations.

Seborrheic dermatitis has a genetic predisposition; hormones, nutritional status, infection, and emotional stress influence its course. There are remissions and exacerbations of this condition, which should be explained to the patient.

(Test continues on p. 1258)

Care of Patients With Dermatoses (Abnormal Skin Conditions)

Nursing Interventions	*Rationale*	*Expected Outcomes*

Nursing Diagnosis: Potential alteration in skin integrity related to changes in barrier function of skin

Goal: Maintenance of skin integrity

Changes Related to Trauma

1. Protect healthy skin from maceration (excessive hydration of stratum corneum) when applying wet dressings.		• Patient maintains skin integrity • Absence of maceration • No signs of thermal injury • Absence of infection • Patient applies prescribed topical medication • Takes prescribed medication on schedule
2. Remove moisture from skin by blotting gently and avoiding friction.	2. Friction and maceration play a major role in some skin diseases.	
3. Guard carefully against risks of thermal injuries from excessively hot wet dressings and from subtle heat injuries (heating pads, radiators).		
4. Advise patient to use sun-screening agents	4. Many cosmetic problems and virtually all cutaneous malignancies can be attributed to chronic skin damage.	

Changes From Infection (Related to Entry of Organisms Through Break in Skin)

1. Have a high index of suspicion for an infection in patients with compromised immune systems.	1. Any condition that compromises the immune status increases the risk of cutaneous infection.
2. Instruct the patient clearly and in detail about the therapeutic regimen.	2. Effective patient education is dependent on the interpersonal skills of the health professionals and in giving clear instructions reinforced through written instructions.
3. Apply intermittent wet dressings to reduce intensity of inflammation.	3. A wet dressing produces evaporative cooling, causing constriction of superficial cutaneous vessels and thereby decreasing erythema and serum production. Wet dressings help in debridement of vesicles and crusts and control inflammatory processes.
4. Provide tub baths and soaks.	4. Loosens exudates and scales.
5. Administer prescribed antimicrobial.	
6. Use topical medications containing corticosteroids as prescribed and as indicated. • Observe lesion periodically for changes in response to therapy. • Instruct the patient about possible ill effects of long-term use of fluorinated topical steroids.	6. Corticosteroids have an anti-inflammatory action, resulting in part from their ability to induce vasoconstriction of the small vessels in the upper dermis. • Extensive prolonged use of corticosteroids can lead to adrenal suppression.
7. Advise patient to stop using any skin agent that makes the problem worse.	7. A contact allergic reaction may develop from any ingredient in the medication.

(continued)

Nursing Interventions	Rationale	Expected Outcomes

Nursing Diagnosis: Disturbance in self-image related to unsightly skin appearance

Goal: Development of increasing self-acceptance.

1. Assess patient for disturbance of self-image (avoidance of eye contact, self-negating verbalizations, expression of disgust about skin condition).	1. Disturbance of body image may accompany any disease or condition that is apparent to the patient. An impression of one's own body has an effect on self-concept.	• Patient develops increasing acceptance of own body. • Follows through and participates in self-care measures • Reports feeling in control of situation
2. Identify psychosocial stage of development.	2. There is an interaction among development stage, self-image, and the patient's reaction and interpretation of skin condition.	• Gives self positive reinforcement • Verbalizes a more healthy self-regard. • Appears less self-conscious; is not afraid to socialize and be seen by others
3. Provide opportunity for expression. Listen, in an open, nondefensive way to expressions of grief/anxiety about changes in body image.	3. The patient needs the experience of being heard and understood.	• Uses concealing and high-lighting techniques to enhance appearance
4. Find out what the patient worries about and fears. Assist anxious patient to improve insight and identify and cope with problems.	4. This gives health personnel opportunity to neutralize undue anxiety and restore reality to the situation. Fear is an element destructive to adaptation.	
5. Support patient's efforts to improve body image (participation in skin treatments; grooming).		
6. Help patient toward self-acceptance.		
7. Encourage socialization with others.		
8. Advise patient of available cosmetic measures to conceal disfiguring conditions.		

Nursing Diagnosis: Alteration in comfort (itching) related to skin lesions

Goal: Relief of discomfort

1. Examine area of involvement.
  a. Attempt to discover cause of discomfort.
  b. Record observations in detail, using descriptive terminology.
  c. Be aware that *sudden* onset of generalized rash may indicate drug allergy.
	b. An accurate description of a cutaneous eruption is necessary for diagnosis and treatment. Many skin conditions appear similar but have different etiologies. Cutaneous inflammatory response may be muted in the elderly.	• Patient achieves relief of discomfort.
		• Verbalizes that itching has been relieved
		• Demonstrates absence of skin excoriation and scratch marks
		• Complies with prescribed treatment
		• Keeps skin hydrated and lubricated
		• Demonstrates intact skin; skin regaining healthy appearance

2. Control environmental and physical factors.
  a. Keep humidity about 60 percent; use a humidifier.
  b. Maintain a cool environment.
  c. Use mild soap (Dove) or soap made for sensitive skin (Neutrogena; Aveeno)
  d. Remove excess clothing or bedding.
  e. Wash bed linens and clothing with mild soap.
	2. Itching is aggravated by heat, chemicals, and physical irritants.
	  a. At low humidity, the skin loses water.
	
	  c. These contain no detergents, dyes, or hardening agents.	

(continued)

Nursing Interventions	*Rationale*	*Expected Outcomes*

Nursing Diagnosis: Alteration in comfort (itching) related to skin lesions

Goal: Relief of discomfort

f. Stop repeated exposures to detergents, cleansers, and solvents.	f. Any insult that removes water, lipids, or protein from the epidermis alters the barrier function of the skin.	
3. Use skin-care measures to maintain skin integrity.	3. The skin is an important barrier that must be maintained intact in order to function properly.	
a. Provide tepid cooling baths or cool dressings for itching.	a. Gradual evaporation of water from dressings cools the skin and relieves pruritus.	
b. Treat dryness (xerosis) as prescribed.	b. Dry skin can produce areas of dermatitis with redness, itching, scaling, and in more severe forms swelling, blistering, cracking, and weeping.	
c. Apply skin lotion/cream immediately after bathing.	c. Effective hydration of the stratum corneum prevents compromise of the barrier layer of the skin.	
d. Keep nails trimmed.	d. Trimming decreases skin damage from scratching.	
e. Apply prescribed topical therapy.		
f. Help the patient accept the prolonged treatment that some conditions require.		
g. Advise the patient to refrain from using salves/lotions that are commercially available.	g. The patient's problem may be caused by irritation or sensitization from self-medication.	

Nursing Diagnosis: Sleep pattern disturbance related to pruritus

Goal: Achievement of restful sleep

1. Prevent and treat dry skin.	1. Nocturnal pruritus interferes with normal sleep.	• Patient achieves restful sleep.
a. Advise patient to keep bedroom well ventilated and humidified.	a. Dry air will make skin feel scratchy. A comfortable environment promotes relaxation.	• Reports relief of itching • Maintains appropriate environmental conditions
b. Keep skin moisturized.	b. This prevents water loss. Dry, itchy skin can usually be controlled but not cured.	• Avoids caffeine in late afternoon/evening • Identifies measures to promote sleep • Experiences satisfactory rest/sleep pattern

(continued)

Management

Because there is no known cure for seborrhea, the objective of therapy is to control the disorder and allow the skin to repair itself. Seborrheic dermatitis of the body and face may respond to a topically applied corticosteroid cream, which allays the secondary inflammatory response. However, this medication should be used with caution on the eyelids, because it can induce glaucoma in predisposed persons. Patients with seborrheic dermatitis may develop a secondary *Candida* yeast infection in body creases or folds. To avoid this, patients should be advised to ensure maximum aeration of the skin

Nursing Interventions	*Rationale*	*Expected Outcomes*

Nursing Diagnosis: Sleep pattern disturbance related to pruritus

Goal: Achievement of restful sleep

c. Bathe/shower only as absolutely necessary if skin is excessively dry. Use no soap or only mild soap. Apply skin lotion/cream immediately after bathing while skin is damp.	c. This will trap some of the water absorbed into the skin surface during bathing.	
2. Advise patient of the following measures that may be helpful in promoting sleep:		
a. Keep a regular schedule for sleeping. Go to bed at the same time; get up at same time.	a. Regularity of sleep schedule is important in maintaining sleep hygiene.	
b. Avoid caffeinated drinks late in the evening.	b. Caffeine has peak effect 2–4 hours after being consumed.	
c. Exercise regularly.	c. Exercise appears to have beneficial sleep effect if done in late afternoon.	
d. Use a bedtime routine or ritual.	d. This eases transition from wakefulness to sleep.	

Nursing Diagnosis: Knowledge deficit about skin care and methods of treating skin ailment

Goal: Understanding of skin care

1. Determine what the patient knows (understands and misunderstands) about the condition.	1. Assessment of what patients know and how they perceive the present problem is part of nursing assessment.	• Patient acquires understanding of skin care.
2. Keep the patient informed; correct misconceptions/misinformation.	2. Patients need to have a sense that there is something they can do. Most patients benefit from explanations and reassurance.	• Follows treatment as prescribed and can verbalize rationale for measures taken
3. Demonstrate application of prescribed therapy (wet compresses; topical medication).		• Carries out prescribed baths, soaks, wet dressings
4. Advise the patient to keep skin moist and flexible with hydration and application of skin cream/lotion.	4. The stratum corneum needs water to stay flexible. Application of skin cream/lotion to damp skin prevents dry, rough, cracked, and scaly skin.	• Uses topical medication appropriately • Understands importance of nutrition to skin health
5. Encourage the patient to attain a healthy nutritional status.	5. The appearance of the skin reflects a person's general health. Skin changes may be a feature of abnormal nutrition.	

and to cleanse intertriginous areas carefully. Patients with persistent candidiasis should be evaluated for diabetes.

The mainstay of dandruff treatment is proper shampooing, which should be done frequently (daily or at least 3 times weekly) with medicated shampoos. Two or three different types of shampoo should be used in rotation to prevent the seborrhea from becoming resistant to a particular shampoo. Leave the shampoo on at least 5 to 10 minutes. As the problem gets better, the treatment can be less intense. Antiseborrheic shampoos include those containing selenium sulfide suspension, zinc pyrithione shampoos, salicylic acid sulfur shampoos, and tar shampoos that contain sulfur and salicylic acid.

Nursing Interventions: Patient Education

A person with seborrheic dermatitis is advised to remove external irritants and to avoid excess heat and perspiration, because rubbing and scratching will prolong the disorder. To avoid secondary infections, the patient should air the skin and keep skin folds clean and dry.

Instructions on the use of medicated shampoo are reinforced for those with dandruff that requires treatment.

The patient is cautioned that seborrheic dermatitis is a chronic problem that tends to wax and wane. The goal is to keep it under control. Patients need to be encouraged to adhere to the treatment program. Those who become discouraged and disheartened by the effect on body image should be treated with sensitivity and an awareness of their need to express their feelings.

Acne Vulgaris

Acne vulgaris is a common disorder of the sebaceous (oil) glands and their hair follicles (pilosebaceous follicles). It is characterized by the presence of closed comedones (whiteheads), open comedones (blackheads), papules, pustules, nodules, and cysts. The outbreaks occur most readily on the face and back, where the sebaceous follicles are more numerous.

Acne is the most commonly encountered skin condition affecting an estimated 85% of the population between 12 and 35 years of age. It becomes more marked at puberty and during adolescence, perhaps because at this age certain endocrine glands of the body that influence the secretions of the sebaceous glands are functioning at peak activity. It may persist well into adulthood. The etiology of acne appears to be multiple, reflecting an interplay of genetic, hormonal, and bacterial factors.

Pathogenesis

During childhood, the sebaceous glands are small and virtually nonfunctioning. These glands are under endocrine control, especially the androgens. During puberty, the presence of androgen stimulates the sebaceous glands, causing them to enlarge and to secrete a natural oil, *sebum,* which rises to the top of the hair follicle and flows out onto the skin surface. In adolescents who develop acne, androgenic stimulation produces a heightened response in the sebaceous glands. Acne occurs when the pilosebaceous ducts through which the sebum flows become plugged, resulting in an accumulation of the sebaceous material that plugs the duct. This accumulation of material forms comedones.

Clinical Manifestations

The initial lesions of acne are comedones. *Closed comedones* ("whiteheads") are obstructive lesions formed from impacted lipids or oils and keratin that plug the dilated follicle. Whiteheads are small, whitish papules with minute follicular openings that generally cannot be seen. These closed comedones may evolve into *open comedones*, in which the contents of the ducts are in open communication with the external en-

vironment. Open comedones are termed "blackheads." The color of the blackhead is *not* due to dirt but to an accumulation of lipid, bacterial, and epithelial debris that obstructs the flow of sebum.

Although the exact cause is not known, some closed comedones may rupture and result in an inflammatory reaction due to the leakage of follicle contents (sebum, keratin, bacteria) into the dermis. This inflammatory response may result from the action of certain skin bacteria, such as *Propionibacterium acnes,* that live in the hair follicles and break down the triglycerides of the sebum into free fatty acids and glycerin. The resulting inflammation is seen clinically as papules, pustules, nodules, cysts, or abscesses.

Management

The goals of management are to reduce colonization by the bacteria, decrease sebaceous gland activity, prevent the follicles from becoming plugged, reduce inflammation, combat secondary infection, minimize scarring, and eliminate factors that may predispose to acne. The therapeutic regimen depends on the type of lesion (comedonal, papular, pustular, cystic). A combination of therapies may be tried.

Topical Therapy

Benzoyl Peroxide. *Benzoyl peroxide* preparations are widely used because they produce a rapid and sustained reduction of inflammatory lesions. They also have an antibacterial effect by suppressing *Propionibacterium acnes.* They depress sebum production and lead to the breakdown of the comedone plugs. Initially, benzoyl peroxide causes redness and scaling, but generally the skin adjusts quickly to its use. Usually the patient applies a gel preparation of benzoyl peroxide once daily. In many instances this will be the only treatment needed. Benzoyl peroxide is available over the counter and by prescription.

Vitamin A Acid. Topically applied *vitamin A acid* is used to clear the keratin plugs from the pilosebaceous ducts. Vitamin A acid speeds up the cellular turnover, forces out the comedones, and prevents occurrence of new comedones. Thus it is effective in the treatment of comedonal acne. However, the patient should be informed that symptoms may worsen during early weeks of therapy because inflammation may occur during the process. Erythema and peeling are also a frequent result. Improvement may take up to 8 to 12 weeks. Some patients cannot tolerate this therapy. The patient is cautioned against sun exposure while using this topical medication because it may cause an exaggerated sunburn. Package insert directions are to be followed implicitly.

Topical Antibiotics. The use of *topically applied antibiotics* for the treatment of acne has become widespread. Topical antibiotics suppress the growth of *P. acnes;* reduce skin-surface free fatty acid levels; decrease comedones, papules, and pustules; and do not have systemic side-effects. Topical preparations containing clindamycin, erythromycin, or tetracycline hydrochloride are frequently used.

Systemic Therapy

Systemic Antibiotics. Oral antibiotics given in small doses over a long period are very effective in the treatment of patients with moderate and severe acne, especially when the acne is inflammatory and results in pustules, abscesses, and scarring. Therapy may be continued for months to years. The patient is advised to take tetracycline at least 1 hour before or 2 hours after meals, because the drug is poorly absorbed with food. Side-effects of tetracyclines include photosensitivity, nausea, diarrhea, vaginitis in women, and cutaneous infection in either sex. (In some women, broad-spectrum antibiotics may suppress normal vaginal bacteria and predispose the patient to candidiasis, a fungal infection.)

Oral Retinoids. Synthetic vitamin A compounds (*retinoids*) are being used with dramatic results in patients with nodular cystic acne that is unresponsive to conventional therapy. One compound is *isotretinoin,* which is also used for active inflammatory papular pustular acne that has a tendency to scar. Isotretinoin causes a reduction in sebaceous gland size and inhibits sebum production. It also causes the epidermis to shed (*epidermal desquamation*), thereby unseating and expelling existing comedones. The most common side-effect, experienced by almost all patients, is *cheilitis* (inflammation of the lips). Drying and chapping of the skin and mucous membranes are also frequently encountered. These changes are reversible with the withdrawal of the medication. Most importantly, isotretinoin is teratogenic in humans, meaning that it can have an adverse effect on a fetus. Therefore, contraceptive measures for females of childbearing age are obligatory during treatment and for about 4 to 8 weeks thereafter. Patients are also cautioned not to take vitamin A supplements while on this drug, to avoid additive toxic effects.

Hormone Therapy. Estrogen therapy (progesterone–estrogen preparations) has been found to suppress sebum production and reduce skin oiliness. It is usually reserved for young women when the acne begins somewhat later than usual and tends to flare at certain times in the menstrual cycle, which is often irregular. Estrogen in the form of estrogen-dominant oral contraceptive compounds may be given on a prescribed cyclic regimen. Estrogen is not given to males because of undesirable side-effects.

Surgical Treatment

Surgical treatment of acne consists of comedo extraction, injections of steroids into the inflamed lesions, and incision, and drainage of large, fluctuant, nodular cystic lesions. *Cryosurgery* (freezing with liquid nitrogen) may be used for nodular and cystic forms of acne. Patients with deep scars may be treated with deep abrasive therapy (*dermabrasion,* p. 1289), in which the epidermis and some superficial dermis are removed down to the level of the scars.

Comedo Extraction. Comedones may be removed with a comedo extractor. The site is first wiped with an alcohol sponge. The comedo is nicked with an 18-gauge needle or scalpel blade to incise the follicular opening, widen the port, and facilitate the removal of the comedo. The opening of the extractor is then placed over the lesion, and direct pressure is applied to cause extrusion of the plug through the expressor.

Removal of comedones will leave areas of erythema, which may take several weeks to subside. Recurrence of comedones after extraction is common because part of the comedone frequently remains in the pilosebaceous canal. However, the procedure is of immediate cosmetic benefit and encourages the patient as result of the improvement that occurs.

▶ Nursing Process
The Patient With Acne

▷ Assessment

Virtually all persons will develop an occasional blemish or lesion during adolescence. The nurse, through observation and listening, finds out how patients perceive their skin condition. One young person will view a small blemish as intolerable, while another teenager will regard more extensive involvement as "normal." Adolescents, who are in their formative years of development, are vulnerable and need to be approached with empathy and compassion as they attempt to deal with acne. The nurse keeps this in mind during her assessment and other contacts with them.

When assessing the patient, stretch the skin gently and inspect the lesions. Closed comedones (which are precursors of larger inflammatory lesions) appear as slightly elevated small papules. Open comedones appear flat or slightly raised with a central follicular impaction. Look for and document the presence of inflammatory lesions: papules, pustules, nodules, or cysts.

▷ Nursing Diagnoses

Based on the nursing assessment data, major nursing diagnoses for the patient may include the following:

- Knowledge deficit of cause and treatment of acne
- Disturbance in self-esteem related to embarrassment and frustration over appearance

▷ Planning and Implementation

▷ *Goals:* The major goals of the patient include development of knowledge and understanding of the condition, and development of self-acceptance.

Nursing Interventions

Patient Education and Home Health Care. Before treatment is initiated, patients are counseled and assured that the problem is not related to uncleanliness, dietary indiscretions, masturbation, sexual activity, or any of the other popular misconceptions. Reinforce the concept that acne arises because of a combination of factors, including heredity, large sebaceous glands, and large numbers of *P. acnes* bacteria, all of which are beyond the control of the patient.

When treatment is instituted, it usually takes 4 to 6 weeks or longer for results to be seen. Patients are instructed to wash the face with mild soap and water twice a day to remove the surface oils and prevent obstruction of the oil glands. Caution them to avoid scrubbing the face constantly, since acne is not caused by dirt and cannot be washed away. Mild abrasive soaps and drying agents are prescribed to eliminate the oily feeling that troubles many patients. However, excessive abrasion is to be avoided because it only makes acne worse. It is also important to realize that soap itself can be irritating to the skin. The use of a polyester sponge pad (Buf-Puf) provides the mechanical removal of superficial skin cells (*epidermabrasion*) and may be helpful to some patients. Hair should be kept off the face and shampooed daily if necessary.

All forms of friction and trauma are to avoided: propping the hands against the face, rubbing the face, and wearing tight collars and helmets. Patients are instructed to keep hands away from the face and not to squeeze pimples or blackheads. Squeezing merely worsens the problem, because a portion of the blackhead is pushed down into the skin which may cause the follicle to rupture. Because cosmetics, shaving creams, and lotions can aggravate acne, these substances are best avoided unless the patient is advised otherwise. There is no evidence that a particular food can cause or worsen acne. In general, a nutritious diet is followed.

Patients are counseled that acne is not something that can be cleared up in a short time, and that they must be consistent with treatment *every day*. Reinforce the instruction that they should use the cleansing product prescribed by the physician. Reassure them that most acne medications cause some degree of drying and peeling, although the sudden appearance of diffuse redness and vesicles suggest contact allergy. Continue to clear up misconceptions, because understanding promotes adherence and a better chance of success.

Development of Self-Acceptance. The patient is enrolled as a partner in therapy. It is of great importance that the problems be taken seriously and that the patient be given understanding, reassurance, and support. All facets of the emotional factors involved must be taken into account, including the possibility that acne can become a power struggle between teenager and parents. Stressful situations (*e.g.*, final exams) cause exacerbations. Learning stress reduction techniques may be helpful.

▷ *Evaluation*

▷ *Expected Outcomes*

1. Patient develops increasing understanding of the skin problem
   a. Reviews drawings of obstructive and inflammatory lesions of acne
   b. Reads patient education brochures
   c. Verbalizes that picking and squeezing blemishes/lesions will worsen the condition and may cause scarring
   d. Reads the product information brochure of the prescribed medication
2. Adheres to the prescribed therapy
   a. States he will make a major commitment to required treatment that may take months or years
   b. Verbalizes that he must continue with the treatment when the skin clears
   c. Follows cleansing program
   d. Avoids overcleansing
3. Develops self-acceptance
   a. Avoids mirror-gazing
   b. Identifies someone with whom he can talk over problems
   c. Expresses optimism about outcome of treatment

Infections and Infestations of the Skin

Bacterial Infections (Pyodermas)

Bacterial infections of the skin may be primary or secondary. Primary skin infections originate in previously normal-appearing skin and are usually caused by a single organism. Secondary skin infections arise from a preexisting skin disorder in which several microorganisms may be implicated.

The most common primary bacterial skin infections are impetigo and folliculitis. Folliculitis may lead to furuncles or carbuncles.

Impetigo

Impetigo is a superficial infection of the skin caused by streptococci, staphylococci, or multiple bacteria. The lesions begin as small, red macules, which quickly become discrete, thin-walled vesicles that soon rupture and become covered with a loosely adherent honey-yellow crust (Fig. 48-3). These crusts are easily removed and reveal smooth, red, moist surfaces on which new crusts soon develop. The exposed areas of the body, face, hands, neck, and extremities are most frequently involved. Impetigo is contagious and may spread to other parts of the patient's skin or to other members of the family who touch the patient or use towels that are soiled with the exudate of the lesions.

Although impetigo is seen at all ages, it is particularly common among children living in poor hygienic conditions. Often it appears secondary to pediculosis capitis, scabies, herpes simplex, insect bites, poison ivy, or eczema. In adults,

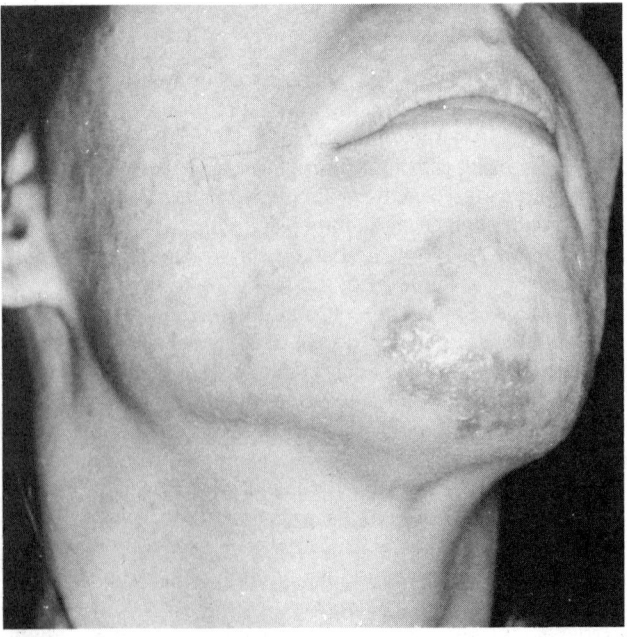

Figure 48-3
Impetigo of the chin. (Courtesy of Mervyn L. Elgart, M.D.)

ill health, poor hygiene, and malnutrition may predispose to impetigo.

Bullous impetigo, a superficial infection of the skin caused by *Staphylococcus aureus,* is characterized by the formation of bullae from original vesicles. The bullae rupture, leaving a raw, red area.

Management. Systemic antibiotic therapy is the usual treatment. It is used to reduce contagious spread, treat deep infection, and prevent acute glomerulonephritis, which has been known to occur as an aftermath of streptococcal skin diseases. In nonbullous impetigo, benzathine penicillin or oral penicillin may be given. Bullous impetigo is treated with a penicillinase-resistant penicillin (cloxacillin, dicloxacillin).

An antiseptic preparation (povidone-iodine [Betadine]; chlorhexidine [Hibiclens]) may be used to cleanse the skin in the vicinity of the infection to prevent spread.

The lesions are soaked or washed with soap solution to remove the central site of bacterial growth and to give the topical antibiotic an opportunity to reach the infected site. After the crusts are removed, a topical medication (*e.g.,* neomycin, bacitracin) is applied. Topical treatment must be done several times a day. Gloves should be worn when care is given to these patients.

Patient Education and Home Health Care. The patient and family should be instructed to bathe at least once daily with bactericidal soap. Cleanliness and good hygienic practices help prevent the spread of the lesions from one skin area to another and from one person to another. Each person should have a separate towel and washcloth. Since impetigo is a contagious disorder, an infected child should be kept away from other children.

Folliculitis, Furuncles, and Carbuncles

Folliculitis refers to a staphylococcal infection that arises within the hair follicles. Lesions may be superficial or deep. Single or multiple papules or pustules appear close to the hair follicles. Folliculitis is commonly seen in the beard area of men who shave and on women's legs.

Pseudofolliculitis barbae ("shaving bumps") is an inflammatory reaction on the face of curly-haired males caused by ingrowing hairs that pierce the skin and cause an irritative reaction. Curly hair has a curved root that grows at a more acute angle. This is a common problem in black males but may also occur in others. The initial treatment is to avoid shaving and grow a beard. If this is not possible, a handbrush may be used over the facial area to dislodge the hairs mechanically. If the patient must shave, a depilatory cream may be useful.

A furuncle (boil) is an acute inflammation arising *deep* in one or more hair follicles and spreading into the surrounding dermis. It is a deeper form of folliculitis. (*Furunculosis* refers to multiple or recurrent lesions.) Furuncles may occur anywhere on the body but are more prevalent in areas subjected to irritation, pressure, friction, and excessive perspiration, such as the back of the neck, the axillae, or the buttocks.

A furuncle may start as a small, red, raised, painful "pimple." Frequently, the infection progresses and involves the skin and subcutaneous fatty tissue, causing tenderness, pain, and surrounding cellulitis. The area or redness and induration represents an effort of the body to keep the infection local-

ized. The bacteria (usually staphylococcus) produce necrosis of the invaded tissues, followed in a few days by the characteristic pointing of a boil. When this occurs, the center becomes yellow or black, and the boil is said popularly to have "come to a head."

A carbuncle is an abscess of the skin and subcutaneous tissue representing an extension of a furuncle that has invaded several follicles and is larger and more deep-seated. It is usually caused by a staphylococcal infection. Carbuncles appear most commonly in areas in which the skin is thick and inelastic. The back of the neck and the buttocks are common sites. In carbuncles, the extensive inflammation frequently is not associated with a complete walling off of the infection, so that absorption occurs, resulting in high fever, pain, leukocytosis, and even extension of the infection to the bloodstream.

Furuncles and carbuncles are more apt to occur in patients with underlying systemic diseases, such as diabetes or hematologic malignancies, and those receiving immunosuppressive therapy for other diseases.

Management. In the treatment of staphylococcal infections, it is important not to rupture or destroy the protective wall of induration that has localized the infection. Therefore, the boil or pimple should never be squeezed.

The follicular disorders (folliculitis, furuncles, carbuncles) are usually caused by staphylococci. If the immune system is impaired, the causative organisms may be gram-negative bacilli.

Systemic antibiotic therapy, selected by sensitivity study, is generally indicated. Intravenous infusions, fever sponges, and other supportive modalities are indicated for the very ill and toxic patient. Warm, moist compresses increase vascularization and hasten resolution of the furuncle or carbuncle. The surrounding skin is cleansed gently with antibacterial soap, and an antibacterial ointment is applied to prevent spillage and seeding of the bacteria in the event that the lesion ruptures or is incised.

When the pus has localized and is fluctuant (moving in palpable waves), a small incision with a scalpel will speed resolution by relieving the tension and ensuring a direct evacuation of the pus and slough. The patient is instructed to keep the draining lesion covered with a dressing. Soiled dressings should be wrapped in paper and burned. Nursing personnel should carefully follow isolation precautions in order to avoid becoming staphylococcus carriers. Disposable gloves should be worn when caring for these patients.

Special precautions must be taken with boils on the face, for the skin area drains directly into the cranial venous sinuses. Sinus thrombosis, with fatal pyemia, has been known to develop after manipulation of a boil in this location.

Bed rest is advised for patients who have boils on the perineum or in the anal region, and a course of systemic antibiotic therapy is indictated to control the spread of the infection.

Patient Education. To prevent and control staphylococcal skin infections (boils, carbuncles), the staphylococcus must be eliminated from the skin and environment. Efforts must be made to increase the patient's resistance and provide a hygienic environment. If lesions are actively draining, the mattress and pillow should be covered with plastic material and wiped off with disinfectant daily; the bed linens, towels, and clothing should be laundered after each use; the patient should shower and shampoo with an antibacterial soap and shampoo for an indefinite period. The prescribed antibiotic should be taken for the full length of time as directed.

Viral Infections

Herpes Zoster (Shingles)

Herpes zoster (shingles) is an inflammatory viral condition in which the virus produces a painful vesicular eruption along the distribution of the nerves from one or more posterior ganglia. It is caused by the varicella virus, commonly known as varicella-zoster virus, which is a member of a group of DNA viruses. (The viruses of chicken pox and zoster are indistinguishable; hence the name varicella-zoster). It is assumed that herpes zoster represents a reactivation of latent varicella (chicken pox) virus and reflects a lowered immunity. After a case of chicken pox runs its course, it is believed that the varicella-zoster viruses responsible for the outbreak lie dormant inside nerve cells near the brain and spinal cord. Later, when these sleeping viruses are reactivated, they travel by way of the peripheral nerves to the skin. There, the viruses multiply, creating a red rash of small fluid-filled blisters. About 10% of adults get shingles during their lifetime, usually after the age of 50. There is an increased frequency of herpes zoster in patients with weakened immune systems and malignancies, especially the leukemias and the lymphomas.

Clinical Manifestations. The eruption is generally accompanied or preceded by pain, which may radiate over the entire region supplied by the nerves. The pain may be burning, lancinating (tearing; sharply cutting), stabbing, or aching. In some patients the pain is absent. Some itching and tenderness may occur over the area. At times malaise and gastrointestinal disturbances precede the eruption.

The patches of grouped vesicles appear on the red and swollen skin. The early vesicles contain serum and later become purulent, rupture, and form crusts. The inflammation is usually unilateral, involving the thoracic, cervical, or cranial nerves in a bandlike configuration. The blisters are usually confined to a narrow region of the face or trunk. The clinical course varies from 1 to 3 weeks. If an ophthalmic nerve is involved, the patient may have a painful eye. Inflammation and a rash on the trunk may cause pain at the slightest touch. The healing time varies between 7 and 26 days.

Herpes zoster in healthy adults is usually localized and benign. However, in immunosuppressed patients, the disease may be severe and the clinical course acutely disabling.

Management. The goals of management are to relieve the pain and to reduce or avoid complications. These include infection, scarring, and postherpetic neuralgia and eye complications.

The pain is controlled with analgesics, because adequate pain control during the acute phase will help prevent persistent pain patterns.

Systemic corticosteroids are given to patients over age 50 to reduce the incidence and duration of postherpetic neuralgia (persistent pain of affected nerve following healing). Healing is usually more rapid in those who have been treated with steroids. Triamcinolone in saline, injected subcutaneously under painful areas, is effective. There is some evidence

that infection is arrested if oral acyclovir is given within 24 hours of the appearance of the eruption. Intravenous acyclovir, if started early, is effective in significantly reducing the pain and halting the progression of the disease. Another antiviral drug, vidarabine, may also be tried.

If the eye is involved, the patient is referred to an ophthalmologist, because keratitis, uveitis, ulceration, and blindness may occur.

A susceptible person can acquire chicken pox through contact with the infective vesicular fluid of a zoster patient. A person with previous history of chicken pox is immune and thus not at risk of infection after exposure to zoster patients. In older persons, the pain from herpes zoster may persist as postherpetic neuralgia for months after the skin lesions disappear.

Patient Education and Home Health Care. The nurse assesses the patient's discomfort and response to medication, and works collaboratively with the physician to make necessary adjustments. The patient is taught how to apply wet dressings or medication to the lesions and to follow proper hand washing techniques to avoid spreading the herpes zoster virus.

Diversionary activities, such as television or crafts, and relaxation techniques are encouraged to assure restful sleep—all of which help to alleviate discomfort.

Because so many of these patients are elderly, a caregiver may be required to assist with dressings. Relatives, neighbors, or a community nurse may need to help with dressing changes and food preparation for patients who are unable to care for themselves or prepare nourishing meals. Emphasize to the patient that vitamin C is necessary to help the lesions heal.

Mycotic (Fungal) Infections

The fungi, tiny representatives of the plant kingdom that feed on organic matter, are responsible for a variety of common skin infections. In some cases, they affect only the skin and its appendages (*i.e.*, hair and nails), but in others, the internal organs are involved. In the latter instance, fungal disease may be so serious as to constitute a threat to life. Superficial infections, on the other hand, rarely cause temporary disability and respond readily to treatment. Secondary infection with bacteria or *Candida* or both may occur.

To obtain material for diagnosis, the lesion is cleaned and a scalpel is used to remove scales from the margin of the lesion. The scales are dropped onto a slide to which potassium hydroxide has been added. The diagnosis is made by examining the infected scales microscopically and by isolating the organism in culture.

Wood's light induces fluorescence of a specimen of infected hair and may be helpful in diagnosing some cases of tinea capitis.

Tinea Pedis (Ringworm of the Feet; Athlete's Foot)

Tinea pedis, the most common fungal infection, is a superficial infection that affects the soles of the feet or the space between the toes. It may be acute or chronic in nature. As an acute infection, it is characterized by the appearance of inflamed vesicles. As a chronic condition, it is manifested as a scaly, dusky or reddened rash. The toenails may or may not be affected; if involved, they are apt to be discolored, brittle, and heaped-up. As a rule, there is moderate to severe itching. Lymphangitis and cellulitis may be seen occasionally when bacterial superinfection occurs. Sometimes a mixed fungal, bacterial, and yeast infection occurs.

Preventive Measures and Patient Education. Because footwear provides a hospitable environment for fungi, the causative fungi may be in the shoes and socks. Because moisture encourages the growth of fungi, the patient is instructed to keep the feet as dry as possible, including the areas between the toes. Small pieces of cotton can be placed between the toes at night to absorb moisture. Socks should be made of absorbent cotton, and hosiery should have cotton feet, since synthetic material does not absorb perspiration as well as cotton. For persons whose feet perspire excessively, perforated shoes permit better aeration of the feet. Plastic or rubber-soled footwear should be avoided. Talcum powder or antifungal powder applied twice daily helps to keep the feet dry. The shoes should be alternated so that they may dry completely before they are worn again.

Management. During the acute (vesicular) phase, soaks of Burow's solution, saline, or potassium permanganate are used to remove the crusts, scales, and debris and to reduce the inflammation. Topical antifungals (miconazole; clotrimazole) are applied to the infected areas. Topical therapy is continued for several weeks, as there is a high rate of recurrence. Clinical and laboratory examinations are done to confirm the causative agent and indicate the treatment. An antifungal agent, griseofulvin, is given orally if there is an extension of the infection or resistance to topical therapy.

Tinea Capitis (Ringworm of the Scalp)

Ringworm of the scalp is a contagious fungal infection of the hair shafts and a common cause of hair loss in children. *Microsporum* and *Trichophyton* species are the dermatophytes (cutaneous fungi) that infect hair. Clinically, one or several round patches of redness and scaling are present. Small pustules or papules may be seen at the edges of such patches. As the hairs in the affected areas are invaded by the fungi, they become brittle and often break off at or near the surface of the scalp, resulting in areas of baldness. Most cases of tinea capitis heal without scarring, so the hair loss is only temporary. Sometimes a boggy swelling resembling a furuncle occurs in an area of involvement; this lesion is known as a *kerion.*

A second form of ringworm caused by *Trichophyton tonsurans* has become prominent in the inner city. It presents as a scaling dermatitis, similar to seborrhea. The skin may be slightly red and scaly, and there are broken-off hairs.

Diagnostic Evaluation. When fungi invade and interact with the superficial layers of the hair shaft, the infected hairs produce a yellow green fluorescence when irradiated by Wood's light. However, infection by the *Trichophyton* species is nonfluorescent.

Management. Griseofulvin, an antifungal agent, is given to patients with tinea capitis. Side-effects of griseofulvin include photosensitivity, headache, skin eruptions, and gastrointestinal disturbances. Topical agents are not effective as a cure because the infection occurs within the hairshaft and below the surface of the scalp. However, topical agents are often used to inactivate organisms already on the hair. This diminishes contagiousness and eliminates the need to clip the hair, which is cosmetically unappealing and only adds to the patient's embarrassment. Infected hairs break off anyway, and noninfected ones may be left in place. The hair should be shampooed 2 to 3 times weekly, and a topical antifungal preparation should be applied to reduce dissemination of the organisms.

Patient Education and Home Health Care. Because the disease is contagious, the patient and family should be advised to set up a hygienic regimen for home use. Each person should have a separate comb and brush and should avoid exchanging headgear. All infected members of the family and household pets must be examined because familial infections are relatively common.

Tinea Corporis (Ringworm of the Body)

Tinea corporis or tinea circinata is ringworm of the body. It begins as an erythematous (red) macule advancing to rings of vesicles with central clearing. The lesions appear in clusters, usually on the exposed areas of the body. These may extend to the scalp, hair, or nails. As a rule, there is an elevated border consisting of small papules or vesicles. Coalescence of individual rings may result in large patches with bizarre scalloped borders. Ringworm of the body may cause intense itching. A frequent cause is the presence of an infected pet in the home.

Management. Topical antifungal medication may be applied to small areas. Griseofulvin is used in extensive cases. Side-effects of griseofulvin include photosensitivity, skin rashes, headache, and nausea. Ketoconazole, an antifungal agent, shows real promise in patients with chronic fungal (dermatophyte) infections, including those resistant to griseofulvin.

Patient Eduation. The patient is instructed to use a clean towel and washcloth daily. All areas and skin folds that retain moisture must be dried thoroughly, because fungal infections are fostered by heat and moisture. Clean cotton clothing should be worn next to the skin.

Tinea Cruris (Ringworm of the Groin)

Tinea cruris ("jock itch") is ringworm infection of the groin, which may extend to the inner thighs and buttock area. It is commonly associated with tinea pedis. It occurs most frequently in young joggers, obese persons, and those who wear tight underclothing. The infection starts with small, red, scaly patches and extends to form circinate (circular) plaques with elevated scaly or vesicular borders. Itching is usually present.

Mild infections may be treated with topical medication such as clotrimazole, miconazole, or haloprogin for at least 3 to 4 weeks to ensure complete eradication of the infection. Oral griseofulvin may be required for more severe infections.

Patient Education and Home Health Care. Heat, friction, and maceration (from sweating) predispose to the infection. The patient is instructed to avoid as far as possible excessive heat and humidity, nylon underwear, tight-fitting clothing, and the prolonged wearing of a wet bathing suit. Concomitant tinea pedis must be treated to minimize reinfection. The groin area should be cleansed, dried thoroughly, and dusted with a topical antifungal agent (tolnaftate [Tinactin]) as a preventive measure, since the infection is apt to recur.

Tinea Unguium (Onychomycosis)

Tinea unguium (ringworm of the nails) is a chronic fungal infection of the toenails or, less commonly, the fingernails, and is usually caused by *Trichophyton* species (*T. rubrum*, *T. mentagrophytes*) or *Candida albicans*. It is usually associated with longstanding fungal infection of the feet. The nails become thickened, friable (easily crumbled), and lusterless. In time, debris accumulates under the free edge of the nail, and ultimately the nail plate becomes separated. The nail may be destroyed.

Management. Griseofulvin is usually given orally for 6 months to a year when the fingernails are involved. Of course, griseofulvin is not of value in treating candidal infections; these must be treated topically with amphotericin-B lotion, miconazole, clotrimazole, nystatin, or other preparations. These products penetrate poorly, and the infections are difficult to treat. Response to griseofulvin in fungal infections of the toenails is poor at best. Toenails are slow-growing organs, with growth from the matrix of the nail to its free edge taking 130 to 160 days (4½ to 5½ months). Therefore, medications have to be used for a year or more, with only a limited chance of cure. Frequently, when the treatment is stopped the infection returns.

Parasitic Skin Diseases

Pediculosis (Infestation by Lice)

Lice infestation affects persons of all ages. Three varieties of lice infest humans: *Pediculus humanus capitis* (head louse); *Pediculus humanus corporis* (body louse); and *Phthirus pubis* (pubic, or "crab," louse). Lice are termed *ectoparasites* because they live on the outside of the host's body. They depend on the host for their nourishment, feeding on human blood approximately 5 times a day. They inject their digestive juices and excrement into the skin, which causes severe itching.

Pediculosis Capitis

Pediculosis capitis is an infestation of the scalp by the head louse, *Pediculus humanaus capitis*. The female head louse lays her eggs (nits) close to the scalp. The nits become firmly attached to the hair shafts with a tenacious substance. The young lice hatch in about 10 days and reach maturity in 2 weeks. Head lice are found most commonly along the back of the head and behind the ears. The eggs are visible to the naked eye as silvery, glistening oval bodies that are difficult to remove from the hair. The bite of the insect causes *intense itching*, and the resultant scratching often leads to secondary bacterial infection with pustules, crusts, matted hair, impetigo, and furunculosis. The infestation is more common in children and people with long hair. Head lice may be transmitted by direct physical contact or indirectly by the use of infested combs, brushes, wigs, hats, and bedding.

Management. Treatment involves washing the hair with a shampoo containing lindane (Kwell) or pyrethrin compounds with piperonyl butoxide (RID or R&C Shampoo). The patient is instructed to shampoo the scalp and hair according to the product directives. After the hair is rinsed thoroughly, it is combed with a fine-toothed comb that is dipped in vinegar to remove any remaining nits or nit shells freed from the hair shafts. These are extremely difficult to remove and may have to be picked off by the fingernails, one by one (thus, the term "nit picking"). All articles, clothing, towels, and bedding that might have lice or nits should be washed in hot water (at least 54°C [130°F]) or dry-cleaned to prevent reinfestation. Upholstered furniture, rugs, and floors should be vacuumed frequently. Combs and brushes are also disinfected with the shampoo. All family members and close contacts are treated.

Complications such as severe pruritus, pyoderma (pus-forming infection of the skin), and dermatitis are treated with antipruritics, systemic antibiotics, and topical corticosteroids.

Patient Education. The patient is reassured that head lice infestation may happen to anyone and is not a sign of uncleanliness. This condition spreads rapidly, so treatment must be started immediately. Control of school epidemics may be helped by having all of the students shampoo their hair on the same night. Students should be warned not to share combs, brushes, or hats. Each family member should be inspected for head lice daily for at least 2 weeks. The patient should be instructed that Kwell may be toxic when not used properly.

Pediculosis Corporis and Pediculosis Pubis

Pediculosis corporis is an infestation of the body by the body louse, *Pediculus humanus corporis*. This is a disease of the unwashed, usually "street people" who do not change their clothing. The body louse lives chiefly in the seams of underwear and clothing, to which it clings as it pierces the skin with its proboscis. Its bites cause characteristic minute hemorrhagic points. Widespread excoriation may appear as a result of intense itching and scratching, especially on the trunk and neck. Among the secondary lesions produced are parallel linear scratches and a slight degree of eczema. In longstanding cases, the skin may become thickened, dry, and scaly, with dark pigmented areas. The areas of the skin chiefly involved are those that come in closest contact with the underclothing (*i.e.*, the neck, trunk, and thighs). The lice may be seen even in the seams of the clothing, so the clothing and bedding must be laundered or dry-cleaned to destroy the parasite and its eggs. A shower should be taken and precautionary methods followed to prevent reinfestation.

Complications, such as severe pruritus, pyoderma (pus-forming infection of the skin), and dermatitis are treated with antipruritics, systemic antibiotics, and topical corticosteroids. It is important to remember that body lice are capable of transmitting epidemic disease in humans, namely rickettsial disease (epidemic typhus, relapsing fever, and trench fever). The causative organism may be in the gastrointestinal tract of the insect and may be excreted on the skin surface of the infested person.

Pediculosis pubis, infestation by *Phthirus pubis* ("crab louse"), is an extremely common problem that is generally localized in the genital region and transmitted chiefly by sexual contact.

Reddish brown "dust" from the excretions of the insects may be found in underclothing. Lice may also infest the hairs of the chest, axillary hair, beard, and eyelashes. Grayblue macules may sometimes be seen on the trunk, thighs, and axillae as a result of either the reaction of the insects' saliva with bilirubin (converting it to biliverdin) or an excretion produced by the salivary glands of the louse. The pubic crease should be examined with a magnifying glass to detect the presence of *Phthirus pubis* crawling down a hair shaft, or nits cemented to the hair or at the junction with the skin. Itching is the most common symptom, particularly at night. Infestation by pubic lice may coexist with other sexually transmitted diseases (gonorrhea, candidiasis, syphilis).

Management and Patient Education. The patient is instructed to bathe with soap and water. Then either lindane (Kwell) or malathion in isopropyl alcohol (Prioderm lotion) is applied to affected areas of the skin and to hairy areas, according to the product information directives. An alternate topical therapy is a pyrethrin-based pediculicide (RID, which is an over-the-counter preparation) or 0.03% copper oleate (Cuprex). If the eyelashes are involved, petrolatum may be thickly applied twice daily for 8 days, followed by mechanical removal of any remaining nits.

All sexual contacts and family members must be treated. The patient and partner(s) must also be scheduled for a workup for coexisting sexually-transmitted disease. All clothing and bedding should be machine-washed or dry-cleaned.

Scabies

Scabies is an infestation of the skin by the itch mite, *Sarcoptes scabiei*. The disease may be found in poor persons living under substandard hygienic conditions, but it is also common in very clean individuals. It is often found among the sexually active. However, infestations are not dependent on sexual activity, because the mites frequently involve the fingers, and hand contact may produce infection. In children, overnight stays with friends or the exchange of clothes may be a source of infection. Health care personnel who have prolonged "hands on" physical contact with an infected patient may likewise become infected.

The adult female burrows into the superficial layer of the skin and remains there for the rest of her life. With her jaws and the sharp edges of the joints of her forelegs, the mite extends the burrow, laying 2 to 3 eggs daily for up to 2 months. She then dies. The larvae (eggs) hatch in 3 to 4 days, and progress through larval and nymphal states to form adult mites in about 10 days.

Clinical Manifestations. It takes approximately 4 weeks from the time of contact for the patient's symptoms to appear. The patient complains of severe itching caused by a delayed type of immunological reaction to the mite or its fecal pellets. During examination, the patient is asked where the itch is most severe. A magnifying glass and a penlight are held at an oblique angle to the skin while a search is made for the small, raised burrows. The burrows may be multiple, straight or wavy, brown or black, threadlike lesions, most commonly observed between the fingers and on the wrists.

Other sites are the extensor surfaces of the elbows, the knees, the outer borders of the feet, the points of the elbows, around the nipples, in the axillary folds, under pendulous breasts, and in or near the groin or gluteal fold, penis, or scrotum. Red pruritic eruptions usually appear between adjacent skin areas. The burrow, however, is not always seen. Any patient with a rash may have scabies.

One classic sign of scabies is the increased itching that occurs at night, perhaps because the increased warmth of the skin has a stimulating effect on the parasite. Also, hypersensitivity to the organism and its products of excretion may contribute to the itching. If the infection has spread, other members of the family and close friends will also complain of itching about a month later.

Secondary lesions are quite common and include vesicles, papules, excoriations, and crusts. Bacterial superinfection may result from constant excoriation of the burrows and papules.

The diagnosis is confirmed by recovering *Sarcoptes scabei* or the mites' by-products from the skin. A sample of superficial epidermis is scraped off the top of the burrows or papules with a small scalpel blade. The scrapings are placed on a microscope slide and examined through a low-powered microscope to demonstrate the presence of any stage of the mite (adult, eggs, egg casings, larva, nymph) and fecal pellets.

Patient Education. The patient is instructed to take a warm, soapy bath or shower to remove the scaling debris from the crusts and then to dry thoroughly and allow the skin to cool. Then a scabicide, such as lindane (Kwell) or crotamiton (Eurax cream and lotion), is applied thinly to the entire skin from the neck down, sparing only the face and scalp (which are not affected in scabies). The medication is left on for 12 to 24 hours, after which the patient is instructed to wash thoroughly. One application is usually curative. The patient should wear clean clothing and sleep between freshly laundered bed linens. All bedding and clothing should be washed in very hot water.

After the treatment is completed, a bland ointment may be applied because the solution may be irritating to the skin. The hypersensitivity state does not cease upon destruction of the mites. Itching may remain a troublesome problem for a few days or weeks because itching is a manifestation of hypersensitivity, particularly in atopic (allergic) persons. However, this is not a sign that the treatment has failed. The patient is instructed *not* to apply more scabicide (as this will cause more irritation and increased itching) and *not* to take frequent hot showers (as this dries the skin and produces itching).

All family members and close contacts should be treated simultaneously to eliminate the mites. If scabies is sexually transmitted, the patient may require treatment for coexisting sexually-transmitted disease. Scabies may also coexist with pediculosis.

Gerontological Considerations. Although the older patient itches severely, the vivid inflammatory reaction seen in younger people is usually absent. Scabies may not be recognized in the elderly, and the itching may erroneously be attributed to the dry skin of old age or anxiety.

For patients in extended care facilities, health care personnel should wear gloves when providing hands-on care for a patient suspected of having scabies until the diagnosis is confirmed and treatment accomplished. No special precautions need be taken when handling the bedding or clothing of these patients.

Contact Dermatitis

Contact dermatitis (dermatitis venenata) is an inflammatory reaction of the skin to physical, chemical, or biologic agents. The epidermis is damaged by repeated physical and chemical irritations. Contact dermatitis may be of the primary irritant type, in which a nonallergic reaction results from exposure to an irritating substance, or it may be allergic in nature (*allergic contact dermatitis*), resulting from exposure of sensitized persons to contact allergens. (Allergic dermatoses are discussed in Chap. 46.) Common causes of *irritant contact dermatitis* are soaps, detergents, scouring compounds, industrial chemicals, and the like. Predisposing factors include extremes of heat and cold, frequent immersion in soap and water, and a preexisting skin disease.

Clinical Manifestations

The eruptions begin at the point at which the causative agent contacts the skin. The first reactions include itching, burning, and erythema, followed soon by edema, papules, vesicles, and oozing or weeping. In the subacute phase, these vesicular changes are less marked and alternate with crusting, drying, fissuring, and peeling. If repeated reactions occur, or if the patient continually scratches the skin, thickening of the skin (*lichenification*) and pigmentation (*coloration*) occur. Secondary bacterial invasion may follow.

Management

The objectives of management are to rest the involved skin and protect it from further damage. The distribution pattern of the reaction is determined in order to differentiate between allergic contact dermatitis and the irritant type. A detailed history is obtained. Then the offending irritant is identified and removed. Local irritation should be avoided, and soap is not generally used until healing occurs.

There are innumerable preparations advocated for the relief of dermatitis. In general, a bland, unmedicated lotion is used for small patches of erythema. Cool, wet dressings also are applied over small areas of vesicular dermatitis. Finely cracked ice added to the water often enhances its antipruritic effect. Wet dressings usually help clear the oozing eczematous lesions. Then a thin layer of cream or ointment containing one of the steroids may be used. Medicated baths at room temperature are prescribed for larger areas of dermatitis.

In more widespread conditions, a short course of systemic steroids may be prescribed. This can diminish the course of a severe disease considerably.

Patient Education and Home Health Care.

The patient is instructed as follows:

- Study the pattern of your dermatitis (location on the skin) and think about things that have touched your skin and may have caused the problem.

- Try to avoid contact with these materials.
- Avoid heat, soap, and rubbing, all of which are external irritants.
- Avoid topical medications except when specifically prescribed.
- Wash the skin thoroughly immediately after exposure to irritants or antigens.
- When gloves are used for washing dishes, use cotton-lined gloves but do not wear them more than 15 to 20 minutes at a time.

The instructions should be followed for at least 4 months after the skin appears to be completely healed, because the resistance of the skin is lowered.

Noninfectious Inflammatory Dermatoses

Psoriasis

Psoriasis is a chronic inflammatory disease of the skin in which the production of epidermal cells occurs at a rate that is approximately 6 to 9 times faster than normal. The cells in the basal layer of the skin divide too quickly, and the newly formed cells move so rapidly to the skin surface that they become evident as profuse scales or plaques of epidermal tissue. The psoriatic epidermal cell may travel from the basal cell layer of the epidermis to the stratum corneum (skin surface) and be cast off in 3 to 4 days, which is in sharp contrast to the normal 26 to 28 days. As a result of the increased number of basal cells and rapid cell passage, the normal events of cell maturation and growth cannot take place. This abnormal process does not allow formation of the normal protective layers of the skin.

Psoriasis, one of the most common skin diseases, affects approximately 2% of the population. There appears to be a hereditary defect that causes overproduction of keratin. The primary defect is unknown. A combination of specific genetic makeup and environmental stimuli may trigger the onset of the disease. There is some evidence that the cell proliferation is mediated by the immune system. Periods of emotional stress and anxiety aggravate the condition, and trauma, infections, and seasonal and hormonal changes are trigger factors. The onset may occur at any age, but is most common between the ages of 10 and 35 years. Psoriasis has a tendency to improve and then recur throughout life.

Clinical Manifestations

The lesions appear as red, raised patches of skin covered with silvery scales. The scaly patches are formed by the build-up of living and dead skin that results from the vast increase in rate of skin-cell growth and turnover (Fig. 48-4). If the scales are scraped away, the dark red base of the lesion is exposed, producing multiple bleeding points. These patches are not moist and may or may not itch. The lesions may remain small, giving rise to the term "guttate psoriasis." Usually, the lesions enlarge slowly, but after many months they

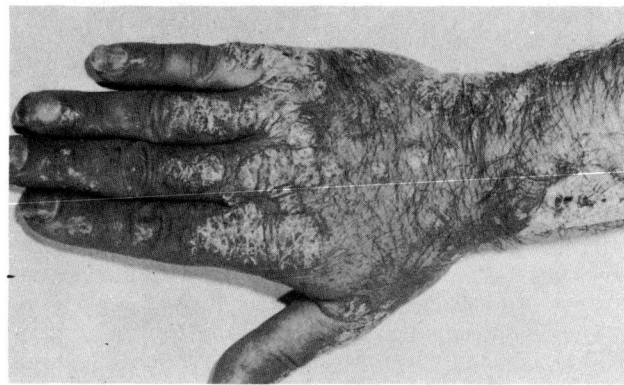

Figure 48-4
Psoriasis of the hand. (Sauer GC. Manual of Skin Diseases. Philadelphia, JB Lippincott.)

coalesce, forming extensive irregularly shaped patches. Psoriasis may range from a cosmetic source of annoyance to a physically disabling and disfiguring affliction. Particular sites of the body tend to be affected by this ailment; they include the scalp, the area over the elbows and knees, the lower part of the back, and the genitalia. Psoriasis also appears on the extensor surfaces of the arms and legs, on the scalp and ears, and over the sacrum and the intergluteal fold. Bilateral symmetry is a feature of psoriasis. In approximately one quarter to one half of the patients, the nails are involved, with pitting, discoloration, crumbling beneath the free edges, and separation of the nail plate. When psoriasis occurs on the palms and soles, it can cause pustular lesions. The disease may be associated with arthritis of multiple joints, causing a crippling disability. The relationship between arthritis and psoriasis is not understood. Another complication is an exfoliative psoriatic state in which the disease progresses to involve the total body surface.

Psychological Considerations

Psoriasis may cause despair and frustration for the patient; observers may stare, comment, ask embarrassing questions, or even avoid the person. The disease can eventually exhaust the patient's resources, interfere with his job, and make life miserable in general. Teenagers are especially vulnerable to the psychological effects of this ailment. Many a teenager's personality has been scarred by the occurrence of such a disfiguring disease at a stage of life when appearance is all-important. The family, too, is affected, since time-consuming treatments, messy salves, and constant shedding of scales disrupt home life and cause resentment. In many cases, the patient's frustrations are expressed through hostility directed at health care personnel.

Management

The goals of management are to reduce the rapid turnover of epidermis and to promote resolution of the psoriatic lesions. Thus, the goal is limited to control of the problem, because there is no known cure.

The therapeutic approach should be one that the patient understands; it should be cosmetically acceptable and not too disruptive of life-style. It will involve the commitment of time and effort by the patient and possibly the family.

First, any precipitating or aggravating factors are removed. Then an assessment is made of life-style, since psoriasis is significantly affected by stress. The patient must also be advised that treatment of a severe psoriasis can be time-consuming, expensive, and esthetically unappealing at times.

Therapy can be divided into three types: topical, intralesional, and systemic.

Topical Therapy. Topically applied agents are given to slow down the overactive epidermis without affecting other tissues. Medications include such agents as tar preparations, anthralin, salicylic acid and corticosteroids. These therapies seem to act by suppressing *epidermopoiesis* (creation of epidermal cells).

Tar is formulated as lotions, ointments, pastes, creams, and shampoos. Tar baths or tar preparations may retard and inhibit the rapid growth of psoriatic tissue. This aspect of therapy may be combined with carefully graded doses of ultraviolet-B light, which produces radiation in wavelengths between 280 and 320 nm. Ultraviolet-B light seems to potentiate the action of tar. The tar is partially removed prior to ultraviolet light exposure to allow maximum transmission of light. During this phase of treatment, the patient is advised to wear goggles and to protect the eyes. Using a timer will prevent the danger of severe burns due to overexposure to the light rays. A daily tar shampoo followed by an application of steroid lotion may be used for scalp lesions. The patient is also taught to remove excess scales by scrubbing with a soft brush while bathing.

Anthralin preparations (a distillate of crude coal tar) are useful for thick and resistant psoriatic plaques. The patient is instructed to apply anthralin medication with a tongue blade or gloved fingers, taking special care not to cover normal skin. The hands must be washed after the medication is handled, because a chemical conjunctivitis can be produced if the patient touches the eyes while medication is still on the hands. Anthralin stains badly and should be covered in some way (gauze dressings, stockinette, old pajamas) when applied. The preparation is left on the skin for 8 to 12 hours.

Topical Steroids. Topical steroids may be applied for their anti-inflammatory activity. Once the medication is applied, the area is covered with an occlusive plastic film dressing to enhance drug penetration and soften the scaly plaques. Tape that is impregnated with steroid medication may be used in patients with relatively few but resistant psoriatic plaques. However, once the steroid treatment is stopped, the psoriasis may quickly reappear (rebound phenomenon) and, in some instances, be more extensive than the original lesions.

Occlusive Dressings. Some patients will require occlusive dressings over the entire body. For the hospitalized patient, large plastic bags may be used—one for the upper body (with holes cut out for the head and arms) and one for the lower part (with holes for the legs). This leaves only the extremities to wrap. In some dermatologic units, large rolls of tubular plastic are used (such as the kind that dry-cleaners place over clean clothes). However, when these substances are used, *it is important to check for flammability*. Some of these thin, plastic films will burn slowly (if touched by a lighted cigarette), whereas others will burst rapidly into flame and may cause severe injury. The patient should be cautioned not to smoke while wrapped in these dressings.

In patients being treated at home, a plastic vinyl jogging suit may be purchased. The medication is applied and the suit simply put over it. The hands can be wrapped in gloves, the feet in plastic bags, and the head in a shower cap. The suit can be machine-washed, making a difficult task much easier.

Intralesional Therapy. Intralesional injections of triamcinolone acetonide directly into highly visible or isolated patches of psoriasis are highly effective and seldom produce side-effects.

Systemic Therapy. Systemic cytotoxic preparations, such as methotrexate, have been used in treating extensive psoriasis that fails to respond to other forms of therapy. Methotrexate appears to function by inhibiting DNA synthesis in epidermal cells, therefore reducing the turnover time of the psoriatic epidermis. However, the drug can be very toxic, especially to the liver, which can suffer irreversible damage. Thus, laboratory studies must be monitored to ensure that the hepatic, hematopoietic, and renal systems are functioning adequately.

The patient should avoid drinking alcohol while on methotrexate, because this increases the possibility of liver damage. The drug is teratogenic (producing physical defects in the fetus) in pregnant women.

Oral Retinoids. Oral retinoids (synthetic derivatives of vitamin A and its metabolite, vitamin A acid) modulate the growth and differentiation of epithelial tissue and thus show great promise in treating the patient with severe psoriasis.

Another drug currently being used is hydroxyurea (Hydrea), which inhibits cell replication by affecting DNA synthesis. The patient is monitored for signs and symptoms of bone marrow depression.

Photochemotherapy (Psoralen Ultraviolet-A Light Therapy; PUVA Therapy). A treatment for severely debilitating psoriasis is PUVA (psoralen and ultraviolet-A) therapy, which involves the patient taking a photosensitizing drug (usually 8-methoxypsoralen) in a standard dose with subsequent exposure to long-wave ultraviolet light when peak drug plasma levels are obtained. Although the mechanism of action is not completely understood, it is assumed that there is an interaction between the psoralen molecule and light energy, resulting in decrease in cellular proliferation. PUVA is not without its hazards; it has been associated with long-term risks of skin cancer, cataracts, and premature aging of the skin.

PUVA therapy requires that psoralen be taken orally, followed in 2 hours by irradiation with high-intensity long-wave ultraviolet light (UVA). (Ultraviolet light is the portion of the electromagnetic spectrum containing wave lengths from 180 nm to 400 nm.) The PUVA unit consists of a light cabinet containing high-output blacklight lamps and an external reflectance system. The exposure time is calibrated according to the specific unit in use and the anticipated tolerance of the patient's skin. The patient is usually treated 2 to 3 times a week until the psoriasis clears. An interim period of 48 hours between treatments is necessary, because it takes this long for any PUVA burns to become evident. The patient is then placed on a maintenance program. Once little or no disease is present, less potent therapies are used to keep minor flare-ups under control.

Patient Education During PUVA Therapy. PUVA treatment produces photosensitization, which means that the patient is sensitive to the sun until methoxsalen has been ex-creted from the body (about 6 to 8 hours). Therefore, exposure to the sun must be avoided at this time. If exposure is unavoidable, the skin must be protected with sunscreen and clothing. Gray- or green-tinted wraparound sunglasses should be worn to protect the eyes during and after treatment. Ophthalmologic examinations are carried out on a regular basis. Nausea, which may be a problem in some patients, is lessened when methoxsalen is taken with food. Lubricants and bath oils may be used to help remove scales and prevent excess dryness. No other creams or oils are to be used except on areas that have been shielded from ultraviolet light. Contraceptives should be used by sexually active women of reproductive age, as the teratogenic risk of PUVA has not been established. The patient must remain under constant and careful supervision and is encouraged to look for unusual changes in the skin.

▶ Nursing Process
The Patient With Psoriasis

▷ Assessment

The nursing assessment focuses on how the patient is functioning with the skin condition, the appearance of the "normal" skin, and the appearance of the skin lesions. (See Clinical Manifestations, above.) The major manifestations to note are red, scaling papules that coalesce to form oval, well-defined plaques. Silvery white scales are also present. Adjacent skin areas reveal red, smooth plaques with a macerated surface. Examine the areas especially favored by psoriasis: elbows, knees, scalp, gluteal cleft, fingers, and toenails (for small pits).

▷ Nursing Diagnoses

Based on the nursing assessment data, major nursing diagnoses for the patient may include the following:

- Knowledge deficit of the disease process and treatment
- Impairment of skin integrity related to diminished protective function of the stratum corneum
- Disturbance in body image related to embarrassment over appearance and self-perception of uncleanliness
- Potential sexual dysfunction related to visible red and scaling lesions

▷ Planning and Implementation

▷ *Goals:* The major goals of the patient may include acquisition of knowledge about psoriasis and its treatment, and achievement of smoother skin with control of lesions.

Nursing Interventions

Patient Education. The patient is told with sensitivity that at the present time there is no permanent cure for psoriasis, that lifetime management is necessary, but that the condition can usually be cleared and controlled. Review what psoriasis is and that the method by which the patient's skin replenishes itself is abnormal. The factors that provoke psoriasis are reviewed: any irritation or injury to the skin (cut, abrasion, sunburn), any current illness (*e.g.*, pharyngeal infection), and emotional stress. Emphasize that repeated trauma to the skin as well as an unfavorable environment (cold) and any drug (lithium, beta blockers, indomethacin) may exacerbate psoriasis. The patient should be advised not to pick or scratch the psoriasis areas to avoid injuring the skin. In addition, any topical irritant or allergy-producing substance is to be avoided. The patient should report to the physician any infection especially a streptococcal sore throat, that appears to aggravate the psoriasis. The patient is cautioned about taking any medication, as some drugs may worsen a mild psoriasis. It is also important to emphasize the need for a balanced life, including recreation, exercise, and rest.

Keep the skin from drying out, because dry skin causes psoriasis to worsen. Too frequent washing produces more soreness and scaling. Water should not be too hot, and the skin is dried by patting with a towel rather than vigorous rubbing. Emollients have a moisturizing effect by providing an occlusive body film on the skin surface so that normal water loss through the skin is halted, allowing the trapped water to hydrate the stratum corneum. A bath oil or emollient cleansing agent can give comfort to sore and scaling skin. Softening the skin can prevent fissuring. (See also Nursing Care Plan 48-1, p. 1256.)

Successful treatment of psoriasis takes persistence and patience because treatment is constant, interminable, and expensive. Some patients spend 2 or more hours daily in applying medications and carrying out other cosmetic efforts. The patient is taught to use topical therapy appropriately. A therapeutic alliance with health care professionals should be educative and supportive, and should help the patient move toward self-acceptance. Mental health professionals can ease emotional strain and give recognition and support. Belonging to a support group helps patients acknowledge that they are not alone in experiencing life adjustments in response to a visible, chronic disease. The National Psoriasis Foundation publishes periodic bulletins and reports updating new and relevant developments about this condition. (See Bibliography for the address.)

▷ *Evaluation*

▷ *Expected Outcomes*

1. Patient acquires knowledge and understanding of psoriasis.
   a. Describes psoriasis and the prescribed therapy
   b. Verbalizes that trauma, infection, and emotional stress may be trigger factors
2. Achieves smoother skin and control of lesions
   a. No new lesions appear.
   b. Keeps skin lubricated and soft.
3. Adheres to the therapeutic regimen
   a. Maintains control with appropriate therapy
   b. Demonstrates proper application of topical therapy

Exfoliative Dermatitis

Exfoliative dermatitis is a serious condition characterized by a progressive inflammation in which erythema and scaling often occur in a more or less generalized distribution. It may be associated with chills, fever, prostration, severe toxicity, and an itchy scaling of the skin. There is a profound loss of stratum corneum (outermost layer of the skin), which causes capillary leakage, hypoproteinemia, and negative nitrogen balance. The iron loss from the skin produces anemia. Thus, exfoliative dermatitis has a marked effect on the entire body.

Exfoliative dermatitis has a variety of causes. It is considered to be a secondary or reactive process to an underlying skin or systemic disease. It may appear as a part of the lymphoma group of diseases, and may actually precede the appearance of lymphoma. It also appears as a severe reaction to a wide number of drugs, including penicillin and phenylbutazone.

This condition starts acutely as either a patchy or a generalized erythematous eruption accompanied by fever, malaise, and, occasionally, gastrointestinal symptoms. The skin color changes from pink to dark red; then, after a week, the characteristic exfoliation (scaling) begins, usually in the form of thin flakes that leave the underlying skin smooth and red, new scales forming as the older ones exfoliate (cast off). Hair loss may accompany this disorder. Relapses are the rule. The systemic effects include high-output congestive heart failure, intestinal disturbances, breast enlargement (gynecomastia), elevated levels of uric acid in the blood (hyperuremia), and temperature disturbances.

Management. The objectives of management are to maintain fluid and electrolyte balance and to prevent intercurrent or cutaneous infection. The treatment is individualized and supportive, and depends on the cause. The patient is hospitalized and placed on bed rest. All drugs that may be implicated are stopped. A comfortable room temperature should be maintained, since the patient does not have normal thermoregulatory control because of fluctuations in temperature due to vasodilatation and evaporative water loss. The fluid and electrolyte balance must be maintained, since there is considerable water and protein loss from the skin surface. Plasma expanders may be indicated.

Continual nursing assessment is carried out to detect intercurrent and cutaneous infection. The erythematous, moist skin is receptive to infection and becomes colonized with pathogenic organisms, which produce more inflammation. Antibiotics are given if infection is present, and are selected on the basis of culture and sensitivity.

- Watch for signs and symptoms of congestive heart failure, because hyperemia and increased cutaneous blood flow can produce a cardiac failure of high output origin.

Hypothermia may also occur as increased skin blood flow, coupled with increases in water loss through the skin, leads to heat loss by radiation, conduction, and evaporation.

As in any acute dermatitis, topical therapy is used to give symptomatic relief. Soothing baths, compresses, and lubrication with emollients are used to treat the extensive dermatitis. The patient is likely to be extremely irritable because of the severe itching. Oral or parenteral steroids may be given when the disease is not controlled by more conservative therapy. When a specific cause is known, more specific therapy may be used.

Patient Education. The patient is advised to avoid all irritants in the future, particularly drugs.

Pemphigus Vulgaris

Pemphigus vulgaris is a serious disease of the skin characterized by the appearance of bullae (blisters) of various sizes

(1 cm–10 cm) on apparently normal skin (Fig. 48-5) and mucous membranes (mouth, vagina).

Available evidence indicates that pemphigus is an autoimmune disease. (See Chap. 45.) Genetic factors may also play a role in its development. The disorder usually occurs in middle and late adult life.

Clinical Manifestations. The majority of patients initially present with oral lesions appearing as irregularly-shaped erosions that are painful, bleed easily, and heal slowly. The skin bullae enlarge, rupture, and leave large, painful eroded areas that are accompanied by crusting and oozing. A characteristic offensive odor emanates from the bullae and the exuding serum. There is blistering or sloughing of uninvolved skin when minimal pressure is applied (Nikolsky's sign). The eroded skin heals slowly, so that eventually huge areas of the body are involved. Bacterial superinfection is common.

Diagnostic Evaluation. A biopsy specimen from the blister and surrounding skin will demonstrate *acantholysis* (separation of epidermal cells from each other because of damage to or an abnormality of the intracellular substance). Circulating antibodies (pemphigus antibodies) may be demonstrated by immunofluorescent studies of the patient's serum.

Management. The goals of therapy are to bring the disease under control as rapidly as possible, to prevent loss of serum and the development of secondary infection, and to promote reepithelialization of the skin.

Corticosteroids (prednisone) are administered in large doses to control the disease and keep the skin free of blisters. The high dosage level is maintained until remission is apparent. Prednisone is given with or immediately after a meal and may be accompanied by an antacid as prophylaxis against gastric complications. Essential to the patient's therapeutic management are daily evaluations of body weight, measurement of blood pressure, testing of blood for glucose, and recording of fluid balance. (High-dosage corticosteroid therapy has its own serious toxic effects.)

Immunosuppressive agents (azathioprine; cyclophosphamide; gold) may be given to help control the disease and

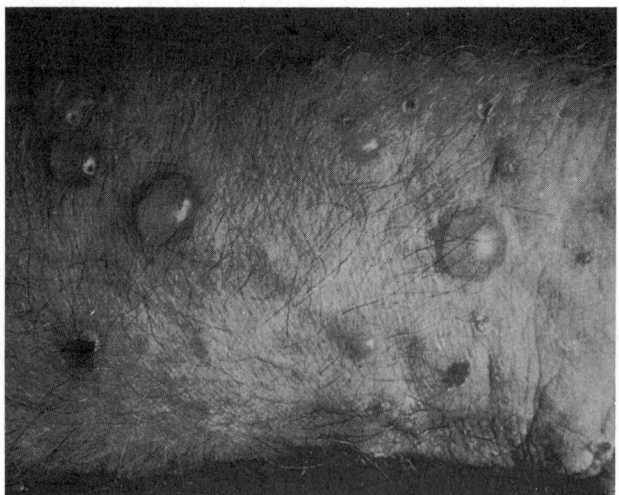

Figure 48-5
Pemphigus vulgaris bullae on the wrist. (Sauer GC. Manual of Skin Diseases. Philadelphia, JB Lippincott.)

reduce the steroid dose. *Plasmapheresis* (reinfusion of specially treated plasma cells) temporarily decreases the serum level of antibodies and has been used with variable success.

▶ Nursing Process
The Patient With Pemphigus

▷ Assessment

Because patients with pemphigus are invariably hospitalized at one time or another during exacerbations of the disease, the nurse soon discovers that pemphigus is perhaps the most debilitating skin disease of all. The constant misery of the patient and foul smell of the lesions make effective assessment and nursing management a challenge.

Disease activity is monitored clinically by examining the skin for the appearance of new blisters, which are usually tense and not easily broken. Look at the scalp, chest, and adjacent skin areas for blistering. Particular attention is given to assessing for signs and symptoms of infection.

▷ Nursing Diagnoses

Based on nursing assessment data, major nursing diagnoses for the patient may include the following:

- Alteration in oral mucous membranes related to blistering and erosions
- Alteration in skin integrity related to ruptured bullae and denuded areas of the skin
- Potential fluid and electrolyte imbalance related to loss of tissue fluids
- Anxiety and ineffective coping related to appearance of the skin

Possible complications that might develop include opportunistic infections, psychosis, and hyperglycemia.

▷ Planning and Implementation

▷ **Goals:** The major goals of the patient may include relief of discomfort from oral lesions, achievement of skin healing, fluid and electrolyte balance, avoidance of infection, reduction in anxiety, and an improvement in coping capacity.

Nursing Interventions

Relieving Oral Discomfort. The patient's entire oral cavity may be affected with erosions and denuded surfaces. A necrotic slough may develop over these areas, adding greatly to the patient's misery and interfering with food intake. Weight loss and hypoproteinemia may thus result. Meticulous oral hygiene is important to keep the oral mucosa clean and allow for regeneration of epithelium. Prescribed mouth washes are used to rinse the mouth of debris. This is done frequently to soothe ulcerative areas. Commercial mouth washes are avoided. The lips are kept moist with lanolin, petrolatum, or lip balm. Cool mist therapy is helpful to humidify environmental air.

Cool, nonirritating fluids (*e.g.*, grape or apple juice) are encouraged to maintain hydration. Small, frequent feedings of high-protein, high-calorie foods (Ensure®; Sustacal®; egg-nogs; milkshakes) will help maintain nutritional status. Parenteral nutrition is considered if the patient is unable to eat.

Secondary infection may be associated with offensive odor from oral lesions. *Candida albicans* of the mouth is frequently seen in patients on high-dose steroid therapy. The oral cavity should be inspected daily and any changes noted and reported. Oral lesions are slow to heal.

Control of Infection. The patient is susceptible to infection because the barrier function of the skin is compromised. Bullae are also susceptible to infection, and septicemia may follow.

The skin is kept clean to eliminate debris and dead skin and to prevent infection.

Infection is the leading cause of death. Particular attention is given to assessing the patient for signs and symptoms of local and systemic infection. Be suspicious of trivial complaints or minimal changes, because steroids mask or alter typical signs and symptoms of infection. The vital signs are taken and temperature fluctuations monitored. The patient is observed for chills, and all secretions and excretions are monitored for suspicious changes. Results of culture and sensitivity tests are followed. Antimicrobials are administered as prescribed, and response to treatment is noted. Health care personnel should employ effective hand washing techniques. Environmental contamination is avoided as much as possible by having the housecleaning personnel dust with a damp cloth and wash the floor with a wet mop.

Skin Care. Cool, wet dressings or baths are protective and soothing. Patients with large areas of blistering have a characteristic odor that is lessened when secondary infection is controlled. Potassium permanganate baths help keep the areas from becoming infected and to some extent precipitate some of the protein that oozes through the open skin. They also have deodorant properties. The potassium permanganate crystals should be thoroughly dissolved, as undissolved crystals can burn the skin. Following the bath, the patient is dried carefully and dusted liberally with talcum powder, which enables the patient to move freely in bed. Fairly large amounts are necessary to keep the patient from sticking to the sheets. Tape should never be used on the skin because it may produce more blisters.

The nursing management of patients with bullous skin conditions is similar to that of patients with extensive burns (see Chap. 49).

Achieving Fluid and Electrolyte Balance. Extensive denudation of the skin leads also to fluid and electrolyte imbalance. There is significant loss of tissue fluids, and therefore of sodium chloride. This salt loss is responsible for many of the constitutional symptoms associated with the disease, and is combated with administration of saline infusions.

A large amount of protein and blood is lost from the denuded skin areas. Blood or component therapy may be prescribed to maintain the blood volume as well as the hemoglobin and plasma protein concentrations. The patient is encouraged to attain adequate oral fluid intake. Serum albumin and protein levels are monitored.

Reducing Anxiety. Critical to the nursing management of the patient with pemphigus is the development of a trusting relationship. One has to enter the world of the patient to create such a relationship. This encompasses the way the nurse listens, interacts, and demonstrates a warm and caring concern. The patient has legitimate concerns that may be reduced when the health team shows appropriate concern. The patient is allowed free expression of anxieties, discomfort, and feelings of hopelessness. This is necessary for specific reassurance to be more effective.

Attention to the psychological needs of this patient require being available, giving expert nursing care, and educating the patient and the family. This provides support from which the patient gains strength. Arranging for a family member/significant other to spend more prolonged periods of time with the patient can be supportive. When patients receive information about the disease and its treatment, uncertainty is reduced and the patients' capacity to act on their own behalf is enhanced.

If the patient continues to exhibit fear, anxiety, and depression, a referral for psychological counseling may be helpful.

Patient Education. The disease can be characterized by recurrent relapses that require continuing therapy to maintain clinical control. Regular monitoring for the side-effects of corticosteroids is necessary. Long-term administration of immunosuppressive drugs is associated with increased risk of cancer. The patient is to report for health-care follow-up regularly.

▷ *Evaluation*

▷ *Expected Outcomes*

1. Patient achieves relief from pain of oral lesions.
   a. Identifies therapies that reduce pain
   b. Uses mouth washes and anesthetic–antiseptic aerosol mouth spray
   c. Drinks chilled fluids at 2-hour intervals
2. Achieves skin healing
   a. States purpose of therapeutic regimen
   b. Cooperates with soaks/bath regimen
   c. Reminds personnel to use liberal amounts of powder on sheets
3. Attains fluid and electrolyte balance
   a. Keeps input record to assure adequate fluid intake
   b. Verbalizes an understanding of the necessity of intravenous infusion therapy
   c. Reports that urine output is within normal limit
   d. Has serum chemistries within normal limits
4. Is free of infection
   a. Cultures from bullae, skin, and orifices are negative for pathogenic organisms.
   b. Shows signs that skin is clearing.

Toxic Epidermal Necrolysis (TEN)

Toxic epidermal necrolysis (TEN) is a severe, potentially fatal skin disease. Its etiology is unknown, but it is probably linked to the immune system as a reaction to drug ingestion or possibly secondary to a viral infection. Antibiotics, barbiturates, hydantoins, butazones, and sulfonamides are the drugs most frequently implicated. TEN is characterized by initial signs of conjunctival burning or itching, cutaneous tenderness, fever, headache, extreme malaise, and myalgias. These signs are followed by rapid onset of erythema, involving much of the skin surface. Large, flaccid bullae develop in some areas, while in other areas large sheets of epidermis are shed, exposing the underlying dermis. Fingernails, toenails, eyebrows, and eyelashes may all be shed along with the surrounding epidermis. The skin is excruciatingly tender, and the loss of skin leaves a weeping surface similar to that of a second-degree burn. The patient with TEN is severely ill. High fever, tachycardia, and extreme weakness and fatigue are seen, perhaps as a result of the process of epidermal necrosis, increased metabolic needs, and possible gastrointestinal and respiratory mucosal sloughing. (The mucosa can have an injury similar to that of the skin.)

The major cause of death is infection, and the most common sites of infection are the skin and mucosal surfaces, lungs, and blood. The organisms most frequently recovered are *Staphylococcus aureus, Pseudomonas, Klebsiella, Escherichia coli, Serratia,* and *Candida.* The patient is monitored for ophthalmologic complications to avoid keratoconjunctivitis. Hypertrophic scarring of the skin is not unusual.

Frozen histologic studies of peeled skin from a fresh lesion of TEN and cytodiagnosis of collections of cellular material from a freshly denuded area are diagnostic procedures used.

Management

The goals of treatment are control of fluid and electrolyte balance and prevention of death from infection. Supportive care is the mainstay of treatment.

All nonessential drugs are stopped immediately. It is desirable that the patient be treated in a regional burn center because aggressive treatment similar to that of a severe burn is required. Skin loss may approximate 100% of the total body surface area. Cultures are taken of the nasopharynx, eyes, ears, blood, urine, skin, and unruptured blisters to determine the presence of pathogenic organisms. Intravenous infusions are started to maintain fluid and electrolyte balance. However, because an indwelling intravenous catheter may result in infection, fluid replacement is carried out by nasogastric tube and orally as soon as possible.

Protecting the skin with topical agents is paramount. A variety of topical antibacterial agents are used to prevent wound sepsis, including silver nitrate solution, nitrofurazone, and polymyxin. Temporary biological dressings (pigskin; amniotic membrane) or plastic semipermeable dressings (Vigilon) may be used to reduce pain, decrease evaporative losses, and prevent secondary infection while awaiting reepithelialization.

▶ Nursing Process
The Patient With Toxic Epidermal Necrolysis

▷ Assessment

A careful inspection of the skin is made, with emphasis on its appearance and extent of involvement. The "normal" skin is closely observed to determine if new areas of blistering are developing. Skin seepage is monitored for amount, color, and odor. An inspection of the oral cavity for blistering and

erosive lesions is carried out daily. The patient's ability to drink fluids is determined.

The patient's vital signs are monitored, with special attention given to the presence and character of fever and the respiratory rate, depth, rhythm, and cough. The character and amount of respiratory secretions are noted. Urine volume, specific gravity, and color are monitored. The intravenous insertion sites are inspected for local signs of infection. The patient's height is noted, and daily weight checks are made.

The patient is asked about fatigue and pain. An attempt is made to evaluate the patient's level of anxiety. The nurse asks what the patient usually does to handle anxious feelings. The patient's basic coping mechanisms, which may be altered because of acute illness, are evaluated.

▷ Nursing Diagnoses

Based on all the assessment data, major nursing diagnoses for the patient may include the following:

- Impaired tissue integrity (oral and skin) related to epidermal shedding
- Fluid volume deficit and electrolyte losses related to loss of fluids from denuded skin
- Potential alteration in body temperature related to heat loss secondary to skin loss
- Pain related to raw, denuded skin, oral lesions, and possible infection
- Anxiety related to the appearance of skin and fear for survival

▷ Planning and Implementation

▷ *Goals:* The major goals of the patient may include achievement of skin and oral tissue healing, attainment of fluid balance, prevention of heat loss, relief of pain, and lessening of anxiety.

Nursing Interventions

Skin Care. The local care of the skin is a nursing challenge. The skin denudes easily, even when the patient is lifted and turned. It may be necessary to place the patient on a circular turning frame.

Secondary infection can be introduced through the damaged skin surface, which also has a compromised blood supply. Strict isolation techniques are employed to reduce the chances of secondary skin infection. Aseptic techniques are used during treatments of denuded skin.

The nurse applies the prescribed topical agents that reduce the bacterial population of the wound surface. Warm compresses, if prescribed, should be applied *gently* to raw areas. The topical antibacterial agent may be used in conjunction with hydrotherapy in a tank, bathtub, or shower. The hydrotherapy aids in débridement (removal of foreign material and devitalized tissue), reduces pain, and provides a form of physical therapy. The nurse's role is that of monitoring during the treatment and encouraging the patient to exercise the extremities during this hydrotherapy.

The painful oral lesions make oral hygiene difficult. Careful oral hygiene is practiced to keep the oral mucosa clean. Prescribed mouth washes are frequently used to rinse the mouth of debris and soothe ulcerative areas. The oral cavity is inspected daily, and any changes are noted and reported. Local applications of petrolatum (or prescribed ointment) are used on the lips.

Attaining Fluid Balance.   The vital signs, urine output, and sensorium are observed for signs of hypovolemia. Mental changes from fluid and electrolyte imbalance or sensory overload or deprivation may be manifested. The results of laboratory tests are evaluated, and abnormal results are reported. It is desirable that the patient is weighed daily, using a bed scale if necessary.

The nurse regulates intravenous fluids at appropriate rates and assesses for systemic (overinfusion or underinfusion) and local (infection) complications. An indwelling intravenous catheter may result in septicemia, so fluid replacement is carried out by a feeding tube, and orally as soon as possible. Oral lesions may result in dysphagia, making tube feeding or even hyperalimentation therapy necessary.

Preventing Heat Loss.   A patient with TEN is prone to chilling. Dehydration may be worsened by exposure of denuded skin to a continuous current of warm air. The patient is usually conscious of room temperature changes. As in caring for a burn patient, the use of cotton blankets, ceiling-mounted heat lamps, or heat shields is useful in maintaining the patient's body temperature. The nurse should work rapidly and efficiently when large wounds are exposed for wound care in order to minimize shivering and heat loss. The patient's temperature is carefully monitored.

Relieving Pain.   The patient is assessed for the presence and character of pain, behavioral responses, and any factors that influence the pain. The prescribed analgesics are administered, and the nurse observes for pain relief, any side-effects, and the activity of the patient. It is wise to administer analgesics before painful treatments. Proper explanations and speaking soothingly to the patient during treatments can alleviate the anxiety that may worsen pain. Emotional support and reassurance and providing measures to promote rest and sleep are essential in achieving pain control. As the pain diminishes and the patient has more physical and emotional energy, self-management techniques for pain relief, such as progressive muscle relaxation and imagery, may be taught.

Lessening Anxiety.   It is well to remember that the lifestyle of TEN patients has been abruptly changed to one of complete dependence. Assessment of their emotional state may reveal anxiety, fear of dying, and depression. Patients can be reassured that these reactions are normal. They need nursing support, honesty, candor, and some hope that things can get better. They are encouraged to express their feelings to someone with whom they have developed a trusting relationship. Listening to their concerns and being readily available with skillful and compassionate care are anxiety-relieving interventions.

Emotional support by a psychiatric nurse, chaplain, psychologist, or psychiatrist may be invaluable for providing coping methods during the long period of recovery.

▷ *Evaluation*

▷ *Expected Outcomes*

1. Patient achieves increasing skin and oral tissue healing.

   a. Skin reveals larger areas of healing.
   b. Patient is able to swallow fluids.
2. Attains fluid balance
   a. Laboratory reports are within normal range.
   b. Urine volume and specific gravity are within acceptable range.
3. Attains thermoregulation.
4. Reports lessening of intensity of pain
5. Appears less anxious
   a. Discusses concerns freely
   b. Sleeps at longer intervals

Ulcers and Tumors of the Skin

Ulcerations

The superficial loss of surface tissue due to death of the cells is called an ulceration. A simple ulcer, such as is found in a small, superficial, second-degree burn, tends to heal by granulation if kept clean and protected from injury. If it is exposed to the air, the serum that escapes will dry and form a scab, under which the epithelial cells will grow and cover the surface completely. Certain diseases cause characteristic ulcers—tuberculous ulcers and syphilitic ulcers are examples.

Ulcers Due to a Deficient Arterial Circulation.   Ulcers related to problems with arterial circulation are seen in patients with peripheral vascular disease, arteriosclerosis, Raynaud's disease, and frostbite. In these patients, the treatment of the ulceration must be carried out in conjunction with the treatment of the arterial disease. The danger is from secondary infection. Frequently, amputation of the part is the only effective therapy.

Pressure Sores.   Pressure sores (decubitus ulcers) result from continuous pressure on a particular area of the skin (see p. 222).

Tumors of the Skin

Cysts

Cysts of the skin are epithelium-lined cavities containing fluid or solid material.

Epidermal cysts (epidermoid) occur frequently and may be described as slow-growing, firm, elevated tumors found most frequently on the face, neck, upper chest, and back. Removal of the cysts provides cure.

Pilar cysts (trichilemmal cysts), originally called sebaceous cysts, are most frequently found on the scalp. They apparently originate from the middle portion of the hair follicle and from the cells of the outer root sheath. The treatment is surgical removal.

Benign Tumors

Seborrheic Keratoses.   These tumors are benign, wart-like lesions of varying size and color, ranging from light tan to black. They are usually located on the face, shoulders, chest, and back and are the most common skin tumors seen in middle-aged and elderly persons. They may be cosmetically unacceptable to the patient, and a black keratosis may be erroneously diagnosed as malignant melanoma. The treatment is removal of the tumor tissue by excision, electrodesiccation, and curettage, or the application of carbon dioxide or liquid nitrogen.

Actinic keratoses are premalignant skin lesions that develop in chronic sun-exposed areas of the body. They appear as rough, scaly patches with underlying erythema. An estimated 10% to 20% of these lesions gradually transform into invasive squamous cell carcinoma.

Verrucae (Warts).   Warts are common benign skin tumors caused by infection with the human papilloma virus that belongs to the DNA virus group. All age groups may be affected, but the condition occurs most frequently between the ages of 12 and 16. Warts come in many varieties.

As a rule, warts are asymptomatic, except when they occur on weight-bearing areas, such as the soles of the feet. They may be treated with locally applied liquid nitrogen, salicylic acid plasters, electrodesiccation, or the application of cantharidin.

Venereal Warts.   Warts occurring on the genitalia and perianal areas are known as *condyloma acuminata* and have been shown to be sexually transmitted. These are treated with podophyllin in tincture of benzoin, which is applied to the wart and washed off later. Other treatment modalities include liquid nitrogen, cryosurgery, electrosurgery, and curettage.

Angiomas (Birthmarks).   Birthmarks are benign vascular tumors involving the skin and the subcutaneous tissues. They may occur as flat, violet red patches (port-wine angiomas) or as raised, bright red nodular lesions (strawberry angiomas). The latter have a tendency to involute spontaneously. Port-wine angiomas, on the other hand, usually persist indefinitely. Most patients use masking cosmetics (Covermark) to camouflage the defect. The argon laser is being used on various angiomas with some success.

Pigmented Nevi (Moles).   Moles are common skin tumors of various sizes and shades, ranging from yellowish brown to black. They may be flat, macular lesions or elevated papules or nodules that occasionally contain hair. The great majority of pigmented nevi are harmless lesions. However, in rare cases, malignant changes supervene and a melanoma develops at the site of the nevus. Some authorities feel that all congenital moles should be removed, since these may have a higher incidence of malignant change. Nevi that show change in color or size or become symptomatic (itch) or develop notch borders should be removed to determine if malignant changes have occurred. Moles that occur in unusual places should be examined carefully for any irregularity and for notching of the border and variation in color. (Early melanomas may frequently show some redness and irritation and areas of bluish pigmentation where the pigment-containing cells have become deeper in the skin.) Nevi larger than 1 cm should be examined carefully. Excised nevi should be examined histologically.

Keloids.   Keloids are benign overgrowths of fibrous tissue at the site of a scar or trauma. They appear to be more common among black persons. Keloids are asymptomatic but may cause disfigurement and cosmetic concern. The treatment, which is not always satisfactory, consists of surgical excision, intralesional corticosteroid therapy, and radiation.

Dermatofibroma.   A dermatofibroma is a common benign tumor of connective tissue that occurs predominantly on the extremities. It is a firm, dome-shaped papule or nodule that may be skin-colored or a pinkish brown hue. Excisional biopsy is the recommended method of treatment.

Neurofibromatosis (von Recklinghausen's Disease). Neurofibromatosis is a hereditary condition manifested by pigmented patches (café au lait macules), axillary freckling, and cutaneous neurofibromas that vary in size. Developmental changes may occur also in the nervous system, muscles, and bone. Malignant degeneration of the neurofibromas is found in 2% to 5% of the patients.

Cancer of the Skin

Skin cancer is the most common form of cancer in the U.S. If it continues at the present rate, an estimated one of seven Americans will develop skin cancer. Because the skin is accessible to direct visualization, skin cancer is readily detected and is the most successfully treated type of cancer.

Causes and Prevention

The sun is the leading cause of skin cancer; incidence is related to the total amount of exposure to the sun. Sun damage is cumulative, and harmful effects may be severe by the age of 20. The increase in skin cancer is probably due to changing life-styles and emphasis on sunbathing and related activities. Protective measures should be started in childhood and carried on throughout life. Persons who do not produce sufficient melanin pigment in the skin to give protection to underlying tissue are very susceptible to sun damage; those at greatest risk are fair, blue-eyed, red-haired persons of Celtic ancestry or persons with ruddy or light complexions, as well as those who suffer prolonged sunburn and do not tan. Others at risk are outdoor workers, such as farmers, sailors, fishermen, and people who are exposed to the sun over a period of time. Elderly persons with sun-damaged skin are also at risk, as are persons who have had a history of x-ray treatment for acne or benign skin lesions. Workers exposed to certain chemical agents (arsenic, nitrates, coal, tar and pitch, oils and paraffins) are also included in the risk group. People who have scars due to severe burns may develop skin cancer 20 to 40 years later. Squamous cell cancer can develop in areas of chronic draining osteomyelitis. Neoplastic changes can develop in chronic fistulae. Chronic ulcers of the lower extremity may be the site of origin of skin cancer. In fact, any condition causing scarring or chronic irritation may lead to cancer. Immunosuppressed patients have an increased incidence of malignant skin tumors. Genetic factors are also involved.

Types of Skin Cancer

The most common types of skin cancer are basal cell carcinoma, squamous cell (epidermoid) carcinoma, and malignant melanoma.

Basal cell carcinomas arise from the basal cell layer of the epidermis or the hair follicles. This is the most common type of skin cancer. It generally appears on the sun-exposed areas of the body, and is more prevalent in regions where the population is subjected to intense and extensive exposure to the sun. The incidence is proportional to the age of the patient (average age of 60) and the total amount of sun exposure, and is inversely proportional to the amount of melanin pigment in the skin.

Basal cell carcinoma usually presents as a small, waxy nodule with rolled, translucent, pearly borders; telangiectatic vessels may be present. As it grows, it undergoes central ulceration and sometimes crusting (Fig. 48-6). The tumors appear most frequently on the face between the hairline and the upper lip. Basal cell carcinoma is characterized by invasion and erosion of contiguous (adjoining) tissues, but it rarely metastasizes. However, a neglected basal cell carcinoma can account for the loss of a nose, an ear, or a lip. Other lesions of this disease may appear as shiny, flat, gray, or yellowish plaques.

Squamous cell carcinoma is a malignant proliferation arising from the epidermis. Although it usually appears on sun-damaged skin, it may arise from normal skin or from preexisting skin lesions. It is of greater concern than basal cell carcinoma because it is a truly invasive carcinoma. The lesions may be primary, arising both on the skin and mucous membranes, or may develop from a precancerous condition, such as actinic keratosis (lesions occurring in sun-exposed areas), leukoplakia (premalignant lesion of the mucous membrane), or scarred or ulcerated lesions. It appears as a rough, thickened, scaly tumor that may be asymptomatic or may involve bleeding (Fig. 48-7). The border of the lesion may be wider, more infiltrated, and more inflammatory than that of basal cell carcinoma. Secondary infection can occur. Exposed areas, especially of the upper extremities and of the face, lower lip, ears, nose, and forehead, are common sites.

Skin cancer is diagnosed by biopsy and histological evaluation.

The incidence of metastases is related to the histologic type and the level or depth of invasion. Usually, tumors arising in sun-damaged areas are less invasive and rarely cause death, whereas squamous cell carcinoma arising without a history

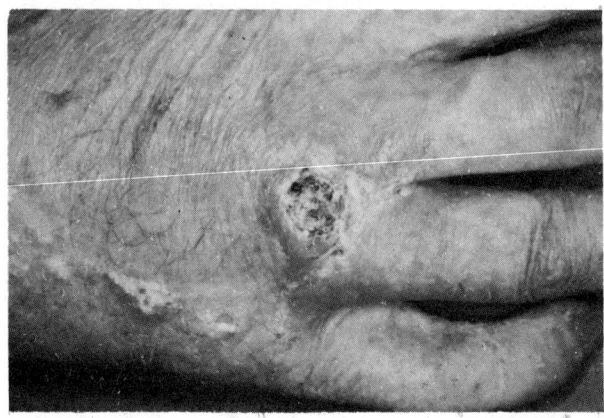

Figure 48-7
Squamous cell carcinoma. (Courtesy of Mervyn L. Elgart, M.D.)

of sun or arsenic exposure or scar formation appears to have a greater chance of metastatic spread. The patient should be evaluated subsequently for regional lymph node metastases.

Management of Basal Cell and Squamous Cell Carcinomas

The goal of treatment is to eradicate or completely destroy all the tumor. The method of treatment depends on the tumor location, cell type (location and depth), cosmetic desires of the patient, history of previous treatment, whether or not the tumor is invasive, and the presence or absence of metastatic nodes.

The usual methods of treatment of both basal cell carcinoma and squamous cell carcinoma are curettage and electrodessication (destruction of tissue with heat produced by electricity), surgical excision, cryosurgery, radiation therapy, and microscopically controlled chemosurgery.

Curettage Followed by Electrodesiccation. Curettage is carried out by excising the skin tumor by scraping its surface with a curette; electrodesiccation is then applied to achieve hemostasis and to destroy any viable malignant cells at the base of the wound or along its edges. It is useful for small lesions (smaller than 1–2 cm [0.4–0.8 inch] in diameter). This method takes advantage of the fact that the tumor in each instance is softer than surrounding skin and therefore can be outlined by a curette, which "feels" the extent of the tumor. The tumor is removed and the base cauterized. The process is repeated three times. Usually, healing occurs within a month.

Surgical Excision. Wide surgical excision may be necessary. The adequacy of excision is verified by microscopic study of sections of the specimen. Such a histologic study of excised tissue shows whether or not the margins are free of tumor. Skin grafting may be necessary if primary closure is not possible.

Radiation Therapy. Radiation therapy is frequently done for cancer of the eyelid, the tip of the nose, and areas in or near vital structures (*e.g.,* facial nerve). It is reserved for older patients, because x-ray changes may be seen after 5 to 10 years and malignant changes in scars may be induced by x-rays 15 to 30 years later.

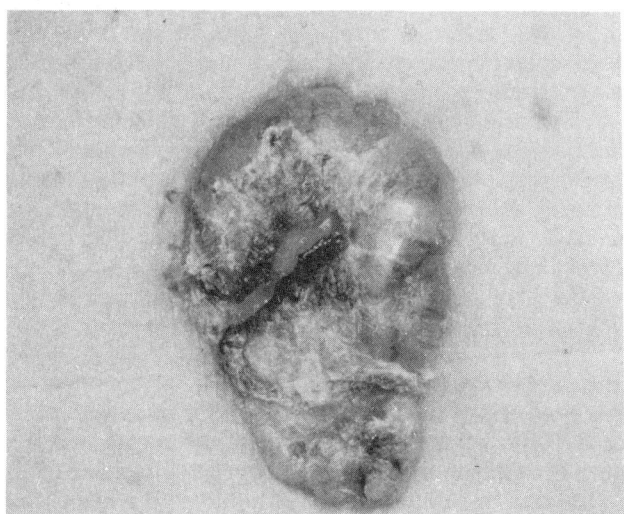

Figure 48-6
Basal cell carcinoma. (Courtesy of Mervyn L. Elgart, M.D.)

The patient should be informed that the skin may become red and blistered. A bland skin ointment (prescribed by the physician) may be applied to relieve discomfort. The patient should also be cautioned against exposure to the sun.

Cryosurgery. Cryosurgery employs deep freezing to destroy the tumor tissue selectively. A thermocouple needle apparatus is inserted into the skin, and liquid nitrogen is directed to the center of the tumor until a temperature of $-50°C$ is reached at the tumor base. The tumor tissue is frozen, allowed to thaw, and then refrozen. The site thaws naturally and then becomes gelatinous and heals spontaneously. Swelling and edema follow the freeze. The appearance of the lesion varies. Normal healing may take 4 to 6 weeks, occurring faster in areas with a good blood supply.

Microscopically Controlled Surgery (Chemosurgery). Chemosurgery combines the use of topically applied chemicals and serial surgical excisions of tumors layer by layer. Immediate microscopic examination is made of frozen sections for evidence of cancer cells. This procedure may be repeated until the specimens are cancer-free and all peripheral extensions of the tumor are eradicated. Chemosurgery is useful for recurrent tumors or for infiltrating tumors whose margins cannot be determined.

Nursing Management

Because many skin cancers are removed by excision, patients are treated in outpatient surgical units. The role of the nurse is that of teaching the patient postoperative self-care activities.

The wound is usually (but not always) covered with a dressing to protect the site from physical trauma, external irritants, and contaminants. The patient is advised when to report for a dressing change or is given written information on how to change dressings—including what type of dressing to purchase, how to remove dressings and apply fresh ones, and the importance of hand washing before and after the procedure.

The patient is advised to watch for excessive bleeding and dressings so tight that circulation is compromised. If the lesion is in the perioral area, the patient is instructed to drink liquids through a straw and limit excess talking and facial movement.

After the sutures are removed, an emollient cream may be used to help reduce dryness. Sunscreens over the wound to prevent postoperative hyperpigmentation are advised if the patient spends time outdoors.

Patient Education. The follow-up treatment should be regular, including palpation of the adjacent nodes. The following points of emphasis should be made part of patient education:

1. Do not try to tan if your skin burns easily, never tans, or tans poorly.
2. Avoid unnecessary exposure to the sun, especially during times when ultraviolet radiation light is most intense (10 AM to 3 PM).
3. *Do not become sunburned.*
4. Apply a protective sunscreen if you must be in the sun; sunscreens block out harmful sunrays.
   a. Sunscreens are rated in strengths from 4 (weakest) to > 15 (ultra sun protection). This number is called SPF (solar protection factor) and is printed on the bottle. Use a sunscreen with a SPF of 15.
   b. Water-resistant sunscreens should probably be reapplied after swimming or during prolonged sunbathing.
   c. Oils applied before or during sunning do *not* protect against sunburn or sun damage.
5. Use a lip balm that contains a sunscreen with the highest SPF number.
6. Wear appropriate protective clothing (*e.g.*, broad-brimmed hat, long-sleeved clothing). However, clothing does not provide complete protection, as up to 50% of the sun's damaging rays can go through clothes. Ultraviolet rays also penetrate clouds.
7. Do not use sun lamps for indoor tanning; avoid commercial tanning booths.
8. Have moles treated that are accessible to repeated friction and irritation.
9. Watch for indications of potential malignancy in moles (*e.g.*, increase in size, ulceration, bleeding, or serous exudation).
10. Have follow-up evaluation throughout lifetime. Watch for development of new lesions. (There is also an incidence of internal malignancy associated with squamous cell cancer.)
11. Caution your children and grandchildren, especially those with fair skin, to avoid excessive exposure to the sun and to use sunscreen so as to prevent later skin cancers.

Malignant Melanoma

A malignant melanoma is a malignant neoplasm in which atypical *melanocytes* (pigment cells) are present in both the epidermis and the dermis (and sometimes the subcutaneous cells). It can occur in one of several forms: superficial spreading melanoma, lentigo-maligna melanoma, nodular melanoma, and acral-lentiginous melanoma. These types have certain clinical and histologic features as well as different biological behaviors. Most melanomas derive from cutaneous epidermal melanocytes, but some appear in preexisting nevi (moles) in the skin or develop in the uveal tract of the eye. Melanomas frequently appear simultaneously with cancer of other organs.

The incidence of melanoma has doubled during the past few decades, a rise that is probably related to increased recreational sun exposure. The incidence of melanoma is increasing faster than that of almost any other cancer, and the mortality rate is increasing faster than that of any other cancer except lung cancer.

Clinical Manifestations

The *superficial spreading melanoma* occurs anywhere on the body and is the most common form of melanoma. It usually affects persons of middle age, and occurs most frequently on the trunk and lower extremities. The lesion tends to be circular with irregular outer portions. The margins of the lesion may be flat or elevated and palpable (Fig. 48-8). This type of melanoma may appear in a combination of colors,

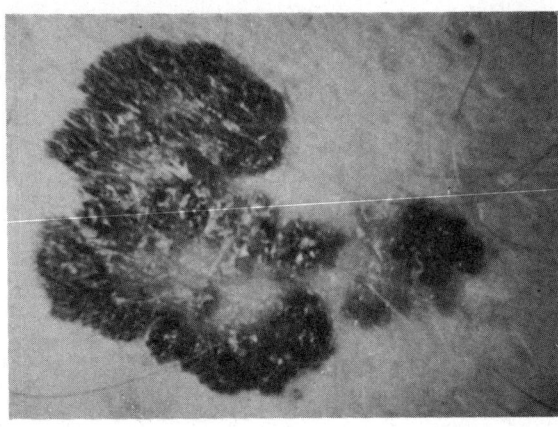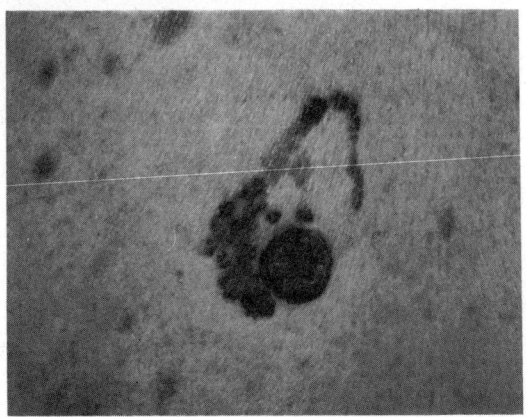

Figure 48-8
Malignant melanoma. (*Left*) Superficial melanoma. (*Right*) Nodular melanoma. (Courtesy of Mervyn L. Elgart, M.D.)

with hues of tan, brown, and black mixed with gray, bluish black, or white. Sometimes there is a dull pink rose color in a small area within the lesion.

The *lentigo-maligna melanomas* are slowly evolving pigmented lesions that occur on exposed skin areas, especially of the head and neck, in elderly people. They first appear as tan, flat lesions, and in time undergo changes in size and color.

The *nodular melanoma* is a spherical, blueberrylike nodule with a relatively smooth surface and relatively uniform blue black color (Fig. 48-8). It may be dome-shaped with a smooth surface. It may have other shadings of red, gray, or purple. Sometimes nodular melanomas appear as irregularly shaped plaques. The patient may describe this as a "blood blister" that fails to resolve. A nodular melanoma invades directly into subjacent dermis (vertical growth), and hence has a poorer prognosis.

Acral-lentiginous melanoma are a form of melanoma that occurs in areas not excessively exposed to sunlight and where hair follicles are absent. They are found on the palms of the hands, soles, nail beds, and mucous membranes in black and other dark-skinned persons. These melanomas appear as irregular pigmented macules, which develop nodules. They may become invasive early.

An excision biopsy specimen is taken to gain histologic information on the type, level of invasion, and thickness. In addition, the patient is thoroughly examined to determine the extent of the disease.

Prognosis

The prognosis is related to the depth of dermal invasion and the thickness of the lesion. The deeper and thicker the melanoma, the greater the likelihood of metastases. If the melanoma is growing radially (horizontally) and is characterized by peripheral growth with minimal or absent dermal invasion, the prognosis is favorable. When the melanoma progresses to the vertical growth phase (dermal invasion), the prognosis is poor. The presence of ulceration correlates with a poor prognosis. Malignant melanoma can spread through both the bloodstream and the lymphatic routes, and can metastasize

to every organ of the body. Melanomas of the trunk appear to have a poorer prognosis than those of other sites, perhaps because the network of lymphatics in the trunk permits metastasis to regional nodes.

Causes and Persons at Risk

The etiology is unknown, but ultraviolet rays are strongly suspected. In general, at greatest risk are patients with fair complexions, blue eyes, red or blonde hair, and freckles. These persons synthesize melanin more slowly. Persons of Celtic or Scandinavian origin are at greater risk. Persons who burn and do not tan are also at risk. In areas where sunlight is intense, there is a disproportionate increase in incidence. Older Americans retiring to the Southwestern sunbelt appear to have a higher incidence. Others at risk have had a melanoma in the past, have a family history of melanoma, have giant congenital nevi, or have a significant history of severe sunburn.

Up to 10% of melanoma patients are members of melanoma-prone families who have multiple changing moles (dysplastic nevi) that are susceptible to malignant transformation. Persons with *dysplastic nevus syndrome* have been found to have unusual moles, larger and more numerous moles, lesions with irregular outlines, and pigmentation located all over the skin. Microscopic examination of dysplastic moles shows disordered, faulty growth.

Management

The therapeutic approach to the treatment of malignant melanoma depends on the level of invasion and the measurement of thickness.

Surgery. Small superficial lesions are treated by local excision. Deeper lesions require wide local excision and coverage with a skin graft. This is the primary mode of treatment at this time. A regional node dissection may be done.

Regional Perfusion for Melanoma of the Extremities. The regional perfusion method consists of isolating an anatomical region (*e.g.*, the leg) by mechanically controlling its arterial inflow and venous outflow. A chemotherapeutic agent is perfused directly into the area that contains the melanoma. This approach allows delivery of a high concentration of cytotoxic drugs while avoiding systemic toxic effects of these higher doses. Regional perfusion can achieve excellent control of metastases and the primary tumor itself, especially when used in combination with surgical excision of the primary lesion and with regional lymph node dissection.

Immunotherapy. The term *immunotherapy* encompasses treatment methods that modify not only immune but other biological responses to cancer. There have been some encouraging results with several new forms of immunotherapy (interleukins; interferons; monoclonal antibodies directed against melanoma antigens). Research continues to define an effective systemic therapy.

▶ Nursing Process
The Patient With Malignant Melanoma

▷ Assessment

An assessment of the patient with malignant melanoma is based on the history and symptomatology. Ask specifically about pruritus, tenderness, and pain, which are *not* features of a benign nevus. Question the patient about changes in preexisting moles or the development of a new pigmented lesion. Have a high index of suspicion for persons at risk.

Use a magnifying lens in good lighting to look for *irregularity* and *changes* in the mole. Signs that suggest malignant changes include the following:

1. *Variegated color*
   - Colors that may indicate malignancy in a brown or black lesion are shades of red, white, and blue; shades of blue are considered ominous.
   - White areas within a pigmented lesion are suspicious.
   - Some malignant melanomas are not variegated but uniformly colored (bluish-black; bluish gray; bluish red).

2. *Irregular border*
   - Look for angular indentation or notch in the border of the mole.

3. *Irregular surface*
   - Look for uneven elevations of the surface; irregular topography may be palpable or visible. The change in the surface may be from smooth to scaly.
   - Some nodular melanomas have a smooth surface.

The common sites of melanomas are the skin of the back, the legs (especially in women), between toes and on the feet, face, scalp, fingernails, and backs of hands. In black persons, melanomas are most apt to occur in the less pigmented sites: palms, soles, subungual areas, and mucous membranes.

The diameter of the mole is measured, because melanomas are often larger than 6 mm. Satellite lesions (those situated near the mole) are noted.

▷ Nursing Diagnoses

Based on the nursing assessment data, major nursing diagnoses for the patient may include the following:

- Pain related to surgical excision and grafting
- Anxiety and depression related to possible life-threatening consequences of melanoma
- Potential for recurrence

▷ Planning and Implementation

▷ *Goals:* The major goals of the patient may include relief of pain and discomfort, reduction of anxiety, and absence of recurrence.

Nursing Interventions

Relief of Pain and Discomfort. Surgical removal of melanoma in different locations (head and neck, eye, trunk, abdomen, extremities, central nervous system) presents different challenges, taking into consideration the removal of the primary melanoma, the intervening lymphatics, and the lymph nodes to which metastases may spread. Nursing management of the patient having surgery in these regions is discussed in the appropriate chapters.

Nursing intervention following surgery for a malignant melanoma centers on promoting comfort, because wide excision surgery may be necessary. A split-thickness skin graft is done when large defects are created by surgical removal of a melanoma. Anticipating the need for and giving appropriate analgesic medication are part of the nursing function.

Reduction of Anxiety. Psychological support is essential when mutilative surgery is done. Support includes allowing patients to express feelings about the seriousness of this cutaneous neoplasm, understanding their anger and sadness, and conveying understanding of these feelings. During the period the diagnosis is being made and the tumor is classified by type and depth, the nurse answers questions, clarifies information, and helps clear up misconceptions. Learning that they have a melanoma can cause patients considerable fear and anguish. Pointing out patients' resources, past effective coping mechanisms, and social support systems helps them to cope with the problems associated with diagnosis, treatment, and continuing follow-up.

Patient Education. The best hope of controlling the disease lies in the education of patients regarding the *early* signs of melanoma. Patients are taught to examine their skin monthly in an orderly manner, including scalp examination (Fig. 48-9). The following are points to stress in patient education:

1. Use a full-length mirror and a small hand mirror to aid in examination.
2. Learn where moles and birthmarks are located.
3. Inspect all moles and other pigmented lesions; report to the physician/clinic immediately moles that *change* colors, enlarge, become raised or thicker, itch, or bleed.
4. Have a physician examine your skin at least twice yearly. A person who has had a malignant melanoma should have lifelong follow-up. A person developing a

malignant melanoma has a higher risk of developing a second one.

A key factor in development of malignant melanoma is exposure to sunlight. See page 1278 for preventive measures.

▷ *Evaluation*

▷ *Expected Outcomes*

1. Patient experiences relief of pain and discomfort.
   a. States pain has lessened and is diminishing
   b. Exhibits healing of surgical scar with no evidence of heat, redness, or swelling
2. Achieves reduction of anxiety
   a. Ventilates fears and fantasies
   b. Asks questions about medical condition
   c. Requests repetition of facts about melanoma
   d. Identifies family member or significant other for positive reinforcement
3. Demonstrates an understanding of the means for detecting melanoma
   a. Demonstrates how to conduct self-examination of skin on a monthly basis
   b. Verbalizes the following danger signals of melanoma: change in size of mole, color of mole, mole surface, shape or outline of mole, or skin around mole
   c. Recalls measures to protect self from sun

Metastatic Skin Tumors

The skin is an important, although not a common, site of metastatic cancer. All types of cancer may metastasize to the skin, but carcinoma of the breast is the primary source of cutaneous metastases in women. Cancer of the large intestine, ovaries, and lungs are other sources. In men, the primary site is most commonly the lungs, large intestine, oral cavity, kidneys, or stomach. Skin metastases from melanomas are found in both sexes. The clinical appearance of metastatic skin lesions is not distinctive, except perhaps in some cases of breast cancer in which diffuse, brawny hardening of the skin of the involved breast is seen ("cancer en cuirasse"). In most instances, metastatic lesions occur as multiple cutaneous or subcutaneous nodules of varying size that may be skin-colored or show different shades of red.

Dermatologic and Plastic Reconstructive Surgery

The word "plastic" comes from a Greek word meaning "to form." Plastic or reconstructive surgery is done to reconstruct or alter congenital or acquired defects in order to restore or improve the body's form and function. (Often the terms *plastic* and *reconstructive* are used interchangeably). This type of surgery includes the closure of wounds, removal of skin tumors, repair of soft tissue injuries or burns, correction of deformities of the breast, and repair of cosmetic defects. Fre-

quently, plastic surgery is done primarily for aesthetic and cosmetic improvement, but it is applicable to many parts of the body and to numerous structures, such as bone, cartilage, fat, fascia, mucous membrane, muscle, nerve, and cutaneous structures. Bone inlays and transplants for deformities and nonunion can be done; muscle can be transferred; nerves can be reconstructed and spliced; and cartilage can be replaced. Last, but as important as any of these measures, is the reconstruction of the cutaneous tissues around the neck and the face; this is usually referred to as *aesthetic* or *cosmetic surgery*.

Wound Coverage: Grafts and Flaps

Skin Grafts

Skin grafting is a technique in which a section of skin is detached from its own blood supply and transferred as free tissue to a distant (recipient) site. Skin grafting can be used to repair almost any type of wound, and is the most common form of reconstructive surgery. In dermatology, skin grafts are commonly used to repair defects that result from excision of skin tumors, to cover areas denuded of skin, and to cover wounds in which insufficient skin is available to permit wound closure. They are also used when primary closure of the wound increases risk of complications or when primary wound closure will interfere with function.

Skin grafts may be classified as autografts, allografts, or xenografts. *Autografts* are grafts done with tissue transplanted from the patient's own skin. *Allografts* involve the transplant of tissue from one individual to another individual of the same species. These grafts are also called *allogenic* or *homograft*. A *xenograft* or *heterograft* involves the transfer of tissue from another species.

Grafts are also referred to by their thickness. A skin graft may be split-thickness (thin, intermediate, or thick) or full-thickness, depending upon the amount of dermis included in the specimen. A split-thickness graft can be cut at varying thicknesses, and is commonly used to cover large wounds or defects for which a full-thickness graft or flap is impractical (Fig. 48-10, p. 1284). A full-thickness graft consists of epidermis and the entire dermis without the underlying fat. It is used to cover wounds that are too large to close directly.

Application of the Graft. A graft is obtained by a variety of instruments: razor blades, skin-grafting knives, electric- or air-powered dermatomes, or drum dermatomes. The skin graft is taken from the "donor" or "host" site and applied to the wound/ulcer site, called the "recipient" site or "graft bed."

For a graft to survive and be effective, certain conditions must be met: (1) the recipient bed must have an adequate blood supply so that normal physiologic function can resume; (2) the graft must be in close contact with its bed (to avoid accumulation of blood or fluid); (3) the graft must be fixed firmly (immobilized) so that it remains in place on the recipient site; and (4) the area must be free of infection.

The graft, when applied to the recipient site, may or may not be sutured in place. It may be slit and spread apart to cover a greater area. The process of revascularization and reattachment of a skin graft to a recipient bed is referred to as a "take."

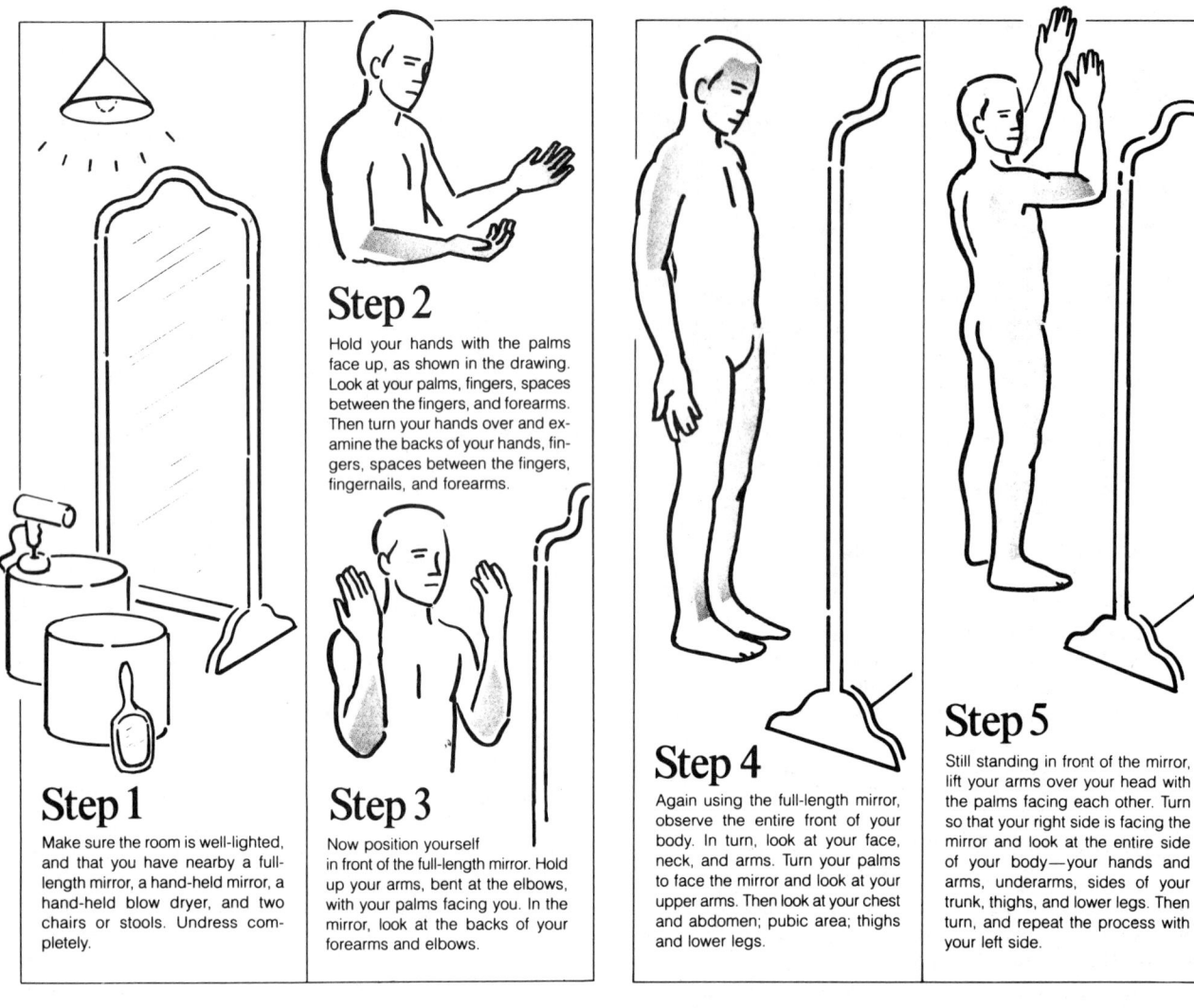

Step 1

Make sure the room is well-lighted, and that you have nearby a full-length mirror, a hand-held mirror, a hand-held blow dryer, and two chairs or stools. Undress completely.

Step 2

Hold your hands with the palms face up, as shown in the drawing. Look at your palms, fingers, spaces between the fingers, and forearms. Then turn your hands over and examine the backs of your hands, fingers, spaces between the fingers, fingernails, and forearms.

Step 3

Now position yourself in front of the full-length mirror. Hold up your arms, bent at the elbows, with your palms facing you. In the mirror, look at the backs of your forearms and elbows.

Step 4

Again using the full-length mirror, observe the entire front of your body. In turn, look at your face, neck, and arms. Turn your palms to face the mirror and look at your upper arms. Then look at your chest and abdomen; pubic area; thighs and lower legs.

Step 5

Still standing in front of the mirror, lift your arms over your head with the palms facing each other. Turn so that your right side is facing the mirror and look at the entire side of your body—your hands and arms, underarms, sides of your trunk, thighs, and lower legs. Then turn, and repeat the process with your left side.

Figure 48-9
Technique for self-examination of the skin. (Courtesy of American Cancer Society.)

After a skin graft is put in place, the graft may be left exposed (in areas that are impossible to immobilize) or covered with a light dressing or a pressure dressing, depending on the area.

Patient Education and Home Health Care. The patient is instructed to keep the affected part immobilized as much as possible. For a facial graft, strenuous activity must be avoided. A graft on the hand or arm may be immobilized with a splint. When a graft is placed in a lower extremity, the part is kept elevated because the new capillary connections are fragile and excess venous pressure may cause rupture. When ambulation is permitted, the patient wears an elastic stocking to counteract venous pressure.

The patient or family member is instructed to inspect the dressing daily. Unusual drainage or an inflammatory reaction around the wound margin suggests infection and should be reported to the physician. Any fluid, purulent drainage, blood, or serum that has collected will be gently evacuated by the surgeon, because this material would cause the graft to separate from its bed.

When the graft appears pink, it apparently is vascularized. After 2 to 3 weeks, mineral oil or a lanolin cream is massaged into the wound to moisten the graft and stimulate circulation. Because there may be loss of feeling or sensation in the grafted area for a prolonged period, the application of heating pads and exposure to sun are avoided.

Donor Site for Skin Grafting

Selection Criteria. The donor site is selected with several criteria in mind: (1) to obtain the closest possible color match in keeping with the amount of skin graft required, (2) to match the texture and hair-bearing qualities, (3) to obtain the thickest possible skin graft without jeopardizing the healing process of the donor site (Fig. 48-11), and (4) to consider the cosmetic effects of the donor site after healing, so that it is in an inconspicuous location.

Donor Site Care. Detailed attention to the donor site is just as important as the care of the recipient area. The donor site heals by reepithelialization of the raw, exposed dermis. Usually a single layer of nonadherent fine-mesh gauze is placed directly over the donor site. Absorbent gauze dressings

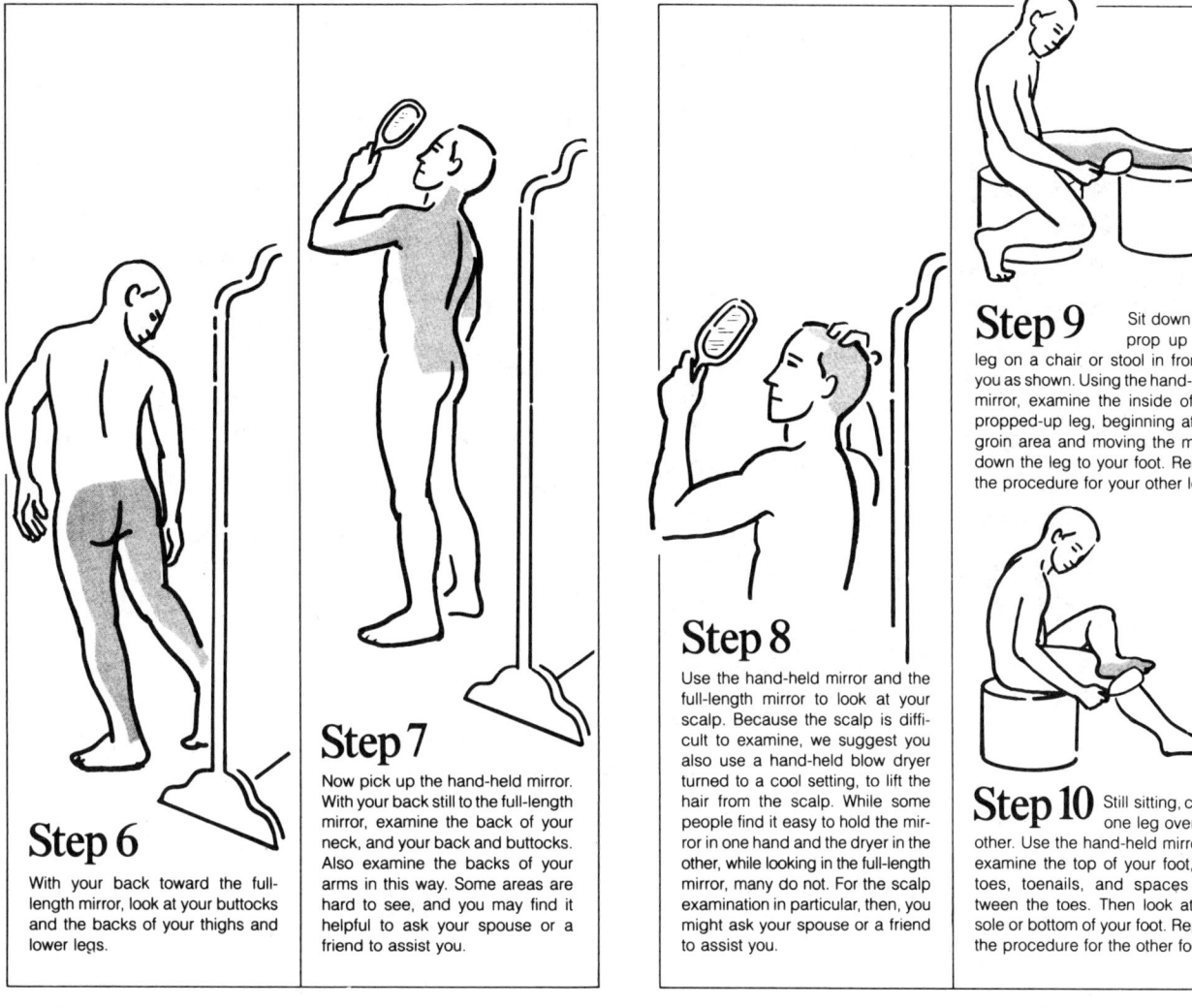

Step 6

With your back toward the full-length mirror, look at your buttocks and the backs of your thighs and lower legs.

Step 7

Now pick up the hand-held mirror. With your back still to the full-length mirror, examine the back of your neck, and your back and buttocks. Also examine the backs of your arms in this way. Some areas are hard to see, and you may find it helpful to ask your spouse or a friend to assist you.

Step 8

Use the hand-held mirror and the full-length mirror to look at your scalp. Because the scalp is difficult to examine, we suggest you also use a hand-held blow dryer turned to a cool setting, to lift the hair from the scalp. While some people find it easy to hold the mirror in one hand and the dryer in the other, while looking in the full-length mirror, many do not. For the scalp examination in particular, then, you might ask your spouse or a friend to assist you.

Step 9

Sit down and prop up one leg on a chair or stool in front of you as shown. Using the hand-held mirror, examine the inside of the propped-up leg, beginning at the groin area and moving the mirror down the leg to your foot. Repeat the procedure for your other leg.

Step 10

Still sitting, cross one leg over the other. Use the hand-held mirror to examine the top of your foot, the toes, toenails, and spaces between the toes. Then look at the sole or bottom of your foot. Repeat the procedure for the other foot.

Figure 48-9 (cont'd.)

are then placed on top to take up blood or serum from the wound. A membrane dressing may be used (Op-Site), and provides certain advantages: it is transparent and allows the wound to be checked without disturbing the dressing, it permits the patient to shower without fear of saturating the dressing with water, and it is virtually painless.

After healing, the patient is instructed to keep the donor site soft and pliable with cream (lanolin; olive oil). Extremes in temperature, external trauma, and sunlight are to be avoided for both donor sites and grafted areas because these areas are sensitive, especially to thermal injuries.

Flaps

Another form of wound coverage may be provided by flaps. A *flap* is a segment of tissue that has been left attached at one end (called a *base* or *pedicle*) while the other end has been moved to a recipient area. It is dependent for its survival on functioning arterial and venous blood supplies and lymphatic drainage in its pedicle or base. A flap differs from a graft in that a portion of the tissue is attached to its original site and retains its blood supply. (An exception is the free flap, described below). Flaps may consist of skin, mucosa, muscle, adipose tissue, omentum, and bone. They are used for wound coverage and provide bulk, especially when bone, tendon, blood vessels, or nerve tissue is exposed. Flaps are used to repair defects caused by congenital deformity, trauma, or tumor ablation in an adjacent part of the body.

Flaps have the advantage of offering the best aesthetic solution because a flap retains the color and texture of the donor area, is more apt to survive than a graft, and can be used to cover nerves, tendons, and blood vessels. However, a series of operations are usually required to move a flap. The major complication is necrosis of the pedicle or base due to failure of the blood supply.

Free Flaps. A striking advance in reconstructive surgery is the use of *free flaps* or *free-tissue transfer*, achieved by means of microvascular techniques. A free flap is completely severed from the body and transferred to another site, and receives early vascular supply from microvascular anastomosis

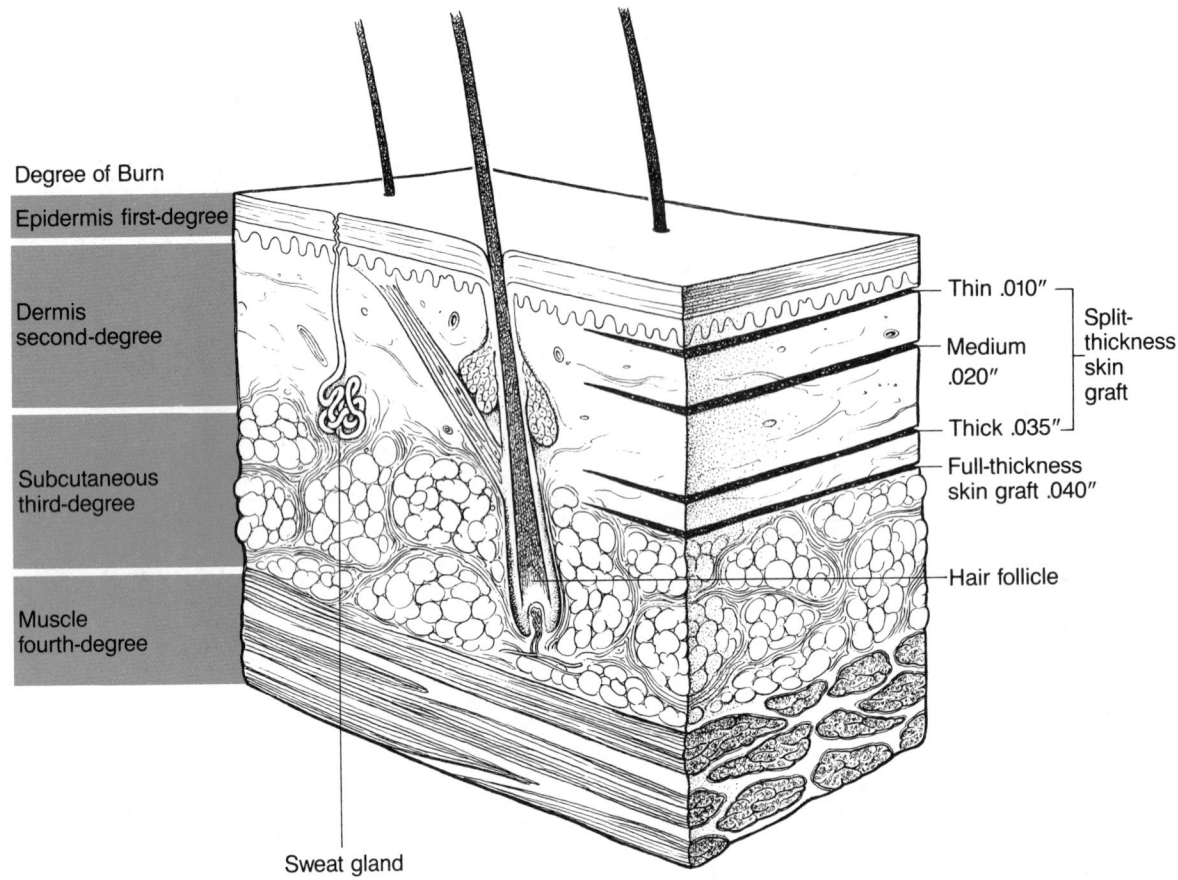

Degree of Burn

Epidermis first-degree

Dermis second-degree

Subcutaneous third-degree

Muscle fourth-degree

Thin .010″ ⎤
Medium .020″ ⎬ Split-thickness skin graft
Thick .035″ ⎦

Full-thickness skin graft .040″

Hair follicle

Sweat gland

Figure 48-10
Layers of skin showing split-thickness graft.

with vessels at the recipient site. Thus the procedure is generally done in one step, eliminating a series of operations to move the flap. Microvascular surgery has opened an era that allows surgeons of differing specialties to use a variety of donor sites for tissue reconstruction.

Fascial, Cartilage, and Bone Transplants

Transplants of fascial or muscle tissue have numerous uses. The tissue is usually obtained from the fascia lata of the thigh, and is adaptable for use as suture material, for repair of hernia defects, and for replacement of tendon loss. Cartilage transplantation may be immediate and direct, taken from the costal cartilages and transferred to the nose. Bone grafts demand careful aseptic technique and rigid fixation in their new site. They may be taken from the crest of the tibia, the upper border of the iliac bone, or a rib. All donor areas should receive the same careful treatment given any other surgical wound.

Management of the Patient With Facial Reconstructive Surgery

Reconstructive procedures on the face are designed to suit the individual patient and to repair deformities or restore nor-

mal function as much as possible. They may vary from closure of small defects to complicated procedures involving implantation of prosthetic devices to conceal a large defect or replace a lost part of the face (*e.g.*, nose reconstruction, ear reconstruction; resection of the mandible). Each surgical solution is custom-tailored and involves a variety of incisions, flaps, and grafts.

In correcting a primary defect, the surgeon may have to create a secondary defect. Although the operation may restore some function, such as eating or talking, the cosmetic or esthetic results are sometimes limited. The original appearance of a patient with severe damage to soft tissue and bone structure can seldom be restored. Multiple surgical procedures may be required. The process of facial reconstruction is often slow and tedious.

▶ *Nursing Process*
The Patient With Facial Reconstructive Surgery

▷ *Assessment*

The face is a part of the body that every person desires to keep at its best or improve because most human interactions center on the face. When the face loses its appearance and

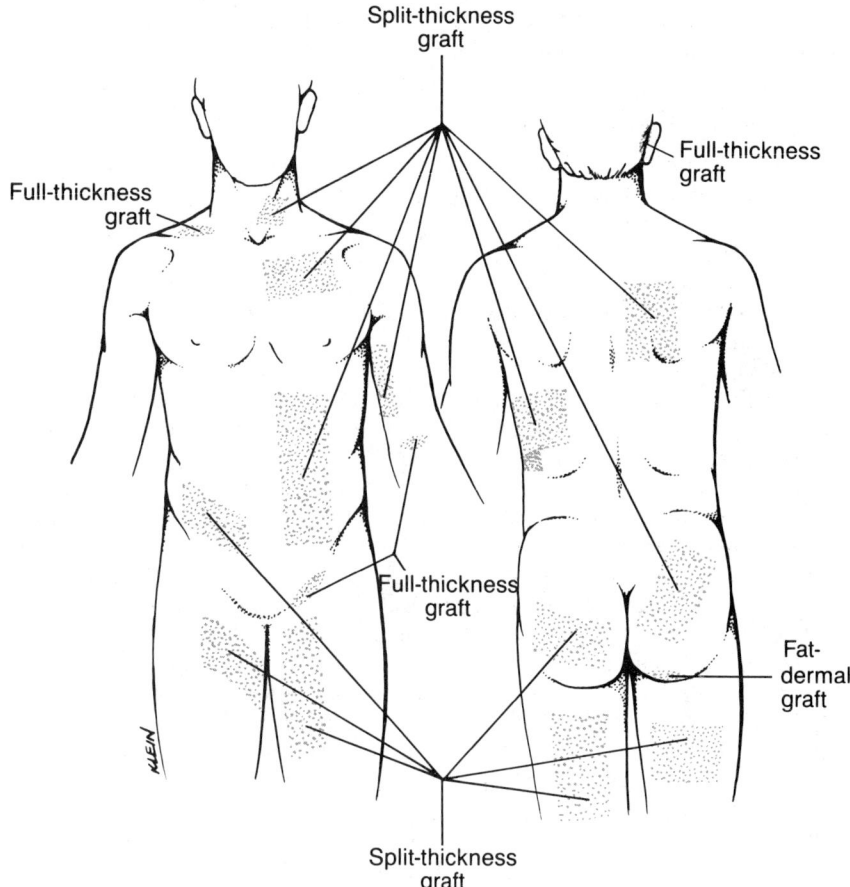

Split-thickness
graft

Full-thickness
graft

Full-thickness
graft

Full-thickness
graft

Fat-
dermal
graft

Split-thickness
graft

Figure 48-11
Commonly employed sites for donor
areas of skin grafts. (Converse JM and
Brauer RA. Reconstructive Plastic
Surgery. Philadelphia, WB Saunders.)

function (*e.g.*, by accident or cancer), an emotional reaction occurs. Changes in appearance frequently cause anxiety and depression. Patients with facial changes frequently mourn for the lost part, suffer a loss of self-esteem due to reactions or rejection by others, and withdraw and isolate themselves. Health care personnel can legitimize these emotions by acknowledging that anxiety and depression are appropriate for what the patient is experiencing.

In addition to assessing emotional responses, the nurse identifies strengths as well as usual coping mechanisms to determine how the patient will handle the surgical procedure. Any area in which the patient and family will need extra support is also highlighted.

Preoperative Nursing Management

The patient is prepared as thoroughly as possible for the extent of disfigurement and improvement that can be anticipated. The nurse is in a better position to reinforce factual information and clarify misconceptions when the surgeon has fully informed the patient about the procedure, the functional defects that may result, the possible need for a tracheostomy and/or other prosthesis, and the necessity for additional surgery.

Preoperative teaching also includes an explanation of intravenous feedings, the use of a nasogastric tube to allow gastric decompression and prevent vomiting, and the frequent and lengthy dressing periods that may be necessary to care for wounds, flaps, and skin grafts. Extra time is needed when presenting this information to anxious patients because they may not listen, may not comprehend, or may distort what is being said.

▷ Nursing Diagnoses

Based on the nursing assessment data, major nursing diagnoses for the patient may include the following:

- Ineffective airway clearance related to tracheobronchial secretions
- Alteration in comfort (pain) related to facial edema and effects of procedure
- Potential alteration in nutrition (less than body requirements) related to changed physiology of oral cavity, dribbling, impairment of chewing and swallowing, excision surgery affecting the tongue
- Impaired verbal communication related to trauma/surgery producing anatomical and physiological abnormalities of speech
- Alteration in self-image related to disfigurement
- Alteration in family process related to grief reaction and disruption of family life

▷ Planning and Implementation

▷ *Goals:* The major goals of the patient may include maintenance of a patent airway and pulmonary function, achievement of increased comfort, attainment and maintenance of adequate nutritional status, development of some form of effective communication, reinforcement of positive self-concept, and achievement of effective family coping.

Nursing Interventions

Maintaining Airway and Pulmonary Function. The immediate postoperative concern following facial reconstruction is maintenance of an adequate airway. If the patient has regained consciousness, mental confusion with combative anxious behavior is a sign of anoxia. Sedatives or narcotics are not given in this situation as they may impair oxygenation. If the patient shows signs of restlessness, the airway is carefully inspected to see if there is laryngeal edema or accumulation of tracheobronchial mucus. Secretions are suctioned as necessary until the patient can manage the secretions without help. If a tracheostomy is used, suctioning is done with a sterile technique to prevent infection and cross-contamination. (See p. 432 for care of the patient with a tracheostomy.)

Achieving Comfort. Edema of the face is uncomfortable and is a consequence of this type of surgery. The patient's head and upper torso are kept slightly elevated (according to stability of blood pressure readings) to help reduce facial edema. Suction catheters attached to closed drainage may be in place to keep the tissues in close apposition and to remove serous discharge. If extensive reconstruction has been performed, sandbags ⅔ filled with sand and ⅓ filled with rice (easier to mold) are used to help keep the patient's head in the desired position.

Mild doses of analgesics as prescribed will usually control pain. If bone grafts have been taken for reconstruction, there can be considerable pain in the donor area. Pain may be more severe if secondary infection occurs, a complication that may be minimized if frequent oral hygiene is practiced. Inspect the mouth to note the location of sutures so that they are not accidently disturbed during the cleansing process. The mouth is cleansed according to the type of surgery. Loose clots may be removed by gentle swabbing. The patient is advised not to loosen clots with the tongue, as this may provoke fresh bleeding.

If the patient has head and neck cancer with increasing levels of pain, more sophisticated modalities of nursing management will be required. (See Chap. 15, The Person Experiencing Pain.)

Maintaining Adequate Nutrition. After oral and pharyngeal edema have diminished, the incisional areas and flaps are healed, and the patient is able to swallow saliva, fluids may be offered, followed gradually by soft foods. If the patient cannot eat enough to satisfy nutritional needs, enteral alimentation (infusion of nutrients, water, and vitamins into the stomach or proximal small intestine via tube) is employed. The formula strength and the feeding rate are gradually increased until the desired daily kcal are attained. (See p. 759 for nursing management of the patient requiring enteral feedings.) Patients who have had radical operations for large, encroaching neoplasms will literally have to learn to eat again. Positive nutrition is reflected in weight gain, and nutritional status is monitored by daily checks of weight and periodic checks of serum protein and electrolyte levels.

Enhancing Communication. Communication problems can present a major difficulty, and may range from little or no problem to loss of oral speech. Some tumors and trauma require aggressive surgical treatment that involves the larynx, tongue, and mandible. Paper, pen or pencil, and a firm writing surface should be provided. If the patient cannot write, a pictograph board may be used.

The family may become frustrated by the patient's inability to communicate. The patient soon senses this, and both parties withdraw. Allowing the family to vent their feelings and fears (away from the patient) is supportive.

Improving Self-Concept. Success in rehabilitation of the patient undergoing reconstructive surgery is determined in no small measure by the relationship among the patient, nurse, physician, and other personnel. Mutual trust, respect, and clear lines of communication are essential for an effective relationship. Unhurried visits provide emotional reassurance and support. Giving attention to the details of care brings physical and emotional relief and release.

Often the kinds of dressings that have to be worn, the unusual positions that have to be maintained, and the temporary incapacities that must be experienced can be upsetting to the most stable person. Honest praise for the patient's coping and fortitude reinforces self-respect. If prosthetic devices are to be used, the patient is taught how to use and care for them in order to gain a sense of greater independence. Once involved in self-care activities, the patient may feel new control over what was previously an overwhelming situation.

Patients with a severe disfigurement are encouraged to socialize in the hospital to experience the reactions of others in a more protected environment. Gradually they can widen this sphere of contact. Every effort is made to cover or mask defects. Patients may require support by members of the mental health team to accept their changed appearance.

Helping Family Coping. The family is informed about the patient's appearance following surgery, the presence of supportive equipment, and how the equipment aids in recovery. It is helpful to join the family for a few minutes during their first postoperative visit to help them cope with the changes they will see.

A major nursing task is to support the family in their decision to participate (or not to participate) in the patient's treatment. Nursing interventions also include helping the family members communicate by suggesting techniques for reducing anxiety and stress and promoting problem-solving and decision-making. These activities encourage nurturance and growth of family members.

▷ Evaluation

▷ *Expected Outcomes*

1. Patient maintains patent airway.
   a. Demonstrates respiratory rate within normal limits
   b. Has normal breath sounds
   c. Has no signs of choking or aspiration
2. Is free of complications
   a. Demonstrates vital signs within normal limits
   b. Undergoes normal wound healing
   c. Is free of signs of infection
3. Achieves increasing comfort
   a. Reports decreasing pain
   b. Demonstrates lessening facial edema
   c. Adheres to oral hygiene regimen to prevent infection/subsequent pain

4. Communicates effectively
   a. Uses appropriate aids to enhance communication
   b. Interacts with health team members and family/support persons
5. Develops positive self-image
   a. Expresses positive feelings about surgical changes
   b. Has appropriate eye contact and attention span
   c. Demonstrates increasing independence in self-care activities
   d. Uses prosthetic devices independently (when appropriate)
   e. Verbalizes plans for resumption of pre-illness activities (*e.g.*, work, recreational)
6. Family copes with situation.
   a. Demonstrate lessening anxiety and conflict among family members
   b. Verbalize what to expect

Laser Treatment of Cutaneous Lesions

Lasers are devices that amplify or generate highly-specialized rays of potent light. They are capable of mobilizing immense heat and power when focused at close range, and are a valuable tool in surgical procedures. Two types of lasers, the argon laser and carbon-dioxide laser, have application in dermatologic surgery.

Argon Laser

The argon laser produces a blue green light that is absorbed by vascular tissue and hence is useful in treating vascular lesions: port-wine stains, telangiectasias, vascular tumors, and pigmented lesions. The argon beam passes through the overlying skin and reaches the pigmented layer of the skin, causing protein coagulation in this area. An immediate effect is that tiny blood vessels under the skin are coagulated, causing the area to turn a much lighter color. A crust forms within a few days, persisting about 2 weeks.

Patient Education and Home Health Care. Cold compresses are usually applied over the treatment area for approximately 6 hours to minimize edema, exudate, and loss of capillary permeability. The patient is advised that there may be swelling of the treated area, and to avoid picking at the crust. Antibiotic ointment is applied sparingly until the crust separates. Makeup is not applied until after the wound has healed. Sun exposure over the treated area is avoided to prevent the development of hypopigmentation, and a sunscreen is to be used when exposure is unavoidable.

Carbon-Dioxide Laser

The carbon-dioxide laser emits light in the infrared spectrum that is absorbed at the skin surface because of the high water content of the skin and the long wavelength of the CO_2 light. As the laser beam strikes human tissue, it is absorbed by the intra- and extracellular water, which vaporizes, destroying the tissue. The CO_2 laser is a precise surgical instrument for use in vaporizing and excising tissue with minimal tissue damage. Because of the ability of the beam to seal blood and lymphatic vessels, it creates a dry surgical field that makes many procedures easier and quicker. It is useful for removal of epidermal nevi, tattoos, certain warts, and the like. Incisions made with the laser heal in much the same way as those made by a scalpel.

Patient Education and Home Health Care. The wound is covered with antibacterial ointment and a nonstick dressing. The patient is instructed to keep the wound dry and apply the prescribed ointment and dressing. After reepithelialization is complete, the dressing is removed. A steroid ointment may be prescribed at this stage to reduce chances of hypertrophic scarring.

Aesthetic Surgery

Rhytidectomy (face lift) is an operation on the face to remove soft-tissue folds and minimize cutaneous wrinkles. It is done to improve and create a more youthful appearance.

Psychological preparation requires that the person recognize the limitations of surgery and that miraculous rejuvenation will not occur. The patient is informed that the face may appear bruised and swollen after the dressings are removed, and that several weeks may pass before the edema subsides.

The procedure is done under local or general anesthesia, and the outpatient setting has become an increasingly popular site for the surgery. The incisions are placed in areas of concealment (natural skin folds and creases and areas hidden by hair). The loose skin, separated from underlying muscle, is pulled upwards and backwards. Excess skin that overlaps the incision line is removed. More recently, liposuction-assisted rhytidectomy is being done, in which fat is suctioned via a cannula through a small incision.

Patient Education. The patient is encouraged to rest quietly for the first 2 postoperative days until the dressings are removed. The head of the bed is elevated and neck flexion is discouraged to avoid compromising the circulation in the cervical (neck) flap. There is some degree of tightness of the face and neck due to pressure created by the newly-tightened muscles, fascia, and skin. Analgesics may be prescribed for discomfort. A liquid diet may be given by means of straws, and a soft diet is permitted if chewing is not too uncomfortable.

When the dressings are removed, the skin is gently cleansed of crusting and oozing and coated with the prescribed topical ointment. The matted hair may be combed with warm water and a wide-tooth comb.

The patient is advised not to lift or bend for 7 to 10 days because this activity may increase edema and provoke bleeding. Activities are gradually increased. When all sutures are removed, the hair may be shampooed and blown dry with *warm*, not hot, air to avoid burning the ears, which may be numb for a period of time. Sudden pain indicates that blood is accumulating underneath the skin flaps, and should be reported to the surgeon immediately. Complications include sloughing of the skin, deformities of the face and neck, and partial facial paralysis. Cigarette smoking has been implicated as a cause of skin slough in some patients.

The effects of a face lift will not stop the aging process. With time, the tissues drift downward. Some patients have two or more face lifts.

Rhinoplasty

Rhinoplasty is an operation designed to alter the shape of the nose. There are many variations of the procedure, and the operation is tailored to the specific nose. The patient may request that the nose be made narrower, that the tip be thinned, or that a hump be removed. If the function of the nose is altered, the term *nasal reconstruction* is used. Nasal reconstruction is usually done for developmental and traumatic deformities.

Rhinoplasty is done through intranasal incisions under local or general anesthesia. Following the operation, packing may or may not be placed inside the nose.

Patient Education. The patient is advised to rest sitting upright and reminded not to touch, pick, or blow the nose in order to avoid bleeding. Chewing may be uncomfortable for a time, and liquids are advised. Some degree of bruising may be noted. Due to swelling inside the nose, the patient will have symptoms of a head cold. This is to be expected.

Complications include unexpected bleeding, hematoma, and infection (rare).

Blepharoplasty

Blepharoplasty is an aesthetic operation designed to remove skin or fat from the upper or lower eyelids. The goal is restoration of the eyelids for a more youthful appearance. The procedure may be combined with a face lift. Although it is effective in tightening the eyelid skin and eliminating or reducing fat pads around the eye, blepharoplasty does not eliminate fine wrinkles, laugh lines, age lines, or pigmentation around the eyes.

The procedure is done in an outpatient/hospital/ambulatory care facility under local or general anesthesia. The incisions are made in the upper lid crease line and in the lower lid immediately below the eyelashes.

Patient Education and Home Health Care. The following are teaching points applicable to most patients:

* Considerable eyelid swelling can be expected within 24 hours, and may last up to 3 weeks. Sleeping with the head elevated will help to diminish swelling.
* Ice compresses may be applied (with approval by the surgeon) to the eyelids for 20 minutes, 3 to 4 times daily, to reduce postoperative swelling and ecchymoses and to provide a soothing effect. (This self-care activity also serves to distract the patient from the discomfort.) Warm compresses are applied after 48 hours to hasten resolution of bruising.
* During the early postoperative period, the lashes are cleansed with cotton-tipped applicators moistened with clear water or prescribed solution.
* A sunscreen should be used after healing because sun-damaged skin wrinkles more easily. Usually there are no contraindications to the application of eye cosmetics after sutures are removed.
* Complications include spontaneous bleeding, which may result in a hematoma and require surgical drainage. The patient is advised to contact the surgeon immediately if

bleeding occurs. *Epiphora* (excessive tearing) and *ectropion* (pulling-down of lower eyelid) may occur.

Chemical Face Peeling

Chemical face peeling involves the application of a chemical mixture to the face for the purpose of causing superficial destruction of the epidermis and the upper layers of the dermis. It is used to treat fine wrinkles and superficial blemishes. It is not a substitute for face lifting.

Pretreatment medication (analgesic and tranquilizer) is designed to control pain and apprehension. Prior to surgery, the skin is cleansed thoroughly and any soap and oily residue are removed with ether or acetone wipes. A phenol-based chemical in an oil–water emulsion is frequently used in the procedure because it causes a controlled, predictable chemical burn. The chemical is carefully applied in a systematic manner to the face with cotton-tipped applicators. The patient will experience a burning sensation at this time. A mask of waterproof adhesive may then be applied directly to the skin and molded closely to the contours of the face, thereby acting as an occlusive dressing that increases the chemical penetration and action. Some surgeons feel that equally good results can be obtained without occlusive tape. After the tape mask is applied, the burning sensation returns. Frequent small doses of analgesics and tranquilizers are given to keep the patient as comfortable as possible.

Nursing Interventions

After 6 or 8 hours, the face becomes edematous and the eyelids often swell shut. The patient should be reassured that this reaction is normal. Caution the patient to move the mouth as little as possible so that the tape stays adherent to the skin. The head of the bed is elevated, and liquids are administered through a straw.

By the second day, the patient may feel moisture under the dressings as serous exudate seeps from the chemically-treated skin.

Most of the burning pain usually subsides after the first 12 to 24 hours. The dressings are removed after 48 hours, exposing skin similar to that of a second-degree burn. The patient may become alarmed by the appearance of the skin, and should be reassured again. After the tape mask is removed, some surgeons dust the treated skin surface with thymol-iodide powder because of its drying and bacteriostatic effects. The powdered surface is left open and dry for a period of time, during which a thin, yellow brown crust forms. Some type of ointment is prescribed to cover the face in order to soften and loosen the crust. After several days, the patient is advised to wash the face with lukewarm water and to lubricate the face with an ointment between washings.

Patient Education and Home Health Care. Reinforce the physician's explanations that the redness of the skin gradually decreases over the next 4 to 12 weeks. Although a line between treated and untreated skin may be noted, makeup is usually permitted after the first few weeks. The patient is cautioned to avoid direct or reflected sunlight, as the treatment has reduced the natural protection from sun of the skin. The skin will probably never tan normally again. Blotchy pigmentation can occur if sunlight is not avoided.

Dermabrasion

Dermabrasion (skin planing) is a form of skin abrasion used to correct acne scarring, aging, and sun-damaged skin. A special instrument (motor-driven wire brush, diamond-impregnated disk, serrated wheel) is used in the procedure. The epidermis and some superficial dermis is removed, while enough of the dermis is preserved to allow reepithelialization of the dermabraded areas. Results are best in the face because it is rich in intradermal epithelial elements.

Patient Instruction and Preparation. The primary reason for undergoing dermabrasion is to improve appearance. The surgeon explains to the patient what can be expected from dermabrasion. The patient should also be informed about the nature of the postoperative dressing, what discomfort may be experienced, and how long it will be before the tissues look normal. Dermabrasion may be carried out in the office, the operating room, or an outpatient setting. It is done under local or general anesthesia. During the procedure, some dermatological surgeons use refrigerant anesthetics to turn the skin into a numb, solid mass of rigid tissue and to provide a momentarily bloodless surgical field. During and after planing, the area is irrigated with copious amounts of saline solution to remove debris and allow the surgeon to see the area. A dressing impregnated with ointment is usually applied to the abraded surface.

Patient Education and Home Health Care. The nurse instructs the patient about the aftereffects of the surgery. Edema occurs during the first 48 hours and may cause the eyelids to close. The patient should elevate the head of the bed to hasten fluid drainage. Erythema occurs, and can last for weeks or months. After 24 hours, the dressing may be removed (upon physician directives). When the serum oozing from the skin begins to gel, the patient applies the prescribed ointment to the face several times a day to prevent hard crusting and to keep the abraded areas soft and flexible. Clear water cleansing/soaking of the face is started with physician approval to remove crusts from the healing skin.

The patient is advised to avoid extreme cold and heat and excessive straining or lifting, which may bruise delicate new capillaries. Direct or reflected sunlight is avoided for 3 to 6 months, and a sunscreen should be used.

Body Contouring Surgery

Suction lipectomy is the removal of localized deposits of fat by suction after small incisions are made through the skin. It is done to reduce the volume of localized fat deposits and improve the contour of the body. A cannula is inserted through the skin incision into the fatty tissue, and fat is aspirated through the suction tube as the cannula is removed. The procedure is done most often on the abdomen, hips, buttocks, and thighs. Intraoperatively, blood is removed with fat and therefore blood loss is directly proportional to the size of the area being treated.

Suction lipectomy is more successful in younger persons because they have greater skin elasticity and better potential for the aspirated areas to contract smoothly. Aging and flabbiness impose limitations.

Patient Education and Home Health Care. The nurse advises the patient that there is minimal postoperative pain and discomfort, although bruising may be seen in the aspirated areas, and that a rapid recovery can be anticipated. The dressings over the area are to be kept dry. A compression garment or bandages aid in the reduction of edema. The patient is advised that full improvement may not be apparent for several months.

Potential complications include hypovolemia, infection, and failure of the skin to shrink adequately over the treated areas, which leaves irregular waves or depressions on the skin that can mar the aesthetic effect.

Tissue Expanders

A new trend in plastic and reconstructive surgery is the use of tissue expanders to produce tissue growth through stretch and molding techniques (Fig. 48-12). Skin has the ability to increase in surface area (expand) when mechanically stimulated from beneath by an enlarging mass. (This occurs naturally during pregnancy).

An inflatable expander is implanted beneath subcutaneous tissue and can be stretched by injections of fluid to produce an enlargement in the area of overlying skin and

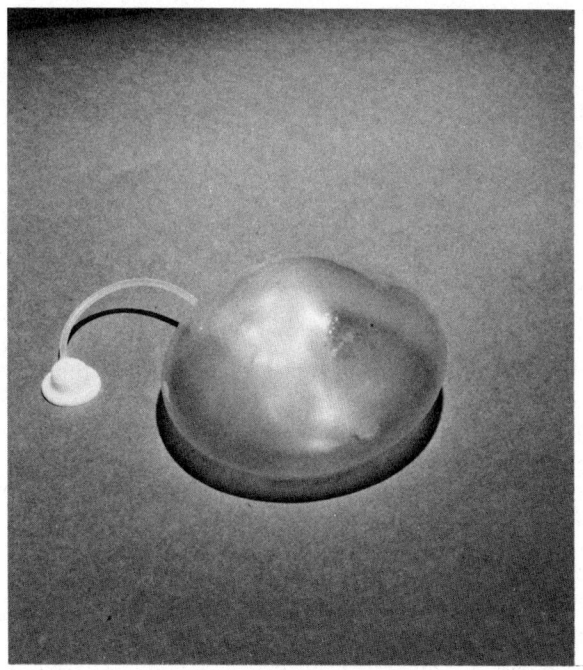

Figure 48-12
A round tissue expander, one of several types available. The expander is implanted to produce tissue growth in order to provide tissue of similar color and texture for reconstructive surgery. (Courtesy of Cox-Uphoff International.)

subcutaneous tissue. When the desired expansion is obtained, the expander is removed. Tissue expanders are used in breast reconstruction, for repair of tissue defects, and to facilitate the development of soft-tissue flaps in areas in which such flaps are not readily available.

Potential problems include compression and functional compromise of structures such as nerves and arteries.

Hair Disorders

Growth Cycle of Hair

Human scalp hair constantly renews itself and progresses through different phases of growth. Hair grows during the *anagen* (growth) phase, which may last 3 to 5 years (an average of 4 years). Approximately 90% of the hairs on the scalp are in this anagen phase. Hair grows at the rate of approximately 1 cm per month.

The second phase, *catagen* phase, lasts 1 to 2 weeks. The blood supply to the hair root slowly diminishes, the hair root becomes smaller, and the cells in the papilla slowly stop dividing.

The final phase is the *telogen* (end of growth) phase, lasting 4 to 6 months. The hair which only has a superficial root, pulls out easily when it is combed or brushed, or it is forced out of the scalp when a new hair, growing in the same follicle, enters the anagen phase. Thus, hair naturally falls out, with an average of 65 to 80 hairs being shed each day.

Alopecia

Alopecia is loss of hair or baldness. It may occur due to illness, drug therapy, hormonal imbalance, or nutritional problems. In these events, it usually can be reversed when the underlying disorder is corrected. Other causes include excessive traction on the hair (from braiding too tightly), excessive use of dyes, straighteners, and oils, fungus infection of the scalp, and moles or cancer on the scalp.

The most common cause of alopecia is male pattern baldness, affecting more than half of the male population. This is believed to be caused by a combination of factors including heredity, increasing age, and androgen (male hormone) levels. (The presence of androgen is necessary for male pattern baldness to develop.) The pattern of hair loss begins with receding of the hairline in the frontal-temporal area, and progresses to gradual thinning and complete loss of hair over the top of the scalp and crown.

Management

There are literally hundreds of over-the-counter products claiming to grow hair or prevent hair loss. Most, if not all, of these products are not effective. Search continues for a suitable antiandrogen to prevent hair loss.

Topical minoxidil is currently receiving a great deal of publicity as a method for treating baldness. The medication is applied to the scalp twice daily. It stimulates hair growth in some men with male pattern baldness, presumably by increasing the blood supply to the scalp. Hair growth is only maintained while treatment continues.

Natural-appearing hair pieces have been developed that allow the wearer to feel more attractive.

Hair Transplantation Surgery. Hair transplantation surgery (hair replacement surgery) involves transplanting hair-bearing skin from the sides and posterior portions of the scalp to recipient spaces in the bald areas. This redistributes the patient's remaining hair as naturally and evenly as possible over the bald scalp area, and is accomplished by punch grafting, scalp reduction, or the use of flaps of various kinds.

Punch grafting is the transplantation of small plugs of hair-bearing scalp from the uninvolved areas at the back and side of the head to the bald areas. It is done in 4 or more sessions, 1 to 2 months apart, and is an office outpatient procedure.

Scalp reduction is a surgical procedure in which the bald portion of the scalp is reduced by staged surgical excisions. It is usually the procedure of choice for baldness of the vertex (top of head) and anterior vertex regions.

Hair-bearing *flaps* can be transposed from adjacent areas into bald areas. This procedure may be performed in several stages over a period of several months. With the use of flaps, 200 to 250 hairs per square centimeter, about normal density, can be transferred. Thus hair is obtained instantly as soon as the flap is rotated over the bald area. (Flaps are discussed on p. 1283.)

Infection and bone necrosis can occur in scalp operations.

Bibliography

Books

Aldhizer TG, Krop TM, and Dunn JW. The Doctor's Book on Hair Loss. Englewood Cliffs, Prentice-Hall, 1983.

Baker TJ and Gordon HL. Surgical Rejuvenation of the Face. St Louis, CV Mosby, 1986.

Balch CM and Milton GW. Cutaneous Melanoma. Philadelphia, JB Lippincott, 1985.

Blitzer A et al. Rehabilitation of the Head and Neck Cancer Patient. Springfield, Charles C Thomas, 1985.

Burton JL. Essentials of Dermatology, 2nd ed. New York, Churchill Livingstone, 1985.

Dagher FJ (ed). Cutaneous Wounds. Mt Kisco, Futura Publishing, 1985.

DeLauney WE and Land WA. Principles and Practice of Dermatology. Sydney, Butterworths, 1984.

Dobson RL and Abele DC. The Practice of Dermatology. New York, Harper & Row, 1985.

Epstein E. Regional Dermatology: A System of Diagnosis. New York, Grune & Stratton, 1984.

Fisher JC, Guerrerosantos J, and Gleason M. Manual of Aesthetic Surgery. New York, Springer-Verlag, 1985.

Fitzpatrick TB et al. Dermatology in General Medicine, 3rd ed, Vol 1 and 2. New York, McGraw-Hill, 1987.

Flowers FP and Krusinski PA. Dermatology in Ambulatory and Emergency Medicine: A Clinical Guide With Algorithms. Chicago, Year Book Medical Publishers, 1984.

Fry L. Dermatology: An Illustrated Guide, 3rd ed. Boston, Butterworths, 1983.

Fry L and Cornell MNP. Dermatology. Boston, MTP Press, 1985.

Fry L (ed). Skin Problems in the Elderly. New York, Churchill Livingstone, 1985.

Gilchrest BA. Skin and Aging Processes. Boca Raton, Florida, CRC Press, 1984.

Goin JM and Goin MK. Changing the Body: Psychological Effects of Plastic Surgery. Baltimore, Williams & Wilkins, 1981.

Habif TP. Clinical Dermatology. St Louis, CV Mosby, 1985.

Kemble JVH and Lamb BE. Plastic Surgical and Burns Nursing. Philadelphia, Baillière Tindall, 1984.

Landow RK. Handbook of Dermatologic Treatment. Greenbrae, California, Jones Medical Publishers, 1983.

Lowe NJ. Practical Psoriasis Therapy. Chicago, Year Book Medical Publishers, 1986.

McFarland GK and Wasli EL. Nursing Diagnoses and Process in Psychiatric Mental Health Nursing. Philadelphia, JB Lippincott, 1986.

McQuarrie DG et al. Head and Neck Cancer. Chicago, Year Book Medical Publishers, 1986.

Moschella SL and Hurley HJ. Dermatology: Vols 1 and 2, 2nd ed. Philadelphia, WB Saunders, 1985.

Norwood OT and Shiell RC. Hair Transplant Surgery, 2nd ed. Springfield, Charles C Thomas, 1984.

Orkin M and Maibach HI. Cutaneous Infestations and Insect Bites. New York, Marcel Dekker, 1985.

Ratz JL. Lasers in Cutaneous Medicine and Surgery. Chicago, Year Book Medical Publishers, 1986.

Regnault P and Daniel RK. Aesthetic Plastic Surgery. Boston, Little, Brown & Co, 1984.

Rosen T, Lanning MB, and Hills MJ. The Nurses' Atlas of Dermatology. Boston, Little, Brown & Co, 1983.

Roses DF and Harris MN. Malignant Melanoma. In Nealon TF Jr. Management of Patient With Cancer, pp 40–91. Philadelphia, WB Saunders, 1986.

Sauer GC. Manual of Skin Diseases, 5th ed. Philadelphia, JB Lippincott, 1985.

Stegman SJ and Tromovitch TA. Cosmetic Dermatologic Surgery. Chicago, Year Book Medical Publishers, 1984.

Thiers BH and Dobson RL. Pathogenesis of Skin Disease. New York, Churchill Livingstone, 1986.

Vallis CP. Hair Transplantation for the Treatment of Male Pattern Baldness. Springfield, Charles C Thomas, 1982.

Verbow JL. Dermatological Surgery. Boston, MTP Press, 1986.

Webster MHC and Soutar DS. Practical Guide to Free Tissue Transfer. Boston, Butterworths, 1986.

Zacarian SA. Cryosurgery. St Louis, CV Mosby, 1985.

Articles

Assessment and Treatment

Alexander-Williams J. Pruritus ani. Postgrad Med 1985 Jan; 77(1):56–59, 62, 65.

Bergfeld WF. Cutaneous signs of internal malignancy. Postgrad Med 1986 Feb 15; 79(3):75–80.

Dangel RP. Pruritus and cancer. Oncol Nurs Forum 1986 Jan/Feb; 13(1):17–21.

Fenske NA and Cohen LE. The dermatologic exam. Emerg Clin North Am 1985 Nov; 3(4):643–658.

Gilchrest BA. Age-associated changes in the skin. J Am Geriatr Soc 1982 Feb; 30(2):139–143.

Norris J and Kunes-Connell M. Self-esteem disturbance. Nurs Clin North Am 1985 Dec; 20(4):745–761.

Weston W. Topical corticosteroids in dermatologic disorders. Hosp Pract 1984 Jan; 19(1):159–178.

Acne

Jowett S and Ryan T. Skin disease and handicap: An analysis of the impact of skin conditions. Soc Sci Med 1985; 20(4):425–429.

Orfanos CE et al. Current developments of oral retinoid therapy with three generations of drugs. Curr Probl Dermatol 1985; 13:33–49.

Shalita AR (ed). Symposium on acne. Derm Clin 1983 July; 1(3):33–413.

Alopecia

Birnbaum PS and Arndt KA. Alopecia: Common and uncommon. Hosp Pract 1986 May 30; 21(5A):19, 23, 26–27.

Kabaker SS et al. Tissue expansion in the treatment of alopecia. Arch Otolaryngol Head Neck Surg 1986 July; 112(7):720–725.

Storer JS et al. Review: Topical minoxidil for male pattern baldness. Am J Med Sci 1986 May; 291(5):328–333.

Stough DB, Mendoza F, and Freilich IW. Surgical procedures for the treatment of baldness. Cutis 1986 May; 37(5):362–365.

Blistering Diseases

Ahmed AR. Pemphigus vulgaris: Clinical features. Derm Clin 1983 Apr; 1(2):171–177.

Bystryn J-C. Adjuvant therapy of pemphigus. Arch Dermatol 1984 July; 120(7):941–951.

Chu AC. Bullous dermatoses. Curr Top Pathol 1985; 74:225–270.

Edlich RF et al. Toxic epidermal necrolysis. Compr Ther 1986 May; 12(5):43–49.

Flowers FP and Sherertz EF. Immunologic disorders of the skin and mucous membranes. Med Clin North Am 1985 July; 69(4):657–673.

Kamanabroo D, Schmitz-Landgraf W, and Czarnetzki BM. Plasmapheresis in severe drug-induced epidermal necrolysis. Arch Dermatol 1985 Dec; 121(12):1548–1549.

Lever WF and Schaumberg-Lever G. Treatment of pemphigus vulgaris. Arch Dermatol 1984 Jan; 120(1):44–47.

Levine N. Management of life-threatening dermatoses. Emerg Clin North Am 1985 Nov; 3(4):747–763.

Lynch DP. Ulcerations of the tongue. Postgrad Med 1984; 75(4):191–203.

Management of toxic epidermal necrolysis. Lancet 1984 Dec 1; 2(8414):1250–1252.

Merot Y and Saurat JH. Clues to pathogenesis of toxic epidermal necrolysis. Int J Dermatol 1985 Apr; 24(3):165–168.

Rayle RT. 5 nursing lessons from a patient with T.E.N. Am J Nurs 1986 May; 86(5):300–302.

Singer KH et al. Pathogenesis of autoimmunity in pemphigus. Annu Rev Immunol 1985; 3:87–108.

Cancer of the Skin; Melanoma

Callen JP and Allegra JC. Cutaneous oncology. Med Clin North Am 1986 Jan; 70(1):1–209.

Evans JF and Miller OF. Malignant melanoma and its precursors. Postgrad Med 1986 Feb; 79(2):215–222.

Fraser MC and McGuire DB. Skin cancer's early warning system. Am J Nurs 1984 Oct; 84(10):1232–1236.

Friedman RJ, Rigel DS, and Kopf AW. Early detection of malignant melanoma. CA 1985 May/June; 35(3):130–151.

Krementz ET. Regional perfusion: Current sophistication. What next? Cancer 1986 Feb 1; 57(3):416–437.

Minton JP. The staging and surgical management of primary malignant melanoma. Cancer Treat Res 1984; 21:1–59.

Pathak MA. Sunscreens: Topical and systemic approaches for the prevention of acute and chronic sun-induced skin reactions. Dermatol Clin 1986 Apr; 4(2):321–334.

Stegman SJ. Basal cell carcinoma and squamous cell carcinoma: Recognition and treatment. Med Clin North Am 1986 Jan; 70(1):95–107.

White MJ and Polk HC Jr. Therapy of primary cutaneous melanoma. Med Clin North Am 1986 Jan; 70(1):71–87.

Zitelli JA. Mohs surgery. Int J Dermatol 1985 Nov; 24(9):541–548.

Infestations and Infections

Balfour HH. Acyclovir therapy for herpes zoster: Advantages and adverse effects. JAMA 1986 Jan 17; 255(3):387–388.

Hallal JC. Understanding herpes zoster and relieving its discomfort. Geriatr Nurs 1985 Mar/Apr; 6(2):74–78.

Leyden JJ. Infection in the immunocompromised host. Arch Dermatol 1985 July; 121(7):855–857.

Orkin M and Maibach HI. Modern aspects of scabies. Curr Probl Dermatol 1985; 13:109–127.

Potter B. Skin diseases: Current concepts, therapy. 5. Virus infections. Indiana Med 1985 Nov; 78(11):1004–1006.

Stawiski MA. Insect bites and stings. Emerg Clin North Am 1985 Nov; 3(4):785–808.

Psoriasis

Anderson PC. Psoriasis. Postgrad Med 1986 Apr; 79(5):185–190.

Morrow NC. Printed information for patients receiving PUVA therapy. J Clin Hosp Pharm 1984 Dec; 9(4):333–340.

Muller SA and Perry HO. The Goeckerman treatment in psoriasis: Six decades of experience at the Mayo Clinic. Cutis 1984 Sept; 34(3):265–268.

Watson A. The treatment of psoriasis. Aust Fam Physician 1985 Oct; 14(10):1082–1083.

Weinstein GD and Voorhees JJ (eds). Symposium on psoriasis. Dermatol Clin 1984 July; 2(3):357–515.

Surgery

Barratt GE and Koopmann CF Jr. Skin grafts: Physiology and clinical considerations. Otolaryngol Clin North Am 1984 May; 17(2):335–351.

Dixon JA and Gilbertson JJ. Cutaneous laser therapy. West J Med 1985 Dec; 143(6):758–763.

Farrior RT. Dermabrasion in facial surgery. Laryngoscope 1985 May; 95(5):534–545.

Halbal MB. Prevention of postoperative facial edema with steroids after facial surgery. Aesthetic Plast Surg 1985; 9(7):69–71.

Levine MR. Prevention and management of complications of blepharoplasty. Facial Plast Surg 1984 Summer; 1(4):311–321.

Macgregor FC (ed). Symposium on social and psychologic considerations in plastic surgery. Clin Plast Surg 1982 July; 9(3):281–395.

Mangan M. Patient education with tissue expanders. Plast Surg Nurs 1986 Summer; 6(2):76–78.

Markland A. Nursing care of the suction lipectomy patient. Plast Surg Nurs 1984 Summer; 4(2):44–46.

Nahai F and Mathes SJ. Musculocutaneous flap or muscle flap and skin grafts. Ann Plast Surg 1984 Feb; 17(7):199–203.

Noe JM and Olbricht SM. Lasers in plastic surgery. Adv Plast Reconstr Surg 1986; 2:147–191.

Rees TD, Liverett DM, and Guy CL. The effect of cigarette smoking on skin-flap survival in the face-lift patient. Plast Reconstr Surg 1984 June; 73(6):911–915.

Seaton C and Dempsey P. Suction lipolysis: A personal perspective. Plast Surg Nurs 1984 Summer; 4(2):47–49.

Trimble JR. Skin grafting as an office procedure in dermatology. Dermatol Clin North Am 1984 Apr; 2(2):251–270.

Agencies and Sources of Information

American Cancer Society, Inc., 90 Park Avenue, New York, NY 10016.

National Institute of Arthritis and Musculoskeletal and Skin Diseases, National Institutes of Health, Bethesda, MD 20892.

National Psoriasis Foundation, 6415 S.W. Canyon Court, Suite 200, Portland, OR 97221.

Skin Cancer Foundation, 575 Park Avenue South, New York, NY 10016.

Management of Patients With Burn Injury

Approximately 2,000,000 people experience burn injury in the United States annually. Of this group, 200,000 require outpatient treatment and 75,000 are hospitalized. About 12,000 people die from burns and related inhalation injuries. More than half of burn injuries leading to hospital admissions could have been prevented. Nurses can play an active role in preventing fires and burns by teaching prevention concepts and promoting legislation related to the use of smoke detectors, space heaters, and fire-retardant fabrics.

Young children and the elderly are at particularly high risk for burn injury. Adolescent males and men of working age also are burned more frequently than would be expected by their representation in the total population. Most burn injuries occur in the home or in the immediate vicinity. Cooking, heating, or use of electrical appliances is usually involved. Industrial settings also account for a large number of burn injuries.

The National Institute for Burn Medicine, which collects statistical data from burn centers throughout the U.S., notes that most patients (75%) are victims of their own actions. Scalds in toddlers, match play in school-age children, electrical injury in adolescent males, and cigarette smoking and alcohol use in adults all contribute to this fact and are prime targets for burn prevention.

There are four major goals relating to human burns:

1. Prevention
2. Institution of lifesaving measures for the severely burned person
3. Prevention of disability and disfigurement through early, specialized, individualized treatment
4. Rehabilitation of the individual through reconstructive surgery and rehabilitative programs

Pathophysiology of Burns

Burns are caused by a transfer of energy from a heat source to the body. Heat may be transferred through conduction or electromagnetic radiation. Burns can be categorized as thermal, radiation, electrical, or chemical. Tissue destruction results from coagulation, protein denaturation, or ionization of cellular contents. The skin and the mucosa of the upper airways are the most common sites of tissue destruction. Deep tissues, including the viscera, can be damaged by electrical burns or through prolonged contact with the burning agent.

The depth of the injury depends on the temperature of the burning agent and the duration of contact with the agent. For example, in the case of scald burns, hot tap water at a temperature of 68.9°C (156°F) may in the course of 1 second result in a burn that destroys both epidermis and dermis (full-thickness injury). Within 15 seconds of exposure to hot water at 56.1°C (133°F), a similar full-thickness injury will occur.

The first effect a burn has is to produce a dilatation of the capillaries and small vessels in the area of the burn, thus increasing capillary permeability. Plasma seeps out into the surrounding tissues, producing blisters and edema. The type, the duration, and the intensity of the burn affect the amount and duration of the fluid loss.

Generally, the fluid leak occurs in greatest magnitude over the first 24 to 36 hours postburn, peaking by 12 hours postinjury. In major burns, capillary leaking continues in small amounts for several weeks. This capillary leak is not confined to the burn area alone when the burns involve more than 30% of the body surface. Rather, edema occurs throughout the body.

- One of the first steps in the management of burns is to provide fluid replacement therapy.

With a burn, plasma, proteins, and electrolytes are lost from the vascular compartment and move to the interstitial compartment. However, red blood cells usually remain in the vascular compartment, which results in an increase in blood viscosity, hematocrit, and hemoglobin in the early hours postburn.

The fluid loss following a burn results in reduced fluid volume in the vascular system and a fall in blood pressure and cardiac output. The response of the sympathetic nervous system to this burn shock is an increase in peripheral resistance, reflected in decreased pulse pressure and an increase in pulse rate. Prompt fluid resuscitation allows blood pressure to stay in the low normal range.

As the capillaries begin to regain their integrity, 48 to 72 hours postburn, fluid returns to the vascular compartment and the patient moves into the acute stage of burn care. As fluid is reabsorbed from the interstitial tissue into the vascular compartment, blood volume increases. An extra strain is placed on the heart and, if renal function is adequate, urinary output is greatly increased. Diuresis continues for several days to 2 weeks, with a loss of body weight. During this period, the patient is at risk for fluid overload and may require cardiotonic drugs and diuretics to support circulatory function and prevent congestive heart failure. Fluid restriction may be needed to prevent pulmonary edema.

Fluid, Electrolyte, and Blood Needs

Evaporative fluid loss through the burn wound may reach 3 to 5 liters or more per 24-hour period. The need for water replacement can be measured by monitoring serum sodium and potassium; a sodium reading higher than the normal level of 140 to 144 mEq/liter (140–144 mmol/L) suggests the need

for water. More frequently, *serum hyponatremia* (sodium below 132 mEq/liter [132 mmol/L]) occurs between the third and the tenth day with rapid movement of fluid from the burned area.

Hypokalemia may occur at this time unless adequate oral intake of food and fluids is possible; the patient may need as much as 80 to 100 mEq per day of potassium.

Other indications helpful in determining water replacement needs are urinary output and weight loss, which should not exceed 1 kg per day. If the patient is not able to stand on a scale at the bedside, a bed scale is used.

At the time of burn injury, some red blood cells may be destroyed and others damaged, resulting in anemia. Blood loss during operative procedures, wound care, diagnostic studies, and infection resulting in hemolysis further contribute to anema. (Abnormalities in coagulation, including a decrease in platelets [thrombocytopenia] and prolonged clotting and prothrombin times occur with burn injury.) Blood transfusions are required periodically to maintain hemoglobin above 10 gm/dl (1.55 mmol/L) and hematocrit above 30 vol % (volume fraction: 0.3).

Pulmonary Pathophysiology

Pulmonary pathophysiology frequently accompanies burn injury and falls into four categories: carbon monoxide poisoning, smoke inhalation, upper airway injury, and restrictive defects. Carbon monoxide intoxication and smoke inhalation are the leading causes of death in fire victims. It is estimated that at least 50% of these deaths could have been prevented by such devices as smoke detectors.

Carbon monoxide is a prominent cause of inhalation injury. The pathophysiologic effects are due to tissue hypoxia. Carbon monoxide combines with hemoglobin to form carboxyhemoglobin, which competes with oxygen for available hemoglobin-binding sites. The affinity of hemoglobin for carbon monoxide is 200 times greater than for oxygen. Decreased oxygen in the area of the fire and added effects of smoke poisoning contribute to carbon dioxide poisoning.

Smoke inhalation injury results from noxious chemicals formed in the burning process (particularly organic compounds such as plastics); these chemicals include hydrogen cyanide, hydrochloric acid, sulfuric acid, halogens, and benzene. Smoke inhalation causes loss of ciliary action and severe mucosal edema. In the lungs, surfactant activity is reduced, which results in atelectasis. Expectoration of carbon particles with sputum may occur. In a few hours, sloughing of the tracheobronchial mucosa may occur, and the patient may cough up mucopurulent material.

Upper airway injury occurs from the effects of heated air or steam and noxious chemical gases on the structures of the upper airway. These cause an inflammatory reaction, with edema and airway obstruction possible at any time during the first 48 hours postinjury.

Restrictive defects arise from burns. Full-thickness burns encircling the neck and thorax result in edema of great magnitude. Edema may compress the trachea and occlude the airway. Chest excursion may be greatly restricted, resulting in a decreased tidal volume. Fluid shifts from the vascular compartment to the interstitial tissue affect the lung parenchyma and may result in decreased lung compliance, non-cardiogenic pulmonary edema, and signs and symptoms of adult respiratory distress syndrome.

Pulmonary abnormalities are not always immediately apparent. More than half of burn victims with pulmonary involvement do not initially demonstrate pulmonary signs and symptoms. Airway obstruction may occur very rapidly or may take hours to develop. Decreased lung compliance, decreased PaO$_2$, and respiratory acidosis may occur gradually.

Indicators of possible pulmonary damage include the following:

1. A history indicating that the burn occurred in an enclosed area
2. Burns of the face, neck, or areas around the mouth
3. Singed nasal hair
4. Hoarseness, voice change, dry cough, sooty sputum
5. Bloody sputum, labored respiration, erythema, and blisters of the oral or pharyngeal mucosa

Diagnosis of inhalation injury is an important priority for many burn victims. Blood carbon monoxide levels, arterial blood gases, and bronchoscopy are frequently used to aid diagnosis in the early postburn period. Xenon lung scans are another adjunct to diagnosis of injury that interferes with air flow in small airways. Pulmonary function studies may also be useful in diagnosing decreased lung compliance or obstruction of air flow.

Other Systemic Effects of Burns

The immunologic defenses of the body are greatly altered by burn injury. The obvious loss of skin integrity is compounded by abnormal inflammatory factors, altered levels of immunoglobulins and serum complement, and a reduction in lymphocytes (*lymphocytopenia*). Loss of skin also results in an inability to regulate body temperature adequately, and burn patients may manifest low body temperatures in the early hours postburn. As hypermetabolism resets core temperatures, burn patients become hyperthermic for much of the postburn period, even in the absence of infection and its effect in producing fever.

Decreased peristalsis and bowel sounds are manifestations of paralytic ileus resulting from burn trauma. Gastric distention and nausea may lead to vomiting unless gastric decompression is initiated. Gastric bleeding may be manifested through occult blood in the stool, regurgitation of coffee-ground material from the stomach, or definite signs of bloody vomitus. These signs provide evidence of gastric or duodenal erosion.

Extent of Burns and Local Response

Burn Depth

Burns are classified according to the depth of tissue destruction, and are identified as superficial partial-thickness injuries, deep partial-thickness injuries, or full-thickness injuries. Corresponding descriptive terms are first-degree, second-degree, and third-degree.

The local response to burn injury is dependent on the depth of tissue destruction.

- In a *superficial partial-thickness (first-degree) injury,* the epidermis is destroyed or injured and a portion of the dermis may be injured. The wound may be painful and may appear red and dry, as in the case of sunburn, or it may be blistered.
- A *deep partial-thickness (second-degree) injury* involves destruction of the epidermis and upper layers of the dermis, and injury to deeper portions of the dermis. The wound is painful, appears red, and weeps fluid. Blanching of the burned tissue is followed by capillary refill; hair follicles remain intact.
- A *full-thickness (third-degree) injury* involves total destruction of epidermis and dermis and, in some cases, underlying tissues as well. The color of the wound varies widely. The burn is painless, due to destruction of nerve fibers, and has a leathery appearance.

Table 49-1 describes these wounds in detail.

Although partial-thickness wounds may heal by spontaneous reepithelialization, a skin graft is frequently required to close the wound. The wound may be quickly colonized by pathogenic bacteria. When a conservative approach to wound care is used, large amounts of dead tissue (*eschar*) are left on the wound for several weeks. After the eschar is removed or sloughs off naturally, the burn wound must heal by secondary intention, which increases repair time as fibroblasts, new capillaries, and collagen fibers form. During this period, the wound is susceptible to infection because the devitalized tissue on the wound serves as a culture medium for prolific bacterial growth.

In determining the depth of a burn, it is important to identify the following factors:

- The causative agent, such as flame or a scalding liquid
- The temperature of the burning agent
- The duration of contact with the agent
- The thickness of the skin

The presence of hemoglobin and myoglobin in the urine suggests deep burns. The depth and extent of the burn are considered in determining the appropriate site for treatment (Table 49-2).

Intravenous fluorescein may be used to determine the functional circulation in the skin and, in that way, differentiate between full-thickness, deep dermal, and superficial burns. Burn wound biopsy and histologic examination also indicate the depth of tissue destruction.

Extent of Surface Area Burned

Rule of Nines. An estimation of the total body surface area (BSA) involved as a result of a burn is simplified by using the Rule of Nines (Fig. 49-1). The Rule of Nines measures the percentage of the body burned by dividing the body into multiples of nine. The initial evaluation is made upon arrival at the hospital and revised on the second and third postburn days, because the demarcation usually is not clear until then.

Berkow Method. A more reliable method of estimating the extent of burned surface area is provided by use of the Berkow method, which is based on Lund and Brower's recognition that the percentage of body surface area of various

TABLE 49-1
Evaluation of Depth of a Burn

Cause of Burn	Skin Involvement	Symptoms	Appearance	Course
Superficial (First Degree)				
Sunburn Low-intensity flash	Epidermis	Tingling Hyperesthesia Painful Soothed by cooling	Reddened; blanches with pressure Minimal or no edema	Complete recovery within a week Peeling
Partial-Thickness (Second Degree)				
Scalds Flash flame	Epidermis and part of dermis	Painful Hyperesthesia Sensitive to cold air	Blistered, mottled red base; broken epidermis; weeping surface Edema	Recovery in 2 to 3 weeks Some scarring and depigmentation Infection may convert to third-degree.
Full-Thickness (Third Degree)				
Fire Prolonged exposure to hot liquids	Epidermis, entire dermis, and sometimes subcutaneous tissue	Painless Symptoms of shock Hematuria and hemolysis of blood likely	Dry; pale white or charred Broken skin with fat exposed Edema	Eschar sloughs Grafting necessary Scarring and loss of contour and function

anatomical parts, especially the head and legs, changes with growth. By dividing the body into very small areas and providing an estimate of the proportion of body surface area accounted for by such body parts, one is able to obtain a very reliable estimate of total surface area involved. This is helpful in estimating fluid requirements and determining prognosis and surgical intervention (Figure 49-2).

Survival Prediction.   The best survival rate occurs in children and young adults, ages 5 to 40 years. In this group, burns of about 60% of the body have a mortality rate of 50%. A burn of more than 20% of the body endangers life. Table 49-3 gives a clear picture of the effects of age and percent of body burned on survival rate.

Prognosis depends on the depth and extent of the burn, as well as on the condition and age of the patient.

Stages of Burn Care

The pathophysiology and management of a burn can be divided into three stages. Although priorities exist for each of the stages, it is imperative to remember that these stages overlap, and that assessment and management of specific problems and complications are *not* limited to these stages but take place throughout the course of burn care.

The three stages and the priorities for care are summarized in Table 49-4.

Stage I: Immediate/Emergent Phase

Emergency Management

On-the-Scene Care

- *When clothes catch on fire*, the flames can be extinguished if the victim falls to the floor or ground and rolls ("drop and roll"); anything available to smother the flames, such as a blanket, rug, or coat, may be used. Standing still would force the victim to breathe flames and smoke, and running would fan the flames.
- After the flames are extinguished, the burned area and adherent clothing are soaked with cold water, briefly, to allow the wound to cool to normal body temperature. Although adherent clothing may be left in place, other clothing and all jewelry should be removed to allow for assessment and to prevent constriction secondary to rapidly developing edema.
- Once a burn has been sustained, the application of cold is the best first-aid measure. Soaking the burn area intermittently in cool water or applying cold towels gives immediate and striking relief from pain and restricts local tissue edema and damage. However, one should not ap-

TABLE 49-2
Types of Burn Injury and Recommended Treatment Site

Type of Injury	Definition/Description	Recommended Treatment Site
Minor Burn Injury	*2nd-degree* (partial-thickness) —less than 15% in adults	Hospital emergency department B (basic level)
	3rd-degree (full-thickness) —less than 2%	
Moderate Uncomplicated Burn Injury	*2nd-degree* (partial-thickness) —15–25% in adults —10–20% in children or elderly	Burn program or burn unit/center I (intermediate level)
	3rd-degree (full-thickness) —less than 10%	
Major Burn Injury	*2nd-degree* (partial-thickness) more than 25%	Burn unit/center A (advanced level)
	3rd-degree (full-thickness) more than 10%	
	Smaller burns at extremes of age (<2 or >60 years)	
	Burns involving face, hands, feet, perineum	
	Burns with inhalation injury	
	Electrical burns	
	Burns with other trauma or illness	

(Data from Specific Optimal Criteria for Hospital Resources for Care of Patients with Burn Injury. American Burn Association.)

Percent (%) refers to percent of body surface area (BSA) burned.

ply ice directly to the burn or use cold soaks or dressings for an extended period of time; such a procedure may worsen the burn and lead to hypothermia in patients with large burns.

- The burn should also be covered as quickly as possible to minimize bacterial contamination and decrease pain by preventing air from coming into contact with the injured surface. Sterile dressings are best, but any clean, dry cloth can be used as an emergency dressing.
- Ointments and salves are not used. In fact, other than the dressing, no medication or material should be applied to the burn wound.
- *Chemical burns,* which result from contact with a corrosive material, are irrigated immediately. Most chemical laboratories have a high-pressure shower for such emergencies; if such an injury occurs at home, all areas of the body that have come in contact with the chemical should be rinsed for several minutes in a shower or other source of continuously running water.
- If a chemical gets in or near the eyes, the eyes should be flushed with cool, clean water for a period of 15 to 20 minutes.

Airway, Breathing, Circulation. Although the local effects of a burn are the most evident, the systemic effects pose a greater threat to life. Therefore, it is important to remember the ABCs of all trauma care during the early postburn period:

- *A*irway
- *B*reathing
- *C*irculation

Breathing must be assessed and a patent airway established immediately during the initial minutes of emergency care. Many burn victims sustain some degree of concomitant pulmonary dysfunction, as previously described.

- Immediate therapy is directed toward establishing an airway, possibly through oropharyngeal suctioning followed by the administration of 100% oxygen. If such a high concentration of oxygen is not available under emergency conditions, oxygen by mask or nasal prongs is given initially.

In mild cases, inspired air is humidified and the patient is encouraged to cough so that secretions can be suctioned. For more severe situations, it is necessary to remove secretions by bronchial suctioning and to administer bronchial dilators and mucolytic agents.

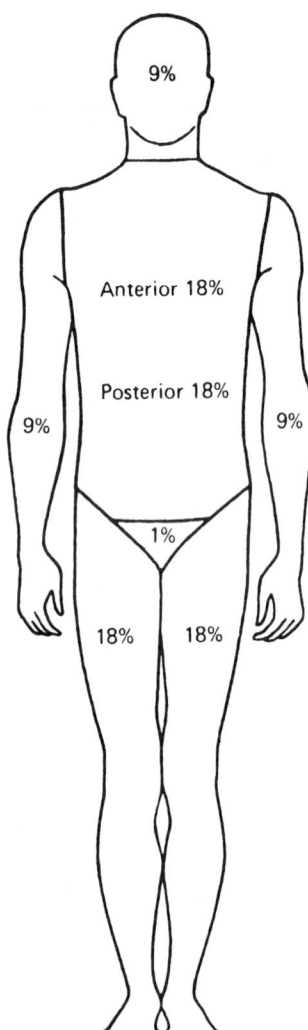

Figure 49-1
The Rule of Nines for estimating the percentage of body burns in the adult.

- When edema of the airway is present, it may be necessary to intubate the patient. Hyperinflation hourly with an Ambu-bag helps to prevent atelectasis. Continuous positive airway pressure and mechanical ventilation may also be required.

Authorities differ on the administration of antibiotics. Gram stains of the sputum will help in determining antibiotic use; if gram-positive organisms and large numbers of neutrophils are present, penicillin or penicillinase-resistant antibiotics are given. Usually, steroids are not given because their disadvantages outweigh advantages. Meticulous aseptic technique in all aspects of tracheal care is required in this infection-prone patient.

The circulatory system must also be assessed quickly. Apical pulse and blood pressure are monitored frequently. Tachycardia and slight hypotension are expected in the untreated patient early postburn.

Prevention of Shock. Prevention of shock in a person with a major burn is imperative. Therefore, intravenous fluid therapy is initiated promptly.

- *Nothing* should be given by mouth, and the patient should be placed in a position that will prevent aspiration of vomitus, since nausea and vomiting often occur as a result of paralytic ileus resulting from the stress of injury.
- In *rare* instances in which definitive care is markedly delayed, an effective first-aid measure is to give fluids to drink to the conscious patient who can tolerate them. To a quart of water (1 liter), add 1 teaspoon (3 gm) of salt and a half teaspoon (1.5 gm) of soda bicarbonate. (Salt provides sodium, and soda bicarbonate helps to combat acidosis.)

Usually, an emergency medical technician (EMT) or ambulance or fire personnel will take steps to cool the wound, establish an airway, supply oxygen, and start an IV line.

Emergency Room Management

The victim is transported to the nearest emergency department. The hospital and physician are alerted that the victim is on the way. Thus, lifesaving measures can be initiated immediately by a trained team, with no time lost.

After adequate respiratory and circulatory status have been established, attention is directed to the burn wound itself. All smoldering clothing and jewelry are removed. Flushing of chemical burns with water is continued. The patient is checked for the presence of contact lenses; these are removed immediately if chemicals have contacted the eyes or if facial burns have occurred. It is important to validate the history of the burn scenario provided by the paramedics, and to assess the patient for cervical neck fracture or head injury if an explosion, a fall, a jump, or an electrical injury has occurred.

Assessment of the extent of body surface area burned and the depth of the burn is carried out by the physician and nurse. Full- and partial-thickness burns are noted and documented on burn assessment diagrams (Figs. 49-1 and 49-2). These assessments are performed after soot and debris have been gently cleansed from the burn wound. Assessment is repeated frequently during the course of burn wound care.

Overview of Immediate Patient Care

When the patient is admitted to the hospital, clothes are carefully removed, weight and height are recorded, and the patient is placed on or between sterile or pathogen-free (freshly laundered) sheets. Because this patient is usually frightened and may be in emotional shock, those in attendance should demonstrate concern. Reassurance and support are provided and explanations are given when necessary. If the patient wants to see a spiritual advisor, one should be notified.

TABLE 49-3
Survival Rate in Relation to Age and Percentage of Burn

Age	Percent of Body Burned	Survival	Mortality
5 and under	50%	66%	34%
5–40	50%	80%	20%
40–60	50%	51%	49%
Over 60	50%	9%	91%

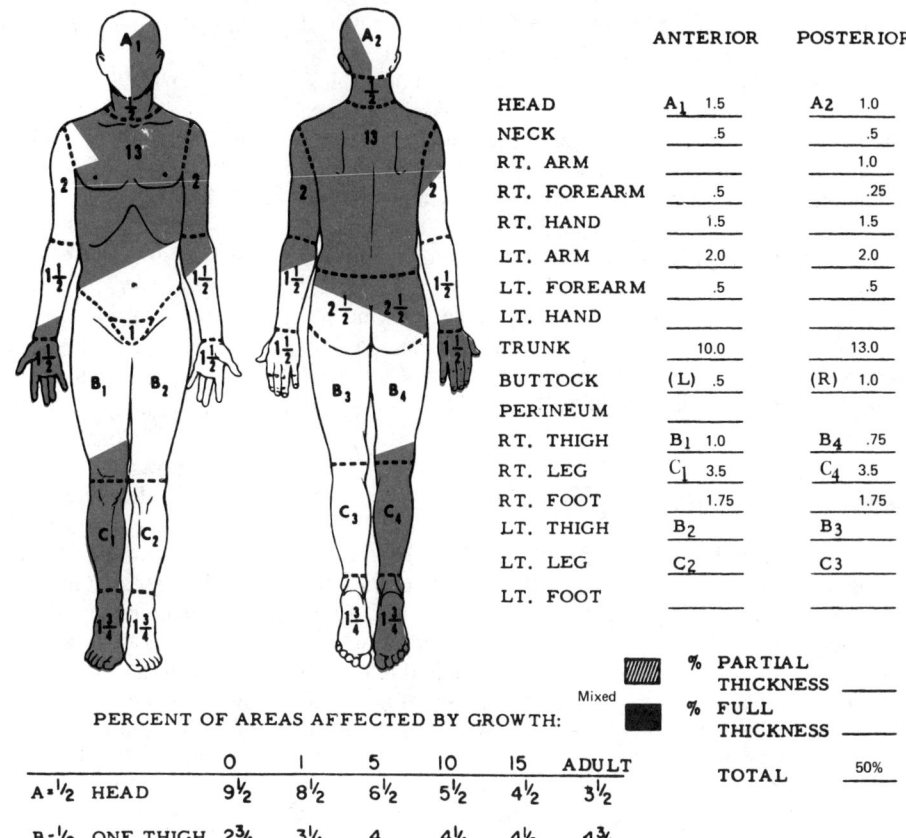

	ANTERIOR		POSTERIOR	
HEAD	A_1	1.5	A_2	1.0
NECK		.5		.5
RT. ARM				1.0
RT. FOREARM		.5		.25
RT. HAND		1.5		1.5
LT. ARM		2.0		2.0
LT. FOREARM		.5		.5
LT. HAND				
TRUNK		10.0		13.0
BUTTOCK	(L)	.5	(R)	1.0
PERINEUM				
RT. THIGH	B_1	1.0	B_4	.75
RT. LEG	C_1	3.5	C_4	3.5
RT. FOOT		1.75		1.75
LT. THIGH	B_2		B_3	
LT. LEG	C_2		C_3	
LT. FOOT				

PERCENT OF AREAS AFFECTED BY GROWTH:

Mixed

% PARTIAL THICKNESS ____

% FULL THICKNESS ____

TOTAL ____ 50%

		0	1	5	10	15	ADULT
A = 1/2	HEAD	9½	8½	6½	5½	4½	3½
B = 1/2	ONE THIGH	2¾	3¼	4	4¼	4½	4¾
C = 1/2	ONE LEG	2½	2½	2¾	3	3¼	3½

Figure 49-2
Burn Evaluation Chart–estimation of percent body burns. (Courtesy of Crozer-Chester Medical Center.)

Careful attention must be given to aseptic technique. Attending personnel wear masks, caps, and gowns; sterile gloves are worn when the burn area is handled. The physician evaluates the patient's general condition, assesses the burn, determines the priorities, and directs the individualized plan of treatment, which is divided into systemic management and local care of the burned area.

Photographs may be taken of the burn areas at this time and periodically throughout the treatment. In this way, the progress of healing may be determined quickly. Such evidence is invaluable in insurance claims and courts of law.

Environment Preparation. When a bed is prepared for a burn patient, the mattress is completely covered with a plastic sheet, which is covered in turn with a sterile bottom

TABLE 49-4
Stages of Burn Care

Stage	Duration	Priorities
I	From onset of injury to completion of fluid resuscitation	• First-aid • Prevention of shock • Prevention of respiratory distress • Wound assessment and initial care • Detection and treatment of concomitant injuries
II	From beginning of diuresis to near completion of wound closure	• Wound care and closure • Prevention and treatment of complications, including infection • Nutritional support
III	From major wound closure to return to individual's optimal level of physical and psychosocial adjustment	• Prevention of scars and contractures • Physical, occupational, and vocational rehabilitation • Functional and cosmetic reconstruction • Psychosocial counseling

sheet. Sterile Microdon sheeting (3M Company) on top of this bedding prevents the patient from sticking to the sheets as a result of the oozing of exudate from the burn. Caps, masks, and sterile gowns and gloves are available for those attending the patient. The equipment most likely to be required should be in the room, including intravenous therapy equipment, with polyethylene central venous catheters and fluids (*e.g.,* plasmanate and lactated Ringer's solution); blood withdrawal syringes, needles, and tubes; catheterization tray and drainage equipment; urine testing devices; tracheostomy set; intubation equipment; venesection set; suction and oxygen therapy equipment; fresh, pathogen-free linens; overbed cradle; and side rails. The particular procedure to be followed in wound care determines additional needs.

Transfer to a Burn Center

If the patient is to be transported to a burn center, the following measures are instituted prior to transfer: a secure IV line is in place, with fluid infusing at the rate required to attain urine output of at least 30 ml per hour; a patent airway is ensured; adequate pain relief is administered; and adequate peripheral circulation in the burned extremities is established. Wounds are covered with sterile, dry dressings and the patient is kept comfortably warm.

Management of Fluid Derangement and Shock

Next to handling respiratory difficulties, the most urgent need is to replace lost fluid and to prevent irreversible shock (Table 49-5).

Therefore, immediate management of the burn patient includes the following:

- An intravenous route is established, preferably through an unburned area.
- Blood specimens are drawn for hematocrit, electrolyte, and blood gas determinations, and for typing, cross-matching, and screening. These parameters must be followed closely in the immediate postburn (resuscitation) period.
- An indwelling urinary catheter is inserted so that urine volume and specific gravity can be monitored hourly. The amount of urine first obtained is recorded, because it may assist in determining the extent of renal function. It should also be tested for hemoglobin. Urine volumes of less than 30 ml per hour (10 ml in children) are reported.
- The patient's vital signs are monitored at frequent intervals: temperatures above 38.3°C (101°F) or below 36.1°C (97°F) are reported.

TABLE 49-5

Water and Electrolyte Changes in the Emergent Phase of Burn Care (First 48 Hours After Major Burns)

Fluid Accumulation Phase (Shock Phase)
Plasma → Interstitial Fluid (Edema at Burn Site)

Observation	*Explanation*
Generalized dehydration	Plasma leaks through damaged capillaries.
Reduction of blood volume	Brought about by plasma loss, fall of blood pressure, and diminished cardiac output
Decreased urinary output	Secondary to: Fluid loss Decreased renal blood flow Sodium and water retention caused by increased adrenocortical activity (Hemolysis of red blood cells, causing hemoglobinuria and myonecrosis or myoglobinuria)
Potassium excess	Massive cellular trauma causes release of K^+ into extracellular fluid (ordinarily, most K^+ is intracellular).
Sodium deficit	Large amount of Na^+ is lost in trapped edema fluid and exudate and by shift into cells (ordinarily, most Na^+ is extracellular).
Metabolic acidosis (base bicarbonate deficit)	Loss of bicarbonate ions accompanies sodium loss.
Hemoconcentration (elevated hematocrit)	Liquid blood component is lost into extravascular space.

(Adapted from Metheny NM and Snively WD. Nurses' Handbook of Fluid Balance. Philadelphia, JB Lippincott)

Fluid Replacement

There is no known way to stop movement of fluid into the interstitial spaces, but replacement of fluids is possible. The physician calculates the projected fluid requirements for the first 24 hours by evaluating the patient's burn injury. Some combination of fluid categories may be appropriate: (1) *colloids*—whole blood, plasma, and plasma expanders; and (2) *electrolytes*—physiologic sodium chloride, Ringer's solution, Hartmann's solution.

Formulas have been developed for estimating fluid loss based on the estimated percentage of body surface area burned and the weight of the patient. These are individualized to meet the requirements of each patient. The various formulas are discussed in the following paragraphs and summarized in Chart 49-1.

The Consensus Formula. At the NIH Consensus Development Conference in Supportive Therapy in Burn Care in November 1978, it was agreed that salt and water are essential requirements of burn patients, but that colloid may or may not be useful during the first 24 to 48 hours postburn.

The consensus formula provides for the volume of balanced salt solution to be administered in the first 24 hours in a range of 2 to 4 ml per kilogram per percent burn. The volume should be started at the lower level of this range, as the overall goal of fluid therapy is to maintain vital organ function at the least immediate or delayed physiological cost.

Generally, 2 ml per kilogram per percent burn of lactated Ringer's solution may be used for adults, while children may require 3 ml per kilogram per percent burn. As with the other formulas, half of the calculated total should be given over the first 8 hours postburn, and the other half given over the next 16 hours. The rate and volume of the infusion must be regulated according to the patient's response.

Studies have demonstrated that with large burns there is a failure of the sodium–potassium pump at the cellular level. Thus, persons with very large burns may need proportionately more milliliters of fluid per percent burn than those with smaller burns.

Fluid Replacement Example:
70-kg patient with 50% body surface area (BSA) burn

1. Consensus formula: 2 to 4 ml/kg/% BSA
2. Calculate $2 \times 70 \times 50 = 7000$ ml/24 hours
3. Plan to administer: First 8 hours = 3500 ml = 437 ml/ hour; next 16 hours = 3500 ml = 219 ml/hour

The Evans Formula. According to the Evans formula, second- to third-degree burns totaling more than 50% BSA are calculated on the basis of 50% BSA.

1. *Colloids* (blood, plasma, dextran): 1 ml × kg body weight × % BSA burned
2. *Electrolytes* (saline): 1 ml × kg body weight × % BSA burned
3. *Glucose* (5% in water): 2000 ml (for insensible losses)

A maximum of 10,000 ml of total fluids is given in a 24-hour period. One half of the calculated fluid is given in the first 8 hours postburn; the remainder is spread evenly over the next 16 hours.

On the second postburn day, the patient receives one half of the colloid, one half of the electrolyte, and all of the insensible replacement.

Chart 49-1
Guidelines and Formulas for Fluid Replacement in Burn Patients

Consensus Formula

Lactated Ringer's solution (or other balanced salt solution): 2–4 ml × kg body weight × % body surface area (BSA) burned. Half to be given in first 8 hours; second half to be given over next 16 hours

Evans Formula

1. *Colloids:* 1 ml × kg body weight × % BSA burned
2. *Electrolytes (saline):* 1 ml × kg body weight × % BSA burned
3. *Glucose (5% in water):* 2000 ml for insensible loss
   Day 1: Half to be given in first 8 hours; second half over next 16 hours
   Day 2: Half of previous day's colloids and electrolytes; 2000 ml for insensible fluid replacement

Brooke Army Formula

1. *Colloids:* 0.5 ml × kg body weight × % BAS burned
2. *Electrolytes (lactated Ringer's solution):* 1.5 ml × kg body weight × % BSA burned
3. *Fluids:* Same as Evans formula
   Day 1: Same as Evans formula
   Day 2: Half of colloids; half of electrolytes; all of insensible fluid replacement

Parkland/Baxter Formula

Lactated Ringer's solution: 4 ml × kg body weight/% BSA burned. One third to be given in first 8 hours; two thirds to be given over next 16 hours

Hypertonic Saline

Concentration solutions of NaCl and lactate with concentration of 300 mEq of sodium, administered at a rate sufficient to maintain a desired urinary output volume. *Goal:* Increase serum sodium level and osmolality to reduce edema and lung complications.

The Brooke Army Hospital Formula. This formula differs from the Evans formula only in that the colloid fraction is reduced from 1 ml to 0.5 ml and the electrolyte fraction is increased from 1 ml to 1.5 ml. Instead of saline, the electrolyte preferred is lactated Ringer's solution because of its lower chloride content.

On the second postburn day, the patient receives one half of the colloid, one half of the electrolyte, and all insensible replacement.

The Parkland or Baxter Formula. The patient is given 4 ml of lactated Ringer's solution per kilogram body weight per percent BSA burned. One third is given in the first 8 hours, and the rest over the next 16 hours.

Hypertonic Saline. This method utilizes concentrated solutions of sodium chloride and lactate, so that the resulting solution has a concentration of 300 mEq of sodium. It is administered at a rate sufficient to maintain a desired urinary output. The rate is *not* usually increased during the first 8 hours postburn. The major therapeutic effects are a result of the sustained hypernatremia and the increase in serum osmolality that occur. Edema is reduced and lung complications from fluid loading are decreased.

Remember: Formulas are a guide. Patient response is the primary determinant of actual fluid therapy, and must be assessed at least hourly.

Fluid Therapy

The amount and speed of fluid given through an indwelling plastic vein cannula are gauged by the urinary output and the blood pressure and pulse rate. Urine flow from an indwelling catheter should be maintained at 30 to 70 ml per hour. This means that the flow from the indwelling catheter must be collected, measured, and recorded every hour. Pulse rate should be lower than 110 per minute.

These parameters are far more important in resuscitation than any formula. Indeed, the patient's individual response *is* the "formula."

- The following observations must be reported:

   1. The presence of hematuria
   2. Urine output below 30 ml per hour—this suggests an inadequate rate of fluid resuscitation.
   3. Urine output above 100 ml per hour, which may precede pulmonary edema or imminent water intoxication (suggested by the following signs: tremor, twitching, nausea, diarrhea, salivation, and disorientation)
   4. Blood pressure below 90/60

If all extremities are burned, blood pressure determination may become difficult. A sterile dressing applied under the blood pressure cuff will protect the wound from contamination. A Doppler (ultrasound) device, an electronic blood pressure device, or other noninvasive means of monitoring may be helpful. An arterial catheter is used in severe burns for blood pressure measurement and accessibility for collection of specimens for measuring blood gases.

The Doppler is a useful tool in monitoring peripheral pulses. A more sophisticated method of determining tissue pressure levels to permit early intervention in the event of compartment syndrome is the use of the Wick catheter, connected to a transducer.

Additional gauges of the fluid requirements include hematocrit and hemoglobin determinations. Blood samples for these examinations and for the determination of electrolyte balance are withdrawn at frequent intervals. If the hematocrit and hemoglobin determinations decrease, or if the urinary output is more than 50 ml of urine per hour, the speed of flow of the intravenous solution may be decreased.

Although not responsible for calculating the patient's fluid requirements, the nurse needs to know the maximal amount of fluid the patient should receive. Infusion pumps and rate controllers are a useful adjunct to the correct delivery of a complex regimen of prescribed intravenous fluids. With the addition of piggy-back IVs for antibiotic infusion and hyperalimentation, monitoring intravenous therapy is a major nursing responsibility.

▶ Nursing Process
Burn Care During
the Immediate/Emergent Phase

▷ Assessment

Assessment data obtained by pre-hospital providers are shared with the physician and nurse in the Emergency Department.

Nursing assessment in the emergent stage of burn injury focuses on the major priorities for assessment of any trauma patient, with the wound as a secondary consideration.

If a patent airway and spontaneous respirations are noted, the nurse looks further for signs of inhalation injury.

Apical, carotid, and femoral pulses are checked. Cardiac monitoring is useful if there is a history of cardiac disease, electrical injury, or respiratory problems, or if the pulse is dysrrhythmic and the rate is abnormally slow or rapid.

Vital signs are checked frequently using a Doppler or Dynamapp device, as increasing edema makes cuff pressures difficult to detect. Signs of hypovolemia are reported to the physician. Peripheral pulses are checked hourly on burned extremities. As edema increases in circumferential burns, pressure on small blood vessels and nerves in distal extremities causes obstruction to blood flow and ischemia. The physician may need to perform an *escharotomy* (surgical incision into the eschar) to relieve the constricting effect of the burned tissue.

Large-bore intravenous lines and an indwelling urinary catheter are inserted, and the nurse's assessment includes monitoring of fluid intake and output. Urine output is usually an excellent indicator of circulatory status; it is monitored constantly and measured hourly. Urine specific gravity, *p*H, glucose, acetone, protein, and hemoglobin levels are assessed periodically.

A burgundy color of the urine may indicate the presence of hemochromogen and myoglobin in the urine as a result of deep muscle damage from deep burns associated with electrical injury or prolonged contact with flames. Glucosuria is a common finding in the early hours postburn, due to the body's response to this stressful event.

Nursing assessment includes reviewing results of laboratory and radiologic tests. Although chest x-ray and arterial blood gases may be normal initially, changes will often occur with time and progression of inhalation injury. It is essential to note the presence of increased hoarseness, stridor, abnormal respiratory rate and depth, or mental changes caused by hypoxia. These may signal the need for intubation, mechanical ventilation, or escharotomy to relieve constriction from circumferential chest burns.

Body temperature, body weight, history of preburn weight, allergies, tetanus immunization, past medical and surgical problems, current illnesses, and use of medication are assessed. A head-to-toe assessment is performed, looking for signs and symptoms of concomitant illness or injury.

Assessment of the burn wound continues, using anatomical diagrams described previously. In addition, the nurse works with the physician to assess the depth of the wound, noting areas of full- and partial-thickness injury.

The neurological assessment focuses on the patient's level of consciousness, psychological status, and behavior. The patient's understanding of the injury and treatment, and that of the family or significant others is assessed.

▷ Nursing Diagnoses

Based on assessment data, clinical manifestations, and laboratory data, nursing diagnoses in the emergent (immediate) postburn stage may include the following:

- Impaired gas exchange related to carbon monoxide poisoning, smoke inhalation, and upper airway obstruction
- Ineffective airway clearance related to edema and effects of smoke inhalation
- Impaired ventilation related to edema
- Fluid volume deficit related to increased capillary permeability and evaporative fluid loss from burn wound
- Decreased cardiac output related to fluid shifts and hypovolemic shock
- Inadequate tissue perfusion related to peripheral burn wound edema and circumferential full-thickness burns
- Potential for altered body temperature: hypothermia related to loss of skin microcirculation and open wounds
- Altered gastric integrity and function related to stress response and burn shock

▷ Planning and Implementation

▷ *Goals:* The major goals of the patient may include maintenance of a patent airway, ventilation, and tissue oxygenation; establishment of optimal fluid and electrolyte balance and perfusion of vital organs; maintenance of normal body temperature; and relief of gastrointestinal dysfunction.

Nursing Interventions

Maintaining Oxygenation. Assessment for signs of upper airway obstruction or a compromised lower airway is an essential nursing activity. Aggressive pulmonary measures—including turning, coughing, deep breathing, periodic forceful expiration using spirometry, and tracheal suction as needed—are particularly important in the burn patient with inhalation injury. Proper positioning to decrease the work of breathing and promote optimal chest expansion and providing humidified oxygen or mechanical ventilation may further decrease metabolic stress and ensure adequate tissue oxygenation. The nurse reports promptly to the physician any signs of respiratory compromise resulting from edema, and prepares to assist with naso- or endotracheal intubation, tracheotomy, or escharotomy as required. Asepsis is maintained to prevent contamination of the respiratory tract and infection that increases metabolic requirements.

Establishing Fluid and Electrolyte Balance. Rapid fluid shifts and losses during the early postburn period require that nurses frequently assess vital signs and urinary output, as well as central venous pressure, pulmonary artery pressure, and cardiac output if required. Intravenous fluids are provided as prescribed, and may need to be titrated with urinary output. Meticulous documentation of intake and output and daily weight is required. The patient must be monitored for early signs of hypovolemic and septic shock or fluid overload, including altered mental status, change in respirations, and hemodynamic parameters.

The extremities are assessed carefully, particularly if burns are circumferential, to detect compromised circulation resulting from increased edema or a constricting effect of eschar formation in full-thickness burns. Placing the affected extremities in an elevated position may be indicated to help reduce edema.

Maintaining Normal Body Temperature. Burn patients are prone to chilling and hypothermia because a loss of the skin microcirculation in the burned areas decreases the patient's ability to retain body heat. The room temperature is adjusted according to the patient's needs. An environment that is too warm may cause fluid loss through perspiration, and in addition may promote bacterial growth. Overcooling of a room, which can easily occur when staff members turn on air conditioners to keep themselves comfortable, will chill the patient and increase metabolic demands. A patient who is allowed to control ambient temperature will select a temperature of approximately 32.2°C to 32.8°C (90°–91°F). Cotton blankets, ceiling-mounted heat lamps, and aluminum-coated "space" blankets are helpful in maintaining the patient's comfort. Heat shields with sensors and blanket-draped bed cradles to deflect drafts are also useful. An efficient approach to removing dressing and caring for the wound shortens the time during which patients are exposed to the ambient temperature and reduces shivering and metabolic stress.

Due to episodes of bacteremia and septicemia, fever is also common in burn patients. A resetting of core body temperature in severely burned persons causes them to have a body temperature a few degrees higher than normal for several weeks postburn in some cases. Bacteremia and septicemia also cause fever in many patients. Acetaminophen and hypothermia blankets may be required to keep body temperature in a range of 37.2° to 39.4°C (99°–103°F) and to reduce metabolic stress.

Alleviating Gastrointestinal Disturbances. Gastric dilatation and paralytic ileus frequently occur in the early postburn period, and are indicated by nausea and distention. A nasogastric tube is inserted early in the treatment to prevent vomiting and aspiration of gastric contents into the lungs. The tube is connected to low intermittent suction until bowel sounds return.

When oral alimentation is initiated after the immediate or emergent burn phase, oral fluids should be administered slowly. The patient's tolerance is noted and, if vomiting and distention do not occur, fluids may be increased gradually and the patient advanced to a normal diet or tube feedings.

Severely burned patients are prone to gastric and duodenal ulcers. Gastric pH should be assessed regularly in the patient with a nasogastric tube and maintained at a level less acidic than usual through antacid therapy. Histamine blockers such as cimetidine or ranitidine (Zantac) are administered as prescribed to prevent gastric erosion and the formation of bleeding ulcers.

▷ Evaluation

▷ *Expected Outcomes*

The major outcomes expected for the burn patient in the Immediate/Emergent phase include the following:

1. Patient maintains patent airway, adequate ventilation, and oxygenation.

  a. Breathes spontaneously with adequate tidal volume
  b. Is free of dyspnea or shortness of breath
  c. Exhibits respiratory rate between 12 and 20
  d. Has pulmonary function parameters within normal limits
  e. Lungs sound clear on auscultation.
  f. Chest x-ray is normal.
  g. Is free of cerebral signs of hypoxia.
  h. Arterial blood gases are within normal limits.
  i. Respiratory secretions are minimal, colorless, and thin.
  j. Uses humidifed oxygen as prescribed.
  k. Coughs and breathes deeply hourly
2. Regains optimal fluid and electrolyte balance and perfusion of vital organs
  a. Intake, output, and body weight correlate with pattern of physiologic pathology and expected results of therapy.
  b. Serum electrolytes are within normal limits.
  c. Urine output is between 0.5 ml/kg and 1.0 ml/kg/hour.
  d. Blood pressure is higher than 90/60.
  e. Heart rate is lower than 110/minute.
  f. Heart is in sinus rhythm.
  g. Sensorium is clear.
  h. Patient is free of thirst.
  i. Shows normal reflexes and muscle tone indicative of electrolyte balance
  j. BUN and creatinine are normal.
  k. Urine is clear yellow; protein, sugar, acetone, pH, and specific gravity are within normal limits.
  j. Hemoglobin and hematocrit are normal.
  k. Patient is free of paresthesias or symptoms of ischemia of nerves and muscles (compartment syndrome).
3. Demonstrates acceptable body temperature
  a. Body temperature is in range of 36.0°C to 38.3°C (97°–101°F).
  b. Patient reports comfort without chills or shivering.
4. Achieves normal gastrointestinal function
  a. Bowel sounds are normal.
  b. Gastric aspirate is normal, with no indication of blood present.
  c. Tolerates oral or nasogastric feedings.
  d. Stools negative for occult blood
  e. Reports absence of abdominal pain or feeling of abdominal fullness or bloating
  f. Exhibits no abdominal distention on palpation

Care of the patient during this emergent or immediate phase of burn care is delineated in Nursing Care Plan 49-1.

Stage II: Intermediate/Acute Phase

General Care Considerations

The intermediate phase of burn care follows the immediate phase of burn care, and begins 48 to 72 hours after the burn injury. During this phase, continued attention is directed toward assessment and maintenance of respiratory and circulatory status, fluid and electrolyte balance, and gastrointestinal function. Burn wound care, however, is also a major focus of this stage.

Airway obstruction as a result of upper airway edema can take as long as 48 hours to develop. Changes in x-rays and blood gases may be noted as the effects of resuscitative fluid and the chemical reaction of smoke ingredients with lung tissues become apparent. The physician uses the patient's arterial blood gases and other parameters to determine the need for intubation, tracheostomy, or mechanical ventilation.

As capillaries regain their integrity, in 48 hours or more postburn, and fluid moves from the interstitial to the vascular compartment, diuresis begins (Table 49-6, p. 1308). If cardiac or renal function is not adequate, fluid overload occurs and symptoms of congestive heart failure may result. Detection of early signs allows for early intervention and careful titration of fluid intake. Cardiotonic drugs and diuretics may also be necessary at this time to prevent congestive heart failure.

Cautious administration of fluids and electrolytes continues during this phase of burn care because of the shifts in fluid from interstitial to vascular compartments, losses of fluid from large burn wounds, and the patient's physiological responses to the burn injury. If blood transfusions are necessary to treat blood loss and anemia, the patient is monitored closely for a possible transfusion reaction.

Central venous, peripheral arterial, Swan-Ganz, or thermal-dilution catheters may be required for monitoring venous and arterial pressures, pulmonary wedge pressures, or cardiac output. Generally, however, invasive lines are avoided unless absolutely necessary because they provide an additional portal for infection in this already greatly compromised patient.

Infection is the major cause of death in patients who have survived the first few days following extensive burns. The infection begins within the burn site and then is carried into the bloodstream. Because of the danger of infection, cultures are taken of the burn wound on admission and twice weekly to monitor colonization of the wound by microbial organisms. A major part of the nurse's role during this and other phases of burn care is detection and prevention of infection. Several parenteral antimicrobial agents may be used to treat or prevent infection and sepsis. It is important that these medications be given as scheduled to maintain proper blood concentrations.

The Burn Wound

The burn wound is unique among surgical wounds because it involves a large amount of dead tissue (eschar) that remains in place for a prolonged period of time. It is rapidly colonized by pathogenic bacteria, exudes large quantities of water, protein, and electrolytes, and frequently requires that tissue be mobilized through skin grafting from another part of the body to achieve permanent closure.

Threat of Infection

Despite aseptic precautions and the use of topical antibacterial agents, the burn wound represents an excellent medium for bacterial growth and proliferation. Bacteria such as *Staphylococcus, Proteus, Pseudomonas, Escherichia coli,* and *Klebsiella* enterobacteria find optimal conditions for growth

(Text continues on p. 1308)

Care of the Patient During the Emergent/Immediate Phase of Burn Care

| *Nursing Interventions* | *Rationale* | *Expected Outcomes* |

Nursing Diagnosis: Alterations in gas exchange and airway clearance

Goal: Assure patent airway and adequate respiratory function

1. Maintain patent airway through proper positioning, removal of secretions, and artificial airway if indicated.	1. Assures patent airway	• Patient breathes spontaneously. • Is free of dyspnea or shortness of breath • Exhibits respiratory rate between 12 and 20 • Has pulmonary function parameters within normal limits • Shows lungs clear on auscultation • Is free of cerebral effects of hypoxia • Has arterial blood gases within normal limits • Exhibits respiratory secretions that are minimal, colorless, and thin
2. Provide humidified oxygen through appropriate mode.	2. Provides humidity to injured tissues and adequate oxygen supply	
3. Assess breath sounds and respiratory rate, rhythm, and depth, chest excursion, and signs of hypoxia.	3. Provides baseline for further assessment and evidence of increasing respiratory compromise	

4. Observe for the following:
   a. Erythema or blistering of lips or buccal mucosa
   b. Singed nares
   c. Burns of face, neck, or chest
   d. Increasing hoarseness
   e. Soot in sputum or tracheal tissue in respiratory secretions
	4. Indicate injury to respiratory tree and/or risk of respiratory dysfunction	

5. Monitor arterial blood gases.	5. Increasing P_{CO_2} and decreasing P_{O_2} may indicate need for mechanical ventilation.	
6. Monitor patient on mechanical ventilation; check settings and patient responses as determined by arterial blood gases.	6. Respiratory dysfunction/pulmonary obstruction changes may occur quickly or gradually.	
7. Encourage patient to turn, take deep breaths, cough, and use incentive spirometry; suction as needed.	7. Reduces risk of atelectasis and promotes removal of increased secretions	

Nursing Diagnosis: Alterations in fluid and electrolyte balance

Goal: Restore optimal fluid and electrolyte balance; maintain perfusion of vital organs and adequate circulation to extremities

1. Observe vital signs (including central venous pressure or pulmonary artery pressure, if indicated), urine output, and signs of hypovolemia or fluid overload.	1. Hypovolemia is a major risk immediately after the burn injury; as mobilization of fluid occurs, there is increased risk of fluid overload and congestive heart failure.	• Patient shows intake, output, and body weight that correlate with pattern of physiologic pathology and expected results of therapy. • Has serum electrolytes within normal limits • Exhibits urine output between 0.5 ml/kg/hour and 1.0 ml/kg/hour • Has blood pressure higher than 90/60 • Shows heart rate less than 110/minute • Exhibits clear sensorium • Is free of excessive thirst • Shows normal reflexes and muscle tone indicative of electrolyte balance
2. Monitor urine output at least hourly and weigh patient daily.	2. Provides information about renal perfusion, adequacy of fluid replacement, and fluid requirement and fluid status	
3. Monitor mental status and sensorium.	3. Provides information about adequacy of cerebral perfusion and oxygenation	
4. Maintain IV lines and regulate fluids at appropriate rates, as prescribed.	4. Adequate fluids are necessary to maintain fluid and electrolyte status and adequate perfusion of vital organs.	

(continued)

Nursing Interventions	*Rationale*	*Expected Outcomes*

Nursing Diagnosis: Alterations in fluid and electrolyte balance

Goal: Restore optimal fluid and electrolyte balance; maintain perfusion of vital organs and adequate circulation to extremities

5. Observe for symptoms of deficiency or excess serum sodium, potassium, calcium, phosphorus, and bicarbonate. Note results of laboratory tests, and report abnormal values to physician.	5. Rapid shifts in fluid and electrolyte status are possible in the postburn period.	
6. Elevate head of patient's bed and elevate burned extremities.	6. Promotes venous return	

Nursing Diagnosis: Potential for infection

Goal: Absence of infection and sepsis

1. Use asepsis in all aspects of patient care:
   a. Careful hand washing with antibacterial cleansing agent before and after patient care
   b. Wear isolation gown or plastic apron for patient contact.
   c. Cover hair and use mask when patient's wounds are exposed or during sterile procedures.
   d. Use clean or sterile gloves in patient care.
   e. Use aseptic technique for wound care and invasive procedures.
   f. Change IV lines and tubing and other equipment as recommended.
	1. Minimizes risk of cross-contamination and spread of bacterial contamination	• Patient is free of signs of local or systemic infection.
		• Has negative blood cultures
		• Has negative wound, sputum, and urine cultures

2. Administer antibiotics and topical antibacterial agents as prescribed.	2. An adequate concentration of the agent is necessary to treat or prevent infection effectively.	
3. Assess wounds daily for local signs of infection: swelling and redness, purulent drainage, discoloration, loss of grafts.	3. Indicative of bacterial contamination and infection	
4. Observe mental status, respiratory rate, bowel sounds.	4. Decreased mentation and peristalsis and increased respiratory rate are early signs of septicemia.	
5. Assess for increased pulse, decreased BP, changes in urine output, facial flushing, fever.	5. These are later signs of septicemia.	
6. Provide adequate nutrition.	6. Adequate nutrition is essential for immunologic response (functioning of white blood cells and lymphocytes) and healing.	
7. Assist with or promote optimal personal hygiene: *e.g.*, daily cleaning of unburned areas, meticulous care of teeth and mouth, shampooing hair.	7. Reduces bacterial contamination from areas adjacent to burn	

(continued)

Nursing Interventions	*Rationale*	*Expected Outcomes*

Nursing Diagnosis: Altered body temperature: hypothermia

Goal: Maintenance of adequate body temperature

1. Provide a warm environment through use of heat shield, space blanket, heat lights, blankets, or thick dressings.	1. Minimizes evaporative heat loss	• Patient demonstrates acceptable body temperature, in range of 36.1°C (97°F) to 38.3°C (101°F). • Exhibits no shivering • States room temperature is not too warm or too cold
2. When wounds must be exposed for wound care, work quickly.	2. Minimizes heat loss through the burn wound	
3. Monitor rectal temperature.	3. Allows frequent assessment of body temperature	
4. Administer antipyretics for elevated body temperature as prescribed.	4. Reduces metabolic stress	

Nursing Diagnosis: Alteration in gastrointestinal function

Goal: Relief of gastrointestinal dysfunction

1. Maintain nasogastric tube on low intermittent suction until bowel sounds return.	1. Burn injury often produces paralytic ileus, which results in gastric and abdominal distention; nasogastric suction removes gastric secretions and prevents vomiting.	• Patient exhibits bowel sounds. • Shows normal gastric aspirate; no bleeding • Tolerates oral or nasogastric feedings • Has negative stools for occult blood
2. Auscultate for bowel sounds every 4 hours.	2. Absent bowel sounds and decreased peristalsis may indicate paralytic ileus, obstruction, or sepsis.	
3. Prior to tube feedings, aspirate stomach contents to check for residual amount and *p*H of gastric contents.	3. Large residual volume of gastric contents indicates inadequate absorption; low *p*H indicates need for histamine blockers or antacids.	
4. Administer histamine blockers and/ or antacids as prescribed.	4. Reduces risk of gastric ulceration common in burn patients	
5. Test stools and gastric aspirate contents for occult bleeding.	5. May indicate presence of gastric or duodenal ulcer	

Nursing Diagnosis: Alteration in comfort: pain and anxiety

Goal: Reduction in pain and anxiety

1. Assess patient for pain, and differentiate from hypoxia.	1. Assessment of pain provides baseline for evaluating pain relief measures.	• Patient shows that comfort level permits adequate rest and active participation in required activities. • Requires analgesics primarily prior to dressing changes and potentially painful treatments
2. Administer narcotic analgesics intravenously as prescribed.	2. Intravenous administration is necessary because of altered absorption and circulation resulting from the burn.	
3. Introduce relaxation techniques, imagery, or other adjuncts to analgesics.	3. Relaxation and imagery complement analgesia and reduce anxiety.	
4. Provide emotional support and reassurance.	4. Emotional support and reassurance are essential to reduce extreme fear and anxiety resulting from burn injury, treatments, and outcomes.	
5. Give honest information regarding status and medical care required for optimal response.	5. Promotes trust needed for patient's emotional well-being and acceptance of painful treatments	

TABLE 49-6
*Water and Electrolyte Changes in the Intermediate/Acute Phase of Burn Care
(Beginning 48 Hours After Major Injuries)*

Fluid Remobilization Phase (State of Diuresis)
Interstitial Fluid → Plasma

Observation	*Explanation*
Hemodilution (decreased hematocrit)	Blood cell concentration is diluted as fluid enters the vascular compartment; loss of red blood cells destroyed at burn site.
Increased urinary output	Fluid shift into intravascular compartment, increases renal blood flow, and causes increased urine formation.
Sodium deficit	With diuresis, sodium is lost with water; existing serum sodium is diluted by water influx.
Potassium deficit (occurs occasionally in this phase)	Beginning on the fourth or fifth postburn day, K^+ shifts from extracellular fluid into cells.
Metabolic acidosis	Loss of sodium depletes fixed base; relative carbon dioxide content increases.

(Adapted from Metheny NM and Snively WD. Nurses' Handbook of Fluid Balance. Philadelphia, JB Lippincott.)

within the burn. The burn eschar is a nonviable crust with no blood supply, so that polymorphonuclear leukocytes and antibodies, even systemic antibiotics, cannot reach the area. Phenomenal numbers of bacteria—over one billion per gram of tissue—may appear and subsequently spread to the bloodstream or release their toxins, which reach distant sites.

During the time in which the burn wound is healing through spontaneous reepithelialization or being prepared for skin grafting, it must be protected from burn wound sepsis. Burn wound sepsis has four key characteristics:

1. 10^5 bacteria/gram of tissue
2. Inflammation
3. Sludging and thrombosis of dermal blood vessels
4. Clinical symptoms of sepsis

The primary source of bacterial infection appears to be the patient's own intestinal tract. A major secondary source is the environment. Antibiotics seldom are given prophylactically today because of the tendency to promote resistant strains—except in patients with suspected respiratory injury. Sensitivity to antibiotics should be determined prior to administration. The choice of antibiotics for sepsis is based on the strains present in the patient's hospital unit. The antibiotics chosen should be effective against *Staphylococcus aureus* and *Pseudomonas*. Serum antibiotic levels are monitored for maximal effectiveness and minimal toxicity. Combination drug regimens may be helpful.

Localized infection must be identified and eliminated. A prime objective is to guard against resistance to antibiotics by maintaining strict isolation precautions.

- A mask and sterile gloves are worn while caring for the patient with extensive burns, in order to prevent infection. Aseptic technique, with cap and gown, is used when caring directly for burn wounds.

Because burns are contaminated wounds, adequate tetanus prophylaxis is given. If the patient has been immunized or has had no booster dose in the preceding 4 years, a booster dose of adsorbed tetanus toxoid is administered. If the patient has never had immunizing toxoid, then tetanus immune globulin (TIG) should be given. The extent of the burn and the environment in which the injury occurred are taken into consideration. If the patient was rolled on the earth or has been lying on the earth, the danger of tetanus is increased.

Wound Care

Wound care includes cleansing and débridement, application of topical or subeschar antimicrobial agents, and dressings. Gauze, biologic, biosynthetic, and synthetic materials may be used. Split-thickness skin grafts are required to close full-thickness and deep partial-thickness wounds.

Wound Cleansing

A variety of measures can be taken to cleanse the burn wound. Total immersion hydrotherapy is done in some settings; bedside baths are done in others; and some use a procedure in which the patient is suspended on a vinyl stretcher over a tub and showered. A walk-in bath, a tub, or a whirlpool may be used. The agitation in the whirlpool aids in cleansing and gently massaging the tissues. Because of the high risk of infection and sepsis, plastic liners are used in hydrotherapy equipment to prevent cross-contamination. Tap water alone, saline, or antiseptic solutions such as dilute iodine preparations may be used.

The temperature of the bath is maintained at 37.8°C (100°F), and the temperature of the room should be between 26.6°C and 29.4°C (80°–85°F).

During the bath, the patient should be encouraged to carry out as much activity as possible. Hydrotherapy provides an excellent medium for exercising the extremities and cleaning the entire body. When the patient is removed from the tub following the bath, any residue adhering to the body can be washed away with a spray or shower of clear water.

Hydrotherapy should be limited to a 20- to 30-minute period to prevent chilling and additional metabolic stress.

Unburned areas including the hair must be washed regularly as well. At the time of wound cleansing, all skin is examined for any hints of skin redness, breakdown, or local infection. Hair in and around the burn area may be clipped short. Intact blisters may be left if they are clean and do not interfere with joint function.

Wound cleansing is usually done at least daily in wound areas that are not undergoing surgical intervention. When the eschar begins to separate from the viable tissue beneath, approximately 1½ to 2 weeks postburn, more frequent cleansing and débridement may be in order.

Following tubbing, wounds are gently patted dry with sterile towels and the prescribed method of wound care is employed. Physician preferences, the skill level of nursing staff, and resources in terms of number of personnel, supplies, and time must be considered in choosing the best method for a given patient. Whatever the method, the goal is to protect the wound from overwhelming proliferation of pathogenic organisms and invasion of deeper tissues until either spontaneous healing or skin grafting can be achieved. Patient comfort and ability to participate in the prescribed method of treatment are also important considerations.

Exposure vs. Occlusive Dressing

Conscientious management of the burned area is of vital importance. When nonviable loose skin is removed, aseptic conditions must be established. Borderline normal skin near the burn wound is shaved to prevent possible contamination from hair follicles.

A variety of approaches are used to meet the goals of promoting protection, comfort, adequate cleansing and débridement, minimization of infection, and eventual healing of the burn wound. These methods include the exposure (open) method and the occlusive dressing (semi-open/semi-closed) method, which incorporates dressing change once or twice daily and application of a topical antibacterial agent.

Exposure Method

The objective of this method is to control bacterial colonization by exposing the wound to light and maintaining a cool environment. This method is most frequently used to treat burns of the face, neck, perineum, and extensive areas of the trunk. Exposing a burn to the drying effect of air allows the exudate to dry and form a hard crust in about 3 days; this protects the wound. In a second-degree burn, regeneration of skin beneath the crust takes 2 to 3 weeks, at which time the eschar falls off. In a third-degree burn, no epithelialization occurs beneath the eschar. In the untreated burn, the eschar usually separates in 2 to 3 weeks.

The success of the exposure method depends on keeping the immediate environment free of organisms. Some practitioners maintain that everything coming in contact with the patient must be sterile. Linens are sterile; those who come in direct contact with the patient wear masks, sterile gowns, and gloves; visitors are instructed to wear gowns and masks and not to touch the bed or hand the patient anything. Other practitioners maintain a clean environment and rely on the efficiency of the topical antibacterial agents to limit burn wound infection.

A cradle may be placed over the patient to prevent sheets from coming in contact with the burn area, to minimize the effects of air currents to which a burn patient is unusually sensitive, and to provide some form of covering.

The use of a sterile "burn pack" facilitates the care of this patient; it may contain sheets, pillowcases, washcloth, bath blanket, loin cloth, halter, and perhaps a gown and mask for the attendant.

When linens are changed, care must be taken not to pull on those parts of the sheet that are adhering to the burn area. Sterile saline may be used to wet the area so that the sheet may be freed gently. Turning is encouraged to prevent pneumonia and contractures and to promote circulation. The patient may prefer to do this without assistance.

The preferred range of humidity in the room is between 40% and 50%. The patient must be kept comfortably warm.

The advantages of the exposure method are (1) there are no painful dressing changes, (2) less equipment is used, (3) infection can be detected early, and (4) large numbers of patients can be treated, making this method particularly suitable for disaster situations.

Disadvantages of this method are (1) it is often not suitable for burns of the hands and feet because proper alignment and elevation are difficult to maintain, (2) it is unsuitable when the patient must be transported any distance, as from a rural area to a burn center; (3) it is less effective when other injuries exist that require the patient to be turned frequently, and (4) it may cause additional metabolic stress unless the patient's body temperature can be adequately maintained by controlling the immediate environment. Bandaging would be preferable in these instances.

Occlusive (Pressure) Dressings

Occlusive dressings are used primarily for burns of the feet and hands. Fine-mesh gauze impregnated with a topical antimicrobial agent is applied lightly to the cleansed burn area and an appropriate dressing is applied. The dressing may consist of sterile, absorptive, fluffed or washed gauze placed in such a way that the material does not clump together.

Precautions are taken to prevent two body surfaces from touching, such as fingers or toes, ear and scalp, the areas under the breast, any point of flexion, or between the genital folds. Functional body alignment positions are maintained; thus, the fingers and thumb curve over fluffed gauze or a bandage roll, the foot is positioned to avoid pronation and dropfoot, and support is placed under the knees.

Some physicians fix the loose gauze in place with an elastic bandage or stockinette; others apply abdominal pads before applying the conforming bandage. Another fixation bandage is elastic, tubular, woven netting, which is a light, conforming overdressing available in many sizes (Fig. 49-3). Evenly-distributed pressure is desired, with no constriction to hinder circulation. Circulation is checked every 3 or 4 hours by noting pulse, color, warmth, and symptoms of paresthesia. Having the tips of fingers or toes exposed provides areas where circulation can be easily checked.

Topical Antibacterial Therapy

There is general agreement that some form of antibacterial therapy applied to the burn wound is the best method of local care in extensive burn injury. Topical antibacterial therapy does not sterilize the burn wound, but simply reduces the

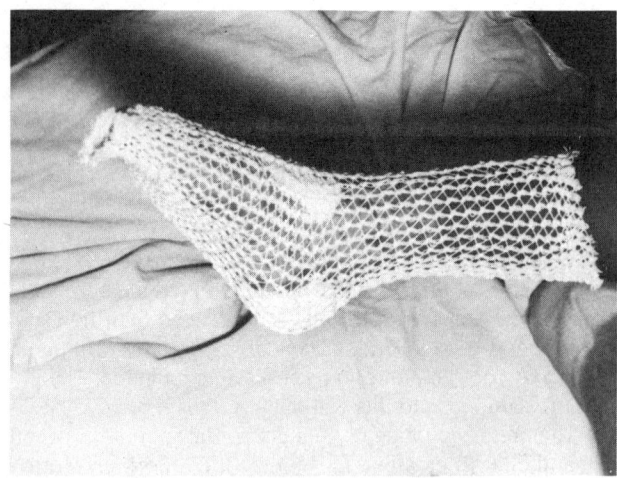

Figure 49-3

Use of tubular mesh overdressing to hold gauze covering in place. Once a wound has been cleansed and débrided, a fine gauze impregnated with a topical antibacterial cream (silver sulfadiazine or mafenide) is applied in one layer. The gauze is cut to fit the wounds only and does not overlap onto unburned skin. The tubular overdressing, holding the gauze in place, is available in several sizes and is elasticized in order to facilitate application to all parts of the body. (Courtesy of Shriners Hospitals for Crippled Children, Burns Institute, Galveston, Texas.)

number of bacteria so that the overall microbial population can be controlled by the body host defense mechanisms. Topical therapy buys time during which vigorous efforts must be made to convert the open, dirty wound to a closed, clean one.

No single agent is universally effective. Use of different agents at different times in the postburn period may be necessary. Effectiveness may decrease over time. Before the topical agent is reapplied, the previously-applied topical agent is thoroughly removed. The nurse should be aware of the length of time the topical agents are effective and the prescribed concentration of each agent. The number of times the dressings are changed and soaked is planned to promote optimal therapeutic use of the topical agent.

Bacteriologic cultures are required to monitor the effect of topical medications. Swab cultures or surface cultures (gauze capillarity) may be used. The procedures are noninvasive, simple, and painless but resulting data apply only to the area sampled. Wound biopsy cultures (invasive) may be required for quantitative sampling. Systemic antibiotics are used sparingly but are essential for pulmonary or other concomitant infections.

Criteria for topical agents include the following: (1) the agent is effective against gram-negative organisms, *Pseudomonas aeruginosa, Staphylococcus aureus,* and even fungi; (2) it is clinically effective; (3) it penetrates the eschar but is not systemically toxic; (4) it does not lose its effectiveness, thereby permitting another infection to develop; (5) it is cost-effective, available, and acceptable to the patient; and (6) it is inexpensive and easy to apply, minimizing nursing care time.

Silver Sulfadiazine (Silvadene)

Silver sulfadiazine, a popular topical medication used in this method of burn treatment, is synthesized by reacting silver nitrate with sodium sulfadiazine. It is available as a water-soluble cream in concentrations of 1%, and is highly effective against gram-negative bacteria. It is more effective when the total burn area involves less than 60% of the body surface area.

Evidence indicates that the *Pseudomonas* cells may split the agent so that silver is bound but sulfadiazine is released. This binding action may account for the potent inhibition of bacterial growth.

Compared with mafenide acetate and other antibacterial agents, silver sulfadiazine is more effective in controlling infection, causes no pain on application, does not disturb acid–base balance, electrolytes, or renal function, allows regeneration of epithelium to progress unhindered, and does not stain. Liberal amounts are applied topically with a gloved hand or on impregnated gauze rolls.

The medicated burn area can be left open or covered with a dressing. When silver sulfadiazine is applied to dermal burns, a proteinaceous gel (several millimeters thick) forms on the wound surface; after 72 hours, this pseudoeschar can be removed easily.

It has been reported that a significant number of gram-negative bacilli can become highly resistant to sulfadiazine as a result of protracted use of this agent.

Silver Sulfadiazine–Cerium Nitrate.   Cerium (a lanthanide element) has been incorporated into silver sulfadiazine to enhance its clinical effectiveness. A combination of just under 1% of silver sulfadiazine and 2.2% of cerium nitrate provides a thin cream that can be applied topically. It appears to be most effective against gram-negative bacteria and has been credited with lowering mortality rates. Occasionally, methemoglobinemia has been noted; however, on the whole it seems effective and safe.

Cerium Nitrate Solution.   Cerium nitrate solution (1.74%) can be used alone or in conjunction with the combination silver sulfadiazine–cerium nitrate cream as a wet soak to enhance the effectiveness of the antibacterial action of these agents. It must be rewet every 4 hours and applied with a bulky dressing for maximal effectiveness and to assist in maintaining the patient's body temperature at optimal levels. A dry top covering, such as a layer of stockinette or cotton bath blanket, helps to reduce evaporative heat loss.

Silver Nitrate Solution (0.5% Aqueous Solution)

Silver nitrate is an effective agent in preventing eschar contamination, particularly in burn injuries involving up to 40% or 50% of the body surface area. However, since the drug is unable to penetrate the eschar, infection can occur in the subeschar region. Because of this possibility, it is necessary to inspect the wound frequently and débride as necessary.

The treatment begins soon after the patient reaches the hospital. The wounds are cleansed, and then covered with gauze dressings thoroughly soaked with 0.5% silver nitrate solution. Concentrations above 1% produce tissue necrosis, whereas those below 0.5% are ineffective antiseptically.

These dressings are kept wet with the silver nitrate solution, which is applied by means of bulb syringes. Dressings are composed of 6 to 8 layers of four-ply gauze applied wet and held in place with bandages of bias-cut wide stockinette or gauze bandage. The gauze of the dressing *should not contain cotton between the layers,* because this interferes with the efficient action of the silver nitrate solution and causes the dressing to stick to the wound. Catheters may be incorporated into the thick dressings to permit saturation every 2 to 4 hours.

The patient is covered with one or two dry sheets and a dry cotton blanket. These dry layers prevent or reduce the heat loss produced by vaporization from the wet dressings and from the burned surface. When the coverings become moist, they are changed. The dressings are changed 2 or 3 times daily.

The use of 0.5% silver nitrate solution dressings is not without danger, because electrolytes, especially sodium and potassium, are withdrawn from the body fluids and pass into the dressings impregnated with silver nitrate solution. The withdrawal of sodium may occur very rapidly, especially in patients with extensive burns and in children, producing an acute electrolyte imbalance.

- In the early phases of the burn treatment, blood must be drawn at frequent intervals to determine sodium, chloride, potassium, and calcium levels. These electrolytes must be replaced, usually by the intravenous administration of Ringer's lactate solution.

Once the patient can take a normal diet, salt is added to the diet. Hypocalcemia is treated by the addition of calcium lactate or gluconate to the diet (usually within a few days postburn), and potassium depletion by the administration of potassium gluconate elixir. Deficits in these constituents of the blood electrolytes naturally are more marked in more extensive burns (comprising 50% to 80% of the body surface).

The silver nitrate solution has the disadvantage of turning black in the sunlight. This means that everything touched by the solution is stained black, including clothes, hands, floors, and other objects. The nurse attending a patient being treated with silver nitrate solution must wear rubber gloves, as a protection against the silver nitrate stains. (Such stains may be prevented by applying an organic iodine preparation, such as Wescodyne or Betadine solutions, to objects that have come in contact with the silver solution and then rinsing them in water.) Stain-resistant floor and wall coverings are available, but such materials increase the cost of care.

Mafenide Acetate (Sulfamylon Acetate)

Mafenide acetate (10%) in cream form with a hydrophilic base diffuses rapidly through the burned skin and eschar and is effective against a broad range of gram-positive and gram-negative organisms in the subeschar area. It is limited in use to the treatment of localized invasive burn wound sepsis caused by organisms sensitive to this agent.

The cream is applied in a thick (3 to 4 mm) layer (Fig. 49-4), once or twice daily; a fine mesh gauze may be applied in strips directly to the burn and changed daily or washed off in a whirlpool bath.

Although it is relatively nontoxic, mafenide acetate is a strong carbonic anhydrase inhibitor and may adversely affect the blood *p*H level, causing a reduction of the renal tubular buffering mechanism. With continued use, severe metabolic acidosis may occur, making it necessary to monitor the respiratory rate, blood gases, and *p*H. Chest x-rays also may be justified because of possible pulmonary failure. The occurrence of these problems may require use of mafenide to be discontinued.

Another disadvantage of this form of treatment is the burning pain experienced by the patient for a few minutes following application of the cream. Thus, analgesics may be required before the ointment is applied. Another problem is that eschar separates very slowly, thereby delaying skin grafting unless the eschar is aggressively débrided.

Other Topical Agents

Povidone iodine ointment (10%) and *Betadine solution* are effective against a wide variety of gram-negative and gram-positive organisms as well as yeasts, fungi, and viruses. These dressings are usually changed every 6 hours. Iodine preparations may be painful to patients when first applied. Some patients are allergic to iodine. Iodine also has the property of staining bed linens.

Gentamicin sulfate is a bactericidal aminoglycoside available in a 0.1% cream for topical use. It is useful for short

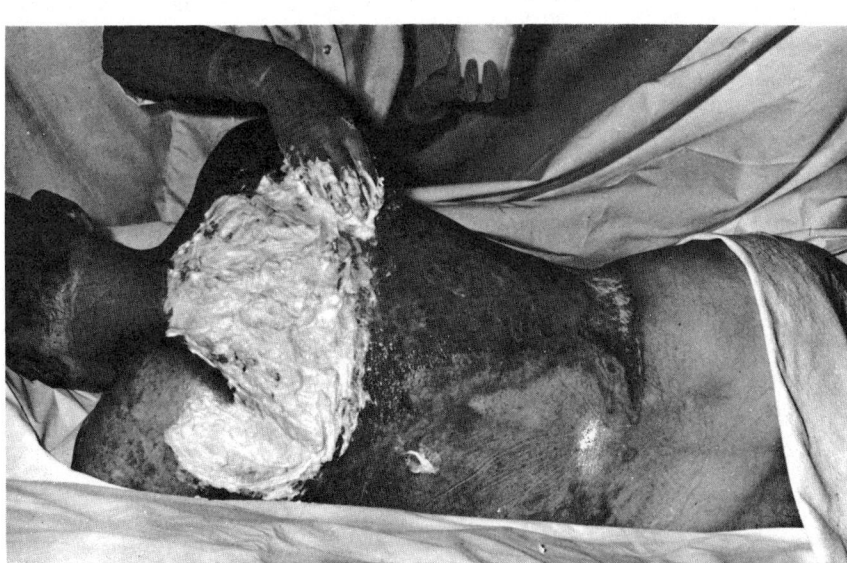

Figure 49-4
Photograph of back of patient with deep second-degree burn being treated with Sulfamylon. The Sulfamylon cream is put on in a thick layer with the gloved hand. (Artz CP and Mancrief VA. The Treatment of Burns. Philadelphia, WB Saunders.)

periods of time in small areas of invasive infection. Superinfection with resistant bacterial strains has been reported, indicating the need for very careful monitoring when this agent is used.

Dressing Changes

Dressings are changed in the patient's unit, hydrotherapy room, or treatment area approximately 20 minutes after the administration of an analgesic. They may also be changed in the operating room after the patient is anesthetized. A mask, hair cover, disposable plastic apron or cover gown, and gloves are worn by health care personnel when removing the dressings. The outer dressings are slit with blunt scissors, and the soiled dressings are removed and disposed of following established procedures for contaminated materials.

Dressings that adhere to the wound can be removed more comfortably if they are moistened with saline or if the patient is allowed to soak for a few moments in the tub. The remaining dressings are *carefully* and *gently* removed with forceps and/or gloved hands. The wounds are then cleansed and débrided to remove debris, any remaining topical agent, exudate, and devitalized skin. Sterile scissors and forceps may be employed to trim loose eschar and encourage separation of devitalized skin. During this procedure, the wound and surrounding skin are carefully inspected. The color, odor, size, exudate, signs of reepithelialization, and character of the eschar and any changes from the previous dressing change are noted. Because wound care procedures, particularly tubbing, are metabolically stressful, the patient is assessed for signs of chilling, fatigue, changes in hemodynamic status, and pain unrelieved by predressing analgesics or relaxation techniques.

Following wound cleansing, the burned areas are patted dry and the prescribed topical agent is applied. Usually coarsemesh gauze is applied to areas that are being débrided in the early weeks postburn. Fine-mesh gauze is useful for granulating wounds. A light dressing is used over joint areas to allow for motion (unless the patient has undergone grafting of the area and motion is contraindicated) and over areas for which a splint has been designed to conform to the body contour for proper positioning.

Multiple layers of gauze are used to create a bulky dressing for use with topical solutions to retain the topical agent at proper concentration on the wound surface. They are remoistened approximately every 4 hours. A dry top layer is essential to prevent evaporative heat loss.

Close communication and cooperation among the surgeon, nurse, and other health team members are essential for optimal burn wound care. Different wound areas on a given patient may require a variety of wound care techniques. Use of a diagram, updated daily by the nurse responsible for wound care, helps to inform all concerned about the latest wound care procedures in use for a given patient. Diagrams posted at the bedside are also useful to inform staff of the current prescription for splints to be applied over dressings and the exercise regimen to be followed before dressings are reapplied.

Débridement

Débridement is another facet of burn wound care. This technique has two aims:

- To remove tissue contaminated by bacteria and foreign bodies, thus protecting the patient from invasive infection
- To remove devitalized tissue or burn eschar in preparation for grafting and wound healing

After partial- and full-thickness burns, bacteria that are present at the interface of the burned tissue and the viable tissue underneath gradually liquefy the collagen fibrils that hold the eschar in place for the first week or two postburn. This occurs due to the action of proteolytic and other natural enzymes.

With *natural débridement,* the dead tissue separates from the underlying viable tissue spontaneously. Use of antibacterial topical agents, however, tends to slow down this natural process of eschar separation. It is often advantageous to the patient to speed this process through other means, and thus reduce the time during which bacterial invasion and other iatrogenic problems may arise.

Mechanical débridement involves the use of surgical scissors and forceps to separate and remove the eschar. This technique can be performed by physicians or experienced nurses and physical therapists, and is usually done with daily dressing changes and wound cleansing procedures. Débridement by this means is carried out to the point of pain and bleeding. Hemostatic agents or pressure can be used to stop small-vessel bleeding.

Dressings are also helpful as débriding agents. Coursemesh dressings applied dry or wet-to-dry (applied wet and allowed to dry) will slowly débride the wound of exudate and eschar when they are removed. Topical enzymatic agents such as sutilains (Travase), a proteolytic enzyme derived from *Bacillus subtilis* and supplied in a petrolatum base, can also be helpful in débriding burn wounds. Because such agents are not antibacterial in themselves, they should be used in conjunction with topical antibacterial therapy to protect the patient from bacterial invasion.

Surgical débridement employs the use of either primary excision of the full thickness of the skin down to the fascia or the shaving of burned skin layers gradually down to freely bleeding, viable tissue. This may be initiated a few days postburn, or as soon as the patient is hemodynamically stable and edema has decreased. The wound is then covered immediately by a skin graft or dressing. A temporary biologic dressing or biosynthetic dressing is used until a skin graft can be applied during a subsequent operation.

The use of excision is increasing in many burn centers, although it must be used selectively, particularly with large burns, for the following reasons. The procedure carries with it high risk due to extensive blood loss (as much as half a pint of blood per percent of body surface area excised) and lengthy operative and anesthesia time. However, when used, excision results in shorter hospital stays and may decrease potential complications from invasive burn wound sepsis.

Grafting the Burn Wound

If wounds are deep or large, spontaneous re-epithelialization is not possible. Therefore, a skin transplant or graft using the patient's own skin (autograft) is required. Priority areas for skin grafting include the face, for cosmetic and psychological reasons; the hands, because the sooner they can be used the sooner the patient can participate in self-care (which also has psychological benefits); and the feet and other areas that involve joints. Grafting permits earlier functional ability and reduces the development of contractures. When burns are very extensive, the chest and abdomen may be grafted first to reduce the extent of the burn surface.

During wound healing, granulation tissue develops. It fills the space created by the wound, creates a barrier to bacteria, and serves as a bed for epithelial cell growth.

Richly vascular granulation tissue is pink, firm, shiny, and free of exudate and debris. It should have a bacterial count of fewer than 100,000 per gram of tissue in order to optimize graft take. A preoperative culture to rule out *Streptococcus* is mandatory before autografting, because enzymes of these bacteria can dissolve a graft or lead to failure of the graft.

Types of Autograft

Autografts can be split-thickness, full-thickness, or pedicle flaps. The last two types are more commonly used for reconstructive surgery, months or years after the initial injury. Full- and split-thickness autografts can be applied in sheets or in postage-stamp pieces, or they can be expanded by meshing so that, for a given amount of donor site area, an area 1½ to 9 times greater can be covered.

Use of split-thickness grafts allows the remaining donor site to retain sweat glands and hair follicles, and allows for rapid healing.

Skin expanders, which enable the surgeon to cut tiny slits into a sheet of donor skin, make it possible to cover large areas of total body surface area with smaller amounts of donor skin. Expanded grafts cling to the recipient bed more easily than sheet grafts, and prevent the accumulation of blood, serum, air, or purulent material under the graft.

If blood, serum, air, fat, or necrotic tissue lies between the recipient bed and the graft, there may be either partial or total loss of the graft. Infection and mishandling of the graft, as well as trauma occurring during dressing changes, account for most other instances of graft loss.

Care of Patients With Autografts

Occlusive dressings are often used after grafting to immobilize the grafts. Homografts, heterografts, or synthetic dressings may also be used to protect the grafts (see below). The graft may be left open, using nylon tulle to immobilize it while affording close observation of the graft's progress.

The first dressing change is usually performed by the surgeon 3 to 5 days postoperatively, or earlier if purulent drainage or a foul odor is noted. If the graft is dislodged, sterile saline compresses will help prevent drying of the graft until the physician reapplies it. The patient begins exercise 7 to 10 days after grafting.

Care of Donor Site

A gauze dressing is applied during the operative period to maintain pressure and stop any oozing. The donor site may be treated with a single layer of petrolatum gauze or saline gauze left in place. The wound is kept dry and open to air when the compression dressing, applied in the operating room, is removed, 4 to 6 hours postoperatively. The wound will start to reepithelialize, beginning at the wound margins—a process that is usually completed within 7 to 10 days.

Biologic Dressings

Biologic dressings consist of homografts (or allografts) and heterografts (or xenografts). *Homografts* involve skin obtained from living or recently deceased humans. *Heterografts* consist of skin taken from animals (usually pigs). *Amnion* from the human placenta may also be used as a biologic dressing.

Homografts tend to be the most expensive biologic dressings. They are available from several skin banks in various regions of the country. Homograft is available in both fresh and cryo-preserved forms, and is considered by most surgeons to provide the best infection control of all the biologic or biosynthetic dressings available.

Amnion is low in cost and is readily available to hospitals, which obtain and process it in cooperation with obstetrical services. Pigskin is available from a number of commercial suppliers. It is available fresh, frozen, or lyophilized for longer shelf-life. Pigskin impregnated with a topical antibacterial such as silver sulfadiazine is also available.

Biologic dressings can be used for several purposes. In a large burn, biologic dressings can be lifesaving by providing temporary wound closure until autografting is complete. They provide immediate coverage for clean, superficial burns, and decrease the wound's evaporative water loss and protein loss. They decrease pain by protecting nerve endings, and are an effective barrier to water and bacteria. When applied to superficial partial-thickness wounds, they appear to speed the healing process.

Biologic dressings protect new granulation tissue when the burn eschar separates unevenly, leaving islands of firmly-attached eschar within the granulation tissue. They protect the granulation tissue during completion of wound débridement or while waiting for donor sites to heal and be reused. This is common in patients with large areas of burn and little remaining normal skin suitable for donor sites.

Biologic dressings are used to débride untidy wounds after eschar separation. With each biologic dressing change, débridement takes place. Once the biologic dressing appears to be "taking," or adheres to the granulating surface with a minimum of underlying exudation, the patient is ready for permanent placement of the patient's own skin, an autograft. Another major use of these dressings is temporary coverage of wounds following excision while awaiting autografting.

Biologic materials can be left open or covered. They are usually changed every 2 to 5 days to avoid systemic and local signs of rejection phenomena.

Biosynthetic and Synthetic Wound Coverings

Problems with availability, sterility, and cost have prompted the search for synthetic skin substitutes, which may eventually replace biologic dressings as temporary wound coverings. The most widely used currently is Biobrane, a knitted, elastic, flexible nylon fabric that is bonded to a thin Silastic semipermeable membrane coated with products of dermal collagen. The material is semitransparent and sterile. It has an indefinite shelf-life and is less costly than homograft or pigskin.

Biobrane adheres to a fresh wound surface as well as does human allograft or homograft. Generally, adherence to the wound surface has been shown to correlate directly with low bacterial counts. Frequent dressing changes until adherence occurs will lower the bacterial count, as they do with allograft. When the Biobrane dressing adheres to the wound, as in the "take" of an allograft without vascularization, the wound remains stable and the Biobrane is left in place for periods of 3 to 4 weeks.

Biobrane dressings readily adhere to donor sites, and will remain until spontaneous epithelialization and wound healing occur. Biobrane can be laid on top of wide-meshed autograft to protect the wound until the autograft epithelium grows out to close the interstices. The Biobrane gradually separates and is trimmed, leaving a healed wound.

Potentially the most important use of Biobrane is for intermediate or long-term closure of a surgically excised wound until an autograft becomes available. Just as with biologic dressings, Biobrane should not be used over grossly contaminated or necrotic wounds. Removal of Biobrane after several weeks is similar to but easier than removal of vascularized allograft, and leaves a bleeding granulation bed which readily accepts autograft.

There are a number of other synthetic dressings available for burn wound care. Op-Site, a thin, transparent, extremely elastic material can be used to cover clean partial-thickness wounds and donor sites. This dressing is occlusive and waterproof, yet permeable to moisture vapor and air. This permeability still provides for protection from microbial contamination, and also allows the exchange of gases that occurs much more quickly in a moist environment. Other synthetic dressings used for burn wounds include Tegaderm, N-TER-FACE, Vigilon, Duo-Derm, and Aquaphor.

Artificial skin was developed in Boston in 1979. Its use is still investigational in several burn centers around the country. It is composed of two main layers. The inner layer corresponds to the human dermis, and is a mixture of a protein from cowhide and a complex carbohydrate derived from shark cartilage. The top layer, equivalent to epidermis, is made by bonding a viscous plastic onto the cowhide–shark sheet.

The artificial dermis breaks down as new natural tissue forms. The plastic top layer acts as a protective covering. Beginning as early as 10 days after the artificial skin graft, postage-stamp patches of plastic are peeled away and replaced by slivers of the patient's own epidermal tissue. At the present time, artificial skin does not permanently take the place of the patient's own skin.

Pain Management

The outstanding features of burn pain are its intensity and long duration. Necessary wound care carries with it pain that is anxiety-producing in its anticipation and profound when experienced.

In a typical burn pain trajectory, there are many peaks and valleys. The primary pain from the burn itself is very intense in the initial acute postburn phase. This primary pain gradually subsides, but for weeks thereafter, until the skin heals or skin grafts are applied and "take," the pain level remains high because of treatment-induced pain. Wound cleansing, dressing change, débridement, and physical therapy are often done simultaneously or serially, inflicting intense pain. Even when grafts are applied, making the burn site more comfortable, donor sites are created and may be exquisitely painful for several days. Discomfort related to tissue healing, such as itching, tingling, and tightness of contracting skin and joints, further adds to the duration if not the intensity of pain over many weeks or months.

Because pain cannot be eliminated short of complete anesthesia, the goal is to minimize the pain through analgesia before the patient faces wound care procedures. With adequate staff working gently, swiftly, and skillfully, the duration of pain from wound care can be shortened. Bolus doses of morphine or meperidine (Demerol) are often used. Ketamine anesthesia administered intravenously is also used for some wound care procedures in burn units.

Patient-controlled analgesia, using continuous morphine drips at 2–3 mg/hr, and/or sustained-release oral morphine, given every 12 hours with an additional bolus dose prior to wound care, have been found to be helpful for burn patients. Self-administered nitrous oxide also helps to make dressing changes more tolerable for those patients who have sufficient hand function to hold a mask to their faces intermittently during dressing changes.

Early surgical excision with grafting under anesthesia is perhaps the best way to reduce the overall pain experience for burn patients.

Disorders of Wound Healing

Disorders of wound healing in the burn patient result from excessive abnormal healing or inadequate new tissue formation. Hypertrophic scarring and keloid formation are the result of excessive, abnormal healing.

Scars. Hypertrophic scars and wound contractures are more likely to occur if the initial burn injury extends below the level of the deep dermis. Healing of these deep wounds results in the replacement of normal integument with highly metabolically active tissues lacking the normal architecture of the skin. In the collagen layer beneath the epithelium, many fibroblasts gradually proliferate. Myofibroblasts, cells that have the ability to contract, are also present in immature wounds. As these elements contract, the collagen fibers, which normally are laid down in flat bundles, tend to form a wavy pattern. Eventually the collagen bundles take on a supercoiled appearance and collagen nodules develop. The scar becomes very red (due to its hypervascular nature), raised, and hardened.

The wound is in a dynamic state for 1½ to 2 years postburn. If appropriate measures are instituted during this active period, the scar tissue loses its redness and softens. The application of elastic pressure garments induces loosening of collagen bundles and encourages parallel orientation of the collagen to the skin surface with the disappearance of the dermal nodules (Fig. 49-5). With the application of pressure, there is a restructuring of the collagen and a decrease in vascularity and cellularity.

Hypertrophic scarring may cause severe contracture across involved joints. However, these scars are limited to the area of injury and will gradually regress over time.

Keloids. In other patients, a large heaped-up mass of scar tissue develops and may extend beyond the wound surface. It is called a *keloid*. Keloids tend to be found in darkly pigmented persons, grow outside of wound margins, and are more likely to recur after surgical excision.

Failure to Heal. Failure of the wound to heal may be related to many factors, including infection and inadequate nutrition. A serum albumin below 2 gm/dl (20 g/L) is frequently a factor in impaired healing in the burn patient.

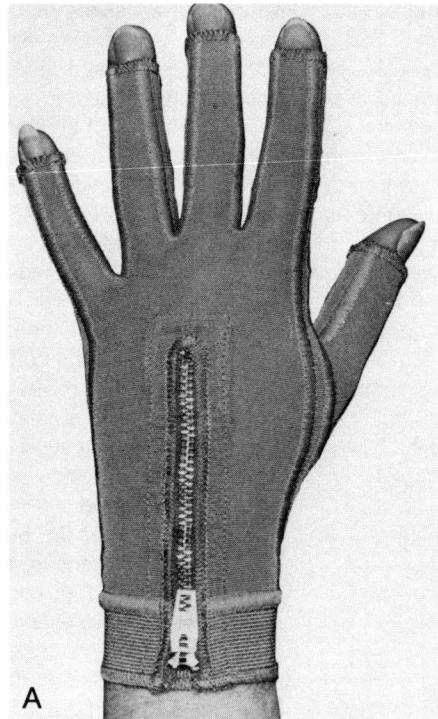
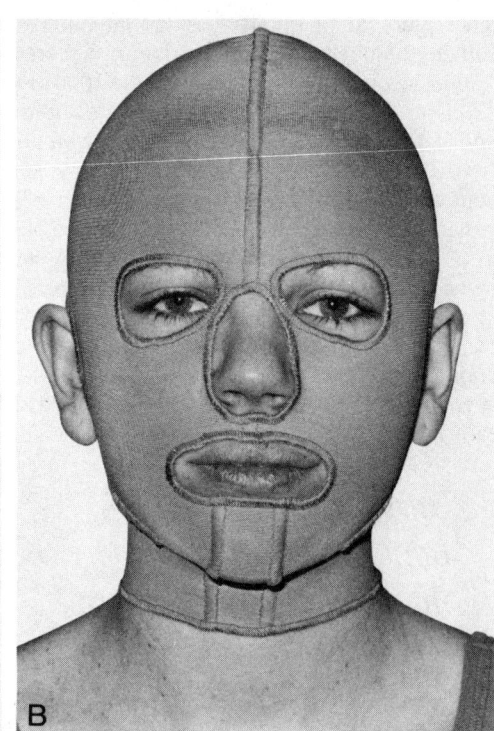

Figure 49-5
Elastic pressure garments. Application of pressure garments prevents hypertrophic burn scarring. (*A*) Elastic pressure glove. (*B*) Elastic pressure face mask. (Pictures provided by Jobst Institute, Inc, Box 653, Toledo, Ohio 43694.)

Contractures. Contractures are another concern as wounds heal. The burn wound will shorten because of the force exerted by the fibroblasts and the flexion of muscles as a natural part of wound healing. An opposing force in the form of splints, traction, and purposeful movement and positioning must be used to counteract deformity caused by this process in burns that occur across joints.

Much of the long-term care of healed burns will be carried out by the patient and significant others at home. Patients commonly leave the hospital with small areas of clean, open wounds that are slowly healing. These areas should be washed daily with mild soap and water, and the prescribed topical agent or dressing applied. Healed areas that are prone to hypertrophic scarring require the use of pressure garments. The physical therapist or a representative of the manufacturer of elastic pressure garments measures the patient for correct fit. While awaiting the arrival of the garment, soft, tubular, knit elastic pressure bandages can be used to help to desensitize the patient's skin, protect healing areas, provide pressure, and promote venous return. Patients must be educated to the need for lubrication and protection of the healing skin and the necessity of wearing pressure garments for at least a year after the injury.

Nutritional Support

Hypermetabolism persists after burn injury until wounds are closed. The goal of nutritional support is to put the patient in a state of positive nitrogen balance. The nutritional support required is based on the patient's preburn status and the extent of total body surface area burned.

A number of formulas exist for estimating the daily metabolic expenditure and caloric requirements of burn patients. Protein requirements may range from 3.0 gm of protein per kilogram of body weight every 24 hours to as much as 25% of total energy needs. Lipids are included in the nutritional support of every burned patient because of their importance for wound healing, cellular integrity, and absorption of fat-soluble vitamins. Carbohydrates are included to meet caloric goals as high as 5000 calories per day and to spare protein, essential for wound healing.

Current research is bringing about rapid changes in specific guidelines for estimating energy expenditure during various phases of postburn recovery. The proportions of fat, protein, and carbohydrate are carefully planned for maximal utilization. Overfeeding can also be detrimental. Therefore, a dietitian familiar with current concepts in nutrition for burn patients should be consulted for all patients with major burns.

As soon as gastrointestinal function returns after the patient's condition stabilizes, nutritional support begins. The enteral route is preferred, and many burn patients will tolerate oral fluids and food. In patients with large burns, tube feeding may be employed to ensure a certain number of calories perday. In this case, a meal tray and high-protein, high-calorie snacks and fluids may be offered as a supplement to the essential tube feedings. A diet containing semi-solid or solid food is usually begun toward the end of the first week, when the patient's tolerance for food improves.

Patients lose a great deal of weight in the process of recovering from severe burns. Reserve fat deposits are tapped during the recovery, fluids have been lost, and calorie intake may have been limited. Because burns cause low resistance to infection and disease, the nutritional state must be improved even though the patient has a poor appetite and is still weak.

Indications for intravenous parenteral nutrition include weight loss greater than 10% of normal body weight, inadequate intake of enteral nutrition due to clinical status, prolonged wound exposure, and malnutrition or debilitated condition prior to injury. The risk of infection of the central catheter required by this method must be considered. While solutions commonly used may provide 1000 or more calories per liter, they are deficient in fatty acids. Therefore, intravenous fat solutions will also have to be given periodically.

Ulcers of the gastric or duodenal mucosa are a common complication of burn injury (Curling's ulcer). This condition is manifested by hemorrhage, detected in the bloody contents from nasogastric suction or in the stool. A sudden drop in hemoglobin concentration may be diagnostic even before the hemorrhage is evident. Gastric surgery may be indicated. Use of histamine blockers (ranitidine [Zantac]) continues during this phase to prevent this serious problem. Small, frequent feedings and antacids are also included in the patient's care.

▶ Nursing Process
Burn Care During the
Intermediate/Acute Phase

▷ Assessment

Continued assessment of the burn patient during the early weeks following the burn focuses on hemodynamic alterations, the process of wound healing, and detection of complications. Vital signs, including apical pulse, are assessed frequently.

Continued assessment of peripheral pulses is essential for the first few days postburn while edema continues to increase, potentially damaging peripheral nerves and restricting blood flow. Observation of the ECG may give clues to dysrhythmias that result from potassium imbalance, preexisting cardiac disease, or sequelae of electrical injury or burn shock.

The patient is assessed for fluid overload and congestive heart failure because of the mobilization of fluid and shifts from the interstitial to the vascular compartment. The neck veins are assessed for fullness and arterial, wedge, and central

venous pressures are monitored closely. The patient's respiratory status is monitored closely for increased difficulty in breathing, change in respiratory pattern, and appearance of adventitious sounds.

Assessment of the patient's respiratory status is also important because it is frequently at this stage that signs and symptoms of injury to the respiratory tract become apparent. As described previously, decreased breath sounds, wheezing, tachypnea, stridor, and sputum tinged with soot or in some cases containing sloughed tracheal tissue are among the many possible findings that can be auscultated or observed. Patients on mechanical ventilation must be assessed for decrease in tidal volume and lung compliance.

Assessment of residual volumes and pH of gastric fluid of the patient with a nasogastric tube is also important and gives clues to early sepsis or the need for antacid therapy. Evidence of blood in gastric fluid or stool should also be noted and reported.

Assessment of the burn wound is a daily activity that requires an experienced eye, hand, and nose. Some of the characteristics of the wound that are assessed include the size, color, odor, presence of eschar or exudate, presence of abscess formation under the eschar, presence of *epithelial buds* (small pearllike clusters of cells on the wound surface), bleeding, nature of granulation tissue, progress of grafts and donor sites, and quality of the surrounding skin. Any rapid changes in the wound are reported to the physician, because they often indicate burn wound or systemic sepsis and require immediate intervention.

The signs of systemic sepsis are listed in Table 49-7. Some are rather subtle and require a high index of suspicion and very close monitoring of changes in the patient's mental status, gradually increasing gastric residual volumes, and increasing respiratory rate. As with many observations of the burn patient, one needs to look for patterns or trends in the data.

Other ongoing assessments significant in burn care include daily patient weights, records of caloric intake, assessment of general hydration, and serum electrolyte, hemoglobin, and hematocrit levels. Weekly audiometry may be

TABLE 49-7
Clinical Features of Septic Shock*

Early Stage	Middle Stage	Late Stage
Vital Signs	*Vital Signs*	*Vital Signs*
Full, bounding pulse	Rapid pulse	Markedly increased pulse; weak, thready pulse
Normal or increased blood pressure	Decreased blood pressure	
Increased pulse pressure		Falling blood pressure
		Decreased pulse pressure
Hyperdynamic State	*Normodynamic State*	*Hypodynamic State*
Increased cardiac output	Decreased cardiac output	Marked fall in cardiac output
Increased urinary output	Falling urinary output or renal failure	Renal failure
Hyperthermia		Pale, moist, cool skin
Warm, dry, flushed skin		
Restlessness		

* Signs and symptoms may be variable and nonspecific.

indicated for patients on long-term ototoxic antibiotics. Careful attention must also be paid to signs or reports of pain related to deep muscle ischemia in patients with electrical burns. The nurse is alert to signs of necrosis of visceral organs injured by electricity and of hemorrhage from blood vessels adjacent to areas of surgical exploration and débridement in patients with serious electrical burns.

▷ Nursing Diagnoses

Based on the assessment data, nursing diagnoses in the intermediate/acute stage of burn care may include the following:

- Potential for fluid volume excess related to resumption of capillary integrity and fluid shift from interstitial to vascular compartment
- Potential for infection related to loss of skin barrier and dysfunctional host defense mechanisms
- Alteration in nutrition: less than body requirements related to hypermetabolism
- Impaired skin integrity related to thermal injury
- Alteration in comfort: pain, itching, and skin and joint tightness related to exposed nerves and wound healing
- Impaired physical mobility related to burn wound edema, pain, and joint contractures

▷ Planning and Implementation

▷ *Goals:* The major goals of the patient may include restoration of normal fluid balance, absence of infection, attainment of anabolic state and normal weight, improved skin integrity, reduction of pain and discomfort, and achievement of optimal physical mobility.

Nursing Interventions

Restoring Normal Fluid Balance. To reduce the risk of fluid overload and congestive heart failure, the nurse closely monitors the patient's intravenous and oral fluid intake, using intravenous infusion pumps to minimize the risk of inadvertent rapid infusion of fluids. To monitor changes in fluid status, careful intake and output records are kept and the patient is weighed daily. Changes in arterial, wedge, and central venous pressures, as well as in blood pressure and pulse rate, are reported to the physician. Cardiotonics and diuretics may be prescribed to promote increased urine output. The nurse's role is to administer these medications as prescribed and to observe the patient's response to them.

Increased difficulty with respiration is reported promptly to the physician. In the meantime, the patient is positioned comfortably, with the head of the bed raised (if not prohibited by other treatments or burn injuries) to promote lung expansion and gas exchange.

Preventing Infection. Aside from monitoring fluid requirements and providing constant care, the nurse is responsible for providing a clean and safe environment and for closely scrutinizing the wound in order to detect early manifestations of infection.

Aseptic technique is used for wound care procedures and for any invasive procedures such as insertion of intravenous lines, urinary catheters, or tracheal suctioning. The nurse protects the patient from sources of cross-contamination, including other patients, staff members, visitors, and equipment. Antibiotics must be administered on schedule to maintain appropriate blood levels. Wound and blood cultures are obtained as prescribed, and results of significance are reported to the physician immediately. The nurse also maintains a constant vigil for early signs of septicemia and promptly intervenes, including administering prescribed intravenous fluids and antibiotics to prevent septic shock, a complication with a high mortality rate.

Tube feeding reservoirs and drainage containers are changed regularly. Visitors are screened to prevent the introduction of pathogens to the severely immunocompromised burn patient. Barrier gowns or disposable aprons are worn when working at the bedside and changed when leaving the room. When wounds are exposed or central intravenous catheters inserted, hair covers, masks, and sterile gloves are required. The simple act of effective hand washing prior to and following each patient contact is also an essential component of nursing care.

Maintaining Adequate Nutrition. The nurse works closely with the dietitian to plan a diet that is high in protein and calories and acceptable to the patient. Family members may be encouraged to bring nutritious favorite foods to the hospital in consultation with the dietitian. Sandwiches made with peanut butter, meat, and cheese and milkshakes may be offered as snacks between meals and late in the evening. Caloric intake must be documented.

If caloric goals cannot be met by oral feeding, a nasogastric tube is inserted and utilized for continuous or bolus feedings of specific formulas. The volume of residual gastric secretions should be checked to ensure absorption. Parenteral hyperalimentation may also be required, and provides the nurse with a new challenge in making frequent assessments related to the expected and untoward effects of this therapy.

Patients should be weighed each day and a graph of their weight maintained. This can be used to help patients set goals for their own nutritional intake and to monitor weight loss and gain. Ideally, the patient will lose no more than 5% of preburn weight if aggressive nutritional management is employed. Vitamins A and D, trace elements such as copper and zinc, and fatty acid supplements may also be required, particularly for patients receiving parenteral nutritional support.

The patient who is experiencing anorexia requires encouragement and considerable support from the nurse to increase food intake. The patient's surroundings should be as pleasant as possible during meals. Catering to food preferences and offering snacks high in proteins and vitamins are ways of tempting a person to gradually increase intake.

Improving Skin Integrity Through Wound Care. Wound care is often the single most time-consuming element of burn care after the emergent period has passed. The surgeon will prescribe the desired topical antibacterial agents and specific biologic, biosynthetic, or synthetic wound coverings, and plan for surgical excision and grafting. The nurse has an opportunmity to make astute assessments of wound status, to use creative approaches to wound dressing, and to support the patient during the emotionally distressing and very painful experience of wound care.

The nurse frequently serves as the coordinator of the complex aspects of wound care and dressing changes for the patient. Nursing functions include assessing and recording any changes or progress in wound healing and keeping all members of the health care team informed of changes in the patient's burn wounds and in the treatment regimen. The nurse also assists the patient and family through instruction, support, and encouragement to take an active part in dressing changes and wound care when appropriate. Home care needs are anticipated early in the course of burn management, and the strengths of the patient and family are assessed and used in preparing for eventual discharge and home care.

Relieving Pain and Discomfort. Pain is more severe in second-degree burns than in third-degree burns, because the nerve endings are destroyed in a third-degree burn. Exposed nerve endings are sensitive to cool, moving air; therefore, a sterile covering can help to reduce pain.

- Symptoms of restlessness and anxiety, often attributed to pain, may actually be due to hypoxia. Therefore, careful respiratory assessment is essential before giving analgesics in the early postburn period. Intravenous morphine or other narcotics are prescribed as needed, but large doses are avoided because of the danger of respiratory depression and the possibility of masking other symptoms. Subcutaneous or intramuscular routes are dangerous because of impaired circulation.

Nursing interventions such as teaching the patient relaxation techniques, giving the patient some control over wound care and analgesia, and providing frequent reassurance are helpful. Imagery has been used effectively to moderate patients' perception of and responses to pain. Hypnosis, biofeedback, and behavioral modification have also been used successfully by staff experienced in these modalities. Minor tranquilizers are administered in conjunction with analgesics as prescribed. Frequent assessment of pain and discomfort is essential.

The nurse works quickly to complete treatments and dressing changes in order to reduce pain and discomfort. She encourages the patient to use analgesic medications before painful procedures, and assesses their effectiveness in making the pain and discomfort more tolerable.

Healing burn wounds are often described by patients as "itchy" and "tight." Oral antipruritic agents, a cool environment, frequent lubrication of the skin with water or silica-based lotion, exercise and splinting to prevent skin contracture, and diversional activities are helpful in promoting comfort in this phase.

Promoting Physical Mobility. An early priority is to prevent complications resulting from immobility. Deep breathing, turning, and proper repositioning are essential nursing practices to prevent atelectasis and pneumonia, to control edema, and to prevent pressure sores and contractures. These interventions are modified to meet the individual patient's needs. Air-fluidized beds and rotation beds may be useful. Early ambulation is encouraged.

Whenever the lower extremities are involved, elastic pressure bandages should be applied before the patient is placed in an upright position.

The burn wound is in a dynamic state for a year or more after wound closure. During this time, aggressive efforts must be made to prevent contracture and hypertrophic scarring of the wound area. Both passive and active range-of-motion exercises are initiated from the day of admission, and are continued after grafting within prescribed limitations.

Splints or functional devices may be applied to extremities for contracture control. The nurse monitors for signs of vascular insufficiency and nerve compression.

▷ *Evaluation*

▷ *Expected Outcomes*

1. Patient achieves optimal fluid balance.
   a. Intake, output, and body weight correlate with expected pattern.
   b. Vital signs and arterial, wedge, and central venous pressures remain within designated limits.
   c. Exhibits no respiratory distress; is able to recline flat without increased respiratory distress.
   d. Lungs are clear to auscultation.
   e. Demonstrates increased urine output in response to diuretics and cardiotonics.
   f. Receives intravenous and oral fluids as prescribed
   g. Exhibits no increase in neck vein distention
   h. Heart rate is lower than 110/min and in normal sinus rhythm.
2. Patient is free of pathogenic organisms.
   a. Has no signs of local or systemic infection
   b. Blood cultures are negative.
   c. Patient exhibits negative wound, sputum, and urine cultures.
3. Demonstrates anabolic nutritional status; normal weight
   a. Gains weight daily after initial loss due to fluid diuresis and NPO status
   b. Has no signs of protein, vitamin, or mineral deficiencies
   c. Meets required nutritional needs entirely by oral intake
   d. Consumes diet high in carbohydrate and protein
   e. Participates in selection of diet with prescribed nutrients
   f. Exhibits normal serum protein levels
4. Majority of wounds are closed; small, open wounds are clean and healing; scars are minimal.
   a. Skin is generally intact and free of infection, signs of pressure, and trauma.
   b. Open wound areas are pink, reepithelializing, and free of infection.
   c. Donor sites are clean and reepithelializing.
   d. Healed wounds feel soft and smooth.
   e. Skin is lubricated and elastic, with no scales or other signs of dryness.
   f. Skin pigmentation is near normal preburn color.
5. Patient experiences minimal pain, itching, or skin tightness.
   a. Requests analgesics only for specific wound care procedures or physical therapy activities
   b. States pain is minimal when assessed
   c. Gives no physiological or nonverbal cues that pain is moderate or severe
   d. Uses pain control measures such as nitrous oxide, relaxation techniques, and imagery to assist with coping with pain
   e. Is able to sleep without being disturbed by pain or itching

Care of the Patient During the Intermediate/Acute Phase of Burn Care

Nursing Interventions	*Rationale*	*Expected Outcomes*

Nursing Diagnosis: Potential infection of burn wound and burn wound sepsis

Goal: Reduce risk of burn wound sepsis

1. Wash hands prior to all patient contacts.	1. Minimizes risk of cross-contamination	• Patient exhibits clean, small, open wounds.
2. Assess for early signs of shock and sepsis.	2. Enables detection of signs of shock, so that treatment can be initiated	• Exhibits open wound areas that are pink, reepithelializing, and free of infection
3. Prevent pressure on wounds.	3. Minimizes trauma and ensures adequate perfusion to burn wounds	• Shows clean reepithelializing donor sites
4. Apply topical antibacterials as prescribed.	4. Promotes adequate antibacterial effects of topical agents	• Exhibits negative burn wound cultures
5. Prevent cross-contamination.	5. Reduces risk of bacterial colonization	
6. Remove possible reservoirs of infection.	6. Reduces or eliminates sources of bacteria and contamination	
7. Utilize barrier gowns, gloves, masks, and hair covers when wounds are exposed or when in direct contact with patient or bed.	7. Minimizes contamination of wound by normal or pathogenic bacteria from health care providers	

Nursing Diagnosis: Impaired skin integrity related to open burn wounds

Goal: Improved skin integrity and wound healing

1. Cleanse wound and rest of body, including hair, daily.	1. Reduces potential bacterial contamination, a common cause of impaired wound healing	• Patient demonstrates that majority of wounds are closed.
2. Apply topical antibacterial agents and dressing as prescribed.	2. Reduces bacterial colonization and promotes healing	• Has completed or nearly completed skin grafting
3. Prevent pressure, infection, and mobilization of autografts.	3. Avoids trauma of grafts necessary for wound closure	• Shows over 80% of body covered with intact skin
4. Provide donor site care.	4. Promotes healing of donor site	
5. Observe and report any signs of poor graft take or loss of skin integrity after healing.	5. Grafted or healed burn wounds are susceptible to trauma.	
6. Provide adequate nutritional support.	6. Adequate nutrition is essential for normal granulation and healing.	

(continued)

---

    f. Does not scratch skin
    g. Reports skin is comfortable, with no itching or tightness
6. Demonstrates optimal physical mobility
    a. Improves range of motion of joints daily
    b. Demonstrates pre-morbid range of motion of all joints
    c. Has no signs of periarticular calcification
    d. Participates in activities of daily living as desired

Nursing care of the patient in the intermediate/acute phase of burn management is further discussed in Nursing Care Plan 49-2.

Stage III: Long-Term/Rehabilitation Phase

Although longer-term aspects of burn care are discussed last, it is important to remember that attention to them begins *immediately* after the burn has occurred—as early as the immediate postburn phase.

In the aftermath of the acute stages of illness, the burn victim now increasingly focuses on the changes in self-image and the alterations in life-style that may be required. Reconstructive surgery to improve cosmetic and functional results

(Text continues on p. 1322)

Nursing Care Plan 49-2 *(continued)*

Nursing Interventions	Rationale	Expected Outcomes

Nursing Diagnosis: Pain and discomfort related to painful burn wound, treatments, debridement, and surgical interventions

Goal: Relief of pain and discomfort

Nursing Interventions	Rationale	Expected Outcomes
1. Assess patient's pain carefully.	1. Provides baseline for assessment of pain relief measures	• Patient obtains relief of pain.
2. Offer analgesics and relaxation breathing, transcutaneous nerve stimulator, or other appropriate measures.	2. Provides multiple interventions that offer relief of pain and anxiety related to fear of pain	• Requests analgesics only occasionally, and specifically for muscle and joint pain
3. Assess and document patient's response to interventions.	3. Allows alteration of ineffective pain relief measures and use of those that are effective	• Verbally reports minimal pain • Is free of physiological and nonverbal indicators of moderate or severe pain
4. Assist patient with appropriate means of expressing pain.	4. Allows/encourages patient to express extended pain and discomfort that accompany repeated painful treatments	
5. Educate patient about the usual pain trajectory in burn recovery.	5. Reduces fear of the unknown, and may provide some measure of control to the patient	

Nursing Diagnosis: Altered nutrition: less than body requirements

Goal: Improved nutritional status

Nursing Interventions	Rationale	Expected Outcomes
1. Provide high-calorie, high-protein diet by appropriate route.	1. Provides nutrients for healing and to meet increased metabolic requirements for calories	• Patient demonstrates optimal nutritional status.
2. Administer parenteral hyperalimentation according to hospital protocol.	2. May be necessary to provide adequate nutrition to anorexic patient	• Demonstrates daily weight gain (by weight curve)
3. Give supplemental vitamins and minerals as prescribed.	3. Necessary for normal healing and function	• Is free of signs of protein, vitamin, or mineral deficiencies • Has increasing energy level
4. Weigh patient daily; record in graphic form.	4. Provides record of trends in weight	• Meets required nutritional needs by oral intake entirely
5. Report intolerance manifested by abdominal distention, diarrhea, osmotic diuresis, dehydration.	5. May indicate abnormal gastrointestinal function or need for alteration in dietary prescription	• Exhibits normal serum protein levels

Nursing Diagnosis: Alteration in body image related to burn wound and changes in role and life-style

Goal: Improved body image and acceptance of alterations required as a result of burn injury

Nursing Interventions	Rationale	Expected Outcomes
1. Assess patient's readiness to express feelings regarding alteration in body image or life-style.	1. Helps to determine patient's awareness of effects of burn injury and ability to begin to deal with these changes	• Patient has realistic concept of changes in body image and alterations required in daily activities as a result of burn injury.

(continued)

Nursing Interventions	*Rationale*	*Expected Outcomes*

Nursing Diagnosis: Alteration in body image related to burn wound and changes in role and life-style

Goal: Improved body image and acceptance of alterations required as a result of burn injury

2. Provide opportunity for expression of thoughts and feelings.	2. Allows patient to express and verbalize feelings regarding burn injury, its effects, and outcomes	• Verbalizes an accurate description of alterations in body image postburn
3. Maintain positive but honest approach in responding to questions.	3. Encourages patient to voice concerns and ask questions in a trusting atmosphere	• Discusses changes in life-style and daily activities that may be required postdischarge
4. Utilize significant others, counselors, and appropriate resource persons to help patient cope.	4. Provides multiple sources of support and increases chances of their success	• Demonstrates interest in resources that may be able to positively affect cosmetic and functional results of injury
5. Support effective premorbid coping mechanisms.	5. Encourages patient to use familiar coping mechanisms that have been successful in the past	• Is free of withdrawal and depression

Nursing Diagnosis: Immobility related to possible development of flexion contractures and muscle atrophy

Goal: Increased mobility and participation in activities of daily living

1. Position patient carefully to prevent flexed position in burned areas.	1. Reduces risk of flexion contractures	• Patient demonstrates range of joint motion that approaches preburn range.
2. Implement range-of-motion exercises several times daily.	2. Minimizes muscle atrophy	• Shows joint motion that permits activities of daily living
3. Assist with ambulation.	3. Encourages increased mobility and use of muscles	• Improves range of motion of contracted joints daily
4. Utilize splints and exercise devices recommended by occupational and physical therapists.	4. Encourages activity while maintaining proper position of joints	• Is free of periarticular calcification
5. Encourage self-feeding and turning and moving in bed.	5. Encourages independence and self-care while encouraging activity and exercise	

Nursing Diagnosis: Deficit in knowledge about surgical procedures and postoperative course

Goal: Increased knowledge about procedures and own role in them

1. Review surgical procedures and postoperative course with patient and family.	1. Prepares patient for procedures and own role in them	• Patient verbalizes understanding of treatments and surgical procedures and participates appropriately in care.
2. Explore patient's previous experience with hospitalization and surgery.	2. Provides basis for explanations and indication of patient's expectations	• Expresses concerns about surgery and treatments with health team and family
3. Tailor information given to patient's questions and nonverbal cues to anxiety level.	3. Promotes adequacy of explanations to patient without excessively increasing anxiety level	• Describes surgical procedures and treatments accurately
4. Define expectations of required patient participation for optimal results.	4. Provides specific directions and goals for patient	• Cooperates with required positioning

may be needed. Counseling, both psychological and vocational, may be valuable. Significant others will also need support and guidance in assisting the patient in returning to optimal health.

Follow-up care planned by the burn team will be necessary. In the case of children, such follow-up care is needed for many years. Preparations for this reality should begin during the earlier stages of care. It is a great challenge to the health care team to prepare a person for independent functioning after such a major traumatic event.

A program including elastic pressure garments, splints, and exercise under the supervision of an experienced physiatrist and physical and occupational therapy team is recommended for optimal functional and cosmetic results. As the inpatient phase of burn recovery gets shorter and shorter, much of the rehabilitation of the burn patient takes place on an outpatient basis or in a rehabilitation center.

Focus on maintaining fluid and electrolyte balance and improving nutritional status continues. The fluid and electrolyte changes that occur in the long-term or rehabilitative phase of care are described in Table 49-8.

▶ *Nursing Process*
Burn Care During Long-Term/ Rehabilitation Phase

▷ *Assessment*

Information about the patient's educational level, cultural background, religion, previous dietary habits and preferences,

TABLE 49-8
*Water and Electrolyte Changes in the Long-Term/
Rehabilitation Phase of Burn Care*

Observation	Explanation
Calcium deficit	Calcium may be immobilized at the burn site in the slough and early granulation phase of burns; symptoms of calcium deficit occur rarely.
Potassium deficit	Extracellular K^+ moves into the cells, leaving a deficit of K^+ in the extracellular fluid.
Negative nitrogen balance (present for several weeks following burns)	Secondary to: Stress reaction Immobilization Inadequate protein intake Protein losses in exudate Direct destruction of protein at burn site
Sodium deficit	

(Adapted from Metheny NM and Snively WD. Nurses' Handbook of Fluid Balance. Philadelphia, JB Lippincott.)

and self-concept is obtained early in the care of the burn patient. Other important information areas for assessment include the patient's occupational history and preference for leisure activities, family interactions, and communication with significant others by both the patient and family members.

The patient's mental status, emotional response to the injury and hospitalization, level of intellectual functioning, previous hospitalizations, response to pain and pain relief measures, and sleep pattern are also essential components of a comprehensive assessment. Information about general self-concept and how the patient has coped with stressful situations in the past will be valuable in addressing emotional needs.

Ongoing assessments related to rehabilitation goals include range of motion of affected joints, functional abilities in activities of daily living, early signs of skin breakdown from splints or positioning devices, evidence of neuropathies, activity tolerance, and quality of healing skin. The patient's participation in care and ability to demonstrate self-care in such areas as ambulation, feeding, wound cleansing, and application of pressure wraps are also documented on a regular basis.

In addition to the assessment parameters identified above, many of which apply to all patients with major burns, specific complications and treatments require specific assessments. For example, the patient undergoing primary excision requires postoperative assessment; the patient receiving nutritional support requires continuous monitoring of metabolic response to parenteral hyperalimentation.

Recovery from burn injury involves every system of the body, so assessment of the burn patient must be comprehensive and continuous. Specific parameters may take priority during one phase and be less important in another. Understanding the physiologic and pathologic processes that underlie the injury and the body's response to it provides a basis for early detection of significant signs and symptoms. Early detection leads to early intervention and enhances potential for optimal patient outcomes.

▷ *Nursing Diagnoses*

Based on the assessment data, nursing diagnoses in the long-term or rehabilitation phases of burn care may include the following:

- Activity intolerance related to metabolic demands, pain, muscle wasting
- Knowledge deficit related to inexperience with burn injury and need for continuing care of burn wounds and healing skin
- Ineffective individual coping related to fear and anxiety, grieving, and forced dependence on health care providers
- Disturbance in self-concept related to altered body image, self-esteem, role performance, and personal identity

▷ *Planning and Implementation*

▷ *Goals:* The major goals of the patient may include increased participation in activities of daily living, increased understanding of injury, treatment, and planned follow-up care, use of appropriate coping strategies, and adaptation and adjustment to alterations in self-concept and life-style.

Nursing Interventions

Promoting Rest. Nursing interventions that must be carried out according to a set regimen and the pain that accompanies movement each take their toll on burn patients. They may become confused and disoriented and lack the energy to participate optimally in their own care. The nurse must plan the care for each patient in a manner that permits some unbroken periods for sleep. A good time for planned patient rest is after the stress of dressing changes and exercise, while pain interventions may still be effective. This plan must be communicated to family members and other care providers. Hypnotics given in the evening, as prescribed, may promote sleep at night. Because burn patients frequently have nightmares related to the situation in which the burn occurred, the nurse listens to and reassures the patient when such nightmares, or other fears and anxieties about the outcome of the injury, cause insomnia.

Planning Activity. Reduction of metabolic stress by relieving pain, preventing chilling, and promoting physical integrity of all body systems will help the patient to conserve energy for therapeutic activities and wound healing. The nurse incorporates physical therapy exercises in the patient's care to prevent muscular atrophy and maintain the mobility required for daily activities. A gradual increase in the patient's activity tolerance, strength, and endurance will occur if activity is planned for time periods of increasing duration. Fatigue, fever, and pain tolerance are monitored and used to determine the amount of activity to be encouraged on a daily basis. Scheduling activities such as family visits, recreational or play therapy, listening to the radio, or walking to the patient lounge can provide diversion, improve a patient's psychological outlook, and increase tolerance for physical activity as well.

Patient Education. Patients will be better able to participate in their care if they are aware of the consequences of the injury, the goals of planned treatment and their role in ongoing care. This education begins in the Emergency Department and continues throughout rehabilitation. Families are included in planning and carrying out care to the extent allowed by their interest and ability and a patient's needs.

Strengthening Coping Strategies. Depression, regression, and manipulative behavior are common coping mechanisms used by burn patients. Withdrawal from participation in required treatments and regression must be viewed with an understanding that such behavior helps the patient cope with an enormously stressful event. Much energy goes into maintaining vital physical functions and wound healing in the early weeks postburn, leaving little emotional energy for coping in a mature and effective manner. Nurses can assist patients to develop effective coping strategies through setting specific expectations for behavior, promoting truthful communication to build trust, helping patients practice appropriate strategies, and giving positive reinforcement when appropriate. Family members must also be informed about the behavioral patterns that may occur so they will not be hurt by unexpected patient behavior and so they can reinforce the health team's approaches to the patient.

Patients are very dependent on health team members during the long period of acute illness. However, even when physically unable to contribute much to self-care, they can be included in decisions regarding care and encouraged to assert their individuality in terms of preferences and recognition of their unique identities. As patients improve in mobility and strength, the nurse works with them to set realistic expectations for self-care, including self-feeding, assistance with wound care procedures, exercise, and planning for the future. Many patients respond positively to the use of contractual agreements and other strategies that recognize their independence and their specific role as part of the health care team moving toward the goal of self-care.

Burn patients frequently suffer profound losses. These include not only their own previous body image due to disfigurement, but also losses of personal property, their homes, their loved ones, and their ability to perform in their occupations. They must grieve for these losses without benefit of the anticipatory grieving that a patient approaching elective surgery or a person dealing with the terminal illness of a loved one goes through. In addition to being available as a listener and counselor, the nurse can refer patients to a support group, such as those usually available at regional burn-centers or through organizations such as the Phoenix Society. Through participation in such groups, patients will meet others with similar experiences and learn to develop coping strategies to help them deal with their losses.

Assisting With Psychological Adjustments. As care progresses, the burn victim becomes aware of daily improvement and begins to exhibit basic concerns: Will I be disfigured? How long will I have to be in the hospital? What about my job and family? Will I ever be independent again? How can I pay for my care? Was this the result of my carelessness? As the patient expresses such concerns, the nurse should take time to listen and be encouraging.

Aside from showing signs of fear, the patient frequently gives vent to angry feelings. At times the anger may be directed inward because of a sense of guilt—perhaps for causing the fire, or even for surviving when loved ones perished; or the anger may reach outward toward those who escaped unharmed or even to those who are now providing care. One way to help the patient handle these emotions is to find someone to whom the patient can vent feelings without fear of retaliation. A nurse, social worker, or clergy member who is not involved in direct care activities may fill this role successfully.

A major responsibility of the nurse is to constantly assess the patient's psychosocial reactions. Why is the patient fearful? Is it fear of losing control of bodily care, or of sanity itself? Is it fear of rejection by family and loved ones? Is it fear of being unable to cope with pain, or physical appearance? Is it concern about sexual function? Being aware of these anxieties and understanding the basis of the patient's fears will enable the nurse to provide support and to cooperate with other members of the health care team in developing a plan to help the patient handle these feelings.

Improving Self-Concept. When caring for burn patients, the nurse needs to be aware that there are prejudices and misunderstandings in our society about those who differ from "the norm." Opportunities available to others are often denied to those who are disfigured, including social participation, means of employment, prestige, various roles, and status. It is the disfigured persons who must show others who they are, how they function, and how they want to be treated.

The nurse can help patients practice their responses to people who may stare or inquire about their injury once they are discharged from the hospital. The nurse can build self-esteem in patients by recognizing their uniqueness through small gestures such as planning for a birthday cake for a patient, combing the patient's hair before visiting hours, sharing information on the availability of a cosmetician to enhance appearance, and teaching the patient to direct attention away from a disfigured body toward the self within. Consultants such as psychologists, social workers, vocational counselors, and teachers are valuable participants in the care of burn patients during rehabilitation.

▷ *Evaluation*

▷ *Expected Outcomes*

1. Patient demonstrates activity tolerance required for desired daily activities.
   a. Obtains sufficient sleep each 24 hours
   b. Reports no nightmares or sleep disturbances
   c. Shows gradually increasing tolerance and endurance in physical activities
   d. Is able to concentrate in conversations
   e. Has energy available to sustain desired daily activities
2. Demonstrates knowledge of self-care and follow-up care required
   a. Describes surgical procedures and treatments accurately
   b. Verbalizes detailed plan for follow-up care
   c. Demonstrates ability to do wound care and exercise
   d. Returns to clinic and physical/occupational therapy appointments as scheduled
   e. Lists resource people and agencies to contact for specific problems
3. Uses appropriate coping strategies to deal with postburn problems
   a. Verbalizes reactions to burns, therapeutic procedures, losses
   b. Identifies coping strategies used previously in stressful situations
   c. Accepts dependency on health care providers during acute illness
   d. Demonstrates denial, anger, regression, and depression in pattern common to postburn illness
   e. Verbalizes realistic view of problems consequent to burn injury and plans for future
   f. Cooperates with health care providers in required therapy
   g. Asks relevant questions regarding burn injuries and outcomes
   h. Participates in decision-making regarding care
   i. Demonstrates interest in resources that may be able to positively affect cosmetic and functional results of injury
4. Adapts and adjusts to alterations in self-concept and life-style
   a. Verbalizes an accurate description of alterations in body image postburn
   b. Discusses changes in life-style and daily activities that may be required after discharge
   c. Adapts to and accepts appearance
   d. Utilizes cosmetics, wigs, and prostheses as desired to achieve acceptable appearance

   e. Socializes with significant others, peers, and usual social group
   f. Seeks and gains employment or return to role in family, school, or community as contributing member
   g. Is free of withdrawal and depression
   h. Resolves grief over losses resulting from burn injury and circumstances surrounding injury (*e.g.*, death of others; damage to house; other property)
   i. States realistic objectives for plastic surgery, further medical intervention and results
   j. States abilities and goals that can be achieved
   k. Has hopeful attitude toward future

Nursing care of the patient during long-term/rehabilitation phase is discussed in Nursing Care Plan 49-3.

Home Care and Follow-Up

As hospital stays become shorter, outpatient and home care of burn patients takes on increasing importance. Patients and families must gradually be educated during the course of the hospital stay to care for the burn wound by active participation in this process as early as possible. Looking at the wound and touching the wound may be difficult and even frightening to some family members and patients. However, with encouragement and support, the majority of patients can handle follow-up wound care with little need for professional care on a daily basis.

Follow-up care for the burn patient is carefully planned by all disciplines involved in the patient's care prior to hospital discharge. The nurse is responsible for coordinating the care needed to achieve a holistic approach. Many patients require outpatient physical and/or occupational therapy, often several times per week. Information related to specific exercises, use of elastic pressure garments, and splints is fully reviewed with both the patient and responsible significant others. Written instructions are also provided.

A referral to the patient's regular physician is required for continuing care of any preexisting or new medical problems.

Patients who receive care in a burn center usually return to a burn clinic periodically for evaluation of their status by the burn team, modification of home care instructions, and planning for reconstructive surgery. Others will be followed by the general or plastic surgeon who cared for them during hospitalization. Other patients require the services of a rehabilitation center and may be transferred to such a facility for aggressive rehabilitation prior to going home.

Some persons, particularly those without competent family members or friends available to help, will need referral to a community health nurse who can provide assistance with wound care and exercises at home. Patients with severe or long-lasting depression or difficulty adjusting to their social and/or occupational roles may require referral to a psychologist, psychiatrist, or vocational counselor.

There are a number of burn patient support groups and other organizations located throughout the United States that offer services for burn victims. They provide caring persons (often recovered burn victims) who can visit a burn patient in the hospital or home or telephone a patient or family periodically to provide support and counseling about skin care,

Care of the Patient During the Long-Term/Rehabilitation Phase of Burn Care

Nursing Interventions	Rationale	Expected Outcomes

Nursing Diagnosis: Ineffective individual coping related to increased emotional and physical dependence on others

Goal: Improved coping and increased independence

1. Be alert for verbal and nonverbal cues of patient regarding rehabilitation and adaptation to altered self-image.	1. Provides information about patient's understanding, awareness, and acceptance of changes in body image and life	• Patient achieves emotional and physical independence.
2. Assist patient to set achievable short-term goals for increased independence in activities of daily living.	2. These are often easier to identify and to meet than long-term goals that seem unrealistic and unachievable to the patient.	• Participates fully in activities of daily living
3. Provide positive feedback and support.	3. Encourages continued progress toward independence	• Is equipped with and knowledgeable about use of prostheses or assistive devices
4. Consult with appropriate health team members for assistance with regressive behavior.	4. Utilizes knowledge and expertise of others	• Verbalizes realistic view of self and plans for future
5. Assist with physical and occupational therapy as outlined by physical medicine staff.	5. Provides assistance to the patient while encouraging independence	• Reports ability to participate in family, social, and vocational spheres

Nursing Diagnosis: Discomfort related to skin tightness, dryness, and itching

Goal: Relief of discomfort and achievement of soft, lubricated, comfortable skin

1. Assist patient with application of cocoa butter, Nivea, or other cream to healed wounds several times daily.	1. Lubricates and softens the skin	• Patient exhibits soft, comfortable, lubricated skin.
2. Use mild soap for daily bathing.	2. Avoids use of harsh, drying soaps	• Demonstrates no evidence of scratching of skin
3. Maintain cool, comfortable environment.	3. Minimizes discomfort and itching	• Is able to sleep without being disturbed by itching
4. Administer antipruritic medication.	4. Prevents or minimizes itching	• Reports minimal or no itching
5. Recommend white, cotton underwear under street clothing.	5. Avoids direct contact of skin with irritating dyes in clothes	• Skin feels soft and smooth.
		• Patient demonstrates no scales or dryness.

(continued)

use of cosmetics, and problems related to psychosocial adjustment. Such organizations, and many regional burn centers, sponsor group meetings and social functions at which outpatients are welcome. Some also provide school reentry programs and are active in burn prevention activities.

Gerontological Considerations

Burns in the elderly are often associated with much greater morbidity and mortality than those in younger patients. Reduced mobility, changes in vision, and decreased sensation in the feet and hands associated with the older age group are significant factors related to the inability of a person to avoid a preventable burn injury. Furthermore, thinning and loss of elasticity of the skin in the elderly predisposes them to a deeper injury from a thermal insult that might cause a less severe burn in a younger person.

Chronic illnesses decrease the aged person's ability to withstand the multi-system stresses of burn injury. Decreased function of the cardiovascular and renal systems and lung disease increase the need for very close observation of elderly patients with even relatively small burns during the emergent and acute phases. Acute oliguric renal failure is much more common than in those under 40 years of age. The margin of difference between hypovolemia and fluid overload is very small. Suppressed immunologic response, a high incidence of malnutrition, and inability to withstand metabolic stressors

Nursing Interventions	Rationale	Expected Outcomes

Nursing Diagnosis: Inactivity related to pain on exercise, limited joint mobility, fatigue, and low endurance

Goal: Increased activity and independence

Nursing Interventions	Rationale	Expected Outcomes

1. Relieve pain:
  a. Assess and document pain.
  b. Utilize analgesics, transcutaneous nerve stimulator, relaxation therapy, or other appropriate nursing interventions prior to exercise periods.
	1. Permits evaluation of baseline of pain and pain's contribution to inactivity.	• Patient exhibits no pain.
		• Requests no analgesics
		• Reports no pain on exercise
		• Is able to sleep without being disturbed by pain
		• Achieves activity tolerance and endurance consistent with desired levels
		• Participates in activities of daily living as desired
		• Has stamina required for usual activities
		• Obtains optimal joint mobility
		• Has normal range of motion in all joints

2. Increase activity tolerance and endurance	2. Promotes pain relief while encouraging exercise and activity	
3. Collaborate with physical and occupational therapists to plan for exercise requiring gradually increasing energy levels.	3. Helps to identify graded increases in exercise and activity within patient's current limitations	
4. Plan daily activities to maximize energy required for specific treatments in which patient must actively participate.	4. Promotes conservation of energy for its expenditure on required tasks and activities	
5. Plan care to provide rest period during day and 8 hours of sleep during night.	5. Encourages rest to decrease fatigue and increase exercise tolerance level	
6. Promote full range of joint motion.	6. Exercises affected joints and minimizes the risk of flexion contractures	
7. Encourage patient to follow exercise schedule planned by physical therapists.	7. Permits exercise while maintaining position of joints needed to prevent flexion contractures	
8. Apply splints as prescribed to reduce contractures. Administer analgesics if required prior to major physical therapy treatments.	8. Minimizes pain and discomfort during physical therapy treatments, and encourages full participation in exercises and treatments	
9. Utilize creative approaches to encourage patient to move joints in activities of daily living and self-care activities.	9. Promotes exercise while maintaining patient's independence	

(continued)

such as a cold environment further compromise the elderly person's ability to respond to burn injury.

Eschar separation in full-thickness burns is often delayed in the elderly. Because older persons are frequently poor risks for operative excision, prolonged hospitalization and immobilization and associated nosocomial problems may ensue.

Nursing assessment of the elderly should include particular attention to pulmonary function, response to fluid resuscitation, and signs of mental confusion or disorientation. A careful history of preburn medications and preexisting illnesses is essential. Nursing care promotes early mobilization, aggressive pulmonary care, and attention to reducing the potential for breakdown of normal skin. Because of lowered host resistance, the danger of burn wound sepsis and systemic septicemia is not only increased but also most likely to be lethal in the elderly. Fever may not be present in the elderly to signal such events. Therefore, surveillance for other signs of infection becomes even more important.

For stable patients, early operative intervention may be preferred to remove eschar and to facilitate wound covering with biologic dressings or autograft before infection and other problems cause deterioration of the patient. Rehabilitation takes into account preexisting functional abilities and problems such as arthritis and low activity-tolerance. Lack of significant others available and able to provide home care is

► **Nursing Care Plan 49-3** *(continued)*

Nursing Interventions	*Rationale*	*Expected Outcomes*

Nursing Diagnosis: Inappropriate grieving and depression related to inability to cope with alterations in appearance, life-style, body image, and self-image

Goal: Reduction of grieving and depression to an appropriate level

1. Employ concepts of psychiatric nursing to explore and improve depressed affect.	1. Interaction and communication skills are necessary to assist the grieving, depressed patient.	• Patient returns to preburn or better level of social and vocational functioning.
2. Help patient employ short-term goals and a "one day at a time" philosophy.	2. Short-term goals are easier to identify and achieve than long-term goals that seem unachievable to the grieving, depressed person.	• Socializes with significant others, peers, usual social group
3. Recognize need for grieving over losses.	3. Provides for a normal grief response to injury	• Is able to seek and gain employment or return to role in school or community as contributing member of the group
4. Have patient talk with other patients who are making good progress after similar injury.	4. Provides encouragement and a model for patient	• Has adapted to and resolved grief over losses resulting from burn injury and circumstances surrounding the injury (*e.g.,* death of others involved; damage to house, other property)
5. Obtain psychiatric consultation and administer prescribed mood elevators if depression lasts abnormally long.	5. Additional intervention may be necessary to help the patient cope with losses while continuing activity without jeopardizing progress and recovery.	• Has hopeful attitude toward the future
6. Explain that depression is a normal sequela of major trauma, but is relieved with general improvement in health.	6. Communicates that the patient's response is normal and is likely to abate as physical condition improves.	

Nursing Diagnosis: Alteration in skin integrity related to hypertrophic scarring

Goal: Prevention of hypertrophic scarring and achievement of optimal cosmetic result

1. Apply elastic bandages or pressure garments over healed areas prone to scarring.	1. These measures restructure the collagen and decrease vascularity and cellularity of the burned area, thus reducing hypertrophic scarring.	• Patient achieves optimal cosmetic results.
2. Instruct patient in proper use and care of elastic garments for optimal results.	2. Provides information for patient to use correctly to promote the optimal result	• Adapts to and accepts appearance
3. Provide information and referral for use of cosmetics and other aids to minimize impact of burn wounds.	3. Provides other resources and aid for the patient and improves body image	• Utilizes cosmetics, wigs, prostheses as desired to achieve acceptable appearance
		• Has met plastic surgery goals
		• Exhibits minimal hypertrophic scarring
		• States interest in acquiring information about cosmetics and other aids

common. It is imperative that social services and community nursing services be contacted to provide for optimal care upon hospital discharge.

Bibliography

Books

Bayley EW and Martin MT (eds). A Curriculum for Basic Burn Nursing Practice, 4th ed. Galveston, Texas: University of Texas Medical Branch and Shriners Burns Institute for the American Burn Association, 1985.

Bernstein NR and Robson MC. Comprehensive Approaches to the Burned Person. New Hyde Park: Medical Examination Publishing Co, 1983.

DiGregorio VR (ed). Rehabilitation of the Burn Patient. New York, Churchill Livingstone, 1984.

Fisher SV and Helm P. Comprehensive Rehabilitation of Burns. Baltimore, Williams & Wilkins, 1984.

Heimbach D and Engrav LH. Surgical Management of the Burn Wound. New York, Karger, 1985.

Mannon JM. Caring for the Burned. Springfield, Illinois, Charles C Thomas, 1985.

Salisbury RE, Newman NM, and Dingaldein GP. Manual of Burn Therapeutics. Boston, Little, Brown & Co, 1983.

Wachtel TL, Kahn V, and Frank HA (eds). Current Topics in Burn Care. Rockville, Maryland, Aspen Systems, 1983.

Zander H and Stehling L. The Burn Patient: Anesthetic Management and Immediate Care. Chicago, Year Book Medical Publishers, 1984.

Articles*

Abshagen D. Topical agents and emergency care for minor burn injuries. J Emerg Nurs 1984 Nov/Dec; 10(6):325–331.

Baxter CR, Burke JF, Curreri PW, and Heimbach D. Excisional therapy in burn injury: Who—when—how? J Burn Care and Rehab 1984 Nov/Dec; 5(6):430–437.

Bayley EW. Nursing education in a burn unit. Crit Care Quart 1984 Dec; 7(3):63–72.

Boswick JA (ed). Burns. Surg Clin North Am 1987 Feb; 67(1):1–189.

Brinkerhoff CE. DIC: Implications for clinical nursing in a pediatric burn population. Crit Care Quart 1984 Dec; 7(3):8–18.

Bruce GL and Ingersoll GL. Critical care orientation of burn nurses. Crit Care Quart 1984 Dec; 7(3):79–84.

Burke JF. Observation on the development of an artificial skin. J Trauma 1983 July; 23(7):543–551.

Cardany CR et al. Influence of hydrotherapy and antiseptic agents on burn wound bacterial contamination. J Burn Care and Rehab 1985 May/June; 9(3):230–232.

Cooke SS. Major thermal injury—the first 48 hours. Crit Care Nurs 1986 Jan/Feb; 6(1):55–63.

Cuzzell JZ. The politics of burn care. Am J Nurs 1986 Feb; 86(2):194–195.

Deitch EA et al. Hypertrophic burn scars: Analysis of variables. J Trauma 1983 Oct; 23(10):895–898.

Desai MH. Inhalation injuries in burn victims. Crit Care Quart 1984 Dec; 7(3):1–7.

Dyess DL, Jurkovich GJ, Luterman A, and Curreri PW. Inhalation injuries. Curr Concepts in Trauma Care 1985 Fall; 8(3):4–8.

Engeman SA. The burned patient. AORN J 1985 July; 40(1):36–41.

Frank DH, Wachtel T, Frank HA, and Sanders R. Comparison of Biobrane, porcine, and human allograft as biological dressings for burn wounds. J Burn Care and Rehab 1983 May/June; 4(3):186–190.

Freeman J. Nursing care of the patient with a burn injury. Crit Care Nurs 1984 Nov/Dec; 4(6):52–68.

Gonzales E. Psychosocial adjustment of children following hospitalization for acute burns. J Burn Care and Rehab 1984 Mar/Apr; 5(2):138–142.

Herndon DN et al. Treatment of burns. Curr Probl Surg 1987 June; 24(6):347–397.

Hurt RA. More than skin deep: Guidelines on caring for the burn patient. Nursing '85 1985 June; 15(6):55–57.

Ireton CS, et al. Do changes in burn size affect measured energy expenditure? J Burn Care and Rehab 1985 Sept/Oct; 6(5):419–421.

Jackson S. Dealing with burns. RN 1984 Oct; 45(10):35–39.

Jacoby F. Care of the massive burn wound. Crit Care Quart 1984 Dec; 7(3):44–53.

Jensen LL and Parshley PF. Postburn scar contractures: Histology and effects of pressure treatment. J Burn Care and Rehab 1984 Mar/Apr; 5(2):158–162.

Jensen TG, Long JM, Dudrick SA, and Johnston DA. Nutritional assessment of postburn complications. J Am Diet Assoc 1985 Jan; 85(1):68–72.

Johnson CL and Cain V. The rehabilitation guide. Am J Nurs 1985 Jan; 85(1):48–50.

* Note: Also see all issues of The Journal of Burn Care and Rehabilitation and BURNS—The Journal of the International Society for Burn Injuries.

Judge C, May SR, and DeClement FA. Control of hypertrophic scarring in burn patients using tubular support bandages. J Burn Care and Rehab 1984 May/June; 5(3):221–224.

Kavanaugh C. A new approach to dressing change in the severely burned child and its effect on burn-related psychopathology. Heart Lung 1983 Nov/Dec; 12(6):612–619.

Kibbee E. Burn pain management. Crit Care Quart 1984 Dec; 7(3):54–62.

Luterman A, Adams M, and Curreri PW. Nutritional management of the burn patient. Crit Care Quart 1984 Dec; 7(3):34–42.

Marvin J. Planning home care for burn patients. Nursing '83 1983 Aug; 13(8):65–67.

Nadel E and Kozerefski PM. Rehabilitation of the critically ill burn patient. Crit Care Quart 1984 Dec; 7(3):19–33.

Nichter LS et al. Injuries due to commercial electric current. J Burn Care and Rehab 1984 Mar/Apr; 5(2):124–137.

Park R. Anesthesia for the burned patient. AORN J 1984 July; 40(1):42–47.

Perdue GF and Hunt JL. Cold injury: A collective review. J Burn Care and Rehab 1986 July/Aug; 7(4):331–342.

Pruitt BA and Levine NS. Characteristics and uses of biological dressings and skin substitutes. Arch Surg 1984 Mar; 119(3):312–322.

Quay N and Alexander L. Preparation of burned children and their families for discharge. J Burn Care and Rehab 1983 July/Aug; 4(4):288–290.

Ragiel CA. The impact of critical injury on patient, family, and clinical systems. Crit Care Quart 1984 Dec; 7(3):73–78.

Robertson KE, Cross PJ, and Terry JC. Burn care. Am J Nurs 1985 Jan; 85(1):29–47.

Robson M et al. Synthetic burn dressings: Roundtable discussion. J Burn Care and Rehab 1985 Jan/Feb; 6(1):29–47.

Ruberg RL. Advances in Burn Care. Clin Plast Surg 1986 Jan; 13(1):entire issue.

Saffle JR et al. Use of indirect calorimetry in the nutritional management of burned patients. J Trauma 1985 Jan; 25(1):32–39.

Shires GT and Black E. Proceedings of Conference on Frontiers in Understanding Burn Injury. J Trauma 1984 Sept (Suppl); 24(9):entire issue.

Surveyor JA and Clougherty DM. Burn scars: Fighting the effects. Am J Nurs 1983 May; 83(5):746–751.

Wachtel TL et al. A semi-closed method of burn wound dressing. J Burn Care and Rehab 1984 Mar/Apr; 5(2):158–162.

Wright PC. Fundamentals of acute burn care and physical therapy. Phys Ther 1984 Aug; 64(8):1217–1231.

Agencies

Alisa Ann Ruch Burn Foundation, 20944 Sherman Way, Suite 115, Canoga Park, CA 91303. *Phone:* (818) 883-7700.

American Burn Association, c/o Thomas L. Wachtel, M.D., Sec. 1130 E. McDowell, B-2, Phoenix, AZ 85006.

Burn Foundation, 1311 Chancellor Street, Philadelphia, PA 19107. *Phone:* (215) 735-4050.

Good Samaritan Hospital, 1130 East McDowell Road, Suite B-2, Phoenix, AZ 85006. *Phone:* (602) 239-2391.

National Institute for Burn Medicine, 909 East Ann Street, Ann Arbor, MI 48104. *Phone:* (313) 769-9000.

Northern California Burn Council, % Andrew Maguire, Director, Trauma Foundation, Trauma Center, Building 1, San Francisco General Hospital, San Francisco, CA 94110. *Phone:* (415) 821-5135.

Phoenix Society, 11 Rust Hill Road, Levittown, PA 19056. *Phone:* (215) 946-4788.

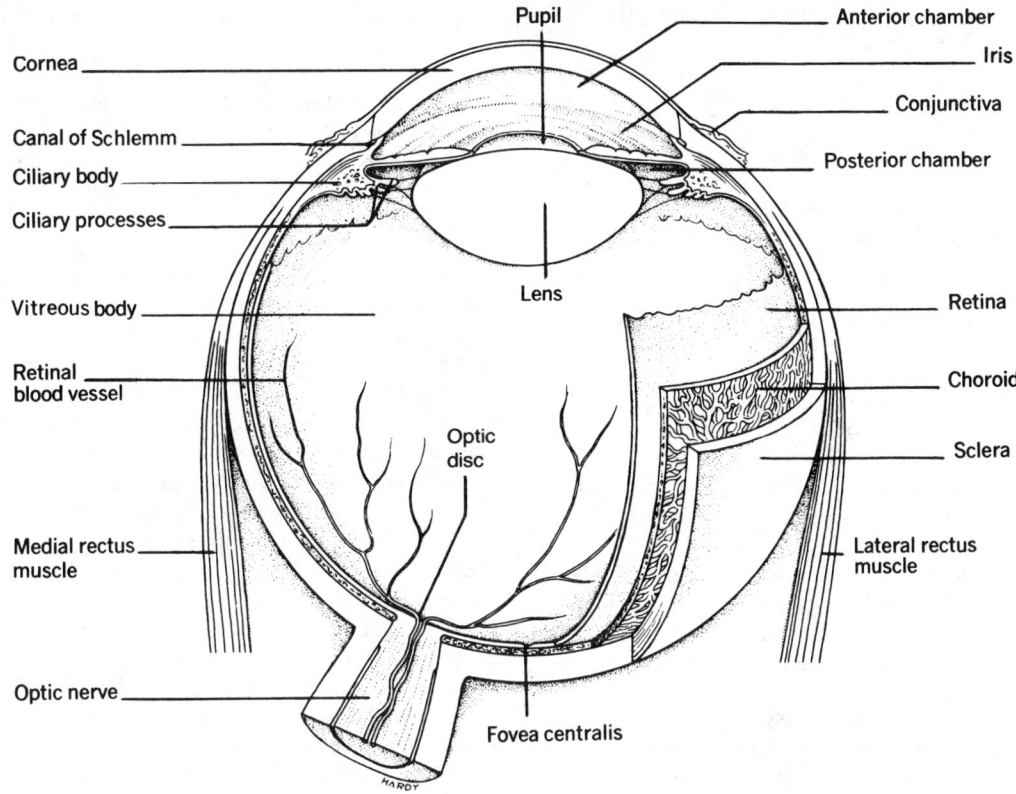

Figure 50-1
Transverse section of eye. (Chaffee EE and Greisheimer EM. Basic Physiology and
Anatomy. Philadelphia, JB Lippincott.)

ical components: the nucleus, the cortex, and the capsule. The nucleus is located in the central zone and is surrounded by a thick layer of softer cortical material, which in turn is enveloped by a thin transparent elastic capsule. The lens is capable of being modified to varying degrees of convexity by the contraction and the relaxation of the ciliary muscles, or zonules ("guy wires"). This adjustment in vision is referred to as *accommodation.*

The cavity within the eye is divided by the lens into two parts. The posterior part contains a jelly-like, translucent substance called the *vitreous humor,* which is the chief factor in maintaining the form of the eyeball. The anterior part contains a clear, watery fluid, the *aqueous humor,* which is secreted by the ciliary processes. It bathes the anterior surface of the lens, escapes at the pupil, and enters the space between the iris and the cornea, known as the *anterior chamber.* Finally, it is drained from the eye through lymph channels (the canal of Schlemm) located at the junction of the iris and the sclera.

Appendages. The *eyelids* are the protective coverings of the eye. Lining the lids and entirely covering the anterior part of the eye is a highly sensitive membrane, the *conjunctiva,* the surface of which is kept moist by a constant flow of lacrimal fluid tears. This fluid is excreted from the *lacrimal gland,* which is located in the upper and outer part of the orbit. It flows downward and inward across the eye and drains into tiny channels (lacrimal puncta). These channels conduct the

fluid to the lacrimal sac and duct, which pass downward and outward and open into the nasal cavity beneath the inferior turbinate bone.

Gerontological Considerations

As a person ages, vision becomes less efficient. The pupil becomes less responsive to light owing to sclerosis of the pupillary sphincter, which results in a decrease in pupil size. The lens becomes more opaque, and the visual field decreases, making peripheral vision more difficult. Eyes adapt to darkness less rapidly; therefore, vision at night or in dimly lit areas is less clear than in younger people. With advancing years, there is a slowing in the process of accommodation as the lens gradually loses its elastic nature and becomes a relatively solid mass. When the lens becomes almost totally nonaccommodating, the condition is called *presbyopia.* Ciliary muscles with time also become less flexible and functional. Since near vision requires the greatest work by the ciliary muscles, near vision is compromised earliest, a condition that requires the wearing of reading glasses, bifocal lenses, and even trifocal lenses.

The vitreous begins to have a clumping of collagen materials; such clumping is referred to as "floaters," which may be apparent in the field of vision. The retina shows fewest changes with aging, except for the macula. The macula is a minute area in the center of the retina that is especially capable of detailed and acute vision. Very small sclerotic changes in the macula will result in impaired vision.

Eye Care Specialists

The importance of adequate eye examinations cannot be emphasized too strongly. Too often we find patients using a pair of glasses that belonged to a relative or was purchased at the local variety store.

The care of the eye is undertaken by four groups of specialists:

1. The *oculist,* the *ophthalmologist,* or the *ophthalmic physician* is a medical doctor who is skilled in the treatment of all conditions and diseases of the eye. Training and experience enable this physician to make a more thorough and complete examination of the eye for refractive errors and other changes.
2. The *optician* is not a physician but is concerned with grinding, mounting, and dispensing lenses.
3. The *optometrist* is licensed to examine the eyes and related structures to determine the presence of vision problems, eye diseases, or other abnormalities and to prescribe and adapt lenses or other optical aids.
4. The *ocularist* is a technician who makes artificial eyes and other prostheses used in ophthalmology.

Examination of the Eye and Assessment of Vision

Examination of the eye is an essential component of the physical examination, not only because of the importance of the function of the eye to the well-being of the patient, but also because the eye is reflective of many facets of the general state of health. The retina, which may be viewed with the ophthalmoscope, is the only site in the human body where a vascular bed may be examined directly. Diseases such as hypertension and diabetes, both exceedingly common in the population, produce changes that are readily observable. The pupil may be said to be a window to the human microcirculation.

Visual Acuity.   Formal testing of visual acuity is a part of the data base of every patient. Testing of visual acuity is accomplished by means of an eye chart placed 6 meters (20 feet) from the patient. If space is lacking, an inverted eye chart may be placed directly behind the patient's head, and a mirror placed 3 meters (10 feet) from the patient. The patient is instructed to cover one eye with a card, to keep both eyes open, and to read each line of the chart until he is no longer able to distinguish the details for a given size of print. If the patient wears glasses, his acuity should be assessed with and without corrective lenses.

Illiteracy may be circumvented by the use of charts that display the letter "E" in four different positions. This enables one to assess the vision of children as young as 5 years of age.

Visual acuity is expressed in a ratio that relates what the patient *should* see at 20 feet to what the patient *can* see at 20 feet. Acuity of 20/50 means that the patient can see at 20 feet what he should see at 50 feet; 20/200, the boundary of legal blindness, indicates that the patient can see at 20 feet what he should be able to see at 200 feet. Such patients can only discern with accuracy the large letter at the top of the chart. The patient whose visual acuity is less than 20/20 when corrected by his or her own glasses should be referred to an ophthalmologist.

Near vision is not routinely assessed unless the patient is complaining of difficulty in reading at close range or is over age 40. After age 40, the lens may become rigid and incapable of accommodating its shape to close-range vision (presbyopia). Having a patient read newsprint at a distance of 30.5 cm (12 inches) provides a general screening for this disorder. Patients who experience difficulty with this examination are referred to an ophthalmologist.

External Evaluation of the Eye.   The external structures of the eye are assessed primarily by inspection. These structures include the eyebrow, eyelid, eyelashes, lacrimal apparatus, conjunctiva, cornea, anterior chamber, iris, and pupil. The examination begins with an assessment of the position and alignment of the eyes. The eyebrows are observed for the quantity and distribution of the hair. The positioning of the lids in relationship to the eyeballs is noted. With the eyes open, no sclera should be visible above the corneas. *Ptosis* (drooping of the lid) may be due to lid edema, muscle weakness, congenital defect, or involvement of the third cranial nerve. The lids are also inspected for color, swelling, lesions, and the presence and direction of eyelash growth. Common abnormalities of the lids are discussed later in this chapter.

The region of the lacrimal gland in the upper lateral orbit is inspected. If enlargement is suspected, the upper lid can be everted to expose the lacrimal gland for further inspection. Next, the lacrimal apparatus is inspected for swelling. Obstruction or inflammation of the nasolacrimal duct can often be identified by pressing on the medial aspect of the lower lid just inside the orbital rim. The area is palpated for tenderness, and regurgitation of fluid from the puncta is watched for.

The sclera and bulbar conjunctiva are inspected concurrently. The lids are separated by placing the index finger on the patient's upper orbital rim and the thumb on the lower rim. As the lids are separated, the patient is instructed to look up, down, and to each side. Small capillaries are normally visible in the conjunctiva, and the white, fibrous sclera is normally clearly visible. In blacks, however, the sclera is often yellowish and is a normal finding, not be confused with jaundice. The palpebral conjunctiva of the lower lid is readily inspected by having the patient look upward while the lower lid is gently everted.

To inspect the cornea and anterior chamber for opacities, the examiner shines a light from a penlight held at an oblique angle. Normally, the cornea is smooth and transparent. Irregularities are often detected by defects in the light reflection through the cornea. Shadows cast on the iris may be indicative of a corneal lesion or forward displacement of the anterior chamber. The iris is inspected for continuity and unusual markings.

The pupils are normally round, regular, and equal in diameter and their reaction to light. Although a small percentage of the population may have unequal pupils that may be considered normal, the phenomenon is sufficiently unusual that it should lead to thorough examination in order to ascertain that the inequality is not due to central nervous system (CNS) disease. When confronted with light, the normal pupil promptly constricts in a regular concentric fashion. The un-stimulated opposite pupil constricts as well. This pupillary reaction is assessed by instructing the patient to focus on a distant object while the examiner shines a bright light on each pupil, in turn.

Constriction of the stimulated pupil is called the *direct light reflex,* whereas constriction of the opposite pupil is termed *consensual light reflex.* Exploration of this phenomenon allows one to separate damage to the optic nerve from blindness owing to more central disease. Direct light stimulation of the nerve-damaged eye results in neither a direct nor a consensual light reflex. Stimulation of the uninvolved eye, however, results in consensual constriction of the pupil of the damaged eye, since the consensual reflex is not dependent on transmission through the optic nerve.

Pupillary reaction to accommodation (adjustments that occur when vision is shifted from near to far objects or vice versa) is best observed by asking the patient to focus on an object in the distance and then at the examiner's finger, which is positioned 7.5 to 12.5 cm (3 to 5 inches) from the patient's nose. A normal response is for the pupils to constrict as the eyes converge and focus on the examiner's finger.

Autonomic disease due to CNS syphilis or to diabetes may result in a pupil that is incapable of responding to light but retains its capacity to respond to accommodation. Such a pupil is known as an *Argyll Robertson pupil.*

Ocular Tension. An increase in intraocular tension is the cardinal manifestation of glaucoma, a disease responsible for more than one fifth of the blindness seen in the United States. A general determination of intraocular pressure can be made by applying gentle finger pressure over the sclera of the closed eye. The tips of both forefingers are placed on the closed upper lid. One finger gently presses inward while the adjacent finger senses the amount of pressure exerted against it. Some examiners then compare the tension "felt"

or perceived in the patient's eye to their own. At best, this maneuver is a general estimation. When a more accurate measurement must be relied on, tonometry is indicated.

Assessment of Extraocular Muscles. The extraocular muscles (Fig. 50-2) are six small muscles attached to each eye. They are innervated by three of the cranial nerves. Synergistic (correlated) action of the extraocular muscles of both eyes results in parallel gaze. Although the mechanism by which this takes place is highly complex, and analysis of abnormality requires physician consultation, this assessment can be done by the nurse.

Parallel alignment of the eyes may be easily detected by shining a light directly into the face while the patient is staring at the light source. The light should be reflected from the pupils of both eyes identically. Light reflexes that vary from one pupil to the other indicate disturbance in parallax vision. In spite of normal alignment of both eyes when they function together, the tendency of either eye to drift to the nasal or temporal side (and the necessity to involuntarily compensate for this with effort) may be assessed by the *cover test.* One eye is covered by a card or by the hand of the examiner, and the patient is asked to focus the free eye on a stationary object, while keeping the covered eye open. The card or hand is abruptly removed from the covered eye, which is then observed for any abnormal movement. If the eye, when uncovered, has drifted to the temporal side, it will snap back into alignment when the cover is removed. Conversely, if it has drifted to the nasal side, the reverse phenomenon will occur. The tendency of an eye to drift, when covered, to the temporal side is called an *exophoria;* a tendency of an eye to drift to the nasal side is called an *esophoria.*

Integrity of the nervous control of the muscles of the eye may be assessed by directing the patient to move his eyes in the six cardinal positions of gaze (Fig. 50-2) while following an object. The object is moved laterally to either side along the horizontal axis and then along two oblique axes, each of which makes a 60-degree angle with the horizontal. Each of the cardinal positions of gaze represents the function of one of the six extraocular muscles attached to each eye. If *diplo-*

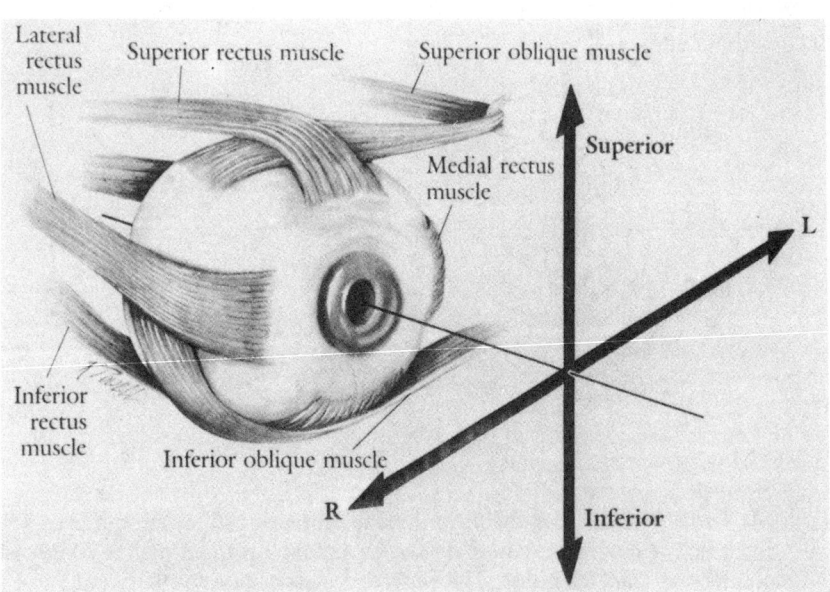

Figure 50-2
The extraocular muscles and their insertions onto the right eye. The arrows and the line to the pupil indicate the six cardinal positions of gaze. (Gittinger JW Jr. Ophthalmology. Boston, Little, Brown & Co, 1984.)

pia, or double vision, develops during the transition to any one of the cardinal positions of gaze, the examiner has an indication that one or more of the extraocular muscles are failing to function properly.

When extraocular movements are checked, the eye is observed for *nystagmus,* an irregular jerking movement of the eyes as gaze is shifted to a lateral position. Nystagmus has two components: a quick component in one or the other direction, and a slower subsequent component that brings the eye back to the intended postion. However, nystagmus on extreme lateral gaze is a normal finding and can be avoided by not placing the object too far laterally beyond binocular gaze. A number of conditions cause nystagmus. Although many of these conditions are benign, others may reflect severe pathologic processes.

Assessment of Field of Vision. Although the visual field (Fig. 50-3) may be assessed with a high degree of precision by an ophthalmologist, a rough estimate may be made in the office or at the patient's bedside when the examiner is concerned with any general disturbance of the visual field. Such a circumstance may arise, for example, in assessing the patient with a stroke. Such patients commonly lose one fourth or one half of the visual fields of both eyes.

A simple and reliable method of testing the fullness of the visual field is direct confrontation. The examiner and patient sit directly facing each other at a distance of 60 cm (2 feet). The patient is instructed to cover one eye with a card while looking directly at the examiner's nose. The examiner in turn covers one eye as a method of comparison. If the patient has covered his left eye, for instance, the examiner covers her right eye. The examiner then takes an object (pen, finger) in her right hand and moves it along a plane halfway between the examiner and the patient. The nasal, temporal upward, and downward fields are assessed by bringing the object into view from various peripheral points. During each maneuver, the patient informs the examiner the moment he is able to see the object. In order to test the nasal fields of gaze for the same eye, the examiner switches the object from the right hand to the left hand. The entire procedure is reversed for an assessment of the fields of the left eye. When confrontation testing reveals decreases in visual fields, or "blind spots," the patient is referred immediately to an ophthalmologist for further evaluation.

Ophthalmoscopy. The internal eye is referred to as the *fundus* and comprises the retina, optic disc, macula, and retinal vessels. It is visualized with the aid of an instrument called an *ophthalmoscope.* With practice and repetition, the nurse can become proficient in the use of the ophthalmoscope. The ophthalmoscope is an instrument that projects light through a prism and bends the light at 90 degrees, allowing the observer to view the retina through a lens in such a way that the line of vision is parallel to the bent ray of light. A number of lenses are available and are arranged on a wheel so that they may be chosen by rotating the wheel with the index finger without interrupting the inspection. The standard ophthalmoscope contains an array of gadgetry that includes grids, slits, filters, and the like—none of which are particularly useful. The small, unfiltered aperture is appropriate and most useful for standard ophthalmoscopy.

In order to avoid a confrontation of noses, the right eye of the patient is examined with the right eye of the examiner, the left eye of the patient with the left eye of the examiner (See Fig. 50-4*A*). The room is darkened so that the pupil will be dilated. The patient is instructed to hold the eyes still and focus on a real or imaginary distant object. The ophthalmoscope is gripped firmly in the hand, with the index finger resting on the lens wheel. The head of the ophthalmoscope is braced within the angle made by the brow and the nose. The lens chosen for initial inspection should be the one labeled zero unless the examiner is knowingly correcting his or her own defect in visual acuity. If the examiner wears glasses, it may be better to remove the glasses and become familiar with which lens is analogous to zero for the examiner with 20/20 vision; or, the examiner may prefer to keep the glasses on and use a zero lens setting. Provided that the patient has 20/20 vision, the zero lens should enable the examiner to obtain a precise focus on the retina. If the retina is out of focus, the lens wheel is rotated until it is brought into focus. The choice of a lens labeled with a red numeral implies that one is focusing farther away than normal; the choice of a

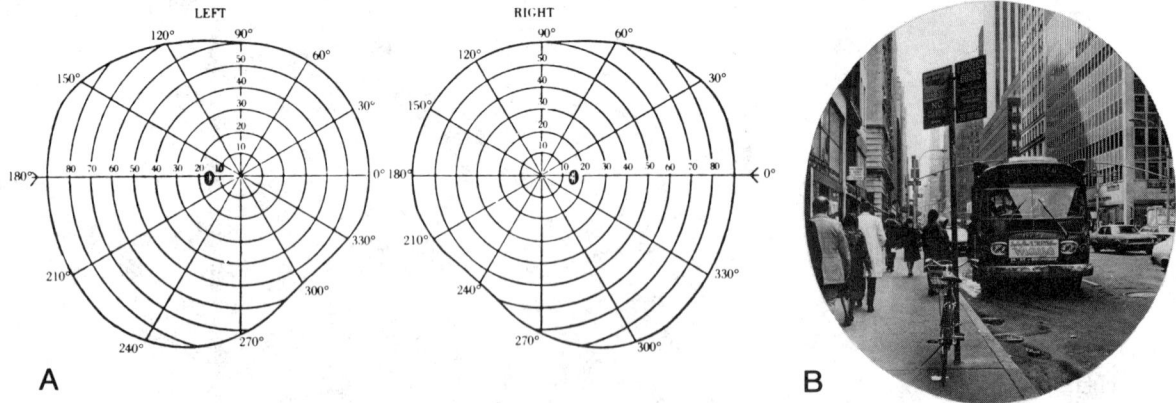

Figure 50-3
(*A*) Visual field charts showing peripheral vision of 180° with both eyes. (*B*) Photograph representing a street scene as viewed by a person with normal or 20/20 vision. (Photo courtesy of The Lighthouse, The New York Association for the Blind.)

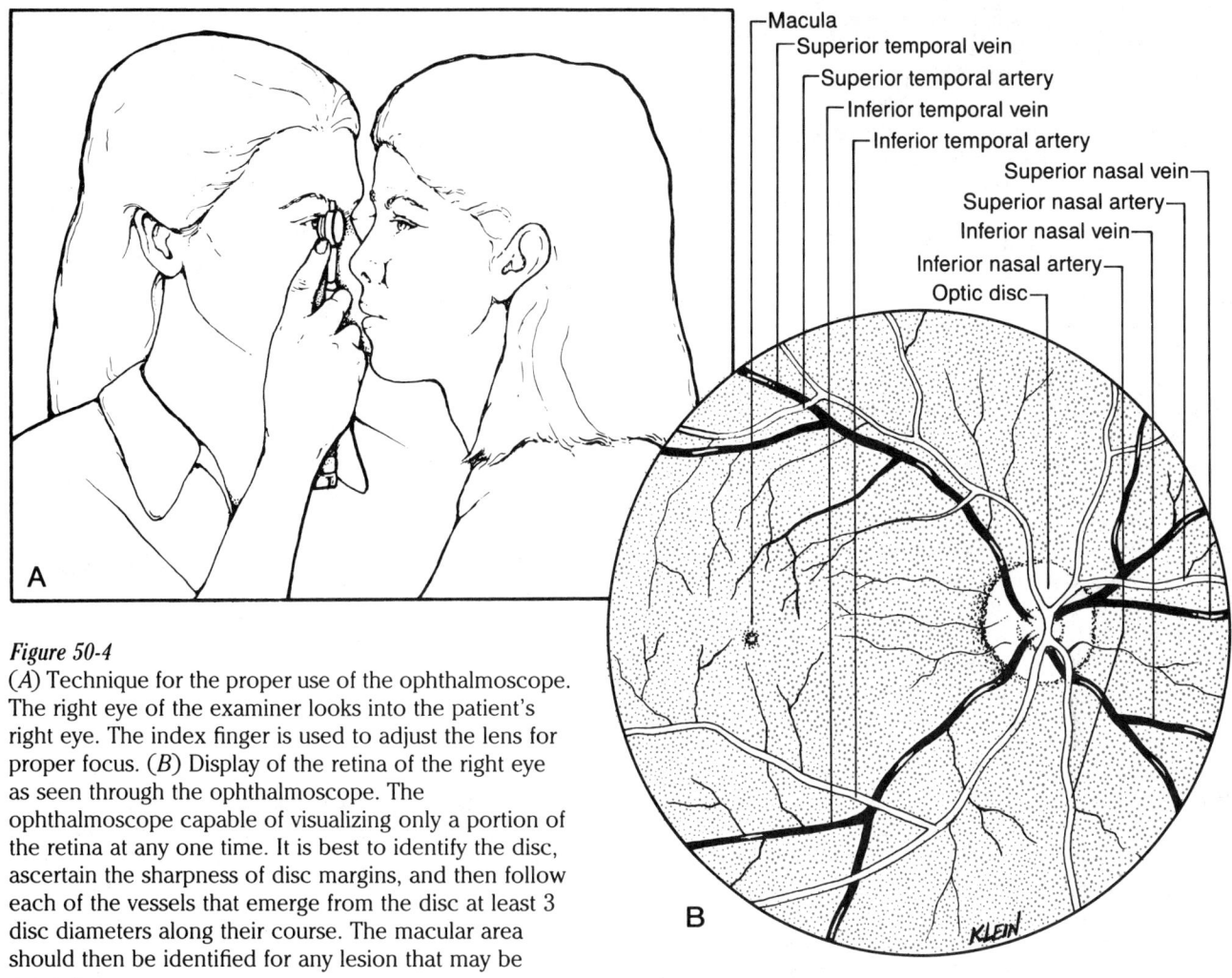

Macula
Superior temporal vein
Superior temporal artery
Inferior temporal vein
Inferior temporal artery
Superior nasal vein
Superior nasal artery
Inferior nasal vein
Inferior nasal artery
Optic disc

Figure 50-4
(*A*) Technique for the proper use of the ophthalmoscope. The right eye of the examiner looks into the patient's right eye. The index finger is used to adjust the lens for proper focus. (*B*) Display of the retina of the right eye as seen through the ophthalmoscope. The ophthalmoscope capable of visualizing only a portion of the retina at any one time. It is best to identify the disc, ascertain the sharpness of disc margins, and then follow each of the vessels that emerge from the disc at least 3 disc diameters along their course. The macular area should then be identified for any lesion that may be present.

lens labeled with a black numeral implies that one is focusing nearer to the examiner. The examiner will choose lenses among the red series for patients who are *hyperopic* (farsighted) and lenses in the black series for patients who are *myopic* (nearsighted).

With the room in darkness, the patient appropriately gazing into the distance, and the ophthalmoscope properly positioned within the cradle of the brow and nose, the examiner may now approach the patient. The examiner stands approximately 37.5 cm (15 inches) from the patient and about 15 degrees lateral to the patient's gaze. When the light is focused on the pupil, the retina will glow red through the dilated pupil opening. This is known as the *red reflex*. The examiner then approaches the patient until her forehead touches her left hand, which she has placed on the patient's forehead (Fig. 50-4*A*). At this point, provided that the proper lens has been selected, the retina should be in focus, and the venules and arterioles that course through the retina are readily apparent (Fig. 50-4*B*). In scanning the surface of the retina, it is important that the examiner hold the scope firmly and move her head rather than the instrument.

The examiner should first focus on the optic disc. In the event that the disc is not in view when the retina is first visualized, the veins that are within the field of vision should

be followed down their tributaries toward the disc from which the arterioles emerge and the venules enter. This is analogous to following the limbs of a tree until one sees the trunk. The optic disc is examined for size, shape, color, and the sharpness of its margin. The disc is circular and yellowish pink. The margin is sharp and occasionally surrounded by a rim of dark pigment (choroidal crescent). One must become familiar with what is regarded as a normal-sized disc. In the center of the disc there is frequently a small physiologic cup into which the central vein of the retina recedes. To focus on the base of this cup accurately, one may have to choose another lens in the direction of the red sequence. A deep cup is seen in glaucoma. Edema of the optic disc with concomitant blurring of the disc margin is seen with increases in cerebrospinal fluid pressure. The disc becomes pink, and accurate focus may require shifting to a lens in the direction of the black sequence. This is termed *papilledema*. *Optic atrophy* is characterized by extreme pallor of the disc and reduction of its size.

The remainder of the retina is now examined. Abnormalities may be precisely located for other observers by using a standard nomenclature that makes reference to an imaginary clock face and by referring to the diameter of the disc to delineate distance. Thus, a hemorrhage may be noted to be one half of the disc diameter in size, located 2 disc diameters away from the disc margin at 2 o'clock. Another observer is then able to replicate this finding.

The examiner now follows each of the major vessels from the margin of the disc. The arterioles are lighter in color and narrower than the venules. Under normal circumstances, arterioles are two thirds to four fifths the diameter of veins. The walls of the vessels are essentially transparent, and what is being observed is the blood column itself. The size and character of the arteriovenous crossings is noted, as well as any lesions in the retina. The retinal changes associated with diabetes are quite distinctive and are discussed in Chapter 36.

Lastly, the macular area of the retina is visualized by having the patient look directly at the light source. This causes the patient slight discomfort and tearing and provides the examiner with only a brief second or two during which to inspect the small, circular, red area of the macula. The glistening reflection of its center is called the *fovea centralis retinae*. Any edema, hemorrhages, or lesions are noted and brought to the attention of an ophthalmologist.

All of the techniques that have been discussed for the examination of the eye will not be performed on every patient. Routinely, one inspects the conjunctiva, the cornea, and the pupil and assesses extraocular motion. Ophthalmoscopic examination is a part of every reasonably complete physical examination. Although visual acuity is a part of the data base, it need not be assessed more often than once every year or two, except in the elderly.

Letter Chart/Microprocessor. The most widely accepted method of screening for visual problems is the letter chart (Snellen). However, its accuracy is limited. A *BVAT (Mentor) microprocessor* produces an E of 30 different sizes on a television monitor. A computer monitors the responses the patient makes with a hand-held response box. A computer printout provides the mean visual acuity and standard deviation computed from 20 trials. The time required is about 8 minutes.

Echography. In echography (ultrasound, ultrasonography), high-frequency pulses of ultrasound are emitted from a small probe placed on the eye. After striking the ocular tissues, the sound energy is reflected to the probe, which, in turn, is displayed on an oscilloscope. Two primary types of ultrasound are used in ophthalmology:

A-scan—Oscilloscopic reflection is a vertical deflection from the baseline (one-dimensional).
B-scan—Oscilloscopic reflections are lines or dots (two-dimensional).

When used jointly, over 100 lesions or groups of lesions may be detected and differentiated in the orbital and periorbital region. Measurements for intraocular lenses can be done by ultrasound and analyzed by computer; this enables the surgeon to determine lens power for an implant and postoperative refractive power.

This procedure is painless but requires the instillation of topical anesthetic eyedrops. After the examination, the patient is cautioned not to rub his eyes, since corneal lesions may occur.

Endothelial Cell Counter. An endothelial cell counter is a photographic instrument that produces very high resolution, revealing subtle details of endothelial cell morphology: cell size, shape, cell population density, nature of cell boundary, and presence of intercellular bodies and pathologic processes. This is a valuable test preoperatively because if a compromised endothelium is observed, it may suggest an increased risk of postoperative complications.

Refractive Errors

Vision is made possible by the passage of rays of light from an object through the cornea, the aqueous humor, the lens, and the vitreous humor to the retina. In the normal eye, rays coming from an object at a distance of 6 meters or more are brought to a focus on the retina by the lens while perfectly at rest.

Types of Refractive Errors. Due to abnormalities in the eye structure or in the lens structure, defective vision may occur because objects are not focused correctly on the retina. If the rays of light are brought to a focus in front of the retina, the condition is referred to as *myopia* (nearsightedness); if the rays are focused behind the retina, the condition is called *hyperopia* or *hypermetropia* (farsightedness) (Fig. 50-5). In such conditions, glass lenses are prescribed. These, in association with the lenses of the eye, will correct the fault and restore a normal focus at the retina.

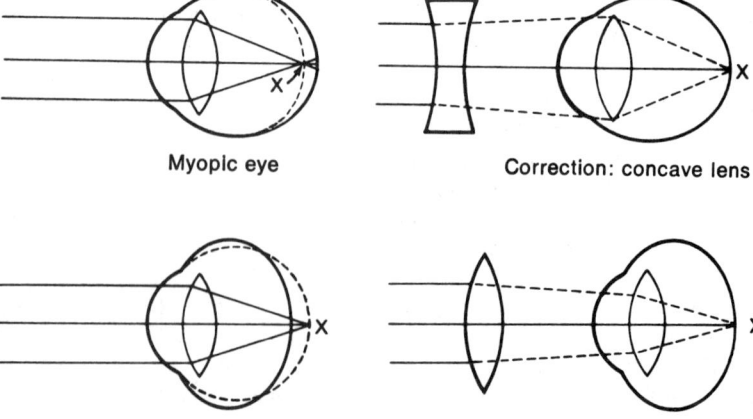

Figure 50-5
Myopia and hypermetropia. (Brunner LS and Suddarth DS. The Lippincott Manual of Nursing Practice, 4th ed. Philadelphia, JB Lippincott, 1986.)

Rays from objects situated at shorter distances (less than 6 meters) require a "stronger" lens to focus them on the retina. This is brought about by a contraction of the ciliary muscle that relaxes the lens capsule and causes the lens to become more convex. This function, as mentioned earlier, is called *accommodation*. By means of accommodation, objects at different distances from the eye may be seen distinctly. With increasing age, the elasticity of the lens decreases, so that accommodation for near vision is not complete, a condition called *presbyopia*. This explains why it is so common to see older people reading a paper while holding it at arm's length. "Reading glasses" may be prescribed for these patients to enable them to focus rays from near objects to the retina.

In the case of presbyopia, two different types of lenses may be used (bifocals), one for far distance and one for near vision and reading. Trifocal lenses are also available; these add a third dimension that gives sharp focus in the 68- to 127-cm (27- to 50-inch) range. Lenses are prescribed for use in eyeglasses, or the lens may be applied directly to the surface of the eye (contact lens).

Astigmatism results from uneven curvature of the cornea—instead of curving equally in all directions the cornea is shaped somewhat like the bowl of a spoon. Two foci thus occur instead of one, and, as a consequence, the patient is unable to focus horizontal and vertical rays on the retina at the same time. These defects may be corrected with lenses called cylinder lenses. A patient may be myopic or hyperopic and also have astigmatism. In such a situation a compound spherocylinder is prescribed by the optician.

Assessment of Refractive Errors. The strength and type of lens that will overcome refractive errors are determined by means of a *retinoscope*, which measures the refractive error. On the basis of this examination, an appropriate corrective lens is selected and then further refined by having the patient read letters on the Snellen chart through several different lenses.

Automated refractors, which rely on photoelectric devices sensitive to light, may also be used. The patient sits in front of the instrument and is instructed to look steadily at a target. A printout on a card or graph indicates the refractive error to be corrected. Other types of automated refractors require the patient to make focusing adjustments by turning a knob. See Chart 50-1, Abbreviations and Terms Used in Ophthalmology.

Contact Lenses

More and more people are wearing contact lenses as a means of correcting refractive errors. Better techniques for measuring the eye and improved methods for supervising and instructing those who wish to wear the lenses have increased the appeal of such lenses. They are particularly effective in certain occupations and are desirable for cosmetic reasons. However, not everyone can wear contact lenses; therefore, all potential candidates should be thoroughly screened by an ophthalmologist. (See Table 50-1, Types of Corrective Lenses.)

Medical conditions in which corneal lenses are recommended included absence of lens (*aphakia*), absence of iris (*aniridia*), congenital absence of pigment, myopia and hyperopia, some types of astigmatism, cone-shaped deformity of the cornea (*keratoconus*), and turned-in eyelashes. Contraindications include allergic and inflammatory conditions (such as chronic blepharoconjunctivitis, corneal infection, iritis, uveitis), *epiphora* (abnormal overflow of tears), severe exophthalmus, pterygium, or local neoplasm.

Contact lenses are usually not recommended for people who do not require full-time visual correction or lack sufficient manual dexterity to insert and remove lenses. Contact lenses are available in either hard or soft form. The hard lens was introduced in the early 1960s, the soft lens in the late 1960s.

Chart 50-1
Abbreviations and Terms Used in Ophthalmology

OD or RE (oculus dexter)—right eye
OS or LE (oculus sinister)—left eye
OU or O_2 (oculi unitas)—both eyes together

D (diopter)—unit of measurement of strength or refractive
    power of lenses. (A 1-diopter lens brings parallel light rays
    to a focus at 1 meter from the lens.)

HT (hypertropia)—upward deviation of one eye
ST (esotropia)—inward deviation of one eye ("crossed eyes")
XT (exotropia)—outward deviation of one eye ("wall eyes")

+ plus or convex
− minus or concave

ECCE—extracapsular cataract extraction
ICCE—intracapsular cataract cryoextraction
PMMA—polymethylmethacrylate (synthetic used in IOLs)
IOL—intraocular lens
EOM—extraocular muscles

Hyperopia, hypermetropia—farsightedness
Myopia—nearsightedness
Diplopia—seeing one object as two ("double vision")

Ectropion—turning out (eversion) of eyelid
Entropion—turning in of eyelid

Ptosis—drooping of upper lid
Epiphora—excessive production of tears
Hemianopia—blindness of one half the field of vision
Photophobia—abnormal sensitivity to light
Presbyopia—lessening of power of accommodation due to aging
    process

When properly fitted, contact lenses "float" on the fluid layer of the eyeball and are held loosely in place by the capillary attraction of the tears and the upper lid. The lens moves with the eye and is centered over the cornea.

Contact lenses have many advantages over framed lenses; they do not steam up when the wearer goes from the cold outside to a warm room; they are automatically cleaned with each blink of the eyelid; they can be worn safely during sports; they eliminate the need for less attractive lenses; they provide increased peripheral vision; and they do not break easily.

However, there are certain disadvantages and dangers in wearing contact lenses: contact lenses may be more expensive than framed lenses; solutions used to clean the lenses are costly; the adjustment period in learning to use them properly is longer; contact lenses can be lost easily, such as down the sink drain or in a swimming pool; and in the event of a chemical splash to the eye, the chemical agent may seep beneath the lens and cause extensive damage before the contact lens can be removed. Some types of contact lenses can result in injury to the cornea if the lenses are worn for an extended period of time.

Hard Lenses. Hard lenses are a form of plexiglass called polymethylmethacrylate (PMMA). They are nonporous, do not absorb water, and cover only the central area of the cornea. Oxygen exchange to the cornea can develop and lead to discomfort if the lenses are worn too long (8 to 12 hours).

When fitting hard lenses, the ophthalmologist usually instills fluorescein into the eye in order to identify changes that occur in the formation of tear film as the lid blinks. However, fluorescein cannot be used with soft lenses because the dye stains the lenses permanently. To offset microbial contamination, special procedures are used to disinfect soft lenses while they are stored during the night.

Soft Lenses. Soft contact lenses are made of polymer gel, although new formulations are being tested as soft lenses grow in popularity. They are porous, water-absorbent, hydrophilic, soft, and flexible.

Soft lenses have certain advantages over hard lenses. They are comfortable from the start and can be worn up to 18 hours a day. They are effective for those who participate in sports, except for swimming. Since these lenses absorb pool chemicals and ocean salt, they should not be worn while swimming unless goggles and a mask are used. If they are worn only occasionally, rather than daily, the wearer will not lose his tolerance to them, as is the case with hard lenses. Finally, it is easier to switch from soft lenses to eyeglasses than from hard lenses to eyeglasses.

Soft lenses are inserted by placing the lens on the inferior conjunctiva while drawing the lower lid downward. With the release of the lid, the wearer then rolls his eye around or massages the eye through the closed lid to position the lens on the cornea. To remove, the lens is grasped between the clean thumb and forefinger.

Gas-Permeable Lenses. Gas-permeable lenses are made of cellulose acetate butyrate (CAB). FDA-approved CAB lenses are usually heat-tempered, which results in a harder, scratch-resistant surface and permits good optic use without affecting gas permeability. These lenses result in fewer problems from lens warpage and flattening.

Extended-Wear Lenses. Extended-wear lenses are highly permeable plastic lenses that are thinner and more pliable than ordinary soft or hard contact lenses and can be worn continuously for weeks or months. They are more expensive than the usual soft contact lenses but are not completely trouble free. Extra fitting time is necessary, and the lenses may no longer be worn if certain conditions develop. Such conditions include microprotein accumulation on the anterior lens surface (soft lens spoilage) and corneal revascularization.

Spoilage or deterioration of soft contact lenses is due to extraneous deposits, physical and chemical changes in the lens material, and microbial invasion. This includes soft lenses of acrylic origin, vinyl origin, and silicone. Removal of encrusted deposits leaves surface irregularities and matrix defects; these lenses should be discarded. At present, no soft contact lenses are completely "safe" for extended wear.

Flexible-Wear Lenses. Flexible-wear lenses are gaining in popularity over extended-wear lenses since fewer complications occur. These newer lenses need not be inserted and removed daily or cleaned on a daily basis. They are permeable enough to wear for extended periods. However, to avoid problems, it is advisable to remove the lenses at night and limit extended wear to special occasions.

For a comparison of the various types of corrective lenses, refer to Table 50-1.

Complications. The improper use of contact lenses (both hard and soft) can cause corneal abrasions, ulcerations, and infection, which result from poorly fitted lenses, improper technique in applying or removing the lenses, poor technique in cleansing the lens, and insufficient tear circulation under the lenses.

Patient Education. Although the advantages of contact lenses outweigh the disadvantages, precautions and safeguards must be understood by the nurse, the wearer, and his employer. The contact lens must be regarded as a medical prosthesis, not a cosmetic device.

Care and precaution must be given to any medical prosthesis, and this certainly applies to contact lenses:

1. Wash hands thoroughly before touching the lenses, whether applying them or removing them.
2. Cleanse lenses only with the recommended sterile solution (noncaustic).*
3. Keep the storage kit clean.
4. Do not wear lenses beyond the prescribed time.
5. Do not sleep with contact lenses in place; to do so may cause abrasion and erosion of the corneal epithelium. (Exception: extended wear lenses)
6. Do not wet lenses with saliva before insertion; this can cause infection.
7. Restrict the wearing of contact lenses, in order to avoid potential corneal abrasions, if the following signs are present: photophobia., dryness, excessive burning, tearing.
8. Follow the physician's recommendations concerning eye makeup. Some ophthalmologists discourage pa-

---

* Some individuals are sensitive to thimerosal, a preservative in cleaning solutions that causes the eyes to sting when the lenses are inserted. Recommendation: Soak lenses in distilled water *or* use Pliagel (USA), a thimerosal-free solution, or Solusol (Canada).

TABLE 50-1
Types of Corrective Lenses

Durability	Advantages	Disadvantages
Eyeglasses (Spectacles)		
Excellent	Excellent vision correction	Fogging in cool weather
New styles may suggest change	Easily cared for	Some cosmetic objections
		Unsuitable for certain activities: sports, some occupational drawbacks
		May need to be replaced more frequently than soft contact lenses
Hard Contact Lenses		
With care, may last for 15–20 years	Excellent vision correction	Uncomfortable for some
	Usually less costly than other types	Require period of adaptation
	Effective for persons with astigmatism	Possibility of eventual intolerance
		May "pop" out of position
Soft Contact Lenses		
May require more frequent replacement (usually replaced 1–3 years)	More comfortable than hard lenses	Require time daily for sanitization
	Can be worn longer than hard lenses	Greater risk of eye irritation and infection
		Not as effective for astigmatism
		Possibility of eventual intolerance
Gas-permeable Lenses		
Usually last longer than soft lenses but not as long as hard lenses	More comfortable than hard lenses	Eventual intolerance
	Many claim more effective vision than with soft lenses	May be more costly
Extended-wear Lenses		
Most fragile of all lenses	Provide corrected vision around the clock	Expensive
May have to be replaced every 6 months or more often	May be left in place for 2 weeks at a time	More frequent visits to "eye" physician
		Risk of corneal injury
		May not correct vision as well
		Possibility of eventual intolerance

tients from wearing eye makeup. Some advise applying mascara after lenses are in position.

9. Keep chemicals such as soaps, lotions, and creams away from lenses, since they may adversely affect the lens; instruct the wearer to keep his eyes tightly closed when applying hair perfume and deodorant sprays. Stay away from areas where household sprays are used.

10. Have an ophthalmologic examination every 6 months to ensure proper fit and to check corneal integrity.

11. With the expansion of available products, it is important to check with the ophthalmologist before changing types of lenses or disinfecting solutions.

Removal of Contact Lenses. Many types of contact lenses are designed to be worn only while the person is awake and fully conscious (exception: extended-wear lenses). They should be removed as a safety measure if the wearer is incapacitated due to accident, sickness, or other cause. In emergency situations, the following directives should be followed:

1. Determine whether the patient is wearing contact lenses. If he is conscious or semiconscious, ask him directly, since he may be able to indicate that he is wearing contact lenses. He may even be able to remove the lenses by himself or with assistance, depending, of course, on his condition. If the patient is unconscious, check "Medic-Alert" tag, driver's license, and other identification cards that may reveal that the patient wears contact lenses. Look for observable indications that contact lenses are being worn by gently separating the patient's eyelids. Shining a light (preferably a small penlight) on the eye from the side will help.

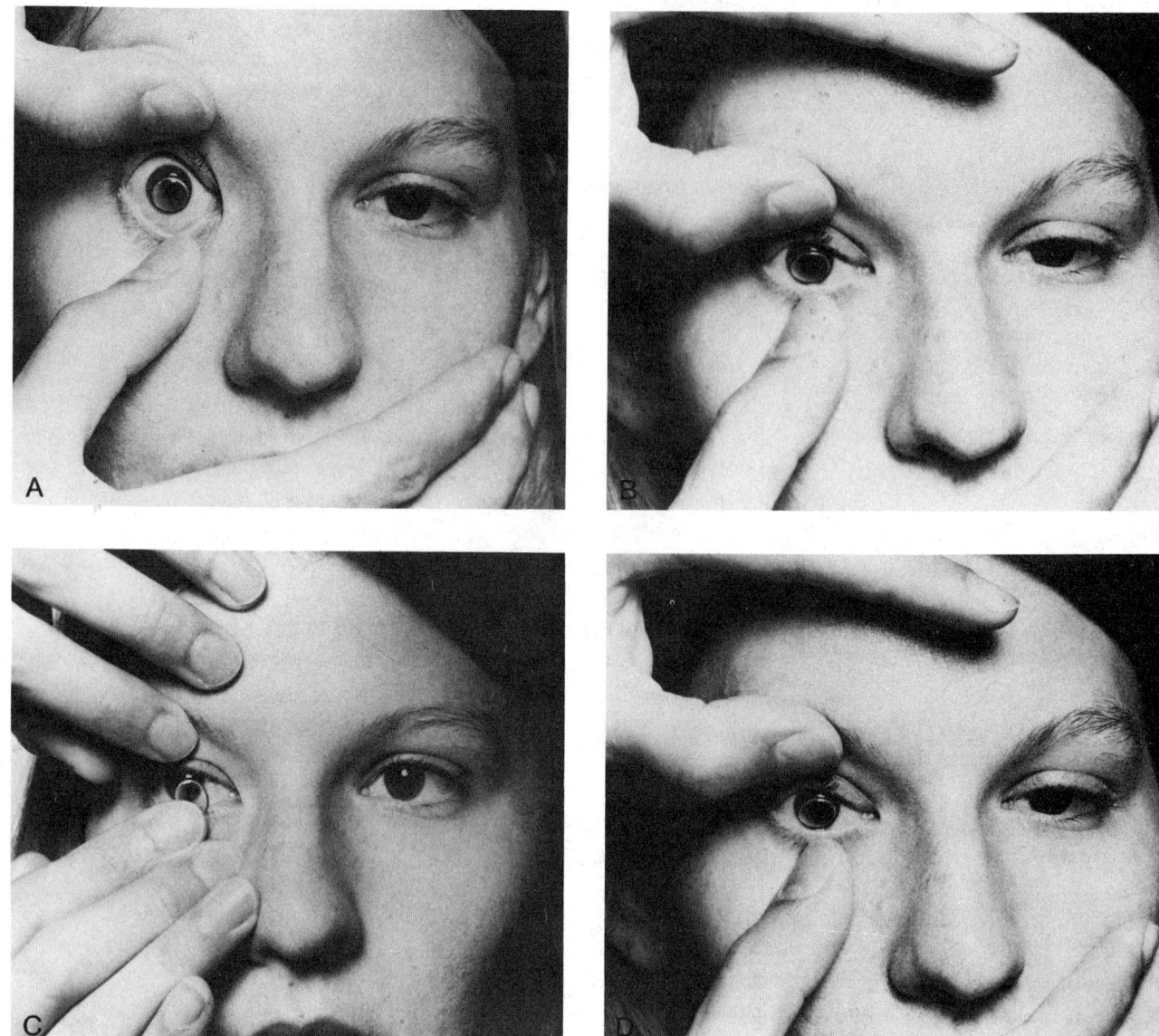

Figure 50-6

Removal of contact lenses. *Primary Stages in Hard Lens Removal:* (*A*) After the eyelids have been separated and the hard contact lens has been correctly positioned over the cornea, widen the eyelid margins beyond the top and bottom edges of lens. (*B*) After the lower eyelid margin has been moved near the bottom lens edge and then the upper eyelid margin has been moved near the top lens edge, you are ready to move under the bottom edge of the lens by pressing slightly harder on the lower eyelid while moving it upward. (*C*) After the lens has tipped slightly, move the eyelids toward one another; this causes the lens to slide out between the eyelids.

Possible Lens Positions: (*D*) Directly over the cornea. This normal wearing position of a contact lens is also the correct position for removing it. If the lens cannot be removed, however, slide it onto the sclera. (*E*, p. 1341) On the sclera only. Here the lens can remain with relative safety until experienced help is available; other white areas of the eye to the side or above the cornea might also be used. If the lens is to be removed, however, slide it to a position directly over the cornea. (*F*, p. 1341) On both the cornea and the sclera. A lens in this position—or a similar one anywhere around the periphery of the cornea—should be moved as soon as possible. If the lens is to be removed, slide it to a position directly over the cornea; if the lens cannot be removed immediately, slide it onto the sclera.

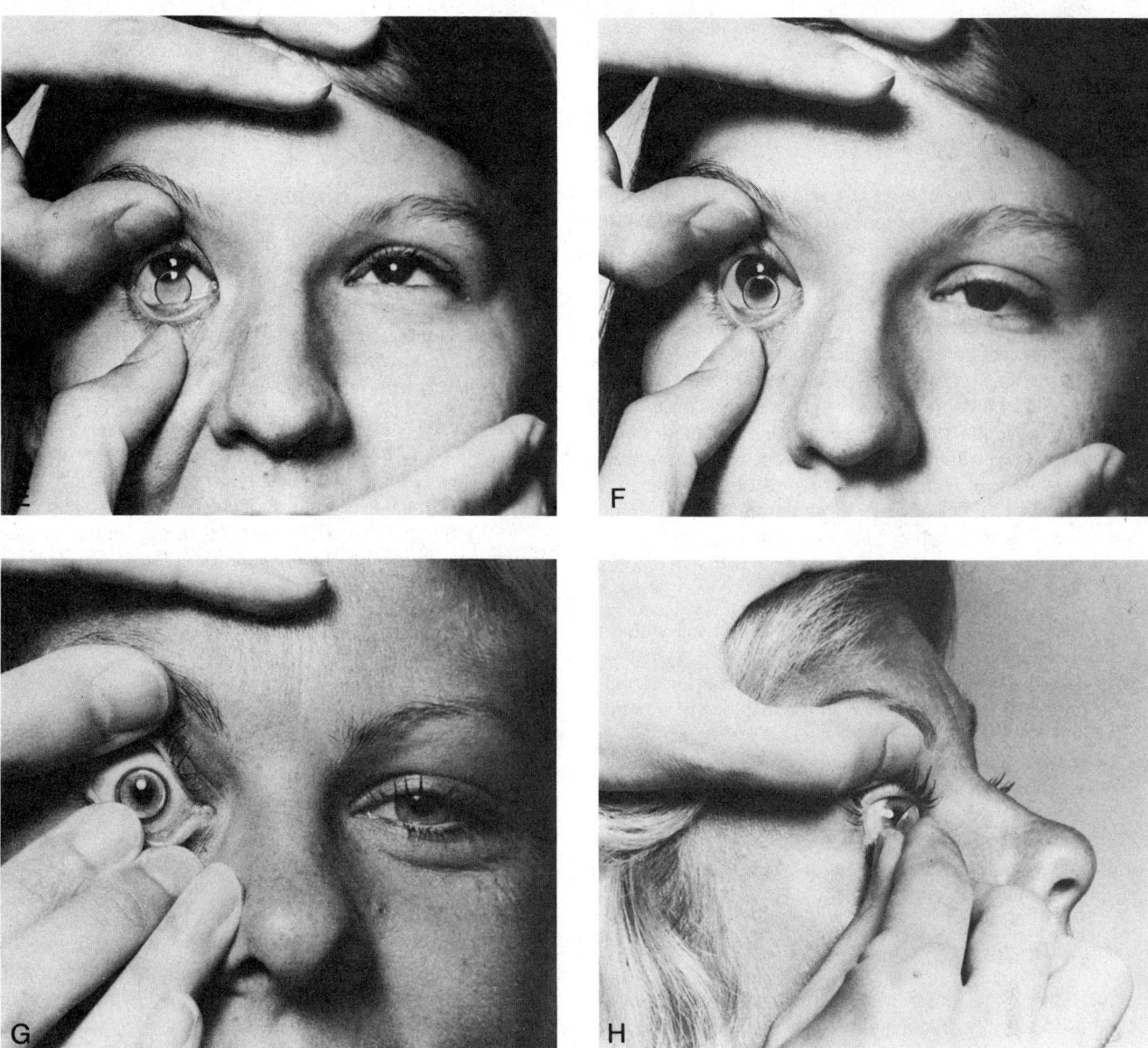

Figure 50-6 (continued)

Soft Contact Lens Removal: (*G*) With clean hands, pull down the lower lid with the middle finger and place the index fingertip on the lower edge of the lens. Slide the lens down to the white part of the eye. (*H*) Compress the lens lightly between the thumb and index finger. Bring thumb and index finger together in a "pinching" motion, causing the lens to double-up between fingers and allowing air underneath. Remove the lens from the eye. (Courtesy of American Optometric Association.)

2. Remove the patient's contact lenses if he cannot do so himself. With clean hands, position one thumb on the upper eyelid and one thumb on the lower eyelid, with thumbs near the margin of each eyelid. Separate the eyelids. A visible lens should slide easily with a gentle movement of the eyelids (Fig. 50-6*A*–*C*). If the lens does not drop out easily, observe for possible lens position and follow instructions given in Figure 50-6*D*–*F* for removal of the lens. Remember that force should not be used. If the lens is seen but cannot be re-

moved, gently slide it onto the sclera, where it can remain with relative safety until experienced help is available.

If the patient is wearing soft contact lenses, it is best to wait until someone experienced in removing these types of lenses is available to lend assistance. If flexible lenses are left in place for many hours, they will do little harm. However, if the emergency is such that they must be removed, then the steps described in Figure 50-6*G, H* should be followed.

Eye Safety: Precautions, First Aid, Treatment

Trauma to the Eye

The prevention of eye injuries is a phase of child and adult education that cannot be emphasized too strongly. Children need to be reminded frequently of the dangers of sticks, arrows, darts, BB guns, "sparklers," sling shots, rubber bands, and even harmless-looking toys. Precautions that should be taken when power tools are used need to be explained, along with the reasons protection is necessary from very bright lights, the sun shining on the snow, chemical fumes, sprays, and flying chips of wood. The use of goggles gives protection against most foreign bodies, but specially designed safety goggles or glasses with impact-resistant lenses are preferable if there is danger of flying metal or wood objects that may break the glass. Elderly people or those unsure of their footing need safeguards where there is a possibility of injury.

General measures in caring for patients with eye injuries may include the following:

- Obtain a history of the injury first, then consult with an ophthalmologist immediately.
- Irrigate the eye with saline solution; however, note that irrigations may be dangerous in the instance of a penetrating eye injury.
- Stain the front surface of the eye with sterile fluorescein paper (Fluor-I-Strip), which uses the yellowish green dye to detect abrasions and ulcers.
- Irrigate the eye again.
- Evaluate the injury and manage as prescribed.
- Employ follow up care.

Foreign Bodies

Foreign bodies (*e.g.,* dust, cinders) frequently cause considerable discomfort by irritating the sensitive conjunctiva. If the foreign body has been in the eye only a short time, it may be removed by a nurse. One way to detect foreign particles in the eye is to have the patient close his eyes, then darken the room and gently place a penlight on the lid. The foreign particle will show up as a black shadow. The lower lid is everted, the patient instructed to look up, and the lower half of the conjunctival sac examined. If the particle is not found, the upper eye is examined by everting the upper lid. The examiner stands in front of the patient and instructs him to look down at his feet. The lashes are grasped between the thumb and fingers of one hand, and a matchstick, an applicator, or a toothpick is placed across the upper part of the lid. The lashes are pulled downward and forward, away from the eye, as the applicator is pressed downward, gently. The foreign body may be removed by touching it gently with a small applicator tipped with cotton and moistened in saline solution.

If this method is unsuccessful, or if the offending particle has been in the eye for a considerable time, no attempt should be made to remove it. It may have become embedded in the cornea, and there is considerable danger of serious injury if removal is attempted by unskilled hands. The ophthalmologist usually requires local anesthesia, a hand lens, fluorescein, an eye spud, normal saline for irrigating the eye, and, as a prophylaxis against infection, an antibiotic solution to instill after the offending particle is removed. If the particle is known to be a metal, the physician may use a magnet to remove it.

Acid and Alkali Burns

Careless use of hair sprays and other spray-on products has increased the incidence of chemical burns of the eye.

- Whenever acid or alkali gets on the lids or in the eye, an emergency exists, requiring that immediate action be taken. *In such an instance, the lids, the conjunctiva, and the cornea must be flushed copiously.*

The easiest and quickest way to flush the eye is to have the patient hold his head under a faucet and allow the water to run over the eye and wash it out. However, it is more satisfactory to flush the eye with a syringe, if available, taking care not to contaminate the other eye if it has not already been contaminated. Continuous flushing for at least 15 minutes is desirable. Plain tap water is adequate under such circumstances.

Actinic Trauma

Ultraviolet rays may damage the cornea as a result of excessive sunlight, snow blindness, and the use of a welder's arc ("welder's flash") or a sun lamp. Treatment consists of instilling anesthetic drops and patching both eyes.

Contusions and Hematoma ("Black Eye")

Trauma to the eye frequently results in hemorrhage. The bleeding that enters the loose tissues of the orbit spreads rapidly, discoloring the lids and surrounding skin. In itself, the injury is not too serious, but frequently it is frightening to patients because the discoloration and swelling is so prominent. The bleeding usually stops spontaneously, but it may be reduced and the swelling lessened by the application of cold compresses. Absorption of the blood may be hastened after the first 24 hours by the use of warm compresses applied 15 minutes at a time at intervals throughout the day. Drugs are now available to help hasten absorption of hematomas.

Corneal Abrasions

Lacerations of the cornea can be detected after being stained with sodium fluorescein (Fluor-I-Strip). A blue penlight more clearly identifies the abrasion than a white light.

Usually, a local anesthetic and antibacterial drops are administered, and an eye patch is applied for 24 to 36 hours. Self-administration of a local anesthetic is discouraged, since it may delay the diagnosis of complications and may even lead to further injury. The patient is instructed to keep the eyes at rest to promote comfort and facilitate the healing process. The danger to be guarded against with an abrasion is the development of a corneal ulcer. Therefore, if there is no improvement after 24 hours, an ophthalmic consultation is desirable.

Lacerations

Lacerations of the eyelids are serious because the lids become scarred and are unable to close. Injuries to the lids are treated in the same way as any other wound, but an ophthalmologist usually is requested to care for them.

Lacerations of the eyeball are more serious because visual defects may result. Since more extensive injuries may endanger the entire eye, such injuries are referred invariably to the ophthalmologist for appropriate care. Injuries of this type may entail transplantation of conjunctival flaps to prevent leakage of ocular fluids, excision of the prolapsed iris, and, in severe injuries, even removal of the eye.

Nursing Care of Patients With Eye Disorders

Preventive Care

The eye is such an important organ that its care and protection are major considerations from the day of birth. The nurse, as an important member of the health team and as a teacher and a practitioner of sound health habits, can provide excellent health education in eye care and in the prevention of eye diseases.

Sound principles of safe care need to be stressed at an early age. Such problems as headache, dizziness, tiredness after close eye work, ("the letters run together"), and scratchy or itchy eyes should be checked by a health care practitioner. Also significant are inflamed or watery eyes; red-rimmed, encrusted, or puffy lids; recurring sties; crossed eyes; and unequal pupils. Unusual behavior should also be noted, such as holding a book too close, frowning, blinking, squinting, rubbing the eyes, and failing in school or study work.

Faulty diet may account for the onset of many eye disorders. For instance, deficiencies of vitamins A and B may cause changes in the retina, the conjunctiva, and the cornea.

The importance of eye care has been recognized by industries that require workers to wear protective devices in activities that pose a danger of injury from foreign objects. Safety glasses should be worn when the task at hand requires it. Eyes should be protected from bright sun, sun lamps, ultraviolet rays, and hair spray. In the home, ammonia and alkali products, such as lye, present a particularly dangerous hazard for both children and adults and should be stored in safe places out of reach and used with care.

Eyes need to rest after being used for close work for a period of time. Occasionally glancing out the window or around the room provides relaxation.

The importance of adequate and well-placed light in preventing eyestrain is essentially no longer a medical problem but one of general, industrial, and social concern.

With many eye conditions, the medical management of patients has changed drastically in recent years and has resulted in less frequent need for hospitalization. For example, a patient with a cataract no longer needs to stay in the hospital for several days, and extended bed rest, which can result in sensory deprivation and a feeling of losing contact with the world, is no longer required. Cataract surgery and many other ophthalmic operations are performed in "day surgery" units, thus allowing the patient to return home on the same day as the surgery. The result has been a reduced incidence of complications. On the other hand, such brief contact by the nurse with the patient or family allows only a short time for observation, assessment, goal determination, nursing interventions, and patient evaluation. Therefore, any teaching sessions or demonstrations of self-care procedures must be done in such a way as to ensure that the patient and family understand their responsibilities for self-care and can recognize those signs and symptoms that may require professional consultation and intervention. Although outpatient surgery is common for some eye disorders, many eye problems do require more prolonged hospital care.

General Management Modalities

Eye Drops

Various drug solutions are inserted into the eyes in the treatment of nearly every kind of eye disorder (Table 50-2).

(Text continues on p. 1346)

TABLE 50-2
Medications Used Frequently in Eye Conditions

Medication	Action
Local Anesthetics	
Tetracaine hydrochloride, 0.25%	Commonly used topical anesthetic
	Anesthesia produced in 5 to 9 minutes
Hexylcaine hydrochloride, 1% to 2%	Effective in 5 to 10 minutes; lasts 60 minutes
Proparacaine hydrochloride, 0.5%	More rapid in action
	Less discomfort during instillation; effective topically
Procaine hydrochloride, 1% and 2%	Commonly used for injection in eye surgery
	Lasts 30 to 45 minutes
Lidocaine hydrochloride, 1% to 2%	Some favor this over procaine because its action is more rapid.

(continued)

TABLE 50-2 (continued)

Medication	Action
Antimicrobial and Chemotherapeutic Agents	
Neomycin sulfate with polymyxin and bacitracin (Neosporin)	Broad-spectrum, ointment or solution Only disadvantage is its allergenic nature (allergy is to neomycin)
Penicillin	Primarily used in newborns in ointment form Occasionally used for intraocular infection Primarily reserved for systemic use
Sodium methicillin	Used for penicillinase-producing organisms
Bacitracin, 500 units/g ointment	Good as a penicillin substitute for local eye uses against gram-positive organisms
Erythromycin, 1% ointment	Effective as a penicillin substitute against resistant staphylococcal organisms

Sulfonamides:
    Sulfisoxazole, 4% solution or ointment
    Sulfacetamide sodium
	Used in treatment of conjunctivitis; sometimes effective against larger viruses

Dyes	
(For corneal staining to detect superficial abrasions)	
Fluorescein sodium	*Note:* Because *Pseudomonas aeruginosa,* highly pathogenic for corneal tissues, grows well in fluorescein solutions, the sterile single-dose containers or sterile Kimura fluorescent papers are recommended.
Rose bengal, 1% and 2%	Selective dye to stain conjunctiva; mucous shreds stain more brillantly than with fluorescein.
Carbonic Anhydrase Inhibitor	
(Carbonic anhydrase is an enzyme present in body tissues. In the ciliary body, it is directly involved in the production of aqueous humor.)	
Acetazolamide	A sulfonamide used as a diuretic and also effective in decreasing production of aqueous humor by ciliary body in glaucoma
Dichlorphenamide	Because of side-effects (gastric distress, shortness of breath, acidosis, tingling of extremities, dermatitis, ureteral stones), it is prescribed cautiously for selected patients.
Sympathomimetic Drugs	
(Used primarily for mydriasis and occasionally as vasoconstrictors)	
Phenylephrine hydrochloride, 2.5% to 10%	Action lasts 3 hours.
Hydroxyamphetamine hydrobromide ophthalmic solution, 1%	Action lasts 3 hours; useful in those with allergy toward phenylephrine
Epinephrine hydrochloride, 1:1,000; 0.5%, 1%, and 2%	Lowers intraocular pressure in open-angle glaucoma (inhibits aqueous production)
Parasympathomimetic Drugs	
(Used as miotics for controlling intraocular pressure in glaucoma)	
Group 1—Act Directly on Myoneural Junction Pilocarpine hydrochloride, 0.5% to 6.0%	Drug of choice in glaucoma Action lasts 4 to 8 hours
Carbachol, 1.5% to 3%	Used if pilocarpine is ineffective

(continued)

TABLE 50-2 *(continued)*

Medication	Action
Parasympathomimetic Drugs	
Group II—Cholinesterase Inhibitors	
Physostigmine salicylate, 0.25% and 0.5%	Action lasts 6 to 8 hours
	Because it is allergenic, unstable, and short in its action, it is gradually being replaced by echothiophate.
Echothiophate iodide, 0.06%, 0.125%, and 0.25%	Water soluble
	Causes less local irritation
Isoflurophate 0.025% ophthalmic ointment; 0.1% ophthalmic solution	Oil-soluble miotic
	May produce side-effects; watch for vomiting, diarrhea, tenesmus.
Parasympatholytic Medications	
(Used as mydriatics to facilitate ophthalmoscopic examination and for mydriasis and cycloplegia in refraction and in treatment of uveitis)	
Mydriatics	
Epinephrine, 1% to 2%	Action lasts 12 hours.
Eucatropine hydrochloride, 5%	Short-lived action
	Can dilate pupil without affecting accommodation
Cycloplegics	
Homatropine hydrobromide, 2% and 5%	A popular drug for cycloplegic refraction
	Action lasts 24 to 36 hours.
	Allergic reactions rare
Scopolamine hydrobromide, 0.2% to 0.5%	Used in children's refraction
	Used in treating uveitis
	Because of low allergic reaction, it is preferred to atropine.
	May cause dizziness and disorientation in older persons
Atropine sulfate, 0.25%, 0.5%, 1%, and 2%	Most powerful of this group
	Action lasts 10 to 14 days, during which time eyes must be protected from bright light.
	Used in treating uveitis
	Used in refraction of children
	Contraindicated in narrow-angle glaucoma
	5% of persons are sensitive to it (symptoms: difficulty in swallowing; dizziness; flushed skin with circumoral pallor; rapid, full pulse; delirium).
Cyclopentolate hydrochloride, 0.5% and 1%	Action is less than 24 hours.
	Very popular drug for cycloplegic refraction
Tropicamide, 0.5% and 1%	Newer, shorter acting—lasts 6 hours
Adrenal Corticosteroids	
(Effective in treating inflammatory conditions of the eye: uveitis, episcleritis, chemical burns. Decreases vascularization and scarring following burns, trauma, and severe inflammation)	
Cortisone acetate, 0.5% to 2.5% suspension; 1.5% ointment	Least expensive
Hydrocortisone, 0.5% to 2.5% suspension; 1.5% ointment	Greater potency than cortisone, so it can be used in lower concentrations
Prednisone, prednisolone, dexamethasone, and betamethasone	These are thought to be more potent than hydrocortisone

Note: Corticosteroids are highly dangerous when used in the presence of herpes simplex keratitis. The patient should definitely be under the care of an ophthalmologist with these medications. All steroids are now known to produce glaucoma in certain predisposed patients. Use of steroids locally or systemically must be carefully supervised.

Before drops are instilled, it is important to see that the correct drug is being given. Some drugs (*e.g.*, miotics and mydriatics) act in exactly opposite ways (Fig. 50-7). Therefore, if one of these drugs is indicated in the treatment of a certain eye disease, the other is contraindicated. It may seem needless to emphasize this warning, but experience has taught how easy it is to pick up the wrong bottle from a tray containing similar vials when the room is dimly lighted.

In addition, the solution should be checked for color changes or sedimentation, which indicates that the solution be discarded. Patients especially are warned to avoid using medication of any kind if it has been in the medicine cabinet at home for months or years. Of course, the use of small, sterile, disposable containers has helped reduce this problem and has also eliminated the need for a separate dropper.

Instillation.   Before the medication is instilled into the eyes (Fig. 50-8*A*), the lids and the lashes are cleansed. Then the head of the patient is tilted backward and inclined slightly to the side, so that the solution will run away from the tear duct. This latter precaution is especially necessary when toxic solutions, such as atropine, are employed, because absorption of the excess drug by way of the nose and the pharynx may lead to toxic symptoms. In most patients, it is well to press the inner angle of the eye after instilling the drops to prevent the excess solution from entering the nose.

- The lower lid is depressed with the fingers of the left hand, the patient is told to look upward, and the solution is dropped on the everted lower lid.

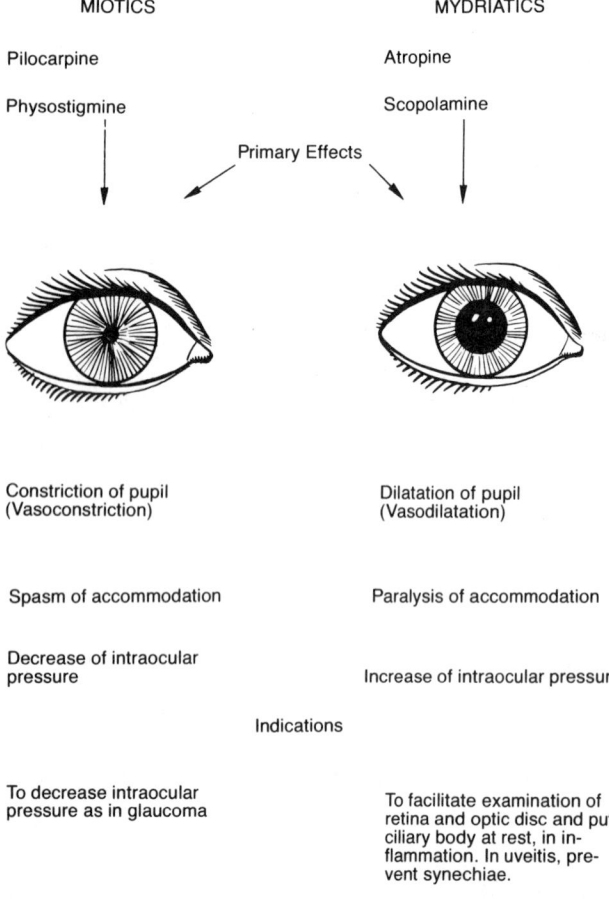

MIOTICS

Pilocarpine

Physostigmine

MYDRIATICS

Atropine

Scopolamine

Primary Effects

Constriction of pupil
(Vasoconstriction)

Dilatation of pupil
(Vasodilatation)

Spasm of accommodation

Paralysis of accommodation

Decrease of intraocular
pressure

Increase of intraocular pressure

Indications

To decrease intraocular
pressure as in glaucoma

To facilitate examination of
retina and optic disc and put
ciliary body at rest, in inflammation. In uveitis, prevent synechiae.

Figure 50-7
Effects and indications of miotics and mydriatics.

- *Care must be taken that the pipette does not touch any part of the eye or the lids, to guard against contamination of the dropper and injury to the eye.*
- After the drops (one or two at most) are placed in the eye, the lid is released and any excess fluid is sponged gently from the lids and the cheeks with sterile cotton.
- After the medication is instilled, the patient is instructed to close his eyes *gently* and keep them closed for 3 to 5 minutes. Patients often have a tendency to "squeeze" their eyes closed, thereby expelling the medication. When the lids are kept closed as directed, the pumping action of the eyelids (to remove fluids from the eye) is stopped. This keeps the medication on the eye longer.
- If the dropper has not been contaminated, it may be replaced in the bottle, but it is to be used only for this patient

Ointments

Ointments of various kinds are used frequently in the treatment of inflammatory diseases of the lids, the conjunctiva, and the cornea. Those prescribed most commonly are sulfonamides, bacitracin, neomycin, chloramphenicol, steroids, and various combinations.

Ointments are applied best by gently pulling down the lower lid and expressing a small amount of the ointment from the tube onto the conjunctiva of the lower lid. Care is taken not to touch the eye or the eyelid with the tube. The lid then may be massaged gently in such a way as to distribute the drug over the eyeball (Fig. 50-8*B*).

Ocular Irrigations

Ocular irrigations are indicated in treating various inflammations of the conjunctiva, in preparing the patient for eye surgery, and in removing inflammatory secretions. They are also used for their antiseptic effect. The fluid to be employed depends on the condition present and is warmed before being used. The irrigating apparatus is simple, consisting of a commercially prepared irrigating bottle containing sterile isotonic ophthalmic solution (Blinx, Dacriose) and a small, curved basin and cotton for catching the fluid and the secretions.

- The patient lies flat on his back or sits with the head tilted backward and inclined slightly toward the side to be treated. The basin may be held by the patient, if he is sitting, or so placed that when he is lying down it will catch the fluid as it runs from the eye. The nurse stands in front of the patient. The patient's clothing and the bed are protected with bed-saver pads.
- After the lids are carefully cleansed to remove dust, secretions, and crusts, the lids are held open with the thumb and the fingers of one hand and the eye flushed gently, directing the stream way from the nose. The fluid is never directed toward the nose because of the danger that it may spill over into the other eye. The procedure is continued until the eye is entirely free of secretions.
- It must be remembered that very little force is to be used because of the danger of injury. For the same reason, and to prevent contamination, no part of the irrigator should touch the eye, the lid, or the lashes.
- When the irrigation has been completed, the eye and the cheek are dried gently with cotton.

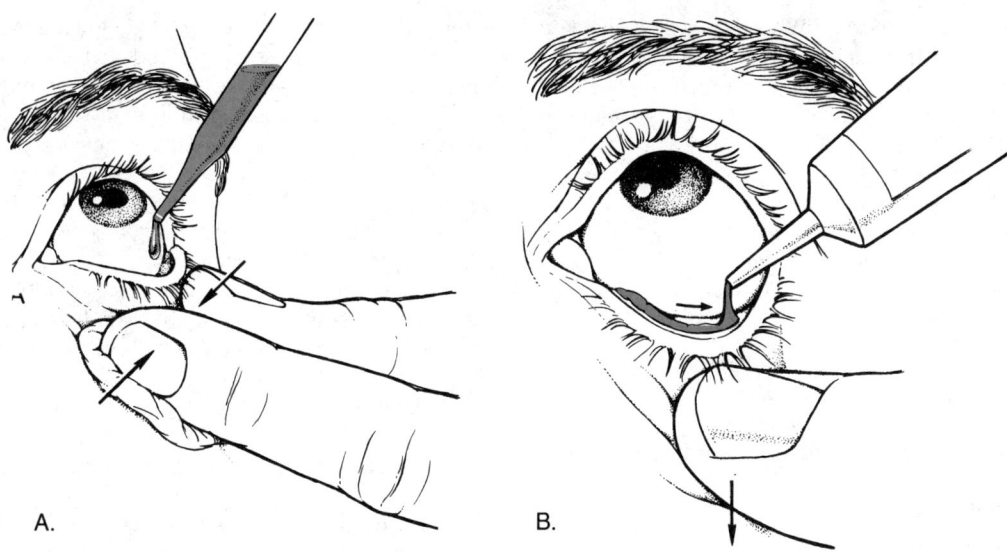

Figure 50-8
Instillation of eye drops. (*A*) When instilling eye drops, instruct the patient to look
upward, then lightly pinch the lower lid to form a receptacle for the dropped medication.
(*B*) In applying ointment, instruct the patient to look upward, then depress the lower lid
and gently squeeze ointment along the everted lid, beginning at the inner canthus (close
to the nose) and then moving outward.

Continuous Irrigation of the Eye. Continuous irrigation is indicated in chemical burns, resistant corneal ulcers,
uveitis, socket infections after enucleation, or conditions in
which constant medication or debridement is indicated. Prior
to irrigation, proparacaine is instilled as a local anesthetic.

Warm Wet Compresses. Heat relieves pain and increases the circulation, thereby promoting absorption and
reducing tension in the eye. It is especially valuable for conjunctivitis accompanied by excessive secretions. Heat is best
applied in the form of compresses composed of seven or
eight layers of gauze or cotton just large enough to cover
the eye.

- A towel is used to cover the chest. The skin of the lids
  and the adjacent cheek may be anointed with cold cream
  or petrolatum.
- The compresses then are moistened in a basin of water
  or any other prescribed solution that has been heated.
- The fluid, which should be kept at a temperature between
  46°C to 49°C (115°F to 120°F), is expressed or squeezed
  from the pad, and the compress, after being tested for
  temperature on the back of the hand, is placed gently
  over the closed lids.
- The pads are changed every 30 to 60 seconds for 10 to
  15 minutes, and the application is repeated every 2 or 3
  hours.
- At the completion of the period of application, the lids
  are dried gently with cotton.
- New pads are used for each application and, if the eyes
  have a purulent secretion, the compresses are applied
  to one eye at a time, the solution and the basin being
  changed between applications in order not to carry infection from one eye to the other.

Cold Compresses. Cold causes a capillary constriction
that tends to reduce the amount of secretion and relieve pain

during the early stages of acute inflammatory conditions of
the conjunctiva. Cold compresses are useful in relieving itching due to allergic conjunctivitis.

- Cold compresses are never used in the treatment of inflammations of the eye (iritis, keratitis), because cold,
  by constricting the capillaries, interferes with the nutrition
  of the cornea.

The patient is positioned comfortably. An absorbent
towel is placed around the neck in bib fashion to absorb any
droplets. Gauze compresses with cotton filler or a clean
washcloth are moistened and placed in a clean bowl of floating ice and a small amount of water.

The compresses are wrung out thoroughly and applied
gently to the closed eye. Compresses are changed as they
become warm. The procedure is continued for about 15 minutes and repeated every 2 to 3 hours.

▶ *Nursing Process*
Overview of Patients With
Eye Problems

▷ *Assessment*

An initial nursing history is taken to determine the patient's
primary problem, such as difficulty in reading, blurred vision,
a burning sensation in the eyes, "watering of the eyes," double
vision, spots, and isolated areas of lost vision (scotomas, itching, myopia, or hyperopia). The nurse should determine
whether the problem is in one or both eyes and how long
the patient has had this difficulty.

It is also important to ascertain the patient's general ocular condition or status: Does he wear glasses, contact lenses,

or other vision assistive devices? When were they checked last? Is he under the regular care of an ophthalmologist? When was his last eye check-up? Was his eye pressure checked? Does he have difficulty seeing (focusing) at close range or at a distance? Does he have problems reading or watching television? What about problems differentiating colors or problems with lateral or peripheral vision? Has the patient had any past eye trauma or eye infections? If so, when? What eye problems exist in the patient's family?

A pertinent past ocular history is essential. What past illnesses has the patient had?

> Childhood: strabismus, amblyopia, injuries?
> Adult: glaucoma, cataract, eye trauma, refractive errors—how corrected? Any previous eye surgery? Hypertension, diabetes, thyroid disorders, sexually transmitted diseases, allergies, cardiovascular and collagen diseases?
> Family illnesses: Is there a history of eye disorders in parents or grandparents?

The client's understanding of eye care and treatment is elicited in order to determine misconceptions or misinformation that can be corrected early.

▷ *Nursing Diagnoses*

Based on the nursing assessment data, the patient's major nursing diagnoses may include the following:

- Alteration in comfort (pain) related to injury of or pressure in the eye
- Fear and anxiety related to impaired vision and potential for further loss of sight
- Alteration in visual sensory perception related to ocular trauma, inflammation, infection, tumor, or degeneration
- Self-care deficit related to impaired vision and limited knowledge regarding eye care
- Social isolation related to limited ability to participate in recreational and social activities secondary to impaired vision

▷ *Planning and Implementation*

▷ *Goals:* The major goals of the patient may include relief of pain, control of anxiety, prevention of further visual deterioration and acceptance of treatment, accomplishment of self-care activities including medication administration, and avoidance of social isolation and participation in diversional activities.

Nursing Interventions

Providing Eye Care. Regardless of the cause of a visual problem, measures can be initiated in an attempt to control as well as prevent further progression of deterioration. This can be accomplished by putting the eye at rest, restricting activities, wearing dark glasses, or instilling a prescribed local anesthetic. If the problem is related to an infection, an antibiotic or antimicrobial medication may be prescribed as eyedrops.

Relieving Pain and Anxiety. Pain may be due to trauma, such as a scratched cornea or increasing pressure within the eye. An eye patch will help to limit eye movement. However, it must be remembered that the uncovered eye should also rest because eyes move in synchrony.

Because light causes pain in many eye conditions, and because the eyes should be rested as much as possible before and after an operation to facilitate the healing process, it is best to maintain subdued lighting in the room. If those assisting the patient need light to carry out their activities, then dimmed artificial lights may be used.

Prescribed analgesics and antibiotics will help to control discomfort. Avoiding emotional disturbances and physical stresses promote relaxation, which in turn helps to relieve pain.

Following a physical examination and diagnostic studies, a diagnosis is determined; anxieties are frequently lessened when a specific treatment plan to correct the problem is in place.

Dealing With Sensory Deprivation. When the eyes are bandaged, distortions in perception can occur, such as "eye-patch delirium," inappropriate behavior, loss of position sense, and a sensation of floating. Often these problems are magnified and become frightening and upsetting. One way to assist the patient in overcoming these unsettling feelings is to reorient him constantly to reality and offer reassurance, explanations, and understanding. Anyone entering the patient's room should speak and identify himself so as not to startle the patient.

Preoperative Nursing Management. The preparation of the patient for an ophthalmic operation must be carried out with scrupulous care so that complications are minimized, comfort is achieved, and delay is minimized. The type of anesthesia often determines how the patient is prepared. For example, if the anesthetic is general, the lower intestinal tract is evacuated the morning of the operation and only a liquid diet is given after that. Before the eyes are prepared for surgery, the patient's hair is covered with a cap and the face is cleansed. If the eyelashes are to be cut, the scissors are coated lightly with petrolatum so that the lashes adhere to the scissors and do not fall into the eye. An antibiotic is usually instilled as prescribed prior to surgery, while the patient is awake. The patient is encouraged to mention any of his concerns so that they may be addressed before surgery.

Postoperative Nursing Interventions. Following surgery in which both eyes are bandaged, the patient is placed in bed in a supine position with a small pillow under his head. Pillows may be placed on each side of the head to keep it still, and side rails may be set in place to give the patient a sense of security. The patient is provided with a nurse-call system and instructed to ask for help rather than move or strain in an attempt to be self-sufficient.

If a local anesthesia is used during the operation, the patient is usually ambulatory in a few hours after surgery.

The ophthalmologist is notified immediately if the patient has excessive pain or if the dressings are disturbed.

- Morphine is never given to ophthalmic patients unless it is certain that vomiting will not injure the eye.

Diversional or recreational therapy is important but should be of such a nature that the eyes are not fatigued in any way. Even the patient's environment is an important consideration. Light is regulated so that it is not bright and does not produce a glare.

Enhancing Self-Care Activities. The patient is encouraged to carry out as much self-care as possible in order to promote a feeling of self-sufficiency. Nursing assistance is given as needed. A patient who cannot see is assisted with eating, but if he is accustomed to feeding himself, he is encouraged to do so. Proper elimination is promoted by proper diet, stool softeners, or enemas, as prescribed. Ambulatory patients are to have a daily rest period in the afternoon. Ophthalmic patients are not to read, smoke, or shave unless given permission by the physician. They must be cautioned against rubbing their eyes or wiping them with a soiled handkerchief. All patients receiving dilating medications should wear dark glasses.

Medication bottles and instructions should be labeled in large letters and kept and used where there is plenty of light. Before the patient uses any medication he must wash his hands. When instilling eye drops, the patient is supervised so that he develops a technique specific to his needs. He may find it convenient to rest the base of the hand that is holding the medicine dropper against his forehead. With his other hand, he can lightly pinch the lower lid to form a V-trough to catch the eye drop.

Promoting Coping Mechanisms and Diversional Activities. The mental anxiety frequently experienced by the ophthalmic patient requires as much consideration as his physical condition. A person's dependence on sight is emphasized when one faces a temporary or possible permanent loss of this vital sense. Worry, fear, and depression are common reactions in addition to tension, resentment, anger, and rejection. By encouraging the patient to express his feelings, the nurse may discover the basic problems involved and can then take steps to alleviate them.

The patient should be encouraged to have visitors and to socialize. Depending on his interests and preferences, suggestions can be made for diversional and interesting activities. When permissible, the radio and occupational therapy may be used to keep the patient's mind occupied. Although it is important not to be oversolicitous, showing interest, empathy, and understanding enhances the patient's sense of well-being. Because of differences of personality, the approaches in overcoming the anxiety of individual patients vary. When permanent blindness is apparent, re-education may be done by specially trained personnel or similarly afflicted persons.

▷ *Evaluation*

▷ *Expected Outcomes*

1. Patient experiences less pain.
   a. Takes prescribed medication to counteract irritant, to rest the eyes, and to attack the cause of the infection; also takes medication (sedation) for body relaxation.
   b. Applies prescribed cold or warm compresses depending on the situation.
   c. Reduces eye activity by applying appropriate eye dressing and resting.
   d. Protects eye from additional injury by using a protective shield.
2. Shows evidence of calmness and absence of anxiety.
3. Accepts treatment regimen and carries out recommendations.

   a. Washes his hands before using eye drops and taking medications.
   b. Reports any untoward signs such as accumulation of granulations, watering of eyes, and pain.
   c. Reduces eye activity by using an eye patch.
   d. Keeps a diary about his progress and jots down questions to ask when he next visits his physician.
4. Practices self-care activities effectively.
   a. Demonstrates how he manages treatments; forms a V-trough in lower lid to receive eye drops.
   b. Cleans lenses effectively as taught.
   c. Lists safety measures to prevent falls such as being aware of loose carpeting and cluttered steps.
   d. Describes proper lighting for reading and hand crafts.
5. Participates in diversional and social activities.

Conditions of the Eyelids

Blepharitis. Blepharitis, or inflammation of the eyelids, is a common disorder that can be controlled through cleanliness and the prevention of excessive dryness. Since blepharitis is frequently associated with seborrhea (excessive oiliness of the skin), attempts are made to keep the scalp clean. Daily cleaning of the eyelids by rubbing them gently with a clean, wet washcloth helps to remove scales. Usually, an anti-infective ointment is prescribed, such as steroid–sulfa drops, to be applied to the lid margin twice a day. For pure staphylococcal blepharitis, local application of antibiotic solutions and moist heat is helpful.

Sty (External Hordeolum). A sty is an infection of the Zeis glands or Moll's glands that empty at the free edge of the eyelid. When a sty develops, this area becomes swollen, red, tender, and painful. Frequently, an eyelash will be found in the center of the yellow point that appears. Warm compresses applied in the early stage hasten the pointing of the abscess. Removal of the central lash often is followed by drainage of pus, but incision is necessary if resolution does not begin within 48 hours. An antibiotic instilled into the conjunctival sac hastens control of the infection.

Chalazia. A chalazion is a cyst of the meibomian glands. It appears as a small, hard, painless lump in the lid and usually occurs secondary to infection of the gland, which results when the opening on the lid margin becomes plugged. Occasionally, such a cyst may become infected. When this occurs, warm compresses are used; an incision and drainage also may be necessary. Incision and drainage (or excision of the cyst) are indicated if the mass distorts vision, causes astigmatism, or becomes a cosmetic blemish. Another method of treatment being used by some ophthalmologists is to inject steroids directly into the chalazion.

Trachoma. Trachoma is a chronic, highly communicable disease of the conjunctival and corneal epithelium. It is one of the most common diseases of humans and affects about 15% of the world's population. It is the greatest single cause for progressive loss of sight in the world. Trachoma is common in Asian countries and in countries around the Mediterranean Sea, particularly Egypt. In the United States, it is rare except among American Indians and Mexicans in the southwest.

Assessment and Clinical Manifestations. The principal symptoms are mild itching and irritation. After an acute inflammatory process, follicles appear on the conjunctiva. Blurring of vision and increasing discomfort occur. The upper palpebral conjunctiva are affected.

The progress of the disease has been classified into four stages: in stage I (incipient trachoma), immature follicles are present, especially in the upper tarsal conjunctiva. At the top of the cornea there is incipent pannus (abnormal vascularization). Stage II (established trachoma) consists of two types—type A and type B. In type A, follicular hypertrophy is predominant, while in type B, papillary hypertrophy is predominant ("acute trachoma"). In stage III, early conjunctival scarring is observed as fine, white lines; corneal pannus also increases. In stage IV, smooth scarring of the tarsal conjunctiva occurs and vascular pannus becomes inactive. Secondary bacterial conjunctivitis increases the hazard of corneal ulceration, and this in turn leads to blindness.

Management. Trachoma is spread by direct contact; therefore, personal cleanliness is a key factor in prevention. Isolating known cases and initiating antibiotic therapy early may help control the disease. If untreated, it will last for months or years. Medical treatment consists of a 3- to 4-week course of tetracycline or erythromycin. The World Health Organization is making great strides in eliminating this curable disease.

Inflammations of the Eye

Conjunctivitis. Conjunctivitis, or inflammation of the conjunctiva, may result from bacterial, viral, and rickettsial infections or from allergy, trauma, or chemical injury.

No matter what the cause, the symptoms are similar: redness, pain, swelling, and lacrimation. The amount and the nature of discharge depend on the offending organisms; for instance, the pneumococcus and the gonococcus cause an abundant purulent discharge.

Frequent saline irrigations are required to remove the discharge. Warm compresses are recommended to be applied for 15 minutes three or four times a day. Ointments such as sulfacetamide or gentamicin or chloramphenicol drops or ointment may be instilled to clear the infection in 1 to 3 days. Untreated, the infection usually subsides in 7 to 10 days. Precautions must be taken to prevent dissemination of infection to the other eye, as well as to other people. Hands should be kept clean when treating the eye; individual clean washcloths and towels should be used.

Uveitis. Uveitis is a general term for inflammatory conditions of the uveal tract (iris, ciliary body, choroid), which may be due to a number of causative agents. *Anterior uveitis* refers to *choroiditis* and *chorioretinitis; panuveitis* involves the entire uveal tract. Uveitis (iritis) is usually unilateral and is characterized by pain, photophobia, blurring of vision, redness (circumcorneal flush), and a constricted pupil.

Some authorities prefer to classify the various forms of uveitis as granulomatous and nongranulomatous. In some aspects, the two forms are similar, but in others there occurs a significant difference (Table 50-3).

Complications and sequelae may result if uveitis is not treated. Adhesions may develop, impeding aqueous outflow

TABLE 50-3

Comparison Between Granulomatous and Nongranulomatous Uveitis

Granulomatous	Nongranulomatous
Location	
Any portion of uveal tract, but predilection for posterior part	Anterior portion; iris, ciliary body
Onset	
Insidious	Acute
Pain	
None or minimal	Marked
Circumcorneal Flush	
Slight	Present
Photophobia	
Slight	Marked
Course	
Chronic	Acute
Prognosis	
Fair to poor	Good
Sometimes	Common

at the anterior chamber angle and causing glaucoma. If adhesions hinder the flow of aqueous humor from the posterior to the anterior chamber, cataracts may develop. Even retinal detachment may occur as a result of traction exerted on the retina by vitreous strands.

Management. Treatment is directed to the specific type of involvement. For granulomatous uveitis, atropine is used to reduce the likelihood of adhesions. Anti-infective chemotherapy may be initiated, and if the response is not favorable, it is followed with corticosteroids. Medications for comfort and relief of pain are also prescribed. Intraocular tension should be monitored regularly on all patients with uveitis especially when topical ophthalmic steroids are used.

Nongranulomatous uveitis is also treated with atropine to keep the pupil dilated. Local, and possibly systemic, steroids may be required.

Nongranulomatous uveitis subsides with treatment in a few weeks. Granulomatous uveitis may last months and even years in spite of treatment.

Sympathetic Ophthalmia. Sympathetic ophthalmia is a severe granulomatous bilateral uveitis that may occur from 1 week to several years after an eye injury. Fortunately, this is a rare condition, but it may be suspected when there is a history of a penetrating eye injury in one eye (exciting eye) and the patient complains of photophobia, blurring vision, and infection in the other eye (sympathizing eye).

Medical management is directed in one of two ways: corticosteroids are administered both locally and systemically, while atropine is given locally. This treatment has been proven effective. The other, more radical procedure is preventive enucleation or removal of the severely injured eye before sympathetic ophthalmia develops. This decision is a difficult one; often, a patient can think more clearly and reach a satisfactory decision if he has the time and opportunity to express his thoughts and feelings about the operation. In such a case, it helps to understand the nature of the problem, the patient's ability and condition, and the desired goals. Untreated, the disease progresses to bilateral blindness.

Pterygium. Pterygium is an abnormal triangular fold of membrane that extends onto the cornea from the white of the eye; it always occurs toward the nose. It is thought to be caused by chronic irritation, as from dust or wind. Surgical intervention prevents its growth and protects against loss of vision. In some eye clinics, surgery is followed by β-radiation therapy, which helps to prevent recurrence of pterygium. Patients often erroneously refer to pterygium as a cataract.

Corneal Disorders

Corneal Ulcers

Inflammation of the cornea (*keratitis*) with loss of corneal tissue results in corneal ulcer. The inflammatory reaction often spreads deeper to the iris (*iritis*), resulting in the formation of pus, which collects as a white or yellow deposit behind the cornea (*hypopyon*). If the ulceration perforates, the iris may prolapse through the cornea or other serious complications may follow.

Because the cornea is so important to vision, any ulceration must be considered a most serious condition. Scarring or performation due to corneal ulceration is a major cause of blindness; 10% of all blindness is caused by corneal ulcers (6% in the United States). The healing of all but the most superficial ulcers is attended with some degree of opacity of the cornea and, therefore, with some diminution of vision.

The symptoms of corneal ulceration are pain, marked photophobia, and increased lacrimation. The eye usually appears somewhat injected or "bloodshot." See Table 50-4.

Management. Prevention is much simpler and easier than cure. Therefore, prompt removal of foreign bodies and early treatment of scratches and infections may prevent the occurrence of a corneal ulcer.

Dark glasses are provided to relieve the photophobia. Mydriatics are given at frequent intervals. Optical anesthetics may be used to relieve pain. Fluorescein generally is used to outline the ulcers before the healing solutions are applied. Antibiotic solutions and chemotherapeutic agents are prescribed for the specific type of infection, since the microorganism may be bacterial, viral, or fungal.

Corneal Transplantation (Keratoplasty)

A keratoplasty in which the damaged cornea is replaced with a transplanted cornea may be done to repair a corneal opacity

(scar), keratoconus, or chemical burn of the eye. The circular segment of cornea removed from the patient must be exactly matched and replaced by a similar segment of cornea from a donor eye (Fig. 50-9). For best results, the graft should be removed within 8 to 10 hours following the death of the donor (to prevent softening of the cornea) and transplanted within 2 days.*

The graft may be a *penetrating graft* (including all layers of the cornea) or a *lamellar graft* (involving only the outer layers of the cornea). The lamellar graft, popular in the past, is gradually being replaced by the penetrating graft.

Preoperative Nursing Interventions. Since keratoplasty is elective surgery, the patient is probably aware of the nature of the operation and is no doubt optimistic about the likelihood of improved vision. The nurse, nevertheless, must allow time for the expression of concerns or questions that the patient may still have. Psychological and cultural concerns regarding the disability may have to be explored before the patient is in optimal condition for surgery. Physically, the patient should be free from respiratory or eye infections in order to promote postoperative healing.

Intraoperative Procedure. Usually, a transplant is done under local anesthesia and takes 1 to 2 hours. The instrument used, a trephine, has an end that resembles a cookie cutter in the size needed to remove the desired circular area of cornea. The trephine is placed over the opacity, and the cornea is removed. The same instrument is used to remove the donor cornea so that the graft is a perfect fit. Ultrafine sutures are placed evenly to create a tight seal; this is done with the use of an operating microscope.

Postoperative Nursing Interventions. Goals for postoperative patient care are (1) to monitor for and avoid activities that will cause an elevation of intraocular pressure as well as pressure on the operated eye, (2) to rest the eye so that healing progresses smoothly, and (3) to institute measures that will prevent infection of the eye.

Elevated intraocular pressure constricts the vascular supply and can cause retinal atrophy or damage to the graft. To prevent pressure from increasing within the eye, the nurse must be cognizant of those activities that can elevate pressure (sneezing, coughing, straining during defecation, or lifting heavy objects). Loss of aqueous humor through the suture line by increased pressure could cause dislocation of the newly transplanted cornea, prolapse of the iris, adhesions of the iris to the cornea, or malformation of the anterior chamber. To avoid these problems, when the patient is transferred from the operating table to the bed or stretcher, adequate personnel are required to move him horizontally in one smooth shift, giving adequate support to his head. Intraocular pressure can be measured by sensitive electronic applanation tonometers. If the pressure is elevated, pharmacologic control can be achieved with such drugs as acetazolamide, which inhibits the production of aqueous humor.

Healing is slow because the cornea is avascular, which also increases the possibility of infection. Thus, meticulous sterile technique is followed in dressing changes to protect the susceptible corneal epithelium from infection. Another

---

* The Eye-Bank Association of America, 6560 Fannin, Houston TX 77030, was founded in 1945. Eyes have been donated from persons all over the country and distributed to qualified ophthalmologists throughout the United States.

TABLE 50-4
Assessment of Acute Eye Conditions

Acute Conjunctivitis	Acute Iritis (Anterior Uveitis)	Acute Glaucoma (Closed-Angle)	Corneal Ulcer or Trauma
Incidence			
Very common	Common	Not common	Common
Vision			
Normal	Some blurring	Marked blurring	Blurred (usually)
Pain			
None	Moderate	Severe	May have pain
Intraocular Pressure			
Normal	Normal or low	Elevated	Normal
Cornea			
Clear	Clear	Steamy	May have abrasion, foreign body, or ulcer
Ocular Discharge			
Moderate to copious	None	None	Watery and perhaps purulent
Pupillary Response to Light			
Normal	Weak	Weak	Normal
Pupil Size			
Normal	Small	Dilated	Normal or small
Conjunctival Vessels Dilated			
Yes	Mostly circumcorneal	Yes	Yes
Prognosis			
Self-limited; 3 to 5 days	Good with treatment	Poor without proper treatment	Poor without proper treatment

means of reducing the chance for infection is to provide the patient with soft contact lenses which protect the suture line. This is particularly effective in patients who have chemical burns. To prevent herpes simplex infection, the administration of antiviral agents may be indicated.

Radial Keratotomy

Radial keratotomy (Fig. 50-10) is a procedure designed to correct myopia (nearsightedness) and astigmatism. It is performed under topical anesthesia, using proparacaine; hypnotic suggestion can be used to supplement this anesthetic. Incisions are made into the cornea. In earlier forms of the operation, the pattern of the incisions resembled bicycle spokes (usually 8 or 16). More recent procedures use fewer incisions. In the United States, the initial number of incisions was 16; now most surgeons use 8 or 4 incisions. The patterns and depth of the incisions vary with the surgeon. Following the incisions, pressure from the intraocular fluid stretches the

radial cuts to distort the cornea into a flatter shape, thereby improving the myopia. The surgery usually takes about 30 minutes and can be performed on an outpatient basis.

The procedure continues to be studied as more data are collected on the outcome and effects of the surgery. Ongoing studies such as PERK (Prospective Evaluation of Radial Keratotomy) provide additional information on the safety and temporary sequelae of the procedure, control of wound healing, and possible complications.

Retinal Disorders

Detached Retina

A retinal detachment occurs when the sensory retina separates from the pigment epithelium of the retina. The retina is that

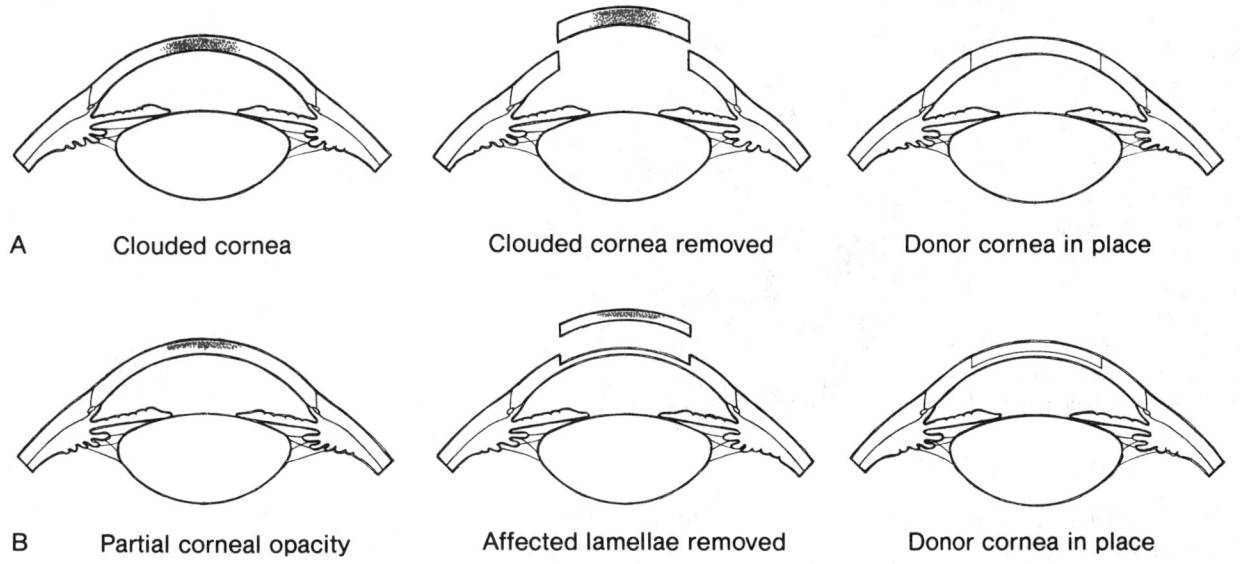

A   Clouded cornea   Clouded cornea removed   Donor cornea in place

B   Partial corneal opacity   Affected lamellae removed   Donor cornea in place

Figure 50-9
Corneal transplantation (keratoplasty). (*A*) Penetrating keratoplasty: a full-thickness (7-mm to 8-mm) disc is removed from the host and replaced with a matching full-thickness button from the donor. (*B*) Lamellar keratoplasty: a thin layer of corneal tissue is excised from the host eye. Stroma and entire endothelium are spared.

layer of the eye that perceives light and transmits impulses from its nerve cells to the optic nerve. When a tear or rip occurs in the retina, vitreous humor and transudate seep out between the rods and cones of the retina and the pigment epithelium. Tears or holes in the retina may occur suddenly or slowly, as a result of trauma or degeneration. It may also result from hemorrhage, exudation, or tumor in front of or behind the retina. Studies have shown that approximately 6% of the population have small holes or tears in the retina. Aging weakens these spots.

The most frequent type of retinal detachment is *rhegmatogenous* (induced by a rip or tear), which occurs in 1 in 20,000 people. *Tractional* retinal detachment may occur in patients with diabetes or other vasculopathies that cause an abnormal bonding of vitreous membrane to the internal surface of the retina. *Exudative* retinal detachment arises from choroidal tumors.

Assessment and Clinical Manifestations. The usual symptoms include flashes of light and blurred or "sooty" vision that is sudden in onset; the patient may have the sensation of particles moving in his line of vision. These floating particles consist of retinal cells and blood that are released at the time of the tear and cast shadows on the retina as they drift by. Definite areas of vision may be blank (Fig. 50-11), and in a few days the patient may have the sensation of a veil coming up or down in front of the eye, finally resulting in loss of vision. To diagnose the condition, the pupils are fully dilated and the eye is examined by slit lamp and ophthal-

Figure 50-10
Technique for keratotomy.
(*A*) Incisions (8) are made from the edge of the cornea toward its center. (*B*) Lateral view of the cornea, showing its shape in a patient with myopia.
(*C*) Following keratotomy, the cornea is flatter.

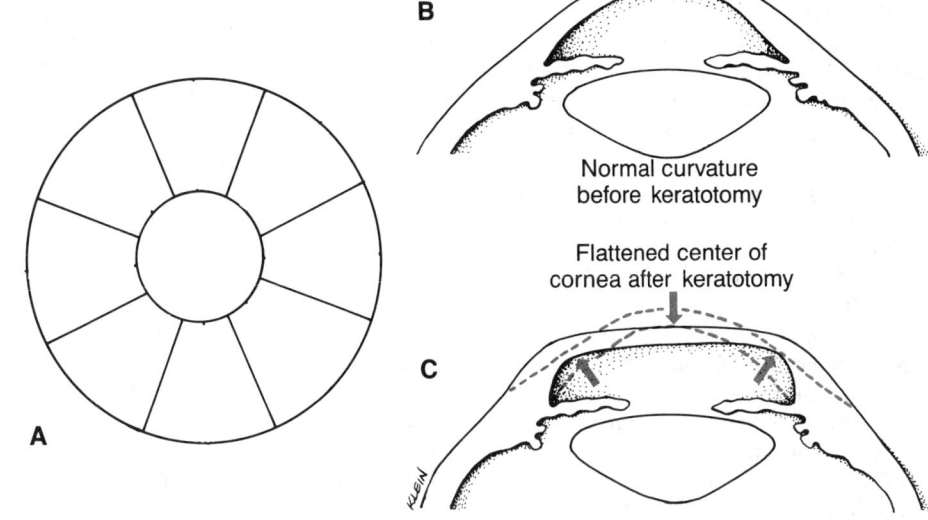

B

Normal curvature
before keratotomy

Flattened center of
cornea after keratotomy

C

A

Figure 50-11
Retinal detachment, shown here in the active stage. There are many causes for detachment, but the hole or tear allows fluid to lift the retina from its normal position. This elevated retina causes a field or vision defect, seen as a dark shadow in the peripheral field. It may be above, or below as illustrated. (Photo courtesy of The Lighthouse, The New York Association for the Blind.)

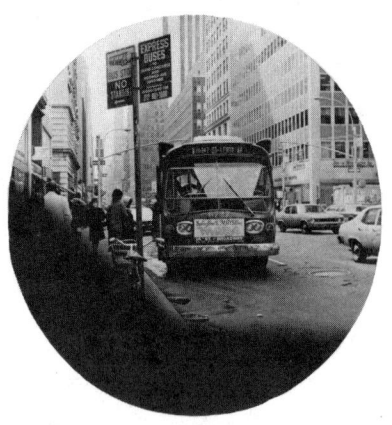

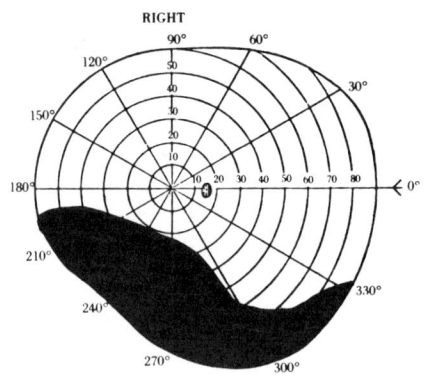

moscope. A determination of visual fields and ultrasonography may also be required.

Conservative Management. The suddenness of the incapacity creates confusion and apprehension in most patients, as well as a fear of blindness. Usually, it means that the person must abandon his business or activity, with little or no time to make plans. The patient is treated with rest immediately. The eye is bandaged in the hope that the retina will fall back into place as much as possible before surgery and thus facilitate the retina's adhering to the choroid. Specific positioning, whether sitting or lying flat or on one side, will be requested by the ophthalmologist. This is determined by the location of the tear. An intraocular air or gas bubble may be injected to facilitate adherence. Again, the physician will recommend the position that the patient is to maintain, so that maximum adherence of the retina to the choroid is achieved. Sedation and tranquilizing drugs may keep the patient comfortable and quiet.

Surgical Intervention

The objective in surgical treatment is to create a scar that seals the retina to the choroid as it heals. Such treatment may be accomplished in one of several ways: photocoagulation, cryosurgery, electrodiathermy, or scleral buckling.

Photocoagulation makes use of a strong beam of light (from a carbon-arc source) that is directed through the dilated pupil to form a small burn, causing a choroid retinal inflammatory exudate. The *laser beam* (light amplification by stimulated emission of radiation) can be used in photocoagulation. This method of treatment is used for limited retinal detachments and also may be used after operation to reattach small areas.

In *cryosurgery*, a supercooled probe is applied to the sclera, causing minimal damage; the choroid, pigment epithelium, and retina adhere as a result of the scarring. The advantage of this method over diathermy is the reduced damage to the sclera.

In *electrodiathermy*, an electrode needle is passed through the sclera, allowing the subretinal collection of fluid to escape. Because an exudate forms from the choroid, the torn retina adheres to the choroid, which in turn adheres to the sclera. This method is being replaced by cryosurgery.

In *scleral buckling*, the idea is to shorten the sclera to enhance contact between the choroid and retina (Fig. 50-

12). After the subretinal fluid is withdrawn, the detachment is treated by one of the methods described above. The treated area is then indented to "buckle" inward toward the vitreous humor.

Postoperative Management

Both eyes are bandaged, and the patient may be kept in bed as directed. This routine varies with the surgical procedure; patients with scleral buckling operations are permitted out of bed much sooner than those who have undergone diathermy. During and following cryotherapy, the patient may experience periocular ache similar to the effect one gets sometimes from eating ice cream; usually this discomfort is controlled with an analgesic.

Precautions are taken to prevent the patient from bumping his head, which could dislodge the retina from the desired position. After a gradual resumption of function, the patient may resume usual activities in 3 to 5 weeks.

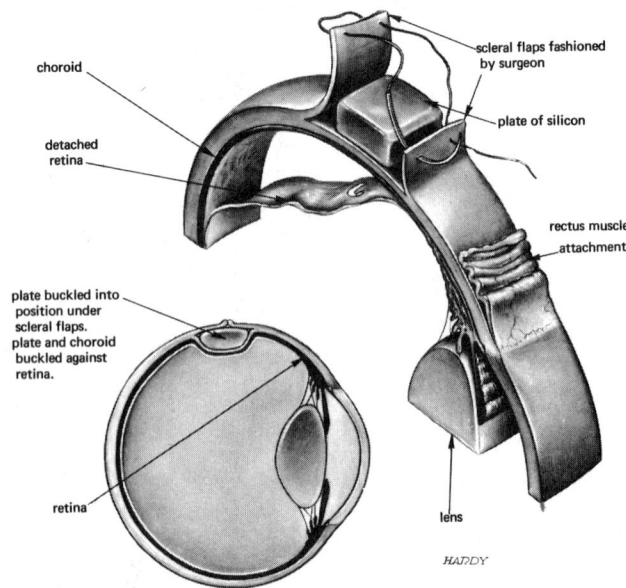

Figure 50-12
Scleral buckling for detached retina. (Ethicon, Inc.)

The psychological nursing care of this patient is of major importance. Diversion that is relaxing is desirable, such as conversation, listening to music, having someone read a favorite book, and so forth.* These patients become depressed easily; therefore, every attempt should be made to prevent this reaction.

At the time of discharge, the nurse should be sure that the patient understands all instructions for post-hospital care and follow-up visits.

Prognosis. If retinal detachment is not treated, further detachment and eventual blindness will occur. About 90% of patients can be cured with treatment. Some patients may require a second operation, which may be performed 10 to 14 days after the first one. Twenty percent of all detachments are or will become bilateral.

Senile Macular Degeneration

Senile macular degeneration (SMD) is a degeneration of the retina that increases in incidence with age. Normally the retina is closely adherent to the pigment epithelium, which is next to Bruch's membrane. Underneath Bruch's membrane are the minute capillaries. The complicated process of degeneration may reveal a defect in Bruch's membrane that permits fluid and a capillary to push through the defect and the pigment epithelium, resulting in a subretinal hemorrhage. Usually the hemorrhage and subsequent scar occur at the most vulnerable part of the retina, the macula. (The *macula* is an oval area of the retina that is devoid of blood vessels and appears darker than the surrounding retina on the posterior eye.)

Gradual progression of the deterioration occurs over months or years until the macula is destroyed. Central vision is affected so that reading becomes impossible. Peripheral vision permits a measure of orientation and allows ambulation in familiar areas.

Management. Light rays from an argon laser are focused on the tiny involved area of the retina (away from the macula) to seal abnormal blood vessels, thereby preventing further fluid leakage (photocoagulation). The success rate is remarkable in patients who are treated early. Success depends on the location of the neovascular membranes. Argon laser photocoagulation on vessels closer than 200 μm to the center of the fovea (the center of the macula) is not successful. Clinical trials using other kinds of lasers are being studied.

The nurse recognizes that this condition causes the patient to be anxious and depressed. If the condition is treated early, the patient is helped. Most often the patient is seen after considerable deterioration has taken place. He needs to be reassured that although his central vision is affected, he can still manage activities of daily living in an independent manner. Measures to combat his depression are in order. When he is unable to read or watch television, he can continue to be "in contact" with his radio and friends.

Cataracts

A cataract is an opaque (nontransparent) area of the crystalline lens or its capsule. Occasionally, it occurs at birth

* Recordings of books may be obtained from the public library or local association for the blind.

(congenital cataract) or in younger people as a result of trauma or disease, but most commonly it occurs in adults past middle age (senile cataract).

Pathophysiology. The normal lens is a clear, transparent, button-like structure lying in back of the iris; it possesses strong refractive powers. The lens consists of three anatomical components. In the central zone is the *nucleus,* peripherally is the *cortex,* and surrounding both is a *capsule.* With aging, the nucleus takes on a yellowish brown hue. Surrounding opacities are spokelike white densities occurring anteriorly and posteriorly to the nucleus. Opacity of the posterior capsule is the most significant form of cataract—it looks like frost on a window.

Physical and chemical changes may produce a loss of transparency of the lens. Changes in the multiple fine fibers (zonules) that extend from the ciliary body to the outer circumference of the lens, for example, may cause a distortion of the image. A chemical change in lens protein may cause coagulation, thereby producing cloudy vision by blocking the passage of light to the retina. Cataracts may be caused by aging, trauma, or radiation or as a result of certain diseases. One theory postulates that a breakdown in normal lens protein occurs with an influx of water into the lens. This process disrupts the tight lens fibers and interferes with the transmission of light. Another suggestion is that an enzyme plays a part in protecting the lens from degeneration. It decreases with aging and is absent in many patients with cataracts.

Clinical Manifestations. Because the rays of light entering the eye must pass through the pupil and the lens to reach the retina, any opacity in the lens behind the pupil will produce alterations in vision. Objects may seem distorted, blurred, or hazy. The patient may describe it as a "film" over the eye or "looking through a fog" (Fig. 50-13). In bright light, a cataract tends to scatter the light, causing an unpleasant glare. The patient experiences no pain, and visual loss is usually gradual.

In time, the degenerative processes cause more opacification of the lens until the opacity becomes complete. Ordinarily, the lens is not visible; however, when a cataract develops, the pupil, which is normally black, becomes gray, and later milky white. A cataract usually develops in one eye first. Later, one begins to develop in the other eye.

Diagnostic Evaluation. In addition to the usual eye tests, keratometry, and slit lamp and ophthalmoscopic examination, A-scan ultrasound (echography) and the endothelial cell counter are particularly useful diagnostic tools. With an endothelial cell count of 2000 cells/mm², the patient is a good candidate for phacoemulsification and insertion of an intraocular lens.

Management

The affected lens may be removed by one of two methods: intracapsular extraction or extracapsular extraction (Fig. 50-14).

Intracapsular Extraction. Intracapsular extraction is the removal of the nucleus, cortex, and capsule as one unit. When difficulty is experienced in freeing the capsule of its zonules, a fibrinolytic and proteolytic enzyme, α-chymotrypsin, is injected into the anterior chamber under the iris. The lytic action is completed in 2 or 3 minutes and allows the lens to be extracted more easily.

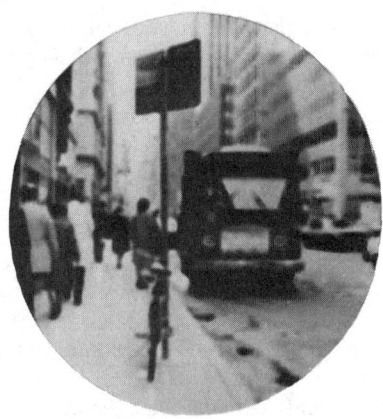

Cataract Diminished acuity from an opacity of the lens. The field of vision is unaffected. There is no scotoma, but the person has an overall haziness of the view, particularly in glaring light conditions.

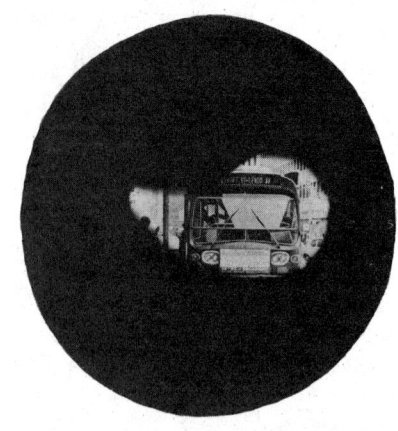

Glaucoma Advanced glaucoma involves loss of peripheral vision but the individual still retains most of his central vision.

Figure 50-13
Effects of cataract and glaucoma on vision. Photographs representing the eye diseases are done as if the camera were the right eye. (Photos courtesy of The Lighthouse, The New York Association for the Blind.)

Frequently in intracapsular extraction, a cryoprobe is used. *Cryosurgery* is a surgical technique in which freezing temperatures are used. All cryosurgical instruments operate on the principle that a cold metal adheres to a moist object. A thin, pencil-like instrument with a metal-probe tip (straight or curved) is activated so that the temperature of the tip ranges from −30°C to −40°C. The cryosurgical instrument is placed directly on the lens capsule. An ice ball forms in seconds, causing the capsule to adhere to the probe. A gentle upward and then sideward force frees and delivers the lens. The corneal flap is sutured back in place.

Extracapsular Extraction.   Extracapsular extraction is the removal of the nucleus, cortex, and only the anterior capsule. The posterior capsule is left intact. Often extracapsular extraction is done by *phacoemulsification.* This is the removal of the lens by a mechanized instrument that is composed of three systems: irrigation, ultrasonic vibration, and aspiration. As the titanium tip of the instrument vibrates 30,000 times per second, the lens is broken up into minute particles, which are then aspirated. The procedure is generally done under local anesthesia with the use of a microscope.

When the lens is removed, the eye is referred to as

Figure 50-14
Basic surgical techniques for cataract removal are the extracapsular method (*B*) and the intracapsular method (*C*), with normal eye anatomy shown in (*A*). During extracapsular extraction, the contents of the lens are removed but the posterior capsule is left intact, leaving a good site for attachment of an intraocular lens. During intracapsular extraction, both the lens contents and the capsular bag are removed entirely and an intraocular lens must be placed in the anterior chamber. The extracapsular method, perceived as safer and less prone to complications, is now the more popular. (Reproduced with permission from Patient Care, August 15, 1986. Copyright © 1986, Patient Care Communications, Inc., Darien, Connecticut. Artist: Paul J. Singh-Roy. All rights reserved.)

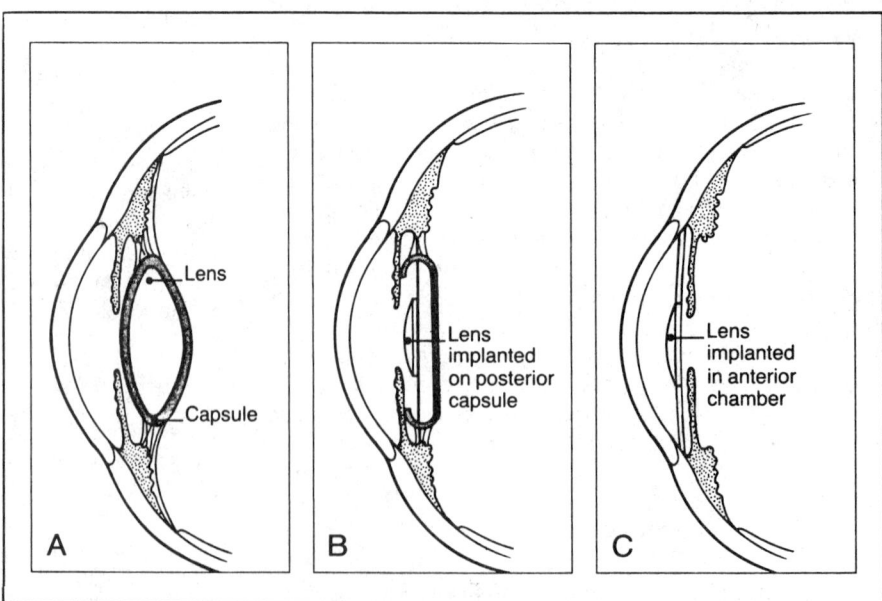

aphakic (lacking the lens) and has no accommodative power. Refractive ability is almost totally gone. Aphakia is corrected by thick eyeglasses, contact lenses, or an implanted intraocular lens. The thick eyeglasses have disadvantages, including an adjustment period that can be frustrating. Contact lenses are more effective, but they require manual dexterity to insert and remove. This kind of skill may be a problem for an older person. Far more popular and successful in its effectiveness is the use of the intraocular lens implant, which is incorporated at the time of lens extraction.

An *intraocular lens implant (IOL),* of which there are over 400 styles, is a prosthetic lens usually made of polymethylmethacrylate (PMMA) that is slipped into the vacated lens pocket and attached to surrounding tissues in an anatomically correct position. The chief advantage of this procedure is the minimal distortion in the size or shape of the image. The operation can be done under local anesthesia and can be completed in less than an hour.

More recent IOLs have built-in protection against ultraviolet light damage (a controversial complication) and contain a coating to reduce risk of damage to the cornea. Some of the newer types of IOLs can be folded or compressed before insertion to reduce the size of the incision through which it is slipped into place. A type of rubber may be used in the future, since it more closely resembles a natural lens. Enzymes are also being studied as a means of emptying the capsular area, followed by the injection of a substance that could function as a lens when it gels or semi-hardens.

In summary, the most successful type of surgery currently for a senile cataract is an implant following extracapsular cataract extraction with an intact posterior capsule. This membranous capsule supported the patient's own lens, and it now supports the artificial lens implant.

▶ Nursing Process
The Patient Undergoing Surgery for Cataract Removal

▷ *Assessment*

The nursing history of the patient with a cataract will focus on how the cataract has affected his life-style. Questions to be asked include the following: Describe how your vision has become impaired? How long have you noticed this change? What activities has your altered visual acuity affected (such as shopping in a store, watching television, driving a car, or close work such as hand crafts)?

What has the physician told you about treatment? Do you understand the nature of the proposed surgery? The nurse should elicit misconceptions and the psychological/sociological impact.

▷ *Nursing Diagnoses*

Based on the assessment data the nursing diagnoses for a patient undergoing surgery for cataract removal may include the following:

- Fear/depression related to sensory impairment and lack of understanding of the procedure

- Potential for trauma (preoperative) related to increasing vulnerability to injury/attack
- Potential for postoperative complications related to recent surgical intervention
- Visual sensory perception alteration related to adjustment to new lens

▷ *Planning and Implementation*

▷ *Goals:* The patient's major goals may include reduction of emotional stress, fear, and depression; prevention of ocular injury; avoidance of complications; and adjustment to altered visual status.

Preoperative Nursing Interventions

Reducing Preoperative Anxiety. Because this particular surgery can be performed safely on elderly persons, even those in their 90s, the nurse is in a position to dispel the belief that the patient may be "too old" for the procedure. Likewise, it is no longer necessary to lie immobile for days following surgery; one does not have to wait for treatment until the cataract is mature; thick eyeglasses are not the only means of assisting vision after cataract surgery. "Same-day" surgery has made all this possible. In the United States, more than 70% of all cataract surgery is performed in day-care settings. Clients can be encouraged that significant progress has been made that permits improved vision with minimal discomfort.

The nurse should be sure the patient understands the nature of surgery before he signs the "informed consent" form. He should know that it will be several weeks before the best visual result is realized. Usually the lens selected is designed to leave the patient slightly myopic since this facilitates reading vision. For distance vision, a pair of glasses may be required.

The patient is informed that a local anesthetic will be given in the operating room and that the injection may be uncomfortable at first but that this discomfort will abate quickly. The surgeon may converse with him during the procedure.

Further instruction includes such details as what to expect in the operating room: quiet conversation among the members of the surgical team, sounds of equipment being used, and frequent blood pressure checks. The patient needs to understand the importance of lying still during the procedure. After the operation, he is not to bend forward for extended periods of time. Lifting and strenuous activities are to be avoided. He is to report any pain, eye discharge, increased redness, or swelling around the eye.

Preventing Injury. Because of increasing impaired vision, the person with a cataract has a tendency to limit his activities and reduce his venturing out in the community. When he does, his hesitating steps make him more vulnerable to being pushed, shoved, or even attacked. To prevent bodily injury and additional ocular injury, it is important for the patient and his family to seek medical attention.

When he is to have surgery if he is hospitalized overnight, the patient is oriented to his room so that he will be familiar with his environment. In this way, he will avoid bumping into furniture or doors before and after surgery when his eye is bandaged.

Preoperative teaching stresses those activities and restrictions he will experience after the operation as well as what position he will be expected to maintain if he is kept in bed. He should know his eye will be patched, and he probably will require assistance when eating or going to the bathroom.

In some clinics a facial scrub is recommended the evening before and the morning of surgery in order to reduce pathogens and postoperative infection. Eyelashes may be cut using scissors with blades coated with petrolatum to which the lashes will adhere and not enter the patient's eye.

Preoperative Preparation.   Usually a sedative is prescribed the night before surgery and a clear liquid breakfast is taken the morning of the operation, depending on the time of day that the operation is scheduled. Preoperative medications in step-up fashion may be given in the morning, including a sedative, narcotic, and tranquilizer. Eye medications may include antibiotics, a topical mydriatic (which facilitates removal of the cataract when the pupil is dilated), and cycloplegic (to paralyze the muscles of accommodation). Medications may also be given to lower intraocular pressure (osmotic agents or carbonic anhydrous inhibitors). The patient should be informed of the possible diuretic action of these drugs.

In some clinics in the immediate preoperative period oculocompression (Honan balloon) is applied to soften the eye and enhance the spread of local anesthesia. Monitoring is done to maintain adequate pressure but not so much as to produce potential optic nerve decompensation.

Postoperative Nursing Interventions

Avoiding Complications.   Major goals of postoperative care of the cataract patient (excluding phacoemulsification) are to prevent hemorrhage and stress on the sutures. The eye is kept bandaged for 1 day, and an eye shield is worn over the dressing to protect the eye from injury. Only the operated eye is covered.

Atropine may be instilled postoperatively as prescribed to relieve pain. Pain is usually slight after cataract extraction, but should it become severe, the surgeon is to be notified since severe pain may be a symptom of a serious complication, such as hemorrhage.

Liquid diet is supplemented with custards, junkets, and gelatin. A soft or regular diet is resumed when desired. The effects of sensory deprivation can be minimized if the patient is kept interested in diversional activities, such as the radio,

---

Chart 50-2
Patient Education for Self-Care Following Cataract Surgery

Note: To be reviewed with patient or caregiver. Print directions in large letters using felt-tipped pen for strong contrast.

Activity Limitations

Permissible

- Watch television; read if necessary—use moderation.
- Do everything in moderation.
- At first "sponge baths"—later use tub or shower (with assistance).
- Wash hair in about 2 weeks; do not bend over sink or tub; tilt head slightly backward.
- Sleep with protective eyeshield (3 weeks); lie on back or side, not stomach.
- Sedentary activities—2 weeks.
- Wear sunglasses if soothing.

Avoid

- Rubbing the eyes; squeezing eyelids
- Straining at bowel movement
- Getting soap near eyes
- Lifting anything over 15 to 20 pounds
- Sexual relations until _____ (date)
- Driving, if possible
- Bending head down below waist; bend knees only and keep back straight to pick up something from the floor.

Medications and Eye Care

- Wash hands before and after instilling eye medications.
- Clean around eye with sterile cotton balls or gauze sponges moistened with sterile water (Eye Stream); wipe lid gently from inner corner to outer corner.
- To instill eye drops, be seated and tilt head back; gently pull down lower lid margin.
- At follow-up visit, take all eye medications so that dosages can be checked and adjusted.

Report Unusual Signs and Symptoms

- Eye pain in and around eyes
- Changes in visual acuity, blurring diplopia, a film over visual field, light flashes, showers of spots before eyes
- Persistent headaches
- Inflammation, discharge from eyes

"talking books," or visitors. Any signs of decreased vision may be due to hemorrhage, infection, corneal edema, or corneal scarring and must be reported.

Complications following an intraocular lens implant may occur at any time, even years later. Any visual changes must be reported, including loss of corneal clarity, bleeding, retinal detachment, and signs of glaucoma.

Patient Education.   Teaching points emphasized by the nurse are summarized in Chart 50-2.

▷ *Evaluation*

▷ *Expected Outcomes*

1. Patient copes with psychosocial adjustment required to treat a cataract.

   Preoperatively:

   a. Accepts the progressive nature of cataract development and the need to have the treatment.
   b. Discusses his condition and the need for surgery
   c. Asks direct questions relating to mobility during the postoperative phase

   Postoperatively:

   a. Describes activities that he can or cannot do immediately following surgery.
   b. Participates in stress-relieving experiences.
   c. Relates a positive attitude that reveals optimistic thinking.
2. Prevents ocular injury
   a. Limits eye activity before and immediately after surgery.
   b. Adheres to proper head positioning until instructed to elevate and move head.
   c. Avoids bending at the waist for prescribed number of days/weeks.
   d. Takes precautions to avoid colds (sneezing, coughing) and lifting in order keep ocular pressure from rising.
3. Takes precautions to avoid complications
   a. Recites the precautions he must take to ensure optimum vision.
   b. Keeps fingers and tissue wipes away from eye (it is expected eye will tear, blur, or itch because of reaction to sutures).
   c. Asks for sunglasses when eye patch is removed (because of sensitivity to light).
   d. Washes hands before and after treating eye.
   e. Instills eye drops as prescribed and as taught.
   f. Demonstrates effective technique in keeping periorbital area clean, including eyelashes.
4. Adjusts to altered visual status.
   a. Adapts to the changes required, such as using eyeglasses or contact lenses.
   b. Indicates the range of vision possibilities with his "new lenses."
   c. Describes the widened scope of activities that he can now pursue.
   d. Relates an understanding of the need for follow-up visits to the physician and ophthalmologist.

Care of the patient with a cataract is outlined in Nursing Care Plan 50-1, pp. 1360–1361.

Glaucoma

Glaucoma is a condition characterized by increased tension or pressure within the eye causing progressive structural or functional damage to the eye. If unchecked, it may lead to blindness. Medication will not cure glaucoma but can keep it under control. Surgery is often curative.

Classification.   The following is a simplied classification of glaucoma:

1. Adult primary glaucoma
   a. Open angle (chronic simple, simple)
   b. Closed angle (narrow angle, angle-closure)
2. Congenital glaucoma—see pediatric or ophthalmology texts.
3. Secondary glaucoma—this is related to such conditions as trauma, aphakia, iritis, tumor, and hemorrhage

Adult Primary (Open Angle) Glaucoma

The cause of primary glaucoma is unknown. Some evidence indicates that chronic simple glaucoma, the most common form, is inherited. This disorder is the second most common cause of blindness in the United States. In view of the fact that about 1 million Americans have undiagnosed glaucoma, health care professionals have a responsibility to encourage annual eye checkups, because *early detection could substantially reduce the incidence of blindness from glaucoma.*

Pathophysiology.   The total volume and pressure of intraocular fluid is regulated by the balance between the formation and reabsorption of aqueous humor. Ordinarily, the pressure-regulating mechanism maintains an almost constant balance throughout life. The exact action of this mechanism is not known; however, pathologic changes at the iridocorneal angle prevent the usual outflow of aqueous humor through the *trabecular meshwork* (connective tissue with perforations that permit fluid to pass through) to a tubular structure, the *canal of Schlemm,* and into the venous system. As a result, intraocular pressure is increased (Fig. 50-15, p. 1362). Early detection of increased ocular pressure (22 to 30 mm Hg) does not necessarily mean that the patient will develop frank glaucoma.

Apparently, both physical and emotional factors are involved in increasing pressure within the eye. The underlying mechanism is episcleral (overlying the sclera) venous pressure engorgement transmitted by the Valsalva phenomenon. That is, intraocular pressure increases when the patient exerts energy, as in climbing the stairs, bending over to pick up an object, sneezing, or even turning the head suddenly. It also occurs in relation to emotional upsets (*e.g.,* apprehension about the nature of prognosis of surgery may cause an increase in pressure).

Clinical Manifestations

Symptoms are insidious and develop slowly. The patient may have mild discomfort, such as a tired feeling in the eye, trouble in focusing, and headache. Impairment of peripheral vision occurs long before any effects on central vision are noted. The patient may become aware of peripheral visual impairment by bumping into things that he did not see at his side.

Nursing Care Plan 50-1

Care of the Patient With a Cataract

Nursing Interventions	Rationale	Expected Outcomes

Nursing Diagnosis: Fear/depression related to sensory impairment and lack of understanding

Goal: Reduction of emotional stress, fear, and depression; acceptance of surgery

1. Determine patient's concerns; encourage conversation and allay fears.	1. When the patient finds answers to his fears, he is more likely to accept treatment willingly.	• Tells of feeling better now that he understands more of the plan of treatment
2. Begin rehabilitation measures as soon after admission as possible:	2. Early understanding of the total plan facilitates patient cooperation in each phase of that plan.	• Reviews the projected plan with his spouse
a. Have him explain how he administers his eyedrops; correct any problems.		• Demonstrates correct method of instilling eyedrops
b. Review overall program of events so that in general he knows what to expect.		• Practices how to close his eyes without squeezing the lids
3. Orient patient to his new surroundings.	3. Familiarity with surroundings helps allay fears.	• Asks questions about the various preoperative preparatory measures
4. Instruct the patient about the medications he is to have prior to surgery, the dietary limitations, and physical preparation.	4. Being a knowledgeable participant in preoperative preparation will assist him in relaxing with understanding.	• Relaxes comfortably with soft music on the radio

Nursing Diagnosis: Potential for trauma (preoperative) related to increasing vulnerability to injury/attack

Goal: Prevention of ocular injury/infection

1. Inform the patient that insidious changes take place as the cataract develops that diminishes vision.	1. Preparation of the patient to understand his limitations will help him to avoid accidents.	• Elects to give up driving his car because of peripheral vision changes
		• Uses a cane for added support when walking
		• Ensures that corridors and stairways are well lighted

(continued)

Driving a car may be a hazard to others because of an inability to see pedestrians or vehicles approaching from the side. The patient may also note halos around lights.

Diagnostic Evaluation and Measurement of Intraocular Pressure

An increase in intraocular pressure or hardening of the eyeball may be noted with the fingers, but more accurately it is measured by means of tonometry, tonography, and peripheral vision testing. *Tonometry* is a simple and painless test in which the patient tilts his head back and looks to the ceiling (Fig. 50-16). The cornea of the eye is anesthetized with a drop of 0.5% proparacaine. The sterile footplate of the tonometer is placed on the cornea, and a small pressure is applied to the central plunger, causing the central cornea to be displaced inward. Pressure within the eye exerts a force that moves an indicator. A normal reading is 11 to 22 mm Hg.

Electronic tonometry measures the force required to flatten the central cornea (by air, using an applanation tonometer). In this method the instrument does not touch the eye. Applanation tonometry is more sensitive in measuring eye pressure than the Schiotz tonometer described above and is performed with a sophisticated and expensive instrument.

Gonioscopy is the direct visualization of the anterior chamber angle. Local anesthesia is used. The examiner places a goniolens over the cornea. Sterile saline solution is injected

Nursing Interventions	*Rationale*	*Expected Outcomes*

Nursing Diagnosis: Potential for trauma (preoperative) related to increasing vulnerability to injury/attack

Goal: Prevention of ocular injury/infection

2. Impress on the patient his vulnerability when walking alone along the street when it is poorly lighted.	2. The risks an elderly person with impaired vision might sustain include potential for falling, stumbling, and being attacked.	• Tells of his decision to be accompanied by someone when it is necessary to leave his home

Nursing Diagnosis: Potential postoperative complications related to recent surgical intervention

Goal: Avoidance of complications

1. Reduce conjunctival bacterial count by using aseptic technique in eye treatments and broad-spectrum antibiotics as prescribed.	1. Minimizing opportunities for infection will enhance the healing process.	• Adheres to appropriate treatment measures including avoidance of touching eyes with fingers
2. Prevent tension on the suture line by avoiding stressful causes such as bending at the waist and coughing forcefully.	2. Bending at the waist, lifting heavy objects, and strong sneezing or coughing produce increased pressure and strain on the eye.	• Avoids stressful movements; controls the force of sneezing or coughing.

Nursing Diagnosis: Visual sensory alterations related to adjustment to new lens

Goal: Adjustment to altered visual status

1. Encourage patient to become independent.
  a. Teach him to increase his activities gradually.
  b. Walk with him when he gets out of bed.
	1. Nursing support provides opportunity for determining current limitations and how they can be overcome.	• Rises from his bed slowly and maneuvers carefully
		• Avoids straining his eyes by limiting his reading and watching of television

2. Refer patient to appropriate agencies if home assistance is needed.	2. Resources are available for home health services, escort services, and companion services.	• Calls community nursing agency for their suggestions in meeting some of his needs
3. Teach patient what signs and symptoms need to be heeded and reported.	3. An understanding of possible occurrences that require professional assistance will permit early attention and avoidance of severe complications.	• Relates the signs that need to be reported to a member of the health care team should such signs occur

between the cornea and the lens. The examiner uses a microscope and illuminating source to view the contents of the anterior chamber, particularly the anterior chamber angle.

Management

Treatment depends on the stage of the condition, the degree of the reduced angle between the iris and the cornea, the response to medication, and the reliability of the patient in adhering to the regimen. In general, pharmacotherapy can keep the condition under control.

    Pharmacotherapy.   Primary (open-angle) glaucoma is often treated by one or a combination of the following medications:

• Miotics, such as pilocarpine, increase outflow of aqueous humor.
• Timolol maleate (Timoptic), a β-adrenergic receptor blocking agent, is popular for the treatment of primary open-angle glaucoma, aphakic glaucoma, and, in selected patients, secondary glaucoma. It appears to be better tolerated than previously used drugs. When applied topically, timolol decreases production of aqueous humor and reduces intraocular pressure for as long as 24 hours. Pupillary size is not changed, and the tone of the ciliary body is not altered; hence, this medication does not interfere with vision. In some patients, timolol may cause palpitations and tachycardia and the nurse must be alert for these manifestations.

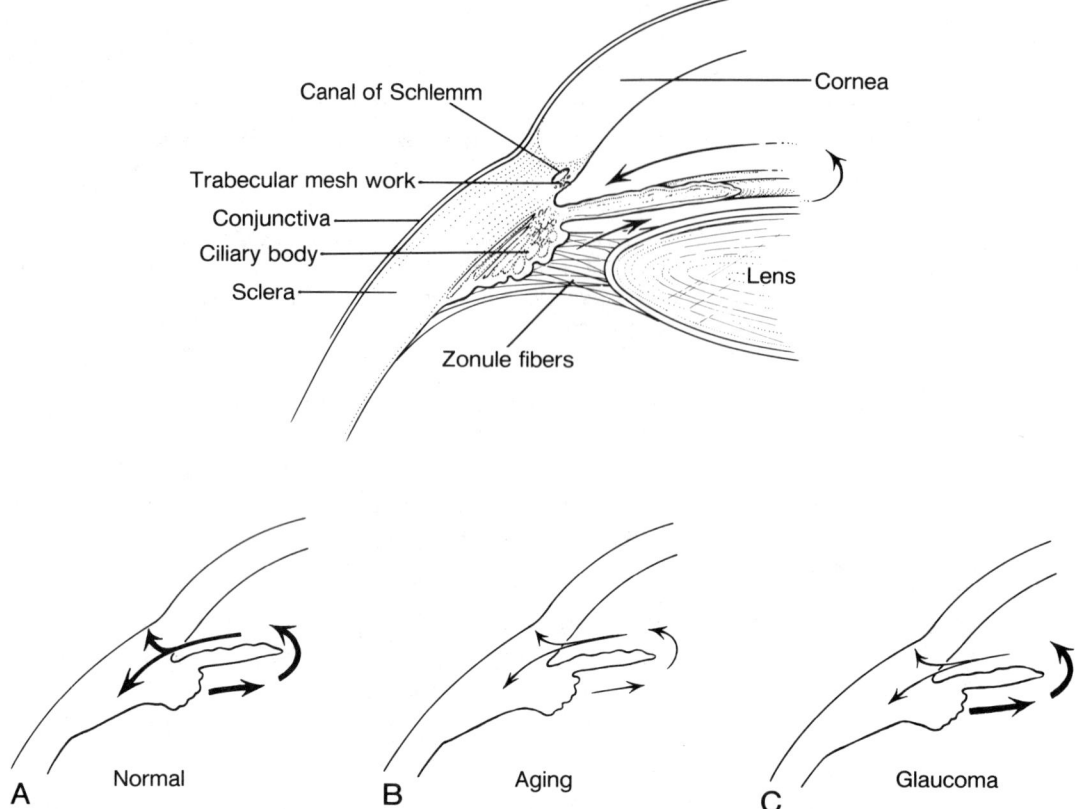

Figure 50-15

Effects of aging and of glaucoma on secretion of aqueous humor. Normal anatomy is identified in the upper illustration. (*A*) Arrows indicate the secretion of aqueous humor from the ciliary body to the posterior chamber, through the pupil into the anterior chamber, and out through the trabecular meshwork to the canal of Schlemm and then into the venous system. (*B*) The same pathway is followed in the aging person, except that the amount of fluid is less. (*C*) In glaucoma, more fluid enters the anterior chamber than leaves it. This accounts for hardness of the eyeball due to the increase of pressure.

Drug dosage of timolol is usually one drop twice a day. Occasionally, mild eye irritation or brief blurring of vision occurs with timolol. This medication is prescribed with caution for patients who may have adverse effects from systemic use of β-adrenergic receptor blocking agents (such as patients with asthma, heart block, or heart failure).

- Carbonic anhydrase inhibitors, such as acetazolamide (Diamox), can decrease the production of aqueous humor.
- Anticholinesterases, such as echothiophate iodide (Phospholine Iodide) or demecarium bromide (Humorsol), can facilitate the outflow of aqueous humor.
- Epinephrine drops decrease production of aqueous humor and promote its outflow from the eye.

Surgical Management

Surgical treatment may consist of corneal trephining, trabeculectomy, or laser or argon laser trabeculoplasty.

Corneal Trephining and Trabeculectomy. In corneal trephining, the surgeon uses a circular knife to make a small opening at the junction of the cornea and the sclera through which aqueous humor can drain. The opening is permanent and is usually covered by a flap of conjunctiva. In trabeculectomy, a small fistula or opening is made into the anterior chamber at the junction (limbus) of the cornea and sclera, allowing aqueous humor to flow into the subconjunctival space.

Nursing Considerations. One major risk in these surgical procedures is endophthalmitis, an inflammation of the internal structure of the eye due to infection. To prevent infection, meticulous care must be taken when administering eye medications or when touching the eyes.

Since the patient has undergone surgery in which general anesthesia is usually required, the nurse must monitor vital signs and the intravenous infusions and provide comfort measures and pain control as the patient emerges from the anesthesia. To prevent blood from entering the anterior chamber following a trabeculectomy, the patient's head is elevated or the patient is placed in a sitting position as soon as possible following recovery from anesthesia. An eye shield is worn during the hospital stay. At the time of discharge, the patient is instructed to wear the eye shield at night for 3 to 4 weeks.

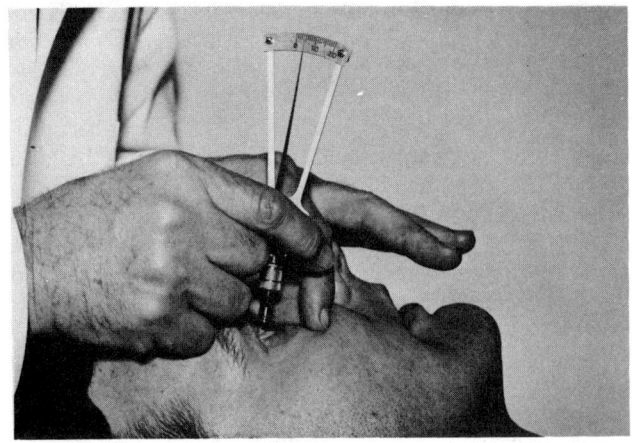

Figure 50-16
Tonometry. After a local anesthetic is instilled into the eye, the Schiotz tonometer is gently rested on the eyeball, the indicator measures the ocular tension in millimeters of mercury. (Courtesy of F. H. Roy, M.D.)

Laser Trabeculoplasty or Argon Laser Trabeculoplasty. In these two procedures, referred to as LTP or ALT, a narrow laser beam (usually blue-green argon) is focused on the trabecular meshwork of an open angle, resulting in a nonpenetrating burn that changes the meshwork pattern and facilitates drainage of the aqueous humor. Laser trabeculoplasty is a painless outpatient procedure that may have to be done several times to lower eye pressure. Meanwhile the patient continues using his eye drop prescription and possibly steroid eye drops to control inflammation. With primary open-angle glaucoma, the success rate of this procedure is about 80%; it is less effective with other types of glaucoma.

Acute Closed-Angle Glaucoma

Acute closed-angle glaucoma is the sudden building up of intraocular pressure (within ½ to 1 hour) due to a complete blockage of the filtering angle caused by a bunching up of the iris (Fig. 50-17*B*). This is an emergency situation, which, if left untreated, may lead to blindness. *Note:* Acute closed-angle glaucoma may be precipitated in patients who have narrow anterior chamber angles by administering anticholinergic drugs such as atropine and scopolamine.

Clinical Manifestations

When pressure increases rapidly, severe pain occurs in and around the eye (periocular). Artificial lights appear to have a rainbow around them, and vision becomes cloudy or blurred. The eye is red and the cornea is steamy; nausea and vomiting, as well as pupil dilatation may be noted. Intraocular pressure is elevated; as the pressure rises, the retinal artery is compressed, reducing nutrition to the eye. This can cause retinal and corneal atrophy.

Diagnostic Evaluation

Intraocular pressure is measured, and the angle between the involved cornea and the iris is observed with a gonioscope. Pressure above 22 mm Hg is suggestive of an early form of glaucoma. A tight or closed angle condition causes the pressure to increase in excess of 50 mm Hg.

Management

Treatment is principally surgical and is discussed below. However, prior to surgery, medications may be requested by the ophthalmologist. Miotic drugs will cause the pupil to con-

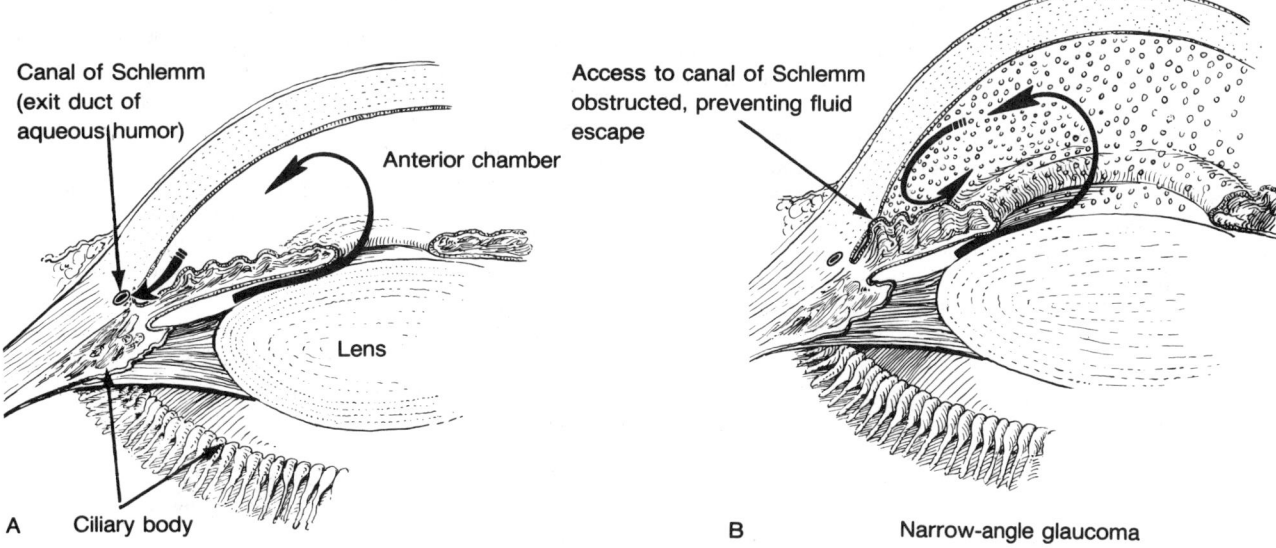

Canal of Schlemm
(exit duct of
aqueous humor)

Anterior chamber

Lens

A   Ciliary body

Access to canal of Schlemm
obstructed, preventing fluid
escape

B   Narrow-angle glaucoma

Figure 50-17
Obstruction of flow of aqueous fluid in glaucoma. (*A*) Normal flow of aqueous fluid through canal of Schlemm. (*B*) Obstruction to the flow of fluid, causing closed-angle glaucoma. (Lechliger M and Moya F. Introduction to the Practice of Anesthesia, 2nd ed. New York, Harper & Row.)

tract and the iris to draw away from the cornea, thus allowing the aqueous humor to drain through the lymph spaces into the canal of Schlemm. Pilocarpine or timolol maleate (Timoptic) may also be prescribed. Dosage and frequency of drops are regulated to meet individual requirements.

Carbonic anhydrase inhibitors restrict the action of the enzyme that is necessary to produce aqueous humor. Acetazolamide is an example of such an agent. Decreased production of aqueous humor aids in improving some patients' conditions before surgery and may control intraocular tension in other patients to such an extent that surgery may not be necessary.

Ordinary USP glycerin given orally reduces intraocular pressure through the mechanism of osmotic balance exchange. Glycerol 50% also administered orally has a high osmotic pressure; it withdraws fluid from the eye through the membrane and lowers pressure. Mannitol 20% may be used intravenously.

Surgical Management

For surgical intervention, an incision is made through the cornea so that a portion of the iris may be drawn out and excised (*peripheral iridectomy*). An iridectomy prevents the iris from bulging forward to crowd the chamber angle and permits drainage of aqueous humor from the anterior chamber, thereby reducing intraocular tension. With surgery there is a risk of hemorrhage and infection that must be monitored by the nurse.

Argon laser beam surgery is an alternative treatment; it burns the iris and has the same effect as an iridectomy. This is often a preferred treatment because it avoids an incision, is relatively painless, and is done under topical anesthesia on an outpatient basis.

About 30 minutes before laser treatment, pilocarpine eye drops are administered to prevent further iris contraction. Proparacaine is applied topically to permit placement of a fundus contact lens (this keeps the lid open during the treatment). There is little discomfort during the delivery of laser beams. The patient will be seated during the treatment, resting his chin in a chin rest as the ophthalmologist instructs him to focus on a fixed point.

Following treatment there may be headache and blurring of the vision, which disappears after 24 hours. Discomfort is controlled with an analgesic. Topical steroids may be prescribed to reduce inflammation. An eye patch may be comfortable for a few hours. The patient is instructed to have someone drive him home after the treatment. If necessary, these treatments are repeated in 1 or 2 weeks.

▶ Nursing Process
The Patient With Glaucoma

▷ Assessment

The nursing history is important in evaluating the patient with glaucoma because there are several kinds of glaucoma with differing symptoms. Also it is common knowledge that untreated glaucoma can lead to blindness. All patients need to be aware of the seriousness of the condition. Through a nurs-

ing history, the nurse is able to determine the patient's understanding about glaucoma and his awareness that with conscientious adherence to the treatment plan this condition can be controlled.

The nurse determines how long the patient has had glaucoma and what he understands about the problem. Does he have mild or extensive discomfort, difficulty focusing, problems with peripheral vision, cloudy or blurred vision, or halos around lights? Does he have frequent headaches, nausea, and vomiting? Are his eyes red? Is there a steamy cornea and signs of infection? Does he complain that the eyeball feels hard or is painful?

▷ Nursing Diagnoses

Based on the assessment data, the patient's major nursing diagnoses may include the following:

- Alteration in visual sensory perception related to progressive nature of glaucoma
- Alteration in comfort; pain related to increasing pressure within the eye
- Anxiety/fear related to possible or actual loss of vision
- Self-care deficit related to impaired vision
- Potential social isolation related to fear of injury which may further complicate his visual problem

▷ Planning and Implementation

▷ *Goals:* The major goals of the patient may include control of the condition of glaucoma by whatever means are necessary, relief of pain and discomfort, realistic adaptation to treatment measures and reduction of anxieties, resumption of responsibility for his own care to the best of his ability, and participation in social activities within the constraints of his limitations.

Nursing Interventions

Relieving Pain. Early in the onset of glaucoma there is little discomfort, but as the condition progresses, with degenerative changes of the trabecular meshwork, more fluid enters the anterior chamber than leaves. Fluid accumulation "hardens" the eye and exerts pressure on the optic nerve, which causes discomfort. The patient is reminded that relief can be obtained by conscientiously using the prescribed eye drops. The technique in using these drops may need to be reviewed for effectiveness. Any habits that might cause an infection must be corrected.

Since emotional upsets, anger, fear, or excitement can cause increased intraocular pressure, emotional stress needs to be minimized. Therefore, maintaining a calm atmosphere can help to keep eye discomfort under control. Excessive straining or lifting is also to be avoided.

The patient is cautioned to use only the medication prescribed; if he accidentally uses the wrong eye drops, it could have adverse effects.

Promoting Self-Care Measures. Support systems are important for the patient with glaucoma. He and his family should be aware of the necessity of administering eye medications regularly. Although this will not cure the problem, it will keep it under control. He is told of the side-effects of his medication, and his ability to read labels, particularly those of his medications, is checked. The nurse discusses with him the nature of all treatments and the role he plays in keeping his condition under control. She encourages his questions and anticipates his fears so that they can be addressed.

When vision is blurred, there is a tendency not to be as particular about one's appearance. All who contact this patient can encourage him to use all his resources and can compliment him when he does well. He is encouraged to maintain proper eating habits and to participate in activities that he enjoys.

The patient is assisted in modifying his environment so that it will be safe; light fixtures can be placed where they will do the most good. Advice to suit a patient's particular needs in caring for himself can be individualized, and assistance can be provided if he is unable to manage his own care.

Patient Education and Home Health Care. Ineffective coping related to knowledge deficit can be averted by teaching and repeating the basic fundamentals of care. The need to be consistent in administering eye medications must be reemphasized even though the patient may feel all right and see no need to continue (nor even note any benefit). The nurse can discuss with him the need for periodic checkups with his ophthalmologist and can review his life-style and assist him in making adaptations if necessary.

Although glaucoma cannot be cured, it can be controlled to a great extent. Whether the patient has had surgery or not, certain limitations must be set.

Activities that may increase intraocular pressure and should be avoided are

- Excessive fluid intake
- Use of antihistamines or sympathomimetic medications without proper medical supervision

A *recommended activity* is carrying a card or Medic Alert tag indicating that the individual has glaucoma.

Eye drops are an essential part of the treatment of a patient with glaucoma. It is imperative that fresh eye drops be used and that they be administered consistently.

Promoting Social Activities. The patient is encouraged to contact family, relatives, or friends to be available when he needs company or assistance. If arrangements can be made to have someone accompany him when shopping in order to read labels on the shelves and carry heavier packages, this can be of significant help. Whatever can be suggested to prevent isolation will help to keep his condition under control; brooding, worry, and isolation will aggravate his problem by increasing intraocular pressure.

▷ *Evaluation*

▷ *Expected Outcomes*

1. Patient reports that pain and discomfort are relieved/controlled.
   a. Uses prescribed eyedrops regularly, with proper technique.
   b. Avoids or manages stress.
   c. Avoids straining or lifting.
2. Increases self-care skills.
   a. Makes use of family support systems.
   b. Maintains personal grooming.
   c. Takes part in modifying the environment for safety and efficiency.
3. Maintains social contacts with family and friends.

Gerontological Considerations

Most patients with glaucoma are in the older age-group. Often dimming vision is accepted as part of the aging process and medical assistance is not sought. Therefore, as part of the physical examination of anyone over age 65, tonometry should be recommended and eye pressure periodically checked thereafter. The major problem of patients with glaucoma is the tendency to stop taking eye drops, claiming "it doesn't help." However, it keeps glaucoma from worsening. To stop medication means that glaucoma will continue insidiously until the patient is blind. Other problems of aging such as arthritis, aloneness and depression, constipation (straining on defecation), and potential for falling/accidents have a direct affect on glaucoma.

Blindness or Near Blindness

Telescopic eyeglasses and magnifying glasses are easily accessible aids that can be recommended by the nurse for those who have exhausted conventional prescribed lenses.

Mobility aids are probably the most basic need for the visually impaired. One needs reassurance that he can move safely from one place to the next. Only about 1% of the blind use guide dogs—probably the reason is that most sightless persons are over age 65, and they are less trusting of dogs and may even have difficulty keeping up with them. The most useful aid is a long, lightweight cane that very subtly provides accurate information by simple maneuvers and ensures that the next step is safe in a small, limited area. Overhead hazards are not detected, however.

Other aids are available to supplement the cane in enlarging the world of the visually impaired person. A flashlight eye sonar device (Morvat Sensor*) emits ultrasound waves that bounce back from objects up to 3.66 meters (4 yards) away. A Sonicguide* has its transmitter and receivers built into an eyeglass frame. An earphone piece converts sound into a different pitch, loudness, and tone. The lower the pitch, the closer the object. Quality of tone enables the wearer to distinguish surface characteristics—glass, concrete, or wooden walls. Interpretation can be a problem. Recent research is attempting to use the sonar focusing element in the Polaroid camera into a mobility device that minimizes sonic confusion.

Laser canes are also available. A particular model sends out three beams: straight ahead, at head level, and in front of the feet. When an object crosses a beam, the user is warned by hearing a buzzing sound. Such sophisticated devices unfortunately are expensive at present.

For reading (work, study, leisure), a portable electronic magnifying system is available. In this system, one moves a small hand-held camera across the page and then views on

---

* Sensory Aids Corporation, Bensenville, Illinois.

a display screen a bright magnified image of the text (View-scan by Wormald).

Additional aids are telescopic lenses (Honey Bee lens†, a bug-eyed arrangement), glasses combined with mirrors, nightscopes, closed-circuit TV cameras, and fiberoptic systems. By being aware of these possibilities, the nurse is able to recommend invaluable aids to the person with such a need.

Enucleation

Removal of the eyeball, enucleation, is necessitated by a variety of factors, including trauma that forces the contents of the globe to escape, infections, and other injuries that threaten to lead to sympathetic ophthalmia (see p. 1350). During the removal of the eye, muscles are cut as close to the globe as possible. These muscles are approximated with sutures over a plastic prosthesis, thereby providing the means for coordinated motion of the prosthesis with the patient's real eye. A plastic, gold, or Teflon ball is placed in the area of the removed eyeball to form a stump on which the ocularist fixes the prosthesis (artificial eye). This prosthesis is colored to match the patient's eye. In successful cases, it is difficult to distinguish the prosthesis from the normal eye.

In certain cases, the sclera can be retained and the rest of the contents of the eye "scooped" out; this procedure is known as *evisceration*. The main advantage of evisceration is that it provides better motion to the artificial eye. The disadvantage is that sympathetic ophthalmia may occur.

Exenteration is usually performed in advanced malignancy or severe war injuries. In this procedure, the eyelids, the eyeball, and all contents of the orbit are removed, down to the bone. This operation is *very* disfiguring, and although the ocularist may attempt to build a prosthesis, it very often appears rather poor and unlifelike. These patients usually wear a black patch.

The Newly Blind

The number of blind people in the world is estimated at 28 million, only 6% of whom live in the developed countries. There are about 550,000 legally blind persons in America, and 1.5 million who are severely visually impaired. Of the newly blind cases, it is known that a significant number could have been prevented with our present knowledge.

When a patient has marked visual impairment or is newly blind, he needs a great deal of help in making a healthy adjustment. For the most part, this help is entrusted to those skilled in such rehabilitation. However, a nurse can follow certain practices when caring for such a patient.

The nurse recognizes that there are stages through which this person moves:

1. *Denial*—Do not discredit this phase of the sightless person's experience, since it is a stage through which the person must go.

† Vision, New York, New York.

2. *Value changes*—adapting to aids that he thought he would never use
3. *Independence–dependence conflict*—attempting to accept his place without becoming completely dependent
4. *Coping with stigma*—This person must adjust to unfortunate stigma that is so prevalent among the sighted toward the sightless, such as they are "helpless," "unemployable," "completely dependent," or "depressed."
5. *Learning to communicate* in social settings without visual cues

Goals. The major goals for the patient are to accept the sightless or nearly sightless condition:

1. Adaptation to the use of auxiliary aids
2. Acceptance of his new visual role without becoming completely dependent
3. Continuing with physical self-care
4. Coping with the social climate and stigmata that are prevalent
5. Learning to communicate without visual clues
6. Adherence to the prescribed therapeutic regimen

Nursing Interventions

The nurse is able to assist the patient in several ways: (1) patient teaching, (2) patient support, (3) patient care, and (4) collaboration with the physician.

Patient teaching is done to familiarize the patient with the anatomy of the eye and its function. By monitoring what the physician has told the patient relative to diagnosis, anticipated treatment, and prognosis, the nurse is able to reinforce this information, answer questions, provide support, and relay back to the ophthalmologist the reaction of the patient and his family. If information is withheld, such as little hope for recovery of vision, this will interfere with the patient's adjustment and rehabilitation. The nurse is often helpful in determining when the time is right for conveying such information. Fears are to be described because they can unearth misinformation. Frequently, self-imposed limitations are more restricting than physical disabilities, such as blindness. Even attitudes and beliefs of the nurse can have a direct or indirect effect on the patient. Such attitudes need to be confronted so that only genuine feelings are transmitted. A positive attitude by those who care for patients will affect the patient's self-esteem and body image in a beneficial way.

A blind person should always be treated with the dignity accorded any other person. Expressions of pity are to be avoided. The patient can be kept from becoming discouraged by seeing to it that he has someone with whom he can talk or that he has some other form of diversion, such as the radio. He can be helped to overcome his feeling of awkwardness as he performs simple activities.

If he is allowed out of bed, the blind person should survey his room by walking around and touching the furniture. Thereafter, the nurse should be sure that the furniture remains in the same position. Never leave a door half open; it should be either open or shut. When walking with a blind person, allow him to follow you by lightly touching your elbow, do not push him ahead of you. When he walks alone, he should learn to use a lightweight walking stick to warn him of obstacles.

Personal appearance is a significant part of the patient's care. He should be allowed to dress by himself; a woman even can learn to fix her hair and use cosmetics. Activities such as table etiquette and writing can be acquired with practice.

Familiarity with resources that are available to help the patient is a nursing responsibility. When a patient is declared legally blind, he should be referred to the state blindness agency. A directory of agencies serving the visually handicapped in the United States is available from the American Foundation for the Blind. In most states, the only way to obtain rehabilitation training is through a state agency for the blind. Other resources are "Seeing Eye," and state libraries for the blind, which provide prerecorded magazines and books, Talking Book machines, and cassettes.

Interesting and effective aids are devices that "talk," such as clocks, calculators, thermometers, and scales. There also is an optical scanner that when passed over lines of text in a book send signals to a computer (programmed to recognize letters) that turns them into words and pronounces them. Another similar device scans words and records the shape of letters, which are then converted into vibrations felt by the fingertips of the user.

Technology continues to provide devices that are becoming available and useful in expanding the world of the sightless.

Bibliography

Books

Boyd-Monk H. Nursing Care of the Eye. East Norwalk, Connecticut, Appleton & Lange, 1987.

Doxanas MT and Anderson RL. Clinical Orbital Anatomy. Baltimore, Williams & Wilkins, 1984.

Emery JM and McIntyre DJ. Extracapsular Cataract Surgery. St Louis, CV Mosby, 1983.

Engelstein JM (ed). Cataract Surgery. New York, Grune & Stratton, 1984.

Fraunfelder FT and Roy FH. Current Ocular Therapy, 2nd ed. Philadelphia, WB Saunders, 1985.

Gittinger JW Jr. Ophthalmology. Boston, Little, Brown & Co, 1984.

Jaffe NS. Cataract Surgery and Its Complications, 3rd ed. St Louis, CV Mosby, 1983.

Jakobiec FA and Sigelman L. Advanced Techniques in Ocular Surgery, Philadelphia, WB Saunders, 1984.

Koch DD et al. Adverse Effects of Contact Lens Wear: An Atlas for the Ophthalmic Practitioner. Thorofare, New Jersey, Charles B Slack, 1983.

Luntz MH, Harrison R, and Schenker HI. Glaucoma Surgery. Baltimore, Williams & Wilkins, 1984.

Mackety CJ. Perioperative Laser Nursing: A Practical Guide. Thorofare, New Jersey, Charles B Slack, 1984.

Pavan-Langston D. Manual of Ocular Diagnosis and Therapy, 2nd ed. Boston, Little, Brown & Co, 1985.

Smith JF and Machazel DP. Ophthalmologic Nursing. Boston, Little, Brown & Co, 1980.

Spoor TC (ed). Medical Management of Ocular Diseases. Thorofare, New Jersey, Charles B Slack, 1984.

Trokel SL. YAG Laser Ophthalmic Microsurgery. Norwalk, Connecticut, Appleton-Century-Crofts, 1983.

Tuttle DW. Self-esteem and Adjusting With Blindness. Springfield, Illinois, Charles C Thomas, 1984.

Vaughan D and Asbury T. General Ophthalmology. Los Altos, California, Lange Medical Publications, 1983.

Wybar K and Muir MK. Ophthalmology, 3rd ed. Philadelphia, WB Saunders, 1983.

Yanoff M. Ocular Pathology, 2nd ed. Philadelphia, JB Lippincott, 1985.

Articles

General Articles

Boyd-Monk H. Cardinal positions of gaze. Nurs '86 1986 Feb; 16(2):25–26.

Brown GC. Retinal vascular diseases. Occup Health Nurs 1983 Aug; 31(8):17–20.

Dean AF. The aging surgical patient: Historical overview, implications, and nursing care. Periop Nurs Q 1987 Mar; 3(1):1–7.

Fyfe J and Ellerbroek D. Colour vision defects and the school nurse. Nurs Times 1984 June 27; 80(26):48–49.

Giarratana CM. Reach out . . . reach out and touch Henry. Nurs '84 1984 Feb; 14(2):47–48.

Kirn TF. Simple techniques and eye drop penetration. JAMA 1987 Feb 27; 257(8):1027–1028.

McIntyre DJ. Ambulatory ophthalmic surgery in the Medicare age group. Geriatr Ophthalmol 1986 Mar/Apr; 2(2):42–44.

Roberts AM and Leibowitz HM. Corticosteroid therapy of ophthalmologic disease. Hosp Pract 1984 Feb; 19(2):181–196.

Schneider HA and Easterlin MN. Trachoma: Ophthalmic crisis of the third world. J Ophthalmol Nurs Tech 1984 Jan/Feb; 3(1):11–12.

Schremp PS. Discharge instructions: Providing continuity of care of ophthalmic patients. J Ophthalmol Nurs Tech 1985 Mar/Apr; 4(2):30–33.

Schultz PJ and Fortin SL. Corneal transplant. J. Ophthalmol Nurs Tech 1986 Jan/Feb; 5(1):4–7.

Sheehan KM. Ophthalmic plastic and reconstructive surgery. Today's OR Nurse 1985 Jan; 7(1):12–16.

Todd B. Using eye drops and ointments safely. Geriatr Nurs 1983 Jan/Feb; 4(1):53, 56–57.

Assessment

Bensinger RE. Precautions RE. Precautions in dilating pupils. J Ophthalmol Nurs Tech 1984 Jan/Feb; 3(1):19–21.

Boyd-Monk H. How to use a direct ophthalmoscope. Occup Health Nurs 1983 Aug; 31(8):13–16.

Budassi SA. Ophthalmic examinations. JEN 1984 Mar/Apr; 10(2):112–114.

Garber N. Testing monocular vision loss. J Ophthalmol Nurs Tech 1986 Jan/Feb; 5(1):20–23.

Gittner C. Imaging the eye. Biomed Commun 1984 June; 12(3):31–33.

Jennings BA. The Nd:YAG. J Ophthalmol Nurs Tech 1985 Jan/Feb; 4(1):16–21.

Lawyer TH Jr. Guide to the neuro-ophthalmologic evaluation. Hosp Med 1984 Feb; 20(2):93–103.

Ledford JK. Saving time: Efficiency in the routine ophthalmic exam. J Ophthalmol Nurs Tech 1985 Jan/Feb; 4(1):33–35.

Parker P. Testing single binocular fields. J Ophthalmol Nurs Tech 1986 Jan/Feb; 5(1):8–11.

Rakow PL. Insight into keratometry. J Ophthalmol Nurs Tech 1985 Jan/Feb; 4(1):38–40.

Eye Medications

Seale D. Intraocular injectable miotics. J Ophthalmol Nurs Tech 1983 Aug; 2(3):118–119.

Contact Lenses

Forstot SL and Ellis PP. Identifying and managing contact lens emergencies. ER Rep 1982 Apr 5; 3(7):35–38.

Goldstein J. Contact lens care products. J Ophthalmol Nurs Tech 1987 Mar/Apr; 6(2):70–72.

Harris MD and Rager TM. Learning about contact lenses. In Nursing Photobook, Helping Geriatric Patients, pp 118–121. Springhouse, Pennsylvania, Intermed Communications, 1983.

Horowitz TH and Kracher GP. Guidelines to observe in extended-wear lenses. J Ophthalmol Nurs Tech 1983 Aug; 2(3):124–125.

Rakow PL. Soft lens selection: The key to success. J Ophthalmol Nurs Tech 1983 May; 2(2):89–90.

Rakow PL. Using contact lenses as a tool for understanding. J Ophthalmol Nurs Tech 1983 Aug; 2(3):130–131.

Rakow PL. A closer look at Septicon (to distinct contact lenses). J Ophthalmol Nurs Tech 1983 Nov; 2(4):182–183.

Rakow PL. What's new in contact lenses. J Ophthalmol Nurs Tech 1985 Mar/Apr; 4(20):14–20.

Rakow PL. Tinted lenses—shades of tomorrow. J Ophthalmol Nurs Tech 1986 Jan/Feb; 5(1):32–33.

Refraction

Waring GE III. Refractive keratoplasty. Res Staff Physician 1985 May; 31(5):2–33.

Eye Conditions

Infection

Boyd-Monk H. Conjunctivitis. Nurs '82 1982 Nov; 12(11):67.

Bucci FA Jr, Savia PV and Mauriello JA. Herpes zoster ophthalmicus. Am Fam Physician 1987 Mar; 35(3):121–128.

Greiner JV et al. Effects of eye rubbing in the conjunctiva as a model of ocular inflammation. Am J Ophthalmol 1985 July; 100(1):45–50.

Leopold IH. Update on antibiotics in ocular infections. Am J Ophthalmol 1985 July; 100(1):134–140.

Stoer P and Osman J. Assessing ophthalmic signs in patients with AIDS. J Ophthalmol Nurs Tech 1985 Nov/Dec; 4(6):6–10.

Trauma

Born CP. Ocular injuries—treat or refer? Postgrad Med 1983 Feb; 73(2):311–317.

Mador C et al. Ocular trauma and the impact of sudden vision loss. Ophthalmol Nurs Forum 1985; 1(1):2–7.

Sanke RF. Blunt ocular trauma. Am Fam Physician 1984 Feb; 29(2):159–164.

Tumulty G and Rester MM. Eye trauma. Am J Nurs 1984 June; 84(6):740–744.

Cataract

Alcantara N, Cooper V, and Macisic M. A holistic approach to extracapsular lens extraction. Today's OR Nurse 1984 Mar; 6(3):16–22.

Allopurinol suspected of causing cataracts. Am J Nurs 1983 Apr; 83(4):590.

Applegate WB et al. Impact of cataract surgery with lens implantation on vision and physical function in elderly patients. JAMA 1987 Feb 27; 257(8):1064–1066.

Aquavella JV et al. Cataract surgery: Who's a candidate? Patient Care 1986 Aug 15; 20(13):46–81.

Burlew JA. The art of nursing a patient through a cataract experience. J Ophthalmol Nurs Tech 1983 Feb; 2(1):15–17.

Carver JA. Cataract care made plain. Am J Nurs 1987 May; 87(5):626–630.

Cataract surgery. Nurs '83 1983 Apr; 13(4):65–69.

Easterlin MN and Schneider HA. Calculating intraocular lens power. J Ophthalmol Nurs Tech 1985 Jan/Feb; 4(1):6–8.

Freunfelder F et al. Cataracts associated with allopurinol therapy. Am J Ophthalmol 1982 Aug; 94(2):137–140.

Hussey LCT. Intraocular lens implant. AORN J 1984 Apr; 39(5):880–891.

Jaffe NS. The current status of intraocular lenses. Geriatr Ophthalmol 1985; 1(1):37–46.

Mackety C. Posterior capsulectomy with the Nd:YAG laser. Today's OR Nurse 1985 Aug; 7(8):12–17.

Maitchouk IF. Trachoma and cataract: Two WHO targets. Int Nurs Rev 1985 Jan/Feb; 32(259):23–25.

Sheets JH. The perfect cataract operation. Cataract 1985 June; 2(6):12–17.

Sliney DH. Ultraviolet radiation and the cataract patient. Cataract 1985 June; 2(6):20–24.

Smith JF. The patient having cataract surgery. J Ophthalmol Nurs Tech 1984 May/June; 3(3):124–126.

Smith S. Day-care cataract surgery. J Ophthalmol Nurs Tech 1987 Mar/Apr; 6(2):50–56.

Stark LA. Treating vision loss. Today's OR Nurse 1984 Mar; 6(3):8–10, 13, 44.

Stec J and Wolfe CP. Cataracts. Cataract 1984 May/June; 3(3):130–131.

Zack PL and Smirnow IH. IOL implantation. Today's OR Nurse 1983 Mar; 5(1):12–16, 18, 68–69.

Glaucoma

Bensinger RE. Precautions in dilating pupils. J Ophthalmol Nurs Tech 1984 Jan/Feb; 3(1):19–21.

Borders CR (ed). Glaucoma: Preventing diagnostic misses. Patient Care 1984 Sept 15; 18(15):16–51.

Boyd-Monk H and Starita RJ. Surgical intervention to stop glaucoma. J Ophthalmol Nurs Tech 1985 May/June; 4(3):12–30.

Easterlin MN and Schneider HA. Acute angle closure glaucoma following surgery. AORN J 1984 May; 39(6):992–995.

Fellman RL et al. ALT: Argon laser trabeculoplasty following failed trabeculectomy. J Ophthalmol Nurs Tech 1986 Mar/Apr; 5(2):65–68.

Jindra LF. Closed-angle glaucoma: Diagnosis and management. Hosp Pract 1984 Mar; 19(3):114–119.

Laser trabeculoplasty for open-angle glaucoma. Med Lett Drugs Ther 1984 May 25; 26(662):52–53.

McKenney M. Learning about glaucoma. In Nursing Photobook: Carrying Out Special Procedures, pp 48–55. Springhouse, Pennsylvania, Intermed Communications, 1983.

McKenney M. Special tests (glaucoma). In Nursing Photobook: Carrying Out Special Procedures, pp 48–55. Springhouse, Pennsylvania, Intermed Communications, 1983.

Resler MM and Tumulty G. Glaucoma update. Am J Nurs 1983 May; 83(5):752–756.

Tumulty G and Resler MM. Managing glaucoma using argon laser therapy. J Ophthalmol Nurs Tech 1985 Jan/Feb; 4(1):9–15.

Keratotomy

Boyd-Monk H. A fortunate accident—radial keratotomy. Today's OR Nurse 1984 Mar; 6(3):25–26, 31.

Dodge DC. Radial keratotomy. AORN J 1985 Aug; 42(2):214–221.

Easterlin MN and Schneider HA. A conservative approach to radial keratotomy. J Ophthalmol Nurs Tech 1985 Mar/Apr; 4(2):21–25.

Salz JJ. Improving the results of radial keratotomy. J Refract Surg 1985 Sept/Oct; 1(4):167–172.

Keratoplasty

Smith JF. Nursing care of the patient having penetrating keratoplasty. J Ophthalmol Nurs Tech 1984 July/Aug; 3(4):160–164.

Waring GO. Review: The changing status of radial keratotomy for myopia: I and II. J Refract Surg 1985 May/June; 1(2):81–86; July/Aug; 1(3):119–137.

Whitton S. Penetrating keratoplasty: The gift of sight. Today's OR Nurse 1983 Jan; 5(1):21.

Retina

Boyd-Monk H. Retinal detachment and vitrectomy: Nursing care. Nurs Clin North Am 1981 Sept; 16(3):433–450.

Brown GC. Retinal vascular diseases. Occup Health Nurs 1983 Aug; 31(8):17–20.

Glover SF. Scleral buckling: A fight for sight. Today's OR Nurse 1986 Jan; 8(1):8–12.

Glover SF. Update on scleral buckling: A fight for sight. J Ophthalmol Nurs Tech 1986 Jan/Feb; 5(1):24–29.

Other Eye Conditions

Laibovitz RA. The vitreous and vitreous floaters. Postgrad Med 1984 Apr; 75(5):6.

Marta M. A guide to the posterior vitrectomy. Today's OR Nurse 1983 Mar; 5(1):26–29, 69.

Kinash RG and Fulton NJ. Essential blepharospasm and implications for nursing. 1985 July/Aug; 10(5):26–29.

Shock D. Ischemic optic neuropathy. Postgrad Med 1983 Dec; 74(6): 74–75.

Smith JF. Why a single piece of advice may save your corneal transplant sight. RN 1982 Aug; 45(8):66–68.

Vision Loss—Blindness

Blank HR. Sexuality in the blind. Med Aspects Human Sexuality 1982 June; 16(6):137–140.

Harris MD and Lager TM. Learning about eye implants and prosthesis. In Nursing Photobook: Helping Geriatric Patients, pp 122–124. Springhouse, Pennsylvania, Intermed Communications, 1983.

Margo C and Brown B. Adjustment to visual loss. JAMA 1982 Sept 10; 248(10):1231–1232.

Steffee DR et al. More than a touch (communicating with a blind and deaf patient). Nurs '85 1985 Aug; 15(8):36–39.

Agencies

American Association of Ophthalmology, 1100 17th. Street, NW, Washington, DC 20036.

American Council of the Blind (ACB), 1211 Connecticut Avenue, NW, Washington, DC 20036.

American Foundation for the Blind, 15 West 16th. Street, New York, New York 10011.

American Optometric Association (AOA), 243 Lindbergh Boulevard, St. Louis, Missouri 63141.

American Society of Ophthalmic Registered Nurses, Inc. (ASORN), P.O. Box 3030, San Francisco, California 94119.

Better Vision Institute Inc. (BVI), 230 Park Avenue, New York, New York 10017.

Contact Lens Society of America (CLSA), 40507 National Building, Lexington, Kentucky.

Eye-Bank Association of America (EBAA), 6560 Fannin, Houston, Texas 77030.

Leader Dogs for the Blind, 1039 Rochester Road, Rochester, Michigan 48063.

National Association for Visually Handicapped (NAVH), 305 E. 24th Street, New York, New York 10010.

National Braille Association (NBA), 654 A Goodwin Avenue, Midland Park, New Jersey 07432.

National Federation of the Blind (NFB), 1800 Johnson Street, Baltimore, Maryland 21230.

National Society to Prevent Blindness (NSPB), 79 Madison Avenue, New York, New York 10016.

Recording for the Blind (RFB), 215 East 58th. Street, New York, New York 10022.

Seeing Eye (SE), P.O. Box 375M, Washington Valley Road, Morristown, New Jersey 07960.

Chapter 51

Assessment and Management of Patients With Hearing Problems and Ear Disorders

The ear is a very complex sense organ with a dual function—hearing and the maintenance of equilibrium (Fig. 51-1). The early detection and the accurate diagnosis of ear and hearing disorders are important in both children and adults. Among those who take an important part in the diagnosis of auditory disorders are pediatricians, otolaryngologists, psychiatrists, neurologists, psychologists, speech pathologists, educators, and audiologists. Before a child can speak, he must first be able to hear and then to interpret what he hears. Disorders due to birth injury, bacterial and viral infections in childhood, toxic drug effects, damage to the ear by noise, and changes in the ear as the result of aging are only a few of the problems that require assessment, treatment, and rehabilitation.

Assessment of Hearing Ability

Examination of the Ear

The ear is examined primarily by inspection and palpation and by assessing the external and middle ear. Auditory acuity is also a vital part of this examination and is included in every physical examination.

Auditory Acuity. A general estimation of the patient's hearing is effectively screened by assessing the patient's ability to hear a whisper or the ticking of a watch. One ear is tested at a time. In order to exclude the opposite ear from the testing, the examiner cups the opposite ear with the palm of the hand and produces a masking sound by moving the hand to and fro. At a distance of 30.5 to 61 cm (1 to 2 feet) from the unoccluded ear and out of visual range of the patient, the examiner whispers three or four numbers. A soft whisper can be produced if the examiner begins to whisper after a full exhale. In a quiet room, the patient with normal acuity can correctly repeat the numbers whispered. This procedure is done for each ear. If a ticking watch is used, the examiner holds the watch at a distance of 7.5 cm (3 inches) from the auricle. Because the watch produces a higher-pitched sound than the whispered voice, it is less reliable and is not used as the sole means of assessing auditory acuity.

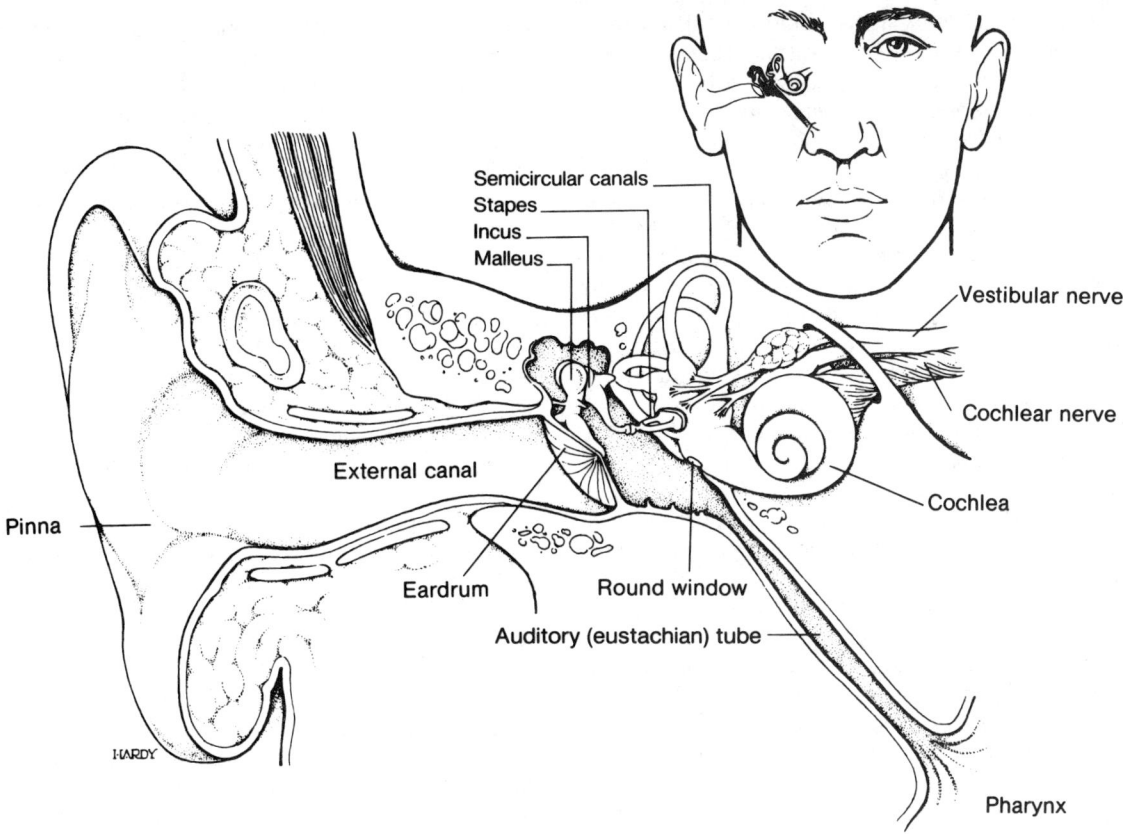

Figure 51-1
Anatomy of the ear.

Hearing normally occurs over two pathways. The sounds that are transmitted by way of the air-filled external and middle ear travel by way of *air conduction*. The sounds transmitted through bone directly to the inner ear travel by means of *bone conduction*. In the normal person, air conduction is the more efficient pathway.

Hearing loss may be one of two types. The first type is a *conductive loss* and usually results from an external ear disorder, such as cerumen impaction, or middle ear disorders, such as otitis media or perforated tympanic membrane. In such instances, the transmission of sound by air to the inner ear, where it is converted to a neural impulse, is blocked. The second type of loss is a *sensorineural, or perceptive,* loss and involves damage to the eighth cranial nerve. These losses may be distinguished through the use of a tuning fork specifically selected for frequencies within the conversational voice range (512 or 1024 cycles per second [cps]).

The *Weber test* uses bone conduction to test lateralization of sound. The tuning fork is set in motion by grasping it firmly by its stem and tapping it lightly between the index finger and thumb. The surface of a knuckle can also be used. It is then placed on the top of the patient's head or in the middle of the forehead. The patient is asked if he can hear a sound. Where does he perceive the sound (one ear? both ears?)? If there is a conductive deficit (cerumen plug [wax], otitis media) in one ear, the sound will be heard better in the poor ear. This is because obstruction in the ear canal or middle ear obliterates the room noise, thus enhancing bone conduction. However, if a sensorineural loss exists, the sound will not be perceived in the ear with the deficit. Instead, the sound lateralizes to the good ear.

In the *Rinne test*, the base of a vibrating tuning fork is placed on the mastoid process of the temporal bone until the patient can no longer hear it. The examiner quickly places the vibrating fork 2.5 cm (1 inch) from the opening of the auditory canal. Under normal circumstances, the patient will continue to perceive the sound, demonstrating that air conduction lasts longer than bone conduction.

In conductive hearing loss, however, bone conduction exceeds air conduction. That is, once bone conduction through the temporal bone has died out, the patient is unable to hear the fork through the usual conductive mechanism. In contradistinction, nerve deafness permits sound to be conducted by air better than by bone, although both are conducted poorly and all sound may be perceived to be distant and faint. Use of the Weber and Rinne tests in concert enables one to distinguish conductive loss from nerve loss when hearing is impaired. These tests are not necessarily a part of the usual physical exmination but will be useful if the patient reports hearing deficit or if the examiner detects an inability of the patient to perceive such sounds as a ticking watch or a whispered voice.

External Ear. Inspection of the external ear is a simple procedure and is often overlooked. The auricle and surrounding tissues are carefully inspected for deformities, lesions, or discharges. Movement of the auricle, specifically the tragus, does not normally elicit pain. If this maneuver is painful, acute external otitis is suggested. Tenderness in the area of the mastoid may indicate mastoiditis or inflammation of the posterior auricular node. Occasionally, sebaceous cysts and tophi (subcutaneous uric acid deposits) may be present on the pinna. A flaky scaliness on or behind the auricle usually indicates seborrheic dermatitis and may be present on the scalp and facial structures as well.

Otoscopic Examination. Proper inspection of the ear canal and eardrum (tympanic membrane) requires that the canal be free of cerumen. If the membrane cannot be visualized because of wax, the ear canal may be gently irrigated with warm tap water. In the event that firmly adherent cerumen is present, a small amount of mineral oil or an analogous commercial preparation may have to be instilled within the ear canal and the patient instructed to return for subsequent removal of the wax and inspection of the ear. The use of a cerumen spoon for wax removal is reserved for physicians and nurses with specialized training because of the danger of perforation of the tympanic membrane. Cerumen buildup demands attention because it is a common cause of hearing deficit and local irritation.

To examine the ear canal and tympanic membrane, the patient's head is tipped away from the examiner. The auricle is grasped firmly and pulled upward, backward, and slightly outward (Fig. 51-2). This straightens the canal for better visualization. The largest speculum that the canal will accommodate is selected and is guided gently down into the canal and slightly forward. The distal portion of the canal is bony and covered by a sensitive layer of epithelium. Here the pressure of the speculum may be painful.

Any discharge, inflammation, or foreign body in the ear canal is noted. The tympanic membrane is pearl grey and positioned obliquely at the base of the ear canal. The examiner identifies its landmarks: the *pars tensa* and cone of light, the umbo, the manubrium of the malleus, and its short process, if visible (Fig. 51-3). A slow movement of the speculum allows further visualization of the malleolar folds and periphery. The position and color of the membrane, as well as any unusual markings or deviation in the cone of light, are noted.

A "retracted eardrum" occurs when there is increased pressure (blocked auditory tube) in the middle ear. This is apparent as the malleus appears shorter and angled backward and as the short process becomes more prominent. Often, the cone of light is broken or absent. Occasionally, air bubbles or a fluid level line may be visible through the tympanic membrane, which suggests serous otitis media. Several dilated blood vessels along the manubrium is a normal finding, not to be confused with the generalized hyperemic membrane of purulent otitis media. All abnormalities are brought to the attention of a physician.

Audiogram

In the detection of deafness, the audiometer is the single most important diagnostic instrument. Audiometric testing is of two kinds: (1) *pure-tone audiometry,* in which the sound stimulus consists of a pure or musical tone (the louder the tone before the patient perceives it, the greater the hearing loss; the unit of measure of loudness or intensity of sound is

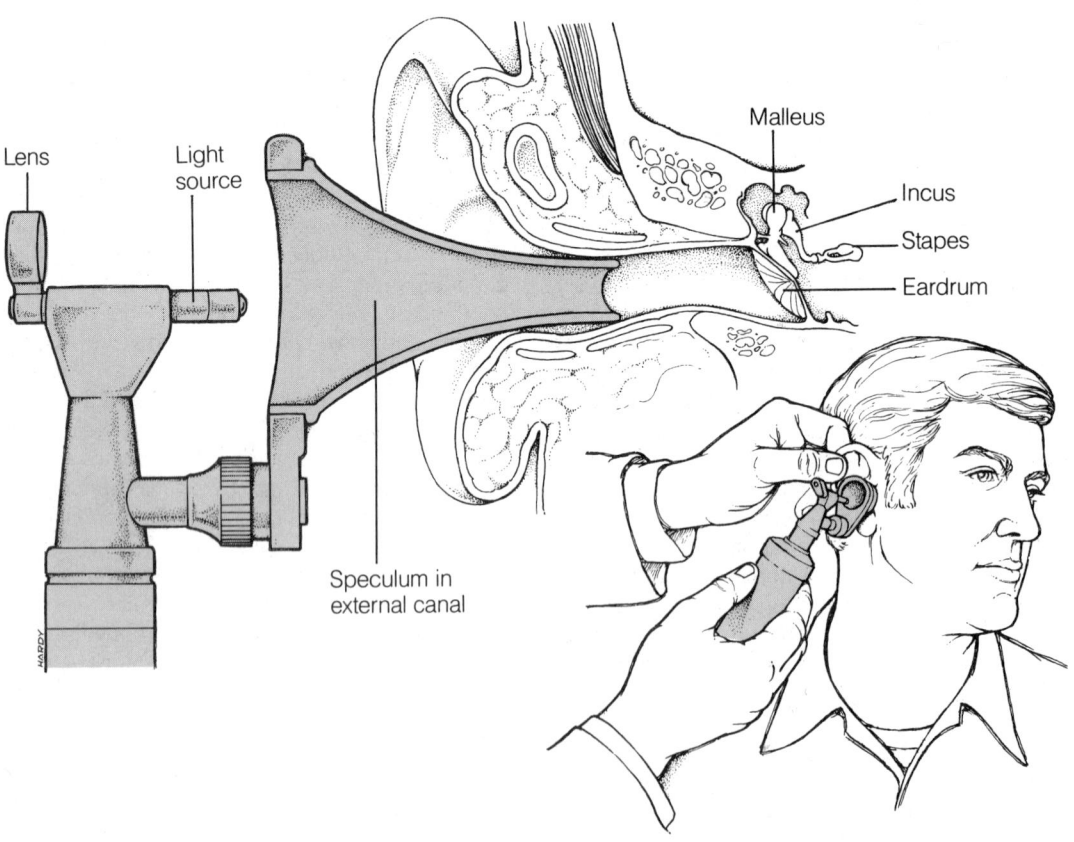

Figure 51-2
Technique for using the otoscope. (See text.)

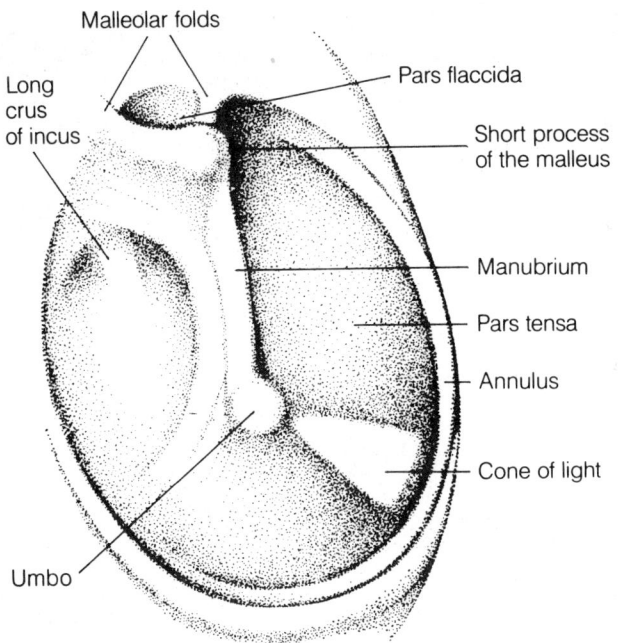

Figure 51-3
Display of the right eardrum as it would be visualized through the otoscope.

the decibel [dB]; and (2) *speech audiometry*, in which the spoken word is used to determine the ability to understand and discriminate sounds.

For accuracy, audiometric tests are done in a soundproof room. The patient wears earphones and is instructed to signal when he hears the tone and again when he no longer hears it. When the tone is applied directly over the external auditory opening, air conduction is measured. When the stimulus is applied to the mastoid bone, thereby bypassing the conductive mechanism, nerve conduction is tested.

The normal human ear perceives sounds ranging from 20 to 20,000 cps; however, only the frequencies from 500 to 2000 cps are important in understanding everyday speech. Clinically, this range is referred to as *speech range*. The critical level of loudness is around 30 dB. In treating patients surgically to improve hearing loss, the aim is to improve the hearing level to 30 dB or better within the speech frequencies (Figs. 51-4 and 51-5).

Gerontological Considerations

With aging, changes occur in the ear that eventually lead to hearing deficits. Not much change occurs in the external ear except that cerumen tends to become harder and there is a greater chance of impaction. In the middle ear, the tympanic membrane may atrophy or sclerose. The inner ear changes with a degeneration of cells at the base of the cochlea. This is manifested by a loss in the ability to hear high-frequency sounds followed in time by the loss of middle and lower frequencies. The term *presbycusis* is used to describe this progressive hearing loss.

Early signs of hearing loss may be tinnitus, increasing inability to hear at group meetings, a need to turn up the volume of the television, and so on. Presbycusis may progress rapidly over a few years or slowly over a decade.

Other factors affect hearing in the elderly, such as life-long exposure to loud noises such as the noise caused by jets, guns, and heavy machinery in the workplace. Also certain drugs, such as streptomycin, neomycin, and even aspirin, may have an ototoxic effect because renal changes in the older person result in delayed drug excretion. Psychogenic factors and other diseases (*e.g.*, diabetes) are also partially responsible for sensory changes.

Figure 51-4
An audiogram presents a graphic outline of the person's hearing as measured by tones of different pitches ranging from 125 through 8000 cycles per second (cps or Hz). This audiogram of the right ear shows a conductive loss. Thresholds for these different tones as heard by air and bone conduction are plotted. The information is important for determining the type of hearing loss. Also, by testing through the critical speech range (approximately 300 to 3000 cps), one can predict how much difficulty there may be in hearing and understanding speech. The code box to the right indicates the signs used on the chart. (Dayal VS. Clinical Otolaryngology. Philadelphia, JB Lippincott, 1981.)

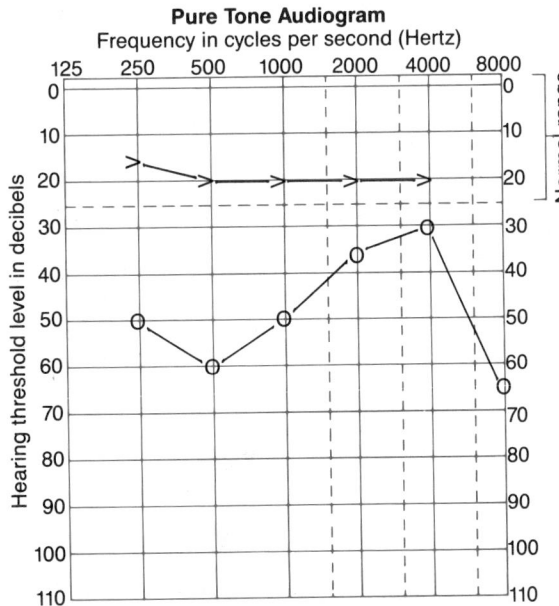

Ear	Air		Bone	
	Un-masked	Masked	Un-masked	Masked
R	O---O	Δ---Δ	]---]	>--->
L	x---x	□---□	[---[	<---<

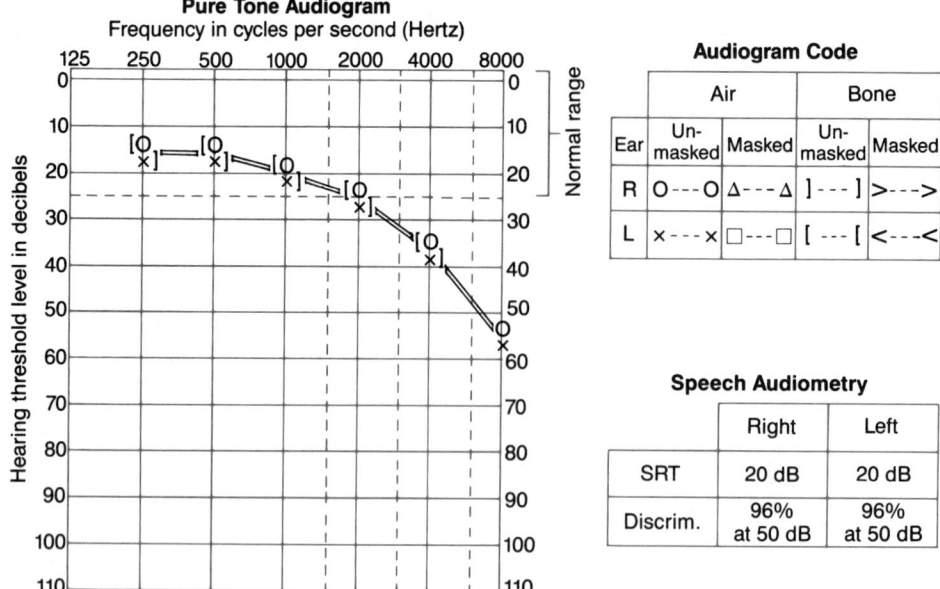

Pure Tone Audiogram

Figure 51-5
Audiogram of right ear shows a sensorineural hearing loss. In this audiogram, speech tests used are speech reception threshold (SRT) and speech discrimination. If the ability of this patient to understand speech is poor, a hearing aid will be of little or no benefit to him, nor will he benefit from reconstructive surgery to correct the conductive hearing loss. (Dayal VS. Clinical Otolaryngology. Philadelphia, JB Lippincott, 1981.)

Hearing impairment should not be assumed to be a normal consequence of aging and thus ignored. When a problem occurs, an audiometric evaluation should be done. Hearing aids are not to be invested in without a medical referral. Even with the best of medical care, the older person will have to learn to adjust to varying degrees of hearing deficit. Part of gerontological care is recognizing emotional reactions such as (1) being suspicious of others because of an inability to hear adequately, (2) frustration and anger with repeated unsuccessful attempts revealed by "I didn't get what you said," and (3) feeling insecure because of the inability to hear the telephone or alarms. Hearing aids help to a certain point, but hearing problems in the elderly are often compounded by difficulty in discriminating speech. As a result, hearing aids frequently are not used.

By understanding what type of hearing loss this patient has, the nurse will more successfully be able to relate to him. Trying to speak in a loud voice to a person who cannot adequately hear high-frequency sounds will only make matters worse. Talking into the least impaired ear, using sign language, gestures, and facial expressions may help.

Noise and Its Effect on Hearing

One of the waste products of the 20th century is noise (unwanted and unavoidable sound). The sheer volume of noise that surrounds us daily has grown from a simple annoyance into a potentially dangerous source of physical and psychological damage.

In terms of physical impact, loud, persistent noise can cause constriction of peripheral blood vessels, alterations in blood pressure and heart rate (because of increased output of adrenalin), disturbances in equilibrium, and increased gastrointestinal activity. Additional research is required to answer many questions regarding the overall effects of noise on the human body. However, one thing seems beyond dispute—a quiet environment is more conducive to peace of mind. A person who is ill will feel more at ease when noise is kept to a minimum.

Sound Intensity and Frequency. Scientists measure sound *intensity* (pressure exerted by sound) in decibels (dB). For example, the shuffling of papers in quiet surroundings represents about 15 dB, a low conversation, 40 dB, and a jet plane 100 feet away about 140 dB. Sound above 80 dB begins to grate harshly on the human ear.

Over the past several decades, the loudest sounds to which humans are exposed have grown from 120 dB (the roar of a small, two-engine prop plane) to 150 dB (the blast of a giant, four-engine jet). Experiments have shown that 160 dB is lethal for small fur-bearing animals. Research at many universities shows that exposure to noise of 90 dB or more can cause the skin to flush, the stomach muscles to constrict, and tempers to be short.

Frequency refers to the number of sound waves emanating from a source per second—cycles per second (cps or Hz). *Pitch* is the term used to describe frequency; a tone with 100 cps is considered low pitch; a tone of 10,000 cps is considered high pitch. Generally, a young adult can distinguish frequencies from 16 to 20,000 cps.

Hearing Loss

Psychosocial Considerations

Impairment of hearing may cause changes in personality and attitude, in the ability to communicate, in the awareness of surroundings, and even in the ability to protect oneself. In a classroom, a student with impaired hearing may show disinterest, inattention, and failing grades. A women at home may think the "world is dead" because she no longer can hear the clock chime, the refrigerator hum, the birds sing, or the traffic pass. A pedestrian may attempt to cross the street at the wrong time because of failure to hear an approaching car. The person with a hearing loss may miss parts of a conversation and may believe that people are talking about him. Many people are not even aware that their hearing is gradually becoming impaired.

More than 20 million people in the United States suffer from some form of hearing loss. Approximately 90% of these people can be helped through medical or surgical measures or with a hearing aid. The nurse and the family physician play a major role in diagnosing hearing loss and guiding patients toward some type of assistance. Although some hearing difficulty may be due to impacted cerumen (wax), which is readily treated, proper assessment is best done by an otologist.

The *otologist* is a physician who specializes in the diagnosis and treatment of problems of the ear. An *otolaryngologist* is a physician who specializes in problems relating to the ear, nose, and throat. An *audiologist* is a person who specializes in nonmedical evaluation and rehabilitation of hearing disorders.

The symptoms of hearing loss are varied, complex, and often subtle, as is indicated in the danger signals listed in Chart 51-1.

The signs of significant ear disease that require referral to an otolaryngologist have been identified by the National Hearing Aid Society (NHAS):

1. Visible congenital or traumatic deformity of the ear
2. Active drainage from the ear within the previous 90 days
3. Sudden or rapidly progressive hearing loss
4. Acute or chronic dizziness or tinnitus
5. Unilateral hearing loss of sudden or recent onset
6. Significant air–bone gap (which can be recognized only from hearing tests)
7. Visible evidence of cerumen accumulation or a foreign body in the ear canal
8. Pain or discomfort in the ear

Not infrequently, a person with a hearing loss refuses to seek medical attention; because of fear that hearing loss is a sign of advancing age, many people refuse to wear a hearing aid for this reason. Others feel self-conscious when they do wear an aid. These attitudes and behaviors should be taken into account when counseling patients who need hearing assistance.

Classification of Hearing Loss

Conductive Loss.   Conductive hearing loss results from an impairment of the outer ear, middle ear, or both. The inner ear is not involved in this type of loss; it can analyze clearly the sounds that come to it. Correction of the problem may be all that is necessary to treat and improve this type of impairment (see Fig. 51-6 and pp. 1376–1379). If the problem cannot be corrected, the patient benefits greatly from a hearing aid, because in most instances he requires only amplification of sounds.

Sensorineural (Perceptive) Loss.   A disease of the inner ear or nerve pathways produces a type of hearing loss in

---

Chart 51-1
Symptoms of Hearing Loss

Speech deterioration—If a person slurs his words or drops word endings, or if speech is "flat" sounding, he may not be hearing correctly! The ears guide the voice, both in loudness and pronunciation.

Fatigue—If a person tires easily when listening to conversation or to a speech, fatigue may be the result of straining to hear. Under these circumstances, he may become irritable or "touchy" very easily.

Indifference—It is easy for a person to become depressed and disinterested in life in general when he can't hear what others are saying.

Social withdrawal—Not being able to hear what is going on around him causes the hard of hearing person to withdraw from situations that might prove embarrassing.

Insecurity—Lack of self-confidence and fear of mistakes create a feeling of insecurity in many hard of hearing persons. No one likes to "say the wrong thing" or do something that might tend to make him look foolish.

Indecision-Procrastination—Loss of self-confidence makes it increasingly difficult for a hard of hearing person to make decisions.

Suspiciousness—Because he often hears only part of what is being said, the hard of hearing person may suspect that others are talking about him or that portions of the conversation relating to him are deliberately spoken softly so that he will not hear them!

False pride—The hard of hearing person wants to conceal his hearing loss. Consequently, he often pretends he is hearing when he actually isn't.

Loneliness and unhappiness—Although everyone wishes for quiet now and then, *enforced* silence can be boring and even somewhat frightening. People with a hearing loss often feel "left out of things."

Tendency to "hog" the conversation—Many hard of hearing people tend to dominate the conversation, knowing that as long as it is centered on them and they can control it they are not so likely to be embarrassed by some mistake.

(Courtesy of Maico Hearing Instruments.)

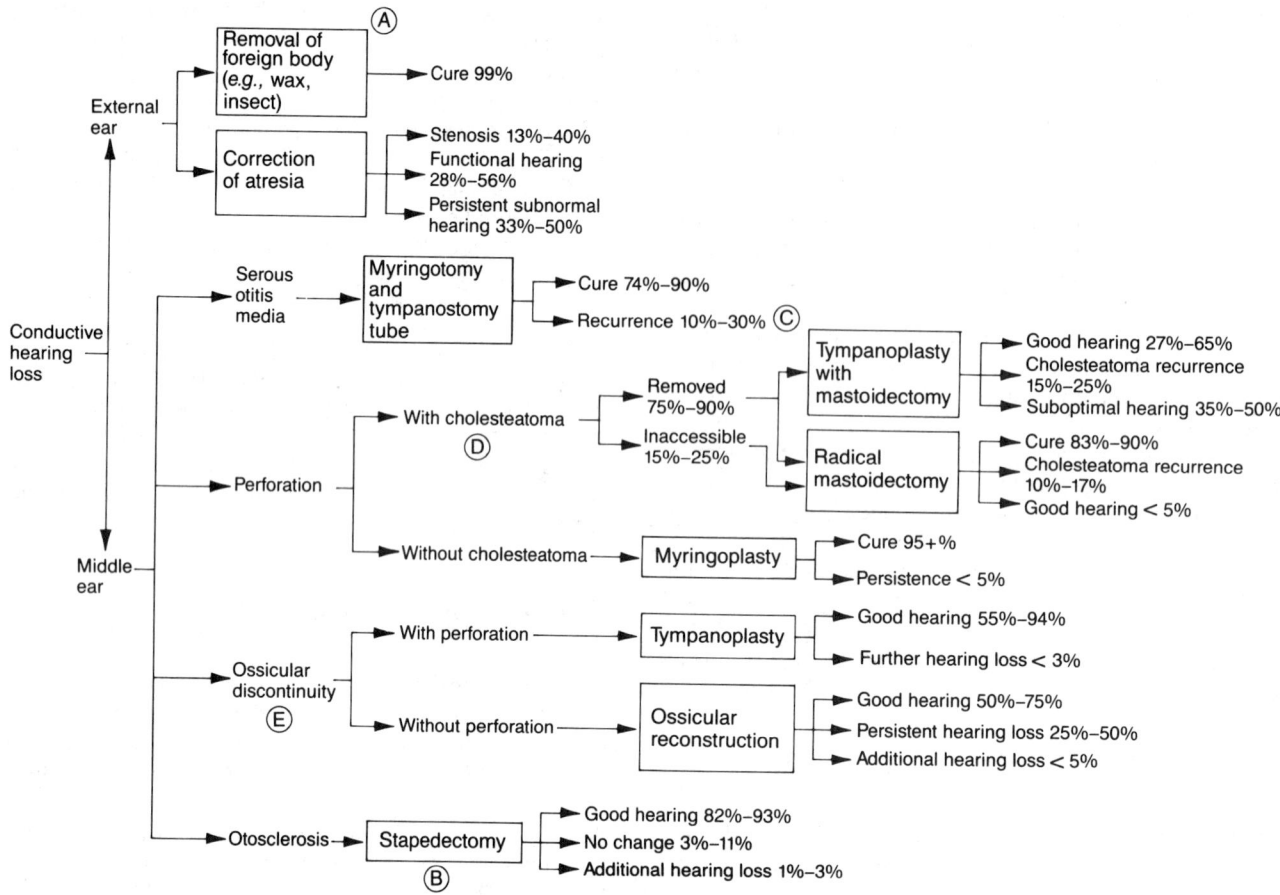

Figure 51-6

Conductive hearing loss. When a patient presents with this problem, the above flow chart indicates how the diagnosis determines the management of the patient and further predicts the outcome. (Jafek BW and Balkany TJ. Conductive hearing loss. In Eiseman B. Prognosis of Surgical Disease. Philadelphia, WB Saunders, 1980.)

which sensitivity to and discrimination of sounds are impaired. Sounds may be conducted properly through the external and middle ear but are not analyzed correctly in the inner ear. Because of poor sensitivity to sound, hearing aids are not as helpful as they are to those with conductive loss. However, a hearing aid should not be ruled out until the patient's hearing is evaluated in relation to hearing aids, that is, until a variety of aids are tested against the patient's hearing loss.

Combined Hearing Loss. A combined hearing loss indicates that the patient has both a conductive and sensorineural loss.

Psychogenic Hearing Loss (Nonorganic, Functional). Hearing loss of this type is unrelated to detectable structural changes in the hearing mechanisms. Usually, it is a manifestation of an emotional disturbance, and the loss is frequently total. *Malingering* is similar to psychogenic hearing loss, except that in this instance the patient really does hear.

Rehabilitation

It is important to classify the kinds of hearing impairment so that rehabilitative efforts can be directed at meeting a partic-

ular need. The Conference of Executives of American Schools for the Deaf proposed the following classification based on (1) time of onset of hearing loss and (2) functional status of hearing:

1. The deaf—those in whom the sense of hearing is nonfunctional for ordinary purposes of life. This general group is made up of two distinct classes:
   a. The congenitally deaf—those who lose hearing before speech is developed.
   b. The adventitiously deaf—those who are born with normal hearing but then suffer some illness or accident that causes their hearing to become nonfunctional
2. The hard of hearing—those in whom hearing, although defective, is serviceable with or without a hearing aid

Hearing Aids

A hearing aid is an instrument through which sounds, both speech and environmental, are received by a microphone, converted into electrical signals, amplified, and reconverted to acoustical signals. A hearing aid is not a new ear. It is as its name implies, only an aid to hearing. Many aids available for nerve deafness depress the low tones and give better hearing for the high tones. Whether a person would benefit by a hearing aid can best be determined by an otologist in conjunction with an audiologist. When the hearing loss is more than 30 dB in the range of 500 to 2000 cps in the better ear, a patient may benefit (but not with certainty) from a hearing aid. A variety of aids are available; the problem is to select the best aid for the individual patient (Table 51-1). Even this does not ensure optimal benefit from such an instrument. Psychological factors, such as vanity, may be involved, as well as other types of sensitivity.

The patient needs to know that the aid will not restore hearing to the level of the person with normal hearing but will improve it in the range of 300 to 3500 cps (range of primary speech).

A hearing aid makes speech louder, but it does not always make it clear enough for the deaf person to understand what is said. The wearer must experiment and adjust the controls for optimal results. He needs to recognize that he will never hear what others cannot hear, nor will he hear as well as one who has no hearing impairment. It may be necessary to receive auditory training and lessons in speech reading (lip reading) in order to make the new hearing aid effective. With such assistance, this person can learn to interpret sounds and use advantageously whatever hearing remains. Speech reading can help fill in the gaps of those words that might be missed. In auditory training, speech discrimination and listening skills are emphasized. The otologist, nurse clinician, or the hearing center can direct the patient to such classes.

A problem with most hearing aids is that background noise is also amplified, which may be distressing to the wearer. Binaural aids (*i.e.*, one for each ear) may be indicated. Such aids can be concealed in the arms of specially made eyeglasses, as may a single aid.

FDA Regulations. In August 1977, the Food and Drug Administration (FDA) established regulations on hearing aids to protect the health and safety of people with hearing impairments.

1. A medical evaluation of the impairment by a licensed physician (preferably one specializing in diseases of the ear) must be obtained within 6 months prior to the purchase of a hearing aid.
   a. Such a written statement from a physician, however, may be waived by the client (a fully informed adult 18 years of age or older) on signing a document.
   b. Children must be evaluated by a physician.
2. Hearing aid dispensers are required to refer prospective users to physicians if any of the eight specified otologic conditions are evident.
3. *A user instructional brochure* is to accompany every hearing aid device. In this brochure, the following information is presented:
   a. Proper use and maintenance of the device described.
   b. Good health practice requires a medical evaluation before purchasing a hearing aid.
   c. Any of the designated otologic conditions should be investigated by a physician before client purchases an aid.
4. Medical evaluation is required to ensure appropriate medical diagnosis and care.

Care of a Hearing Aid. A hearing aid must be cared for carefully. The ear mold, which is the only part of the instrument that may be washed, is washed in soap and water every day, and the cannula is cleansed with a small applicator or pipe cleaner. The mold must be dry before it is snapped into the receiver. The transmitter usually is worn off the body—behind the ear or in the frame of eyeglasses. A spare battery and cord should be carried by the wearer at all times. (This is suggested, but most patients do not do it.)

When a hearing aid is not functioning properly, the following steps should be taken: (1) note whether the on–off switch is on, (2) check the positioning of the batteries, (3) try a new battery, (4) examine the cord for breaks and whether it is plugged in correctly, and (5) examine the ear mold for

TABLE 51-1
Types of Hearing Aids

Site/Range of Hearing Loss	Advantages	Disadvantages
Body (40–110 dB)	Separation of receiver and microphone prevents acoustic feedback, allowing high amplification	Bulky; requires long wire, which may be cosmetically displeasing; some loss of high-frequency response
Behind the ear (25–80 dB)	Cosmetically good because easily hidden by hair; comfortable; no long wires	Proximity of microphone and receiver limits the amount of amplification because of feedback
In the ear (25–55 dB)	Smallest; most easily concealed	Very close proximity of amplifier and microphone and size limitations on power make aid suitable only for mild to moderate losses
Eyeglasses (25–70 dB; greater range with special modifications)	Conceals most of the aid with frame of glasses; allows wires separating microphone and receiver to be hidden within glasses	Requires wearing glasses, usually with bulky, stylistically limited frame

(Sataloff RT. Choosing the right hearing aid. Hosp Pract 1981 May; 16[5]:32E.)

Chart 51-2
Hearing Aid Problems

Whistling Noise

Loose ear mold:
   Improperly made
   Improperly worn
   Worn out
Improper aid selection:
   Too much power required in aid with inadequate separation
      between microphone and receiver
   Open mold used inappropriately

Inadequate Amplification

Dead batteries
Wax in ear
Wax or other material in mold
Wires or tubing disconnected from aid
Aid turned off or volume too low
Improper mold
Improper aid for degree of loss

Pain From Mold

Improperly fitted mold
Ear skin or cartilage infection
Middle ear infection
Ear tumor
Unrelated causes:
   Temporomandibular joint
   Throat or larynx
   Other

(Sataloff RT: Choosing the right hearing aid. Hosp Pract 1981 May; 16[5]:32A.)

cleanliness (see Chart 51-2). If the aid still will not work, notify the local service agency. Meanwhile, if the unit requires days to repair, the agency from whom it was purchased may lend an aid, or one may be borrowed from the local Chapter of the American Hearing Society.

Hearing Guide Dogs

Specially trained dogs are available to assist the person with hearing loss.* At home, the dog reacts to the sound of a telephone, a doorbell, an alarm clock, a baby's cry, a knock at the door, a smoke alarm, or an intruder. The dog does not bark but jumps on the person, thereby alerting him; the dog then runs to the source of the noise. In public, the dog positions himself between the person with a hearing problem and any potential hazard that the person cannot hear, such as an oncoming vehicle or a hostile person.

The dog wears an orange collar, and the person carries a certification card that reads: "The dog has been professionally trained by Hearing Dog Inc. in auditory awareness to serve its hearing-impaired master. Therefore, as with guide dogs for the blind, this dog shall accompany its master at all times."

In many states, a hard of hearing person with a certified hearing guide dog is legally permitted access to public transportation, public eating places, and stores, including grocery markets.

* International Hearing Dog Inc., Henderson, Colorado, provides trained dogs after 3 months of training. Only persons who live alone are eligible to apply for such a dog.

Communication With a Person Who Has a Hearing Impairment

Terry and co-workers offer the following suggestions for better communication with deaf persons whose speech is difficult to understand†:

1. Devote full attention to what the person is saying. Look and listen—do not try to give attention to another task while listening.
2. Engage him in conversation when it is possible for you to anticipate his replies. This will enable you to become accustomed to any peculiarities in speech patterns.
3. Try to catch the essential context of what is being said; you can often fill in the details from context.
4. Do not try to appear as if you understand when you do not.
5. If you cannot understand at all or have serious doubt about your ability to understand what is being said, have the person write his message rather than risk misunderstanding. Having him repeat his message in speech, after you know its content, will also aid you in becoming accustomed to his pattern of speech.

Suggestions for better communication with a deaf person who lip-reads are as follows:

1. When speaking, always face the person as directly as possible.

† Terry FJ et al. Rehabilitation Nursing. St Louis, CV Mosby.

2. Make sure your face is as clearly visible as possible; locate yourself so that your face is well-lighted; avoid being silhouetted against strong light; do not obscure that person's view of your mouth in any way; avoid talking with any object held in your mouth.
3. Be sure the patient knows the topic or subject of your verbal expression before going ahead with what you plan to say—this will enable him to use contextual clues in his lip-reading.
4. Speak slowly and distinctly, pausing more frequently than you would normally.
5. If you question whether the patient has understood some important direction or instruction, check to be certain that he has the full meaning of your message.
6. If for any reason your mouth must be covered (as with a mask) and you must direct or instruct the patient, there is no alternative but to write the message for him.

Problems of the External Ear

The auricle or external ear, which varies in size, shape, and position on the head, aids in the collection of sound waves and their passage into the external auditory canal. The *external auditory canal* is a skin-lined tube that ends at a disclike structure, the tympanic membrane (eardrum), which is also lined with skin. The skin of the canal contains highly specialized glands that secrete a brown, waxlike substance called *cerumen* (ear wax). The ear's self-cleaning mechanism moves skin debris and cerumen to the outer part of the ear. The cerumen seems to have antibacterial properties and serves as a protection for the skin.

Otalgia is pain in the ear (earache). Because the ear is innervated by a rich nerve supply (cranial nerves V, VII, IX and X and the second and third cervical nerve roots) the skin is extremely sensitive. Otalgia is a symptom that can arise from irritation from a number of conditions, including referred pain from disorders of the larynx or pharynx.

Infections (External Otitis)

Bacterial or fungal infections may result from an abrasion of the ear canal or from swimming in contaminated water; they appear more commonly during the summer. Such infections are painful.

The goals of management are directed toward relieving the discomfort, reducing the swelling in the ear canal, and eradicating the infection. Even touching or moving the auricle increases pain. (In a middle ear infection, movement of the auricle does not increase pain.) Aspirin, codeine, and applications of heat provide comfort. If the tissues are edematous, it may be necessary to insert a wick of cotton gently through the canal to the eardrum so that liquid medications (such as Burow's solution [5% aluminum acetate] or antibiotics) may be introduced. Later, these medications may be given by dropper at room temperature. Such medications usually are combinations of antibiotics and agents to soothe the inflamed membranes. Systemic antibiotic therapy may also be required. Patients are also reminded to avoid self-cleaning of the ear (cotton-tipped applicators are not to be used).

Another precaution is for the patient to avoid swimming or allowing water to enter the ear when shampooing or showering. Those prone to "swimmer's ear" should wear specially fitted ear plugs made from plastic material molded to exact measure. The procedure for drying ears with 70% isopropyl alcohol after swimming or showering is as follows:

1. Tilt or shake head to get out as much water as possible.
2. Instill a dropperful of alcohol in ear.
3. Tilt head to drain alcohol.
4. Set hair dryer at *low* volume and heat; blow air gently into ear canal until ear feels dry.

The chronic form of external otitis is often due to a dermatosis such as psoriasis, eczema, or seborrheic dermatitis. Even allergic reactions to hair spray, hair dye, and permanent wave lotions can cause dermatitis, which clears when the offending agent is removed.

Furuncle of the External Canal

Infections of the skin and the subcutaneous tissue of the external canal usually result in a great deal of pain in the affected ear. There may be fever, severe headache, and enlargement of the local lymph nodes. This disorder may be mistaken for mastoid infection. The early administration of antibiotics and application of hot packs usually result in resolution of the furuncle. Incision and drainage are rarely done since such measures may result in perichondritis or chondritis. It is better for the furuncle to localize (point) and open spontaneously or resolve by itself.

Cerumen in the Ear Canal

Ear wax normally accumulates in the ear in varying degrees and color. Although it does not ordinarily need to be removed, on occasion it may become impacted, causing *otalgia* (earache) and hearing difficulties. Attempts to clear the external auditory canal with matches, hair pins, and other implements are dangerous, since trauma to the skin may result in infection or damage to the eardrum.

Management. Wax deposits may be softened by instilling a few drops of warmed glycerin, mineral oil, or acetic acid (0.5%) solution. Other ceruminolytic agents, such as peroxide in glyceryl (Debrox), are available. However, these compounds may cause an allergic reaction in the form of a dermatitis. If the wax deposits cannot be dislodged by this method, the cerumen may be removed by a physician with a cerumen spoon used under magnification. As a last resort, the ear canal may be irrigated, although this mode of treatment is the least preferred because (1) it may cause discomfort; (2) it is messy; (3) it may cause vertigo if the temperature of the solution is higher or lower than room temperature; (4) it tends to macerate the skin, increasing the possiblity of an external otitis; and (5) it could permit fluid to enter and contaminate the middle ear if the tympanic membrane is perforated.

Foreign Bodies in the External Canal

Small objects are at times inserted into the ear, usually by young children. Such objects may be nonirritating and remain for years without symptoms.

An insect in the ear may be disturbing but can be easily managed by instilling oil drops that smother the insect and allow it to be floated or flushed out. However, *vegetable foreign bodies have a tendency to swell, so irrigation is contraindicated*. Attempts at removal may be dangerous in unskilled hands, because the object may be pushed completely into the bony portion of the canal, lacerating the skin of the canal and perforating the eardrum. Serious infections of the middle ear and the mastoid, with ensuing deafness, may result.

Irrigation of the External Auditory Canal

Irrigation of the ear canal is used less frequently today than in the past. When it is used, the purposes are (1) to carry out the caloric test for labyrinthine function, (2) to facilitate surgery on the external ear, and (3) to remove impacted cerumen (done by the physician).

The solutions for irrigating the ear should be at a temperature of about 40.6°C to 43.3°C (105°F–110°F). Solutions that are too hot or too cold or are used with too much force may cause pain or dizziness. The patient may sit or lie with his head tilted toward the side of the affected ear. The curved basin can be supported under the ear to catch the solution. To be effective, the fluids must reach the eardrum. To achieve this end, the auricle is pulled upward and backward in order to straighten the external auditory canal. (In chidlren, this canal may be straightened by pulling the auricle down and back.) Extreme gentleness is used, and care must be taken that the fluid has free exit so that it is not driven into the middle ear. After the irrigation, the external opening is plugged lightly with sterile cotton, which is changed when necessary. After the procedure, the patient is instructed to lie on the affected ear so that gravity facilitates drainage.

- Note: *If injury to the tympanic membrane is suspected, irrigation should not be performed.*

Problems of the Middle Ear

The middle ear, with its ossicles and ligaments and their connection to the eardrum, is vital to the function of hearing. The middle ear connects with the posterior portion of the nose by means of the auditory tube; thus, equal air pressure is maintained on both sides of the eardrum. The tube, which is normally closed, opens by action of the muscles of the palate on yawning or swallowing. The tube serves as a drainage channel for normal and abnormal secretions of the middle ear and equalizes pressure in the middle ear to that of the atmosphere. When the membrane of this tube is inflamed, it offers an easy passage for infection into the middle ear.

Sound waves transmitted by the eardrum to the ossicles of the middle ear are transferred to the *cochlea*, the organ of hearing, lodged in the labyrinth or inner ear. An important ossicle is the stapes, which rocks on its posterior portion, not unlike a piston, and sets up vibrations in fluids contained in the labyrinth. The fluid waves cause the basilar membrane in which the hair cells of the organ of Corti rest to move in a wavelike manner. The waves set up electrical currents that stimulate the various areas of the cochlea. The hair cell sets up a neural impulse that is encoded and then transferred through the auditory cortex in the brain, where it is decoded into a sound message.

Trauma to the Tympanic Membrane (Perforation)

Permanent perforation of the tympanic membrane occurs most frequently as a result of vehicular accidents with skull fracture. The next most frequent cause is infection; perforations of the eardrum membrane that fail to heal are often the end result of acute or chronic suppurative otitis media. Traumatic damage may also result from the blast effects of high explosives or from intense compression caused by a severe blow on the ear, which can rupture the eardrum. The eardrum may also be burned by a spark (red-hot slag) from a welder's equipment.

Less frequently, perforation is caused by foreign objects, water, burns of the face that include the external ear and the eardrum membrane, postmyringotomy defects, scuba diving, and accidental or deliberate blows to the face. Perforations may also occur when people use cotton-tipped applicators to clean their ears. A person may insert one into the external ear pushing the applicator deeper into the ear. Or the tip may be bumped and pushed into the canal. Either occurrence may result in severe destruction of the eardrum, ossicles, and even the inner ear. Thus, all attempts to clean the ear with applicator sticks must be discouraged.

Management. Most accidental perforations of the eardrum membrane heal spontaneously. Some persist because of the growth of scar tissue over the edges of the perforation, thus preventing extension of the epithelial areas across the margins and final healing.

- In suspected traumatic perforations, warn the patient against irrigating the ear. Cleanse the outer ear carefully with sterile cotton, but leave the ear canal alone until an otologist can aspirate blood and inspect the eardrum for evidence of perforation.

If the patient has sustained a head injury, he is kept under observation to detect any evidence of cerebrospinal fluid otorrhea, such as clear, watery drainage. Such fluid can be checked in the laboratory to determine whether its source is the cerebrospinal canal.

Middle Ear Effusion (Serous Otitis Media)

Secretory Otitis Media. Since this condition is found primarily in children, the reader is directed to pediatric nursing texts.

Aerotitis Media. *Aerotitis media* is a form of serous otitis media in which fluid or air is trapped in the middle ear due to sudden descent in an airplane (barotrauma). The condition usually lasts a short time, but it may continue for days. For this reason, many people avoid flying when they have an upper respiratory tract infection. Preventive measures to be taken by flight passengers are to chew gum, suck on hard candy, yawn, or swallow several times during the descent of the plane. Those flying should be taught to inflate their ears by the so-called Valsalva method. In this technique, the nostrils are held tightly, and the ears are inflated by vigorous blowing; thus, pressure in the middle ear is equalized to relieve annoying symptoms.

Acute Otitis Media (Infection of the Middle Ear)

Acute otitis media is an acute infection (or abscess) of the middle ear (Table 51-2). The essential cause of acute otitis media is the entrance of pathogenic bacteria into the normally sterile middle ear when the resistance is lowered or when the virulence of the organism is great enough to produce inflammation. Bacteria commonly found, in the order of importance, are *Streptococcus pneumoniae, Staphylococcus,* and *Hemophilus influenzae.* The mode of entry of the bacteria in most patients is spread by way of the auditory canal or the eustachian tube during the indiscriminate use of nose drops or nasal douching, forcible blowing of the nose, or sneezing; in rare cases, infection may occur after fracture of the skull.

Clinical Manifestations. The symptoms of otitis media may vary with the severity of the infection and may be either very mild and transient or very severe and fraught with serious complications. Pain in and about the ear is the first symptom. It may be intense and is relieved after spontaneous perforation of the eardrum or after myringotomy (see below). Fever varies and in severe cases may range between 40.0°C and 40.6°C (104°F–105°F). Deafness, ear noises, headache, loss of appetite, nausea, and vomiting are other symptoms.

Management. The end results of otitis media depend on the virulence of the bacteria, the efficiency of the therapy, and the resistance of the patient. With early and appropriate wide-spectrum antibiotic therapy, otitis media may clear with healing with no serious sequelae.

It is important to note that symptoms may be masked by the antibiotic therapy and that during the course of treatment

TABLE 51-2
Clinical Features of Acute Diffuse External Otitis and Acute Otitis Media

Feature	External Otitis	Otitis Media
Pain	Persistent	Subsides in 6 to 9 hours
	Aggravated by moving jaw	Relieved immediately if tympanic membrane ruptures
		Aggravated by swallowing, belching
Tenderness	Prominent	Absent
Systemic symptoms	Usually absent	Fever, rhinitis, sore throat
Hearing loss	Conductive type	Conductive type
Swelling of ear canal	Prominent	Absent
Discharge	Foul odor	No odor
	Blue pus, never profuse	
Tympanic membrane	Inflamed but intact	May be perforated
	No middle ear fluid	Fluid in middle ear

(Farmer HS. A guide for the treatment of external otitis. Am Fam Physician 1980 June; 21[6]:98. Published by the American Academy of Family Physicians.)

of an acute middle ear infection, symptoms such as headache, slow pulse, vomiting, and vertigo are all significant and should be recorded for evaluation by the otologist. The appropriate antibiotic, often determined by culture and sensitivity tests, is important to the prognosis for eventual cure.

The condition may become subacute, with persistent purulent discharge from the ear. Healing may take place with permanent deafness.

Perforation as the result of rupture of the eardrum may persist and develop into a chronic form of otitis media. Secondary complications, with involvement of the mastoid, and other serious intracranial complications, such as meningitis or brain abscess, may result.

Myringotomy. In a myringotomy, an incision is made into the posterior or inferior aspect of the tympanic membrane for draining purposes in order to relieve pressure and to drain pus from middle ear infection. In mild cases treated early, myringotomy may not be necessary. However, if pain persists, this procedure is important for promoting surgical drainage. It also offers a ready means of identifying the type of organism present to test its sensitivity to chemotherapeutic agents.

An incision is made in the posteroinferior aspect of the tympanic membrane. Even though a sweeping incision is made to relieve pressure and pus from a middle ear infection, the incision heals rapidly and hearing is not impaired. This procedure is now performed much less frequently than it was before the advent of antibiotic therapy. Usually, when myringotomy is done, a plastic tube is inserted through the eardrum.

Chronic Otitis Media

Chronic otitis media results from repeated attacks of otitis media causing persistent perforation of the eardrum. It is due to particular virulence of the infecting organisms or to bacterial resistance to antibiotic therapy. The chronically infected ear is characterized by persistent or recurrent purulent discharge, with or without pain, and varying degrees of deafness, usually conductive or mixed. Most chronic otitis media begins in childhood and may persist to adult life.

Classification. Chronic suppurative middle ear infection has been classified into five groupings, as indicated in Table 51-3.

Clinical Manifestations. The symptoms of chronic otitis media may be minimal, with varying degrees of deafness and the presence of a persistent or intermittent foul-smelling discharge of variable quantity. Pain may or may not be present. Symptoms such as sudden facial paralysis, unusually profound deafness or dizziness, onset of headache with dizziness, and stiff neck may herald a beginning meningitis or brain abscess or erosion into the semicircular canals. The diagnosis is corroborated by the physical findings, but, in addition, x-ray films of the mastoid usually show pathologic changes.

Management. Local treatment consists of (1) careful cleansing of the ear, (2) instillation of antibiotic drops or application of antibiotic powder, and (3) x-ray study. Tympanoplastic procedures may be required early to prevent further damage to hearing and more serious complications.

Mastoiditis and Mastoidectomy

Mastoiditis is an inflammation of the mastoid resulting from an infection of the middle ear; if it is untreated, osteomyelitis may occur. Symptoms are pain and tenderness behind the

TABLE 51-3
Classification of Chronic Otitis Media

Type	Specific Condition	Involvement	Manifestation
I	Chronic otitis media simplex	Central perforation of the tympanic membrane	Mucoid serous discharge
II	Chronic otitis media with cholesteatoma*	Usually, attic perforation (posterior superior part of eardrum) With or without perforation	Usually, odorous discharge
III	Chronic adhesive otitis media	Marked retraction of tympanic membrane	No discharge Marked hearing loss
IV	Chronic otitis media with tympanosclerosis	Tympanosclerosis, a degenerative process in eardrum and middle ear Plaque of amorphous connective tissue	Severe hearing loss No discharge
V	Chronic serous otitis media	If untreated or neglected, may result in severe deafness, chronic adhesive otitis media, cholesteatoma,* or tympanosclerosis	Repeated bout of serous or fluid ear

* Cholesteatoma is due to the ingrowth of the skin of the external ear canal (squamous epithelium) into the middle ear. The skin from the external canal forms the outer sac, which fills with degenerated skin and sebaceous material. The sac is attached to the structures of the middle ear and mastoid and produces changes by pressure necrosis.

(Woodrow D. Schlesser, M.D., personal communication.)

ear, discharge from the middle ear, and swelling of the mastoid. Usually, this is successfully treated with antibiotics and occasionally myringotomy.

When there is recurrent or persistent tenderness, fever, headache, and discharge from the ear, it may be necessary to remove the mastoid process (mastoidectomy).

Preoperative Management. Aside from general preoperative preparation of the patient, the postauricular or endaural area (whichever is selected as the incision site) is cleansed thoroughly. If the site is postauricular, hair is clipped about 3 cm around the back of the ear. To keep hair out of the operative field, a water-soluble jelly (KY jelly) may be applied to the hairline in the operative room or a commercially available plastic drape with a small, central hole to expose the operative site may be used. (The edge of the hole adheres to the skin with adhesive.)

During the operation, the infection is removed completely from the mastoid process by removing the mastoid cells, and the middle ear is drained (myringotomy), thus preventing spread of the infection to surrounding structures. The middle ear can be saved from further damage, and possible permanent hearing loss can be prevented.

Postoperative Management. Analgesics usually are indicated after the operation and during the first postoperative days to control pain and restlessness. Fluids are given freely when the anesthetic reaction clears. The mastoid is drained by means of a small Teflon drain. The bulky mastoid dressing is changed in 4 or 5 days when sutures are removed; a smaller dressing is applied and changed by the patient as required if drainage is still present. Antibiotics are continued for several days.

A possible complication after mastoidectomy is facial paralysis due to possible erosion of the bone that protects the facial nerve. The nurse may be the first to note this serious indication of facial nerve inflammation or injury. The patient shows immobility of the side affected, so that the eye cannot be closed and the mouth droops. He is unable to drink without

water dripping from the mouth, and he is unable to whistle. When the patient attempts to speak or grimace, the facial paralysis is more pronounced, due to the immobility of the paralyzed side. Any evidence of facial paralysis is reported immediately to the otologist. The patient may be taken back to the operating room, the wound opened, and repair of the facial nerve done at once. Other possible complications are meningitis or brain abscess.

Tympanoplasty

Tympanoplasty denotes a number of reconstructive operations on middle ear structures that have become diseased or are congenitally deformed (Table 51-4). Using an illuminated binocular microscope, the otologist is able to visualize and reconstruct defective conductive mechanisms to maintain or improve hearing. Chemotherapy or antibiotics maintain an infection-free area so that healing is promoted.

Physiologic Principles Underlying Sound Conduction. The conductive function of the eardrum and the ossicles transforms sound waves from airborne vibrations to mechanical stimulation of the endolymphatic fluids. The prevailing physiologic concept holds that the ratio of the large tympanic membrane to the smaller oval window, combined with the lever action of the ossicles, transforms stimuli from the ear to the inner ear fluids with great increase in force. Obviously, defects in the tympanic membrane or interruption of the ossicular chain will disturb that mass relationship to the oval window and will cause a loss of the sound–pressure ratio, resulting in hearing loss.

The functional physiology of the round and oval windows plays in important role as well. The oval window is bordered by the annular ligament, and the unimpeded motility of the stapedial footplate receives impulses transmitted by the incus and the malleus from the eardrum membrane. The round window, opening on the opposite side of the cochlear duct, permits motion of the endolymphatic fluids with sound wave

TABLE 51-4
Tympanoplastic Procedures

Type	Damage of Middle Ear	Methods of Repair
I	Perforated tympanic membrane with normal ossicular chain	Closure of perforation; same as myringoplasty
II	Perforation of tympanic membrane with erosion of malleus	Closure with graft against incus or remains of malleus
III	Destruction of tympanic membrane and ossicular chain *but with* intact and mobile stapes	Graft contacts normal stapes; also gives sound protection to round window
IV	Similar to type III, but head, neck, and crura of stapes missing; footplate mobile	Mobile footplate left exposed; air pocket between round window and graft provides sound protection for round window
V	Similar to type IV plus *fixed* footplate	Fenestra in horizontal semicircular canal; graft seals off middle ear to give sound protection for round window

(DeWeese DD and Saunders WH. Textbook of Otolaryngology, 6th ed. St. Louis, CV Mosby, 1982.)

stimulation. With the normally intact eardrum membrane, sound waves stimulate the oval window first, and a lag occurs before the terminal effect of the stimulus reaches the round window. This phase lag, normally present with an intact eardrum, is changed by a perforation of the eardrum that is large enough to allow sound waves to impinge on both the round and oval windows simultaneously. This effect cancels the lag and prevents the maximal effect of labyrinth fluid motility and its subsequent effect in stimulating the hair cells in the organ of Corti. The result is a reduction in hearing ability.

Pathophysiology. Pathologic sequelae vary after otitis media, with minimal or large defects remaining in the tympanic membrane. In protracted or virulent infections, necrotic involvement of the ossicles may occur. Impairment of freedom of motion of one or all parts of the ossicular chain may occur as a result of fibrosis or necrosis. The malleus commonly is involved, the handle being lost by osteonecrosis as the perforation in the eardrum enlarges. The lenticular process of the incus often is involved because of its tenuous blood supply. Osteonecrosis may involve the entire ossicular chain, so that the stapedial footplate is the only portion remaining. The oval and round windows may be impeded functionally by granuloma, polyps, and fibrous or bony plaques. Otosclerosis may exist along with the pathologic sequelae of otitis media. Obstruction of the tympanic orifice of the auditory tube by pathologic tissue deposits or fibrotic stenosis may result in dysfunction of this structure.

Procedures. Tympanoplasty is performed to reestablish two functions of the middle ear: (1) the transformer action and (2) sound protection for the round window.

Originally, five types of tympanoplastic procedures were

described (Table 51-4). Since then, modifications and innovations have been devised. In the original procedures of types I, II, and III, both of the above objectives were achieved; however, with types IV and V, only sound protection was provided for the round window. Variations of these operations are being done with the following innovations: incus interposition and prosthetic replacement.

Incus interposition is a procedure in which the incus is detached from the malleus, diseased segments of the incus are removed, and the remains of the incus are balanced on the head of the stapes; the contact is maintained with pieces of Gelfoam.

Homologous tympanic membrane, including annulus and malleus, may be taken from a cadaver and used in place of a fascial graft. Other prostheses may include tragal cartilage or a piece of shaped cortical bone from the patient's own mastoid.

Tympanoplasty, Type I (Myringoplasty)

Indications and Management. Myringoplasty is a plastic surgical procedure designed to close perforations of the tympanic membrane. The operation has dual goals: (1) to create a closed middle ear cavity by graft over the perforation and (2) to improve hearing.

The most important advantage of the closed tympanic membrane is the avoidance of the risk of contamination of the middle ear during bathing, swimming, or diving. Thus, the reactivation of a chronic otitis media or mastoiditis may be prevented. Dramatic improvement in hearing may result from closure of a perforation if there is no involvement of the ossicles. The probability of improved hearing after closure of the eardrum membrane can be prognosticated to some degree by an audiometric study with evaluation of the air–bone conduction levels. Preoperative testing, with and without a patch prosthesis over the perforation, usually provides a fairly accurate estimate of the degree of hearing levels. Temporary patching of the defect with glazed paper, latex, or a cotton collodium disc should be a routine maneuver during the preliminary examination of the patient. When the patching of a perforation of the eardrum is not followed by audiometric improvement, one must consider involvement of the ossicular chain. During the surgical repair of a perforation, a careful inspection of the middle ear contents, with particular attention to the continuity of the ossicles, is important.

Contraindications. Medical or surgical closure of perforations of the eardrum in the presence of an active infection usually is contraindicated. In chronic disease of the middle ear with malfunction of the auditory canal (eustachian tube), and therefore inadequate drainage from the middle ear (the only avenue for egress of discharges), surgery is contraindicated. Involvement of the nasopharynx because of chronic infectious discharge from sinusitis or allergy, plus a history of acute exacerbations of otitis media, is an obvious contraindication.

Postoperative Management. An antibiotic is administered routinely for at least 5 days after surgery. The dressing is left undisturbed except for the external bandage, which may be changed if it becomes soiled from bleeding. The gauze strip is removed from the canal on the seventh day; the Gelform is left undisturbed. No suction or probing is carried out at this time.

About the 20th day, capillary suction can be used carefully to remove the Gelfoam or crusted debris. Gentle inflation may be carried out to test the efficiency of the closure of the perforation by the graft.

The patient is seen at 5-day intervals and is instructed to avoid contaminating the ear by shampooing or showering. Antibiotics are given for 5 days, but may be continued if there is evidence of complicating respiratory infection. An antihistamine with an ephedrine derivative is used routinely for 1 month postoperatively. In those patients with known seasonal or perennial rhinologic allergy, an antihistamine is continued.

Tympanoplasty, Types II to V and Modified Versions

Tympanoplasty may be done by various techniques. Either the postauricular or the endaural approach is used. Skin grafts have been replaced by fascial grafts. The operation may be done in one or two stages. When done in two stages, the first is performed to clear the infection or remove cholesteatoma, and the second stage is directed to mechanical correction of the deficient sound transmission system.

Preoperative Care. The bacterial flora in all patients is studied by culture and sensitivity tests. In those whose treatment is accompanied by the parenteral administration of an appropriate antibiotic, the postoperative morbidity is reduced. Topical and systemic antibiotic treatment should precede surgery when there is continuous or frequent discharge.

Operative Procedure. Part of the tympanoplastic procedure includes restoring the continuity of the sound mechanism, when it is involved. Ossicular interruption is most frequent in otitis media, but problems of reconstruction occur with malformations of the middle ear and ossicular dislocations due to head injuries.

Polyethylene tubing, stainless steel wire, bone, and cartilage have been used as replacements, either to use the remaining parts of the ossicles or to create a columella (little column) effect for the transmission of impulses from the tympanic graft to the oval window.

A two-stage procedure may be necessary—the first for the surgical eradication of all pathology and the establishment of a healed, dry middle ear and the second for the reconstructive process. The ear should remain dry for 2 or 3 months before the second stage for the exploration of the window niches and the restoration of a conductive mechanism. Remaining parts of the ossicular chain may be repositioned to establish impulse transmission to the oval window.

Postoperative Care. Outer dressings may be reinforced if soiled with blood or drainage, but the inner dressing is undisturbed.

The patient must be assisted the first time out of bed since dizziness and nystagmus are typical reactions. Medications to combat vertigo and nausea may be prescribed. The patient is cautioned to avoid blowing his nose or wetting the dressings during bathing. Eventually, he will be permitted to resume showering and swimming.

Clinical Results. Patients with a lengthy history of disease may regain as much hearing as those with less protracted infections. In the patient whose otitis media has been healed and whose ear has remained dry for a lengthy period, hearing improvement may be marked after tympanoplasty. Younger patients achieve better results than older patients. The simpler the surgery, the better the chance for hearing gain; this, of course, relates directly to the functional integrity of the os-

sicular chain and the efficiency of the newly created tympanic covering.

Continued research is being done to improve tympanoplasty procedures. In some instances, clinical failures have been due to infection, poor technique, and tissue rejection of graft or prosthesis.

Otosclerosis

Otosclerosis, or otospongiosis, is the term applied to a form of progressive deafness caused by the formation of new, abnormal spongy bone in the labyrinth that eventually locks the stapes in a fixed position (clinical otosclerosis) and prevents sound transmission because the stapes is unable to vibrate and carry the stimulus of the vibrating malleus and incus to the inner ear fluids.

Etiology. The cause of the condition is unknown, but it occurs most commonly in women, beginning after puberty, and it has a hereditary basis.

The condition, which involves both ears but unequally, begins with insidious loss of hearing and a ringing or buzzing. The patient gives a history of slowly progressive hearing loss without middle ear infection. Sound transmission by air as tested with a tuning fork is markedly reduced, while intensification of sound is noted by placing the tuning-fork handle over the mastoid and recording the marked difference in hearing between air and bone. The bone conduction is far better than air conduction, which is the reverse of normal. Of all the tests, the diagnosis is evident from the findings of audiometry.

Stapedectomy. There is no known medical treatment for this form of deafness other than the help offered by amplification with an electric hearing aid or, preferably, a stapedectomy. A stapedectomy involves removing the otosclerotic lesion at the footplate of the stapes and creating a suitable implant with a prosthesis to replace this portion of the conductive mechanism (Fig. 51-7).

Microsurgery. The otologic binocular microscope is of distinct value in this operation. To bridge the gap between the incus and the inner ear, Schuknecht uses steel wire and fat implant, whereas House's technique employs Gelfoam and prefabricated stainless steel wire (two popular procedures). Kos uses wire and a segment of a vein as a plug in the oval window, and Shea advocates a vein graft with polyethylene tubing.

Nursing Management. See the following Nursing Process section.

▶ Nursing Process
The Patient Undergoing Ear Surgery

▷ Assessment

The nursing history will reveal a description of the ear problem, for example, earache, discharge, and hearing loss. When discomfort is apparent, gentleness is necessary when touching the ear, such as is required in using an otoscope speculum. The auricle is slowly lifted upward, outward, and backward with one hand while introducing the otoscope with the other. Swelling, redness, lesions, drainage, and odor of any discharge are noted. One ear is compared with the other. The

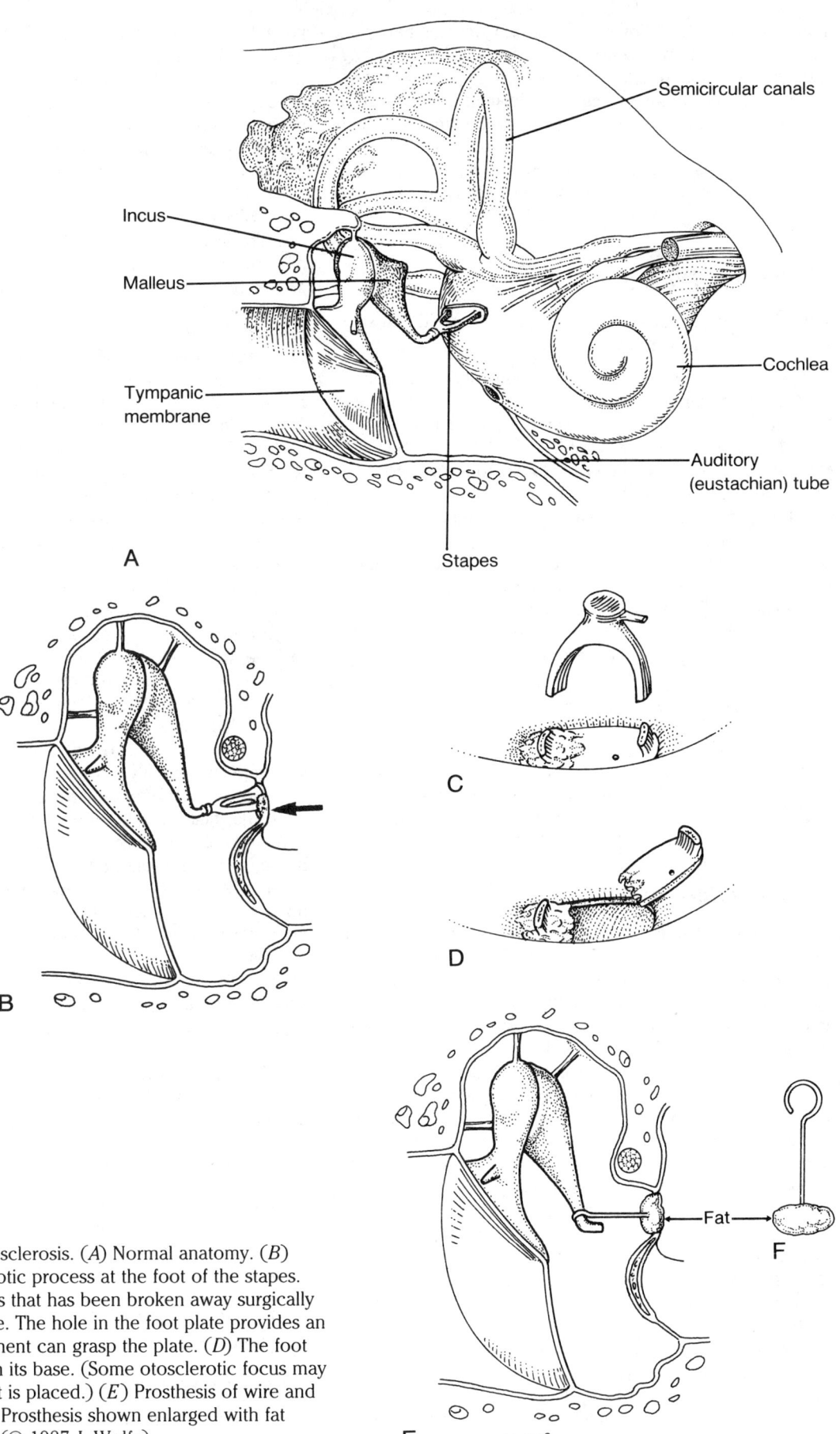

Figure 51-7
Stapedectomy for otosclerosis. (*A*) Normal anatomy. (*B*)
Arrow points to sclerotic process at the foot of the stapes.
(*C*) Blow-up of stapes that has been broken away surgically
from its diseased base. The hole in the foot plate provides an
area where an instrument can grasp the plate. (*D*) The foot
plate is removed from its base. (Some otosclerotic focus may
remain over which fat is placed.) (*E*) Prosthesis of wire and
fat is positioned. (*F*) Prosthesis shown enlarged with fat
attached to one end. (© 1987 J. Wolfe)

patient is asked the following questions: How long have you had the problem? What have you tried in treating yourself? Can you relate your problem to some episode (such as getting water in the ear during swimming, cleaning the ear with a cotton-tipped applicator, recalling an insect entering the ear canal, being exposed to a sudden loud noise)? The nurse asks about other physical problems and determines what medications the patient is taking specifically for the ear problem as well as all other medications being used.

▷ *Nursing Diagnoses*

Based on the assessment data the patient's major nursing diagnoses may include the following:

- Anxiety related to lack of knowledge about the anticipated operation
- Alteration in comfort: nausea/vomiting related to stimulation of the vomiting center
- Potential for injury related to falls due to vertigo resulting from disturbance of the labyrinth
- Potential for infection related to contamination of the operated area
- Altered auditory sensory perception related to hearing loss preoperatively and temporary interference with sound transmission (dressings, blood, drainage, packing)
- Knowledge deficit of the nature of the operation, protocol, and expectations postoperatively

▷ *Planning and Implementation*

▷ *Goals:* The major goals of the patient may include reduction of anxiety and acquisition of knowledge, freedom from discomfort (pain, nausea, and vomiting), prevention of infection and absence of injury, improved hearing/minimal hearing loss, and knowledge regarding follow-up care.

Nursing Interventions

Reducing Anxiety. The nurse reinforces information the surgeon has already discussed with the patient regarding the nature of the anesthesia, the location of incision, and the expected surgical results. Before the operation the patient is informed that in the immediate postoperative period, he will probably be expected to rest quietly for the first 24 hours in order to prevent dislodgement of the prosthesis. Collaboration with the otologist will determine whether the patient may turn on his side and which side is desirable. Sudden movement of the head is undesirable for the same reason; therefore, sneezing and coughing are to be avoided. If sneezing and coughing are unavoidable, the patient is instructed to open the mouth and sneeze or cough as gently as possible. Blowing the nose, straining during defecation, and bending at the waist must also be avoided. All motions are to be performed slowly. If the patient becomes nauseated, the physician should be notified so that an antiemetic or anti–motion sickness medication can be prescribed.

Relieving Pain and Discomfort. Pain may last for several hours postoperatively; therefore, it is desirable to administer the prescribed narcotic analgesic.

Vertigo occurs because the semicircular canals and vagus nerve were manipulated and stimulated during surgery. Anti–motion sickness drugs are administered as prescribed. The patient's position is changed slowly and he is encouraged to move slowly when moving any part of the body. Side rails are kept in place to prevent the patient from falling should he experience vertigo or disturbances in equilibrium. The nurse monitors the patient for effects of the medication to see if the desired results have been obtained. Later, she assists the patient with ambulation. He should avoid looking down while walking.

Preventing Infection. Measures are initiated to prevent infection in the operated ear. Prophylactic antibiotics are given as prescribed. Visitors with an upper respiratory tract infection should be discouraged. Aseptic technique is required when changing dressings. The patient is told not to touch his dressings to prevent contamination and to avoid getting his ear or dressings wet when washing his face since wet fibers act as a wick in transmitting contaminants. No shampoos are permitted until the physician determines that their use is safe. The patient is reminded not to blow his nose or sneeze since such actions may force organisms through the auditory canal to the middle ear. Any signs of infection such as temperature elevation and the presence of purulent, foul-smelling drainage are observed for, and the white blood cell count is monitored for elevation, which would be indicative of possible infection. The nurse reports patient complaints of increasing ear pressure or pain and should be alert for evidence of facial paralysis: drooping of mouth on operative side, altered taste, drooling when drinking, and excessive mouth dryness. Loss of taste or facial weakness should also be reported since these signs may suggest trauma to the seventh cranial nerve.

Should facial nerve damage occur, fluid intake is increased. If drooling occurs, a straw is used and frequent mouth care is provided. The patient must be reassured that these symptoms will usually resolve.

Improving Communication. The patient must be advised that hearing in the operated ear will be reduced for several weeks due to edema, accumulation of drainage or blood, and dressings or packing. Thus measures to improve communication are initiated, such as reducing environmental noise, facing the patient when speaking, speaking louder and more slowly than usual, speaking into the better ear, providing good lighting if the patient relies on lip reading, and using nonverbal clues such as facial expression, pointing, gestures, and other forms of communication. Family members or significant others must be instructed regarding effective practices so they may communicate successfully with the patient.

Patient Education for Self-Care at Home. The patient is usually discharged in 1 or 2 days and may require assistance at home.

To Prevent Dislodgment of Prosthesis:

- Avoid blowing nose and sneezing during the first week. This will protect tympanic membrane (eardrum) from air pressure changes.
- Avoid sudden rapid movements and even high elevations for at least 1 month.
- Do not bend at the waist or strain on defecation. Do not lift heavy objects.

To Prevent Infection in the Ear:

- Do not touch dressings unnecessarily.
- Change dressings as instructed.
- Do not wash hair for 10 to 14 days.

- Do not shower or swim for 6 weeks to prevent water from entering the ear.
- Cover the ear when outside.
- Avoid people with colds.
- Report any unusual signs and symptoms.

▷ *Evaluation*

▷ *Expected Outcomes*

1. Patient verbalizes lessened anxiety and can explain the reasons and methods of his care/treatment.
   a. Shares knowledge with family about treatment protocol.
   b. Tells nurse he can accept results of surgery and even adjust to temporary impairment, if necessary.
   c. Describes treatment he had and the time frame he will follow in recovery phase.
   d. Shows the home care plan he formulated with the nurse with regard to rest periods, medication, and activities permitted and restricted.
2. Is free of discomfort and complications.
   a. Says he is no longer experiencing dizzy spells.
   b. Reports no taste distortion or mouth dryness.
   c. Lists ways to prevent dislodging prosthesis.
   d. Can recite symptoms of possible complications that are to be reported to health care person.
   e. Lists methods for preventing ear infections as taught.
3. Has no infection/injury.
   a. Avoids falls by environmental modification (lights on at night; no clutter on steps).
   b. Practices acceptable technique when changing dressings.
   c. Is afebrile on hospital discharge.
   d. Postpones showers and shampoos as advised.
4. Demonstrates improved hearing.
   a. Verbalizes that he hears sounds he was unable to hear before treatment.
   b. Expresses pleasure about progressive hearing gain noticed from day to day.
5. Understands (as confirmed by conversation) what is expected of him in self-care/follow-up care.
   a. Reiterates limitations in activities and for how long regarding showering, swimming, lifting, and air flights.
   b. Demonstrates how to move when getting in and out of bed.
   c. Lists symptoms that should be reported to health care personnel.
   d. Shows appointment card for follow-up date and place; tells nurse that he intends to be there.

Problems of the Inner Ear

Body balance is maintained by the cooperation of muscles, joints, tendons, visceral senses, eyes, and inner ear or vestibular apparatus. The last is the most important in this function. The inner apparatus of the ear provides feedback regarding the movements and the position of the head in space, co-ordinates all body muscles, and positions the eyes during rapid motion or head movement.

The vestibular apparatus consists of the utricle, the saccule, and the semicircular canals, of which there are three in each ear. Each canal lies in a plane at right angles to the others, with the entire apparatus grouped in working pairs for this complex function. The mechanism of action of the semicircular canals may be likened to the cochlea or organ of hearing. Here, also, fluids are set in motion by head or body movement, which in turn stimulate extremely delicate nerve fibers that transmit messages as electrical impulses along the nerve to centers in the brain, where they are interpreted.

Motion Sickness

Motion sickness is a disturbance of equilibrium caused by constant motion, such as occurs aboard a ship or boat, riding on a merry-go-round or swing, or even riding a distance in the back seat of a car. Symptoms are dizziness, nausea, and frequently vomiting. These manifestations may persist several hours after the stimulation stops. Dimenhydrinate (Dramamine), scopolamine, and other antivertiginous drugs (drugs that prevent and treat dizziness and motion sickness) are helpful in providing some relief. Some side-effects may be experienced, such as dry mouth, cycloplegia, and drowsiness. These complications are reduced by using a disc (Transderm-V) in which scopolamine has been incorporated. The disc is applied to the skin, usually in back of the ear, for 4 to 16 hours before embarking on a long trip and left there for 3 days, if necessary. Dry mouth may develop, which can be relieved with lozenges.

Endolymphatic Hydrops (Ménière's Disease)

Ménière's disease is an innner ear problem stemming from a labyrinthine dysfunction, the cause of which has not been definitely established. Many theories have been advanced, such as abnormal hormonal and neurochemical influences on the blood flow to the labyrinth, electrolyte disturbance within labyrinthine fluids, or an allergic reaction. Some attribute impairment of the microvasculature of the inner ear to abnormal metabolites (sugar, insulin, triglycerides, and cholesterol) in the bloodstream.

Clinical Manifestations. Ménière's disease is most frequently characterized by the presence of a triad of symptoms: paroxysmal whirling vertigo (with nausea and vomiting), tinnitus, and neurosensory hearing loss. Some add a fourth manifestation, that of a sense of pressure in the ear. At the onset of the condition, perhaps only one or two of these symptoms are manifested; however, the disease is not diagnosed as Ménière's syndrome until all three signs are present (Fig. 51-8).

Vertigo, the outstanding symptom of Ménière's disease, occurs as a sudden attack, appearing at irregular intervals and possibly persisting for several hours. Early in this condition, weeks or months pass between attacks, but the time is gradually reduced so that they may be experienced every 2 to 3 days. Usually, only one ear is involved. Nystagmus and

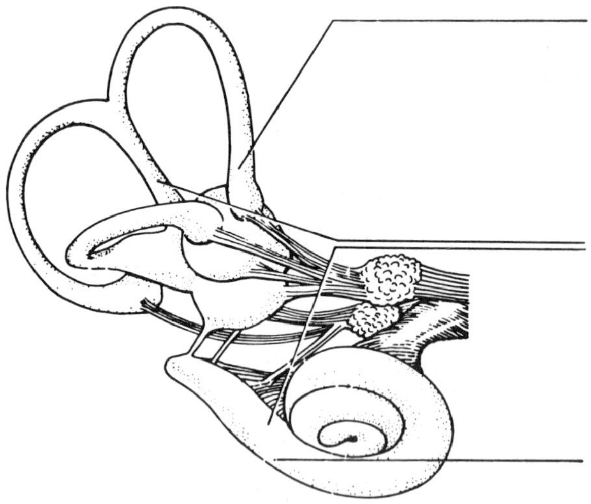

	TYPE	**SYMPTOMS AND SIGNS**

Endolymphatic hydrops of the vestibular variety

- dizziness only episodic
- reduced vestibular response or total lack of response in affected ear
- no cochlear symptoms
- no objective hearing loss
- may eventually develop cochlear symptoms and signs

True endolymphatic hydrops

Clinical triad of typical Ménière's disease present
1. Episodic vertigo
2. Fluctuating neurosensory hearing loss
3. Tinnitus

Endolymphatic hydrops of the cochlear variety

Symptoms and signs confined to cochlear portion of labyrinth
- fluctuating hearing loss
- sense of fullness in ear
- tinnitus
- neurosensory hearing loss demonstrated on testing
- no dizziness
- normal vestibular labyrinthine tests
- may eventually develop vestibular symptoms and signs

Figure 51-8
A practical classification of Ménière's disease.

ataxia may also be apparent. *Tinnitus* is characteristically a low, fluctuating, buzzing sound in the ears. It is often louder preceding and during an attack. Sensorineural loss applies to low tones and usually occurs in only one ear. It gets progressively worse and may cause severe cochlear damage if untreated.

Diagnostic Evaluation.   Because Ménière's disease simulates signs and symptoms of acoustic neuroma and other cerebellopontine angle tumors, careful diagnostic evaluation is required, including an audiogram, head scan, and allergy evaluation. Early in the condition patients are evaluated for glucose tolerance and for abnormal insulin levels. If results are abnormal, these patients are regarded as prediabetic and are managed by a controlled-carbohydrate weight-reduction diet.

Electronystagmography (ENG) is the preferred test; it measures the electropotential of the eye movements when nystagmus is produced and provides a graphic record of labyrinthine function.

Auditory Dehydration Test.   Endolymphatic hydrops is reputed to be verified when a hearing gain occurs after the intake of hyperosmolar substances (glycerin and urea). The patient eats a light breakfast about 2 hours before the test. A baseline audiogram is done, and a serum osmolality value is obtained. Then the patient drinks the prescribed amount of the hyperosmolar substance usually mixed with unsweetened fruit juice. Serum osmolalities are taken hourly after an audiogram and measured on an osmometer. A positive audiometric fluctuation at any hour constitutes a positive test.

Management

The goals of treatment are to eliminate vertigo and improve or stabilize the patient's hearing. This is accomplished by a combination of methods done early in the disease in order to avoid severe hearing loss. For an acute attack, the patient is permitted to assume whatever position is most comfortable. Usually, an intravenous line is started to permit the administration of medications such as diazepam (Valium), which is given slowly to control vertigo. Vital signs and the patient's condition are monitored. On occasion, a rectal suppository of dimenhydrinate may be prescribed. Other oral antivertiginous drugs may be prescribed.

Three-fourths of the patients respond to the treatment of a salt-free diet (Chart 51-3) and a diuretic. If there is an immediate favorable reaction to this regimen, it is continued for 2 or 3 months before the amount of diuretic (urea) is gradually decreased. The patient, however, never returns to the full use of salt. Food allergy is investigated and may require that certain elements be eliminated from the diet.

Vasodilating drugs, such as nicotinic acid, tolazoline hydrochloride (Priscoline), and methantheline bromide (Banthine), improve tinnitus.

For patients with a history of allergy (about 5% of these patients), relief may be obtained from chlorpheniramine. Vestibular suppressants such as diazepam, meclizine, or other anti–motion sickness drugs may be helpful. Stimulants and vasoconstrictors such as coffee, tobacco, decongestants, and alcohol are eliminated during periods of exacerbation. Chlor-

Nursing Interventions	*Rationale*	*Expected Outcomes*

Nursing Diagnosis: Self-care deficit related to labyrinth dysfunction and frequent necessity to assume the recumbent position

Goal: Ability to care for self

3. Encourage patient to care for bodily needs when free of attacks.	3. Since attacks may vary from occurring every few minutes to several hours and all day, spacing activities is advisable.	• Is free of nausea and vomiting.
4. Review Furstenberg diet with patient.	4. This is an effective diet because of the restriction of sodium.	
5. Offer liquids; if these are not tolerated, an IV line will be started.	5. Fluids are needed to prevent dehydration.	

Nursing Diagnosis: Anxiety related to the often disabling effects of attacks of Ménière's disease and concern about progressive hearing loss

Goal: Freedom from worry and acceptance of outcome of treatment

1. Provide comfort measures and avoid any stress-producing activities.	1. Stressful situations apparently exacerbate the severity of the disease.	• Avoids upsetting encounters and verbalizes the relationship between these and his ear problem.

Nursing Diagnosis: Altered sensory perception (hearing loss) related to labyrinthe dysfunction and the outcome of treatment (including surgery)

Goal: Improved hearing and freedom from complications

1. Assist patient in preparing for auditory dehydration test.	1. This reveals whether the patient in fact has Ménière's disease; hearing gain is a positive interpretation.	• Accepts the preparation for this test and tells that he knows he will have several audiometric and blood tests during the examination
2. Prepare the patient for surgery if this is indicated.	2. Endolymphatic sac surgery or other more extensive surgical procedure may be done to relieve symptoms. Only a small number of patients require surgery; most find relief from conservative measures.	• Expresses hope that surgery may help, however recognizes that some hearing loss may result
3. In addition to postoperative care required following the specific kinds of anesthesia, observe for potential complications.	3. If the subarachnoid space was entered, the nurse is alert for signs of possible complications: infection, increased loss of hearing, spinal fluid leakage, speech paralysis.	• Demonstrates no postoperative complications; absence of symptoms of infection; exhibits normal speech
4. Expect dizziness and nausea following labyrinthectomy. Assist the unsteady patient as required.	4. Patients may take months to recover their equilibrium following destructive procedures.	• Conducts a dialogue with the nurse and otologist to develop an understanding of what to expect postoperatively
5. Arrange for psychosocial and family support if results are poor and hearing is lost.	5. This patient has experienced much discomfort with this medical diagnosis and needs all the support he can get.	• Learns to read lips, "just in case"
6. Direct the patient to the proper hearing aid service as recommended by the surgeon.	6. Some improvement in hearing may be realized with a hearing aid (obviously from the other ear).	• Indicates that the recovery process is slow and that patience is required
		• Responds positively to support systems and modifies his life-style

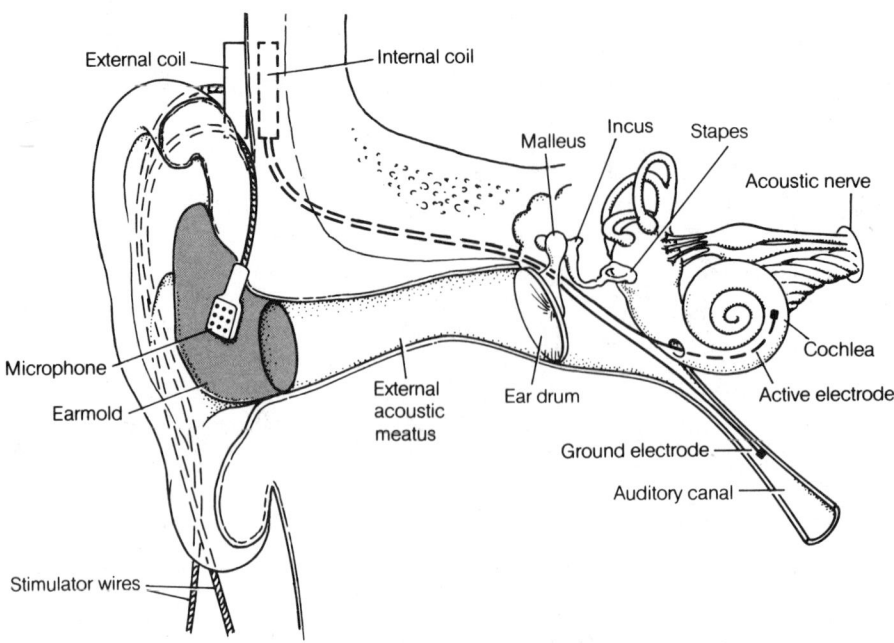

Figure 51-9
The cochlear implant. The internal coil has a stranded electrode lead. The electrode is inserted through the round window into the scala tympani of the cochlea. The external coil (the transmitter) is held in alignment with the internal coil (the receiver) by a magnet. The microphone receives the sound. The stimulator wire receives the signal after it has been filtered, adjusted, and modified so that the sound is at a comfortable level for the patient. Sound is passed by the external transmitter to the inner coil receiver by magnetic conduction and is then carried by the electrode to the cochlea.

other methods. The House 3M Cochlear Implant system was granted FDA approval in 1984 (Fig. 51-9).

The process includes an otologic history, physical examination, and audiologic assessment. A determination is made as to whether the candidate would do better with properly fitted powerful hearing aids or the cochlear implant. Some patients do best when a hearing aid is used in the ear with the least impairment and with the implant in the other ear.

The surgical procedure involves a mastoidectomy and the opening of the facial recess to permit access for the placement of the electrode into the scala tympani of the cochlea. Surgery takes about 1½ hours; after 2 months of recuperation, the patient is fitted with the external portion of the device. The patient carries the signal processor, approximately the size of a small cigarette package (3½ × 2 × ¾ inches) which uses mercury batteries that last about 3 weeks.

During rehabilitation, the patient learns about the use and care of the implant, determines the appropriate settings for the signal processor, and attends an auditory training program. These sessions are an important part of the whole process to ensure that the implant is used and that the person has made progress in differentiating sounds. Although clearly spoken word sounds will not be heard, the patient is able to differentiate between one kind of sound and another—such as the difference between the doorbell and the telephone.

Continued development of this device, the input of patients who are using it, and the dedication of researchers will undoubtedly lead to greater advancements in this facet of care.

Bibliography

Books

Alberti PW and Ruben RJ. Otologic Medicine and Surgery. New York, Churchill Livingstone, 1985.

Ballenger JJ. Diseases of the Nose, Throat, Ear, Head and Neck. Philadelphia, Lea & Febiger, 1985.

Carcio H. Manual of Health Assessment. Boston, Little, Brown & Co, 1985.

DeWeese DD and Saunders. WH. Textbook of Otolaryngology, 6th ed. St Louis, CV Mosby, 1982.

Feldman A. Hearing Conservation in Industry. Baltimore, Williams & Wilkins, 1985.

Gates GA. Current Therapy in Otolaryngology—Head Neck Surgery. St Louis, CV Mosby, 1984.

Hodgson W. Hearing and Assessment and Use in Audiologic Habilitation. Baltimore, Williams & Wilkins, 1986.

Karmody CS. Textbook of Otolaryngology. Philadelphia, Lea & Febiger, 1983.

Lucenti FE and Sobol SM. Essentials of Otolaryngology. New York, Raven Press, 1983.

Meyerhoff WC. Diagnosis and Measurement of Hearing Loss. Philadelphia, WB Saunders, 1984.

Miglets AW et al. Atlas of Ear Surgery, 4th ed. St Louis, CV Mosby, 1986.

Saunders WH et al. Nursing Care in Eye, Ear, Nose and Throat Disorders, 4th ed. St Louis, CV Mosby, 1979.

Thaller S. Otolaryngology. Baltimore, Williams & Wilkins, 1985.

Articles

(Asterisks indicate nursing research articles.)

General Articles

Advances in inner ear research. AORN J 1984; 39(2):202–204.

Bernardini L. Effective communication as an intervention for sensory deprivation in the elderly client. Top Clin Nurs 1985 Jan; 6(4):72–81.

Epstein GH and Sataloff RT. Biologic and nonbiologic materials used in otologic surgery. Otolaryngol Clin North Am 1986 Feb; 19(1):45–53.

Graham GH and Kemink JL. The wet ear. Otolaryngol Clin North Am 1986 Feb; 19(1):39–44.

Harner SG. Peripheral labyrinthe causes of dizziness. Postgrad Med 1987 Mar; 8(4):251–258.

Hart CW. Vertigo: Medical treatment. In Gates GA (ed). Current Therapy in Otolaryngology—Head and Neck Surgery 1984–1985. St Louis, CV Mosby, 1984.

Knudsen JF. Noise-induced hearing loss. Med Times 1986 Jan; 114(1):27–31.

Lewis JS. Cancer of the ear. CA 1987 Mar/Apr; 37(2):78–87.

McDonald TJ. Otolaryngology 1947–1987. Postgrad Med 1987 Mar; 81(4):179–191.

McDonald TJ. Twenty questions about middle ear fluid and ventilation tubes. Postgrad Med 1987 Mar; 8(4):239–246.

Neely JG. Mechanisms of hearing: Cochlear physiology. Ear Nose Throat J 1985 June; 64(6):40–68.

Ortiz-Armenta LA et al. Surgical treatment of vertigo. Ear Nose Throat J 1986 June; 65(6):46–61.

Wiet RJ, Monsell EM, and Hotaling AJ. Hearing and balance disorders. Postgrad Med 1985 Jan; 17(1):119–130.

Assessment

Barbour PJ. A neurologist's approach to a patient with hearing impairment. Otolaryngol Clin North Am 1985 May; 18(2):207–221.

Bower FN and Patterson J. A theory-based nursing assessment of the aged. Top Clin Nurs 1986 Apr; 8(1):22–32.

Hoffman SR. Evaluation of hearing loss in adults. Hosp Med 1984 Sept; 20(9):197–226.

Iadarola G and Kerrigan MB. Do you hear what I hear? AORN J 1986 Feb; 43(2):478–483.

Malkiewicz J. How to assess the ears and test hearing acuity. RN 1982 Mar; 45(3):56–63.

O'Flaherty KP, Miller MH, and Rose RM. A re-evaluation of the conventional approach to hearing aid evaluations. Ear Nose Throat J 1985 Nov; 64(11):11–24.

Thomas PD et al. Hearing acuity in a healthy elderly population: Effects on emotional, cognitive and social status. J Gerontol 1983 Mar; 38(3):321–325.

Webster DB, Packer DJ, and Webster M. Functional anatomy of the external and middle ear. Ear Nose Throat J 1985 June; 64(6):8–18.

Hearing Devices

Dreyfus PA. Buying a hearing aid with ear appeal. Money 1986 Feb; 15(2):149.

McKenna EL Jr. Counseling the hearing aid user and his family. Bryn Mawr Hosp Bull 1984 Winter; 6(2):38–39.

O'Flaherty KP, Miller MH, and Rose RM. A re-evaluation of the conventional approach to hearing aid evaluations. Ear Nose Throat J 1985 Nov; 64(11):11–24.

*Magilvy JK. Quality of life of hearing-impaired older women. Nurs Res 1985 May/June; 34(3):140–144.

Sataloff RT. Sensorineural hearing loss. Otolaryngol Clin North Am 1986 Feb; 19(1):3–37.

Teitelman R. Beyond hearing aids. Forbes 1984 Dec 3; 134(13):226, 230.

Hearing Problems and Conditions

Bell DN. Otitis externa. Postgrad Med 1985 Sept 1; 78(3):101–106.

Koegel L. Ototoxicity: A contemporary review of aminoglycosides, loop diuretics, acetylsalicyclic acid, quinine, erythromycin, and cisplatinum. Am J Otol 1985 Mar; 6(3):194–195.

Olsen WO. Presbycusis. Postgrad Med 1984 Sept 1; 76(3):189–198.

Stapedectomy

McGee TM. Stapedial otosclerosis. In Gates GA (ed). Current Therapy in Otolaryngology—Head and Neck Surgery 1984–1985. St Louis, CV Mosby, 1984.

Hanson C and Roffo F. Comprehensive care of patient undergoing stapedectomy for otosclerosis. Periop Nurs Q 1985 June; 1(2):21–27.

Ménière's Disease

Boles R. Ménière's disease: Medical management. In Gates GA (ed). Current Therapy in Otolaryngology—Head and Neck Surgery 1984–1985. St Louis, CV Mosby, 1984.

Imoto T and Stahle J. Glycerin and urea tests in Ménière's disease. Otolaryngol Clin North Am 1983 Feb; 16(1):37–48.

Maddox HE III. Medical treatment of Ménière's disease compared to early sac surgery. Otolaryngol Clin North Am 1983 Feb; 16(1):129–133.

Wiet RJ. Case selection in surgery for Ménière's disease. Otolaryngol Clin North Am 1983 Feb; 16(1):115–121.

Cochlear Implant

Alpiner JG. Rehabilitation concepts with the cochlear implant. Otolaryngol Clin North Am 1986 May; 19(2):259–265.

Chasse PS. Hope of hearing. Today's OR Nurse 1983 Oct; 5(8):14–16.

Clark GM. The University of Melbourne/Cochlear Corporation (Nucleus) program. Otolaryngol Clin North Am 1986 May; 19(2):329–354.

Cochlear implants. Med Lett Drugs Ther 1985 June 5; 27(689):51–52.

Farrar CL, Mangham CA, and Kuprenas SV. The cochlear prosthesis. Postgrad Med 1984 Nov 15; 76(7):73–76.

FDA approval opens US market for "bionic ear." Res Dev 1986 Jan; 33.

House WF and Berliner KI. Safety and efficacy of the House/3M cochlear implant in profoundly deaf adults. Otolaryngol Clin North Am 1986 May; 19(2):275–286.

Maddox HE and Porter TH. Who is a candidate for cochlear implantation? Otolaryngol Clin North Am 1983 Feb; 16(1):249–255.

Rupp RR and Jackson PD. Primary care for the hearing impaired: A changing picture. Geriatrics 1986 Mar; 41(3):75–80.

Yin L and Segerson DA. Cochlear implants: Overview of safety and effectiveness. Otolaryngol Clin North Am 1986 May; 19(2):423–433.

Agencies

Alexander Graham Bell Association for the Deaf, Inc., 3417 Volta Place, NW, Washington, DC 20007.

American Academy of Facial Plastic and Reconstructive Surgery, 1101 Vermont Ave, NW, Suite 304, Washington, DC 20005.

American Speech-Language-Hearing Association, 10801 Rockville Pike, Rockville, Maryland 20852.

American Tinnitus Association, PO Box #5, Portland, Oregon 97207.

National Association for Hearing and Speech Action, 10801 Rockville Pike, Rockville, Maryland 20852.

National Association for the Deaf, 814 Thayer Avenue, Silver Spring, Maryland 20910.

National Hearing Aid Society (NHAS), 20361 Middlebelt, Livonia, Michigan 48152.

National Hearing Association (Deaf) (NHA), Butterfield Ridge Office Center, 1430 Branding Lane, Suite 122, Downers Grove, Illinois 60515.

The Deafness Research Foundation, 55 East 34th. Street, New York, New York 10016.

Self-Help for Hard of Hearing People (DEAF) (SHHH), 7800 Wisconsin Avenue, Bethesda, Maryland 20814.

Chapter 52

Assessment of Neurologic Function

Physiologic Overview

The nervous system consists of the brain, the spinal cord, and the peripheral nerves. Its function is to control and to coordinate cellular activities throughout the body. It controls these activities through the transmission of electrical impulses. These impulses are routed by way of nerve fibers and nerve pathways that are direct and continuous. The responses elicited are practically instantaneous because changes in electrical potential transmit the signals.

The Brain

The brain is divided into the cerebrum, brain stem, and cerebellum. It is enclosed in a rigid, bony box—the skull, or cranium. At the base of this box is the *foramen magnum,* an opening through which the spinal cord forms a continuous connection with the brain (Fig. 52-1). The brain has three coverings: (1) the *dura,* the outer covering of dense fibrous tissue that closely hugs the inner wall of the skull; (2) the *arachnoid,* a very delicate membrane beneath the dura mater; and (3) the *pia mater,* a layer of delicate connective tissue that adheres closely to the brain and the spinal cord.

The *brain stem* from the top down consists of the midbrain, the pons, and the medulla oblongata.

The *cerebrum* is divided into two hemispheres and consists of four lobes: frontal, parietal, temporal, and occipital (Fig. 52-2). The cerebrum is the largest part of the brain. On its surface, or cortex, are located the "centers" from which motor impulses are carried to the muscles and to which sensory impulses come from the various sensory nerves.

The *midbrain* connects the pons and the cerebellum with the cerebral hemispheres. The *cerebellum* is located below and behind the cerebrum. Its function is the control or the coordination of muscles and equilibration.

The *pons* is situated in front of the cerebellum between the midbrain and the medulla and is a bridge between the two halves of the cerebellum as well as between the medulla and the cerebrum.

The *medulla oblongata* transmits motor fibers from the brain to the spinal cord and sensory fibers from the spinal

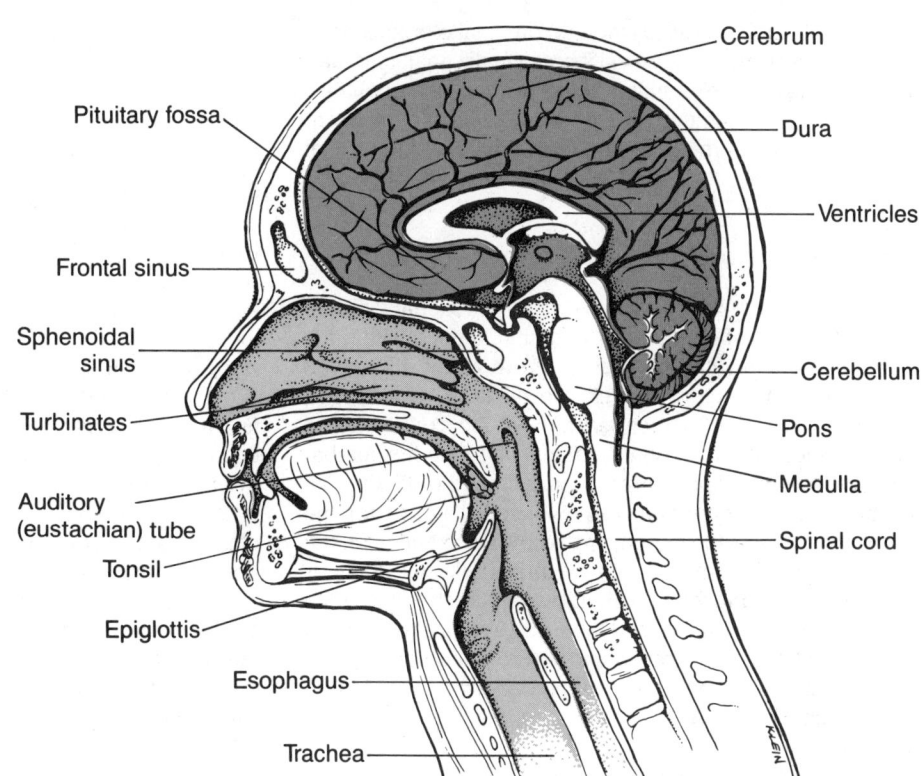

Figure 52-1
Cross-sectional view showing the anatomical position and the relation of structures of the head and the neck.

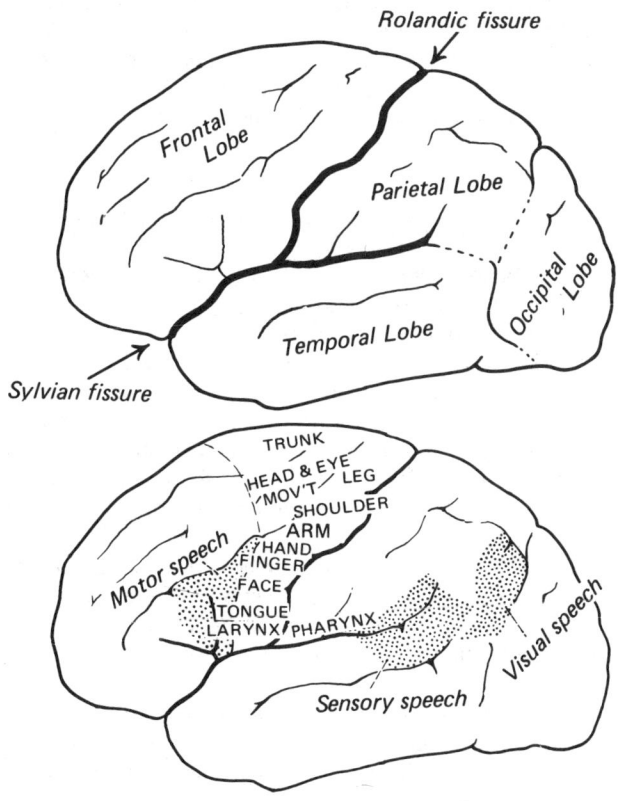

Figure 52-2
(*Top*) Diagrammatic representation of the cerebrum, showing relative locations of various lobes of the brain and the principal fissures. (*Bottom*) Diagrammatic representation of cerebral localization for motor movements of various portions of the body.

cord to the brain. The majority of these fibers cross, or decussate, at this level. The pons also contains important centers controlling heart, respiration, and blood pressure and is the site of origin of the fifth, sixth, seventh, and eighth cranial nerves.

There are two glands present in the brain: the pituitary and the pineal. The pituitary gland is frequently approached surgically. It lies at the base of the brain in a bony fossa termed the *sella turcica*, just posterior to the optic chiasm, on which it may press when the gland is enlarged.

Cerebral Cortex. Although the cells in the cerebral cortex are quite similar in appearance, their functions vary widely, depending on their geographic location. The topography of the cortex in relation to certain of its specific functions is shown in Figure 52-2. The posterior portion of each hemisphere (*i.e.*, the occipital lobe) is devoted to all aspects of visual perception. The lateral region, or temporal lobe, incorporates the auditory center. The mid-central zone, or parietal zone, posterior to the fissure of Rolandi, is concerned with sensation; the anterior portion is concerned with voluntary muscle movements. The large, uncharted area beneath the forehead (*i.e.*, the frontal lobes) contains the association pathways that determine emotional attitudes and responses and contributes to the formation of thought processes. Damage to the frontal lobes as a result of trauma or disease is by no means incapacitating from the standpoint of muscular control or coordination but has a decided effect on the person's personality, as reflected by basic attitudes, sense of humor and propriety, self-restraint, and motivations.

Internal Capsule, Pons, and Medulla. Nerve fibers from all portions of the cortex converge in each hemisphere and make their exit in the form of tight bundles known as the "internal capsule." Having entered the pons and the medulla, each bundle crosses the corresponding bundle from the opposite side. Some of these axons make connections with axons from the cerebellum, basal ganglia, thalamus, and hypothalamus; some connect with the cranial nerve cells. Other fibers from the cortex and the subcortical centers are channeled through the pons and the medulla into the spinal cord.

The Spinal Cord and Its Connections

The spinal cord, a direct continuation of the medulla oblongata, is that part of the nervous system contained within the vertebral column (Fig. 52-3). It is a cord about 45 cm (18 inches) long and approximately the thickness of a finger, extending from the foramen magnum of the skull, where it is continuous with the medulla oblongata, to the first lumbar vertebra, where it tapers off into a fine thread of tissue. The spinal cord is an important center of reflex action for the body and contains the conducting pathways to and from the higher centers in the cord and the brain. Like the brain, it consists of gray and white matter, but, although in the brain the gray matter is external and the white internal, in the cord the gray matter is in the center and is surrounded on all sides by the white fibers, both those of sensory tracts running up to the brain and those of motor fibers coming down from the brain.

Gray Matter.   The gray matter is shaped like two pairs of horns, the anterior horn and the posterior horn. The cord gives off 31 pairs of spinal nerves. Each is formed by the union of two roots, an anterior or motor root and a posterior or sensory root on which is the sensory ganglion. These two roots unite to form one spinal nerve. As a result, all the spinal nerves are mixed. Those leaving the right side of the cord supply the muscles, the skin, and the organs on the right side of the body; those of the left side supply the corresponding muscles on that side of the body.

Cerebrospinal Fluid

Within each cerebral hemisphere is a central cavity, the lateral ventricle, which is filled with clear cerebrospinal fluid. This fluid is extracted from the blood as it circulates through the capillaries of the choroid plexus. It then passes through well-defined channels from the lateral ventricles through narrow, tubular openings to the third and the fourth ventricles. From this narrow cavity it escapes to the subarachnoid space to bathe the entire surface of the brain and the spinal cord. The cerebrospinal fluid normally is absorbed by the large venous channels of the skull and along the spinal and the cranial nerves.

Cerebrospinal fluid is clear and colorless and has a specific gravity of 1.007. The average patient's ventricular and subarachnoid systems contain about 150 ml of this fluid. The organic and inorganic contents of the cerebrospinal fluid are very similar to that of the plasma; however, their concentration is somewhat different.

Disease produces changes in the composition of the cerebrospinal fluid. Determinations of the protein content and the quantity of glucose and chloride present constitute the chief chemical examinations. In a state of health, there are a minimal number of white cells and no red cells in the spinal fluid. Cerebrospinal fluid is also tested for immunoglobulins.

Pathophysiology

Vision and Cortical Blindness

There is a definite area in the rear of each hemisphere where the fibers of the corresponding optic nerve end. It is by means of these receiving cells that vision is possible. The eyes may be normal and the optic nerve perfect, but if these cells in one hemisphere are diseased, the person is half-blind and has cortical blindness. He cannot see to one side of the midline. He sees only half of any object. This is known as *hemianopsia* (half-blindness).

Cortical blindness of one optic area (*i.e.*, of the posterior tip of one cerebral hemisphere) always affects both eyes equally. Total blindness in one may be due to disease of that eye itself or to disease of its optic nerve. Just behind the two eyes, however, the two optic nerves become confluent (the chiasm), then again become separate and continue to the brain as two optic tracts.

In each of these tracts is just half of each optic nerve, so that if one tract is injured, there is blindness of exactly one half of each retina. For example, if the right tract is injured, the patient is blind on the right half of each retina, so that with either eye he can see nothing to his left but will see perfectly to his right. If the cortical optical area of the hemisphere to which that tract runs is destroyed, this same form of hemianopsia occurs.

The pituitary gland is located just beneath the chiasm; a tumor of this gland often disturbs the chiasm and produces blindness of both inner halves of the retinas, since it is only the fibers in the nasal halves of the optic nerves that cross. In many cases of blindness, it is thus possible to locate the disorder.

Motor Controls: Paralysis and Dyskinesia

A vertical band of cortex on each cerebral hemisphere governs the voluntary movements of the body. This region, known as the "motor cortex," can be located accurately.

We know the exact location of the cell in which originate the voluntary movements of the muscles of the face, the thumb, the hand, the arm, the trunk, or the leg. Before a person can move a muscle, these particular cells must send the stimulus down along their fibers. If these cells are stimulated with an electric current, the muscles they control will contract.

En route to the pons, as described previously, the motor fibers converge into a tight bundle known as the *capsule*. A comparatively small injury to the capsule causes paralysis in more muscles than does a much larger injury to the cortex itself.

The brain is like a telephone station, in which one blow of an ax can sever all the wires at the point where they leave the building, but a similar blow on the switchboard would sever only a few.

The ordinary cause of a stroke, followed by paralysis of one half of the body (hemiplegia), is usually a small hemorrhage from a blood vessel in the capsule. A much larger hemorrhage nearer to or in the cortex might paralyze one extremity, but hardly half of the body. Hemiplegia may be due to the rupture of a microaneurysm of a tiny artery running to

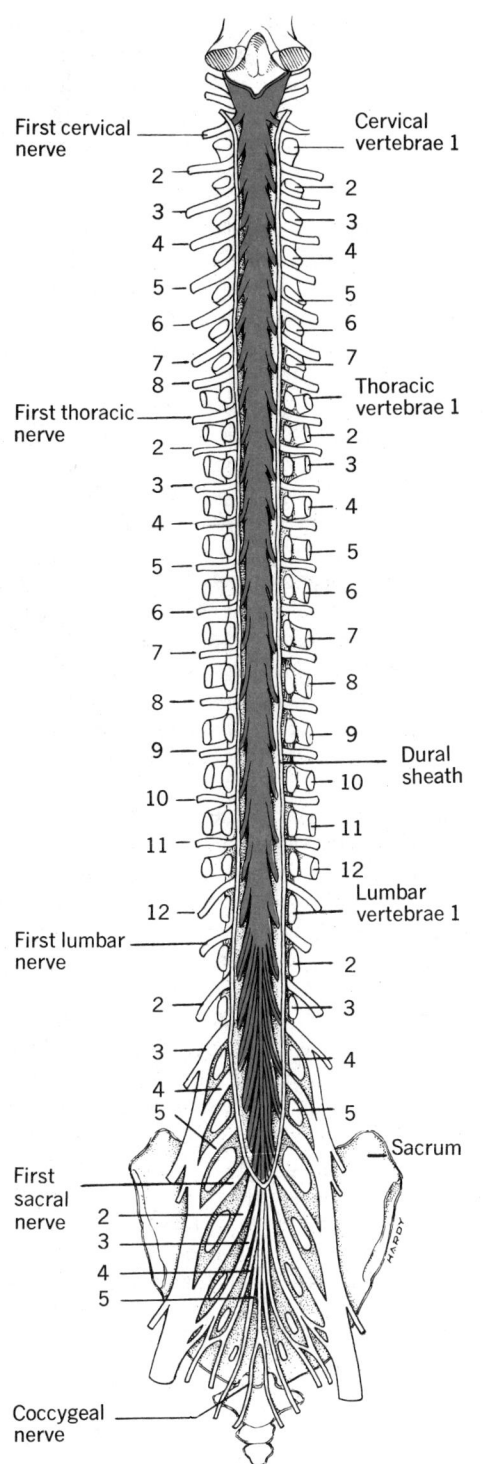

Figure 52-3
Spinal cord lying within the vertebral canal; spinous processes and laminae have been removed; dura and arachnoid have been opened. Spinal nerves are numbered on the left side; vertebrae are numbered on the right side. (Chaffee EE and Greisheimer EM. Basic Physiology and Anatomy, 4th ed. Philadelphia, JB Lippincott.)

the internal capsule or to the plugging of this artery by a thrombus or an embolus, and the subsequent death of the fibers that it supplies with blood.

Immediately after a stroke, one half of the body, as a rule, is paralyzed. Then, gradually, the person recovers the use of certain muscles, usually those of the leg, often those of the upper arm, least often those of the hand. Although the hemorrhage actually destroys the fibers of only a few nerves, it temporarily injures all those in its surrounding area, perhaps by the pressure of the escaped blood or by the edema. As the swelling from the hemorrhage diminishes, these latter fibers resume their function, but those actually destroyed never do.

Within the medulla, the motor axons from the cortex form two well-defined bands known as the *corticospinal* or *pyramidal tracts*. Here the majority of these fibers cross (or decussate) to the opposite side, continuing thereafter as the "crossed pyramidal tract." The remaining fibers then enter the spinal cord on the original side as the "direct pyramidal tract," each fiber in this tract finally crossing to the opposite side of the cord near the point of termination and coming to an end within the gray matter comprising the anterior horn on that side, in close proximity to a motor nerve cell. Fibers of the crossed pyramidal tract terminate within the anterior horn and make connections with anterior horn cells on the same side. All of the motor fibers of the spinal nerves represent extensions of these anterior horn cells, with each of these fibers communicating with only one particular muscle fiber.

Thus, each muscle fiber is under voluntary control through a combination of two nerve cells. One is located in the motor cortex, its fiber in the direct or crossed pyramidal tract, and the other is located in the anterior horn of the spinal cord, its fiber running to the muscle. The former is referred to as the *upper motor neuron;* the latter, as the *lower motor neuron.* Every motor nerve serving a muscle is a bundle comprised of several thousand lower motor neurons.

Several motor nerve tracts, other than the corticospinal, are contained in the spinal cord. Some represent the pathways of the so-called extrapyramidal system, establishing connections between the anterior horn cells and the automatic control centers located in the basal ganglia and the cerebellum. Others are components of reflex arcs, forming synaptic connections between anterior horn cells and sensory fibers that have entered adjacent or neighboring segments of the cord.

Motor Paralysis. Paralysis of a muscle may be due to pathologic changes in either the upper or the lower motor neuron. If a motor nerve is cut somewhere between the muscle and the spinal cord, the muscle becomes paralyzed, and the person is not able to move it. Furthermore, it takes no part in reflex movements. Moreover, this muscle becomes limp and wastes away; that is, it atrophies due to disuse. The injury to the spinal nerve trunk may heal, and the patient may regain the use of the muscles that it supplies. However, if the anterior horn motor nerve cells are destroyed, the nerve cannot regenerate, and that muscle never will be useful again. This is what occurs in anterior poliomyelitis.

If the upper motor neuron is destroyed, a different condition exists in the muscle. It is paralyzed as far as voluntary movement is concerned but not necessarily for reflex (involuntary) movements, because these originate in the nerve cells in the cord or the medulla. The muscle does not atrophy, and it will not become limp; on the contrary, it remains permanently more tense than normal. This paralysis seldom affects a part of one muscle, one single muscle, or only a few muscles; it usually affects a whole extremity, both extremities, or an entire half of the body.

A good illustration of this form of paralysis is the spastic (stiff) paralysis of those infants who during birth receive some mechanical injury that may have caused the rupture of a subdural blood vessel. The long-continued pressure of the escaped blood may injure large areas of cortex; hence, these children are frequently mentally retarded. Many have convulsions. When such a child begins to walk, the legs and the arms are stiff. During life, movements are awkward, stiff, and weak. Since those muscles that draw the feet and the knees toward each other (the adductor muscles) are naturally stronger than those that spread those extremities apart (the abductor muscles), these patients walk by a cross-legged progression, called also the *scissors gait;* that is, in each step the leg is moved not only forward but is also swung round across the front of the other. When both legs are paralyzed, the condition is called *paraplegia;* and when the arm and the leg on the same side are paralyzed, the term *hemiplegia* is used. Paralysis of all four extremities is *quadriplegia.*

A common illustration of upper motor neuron paralysis is hemiplegia. If a hemorrhage, an embolus, or a thrombus destroys the fibers from the motor area in the internal capsule, the arm and the leg of the opposite side promptly become stiff and more or less paralyzed, and the reflexes are exaggerated. Another illustration of upper neuron disease is seen in adults with spastic paraplegia, a chronic stiffness of both legs due to a gradual degeneration of the fibers in the pyramidal tract. The person so afflicted walks stiffly, as though wading through water, the knees always touching each other and the feet scarcely raised from the ground (the spastic gait).

Both an upper and a lower motor neuron paralysis may result from an injury that crushes the spinal cord, a type of injury that is all too common. A person diving into too-shallow water, for example, strikes his head and "breaks" his neck. That is, at one point the vertebrae are no longer in line, and the cord is badly crushed at the point of the dislocation. Knuckling of the backbone due to tuberculosis may accomplish the same thing, only more slowly. The result of such crushing of the cord leads to a rigid paralysis on both sides of all muscles whose nerves leave the cord below the crushed spot. Flaccid paralysis also occurs in those muscles whose motor nerve fibers come from cells in the crushed area. There also will be insensibility of the skin below the crushed area, since the sensory fibers from below the injury no longer reach the brain. Tumors of the cord ultimately cause this same picture. At first, only that part of the cord directly involved is disturbed, but as the tumor grows, it may completely crush the cord.

Extrapyramidal Motor Controls. The smoothness, the accuracy, and the strength that characterize the muscular movements of a normal person are attributable to the influence of the cerebellum and the basal ganglia.

The cerebellum (see Fig. 52-1), nestled beneath the posterior lobe of the cerebrum, chief assistant to the higher motor centers in the cerebral cortex, is responsible for coordinating, balancing, timing, and synergizing with precision all muscular movements that originate in those centers. Through the agency of the cerebellum, the contractions of opposing muscle groups are adjusted in relation to each other to maximal mechanical advantage; muscular contractions can be sustained evenly at the desired tension and without significant fluctuation, and reciprocal movements can be reproduced at high and constant speed, in stereotyped fashion, and with relatively little effort.

The basal ganglia are masses of gray matter in the midbrain beneath the cerebral hemispheres. These border or project into the lateral ventricles and lie in close apposition to the internal capsule. It is their function to control habitual or automatic acts and to maintain a "postural background" against which voluntary movements are performed. These ganglia, aided by their connections with the organs of special sense, keep the contractile tone of every muscle in the trunk and the extremities in a constant state of adjustment, so that a person is able to keep his balance regardless of the posture of his body, in darkness as well as in light and irrespective of the status underfoot. Moreover, thanks to this control station, the person is equipped to react swiftly, appropriately, and automatically to any smell, sight, or sound that demands an immediate response.

Dyskinesias. Loss of cerebellar function, which may occur as a result of intracranial injury, hemorrhage, abscess, or tumor, results in muscular flabbiness, weakness, and fatigue. The patient exhibits a coarse involuntary tremor that increases in intensity in association with voluntary movements. He is unable to control his movements accurately or to coordinate his muscles efficiently or smoothly, every act being performed in disjointed fashion, according to stages, or "by the numbers." He is incapable of performing alternating movements with speed or uniformity, a characteristic of cerebellar disease called *adiadochokinesis.* When he walks, he staggers, lurching from side to side as though intoxicated, feet wide apart, but steps short and not stamping (*i.e.,* with the vertiginous, reeling gait of cerebellar ataxia).

Destruction or dysfunction of the basal ganglia does not lead to paralysis but to muscular rigidity, with consequent disturbances of posture and movement. Such patients are afflicted by a tendency to display involuntary movements. These may take the form of coarse tremors. characterized by approximately six oscillations per second; *athetosis,* namely, movement of a slow, squirming, writhing, twisting type; or *chorea,* marked by spasmodic, purposeless, and grotesque motions of the trunk and the extremities, and facial grimacing. Clinical syndromes based on lesions involving the basal ganglia include parkinsonism (see p. 1477); Huntington's disease (see p. 1481); Wilson's disease, or hepatolenticular degeneration; and spasmodic torticollis.

Sensory Pathways and Disturbances

The Thalamus. The thalamus, a major receiving and communication center for the afferent sensory nerves, is a large and complicated structure located in the midbrain. It lies in close relation to the third ventricle, forming its lateral wall, and to the lateral ventricle, forming its floor, and is in close proximity to the basal ganglia and adjacent to the internal capsule. To the thalamus may be attributed the vague awareness of sensations described as "feelings" of pleasure, discomfort, or pain. Moreover, it is responsible for the routing of all sensory stimuli to their many destinations, including the cerebral cortex, which receives them and translates them automatically into appropriate responses.

Sensory Pathways. The transmission of sensory impulses from their points of origin to their cerebral destinations involves three neuron relays; moreover, there are three major pathways by which they may be routed, depending on the type of sensation that is registered. Specific knowledge regarding these paths is of great importance from the standpoint of neurologic diagnoses, being indispensable for the accurate localization of brain and cord lesions in many patients.

The axon of the nerve in which the sensory impulse originates enters the spinal cord by way of the posterior root. Axons conveying sensations of heat, cold, and pain immediately enter the posterior gray column of the cord, where they make connections with the cells of secondary neurons. Pain and temperature fibers cross immediately to the opposite side of the cord and course upward to the thalamus. Fibers carrying sensations of touch, light pressure, and localization do not connect immediately with the second neuron but ascend the cord for a variable distance before entering the gray matter and completing this connection. The axon of the secondary neuron crosses the cord and proceeds upward to the thalamus.

The third category of sensation, produced by stimuli arising from muscles, joints, and bones, includes position sense and vibratory sense. These stimuli are conveyed, uncrossed, all the way to the brain stem by the axon of the primary neuron. In the medulla, synaptic connections are made with cells of the secondary neurons, whose axons then cross to the opposite side and proceed to the thalamus.

Sensory Losses. Severance of a sensory nerve results in total loss of sensation in its area of distribution. Transection of the spinal cord yields complete anesthesia below the level of injury. Selective destruction or degeneration of the posterior columns of the spinal cord, a characteristic of combined system disease, is responsible for a loss of position sense in segments distal to the lesion, unaccompanied by loss of touch, pain, or temperature perception. Such people, unless they look, cannot tell where their feet are or in what direction they are pointing. Moreover, they cannot perceive vibrations in the affected area. A lesion, such as a cyst, in the center of the cord causes dissociation of sensation, that is, loss of pain at the level of the lesion. This is explainable on the basis of the fact that the fibers carrying pain and temperature cross the cord immediately on entering; thus, any lesion that divides the cord longitudinally divides these fibers likewise. Other sensory fibers ascend the cord for variable distances, some even to the medulla itself, before crossing, thereby bypassing the lesion and avoiding destruction.

Dysesthesias. Irritative lesions affecting the posterior spinal nerve roots may cause intermittent severe pains that are referred to their areas of distribution. This phenomenon explains the pains of tabes dorsalis. The sensation of tingling of the fingers and the toes constitutes a prominent symptom of combined systems disease, presumably due to degenerative changes in the sensory fibers that extend to the thalamus (*i.e.,* belonging to the spinothalamic tract).

Autonomic Nervous System

The contractions of muscles that are not under voluntary control, including the heart muscle, the secretions of all digestive and sweat glands, and the activity of certain endocrine organs as well, are controlled by a major component of the nervous system known as the autonomic nervous system. The term *autonomic* refers to the fact that the operations of this system are independent of the desires and the intentions of the person. It is not subject to his will; that is, it is in a sense autonomous.

To the extent that it is not subject to regulation by the cerebral cortex, the autonomic nervous system resembles the extrapyramidal systems that are centered in the cerebellum and the basal ganglia. However, in other respects it is unique. First, its regulatory effects are exerted not on individual cells but on large expanses of tissue and on entire organs. Second, the responses that it elicits do not appear instantaneously, but only after a lag period, and they are sustained far longer than other neurogenic responses, a type of response that is calculated to ensure maximal functional efficiency on the part of receptor organs, such as the blood vessels and the hollow viscera.

The quality of these responses is explained by the fact that the autonomic nervous system transmits its impulses only partly by way of nerve pathways, the remainder of the route being serviced by chemical mediators, resembling in this respect the endocrine system. Electrical impulses, conducted through nerve fibers, stimulate the formation of specific chemical agents at strategic locations within the muscle mass, the diffusion of these chemicals being responsible for the contraction.

The Hypothalamus. Overall supervision of the autonomic nervous system is considered a function of the hypothalamus. The hypothalamus is a portion of the diencephalon (interbrain) located immediately beneath and lateral to the lower portion of the wall of the third ventricle. It includes among its components the optic chiasm; the tuber cinereum; the pituitary stalk, which originates from the latter; and the pituitary gland itself. Large cell groups in adjacent portions of the hypothalamus have been assigned the role of the probable centers of autonomic regulation. These centers are richly endowed with connections linking the autonomic system with the thalamus, the cortex, the olfactory apparatus, and the pituitary gland. Here reside the mechanisms for the control of visceral and somatic reactions that were designed originally for defense or attack, but in man these are associated with his emotional states (*i.e.,* his fears, anger, anxiety); for the control of metabolic processes, including fat, carbohydrate, and water metabolism; for the regulaton of body temperature, arterial pressure, and all muscular and glandular activities of the gastrointestinal tract; for control of the genital functions; and for the sleep rhythm. The close proximity, histologic similarity, and multiple connections between the pituitary gland, master gland of the endocrines, and this portion of the brain suggest that here may be located the supreme headquarters of the endocrine and autonomic nervous systems, commanding all vital processes.

Sympathetic and Parasympathetic Nervous Systems

The autonomic nervous system comprises two divisions that are anatomically and functionally distinct, referred to as the sympathetic and the parasympathetic nervous systems. The majority of the tissues and the organs under autonomic control are innervated by both systems. Sympathetic stimuli are mediated by norepinephrine, and parasympathetic impulses are mediated by acetylcholine. These chemicals produce opposing and mutually antagonistic effects, as indicated in Table 52-1.

Sympathetic Nervous System. Sympathetic neurons are located in the thoracic and the lumbar segments of the spinal cord; their axons, called *preganglionic fibers*, emerge by way of all anterior nerve roots from the eighth cervical or first thoracic segment to the second or third lumbar segment, inclusive. A short distance from the cord these fibers diverge to join a chain composed of 22 linked ganglia that extends the entire length of the spinal column, flanking the vertebral bodies on both sides. Some form multiple synapses with nerve cells within the chain. Others traverse the chain without making connections or losing continuity to join large "preverte-

TABLE 52-1
Comparison of Parasympathetic and Sympathetic Effects on Specific Organs and Tissues

Organ or Tissue	Parasympathetic Effects	Sympathetic Effects
Vessels		
Cutaneous		Constriction
Muscular		Variable
Coronary	Constriction	Dilatation
Salivary gland	Dilatation	Constriction
Buccal mucosa		Dilatation
Pulmonary	Variable	Variable
Cerebral	Dilatation	Constriction
Of abdominal and pelvic viscera		Constriction
Of external genitalia	Dilatation	Constriction
Heart	Inhibition	Acceleration
Eye		
Iris	Constriction	Dilatation
Ciliary muscle	Contraction	Relaxation
Smooth muscle of orbit and upper lid		Contraction
Bronchi	Constriction	Dilatation
Glands		
Sweat		Secretion
Salivary	Secretion	Secretion
Gastric	Secretion	Inhibition?
		Secretion of mucus
Pancreatic		
Acini	Secretion	
Islets	Secretion	
Liver		Glycogenolysis
Adrenal medulla		Secretion
Smooth Muscle		
Of skin		Contraction
Of stomach wall	Contraction (predominantly)	Inhibition (predominantly)
Of small intestine	Increased tone and motility	Inhibition
Of large intestine	Increased tone and motility	Inhibition
Of bladder wall (detrusor muscle)	Contraction	Inhibition
Of trigone and sphincter	Inhibition	Contraction
Of uterus, pregnant	None	Contraction
Of uterus, nonpregnant	None	Inhibition

(Best CH and Taylor NB. Physiological Basis of Medical Practice, 6th ed. Baltimore, Williams & Wilkins.)

bral'' ganglia in the thorax, the abdomen, or the pelvis or one of the ''terminal'' ganglia in the vicinity of an organ, such as the bladder or the rectum. Postganglionic nerve fibers originating in the sympathetic chain rejoin the spinal nerves that supply the extremities and are distributed to blood vessels, sweat glands, and smooth muscle tissue in the skin. Postganglionic fibers from the prevertebral plexuses (*i.e.,* the cardiac, pulmonary, splanchnic, and pelvic plexuses) supply structures in the head and the neck, the thorax, the abdomen, and the pelvis, respectively, having been joined in these plexuses by fibers from the parasympathetic division.

The adrenals, the kidneys, the liver, the spleen, the stomach, and the duodenum are under the control of the giant celiac plexus, familiarly known as the ''solar plexus.'' This receives its sympathetic nerve components by way of the three splanchnic nerves, composed of preganglionic fibers from nine segments of the spinal cord (*i.e.,* T4 to L1), and is joined by the vagus nerve, representing the parasympathetic division. From the celiac plexus, fibers of both divisions travel along the course of blood vessels to their target organs.

Parasympathetic Nervous System. The preganglionic nerve cells of the sympathetic division, as described above, are consolidated in consecutive segments of the cord, from C7 to L1 or L2. Those of the parasympathetic system, on the other hand, are located in two sections, one in the brain stem and the other from spinal segments below L2. On this account, the parasympathetic system is referred to as the ''craniosacral'' division, as distinct from the ''thoracolumbar'' division of the autonomic nervous system.

The cranial parasympathetics arise from the midbrain and the medulla oblongata. Fibers from cells in the midbrain travel with the third oculomotor nerve to the ciliary ganglia, where postganglionic fibers of this division are joined by those of the sympathetic system. Forming the ciliary nerve, these innervate the ciliary muscles of the eye to control the caliber of the pupil. Parasympathetic fibers from the medulla travel with the seventh (facial), ninth (glossopharyngeal), and tenth (vagus) cranial nerves. Those from the facial nerve end in the splenopalatine ganglion, from which emanate the fibers that innervate the lacrimal glands, the ciliary muscle, and the sphincter of the pupil. Those from the glossopharyngeal nerve innervate the parotid gland. The vagus nerve carries preganglionic parasympathetic fibers without interruption to the organs that it innervates, joining ganglion cells within the myocardium and within the walls of the esophagus, the stomach, and the intestine.

Preganglionic parasympathetic fibers from the anterior roots of the sacral nerves coalesce to become the pelvic nerves, consolidate and regroup in the pelvic plexus, and terminate around ganglion cells in the musculature of the pelvic organs. These innervate the colon, the rectum, and the bladder, inhibiting the muscular tone of the anal and the bladder sphincters and dilating the blood vessels of the bladder, the rectum, and the genitalia.

The vagus, splanchnic, pelvic, and other autonomic nerves carry impulses generated in the viscera to the dorsal nucleus of the vagus, where connections are made with efferent parasympathetic neurons, forming a series of reflex arcs. These provide the basis for self-regulation, a cardinal feature of the autonomic nervous system, and one reason for ''autonomy.''

Autonomic Functions and Dysfunctions. A detailed listing of the effects produced by the two divisions of the autonomic nervous system is supplied in Table 52-1. This listing provides impressive evidence of the scope and the importance of autonomic activity in relation to all bodily functions and from the standpoint of survival itself. Both sympathetic and parasympathetic divisions are in a constant state of activity, the activity of each relative to the other being one of controlled opposition, with a delicate balance maintained between the two at all times.

Sympathetic Syndromes. Certain syndromes are distinctive of diseases of the sympathetic nerve trunks. Among these are dilatation of the pupil of the eye on the same side as a penetrating wound of the neck (evidence of disturbance of the cervical sympathetic cord); temporary paralysis of the bowel (indicated by the absence of peristaltic waves and the distention of the intestine by gas) following fracture of any one of the lower dorsal or upper lumbar vertebrae with hemorrhage into the base of the mesentery; and the marked variations in pulse rate and rhythm that often follow compression fractures of the upper six thoracic vertebrae.

The Neurologic Examination

The neurologic examination is a sophisticated and subtle process, comprising a large number of tests of highly specialized function. Although the neurologic examination is limited in most instances to a simple screening, it is necessary for the examiner to be able to conduct a thorough neurologic assessment when the history or other physical findings warrant it.

A neurologic assessment is divided into five components: cerebral function, cranial nerves, motor system, sensory system, and reflex status. As in other facets of the physical assessment, the neurologic examination follows a logical sequence and is pursued from higher levels of cortical function through to a determination of the integrity of peripheral nerves.

Much of the patient's neurologic function is assessed during the history and during the routine of the earlier parts of the physical examination. One can learn much about speech patterns, mental status, gait, stance, motor power, and coordination. The simple act of shaking a patient's hand as he enters the room conveys an enormous amount of information to the alert observer.

Cerebral Function

Cerebral abnormalities may cause disturbances in communication, in intellectual functioning, and in patterns of emotional behavior. Adequate cerebral functioning is determined by assessing the patient's *mental status*. The examiner observes the patient's appearance and behavior, noting the patient's dress, grooming, and personal hygiene. Observation of posture, gestures, movements, facial expressions, and motor activity often provides important information about the patient's attitude. The manner of speech and the patient's level of consciousness are also observed: Is his speech clear and coherent? Is he alert and responsive, or drowsy and stuporous?

Intellectual function is tested when doubts exist about the patient's intellectual competence. Often, patients in a toxic state or those who have destruction of frontal cortex appear superficially normal until or unless one or more tests of integrative capacity are performed. First, the examiner determines whether the patient is oriented to time, place, and person. Does the patient know what day it is, what year it is, or who is the president of the United States? Is the patient aware of where he is? Is the patient aware of who you are and of his purpose for being in the room? Is the capacity for immediate memory intact? A person with an average IQ is able to repeat seven digits without faltering and is able to recite five digits backward. The examiner might ask the patient to count backward from 100, or to subtract 7 from 100, then 7 from that, then 7 from that, etc. The capacity to interpret well-known proverbs is a test of even higher intellectual function (abstract reasoning). Does the patient know what is meant by "the early bird catches the worm?"

It is important to determine the patient's thought content as it emerges during the course of the interview. Are his thoughts spontaneous, natural, and clear? Are his ideas relevant and coherent? Does he have any fixed ideas, illusions, or preoccupations? What are his insights into these thoughts? Preoccupation with death or morbid events, evidence of hallucinations, and paranoid ideation are all important and require further evaluation.

An assessment of cerebral functioning also includes the patient's emotional status. Is the patient's affect natural and even, or is he irritable and angry, anxious, apathetic, or euphoric? Does his mood fluctuate normally, or does he unpredictably swing from joy to sadness during the interview? Is his affect appropriate to his words and thought content? Are his verbal communications consistent with his nonverbal communications?

The examiner may now look at more specific areas of higher cortical function. *Agnosia* is the inability to interpret or recognize objects seen through the special senses. The patient may see a pen but not know what it is called or what to do with it. He may even be able to describe it but not to interpret its function. The patient may experience auditory or tactile agnosia, as well as visual agnosia. Each of the dysfunctions implicates a different part of the cortex.

To screen for agnosia, the examiner tests the patient's cortical sensory interpretation. The patient is shown a familiar object and asked to identify it by name. Next, he is confronted with a familiar sound (bell) and asked to identify its source. Tactile interpretation is easily assessed by placing a familiar object (key, coin) in the patient's hand and having him identify it while his eyes are closed.

An assessment of cortical motor integration is carried out by asking the patient to perform a skilled act (throw a ball, move a chair). Successful performance hinges on the person's ability to understand the activity desired. He must also have normal motor strength. Failures signal cerebral dysfunction.

Lastly, language function is assessed. The normal person is able to understand and communicate in spoken and written language. Does the patient answer questions relevantly? Can he read a sentence from a newspaper and explain its meaning? Can he write his name or copy a simple figure that the examiner has drawn? A deficiency in language function is called *aphasia*.

Interpretation of neurologic abnormalities is a highly sophisticated and technical process. It is the obligation of the examiner to record and report what is found. Analysis and the conclusions that may be drawn from these findings will

usually depend on the physician's extensive knowledge of neuroanatomy, neurophysiology, and neuropathology.

Examination of the Cranial Nerves

There are 12 pairs of cranial nerves that emerge from the undersurface of the brain. They are designated by the Roman numerals I to XII, according to the order of their placement. The cranial nerves are often assessed during a complete head and neck examination. These nerves, their functions, and the tests for their measurement are outlined in Table 52-2.

Examination of the Motor System

The motor system is quite complex, and the end result of motor function is a synthesis of the integrity of the corticospinal tracts, the extrapyramidal system, and cerebellar function. A motor impulse traverses two neurons. The *upper motor neuron* begins in the cortex of the opposite side of the brain, descends through the internal capsule, crosses to the opposite side in the brain stem, descends through the corticospinal tract, and synapses with the *lower motor neuron* in the cord. The lower motor neuron receives the impulse in the posterior part of the cord and runs to the myoneural junction. The other two systems, the extrapyramidal system and the cerebellar system, act as modifiers.

A thorough examination of the motor system includes an assessment of muscle size, muscle tone, muscle strength, coordination, and balance. The patient is instructed to walk across the room while the examiner notes his posture and gait. The muscles are inspected, and palpated if necessary, for their size and symmetry. Any evidence of atrophy or involuntary movements (tremors, tics) is noted. Muscle tone is evaluated by palpating various muscle groups at rest and during passive movement. The resistance to these movements is noted. Abnormalities in tone include spasticity, rigidity, or flaccidity.

Muscle strength is tested by ascertaining the patient's ability to flex or extend his extremity against resistance. The function of an individual muscle or group of muscles is evaluated by placing the muscle at a disadvantage. The quadriceps, for example, is a powerful muscle responsible for straightening the leg. Once the leg is straightened, it is exceedingly difficult for the examiner to flex the knee. On the other hand, if the knee is flexed, and the patient is asked to straighten the leg against resistance, a more subtle disability can be brought out. It is critically important to compare the two sides if one is looking for minor degrees of disability.

Some authorities advocate the use of a five-point scale for strength of motor power. A five would indicate full power of contraction; a four would indicate fair, but not full, strength; a three would imply just sufficient strength to overcome the force of gravity; a two indicates the ability to move but not to overcome the force of gravity; a one indicates minimal contractile power; a zero implies no contraction whatsoever.

Assessment of motor power can be as restricted or detailed as the examiner wishes. One may quickly test the strength of the proximal muscles of the upper and lower extremities, comparing the two. The motor capacity of the finer muscles that control the function of the hand and of the foot can then be assessed.

Cerebellar influence on the motor system is reflected in balance control and coordination. Coordination in the hands

TABLE 52-2
Cranial Nerves

Cranial Nerve	Function	Clinical Examination
CN I (olfactory)	Sense of smell	With his eyes closed, the patient identifies familiar odors (coffee, tobacco). Each nostril is tested separately.
CN II (optic)	Visual acuity	Snellen eye chart Visual fields Funduscopic examination
CN III (oculomotor) CN IV (trochlear) CN VI (abducens)	Cranial nerves III, IV, and VI function in the regulation of eye movements; CN III also innervates the levator muscle of the eyelid, the constrictor muscle of the pupil, and the ciliary muscle, which controls accommodation.	Test for ocular rotations, conjugate movements, nystagmus. Test for pupillary reflexes, and inspect eyelids for ptosis.
CN V (trigeminal)	Facial sensation	Have patient close his eyes. Touch cotton to forehead, cheeks, and jaw. Opposite sides of face are compared. Sensitivity to superficial pain is tested by using a safety pin. Alternate between the sharp point and the dull end. Patient reports "sharp" or "dull" with each movement. If responses are incorrect, test for temperature sensation. Test tubes of cold and hot water are used alternately.
	Corneal reflex	While the patient looks up, lightly touch a wisp of cotton against the temporal surface of each cornea. A blink and tearing is a normal response.
	Mastication	Have the patient clench his jaw and move it from side to side. Palpate the masseter and temporal muscles, noting strength and equality.
CN VII (facial)	Facial muscle movement	Observe for symmetry while the patient performs facial movements: smiles, whistles, elevates eyebrows, frowns, tightly closes eyelids against resistance (examiner attempts to open them). Observe face for flaccid paralysis (shallow nasolabial folds).
	Taste: anterior two thirds of tongue	Patient extends his tongue. His ability to discriminate between sugar and salt is tested.
CN VIII (vestibulocochlear)	Hearing and equilibrium	Whisper or watch-tick test Test for lateralization (Weber) Test for air and bone conduction (Rinne)
CN IX (glossopharyngeal)	Taste: posterior third of tongue	Assess patient's ability to discriminate between sugar and salt on posterior third of the tongue.
CN X (vagus)	Pharyngeal contraction	Depress a tongue blade on posterior tongue, or stimulate posterior pharynx to elicit gag reflex.
	Symmetrical movement of vocal cords.	Note any hoarseness in voice.
	Symmetrical movement of soft palate	Have patient say "ah." Observe symmetrical rise of uvula and soft palate.
CN XI (spinal accessory)	Movement of sternocleidomastoid and trapezius muscles	Palpate and note the strength of the trapezius muscles while the patient shrugs his shoulders against resistance.
		Palpate and note the strength of each sternocleidomastoid muscle as the patient turns his head against opposing pressure of the examiner's hand.
CN XII (hypoglossal)	Movement of the tongue	While the patient protrudes his tongue, any deviation or tremors are noted. The strength of the tongue is tested by having the patient move his protruded tongue from side to side against a tongue depressor.

and upper extremities is tested by having the patient perform *rapid, alternating movements* and *point-to-point testing*. First, the patient is instructed to pat his thigh as fast as he can with his hand. Each hand is tested separately. Then, he is instructed to turn his hands from a supine to a prone position as rapidly as possible. Lastly, he is asked to touch each of his fingers with his thumb in a consecutive motion. Speed, symmetry, and degree of difficulty are noted.

Point-to-point testing is accomplished by having the patient touch the examiner's extended finger and then his own nose. This is repeated several times. This assessment is then carried out with the patient's eyes closed.

Coordination in the lower extremities is tested by having the patient run his heel down the anterior surface of his tibia. Each leg is tested in turn. Inability to perform these maneuvers is referred to as *ataxia*. The presence of ataxia or tremors (rhythmic, involuntary movements) during these movements suggests cerebellar disease.

It is not necessary to carry out each of these assessments for coordination. During a routine examination, it is advisable to perform a simple screening of the upper and lower extremities by having the patient perform either rapid, alternating movements or point-to-point testing. When abnormalities are observed, a more thorough examination is indicated.

The *Romberg test* is a screening measurement for balance. The patient stands with his feet together, arms extended in front of him, and eyes closed. The examiner stands close to the patient and reassures him that he will be supported if he begins to lose his balance. Slight swaying is normal. Additional cerebellar tests for balance in the ambulatory patient include hopping in place, alternating knee bends, and heel-to-toe walking.

Examination of the Reflexes

The motor reflexes are involuntary contractions of muscles or muscle groups in response to abrupt stretching near the site of the muscle's insertion. The tendon is struck directly with a reflex hammer, or indirectly by striking the examiner's thumb, which is placed firmly against the tendon. In testing the reflexes, we are examining involuntary reflex arcs that depend on the presence of afferent stretch receptors, spinal synapses, efferent motor fibers, and a variety of modifying influences from higher levels. Common reflexes that may be tested include the biceps, the brachioradialis, the triceps, the patellar, and the ankle (or Achilles) reflexes (Fig. 52-4).

A reflex hammer is used to elicit a deep tendon reflex. The stem of the hammer is held loosely between thumb and index finger, allowing a full swinging motion. The wrist motion is similar to that used during percussion. The extremity is positioned so that the tendon is slightly stretched. This requires a sound knowledge of the location of muscles and their tendon attachments. The tendon is then struck briskly and the response compared with the corresponding reflex on the opposite side of the body. Wide variation in reflex response may be considered normal. However, it is more important that the reflexes be symmetrically equivalent. When the comparison is made, both sides should be equivalently relaxed and each tendon struck with equal force.

Valid findings depend on several factors: proper use of the reflex hammer, proper positioning of the extremity, and a relaxed patient. If the reflexes are symmetrically diminished or absent, the examiner may use a technique called *rein-*

forcement to increase reflex activity. This involves the isometric contraction of other muscle groups. If lower extremity reflexes are diminished or absent, the patient is instructed to lock his fingers together and pull in opposite directions. Having the patient clench his jaw or press his heel against the floor or examining table may likewise elicit more reliable biceps, triceps, or brachioradialis reflexes.

The absence of reflexes is significant, although ankle jerks (Achilles reflex) may be absent in older people.

Reflex responses are often graded on a 0 to 4+ scale:

4+—brisk, hyperactive
3+—more brisk than normal
2+—normal
1+—less than normal, slow response
0 —no response

As was previously mentioned, scale ratings are highly subjective. When used, the findings are recorded as a fraction, indicating the scale range (*e.g.,* 2+/4+). Some examiners prefer to use the terms "present," "absent," and "diminished" when describing reflexes.

The *biceps reflex* is elicited by striking the biceps tendon of the flexed elbow. The examiner supports the forearm with one arm while placing the thumb against the tendon and striking the thumb with the reflex hammer. Note the normal flexion at the elbow and the contraction of the biceps.

To elicit a *triceps reflex*, the patient's arm is flexed at the elbow and positioned in front of the chest. The examiner supports the patient's arm and identifies the triceps tendon by palpating 2.5 to 5 cm (1 to 2 inches) above the elbow. A direct blow on the tendon normally produces contraction of the triceps muscle and extension of the elbow.

With the patient's forearm resting on the lap or across the abdomen, the *brachioradialis reflex* is assessed. A gentle strike of the hammer 2.5 to 5 cm (1 to 2 inches) above the wrist results in flexion and supination of the forearm.

The *patellar reflex* is elicited by striking the patellar tendon just below the patella. The patient may be in a sitting or a lying position. If the patient is supine, the examiner supports the legs to facilitate relaxation of the muscles. Contraction of the quadriceps and knee extension are normal responses.

To facilitate an *ankle reflex*, the foot is dorsiflexed at the ankle and the hammer strikes the stretched Achilles tendon. This reflex normally produces plantar flexion. If the examiner experiences difficulty with the ankle reflex and suspects that the patient is unable to relax, the patient is instructed to kneel on a chair or similar elevated, flat surface. This position places the ankles in dorsiflexion and reduces any muscular tension in the gastrocnemius. The Achilles tendons are struck in turn, and plantar flexion is usually demonstrated.

When reflexes are exceedingly hyperactive, a phenomenon called *clonus* may be elicited. If the foot is abruptly dorsiflexed, it may "chatter" for two or three beats before it settles into a position of rest. Occasionally, in central nervous system (CNS) disease, this activity will persist, and the foot will not come to rest while the tendon is being stretched but will persist in repetitive activity. The unsustained clonus associated with normal but hyperactive reflexes is not considered pathologic. Sustained clonus always indicates the presence of CNS disease and requires evaluation by a physician.

Certain superficial reflexes may be elicited by scratching the skin of the abdominal wall, or the inside of the thigh in men. The former results in involuntary contraction of the ab-

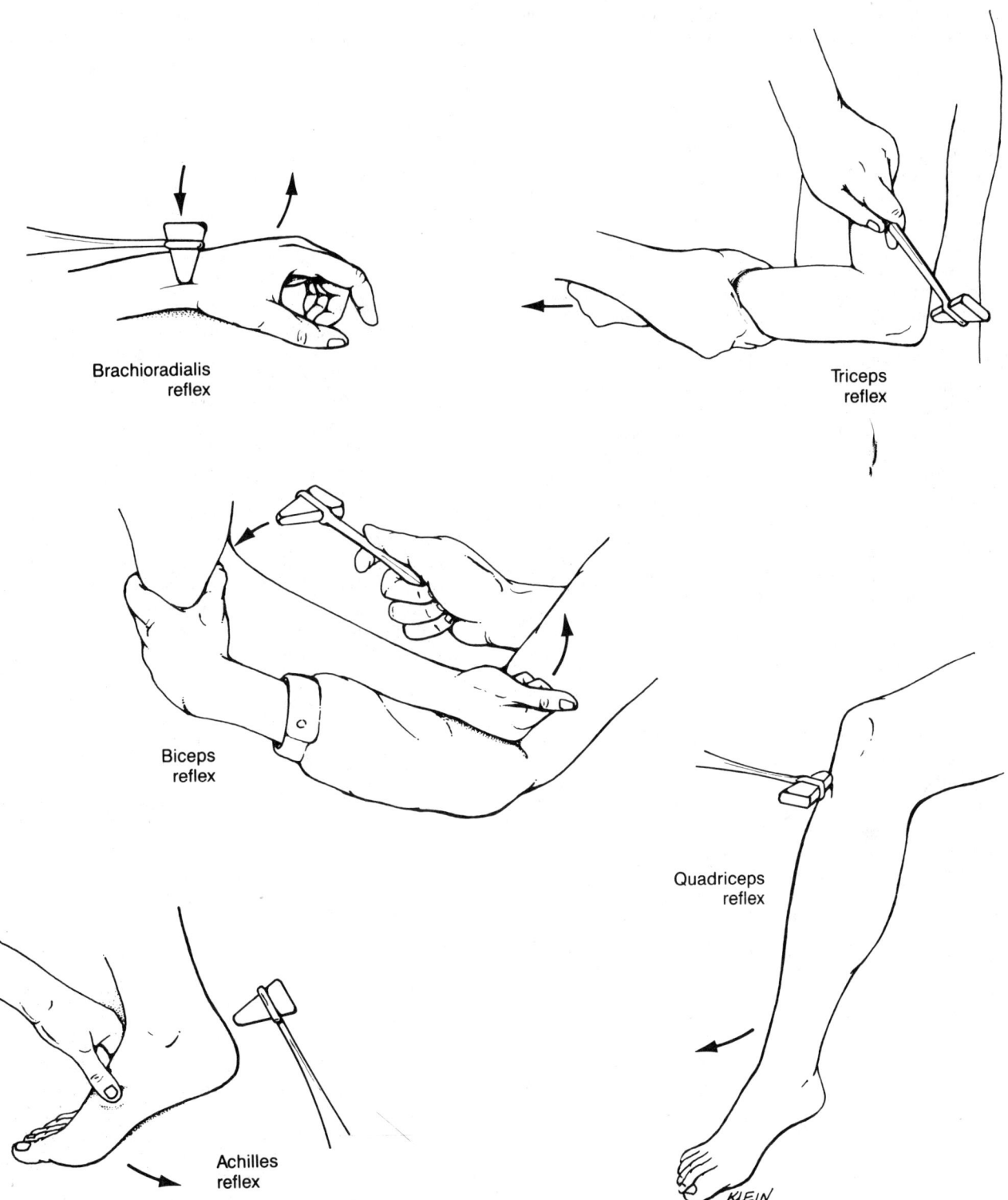

Figure 52-4

The proper technique for eliciting the major tendon reflexes. The tendon can be struck *directly* with the reflex hammer or *indirectly* by striking the examiner's thumb, which is placed on the tendon. Arrows indicate the normal extremity motion expected.

dominal muscles, and the latter results in retraction of the scrotum. Although interesting phenomena, they have little clinical significance.

A well-known reflex, indicative of CNS disease afflicting the corticospinal tracts, is the *Babinski response*. If the lateral aspect of the sole of the foot is stroked, in normal people the toes will contract and be drawn tightly together. In patients with CNS disease of the motor system, the toes will fan out and be drawn back. This is normal in newborns but represents serious pathology in the adult. There are a variety of described reflexes that convey similar information. Many of them are interesting but not particularly informative.

Sensory Examination

The sensory system is even more complex than the motor system because sensory modalities are carried in different tracts, located in different portions of the cord. Remember that the sensory examination is largely subjective and requires the cooperation of the patient. It is recommended that the examiner become familiar with dermatomes that represent the distribution of the peripheral nerves that ramify from the spinal cord. Most sensory deficits result from peripheral neuropathy and will follow anatomical dermatomes. Exceptions to this include major destructive lesions of the brain; loss of sensation, which may affect an entire side of the body; and the neuropathies associated with alcoholism, which occur in a glove and stocking distribution.

Assessment of the sensory system involves tests for tactile sensation, superficial pain, vibration, and proprioception. Throughout the sensory assessment, the patient's eyes are closed. The cooperation of the patient is encouraged by simple directions and reassurance that the examiner will not hurt the patient.

Tactile sensation is assessed by lightly touching a cotton wisp to corresponding areas on each side of the body. The sensitivity of proximal parts of the extremities are compared to distal parts.

Pain and temperature sensation are carried together in the lateral part of the cord. Thus, it is not necessary to test for temperature sense in most circumstances. Superficial pain is assessed by determining the patient's sensitivity to pinprick. The sharp and dull ends of a safety pin are alternately applied to symmetrical areas of the body. The patient is asked to differentiate between a sharp and dull sensation.

The pin is applied with equal intensity at all times, and the two sides are tested symmetrically.

Vibration and proprioception (the subjective sense of joint position) are carried together in the posterior part of the cord. Vibration may be evaluated through the use of a low-frequency (128 or 256 cycles per second) tuning fork. The handle of the vibrating fork is placed against a bony prominence and the patient is asked whether he feels a buzz. He is instructed to signal the examiner when the buzz ceases. If the patient does not perceive the vibrations at the distal bony prominences, the examiner progresses upward with the tuning fork until the vibrations are felt. As with all measurement of sensitivity, side-to-side comparison is made.

Position sense may be determined by asking the patient to close his eyes and indicate, as the toes are moved, in which direction movement has taken place. Vibration and position sense are often lost together, frequently in circumstances where all others remain intact.

Having tested peripheral sensation, one now asks whether *integration of sensation* in the brain is being carried out properly. This may be done by testing two-point discrimination. That is, if the patient is touched with two sharp objects simultaneously, are they perceived as two or as one? If a patient is touched simultaneously on opposite sides of the body, he should normally recognize that he has been touched in two places. If he recognizes only one, the one not recognized is said to demonstrate *extinction*. A good test of higher cortical sensory ability is that of *stereognosis*. The patient is instructed to close his eyes and identify a variety of objects (keys, coins, etc.) that are placed in his hand by the examiner.

Gerontological Considerations in Neurologic Assessment

The nervous system in older adults is vulnerable to general systemic illness and readily affected by dysfunctions of other organ systems. In addition, a number of neurologic alterations occur with the aging process: sluggishness of pupil response to light, diminished or absent Achilles reflexes, loss of strength, and some muscle wasting. Loss of neurons occurs in selected layers and regions of the cerebral cortex. Another characteristic of the aging nervous system is slowing of nerve conduction. Thus, a little more time is required to obtain a history of neurologic dysfunction and its associated symptoms when an older person is being assessed.

Mental status is evaluated while the history is obtained, and areas of judgment, intelligence, memory, affect, mood, orientation, speech, and grooming are assessed. Changes in mental status may be discerned by family members who bring the patient to the health care setting. Drug toxicity should always be suspected as an etiologic factor when the patient has a change in mental status. Delirium (mental confusion, usually with delusions and hallucinations) is seen in elderly patients who have underlying CNS damage or are experiencing an acute condition such as infection or dehydration. Dementia (deterioration of intellectual function) may be reversible and treatable (as in drug toxicity or thyroid disease) or chronic and irreversible. Depression may produce impairment of attention and memory.

Common neurologic problems of the aged include headache, low back pain, dizziness, weakness, and falling.

Diagnostic Tests and Procedures

Imaging Procedures

Computed Tomography (CT) Scanning. Computed tomography makes use of a narrow beam of x-ray to scan the head in successive layers. The images that are produced provide cross-sectional views of the brain, with distinguishing differences in tissue densities of the skull, cortex, subcortical structures, and ventricles. A computer printout is obtained of the absorption values of the tissues in the plane that is being scanned. The data are transformed into an image through a series of complex equations. Therefore, the brightness of each portion or "slice" of brain in the final image is proportional to the degree to which it absorbs x-ray. The image is displayed on an oscilloscope or TV monitor and is photographed.

Lesions within the brain are seen as variations in tissue density differing from the surrounding normal brain tissue. Abnormalities of tissue indicate possible tumor masses, brain infarction, displacement of the ventricles, and cortical atrophy.

CT scanning is usually done first without contrast material and then with intravenous contrast enhancement. The patient lies on an adjustable table, with his head held in a fixed position, while the scanning system rotates around the head. (The patient is used as the axis, and the machine is rotated around this axis, resulting in a cross-cut image). The patient must lie with the head held perfectly still and with a careful effort not to talk or move the face, since head motion may cause considerable distortion of the image.

Computed tomography is the most revolutionary development in neurologic diagnosis in this century. It is noninvasive, painless, and has high degree of sensitivity for detecting lesions.

Positron Emission Tomography (PET). Positron emission tomography is a computer-based nuclear imaging technique that can produce pictures of actual organ functioning. The patient either inhales a radioactive gas or is injected with a radioactive substance that emits positively charged particles. When these positrons combine with negatively charged electrons (normally found in the body's cells), the resultant gamma rays can be detected by a scanning device. In the scanning equipment, detectors are arranged in a ring and produce a series of two-dimensional views at various levels of the brain. This information is integrated into a computer and reveals a composite picture of the brain at work.

Positron emission tomography permits the measurement of blood flow, tissue composition, and brain metabolism. The brain is one of the most metabolically active organs, consuming 80% of the glucose the body uses. PET measures this activity in specific areas of the brain and is able to detect changes in glucose use. This test is useful in showing metabolic changes in the brain (Alzheimer's disease), in locating lesions (brain tumor, epileptogenic lesions), in identifying blood flow and oxygen metabolism in stroke patients, in evaluating new therapies for brain tumors, as well as in revealing biochemical abnormalities associated with mental illness.

Single Photon Emission Computed Tomography. Single photon emission computed tomography (SPECT) is a three-dimensional imaging technique using nuclear medicine procedures that employ radionuclides and instruments that emit and detect (respectively) single photon. Gamma photons are emitted from a radiopharmaceutical in the patient and are detected by a rotating gamma camera or cameras; and the image is sent to a minicomputer. This approach allows viewing behind overlying structures or background, which greatly increases the contrast between normal and abnormal tissue. It is relatively inexpensive and patient participation time is similar to that of CT scanning.

SPECT is useful in detecting the extent and location of abnormally perfused areas of the brain, thus allowing detecting, localizing, and sizing of stroke (before it is visible by CT), localizing seizure foci in epilepsy, and evaluating brain perfusion before and after neurosurgical procedures.

Magnetic Resonance Imaging (MRI). Magnetic resonance imaging relies on magnets and computers to produce images of different areas of the body (Fig. 52-5). A magnetic field surrounds the patient and causes hydrogen atoms in the body to line up in a certain fashion. When the atoms move back to their original places a signal is released that is processed by a computer. In CNS conditions, MRI has the potential for identifying cerebral pathology earlier and more clearly than other diagnostic tests. It can provide information about the chemical changes within cells, thus allowing the

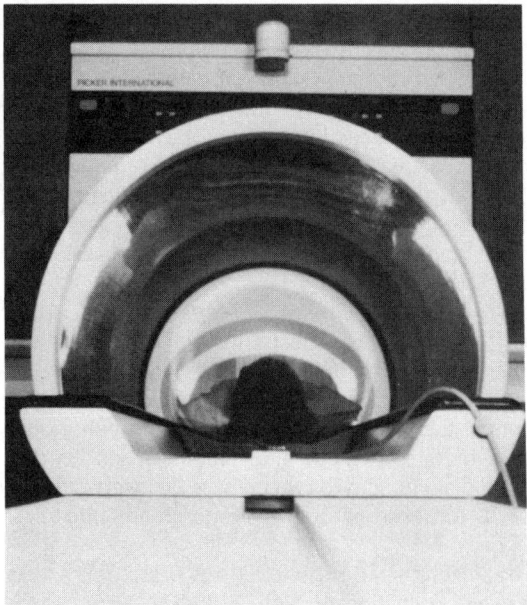

Figure 52-5
Magnetic resonance imaging (MRI). In central nervous system conditions, MRI has the potential for identifying cerebral pathology earlier and more clearly. (Courtesy of National Institutes of Health.)

physician to monitor a tumor's response to treatment. It does not require ionizing radiation.

Before the test the patient must remove all metallic objects (jewelry, including wedding ring and watch) from his person, as well as credit cards which the magnetic field can erase. The patient will lie on a flat platform that will be moved into a tube containing the magnet. Nothing will be felt during the scanning process, but he will hear the thumping of the sound of the magnetic coils as the magnetic field is being pulsed. Throughout the scan the patient can talk to and hear the staff by means of a microphone placed in the scanner.

Cerebral Angiography

Cerebral angiography is an x-ray study of the cerebral circulation following injection of contrast material into a selected artery. Cerebral angiography is a valuable tool for investigating vascular disease, aneurysms (dilation of a segment of a blood vessel), and arteriovenous malformations. It is frequently done prior to craniotomy.

The majority of cerebral angiograms are done by threading a catheter through the femoral artery in the groin and up to the desired vessel. The procedure may also be accomplished by direct puncture of the carotid/vertebral artery or by retrograde injection of contrast medium into the brachial artery.

Patient Preparation. The patient should be well hydrated, and clear liquids are usually permitted up to the time of the study. Before going to the radiology department, the patient is requested to void. The locations of the appropriate peripheral pulses are marked with a felt-tip pen. The patient is informed that he should try to remain immobile during the film sequence and that a brief feeling of warmth in the face, behind the eyes, or in the jaw, teeth, tongue, and lips and a metallic taste are likely to be expected.

After the groin is shaved and prepared, a local anesthetic is used for patient comfort and for reduction of arterial spasm. A catheter is introduced into the femoral artery, flushed with heparinized saline, and filled with contrast material. Under fluoroscopic guidance, the catheter is advanced to the appropriate vessel(s). During injection of the contrast medium, x-rays are made of the arterial and venous phases of circulation through the brain.

Postprocedure Nursing Management. In some instances, patients may experience major or minor arterial block due to embolism, thrombosis, or hemorrhage, producing a neurologic deficit. Signs of such an occurrence include alterations in the level of responsiveness and consciousness, weakness on one side of the body, motor or sensory deficits, or speech disturbances. It is necessary to observe the patient repeatedly for these signs and to report them immediately if they occur.

The injection site is observed for hematoma formation (a localized collection of blood), and an ice cap may be applied intermittently to the puncture site to relieve swelling and discomfort. Since a hematoma at the puncture site or embolization to a distant artery will affect the peripheral pulses, these signs are monitored frequently. The color and temperature of the involved extremity are also noted as a means of detecting possible embolism.

Myelography

A myelogram is an x-ray of the spinal subarachnoid space taken after an opaque medium or air is injected into the spinal subarachnoid space through a spinal puncture. It outlines the spinal subarachnoid space and shows any distortion of the spinal cord or spinal dural sac caused by tumors, cysts, herniated intervertebral discs, or other lesions.

After the contrast medium is injected, the head of the table is tilted down and the course of the contrast medium is observed radioscopically. The contrast medium may be water soluble or oil based. Metrizamide is a water-soluble contrast agent that is absorbed by the body and excreted by the kidneys. It does not have to be removed via the needle route from the spinal canal because it is highly soluble and clears relatively quickly from the cerebrospinal fluid. Side-effects include headache, which is most probably due to CNS irritation by the metrizamide.

If iophendylate (Pantopaque), an oil-based iodine compound, is used for meylography, the radiologist may remove it by syringe and needle aspiration. The patient may complain of sharp pain down the leg during aspiration if a nerve root is affected. This is remedied by rotating the needle point or adjusting the depth of the needle.

Nursing Management. Since most patients have some misconceptions about this procedure, the nurse can answer questions and clarify the explanation offered by the physician. The patient should be aware that the x-ray table may be tilted in varying positions during the study. The meal that would normally be eaten prior to the procedure is omitted. The patient may be given a light sedative to help cope with a rather lengthy test.

Following myelography, when a water-soluble medium has been used, the patient lies in bed with the head of the bed elevated 15 to 30 degrees to reduce the rate of upward dispersion of the medium. The patient may be ambulatory or remain in bed per the physician's request.

Following a procedure in which an oil-based medium has been used, the patient should lie in a recumbent position for the amount of time specified by the physician (usually 12 to 24 hours) to reduce cerebrospinal fluid leakage and decrease the frequency of headache. Usually, he is permitted to turn from side to side.

The patient is encouraged to drink liberal amounts of fluid for rehydration and replacement of cerebrospinal fluid and to decrease the incidence of post–lumbar puncture headache. The blood pressure, pulse, respiratory rate, and temperature are monitored, as well as the patient's ability to void. Other untoward signs to watch for include fever, stiff neck, photophobia (sensitivity to light), or signs of chemical or bacterial meningitis.

Lumbar Epidural Venography

In lumbar epidural venography, a catheter is inserted percutaneously into the femoral vein and guided into the ascending lumbar vein or internal iliac veins. The contrast medium is injected to fill the epidural veins overlying the disc spaces and to opacify the epidural venous plexus. The procedure may be useful in the diagnosis of herniated lumbar discs that are not demonstrated by myelography. It reveals deviation or compression of the epidural veins due to a herniated disc or tumor. The procedure is relatively easy to perform, well tolerated, fairly painless, and not associated with arachnoiditis. Lumbar epidural venography and myelography may be done as complementary diagnostic studies. Following the test, the site is observed for evidence of hematoma formation.

Radionuclide Imaging Studies (Brain Scan)

Radionuclide imaging is based on the principle that a radiopharmaceutical may diffuse through the blood–brain barrier at a point where it has been disrupted and collect in abnormal cerebral tissue. (Normal brain tissue is relatively impermeable.) There is increased uptake of radioactive material at the site of pathology.

In this procedure, the patient is given an intravenous injection of a radiopharmaceutical. The radioactivity subsequently transmitted through the skull is traced by a scanner that prints out a picture, or a gamma camera is used to monitor the passage of the radiopharmaceutical through the cerebral circulation to gain information about cerebral blood flow.

Brain scanning is particularly useful in evaluating vascular lesions of the brain and meninges and in locating vascular neoplasms and brain tumors. It is useful in the early detection and evaluation of stroke, abscess, and follow-up of surgical or radiation therapy of the brain. Newer techniques permit the evaluation of cerebral circulation during the brain scan. However, CT scanning is replacing traditional radioisotope scanning.

Sonography and Echoencephalography

Sonography is the application of ultrasound to the body. *Echoencephalography* is the recording of echoes from the deep structures within the skull by means of ultrasound (high-frequency sound waves). Ultrasonic transducers are positioned over specified areas of the head, while echoes are transcribed into images. Echoencephalography is a rapid and useful technique to determine the position of midline structures of the brain and the distance from the midline to the lateral ventricular wall or the third ventricular wall. Therefore, it is done to detect a shift of the cerebral midline structures caused by subdural hematoma, intracerebral hemorrhage, massive cerebral infarction, and neoplasms. It is useful in the evaluation of hydrocephalus, since it can detect dilation of the ventricles.

The nurse may explain that this is a noninvasive test, and that some type of water-soluble jelly is used to eliminate the air gap between the hand-held transducer and the patient's head.

Air Studies

The cerebrospinal fluid spaces in and around the brain may be seen in x-ray examination when the fluid is replaced with a gas. This is based on the principle that gas, replacing the fluid within the ventricular and subarachnoid systems, serves as a contrast medium, because air is less dense than fluid to roentgen rays. The cerebrospinal fluid may be partially replaced with air through *pneumoencephalography* and *ventriculography*.

Pneumoencephalography is a diagnostic procedure in which air or gas is instilled through a lumbar puncture as a means of demonstrating the ventricular system and subarachnoid space overlying the hemispheres and basal cisterns. A small amount of cerebrospinal fluid is removed and an equal amount of air injected. A special chair allows the patient to be rotated in all directions so that air may be placed selectively in the desired cavities. Films are then taken and studied.

A ventriculogram is an x-ray taken of the lateral ventricles following withdrawal of cerebrospinal fluid and injection of air or gas into the lateral ventricles through openings in the skull.

- These procedures are used infrequently since the advent of computed tomography.

Electrophysiologic Tests

Electroencephalography (EEG)

An electroencephalogram represents a record of the electrical activity generated in the brain and obtained through electrodes applied on the scalp surface or through microelectrodes placed within the brain tissue. It provides physiologic assessment of cerebral activity. EEG is a useful test for diagnosing seizure disorders such as the epilepsies and is a screening procedure for coma or organic brain syndrome. It also serves as an indicator of brain death. Tumors, abscesses, brain scars, blood clots, and infection may cause electric changes to differ from normal patterns of rhythm and rate.

Electrodes are arranged on the scalp to record the electrical activity in various regions of the head. The amplified activity of the neurons is recorded on a continuously moving paper sheet; this record is the encephalogram (Fig. 52-6). For a baseline recording, the patient lies quietly with his eyes closed. Then he may be asked to hyperventilate for 3 to 4 minutes and then to look at a bright, flashing light for photic stimulation. These are activation procedures done to evoke abnormal electrical discharges, especially seizure potentials. A sleep EEG may be recorded following sedation because some abnormal brain waves are seen only when the patient is asleep. If the epileptogenic area is inaccessible to the conventional scalp electrodes, nasopharyngeal electrodes may be used.

Depth recording of EEG is done by introducing electrodes stereotactically into a target area of the brain as dictated by the patient's seizure pattern and scalp EEG. It is used to select

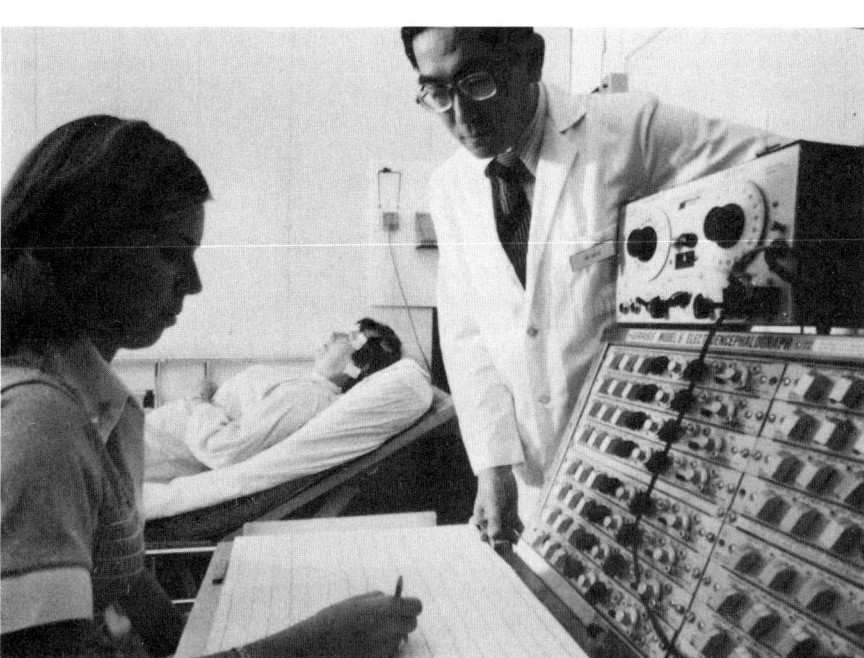

Figure 52-6
Neurologist and EEG technician checking the patient's electroencephalogram, which is a valuable diagnostic instrument in epilepsy and other neurologic disorders. (Courtesy of National Institute of Neurological and Communicative Disorders and Stroke.)

patients who may benefit from surgical excision of epileptogenic foci.

Patient Preparation. Tranquilizers and stimulants may be withheld 24 to 48 hours before an EEG, since these medications can alter the EEG wave patterns or mask the abnormal wave patterns of seizure disorders. Coffee, tea, or cola drinks are omitted in the meal before the test because of their stimulating effect. However, the meal is not omitted because an altered blood sugar level can also cause changes in the brain wave patterns.

The patient is informed that the EEG will take 45 to 60 minutes or longer if a sleep EEG is performed. At the same time, the patient is assured that the procedure will not cause an electric shock and that the EEG is a test, not a form of treatment.

Evoked Potential Studies

Evoked potential studies evaluate the changes and responses in brain waves recorded from scalp electrodes that are evoked (elicited) by the introduction of an external stimulus. Evoked changes are detected with the aid of computerized devices that extract the signal, display it on an oscilloscope, and store the data on magnetic tape or disc. These studies are based on the concept that any insult or dysfunction that can alter neuronal metabolism or disturb membrane function may change evoked responses in brain waves. In neurologic diagnosis they reflect conduction times in the peripheral nervous system. In clinical practice, the visual, auditory, and somatosensory systems are most often tested.

In *visual evoked responses* the patient looks at a visual stimulus (flashing light, checkerboard pattern on a screen). The average of several hundred stimuli is recorded by EEG leads placed over the occiput. The transit time from the retina to the occipital area is measured using computer averaging methods.

To measure *auditory evoked responses* an auditory stimulus (repetitive auditory click) is given and the transit time up the brain stem into the cortex is measured. Specific lesions in the auditory pathway will modify or delay the response.

In *somatosensory evoked responses* the peripheral nerves are stimulated (electrical stimulation through skin electrodes) and the transit time up the spinal cord to the cortex is measured and recorded from scalp electrodes. This test is used to detect a deficit in spinal cord conduction and to monitor cord function during operative procedures.

There is no specific patient preparation other than reassurance and encouragement of relaxation. The patient is advised to remain perfectly still throughout the recording in order to prevent artifacts (potentials not generated by the brain) that interfere with the recording and interpretation of the test.

Electromyography (EMG)

An electromyogram is obtained by introducing needle electrodes into the skeletal muscles in order to study changes in the electrical potential of the muscles and the nerves leading to them. The electrical potentials are shown on an oscilloscope and amplified by a loudspeaker so that both the sound and appearance of the waves can be analyzed and compared simultaneously. EMGs are useful in determining the presence of a neuromuscular disorder and myopathies. They help to distinguish weakness due to neuropathy (functional or pathologic changes in the peripheral nervous system) from weakness due to other causes.

No special patient preparation is required. The patient is told that he will experience a sensation similar to that of an intramuscular injection as the needle is inserted into the muscle. The muscles examined may ache for a short time following the procedure.

Nerve Conduction Studies

Nerve conduction studies are performed by stimulating a peripheral nerve at several points along its course and recording the muscle action potential or the sensory action potential that results. Surface or needle electrodes are placed on the skin over the nerve to stimulate the nerve fibers. This test is useful in the study of peripheral nerve neuropathies.

Special Procedures

Lumbar Puncture and Examination of Cerebrospinal Fluid

A lumbar puncture is carried out by inserting a needle into the lumbar subarachnoid space in order to withdraw cerebrospinal fluid for diagnostic and therapeutic purposes. The purposes are to obtain spinal fluid for examination, to measure and relieve spinal fluid pressure, to determine the presence or absence of blood in the spinal fluid, to detect spinal subarachnoid block, and to administer antibiotics intrathecally in certain cases of infection.

The needle is usually inserted into the subarachnoid space between the third and fourth lumbar interspace. Since the spinal cord divides into a sheaf of nerves at the first lumbar vertebra, the needle is inserted below the level of the third lumbar vertebra (Fig. 52-7) to prevent the spinal cord from being punctured.

A successful lumbar puncture requires that the patient be relaxed, since an anxious patient may become tense, thereby causing an increase in the pressure reading. The normal range of spinal fluid pressure with the patient in a lateral recumbent position is 70 to 200 mm H_2O. Pressures over 200 mm H_2O are considered abnormal. A lumbar puncture may be quite dangerous in the presence of an intracranial mass lesion, because when pressure is released the intracranial contents may herniate.

A lumbar manometric test (Queckenstedt test) may be performed by compressing the jugular veins on each side of the neck during the lumbar puncture. The increase in the pressure caused by the compression is noted. Then the pressure is released and pressure readings are made at 10-second intervals. In normal people, the cerebrospinal fluid pressure rises rapidly in response to compression of the jugular veins and returns quickly to normal when the compression is released. A slow rise and fall in pressure indicates a partial block due to a lesion compressing the spinal subarachnoid pathways. If there is no pressure change, a complete block is indicated. This test is not done if an intracranial lesion is suspected.

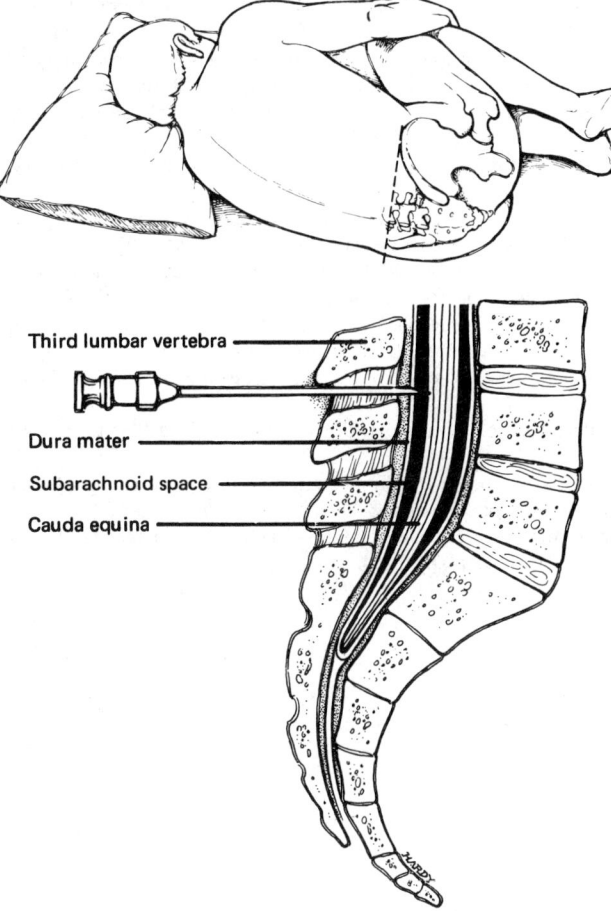

Figure 52-7
Technique of lumbar puncture. The interspaces between L3 and L5 are just below the line connecting the anterior-superior iliac spines.

Nursing Support. During the initial explanations, the patient should be assured that inserting a needle into the spine will not result in paralysis. Prior to the lumbar puncture, the bladder and bowel should be emptied. The patient is placed on his side with his back toward the physician. The thighs and head are flexed as much as possible to increase the space between the spinous processes of the vertebrae and afford easier entry into the subarachnoid space. A pillow fixed between the legs will prevent the upper leg from rolling forward. A small pillow is placed under the patient's head so that the spine is maintained in a horizontal position. The nurse may assist the patient to maintain the position in order to avoid sudden movement, which can produce a traumatic (bloody) tap. During the procedure, the patient is instructed to breathe normally since hyperventilation may lower an elevated pressure. Following the procedure, the patient is asked to remain prone (on abdomen) for 3 hours to allow the tissue surfaces along the needle track to come together (to prevent cerebrospinal fluid leakage). A liberal fluid intake is encouraged.

Examination of the Cerebrospinal Fluid. Spinal fluid should be clear and colorless. Bloody spinal fluid may indicate cerebral contusion, laceration, or subarachnoid hemorrhage. Usually, specimens are sent to the laboratory for cell count,

culture, and chemical analysis. The specimens should be sent immediately, since changes will take place and alter the result if the specimens are allowed to stand. (See Appendix for the normal values of cerebrospinal fluid.)

Post–Lumbar Puncture Headache. A post–lumbar puncture headache, ranging from mild to severe, may appear in a few hours to several days following the procedure. This is the most frequently encountered complication occurring in 11% to 25% of patients. It is a throbbing bifrontal or occipital headache, dull and deep in character, that is particularly severe when the patient sits or stands upright but lessens or disappears when he lies down in a horizontal position.

The cause of this unpleasant complication is the leakage of spinal fluid at the puncture site. The fluid continues to escape into the tissues by way of the needle tract from the spinal canal. It is then absorbed promptly by the lymphatics, never having accumulated in sufficient volume to be detected. As a result of this leak, the supply of cerebrospinal fluid in the cranium is depleted to a point at which it is insufficient to maintain proper mechanical stabilization of the brain. This leakage of spinal fluid allows settling of the brain when the patient assumes an upright position. This produces tension and stretching of venous sinuses and pain-sensitive structures. Both traction and pain are lessened and the leakage reduced when the patient lies down.

The post puncture headache is usually managed by bed rest, analgesics, and hydration. If the postpuncture headache persists, the epidural blood patch technique may be used. Blood is withdrawn from the patient's antecubital vein and injected into the epidural space, usually via the site of the previous spinal puncture. The rationale is that the blood acts as a gelatinous plug to seal the hole in the dura, thus preventing continuing loss of cerebrospinal fluid.

The lumbar puncture headache may be avoided if a needle with a small gauge is used and if the patient is encouraged to remain prone following the procedure. When large volumes of fluid are collected (>20 ml), the patient is positioned prone for 2 hours, then flat in a side-lying position for 2 hours, and then supine or prone for 6 more hours. Keeping the patient flat overnight may reduce the incidence of headaches.

Other complications of a spinal puncture include herniation of the intracranial contents, traumatic complications, spinal epidural abscess, spinal epidural hematoma, and meningitis.

Bibliography

Books

Chusid JG. Correlative Neuroanatomy and Functional Neurology. Los Altos, California, Lange Medical Publications, 1985.

Darby JK. Speech and Language Evaluation in Neurology: Adult Disorders. New York, Grune & Stratton, 1985.

Davis RL and Robertson DM. Textbook of Neuropathology. Baltimore, Williams & Wilkins, 1985.

Massey WE, Pleet AB, and Scherokman BJ. Diagnostic Tests in Neurology. Chicago, Year Book Medical Publishers, 1985.

Mitchell PH et al. Neurological Assessment for Nursing Practice. Reston, Virginia, Reston Publishing Co, 1984.

Pallett PH and O'Brien MT. Textbook of Neurological Nursing. Boston, Little, Brown & Co, 1985.

Rosenberg RN et al. The Clinical Neurosciences. New York, Churchill Livingstone, 1983.

Ross RT. How To Examine The Nervous System, 2nd ed. New York, Medical Examination Publishing Co, 1985.

Rudy EB. Advanced Neurological and Neurosurgical Nursing. St Louis, CV Mosby, 1984.

Scheinberg LC, Giesser BS, and Schaumburg HH. The Neurology Handbook. New Hyde Park, New York, Medical Examination Publishing Co, 1983.

Strub RL and Black FW. The Mental Status Examination in Neurology, 2nd ed. Philadelphia, FA Davis, 1985.

Swanson PD. Signs and Symptoms in Neurology. Philadelphia, JB Lippincott, 1984.

Vogt G, Miller M, and Esluer M. Mosby's Manual of Neurological Care. St Louis, CV Mosby, 1985.

Walsh TJ. Neuro-Ophthalmology: Clinical Signs and Symptoms. Philadelphia, Lea & Febiger, 1985.

Articles

Anderson MS. My head hurts. Nurs '84 1984 Sept; 14(9):34–41.

Berlin RM et al. Psychiatric symptomatology in an outpatient neurology clinic. J Clin Psychiatry 1983 June; 44(6):204–206.

Bernick C and Stern LZ. Neurologic complaints of the elderly: The challenge of diagnosis. Postgrad Med 1985 June; 77(8):124–133.

Cammermeyer M. A growth model of self-care for neurologically impaired people. J Neurosurg Nurs 1983 Oct; 15(5):299–305.

Gerard G and Rossi DR. Nuclear magnetic imaging of the brain. Hosp Pract 1984 July; 19(7):143–156.

Gorelick PB and Biller J. Lumbar puncture. Postgrad Med 1986 June; 79(8):257–268.

Hendrickson S. Psychological care of the patient with neurological dysfunction. J Neurosurg Nurs 1984 Aug; 16(4):202–207.

Hickey JV and McKenna JE. Effective discharge planning and the neurosurgical nurse. J Neurosurg Nurs 1984 Apr; 16(2):101–106.

Keating JW Jr, Numaguchi Y, and Robertson HJ. Neuroimaging of the spine. Neurol Clin 1984 Nov; 2(4):797–821.

Long DM. Aging in the nervous system. Neurosurgery 1985 Aug; 17(2):348–354.

Malden M. Chronic neurologic disease. Postgrad Med 1984 Dec; 76(8):101–104, 109.

Price MB and DeVroom HL. A quick and easy guide to neurological assessment. J Neurosurg Nurs 1985 Oct; 17(5):313–320.

Walker MD, Research issues in positron emission tomography. Ann Neurol 1984; 15(suppl):S1–S204.

Chapter 53

Management of Patients With Neurologic Dysfunction

Scope of Neurologic Nursing

Neurologic illness is the principal cause of chronic disease in our society. The final common pathway of many neurologic disorders is musculoskeletal dysfunction. These patients are prone to deconditioning that increases functional losses from weakness, immobility, impaired postural reflexes, painful joints, and attitudinal depression of the patient and his family.

A damaged brain cannot be completely restored. Neurologic tissue that has been injured by trauma or bleeding cannot tolerate much compression by blood clot or edema. The resultant pressure on neighboring tissue may displace vital centers or disrupt the function of adjacent tissue. Paralysis, coma, and chronic pain are frequently seen after central nervous system (CNS) injury. Many brain diseases are manifested by disorders in behavior. Experience in neurologic outpatient clinics suggest a high incidence of psychiatric disorders in this group of patients. Recovery is slow and unpredictable. Neurologic problems change over a period of time and affect every aspect of living.

Neuroscience nursing has become a specialty and requires an understanding of neuroanatomy, neurophysiology, neurodiagnostic testing, critical care nursing, and rehabilitation nursing. In addition to ongoing assessment of the patient's neurologic function and health needs, the nurse's role is to help the patient identify problems, set mutual goals, direct a course of action, use appropriate nursing interventions (including teaching, counseling, and coordinating activities), and evaluate the outcomes of care.

Although sometimes the patient's body may be damaged, his brain impaired, his vision and speech changed, and his self-esteem diminished, the nurse and health care team can take a fresh look, redefine problems, suggest other options, and help the patient gain control, while tapping all available educational and support resources. There are great rewards in this type of nursing. The goals of helping the patient achieve as high a level of function as possible and the enhancement of the quality of life for the patient and family may be realized.

Nursing Process Overview

Assessment

The patient with a neurologic dysfunction undergoes a thorough neurologic examination that is described in Chapter 52, Assessment of Neurologic Function. The neurologic examination involves tests of several major areas of functioning, including cerebral, cranial nerve, motor system and sensory system function, and reflex responses. The patient's movements are observed, and he is questioned about changes in sensation. When assessing the patient's neurologic dysfunction, the nurse observes his level of alertness and determines whether there is a disturbance of consciousness. Alterations in the patient's mental and emotional status are elicited. Cognitive function is tested by determining if the patient is oriented to person, place, and time. Intellectual functions are evaluated by asking questions of general knowledge, ascertaining reasoning ability, and assessing recent and remote memory. An assessment is also made of the person's language abilities. Loss of function and certain alterations in function indicate deterioration and are reported to the physician. These indices are described further in the discussions of specific types of neurologic dysfunctions that follow.

Potential Nursing Diagnoses of Patients With Neurologic Dysfunction

There is no known cure for a large number of neurologic illnesses. The nursing goal is to help the patient to adapt to his dysfunction and continue with his life in as meaningful a way as possible. Nursing interventions include knowing and accepting the patient's self-protective responses, providing information, helping the patient set achievable goals, reinforcing positive coping skills, and offering ongoing support.

Many patients with neurologic conditions face a wide range of possible nursing diagnoses, including the following:

Ineffective breathing pattern
Impaired swallowing
Potential impairment of skin integrity
Impaired physical mobility
Self-care deficits
Alteration in comfort: pain
Alterations in oral mucous membranes
Impaired tissue integrity: cornea
Alteration in nutrition: less than body requirements
Alteration in urinary and bowel elimination
Alteration in thought processes
Sexual dysfunction
Ineffective individual coping
Alteration in family processes

Nursing Interventions

Managing Impaired Breathing.   Patients with neuromuscular disorders such as Guillain-Barré syndrome, myasthenia gravis, and demyelinating diseases may have weakness of the diaphragm, intercostal muscles, and accessory muscles of respiration that compromises ventilation. When the diaphragm is paralyzed the patient is in danger while sleeping,

when hypoventilation may be particularly severe. Additionally, the patient's inability to breathe deeply and cough results in increased secretions. The end result may be respiratory inefficiency and failure.

Nursing interventions include monitoring the adequacy of alveolar ventilation by frequent measurements of the respiratory rate, vital capacity, and inspiratory force. Measures to promote chest expansion include elevating the head of the bed 30 degrees and working with the respiratory therapist in assessing the effectiveness of incentive spirometry and positive-pressure breathing. If the disorder appears to be progressing (increasing respiratory rate; vital capacity < 15 ml/kg of body weight; or inspiratory force less than −25 cm H_2O), the patient may require intubation and mechanical ventilation. In many instances the neuromuscular weakness is reversible, but the patient often requires prolonged ventilatory support.

In patients with depressed states of consciousness, a common cause of airway obstruction is the posterior displacement of oropharyngeal soft tissue structures; the tongue becomes flaccid and falls back against the posterior pharyngeal wall. An immediate nursing intervention is to extend the patient's head and/or elevate the mandible. It may be necessary to insert an oropharyngeal tube or airway. Placing the patient on his side allows the tongue to fall to the side and away from the back of the pharynx.

Managing Swallowing Problems.   Neurologic disorders that impair breathing often cause swallowing dysfunctions. These patients are at risk of aspiration of secretions or regurgitated gastric contents. The awake patient is observed for paroxysms of coughing or nasal regurgitation when swallowing liquids. The patient with impaired swallowing, laryngeal, and cough reflexes is placed in a lateral position. Respiratory function may be improved by clearing the obstructed airway by means of suctioning and by correcting the hypoxia by immediate ventilation. Patients with swallowing dysfunctions may require nasogastric tube feedings to prevent aspiration and ensure adequate nutrition. The nurse's responsibilities are to place the patient in an upright position, to check the position of the tube before feeding or to check the cuff of the endotracheal tube before feeding, and to give the tube feeding slowly.

Maintaining Skin Integrity.   Special nursing challenges arise when the patient is paralyzed and has sensory disturbances and/or altered mental status (confusion, depression, stupor, or coma). Patients with chronic neurologic conditions usually have some physical defect and are at high risk for pressure sores. Prevention is the hallmark of management. For the patient with impaired neurologic function, this includes inspecting one's skin for signs of pressure, having properly fitted wheelchair cushions, and wearing a wrist watch with a buzzer alarm (for auditory cueing) as a reminder to shift position to relieve pressure. An additional discussion of the prevention of pressure sores is presented on p. 222.

Promoting Physical Mobility.   Any paralyzed extremity deserves careful attention. Care must be taken to see that the patient does not lie on the extremity too long and that the circulation to the part is not impeded. To prevent contractures, the nurse ensures that the patient is positioned correctly and that the joints are moved either actively or passively through their range of motion several times daily.

Muscle weakness (lack of strength) is seen in clinical conditions that have resulted from lesions of the cortex, brain stem, spinal cord, anterior horn cells, peripheral nerve, neuromuscular junction, or muscle. In general, therapeutic exercises are carried out to increase strength. In some neuromuscular conditions the patient should not work to the point of fatigue because weakness will occur from overuse. Patients with neurologic conditions have increased energy demands resulting from motor involvement, the secondary effects of deconditioning, and the emotional stress of living with a disability.

Promoting Self-Care Ability. An impairment of neuromuscular function can interfere with activities that are necessary for caring for personal needs. The nurse, working collaboratively with other rehabilitation team members, evaluates the patient's joint range of motion, sensation, muscle strength, endurance, and coordination as well as his ability to learn. The patient is taught self-care skills and compensatory techniques to enhance his abilities. This is discussed on pp. 230–231.

Relieving Discomfort. As in any other condition, the nursing assessment of the patient with a neurologic dysfunction who is complaining of pain focuses on how the patient is functioning. The nurse works with the patient to elicit the location of the pain, its distribution, the degree of limitation, and its adverse effects on the patient's life. She listens to the patient's description of pain and what makes it better or worse. Patients with chronic pain from neurologic conditions become depressed and anxious and are subject to insomnia. In addition, they usually limit their activities because of the pain, which causes a generalized loss of strength.

Nursing interventions include establishing a trusting relationship with the patient, teaching the patient about pain and its relief, decreasing noxious stimuli, providing distraction from pain, being with the patient, and using assistance from other professionals. The nurse administers the prescribed pharmacologic agent and monitors the patient's response. Nursing interventions also include appropriate reassurance to relieve the anxiety that pain produces. Maximum function within the framework of the patient's disability is encouraged. Explanations may be given of the deleterious effects of prolonged inactivity.

A patient with neuromuscular dysfunction is at risk for painful contractures because as he lies in bed his feet drop into plantar flexion and his knees and hips flex. Fibrous tissue stiffening within muscles occur, and painful spasticity accentuates the problem. Prevention is the key to this type of pain by range of motion exercise of each joint on a daily basis. Encouraging the patient to participate in self-care is important.

Specific nursing interventions for the relief of pain and discomfort are found in the sections on headache, intracranial and spinal surgery, head injuries, and the neurosurgical relief of pain.

Mouth Care. The unconscious patient is at risk of developing parotitis (inflammation of the parotid gland) if the mouth is not kept clean. The condition of the patient's oral mucous membranes is checked often, because buccal structures tend to become exceedingly dry after a short period of mouth-breathing. The lips, tongue, and gums are cleansed and lubricated at frequent intervals, and the patient's fluid intake is maintained at an adequate level.

Eye Care. When facial paralysis, from any cause, makes it impossible for the patient to shut his eyes, or the patient has an inefficient corneal reflex, the cornea is left exposed, which can lead to keratitis and corneal ulceration. Gentle cleansing of the eyelids with warm water or normal saline every few hours will remove discharge and debris. Artificial tears may be instilled when prescribed. An eye shield or patch is worn when necessary. The nurse inspects the eyes regularly for signs of inflammation. Patients who are conscious and able can administer their own eye care with proper instruction and supervision.

Maintaining Adequate Nutrition. Patients with neuromuscular dysfunction are at risk for nutritional disorders. Depression, so commonly encountered in patients with neurologic conditions, may suppress the appetite. Nutritional problems also arise if there is impairment of chewing and swallowing.

Some patients will require gastrostomy feedings, usually ingesting foods that have been prepared in a food blender. The blenderized meal is tolerated well, since the patient's gastrointestinal tract is accustomed to this type of diet. In addition to initiating a referral to the dietitian for nutritional counseling, the nurse works with the occupational therapist to obtain eating utensils that assist the patient to compensate for a physical disability.

Managing Urinary and Bowel Elimination. Many patients with CNS disease initially or eventually, temporarily or permanently, exhibit urinary and fecal incontinence. The hygienic care of patients with incontinence is an important nursing priority.

The management of bladder disturbances due to a lesion of the nervous system is discussed on p. 1014. The management of urinary incontinence from other causes is discussed p. 1014. Promotion of a bowel training program is described on p. 238.

Supporting Cognitive Function. Some patients with brain tumors, head injuries, and strokes, for example, experience cognitive impairment characterized by deficits in memory and/or abstract thinking, judgment, and intellectual performance. This profoundly affects not only the patient but also the caregiver and the family.

In general, the nurse counsels the family to create a stable, dependable environment, to minimize confusion, to provide sensory cues, to give information simply and in a positive manner, and to readjust tasks to fit the patient's level of functioning. When the patient becomes agitated and manifests undesirable behavior, the use of motor distraction (giving him something to hold) and reducing environmental stimulation (turning off the television) can be effective. Management of patients with brain damage involves a combination of psychiatric nursing skills and neuroscience nursing skills.

Managing Sexual Dysfunction. Sexual dysfunction may be due to a lesion in the neural pathways in which there is loss of erection, lubrication, ejaculation, or emission. The nurse can allow expression of beliefs and feelings; sexual counseling by one skilled in sexual counseling of the disabled can be initiated. (see p. 239).

Promoting Effective Coping. Patients with neurologic dysfunctions are faced with multiple stresses; serious and often unpredictable outcomes; assault of self image; and, in many instances, a long-term illness. The patient and his family experience reactive responses to the crisis of diagnosis and prolonged treatment. The patient may react to these stresses with a mix of psychological responses, including regression, depression, anger, denial, and anxiety.

Supporting Family Functioning. The family faces the disruption of illness, which means an alteration in life-style, role changes, and possible intrafamilial conflicts. Denial or nonacceptance by the family can produce enormous strains on its individual members. The family will require time to deal with their feelings of powerlessness, ambivalence, anger, and guilt. They should be included and educated about the patient's therapy, understand the nature of the neurologic dysfunction and the meaning of remissions and exacerbations, and have some awareness of present and future changes.

Commonly encountered nursing diagnoses, nursing interventions and rationales, and expected outcomes of the patients with impaired neurologic function are summarized in Nursing Care Plan 53-1 (pp. 1418–1421).

Special Problems of Patients With Neurologic Dysfunction

The Patient With Increased Intracranial Pressure

Pathophysiology

Intracranial pressure (ICP) is the result of the amount of brain substance, intracranial blood volume, and cerebrospinal fluid (CSF) within the skull at any one time. The normal ICP varies depending on the position of the patient and is considered to be less than or equal to 15 mm Hg.

The rigid cranial vault contains brain (1400 g), blood (75 ml), and CSF (75 ml). The volume and pressure of these three components are usually in a state of equilibrium. Since there is limited space for expansion within the skull, an increase of any one of these components causes a change in the volume of the other, by either displacing or shifting CSF, increasing the absorption of CSF, or decreasing cerebral blood volume. Under normal circumstances, minor changes in blood volume and CSF volume occur constantly when there are changes in intrathoracic pressure (coughing, sneezing, straining), posture, and blood pressure and fluctuations in arterial blood gas levels.

Pathologic conditions such as head injury, stroke, inflammatory lesions, brain tumor, or intracranial surgery have a negative influence on the relationship between intracranial volume and pressure. Increased ICP may significantly reduce cerebral blood flow. The resultant ischemia stimulates the vasomotor centers, and the systemic pressure rises to maintain cerebral blood flow. Usually this is accompanied by a slow bounding pulse and respiratory irregularities. These changes in blood pressure, pulse, and respiration are of importance clinically because they are clues to the existence of increased ICP. The ultimate effect of raised ICP is cerebral ischemia. The brain is very vulnerable to ischemia and generally will not recover function if it is subjected to more than 3 to 5 minutes of complete ischemia.

The concentration of carbon dioxide in the blood and in brain tissues also has a role in the regulation of cerebral blood flow. A rise in Pco_2 causes the cerebral blood vessels to dilate, leading to increased cerebral blood flow and increased ICP, while a fall in Pco_2 has a vasoconstrictor effect. Decreased venous outflow may also increase cerebral blood volume, thus raising ICP.

Cerebral swelling or edema occurs when there is an increase in the water content of the CNS. Certain brain tumors are associated with the development of large quantities of water. Even a small tumor may create a great increase in ICP.

Although an elevated ICP is most commonly associated with head injury, an elevated pressure may be seen as a secondary effect in a variety of other conditions: brain tumors, subarachnoid hemorrhage, and toxic and viral encephalopathies.

Thus, increased ICP is the summation of a number of physiologic processes. Increased ICP from any cause affects cerebral perfusion and produces distortion and shifts of brain tissue.

Clinical Manifestations

When ICP increases to the point where the brain's ability to adjust has reached its limits, neural function is impaired and may be expressed by changes in the level of consciousness and by abnormal respiratory and vasomotor responses.

The level of responsiveness/consciousness is the most important measure of the patient's condition.

- The earliest sign of increasing ICP is *lethargy*. Watch for slowing of speech and a delay in response to verbal suggestions.

Any sudden change in condition, such as shifting from quietness to restlessness (without apparent cause), shifting from orientation to confusion, or increasing drowsiness, has neurologic significance. These signs may result from compression of the brain due to either swelling from hemorrhage or edema or an expanding intracranial lesion (hematoma or tumor) or a combination of both.

As pressure increases, the patient may react only to loud auditory or painful stimuli. At this stage, serious impairment of brain circulation is probably taking place and immediate surgical intervention may be required. If the stupor deepens, the patient responds to painful stimuli by moaning but may not attempt to withdraw. As the condition worsens, the extremities become flaccid and reflexes are absent. The jaw sags and the tongue becomes flaccid, producing inadequate respiratory exchange. When the coma is profound, with the pupils dilated and fixed and the respirations impaired, a fatal outcome is usually inevitable.

Management

- Increased ICP constitutes a true emergency and must be treated promptly. As pressure rises, the brain substance is compressed. Secondary phenomena caused by circulatory impairment and edema may lead to death.

The immediate management for relief of increased ICP is based on reducing the size of the brain by decreasing brain edema, lowering the volume of CSF or decreasing blood volume. These goals are accomplished by administering osmotic diuretics, restricting fluids, draining CSF, hyperventilating the patient, controlling fever, and reducing cellular metabolic demands.

Osmotic diuretics (mannitol, glycerol) may be given to dehydrate the brain and reduce cerebral edema. They act by drawing water across intact membranes, thereby reducing the volume of brain and extracellular fluid. An indwelling catheter is usually inserted into the bladder for the management of the ensuing diuresis.

Steroids (such as dexamethasone) help reduce edema surrounding brain tumors when a brain tumor is the cause of increased ICP.

CSF drainage is frequently employed since the removal of even a small amount of CSF may dramatically reduce ICP and restore cerebral perfusion pressure.

Hyperventilation (with a volume ventilator) produces respiratory alkalosis, which in turn causes cerebral vasoconstriction. The result of this action is a reduction in cerebral blood volume and lowering of ICP. It is considered a short-term means of control.

Temperature control is aimed at preventing an elevation of temperature, since fever increases cerebral metabolism and the rate at which cerebral edema forms. Cardiac output is monitored if measures are taken to reduce the patient's temperature.

Reducing cellular metabolic demands may also be accomplished through the administration of high doses of barbiturates when the patient is not responsive to conventional treatment. The mechanism by which barbiturates decrease ICP and protect the brain is uncertain, but the resultant comatose state is thought to reduce metabolic requirements of the brain, thus giving it some protection.

- The patient receiving high doses of barbiturates experiences loss of all neurologic clinical parameters. Barbiturates are significant cardiorespiratory depressants. Thus, prolonged barbiturate anesthesia requires a high level of nursing surveillance and support, since the patient is totally dependent and vulnerable to many complications. The patient is placed in the intensive care unit, and the following parameters are monitored: ICP, electroencephalogram (EEG), arterial pressures, and blood and serum barbiturate levels.

▶ Nursing Process
The Patient With Increased Intracranial Pressure

▷ Assessment

The Glasgow Coma Scale uses as criteria three types of behavior by which the patient's level of responsiveness is judged: eye opening, motor responses, and verbal performance. The nursing assessment for determining the level of the patient's responsiveness can be organized on these levels. In order to provide all health care personnel with information on the baseline condition and the patient's present status, a neurologic observation record is kept of the following points of assessment:

1. Eye opening
   a. Opens eyes spontaneously
   b. Opens eyes when spoken to
   c. Opens eyes when painful stimulus is applied
   d. Does not respond
2. Verbal response: response to commands
   a. Answers questions readily and correctly; can perform a requested maneuver
   b. Shows delayed response
   c. Engages in confused conversation and inappropriate speech
   d. Responds only to loud voice
   e. Does not respond
3. Observation of motor responses (to painful stimuli)
   a. Obeys verbal commands; changes position
   b. Localizes pain
   c. Withdraws from pain by means of flexion
   d. Exhibits abnormal flexion
   e. Exhibits abnormal extension
   f. Does not respond

Subtle Changes. Restlessness, headache, forced breathing, purposeless movements, and mental cloudiness may be early clinical indications of rising ICP.

Changes in Vital Signs. Alterations in vital signs may be a late sign of increased ICP.

- As the ICP increases, the pulse rate and respiratory rate are slowed and the blood pressure and temperature rise. Special signs to look for are arterial hypertension, bradycardia, and respiratory irregularity; the development of any of these signs warrants further investigation. Cheyne-Stokes breathing (rhythmic waxing and waning of rate and depth of respirations alternating with brief periods of apnea) and ataxic breathing (irregular breathing with a random sequence of deep and shallow breaths) are frequently seen respiratory irregularities.

The vital signs of the patient compensate as long as the major circulation of the brain is preserved. If, as a result of brain compression, the major circulation begins to fail, the pulse and respirations become rapid and the temperature usually rises but does not follow a consistent pattern. The pulse pressure (the difference between the systolic and the diastolic pressure) widens; this is considered a serious development. Immediately preceding this reversal of clinical responses there is usually a period of rapid fluctuations in the pulse, varying from a slow rate to a rapid one. Surgical intervention is indicated or death will ensue.

- The vital signs may not always be altered, even in the event of increased ICP. The patient is assessed for changes in the level of responsiveness and for the presence of shock; these manifestations aid in evaluation.

Headache. The headache is constant, increasing in intensity, and aggravated by movement or straining.

Pupillary Changes. Increasing pressure or an expanding clot can displace the brain against the oculomotor or optic nerves, producing pupillary changes.

(Text continues on p. 1422)

Care of the Patient With Impaired Neurologic Function

Nursing Interventions	*Rationale*	*Expected Outcomes*

Nursing Diagnosis: Ineffective breathing pattern related to neurogenic pulmonary dysfunction (head trauma, intracranial pressure variations)

Goal: Attain/maintain effective respirations

1. Evaluate the abnormal breathing pattern.
  a. Auscultate lungs.
  b. Assess ventilatory status and ability to clear airway.
	1. Respiratory function is impaired in the presence of abnormal breathing patterns if there are prolonged periods of apnea (Cheyne-Stokes respiration; ataxic breathing) or if the work of breathing is associated with elevated oxygen consumption (hyperthermia; central neurogenic hyperventilation)	• Exhibits improved respiratory status
		• Shows adequate ventilatory function
		• Has blood gas values within acceptable range
		• Absence of crackles
		• Verbalizes signs and symptoms of early respiratory impairment

2. Prepare for ventilatory support for management of respiratory dysfunction.	2. Ventilatory support maintains the patency of the airway, helps ensure adequate oxygen uptake in the lungs, prevents carbon dioxide retention, and decreases the work of breathing.	
a. Controlled mechanical ventilation—usually employed with severe head trauma.		
b. Intermittent mandatory ventilation—allows progressive transition from mandatory ventilation by the ventilator to spontaneous breathing.	b. Adequate gas exchange is essential to maintain intracranial homeostasis as near normal as possible.	
c. Continuous positive airway pressure (CPAP)—used when patient has inadequate alveolar ventilation and when intubation is necessary for airway control and positive airway.	c. Positive airway pressure is used to prevent alveolar-collapse.	

Nursing Diagnosis: Impaired swallowing related to cranial nerve involvement and muscle weakness

Goal: Regain/develop ability to swallow within limits imposed by neurologic dysfunction

1. Assess patient's ability to handle his secretions; position upright with neck slightly flexed.	1. Patients with drooling and swallowing deficits are at risk for aspiration.	• Secretions are managed; aspiration is avoided.
2. Suction as necessary, using great care.	2. Care is needed because suctioning can raise intracranial pressure.	
3. Ensure adequate hydration.	3. Adequate hydration loosens pulmonary secretions and helps replenish fluid losses.	

(continued)

Nursing Interventions	*Rationale*	*Expected Outcomes*

Nursing Diagnosis: Potential impairment of skin integrity related to neurologic impairment (inability to shift position, immobility, motor paralysis, decreased sensory awareness, abnormal posture secondary to spasticity)

Goal: Attain and maintain a healthy, intact skin

1. Monitor for signs of pressure, especially on weight-bearing areas.	1. Excessive pressure is the initiating factor for pressure sores. Pressure causes tissue damage by closure of blood vessels, resulting in ischemic necrosis.	• Has healthy appearing, intact skin • Monitors self for pressure areas • Adheres to turning and positioning schedule
2. Check for signs and symptoms of pressure (redness, warmth, tenderness, edema) after change in position.	2. Pressure sores are encountered on weight-bearing areas in different positions	
3. Use interventions to relieve pressure (reposition every 2 hours; use cushions, mattress; establish turning schedule).	3. Skin and subcutaneous compression, blood flow obstruction, and tissue ischemia are relieved. Cushions and mattress provide greater pressure distribution.	
4. Teach patient to inspect for potential pressure areas.		

Nursing Diagnosis: Impaired physical mobility related to central nervous system deficit/injury, weakness, and fatigue

Goal: Gain mobility within limits imposed by neurologic dysfunction

1. Determine activity level.		• Demonstrates improving joint mobility
2. Initiate passive/active range of motion; teach family these techniques. Maintain a functional range of motion for all joints.	2. Passive range of motion helps prevent painful contractures. ROM exercises maintain muscle length and joint flexibility, help stimulate circulation, and give the patient sensory feedback.	• Absence of contractures • Caregiver demonstrates ability to give range of motion exercises. • Uses adaptive equipment
3. Instruct patient in self-range of motion and transfer techniques.		
4. Use safety precautions when teaching patient transfer techniques.	4. Patients with lower extremity paralysis should be trained as wheelchair travelers.	
5. Work collaboratively with physical and occupational therapists to activate the patient. (See Chapter 14, *Principles and Practices of Rehabilitation.*)	5. Many neurologic lesions cause mental dulling and loss of initiative. Loss of muscle strength occurs quickly. It takes deliberate stimulation and cooperative action by the health care team to prevent deterioration.	

(continued)

Nursing Interventions	*Rationale*	*Expected Outcomes*

Nursing Diagnosis: Self-care deficits related to neuromuscular impairment, unilateral neglect, inattention, confusion, cognitive and perceptual dysfunction

Goal: Achieve self-care within limits of neurologic dysfunction

1. Assess patient's ability to perform activities of daily living (ADL).	1. The long range goal is maximal independence in as many self-care activities as possible. ADL should be within the patient's functional limitations.	• Functions as independently as possible within limitations imposed by neurologic dysfunction • Identifies goals for self-care • Shows beginning ability to perform self-care
2. Help patient identify small achievable goals.		
3. Explain and demonstrate specific ADL skills.		
4. Discuss and demonstrate adaptive equipment.		
5. Encourage patient and show him extent of his progress on ADL record.	5. Encouragement helps patient gain confidence and feelings of self-worth.	

Nursing Diagnosis: Social isolation related to limits imposed by neurologic dysfunction

Goal: Participate in social relationship(s) and social system

1. Determine pre-illness activities and coping skills.	1. Neurologic impairment increases vulnerability to loneliness and social isolation. A restricted environment causes sensory and social deprivation.	• Seeks diversional activities • Working with occupational therapist • Continues with social contacts via the telephone • Has materials/phone numbers of support persons and groups
2. Listen for expressions that may indicate underlying loneliness, fear, sadness, boredom, dread; observe behavior indicating the presence of these feelings.	2. Social isolation can be used (inappropriately) to protect from loss of self-esteem, rejection, and feelings of worthlessness. Human companionship is essential for physical and emotional well-being.	
3. Encourage patient to discuss his problems with a confidant.	3. Good relationship with a confidant may help reduce psychological stress.	
4. Help patient develop social network.	4. Through interactions the patient attains/maintains internal and external harmony and balance.	
5. Encourage individual and group counseling, joining mutual self-help group, and participation in church, civic, and social groups.	5. These can be growth-producing interactions.	

Nursing Diagnosis: Alteration in comfort (pain) related to damage of neuronal structures, stimulation of pain receptors, compression or infiltration by tumor; stretching or compression of nerve roots, consequences of therapy (surgery, radiation, chemotherapy)

Goal: Achieve relief of pain

1. Assess for pain, including history of pain experience and evaluation of physical and psychosocial factors.		• Achieving relief of pain • Identifies factors and situations that induce and relieve pain

(continued)

Nursing Interventions	*Rationale*	*Expected Outcomes*

Nursing Diagnosis: Alteration in comfort (pain) related to damage of neuronal structures, stimulation of pain receptors, compression or infiltration by tumor; stretching or compression of nerve roots, consequences of therapy (surgery, radiation, chemotherapy)

Goal: Achieve relief of pain

2. Encourage verbalization of fears and concerns.	2. Anxiety, depression, and sleeplessness commonly accompany pain.	• Uses measures to prevent pain
3. Give prescribed pain medication for acute pain	3. The management of *acute* neurologic pain usually requires drug therapy.	• Sleeps during most of night • Appears more relaxed
4. Instruct patient in pain-relieving techniques (relaxation training, biofeedback, cognitive training).	4. The management of pain from neurologic causes requires a multidisciplinary approach that includes analgesic drug therapy; behavioral techniques; neurosurgical procedures (placement of epidural, intrathecal, and intraventricular catheters for narcotic drug delivery), and supportive care. Behavioral methods aim at promoting an increased sense of control by reducing the helplessness and hopelessness.	

Nursing Diagnosis: Alteration in family processes related to uncertainty, changes in family member's (patient's) ability to function, preexisting interpersonal problems, and inadequate financial resources

Goal: Family members gain control over their lives

1. Assess family strengths as a family unit, signs of stress, interactions with patient, and interactions with one another.	1. Family needs can be met using a collaborative approach, building on each members strengths. An enabling family provides support, maintains patient's valued role, involves patient in decision making and encourages adherence to the therapeutic program.	• Demonstrate increasing ability to cope with situation • Demonstrate a more optimistic outlook • Maintain ongoing positive contact with patient • Able to accurately describe patient's condition • Demonstrate increasing ability to assist in patient's care when appropriate • Seek support through counseling when necessary • Use appropriate referrals and community resources
2. Provide opportunity for verbalization of concerns and fears.		
3. Acknowledge their fears; convey hope. Give accurate information. Model appropriate behavior when interacting with patient/family.	3. Information is essential for problem solving.	
4. Reassure family that health care professionals are accessible.		
5. Encourage family to obtain adequate rest and sleep.	5. Sleep deprivation causes mood disturbances, irritability, and cognitive impairment.	
6. Make appropriate referrals for financial service and psychological counseling.	6. Some families may be alienated, overprotective, neglectful, punitive, and withdrawn. Family may need assistance in deciding when and where to ask for help.	
7. Arrange for contact with other patients/families/support groups.	7. Contact with others offers opportunity for exchange of information, attention, and support.	

- The pupils are periodically inspected with a penlight to evaluate size, configuration, and reaction to light. Both eyes are compared for similarities or differences.
- Gaze is evaluated as to whether it is conjugate (paired; working together) or dysconjugate.
- The ability of the eyes to abduct (cranial nerve function) and adduct (cranial nerve function) is assessed.
- The retina and optic nerve are inspected for hemorrhage and papilledema.

Vomiting.   Vomiting is recurrent and may be projectile.

Clinical assessment is not always a reliable guide in recognizing increased ICP, especially in comatose patients. In certain situations, ICP monitoring is an essential part of management (see p. 1423).

▷ *Nursing Diagnoses*

Based on the assessment data, the patient's major nursing diagnoses may include the following:

- Alteration in cerebral tissue perfusion related to the effects of increased ICP
- Ineffective breathing patterns related to neurologic dysfunction (brain stem compression, structural displacement)
- Ineffective airway clearance related to accumulation of secretions secondary to depression of level of responsiveness
- Potential fluid volume deficit related to dehydration procedures
- Alteration in urine and bowel elimination related to effects of medication, indwelling urethral catheter, and diminished fluid/food intake.
- Potential for infection related to ICP monitoring system (intraventricular catheter)

Other relevant nursing diagnoses could include impaired tissue integrity (oral mucous membranes) related to mouth-breathing, absence of pharyngeal reflex, and inability to ingest fluids; potential of impairment of skin integrity related to immobility and constraints imposed by ICP monitoring system; impaired tissue integrity (cornea) related to diminished or absent corneal reflex; and alteration in family process related to crisis situation. (These diagnoses are discussed in the sections on the patient undergoing intracranial surgery, p. 1453, and the patient with a head injury, p. 1501.)

▷ *Planning and Implementation*

▷ *Goals:*   The goals of the patient may include achievement of cerebral tissue perfusion through reduction in ICP, normalization of respiration, achievement of airway clearance, restoration of fluid balance, normal urine and bowel elimination, and absence of infection.

Nursing Interventions

Achieving Cerebral Tissue Perfusion.   In addition to ongoing nursing surveillance, the following nursing strategies may be employed to eliminate factors contributing to the elevation of ICP:

- The patient is monitored for bradycardia and a rising blood pressure, which are signs of increasing ICP.
- Any activity interfering with venous drainage of blood from the head will raise jugular venous pressure and with it, ICP.

> The patient's head is kept in a neutral (midline) position, which is maintained with the use of a cervical collar if necessary.
> Slight elevation of the head is maintained to aid in venous drainage unless otherwise prescribed.
> Extreme rotation of the neck and flexion of the neck are avoided because compression or distortion of the jugular veins increases ICP.

- Extreme hip flexion is avoided because this position causes an increase in intraabdominal and intrathoracic pressures, which can produce a rise in ICP.
- The Valsalva maneuver, which can be produced by straining at defecation or even moving in bed, is to be avoided. The patient can be instructed to exhale (which opens the glottis) while being moved or turned passively.
- Isometric muscle contractions are also contraindicated, since they raise the systemic blood pressure and hence the ICP.
- Relatively minor changes in the patient's position may significantly affect ICP. If monitoring parameters demonstrate that turning the patient raises his ICP, rotating beds and turning sheets may be used and the patient's head may be held in the nurse's hands during turning to minimize the stimuli that increase ICP.
- Before suctioning is instituted, the patient should be hyperventilated with a resuscitator bag attached to 100% oxygen. Suction should not last longer than 15 seconds.
- Nursing activities that raise ICP should be avoided if possible. Spacing the occurrence of nursing interventions may prevent transient increases in ICP.
- During nursing interventions the ICP should not rise above 25 mm Hg and should return to baseline levels within 5 minutes.
- Emotional stress and frequent arousal from sleep are to be avoided. A calm atmosphere is maintained. Environmental stimuli (noise, conversation) should be minimal.
- Abdominal distention, which increases intra-abdominal, intrathoracic, and intracranial pressure, should be noted. Enemas and cathartics are avoided if possible.

Attaining Normal Respiratory Pattern.   The nurse monitors the patient constantly for respiratory irregularities. Increased pressure on the frontal lobes or deep midline structures may result in Cheyne-Stokes respirations, while pressure in the midbrain may cause hyperventilation. When there is involvement of the lower portion of the brain stem (the pons and medulla), respirations become irregular and eventually cease.

When hyperventilation therapy is used to reduce ICP (by causing cerebral vasoconstriction and a decrease in cerebral blood volume), the nurse collaborates with the respiratory therapist in monitoring the $PaCO_2$, which is usually maintained between 20 and 25 mm Hg.

- A neurologic observation record (see p. 1500) is kept and all observations are made in relation to the patient's baseline condition. Repeated assessments of the patient are made (sometimes minute by minute) so that improvement or deterioration may be noted immediately. If the patient's condition deteriorates, preparations are made for surgical intervention.

Achieving Airway Clearance. The patency of the airway is assessed. If secretions are obstructing the airway, they may be suctioned with care, because transient elevations of ICP occur with suctioning. It may be necessary to oxygenate the patient before and after suctioning to maintain adequate oxygenation. Hypoxia caused by poor oxygenation leads to poor cerebral perfusion. Coughing is discouraged because coughing and straining also increase ICP. The lung fields are auscultated at least daily to determine the presence of adventitious sounds or any areas of congestion. Elevating the head of the bed may also aid in clearing secretions as well as improving venous drainage of the brain.

Attaining Fluid Balance. The administration of various dehydrating agents is part of the treatment protocol. Corticosteroids are used to reduce cerebral edema; also, fluids may be restricted. All of these treatment modalities promote the development of dehydration.

The patient's skin turgor, mucous membranes, and urine osmolality are monitored for signs of dehydration. If fluids are given intravenously, the nurse makes sure that they are given at a slow to moderate rate with a drip-monitoring device to prevent too rapid administration. In the patient receiving mannitol, the nurse observes for the possible development of congestive heart failure and pulmonary edema due to the ability of mannitol to shift fluid from the intracellular compartment to the intravascular system.

Patients undergoing dehydrating procedures require careful oral hygiene because dehydration is associated with mouth dryness. Frequent rinsing of the mouth, lubrication of the lips, and removal of encrustations will relieve dryness and promote comfort.

Attaining Normal Urine and Bowel Elimination. The urine is tested for specific gravity and monitored for glucose. A complication of steroid therapy is hyperglycemia. Patients receiving osmotic therapy frequently have an indwelling urethral catheter. The nurse observes for suppurative drainage and encrustation around the area where the catheter enters the urinary meatus, maintains the patency of the catheter and an unobstructed flow of urine by proper positioning of the tubing and drainage bag, uses measures to prevent cross-contamination (*e.g.*, hand washing, keeping infected patients separate from other patients), and monitors urine for the presence of infection (fever; cloudy, bloody, or odoriferous urine).

The patient's lower abdomen is inspected for signs of bowel distention and the area is auscultated for bowel sounds. Usually the stools are tested for blood if the patient is on high doses of steroids because gastrointestinal bleeding is a complication of this therapy. The patient is cautioned to avoid straining while having a bowel movement because the Valsalva maneuver can increase ICP.

Preventing Infection. The nurse is aware that infection is the greatest risk of ICP monitoring with an intraventricular catheter. Most health care agencies have written protocols for managing these systems, and strict adherence to these guidelines should be observed.

The dressing over the ventricular catheter should be kept dry since a wet dressing is conducive to bacterial growth. Aseptic technique is used when managing the system and changing the ventricular drainage bag. The drainage system is also checked for loose connections since they cause leaking and contamination of the system and cerebrospinal fluid (CSF) as well as inaccurate readings of ICP. The patient is monitored for signs and symptoms of meningitis: fever, chills, nuchal (neck) rigidity, and increasing or persisting headache.

▷ *Evaluation*

▷ *Expected Outcomes*

1. Patient achieves improved cerebral tissue perfusion.
   a. Becomes increasingly oriented to time, place, and person.
   b. Follows verbal commands; answers questions correctly.
2. Attains normal respirations.
   a. Breathes in a normal pattern.
   b. Attains/maintains arterial blood gas values within acceptable range.
3. Is free of excessive airway secretions.
4. Attains improved fluid balance.
   a. Takes fluids orally.
   b. Has urine osmolality within acceptable range.
5. Attains normal urine and bowel elimination.
6. Has no sign of infection.
   a. Has no fever.
   b. Has normal ventricular drainage system.

Monitoring Intracranial Pressure

ICP monitoring is the recording of the pressure exerted within the skull by the brain, cerebral blood, and CSF. The volume of any of these elements can expand as a result of tumor, trauma, edema, bleeding, cerebral vessel dilatation, and so on. ICP monitoring provides a continuous reflection of the intracranial state.

The purposes of ICP monitoring are to (1) identify increased pressure early in its course (before cerebral damage occurs), (2) quantitate the degree of abnormality, (3) initiate appropriate treatment, (4) have access to CSF for sampling and drainage, and (5) evaluate the effectiveness of treatment.

ICP is not in a steady state but fluctuates, as indicated by waves of high pressure and troughs of relatively normal pressure. These waves have been classified as A waves (plateau waves), B waves, and C waves (Fig. 53-1). The *plateau waves* (*A waves*) are transient, paroxysmal, recurring elevations of ICP that may last from 5 to 20 minutes and range in amplitude between 50 and 100 mm Hg. Plateau waves have clinical significance and indicate vascular volume changes within the intracranial compartment that are beginning to compromise cerebral perfusion. They may increase in amplitude and frequency, reflecting cerebral ischemia and brain damage that can occur before overt signs and symptoms of raised ICP are seen clinically. This is especially true in the unconscious patient. Rapid variations of pressure waves may also indicate a potentially serious intracranial situation. Therefore, ICP monitoring provides a more objective evaluation of early or changing trends of ICP than other forms of observation.

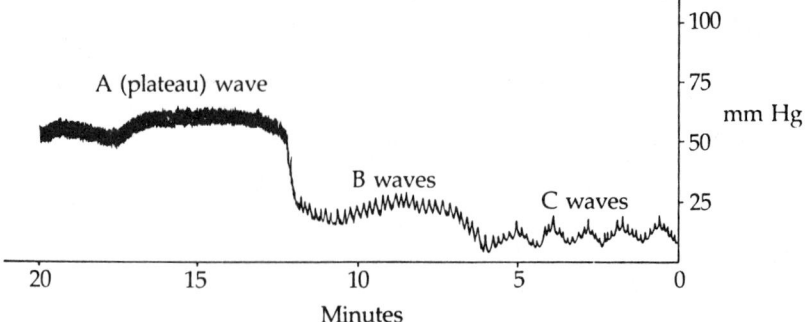

Figure 53-1
Intracranial pressure waves. Composite
diagram of A (plateau) waves, B waves, and
C waves. (Holloway NM. Nursing the
Critically Ill Adult, 2nd ed. Menlo Park,
California, Addison-Wesley, 1984.)

B waves are of shorter duration (½ to 2 minutes) with smaller amplitude (up to 50 mm Hg). They have less clinical significance but if seen in "runs" in a patient with depression of consciousness may precede the appearance of A waves.

C waves are small, rhythmic oscillations with frequencies of approximately six per minute. They appear to be related to rhythmic variations of the systemic arterial blood pressure.

Monitoring Devices

ICP is monitored by measuring CSF pressure within the lateral ventricle, the subarachnoid space, and the epidural space. A large number of devices are available that monitor ICP by means of sensors or transducers that are either connected to an intraventricular catheter or implanted in the skull (Fig. 53-2). The three main types are the intraventricular catheter, subarachnoid screw (or bolt), and epidural pressure recording devices.

Ventricular Catheter Monitoring. Ventricular catheter monitoring (Fig. 53-2) is the insertion of a fine catheter into a lateral ventricle, using either a twist drill or burr hole opening. It is connected by way of a fluid-filled system to a transducer. In addition to obtaining continuous ICP recordings, the ventricular catheter allows for drainage of CSF, particularly during acute rises in pressure.

This method of monitoring is useful in patients with infratentorial brain tumors and aneurysms. Also, continuous drainage of ventricular fluid under pressure control is an effective method of treating intracranial hypertension. Another advantage of an indwelling ventricular catheter is the route it provides for the intraventricular administration of drugs and the instillation of air or contrast medium for ventriculography. Complications include ventricular infection, meningitis, ventricular collapse, and problems with the monitoring system.

Subarachnoid Screw. The subarachnoid screw (or bolt) is a hollow screw that is inserted through the skull and dura mater to the cranial subarachnoid space (Fig. 53-2). It has the advantage of not requiring a ventricular puncture. The subarachnoid screw is inserted through a small twist drill hole in the skull under local anesthesia; it is attached to a pressure transducer, and the output is recorded on an oscilloscope for continuous monitoring. The hollow screw technique is useful in patients with head trauma and those with supratentorial brain tumors. It has the additional advantage of avoiding complications from brain shift and small ventricle size. Complications include blockage of the screw by clot and/or brain substance, which leads to loss of pressure tracing.

A disposable stopcock network is used for both the ventricular catheter and hollow screw monitoring systems to connect the patient to a pressure transducer and display system. The network contains a three-way stopcock attached to the screw or ventricular catheter, a nondistensible saline-filled tubing leading from one outlet of the three-way stopcock to a manifold containing the pressure transducer. The pressure transducer transmits a waveform through the electrical circuitry to a display system for continuous monitoring. The system is flushed with sterile saline at varying time intervals to keep the device patent.

Epidural Monitoring. Another method of ICP monitoring is implantation of a miniature transducer in the epidural space, usually through a burr hole in the skull. One type of epidural ICP monitoring mode is the pneumatic flow sensor and monitor that works on a nonelectrical basis. This pneumatic epidural monitoring system has a low incidence of infection and complications and appears to "read" pressures accurately. Calibration of the system is maintained automatically, and abnormal pressure waves trigger an alarm system.

Clinical Implications

ICP is expressed by ventricular fluid pressures that normally fluctuate in the range of 0 to 10 mm Hg (110 to 140 mm H_2O). Sustained elevations above 15 mm Hg (200 mm H_2O) are generally considered abnormal.

Nursing Implications of ICP Monitoring

The trend of ICP measurements over time is an important indication of the underlying state of the patient. However, the measurement of ICP is only one parameter of patient assessment. Repeated neurologic checks and clinical examination are important.

Strict aseptic techniques are used when handling any part of the monitoring system. The insertion site is inspected for signs of infection. The patient's temperature, pulse, and respirations are closely monitored for systemic signs of infection. All connections and stopcocks are checked for leaks because small leaks can distort pressure readings.

When recording the ICP, the transducer is zeroed at a particular reference point on the patient's head. (CSF pressure is very dependent on the patient's position.) For subsequent pressure readings, the patient's head should be in the same position relative to the transducer.

Whenever technology is associated with patient management, the nurse must be certain that the technology remains functioning. The most important concern is that there is a patient attached to the technology. Talking in a soothing tone and stroking the patient's hand or cheek may be helpful in reducing emotional stress.

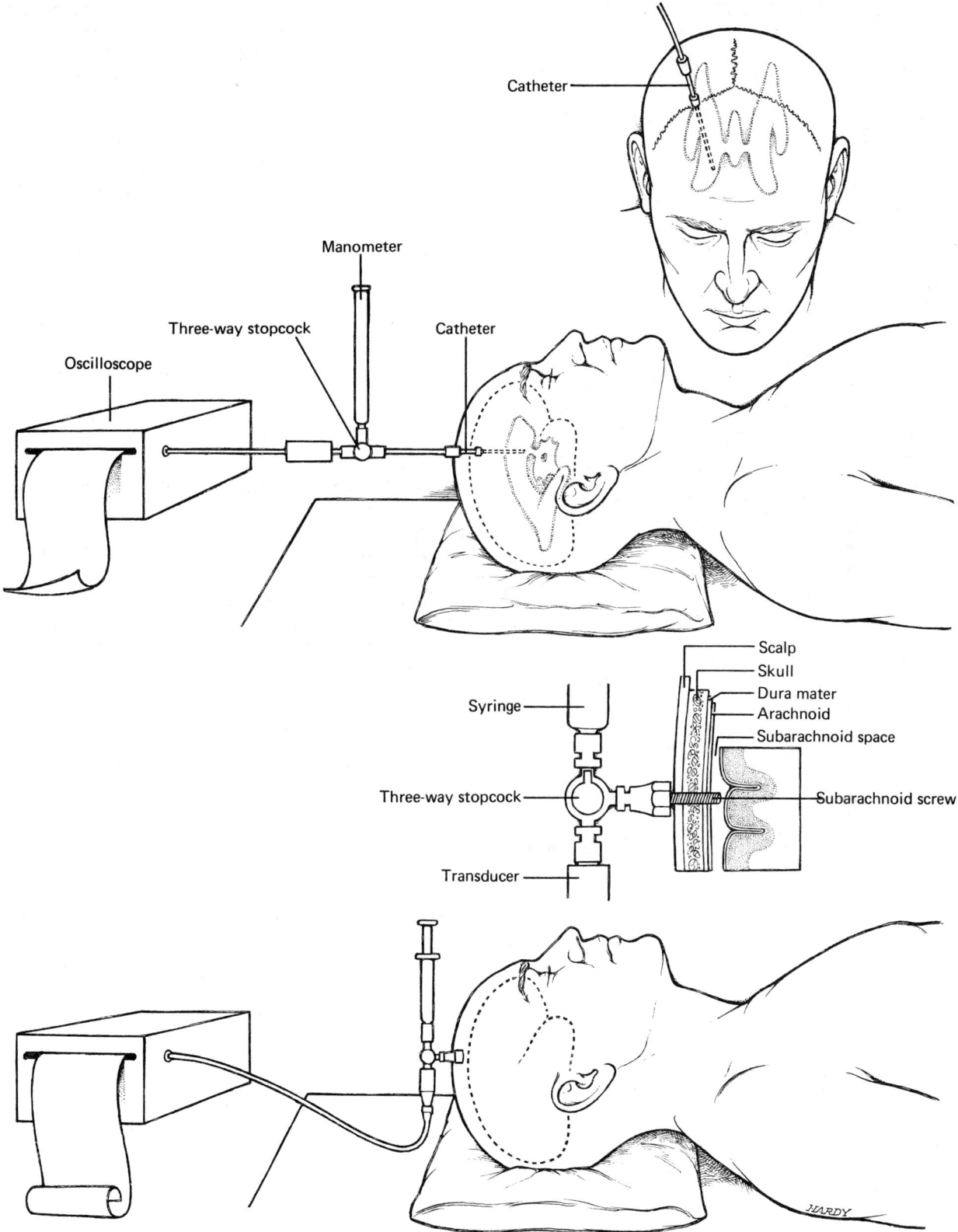

Figure 53-2
Intracranial pressure monitoring. (*Top*) Ventricular catheter. (*Center*) Subarachnoid or hollow screw. (*Bottom*) Monitoring system connected to pressure transducer and display system.

Other Monitoring Modalities (Electrophysiologic Monitoring)

Evoked potential monitoring (electrical potentials produced by nerve tissue in response to external stimulation) is useful for following the course of a patient in drug-induced coma or in any condition in which clinical examination is unreliable. Special EEG recording devices are useful in evaluating some forms of abnormal EEG activity. The major nursing responsibility is ensuring that the electrodes are not displaced during patient care interventions.

Hyperthermia

Because of damage to the heat-regulating center in the brain or severe intracranial infection, neurologic and neurosurgical patients often develop very high temperatures. Such temperature elevations must be controlled, because the increased metabolic demands by the brain will overburden brain circulation and oxygenation, resulting in cerebral deterioration. Persistent hyperthermia is indicative of brain stem damage and has a poor prognosis. It has been shown that body temperatures well below normal decrease cerebral edema, reduce the quantity of oxygen and metabolites required by the brain, and protect the brain from continued ischemia. Also, the collateral circulation in the brain may be able to provide an adequate blood supply to the brain if the body metabolism can be lowered. Hyperthermia is also seen in the neurologically impaired patient with CNS, respiratory, urinary, and wound infections. Drug reactions may also be the cause.

Nursing Considerations. The induction and maintenance of hypothermia is a major clinical procedure and requires knowledge and skilled nursing observation and management. It is desirable to begin treatment before the patient's temperature gets too high.

- All bedding over the patient should be removed (with the possible exception of a light sheet or loin cloth).
- Repeated doses of aspirin or acetaminophen may be given as prescribed.
- Alcohol or cool water sponging and an electric fan blowing over the patient to increase surface cooling are also helpful.
- The use of the hypothermia blanket and equipment is usually effective in controlling neurogenic hyperthermia.

The Unconscious Patient

Unconsciousness is a condition in which there is a depression of cerebral function, ranging from stupor to coma. In *stupor*, the patient shows symptoms of annoyance when stimulated by something unpleasant, such as a pinprick or loud clapping of hands. He may draw back or make facial grimaces or unintelligible sounds. *Coma* is a clinical state of unconsciousness in which the patient is unaware of himself and his environment. *Akinetic mutism* is a state of unresponsiveness to the environment in which the patient makes no movement or sound but sometimes has his eyes open. A *persistent vegetative state* is one in which the patient is described as wakeful but devoid of conscious content, without cognitive or effective mental function.

The causes of unconsciousness may be neurologic (head injury, stroke), toxicologic (drug overdose, alcohol intoxication), or metabolic (hepatic or renal failure).

Diagnostic Evaluation

Laboratory tests that may be helpful in diagnosing the cause of unconsciousness include tests for blood sugar, electrolytes, blood urea nitrogen, osmolality, calcium, prothrombin time, serum ketones, and arterial blood gases.

Management

The first priority is assessment and stabilization of the airway to ensure respiration and ventilation. The circulatory status (carotid pulse, heart beat, blood pressure) is checked because perfusion of the brain depends on the ability of the heart to maintain adequate cardiac output. An intravenous line is established and dextrose in water is administered to prevent hypoglycemia, which causes an altered mental status and CNS damage.

Oxygen may be administered until the cause of unconsciousness or the arterial blood gas measurements are known. Usually an indwelling catheter is inserted.

The neurologic examination is repeated frequently to determine whether the cause of coma is increased ICP or metabolic encephalopathy (reaction of brain in response to generalized change in the metabolism of the brain or in its extracellular environment) due to acidosis, drug overdose, or toxic exposure. Specific therapies are administered for increased ICP and metabolic abnormalities.

▶ Nursing Process
The Unconscious Patient

▷ Assessment

The level of responsiveness (consciousness) is assessed by evaluating eye opening responses, verbal responses, and motor responses to a command or painful stimulus. These measurements are assessed and graded using the Glasgow Coma Scale rating (see p. 1499). The pupils are evaluated as to size, equality, and reaction to light. In addition, the movement of the eyes is noted. Facial symmetry, swallowing reflexes, and deep tendon reflexes are elicited. If the patient is not obeying commands, motor response is tested by applying a painful stimulus (firm but *gentle* pressure) on the supraorbital notch or to the nailbed or by squeezing a muscle. If the patient attempts to push away or withdraw, the response is recorded as purposeful or appropriate. An inappropriate or nonpurposeful response is random and aimless. The unconscious patient with severely impaired cerebral function may respond to a stimulus with *decorticate posturing* (arms flexed, adducted, and internally rotated and legs in extension) or *decerebrate posturing* (extremities extended and reflexes exaggerated); see Chart 53-1. Absence of movement is the lowest level of response.

Body functions (circulation, respiration, elimination, fluid and electrolyte balance) are examined in a systematic manner. If the patient is comatose and localized signs are observed, it is assumed that neurologic disease is present until proved otherwise. If the patient is comatose and a pupillary light reflex is preserved, a toxic or metabolic disorder is suspected.

Important signs to evaluate in assessing the unconscious patient are noted in Chart 53-1 and on p. 1499 in the section on the assessment of the patient with a head injury.

▷ *Nursing Diagnoses*

Based on the assessment data, the patient's major nursing diagnoses may include the following:

- Ineffective airway clearance related to inability to clear respiratory secretions
- Potential fluid volume deficit related to inability to ingest fluids
- Alteration in oral mucous membranes related to mouth-breathing, absence of pharyngeal reflex, and inability to ingest fluids
- Potential impairment of skin integrity related to immobility or restlessness
- Impaired tissue integrity of cornea related to diminished/absent corneal reflex
- Ineffective thermoregulation related to damage to hypothalamic center
- Alteration in urinary elimination (incontinence or retention) related to the unconscious state
- Alteration in bowel elimination (diarrhea and/or constipation) related to the unconscious state
- Alteration in family process related to sudden crisis of unconsciousness

▷ *Planning and Implementation*

▷ *Goals:* The goals of care during the unconscious period may include maintenance of a clear airway, attainment of fluid volume balance, achievement of intact oral mucous membranes, maintenance of normal skin integrity, absence of corneal irritation/keratitis, attainment of thermoregulation, absence of urinary retention and infection, absence of diarrhea/fecal impaction, and maintenance of intact family/support system.

The quality of nursing care given an unconscious patient may literally mean the difference between life and death, since the patient's protective reflexes are impaired. The nurse must assume responsibility for the patient until the basic reflexes return (coughing, blinking, and swallowing) and the patient becomes conscious and oriented. Thus, the major nursing goal is to assume these protective reflexes for the patient until he is aware of himself and can function consciously.

Nursing Interventions

Maintaining the Airway. The most important consideration in the management of the unconscious patient is establishment of an adequate airway and ventilation. Circulation to the brain must be ensured. Obstruction of the airway is a risk facing the unconscious patient, since the epiglottis and tongue may relax, occluding the oropharynx, or the patient may inhale vomitus or nasopharyngeal secretions.

- The patient is positioned in a lateral or semiprone position, which permits the jaw and tongue to fall forward and thus facilitates drainage of secretions. *An unconscious patient must not be allowed to remain on his back.*

The accumulation of secretions in the pharynx presents a serious problem that demands intelligent and conscientious management. Since the patient is unable to swallow and lacks pharyngeal reflexes, these secretions must be removed to eliminate the danger of aspiration.

- Elevating the head of the bed to a 30-degree angle helps prevent aspiration of secretions.
- Suction is employed to remove secretions from the posterior pharynx and upper trachea. With the suction turned *off*, a whistle-tip catheter is lubricated with a water-soluble lubricant and maneuvered to the desired level. Then the suction is turned on (negative pressure) while the aspirating catheter is withdrawn with a twisting motion of the thumb and forefinger. This twisting maneuver prevents the suctioning end of the catheter from irritating the tracheal or pharyngeal mucosa, since irritation increases secretions and produces mucosal bleeding.
- The chest is auscultated periodically for crackles, rhonchi, or absence of breath sounds.

Attaining Fluid and Nutritional Balance. The patient is assessed for hydration status; the mucous membranes are examined, and the skin is evaluated for tissue turgor. The fluid needs of this patient are initially met by giving the required fluids intravenously and then by nasogastric or gastrostomy feedings.

- Intravenous solutions and blood transfusions for patients with intracranial conditions must run in slowly. If given too rapidly, they may increase the ICP. The quantity of fluids administered may be limited to minimize the possibility of producing cerebral edema.
- Fluids should never be given by mouth to the patient who cannot swallow. One way of testing to see whether the patient is able to swallow without choking is to give him a wet swab to suck.
- A nasogastric tube may be passed so that the patient can be given liquid and blenderized feedings.

Maintaining Healthy Oral Mucous Membranes. The patient's mouth is inspected for dryness, inflammation, and the presence of crusting. The unconscious patient requires conscientious oral care because there is a risk of parotitis if the mouth is not kept scrupulously clean. The mouth is cleansed with a gauze-covered tongue blade and rinsed carefully to remove secretions and crusts and to keep the membranes moist. A thin coating of petrolatum on the lips prevents drying, cracking, and the formation of encrustations.

Maintaining Skin Integrity. Preventing skin breakdown requires continuing nursing assessment and intervention. Special attention is given to unconscious patients because they are insensitive to external stimuli. This includes avoiding pressure, which can cause necrosis of the skin, by a regular schedule of turning. Turning also provides kinesthetic (sensation of movement), proprioceptive (awareness of position), and vestibular (equilibrium) stimulation. After turning,

Chart 53-1
Nursing Assessment of the Unconscious Patient

Examination	Clinical Assessment	Clinical Significance
Level of responsiveness or consciousness	Eye opening; verbal and motor responses; pupils (size, equality, reaction to light)	Obeying commands is a favorable response and demonstrates a return to consciousness.
Pattern of respiration	Cheyne-Stokes respiration	Disturbances of regulating center of brain may result in various respiratory patterns. Lesions deep in both hemispheres; area of basal ganglia and upper brain stem
	Hyperventilation	Suggests onset of metabolic problem
	Ataxic respiration with irregularity in depth/rate	Ominous sign of damage to medullary center
Eyes Pupils (size, equality, reaction to light)	Equal normally reactive pupils	Shows that coma is toxic or metabolic in origin
	Equal or unequal diameter	Localizing sign
	Progressive dilatation	Indicates increasing intracranial pressure
	Fixed dilated pupils	Indicate injury at level of midbrain

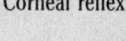
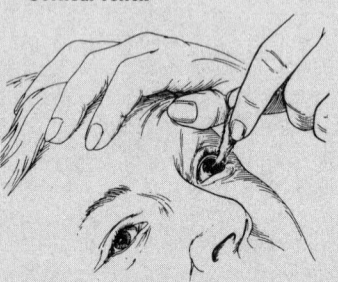

Eye movements	Normally eyes should move from side to side	Functional and structural integrity of brain stem is assessed by inspection of extraocular movements; usually absent in deep coma
Corneal reflex	When cornea is touched with a wisp of clean cotton, blink response is normal	Tests cranial nerves V and VII; localizing sign if unilateral; absent in deep coma
Facial symmetry	Asymmetry (sagging, decrease in wrinkles)	Sign of paralysis
Swallowing reflex	Drooling versus spontaneous swallowing	Absent in coma Paralysis of cranial nerves X and XII
Neck	Stiff neck	Subarachnoid hemorrhage, meningitis
	Absence of spontaneous neck movement	Fracture or dislocation of cervical spine
Response of extremity to noxious stimuli	Firm pressure on a joint of the upper and lower extremity	Asymmetrical response in paralysis
	Observe spontaneous movements	Absent in deep coma

(continued)

the patient is carefully repositioned to prevent ischemic necrosis over pressure areas. Dragging the patient up in bed must be avoided since this creates a shearing force and friction on the skin surface.

Maintaining correct body position is important; equally important is passive exercise of the extremities so that con-

tractures are prevented. The use of a footboard aids in the prevention of footdrop and eliminates the pressure of bedding on the toes. Trochanter rolls supporting the hip joints keep the legs in good position (see p. 219). The arm should be in abduction, the fingers lightly flexed, and the hand in a position of slight supination.

Chart 53-1 (continued)

Examination	Clinical Assessment	Clinical Significance
Deep tendon reflexes	Tap patellar and biceps tendons	Brisk response may have localizing value Asymmetrical response in paralysis Absent in deep coma
Pathologic reflexes	Firm pressure with blunt object on sole of foot moving along lateral margin and crossing to the ball of foot	Flexion of the toes, especially the great toe, is normal except in newborn Dorsiflexion of toes (especially great toe) indicates contralateral pathology of corticospinal tract (Babinski reflex) Localizing signs
Abnormal posture	Observation for posturing (spontaneous or in response to noxious stimuli) Flaccidity with absence of motor response Decorticate posture (flexion and internal rotation of forearms and hands; see *A* below) Decerebrate posture (extension and external rotation; see *B* below)	Deep extensive brain lesion Seen with cerebral hemisphere pathology and in metabolic depression of brain function Decerebrate posturing indicates deeper and more severe dysfunction than does decorticate posturing; implies brain stem pathology; poor prognostic sign

A   B

Muscle tone	Flexor or extensor rigidity or extremity flaccidity	Indicates paralysis

Maintaining Corneal Integrity. Some unconscious patients lie with their eyes open and have inefficient or absent corneal reflexes. The cornea is likely to become irritated or scratched, leading to keratitis and corneal ulcers.

The eyes may be cleansed with cotton balls moistened with sterile normal saline to remove debris and discharge. It may be necessary to instill artificial tears every 2 hours. (This is an interdependent action requiring consultation with the physician.) Often, periocular edema (swelling around the eyes) occurs following head surgery. Cold compresses may be prescribed, and care must be exerted to avoid contact with the cornea.

Attaining Thermoregulation. High fever in the unconscious patient may be caused by infection of the respiratory tract or urinary tract, drug reactions, or damage to the hypothalamic temperature-regulating center. A slight elevation of temperature may be caused by dehydration. The temperature of the environment is determined by the patient's condition. An elevated body temperature would call for a minimum amount of bedding—a sheet or perhaps only a loin cloth.

The room may be cooled to 18.3°C (65°F). However, if the patient is older and does not have an elevation of temperature, a warmer atmosphere is needed. Regardless of the temperature, the air should be fresh and free from odors.

- The body temperature of an unconscious patient never is taken by mouth. Rectal temperature is preferred to the less accurate axillary temperature.

Hyperpyrexia is treated by measures described on p. 1526.

Preventing Urinary Retention. The unconscious patient is either incontinent or has urinary retention. The patient's bladder is palpated at intervals to determine whether urinary retention is present, since a full bladder may be an overlooked cause of incontinence. If there are signs of urinary retention, initially an indwelling catheter attached to a closed drainage system is inserted. Since the catheter is a major cause of urinary infection, the patient is observed for fever and cloudy urine. The area around the urethral orifice is inspected for suppurative drainage. The urinary catheter is usually removed when the patient has a stable cardiovascular system and if no problems with diuresis, sepsis, or voiding dysfunction existed before the onset of coma. Although many comatose patients will urinate spontaneously after catheter removal, the patient's bladder should be periodically palpated for urinary retention. An external penile catheter (condom catheter) for the male patient and absorbent pads for the female patient can be used for the unconscious patient who can urinate spontaneously, although involuntarily. As soon as consciousness is regained, a bladder training program is initiated.

Promoting Bowel Function. Abdominal distention is evaluated by listening for bowel sounds and measuring the girth of the abdomen with a tape measure. There is a risk of diarrhea from infection, antibiotics, and hyperosmolar fluids. Frequent loose stools are also an indication of fecal impaction. Commercial fecal collection bags are available for patients with fecal incontinence.

Immobility and lack of dietary fiber may cause constipation. The nurse monitors the number and consistency of bowel movements and performs a rectal examination for signs of fecal impaction. The patient may require an enema every other day to empty the lower colon. However, enemas may be contraindicated if the Valsalva maneuver increases a compromised intracranial pressure. A glycerin suppository stimulates bowel emptying. Stools softeners may be prescribed and can be given with the tube feedings.

Supporting the Family. The family of the unconscious patient may be thrown into a sudden state of crisis and go through the process of high anxiety, denial, anger, remorse, grief, and reconciliation. In order to assist family members to mobilize their own adaptive capacities, the nursing personnel can reinforce and clarify information about the patient's condition, permit the family to be involved in the care of their loved one, and listen and encourage ventilation of feelings and concerns while supporting them in their decision-making process concerning post-hospitalization management and placement.

Other Nursing Interventions

Safety. For the protection of the patient, padded siderails should be provided. Every measure that is available and appropriate for calming and quieting the disturbed patient should be carried out. Any form of restraint is likely to be countered by resistance, whether the patient is fully conscious or not, and fury so incited may lead to self-injury or to a dangerous increase in ICP.

Promoting Sensory Stimulation. Continuing sensory stimulation is provided to help overcome the profound sensory deprivation of the unconscious patient. Efforts are made to maintain the sense of daily rhythm by keeping the usual day and night patterns for activity and sleep. The nurse touches and talks to the patient and encourages family members and friends to do the same. Communicating with the patient is extremely important and includes touching him and spending enough time with him to become perceptive of his needs. It is also important to avoid making any negative comments about the patient's status or prognosis in his presence. The patient is periodically oriented to time and place. Sounds from the patient's home and workplace may be introduced by means of a tape recorder. In addition, family members can read to the patient from a favorite book and may suggest radio and television programs that he previously enjoyed as a means of enriching the environment and providing meaningful input.

Attaining Self-Care. The unconscious patient is dependent on the nursing staff for all his activities of daily living. As soon as consciousness returns, the nurse begins to teach, support, encourage, and supervise these activities until the patient gains independence. (See Activities of Daily Living, p. 230.)

A summary of the nursing management of the unconscious patient is found in Nursing Care Plan 53-2.

▷ Evaluation

▷ Expected Outcomes

1. Patient maintains clear airway.
   a. Has no crackles on lung auscultation.
2. Attains/maintains adequate fluid status.
   a. Has no clinical signs of dehydration.
   b. Demonstrates normal range of serum electrolytes.
3. Attains/maintains healthy oral mucous membranes.
   a. Has moist and intact oral mucosa.
4. Maintains normal skin integrity.
5. Has no cornea irritation.
6. Attains/maintains thermoregulation.
   a. Temperature within acceptable range.
   b. Skin of normal temperature and texture.
7. Has no urinary retention.
8. Has no diarrhea/fecal impaction.
9. Family members coping with crisis.
   a. Verbalize fears and concerns.
   b. Participate in patient's care.
   c. Provide sensory stimulation through talking and touching.

Aphasia

Aphasia is a disturbance of language function resulting from injury or disease of the brain centers. It may involve impairment of the ability to read and write as well as to speak, listen, calculate, comprehend, and understand gestures (Chart 53-2, p. 1438). Nearly 1 to 1.5 million adults in this country have a chronic disabling aphasia. The major causes are stroke, head injury, and brain tumor. An estimated 20% of stroke patients develop aphasia. The number of aphasic patients is growing since more stroke patients are surviving.

The cortical area that is responsible for integrating the myriad association pathways required for the comprehension and formulation of language measures little more than a square inch in extent. The principal speech center, called *Broca's area,* is located in a convolution adjoining the middle cerebral artery. Here are stored the combinations of muscular movements necessary to speak each word. They are not the cells that govern the muscles of speech; these cells are in the motor area itself. Each word requires for its utterance a combination or sequence of combinations of muscular contractions. Not only must the muscles of the vocal cords contract, but also those of the throat, the tongue, the soft palate, the lips, and the chest wall. These combinations are stored in the cells of Broca's convolution. They direct the cells of the motor area, which make the muscles contract at the proper time and with the proper force.

Broca's area is so near the left motor area that a disturbance in the motor area often affects the speech area. This is the reason that so many patients paralyzed on the right side (due to damage or injury to the left side of the brain) are unable to speak, whereas in those paralyzed on the left side, speech disturbances are less common. Some patients are not affected, but these usually are left-handed persons whose speech area is located on the right hemisphere.

▶ Nursing Process
The Patient With Aphasia

▷ Assessment

The speech–language pathologist in cooperation with the neurologist determines the communication abilities of the patient. Information is obtained regarding the patient's pre-illness speech–language skills and interests. Formalized, standardized tests and observational methods are used to evaluate comprehension, mathematical, reading, and residual language skills.

The nursing assessment of the aphasic patient includes *listening* to him, asking him to follow simple directions (*i.e.,* "pick up the book"), and observing him cope with his dysfunction.

▷ Nursing Diagnoses

Based on the assessment data, the patient's major nursing diagnoses may include the following:

- Disturbance in self-concept related to loss of ability to communicate

- Impaired communicative behavior related to brain damage
- Ineffective family coping related to sudden disruption in life-style and lack of understanding of brain damage and how to help the patient

▷ Planning and Implementation

▷ **Goals:** The major goals of the patient may include development of a more positive self-concept, improved communication abilities, and improved family coping.

Nursing Interventions

Developing a Positive Self-Concept. A patient with aphasia should be given as much psychological security as possible. The same manner is used with this patient as with a young child learning to speak. At the same time, the patient is treated as an adult. A kind, unhurried manner combined with encouragement, patience, and a willingness to invest time are required. Relearning speech and language skills may take several years.

An aphasic person may become very depressed because of the inability to talk to others. Not being able to talk on the telephone or answer a question or being excluded from conversation causes suppressed anger, frustration, fear of the future, and a sense of hopelessness.

The nurse must accept the patient's behavior, relieve his embarrassment, and give support by assuring him that there is nothing wrong with his intelligence and that she realizes he knows what he wants to say. The environment should be relaxed and permissive, and the patient should be encouraged to socialize with family and friends. The typical aphasic person has almost an obsession with orderliness. Thus, nurses and family members should return items in the room to their proper place.

Improving Communication Abilities. It is essential that aphasic patients be guided in their efforts to improve their communication skills. Listening skills as well as speaking skills are emphasized in the rehabilitation program.

Increasing Auditory Stimulation. First the patient is encouraged to *listen.* Speaking is thinking out loud, and the emphasis is on *thinking.* The patient must think and sort out incoming messages and formulate a response. Listening requires mental effort; yet the patient must struggle against mental inertia and needs time to organize an answer.

In working with the aphasic patient, the nurse must remember to *talk* to the patient while caring for him. This provides social contact for the patient.

- It is best to face the patient and establish eye contact, at the same time speaking in a normal manner but in short phrases, pausing between phrases. The emphasis here is on ensuring that the patient understands what is being said.
- Conversation should be confined to practical and concrete matters and supplemented with gestures, pictures, and objects.
- As the patient handles and uses the object, the word should be stated; it helps when words are matched with actions.

(Text continues on p. 1438)

Care of the Unconscious Patient

Nursing Interventions	*Rationale*	*Expected Outcomes*

Note: The basic nursing principles underlying the care of an unconscious patient are applicable to any unconscious patient, regardless of the clinical cause. There are two major threats to the patient: (1) the disease or trauma that produced unconsciousness and (2) the threat of the unconscious state. The primary problem is that the patient's normal protective reflexes are impaired. The nursing goal is to assume these protective mechanisms for the patient until he is aware of himself and can function in his environment

Nursing Diagnosis: Ineffective breathing related to unconscious state

Goal: Attainment of normal breathing

1. Establish and maintain an adequate airway, respiratory exchange, and circulation.
   a. Place the patient in a three-fourths prone position or in a lateral position with his head turned to one side. (In the event of increased intracranial pressure, the head of the bed may be elevated as prescribed.)
   b. Note the respiratory rate and pattern.

   c. Insert oral airway if tongue is paralyzed or is obstructing the airway.

   d. Start oxygen and other therapies as prescribed.
   e. Keep the airway free of secretions by efficient suctioning.

   f. Prepare for insertion of cuffed endotracheal tube if patient's condition requires (inefficient cough reflex, respiratory failure).

1. Inadequate respiratory exchange promotes carbon dioxide retention, which can produce diffuse cerebral edema. Airway obstruction will aggravate cerebral swelling and may be a cause of continuing or deepening unconsciousness.

   b. The respiratory pattern reflects activity throughout the brain and spinal cord. Disordered respiration is an indication of brain dysfunction; prompt initiation of respiratory support is indicated.
   c. A noisy airway is an obstructed airway. (An obstructed airway increases intracranial pressure.) The use of an oropharyngeal airway is considered a short-term measure.

   e. With the absence of the cough and swallowing reflexes, secretions rapidly accumulate in the posterior pharynx and upper trachea and can pave the way to fatal respiratory complications.
   f. Endotracheal intubation is more effective in permitting positive-pressure ventilation. The cuffed tube seals off the digestive tract, thus preventing aspiration, and allows efficient removal of tracheobronchial secretions.

- Attains normal breathing
- Respirations quiet and appear effortless
- Absence of excessive respiratory secretions
- Respirations within normal range
- Peripheral pulses are of normal amplitude
- Has blood pressure within acceptable range for condition
- Has less than 50 ml of gastric aspirate before NG feeding

(continued)

Nursing Interventions	*Rationale*	*Expected Outcomes*

Nursing Diagnosis: Ineffective breathing related to unconscious state

Goal: Attainment of normal breathing

g. Use humidified oxygen, positive-pressure assisted breathing techniques, or mechanical ventilation when there is indication of impending respiratory failure.

g. When arterial blood gas measurements reveal that patient has insufficient ventilation and gas exchange, respiratory failure may quickly ensue.

h. Evaluate pulses (radial, carotid, apical, pedal): measure blood pressure.

h. These are a measure of circulatory adequacy/inadequacy and give clues to the cause of the unconscious states.

i. Assist with passage of a nasogastric (NG) tube. (The cuffed endotracheal tube should be in place before passage of NG tube).

i. Aspiration of gastric contents is common in unconscious patients secondary to the loss of protective pharyngeal reflexes, decreased gastric motility, and regurgitation. An NG tube permits suctioning of stomach contents and provides a route for oral feeding.

j. Assess cardiac functioning.

j. The ECG may indicate an acute myocardial infarction accompanied by a cerebral embolism as the cause of the unconscious state.

k. Assist with diagnostic tests (blood, urine, nasogastric aspirate).

k. Blood is drawn for glucose determinations and toxicology screening.

Nursing Diagnosis: Alteration in cerebral tissue perfusion related to unconscious state

Goal: Achievement of cerebral tissue perfusion to maintain cerebral homeostasis

1. Maintain a constant assessment of patient's level of consciousness and changes in responsiveness.

1. The level of consciousness is the most sensitive indicator of improvement or deterioration. Unconscious patients can deteriorate rapidly from numerous clinical causes.

• Beginning to open eyes, responds to commands
• Pupils of normal size, equality, and reaction
• Appears more alert, less restless
• Moves extremities appropriately in response to commands or noxious stimuli
• Vital signs within acceptable limits

2. Record the patient's exact reactions: eye opening, verbal response, movements, and quality of speech. Describe the stimuli required to elicit the patient's responses.

2. The Glasgow Coma Scale depicts these modes of behavior. An unconscious patient is unable to obey commands or utter recognizable words.

3. Examine pupils of eyes for size, shape, and reaction to light.

3. Pupillary abnormalities are important in localizing the cause of unconsciousness.

4. Assess movements of extremities in response to verbal commands or painful stimulus.

4. No response or a delayed or unequal response is an unfavorable clinical sign. Obeying commands is a favorable response and indicates a return to consciousness.

(continued)

Nursing Interventions	*Rationale*	*Expected Outcomes*

Nursing Diagnosis: Alteration in cerebral tissue perfusion related to unconscious state

Goal: Achievement of cerebral tissue perfusion to maintain cerebral homeostasis

5. Evaluate the progression of vital signs:
   a. Know the patient's baseline (initial) vital signs, and alert the physician if there are significant fluctuations of blood pressure and instability of the pulse and respiratory cycles.
   b. Take blood pressure readings, pulse, respiratory rate and patterns, and temperature at frequently specified intervals until there is clinical evidence of stabilization.

a. Fluctuations of vital signs indicate a change in intracranial homeostasis. Monitoring of vital signs is also essential to detect hidden bleeding.

b. Taking and recording of temperature is mandatory since temperature-regulating mechanisms may be impaired. Hyperthermia is an unfavorable prognostic sign. The systolic blood pressure must be adequate to maintain cerebral perfusion pressure. Brain injury can both elevate and depress blood pressure. A slow pulse, rising blood pressure, and slowing respirations are associated with cerebral compromise.

Nursing Diagnosis: Alteration in fluid volume deficit (potential deficit) related to inability to ingest oral fluids secondary to unconscious state

Goal: Maintain fluid balance

1. Observe for signs of overhydration or dehydration. Administer intravenous fluids as indicated.

1. Serial laboratory electrolyte evaluations are made when the patient is maintained on intravenous fluids to ensure proper balance.

- Laboratory evaluations within acceptable range
- Normal skin turgor

Nursing Diagnosis: Alteration in nutritional status (less than required) related to unconscious state

Goal: Meet nutritional requirements

1. Prepare for nasogastric feedings.

1. Feeding through a gastric tube ensures better nutrition than does intravenous feeding. Paralytic ileus is fairly frequent in unconscious patients and a nasogastric tube assists in gastric decompression.

- Taking NG feedings well
- No evidence of aspiration

   a. Insert gastric tube through nose into stomach.
   b. Aspirate the stomach before each feeding.

b. If aspirated residual exceeds 50 ml, the patient may be developing an ileus. Gastric distention and vomiting may result.

(continued)

Nursing Interventions	*Rationale*	*Expected Outcomes*

Nursing Diagnosis: Alteration in nutritional status (less than required) related to unconscious state

Goal: Meet nutritional requirements

c. Elevate the patient's head and thorax and give 100 to 150 ml blenderized feeding slowly. Give small amount at first and gradually increase until 400 to 500 ml is given at each feeding.	c. Elevation of the patient's head before, during, and after feeding reduces likelihood of esophageal reflux, regurgitation, and aspiration.	
d. Give 2000 to 2500 ml of fluid through the tube daily.	d. An unconscious patient requires adequate fluids daily. High-protein feedings can produce a solute diuresis that will produce dehydration and hyperosmolar coma unless enough fluid intake is ensured. Fever, excessive sweating, or fluid loss elsewhere in the body increases fluid reqirements.	
e. Rinse the tube with water after each feeding. Keep tube feeding refrigerated.		
2. Prepare for gastrostomy or hyperalimentation if patient is expected to remain comatose for an indefinite period.	2. Prolonged nasogastric intubation can cause esophagitis (from gastric reflux) and erosion of the nasal septum.	

Nursing Diagnosis: Alteration in bladder elimination (incontinence) related to unconscious state

Goal: Attain/maintain bladder continence as soon as possible

1. Observe the patient for indications of an overdistended bladder.	1. Most unconscious patients are incontinent but empty their bladders regularly.	• Absence of bladder distention • Absence of skin breakdown
a. Use external sheath catheter (condom catheter) for male patient and indwelling catheter for female patient if skin maceration becomes a problem.		
b. Send urine culture to laboratory at specified intervals.	b. Culture can detect urinary infection.	

Nursing Diagnosis: Alteration in bowel elimination (constipation and/or diarrhea) related to unconscious state

Goal: Attainment of bowel continence

1. Watch for constipation and/or diarrhea.	1. Constipation results from immobilization and lack of dietary fiber. Diarrhea occurs from infection, antibiotics, hyperosmolar feedings, and fecal impaction.	• Has soft, formed stool
2. Place patient on bowel program (p. 238) as soon as possible.		

(continued)

Nursing Care Plan 53-2 *(continued)*

Nursing Interventions	*Rationale*	*Expected Outcomes*

Nursing Diagnosis: Potential impairment of skin integrity related to immobility or restlessness

Goal: Maintenance of normal skin integrity

1. Keep the skin clean, dry, and free of pressure.	1. Comatose patients are susceptible to the formation of pressure sores. All of these activities are to prevent formation of pressure sores on pressure-sensitive areas.	• Absence of skin breakdown • Skin appears healthy with normal turgor.
2. Turn patient frequently.	2. To relieve pressure	
3. Lubricate skin with emollient lotions.	3. Prevents irritation from sheet, dryness, chafing, and cracking.	
4. Inspect pressure areas for evidence of skin redness and breakdown.	4. See p. 222 for other preventive measures for pressure sores.	
5. Clip patient's fingernails to prevent skin excoriation by accidental or reflex scratching.		

Nursing Diagnosis: Potential impaired tissue integrity (cornea) related to unconscious state

Goal: Preservation of sight

1. Protect the eye from corneal irritation.
  a. Make sure patient's eye is not rubbing against the bedding.
  b. Routinely inspect size of pupils and condition of eyes using a penlight.
  c. Irrigate eyes with prescribed solution and instill ophthalmic drops or ointment in each eye.
  d. Seal eyelids shut with plastic tape or prepare for temporary tarsorrhaphy (suturing of eyelids in closed position) if unconscious state is prolonged.
	1. The cornea functions as a shield. If the eyes remain open for long periods, corneal drying, abrasion, and secondary infection and ulceration are apt to result.
	
	  c. Removes discharge and helps prevent glazing and corneal ulceration.
		• Eyes appear normal; absence of redness, purulent drainage, or signs of irritation or infection

(continued)

Nursing Interventions	*Rationale*	*Expected Outcomes*

Nursing Diagnosis: Potential for injury related to occurrence of seizures and restlessness

Goal: Protection from injury

1. Protect the patient from self-injury.
  a. See p. 1489 for nursing interventions.
  b. Observe the patient during the seizure and record observations.
  c. Give prescribed anticonvulsant medications via nasogastric tube.
2. Give nursing support as the patient's changing condition indicates. Be aware of the varying phases of restlessness.
 	
  a. Have adequate lighting in the room to prevent hallucinations in the patient who is regaining consciousness.
  b. Pad side rails, apply mitts or boxing gloves.
  c. Avoid oversedating the patient.
	1. A patient with head trauma is a potential candidate for seizures.
	
	2. A certain degree of restlessness may be favorable as it may indicate the patient is regaining consciousness. However, restlessness is quite common in cerebral hypoxia or when there is a partially obstructed airway, distended bladder, overlooked bleeding, or fracture; it may be a manifestation of brain injury.
	  b. To prevent injury
	
	  c. Sedatives and narcotics depress the level of responsiveness, which is a guide to clinical assessment. Certain drugs affect pupillary size and reaction, which are important signs.
		• No evidence of injury or trauma
		• No undue restlessness noted

Nursing Diagnosis: Sensory-perceptual deficit related to unconsciousness

Goal: Promotion of sensory stimulation

1. Provide for environmental enrichment and social contacts.
  a. Direct conversation to the patient; encourage family to talk to the patient.
  b. Arouse patient; touch him; stimulate his senses.
  c. Introduce sounds from the patient's home and work environment via a tape recorder to "normalize" the environment.
2. Give the patient an explanation of what has happened during the period of unconsciousness. Permit him to question and talk about the experience of unconsciousness.
	1. Introducing meaningful sounds stimulates the cortical levels.
	  a. Attempting to stimulate the patient's senses helps overcome sensory deprivation.
	
	  c. Know the patient's preferences in music, radio, TV, and patterns of daily living.
	
	2. This will help the patient to cope with anxieties, mobilize psychological defenses, and promote psychological recovery.
		• Family visiting and interacting with patient
		• Family initiate reading-aloud session; have planned television/radio sessions taking into consideration patient's previous interests
		• Asks questions and listening to responses

Chart 53-2
Glossary of Selected Terms Relating to Aphasia*

Acalculia; dyscalculia—difficulty in dealing with mathematical processes or numerical symbols in general

Agnosia—failure to recognize familiar objects perceived by the senses

   Auditory agnosia—inability to recognize significance of sounds

   Color agnosia—inability to recognize differences in color

   Tactile agnosia—inability to recognize familiar objects by touch or feel

   Visual object agnosia—inability to recognize objects; visual acuity may or may not be intact

Agraphia; dysgraphia—disturbances in writing intelligible words

Alexia; dyslexia—difficulty in reading

Anomia; dysnomia—difficulty in selecting appropriate words, particularly nouns

Apraxia—inability to perform previously learned purposeful motor acts on a voluntary basis

   Verbal apraxia—difficulty in forming and organizing intelligible words although the musculature is intact

Dysarthria—defects of articulation due to neurologic causes

Hemianopia—blindness of one half of the field of vision in one or both eyes

Paraphasia—a frequently observed characteristic in many aphasic patients; uses wrong words, word substitutions, grammatical errors, faults in word usage; may be observed in both oral and written language

Perseveration—continued and automatic repetition of an activity or word or phrase that is no longer appropriate

* The prefix *a* means "without" or "absence." The prefix *dys* refers to "difficulty" or "disordered." These prefixes are frequently used interchangeably in these conditions.

- Consistency is important and the same wording and gestures are used each time instructions are given and questions are asked.
- Since the patient is easily fatigued and distracted, extraneous noises and sounds must be kept at a minimum since the patient cannot sort out messages when there is too much noise and confusion in the environment.

Restoring Speech. When the patient attempts to communicate, the nurse should make a real effort to understand him and to treat him as an intelligent adult. It is important to behave in a way that shows acceptance of the patient as a worthwhile person. The patient should never be forced to correct his mistakes since this merely adds to his tension, nor should the nurse rush to finish sentences for him. During periods of emotional lability, the patient should be approached in a calm, accepting, and deliberate manner since frustration and depression are frequent reactions to the inability to communicate. Because speech that is motivated by emotions usually comes first (*i.e.*, swearing), the content of this speech should be ignored by the nursing personnel.

Patients with aphasia must be stimulated both internally and externally to action. Therapy is based on a recognition of the patient's needs, *previous* interests, drives, and motivation. If the patient's speech is unintelligible or filled with jargon, his gestures may offer a clue to his intent.

- Continue to listen to him.
- Nod and make neutral statements occasionally.

When appropriate, shift the topic to gain another point of interest and frame of reference.

The environment should provide sensory input, with auditory stimulation supplemented with visual stimulation. Reading is encouraged for a few minutes at a time, and the patient can look at pictures while another person talks about them. Games stimulate the mind and help organize the thoughts. The nurse can try to elicit responses from the patient, asking him to nod his head if he understands. Every correct response should be reinforced. For more relaxed forms of communication, the television, radio, electronic games, and tape recorder can be used.

Helping the Family Cope. Helping the family cope with irrevokable changes in their life-style is accomplished by talking about the stroke/head injury, acknowledging the changes that have occurred, focusing on the patient's abilities, and informing them of support systems. The attitude of the family is an important factor in helping the patient adjust to this deficit. Family members are encouraged to act naturally and treat the patient in the same manner as before his illness. They should be aware that the patient's ability to speak may vary from day to day and that fatigue will have an adverse effect on speech. They should also be aware that the patient may strike out verbally when his emotional controls are lowered. The patient is likely to become very frustrated. Tears and laughter may flow without apparent cause, and frequent mood shifts are encountered.

Support groups such as Stroke Clubs and group therapy for aphasic patients can help in the socialization and motivation of the patient as well as aid in the relief of anxiety and tension. The strain of the constant adjustment to the patient's illness, demands, and needs, as well as the financial drain and the change in life-style, can produce explosive pressures on the family. Members of the family actually go through a period of mourning. In addition to the family learning as much as possible about the support of the patient with aphasia, they should also be counseled to continue a life of their own and to seek the aid of a social worker, clergyman, or psychologist if they need additional help in dealing with their frustrations and pressures. (See bibliography at end of chapter for resources for patients with aphasia.)

▷ *Evaluation*

▷ *Expected Outcomes*

1. Patient demonstrates improvement in self-concept.
   a. Participates in decision making.
   b. Returns to a few former activities.
   c. Attends support group.
2. Communicates with others according to his ability/disability.
   a. Practices relaxation techniques.
   b. Attempts to read aloud; repeats words.
3. Family members improve coping abilities.
   a. Include patient in activities and social affairs.
   b. Demonstrate an encouraging attitude toward patient.
   c. Modify their expectations of patient.
   d. Continue to pursue their own interests.

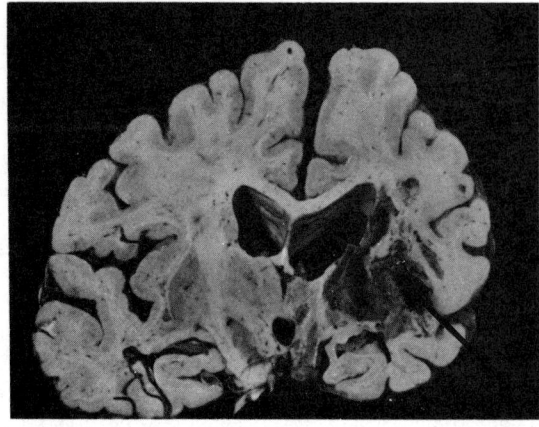

Figure 53-3
Impairment of cerebral circulation leading to a stroke. The arrow points to the area of cerebral infarction. (Armed Forces Institute of Pathology: Neg. No. 55-13956.)

Neurologic Deficits Due to Cerebrovascular Disease

Cerebrovascular disease refers to any functional abnormality of the CNS caused by interference with the normal blood supply to the brain. The pathology may involve an artery, a vein, or both, when the cerebral circulation becomes impaired as a result of partial or complete occlusion of a blood vessel or hemorrhage resulting from a tear in the vessel wall. The blood vessel most frequently associated with cerebrovascular disease is the internal carotid artery.

Vascular disease of the CNS may be caused by arteriosclerosis (most common), hypertensive changes, arteriovenous malformations, vasospasm, inflammation, arteritis, or embolism. As a result of vascular disease, blood vessels lose their elasticity, become hardened, and develop atheromatous deposits, or plaques, which may be the source of an embolus. The lumen of the vessel may gradually close, causing impairment of cerebral circulation and ischemia of the brain. If cerebral ischemia is transient, there is usually no lasting neurologic deficit. However, occlusion of a large vessel produces cerebral infarction (Fig. 53-3). The vessel may rupture and produce hemorrhage.

Stroke (Cerebrovascular Accident)

A stroke is a sudden loss of brain function resulting from a disruption of the blood supply to a part of the brain. Frequently, it is the culmination of cerebrovascular disease of many years standing.

Stroke is the primary neurologic problem in the United States and in the world. Although preventive efforts have brought about a steady decline in the incidence in the past decade, stroke is the third ranking cause of death, striking over 510,000 people annually in this country with an overall mortality rate of 18% to 37% for the first stroke and as high as 62% for subsequent strokes. At least two thirds of those surviving have some degree of permanent disability.

Causes of Stroke

A stroke is usually brought on by one of four events: (1) thrombosis (a blood clot within a blood vessel of the brain or neck), (2) cerebral embolism (a blood clot or other material carried to the brain from another part of the body), (3) ischemia (decrease of blood flow to an area of the brain), and (4) cerebral hemorrhage (rupture of a cerebral blood vessel with bleeding into the brain tissue or spaces surrounding the brain). The result is an interruption in the blood supply to the brain, causing temporary or permanent loss of movement, thought, memory, speech, or sensation.

Cerebral Thrombosis. Cerebral arteriosclerosis and slowing of the cerebral circulation are major causes of cerebral thrombosis, which is the most common cause of stroke.

Headache is rather uncommon at the onset of cerebral thrombosis. Some patients may experience dizziness, mental disturbances, or convulsions, and some may have an onset indistinguishable from that of intracerebral hemorrhage or cerebral embolism. In general, cerebral thrombosis does not develop abruptly, and a transient loss of speech, hemiplegia, or paresthesias in one half of the body may precede the onset of a severe paralysis by a few hours or days.

Cerebral Embolism. Pathologic abnormalities of the left side of the heart, such as infective endocarditis, rheumatic heart disease, and myocardial infarction, as well as pulmonary infections, are the sites where emboli originate. It is possible that the insertion of a prosthetic heart valve may precipitate a stroke since there seems to be an increased incidence of embolism following this procedure. The incidence of stroke following this procedure can probably be reduced with postoperative anticoagulant therapy. Pacemaker failure, atrial fibrillation, and cardioversion for atrial fibrillation are other possible causes of cerebral emboli and stroke.

The embolus usually lodges in the middle cerebral artery or its branches, where it disrupts the cerebral circulation.

- Sudden onset of hemiparesis or hemiplegia with or without aphasia or loss of consciousness in a patient with cardiac or pulmonary disease is characteristic of cerebral embolism.

Cerebral Ischemia.   Cerebral ischemia (insufficiency of the blood supply to the brain) is due mainly to atheromatous constriction of the arteries supplying the brain. The most common manifestation is transient ischemic attacks (see p. 1448).

Cerebral Hemorrhage.   In the Framingham Study on Heart Disease and Stroke, which covered 24 years of study, hemorrhage was found to be the mechanism of stroke in 15% of the patients. Hemorrhage may occur outside the dura mater (extradural hemorrhage), beneath the dura mater (subdural hemorrhage), in the subarachnoid space (subarachnoid hemorrhage), or within the brain substance (intracerebral hemorrhage).

Extradural Hemorrhage.   Extradural hemorrhage (epidural hemorrhage) is a neurosurgical emergency that requires urgent care. It usually follows skull fracture with a tear of the middle artery or other meningeal artery. If the patient is not treated within hours following the accident, he has very little chance of survival. (This is discussed in the section on head injury on p. 1497.)

Subdural Hemorrhage.   Subdural hemorrhage (excluding the acute subdural) is basically the same as an epidural hemorrhage, except that in subdural hematoma usually a bridging vein is torn. Thus, a longer period of time (longer lucid interval) is required for the hematoma to form and cause pressure on the brain. (This is discussed in the section on head injury on p. 1498.)

Subarachnoid Hemorrhage.   Subarachnoid hemorrhage (hemorrhage occurring in the subarachnoid space) may occur as a result of trauma or hypertension, but the most common cause is a leaking aneurysm in the area of the circle of Willis and congenital arteriovenous malformations of the brain. Any artery within the brain can be the site of an aneurysm. (The treatment of intracranial aneurysms is discussed on p. 1472.)

Intracerebral Hemorrhage.   Hemorrhage or bleeding into the brain substance is most common in patients with hypertension and cerebral atherosclerosis, since degenerative changes due to these diseases usually cause rupture of the vessel. The bleeding is usually arterial and occurs particularly around the basal ganglia. Intracerebral hemorrhage may also be due to certain types of arterial pathology, presence of brain tumor, and the use of medications (oral anticoagulants, amphetamines, and a variety of addictive drugs). The clinical picture and the prognosis depend mainly on the degree of hemorrhage and brain damage. Occasionally, the bleeding ruptures the wall of the lateral ventricle and causes intraventricular hemorrhage, which is frequently fatal.

Usually, the onset is abrupt, with severe headache. As the hematoma enlarges, a more pronounced neurologic deficit occurs in the form of decreased alertness and abnormalities in the vital signs. If the bleeding is limited or develops gradually, there may be no significant pressure effects. On the other hand, the full deficit may evolve in a matter of hours. A marked reduction in consciousness (stupor/coma) in the early phase of the bleeding episode usually has an ominous prognosis.

The treatment of intracerebral hemorrhage is controversial. If the hemorrhage is small, the patient is treated conservatively and symptomatically.

- The blood pressure is carefully lowered with antihypertensive drugs. The patient's neurologic deficit may worsen if the blood pressure is dropped too low or lowered too rapidly. The most effective form of treatment is the prevention of hypertensive vascular disease.

Risk Factors and Prevention of Stroke

Prevention of stroke is the best possible approach. Steps are taken to alter those factors and human conditions that predispose certain people to stroke or increase their risk of having a stroke.

- Control of hypertension, the major risk factor, is the key to prevention of stroke.
- Patients with cardiovascular disease (rheumatic heart disease, rhythm abnormalities [particularly atrial fibrillation], congestive heart failure, left ventricular hypertrophy) are at increased risk since cerebral embolism may originate in the heart.
- A high normal hematocrit level is related to an increased incidence of cerebral infarction.
- Diabetes is associated with accelerated atherogenesis.
- There appears to be an increased risk of stroke among women taking oral contraceptives, which is enhanced by coexisting hypertension, age over 35 years, cigarette smoking, and high estrogen levels.
- An excessive or prolonged fall of blood pressure following shock, hemorrhage, surgery, diagnostic procedures, and ingestion of certain drugs may cause general cerebral ischemia. In these instances, the patient requires careful monitoring.
- Drug abuse is a cause of stroke, particularly in adolescents and young adults.
- In younger persons, attention should be directed at controlling blood lipids (particularly cholesterol), blood pressure, cigarette smoking, and obesity.
- There appears to be a link between alcohol consumption and stroke.

Clinical Manifestations

A stroke causes a wide variety of neurologic deficits depending on the location of the lesion (which vessels are obstructed), the size of the area of inadequate perfusion, and the amount of collateral (secondary or accessory) blood flow. The damaged brain cannot be fully restored.

Motor Loss.   Stroke is a disease of the upper motor neurons and results in loss of voluntary control over motor movements. Since the upper motor neurons decussate (cross), a disturbance of voluntary motor control on one side of the body may reflect damage to the upper motor neurons on the opposite side of the brain. The most common motor dysfunction is hemiplegia (paralysis of one side of the body) due to a lesion of the opposite side of the brain. Hemiparesis, or weakness of one side of the body, is another sign.

In the early stage of stroke, the initial clinical feature may be flaccid paralysis and loss or decrease in the deep tendon reflexes. When these deep reflexes reappear (usually by 48 hours), increased tone is observed along with spasticity (abnormal increase in muscle tone) of the extremities on the affected side.

Communication Loss.   Other brain functions affected by stroke are language and communication. Dysfunction in these areas may be manifested by

- *Dysarthria* (difficulty in speaking), as demonstrated by poorly intelligible speech caused by paralysis of the muscles responsible for producing speech
- *Dysphasia* or *aphasia* (defective speech or loss of speech), which is mainly expressive or receptive
- *Apraxia* (inability to perform a previously learned action), as may be seen when a patient picks up a fork and attempts to comb his hair with it

(The nursing management of aphasia is discussed on p. 1431.)

Perceptual Disturbances.   Perception is the ability to interpret sensation. Visual perceptual dysfunctions are due to disturbances of the primary sensory pathways between the eye and visual cortex. *Homonymous hemianopia* (loss of half of the visual field) may occur from stroke and may be temporary or permanent. The affected side of vision corresponds to the paralyzed side of the body. The patient's head turns away from the affected side of his body, and he tends to neglect that side and the space on that side. In such instances the patient will not be able to see food on half of the tray; only half of the room will be visible.

To assess for hemianopia, the nurse requests the patient to look at her face. The nurse's examining finger is placed about 30 cm (12 inches) from the patient's ear on the unaffected side and is moved inward toward his field of vision. Inability to detect movement on one or both sides suggests visual neglect and hemianopia. This decreased field of vision must be kept in mind during all rehabilitation procedures. Personnel should approach the patient on the side where visual perception is intact. All visual stimuli (clock, calendar, television) should be placed on this side. The patient can be taught to turn his head in the direction of the defective visual field in order to compensate for this loss. The nurse should make eye contact with the patient and draw his attention to his affected side by encouraging him to move his head. Increasing the natural or artificial lighting in the room and providing his eyeglasses are important in increasing vision.

Disturbances in visual-spatial relationships (perceiving relationship of two or more objects in spatial areas) are frequently seen in patients with left hemiplegia. The patient may not be able to dress himself due to his inability to match his clothing to his body parts. To assist this patient, the nurse can take steps to keep his environment organized and uncluttered since the patient with a perceptual problem is easily distracted. He is told to "slow down" and gently reminded where an object is located.

Sensory losses from stroke may take the form of slight impairment of touch or be more severe with loss of proprioception (inability to perceive position and motion of body parts) as well as difficulty in interpreting visual, tactile, and auditory stimuli.

Impairment of Mental Activity and Psychological Effects.   If damage has occurred to the frontal lobe, then learning capacity, memory, or other higher cortical intellectual functions may be impaired. Such dysfunction may be reflected in a limited attention span, difficulties in comprehension, forgetfulness, and a lack of motivation, which cause these patients to encounter frustrating problems in their rehabilitation programs. Depression is a natural response to such a catastrophic illness. Other psychological problems are myriad and are manifested by emotional lability, hostility, frustration, resentment, and noncooperation.

Bladder Dysfunction.   Following a stroke the patient may have transient urinary incontinence due to confusion, inability to communicate his needs, and inability to use the urinal/bedpan because of impaired motor and postural controls. Occasionally, following a stroke the bladder becomes atonic with impaired sensation in response to bladder filling. Sometimes control of the external urinary sphincter is lost or diminished. During this period, intermittent catherization with sterile technique is carried out. When muscle tone increases and deep tendon reflexes return, bladder tone increases and spasticity of the bladder may develop. Because the patient's sense of awareness is clouded, persistent urinary incontinence or urinary retention may be symptomatic of bilateral brain damage. Continuing bladder and bowel incontinence may reflect extensive neurologic damage.

Management of the Acute Phase of a Patient With Stroke

A patient who is in deep coma on admission to the hospital is considered to have a poor prognosis. Conversely, a fully conscious patient faces a more favorable outcome. The acute phase usually lasts 48 to 72 hours. The principles underlying the management of the unconscious patient are summarized on page 1426. Maintaining the airway and adequate ventilation are priorities in the acute phase.

Medical treatment for the patient with acute stroke may include antiedema agents (dehydrating agents) to reduce cerebral edema, which reaches maximum levels 3 to 5 days after cerebral infarction. Anticoagulants may be given to prevent further development or propagation of the thrombosis or embolization from elsewhere in the cardiovascular system. Antiplatelet drugs may be given since platelets play a major role in thrombus formation and embolization.

Treatment is also aimed at improving cerebral blood flow and metabolism.

- A patent airway and circulation to the brain are maintained.
- Adequate oxygenation of blood to the brain is necessary to minimize cerebral damage. Brain function is absolutely dependent on available oxygen being delivered to the neuronal tissues. The blood pressure and cardiac output must be maintained to sustain cerebral blood flow, and hydration (intravenous fluids) must be ensured to reduce blood viscosity and improve cerebral blood flow. Oxygen therapy, if necessary, should be given at an adequate perfusion pressure.
- The patient is placed in a lateral or semiprone position with the head of the bed slightly elevated to lower cerebral venous pressure.
- Endotracheal intubation and mechanical ventilation are necessary for patients with massive stroke since respiratory arrest is usually the life-threatening factor in this situation.
- The patient is monitored for pulmonary complications (aspiration, atelectasis, pneumonia), which may be due to loss of airway reflexes, immobility, or hypoventilation.
- The heart is examined for abnormalities in size, rhythm, and signs of congestive failure.

  A dysrhythmia may have caused a cerebral embolus and must be corrected.

Cerebral embolism may occur following myocardial infarction or atrial fibrillation or may originate from a prosthetic heart valve.

The blood pressure is not allowed to drop precipitously since brain ischemia or myocardial ischemia may result.

► Nursing Process
The Patient With a Stroke

▷ Assessment

A neurologic flow sheet is maintained to reflect the following nursing assessment parameters:

1. A change in the level of responsiveness as evidenced by movement, resistance to changes of position, and response to stimulation; orientation to time, place, and person
2. Presence or absence of voluntary or involuntary movements of the extremities; the tone of the muscles; the body posture and the position of the head
3. Stiffness or flaccidity of the neck
4. Eye opening, the comparative size of the pupils and pupillary reactions to light, and ocular position
5. The color of the face and the extremities; the temperature and the moisture of the skin
6. The quality and the rates of pulse and respiration; the body temperature and the arterial pressure
7. The ability to speak
8. The volume of fluids ingested or administered and the volume of urine excreted each 24 hours

When the patient begins to regain consciousness, signs of extreme fatigue and confusion will be apparent as a result of the cerebral edema that follows a stroke. To offset any anxiety, efforts should be made at frequent intervals to orient the patient to time and place and to reassure him that he has not lost his mind.

If the lesion occurs in the dominant hemisphere the patient will most likely also have aphasia. A nondominant hemispheric lesion may result in apraxia (inability to perform previously learned movements).

After the acute phase the nurse assesses the following functions: mental status (memory, attention span, perception, orientation; affect, speech/language), sensation/perception (usually patient has decreased awareness of pain and temperature); motor control (upper and lower extremity movement); bladder function.

Nursing assessment continues to focus on the impairment of function in the patient's daily activities since the quality of life after stroke is closely related to the patient's functional status.

▷ Nursing Diagnoses

Based on the assessment data, the patient's major nursing diagnoses may include the following:

- Impaired physical mobility related to hemiparesis, loss of balance and coordination, spasticity, and brain injury
- Alteration in comfort (painful shoulder) related to hemiplegia and disuse
- Self-care deficits (hygiene, toileting, transfers, feeding) related to stroke sequelae
- Alteration in urinary elimination (incontinence) related

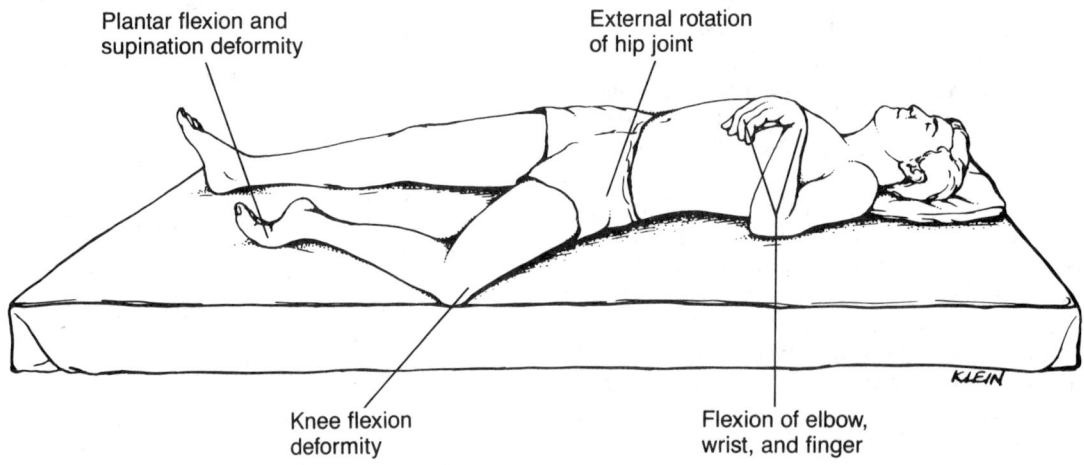

Plantar flexion and supination deformity

External rotation of hip joint

Knee flexion deformity

Flexion of elbow, wrist, and finger

Figure 53-4
Hemiplegic deformities. The involved leg immediately falls into external rotation. The knee almost invariably flexes. As soon as knee flexion occurs, abduction of the upper leg follows. The foot falls into plantar flexion, so that there is always a footdrop and a shortening of the Achilles tendon. This position of the leg is assumed whether the leg is flaccid or spastic. The arm of the affected side is held against the body. Often, a flail arm is placed across the body for convenience in handling the patient, but if spastic, the elbow flexes to about 90 degrees. With the arm across the body, the wrist is dropped. If the arm is spastic, the fingers curl into a fist, with the thumb adducted and flexed under the fingers. (After Covalt NK. Preventive technics of rehabilitation for hemiplegic patients. GP 17:131.)

Figure 53-5
Positioning for a patient following a stroke. (Dark side of pajamas represents affected or hemiplegic side.)

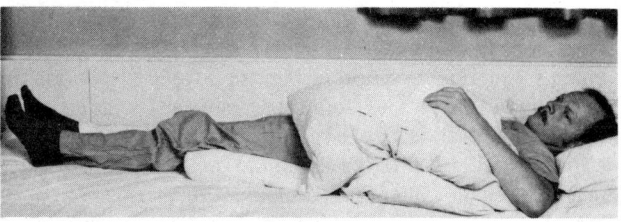

1. A pillow is placed in the axilla to prevent adduction of the affected shoulder. Pillows are placed under the arm, which is in a slightly flexed position with each joint positioned higher than the preceding one.

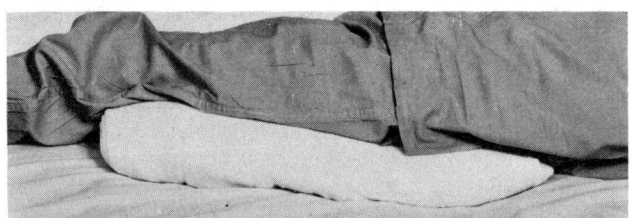

2. The trochanter roll should extend from the crest of the ilium to the midthigh, since the hip joint lies between these two points. The trochanter roll acts as a mechanical wedge under the projection of the greater trochanter and prevents the femur from rolling.

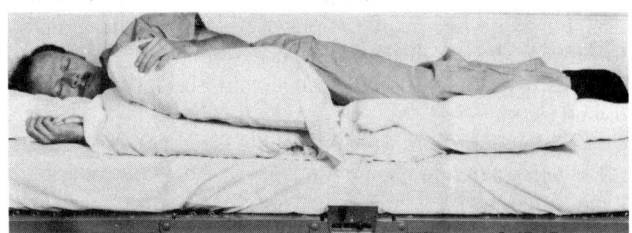

3. Lateral or side-lying position. The patient should be turned on his unaffected side. The upper thigh should not be acutely flexed.

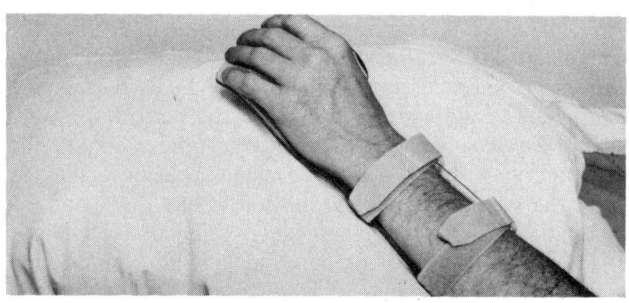

4. A volar resting splint may be used to support the wrist and hand if the upper extremity is flaccid.

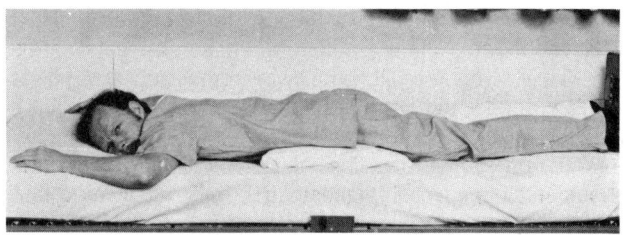

5. Prone position. A pillow is placed under the pelvis to help promote hyperextension of the hip joints, which is essential for normal gait. Note position of arms.

to flaccid bladder, detrusor instability, confusion, difficulty in communicating
· Alteration in thought processes related to brain damage, confusion, inability to follow instruction
· Impaired verbal communication related to brain damage
· Alteration in family processes related to catastrophic illness and caregiving burdens

▷ *Planning and Implementation (Rehabilitation Phase)*

Although rehabilitation begins on the day the patient has the stroke, the process is intensified during the convalescent phase and requires a coordinated team effort. The team has to know what the patient was like before this catastrophic illness: what he was able to do, his mental and emotional state, behavioral characteristics, and activities of daily living.

▷ *Goals:* The major goals of the patient (and family) may include improvement of mobility, avoidance of shoulder pain,

achievement of self-care, attainment of bladder control, improvement of thought processes, achievement of some form of communication, and restoration of family functioning.

Nursing Interventions
Improving Mobility: Preventing Deformities

A hemiplegic patient has unilateral paralysis. When control of the voluntary muscles is lost, the strong flexor muscles exert control over the extensors. The arm tends to adduct (adductor muscles are stronger than abductors) and to rotate internally. The elbow and the wrist tend to flex, the affected leg tends to rotate externally at the hip joint and flex at the knee, while the foot at the ankle joint supinates and tends toward plantar flexion (Fig. 53-4).

Positioning. Correct positioning in bed is of prime importance (Fig. 53-5) in order to prevent contractures, relieve pressure, assist in maintaining good body alignment, and prevent compressive neuropathies, especially of the ulnar and peroneal nerves. A bed board under the mattress provides firm support for the body. The patient should remain flat in bed except when engaged in activities of daily living. Maintaining the upright position in bed for extended periods of time is one of the greatest contributors to hip flexion deformity. A footboard may be used at intervals during the flaccid period following a stroke to keep the feet at right angles to the legs when the patient is in a supine (dorsal) position. This prevents footdrop and the heel cords from shortening as a result of contracture of the gastrocnemius muscles. As soon as spasticity develops, a footboard is generally not used because it may worsen spasticity and a plantar flexion deformity. If the affected extremity is spastic, a bed cradle is used to keep the bedding off the extremity.

Because flexor muscles are stronger than extensor muscles, it may be necessary to apply a posterior splint at night to prevent flexion of the affected extremity. The posterior splint is used only at night to maintain correct positioning during sleep.

To prevent external rotation at the hip joint, a trochanter roll is used, extending from the crest of the ilium to the mid thigh, since the hip joint lies between these two points (Fig. 53-5B). A sandbag applied at the side of the leg will not prevent external rotation inasmuch as this motion originates in the ball and socket joint of the hip. The knee has no such rotating function. The trochanter roll acts as a mechanical wedge under the projection of the greater trochanter and prevents the femur from rolling.

To prevent adduction of the affected shoulder, a pillow is placed in the axilla when there is limited external rotation (Fig. 53-5A). This keeps the arm away from the chest. A pillow is placed under the arm, and the arm is placed in a neutral (slightly flexed) position, with each joint positioned higher than the preceding one. Thus, the elbow is higher than the shoulder and the wrist is higher than the elbow. The elevation of the arm helps to prevent edema and the resultant fibrosis that will prevent normal range of motion if the patient regains control of the arm.

The fingers are positioned so that they are barely flexed. The hand is placed in slight supination (palm faces upward), which is its most functional (*i.e.,* useful) position. If the upper extremity is flaccid, a volar resting splint can be used to support the wrist and hand in a functional position. If the upper extremity is spastic, a hand roll is *not* desirable because it stimulates the grasp reflex. In this instance a dorsal wrist splint is useful in allowing the palm to be free of pressure. Every effort is made to prevent hand edema.

Changing Positions. The patient's position should be changed every 2 hours. To place a patient in a lateral (side-lying) position, a pillow is placed between the legs before the patient is turned. The upper thigh should not be acutely flexed. The patient may be turned from side to side, but the amount of time spent on the affected side should be limited because of impaired sensation. However, lying on the affected side is thought to increase the patient's awareness of the side and allows use of the unaffected hand.

If possible, it is desirable to place the patient in a prone position for 15 to 30 minutes several times a day. A small pillow or a support is placed under the pelvis, extending from the level of the umbilicus to the upper third of the thigh (Fig. 53-5E). This helps to promote hyperextension of the hip joints, which is essential for normal gait and helps prevent knee and hip flexion contractures. The prone position also helps to drain bronchial secretions and prevents contractural deformities of the shoulders and knees.

Retraining the Affected Extremities

Exercise. The affected extremities are exercised passively and put through a full range of motion four to five times a day to maintain joint mobility, to regain motor control, to prevent development of a contracture in the paralyzed extremity, to prevent further deterioration of the neuromuscular system, and to enhance circulation. Exercise is helpful in the prevention of venous stasis, which may predispose to thrombosis and pulmonary embolus.

Repetition of an activity forms new pathways in the CNS and therefore encourages new patterns of motion. At first, the extremities are usually flaccid. If tightness occurs in any area, the range of motion exercises should be done more frequently. (See p. 218 for techniques of range of motion exercises.) Signs to watch for include shortness of breath, chest pain, cyanosis, and increasing pulse rate during the exercise period.

Frequent short periods of exercise always are preferred to longer periods at infrequent intervals. *Regularity* in exercise is most important. Improvement in muscle strength and maintenance of range of motion can be achieved only through daily exercise.

The patient is encouraged and reminded to exercise the unaffected side at intervals throughout the day. It is well to work out a written time schedule that can be used to remind the patient of the exercise activities. The nurse has the responsibility of supervising and supporting the patient during these activities. The patient can be taught to put the unaffected leg under the affected one to move it when turning and exercising. Flexibility, strengthening, coordination, endurance, and balancing exercises prepare the patient for ambulation and give the patient a goal. Quadriceps muscle setting and gluteal setting exercises are started early to improve the muscle strength needed for walking. These are done at least five times daily for 10 minutes at a time.

Quadriceps Setting. The patient is instructed to contract the quadriceps muscle (on the anterior portion of the thigh) while raising the heel and pushing the popliteal space against the mattress. The muscle contraction is held until the count of 5, then relaxed until the count of 5. Repeat. This exercise is performed by each extremity.

Gluteal Setting. Gluteal setting is done in the following manner: contract or "pinch" the buttocks together until the count of 5; relax until the count of 5; repeat.

Biofeedback. Electromyographic biofeedback is being used in neuromuscular re-education for improving muscle strength and reducing spasticity.

Preparing for Ambulation

As soon as possible, the patient is assisted out of bed. Usually, when hemiplegia has resulted from a thrombosis, an active rehabilitation program is started as soon as the patient regains consciousness, whereas a patient who has had a cerebral hemorrhage cannot participate actively until all evidence of bleeding is gone.

Sitting Balance. A hemiplegic patient tends to lose his sense of balance and needs to learn to maintain balance in a sitting position before learning to balance himself in the standing position.

- Before the patient attempts to rise from a recumbent position, blood pressure should be checked since orthostatic hypotension may occur. A fall in blood pressure may further damage the ischemic area.
- To develop sitting balance, the head of the bed is raised to an upright position and the patient is instructed to hold the bedrail with his good hand.

The patient is then helped to come to a sitting position on the edge of the bed. This may be achieved in the following manner:

1. Adjust the bed to the low position.
2. Instruct the patient to place the strong leg beneath the weak leg and lift it toward the side of the bed.
3. Instruct the patient to press the strong elbow that is flexed to a 90-degree angle into the mattress and come to a sitting position by transferring weight to the forearm and then to the hand, while lifting the uninvolved leg with the strong leg over the edge of the bed. The force of gravity, set in motion by pushing against the hand and moving the legs, is sufficient to pivot the patient's torso on the buttocks.
4. Extend the patient's strong arm with his hand flat on the bed behind him to assist in balancing.
5. Stand in front of the patient to observe and, if necessary, help him to maintain this posture.

- A change in color, shortness of breath, increasing pulse rate, or profuse perspiration is an indication that the patient should be placed in bed again. The sitting time is increased as rapidly as the patient's condition permits.

Standing Balance. As soon as the patient is able to balance while sitting, he is taught standing balance. He should wear walking shoes with a strong shank for all ambulation activities. A tape on the shoe or colored shoelaces will help identify the affected foot and leg if the patient is having perceptual problems.

- Seat the patient on the edge of the bed, and place a straightback chair on each side of him (Fig. 53-6). If the patient lacks strength to grasp and to push the chair with his affected hand, the hand can be comfortably tied to the top of the chair. This stabilization gives the patient greater support.
- Help the patient to come to a standing position by supporting his lower back with your hands and positioning your knees on the outside of the patient's knees. This will give the patient maximum support in the standing position and will prevent his knees from buckling. The patient should be reminded to lean forward when he comes from a sitting to a standing position. The patient's arms must be left free for balance and support.
- Stand behind the patient and stabilize him at his waist.

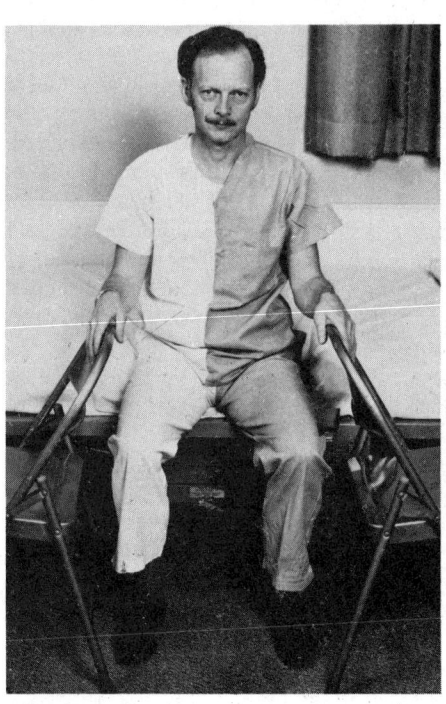 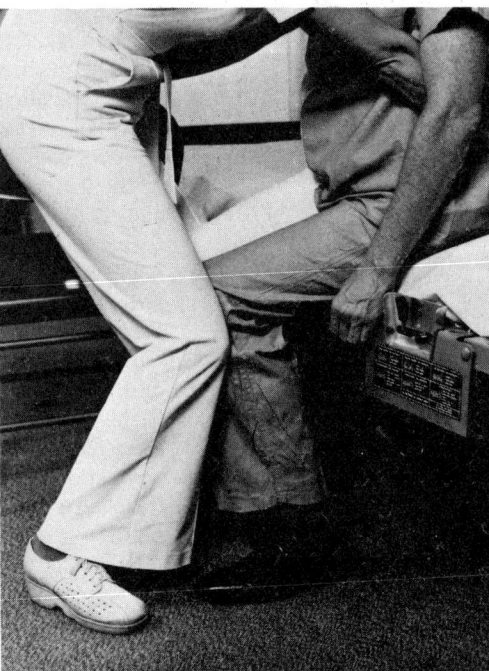 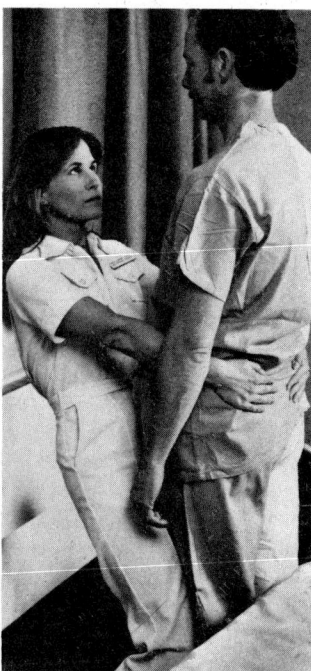

Figure 53-6
Getting the patient out of bed following a stroke. (*Left*) Place the bed in the low position so that the patient's feet are resting on the floor. Observe the patient's reaction and increase the sitting time as rapidly as the patient's condition permits. (*Center*) Getting ready to rise to a standing position. Positioning the nurse's knees on the outside of the patient's knees will prevent the patient's knees from buckling. (*Right*) Stabilizing the patient as he assumes a standing position. Note that the nurse is (1) stabilizing the patient's lower back and knees and (2) assessing his reaction to standing. (Courtesy of Washington Adventist Hospital; Glenn Dalby, photographer.)

Place a waistband or a belt (a scultetus binder can serve as a waistband) around the patient's waist and grasp it for patient support.

- Dizziness, pallor, and an increasing pulse rate indicate that the patient should be permitted to rest in a sitting position. If the symptoms continue, the patient should be put back in bed. With repeated effort, the patient will tolerate this activity for longer periods.
- Have the patient practice standing and shifting weight from one leg to another.
- After the patient learns to sit and stand, a portable commode is used instead of the bedpan.

If the patient has difficulty in achieving standing balance, a tilt table will help him assume an upright position. This will help the patient in weight-bearing, provide a sense of being upright, and increase endurance in the upright position. There should be frequent periods of standing before walking is started.

Walking.   The patient is usually ready to walk as soon as standing balance is achieved. Parallel bars are useful when the patient first starts to walk. A chair or wheelchair should be readily available in the event of sudden fatigue or vertigo. The following method is one way to ambulate the patient:

1. Instruct the patient to stand between the parallel bars or beside one rail with his weight evenly distributed on both feet and his strong arm on the rail about 10 cm (4 inches) in front of his body.
2. Have the patient shift the weight to the strong leg and advance the involved leg while pushing *down* on the rail.
3. The patient then shifts the weight to the weak leg. (If the patient has poor muscle tone and cannot advance his involved leg, functional electrical stimulation may be used. Stimulating muscles electrically may increase strength, reverse atrophy, and enhance voluntary control.)
4. Encourage the patient to look at his feet occasionally since proprioceptive loss may accompany hemiplegia.

The training periods for ambulation should be short and frequent. As the patient gains in strength and confidence, he can begin to walk with an adjustable aluminum cane. Generally a three- or four-prong cane provides a more stable support in the early phases of this training program.

Orthotic devices (braces) may be necessary to give adequate joint support and stability. An ankle–foot orthosis of lightweight thermoplastic material will provide ankle and knee stability. If the patient's knee tends to buckle, a small rubber cushion placed in the heel of the shoes will decrease the impact of the heel striking the floor as the patient walks. A small lift on the opposite shoe is helpful if the patient drags the affected leg. After a period of time has elapsed the patient is evaluated to determine if he needs to be fitted with a short or a long leg brace.

Wheelchair.   If the patient needs a wheelchair, the folding type with hand brakes is the most practical since it allows the patient to manipulate the chair. The chair should be low enough so that the patient can propel it with the uninvolved foot and narrow enough to permit it to be used in the home. To propel the wheelchair, the patient places the strong hand on the hand rim and the stronger foot on the floor to guide and direct the chair.

When the patient is transferred from the wheelchair, the brakes are applied on both sides of the chair. The technique a patient uses for transferring from a wheelchair placed on his unaffected side is as follows:

- Lift the foot pedals out of the way and move forward in the chair, placing weight on the strong leg.
- Push up with the strong arm and foot.
- Place most of the weight on the strong leg while keeping the weak knee locked.
- Pivot in the direction of the stronger leg; bring weak leg over to stronger leg. Maintain standing position for a few minutes.
- Lower body into wheelchair gradually, using strong arm and leg.

Wheelchair mobility provides greater independence in self-care activities. When a permanent wheelchair is needed, it is ordered with specific instructions for the individual patient.

Preventing Shoulder Pain

Up to 70% of stroke patients suffer from severe pain in the shoulder that prevents them from learning new skills, since shoulder function is essential in achieving balance and performing transfers and self-care activities. Three problems can occur: painful shoulder, subluxation of the shoulder, and shoulder–hand syndrome.

A flaccid shoulder joint may be overstretched by the use of excessive force in turning the patient or from overstrenuous arm and shoulder movement. To prevent *shoulder pain*, the nurse should never lift the patient by the flaccid shoulder or pull on the affected arm or shoulder. If the arm is paralyzed, *subluxation* (incomplete dislocation) at the shoulder can occur from overstretching of the joint capsule and musculature by the force of gravity when the patient sits or stands in the early stages following a stroke. This results in severe pain. *Shoulder–hand syndrome* (painful shoulder and generalized swelling of the hand) can cause a frozen shoulder and ultimate atrophy of subcutaneous tissues. When a shoulder becomes stiff it is usually more painful.

These problems can be prevented by proper patient movement and positioning. The flaccid arm is positioned on a table or pillows while the patient is seated. Some authorities advocate a properly worn sling when the patient first becomes ambulatory to prevent the paralyzed upper extremity from dangling without support. Range of motion exercises are important in preventing painful shoulder. Overstrenuous arm movements are avoided. The patient is instructed to interlace his fingers, place his palms together, and push his clasped hands slowly forward to bring the scapulae forward. He then raises his hands above his head. This is repeated throughout the day. The patient is instructed to flex the affected wrist at intervals and move all the joints of the affected fingers. He is encouraged to touch, stroke, rub, and look at his hands. Pushing the heel of the hand firmly down on a surface is useful. Elevation of the arm and hand is also important in preventing dependent edema of the hand.

Achieving Self-Care

As soon as the patient is able to sit up, he is encouraged to assist in his personal hygiene. He is helped to set realistic goals and, if feasible, a new task is added daily. The first step is to have the patient carry out all self-care activities on the unaffected side. Such activities as combing the hair, brushing the teeth, shaving with an electric razor, bathing, and eating can be carried out with one hand and are suitable for self-care. Although the patient may feel awkward at first, the various motor skills can be learned by repetition and the unaffected side will become stronger with use. The nurse must be sure that he does not neglect his affected side. Assistive devices will help make up for some of the patient's deficits. A small towel is easier to control while drying after bathing, and boxed paper tissues are easier to use than a roll of toilet tissue.

Dressing Activities. The patient's morale will improve if ambulatory activities are carried out while he is fully dressed. The family is instructed to bring in clothing that is preferably a size larger than that normally worn. Clothing fitted with front or side fasteners or Velcro closures is the most suitable. The patient has better balance if most of the dressing activities are done in a seated position.

The clothing is placed on his affected side in the order in which the garments are to be put on. Using a large mirror while dressing will help make the patient aware of what he is putting on his affected side. Each garment is put on the affected side first. The patient has to make many compensatory movements when dressing that can produce fatigue and painful twisting of the intercostal muscles. He will require support and encouragement to prevent overfatigue and discouragement. Even with intensive training, not all patients are able to achieve independence in dressing skills.

Attaining Bladder Control. Most stroke patients have bladder problems in the early stage, but bladder control is usually quickly regained. The patient's voiding pattern is analyzed and the urinal/bedpan offered on this pattern or schedule. The upright posture and standing position is helpful for male patients during this aspect of rehabilitation. (See also p. 238 for a bladder retraining program.)

Improvement of Thought Processes. Following a stroke the patient may have problems with cognitive, behavioral, and emotional deficits related to brain damage. However, in many instances there can be considerable recovery of functioning because not all areas are equally damaged; some remain more intact and functional than others.

After assessment procedures that delineate and describe the patient's problems, the neuropsychologist, interacting when possible with the psychologist, psychiatrist, nurse, and other professionals, structures a training program using cognitive-perceptual retraining, visual imagery, reality orientation, and cueing procedures to compensate for losses.

The role of the nurse is supportive. The nurse reviews the results of neuropsychologic testing, observes the patient's performance and progress, gives positive feedback, and, most important, conveys an attitude of confidence and hopefulness. Interventions capitalize on the patient's strengths and what he can still do, while attempting to improve performance of affected functions. Other interventions are similar to those for improvement of cognitive functioning following a head injury (see p. 1503).

Achieving Communication. Dysphasia impairs the patient's ability to communicate both in understanding what is being said and in the ability to express himself. The speech–language pathologist assesses the communication needs of the stroke patient, describes the precise deficit, and suggests the best overall method of communication for the patient.

There are many language intervention strategies for the adult aphasic person, and the program is individually tailored. Goals are established with the patient, and he is expected to take an active part.

Nursing interventions include doing everything possible to make the atmosphere conducive to communication. This includes being sensitive to the patient's reactions and needs and reacting to them in an appropriate manner, always keeping in mind that the patient is treated as an adult. The nurse lends strong moral support and understanding to allay anxiety. A consistent schedule, routines, and repetitions help the patient to function in spite of significant deficits. He may be given a written copy of his schedule, a folder of personal information (birth date, address, names of relatives), checklists, and an audiotaped list to help his memory and concentration. Reviewing an album of snapshots with him can be stimulating. Surrounding the patient with familiar objects and caring people is reassuring.

When talking with the patient, the nurse must make sure she has his attention, must speak slowly, and must keep the language of instruction consistent. One instruction is given at a time, and time is allowed for the patient to process what has been said. The use of gestures may enhance comprehension. Other nursing strategies for helping the aphasic patient are found on page 1431.

Improving Family Coping Through Health Teaching. Members of the patient's family play an important role in the patient's recovery. Some type of counseling and support system should be available to them to prevent the care of the patient from taking a significant toll on their health and interfering too radically with their life-style. Respite care, which is planned short-term care to ease the burden of the family in providing continuous 24-hour care, may be available from an adult day care center. Some hospitals also offer weekend respite care.

Family coping is also facilitated by involving others in the patient's care, stress management techniques, and maintenance of personal health.

The family may have difficulty in accepting the patient's disability and may be unrealistic in their expectations. They are given advice concerning the expected outcomes of the patient's stroke and are counseled to avoid doing for the patient those things that he can do for himself. They are assured that their loving and warm interest is part of the patient's therapy. The family needs to be informed that the rehabilitation of the hemiplegic patient requires many months and that progress may be slow. The gains made by the patient during hospitalization must be maintained. All should approach the patient with a supportive and optimistic attitude focusing on the abilities that remain.

Most relatives of stroke patients have problems with the emotional aspects of care. The family should be prepared to expect occasional episodes of emotional lability. The patient may laugh or cry easily. He may be irritable and demanding or depressed and confused. The nurse can explain to the family that the patient's laughing does not necessarily mean he is glad nor does crying mean that he is sad and that emotional lability usually improves with time.

Home Health Care. Some of the patient's emotional problems are related to speech dysfunction. A *speech therapist* coming to the home allows the family to be involved and gives them practical instructions to help the patient between speech therapy sessions.

The family is advised that the patient will tire easily, will become irritable and upset by small events, and is apt to show less interest in things. Since a stroke frequently occurs in the later stages of life, there is the possibility of intellectual decline related to dementia.

Asking the patient what he would like to do gives insight into establishing new goals. Depression is a common and serious problem in the post-stroke patient. The nurse can discuss this event with the physician because antidepressant therapy may help if depression dominates the patient's life. As progress is made in the rehabilitation program, some problems will diminish. The family can help by continuing to support the patient and giving honest praise for progress that is made.

The *occupational therapist* makes a home assessment and recommends modifications to help the patient to become more independent. A shower is more convenient than a tub for the hemiplegic patient, since most patients do not gain sufficient strength to get up and down from a tub. Sitting on a stool of medium height with rubber suction tips will permit him to wash with greater ease. A long-handled bath brush with a soap container is helpful to the patient who has only one functional hand. If a shower is not available, a stool may be placed in the tub and a portable shower hose attached to the faucet. Handrails may be attached beside the bathtub and the toilet. There are numerous self-help devices on the market that can assist the patient in the activities of daily living. Community-based "stroke clubs" give the patient a feeling of belonging and fellowship with others who have similar problems. He is encouraged to continue with hobbies, avocational interests, and contact with friends to prevent social isolation.

Sexual Function. Sexual functioning can be profoundly altered by disability. A stroke is such a catastrophic illness that the patient often experiences loss of self-esteem and value as a sexual being. Although research in this area of stroke management is limited, it appears that post-stroke patients believe that sexual function is important but most experience sexual dysfunction following stroke (see Sexuality and the Disabled, p. 239).

All nurses coming in contact with the patient, whether as members of the hospital health care team, community health nurses, or office or occupational health nurses should encourage the patient to *keep active*, faithfully adhere to the exercise program, and confidently continue to remain as self-sufficient as possible.

▷ *Evaluation*

▷ *Expected Outcomes*

1. Patient achieves improved mobility.
   a. Avoids deformities; absence of contractures and footdrop.
   b. Participates in prescribed exercise program.
   c. Achieves sitting balance.
   d. Increases walking time.
   e. Uses unaffected side to compensate for loss of function of hemiplegic side.
2. Has no complaints of shoulder pain.
   a. Demonstrates shoulder mobility.
   b. Elevates arm and hand at invervals.
   c. Exercises shoulder; no evidence of hand edema.

3. Achieves self-care.
   a. Is able to do hygienic care.
   b. Uses adaptive equipment.
4. Attains bladder continence.
5. Participates in cognitive improvement program (see Head Injury, p. 1503).
6. Demonstrates improved communication (see Aphasia Evaluation, p. 1439).
7. Family members demonstrate a positive attitude and coping mechanisms.
   a. Encourage patient in exercise program.
   b. Take an active part in rehabilitation process.
   c. Help patient set new goals.

Transient Ischemic Attacks

A transient ischemic attack (TIA) is a transient or temporary episode of neurologic dysfunction commonly manifested by a sudden loss of motor, sensory, or visual function, lasting a few seconds or minutes but no longer than 24 hours. Complete recovery usually occurs between attacks. A transient ischemic attack may serve as a warning of impending stroke, which has its greatest incidence in the first month after the first attack. The cause of this clinical entity is a temporary impairment of blood flow to a specific region of the brain due to a variety of reasons, including atherosclerosis of the vessels supplying the brain, obstruction of cerebral microcirculation by a small embolus, a fall in cerebral perfusion pressure, cardiac dysrhythmias, and so on.

The most common sites of atherosclerosis in the extracranial arteries are located at the bifurcation of the common carotid and at the origin of the vertebral arteries. Among the intracranial arteries, the middle cerebral artery is the most common location of atherosclerosis.

Clinical Manifestations

The classic symptom of carotid artery disease is *amaurosis fugax* (fleeting blindness) occurring without warning in which there is sudden, painless loss of vision of one eye or dimming or graying out of the field of vision of one eye. This is suggestive of retinal ischemia due to insufficiency of the homolateral ophthalmic or carotid artery. If the ischemia occurs in the vertebral basilar system, vertigo, diplopia, disturbances of consciousness, and various signs of motor and sensory impairment may occur.

Diagnostic Evaluation

A *bruit* (abnormal sound heard on auscultation) may be heard over the carotid artery. There are diminished or absent carotid pulsations in the neck.

Carotid phonoangiography may be done, which provides auscultation, direct visualization, and photographic recording of carotid bruits. *Oculoplethysmography* (OPG) measures pulsation in blood flow through the ophthalmic artery. *Carotid angiography* visualizes intracranial and cervical vessels.

Digital subtraction angiography is being used with increasing success to define carotid artery obstruction and provide information on patterns of cerebral blood flow.

Management

Patients who are not candidates for surgical intervention may be placed on anticoagulant therapy in order to prevent future attacks and a possible massive cerebral infarction. Platelet-inhibiting drugs (particularly aspirin) are useful in decreasing the occurrence of cerebral infarction in patients who have experienced multiple TIAs.

Surgical intervention procedures in common use are endarterectomy (see below) and angioplasty in which a balloon on a catheter is inserted in the artery to break up the plaque and dilate the artery.

Carotid Endarterectomy. A carotid endarterectomy is the removal of an atherosclerotic plaque(s) or thrombus from the carotid artery to prevent stroke in patients with occlusive disease of the extracranial cerebral arteries. (The majority of ischemic strokes are associated with lesions of the extracranial arteries.)

- Following endarterectomy, a neurologic flow sheet is kept to maintain close assessment of the patient's neurologic status. The neurosurgeon is notified immediately if the patient develops a neurologic deficit. Formation of a thrombus at the site of endarterectomy can be suspected if there is a sudden increase in neurologic deficit(s), such as weakness on one side of the body. The patient should be prepared for reoperation.
- The primary complications of carotid endarterectomy are stroke, cranial nerve injuries, infection/hematoma of the wound, and carotid artery disruption.
- It is important to maintain adequate blood pressure levels in the immediate postoperative period. Hypotension is avoided to prevent cerebral ischemia and thrombosis.
- Excessive hypertension may precipitate cerebral hemorrhage. Edema, hemorrhage in the operative wound, or disruption of the arterial reconstruction may also result from excessive hypertension. Sodium nitroprusside is commonly used to bring the blood pressure to previous levels.
- Difficulty in swallowing, hoarseness, or other signs of cranial nerve dysfunction must be assessed. Some swelling in the neck following surgery is expected. However, swelling and hematoma formation, if large enough, can obstruct the patient's airway. A tracheostomy set must be available.
- Close cardiac monitoring is necessary since these patients have a high incidence of coronary artery disease.
- Long-term complications include recurrent stroke and myocardial infarction.

Neurosurgical Treatment of Pain

The management of long-term pain requires a multidisciplinary approach. (The reader is referred to Chap. 15 for a discussion of the basic theories of the psychophysiology of pain and its management.)

Intractable pain refers to pain that cannot be relieved satisfactorily by drugs without causing drug addiction or incapacitating sedation. Such pain usually is the result of malignancy (especially of the cervix, bladder, prostate, and lower bowel), but it does occur in many other conditions, such as post-herpetic neuralgia, trigeminal neuralgia, spinal cord arachnoiditis, and uncontrollable ischemia and other forms of tissue destruction.

Neurosurgical methods available for pain relief include (1) stimulation procedures (intermittent electric stimulation of a tract or center to inhibit the transfer of pain information, (2) administration of intraspinal opiates, and (3) interruption of the tracts conducting the pain between the periphery and the cerebral integration centers. The latter are destructive or ablative procedures.

Stimulation Procedures

Electrical stimulation or neuromodulation is a method of suppressing pain by applying controlled low-voltage electrical pulses to the different parts of the nervous system. Electrical stimulation is thought to relieve pain by preventing messages from reaching the brain by blocking small afferent fiber input at the dorsal horn or by stimulating the release of endogenous opiates (natural pain-relieving peptides). This pain-modulating technique is administered by many modes. At the present time transcutaneous electrical nerve stimulation and dorsal column stimulation are the procedures most frequently done. In addition there are also brain stimulators in which stimulating electrodes are implanted in the periventricular area of the posterior third ventricle, allowing self-stimulation of the periventricular gray area to produce analgesia.

Transcutaneous Electric Nerve Stimulation (TENS)

Transcutaneous electric nerve stimulation (TENS) is the passage of small electrical currents through the skin for the purpose of controlling pain. The stimulating electrodes are placed over the site of pain or along the course of the major peripheral nerves innervating the area or over the peripheral plexus. The patient operates the amplitude control until stimulation, detected by a vibration, buzzing, or tapping sensation, is felt within the deeper tissue. The amplitude is increased slowly until the sensation is perceived at the site or origin of pain and/or along radiating pathways. The patient controls the amplitude, frequency, and duration of stimulation. It appears very useful to the well-instructed patient in the early management of acute pain as well as for the patient with chronic pain. It is best used as an adjunct to a comprehensive rehabilitation program for relief and elimination of pain.

Patient Education for TENS. The patient is given the instruction booklet provided by the manufacturing company that explains care of the skin, electrodes, and generator. The skin is cleansed and electrode gel is applied to the electrodes, which are then placed over the nerves that serve the painful area. The electrodes are secured with hypoallergenic tape. The major problem of transcutaneous electric nerve stimulation is skin irritation from the tape (from mechanical stresses created by shearing forces between tape and skin), gels, or electrodes. The patient is advised to keep a record evaluating the effectiveness of TENS. If there is a progression of pathology (as in advanced cancer), changes in amplitude, and so on may be adjusted.

Dorsal Column Stimulation (DCS)

Dorsal column stimulation (DCS) is a technique used for the relief of chronic intractable pain in which a surgically implanted device allows the patient to apply pulsed electrical stimulation to the dorsal aspect of the spinal cord to block pain impulses. (The largest accumulation of afferent fibers is found in the dorsal column of the spinal cord.)

The dorsal column stimulation unit consists of a radiofrequency stimulation transmitter, a transmitter antenna, a radiofrequency receiver, and a stimulation electrode. The battery-powered transmitter and antenna are worn externally while the receiver and electrode are implanted. A laminectomy is performed above the highest level of pain input, and the electrode is placed in the epidural space over the posterior column of the spinal cord. (The placement of the stimulating systems is varied.) The subcutaneous pocket is constructed over the clavicular area or some other site for placement of the receiver. The two are connected by a subcutaneous tunnel.

Postoperative Nursing Management. The postoperative nursing management is similar to that following a laminectomy. The patient is assessed for evidences of paraplegia, quadriplegia, and urinary incontinence. The extremities are evaluated for movement. Leakage of CSF at the laminectomy site is also checked since the dura is opened during surgery. The implant site is checked for signs of infection. As soon as the patient is fully alert, the dorsal column stimulation system may be tested, although initial testing may not be accurate because a bandage may cover the receiver site. Complications include infection, cord trauma, CSF leakage, and pain around the implantation site.

Patient Education and Home Health Care. The patient is given the manufacturer's booklet to become acquainted with the system. Proper skin care is taught as well as the method for attaching the antenna to the skin, connecting the transmitter, and adjusting the settings. Different stimulation frequencies should be tried to determine which one gives the best pain relief. A record is to be kept of the stimulation used. The patient is also instructed to keep several batteries in reserve. (Battery life depends on the extent of use.) The transmitter and antenna are cleaned according to the manufacturer's directions.

Percutaneous Epidural Neurostimulation

Percutaneous epidural neurostimulation is a method of neurostimulation in which electrodes are inserted percutaneously into the spinal epidural space. It appears effective in treating arachnoiditis and postamputation neuroma.

Deep Brain Stimulation

Deep brain stimulation is done for very special pain problems when the patient does not respond to the usual techniques of pain control. With the patient under local anesthesia electrodes are introduced through a burr hole and inserted into a selected site in the brain, depending on the location or type of the patient's pain. After the effectiveness of stimulation is confirmed, the implanted electrode is connected to a radiofrequency device or pulse generator system operated by external telemetry.

Immediate postoperative complications include infection and transient neurologic deficits following insertion of the electrodes. Failure of the stimulating system and development of tolerance may occur later. Nursing interventions include teaching the patient and family about the system, encouraging the patient to keep a record of amplitude and frequency settings and the relief obtained, and monitoring for complications.

Intraspinal Opiates

Opiate receptors have been demonstrated not only in the brain but also in the substantia gelatinosa of the spinal cord. These receptors can combine with locally administered opiates (morphine) injected epidurally or intrathecally to produce long-lasting pain relief with little or no blunting of the patient's level of responsiveness and no losses of sensory, motor, or sphincter function.

There are numerous techniques employed, but most include placing a catheter in the epidural or subarachnoid space via a spinal needle and inserting the catheter as near as possible to the spinal segment where the pain is projected. Small doses of preservative-free morphine diluted in saline are injected into the system at 6- to 24-hour intervals. If the patient requires long-term management, an implantable programmable pump is used.

Following the procedure the patient is evaluated for the degree of pain relief, which ranges from good to excellent. The puncture site is examined for evidence of infection.

With this method the patient may be at home. The necessary dose of drug is small, the patient's mind is clear, and he is usually able to function at a relatively high level. He may complain of generalized itching and urinary retention (self-limited) for several days. With long-term use there can be tolerance buildup and mechanical failure (catheter obstructed, dislodged, broken) of the application system. If the patient has rapid tumor growth, the dosage of morphine is increased, but the doses needed are low in comparison to that required for systemic administration for intractable pain.

Destructive or Ablative Procedures

Pain-conducting fibers can be interrupted at any point from their origin to the cerebral cortex. There is destruction of some part of the nervous system that can result in varying amounts of neurologic deficit and incapacity. In time, pain usually returns as a result of either regeneration of axonal fibers or the development of alternative pain pathways.

Cordotomy

Cordotomy is the division of certain tracts of the spinal cord. It may be performed percutaneously, by the open method after laminectomy, or by other techniques.

Percutaneous cordotomy uses radiofrequency currents to produce lesions in the anterolateral surface of the spinal cord. With the patient under local anesthesia, a needle is inserted into the neck below and behind the mastoid process. It is guided into the spinal cord under x-ray control, and then an electrode is inserted through it. By means of radiofrequency currents, a lesion is made at the desired spinal cord level.

Verification of electrode placement is determined by the patient's response to stimulation. The procedure is tolerated by wasted and debilitated patients.

An *open cordotomy* is the surgical division of the anterolateral columns of the spinal pain fibers high in the thoracic or cervical region. This procedure interrupts or destroys conduction of pain and temperature sense, while touch and position sense are preserved. The cord is exposed by laminectomy. Cordotomy is used most frequently in controlling the severe pain of terminal cancer, especially of the thorax, abdomen, or lower extremities. Since a significant percentage of cordotomies lose their effectiveness in 1 to 5 years, the procedure is used for pain associated with conditions in which survival time is limited.

Postoperative Nursing Management. The principles of nursing management following a laminectomy are applicable in the postoperative and rehabilitation requirements of this patient (see p. 1518). Following a cordotomy, the patient may be kept flat for the prescribed time period, because there is less tension on the incision when this position is assumed. A patient with a thoracic cordotomy may be turned to the prone position. In instances of a cervical incision, pillows should not be used when the patient is in a supine position. Trauma to the surgical site is eliminated when the neck is kept in a neutral position. The patient is turned as a unit ("log" fashion) by two persons using a turning sheet to avoid twisting the body and putting pressure on the incision.

Assessment for Complications. The patient is watched for respiratory complications, as well as for signs of fatigue and weakening of the voice. The patient may ventilate adequately while awake but may experience progressive hypercarbia and hypoxia while asleep. Therefore, arterial blood gases are monitored, and assisted mechanical ventilation is initiated when required.

Since hemorrhage may result in motor and sensory loss, the motion, strength, and sensation of each extremity must be tested every few hours (or more frequently if necessary) during the first 48 hours postoperatively. If hemorrhage is indicated, immediate surgical intervention is imperative. Because the patient has no sense of temperature, the skin should be felt at intervals to ascertain any changes in temperature. Since pressure sores may develop without the patient realizing it, the patient is taught to inspect his skin using a hand mirror to view the hard-to-see areas. Urinary retention may be encountered. There is usually a slow return to normal voiding, but this cannot be guaranteed. If there is permanent loss of urinary control from a high cervical procedure, a bladder training program is started.

Rhizotomy

Rhizotomy is the surgical division of the spinal roots and is used in controlling severe chest pain of lung cancer and for pain relief in head and neck malignancies.

Since many patients with metastatic malignancies may not be able to tolerate an open rhizotomy, a *percutaneous rhizotomy* may be done, whereby a radiofrequency current is used to selectively coagulate the pain fibers, while the fibers concerned with touch and proprioception are preserved.

A *chemical rhizotomy* is one in which alcohol, phenol, or a mixture of drugs is injected into the subarachnoid space. The medication is maneuvered over the affected nerve roots by tilting the patient to the desired level. This renders the sensory nerve roots functionless. The patient's perception of pain is absent, but the motor nerve roots are usually not affected.

Psychosurgical Approaches

The purpose of psychosurgical procedures is to alter the patient's response to pain. A *thalamotomy* is the destruction (either unilateral or bilateral) of the specific cell groups within the thalamus. Burr holes are made in the skull, electrodes are placed in the target area by stereotaxic techniques, and a radiofrequency current is then directed through the electrodes to create the lesion. This procedure represents the highest level in the CNS in which pain pathways can be interrupted and is usually done for malignancy of the head and neck.

Cingulumotomy is a unilateral or bilateral interruption of the anterior cingulate bundle in the frontal lobe of the brain. It is accomplished either by an open or stereotaxic approach. It tends to modify the patient's affective reaction to pain.

The Patient Undergoing Intracranial Surgery

In recent years, certain technological advances have helped to refine existing neurologic procedures and develop newer ones. Superior neuroradiologic techniques have made it possible to localize intracranial lesions. Improved illumination and magnification have made it possible to obtain a three-dimensional view of the field of operation. Lasers enable neurosurgeons to remove tumors precisely with minimal trauma to surrounding tissue, which is of utmost importance in neurosurgery. It is possible to coagulate vessels adjacent to structures without causing injury to the structures themselves. Microsurgical instruments allow delicate tissue to be separated without trauma. Ultrasonic dissecting systems permit rapid and gentle removal of certain brain and spinal cord tumors with amazing precision. Probes placed deep into brain tissue can be used for application of interstitial radiation, hyperthermia, or chemotherapy to formerly inaccessible lesions. Suture material smaller than a strand of human hair permits very small nerves and vessels to be sutured and anastomosed.

Surgical Approaches

A *craniotomy* is the surgical opening of the skull to gain access to intracranial structures. This procedure is done to remove a tumor, relieve ICP, evacuate a blood clot, and control hemorrhage. The skull is opened by making a bony flap that is replaced following surgery and fixed in position by periosteal or wire sutures. In general, two approaches are used: (1) above the tentorium (supratentorial craniotomy) into the supratentorial compartment and (2) below the tentorium into the infratentorial (posterior fossa) compartment (Fig. 53-7).

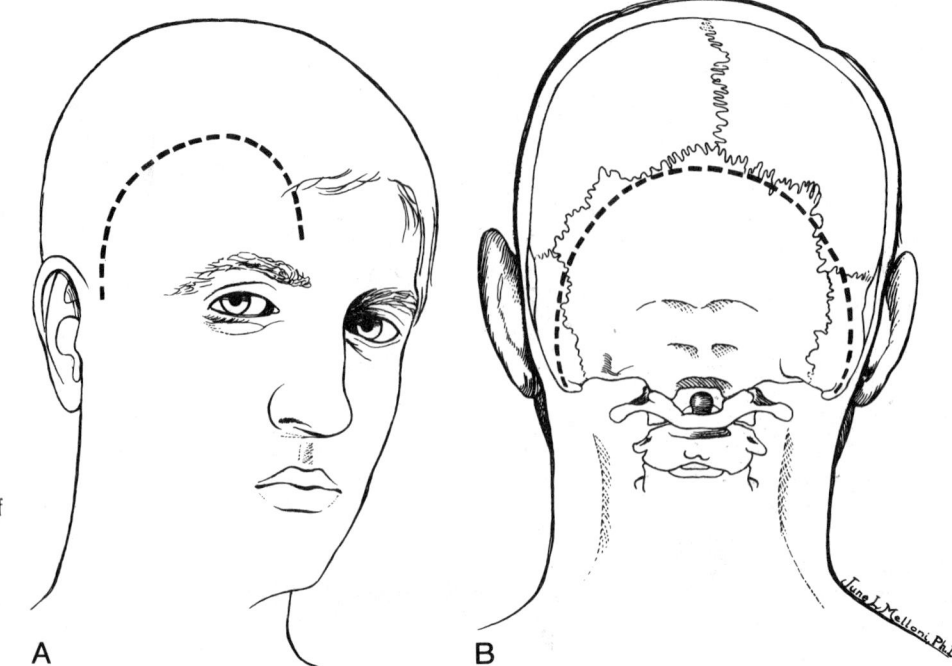

Figure 53-7
Surgical approaches for craniotomy (surgical opening of the cranial cavity). The dotted lines indicate scalp incisions. (*A*) Supratentorial approach. (*B*) Infratentorial approach. See text, p. 1451.

A

B

The intracranial structures may be approached through *burr holes* (Fig. 53-8), which are circular openings made in the skull by either a hand drill or an automatic craniotome (which has a self-controlled system to stop the drill when the bone is penetrated). Burr holes are made for exploration or diagnosis. They may be used to determine the level of brain tension and the size and position of the ventricles. They are also a means of evacuating an intracranial hematoma or abscess, making a bone flap in the skull, and allowing access to the ventricles for decompression purposes, ventriculography, or shunting procedures.

Other cranial procedures include *craniectomy* (an excision of a portion of the skull) and *cranioplasty* (repair of a cranial defect by means of a plastic or metal plate).

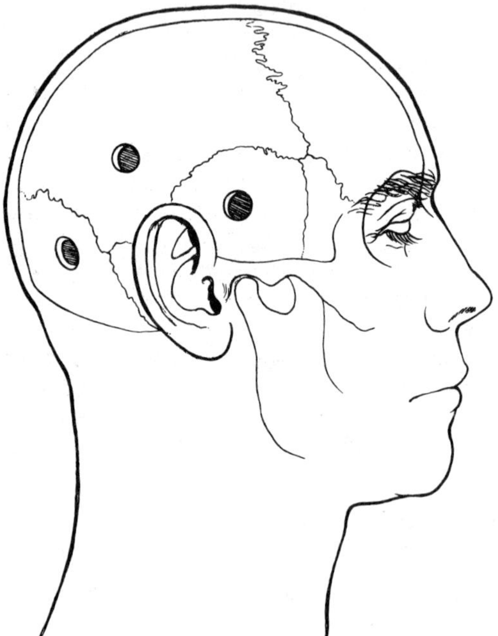

Diagnostic Evaluation

Preoperative diagnostic procedures may include computed tomography (CT scanning) to demonstrate the lesion and reveal the degree of surrounding brain edema, the ventricular size, and the displacement. Magnetic resonance imaging (MRI) provides information similar to that of the CT scan with the additional advantage of examining the lesion in other planes. Cerebral angiography may be used to study the tumor blood supply or give information about vascular lesions.

Preoperative Management

Usually patients are placed on anticonvulsant medication (phenytoin) before surgery to reduce the risk of postoperative seizures. Preoperative steroids (dexamethasone) are introduced before surgery to reduce cerebral edema. Fluids may be restricted. A hyperosmotic agent (mannitol) and a diuretic (furosemide) may be given intravenously immediately before (and sometimes during) surgery if the patient tends to retain water, as many do who have intracranial dysfunction. An indwelling urethral catheter is inserted before the patient is taken to the operating room to drain the bladder during the administration of diuretics and measure urinary output and for periodic measurements of urine specific gravity and sugar.

The scalp is shaved immediately prior to surgery so that any resultant superficial abrasions will not have time to become infected. Most patients find this alteration in their ap-

Figure 53-8
Burr holes may be used in neurosurgical procedures for making a bone flap in the skull, for aspiration of a brain abscess, or to evacuate a hematoma.

pearance very distressing. Reassuring the patient that his head will be covered with a head dressing after surgery will help him cope. He may be given diazepam preoperatively to allay anxiety.

Postoperative Management

An arterial line and a central venous pressure (CVP) line may be in place for blood pressure monitoring and CVP measurements. Oxygen is usually administered. Drug therapy for cerebral edema includes the administration of mannitol, which increases serum osmolality and drains free water from areas of the brain (with an intact blood–brain carrier). The fluid is then excreted by osmotic diuresis. Dexamethasone may be administered intravenously every 6 hours for 24 to 72 hours and then tapered.

Acetaminophen is usually given for temperature over 99.6°F (37.5°C) and for pain. There will be a certain amount of headache following craniotomy, which is mostly attributed to stretching or irritation of the nerves of the scalp that occurs during operation. Codeine, given parenterally, is usually sufficient to relieve headache. Anticonvulsant medication (phenytoin, diazepam) is given to patients who have undergone supratentorial craniotomy because of the high risk of epilepsy following supratentorial neurosurgical procedures. Serum levels are monitored to keep the drug within therapeutic range.

Ventricular catheters, or some type of drainage, are frequently inserted in patients undergoing surgery for tumors of the posterior fossa. These catheters are connected to an external drainage bottle. The patency of the catheter is noted by the pulsations of the fluid in the tubing. In addition, the degree of ICP can be determined by the height of the fluid level in the tube above the level of the ventricle. The catheter is removed when the ventricular pressure is normal. The neurosurgeon should be notified if at any time the catheter appears to be obstructed.

Ventricular shunting is sometimes done before certain operations to control intracranial hypertension, particularly in patients with posterior fossa tumors.

▶ Nursing Process
The Patient Undergoing Intracranial Surgery

▷ Preoperative Assessment/Preparation

Proper assessment of the postoperative status of the patient requires an awareness of the patient's signs and symptoms so that a comparison may be made between the preoperative and postoperative conditions. Included in this assessment are evaluation of the level of responsiveness/consciousness and the presence of any neurologic deficits. Observations of paralysis, visual dysfunction, alterations in personality or speech, and bladder and bowel disturbances are made. Motor function of the hands can be tested by the hand grip. Observations of leg movement should be especially noted if the patient is not ambulatory.

If there is paralysis of the extremities, trochanter rolls are applied to both extremities, and the feet positioned against a footboard. Patients who have speech difficulties, failing vi-

sion, and hearing loss are a challenge to the nurse's ingenuity. If the patient is aphasic, writing materials or picture and word cards showing the bedpan, glass of water, blanket, and so on may be supplied to help improve communication. If the patient is able to ambulate, he is encouraged to do so in a quiet, unhurried way.

The emotional preparation of the patient is also important, including informing him of postoperative expectations. The large head dressing applied following surgery may impair his hearing ability temporarily. He will have difficulty seeing if his eyes are swollen shut. If he has a tracheostomy or endotracheal tube, he will be unable to talk. Thus, an alternate method of communication should be developed before surgery.

The patient may not realize that he is about to undergo surgery. Even so, encouragement and attention to his needs usually will reinforce his confidence. Whatever the state of awareness of the patient, the family needs reassurance and consideration, since they recognize the seriousness of a brain operation.

▷ Postoperative Assessment

Postoperative nursing monitoring of the patient having intracranial surgery is done minute by minute and/or hour by hour depending on his clinical status. Assessment of respiratory status is essential because small degrees of hypoxia can aggravate cerebral ischemia. The respiratory rate and patterns of respiration are monitored, and arterial blood gas values are reviewed. Fluctuations of the patient's vital signs are carefully watched for because they indicate increased ICP. The patient's rectal temperature is taken at intervals to evaluate for hyperthermia that may result from damage to the hypothalamus, which regulates body temperature.

Neurologic checks are made frequently to detect increased ICP resulting from edema or bleeding following intracranial surgery. A change in the level of responsiveness/consciousness may be the first sign of increasing ICP. Assessment of neurologic status includes determining the level of responsiveness/consciousness, eye signs, motor response, and vital signs. The nurse carefully observes for the insidious development of any neurologic deficit, such as diminished response to stimuli, speech problems, difficulty in swallowing, weakness or paralysis of an extremity, visual changes (diplopia, blurred vision), and paresthesias. The patient is observed for restlessness, which may reflect a return to consciousness or be due to pain, confusion, an obstructed urinary drainage system, or other stimuli. Any evidence of seizure activity is reported immediately.

The patient's head dressing is inspected to determine the presence of bleeding and CSF drainage. In patients undergoing transsphenoidal surgery, the nasal packing is checked for signs of bloody or CSF drainage.

The intravenous infusion drip rate monitoring device is checked to see that it is working properly to prevent uncontrolled infusion. The infusion site is observed for redness, pain, swelling, or purulent drainage.

Patient positioning depends on the surgical approach used. However, the patient's neck should be in a straight line because neck flexion may interfere with cerebral drainage.

The nurse is always alert to the development of complications (p. 1457), and all assessment is carried out with these problems in mind.

(Text continues on p. 1456)

Chart 53-3
Summary: Nursing Management of the Patient Having Intracranial Surgery

Postoperative Interventions

Nursing Diagnosis: Potential for ineffective breathing pattern related to postoperative cerebral edema
Goal: Achievement of adequate respiratory function
1. Establish proper respiratory exchange and adequate brain oxygenation to eliminate systemic hypercarbia and hypoxia, which increase cerebral edema.
   a. Place the patient in a lateral or a semiprone position to facilitate respiratory exchange until consciousness returns, unless contraindicated.
   b. Employ tracheopharyngeal aspiration cautiously to remove secretions; suctioning can raise intracranial pressure.
   c. Maintain patient on controlled ventilation if prescribed to maintain normal ventilatory status; monitor arterial blood gas results to determine respiratory adequacy.
   d. Elevate the head of the bed 30.5 cm (12 inches) after patient is conscious to aid venous drainage of the brain.
   e. See that the patient has nothing by mouth until an active coughing and swallowing reflex is demonstrated; this prevents regurgitation.
   f. Ensure cardiovascular stability.
Potential Complication: Brain edema secondary to intracranial surgery
Goal: Prevention of brain edema
1. Assess patient's level of responsiveness/consciousness; the diminution of the level of consciousness may be the first sign of increased intracranial pressure.
   a. Eye opening (spontaneous, to sound, to pain); pupillary reactions to light
   b. Response to commands
   c. Assessment of spinal motor reflexes (pinch Achilles tendon, arm, or other body site)
   d. Observation of patient's spontaneous activity
2. Keep a neurologic flow sheet for sequentially assessing and documenting neurologic status, fluid administration, therapeutic agents, and laboratory data.
3. Evaluate for signs and symptoms of increasing intracranial pressure, which can lead to ischemia and further impairment of brain function.
   a. Assess patient minute by minute, hour by hour, for:
      1) Diminished response to stimuli
      2) Fluctuations of vital signs
      3) Restlessness
      4) Weakness and paralysis of extremities
      5) Increasing headache
      6) Changes or disturbances of vision; pupillary changes
   b. Modify nursing management to prevent further increases in intracranial pressure. (See p. 1422).

4. Control postoperative cerebral edema as prescribed.
   a. Give steroids and osmotic dehydrating agents when prescribed in postoperative period to reduce brain swelling.
   b. Monitor fluid intake; basic fluid requirements are usually precisely met; care is taken not to overload the patient.
   c. Maintain a normal temperature during the postoperative period. Temperature control may be lost in certain neurologic states, and fever increases the metabolic demands of the brain.
      1) Take rectal temperature at specified intervals. Assess temperature of extremities, which may be cold and dry due to paralysis of heat-losing mechanisms (vasodilation and sweating).
      2) Employ measures as prescribed to reduce excessive fever when present: ice bags to axillae and groin; tepid or cool water sponges; hypothermia blanket. Use ECG monitoring to detect dysrhythmias during hypothermia procedures.
   d. Employ hyperventilation when prescribed (results in respiratory alkalosis, which causes cerebral vasoconstriction and reduces circulation, which therefore reduces intracranial pressure).
   e. Elevate head of bed to reduce intracranial pressure and facilitate respirations.
   f. Avoid excessive stimuli.
   g. Use intracranial pressure monitoring if patient is at risk for intracranial hypertension.
Nursing Diagnosis: Potential alteration in fluid volume related to intracranial pressure or diuretics
Goal: Attainment of fluid and electrolyte balance
1. Monitor for polyuria especially during first postoperative week; diabetes insipidus may develop in patients with lesions around the pituitary or hypothalamus
   a. Take urinary specific gravity readings at intervals.
   b. Monitor serum and urinary electrolyte levels.
2. Evaluate patient's electrolyte status, since following certain major procedures patients have a tendency to retain water and sodium.
   a. Early postoperative weight gain indicates fluid retention; a greater than estimated weight loss indicates negative water balance.
   b. Loss of sodium and chlorides will produce weakness, lethargy, and coma.
   c. Low potassium will cause confusion and decreased level of responsiveness.
3. Weigh patient daily; keep intake and output record.

(continued)

Chart 53-3 *(continued)*

Postoperative Interventions

4. Give prescribed intravenous fluids with care—rate and composition depend on fluid deficit, urine output and composition, and blood loss.
   Fluid intake and fluid losses should remain relatively equal.

Nursing Diagnosis: Alteration in sensory perceptions (visual/auditory) related to periorbital edema and head dressings

Goal: Compensate for sensory deprivation

1. Perform supportive measures until the patient is able to care for himself.
   a. Change position as indicated; be aware that position changes can increase intracranial pressure.
   b. Give prescribed analgesics that do not mask the level of responsiveness (codeine).
2. Employ prescribed measures to relieve signs of periocular edema.
   a. Lubricate eyelids and around eyes with petrolatum.
   b. Apply light, cold compresses over eyes at specified intervals.
   c. Watch for signs of keratitis if cornea has no sensation.
3. Put extremities through range of motion exercises.
4. Evaluate and support patient during episodes of restlessness.
   a. Evaluate for airway obstruction, distended bladder, meningeal irritation from bloody cerebrospinal fluid.
   b. Pad patient's hands and bed rails to protect him from injury.
5. Reinforce blood-stained dressings with sterile dressing; blood-soaked dressings act as a culture medium for bacteria.
6. Orient patient frequently to time, place, and person.

Monitoring the Patient for Complications

1. *Intracranial hemorrhage*
   a. Postoperative bleeding may be intraventricular, intracerebellar, subdural, or extradural.
   b. Watch for progressive impairment of state of responsiveness and other signs of increasing intracranial pressure.
   c. Prepare deteriorating patient for reoperation and evacuation of hematoma.
2. *Increased intracranial pressure; cerebral edema* (see p. 1416)
3. *Epilepsy* (There is a greater risk with supratentorial operations.)
   a. Administer prescribed anticonvulsants; monitor anticonvulsant blood levels.
   b. Watch for status epilepticus, which may occur after any intracranial operation.

4. *Infections*
   a. Urinary tract infections
   b. Pulmonary infections related to aspiration secondary to depressed level of responsiveness; may result in atelectasis and bronchopneumonia
   c. CNS infections (postoperative meningitis, cerebrospinal fluid shunt infection)
   d. Wound infections/septicemia
5. *Venous thrombosis*
6. *Leakage of cerebrospinal fluid*
   a. Differentiate between cerebrospinal fluid and mucus.
      1) Collect fluid on Dextrostix; if cerebrospinal fluid is present, the indicator will have a positive reaction since cerebrospinal fluid contains sugar.
      2) Assess for moderate elevation of temperature and mild neck rigidity.
   b. Caution patient against nose blowing or sniffing.
   c. Elevate head of bed as prescribed.
   d. Assist with insertion of lumbar subarachnoid drainage catheter that is placed to lower spinal fluid pressure.
      1) Ventricular catheters may be inserted in the patient undergoing surgery of the posterior fossa (ventriculostomy); the catheter(s) is connected to a closed reservoir system.
      2) Give antibiotics as prescribed.
7. *Gastrointestinal ulceration;* monitor for signs and symptoms of hemorrhage, perforation, or both (probably caused by stress response).

Evaluation

Expected Outcomes

1. Demonstrates normal breathing pattern
   a. Absence of crackles
   b. Demonstrates active swallowing and coughing reflexes
2. Demonstrates improved neurologic function
   a. Opens eyes on request
   b. Obeys commands
   c. Has appropriate motor responses
   d. Shows increasing alertness
3. Attains/maintains fluid balance
   a. Takes fluids orally
   b. Maintains weight within expected range
4. Compensates for sensory deprivation
   a. Makes needs known
   b. Demonstrates improvement of vision
5. Reveals absence of complications
   a. No evidence of increased intracranial pressure
   b. No evidence of rhinorrhea, otorrhea, or spinal fluid seepage
   c. Absence of fever
   d. No evidence of inflammation/infection around wound
   e. Absence of seizures

▷ *Nursing Diagnoses*

Based on the assessment data, the patient's major nursing diagnoses following intracranial surgery may include the following:

- Alteration in cerebral tissue perfusion related to cerebral edema.
- Potential ineffective thermoregulation related to damage to the hypothalamus, dehydration, and infection
- Alteration in fluid and electrolyte balance related to possible metabolic/hormonal dysfunction
- Sensory-perceptual alterations (visual, auditory, possibly speech) related to periorbital edema, head dressing, endotracheal tube, and effects of intracranial pressure
- Potential for infection (intracranial and other) related to neurosurgical procedure (brain exposure; bone exposure, removal and replacement; wound hematomas)
- Potential pulmonary infection related to hypoventilation, aspiration, and immobility
- Disturbance in self-concept: body image related to change in appearance and/or physical disabilities

Other nursing diagnoses may include impaired verbalization (dysphasia) related to insult to brain tissue and potential impairment of skin integrity related to immobility, pressure, and incontinence. There may be impaired physical mobility related to a neurologic deficit secondary to the neurosurgical procedure.

▷ *Planning and Implementation*

▷   *Goals:*   The major goals of the patient may include achievement of neurologic homeostasis to improve cerebral tissue perfusion, achievement of thermoregulation, achievement/maintenance of fluid and electrolyte balance, ability to cope with sensory deprivation, avoidance of intracranial infection, avoidance of pulmonary infection, and restoration of confidence concerning body image. A summary of the nursing management of the patient having intracranial surgery is on pages 1454 and 1455.

Nursing Interventions

Achieving Neurologic Homeostasis.   Attention to the respiratory status is essential because even slight deficiencies in oxygen supply (hypoxia) can aggravate cerebral ischemia. Nursing assessment and monitoring will affect the clinical course. The endotracheal tube is left in place until the patient shows signs of awakening and is breathing spontaneously as evaluated clinically and by arterial blood gas analysis. Secondary brain damage can result from impaired cerebral oxygenation.

Cerebral edema is an increase in the water content of brain tissue leading to an increase in brain volume. Some degree of brain edema occurs following brain surgery, which tends to be maximal 24 to 36 hours postoperatively. This is why there may be a slump in the patient's level of responsiveness on the second postoperative day. The control of cerebral edema is discussed on page 1416. The nursing strategies employed to eliminate factors contributing to the elevation of ICP are found on page 1422. Intraventricular drainage is carefully monitored, using strict asepsis if any part of the system is handled.

The vital signs and neurologic checks (level of responsiveness, pupillary and motor responses) are made every 15 minutes to 1 hour and recorded. Extreme head rotation is avoided, as this raises ICP. Following a supratentorial operation, the patient is placed on his back or side (unoperated side if a large lesion was removed) with one pillow under his head. The head of the bed may be elevated 20 to 30 degrees according to the level of the ICP and the neurosurgeon's directives. (Usually, the patient is kept in relatively the same position as during the operation.) Following a posterior fossa operation (infratentorial), the patient is kept flat on his side (off his back) with his head on a small, firm pillow. He may be turned on either side, but his head should not be flexed on his chest. When the patient is being turned, his body should be turned as a unit to prevent strain on the wound and possible tearing of the sutures.

The patient's position is changed every 2 hours and skin care is given frequently. If the position is changed too frequently, the intracranial monitoring equipment will be disrupted. A turning sheet from the head to the mid-thigh level will make it easier to move the patient.

Temperature Regulation.   Moderate levels of fever can be expected after intracranial operations due to reaction of blood at the operative site or in the subarachnoid. Injury to the hypothalamic centers that control heat-conserving mechanisms can occur during surgery. High fever is treated vigorously to combat the effect of increasing temperature on brain metabolism and function. Nursing interventions include taking the temperature at specified intervals and employing measures to reduce excessive fever: removing blankets, applying ice caps to axillae and groin areas, administering tepid to cold sponges, allowing a fan to blow on the patient to increase surface cooling, and using a hypothermia blanket as directed.

Conversely, hypothermia may be seen following lengthy neurosurgical procedures. Therefore, frequent measurements of rectal temperature are necessary.

Maintaining Fluid and Electrolyte Balance.   The postoperative fluid regimen depends on the type of neurosurgical procedure and is calculated on an individual basis. The volume and composition of fluids are adjusted according to daily electrolyte determinations and intake and output.

Electrolyte imbalance, particularly sodium imbalance, may contribute to the development of brain edema. Sodium retention is observed in the immediate postoperative period in certain intracranial operations. Serum and urine electrolytes, blood urea nitrogen, blood glucose, weight, and clinical status are monitored. The intake and output are measured in view of losses incurred from fever, respiration, and ventricular/spinal drainage. Fluids may have to be restricted in patients with cerebral edema.

Oral fluids are usually resumed in a short period, and the body's own homeostatic mechanisms regulate electrolyte balance. However, some patients with posterior fossa tumors may have impaired swallowing, and fluids may have to be administered by way of alternate routes.

Patients having surgery for brain tumors may be on large doses of corticosteroids and thus may have a tendency to develop hyperglycemia. Urine sugar determinations are made every 4 hours in this event.

Following surgery in and around the pituitary gland and hypothalamus, the patient may develop symptoms of diabetes insipidus, which is characterized by excessive urinary output.

The urine specific gravity is measured hourly, and fluid intake and output charts are kept and evaluated.

The syndrome of inappropriate secretion of antidiuretic hormone (SIADH) resulting in water retention with hyponatremia and serum hypo-osmolality, occurs in a wide variety of CNS dysfunction (brain tumor, head trauma) causing fluid and electrolyte disturbances. Nursing management of this syndrome requires careful intake and output measurements, specific gravity determinations of urine, and monitoring of serum and urine electrolyte studies, while following directives for fluid restriction. This syndrome is usually self-limiting.

Coping with Sensory Deprivation. Periorbital edema is a common consequence of intracranial surgery since fluid drains into the dependent periorbital areas when the patient has been positioned in a prone position during surgery.

When drainage catheters are not used, a hematoma frequently forms under the scalp and spreads down to the orbit, producing an area of ecchymosis (black eye). Sometimes the eyes cannot be opened for a few days due to edema of the eyelids.

Preoperatively the patient is warned that one or both eyes may close temporarily after operation. The head-up position and cold compresses over the eyes help reduce the edema. However, if it worsens significantly, it may indicate a postoperative clot is developing or there is increasing ICP and poor venous drainage. The surgeon is then notified. Health care personnel should announce their presence when entering the room to avoid startling the patient.

Preventing and Managing Intracranial and Other Infections. There is an increased risk for infection for patients who undergo lengthy intracranial operations, for those with external ventricular drains left *in situ* longer than 48 to 72 hours, and for those with neurosurgical procedures in the region of the third ventricle of the hypothalamus. A CSF leak carries the threat of infection and meningitis.

An early rise in temperature after surgery may be due to the reaction to blood at the operative site. This usually resolves in a few days.

The incision site is monitored for evidence of redness, tenderness, bulging, separation, or foul odor. The dressing is often stained with blood in the immediate postoperative period. It is important to reinforce the dressing with sterile pads so that contamination and infection may be avoided. (Blood is an excellent culture medium for bacteria.) If the dressing is heavily stained or displaced, it should be reported immediately. (A drain is sometimes placed in the craniotomy wound to facilitate drainage.)

Following suboccipital operations, CSF may leak through the wound. This complication is dangerous because of the possibility of meningitis. Any sudden discharge of fluid from a cranial or spinal wound is reported at once since a massive leak requires direct surgical repair. Attention should be paid to the patient complaining of a salty taste in his mouth since this can be due to CSF fluid trickling down his throat. He is warned against coughing, sneezing, or nose blowing, which may cause CSF leakage by creating pressure on the operative site.

Other causes of infection in the patient having intracranial surgery are similar to those of other postoperative patients: reactions to drugs, phlebitis/deep vein thrombosis, and urinary tract infections.

Preventing and Managing Pulmonary Infections. Neurosurgical patients are at risk for pulmonary infections because of immobility, immunosuppression, decreased levels of awareness, and fluid restriction. Immobility compromises the respiratory system by causing pooling and stasis of secretions in dependent areas and the development of atelectasis. Underhydrated patients may be more vulnerable to atelectasis as a result of inability to expectorate thickened secretions. Pneumonia is frequently seen in neurosurgical patients, possibly related to aspiration.

The patient is observed for signs of respiratory infection: rise in temperature, increase in pulse rate, and changes in respirations. The lungs are auscultated for decreasing breath sounds.

Nursing interventions include repositioning the patient every 2 hours to mobilize secretions and prevent stasis; encouragement of yawning, sighing, deep breathing, and coughing to open up collapsed alveoli; and suctioning secretions that cannot be raised by cough. It is well to remember that coughing and suctioning raise ICP. Humidification of the air may be helpful. The nurse works interdependently with the respiratory therapist to monitor the effects of pulmonary physical therapy.

Assessing for Postoperative Complications

Complications that may develop within hours following surgery include intracranial bleeding/hematoma, cerebral edema, and water intoxication.

- A drop in blood pressure, a fast pulse and respiration, and a pale and cold body are usually manifestations of hypovolemic shock following long operations. This type of shock is best treated by blood transfusion.
- Conversely, an increase in blood pressure and decrease in pulse with respiratory failure may indicate increased ICP.
- An accumulation of blood deep to the bone flap (extradural, subdural, intracerebral) may pose a threat to life. A clot must be suspected in any patient who does not waken as expected or whose condition deteriorates. An intracranial hematoma is suspected if the patient has any new postoperative neurologic deficits (especially a dilated pupil on the side of surgery). In these events the patient is returned to the operating room immediately for evacuation of the clot if it is believed to be significant.
- Cerebral edema, infarction, metabolic disturbances, and hydrocephalus are conditions that may simulate the clinical manifestations of a clot.

Aside from the immediate postoperative complications, other complications may occur during the first 2 weeks or later and may endanger the patient's recovery. The most important of these are thromboembolic complications (deep vein thrombosis, pulmonary embolism), pulmonary infection, urinary infection, and pressure sores. The majority of these complications may be avoided by frequent change of position, adequate suctioning of secretions, observation and auscultation for pulmonary complications, observation for urinary complications, and skin care.

Postoperative Seizures. Epilepsy may be a complication following any intracranial neurosurgical procedure. Preventing seizures is essential to avoid further cerebral edema. Giving the prescribed anticonvulsant medication prior to and immediately following the operation may prevent the appearance of seizures in subsequent months and years. Status epilepticus (occurrence of prolonged seizures without recovery of consciousness in the intervals between seizures) may occur after craniotomy and may also be related to the development of complications (hematoma, ischemia). The management of status epilepticus is found on page 1494.

General Postoperative Interventions. Patients without complications are ambulated with assistance as soon as possible, while those with depressed levels of responsiveness will require nursing management similar to that for the unconscious patient (p. 1432). Postneurosurgical patients with motor deficits will require nursing management similar to that following a stroke (p. 1442). Those with postoperative intellectual and speech impairment require psychological evaluation, speech therapy, and rehabilitation. The nurse works collaboratively with these health care professionals to achieve as complete a rehabilitation of the patient as is possible.

Achieving Self-Acceptance. The patient is encouraged to verbalize his feelings and frustrations about his changed appearance. Nursing support is based on the patient's right to feelings and their expression. Factual information may need to be provided if the patient has misconceptions about puffiness about the face, periorbital bruising, and hair loss. Attention to grooming, the use of his own clothing, and covering the head with a turban (and ultimately a wig until hair growth occurs) are encouraged. Social interaction with close friends, family, and hospital personnel may increase his sense of self-worth.

It takes time for the acquisition of a good self-concept. As the patient begins to take more responsibility for self-care and participates in more experiences, he gains a sense of control and personal competence. The patient's family and social support system can help sustain him until adaptation is fully made.

Patient Education and Home Health Care. The convalescence at home of a neurosurgical patient depends on the extent of the procedure and the success with which it was carried out. The family is made aware of the patient's strengths as well as limitations and their part in promoting his recovery. Since remembering to take the anticonvulsant medication is a priority, the patient/family are advised to have a check-off system to make sure the medication is taken. The patient may need to be accompanied while walking if he has sudden attacks of dizziness or seizures.

Usually the patient does not have any dietary restrictions unless there is another health problem requiring a special diet. He may take a shower or tub bath but should avoid getting his scalp wet until all the sutures have been removed. A clean scarf or cap may be worn until a wig or hairpiece is purchased. If skull bone has been removed the neurosurgeon may advocate a protective helmet.

Following a craniotomy the patient is usually more sensitive to loud noises. Television noise can be very irritating to the convalescing person. If the patient is aphasic, speech therapy may be necessary. This is likely to become a long-term and time-consuming project. It demands great patience and continuing encouragement on the part of all who are working with the patient.

When tumor, injury, or disease is of such a nature that the prognosis is poor, care is directed toward making the patient as comfortable as possible. With return of the tumor or cerebral compression, the patient becomes less alert and aware. Other possible sequelae include paralysis, blindness,

and seizures. If the family is not able to give this type of care, the community health nurse and social worker plan together with the family in making arrangements for additional home health care or in placing the patient in an extended-care or hospice facility. (See also Cerebral Metastases, p. 1468.)

▷ *Evaluation*

▷ *Expected Outcomes*

1. Patient achieves neurologic homeostasis/improved cerebral tissue perfusion.
   a. Opens eyes on request; utters recognizable words progressing to normal speech.
   b. Obeys commands with appropriate motor responses.
2. Attains thermoregulation.
3. Attains fluid and electrolyte balance.
   a. Demonstrates serum chemistries within acceptable limits for a patient undergoing intracranial surgery.
   b. Complies with fluid restriction.
4. Copes with sensory deprivation.
5. Has no intracranial infection.
6. Has no pulmonary infection.
7. Demonstrates an improving self-concept.
   a. Pays attention to grooming.
   b. Visits and interacts with others.

Transsphenoidal Surgery

Pituitary tumors (which represent 10% to 20% of all intracranial tumors) may be treated by surgery or irradiation. Surgical removal may be carried out through an open craniotomy (usually transfrontal) or by the transsphenoidal approach. The choice is determined by anatomical considerations and the extent and nature of the pathologic process.

Tumors located within the sella turcica and small adenomas of the pituitary can be removed by way of the transsphenoidal approach (Fig. 53-9). The incision is made beneath the upper lip, and entry is then gained successively into the nasal cavity, sphenoidal sinus, and sella turcica. Although the initial opening may be made by an otorhinolaryngologist, the neurosurgeon completes the opening into the sphenoidal sinus and exposes the floor of the sella. Microsurgical techniques provide improved illumination, magnification, and visualization so that nearby vital structures can be avoided.

This approach, which is being used with greater frequency, offers direct access to the sella with minimal risk of trauma and hemorrhage. It avoids many of the risks of craniotomy, and the postoperative discomfort is similar to that of other transnasal operations. It is also used for pituitary ablation (removal) in patients with disseminated breast or prostatic cancer.

Preoperative Evaluation

The preoperative workup includes a series of endocrine tests, rhinologic evaluation (to assess status of the sinuses and nasal cavity), and neuroradiologic studies. Funduscopic examination and visual field determinations are done, since the most serious effect of pituitary tumor is localized pressure on the optic nerve or chiasm. In addition, the nasopharyngeal se-

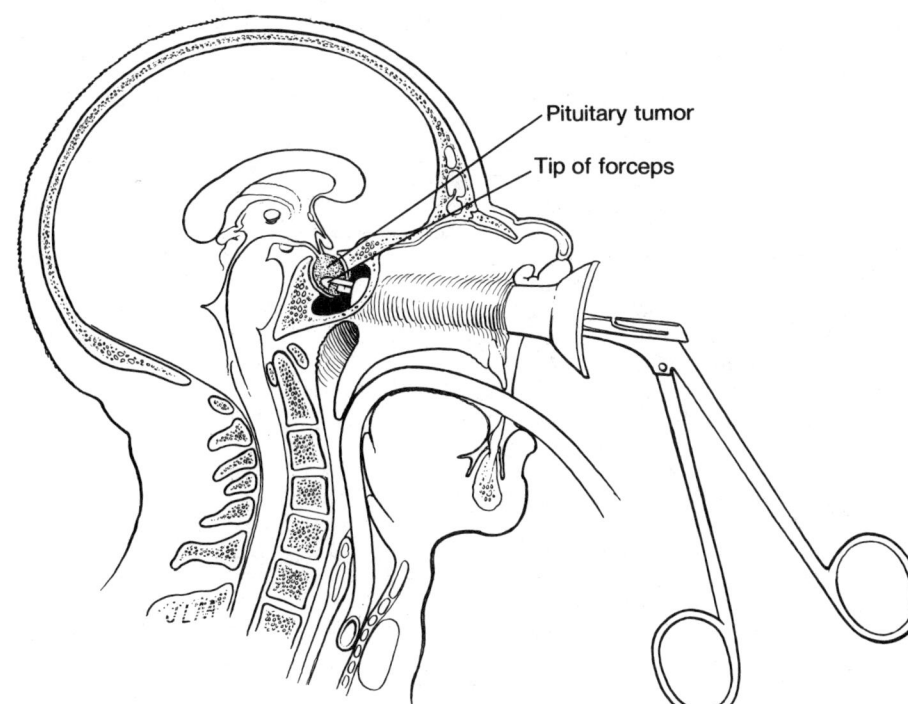

Pituitary tumor

Tip of forceps

Figure 53-9
Transsphenoidal approach to the pituitary. A special nasal speculum is used to view the sinus cavity. After the dura is opened, the tumor is removed using microcurettes or other specially designed instruments.

cretions are cultured because a sinus infection is a contraindication to an intracranial procedure through this approach. Cortisone may be given preoperatively and postoperatively (since the source of ACTH is removed). Antibiotics may or may not be administered prophylactically. Deep breathing is taught preoperatively. The patient is instructed that vigorous coughing and sneezing may cause a CSF leak after surgery. He is instructed to apply pressure on the inner aspect of both sides of the nose to control sneezing.

Postoperative Management

Because there has been disruption of the oral and nasal mucous membranes, management focuses on preventing infection and promoting healing. Medications given to the patient include antimicrobials (which are continued until the nasal packing is removed), cortisone, analgesics for discomfort, and agents for the control of diabetes insipidus, when necessary.

The nasal packing is removed in 24 hours to several days. The area around the nares is cleaned with the prescribed solution to dissolve crusted blood and moisten the mucous membranes.

Postoperative Nursing Interventions

The vital signs are taken to monitor hemodynamic, cardiac, and ventilatory status. Because of the anatomical proximity of the pituitary gland to the optic chiasm, visual acuity is checked at regular intervals. One method is to ask the patient to count the number of fingers held up by the nurse. Evidence of decreasing visual acuity suggests an expanding hematoma.

The major discomfort of the patient is related to the nasal packing and to mouth dryness and thirst from mouth-breathing. Oral care is provided every 4 hours or more frequently. Usually, the patient's teeth are not brushed until the incision

above the teeth has healed. The use of warm saline mouth rinses, dental floss, and occasionally a cool mist vaporizer is helpful. Petrolatum is soothing when applied to the lips. A room humidifer assists in keeping the patient's mucous membranes moist.

The head of the bed is raised to decrease pressure on the sella turcica and to promote normal drainage. The patient is cautioned against blowing his nose or engaging in any activity that raises ICP, such as bending over or straining during urination or defecation.

The intake and output are measured as a guide to fluid and electrolyte replacement. The urinary specific gravity is measured after each voiding. The patient's daily weight is monitored. Fluids are generally given when nausea ceases, and the patient then progresses to a regular diet.

Complications

Manipulation of the posterior pituitary gland during operation may produce transient diabetes insipidus of several days' duration that is treated with vasopressin. Occasionally, there is more persistent diabetes insipidus. Other complications include CSF leakage, postoperative meningitis, and inappropriate secretion of antidiuretic hormone (SIADH).

The patient is advised to have a room humidifier when he returns home. This keeps the membranes moist and soothes irritation. Keeping the head of the bed elevated for at least 2 weeks after surgery is helpful.

Bibliography

Books

Ashworth B and Saunders M. Management of Neurological Disorders, 2nd ed. Boston, Butterworths, 1985.

Bannister R. Brain's Clinical Neurology, 6th ed. New York, Oxford University Press, 1985.

Barnett HJM et al. Stroke: Pathophysiology, Diagnosis and Management. New York, Churchill Livingstone, 1986.

Bray GP and Clark GS. A Stroke Family Guide and Resources. Springfield, Illinois, Charles C Thomas, 1984.

Chusid JG. Correlative Neuroanatomy and Functional Neurology. Los Altos, California, Lange Medical Publications, 1985.

Davies PM. Steps to Follow: A Guide to the Treatment of Adult Hemiplegia. New York, Springer-Verlag, 1985.

Dickson S (ed). Communication Disorders: Remedial Principles and Practices, 2nd ed. Glenview, Illinois, Scott, Foresman, 1984.

Dyck P (ed). Stereotactic Biopsy and Brachotherapy of Brain Tumors. Baltimore, University Park Press, 1984.

Eastcott HHG. Color Atlas of Operations on the Internal Carotid Artery. Oradell, New Jersey, Medical Economics Books, 1984.

Eisenson J. Adult Aphasia, 2nd ed. Englewood Cliffs, New Jersey, Prentice-Hall, 1984.

Fein JM and Flamm ES. Cerebrovascular Surgery. New York, Springer-Verlag, 1985.

Friedberg SR. The neurosurgeon's approach to pain. In Aronoff GM. Evaluation and Treatment of Chronic Pain, pp 319–331. Baltimore, Urban & Schwarzenberg, 1985.

Frost EAM. Clinical Anesthesia in Neurosurgery. Boston, Butterworths, 1984.

Halstead LS, Grabois M, and Howland CA. Medical Rehabilitation. New York, Raven Press, 1985.

Heldick-Smith M. Neurological Problems in the Elderly. Philadelphia, Baillière Tindall, 1985.

Henning RS and Jackson DL. Handbook of Critical Care Neurology and Neurosurgery. New York, Praeger Scientific, 1985.

Henry GL and Little N. Neurologic Emergencies: A Symptom-Oriented Approach. New York, McGraw Hill, 1985.

Hintgen TL and Mueller PB. Communicating with Aphasic Adults: A Guide for Families and Caregivers. Springfield, Illinois, Charles C Thomas, 1983.

Hooper CR and Dunkle RE. The Older Aphasic Person. Rockville, Maryland, Aspen Systems Corp, 1984.

Illis LS, Sedgwick EM, and Glanville HJ. Rehabilitation of the Neurological Patient. Boston, Blackwell Scientific, 1982.

Kaplan PE and Cerullo LJ. Stroke Rehabilitation. Boston, Butterworths, 1986.

Liechty RD and Soper RT. Neurological Surgery. In Nishioka H (ed). Synopsis of Surgery. St Louis, CV Mosby, 1985.

Lubbock G. Stroke Care: An Interdisciplinary Approach. Boston, Faber & Faber, 1983.

Lundgren J. Acute Neuroscience Nursing: Concepts and Care. Boston, Jones & Bartlett, 1986.

Mohr JP. Manual of Clinical Problems in Neurology. Boston, Little, Brown, 1984.

Neurologic Disorders, Springhouse, Pennsylvania, Springhouse Corp, 1984.

Pallett PJ and O'Brien MT. Textbook of Neurological Nursing. Boston, Little, Brown & Co, 1985.

Pearlman AL and Collins RC. Neurological Pathophysiology. New York, Oxford University Press, 1984.

Regan PA (ed). Teaching Guides for Patients with Neurologic Disorders. Reston, Virginia, Reston Publishing Co, 1984.

Rudy EB Advanced Neurological and Neurosurgical Nursing. St Louis, CV Mosby, 1984.

Ruskin A. Section I Stroke. Current Therapy in Physiatry, Physical Medicine and Rehabilitation, pp 5–81. Philadelphia, WB Saunders, 1984.

Samuels MA. Manual of Neurologic Therapeutics. Boston, Little, Brown Co, 1986.

Skinner PH and Shelton RL. Speech, Language and Hearing: Normal Processes and Disorders, 2nd ed. New York, John Wiley & Sons, 1985.

Smith G and Covino BG. Acute Pain. Boston, Butterworths, 1985.

Smith RR (ed). Stroke and the Extracranial Vessels. New York, Raven Press, 1984.

Spetzler RF et al. Cerebral Revascularization for Stroke. New York, Thieme-Stratton, 1985.

Tindall GT, Barrow DL, and Martin JB. Disorders of the Pituitary. St Louis, CV Mosby, 1986.

Toole JF. Cerebrovascular Disorders, 3rd ed. New York, Raven Press, 1984.

Umphred DA. Neurological Rehabilitation. St Louis, CV Mosby, 1985.

Vogt G, Miller M, and Esluer M. Mosby's Manual of Neurological Care. St Louis, CV Mosby, 1985.

Wade DT et al. Stroke: A Critical Approach to Diagnosis, Treatment and Management. London, Chapman & Hall, 1985.

Wall PD and Melzack R. Textbook of Pain. New York, Churchill Livingstone, 1984.

Wilkins RH and Rengachary SS. Neurosurgery. New York, McGraw-Hill, 1985.

Youmans JR (ed). Neurological Surgery. Philadelphia, WB Saunders, 1982.

Articles

(Asterisks indicate nursing research articles.)

Care of the Neurosurgical Patient

Boortz-Marx R. Factors affecting intracranial pressure: A descriptive study. J Neurosurg Nurs 1985 Apr; 17(2):89–94.

Bunt TJ and Haynes JL. Carotid endarterectomy. Am Surg 1985 Feb; 51(2):61–69.

Cammermeyer M. A growth model of self-care for neurologically impaired people. J Neurosurg Nurs 1983 Oct; 15(5):299–305.

Cerullo LJ and Burke LP. Use of the laser in neurosurgery. Surg Clin North Am 1984 Oct; 64(5):995–1000.

Diaz FG. Extracranial-intracranial bypasses J Vasc Surg 1985 Jan; 2(1): 224–236.

Gruca JK. Oncology rehabilitation. Rehabil Nurs 1984 May/June; 9(3): 27–30.

Hendrickson S. Psychological care of the patient with neurological dysfunction. J Neurosurg Nurs 1984 Aug; 16(4):202–207.

Hickey JV and McKenna JE. Effective discharge planning and the neurosurgical nurse. J Neurosurg Nurs 1984 Apr; 16(2):101–106.

Kennedy DW et al. Transsphenoidal approach to the sella: The Johns Hopkins experience. Laryngoscope 1984 Aug; 94(8):1066–1071.

Kruger LB. Complications of transsphenoidal surgery. J Neurosurg Nurs 1985 June; 17(3):179–183.

Landolt AM (ed). Complications in neurosurgery. Prog Neurol Surg 1984; 1:1–164.

Lee KJ, Goodrich I, and Pensak M. Pituitary surgery: Current status, including transsphenoidal surgery. Am J Otolaryngol 1984 Nov/Dec; 5(2):138–150.

Lusby RJ and Wylie EJ. Complications of carotid endarterectomy. Surg Clin North Am 1983 Dec; 63(6):1293–1302.

McCash AM. Meeting the challenge of craniotomy care. RN 1985 July; 48(6):26–33.

Myers DL and Sataloff RT. Spinal fluid leakage after skull base surgical procedures. Otolaryngol Clin North Am 1984 Aug; 17(3):601–612.

*Resio MJ. Nursing diagnosis: Alteration in oral/nasal mucous membranes related to trauma of transsphenoidal surgery. J Neurosci Nurs 1986 June; 18(3):112–115.

Robertson JB. Carotid endarterectomy. Neurol Clin 1985 Feb; 1(1):119–129.

Rovit RL, Murali R, and Rosiello A. Management of patients following brain tumor surgery: I, II. Contemp Neurosurg 1986; 8(10):1–6; 8(11):1–6.

Thames B and Luedtke M. Trends in neurosurgery. Today's OR Nurse 1984 Dec; 6(12):20–32.

Watson CA, Ross JE, and Ramsey M. Identification of neurosurgical patients susceptible to pulmonary infection. J Neurosurg Nurs 1983 June; 16(3):123–127.

Intracranial Pressure and Intracranial Pressure Monitoring

Boortz-Marx R. Factors affecting intracranial pressure: A descriptive study. J Neurosurg Nurs 1985 Apr; 17(2):89–94.

Gaab MR and Heissler HE. ICP monitoring. Crit Rev Biomed Eng 1984; 11(3):189–250.

Hinkle JL. Treating traumatic coma. Am J Nurs 1986 May; 86(5):551–556.

Horner AJ and Mechsner WK. Bedside insertion of ICP monitoring devices. Crit Care Nurse 1985 July/Aug; 5(4):21–27.

Landy HJ et al. An improved subarachnoid screw for intracranial pressure monitoring. J Neurosurg 1984 Sept; 61(3):606–608.

Levin AB, Kahn AR, and Bahr DE. Epidural intracranial pressure monitoring: A new system. Med Instrum 1983 July/Aug; 17(4):293–296.

Marcotty SF and Levin AB. A new approach in epidural intracranial pressure monitoring. J Neurosurg Nurs 1984 Feb; 16(1):54–59.

Mitchell PH. Decreased adaptive capacity, intracranial: A proposal for a nursing diagnosis. J Neurosci Nurs 1986 Aug; 18(4):170–175.

Quandt CM and de los Reyes RA. Pharmacologic management of acute intracranial hypertension. Drug Intell Clin Pharm 1984 Feb; 18(2):105–112.

Robinet K. Increased intracranial pressure: Management with an intraventricular catheter. J Neurosurg Nurs 1985 Apr; 17(2):95–104.

Shields CB, McGraw P, and Garretson HD. Accurate intracranial pressure monitoring. Neurosurgery 1984 May; 14(5):592–593.

Villanueva PA. Simplified technique for subdural pressure monitoring: Technical note. Neurosurgery 1985 Feb; 16(2):238–240.

Pain

*Dolphin NW. Neuroanatomy and neurophysiology of pain: Nursing implications. Int J Nurs Stud 1983; 20(4):255–263.

Foley KM. The treatment of cancer pain. N Engl J Med 1985 July 11; 313(2):84–95.

Jacobson LJ. Intrathecal and extradural narcotics. Adv Pain Res Ther 1984; 4:199–236.

Krames ES et al. Continuous infusion of spinally administered narcotics for the relief of pain due to malignant disorders. Cancer 1985 Aug 1; 56(3):696–702.

Kumar K and Wyant GM. Deep brain stimulation for alleviating chronic intractable pain. Can J Surg 1985 Jan; 28(1):20–22.

Malone BT, Beye R, and Walker J. Management of pain in the terminally ill by administration of epidural narcotics. Cancer 1985 Jan 15; 55(2):438–440.

Moore DE and Blacker HM. How effective is TENS for chronic pain? Am J Nurs 1983 Aug; 83(8):1175–1177.

Onofrio BM. Treatment of chronic pain of malignant origin with intrathecal opiates. Clin Neurosurg 1983; 31:304–315.

Pagni CA. Role of neurosurgery in cancer pain: Reevaluation of old methods and new trends. Adv Pain Res Ther 1984; 7:603–629.

Penn RD. Drug pumps for treatment of neurologic diseases. Neurol Clin 1985 May; 3(2):439–451.

Richardson DE. Intracranial stimulation for the control of chronic pain. Clin Neurosurg 1983; 31:316–322.

Siegfried J, Kühner A, and Sturm V. Neurosurgical treatment of cancer pain. Recent Results Cancer Res 1984; 89:146–156.

Spross JA. Cancer pain and suffering: Clinical lessons from life, literature and legend. Oncol Nurs Forum 1985 July/Aug; 12(4):23–31.

Taylor AG. How effective is TENS for acute pain? Am J Nurs 1983 Aug; 83(8):1171–1174.

Wang JK. Intrathecal morphine for intractable pain secondary to cancer of pelvic organs. Pain 1985 Jan; 21(1):99–102.

Williams AE. Deep brain stimulation—A contemporary methodology for chronic pain. J Neurosurg Nurs 1984 Feb; 16(1):1–9.

Yablonski-Peretz T et al. Continuous epidural narcotic analgesia for intractable pain due to malignancy. J Surg Oncol 1985 May 1; 29(1):8–10.

Zenz M. Epidural opiates for the treatment of cancer pain. Recent Results Cancer Res 1984; 89:107–114.

Stroke

Ahlsiö B et al. Disablement and quality of life after stroke. Stroke 1984 Sept/Oct; 15(5):886–890.

Alkalay L and Wasserman M. Cerebrovascular accidents: Care and rehabilitation. Practitioner 1983 Mar; 227(1377):469–473.

*Axelsson K, Norberg A, and Asplund K. Eating after a stroke—towards an integrated view. Int J Nurs Stud 1984; 21(2):93–99.

Bunt TJ and Haynes JL. Carotid endarterectomy. Am Surg 1985 Feb; 51(2):61–69.

Field D, Cordle CJ, and Bowman GS. Coping with stroke at home. Int Rehabil Med 1983; 5(2):96–100.

Golper LAC. Clinical procedures with communicatively impaired stroke victims. Stroke 1984 Nov/Dec; 15(6):1077–1080.

Gorelick PB. Alcohol and stroke. Curr Concepts Cerebrovasc Dis Stroke 1986 Sept/Oct; 21(5):21–25.

Grotta JC et al. Does platelet antiaggregant therapy lessen the severity of stroke? Neurology 1985 May; 35(5):632–636.

Howard G et al. Factors influencing return to work following cerebral infarction. JAMA 1985 Jan 11; 253(2):226–232.

Johnson VM and Keister M. Early rehabilitation for stroke: A new look. Arch Phys Med Rehabil 1984 Aug; 65(8):437–441.

Kase CS. Intracerebral hemorrhage: Common nonhypertensive causes. Curr Concepts Cerebrovasc Dis Stroke 1985 July/Aug; 20(4):19–24.

Kelly JF and Winograd CH. A functional approach to stroke management in elderly patients. J Am Geriatr Soc 1985 Jan; 33(1):48–60.

Kistler JP, Ropper AH, and Heros RC. Therapy of ischemic cerebral vascular disease due to atherothrombosis. N Engl J Med 1984 July 12; 311(2):100–105.

Konikow NS. Alterations in movement: Nursing assessment and implications. J Neurosurg Nurs 1985 Feb; 17(1):61–65.

Kuller LH and Sutton KC. Carotid artery bruits: Is it safe and effective to auscultate the neck? Stroke 1984 Nov/Dec; 15(6):944–947.

Liang MH et al. Management of functional disability in homebound patients. J Fam Pract 1983 Sept; 17(3):429–435.

Longstreth WT and Swanson PD. Oral contraceptives and stroke. Stroke 1984 July/Aug; 15(4):747–750.

Loustau A and Lee KA. Dealing with the dangers of dysphagia. Nurs '85 1985 Feb; 15(2):47–50.

Lusby RJ and Wylie EJ. Complications of carotid endarterectomy. Surg Clin North Am 1983 Dec; 63(6):1293–1302.

Management of stroke: 12 hours to 2 months. Drug Ther Bull 1985 Feb 11; 213(3):9–12.

Mumma CM. Perceived losses following stroke. Rehabil Nurs 1986 May/June; 11(3):19–24.

Ozuna J. Alterations in mentation: Nursing assessment and intervention. J Neurosurg Nurs 1985 Feb; 17(1):66–79.

Rivera VM. Stroke: A guide to differential diagnosis and prevention. Postgrad Med 1985 Mar; 77(4):81–88.

Rizk TE et al. Arthrographic studies in painful hemiplegic shoulders. Arch Phys Med Rehabil 1984 May; 65(5):254–256.

Robinson RG, Lipsey JR, and Pearlson GD. The occurrence and treatment of poststroke mood disorders. Compr Ther 1984 Sept; 10(9):19–24.

Rottkamp BC. A holistic approach to identifying factors associated with an altered pattern of urinary elimination in stroke patients. J Neurosurg Nurs 1985 Feb; 17(1):37–44.

Ruskin AP. Understanding stroke and its rehabilitation. Stroke 1983 May/June; 14(3):438–442.

Sage JI. The use and overuse of heparin in therapeutic trials. Arch Neurol 1985 Apr; 42(4):315–317.

Scherokman BJ and Hallenbeck JM. Management of acute stroke. Am Fam Physician 1985 Mar; 31(3):190–199.

Sundt TM et al. Results, complications, and follow-up of 415 bypass operations for occlusive disease of the carotid system. Mayo Clin Proc 1984 Apr; 60(4):230–240.

Sutherland GR and Barr HWK. Postoperative complications following carotid endarterectomy and their management. Int Anesthesiol Clin 1984 Fall; 22(3):165–173.

Taylor JW. Nursing management of stroke: I. Acute care. Cardiovasc Nurs 1985 Jan/Feb; 21(1):1–5.

Wald ME. Cerebral thrombosis: Assessment and nursing management of the acute phase. J Neurosci Nurs 1986 Feb; 18(1):36–38.

Wolf, PA, Kannel WB, and Verter J. Current status of risk factors for stroke. Neurol Clin 1983 Feb; 1(1):317–343.

Wyness MA. Perceptual dysfunction: Nursing assessment and management. J Neurosurg Nurs 1985 Apr; 17(2):105–110.

Yarnell P. Stroke rehabilitation. Curr Concepts Cerebrovasc Dis Stroke 1986 May/June; 21(3):9–13.

Unconscious Patient/Coma

Allan D. Glasgow Coma Scale. Nurs Mirror 1984 June; 158(23):32–34.

Bates D. Predicting recovery from medical coma. Br J Hosp Med 1985 May; 33(5):276–280.

Cameron-Barry J et al. Overcoming acute complications in the unconscious patient. Nurs '84 1984 May; 14(5):42–45.

Chang G. Emergency evaluation of the comatose patient. Hosp Pract 1984 Jan; 19(1):182–183, 186.

Crigger NJ and Strickland CC. Selecting a nursing diagnosis for changes in consciousness. Dimens Crit Care Nurs 1985 May/June; 4(3):156–163.

Fitzgerald FT, Tierney LM, and Wall SD. The comatose patient. Postgrad Med 1983 July; 74(1):207–215.

Hahn AL. Stupor and coma: A clinical approach. Geriatrics 1983 July; 38(7):65–67; 71–73.

Hinkle JL. Treating traumatic coma. Am J Nurs 1986 May; 86(5):551–555.

Levy DE et al. Predicting outcome from hypoxic-ischemic coma. JAMA 1985 Mar 8; 253(10):1420–1426.

Marrubini MB. Classification of coma. Intensive Care Med 1984; 10(5):217–226.

Miller BL and McIntyre HB. Evaluation of the comatose patient. Primary Care 1984 Dec; 11(4):693–706.

RN Master care plan: The patient in a coma. RN 1985 Apr; 48(4):33.

Scherer P. Assessment: The logic of coma. Am J Nurs 1986 May; 86(5):541–550.

Stolarik A. What the comatose patient can tell you. RN 1985 Apr; 48(4):26–33, 66.

Wong J, Wong S, and Dempster IK. Care of the unconscious patient: A problem-oriented approach. J Neurosurg Nurs 1984 June; 16(3):145–150.

Wyndaele JJ. Micturition in comatose patients. J Urol 1986 June; 135(6):1209–1211.

Agencies and Sources of Information

Aphasia and Stroke

National Institute of Neurological and Communicative Disorders and Stroke, National Institutes of Health, Bethesda, Maryland 20892.

American Speech-Language-Hearing Association, 10801 Rockville Pike, Rockville, Maryland 20852.

American Heart Association, 7320 Greenville Avenue, Dallas, Texas 75231.

National Easter Seal Society, 2023 West Ogden Avenue, Chicago, Illinois 60612.

The Stroke Foundation, 898 Park Avenue, New York, New York 10021.

Will Rogers Institute, 785 Mamaroneck Avenue, White Plains, New York 10605.

Pain

A directory of pain clinics is available from The American Society of Anesthesiologists, 515 Busse Highway, Park Ridge, Illinois 60068.

Chapter 54

Management of Patients With Neurologic Disorders

Headache

Possibly the most common of all human afflictions is headache or *cephalgia* ("condition of head pain"). Headache may arise from a variety of sources due to a variety of mechanisms, such as vascular spasms caused by muscle contraction or inflammation of pain-sensitive structures inside or outside the skull. Most headaches are not caused by structural diseases but are a symptom of the patient's problems in coping with or adapting to a life situation.

Assessment

The physical examination includes a careful history, a physical assessment of the head and neck, a neurologic examination of the cranial nerves, evaluation of the size and reactions of the pupils, a funduscopic examination of the eyes, and a test of motor and sensory systems. For patients with abnormalities on the neurologic examination, computed tomography is employed to detect underlying causes such as tumors, aneurysms, and displacements of the ventricular system. Other diagnostic tests are indicated for patients with persisting or disabling pain.

When data are obtained for the nursing history, patients should be given a chance to describe their headache *in their own words* as related to the following questions:

- How old were you when these headaches started? Under what circumstances did they start?
- What is the location? Is it unilateral or bilateral? Does it radiate?
- What is the quality—dull, aching, steady, boring, burning, intermittent, continuous, paroxysmal?
- How many headaches occur during a given time?
- Are there any precipitating factors (environmental, such as sunlight and weather change; foods; exertion, other)?
- What makes the headache worse (coughing, straining)?
- What time (day/night) does it occur?
- Are there any associated symptoms (facial pain, lacrimation, scotomas (blind spots in field of vision)?
- What usually relieves the headache (aspirin, ergot preparation, food, heat, rest, neck massage)?
- Is there nausea, vomiting, weakness, numbness in the extremities?
- Does the headache interfere with your daily activities?
- Do you have any allergies?
- Do you have insomnia, poor appetite, loss of energy?
- Is there a family history of headache? "sick" headache?
- What is the relationship of the headache to the life-style: physical/emotional stress?
- What is your medication history?

Vascular Headaches

Vascular headaches result from dilation, compression, edema, or inflammation of the intracranial or extracranial arteries.

Migraine

Migraine is a symptom-complex characterized by periodic unilateral (or generalized) attacks of severe headache. The cause of migraine has not been clearly demonstrated, but it is primarily a vascular disturbance that occurs more commonly in women, the highest incidence being reached during hormonally active reproductive years. A positive family history is present in 90% of patients with migraine.

Clinical Manifestations and Pathophysiology. A "preheadache" phase or an "aura" (warning sign) may occur, forewarning the patient of an impending attack and providing enough time to take the prescribed medication in order to avert a full-blown attack. The aura may be in the form of visual, sensory, or motor symptoms. These sensations preceding the headache are described at times as "scintillating scotomata" or "visual field defects," and are attributed to vasoconstriction and ischemia within the cerebral cortex and possibly also in the retina. Other neurologic phenomena preceding the attacks include paresis of an extremity, aphasia, or confusion.

The cerebral symptoms and signs of migraine are the results of cortical ischemia of varying degree. The typical attack begins with vasoconstriction affecting the arteries of the scalp and certain cerebral or retinal vessels. The patient appears pale and may experience sensory, motor, and mood

disturbances. Extracranial and intracranial blood vessels dilate, causing pain and discomfort. Studies suggest that the dilated artery becomes hyperpermeable and that sterile local inflammatory reactions occur in the vicinity of the painful, dilated arteries. It is proposed that vasoactive substances (histamine, serotonin, plasmokinins) participate in this sterile inflammatory reaction.

The pain begins in the areas around the eyes (supraorbital, retro-orbital) or the temples. It starts on one side and increases in such intensity that the patient is prostrated, frequently with nausea and vomiting. The attack may last 2 hours to several days. Sleep tends to relieve the symptoms.

Management of Acute Attack. The objective of management during an acute attack is to prevent the painful dilation of cranial vessels. Ergotamine preparations (taken orally, sublingually, subcutaneously, intramuscularly, by rectum, or by inhalation) may be effective in aborting the headache if taken *early* in the migraine process. Ergotamine tartrate acts on smooth muscle, causing prolonged constriction of the cranial blood vessels. Each patient's dosage is titrated according to individual needs. Side-effects include aching muscles, paresthesias, nausea, and vomiting. During the acute attack, the patient may find relief by lying quietly in a darkened room with the head slightly elevated. Drinking black coffee may also be helpful in counteracting the attack. Symptomatic therapy for migraine includes analgesics, sedatives, and antianxiety agents.

Management Between Attacks. Methysergide is an effective prophylactic agent in preventing frequent and severe migraine attacks. It is thought to inhibit or block the effects of serotonin, a substance possibly involved in the mechanism of vascular headaches. Troublesome side-effects include abdominal discomfort, muscle cramps, edema, numbness, tingling of extremities, and depression. There should be a medication-free interval after every 6-month course of treatment because of the potential complication of retroperitoneal fibrosis and pleuropulmonary and cardiac fibrosis.

Beta-blocking drugs, like propranolol, stop the activities of beta receptors—cells in the heart and brain that control the dilation of blood vessels. The ability of beta blockers to halt the dilation of blood vessels in the brain is believed to be a major reason for their antimigraine action. Cyproheptadine hydrochloride (Periactin), which is an antagonist to serotonin and histamine, reduces the severity of pain in some patients and also prevents headache.

Antidepressants, barbiturates, and tranquilizers may help the patient to cope with stress. Because of the diversity of treatment for migraine, the patient must be treated on an individual basis and followed closely.

Nursing Interventions/Patient Education. The first step in assessing the problem is to review the findings of the physical examination and the neurologic evaluation. A survey of social, environmental, and personality factors is helpful. Although there is a wide variation in the personality types of those who are subject to migraine, there is evidence that the hard-driving, somewhat compulsive perfectionist is most vulnerable to this condition.

Patients can be helped to develop insight into their feelings, behavior, and conflicts and to make the necessary modifications in life-style on the basis of these analyses. Regular periods of exercise and relaxation are suggested, and any offending or provoking factors (allergens, fatigue, foods, environmental stresses) are removed or reduced in order to obtain relief.

Certain foods containing tyramine, monosodium glutamate, milk products, or nitrite (aged cheese, chocolate, many processed foods) may trigger headaches. Potential headache-causing substances should be avoided. Long intervals between meals should also be avoided. Advise the patient to awaken at the same time each day, as disruption in the normal sleeping pattern provokes a migraine in many patients. Birth control pills will increase the frequency and severity of the attacks in some women.

A record may be kept of the circumstances surrounding the attack (*e.g.*, activities, food, feelings) to determine if there is a pattern to the migraine episodes. If so, a change in the pattern may help avoid the attacks.

The National Migraine Foundation* provides a list of clinics in the U.S. and the names of physicians in specific areas who specialize in headache and who are members of the American Association for the Study of Headache.

Cluster Headache

Cluster headaches are another severe form of vascular headache. They are seen most frequently in men. The attacks come in "clusters" or groups, with excruciating pain localized in the eye and orbit and radiating to the facial and temporal regions. The pain is accompanied by watering of the eye and nasal congestion. Each attack lasts from 15 minutes to 2 hours and may have a crescendo–decrescendo pattern.

One theory is that this type of headache is due to dilatation of orbital and nearby extracranial arteries. Cluster headaches may be precipitated by alcohol, nitrites, vasodilators, and histamines. Eliminating these factors helps in preventing the headaches. Cluster headache responds to vasoconstricting agents (ergotamine tartrate). The serotonin antagonist methysergide and the beta-blocker propranolol may also give relief. Chlorpromazine may also be effective. Inhalation of 100% oxygen eases the pain of cluster headache by reducing blood flow to the brain.

Cranial Arteritis

Inflammation of the cranial arteries is characterized by a severe headache localized in the region of the temporal arteries. The inflammation may be generalized, in which cranial arteritis is part of a vascular disease, or of a focal type, in which only the cranial arteries are involved. Cranial arteritis is a cause of headache in the older population, reaching its greatest incidence in those over age 70.

Often the disease begins with general manifestations, such as fatigue, malaise, weight loss, and fever. Clinical manifestations associated with inflammation (heat, redness, swelling, tenderness, or pain over the involved artery) are usually present. Sometimes a tender, swollen, or nodular temporal artery is visible. Visual problems are caused by ischemia of the involved structures.

Cranial arteritis is thought to represent an immune vasculitis in which immune complexes are deposited within the walls of affected blood vessels, producing vascular injury and

---

* 15252 Western Avenue, Chicago, Illinois 60625.

inflammation. The involved artery may be biopsied to confirm or refute diagnosis.

Treatment consists of early administration of a corticosteroid drug to prevent the possibility of loss of vision due to vascular occlusion or rupture of the involved artery. The patient is instructed not to stop the medication abruptly because this can lead to relapse. Analgesic agents are given for comfort.

Tension Headache (Muscle Contraction Headache)

Emotional or physical stress may cause contraction of the muscles in the neck and scalp, resulting in tension headache. The headache may be characterized by a steady, constant feeling of pressure that usually begins in the forehead, the temple, or the back of the neck. It is often bandlike or may be described as "a weight on top of my head." Tension headaches tend to be more chronic than severe and are probably the most common type of headache. The patient needs reassurance that the headache is not due to a brain tumor. This is a common unspoken fear. Symptomatic relief may be obtained by local heat, massage, analgesics, antidepressants, and muscle relaxants.

Nursing Interventions

A discussion of the patient's problems (instead of the headache) can be very helpful. To obtain long-term relief, the person needs to understand the source of any emotional conflicts and attempt to change or adapt to stressful and anxiety-producing situations. This requires supportive counseling and education, including biofeedback and relaxation techniques. (Cognitive restructuring teaches people to change their attitudes to stress.)

The nurse's role is one of supportive care during physical or emotional distress, listening, giving instructions, and positive reinforcement so that a beneficial outcome will be achieved. "Use moderation in all things" is appropriate counseling.

Brain Tumors

A brain tumor is a localized intracranial lesion that occupies space within the skull and tends to cause a rise in intracranial pressure. In adults, the majority of brain tumors originate from *glial cells*. (Glial cells generally make up the structure and support system of the brain and spinal cord.) The highest incidence of brain tumors in adults occurs in the fifth, sixth, and seventh decades, and the majority of these are *supratentorial* (above the covering of the cerebellum) in location. Brain tumors rarely metastasize outside the central nervous system but cause death by impairing vital functions, either by direct involvement or by increasing intracranial pressure.

Classification

Brain tumors may be classified into several groups: (1) those arising from the coverings of the brain, such as the dural meningioma; (2) those developing in or on the cranial nerves, best exemplified by the acoustic neuroma and the optic nerve spongioblastoma polare; (3) those originating in the brain tissue, such as the various gliomas; and (4) metastatic lesions originating elsewhere in the body. (See Chart 54-1.) The major concerns are the location and the histological character of the tumor. Tumors may be benign or malignant. However, because a benign tumor may occur in a vital area, it may have effects as serious as those of a malignant tumor.

Specific Tumors

Gliomas. The malignant glioma is the brain neoplasm most frequently seen. Usually, these tumors cannot be totally removed because they spread by infiltrating into the surrounding neural tissue.

Pituitary Adenomas. The *pituitary gland*, also called the *hypophysis*, is a relatively small gland located in the sella turcica. It is attached to the hypothalamus by a short stalk (hypophyseal stalk) and is divided into two lobes: the anterior (adenohypophysis) and the posterior (neurohypophysis). The anterior lobe secretes growth hormone (GH), adrenocorticotrophic hormone (ACTH), thyroid-stimulating hormone (TSH), prolactin and the gonadotropic hormones, follicle-stimulating hormone (FSH), and luteinizing hormone (LH).

Chart 54-1
Classification of Brain Tumors

Tumors Originating in the Brain Tissue
Gliomas—infiltrating tumors that may invade any portion of the brain; most common type of brain tumor
  Astrocytomas (grades 1 and 2)
  Glioblastomas (grades 3 and 4 astrocytomas)
  Ependymomas
  Medulloblastomas
  Oligodendrogliomas
  Colloid cysts
  } Subclassified according to cell type

Tumors Arising From Covering of Brain
Meningioma—encapsulated, well-defined, growing outside the brain tissue; compresses rather than invades brain

Tumors Developing in or on the Cranial Nerves
Acoustic neuroma—derived from sheath of acoustic nerve
Optic nerve spongioblastoma polare

Metastatic Lesions
Most commonly from lung and breast

Tumors of the Ductless Glands
Pituitary
Pineal

Blood Vessel Tumors
Hemangioblastoma
Angioma

Congenital Tumors

The posterior pituitary stores and releases antidiuretic hormone (vasopressin) and oxytocin.

Pituitary tumors may cause symptoms due to mass (pressure) effects on adjacent structures or to hormonal effects (hyperfunction or hypofunction) of the pituitary. The mass effects of adenomas of the pituitary gland are caused by pressure on the optic nerves, optic chiasm, or optic tracts, or on the hypothalamus or the third ventricle when the tumors invade the cavernous sinuses or expand into the sphenoid bone. These pressure effects produce headache, visual dysfunction, hypothalamic disorders (*e.g.*, of sleep, appetite, temperature, emotions), increased intracranial pressure, and enlargement and erosion of the sella turcica.

Functioning pituitary tumors can produce one or more hormones normally produced by the anterior pituitary. These hormones may cause prolactin-secreting pituitary adenomas (prolactinomas), growth hormone-secreting pituitary adenomas that produce acromegaly in adults, and ACTH-producing pituitary adenomas that give rise to Cushing's disease. Adenomas secreting TSH or FSH-LH occur infrequently, while adenomas that produce both growth hormone and prolactin are relatively common.

The female patient whose pituitary gland is secreting excessive quantities of prolactin will present with amenorrhea and/or *galactorrhea* (excessive or spontaneous flow of milk). Male patients with prolactinomas may present with impotence and hypogonadism.

Acromegaly, caused by excess growth hormone, produces enlargement of the hands and feet, distortion of the facial features, and peripheral nerve entrapment syndromes.

The clinical features of Cushing's disease, a condition associated with prolonged overproduction of cortisol, include a form of obesity with redistribution of fat to the facial, supraclavicular, and abdominal areas, hypertension, purple striae and ecchymoses, osteoporosis, glucose intolerance, and emotional disorders.

The majority of pituitary adenomas are treated by transsphenoidal microsurgical removal (see p. 1458), while the remainder of tumors that cannot be removed completely are treated by radiation.

Angiomas. Brain angiomas (masses composed largely of abnormal blood vessels) are found either in or on the surface of the brain. Some persist throughout life without causing symptoms; other give rise to symptoms of brain tumor. Occasionally, the diagnosis is suggested by the presence of another angioma somewhere in the head or by a *bruit* (an abnormal sound) audible over the skull. Since the walls of the blood vessels in angiomas are thin, a cerebral vascular accident (stroke) frequently occurs. In fact, cerebral hemorrhage in persons under 40 years of age should suggest the possibility of an angioma.

Acoustic Neuroma. An acoustic neuroma is a tumor of the eighth cranial nerve, the nerve of hearing and balance. It usually arises just within the internal auditory meatus, where it frequently expands before filling the cerebellopontine recess.

An acoustic neuroma may grow slowly and attain a considerable size before it is correctly diagnosed. The patient usually experiences loss of hearing, tinnitus, and episodes of vertigo and staggering. As the tumor becomes larger, painful sensations of the face may occur on the same side as a result of the tumor's compressing the fifth cranial nerve.

With improved radiologic techniques and the use of the

operating microscope and microsurgical instrumentation, even large tumors can be removed through a relatively small craniotomy.

Clinical Manifestations

Brain tumors produce clinical manifestations when they cause increased intracranial pressure or produce localizing symptoms and signs as a result of the tumor interfering with specific regions of the brain.

Increasing Intracranial Pressure Symptoms. Symptoms of increased intracranial pressure (ICP) are caused by a gradual compression of the brain due to the growth of the tumor. The effect is to disrupt the equilibrium that exists between the brain, the cerebrospinal fluid, and the cerebral blood—all located within the skull. As the tumor grows, adjustment may occur through compression of intracranial veins, through reduction of cerebrospinal fluid volume (by increased absorption or decreased production), through a modest decrease of cerebral blood flow, and through reduction of intra- and extracellular brain tissue mass. When these compensatory mechanisms fail, the patient develops signs and symptoms of increased intracranial pressure.

The most common symptoms produced by this pressure are headache, vomiting, *papilledema* (choked disc or edema of the optic nerve) with associated blurring of vision and diplopia, and stupor. Headache, though not always present, is most common in the early morning and is made worse by coughing, straining, or sudden movement. It is thought to be caused by the tumor's invading, compressing, or distorting the pain-sensitive structures or by the edema that accompanies the tumor.

Headaches are usually described as deep or expanding or as dull but unrelenting. Frontal tumors usually produce a bilateral frontal headache; pituitary gland tumors produce pain radiating between the two temples (bitemporal); in cerebellar tumors the headache may be located in the suboccipital region at the back of the head.

Vomiting, seldom related to food intake, is usually due to irritation of the vagal centers in the medulla. If the vomiting is of the forceful type, it is described as "projectile" vomiting.

Papilledema (edema of the optic nerve) is present in a larger percentage of patients and can lead to impaired vision.

Localizing Symptoms. Localizing symptoms occur when specific regions of the brain are disrupted, resulting in locally referable signs, such as sensory and motor abnormalities, visual alterations, and convulsive seizures.

Because the functions of the different parts of the brain are known, the location of the tumor can be determined, in part, by identifying functions that are affected by the presence of the tumor. For example, a tumor of the motor cortex manifests itself by causing convulsive movements localized to one side of the body, spoken of as *Jacksonian seizures.* Tumors of the occipital lobe cause blindness in half of each eye (*hemianopsia*) by involving the centers of the tracts for vision of one side of the brain. Tumors of the cerebellum cause dizziness, a staggering gait with a tendency to fall toward the side of the lesion, marked muscle incoordination, and *nystagmus* (rhythmical vibration of the eyeballs). Tumors of the frontal lobe frequently produce personality disorders, changes in emotional state and behavior, and a disinterested mental attitude. The patient often becomes extremely untidy and careless and may use obscene speech.

Personality changes, confusion, speech dysfunction, and disturbances of gait appear to be seen more frequently in elderly patients with intracranial tumors. The most frequent tumor types in the elderly are meningiomas, glioblastomas, and cerebral metastases from other sites.

Tumors of the cerebellopontine angle usually originate in the sheath of the acoustic nerve and give rise to a sequence of symptoms that is the most characteristic of all brain tumor symptomatology. First, tinnitus and vertigo appear, soon followed by progressive nerve deafness (eighth nerve dysfunction); next, there are numbness and tingling of the face and the tongue (due to involvement of the fifth nerve); still later, weakness or paralysis of the face develops (seventh nerve involvement); and finally, since the enlarging tumor presses on the cerebellum, abnormalities in motor control may be present.

Many tumors are not so easily localized, because they lie in the so-called *silent areas* of the brain (*i.e.*, areas where functions are not definitely determined).

The *progression* of the signs and symptoms is important, because it indicates tumor growth and expansion.

Diagnostic Evaluation

The history of the illness and the manner in which the symptoms evolved are important. A neurologic examination indicates the areas of the central nervous system involved. To assist in the precise localization of the lesion, a battery of tests is performed. Computed tomography (CT) will give specific information concerning the number, size, and density of the lesion(s) and the extent of secondary cerebral edema. It also provides information about the ventricular system. The use of CT has resulted in the detection of smaller lesions. Computer-assisted stereotactic (three-dimensional) biopsy is being used to diagnose deep-seated brain tumors and to provide a basis for treatment and prognostic information. Cerebral angiography provides visualization of cerebral blood vessels and can localize most cerebral tumors.

A brain scan may be valuable, since an abnormal amount of radioactive material will accumulate in the area of the tumor and can be localized with a scintillation counter. An electroencephalogram can detect abnormal brain waves in regions occupied by the tumor and can enable evaluation of temporal lobe seizures. Echoencephalography can show whether certain structures have been displaced from the midline by a lesion in one hemisphere. Pneumoencephalography provides critical information in selected patients.

Cytologic studies of the cerebrospinal fluid may be done to detect malignant cells, because tumors of the central nervous system are capable of shedding cells into the cerebrospinal fluid.

Management

An untreated brain tumor ultimately leads to death, either from increasing intracranial pressure or from the brain damage it causes. Patients with possible brain tumor should be investigated and treated as soon as possible before irreversible damage occurs.

The objective of management is to remove all of the tumor or as much as possible without increasing the neurologic deficit (paralysis, blindness) or to achieve relief by partial tumor removal and by decompression, radiation, chemotherapy, or a combination of these. The majority of patients with brain tumors undergo a neurosurgical procedure, when possible, followed by radiation therapy and/or chemotherapy when indicated. Corticosteroids are highly effective in combating cerebral edema, thus allowing for a thorough diagnostic workup and a carefully planned surgical approach. (Also, appropriate dosages of corticosteroids treat postoperative swelling and facilitate a smoother, more rapid recovery.) In general, patients with meningiomas, acoustic neuromas, cystic astrocytomas of the cerebellum, colloid cyst of the third ventricle, congenital tumors such as dermoid cyst, and some of the granulomas can be cured by surgical removal of the tumor. A complete extirpation (removal) of the infiltrating gliomas is not possible. In these patients, the treatment consists of biopsy to establish the diagnosis; partial removal; decompression (relief of increased intracranial pressure) if necessary; and radiation therapy. Certain chemotherapeutic agents combined with radiation therapy are also being used. More recently, deep-seated brain tumors have been removed using the carbon dioxide laser with CT scanning and stereotactic techniques.

Intravenous autologous bone marrow transplantation is being investigated as a possible new technique because it has the potential to "rescue" the patient from the marrow toxicity associated with high dosages of drugs and radiation. A fraction of the patient's bone marrow is aspirated, usually from the iliac crest, and stored. The patient is exposed to large doses of chemoradiotherapy for the purpose of destroying large numbers of malignant cells. The patient's marrow is then reinfused intravenously after chemoradiotherapy is completed.

Radioisotopes (^{125}I) are being implanted directly into the brain tumor to permit high total doses of radiation to the localized tumor. With the use of sophisticated three-dimensional guidance systems with CT monitoring and computer graphics, the tumor can be visualized and interstitial radioisotopes precisely implanted (*brachytherapy*). This helps avoid radiation toxicity to the surrounding normal brain.

Newer drugs are continually being evaluated, and there is hope that these will eventually be more successful.

Nursing Interventions

The patient with a brain tumor may have problems with aspiration related to cranial nerve dysfunction. Preoperatively, the gag reflex and ability to swallow are evaluated. Before neurosurgery these needs are addressed by placing the patient upright to eat, offering a semisoft diet, and having suction readily available.

The problems of increased intracranial pressure caused by the tumor mass are reviewed on page 1416. The nurse performs neurologic checks, monitors vital signs, maintains a neurologic flow record, spaces nursing interventions to prevent rapid increase in ICP, and reorients the patient when necessary to person, time, and place. Patients with changes in cognition caused by the lesion will require frequent reorientation and the use of orienting devices (personal possessions, photographs, lists, clock), supervision of and assistance with self-care, and ongoing monitoring and intervention for prevention of injury. Patients with seizures are carefully monitored.

Motor function is checked at intervals because specific motor deficits may be involved, depending on the tumor's location. Sensory disturbances are assessed. The patient's speech function is evaluated. Eye movement and pupillary size and reaction may be affected by cranial nerve involvement.

The major treatment of brain tumor is surgery. The nursing process applied to the patient undergoing neurosurgery is found on page 1453.

Cerebral Metastases

A significant number of patients suffer central nervous system complications as a result of systemic cancer and neurologic deficits caused by cerebral metastases. Cancer of the lung commonly metastasizes to the brain, as do tumors of the breast, kidney, prostate gland, uterus, thyroid, skin (melanoma), and gastrointestinal tract.

Neurologic symptoms and signs include headache, disturbances of gait, deterioration of vision, personality changes, altered mentation (memory loss and confusion), focal weakness, paralysis, aphasia, and seizures. These problems can be devastating to both patient and family.

Management

The treatment is palliative and involves eliminating or reducing serious symptomatology. Bear in mind that, even when palliation is the goal, distressing signs and symptoms can be resolved, thereby improving the quality of life that remains. Patients with intracerebral metastases who are not treated have a steady downhill course with a very limited survival time.

The therapeutic approach includes radiation therapy, which is the foundation of treatment; surgery (usually for a single intracranial metastasis); chemotherapy; or a combination of these methods. Adrenocorticosteroid hormones may be helpful in relieving headache and alterations of consciousness. It is thought that adrenocorticosteroids (dexamethasone, prednisone) reduce inflammatory reaction around the metastatic deposits and decrease the edema surrounding them. Other drugs include osmotic agents (mannitol, glycerol) to decrease the water content of the brain, which leads to a decrease in intracranial pressure. Anticonvulsant drugs (phenytoin) are used to prevent and treat seizures. There have been encouraging results with nitrosourea compounds.

If the patient has severe pain, morphine can be infused into the epidural or subarachnoid space via a spinal needle and insertion of a catheter as near as possible to the spinal segment where the pain is projected. Small doses of morphine are injected into the system at prescribed intervals. (See p. 256.)

▶ Nursing Process
The Patient With Cerebral Metastases or Incurable Brain Tumor

▷ Assessment

The nursing assessment focuses on how the patient is functioning, moving and walking, adapting to weakness/paralysis, visual loss, and speech loss, and dealing with seizures.

A dietary history is taken to find out dietary intake and food intolerances and preferences. Anthropometric measurements will confirm the loss of subcutaneous fat and lean body mass. Biochemical measurements (albumin, transferrin, total lymphocyte count, creatinine index, and urinary tests) are reviewed to assess the degree of malnutrition, impaired cellular immunity, and electrolyte balance.

Cachexia (weak and emaciated condition) is seen in patients with metastases and is characterized by anorexia, pain, weight loss, altered metabolism, muscle weakness, malabsorption, and diarrhea. The patient may have altered taste sensation secondary to dysphagia, weakness, and depression. Smell distortions and diminution of smell (*anosmia*) frequently occur among these patients.

Assessment is made for symptoms that cause distress to the patient, including pain, respiratory problems, problems with elimination and urination, disturbances in sleep, and impairment of skin integrity, fluid balance, and temperature regulation. These problems may be caused by tumor invasion, compression, or obstruction.

The nurse may discuss with the social worker the impact of the patient's illness on the family in terms of home care, altered relationships, financial problems, time pressures, and intrafamily problems. This information is important in helping family members strengthen their coping skills.

▷ *Nursing Diagnoses*

Based on the assessment data, the patient's major problems may include the following:

- Self-care deficits related to loss/impairment of motor and sensory function and decreased cognitive abilities
- Alteration in nutrition—less than body requirements related to cachexia due to treatment and tumor effects, decreased nutritional intake, and malabsorption
- Anxiety related to fear in anticipation of death, uncertainty, change in appearance, discontinuity in life-style
- Potential alterations in family processes related to anticipatory grief and the burdens imposed by the care of the person with a terminal illness.

Other nursing diagnoses of the patient with cerebral metastases may include alteration in comfort (pain) related to tumor compression; impaired gas exchange related to dyspnea; alteration in bowel elimination (constipation) related to decreased fluid and dietary intake and medications; alteration in urinary elimination patterns related to reduced fluid intake, vomiting, and reactions to medications; sleep pattern disturbances related to discomfort and fear of dying; impairment of skin integrity related to cachexia, poor tissue perfusion, and decreased mobility; potential or actual fluid volume deficit related to fever, vomiting, and low fluid intake; impaired thermal regulation related to hypothalamic involvement, fever, and chills. The reader is referred to Chapter 16 for appropriate assessment and nursing interventions for these conditions.

▷ *Planning and Implementation*

▷ *Goals:* The goals of the patient may include compensating for self-care deficits, attaining improved nutrition, relief of anxiety, and enhancing of family coping skills.

Nursing Interventions

Compensating for Self-Care Deficits. The patient may have difficulty in participating in goal-setting as the tumor metastasizes and affects mental capabilities. Work with the family in keeping the patient mobile and at the highest level of functioning possible. Increasing assistance with self-care activities will be required. The patient with cerebral metastasis (and the family) lives with uncertainty. Encourage them to plan for each day and make that day count. The tasks and challenges are to assist the patient to find useful coping mechanisms, adaptations, and compensations in solving problems that arise. This helps patients maintain some sense of control even though they may be in a marginal state. An individualized exercise program will help maintain strength, endurance, and range of motion. Eventually referral may have to be made for home health care assistance.

Improving Nutrition. Patients with nausea, vomiting, breathlessness, and pain are disinterested in eating. These symptoms must be managed or controlled by assessment, planning, and appropriate nursing and medical interventions.

The nurse teaches the family optimum positioning of the patient for comfort during meals. The timing of meals is important. Food is offered when the patient is more rested and in less distress from pain or effects of treatment. The patient needs to be clean, comfortable, and free of pain, with an environment that is as attractive as possible. This requires planning to minimize offensive sights, sounds, and odors. Oral hygiene helps to improve oral intake. The family is taught to keep a daily weight chart. It may be necessary to record the quantity of food eaten to determine the daily calorie count. Nursing ingenuity is called for to make food more palatable, provide enough fluids, and increase opportunities for socialization. This involves communication and interaction with the dietician, physician, patient, and family.

Dietary supplementation, as preferred by the patient, can be encouraged to take care of increased caloric needs. If the patient refuses to eat the foods needed, it may be wise to offer whatever diet will be accepted.

When the patient shows marked deterioration as a result of tumor growth and effects, some other form of nutritional support (tube feeding, total parenteral nutrition) may be used. Nursing interventions include assessment to ensure vein integrity, monitoring the insertion site for infection, checking infusion rate, keeping intake and output records, and changing IV tubing and feeding. These techniques can be taught to the caregivers at home. There are programs available for home parenteral nutrition.

The quality of life for the patient may serve to guide in the selection, institution, and maintenance of nutritional support. The patient may become weary with all the urging to eat and the discussions about food, and may not desire aggressive nutritional intervention. This is a real dilemma. The subsequent course of action should be ethical, and humane, taking into consideration the wishes of the patient and family.

Relieving Anxiety. Persons with cerebral metastases may be restless, with changing moods that may include intense depression, euphoria, paranoia, severe anxiety, and a sense of impending doom. The response of patients to terminal illness reflects their pattern of reaction to other crisis situations. Serious illness imposes additional strains that often bring other unresolved problems to light. Learning to use patients' own coping strategies to help them deal with their feelings can be very beneficial. This requires experience and sensitivity to the patients' stated concerns.

Patients need the opportunity to exercise some control over their situation. A sense of intellectual mastery can be gained as they learn to understand the disease and its treatment, and how to deal with their feelings. The presence of family, friends, clergy, and health professionals may be supportive. Support groups such as Make Today Count may provide a feeling of support and strength through bonding.

Time spent with patients is helpful. Give them time to talk and to communicate their worries. Communication has been called the "final comfort." Sponsoring open communication and acknowledging fears is therapeutic. Touch is also a form of communication. These patients need assurance of the continuation of the relationship with the nurse and that they will not be abandoned. Life becomes more endurable when others share in the experience of dying.

If a patient's emotional reactions are very intense or prolonged, additional help from a member of the clergy, social worker, mental health professional, occupational therapist, or recreational therapist may be in order.

Enhancing Family Coping. The family needs to be reassured that their loved one is receiving optimal care and that attention will be paid to the patient's changing symptoms and to their problems. When the patient can no longer engage in self-care, the family is helped with the essentials of the patient's physical care and assisted in finding support systems (social worker, home health aid, community nurse, hospice care). The nursing goal is to keep their anxiety at manageable levels.

▷ *Evaluation*

▷ *Expected Outcomes*

1. Patient engages in self-care activities as long as possible.
   a. Uses assistive devices
   b. Accepts assistance
2. Demonstrates some improvement in nutritional status
   a. Shows no additional weight loss
   b. Has increased calorie intake
3. Appears less anxious
   a. Seems less restless and is sleeping better
   b. Talking about concerns
4. Family members seek help as needed.
   a. Demonstrate ability to bathe, feed, and care for patient
   b. Express feelings and concerns to appropriate health professionals

Intracranial Infection: Brain Abscess

A brain abscess is a collection of pus within the substance of the brain itself. It may occur by *direct invasion of the brain* from intracranial trauma or surgery; by *spread of infection from nearby sites* such as the sinuses, ears, and teeth (paranasal sinus infections, otitis media, dental sepsis); or by *spread of infection from other organs* (lung abscess, infective endocarditis). Brain abscess is a complication encountered increasingly in patients whose immune systems have been suppressed through either therapy or disease. To prevent brain

abscesses, otitis media, mastoiditis, sinusitis, dental infections, and systemic infections should be treated promptly.

Assessment

Clinical Manifestations. The clinical manifestations of a brain abscess result from alterations in intracranial dynamics (edema, brain shift), infection, or the location of the abscess. Headache, usually worse in the morning, is the patient's most continuing symptom. Vomiting is also common. Focal neurologic signs (weakness of an extremity, decreasing vision, seizures) may occur, depending on the site of the abscess. There may be a change in the patient's mental alertness as reflected in lethargic, confused, irritable, or disoriented behavior. Fever may or may not be present.

Diagnostic Evaluation. Repeated neurologic examinations and continuing assessment of the patient are necessary to determine accurately the location of the abscess. Computed tomography is invaluable in showing the site of the abscess, following the evolution and resolution of suppurative lesions, and determining the optimum time for surgical intervention.

Management

The goal of management is to eliminate the abscess. Brain abscess is treated with antimicrobial therapy and surgery. Antimicrobial treatment is given to eliminate the causative organism or reduce its virulence. Large intravenous doses are usually prescribed preoperatively to penetrate brain tissue and brain abscess. The therapy is continued postoperatively. Corticosteroids may be given if the patient shows evidence of an increasing neurologic deficit to help reduce the inflammatory cerebral edema.

Anticonvulsant medications (phenytoin, phenobarbital) may be given as a prophylaxis against seizures.

Multiple abscesses may be treated with appropriate antimicrobial therapy alone, with close monitoring by CT scans.

Surgical Approach

The definitive treatment of a brain abscess is usually surgical intervention either to aspirate or to excise the abscess. Pus may be evacuated by a needle or catheter that is placed through burr holes into the abscess cavity. An alternative is a craniotomy, in which a bone flap is cut and elevated to allow access to the brain so that the abscess can be excised. Following surgery, serial CT scans are done to see if the infection has been eradicated.

Complications. Neurologic deficits following treatment of brain abscess include hemiparesis, seizures, visual defects, and cranial nerve palsies because of possible interference with brain tissue. Relapse is common, with a high mortality rate.

Preoperative Nursing Interventions. A neurologic flow chart is maintained, and the patient is monitored closely for signs and symptoms of increased intracranial pressure (p. 1416), which may result suddenly from cerebral edema caused by a rapidly growing abscess. This increased pressure may limit further blood flow to the brain, leading to brain damage. Secondary compression of the midbrain and brain stem can quickly lead to coma and death.

Postoperative Nursing Interventions. The patient who has undergone a craniotomy to remove an abscess receives the type of nursing care described on page 1453 (Care of the Patient Undergoing Intracranial Surgery). An essential part of this care is to monitor the patient for increased intracranial pressure, to detect signs of brain herniation, brain stem compression, and cerebral ischemia.

Following surgery, drainage may be copious. Dressings are reinforced as soon as they become moist, and strict aseptic technique is maintained. The patient usually is advised to lie on the operative side to promote drainage.

The prescribed antimicrobial agents are administered on an exact time schedule because *meningitis is an ever-present danger*. These patients must be watched carefully for retraction (drawing back) of the head, stiffness of the neck, headache, chills, sweats, and any other symptoms suggestive of postoperative meningitis.

Patient Education and Home Health Care. The family is advised that residual infection may flare again after an abscess has been aspirated, and that when this occurs, surgical removal of the abscess is sometimes required. Antimicrobial agents may be prescribed for several weeks after the patient returns home. The nurse helps the patient devise a check-off system to make sure that the medication is taken exactly as prescribed. It is important also that the patient remember to take the prescribed anticonvulsant medication daily for an indefinite period of time, because epilepsy is a complication of brain abscess.

Intracranial Aneurysms (Rupture of Intracranial Aneurysm With Subarachnoid Hemorrhage)

An intracranial (cerebral) aneurysm is a dilation of the walls of a cerebral artery (Fig. 54-1). An aneurysm may be due to atherosclerosis, resulting in a defect in the vessel wall with subsequent weakness of the wall; a congenital defect of the vessel wall; hypertensive vascular disease; head trauma; or advancing age. The cerebral arteries most commonly affected by an aneurysm are the internal carotid, anterior cerebral, anterior communicating, and middle cerebral arteries. A small percentage develop in the vertebrobasilar territory. Multiple cerebral aneurysms are not uncommon.

Pathophysiology

Symptoms are produced when the aneurysm enlarges and presses on nearby cranial nerves or brain substance, or more drastically, when the aneurysm ruptures, causing *subarachnoid hemorrhage* (hemorrhage into the cranial subarachnoid space). Normal brain metabolism is disrupted by the brain being exposed to blood; by an increase in intracranial pressure resulting from the sudden entry of blood into the subarachnoid space, which compresses and injures brain tissue; or by ischemia of the brain resulting from the reduced perfusion, pressure, and vasospasm that frequently accompany subarachnoid hemorrhage.

In addition to aneurysms, other causes of subarachnoid hemorrhage include arteriovenous malformations, tumors, trauma, blood dyscrasias, and unknown causes.

Clinical Manifestations

Rupture of the aneurysm usually produces a sudden, unusually severe headache and often loss of consciousness for a variable period of time. There may be pain and rigidity of the back of the neck and spine due to meningeal irritation. Visual disturbances (visual loss, diplopia, ptosis) occur when the aneurysm is adjacent to the oculomotor nerve. Tinnitus, dizziness, and hemiparesis may also occur.

At times, an aneurysm will "leak" blood, leading to the formation of a clot that seals the site of rupture. In this instance, the patient may show little neurologic deficit, or there

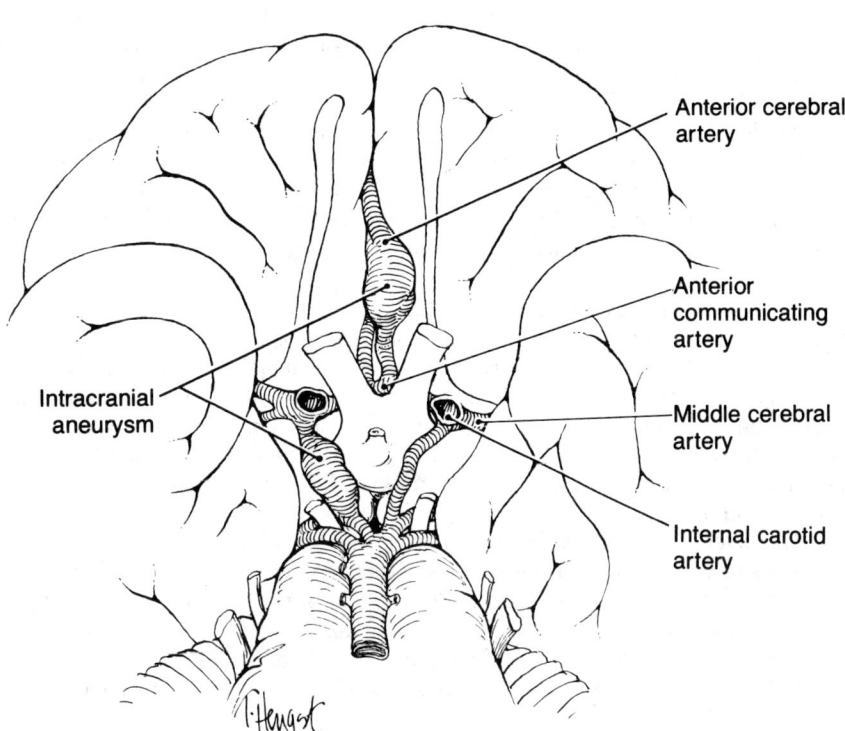

Figure 54-1
Intracranial aneurysm.

Anterior cerebral artery

Anterior communicating artery

Middle cerebral artery

Internal carotid artery

Intracranial aneurysm

may be severe bleeding, resulting in cerebral damage followed rapidly by coma and death. The mortality rate corresponds to the level of consciousness and neurologic deficit, but there is a high *immediate* mortality rate. Prognosis depends on the neurologic condition of the patient, age, associated diseases, and the extent and location of the aneurysm. Subarachnoid hemorrhage from an aneurysm is truly a catastrophic event.

Diagnostic Evaluation

The diagnosis is confirmed by CT scanning; lumbar puncture, which reveals blood in the cerebrospinal fluid; and cerebral angiography, which shows the location and size of the aneurysm and gives information about the affected vessel, adjoining vessels, and vascular branches.

Management

The goals of treatment are to allow the brain to recover from the initial insult (bleeding), to prevent or minimize the risk of rebleeding, and to prevent or treat other complications. These include rebleeding; cerebral vasospasm resulting in cerebral ischemia; acute hydrocephalus, which results when intraventricular blood obstructs the pathway for cerebrospinal fluid; epilepsy; and psychiatric and psychological problems.

Management consists of bed rest with sedation to prevent agitation and stress, management of the vasospasm, and surgical or medical treatment to prevent rebleeding.

Vasospasm. The development of cerebral vasospasm (narrowing of the lumen of the involved cranial blood vessel) is a serious complication of subarachnoid hemorrhage and often is correlated with a poor clinical condition and prognosis. The mechanism responsible for the spasm is not clear, but the occurrence of vasospasms correlates with increasing amounts of blood in the subarachnoid cisterns and cerebral fissures, as visualized by CT scan. Vasospasm leads to increased vascular resistance, which impedes cerebral blood flow and causes brain ischemia and infarction. The signs and symptoms exhibited by the patient reflect the areas of the brain involved. Vasospasm is often heralded by a worsening headache, a decrease in level of responsiveness (confusion, lethargy, disorientation), or the appearance of a new focal neurologic deficit (aphasia, hemiparesis [partial paralysis affecting one side of the body]). Vasospasm frequently occurs within the fourth to twelfth day following the initial hemorrhage. It is during this time that the clot undergoes the lytic process (dissolution), and this increases the chances of rebleeding.

It is felt by many neurosurgeons that early operation to clip the aneurysm will prevent rebleeding, and that the removal of blood from the basal cisterns around the major cerebral arteries may prevent the development of vasospasm. In addition, the intravenous administration of the calcium blocker nimodipine during the critical time in which vasospasm may develop may offer protection against delayed ischemic deterioration.

Increased Intracranial Pressure. An increase in intracranial pressure almost always follows a subarachnoid hemorrhage, probably due to disturbed circulation of cerebrospinal fluid (CSF) caused by blood in the basal cisterns. If the patient shows evidence of deterioration from increased intracranial pressure (due to cerebral edema, herniation, hydrocephalus, or vasospasm), CSF drainage is instituted by lumbar puncture or ventricular catheter drainage, and mannitol is given to reduce intracranial pressure. When mannitol is used as a long-term measure to control intracranial pressure, dehydration and disturbances in electrolyte balance (hyponatremia/hypernatremia; hypokalemia/hyperkalemia) may occur. Mannitol acts by osmotically pulling water out of the brain as well as by reducing total body water through diuresis. The patient is monitored for signs of dehydration and for rebound elevation of intracranial pressure.

If surgery is delayed or contraindicated, antifibrinolytic agents (aminocaproic acid; tranexamic acid) may be administered to delay or prevent dissolution of the clot at the site of the aneurysmal rupture.

Systemic Hypertension. Sudden systemic hypertension is guarded against. If blood pressure is elevated, antihypertensive therapy (nitroprusside) may be prescribed. Constant blood pressure monitoring by arterial line is carried out to avoid a precipitous drop in blood pressure, which can produce brain ischemia. Because seizures cause blood pressure elevation, anticonvulsant agents are administered prophylactically. Stool softeners prevent straining, which can elevate the blood pressure.

Analgesics (codeine; acetaminophen) may be prescribed for head and neck pain. The patient is fitted with graded pressure elastic stockings to prevent deep vein thrombophlebitis, a threat to any patient who is on bed rest.

Nursing Interventions

The patient is monitored continually for neurologic deterioration occurring from recurrent bleeding, increasing intracranial pressure, or vasospasm. A neurologic flow record is kept. The blood pressure, pulse, level of responsiveness (an indicator of cerebral perfusion), pupillary responses, and motor function are checked hourly. The respiratory status is watched as reduction in PO_2 in brain areas with impaired autoregulation increases the chances of a cerebral infarction. Any changes are reported immediately.

The patient is placed on immediate and absolute bed rest in a quiet, nonstressful setting because activity, pain, and anxiety elevate the blood pressure, which increases the risk of bleeding. Visitors, except for family, are restricted.

The head of the bed is elevated moderately to provide venous drainage and decrease intracranial pressure. However, some neurologists prefer that the patient remain flat to increase cerebral perfusion.

Any activity that suddenly increases the blood pressure or obstructs venous return is avoided. This includes the Valsalva maneuver, straining, forceful sneezing, pulling up in bed, acute flexion or rotation of the head and neck (which compromises the jugular veins), and cigarette smoking.

Any activity requiring exertion is contraindicated. The patient is instructed to exhale through the mouth during voiding or defecation to decrease strain. Dim lighting is helpful, since *photophobia* (visual intolerance of light) is common. Coffee and tea, unless decaffeinated, are usually eliminated. Appropriate reassurance helps relieve the patient's fears and anxiety. The family also requires information and support.

The patient is prepared for surgical intervention as soon as his condition is deemed suitable. The nursing management of the patient following a craniotomy is found on page 1453.

Surgical Management

The goal of surgery is to prevent further bleeding. This is done by isolating the aneurysm from its circulation or by strengthening the arterial wall. An aneurysm may be treated by excluding it from the cerebral circulation by means of a ligature or a clip across its neck (Fig. 54-2). If this is not anatomically possible, the aneurysm can be reinforced by wrapping it with plastic, muscle, or some other substance. An extracranial–intracranial arterial bypass may be done to establish collateral blood supply in order to allow surgery on the aneurysm. Alternatively, an extracranial method may be used, whereby the carotid artery is occluded in the neck in order to reduce pressure within the blood vessel (*carotid endarterectomy*, see p. 1449). Following ligation of the carotid artery, there is some risk of cerebral ischemia and sudden hemiplegia because during the operative procedure there is a temporary occlusion of the blood supply to the brain (unless a temporary inlying bypass shunt is used). In anticipation of these complications, measurements of cerebral blood flow and internal carotid pressure may be taken in order to identify those patients who are at risk for postoperative ischemic episodes.

Other postoperative complications include the appearance of psychological symptoms (disorientation, amnesia, Korsakoff's syndrome, personality impairment), intraoperative embolization, postoperative internal artery occlusion, water and electrolyte disturbances (from dysfunction of the neurohypophyseal system), and gastrointestinal bleeding. (The management of the patient following intracranial surgery is discussed on pp. 1453–1458.)

Multiple Sclerosis

Multiple sclerosis (MS) is a chronic, frequently progressive disease of the central nervous system characterized by the occurrence of small patches of demyelination in the brain and spinal cord. (*Demyelination* refers to the destruction of myelin, the fatty and protein material that ensheathes certain nerve fibers in the brain and spinal cord.) Demyelination results in a disorder in the transmission of nerve impulses.

The cause of multiple sclerosis is not known. Research evidence suggests that myelin damage is the primary event, and that it results from a viral infection early in life that becomes apparent as an immune process later in life. Although some form of viral infection may be the initiating mechanism, a defective immune response probably plays a major role in the pathogenesis of multiple sclerosis.

Epidemiologic findings indicate that MS is more common in people living in the northern latitudes. It is one of the most disabling neurologic diseases of young adults (20 to 40 years of age) in this country, affecting twice as many women as men. Its occurrence when patients are young increases the medical, psychological, social, and economic problems encountered by both patient and family.

Pathophysiology

In multiple sclerosis, the demyelination is scattered irregularly throughout the central nervous system (Fig. 54-3). In time, myelin peels off the axis cylinders, and the axons themselves degenerate. The plaques or patches in the involved areas become sclerosed, interrupting the flow of nerve impulses and resulting in a variety of manifestations, depending on which nerves are affected. The areas most frequently affected are the optic nerves, chiasm, and tracts, the cerebrum, the brain stem and cerebellum, and the spinal cord.

Clinical Manifestations

The signs and symptoms of MS are varied and multiple, reflecting the location of the lesion (plaque) or combination of lesions. The symptoms most commonly reported are fatigue, weakness, numbness, difficulty in coordination, and loss of balance. About 75% of patients in one survey had visual disturbances due to lesions in the optic nerves or their connections: blurring of vision, patchy blindness (*scotoma*), or total blindness. Spastic weakness of the extremities and loss of the abdominal reflexes are due to involvement of the main motor pathways (*pyramidal tracts*) of the spinal cord. Disruption of the sensory axons may produce sensory dysfunction. Cognitive and psychosocial problems may reflect frontal and/or parietal lobe involvement. Involvement of the cerebellum and/or basal ganglia can produce *ataxia* (im-

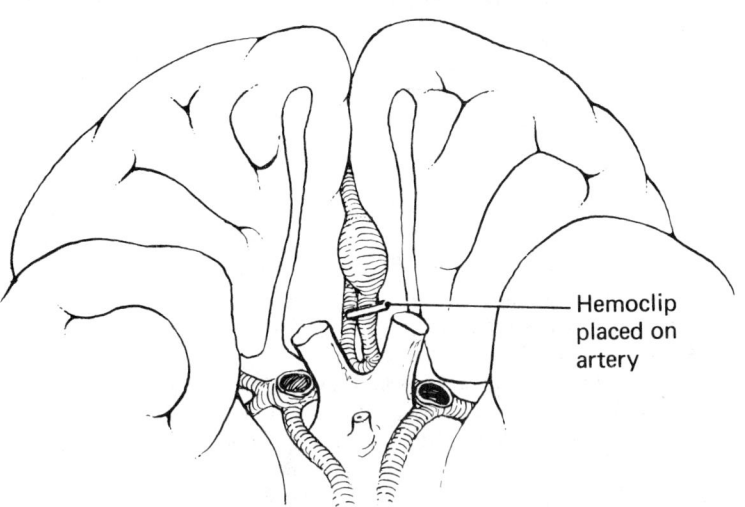

— Hemoclip placed on artery

Figure 54-2
Cerebral aneurysm isolated by means of a hemoclip.

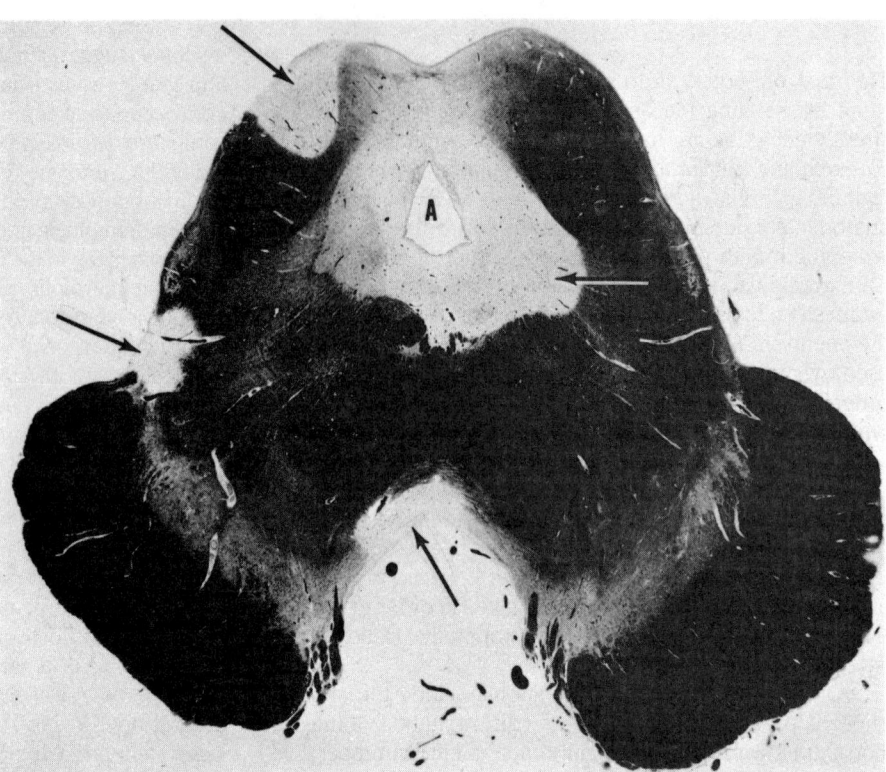

Figure 54-3
Cross section from the midbrain (enlarged approximately three times) of a patient with chronic MS. Specimen stained to show myelin (*black*). The four white areas indicated by the arrows are typical plaques in which the myelin has been destroyed. The plaque to the right of the aqueduct (A) impinges upon periaqueductal gray matter. The nerve fibers in these plaques have lost their myelin sheaths, and as a consequence, conduction of stimuli in these areas would be impeded or lost. (Courtesy of Cedric S. Raine, M.D., Professor of Pathology [Neuropathology] and Neuroscience, Albert Einstein College of Medicine of Yeshiva University.)

paired coordination of movements) and tremor. Emotional hyperexcitability and inappropriate euphoria result from loss of the control connections between the cortex and the basal ganglia. Bladder, bowel, and sexual problems also occur if the process involves the cord pathways connected with the pontine micturition center and the sacral plexus.

Secondary manifestations are related to complications: urinary tract infections, rectal distention, pressure sores, contracture deformities, dependent pedal edema, pneumonia, and reactive depressions. Tertiary problems (emotional, social, marital, economic, vocational) may result as a consequence of the disease.

Multiple sclerosis is characterized by exacerbations (the appearance of new symptoms and worsening of existing ones) and remissions (periods in which symptoms decrease or disappear). Relapses are often associated with periods of emotional and physical stress. However, as evidenced by CT scanning, many plaques do not produce serious symptoms and many patients are not seriously incapacitated but have long periods of remission between episodes. There is evidence that remyelination occurs in some patients.

Diagnostic Evaluation

Electrophoresis study of the cerebrospinal fluid usually reveals the presence of *oligoclonal banding* (several bands of IgG), reflecting immunoglobulin abnormalities. In fact, abnormal IgG antibody appears in the CSF of up to 95% of patients with MS. Evoked potential studies are carried out to help define the extent of the disease process and monitor changes. CT scans may reveal cerebral atrophic changes. Magnetic resonance imaging has become a primary diagnostic tool for visualizing small plaques and for evaluating the course of the disease and effect of the treatment. Underlying bladder dys-

function is diagnosed by urodynamic studies. Neuropsychologic testing may be indicated to show cognitive impairment. A sexual history helps to identify specific areas of concern.

Management

At this time there is no cure for MS, but an individualized, organized, and rational treatment program can relieve the patient's symptoms and provide continuing support. Many patients with MS are in stable condition and only require intermittent treatment aimed at controlling symptoms, while others experience steady progression of their disease.

Corticosteroids or adrenocorticotrophic hormone (ACTH) is used as an antiedema and anti-inflammatory agent that may improve the nerve conduction. Since it is possible that immune mechanisms may be a factor in the pathogenesis of MS, a number of pharmacologic agents are being tried to modulate the immune response and reduce the rate at which the disease progresses and the frequency and severity of the exacerbations. These drugs include azathioprine, cyclophosphamide, and interferon.

Baclofen is the current drug of choice for spasticity. Patients with severe spasticity and contractures may require nerve blocks and surgical intervention to prevent further disability.

Management of bladder and bowel control are among the patient's most difficult problems. Generally, bladder symptoms fall into the following categories: (1) inability to store urine (hyperreflexic; uninhibited); (2) inability to empty the bladder (hyporeflexic; hypotonic); and (3) a mixture of both types. While a variety of drugs are employed to treat these problems, intermittent self-catheterization is an effective treatment of bladder dysfunction. Often urinary tract infection is superimposed on the underlying neurologic dysfunction.

Ascorbic acid may be given to acidify the urine, making bacterial growth less likely. Antimicrobial drugs are given when appropriate.

▶ Nursing Process
The Patient With Multiple Sclerosis

▷ Assessment

Nursing assessment is carried out with an awareness of actual and potential problems associated with the disease, including neurologic problems, secondary complications, and the consequences of the disease on the patient and family. Watch movements and walking to determine if the patient is in danger of falling. Observe the patient functioning when well rested and when fatigued. Ask what are the major problems: Weakness? spasticity? visual impairment? incontinence? How has this condition affected his life-style? How well is the patient coping? What would the patient like to do better?

▷ Nursing Diagnoses

Based on all the assessment data, the patient's potential nursing diagnoses may include the following:

- Impaired physical mobility related to weakness, muscle paresis, spasticity
- Potential for injury related to sensory and visual impairment
- Alteration in urinary and bowel elimination related to spinal cord dysfunction
- Alteration in thought processes (loss of memory, dementia, euphoria) related to cerebral dysfunction
- Potential sexual dysfunction related to spinal cord involvement and/or psychological reactions to condition
- Impaired home maintenance management related to physical, psychological, and social problems imposed by MS

▷ Planning and Implementation

▷ *Goals:* The patient's major goals may include promotion of physical mobility, avoidance of injury, achievement of bladder and bowel continence, improvement of cognitive dysfunction, adaptation to sexual dysfunction, and development of coping strengths.

Nursing Interventions

An individualized program of physical therapy, rehabilitation, and education is combined with emotional support. The nursing framework focuses also on the social and psychological problems of the person with chronic disease.

Promoting Physical Mobility. Relaxation and coordination exercises promote muscle efficiency for the person with MS. Progressive resistive exercises are used to strengthen weak muscles, because diminishing muscle power is a significant problem for these patients. The patient is encouraged to work up to the point just short of fatigue. Vigorous physical exercise is *not* advisable, because it raises the body temperature and may aggravate symptoms. Prolonged exercise that

tires an extremity may cause paresis, numbness, or incoordination. The patient is advised to take frequent short rest periods, preferably lying down. Extreme fatigue may be a contributing factor in exacerbation of symptoms.

Walking exercises improve the gait, particularly when there is loss of position sense of the legs. If certain muscle groups are irreversibly affected, other muscles can be trained to take over their actions.

Muscle spasticity is common and, in its later stages, is characterized by severe adductor spasm of the hips with flexor spasm of the hips and knees. If this is not relieved, fibrous contractures of these joints with resultant pressure sores over the sacrum and hips (due to inability to properly position the patient) will occur. Warm packs may be beneficial, but hot baths should be avoided. Daily exercises for muscle stretching are prescribed to minimize joint contractures. Special attention is given to hamstrings, gastrocnemius muscles, hip adductors, biceps, and wrist and finger flexors. Muscle spasticity is common and interferes with normal function. A stretch-hold–relax routine is helpful for relaxing and treating muscle spasticity. Swimming and stationary bicycling are useful, while progressive weight-bearing will relieve spasticity in the legs. The patient should not be hurried in any of these activities because hurrying increases spasticity.

Preventing Injury. If motor dysfunction causes problems of incoordination and clumsiness, or if ataxia is apparent, the patient is at risk for falling. To overcome this disability, the patient is taught to walk with feet wide apart in order to widen the base of support and increase walking stability. If there is loss of position sense, the patient is taught to watch the feet while walking. Gait training may require aids (walker, cane, braces, crutches, parallel bars) and physical therapy. If the gait remains inefficient, a wheelchair may be the solution. The occupational therapist is a valuable resource person in suggesting and securing aids to promote independence. If incoordination is a problem, and tremor of the upper extremities occurs when voluntary movement is attempted (*intention tremor*), weighted bracelets or wrist cuffs are helpful. The patient is trained in transfers and activities of daily living.

Since sensory loss may occur in addition to motor loss, pressure sores are a continuing threat to skin integrity. Confinement to a wheelchair compounds the threat. (See pp. 222–230 for a discussion of the prevention and treatment of pressure sores.)

Promoting Bladder and Bowel Control. The patient with urinary frequency, urgency, or incontinence requires special support. The sensation of the need to void must be heeded immediately, so the bedpan or urinal should be readily available. A voiding time schedule is set up (every 1½–2 hours initially, with gradually lengthening of the time intervals). The patient is instructed to drink a measured amount of fluid every 2 hours and then attempt to void 30 minutes after drinking. An alarm clock may be set for the patient who does not have enough sensation to warn of the need to empty the bladder. The nurse encourages the patient to take the prescribed drugs to treat bladder spasticity, as this allows greater independence.

If the female patient has permanent urinary incontinence, urinary diversion procedures are considered. The male patient may wear a condom appliance for urine collection.

Bowel problems include constipation, fecal impaction, and incontinence. Adequate fluids, dietary fiber and a bowel-training program are effective in solving these problems. (See p. 238.)

Improving Sensory and Cognitive Function. Measures may be taken if optic and speech defects occur (the cranial nerves relating to sight and speech are affected by MS). An eye patch or an eyeglass occluder may be used to block visual impulses of one eye when the patient has *diplopia* (double vision). Prism glasses may be helpful for the bedridden patient. When the vision begins to fail, painting the cane tip and shoe tips with fluorescent paint helps. Persons with any physical limitations preventing them from reading regular print materials are eligible for the free talking book services of the Library of Congress (address at end of chapter).

When the cranial nerves controlling the mechanisms of speech are involved, *dysarthrias* (defects of articulation) marked by slurring, low volume of speech, and difficulties in phonation are seen. There are problems with shallow breathing and low breath pressure. A speech-language pathologist teaches the patient, family, and health team members about communication problems and the use of compensatory techniques.

MS imposes numerous stresses on the patient and family. Cognitive impairment may occur early in the disease. Embarrassing and humiliating symptoms may result in "inappropriate" responses by the patient. As there may be organic changes in the brain, MS patients may be forgetful and easily distracted and may exhibit emotional lability. Patients adapt to illness in a variety of ways which may include denial (with euphoria), depression, withdrawal, and hostility. MS patients frequently conceal their emotions behind a smiling or flat, unsmiling mask. Compassion and significant emotional support are required to help patients adapt to a new self-image and cope with the disruption in their lives. Help the patient set meaningful and realistic short-term goals to achieve a sense of purpose. Encourage the patient to remain in the mainstream of life as much as possible and to keep up social interests and activities. Hobbies may help the patient's morale and provide satisfying interests when the disease has progressed to the stage in which normal activities cannot be pursued.

The family should be made aware of the nature and degree of cognitive impairment. The environment is kept structured, and lists and other memory aids are used to help the patient move ahead in the daily routine.

Strengthening Coping Mechanisms. The family faces almost overwhelming frustrations and problems. Multiple sclerosis strikes individuals who are in the developmental stage of life concerned about career and family responsibilities. Family conflict, disintegration, separation, and divorce are not uncommon. Often very young family members assume the responsibility of caring for a disabled parent. Nursing interventions in this area include alleviating stress and making appropriate referrals for counseling and support to moderate the adverse effects of dealing with chronic illness.

The nurse, mindful of these complex problems, initiates home care through several channels and coordinates a network of services: social services, speech therapy, physical therapy, homemaker services, and the like. To nurture the patient's coping strengths, give as much information as possible. People who live with chronic illness need an updated list of aids and resources that are available.

Coping through problem-solving involves helping the patient define the problem and develop alternatives for its management. Careful planning, staying flexible, and maintaining a hopeful attitude are useful for psychological and physical adaptation.

Encouraging Self-Care. MS can affect every facet of daily living. Once certain abilities are lost, they are almost impossible to regain. Physical abilities may vary from day to day. Modifications that allow continuance of self-care activities should be sought (raised toilet seat, bathing helps, telephone modifications, long-handled comb, tongs, modified clothing). Physical and emotional stresses should be avoided as much as possible, since these worsen symptoms and impair performance. Exposure to heat appears to increase fatigue, and fatigue lessens motor power. Air-conditioning in at least one room is recommended. Exposure to extreme cold may increase spasticity. The patient must remain under continuing medical supervision.

Encourage the patient to contact the local chapter of the National Multiple Sclerosis Society for services, publications, and contact with other MS patients. Local chapters give direct services to patients. Through group participation, the patient has an opportunity to identify with others having similar problems, gain relief and release, and learn self-help methods in a social environment.

Adapting to Sexual Dysfunction. MS patients and their partners face problems that interfere with sexual activity, arising not only as a direct consequence of nerve damage, but also from psychological or related reactions to the disease. Easy fatigability, conflicts arising from dependency and depression, emotional lability, and loss of self-esteem and feelings of self-worth compound the problem. Erectile and ejaculatory disorders in males and orgasmic dysfunction and adductor spasms of the thigh muscles in females can make intercourse difficult or impossible. Bladder and bowel incontinence and urinary tract infections add to the difficulties.

An experienced sexual counselor will help bring into focus the patient's and/or partner's sexual resources and suggest relevant information and supportive therapy. Sharing and communicating feelings, planning for sexual activity (to counteract fatigue), exercising different sexual options, and demonstrating a willingness to experiment may open up a wide range of sexual enjoyment and experiences.

▷ *Evaluation*

▷ *Expected Outcomes*

1. Patient adapts to impaired mobility and spasticity.
   a. Participates in gait-training and rehabilitation program
   b. Establishes a balanced program of rest and exercise
   c. Uses assistive devices
   d. Identifies measures to conserve energy; arranges schedule to accommodate periods of higher energy levels
2. Avoids injury
   a. Uses visual cues to compensate for decreased sense of touch/position
   b. Asks for assistance when necessary
3. Attains/maintains improved bladder and bowel control
   a. Monitors self for urine retention
   b. Knows the signs and symptoms of urinary tract infection

  c. Maintains adequate fluid and fiber intake
  d. Shows no fecal soiling
  4. Compensates for cognitive dysfunction
    a. Uses lists to compensate for memory losses
    b. Discusses problems with trusted advisor-friend
    c. Substitutes new activities for those that have been given up
  5. Demonstrates improvement of coping strengths
    a. Maintains sense of control
    b. Makes plans to redesign life-style
    c. Verbalizes desire to pursue goals and developmental tasks of adulthood
  6. Adapts to sexual dysfunction
    a. Is able to discuss problem with appropriate health professional

Parkinson's Disease

Parkinson's disease is a progressive neurologic disorder affecting the brain centers that are responsible for control and regulation of movement. It is characterized by *bradykinesia* (slowness of movement), tremor, and muscle stiffness or rigidity.

Pathophysiology. The major lesion appears to result in a loss of pigmented neurons, particularly those in the substantia nigra of the brain (Fig. 54-4). (The *substantia nigra* is a collection of midbrain nuclei that project fibers to the corpus striatum.) One of the major neurotransmitters in this area of the brain, and in other parts of the central nervous system, is dopamine, which has an important inhibiting func-

tion in the central control of movement. Although dopamine normally exists in high concentration in certain parts of the brain, in Parkinson's disease it is depleted in the substantia nigra and the corpus striatum. Depletion of dopamine levels in the basal ganglia is associated with bradykinesia, rigidity, and tremors.

Regional cerebral blood flow is reduced in patients with Parkinson's disease, and there is a high prevalence of dementia. Biochemical and pathologic data suggest that demented patients with Parkinson's disease may have coexistent Alzheimer's disease.

In the majority of patients, the cause of the disease is unknown. Arteriosclerotic parkinsonism is seen more frequently in older age groups. It may follow encephalitis, poisoning or toxicity (manganese, carbon monoxide), or hypoxia, or may be drug-induced.

The disease most frequently attacks persons in their 50s and 60s and is the second most common neurologic disorder of the elderly.

Clinical Manifestations. The chief manifestations of Parkinson's disease are impaired movement, muscular rigidity, tremor, muscle weakness, and loss of postural reflexes. Early signs include a stiffening of the extremities and a wax-like rigidity in the performance of all movements. The patient has difficulty in initiating, maintaining, and performing motor activities, and experiences some delay in carrying out normal activity.

As the disease progresses, the tremor begins, frequently in one hand and arm, then the other, and later in the head, although the tremor may remain unilateral (Fig. 54-5). The tremor is characteristic: it is a slow, turning motion (pronation–supination) of the forearm and the hand, and a motion of the thumb against the fingers as if rolling a pill between the fingers. It increases when the patient is concentrating or feeling anxious.

Other characteristics of the disease affect the face, stature, and gait. There is loss of normal arm swing. Eventually, the rigid extremities become definitely weaker. Since there is limited movement in the muscles, the face has so little expression that it is said to be masklike (with infrequency of blinking), a feature that can be recognized at a glance.

There is a loss of postural reflexes, and the patient stands with head bent forward and walks as if in danger of falling forward. Difficulty in pivoting and loss of balance (either forward or backward) may lead to frequent falls.

Frequently, these patients show signs of depression, and it has not been established whether the depression is a reaction to the disorder or related to a biochemical abnormality. Mental manifestations may appear in the form of cognitive, perceptual, and memory deficits. A number of psychiatric manifestations (personality changes, psychosis, dementia, acute confusion) are particularly common among the elderly. Complications from immobility (pneumonia, urinary tract infection) and the consequences of falls and accidents are major causes of death.

Diagnostic Evaluation. Early diagnosis of Parkinson's disease can be difficult, as the patient can rarely pinpoint when symptoms started. Often someone close to the patient notices a change such as stooped posture, a stiff arm, a slight limp, or tremor. Handwriting changes may be an early diagnostic clue. A diagnosis of Parkinson's disease can usually be made with certainty when there is evidence of tremor,

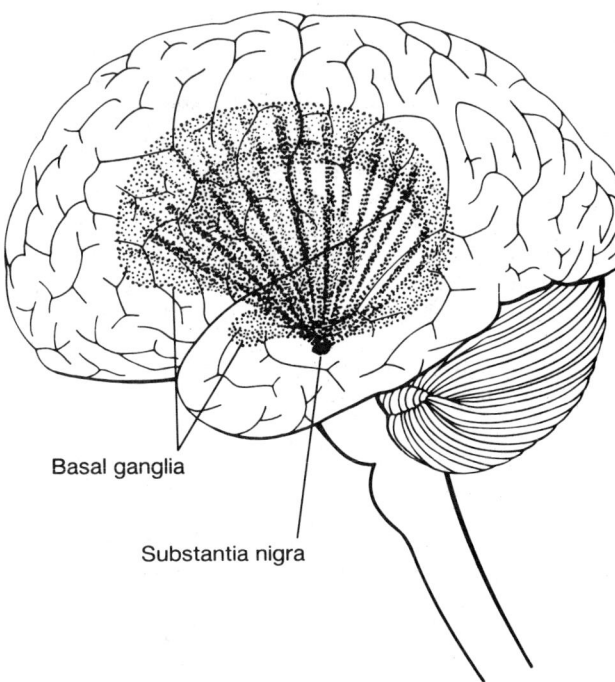

Basal ganglia

Substantia nigra

Figure 54-4
The loss of dopamine nerve cells from the brain's substantia nigra is thought to be responsible for the symptoms of parkinsonism. (Courtesy of National Institutes of Health.)

CLINICAL FEATURES

Head bent forward

Tremors of the head

Mask-like facial expression

Drooling

Rigidity

Stooped posture

Weight loss

Akinesia
(absence or poverty
of normal movement)

Tremor

Loss of postural reflexes

Bone demineralization

Shuffling and propulsive gait

NURSING MANAGEMENT

Drug therapy

Rehabilitation

Patient and family education

Warm baths and massage
to relax muscles

Specific drug therapy

Bowel routine

Self-help devices to meet daily needs
Raised toilet seat
Long-handle comb and razor

Exercise to loosen joint structures

Range of motion exercises
to prevent deformities

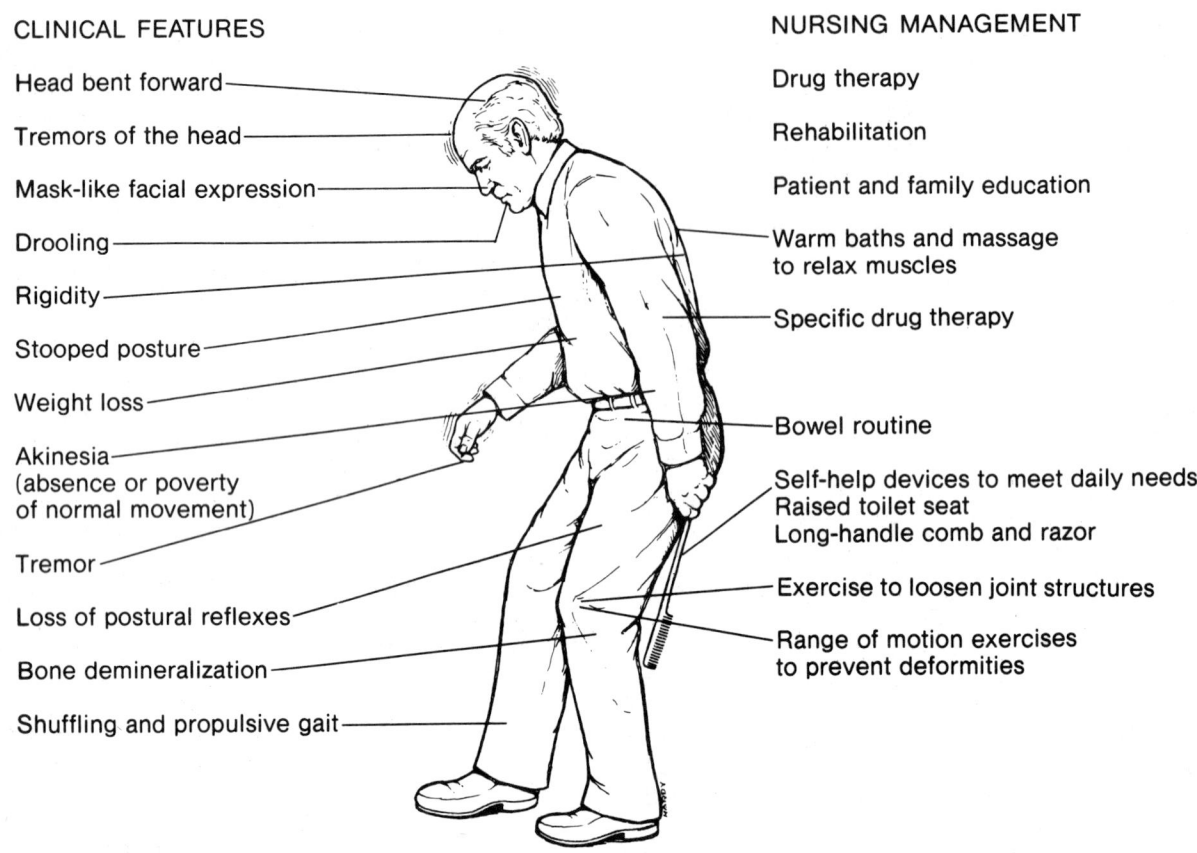

Figure 54-5
Clinical manifestations and nursing management of the patient with parkinsonism.

rigidity, and bradykinesia (abnormally slow movements). The results of the patient's history and neurologic examination are carefully evaluated.

Management

The goal of treatment is to enhance dopamine transmission. Drug therapy includes antihistamines, anticholinergics, amantadine, and levodopa. Many of these drugs cause psychiatric side-effects in the elderly.

Antihistamine Drugs. Antihistamine drugs have mild central anticholinergic and sedative effects, and may be helpful in allaying tremors.

Anticholinergic Therapy. Anticholinergic drugs (trihexyphenidyl, procyclidine, and benztropine mesylate) are effective for controlling the tremor and rigidity of parkinsonism. These drugs may be used in combination with levodopa. They counteract the action of acetylcholine in the central nervous system. Side-effects of these drugs include blurred vision, flushing, rash, constipation, urinary retention, and acute confusional states. Intraocular pressure is closely monitored because these drugs are contraindicated in patients with narrow-angle glaucoma. Patients with prostatic hyperplasia are watched for signs of urinary retention.

Amantadine Hydrochloride. Amantadine hydrochloride (Symmetrel), an intiviral agent, is used early in the treatment of Parkinson's disease to reduce rigidity, tremor, and bradykinesia. It is thought to act by releasing dopamine from

the nigrostriatal nerve terminals. Adverse reactions include psychiatric disturbances (mood changes, confusion, hallucinations), nausea, epigastric distress, headache, and visual impairment.

Levodopa Therapy. Levodopa, though not a cure, is currently the most effective agent for the treatment of Parkinson's disease. It is presumably converted to dopamine in the basal ganglia to relieve the patient's symptoms.

The beneficial effects of levodopa are most pronounced in the first few years of treatment. Benefits to the patient begin to wane and adverse side-effects become more severe with the passage of time. Confusion, hallucinations, depression, and sleep alterations are associated with prolonged use of the drug. The patient may experience an "on–off" reaction in which sudden periods of near immobility ("off effect"), lasting minutes to hours, are followed by a sudden return of effectiveness ("on effect"). *Dyskinesias* (abnormal involuntary movements) are fairly common side-effects, and include facial grimacing, rhythmic jerking movements of the hands, head bobbing, chewing and smacking movements, and involuntary movements of the trunk and extremities. This is probably due to the body's failure to readjust properly to the disappearance of dopamine. One method of dealing with on–off fluctuations is to give a "drug holiday" by taking the patient off the drug. This requires hospitalization and expert medical and nursing care.

Levodopa is usually given in combination with a decarboxylase inhibitor, carbidopa, which allows a greater concentration of levodopa to reach the brain and decrease the peripheral side-effects.

Dopamine-Agonist-Ergot Derivatives. These agents (bromacriptine) are thought to be dopamine receptor agonists, and are useful when added to levodopa and in patients experiencing "on–off" reactions to smooth out clinical fluctuations.

Antidepressant Drugs. Tricyclic antidepressants may be given to alleviate the depression that is so commonly present.

Surgical Intervention. In some patients with disabling tremor or with severe levodopa-induced dyskinesia, surgery may be considered. Although surgery provides a certain amount of relief in selected patients, it does not alter the course of Parkinson's disease or assure permanent improvement. The purpose of the surgery is to destroy a part of the thalamus (*stereotaxic thalamotomy*) in order to relieve certain types of excessive muscle contraction.

The stereotaxic technique allows the neurosurgeon to position precisely and localize a small target deep within the brain. Special guiding instruments and rapid x-rays are used to place an electrode or freezing probe with pinpoint precision in the target area of the brain. A lesion is then created at that point.

▶ Nursing Process
The Patient With Parkinson's Disease

▷ Assessment

The nursing history and assessment focus on how the disease has affected the patient's activities and functioning abilities. Observe what the patient can do and what changes in function occur throughout the day. Watch responses following the administration of medications. Ask what the patient would like to do better. The following questions may be asked:

- Do you have leg or arm stiffness?
- Have you experienced any irregular jerking of your arms or legs?
- Have you ever been "frozen" or rooted to the spot and unable to move?
- Does your mouth water excessively?
- Have you (or others) noticed yourself grimacing or making faces or chewing movements?
- What specific activities do you have difficulty doing?

During this process, observe the patient roll over in bed, get out of bed, get out of a chair, walk, drink, and eat.

▷ Nursing Diagnoses

Nearly every patient with a movement disorder has some functional alteration and may have some type of behavioral dysfunction. Based on the assessment data, the patient's major nursing diagnoses may include the following:

- Impaired physical mobility related to muscle rigidity and weakness
- Self-care deficits (eating, drinking, dressing, hygiene) related to tremor and motor disturbance

- Alteration in bowel elimination related to medication and reduced activity
- Alteration in nutrition—less than body requirements related to tremor, slowness in eating, difficulty in chewing and swallowing
- Impaired verbal communication related to decreased speech volume, slowness of speech, inability to move facial muscles
- Impaired social interaction related to depression and dysfunction due to disease progression

Other nursing diagnoses may include sleep pattern disturbances, knowledge deficit, alteration in thought processes, and ineffective family coping.

▷ Planning and Implementation

▷ *Goals:* The patient's goals may include improvement of mobility, attainment of independence in activities of daily living, achievement of adequate bowel elimination, attainment and maintenance of satisfactory nutritional status, achievement of communication, and development of positive coping mechanisms.

Nursing Interventions

Improving Mobility: Exercise. A progressive program of daily exercise will increase muscle strength, improve coordination and dexterity, reduce muscular rigidity, and prevent contractures that occur when muscles are not used. Walking, riding a stationary bicycle, swimming, and gardening are all exercises that help maintain joint mobility. Stretching exercises (stretch–hold–relax) will help loosen the joint structures. Postural exercises are important to counter the tendency of the head and neck to be drawn forward and down. Special walking techniques must also be learned to offset the shuffling gait and the tendency to lean forward.

The patient may also walk off balance because of the rigidity of the arms. (Arm swinging is necessary in normal walking.) The patient is taught early in the course of the disease to concentrate on walking erect, to watch the horizon, and to use a broad-based gait (*i.e.*, walking with the feet separated). A conscious effort must be made to swing the arms and raise the feet while walking and to use a heel–toe, heel–toe gait in fairly long strides. Advise the patient to practice walking to marching music or the sound of a ticking metronome, because this provides sensory reinforcement. Breathing exercises while walking help to move the rib cage and transport oxygen to poorly-aerated parts of the lungs. Frequent rest periods aid in preventing frustration and fatigue.

Warm baths and massage in addition to passive and active exercises help relax muscles and relieve painful muscle spasms that accompany rigidity.

Enhancing Self-Care Activities. Teach, support, and supervise the patient during activities of daily living. (See Chapter 14, p. 230, for rehabilitation techniques.)

Environmental modifications are necessary to compensate for functional disabilities. These patients have difficulty turning in bed and getting in and out of bed. Bedside rails or a rope tied to the foot of the bed will provide assistance in pulling up without help.

Promoting Bowel Elimination. A patient with parkinsonism may have severe problems with constipation. Among the factors causing this condition are weakness of the muscles used in defecation, lack of exercise, an inadequate fluid intake, and decreased autonomic nervous system activity. The drugs used for the treatment of the disease also inhibit normal intestinal secretions. A regular bowel routine may be established by encouraging the patient to follow a regular time pattern, consciously increase fluid intake, and eat foods with a moderate fiber content. A raised toilet seat is a useful device to facilitate toilet activities, since the patient has difficulty in changing from a standing to a sitting position.

Assuring Adequate Nutrition. These patients have a problem in maintaining their weight. They become embarrassed by their slowness and untidiness in eating. Their mouths are dry from the medications, and they experience difficulty in chewing and swallowing. Persons with Parkinson's disease are "silent aspirators" with decreased cough reflexes. They are not aware that they are aspirating, and may develop bronchopneumonia. Some patients have saliva build-up due to a slow rate of swallowing. Because of problems in eating, they eventually show a considerable weight loss, and demineralization starts in the bones as a result of malnutrition. This gives rise to the added threat of fractures occurring if the patient falls.

Swallowing disorders are also due to tongue tremor, hesitancy in initiating swallowing, difficulty in shaping food into a bolus, and disturbances in pharyngeal motility. To offset these problems, the patient should sit in an upright position during mealtime. A semisolid diet with thick liquids is easier to swallow than solids and thin liquids. Thin liquids should be avoided. It is helpful for patients to think through the swallowing sequence. Teach them to place the food on the tongue, close lips and teeth, lift the tongue up and then back, and swallow. Tell them to make an effort to chew first on one side of the mouth and then on the other. To control the build-up of saliva, remind them to hold the head upright and make a conscious effort to swallow. Massaging the facial and neck muscles before meals may be beneficial.

An electrical warming tray will keep food hot and permit the patient to rest during the prolonged time that it takes to eat. Special utensils will also assist at mealtime. A plate that is stabilized, a nonspill cup, and specially constructed eating utensils are useful self-help devices. Supplementary feedings will augment caloric intake. Monitoring weight on a weekly basis will indicate whether caloric intake is sufficient.

Improving Communication. Speech disorders are present in the majority of patients with Parkinson's disease. Their low-pitched, monotonous, soft speech requires that they make a conscious effort to speak slowly, with deliberate attention to what they are saying. Remind patients to face the listener, exaggerate the pronunciation of words, and speak in short sentences. Encourage them to take a few deep breaths before speaking.

A speech–language pathologist may be helpful in designing speech improvement exercises and assisting health care personnel to develop a method of communication to meet the patient's needs. Having the patient speak into a tape recorder periodically is useful in monitoring the patient's progress. A small electronic amplifier is helpful if the patient has difficulty in being heard.

Developing Positive Coping Abilities. Faithful adherence to an exercise and walking program helps to delay the progress of the disease. Encouragement and reassurance can be given by praising the patient for perseverance and pointing out that activities are being maintained through active participation. A combination of physiotherapy, psychotherapy, drug therapy, and sociotherapy may be necessary to help combat the depression that so often accompanies this condition.

Patients with Parkinson's disease often feel embarrassed, apathetic, inadequate, bored, and lonely. These feelings may be due, in part, to physical slowness and the great effort that even small tasks require. Help patients set achievable goals (*e.g.,* improvement of mobility). Since parkinsonism tends to lead to withdrawal and depression, patients must be *active* participants in their therapeutic program, including social and recreational events. There should be a planned program of activity throughout the day to prevent too much daytime sleeping as well as disinterest and apathy.

Every effort should be made to encourage patients to carry out the tasks involved in coping with their own daily needs and to retain independence. "Doing things" for the patient merely to save time runs contrary to this basic goal of improvement of coping abilities.

Patient Education and Home Health Care. The need for information about Parkinson's disease is ongoing as adaptations and concessions are made to the illness. Every effort is made to explain the nature of the disease and its management in order to offset anxieties and fears that may be as disabling as the disease itself. The American Parkinson's Disease Foundation publishes booklets and a newsletter for patient education.

The family is under considerable stress from living with a disabled member. Giving them information about treatment and care prevents many unnecessary problems. The caregiver is included in the plan. Counsel the caregiver to learn stress reduction techniques, to include others in the care-giving process, to obtain periodic relief from responsibilities, and to have a yearly health assessment. Giving family members "permission" to express feelings of frustration, anger, and guilt is often helpful to them.

▷ *Evaluation*

▷ *Expected Outcomes*

1. Patient strives toward improved mobility.
   a. Participates in exercise program daily
   b. Avoids hurrying
   c. Walks with wide base of support; exaggerates arm swinging when walking
   d. Takes prescribed medications faithfully
2. Progresses toward self-care
   a. Plans for and allows time for self-care
   b. Uses self-help devices
3. Attains improved nutritional status
   a. Swallows without choking
   b. Takes time while eating
4. Achieves a method of communication
   a. Communicates needs
   b. Practices speech exercises
5. Copes with effects of Parkinson's disease
   a. Sets realistic goals
   b. Demonstrates persistence in meaningful activities
   c. Verbalizes feelings to appropriate person

Huntington's Disease

Huntington's disease (HD) is a chronic, progressive, hereditary disease of the nervous system that results in progressive involuntary choreiform (dancelike) movement and dementia. It affects men and women of all races. Because it is transmitted as an autosomal dominant genetic disorder, each child of a parent with Huntington's disease has a 50% risk of inheriting the illness. A marker for the gene linked to HD has recently been identified. This may, in the future, provide a predictive test for those at risk.

Pathophysiology

The basic pathology involves premature death of cells in the basal ganglia, the region deep within the brain involved in the control of movement. There is also loss of cells in the cortex, which is associated with thinking, memory, perception, and judgment. Research suggests that the disease may be related to a lack of important brain chemicals (gamma-aminobutyric acid [GABA] and acetylcholine [ACh]) that inhibit nerve action. Onset usually occurs between the ages of 35 and 45; the patient slowly progresses toward death in 10 to 15 years. Approximately 10% of victims are children.

Clinical Manifestations

The most prominent clinical features of the disease are abnormal involuntary movements (*chorea*), intellectual decline, and, often, emotional disturbance. As the disease progresses, a constant writhing, twisting, uncontrollable movement may involve the entire body. These motions are devoid of purpose or rhythm, although patients may try to turn them into purposeful movement. All of the body musculature is involved. Facial movements produce tics and grimaces. Speech is affected, becoming slurred, hesitant, often explosive, and eventually unintelligible. Chewing and swallowing are difficult and there is a constant danger of choking and aspiration. Like speech, the gait becomes disorganized to the point that ambulation eventually is impossible. Although independent ambulation should be encouraged for as long as possible, a wheelchair is usually necessary at some point. (Eventually, the patient is confined to bed, as the chorea interferes with walking, sitting, and all activities.) Control of bladder and bowel is lost. Likewise, the sensorium is usually involved. There is progressive intellectual impairment, although the patient is generally aware that the disease is responsible for the myriad dysfunctions that are occurring.

The mental and emotional changes may be more devastating to the patient and family than the abnormal movements. Patients may be nervous, clumsy, irritable, or impatient. Particularly in the early stages of the illness, patients are subject to uncontrollable fits of anger; profound, often suicidal depression; apathy; or euphoria. Judgment and memory are impaired. Hallucinations, delusions, and paranoid thinking may even precede the appearance of disjointed movements. Emotional symptoms often become less acute as the disease progresses, although dementia eventually ensues. Despite a ravenous appetite, often for sweets, patients usually become emaciated and exhausted. Eventually, patients succumb from heart failure, pneumonia, or infection, or die as a result of a fall or choking.

Management

Although no treatment halts or reverses the underlying process, several methods of management have fairly good palliative action. The phenothiazines, butyrophenones, and thioxanthenes, which predominantly block dopamine receptors, improve the chorea in many patients. Chorea is also lessened by reserpine (acts by depleting presynaptic dopamine) and tetrabenazine (reduces dopaminergic transmission).

The patient's motor signs must be assessed and evaluated on a continuing basis so that optimal therapeutic drug levels may be reached. *Akathisia* (motor restlessness) in the overmedicated patient is a danger because it may be mistaken for the restless fidgetiness of the illness and consequently be overlooked.

In certain types of the disease in which hypokinetic motor impairment resembles parkinsonism, some benefit may be obtained from antiparkinsonism therapy (see p. 1478). Patients who have emotional disturbances, particularly depression, may be helped by antidepressant medications. The threat of suicide is always present. Psychotic symptoms usually respond to antipsychotic drugs. Psychotherapy aimed at allaying anxiety and reducing stress may be beneficial. It is imperative that nurses look beyond the disease to focus on the patient's needs and capabilities (Chart 54-2).

Patient and Family Teaching. A program combining medical, psychological, social, occupational, speech, and physical rehabilitation services is needed to help the patient and family cope with this severely disabling illness. More than most disorders, Huntington's disease exacts enormous emotional, physical, social, and financial tolls on every member of the patient's family. Entire families often live under a heavy burden of uncertainty, anxiety, and guilt. Not only is genetic counseling crucial, but patients and their families also require access to long-term psychological counseling, marriage counseling, and emotional, financial, and legal support. Regular follow-up helps to allay fear of abandonment. Some form of home care assistance, work and recreation day centers, respite care, and eventually skilled long-term care is necessary to help the patient and family cope with the constant strain of the illness. Although nothing can stop the relentless progress of the disease, families who have had supportive care have benefitted tremendously.

Voluntary health organizations are major aids to families and have been largely responsible for bringing the illness to national attention. The Huntington's Disease Foundation of America (see Bibliography for address) is oriented toward helping patients and their families by providing information, referrals, family and public education, and support for research.

Alzheimer's Disease

Alzheimer's disease, or senile dementia of the Alzheimer's type, is a chronic, progressive, and deteriorative brain disorder

Chart 54-2
The Challenges of a Patient With Huntington's Disease

Problem/Challenge	*Nursing Interventions*
Constant movement Skin excoriation Abrasions or pressure sores Falls	Pad the sides and head of the bed; ensure that the patient can see over the sides of bed. Use lamb's wool padding for heel and elbow protection. Keep the skin meticulously clean. Apply emollient cleansing agent and skin lotion frequently. Use *soft* sheets and bedding. Have patient wear football or other padding. Encourage ambulation with assistance to maintain muscle tone. Tie the patient (only if absolutely necessary) in bed or chair with padded protective devices, making sure that they are loosened frequently. Remove objects that the patient can trip over.
Feeding Constant movement Difficulty in chewing or swallowing Choking/Aspiration Malnutrition/Emaciation Dehydration	Give phenothiazines before meals; it appears to calm some patients. Use a warming tray. Talk to the patient before mealtime to promote relaxation; use mealtime for social interaction. Give your undivided attention. Help the patient enjoy the mealtime experience. Learn the position that is best for *this* patient. Keep patient as close to upright as possible while feeding. Stabilize patient's head gently with one hand while feeding. Show the food and tell the patient what the foods are (*e.g.,* whether hot or cold). Encircle the patient with one arm and get as close as possible to provide stability and support. Use pillows and wedges for additional support. Do not interpret stiffness, turning away, or sudden turning of the head as rejection; these are uncontrollable choreiform movements. In feeding, use a long-handled spoon (iced-tea spoon). Place spoon on middle of tongue and exert slight pressure. Place bite-size food between teeth. Serve stews, casseroles, thick liquids; avoid too many milk drinks (produces mucus). Disregard "messiness." Treat the person with dignity. *Wait* for the patient to chew and swallow before introducing another spoonful. Make sure that bite-sized food is small. Give between-meal feedings. Constant movement burns more calories. Patients are often voracious, particularly for sweets.

(continued)

accompanied by profound effects on memory, cognition, and ability for self-care. Approximately 4% of the population over 65 is affected, and the prevalence reaches 20% by age 80. It is one of the most feared disorders of modern times because it has catastrophic consequences for the victim and family, who experience what has been termed an "endless funeral."

The cause of Alzheimer's disease remains unknown. A variety of factors that may contribute to the development of the disease have been suggested, including age; familial, genetic, and chromosomal factors; metabolic abnormalities; and perhaps a virus.

Possible risk factors include the occurrence of either dementia or Down's syndrome in other family members, birth to a mother older than 40, and head trauma with loss of consciousness.

Pathophysiology. Available evidence indicates that a number of neuronal systems are involved in this disease. The distinguishing microscopic feature is an accumulation of *neurofibrillary tangles* (abnormal tangled fibers) and the occurrence of *senile plaques* (round or ovoid structures composed of destroyed dendrites and synapses that are imbedded in a central amyloid core) in the brains of patients with Alzheimer's

Chart 54-2 (continued)

Problem/Challenge	Nursing Interventions
	Use *blenderized meals* if patient cannot chew; do not give the same strained baby foods; gradually introduce increased textures and consistencies to the diet.
	For swallowing difficulties:
	Apply gentle deep pressure around the patient's mouth.
	Rub fingers in circles on the patient's cheeks.
	Rub fingers simultaneously down each side of the patient's throat.
	Know the Heimlich maneuver (to be used in the event of choking).
Psychological support and communication Grimacing Unintelligible speech	Approach from the front and avoid startling the patient.
	Respect the patient as a fellow human being with rights and needs.
	Use eye contact. Touch the patient.
	Talk, even though the patient may not be able to answer.
	Read to the patient.
	Employ biofeedback and relaxation therapy to reduce stress.
	Use speech and language therapy to help maintain and prolong communication abilities.
	Try to devise a communication system, perhaps using cards with words or pictures of familiar objects, before verbal communication becomes too difficult.
	Patients can indicate correct card by hitting it with hand, grunting, or blinking the eyes.
	Learn how this particular patient expresses needs and wants—particularly nonverbal messages (widening of eyes, responses).
	Patients can understand even if unable to speak. Do not isolate patients by ceasing to communicate with them.
Progressive intellectual impairment and emotional disturbance	Have a clock, calendar, and wall posters in view.
	Interact with the patient in a *creative* manner.
	Use every opportunity for one-to-one contact.
	Use music for relaxation.
	Reorient the patient after awakening.
	Have the patient wear an identification bracelet with name, telephone number, and "memory impaired" on it.
	Keep the patient in the social mainstream.
	Recruit and train volunteers for social interaction. Set a good example.
	Do not abandon a patient because the disease is eventually terminal. Patients are *living* until the end.

disease. There is a marked loss of nerve cells from the cerebral cortex. The cell death is accompanied by a corresponding reduction in blood flow in the brain. Research scientists report that there is evidence of a significant and progressive decrease in the activity of the enzyme choline acetyltransferase in the brain tissue. Choline acetyltransferase is a crucial ingredient in the chemical process that produces *acetylcholine*, a neurotransmitter involved in learning and memory.

Clinical Manifestations. While the onset may be insidious, family members usually notice that the patient has significant forgetfulness and memory impairment. Gradually there is deterioration of higher cognitive function, with loss of ability to read, to write, to calculate, and even to communicate intelligently. Personality changes may be marked. In time disorders of motor function, including disorders of gait, occur.

The family, who are the "other victims" of this dementing illness, report that the patient's restlessness, neglect of self-care, confusion, urinary incontinence, falls, and episodes of rage are particularly troublesome burdens.

Diagnostic Evaluation. At this time Alzheimer's disease can only be confirmed with certainty by microscopic examination of neural tissue, usually at autopsy. CT scans in some patients demonstrate progressive reduction in brain volume (atrophy) in excess of that occurring in normal aging. Positron emission tomography (PET) reveals decreased regional metabolism of glucose and oxygen and decreased blood flow in cortical areas. Serial evaluations of neuropsychological testing provide information on the rate of deterioration.

Probable Alzheimer's disease diagnosis is based on clinically determined progressive dementia (confirmed by neuropsychologic tests), two or more cognitive deficits, progressive worsening of memory or other cognitive functions, no disturbances of consciousness, and absence of systemic disorders or other brain disorders that could cause progressive deficits in memory and cognition.

Nursing Process. The nursing process applied to the management of the patient with Alzheimer's disease is found in Chapter 11.

Neuromuscular Diseases

Myasthenia Gravis

Myasthenia gravis is a disorder affecting the neuromuscular transmission of the voluntary muscles of the body; it is characterized by excessive weakness and fatigability of muscle function. It affects younger women; men who develop the disease do so later in life.

Pathophysiology. The basic abnormality in myasthenia gravis is a defect in the transmission of impulses from nerve to muscle cells due to loss of available or normal receptors on the postsynaptic membrane of the neuromuscular junction. Myasthenia gravis is considered an autoimmune disease in which antibodies directed against acetylcholine receptor (AChR) impair neuromuscular transmission.

Clinical Manifestations. The disease is characterized by *extreme muscular weakness* and easy fatigability, which generally is worse after effort and is relieved by rest. Patients with this disease tire on such slight exertion as combing the hair, chewing, and talking, and must stop for rest. Symptoms vary according to the muscles affected. Symmetrical muscles are involved, first and foremost those innervated by cranial nerves. Because of the involvement of the ocular muscles, *diplopia* (double vision) and *ptosis* (drooping of the eyelids) are early symptoms. The patient has a sleepy, masklike expression because the facial muscles are affected. Laryngeal involvement produces a *dysphonia* (voice impairment) in the form of a nasal sound of the voice or difficulty in articulation. Weakness of the bulbar muscles causes problems with chewing and swallowing and presents a danger of choking and aspiration. Approximately 15% to 20% of patients complain of weakness of arm and hand muscles and, less commonly, of leg muscle weakness, which makes the patient subject to falls.

- *Progressive weakness of the diaphragm and intercostal muscles may produce respiratory distress or myasthenic crisis, which is an acute emergency.*

Diagnostic Evaluation. The signs and symptoms of myasthenia gravis are sometimes so striking that a presumptive

diagnosis can be made on the basis of the patient's history and physical examination. An injection of edrophonium (Tensilon), a drug that facilitates the transmission of nerve–muscle messages, is used to confirm the diagnosis. Within 30 seconds of an intravenous injection of edrophonium, most patients will improve substantially, but only temporarily. Improvement in muscle strength following administration of this agent usually confirms the diagnosis of myasthenia. Demonstration of the antiAChR antibodies in the serum is found in nearly 90% of patients with myasthenia gravis.

Electromyography (EMG) is used to measure the electrical potential of muscle cells.

Management

Management of myasthenia gravis is directed at improving remaining function through the administration of anticholinesterase medications, reducing antibodies, and removing circulating antibodies. Therapy includes anticholinesterase drugs and immunosuppressive therapy, including plasmapheresis, and thymectomy.

Anticholinesterase drugs act by increasing the relative concentration of available acetylcholine in the neuromuscular junction. They are given to increase the response of the muscles to nerve impulses and to improve strength. However, these provide only symptomatic relief.

Drugs in current use include pyridostigmine bromide (Mestinon), ambenonium chloride (Mytelase), and neostigmine bromide (Prostigmin). Most patients prefer pyridostigmine because it produces less marked side-effects. The dosage is increased gradually until maximal benefits are obtained (additional strength, less fatigue), although normal muscle strength may not be achieved and the patient may have to adapt to some disability. Anticholinesterase medications are given with milk, crackers, or other buffering substances. Their side-effects include abdominal cramps, nausea, and vomiting. Small doses of atropine, given once or twice daily, may ameliorate or prevent these side-effects. Other side-effects of anticholinesterase therapy include adverse effects on skeletal muscles, such as fasciculations (fine twitching), spasm, and weakness. The effects on the central nervous system include irritability, anxiety, insomnia, headache, dysarthria, syncope, convulsions, and coma. Increased salivation and lacrimation, increased bronchial secretions, and moist skin may also be noted.

- The nursing (and patient) priority is to give the drug prescribed according to an exact time schedule in order to control the patient's symptoms. *Any delay in drug administration may result in the patient's losing the ability to swallow.* Watch for an increase in muscle weakness within 1 hour after the patient takes the anticholinesterase drug, and be particularly alert for signs of respiratory distress.

After the initial medication doses have been adjusted, the patient learns to take the medication according to his needs and time plan. Further adjustments may be necessary in the presence of physical or emotional stress and intercurrent infection.

Immunosuppressive Therapy. Immunosuppressive therapy is directed toward reducing the production of antireceptor antibody or its direct removal by plasma exchange (explained below). Included in immunosuppressive therapy are corticosteroids, plasmapheresis, and thymectomy. Corticosteroid therapy may benefit the patient with severe generalized myasthenia. Steroids exert their effect by suppressing the patient's immune response, thus decreasing the amount of blocking antibody. The anticholinesterase dosage is lowered while the patient's ability to maintain effective respirations and to swallow is monitored. The steroid dosage is gradually increased and the anticholinesterase medication is slowly reduced. Prednisone, taken on alternate days to lower the incidence of side-effects, appears to be successful in suppressing the disease. Sometimes the patient will show a marked decrease in muscle strength right after steroid therapy is started, but this is usually only temporary. The patient is given a tap bell to use in emergency situations.

Plasma Exchange. Plasma exchange is a technique that permits selective removal of the patient's plasma and plasma components. The remaining cells are reinfused into the patient. Plasma exchange produces a temporary reduction in the titer of circulating antibodies. This process has caused remarkable improvement in some patients, but does not treat the underlying abnormality (production of antireceptor antibody) over the long term.

Surgical Management

The thymus in myasthenia gravis patients seems to be involved in the process of AChR antibody production. *Thymectomy* (surgical removal of the thymus) causes substantial remission of the disease, especially in patients with tumor or hyperplasia of the thymus gland. Thymectomy is carried out through the sternum because the entire thymus must be removed.

It is felt that thymectomy *early* in the course of the disease is specific therapy, as it prevents formation of antireceptor antibodies. Following surgery, the patient is monitored in an intensive care unit; special attention is given to ventilatory function.

Myasthenic Crisis

Myasthenic crisis is the sudden onset of muscular weakness in patients with myasthenia. It may be manifested by sudden respiratory distress and an inability to swallow or speak. Weakness of respiratory, laryngeal, pharyngeal, and bulbar musculature causes respiratory depression and airway obstruction as well as cerebral hypoxia with its attendant sequelae of central nervous system injury and death.

Myasthenic crisis may result from progression of the disease, emotional upset, systemic infections, certain drugs, surgery, or trauma, or it may be brought about by ACTH therapy.

Cholinergic crisis occurs from overmedication with anticholinesterase drugs, which release too much acetylcholine at the neuromuscular junction. *Brittle crisis* occurs when the receptors at the neuromuscular junction become insensitive to anticholinesterase medication. It is not controlled by increasing or decreasing anticholinesterase therapy.

Recognition and Management of Myasthenic Crisis

Respiratory distress combined with varying signs of dysphagia (difficulty in swallowing), dysarthria (difficulty in speaking), eyelid ptosis, and diplopia are symptoms of impending crisis.

- Providing adequate ventila
  dence in the immediate ma
  myasthenic crisis.
- The patient is suctioned, bec
  problem. Arterial blood is (
  analysis. Endotracheal intul
  tilation may be needed (se
  placed in an intensive care u
  since this condition is marl
  fluctuations.

Intravenous edrophonium (Tensilon) is given to differentiate the type of crisis. It improves the condition of the patient in myasthenic crisis, temporarily worsens that of the patient in cholinergic crisis, and it unpredictable in brittle crisis. If the patient is in true myasthenic crisis, neostigmine methylsulfate (Prostigmin) is administered intramuscularly or intravenously.

If the edrophonium (Tensilon) test is uncertain or there is increasing respiratory weakness, all anticholinesterase drugs are withdrawn and atropine sulfate is given to reduce excessive secretions.

Other supportive measures include the following:

- Monitor arterial blood gases, serum electrolytes, input and output, and daily weight
- If the patient is unable to swallow, feed by way of nasogastric tube (200 ml at a time). (Postural drainage should not be done for half an hour after feeding.)
- Avoid use of sedatives and tranquilizing drugs, since these agents aggravate hypoxia and hypercapnia and can cause respiratory and cardiac depression.

Nursing Interventions During Myasthenic Crisis

In a patient with diminishing ventilatory capacity, the nurse assesses respiratory rate, depth, and breath sounds and studies the results of pulmonary function tests (tidal volume, vital capacity, inspiratory force) at very frequent intervals to detect pulmonary problems before changes in arterial blood gas levels become clinically apparent. When there is severe weakness of abdominal, intercostal, and pharyngeal muscles, the patient is unable to cough and breathe deeply or clear secretions. Chest physical therapy, including postural drainage to mobilize secretions and suctioning to remove secretions, may have to be done frequently.

The patient with insufficient air exchange will experience anxiety sometimes bordering on panic. This is compounded by an inability to communicate verbally and by a tendency to choke. Acknowledging the patient's fears can give assurance that the nurse understands the concerns. The patient gains some sense of control through skilled care and the calm support of the nurse.

The weakened speech muscles in patients in myasthenic crisis interfere with communication. Techniques for improving communication include listening to patients; repeating what they have tried to communicate, to clarify and verify information; and asking patients to blink eyes or wiggle fingers or toes for "yes" and "no" answers. After the period of myasthenic crisis has resolved, patients are usually able to make their needs known.

...d ability to chew and swallow may result in ...d aspiration. The patient is assessed for drooling, ...tion through the nose, and choking while attempting ...allow. Standby suction should be available. Encourage ...t before meals to lessen muscle fatigue. Place the patient in an upright position with neck slightly flexed to facilitate swallowing. Soft foods in gravy or sauces appear to be swallowed more easily than liquids. If the patient is taking an anticholinesterase agent, the nurse makes sure it is given one hour before mealtime to ensure maximum muscle strength. Because muscles of mastication may be stronger in the morning, the calorie intake can be increased at breakfast. The patient is encouraged to rest after eating.

Impaired vision results from ptosis of one or both eyelids, decreased eye movement, or double vision. Nursing interventions to help the patient cope include taping the eyes open for short intervals, instilling artificial tears to prevent corneal damage when eyelids do not close completely, placing a patch over one eye when double vision is a problem, and/or keeping the patient informed while giving care.

Indicating that the crisis should pass and that the patient will not be left alone may help to make the situation bearable.

Patient Education and Home Health Care. The patient's goal is improvement of strength and endurance. To be a participant in treatment the patient should learn the basic facts about anticholinergic drugs—their action, timing, dosage adjustment, symptoms of overdose, and toxic effects. Stress the importance of taking the medication on time. Encourage the patient to keep a diary to determine fluctuation of symptoms and to know when the medication is wearing off.

There are a number of drugs that aggravate myasthenia gravis, and the patient is advised to consult with the physician before taking any new medications, including certain antibiotics, cardiovascular drugs, anticonvulsant and psychotrophic drugs, morphine, quinine and related agents, beta blockers, and the like. Novocain should be avoided, and the patient's dentist so advised.

Mealtimes should coincide with the peak effects of anticholinesterase if the patient has difficulty in swallowing. If choking occurs frequently, blenderized food may be easier to swallow. Standby suction should be available at home. Gastrostomy feedings may be necessary.

If diplopia occurs, wearing an eye patch over one eye (alternating from side to side) is useful. Applying a thin adhesive tape over the upper eyelid helps relieve ptosis. Sunglasses will diminish the effects of bright light that frequently increase eye problems.

Certain factors may increase weakness and precipitate a myasthenic crisis: emotional upset, infections (particularly respiratory infections), vigorous physical activity, and exposure to heat (hot baths, sun bathing) and cold. These situations should be avoided. To avoid the risk of fatigue, it is best to rest *before* becoming too tired. A cervical collar is useful for patients with weak neck muscles. Adaptive or self-help devices are available and are useful in helping the patient handle the disease more effectively and to live as full a life as possible. The patient is also advised to wear an identification bracelet.

The Myasthenia Gravis Foundation has materials written for both lay and professional readers, available upon request (see Bibliography for address).

Amyotrophic Lateral Sclerosis

Amyotrophic lateral sclerosis (ALS, Lou Gehrig's disease) is a disease of unknown cause in which there is a loss of motor neurons (nerve cells controlling muscles) in the anterior horns of the spinal cord and the motor nuclei of the lower brain steam. As these cells die, the muscle fibers that they supply undergo atrophic changes. The degeneration of the neurons may occur in both the upper and lower motor neuron systems.

ALS affects more men than women, with onset occurring usually in the fifth or sixth decade. In this country, it is often referred to as "Lou Gehrig's disease" after the famous ballplayer who died from it.

Clinical Manifestations. The clinical manifestations of ALS depend on the location of the affected motor neurons, since specific neurons activate specific muscle fibers. The chief symptoms are progressive muscle weakness, atrophy, and fasciculations (twitching). Loss of motor neurons in the anterior horns of the spinal cord results in progressive weakness and atrophy of the muscles of the arms, trunk, or legs. Spasticity is usually present, and the stretch reflexes become brisk and overactive. Usually the anal and bladder sphincters are not affected because the spinal nerves that control muscles of the rectum and urinary bladder are preserved. In approximately 25% of patients, weakness starts in the musculature supplied by the cranial nerves and there is difficulty talking, swallowing, and ultimately breathing. When the patient ingests liquids, the soft palate and upper esophageal weakness cause the liquid to be regurgitated through the nose. Weakness of the posterior tongue and palate impairs the ability to laugh, cough, or even blow the nose. When bulbar muscles are impaired, there is progressive difficulty in speaking and swallowing, and choking becomes a problem. The voice assumes a nasal sound and speech articulation becomes so disrupted that the patient is unintelligible. Some emotional lability may be present, but intellectual function is not impaired. Eventually respiratory function is compromised.

The prognosis generally is based on the area involved and the speed with which the disease progresses. Usually the patient dies from a secondary cause such as pneumonia. While 50% of patients with ALS die in approximately 3 years, 20% survive beyond 5 years, 10% survive beyond 10 years, and up to 20% experience plateaus for extended periods, and the eventual permanent arrest of the disease.

Diagnostic Evaluation. ALS is diagnosed on the basis of the signs and symptoms, because no clinical or laboratory tests are specific for this disease. Electromyographic studies of the affected muscle indicate reduction in the number of motor units.

Management

No specific treatment for ALS is available. Symptomatic treatment and rehabilitative measures are employed to support the patient and improve the quality of life. Baclofen or diazepam may be useful for patients troubled by spasticity, since spasticity causes pain and interferes with self-care. Quinine therapy may be prescribed for painful muscle cramps. High doses of thyrotropin-releasing hormone, a naturally occurring hormone produced by the brain and found in the motor neurons of the spinal cord, are being used investigationally to improve function. Interferon, a compound that appears to stimulate the body's defense system, is another investigational drug. A patient experiencing problems with aspiration and swallowing may require nasogastric or gastrostomy feedings. A cervical *esophagostomy* (opening into the esophagus) may be done to bypass the larynx and prevent aspiration.

Mechanical ventilation is considered when alveolar hypoventilation develops. The decision for the use of life support measures is made by the patient and family. Patients who decide against ventilation therapy may consider making a "living will" to preserve their autonomy.

▶ *Nursing Process*
The Patient With Amyotrophic Lateral Sclerosis

▷ *Assessment*

The focus of the nursing assessment is on determining how ALS is affecting the patient's functioning. Ongoing assessment is directed at detecting incipient respiratory difficulties. A history of present eating habits is obtained. Find out what foods the patient can manage. Inspect the facial muscles for bilateral weakness. Offer a glass of water and watch the patient drink. Observe for incomplete lip closure, poor head position, pooling of secretions, difficulty in swallowing, choking, and regurgitation of fluids through the nose. Look for loss of tongue coordination, which causes difficulty in moving solids back towards the pharynx. Speech abnormalities also indicate oral or palatal dysfunction.

Ask the patient to cough, clench the jaw, and hold a breath. Observe for wasting of musculature. Watch the patient perform self-care, if able. See if the patient can turn a page of a book.

▷ *Nursing Diagnoses*

Based on all the assessment data, the patient's major nursing diagnoses may include the following:

- Impaired physical mobility related to muscle weakness and wasting
- Inadequate nutritional intake related to inability to chew and swallow
- Impaired communication related to disturbance in muscular control of speech mechanisms
- Potential respiratory failure related to impaired intercostal, thoracic, and diaphragmatic muscle function/bulbar paralysis with aspiration/asphyxiation
- Ineffective family coping related to overwhelming physical and emotional demands imposed by the disease

▷ *Planning and Implementation*

▷ *Goals:* The patient's goals may include compensation for muscle weakness and wasting, improvement of nutritional intake, development of an alternative communication system, and recognition of and dealing with respiratory dysfunction.

The family's goals are adaptation to and coping with prolonged illness.

Nursing Interventions

Compensating for Muscle Weakness and Atrophy. An important nursing goal is to assist the patient in maximizing independence. The patient should remain active as long as possible without tiring the involved muscles. Active exercises and range-of-motion exercises help to strengthen uninvolved muscles and maintain muscle power at optimum levels. Stretching exercises (stretch–hold–relax) are beneficial. Exercise is stopped short of fatigue. Such devices as ankle–foot orthoses for patient with weak dorsiflexors, (which impair dorsiflexion of the ankle) help keep the patient mobile. Hand splints can provide a stronger grip and more effective use of the hand, while other devices to support weakened extremities or neck muscles can maintain optimum joint position.

As the muscles grow weaker, the patient may use a wheelchair for activities outside the house. Assistive devices are used to help the patient function independently for as long as possible. Offer instructions in energy conservation and work-simplification methods. When the illness has progressed to the point where the patient is confined to a wheelchair, an electrically-powered model can be used. At this stage, the prevention of contractures is important. When the patient becomes dependent, a mechanical lift for bed, toilet, and tub transfers will be needed, and special instructions will have to be given to the family concerning the best way to position the patient for the greatest comfort. (See p. 222 for prevention of pressure sores.)

Improving Nutritional Intake. Nutrition is very important, especially in the patient with progressive bulbar involvement that affects the swallowing mechanism and causes choking and difficulty in swallowing and speaking. Aspiration is a constant danger. Standby suction should be available. Encourage the patient to rest before meals to alleviate muscle fatigue, which increases swallowing difficulty. The patient is placed in an upright position with his neck slightly flexed to facilitate swallowing, and should remain in the upright posture for 15 to 30 minutes after eating. Foods with consistency (soft foods in gravy) seem to be more easily swallowed than liquids. Weakened swallowing muscles allow fluid and food to become entrapped in the throat. Avoid "washing down" solid foods with liquids, as this may cause choking and aspiration. The family is taught procedures for dislodging food in the event of choking. A soft cervical collar is useful if the patient has difficulty holding the head erect.

Improving Communication. The patient will require an alternate communication system as the disease relentlessly progresses and speech is lost. Practical methods can be selected by a speech–language pathologist to maximize the patient's remaining potential for speech. For patients who can use their hands, small computers are available with artificial speech articulation. A pointer held in the teeth may be used with a picture or word chart. There are ingenious high-tech instruments that can assist ALS patients to speak through a computer's synthesizer by moving the muscles of the eyebrows. A predetermined code using eye blinks for "yes" and "no" may eventually be the patient's only means of communication.

Assuring Respiratory Function. Central respiratory drive may be reduced during sleep, causing restless sleep, multiple awakenings, and daytime drowsiness. The most serious complication in the later stages of the disease is respiratory dysfunction, because all muscles involved in breathing may be affected. The patient with ALS should be evaluated periodically with pulmonary function testing. Techniques to enhance pulmonary function include upright positioning, breathing exercises, suctioning of excessive secretions, chest physical therapy, and the use of incentive spirometry. Decisions about whether or not to use assisted ventilation are based on respiratory assessment and patient desire. Improved technology and lightweight portable units have made the home use of positive pressure ventilators more practical.

Promoting Family Coping and Home Health Care. The patient and family facing this cruel affliction need compassionate caring and support. It is often agonizing to discuss this disease with them, but information about the disease and the teaching of nursing procedures and comfort measures are essential for the management of the patient in the home care setting. The family will require ongoing assistance and supervision. Professionals can help in making practical suggestions and in giving information about home health care products and equipment, services, and support groups. Arranging for respite care for the family and providing emotional support and reliable back-up in the event of emergencies are part of caring for the caregivers. It is desirable that a social worker/counselor support the patient and family throughout the course of the illness. This helps keep stress within manageable limits.

The ALS Association has broad programs of research funding, patient and clinical services, patient information and support, and medical and public information (see Bibliography for address). The ALS Association Quarterly Newsletter is filled with practical information.

▷ *Evaluation*

▷ *Expected Outcomes*

1. Patient copes with impaired mobility.
   a. Family uses mechanical lift, wheelchair, and other aids.
   b. Patient maintains interest in reading and in listening to "talking books" and tapes as a means of diversion.
2. Attempts to maintain nutritional status
   a. Avoids empty calories
   b. Chooses food that he is able to swallow
3. Uses alternative communication system
   a. Seeks direction from speech–language pathologist
   b. Reviews information about computer programs
4. Is aware of danger of respiratory failure
   a. Family members can verbalize symptoms and signs of respiratory dysfunction.
   b. Patient and family know treatment options
5. Family members use coping mechanisms.
   a. Have adequate backup system of trained family, friends, health professionals
   b. Use community and other resources appropriately

The Muscular Dystrophies

The muscular dystrophies are a group of chronic muscle disorders characterized by progressive weakening and wasting of the skeletal or voluntary muscles. Most of these diseases are inherited.

The pathologic features include muscle fiber necrosis, variation in muscle fiber size, cellular reaction, increased internal nuclei, and replacement of muscle tissue by connective tissue.

The common characteristics of these diseases include varying degrees of muscle wasting and weakness; abnormal elevation in serum creatine phosphokinase, indicating a leakage of muscle enzymes; a myopathic electromyographic pattern; and myopathic findings on muscle biopsy. The differences center around the pattern of inheritance, the muscles involved, the age of onset, and the rate of progression.

Management

There is no specific treatment at this time for the muscular dystrophies. The objectives of supportive management are to keep the patient as active and functioning as normally as possible and to minimize functional deterioration. A therapeutic exercise program is prescribed for the individual patient to prevent muscle tightness, contractures, and disuse atrophy. Night splints and stretching exercises are used to delay contractures of the joints, especially the ankles, knees, and hips. Braces may compensate for muscle weakness.

Spinal deformity is a severe problem. Weakness of trunk muscles and spinal collapse occur almost routinely in patients with severe neuromuscular disease. In the battle against spinal deformity, the patient is fitted with an orthotic jacket to improve sitting stability and reduce trunk deformity. This measure also supports cardiovascular status. In time, spinal fusion is performed to maintain spinal stability. Other surgical procedures may be carried out to correct deformities.

Compromised pulmonary function may be due either to progression of the disease or to deformity of the thorax secondary to severe scoliosis. Intercurrent illnesses, upper respiratory infections, and fractures from falls must be vigorously treated in a way that minimizes immobilization, since joint contractures will become worse if the patient's activities are restricted more than usual. Aside from muscle weakness and contractures, a variety of other difficulties may be manifested in relation to the underlying disease. Dental and speech problems may result from weakness of the facial muscles, which makes it difficult to attend to dental hygiene and to speak coherently. Additional problems may affect the gastrointestinal tract, resulting in gastric dilatation, rectal prolapse, and fecal impaction. Finally, cardiomyopathy appears to be a common complication in all forms of muscular dystrophy.

Because of the genetic nature of this disease, parents and siblings of the patient are advised to seek genetic counseling. The Muscular Dystrophy Association works to combat neuromuscular disease through scientific research, programs of patient services and clinical care, and professional and public education (see Bibliography for address).

Nursing Interventions and Home Health Care

The goals of the patient and the nurse are to maintain function at optimal levels and to enhance the quality of life. This is accomplished, in part, by attending to the patient's physical requirements, which are considerable, without losing sight of emotional needs. The patient and family are made to feel actively involved in decision making.

Both the neuromuscular disease and the associated deformities may progress in adolescence and adulthood. Self-help devices can assist in achieving a greater degree of independence. Additional self-help devices become necessary as more muscle groups become affected. The patient is encouraged to continue with range-of-motion programs to prevent contractures, which are particularly disabling. The family is taught to monitor the patient for respiratory problems.

Practical adaptations must be made to cope with the effects of chronic neuromuscular disability. To maximize functional independence, the patient at various stages of the disease may require a manual or an electric wheelchair, gait aids, upper and lower extremity and spinal orthoses, seating systems, bathroom equipment, lifts, ramps, and additional ADL aids. This requires a team approach. The home health nurse assesses how the patient and family are managing, makes referrals, and coordinates the activities of the physical therapist, occupational therapist, and social services.

Of great concern to the patient are the issues surrounding the threat of increasing disability. The patient is faced with a drawn-out, progressive loss of powers, leading eventually to death. Helplessness and powerlessness are central in the course of prolonged illness. Each functional loss involves a period of grieving and mourning. The patient's coping mechanisms are analyzed for signs of depression, prolonged anger, bargaining, or denial. A psychiatric nurse clinician or other mental health professional is invaluable in helping the patient cope and adapt to chronic disease. By understanding and providing for the physical and psychological needs of the patient and family, the nurse can communicate strength to the patient and help provide a hopeful, supportive, and nurturing environment.

Convulsive Disorders

Seizures

Seizures are episodes of abnormal motor, sensory, autonomic, or psychic activity (or a combination of these) as a consequence of sudden excessive discharge from cerebral neurons. A part or all of the brain may be involved. The seizures are usually sudden and transient.

The causes are varied and are classified as idiopathic (genetic, developmental defects) and acquired. Among the causes of acquired seizures are hypoxemia of any cause, including vascular insufficiency, fever (childhood), head injury, hypertension, central nervous system infections, metabolic and toxic conditions (*e.g.*, renal failure, hyponatremia, hypocalcemia, hypoglycemia, pesticides), brain tumor, drug withdrawal, and allergies. Stroke and cerebral metastasis are the leading causes of seizures in the elderly.

Often there is memory loss for the convulsive episode and for a short time thereafter. Brain damage may occur when seizures are severe or prolonged. The patient is at risk for hypoxia, vomiting, and pulmonary aspiration or persistent metabolic abnormalities.

The immediate therapeutic goal is to control the seizure, and the long-term goal is to seek out and control the cause.

Nursing Assessment During a Seizure

A major responsibility of the nurse is to observe and to record the sequence of symptoms. The nature of the seizure usually indicates the type of treatment that is employed. Before and during an attack, the following should be noted:

1. Description of the circumstances before the attack (visual stimuli, auditory stimuli, olfactory stimuli, tactile stimuli, emotional or psychic disturbances, sleep, hyperventilation)
2. The first thing the patient does in an attack—where the movements or the stiffness starts, position of the eyeballs and the head at the beginning of the attack. This information gives clues as to the location of the epileptogenic focus in the brain. (In recording, always state whether or not the beginning of the attack was observed.)
3. The type of movements of the part involved
4. The parts involved. (Turn back bedding and expose patient.)
5. The size of both pupils. Are the eyes open? Did the eyes/head turn to one side?
6. Whether or not automatisms (involuntary motor activity such as lip smacking or repeated swallowing) were observed
7. Incontinence of urine or feces
8. Duration of each phase of the attack
9. Unconsciousness, if present, and its duration
10. Any obvious paralysis or weakness of arms or legs after the attack
11. Inability to speak after the attack
12. Movements at the end of the seizure
13. Whether or not the patient sleeps afterward
14. Whether or not the patient was confused following the attack

Nursing Management During a Seizure

During a convulsive seizure, the nursing goal is to prevent injury to the patient. This includes not only physical support, but psychological support as well.

- Provide privacy and protect the patient from curious onlookers. (The patient who has an *aura* [warning of an impending seizure] may have time to seek a safe place.)
- Ease the patient to the floor, if there is enough time.
- Protect the head with a pad to prevent injury (from striking a hard surface).

- Loosen constrictive clothing.
- Push aside any furniture that may be struck by the patient during the attack.
- If the patient is in bed, remove the pillows.
- If an aura precedes the seizure, insert a handkerchief between the teeth to reduce the possibility of the tongue or cheek being bitten. *Do not attempt to pry open jaws that are clenched in a spasm to insert a mouth gag.* Broken teeth and injury to the lips and tongue may result from such an action.
- No attempt should be made to restrain the patient during the seizure, since muscular contractions are strong and restraint can produce a fracture.
- If possible, place the patient on one side with head flexed forward which permits the tongue to fall forward and facilitates drainage of saliva and mucus.
- After the seizure, keep the patient turned on one side to prevent aspiration. Make sure the airway is adequate.
- There is usually a period of confusion following epileptic attacks.
- The patient, upon awakening, should be reoriented to the environment.
- If the patient experiences severe excitement following a seizure (postictal), try to handle the situation with calm persuasion and gentle restraint.

The Epilepsies

The epilepsies are a symptom-complex of several disorders of brain function characterized by recurring seizures. There may be associated loss of consciousness, excess or loss of muscle tone or movement, and disturbances of behavior, mood, sensation, and perception. Thus, epilepsy is not a disease, but a symptom.

The basic problem is thought to be an electrical disturbance (dysrhythmia) in the nerve cells in one section of the brain, causing them to give off abnormal, recurring, uncontrolled electrical discharges. The characteristic epileptic seizure is a manifestation of this excessive neuronal discharge.

Incidence. An estimated 1% of the population (more than 2 million people) in the United States have epilepsy, with approximately 100,000 new patients diagnosed each year. There has been an increasing incidence of this condition, probably due to a number of factors. Improved obstetric and pediatric care salvages babies who experience respiratory, circulatory, and other distress during delivery; these persons are predisposed to intermittent seizures. The improved medical, surgical, and nursing management of patients with head injuries, brain tumors, meningitis, and encephalitis saves those whose conditions may produce cerebral changes with resultant seizures. Also, advances in electroencephalography have aided in the identification of patients with epilepsy. Education has served to enlighten the general public and has lessened the stigma associated with the condition, so that more persons are more willing to admit that they have epilepsy.

Altered Physiology. Messages from the body are carried by the neurons (nerve cells) of the brain by means of discharges of electrochemical energy that sweep along them. These impulses occur in bursts whenever a nerve cell has a task to perform. Sometimes certain of these cells or groups

of cells continue firing after a task is finished. It is as if a switch sticks in the "on" position until the power source runs down, and then closes to allow recharge. During the period of unwanted discharges, parts of the body controlled by the errant cells may perform erratically. Resultant discomfort and dysfunction range from mild to incapacitating, and usually cause unconsciousness. When these uncontrolled, abnormal discharges happen repeatedly, a person is said to have epilepsy. The erratic physical movements are called "seizures."*

Causes. No one knows what makes brain cells in some people cause epilepsy. Scientists have produced seizures in experimental animals through surgical injury or chemical or electrical stimulation. Epilepsies often follow birth trauma, asphyxia neonatorum, head injuries, some infectious diseases (bacterial, viral, parasitic), toxicity (carbon monoxide and lead poisoning), circulatory problems, fever, metabolic and nutritional disorders, and drug or alcohol intoxication. They are also associated with brain tumors, abscesses, and congenital malformations. In most cases of epilepsy the cause is unknown (idiopathic). There is evidence that susceptibility to some types may be inherited. Epilepsy strikes before the age of 20 in more than 75% of patients.

The epilepsies have little to do with intelligence in most cases. Persons with epilepsy who do not have other brain or nervous system disabilities will fall within the same intelligence ranges as does the overall population. Epilepsy is not synonymous with mental retardation or illness. However, many who are retarded because they have serious neurologic damage often have epilepsy too, thus pulling the mean IQ for all epilepsy victims below that of the so-called normal range.

Prevention of Epilepsy. A full-scale attack incorporating a wide range of measures must be mounted for the prevention of epilepsy. Since the infants of epileptic mothers who take certain antiepileptic medications are at risk, these women need careful monitoring, including blood studies to detect the level of antiepileptic drugs taken throughout pregnancy. High-risk mothers (teenagers, women with histories of difficult deliveries, drug addicts, those with diabetes and hypertension) should be identified and supervised closely during pregnancy because brain lesions or injury that ultimately causes epilepsy may occur to the fetus during pregnancy and delivery.

Childhood infections (measles, mumps, bacterial meningitis) should be controlled with appropriate vaccination. Lead poisoning is another preventable cause of epilepsy. Parents with a child who has had a febrile convulsion should be taught fever-regulating techniques (cool sponging, antipyretic medications).

Head injury is one of the main causes that can be prevented. Through highway safety programs and occupational safety precautions, not only can lives be saved, but the possible development of epilepsy from head injury can be prevented.

Screening programs to detect children with seizure disorders at an early age and seizure prevention programs with the judicious use of antiepileptic medications and modification of life-style are part of this prevention plan.

---

* Adapted from a report of the National Institute of Neurological Disease and Stroke.

Clinical Manifestations. Depending on the location of the discharging neurons, seizures may range from a simple staring spell to prolonged convulsive movements with loss of consciousness. The variations in seizures have been classified internationally according to the area of the brain involved, and have been identified as partial, generalized, and unclassified. *Partial* seizures are focal in origin and affect only part of the brain. *Generalized* seizures are nonspecific in origin and affect the entire brain simultaneously. *Unclassified* seizures are so termed because of incomplete data. (See Chart 54-3 for the international classification of seizures.)

The initial pattern of the seizures indicates the region of the brain in which the attack originates. Also, it is important to determine if the patient has had an *aura* (premonitory or warning sensation before an epileptic seizure), which may indicate the origin of the seizure (*e.g.,* seeing a flashing light may indicate the seizure originated in the occipital lobe).

In *simple partial seizures,* only a finger or hand may shake, or the mouth may jerk uncontrollably. The person may speak nonsense, may be dizzy, and may experience unusual or unpleasant sights, sounds, odors, or tastes, but without loss of consciousness.

In *complex partial seizures,* the person either remains motionless or moves automatically but inappropriately for time and place, or may experience excessive emotions of fear, anger, elation, or irritability. Whatever the manifestations, the person does not remember the episode when it is over.

Generalized seizures, more commonly referred to as *grand mal seizures,* involve both hemispheres of the brain, causing both sides of the body to react. There may be intense rigidity of the entire body followed by jerky alternations of muscle relaxation and contraction (generalized tonic–clonic contraction). The simultaneous contractions of the diaphragm and chest muscles may produce a characteristic "epileptic cry." Often the tongue is chewed, and stools and urine may be passed involuntarily. After 1 or 2 minutes, the convulsive movements begin to subside; the patient relaxes and lies in deep coma, breathing noisily. The respirations at this point are chiefly abdominal. In the postictal state (after the seizure), the patient is often confused and hard to arouse, and may sleep for hours. Many patients complain of headache or sore muscles.

Diagnostic Evaluation. The diagnostic assessment is aimed at determining the *type* of seizures, their frequency and severity, and the factors that precipitate them. A development history is taken, including events of pregnancy and childbirth, to seek evidence of preexisting injury. A search is made for illnesses or head injuries that may have affected the brain. In addition to a physical and neurologic examination, diagnostic examinations include biochemical, hematologic, and serologic studies. Computed tomography is used to detect lesions in the brain, focal abnormalities, cerebrovascular abnormalities, and cerebral degenerative changes.

The *electroencephalogram* (*EEG*) furnishes diagnostic evidence in a substantial proportion of patients with epilepsy and aids in classifying the type of seizure. Abnormalities in the EEG usually continue to be apparent between attacks, or, if concealed, may be brought out by hyperventilation or during sleep. In addition, microelectrodes can be inserted deep in the brain to probe the action of single brain cells. It should be noted, however, that some persons with seizures may have normal EEGs, whereas persons who have never had seizures may have abnormal EEGs. Telemetering and computer equipment developed by space technology are used to take and store electroecephalographic readings on computer tapes while patients pursue their normal activities. Videorecording of seizures taken simultaneously with EEG telemetry is useful in determining the type of seizure as well as its duration and magnitude. This type of intensive monitoring is revolutionizing the treatment of severe epilepsy in this country.

Management

The management of epilepsy is planned according to a long-range program, one that is tailored to meet the special needs of each patient and not just to manage and prevent seizures. There is no simple solution, since some forms of epilepsy arise from brain damage and others depend on alterations of brain chemistry.

Drug Therapy. Many antiepileptic drugs are available to control seizures, although the mechanisms of their actions are still unknown. The objective of drug therapy is to achieve seizure control with minimal side-effects. Drug therapy is a form of control, not cure. The drug is selected according to

---

Chart 54-3
International Classification of Seizures

Partial Seizures (seizures beginning locally)

1. Simple partial seizures (with elementary symptomatology, generally without impairment of consciousness)
   A. With motor symptoms
   B. With special sensory or somatosensory symptoms
   C. With autonomic symptoms
   D. Compound forms
2. Complex partial seizures (with complex symptomatology, generally with impairment of consciousness)
   A. With impairment of consciousness only
   B. With cognitive symptomatology
   C. With affective symptomatology
   D. With psychosensory symptomatology
   E. With psychomotor symptomatology (automatisms)
   F. Compound forms
3. Partial seizures secondarily generalized

Generalized Seizures (bilaterally symmetrical, without local onset)

1. Tonic–clonic seizures
2. Tonic seizures
3. Clonic seizures
4. Absence seizures
5. Atonic seizures
6. Myoclonic seizures (bilaterally massive epileptic)
7. Infantile spasms

the type of seizure being treated and the effectiveness and safety of the drug. If properly prescribed and taken, these drugs will result in seizure control in 50% to 60% of patients with recurring seizures, and in partial control in another 15% to 35%. The condition of approximately 15% to 35% of patients will not be improved by any drugs currently available.

Usually, treatment is started with a single drug. The starting dose and the rate at which the dosage is increased depend on whether or not side-effects develop. The drug levels are monitored in the blood, since the rate of drug absorption varies among people. Changing to another drug may be necessary if seizure control is not achieved or when toxicity makes it impossible to increase the dosage. The drug may have to be adjusted because of intercurrent illness, weight gain, or increases in stress. Sudden withdrawal of antiepileptic medication can cause seizures to occur with greater frequency or can precipitate the development of status epilepticus (see p. 1494).

The side-effects of these medications may be divided into three groups: (1) idiosyncratic or allergic disorders, which present primarily as skin reactions; (2) acute toxicity, which may be manifested when the drug is initially prescribed; or (3) chronic toxicity, which occurs late in the course of drug therapy. The manifestations of drug toxicity are variable, and any organ system may be involved. Periodic physical examinations and laboratory tests are done on patients receiving drugs known to have toxic effects on the hematopoietic, genitourinary, or hepatic systems. Table 54-1 summarizes the antiepileptic drugs in current use.

Surgery for Epilepsy. Surgery is indicated for patients whose epilepsy results from intracranial tumors, abscess, cysts, or vascular anomalies.

TABLE 54-1
Major Antiepileptic Drugs

Generic Name	Dose-Related Side-Effects	Toxic Effects
Carbamazepine	Dizziness; drowsiness Unsteadiness; nausea and vomiting Diplopia; mild leukopenia	Severe skin rash Blood dyscrasias Hepatitis
Primidone	Lethargy; irritability Diplopia; ataxia Sexual impotence	Skin rash
Phenytoin	Drowsiness; ataxia Visual problems Hirsutism Gingival hyperplasia	Severe skin reaction Peripheral neuropathy
Phenobarbital	Sedation; irritability Diplopia Ataxia	Skin rash
Ethosuximide	Nausea and vomiting Headache Gastric distress	Skin rash Blood dyscrasias Hepatitis Lupus
Valproate	Nausea and vomiting Weight gain Loss of hair	Skin rash Blood dyscrasias Nephritis Hepatotoxicity

Patient Counseling

1. Take medication daily to keep the amount of drug in the body constant to prevent seizures.

2. Report to the lab for blood sampling before taking morning medication when testing is prescribed.

3. Do not stop taking the drug abruptly; sudden withdrawal of medication may cause seizures.

4. Avoid activities that require alertness and coordination until after the effects of the drug have been evaluated.

5. Maintain oral hygiene and have regular dental care.

6. Carry a personal identification card stating the name of the drug you are taking.

Some patients have intractable seizure disorders that do not respond to drug therapy. There may be a focal atrophic process secondary to trauma, inflammation, stroke, or anoxemia. If the seizures originate in a reasonably well-circumscribed area of the brain that can be excised without producing significant neurologic deficits, the removal of the epileptogenic focus generating the seizures seems to give long-term control and improvement. This type of neurosurgery has been aided by several modern advances, including microsurgical techniques, depth electroencephalography, improved illumination and hemostasis, and the introduction of neuroleptanesthetic drugs (droperidol and fentanyl). These techniques, combined with local infiltration of scalp incisions, enable the neurosurgeon to perform surgery on an alert and cooperative patient. With special testing devices, electrocortical mapping, and the patient's response to stimulation, the boundaries of the epileptogenic focus are determined. Any abnormal epileptogenic cortex (*i.e.,* abnormal area of the brain) is then removed.

▶ *Nursing Process*
The Patient With Epilepsy

▷ *Assessment*

The nurse serves as an historian and observer to elicit information about the patient's seizure history. Find out if the patient knows the factors or events that precipitate the seizures. Ask about alcohol intake. Find out how epilepsy has interfered with life-style. Does the patient have a recreational program? Social contacts? Is work a positive experience? What coping mechanisms are used? What are the limitations imposed by the seizure disorder?

Observation and neurologic nursing assessment during and after a seizure are important for determining the type of seizure and its management.

▷ *Nursing Diagnoses*

Based on the assessment data, the patient's major nursing diagnoses may include the following:

- Fear related to concern about the ever-present possibility of having seizures
- Social isolation related to stresses imposed by epilepsy
- Deficit in knowledge about epilepsy and its control
- Potential for injury during seizures

▷ *Planning and Implementation*

▷ *Goals:* The major goals of the patient may include maintenance of control of seizures, achievement of a satisfactory psychosocial adjustment, and acquisition of knowledge and understanding about the condition. The long-term goal is to achieve a satisfactory life adjustment.

Nursing Interventions

Control of Seizures. The complete cooperation of the patient and family is of the utmost importance. They must have confidence in the value of the regimen that is prescribed. It must be emphasized that the prescribed antiepileptic drug must be taken on a continuing basis and that the medicine is not a habit-forming "dope." It may be taken without fear, for many years if necessary, if the patient is under health supervision and following instructions faithfully.

Explain that the control of seizures depends in part on the patient's understanding and cooperation. Life-style and environment are examined to determine whether certain factors precipitate the seizures: emotional disturbances, new environmental stresses, onset of menstruation in female patients, or fever. The patient is encouraged to follow a regular and moderate routine in life-style, diet (avoiding excessive stimulants), exercise, and rest. (Sleep deprivation may lower the patient's threshold to seizures.) Moderate activity is good therapy, but excessive expenditure of energy is to be avoided. Some patients need to avoid photic stimulation (bright flickering lights, television watching). Wearing dark glasses or covering one eye may help control this problem. Tension states (anxiety, frustration) induce seizures in some patients. Classes in stress management may be of value. Because seizures are known to follow alcohol intake, alcoholic beverages are restricted. All in all, the best therapy is to follow the therapeutic program.

Improving Coping Mechanisms. It has been noted that the social, psychological, and behavioral problems frequently accompanying epilepsy can be more of a "handicap" than the actual seizures. Epilepsy imposes feelings of fear, alienation, depression, and uncertainty. The patient must cope with the constant fear of a seizure and its embarrassing consequences. Children with epilepsy may be ostracized and excluded from school and peer activities. These problems are compounded in the teen years and add to the challenges of dating, not being able to drive, and "being different." Adults face all of these problems plus the burden of finding employment, decisions concerning marriage and childbearing, noninsurability, stigma of all kinds, and legal barriers. Alcohol may complicate matters. The burden on the family is great, and family problems run the gamut of outright rejection to overprotection. As a result of all these factors, many persons with epilepsy have psychological and behavioral problems.

Counseling is a must for helping the individual and the family to understand the condition and the limitations imposed by it. Social and recreational opportunities are necessary for good mental health. Some persons are not able to cope with epilepsy; others have psychological problems resulting from brain damage. Those with seizures originating in the temporal lobes of the brain (areas controlling thought and emotions) have particular mental problems. Symptoms of schizophrenia and impulsive or irritable behavior may be due to brain damage associated with temporal lobe seizures. These patients require comprehensive mental health services.

Patient Education. Of all the services that are contributed by the nurse in the care of the person with epilepsy, perhaps the most valuable are efforts to reorient the attitude of the patient and family to the disease itself.

For the observer, an epileptic seizure is a terrifying or a repulsive spectacle; thus, for the person who has them, every seizure is inevitably a source of humiliation and shame. This in turn breeds anxiety, depression, hostility, secrecy, and deceit, to which the public reacts with abhorrence, and the like, and the vicious cycle is complete. The reaction of shame and the recourse to deceit are not confined merely to persons with epilepsy, but extend to their families as well.

In order to escape from this vicious cycle, patients who have epilepsy, their families, and the public at large need facts. These are the facts: Epilepsy is not a mysterious disease; it does not reflect the supernatural. It is not a stigma. Epilepsy is no more disgraceful than diabetes, pernicious anemia, or hyperthyroidism. It is not a form of insanity. It does not tend to get worse with time. It can be controlled effectively. It should not keep the adult from work. *Activity tends to inhibit, not stimulate, epileptic seizures.* Some 50% to 60% of patients with epilepsy now may have their symptoms controlled.

Enlightenment of the public will give new hope to those facing centuries-old prejudices. Continuing encouragement should be given patients to mobilize their inner resources to overcome feelings of inferiority and self-consciousness resulting from seizures. The licensing of persons with epilepsy to drive automobiles varies from state to state. The patient with epilepsy should carry an emergency medical identification card in wallet or purse or wear an identification bracelet around the wrist.

Hereditary transmission of epilepsy has not been proved. The matter of marriage and children must be decided on an individual basis, but this right should not be denied to persons with epilepsy merely because they have the disease. However, genetic counseling is advised.

Resources for Patients. Since epilepsy is a long-term disorder, the continuous use of expensive medications may present a sizable burden to the patient and family. The Epilepsy Foundation of America offers a mail order program to provide medications at minimum cost and access to life insurance. This organization serves as a referral source through which a person with epilepsy may reach special services (see Bibliography for address).

For many, employment problems still remain the greatest handicap of epilepsy. Studies have demonstrated that the person with epilepsy who is properly placed in work has a satisfactory job performance. The director of each State Vocational Rehabilitation agency can provide information about vocational rehabilitation. The Epilepsy Foundation of America has developed a training and placement service. If the individual's seizures are not well-controlled, information about sheltered workshops or home employment programs may be obtained.

Counseling and job training are provided for qualified persons through the Veterans' Administration. The U.S. Civil Service Commission now grants government jobs to individuals if seizures are controlled and the person is otherwise qualified. The Rehabilitation Act helped to end job discrimination of the handicapped. Private firms are becoming enlightened, and the number of employers who knowingly hire persons with epilepsy is increasing.

The Commission for the Control of Epilepsy and Its Consequences makes recommendations covering all aspects of the problem of epilepsy in the U.S.—social, legal, scientific, economic, and humanitarian. Epilepsy International sponsors international congresses, publishes *Epilepsia* (the international journal on epilepsy), and has ongoing projects of international significance.

Persons who have uncontrollable seizures and psychological and social maladaptation with other overwhelming problems can be referred to comprehensive epilepsy centers where continuous television and EEG monitoring, specialized treatment, and rehabilitation services are available.

▷ *Evaluation*

▷ *Expected Outcomes*

1. Patient maintains control of seizures.
   a. Complies with drug regimen
   b. Verbalizes the need to take prescribed antiepileptic drug; can relate the hazards of drug stoppage
   c. Recalls the side-effects of drugs
   d. Has laboratory appointment following hospital discharge for serum level determination of antiepileptic drug
   e. Avoids factors/situations that may precipitate seizures (flickering light, hyperventilation)
   f. Follows a healthful life-style by
      (1) Getting enough sleep
      (2) Eating meals at regular times to avoid hypoglycemia
   g. Wears an identification bracelet
2. Strives to improve psychosocial adjustment
   a. Identifies "significant other" with whom to talk
   b. Is able to discuss feelings
   c. Relates rights under Federal law
   d. States knowledge that job counseling/job placement services are available
3. Gains knowledge and understanding of epilepsy
   a. Reads pamphlets/books about epilepsy
   b. Answers majority of questions about epilepsy correctly

Status Epilepticus

Status epilepticus (acute prolonged seizure activity) is a series of generalized convulsions that occur without full recovery of consciousness between attacks. The term has been broadened to include continuous clinical or electrical seizures lasting at least 30 minutes, even without impairment of consciousness. It is considered a major medical emergency. Status epilepticus produces cumulative effects. Vigorous muscular contractions impose a heavy metabolic demand and can interfere with respirations. There is some respiratory arrest at the height of each seizure that produces venous congestion and hypoxia of the brain. Repeated episodes of cerebral anoxia and swelling may lead to irreversible and fatal brain damage.

Common factors that precipitate status epilepticus include withdrawal of antiepileptic medication, fever, and intercurrent infection.

Management. The goals of treatment are to stop the seizures as quickly as possible, to ensure adequate cerebral oxygenation, and to maintain the patient in a seizure-free state. An airway and adequate oxygenation are established. If the patient remains deeply unconscious, a cuffed endotracheal tube is inserted. Intravenous diazepam is given slowly in an attempt to halt seizures immediately. Other antiepileptic drugs (phenytoin, phenobarbital) are given as prescribed after diazepam is administered to maintain a seizure-free state, because the anticonvulsant effect of diazepam is short-lived.

An intravenous line is established and kept open to monitor electrolytes, blood urea, and glucose. EEG monitoring may be useful in determining the nature of epileptogenic activity. Of course, vital and neurologic signs are monitored on a continuing basis. An intravenous infusion of dextrose is given if hypoglycemia has caused the seizure. If initial treatment is unsuccessful, general anesthesia with a short-acting barbiturate may be used.

As soon as control of seizures is achieved, serum concentration of the antiepileptic drug is measured, since a low level will suggest that the patient was not taking the medication or that the dosage was too low. Patients recovering from status epilepticus may die within a few days from cardiac involvement or respiratory depression. There is also the potential for postictal (after a seizure) cerebral swelling.

Nursing Interventions. The nurse provides ongoing assessment and monitoring of respiratory and cardiac function. There may be delayed depression of respiration and blood pressure induced by the medications given to halt the seizures. Nursing assessment also includes monitoring the seizure type and the general condition of the patient.

The patient is moved to the semiprone position, if possible, to assist in draining pharyngeal secretions. Standby suction equipment must be available because there is danger of aspiration. The intravenous line is closely watched, since it may become dislodged during seizures.

A person with epilepsy who is receiving long-term anticonvulsant therapy has a significant incidence of fractures resulting from bone disease. Chronic treatment with anticonvulsant drugs leads to a combination of osteoporosis, osteomalacia, and hyperparathyroidism. Thus, during seizures the patient is protected from injury with padded side rails and is kept under constant observation. No effort should be made to restrain movements. The patient having seizures can inadvertently injure attending persons, so nurses should take care to protect themselves. Other nursing interventions for the person having seizures are discussed on page 1489.

Head Injuries

Injuries to the head encompass trauma to the scalp, skull, and brain. Head injuries are among the most frequent and serious neurologic disorders, and have reached epidemic proportions as a result of traffic accidents. An estimated 100,000 persons die annually from head injuries, and more than 700,000 have injuries severe enough to require hospitalization. Of this group, between 50,000 and 90,000 people a year are left with intellectual or behavioral deficits that preclude their return to normal life. Two-thirds of these are below the age of 30, with males outnumbering females. Detectable blood alcohol levels have been found in more than 50% of head-injured patients treated in emergency departments. At least half of all severely head-injured patients have significant injuries to other parts of the body. Hypovolemic shock in a head-injured patient is usually due to injuries to other parts of the body.

Scalp and Skull Injuries

Scalp Injury

Because of its many blood vessels, the scalp can bleed profusely when injured. Scalp wounds are also a portal of entry for intracranial infections. Trauma may result in an abrasion ("brush wound"), contusion, laceration, or avulsion. An injection of procaine makes it easier for the wound to be cleaned and treated. The area is irrigated to remove foreign material and minimize the chance of infection before lacerations are closed.

Skull Injury—Fractures of the Skull

A skull fracture is a break in the continuity of the skull caused by trauma (Fig. 54-6). It may occur with or without damage to the brain. The presence of a skull fracture usually means that there was considerable force upon impact. Skull fractures are classified as open or closed. In an *open* fracture, the dura is torn, and in a *closed* fracture, the dura is not torn.

Clinical Manifestations. The symptoms, aside from those of the local injury, depend on the amount and the distribution of brain injury. Pain, persistent or localized, usually suggests that a fracture is present. Fractures of the cranial vault produce swelling in the region of the fracture, and for this reason an accurate diagnosis cannot be made without an x-ray. Fractures of the base of the skull frequently produce hemorrhage from the nose, the pharynx, or the ears, and blood may appear under the conjunctivae. An area of *ecchymosis*, or bruising, may be seen over the mastoid. The escape of cerebrospinal fluid from the ears (*cerebrospinal fluid otorrhea*) and the nose (*cerebrospinal rhinorrhea*) suggests skull fracture. Bloody spinal fluid, if present, suggests brain laceration or contusion.

Diagnostic Evaluation. Although a rapid physical examination and evaluation of the neurologic status will reveal the more obvious brain injuries, the less apparent abnormalities found in head injuries may be detected by cranial computed tomography, which can differentiate subtle changes in the degree to which the soft tissue absorbs x-ray. It is accurate and safe in showing the presence, nature, location, and extent of the lesion as well as in revealing cerebral edema, contusion, intracerebral or extracerebral hematoma, subarachnoid and intraventricular hemorrhage, and late traumatic changes (infarct, hydrocephalus).

If computed tomography is not available, cerebral angiography will demonstrate the presence of supratentorial, extracerebral, and intracerebral hematomas and cerebral contusion. Lateral and anteroposterior views of the skull are obtained.

Management. In general, nondepressed skull fractures usually do not require surgical treatment, but close observation of the patient is essential.

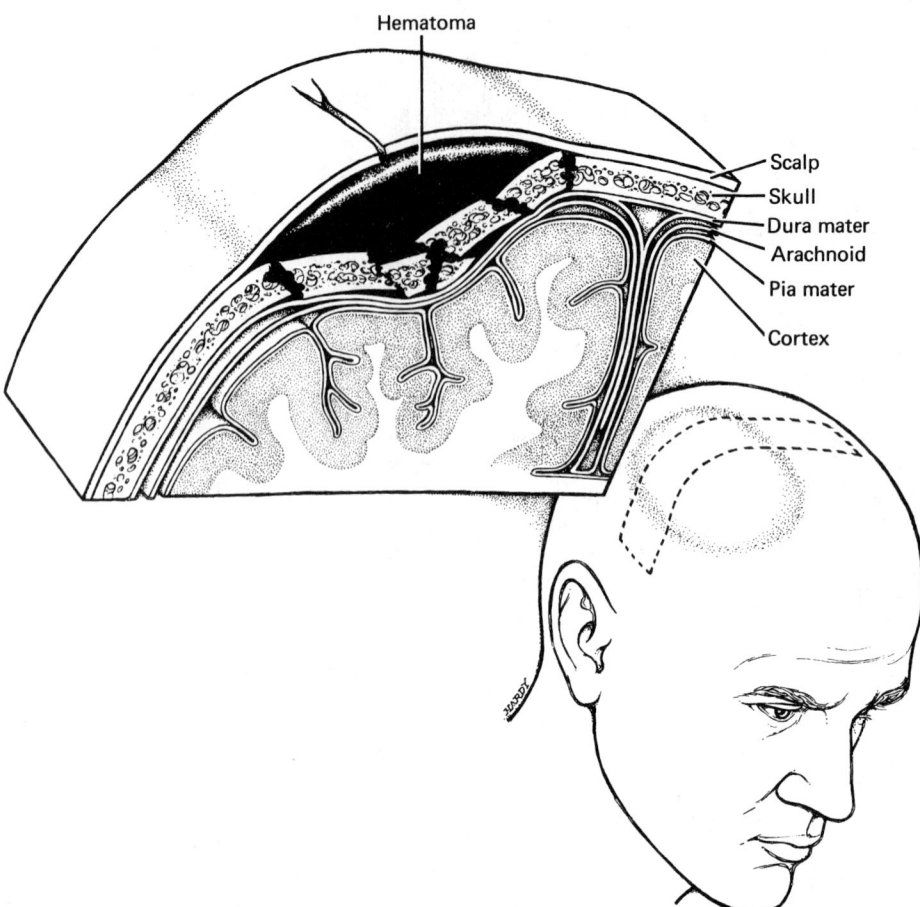

Figure 54-6
Depressed fracture of the skull.

For depressed skull fractures, surgery is indicated. The scalp is shaved and cleansed and the fracture exposed. The skull fragments are elevated and the area is débrided. Closure of the dura is carried out if possible, and the wound is closed. Large defects in the skull can be repaired later with metallic or plastic plates if necessary. In instances of a clean wound and an intact dura, the elevated fragments can be replaced, making a later cranioplasty unnecessary. Penetrating wounds require surgical débridement to remove foreign bodies and devitalized brain tissue and to control hemorrhage. Antibiotic treatment is immediately instituted, and blood transfusions are made available.

Fractures of the base of the skull are serious because they are usually open (involving the paranasal sinuses or middle or external ear) and the possibility of leakage of cerebrospinal fluid and meningitis is always present. The nasopharynx and the external ear should be kept clean, and usually a plug of sterile cotton is placed in the ear to absorb discharges.

Brain Injury

The most important consideration in any head injury is whether or not the brain has been injured. Even "minor" injury can cause permanent brain damage. The brain is unable to store oxygen and glucose to any significant degree. The cerebral cells need an uninterrupted blood supply for oxygen and nutrients. The brain dies when its blood supply is interrupted for only a few minutes; there is no regeneration of damaged neurons.

Serious brain injury may occur following blows or injuries to the head, with or without fracture of the skull, that produce contusions, laceration, and hemorrhage of the brain.

Concussion. A cerebral concussion following a head injury is a temporary loss of neurologic function from which there is complete recovery. A concussion generally involves a period of unconsciousness lasting from a few seconds to a few minutes. The jarring of the brain may be so slight as to cause only dizziness and spots before the eyes (spoken of as "seeing stars"), or there may be complete loss of consciousness for a time. If the brain tissue in the frontal lobe is affected, the patient may exhibit bizarre irrational behavior, whereas disruption of brain tissue in the temporal lobe can produce temporary amnesia or disorientation. Continuing amnesia is regarded as a severe concussion.

The treatment of concussion is to observe the patient for headache, dizziness, irritability, and anxiety (*postconcussional syndrome*), which may follow this type of injury. Giving the patient information, explanations, and encouragement may reduce some of the problems of postconcussional syndrome.

The patient is discharged from the hospital in a relatively short time after a head injury, the family is instructed to look for the following signs and to notify the physician or clinic or bring the patient back to the Emergency Department if they occur: difficulty in awakening, difficulty in speaking, confusion, severe headache, vomiting, pulse change, development of unequal pupils, or weakness of one side of the body.

The patient is advised to resume normal activities slowly.

Contusion. A cerebral contusion is a more severe cerebral injury in which the brain is bruised, with possible surface hemorrhage. The patient will be unconscious for a considerable period. The symptoms, as would be expected, are more marked. The patient may lie motionless, the pulse will be feeble, the respiration shallow, and the skin cold and pale. Often there is involuntary evacuation of the bowels and the bladder. The patient may be aroused with effort but soon slips back into unconsciousness. The blood pressure and the temperature are subnormal, and the picture is somewhat similar to that of shock.

In general, persons with diffuse injury who have abnormal motor function, abnormal eye movements, and raised intracranial pressure have a poor outcome. On the other hand, the patient may recover consciousness completely and perhaps pass into a stage of cerebral irritability.

In the stage of cerebral irritability, the patient is no longer unconscious but, on the contrary, is easily disturbed by any form of stimulation, noises, light, and voices, and may become hyperactive at times. Gradually, the pulse, respirations, temperature, and other body functions return to normal. However, recovery is not complete at once. Residual headache and vertigo are common, and often impaired mentality or epilepsy occurs as a result of irreparable cerebral damage.

Intracranial Hemorrhage

The most common serious results of brain injuries are *hematomas* (collections of blood) that develop within the cranial vault (Fig 54-7). The hematoma is referred to as epidural, subdural, or intracerebral, depending on its location. The main effects are frequently delayed until the hematoma is large enough to cause distortion and herniation of the brain and increased intracranial pressure. *The signs and symptoms of brain ischemia resulting from compression caused by a hematoma are variable and depend on the speed with which vital areas are encroached upon and/or the changes that involve the underlying brain.* In general, a small hematoma that develops rapidly may be fatal, while a more massive hematoma that develops slowly may allow the patient to adapt.

Epidural Hematoma (Extradural Hematoma or Hemorrhage)

Following a head injury, blood may collect in the epidural (extradural) space between the skull and the dura. This often

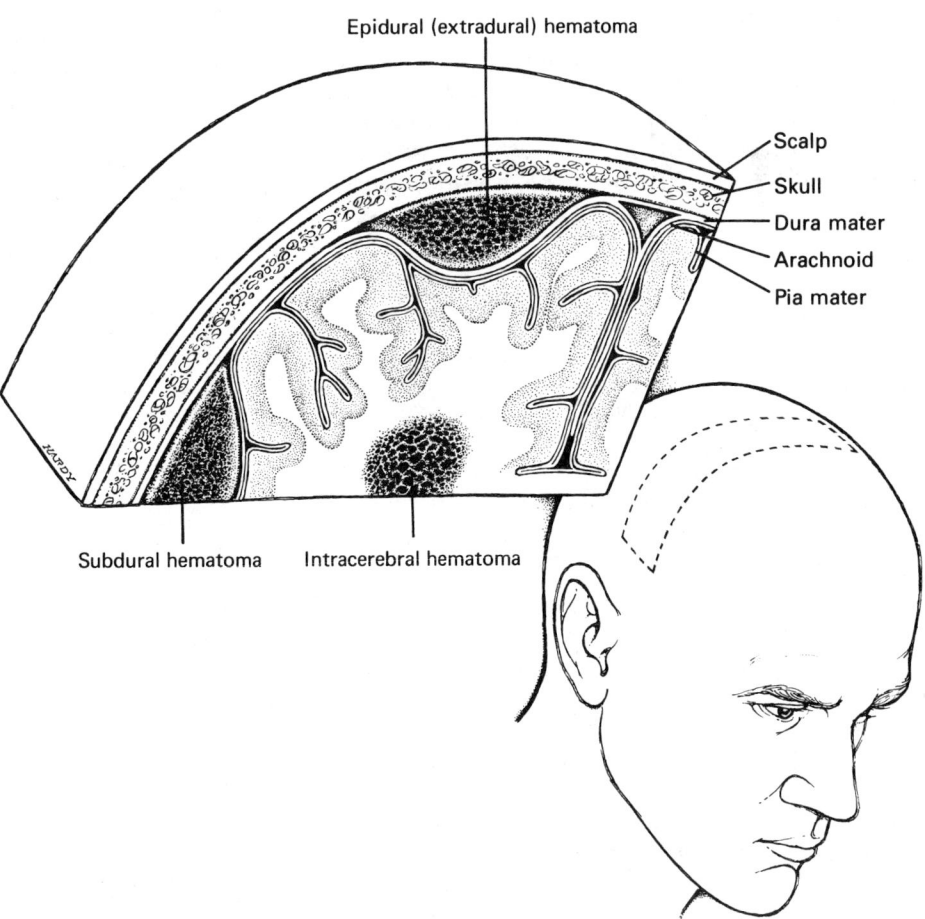

Figure 54-7
Diagrammatic views showing epidural, subdural, and intracerebral hematomas.

results from fractures of the skull that cause rupture or laceration of the middle meningeal artery, which runs between the dura and the skull; hemorrhage from this artery causes pressure on the brain.

More frequently, bleeding sites along the fracture line produce acute hematomas. Epidural hematomas occur most frequently in the temporal area.

The symptoms are caused by the expanding hematoma. There is usually a momentary loss of consciousness at the time of injury, followed by an interval of apparent recovery (lucid interval). A lucid interval is not always present with an epidural hematoma, although it may occur with a subdural hematoma. During the lucid interval, compensation for the expanding hematoma takes place by rapid absorption of cerebrospinal fluid and decreased intravascular volume, which maintains a normal intracranial pressure. When these mechanisms can no longer compensate, even a small increase in the volume of the blood clot will produce a marked elevation of intracranial pressure. Then, often suddenly, signs of compression appear (usually deterioration of consciousness and signs of focal neurologic deficits such as dilation and fixation of a pupil or paralysis of an extremity), and the patient deteriorates rapidly.

Management. An epidural hematoma is considered an extreme emergency, since marked neurologic deficit or even cessation of breathing may occur within minutes. The treatment consists of making openings through the skull (*burr holes*), removing the clot, and controlling the bleeding point.

Subdural Hematoma

A subdural hematoma is a collection of blood between the dura and the underlying brain, a space normally occupied by a film of fluid. The most common cause is trauma, but it may also occur in various bleeding diatheses and aneurysms. A subdural hemorrhage is more frequently venous in origin and is attributed to the rupture of small vessels that bridge the subdural space.

A subdural hematoma may be acute, subacute, or chronic, depending on the size of the involved vessel and the amount of bleeding present. Usually, the patient is comatose, and the clinical signs are similar to those of epidural hematoma. A rising blood pressure with slowing of pulse and respirations indicates a rapidly increasing hematoma. Older patients are more apt to demonstrate delirium.

The mortality rate for patients with acute subdural hematomas is high, because frequently there is associated brain damage.

If the patient can be transported rapidly to the hospital, an immediate craniotomy is performed to open the dura, allowing for the solid subdural clot to be evacuated. Successful outcome also depends on the control of intracranial pressure and careful monitoring of respiratory function (see The Patient Undergoing Intracranial Surgery, p. 1453).

Chronic subdural hematoma imitates other conditions and may be mistaken for a stroke. In fact, it has been termed "the great imitator." Symptoms may appear weeks after what may have seemed to be a minor injury. The bleeding is less profuse and there is compression of the intracranial contents. The blood within the brain changes in character in 2 to 4 days, becoming thicker and darker. In a few weeks, the clot breaks down and has the color and consistency of motor oil. Eventually, calcification or ossification of the clot takes place. The brain adapts to this foreign body invasion, and the patient's clinical signs and symptoms fluctuate. There may be severe headache, which tends to come and go; alternating focal neurologic signs; personality changes; mental deterioration; and focal convulsions. Unfortunately, the patient may be labeled "neurotic" or "psychotic" if the cause of the symptoms is overlooked.

The treatment of chronic subdural hematoma consists of surgically evacuating the clot by suctioning or irrigating the area. The procedure may be carried out through multiple burr holes, or a craniotomy may be performed for a sizable subdural mass lesion that cannot be drained through burr holes.

Intracerebral Hemorrhage/Hematoma

Intracerebral hemorrhage is bleeding into the substance of the brain. It is commonly seen in head injuries in which force is exerted to the head over a small area (missile injuries; stab injury). These hemorrhages within the brain may also result from systemic hypertension which causes degeneration and rupture of a vessel, from rupture of a saccular aneurysm, from vascular anomalies, from intracranial tumors, from systemic causes including bleeding disorders such as leukemia, hemophilia, aplastic anemia, and thrombocytopenia, and from complications of anticoagulant therapy.

There may be an insidious development with the onset of neurologic deficits followed by headache. Medical therapy involves careful administration of fluids and electrolytes, antihypertensive medications, control of intracranial pressure, and supportive care. Surgical intervention via craniotomy or craniectomy permits removal of the blood clot and provides opportunity for control of the sites of hemorrhage. Physicial therapy is usually required for the rehabilitation of these patients.

General Approach to Head Injuries

Clinical Manifestations

Brain trauma may affect every system of the body. The clinical manifestations of brain injury include disturbances of consciousness, confusion, pupillary abnormalities, sudden onset of neurologic deficits, and changes in vital signs. There may be visual impairment, hearing impairment, sensory dysfunction, spasticity, headache, vertigo, movement disorders, seizures and many other effects. The presence of hypovolemic shock alerts to the possibility of multisystem injury, because CNS injury alone is not apt to produce shock.

Diagnostic Evaluation

The initial physicial and neurologic examinations are the baseline upon which all future examination comparisons are made. Computed tomography is the primary neuroimaging diagnostic tool, and is useful in the evaluation of soft tissue injuries.

Management

A person with a head injury is presumed to have a cervical spine injury until proven otherwise. The patient is transported from the scene of accident on a board, with head and neck maintained in alignment with the axis of the body. Slight traction should be maintained on the head.

The initial brain injury is not amenable to treatment, and all therapy is directed towards the preservation of brain homeostasis and prevention of secondary brain damage. This includes stabilization of cardiovascular and respiratory function to maintain adequate cerebral perfusion. Hemorrhage is stopped, hypovolemia is corrected, and blood gas tensions are maintained at their physiologic values.

As the damaged brain swells with edema, a rise in intracranial pressure can be expected and requires aggressive treatment. Increased intracranial pressure is managed by avoiding hypoxia; administering mannitol, which reduces brain water by osmotic dehydration; hyperventilation; the use of steroids; a head-up position in bed; monitoring of intracranial pressure; and possibly neurosurgical intervention. Surgery is required for evacuation of blood clots, débridement and elevation of depressed fractures of the skull, suture of severe scalp lacerations, and insertion of devices to monitor intracranial pressure.

Drainage of cerebrospinal fluid from the nose (*cerebrospinal rhinorrhea*) and ears (*cerebrospinal fluid otorrhea*) may indicate a basal skull fracture. To determine whether a fluid discharge is spinal rhinorrhea or otorrhea, the area is blotted with sterile gauze. If the discharge is bloody (which is readily observed), a red spot forms on the gauze, but if the discharge also contains cerebrospinal fluid, a clear wet halo encircles the blood spot.

A sterile cotton pad may be taped loosely under the nose or against the ear to collect the draining fluid. The patient who is conscious is cautioned against sneezing or blowing the nose. The head is usually elevated 30 degrees to reduce intracranial pressure and promote spontaneous closure of the leak. (Some neurosurgeons prefer that the bed be kept flat). Persistence of spinal fluid rhinorrhea or otorrhea usually requires surgical intervention.

Treatment also includes ventilatory support, prevention of seizures, and maintenance of fluid, electrolyte, and nutritional balance. Patients with severe head injury who are in coma are intubated and placed on mechanical ventilation to control and protect the airway. Controlled hyperventilation also induces hypocapnia, which causes vasoconstriction, lowers cerebral blood flow, and decreases cerebral blood volume.

Because seizures are common after head injury and can cause secondary brain damage from hypoxia, anticonvulsant therapy may be started.

If the patient is very agitated, chlorpromazine may be prescribed to quiet the patient without deepening the consciousness level. A nasogastric tube may be inserted, since reduced gastric motility and reverse peristalsis are associated with head injury, making regurgitation common in the first few hours.

▶ Nursing Process
The Patient With a Head Injury

▷ *Assessment*

The nursing (or medical) history may include the following questions:

At what time did the injury occur?
What caused the injury? A high velocity missile? An object striking the head? A fall?
What was the direction and force of the blow?
Was there a loss of consciousness? What was the duration of the unconscious period? Could the patient be aroused? (A history of unconsciousness or amnesia after a head injury indicates a significant degree of brain damage, while subsequent changes can reflect recovery or indicate the development of secondary brain damage.)

Assessing the Level of Responsiveness/Consciousness. The level of consciousness/responsiveness is constantly assessed because an alteration in the level of consciousness will precede all other changes in vital and neurologic signs. A practical means of monitoring changes in the level of consciousness is the Glasgow Coma Scale, which is based on three aspects of the patient's behavior: eye opening, verbal responses, and motor responses to a verbal command or painful stimulus. These elements are further subdivided into different levels of response, and the best responses the patient makes to predetermined stimuli are recorded as follows:

Eyes Open:	
Spontaneously	4
To speech	3
To pain	2
No response	1
Best Motor Response:	
Obeys	6
Localizes pain	5
Withdraws	4
Abnormal flexion	3
Extends	2
Nil	1
Verbal Response	
Oriented	5
Confused conversation	4
Inappropriate words	3
Incomprehensible sounds	2
Nil	1

Total: 3–15

Each response is given a number (high for normal and low for impaired), and the summation of these figures gives an indication of the severity of coma and a prediction of possible outcome. The lowest score is 3 (least responsive), and the highest is 15 (most responsive). In general, a score of 4 or 5 indicates the patient is deeply comatose, a score of 6 to 10 shows intermediate disturbance of consciousness, and a score of more than 10 approaches a conscious state.

Figure 54-8 is a neurological observation chart incorporating the Glascow Coma Scale, vital signs, pupillary size and reactivity, and extremity movement and strength, which provides a comprehensive record of the patient's neurologic status at any given point in time.

Monitoring Vital Signs. Although deterioration of the patient's level of consciousness is the most sensitive neurologic indication of impending danger, vital signs are monitored at frequent intervals to assess the intracranial state.

- Signs of increasing intracranial pressure include slowing of the pulse, increasing systolic pressure, and widening pulse pressure.
- If brain compression encroaches upon cerebral circulation, the vital signs tend to be reversed—the pulse and respiration become rapid, and the blood pressure may

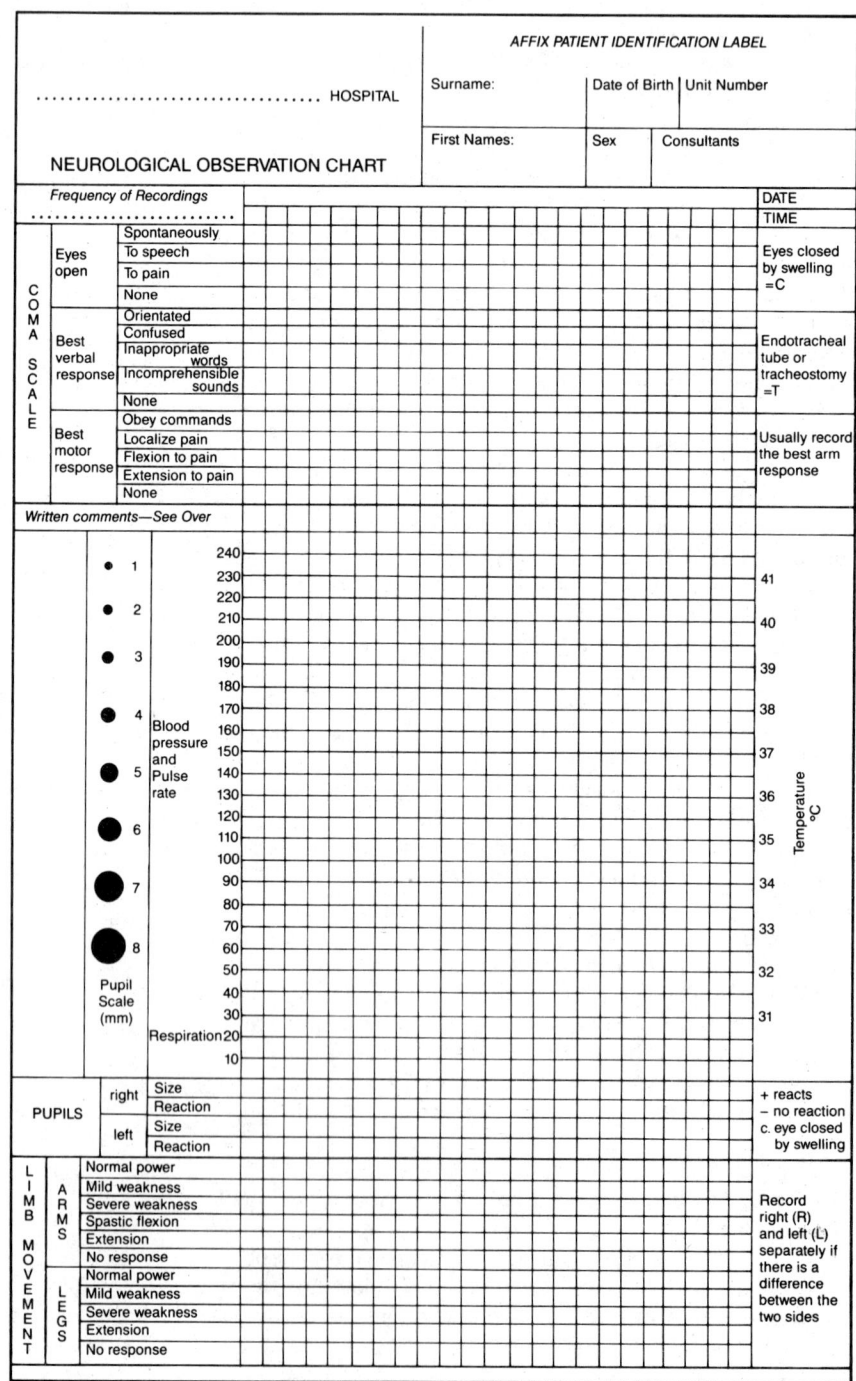

Figure 54-8
Example of neurological observation chart that includes the Glasgow Coma Scale. (Reproduced by courtesy of Butterworth and Company, London, from Campkin and Turner, Neurosurgical Anaesthesia and Intensive Care.)

fall. This is an ominous development, as is a rapid fluctuation of vital signs.

- A rapid rise in body temperature is regarded as unfavorable, because hyperthermia increases the metabolic demands of the brain. The temperature is kept below 38°C (100.4°F).
- Tachycardia and arterial hypotension may indicate that bleeding is occurring somewhere in the body.

Motor Function. Motor function is checked frequently by observing spontaneous movements, asking the patient to raise and lower the extremities, and comparing the power of the hand grip at various times. Notice whether one extremity is moved less frequently than the other.

- If the patient does not demonstrate spontaneous movement, determine responses to painful stimuli. Abnormal responses (lack of motor response; extension responses) carry a poorer prognosis.
- Also determine the patient's ability to speak, and note the quality of speech. The capacity to speak indicates a high level of brain function.

Eye Signs

- Determine whether the patient is opening his eyes.
- The size of the pupils and their reaction to light are evaluated. A unilaterally dilated and poorly responding pupil may indicate a developing hematoma with subsequent pressure on the third cranial nerve due to shifting of the brain. If both pupils become fixed and dilated, overwhelming injury and intrinsic damage to the upper brain stem usually are indicated.

Assessment for Complications

Deterioration in the patient's condition may be due to an expanding intracranial hematoma and progressive brain engorgement or edema. Other complications following traumatic head injuries include systemic infections (pneumonia, urinary tract infection, septicemia) and neurosurgical infections (wound infection, osteomyelitis, meningitis, ventriculitis, brain abscess).

Following injury, these patients may develop focal nerve palsies such as *anosmia* (lack of sense of smell) or eye movement abnormalities and focal neurologic deficits such as aphasia, memory defects, and posttraumatic seizures/epilepsy. Patients may be left with organic psychosocial deficits (impulsiveness, emotional lability, or uninhibited, aggressive behaviors) and, as a consequence of the impairment, lack insight into their emotional responses.

▷ Nursing Diagnoses

Based on all the assessment data, the patient's major nursing diagnoses may include the following:

- Ineffective airway clearance and ventilation related to hypoxia
- Fluid volume deficit related to disturbances of consciousness and hormonal dysfunction
- Alteration in nutrition, less than body requirements, related to metabolic changes and fluid restriction
- Potential for violence (self-directed and directed to others) related to disorientation, restlessness, and brain damage
- Alteration in thought processes (deficits in intellectual function, communication, memory, information processing) related to results of head injury
- Potential ineffective family coping related to unresponsiveness of patient, unpredictability of outcome, prolonged recovery period, and patient's residual physical and emotional deficit

The nursing diagnoses for the unconscious patient (p. 1427) and the patient with increased intracranial pressure (p. 1422) also apply.

▷ Planning and Implementation

▷ **Goals:** The patient's goals may include attainment of a patent airway, achievement of fluid and electrolyte balance, achievement of adequate nutritional status, prevention of injury, improvement of cognitive function, and accomplishment of effective family coping behaviors.

Nursing Interventions

As soon as the initial assessment and diagnostic tests are made, a neurologic flow record is started and maintained (see Fig 54-8). Chart 54-4 is a flow chart including ongoing nursing assessments, priorities for nursing interventions, and anticipatory and rehabilitation nursing of the patient with a head injury.

Maintaining the Airway. One of the most important nursing goals in the management of the patient with a head injury is to establish and maintain an adequate airway. The brain is extremely sensitive to hypoxia, and a neurologic deficit can worsen if the patient is hypoxic. Therapy is directed toward maintenance of adequately oxygenated circulation so that there will be a supply of oxygenated blood to the brain to preserve cerebral function. An obstructed airway causes CO_2 retention and hypoventilation, which produce cerebral engorgement and increases intracranial pressure.

Therapeutic and nursing activities to ensure an adequate exchange of air are summarized on page 1427 and include the following:

- Keep the unconscious patient in a semiprone or prone position, with the head of the bed elevated about 30 degrees to decrease intracranial venous pressure.
- Establish effective suctioning procedures. (Pulmonary secretions produce coughing and straining, which increase intracranial pressure.)
- Guard against aspiration and respiratory insufficiency.
- Monitor arterial blood gases to assess adequacy of ventilation. (The goal is to keep blood gases within normal range to ensure adequate cerebral blood flow.)
- Monitor the patient who is on mechanical ventilation.

Fluid and Electrolyte Balance. Brain damage can produce metabolic and hormonal dysfunctions. The monitoring of serum electrolyte concentrations is important, especially in patients receiving osmotic diuretics, those with inappropriate antidiuretic hormone secretion, and those with posttraumatic diabetes insipidus.

Chart 54-4
The Patient With a Head Injury

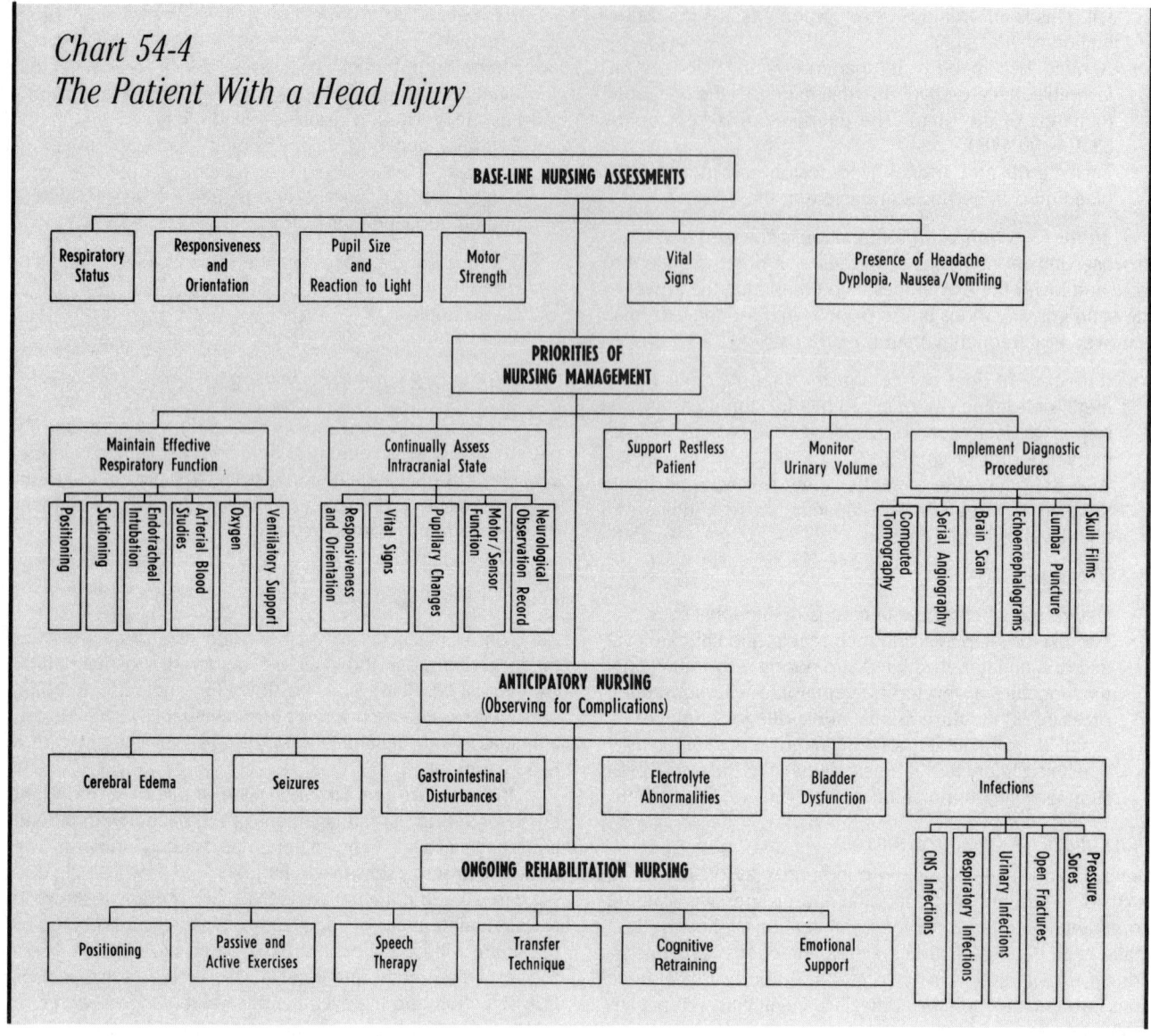

- Serial studies of blood and urine electrolytes and osmolality are carried out, since head injuries may be accompanied by disorders of sodium regulation. Sodium retention may last several days, followed by sodium diuresis. Watch for lethargy, confusion, and convulsions due to electrolyte imbalance.
- Endocrine dysfunctions are evaluated by monitoring serum electrolytes, glucose values, and input and output records.
- Urine is tested regularly for sugar and acetone.
- A record of daily weight is kept, especially if the patient has hypothalamic involvement and must be watched for the development of diabetes insipidus.

Ensuring Adequate Nutrition.   Head injury results in metabolic changes that increase calorie consumption and nitrogen excretion. Steroid therapy also increases the catabolic state. As soon as the patient's condition has stabilized, nasogastric feedings are started unless there is discharge of cerebrospinal fluid from the nose (*cerebrospinal rhinorrhea*).

Small, frequent feedings lessen the possiblity of vomiting and diarrhea. Elevating the head of the bed and aspirating the tube before feeding (for evidence of residual feeding in the stomach) are measures used to prevent distention, regurgitation, and aspiration. A continuous drip infusion or controlling pump may be used to regulate the feeding. The principles and technique of nasogastric feedings are discussed on page 759. The feeding tube is usually retained until the swallowing reflex returns.

Preventing Injury.   As the patient emerges from coma, there is a period of lethargy and stupor followed by a period of agitation. Each stage is variable, depending on the individual, the depth and duration of coma, and the patient's age. The patient emerging from a coma may become increasingly agitated toward the end of the day. Restlessness may be due to hypoxia, fever, pain, or a full bladder. It may indicate injury of the brain, but is also a sign that the unconscious patient is regaining consciousness. (Some restlessness may be beneficial because the lungs and extremities are exercised.) Agitation may also be due to annoyance from an indwelling urinary catheter, intravenous lines, restraints, and repeated neurologic checks.

- Make sure that the patient's airway is adequate and the bladder is not distended. Likewise, bandages and casts should be checked for constriction.
- To protect the patient from self-injury and dislodging of body tubes, siderails are padded and the patient's hands may be wrapped in mitts. Restraints should be avoided when possible because straining against them can increase intracranial pressure.
- Restlessness should not be controlled with narcotics, because these substances depress respiration, constrict the pupils, and alter the level of the patient's responsiveness.
- The use of a floor bed (floor mattresses surrounded by a "wall" of mattresses) allows freedom of movement and promotes patient safety.
- Environmental stimuli should be kept to a minimum by keeping the room quiet, limiting visitors, speaking calmly, and providing frequent orientation information (*e.g.*, saying where the patient is and what is being done).
- Adequate lighting may prevent visual hallucinations.
- The patient's sleep–wake cycles should not be interrupted.
- Lubricate the skin with oil or emollient lotion to prevent irritation due to rubbing against the sheet.
- If incontinence is a problem, an external sheath catheter may be used on the male patient. Since prolonged use of an indwelling catheter inevitably produces infection, the patient may be placed on an intermittent catheterization schedule.

Improving Cognitive Functioning. Although many brain-damaged victims survive because of resuscitative and supportive technology, they frequently sustain significant mental sequelae that may not be noticed during the acute phase of injury. Cognitive impairment includes memory deficits, decrease in ability to focus and sustain attention to a task (easily distracted), reduced ability to process information, and slowness in thinking, perceiving, communicating, reading, and writing. An estimated 25% to 38% of these persons develop psychiatric problems. Such psychosocial, behavioral, and emotional impairments are devastating to the family as well as to the patient.

These problems require collaboration among many disciplines. A *neuropsychologist* (specialist in evaluating and treating cognitive problems) plans a program and initiates therapy or counseling that is designed to help the patient reach maximum potential. Cognitive rehabilitation activities are directed at redeveloping the patient's ability to devise new problem-solving strategies. The retraining is carried on over an extended time period, and includes the use of computer training programs, video games, sensory stimulation and reinforcement, behavior modification, and reality orientation. Assistance from many disciplines is necessary during this phase of recovery. Intellectual ability may not improve after a period of time, but social and behavioral aspects may improve.

The nurse needs to be aware that there are fluctuations in the orientation and memory of such patients. They are easily distracted. If they are pushed to a level greater than their impaired cortical functioning will allow, symptoms of fatigue and stress (headache; dizziness) will be noted.

Patient and Family Education. Serious head injury can produce a great deal of prolonged stress in the family because of the patient's physical and emotional deficits, the unpredictable outcome, and altered family relationships. Families report difficulties in dealing with changes in temperament, behavior, and personality. These are associated with disruption in family cohesion, loss of leisure pursuits, and loss of work capacity, as well as the social isolation and entrapment of the caretaker. The family may experience such feelings as anger, grief, guilt, and denial in recurring cycles.

Ask the family how the patient is different at this time. What has been lost? What is most difficult about coping with this situation? Helpful interventions include providing family members with accurate and honest information, and encouraging them to continue to set well-defined, mutual, short-term goals. Family counseling helps deal with overwhelming feelings of loss and helplessness and gives guidance to the management of inappropriate behaviors. Support groups are available to provide a forum for sharing problems, developing insight, referring information, networking, and gaining assistance in maintaining realistic expectations and hope.

The National Head Injury Foundation serves as a clearinghouse for information and resources for patients with head injuries and their families, including specific information on coma, rehabilitation, behavioral consequences of head injury, and family issues. This organization can provide names of facilities and professionals who work with persons with head injuries and can assist families in organizing local support groups.

The patient is encouraged to continue the rehabilitation program after discharge, since improvement in status may continue up to 3 or more years following injury. Headache may be the most reliable guide to recovery. A second pillow or backrest at night may be helpful to alleviate some head discomfort.

Because posttraumatic seizures occur frequently, anticonvulsants may be prescribed for 1 to 2 years following injury. The patient is encouraged to return to normal activities gradually.

▷ *Evaluation*

▷ *Expected Outcomes*

1. Patient attains/maintains effective airway clearance, ventilation, and brain oxygenation.
   a. Achieves normal blood gas values
   b. Has normal breath sounds on auscultation
   c. Coughs up secretions
2. Achieves satisfactory fluid and electrolyte balance
   a. Demonstrates serum electrolytes within normal range
   b. Has no clinical signs of dehydration or overhydration
3. Attains adequate nutritional status
   a. Has less than 50 ml of aspirate in stomach before each tube feeding
   b. Is free of gastric distention and vomiting
   c. Shows minimal weight loss

4. Avoids injury
   a. Shows lessening agitation and restlessness
   b. Is oriented to time, place, and person
5. Shows cognitive progression
   a. Demonstrates lessening of inappropriate behaviors
   b. Shows improved memory
   c. Verbalizes realistic plans
6. Family members demonstrate adaptive coping mechanisms.
   a. Have joined support group
   b. Are willing to identify problem areas
   c. Share their feelings with appropriate health-care personnel

Spinal Cord Injury

Spinal cord injury is a major health problem affecting 150,000 to 500,000 persons in this country, with an estimated 10,000 new injuries occurring each year. Half of these injuries result from motor vehicle accidents; most of the others occur from falls, sporting and industrial accidents, and gunshot wounds. Two thirds of the victims are 30 years of age or younger. The estimated total annual cost of these injuries exceeds $2 billion a year. There is a high frequency of associated injuries and medical complications. The vertebrae most frequently involved in spinal cord injuries are the fifth, sixth, and seventh cervical (neck), the twelfth thoracic, and the first lumbar vertebrae. These vertebrae are the most susceptible because there is a greater range of mobility in the vertebral column in these areas.

Prevention. To prevent this devasting and catastrophic injury, the following steps should be taken: (1) reduction in driving speed, (2) use of a seat belt/shoulder harness, (3) wearing of helmets by motorcyclists, (4) educational programs directed against driving while intoxicated, (5) water safety instruction, (6) prevention of falls, and (7) use in sports of protective devices and proper coaching techniques. Paramedical personnel are taught the importance of properly removing a car-crash victim from a motor vehicle and of following proper methods in transporting the victim to a hospital emergency department in order to avoid further and possibly permanent damage to the spinal cord.

Pathogenesis. Damage to the spinal cord ranges from transient concussion (from which the patient fully recovers) to contusion, laceration, and compression of the cord substance (either alone or in combination) to complete transection of the cord (which renders the patient paralyzed below the level of the injury). When hemorrhage occurs in the area of the spinal cord, the blood may seep into the extradural, subdural, or subarachnoid spaces of the spinal canal. Immediately after a contusion or tear injury, the nerve fibers begin to swell and disintegrate. Blood circulation to the gray matter of the spinal cord is curtailed. Not only is there injury to the spinal cord vasculature, but there also appears to be a pathogenic process responsible for the progressive damage of the acute spinal cord injury. A secondary chain of events produces ischemia, hypoxia, edema, and hemorrhagic lesions, which in turn result in destruction of myelin and axons.

These secondary reactions, believed to be the principal causes of spinal cord degeneration at the level of injury, are

now thought to be reversible 4 to 6 hours after injury. Therefore, if the cord has not suffered irreparable damage, some method of *early* treatment is needed to prevent partial damage from developing into total and permanent damage. Dexamethasone, given as an anti-inflammatory agent; mannitol, given to decrease edema; and dextran, given to prevent the blood pressure from dropping and to improve capillary blood flow, are being investigated. Naloxone, a drug that has shown promise in treating animal models of spinal cord injury, has minimal side-effects and may promote neurologic improvement in humans. The effectiveness of using cooling techniques or hypothermia perfusion on the injured area of the spinal cord to counteract the autodestructive forces that follow this type of injury is being studied. The use of high-dosage steroids to maintain the vascular integrity of the cord following acute injury is viewed as promising by researchers.

Emergency Management

The immediate management of the patient at the scene of the accident is critical, because improper handling can cause further damage and loss of neurologic function. Any victim of a motor vehicle or diving accident, a contact sport injury, falls, or any direct trauma to the head and neck should be suspected of having a spinal cord injury until such an injury is ruled out.

- At the scene of the accident, the victim should be immobilized on a spinal (back) board, with head and neck in a neutral position, to prevent an incomplete injury from becoming complete.
- One member of the team should assume control of the patient's head to prevent flexion, rotation, or extension.
- Place each hand on either side of the head about at the ear to maintain traction and alignment while a spinal board or cervical immobilizing device is applied.
- At least four persons should slide the victim carefully onto a board for transfer to the hospital. Any twisting movement may irreversibly damage the spinal cord by causing a bony fragment of the vertebra to cut into, crush, or sever the cord completely.

It is desirable that the patient be referred to a regional spinal injury or trauma center because of the multidisciplinary personnel and support services required to counteract destructive changes that occur in the first few hours after injury.

Tranferring the Patient. During treatment in the emergency and x-ray departments, the patient is kept on the transfer board. The transfer of the patient to a bed presents a definite nursing problem.

- The patient must always be maintained in an extended position. No part of the body should be twisted or turned, nor should the patient be allowed to assume a sitting position.

The patient should be placed on a Stryker frame when transfer to a bed is planned. Later, if it proved that there is no cord injury, the patient always can be moved to a conventional bed without harm; the reverse, however, is not true. If a Stryker frame is not available, the patient should be placed on a firm mattress with a bedboard under it. The patient may be transferred from the board to the Stryker frame in the following manner:

- The board on which the patient is strapped is placed directly on the posterior frame.
- Unstrap the patient from the board, but do not remove the head strappings.
- Place a blanket roll between the legs.
- Place the anterior frame in position, and secure the frame straps.
- Turn the frame so that the patient is in the prone position.
- Remove the frame straps and the posterior frame. Remove the head strapping with care. Then remove the transfer board.

Clinical Manifestations

If conscious, the patient will probably complain of acute pain in the back or neck, which may radiate along the involved nerve. Often the patient will speak of fear that the neck or back is broken. *The consequences of spinal cord injury depend on the level of injury of the cord* (Fig. 54-9). *Neurologic*

level refers to that lowest level at which sensory and motor functions are normal. There is total sensory and motor paralysis below the neurologic level, loss of bladder and bowel control (usually with urinary retention and bladder distention), loss of sweating and vasomotor tone below the neurologic level, and marked reduction of blood pressure from loss of peripheral vascular resistance.

Respiratory problems are related to compromised respiratory function, the severity of which depends on the level of injury. The muscles contributing to respiration are the abdominals, intercostals (T1–T11), and the diaphragm. In high cervical cord injury, acute respiratory failure is the leading cause of death.

Diagnostic Evaluation

A detailed neurologic examination is performed. Radiographic examination (lateral cervical spine x-rays and CT scanning) is carried out. A search is made for other injuries because

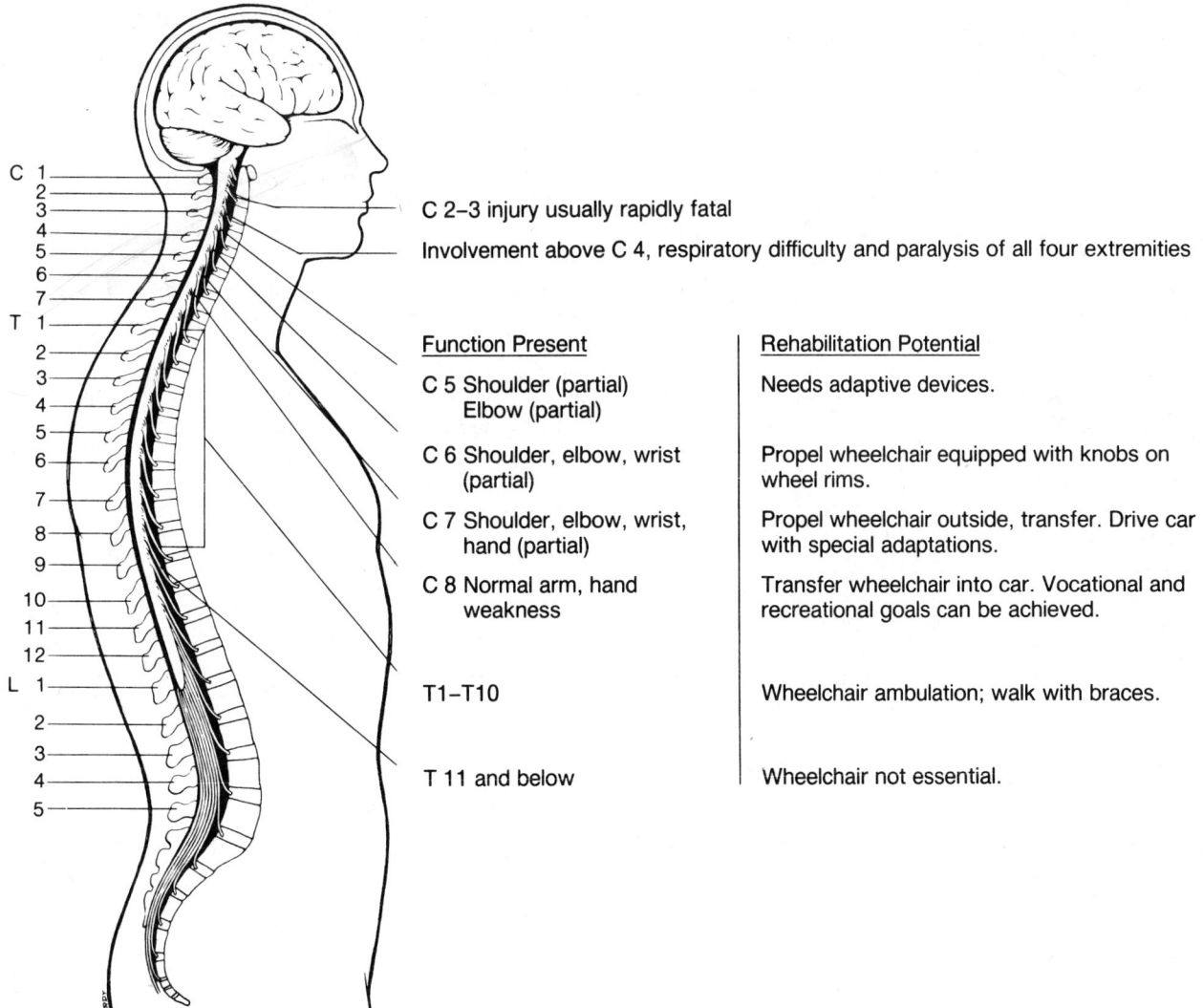

C 2–3 injury usually rapidly fatal

Involvement above C 4, respiratory difficulty and paralysis of all four extremities

Function Present	Rehabilitation Potential
C 5 Shoulder (partial) Elbow (partial)	Needs adaptive devices.
C 6 Shoulder, elbow, wrist (partial)	Propel wheelchair equipped with knobs on wheel rims.
C 7 Shoulder, elbow, wrist, hand (partial)	Propel wheelchair outside, transfer. Drive car with special adaptations.
C 8 Normal arm, hand weakness	Transfer wheelchair into car. Vocational and recreational goals can be achieved.
T1–T10	Wheelchair ambulation; walk with braces.
T 11 and below	Wheelchair not essential.

Figure 54-9
Sequelae of spinal cord injury and rehabilitation challenges. (The vertebrae are numbered on the left side of the drawing and the spinal nerves are numbered on the right.)

spinal trauma is associated with multiple injuries, commonly affecting the head and chest. Continuous ECG monitoring may be indicated, because *bradycardia* (slow heart rate) and *asystole* (cardiac standstill) are common in acute cervical injuries.

Management of Cervical Spine Injuries (Acute Phase)

The goals of management are to prevent further spinal cord injury and to observe for symptoms of progressive neurologic deficits.

The patient is resuscitated as necessary, and oxygenation and cardiovascular stability are obtained. High-dose steroids may be administered to counteract cord edema. Oxygen is administered to maintain a high arterial PO$_2$, because anoxemia can create or worsen a neurologic deficit of the spinal cord. If endotracheal intubation is necessary, extreme care is taken to avoid flexing or extending the neck, which can result in worsening the injury. *Diaphragm pacing* (electrical stimulation of the phrenic nerve) may be considered for the patient with a high cervical lesion.

Management of cervical spinal injury requires *immobilization*, and *reduction* of dislocations (restoration of normal position), and *stabilization* of the vertebral column. To reduce the fracture dislocation and maintain alignment of the cervical spine, some form the skeletal traction such as skeletal tongs/calipers or the halo-vest technique is used (Fig. 54-10). A variety of skeletal tongs are available, all of which involve fixation in the skull in some manner. The Gardner-Wells tongs require no predrilled holes in the skull. Crutchfield and Vinke tongs are inserted through holes made with a special drill under local anesthesia.

Traction is applied to the tongs by weights, the amount depending on the patient's size and the degree of fracture displacement. The traction force is exerted along the longitudinal axis of the vertebral bodies, with the neck in a neutral position. Then the traction is gradually increased by the addition of more weights. As the amount of traction is increased, the spaces between the intervertebral discs widen, and the vertebrae slip back into position. Reduction usually takes place after correct alignment has been regained. Once reduction is achieved, as verified by cervical spine films and neurologic examination, the weights are gradually removed until the amount of weight needed to maintain the alignment is obtained. The weights should hang free so as not to interfere with the traction. The patient is placed on a turning frame if one is available. (See p. 1504 for a method of transfer to the turning frame.) Some neurosurgeons do not advocate the use of the circOlectric bed for spinal injuries because excessive pressure is placed on the fracture when the patient is turned in a vertical fashion.

A halo device may be used initially with traction or may be applied following removal of the skull tongs. It consists of a stainless steel "halo ring" that is fixed to the skull by 4 pins. The ring is attached to a removable halo vest, which suspends the weight of the unit circumferentially around the chest. A metal frame connects the ring to the chest. Halo devices afford immobilization of the cervical spine while allowing early mobilization.

Surgical Intervention

If the patient's deformities cannot be reduced by traction, or if there is significant instability of the cervical spine, or if the patient's neurologic status is deteriorating, surgery is performed to reduce the spinal fracture or dislocation and/or decompress the cord.

A *laminectomy* (excision of the posterior arches and spinous processes of a vertebra) may be indicated in the presence of progressive neurologic deficit, suspicion of epidural hematoma, or penetrating injuries that require surgical débridement, or to permit direct visualization and exploration of the cord. (The care of the patient following a laminectomy is discussed on p. 1518).

Management of Spinal Shock

Spinal shock represents a sudden depression of reflex activity in the spinal cord (*areflexia*) below the level of injury. In this condition, the muscles innervated by the part of the cord segment situated below the level of the lesion become completely paralyzed and flaccid, and the reflexes are absent. The blood pressure falls, and the parts of the body below the level of the cord lesion are paralyzed and without sensation. With injuries to the cervical and upper thoracic spinal cord, the innervation to the major accessory muscles of respiration is lost and respiratory problems develop: decreased vital capacity, retention of secretions, increased PCO$_2$, decreased PO$_2$, hypoxia, respiratory failure, and pulmonary edema. The reflexes that initiate bladder and bowel function likewise are affected. (The management of the patient with a neurogenic bladder—*i.e.*, a bladder disturbance due to a lesion of the central nervous system—is discussed on p. 1014.) Bowel distention and paralytic ileus caused by depression of the reflexes may be treated with intestinal decompression. The patient does not perspire on the paralyzed portions of his body, since sympathetic activity is blocked, so he must be watched carefully for an abrupt onset of fever. (Hyperthermia is treated as outlined on p. 1426.)

- The patient's body defenses are supported and maintained until spinal shock abates and the system has recovered from the traumatic insult (3–6 weeks). Special attention must also be directed to the respiratory system. There may not be enough intrathoracic pressure for the patient to cough effectively. Chest physical therapy is used to help clear pulmonary secretions.

▶ Nursing Process
The Patient With Spinal Cord Injury

▷ Assessment

The breathing pattern is observed, the strength with which the patient coughs is assessed, and the lungs are auscultated because paralysis of abdominal and respiratory muscles diminishes coughing and makes it difficult to clear bronchial and pharyngeal secretions. Ventilation is also affected when these muscles decrease the ventilatory excursion of the chest.

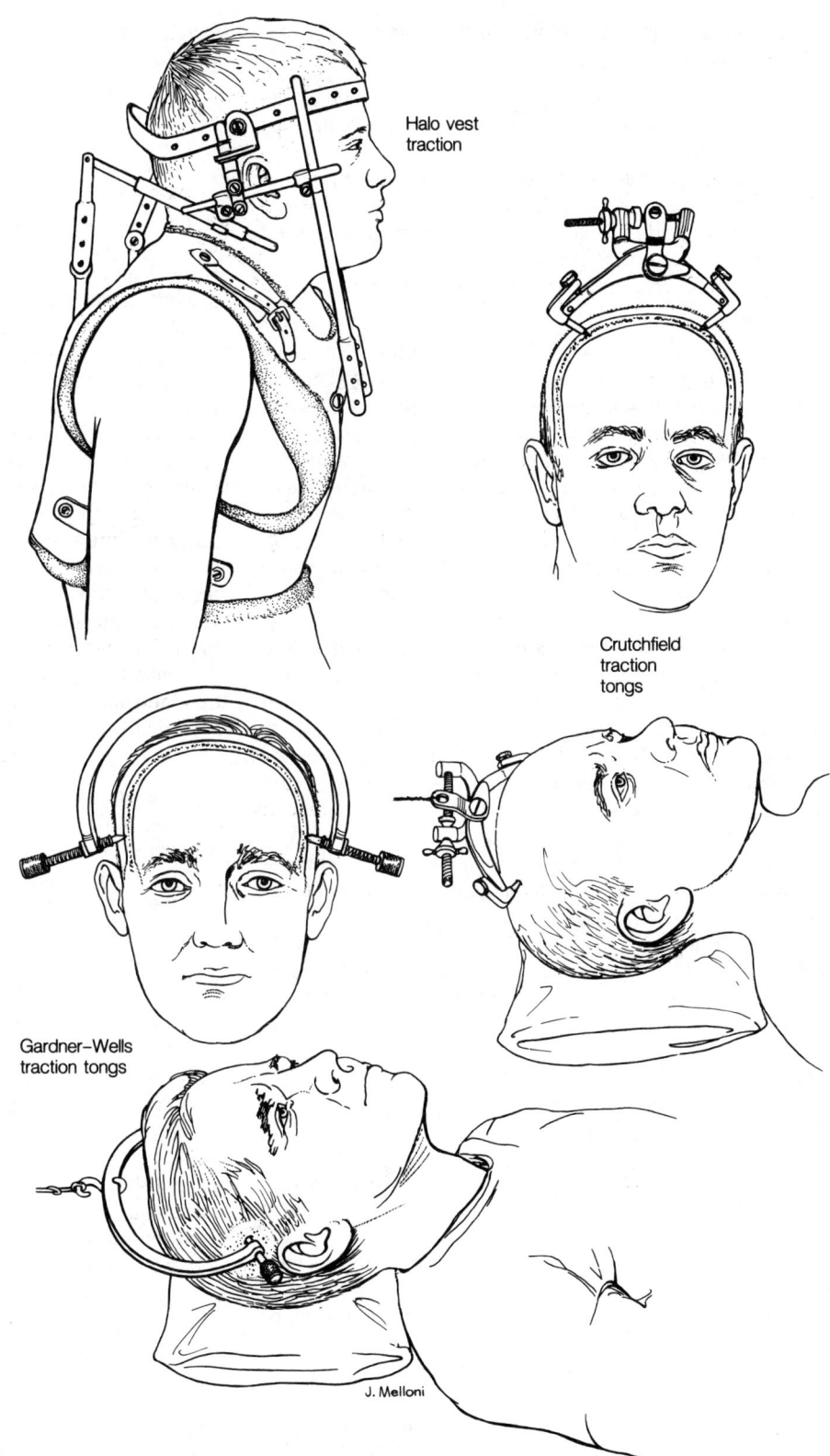

Halo vest traction

Crutchfield traction tongs

Gardner–Wells traction tongs

J. Melloni

Figure 54-10
Methods of cervical traction.
(Brunner LS and Suddarth DS. The Lippincott Manual of Nursing Practice, 4th ed. Philadelphia, JB Lippincott, 1986.)

The patient is monitored constantly for any changes in motor or sensory function and symptoms of progressive neurologic damage. It may be impossible in the early stages of cord injury to determine whether the cord has been transected, because signs and symptoms of cord edema are indistinguishable from those of cord transection. Edema of the spinal cord may occur with any severe cord injury, and may further compromise spinal function.

Motor and sensory function is determined by careful neurologic examination. These findings are recorded so that changes in or progression from the baseline neurologic status can be evaluated accurately.

- Motor ability is tested by asking the patient to spread the fingers, squeeze the examiner's hand, and move the toes or turn the feet.
- Sensation is evaluated by pinching the skin or pricking it with a pin, starting at the shoulder level and working down both sides of the extremities. The patient is asked where the sensation is felt.
- Any decrease in neurologic function is reported immediately.

The patient is also assessed for the presence of spinal shock, in which there is complete loss of all reflex, motor, sensory, and autonomic activity below the level of the lesion. This causes bladder distention from paralysis of the bladder. The area over the bladder is palpated for signs of urinary retention and overdistention of the bladder. Further assessment is made for gastric dilatation and ileus due to an atonic bowel, a result of autonomic disruption.

Temperature is monitored because the patient may have periods of hyperthermia as a result of alteration in temperature control due to autonomic disruption.

Assessment for Complications. In addition to watching for respiratory complications (respiratory failure; pneumonia) and *autonomic hyperreflexia* (which is characterized by pounding headache, profuse sweating, nasal congestion, piloerection [gooseflesh], bradycardia, and hypertension [see p. 1510]), constant surveillance is maintained for signs and symptoms of pressure sores and infection (urinary; respiratory; local infection at the pin sites).

Deep vein thrombosis with pulmonary embolism is a common complication of immobility; its clinical manifestations include anxiety, shortness of breath, and changes in blood gas values. Thigh and calf measurements are made daily. The patient is prepared for venography if there is a significant increase in the circumference of one extremity.

Nursing Diagnoses

Based on all the assessment data, the patient's major nursing diagnoses may include the following:

- Ineffective breathing patterns related to weakness/paralysis of abdominal and intercostal muscles and inability to clear secretions
- Impaired physical mobility related to motor and sensory impairment
- Potential impairment of skin integrity related to immobility, sensory loss
- Urinary retention related to inability to void spontaneously
- Alteration in bowel elimination, constipation, related to presence of atonic bowel as a result of autonomic disruption
- Alteration in comfort related to prolonged immobility

▷ Planning and Implementation

▷ *Goals:* The patient's goals may include improvement of breathing pattern, improvement of mobility, achievement of skin integrity, relief of urinary retention, improvement of bowel function, and promotion of comfort.

Nursing Interventions

Assuring Adequate Breathing. Possible impending respiratory failure is detected by observing the patient, measuring vital capacity, and monitoring arterial blood gas values. Early and vigorous attention to clearing bronchial and pharyngeal secretions can prevent retention of secretions and resultant atelectasis. Suctioning may be indicated, but caution must be employed during suctioning because this procedure can stimulate the vagus nerve, producing bradycardia, which can result in cardiac arrest. If the patient cannot cough effectively due to decreased inspiratory volume and inability to develop sufficient expiratory pressure, chest physical therapy may be indicated. Specific breathing exercises are supervised by the nurse to increase strength and endurance of inspiratory muscles, particularly the diaphragm. The nurse also ensures proper humidification and hydration to prevent secretions from becoming viscid and difficult to cough up. Signs of respiratory infection (cough, fever, dyspnea) are watched for. Smoking is discouraged because it increases bronchial and pulmonary secretions and damages cilia.

Improving Mobility. Proper body alignment is maintained at all times. The patient is placed in the dorsal or supine position as follows:

- The feet are positioned against a padded footboard to prevent footdrop. There should be a space between the end of the mattress and the footboard to allow free suspension of the heels. A wooden block on either end of the mattress prevents the mattress from pushing against the footboard.
- Trochanter rolls are applied from the crest of the ilium to the midthigh of both extremities to prevent external rotation of the hip joints.

Patients with lesions above the midthoracic level have loss of sympathetic control of peripheral vasoconstrictor activity, leading to hypotension. These patients may tolerate changes in position poorly, and will require monitoring of blood pressure when positions are changed. Usually the patient is turned every 2 hours. If not on a turning frame, the patient should not be turned unless the physician has said to do so. Directives for turning a patient not on a Stryker frame are found in Chart 54-5. Take adequate time while turning the patient, maintaining a gentle, firm, and steady touch.

Contractures develop rapidly in association with immobility and muscle paralysis. Atrophy of the extremities will result from disuse. To avoid these complications, passive range-of-motion exercises may be prescribed within 48 to 72 hours after injury. These exercises preserve joint motion and stimulate circulation. A joint that is immobilized too long becomes fixed as a result of contractures of the tendon and joint capsule. Toes, metatarsals, ankles, knees, and hips should be put through a full range of motion at least 4, and ideally 5, times daily. Range-of-motion exercises can prevent many complications.

Maintaining Skin Integrity. Because the patient with a spinal cord injury is immobilized and has loss of feeling, there is an ever-present, life-endangering threat of pressure

Chart 54-5
Turning the Patient
With Crutchfield Tongs
(Not on Stryker Frame)

If Crutchfield tongs are used and the patient is not on a Stryker frame, a directive from the physician must be obtained before the patient is turned. The patient's head *should never be flexed*, either forward or laterally, and at all times should be kept in a direct line with the axis of the cervical spine.

To Turn the Patient

- Three persons should turn the patient in a logrolling fashion, making sure that the shoulder turns with the head and the neck. One nurse should support the head; the second nurse or attendant, the shoulders; and the third person, the hips and the legs.
- The nurse supporting the head gives the commands for turning.
- Place a pillow between the legs of the patient to prevent the upper leg from slipping forward and jarring the patient's head.
- Place a pillow longitudinally on the chest, with the patient's upper arm resting on it. The pillow prevents the shoulder from sagging and pulling on the neck as the patient is turned.
- As the patient is turned in a logrolling fashion, the traction should be moved carefully to keep it in a direct line with the cervical spine. The patient's position should be adjusted so that the traction, the patient's head, and the cervical spine are in correct alignment.
- While the nurse still supports the head in the lateral position, a small pillow is placed under the head to maintain cervical alignment.

sores. In areas of local tissue ischemia where there is continuous pressure and where the peripheral circulation is inadequate as a result of the spinal shock and recumbency, pressure sores have been known to develop within 6 hours. The most common sites are over the ischial tuberosity, the greater trochanter, and the sacrum.

- The patient's position is changed at least every 2 hours. Turning not only aids in the prevention of pressure sores, but also prevents the pooling of blood and tissue fluid in the dependent areas.

Careful inspection of the skin is made each time the patient is turned. Check the skin over the pressure points for redness, the perineum for soilage, and the catheter for drainage, and assess for general alignment and comfort.

- Every few hours the patient's skin should be washed with a mild soap, rinsed well, and *blotted* dry. Pressure-sensitive areas should be kept well-lubricated and soft with

bland cream or lotion. Massage should be done gently with a circular motion.
- The patient must know the danger of pressure sores and accept responsibility for prevention. (See p. 222 for other aspects of the prevention of pressure sores.)

Promoting Urinary Elimination. Immediately after a spinal cord injury, the urinary bladder becomes atonic and cannot contract by reflex activity. Urinary retention is the immediate result of spinal cord injury. Because the patient has no sensation of bladder distention, overstretching of the bladder and detrusor muscle may occur and delay the return of bladder function.

Intermittent catheterization is carried out to avoid overstretching and infection. If this is not feasible, and indwelling catheter is inserted. At an early stage, family members are shown how to carry out the procedure and encouraged to participate in this facet of care, because they will be involved in long-term follow-up and must be able to recognize complications so that treatment can be instituted.

The patient is taught to note and write down fluid intake, voiding pattern, amounts of residual urine following catheterization, quality of urine, and any "unusual" feelings that may be occurring. The management of a neurogenic bladder is discussed in detail on page 1014.

Improving Bowel Function. Immediately after spinal cord injury, the patient usually has a paralytic ileus due to neurogenic paralysis of the bowel. The nurse monitors the patient's reactions to gastric intubation, which is prescribed to relieve gastric distention and prevent aspiration.

Bowel activity usually returns within the first week. As soon as bowel sounds are heard via auscultation, the patient is given a high-calorie, high-protein, and high-fiber diet with the amount of food gradually increased. The nurse administers the prescribed stool softener to counteract the effects of immobility and pain medications. A bowel program is instituted as early as possible (see p. 238).

Promoting Comfort. When skull tongs or calipers are in place, the patient's skull is assessed for signs of infection, including drainage around the tongs. The back of the head is checked periodically for signs of pressure and is massaged at intervals, with care being taken not to move the neck. The hair around the tongs is shaved to facilitate inspection. Avoid probing under encrusted areas.

Halo Traction. The patient may experience a slight headache or discomfort around the skull pins for several days after the pins are inserted. The patient may not initially appreciate the rather startling appearance of this apparatus, but can readily adapt to it because the device provides comfort for the unstable neck. The patient may complain of being "caged in" and of noise created by any object coming in contact with the steel frame, but can be reassured that adaptation to such annoyances will occur.

The areas around the pin sites are cleansed daily and observed for redness, drainage, and pain. Observe for any loosening of the pins, which is apt to contribute to infection. If one of the pins becomes detached, stabilize the patient's head in a neutral position while another person notifies the neurosurgeon. A torque screwdriver should be readily available in case the screws on the frame need tightening.

The skin under the halo vest is inspected for excessive

perspiration, redness, and skin blistering, especially on the bony prominences. The vest is opened at the sides to allow the patient's torso to be washed. Do not allow the liner of the vest to become wet, because dampness will cause skin problems. Avoid putting powder inside the vest, because this may contribute to the development of pressure sores.

Promoting Ambulation. For patients with a cervical fracture without neurologic deficit, reduction in traction followed by rigid immobilization for approximately 16 weeks will restore skeletal function with most patients. These patients will be allowed to move gradually to an erect position. Anticipate that a four-poster neck brace or molded collar will be applied when the patient is mobilized after traction is removed.

The rehabilitation of the patient with a permanent spinal cord injury, *i.e.*, the paraplegic patient, is discussed in the next section.

▷ *Evaluation*

▷ *Expected Outcomes*

1. Patient demonstrates improvement in breathing.
   a. Has no evidence of respiratory infection
   b. Is able to clear secretions
2. Is able to move within limits of the dysfunction
   a. Understands turning schedule; reminds health care personnel of it
   b. Explains importance of exercise program
3. Shows no skin breakdown
4. Regains urinary elimination
   a. Shows no signs of urinary infection
   b. Monitors own intake and output
5. Regains bowel elimination capacity
6. States that he has no discomfort
   a. Shows no redness/drainage around skull pins
   b. Makes plans for the future

The Paraplegic Patient

Paraplegia refers to loss of motion and sensation in the lower extremities and all or part of the trunk as a result of damage to the thoracic or lumbar spinal cord or to the sacral root. It most frequently follows trauma due to accidents and gunshot wounds, but may be the result of spinal cord lesions (intervertebral disc, tumor, vascular lesions), multiple sclerosis, infections and abscesses of the spinal cord, and congenital defects.

Diagnostic Evaluation

Evaluation includes the observations and studies performed for the patient with a spinal cord injury: full neurologic examination, x-ray studies, and ECG monitoring.

Management

The patient faces a lifetime of great disability, requiring ongoing follow-up and care and the expertise of a number of health professionals, including the physician, physiatrist, rehabilitation nurse, occupational therapist, physical therapist, psychologist, social worker, rehabilitation engineer, and vocational counselor at different times as the need arises. As the years go by, these patients also have the same medical problems as others in the aging population. Additionally, they face the threat of complications associated with paraplegia. Usually the patient is encouraged to attend a spinal clinic when problems arise. Lifetime care includes assessment of the urinary tract at prescribed intervals, because there is likelihood of continuing alteration in detrusor and sphincter function and the patient is prone to urinary tract infections.

Management includes observing and caring for any alteration in physiological status and psychological outlook, and the prevention and management of complications.

Complications

Autonomic Dysreflexia. Autonomic dysreflexia (autonomic hyperreflexia) is an acute emergency that occurs as a result of exaggerated autonomic responses to stimuli that are innocuous in normal individuals. This syndrome is characterized by severe, pounding headache with paroxysmal hypertension, profuse sweating (most often of the forehead), nasal congestion, and bradycardia. It occurs among patients with cord lesions above the T6 level (the sympathetic visceral outflow level), generally after spinal shock has subsided. The sudden rise in blood pressure may cause a rupture of one or more cerebral blood vessels or lead to an increase in intracranial pressure. A number of stimuli may trigger this reflex: distended bladder (the most common cause), distended bowel, stimulation of the skin (tactile, pain, thermal stimuli), or distention or contraction of the visceral organs, especially the bowel (from constipation, impaction). Since this is an emergency situation, the objective is to remove the triggering stimulus and to avoid the possibly serious complications.

The following measures are carried out:

- Place the patient in a sitting position to lower the blood pressure.
- Drain the bladder via the catheter. If the catheter is not patent, irrigate it with a small amount of irrigating solution or insert another catheter.
- After the symptoms subside, the rectum is examined for a fecal mass. If one is present, dibucaine ointment is inserted 10 to 15 minutes before the mass is removed, since visceral distention or contraction can cause autonomic dysreflexia.
- Any other stimulus that can be the triggering event, such as an object on the skin or a draft of cold air, must be removed.
- If these measures do not relieve the patient's hypertension and excruciating headache, a ganglionic blocking agent (hydralazine hydrochloride [Apresoline]) is prescribed and given slowly by vein.
- The patient's chart should tagged with an allergic marker.
- Instruct the patient in prevention and management measures.

Any patient with a lesion above the T6 segment should be informed that such an episode is possible and may even occur many years after the initial injury.

Other Complications of Paraplegia. Other long-term complications of paraplegia include bladder and kidney infections (which are discussed under Neurogenic Bladder, p. 1014), pressure sores with complications of sepsis, osteomyelitis, fistulas, and depression. Flexor muscle spasms may be particularly disabling. *Heterotopic ossification* (overgrowth of bone) occurs in 20% to 40% of spinal cord injury patients in the hips, knees, shoulders, and elbows. This complication can produce a loss of range of motion. The nursing role is that of emphasizing the need for vigilance in self-assessment and care.

▶ Nursing Process
The Patient With Paraplegia

▷ Assessment

Patients with paraplegia have experienced varying degrees of loss of motor power, deep and superficial sensation, vasomotor control, bladder and bowel control, and sexual function. They are faced with threats of dysfunction related to paraplegia including mobility, skin breakdown and pressure sores, recurring urinary infection, contractures, and psychosocial problems. Nurses in any health care setting must be cognizant of these potential problems in the lifetime management of these persons. Assessment focuses on the patient's general condition, observation for complications, and determining how the patient is managing at this particular point in time.

Psychosocial Assessment. It is usually some time before these patients comprehend the magnitude of their disability. They may go through stages of adjustment, including shock and disbelief, denial, depression, grief, and acceptance. During the acute phase of the injury, denial can be a protective mechanism to shield patients from the overwhelming reality of what has happened. As they realize the finality of paraplegia (or quadriplegia), the grieving process may be prolonged and all-encompassing because of the awareness of "what will never be." A period of depression follows as the patient experiences a loss of self-esteem in areas of self-identity, sexual functioning, and social and emotional roles. Self-esteem is related to being strong, loved, and lovable—all of which are threatened.

▷ Nursing Diagnoses

Based on all the assessment data, the major nursing diagnoses of the patient with paraplegia may include the following:

- Immobility related to inability to walk
- Impairment of skin integrity related to permanent sensory loss and immobility
- Alteration in patterns of urinary elimination—retention related to level of spinal cord injury
- Alterations in bowel elimination related to effects of spinal cord disruption
- Sexual dysfunction related to neurologic dysfunction
- Ineffective individual coping related to impact of dysfunction on daily living

▷ Planning and Implementation

▷ *Goals:* The goals for the patient may include attainment of some form of mobility, maintenance of healthy, intact skin, achievement of bladder management without infection, achievement of bowel control, achievement of sexual expression, and strengthening of coping mechanisms.

▷ Nursing Interventions

The patient requires extensive rehabilitation, which will be less difficult if appropriate nursing management has been carried out during the acute phase of the injury or illness. (See the management of spinal cord injuries, p. 1506). The nursing care is one of the determining factors in the success of the rehabilitation program. The main objective is for the patient to live as independently as possible in the home community.

Achieving Mobility.

Weight-Bearing Activities. A patient with complete severance of the cord can begin weight-bearing early, because no further damage can be incurred. The sooner muscles are strengthened, the less is the chance they will atrophy (disuse atrophy). The earlier the patient is brought to a standing position, the less opportunity there will be for osteoporotic changes to take place in the long bones. Weight-bearing also reduces the possibility of urinary infections and formation of renal calculi and enhances many other metabolic processes.

Exercise Program. The unaffected parts of the body are built up to optimal strength to enable the patient to ambulate with braces and crutches. The muscles of the hands, arms, shoulders, chest, spine, abdomen, and neck must be strengthened, since the patient must bear full weight on these muscles. The triceps and the latissimus dorsi are important muscles used in crutch walking. The muscles of the abdomen and the back also are necessary for balance and the maintenance of the upright position.

To strengthen these muscles, the patient can do "push-ups" when in a prone position and "sit-ups" when in a sitting position. Extending the arms while holding weights (traction weights can be used) also develops muscle strength. Squeezing rubber balls or crumbling newspaper promotes hand strength.

Through the encouragement of all of the members of the rehabilitation team, the patient develops the increased exercise tolerance needed for gait training and ambulation activities.

Managing Postural Hypotension. Because vasomotor tone is lacking in the lower extremities, the patient may become hypotensive when placed in an upright position. Profound postural hypotension is seen in all patients with lesions above the midthoracic level. Postural hypotension results because the reflex arcs that normally produce vasoconstriction in the upright position have been interrupted. There is pooling of blood in the peripheral veins and splanchnic bed from lack of muscle tone and poor skin turgor. Reduced venous return to the heart, orthostatic hypotension, and decreased cerebral blood flow also occur.

To counteract this problem, a tilt table may be used to help the patient overcome vasomotor instability and tolerate the upright posture. Other possible measures include using elastic stockings to facilitate venous return in the legs and applying an abdominal binder to alleviate the pooling of blood in the abdominal area.

When a tilt table is used, gradually elevate the patient to an upright position. At first the patient may be able to tolerate only an elevation of 45 degrees (or less), but gradually the angle of elevation is increased. Observe closely for signs of intolerance, including nausea, perspiration, pallor, dizziness, and syncope. Blood pressure is taken before the patient is allowed up and when positioned on the tilt table, since periods of recumbency also favor the development of orthostatic hypotension.

If no tilt table is available, a high-back reclining wheelchair with extension leg rests may be used. To overcome the effects of hypotension, the backrest is raised slowly and the leg rests are lowered gradually over a period of 7 to 10 days. While in the wheelchair, the patient may experience dizziness, tachycardia, hypotension, and blackouts. If dizziness develops, the brakes should be placed in the "on" position and the wheelchair tilted back for several minutes. If hypotension is prolonged, cerebral anoxia with the possibility of a cerebrovascular accident is a distinct threat and must be avoided.

Mobilization. When the spine is stable enough to allow the patient to assume an upright posture, mobilization activities are initiated. A brace or vest may be used, depending on the level of the lesion. Braces and crutches enable some patients to ambulate for short distances and even to drive manually-operated automobiles. Crutch ambulation in paraplegics requires high energy expenditure. Modern technological developments, such as motorized wheelchairs and specially equipped vans, are contributing to the greater independence and mobility of patients with high-level spinal cord injuries.

A major goal of nursing management is to help these patients overcome their sense of futility and to encourage them in the emotional adjustment that must be made before they are willing to venture into the "outside world." To achieve this goal, it is important to realize that an excessively sympathetic attitude may cause patients to develop an overdependence that defeats the purpose of the entire rehabilitation program.

Teach and help when necessary, but do not take over activities that patients can do for themselves with a little effort. This type of nursing care more than repays itself in the satisfaction of seeing a completely demoralized and helpless patient begin to find meaning in a newly-emerging life-style.

Achieving Healthy Skin. Because paraplegic patients spend a great portion of their lives in a wheelchair, pressure sores are ever-present threat, causing sickness and loss of time and money. Contributing factors are permanent sensory paralysis and loss of sensation over pressure areas, immobility that makes pressure relief a problem, trauma from bumps (against the wheelchair, toilet, or whatever) that cause unperceived abrasions and wounds, loss of protective function of the skin from excoriation and maceration due to excessive sweating and possible urine and fecal incontinence, and poor general health (anemia, edema, malnutrition) leading to poor tissue perfusion.

The prevention and management of pressure sores are discussed in detail in the rehabilitation chapter on pages 222–230 and under the care of the patient with a spinal cord injury, pages 1508–1509.

The person with paraplegia must take responsibility for monitoring his skin condition. This involves relieving pressure and avoiding holding any position for longer than 2 hours, in addition to seeing that the skin receives meticulous attention

and cleanliness. The patient is taught that sores develop over bony prominences exposed to unrelieved pressure in the lying and sitting positions. The most vulnerable areas are pointed out, and the patient is instructed to use mirrors to inspect these areas morning and night, observing for redness, slight edema, or any abrasions. While in bed the patient should turn at 2-hour intervals and then inspect the skin again for redness that does not fade on pressure. The foundation sheet should be checked for wetness and for creases.

The patient is taught to relieve pressure in the wheelchair by doing pushups, leaning from side to side to relieve ischial pressure, and tilting forward while leaning on a table. Each person requires a wheelchair cushion prescribed to meet individual needs, which may change in time with changes in posture, weight, and skin tolerance. A referral can be made to a rehabilitation engineer who can measure pressure levels while the patient is sitting and then tailor the cushion and other necessary aids and appliances to this patient's needs.

The diet for the patient with paraplegia should be high in protein, vitamins, and calories to ensure minimal wasting of muscle, well-functioning kidneys, and the maintenance of healthy skin.

Achieving Bladder Management. The effect of the spinal lesion on the bladder depends on the level of the cord injury, degree of cord damage, and length of time after injury. A patient with paraplegia usually has either a reflex or a nonreflex bladder, which are discussed under Neurogenic Bladder on page 1014. Both problems increase the risk of urinary tract infection.

The nurse emphasizes the importance of maintaining an adequate flow of urine by encouraging the drinking of approximately 2.5 liters of liquids daily, emptying the bladder frequently so there is minimal residual urine, and giving attention to personal hygiene because infection of the bladder and kidneys almost always occurs by the ascending route. The perineum is to be kept clean and dry and attention given to perianal skin after defecation. Underwear should be cotton (more absorbent) and changed at least daily.

If an external catheter (condom catheter) is used, the sheath is removed nightly; the penis is cleansed to remove urine and dried carefully because warm urine on the periurethral skin promotes growth of bacteria. Attention is also given to the collection bag. The nurse emphasizes the importance of monitoring for indications of urinary tract infection: cloudy urine or *hematuria* (blood in the urine), fever, chills, or flank pain.

The female patient who cannot achieve reflex bladder control or self-catheterization may need to wear pads or waterproof undergarments. Surgical intervention may be necessary in the form of some type of urinary diversion procedure.

Achieving Bowel Control: Bowel Training Program. The objective of a bowel training program is to establish bowel evacuation through reflex conditioning. This technique is described on page 238. If a cord injury occurs above the sacral segments or nerve roots and there is reflex activity, the anal sphincter may be massaged to stimulate defecation. (If the cord lesion involves the sacral segment or nerve roots, anal massage is not done because the anus may be relaxed and lack tone. Massage is also contraindicated if there is spasticity of the anal sphincter.) The anal sphincter is massaged by inserting a gloved finger (which has been adequately lubricated) 2.5 to 3.7 cm (1–1½ inches) into the rectum and moving it in a circular motion or from side to side. It will soon become apparent which area triggers the defecation response. This procedure should be done at the same time (usually every 48 hours) after a meal and at a time that will be convenient for the patient upon returning home. The patient is also taught the symptoms of impaction (frequent loose stools; constipation) and cautioned to watch for the development of hemorrhoids. A diet with sufficient fluids and fiber is essential to a bowel training program.

Finding Sexual Expression.   Most patients with cord injury can have some form of meaningful sexual relationship, although some modifications will have to be made to cope with anxiety. The patient and partner will benefit from counseling on the range of sexual expression possible, special techniques, positions, exploration of body sensations offering sensual feelings, and urinary and bowel hygiene as related to sexual activity. Penile prostheses are available for men with erectile failure. Sexual education and counseling services are being included in the rehabilitation services at spinal centers. Small group meetings in which the patients can share their feelings, receive information, and discuss sexual concerns and practical aspects are helpful in producing effective attitudes and adjustments.

Strengthening Coping Mechanisms.   The impact of the full realization of their disability and loss becomes marked when patients return home. Each time something new enters their life (*e.g.*, a new relationship, going to work), they are reminded anew of their limitations. Grief reactions and depression are frequently encountered.

To be able to work through this depression, patients must be able to see some hope for relief in the future. Thus, they are guided toward a sense of confidence in their ability to achieve self-care and relative independence. The role of the nurse ranges from caretaker during the acute phase to teacher, counselor, and facilitator as patients gain mobility and independence.

Adjustment to the disability leads to the development of realistic goals for the future, making the best of those abilities that are left intact and reinvesting in other activities and relationships. Rejection of the disability will cause self-destructive neglect and noncompliance with the therapeutic program. This leads to more frustration and depression. Crises for which interventions may be sought include social, psychological, marital, sexual, and psychiatric problems. The family usually requires counseling, social services, and other support systems to help them cope with the changes that will be made in their life-style and socioeconomic status. (The psychological implications of a disability are discussed also on p. 216.)

Patient Education and Home Health Care.   Patients with a spinal injury are at special risk during the first few weeks after their return home. Urinary infections and deconditioning resulting in contractures may appear and require rehospitalization. For the rest of their lives, patients are at risk of developing pressure sores which pose a serious threat to life. To avoid these complications, the patient and a family member are taught skin care, catheter care, range-of-motion exercises, and other care techniques while the patient is still in the hospital. The teaching is reinforced during home visits by the home care nurse. Environmental modifications are made and specialized equipment is purchased before the patient comes home. Other complications during the extended care period may include lower extremity edema, ankle and feet contractures, pain, and alcohol abuse.

The community health nurse provides continuing follow-up evaluation to reinforce previous teaching and to determine if further physical help is needed. The patient's self-esteem and body-image perceptions may be very low at this time.

It has been shown that persons with high levels of social support who are satisfied with their social contacts and feel that they have high levels of control generally report feelings of well-being despite the presence of a major disability. Thus it behooves the nurse to assess and promote further development of the support system of each patient.

The local counselor for the Division of Vocational Rehabilitation works with the patient with respect to job placement or additional educational or vocational training.

The patient requires continuing, lifelong follow-up by the physician, physical therapist, and other rehabilitation team members, because the neurologic deficit is permanent and new problems can erupt that require prompt attention before they take their toll in additional physical impairment, time, morale, and money.

▷ *Evaluation*

▷ *Expected Outcomes*

1. Patient attains some form of mobility.
2. Maintains healthy, intact skin
3. Achieves bladder control, absence of urinary tract infection
4. Achieves bowel control
5. Reports sexual satisfaction
6. Shows improved adaptation to environment and others

Intraspinal Tumors

Tumors within the spine are classified according to their anatomic relation to the spinal cord. They include *intramedullary* lesions (within the spinal cord); *extramedullary–intradural* lesions (within the subarachnoid space), and *extradural* lesions (outside the dural membrane). Tumors that occur within the spinal cord or exert pressure on it cause symptoms ranging from weakness and loss of reflexes above the tumor level and localized or shooting pains, to progressive loss of motor function and paralysis. Usually, sharp pain occurs in the area that is innervated by the spinal roots that arise from the cord in the region of the tumor. In addition, increasing paralysis develops below the level of the lesion.

The diagnosis is made by neurologic examination and myelography in combination with CT scanning.

Preoperative Management

The patient is assessed for weakness, muscle wasting, spasticity, and sensory or sphincter disorders. A search is made for potential pulmonary problems, especially if a cervical tumor is present. The patient is also evaluated for coagulation deficiencies. Ask about aspirin intake because this may create problems with hemostasis. Breathing exercises are taught and demonstrated preoperatively.

Surgical Management

The removal of the tumor is usually desired but not always feasible. The goal is to remove as much tumor as possible while sparing intact portions of the spinal cord. Microsurgical techniques have improved the prognosis for surgical treatment of intramedullary tumors. The prognosis is related to the degree of neurologic impairment at the time of surgery, the speed of occurrence of symptoms, and the tumor's origin. Patients with large neurologic deficits before surgery usually do not make significant functional recovery following successful tumor removal.

Other treatment modalities include subtotal removal of the tumor, decompression of the spinal cord, chemotherapy, and radiation therapy.

If the patient has epidural spinal cord compression resulting from metastatic cancer (from breast, prostate, or lung), high-dose dexamethasone combined with radiation therapy appears to be effective in relieving pain.

Postoperative Nursing Interventions

The nursing management is similar to that following disc surgery (see p. 1518). Watch for any increase in neurologic deterioration. A sudden onset of neurologic deficit is a sinister sign. It may be due to vertebral collapse associated with spinal cord infarction. Neurologic checks are made, with emphasis on evaluating arm and leg movement, strength, and sensation. Sensory function is checked by pinching the skin on the arms, legs, and trunk to determine if there is loss of feeling and, if so, at what level. Vital signs are monitored at intervals. If the tumor was in the cervical area, there is always the possibility of postoperative respiratory compromise. Chest movement is observed for symmetry and abdominal breathing, and the chest is auscultated for abnormal breath sounds. In the instance of a high cervical lesion, the endotracheal tube is left in place until respiratory function is assured. Deep breathing and coughing are encouraged.

The area over the patient's bladder is palpated for urinary retention. Incontinence may be present. Urinary dysfunction usually implies significant decompensation of spinal cord function. An intake and output record is maintained. Additionally, the bowel area is auscultated for bowel sounds.

The prescribed pain medication should be given in adequate amounts and at appropriate intervals to relieve pain and prevent its recurrence. Pain is the hallmark of spinal metastasis. Patients with sensory root involvement or vertebral collapse may suffer excruciating pain.

The bed is usually kept flat. The patient is turned as a unit, keeping shoulders and hips aligned. The back is kept straight. The side-lying positon is usually the most comfortable because it avoids pressure on the wound. A pillow is placed between the knees of the patient in a side-lying position, and extreme knee flexion is avoided.

Staining of the dressing may indicate leakage of cerebrospinal fluid. Any CSF leakage from the area of operation may lead to disastrous infection or to an inflammatory reaction in the surrounding tissues that can cause severe pain in the postoperative period.

Patient Education

Patients with residual sensory involvement are cautioned about the dangers of extremes in temperature. They should be alert to the dangers of heating devices (*e.g.*, space heaters, fireplaces). The patient is taught to check skin integrity daily.

A patient who has impaired motor function related to motor weakness or paralysis may require training in activities of daily living and an ambulatory aid such as a cane or walker.

Herniation or Rupture of an Intervertebral Disc

The intervertebral disc is a cartilaginous plate that forms a cushion between the vertebral bodies. This tough, gristlelike material is incorporated in a capsule. A ball-like condensation in the disc is called the *nucleus pulposus*. In herniation of the intervertebral disc (ruptured disc), the nucleus of the disc protrudes into the annulus (the fibrous ring around the disc), with subsequent nerve compression. Protrusion or rupture of the nucleus pulposus is usually preceded by degenerative changes that occur with aging. Loss of protein polysaccharides in the disc decreases the water content of the nucleus pulposus. The development of radiating cracks in the annulus weakens resistance to nucleus herniation. Following trauma (falls, accidents, and repeated minor stresses, such as lifting), the cartilage may be injured.

In most patients, the immediate symptoms of trauma are short-lived, and those resulting from injury to the disc do not appear for months or years. Then, with degeneration in the disc, the capsule pushes back into the spinal canal, or it may rupture and allow the nucleus pulposus to be pushed back against the dural sac or against a spinal nerve as it emerges from the spinal column (Fig. 54-11). This sequence produces pain due to pressure in the area of distribution of the involved nerve endings. Continued pressure may produce degenerative

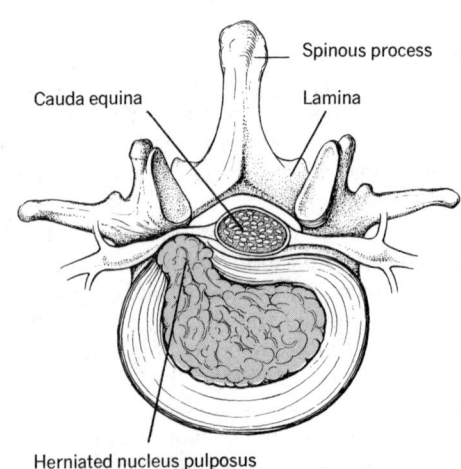

Figure 54-11
Ruptured vertebral disc. (Chaffee EE and Greisheimer EM. Basic Physiology and Anatomy, 3rd ed. Philadelphia, JB Lippincott.)

changes in the involved nerve, such as changes in sensation and reflex action.

Clinical Manifestations. A herniated disc with accompanying pain may occur in any portion of the spine: cervical, thoracic (rare), or lumbar. The clinical manifestations depend on the location, the rate of development (acute or chronic), and the effect on the surrounding structures.

Diagnostic Evaluation. A myelogram usually demonstrates the area of pressure and localizes the herniation of the disc. Computed tomography scans may identify small disc protrusions. Magnetic resonance imaging is complementary to CT scans. A neurologic examination is carried out to determine if there is reflex, sensory, or motor impairment from root compression. Electromyography may be used to localize the specific spinal nerve roots involved.

Management. Herniations of the cervical and the lumbar discs occur most commonly and these are usually managed conservatively. The specific conservative management and surgical interventions for each form of herniation will be discussed in detail.

Disc Surgery. In general, surgical excision of a herniated disc is done when there is evidence of a progressing neurologic deficit (muscle weakness and atrophy, loss of sensory and motor function, loss of sphincter control) and continuing pain and sciatica that are unresponsive to conservative management. The goal of surgical treatment is to relieve pressure on the nerve root in order to relieve pain. Microsurgical techniques are making possible the precise removal through a small incision of only that amount of tissue that is absolutely necessary. This approach better preserves the integrity of normal tissue and imposes less trauma on the body. During these procedures, spinal cord function can be monitored electrophysiologically.

To achieve the goal of pain relief, several operative techniques are employed, depending on the type of disc herniation, operative morbidity, and overall results of surgery:

- *Discectomy*—removal of herniated or extruded fragments of intervertebral disc
- *Laminectomy*—removal of the lamina to expose the neural elements in the spinal canal; allows the surgeon to inspect the spinal canal, identify and remove pathology, and relieve compression of the cord and roots.
- *Laminotomy*—division of the lamina of a vertebra
- *Discectomy with fusion*—a bone graft (from iliac crest/bone bank) is used to fuse the vertebral spinous process; the object of spinal fusion is to bridge over the defective disc in order to stabilize the spine and reduce the rate of recurrence.

Surgeries for herniated cervical disc and lumbar disc are discussed in detail in the sections that follow.

Herniation or Rupture of a Cervical Intervertebral Disc

The cervical spine is subjected to stresses that result from disc degeneration (from aging, occupational stresses) and *spondylosis* (degenerative changes occurring in disc and adjacent vertebral bodies). Cervical disc degeneration may lead to lesions that can cause damage to the spinal cord and its roots.

A cervical disc herniation usually occurs at the C5–C6 and C6–C7 interspaces. Pain and stiffness may occur in the neck, the top of the shoulders, and the region of the scapulae. Sometimes patients interpret these signs as symptoms of heart trouble or bursitis. Pain may also occur in the upper extremities and head, accompanied by paresthesia and numbness of the upper extremities. The diagnosis is usually confirmed by cervical myelography.

Management

The goals of treatment are (1) to rest and immobilize the cervical spine to give the soft tissues time to heal, and (2) to reduce inflammation in the supporting tissues and the affected nerve roots in the cervical spine. Bed rest (usually 2 weeks) is important, since it eliminates the stress of gravity and frees the cervical spine from having to support the weight of the head. It also reduces inflammation and edema in soft tissues around the disc, relieving pressure on the nerve roots. Proper positioning on a firm mattress may bring dramatic relief from pain.

The cervical spine may be rested and immobilized by a cervical collar, cervical traction, or a brace. A collar allows maximal opening of the intervertebral foramina and holds the head in a neutral or slightly flexed position. The patient may have to wear the collar 24 hours a day during the acute phase. The skin site under the collar is inspected for irritation. When the patient is free of pain, cervical isometric exercises are started to strengthen the muscles in the neck.

Cervical traction is accomplished by means of a head halter attached to a pulley and weight. It increases vertebral separation and thus relieves pressure on the nerve roots. The head of the bed is elevated to provide countertraction. If the skin becomes irritated, the halter can be padded. Experience has shown that a male patient may suffer more skin irritation if he shaves; the beard offers a natural form of padding.

Hot, moist compresses (for 10–20 minutes) applied to the back of the neck several times daily will increase blood flow to the muscles and help to relax the spastic muscles, as well as the patient. Analgesics are given during the acute phase to relieve pain, and sedatives may be administered to control the anxiety often associated with cervical disc disease. Muscle relaxants are administered to interrupt the cycle of muscle spasm and to allow for patient comfort. Anti-inflammatory drugs (aspirin, phenylbutazone [Butazolidin], oxyphenbutazone [Tandearil]) or steroids are given to treat the inflammatory response that usually occurs in the supporting tissues and affected nerve roots. Occasionally, an injection of a corticosteroid drug into the epidural space may be tried as a means of relieving radicular pain. Food and antacids are given with anti-inflammatory agents to prevent gastrointestinal irritation. Periodic blood evaluations should be carried out to detect the development of blood dyscrasias because hematologic toxicity to phenylbutazone can occur.

Surgical Management

Surgical excision of the herniated disc may be necessary when there is a significant neurologic deficit, progression of a neurologic deficit, evidence of cord compression, or pain that either fails to improve or worsens. A cervical discectomy, with or without fusion, may be done to alleviate symptoms.

In the cervical area, an anterior approach may be used through a transverse incision in the neck to remove disc material that has herniated into the spinal canal and foramina, or a posterior approach may be used at the desired level of the cervical spine.

Potential Postoperative Complications

Potential complications for the anterior approach include carotid or vertebral artery injury, recurrent laryngeal nerve dysfunction, esophageal perforation, and airway obstruction. Complications of the posterior approach include damage to the nerve root or to the spinal cord due to retraction or contusion of either of these structures, resulting in weakness of muscles supplied by the nerve root or cord.

▶ Nursing Process
The Patient Undergoing a Cervical Discectomy

▷ Assessment

The patient is asked about past injuries to the neck (whiplash) because unresolved trauma may cause persistent discomfort, pain, and tenderness and the development of arthritis in the injured joint of the cervical spine. Assessment of the patient's problems includes determining the onset, location, and radiation of pain, paresthesias, limited movement, and diminished function of the neck, shoulders, and upper extremities. Determine whether or not the symptoms are bilateral because, with large herniations, bilateral symptoms may be due to cord compression. Examination of the area around the cervical spine includes palpation to assess muscle tone and tenderness.

Range of motion in the neck and shoulders is evaluated. The patient is also queried about any health problems that may influence the postoperative course. The nurse determines the patient's need for information about the operative procedure and reinforces what has been explained by the physician. Strategies that have been used in the past for pain management are elicited.

Postoperative Assessment. Assessment includes monitoring the blood pressure and pulse for evaluation of the cardiovascular status. The patient is evaluated for bleeding that is manifested by the complaint of excessive pressure in the neck or severe pain in the incisional area. The dressing is inspected for serosanguineous drainage, which suggests a dural leak. In this event, meningitis is a threat. A complaint of headache requires careful evaluation. Neurologic checks are made for upper and lower extremity weakness because cord compression may produce rapid or delayed onset of paralysis. Throughout the postoperative course, the vital signs are monitored frequently to detect any signs of respiratory difficulty. Occasionally, during surgery, the recurrent laryngeal nerve may be injured by retractors, resulting in hoarseness and inability to cough effectively. The elimination of pulmonary secretions then becomes a problem requiring chest physical therapy. One sign to watch for following an anterior cervical discectomy is a sudden return of radicular (spinal nerve root) pain, which may indicate that the spine has become unstable.

▷ Nursing Diagnoses

Based on all the assessment data, the patient's major nursing diagnoses may include the following:

- Alteration in comfort—pain related to the surgical procedure
- Alteration in mobility related to postoperative surgical regimen
- Deficit in knowledge about the postoperative course and home care management

Other nursing diagnoses (which may be encountered in any surgical patient) may include preoperative anxiety and a number of postoperative concerns, as follows: alteration in bowel elimination related to the procedure; urinary retention related to dehydration and the operative procedure; self-care deficits related to neck orthosis; and sleep pattern disturbance related to disruption in life-style.

▷ Planning and Implementation

▷ *Goals:* The goals of the patient may include achievement of comfort, attainment of improved mobility, and increased knowledge and self-care ability

Nursing Interventions

Pain Relief. The patient may be kept flat in bed for 12 to 24 hours. If the patient has had a bone fusion in which bone has been removed from the iliac crest, considerable pain may be experienced. Nursing interventions consist of monitoring the donor site for hematoma formation, giving the prescribed postoperative analgesic according to the patient's needs, positioning for comfort, and reassuring the patient that the pain can be controlled. If the patient experiences a sudden reappearance of radicular pain, extrusion of the graft may have occurred, a situation requiring reoperation and surgical repositioning of the graft.

Usually the major complaint of the patient is a sore throat, hoarseness, or dysphagia that may be related to temporary edema. These complaints may be relieved by throat lozenges, voice rest, and room humidification. A blenderized soft diet may be given if the patient is experiencing some dysphagia.

Improving Mobility. A cervical *neck orthosis* (neck collar) is usually worn following the procedure, which contributes to limited neck motion and altered mobility. Patients are taught to turn the body instead of the neck when looking from side to side. The neck should be kept in a neutral (midline) position. Patients are assisted during positional changes, making sure that head, shoulders, and thorax are aligned during turning. When assisting a patient to a sitting position, the nurse provides support behind the neck and shoulders. Patients should wear shoes when ambulating to increase stability.

Patient Education and Home Health Care. The neck orthosis is usually worn for about 6 weeks. Patients are cautioned against flexing, extending, or rotating the neck in any extreme manner while stretching, exercising, or working. While sleeping, the prone position should be avoided. The head is to be kept in a neutral position. Patients should be cautioned not to prop themselves up in bed with several pillows, because this produces unwanted neck flexion.

Patients are advised to monitor themselves for signs and symptoms of infection: fever, wound drainage, or increased pain. If any of these appear, medical attention should be sought.

Sitting or standing for more than 30 minutes can induce considerable neck strain. Advise patients to alternate tasks in which the body does not move (*e.g.*, reading) with tasks that require greater body movement. Long automobile rides should generally be avoided, because vibration associated with such trips has an adverse effect on the spine. Patients are instructed to report for reevaluation at prescribed intervals to document the disappearance of old symptoms and for examination of range of motion of the neck.

▷ *Evaluation*

▷ *Expected Outcomes*

1. Patient achieves increasing comfort.
   a. Is able to get out of bed
   b. States that pain is lessening
2. Attains improved mobility
   a. Walks in hallway
   b. Turns body when looking in a lateral direction
3. Acquires knowledge for self-care
   a. Asks questions; gives positive feedback
   b. Knows the signs and symptoms that are reportable

Herniated Lumbar Disc

The majority of lumbar disc herniations occur at the L4–L5 or the L5–S1 interspaces. A lumbar disc produces low back pain accompanied by varying degrees of sensory and motor impairment. The patient complains of low back pain with muscle spasms, which is followed by radiation of the pain into one hip and down into the leg (*sciatica*). Pain is aggravated by actions that increase intraspinal fluid pressure (bending, lifting, straining, as in sneezing and coughing) and is usually relieved by bed rest. There is usually some type of postural deformity, since pain causes an alteration of the normal spinal mechanics. If the patient lies on the back and attempts to raise a leg in a straight position, pain will radiate into the leg because this maneuver (*straight-leg raising test*) stretches the sciatic nerve. Additional signs include muscle weakness, alterations in tendon reflexes, and sensory loss.

Diagnostic Evaluation

The diagnosis of lumbar disc disease is based on the history and physical findings and the use of imaging techniques, myelography, and/or CT scanning. Dynamic studies, such as lateral bending and flexion–extension of the spine, are used to enhance the value of the myelogram.

Management

The objectives of treatment are to relieve the pain and slow the progression of the disease and to increase the functional ability of the patient. Bed rest on a firm mattress (to limit spinal flexion) is encouraged to reduce the weight load and gravitational forces, thereby freeing the disc from stress. The patient is allowed to assume a comfortable position; usually,

a semi-Fowler's position with moderate hip and knee flexion to relax the back muscles is most satisfactory. While in the side-lying position, a pillow is placed between the legs. To get out of bed, the patient lies on his side while pushing up to a sitting position.

Since muscle spasm is prominent during the acute phase, muscle relaxants are used. Anti-inflammatory drugs and systemic steroids may be administered to counter the inflammation that usually occurs in the supporting tissues and the affected nerve roots. Moist heat and massage help to relax spastic muscles and produce a sedating effect on the patient. See also Nursing Process: The Patient With Low Back Pain, Chapter 58, for nursing interventions.

Chemonucleolysis. Chemonucleolysis (nonoperative chemical removal of displaced lumbar disc material) is a method of treating a protruding lumbar disc accompanied by root irritation. The procedure consists of injecting chymopapain (Discase) into the diseased disc. Chymopapain is an enzyme derived from the papaya plant; it has a proteolytic action that dissolves all or part of the nucleus pulposus, reducing the pressure of the adjacent nerve roots and thus alleviating pain.

Chemonucleolysis is used for patients with low back pain and sciatica who have not responded to conservative measures. It is not considered an alternative to surgical removal of a free disc fragment, nor is it used in situations in which there is progressive neurologic deficit with paralysis and impaired bowel and urinary function.

Chymopapain may induce an immediate systemic reaction (anaphylaxis), and the health care team should anticipate the event by being on the alert for such a reaction, detecting it immediately, and having appropriate equipment available (epinephrine, intravenous fluids, endotracheal tubes).

If there are no complications and the neurologic examination reveals no abnormal findings, the patient is allowed to go home as soon as it is possible to walk without difficulty and void spontaneously. Back pain that occurs as a result of the injection is alleviated with oral analgesics.

Surgical Management

In the lumbar region, surgical treatment includes lumbar disc excision through a posterolateral laminotomy and the newer techniques of microdiscectomy and percutaneous discectomy.

Microdiscectomy incorporates the use of the operating microscope to visualize the offending disc and compressed nerve roots; it permits a smaller incision (2.5 cm [1 inch]) and minimal blood loss, and takes about 30 minutes of operating time. Generally it involves a shorter hospital stay, and the patient makes a more rapid recovery.

Percutaneous discectomy is an alternative treatment for herniated intervertebral discs of the lumbar spine at the L4–L5 level. One approach in current use is through a 2.5-cm (1-inch) incision just above the iliac crest. A tube, trocar, or cannula is inserted under x-ray guidance through the retroperitoneal space to the involved disc space. Specially-lengthened instruments are used to remove the disc. The operating time is approximately 15 minutes. Blood loss and postoperative pain are minimal, and the patient is generally discharged within 2 days after surgery.

The disadvantage of this procedure involves the possibility of damage to structures located in the surgical pathway.

Preoperative Nursing Management

Most patients fear surgery on any part of the spine, and therefore need assurance (that surgery will not "weaken" the back) and explanations all along the way. When data are being collected for the nursing history, any complaints of pain, paresthesia, and muscle spasm are recorded in order to have a baseline for comparison after surgery. Preoperative assessment should also include an evaluation of movement in the extremities as well as bladder and bowel function. To facilitate the postoperative turning procedure, the patient is taught to turn as a unit (logrolling), as part of the preoperative preparation. Other facets of the postoperative regimen that should be practiced before the operation are deep-breathing, coughing, and muscle-setting exercises, which will help maintain muscle tone.

Postoperative Nursing Management

Following lumbar disc excision, the vital signs are checked frequently and the wound is inspected for evidence of hemorrhage, because vascular injury is a complication of disc surgery. Since postoperative neurologic deficits may occur from nerve root injury, the sensation and motor power of the lower extremities are evaluated at specified intervals, along with the color and temperature of the legs and sensation of the toes. Another important sign to check for is possible urinary retention.

Most patients walk to the bathroom the same day (the day of surgery), and all but a few are home by the second postoperative day. They are instructed in how to turn in bed (see below) and taught an exercise routine. Sitting is discouraged except for defecation.

To position the patient, a pillow is placed under the head, and the knee rest is elevated slightly, since slight knee flexion relaxes the muscles of the back. When the patient is lying on one side, however, extreme knee flexion must be avoided. The patient is encouraged to move from side to side to relieve pressure, but is first reassured that no injury will result from moving. When the patient is ready to turn, the bed is placed in a flat position and a pillow is placed between the legs. Turning is done with the body as a unit (logrolling), without twisting the back.

To get out of bed, the patient lies on one side while pushing up to a sitting position. At the same time, a second person eases the patient's legs over the side of the bed. Coming to a sitting or standing posture is accomplished by one long, smooth motion.

In cases requiring discectomy with fusion, the patient will have an additional wound if bone fragments are taken from the iliac crest or fibula to serve as wedges in the spine. The recovery period is somewhat slower than those patients who have undergone removal of the ruptured portion of the disc without a spinal fusion, because bony union must take place.

Complications of Disc Surgery

A person having a disc procedure at one level may have degenerative process at other levels of the vertebral column. A herniation relapse may occur at the same level or elsewhere, so that the patient is apt to become a candidate for another disc procedure. *Arachnoiditis,* (inflammation of the arachnoid membrane) may occur after operation (and after myelography); it involves an insidious onset of diffuse, frequently burning pain in the lower back, radiating into the buttocks. Disc excision can leave adhesions and scarring around the spinal nerves and dura, which then produce inflammatory changes that can create chronic neuritis and neurofibrosis. Disc surgery may relieve pressure on the spinal nerves, but it does not reverse the effects of neural injury and scarring and the pain that ensues.

Failed disc syndrome (recurrence of sciatica after lumbar discectomy) remains a common cause of disability.

Patient Education and Home Health Care

The patient is advised that, since it takes up to 6 weeks for the ligaments of the muscles to heal, activity is to be gradually increased up to the point of tolerance. Excessive activity may result in spasm of the paraspinal muscles.

Activities that produce flexion strain on the spine (*e.g.,* driving a car) should be avoided until healing has taken place. Heat may be applied to the back to soothe and relax muscle spasm and help absorb exudates in the tissues. Scheduled rest periods are important. Usually, the patient is advised to avoid heavy work for 2 to 3 months after surgery. Exercises are prescribed to strengthen the abdominal and erector spinal muscles. A back brace or corset may be necessary if back pain persists. (See also patient education for low back pain, Chap. 58.)

Cranial Nerve Disorders

There are 12 pairs of cranial nerves that emerge from the lower surface of the brain and pass through the *foramina* (openings) in the skull. They are classified as motor, sensory, and mixed nerves. The cranial nerves are numbered in the order in which they arise from the brain. The names of the cranial nerves suggest their primary function or some anatomical characteristic. Most cranial nerves originate in the brain stem and innervate the head, neck and special organs.

The cranial nerves are examined separately and in sequence (see p. 1402). Some cranial nerve deficits can be detected by observing the patient's face, eye movements, speech, and swallowing. Electromyography is used to investigate motor and sensory dysfunction. Magnetic resonance imaging produces excellent images of the cranial nerves and brain stem.

Since the brain stem and cranial nerves control vital motor, sensory, or autonomic functions of the body, they may be involved in conditions arising primarily within these structures or in secondary extension from adjacent disease processess. The following discussions will center on trigeminal neuralgia, a condition affecting the fifth cranial nerve, and on Bell's palsy, caused by involvement of the seventh cranial nerve.

An overview of disorders that may affect each of the cranial nerves, including clinical manifestations and nursing interventions, is presented in Table 54-2 and the cranial nerves are illustrated in Figure 54-12.

TABLE 54-2
Disorders of Cranial Nerves

Disorder	Clinical Manifestations	Nursing Interventions
Olfactory Nerve I		
Head trauma Intracranial tumor Intracranial surgery	Unilateral or bilateral anosmia (temporary or persistent) Diminished taste for food	Assess for CSF rhinorrhea if patient has sustained head trauma.
Optic Nerve II		
Optic neuritis (MS) Increased intracranial pressure Pituitary tumor	Lesions of optic tract produce homonymous hemianopia.	Assess level of visual acuity. Restructure environment to prevent accidents. Teach patient to accommodate for visual loss.
Oculomotor Nerve III *Trochlear Nerve IV* *Abducens Nerve VI*		

Vascular
  Brain stem ischemia
  Hemorrhage/infarct
Neoplasm
Trauma
Infection
	Dilation of pupil with loss of light reflex
	  on one side
	Impairment of ocular movement
	Diplopia
	Gaze palsies
	Ptosis of eyelid
		Assess extraocular movement and for
		  nonreactive pupil.

Trigeminal Nerve V		

Trigeminal neuralgia
Head trauma
Cerebellopontine lesion
Sinus tract tumor/metastatic disease
Compression of trigeminal root by tumor
	Pain in face
	Facial membrane
	Diminished/loss of corneal reflex
	Chewing dysfunction
		Assess for pain and triggering mechanisms for
		  pain.
		Assess for difficulty in chewing.
		Discuss trigger zones and pain precipitants
		  with patient.
		Ensure good oral hygiene.
		Educate patient about medication regimen.

Facial Nerve VII		

Bell's palsy
Facial nerve tumor
Intracranial lesion
Herpes zoster
	Facial dysfunction; weakness and
	  paralysis
	Hemifacial spasm
	Diminished/absent taste
		Recognize facial paralysis as emergency; refer
		  for treatment as soon as possible.
		Teach protective care for eyes.
		Select easily chewed foods; patient should eat
		  and drink from unaffected side of mouth.
		Emphasize importance of oral hygiene.
		Provide emotional support for changed
		  appearance of face.

Vestibulocochlear Nerve VIII		

Tumors/acoustic neuroma
Vascular compression of nerve
Meniere's syndrome
	Tinnitus
	Vertigo
	Hearing difficulties
		Assess pattern of vertigo.
		Provide for safety measures to prevent falls.
		  Patient should obtain balance before
		    ambulating.
		  Caution patient to change positions slowly.
		  Assist with ambulation.
		  Encourage use of ADL aids.

Glossopharyngeal Nerve IX		

Glossopharyngeal neuralgia from
  neurovascular compression of IXth
  and Xth nerves
	Pain at base of tongue
	Difficulty in swallowing
	Loss of gag reflex
		Assess for paroxysmal pain in throat,
		  decreased or absent swallowing, gag and
		  cough reflexes.

(continued)

TABLE 54-2 (continued)

Disorder	Clinical Manifestations	Nursing Interventions
Glossopharyngeal Nerve IX		
Trauma Inflammatory conditions Tumor Vertebral artery aneurysms	Palatal, pharyngeal, and laryngeal paralysis	Monitor for dysphagia, aspiration, nasal dysarthric speech. Position patient upright for eating or tube feeding.
Vagus Nerve X		
Spastic palsy of larynx; bulbar paralysis; high vagal paralysis Guillain-Barré syndrome Carotid endarterectomy Vagal body tumors Nerve paralysis from malignancy, surgical trauma	Voice changes (temporary or permanent hoarseness) Vocal paralysis Dysphagia	Assess for airway obstruction/provide airway management. Prevent aspiration. Support patient having voice reconstruction procedures.
Spinal Accessory Nerve XI		
Spinal cord disorder Amyotrophic lateral sclerosis Trauma Guillain-Barré syndrome	Drooping of affected shoulder with limited shoulder movement Weakness/paralysis of head rotation, flexion, extension; shoulder elevation	Support patient undergoing diagnostic tests.
Hypoglossal Nerve XII		
Medullary lesions Amyotrophic lateral sclerosis Polio and motor system disease may destroy hypoglossal nuclei. Multiple sclerosis Trauma	Abnormal movements of tongue Weakness/paralysis of tongue muscles Difficulty in talking, chewing, and swallowing	Observe swallowing ability. Observe speech pattern. Be aware of attendant swallowing/vocal difficulties. Prepare for alternate feeding methods (tube feeding) to maintain nutrition.

Trigeminal Neuralgia (Tic Douloureux)

Trigeminal neuralgia is a condition of the fifth cranial nerve characterized by an explosive onset of pain similar to an electric shock or a lancinating burning sensation in the area distributed by one or more branches of the trigeminal nerve. The pain ends as abruptly as it starts. Each pain episode can be described as stabbing and explosive and produces contraction of some of the facial muscles, such as a sudden closing of the eye or a twitch of the mouth; hence the name *tic douloureux* (painful twitch). The etiology is not certain, but chronic compression or irritation of the trigeminal nerve or degenerative changes in the Gasserian ganglion are suggested causes. Some investigators believe that the condition may be due to vascular pressure from structural abnormalities (loop of an artery) encroaching upon the trigeminal nerve, Gasserian ganglion, or root entry zone.

Early attacks, appearing most often in the fifth decade of life, are usually mild and brief. Pain-free intervals may be measured in terms of minutes, hours, days, or longer. With advancing years, the painful episodes tend to become more and more frequent and agonizing. The patient lives in constant fear of attacks.

The pain of this neuralgia is felt in the skin, not in the deeper structures, but it is more severe at the peripheral areas of distribution of the affected nerve, notably over the lip, the chin, the nostrils, and in the teeth. Paroxysms are aroused by any stimulation of the terminals of the affected nerve branches, such as washing the face, shaving, brushing the teeth, eating, and drinking. A draft of cold air and direct pressure against the nerve trunk may also cause pain. Certain areas are called *trigger points*, since the slightest touch immediately starts a paroxysm. To avoid stimulating these areas, patients with trigeminal neuralgia try not to touch or wash their faces, shave, chew, or do anything else that might cause an attack. Behavior of this type is a clue to diagnosis.

Management

The antiepileptic drugs carbamazepine (Tegretol) and phenytoin (Dilantin), by reducing the transmission of impulses at certain nerve terminals, will relieve pain in most patients. Carbamzepine is taken with meals, in dosages gradually increased until relief is obtained. Side-effects include nausea, dizziness, drowsiness, and hepatic dysfunction. The patient's blood is monitored for bone marrow depression. Phenytoin also produces such side-effects as nausea, dizziness, somnolence, ataxia, and skin allergies.

When medication fails to provide pain relief, a number of surgical options are available, as described in the following paragraphs. Patients should participate in choosing the procedure that best suits their health status.

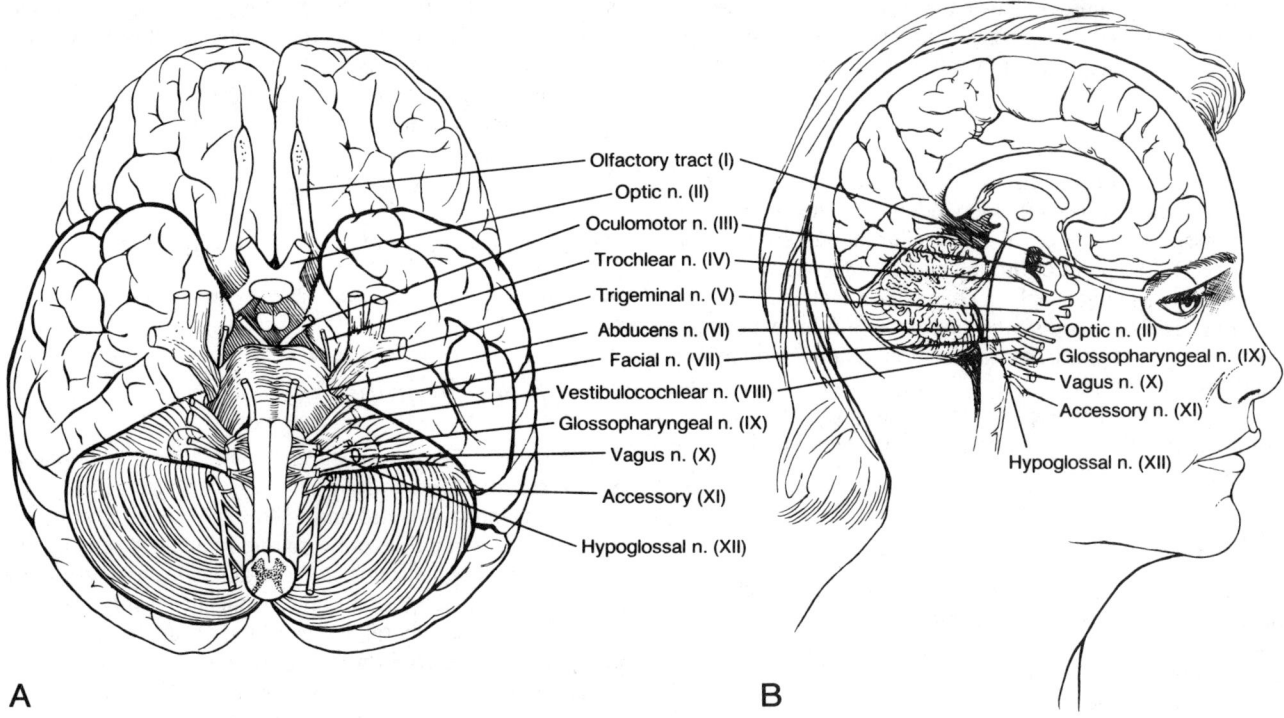

Figure 54-12
The cranial nerves. (*A*) Inferior view of the brain showing the cranial nerves. (*B*) Lateral view of the brain showing a schematized version of the cranial nerves.

Alcohol injection of the Gasserian ganglion and peripheral branches of the trigeminal nerve will relieve pain for several months. However, the pain returns after the nerve regenerates.

Percutaneous Radiofrequency Trigeminal Gangliolysis. Percutaneous radiofrequency interruption of the Gasserian ganglion, whereby the small unmyelinated and thinly-myelinated fibers that conduct the pain are thermally destroyed, is becoming the surgical procedure of choice for trigeminal neuralgia.

Under local anesthesia, the needle is introduced through the cheek on the affected side. Under fluoroscopic control, the needle electrode is guided through the foramen ovale into the Gasserian ganglion. The division of the Gasserian ganglion (mandibular, maxillary, and ophthalmic) are encountered sequentially. The nerve is stimulated with a small current, while the patient is awake. The patient then reports when a tingling sensation is felt. When the electrode needle is in the desired position, the patient is anesthetized briefly and a radiofrequency current (heating current to destroy the nerve) is passed in a controlled manner to thermally injure the trigeminal ganglion and rootlets. The patient is then awakened from the anesthetic and examined for sensory deficits. Repeat lesions may be produced until the desired effect is achieved. The operative procedure takes less than 1 hour and gives permanent pain relief in most patients. Touch and proprioceptive functions are left intact.

Microvascular Decompression of the Trigeminal Nerve. An intracranial approach can be used to decompress the trigeminal nerve, since tic douloureux may be caused by vascular compression of the entry zone of the trigeminal root by an arterial loop and occasionally by a vein. With the aid of an operating microscope, the artery loop is lifted from the nerve in order to relieve the pressure, and a small prosthetic device is inserted to prevent recurrence of impingement on the nerve. This procedure relieves facial pain while preserving normal sensation. It is a major procedure, involving a craniotomy. The postoperative management is the same as for any intracranial operation (see p. 1453).

Nursing Interventions

Preoperative management of a patient with trigeminal neuralgia includes recognizing that certain factors may aggravate excruciating facial pain, such as food that is too hot or too cold or jarring the bed. Even washing the face, combing the hair, or brushing the teeth may produce acute bouts of pain. The nurse can lessen these discomforts in a variety of ways— by using cotton pads and room-temperature water to wash the patient's face, instructing the patient to rinse the mouth after eating when tooth brushing causes pain, and doing personal hygiene during pain-free intervals. The patient is advised to take food and fluids at room temperature, chew on the unaffected side, and ingest soft foods when maintenance of nutrition is a problem. The nurse is aware that anxiety, depression, and insomnia often accompany chronic painful conditions and uses appropriate interventions and referrals.

Bell's Palsy

Bell's palsy (facial paralysis) is due to peripheral involvement of the seventh cranial nerve on one side, which results in weakness or paralysis of the facial muscles. The etiology is unknown, although possible causes may include vascular ischemia, viral disease (herpes simplex, herpes zoster), autoimmune disease, or a combination of all of these factors.

Pathophysiology

Bell's palsy is considered by some to represent a type of pressure paralysis. The inflamed, edematous nerve becomes compressed to the point of damage, or its nutrient vessel is occluded to the point of producing ischemia necrosis of the nerve within its long canal—a channel in which the fit at best is very snug. There is distortion of the face from paralysis of the facial muscles; increased lacrimation (tearing); and painful sensations in the face, behind the ear, and in the eye. The patient may experience speech difficulties and may be unable to eat on the affected side because of relaxation of the facial muscle.

Management

The objectives of treatment are to maintain the muscle tone of the face and to prevent or minimize denervation. The patient should be reassured that no stroke has occurred and that spontaneous recovery occurs within 3 to 5 weeks in the majority of patients.

Steroid therapy (prednisone) may be given to reduce inflammation and edema, which in turn reduces vascular compression and permits restoration of blood circulation to the nerve. Early administration of the drug appears to diminish the severity of the disease, relieve the pain, and help prevent or minimize denervation.

Face pain is controlled with analgesics. Heat may be applied to the involved side of the face to promote comfort and the flow of blood through the muscles.

Electrical stimulation may be applied to the face to prevent atrophy of the muscles. Although most patients recover with conservative treatment, surgical exploration of the facial nerve may be undertaken in patients who are suspected of having a tumor or for surgical decompression of the facial nerve and for surgical rehabilitation of a paralyzed face.

Patient Education and Home Health Care

While the paralysis lasts, the involved eye must be protected. Frequently, the patient's eye does not close completely, and the blink reflex is diminished so that the eye is vulnerable to dust and foreign particles. Corneal irritation and ulceration are a major threat to this patient. Sometimes there is an overflow of tears down the cheek (*epiphora*) from keratitis caused by drying of the cornea and absence of the blink reflex. The laxity of the lower lid alters the proper drainage of tears. To counter these problems, the eye should be covered with a protective shield at night. However, the eye patch may abrade the cornea, since there is some difficulty in keeping the partially-paralyzed eyelids closed. The application of eye ointment at bedtime will cause the eyelids to adhere to one another and remain closed during sleep. The patient can be taught to close the paralyzed eyelid manually before going to sleep. Wrap-around sunglasses or goggles are worn to decrease normal evaporation from the eye.

If the nerve is not too sensitive, the face may be massaged several times daily to maintain muscle tone. The technique

is to massage the face with a gentle upward motion. Facial exercises, such as wrinkling the forehead, blowing out the cheeks, and whistling, may be performed with the aid of a mirror and are intended to prevent muscle atrophy. The face should be kept warm.

Disorders of the Peripheral Nervous System

Peripheral Neuropathies

A peripheral neuropathy is a disorder affecting the peripheral motor, sensory, or autonomic nerves. Peripheral nerves, by connecting the spinal cord and brain to all other body organs, transmit motor impulses outward and relay back sensory impulses to encode sensation in the brain. A *mononeuropathy* affects a single peripheral nerve, while the involvement of multiple single peripheral nerves or their branches is termed *multiple mononeuropathy* or *mononeuritis multiplex. Polyneuropathies* are characterized by bilaterally symmetrical disturbance of function, usually beginning in the feet and hands. (Most nutritional, metabolic, and toxic neuropathies take this form.)

The most common causes of peripheral neuropathy are diabetes, alcoholism, and occlusive vascular disease. Many bacterial and metabolic toxins and exogenous poisons also affect the structure and function of the peripheral nerves. Due to the growing use of chemicals in industry, agriculture, and medicine, the number of substances known to cause peripheral neuropathies is increasing. In the developing countries, leprosy is a major cause of severe nerve disease because *Mycobacterium leprae* invade the peripheral nervous system.

The major symptoms of peripheral nerve disorders are loss of sensation, muscle atrophy, weakness, diminished reflexes, pain, and paresthesia (tingling, prickling) of the extremities. The patient frequently describes some part of the extremity as "numb." Autonomic features include decreased or reduced sweating, orthostatic hypotension, nocturnal diarrhea, tachycardia, impotence, and atrophic skin and nail changes.

Peripheral nerve disorders are diagnosed by electromyography and the recording of the nerve and muscle responses evoked when electrical stimulation is applied to a nerve.

Mononeuropathy

Mononeuropathy is limited to a single peripheral nerve and its branches. It arises when the trunk of the nerve is compressed or entrapped (as by carpal tunnel syndrome, Chap. 58); traumatized, as when bruised by a blow, or overstretched, as in cases of dislocation of a joint; punctured by a needle used to inject a drug, or damaged by the drugs thus injected; or inflamed because an adjacent infectious process extends to the nerve's trunk. Mononeuropathy is frequently seen in the patient with diabetes.

Pain is seldom a conspicuous symptom of mononeuropathy due to trauma, but in patients with complicating inflammatory conditions, such as arthritis, this feature is prominent. Such pain is increased by all body movements that tend to stretch, strain, or cause pressure on the injured nerve, and by all sudden jarrings of the body, such as those incident to coughing and sneezing. The skin in the areas supplied by nerves that are injured or diseased may become reddened and glossy; its subcutaneous tissue may become edematous, and the nutrition of the nails and the hair in this area defective. Chemical injuries to a nerve trunk, such as those caused by drugs injected into or near it, often are permanent.

Management. The objective of treatment of mononeuropathy is to remove the cause if possible, such as by freeing the compressed nerve. Local steroid injections may lessen inflammation, resulting in less pressure on the nerve. Pain may be relieved by aspirin or codeine.

Causalgia

Causalgia (Greek word for heat and pain) refers to the group of symptoms and signs that follow peripheral nerve injuries. The nerves most often affected, in order of frequency, are the median, the ulnar, the radial, and the internal and external popliteals.

The chief symptom of causalgia is severe burning pain along the course of the injured nerve. The pain may be described as "hot," "burning," "stabbing," or "crushing." This is more or less persistent, but becomes severe following such physical stimuli as the contact of clothes. The skin over the affected extremity becomes hot, shiny, and, at times, swollen; it shows abnormalities in sweating, and eventually undergoes atrophic changes involving the nails also. The patient holds the extremity quiet, since each movement tends to increase the pain.

Sympathetic nerve blocks, repair of local nerve lesions, and aggressive physical therapy are part of the treatment program. Experience with battle casualties revealed that active and passive exercises with very early mobilization appeared to reduce the incidence of causalgia following wounds of the extremities.

Guillain-Barré Syndrome (Polyradiculoneuritis)

Guillain-Barré syndrome is a clinical syndrome of unknown cause involving the peripheral and cranial nerves. In the majority of patients, the syndrome is preceded by an infection (respiratory or gastrointestinal), 1 to 4 weeks before the onset of neurologic deficits. In some instances, it has occurred following vaccination or surgery. It may be due to a primary viral infection, an immune reaction, some other process, or a combination of processes. One hypothesis is that a viral infection induces an autoimmune reaction that attacks the myelin of the peripheral nerves. (*Myelin* is a substance that surrounds or ensheaths the axons of certain nerves and plays an important role in the transmission of nerve impulses.)

Proximal portions of the nerves tend to be affected most often, and the nerve roots within the subarachnoid space are commonly involved. Autopsy findings have revealed inflammatory edema and demyelination with some lymphocytic infiltration that is especially prominent in the spinal nerve roots.

Clinical Manifestations

There is variation in the mode of onset. The initial neurologic symptoms are *paresthesia* (tingling and numbness) and muscle weakness of the legs, which may progress to the upper extremities, trunk, and facial muscles. Muscle weakness may be followed quickly by complete paralysis. The cranial nerves are frequently affected, leading to paralysis of the ocular, facial, and oropharyngeal muscles and thus causing marked difficulty in talking, chewing, and swallowing. Autonomic dysfunction frequently occurs and takes the form of overreactivity or underreactivity of the sympathetic or parasympathetic nervous systems, as manifested by disturbances of heart rate and rhythm, blood pressure changes (transient hypertension; orthostatic hypotension), and a variety of other vasomotor disturbances. There may be severe and persistent pain in the back and calves of the legs. Frequently the patient exhibits loss of position sense as well as diminished or absent tendon reflexes. Sensory changes are manifested by paresthesias.

The majority of patients make a full recovery over several months to a year, but about 10% are left with a residual disability.

Diagnostic Evaluation

The spinal fluid shows an increased protein concentration with a normal cell count. Electrophysiologic testing demonstrates marked slowing of nerve conduction velocity.

Management

Guillain-Barré syndrome is considered a medical emergency, and the patient is managed in an intensive care unit. A patient with respiratory problems will require mechanical ventilation, sometimes for prolonged periods. *Plasmapheresis* (plasma exchange), which produces a temporary reduction in circulating antibodies, may be used in the severely affected and deteriorating patient to limit the deterioration and demyelination. Continuous ECG monitoring may be required because of possible alteration in heartbeat. Cardiac dysrhythmias associated with autonomic abnormalities are treated with propranolol to prevent tachycardia and hypertension. Atropine may be administered to avoid episodes of bradycardia during endotracheal suctioning and physical therapy.

▶ Nursing Process
The Patient With Guillain-Barré Syndrome

▷ Assessment

Careful and continuing assessment of respiratory function is essential because respiratory insufficiency and failure due to weakness or paralysis of the intercostal and diaphragm muscles may develop *quickly*. In fact, this is the main threat to life. The patient's vital capacity is monitored around the clock to anticipate respiratory insufficiency. A decreasing vital capacity along with weakness of the muscles used in swallowing, which causes difficulty in coughing and swallowing, indicates deterioration of respiratory function. Signs to watch for are breathlessness while talking, shallow and irregular breathing, increasing pulse rate, use of accessory muscles while breathing, and any *change* in the respiratory pattern.

Because the diaphragm is the prime muscle of inspiration, observe for paradoxical inward movement of the upper abdominal wall while the patient is in a supine position. This is a sign of weakness and impending paralysis of the diaphragm.

Assessment for Complications. Assessment for complications of the patient with Guillain-Barré syndrome involves constant monitoring for the life-threatening problem of acute respiratory failure. Other complications include cardiac dysrhythmias, which necessitate ECG monitoring and observing the patient for signs of deep venous thrombosis and pulmonary embolism, ever-present threats to any immobilized and paralyzed patient.

▷ Nursing Diagnoses

Based on the assessment data, the patient's major diagnoses may include the following:

- Ineffective breathing pattern related to rapidly progressive weakness and impending respiratory failure
- Impaired physical mobility related to paralysis
- Alteration in nutrition, less than body requirements, related to inability to swallow which is secondary to cranial nerve dysfunction
- Impaired verbal communication related to cranial nerve dysfunction
- Fear related to loss of control and paralysis

▷ Planning and Implementation

▷ *Goals:* The major goals of the patient may include attainment of respiratory function and spontaneous breathing, achievement of mobility, accomplishment of normal nutrition, achievement of communication, and resolution of fear.

Nursing Interventions

Ensuring Respiratory Function. The patient with Guillain-Barré syndrome is absolutely dependent on nursing surveillance and care for recovery. Artificial ventilation will probably be required if serial measurements of the patient's vital capacity show progressive deterioration, indicating worsening of respiratory muscle power. A particularly dangerous situation occurs when the patient has difficulty in coughing and swallowing, which may cause aspiration of saliva and precipitate acute respiratory failure. The management of the patient requiring mechanical ventilation is a team effort and is discussed in Chapter 22. Chest physical therapy is usually indicated if crackles are heard upon auscultation.

Promoting Mobility. The paralyzed extremities are supported in functional positions and given passive range-of-motion exercises at least twice daily. The nurse works with the physical therapist to prevent contracture deformities by using careful positioning and range-of-motion exercises. Deep venous thrombosis and pulmonary embolism are threats to the paralyzed patient, who is unable to move his extremities.

Nursing interventions include ensuring adequate hydration, assisting with physical therapy, and administering the prescribed heparin regimen.

A paralyzed person has the potential to develop compression neuropathies, most often of the ulnar and peroneal nerves. Padding may be placed over the elbows and head of the fibula to prevent this problem. The prevention of pressure sores is a major nursing challenge. For severely paralyzed patients, the principles of nursing management of the unconscious patient (p. 1426) may be applied, although these patients are in full possession of their mental faculties.

When recovery begins to take place, these patients may experience orthostatic hypotension (from autonomic dysfunction) and will probably require the use of a tilt table to help them assume an upright posture.

Establishing Normal Nutrition. Attention is paid to adequate nutrition and prevention of muscle wasting. Paralytic ileus may result from insufficient parasympathetic activity. In this event, intravenous feedings are prescribed by the physician and monitored by the nurse until bowel sounds are heard. If the patient is unable to swallow, nasogastric tube feedings may be prescribed (see p. 759). When the patient can swallow normally, oral feeding is gradually resumed.

Improving Communication. Because of paralysis, tracheostomy, and intubation, the patient is unable to talk, laugh, or cry, and thus has no outlet for emotional expression. These problems are compounded by boredom, dependency, ioslation, and frustration. To establish some form of communication, lip reading and the use of picture cards, combined with a system of blinking the eyes to indicate "yes" or "no," may be tried. If the patient remains on the ventilator for a prolonged period, a referral to a speech-language pathologist may be made. Diversional therapy (television, cassette tapes, visits from the family) can alleviate some of the frustrations that are encountered.

Relieving Anxiety and Fear. Involving the family/friends with selected patient care activities, reading aloud, and the like will reduce the sense of isolation of patients. Nursing interventions that are helpful in increasing patients' sense of control (and hence reduction of fear) include giving them information about their condition, emphasizing a positive appraisal of their coping resources, involving them in relaxation exercises and distraction techniques, and giving positive feedback. The attitude and atmosphere created by the nurse, physical therapist, and occupational therapist are important. Giving high-level nursing care, explanations, and reassurance will help patients gain some control over their situation.

Patient Education. After discharge from the hospital, patients are encouraged to continue with the exercise program. A walker may be required for ambulation. Patients are cautioned about avoiding fatigue and overworking muscles. "Take one day at a time" is good advice when the patient feels overwhelmed with problems of fatigue. The Guillain-Barré support group offers emotional support and information booklets.

▷ Evaluation

▷ *Expected Outcomes*

1. Patient attains spontaneous breathing and normal respiratory function.

a. Has vital capacity within normal range

b. Has been weaned from mechanical ventilation

2. Shows increasing mobility

a. Is able to move all extremities

b. Is working on ambulation techniques

3. Demonstrates ability to swallow

a. Expresses desire for food

b. Is taking oral fluids and food

4. Demonstrates recovery of speech

a. Is talking without undue breathlessness

b. Can make wants known

5. Shows lessening fear

a. Patient is sleeping at longer intervals.

b. Appears more relaxed; does not appear anxious

Bibliography

Books

Adamovich BB, Henderson JA, and Auerbach S. Cognitive Rehabilitation of the Closed Head Injured Patient. San Diego, College Hill Press, 1985.

Aird RB, Masland RL, and Woodbury DM. The Epilepsies: A Critical Review. New York, Raven Press, 1984.

Albuquerque EX and Eldefrawi AT. Myasthenia Gravis. New York, Chapman & Hall, 1983.

Bailey RW et al. The Cervical Spine. Philadelphia, JB Lippincott, 1983.

Bannister Sir R. Brain's Clinical Neurology, 6th ed. New York, Oxford University Press, 1985.

Bedbrook GM. Lifetime Care of the Paraplegic Patient. New York, Churchill Livingstone, 1985.

Blumer D. Psychiatric Aspects of Epilepsy. Washington, DC, American Psychiatric Press, 1984.

Bromley I. Tetraplegia and Paraplegia. New York, Churchill Livingstone, 1985.

Brooks N. Closed Head Injury. New York, Oxford University Press, 1984.

Charness A. Stroke/Head Injury: A Guide to Function Outcomes in Physical Therapy Management. Rockville, Aspen Systems, 1986.

Cummings JL. Clinical Neuropsychiatry. New York, Grune & Stratton, 1985.

Duvoisin RC. Parkinson's Disease: A Guide for Patient and Family, 2nd ed. New York, Raven Press, 1984.

Edelstein BA and Couture ET. Behavioral Assessment and Rehabilitation of the Traumatically Brain-Damaged. New York, Plenum Press, 1984.

Graham J. Multiple Sclerosis: A Self-Help Guide to its Management. New York, Thorsons Publishers, 1984.

Hallpike JF et al. Multiple Sclerosis: Pathology, Diagnosis, and Management. London, Chapman & Hall, 1983.

Hanak M and Scott A. Spinal Cord Injury: An Illustrated Guide for Health Professionals. New York, Springer-Verlag, 1983.

Henning RJ and Jackson, DL. Handbook of Critical Care Neurology and Neurosurgery. New York, Praeger Scientific, 1985.

Hickey JV. The Clinical Practice of Neurological and Neurosurgical Nursing, 2nd ed. Philadelphia, JB Lippincott, 1986.

Hopkins A. Epilepsy: The Facts, 2nd ed. New York, Oxford University Press, 1984.

Katz RI. "Neurologic disease and sexual function." In Farber M. Human Sexuality: Psychosexual Effects of Disease, pp 264–273. New York, Macmillan, 1985.

Laidlaw MV and Laidlaw J. People with Epilepsy. New York, Churchill Livingstone, 1984.

Matthews B. Multiple Sclerosis: The Facts, 2nd ed. New York, Oxford University Press, 1985.

Oosterhuis HJGH. Myasthenia Gravis. New York, Churchill Livingstone, 1984.

Pallett PJ and O'Brien MT. Textbook of Neurological Nursing. Boston, Little, Brown & Co, 1985.

Pensis NT and Maloney MA. Mealtimes for People with Handicaps. Springfield, Illinois, Charles C Thomas, 1983.

Raimond J and Taylor JW. Neurological Emergencies: Effective Nursing Care. Rockville, Maryland, Aspen Systems, 1986.

Rose FC (ed). Research Progress in Motor Neuron Disease. London, Pitman, 1984.

Rudy EB. Advanced Neurological and Neurosurgical Nursing. St Louis, CV Mosby, 1984.

Schneider JW and Conrad P. Having Epilepsy: The Experience and Control of Illness. Philadelphia, Temple University Press, 1983.

Sengupta RP and McAllister VL. Subarachnoid Haemorrhage. New York, Springer-Verlag, 1986.

Simons AF (ed). Multiple Sclerosis: Psychological and Social Aspects. London, W Heinemann Medical Books, 1984.

Solomon GE, Kutt H, and Plum F. Clinical Management of Seizures, 2nd ed. Philadelphia, WB Saunders, 1983.

Sugarman GI. Epilepsy Handbook: A Guide to Understanding Seizure Disorders. St Louis, CV Mosby, 1984.

Swift-Bandini N. Manual of Neurological Nursing, 2nd ed. Boston, Little, Brown & Co, 1982.

Vogt G, Miller M, and Esluer M. Mosby's Manual of Neurological Care. St Louis, CV Mosby, 1985.

Walker MD (ed). Oncology of the Nervous System. Boston, Nijoff, 1983.

Woll NM (ed). Nursing Spinal Cord Injuries. Totowa, New Jersey, Rowman & Allanheld, 1984.

Zejdlik CP. Management of Spinal Cord Injury. Monterey, California, Wadsworth Health Sciences Division, 1983.

Articles

(Asterisks indicate nursing research articles.)

Amyotrophic Lateral Sclerosis

Azar I. The response of patients with neuromuscular disorders to muscle relaxants: A review. Anesthesiology 1984 Aug; 61(2):173–187.

Beebe WK and Gomez K. Amyotrophic lateral sclerosis. Home Healthc Nurse 1985 May/June; 3(3):8–17.

Campbell MJ and Enderby P. Management of motor neuron disease. J Neurol Sci 1984 Apr; 64(1):65–71.

Charles RA. Coping with life on a portable ventilator. Home Healthc Nurse 1984 Mar/Apr; 3(2):27–30.

Engel WK, Nicoloff JT, and Siddique T. Effect on weakness and spasticity in amyotrophic lateral sclerosis of thyrotropin-releasing hormone. Lancet 1983 July 9; 2(8341):73–75.

Festoff BW, Perurena OH, and Singer PA. "Untreatable" neuromuscular disease. J Kans Med Soc 1983 June; 84(6):312–316.

*Garyfallia L et al. Vying for a winning postion: Management style of the chronically ill. Res Nurs Health 1984; 7:181–188.

Ho L and Connors J. Amyotrophic lateral sclerosis. Can Nurse 1983 Mar; 79(3):35.

*Hoskins LM et al. Nursing diagnosis in the chronically ill: Methodology for clinical validation. ANS 1986 Apr; 8(3):80–89.

Rabin D. Practical tips for patients with A.L.S. Nursing '86 1986 Feb; 16(2):47–49.

Rabin PL. Credo for creeping paralysis. JAMA 1983 May 20; 249(19):2649–2650.

Rowland; LP. Looking for the cause of amyotrophic lateral sclerosis. N Engl J Med 1984 Oct 11; 311(15):979–981.

Slowie LA, Paige MS, and Antel JP. Nutritional considerations in the management of patients with amyotrophic lateral sclerosis. J Am Diet Assoc 1983 July; 83(1):44–47.

Splaingard ML et al. Home negative pressure ventilation: Report of 20 years experience in patients with neuromuscular disease. Arch Phys Med Rehabil 1985 Apr; 66(4):239–242.

Welnetz K. Maintaining adequate nutrition and hydration in the dysphagic ALS patient. Can Nurse 1983 Mar; 79(3):30–34.

Spinal Cord Injuries

Bedbrook G et al. Preventive measures in the tertiary care of spinal cord injured people. Paraplegia 1985 Apr; 23(2):69–77.

Bell JA and Hannon K. Pathophysiology involved in autonomic dysreflexia. J Neuroscience Nurs 1986 Apr; 18(2):86–88.

Collins WF. A review of treatment of spinal cord injury. Br J Surg 1984 Dec; 71(12):974–975.

Donovan WH and Dwyer AP. An update on the early management of traumatic paraplegia (Nonoperative and operative management). Clin Orthop 1984 Oct; 189:12–21.

Earnhardt JR and Frye BA. Understanding autonomic dysreflexia. Rehabil Nurs 1984 Mar/Apr; 9(2):28–30.

*Ferington FE. Personal control and coping effectiveness in spinal cord injured persons. Res Nurs Health 1986; 9:257–265.

Flamm ES et al. A phase I trial of naloxone treatment in acute spinal cord injury. J Neurosurg 1985 Sept; 63(3):390–397.

Friedman-Campbell M and Hart CA. Theoretical strategies and nursing interventions to promote psychosocial adaptation to spinal cord injuries and disability. J Neurosurg Nurs 1984 Dec; 16(6):335–342.

Graham PM. Bridge building—Linking a spinal cord unit to a skilled nursing facility. Rehabil Nurs 1985 Sept/Oct; 10(5):22–25.

Howlett M and Stevens J. Recognizing the symptoms of autonomic dysreflexia. Can Nurse 1985 May; 81(5):40–41.

McGuire TJ and Kumar VN. Autonomic dysreflexia. Postgrad Med 1986 Aug; 80(2):81–89.

Perry J. Rehabilitation of the neurologically disabled patient: Principles, practice, and scientific basis. J Neurosurg 1983 June; 58(6):799–816.

Schulz R and Decker S. Long-term adjustment to physical disability: The role of social support, perceived control, and self-blame. J Pers Soc Psychol 1985 May; 48(5):1162–1172.

Stanton GM. A needs assessment of significant others following the patient's spinal cord injury. J Neurosurg Nurs 1984 Oct; 16(5):253–256.

Thiyagarajan C and Silver JR. Aetiology of pressure sores in patients with spinal cord injury. Br Med J 1984 Dec 1;289(6457):1487–1490.

Toth LL. Spasticity management in spinal cord injury. Rehabil Nurs 1983 Jan/Feb; 8(1):14–17.

*Wells P and Geden E. Paraplegic body-support pressure on convoluted foam, waterbed, and standard mattress. Res Nurs Health 1984; 7: 127–133,

Aneurysms/Brain Tumors

Benson CA and Harris AA. Acute neurologic infections. Med Clin North Am 1986 Sept; 70(5):987–1011.

Cascino TL. Treatment of patients with brain tumors. Mayo Clin Proc 1985 Apr; 60(4):279–280.

Chase M and Whelan-Decker E. Nursing management of a patient with a subarachnoid hemorrhage. J Neurosurg Nurs 1984 Feb; 16(1): 23–29.

Gruca JK. Oncology rehabilitation. Rehabil Nurs 1984 May/June; 9(3): 27–30.

Horner TG. Management of vasospasm from ruptured intracranial aneurysms with induced hypotension. Indiana Med 1985 May; 78(5): 367–377.

Houston CS. Intracranial aneurysms: Diagnosis, treatment, and nursing implications. Periop Nurs Q 1985 June; 1(2):39–48.

Kaplan K. Brain abscess. Med Clin North Am 1985 Mar; 69(2):345–360.

Kassell NF et al. Cerebral vasospasms following aneurysmal subarachnoid hemorrhage. Stroke 1985 July/Aug; 16(4):562–572.

Kee DB Jr and Wood JH. Current concepts in the diagnosis and management of brain metastasis. J Med Assoc Ga 1983 Feb; 72(2):127–132.

Kessinger A. High dose chemotherapy with autologous bone marrow rescue for high grade gliomas of the brain: A potential for improvement in therapeutic results. Neurosurgery 1984 Nov; 15(5):747–750.

Kim LYS and Tew JM Jr. Saccular aneurysms, subarachnoid hemorrhage, and the timing of surgery. Heart Lung 1985 Jan; 14(1):68–74.

Lamb S and Gutin PH. Interstitial radiation for treatment of primary brain tumors using the Brown-Roberts-Wells stereotaxic system. J Neurosurg Nurs 1985 Feb; 17(1):22–29.

Ljunggren B et al. Cognitive impairment and adjustment in patients without neurological deficits after aneurysmal SAH and early operation. J Neurosurg 1985 May; 67(5):673–679.

Longstreth WT et al. Risk factors for subarachnoid hemorrhage. Stroke 1985 May/June; 16(3):377–385.

McCool JA. In memory of a brain tumour. Br Med J 1985 Jan 26; 290(6464):296–297.

Mitchell SK and Yates RR. Cerebral vasospasm: Theoretical causes, medical management, and nursing implications. J Neurosci Nurs 1986 Dec; 18(6):315–324.

Moseley JR. Alterations in comfort. Nurs Clin North Am 1985 June; 20(2): 427–438.

Muizelaar JP and Becker DP. Improving outcome of aneurysmal subarachnoid hemorrhage. Va Med 1985 June: 112(6):374–379.

Nishioka H et al. Cooperative study of intracranial aneurysms and subarachnoid hemorrhage: A long-term prognostic study. Arch Neurol 1984 Nov; 41(11):1142–1146.

Oertel LB. The dilemma of cerebral vasospasm treatment. J Neurosurg Nurs 1985 Feb; 17(1):7–13.

Rosenblum MV and Wilson CB (eds). Brain tumor therapy. Prog Exp Tumor Res 1984; 28:1–254.

Rosenwasser RH, Buchheit WA, and Truex RC. Management of subarachnoid hemorrhage. Penn Med 1984 Dec; 87(12):72, 74.

Salcman M. The morbidity and mortality of brain tumors. Neurol Clin 1985 May; 3(2):229–257.

Wilson CB and Gutin PH. New therapeutic approaches for brain tumor. Cancer 1984 Dec 1; 54(11 Suppl):2702–2705.

Epilepsy

Barry K and Teixeira S. The role of the nurse in the diagnostic classification and management of epileptic seizures. J Neurosurg Nurs 1983 Aug; 15(4):243–249.

Conomy JP. Management of patients with intractable seizures. Postgrad Med 1985 Feb 15; 77(3):138, 140, 142.

Jabbari B. Management of epileptic seizures in adults. Am Fam Physician 1985 June; 31(6):162–172.

Peterson GM, McLean S, and Millingen KS. A randomised trial of strategies to improve patient compliance with anticonvulsant therapy. Epilepsia 1984 Aug; 25(4):412–417.

Scott AK. Management of epilepsy. Br Med J 1984 Mar 31; 288(6422): 986–987.

Spencer DD and Spencer SS. Surgery for epilepsy. Neurol Clin 1985 May; 3(2):313–330.

Head Injury

Anderson BJ. A theoretical protocol for nutritional maintenance in head-injured patients. J Neurosurg Nurs 1984 Feb; 16(1):50–53.

Black DW. Subdural hematoma. Postgrad Med 1985 July; 78(1):107–123.

Brigman C, Dickey C, and Zegeer LJ. The agitated aggressive patient. Am J Nurs 1983 Oct; 83(10):1408–1412.

Elliott J and Smith DE. Meeting family needs following severe head injury: A multidisciplinary approach. J Neurosurg Nurs 1985 Apr; 17(2): 111–113.

Giannotta SL. High dose glucocorticoids in the management of severe head injury. Neurosurgery 1984 Oct; 15(4):497–501.

Hendrickson S. Psychological care of the patient with neurological dysfunction. J Neurosurg Nurs 1984 Aug; 16(4):202–207.

Lillehei K and Hoff JT. Advances in the management of closed head injury. Ann Emerg Med 1985 Aug; 14(8):789–795.

*Parsons LC and Shogan JSO. The effects of endotracheal suctioning/manual hyperventilation procedure on patients with severe closed head injuries. Heart Lung 1984 July; 13(4):372–380.

*Parsons LC, Peard ALS, and Page MC. The effects of hygienic interventions on the cerebrovascular status of severe closed head injured persons. Res Nurs Health 1985 Jan; 8(2):173–181.

Schaffer L, Kranzler C, and Siqueira EB. Aspects of evaluation and treatment of head injury. Neurol Clin 1985 May; 3(2):259–273.

Huntington's Disease

Bird SJ. Presymptomatic testing for Huntington's disease. JAMA 1985 June 14; 253(22):3286–3289.

Leopold NA and Kagel MC. Dysphagia in Huntington's disease. Arch Neurol 1985 Jan; 42(1):57–60.

Mann SH. Practical management strategies for families with demented victims. Neurol Clin 1986 May; 4(2):469–478.

Myers RH, Schoenfeld M, and Bird ED. Huntington's disease: Genetics, chemical pathology, and management. Prog Med Genet 1985; 6: 91–122.

Sands RG. Social work with victims of Huntington's disease. Soc Work Health Care 1984 Summer; 9(4):63–71.

Shoulson I. Huntington's disease. Neurol Clin 1984 Aug; 2(3):515–526.

Simpson JM. Neurological disorders with autosomal dominant transmission. J Neurosurg Nurs 1984 Oct; 16(5):262–269.

Small O. Huntington's chorea. Nurs Times 1986 Apr 9; 82(15):32–33.

Intervertebral Disc

Apfelbach H. Technique for chemonucleolysis. Today's OR Nurse 1984 Jan; 6(1):20–25.

Bosacco SJ and Berman AT. Surgical management of lumbar disc disease. Radiol Clin North Am 1983 June; 21(2):377–393.

Chymopapain administration procedures modified. FDA Drug Bull 1984 Aug; 14(2):14–15.

Devoti AL. Lumbar laminectomy: Diagnosis to discharge. J Neurosurg Nurs 1983 Jan; 15(3):140–143.

Fisher RG. Injection therapy for herniated disks. Postgrad Med 1984 June; 75(8):66–68; 74–79.

Fraser RD. Chymopapain for the treatment of intervertebral disc herniation. Spine 1984 Nov/Dec; 9(8):815–818.

Friedman WA. New techniques for treatment of disk disease. Geriatrics 1984 Aug; 39(8):41–53.

Gentry LR et al. Chymopapain chemonucleolysis: CT changes after treatment. AJR 1985 Aug; 145(2):361–369.

Javid MJ. Efficacy of chymopapain chemonucleolysis. J Neurosurg 1985 May; 62(5):662–666.

Kranzler LI, Schaffer L, and Siqueira EB. Recent advances in the treatment of ruptured lumbar intervertebral disks. Neurol Clin 1985 May; 3(2): 405–416.

Maroon JC and Abla A. Microdiscectomy versus chemonucleolysis. Neurosurgery 1985 May; 16(5):644–649.

Mims BC. Back surgery: Helping your patient get through it. RN 1985 May; 48(5):26–32.

Onik G et al. Percutaneous lumbar discectomy using a new aspiration probe. AJR 1985 June; 144(6):1137–1140.

Shields CB and Arpin EJ. Update on chymopapain. Neurol Clin 1985 May; 3(2):393–403.

Multiple Sclerosis

Belohorec A and Kikuchi JF. How do you mother when you are disabled? Can Nurs 1985 Mar; 81(3):32–35.

Carpenito LJ. Acutal, potential, or possible. Am J Nurs 1985 Apr; 85(4): 458.

Cook CV and Bass BH. Nursing care of the multiple sclerosis patient with cyclophosphamide. Can Nurse 1985 Mar; 81(3):36–38.

Delisa JA et al. Multiple sclerosis: Part I. Common physical disabilities and rehabilitation. Am Fam Physician 1985 Oct; 32(4):157–163.

Farrell MA et al. Oligoclonal bands in multiple sclerosis. Neurology 1985 Feb; 35(2):212–218.

Frankel D. Long-term care issues in multiple sclerosis. Rehabil Lit 1984 Sept; 45(9–10):282–285.

Giesser B. Multiple sclerosis: Current concepts in management. Drugs 1985 Jan; 29(1):88–95.

Gonor SE, Carroll DJ, and Metcalfe JB. Vesical dysfunction in multiple sclerosis. Urology 1985 Apr; 25(4):429–431.

Graham OC and Carico J. The primary nurse as a caregiver in a neurology research setting. J Neurosurg Nurs 1985 Aug; 17(4):260–268.

Gulick EF. Multiple sclerosis: The nurses' role using a self-care framework. J Community Health Nurs 1984; 1(4):247–255.

Halligan FR and Reznikoff M. Personality factors and change with multiple sclerosis. J Consult Clin Psychol 1985 Aug; 53(4):547–548.

Halper J. Multiple scherosis and self-help: New roles for nursing. J Community Health Nurs 1984; 1(3):153–157.

Holland NJ, Wiesel-Levison P, and Madonna MG. Community care of the patient with multiple sclerosis. Rehabil Nurs 1984 Nov/Dec; 9(6):18–20.

Jacobs L et al. Intrathecal interferon in the treatment of multiple sclerosis. Arch Neurol 1985 Sept; 42(9)841–847.

Kirschner HS et al. Magnetic resonance imaging and other techniques in the diagnosis of multiple sclerosis. Arch Neurol 1985 Sept; 42(9): 859–863.

Larocca N et al. Factors associated with unemployment of patients with multiple sclerosis. J Chronic Dis 1985; 38(2):293–210.

Levine AM. Management of multiple sclerosis. Postgrad Med 1985 Apr; 77(5):121–127.

Lewis SM. Therapeutic swimming: A different kind of nursing. J Nurs Educ 1985 Mar; 24(3):125.

Patterson MB and Foliart R. Multiple sclerosis: Understanding the psychologic implications. Gen Hosp Psychiatry 1985 July; 7(3):234–238.

Paulley JW. Psychosomatic aspects of multiple sclerosis. Adv Psychosom Med 1985; 13:85–110.

Peters LC and Esses LM. Family environment as perceived by children with a chronically ill parent. J Chronic Dis 1985; 38(4):301–308.

Rao SM et al. Chronic progressive multiple sclerosis. Arch Neurol 1985 July; 42(7):678–682.

Sadovnick AD and Baird PA. Reproductive counselling for multiple sclerosis patients. Am J Med Genet 1985 Feb; 20(2):349–354.

Samonds RJ and Cammermeyer M. The patient with multiple sclerosis. Nursing '85 1985 Sept; 15(9):60–64.

Schweitzer SF. Immunosuppressive treatment of multiple sclerosis. J Neurosurg Nurs 1985 Aug; 17(4):256–259.

Symposium on multiple sclerosis. Neurol Clin 1983 Aug; 1(3):573–782 (entire vol).

van den Noort S. Immunosuppressant treatment in multiple sclerosis. Clin Neuropharmacol 1985 Mar; 8(1):58–63.

VanderPlate C. Psychological aspects of multiple sclerosis and its treatment: Toward a biopsychosocial perspective. Health Psychol 1984: 3(3):253–272.

*Young FK and Brooks BR. Patient teaching manuals improve retention of treatment information: A controlled clinical trial in multiple sclerosis. J Neuroscience Nurs 1986 Feb; 18(1):26–28.

Ziporyn T. Magnetic resonance "sees" lesions of multiple sclerosis. JAMA 1985 Feb 15; 253(7):949–951.

Myasthenia Gravis

Adams SL, Mathews J, and Grammer LC. Drugs that may exacerbate myasthenia gravis. Ann Emerg Med 1984 July; 13(7):532–538.

d'Empaire G et al. Effect of prethymectomy plasma exchange on postoperative respiratory function in myasthenia gravis. J Thorac Cardiovasc Surg 1985 Apr; 89(4):592–596.

Engel AG. Myasthenia gravis and myasthenic syndromes. Ann Neurol 1985 Nov; 16(5):519–534.

Kess R. Suddenly in crisis—Unpredictable myasthenia. Am J Nurs 1984 Aug; 84(8):994–998.

Lisak RP. Plasma exchange in neurologic disease. Arch Neurol 1984 June; 41(6):654–657.

Noroian EL. Myasthenia gravis: A nursing perspective. J Neuroscience Nurs 1986 Apr; 18(2):74–80.

Riggs JE. Adult-onset muscle weakness. Postgrad Med 1985 Sept; 78(3): 217–226.

Schoenfeld Y and Schwartz RS. Immunologic and genetic factors in autoimmune diseases. N Engl J Med 1984 Oct 18; 311(16):1019–1029.

Sellman MS and Mayer RF. Weakness and "tiredness": When to suspect myasthenia gravis. Geriatrics 1985 Jan; 40(1):92–112.

Parkinson's Disease

Bulpitt CJ et al. The symptoms of patients treated for Parkinson's disease. Clin Neuropharmacol 1985 June; 8(2):175–183.

Burton K and Calne DB. Pharmacology of Parkinson's disease. Neurol Clin 1984 Aug; 2(3):461–472.

Cummings JL. Psychosomatic aspects of movement disorders. Adv Psychosom Med 1985; 13(1):111–132.

Dakof GA and Mendelsohn GA. Parkinson's disease: The psychological aspects of a chronic illness. Psychol Bull 1986 May; 99(3):375–387.

Feldman RG. Parkinson disease: Individualizing therapy. Hosp Pract 1985 Jan 15; 20(1):80A–80FF.

Fonda D. Parkinson's disease in the elderly: Psychiatric manifestations. Geriatrics 1985 Apr; 40(4):109–112.

Friedman JE. "Drug holidays" in the treatment of Parkinson's disease. Arch Intern Med 1985 May; 145(5):913–915.

Gever LN. Anticholinergics. Nursing '84 1984 Sept; 14(9):64.

Globus M, Mildworf B, and Melamel E. Cerebral blood flow and cognitive impairment in Parkinson's disease. Neurology 1985 Aug; 35(8):1135–1139.

Greer M. Recent developments in the treatment of Parkinson's disease. Geriatrics 1985 Feb; 40(2):34–41.

*Knafl KA and Deatrick JA. How families manage chronic conditions: An analysis of the concept of normalization. Res Nurs Health 1986; 9:215–222.

Laitinen LV. Brain targets in surgery for Parkinson's disease. J Neurosurg 1985 Mar; 62(3):349–351.

Lang AE. Treatment of Parkinson's disease with agents other than levodopa and dopamine agonists: Controversies and new approaches. Can J Neurol Sci; 1984 Feb; 11(1 Suppl):210–220.

Lannon MC et al. Comprehensive care of the patient with Parkinson's disease. J Neurosci Nurs 1986 June; 18(3):121–131.

Legg NJ. Parkinson's disease: Course and Management. Practitioner 1983 Mar; 227(1377):375–379.

Lieberman AN. Parkinson's disease. Compr Ther 1986 Mar; 12(3):25–29.

Mayeux R. Behavioral manifestations of movement disorders. Neurol Clin 1984 Aug; 2(3):527–540.

Nanton V. The consequences of Parkinson's disease—Needs, provisions, and initiatives. J R Soc Health 1985 Apr; 105(2):52–54.

Robbins JA, Logemann JA, and Kirshner HS. Swallowing and speech production in Parkinson's disease. Ann Neurol 1986 Mar; 19(3):283–287.

Peripheral Nervous System Condition

Cramer FE. First: Make the patient a believer (Guillain-Barré). Nursing '84 1984 July; 14(7):36–38.

Edwards R. Maternal Guillain-Barré syndrome. J Neurosurg Nurs 1984 Dec; 16(6):306–312.

Koski CL, Khurana R, and Mayer RF. Guillain-Barré syndrome. Am Fam Physician 1986 Sept; 34(3):198–210.

Miller RG. Acute vs. chronic compressive neuropathy. Muscle Nerve 1984 July/Aug; 7(6):427–430.

Ropper AH. Severe acute Guillain-Barré syndrome. Neurology 1986 Mar; 36(3):429–432.

Sunderrajan EV and Davenport J. The Guillain-Barré syndrome: Pulmonary-neurologic correlations. Medicine 1985 Sept; 64(5):333–341.

Trigeminal Neuralgia

Editorial. Management of trigeminal neuralgia. Lancet 1984 Mar 24; 1(8378):662–663.

Fromm GH, Terrence CF, and Maroon JC. Trigeminal neuralgia: Current concepts regarding etiology and pathogenesis. Arch Neurol 1984 Nov; 41(11):1204–1207.

Management of trigeminal neuralgia. Drug Ther Bull 1983 Dec 16; 21(25):97–99.

Sweet WH. The treatment of trigeminal neuralgia (tic douloureux). N Engl J Med 1986 July 17; 415(3):174–177.

Tew JM Jr and Van Lovern H. Surgical treatment of trigeminal neuralgia. Am Fam Physician 1985 May; 31(5):143–150.

Zorman G and Wilson CB. Outcome following microsurgical vascular decompression or partial sensory rhizotomy in 125 cases of trigeminal neuralgia. Neurology 1984 Oct; 34(10):1362–1365.

Post-Polio Syndrome

Dalakas MC. A long-term follow-up study of patients with post-poliomyelitis neuromuscular symptoms. N Engl J Med 1986 Apr 10; 314(15):959–963.

Holman KG. Post-polio syndrome. Postgrad Med 1986 June; 79(8):44–53.

Raymond CA. Decades after polio epidemics, survivors report new symptoms. JAMA 1986 Mar 21; 255(11):1397–1404.

Twist DJ and Ma DM. Physical therapy management of the patient with post-polio syndrome. Phys Ther 1986 Sept; 66(9):1403–1406.

Agencies and Sources of Information

Governmental

Division for the Blind and Physically Handicapped, Library of Congress, Washington, DC 20542.

National Institute of Neurological and Communicative Disorders and Stroke, National Institutes of Health, Bethesda, MD 20892.

Voluntary

American Cancer Society, 90 Park Avenue, New York, NY 10016.

American Parkinson Disease Association, 116 John Street, New York, NY 10038.

American Speech–Language–Hearing Association, 10801 Rockville Pike, Rockville, MD 20852.

Amyotrophic Lateral Sclerosis Association, 15300 Ventura Boulevard, Suite 315, PO Box 5951, Sherman Oaks, CA 91403 and 185 Madison Avenue, Suite 1001, PO Box 2130, New York, NY 10016.

Epilepsy Foundation of America, 4351 Garden City Drive, Landover, MD 20785.

Guillain-Barré Syndrome Support Group, PO Box 262, Wynnewood, PA 19096.

Hereditary Disease Foundation, 9701 Wilshire Bouldevard, Suite 1204, Beverly Hills, CA 90212.

Huntington's Disease Foundation of America, 250 West 5th Street, Suite 2016, New York, NY 10019.

Muscular Dystrophy Association, 810 Seventh Avenue, New York, NY 10019.

Myasthenia Gravis Foundation, 15 East 26th Street, New York, NY 10010.

National Easter Seal Society, 2023 West Ogden Avenue, Chicago, IL 60612.

National Head Injury Foundation, P.O. Box 567, Framingham, MA 01701.

National Migraine Foundation, 15252 Western Avenue, Chicago, IL 60625.

National Multiple Sclerosis Society, 205 East 42nd Street, New York, NY 10017.

National Parkinson Foundation, 1501 N.A. Ninth Avenue, Miami, FL 31316.

National Spinal Cord Injury Association, 369 Elliot Street, Newton Upper Falls, MA 02164.

Paralyzed Veterans of America, 4350 East-West Highway, Suite 900, Bethesda, MD 20814.

Parkinson's Disease Foundation, William Black Medical Research Building, Columbia University Medical Center, 640 West 168th Street, New York, NY 10032.

Nursing Research Profile for Unit XIV

Eye and Ear Nursing

Overview

Nursing research studies on the care of patients with eye and ear problems have been very few but predictably will increase in the future because of the increase in day surgery and the aging population. How well the patient is prepared for treatment both physically and psychologically is important both before and after treatment regimens. Since greater responsibility for self-care is currently being placed on the patient, education of the patient and his supporters is increasingly important to prevent discomfort and complications.

Two studies are presented, one relating to day-care eye surgery and the other to the patient with hearing loss in later life. The need for additional nursing research in these areas is apparent, since so little has been done.

▷ *Smith S. Day-care cataract surgery: The patient's perspective. J Ophthalmol Nurs Tech 1987 Mar/Apr; 6(2):50–55.*

It is estimated that 85% of the population will have some form of clouding of the lens by the time they reach 80 years of age. Currently the number of cataract extractions in people over 65 is increasing and exceeds the current growth in the aging population. Reasons for the increase appear to be the following: (1) advances in technology, medications, and anesthesia; (2) increased demand; (3) increased consumer satisfaction with intraocular lenses; and (4) shorter stay in the hospital for cataract surgery.

The two major trends affecting nursing care are the increasing number of persons undergoing cataract surgery (especially elderly people) and the decreased hospital stay.

The purpose of the study was to determine the patient's and family members' perceptions of day-care surgery and their ability to manage at home postoperatively. The study included only those clients who were at low risk and had potential for a successful day-care experience. Chosen were 9 women and 8 men ranging in age from 26 to 72 (most in their 60s) whose conditions were not complicated by glaucoma, diabetes, dislocated lens, *etc.* Elements of preoperative preparation included the following:

1. Surgeon met with patient for the purpose of describing the types of correction and potential visual outcome.
2. Pamphlets and literature (large print) were provided.
3. Hospital routines and expectations were discussed.
4. One week preoperatively, patient attended the hospital clinic for laboratory and preoperative tests. Written instructions were given about the perioperative period.
5. Medications were prescribed (chloramphenicol preoperatively).
6. Arrangements were made for a home-care nurse to visit, teach, and demonstrate procedures (administration of eye drops, application of eye shield, *etc.*).

Nursing Implications.   Although the group studied was small, pertinent conclusions about nursing care could be drawn:

- A family member should be present at teaching sessions (more than one session in advance of surgery).

- Provide opportunity to practice eye drop administration in a normal eye prior to surgery.
- Emphasize the need to agitate the eye drop bottle if this is pertinent.
- Provide a nurse/patient relationship that is conducive to the patient's expressing feelings and asking questions.
- Encourage the presence of a support person at home to assist the patient.

▷ *Magilvy JK. Experiencing hearing loss in later life: A comparison of deaf and hearing-impaired older women. Res Nurs Health 1985 Dec; 8(4):347–353.*

The purpose of the Magilvy study was to determine differences in the effect of hearing loss in women between the ages of 54 and 96, comparing those who had severe hearing loss prior to age 19 with those who had a later onset of hearing loss. Another objective was to learn whether different approaches should be used by health care providers with these two groups. The prevocationally deaf women experienced problems in communicating with the hearing world. Women whose hearing loss occurred in later years showed the greatest emotional difficulty.

A variety of anecdotes are presented which in themselves have nursing implications worth reviewing.

Nursing Implications. Since Americans over age 60 represent more than 15% of the total population, nurses will be caring for increasing numbers of elderly persons with hearing deficits. Because of broad differences in the hearing-impaired, the nurse will need to provide extra time and use a creative approach to facilitate communication and develop effective nursing interventions (*e.g.*, a sign language interpreter may be required to ensure accurate history taking). Patience and flexibility are necessary with hearing-impaired persons. The slowing effects of aging must also be recognized.

Neuroscience Nursing

Overview

Research in neuroscience nursing has mainly focused on nursing considerations, management, and implications for patients with head and spinal cord injuries, stroke, and multiple sclerosis. Certainly these are catastrophic events for the patient which require intensive nursing management. The effects of nursing interventions on intracranial pressure have been identified in several studies. Some studies of the concerns of families of these patients have been undertaken. Investigation of neurologic problems should continue to yield important implications for future nursing practice and research.

▷ *Ferington FE. Personal control and coping effectiveness in spinal cord injured persons. Res Nurs Health 1986 Sept; 9(3):257–265.*

The Ferington study was done to explore the relationship between varying conditions of control and depression in hospitalized spinal cord injured persons. Control was conceptualized at three levels: the participants' preference to control, their generalized expectation for control, and their perceptions of options to control. Depression was used as an indi-

cator of the level of coping effectiveness. Trait anxiety was selected as an indicator of participant style in responding to threat. Demographic data (age, socioeconomic status, ethnicity, duration of injury) were indicated as possible correlates of the variables of interest.

One hundred and four spinal cord injured males participated in the study, which used a variety of instruments to measure depression, trait anxiety, locus of control, and interpersonal relations. Personal interviews were also conducted.

The hypothesis that locus of control orientation (internal or external) is positively related to depression was supported. High levels of perceived control were associated with low levels of depression in those participants with a high preference for control (both internally and externally oriented). Depression scores were unrelated to perceived control for those without such a preference. Findings indicated that the significance of having control is an individual matter.

Nursing Implications. Control may not have an inherent coping value in some persons. Not all patients may wish to participate in a decision-making process. Some persons have limited capacity to exercise control options. The nurse will need to develop assessment tools to determine which patients will benefit from participating in their own care.

▷ *Hendrickson SL. Intracranial pressure changes and family presence. J Neurosci Nurs 1987 Feb; 19(1): 14–17.*

The Hendrickson study investigated the association between family visits and fluctuations in intracranial pressure (ICP) in 24 patients who were undergoing ICP monitoring with ventriculostomies or Richmond bolts. Each patient's ICP was recorded every 15 minutes around the clock and every 5 minutes while a family member was present. These records provided over 10,000 raw data points. A time series quasi-experimental design was used for data analysis.

In 7 patients the family had a positive effect on ICP, manifested clinically by a decrease in ICP ranging from 1.41 mm Hg to 4.24 mm Hg. In 11 instances the presence of family was recorded as nonsignificant, with decreases in ICP between 1.57 mm Hg to 0.03 mm Hg. Six instances of rising ICP (0.03 mm Hg to 0.90 mm Hg) were deemed statistically nonsignificant.

Nursing Implications. While it is known that certain nursing interventions are associated with an increased intracranial pressure, this study reflects nursing's growing concern with controlling the environment to produce positive changes in the patient's health status. It would be useful to investigate the effects on ICP fluctuations of touch, soothing voice, and presence by the bedside of the family for a longer period.

▷ *Mumma CM. Perceived losses following stroke. Rehabil Nurs 1986 May/June; 11(3):19–24.*

The Mumma study was an exploratory, cross-sectional survey to describe losses following a stroke as perceived by patients and their spouses. Sixty middle-aged and older couples in which one person had suffered a stroke were interviewed. Data were collected by semistructured interviews using structured scales and open-ended questions.

Three major categories of loss emerged from content analysis of responses about perceived loss: (1) activities, (2) abilities and characteristics, and (3) independence. The loss mentioned most frequently by both male and female respondents was mobility. The top two losses reported by both male and female spouses were the same—traveling and independence. Patients with right-brain damage missed their independence and mobility, while patients with left-brain damage missed mobility and driving. The losses identified by spouses of persons with both right-brain and left-brain damage were independence and social life. Patients with left-brain damage and their spouses identified communication among their top five losses.

Nursing Implications. Many older people look forward to traveling after retirement. A stroke is a catastrophic event that thwarts plans and forces those involved to come to terms with various losses. During the rehabilitation phase, the nurse may examine what the patient's premorbid goals were and how he or she can adapt to and live with the limitations of physical disability. Since over time patients and their spouses become more aware of disability-related limitations, an effective nursing intervention may be to encourage them to join a support group as soon as possible. Periodic respite care for the patient may be considered preventive health care for the spouse. More research in the area of support for the caregiver seems to be indicated.

▷ *Parsons LC and Wilson MM. Cerebrovascular status of severe closed head injured patients following passive position changes. Nurs Res 1984 Mar/Apr; 32(2): 68–75.*

The Parsons and Wilson study of 18 severely head-injured patients evaluated the effects of six passive position changes on cerebrovascular status. Changes in mean arterial blood pressure, mean intracranial pressure, cerebral perfusion pressure, and heart rate were monitored. The patient was informed that the nurse planned to change his position. An observer recorded baseline measurements of the physiologic variables, the highest displayed value of each variable with position change, and recovery values 1 minute after the completion of position change.

The position changes were standardized as follows: (1) turning side to back, extension of lower extremities; (2) turning back to side, flexion of upper and lower extremities; (3) range of motion exercise of upper and lower extremities; (4) head rotation to the right or left; (5) elevation of head of the bed greater than 35°; and (6) lowering the head of the bed from 35° to 0°.

Over 200 observations of the effects of position changes on the above physiologic variables that were recorded and analyzed showed that all position changes (with the exception of raising the head of the bed) produced changes in the heart rate, mean arterial blood pressure, mean intracranial pressure, and cerebral perfusion pressure. However, these changes were usually transient and showed return toward baseline value 1 minute after the intervention measures.

Although the sample was nonrandomized, the study did indicate that passive positional changes are safe if the resting mean intracranial pressure is ≤15 mm Hg.

Nursing Implications. This study lends credence to the importance of not grouping nursing activities together in order to prevent episodic increases in intracranial pressure in patients with head injuries. It would also be interesting to note whether very slow changes in position would make a

difference. This study underscores the importance of physiologic monitoring of patients with severe closed head injuries in defining safe limits for turning and other interventions.

▷ *Young FK and Brooks BR. Patient teaching manuals improve retention of treatment information—A controlled clinical trial in multiple sclerosis. J Neurosci Nurs 1986 Feb; 18(1):26–28.*

Studies have shown that increased or better teaching is an effective way to improve patients' medication knowledge and compliance. In the Young and Brooks study, patients in the Johns Hopkins University Multiple Sclerosis Clinic were prescribed alternate-day steroid medications as a treatment for motor dysfunction caused by their disease. The clinical nurse specialist and physician each met with the patient to explain how the drug was to be taken, physiologic effects, potential side-effects, and potential danger signs. The session was followed by a written pretest of the orally imparted information. Subsequently it was noted that many patients did not take the medication as prescribed.

A written informational booklet on steroids was developed for patients. A study was designed to determine whether the written booklet would result in greater retention of information about alternate-day steroids. Patients were randomly assigned to groups, with alternate patients going into experimental or control groups. The experimental group received oral instructions from the nurse and physician and were given the patient information booklet. The control group received oral instructions only.

After 1 month a written posttest was given. Patients who received the written instructional booklet showed a significant increase in retained knowledge about their medication.

Nursing Implications. The problem of following medication and treatment instructions is not unique to persons with multiple sclerosis. It appears that patients who receive both oral and written information have a better understanding of the treatment regimen. Nurses may work with pharmacists, health science writers, and others to develop written informational booklets on medications. This is a large order, but it should reap benefits in improved patient education and compliance and fewer untoward reactions to medications.

Additional Studies

Axellson K, Norberg A and Asplund K. Relearning to eat late after a stroke by systematic nursing intervention: A case report. J Adv Nurs 1986 Sept; 11(5):553–559.

Bell TN. Nurses' attitudes in caring for the comatose head-injured patient. J Neurosci Nurs 1986 Oct; 18(5):279–289.

Boortz-Marx R. Factors affecting intracranial pressure: A descriptive study. J Neurosurg Nurs 1985 Apr; 17(2):89–94.

Bronstein K et al. The Stroke Data Bank Project: Implications for nursing research. J Neuroscience Nurs 1986 June; 18(32):132–134.

Dai Y-T. Health beliefs and compliance with a skin care regimen. Rehabil Nurs 1987 Jan/Feb; 12(1):13–16.

Ende RM. The significance of selected variables in laminectomy length of stay. J Neurosci Nurs 1986 June; 18(3):150–152.

Evans RL, Becker V and Stone BW. Identifying social needs of patients with neuromuscular disorders. Rehabil Nurs 1982 Sept/Oct; 7(4): 21–25; 45.

Hinkle JL et al. Restoring social competence in minor head-injury patients., J Neurosci Nurs 1986 Oct; 18(5):268–271.

Holland NJ, Francabandera F and Wiesel-Levison P. International scale for assessment of disability in multiple sclerosis. J Neurosci Nurs 1986 Feb; 18(1):39–44.

Holland NJ, Wiesel-Levison P and Madonna MG. Rehabilitation research: Pathophysiology and management of neurogenic bladder in multiple sclerosis. Rehabil Nurs 1985 Jul/Aug; 10(4):31–33.

Hooker EZ. Problems of veterans spinal cord injured after age 55: Nursing implications. J Neurosci Nurs 1986 Aug; 18(4):188–195.

Keller E and Bzdek VM. Effects of therapeutic touch on tension headache pain. Nurs Res 1986 Mar/Apr; 35(2):101–106.

Lewis NA. Functional gains in CVA patients: A nursing approach. Rehabil Nurs 1986 Mar/Apr; 11(2):25–27.

Madonna MG, Holland NJ and Wiesel-Levison P. The value of physical therapy in improving gait in multiple sclerosis: A research design. Rehabil Nurs 1985 Sept/Oct; 10(5):32–34.

Markin DA. Preoperative concerns of the patient undergoing craniotomy. J Neurosci Nurs 1986 Oct; 18(5):275–278.

Myco F. Stroke and its rehabilitation: The perceived role of the nurse in medical and nursing literature. J Adv Nurs 1984 Dec; 9(5):429–439.

Parsons LC, Peard ALS and Page MC. The effects of hygiene interventions on the cerebrovascular status of severe closed head injured persons. Res Nurs Health 1985 June; 8(2):173–181.

Rudy EB et al. The relationship between endotracheal suctioning and changes in intracranial pressure: A review of the literature. Heart Lung 1986 Sept; 15(5):488–494.

Snyder M. Stressor inventory for persons with epilepsy. J Neuroscience Nurs 1986 Apr; 18(2):71–73.

Wells P and Geden E. Paraplegic body-support pressure on convoluted foam, waterbed, and standard mattresses. Res Nurs Health 1984 June; 7(2):127–133.

Musculoskeletal and Locomotion Problems

Unit XV

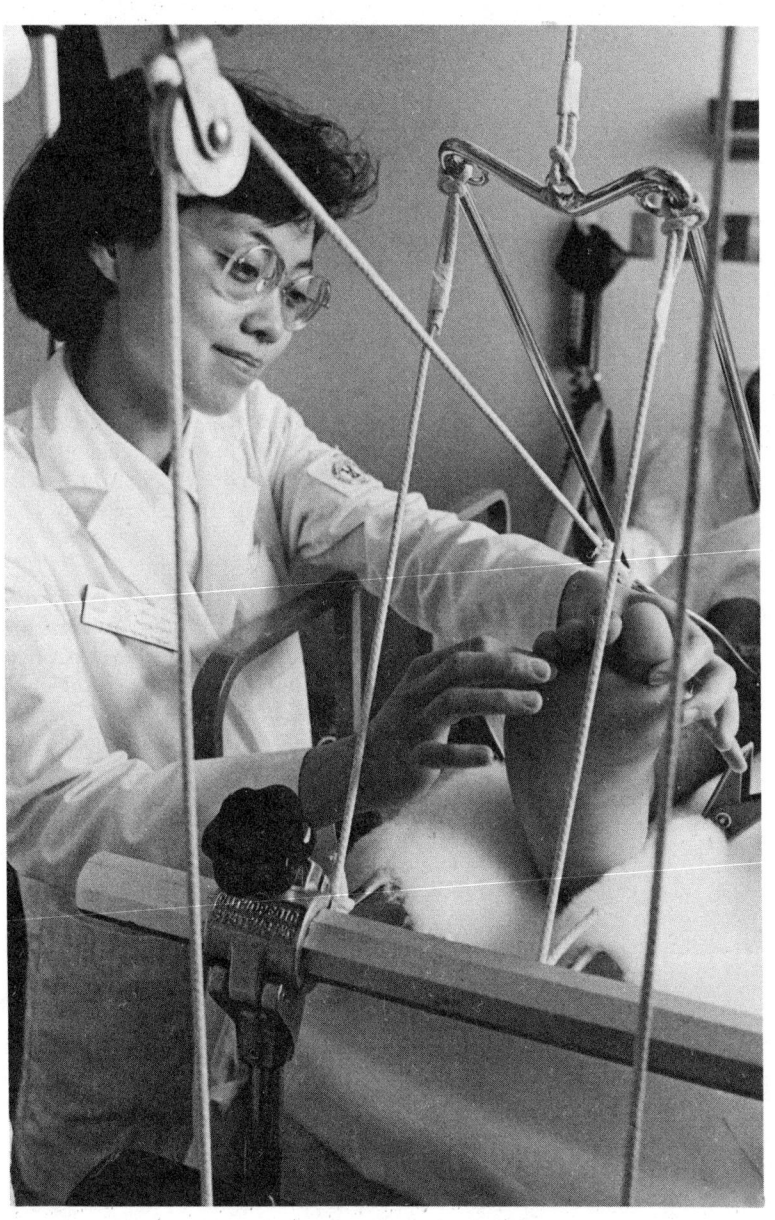

Chapter 55

Assessment of Musculoskeletal Function

The musculoskeletal system includes the bones, joints, muscles, tendons, ligaments, and bursae of the body. The occurrence of problems associated with these structures is very common and affects all age groups. Problems with the musculoskeletal system are generally not life-threatening, but they have a significant impact on one's productivity and financial situation. Problems associated with the musculoskeletal system will be encountered by the nurse practicing in any field of nursing and during daily living experiences.

Physiologic Overview

The musculoskeletal system is collectively the largest organ system in the body. Bony structures and connective tissue account for approximately 25% of the body weight, and muscle accounts for approximately 50% of the body weight. The health and functions of the musculoskeletal system are interdependent with the rest of the body systems.

The functions of the musculoskeletal system include protection, support, locomotion, mineral storage, hematopoiesis, and heat production. The bony structure provides protection for vital organs, including the brain, heart, and lungs. The bony skeleton supports body structures by providing a strong and sturdy framework. The muscles attached to the skeleton allow the body to move. Calcium, phosphorus, and magnesium are among the minerals deposited and stored in the bone matrix. The red bone marrow located within the bone cavity is responsible for the production of red and white blood cells. Muscle contracton results in mechanical action for movement as well as heat production to maintain body temperature.

The Skeletal System

Anatomy of the Skeletal System. There are 206 bones in the human body, divided into four categories: *long bones* (*e.g.,* the femur), *short bones* (*e.g.,* the tarsals), *flat bones* (*e.g.,* the sternum), and *irregular bones* (*e.g.,* the vertebrae). The shape and construction of a specific bone are determined by its function and the forces exerted on the bone.

Bones are constructed of *cancellous* (trabecular or

spongy) or *cortical* (compact) bone tissue. Long bones are shaped like rods or shafts with rounded ends. The shaft, or *diaphysis,* is primarily cortical bone. The ends of the long bones are called *epiphyses* and are primarily cancellous bone. The *epiphyseal plate* separates the epiphyses from the diaphysis and is the center for longitudinal growth in children. In the adult, it is calcified. The ends of long bones are covered by articular cartilage at the joints. Long bones are constructed for weight-bearing and movement.

Short bones consist of cancellous bone covered by a layer of compact bone.

Flat bones are important sites for *hematopoiesis* (formation of blood), and frequently provide vital organ protection. They are made of cancellous bone layered between compact bone.

Irregular bones have unique shapes related to their function. Generally, irregular bone makeup is similar to that of flat bones.

Bone is composed of cells, protein matrix, and mineral deposits. The cells are of three basic types—osteoblasts, osteocytes, and osteoclasts. *Osteoblasts* are involved in bone formation by secreting *bone matrix.* The matrix is 98% collagen and 2% ground substances (glucosamine glycans [acid polysaccharides] and proteoglycans). The matrix is a framework in which inorganic mineral salts are deposited. *Osteocytes* are mature bone cells involved in homeostatic bone functions and are located in *osteons* (bone matrix units). *Osteoclasts* are multinuclear cells involved in bone destruction, resorption, and remodeling.

The osteon is the microscopic functioning unit of mature bone. The center of the osteon contains a capillary. Around the capillary are circles of bone matrix called *lamellae.* Within the lamellae are *osteocytes* (mature, living bone cells). They are nourished by processes extending into tiny *canaliculi* (canals that communicate with the blood vessel). The size of the osteon is limited by the nutritional supply. Bone cells and their nourishing blood vessel must be less than 0.1 mm apart.

Covering the bone is a dense, fibrous membrane known as the *periosteum.* The periosteum functions in the nutrition and growth of bone, and provides for the attachment of tendons and ligaments. The periosteum contains nerves, blood vessels, and lymphatics. The layer closest to the bone contains osteoblasts, which are bone-forming cells.

Endosteum is a thin, vascular membrane covering the marrow cavity of long bones and the spaces in cancellous bone. *Osteoclasts,* which dissolve away bone to maintain the marrow cavity, are located near the endosteum and in *Howship's lacunae* (indentations on bone surfaces).

Bone marrow is a vascular tissue located in the medullary (shaft) cavity of long bones and in flat bones. Red bone marrow is responsible for the production of red and white blood cells. In the adult, the red bone marrow in the long bone cavity is replaced mostly by fatty, yellow marrow. Red bone marrow in the adult is located mainly in the sternum, ilium, vertebrae, and ribs.

Bone tissue is well vascularized. Periosteal vessels connect with bone tissue through minute *Volkmann canals.* In addition, nutrient arteries penetrate the periosteum and enter the medullary cavity through *foramina* (small openings). Nutrient arteries supply blood to the marrow and bone. The venous system may accompany arteries or may exit independently.

Bone Formation. Bone begins to form long before birth. The process by which intercellular material is formed and hardening minerals are deposited into the bone is known as *ossification.* There are two basic models of ossification: intramembranous and endochondral. *Intramembranous ossification,* in which bone develops within membrane, occurs in the bones of the face and skull. Therefore, when the skull heals, it is by fibrous union. The other kind of bone formation is known as *endochondral ossification,* in which a cartilage model exists and is resorbed and replaced by bone. Most bones in the body are formed and healed by endochondral ossification.

The exact mechanism by which ossification occurs is unknown. The cell mitochondria probably play a vital role in the formation of microcrystallites, which are deposited in the matrix as precursors of larger mineral deposits. The ground substances may be the stimulus for the deposition of crystals. In addition, a specific charge may occur on the collagen fibers that initiate the crystal formation and electrostatically hold the crystals, once formed, in place. Actively growing bone is electronegative. More than 99% of the total body calcium is present in the bones. Other minerals deposited within the bone matrix include sodium, magnesium, fluoride, and carbonate.

Bone Maintenance. Bone is a dynamic tissue in a constant state of turnover (resorption and reforming). Calcium in bone in an adult is replaced at the rate of about 18% a year. The important regulating factors that determine the balance between bone formation and bone resorption include local stress, vitamin D, parathyroid hormone, calcitonin, and circulation.

Local stress (weight-bearing) acts to stimulate local bone resorption and formation and can result in extensive remodeling. In this way, deformed bones may tend to straighten out. This phenomenon also explains why important weight-bearing bones are thick and strong. When weight-bearing or stress is prevented, as in prolonged bed rest, calcium is lost from the bone. If the stress on the bone is excessive, bone necrosis will occur.

Vitamin D functions to increase the amount of calcium in the blood by promoting absorption of calcium from the gastrointestinal tract and accelerating mobilization of calcium from the bone.

Parathyroid hormone and calcitonin are the major hormonal regulators of calcium homeostasis. Parathyroid hormone regulates the concentration of calcium in the blood, in part by promoting movement of calcium from the bone. Excessive mobilization of calcium due to excess parathyroid hormone results in demineralization of the bone and formation of bone cysts. Calcitonin, from the thyroid gland, increases the production of bone.

Blood supply to the bone also affects bone formation. With diminished blood supply or *hyperemia* (congestion), osteogenesis is reduced and the bone becomes osteoporotic. Bone necrosis occurs when the bone is deprived of blood.

The Articular System

The bones of the body are joined together at *joints* or *articulations* that allow for a variety of movements. Regardless of the amount of movement possible, the junction of two or more bones is called a joint. There are three basic kinds of joints: synarthrosis, amphiarthrosis, and diarthrosis joints (also called synarthroses, amphiarthroses, and diarthroses). *Synarthrosis joints* are immovable, as exemplified by the skull sutures. *Amphiarthroses*, such as the vertebral joints and symphysis, allow some limited motion. The bones are separated by fibrous cartilage. *Diarthroses*, like the elbow, are freely-movable joints. Synovial fluid lubricates the movement of diarthroses (or synovial) joints.

At a typical movable joint, the ends of the articulating bones are covered with a smooth hyaline cartilage. The articulating bones are surrounded by a tough, fibrous sheath, the *joint capsule*. The capsule is lined with a membrane, the *synovium*, which secretes the lubricating and shock-absorbing synovial fluid into the joint capsule. Therefore, the bone surfaces do not come in direct contact. In some synovial joints, fibrocartilage discs are located between the articular cartilage surfaces. They provide shock absorption. In some joints, such as the knee, interosseous ligaments, which add strength to the joint, are found within the capsule.

Ligaments (fibrous connective tissue bands) bind the articulating bones together. Ligaments and muscle tendons, which pass over the joint, provide joint stability.

Movable joints are of several different kinds.

- *Ball and socket joints*, best exemplified by the hip or the shoulder, permit full freedom of movement.
- *Hinge joints* permit bending in one direction only, and are best exemplified by the elbows and knees.
- A *saddle joint* allows movement in two planes at right angles to each other. The joint at the base of the thumb is a saddle, biaxial joint.
- The *pivot joint* is characterized by the articulation between the radius and the ulna. It permits rotation for such activities as turning a doorknob.
- *Gliding joints* allow for limited movement in all directions and are located at the joints of carpal bones in the wrist.

Bursae are additional structures associated with some joints. A bursa is a sac filled with synovial fluid that is located at a point of friction. Bursae are generally found cushioning the movement of tendons, ligaments, and bones at the elbow, shoulder, knee, and other joints.

The Skeletal Muscle System

Anatomy of Skeletal Muscles. Skeletal (striated) muscles are involved in body movement, posture, and heat-production functions. Muscles are attached by *tendons* (cords of fibrous connective tissue) or *aponeuroses* (broad, flat sheets of connective tissue) to bones, connective tissue, other muscles, soft tissue, or skin. Muscles contract to bring the two points of attachment closer together. Muscles vary in shape and size according to the activity for which they are responsible. Muscles develop and are maintained when actively used. Age and disuse cause loss of muscular function as fibrotic tissue replaces the contractile muscle tissue.

The muscles of the body are composed of parallel groups of muscle cells (*fasciculi*) encased in fibrous tissue called *epimysium* or *fascia*. The more fasciculi contained in a muscle, the more precise the movements.

The speed of the muscle contraction is variable. *Myoglobulin*, a hemoglobinlike protein pigment, is present in striated muscle cells and transports oxygen from the blood

capillaries to the muscle cell mitochondria for cellular metabolic needs. Muscles containing large quantities of myoglobulin (*red muscle*) have been observed to contract slowly and powerfully (*e.g.*, respiratory and postural muscles). Muscles containing little myoglobulin (*white muscles*) contract quickly and for extended periods of time (*e.g.*, extraocular eye muscles). Most body muscles contain both red and white muscle fibers.

Each muscle cell (also referred to as a *muscle fiber*) contains *myofibrils*, which in turn are composed of a series of *sarcomeres*, the actual contractile units of skeletal muscle. The components of the sarcomeres are known as thick and thin filaments. The thin filaments are composed mainly of a protein known as actin. The thick filaments are composed mainly of myosin, another protein material.

Skeletal Muscle Contraction. Contraction of a muscle is due to the contraction of each of its component sarcomeres. The contraction of a sarcomere is due to interactions between the myosin in the thick filaments and the actin in the thin filaments, brought about by a local increase in the calcium ion concentration. The thick and thin filaments slide across one another. When calcium concentration in the sarcomere subsequently falls, the myosin and actin filaments cease to interact and the sarcomere returns to its original resting length (relaxation). Interaction between actin and myosin does not occur in the absence of calcium.

Muscle fibers contract in response to electrical stimulation. When stimulated, muscle cells generate an action potential in a manner similar to that described for nerve cells. These action potentials propagate along the muscle cell membrane and lead to the release in the muscle cell of calcium ions that are stored in specialized organelles called the *sarcoplasmic reticulum*. The calcium allows the interaction of actin and myosin in the sarcomere. Very shortly after the muscle cell membrane is depolarized, it recovers its resting membrane voltage. Calcium is rapidly removed from the sarcomeres by active reaccumulation in the sarcoplasmic reticulum, and the muscle relaxes.

Depolarization of the muscle cells normally occurs in response to a stimulus delivered by a nerve cell. The communication between the nerve cell and the muscle cell takes place at the motor end plate. The neurons that control the activity of skeletal muscle cells are called *lower motor neurons*, which originate in the anterior horn of the spinal cord.

Energy is consumed during muscle contraction and relaxation. The rate of energy used by skeletal muscle varies; it increases markedly during exercise. The source of energy for the muscle cells is adenosine triphosphate (ATP) that is generated through cellular oxidative metabolism. Creatine phosphate, also present in muscle cells, functions as a second reservoir of metabolic energy; it can be converted to ATP when necessary. At low levels of activity, the skeletal muscle synthesizes ATP from the oxidation of glucose to water and carbon dioxide. During periods of high activity, when sufficient oxygen may not be available, glucose is metabolized primarily to lactic acid. Although ATP is generated during production of lactic acid, the process is inefficient compared with that of oxidative pathways. Therefore, increased amounts of glucose are required and are supplied by muscle glycogen. *Glycogen* is a starch that is produced from glucose, stored in the cells during periods of rest, and utilized during periods of activity. Muscle fatigue is thought to be caused by a rapid rate of work of the muscle, resulting in depletion of glycogen and energy stores and accumulation of lactic acid. As a result, the cycle of muscle contraction and relaxation cannot continue.

During muscle contraction, the energy released from ATP is not completely utilized by the contractile apparatus. This excess energy is dissipated in the form of heat. During isometric contraction, almost all the energy is released in the form of heat; during isotonic contraction, some of the energy is expended in mechanical work. In some situations, such as shivering, the need for generation of heat is the primary stimulus for muscle contraction.

Muscle Status. The contraction of muscle fibers can result in either isotonic or isometric contraction of the muscle. In *isometric contraction,* the length of the muscles remains constant, but the force generated by the muscles is increased. An example of this is when one pushes against an immovable wall. *Isotonic contraction,* on the other hand, is characterized by shortening of the muscle with no increase in tension within the muscle. An example of this is flexion of the forearm. In normal activities, many muscle movements are a combination of isometric and isotonic contraction. For example, during walking, isotonic contraction results in shortening of the leg and, during isometric contraction, the stiff leg pushes against the floor.

Relaxed muscles demonstrate a state of readiness to respond to contraction stimuli. This state of readiness is known as *muscle tone* (tonus), and is due to the maintenance of some of the muscle fibers in a contracted state. Sense organs in the muscles (*muscle spindles*) monitor muscle tone. Muscle tone is found to be minimal during sleep and increased when anxious. In lower motor neuron destruction (*e.g.,* polio), the denervated muscle becomes *atonic* (soft and flabby) and atrophies. A muscle that has less than normal tonus is known as *flaccid. Spastic* describes the muscle with greater than normal tonus.

Muscle Actions. Muscles accomplish movement only by contraction. They cannot push. Through the coordination of muscle groups, the body is able to perform a wide variety of movement. The *prime mover* is the muscle that causes a particular motion. The muscles assisting the prime mover are known as *synergists.* The muscle causing movement opposite to that of the primary mover is known as the *antagonist.* The antagonist must relax to allow the prime mover to contract, producing motion. For example, when contraction of the biceps causes flexion of the elbow joint, the biceps is the prime mover and the triceps is the antagonist. With muscle paralysis, a person may be able to retrain functioning muscles within a synergistic group to coordinate in such a way as to effect the needed movement. Secondary movers then become the primary mover.

The body movements that muscle contractions can produce are many. *Flexion* is characterized by bending at a joint (*e.g.,* elbow). The opposite movement is *extension* or straightening at a joint. *Abduction* is the action of moving away from the midline of the body. To move toward the midline is *adduction. Rotation* describes turning around a specific axis (*e.g.,* shoulder joint). *Circumduction* is the conelike movement of the thumb. Special body movements include *supination* (turning the palm up), *pronation* (turning the palm down), *inversion* (turning the sole of the foot inward), *eversion* (the opposite of inversion), *protraction* (the jaw is pulled forward), and *retraction* (the jaw is pulled backward).

Exercise, Disuse, and Repair. Muscles need to be exercised to maintain function and strength. When a muscle is repeatedly caused to develop maximum or close to maximum tension over a long period of time, as in regular exercise with weights, the cross-sectional area of the muscle increases (hypertrophies). This is due to an increase in the size of individual muscle fibers without an increase in the number of muscle fibers. Hypertrophy will persist only if the exercise is continued.

The opposite phenomenon occurs with disuse of muscle over a long period of time. The decrease in the size of a muscle is called *atrophy.* Bed rest and immobility will cause loss of muscle mass and strength. When immobility is due to a treatment mode (*e.g.,* casting or traction), the patient can decrease the effects of immobility by isometric exercise of the muscles of the immobilized part. Quadriceps exercises (tightening the muscles of the thigh) and gluteal setting exercises (tightening of the muscles of the buttocks) help maintain the larger muscle groups that are important in ambulation. Active and weight-resistant exercises of uninjured parts of the body prevent degeneration.

When muscles are injured, they need rest and immobilization until tissue repair occurs. The healed muscle then needs progressive exercise to resume its preinjury functional state.

Gerontological Considerations

Multiple changes in the musculoskeletal system occur with aging. Bone mass peaks at about age 35, after which there is a universal gradual loss of bone. Numerous metabolic changes, including menopausal withdrawal of estrogen and decreased activity, contribute to the loss of bone mass (*osteoporosis*). Women lose more bone mass than men. By the age of 75, the average women has lost 25% of her cortical (compact) bone and 40% of her trabecular (cancellous) bone. Additionally, bones change in shape and have reduced strength. If fractured, fibrous tissue develops more slowly in the aged.

In the elderly, the ability of the collagen structures to absorb energy is reduced. This contributes to the development of osteoarthritis. The articular cartilage degenerates in weight-bearing areas and has a reduced ability to heal.

Likewise, muscle strength is diminished. There is an actual loss in the number of muscle fibers due to myofibril atrophy, which begins in the fourth decade.

Many of the effects of aging can be overcome if the body is kept healthy and active.

Remote musculoskeletal problems for which the patient has compensated may become new problems with age-related changes. For example, patients who have recovered from polio and who have been able to function normally by using synergistic muscle groups may discover increasing incapacity. They have a reduced compensatory ability.

Physical Assessment

An examination of the musculoskeletal system ranges from a basic assessment of functional capabilities to sophisticated physical examination maneuvers that facilitate diagnosis of specific muscle and joint disorders. The nurse examiner's assessment is primarily a functional evaluation. Techniques of inspection and palpation are employed to evaluate the patient's posture and gait, joint function, bone stability, muscle integrity and strength, and ability to perform activities of daily living.

The musculoskeletal assessment is commonly integrated into the routine progression of the physical examination. This system relates closely to the neurologic and cardiovascular systems, and thus all three assessments are often carried out together. The basis of the assessment is a comparison of symmetrical regions of the body. The extent of the assessment depends on the patient's physical complaints, health history, and any physical clues detected by the examiner that warrant further exploration.

When specific symptoms or physical findings of musculoskeletal dysfunction are apparent, the examination is carried out and carefully documented and the information is shared with a physician, who may decide that a more extensive examination and diagnostic workup are necessary.

Gait Assessment. An assessment of gait is done by having the patient walk normally for a short distance away from the examiner. The examiner observes the gait for smoothness and rhythm. Any unsteadiness or irregular movements (frequently noted in elderly patients) are considered abnormal. When a limping motion is noted, it is most likely due to painful weight-bearing. In such instances, the patient can usually pinpoint the area of discomfort, thus guiding a further examination. When one extremity is shorter than another, a limp may also be observed as the patient's pelvis drops downward on the affected side with each step. Paralysis in the lower extremities results in a variety of gaits. These gaits are associated with such neurologic disorders as Parkinson's disease, and stroke.

Joint Assessment. The joints are evaluated for their size and range of motion, and for the strength of the muscles that flex and extend the joints. The examiner is familiar with the normal range of motion of major joints, and focuses on specific joints if functional loss is apparent. Most persons are able to hyperextend all joints. If the maximum extension of a joint still reveals some residual degree of flexion, the range of motion is said to be limited.

In the event that joint motion is compromised, or that the joint is painful, the joint is examined for the presence or absence of fluid within its capsule (*effusion*) and for an increase in temperature that might reflect active inflammation. An effusion is suspected when the joint is swollen in size and the normal bony landmarks are obscured. The most common site for joint effusion is in the knee. If a small amount of fluid is present in the joint spaces beneath the patella, it may be identified by the following maneuver. The examiner firmly milks the medial and lateral aspects of the extended knee in a downward motion. This displaces any fluid downward. As pressure is exerted against the medial or lateral side, the examiner observes the opposite side for a bulge below the patella. When larger amounts of fluid are present, the patella becomes elevated from the femur during knee extension. If the patella bounces back when tapped firmly against the femur, a "click" may be palpable. This is a test for *ballottement* of the patella. When inflammation or fluid is present in a joint, physician consultation is indicated.

Passive movement of the joint may produce an audible crunching sound, called *crepitus*. Crepitus may be palpable as well.

Joints and the tissues surrounding them are examined for nodule formation. Rheumatoid arthritis, gout, osteoarthritis, and rheumatic fever all produce characteristic nodules that are diagnostic of the disease. The subcutaneous nodules of rheumatoid arthritis are soft and occur within and along tendons that provide extensor function to the joints. Usually, involvement of the joints assumes a symmetrical pattern. The nodules of gout are hard and lie within and immediately adjacent to the joint capsule itself. Frequently, they rupture, exuding white uric acid crystals onto the skin surface. The nodules of osteoarthritis are hard and painless and represent bony overgrowth that has resulted from destruction of the cartilaginous surface of bone within the joint capsule. These are frequently seen in older adults.

Atrophy of muscle results from disuse and from neurologic damage. Thus, the muscles that provide function to a diseased joint will atrophy when the joint is kept passive to avoid the pain that may arise from moving it. This is dramatically seen in rheumatoid arthritis of the knees, in which the quadriceps muscle may atrophy in a very dramatic way. Often, the size of a diseased joint is exaggerated by the atrophy of muscles proximal and distal to that joint.

Examination of the Spine. Inspection of the spine is carried out with the patient's gown open to expose the entire back, buttocks, and legs. The examiner stands behind the patient, noting any differences in the height of the shoulders or iliac crests. The gluteal folds are normally symmetrical. Shoulder and hip symmetry, as well as the straight line of the vertebral column, are inspected with the patient erect and bending forward (*flexion*).

The normal curvature of the spine is convex through the thoracic portion and concave through the cervical and lumbar portions. The concavity of the lumbar spine is referred to as *lumbar lordosis* and is normal. Excessive curvature of the thoracic spine is called *kyphosis*. Deviation of the spine to the left or right is termed *scoliosis*. Kyphosis and scoliosis may result from damage to the paraspinal musculature in poliomyelitis or from disease of the vertebral column, as may be seen in tuberculosis.

Diagnostic Evaluation

Radiologic Procedures

X-rays are important in evaluating patients with musculoskeletal disorders. Bone films determine bone density, texture, erosion, and changes in bone relationships. Multiple x-ray views are needed for full assessment of the structure being examined. X-ray of the cortex of the bone reveals widening, narrowing, and any signs of irregularity. Joint x-rays will reveal the presence of fluid, irregularity, spur formation, narrowing, and changes in the joint structure.

Laminography or *tomography* shows in detail a specific plane of involved bone.

Computed tomography can be useful in orthopedic diagnosis by revealing tumors of the soft tissue or injuries to the ligaments or tendons. It is helpful in identifying the location and extent of fractures in areas difficult to define (*e.g.,* the acetabulum).

Myelography, the injection of contrast medium into the subarachnoid space of the lumbar spine, is carried out to determine disc herniation, *spinal stenosis* (narrowing of the spinal canal), or the site of a tumor. This technique is discussed on page 1408.

Discography is a study of the intervertebral discs in which a contrast medium is injected into the disc and its distribution is noted.

Arteriography is a study of the arterial system. A radiopaque contrast medium is injected into the selected artery, and serial films are taken of the supplied arterial system. It is useful for determining arterial perfusion and aids in determining the amount of extremity that needs to be amputated.

Arthrography is the injection of a radiopaque substance or air into the joint cavity in order to outline soft tissue structures and the contour of the joint. The joint is put through its range of motion while a series of radiographs are taken. Arthrography is useful in identifying acute or chronic tears of the joint capsule or supporting ligaments of the knee, shoulder, ankle, hip, or wrist. (If a tear is present, the contrast medium will leak out of the joint and show on x-ray.)

Other Studies

An *arthrocentesis* is carried out to obtain synovial fluid for purposes of examination. A needle is inserted into the joint, and fluid is then aspirated. Since this procedure has the potential for introducing bacteria into the joint, aseptic techniques must be followed. Following aspiration, no special precautions are necessary.

Normally, synovial fluid is clear, pale, straw-colored, and scanty in volume. The fluid is examined grossly for volume, color, clarity, viscosity, and formation of mucin clot. It is examined microscopically for cell count, cell identification, Gram's stain, and formed elements. Examination of synovial fluid is helpful in the diagnosis of rheumatoid arthritis and other inflammatory arthropathies, and will reveal the presence of *hemarthrosis* (bleeding into the joint cavity), which suggests trauma or a tendency to bleed.

Arthroscopy is an endoscopic procedure that allows direct visualization of a joint. The procedure is carried out in the operating room, under sterile conditions and following the injection of a local anesthetic into the joint or a general anesthesia. A large-bore needle is inserted and the joint is distended with saline. The arthroscope is introduced and the knee joint visualized, including the synovium, articular surfaces, and joint structures. If an arthrotomy is not indicated, the puncture wound is covered with a sterile Band-Aid and the extremity is wrapped from the midthigh to the midcalf with a compressive wrap that is worn for 24 to 48 hours for support. The joint is kept in extension and elevated to reduce swelling, and neurovascular function is evaluated periodically. The patient is advised to limit activity following the procedure. Complications are rare, but may include infection, hemarthrosis (blood in the joint cavity), thrombophlebitis, stiffness, and delayed wound healing.

A *bone scan* reflects the degree to which the matrix of bone "takes up" a bone-seeking radioactive isotope that is injected into the system. The degree of nuclide uptake is related to the metabolism of the bone. An increased uptake of isotope is seen in primary skeletal disease (osteosarcoma), metastatic bone disease, inflammatory skeletal disease (osteomyelitis), and certain types of fractures.

Thermography measures the degree of heat radiating from the skin surface. It is used to investigate the pathophysiology of inflamed joints (rheumatoid arthritis) and to assess the patient's response to anti-inflammatory drug therapy.

Electromyography provides information on the electric potential of the muscles and the nerves leading to them. The purpose of this procedure is to determine any abnormal physiology involving the motor unit. Needle electrodes are inserted into selected muscles, and responses to electrical stimuli are recorded on an oscilloscope.

Single and dual *photon absorptiometry* are noninvasive tests to determine bone mineral content at the wrist or vertebrae. Osteoporosis may be monitored with this type of densitometry.

Bone biopsy may be done to determine the structure and composition of bone tissue, which may be helpful in diagnosing specific diseases.

Laboratory Studies

Examination of the patient's blood and urine can provide information concerning a primary musculoskeletal problem (*e.g.*, Paget's disease), a developing complication (*e.g.*, infection), baseline information for instituting therapy (*e.g.*, anticoagulant therapy), or response to therapy. The complete blood count will provide information concerning the hemoglobin level (frequently lower after bleeding associated with trauma) and the white blood cell count. Prior to surgery, coagulation studies are done to determine bleeding tendencies, because bone is a very vascular tissue. Blood chemistry studies provide data concerning a great variety of musculoskeletal conditions, including osteomalacia and muscle trauma. Alkaline phosphatase is elevated during fracture healing and in diseases with increased osteoblastic activity (*e.g.*, osteomalacia, osteoblastic bone tumors). Urine calcium levels increase with bone destruction (*e.g.*, metastatic bone tumors, multiple myeloma). Serum calcium levels increase with prolonged immobilization and diseases, including Paget's disease and metastatic cancers. Serum phosphorus levels are inversely related to calcium levels and are diminished in rickets associated with malabsorption syndrome. Serum enzyme levels of CPK and SGOT become elevated with muscle damage.

Nursing Process Considerations

Initially, the patient with a muscoskeletal problem will require support and nursing care during the period of examinations and testing. There will be a need for physical and psychological preparation. Prior to the test, patient education (including what is to be done, why it is being done, and what patient participation is expected) will reduce anxiety and enable the patient to be an active participant in care.

The resulting diagnosis and prescribed treatment regimen will affect the nursing management of the patient. The nursing plan of care will reflect nursing measures that will facilitate the resolution of the patient's problems.

The nursing assessment will enable the nurse to identify the health problems that can be improved by nursing interventions. Actual and potential nursing diagnoses common to patients with musculoskeletal disorders include the following:

- Impaired physical mobility
- Alteration in comfort—pain

- Impairment of skin integrity, actual or potential
- Alteration in bowel elimination—constipation
- Alteration in tissue perfusion—peripheral
- Potential for infection
- Knowledge deficit of the disease process and treatment regimen
- Self-care deficits
- Disturbance in self-concept, body image
- Ineffective individual coping
- Alteration in family process
- Potential sexual dysfunction
- Powerlessness
- Sleep pattern disturbance
- Diversional activity deficit
- Potential for alteration in nutrition—less than body requirements

In collaboration with the patient, health goals and nursing strategies are formulated to achieve the goals and resolve the identified problems.

Bibliography

Books

Arthroscopy of the Knee (Monograph). Pitman, New Jersey, National Association of Orthopaedic Nurses, 1983.

Bates B. A Guide to Physical Examination and History Taking, 4th ed. Philadelphia, JB Lippincott, 1987.

Bellack JP and Bamford PA. Nursing Assessment: A Multidimensional Approach. Monterey, Wadsworth Health Science Division, 1984.

Birnbaum JS. The Musculoskeletal Manual. New York, Academic Press, 1982.

Duthie RB and Bentley G (eds). Mercer's Orthopaedic Surgery, 8th ed. Baltimore, University Park Press, 1983.

Farrell J. Illustrated Guide to Orthopedic Nursing, 3rd ed. Philadelphia, JB Lippincott, 1986.

Holbrook TL. The Frequency of Occurrence, Impact, and Cost of Selected Musculoskeletal Conditions in the United States. Chicago, American Academy of Orthopaedic Surgeons, 1984.

Malasanos L et al. Health Assessment, 2nd ed. St Louis, CV Mosby, 1981.

McRae R. Clinical Orthopaedic Examination, 2nd ed. New York, Churchill Livingstone, 1983.

Nelson CL and Dwyer AP (eds). The Aging Musculoskeletal System: Physiological and Pathological Problems. Lexington, Massachusetts, Collamore Press, 1984.

Nurse's Reference Library: Diagnostics. Springhouse, Pennsylvania, Intermed Communications, 1981.

Pellino T et al (eds). National Association of Orthopaedic Nurses: Core Curriculum for Orthopaedic Nursing. Pitman, New Jersey, Anthony J Jannetti, 1986.

Photobook: Working with Orthopedic Patients. Springhouse, Pennsylvania, Intermed Communications, 1982.

Rockwood CA and Green DP (eds). Fractures in Adults, 2nd ed. Philadelphia, JB Lippincott, 1984.

Sculco TP (ed). Orthopaedic Care of the Geriatric Patient. St Louis, CV Mosby, 1985.

Turek SL. Orthopedics: Principles and Their Application, 4th ed. Philadelphia, JB Lippincott, 1984.

Articles

Burggraf V and Donlon B. Assessing the elderly, Part 1: System by system. Am J Nurs 1985 Sept; 85(9):974–984.

Dunn BH. Musculoskeletal assessment: Components of the musculoskeletal examination. Orthop Nurs 1982 Nov/Dec; 1(6):33–37.

Dunn BH. Musculoskeletal assessment: Gait assessment. Orthop Nurs 1983 May/June; 1(3):33–36.

Farrell J. Orthopedic pain: What does it mean? Am J Nurs 1984 Apr; 84(4):466–469.

Henderson ML. Assessing the elderly, Part 2: Altered presentations. Am J Nurs 1985 Oct; 85(10):1103–1111.

Jones-Walton P. Orthopedic health promotion: Injury and disability prevention. Orthop Nurs 1984 Nov/Dec; 3(6):35–42.

Kleinstuber M and Reed D. Performing knee arthroscopy under local anesthesia. Today's OR Nurs 1985 Nov; 7(11):22–27.

Kostopoulos MR. Reducing patient falls. Orthop Nurs 1985 Nov/Dec; 4(6):14–15.

Ross DG. Musculoskeletal assessment: The knee. Orthop Nurs 1983 Sept/Oct; 2(5):23–28.

Unbanski PA. The orthopedic patient: Identifying neurovascular injury. AORN J 1984 Nov; 40(11):707–711.

Vanderbeck KA. Getting the facts: A guide to orthopaedic assessment. Orthop Nurs 1984 Sept/Oct; 3(5):31–34.

Agencies

National Institute of Arthritis and Musculoskeletal and Skin Diseases, National Institutes of Health, Bethesda, MD 20892.

Chapter 56

Management Modalities for Patients With Musculoskeletal Dysfunction

Nursing Process Overview

▷ Assessment

The nursing assessment of the patient with musculoskeletal dysfunction includes an evaluation of the impact of the musculoskeletal problem on the patient. The nurse is concerned with assisting persons with musculoskeletal problems to maintain their general health, accomplish their activities of daily living, and manage their treatment modalities. Systemic homeostasis is assured; optimum nutrition is encouraged; and problems related to immobility are prevented. The nurse helps the patient achieve a balance between periods of exercise and rest through an individualized plan of care.

In the initial interview, the nurse obtains a general impression of the patient's status. A general inspection of the body will reveal the existence of any gross deformity, asymmetry of contours or size, swelling, edema, bruising, or breaks in the skin. Observing the patient's posture, movement, and gait will provide information concerning alterations in ability to move, the existence of discomfort, or the presence of involuntary movements (fasciculations or twitches). The nurse will gather information concerning existing concurrent health problems, the patient's perceptions and expectations related to the health problems, and socioeconomic factors that will affect restoration of well-being.

History

The nurse needs to obtain subjective data from the patient concerning the onset of the problem and how it has been managed to this point. The existence of other health problems (*e.g.,* diabetes, heart disease, a cold) needs to be noted for consideration when developing the plan of care. A history of medication use and response to pain medication will aid in designing drug management regimens. Allergies are noted and should include the type of reaction the patient has experienced. The use of tobacco, alcohol, and other drugs should be assessed in order to evaluate the effects of these habits on the patient's needs. Notations of the patient's ability to learn, economic status, and current occupation are needed for discharge planning and for rehabilitation. Additions to the initial interview data will be made as the nurse interacts with the patient. Such data allow for adjustment of the individualized plan of care.

Physical Assessment

Much information about the structure and functioning of the musculoskeletal system can be obtained by physical assessment. The nurse is interested in identifying the functional abilities of the patient and the effects that any disabilities and medical treatment have on the patient's ability to meet his needs effectively. The patient's posture and gait, bone stability, joint function, muscle integrity and strength, and ability to perform activities of daily living are assessed. Any deviations from normal are noted. Throughout the initial assessment, the nurse establishes a baseline for noting and evaluating changes in the person's abilities.

Assessment of Bony Skeleton. The bony skeleton is assessed for deformities and alignment. Abnormal bony growths due to bone tumors may be observed. Shortened extremities, amputations, and body parts out of anatomical alignment are noted. Loss of height occurs with loss of vertebral cartilage in the aged.

Possible common deformities of the spine that may be noted include *scoliosis* (a lateral curving deviation of the spine), *kyphosis* (an increased roundness of the thoracic spine curve), and *lordosis* (swayback; exaggeration of the lumbar spine curve). Kyphosis is frequently seen in the elderly patient.

Abnormal angulation of long bone or motion at points other than joints is frequently indicative of fracture. *Crepitus* (grating sensation) at the point of abnormal motion may also be detected. Movement of bony fragments must be minimized to avoid additional injury.

Assessment of Articular System. The articular system is evaluated by noting joint swelling, nodule formation, deformity, stability, and range of motion. Joint swelling might be noted with arthritis, inflammation, or *effusion* (fluid accumulated in the joint capsule). Rheumatoid arthritis, gout, and osteoarthritis produce characteristic nodules. Hard, painless, overgrowth nodules associated with osteoarthritis are frequently seen in older adults.

Joint deformity may indicate *contracture* (shortening of surrounding joint structures), *dislocation* (complete separation of joint surfaces), *subluxation* (partial separation of articular surfaces), or *disruption of structures* surrounding the joint. Weakness or disruption of joint-supporting structures may result in a joint that is too weak to function as designed and may therefore require external supporting appliances. Range of motion is evaluated both actively (joint is moved by the muscles surrounding the joint) and passively (joint is moved by the examiner).

Range of Motion. Restricted range of motion means that the joint cannot be moved throughout the normal joint range as defined by the American Academy of Orthopedic Surgeons. Precise measurement of range of motion can be made by an instrument known as a *goniometer* (a protractor designed for evaluating joint motion). Limitation in range of motion may be due to skeletal deformity, joint pathology, muscular weakness, contracture of surrounding muscles and tendons, or neurologic denervation.

Feeling the joint while passively moving it will provide information concerning the integrity of the joint. Normally, the joint moves smoothly. A snap or a crack may indicate that a ligament is slipping over a bony prominence. Slightly roughened surfaces, as in arthritic conditions, will result in *crepitus* as the surfaces of the joint are moved across one another.

In elderly persons, limitations of range of motion associated with degenerative joint pathology may reduce their ability to perform activities of daily living.

Assessment of Muscular System. The muscular system is assessed by noting the patient's ability to change position, muscular strength and coordination, and individual muscle size. Muscular weakness of a group of muscles might indicate a variety of conditions, such as polyneuropathy, electrolyte disturbances (particularly potassium and calcium), myasthenia gravis, poliomyelitis, and muscular dystrophy. By palpating the muscle while passively moving the relaxed extremity, the nurse can determine the muscle tone. Muscle strength can be estimated by having the patient perform certain tasks with and without added resistance. For example, the biceps can be tested by requesting the patient to fully extend the arm and then flex it while the nurse applies resistance to prevent the arm from flexing. A simple handshake provides an indication of grasp strength.

Muscle clonus (rhythmic contractions of a muscle) may be elicited in the ankle or wrist by sudden, forceful, sustained dorsiflexion of the foot or extension of the wrist. *Fasciculations* (involuntary twitching of muscle fiber groups) may be observed.

The girth of an extremity must be measured at times to monitor increased swelling due to edema or bleeding into the muscle or to a decrease in size due to atrophy. The unaffected extremity is measured and used as the reference standard. Measurements are to be taken at the maximum circumference of the extremity. It is important that the measurements be at the same location on the extremity and with the extremity in the same position with the muscle at rest. Distance from a specific anatomical landmark (*e.g.,* 10 cm below the medial aspect of the knee for measurement of the calf muscle) should be indicated in the chart so that subsequent measurements are made at the same point. For ease of serial assessment, the point of measurement can be indicated by marking the skin. Variations in size need to be greater than 1 cm to be considered significant.

Assessment of Skin and Peripheral Circulation. In addition to the musculoskeletal system, the nurse must inspect the skin and assess peripheral circulation. Cuts, bruises, skin color, and evidence of decreased circulation or infection can influence nursing management. Feeling the skin can reveal if any areas are warmer or cooler than others and if edema is present. Peripheral circulation is evaluated by assessing peripheral pulses, color, temperature, and capillary refill time.

Subjective Assessment Data. During the interview and physical assessment, the patient may report the presence of pain, tenderness, tightness, and abnormal sensations. This information needs to be noted and assessed.

Pain

Most patients with diseases and traumatic conditions of muscles, bones, and joints experience pain. *Bone pain* is characteristically described as a dull, deep ache that is boring in nature, whereas *muscular pain* is considered sore and aching and is frequently referred to as "muscle cramps." *Fracture pain* is sharp and piercing and is relieved by immobilization.

Sharp pain may also result from *bone infection* with muscle spasm or pressure on a sensory nerve.

Most musculoskeletal pain is relieved by rest. Pain that increases with activity may indicate joint sprain or muscle strain, while steadily increasing pain points to a progression of an infectious process (osteomyelitis), a malignant tumor, or vascular complications. Radiating pain is seen in conditions in which pressure is exerted on a nerve root. Pain is variable, and its assessment and nursing management must be individualized.

Assessment of Pain

- What was the patient doing before the complaint of pain?
- Is the body in proper alignment?
- Is there pressure from traction, bed linen, a cast, or other appliances?
- Is the position of a muscle mass causing tension on the skin at a pin site?
- Is the patient overly tired from lack of sleep, exciting stimuli, or too much activity?
- Can the pain be localized?
- How does the patient describe it?
- What was the manner of onset?
- Is there radiation of pain? If so, in what direction does it occur?
- Is there pain in any other part of the body?
- What is the character of the pain (sharp, dull, boring, shooting, throbbing, cramping)?
- Is it constant?
- What relieves it?
- What makes it worse?

Pain and discomfort are important to the patient and must be managed successfully. Not only is pain exhausting, but if prolonged it can force the patient to become increasingly preoccupied and dependent.

Altered Sensations

Sensory disturbances are frequently associated with musculoskeletal problems. The patient may describe the presence of *paresthesias* (burning or tingling sensations) and numbness. These sensations may be due to pressure on nerves or circulatory impairment. Soft tissue swelling or direct trauma to these structures can impair their function. Assessment of the neurovascular status of the involved musculoskeletal area provides information for management. Loss of function can result from impaired nerves and circulatory structures located throughout the musculoskeletal system.

Assessment of Neurovascular Integrity

- Is the patient experiencing any abnormal sensations or numbness?
- When did this begin? Is it getting worse?
- Is the patient also experiencing pain?
- What is the color of the part distal to the problem? Pale? Dusky? Cyanotic?
- Is there a pulse present distal to the problem?
- Is there rapid capillary refill? (Compress the patient's nail and release. When pressure is released, the color of the nailbed should quickly assume a pink hue.)
- Is the motor component of the nerve intact? Is the patient able to move the innervated part?

- Is edema present?
- Is any constrictive device or clothing causing the nerve or vascular compression?
- Is it relieved by elevation of the affected part or modification of position?

▷ Nursing Diagnoses

Based on the nursing assessment data, the major nursing diagnoses for a patient with musculoskeletal dysfunction may include the following:

- Anxiety related to changes in body integrity
- Knowledge deficit of the therapeutic regimen
- Alteration in comfort related to musculoskeletal disorder
- Impaired physical mobility related to musculoskeletal impairment

▷ Planning and Implementation

▷ *Goals:* The major goals of the patient with musculoskeletal dysfunction may include reduced anxiety, understanding of the therapeutic regimen, relief of discomfort, and improved physical mobility.

Nursing Interventions

Reducing Anxiety. Musculoskeletal problems may be due to an acute traumatic injury or may be of a persistent, recurrent, long-term nature. The psychological and social/economic impact of the problem causes a variety of reactions in these patients. The nurse needs to assist the patient in coping with the problems associated with musculoskeletal dysfunction and the associated therapies.

Most patients with acute musculoskeletal problems are anxious and have pain. They experience a curious mixture of fear and anticipation before definitive therapy begins. People who have long-term disabilities frequently experience repeated reconstructive operations. They are familiar with the routines of the hospital and are concerned with the ultimate outcome of the procedure. Their patience and hope may be limited. Persons with musculoskeletal problems need an understanding, supportive nurse.

Patient Education. One way to aid these patients is to prepare them for the anticipated therapeutic modality. If patients are given information concerning preparatory measures and if they share in this preparation, they will be more inclined to accept the care given. Information about what to expect during and following the therapy will encourage active participation in the therapeutic regimen. When possible, specific information concerning anticipated equipment (*e.g.*, casts, traction), mobilization aids (*e.g.*, trapeze, walker, crutches), exercises (*e.g.*, quadriceps setting, deep breathing), and medications (*e.g.*, analgesics, antibiotics) should be shared with the patient. Cognitive preparation decreases anxiety and alerts patients as to what is expected of them and what is usually involved in recovery. At times patients can practice recuperative activities, such as using a urinal in a recumbent position, before they are immobilized and need to tend to basic bodily functions in unusual positions.

Relieving Pain and Discomfort. Patients who have bone and joint problems frequently experience severe pain.

Often the person who has undergone surgery to correct a foot condition is much more uncomfortable than one who has had extensive abdominal surgery. Narcotics and other pain-relieving measures are given as prescribed, taking into consideration the type and the site of the musculoskeletal problem and the patient's age. In the long-term patient, drug dependence may occur and poses a considerable problem.

Pain may result from associated problems rather than from the primary musculoskeletal problem. When it occurs under restrictive bandages or casts, the blood supply may be diminished and excruciating pain may result. Swelling will occur distal to the constriction. Capillary refill will be diminished, as evidenced by gently squeezing a fingernail or toenail until it blanches, and then releasing pressure and noting the time it takes for the normal color to return. (Color normally returns quickly, within about 3 seconds.) The skin will feel cool to the touch and will appear dusky, pale, or blue. Sensory or motor function may be altered or diminished.

Usually, swelling can be controlled and prevented by elevating the injured part slightly above the level of the heart and intermittently applying an ice pack to the injury for 20 to 30 minutes.

Prolonged pressure over bony prominences (e.g., heel, head of fibula, tibial tuberosity) may cause a burning type of pain. Relieving the pressure is necessary to relieve the pain and prevent further tissue damage.

Muscle spasm is another associated cause of pain. When a muscle is injured, the natural response of the muscle is to contract, thereby splinting and protecting the injured area. Prolonged muscle contraction is painful. Relaxation techniques, traction, or medications may be used to reduce pain from muscle spasm.

Additional information and guidelines to nursing management of the patient with pain are presented in Chapter 15.

Improving Mobility and Patient Rehabilitation. Throughout the treatment period, the nurse is concerned with health maintenance and ultimate restoration of function. The immobility necessitated by some treatment modalities must not result in undue deterioration. Exercise of nonimmobilized muscles and joints helps maintain their strength and function, minimizes cardiovascular deterioration, and prevents disuse osteoporosis. Isometric exercises of immobilized extremities help to maintain muscle strength.

Involvement in activities of daily living (e.g., hygiene, dressing, eating) provides a sense of independence and accomplishment. Coordinating nursing interventions with special therapy approaches (e.g., physical therapy, occupational therapy) makes it easier for the patient to learn and practice the therapeutic regimens. Emphasis is placed on what the patient is able to do within the limits of the treatment modalities.

Before the time of discharge, patients should have explicit instructions that they understand, indicating those activities they may and may not perform. It is not enough to bid them "goodbye, and take it easy." Patients must know any untoward signs and symptoms that should be reported to the physician. They must be aware of the importance of follow-up visits. If they have any difficulties, they ought to know where and how to get help. The nurse has a major part of the responsibility for educating these patients before they leave the hospital (see Chap. 14 Principles of Rehabilitation).

▷ **Evaluation**

▷ *Expected Outcomes*

1. Patient exhibits minimal anxiety.
   a. Appears relaxed and confident in abilities
   b. Utilizes effective coping strategies
   c. Participates in care
2. Relates plan for continued health management
   a. Describes planned treatment regimen
   b. States signs and symptoms to report to physician
   c. Makes appointment for follow-up care
3. Achieves comfort
   a. Controls discomfort with occasional oral medications
   b. Moves with minimal discomfort
   c. Utilizes positioning to increase comfort
4. Demonstrates improved physical mobility
   a. Transfers self independently or with minimal assistance
   b. Participates in activities of daily living
   c. Utilizes mobility aids safely

Management of the Patient in a Cast

A cast is a rigid external immobilizing device that is molded to the contours of the body to which it is applied. The purpose of a cast is to immobilize a body part in a specific position and to apply uniform pressure on encased soft tissue. It may be used to immobilize a reduced fracture, correct a deformity, apply uniform pressure to underlying soft tissue, or provide support and stability for weakened joints. Generally, casts permit mobilization of the patient while restricting movement of some body part.

Types of Casts

The condition being treated influences the type and thickness of the cast applied. Generally speaking, the joints proximal and distal to the area to be immobilized are included in the cast. However, with some fractures, cast construction and molding may allow movement of a joint while immobilizing a fracture (e.g., 3-point fixation in a patellar tendon weight-bearing cast).

Figure 56-1 illustrates some of the common types of cylindrical casts and areas in which pressure problems commonly occur.

Short arm cast—extends from below the elbow to the proximal crease, secured around the base of the thumb. If the thumb is included, it is known as a *thumb spica* or *gauntlet* cast.

Long arm cast—extends from the upper level of the axillary fold to the proximal palmar crease; the elbow usually is immobilized at a right angle

Short leg cast—extends from below the knee to the base of the toes. The foot is at a right angle in a neutral position.

Long leg cast—extends from the junction of the upper

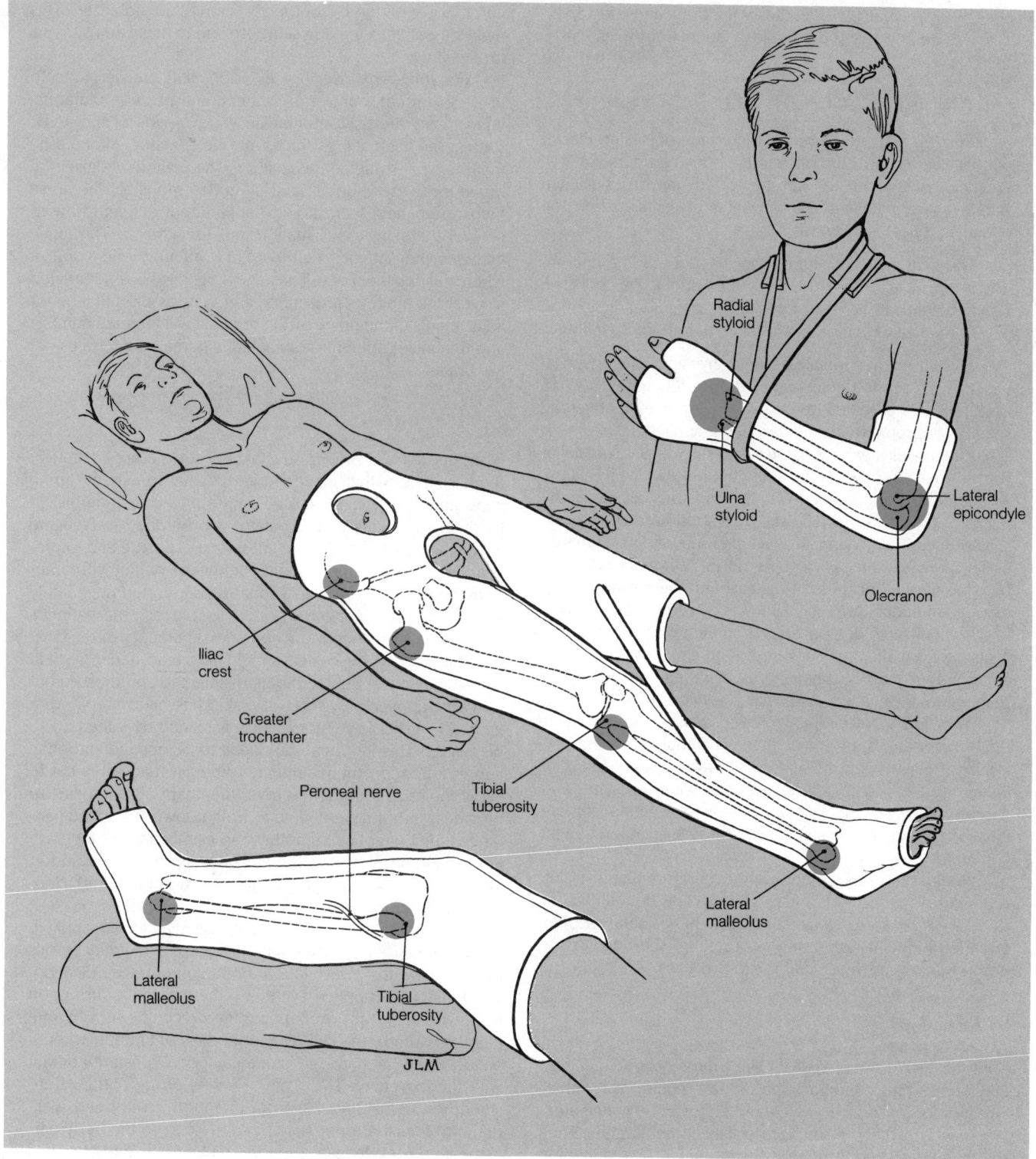

Figure 56-1
Pressure areas in different types of casts. (Brunner LS and Suddarth DS. The Lippincott
Manual of Nursing Practice, 4th ed. Philadelphia, JB Lippincott, 1986.)

and middle third of the thigh to the base of the
toes. The knee may be slightly flexed.
Walking cast—a short- or long-leg cast reinforced for
strength. It might incorporate a walking heel.
Body cast—encircles the trunk

Spica cast—incorporates a portion of the trunk and
one or two extremities (single or double spica cast)

· *Shoulder spica cast*—a body jacket that encloses
the trunk and the shoulder and elbow

- *Hip spica cast*—encloses the trunk and a lower extremity; may be a single or double hip spica cast

Casting Materials

Plaster. The traditional cast is made of plaster. Plaster bandages mold very smoothly to the body contours. Rolls of crinoline are impregnated with powdered, anhydrous calcium sulfate (gypsum crystals). When wet, a crystallizing reaction occurs and heat is given off.

- The heat given off during this reaction can be uncomfortable. Therefore, the water used should be cool. The cast needs to be exposed to allow maximum dissipation of the heat. Most casts are cool after about 15 minutes.

The crystallization produces a rigid dressing. The speed at which the reaction occurs varies from a few minutes to 15 to 20 minutes. The orthopedist will determine what setting speed is appropriate for the cast being applied.

After the plaster has set, the cast is still wet and somewhat soft. It does not have its full strength until dry. While damp, it can be dented if handled with the fingertips instead of the palms of the hand or if allowed to rest on hard surfaces or sharp edges. These dents produce pressure areas on the skin under the cast. The cast requires 24 to 72 hours to dry, depending on the thickness of the cast and the environmental drying conditions. A freshly applied cast should be exposed to circulating air to dry. Covers restrict the escape of moisture. A dry cast is white and shiny, resonant, and odorless as well as firm; a wet cast is gray and dull in appearance, is dull to percussion, feels damp, and has a musty odor.

Nonplaster. Generally referred to as *fiberglass casts*, these water-activated polyurethane materials have the versatility of plaster and the additional advantages of being of lighter weight and increased strength, water-resistant, and durable. They are made of an open-weave, nonabsorbent fabric impregnated with hardeners that reach full rigid strength in minutes.

Nonplaster casts are porous and therefore diminish skin problems. They do not soften when wet, which allows for *hydrotherapy* (use of water for treatment). When wet, they are dried with a hair drier on a cool setting. Thorough drying is important to prevent skin breakdown.

Splints and Braces

Contoured splints of plaster or pliable thermoplastic materials may be used for conditions that do not require rigid immobilization or for those in which swelling may be anticipated. The splints need to provide for adequate immobilization. They should be designed to support the body part in a functional position. The splints must be well padded to prevent pressure, skin abrasion, and skin breakdown. To avoid burns from the exothermic reaction of the plaster, cold water is used to make the splint and the heat is allowed to dissipate before the splint is overwrapped with an elastic bandage. The bandage is applied in a spiral fashion, and the pressure is uniform so that the circulation is not restricted. The circulatory status of the splinted extremity is assessed frequently by the nurse.

When soft immobilizers are used to support an injured body part, rigid immobilization is not achieved. Usually the extremity is wrapped with an elastic bandage and then secured to a padded, contoured, canvas immobilizer. This makes it easier to provide skin care and to make adjustments for swelling.

For long-term use, braces (*orthoses*) are designed to provide support, control movement, and prevent additional injury. They are custom-fitted to various parts of the body, such as the back of leg. Braces may be constructed of plastic materials or of metal and leather. The orthotist adjusts the brace for fit, positioning, and permitted mobility. The nurse helps the patient learn how to apply the brace and how to protect the skin from irritation and breakdown. The nurse assesses the patient's neurovascular integrity and comfort when wearing the brace. The patient needs to be encouraged to wear the brace as prescribed and to be assured that minor adjustments of the brace by the orthotist will increase comfort and minimize problems associated with the long-term use of the brace.

Cast Application

It is important to prepare the patient for the application of the cast. The patient needs to know what to expect during application, and that the casted body part will be immobilized following application. The patient is positioned to facilitate casting and is draped to prevent undue exposure and to prevent the plaster materials from coming in contact with other body parts. The body part should be supported adequately when the cast is applied in order to increase the patient's comfort and maintain reduction and alignment.

The part to be casted should be clean and dry. Skin abrasions, if present, need to be disinfected and dressed before cast application. When the skin has been prepared, a knitted material (*e.g.*, stockinette) is placed over the part to be casted. This knit material needs to be applied smoothly and in a nonconstrictive manner. Enough material is cut to allow the ends to be folded over the nearly finished cast to provide a smooth, padded edge. Soft, nonwoven, rolled padding is then wrapped smoothly and evenly around the part. Extra padding is placed around bony prominences and at nerve grooves (*e.g.*, head of fibula, olecranon process). Nonabsorbent materials are used with nonplaster casts.

When padding is adequate, the casting material is applied. The plaster and nonplaster materials come in bandaging rolls of various widths to facilitate smooth, contoured application. The bandage is applied evenly on the extremity, turn upon turn, with each turn overlapping the preceding turn by one half the width of the roll. The motion is continuous, without pause, while the bandage is maintained in constant contact with the extremity. The turns or layers of the bandage are smoothed and rubbed to form a smooth, solid, and well-contoured cast. Proper shaping of the cast to the body part is required for adequate support. At the joints and at points of anticipated cast stress, additional casting material (splints) is incorporated into the cast for additional strength.

During the application, care is taken to ensure that the body part is immobilized in the desired position. Improper extremity position can result in contracture or malunion of fractures.

To enhance comfort and the patient's ability to participate in activities, the cast must be "finished" properly. The edges need to be smooth and padded to prevent skin abrasion. Full range of motion of joints adjacent to the immobilized part needs to be assured. If necessary, the cast can be trimmed and reshaped with a cast knife or manual cutters to allow for full motion and to eliminate any restriction due to the cast.

Plaster materials that have adhered to the skin during application are removed. If not cleaned off, these will loosen, crumble, and slide underneath the cast, causing discomfort and possible skin breakdown.

▶ Nursing Process
The Patient in a Cast

▷ Assessment

The main concern following the application of a cast is to avoid complications. Experience has taught that any complaint of discomfort must not go unheeded. Two types of complications occur: constriction of circulation and pressure on tissues and bony parts.

Trauma or surgery affecting an extremity will produce swelling as a result of hemorrhage from bone and surrounding tissue and from tissue edema. Vascular insufficiency and nerve compression due to unrelieved swelling can reduce or cut off blood supply to an extremity and result in peripheral nerve damage.

The nurse monitors for pain, swelling, discoloration (paleness or blueness), tingling or numbness, diminished or absent pulses, paralysis, and coldness of the extremity. Signs of circulatory impairment are noted by assessing the toes or fingers of a leg or arm that has recently been placed in a cast. The toes and fingers should be pink in color and warm to the touch. The capillary refill response is another means of assessing circulatory insufficiency. The nail beds and the fleshy pulp of toes/fingers are pressed lightly and then released to check how quickly color returns. The color should return rapidly, indicating good perfusion. A blue tinge to the toes or fingers suggests venous obstruction, while white and cold fingers or toes suggest arterial obstruction. The temperature of the injured extremity is compared with that of the uninjured one, as are the pulses. Nerve status is assessed by asking the patient about sensations in the toes/fingers and ability to move (wiggle) toes/fingers. Inability to move the fingers or toes, pain on extension of the hand or foot, and coldness of an extremity indicate ischemia. If there is swelling, the cast will seem tight.

The pressure of the cast on neurovascular structures and bony structures causes necrosis, pressure sores, and nerve palsies or paralysis, such as may occur when a leg cast damages a peroneal nerve. A severe initial pain over bony prominences is a warning symptom of an impending pressure sore. *Pain decreases when ulceration occurs.* The nurse also monitors for an odor emanating from the cast and observes for drainage on the cast.

Sites most susceptible to pressure on the lower extremity are the heel, malleoli, dorsum of the foot, head of the fibula, and anterior surface of the patella. On the upper extremity, the main pressure sites are located at the medial epicondyle of the humerus and the ulnar styloid (see Fig. 56-1).

▷ Nursing Diagnoses

Based on all the assessment data, the patient's major nursing diagnoses may include the following:

- Alteration in comfort (pain; paresthesias) related to cast pressure
- Alteration in tissue perfusion (peripheral) related to cast pressure
- Potential alteration in skin integrity related to cast pressure
- Impaired physical mobility related to presence of cast
- Knowledge deficit concerning cast management

▷ Planning and Implementation

▷ *Goals:* The goals of the patient may include achievement of comfort, attainment of tissue perfusion, attainment of skin integrity, achievement of mobility, and acquiring knowledge of cast management.

Nursing Interventions

Promoting Comfort, Tissue Perfusion, and Skin Integrity

Although it takes minutes for a cast to harden, it will take 24 to 72 hours for the plaster cast to dry and achieve maximum strength. A moist cast is handled with the palms of the hands and should not rest on a hard surface or sharp edge, which may dent the cast and cause pressure areas. If ice bags are prescribed, they may be applied (⅓ to ½ full) to each side of the cast, making sure that they do not make indentations in the plaster.

The affected extremity is elevated above the level of the heart on cloth-covered pillows to control swelling. The patient is encouraged to wiggle fingers/toes. If any symptom such as blueness/paleness of fingernails/toenails accompanied by pain and tightness, numbness, cold, or tingling sensations occurs, the physician should be notified. The capillary refill response is checked frequently for signs of circulatory impairment.

If the patient complains of pain, analgesics are not given until the cause of pain is determined. The first step in determining the cause is to ask the patient to indicate the exact site of pain.

- *Do not ignore the complaints of pain of the patient in a cast: suspect circulatory complications or a pressure sore.*

If the patient continues to have pain, the cast may be exerting pressure on a nerve, blood vessels, or bony prominences.

- Unrelieved pain, excessive swelling, poor capillary refill response, or inability to move toes/fingers must be reported to the physician immediately to avoid possible paralysis and necrosis.
- If constriction of circulation is suspected, the cast may need to be bivalved (cut in half) to relieve pressure. Bivalving a cast does not disturb the alignment of the fracture.

The procedure for bivalving a cast is as follows:

1. A longitudinal cut is made in the cast, dividing it into two halves.
2. The underlying padding is also cut, since blood-soaked padding may shrink and constrict the circulation.
3. The cast is spread apart sufficiently to relieve constriction.

4. The anterior and posterior parts of the cast may be held together with an elastic compression bandage.
5. After the cast is bivalved, the extremity is elevated until the circulation is restored, swelling diminishes, and pain is relieved.

Another method of checking the cause for discomfort or for viewing a surgical wound is to cut an opening or "a window" in the cast. The orthopedic surgeon carries out this procedure by cutting a small oblong or square piece of the cast, which can be removed and then replaced. After the window is opened, a soft pad is inserted into the opening and the "window" is replaced with tape to prevent the underlying tissue from swelling through the window and forming pressure areas around its margins.

The skin around the cast edges is inspected periodically for signs of irritation. Rough edges of the cast may be covered with tape to protect the skin.

Promoting Mobility

While in a cast, the patient should be taught to tense or contract muscles without moving the joints. The patient may actually forget how to "will" a motion through the central nervous system pathways to the immobilized muscle. Therefore, *isometric muscle contractions* (contracting the muscle without moving the part) may be carried out to prevent atrophy and maintain muscle strength (Chart 56-1). Isometric contractions should be done at least hourly while the patient is awake.

• If the patient has a leg cast, place your hand under the knee and instruct the patient to "push down."

Chart 56-1
Muscle Setting Exercises

Isometric contraction of the muscle maintains muscle mass and strength and prevents atrophy.

Quadriceps-Setting Exercises

• Position patient supine with leg extended.
• Instruct patient to push knee back onto the mattress by contracting the anterior thigh muscles.
• Encourage patient to hold the position for 5 to 10 seconds.
• Let patient relax.
• Repeat exercise 10 times each hour when patient is awake.

Gluteal-Setting Exercises

• Position patient supine with legs extended, if possible.
• Instruct patient to contract muscles of buttocks and abdomen.
• Encourage patient to hold the contraction for 5 to 10 seconds.
• Let patient relax.
• Repeat exercise 10 times each hour when patient is awake.

• If the patient has an arm cast, instruct him to "make a fist."

At times, portable electrical muscle stimulators may have been attached to the skin over large muscles prior to casting. Muscle contractions are electrically stimulated for about 8 hours a day to prevent the development of disuse atrophy.

Every joint that is not immobilized may be exercised. The patient is encouraged to exercise toes/fingers frequently and actively. Encourage the patient to participate in goal-setting and self-care activities. It is important that the patient remain actively involved so that an untoward psychological reaction (*e.g.*, depression) associated with immobility, dependence, and loss of control is avoided.

Patient Education and Home Health Care

When the cast is dry, the patient is instructed as follows:

1. Move about as normally as possible. Avoid excessive use of the injured extremity.
2. Perform the prescribed exercises faithfully.
3. Elevate the casted extremity above heart level frequently to prevent swelling.
4. Keep the cast dry.
   a. Wetness destroys the hardness of plaster casts.
      (1) Do not cover the cast with plastic or rubber, as this causes condensation and wetting of the cast.
      (2) Avoid walking on wet floors or sidewalks.
   b. Fiberglass casts, after being wet, must be dried thoroughly with a hair drier on a cool setting to avoid skin problems.
5. Cushion rough edges of the cast with tape.
6. Report to the physician if the cast breaks; do not attempt to fix it yourself.
7. To clean a cast:
   a. Remove surface soil with a damp cloth.
   b. Stained areas may be touched up with a thin layer of white shoe polish.
8. Do not attempt to scratch the skin under the cast. This may cause a break in the skin and result in the formation of a cast sore. Cool air from a hair drier may alleviate an itch.
9. Note odors about the cast, cast staining areas, warm spots, and pressure spots. Report them to the physician.
10. Report to the physician: persistent pain, swelling that does not respond to elevation, changes in sensation, decreased ability to move exposed fingers/toes, and changes in skin color and temperature.

Removing a Cast

A cast may be removed with a *cast cutter*—an electric saw with a circular blade that oscillates through the plaster. Before the procedure, the patient should be assured that the cast cutter will not cut the body. The usual method of cutting the cast is to bivalve it. The cast is cut by a series of alternating pressures and linear movements of the blade along the line of the cut. If the saw blade is left against the padding too long, the patient will feel a burning sensation on the skin from the rapidly oscillating blade. Be sure to protect the patient's eyes from flying cast particles during the cast-cutting procedure. As a last step, the padding is cut with scissors.

Management of the Patient After the Cast is Removed. Remember when a cast is removed that the part or parts involved have been immobilized for a considerable period of time. When the support and protection of the cast have been removed, stresses and strains are placed on parts that have been at rest. The patient complains of pain and stiffness, often much different from the original injury, and may be depressed and discouraged because the anticipated release from the cast has only added problems to the situation.

To help the patient adjust to this new discomfort, the nurse may support the part so that it is maintained in the same position as when in the cast. A small pillow can be used to support the knee, the lumbar spine, and like body parts. The support is then gradually removed. When the extremity is moved, adequate support must be provided. Exercises are prescribed to redevelop and to increase strength. The patient who has been doing isometric muscle contractions will not have to relearn to contract the muscles and will progress more rapidly with the rehabilitation program.

Once the cast is removed, there will be a considerable amount of desquamated epithelium (dead skin) that may adhere to the skin surface. The skin is washed carefully and blotted dry, and some type of emollient lotion is applied. The patient should be cautioned against rubbing or scratching the skin, which could cause a break in the skin.

Atrophy of the part may be noted, but this disappears gradually with the return of muscle function. Swelling after a cast is removed is common, and is treated by elevating and supporting the tissues with elastic bandages or an elastic stocking.

If a new cast is to be applied, the patient's skin should be washed and dried carefully. The patient will need to be reminded again of the care of wet casts, needed neurovascular observations, and general cast care instructions.

Patient Education After Cast Removal

1. Cleanse the skin gently with bland soap and water. Blot dry.
2. Apply emollient lotion. Avoid scratching the skin.
3. Resume activities and exercise gradually.
4. Control swelling by elevating the extremity above heart level, and use elastic bandages as directed.

▷ *Evaluation*

▷ *Expected Outcomes*

1. Patient maintains adequate circulation to extremity.
   a. Is free of pain
   b. Has normal skin color
   c. Demonstrates skin temperature of injured extremity that is similar to that of uninjured extremity
   d. Achieves satisfactory capillary refill on testing
2. Shows no signs of necrosis, pressure sores, or nerve paralysis
   a. Is free of pain over bony prominences
   b. Demonstrates normal sensory and motor function of injured extremity
   c. Shows no evidence of musty cast odors, cast staining, or warm spots on cast
   d. Exhibits intact skin

3. Appears to have adequate knowledge about therapeutic regimen
   a. Elevates extremity that is in the cast
   b. Exercises according to instructions
   c. Keeps cast dry
   d. Reports any problems that develop
   e. Keeps follow-up clinic or physician appointments

Arm Casts

The patient whose arm is immobilized in a cast must readjust to many routine tasks. The unaffected arm must assume all the upper extremity activities. The patient may experience muscle fatigue due to the additional activities and the weight of the cast. Frequent rest periods are necessary.

To diminish and control swelling when the patient is lying down, the arm is elevated, with each joint positioned higher than the preceding proximal joint (*e.g.*, elbow higher than the shoulder, hand higher than the elbow). When the patient becomes ambulatory, a sling may be used. To minimize venous congestion and edema, the extremity should be higher than the level of the heart. Thus, the patient should be encouraged to remove the arm from the sling frequently and to extend it above the head.

Slings should distribute the supported weight over a large area and not on the back of the neck. Triangular cloth slings, when used, need to be pinned at the sides and not tied with a knot behind the neck, to prevent pressure on cervical spinal nerves.

Circulatory disturbances in the hand may become apparent with signs of cyanosis, swelling, and an inability to move the fingers.

- One serious effect of circulatory constriction in an arm cast is *Volkmann's contracture*, a compartment syndrome (see Fig. 57-5). Contracture of the fingers and wrist occurs as the result of ischemia due to the obstruction of arterial flow to the forearm and hand. The patient is unable to extend the fingers, describes abnormal sensation, and presents signs of diminished circulation to the hand.

  This serious complication can be prevented by nursing surveillance and proper care. Neurovascular checks need to be made frequently. Tissue pressure within muscle compartments may be measured directly, using a manometer setup. Constricting casts and dressings need to be removed and a fasciotomy may be necessary to improve vascular status and prevent permanent damage, which will develop within a few hours if no action is taken.

Leg Casts

The application of a leg cast imposes a degree of immobility on the patient. The leg cast may be a short leg cast, extending to the knee, or a long leg cast, extending to the groin. The fresh cast must be handled in a manner that will not cause denting or disruption.

As with other cast applications, the leg must be assessed for swelling, adequate circulation, and normal nerve function.

The leg is supported on soft pillows above heart level to control swelling. Ice packs may be applied over the fracture site for the first day or two. The circulation is assessed by observing the color, temperature, and capillary refill of the exposed toes. Nerve function is assessed by observing the patient's ability to move the toes and by asking about the sensations in the foot. Numbness, tingling, and burning may be due to peroneal nerve injury from pressure at the head of the fibula.

· Injury to the peroneal nerve as a result of pressure is a common cause of footdrop.

When the cast is dry, the patient is taught how to transfer and ambulate safely with walking aids (*e.g.*, crutches, walker). The gait to be used depends on whether or not the patient's problem allows weight-bearing. If weight-bearing is allowed, the cast will be reinforced to withstand the body weight. A walking heel (a rubber pad) may be incorporated into the bottom of the cast, or the patient may be given a cast boot to wear over the casted foot (Fig. 56-2). Cast boots are preferred to walking heels because they provide a broader support surface and do not disturb the patient's balance or posture by elevating the injured leg.

After ambulation begins, encourage elevation of the cast when the patient is seated. Several times during the day, the patient should lie down, because a sitting position does not promote complete drainage. If the skin has become irritated at the cast edges, moleskin padding may be added.

Cast Brace

A cast brace is a special type of cast in which hinges are incorporated to allow for joint motion while providing adequate alignment and immobilization (Fig. 56-3). Some cast braces are constructed with hinges at the hip, knee, ankle,

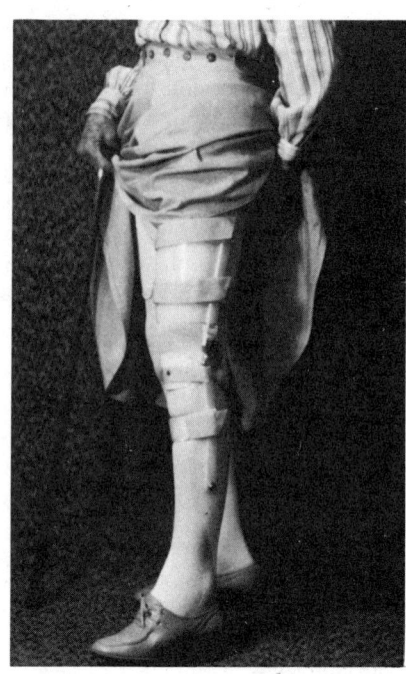

Figure 56-3
A type of cast brace. This molded plastic knee–ankle–foot orthosis with total contact femoral section orthosis is useful when long-term (greater than 6-month) immobilization is required. It is removable by the patient. (Courtesy The University of Texas Health Science Center at Dallas.)

elbow, or wrist. Most frequently, cast braces are used when femoral shaft fractures demonstrate some healing and little thigh swelling. Usually, the patient has been in skeletal traction for a few weeks prior to cast brace application.

The application of a cast brace includes the following: A 10-cm (4-inch) elastic bandage may be applied to the knee area to minimize swelling. A circumferential thigh cast and a short leg walking cast are applied. Hinges (metal or polypropylene) are placed on each side of the knee and incorporated into the cast. They allow flexion movements.

Fracture healing is enhanced with cast braces. Weight-bearing (stress) stimulates bone healing. In addition, the cast brace produces hydraulic pressure on the soft tissues, which facilitates fracture healing.

The patient managed with a cast brace is better able to maintain physiologic homeostasis. Rehabilitation is promoted by maintaining muscle strength and joint mobility. After the cast is dry (about 48 hours for plaster cast braces), the patient can ambulate with crutches, using a three-point gait (see p. 236) progressing from partial to full weight-bearing on the fractured extremity.

Problems that the patient may have after cast brace application include angulation deformity of the fracture site (malalignment of bone resulting in a bend in the bone), edema about the knee, skin breakdown on the thigh as a result of pressure from the edge of the cast, and soiling of the thigh cast. The patient is monitored for excessive swelling, neurovascular problems, and skin breakdown. Since the cast may extend to the groin, measures should be taken to protect this

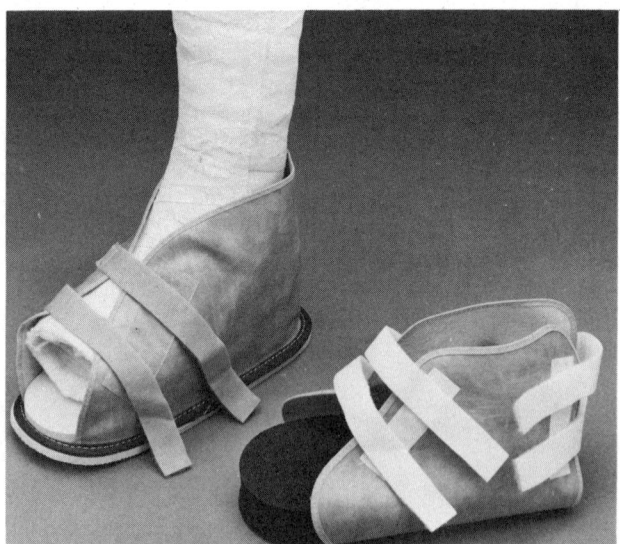

Figure 56-2
Two types of cast boots. (Courtesy Srouse Manufacturing, Inc, Ligonier, Indiana.)

area of the cast from becoming soiled with urine and feces. To promote venous return, the cast brace is elevated when the patient is not walking.

Body or Spica Casts

Casts that encase the trunk (*body cast*) and portions of the trunk and one or two extremities (*spica cast*) require special nursing techniques. Body casts may be used in situations requiring spinal immobility. Hip spicas are used for patients following femoral fractures and some hip joint surgeries. Shoulder spica casts are used for some humeral neck fractures. Patient preparation, turning, and skin and hygienic care are the nurse's concern.

Prepare the patient for the casting procedure by explaining the procedure. This will help reduce the patient's apprehension about being encased in a large cast. Often the patient has been immobilized in traction for weeks, and anticipates recurrence of pain while being moved for casting. Also, the fracture table used for large cast application looks like a torture device. Saying that the patient will be cared for by several people during the application and that support for the injured body will be adequate and as gentle as possible will help to allay fear. Medications for pain and relaxation administered prior to the procedure will help the patient relax, be comfortable, and cooperate during the procedure. Information concerning the casting procedure will help prepare the patient.

Following cast application, the patient needs to be supported by flexible, waterproof pillows until the cast is dry to prevent it from being dented. Inadequate cast support will cause a soft cast to crack or become dented, resulting in subsequent pressure points. The bed receiving the freshly casted patient needs to have firm mattress support. Three pillows placed crosswise on the bed will suffice for the body cast; for a hip spica, one pillow placed crosswise at the waist and two pillows placed lengthwise for the affected leg are necessary. If both legs are involved, two additional pillows are necessary. It is important that the pillows be next to each other, because any spaces in between will allow the damp cast to sag, become weak, and possibly break. It is also important to see that a pillow is not placed under the head and shoulders (of a patient in a body cast) while the cast is drying, since this causes pressure on the chest.

Patients are turned every 2 hours to relieve pressure and to allow the cast to dry. Sufficient personnel (at least three people) are needed when the patient is turned so that the fresh cast can be adequately supported with the palms of the hands. Vulnerable points in the cast are located at the body joints and need to be supported to prevent the cast from cracking. The patient is encouraged to assist in the repositioning by using the trapeze or bedrail. An abduction bar might be incorporated in spica casts to stabilize cast positioning. This bar is NOT to be used as a turning device. Pillows are readjusted so that support is provided and no pressure areas are present. The patient is turned as a unit toward the uninjured side to prevent stress on the cast and twisting of the body within the cast.

The patient is turned to a prone position, twice daily if tolerated, in order to provide postural drainage of the bronchial tree and relieve pressure on the back. A small pillow under the abdomen will be an added comfort measure. Placing a pillow lengthwise under the dorsum of the feet will prevent the toes from being forced into the mattress. Allowing the toes to hang over the edge of the mattress is a welcome change.

Turning the Patient in a Hip Spica Cast
1. The patient is moved with a steady, even, pulling motion to the side of the bed.
2. Pillows are placed along the other side of the bed for cast support.
3. Instruct the patient to assist by using the arm on the involved side to pull the shoulder over when turning.
4. Two nurses are on the side to which the patient is being turned to provide support for the cast while rolling the patient toward them.
5. The third nurse assists in rolling the patient from behind, adjusts the patient's shoulder, and adjusts the pillows.
6. The patient's body should be turned as a unit and positioned comfortably in good alignment.

The skin around the edges of the cast must be inspected frequently for signs of irritation. Some of the area under the cast can be inspected by pulling the skin taut and using a flashlight. Reaching under the cast edges with the fingers allows for removal of cast crumbs and massage of the skin. Accessible skin should be bathed carefully and massaged with an emollient.

The area around the perineum needs to be protected from excreta. If the opening in the cast is inadequate for hygienic care, the nurse needs to see that this part of the cast is adjusted. When the cast is dry, the perineum is covered with a towel and the perineal area of the cast is sprayed with a plastic aerosol spray. Clean, dry, plastic sheeting can be inserted under the cast and brought over the cast edge before each elimination to protect the cast from soiling. Fracture bed pans are easier for hip spica patients to use. Good perineal care is essential.

Cast Syndrome

Patients immobilized in large casts may develop psychological and physiological responses to the confinement. The psychological component of cast syndrome is similar to a claustrophobic reaction. The patient exhibits an acute anxiety reaction characterized by behavioral changes and autonomic responses (*e.g.*, increased respiratory rate, diaphoresis, dilated pupils, increased heart rate, elevated blood pressure). The nurse needs to recognize the anxiety reaction and provide an environment in which the patient feels secure.

The physiological responses to large casts are associated with the imposed immobility. With decreased physical activity, gastrointestinal motility decreases. With accumulation of intestinal gases, pressure increases and actual ileus occurs. The patient has distention, abdominal discomfort, nausea, and vomiting. As with other adynamic ileus situations, the patient is treated conservatively with decompression (nasogastric intubation connected to suction) and intravenous fluid therapy until gastrointestinal motility is restored. If the cast restricts the abdomen, a window needs to be cut in the cast over the abdominal area. Occasionally, the condition will progress to complete obstruction or the bowel may become gangrenous. Then surgical intervention is required.

The nurse needs to be aware of the possible development of cast syndrome in patients with large casts and to provide for its prevention or resolution.

Management of the Patient in Traction

Traction is the application of a pulling force to a part of the body. Traction is used to minimize muscle spasms; to reduce, align, and immobilize fractures; to lessen deformity; and to increase space between opposing surfaces within a joint. Traction must be applied in the desired direction and magnitude to obtain the therapeutic effects. Factors that reduce the effective pull of the traction must be eliminated.

At times, the traction needs to be applied in more than one direction to achieve the desired line of pull. When this is done, part of one of the lines of pull counteracts the other line of pull. These lines of pull are known as the *vectors of force.* The actual resultant pulling force is somewhere between the two lines of pull (Fig. 56-4). The effects of applied traction are evaluated with x-ray, and adjustments may be necessary. As the muscle and soft tissue relax, the amount of weight used may be changed to obtain the desired pulling force.

Types of Traction

Straight or running traction applies the pulling force in a straight line with the body part resting on the bed. Buck's extension traction (Fig. 56-5) and pelvic traction are examples of straight traction.

Balanced suspension traction (Fig. 56-6) supports the extremity (being treated) off the bed and allows for some patient mobility without disruption of the line of pull.

Traction may be applied to the skin (*skin traction*) or directly to the bony skeleton (*skeletal traction*). The mode of application is determined by the purpose of the traction.

Traction can be applied with the hands (*manual traction*). This is a very temporary traction that may be used when applying a cast, giving skin care under foam boots, or adjusting traction apparatus.

Principles of Effective Traction

Whenever traction is applied, the *countertraction* must be considered. Countertraction is the force acting in the opposite direction. (Newton's third law of motion states that for every action there is an equal and opposite reaction.) Generally, the patient's body weight and bed position adjustments supply the needed countertraction.

- Countertraction must be maintained for effective traction.

For traction to be effective in reducing fractures and in providing immobilization, it must be *continuous*. Pelvic and cervical skin tractions are frequently used to reduce muscle spasm and are usually prescribed as an intermittent traction.

- Never interrupt skeletal traction.
- Do not remove weight unless the traction is prescribed intermittently.

Maintain the line of pull. Any factor that might reduce the pull or alter its resultant line of pull must be eliminated.

- The patient is centered in bed and in good body alignment when traction is applied.
- Weights should hang free and not rest on the bed or floor.
- Ropes should be unobstructed in straight alignment.
- Knots in the rope or the footplate do not touch the pulley or the foot of the bed.

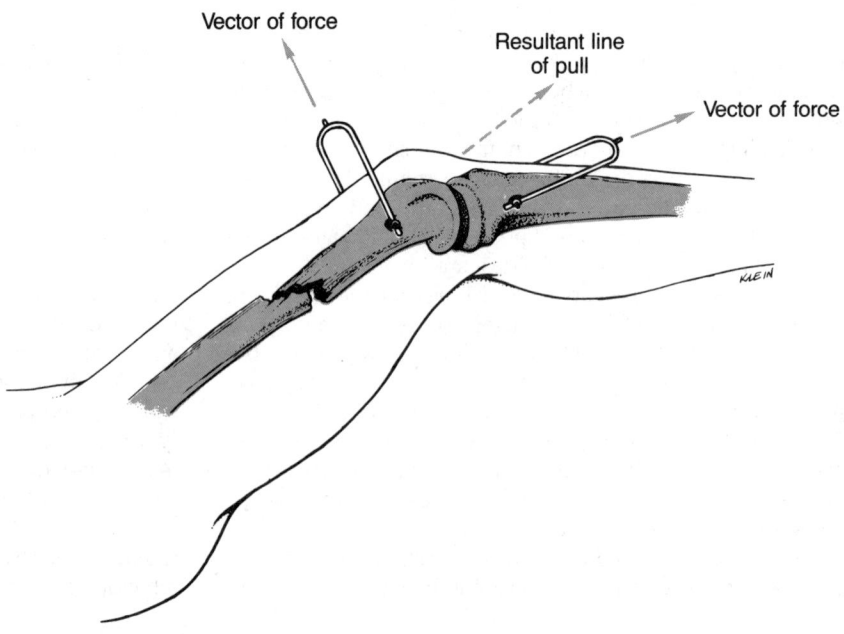

Vector of force

Resultant line of pull

Vector of force

KLEIN

Figure 56-4
Traction may be applied in different directions to achieve the desired therapeutic line of pull. Adjustments in applied forces may be prescribed over the treatment period.

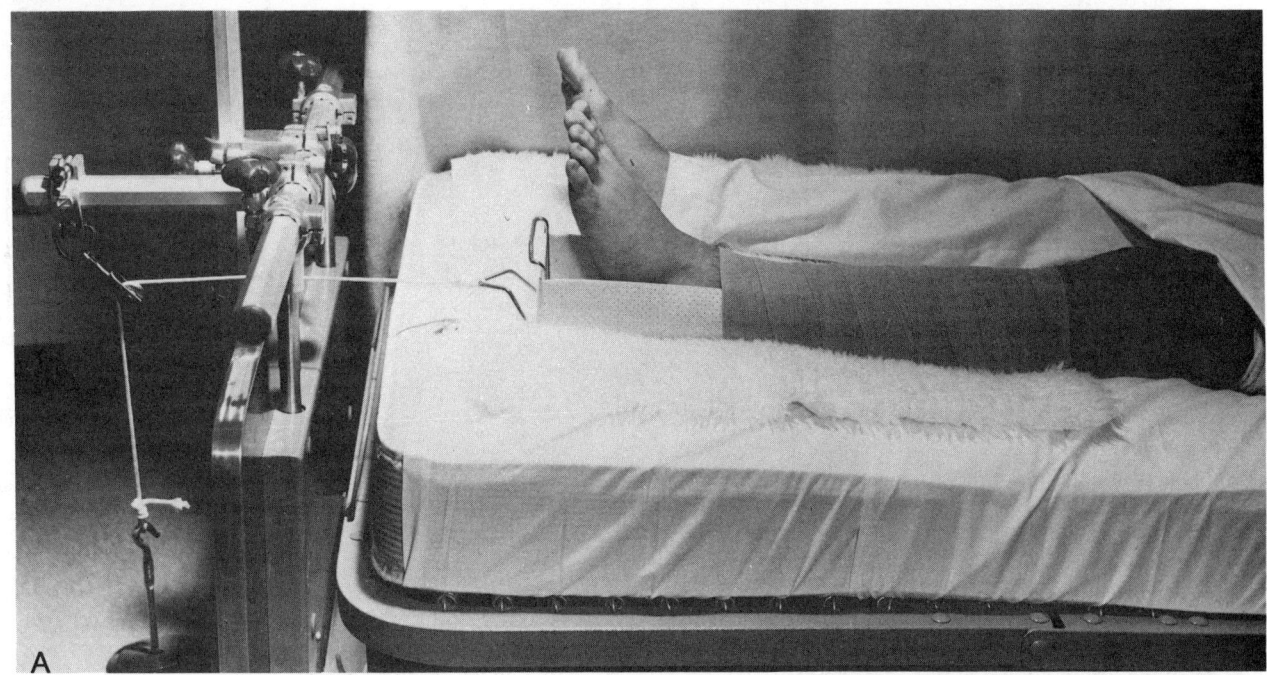

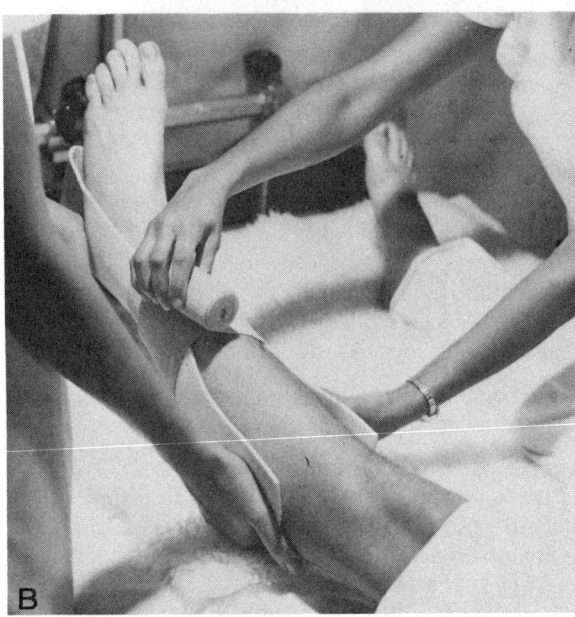

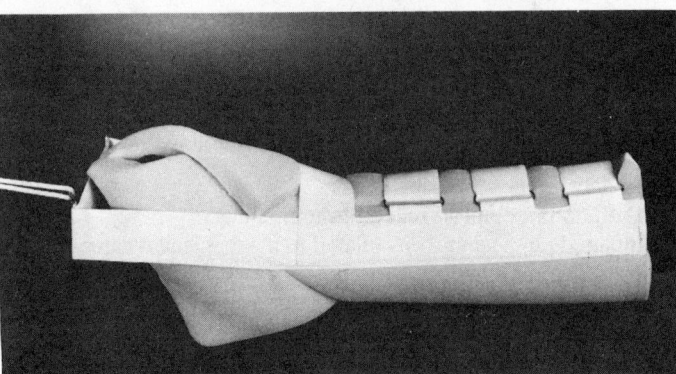

Figure 56-5
Buck's extension. (*A*) Lower extremity in Buck's extension traction. (*B*) Applying elastic bandage for Buck's extension traction. (*C*) Prepadded boot that may be used in Buck's extension. (Photo of boot courtesy of All Orthopedic Appliances.)

- The resultant line of pull should be in line with the long axis of the bone.
- The patient must be helped to maintain a therapeutic position.

▶ *Nursing Process*
The Patient in Traction

▷ *Assessment*

The application of traction results in impaired physical mobility and can be a frightening experience. The equipment looks threatening. The patient's anxiety level needs to be assessed. Additionally, the physiological impact on the patient of the immobilization, the traction device, and the musculoskeletal problem must be considered.

The nurse needs to assess the skin integrity of the extremity to be placed in traction. Its neurovascular status (*i.e.*, color, temperature, capillary refill, edema, pulses, sensations, and ability to move) is assessed, and compared with that of the unaffected extremity. The alignment of the body part in traction must be maintained as prescribed. Systemic assessment is appropriate. A patient may have problems with the skin, respiration, gastrointestinal tract, or urinary tract when immobilized in traction. Development of deep vein thrombosis is assessed by checking for calf tenderness and a positive *Homans's sign* (discomfort in the calf when the foot is forcibly

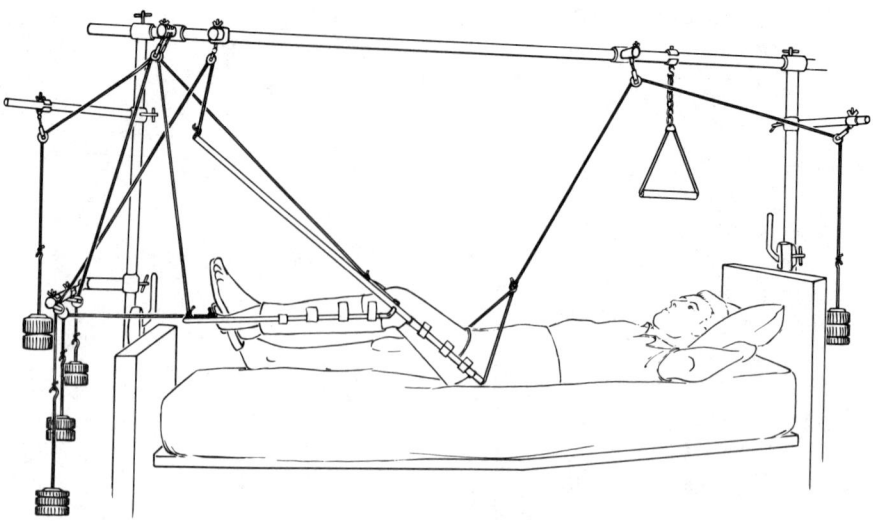

Figure 56-6
Principles of balanced suspension traction with Thomas leg splint. Vertical movement of the patient is permitted as long as resultant line of pull is maintained. In the nursing management of the patient in traction, one has to understand the direction in which the force is operating. Study the line drawing carefully. Notice that the force produced by the weights is changed in direction by the pulleys.

dorxiflexed). Confusion, disorientation, and behavioral problems may develop which are related to confinement in a limited space for an extended period of time.

▷ *Nursing Diagnoses*

Based on the nursing assessment, the patient's major nursing diagnoses related to traction may include the following:

- Anxiety related to health status
- Alteration in comfort related to immobility
- Impaired physical mobility related to mechanical devices restricting mobility
- Knowledge deficit of the treatment regimen
- Self-care deficit related to traction devices

▷ *Planning and Implementation*

▷ *Goals:* The major goals of the patient in traction may include reducing anxiety, increasing comfort, increasing mobility, understanding the rationale for traction interventions, and increasing the ability to perform self-care.

Nursing Interventions

Reducing Anxiety. Prior to the application of any traction, the patient needs to be informed about the procedure, its purpose, and its implications. Talking to the patient about what is being done and why, helps to allay apprehension. After being in traction for a period of time, the patient may react to being confined to a limited space. Frequent visits by the nurse will reduce feelings of isolation and confinement. Family and friends should be encouraged to visit frequently for the same reason. Diversional activities that can be done within the limits of the traction are encouraged.

Increasing Comfort. Because the patient will be immobilized in bed, the mattress needs to be firm and supported with a bed board. Special mattress pads designed to minimize the development of pressure sores should be placed on the bed before application of the traction.

- The patient's skin should be examined frequently for evidence of pressure or friction over bony prominences.

- Pressure on dependent body parts can be relieved by turning and by positioning the patient for comfort within the limits of the traction.
- The bed linens need to be kept wrinkle-free and dry.

The problems associated with immobility that affect other body systems and cause the patient discomfort are minimized through active preventive nursing measures. Deep-breathing exercises that aid in full expansion of the lungs are taught; ankle and foot exercises possible within the limits of the traction decrease venous stasis and the development of deep vein thrombosis; adequate fluid intake ensures urine flow and aids in preventing constipation. The nurse assesses the function of each body system in order to identify alterations in function. The patient is monitored closely for the development of complications associated with immobility.

- Every complaint of the patient in traction is to be investigated immediately.

Improving Mobility Within the Limits of Traction. During traction therapy, the patient needs to exercise non-immobilized muscles and joints to diminish their deterioration due to immobilization. Active motion of all unaffected joints is encouraged. The physical therapist can be consulted to design bed exercises that minimize loss of muscle strength. The nurse needs to encourage and support the patient in exercising. During exercising, the nurse must ensure that traction forces are maintained and that the patient is properly positioned to prevent complications resulting from poor alignment.

Patient Education. The patient must accurately perceive the rationale for the use of traction. The information needs to be repeated and reinforced frequently. With increased understanding of the therapy, patients become active participants in their own health care.

Improving Self-Care. Initially the patient may require much assistance with self-care activities. The nurse will help the patient learn how to provide for such needs as eating, bathing, dressing, and toileting while immobilized in the traction device. Devices such as patient reachers and an overbed trapeze to facilitate self-care may be useful. The patient will feel less dependent and less frustrated and will experience improved self-esteem with resumption of self-care activities.

Some assistance will be required throughout the period of immobility; however, the nurse and the patient can creatively develop routines that will maximize the patient's independence.

▷ *Evaluation*

▷ *Expected Outcomes*

1. Patient's anxiety is reduced.
   a. Patient appears relaxed.
   b. Uses effective coping mechanisms
   c. Expresses concerns and feelings
2. Feels increased comfort
   a. Expresses comfort
   b. Develops no pressure sores
   c. Avoids problems related to immobility
3. Demonstrates increased mobility
   a. Performs prescribed exercises
   b. Uses assistive devices
4. Understands rationale for traction interventions
   a. Describes traction regimen
   b. Participates in plan of care
5. Shows increased ability to perform self-care
   a. Feeds, bathes, dresses, and toilets self with minimal assistance

Specific Traction Applications

Skin Traction

Skin traction is accomplished by a weight pulling on tape, sponge rubber, or plastic materials that have been attached to the skin. Traction on the skin transmits traction to the musculoskeletal structures. However, only limited traction can be applied with skin traction. The amount of weight applied must not exceed the tolerance of the skin. No more than 2 to 3 kg (4.5–7 lbs) of traction can be used on an extremity. Pelvic traction is generally 4.5 to 9 kg (10–20 lbs), depending on the weight of the patient. Therefore, when prolonged or heavy traction weight is necessary, skeletal traction is used rather than skin traction.

Two forms of skin traction used for adults are *Russell's traction* and *Buck's extension traction*.

Russell's Traction. Russell's traction, which may be used for fractures of the tibial plateau, supports the flexed knee in a sling and applies the horizontal pulling force to the lower leg. If prescribed, the leg may be supported by a pillow to assure proper knee flexion and to prevent pressure on the heel.

Buck's Traction. Buck's extension (unilateral or bilateral) is a form of skin traction in which the pull is exerted in one plane when partial or temporary immobilization is desired (see Fig. 56-5*A*). It is used following injuries to the hip while the patient is awaiting surgical fixation.

Before the traction is applied, the skin is inspected for abrasions and circulatory disturbances, since the skin and circulation must be in healthy condition to tolerate the traction. The extremity should be clean and dry before the traction tape or a foam boot is applied (Fig. 56-5*B, C*).

To apply Bucks traction with tape, foam-rubber-padded straps are applied with the foam surface against the skin on each side of the affected leg. A loop of tape about 10 to 15 cm (4–6 inches) long is extended beyond the sole of the foot. The malleoli and proximal fibula are padded with cast padding to prevent pressure sores and skin necrosis. While one person elevates and supports the extremity under the patient's heel and knee, another person wraps the elastic bandage circumferentially over the traction tape, beginning at the ankle and wrapping up to the tibial tubercle. The elastic bandage helps the tape to adhere to the skin and prevents slipping. A spreader is applied to the distal end of the tape to prevent pressure along the side of the foot. A rope is attached to the spreader and passed over a pulley fastened to the end of the bed. Then a weight is attached to the rope. A sheepskin pad is placed under the leg to reduce the friction of the heel against the bed.

Skin and Nerve Pressure. Skin traction can irritate the skin and cause pressure on peripheral nerves. If skin tapes are used, the circumferential wrappings should not impair circulation, but must be firm enough to ensure that the tapes will remain in contact with the skin.

- To detect pressure points in skin traction, the area over the traction tapes should be palpated daily. The area over the Achilles tendon should be inspected several times daily because pressure in this region may occur when skin traction is applied to the leg. Care must be taken to avoid pressure on the peroneal nerve at the point at which it passes around the neck of the fibula just below the knee. Pressure at this point can cause footdrop (see Fig. 56-1). The patient needs to be asked about sensation and requested to move the toes and foot. Dorsiflexion of the foot—"point your toe at your nose"—demonstrates the function of the peroneal nerve. Plantar flexion demonstrates function of the tibial nerve.

  Assess for altered sensation, weakness of dorsiflexion or foot movement, and inversion of the foot, which might indicate pressure on the common peroneal nerve. Any complaint or burning sensation under the traction bandage is investigated immediately.
- When skin traction is applied to the arm, the area around the elbow where the ulnar nerve is located should not be wrapped tightly.
- Sensation and motion need to be assessed.
- Foam boots and wrappings applied around the leg should be removed and the skin inspected 3 times a day.
- A second nurse needs to support the extremity in position during skin inspection and care.
- Special care is given to the back at regular intervals, because the patient maintains a supine position.
- Prevent shearing forces on the skin.

Circulation. Following application of skin traction, the foot or hand is inspected for circulatory difficulties within a few minutes and then every 2 hours.

- Check peripheral pulses and the color, capillary refill, and temperature of the fingers or toes.
- Check for calf tenderness and for a positive Homans's sign for indications of thrombophlebitis.
- Encourage active foot exercise hourly.

Ensuring Effective Traction. To ensure effective traction, observe for wrinkling and slipping of the traction bandage and maintain counteraction. Proper positioning must also be maintained to keep the leg or arm in a neutral position.

The patient should not turn from side to side to prevent bony fragments from moving against one another.

Skeletal Traction

Skeletal traction is applied directly to the bone. This method of traction is used most frequently in the treatment of fractures of the femur, the humerus, the tibia, and the cervical spine. The traction is applied directly to the bone by use of a metal pin or wire (*e.g.,* Kirschner wire, Steinmann's pin) that is inserted through the bone distal to the fracture. Crutchfield or Gardner-Wells head tongs are fixed in the skull to apply traction that immobilizes cervical fractures.

The skeletal traction is applied under surgical asepsis. Patient preparation contributes to the patient's comfort and cooperation during the pinning procedure. Frequently, the skeletal traction is inserted on the patient care unit and not in the surgical suite.

The insertion site is prepared with surgical scrub, such as povidone-iodine. A local anesthetic is administered at the insertion site and periosteum. A small skin incision is made, and the sterile pin or wire is drilled through the bone. The patient feels pressure during this procedure and possibly some discomfort when the periosteum is penetrated.

Following insertion, the pin or wire is attached to the traction bow or caliper. The ends of the wire are covered with corks or tape to prevent injury to the patient. The weights are attached to the bow by a rope–pulley system that exerts the appropriate amount and direction of pull for effective traction. Skeletal traction frequently uses 7 to 12 kg (15–25 lbs) to secure the therapeutic effect. Often the skeletal traction is balanced traction, which supports the affected extremity and facilitates patient independence and nursing care while maintaining effective traction.

The *Thomas splint with the Pearson attachment* is frequently used with skeletal traction in fractures of the femur (see Fig. 56-6). It may be used with skin traction and other balanced suspension apparatus. Because upward traction is required, an overbed frame is utilized. Figure 56-7 shows suspension traction using slings.

The Pin Site.   The wound at the insertion site requires attention. Generally, the site is covered with a sterile dressing. Subsequent care of the pin site is individually prescribed. The area must be kept clean. It is assessed for odor and other signs of infection. The goal is to avoid infection and development of osteomyelitis. Slight serous oozing at the pin site is to be expected. This decreases the bacteria in the pin tract. Crusting is prevented, and the area is kept clean.

- Inspect the pin site daily for signs of inflammation and evidence of infection.

Neurovascular Status.   The skin around the traction device is inspected for signs of circulatory impairment. Neurovascular assessment of the immobilized extremity is conducted at least every 2 hours initially and later several times a day.

Pressure.   Specific pressure points need to be checked for redness and skin breakdown. Pressure areas caused by the traction apparatus may include the ischial tuberosity, popliteal space, Achilles tendon, and heel. The unsupported muscle may cause discomfort due to the tension at the pin.

Often patients use the heel of the good leg to act as a brace when they raise themselves. This digging of the heel into the mattress may cause injury to the tissues; hence, the heel must be massaged and inspected for pressure areas. If patients are unable to raise themselves, the nurse can push down on the mattresss with one hand, leaving space for the other hand to massage the back and bony prominences.

Positioning.   The foot should be positioned to avoid *footdrop* (plantar flexion), inward rotation (*inversion*), or outward rotation (*eversion*). The patient's foot may be supported in a neutral position by orthopedic devices (*e.g.,* foot supports). Frequent active flexion–extension ankle exercises are encouraged.

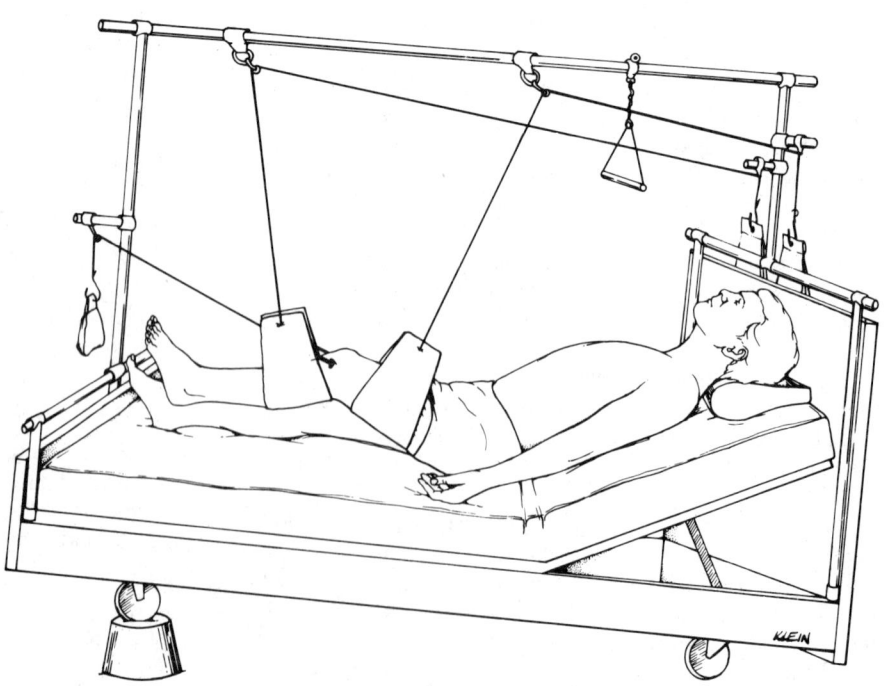

Figure 56-7
A type of balanced suspension traction for the lower extremity. Weights elevate the patient's injured leg which is supported in slings. Skeletal traction is applied.

Maintaining Effective Traction. When traction is being used, the apparatus is checked to see that the ropes are in the wheel groove of the pulleys; that the ropes are not frayed; that the weights hang freely; and that the patient has not slipped down in bed, causing ineffective traction. The knots in the rope are tied securely. Figure 56-8 suggests a secure knot-tying method.

The weights that are applied initially are sufficient to overcome the shortening spasms of the affected muscles. As muscles relax, the traction weight is reduced to prevent fracture distraction and to promote fracture healing.

- *Weights should never be removed from a patient with a fracture unless a life-threatening situation occurs. If the weights are removed, the whole purpose of their use has been defeated.*

Skin Care. When traction frames are used, a trapeze may be suspended overhead within easy reach of the patient. This apparatus is of great help in assisting the patient to move about in bed and on and off bedpans. It is also a help to the nurse in caring for these patients.

The patient's elbows frequently become sore, and nerve injury may occur if most repositioning is done by pushing on the elbows. When a patient is not permitted to turn on one side or the other or on the abdomen, the nurse must make a special effort to provide good back care and to keep the bed dry and free of crumbs and wrinkles. This can be accomplished by having the patient raise the hips from the bed by holding onto the overhead trapeze.

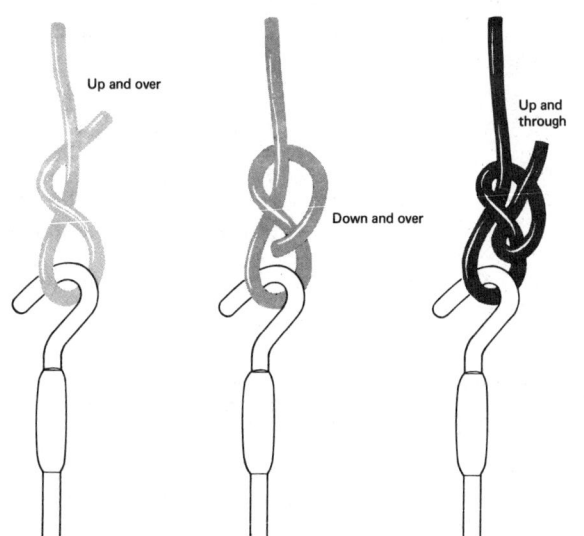

Figure 56-8
Guidelines for traction knot tying. Tying knots correctly is an orthopedic nursing activity essential for the safety of the patient in traction. To save time, follow this simple phrase:

Up and over
Down and over
Up and through

Practice a few times with a traction cord. It is a good idea to secure all knots tightly with adhesive tape. (Courtesy of Zimmer Manufacturing Company.)

Exercise. Patient exercises are valuable in maintaining muscle strength and tone and in promoting circulation. Exercises need to be planned within the therapeutic limits of the traction. Active exercise frequently permitted includes pulling up on the trapeze, flexing and extending the feet, and range-of-motion and weight-resistance exercises for noninvolved joints. The immobilized extremity benefits from isometric exercises. Quadriceps- and gluteal-setting exercises promote the strength of these muscles, which are important in ambulatory stability. Without bed exercises, the patient will lose much muscle mass and strength, and rehabilitation time will be greatly extended.

Development of thrombophlebitis is a real concern for anyone immobilized for a period of time. Daily assessment for the development of deep vein thrombophlebitis is necessary (see p. 650). Antiembolic stockings, dextran, and warfarin may be prescribed to help prevent thrombus formation. Prompt identification and treatment of thrombophlebitis is essential. Ankle exercises and isometric contracting of the calf muscle 10 times an hour decrease venous stasis.

Pin Removal. When x-ray studies demonstrate the presence of callus, skeletal traction is discontinued. The extremity is gently supported while the weights are removed. The pin is cut close to the skin and removed by the physician. Casts or splints are used to support the healing bone.

Summary of Nursing Interventions

When the patient is in traction, the nurse's responsibilities include the following:

1. Assess the neurovascular status of the extremity frequently.
2. Ensure that the ropes and pulleys are freely movable.
3. Maintain continuous traction for effectiveness.
4. Observe for skin irritation around the traction bandage.
5. Assess the patient for signs of infection.
6. Observe for pressure under the sling and equipment and at common pressure points (*e.g.*, ischial tuberosity, popliteal space, heel).
7. Encourage active foot exercises, and use foot supporters as needed.
8. Encourage exercises to minimize deconditioning of the immobilized patient.
9. Involve the patient in care to help avoid the depression and boredom that frequently accompany weeks of traction therapy.

Management of the Patient Undergoing Orthopedic Surgery

Many patients who have musculoskeletal dysfunction need to undergo surgery to correct the problem. Problems that may be corrected by surgery include impaired function due to unstabilized fracture, deformity, or joint disease; necrotic or infected tissue; impaired circulation (*e.g.*, compartment syndrome); and tumors or growths. Frequent surgical procedures include *open reduction with internal fixation* for fractures; *arthroplasty, meniscectomy,* and *joint replacement* for joint problems, *amputation* for severe extremity problems (*e.g.,* gangrene, massive trauma); *bone graft* for joint stabilization, defect-filling, or stimulation of healing; and *tendon transplants* for improvement of motion. The goals of most orthopedic surgery include improving function by restoring motion and stability and relieving pain and disability.

Types of Surgery

Orthopedic surgery falls into the following categories:

Open reduction—the reduction and alignment of the fracture following surgical dissection and exposure of the fracture

Internal fixation—the stabilization of the reduced fracture by the use of metal screws, plates, nails, and pins

Bone graft—the placement of bone tissue (autologous or homologous grafts) to promote healing, stabilization, or replacement of diseased bone

Amputation—the removal of a body part

Arthroplasty—the repair of joint problems through the operating arthroscope (an instrument that allows the surgeon to operate within a joint without a large incision) or through open joint surgery

Meniscectomy—the excision of damaged knee joint fibrocartilage

Joint replacement—the substitution of joint surfaces with metal or plastic materials

Total joint replacement—the replacement of both articular surfaces within a joint with metal or synthetic materials

Tendon transfer—the movement of tendon insertion to improve function

Fasciotomy—the cutting of the muscle fascia to relieve muscle constriction or to reduce fascia contracture

▶ Nursing Process
Preoperative Care of the Patient Undergoing Orthopedic Surgery

▷ Assessment

The nurse assesses the patient for adequate hydration, current medication history, and possible infection.

Adequate hydration is an important goal for orthopedic patients. Immobilization and bed rest contribute to urinary stasis and associated bladder infections and to stone formation. Adequate hydration assures adequate urine flow and helps to prevent the occurrence of urinary tract problems. In order to avoid preoperative dehydration, the nurse assesses the skin, vital signs, urinary output, and laboratory values for evidence of dehydration.

It should be determined whether the patient has undergone previous therapy with corticosteroids. The person with rheumatoid arthritis or chronic pulmonary disease frequently has had steroid medications to control the disease. Steroid therapy, whether current or past, may adversely affect the body's ability to withstand the stress of surgery. The steroid should be given preoperatively as prescribed to assure adequate corticosteroid levels.

The patient may be on other long-term medications, such as anticoagulants, cardiovascular drugs, insulin, and the like. All of these need to be documented and discussed with the surgeon and anesthesiologist.

The patient needs to be asked specifically about the existence of colds, dental problems, urinary tract infections, and other possible loci of infection occurring in the two weeks prior to surgery. Osteomyelitis could develop from spread of infection through the blood stream. In no instance are antibiotics relied on solely to prevent the spread of infection. Permanent disability can result if infection occurs within a bone or joint.

Other areas of preoperative assessment are similar to those for any patient undergoing surgery. The "on-call" preoperative medications are injected into an uninvolved area because tissue absorption is better in a nontraumatized area.

Nursing Diagnoses

Based on the nursing assessment data, the patient's major preoperative nursing diagnoses related to his orthopedic status may include the following:

- Alteration in comfort—pain related to fracture, swelling, or inflammation
- Actual or potential alteration in tissue perfusion (peripheral) related to swelling, constricting devices, impaired venous return
- Alteration in health maintenance related to loss of independence
- Impaired physical mobility related to pain, swelling, and possibly an immobilizing device
- Disturbance in self-concept (body image, self-esteem, role performance) related to impact of musculoskeletal problem

▷ Planning and Implementation

▷ *Goals:* The major goals of the patient before orthopedic surgery may include relief of pain, adequate tissue perfusion, health maintenance, improved mobility, and improved self-concept.

Nursing Interventions

Relieving Pain. Physical, pharmacological, and psychological management techniques to control pain are useful in the preoperative period. Specific methods selected are tailored to the individual patient and prescribed by the physician. Immobilization of a fractured bone or injured, inflamed joint will decrease discomfort. Elevation of a swollen extremity will promote venous return and reduce associated discomfort. Ice, if prescribed, will relieve swelling and directly reduce discomfort by diminishing nerve stimulation. Drugs are frequently prescribed to control the acute pain of musculoskeletal injury and associated muscle spasm. During the immediate preoperative period, the nurse needs to discuss and coordinate administration of analgesic medications with the anesthesiologist and surgeon. Alternative methods of pain control (*e.g.,* distraction, focusing, guided imagery, quiet environment, back rubs) may be used to decrease pain perception.

Promoting Adequate Tissue Perfusion. Trauma, swelling, or immobilization devices may interrupt tissue perfusion. Venous return is promoted by avoiding pressure in the popliteal area and by using antiembolic stockings unless contraindicated. The circulatory status (*i.e.*, color, temperature, capillary refill, pulse, pain, edema, paresthesia) of the extremity must be assessed frequently. If compromised circulation is noted, measures to restore adequate circulation are instituted. The physician is notified promptly, the extremity is elevated, and constricting wraps and casts are released.

Health Maintenance. The nurse needs to assist the patient in activities that will promote health during the perioperative and rehabilitative periods. *Nutritional needs and hydration* are assessed. Generally, nutrition for orthopedic patients is a reflection of their normal eating patterns. It may be appropriate to discuss ways of modifying the diet or to refer the patient to the dietitian. The preoperative fasting regimen is usually tolerated well. If the patient is diabetic, elderly and frail, or the victim of multiple trauma, special provisions may be necessary. Abnormal urinalysis findings and complaint of burning on urination require further investigation prior to surgery. At times patients will decide to limit their fluid intake to minimize the use of a bedpan. A small fracture pan may be more comfortable for the patient to use. The nurse monitors fluid intake and urinary output. The use of an indwelling catheter should be limited to avoid urinary tract infection.

Smoking should be stopped during the preoperative period to facilitate optimum *respiratory function*. Coughing, deep breathing, and use of the incentive spirometer are practiced for improved respiratory function during the postoperative period.

Exercises are taught during the preoperative period. Gluteal-setting and quadriceps-setting isometric exercises are taught for maintenance of the muscles needed for ambulation. Unless contraindicted, isometric contraction of the calf muscles (calf pumping) is practiced to minimize venous stasis and prevent thrombophlebitis. Active range-of-motion exercises of uninvolved joints are encouraged. The patient who will be using ambulatory aids may exercise to strengthen the upper extremities and shoulders. If possible, assistive devices (*e.g.*, trapeze) are used and transfer techniques practiced before surgery.

In order to minimize the chance of infection, meticulous nontraumatizing cleansing of the skin with germicidal soap and water is done the day before surgery and is repeated at the time of surgery. If the operation is elective, the orthopedist may advise the patient to begin the skin cleansing prior to hospitalization.

Improving Mobility. Preoperatively, the patient's mobility is impaired by pain, swelling, and immobilizing devices (*e.g.*, splints, casts, traction). The nurse must gently assist the patient in moving the injured part while providing adequate support. Swollen extremities are elevated and adequately supported with hands and pillows. Pain is controlled before an injured part is moved by splinting it and by administering medication in time to take effect before the injured part is moved. Skin care is provided, especially around pressure points. The use of pressure-reducing devices (*e.g.*, convoluted foam mattress, alternating air mattress) needs to be instituted before surgery for those at risk of skin breakdown. Movement within the limits of therapeutic immobility is encouraged.

Improving Self-Concept. Preoperative orthopedic patients may need assistance in accepting changes in body image, diminished self-esteem, or inability to perform the responsibilities of their life roles. The degree of assistance

required in this area varies greatly, depending on the events preceding hospitalization, the surgery and rehabilitation planned, the temporary or permanent nature of the altered body image, and the extent of changes required in role performance. The nurse promotes a trusting relationship for patients to express concerns and anxieties, and helps them examine their feelings about changes in self-concept. The nurse can clarify any misconceptions patients may have, and help them work through modifications that may be necessary due to alterations in physical capacity and self-concept.

▷ *Evaluation*

▷ *Expected Outcomes*

1. Patient experiences less pain.
   a. States medication is effective in controlling discomfort
   b. Uses multiple approaches to reduce pain
   c. Requests assistance when moving to increase comfort
2. Exhibits adequate tissue perfusion
   a. Demonstrates reduced swelling
   b. Experiences reduced inflammation
   c. Exhibits normal capillary refill
   d. Has palpable peripheral pulses
   e. Has warm skin
   f. Participates in exercise program
3. Promotes health
   a. Eats balanced diet appropriate to meet nutritional needs
   b. Maintains adequate hydration
   c. Abstains from smoking
   d. Practices respiratory exercises
   e. Engages in strengthening and preventive exercises
4. Functions within limits of therapeutic mobility/immobility
   a. Moves with less discomfort
   b. Elevates swollen extremity after transfer
   c. Uses immobilizing devices
   d. Repositions self to relieve skin pressure
5. Expresses positive self-concept
   a. Acknowledges temporary or permanent changes in body image
   b. Discusses role performance changes
   c. Views self as valuable and capable of assuming responsibilities

▶ *Nursing Process*
Postoperative Care of the Patient Undergoing Orthopedic Surgery

▷ *Assessment*

In major orthopedic surgery, *shock* may be a problem, because orthopedic wounds have a tendency to ooze and bleed more than do other surgical wounds. As a result, the nurse must be on the alert for symptoms of shock. A rising pulse rate or slowly-falling blood pressure indicates persistent bleeding or the development of shock. Changes in the respiratory rate or in the patient's color indicate obstruction of respiratory exchange and pulmonary or cardiac complications. Fat embolus (p. 1582) may occur. Thromboembolic disease (p. 649) is one of the most common and most dangerous of all complications occurring in the postoperative orthopedic patient.

Other complications that may occur are similar to those of patients undergoing general surgery, including abdominal distention and wound infection. In addition, elderly men usually have some degree of prostatism and may have difficulty in voiding, so it is important to watch urinary output.

The patient is assessed regularly for the presence of pain. Skeletal trauma and surgery performed on bones, muscles, and joints can produce significant pain.

▷ Nursing Diagnoses

Based on all assessment data, the patient's major postoperative orthopedic nursing diagnoses may include the following:

- Alteration in comfort—pain related to the surgical procedure and immobilization
- Potential for infection related to the surgical procedure
- Impaired physical mobility related to the surgical procedure and presence of immobilizing devices (splints, traction, cast, external fixator)
- Alteration in self-concept (body image, self-esteem, role performance) related to the impact of musculoskeletal problems. (Interventions for this nursing diagnosis have been discussed under the preoperative nursing diagnoses, p. 1559.)

▷ Planning and Implementation

▷ *Goals:* The major goals of the patient after orthopedic surgery may include relief of pain, absence of infection, improved mobility, and restoration of function.

Nursing Interventions

Relieving Pain. Pain can be a limiting factor, and every effort is made to relieve its intensity. The preoperative teaching and exercise programs help the patient know what to expect following surgery. The patient is monitored closely, and the prescribed analgesic is administered before the pain occurs if its onset can be predicted, or at least before it reaches a severe intensity. The nurse can administer the analgesic on a preventive basis as long as the prescribed interval between doses is observed. Eventually, pain should diminish; increased pain suggests that a problem exists and needs to be checked.

Patients may be afraid to move after orthopedic surgery and may therefore maintain a rigid extremity, which can cause painful muscle spasm and guarding. Reassuring patients that they cannot hurt themselves by moving and that some discomfort is normal and to be expected may help patients relax and go forward in their program.

If the dressing becomes too tight and painful, the surgeon must be notified.

Setting realistic goals; motivating for self-care; using relaxation, distraction, and guided imagery techniques; and establishing a relationship with the patient are nursing activities that can be used to help the patient cope with pain.

The nurse also monitors for any evidence of pressure sores, which are a constant threat to any patient who must spend a prolonged period in bed or who is elderly, malnourished, or unable to move without assistance. Turning, washing, blotting dry, and massaging the skin are necessary to avoid this complication as well as to promote comfort.

Monitoring for Potential Infection. Infection is a potential problem following any surgery. It is of particular concern for the postoperative orthopedic patient because of the potential for osteomyelitis. The nurse monitors the patient's vital signs, assesses the appearance of the wound, and notes the character of the drainage. Prompt recognition of the development of an infective process is necessary. Prophylactic systemic antibiotics are frequently prescribed during the perioperative and immediate postoperative period. The nurse assesses the patient's response to these antibiotics. When changing dressings and emptying wound drainage devices, aseptic technique is essential. Patient education concerning reporting of the signs and symptoms of infection, hand washing, and wound care reduces the development of infections.

Improving Mobility and Restoring Function. Some orthopedic operations may require prolonged periods in bed. Bone does not mend as rapidly as soft tissues. Therefore, even when the skin incision is healed, bony structures underneath still need time to repair. This is especially important to remember in surgery of the lower extremities because, in addition to allowing normal movement, bone must be able to bear weight in ambulation. Metal pins, screws, rods, and plates used in internal fixations are not strong enough to support the body's weight and will bend and break if stressed. The stability of the fracture, reduction and fixation, and bone healing are the important considerations in determining the amount of weight-bearing a reduced fracture can tolerate.

The exercise program is tailored to the individual's clinical problem. The goal is to return the patient to the highest level of function in the shortest period of time consistent with the surgical procedure. In the postoperative period, rehabilitation is started by increasing the exercises that have been prescribed and increasing the patient's activities. Usually, some form of walking aid (crutches, walker) is used for postoperative mobility. Within the limits of the patient's weight-bearing tolerance (determined by the type of surgery), the nurse monitors the patient's gait, making sure that it is safe and does not have a potentially destructive pattern. (Crutch walking and using a walker are discussed on pp. 234 and 236.)

Well-balanced diets with adequate protein and vitamins are needed for healthy tissue and wound healing. The patient is placed on a normal diet as soon as possible. However, large amounts of milk should not be given to orthopedic patients who are on bed rest, because this only adds to the calcium pool in the body and requires that more calcium be excreted by the kidneys, which can lead to formation of urinary calculi.

▷ Evaluation

▷ *Expected Outcomes*

1. Patient achieves progressive pain relief.
   a. Utilizes relaxation techniques
   b. Requires decreasing amounts of analgesic medication
   c. Participates in own care

2. Does not develop an infection
   a. Shows no signs or symptoms of wound infection
   b. Has vital signs within normal limits
   c. Shows no purulent drainage
   d. Wound heals without redness, induration, or swelling.
   e. Wound appears to have healed well.
3. Patient attains improved mobility.
   a. Increases independence in position changes
   b. Regains muscle strength and joint mobility
   c. Participates in exercise program
   d. Keeps a progress chart
4. Demonstrates some restoration of function
   a. Assumes increased responsibility for own care
   b. Walks with crutches using prescribed gait

Reconstructive Joint Surgery

At times, the impact of joint disease or deformity will necessitate surgical intervention to relieve pain, improve stability, and improve function. Surgical therapies used for joint disease include excision of damaged and diseased tissue, repair of damaged structures (*e.g.*, ruptured tendon), removal of loose bodies (débridement), immobilizing fusion of a joint (*arthrodesis*), and replacement of all or part of the joint surfaces (*e.g.*, arthroplasty, prosthesis, total joint).

The procedure is selected according to the patient's underlying problem(s), general physical health, impact of joint disability on life, and age. Timing of these procedures is important for gaining maximum function. Surgery should be performed before surrounding muscles become contracted and atrophied and serious structural abnormalities occur. The total patient must be evaluated so that the procedure with the best chance of success and best long-range benefits is selected.

Total Joint Replacement

Patients with severe pain and disability associated with the joint may be selected for total joint replacement. Conditions contributing to joint degeneration include rheumatoid arthritis, osteoarthritis (degenerative joint disease), trauma, and connital deformity. At times, total joint replacement is a salvage procedure due to disruption of the blood supply and subsequent avascular necrosis. Joints frequently replaced include the hip, knee, shoulder, and finger joints (Fig. 56-9). Less frequently, more complex joints (elbow, wrist, and ankle) are replaced.

Most joint replacements consist of metal and high-density polyethylene components. Finger prostheses are generally silastic. The joint implants may be cemented in the prepared bone with methyl methacrylate (a bone-bonding agent), which has properties similar to bone. Loosening of the bone in 5 to 15 years is the most common reason for prosthesis failure. Newer techniques and materials seem to reduce the failure rate. Ingrowth prostheses (porous-coated, cementless, artificial joint components) that allow the patient's bone to grow into and securely fix the prosthesis are being evaluated. It is projected that they will last several times longer than current cemented components. Accurate fitting and the pres-

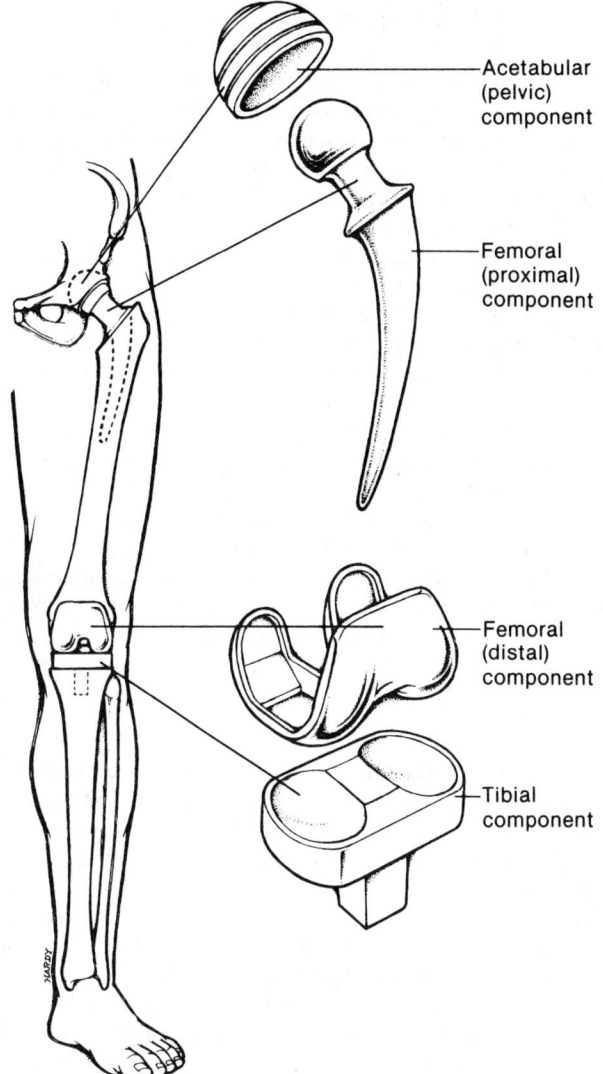

Figure 56-9
Hip and knee replacement.

ence of healthy bone stock with adequate blood supply are important in the use of cementless components.

With total joint replacement, excellent pain relief is obtained in 85% to 90% of patients. Return of motion and function depends on the preoperative soft tissue condition, soft tissue reactions, and general muscle strength. Early failure of total hip replacement is associated with higher levels of activity and prereplacement joint pathology.

Infection is a major concern because it is not always possible to achieve a functional extremity when the reconstruction procedure has to be repeated. Strict surgical asepsis and surgical environment controls are used to diminish surgical infection. Careful preoperative assessment of the patient for loci of infection is necessary. Prophylactic perioperative antibiotics are used. Infection occurs nearly twice as often in patients with rheumatoid arthritis as in those with osteoarthritis. (This may be associated with a deficit in polymorphonuclear leukocyte function observed in many rheumatoid arthritis patients.)

Total Hip Replacement

Total hip replacement is the replacement of a severely damaged hip with an artificial joint. Although a large number of implants are available, most consist of a metal femoral component topped by a spherical ball fitted into a plastic acetabular socket (see Fig. 56-10). Following a successful operation and rehabilitation, the hip is free or nearly free of pain, has good motion, is more stable, and usually permits normal or near normal ambulation.

The operation is usually reserved for patients over 60 with unremitting pain or irreversibly damaged hip joints. The following conditions are amenable to this type of surgery: arthritis (degenerative joint disease, rheumatoid arthritis), femoral neck fractures, failure of previous reconstructive surgery (osteotomy, cup arthroplasty, femoral head replacement), and problems resulting from congenital hip disease.

The procedure is generally an elective one. Assessment of the patient's status and preoperative management are aimed at establishing the patient in an optimal condition for surgery. Any infection 2 to 4 weeks prior to planned surgery may result in postponement of surgery.

Assessment

A complete preoperative evaluation is carried out, with emphasis on cardiovascular, respiratory, renal, and hepatic function because this surgery is done in patients in the older age group. Every effort is made to prevent deep vein thrombosis and pulmonary embolism, the most common cause of postoperative mortality. Obesity, preoperative leg edema, history of deep vein thrombosis, and varicose veins increase the risk of postoperative pulmonary embolism.

Infection is the most feared complication, because it generally means that the implant unit must be removed. A search is made before the operation for any possible source of infection. Preoperative urine cultures may be taken, because urinary tract infection is a likely portal of entry for bacteria. Research suggests that the majority of deep infections are caused by bacteria that are implanted into the wound at the time of surgery, mostly from airborne sources. During operation, there is strict adherence to aseptic principles and the operating area is controlled and made as nearly bacteria-free as possible. Preoperative skin preparation frequently begins a day or two before the surgery. Antibiotics may be administered in loading-dose fashion just prior to surgery or started intraoperatively. (Culture of the hip joint during surgery may be important in identifying and treating subsequent infections. Therefore, antibiotics may not be started until after the culture is obtained.)

Preoperatively, the nurse needs to assess the patient's physiologic parameters and the neurovascular status of the lower extremities. Postoperative assessment data are compared with preoperative data to identify deficits and changes. Nerve palsy can occur during surgery. Absence of peripheral pulses postoperatively may be of concern, unless the pulse was also absent preoperatively.

The home environment is evaluated early. Stair climbing and stooping are to be avoided during the first 3 months following surgery and kept to a minimum for the next 3 months. Modifications of the home environment may need to be made before the patient gets home.

Preoperative Patient Teaching

During the patient interview, the nurse may clarify what the patient can reasonably expect from the surgery, during hospitalization, and during rehabilitation. Establishing rapport early in this process helps patients to become active participants in their care.

Patient education is necessary in relation to coughing and deep breathing, muscle exercises, positioning, turning, and transfer techniques. Coughing and deep-breathing regimens are reviewed and practiced with the patient. The pulmonary complications of atelectasis and pneumonia are frequently seen and may be related to the patient's age, preexisting pulmonary disease, deep anesthesia, minimal activity, and pain medications. Learning how to use the incentive spirometer and intermittent positive pressure breathing equipment before surgery is helpful in maximizing the benefits from these devices and therapy. Isometric contraction of calf muscle and foot and ankle exercises are taught to prevent thrombophlebitis.

The patient is taught about positioning the leg in abduction to prevent dislocation of the prosthesis. The use of abduction splints (Fig. 56-10), wedge pillows, or 2 to 3 pillows between the legs is demonstrated. Review the patient's responsibility in maintaining abduction. Explain and demonstrate the limits for hip flexion (45–60 degrees).

The patient is taught upper extremity strengthening and isometric exercises of the quadriceps and gluteal muscles. When fitted with crutches or a walker, the patient is instructed in a nonweight-bearing gait (no weight-bearing on the affected extremity) to facilitate postoperative ambulation. Instructions are given in how to transfer from the bed to the wheelchair without flexing the hip joints beyond the prescribed limits. Semireclining wheelchairs may be used to help avoid excessive flexion. The use of the overhead frame and trapeze is practiced. When using the fracture bed pan, the patient is instructed not to bear down on the operated hip in flexion when getting on the bed pan, but to flex the unoperated hip and knee and use the trapeze to lift the pelvis onto the pan.

The more familiar the patient is with what will be expected postoperatively, the better the chances of compliance. Practicing activities before surgery facilitates the ability to do them postoperatively, when the patient is less agile.

Postoperative Care

Prior to the patient's return from surgery, the bed should be equipped with a firm mattress and an overbed traction frame

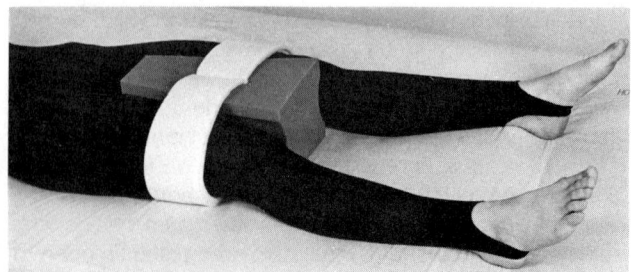

Figure 56-10
An abduction splint may be used after a total hip replacement to prevent dislocation of the prosthesis.

and trapeze. A turning sheet will prove useful. An adequate supply of pillows is needed to ensure proper positioning and comfort.

Positioning. Following surgery, the patient usually is positioned flat in bed with the affected extremity held in abduction by either an abduction splint or pillows to prevent dislocation of the prosthesis. Usually, the patient is not turned until the physician so indicates. At first the patient is turned only 45 degrees on the unoperated side, with the hip kept fully abducted and the entire length of the leg supported by pillows. As the turning routine becomes familiar, the patient is encouraged to assist by using the overbed trapeze but told not to adduct or flex the operated hip. The head of the bed should not be elevated more than 45 degrees to prevent acute flexion of the hip.

Exercise. On the day following surgery, specific exercises are begun and supervised by the physical therapist. A continuous passive motion machine may be used to exercise the joint (Fig. 56-11, p. 1569). The exercises are carried out to increase range of motion and muscle strength in the operated hip and to work toward the goal of independence in ambulation.

Ambulation. When the patient is helped out of bed, usually on the second postoperative day, an abduction splint or pillows are kept between the legs. Once the patient is out of bed, the hip is kept at maximum extension. The procedure for helping the patient out of bed consists of instructing the patient to pivot on the unaffected extremity while the nurse supports the extremity that has the implant. An aged or weakened patient may need to be lifted into a chair by several persons. Active participation of the patient is always encouraged. Frequent short periods of time out of bed are preferred to occasional long periods of sitting.

At first the patient may merely be able to stand because of weakness or light-headedness from orthostatic hypotension. Specific weight-bearing limits are determined by the physician based on the patient's condition, the procedure, and the fixation method. If the patient has an in-growth prosthesis, weight-bearing may not be advocated in order to minimize motion of the prosthesis in the bone. This type of motion can disrupt the bone growth into the prosthesis, causing the prosthesis to loosen and fail.

When ready to ambulate, the patient is taught to use a walker by first advancing the walker and then advancing the involved extremity to the walker, bearing most of the weight on the hands. After mastering ambulation with the walker, the patient progresses to crutch walking and is taught the three-point gait. The patient moves the crutches and involved extremity while supporting his weight on the crutches, and then moves the uninvolved extremity. The choice of ambulatory aids depends on the patient's balance and comfort.

Patient Education. A program of patient education involves teaching how important it is that the hip be maintained in abduction at all times and that stooping be avoided. Until otherwise instructed, the patient should use a pillow between the knees when lying in a supine or side-lying position and when turning. This prevents possible dislocation of the affected hip before the soft tissue has had a chance to heal and adequate muscle control has been restored. The patient is not to sleep on the operated side until directed to do so by the surgeon and, when seated, should keep the operated leg elevated. At no time should the legs be crossed.

Postoperative Complications

Dislocation of the Hip Prosthesis. Dislocation of the prosthesis needs to be recognized and reduced early so that circulatory and nerve damage to the leg does not occur. Dislocation may occur with major moves several days postoperatively or through positioning that exceeds the limits of the prosthesis. The indicators of dislocation are shortening of the leg, inability to move it, malalignment, abnormal rotation, and increased discomfort. If a prosthesis dislocates, the surgeon needs to be notified to reduce and stabilize the hip. As the muscles and joint capsule heal, the chance of dislocation diminishes. Stresses to the new hip joint should be minimal for the first 3 to 6 months.

Positioning and activities that will ensure positioning of the femoral head component in the acetabular cup are essential.

Pain. Pain in the immediate postoperative period is controlled by parenteral narcotics. Injection sites should be rotated, avoiding the operative hip and thigh. Muscle spasm may contribute to the pain experienced. At times the patient will indicate that the degree of postoperative pain is less than that experienced preoperatively, and only moderate amounts of analgesics are needed. By the second or third postoperative day, the pain has generally decreased to the point at which oral analgesics provide relief. Planned administration of an analgesic a half hour prior to exercise sessions may allow increased participation because comfort is increased. Hematomas and edema are controlled, reducing the discomfort associated with pressure caused by the accumulation of fluid. An ice pack to the operative site may be prescribed to reduce edema and bleeding. Portable suction of the wound will decrease fluid accumulation and hematoma formation, which could be a focus of infection. Drainage of 200 to 500 ml in the first 24 hours is expected; by 48 hours postoperatively, the total drainage in 8 hours has decreased to 30 ml or less, and the suction device is then removed.

Thromboembolism. Patients undergoing lower-extremity orthopedic surgery are at high risk for developing deep venous thrombosis. Advancing age, conditions contributing to hemostasis, and immobilization are additional risk factors. The nurse checks the legs daily for calf edema, tenderness, and a positive Homans's sign. (See Chap. 28.) The incidence of deep vein thrombosis in hip and knee reconstruction surgery is 45% to 70%. Of these patients, 20% develop pulmonary emboli, with 1% to 3% being fatal. Therefore, the nurse must institute preventive measures and monitor the patient closely for the development of deep venous thrombosis and pulmonary emboli. Antiembolic elastic stockings, elevation of the foot of the bed, ankle exercises, and early ambulation facilitate circulation. Prophylactic warfarin and dextran may be prescribed, for 7 days or as long as the patient is nonambulatory. Aspirin and low-dose heparin have no apparent prophylactic effect in the orthopedic patient. Measures to promote circulation and decrease venous stasis are priorities for the hip and knee reconstruction patient.

Infection. Infection is the most serious complication following total hip replacement. Deep infection may require removal of the implant. Acute infections may occur within 3 months of surgery, and are associated with progressive superficial infections or draining hematomas. Delayed surgical infections may appear 4 to 26 months following surgery. In-

(Text continues on p. 1568)

Care of the Patient With a Total Hip Replacement

Nursing Interventions	Rationale	Expected Outcomes

Nursing Diagnosis: Alteration in comfort: pain related to total hip replacement

Goal: Relief of pain

Nursing Interventions	Rationale	Expected Outcomes
1. Assess patient for pain.	1. Pain is expected following a surgical procedure due to the surgical trauma and tissue response. Muscle spasms occur following total hip replacements. Immobility causes discomfort at pressure points.	• Patient describes discomfort. • Expresses confidence in efforts to control pain • States pain is reduced • Appears comfortable and relaxed • Uses physical, psychological, and pharmacological measures to reduce discomfort
2. Ask patient to describe discomfort.	2. Pain characteristics may help to determine cause of discomfort. Pain may be due to complication (hematoma, infection, flatus). Pain is an individual experience—it means different things to different people.	
3. Acknowledge existence of pain; inform patient of available analgesics and/or muscle relaxants.	3. Reduces the stress experienced by patient by communicating concern and availability of assistance to help patient deal with the pain	
4. Use pain-modifying techniques. a. Use pain medications.	a. Patient will require parenteral narcotics during the first 24–48 hours, and will then progress to oral analgesics.	
b. Change position within prescribed limits.	b. Use pillows to provide adequate support; relieve pressure on bony prominences.	
c. Modify environment.	c. Interactions with others, distractions, and sensory overload or deprivation may modify pain experience.	
d. Call surgeon if necessary.	d. Surgical intervention may be necessary if pain is due to hematoma or excessive edema.	
5. Evaluate and record discomfort and effectiveness of pain-modifying techniques.	5. Effectiveness of action is based on experience; notations provide data concerning pain experiences, management, and pain relief.	

Potential Complications: Hemorrhage; neurovascular compromise; dislocation of prosthesis; thrombophlebitis; infection related to surgery

Goal: Patient experiences no postoperative complications.

Hemorrhage

Nursing Interventions	Rationale	Expected Outcomes
1. Monitor vital signs, observing for shock.	1. Changes in pulse, blood pressure, and respirations may indicate development of shock. Blood loss and stress of surgery may contribute to development of shock.	• Vital signs stabilize within normal limits. • Amount of drainage decreases • No bright red bloody drainage • Hematology values are within normal limits.

(continued)

Nursing Interventions	*Rationale*	*Expected Outcomes*

Potential Complications: Hemorrhage; neurovascular compromise; dislocation of prosthesis; thrombophlebitis; infection related to surgery

Goal: Patient experiences no postoperative complications.

Hemorrhage

2. Note character and amount of drainage.	2. Within 48 hours, bloody drainage collected in portable suction device decreases to 25–30 ml per 8 hours. Excessive drainage (more than 250 ml in first 8 hours after surgery) and bright red drainage may indicate active bleeding.	
3. Notify surgeon if patient develops shock and/or excessive bleeding.	3. Corrective measures need to be instituted.	
4. Note hemaglobin and hematocrit values.	4. Anemia due to blood loss may develop. Blood replacement therapy may be needed.	

Neurovascular Compromise

1. Assess affected extremity for color and temperature.	1. The skin becomes pale and feels cool with decreased tissue perfusion. Venous congestion may produce cyanosis.	• Color normal • Extremity warm • Normal capillary refill
2. Assess toes for capillary refill response.	2. After compression of the nail, rapid return of pink color indicates good capillary perfusion.	• Moderate edema and swelling; tissue not palpably tense • Pain is controllable.
3. Assess extremity for edema and swelling. Listen to patient complaints of leg tightness.	3. The trauma of surgery will cause swelling and edema. Excessive swelling and hematoma formation can compromise circulation and function.	• No pain with passive dorsiflexion • Normal sensations • No paresthesia • Normal motor abilities • No paresis or paralysis
4. Elevate extremity (keep lower than hip when in chair).	4. Minimizes dependent edema.	• Pulses strong and equal
5. Assess for deep, throbbing, unrelenting pain.	5. Surgical pain can be controlled; pain due to neurovascular compromise is refractory to treatment.	
6. Assess for pain on passive flexion of foot.	6. With nerve ischemia, there will be pain on passive stretch. Additionally, pain may indicate thrombophlebitis—positive Homans's sign.	
7. Assess for sensations and numbness.	7. Diminished pain and paresthesia may indicate nerve damage. Sensation in web between great and second toe—peroneal nerve; sensation on sole of foot—tibial nerve	
8. Assess ability to move foot and toes.	8. Dorsiflexion of ankle and extension of toes indicate function of peroneal nerve. Plantar flexion of ankle and flexion of toes indicate function of tibial nerve.	
9. Assess pedal pulses in both feet. Notify surgeon if diminished neurovascular status is noted.	9. Indicator of extremity circulation Function of extremity needs to be preserved.	

(continued)

Nursing Interventions	Rationale	Expected Outcomes

Potential Complications: Hemorrhage; neurovascular compromise; dislocation of prosthesis; thrombophlebitis; infection related to surgery

Goal: Patient experiences no postoperative complications.

Dislocation of Prosthesis

1. Assess for dislocation of prosthesis (extremity shortens, internally or externally rotated, severe hip pain, patient unable to move extremity)	1. Findings may indicate dislocation of prosthesis.	• Prosthesis not dislocated
2. Notify surgeon of possible dislocation.	2. Joint dislocations compromise neurovascular status and future function of extremity.	
3. Position patient as prescribed.	3. Hip component positioning (femoral component in acetabular component) needs to be maintained.	
4. Use abductor splint or pillows to maintain position and to support extremity.	4. Keep hip in abduction and in a neutral rotation to prevent dislocation.	
5. Support leg and place pillows between legs when patient is turning and side-lying; turn to the unaffected side.		
6. Avoid acute flexion of hip (head of bed at 45°).		
7. Avoid crossing legs.		

Thrombophlebitis

1. Apply thigh-high antiembolitic stockings as prescribed.	1. Antiembolism compression stockings aid in venous blood return and prevent stasis.	• Patient wears thigh-high antiembolism stockings
2. Remove stockings for 20 minutes twice a day and provide skin care.	2. Skin care is necessary to avoid breakdown. Extended removal of stockings defeats purpose of stockings.	• No skin breakdown • Pulses equal and strong • No warmer skin areas • Negative Homans's sign
3. Assess popliteal, dorsalis pedis, and posterior tibial pulses.	3. Pulses indicate arterial perfusion of extremity.	• Patient changes position with assistance and supervision.
4. Assess skin temperature of legs.	4. Local inflammation will increase local skin temperature.	• Participates in exercise regimen • Body temperature normal
5. Assess for Homans's sign every tour of duty.	5. Pain on dorsiflexion of ankle may indicate thrombophlebitis.	• No chest pain; lungs clear to auscultation; no evidence of pulmonary emboli
6. Avoid pressure on popliteal blood vessels from appliances or pillows.	6. Compression of blood vessels diminishes blood flow.	
7. Change position and increase activity as prescribed.	7. Activity promotes circulation and diminishes venous stasis.	
8. Supervise ankle exercises hourly.	8. Muscle exercise promotes circulation.	
9. Monitor body temperature.	9. Body temperature elevates with inflammation.	
10. Assess lung status; encourage coughing, deep breathing, and use of incentive spirometer.	10. Provides for optimal ventilation	

(continued)

Nursing Interventions	*Rationale*	*Expected Outcomes*

Potential Complications: Hemorrhage; neurovascular compromise; dislocation of prosthesis; thrombophlebitis; infection related to surgery

Goal: Patient experiences no postoperative complications.

Wound Infection

1. Monitor vital signs.	1. Temperature, pulse, and respirations elevate in response to infection. (Magnitude of response may be minimal in an elderly patient.)	• Vital signs normal • Well-approximated incision without drainage or excessive inflammatory response
2. Use aseptic techniques for dressing changes and emptying of portable drainage.	2. Avoid introducing organisms.	• Minimal discomfort; no hematoma • Patient tolerates antibiotics.
3. Assess wound appearance and character of drainage.	3. Red, swollen, draining incision is indicative of infection.	
4. Assess complaint of pain.	4. Pain may be due to wound hematoma—a possible locus of infection—that needs to be surgically evacuated.	
5. Administer prophylactic antibiotics if prescribed, and observe for side-effects.	5. Infected prosthesis is to be avoided.	

Nursing Diagnosis: Impaired physical mobility related to enforced bed rest following hip replacement

Goal: Patient achieves pain-free, functional, stable hip joint.

1. Maintain proper positioning of hip joint (abduction, neutral rotation, limited flexion).	1. Prevent dislocation of hip prosthesis.	• Prescribed position maintained • Patient assists in position changes. • Shows increased independence in transfers
2. Instruct and assist in position changes and transfers.	2. Encourage patient's active participation while preventing dislocation.	• Exercises hourly • Participates in progressive ambulation program
3. Instruct and supervise isometric quadriceps and gluteal setting exercises.	3. Strengthens muscles needed for walking	• Actively participates in exercise regimen • Uses ambulatory aids correctly and safely
4. In consultation with physical therapist, instruct and supervise progressive safe ambulation within limitations of weight-bearing prescription.	4. Amount of weight-bearing depends on patient's condition and prosthesis; ambulatory aids are used to assist the patient with nonweight-bearing and partial weight-bearing ambulation.	
5. Offer encouragement and support exercise regimen.	5. Reconditioning exercises can be uncomfortable and fatiguing; encouragement helps patient comply with exercise program.	
6. Instruct and supervise safe use of ambulatory aids.	6. Prevents injury from unsafe use	

(continued)

Nursing Interventions	*Rationale*	*Expected Outcomes*

Nursing Diagnosis: Potential impaired home maintenance management related to total hip replacement

Goal: Patient cares for self at home.

1. Assess home environment for discharge planning.	1. Physical barriers (especially stairs, bathrooms) may limit patient's ability to ambulate and care for self at home.	• Home is accessible for patient at time of discharge. • Patient appears relaxed and develops strategies to deal with identified problems.
2. Encourage patient to express concerns about care at home; explore together possible solutions to the problem.	2. Patient may have special problems that need to be identified and dealt with.	• Personal assistance is available. • Patient demonstrates ability to provide necessary assistance within therapeutic prescription.
3. Assess availability of physical assistance for health care activities.	3. Due to limitation of mobility and limited hip range of motion, patient may require some assistance in routine health care.	• Complies with home care program • Keeps follow-up health care appointments
4. Teach care giver home health care regimen.	4. Understanding of rehabilitative regimen necessary for compliance.	
5. Instruct patient on posthospital care: a. Activity limitations (avoid stressing prosthesis) b. Reinforce exercise instructions. c. Safe use of ambulatory aids d. Wound care e. Measures to promote healing f. Medications, if any g. Potential problems h. Continuing health care supervision and management	5. Lack of knowledge and poor preparation for care at home contribute to patient anxiety, insecurity, and nonadherence to therapeutic regimen.	

fections occurring more than 2 years after surgery are attributed to the spread of infection through the bloodstream from another place in the body.

Classic signs of infection may be present, or the patient may at some time months to years after surgery indicate return of discomfort in the hip, which could mean a late infection. The infection rate of patients having total hip surgery with rheumatoid arthritis is greater than those with osteoarthritis. This may be due to altered immunocompetency that results in an overall lower level of health and resistance. Patients who are diabetic, extremely elderly, obese, or poorly nourished, or who have concurrent infections (*e.g.*, urinary tract infections, dental abscesses) or develop large hematomas, are at higher risk for infection.

Because total joint infections are so disastrous, all efforts are undertaken to minimize their occurrence. Potential sources of infection are scrupulously avoided. A sterile operating room environment is essential, and surgery is conducted in such a way as to minimize trauma and promote wound healing. Prophylactic antibiotics are used. If an indwelling urinary catheter or portable wound suction is used, it is removed as soon as possible to avoid infections. Antibiotic therapy may be continued for 7 to 10 days. Prophylactic antibiotics may be advised if the patient needs any future surgical

instrumentation, such as tooth extraction or cystoscopic examination.

If an infection occurs, antibiotics are used to treat the infection. Management of severe infections may require surgical débridement or removal of the prosthesis. Some patients may be candidates for implantation of a new prosthesis.

Temperature. Monitoring the patient's temperature can provide good clues to the source of the problem. Temperature elevations within the first 48 hours are frequently related to atelectasis or other respiratory problems. Temperature elevations during the next few days are associated with urinary tract infections. Superficial wound infections take about 5 to 9 days to develop. Phlebitis-associated temperature elevations occur during the second and third week.

Other Complications. Other complications of total hip replacement include those associated with immobility, loosening of the prosthesis, *heterotrophic ossification* (formation of bone in the periprosthetic space) and *avascular necrosis* (bone death caused by loss of blood supply). Methods for improved cement fixation, ingrowth prosthesis, and bone grafts are aimed at reducing the chance of prosthesis loosening.

Patient Education and Home Health Care. Before the patient prepares to leave the acute care setting, the nurse provides a thorough teaching program to promote continuity of the therapeutic regimen and work toward full rehabilitation. The patient must accept the responsibility for being the primary rehabilitative resource.

The patient is advised to be faithful in the daily exercise program in order to maintain the functional motion of the hip joint and strengthen the abductor muscles of the hip. It will take time to strengthen and reeducate the muscles.

Ambulatory aids (crutches, walker, or cane) are used for a period of time. When sufficient muscle tone has developed to permit a normal gait without discomfort, the cane may be abandoned. Walking efficiency after total hip replacement is improved because of the acquired painless normal gait. In general, by 3 months the patient is able to resume all routine daily living activities. Frequent walks, swimming, and use of a high rocking chair are excellent for hip exercises. Sexual activities should be carried out in the dependent position for 3 to 6 months to avoid adduction and flexion of the new hip.

At no time should the patient cross the legs or assume positions of acute flexion, more than 90 degrees. Assistance in putting on shoes and socks may be needed. Low chairs are avoided, as well as sitting for more than 30 minutes at a time, to minimize hip flexion and the risk of prosthetic dislocation and to prevent hip stiffness and flexion contracture. Traveling long distances is to be avoided unless frequent changes in position are possible. Other activities to avoid include overexertion, lifting heavy loads, and excessive bending and twisting (lifting, shoveling snow, forceful turning).

Care of the patient with a total hip replacement is outlined in Nursing Care Plan 56-1, pages 1564–1568.

Total Knee Replacement

Total knee replacement surgery is considered for patients who have severe pain and functional disabilities related to joint surfaces destroyed by arthritis (rheumatoid arthritis, osteoarthritis, posttraumatic arthritis) and hemophilia. There are a large variety of metal and acrylic prostheses that are designed to provide the patient with a functional, painless, stable joint. If the patient's ligaments have weakened, a fully constrained (hinged) or semiconstrained prosthesis may be used to provide joint stability. A nonconstrained prosthesis depends on the patient's ligaments for joint stability.

Preoperative Management. Preoperative evaluation and patient education are important for postoperative nursing management. Care is taken to prevent infection. Thigh-high antiembolic stockings are used to help prevent thrombophlebitis.

Postoperative Management. Postoperatively, the knee is dressed with a compression bandage. Ice may be applied to control edema and bleeding. The neurovascular status of the leg is assessed (see p. 1543). Active flexion of the foot is encouraged.

A wound suction drain removes fluid accumulating in the joint. Drainage during the first 8 hours following surgery is about 200 ml; it diminishes to less than 25 ml by 48 hours postoperatively. The drains are then removed by the surgeon.

Frequently the patient's leg is placed on a continuous passive motion (CPM) device (Fig. 56-11) in the postanesthesia area. This device promotes healing by increasing cir-

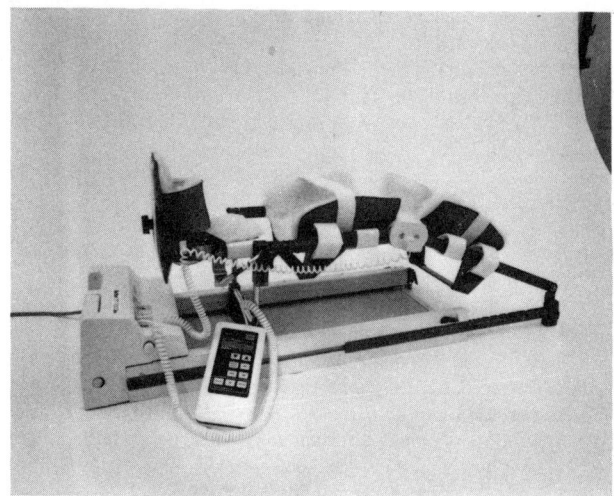

Figure 56-11
Continuous passive motion device used for postoperative total knee arthroplasty patients to facilitate joint range of motion. (Courtesy of Sutter Biomedical Inc.)

culation and movement of the knee joint. The rate and amount of extension and flexion are prescribed. Usually 10 degrees of extension and 50 degrees of flexion are initiated, and progress to 90 degrees of flexion by discharge. The patient is encouraged to use the device most of the time. If satisfactory flexion is not achieved, gentle manipulation of the knee joint under general anesthesia may be done about 2 weeks after surgery.

Efforts are directed at preventing complications (thromboembolism, peroneal nerve palsy, infection). The patient begins nonweight-bearing transfers out of bed on the first postoperative day. Support and elevation of the leg are needed when the patient is out of bed in a chair. The physical therapist supervises exercises for strength and range of motion. Progressive ambulation, using ambulatory aids and within the prescribed weight-bearing limits, is begun within days of the surgery.

Following discharge from the hospital, the patient may continue to use the CPM at home as well as to do physical therapy on an outpatient basis. Late complications that may occur include infection and loosening and wear of prosthetic components. Generally, the patient is able to achieve a pain-free, functional joint and participate more fully in life activities.

Bibliography

Books

Benjamin A and Helal B. Surgical Repair and Reconstruction in Rheumatoid Disease. New York, John Wiley & Sons, 1980.

Brooker A and Schmeisser G. The Orthopaedic Traction Manual. Baltimore, Williams & Wilkins, 1980.

Brunner NA. Orthopedic Nursing: A Programmed Approach. St Louis, CV Mosby, 1983.

Duthie RB and Bentley G (eds). Mercer's Orthopaedic Surgery, 8th ed. Baltimore, University Park Press, 1983.

Epps CH. Complications in Orthopaedic Surgery, 3nd ed. Philadelphia, JB Lippincott, 1986.

Farrell J. Illustrated Guide to Orthopedic Nursing, 3rd ed. Philadelphia, JB Lippincott, 1986.

Gartland J. Fundamentals of Orthopedics, 3rd ed. Philadelphia, WB Saunders, 1979.

Heppenstall R (ed). Fracture Treatment and Healing. Philadelphia, WB Saunders, 1980.

Hilt N and Cogburn S. Manual of Orthopedics. St Louis, CV Mosby, 1981.

Pellino T et al (eds). National Association of Orthopaedic Nurses: Core Curriculum for Orthopaedic Nursing. Pitman, New Jersey, Anthony J Jannetti, 1986.

Photobook: Working with Orthopedic Patients. Springhouse, Pennsylvania, Intermed Communications, 1982.

Pinney EC and Stone EM. Orthopaedic Nursing, 6th ed. London, Bailliere Tindall, 1983.

Powell M (ed). Orthopaedic Nursing and Rehabilitation, 9th ed. Edinburgh, Churchill Livingstone, 1986.

Rakel RE (ed). Conn's 1986 Current Therapy. Philadelphia, WB Saunders, 1986.

Roal R and Hodkinson L. Textbook of Orthopaedic Nursing, 3rd ed. Oxford, Blackwell Scientific, 1980.

Rockwood CA and Green DP (eds). Fractures in Adults, 2nd ed. Philadelphia, JB Lippincott, 1984.

Steward JDM and Hallett JP. Traction and Orthopaedic Appliances, 2nd ed. Edinburgh, Churchill Livingstone, 1983.

Turek, SL. Orthopaedics: Principles and Their Application, 4th ed. Philadelphia, JB Lippincott, 1984.

Webb JT. Notes on Orthopaedic Nursing, 2nd ed. Edinburgh, Churchill Livingstone, 1985.

Articles

General

Aaron RK and Ciombor D. Venous thrombosis in the orthopedic patient. Surg Clin North Am 1983 June; 63(3):529–538.

Cassels CJ. Fundamentals of long bone traction, Part 1. Crit Care Update 1983 Mar; 10(3):36–39.

Celeste SM et al. Identifying a standard for pin site care using the quality assurance approach. Orthop Nurs 1984 July/Aug; 3(4):17–24.

Crutchley C. Trends in orthopedic surgery. Today's OR Nurs 1984 Dec; 6(12):22–24.

Farrell J. Positioning postoperative orthopedic patients. Today's OR Nurs 1984 Oct; 6(12):12–16.

Farrell NA. Cast syndrome. Orthop Nurs 1985 July/Aug; 4(4):61–64.

Gates SJ. Helping your patient on bed rest cope with perceptual/sensory deprivation. Orthop Nurs 1984 Mar/Apr; 3(2):35–38.

Gill KP et al. External fixation: The erector sets of orthopedic nursing. Can Nurs 1984 May; 80(5):29–31.

Goldstone LA et al. A clinical trial of a bead bed system for the prevention of pressure sores in elderly orthopaedic patients. J Adv Nurs 1982 Nov; 7(6):545–548.

Hankin F et al. Bleeding beneath postoperative casts. Orthop Nurs 1983 Jan/Feb; 2(1):27–32.

Harris WH et al. Prophylaxis of deep-vein thrombosis after total hip replacement. J Bone Joint Surg [Am] 1985 Jan; 67(1):57–62.

Jensen JE et al. Nutrition and orthopedic surgery. Nutr Support Serv 1984 Feb; 4(2):27, 30–31, 35.

Johnson-Pawlson J and Koshes R. Exercise is for everyone. Geriatr Nurs 1985 Nov/Dec; 6(6):322–327.

Kelly DJ. The use of fiberglass as reinforcement with plaster casts. Orthop Nurs 1983 Nov/Dec; 2(6):33–36.

Lane PL et al. New synthetic casts: What nurses need to know. Orthop Nurs 1982 Nov/Dec; 1(16):13–20.

McFarland MB. Encircling cast drainage: Is it valuable? Orthop Nurs 1984 Mar/Apr; 3(2):41–43.

Miller MC. Nursing care of the patient with external fixation therapy. Orthop Nurs 1983 Jan/Feb; 2(1):11–15.

Mindell ER. Orthopedic Surgery. JAMA 1985 Oct 25; 254(18):2213–2215.

Moran-Higgins. Perioperative concerns for the patient with osteoporosis. Orthop Nurs 1985 May/June; 4(3):68.

Morse J et al. The patient who falls and falls again: Defining the aged at risk. J Gerontol Nurs 1985 Nov; 11(11):15–21.

Reid H. Plastering in the '80s. Nurs Mirror 1984 Aug 29; 159(7):i–vii.

Searls K et al. External fixation: General principles of patient management. Crit Care Q 1983 June; 6(1):45–54.

Simchen E et al. Multivariate analysis of determinants of postoperative wound infection in orthopaedic patients. J Hosp Infect 1984 June; 5(2):137–146.

Smith C. Nursing the patient in traction. Nurs Times 1984 Apr 18–24; 80(16):36–39.

Sproles KJ. Nursing care of skeletal pins: A closer look. Orthop Nurs 1985 Jan/Feb; 4(1):11–12, 15–20.

Sullivan D. Complications from intraoperative positioning. Orthop Nurs 1985 July/Aug; 4(4):56–57.

Trigueiro M. Pin site care protocol. Can Nurs 1983 Sept; 79(8):24–26.

Voluz JM. Surgical implants; Orthopedic; devices. AORN J 1983 June; 37(7):1341–1349.

Wittert D and Barden R. Deep vein thrombosis, pulmonary embolism, and prophylaxis in the orthopaedic patient. Orthop Nurs 1985 July/Aug; 4(4):27–32.

Total Joint Arthroplasty

Aaron RK. Total joint arthroplasty. Surg Clin North Am 1983 June; 63(3):697–714.

Consensus Conference. Total hip joint replacement in the United States. Bethesda, Maryland, National Institutes of Health, 1982.

Doheny MO. Porous coated femoral prosthesis: Concepts; and care considerations. Orthop Nurs 1985 Jan/Feb; 4(1):43–45.

Engh CA, Hip arthroplasty with a Moore prosthesis with porous coating: A five-year study. Clin Orthop 1983 June; 176:52–66.

Harris W et al. Prophylaxis of deep vein thrombosis after total hip replacement: Dextran and external pneumatic compression compared with 1.2 or 0.3 gm of aspirin daily. J Bone Joint Surg [Am] 1985 Jan; 67-A(1):57–62.

Lotke PA et al. Indications for the treatment of deep venous thrombosis following total knee replacement. J Bone Joint Surg [Am] 1984 Feb; 66(2):202–208.

Lovelock JE et al. Complications of total knee replacement. AJR 1984 May; 142(5):985–992.

Olivo J et al. Total knee arthroplasty: A team approach. Today's OR Nurs 1985 Sept; 7(9):10–17.

Rand JA et al. Management of the infected total joint arthroplasty. Orthop Clin North Am 1984 July; 15(3):491–504.

Sachs BL et al. An improvised passive motion apparatus. Clin Orthop 1985 Apr; 194:205–206.

Strang EL and Johns JL. Nursing care of the patient treated with continuous passive motion following total knee arthroplasty. Orthop Nurs 1984 Nov/Dec; 3(6):27–32.

Stulberg BN et al. Deep-vein thrombosis following total knee replacement. J Bone Joint Surg [Am] 1984 Feb; 66(2):194–201.

Walsh CR and Wirth CR. Total knee arthroplasty: Biomechanical and nursing considerations. Orthop Nurs 1985 Jan/Feb; 4(1):29–34, 70.

Wong S et al. Total hip replacements: Improving post-hospital adjustment. Nurs Manage 1984 July; 15(7):34C–D, 34F–G.

Agencies

Arthritis Foundation, 1314 Spring Street NW, Atlanta, GA 30309.

National Institute of Arthritis and Musculoskeletal and Skin Diseases, National Institutes of Health, Bethesda, MD 20892.

National Scoliosis Foundation, 48 Stone Road, Belmont, MA 02178.

Scoliosis Association, One Penn Plaza, New York, NY 10119.

Chapter 57

Management of Patients With Musculoskeletal Trauma

Injury to one part of the musculoskeletal system usually produces injury or dysfunction of adjacent structures and of structures enclosed or supported by them. If the bones are broken, the muscles cannot function; if the nerves do not send impulses to the muscles, as in paralysis, the bones cannot move; if the joint surfaces do not articulate normally, neither the bones nor the muscles can function properly. Thus, although a fracture primarily affects the bone, it may also produce injury to the muscles surrounding the injured bone and to the blood vessels and the nerves in the vicinity of the fracture.

In the treatment of injury of the musculoskeletal system, support is provided for the injured part until nature has time to heal it. Support may be accomplished by bandages, adhesive strapping, splints, or casts, applied externally. Support may be applied directly to the bone in the form of pins or plates. At times, traction must be applied to correct deformity or shortening.

After the immediate and the painful effects of the injury have passed, consideration must be given to the prevention of fibrosis and the resulting stiffness in the injured muscles and the joint structures. *Active function by the patient is the best form of treatment to guard against this disability.* In some cases, the support applied may permit active function almost from the start. The healing process and recovery of function may be hastened by various forms of physical therapy.

Contusions, Strains, Sprains, and Dislocations

Contusions

A contusion is an injury of the soft tissues, produced by blunt force (*e.g.*, a blow, kick, fall). There is always some bleeding into the injured part (*ecchymosis*), due to the rupture of many small vessels. This produces the well-known discoloration of the skin (bruising), which gradually turns to brown and then to yellow, and finally disappears as absorption becomes complete. When the bleeding is sufficient to cause an appreciable collection of blood, it is called *hematoma*. The local symptoms (pain, swelling, and discoloration) are easily explained.

Management. Treatment consists of elevating the affected part and applying moist or dry cold for the first 24 hours to produce vasoconstriction, which results in decreased bleeding and edema. Application of cold should be intermittent for 20 to 30 minutes. In the recovery phase, moist heat is applied for 20 minutes at a time to promote vasodilatation, absorption, and repair. Elastic bandage wrapped over the contused area controls bleeding and reduces associated swelling.

Strains

A strain is a "muscle pull" due to overuse, overstretching, or excessive stress. Strains are microscopic, incomplete muscle tears with some bleeding into the tissue. The patient experiences gradual soreness or sudden pain and then local tenderness. Pain is experienced with muscle use and isometric contraction.

Management. The injured muscle must be allowed to rest and repair itself. Intermittent ice compresses for the first day followed by intermittent heat provide both comfort and increased circulation to the injured muscle, promoting healing. Elevation and an elastic pressure bandage control any associated edema. Patient education needs to emphasize minimal exercise until healing has taken place, and then gradual progression of activity. Too much exercise too soon will cause restrain and delayed recovery.

Sprains

A sprain is an injury to the ligamentous structures surrounding a joint, caused by a wrench or a twist. The function of a ligament is to maintain stability while permitting mobility. A torn ligament loses its stabilizing ability. As is the case with contusions, blood vessels are ruptured, and ecchymosis and edema occur. The joint is tender and movement of the joint becomes painful. The degree of disability and pain increases during the first 2 to 3 hours after the injury because of the associated swelling and bleeding. To be certain that there is no bone injury, these patients should have an x-ray examination. *Avulsion fracture* (a bone fragment is pulled away by a ligament or tendon) may be associated with sprains.

Management. Sprains are treated initially with cold, elevation, and splinting or cast immobilization. The application of cold reduces the associated pain and causes vasoconstriction, which retards extravasation of blood and the development of edema. Elastic bandages reduce swelling and edema. The part should be elevated and rested.

After 24 hours, mild heat may be applied (15 to 30 minutes, 4 times daily) to promote healing. If the sprain is severe (torn muscle fibers and disrupted ligaments), surgical repair or cast immobilization is necessary so that the joint will not lose its stability. A severe sprain will take about a month to heal, and then active exercise can begin and build gradually.

Joint Dislocations

A dislocation of a joint is a condition in which the articular surfaces of the bones forming the joint are no longer in an-atomical contact. The bones are literally "out of joint." A *subluxation* is a partial dislocation of the articulating surfaces. Traumatic dislocations are orthopedic emergencies, because the associated joint structures, blood supply, and nerves are distorted and severely stressed. *Avascular necrosis* (tissue death due to anoxia and diminished blood supply) and nerve palsy may occur.

Dislocations may be (1) congenital (present at birth, due to some maldevelopment, most often noted at the hip); (2) spontaneous or pathologic, due to disease of the articular or the periarticular structures; and (3) traumatic, due to injury, such as the application of force in such a manner as to produce disruption of the joint.

The signs and symptoms of a traumatic dislocation are (1) pain, (2) change in contour of the joint, (3) change in the length of the extremity, (4) loss of normal mobility, and (5) change in the axis of the dislocated bones.

X-ray films confirm the diagnosis and should be made in every case, because frequently there is an associated fracture.

Management. The part needs to be immobilized while the patient is transported. The dislocation is reduced (*i.e.*, displaced parts brought into normal position), usually under anesthesia. The head of the dislocated bone is manipulated back into the joint cavity. The joint is immobilized by bandages, splints, casts, or traction. It is kept in a stable position. With a stable reduced dislocation, gentle active motion 3 or 4 times a day is begun several days to weeks after reduction. This is to preserve range of motion. The joint is supported between exercise sessions.

Nursing concerns are directed at providing comfort, evaluating the neurovascular status, and protecting the joint during healing. The patient needs to learn how to manage the immobilizing devices and how to protect the joint from reinjury.

Sports Injuries

More and more people are participating in recreational sports. These recreational athletes may push themselves beyond the level of their physical conditioning and incur sports injuries. Injuries to the musculoskeletal system may be of an acute nature (sprains, strains, dislocations, fractures) or may result from gradual overuse (chondromalacia patella, tendinitis, stress fractures). Professional athletes are also susceptible to injury, even though their training is supervised closely to minimize the occurrence of injury and to enhance the development of athletic performance.

Musculoskeletal contusions result from direct falls or blows from sporting equipment. The initial dull pain becomes greater, with edema and stiffness occurring by the next day. Sprains commonly occur in fingers, ankles, and knees. If the ligamentous damage is major, the joint becomes unstable and surgical repair may be required. An avulsion fracture may exist. Strains present with a sharp, stabbing pain from bleeding and immediate protective muscle contraction. Tennis players often suffer calf muscle strains; soccer players experience quadriceps strains; swimmers, weight lifters, and tennis players suffer shoulder strains. *Tendinitis* (inflammation of a tendon) is due to overuse and is seen in tennis players (epicondylar tendinitis), runners and gymnasts (Achilles tendinitis), and runners and basketball players (infrapatellar tendinitis). Meniscal injuries of the knee occur with excessive rotational stress. Dislocations are seen with throwing and lifting sports. Fractures occur with falls. Skaters and bikers frequently suffer Colles's fractures of the wrist when they fall on outstretched arms; ballet dancers and field and track athletes experience metatarsal fractures. Stress fractures occur with repeated bone trauma from activities such as jogging, gymnastics, basketball, and aerobics. The tibias, fibulas, and metatarsals are most vulnerable.

Management. Generally, musculoskeletal injuries need to be recognized and managed early to facilitate healing and to minimize residual disabilities. Basic to the management of most soft-tissue injuries is ICE (*I*ce, *C*ompression, *E*levation). The ice is applied for 20 to 30 minutes every 3 to 4 hours during the first 24 to 48 hours to control swelling and relieve pain. The area is wrapped with an elastic compression bandage to minimize effusion, support the area, and provide comfort. The wrap must not be constricting. Monitoring the neurovascular status of the extremity becomes an important nursing function. The injured extremity is elevated above the heart to control swelling and to promote rest. Depending on the site and the severity of the injury, the extremity may be immobilized and/or surgical intervention may be required. Arthroscopic surgery may be required for meniscus tears and other joint injuries that limit joint function and contribute to articular cartilage wear.

Patients who have experienced a sports-related injury are highly motivated to return to their previous level of activity. Compliance with restriction of activities and resumption of them on a *gradual, progressive* timetable may be a real problem for these patients. They need to be taught how to avoid further injury or new injury. With recurrence of symptoms, they need to learn to diminish the level and intensity of activity to a comfort level and to treat the symptoms (ICE). Activity should be resumed gradually and sensibly. Recovery from sports-related injury can take a few days to 6 or more weeks.

Prevention of sports-related injuries can be achieved by use of appropriate equipment (*e.g.*, running shoes) and by training and conditioning the body. Changes in activities and stresses should occur gradually. The athlete needs to be taught to "tune in" to body symptoms indicating stress and to modify activities in order to minimize injury and to promote healing.

Fractures

A fracture is a break in the continuity of bone and is defined according to type and extent (Fig. 57-1). Fractures occur when the bone is subjected to stress greater than it can absorb. Fractures can be caused by direct blow, crushing force, sudden twisting motion, and even extreme muscle contraction.

While the bone is the part most directly affected, other structures also may be involved, resulting in soft-tissue edema, hemorrhage into the muscles and joints, joint dislocations, ruptured tendons, severed nerves, and damaged blood vessels. Body organs may be injured by the force that caused the fracture or by the fracture fragments.

Types of Fractures

A *complete fracture* involves a break across the entire cross-section of the bone and is frequently displaced (removed

from normal position). In an *incomplete fracture,* the break occurs through only part of the cross-section of the bone.

A *closed fracture* does not produce a break in the skin. An *open fracture* is one that extends through the skin or mucous membrane. Open fractures are graded: Grade I is a clean wound less than 1 cm long; Grade II is a larger wound without extensive soft-tissue damage; and Grade III is the most severe, with extensive soft-tissue damage.

Fractures may also be described according to anatomical placement of fragments—*displaced/nondisplaced fracture.*

The following are specific types of fractures (see Fig. 57-1):

Greenstick—a fracture in which one side of a bone is broken and the other side is bent
Transverse—a fracture that is straight across the bone
Oblique—a fracture occurring at an angle across the bone (less stable than transverse)
Spiral—a fracture twisting around the shaft of the bone
Comminuted—a fracture in which bone has splintered into several fragments
Depressed—a fracture in which fragment(s) is (are) indriven (seen frequently in fractures of skull and facial bones)
Compression—a fracture in which bone has been compressed (seen in vertebral fractures)
Pathologic—a fracture that occurs through an area of diseased bone (bone cyst, Paget's disease, bony metastasis, tumor)
Avulsion—a pulling away of a fragment of bone by a ligament or tendon and its attachment
Epiphyseal—a fracture through the epiphysis

Clinical Manifestations

The clinical manifestations of a fracture are pain, loss of function, false motion, deformity, shortening, crepitation, local swelling, and discoloration. In an open fracture, the bone penetrates through the skin.

1. The *pain* is of a continuous type and increases in severity until the bone fragments are immobilized.
2. Following the break, the part cannot be used and tends to move unnaturally (false motion) instead of remaining rigid as it normally would. The displacement of the fragments in a fracture of the arm or leg causes a deformity (either visible or palpable) of the extremity, detectable when it is compared to the normal extremity. The extremity cannot function properly because normal function of the muscles depends upon the integrity of the bones to which they are attached.
3. In fractures of long bones, there is actually shortening of the extremity because of the contraction of the muscles that are attached above and below the site of the fracture. The fragments may often overlap as much as 2.5–5 cm (an inch or two). The muscle spasm that accompanies fracture is natural splinting to minimize further movement of the fracture fragments.
4. When the extremity is examined with the hands, a grating sensation, called *crepitus*, can be felt due to the rubbing of the fragments one upon the other. (Testing for crepitation can produce further tissue damage.)

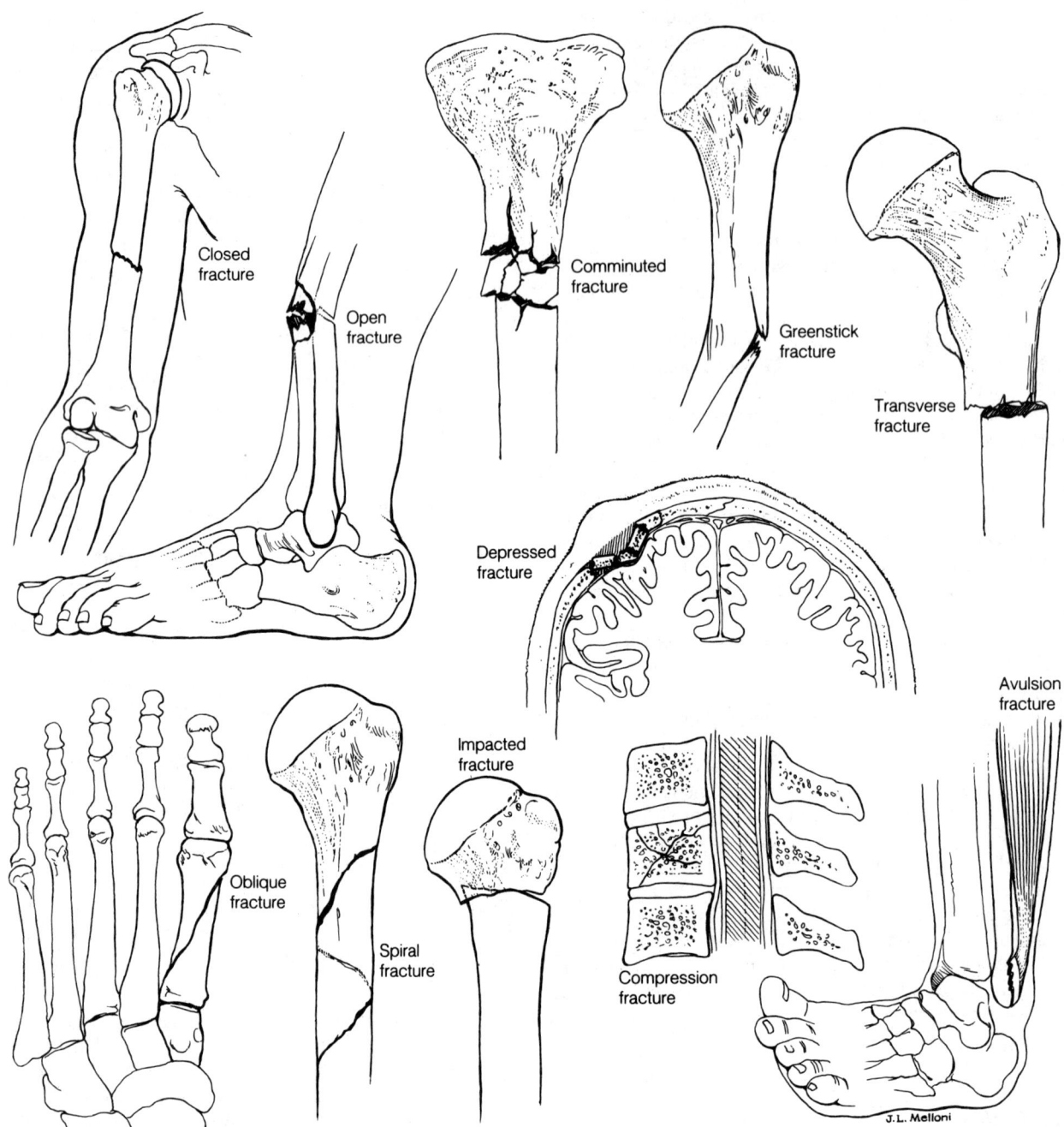

Figure 57-1
Types of fractures. (Brunner LS and Suddarth DS. The Lippincott Manual of Nursing
Practice, 4th ed. Philadelphia, JB Lippincott, 1986.)

5. Localized swelling and discoloration of the skin occur as a result of trauma and hemorrhage that follow a fracture. These signs may not develop for several hours or days following the injury.

All of these signs and symptoms are not necessarily present in every fracture. When there is a linear or fissure fracture, or in cases in which the fractured surfaces are driven together (*impacted fractures*), many of these symptoms do not occur.

The diagnosis of a fracture depends on the symptoms of the patient, the physical signs, and x-ray examination. Usually, the patient reports he sustained an injury to the area.

Emergency Management

The fractured extremity is rendered as immobile as possible *before the patient is moved*. If an injured patient must be removed from a vehicle before splints can be applied, the extremity is supported above and below the fracture site, and traction is applied in accordance with the line of the long axis of the bone to prevent rotation as well as angular motion. Movement of fracture fragments will cause additional pain, soft-tissue damage, and additional hemorrhage. Adequate splinting is essential to prevent damage to the soft tissue by the bony fragments. It must be remembered that the pain associated with a fractured bone is severe, and that the surest way to decrease pain and hemorrhage and prevent possible shock is by preventing movement of the bone fragments and the joints adjacent to the fracture.

Immobilization is established by applying temporary, well-padded splints, which are then firmly bandaged over the clothing. Immobilization of the long bones of the lower extremities may also be accomplished by bandaging the extremities together, with the sound extremity serving as a splint for the injured one. In an upper extremity injury, the arm may be bandaged to the chest, or an injured forearm may be placed in a sling.

The peripheral pulses distal to the injury should be palpated to ensure that circulation has not been compromised and that tissue perfusion is sufficient.

In an *open fracture*, the wound is covered with a clean (sterile) dressing to prevent contamination of deeper tissues. No attempt is made to reduce the fracture, even if one of the bone fragments is protruding through the wound. Splints should be applied as described above.

Immediately following injury, a patient who is in a state of confusion may not be aware of the fracture (*i.e.*, he may walk on a fractured extremity). Therefore, it is important to immobilize that part of the body immediately when a fracture is suspected.

When a patient comes to a hospital suffering from a fracture, a narcotic sufficient to relieve the pain should be given, provided there is not head injury. The intravenous route allows for smaller dosage and prompt action.

Then, with care and gentleness the clothes are removed, first from the uninjured side of the body and then from the injured side. Sometimes the patient's clothing must be cut away on the injured side. The fractured extremity is moved as little as possible to avoid causing more damage.

Physiology of Bone Healing

When the bone is injured, the bone fragments are not merely patched together with scar tissue. The bone regenerates itself.

Stages of Bone Healing

There are several stages in fracture healing: (1) inflammation, (2) cellular proliferation, (3) callus formation, (4) callus ossification, and (5) remodeling into mature bone.

Inflammation. With a fracture, the body response is similar to that of injury elsewhere in the body. There is bleeding, extravasation of blood, and the formation of a fracture hematoma. The area exhibits edema, swelling, inflammation, and pain. The fracture fragment ends become devitalized because of the interrupted blood supply. The injured area is invaded by macrophages (large, white blood cells), which débride the area. The inflammatory stage lasts a couple of days, and resolution of the inflammatory response is characterized by a decrease in pain and swelling.

Cellular Proliferation. Fibrin strands form within the fracture hematoma and adjacent tissue begin to grow into the clot. Revascularization begins. Fibroblasts and osteoblasts (developed from osteocytes, endosteal cells, and periosteal cells) produce collagen and proteoglycans for a collagen matrix at the fracture. Cartilage and fibrous connective tissue

develop. From the periosteum, a collar of growth is in evidence. This is the beginning of an external cartilaginous callus. Minimal micromotion at the fracture site stimulates callus formation and healing. Actively growing bone exhibits electronegative potentials.

Callus Formation. Tissue growth continues and the cartilage collar from each bone fragment grows toward the others until the fracture gap is bridged. The fracture fragments are joined by fibrous tissue, cartilage, and immature fiber bone. An internal callus also develops and invades the remaining blood clot. The shape of the callus and the volume of tissue required to bridge the defect are directly proportional to the amount of bone damage and displacement. It takes 3 to 4 weeks for fracture fragments to be united by cartilage or fibrous tissue. Clinically, the fragments are no longer easily moved.

Ossification. Ossification of the developed callus begins within 2 to 3 weeks postfracture, through the process of endochondral ossification (see Chap. 55—Bone Formation). The mineral deposition continues, and produces a firmly reunited bone. The callus surface continues to be electronegative. With major adult long bone fractures, ossification takes 3 to 4 months.

Remodeling. The final stage of fracture repair consists of removal of any remaining devitalized tissue and reorganization of the new bone into its former structural arrangement. Bone architecture is related to its function. Compact bone and cancellous bone develop according to functional stresses. Depending on the extent of bone modification needed, remodeling may take months to years. Cancellous bone heals and remodels more rapidly than compact cortical bone, especially at points of direct contact. When remodeling is complete, the fracture surface charge is no longer negative.

The progress of bone healing is monitored by serial x-rays. Adequate immobilization is essential until there is radiologic evidence of callus. Progression of the therapeutic regimen (*e.g.*, application of a cast brace to a patient who has had a femur fracture reduced and immobilized by skeletal traction) depends on data indicating fracture healing.

Bone Healing With Fragments Firmly Approximated. When fractures are treated with open rigid fixation techniques, the bony fragments can be placed in direct contact. Motion at the fracture is eliminated. In this situation, the stages of bone healing are modified. Hematoma formation is not essential and is not observed. Little or no external cartilaginous callus develops. Primary bone healing occurs.

Immature bone develops from the endosteum. There is an intensive regeneration of new osteons. The new osteons develop in the fracture line by a process similar to normal bone maintenance. Fracture strength is obtained when the new osteons have become established. With rigid internal fixation, the bone heals through cortical bone remodeling. This process is slower than bone healing by callus formation.

Healing Time of Fractures

Many factors influence the speed with which healing occurs (Chart 57-1). The reduction of the displaced fracture fragments must be accurate and successfully maintained to ensure healing. The affected bone must have an adequate blood supply. The age of the patient and the type of fracture also affect healing time. In general, fractures of flat bones (pelvis, scapula) heal quite rapidly. Fractures at the ends of long bones

Chart 57-1
Factors Affecting Bone Healing

Factors Enhancing Fracture Healing

- Immobilization of fracture fragments
- Maximum bone fragment contact
- Sufficient blood supply
- Proper nutrition
- Exercise—weight-bearing for long bones
- Hormones—growth hormone, thyroid, calcitonin, insulin, vitamins A and D, anabolic steroids
- Electric potential across fracture

Factors Inhibiting Fracture Healing

- Extensive local trauma
- Bone loss
- Inadequate immobilization
- Space/tissue between bone fragments
- Infection
- Local malignancy
- Metabolic bone diseases (*e.g.,* Paget's)
- Irradiated bone (radiation necrosis)
- Avascular necrosis
- Intra-articular fracture (synovial fluid contains fibrolysins, which lyse the initial clot and retard clot formation)
- Age (elderly persons heal more slowly)
- Corticosteroids (they inhibit the repair rate)
- Denervation

where the bone is more vascular and cancellous heal more quickly than do fractures in areas where the bone is dense and less vascular (midshaft). Weight-bearing will stimulate healing of stabilized fractures of the long bones in the lower extremities. In addition, activity minimizes the development of immobility-related *osteoporosis* (a reduction of total bone mass producing porous and fragile bones due to imbalance in homeostatic bone turnover). Table 57-1 shows the approximate immobilization times necessary for union of the most common types of fractures.

If fracture healing is disrupted, the bone union time may be delayed or stopped completely. Factors that may interrupt fracture healing include loss of fracture hematoma by débridement, devitalization of adjacent tissue by inadequate blood supply, extensive space between bone fragments, interposition of soft tissue between bone ends, inadequate fracture immobilization, infection, complications from the treatment, and metabolic problems.

Principles of Fracture Management

The principles of fracture treatment include reduction, immobilization, and regaining of normal function and strength through rehabilitation. (Chart 57-2).

Fracture Reduction and Immobilization

Reduction of a fracture ("setting" the bone) refers to restoration of the fracture fragments into anatomical rotation and alignment as nearly as possible. This is accomplished by closed or open manipulation.

Before fracture reduction, the patient should be prepared for the procedure. Medications for pain relief are administered. The extremity that is to be manipulated should be handled gently to avoid additional damage, elevated to minimize swelling, and gently cleaned before being dressed in a cast or splint.

After the fracture has been reduced, bone fragments must be immobilized or held in correct position and alignment until union has had time to take place. Immobilization may be accomplished by external or internal fixation. Methods of *external fixation* include bandages, casts, splints, continuous traction, pin and plaster technique, or external fixators. *Internal fixation* devices (metal implants) include nails, plates, screws, wires, and rods. These serve as internal splints to hold the fractured bone in alignment while healing takes place.

TABLE 57-1
Approximate Immobilization Time Necessary for Union

Fracture Site	Number of Weeks
Phalanx	3–5
Metacarpal	6
Carpal	6
Scaphoid	10
	(or until x-ray shows union)
Radius and ulna	10–12
Humerus:	
Supracondylar	8
Midshaft	8–12
Proximal (impacted)	3
Proximal (displaced)	6–8
Clavicle	6–10
Vertebra	16
Pelvis	6
Femur:	
Intracapsular	24
Intratrochanteric	10–12
Shaft	18
Supracondylar	12–15
Tibia:	
Proximal	8–10
Shaft	14–20
Malleolus	6
Calcaneus	12–16
Metatarsal	6
Toes	3

(Compere EL et al. Pictorial Handbook of Fracture Treatment, 5th ed. Chicago, Year Book Medical Publishers.)

Chart 57-2
The Treatment of Fractures

Principles of Care in Treating Fractures

1. Restore fracture fragments to their normal anatomical position (reduction).
2. Maintain reduction in place until healing occurs (immobilization).
3. Promote regaining of normal function and strength of the affected part (rehabilitation).

Methods Used to Obtain Fracture Reduction

1. Closed reduction
2. Traction
3. Open reduction

Methods Used to Maintain Fracture Reduction (Fixation)

1. Cast or cast brace
2. Splints
3. Continuous traction
4. Pin and plaster technique
5. Internal fixation devices
   - a. Nails   c. Screws   e. Rods
   - b. Plates   d. Wires
6. External fixation devices
7. Endoprosthetic replacements

Bandages of muslin or elastic are commonly used to immobilize certain fractures. The *Velpeau* bandage is used for fractures of the scapula, clavicle, and humerus (Fig. 57-2). Fractured vertebrae may be splinted with an elastic back-supporting girdle. Splints (plastic or plaster) may be used for temporary or permanent immobilization, especially for fractures of the upper extremity. Any splint that is not molded to the contours of the extremity should be padded well to prevent pressure.

Methods of Fracture Reduction

Several methods are used to obtain reduction of a fracture; the method selected depends on the nature of the fracture. Variations of these methods are carried out, but the underlying principles are the same. Usually, fractures are reduced as soon as possible because tissues may lose their elasticity if infiltrated by edema or hemorrhage. At times, the patient may need anesthesia when a fracture is reduced and immobilized. In most cases, fracture reduction becomes more difficult as the injury begins healing.

Closed Reduction.   In most instances, closed reduction is accomplished by bringing the bone fragments into apposition (ends in contact) by *manipulation* and *manual traction*.

Following the manipulation, x-ray films are taken to determine that the bone fragments are in correct alignment. A cast is usually applied to immobilize the extremity and maintain the reduction. A second person may hold the extremity in the desired position while it is being encased in plaster.

Traction.   Traction may be used to effect fracture reduction and immobilization. Adjustments of the magnitude of traction are made as muscle spasm is overcome. X-rays are used to monitor the fracture reduction and approximation of the bony fragments. As the fracture heals, evidence of callus formation is noted radiologically. When the callus is well established, a cast is frequently used for the immobilization technique. Traction therapy and the nursing management of a patient in traction are discussed more fully on page 1552.

Open Reduction or Open Operation.   Some fractures require an operation or open reduction. The fracture fragments are reduced (put into alignment). Internal fixation devices in the form of metallic pins, wires, screws, plates, nails, or rods may be used to hold the bone fragments in position until solid bone healing occurs. Internal fixation devices may

Figure 57-2
The types of immobilizing dressings used for upper humeral fractures. (*A*) A commercial sling and swathe that permits easy removal of the arm for hygiene and is comfortable on the neck. (*B*) A conventional sling and swathe. (*C*) A stockinette Velpeau and swathe is used when there is an unstable surgical neck component, because this position relaxes the pectoralis major. (Redrawn from Rockwood CA and Green DP. Fractures. Philadelphia, JB Lippincott.)

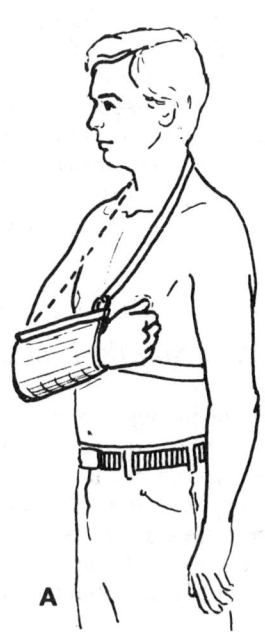
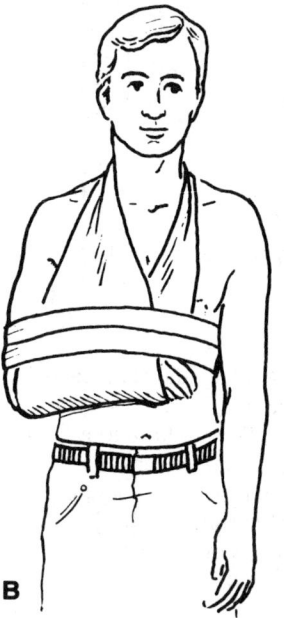
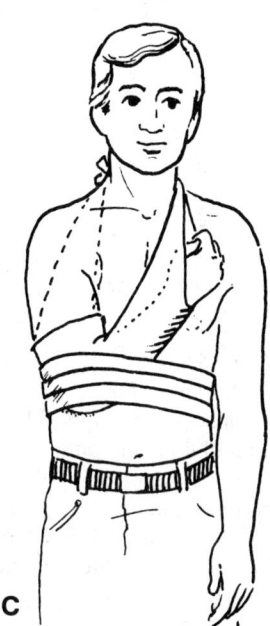

A   B   C

be attached to the sides of bone or inserted through the bony fragments or directly into the medullary cavity of the bone (Fig. 57-3). These devices assure firm approximation and fixation of the bony fragments.

Nursing Management Following Open Reduction. During the immediate postoperative period following open reduction, the nursing management is the same as for any other major surgical procedure (see Chap. 19). If the patient is to be immobilized in traction following surgery, the traction may be applied immediately following surgery in the operating room. Ice to control edema may be prescribed. Neurovascular monitoring is done at frequent intervals. The affected part is elevated.

- Symptoms of pain, pallor, pulselessness, paresthesia, paralysis (the five Ps), or coolness, indicate abnormal circulatory changes or neurologic disturbances.
- The orthopedist should be notified immediately so that

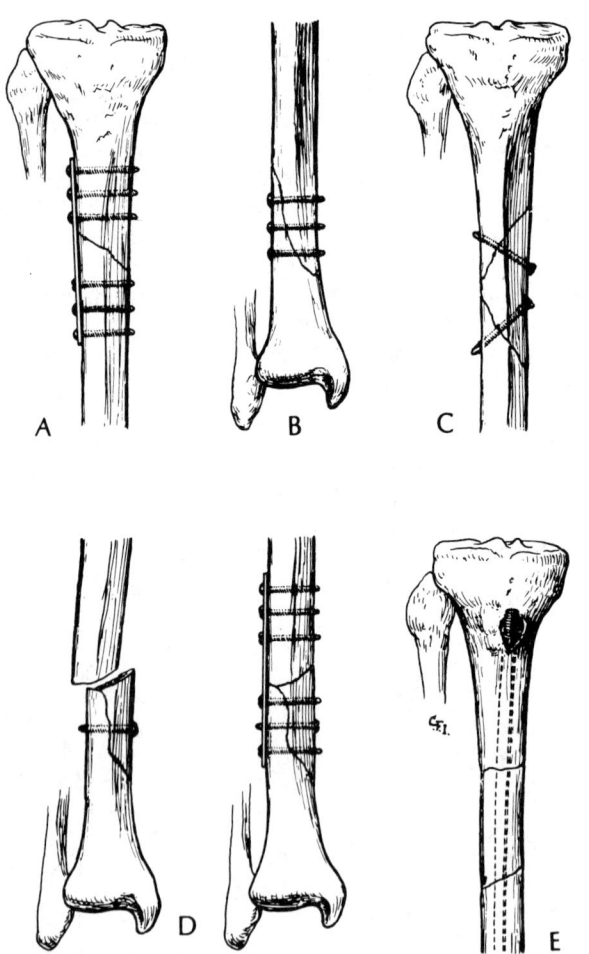

Figure 57-3
Techniques of internal fixation. (*A*) Plate and six screws for a transverse or short oblique fracture. (*B*) Screws for a long oblique or spiral fracture. (*C*) Screws for a long butterfly fragment. (*D*) Plate and six screws for a short butterfly fragment. (*E*) Medullary nail for a segmental fracture. (Smith H. Fractures. In Crenshaw AH [ed]. Campbell's Operative Orthopeadics, Vol 1. St Louis, CV Mosby.)

the dressings may be loosened or the cast bivalved in order to relieve pressure (see p. 1547). Hematoma drainage or fasciotomy may be needed. Dressings should be inspected at regular intervals.

The assessment and management of postoperative pain is an individualized problem. During the immediate postoperative period, narcotics may be prescribed. In general, an elderly patient requires less narcotic than a younger patient. As soon as possible, oral nonnarcotic analgesics should be given as prescribed, since patients who have undergone orthopedic operations may have prolonged musculoskeletal complaints. Restlessness, anxiety, and general discomfort may be relieved by appropriate nursing measures, including reassurance, position changes, and pain modification techniques.

Orthopedic wounds have a tendency to ooze more than other surgical wounds. External muscle dissection frequently produces wounds in which hemostasis is poor. Wounds that are closed while under tourniquet control may bleed when the tourniquet is released in the postoperative period. Drains and portable wound suction are used to minimize blood accumulation and the possibility of infection.

Maintenance of good aseptic technique is essential when caring for patients having bone surgery. *Osteomyelitis* (bone infection) is difficult to treat, and prevention is the objective. Aseptic wound dressing technqiue is necessary. Prevention of wound infections will eliminate that source for subsequent osteomyelitis.

Usually, internal fixation will allow early mobilization of the patient. The actual stability of the fracture fixation determines the amount of movement and stress the extremity can withstand. The surgeon can estimate the degree of stability obtained and will prescribe activity limits. An overbed trapeze is available to assist the patient moving in bed.

Removal of Internal Fixation Devices. Internal fixation devices may be removed after bony union has taken place, but for the majority of patients a device is not removed unless it produces symptoms. Pain and decreased function are the prime indicators that a problem has developed. Such problems may include mechanical failure (inadequate insertion and stabilization); material failure (faulty or damaged internal fixation devices); corrosion of the device, causing local inflammation; allergic response to the metallic alloy used; and osteoporotic remodeling adjacent to the fixation device (stress needed for bone strength is carried by the device, causing a disuse osteoporosis). If the device is removed, the bone needs to be protected from refracture related to osteoporosis, altered bone structure, and accident. Bone remodeling reestablishes the bone's structural strength.

Nursing Care of the Patient With a Simple Fracture

An important objective in treating fractures is to help patients return to their usual activities as rapidly as possible. Weeks to months are required for most fractures to heal. Patients are taught how to control swelling and pain associated with the fracture and soft-tissue trauma. They are encouraged to be active within the limits of the fracture immobilization. Bed rest is kept at a minimum. Exercises are begun to maintain health of unaffected muscles and to increase strength of muscles needed for transferring and using ambulatory aids. Patients are taught how to use these devices safely. Planning is done to help patients modify their home environment as needed and secure personal assistance if necessary. Patient teaching includes self-care, medication information, monitoring for potential problems, and the need for continuing health care supervision. The goal is to return to the prior level of activity, but it may take months for fracture healing and restoration of full strength and mobility.

Nursing Care Plan 57-1 outlines the basic nursing care for the patient who has sustained a simple fracture.

Management of Open Fractures

In an open fracture (one associated with an open wound extending through the skin surface and down to the area of bone injury) there is risk of *infection*—osteomyelitis, gas gangrene, and tetanus. The objectives of management are to minimize the chance of infection of the wound, soft tissue, and bone and to promote healing of soft tissue and bone.

The patient is taken to the operating room, where the wound is cleansed, débrided (foreign matter and devitalized tissue removed) and irrigated. The wound is swabbed for culture and sensitivity studies. Devitalized bone fragments are usually removed. Bone grafting may be done to bridge the defect, provided that the recipient tissue is healthy and able to facilitate union. The fracture is carefully reduced and stabilized by external fixation. Repair of damage to blood vessels, soft tissue, muscles, nerves, and tendons is usually carried out.

Primary closure may not be accomplished because of edema and potential ischemia, restricted wound drainage, and anaerobic infection. A heavily contaminated wound may be left open, dressed with sterile gauze, and not closed until it is clear that infection has been aborted or overcome. Tetanus prophylaxis is given. Usually, intravenous antibiotics are started to prevent or treat serious infection. The wounds are closed by suture or by autogenous skin or flap grafts in 5 to 7 days.

Nursing Care. Upon return from the operating room, the patient is observed for signs of shock because considerable loss of blood usually occurs during surgery. The extremity is elevated to minimize the development of edema. The distal pulses are palpated and neurovascular status is assessed frequently. The temperature is taken at regular intervals, and the patient is observed for signs of infection.

External Fixators

External fixation devices are used to manage open fractures with soft-tissue damage and provide stable support for severe comminuted fractures while permitting active treatment of damaged soft tissue (Fig. 57-4).

Complicated fractures of the humerus, forearm, femur, tibia, and pelvis are managed with external skeletal fixators. The fracture is reduced, aligned, and immobilized by a series of pins inserted in the bone fragments. The pins are maintained in position through attachment to a portable frame. The fixators facilitate patient comfort, early mobility, active exercise of adjacent uninvolved joints, and shortened hos-

pitalization. In addition, complications related to disuse and immobility are minimized.

The fixator is removed when the soft tissue has healed; the fracture may be stabilized by cast or molded orthosis until the bone has healed by callus formation. (Continuous compression at the fracture site with an external fixator for primary bone healing is difficult to achieve.)

Nursing Care. Psychological preparation for application of the external fixator is important. The apparatus looks clumsy and foreign to the patient. Reassurance that the discomfort associated with the device is mild and that early mobility is anticipated aids in the acceptance of the device. Involvement of the patient in the care associated with the fixator after it is applied will also help.

Following application of the external fixator, the extremity is elevated to reduce swelling. The neurovascular status of the extremity is monitored frequently. The injured area and pin sites are checked for signs of infection. Some serous drainage from the pin sites is to be expected. Assess each pin site for redness, drainage, tenderness, pain, and loosening of the pin.

- NEVER adjust the clamps on the external fixator frame.

Pin care to prevent pin tract infection is carried out according to the prescribed routine. Crusts should not form at the pin site, and the fixator must be kept clean.

Isometric and active exercises are encouraged within the limits of tissue damage. The nurse must be alert for potential problems due to pressure by the device on the skin, nerves, or blood vessels, and prevent device-induced injury by covering any sharp points on the fixator or pins. When the swelling has subsided, the patient is mobilized within the limits of any other injuries. Weight-bearing limits need to be prescribed to minimize the chance of pins loosening when stress is applied at the bone-pin interface.

Complications of Fractures

Immediate Complications

The immediate complications following fracture are *shock,* which may be fatal within a few hours after injury; *fat embolism,* which may occur within 48 hours or later; *compartment syndrome,* which may result in permanent loss of extremity function; *infection; thromboembolism* (pulmonary embolism), which may cause death several weeks after injury; and *disseminated intravascular coagulation.*

Shock

Hypovolemic or traumatic shock, resulting from hemorrhage (both external and nonvisible blood loss) and loss of extracellular fluid into damaged tissues, may occur in fractures of the extremities, thorax, pelvis, and spine. Because the bone is very vascular, large quantities of blood may be lost as a result of trauma, especially in femoral and pelvic fractures.

Treatment consists of replacing the depleted blood volume, relieving the patient's pain, providing adequate splinting, and protecting the patient from further injury.

(Text continues on p. 1582)

Care of the Patient With a Simple Fracture

Nursing Interventions	*Rationale*	*Expected Outcomes*

Nursing Diagnosis: Alteration in comfort—pain related to fracture

Goal: Relief of pain

1. Encourage patient to describe type and location of discomfort.	1. Pain and tenderness are expected with fracture and tissue damage; muscle spasms occur in response to injury and immobilization.	• Patient describes discomfort. • Keeps injured extremity elevated • Uses ice during first 24–48 hours • Controls edema; neurovascular status intact
2. Assess patient's discomfort.	2. Pain assessment provides basis for planning nursing interventions.	• Patient utilizes relaxation techniques. • Patient demonstrates methods to control pain and swelling.
3. Utilize measures to control pain: a. Splint and support injured area.	a. Prevents additional injury; minimizes movement of fracture fragments	• Performs active and passive range-of-motion exercises on nonimmobilized joints; changes position frequently
b. Perform position changes gently.	b. Decreases muscle spasms	• Elevates injured extremity
c. Elevate injured extremity above heart level.	c. Controls edema by promoting drainage	• Obtains pain relief
d. Apply ice, if prescribed.	d. Ice decreases pain and controls bleeding and edema.	
e. Monitor swelling and neurovascular status.	e. Edema and bleeding into the traumatized tissues cause discomfort; unrelenting pain may indicate compartment syndrome.	
f. Administer pain medications as prescribed early in pain experience.	f. Oral analgesics provide pain relief following fracture; control techniques are more effective early in pain cycle.	
g. Suggest relaxation techniques.	g. Modifies pain experience	
4. Offer explanation of nursing measures to control pain, swelling, and additional tissue damage.	4. Damaged tissues cause pain; immobilization decreases discomfort from movement of fracture fragments; understanding of cause of pain reduces patient's perception of pain.	
5. Encourage active and passive range-of-motion exercises for nonimmobilized joints; encourage position changes as permitted within limits of immobilizing device.	5. Pressure on bony prominences and disuse contribute to discomfort.	
6. Minimize the time the injured extremity is in dependent position.	6. Swelling will occur in injured tissues when dependent; swelling contributes to discomfort.	

Nursing Diagnosis: Potential for injury related to neurovascular compromise and disuse

Goal: Achievement of uncomplicated healing

1. Assess for the development of neurovascular compromise:
  a. Increasing pain
  b. Cool skin temperature
  c. Increasing swelling
  d. Decreased motor abilities
  e. Abnormal sensations
  f. Diminished capillary refill
	1. Early recognition of circulation and nerve problems due to compartment syndrome is needed to prevent loss of function.	• Neurovascular status distal to fracture is intact.
		• Patient describes signs and symptoms of neurovascular compromise.
		• Shows no evidence of skin breakdown
		• Describes signs and symptoms of skin breakdown

(continued)

Nursing Interventions	Rationale	Expected Outcomes

Nursing Diagnosis: Potential for injury related to neurovascular compromise and disuse

Goal: Achievement of uncomplicated healing

2. Teach the signs and symptoms of neurovascular compromise.	2. Patient education is needed for self care.	• Participates in activities that will minimize diminished muscle function and loss of joint motion
3. Assess for the development of skin breakdown: a. Skin abrasion b. Cast "hot spots" c. Drainage d. Irritation sensations	3. Pressure of casts and appliances can cause skin breakdown.	
4. Teach the signs and symptoms of skin breakdown.	4. Patient education is needed for self-care	
5. Encourage active exercise and range-of-motion exercise of body parts not immobilized.	5. Disuse results in atrophy of muscles and loss of joint motion.	
6. Encourage isometric exercises of immobilized muscles.	6. Patient education is needed for self-care.	

Nursing Diagnosis: Self-care deficit related to disruption of ability to perform activities of daily living

Goal: Patient demonstrates satisfactory adjustment to altered performance of activities of daily living.

1. Encourage patient to express concerns and to discuss injury and problems associated with injury. Listen actively.	1. Fractures result from accidents, which impact on one's ability to perform activities of daily living. Life-style is interrupted. Time loss from employment occurs.	• Patient discusses injury and its impact on life. • Utilizes available resources and coping mechanisms to modify emotional stress • Participates in development of health care plan • Participates in activities of daily living • Demonstrates safe use of treatment modalities and mobilization aids • Patient achieves appropriate level of self-care at home.
2. Support use of coping mechanisms.	2. Sudden disruption of routines and plans requires use of coping mechanisms.	
3. Involve significant others and support services as needed and appropriate.	3. Others can assist patient with activities of daily living.	
4. Modify home environment as necessary.	4. Accommodations for home management of fracture may be necessary.	
5. Engage patient in development of treatment regimen.	5. Patient regains self-control by active participation in treatment plan decisions.	
6. Explain various facets of treatment regimen.	6. Patient education and understanding of rationale increase compliance.	
7. Encourage active participation in activities of daily living within therapeutic limits.	7. Self-esteem is enhanced through self-care activities.	
8. Teach safe use of treatment modalities and mobilization aids. Supervise use to assure safety.	8. Injury from unsafe use of modalities or mobilization aids can be prevented through education.	
9. Evaluate patient's ability to care for self at home: a. Planned treatment regimen b. Recognition of potential problems c. Recognition of unsafe situations d. Continued health supervision	9. Ensures patient's ability to manage fracture at home. Lack of knowledge and poor preparation for self-care at home contribute to anxiety and nonadherence to therapeutic regimen.	

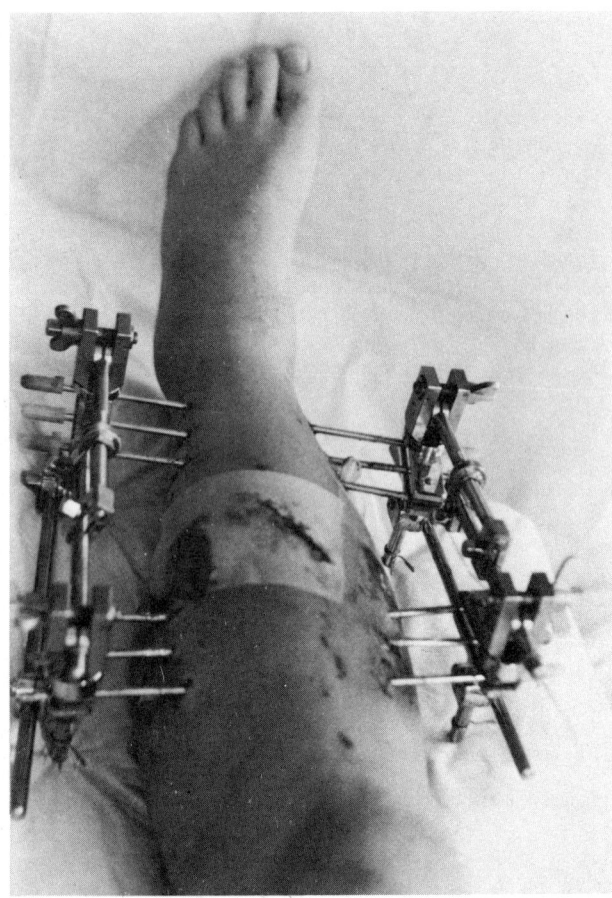

Figure 57-4
External fixation device. Pins are inserted into bone fragments. The fracture is reduced and aligned. The reduction is stabilized by attaching the pins to a rigid portable frame. The device facilitates treatment of soft tissue damaged in complex fracture situations.

Fat Embolism Syndrome

Following fracture of long bones or pelvis, multiple fractures, or crush injuries, fat emboli may develop, especially in the young adult (20–30 years old) male. At the time of fracture, innumerable fat globules may move into the blood because the marrow pressure is greater than the capillary pressure or because catecholamines elevated by the patient's stress reaction cause mobilization of fatty acids and the development of fat globules in the bloodstream. The fat globules combine with platelets to form emboli, which then occlude the small blood vessels that supply the brain, lungs, kidneys, and other organs. The onset of symptoms may occur a few hours after injury to a week after injury, but usually occurs within 48 hours after injury. The onset of symptoms is rapid.

The presenting feature is usually cerebral disturbance manifested by bizarre mental symptoms varying from mild agitation and confusion to delirium and coma that occur in response to hypoxia, which results from the lodging of fat emboli in the brain. In addition, tachycardia is noted.

The respiratory response includes tachypnea, dyspnea, crackles, wheezes, and large amounts of thick, white sputum. Blood gases reveal PO_2 below 60 mm Hg, with an early respiratory alkalosis and later respiratory acidosis. The chest x-ray exhibits a typical "snow storm" infiltrate.

With systemic embolization the patient appears pale. Petechiae are noted in the buccal membranes and conjunctival sacs, on the hard palate, on the fundus of the eye, and over the chest and anterior axillary folds. Free fat may be found in the urine when emboli reach the kidneys.

- Personality changes, restlessness, irritability, or confusion in a patient who has sustained a fracture is an indication that immediate blood gas studies should be done. Occlusion of a large number of small vessels causes the pulmonary pressure to rise, possibly resulting in acute right heart failure. Edema and hemorrhages in the alveoli impair oxygen transport, leading to hypoxia. There is an increase in respiratory rate, precordial chest pain, cough, dyspnea, and acute pulmonary edema.

Management. Immediate immobilization of fractures, minimal fracture manipulation, and adequate support for fractured bones during turning and positioning are measures that may reduce the incidence of fat emboli. Frequently, fat emboli syndrome becomes apparent through subtle changes in the patient's mental status. Monitoring high-risk patients will aid in the early identification of this problem. Prompt institution of respiratory support is essential.

The objectives of management are to support the respiratory system and to correct homeostatic disturbances. Arterial blood gas analysis is done to determine the degree of respiratory impairment, as respiratory failure is the most common cause of death. Respiratory support is provided with oxygen given in high concentrations. Controlled volume ventilation with positive end-expiratory pressure (PEEP) may be employed to decrease and inhibit the formation of pulmonary edema. Steroids may be given to treat the inflammatory lung reaction and to control cerebral edema. Low-molecular-weight dextran may improve pulmonary and capillary flow because of its desludging effect. Heparin may be used for its lipolytic action (breakdown of fat globules), but its anticoagulant effect may cause hemorrhage at the fracture site.

To allay apprehension and decrease pain, morphine may be administered to patients on a ventilator.

Fat emboli are a major cause of death in patients with fractures. Respiratory support must be instituted early. Response to therapy frequently occurs within 48 hours.

Compartment Syndrome

Compartment syndrome is a problem that develops when tissue perfusion in the muscles is less than that required for tissue viability. This can be due to (1) reduction of the muscle compartment size because the enclosing muscle fascia is too tight or a cast or dressing is constrictive, or (2) an increase in muscle compartment contents because of edema or hemorrhage associated with a variety of problems (*e.g.*, ischemia, crush injuries, injection of tissue-destroying (toxic) substances, fractures). The forearm and the leg muscle compartments are involved most frequently. Permanent function can be lost if the situation continues for more than 6 to 8 hours and *myoneural* (muscle and nerve) ischemia and necrosis occur. Volkmann's contracture (Fig. 57-5) is an example of this complication.

The patient complains of deep, throbbing, unrelenting pain, which is not controlled by narcotics. Palpation of the muscle, if that is possible, will reveal it to be swollen and hard. Passive stretching movement of the muscle will cause acute pain. If it does not, the patient's pain may be due to nerve ischemia. Diminished capillary refill, cyanotic nailbeds, paralysis, and paresthesia may be present. The pulse may be obscured by swelling. Usually, major arteries are not occluded by compartment syndrome. The actual tissue pressures can be monitored by inserting a fluid-filled needle or wick catheter into the suspected compartment and determining the pressure via a pressure transducer monitoring setup similar to that used for hemodynamic pressure monitoring. (Normal pressure is up to 22 mm Hg.) Nerve and muscle tissues deteriorate as compartment pressures increase.

Prevention and Management. Compartment syndrome can be prevented by elevating the injured extremity and by applying ice after injury. If it occurs, restrictive dressings must be released, and fasciotomy may be needed if conservative measures have not restored tissue perfusion and relieved pain within an hour.

The extremity is splinted in a functional position, and passive range-of-motion exercises are usually prescribed every 4 to 6 hours. The wound is débrided and closed in 3 to 5 days when the edema has resolved and tissue perfusion has been restored.

Other Immediate Complications

Thromboembolism (discussed on p. 649), *infection* (all open fractures are considered to be contaminated—see p. 1579), and *disseminated intravascular coagulation (DIC)* are other possible complications of fractures. DIC includes a group of bleeding disorders with diverse causes, including massive tissue trauma. Manifestations include ecchymoses, unexpected bleeding after surgery, and bleeding from the mucous membranes, venipuncture sites, and gastrointestinal and urinary tracts. The treatment of DIC is discussed on page 693.

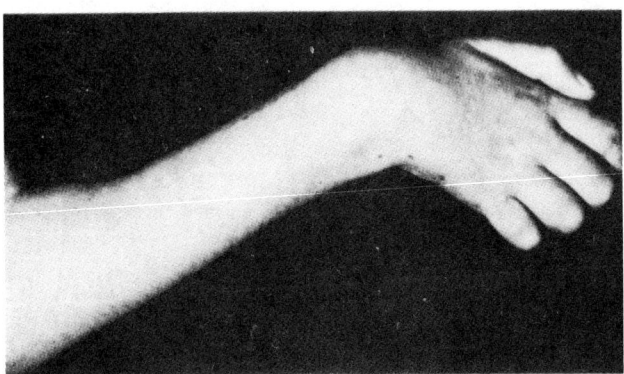

Figure 57-5
The forearm and hand of a patient with late Volkmann's ischemic contracture. (Rockwood CA and Green DP [eds]. Fractures, Vol 1. Philadelphia, JB Lippincott.)

Delayed Complications

Delayed Union and Nonunion. *Delayed union* occurs when healing does not advance at a normal rate for the location and type of fracture. *Nonunion* results from failure of the ends of a fractured bone to unite. The patient complains of persistent discomfort and movement at the fracture site. Factors contributing to union problems include infection at the fracture site; interposition of tissue between the bone ends; inadequate immobilization or manipulation, which disrupts callus formation; excessive space between bone fragments (bone gap); limited bone contact; and restricted blood supply that results in avascular necrosis.

In nonunion, fibrocartilage or fibrous tissue exists between the bone fragments; no bone salts have been deposited. A false joint (*pseudoarthrosis*) often develops at the site of the fracture. Fractures of the middle third of the humerus, of the neck of the femur in elderly people, and of the lower third of the tibia most frequently result in nonunion.

Nonunion may be managed by *bone grafting*. Surgically, the fractured bone fragments are freshened, infection if present is removed, and a bone graft, frequently from the iliac crest, is placed in the bony defect. The bone graft provides a lattice work for invasion by bone cells. Following grafting, rigid immobilization is required.

Electrical Stimulation of Osteogenesis. Osteogenesis in nonunion may be stimulated by electricity, and is approximately as effective as bone grafting. It is not effective with large bone gaps or synovial pseudoarthrosis. The electrical stimulation modifies the tissue environment, enhancing mineral deposition and bone formation.

In some situations, pins that act as cathodes are inserted percutaneously directly into the fracture site, and direct current is passed over the fracture continuously. Direct current methods cannot be used when infection is present.

Another method is noninvasive inductive coupling. Pulsing electromagnetic fields (PEMFs) are delivered to the fracture for 10 to 12 hours a day by an electromagnetic coil implanted in the dressing over the nonunion site (Fig. 57-6). During the electrical stimulation treatment period, rigid fracture fixation with adequate support is needed.

Avascular Necrosis of Bone. *Avascular necrosis* occurs when the bone loses its blood supply and dies. It may follow a fracture (especially of the femoral neck), dislocations, prolonged high-dosage steroid therapy, chronic renal disease, sickle cell anemia and other diseases. The devitalized bone may collapse or reabsorb and be replaced by new bone. The patient develops limitation of movement and pain. X-ray demonstrates calcium loss and structural collapse. Treatment generally consists of attempts to revitalize the bone with bone grafts, prosthetic replacement, or *arthrodesis* (joint fusion).

Fractures of Specific Sites

An injury to the skeletal structure may vary from a simple linear fracture to a severe crushing injury. The therapeutic program is determined by the type and location of the fracture and the degree of involvement of surrounding structures. Maximum functional recovery is the goal of fracture management.

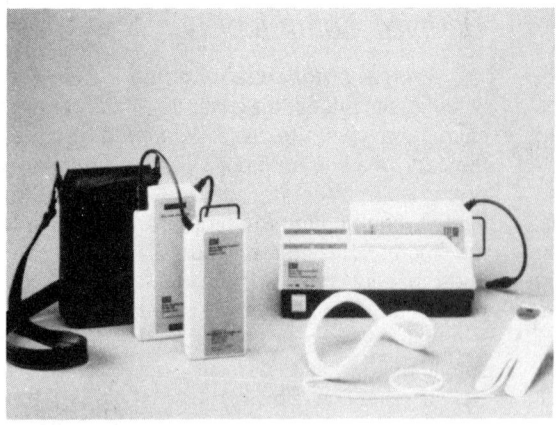

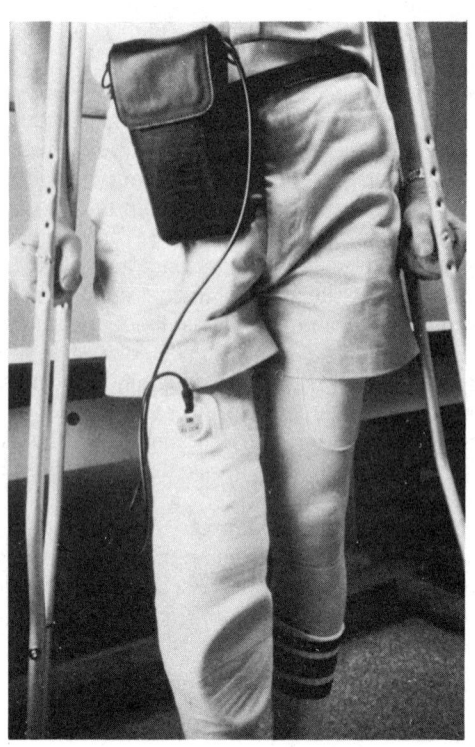

Figure 57-6
Electromagnetic bone-healing stimulator. Pulsed electromagnetic fields generated through coils included in the cast produce bone growth (osteogenesis) at the fracture site. The system is portable and battery powered. The therapy is used for 10 to 12 hours a day (Courtesy of EBI Medical Systems, Inc., Fairfield, New Jersey.)

Fractures of the skull and cervical spine have been considered in Chapter 54 on the management of patients with neurologic disorders. Fracture of the mandible is discussed in Chapter 30.

Clavicle (Collar Bone) Fractures

Fracture of the collar bone is a common fracture that results from a fall or a direct blow to the shoulder. Associated head or cervical spine injuries are seen with these fractures.

The clavicle helps to hold the shoulder upward, outward, and backward from the thorax. Therefore, when the clavicle is fractured, the patient assumes a protective position—slumping the shoulders and immobilizing the arm to prevent shoulder movement. The objective of management is to hold the shoulder in its normal position by means of closed reduction and immobilization.

More than 80% of these fractures occur in the middle or inner two thirds of the clavicle. A modified shoulder spica (clavicular cast) or a figure-of-8 bandage or a commercially available clavicular strap (Fig. 57-7) may be used to pull the shoulders back and hold them in that position. When a clavicular strap is used, the axillae are well padded to prevent a compression injury to the brachial plexus and axillary artery. There should be no restriction of circulatory or nerve function in either arm.

Fracture of the distal third of the clavicle without displacement and ligament disruption is treated with a sling and restricted use of the arm. When a fracture in the distal third is accompanied by a disrupted coracoclavicular ligament, there is displacement and it is more difficult to obtain healing. Open reduction and internal fixation with a Kirschner wire

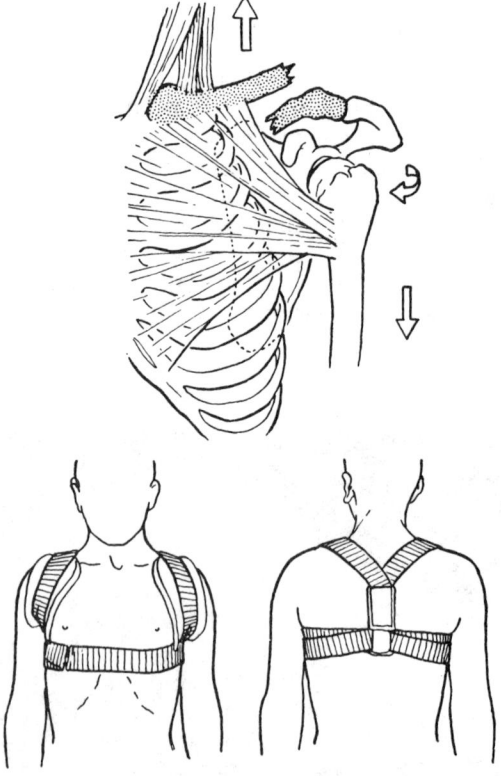

Figure 57-7
Fracture of the clavicle. (*Top*) Anteroposterior view, showing typical displacement of midclavicle fracture. (*Bottom*) Method of immobilization with a clavicular strap. (Hardy JD. Rhoads' Textbook of Surgery. Philadelphia, JB Lippincott.)

are recommended. Immobilization of the shoulder with a Velpeau dressing or a shoulder spica is necessary to ensure that the bone fragments are reduced in proper anatomical alignment.

Complications of clavicular fractures include trauma to the nerves of the brachial plexus, injury to the subclavian vein or artery from a bony fragment, and malunion. Malunion may be a cosmetic problem when low-neckline clothing is worn.

Patient Education and Home Health Care. The patient is cautioned not to elevate the arm above shoulder level until the fracture has united, about 6 weeks, but is encouraged to exercise the elbow, wrist, and fingers as soon as possible. When the patient is able, shoulder exercises (Fig. 57-8) are prescribed to obtain full shoulder motion. Heavy activity is limited for 3 months.

Rib Fractures

Uncomplicated fractures of the ribs occur frequently in adults, and usually result in no impairment of function. However, because fractures of the ribs produce painful respirations, the patient tends to decrease respiratory excursions and refrains from coughing. As a result, tracheobronchial secretions are not coughed up, aeration of the lung is diminished, and a predisposition to pneumonia and atelectasis is created. To help the patient cough and take deep breaths, the nurse may splint the chest with her hands. Intercostal nerve blocks are done to relieve respiratory pain and permit productive coughing.

Chest strapping to immobilize the rib fracture is not usually used, because decreased chest expansion may result in respiratory complications of pneumonia and atelectasis. The pain associated with rib fracture diminishes significantly in 3 or 4 days, and the fracture is healed in 6 weeks.

Other serious problems may result from rib fractures. Multiple rib fractures may lead to a flail chest (see p. 497), while severe rib fractures may result in puncture of the lung with the escape of air into the pleural space (*pneumothorax*) or of blood into the pleural space (*hemothorax*). The management of these patients is discussed on page 497.

Upper Extremity Fractures

Fractures of the Humeral Neck

Fractures of the proximal humerus may occur through either the anatomical or the surgical neck of the humerus. The anatomical neck is located just below the humeral head. The surgical neck is the region below the tubercles. Impacted fractures of the surgical neck of the humerus are seen most frequently in older women following a fall on an outstretched arm. These are essentially nondisplaced fractures. Active middle-aged patients may suffer severely displaced humeral neck fractures with associated rotator cuff damage.

The patient comes for aid with the affected arm hanging limp at the side and supported by the uninjured hand.

Neurovascular assessment of the involved extremity is essential to fully evaluate the extent of injury and possible involvement of the neurovascular bundle (nerves and blood vessels) of the arm.

Many of the impacted fractures of the surgical neck of the humerus do not require reduction. The arm is supported by a sling supplemented by a modified Velpeau bandage. When this sling arrangement is used, a soft pad is placed in the axilla to prevent skin maceration.

In any fracture of the arm, limitation of motion and stiffness of the shoulder occur from disuse. Therefore, *pendulum exercises* are begun as soon as tolerated by the patient. (In

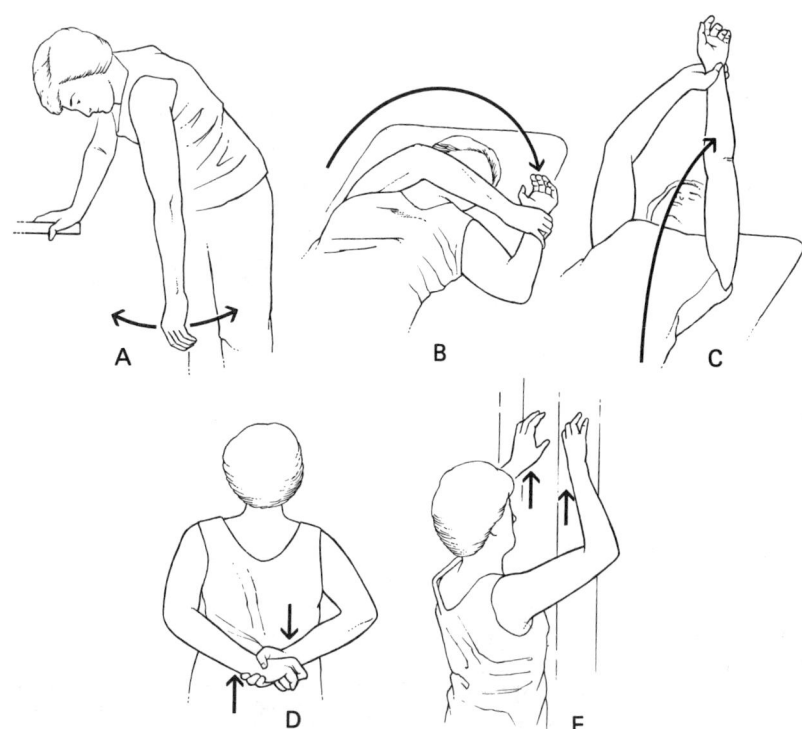

Figure 57-8
Exercises to develop range of motion of shoulder. (*A*) Pendulum exercise. (*B*) External rotation. (*C*) Elevation. (*D*) Internal rotation. In all of these, the unaffected arm is used for power. (*E*) Wall climbing.

pendulum or circumduction exercises, the patient is instructed to lean forward and to allow the affected arm to abduct and rotate [see Fig. 57-8]). Early motion of the joint does not displace the fragments if motion is carried out within the limits imposed by pain.

These fractures require 6 to 8 weeks to heal, and the patient should avoid vigorous activity, such as tennis, for an additional 4 weeks. Residual stiffness, aching, and some limitation of range of motion may persist for 6 or more months.

When a humeral neck fracture is displaced, treatment consists of closed reduction under x-ray control, open reduction, or replacement of the humeral head with a prosthesis. In this type of fracture, there must be a specified period of immobilization before exercises are started.

Fractures of the Shaft of the Humerus

Fractures of the shaft of the humerus are most frequently caused by (1) direct violence that results in a transverse, oblique, or comminuted fracture, or (2) an indirect twisting force that results in a spiral fracture. The nerves and brachial blood vessels may be injured with these fractures. Wrist drop is indicative of radial nerve injury. Initial neurovascular assessment is essential to differentiate between trauma from the injury and complications from treatment.

Frequently, the weight of the arm helps to correct any displacement so that surgery is not required. With oblique, spiral, or displaced fracture that has resulted in shortening of the humeral shaft, a hanging cast may be used. This cast is designed so that its weight provides traction to the arm when the patient is upright, thereby reducing and immobilizing the fracture. The hanging cast must be dependent (allowed to hang free without support), since the weight of the cast is the means by which continuous traction is applied to the long axis of the arm. The patient is advised to sleep in an upright position so that traction from the weight of the cast is maintained constantly.

Problems encountered with this mode of therapy are fracture distraction (pulling fracture fragments too far apart) due to the weight of the cast, and fracture angulation due to excessive fracture motion.

Finger exercises are started as soon as the cast is applied, while pendulum-shoulder exercises are done as directed to provide active movement of the shoulder, thereby preventing adhesions of the shoulder joint capsule. Isometric exercises may be prescribed to prevent muscle atrophy.

After the cast is removed, a sling is applied and exercises of the shoulder, elbow, and wrist are begun. It requires about 10 weeks for humeral fractures to heal when treated with hanging casts.

Elderly patients may not tolerate a cast. A sling and swathe (cloth that secures the supported arm to the trunk; Fig. 57-2) may provide adequate comfort and immobilization. Shoulder exercises may begin in a couple of weeks.

Functional bracing is another form of treatment being used for these fractures. A hanging cast is applied for about 1 week, and then a contoured thermoplastic sleeve is secured in place with Velcro closures around the upper arm. As swelling decreases, the Velcro is tightened, applying uniform pressure and stability to the fracture. Functional bracing allows active use of muscles, shoulder and elbow motion, and good approximation of fracture fragments. The callus that develops is substantial, and the sleeve can be discontinued in about 9 weeks. Shoulder spica casts may be used during early treatment of unstable humerus fractures. Generally, the patient is uncomfortable and feels quite awkward.

Skeletal traction may be appropriate for patients who must remain in bed due to other injuries (Figs. 57-9, 57-10). Active exercises of the hand and wrist are encouraged.

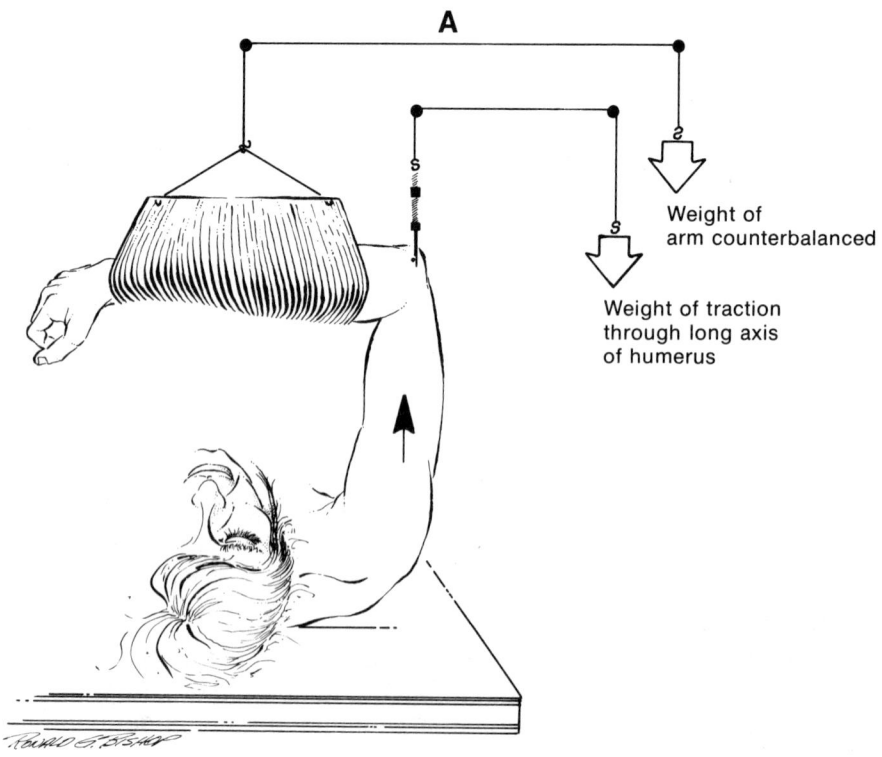

A

Weight of arm counterbalanced

Weight of traction through long axis of humerus

Figure 57-9
Treatment of supracondylar fracture. Over-the-face traction reduces swelling by creating a very effective elevation of the extremity. (Lewis RC. Handbook of Traction, Casting and Splinting Techniques. Philadelphia, JB Lippincott.)

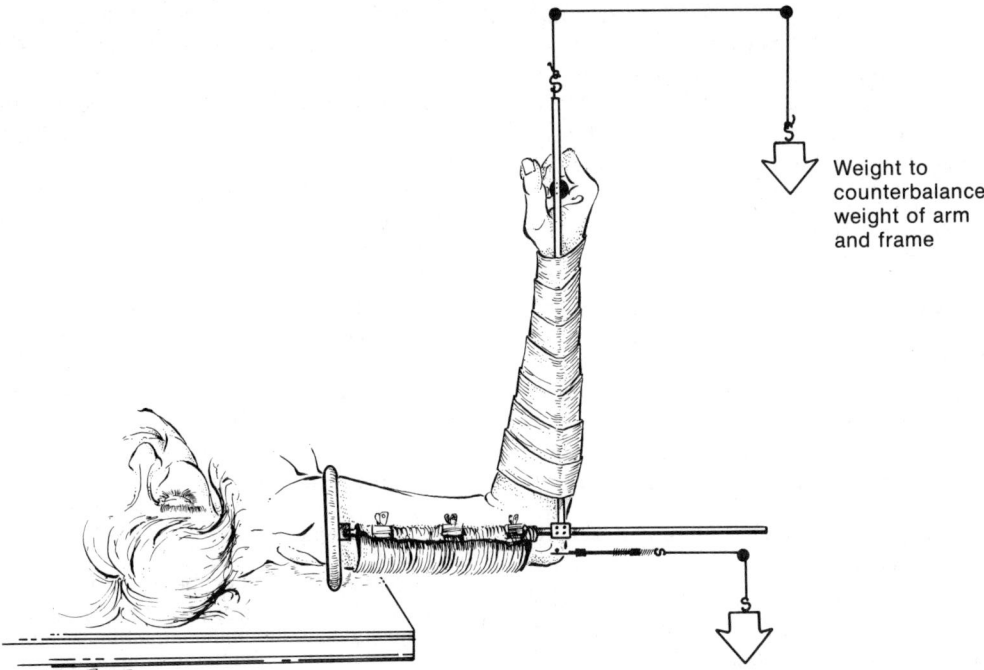

Weight to
counterbalance
weight of arm
and frame

Figure 57-10

Balanced side-arm traction. The arm is passed through the ring, which is then passed up so that it encompasses the shoulder. The upright attachment for the forearm may be moved in either direction to accommodate the length of the humerus. A cloth sling is placed on the horizontal segment to provide a surface on which the arm may rest. The olecranon extends just past the vertical extremity, so that the pin drilled through the olecranon will be clear and allow unimpeded traction. The forearm is placed between the two upright supports, and is usually held there with a circumferentially applied elastic bandage. A rope is attached to the vertical section and is passed through pulleys. A weight is attached to exactly counterbalance the weight of the arm and the frame. Skeletal traction is then applied in the desired amount through the pin in the olecranon. The entire extremity is counterbalanced so that a balanced traction system is created. (Lewis RC. Handbook of Traction, Casting and Splinting Techniques. Philadelphia, JB Lippincott.)

Open fractures of the humeral shaft are frequently treated by external fixators (see p. 1579). Open reduction of a humerus fracture is necessary with evidence of nerve palsy, pathologic fractures, or when other systemic or neurological disease (*e.g.,* Parkinson's disease) would make management with a hanging cast inappropriate.

Fractures at the Elbow

Fractures of the distal humerus result from automobile accidents, from falls on the elbow or the flexed elbow, or by direct blow. These fractures may result in nerve damage from injury to the median, radial, or ulnar nerves. The patient is evaluated for paresthesias and also for signs of compromised circulation in the forearm and hand. The most serious complication of a supracondylar fracture of the humerus is *Volkmann's ischemic contracture*, which results from antecubital swelling or damage to the brachial artery (see Fig. 57-5).

- Observe the hand for swelling, skin color (blueness and blanching of the nailbeds), and temperature, comparing it with the unaffected hand.

- Evaluate the amplitude of the radial pulse. If it weakens or disappears, the orthopedic surgeon must be informed *immediately* because irreversible ischemia may result. Fasciotomy may become necessary.
- Assess for paresthesias (prickling and burning sensations) in the hand, since such signs may indicate nerve injury or impending ischemia. Early treatment is indicated to restore circulation before irreparable damage occurs.
- Encourage the patient to move his fingers frequently.

Prompt reduction is desired. *Hemarthrosis* (blood in the joint) may be aspirated to relieve pain. The articular surfaces may be injured. The goal of therapy is reduction and stabilization of the fracture, followed by controlled active motion when swelling has subsided and healing has begun. If the fracture is not displaced, the arm is immobilized in a cast or posterior splint with the elbow at 45 to 90 degrees of flexion, or the elbow may be supported with a pressure dressing and a sling.

A displaced fracture is usually treated by traction and/or open reduction and internal fixation. Sometimes the bone fragments are excised. Additional external support with a plaster splint is then applied.

Gentle range-of-motion exercise of the injured joint is begun about 1 week after internal fixation and after 2 weeks with nondisplaced closed reduction. Motion aids healing of injured joints by movement of synovial fluid into the articular cartilage. Active exercise of the elbow is carried out when prescribed, as limitation of motion is common unless an intensive rehabilitation program is done.

Radial and Ulnar Fractures

Fractures of the Radial Head. Radial head fractures are common, and are usually produced by a fall on the outstretched hand with the elbow in extension. If blood has collected in the elbow joint (*hemarthrosis*), it is aspirated to relieve pain and allow early range of motion. Immobilization for these undisplaced fractures is accomplished by a sling. Active joint motion may be prescribed as early as 1 to 2 days after injury.

If the fracture is displaced, an open operation is required, with excision of the radial head when necessary. Postoperatively, the arm is immobilized in a posterior plaster splint and sling. The patient is encouraged to carry out a program of active motion of the elbow and forearm when prescribed.

Fractures of the Shafts of the Radius and Ulna. Fractures of the shaft of the bones of the forearm occur most frequently in children. Either the radius, the ulna, or both bones may be broken at any level. Frequently, displacement occurs when both bones are broken.

The forearm has the unique functions of pronation and supination, and those motions must be preserved by good anatomical position and alignment.

If the fragments are not displaced, the fracture is treated by closed reduction with a long arm cast applied from the upper arm to the proximal palmar crease. A loop may be incorporated in the cast near the elbow and a sling pulled through it to prevent the cast from sagging against the forearm.

The circulation, sensation, and motion of the hand are assessed after the cast is applied. The arm is elevated to control edema. Frequent finger flexion and extension are encouraged to reduce edema. Active motion of the involved shoulder is essential. The reduction and alignment are monitored closely by x-ray to ensure adequate immobilization.

The fracture is immobilized for about 12 weeks; during the last 6 weeks the arm may be in a functional forearm brace that allows exercise of the wrist and elbow.

Displaced fractures are managed by open reduction with internal fixation, using a compression plate with screws, intramedullary nails, or rods. The arm is usually immobilized in a plaster splint, cast, or pressure dressing. Open fractures may be managed with external fixation devices. The arm is elevated to control swelling. Neurovascular status is monitored. Elbow, wrist, and hand exercises are begun as permitted by the immobilization device.

Fractures of the Wrist

A fracture of the distal radius (Colles's fracture) is a common fracture and is usually the result of a fall on an open dorsiflexed hand. It is frequently seen in elderly women with osteoporotic bones and weak soft tissues that do not dissipate the energy of the fall. The patient has a deformed wrist with radial deviation, pain, swelling, weakness, limited finger range of motion, and numbness.

Treatment usually consists of closed reduction and immobilization with a cast. For more severe fractures, a Kirschner wire may be inserted or an external fixation device used to maintain reduction.

The wrist and forearm are elevated for 48 hours after reduction. The arm may be suspended from an overhead frame or IV pole.

Swelling of the fingers (from decreased venous and lymphatic return) is watched for and treated actively. Constricting casts and bandages must be released promptly. The median nerve is assessed for function. (Assess sensation by pricking the distal aspect of the index finger, and evaluate motor function by testing the ability to touch the thumb to the little finger). Active motion of the fingers and shoulder is begun on recovery from anesthesia.

The patient is taught to do the following finger exercises to reduce swelling and prevent stiffness:

1. Hold the hand above the level of the heart.
2. Move the fingers from full extension to flexion. Hold and release.
   (Repeat above at least 10 times every half hour when awake).
3. Use the hand in functional activities.
4. Actively exercise the shoulder and elbow.

Fracture of the Hand

Because trauma to the hand can be a complex problem, requiring extensive reconstructive surgery, the reader is referred to specialized books on the hand. The objective of treatment is always to regain maximum function of the hand.

For an undisplaced fracture of the distal phalanx (finger bone), the finger is splinted (for 3 to 4 weeks to relieve pain and to protect the fingertip from further trauma. Displaced fractures and open fractures may require open reduction with internal fixation, using wires or pins.

Neurovascular status of the injured hand is evaluated. Swelling is controlled by elevation of the hand. Functional use of the uninvolved portions of the hand is encouraged.

Lower Extremity Fractures

The objectives of management of a fracture of the lower extremity are (1) to obtain adequate bony union with full length and normal alignment and without rotational or angular deformity, (2) to restore muscle power and joint motion, and (3) to restore the preinjury ambulatory status of the patient.

Special Rehabilitation Nursing Measures

- A fractured lower extremity is not to be placed in a dependent position for prolonged periods, because *edema is a common problem* following all injuries of the lower extremities.
- The patient is encouraged to exercise regularly all joints that do not move the bone fragments.

- The extremity is elevated intermittently when the patient becomes ambulatory to minimize recurrence of edema. It is best for the patient to lie down when elevating the healing leg.
- After the immobilizing device is removed, elastic stockings can be worn to support venous circulation, thus reducing the problem of edema.

Because practically all fractures of the lower extremity require the use of crutches, walker, or cane during convalescence, adjustable equipment should be acquired for the patient. The safe use of these ambulatory aids is discussed in Chapter 14.

Femur Fractures

Fractures of the femur can occur at several sites (Fig. 57-11). When the head, neck, or trochanteric region of the femur is involved, a hip fracture results.

Hip Fractures

There is a high incidence of hip fractures among elderly people because their bones are brittle from osteoporosis and they fall readily from weakness of the quadriceps muscles as well as from general frailty due to age and a sedentary existence. Falls in the elderly also occur because of conditions that produce a decrease in cerebral arterial perfusion (transient ischemic attacks, anemia, emboli, cardiovascular disease, drug effects). Their therapeutic and nursing management is further complicated by associated medical diseases (cardiovascular, pulmonary, renal, and endocrine disorders). Hip fractures are the most frequent cause of traumatic death after the age of 75, occurring more frequently in women with osteoporosis, often after insignificant injuries. A hip fracture is viewed by the patient and the family as a catastrophic event that will make a negative impact on the patient's life-style.

Classification. There are two major types of hip fractures. *Intracapsular fractures* are fractures of the neck of the femur. *Extracapsular fractures* are fractures of the trochanteric region (between the base of the neck and the lesser trochanter of the femur) and the subtrochanteric region.

Fractures of the neck of the femur are more difficult to heal than those of the trochanteric region, because the vas-

cular system supplying blood to the head and the neck of the femur may be damaged with the fracture. The nutrient vessels within the bone may be interrupted, and the bone cells may die. For this reason, nonunion or aseptic necrosis is common in patients with these types of fractures.

Extracapsular intertrochanteric fractures have an excellent blood supply and heal readily. However, there is a fairly high mortality rate following intertrochanteric hip fractures, mainly because the patients are older (ages 70 to 85) and are poorer operative risks. Their conditions are further compromised by the degree of soft-tissue damage that occurs at the time of injury. Added difficulties can be anticipated when the fracture is comminuted and unstable, as is frequently the case.

Clinical Manifestations. Because of the fracture, the leg is shortened, adducted, and externally rotated. The patient may complain of slight pain in the groin or in the medial side of the knee. With most fractures of the femoral neck, the patient is in pain, is unable to move the leg without significant increase in pain, and is able to achieve some comfort with the leg slightly flexed in external rotation. Impacted femoral neck fractures cause moderate discomfort even with movement, may allow the patient to bear weight, and may not demonstrate obvious shortening or rotational changes. With extracapsular femoral fractures, the extremity is significantly shortened, presents external rotation to a greater degree than intracapsular fractures, exhibits muscle spasm that resists positioning of the extremity in a neutral position, and has an associated large hematoma or area of ecchymosis.

The diagnosis of fractured hip is confirmed with x-ray films.

Gerontological Considerations. Many elderly persons are confused, not only as a result of the stress of the trauma and unfamiliar surroundings, but also because of underlying systemic illness. Confusion that develops in some elderly patients may be due to mild cerebral ischemia. Examination of the legs may reveal edema due to congestive heart failure and absent peripheral pulses due to arteriosclerotic vascular disease. Frequently the elderly are taking cardiac or blood pressure medications that need to be continued and monitored. Likewise, chronic respiratory problems may be present and contribute to the possible development of inadequate pulmonary ventilation. Coughing and deep-breathing exercises are encouraged.

Dehydration and poor nutrition may be present. At times elderly persons who live alone are unable to summon help at the time of injury. A day or two may pass before assistance is provided, and as a result dehydration occurs. Dehydration contributes to hemoconcentration and predisposes to thromboembolism problems. Therefore the patient needs to be encouraged to consume adequate fluids and a balanced diet.

Muscle weakness and wasting may have contributed to the fall and fracture. Bed rest and immobility will cause an additional loss. The nurse needs to encourage movement of all joints except the involved hip and knee. Patients are encouraged to use their arms and the overhead trapeze to reposition themselves, thereby improving arm and shoulder strength, which are required for walking with ambulatory aids.

Management. Surgical intervention is carried out as soon as possible after the injury. The preoperative objective is to ensure that the patient is in as favorable a condition as

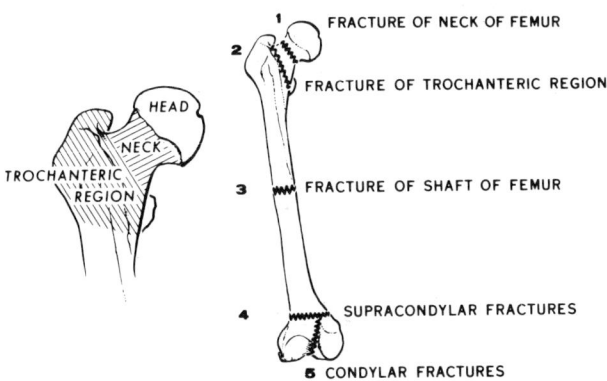

1 FRACTURE OF NECK OF FEMUR
2 FRACTURE OF TROCHANTERIC REGION
HEAD
NECK
TROCHANTERIC REGION
3 FRACTURE OF SHAFT OF FEMUR
4 SUPRACONDYLAR FRACTURES
5 CONDYLAR FRACTURES

Figure 57-11
Sites of fracture of the femur.

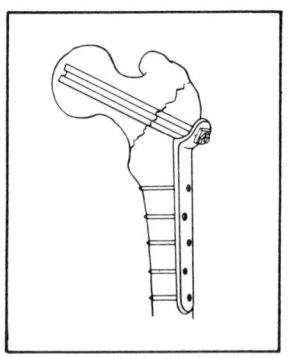

**Smith-Petersen nail
with McLaughlin plate**

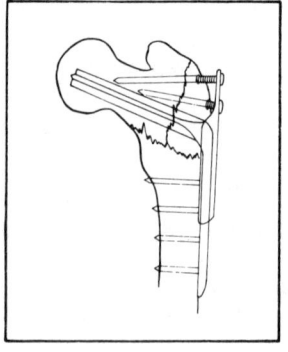

**Jewett nail
with overlay plate**

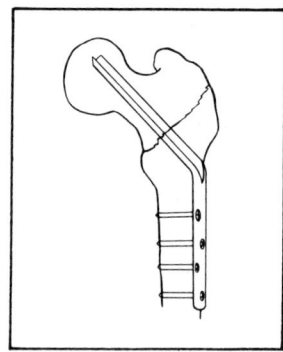

Neufeld nail

Figure 57-12
Examples of internal fixation for trochanteric fractures. In fractures of the femoral neck and trochanteric region, internal fixation is achieved through the use of nails and plates specifically designed for stability and fixation. (Courtesy of Zimmer-USA, Warsaw, Indiana.)

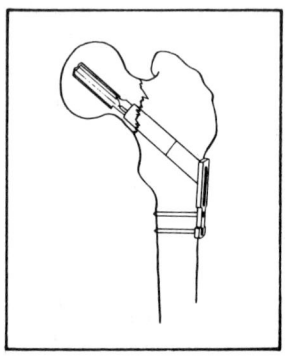

Massie nail assembly

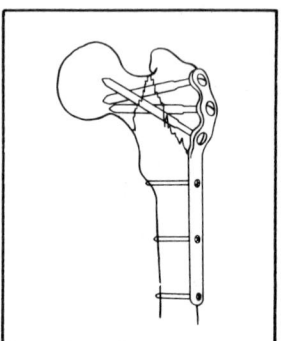

Moe intertrochanteric plate

possible. Displaced femoral neck fractures may be treated as elective emergencies, and reduction and internal fixation are done within 12 to 24 hours after fracture. This is to minimize the effects of diminished blood supply and the development of avascular necrosis.

Temporary skin traction in the form of Buck's extension (see p. 1555) may be applied to reduce muscle spasm, to immobilize the extremity, and to relieve pain. Sand bags or a trochanter roll may be used to control the external rotation.

The goal of surgical treatment of hip fractures is to obtain a satisfactory fixation so that the patient can be mobilized quickly and thereby avoid secondary medical complications. Operative treatment consists of (1) reduction of the fracture and internal fixation, or (2) replacement of the femoral head with a prosthesis (*hemiarthroplasty*).

After general or spinal anesthesia, the femoral neck fracture is reduced under radiographic control, using an image intensifier. A stable fracture is usually fixed with nails, a nail-and-plate combination, multiple pins, or compression screw devices (Figs. 57-12 and 57-13). The choice of fixation device is determined by the fracture site and the preference of the orthopedic surgeon. A Zickel nail is particularly useful with subtrochanteric fractures, permitting earlier weight-bearing (Fig. 57-13). Adequate reduction is important for fracture healing. (The better the reduction, the better the healing.)

Replacement of the head of the femur with a prosthesis is usually reserved for a fracture that cannot be satisfactorily reduced or securely nailed. Some orthopedists prefer this method because nonunion and avascular necrosis of the head are common complications of internal fixation techniques. Salvage of the hip is usually preferred to prosthetic replace-

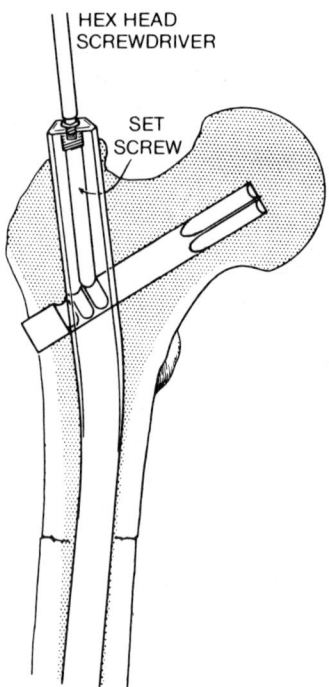

HEX HEAD
SCREWDRIVER

SET
SCREW

Figure 57-13
Zickel nail for subtrochanteric fractures. The triflanged nail is locked in the Zickel rod by a set screw. The Zickel nail fixation controls rotation and maintains alignment, permitting early active hip movement and early progressive weight-bearing ambulation. (Courtesy of Howmedica, Inc.)

ment. Total hip replacement (see p. 1562) may be used in selected patients with acetabular defects.

Postoperative Management. The immediate postoperative care of a patient with a hip fracture is similar in many ways to that for other major surgery patients. However, additional attention is given to preventing secondary medical problems and to early mobilization of the patient so that independent functioning can be restored.

During the first 24 to 48 hours, attention is given to the relief of pain and the prevention of respiratory complications. Hourly foot flexion exercises are encouraged. Intravenous antibiotics are used prophylactically. Hydration, general nutrition, and output are monitored. Activity in bed is encouraged. A pillow is used between the legs to maintain alignment and to provide needed support when turning the patient.

Turning. The patient may be turned on the unaffected extremity by the following method:

- A pillow is placed between the legs to keep the affected leg in an abducted position. Then the patient is turned onto the unaffected side. After initial soreness has gone and the incision has healed, the patient usually may be turned in the same manner on the affected hip.

Exercise. It is important that the patient exercise as much as possible by means of the overbed trapeze. This helps strengthen the triceps and shoulders in preparation for ambulatory activities.

On the second or third postoperative day, the patient is generally fairly comfortable and can transfer to a chair with assistance. On the third day, assisted ambulation can begin. The amount of weight-bearing that can be permitted depends on the stability of the fracture reduction and the location of the fracture. The physician will prescribe the amount of weight bearing permitted and the rate at which the patient can progress to full weight-bearing. Physical therapists will work with the patient on transfers, ambulation, and the safe use of walker and crutches.

Patients with hip fractures can anticipate discharge with the use of an ambulatory aid. Some modifications in the home to permit safe use of walkers and crutches and for the patient's continuing care may be needed.

Complications. Elderly persons who suffer hip fractures are particularly prone to developing complications that may require more vigorous treatment than the fracture itself. In some instances, the shock of the injury may prove fatal. In less drastic responses, shock following this traumatic experience may cause bladder incontinence, although urinary control is usually gradually regained. In general, the routine use of an indwelling catheter is to be avoided. Yet urinary problems may occur. Therefore, the color, odor, and volume of urine are monitored to detect problems such as urinary retention, which is common following orthopedic operations, especially in the elderly. To assure proper kidney function, a liberal fluid intake is important.

As in many postoperative situations, thromboembolism is the most common complication. To prevent thromboembolism, prophylactic anticoagulation therapy is frequently used, along with elastic stockings and ankle exercises. The patient's legs are checked daily for evidence of thrombophlebitis.

Pulmonary complications are also a threat to elderly patients undergoing hip surgery. Deep-breathing exercises, a change of position at least every 2 hours, and the use of an incentive spirometer help to prevent the development of respiratory complications. Breath sounds should be assessed for the development of adventitious or diminished sounds.

Because patients with hip fractures generally have poor circulation and tend to remain in one position, pressure sores frequently develop. Giving proper skin care, especially to the back and heels and under the hips and shoulders, helps relieve the constant pressure. A convoluted foam mattress may provide protection by relieving pressure.

Delayed complications of hip fractures include protrusions of the fixation device through the acetabulum, metal fatigue failure of the device, avascular necrosis of the femoral head (particularly with intracapsular fractures), nonunion, and infection. Infection is suspected if the patient complains of moderate discomfort in the hip and has a mildly elevated temperature and a moderately elevated sedimentation rate.

The nursing management of the patient with a hip fracture is summarized in Nursing Care Plan 57-2.

Fractures of the Shaft of the Femur

Considerable force is required to break the shaft of the femur in adults. Most of these fractures are seen in the young male who has been involved in a vehicular accident or has fallen from a height. Frequently, these patients have associated multiple trauma problems.

The patient presents with an enlarged, deformed, painful thigh. The patient cannot move the hip or the knee. The fracture may be transverse, oblique, spiral, or comminuted. Frequently, the patient is in impending shock, since the loss of 2 to 3 units of blood into the tissues with this fracture is common. An expanding thigh may indicate continued bleeding.

Assessment includes checking neurovascular status of the extremity, especially circulatory perfusion of the foot. (Check popliteal and pedal pulses and toe capillary refill.) A Doppler ultrasound monitoring device may be needed to assess blood flow.

Dislocation of the hip and knee may accompany these fractures. Knee effusion suggests ligament damage and possible instability of the knee joint.

Management. Treatment is begun with skin traction for comfort and to immobilize the fracture so that additional soft-tissue damage does not occur. Generally, skeletal traction (suspension traction with Thomas splint and Pearson attachment or with slings, Bohler-Baum frame, or Neufield roller traction) is used for a while to achieve separation of the fracture fragments (which facilitates the operative procedure) for internal fixation or to achieve reduction and immobilization of the fracture site for subsequent cast bracing (Fig. 57-14), page 1598.

To preserve muscle strength, the patient should exercise the lower leg, foot, and toes on a regular basis. A common complication following fracture of the femoral shaft is restriction of knee motion. Thus, quadriceps-setting exercises should be started early. Active and passive knee exercises are done as soon as possible, depending on the stability of the fracture and knee ligaments. Progressive strengthening exercises for the upper extremities are needed to prepare for ambulation. Continued neurovascular monitoring is needed.

Internal fixation is generally carried out 7 to 10 days after

(Text continues on p. 1598)

Care of the Elderly Patient With a Fractured Hip

Nursing Interventions	*Rationale*	*Expected Outcomes*

Nursing Diagnosis: Alteration in comfort—pain related to fracture, soft-tissue damage, muscle spasm, and surgery

Goal: Relief of pain

1. Encourage patient to describe type and location of pain.	1. Pain is expected following fracture; soft-tissue damage and muscle spasm contribute to discomfort; pain is subjective and is evaluated through description of characteristics and location, which are important for determining cause of discomfort and for proposing interventions. Continuing pain may indicate development of neurovascular problems.	• Patient describes discomfort. • Expresses confidence in efforts to control pain • Expresses little discomfort with position changes • Expresses comfort when fracture is positioned and immobilized • Minimizes movement of extremity prior to reduction and fixation • Uses physical, psychological, and pharmacological measures to reduce discomfort
2. Acknowledge existence of pain; inform patient of available analgesics; record discomfort.	2. Reduces stress experienced by the patient by communicating concern and availability of help in dealing with pain. Notation provides data on pain experience.	• Patient relates a decrease in pain in 24–48 hours after surgery. • Requests pain medications and uses pain relief measures early in pain cycle
3. Handle the affected extremity gently, supporting it with hands and/or pillow.	3. Movement of bone fragments is painful; muscle spasms occur with movement; adequate support diminishes soft-tissue tension.	• States that positioning provides comfort • Appears comfortable and relaxed • Moves with increasing comfort as healing progresses
4. Apply Buck's traction as prescribed. Use trochanter roll.	4. Immobilizes fracture to decrease pain and additional tissue trauma; decreases muscle spasm	
5. Utilize pain-modifying strategies.	5. Pain perception can be diminished by distraction and refocusing of attention.	
a. Modify the environment.	a. Interaction with others, distraction, and sensory overload or deprivation may modify pain experiences.	
b. Administer prescribed pain medications as needed.	b. Analgesics and narcotics reduce the pain; muscle relaxants may be prescribed to decrease discomfort associated with muscle spasm.	
c. Encourage patient to use pain relief measures before pain is "unbearable."	c. Mild pain is easier to control.	
d. Evaluate and record patient's response to medications and pain-reduction techniques.	d. Notation of effectiveness of measures provides basis for future management interventions; early identification of adverse reactions is necessary for corrective measures and care plan modifications.	
e. Call physician if necessary.	e. Change in treatment plan may be necessary.	

(continued)

Nursing Interventions	*Rationale*	*Expected Outcomes*

Nursing Diagnosis: Alteration in comfort—pain related to fracture, soft-tissue damage, muscle spasm, and surgery

Goal: Relief of pain

6. Position for comfort and function.	6. Alignment of body facilitates comfort; positioning for function diminishes stress on musculoskeletal system.	
7. Assist with frequent changes in position.	7. Change of position relieves pressure and associated discomfort.	

Nursing Diagnosis: Potential alteration in thought process related to age, stress of trauma, unfamiliar surroundings, and drug therapy

Goal: Patient remains oriented and participates in decision making.

1. Assess orientation status.	1. Evaluate presenting orientation of patient; confusion may result from stress of fracture, unfamiliar surroundings, coexisting systemic disease, cerebral ischemia, or other factors. Baseline data is important for determining change.	• Patient establishes effective communication. • Demonstrates orientation to time, place, and person • Patient participates in self-care activities. • Remains mentally alert • Avoids episodes of confusion
2. Interview family regarding orientation and cognitive abilities prior to injury.	2. Provides data for evaluation of current findings	
3. Assess patient for auditory and visual deficits.	3. Diminished vision and auditory acuity frequently occurs with aging; glasses and hearing aid may increase patient's ability to interact with environment.	
4. Assist patient with use of sensory aids and interacting with environment.	4. Aids must be in good working order and available for use; nonverbal clues, simple direct statements, and control of environmental distractors facilitate communication.	
5. Orient to and stabilize environment a. Use orientation activities and aids (*e.g.*, clock, calendar, pictures, introduction of self). b. Minimize number of staff working with patient.	5. Short-term memory may be faulty in the elderly; frequent reorientation helps. b. Consistency of caregivers promotes trust.	
6. Give simple explanations of procedures and plan of care.	6. Short-term memory may be faulty.	
7. Encourage participation in hygiene and nutritional activities.	7. Participation in routine activities helps orientation; increases awareness of self.	
8. Provide for safety a. Keep side rails up when in bed b. Use vest restraints, as necessary c. Keep light on at night. d. Have call bell available e. Provide prompt response to requests for assistance.	8. Side rails and vest restraints decrease chance for additional injury from falls; mechanism for securing assistance is available to patient; independent activities based on faulty judgment may result in injury.	
9. Assess mental reponses to medications, especially sedatives and analgesics.	9. Elderly persons tend to be more sensitive to medications; abnormal responses (hallucinations, depression, "hangover") may occur.	

(continued)

Nursing Interventions	*Rationale*	*Expected Outcomes*

Nursing Diagnosis: Potential ineffective individual coping related to injury, anticipated surgery, and dependence

Goal: Patient utilizes effective coping mechanisms to modify stress.

1. Encourage patient to express concerns and to discuss meaning of fractured hip.	1. Verbalization helps patient deal with problems and feelings. Clarification of thoughts and feelings promotes problem-solving.	• Patient describes feelings concerning fractured hip and implications for lifestyle.
2. Support use of coping mechanisms. Involve significant others and support services as needed.	2. Coping mechanisms modify disabling effects of stress; sharing concerns lessens the burden and facilitates necessary modification.	• Uses available resources and coping mechanisms; develops health promotion strategies
3. Contact social services, if needed.	3. Anxiety may be related to financial or social problems; facilitates management of problems associated with continuing care.	• Uses community resources as needed • Participates in development of health care plan
4. Explain anticipated treatment regimen and routines to facilitate positive attitude in relation to rehabilitation.	4. Understanding of plan of care helps to diminish fears of the unknown.	
5. Encourage patient to participate in planning.	5. Participating in care provides for some control of self.	

Potential Complications: Hemorrhage; neurovascular compromise; thrombophlebitis

Goal: Patient experiences no complications.

Hemorrhage

1. Monitor vital signs, observing for shock.	1. Changes in pulse, blood pressure, and respirations may indicate development of shock; blood loss and stress may contribute to development of shock.	• Vital signs stabilized within normal limits • Patient experiences no excessive or bright red drainage.
2. Consider preinjury blood pressure values and management of coexisting hypertension, if present.	2. Necessary for interpretation of current blood pressure determinations	• Exhibits hematology values within normal limits
3. Note character and amount of drainage.	3. Excessive drainage and bright red drainage may indicate active bleeding.	
4. Notify surgeon if patient develops shock and/or excessive bleeding.	4. Corrective measures need to be instituted.	
5. Note hemoglobin and hematocrit values.	5. Anemia due to blood loss may develop; bleeding into tissues following hip fracture may be extensive; blood replacement therapy may be needed.	

Neurovascular Compromise

1. Assess affected extremity for color and temperature.	1. The skin becomes pale and feels cool with decreased tissue perfusion. Venous congestion may cause cyanosis.	• Has normal color and the extremity is warm • Patient demonstrates normal capillary refill response.
2. Assess toes for capillary refill response.	2. After compression of the nail, rapid return of pink color indicates good capillary perfusion.	• Exhibits moderate edema and swelling; tissue not palpably tense • States pain is controllable

(continued)

Nursing Interventions	*Rationale*	*Expected Outcomes*

Potential Complications: Hemorrhage; neurovascular compromise; thrombophlebitis

Goal: Patient experiences no complications.

Neurovascular Compromise

3. Assess extremity for edema and swelling.	3. The trauma of surgery will cause swelling and edema; excessive swelling and hematoma formation can compromise circulation and function; edema may be due to co-existing cardiovascular disease.	• Reports no pain with passive dorsiflexion • Reports normal sensations and no paresthesia • Demonstrates normal motor abilities and no paresis or paralysis • Patient has strong and equal pulses.
4. Elevate extremity.	4. Minimizes dependent edema	
5. Assess for deep, throbbing, unrelenting pain.	5. Surgical pain can be controlled; pain due to neurovascular compromise is refractory to treatment with analgesics.	
6. Assess for pain on passive flexion of foot.	6. With nerve ischemia, there will be pain on passive stretch. Additionally, pain may indicate thrombophlebitis (positive Homans's sign).	
7. Assess for sensations and numbness.	7. Diminished pain and paresthesia may indicate nerve damage. Sensation in web between great and second toe—peroneal nerve; sensation on sole of foot—tibial nerve	
8. Assess ability to move foot and toes.	8. Dorsiflexion of ankle and extension of toes indicate function of peroneal nerve. Plantar flexion of ankle and flexion of toes indicate functioning of tibial nerve.	
9. Assess pedal pulses in both feet.	9. Indicator of extremity circulation	
10. Notify surgeon if diminished neurovascular status occurs.	10. Function of extremity needs to be preserved.	

Thrombophlebitis

1. Apply thigh-high elastic stockings as prescribed.	1. Elastic compression stockings aid in venous blood return and prevent stasis.	• Wears thigh-high elastic compression stockings • Experiences no skin breakdown • Experiences no more warmth than usual in skin areas. • Demonstrates a negative Homans's sign • Changes position with assistance and supervision • Participates in exercise regimen • Patient experiences no chest pain; has lungs clear to auscultation; presents no evidence of pulmonary emboli. • Exhibits no signs of dehydration; has normal hematocrit • Maintains normal body temperature
2. Remove stockings for 20 minutes twice a day and provide skin care.	2. Skin care is necessary to avoid breakdown. Extended removal of stockings defeats purpose of stockings.	
3. Assess popliteal, dorsalis pedis, and posterior tibial pulses.	3. Pulses indicate arterial perfusion of extremity. With coexisting arteriosclerotic vascular disease, pulses may be diminished or absent.	
4. Assess skin temperature of legs.	4. Local inflammation will increase local skin temperature.	
5. Assess for Homans's sign every tour of duty.	5. Pain in calf on dorsiflexion of ankle may indicate thrombophlebitis.	
6. Avoid pressure on popliteal blood vessels from appliances or pillows.	6. Compression of blood vessels diminishes blood flow.	
7. Change position and increase activity as prescribed.	7. Activity promotes circulation and diminishes venous stasis.	
8. Supervise ankle exercises hourly.	8. Muscle exercise promotes circulation.	

(continued)

Nursing Interventions	*Rationale*	*Expected Outcomes*

Potential Complications: Hemorrhage; neurovascular compromise; thrombophlebitis

Goal: Patient experiences no complications.

Thrombophlebitis

9. Assess lung status; promote coughing and deep breathing; encourage use of incentive spirometer.	9. Provides for optimal ventilation. Co-existing respiratory conditions diminish ventilation.	
10. Ensure adequate hydration.	10. Elderly persons may be dehydrated due to low fluid intake, resulting in hemoconcentration.	
11. Monitor body temperature.	11. Body temperature elevates with inflammation (magnitude of response minimal in elderly).	

Nursing Diagnosis: Actual skin impairment related to surgical incision

Goal: Patient achieves wound healing.

1. Monitor vital signs.	1. Temperature, pulse, and respirations elevate in response to infection. (Magnitude of response may be minimal in elderly patients.)	• Patient maintains vital signs within normal range.
2. Employ aseptic dressing changes.	2. Avoid introducing organisms.	• Exhibits well-approximated incision without drainage or excessive inflammatory response
3. Assess wound appearance and character of drainage.	3. Red, swollen, draining incision is indicative of infection.	• Relates minimal discomfort; demonstrates no hematoma
4. Assess complaint of pain.	4. Pain may be due to wound hematoma—a possible locus of infection—which needs to be surgically evacuated.	• Tolerates antibiotics; displays no evidence of osteomyelitis
5. Administer prophylactic antibiotic if prescribed, and observe for side-effects.	5. Osteomyelitis is to be avoided.	

Nursing Diagnosis: Potential alteration in patterns of urinary elimination related to immobility

Goal: Patient maintains normal urinary elimination patterns.

1. Monitor intake and output.	1. Adequate fluid intake ensures hydration; adequate urinary output minimizes urinary stasis.	• Intake and output are adequate; patient exhibits normal voiding patterns.
2. Avoid use of indwelling catheter.	2. Source of bladder infection	• Demonstrates no evidence of urinary tract infection

Nursing Diagnosis: Impaired mobility related to fractured hip

Goal: Patient achieves pain-free, functional, stable hip.

1. Maintain neutral positioning of hip.	1. Prevents stress on fixation	• Patient engages in therapeutic positioning.
2. Use trochanter roll.	2. Minimizes external rotation	• Uses pillow between legs when turning
3. Place pillow between legs when turning.	3. Supports leg; prevents adduction	• Presents no skin breakdown
4. Give skin care, especially to pressure points; use a convoluted foam mattress.	4. Immobility causes pressure at bony prominences; massage and position changes relieve pressure.	• Assists in position changes; shows increased independence in transfers
		• Exercises hourly

(continued)

Nursing Interventions	Rationale	Expected Outcomes

Nursing Diagnosis: Impaired mobility related to fractured hip

Goal: Patient achieves pain-free, functional, stable hip.

5. Instruct and assist in position changes and transfers.	5. Encourage patient's active participation while preventing stress on hip fixation.	• Uses trapeze • Participates in progressive ambulation program
6. Instruct in and supervise isometric, quadriceps- and gluteal-setting exercises.	6. Strengthens muscles needed for walking	• Patient actively participates in exercise regimen.
7. Encourage use of trapeze.	7. Strengthens shoulder and arm muscles necessary for use of ambulatory aids.	• Uses ambulatory aids correctly and safely
8. In consultation with physical therapist, instruct in and supervise progressive safe ambulation within limitations of weight-bearing prescription.	8. Amount of weight-bearing depends on the patient's condition, fracture stability, and fixation device; ambulatory aids are used to assist the patient with nonweight-bearing and partial-weight-bearing ambulation.	
9. Offer encouragement and support exercise regimen.	9. Reconditioning exercises can be uncomfortable and fatiguing; encouragement helps patient comply with the program.	
10. Instruct in and supervise safe use of ambulatory aids.	10. Prevents injury from unsafe use	

Nursing Diagnosis: Potential impaired home maintenance related to fractured hip

Goal: Patient cares for self at home.

1. Assess home environment for discharge planning.	1. Physical barriers (especially stairs, bathrooms) may limit patient's ability to ambulate and care for self at home.	• Home is accessible for patient at time of discharge. • Patient appears relaxed and develops strategies to deal with identified problems.
2. Encourage patient to express concerns about care at home; explore with patient possible solutions to the problem.	2. Patient may have special problems that need to be identified and dealt with.	• Has personal assistance available • Demonstrates ability to provide necessary assistance within therapeutic prescription
3. Assess availability of physical assistance for health care activities.	3. Due to limitation of mobility, patient may require some assistance in routine health care.	• Complies with home care program; keeps follow-up health care appointments
4. Teach caregiver the home health care regimen.	4. Understanding of rehabilitative regimen is necessary for compliance.	

5. Instruct patient in posthospital care.
  a. Activity limitations
  b. Reinforce exercise instructions.
  c. Safe use of ambulatory aids
  d. Wound care
  e. Measures to promote healing (nutrition, wound care)
  f. Medications, if any
  g. Potential problems
  h. Continuing health care supervision and management
	5. Lack of knowledge and poor preparation for care at home contribute to patient anxiety, insecurity, and nonadherence to therapeutic regimen.	

injury. Intramedullary nailing using a Küntscher rod, Schneider rod, or Sampson rod obtains adequate internal fixation, which allows for early mobilization. The active muscle movement is important for increasing blood supply and increasing generated electrical potentials at the fracture site, which enhances healing. A thigh cuff may be used for external support. Dual compression plates may be used, but need external support from a cast brace for stability. Intramedullary implant and compression plates should be removed after 18 months. When plates are being removed, the resultant osteoporosis needs to be considered. Following plate removal, the bone remodels and requires support from a thigh cuff orthosis for several months.

A cast brace is commonly used for fractures of the mid- and distal shaft (*supracondylar*). Two to four weeks after the injury, when pain and swelling have subsided, the patient is removed from skeletal traction and placed in a *cast brace* (see p. 1550). The cast (fracture) brace is a total contact device that holds the reduced fracture. The muscle, through hydrodynamic compression, stabilizes the bone and stimulates healing. Minimal partial weight-bearing is begun and is progressed to full weight-bearing as tolerated. Functional ambulation stimulates fracture healing. The cast brace is worn for 12 to 14 weeks. In management of femoral shaft fractures, a major goal is rapid functional healing with sufficient strength to support the multiple stresses placed on the femur.

An external fixator may be used if the patient has experienced a grade III fracture, has extensive soft-tissue trauma, has lost bone, has an infection, or has hip and tibial fractures also.

Fractures of the Tibia and Fibula

The most common fracture below the knee is a fracture of the tibia (and fibula) that results from a direct blow, falls with the foot in a flexed position, or a violent twisting motion. Fractures of the tibia and fibula often occur in association with each other. The patient presents with pain, deformity, obvious hematoma, and considerable edema. Frequently, these fractures involve severe soft-tissue damage because there is little subcutaneous tissue in the area.

Peroneal nerve functioning needs to be assessed for baseline data. If the nerve is not functioning, the patient is unable to dorsiflex the great toe and has diminished sensation in the first web space. Tibial artery damage is assessed by testing the capillary refill response. Development of an anterior compartment syndrome could occur. (Symptoms include intense pain, paresthesia, pain on passive movement, and diminished capillary refill.) Articular fracture may be complicated by hemarthroses and/or ligament damage.

Most closed tibial fractures are treated with closed reduction and initial immobilization in a long leg-walking or patellar-tendon-bearing cast. Reduction must be relatively accurate in relation to angulation and rotation. The patient attains partial weight-bearing status in 7 to 10 days. A cast (fracture) boot decreases pivoting and rotary stress. This activity decreases edema, increases circulation, and minimizes displacement because of the cast influence on the distribution of forces to the fracture site. The cast is changed to a short leg cast or brace in 3 to 4 weeks, which allows for knee motion. Fracture healing takes 16 to 24 weeks.

Open and comminuted fractures may be treated with

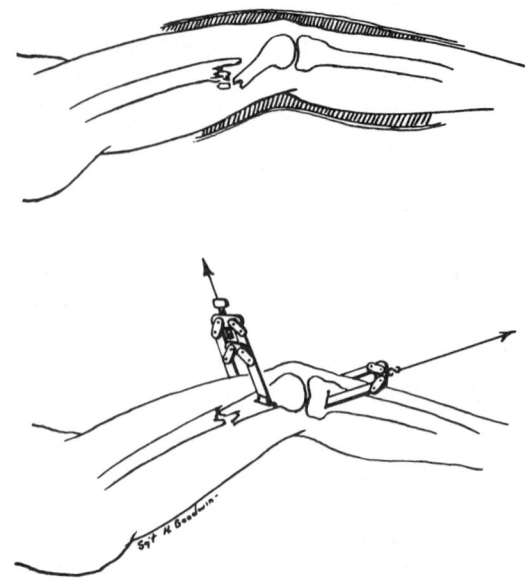

Figure 57-14
Two-wire skeletal traction for fracture of the femur in distal third. (*Top*) Deformity on admission to hospital. (*Bottom*) Adequate reduction when additional wire is inserted in lower femoral fragment and vertical lift is secured. (Hampton OP Jr. Wounds of the Extremities in Military Surgery. St Louis, CV Mosby.)

traction or with an external fixator. The pins-in-plaster technique is used for those situations in which it is hard to maintain reduction. The patient is not allowed to bear weight for about 6 weeks. Intramedullary nails and compression plates may be selected for certain situations. External plaster support is needed with nailing. Compression plates allow for anatomical reduction, early foot and knee motion, and early partial weight-bearing.

As with other lower extremity fractures, the leg should be elevated to control edema. Continued neurovascular evaluation is needed. The development of compartment syndrome requires prompt recognition and resolution or there will be a permanent functional deficit.

Internal Derangement of the Knee

Injury to most joints consists of a tear of the supporting ligaments. In the knee joint, however, there may also be a displacement or tear of the *semilunar cartilages,* which are two crescent-shaped cartilages attached to the edge of the shallow articulating surface of the head of the tibia. They normally move slightly backward and forward to accommodate the change in the shape of the condyles of the femur when the leg is in flexion or extension. In sports and in certain accidents, the body is often twisted with the foot fixed. Since little torsion movement is normally permitted in the knee joint, either the cartilage is torn from its attachment to the head of the tibia or an actual tear or fracture of the cartilage itself occurs.

These injuries leave a loose cartilage in the knee joint that may slip between the femur and the tibia, preventing full extension of the leg. If this happens during walking or running, patients often describe the disability as their "leg giving way" under them. Patients may hear or feel a click in the knee when they walk, expecially when they extend the leg that is bearing weight, as in going upstairs. When the cartilage is attached front and back, but torn loose laterally (bucket-handle tear), it may slide between the bones to lie between the condyles and prevent full flexion or extension. As a result, the knee "locks."

These various types of injury are spoken of as *internal derangements* of the knee joint, and they produce a disturbing disability because the patient never knows when the knee will give trouble. The treatment of this disability is removal of the injured cartilage while preserving normal intra-articular structures. This can be done through an incision into the knee joint or through an operating arthroscope. Arthroscopic surgery is frequently an outpatient procedure, allowing the patient to resume activities in 1 to 2 days and sports in a couple of weeks. The joint function can return to normal.

Postoperative Care. A pressure dressing is applied, and usually a knee immobilizing splint may be used. The leg should be elevated on pillows to minimize edema. The most common complication is an effusion into the knee joint, which produces marked pain. If this occurs, the physician should be notified. Relief can be obtained by loosening the pressure dressing. The physician may need to aspirate the joint to relieve the pressure.

To prevent atrophy of the thigh muscles, these patients are instructed to contract their quadriceps muscles. Additional exercises are given to achieve full function, stability, and strength.

Rupture of the Achilles Tendon

Traumatic rupture of the Achilles tendon is a common occurrence. Sudden contraction of the calf muscle with the foot fixed firmly to the floor may cause snapping of the tendon, generally within the tendon sheath. The patient is acutely aware of the problem because of the pain and inability to plantar flex the foot. Immediate surgical repair usually obtains satisfactory results. Conservative management with a plantar-flexed cast for 6 to 8 weeks can be used.

Fractures of the Thoracolumbar Spine

Fractures of the thoracolumbar spine may involve (1) the vertebral body, (2) the lamina and articulating processes, and (3) the spinous processes or transverse processes. Five percent or fewer of spinal fractures are associated with neurologic deficits. The fractures are generally due to indirect trauma caused by excessive loading, sudden muscle contraction, or excessive motion beyond physiologic limits. Osteoporosis contributes to vertebral body collapse. The T12 to L2 area of the spine is most vulnerable to fracture.

The patient with a spinal fracture presents with acute tenderness, swelling, paravertebral muscle spasm, and possibly change in normal curves or gap between spinous processes. Pain is greater when moving, coughing, or weight-bearing. The most important assessment done initially is to determine if there is injury to the spinal cord and if the fracture is stable or unstable. Immobilization is essential until these determinations are made. With a neurologic deficit, immediate spinal cord decompression with laminectomy and fusion is usually performed.

With a stable spinal fracture, only the anterior structural column (vertebral bodies and discs) or the posterior structural column (neural arch, articular processes, ligaments) has been disrupted. Unstable fractures occur with fracture dislocations, and exhibit disruption of both anterior and posterior structural columns and the potential for neural damage exists.

Stable spinal fractures (due to flexion, extension, lateral bending, and vertical loading) are treated conservatively. The patient is placed on bed rest until the acute pain subsides (days to 2–3 weeks). Analgesics control pain. The patient is monitored for the development of a transient ileus due to associated retroperitoneal hemorrhage. Sitting is avoided until the pain subsides. A spinal brace or plastic thoracolumbar orthosis may be used for support during progressive ambulation and resumption of activities.

With unstable spinal fractures, the patient is placed on a side-to-side turning frame. Within 24 hours, open reduction and fixation with spinal fusion and Harrington or Luque rod stabilization are usually accomplished. The patient is cared for on a turning frame postoperatively. Neurological status is monitored closely during the preoperative and postoperative periods. Progressive ambulation is begun about 2 weeks after surgery, with the patient in a body jacket cast or brace.

Patient education emphasizes good posture, good body mechanics, and, when healing is sufficient, back-strengthening exercises.

Pelvic Fractures

The severity of pelvic fractures varies (Fig. 57-15). Most fractures of the pelvis heal rapidly because the innominate bone (hip bone) is made up mostly of cancellous bone, which has a rich blood supply.

Type I pelvic fractures exhibit no break in the pelvic ring. They include fractures of the coccyx and single ramus of the pubis or ischium bone. Fractures of the coccyx can be disabling, causing pain on sitting and defecation. Treatment includes bed rest, sitz baths, and stool softeners. Other Type I pelvic fractures are treated with bed rest until the discomfort resolves. A bedboard under the mattress is desirable to give more stability. The patient is turned as a unit. Patients with a fractured sacrum should be monitored for bowel sounds and activity.

The most common *Type II* pelvic fracture (single break in the pelvic ring) is the fracture of two ipsilateral rami. Bed rest is utilized, with the addition of a pelvic sling and/or bilateral Buck's traction for slightly displaced fractures. Full activity can be resumed in 10 to 16 weeks.

A double break in the pelvic ring (*Type III* fracture) occurs as a result of automobile accidents, crush injuries, and falls from buildings and scaffolds. General symptoms include deformity, local swelling, ecchymosis, tenderness over the symphysis pubis, anterior iliac spines, iliac crest, sacrum, or coccyx, and inability to bear weight without discomfort. In addition, shock and hemorrhage may occur.

Pelvic fractures are serious because at least two thirds of these patients have significant and multiple injuries. (The care of the patient with multiple injuries is discussed in Chap.

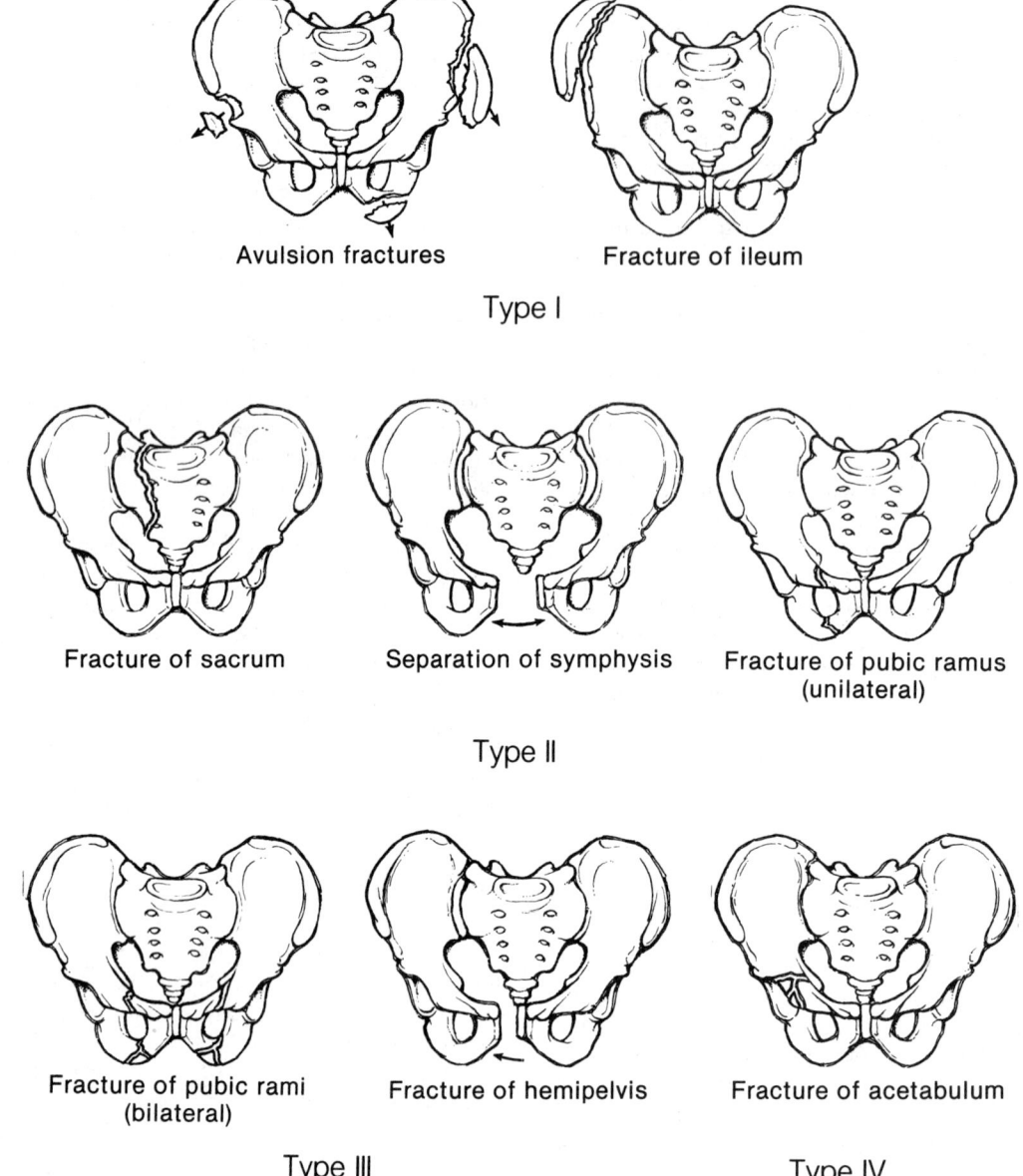

Avulsion fractures   Fracture of ileum

Type I

Fracture of sacrum   Separation of symphysis   Fracture of pubic ramus
(unilateral)

Type II

Fracture of pubic rami   Fracture of hemipelvis   Fracture of acetabulum
(bilateral)

Type III   Type IV

Figure 57-15
Fractures of the pelvis.

60.) Therefore, a high mortality rate accompanies these fractures. Death may ensue from local hemorrhage in view of the rich blood supply to the pelvis and the possibility of massive and hidden bleeding in the retroperitoneal region. Bleeding also arises from the cancellous surfaces of the fracture fragments and the laceration of veins and arteries by bone spicules. There is also the added danger of intra-abdominal hemorrhage from a torn iliac artery. In addition to hemorrhage, the bladder, the urethra, or the intestines may be lacerated, resulting in conditions that can prove to be more serious than the fracture itself. To check for possible damage to the urinary tract, the patient's urine is examined for blood. A cystourethrogram and an intravenous urogram are often done if injury to the urinary tract is suspected. Since

hemorrhage is possible in these injuries, the abdomen is examined for evidence of intra-abdominal hemorrhage with peritoneal lavage. The peripheral pulses of both lower extremities are palpated, because absence of peripheral pulses may indicate the possibility that an iliac artery or one of its branches is torn. The patient is handled carefully and gently to minimize further bleeding and shock. Management of hemorrhage and associated intra-abdominal, thoracic, or cranial injuries has priority over treatment of fractures. Ongoing and continuing nursing assessments are done for injuries to the bladder, rectum, intestines, and intra-abdominal organs.

For fractures that disrupt the pelvic ring or involve weight-bearing areas, skeletal traction to reduce the displacement, lateral recumbent positioning with spica cast, pelvic sling, open reduction with internal fixation, or an external fixator may be used.

When both sides of the pelvis are fractured, a pelvic sling is used to immobilize the pelvis into a single unit so that the patient can move the rest of the body with less pain. The pelvic sling lifts the weight of the pelvis very slightly from the mattress (Fig. 57-16A). The sling may be folded back over the buttocks in order to permit the patient to use the bedpan. (Some orthopedists permit the sling to be loosened for certain nursing care activities if the patient's condition permits.) Since skin care is a problem, sheep skin may be used to line the sling to prevent excoriation. It is necessary to reach under the sling to give skin care.

If separation of the symphysis pubis has occurred, a compression force must be applied. This is obtained by crossing the ropes from the sling to the weights on the opposite side (Fig. 57-16B). The pelvic sling is adjusted to exert a compression effect from side to side to correct the separation of bones. Because the sling exerts pressure over the trochanteric region, the patient may become quite uncomfortable.

Pelvic slings are not used with fractures that have collapsed inward or when the acetabulum is fractured.

Undisplaced fractures of the acetabulum (*Type IV* fractures) are seen following motor vehicle accidents in which the femur is jammed into the dashboard. Open reduction and fixation with multiple screws or direct lateral skeletal traction by insertion of a large trochanter screw into the femoral head is usually necessary. Traction is maintained for 6 weeks, followed by non-weight-bearing for another 6 weeks. Internal fixation permits earlier motion and function.

During the period of immobility, exercises (leg, respiratory, range-of-motion, and strengthening), elastic stockings, and elevation of the foot of the bed to aid venous return are appropriate measures to help diminish the effects of prolonged bed rest. Paralytic ileus may accompany pelvic fractures and immobility. When bony healing has taken place in a pelvic fracture, the patient is mobilized with a method of progressive weight-bearing, usually with crutches.

Amputation

Amputation of an extremity is often necessary as a result of progressive peripheral vascular disease, trauma (crushing injuries, burns, frostbite, electrical burns), congenital deformities, or malignant tumor. Of all these causes, peripheral vascular disease accounts for the majority of amputations of lower extremities.

Amputation is really reconstructive surgery designed to improve the patient's quality of life. It is used to relieve symptoms and to facilitate improved function. If the health care team is able to communicate a positive attitude, the patient will adjust to the amputation and actively participate in the rehabilitative plan.

The loss of an extremity requires major adjustments. The patient's perception of the amputation must be understood by the health care team. The patient must adjust to a permanent change in body image, which must be incorporated in such a way that self-esteem is not lost. Physical mobility

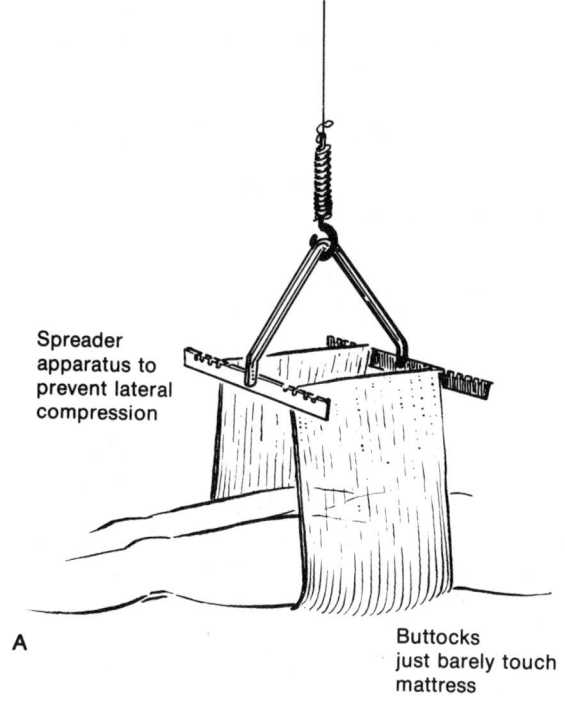

Spreader apparatus to prevent lateral compression

A

Buttocks just barely touch mattress

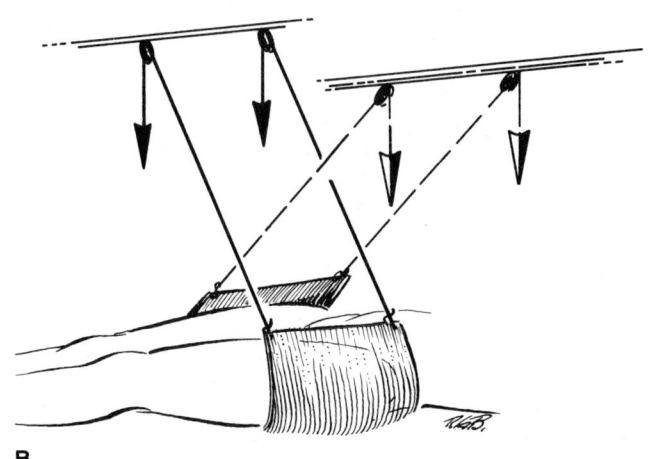

B

Figure 57-16

Pelvic sling suspension for fractures of the pelvis. (*A*) A suspension of the pelvis without an attempt at compression. The sling is suspended by means of a large metal frame, and weight is applied so that the pelvis is largely counterbalanced and becomes, to a certain extent, "weightless." Movement can then occur without moving the pelvic fragments. (*B*) The method for applying compression when there has been separation of the anterior pelvic ring, particularly at the symphysis pubis. This suspension compresses the pelvis from side to side to correct any diastasis that may have occurred. Pain developing at pressure points over the trochanters is unavoidable; it will often limit the duration of time that compression traction is useful. (Lewis RC. Handbook of Traction, Casting and Splinting Techniques. Philadelphia, JB Lippincott.)

and/or ability to perform activities of daily living are altered, and the patient needs to learn how to modify activities and environment to accommodate the use of mobility aids and assistive devices. The rehabilitation team is multidisciplinary (patient, nurse, physician, social worker, psychologist, prosthetist, vocational rehabilitation worker), and helps the patient achieve the highest possible level of function and participation in life activities.

Factors Affecting Amputation

Patients who require amputation are usually either young with severe extremity trauma or tumor, or elderly with peripheral vascular disease. *The young* are generally healthy, heal rapidly, and participate in a vigorous rehabilitation program. Since the amputation is usually the result of an injury, much psychological support is needed in accepting the sudden change in body image and in dealing with the stresses of hospitalization, long-term rehabilitation, and modification of life-style. These patients need time to work through their feelings about their permanent loss. Their reactions are unpredictable and can range from open, bitter hostility to euphoria.

On the other hand, *the elderly* with peripheral vascular disease frequently have concurrent health problems. These cardiovascular, respiratory, or neurological problems may limit their rehabilitation potential. Therapeutic amputations for long-standing problems may relieve a patient of pain, disability, and dependency. These patients have had time to work through some feelings and come to terms with the amputation. Adjusting to the change in body image may be easier. Planning for psychological and physiological rehabilitation can be started prior to the amputation.

Levels of Amputation

Amputation is performed at the most distal point that will heal. The site of amputation is determined by two factors: circulation in the part and the requirements of the prosthesis.

The circulatory status of the extremity is evaluated through physical examination and specific studies. Muscle and skin perfusion are important for healing. Doppler flowmetry, segmental blood pressure determinations, and transcutaneous PO_2 are valuable studies. Angiography may be done, especially if revascularization is considered to be an option. Xenon 133 clearance studies are used in some centers.

For the most part, every attempt is made to preserve as much length as possible and to keep the knee and elbow joints intact. (Fig. 57-17 shows the different levels at which an extremity may be amputated.) Almost any level of amputation can be fitted with a prosthesis.

Energy requirements and resultant cardiovascular demands for mobility increase as the patient progresses from using a wheelchair to a prosthesis or to crutch-walking without a prosthesis. Therefore, careful cardiovascular and nutritional monitoring is essential so that physiological limits and demands can be met.

The amputation of toes and portions of the foot causes minor changes in gait and balance. A *Syme* amputation (modified ankle disarticulation amputation) is done most frequently for extensive foot trauma, and produces a painless,

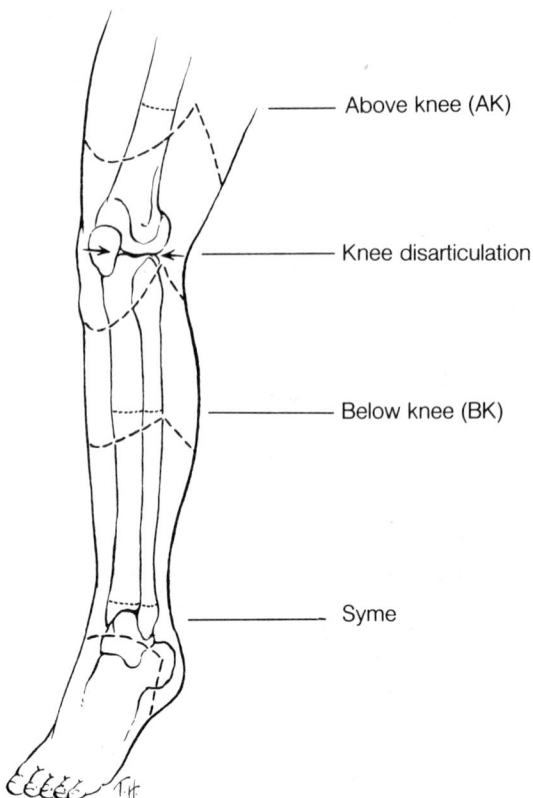

Figure 57-17
Levels of amputation are determined by circulatory adequacy, type of prosthesis, function of the part, and muscle balance.

durable extremity end that can withstand full weight-bearing. Below-knee amputations are preferred to above-knee amputations because of the importance of the knee joint and the energy requirements for walking. Preserving the knee joint of an elderly patient can mean the difference between walking with aids or being confined to a wheelchair. Knee disarticulations are most successful with young, active patients who are able to develop precise control of the prosthesis. When above-knee amputations are done, all possible length is preserved, muscles are stabilized and shaped, and hip contractures are prevented for maximum ambulatory potential. If a hip disarticulation amputation is done, most elderly people must rely on a wheelchair for mobility.

Upper-extremity amputations are performed to preserve the maximum functional length. The prosthesis is fitted early for maximum function.

Management

The major surgical objective is to achieve uncomplicated healing of the amputation wound, resulting in a nontender residual limb (stump) with healthy skin for prosthesis use. The elderly may have slower healing due to preexisting poor nutrition and other health problems. Healing is enhanced by gentle handling of the residual limb, controlling residual limb edema through rigid or soft compression dressings, and using aseptic technique in wound care to avoid infection.

Rigid Cast Dressings. A closed *rigid cast dressing* is frequently used to provide uniform compression, to support soft tissues and thereby control pain, and to prevent contractures. Immediately following surgery, a rigid plaster dressing is applied and is equipped to attach a temporary prosthetic extension (pylon) and an artificial foot. A sterilized residual limb sock is applied to the residual limb. Felt pads are placed over pressure-sensitive areas. Starting from the distal end, the residual limb is wrapped with elastic plaster of paris bandages while firm, even pressure is maintained (Fig. 57-18). Care is taken not to constrict circulation. This rigid dressing technique is used as a means for creating a socket for immediate postoperative prosthetic fitting. The length of the prosthesis is tailored to the individual patient.

The original cast may be left on for 10 to 14 days unless contraindicated by factors such as elevated body temperature, severe pain, or loose-fitting cast. A second cast is then applied, and changed usually 10 to 14 days after the initial cast is changed.

Soft Dressings. When frequent inspection of the residual limb (stump) is desired, a *soft dressing*, with or without compression, may be used. An immobilizing splint may be incorporated in the dressing. Stump (wound) hematomas are controlled to minimize infection.

Staged Amputation. A staged amputation may be used when gangrene and infection exist. Initially, a guillotine amputation is done to remove the dead and septic tissue. The wound is débrided and allowed to drain. The sepsis is treated

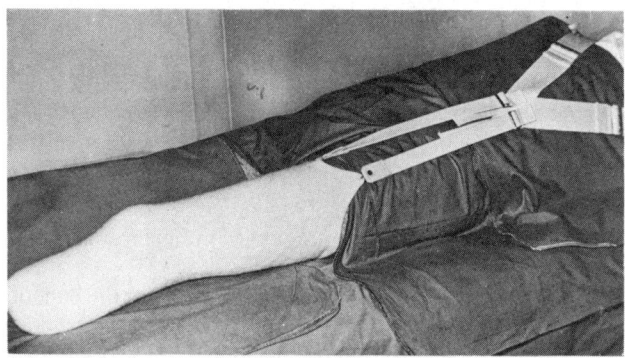

A

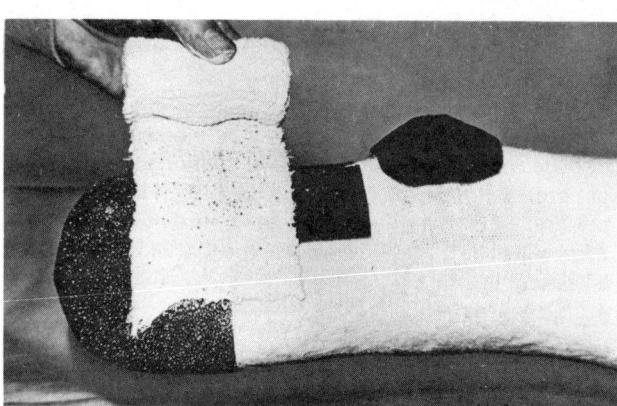

B

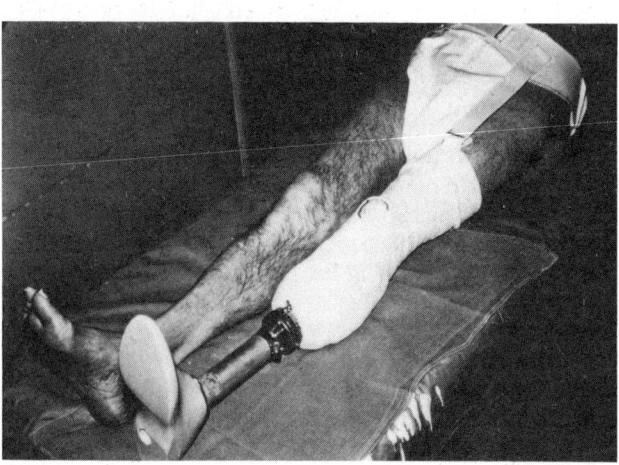

C

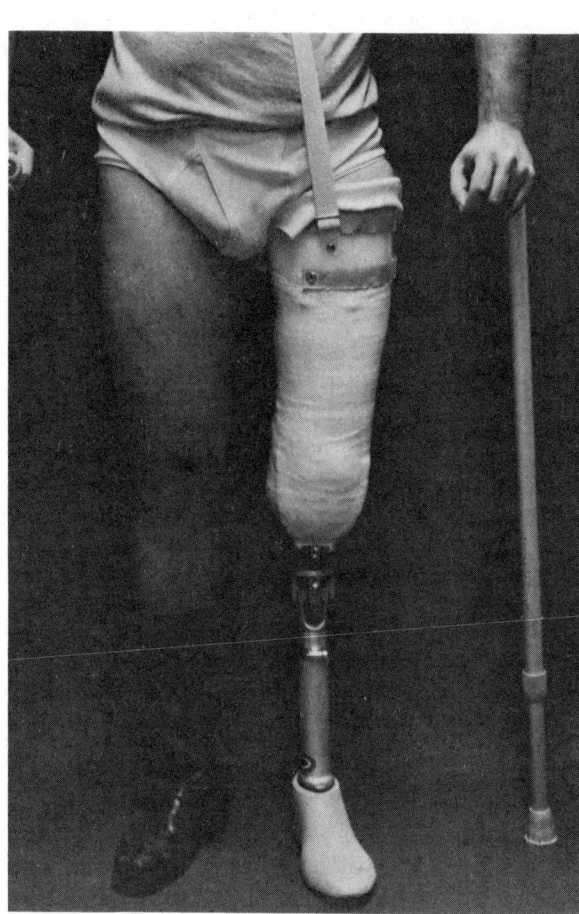

D

Figure 57-18
Immediate prosthetic fitting after amputation. (*A*) Sterile stocking held under firm tension as the rigid dressing is applied. (*B*) Pressure relief pads and distal polyurethane pad in place prior to application of the plaster of paris rigid dressing. (*C*) Complete assembly of components for the immediate postsurgical prosthetic fitting of the above-knee amputee. (Courtesy of the Prosthetics Research Study, Veterans Administration Contract V663P-784.)

with systemic antibiotics. In a few days, when the infection has been controlled and the patient has stabilized, a definitive amputation with skin closure is done.

▶ *Nursing Process*
The Patient Undergoing
an Amputation

▷ *Assessment*

Before surgery, the neurovascular and functional status of the extremity must be evaluated through history and physical assessment (*e.g.*, color, temperature, palpable pulses, hair distribution, condition of skin, responses to positioning, sensations, pain, function). A Doppler (a hand-held ultrasonic instrument) may be used to evaluate arterial blood flow. Limitation of range of motion and presence of hip and knee flexion contractures may affect the function and fit of the prosthesis. The circulatory status and function of the sound extremity are also assessed.

If infection or gangrene exists, the patient may have associated enlarged lymph nodes, fever, and purulent drainage. A culture is taken to determine appropriate antibiotic therapy. If the patient has experienced a traumatic amputation, the function and condition of the residual limb are assessed.

The patient's nutritional status is evaluated and a plan for nutritional care is made when necessary. Frequently, elderly persons are poorly nourished, obese, or on special diets due to concurrent health problems. For wound healing, a balanced diet with adequate vitamins and protein is essential.

Any concurrent health problems (*e.g.*, dehydration, anemia, cardiac insufficiency, chronic respiratory problems, diabetes mellitus) need to be identified and treated so that the patient is in the best possible condition to withstand the trauma of surgery. The use of steroids, anticoagulants, vasoconstrictors, or vasodilators may influence management and wound healing.

An assessment of the patient's psychological status is very important. Determination of the patient's emotional reaction to amputation is essential for nursing care. Grief response to a permanent alteration in body image is appropriate. Even if the amputation decreases pain and increases functioning, major adjustments are needed. Coping will be facilitated by the presence of an adequate support system and professional help.

▷ *Nursing Diagnoses*

Based on the assessment data, the patient's major nursing diagnoses may include the following:

- Alteration in comfort—pain, related to surgery and phantom limb sensation
- Impairment of skin integrity, actual and potential, related to surgical amputation and skin irritation
- Disturbance in self-concept—body image, related to amputation
- Grieving—dysfunctional, related to loss of body part

- Self-care deficit in feeding, bathing, dressing, grooming, and toileting related to loss of body part
- Impaired physical mobility related to loss of extremity

▷ *Planning and Implementation*

▷ *Goals:* The major goals of the patient may be relief of pain and absence of phantom sensations, restoration of intact skin, improvement of self-concept, resolution of grieving process, independence in self-care, and restoration of physical mobility.

Nursing Interventions

Assessing for Complications

Following any surgery, efforts are made to reestablish homeostasis and prevent problems related to surgery, anesthesia, and immobility.

The most threatening problem is massive hemorrhage due to a loosened ligature. The patient is monitored carefully for any signs or symptoms of bleeding. The patient's vital signs are monitored, and suction drainage is observed frequently.

- Immediate postoperative bleeding may develop slowly or take the form of a massive hemorrhage resulting from a loosened ligature.
- A large tourniquet should be in plain sight at the patient's bedside so that, if severe bleeding occurs, the tourniquet can be applied to the residual limb to control the hemorrhage.
- Notify the surgeon promptly in the event of excessive bleeding.

Positioning

Postoperative positioning to prevent development of hip and/or knee contracture is important. According to the surgeon's preference, the residual limb may be placed in an extended position or elevated for a brief period following surgery. If the residual limb is to be elevated, the foot of the bed should be raised.

- The residual limb should not be placed on a pillow because a flexion contraction of the hip may result. A contracture of the next joint above the amputation is a frequent complication.

In a lower extremity amputation, after the first 24 to 48 hours, the patient should be encouraged to turn from side to side and to assume a prone position to stretch the flexor muscles and to prevent flexion contracture of the hip. A pillow may be placed under the abdomen and the residual limb, with the sound foot resting over the edge of the mattress. The legs should remain close together while the patient is in the prone position in order to prevent an abduction deformity. It is important that the patient recognize the value of moving the residual limb. Sitting for prolonged periods should be discouraged.

Relieving Pain and Phantom Limb Sensation

Surgical Pain. Surgical pain is located at the incision and can be readily controlled with analgesics or evacuation of the hematoma or accumulated fluid.

The expression of pain is individual. If the patient has experienced much discomfort prior to surgery, the postoperative pain may be interpreted as minimal and may be controlled effectively by minimal analgesics. On the other hand, the pain may be combined with the expression of grief and alteration of body image, and not modified adequately by analgesics. Severe pain may be due to excessive pressure on a bony prominence or hematoma. The surgeon must be notified and the cause of the discomfort determined. The physician may split the cast and examine the residual limb. Evaluation of the patient's pain and responses to chosen interventions is an integral part of the nurse's management of pain.

Patients who are managed with a cast dressing experience less pain than those with soft dressings. Within a few days, the surgical pain is generally controlled effectively with oral analgesics and pain-modifying techniques.

Phantom Sensations. Amputees also experience phantom pain, in which the patient describes pain or unusual sensation in the part that has been amputated. The sensation creates a feeling that the extremity is present and possibly crushed, cramped, or twisted in an abnormal position. These sensations are real and need to be accepted by the patient and the caregivers.

Phantom sensation will eventually disappear, but while it lasts it can have a disquieting effect on the patient. The pathogenesis of phantom limb phenomena is unknown. However, *keeping the patient active* helps decrease the occurrence of phantom limb pain. Phantom limb pain may occur 2 to 3 months after amputation, and is seen more frequently in above-knee amputations.

When the patients describe phantom pains/sensations, the nurse needs to acknowledge these disquieting feelings and help patients modify their perception of them. Distraction techniques and activity are helpful. TENS (transcutaneous electrical nerve stimulation) may provide relief for some patients.

Muscle Spasms. Muscle spasms may add to the patient's discomfort during convalescence. Changing the patient's position, application of heat, or placing a light sandbag on the residual limb to counteract the muscle spasm may improve the patient's level of comfort.

Early minimal weight-bearing on the residual limb with the pylon attached produces little discomfort.

Promoting Wound Healing

Skin integrity has been altered due to the surgical amputation. Potential healing problems may exist in relation to associated peripheral vascular, nutritional, or other concurrent health problems such as diabetes mellitus. Immobilization and pressure from various aids may contribute to skin breakdown. The prosthesis may cause pressure areas to develop. The nurse assesses the skin for breaks in the skin.

To promote healing of the incision, edema is controlled by means of the cast dressing or compression dressing. This helps to reestablish the circulation and lymph drainage.

- *A most important consideration is that the residual limb remain in the plaster cast socket during the patient's entire hospitalization.* If the cast inadvertently comes off, the residual limb must immediately be wrapped tightly with an elastic compression bandage and the surgeon notified so that another cast can be applied. Excessive edema will develop in a very short time and will result in a delay in rehabilitation.

The residual limb must be handled gently. Whenever the dressing is changed, aseptic technique is required to prevent wound infections and possible osteomyelitis. If a cast dressing is used, the nurse needs to observe for drainage, odor, and increasing discomfort, which may indicate infection or necrosis. These problems should be reported to the surgeon promptly. Systemic indicators of infection need to be monitored.

Residual limb shaping is important for prosthesis fitting. The patient needs to be taught how to wrap the residual limb with elastic dressings. When the incision is healed, the patient is taught to care for the residual limb.

Careful skin hygiene is essential to prevent skin irritation, infection, and breakdown. The residual limb is washed and dried (gently) at least twice daily. The skin is inspected for pressure areas, eczema, and blisters. If present, they must be treated before a major problem develops. Usually, a residual limb sock is worn to absorb perspiration and avoid direct contact between the skin and the prosthetic socket. The residual limb sock is changed daily and must fit smoothly to prevent the irritation caused by wrinkles. The socket of the prosthesis is washed with a mild detergent, rinsed, and dried thoroughly with a clean cloth. The patient is advised that the socket must be thoroughly dry before the prosthesis is applied.

When amputations of the leg have been performed on elderly, debilitated patients, especially those with diabetes and arteriosclerosis, they frequently become incontinent of urine and feces. The dressing and the wound of the residual limb may become soiled. Plastic material secured by a wide adhesive strip about the leg above the dressing has proven to be a good method of protecting the residual limb from becoming soiled.

Enhancing Self-Concept

Although amputation is a reconstructive procedure, it alters the patient's body image. The patient will need to accept the irreversible changes. The nurse establishes a trusting relationship with the patient and communicates acceptance of the patient who has experienced an amputation. The patient and family are encouraged to express and share their feelings concerning the loss of an extremity and to work through the grief process. The patient is encouraged to look at, feel, and then care for the residual limb. Strengths of and resources available to the patient are identified to facilitate rehabilitation. Care is provided to assist the patient to regain the previous level of independent functioning. When patients perceive that others accept them as whole persons and they are able to resume responsibility for self-care, their self-concept improves and changes in body image are accepted. This process may take months.

Resolution of Grieving. The realization that an extremity has been removed may come as a shock even though the patient had been prepared preoperatively. The patient's behavior (*e.g.,* crying, withdrawal, apathy, anger) and expressed feelings (*e.g.,* depression, fear, helplessness) will demonstrate how the patient is beginning to cope with the loss and work through the grieving process. The nurse acknowledges the reality of the loss by listening and providing support.

Acceptance and support of the patient and family through a trusting relationship during all phases of the process will assist them in dealing with the loss. The patient must feel free to express feelings. Support available from family and friends promotes acceptance of the loss. The nurse helps the patient deal with immediate needs and become oriented to realistic rehabilitation goals and future independent functioning.

Attaining Independent Self-Care

Amputation of an extremity affects the patient's ability to care for himself. Encourage the patient to be an active participant in self-care. The patient needs time to accomplish these tasks, and must not be hurried. Practicing an activity with consistent supportive supervision in a relaxed environment will enable the person to learn self-care skills. The patient and nurse need to maintain positive attitudes and minimize fatigue and frustration during the learning process.

Independence in dressing, toileting, and bathing (shower or tub) depends on balance, transfer abilities, and physiological tolerance of the activities. The nurse works with the physical therapist and occupational therapist in teaching and supervising the patient in these self-care activities.

The upper-extremity amputee will have self-care deficits in feeding, bathing, and dressing. Assistance is provided only as needed; the patient is encouraged to learn to do the task without help and to learn how to use feeding and dressing aids for eventual independent activities of daily living. The nurse, therapists, and prosthetist work with the patient to achieve maximum independence.

Promoting Physical Mobility

Exercises. If the amputation is not an emergency procedure, efforts should be made preoperatively to strengthen the upper extremities as well as the trunk and the abdominal muscles. The extensor muscles in the arm and the depressor muscles in the shoulder especially need to be strengthened, since these muscle groups play an important part in crutch walking. The patient may flex and extend the arms while holding weights. Doing push-ups while in a prone position and sit-ups while seated will strengthen the triceps muscles.

In addition, the patient should be taught to crutch walk before the surgical procedure in order to prepare for postoperative mobility.

Postoperatively, range-of-motion exercises (see pp. 218–225) are started early because contracture deformities develop rapidly. Range of motion exercises are carried out to the hip and knee for below-the-knee amputations and to the hip for above-the-knee amputations.

An overhead trapeze can be used by the patient to change position and strengthen the biceps. The triceps, necessary in crutch walking, can be strengthened by pressing the palms against the bed while pushing the body upward (push-up exercises). Exercises such as hyperextension of the residual limb, conducted under the supervision of the physical therapist, also aid in strengthening muscles as well as increasing circulation, reducing edema, and preventing atrophy.

Assessment of body systems (*e.g.*, respiratory, gastrointestinal, genitourinary) for problems associated with immobility (*e.g.*, pneumonia, anorexia, constipation, urinary stasis) is needed, and corrective management is instituted. Avoiding problems associated with immobility and restoring physical activity are necessary for maintenance of health.

Strength and endurance are assessed, and activities are increased gradually in order to prevent fatigue. As the patient progresses to independent use of the wheelchair, ambulation with aids, or ambulation with prosthesis, safety considerations are emphasized. Environmental barriers (*e.g.*, steps, inclines, doors, wet surfaces) are identified, and methods of managing them are practiced. Problems associated with the use of the mobility aids (*e.g.*, pressure on the axilla from crutches, skin irritation of the hands from wheelchair use, residual limb irritation from prosthesis) are identified and managed.

Ambulation. Amputation changes the center of gravity, so the patient may need to practice position changes (*e.g.*, standing from sitting and standing on one foot). A well-fitting shoe with a nonslip sole should be worn. During position changes, the patient should be guarded and possibly stabilized at the waist to prevent falling.

The patient is taught transfer techniques early. When the patient gets out of bed, good posture must be maintained. As soon as possible, the patient may stand between parallel bars or be raised to an upright position on a tilt table to allow extension of the temporary prosthesis to the floor with *minimal* weight-bearing.

- Excessive pressure on the residual limb is to be avoided because it may compromise wound healing.

How soon after surgery the patient is allowed to "touch down" the artificial foot depends on such factors as age and physical status and the condition of the other foot. Patients who are debilitated or have severe diabetes or peripheral vascular disease may not be able to tolerate the degree of pressure required to "touch down" the foot, and thus must wait for a longer period before starting this activity.

The patient usually stands between parallel bars twice daily. As endurance increases, ambulation is started within the parallel bars, but full weight-bearing is not permitted on the amputated side. Crutch walking is started when stable balance is achieved.

While crutch walking, the patient should learn to use a normal gait. The residual limb should move back and forth while the patient is walking with the crutches. To prevent a permanent flexion deformity from occurring, the residual limb should not be held up in a flexed position.

Prosthesis Preparation

Patients who are candidates for prosthesis will be seen by the prosthetist. Effective preprosthetic care is important to ensure proper fitting of the prosthesis. The major problems that can delay the prosthetic fitting during this period are (1) flexion deformities, (2) nonshrinkage of the residual limb, and (3) abduction deformities of the hip. These deformities can be avoided.

The prosthesis socket is custom-molded to the residual limb. Prostheses are designed for specific activity levels and patient abilities. Types of prostheses include hydraulic, pneumatic, biofeedback-controlled, myoelectrically-controlled joints, synchronized joints, and others.

Gait training is continued under the supervision of a physical therapist until optimal gait is achieved. Adjustments of the prosthetic socket are made by the prosthetist to accommodate the residual limb changes that take place during the first 6 months to a year after surgery. A light plaster cast or a tensor bandage is used to limit edema during the times the patient is not wearing the permanent prosthesis.

Residual Limb Shaping and Conditioning. The residual limb must be shrunk and shaped into a conical form to permit accurate measurement and maximum comfort and fit of the prosthetic device. This is done by applying bandages, an elastic residual limb shrinker, or an air splint. The patient or some member of the family can be taught the correct method of bandaging.

Bandaging supports the soft tissue and minimizes the formation of edematous fluid while the residual limb is in a dependent position. The bandage is applied in such a manner that the remaining muscles required to operate the prosthesis are as firm as possible, while those muscles that are not longer useful will atrophy (Fig. 57-19). An improperly applied elastic

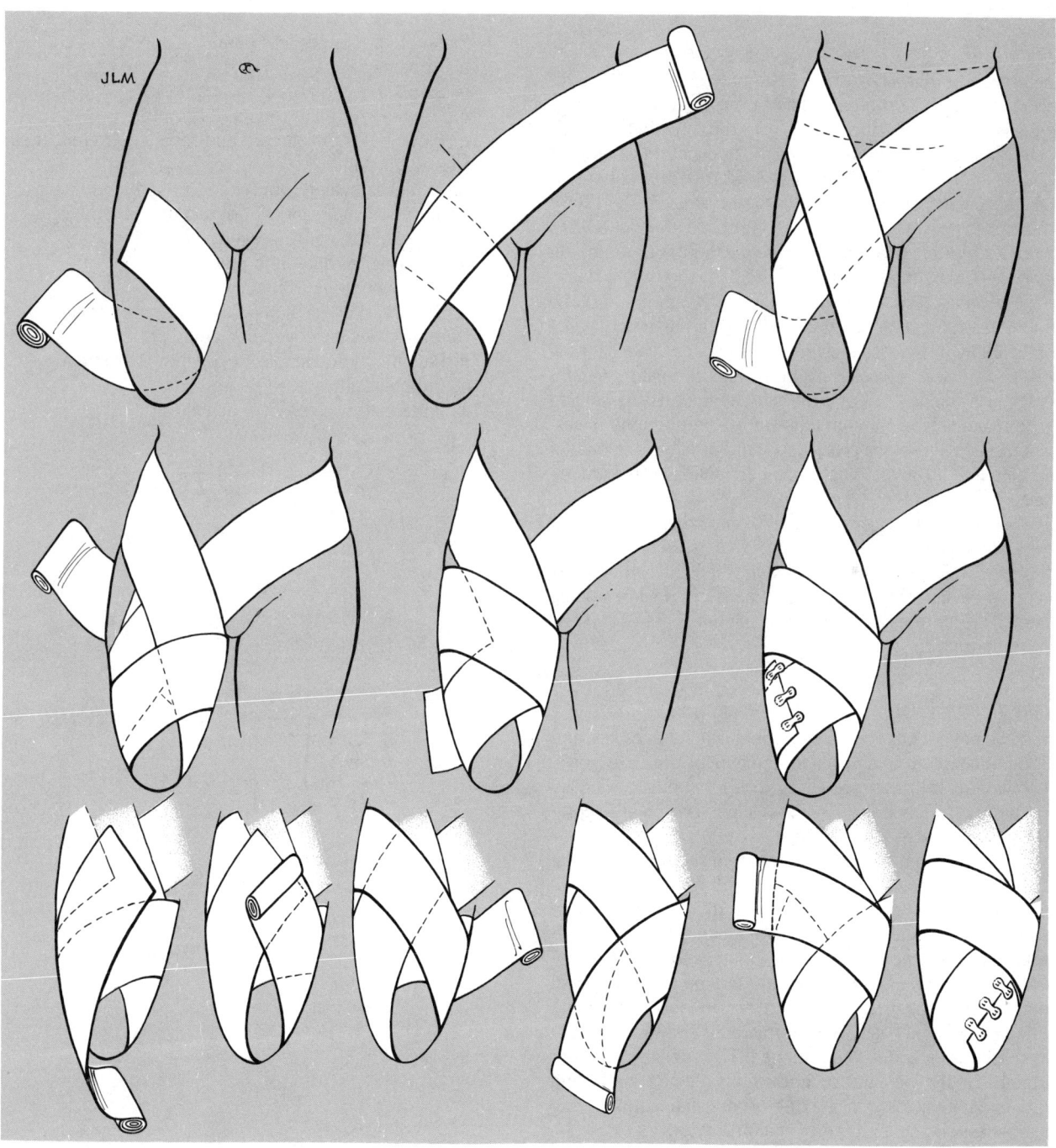

Figure 57-19
Wrapping above-knee residual limb. Elastic bandaging reduces edema and shapes the residual limb in a firm conical form for the prosthesis. (Brunner LS and Suddarth DS. The Lippincott Manual of Nursing Practice, 4th ed. Philadelphia, JB Lippincott, 1986.)

bandage contributes to circulatory problems and a poorly-shaped residual limb.

In order to "toughen" the residual limb in preparation for a prosthesis, activities to condition the residual limb are usually prescribed. The patient begins by pushing the residual limb into a soft pillow, then into a firmer pillow, and finally against a hard surface. The patient is taught to massage the residual limb to mobilize the scar, decrease tenderness, and improve vascularity. Massage is usually started when healing takes place, and is first done by the physical therapist. Skin inspection and preventive care are taught.

Rehabilitation

The complete rehabilitation of an amputee requires the concerted efforts of the entire rehabilitation team. The orthopedic surgeon, the nurse, the physiatrist, the prosthetist (limb maker), the physical therapist, and the occupational therapist all unite their efforts to condition and train the patient to make a satisfactory adjustment to the prosthesis. The establishment of prosthetic clinics has improved the outlook of amputees. With vocational counseling and job retraining where necessary, many of these patients can return to work.

Nonambulatory Amputees. Some patients may not be candidates for a prosthesis. Conditions that may limit a patient's ability to walk with a prosthesis include diabetes mellitus, heart disease, stroke, hypertension, circulatory insufficiency, advancing age, obesity, infections, delayed healing of the residual limb (amputation stump), and peripheral vascular disease. If use of a prosthesis is not possible, the patient can be taught to participate in self-care activities in a wheelchair.

A special wheelchair designed for amputees is advocated for persons who have lost one or both legs. Because of the decreased weight in the front, a regular wheelchair is in danger of tipping backward when an amputee sits in it. In an amputee wheelchair, the rear axle is set back about 5 cm (2 inches) to compensate for this danger.

Home Health Care

When the patient has achieved physiological homeostasis and has demonstrated achievement of major health care goals, rehabilitation will continue either in a rehabilitation facility or at home. Continued support and supervision by the community health nurse are essential.

Prior to the patient's discharge from the acute care facility, the home should be assessed in terms of the patient's continuing care, safety, and mobility. Modifications are made according to the individual patient's needs. An overnight or week-end experience at home may be tried to identify problems that were not identified on the assessment visit. Physical therapy and occupational therapy may continue in the home or on an outpatient basis. Transportation to continuing health care appointments must be arranged. The social service department of the hospital or community agency managing continued health care may be of great assistance in securing personal assistance and transportation services.

During follow-up health visits, the nurse evaluates the patient's physical and psychosocial adjustment. Periodic preventive health assessments are necessary. Frequently, an elderly spouse is unable to provide the assistance required, and

additional help at home is needed. Modifications in the care plan are made on the basis of such findings. Often, the patient and family find involvement in an amputee support group to be of value. Here they are able to share problems, solutions, and resources. Talking with those who have successfully dealt with a similar problem may help the patient develop a satisfactory solution.

▷ *Evaluation*

▷ *Expected Outcomes*

1. Patient experiences less pain
   a. Appears relaxed
   b. States that he feels comfortable
   c. Uses measures to reduce discomfort
   d. Participates in self-care and rehabilitative activites
2. Has intact skin
   a. Achieves healed, nontender, nonadherent scar
   b. Is free of signs and symptoms of infection
   c. Repositions self to prevent pressure sores
   d. Controls residual limb edema
   e. Demonstrates residual limb care
   f. Reports skin problems that need to be treated
3. Demonstrates improved self-concept
   a. Patient acknowledges change in body image
   b. Projects self as a whole person
   c. Participates in self-care activities

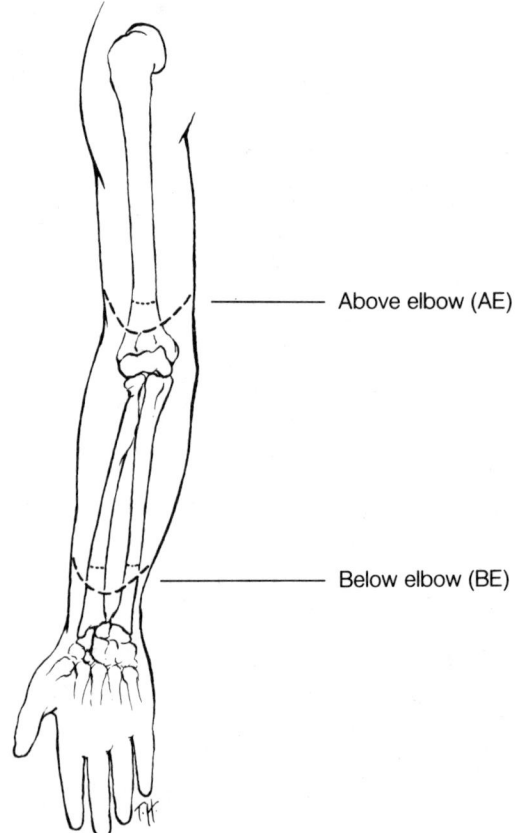

Figure 57-20
Levels of amputation of upper extremity.

d. Demonstrates increasing independence
e. Resumes role-related responsibilities
f. Reestablishes social contacts
g. Demonstrates confidence in abilities
4. Resolves grieving
   a. Expresses grief
   b. Utilizes family and friends to work through feelings
   c. Focuses on future functioning
5. Achieves independent self-care
   a. Maintains balance when sitting and transferring
   b. Demonstrates safe transferring ability
   c. Uses aids and assistive devices to facilitate self-care
   d. Asks for assistance when needed
   e. Verbalizes satisfaction with abilities to perform activities of daily living
6. Achieves maximum independent mobility
   a. Is free of systemic immobility problems
   b. Avoids positions contributing to contracture development

c. Repositions self frequently
d. Demonstrates full active range of motion
e. Uses wheelchair and ambulatory aid safely
f. Achieves functional use of prosthesis
g. Is free of pressure-related problems
h. Increases strength and endurance
i. Overcomes environmental barriers to mobility
j. Uses community services and resources as needed

Upper Extremity Amputations

The loss of an upper extremity can be a greater catastrophe than the loss of a lower extremity, because the upper extremity has such a highly specialized function. The major reasons for upper extremity amputation are severe trauma (acute injury, electrical burns, frostbite), malignant tumors, infection (fulminating gas gangrene, chronic osteomyelitis), and congenital malformations.

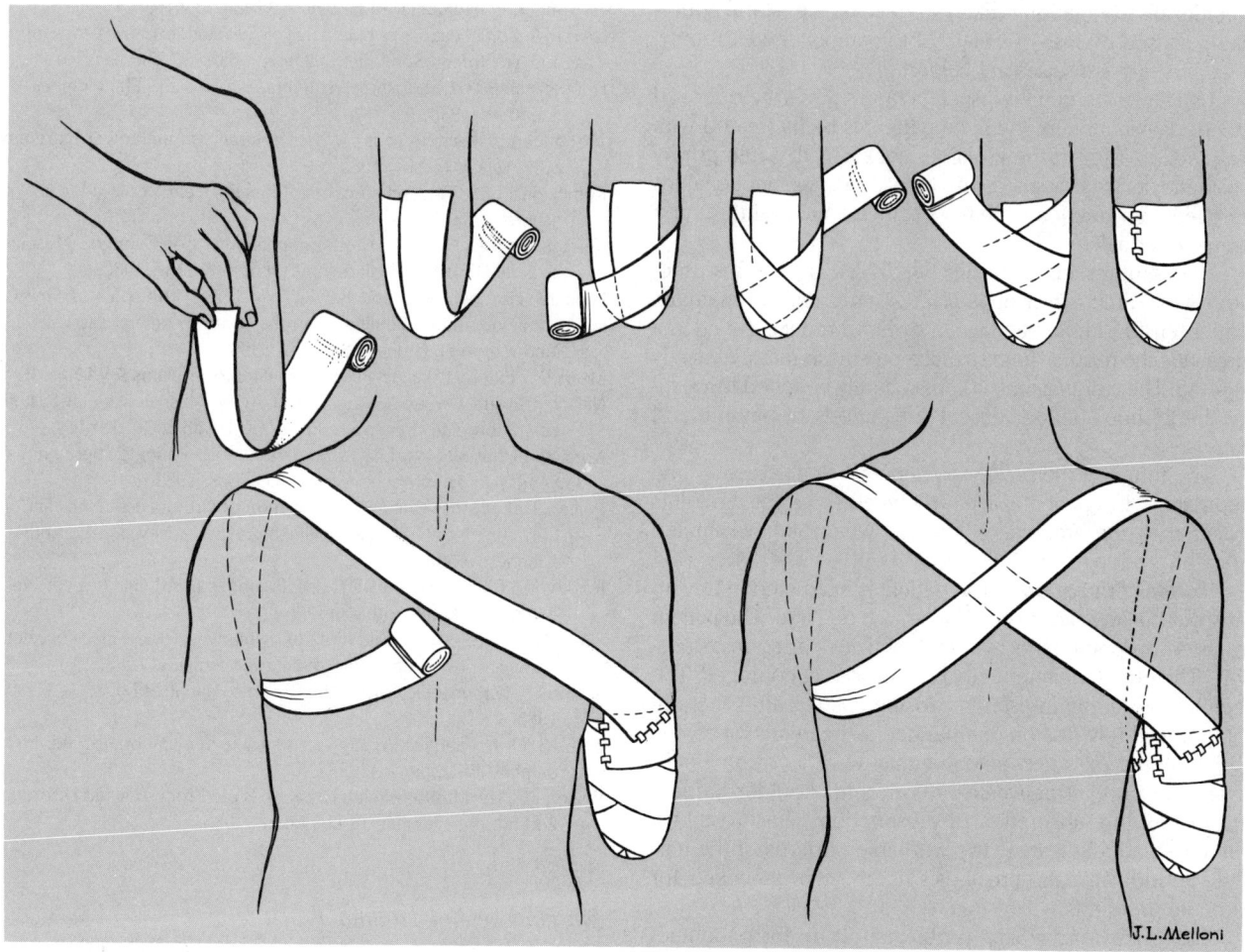

Figure 57-21
Wrapping above-elbow residual limb. An elastic bandage wrapping for an above-the-elbow residual limb minimizes edema and shapes it for a prosthesis. The bandage may need to be secured by wrapping across the back and shoulders. (Brunner LS and Suddarth DS. The Lippincott Manual of Nursing Practice, 4th ed. Philadelphia, JB Lippincott, 1986.)

If time permits (and it usually does *not* with acute trauma), the patient is able to find out about the available prosthetic replacement and one-handed devices that aid independence. Regardless of what assistive devices are available, psychological support is essential to help the patient adapt to changes that will be made in life-style.

The objective of surgery is to conserve as much extremity length as possible, consistent with eradicating the disease process (Fig. 57-20, p. 1608). Following surgery, a rigid plaster dressing with provision for the application of a temporary prosthesis or a compression bandage will be applied. Usually, suction drainage is used to eliminate hematoma and achieve better approximation of tissues. The residual limb may be elevated to control edema.

Residual limb exercises (muscle-setting and joint-mobilizing exercises) are started as soon as tolerated to strengthen the muscles and mobilize the joints. These exercises are usually done under the supervision of the physical therapist. The muscles of both shoulders are exercised, since an upper-extremity amputee uses both shoulders to operate the prosthesis. A patient with an above-the-elbow amputation or shoulder disarticulation is likely to develop a postural abnormality caused by loss of weight of the amputated extremity. Thus, postural exercises are helpful.

Usually, the wound is inspected and sutures are removed 7 to 10 days after surgery. If the patient is being treated with the rigid dressing, a new plaster socket with a temporary prosthetic device is applied. This type of management enables the patient to practice with the prosthesis and be fitted for a permanent device.

If a compression dressing (Fig. 57-21, p. 1609) is used, the residual limb is rewrapped 3 to 4 times daily to maintain proper tension in the bandage in order to reduce the edema and shape the residual limb so that a prosthesis may eventually be fitted. The residual limb is kept securely wrapped throughout the 24-hour period, except for periods of bathing and exercise.

The fitting of the prosthesis depends on the level of the amputation, the patient's age, and whether or not the joints proximal to the amputation site are weak or have limited range of motion.

Patient Education. The patient is instructed in how to carry out the activities of daily living with one arm. The patient is started on one-handed self-care activities as soon as possible. The use of the temporary prosthesis is encouraged. The patient who learns to use the prosthesis soon after the amputation will rely less on one-handed self-care activities.

An upper-extremity amputee may wear a cotton T-shirt to prevent contact between the skin and shoulder harness and to promote absorption of perspiration. The prosthetist will advise about cleaning the washable portions of the harness. Periodically, the prosthesis needs to be checked for potential problems.

Complications. Skin problems occur from contact dermatitis that results from irritants in the prosthetic components and from lack of ventilation and poor skin hygiene. Residual limb contracture or residual limb contour problems may develop. Infection, necrosis of the skin edges, and phantom sensations (feeling that the arm is still present) are other complications. Psychological problems (denial, withdrawal) may be influenced by the type of support the patient receives from the rehabilitation team and by how quickly one-handed

activities and use of prosthesis are taught and learned. Knowing the full options and capabilities available in the various prosthetic devices can give the patient a sense of control over the disability. The patient is not fully rehabilitated until a prosthesis has been fitted and the patient has learned how to use it. Training of this nature is best accomplished in a specialized rehabilitation unit or center.

Bibliography

Books

Arthroscopy of the Knee (monograph). Pitman, New Jersey, National Association of Orthopaedic Nurses, 1983.

Assessment and Fracture Management of the Lower Extremities (monograph). Pitman, New Jersey, National Association of Orthopaedic Nurses, 1984.

Campbell WC and Crenshaw AH (eds). Cambell's Operative Orthopaedics, 7th ed. St Louis, CV Mosby, 1987.

Farrell J. Illustrated Guide to Orthopedic Nursing, 3rd ed. Philadelphia, JB Lippincott, 1986.

Gossling HR and Pillsbury SL (eds). Complications of Fracture Management. Philadelphia, JB Lippincott, 1984.

Green SA. Complications of External Skeletal Fixation: Causes, Prevention, and Treatment. Springfield, Illinois, Charles C Thomas, 1981.

Heppenstall R (ed). Fracture Treatment and Healing. Philadelphia, WB Saunders, 1980.

Jarrett F and Hirsch SA (eds). Vascular Surgery of the Lower Extremity. St Louis, CV Mosby, 1985.

Kempczinski RF. The Ischemic Leg. Chicago, Year Book Medical Publishers, 1985.

Kessler RM and Hertling D (eds). Management of Common Musculoskeletal Disorders. Philadelphia, Harper & Row, 1983.

Leek JC, Gershwin ME, and Fowler WM (eds). Principles of Physical Medicine and Rehabilitation in the Musculoskeletal Diseases. Orlando, Florida, Grune & Stratton, 1986.

Mears DC. External Skeletal Fixation. Baltimore, Williams & Wilkins, 1983.

Nelson CL and Dwyer AP (eds). The Aging Musculoskeletal System. Lexington, The Collarmore Press, DC Heath & Co, 1984.

Nursing Skillbook: Working with Orthopedic Patients. Springhouse, Pennsylvania, Intermed Communications, 1982.

Pellino T et al (eds). National Association of Orthopaedic Nurses: Core Curriculum for Orthopaedic Nursing. Pitman, New Jersey, Anthony J Jannetti, 1986.

Rockwood CA and Green DP (eds). Fractures in Adults, 2nd ed. Philadelphia, JB Lippincott, 1984.

Salter RB. Textbook of Disorders and Injuries of the Musculoskeletal System, 2nd ed. Baltimore, Williams & Wilkins, 1983.

Sculco TP. Orthopaedic Care of the Geriatric Patient. St Louis, CV Mosby, 1985.

Turek S. Orthopaedics: Principles and Their Application, 4th ed. Philadelphia, JB Lippincott, 1984.

Wilson FC. The Musculoskeletal System: Basic Processes and Disorders, 2nd ed. Philadelphia, JB Lippincott, 1983.

Articles

Musculoskeletal Trauma/Fracture

A plan of action for open pelvic fractures. Emerg Med 1983 Feb 28; 15(4):57, 60.

Babayov D et al. Sensorimotor integration therapy for hip fracture and CVA patients. Can J Occup Ther 1985 June; 52(3):133–137.

Barden RM. Osteonecrosis of the femoral head. Orthop Nurs 1985 July/Aug; 4(4):45–51.

Barden RM. Case studies: Treatment of nonunions with electrical bone stimulator. Orthop Nurs 1985 Mar/Apr; 4(2):52.

Bassett CA. The development and application of pulsed electromagnetic fields (PEMFs) for ununited fractures and arthrodesis. Orthop Clin North Am 1984 June; 15(1):61–88.

Black J. Tissue response to exogenous electromagnetic signals. Orthop Clin North Am 1984 Jan; 15(1):15–22.

Brighton CT. The semi-invasive methods of treating nonunion with direct current. Orthop Clin North Am 1984 Jan; 15(1):33–46.

Brocker A. New techniques in fracture management. Surg Clin North Am 1983 June; 63(3):607–628.

Callahan J. Compartment syndrome. Orthop Nurs 1985 July/Aug; 4(4):11–15.

Ceccio CM. Postoperative pain relief through relaxation in elderly patients with fractured hips. Orthop Nurs 1984 May/June; 3(3):11–19.

Celeste SM et al. Identifying a standard for pin site care using the quality assurance approach. Orthop Nurs 1984 July/Aug; 3(4):17–24.

Connolly JF. Pathologic fracture. Emerg Med 1984 June 15; 16(11):61–71.

Connolly JF. The foot . . . fracture pitfalls. Emerg Med 1984 May 15; 16(9):67–78.

Connolly JF. The ankle . . . fracture pitfalls. Emerg Med 1984 Apr 15; 16(7):49–59.

Connolly JF. Tibial fracture. Emerg Med 1984 Mar 15; 16(5):43–53.

Connolly JF. The knee bone and soft tissue . . . fracture pitfalls. Emerg Med 1984 Jan 15; 16(1):205–211.

Connolly JF. Electrical treatment of nonunions: Its use and abuse in 100 consecutive fractures. Orthop Clin North Am 1984 Jan; 15(1):89–106.

Connolly JF. The femur . . . fracture pitfalls. Emerg Med 1983 Dec 15; 15(21):51–61.

Connolly JF. The hip . . . fracture pitfalls. Emerg Med 1983 Nov 15; 15(19):53–61.

Connolly JF. The wrist . . . fracture pitfalls. Emerg Med 1983 Aug 15; 15(14):195–205.

Connolly JF. The forearm . . . fracture pitfalls. Emerg Med 1983 July 15; 15(13):235, 238, 240.

Connolly JF. The humerus . . . fracture pitfalls. Emerg Med 1983 May 15; 15(9):170–181.

Connolly JF. The clavical and shoulder girdle . . . fracture pitfalls. Emerg Med 1983 Mar 15: 15(5):148–155.

Connolly JF. The pelvis . . . fracture pitfalls. Emerg Med 1983 Feb 15; 15(3):183–192.

Daniel WW et al. Elbow injuries: Diagnosis and treatment. Hosp Med 1983 Sept; 19(9):211, 214, 217.

Duerksen JR. Hip fractures: Special considerations in the elderly. Orthop Nurs 1982 Jan/Feb; 1(1):11–19.

Evers JA et al. Dealing with fractures. RN 1984 Nov; 47(11):53–55, 57.

Farrell J. The trauma patient with multiple fractures. RN 1985 June; 48(6):22–25.

Geier KA et al. Electrical bone stimulation for treatment of nonunions. Orthop Nurs 1985 Mar/Apr; 4(2):41–50.

Geier KA et al. Case studies: Treatment of nonunions with electrical bone stimulation: The fully implantable, direct current stimulator. Orthop Nurs 1985 Mar/Apr; 4(2):53.

Genge M. Orthopaedic trauma: Pelvic fractures. Orthop Nurs 1986 Jan/Feb; 5(1):11–19.

Gill KP and Laflamme D. External fixation: The erector sets of orthopedic nursing. Can Nurs 1984 May; 80(5):29–30.

Gille G. Patient care—not injury care . . . fracture and tissue injuries. Emergency 1985 Mar; 17(3):36–39.

Harper A. Initial assessment and management of femoral neck fractures in the elderly. Orthop Nurs 1985 May/June; 4(3):55–58.

Heppenstall BR. The present role of bone graft surgery in treating nonunion. Orthop Clin North Am 1984 Jan; 15(1):113–124.

Hughs JH. Diagnosis: Rib fractures and sequelae. Hosp Med 1983 June; 19(6):65–72.

Hull RD and Raskob GE. Prophylaxis of venous throlbic disease following hip and knee surgery. J Bone Joint Surg [Am] 1986 Jan; 68-A(1):146–150.

Keene JS and Anderson CA. Hip fractures in the elderly: Discharge pre-

dictions with a functional rating scale. JAMA 1982 Aug 6; 248(5):564–567.

Kenzora JE et al. Hip fracture mortality. Clin Orthop 1984 June; 186:45–56.

Laughlin RM and Clancy GJ. Musculoskeletal assessment: Neurovascular examination of the injured extremity. Orthop Nurs 1982 Jan/Feb; 1(1):43–48.

Miller MC. Nursing care of the patient with external fixation therapy. Orthop Nurs 1983 Jan/Feb; 2(1):11–15.

Mindell ER. Orthopedic surgery. JAMA 1985 Oct 25; 254(16):2313–2315.

Montrey JS et al. Thromboembolism following hip fracture. J Trauma 1985 June; 25(6):534–537.

Mubarak SJ and Hargens AR. Acute compartment syndromes. Surg Clin North Am 1983 June; 63(3):539–566.

Nickens HW et al. Toward a hip fracture prevention project . . . national hip fracture prevention demonstration program. Orthop Nurs 1985 May/June; 4(3):52–53.

Nicholas JA and Reilly JP. Orthopedic problems in athletes. Compr Ther 1985 Jan; 11(1):48–56.

Nideffer R. The injured athlete—psychological factors in treatment. Orthop Clin North Am 1983 Aug; 14(4):373–385.

Parkinson M. Repair of a comminuted fracture. Nurs Mirror 1984 Apr 18; 159(16):23–26.

Paterson D. Treatment of nonunion with a constant direct current: A totally implantable system. Orthop Clin North Am 1984 Jan; 15(1):47–60.

Pina M et al. Dextran/aspirin versus heparin/dihydroergotamine in preventing thrombosis after hip fractures. J Bone Joint Surg [Br] 1985 Mar; 67(2):305–309.

Pradka L. Use of the wick catheter for diagnosing and monitoring compartment syndrome. Orthop Nurs 1985 July/Aug; 4(4):17–18.

Preventing fat embolism after fracture . . . a short course of corticosteroids. Emerg Med 1984 Mar 15; 16(5):142–144.

Robinson JE et al. A nail-safe method . . . intramedullary nailing of femoral fractures. Am J Nurs 1985 Feb; 85(2):158–161.

Rockett CP. Case studies: Treatment of nonunions with electrical bone stimulation. Nonunion of the humerus: Use of a semi-invasive technique of electrical bone stimulation. Orthop Nurs 1985 Mar/Apr; 4(2):53–54, 107.

Salmond SW. Trauma and fractures: Meeting your patient's nutritional needs. Orthop Nurs 1984 July/Aug; 3(4):27–33.

Sherman M. Thrombophylaxis with antiembolism stockings. Orthop Nurs 1985 July/Aug; 4(4):33–37.

Simpson EF. Heat, cold, or both. Am J Nurs 1983 Feb; 83(2):271–273.

Spickler LL. Knee injuries of the athlete. Orthop Nurs 1983 Sept/Oct; 2(5):11–19.

Sproles KJ. Nursing care of skeletal pins: A closer look. Orthop Nurs 1985 Jan/Feb; 4(1):11–12, 15–20.

Stevenson RDK. Take no chances with fat embolism . . . grave risk that follows bone fractures. Nursing '85 1985 June; 15(6):58–64.

Thygerson AL. Rib fracture. Emergency 1982 Nov; 14(1):48, 54.

Update on fractures. Fracture repair: Conflicts and consensus, Part 1. Orthop Nurs 1984 Sept/Oct; 3(5):25–29.

Update on fractures. Fracture repair: Conflicts and consensus, Part 2. Orthop Nurs 1984 Nov/Dec; 3(6):43–47.

Urbanski PA. The orthopedic patient: Identifying neurovascular injury. AORN J 1984 Nov; 40(5):707–711.

Wassel AC. Sports medicine: Acute and overuse injuries. Orthop Nurs 1984 Apr/May; 3(2):29–34.

Weber ER et al. Colles fracture: A rational approach to recognition and treatment. Consultant 1985 Jan 30; 25(2):25–33.

Westaby S et al. Management of compound fractures. Nurs Times 1983 May 11–17; 79(19):69–72.

White L et al. Who's at risk? Hip fracture epidemiology report. J Gerontol Nurs 1984 Oct; 10(10):26–28.

Wittert DW and Barden RM. Deep vein thrombosis, pulmonary emboli, and prophylaxis in the orthopaedic patient. Orthop Nurs 1985 July/Aug; 4(4):27–32.

Zarins B and Ciullo J. Acute muscle and tendon injuries in athletes. Clin Sports Med 1983 Jan; 2(1):167–182.

Amputations

Boren AH. Adolescent adjustment to amputation necessitated by bone cancer. Orthop Nurs 1985 Sept/Oct; 4(5):30–32.

Burgess EM. Amputations. Surg Clin North Am 1983 June; 63(3):749–770.

Crowther H. New perspectives on nursing lower limb amputees. J Adv Nurs 1982 Sept; 7(5):453–460.

Dernham P. Phantom limb pain. Geriatr Nurs 1986 Jan./Feb; 7(1):34–37.

Farrell J. Helping the new amputee. Orthop Nurs 1982 May/June; 1(3):18.

Hill SL. Interventions for the elderly amputee. Rehab Nurs 1985 May/June; 10(3):23–25.

Moye CE. Nursing care of the amputee: An overview. Orthop Nurs 1982 May/June; 1(3):11–13.

Rubin G and Fliess D. Devices to enable persons with amputation to participate in sports. Arch Phys Med Rehabil 1983 Jan; 64(1):37–40.

Rutan FM. Preprosthetic program for the amputee. Orthop Nurs 1982 May/June; 1(3):14–17.

Smith AG. Common problems of lower extremity amputees. Orthop Clin North Am 1982 July; 13(3):569–578.

Spross JA and Hope A. Alterations in comfort: Pain related to cancer. Orthop Nurs 1985 Sept/Oct; 4(5):48–52.

Stratmann DT and Donnelly LT. Determination of ideal body weight and nutritional requirements post-amputation. Orthop Nurs 1984 May/June; 3(3):37–40.

Thompson DM et al. Living with an amputation: The helper. Soc Sci Med 1985 Apr; 20(4):319–323.

Agencies

Access for the Handicapped, 1012 14th Street NW, Washington, DC 20005.

American Running and Fitness Association, 2420 K Street NW, Washington, DC 20037.

Amputee in Motion, 5900 Sepulveda Boulevard, Sherman Oaks, CA 91411.

Amputee Shoe and Glove Exchange, 1635 Warwickshire Drive, Houston, TX 77077.

52 Association (Sport Program for Amputees), 441 Lexington Avenue, New York, NY 10017.

National Amputation Foundation, 12–45 150th Street, Whitestone, NY 11357.

National Easter Seal Society, 2023 West Ogden Avenue, Chicago, IL 60612.

National Institute of Arthritis and Musculoskeletal and Skin Diseases, National Institutes of Health, Bethesda, MD 20892.

National Odd Shoe Exchange, R.R. 1, Indianola, IA 50125.

Chapter 58

Management of Patients With Musculoskeletal Disorders

Low Back Pain

Back pain is a major health problem. An estimated 80% of the population will experience low back pain sometime during their lifetime. Impairments of the back and spine are the third leading cause of disability of people in their employment years. The limitations imposed by low back pain on the individual are severe. The economic cost, in terms of loss of productivity, is in the billions of dollars. The number of medical visits resulting from low back pain is second only to those for upper respiratory illnesses.

Low back pain may be caused by a large variety of conditions. Most low back pain is caused by musculoskeletal problems (*e.g.*, acute lumbosacral strain, unstable lumbosacral ligaments and weak muscles, osteoarthritis of the spine, spinal stenosis, intervertebral disc problems, inequality of leg length). Older patients may have back pain associated with osteoporotic vertebral fractures or bone metastasis. Other causes include kidney disorders, pelvic problems, retroperitoneal tumors, abdominal aneurysms, and psychosomatic problems. Most back pain due to musculoskeletal disturbances is aggravated by activity, whereas pain due to other considerations is not influenced by activity.

Obesity, stress, and occasionally depression may contribute to low back pain. Patients with chronic low back pain may develop a dependence on alcohol or analgesics.

Pathophysiology

The spinal column can be considered as an elastic rod constructed of rigid units (vertebrae) and flexible units (intervertebral discs) that are held together by complex facet joints, multiple ligaments, and paravertebral muscles. The unique construction of the back allows for flexibility while providing maximum protection for the spinal cord. The spinal curves absorb vertical shocks from running and jumping. The trunk helps to stabilize the spine. The abdominal and thoracic muscles are important in lifting activities. Disuse weakens these supporting structures. Obesity, postural problems, structural problems, or overstretching of the spinal supports may result in back pain.

The intervertebral discs change in character as the person ages. In the young, the disc is mainly fibrocartilage with a gelatinous matrix. It becomes dense, irregular fibrocartilage in the elderly. Disc degeneration is a common cause of back pain. Lower lumbar discs L4–L5 and L5–S1, are subject to the greatest mechanical stress and the greatest degenerative changes. Disc protrusion (herniated nucleus pulposa) or facet joint changes can cause pressure on nerve roots that leave the spinal canal and results in pain that radiates along the nerve. About 12% of the people with low back pain have herniated nucleus pulposa. (Management of intervertebral disc disease is discussed on p. 1517.)

Clinical Manifestations

The patient's history reveals a complaint of either acute pain (present less than 3 days) or chronic back pain and fatigue. During the initial interview, the location of the pain and whether it radiates along a nerve root (*sciatica*) need to be assessed. If the pain is of musculoskeletal origin, the patient will indicate that movement accentuates the pain.

Physical examination may reveal *paravertebral muscle spasm* (greatly increased muscle tone of the back postural muscles). There is a loss of the normal lumbar lordotic curve and possible spinal deformity. When the patient is examined in a prone position, these muscles relax and any deformity caused by the spasm disappears. The patient's gait, spinal mobility, reflexes, leg length, motor strength, sensory ability, and leg movement (*e.g.*, straight leg raises) are evaluated.

If the patient has some *radiculopathy* (nerve root problem) or chronic back pain, additional studies may be conducted.

Diagnostic Evaluation

An x-ray of the spine reveals the presence of a fracture, a dislocation, an infection, osteoarthritis, or scoliosis. An electromyogram (EMG) and nerve conduction studies are used to evaluate radiculopathies. A myelogram can indicate disc protrusions and nerve root compression, which could cause the pain. In situations that are difficult to diagnose, a *discogram* (in which a small amount of contrast medium in injected into the intervertebral disc) may be used to demonstrate degenerative or ruptured disc. Computed tomography (CT) is being used more frequently to identify precisely the underlying problem. Occult (obscure) soft-tissue lesions adjacent to the vertebral column and precise disc problems can be identified with current tomography techniques. Ultrasound may be used to help diagnose narrow spinal canals. Epidural venograms help to assess lumbar disc disease as evidenced by displacement of epidural veins.

At times, an organic basis for the back pain cannot be identified. The pain becomes chronic (lasting more than 2 months without improvement) and may be due to a reaction to continuing emotional stresses or secondary gains associated with being incapacitated (*e.g*, workman's compensation, easier life-style). Working with these patients is a challenge because major readjustments are coupled with the cure.

Management

Physical Measures. Since most back pain improves with bed rest and inactivity, the patient is confined to bed on a firm, nonsagging mattress. Acute muscle spasms subside in 3 to 7 days. The best position is a modified supine position with slight lumbar flexion (elevate the head of the bed 30 degrees and have the knees slightly flexed; Fig. 58-1) or a lateral position with knees and hips flexed and a pillow between the knees and legs. A prone position is avoided because it accentuates lordosis. Bathroom privileges may be permitted, but all other out-of-bed activities (*e.g.*, answering the phone, checking on the children, general activity due to restlessness) are to be avoided.

Frequently, the patient is unable to comply with a bed rest regimen at home and is hospitalized for "active conservative management." Pelvic traction with 15 to 30 pounds of weight is prescribed. Traction promotes additional lumbar flexion (Fig. 58-2). The patient feels something is being done to alleviate the back pain, and becomes an active participant in care by managing the traction. Bed rest with slight lumbar flexion is encouraged. Bed rest does have the associated side-effects of muscle disuse atrophy and circulatory decompensation, for which the nurse needs to be alert when patient mobilization is begun.

Physical therapy may be utilized to decrease pain and muscle spasm. Forms of therapy used are therapeutic cold, infrared radiant heat, hot moist packs, ultrasound, diathermy, and the whirlpool. If the patient has had previous episodes of back pain, the history of treatment that was successful previously is valuable for selecting the treatment modality. Each treatment mode is matched with the patient. Patients with impaired circulation, diminished sensation, and trauma may not be good candidates for hot packs. Whirlpool therapy may be contraindicated for patients with cardiovascular problems because they are not able to tolerate the associated massive peripheral vasodilatation. Ultrasound produces deep heat, which may increase discomfort due to swelling in the acute stages. Additionally, it is contraindicated if the patient has cancer or bleeding disorders. Gentle soft-tissue massage is useful to decrease muscle spasm and to increase circulation to the tissues.

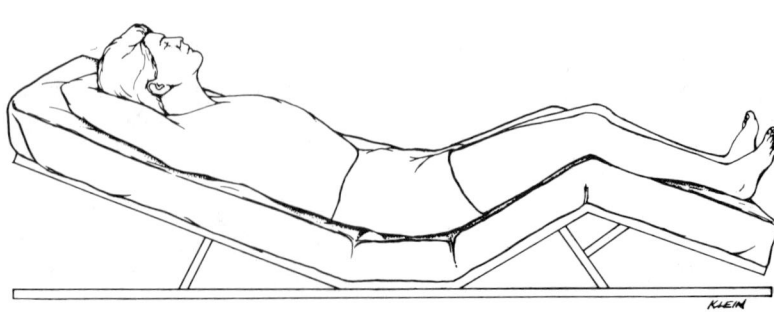

Figure 58-1
Positioning to provide lumbar flexion.

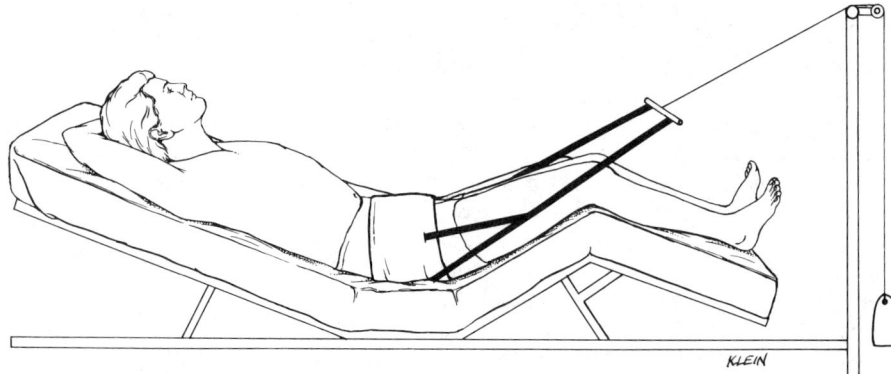

Figure 58-2
Pelvic traction with lumbar
flexion to alleviate low back pain.

Drug Therapy. Acute pain may need to be treated with medications. Narcotic analgesics are required initially to interrupt the muscle spasm pain cycle and to decrease paraspinal muscle spasm. Anti-inflammatory agents, including aspirin and other nonsteroidal anti-inflammatory drugs, are helpful in reducing the pain. Muscle relaxants and tranquilizers will relax the patient and muscles in spasm, thereby providing pain relief. If the patient exhibits nerve root irritation, short-term corticosteroids are used to decrease the inflammatory response of the nerves and to prevent the development of neurofibrosis, which results from ischemic changes. Epidural steroid injections are used for pain relief as well as for diagnostic purposes. Infiltration of paraspinal muscles with local anesthetics may result in relaxation and pain relief.

TENS. Transcutaneous electrical nerve stimulation (TENS) is a portable, noninvasive pain-reduction device that allows the patient to participate in activities comfortably without medication. The unit is thought to afford pain relief by overriding pain input (gate theory of pain control) and stimulating endorphins.

Persons working with the patient need to understand the device and accept its pain relief potential. Electrodes are attached to areas of the body where the patient is able to achieve maximum pain relief. The patient adjusts the stimulator's wave length and intensity to achieve comfort (see also p. 252). Patients who use cardiac pacemakers should not use TENS. Those who operate machinery need to be aware of the potential for accidental shocks. Generally, the patient uses the device for 1 to 2 months and gradually decreases its use as pain subsides and the back strengthens through graduated exercises.

Exercise Program. As the patient achieves comfort at rest, activities can be gradually resumed and an exercise program initiated. *The goal is to increase mobility, muscle strength, and flexibility.* Hyperextension exercises strengthen the paravertebral muscles; flexion exercises increase back movement and strength; and isometric flexion exercises strengthen trunk muscles.

The exercise program is carried out under the direction of the physical therapist and is adapted to the individual patient. The exercise period begins with relaxation.

The nurse needs to encourage patient adherence. Erratic exercising is ineffective. For most exercise programs, it is suggested that the person exercise twice a day, increasing the number of exercises gradually. After months of exercises, the patient may become bored with the routine. Recreational activities that the patient enjoys can be allowed. These activities should not cause excessive lumbar strain, twisting, or discomfort. They may be increased gradually as tolerated. Horseback riding and weight-lifting should be avoided.

Body Mechanics and Posture. The nurse assesses how the patient moves and stands, and engages in patient teaching as needed. However, good body mechanics and posture are essential to avoid recurrence of back pain. Providing the patient with a list of suggestions will help in making these long-term changes. If the patient wears high heels, low heels are suggested.

When sitting, the knees and hips should be flexed, and the knees should be level with the hips or higher to minimize lordosis. The feet should be on the floor. The back needs to be supported. Bending forward for long periods is to be avoided.

If long periods of standing are required, the patient should shift his weight frequently and should rest one foot on a low stool, which decreases lumbar lordosis. The patient can check his posture by looking in a mirror to see if the chest is up and the stomach is tucked in. Locking the knees when standing is to be avoided. Be sure the patient knows the correct way to lift objects—using the strong quadriceps muscles of the thighs and minimal use of weak back muscles. The object should be held as close to the body as possible.

The patient should sleep on one side with knees and hips flexed, or supine with knees supported in a flexed position. Sleeping prone is to be avoided.

It takes about 6 months for a person to readjust postural habits. Practicing these protective and defensive postures, positions, and body mechanics results in natural strengthening of the back and diminishes the chance of a recurrence of back pain.

Additional Therapies. At times, a patient with low back pain will need to undertake a weight-reduction program. Decreasing the body weight will decrease the stresses on the low back. Incorporating weight reduction into the overall supervised plan is important.

Low back supports and braces may be prescribed to limit spinal motion, to correct posture, and to diminish stress on the lower lumbar spine. Long-term use of these devices is discouraged, since they may have the negative effects of promoting disuse muscle atrophy and weakness and decreased muscle elasticity. People with jobs that require heavy lifting may wear wide leather belts (trochanter belts) to decrease the strain on their backs. An individual exercise program is essential so that eventually the needed back support can be supplied by the muscles.

Psychological Considerations

Sometimes low back pain can be a psychosomatic illness or a reaction to environmental and life stresses. Emotional problems resulting from anxiety and stress can evoke muscle spasm, which produces a cycle of anxiety, tension, more spasm, and pain. In some persons, mental conflicts are manifested in physical symptoms. There are psychological components in all illnesses, and chronic pain has an emotional impact. In trying to help the patient, one needs insight into family relationships, environmental variables, and work problems. If the back problem stems from a recent accident, the possibility of pending litigation may be a factor. Psychiatric intervention may be necessary for the patient with chronic depression and low back syndrome.

If the patient has a prolonged recovery and has developed secondary gains associated with the low back disability (*e.g.*, workman's compensation, easier life-style or work load, increased emotional support), a ''low back neurosis'' may develop. Psychotherapy or counseling will be needed to assist the person in resuming a full, productive life. There are pain centers throughout the country that offer help by teaching the patient the significance of pain and the skills and techniques for coping with pain (see p. 257).

▶ Nursing Process
The Patient With Low Back Pain

▷ Assessment

The patient with low back pain is encouraged to describe the discomfort. The onset may have been associated with a specific action (*e.g.*, opening a garage door) or with an activity in which weak muscles were overused (*e.g.*, weekend gardening). Determine if this is a recurrent problem and how it was managed in the past. Information about previous successful pain control helps to plan current management. Descriptions of how this problem occurred and how the patient has dealt with it will suggest areas for patient teaching. Additionally, the patient may indicate how this acute or chronic recurring back problem is affecting his life-style. Information on job and recreational activities will identify areas that need to be modified for back health.

During the interview, the nurse observes the patient's posture, position changes, and gait. Generally, the patient guards his movements, keeping the back as still as possible, and selects a chair for support with arms and a standard seat height. The patient may sit and stand in an unusual position, leaning away from the most painful side, and may ask for assistance when undressing because back movements are uncomfortable.

On physical examination, inspect the spinal curves, pelvic crest, and shoulder symmetry. Palpate the paraspinal muscles, noting spasm and tenderness. Ask the patient to bend forward and laterally, noting any discomfort and limitations in movement. Determine how these limitations in movement will affect activities of daily living. To determine nerve irritation, evaluate the patient for the presence of abnormal sensations (paresthesia, paresis) or back and leg pain with straight-leg raising. (With the patient supine, lift the patient's leg upward with the knee in extension.)

Note if the patient is overweight, as this could contribute to low back pain. A nutritional assessment is appropriate.

▷ Nursing Diagnoses

Based on the assessment data, the patient's major nursing diagnoses may include the following:

- Alteration in comfort—pain in lower back related to musculoskeletal problems
- Impaired physical mobility related to pain, muscle spasms, and decreased flexibility
- Disturbance in self-concept, role performance related to immobility
- Knowledge deficit of body mechanics and back conservation techniques
- Alteration in nutrition—potential for more than body requirements

▷ Planning and Implementation

▷ *Goals:*   The major goals of the patient may include relief of pain, resumption of activities, assumption of usual responsibilities, demonstration of back-conserving body mechanics, and reduction of excess body weight.

Nursing Interventions

Relieving Pain

The patient's description of the acute low back pain and previous pain management techniques assist in planning care. As was indicated earlier, activities and stress must be limited; at times hospitalization is necessary to achieve rest and relaxation. The patient is encouraged to decrease stress on the back by resting in bed. A nonsagging mattress and bedboard are advised. The patient is to lie on one side in a curled position or on the back with his head on a pillow and his legs elevated on a pillow to reduce lordosis. If the patient is hospitalized, the bed can be adjusted to achieve this position (see Fig. 58-1), and intermittent pelvic traction is applied (Fig. 58-2). The patient is positioned to increase lumbar flexion, which reduces compression of the lumbar nerve roots. The head of the bed is elevated as well as the knees.

Analgesic, anti-inflammatory, and anti-spasmodic drugs all play a part in the reduction of pain. The nurse should assess the patient's response to each drug. As the acute pain subsides, medications are reduced as prescribed to decrease dependence on habituating drugs.

Patients can be taught to control and modify the perceived pain through behavior therapies that reduce muscular and psychological stress. Diaphragmatic breathing and relaxation will help reduce muscle tension contributing to low back pain. Diversion of attention from the pain to other activity (*e.g.*, reading, conversation, watching TV) is another method of reducing pain perception. A sophisticated example of diversion is guided imagery, in which the relaxed patient learns to focus on a very pleasant event and thus block the perception of pain.

Physical modalities such as massage and heat or cold increase the circulation to the painful back, relieving congestion and reducing pain. The degree of relief obtained will determine whether therapy should be continued.

Resumption of Activities

As the back pain subsides, self-care activities are resumed to minimize strain on the injured structures. Position changes should be made slowly and carried out with assistance as required. The patient should learn to get out of bed with the least possible amount of discomfort. Twisting and jarring motions are avoided. Activities are gradually increased. The patient is encouraged to alternate lying, sitting, and walking activities and is advised to avoid sitting, standing, and walking for long periods. Planning for recumbent rest periods several times throughout the day is important in minimizing stress on the back.

Coping Strategies

As recovery from an episode of acute low back pain and immobility progresses, the patient may resume former role-related responsibilities. However, if these activities contributed to the development of low back pain, it may be difficult to resume such responsibilities without risking chronic low back pain syndrome with associated disability and depression. The patient may need help in coping with specific stressors and in learning how to control stressful situations. Once people successfully deal with stress, they learn to give themselves positive reinforcement for their success and develop confidence in their abilities to manage other stressful situations.

Dependency is another problem associated with low back pain. Because of the immobility associated with low back pain, the patient will need to depend on others to do various tasks. Dependency may continue beyond physiological needs and become a way to fulfill psychosocial needs. Assisting both patient and support persons in recognizing extended dependency needs helps the patient to identify and cope with the real reason for continued dependency.

Referral to a back clinic or a pain clinic may be needed. These clinics use multidisciplinary approaches to help the patient with the pain and with resumption of role-related responsibilities.

Proper Body Mechanics

Prevention of recurrence of acute low back pain is a major component of nursing care. The patient must be taught how to stand, sit, lie, and lift properly. Prescribed exercises are designed to strengthen abdominal and trunk muscles, to reduce lordosis, and to reduce strain on the back. Long-term adherence to an exercise program is difficult. Improvement of posture and regular use of good body mechanics, along with regular enjoyable exercise activities such as walking, bike riding, or swimming, help to maintain a healthy back.

Patient Education and Home Health Care

Standing

- Avoid prolonged standing and walking.
- When standing for any length of time, rest one foot on a small stool or box to relieve lumbar lordosis.
- Avoid forward-flexion work positions.

Sitting

Stress on the back may be greater in the sitting position than in the standing position.

- Avoid sitting for prolonged periods.
- Sit in a straight-back chair with back well supported. Use a foot stool to position knees higher than hips if necessary.
- Eradicate the hollow of the back by sitting with the buttocks "tucked under."
- Avoid knee and hip extension. When driving a car, have the seat pushed forward as far as possible for comfort.
- Maintain back support.
- Guard against extension strains—reaching, pushing, sitting with legs straight out.
- Alternate periods of sitting with walking.

Lying

- Rest at intervals, because fatigue contributes to spasm of the back muscle.
- Place a firm bedboard under the mattress.
- Avoid sleeping in a prone position.
- When lying on the side, place a pillow under the head and one between the legs, which should be flexed at the hips and knees.
- When supine, use a pillow under the knees to decrease lordosis.

Lifting

- When lifting, keep the back straight and hold the load as close to the body as possible. Lift with the large leg muscles, not the back muscles.
- Squat down while keeping the back straight when it is necessary to pick something off the floor.
- Avoid twisting the trunk of the body, lifting above waist level, and reaching up for any length of time.

Exercise

- *Daily exercise is important in the prevention of back problems.*
- Walking outdoors with progression in distance and pace is recommended.
- Do prescribed back exercises twice daily, increasing exercises gradually.
- Avoid jumping.

Weight Control

Obesity contributes to back strain by stressing the relatively weak back muscles. Exercises are less effective and more difficult to perform. Weight reduction is based on a sound nutritional plan that includes a change in eating habits to maintain desirable weight. Monitoring weight reduction, noting achievement, and continuing encouragement facilitate adherence. Frequently, the back problems resolve as a normal weight is achieved.

▷ **Evaluation**

▷ *Expected Outcomes*

1. Patient experiences relief of pain.
   a. Rests comfortably
   b. Changes positions comfortably
   c. Obtains relief through use of physical modalities, psychological coping techniques, and medications
   d. Avoids drug dependency
2. Demonstrates resumption of self-care activities
   a. Resumes activities gradually
   b. Avoids positions that cause discomfort and muscle spasm

c. Demonstrates decreased dependence on others for self-care
3. Assumes role-related responsibilities
   a. Uses coping techniques to deal with stressful situations
   b. Resumes occupation as low back pain resolves
   c. Resumes full, productive life-style
4. Demonstrates back-conserving body mechanics
   a. Improves posture
   b. Positions self to minimize stress on the back
   c. Demonstrates use of good body mechanics
   d. Participates in exercise program
5. Achieves desired weight
   a. Identifies need to lose weight
   b. Sets realistic goals
   c. Participates in development of weight reduction plan
   d. Complies with weight reduction regimen

Osteoporosis

Osteoporosis is a disorder in which there is a reduction of total bone mass. There is a change in the normal homeostatic bone turnover; the rate of bone resorption is greater than the rate of bone formation, resulting in a reduced total bone mass. The bones become progressively porous, brittle, and fragile. They fracture easily under stresses that would not break normal bone. Osteoporosis frequently results in compression fractures (Fig. 58-3) of the thoracic and lumbar spine, fractures of the neck and intertrochanteric region of the femur, and Colles's fractures of the wrist. Multiple

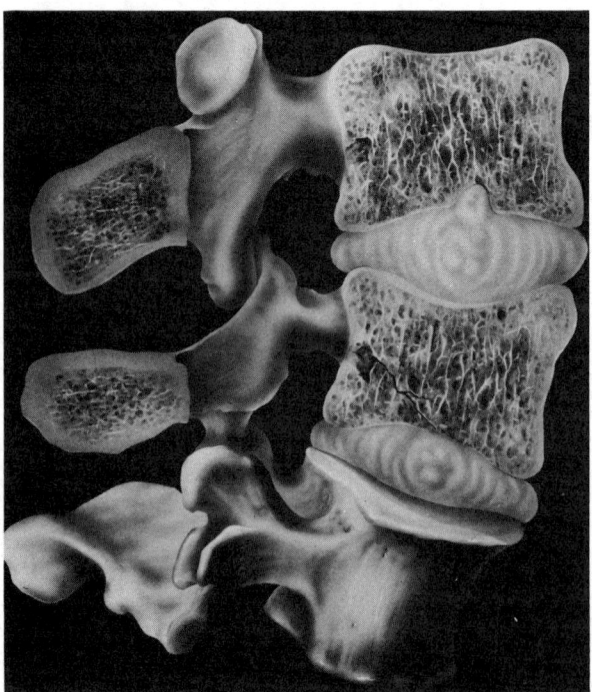

Figure 58-3
Artist's conception of progressive osteoporotic bone loss and compression fractures. (Printed with permission of Ayerst Laboratories, New York, New York.)

compression fractures of the vertebrae result in skeletal deformity (*kyphosis*).

Loss of bone mass is a universal phenomenon associated with aging. Women develop osteoporosis more frequently, earlier, and more extensively than do men. Black women, who have a greater bone mass than white women, experience less osteoporosis. Small-framed, nonobese, white women are at greatest risk for osteoporosis. More than half of all women over the age of 45 show evidence of osteoporosis on x-ray.

Gerontological Consideration

The prevalence of osteoporosis in women over age 75 is 90%. The average 75-year-old woman has lost 25% of her cortical bone and 40% of her trabecular bone. With the aging of the population, the incidence of fractures (1.3 million per year), pain, and disability associated with osteoporosis is rising.

Causes and Pathogenesis

Normal bone remodeling in the adult results in increased bone mass until about age 35. Genetics, nutrition, life-style choices, and physical activity influence the peak bone mass. Age-related loss begins soon after the peak is achieved. The withdrawal of estrogens at menopause and with oophorectomy causes an accelerated bone resorption that continues during the postmenopause years. Men do not experience sudden hormonal changes. In addition, the peak bone mass is greater in men, which contributes to their lower incidence of osteoporosis.

Endogenous (produced by the body) and *exogenous* (from an external source) catabolic agents can cause osteoporosis. Excessive corticosteroids, Cushing's syndrome, hyperthyroidism, and hyperparathyroidism contribute to bone loss. The degree of osteoporosis is related to the length of glucocorticoid therapy. When the therapy is discontinued or the metabolic problem is corrected, the progression of osteoporosis is stopped, but restoration of lost bone mass usually does not occur.

Immobility contributes to the development of osteoporosis. Bone formation is enhanced by the stress of weight and muscle activity. When immobilized by casts, paralysis, or general inactivity, the bone is resorbed faster than it is formed, and osteoporosis occurs.

Nutritional factors contribute to the development of osteoporosis. Dietary calcium and vitamin D must be adequate to maintain bone remodeling and body functions. Vitamin D is necessary for calcium absorption and for normal bone mineralization. Inadequate intake of calcium or vitamin D over a period of years results in decreased bone mass and development of osteoporosis. The recommended daily intake of calcium for an adult is 800 mg. The actual estimated average daily intake is 300 to 500 mg. To compound the situation, elderly persons absorb dietary calcium less efficiently and excrete it more readily through their kidneys. Postmenopausal women and the elderly actually need to consume about 1500 mg of calcium daily. The best source of both calcium and vitamin D is fortified milk.

Coexisting medical conditions (*e.g.,* malabsorption syndromes, lactose intolerance, alcohol abuse, renal failure, liver failure, endocrine disorders) contribute to the development of osteoporosis. Medications (*e.g.,* isoniazid, heparin, tetracycline, aluminum-containing antacids, furosemide, anticonvulsants, corticosteroids, and thyroid supplements) affect calcium utilization and metabolism.

A gradual collapse of a vertebra over a period of time may be asymptomatic and be observed as progressive kyphosis. With the development of kyphosis ("dowager's hump"), there is an associated loss of height (Fig. 58-4). Some postmenopausal women may lose 2.5 to 15 cm (1–6 inches) in height from vertebral collapse. The postural changes result in relaxation of the abdominal muscles and hence a protruding stomach. The deformity may also produce pulmonary insufficiency. Many patients complain of fatigue.

Diagnostic Evaluation

Laboratory studies (*e.g.,* serum calcium, serum phosphate, alkaline phosphatase, urine calcium excretion, urinary hydroxyproline excretion, hematocrit, erythrocyte sedimentation rate) and x-ray films may be conducted to exclude other possible medical diagnoses (*e.g.,* multiple myeloma, osteomalacia, hyperparathyroidism, malignancy) that contribute to bone loss.

Single photon absorptiometry is used to monitor bone mass of the cortical bone in the wrist. Dual photon absorptiometry and computed tomography provide information on bone mass at the spine and hip. These are useful in identifying osteoporotic bone and assessing response to therapy. Osteoporosis is identified on routine x-ray when there has been a 25% to 40% demineralization.

Management

The goals of therapy are to prevent osteoporosis, arrest or slow the process, and relieve the symptoms. Prevention begins with the identification and education of persons at risk. Adequate dietary and/or supplemental calcium, regular weight-bearing exercise, and modification of life-style, if necessary

(*e.g.,* reduced use of caffeine, cigarettes, and alcohol), help to maintain bone mass. Exercise and physical activity are the primary keys to developing high-density bones that are resistant to becoming osteoporotic. An adequate, balanced dietary intake rich in calcium and vitamin D throughout life, with an increased calcium intake beginning in the middle years, protects against skeletal demineralization. Outside activities are encouraged to enhance the body's ability to use sunlight to aid in the production of vitamin D. Elderly persons continue to need sufficient calcium, vitamin D, sunshine, and exercise to minimize the osteoporosis process.

At menopause, estrogen/progesterone replacement therapy may be given to retard bone loss and prevent occurrence of additional fractures. A woman who has had her ovaries removed or has undergone a premature menopause may develop osteoporosis at a fairly young age. Estrogen replacement is considered for this patient. Estrogens decrease bone resorption but do not increase bone mass. Estrogens are not able to diminish the rate of bone loss indefinitely, however, and are of little value in long-term care. Estrogen therapy has been associated with a slightly increased incidence of breast and endometrial cancer. Therefore, during estrogen therapy, the patient must examine her breasts monthly and have a pelvic examination, including a Papanicolaou smear and endometrial biopsy 1 to 2 times a year.

Symptoms of osteoporosis are treated as they occur. Fractures of the wrist and hip are immobilized until healing occurs. Fractures of the vertebrae are treated with bed rest, analgesics, and antispasmodics for days to weeks. Sometimes lumbosacral corsets are used for support. Physical therapy, including intermittent local heat and paraspinous muscle massage, is used for muscle relaxation.

▶ Nursing Process
The Patient With a Spontaneous Vertebral Fracture Related to Osteoporosis

▷ Assessment

Health promotion, identification of people at risk for developing osteoporosis, and recognition of problems associated with osteoporosis form the basis for nursing assessment. The interview includes questions concerning the occurrence of osteoporosis in the family, previous fractures, dietary consumption of calcium, exercise patterns, onset of menopause, and use of steroids. Any symptoms the patient is experiencing such as back pain, constipation, or altered body image are explored.

Physical examination may reveal a fracture, kyphosis of the thoracic spine, or shortened stature. Occasionally problems in mobility and breathing may exist as a result of changes in posture and weakened muscles. Constipation may be present due to inactivity.

▷ Nursing Diagnoses

Based on the assessment data, the major nursing diagnoses for the patient who experiences spontaneous vertebral fracture related to osteoporosis may include the following:

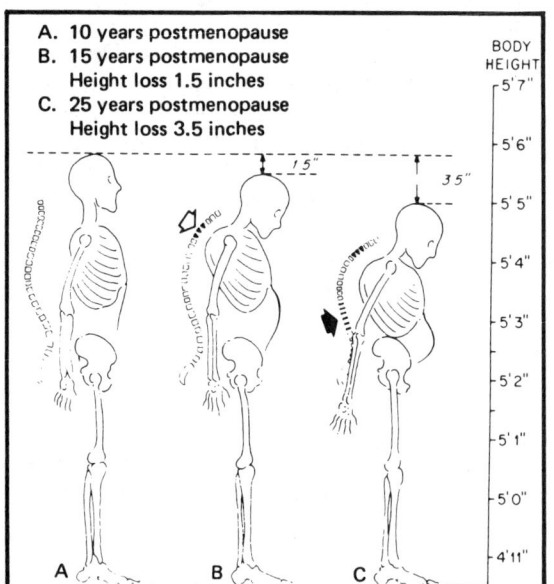

Figure 58-4
Typical loss of height associated with osteoporosis and aging. (Courtesy of Wilson Research Foundation.)

- Alteration in comfort—pain related to fracture and muscle spasm
- Alteration in bowel elimination—constipation related to immobility and/or development of ileus
- Potential for injury—additional fractures related to osteoporotic bone

▷ *Planning and Implementation*

▷ *Goals:* The major goals of the patient may include relief of pain, improved bowel elimination, and absence of additional fractures.

Nursing Interventions

Relief of Pain. Relief of back pain may be accomplished by resting in bed in a supine or side-lying position for several days to a week. The mattress should be firm and nonsagging. Knee flexion increases comfort by relaxing muscles. Intermittent local heat and back rubs afford muscle relaxation. The patient is instructed to move the trunk as a unit, avoiding twisting. Good posture is encouraged, and body mechanics are taught. When the patient is helped out of bed, a lumbosacral corset may be worn for temporary support and immobilization, although such a device is frequently uncomfortable and poorly tolerated by elderly persons. As the patient spends more time out of bed, encourage daily intermittent recumbent rest periods to relieve discomfort and the stress of abnormal posture on weakened muscles.

Oral narcotic analgesics may be needed for the first few days following the onset of back pain. After a few days, non-narcotic analgesics afford relief.

Improved Bowel Elimination. Constipation is a problem related to immobility, medications, and age. Early institution of a high-fiber diet, increased fluids, and the use of stool softeners help to prevent or minimize constipation. If the vertebral collapse involves a T10–L2 vertebra, the patient may develop an ileus. The nurse therefore monitors the patient's intake, bowel sounds, and bowel activity.

Avoiding Additional Fractures. Physical activity is essential to strengthen muscles, prevent disuse atrophy, and retard progressive bone demineralization. Daily activity, preferably outdoors in the sunshine, is necessary. Isometric exercises can be used to strengthen trunk muscles. Walking, good body mechanics, and good posture are encouraged. Sudden bending, jarring, and strenuous lifting are to be avoided.

A balanced diet with adequate calcium, protein, and vitamin D is generally prescribed to slow the rate of bone loss. This would include two or more servings of meat, chicken, or fish or protein equivalent and three glasses of skim or whole vitamin D milk daily. A calcium preparation (calcium carbonate) may be given to add sufficient calcium to the diet, as many older persons frequently suffer from a deficiency in dietary calcium.

When menopause occurs, replacement hormonal therapy slows the development of osteoporosis. Adequate supervision of the woman on hormonal therapy is necessary. This includes patient education in breast examination and regular pelvic examinations, including Pap smear and endometrial biopsy.

Gerontological Considerations. Elderly people fall frequently as a result of environmental hazards, neuromuscular disorders, diminished senses and cardiovascular responses, and responses to drugs. Hazards must be identified and eliminated. Supervision and assistance should be readily available.

The patient and family need to be included in planning for continued care and preventive management regimens. The home environment is assessed for potential hazards (*e.g.*, scatter rugs, cluttered rooms, pets underfoot) and a safe environment is created (*e.g.*, well-lighted staircases with secure hand rails, grab-bars in the bathroom, properly-fitting foot wear).

▷ *Evaluation*

▷ *Expected Outcomes*

1. Patient achieves a reduction in pain.
   a. Experiences pain relief at rest
   b. Experiences minimal discomfort during activities of daily living
   c. Demonstrates diminished tenderness at fracture site
2. Demonstrates normal bowel elimination
   a. Has active bowel sounds
   b. Has regular bowel movements
3. Experiences no new fractures
   a. Maintains good posture
   b. Uses good body mechanics
   c. Consumes balanced diet high in calcium and vitamin D
   d. Engages in weight-bearing exercises (walks daily)
   e. Rests by lying down a couple of times a day
   f. Participates in outside activities
   g. Creates a safe home environment
   h. Accepts assistance and supervision as needed

Osteomalacia

Osteomalacia is a metabolic bone disease characterized by inadequate mineralization of bone. (A similar condition in children is called *rickets.*) In these patients, a large amount of osteoid or remolded bone does not calcify. It is thought that the primary defect is a defective supply of calcium and phosphate from the extracellular fluid to the calcification sites in the bones. As a result of this faulty mineralization, there is softening and weakening of the skeleton, causing pain, tenderness to the touch, and bowing of the bones. In adults, the condition is chronic, and skeletal deformities are not as severe as in children because skeletal growth has been completed.

Pathophysiology

There are a variety of causes of osteomalacia resulting from a generalized disturbance in mineral metabolism. Risk factors for the development of osteomalacia include dietary deficiencies, malabsorption problems, gastrectomy, chronic renal failure, prolonged anticonvulsant therapy (phenytoin, phenobarbital), and insufficient vitamin D (dietary, sunlight).

Osteomalacia may occur as a result of inadequate dietary intake of calcium or phosphate ions, failure of these ions to be absorbed, or excessive loss of these materials from the body.

The malnutrition type (deficiency in vitamin D often associated with poor intake of calcium) is mainly due to poverty, but food faddism and lack of knowledge of nutrition may be factors. It occurs in parts of the world where vitamin D is not added to food and where dietary deficiencies exist and sunlight is scarce.

Gastrointestinal disorders in which fats are inadequately absorbed are likely to produce osteomalacia through loss of vitamin D (along with other fat-soluble vitamins) and calcium, the latter being excreted in the feces in combination with fatty acids. Such disorders include celiac disease, chronic biliary tract obstruction, chronic pancreatitis, and small bowel resections or operative shunts (*gastrectomy*) that involve the small intestine.

Severe renal insufficiency results in acidosis. The available calcium is used to combat the acidosis, and the parathyroid hormone continues to cause a release of skeletal calcium in an attempt to reestablish a physiologic *p*H. During this continual drain of skeletal calcium, bony fibrosis occurs and bony cysts form. Chronic glomerulonephritis, obstructive uropathies, and heavy metal poisoning result in a reduced serum phosphate level and demineralization of bone.

In addition, liver and kidney diseases can produce a lack of vitamin D, as these are the organs that convert vitamin D to its active form. Finally, hyperparathyroidism leads to skeletal decalcification, and thus to osteomalacia, through the promotion of phosphate excretion in the urine.

Gerontological Considerations. In elderly persons who are economically and socially deprived, special attention to a nutritious diet is important. Adequate intake of calcium and vitamin D needs to be assured. Since sunlight is necessary, older people should be encouraged to spend some time in the sun.

Prevention, identification, and management of osteomalacia in the elderly are essential to reduce the incidence of fractures. When osteomalacia is combined with osteoporosis, the incidence of fracture in the elderly increases.

Clinical Manifestations

The most common and distressing symptoms of osteomalacia are bone pain and tenderness. As a result of calcium deficiency, there is usually muscle weakness. The patient develops a waddling or limping gait. In the more advanced disease, the legs become bowed (due to body weight and muscle pull). The softened vertebrae become compressed, thus shortening the patient's trunk and deforming the thorax (*kyphosis*). The sacrum is forced down and forward and the pelvis is compressed laterally. These two deformities explain the characteristic shape of the pelvis that often necessitates cesarean section in pregnant women affected with this disease. Weakness and unsteadiness present a danger of falls and fractures.

Diagnostic Evaluation

On radiography, generalized demineralization of bone is evident. Studies of the vertebrae may reveal compression fracture with indistinct vertebral end plates. Laboratory studies reveal low serum calcium and phosphorus levels and a moderately elevated alkaline phosphatase level. Urine calcium and creatinine excretion is low.

Management

Osteomalacia can be treated with gratifying results on an individualized basis. The underlying cause is corrected as far as possible. Calcium intake is increased. Adequate dietary protein is provided.

Vitamin D is given in the treatment of many forms of osteomalacia. Its various therapeutic actions combine to raise the concentrations of calcium and phosphorus in the extracellular fluid and thus make these ions available for mineralization. If osteomalacia is dietary in origin, a normal diet plus vitamin D is given. If vitamin D deficiency is due to malabsorption, larger doses of vitamin D are required in addition to supplementary doses of calcium. High doses of vitamin D are toxic and enhance the risk of hypercalcemia. Therefore, the patient's serum calcium is monitored.

With malabsorption, the patient may also be treated with ultraviolet irradiation. The patient is encouraged to expose the skin to sunlight, as the ultraviolet portion of sunlight is necessary to transform a cholesterol substance (7-dehydrocholesterol) present in the skin into vitamin D.

Frequently skeletal problems associated with osteomalacia resolve themselves when the underlying disease or nutritional deficiency is adequately treated. Some persistent orthopedic deformities may need to be treated with braces or surgery (osteotomy for long bone deformity).

▶ *Nursing Process*
The Patient With Osteomalacia

▷ *Assessment*

Patients with osteomalacia usually complain of generalized bone pain in the low back and extremities, with an associated tenderness. The description of the discomfort may be vague. The patient may present with a fracture. During the interview, information concerning coexisting diseases (*e.g.*, malabsorption syndrome) and dietary habits is obtained.

On physical examination, skeletal deformities are noted. Spinal deformities and bending deformities of the long bones may give patients an unusual appearance and a waddling gait. Muscular weakness may be present. These patients may be uncomfortable with their appearance.

▷ *Nursing Diagnoses*

Based on the assessment data, the patient's major nursing diagnoses may include the following:

- Alteration in comfort—pain related to bone tenderness and potential fracture
- Disturbance in self-concept—body image related to bowing legs and waddling gait
- Potential nonadherence to therapeutic regimen related to lack of information and understanding

▷ *Planning and Implementation*

▷ *Goals:* The major goals of the patient with osteomalacia may include relief of pain, acceptance of body image, and adherence to the therapeutic regimen.

Nursing Interventions

Relieving Pain. Physical, psychological, and pharmaceutical measures are used to help the patient reduce discomfort. Since the patient has both skeletal pain and tenderness, gentle assistance needs to be provided when changing positions. Frequent position changes will decrease the discomforts from immobility. A convoluted foam mattress and soft pillows will support the body and conform to existing deformities. Diversional activities and focusing attention on conversation, television, and other such distractions will decrease the patient's perception of pain. At times, analgesics will be needed as prescribed to decrease the discomfort. The patient's response to the medications is monitored.

As the condition responds to the therapy, the skeletal discomforts will diminish.

Body Image Adjustment. In an established, trusting relationship, the patient is encouraged to discuss any change in body image and methods for coping with the changes. Accept the patient's self-concept, but help the patient recognize and use existing strengths. The patient is included in planning of care. Being an active participant promotes self-control and improves feelings of self-worth. Interactions with family and friends are encouraged. Social interactions help provide a feeling of being accepted regardless of physical changes.

Patient Education and Home Health Care. Patient education focuses on the cause of osteomalacia and approaches to controlling it. Dietary sources of calcium and vitamin D are taught. Safe use of supplements is reviewed. The need for monitoring of serum calcium levels for therapeutic response is stressed. Measures to prevent injury are discussed with the patient. Long-term monitoring of the patient is appropriate to ensure stabilization or reversal of the osteomalacia process.

▷ ## Evaluation

▷ ### Expected Outcomes

1. Relief of pain and tenderness
   a. Patient reports feeling comfortable.
   b. Experiences no tenderness
   c. Does not experience fracture
2. Shows improved self-concept
   a. Participates in activities of daily living
   b. Demonstrates confidence in abilities
3. Adheres to therapeutic regimen
   a. Consumes therapeutic amount of calcium and vitamin D
   b. Exposes self to sunlight
   c. Has serum calcium level monitored throughout therapy
   d. Keeps follow-up health care appointments

Paget's Disease

Paget's disease (osteitis deformans) is a disorder of increased bone remodeling. A primary proliferation of osteoclasts produces bone resorption followed by a compensatory increase in osteoblastic activity that repairs the bone resorbed. The bone formed is high in mineral content but poorly constructed. This abnormal bone remodeling causes distortion of normal bone anatomy (*i.e.*, enlarged and deformed bones with increasing vascularity). As a result, the structurally weak bone fractures. As the bone turnover continues, a classic mosaic pattern of bone matrix develops. The condition affects single bones, most commonly the lumbosacral vertebrae, skull, pelvic bones, femur, and tibia.

The disease occurs slightly more often in men than in women. The incidence rises with age and is found in 3% to 4% of the population over age 40, increasing to 10% to 15% in the elderly. In 15% to 20% of the cases, a family history has been noted, with sisters and brothers developing the disease. Although a variety of causes have been proposed, a slow virus (not isolated as yet) is currently thought to be the most likely cause.

Clinical Manifestations

The disease is insidious. Most patients with the disease never know they have it. Some patients are asymptomatic but have skeletal deformity. A few patients have symptomatic problems. The condition is most frequently identified when x-rays have been done at a routine physical examination or in the course of workup for another problem. There are sclerotic changes, skeletal deformities (*e.g.*, bowing of femur and tibia, kyphosis, enlargement of the skull) and cortical thickening of the long bones. Bone scans may detect the disease quite early.

In the majority of patients, skeletal deformity involves the skull or long bones. The skull may be thickened and the patient may complain that a hat no longer fits. In well-marked cases of Paget's disease, the cranium is much enlarged, but not the face, which therefore appears small and triangular in shape. Most patients with skull involvement have impaired hearing. Cranial nerve dysfunction may occur due to compression of the nerves. Occasionally, an obstructive hydrocephalus may occur.

The femurs and tibiae tend to bow, producing a waddling gait. The spine is bent foward and is rigid; the chin rests on the chest. The thorax is compressed and immobile on respiration. The trunk is flexed on the legs to maintain equilibrium; the arms, which are bent outward and forward and appear long in relation to the shortened trunk, give the patient an apelike appearance. As a result of the kyphosis and the bowing of the legs, the patient's height may be reduced as much as 30 cm (12 inches).

Pain and tenderness on pressure may be noted in the bones. Such pain, which may be wrongly attributed to old age or arthritis by the patient, may precede the skeletal changes by years. The pain is a mild to moderate, deep, aching pain that increases with weight-bearing if the lower extremities are involved.

There is an increase in skin temperature overlying the bone due to increased vascularity of the bone. Patients with very large, highly vascular lesions may develop a high-output cardiac failure because of the increased vascular bed and metabolic demands.

Diagnostic Evaluation

The serum alkaline phosphatase and the level of urinary hydroxyproline excretion are usually increased, reflecting increased osteoblastic activity. The higher these values, the more active the disease.

Hypercalcemia, hypercalciuria, and nephrolithiasis may occur following fracture and immobilization. Malignant degeneration and osteosarcomas are seen in some patients with Paget's disease.

Management

Usually, no particular treatment is recommended in the patient without symptoms. Pain usually responds to nonsteroidal anti-inflammatory drugs.

Patients with a moderate to severe form of the disease may benefit from suppressive therapy. These patients have severe pain, neurological deficits, or extensive skeletal involvement. At the present time, there are several agents that are potent inhibitors of bone resorption and under certain conditions may permit replacement of diseased bone with normal lamellar bone.

Calcitonin therapy can result in remodeling of the abnormal pagetoid bone into normal lamellar bone. Calcitonin, a polypeptide hormone, retards bone resorption by decreasing the number and availability of osteoclasts. It is used to relieve bone pain and helps alleviate neurologic and biochemical complications. Calcitonin is given subcutaneously. Flushing of the face and nausea are side-effects. These tend to decrease with time or can be managed by taking the drug before bedtime or concurrently with an antihistamine. Treatment lasts for about 3 months.

Disodium etidronate (EHDP), a diphosphonate compound, produces rapid reduction in bone turnover and relief of pain. It also reduces elevated serum alkaline phosphatase and urinary hydroxyproline levels. Food inhibits absorption. Nausea, cramping, and diarrhea may occur and can be alleviated by spacing the doses. Large doses may inhibit fracture healing and may contribute to osteomalacia. Calcitonin and EHDP may be combined and given to patients with very active disease.

Plicamycin (Mithracin), a cytotoxic antibiotic, may be used to control the disease. It is a toxic drug and is reserved for severely affected patients with neurological compromise or for patients who are resistant to other measures. This drug has dramatic effects on pain reduction and on the serum calcium, alkaline phosphatase, and urinary hydroxyproline levels. It is given by intravenous infusion and requires that hepatic, renal, and bone marrow function be monitored during therapy. Clinical remissions may continue for months after the drug is discontinued.

Fractures are managed according to location. Healing does occur if reduction, immobilization, and stability are adequate. Nonunion of a femoral neck fracture requires treatment with an endoprosthesis.

Loss of hearing is managed with hearing aids and communication techniques used with the hearing-impaired person (*e.g.*, lip reading, body language).

Gerontological Considerations

Careful assessment of the patient's complaint of discomfort is necessary. Frequently, elderly persons have discomfort associated with arthritis that may be accentuated by the bone deformities. Also, pain may indicate an impending fracture. The home environment needs to be assessed for safety. Pa-

tient education is needed to help compensate for altered neurologic functioning, thereby preventing falls and reducing the incidence of fracture. Additionally, education concerning medications helps to ensure adherence, reduces side-effects, and prevents adverse reactions.

Musculoskeletal Infections

Osteomyelitis

Osteomyelitis is an infection of the bone. This infection is more difficult to cure than a soft-tissue infection because of the limited blood supply. Osteomyelitis may be a chronic problem affecting quality of life and/or loss of extremity.

The infection may be due to *hematogenous* (blood-borne) spread from other foci of infection (*e.g.*, infected tonsils, boils, infected teeth, upper respiratory infections), erosion of adjacent soft tissue infection (*e.g.*, middle ear infection, infected decubitus or vascular ulcers), or direct bone contamination (*e.g.*, open fracture, gunshot wound, bone surgery). Acute osteomyelitis due to hematogenous spread is seen more frequently in children than in adults. Chronic osteomyelitis is seen more frequently in adults. *Staphylococcus aureus* causes 70% to 80% of bone infections. Other pathogenic organisms frequently found in osteomyelitis include *Proteus, Pseudomonas,* and *Escherichia coli.* There has been an increasing incidence of penicillin-resistant, nosocomial, gram-negative, and anaerobic infections.

Pathophysiology

Osteomyelitis due to hematogenous spread occurs in a bone area where there is lowered resistance, possibly due to subclinical (nonapparent) trauma. It often develops in the long bones of children and vertebrae of adults. Regardless of the source of the infective microbe, the initial response is one of inflammation, increased vascularity, and edema. After 2 or 3 days, thrombosis of the blood vessels occurs in the area and results in ischemia with bone necrosis due to increasing tissue and medullary pressure. The infection extends into the medullary cavity and under the periosteum. Infective pus may spread the infection into adjacent soft tissues and joints. Unless the infective process is controlled early, bone abscess forms.

In the natural course of events, the abscess may point and drain but, more often, incision and drainage are done by the surgeon. The resulting abscess cavity has in its walls areas of dead tissue, as in any abscess cavity; however, dead bone tissue (the *sequestrum*) does not easily liquefy and drain. The cavity cannot collapse and heal as occurs in soft-tissue abscesses. A bone sheath (the *involucrum*) forms and surrounds the sequestrum. Thus, although healing appears to take place, a chronically-infected sequestrum remains that is prone to producing recurring abscesses throughout the life of the individual. This is the so-called *chronic* type of osteomyelitis.

Osteomyelitis may be associated with extension of soft-tissue infection or direct bone contamination. Identification of patients who are at risk is essential. These include poorly nourished, elderly, obese, or diabetic patients, and patients who have rheumatoid arthritis, have been hospitalized for a long time, have required long-term corticosteroid therapy, have had surgery on a joint previously operated on, or have a concurrent sepsis. Other patients at risk are those who have undergone lengthy orthopedic surgery, have prolonged wound drainage, have marginal incisional necrosis or wound dehiscence, or require evacuation of postoperative hematomas.

The onset of an osteomyelitis following orthopedic surgery may occur during the first 3 months (*acute fulminating—stage 1*) and is frequently associated with hematoma drainage or superficial infection. *Delayed onset* (*stage 2*) infections are seen between 4 and 24 months after surgery. *Late onset* (*stage 3*) osteomyelitis is generally due to hematogenous spread and occurs 2 or more years after surgery.

Clinical Manifestations

When the infection is carried by the blood, the onset is usually sudden, occurring often with the symptomatology of septicemia (*e.g.*, chills, high fever, rapid pulse, and general malaise). In children, in whom the disease usually begins as an acute infection of the bone epiphysis (*epiphysitis*), the constitutional symptoms at first may overshadow the local signs completely. As the infection extends from the marrow cavity through the cortex of the bone, it involves the periosteum and the soft tissues, with the extremity becoming painful, swollen, and extremely tender. The patient may describe a constant, pulsating pain that intensifies with movement and is due to the pressure of the collecting pus.

When osteomyelitis occurs from spread of adjacent infection or direct contamination, there is no septicemia symptomatology. The area is swollen, warm, painful, and tender to touch.

Diagnostic Evaluation

With acute osteomyelitis, early x-rays will show only soft-tissue swelling. In about 2 weeks, areas of irregular decalcification, periosteal elevation, and new bone formation will be evident. Blood studies will show elevated leukocytes and an elevated sedimentation rate. Blood cultures and cultures of the abscess are needed for proper antibiotic therapy.

The patient with a chronic osteomyelitis presents with a continuously draining sinus or experiences recurrent periods of pain, inflammation, swelling, and drainage. The low-grade infection thrives in the scar tissue with its reduced blood supply. On x-ray, large, irregular cavities, sequestra, or dense bone formations are seen.

Prevention

Prevention of osteomyelitis is the goal. Treatment of focal infections diminishes hematogenous spread. Management of soft-tissue infections controls erosion to the bone. Careful patient selection and attention to the surgical environment and technique can reduce the incidence of postoperative osteomyelitis.

Prophylactic antibiotics, administered to achieve adequate tissue levels at the time of surgery and for 24 to 48 hours after surgery, are helpful. Aseptic postoperative wound care techniques reduce the incidence of superficial infections and the potential development of an associated osteomyelitis.

Management

The initial goal of therapy is to control and arrest the infective process. Blood cultures and abscess fluid smears and cultures are done to identify the organism and select the best antibiotic. Frequently, the infection is caused by more than one pathogen.

Drug Therapy. Cultures of other loci of infection may be done if hematogenous spread is suspected. Antibiotic therapy is begun immediately, assuming a *Staphylococcus* infection is present that is sensitive to a semisynthetic penicillin. Nafcillin, methicillin, cephalothin, cefazolin, and similar drugs are used parenterally. A sustained high therapeutic blood level of the antibiotic is important. (A bacteriocidal serum level of at least 1 to 8 is desired.) Around-the-clock dosage administration is necessary for 4 to 6 weeks. The aim is to control the infection before the blood supply to the infection diminishes as a result of thrombosis. If necessary, when culture results are obtained, the antibiotic can be replaced by one to which the organism is more sensitive. When the infection appears to be controlled, the antibiotic can be administered orally and so continued for up to 3 months. To enhance absorption of oral antibiotics, these medications should not be administered with food. Suspected regions of pus may be evacuated by needle aspiration.

Surgery. If the patient does not respond to treatment, surgery is carried out whereby the involved bone is exposed, the purulent and necrotic material removed, and the area irrigated directly with sterile physiologic saline solution. A high blood level of antibiotic is maintained.

In chronic osteomyelitis, antibiotics control the infection. Generally it is an adjunctive therapy to surgical débridement. All dead, infected bone and cartilage must be removed before permanent healing takes place. This operation, which is called a *sequestrectomy*, consists of the removal of enough involucrum to enable the surgeon to remove the sequestrum. Often, sufficient bone is removed to convert a deep cavity into a shallow saucer (*saucerization*).

The wound is either closed tightly to obliterate the dead space or packed to be closed later by granulation or possibly by grafting. A closed suction irrigation system may be used to control the hematoma and remove debris. Physiologic saline solution is usually used for 7 to 8 days. The development of superimposed infection may occur with prolonged irrigation.

Saucerization weakens the bone, which then may need stabilization or support from internal or external fixation devices. The débrided cavity may be packed with cancellous bone graft to stimulate healing. With a very large defect, the cavity may be filled with a vascularized bone transfer or *muscle flap* (in which a muscle is moved from an adjacent area with blood supply intact). These microsurgery techniques enhance the blood supply, which facilitates bone healing and eradication of the infection. These surgical procedures may be staged over a period of time to ensure healing. During the postoperative period, measures are taken to ensure adequate circulation (wound suction to prevent fluid accumulation, elevation of the area to promote venous drainage, avoidance of pressure on grafted area), to maintain needed immobility, and to comply with weight-bearing restrictions.

▶ *Nursing Process*
The Patient With Osteomyelitis

▷ *Assessment*

The patient presents with an acute onset of symptoms (*e.g.*, localized pain, swelling, erythema, fever) or recurrent draining of an infected sinus with associated pain, swelling, and low-grade fever. The patient is assessed for risk factors (*e.g.*, older age, diabetes, or long-term steroid therapy) and for previous injury, infection, or orthopedic surgery. The patient will avoid pressure on the area and guard movement. In acute osteomyelitis, the patient will have generalized weakness due to the systemic reaction to the infection.

Physical examination reveals an inflamed, markedly swollen, warm area that is tender. Purulent drainage may be noted. The patient will have an elevated temperature. With chronic osteomyelitis, the temperature elevation may be only minimal, occurring in the afternoon or evening.

Laboratory studies will show an elevated white blood cell count and usually an elevated erythrocyte sedimentation rate. Blood and drainage cultures may be positive. Wound cultures will indicate the causative organisms and sensitivity to various antibiotics. X-rays may be negative until destruction, bone necrosis, and elevation of the periosteum occur.

▷ *Nursing Diagnoses*

Based on the nursing assessment data, the nursing diagnoses for the patient with osteomyelitis may include the following:

- Alteration in comfort—pain related to inflammation and swelling
- Impaired physical mobility associated with positioning, immobilization devices, and weight-bearing limitations
- Knowledge deficit of the home health care program

▷ *Planning and Implementation*

▷ *Goals:* The goals of the patient may include relief of pain, adaptation to mobility limitations, and adherence to the home health care program.

Nursing Interventions

Relieving Pain. The wounds themselves are frequently very painful and must be handled with great care and gentleness. The joints above and below the affected part should be supported and the extremity moved in a smooth manner. The affected part may be immobilized with a splint until the wound has healed. Immobilization decreases pain and muscle spasm.

Elevation reduces swelling and associated discomfort. Warm saline soaks for 20 minutes several times a day may be used to increase circulation to the area. The neurovascular status of the affected extremity is monitored. Techniques for reducing pain perception and pain medications may be useful.

Adapting to Mobility Limitations. Treatment regimens tend to be very restrictive. The patient needs to be taught the rationale for the various therapies and activity restrictions. Full participation within physical limitations is encouraged to promote general well-being.

Patient Education and Home Health Care. Management of osteomyelitis frequently requires wound care and intravenous antibiotic therapy in the home. It is important that the patient and family members understand the antibiotic protocol. Proper education prior to discharge from the hospital and adequate supervision and support systems are important for successful home management of osteomyelitis. The patient must be medically stable and motivated, and the family must be supportive. The home environment needs to be conducive to promotion of health and compliance with the therapeutic regimen.

These patients need to be monitored carefully for the development of additional painful areas or sudden rises in temperature. The patient is instructed to observe for drainage, odor, and increased inflammation. These signs may indicate the extension of the infection or a secondary infection. The wound should be redressed and warm soaks continued.

The general health and nutrition of the patient are monitored and enhanced. Fluids and a balanced diet high in protein, vitamin C, and vitamin D are desired to ensure a positive nitrogen balance and to promote healing.

▷ *Evaluation*

▷ *Expected Outcomes*

1. Patient experiences relief of pain.
   a. Does not complain of pain
   b. Experiences no tenderness in area of previous infection
   c. Experiences no discomfort with movement
2. Functions within prescribed mobility limitations
   a. Participates in self-care activities
   b. Maintains full function of unimpaired extremities
   c. Demonstrates safe use of adaptive and immobility devices
3. Conveys an understanding of the health care program
   a. Takes medications as prescribed
   b. Demonstrates proper wound care
   c. Reports problems promptly
   d. Eats a balanced diet
   e. Keeps follow-up health appointments
   f. Reports increased strength
   g. Reports no elevation of temperature or recurrence of pain, swelling, or other symptoms at the site

Septic (Infectious) Arthritis

Joints can become infected by spread of infection from other parts of the body (*hematogenous spread*) or directly by trauma or surgical instruments. Previous trauma to joints, co-existing arthritis, and diminished host resistance contribute to the development of an infected joint. Gonococci and staphylococci cause most adult joint infections. Prompt recognition and treatment of an infected joint are important because accumulating pus results in *chondrolysis* (destruction of hyaline cartilage), which heals poorly.

Clinical Manifestations. The patient with an acute septic arthritis usually presents with a warm, painful, swollen joint with decreased range of motion. Systemic chills and fever may be present. Assessment for a primary locus of infection (*e.g.*, a carbuncle) should be done. Elderly patients and persons taking corticosteroids or immunosuppressive drugs demonstrate decreased reaction to the infection.

Diagnostic Evaluation. Diagnostic studies include aspiration, examination, and culture of the synovial fluid. Arthrograms may reveal damage to the joint lining. Radioisotope scanning is useful in localizing the process and distinguishing between a joint infection and an overlying cellulitis.

Management. Prompt treatment is essential. Antibiotics, such as nafcillin, cephalosporin, and gentamicin, should be started promptly by intravenous infusion. Penicillin G is used for gonococcal septic arthritis. The parenteral antibiotics are continued until symptoms disappear. Additionally, the synovial fluid is monitored for sterility and decrease in white blood cells.

In addition to prescribing antibiotics, the physician will drain the excessive joint fluid by needle aspiration to remove fluid, exudate, and debris. Occasionally, arthrotomy or arthroscopy is used to drain the joint and to remove dead tissue. The inflamed joint should be supported and put at rest. A splint to immobilize the joint increases the patient's comfort. Codeine may be used to control pain. Nonsteroidal anti-inflammatory drugs may be prescribed after the infection has responded to the antibiotic. Range-of-motion and active exercises are started gradually when the infection subsides. The patient's fluids and nutrition are monitored to promote healing. If septic joints are treated early, recovery of normal function should occur.

The patient is assessed periodically for recurrence. If the articular cartilage was damaged during the inflammatory reaction, joint fibrosis and diminished function may develop.

Bone Tumors

Neoplasms of the musculoskeletal system are of a variety of types. They include osteogenic, chondrogenic, fibrogenic, muscle (rhabdomyogenic), and marrow (reticulum) cell tumors as well as nerve, vascular, and fatty cell tumors. They may be primary or metastatic carcinomas from primary cancers elsewhere in the body (*e.g.*, breast, lung, prostate, kidney). Metastatic bone tumors occur more frequently in older patients.

Benign primary neoplasms of the musculoskeletal system include osteoma, aneurysmal bone cyst, osteoid osteoma, chondroma, osteochondroma, rhabdomyoma, and fibroma. Malignant primary musculoskeletal tumors include osteosarcoma, fibrosarcoma, chondrosarcoma, Ewing's sarcoma, multiple myeloma, rhabdomyosarcoma, and fibrosarcoma. Giant cell tumor (osteoclastoma) is benign for long periods of time; it may invade local tissue, but distant metastasis is not common. Sarcomas originate in connective and supportive tissue.

The presence of a tumor in the bone causes the normal bone tissue to react by *osteolytic* response (bone destruction) or by *osteoblastic* response (bone formation). Some of the bone tumors are common and some are exceedingly rare. Some present no problem, while others rapidly become life-threatening. Some benign tumors have the potential of undergoing malignant transformation.

Clinical Manifestations. Patients with a bone tumor present with a wide range of associated problems. They may be asymptomatic or may have pain (mild and occasional to constant and severe); varying degrees of disability; and, at times, obvious bone growth. Weight loss, malaise, and fever may be present. The tumor may be diagnosed incidentally following pathologic fracture.

Differential diagnosis is based on the history, physical examination, x-rays (including tomograms, bone scans, and arteriography), biochemical assays of the blood and urine (alkaline phosphatase is frequently elevated), and, finally, surgical biopsy for histologic identification (Fig. 58-5). Extreme care is taken during biopsy to prevent seeding and recurrence following excision of the tumor. Radiological studies of the chest are done to determine the presence of lung metastasis. Staging is based on tumor size, grade, and location as well as on metastasis. The treatment regimen is based on findings. The nurse provides support during this diagnostic period.

Management. Management of bone tumors includes surgical excision (ranging from local excision to amputation and disarticulation), radiation when the tumor is radiosensitive, and chemotherapy. Major gains are being made in using wide block excision with restorative grafting technique and chemotherapeutics (preoperative, postoperative, and adjunctive for possible micrometastasis). Survival and quality of life are important considerations in procedures that attempt to save the involved extremity.

Benign Bone Tumors

Benign bone tumors generally are slow-growing and well-circumscribed, present few symptoms, and are not a cause of death.

Osteochondroma is the most common benign bone tumor, and usually occurs as a large projection of bone at the end of long bones (at the knee or shoulder). It develops during growth and then becomes a static bony mass. The cartilage cap of the osteochondroma may undergo malignant transformation following trauma, and a chondrosarcoma may develop.

Echondroma is a common tumor of the hyaline cartilage that develops during the growing years in the hand, ribs, femur, tibia, humerus, or pelvis. Generally, the only symptom is a mild ache. Pathologic fractures may occur.

A painful tumor that occurs in children and young adults is the *osteoid osteoma*. The neoplastic tissue is surrounded by reactive bone formation that assists in its radiologic identification.

Bone cysts are expanding lesions within the bone. *Aneurysmal bone cysts* are seen in young adults, and present with a painful, palpable mass of the long bones, vertebrae, or flat bones. *Unicameral bone cysts* occur in children and cause mild discomfort and possible pathologic fractures of the upper humerus and femur. These may heal spontaneously.

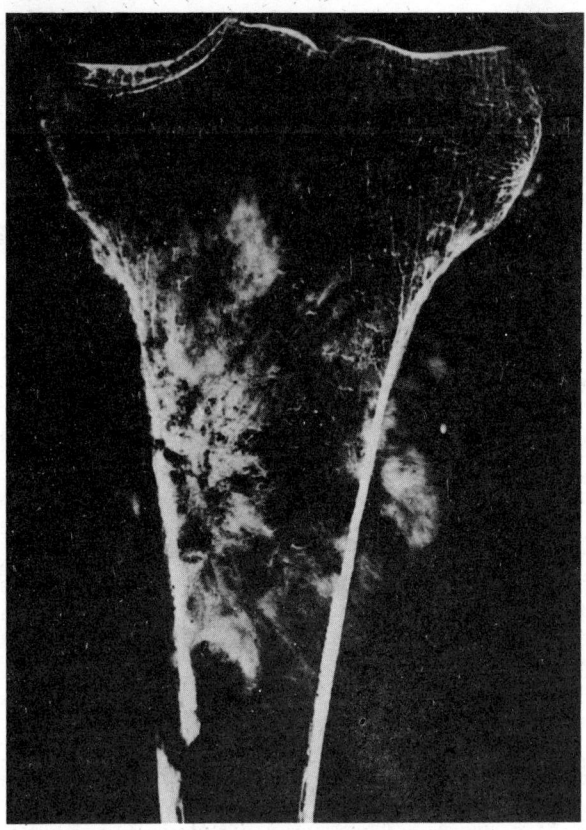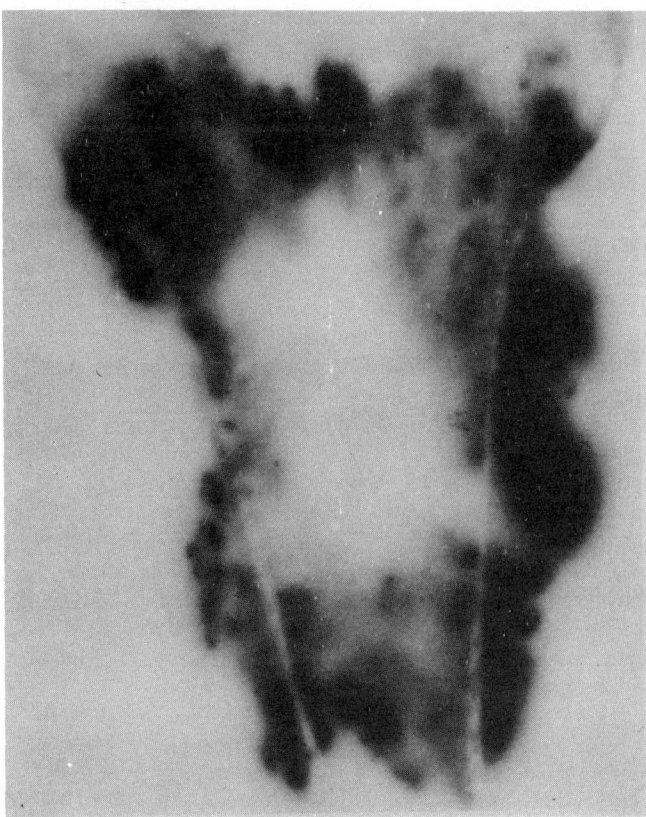

Figure 58-5
Bone scan of a patient with osteosarcoma. (*Left*) X-ray showing osteosarcoma at the proximal end of the tibia. Note the destruction of the normal anatomy of the bone. (*Right*) Contact autoradiograph of the same patient. The patient has received ^{85}Sr intravenously for bone scanning. Note the high uptake (*black areas*) in the peripheral growing margin and the relative lack of uptake centrally. (Armed Forces Institute of Pathology. Negative numbers 67-4-8, 67-4-9.)

Management

The general therapeutic approach to benign bone tumors is to excise completely the tumor tissue and restore the bone continuity with bone grafts. The excised area may be packed with ilium chips to stimulate healing.

Nursing Interventions

The nursing care of a patient who has undergone excision of a bone tumor is similar in many aspects to that for other patients who have skeletal surgery. The operative part should be elevated to control swelling; the neurovascular status of the extremity should be assessed. Generally, the area is immobilized by splints, casts, or elastic bandages until the bone heals. The fluid and electrolyte balance of the patient is monitored. A diet high in protein, with adequate vitamins (especially vitamins C and D) and calcium, is encouraged.

Pain is present both at the surgical and the graft donor sites. Narcotics are prescribed during the early postoperative period. Later, oral, nonnarcotic analgesics are adequate to control discomfort.

Postexcision complications include those associated with immobility, blood loss, and infection. Osteomyelitis is a concern. Prophylactic antibiotics and strict aseptic dressing techniques are used to diminish the occurrence of this dreaded complication. During healing, other infections (*e.g.,* colds) need to be avoided so that hematogenous spread does not result in an osteomyelitis.

Depending on the site of excision, the use of ambulatory aids may be required. An exercise program is designed to restore function. Active participation in exercises and other rehabilitative activities is encouraged.

As the patient prepares to leave the hospital, the nurse provides education concerning continuing care and the medication and exercise regimens. The nurse also encourages needed follow-up medical visits.

Malignant Bone Tumors

Primary malignant bone tumors arise from bone tissue cells (*sarcomas*) or bone marrow elements (*myelomas*). Bone metastasis to the lungs is common. Secondary bone tumors (*carcinomas*) are due to metastasis from breast, prostate, kidney, thyroid, or lung cancers.

Osteogenic Sarcoma. *Osteogenic sarcoma* (osteosarcoma) is the most common and most often fatal primary malignant bone tumor. It is characterized by early hematogenous metastasis to the lungs. The tumor carries a high mortality rate because the sarcoma often has spread to the lungs by the time the patient seeks help.

Osteogenic sarcoma appears most frequently in males in the age group between 10 and 25 and in older persons with Paget's disease or as a sequela of ionizing radiation. It is manifested by pain, swelling, limitation of motion, and weight loss (which is considered an ominous finding). The bony mass may be palpable, tender, and fixed, with an increase in skin temperature over the mass and venous distention. The primary lesion may involve any bone; the most common sites are the distal femur, the proximal tibia, and the proximal humerus.

Chondrosarcoma. Malignant tumors of the hyaline cartilage are called *chondrosarcomas* and are the second most common primary malignant bone tumor. They are large, bulky, slow-growing tumors that affect adults (men more frequently than women). The usual tumor sites include the pelvis, ribs, femur, humerus, spine, scapula, and tibia. Metastasis to the lungs occurs in fewer than half the patients. If these tumors are well differentiated, large block excision or amputation of the affected extremity results in a good survival rate. These tumors may recur.

Giant cell tumors are benign for long periods of time but may invade local tissue and cause destruction. They occur in young adults and are soft and hemorrhagic. Eventually giant cell tumors become malignant and metastasize.

Management

The goal of management is to destroy or remove malignant tissue by the most effective method possible. This requires a multidisciplinary approach, possibly in a cancer treatment center.

Surgical removal of the tumor frequently requires amputation of the affected extremity, with the line of amputation extending through the bone or joint above the bone tumor in order to achieve local control of the primary lesion. (See nursing management of the patient following an amputation, p. 1604.)

Limb-sparing (salvage) procedures remove the tumor and adjacent tissue. The resected portion is replaced by a custom prosthesis, total joint arthroplasty, or bone tissue from the patient or cadaver donor. Soft tissue and blood vessels may need grafting because of the extent of the excision. Complications that may develop include infection, loosening or dislocation of the prosthesis, allograft nonunion, fracture, devitalization of the skin and soft tissues, joint fibrosis, and recurrence of the tumor. Function and rehabilitation following limb salvage depend on reducing the risk of complications and positive encouragement.

Because of the real danger of metastasis with these tumors, combined chemotherapy is started before and continued after surgery in an effort to eradicate micrometastatic lesions. The hope is that combined chemotherapy will have a greater effect at a lower toxicity rate, while reducing resistance to the drugs. There is an improved (60%) long-term survival rate when a localized osteosarcoma is removed and chemotherapy (doxorubicin hydrochloride and cisplatin or methotrexate) is initiated.

Soft-tissue sarcomas are treated with radiation, limb-sparing excision, and adjuvant chemotherapy.

▶ Nursing Process
The Patient With a Primary
Malignant Bone Tumor

▷ Assessment

The patient is encouraged to discuss the problem, and the onset and course of symptoms. During the interview, the nurse notes how the patient and family have been coping with the problem and how the patient has managed the pain. Support during diagnostic studies and therapy is a major nursing concern.

On physical examination, the nurse needs to palpate the mass gently, noting size and associated soft-tissue swelling, pain, and tenderness. Assessment of the neurovascular status and range of motion of the extremity provides baseline data for future comparisons. The patient's mobility and ability to perform activities of daily living are evaluated.

▷ Nursing Diagnoses

Based on the nursing assessment data, the major nursing diagnoses for the patient with a primary malignant bone tumor may include the following:

- Alteration in comfort—pain related to tumor
- Potential for injury—pathological fracture related to tumor and complications of therapy
- Knowledge deficit concerning the therapeutic regimen
- Potential ineffective coping related to perception of disease process and impact on life-style
- Disturbance in self-concept related to loss of body part or role performance
- Potential impaired home management related to alteration in functional abilities and treatment regimen

▷ Planning and Implementation

▷ *Goals:* The patient's goals may include relief of pain, avoidance of injury from fracture or complication of therapy (surgery, chemotherapy, radiation therapy), active participation in the therapeutic regimen, demonstration of effective coping, improvement of self-concept, and demonstration of effective health care at home.

Nursing Interventions

Relieving Pain. Psychological, pharmaceutical, and environmental pain management techniques are useful. The nurse needs to work with the patient in designing the most effective pain management regimen, thereby increasing the patient's control over the pain. The nurse prepares the patient and gives support during painful procedures.

Avoiding Complications.   Assistance is given with position changes and ambulation to prevent stress on the weakened bones. The patient is taught how to use aids safely and how to strengthen unaffected extremities.

The patient is informed of the possible side-effects of the chemotherapeutic drugs. Antiemetics and relaxation techniques reduce the gastrointestinal reaction. Stomatitis is controlled with anesthetic and antifungal mouthwashes. Alopecia is temporary, and hair growth usually resumes after the chemotherapy is discontinued. The patient is taught to avoid persons with colds and infections when the patient's white blood cell count is low. Adequate hydration is essential. With nephrotoxic drugs, diuretics may be prescribed to increase excretion. Specific drugs may be toxic to specific organs (*e.g.*, kidneys, heart, lungs, ears). Laboratory values are monitored to detect abnormalities that may necessitate a change in the treatment regimen. Monitor the functioning of the organs potentially affected.

Additionally, vital signs are watched and other observations are made to assess for the development of complications: thrombophlebitis, pulmonary emboli, infection, contracture, and disuse atrophy.

Patient Education and Home Health Care. Patient and family education is essential. The patient and the family will want to know about the disease process and its diagnostic and management regimens. Cooperation and adherence are based on this understanding. The nurse can most effectively reinforce and clarify information provided by the physician by being present during these physician–patient discussions. Explanation of diagnostic tests, treatments (*e.g.*, wound care), and expected results (*e.g.*, decreased range of motion, numbness, change in body contours) helps the patient deal with the procedures and changes that occur. Include the patient in an assessment of responses to the treatment regimen and scheduling of care. This will increase the patient's understanding of the care.

Preparation for and coordination of continuing health care are begun early as a multidisciplinary effort. Patient education is directed at medication, dressing, and treatment regimens, as well as physical and occupational therapy programs. The safe use of special equipment is taught. The patient and family learn the signs and symptoms of possible complications. The patient is advised to have the phone numbers of persons to contact readily available in case problems arise. Frequently, arrangements are made with a home health care agency for home care supervision. Follow-up appointments are scheduled. Emphasize the need for long-term health supervision to ensure cure or to detect tumor recurrence or metastasis.

Effective Coping. The patient and family must be encouraged to express their feelings honestly. They need to be supported and feel accepted as they come to grips with the impact of the malignant bone tumor. Feelings of shock, despair, and grief are expected. Referral for specific psychological help may be appropriate.

Improved Self-Concept. Independence versus dependence is an issue with the patient who has a malignancy. Lifestyle is dramatically changed, at least temporarily. The family is supported in working through the adjustments that must be made. Changes in body image due to surgery and possibly amputation need to be recognized. Stress the importance of achieving tumor cure, even if it involves a change in body image. Be realistically reassuring about the future and about

resumption of role-related activities. Encourage self-care and socialization. The patient should help plan daily activities. Involvement of the patient and family throughout the treatment process promotes confidence, restoration of self-concept, and a sense of being in control of one's life.

▷ *Evaluation*

▷ *Expected Outcomes*

1. Patient achieves relief of pain.
    a. Experiences no pain at rest, during activities, or at surgical sites
    b. Participates comfortably in activities of daily living
2. Experiences no pathological fracture or injury from therapies
    a. Avoids stress to weakened bones
    b. Manages side-effects of therapies
    c. Reports symptoms of drug toxicity or complications of surgery
    d. Avoids contact with people with colds and infections when white blood cell count is suppressed
3. Demonstrates an understanding of the treatment regimen
    a. Describes problem and management plan
    b. Seeks clarification of information
    c. Participates in self-care activities
4. Demonstrates effective coping
    a. Verbalizes feelings
    b. Identifies strengths and abilities
    c. Makes decisions
5. Demonstrates positive self-concept
    a. Performs self-care activities
    b. Assumes responsibilities
    c. Exhibits confidence in own abilities
6. Demonstrates effective health care at home
    a. Takes prescribed medications
    b. Demonstrates dressing and treatment regimens
    c. Continues physical and occupational therapy programs
    d. Reports occurrence of symptoms of complications
    e. Uses special equipment safely
    f. Schedules follow-up health care appointments
    g. Acknowledges need for long-term health supervision

Metastatic Bone Cancer

Metastatic bone cancer is more common than any primary malignant bone tumor. Tumors arising from tissues other than the bone may invade the bone and produce localized bone destruction, with results that are clinically quite analogous to those occurring in primary bone tumors. Tumors that metastasize to bone most frequently include carcinomas of the kidney, the prostate, the lung, the breast, the ovary, and the thyroid. Metastatic tumors most frequently attack the skull, spine, pelvis, femur, and humerus. Bone scans are useful in diagnostic workup.

A sign of diagnostic importance in patients with metastatic carcinoma of the prostate is an elevation of the serum

TABLE 58-1
Painful Shoulder Syndromes

Syndromes	Clinical Features	Clinical Manifestations	Management
Supraspinatus tendonitis and tenosynovitis	Reaction to mechanical stress and strain plus a degenerative process with traumatic inflammation	Pain in shoulder; "catching" sensation Patient grabs affected shoulder with opposite hand. Night pain; inability to lie on affected side Painful arc beyond 60-degree abduction (as tendons and cuff impinge under coracoacromial arch)	Intermittent heat/cold applications Pendulum exercises Anti-inflammatory medications—salicylates (aspirin) to tolerance Local injection of steroid or anesthetic agent into shoulder joint
Calcific tendonitis	Calcific deposits develop in tendons; causes reaction in overlying bursa. Calcific tendonitis and bursitis often coexist.	Occurs in younger and more active persons Abrupt onset of severe aching pain, 1 to 4 days All shoulder and arm movement is painful. Acute phase followed by pain relief	Infiltration of subacromial area and aspiration of deposit Analgesics for pain Anti-inflammatory agents (aspirin, phenylbutazone, indomethacin) Applications of heat/cold Injection with local anesthetic agent and steroid Operative treatment may be necessary for excision of calcified deposits.
Tears and rupture of rotator cuff	Tears occur at the insertion of rotator cuff into the bone, probably from degenerative changes.	Occur most commonly after age 50 Abrupt shoulder pain in deltoid area Weakness/inability to abduct shoulder "Clicking" sensation felt in shoulder on abduction/rotation	Partial rupture usually responds to conservative management. Infiltration with local anesthetic to relieve pain Confirmation of defect by arthrogram Surgical repair for complete rupture
Bicipital syndromes (lesions on the long head of biceps muscle): tendonitis and tenosynovitis	Long head of biceps is affected by arm and shoulder movement.	Chronic pain in anterolateral area of shoulder associated with muscle spasm and pain in trapezius, scalenus, deltoid	Rest of the extremity Gentle exercises within tolerance Salicylates Heat applications to reduce inflammation Avoid movements that put biceps tendon on stretch.
Bursitis	Almost all cases of subacromial bursitis have preceding tendonitis and tenosynovitis in the rotator cuff, biceps tendon, and sheath or an inflammatory process in bone or joint; the spread of inflammation to bursa is a secondary event.	Deep-seated ache in shoulder Pain upon rotation of arm	Treatment consists of locating and treating the primary process causing the bursitis.

(Adapted from Bateman JE. The Shoulder and Neck. Philadelphia, WB Saunders, 1978.)

acid phosphatase. The first indication of disease in such cases may be a pathologic bone fracture; in later stages, the peripheral blood may show evidence of bone marrow interference. Aspiration or surgical biopsy of the bone tumor can give information as to the primary site if that not known.

The treatment of metastatic bone cancer is palliative, and the therapeutic goal is to relieve the patient's discomfort as much as possible. Internal fixation of pathological fractures minimizes associated disability and pain. At times, large bone metastatic lesions are strengthened by prophylactic internal fixation. The patient is encouraged to be as independent as possible and function as long as possible. Surgery may be indicated in long bone fractures.

Common Problems of the Upper Extremity

Painful Shoulder Syndrome. The structures in and about the shoulder are frequently the sites of painful syndromes. With aging, degenerative alterations occur in all joints, including the articulations that make up the shoulder joint (glenohumeral, sternoclavicular, and acromioclavicular). Pain may arise from supraspinatus tendonitis or bicipital tendonitis, with the inflammation spreading to the tendon sheaths, other tendons and their sheaths (*tenosynovitis*), and the bursa, capsule, synovium, cartilage, bone, and surrounding muscles. Syndromes frequently encountered are listed in Table 58-1.

Patient Education. The nurse provides guidelines for general care and shows the patient how to carry out measures that will promote healing. This involves teaching the patient to do the following:

1. Rest the joint in a position that minimizes stress on the joint structures during the acute phase to prevent further damage and the development of adhesions.
2. Support the affected arm on pillows while sleeping, to keep from rolling over on the shoulder.
3. At first, apply cold intermittently, and then apply heat intermittently, to reduce discomfort and facilitate mobilization. Cold applications help reduce swelling, and heat promotes circulation.
4. Gradually resume motion and use of the joint. Assistance with dressing and other activities of daily living may be needed.
5. Avoid working and lifting above shoulder level or pushing an object against a "locked" shoulder.
6. Do the prescribed daily range-of-motion exercises to strengthen the shoulder girdle and glenohumeral muscle.

"Tennis Elbow." "Tennis elbow" is a chronic painful condition that is due to excessive pronation and supination activities of the forearm (*e.g.*, tennis, sculling, using a screwdriver). The pain characteristically radiates down the extensor (dorsal) surface of the forearm. The patient has a weakened grasp. Most often, relief is obtained by resting the arm in a molded splint, applying moist heat, and taking analgesics. In some instances, local injection of a corticosteroid or procaine

is prescribed. Gentle daily exercises help to prevent elbow stiffness.

Ganglion. A ganglion is a round, firm, cystic swelling, usually near the wrist. It is a collection of gelatinous material near the tendon sheaths and joints. Ganglions develop through defects in the tendon sheath or capsule. Ganglions occur most frequently in women under the age of 50. The ganglion is tender and may cause an aching pain. When a tendon sheath is involved, weakness of the finger occurs.

Carpal Tunnel Syndrome. Carpal tunnel syndrome is an entrapment neuropathy that occurs when the median nerve at the wrist is compressed by a thickened flexor tendon sheath, skeletal encroachment, or soft-tissue mass on the median nerve at the wrist. The patient experiences pain, numbness, paresthesia, and possibly weakness along the median nerve (thumb, first and second fingers). Night pain is common. Rest splints, avoidance of work that requires flexion of the wrist, and cortisone injections may relieve the symptoms. Surgical release of the transverse carpal ligament may be necessary.

Dupuytren's Contracture. Dupuytren's deformity is a slowly progressive contracture of the palmar fascia that causes flexion of the little finger, the ring finger, and frequently the middle fingers, which renders them more or less useless (Fig. 58-6). It is a fairly common abnormality, occurring most frequently in men over age 50 who are of Scandinavian or Celtic origin. It may be caused by an inherited autosomal dominant trait. It starts as a tender nodule of the palmar fascia. The tenderness resolves, and the nodule may not change, or it may progress where the fibrous thickening extends to involve the skin in the distal palm and produces a contracture of the fingers. This condition always starts in one hand, but even-

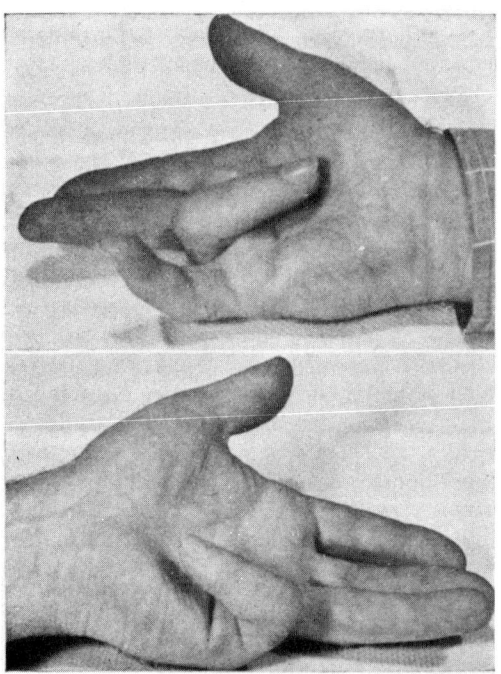

Figure 58-6
Dupuytren's contracture. (Boyes JH. Bunnell's Surgery of the Hand, 5th ed, p 228. Philadelphia, JB Lippincott.)

tually both become deformed symmetrically. Surgery consists of limited palmar and digital fasciectomies that improve function. The recurrence and extension rate is 45% to 80%.

► *Nursing Process*
The Patient Undergoing Surgery of the Hand or Wrist

▷ *Assessment*

Surgery of the hand and wrist is generally an ambulatory surgery procedure. Prior to surgery, the nurse assesses the patient's level and type of discomfort and limitations in function caused by the ganglion, carpal tunnel syndrome, Dupuytren's contracture, or other condition of the hand. Following surgery, the nurse assesses the patient for swelling, neurovascular status, pain, and function. Pain may be related to edema, restrictive bandages, hematoma formation, or surgery.

▷ *Nursing Diagnoses*

Based on the assessment data, the nursing diagnoses for the patient with surgery of the hand or wrist may include the following:

• Alteration in comfort—pain related to inflammation and swelling
• Self-care deficit related to bandaged hands
• Potential for infection

▷ *Planning and Implementation*

▷ *Goals:* The goals of the patient may include relief of pain, improved self-care, and absence of infection.

Nursing Interventions

Relieving Pain. To control swelling, the hand is elevated above heart level with pillows or with an elevating sling or stockinette, which is attached to an IV pole or overhead frame when high elevation is prescribed. If the patient is ambulatory, the arm is elevated in a conventional sling. Ice packs applied intermittently to the surgical area during the first 24 to 48 hours control swelling. Active extension and flexion of the fingers promote circulation and are encouraged, even though movement is limited by the bulky dressing.

Neurovascular checks of the exposed fingers every hour for the first 24 hours are essential for monitoring function of the nerves and perfusion of the hand. Ask the patient to describe the sensations in the hands and to demonstrate finger movement ability. The patient's nerve function is observed carefully preoperatively because this information is needed for interpreting function after surgery. Compromised neurovascular functioning can contribute to pain. Generally, the discomfort can be controlled by oral analgesics. The nurse evaluates the patient's response to the pain medications and to other pain-control measures. Patient education concerning the analgesics is done by the nurse.

Improving Self-Care. During the first few days following surgery, the patient will need assistance with activities of daily living because one hand is bandaged and function is impaired. The patient may need to arrange for assistance with feeding, bathing/hygiene, dressing, grooming and toileting. Within a few days, the patient is able to function with minimal assistance. The pain and swelling are controlled, functional abilities are returning, and the patient has developed skills in one-handed activities of daily living. As rehabilitation progresses, the patient will resume use of the injured hand. Adherence to the therapeutic regimen is emphasized.

Absence of Infection. As with all surgery, there is a potential for infection. The patient is taught to monitor temperature and pulse for elevations that may indicate a possible infection. The patient is instructed to keep the dressing clean and dry. Any drainage, foul odor associated with the dressing, or increased pain and swelling should be reported. Patient education concerning aseptic wound care may be appropriate. The patient may be taking prophylactic antibiotics and need education in relation to these.

▷ *Evaluation*

▷ *Expected Outcomes*

1. Relief of pain
   a. Patient reports increased comfort.
   b. Controls edema through elevation of hand
   c. Experiences no discomfort with movement
2. Improved self-care
   a. Patient secures assistance with activities of daily living during first few days postoperatively
   b. Adapts to one-handed activities of daily living
   c. Uses injured hand functionally
3. Develops no infection
   a. Has temperature and pulse within normal limits
   b. Has no purulent drainage or wound inflammation

Common Foot Problems

Disabilities of the human foot not only develop from poorly-fitting shoes but may be the result of hereditary influence. Probably the foot would cause little pain or disability on its own account if it were not for modern civilization, which disregards the physiology of the foot. Fashion, vanity, and eye appeal, rather than function, are for the most part the determining factors in the design of footwear. The restriction of ill-fitting shoes distorts normal anatomy while inducing deformity and pain.

The discomfort of foot strain can be treated by rest, elevation, physiotherapy, supportive strappings, and orthotic devices. Foot exercises in which active motion occurs will benefit the circulation and help strengthen the feet. Walking in properly-fitting shoes is considered the best form of exercise.

Common Foot Ailments

A *corn* is an area of *hyperkeratosis* (overgrowth of a horny layer of epidermis) produced by pressure from within (the underlying bone is prominent due to congenital or acquired abnormality, commonly arthritis) or by pressure from without (shoes). The usual sites are the lesser toes, mainly the fifth toe, but all toes may be involved.

Corns are treated by soaking and scraping off the horny layer with an instrument, by applying a protective shield or pads, or by surgical removal of the underlying offending osseous structure.

Soft corns are located between the toes and are kept soft by moisture and maceration. Treatment consists of drying the affected web spaces and separating the affected toes. Usually, a podiatrist will be needed to treat the underlying cause.

A *callus* is a discretely thickened area of the skin that has been exposed to persistent pressure or friction. Faulty foot mechanics usually precede the formation of a callus. Treatment consists of eliminating the underlying causes and having the callus pared by a podiatrist if it is painful. A keratolytic ointment may be applied and a thin plastic cup worn over the heel if the callus is on this area. Felt padding with adhesive backing is also used to prevent and relieve pressure. Orthotic devices can be made to remove the pressure from the bony protuberance. The protuberance may be excised.

An *ingrown toenail* (onychocryptosis) is a condition in which the free edge of a nail plate has penetrated the surrounding skin, either laterally or anteriorly. It may be accompanied by secondary infection or granulation tissue. This painful condition is caused by improper self-treatment, external pressure (tight shoes or stockings), internal pressure (deformed toes; growth under the nail), trauma, and infection. Trimming the nails properly can prevent this problem. Active treatment consists of relieving the pain by decreasing the pressure on the surrounding soft tissue by the nail plate. Warm, wet soaks help to drain an infection. A toenail may have to be excised if there is severe infection.

Common Deformities of the Foot

Flatfoot. Flatfoot (pes planus) is a common disorder in which the longitudinal arch of the foot is diminished. It may be due to congenital abnormalities or associated with bone or ligament injury, muscle and posture imbalances, excessive weight, muscle fatigue, poorly-fitting shoes, or arthritis. Symptoms include burning sensation, fatigue, clumsy gait, edema, and pain.

Exercises to strengthen the muscles and to improve posture and walking habits are helpful. A number of foot devices are available to give the foot additional support. Severe flatfoot problems are usually treated by an orthopedic surgeon or a podiatrist.

Hammer Toe. Hammer toe is a flexion deformity of the interphalangeal joint and may involve several toes (Fig. 58-7). The condition is usually an acquired deformity. Tight socks or shoes may push an overlying toe back into the line of the other toes. The toes usually are pulled upward, forcing the metatarsal joints (ball of foot) downward. Corns develop on top of the toes, and tender calluses develop under the metatarsal area. The treatment consists of conservative measures: carrying out manipulative exercises, wearing open-toed sandals or shoes that conform to the shape of the foot, and protecting the protruding joints with pads. Surgical correction is necessary for an established deformity.

Hallux Valgus. Hallux valgus (bunion) is a progressive deformity in which the great toe deviates laterally (Fig. 58-7).

Associated with this is a marked prominence of the medial aspect of the first metatarsal–phalangeal joint, with osseous enlargement of the medial side of the first metatarsal head, over which a bursa may form (secondary to pressure and inflammation). Acute bursitis symptoms include a reddened area, edema, and tenderness. Etiological factors include heredity, narrow shoes, arthritis, and flatfoot.

Treatment depends on the patient's age, the degree of deformity, and the severity of symptoms. If a bunion deformity is uncomplicated, wearing a shoe that conforms to the shape of the foot or one that is molded to the foot to prevent pressure on the protruding portions may be all the treatment that is needed. If not, surgical removal of the bunion and realignment of the toe may be required.

Postoperatively, the patient may have intense throbbing pain at the operative site, requiring rather liberal doses of analgesic medication. The operated food is elevated above the level of the heart to decrease edema and pain. The neurovascular status of the toes is assessed. The duration of immobility and initiation of ambulation depend upon the procedure used. Following surgery, exercises are initiated to flex and extend the toes, since toe flexion is essential in walking. Shoes that do not stress the foot are recommended.

Clawfoot. Clawfoot (pes cavus) refers to a foot with an abnormally high arch (Fig. 58-7). This causes shortening of the foot and increased pressure that produces calluses on the metatarsal area and on the dorsum (bottom) of the foot. Exercises are prescribed to manipulate the forefoot into dorsiflexion and relax the toes. In severe cases, osteotomies are done to reshape the feet.

Morton's Neuroma. Morton's neuroma (plantar digital neuroma; neurofibroma) is a swelling of the third (lateral) branch of the median plantar nerve (Fig. 58-7). The third digital nerve, which is located in the third intermetatarsal space, is most commonly involved. Microscopically, digital artery changes cause an ischemia of the nerve.

The result is a throbbing, burning pain in the foot that is usually relieved when the patient rests. Pain sometimes radiates up the leg. Conservative treatment consists of inserting innersoles, metatarsal bars, and pads designed to spread the metatarsal heads and balance the foot posture. Local injections of hydrocortisone and a local anesthetic may give relief. If these fail, surgical excision of the neuroma is necessary. Pain relief is immediate and permanent.

Other Foot Problems

Several systemic diseases affect the feet. In the case of rheumatoid arthritis, deformities result. Persons with diabetes are prone to develop corns and peripheral neuropathies with diminishing sensation, leading to ulcers over pressure points of the foot. Persons with peripheral vascular disease and arteriosclerosis complain of burning and itching feet with attendant scratching and excoriations. Dermatologic problems commonly affect the feet in the form of fungal infections and plantar warts. The specifics of these problems and others can be found in the discussions of the various dysfunctions covered throughout the text.

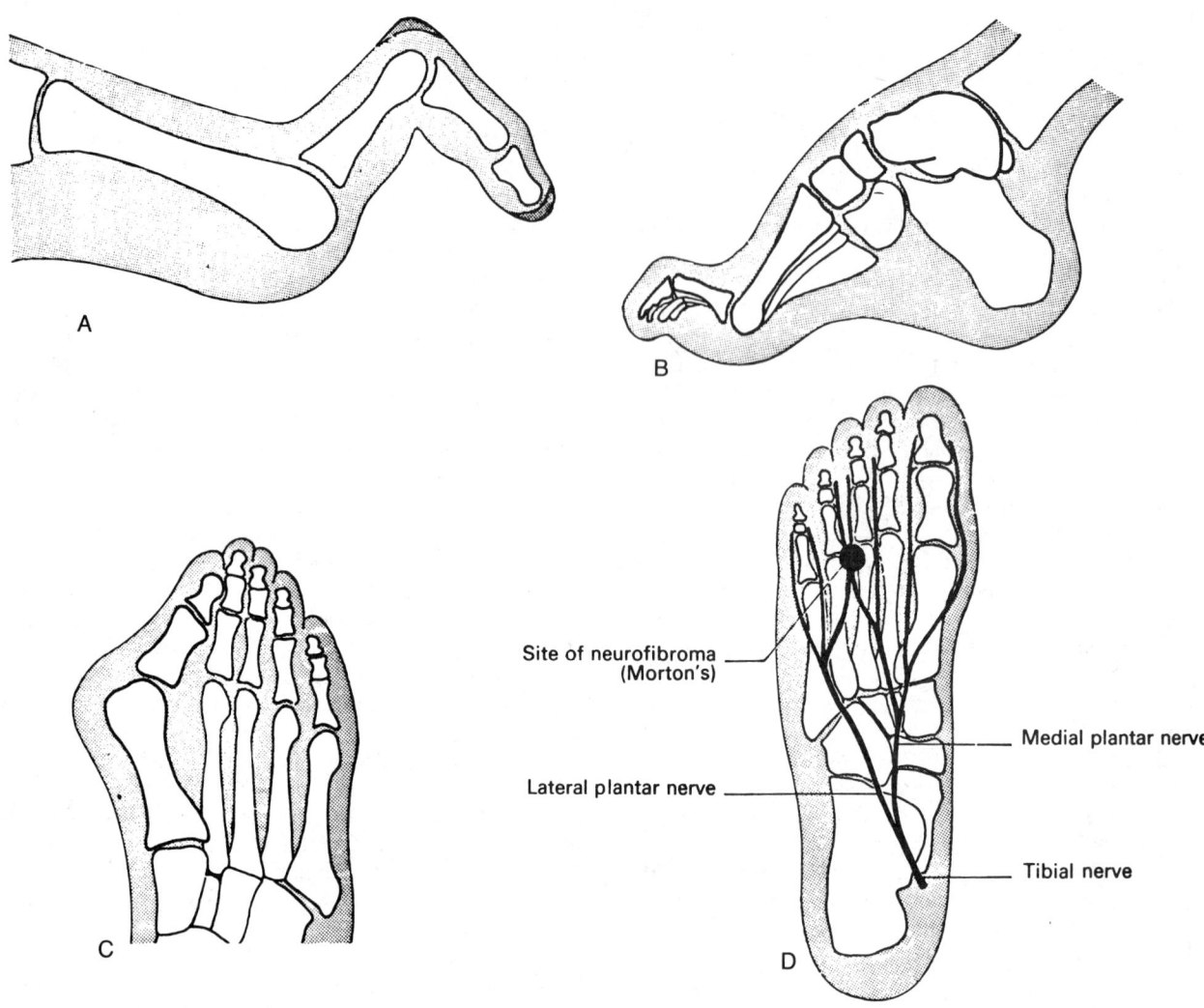

Figure 58-7
Common foot deformities. (*A*) Hammer toe. (*B*) Clawfoot (pes cavus). (*C*) Hallux valgus. (*D*) Site for Morton's neuroma.

▶ *Nursing Process*
The Patient Undergoing Foot Surgery

▷ *Assessment*

Surgery on the foot may be necessary because of a variety of conditions, including neuromas and foot deformities (bunion, hammertoe, clawfoot). Generally, foot surgery is performed on an outpatient basis. The nurse assesses the patient's ambulatory ability and balance and the neurovascular status of the foot prior to surgery. Additionally, assessment of the availability of assistance at home following surgery and the structural characteristics of the home may help in planning for care during the first few days after surgery. These data, in addition to knowledge of the usual management of the problem, are used by the nurse in formulating appropriate nursing diagnoses. Following surgery, the nurse assesses the patient for swelling, neurovascular function, pain, wound status, and mobility.

▷ *Nursing Diagnoses*

Based on the assessment data, the nursing diagnoses for the patient undergoing foot surgery may include the following:

- Alteration in comfort—pain related to inflammation and swelling
- Impaired physical mobility related to the foot immobilizing device
- Potential for infection

▷ *Planning and Implementation*

▷ *Goals:* The goals of the patient may include relief of pain, improved mobility, and absence of infection.

Nursing Interventions

Relieving Pain. Pain experienced by patients who have had foot surgery is related to inflammation and edema. Formation of a hematoma may contribute to the discomfort. To control the swelling, the foot should be elevated on several pillows when the patient is sitting or lying. Ice packs applied for 20 to 30 minutes intermittently during the first 24 to 48 hours after surgery control swelling and provide some pain relief. As activity increases, the patient will find that the dependent positioning of the foot will be uncomfortable. Simply elevating the foot relieves the discomfort. Additionally, oral analgesics may be used to control the pain. The nurse provides the patient with information on the use of these medications.

Neuromuscular checks of the exposed toes every 1 to 2 hours for the first 24 hours are essential to monitor the function of the nerves and the perfusion of the tissues. If the surgery is done on an ambulatory basis, the patient and family need to be taught how to assess for swelling and neurovascular status. Compromised neurovascular function can contribute to the pain experienced.

Improving Mobility. Following surgery, the patient will have a bulky dressing on the foot, protected by a light cast or a special protective boot. Weight-bearing on the foot will be prescribed by the surgeon; it varies according to the procedure and the preference of the surgeon. Some patients are allowed to walk on the heel and progress to weight-bearing as tolerated; others are to be non-weight-bearing. An ambulatory aid may be needed to assist the patient. Choice of the aid depends on the patient's general condition and balance and on the weight-bearing prescription. Safe use of the ambulatory aid must be ensured through adequate patient education and practice prior to discharge. Preoperative instruction and practice with the ambulatory aid are desirable. Problems of moving around the house safely while using the ambulatory aid are discussed with the patient. As healing progresses, the patient will resume ambulation at the previous or an improved level. Adherence to the therapeutic regimen is emphasized.

Absence of Infection. As with all surgery, there is a potential for infection. Since the foot is on or near the floor, care must be taken to protect it from soiling, dirt, and moisture. When bathing, the patient can protect the dressing with a plastic bag secured around it. Additionally, patient instruction concerning aseptic wound care may be appropriate. The patient is taught to monitor temperature and pulse for elevations that could indicate a possible infection. Any such elevations as well as any drainage on the dressing, foul odor, or increased pain and swelling, should be reported. If the patient will be taking prescribed prophylactic antibiotics, education related to these will be needed.

▷ **Evaluation**

▷ *Expected Outcome*

1. Relief of pain
   a. Patient controls edema by elevating foot.
   b. Reports increased comfort
2. Has improved mobility
   a. Uses ambulatory aids safely
   b. Resumes weight-bearing gradually as prescribed
   c. Exhibits diminished disability associated with preoperative condition
3. Develops no infection
   a. Has temperature and pulse within normal limits
   b. Has no purulent drainage or wound inflammation
   c. Keeps dressing clean and dry

Bibliography

Books

Avioli LV (ed). The Osteoporosis Syndrome: Detection, Prevention, and Treatment. New York, Grune & Stratton, 1983.

Birnbaum JS. The Musculoskeletal Manual. New York, Academic Press, 1982.

Calcium: A Summary of Current Research for the Health Professional. Rosemont, Illinois, National Dairy Council, 1984.

Donahoo C and Spickler L (eds). Core Curriculum of Orthopedic Nursing. Atlanta, Orthopedic Nurses' Association, 1980.

Farrell J. Illustrated Guide to Orthopedic Nursing, 3rd ed. Philadelphia, JB Lippincott, 1986.

Finneson B. Low Back Pain, 2nd ed. Philadelphia, JB Lippincott, 1980.

Hadler NM. Medical Management of the Regional Musculoskeletal Diseases. Orlando, Florida, Grune & Stratton, 1984.

Holbrook TL et al. The Frequency of Occurrence, Impact, and Cost of Selected Musculoskeletal Conditions in the United States. Chicago, American Academy of Orthopaedic Surgeons, 1984.

McCarty DJ. Arthritis and Allied Conditions, 10th ed. Philadelphia, Lea and Febiger, 1985.

Nelson CL and Dwyer AP (eds). The Aging Musculoskeletal System. Lexington: The Collarmore Press, DC Heath and Co, 1984.

Osteoporosis. Bethesda, National Institutes of Health Consensus Development Conference Statement. 5(3), 1984.

Pellino T et al (eds). National Association of Orthopaedic Nurses: Core Curriculum for Orthopaedic Nursing. Pitman, New Jersey, Anthony J Jannetti, 1986.

Rodnon GP and Schumacher R (eds). Primer on the Rheumatic Diseases, 8th ed., Atlanta, Arthritis Foundation, 1983.

Rosse C and Clawson DK. The Musculoskeletal System in Health and Disease. Hagerstown, Maryland, Harper & Row, 1981.

Salter RB. Textbook of Disorders and Injuries of the Musculoskeletal System, 2nd ed. Baltimore, Williams & Wilkins, 1983.

Sculco TP. Orthopaedic Care of the Geriatric Patient. St Louis, CV Mosby, 1985.

Turek SL (ed). Orthopaedics: Principles and Their Application, 4th ed. Philadelphia, JB Lippincott, 1984.

Uhthoff HK (ed). Current Concepts of Infections in Orthopedic Surgery. New York, Springer-Verlag, 1985.

White AA and Gordon SI (eds). American Academy of Orthopaedic Surgeons Symposium on Idiopathic Low Back Pain. St Louis, CV Mosby, 1982.

Wilson FC. The Musculoskeletal System: Basic Processes and Disorders, 2nd ed. Philadelphia, JB Lippincott, 1983.

Articles

Low Back Pain

Lehmann TR and Brand RA. Disability in the patient with low back pain. Orthop Clin North Am 1982 July; 13(3):559–568.

Lucas PR. Low back pain. Surg Clin North Am 1983 June; 63(3):515–528.

McCarthy RE. Coping with low back pain through behavioral change. Orthop Nurs 1984 May/June; 3(3):30–35.

Selby D. Conservative care of nonspecific low back pain. Orthop Clin North Am 1983 July; 13(3):427–438.

Taylor SL. Musculoskeletal assessment: Low back pain assessment, part 1—history taking. Orthop Nurs 1983 July/Aug; 2(4):11–16.

Taylor SL. Musculoskeletal assessment: Low back pain assessment, part 2—defining range of motion and terminology. Orthop Nurs 1983 Sept/Oct; 2(5):39–44.

Taylor SL. Musculoskeletal assessment: Low back pain assessment, part 3—the physical examination. Orthop Nurs 1983 Nov/Dec; 2(6):21–27.

Problems of the Upper and Lower Extremities

Bartell L. Bunionectomies. Orthop Nurs 1985 Jan/Feb; 4(1):21–28.

Berger MR. Bunions: An overview. Orthop Nurs 1984 Sept/Oct; 3(5):17–22.

Berger MR. Painful tendon problems of the hand: Trigger thumb, trigger finger, and de Quervain's syndrome. Orthop Nurs 1982 Sept/Oct; 1(5):20–23.

Berger MR. Morton's neuroma. Orthop Nurs 1982 Jan/Feb; 1(1):31–32.

Hill NA. Dupuytren's contracture: Current concepts review. J Bone Joint Surg [Am] 1985 Dec; 67-A(9):1439–1443.

Osteoporosis

Aloia JF. Estrogen and exercise in prevention and treatment of osteoporosis. Geriatrics 1982 June; 37(6): 81–85.

Armann SA and Wells CL. A study of bone loss in ballerinas. Nutr News 1985 Dec; 49(4):16–17.

Beauchamp PJ and Held B. Estrogen replacement therapy: Universal remedy for the post-menopausal woman? Postgrad Med 1984 May; 75(7):42–49.

Chase JA. Spine fractures associated with osteoporosis. Orthop Nurs 1985 May/June; 4(3):31–33.

Chestnut CH III. An appraisal of the role of estrogens in the treatment of postmenopausal osteoporosis. J Am Geriatr Soc 1984 Aug; 32(8): 604–608.

Gleit CJ and Graham BA. The role of calcium and estrogen in osteoporosis. Orthop Nurs 1985 May/June; 4(3):13–18.

Graham BA and Gliet CJ. Osteoporosis: A major health problem in post-menopausal women. Orthop Nurs 1984 Dec; 3(6):19–26.

Gray-Vickrey M. Education to prevent falls. Geriatr Nurs 1984 May/June; 5(3):179–183.

Hallal JC. Osteoporotic fractures exact a toll. J Gerontol Nurs 1985 Aug; 11(8):13–18.

Judd HL et al. Estrogen replacement therapy: Indications and complications. Ann Int Med 1983 Feb; 98(2):195–205.

Lane J and Vigorita V. Osteoporosis. Orthop Clin North Am 1984 Oct; 15(4):711–721.

Liddel DB. An in-depth look at osteoporosis. Orthop Nurs 1985 May/June; 4(3):23–27.

Mindell ER. Orthopedic surgery. JAMA 1985 Oct 25; 254(6):2313–2315.

Parfitt A. Dietary risk factors for age-related bone loss and fractures. Lancet 1983 Nov 19; 2(8360):1181–1185.

Peck WA. Warding off osteoporosis. Patient Care 1985 Jan 15; 19(11):20–49.

Ray R. Symposium: Osteoporosis revisited. Contemp Orthop 1984 Jan; 8(1):127–164.

The role of calcium in health. National Dairy Council Digest 1984; 55(1):1–8.

Todd B. Can osteoporosis be treated? Geriatr Nurs 1985 Nov/Dec; 6(6):359–360.

Torrance C. Boning up on exercise. Nurs Times 1985 Oct 23–29; 81(43):38.

Veninga KS. Osteoporosis: Implications for community health nursing. J Community Health Nurs 1984; 1(4):227–233.

Yeater RA and Martin RB. Senile osteoporosis: The effects of exercise. Postgrad Med 1984 Feb 1; 75(2):147–159.

Osteomalacia/Paget's Disease

Dalinka MK, Aronchick JM, and Haddad JG. Paget's disease. Orthop Clin North Am 1983 Jan; 14(1):1–19.

Doppelt SH. Vitamin D: Rickets and osteomalacia. Orthop Clin North Am 1984 Oct; 15(4):671–696.

Eisman JA and Martin TJ. Osteolytic Paget's disease: Recognition and risks of biopsy. J Bone Joint Surg 1986 Jan; 68(1):112–117.

Huskins DJ. Paget's disease of bone: An update on management. Drugs 1985 Aug; 30(2):156–173.

Johnson CC et al. Review of fracture experience during treatment of Paget's disease of bone with etidronate disodium (EHDP). Clin Orthop Rel Res 1983 Jan/Feb; 172:186–194.

Lane JM (ed). Symposium on metabolic bone disease. Orthop Clin North Am 1984 Oct; 15(4):567–820.

Merkow RL and Lane JM. Current concepts of Paget's disease of bone. Orthop Clin North Am 1984 Oct; 15(4):747–763.

Nugent CA, Gall EP, and Pitt MJ. Osteoporosis, osteomalacia, rickets, and Paget's disease. Primary Care 1984 June; 11(2):353–368.

Ross DG. Paget's disease. Orthop Nurs 1984 May/June; 3(3):41–44.

Stacy-Spencer E. Diagnostic overview: Osteomalacia. Orthop Nurs 1984 July/Aug; 3(4):47.

Wallach S. Treatment of Paget's disease. Adv Int Med 1982; 27:1–43.

Bone and Joint Infections

Arthritis. Am J Nurs 1983 Feb; 83(2):253–262.

Bergers RM, Martin RN, and Streckfuss BL. A home IV antibiotic program. NITA 1985 May/June; 8(3):238–239.

Fitzgerald RH and Kelley PJ (eds). Musculoskeletal sepsis. Orthop Clin North Am 1984 July; 15(3):399–554.

Ho G Jr and Su EY. Therapy for septic arthritis. JAMA 1982 Feb 12; 247(6):797–800.

Sheehan K and Gildea J. Home antibiotic therapy. NITA 1985 Mar/Apr; 8(2):157–159.

Smith DL. Infectious arthritis. Top Emerg Med 1983 July; 5(2):40–45.

Bone Tumors

Berrettoni BA and Carter JR. Mechanisms of cancer metastasis to bone. J Bone Joint Surg [Am] 1986 Feb; 68-A(2):308–311.

Consensus Conference: Limb-sparing treatment of adult soft-tissue sarcomas and osteosarcomas. JAMA 1985 Oct 4; 254(13):1791–1794.

Eilber FR et al. Limb salvage for skeletal and soft-tissue sarcomas. Cancer 1984 June 15; 53(12):2579–2584.

Fedora NL. Fighting for my leg . . . and my life. Orthop Nurs 1985 Sept/Oct; 4(5):39–42.

Fountain MJ. Psychological support for the person experiencing cancer. Orthop Nurs 1985 Sept/Oct; 4(5):33–35.

Gregorcic NJ. Functional abilities following limb-salvage procedures. Orthop Nurs 1985 Sept/Oct; 4(5):24–28.

Kerns LL and Simon MA. Surgical theory, staging, definition, and treatment of musculoskeletal sarcomas. Surg Clin North Am 1983 June; 63(3):671–686.

Lambert MH et al. Soft-tissue sarcoma: Functional outcome after wide local excision and radiation therapy. Arch Phys Med Rehabil 1984 Aug; 65(8):477–480.

Lamphier PC. Primary bone tumors. Orthop Nurs 1985 Sept/Oct; 4(5):17–23.

Matzke KA et al. Case study: Nursing care of a patient with osteogenic sarcoma. Orthop Nurs 1985 Sept/Oct; 4(5):44–47, 69.

Moore TM et al. Symposium: Soft-tissue sarcomas. Contemp Orthop 1984 Apr; 8(4):89–126.

Nirenberg A. The adolescent with osteogenic sarcoma. Orthop Nurs 1985 Sept/Oct; 4(5):11–15.

Piasecki PA and Rodts MF. Bone banking: Its role in skeletal tumor resection Orthop Nurs 1985 Sept/Oct; 4(5):56–60.

Sweetnam R. Osteosarcoma. Br J Hosp Med 1982 Aug; 28(2):112, 116–121.

Agencies

American Brittle Bone Society, 1256 Merrill Drive, Marshalton, PA 19380.

Back Pain Association, 17 Teddington Park, Teddington, Middlesex, TW11 0AB, England.

National Committee on the Treatment of Intractable Pain, P.O. Box 9553, Friendship Station, Washington, DC 20016.

National Easter Seal Society, 2023 West Ogden Avenue, Chicago, IL 60612.

National Institute of Arthritis and Musculoskeletal and Skin Diseases, National Institutes of Health, Bethesda, MD 20892.

Osteogenesis Imperfecta Foundation, P.O. Box 428, Van Wert, OH 45891.

Paget's Disease Foundation, P.O. Box 2772, Brooklyn, NY 11202.

Nursing Research Profile for Unit XV

Orthopedic Nursing

Overview

At this time there is a paucity of nursing research on problems of patients with musculoskeletal conditions. Some locomotion problems have been addressed by nurses concerned with neurologic dysfunctions. The problem of back injuries has received attention. The following studies focus on salient issues and areas for future consideration in the management of patients with orthopedic conditions.

▷ *Crowther H. New perspectives on nursing lower limb amputees. J Adv Nurs 1982 Sept; 7(5):453–460.*

This paper reflects Crowther's research into amputee rehabilitation and a summary of other research findings. There are new perspectives on the psychological and neurological sequelae of amputation, the practical problems of loss of an extremity, and the prosthetic dimension of treatment. Research show that there are a variety of reactions to loss of a leg and that neither denial nor shock are usual following the majority of amputations secondary to vascular disease. The model of sudden and shocking loss is largely incorrect.

The author draws attention to the "unrecognized ordinariness" of patient response, which should become a part of amputee nursing. Patients with amputations have many needs that probably cannot be met in the clinical setting. The nurse could be of great help if she works with the therapists and prosthetists, especially in answering questions that arise as the patient confronts new changes in life-style. Amputation should be regarded as replacement surgery with the uniting of patient and prosthesis as a goal. The author's research revealed that pain and discomfort are underestimated, and that pain is a major characteristic of amputation that continues for many years following surgery.

Nursing Implications. According to one health agency included in the study, adequate control of postoperative pain is thought to prevent the development of phantom pain. Since phantom pain is a universal problem, nurses can address the goal of effective pain control in the postoperative period. Most of the findings from this research can be incorporated into the nursing process.

▷ *Williams MA et al. Reducing acute confusional states in elderly patients with hip fractures. Res Nurs Health 1985 Dec; 8(4):329–337.*

Based on the assumption that idiopathic confusion may be prevented or mitigated by the activities, interpersonal approaches, and environmental manipulations over which nurses may have control, the purpose of this study was to test whether the incidence of confusion in elderly patients with hip fractures and with no prior history of mental impairment could be reduced by specific nursing interventions.

A quantitative method of risk assessment was developed. Subjects from orthopedic units in four acute care community hospitals were selected for the nonintervention phase. The nonintervention sample consisted of 170 subjects with an average age of 78.8 years. The intervention sample had 57 subjects with an average age of 80.6 years. The subjects were over 60, had no validated history of mental impairment and had incurred fracture by trauma.

The incidence of confusion was reduced from 51.5% in the comparison group to 43.9% by conscious, deliberative approaches. Effective interventions appeared to be those that provided orientation and clarification, corrected sensory deficits, and increased continuity of care.

Nursing Implications. Decreasing the incidence of confusion in patients is a true nursing intervention. Since such a large percentage of patients over 60 may exhibit some symptoms of mental impairment when admitted to general hospitals, it would be meaningful to study features of hospitalization that could be altered. A risk assessment for alcoholism should also be considered, because this appears to be a problem in the aging population that has been overlooked.

▷　*Owen BD. Personal characteristics important to back injury. Rehabil Nurs 1986 Jul/Aug; 11(4):12–16.*

Owen's study investigated whether differences in physical, life-style, or lifting-style characteristics could be identified in back-injured and non-back-injured nursing personnel. Sixty-four female nursing personnel participated in the study. Half of the subjects had filed accident reports, indicating back-injury while lifting or transferring patients or equipment, and the other half were non-back injured with no history of low-back pain or injury. A number of data collection instruments were used to identify differences in leg length and abdominal strength and to assess psychological stress. The statistical techniques used were two-way analysis of variance and discriminant analysis.

Results revealed that personal characteristics of individuals are related to low-back injury. Demographic characteristics related to age and length of stay on units requiring frequent lifting of patients or equipment. Personnel whose family members have low back problems seem more likely to be back-injured.

Physical characteristics of nurses who were less apt to be back-injured included greater muscle flexibility, greater proprioceptive ability, and legs that were equal in length.

Nursing personnel whose scores indicated greater vulnerability to the stresses of frustration and overload, and those who spent fewer hours per week in high-energy output exercise, were more apt to be in the back-injured group. The noninjured group smoked an average of 10 cigarettes per day, while the back-injured group smoked an average of 23 cigarettes per day.

In lifting style, the greater the distance the feet were apart during lifting, the less likely were the nursing personnel to be in the back-injured group. The subjects were observed during the lifting and carrying of a 15-pound box. Those who kept the box close to their bodies were less apt to be in the back-injured group.

Nursing Implications. All of these findings have implications for nursing practice. Since a consensus on the correct technique for lifting does not exist at present, further study is indicated. Research is needed because occupational low-back injury is a significant problem in nursing. The author offered some general guidelines important to back injury prevention which may be useful in improving lifting techniques until further research is done.

Other Acute Problems

Unit XVI

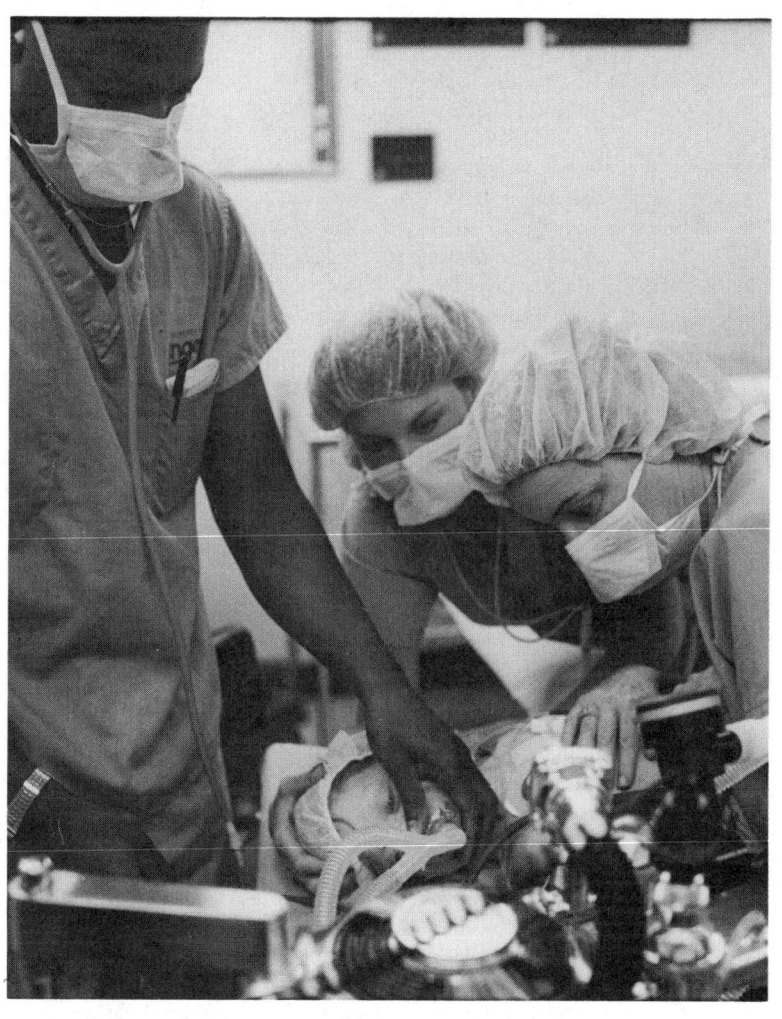

Chapter 59

Management of Patients With Infectious Diseases

The Challenge of Infectious Diseases

An infectious disease is any disease caused by growth of pathogenic organisms in the body. It may or may not be communicable.

Infectious diseases are still the major health problem of the vast majority of people inhabiting the earth. In the developing countries, the principal causes of death are infectious and parasitic diseases. These diseases drain the capabilities of people to work and to learn. The major tropical diseases endemic in many areas are actually increasing in number. New and fearful infectious diseases arising from the tropics in recent years include Lassa, Marburg, and Ebola fevers. The increased number of U.S. citizens traveling abroad has contributed to the resurgence of interest in tropical diseases. The conquering of these diseases is necessary for economic self-sufficiency and national development.

In the industrialized countries, the mortality from infectious diseases has declined dramatically, but these diseases represent the problems most frequently requiring professional attention, accounting for a large portion of the cost of health care. Even in highly developed countries where many diseases have been eliminated, "new" diseases are being introduced by invasive diagnostic techniques, immunosuppressive therapies, and changing cultural, behavioral, and sexual patterns, and by creation of high risk environments such as intensive care units and day care centers. The "new" sexually transmitted diseases (infections caused by *Chlamydia trachomatis*, genital papillomaviruses, *etc.*) have caused epidemics throughout the world; the most awesome problem is the global spread of AIDS (acquired immunodeficiency syndrome). Also, people whose normal host defenses have been compromised are susceptible to organisms that are considered minimally pathogenic. Included in this group are the elderly.

There is an increase in the number of organisms that have developed resistance to a variety of antimicrobials. On the other hand, the advances in modern medicine have led to the development of more antimicrobial drugs, antiviral chemotherapy, and the ability to cultivate viruses in tissue cultures, as well as an increased knowledge about immunity.

The Infectious Process

Epidemiology is the science concerned with the study of the history and occurrence of a disease, along with those factors that may directly or indirectly favor the development of a disease. Table 59-1 provides an overview of infectious diseases, their sources, and their treatment.

A chain of events is necessary for the continual spread of an infectious disease:

- A causative agent
- A reservoir
- A portal or mode of escape
- A mode of transmission
- A mode of entry
- A susceptible host

The chain begins with a *causative agent* or invading organism, which may be bacterial, viral, rickettsial, protozoal, fungal, or helminthic. Infection by each type of organism gives rise to specific reactions in the infected organism.

The second link in the chain is a *reservoir*, a place for the invading organisms to live and multiply. The reservoir is the environment in which the agent is found, whether it be human, arthropod, plant, soil, or inanimate matter; for example, humans are the reservoir for syphilis, soil is the reservoir for tetanus, and animals are the reservoir for brucellosis. In humans, infectious diseases most often arise from contact with infected persons.

The next link is the *mode of escape* (or portal of exit) from the reservoir. Organisms may exit through various body systems, such as the respiratory tract (most common when the reservoir is human), intestinal tract, and genitourinary tract, or through skin lesions. In addition, the agent may escape from the bloodstream or tissues of the host by means of insect bites, hypodermic needles, or surgical instruments.

After the infectious organism has escaped from its reservoir, it is dangerous only if it finds a way of reaching a host. This *mode of transmission* (the next link) may be direct (person-to-person contact, exposure to animal bite, exposure to droplet spray) or indirect (transfer without close contact, usually from an intermediate vehicle, such as water, serum, or contaminated fomites). An example of an organism spread by indirect transmission is the typhoid bacillus, which is able to survive for a long period of time outside the body. Disease may also be transmitted by the vehicle route (contaminated food, water, drugs, blood), by air (droplets), or by vector (arthropod).

The fifth link in the chain is the *mode of entry* of organisms into the human body. This corresponds somewhat to the mode of escape and includes the respiratory tract, gastrointestinal tract, direct infection of mucous membranes, or infection through a break in the skin.

The sixth link in the chain is a *susceptible host*. The presence of an infectious agent does not inevitably produce disease. Whether or not the person becomes ill following the entrance of infectious organisms into the body depends on numerous factors, including the number of organisms to which the host is exposed; the duration of the exposure; the person's age and general physical, mental, and emotional health and nutritional state; the status of the hematopoietic system; the absence of immunoglobulins (or the presence of abnormal immunoglobulins); and the number of T-lymphocytes and their ability to function.

Removing one link in the chain of the infectious process controls infections, which is the purpose of all public health measures.

See Chart 59-1 for a glossary of infectious disease terms.

Principles of Management

Immunity and Immunization

Immunity is the resistance that a person has against disease. Specific immunity to a particular organism implies that an individual either has generated the appropriate antibody in his own body or has received ready-made antibodies from another source. Immunity may be natural (resistance not acquired through previous contact with the infectious agent) or acquired (resistance acquired by the host as a result of previous exposure to the disease). Humoral and cellular immunity are discussed in Chapter 45.

Active Immunization

Active immunization is produced by natural or acquired stimulation, so that the body produces its own antibodies. It may result from clinical or subclinical (inapparent) infection (*e.g.*, the person "gets the disease"). Or it may be produced by administering live or killed microorganisms or their antigens, or inactivated vaccines and toxoids. Modern genetic engineering techniques are being used to develop new vaccines.

Active immunization is the most important and effective tool in preventive medicine. It has been most effective with bacterial exotoxins (diphtherial and tetanus toxoids) and with viruses. Most live-virus vaccines produce antibody responses that consist of prompt (but transient) production of specific immunoglobulins (IgM followed by a sustained production of specific IgG). Live-virus vaccines may produce mild clinical illness, with fever and rash appearing in some patients.

Inactivated vaccines and toxoids give a less complete

(Text continues on p. 1646)

TABLE 59-1
Epidemiology, Therapy, and Control of Communicable Infections

	Infective Organism	Infectious Sources	Entry Site	Method of Spread	Incubation Period	Chemotherapy*	Prophylaxis
Amebiasis	Entamoeba histolytica	Contaminated water and food	Gastrointestinal tract	Patients and carriers; fecal-oral route; oral and sexual contact	Variable	Metronidazole; diloxanide furoate; iodoquinol; chlortetracycline	Detection of carriers and their removal from food handling; plumbing safeguards
Bacillary Dysentery (Shigellosis)	Shigella group	Contaminated water and food	Gastrointestinal tract	Patients and carriers; fecal-oral route	24–48 hours	Ampicillin; chloramphenicol; tetracycline; trimethoprim–sulfamethoxazole	Detection and control of carriers; inspection of food handlers, decontamination of water supplies
Brucellosis	Brucella melitensis and related organisms	Milk, meat, tissues, blood, and absorbed fetuses and placentas from infected cattle, goats, horses, and pigs	Gastrointestinal tract	Ingestion of or contact with infective material	5–30 days (variable)	Tetracycline and streptomycin	Milk pasteurization; control of infection in animals
Chancroid	Haemophilus ducreyi	Human cases and carriers	Genitalia	Direct sexual contact	3–5 days	Erythromycin or trimethoprim–sulfamethoxazole	Effective case-finding and treatment of infection
Chickenpox (Varicella)	Varicella-zoster (V-Z) virus	Human cases	Probably nasopharynx	Probably respiratory droplets	13–17 days	Acyclovir (?)	Varicella-zoster immune globulin (VZIG) primarily for immunocompromised children and certain neonates exposed in utero
Diphtheria	Corynebacterium diphtheriae	Human cases and carriers; fomites; raw milk	Nasopharynx	Nasal and oral secretions; respiratory droplets	2–5 days	Diphtheria antitoxin; penicillin; erythromycin	Active immunization with diphtheria toxoid
Encephalitis, Epidemic (Eastern and Western Equine)	Viruses	Chicken and wild-bird mites; horses	Skin	Mosquitoes	Variable	None	Destroy larvae; eliminate breeding of mosquitoes Eastern equine encephalitis vaccine for those under continued and intensive exposure

Disease	Causative Organism	Reservoir	Portal of Entry	Mode of Transmission	Incubation Period	Therapeutic Agents	Preventive Measures
Gonorrhea	*Neisseria gonorrhoeae*	Urethral and vaginal secretions	Urethral or vaginal mucosa; pharynx; rectum	Sexual activity	2–7 days	Aqueous procaine penicillin G, with probenecid or alternative regimen outlined by Public Health Service	Examination culture; treatment of sexual partners
Granuloma Inguinale	*Calymmatobacterium granulomatis*	Infectious exudate	External genitalia; inguinal and anal region	Direct contact with lesions during sexual activity	Unknown, presumably 8–80 days	Tetracyclines; trimethoprim–sulfamethoxazole	Chemotherapy of carriers and contacts; case-finding and treatment of patients
Infectious Mononucleosis	Epstein-Barr virus	Human cases and carriers	Mouth	Probably oral-pharyngeal route; via blood transfusion in susceptible recipients	2–6 weeks	None	None
Influenza	Virus	Human cases	Respiratory tract	Respiratory	24–72 hours	Amantadine; rimantadine	Influenza virus vaccine
Lymphogranuloma Venereum	*Chlamydia trachomatis*	Human cases	External genitalia; urethral or vaginal mucosa	Sexual intercourse; indirect contact with contaminated articles/clothing	5–21 days	Tetracyclines	Case-finding and treatment of infection
Malaria	*Plasmodium vivax, P. falciparum, P. malariae,* and *P. ovale*	Human cases	Skin	Mosquitoes (*Anopheles*)	Variable, depending on strain	Chloroquine; primaquine; amodiaquine; quinine	Coordinated measures for wide-scale mosquito control; prompt detection and effective treatment of cases; suppressive drugs in malarious areas
Measles	Virus	Human cases	Respiratory mucosa	Nasopharyngeal secretions	8–13 days	None	Measles vaccine
Meningococcal Meningitis	*Neisseria meningitidis*	Human cases and carriers	Nasopharynx; tonsils	Respiratory droplets	2–10 days	Penicillin; ampicillin; chloramphenicol	Meningococcal polysaccharide vaccine for persons at risk; rifampin/sulfadiazine for carriers or contacts

(continued)

TABLE 59-1 (continued)

	Infective Organism	Infectious Sources	Entry Site	Method of Spread	Incubation Period	Chemotherapy*	Prophylaxis
Mumps	Virus	Human cases (early)	Upper respiratory tract	Respiratory droplets	2–3 weeks (avg. 18 days)	None	Live mumps vaccine
Paratyphoid Fever	Salmonella paratyphi A, B, and C, and related organisms	Contaminated food, milk, water	Gastrointestinal tract	Infected feces or rarely urine	7–21 days	Chloramphenicol; ampicillin; trimethoprim–sulfamethoxazole	Control of public water sources, food vendors, food handlers; treatment of carriers
Pneumococcal Pneumonia	Streptococcus pneumoniae	Human carriers; patient's own pharynx	Respiratory mucosa	Respiratory droplets	Variable	Penicillin G; erythromycin	Polyvalent pneumococcal vaccine; control of upper respiratory infections; avoidance of alcoholic intoxication
Poliomyelitis	Polioviruses (types I, II, III)	Human cases and carriers	Gastrointestinal tract	Pharyngeal secretions; fecal-oral	7–14 days	None	Oral polio vaccine (OPV), the live attenuated vaccine containing all three strains of poliovirus—produces long-lasting immunity in most recipients
Rocky Mountain Spotted Fever	Rickettsia rickettsii	Infected wild rodents, dogs, wood ticks, dog ticks	Skin	Tick bites	3–14 days	Tetracyclines; chloramphenicol	Avoidance of tick-infested areas, or wearing of protective clothing in such areas; frequent search for, and prompt removal of, ticks from body; specific vaccination of exposed persons
Rubella (German Measles)	Virus	Human cases	Respiratory mucosa	Nasopharyngeal secretions	14–23 days	None	Rubella virus vaccine; immune globulin (human) given to contacts of rubella; rubella in early stages of pregnancy legally recognized as indication for abortion

Disease	Causative Organism	Reservoir	Portal of Entry	Mode of Transmission	Incubation Period	Treatment	Prevention and Control
Syphilis	*Treponema pallidum*	Infected exudates, body fluids, and secretions (saliva, semen, blood, vaginal secretions)	External genitalia; cervix; mucosal surfaces; placenta	Sexual activity; contact with open lesions; blood transfusion; transplacental inoculation	10–70 days	Penicillin; tetracycline	Case-finding by means of routine serologic testing and other methods; adequate treatment of infected individuals
Tetanus	*Clostridium tetani*	Contaminated soil	Penetrating and crush wounds	Horse and cattle feces	4–21 days (avg. 10 days)	Tetanus immune globulin (human—TIG) and tetanus toxoid; penicillin	Wound debridement; toxoid booster injections for patients previously immunized; tetanus toxoid and tetanus immune globulin (separate sites and separate syringes) for nonimmune persons
Trichinosis	*Trichinella spiralis*	Infected pigs	Gastrointestinal tract	Ingestion of infected pork, undercooked	2–28 days	Steroids; thiabendazole	Regulation of hog breeders; adequate meat inspection; thorough cooking of pork
Tuberculosis	*Mycobacterium tuberculosis*	Sputum from human cases; milk from infected cows (rare in U.S.)	Respiratory mucosa	Sputum; respiratory droplets	Variable	Isoniazid; ethambutol; rifampin; streptomycin; pyrazinamide	Early discovery and adequate treatment of active cases; milk pasteurization
Tularemia	*Francisella tularensis*	Wild rodents and rabbits	Eyes; skin; gastrointestinal tract	Handling infected animals; ingestion of undercooked, infected meat; drinking contaminated water; bites from infected flies, ticks	1–10 days	Streptomycin; tetracyclines; chloramphenicol	Use of rubber gloves when skinning/handling potentially infectious wild animals; avoidance of contact with potentially infected rodents; adequate cooking of wild rabbit dishes; vaccination of hunters, butchers, laboratory workers risking heavy exposure

(continued)

TABLE 59-1 (continued)

	Infective Organism	Infectious Sources	Entry Site	Method of Spread	Incubation Period	Chemotherapy*	Prophylaxis
Typhoid Fever	Salmonella typhi	Contaminated food and water	Gastrointestinal tract	Infected urine and feces	1-3 weeks	Chloramphenicol; ampicillin; sulfatrimethoprim	Decontamination of water sources; milk pasteurization; individual vaccination of high-risk persons; control of carriers.
Typhus, endemic	Rickettsia typhi (mooseri)	Infected rodents	Skin	Flea bites	1-2 weeks	Tetracyclines; chloramphenicol	Delousing procedures; case quarantine
Whooping cough (pertussis)	Bordetella pertussis	Human cases	Respiratory tract	Infected bronchial secretions	Commonly 7 days	Erythromycin; ampicillin	Active immunization with vaccine; case isolation

* Research developments produce changes in drug therapy. The reader is referred to drug brochures and digests to keep abreast of changing dosages and uses.

response after a single injection, and may have to be administered in repeated doses according to a prescribed schedule for long-lasting immunoglobulin response and sustained protection against infection. Following injection with inactivated vaccines and toxoids, there may be a mild local reaction at the site of injection and occasional systemic symptoms of fever, malaise, and headache.

Depending on age and health status, susceptible persons between ages 18 and 24 should be given tetanus and diphtheria toxoids and vaccines against measles, mumps, and rubella. Persons between 25 and 64 should receive a booster dose of tetanus and diphtheria toxoids every 10 years, and susceptible individuals in this group should be given measles, mumps, and rubella vaccines. Persons who are 65 years or older should be given a tetanus and diphtheria toxoid booster every 10 years, influenza vaccine annually, and pneumococcal polysaccharide vaccine one time (if they have not previously received this vaccine). Travelers to developing countries should be given additional appropriate vaccines.

Current recommendations for the administration of vaccines and other biologicals used in the prevention of disease are available from the Advisory Committee on Immunization Practices of the U.S. Public Health Service, Centers for Disease Control, Atlanta, Georgia 30333.

Nursing Considerations.   Before a vaccine is administered, the person is questioned about possible allergies, because some vaccines may contain trace amounts of antibiotics to which some people are allergic. For example, persons with a known allergy to eggs should not receive influenza vaccine because this vaccine is propagated in embryonated chicken eggs.

All vaccines have some side-effects. Immunosuppressed individuals or pregnant women are not usually given live-virus vaccines, and those persons with a febrile illness are not usually vaccinated.

The nurse should be aware that young adults may fall into the "immunization gap" for measles and rubella. Young adults born after 1959 grew up when such vaccines were first licensed but not mandatory. This group may be unprotected and at risk for developing measles and rubella, which may cause different clinical manifestations and complications in adults than in children.

Studies show that members of socially deprived and low-income groups often do not receive the protection of immunization programs; this is a challenge to all health care professionals. A person's acceptance of this type of preventive care may help him to accept other medical services. Nurses, using gentle persuasion, can listen to the fears of such people and teach them the benefits of immunization.

Passive Immunity

Passive immunity provides temporary protection from a disease. It is produced by the injection of serum that contains antibodies that have been formed in another host. The serum is given for immediate but temporary protection against a disease when active immunizing agents are not available (e.g., immune globulin for hepatitis A) or when there is insufficient time for the person to acquire active immunization following exposure to disease. (Passive immunity is not totally satisfactory because of the risk inherent in providing antibodies of one animal to another.)

Chart 59-1
Glossary of Infectious Disease Terms

Antigen—agent that is capable of producing antibodies when introduced into the body of a susceptible person

Antiserum—a serum containing antibodies given to provide immunity against a specific disease; usually regarded as temporary protection

Antitoxin—an antibody that neutralizes a bacterial toxin

Attenuation—the weakening of the toxicity or virulence of an infectious agent

Bacteremia—presence of bacteria in the circulating blood

Bactericidal—lethal or killing to bacteria

Carrier—one who harbors an infectious agent causing a specific disease, although he gives no evidence of having the disease

Case—a particular instance of disease

Communicable—transmissible from person to person, directly or indirectly

Contact—a person known or believed to have been exposed to an infectious disease

Contaminated—persons or objects that have come in contact with infectious agents or materials

Disinfection—destruction (or rendering inert) of pathogenic organisms by chemical or physical means

Endemic—a disease occurring habitually within a given geographic area

Endogenous infection—infection caused by microbes derived from the host's own flora

Epidemic—a disease attacking many people in a community simultaneously

Exanthem—an eruption on the skin

Exogenous infection—infection caused by microbes derived from outside the host

Fomites—inanimate vehicles other than food, milk, water, and air that may harbor or be the means of transmission of organisms

Immune—protected against disease

Incidence—number of new cases of a disease (or event) occurring in a specified time

Incubation period—the development of an infection from the time it gains entry into the body until the appearance of the first signs and symptoms

Infectious—capable of causing infection or disease

Infestation—invasion of body by arthropods, including insects, mites, mosquitoes, and ticks, and by helminths

In vitro—within the test tube

In vivo—within a living body

Morbidity rate—the number of illnesses compared to the population. The rate may be measured in *incidence* or *prevalence: incidence*—the number of cases occurring in the population in a year; *prevalence*—the average number of cases existing in the population.

Mortality rate—the number of deaths compared to the population

Nosocomial infection—infection acquired during hospitalization; not present or incubating at the time of admission to hospital

Pandemic—disease affecting a large portion of the population; extensive epidemic

Pathogenic—disease-producing

Prevalence—ratio of the total number of all individuals who have a disease at a particular time to the population at risk of having the disease

Prodromal—symptoms occurring at the beginning stage of the disease

Prophylaxis—measures taken to prevent disease

Surveillance—dynamic system of collecting, tabulating, analyzing, and reporting data on the occurrence and distribution of disease

Toxin—a poisonous substance produced by bacterial action

Toxoid—a modified toxin capable of stimulating the production of antibodies

Vaccine—a suspension of attenuated or killed microorganisms or their components given to build up an active immunity against an infectious disease

There are several types of preparations in use for passive immunity: standard immune globulin (for general use), special immune serum globulins with a known antibody content for specific illnesses, and animal serums or antitoxins. Products made with animal serum may cause an anaphylaxis-like reaction or serum sickness; therefore, products made with human serum are given whenever possible.

Reporting Communicable Diseases

Incidences of communicable diseases are reported to local public health authorities. This is important in order to keep track of these diseases and initiate investigative or control measures. The local health department forwards the information to the state health department, which transmits weekly reports to the Centers for Disease Control (CDC) in Atlanta, Georgia, where data about communicable and chronic disease are compiled and published in the *Morbidity and Mortality Weekly Report*. This publication provides an up-to-date picture of epidemiologic notes, trends, and reports and feeds back this information to local health departments, people in the field, and others with a need for the information. Thus, the occurrence of any local communicable disease becomes part of a huge network of health surveillance. The CDC operations include epidemiology and disease surveillance, laboratory methods, health education, and organized disease prevention and control programming and training.

The World Health Organization (WHO) receives data about communicable diseases from all countries. Regional epidemiologists keep a careful watch on regional disease trends and disseminate this information to the appropriate people and services within the various countries. Computers are used to help in this rapid dissemination of information.

Controlling Infectious Diseases in the Hospital: Isolation

Isolation precautions are used to prevent the transmission of infectious agents among patients, health care personnel, and visitors. Isolation precautions are used to isolate the infection rather than the patient. Systems for isolation precautions designed by the CDC include Category-Specific Isolation Precautions, in which diseases are grouped by categories, and Disease-Specific Isolation Precautions, in which only the particular precautions for interrupting transmission of the specific disease are recommended.

Isolation precautions may also be established by an individual health agency. The infection control committee of the agency makes the decision about which of the alternative systems of isolation precautions is to be used. Each hospital prepares a manual that includes the specific part of the CDC guideline that pertains to the approach that has been adopted, and incorporates the information into the procedure manual which is distributed to each nursing unit. Standards of practice are evaluated in the light of new information and changing situations. Isolation recommendations are revised periodically.

Techniques for Isolation Precautions

Hand Washing. *Hand washing is the single most important means of preventing the spread of infection.* Hand washing can markedly reduce or eliminate the spread of pathogenic organisms by the hands. Lathering the hands and vigorously rubbing together all lathered surfaces, followed by a thorough rinsing under a stream of water, suspends and rinses away microoganisms. Plain soaps or detergents may be used. Antiseptics are recommended for hand washing when the patient being cared for has been infected with virulent or epidemiologically important microorganisms, especially in intensive care units.

Private Room. A private room is indicated for patients with conditions that are highly infectious (contagious) or those caused by microorganisms that are likely to be virulent when transmitted. A private room is also indicated if the patient has poor hygiene habits that contaminate the environment (*e.g.*, carelessness with excretions). A private room may also be required for patients colonized with microorganisms of special clinical or epidemiologic significance (*e.g.*, multiple resistant bacteria), or for patients whose blood is infective, and if profuse bleeding is likely to expose people in the area to contamination.

Masks, Gowns, and Gloves. Except in patients routinely requiring strict isolation, where masks, gowns, and gloves are uniformly indicated, the health care worker who assigns isolation precautions to the patient has the responsibility in deciding when such precautionary attire is necessary. This decision is based on the likelihood of exposure to infectious material. For example, a nurse who comes in close contact with a patient who is coughing will decide if it is necessary to wear a mask when giving care to the patient. If clothing may become soiled with infectious secretions or excretions, the nurse may decide to wear a gown. If infected materials (excretions, secretions, blood, body fluids) will be touched, gloves are indicated. This approach allows health care workers more responsibility in assuring their own safety and needs.

General Management

The key to management of the infection is identifying the specific organism and instituting specific therapy when available. The drug of choice is usually the most active drug against the pathogenic organism or the least toxic alternative. Supportive therapy includes monitoring the patient's response to therapy; ensuring hydration, fluid balance, and oxygenation; and maintaining constant watchfulness for complications.

▶ Nursing Process
The Patient With an Infectious Disease

▷ Assessment

Many early symptoms of infectious diseases are nonspecific. The illness may begin with malaise and all its attendant sequelae—listlessness, lightheadedness, headache, anorexia, arthralgia. As the disease progresses there is usually fever, although elderly people in general do not have as vigorous a febrile response as younger people, nor will patients who have previously received antibiotics or who are taking immunosuppressive agents exhibit fever.

Other clinical features that are suggestive of infection include chills, myalgia, photophobia, pharyngitis, acute lymphadenopathy, nausea, and vomiting. Since the signs and symptoms associated with infection are a result of the host's inflammatory response as well as the direct response to the pathogen, they can be nonspecific. (The reader is referred to chapters on specific organs or systems for signs and symptoms that suggest infection of a particular organ site.)

In taking the nursing history, it is important to ask the following questions:

- History of fever? Chills? (Abrupt onset of fever is associated with chills.)
- Night sweats? (associated with intermittent fever)
- Back pain? General myalgias? Arthralgias? Headache? (All are commonly associated with fever.)
- Sore throat?
- Diarrhea? (Anyone in family have diarrhea?) Vomiting? Abdominal pain?
- Dysuria? Purulent discharge?
- Evidence of local infection: Redness? Heat? Swelling? Pain?
- Contact with an ill person? His/her secretions/excretions?
- Insect bite? Animal bite? Cat scratch? Exposure to rodents or birds?
- Illness that compromises the body's defenses?
- Medications, especially antibiotics, being taken? Alcohol intake?
- History of sexual practices?
- Travel to or from a developing country?
- Place of work?
- Vaccination history?

While performing the physical examination, look for the manifestations common to many infectious diseases. Observe for breaks in the skin, skin rashes, skin and mucous membrane lesions, productive cough, breathing difficulties, purulent drainage from any site, and lymph node enlargement. Evaluate the nutritional status.

For assessment, the nurse needs to know about specific organisms, where and when they occur, how they can be controlled or eliminated, who is at risk, and some information about the patient's environment. In reviewing the findings, one of the nursing decisions is to determine if the patient is at risk of infecting himself or others.

Gerontological Considerations. Many elderly people with infections develop the typical signs and symptoms. However, infection in those who do not develop these signs and symptoms may come to the attention of the health care provider as a result of other health problems that appear in any illness of the elderly, such as incontinence, confusion, immobility, or falling. Diagnostic evaluation for infection and appropriate therapy are essential so that the underlying infectious condition can be managed along with the presenting problem.

▷ *Nursing Diagnoses*

Ineffective Breathing Patterns. An altered breathing pattern in the patient with an infectious disease may result from the disease itself or occur when the normal respiratory defense mechanisms have become impaired or overwhelmed by microbial assault. Also, patients with impaired cell-mediated immunity are susceptible to bacterial, viral, and fungal pneumonias.

Alteration in Body Temperature. Fever is a common symptom of illness. It may occur as a result of a specific infection or a nosocomial infection related to invasive devices used to monitor and support the patient, or it may be of unknown origin.

Potential Fluid Volume Deficit. Fluid volume deficits in infectious illnesses can result from excessive fever, sweating, and watery diarrhea. Inability to ingest fluids is another cause and can lead to serious dehydration.

Alteration in Integrity of Oral Mucous Membranes. The oral tissues are bathed by the patient's own microbial flora and by other organisms that enter the mouth by way of food, water, and other substances. The normal flow of saliva and the motion of the lips, cheeks, and tongue help maintain the integrity of the oral mucosa. The combination of fever, dyspnea, and inability to ingest fluids and food can cause dryness and cracking of the mucous membranes. Viral infections affect the oral mucosa, beginning as vesicles and rapidly develop into ulcers. The patient receiving chemotherapy may have painful mouth ulcers from the toxic effect of the drug or may be increasingly susceptible to infection. Fungal infection involving the oral mucosa is also found in patients receiving chemotherapy. The treatment of the cause of the oral lesions is individualized, but the problems encountered by the patient, such as oral discomfort, can be relieved by appropriate nursing interventions.

Alteration in Bowel Elimination (Diarrhea). Normal bowel flora plays an important protective role. Anytime the bowel flora is altered (*e.g.*, by taking broad-spectrum antibiotics), diarrhea may ensue. The normal flora of the bowel can be overcome by large numbers of virulent organisms such as occurs in salmonellosis. Diarrhea is a common illness of travelers. Acute-onset diarrhea is caused by a variety of bacterial, parasitic, and viral agents, which will be discussed under the appropriate conditions.

Alteration in Nutrition. A severe and prolonged infection may result in muscle wasting and weight loss, because protein is being catabolized for energy. Patients who have been acutely ill and who have been without protein and calorie intake for several days, or who were malnourished at the onset of their illness, will require extra nutritional support.

Knowledge Deficit. One major goal in the health education of all people is to inculcate a sense of responsibility for their own health and the need to avoid injury to others. Additionally, the person with an infectious disease is taught about his specific disease and the therapeutic regimen, and in some instances is instructed about personal hygiene and the maintenance of the home environment for infection prevention. Patients who have immigrated from developing countries may have diseases that reflect crowding and poor sanitation. This situation will require specific teaching.

Potential for Infection (Spread to Others). When caring for those with infectious diseases, all health care personnel must prevent the spread of infection to others. The types of infection control precautions used are based on the mode of transmission of the disease.

Potential for Social Isolation. The patient with an acute illness may exhibit anxiety and ineffective coping strategies that are related to physiologic and organic disturbances brought about by the illness, the patient's underlying emotional state, the effects of hospitalization (isolation), and negative interaction with health care personnel (*e.g.*, inadequate explanation). These factors can cause a combination of problems, including social isolation.

▷ *Planning and Implementation*

▷ *Goals:* The major goals of the patient may include attainment of normal breathing pattern, attainment of normal body temperature, achievement of fluid balance, achievement of intact and healthy oral mucous membranes, attainment of normal bowel elimination, improvement of nutritional status, acquisition of knowledge about the condition, prevention of the spread of infection, and achievement of social participation.

Nursing Interventions

Attaining a Normal Breathing Pattern. Health care personnel must be aware of which patients are at risk for pulmonary infection and subsequent ineffective breathing patterns. Patients with pre-existing illness (immunosuppression, alcoholism, drug overdose) tend to have impaired lung clearance. Viral infections and hematologic malignancies depress the cellular defenses of the lungs. Pulmonary compliance is decreased in aging patients. Pulmonary infection also occurs as a result of mechanical disruption of pulmonary defenses, as is seen in the patient with endotracheal intubation.

The nurse monitors these high-risk patients for cough, shortness of breath, change in skin color, and altered chest movements. Respiratory rate, depth, and pattern are assessed. The patient's chest is auscultated for breath sounds.

Turning the patient and changing his position help drain secretions and thus reduce the potential for retention of secretions and infection. Yawning, taking deep breaths, and coughing help expand alveolar sacs. If the patient is not able to raise secretions effectively, suctioning is indicated. A high fluid intake (within limits of the patient's cardiac reserve) is encouraged because adequate hydration thins mucus and serves as an effective expectorant. The air may be humidified to loosen secretions and improve ventilation. As soon as his condition permits, the patient is encouraged to ambulate, because this activity helps mobilize secretions and expand the lungs.

If the patient show signs of respiratory insufficiency, arterial blood gas values are obtained and recorded on a flow sheet so that comparisons can be made over time.

Attaining Normal Body Temperature. The patient's temperature, pulse, and respiration are taken at regular intervals to deterine the type of fever (continuous, remittent, or intermittent). These checks also help monitor the severity and duration of the infectious process and the patient's response to therapy. Since not all infected patients have a febrile response, the patient is assessed for signs and symptoms of infection: headache, joint pain, muscle aches, backache, cough, diarrhea, and enlarged lymph nodes.

Oral fluids are encouraged because an adequate fluid intake is important to replace fluid losses due to fever, diaphoresis, dehydration, and dyspnea. Nursing interventions to combat the generalized discomfort that accompanies fever include helping the patient change positions, giving back massages, providing intermittent cool compresses for headache, and encouraging rest to lower metabolic activity. Oral hygiene promotes comfort and may help prevent oral complications, since many bacterial, mycotic, and viral infections affect the oral cavity.

Although fever occurring during infection may be beneficial and may enhance host defenses, there are times when fever may be deleterious; high fever can permanently damage body tissues. Tepid water sponging of the entire body cools the body through evaporation of water.

The aging patient with fever requires special nursing surveillance. Fever increases the heart rate, decreases diastolic filling time, and reduces stroke output. Decreased cardiac output in the elderly may cause reductions in perfusion and in the delivery of oxygen to the brain and kidneys. Many older patients, however, may have serious infections with minimal or no rise in temperature.

Attaining Fluid Balance. The patient is assessed for signs of dehydration: thirst, dryness of mucous membranes, loss of skin turgor, muscle cramping, reduced peripheral pulses, and decreasing urine output. Skin turgor is evaluated by pinching the skin over the sternum, the inner aspects of the thighs, or the forehead. If the patient has a fluid volume deficit, the skin flattens more slowly after the pinch is released. The patient's oral cavity is inspected for dryness, and the tongue is examined for longitudinal furrows. The weight is monitored because changes in weight indicate fluid volume changes. A rapid loss of weight occurs when the total fluid intake is less than the total fluid output. Serum electrolyte values are noted because dehydration produces a deficit of some electrolytes. The nurse also keeps an intake and output record and monitors urine specific gravity. Concentrated scanty urine indicates a lack of fluids. When oliguria (low urine output in relation to fluid intake) is present, urinary specific gravity increases.

Oral administration of fluids is preferable to intravenous administration. Varying the type and temperature of oral fluids is helpful. If the patient is vomiting or critically ill, the nurse administers the prescribed intravenous fluids. Nursing interventions include informing the patient about the procedure, selecting a suitable vein, regulating and maintaining the proper rate of infusion flow, ensuring patient comfort, and monitoring the patient for untoward effects of intravenous therapy.

Mouth Care. Infectious diseases may be accompanied by changes in and lesions of the oral cavity. Inspect the patient's oral cavity for color, signs of infection, bleeding, and the presence of lesions, cracks, or coatings.

The patient is taught the importance of oral hygiene and assisted when necessary. Warm normal saline or warm water rinsing of the mouth removes debris and helps keep the oral mucosa clean and moist. Strong mouthwashes and antiseptic gargles are avoided. Petrolatum, water-soluble jelly, or mineral oil may be applied to cracked, dry lips to keep them soft and moist. Frequent toothbrushing and flossing remove plaque and help prevent gingivitis.

A high-calorie liquid diet is given when ingestion of solid food is difficult because of painful oral lesions. If oral discomfort persists, a topical anesthetic agent may be prescribed. Chewing is important for oral health, and the patient is encouraged to eat as soon as he is able.

Attaining Normal Bowel Elimination. Most of the diarrheal illnesses that occur are mild and self-limiting. Diarrhea may be antibiotic agent colitis, traveler's diarrhea, food- or water-borne diarrhea, or the type of diarrhea seen in immunosuppressed persons. In taking the nursing history, try to determine whether the patient has taken an antibiotic recently, has traveled to a developing country, or is immunosuppressed.

The patient is asked about the number, color, and form of his stools and whether blood and mucus are present. The existence of other clinical manifestations, such as nausea, vomiting, fever, and abdominal pain, is elicited. The number of stools in 24 hours will give a clue in determining how disabling the patient's diarrhea is. In addition, the patient is assessed for signs of dehydration. The patient's intake, output, and weight are monitored and recorded.

An important nursing function is the collection of fecal specimens. Enteric precautions are required, since there is a wide range of viral, bacterial, and parasitic causes of diarrhea. (Negative cultures do not rule out infectious etiology.)

Fluids and electrolytes represent the essential therapy. Oral fluids (oral glucose and electrolyte-containing rehydration solution) are given when the patient is able to tolerate them. Parenteral fluid replacement is necessary if severe dehydration is present.

The patient is instructed to cleanse the perianal area with mild soap and water and blot the area dry after each bowel movement. This promotes comfort and prevents skin excoriation. The perianal area is inspected for signs of skin breakdown.

Enteric precautions are used in the hospitalized patient with infectious diarrhea. Proper hand washing and the practice of good personal hygiene are emphasized. Other nursing interventions include promoting patient comfort and advising rest for the patient who is having frequent bouts of watery diarrhea.

Improving Nutritional Status. An assessment is made of what the patient is actually eating, because the generalized malaise, discomfort, and anorexia that accompany infections may cause a lack of interest in food. Additionally, the patient with fever has increased catabolism and loss of nutrients. The patient's weight is monitored.

A high-calorie, high-protein diet is necessary for patients with fever to replenish energy used by increased metabolism and restlessness. Increased protein is needed to counteract the loss of nitrogen. Increased fluids are necessary to replenish losses due to perspiration and increased respiratory rate.

A referral may be made to the dietitian so that a diet plan can be tailored to the patient's condition and food preferences. The patient is helped to understand that he will require optimum nutrition during and beyond convalescence to replenish nutrient losses associated with an acute infectious disease, even of short duration. The patient is also encouraged to monitor his weight.

Patient Education. Listening to the patient gives the nurse an opportunity to learn what he knows about his illness and treatment and to detect and correct misunderstandings and misinformation.

Brief and focused explanations can be made about the organism and how it is spread, how the illness is treated, the importance of personal hygiene and environmental cleanliness, and the importance of seeking health care promptly in the event of an infectious disease. Knowledge of his specific illness and treatment imparts a sense of control to the patient and helps him become an active participant in his care. The nurse encourages the patient to ask questions because they serve as a guide to topics that need further clarification.

Health care personnel serve as educators in the prevention of infectious diseases. The program of instruction includes teaching about how infectious diseases are spread, methods of avoiding spread, the importance and availability of immunizations, the role of nutrition in health maintenance, and the control of environmental contaminants, insects, rodents, and other animal vectors and reservoirs of human infections.

Preventing the Spread of Infection. Efforts are directed toward controlling the infectious agent at its source. This includes proper hand washing, using a gown when clothing is likely to become soiled with infective secretions or excretions, and using gloves when indicated by the patient's condition (*e.g.,* when excretions, secretions, blood, or body fluids are considered to be infective material). Needles and syringes are handled with extreme caution because it is usually not known whether a patient's blood is contaminated with hepatitis or HIV viruses. Because accidental needle puncture can occur, needles should not be recapped or broken by hand after use. Wastes should also be handled with all due precautions.

Dissemination of infectious droplets can be controlled by teaching the patient to cover his nose and mouth when coughing or sneezing, bagging and labeling used paper tissues according to agency policy, and handling soiled linen as little as possible.

Environmental cleanliness is maintained by damp dusting of furniture and wet vacuuming of floors, and by reducing to a minimum the activity of personnel in the area. The patient's room is ventilated with a system that directs room air to the outside. The door to the room should be kept closed in the case of an infectious disease that can be spread by aerosolized droplets.

Promoting Social Participation. Patients with infectious diseases may experience heightened states of anxiety, fear, and depression. These dysfunctional emotions reduce the patient's ability to cope with his illness.

An assessment is made of how the patient is reacting to his illness. The patient's family or other support system may have a valuable stress-reducing effect on the patient, and

they are encouraged to visit. Ongoing and regular visits by health care personnel demonstrate to the patient that he is cared for. Being available, answering questions, exploring anxieties that prompt questions, and employing empathetic listening can be therapeutic and can relieve the patient's sense of loneliness. Skilled nursing care promotes the patient's well-being. Stress reduction techniques may be useful.

The patient with a sexually transmitted disease requires an understanding and sensitive approach. Fear of AIDS is widespread and particularly devastating to the patient. AIDS patients may be placed in isolation, which makes them feel particularly stigmatized and untouchable. Coping with this illness is extremely stressful. The nurse's compassionate care, which includes providing information about financial and other entitlements and community resources, can fortify the patient. Crisis intervention and mental health services are available and may be appropriate to help the patient and his family begin the process of adaptation.

▷ *Evaluation*

▷ *Expected Outcomes*

1. Patient attains normal breathing pattern.
2. Demonstrates absence of elevated body temperature.
3. Attains fluid balance.
4. Attains/maintains healthy and intact oral mucous membranes.
5. Attains normal defecation pattern.
6. Achieves improved nutritional status.
7. Acquires some understanding of the infectious process.
8. Shows no evidence of spread of infection.
9. Achieves reduction of stress imposed by social isolation.

Nursing Care Plan 59-1 summarizes the care of the patient with an infectious disease.

Sexually Transmitted Diseases (STDs)

Sexually transmitted diseases (STDs) are diseases acquired through sexual activity with an infected person. These diseases include the traditional "venereal diseases" (gonorrhea, syphilis, chancroid, lymphogranuloma inguinale, and lymphogranuloma venereum) and a complex array of infections and clinical syndromes that make up a new generation of STDs, of which the newest and most serious is acquired immunodeficiency syndrome (AIDS).

The term *sexually transmitted disease* has replaced *venereal disease* as the term of choice. Sexually transmitted diseases are the most common infections in the United States and are epidemic in most of the world. Portals of entry of STD microorganisms and sites of infection include the skin and mucosal linings of the urethra, cervix, vagina, rectum, and oropharynx. Over 21 diseases are classifed as sexually transmitted diseases (Table 59-2, p. 1660). This is due to the increasingly varying nature of sexual practices and attitudes, personal mobility, the number of persons reaching the age of sexual activity, the trend toward nonbarrier methods of

(Text continues on p. 1658)

Care of the Patient With an Infectious Disease

Nursing Interventions	*Rationale*	*Expected Outcomes*

Nursing Diagnosis: Ineffective breathing pattern related to an inflammatory/infectious process

Goal: Attainment of normal breathing pattern

1. Be aware of patient at risk for pulmonary infection:
  a. Immunosuppressed; preexisting pulmonary problems
  b. Aged
 	
  c. Immobilized
 	
  d. Decreased level of awareness
 	
  e. Viral infections, hematologic malignancies
  f. Anesthetized; endotracheal intubation
	1. Patients with predisposing illness (immunosuppression, alcoholism, drug overdose), tend to have impaired mechanical lung clearance.
	  b. Pulmonary compliance is decreased in aging.
	  c. Immobility causes increased secretions, promoting atelectasis and producing generalized hypoxia.
	  d. Depression of respiratory centers in medulla and pons have limited responses to breathing reflexes.
	  e. These depress cellular defenses of lung.
	  f. Pulmonary infection occurs from mechanical disruption of pulmonary defenses.
		• Patient attains normal breathing pattern.
		• Performs deep-breathing exercises.
		• Coughs at prescribed intervals.
		• Increases activity tolerance progressively.
		• Chest clear upon auscultation.
		• Respirations regular.

2. Conduct ongoing pulmonary assessment; look for cough, shortness of breath, change in skin color, altered chest movements.
  a. Auscultate for breath sounds.
  b. Assess respiratory rate, depth, and pattern.
  c. Evaluate laboratory data.		

3. Turn patient at least every 2 hours, more frequently if problem develops.	3. Turning and changing position helps drain secretions; drainage of airway secretions reduces potential for retention of secretions and infection.	
4. Encourage patient to cough; suction his secretions if necessary.		
5. Instruct and demonstrate how to yawn, take deep breaths, and cough at prescribed times (hourly, *etc.*)	5. This helps expand alveolar sacs and prevent collapse.	
6. Ambulate patient as soon as condition permits.	6. Ambulation helps mobilize secretions and expands the lungs.	

Nursing Diagnosis: Alteration in body temperature (fever) related to the presence of infection

Goal: Attainment of normal body temperature

1. Take temperature, pulse and respiration at regular intervals.	1. This helps determine the type (continuous, remittent, intermittent) of fever. It also helps monitor the severity and duration of the infectious process.	• Absence of elevated body temperature. • Pulse within normal limits of individual patient. • Patient maintains adequate fluid intake. • Patient appears more comfortable.

(continued)

Nursing Interventions	*Rationale*	*Expected Outcomes*

Nursing Diagnosis: Alteration in body temperature (fever) related to the presence of infection

Goal: Attainment of normal body temperature

2. Monitor for localizing symptoms and physical findings (headache, pain, tenderness; cough, diarrhea, adenopathy).	2. Not all infected patients have a febrile response.	• Absence of chills and sweats.
3. Pay special attention to the aging patient with fever.	3. Older patients may have serious types of infection with minimal or no rise in temperature, or they may be hypothermic. Fever increases the heart rate, decreases diastolic filling time, and decreases stroke output; thus, reduced cardiac output in the elderly may cause unacceptable perfusion and delivery of oxygen to the brain and kidneys.	
4. Encourage increased oral intake of fluids (if permitted).	4. An adequate fluid intake is important to replace insensible losses via sweat and lungs but also to prevent the complications of infection (shock, renal failure).	
5. Lower the body temperature, when fever itself may be deleterious, by tepid water sponging of the entire body.	5. Fever occurring during infection may be beneficial and benefit host defense. Tepid water sponging cools the body by evaporation of water.	
6. Combat generalized discomfort. a. Help patient change position and suggest positions of comfort. b. Encourage frequent oral hygiene. c. Apply cold compresses for headache intermittently. d. Use massage as necessary. e. Encourage the patient to rest and limit physical activity.	b. A large number of bacterial, mycotic, and viral infections may produce oral manifestations. Oral hygiene helps prevent oral complications and promotes comfort. e. Resting lowers the metabolic activity.	

Nursing Diagnosis: Potential fluid volume deficit related to body's response to infectious process (excessive sweating, fever, watery diarrhea)

Goal: Attainment of fluid balance

1. Assess for dehydration (thirst, dryness of mucous membranes, loss of skin turgor, muscle cramping, reduced peripheral pulses, and decreasing urine output).	1. These are signs and symptoms of serious dehydration which can lead to mental obtundation and circulatory collapse.	• Patient attains fluid balance (output approximates intake). • Mucous membranes appear moist; normal skin turgor. • Patient takes adequate amounts of fluids orally. • Serum electrolytes and urine specific gravity within normal limits.
2. Monitor temperature and weight.	2. Fever increases loss of fluids (from perspiration, increased respirations). Changes in weight indicate fluid volume changes.	
3. Monitor serum electrolytes, urine specific gravity, and intake and output.	3. Dehydration produces a deficit of some electrolytes. Concentrated scanty urine indicates lack of fluids; urinary specific gravity increases when oliguria is present.	

(continued)

Nursing Interventions	*Rationale*	*Expected Outcomes*

Nursing Diagnosis: Potential fluid volume deficit related to body's response to infectious process (excessive sweating, fever, watery diarrhea)

Goal: Attainment of fluid balance

4. Ensure adequate hydration in the event of excessive fluid loss through diarrhea or excessive sweating.	4. Oral hydration is preferable, since this can be done at home. Fruit juices contain sugar and potassium; bouillon provides salt.	
5. If patient is critically ill or vomiting, prepare for administration of intravenous fluids (usually dextrose and normal saline) as required.*	5. Glucose facilitates intestinal reabsorption of electrolytes.	

Nursing Diagnosis: Alteration in integrity of oral mucous membranes related to loss of fluids (fever, sweating) and anorexia

Goal: Achievement of intact and healthy oral mucous membranes

1. Inspect oral cavity for color, signs of infection or edema, presence of lesions, cracks, coatings, or bleeding.	1. Infectious organisms can present with intra-oral manifestations.	• Patient attains/maintains healthy and intact oral mucous membranes. • Has no complaints of oral discomfort/pain. • Absence of oral lesions.
2. Emphasize the importance of oral hygiene; assist patient when necessary.		
a. Use oral mouthwashes (warm normal saline, sodium bicarbonate rinses, *etc.*).	a. Rinsing removes debris and helps keep oral mucosa clean, moist, and intact.	
b. Apply petrolatum, water-soluble jelly, or mineral oil to dry, cracked lips.	b. Lubrication of lips keeps them soft, moist, and intact.	
c. Encourage frequent toothbrushing and flossing.	c. Brushing and flossing removes plaque and help prevent gingivitis.	
3. Maintain adequate fluid intake.	3. Hydration is necessary for healthy moist mucous membranes.	
4. Encourage patient to eat (as indicated).	4. Chewing is important for oral health.	

Nursing Diagnosis: Alteration in bowel elimination (diarrhea) related to infectious agent

Goal: Achievement of normal bowel elimination

1. Take a nursing history to determine if patient	1. Most of the diarrheal illnesses that occur are mild and self-limiting. Diarrhea may be antibiotic-agent colitis, traveler's diarrhea, or food or water-borne diarrhea, or it may be present in immunosuppressed or homosexual individuals.	• Patient achieves normal defecation pattern. • Has stools of normal color and consistency. • Absence of cramping and abdominal pain. • Absence of signs and symptoms of dehydration.
a. Has taken an antibiotic recently.		
b. Has traveled to a developing country.		
c. Has other family members with diarrhea.		
d. Is immunosuppressed or homosexual.		

* Interdependent and collaborative nursing functions.

(continued)

Nursing Interventions	*Rationale*	*Expected Outcomes*

Nursing Diagnosis: Alteration in bowel elimination (diarrhea) related to infectious agent

Goal: Achievement of normal bowel elimination

2. Assess patient's signs and symptoms, and assess stools for character and consistency.
   a. Clinical manifestations: Nausea? vomiting? fever? (how long?) abdominal pain?
   b. Stools: Soft? formed? bloody? watery?
	2. Observation of color, form, or presence of blood and mucus in stool may help determine the cause of diarrhea.

3. Assess for severity and intensity of acute diarrhea. Determine how disabling the patient's diarrhea is:
   Number of unformed stools/24 hr:
   Mild illness: 1–3 stools/24 hr
   Moderate illness: 3–5 stools/24 hr
   More severe illness: 6 or more stools/24 hr
	3. Moderate or severe diarrhea is usually of infectious origins.

4. Assess for thirst, dryness of mucous membranes, loss of skin turgor and elasticity, muscle cramps, reduced peripheral pulses, and decreased urine output.	4. These are manifestations of dehydration; severe dehydration leads to mental obtundation and circulatory collapse.
5. Using enteric precautions, collect and send fecal specimens to the laboratory for examination.	5. There is a wide range of viral, bacterial, and parasitic causes of diarrhea in different settings. When the history or fecal leukocyte findings indicate an infectious process, a culture for invasive pathogens is usually done.
6. Offer oral fluids (oral glucose and electrolyte-containing rehydration solution).	6. Fluids and electrolytes represent the essential therapy. Some enteropathogens cause a derangement of fluid and electrolyte balance.
7. Maintain careful surveillance if patient is immunocompromised.	7. In the immunologically compromised patient, infection may not be contained and systemic spread occurs.
8. Cleanse perianal area with mild soap and water after each bowel movement; blot area dry. Inspect for skin breakdown.	8. This promotes comfort and prevents skin excoriation and breakdown.
9. Instruct patient/family in hand washing techniques.	9. Hand washing is the foundation of infection control.
10. Teach patient/family to a. Monitor consistency and number of stools.	a. Acute diarrhea is often self-limited, but if patient does not improve and watery stools continue, re-examination is required. An antimicrobial agent for specific pathogens may be necessary.

(continued)

Nursing Interventions	*Rationale*	*Expected Outcomes*

Nursing Diagnosis: Alteration in bowel elimination (diarrhea) related to infectious agent

Goal: Achievement of normal bowel elimination

b. Monitor weight and intake and output.	b. Weight changes indicate fluid volume changes (loss or gain).	
c. Report to physician/clinic if fever recurs or if patient has persistent or bloody diarrhea.		

Nursing Diagnosis: Alteration in nutrition (less than body requirements) related to metabolic changes from infection and lack of interest in food

Goal: Improvement in nutritional status

1. Perform a nutritional assessment. a. Assess for decrease in food intake; institute a calorie count.	a. Generalized malaise, discomfort, and anorexia accompany infections, causing disinterest in food.	• Patient achieves improved nutritional status. • Increases oral intake. • Verbalizes beginning understanding of nutritional needs following an infectious illness.
b. Monitor progress of fever.	b. With fever there are increases in catabolism and loss of nutrients; the catabolic response and magnitude of loss are proportional to severity and duration of fever.	
c. Monitor weight	c. Any infectious illness causes metabolic and biochemical changes and triggers the stress response, with accompanying hypermetabolism and negative balances of nitrogen, potassium, phosphorus, and magnesium, and consequent weight loss.	
2. Offer high-calorie, high-protein diet; offer small liquid feedings at first, gradually adding foods that are readily digested as tolerated.	2. Sufficient calories are necessary for patients with fever to replenish energy used by increased metabolism and restlessness. Increased protein is required to counteract the loss of nitrogen.	
3. Encourage liberal fluid intake (3000–4000 ml/24 hr); usually fluids that appeal to patient are satisfactory. Educate the patient:	3. Increased fluids are necessary to replenish losses through perspiration, increased respiratory rate, *etc.*	
a. Encourage patient to continue with optimum plan of nutrition during (and beyond) convalescence.	a. It may take several weeks to replenish nutrient losses associated with an acute infection of short duration.	
b. Continue to monitor weight.	b. If infection is severe and prolonged, there will be muscle wasting and weight loss because protein is catabolized for energy.	
c. Take vitamin supplements as prescribed.	c. Fever increases vitamin requirements (B complex vitamins, ascorbic acid, vitamin A). Antibiotics may inferfere with intestinal synthesis of B complex vitamins.	

(continued)

Nursing Interventions	*Rationale*	*Expected Outcomes*

Nursing Diagnosis: Knowledge deficit concerning cause of infection, treatment, and preventive measures

Goal: Acquisition of understanding of infectious process

1. Listen carefully to what the patient says about his illness and treatment.

2. Keep explanations brief and focused about
   a. Organism and how spread.
   b. Where and when occurs.
   c. How treated.
   d. Importance of environmental cleanliness and personal hygiene.
   e. Importance of seeking health care in the event of a febrile illness or skin eruption, *etc.*

3. Allow for opportunities for questions and discussions.

4. Teach the patient and family about
   a. Availability and importance of prophylactic immunization.
   b. Manner in which infectious illnesses are spread and methods of avoiding spread.
   c. Means of preventing the contamination of food and water supplies.
   d. Importance of adequate nutrition and housing.
   e. Knowledge of insect, rodent, and other animal vectors and reservoirs of human infections and the importance of eliminating them.

1. Listening allows for detection and correction of misunderstanding and misinformation.

2. Knowledge of his specific illness and treatment imparts a sense of control and makes future more predictable and manageable as well as makes the patient an active participant in his care. The act of explanation is, in itself, reassuring.

3. The patient's questions can serve as a guide to topics that need clarification.

4. Education can change human behavior and is an effective way of reducing the risk of infection.

- Patient acquires some understanding of infectious process.
- Relates cause of problem and therapy at a level consistent with intellectual and emotional states.
- Gives feedback of knowledge.
- Actively participates in treatment.

Nursing Diagnosis: Potential for infection (spread of infection to others)

Goal: Prevention of spread of infection

1. Prevent spread of infection.

   a. Wash hands immediately after contact with each patient and after every contact with material that may be contaminated and potentially infectious.
   b. Use gown when indicated; use gown once and discard in appropriate receptacle.

1. Control efforts are directed toward controlling the agent at its source.
   a. Hand washing is the most important procedure for preventing infection.

   b. Gowns are indicated when clothes are likely to be soiled with infective secretions/excretions or when patients have infections that, if transmitted in hospitals, frequently cause serious illness (varicella, disseminated zoster).

- No evidence of spread of infection.
- Personnel employ hand washing at appropriate times.
- Personnel use effective isolation techniques that are appropriate for patients known or suspected to be infected.

(continued)

Nursing Interventions	*Rationale*	*Expected Outcomes*

Nursing Diagnosis: Potential for infection (spread of infection to others)

Goal: Prevention of spread of infection

c. Use masks as indicated.	c. In general, masks are used to prevent transmission of infectious agents through the air. If infection is transmitted by large-particle aerosols, masks may be worn by those close to the patient. If infection (small particle aerosols) is transmitted over longer distances, masks are worn by all persons entering the room.
d. Use gloves when indicated by the patient's condition: (1) Disposable single-use gloves are preferable. (2) Use once and discard in appropriate receptacle.	d. Wearing gloves is indicated for touching the excretions, secretions, blood, or body fluids considered to be infective material.
e. Handle needles and syringes with extreme caution. Avoid recapping needles or bending or breaking by hand after use.	e. It is usually not known if the patient's blood is contaminated with hepatitis or HIV viruses. Accidental needle puncture may occur. Caution must be exercised when handling any used needle.
f. Handle wastes with all due precautions.	
g. Control dissemination of infectious droplets. (1) Teach patient to cover his nose and mouth when coughing or sneezing. (2) Bag and label used paper tissues and dispose according to agency policy.	
h. Handle soiled linen as little as possible; avoid shaking bedlinens.	h. This prevents gross microbial contamination of the air and of persons handling the linen.

(continued)

contraception (*e.g.,* the contraceptive pill), and the problem of locating and bringing to treatment the "silent carriers" of these infections. Those at high risk for acquiring STDs are homosexual or bisexual men, sexual partners of infected persons, and those with multiple sex partners. In the developing countries, prostitution is the major reservoir for syphilis, chancroid, and gonorrhea.

Problems and Risk Factors

The problems and complications of STDs are challenging. They frequently exist without causing symptoms. A high incidence of co-infection places individuals with one STD at risk for concurrent infection (*e.g.,* gonorrhea together with chlamydial infection). Although some of the organisms that

Nursing Interventions	*Rationale*	*Expected Outcomes*

Nursing Diagnosis: Potential for infection (spread of infection to others)

Goal: Prevention of spread of infection

i. Maintain environmental cleanliness by requiring damp dusting for furniture, wet vacuuming of floors, washing visible soil from walls as soon as it appears, and reducing to a minimum the activity of personnel in the patient's room.	i. Appropriate cleaning procedures and methods are designed to remove organic material and soil. Individual agency policies can identify whether cleaning, disinfecting, or sterilizing an item is necessary. Items that ordinarily do not touch the patient (or touch only intact skin) rarely, if ever, transmit disease; washing with a detergent may be sufficient.	
j. Ventilate the patient's room properly with a system that directs room air to the outside. Keep the door to the room closed.		

Nursing Diagnosis: Potential for social isolation related to nature of disease

Goal: Achievement of social participation

1. Assess how patient and family communicate.	1. The patient's family/support system has a valuable stress-reducing effect.	• Patient achieves reduction of stress imposed by social isolation.
2. Provide psychosocial support. a. Be available. b. Answer questions. c. Explore anxieties that prompt questions. d. Employ empathetic listening.	2. Ongoing and regular visits by health care personnel can have a valuable stress-reducing effect. Willingness to listen and ability to understand can relieve sense of loneliness.	• Shares feelings and anxieties of alienation. • Recalls previous reactions to stressful events. • Establishes/reinvests in relationships.
3. Integrate a caring relationship in all nursing strategies.	3. Interpersonal relationships and personal support are basic for reduction of stress and social isolation. Self-regulation emerges when isolation and loneliness are relieved.	
4. Suggest ways to relieve boredom; teach stress-reduction techniques.		
5. Employ a nonjudgmental approach to the patient with a sexually transmitted disease.	5. If the patient perceives negative verbal or nonverbal communication, he may feel anxious and guilty, which would interfere with the nurse–patient relationship.	

cause sexually transmitted diseases are sensitive to antimicrobial therapy, other pathogens demonstrate resistance to treatment. Another problem is that certain drugs used in treatment predispose the patient to superinfection. Diseases that occur in genital mucosal areas may also occur in nongenital mucosal areas that are used for sexual activity (*e.g.,* the pharynx).

Populations at Risk

Women. Sexually transmitted diseases are a major health problem of women. Many of these diseases are asymptomatic in women, and the woman has no way of knowing whether she or her sexual partner is infected. Most of the severe complications of STDs are experienced by

TABLE 59-2
Most Important Sexually Transmitted Pathogens and the Diseases They Cause

Pathogens	Disease or Syndrome
Bacterial Agents	
Neisseria gonorrhoeae	Urethritis, epididymitis, cervicitis, proctitis, pharyngitis, conjunctivitis, endometritis, perihepatitis, bartholinitis, amniotic infection syndrome, disseminated gonococcal infection, premature delivery and premature rupture of membranes, salpingitis and related sequelae (infertility, ectopic pregnancy, recurrent salpingitis)
Chlamydia trachomatis	Urethritis, epididymitis, cervicitis, proctitis, salpingitis, inclusion conjunctivitis, infant pneumonia, otitis media, trachoma, lymphogranuloma venereum, perihepatitis, bartholinitis, Reiter's disease, fetal and neonatal mortality
Mycoplasma hominis	Postpartum fever, salpingitis
Ureaplasma urealyticum	Urethritis, chorioamnioitis, low birth-weight
Treponema pallidum	Syphilis
Gardnerella hemophilus vaginalis	Vaginitis
Hemophilus ducreyi	Chancroid
Calymmatobacterium granulomatis	Donovanosis (granuloma inguinale)
Shigella, Campylobacter sp.	Enterocolitis (among homosexual men)
Group B β-hemolytic streptococcus	Neonatal sepsis, neonatal meningitis
Viral Agents	
Herpes simplex virus	Primary and recurrent genital herpes, aseptic meningitis, neonatal herpes with associated mortality or neurologic sequelae, carcinoma of the uterine cervix, spontaneous abortion and premature delivery
Hepatitis B virus	Acute, chronic, and fulminant hepatitis, with associated immune complex phenomena
Cytomegalovirus	Congenital infection: gross birth defects and infant mortality, cognitive impairment (e.g. mental retardation, sensorineural deafness), heterophile-negative infectious mononucleosis, cervicitis, protean manifestations in the immunosuppressed host
Genital wart (papilloma) virus	Condyloma acuminata, laryngeal papilloma in infants, cervical dysplasia
Molluscum contagiosum viruses	Genital molluscum contagiosum
Human T-lymphotropic viruses	Acquired immune deficiency syndrome (AIDS)
Protozoan Agents	
Trichomonas vaginalis	Vaginitis, urethritis, balanitis
Entamoeba histolytica	Amebiasis (sexually transmitted especially among homosexual men)
Giardia lamblia	Giardiasis (sexually transmitted especially among homosexual men)

(continued)

TABLE 59-2 (continued)

Pathogens	Disease or Syndrome
Fungal Agents	
Candida albicans	Vulvovaginitis, balanitis
Ectoparasites	
Phthirus pubis	Pubic louse infestation ("crabs")
Sarcoptes scabiei	Scabies

(Reproduced with permission from the *Annual Review of Public Health*, Vol 6, 1985. Copyright by Annual Reviews, Inc.)

women. Genital herpes may be a precursor of cervical dysplasia and cancer. Pelvic inflammatory diseases (diseases caused by acute ascending genital tract infections) are the most significant complications and may involve more than one infectious organism. Although the costs have been estimated to be millions of dollars annually, the human costs are higher; infertility, ectopic pregnancy, and chronic pelvic pain produce untold misery.

Homosexual Population. Although sexual practices associated with risk of infection may be seen among both homosexuals and heterosexuals, concern for the health of homosexual men is heightened because of the prevalence of AIDS in this population. The majority of cases of AIDS are reported in homosexual or bisexual men. Contact with multiple nonsteady sexual partners is a major risk factor for transmission of any of the STDs. Anal and oral intercourse and other sexual practices that involve direct or indirect contact with feces increase the risk of sexual transmission of enteric infections. The decision of some male homosexuals to conceal their sexual preference has made it difficult to interrupt transmission of disease by tracing and treating sexual contacts. Some male homosexuals do not seek health care because of anxiety and societal attitudes. However, since the AIDS crisis, the male homosexual community is showing a growing awareness of these problems and is promoting health education and disease detection to reduce the risk of infection.

Preventing the Spread of STDs

Emergency departments, outpatient clinics, college health services, and women's health facilities should be equipped to diagnose and treat STDs in order to reduce their spread. Most patients require counseling about the transmission and manifestations of these diseases as well as advice about treatment, follow-up, and the importance of referring sexual contacts for treatment. Women need to be informed that untreated male partners and multiple sex partners increase their risk of developing these infections. The risk of infertility is greater with each subsequent recurrence of pelvic inflammatory disease. The use of barrier methods of contraception (condom, diaphragm with spermicide) reduces the risk of acquiring certain infections.

Adolescents are not always aware of the cause-and-effect relationship between sexual intercourse and STDs. In addition, denial and risk-taking behaviors are often characteristic of adolescents. Therefore, health care personnel should intensity

efforts to reinforce and expand the knowledge of adolescents. Programs designed to help teenagers deal with social and peer pressures may be an alternative approach to prevention of STDs.

Acquired Immunodeficiency Syndrome (AIDS)

Acquired immunodeficiency syndrome (AIDS) is a severe disorder of immunoregulation, an impairment of the body's ability to fight disease. Severe damage imposed on the immune system predisposes the patient to life-threatening infections by opportunistic organisms and to Kaposi's sarcoma and other unusual neoplasms.

A newly recognized retrovirus, designated human immunodeficiency virus (HIV), has been implicated as the causative agent in AIDS. This virus has its greatest effect on a subpopulation of lymphocytes, the T-4 or T-helper cells, which control the body's response to infections caused by bacteria, viruses, protozoans, fungi, and parasites. Epidemiological data suggest that the virus is transmitted through intimate sexual contact, sharing of contaminated needles, and transfusion of blood or blood components. The virus can also be transmitted by an infected mother to her child before, at, or shortly after the time of birth. Persons at risk include sexually active homosexual and bisexual men with multiple partners, intravenous drug abusers, persons with hemophilia, sexual partners of individuals at risk for AIDS, and persons with symptoms and signs suggestive of the appearance of the disease.

AIDS has become a major public health problem in the United States and abroad. Knowledge about the spread, distribution, and natural course of the disease is still evolving. Because AIDS affects the immune system, it is discussed in greater detail in Chapter 45.

Chlamydial Infections

Genital chlamydial infections caused by *Chlamydia trachomatis* are now recognized as the most prevalent and among the most damaging of all STDs seen in the United States. These infections cause inflammation of the urethra and epididymis in men, and inflammation of the cervix with a mucopurulent discharge and an alarming increase in pelvic infections in women. These complications contribute significantly to the increase in the number of women who experience ectopic pregnancies. Chlamydial infections have been linked to infertility in both sexes and have been associated with many other health problems.

Genital Herpes Infections

Genital herpes is among the most common and most psychologically distressing of the STDs. Five to ten million Americans are affected, and the number is growing by almost a million cases annually. Genital herpes is epidemiologically significant because it can be transmitted to the newborn and because of its possible link to genital cancer.

Management of STDs

Primary prevention is the most important aspect of managing STDs because some of these diseases are not readily cured by antibiotics. Infected persons must be promptly identified and given effective available treatment. Recommendations for the treatment of STDs are periodically updated by the Centers for Disease Control. Antibiotic regimens are now fairly well standardized for some infections, although treatment changes as the various pathogens develop resistance to specific drugs.

Since no antimicrobial regimen is 100% effective, all patients require reexamination and retesting after treatment. Follow-up times vary with the disease.

At the present time, hepatitis B is the only STD for which an effective vaccine is available.

Gonorrhea

Gonorrhea is an infection involving the mucosal surface of the genitourinary tract, rectum, and pharynx. It is caused by the gonococcus *Neisseria gonorrhoeae* and is an infectious disease that is transmitted sexually (the exception being gonococcal ophthalmia of the newborn). It may be acquired through sexual intercourse and by orogenital or anogenital contacts between members of the opposite sex as well as members of the same sex.

The worldwide incidence of gonorrhea continues to rise. Factors contributing to the rapid spread of gonorrhea are its short incubation period and the large number of persons, both male and female, harboring the gonococcus who are asymptomatic (silent) carriers. Another factor is the growing trend toward nonbarrier methods of contraception, such as the pill. Barrier methods (condoms and vaginal spermicides) may prevent the spread of some sexually transmitted diseases. Gonococcal infection among homosexual males is becoming a major health problem. In addition, gonorrhea frequently coexists with other sexually transmitted diseases. Another complicating factor is the development of resistance to penicillin, tetracycline, and other antibiotics.

The highest rate of gonorrhea occurs among persons between the ages of 15 and 24, although there is a rapid rise of the disease in teenagers younger than 15 years of age.

Pathophysiology

The gonococcus causes a surface infection, ascending, in almost all cases, by way of the lower genital tract. The primary infection takes place in or near the urethra in males, and in the cervix, urethra, or rectum in females. If drainage is good, the infection subsides spontaneously and clears in the course of a few days or weeks. However, infection of the prostatic urethra in the male and also of the female urethral and vaginal glands predisposes to chronic infection, with occasionally very serious sequelae. Females are apt to contract secondarily a mixed infection of the endometrium and, thereafter, of the uterine tubes, constituting pelvic infection, with resultant pelvic peritonitis. The upward spread of the infection into the reproductive tract is precipitated by such factors as menstruation, douches, and the trauma associated with sexual intercourse or instrumentation.

Clinical Manifestations and Complications

After an incubation period of 2 to 7 days, most men develop dysuria or a urethral discharge, which may be a scanty clear fluid or a purulent copious drainage. The infection may extend to the prostate, seminal vesicles, and epididymis, causing prostatitis, inguinal lymphadenitis, pelvic pain, and fever. Postgonococcal urethritis develops in one fourth to one third of men treated for gonorrhea. Many cases of nongonococcal urethritis are secondary to chlamydial infections. A particularly serious problem is men with asymptomatic infection ("silent clap") who are carriers of gonorrhea. These men are often not discovered by the usual gonorrhea control measures. They remain infected, untreated, and asymptomatic and can infect their sexual partners.

In females, the infection is very frequently silent, so that a large percentage of women are asymptomatic and unaware that they are infected. A small number have vaginal discharge, urinary frequency, and dysuria. The sites most frequently involved are the urethra and cervix. As the endocervical gonococcal infection spreads upward into the reproductive tract, it causes pelvic infection (pelvic inflammatory disease), with endometritis, salpingitis, or pelvic peritonitis. An estimated 10% to 15% of women infected with the gonococcus develop pelvic infection, as evidenced by abdominal pain, fever, and vaginal discharge. There is marked pelvic tenderness on movement of the cervix and uterus during bimanual pelvic examination. Pelvic infection causes adhesions about the pelvic organs and rectum. This is a major direct cause of infertility. It also leads to ectopic pregnancy and chronic pelvic inflammation, the sequelae of which require surgical intervention.

Other Manifestations of Gonorrhea. *Anal manifestations* consist of anal itching and irritation (from erythema and edema of the anal crypts), a sensation of rectal fullness, rectal bleeding or diarrhea, mucus in the stools, and painful defecation. Anorectal gonorrhea is reported in 28% to 55% of homosexual males attending STD clinics.

Oral manifestations may be the result of the direct contact of the infecting organisms with the pharynx, or of their transmission to the oral cavity from infection elsewhere in the body. Although the majority of pharyngeal infections are asymptomatic, the following oral manifestations are seen: sore throat; painful, ulcerative inflammation of the lips; reddened, spongy, and tender gingivae; reddened, dry tongue; and redness and edema of the soft palate and uvula. The oropharynx may be covered with vesicles.

Systemic manifestations may become apparent, since secondary foci of infection may develop in any organ system, causing disseminated gonococcal infection (gonococcal bacteremia). Disseminated gonococcal infection occurs when the gonococci invade the bloodstream from one of the primary sites of infection. The patient presents with tenosynovitis of the small joints and hemorrhagic skin rash. Two to three weeks later, untreated patients will develop septic arthritis, exhibiting hot, red, and swollen joints.

Other systemic complications include gonococcal endocarditis, meningitis, and fulminant gonococcemia.

Assessment

Physical Assessment. The patient is undressed and inspected for lesions, rashes, adenopathy, and urethral, vaginal, and rectal discharges.

Diagnostic Evaluation. There are a variety of ways of identifying gonorrhea through laboratory diagnosis. The gram-negative intracellular diplococci may be found in smears or through direct fluorescent antibody tests, or may be cultured with selective media, such as modified Thayer–Martin (TM) medium or Martin–Lewis (ML) medium. The pharyngeal and anal sites should be cultured in persons who engage in oral or rectal sex; these cultures should be inoculated on separate plates. In the male, specimens may be obtained from the urethra, anal canal, and pharynx depending on the patient's sexual history and orientation. In the female, cultures are collected from the endocervix and anal canal and are inoculated on separate plates. Sterile, disposable gloves are worn by the nurse when obtaining these cultures. As a rule, lubricating jellies are not used for the vaginal examination because they may contain substances that inhibit growth or kill some pathogens. Water is used as the lubricant instead.

See Chart 59-2, Fig. 59-1*D*, for the method of inoculating the culture plate. The *Neisseria* gonococci are very susceptible to environmental changes. If the specimens cannot be transported to the laboratory immediately, they are inoculated on a medium selective for *N. gonorrhoeae* and placed in a sealed bag with a CO_2-generating system (carbon dioxide enhances the growth of all strains of gonococci). This procedure is shown in Figure 59-1*E* and *F.*

Management

The goals of treatment are to eradicate the organism and educate the patient about his condition. These goals are achieved through screening procedures, drug therapy, and patient education.

A group of experts and staff of the Centers for Disease Control recommends treatment regimens that include one of the following for uncomplicated gonorrhea: amoxicillin, ampicillin, aqueous procaine penicillin G, ceftriaxone plus tetracycline, or doxycycline. Amoxicillin, ampicillin, and penicillin (but not ceftriaxone) are accompanied by oral probenecid to increase the serum concentration of the penicillins. New antimicrobials are becoming available which may also prove to be effective.

An important concern in the treatment of gonorrhea is coexisting chlamydial infection, documented in up to 45% of gonorrhea cases when chlamydial cultures are performed. Because chlamydiae are resistant to penicillin, a tetracycline or doxycycline regimen is recommended. Other treatment schedules are available for patients who are allergic to penicillin and for those with penicillin-resistant *N. gonorrhoeae.* The treatment of complications (endocarditis, disseminated gonococcal infection) is individualized.

All patients with gonorrhea should undergo serologic testing for syphilis and be screened for other sexually transmitted diseases at the time of diagnosis. Patients with both gonorrhea and syphilis are given additional treatment, depending on the stage of the disease.

It is imperative that follow-up cultures be obtained from infected sites 3 to 7 days after the treatment is completed since no therapy is 100% effective. In addition, cultures are obtained from the rectum of women who have been treated for gonorrhea.

Each patient is interviewed for names of sexual contacts. Public health programs are geared to trace contacts and prevent further spread, which they accomplish through reporting, diagnosis, treatment, and follow-up. Contacts should be investigated and treated within 10 days. The patient is instructed to avoid reinfection by untreated sexual contacts until those contacts have been treated.

Nursing Interventions

Infected discharge from a patient with gonorrhea can be spread to the eyes from contaminated fingers. When examining a patient or coming in contact with vaginal or urethral discharge, the nurse should wear gloves, avoid touching her face, and practice careful hand washing. Body discharge precautions are used for the patient until 24 hours after appropriate therapy is completed.

If penicillin is administered, the patient is instructed to remain in the clinic or office for 30 minutes following injection to monitor any untoward reaction.

Points to emphasize for patient education are summarized on page 1667.

Syphilis

Syphilis is an acute and chronic infectious multisystem disease caused by *Treponema pallidum* (a spirochete). It is acquired through sexual contact or may be congenital in origin.

T. pallidum is a threadlike, actively motile spirochete 6 to 20 micra long that always produces its effects locally—never at a distance, as through toxins. It is killed quickly by a few minutes' exposure to drying, heat, or air.

A *chancre* (primary sore) in syphilis appears at the site (or sites) where the treponemes entered the body. Because these open, untreated lesions contain spirochetes, the disease can be transmitted through contact with the lesions. In the pregnant woman, the fetus is infected from the mother by way of the placenta. The vast majority of cases are contracted through sexual activity; the danger of transmission is greatest in the early stage of syphilis.

Epidemiology

People known to have syphilis are interviewed and asked to identify their sexual contacts so that these contacts can be

Chart 59-2
Obtaining Culture for Diagnosis of Gonorrhea

Oropharynx Culture

Swab the posterior pharynx and tonsillar crypts with a cotton-tipped applicator.

Cervical Culture

1. Moisten vaginal speculum with warm water. Do not use any other lubricant.
2. Separate labia. Depress the perineum and posterior vaginal wall with the finger of one hand.
3. Gently insert a bivalve vaginal speculum.
4. Remove excessive cervical mucus with a cotton ball held in ring forceps.
5. Insert sterile cotton-tipped swab into endocervical canal (Fig. 59-1A).
   a. Move from side to side in cervix
   b. Allow 30 seconds for absorption of organisms by the swab.

Anal Canal Culture (Rectal Culture)

1. Obtain anal specimen *after* getting cervical specimen.
2. Insert sterile cotton-tipped swab approximately 2.5 cm (1 inch) into the anal canal (Fig. 59-1B).
3. Move swab from side to side in anal canal.
4. Allow 10 to 30 seconds for absorption of organism by the swab.

For Male Patient

Oropharynx Culture

(Same as in women)

Urethral Culture

Use a sterile bacteriologic wire loop or a sterile calcium alginate urethral swab to obtain a specimen from the anterior urethra by gently scraping the mucosa (Fig. 59-1C). Do not insert loop or swab more than 2 cm

Anal Canal Culture

(Same as in women)

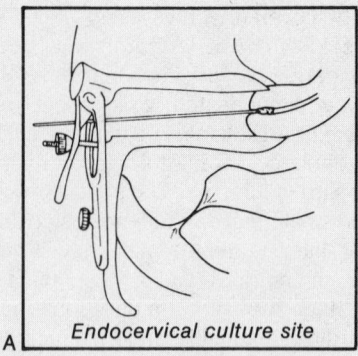

A   *Endocervical culture site*

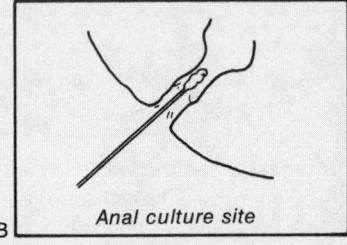

B   *Anal culture site*

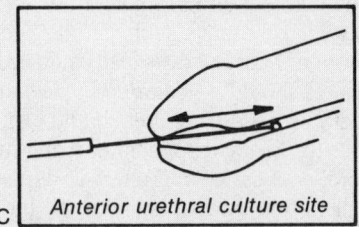

C   *Anterior urethral culture site*

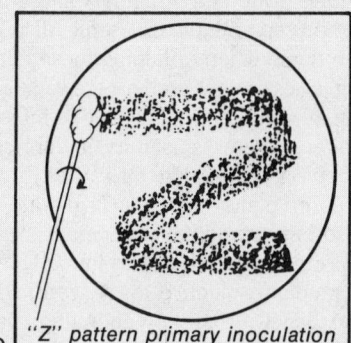

D   *"Z" pattern primary inoculation*

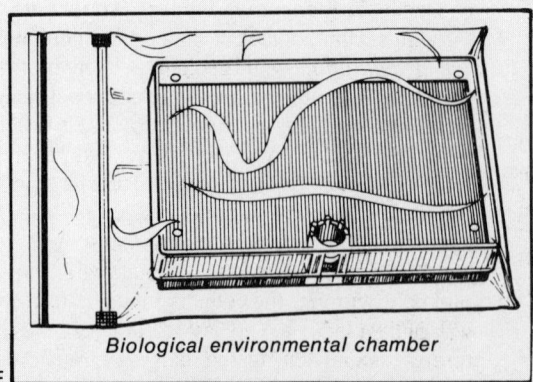

E   *Biological environmental chamber*

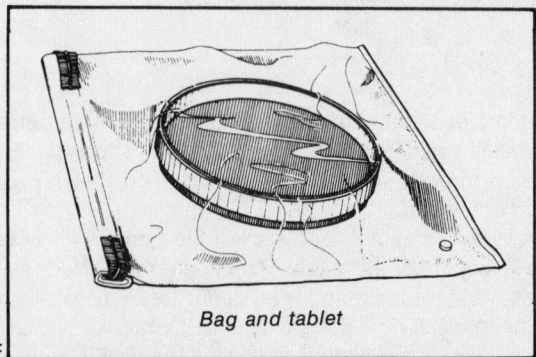

F   *Bag and tablet*

Figure 59-1
Obtaining culture for specimen in diagnosis of gonorrhea. (Criteria and Techniques for the Diagnosis of Gonorrhea. U.S. Public Health Service, Centers for Disease Control.)

examined and treated within a minimal time period. Statistics indicate that syphilis is most prominent among homosexuals, teenagers, young adults, and members of the lower socioeconomic classes.

Each person with syphilis is a potential source for a small outbreak. Studies indicate that each infected individual has an average of three different sexual contacts who are at risk of contracting syphilis. Case reporting of early infectious syphilis is required.

Clinical Manifestations

Syphilis is capable of destroying tissues in almost any organ in the body, resulting in a wide variety of clinical manifestations. Some of the manifestations of syphilis are designated as early and others as late. The time interval between early and late syphilis is about 4 years, during which period the patient develops a partial immunity and an altered tissue response to the spirochete.

Stages of Syphilis

Primary Stage. The incubation period is 10 to 90 days, with an average of 21 days. During the primary (early) stage, which is also the most infectious stage, the chancre (primary sore) appears at the site or sites where the treponemes entered the body: genitalia, anus, rectum, lips, oral cavity, breasts, or fingers (Fig. 59-2). The sites are generally related to the pattern of sexual activity. The typical chancre is an indurated painless nodule that breaks down, forming a shallow ulcer. The lymph nodes draining the ulcer become enlarged, firm, and nontender. Untreated, the primary lesion heals in a few weeks.

Secondary Stage (Stage of Systemic Involvement). Within a few weeks or months, the treponemes have begun to spread throughout the body and a variable systemic illness develops, characterized by low-grade fever, malaise, sore throat, headache, lymphadenopathy, arthralgia, and skin or mucosal rash.

The skin manifestations, which prompt many patients to seek health care, may simulate practically every known skin disease. The rash typically is macular (nonelevated discoloration) or maculopapular (elevated lesions) but can become pustular. It can be anywhere on the body, but often the palms and soles are involved. If untreated, the rash gradually fades. At the same time the hair may drop out, sometimes in patches, giving the scalp a motheaten appearance.

The lesions that appear on the mucous membranes of the mouth and tongue are glistening, slightly elevated, flat, circumscribed patches that are usually covered with a yellowish exudate. These so-called mucous patches contain large numbers of spirochetes. The lesions that develop where skin presses up against itself (about the vagina and anus) take the form of flat wartlike plaques (condylomata); these plaques contain large numbers of spirochetes and are therefore capable of transmitting infection.

Late Syphilis. After the secondary stage, there is a period of latency in which the patient shows no signs or symptoms of syphilis. This stage may last for months or years, and many patients have no further trouble, with or without treatment. Late syphilis is a slowly progressive inflammatory disease that may involve almost any organ. In cardiovascular syphilis, the inflammatory reaction may involve the heart and great vessels, with lesions occurring in the aorta, pulmonary

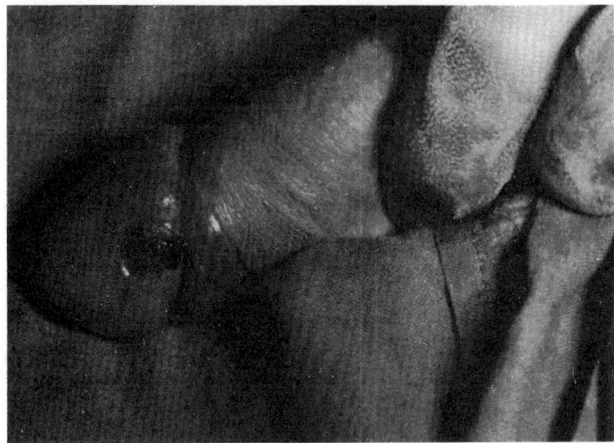

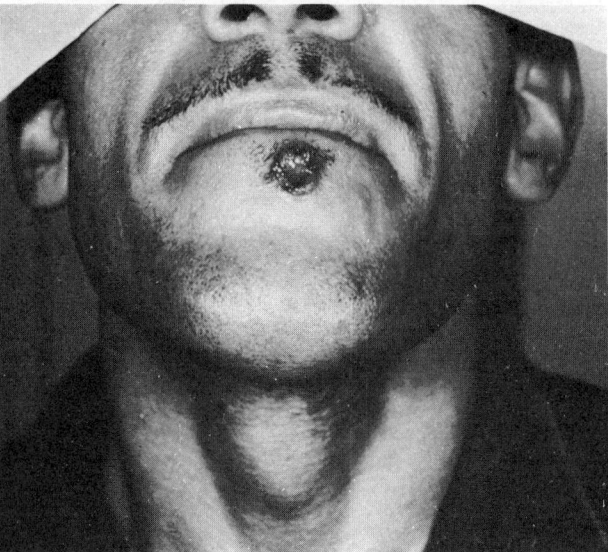

Figure 59-2
(*Top*) Syphilitic chancre on the external surface of the prepuce. (*Bottom*) Primary syphilis: Typical Hunterian chancre on lower lip. (*Top:* Elliott H and Rhyz K. Venereal Diseases: Treatment and Nursing. London, Balliere Tindall. *Bottom:* Syphilis—A synopsis. U.S. Department of Health, Education and Welfare, Public Health Service.)

artery, or great vessels arising from the aorta, resulting in aortitis and aneurysms. In neurosyphilis, disabling lesions occur in the central nervous system, giving rise to a variety of neurologic symptoms. Destructive noninfectious granulomatous lesions of the skin, viscera, bone, and mucosal surfaces, can occur which may impair health and shorten life.

Diagnostic Evaluation

Since syphilis is the great imitator of many diseases, the clinical history and laboratory evaluation are very important. A number of serologic tests are used in the diagnosis and management of syphilis; three are nontreponemal and two are treponemal.

- *Nontreponemal or reagin tests* measure antibodies formed in response to products of tissue destruction (called reagin) in the serum of infected patients. The most widely used are the Venereal Disease Research Laboratory (VDRL) slide flocculation test, the rapid plasma reagin circle card test (RPR-CT), and the automated reagin test (ART). These tests are reliable, simple to perform, and inexpensive.

Treponemal tests are tests to measure specific antibodies to *T. pallidum.* These tests are recommended for patients who have reactive reagin tests and atypical signs of primary or secondary syphilis and for diagnosis of late syphilis. The treponemal tests are the fluorescent treponemal antibody absorption test (FTA-ABS) and the microhemagglutination test (MHA-TP).

Management

The treatment guidelines established by the Centers for Disease Control are updated on a regular basis. The current treatment of all stages of syphilis is administration of antibiotics. Penicillin G benzathine is the drug of choice for early syphilis or latent syphilis of less than 1 year's duration and is given by intramuscular injection at a single session. Patients who are allergic to penicillin are treated with tetracycline.

The optimal treatment schedules for syphilis of greater than 1 year's duration have been less well established than schedules for early syphilis. In general, syphilis of longer duration requires more prolonged therapy.

Although therapy is recommended for established cardiovascular syphilis, antibiotics may not reverse the pathology (loss of elastic tissues in aortic wall) associated with this disease.

Cerebrospinal fluid (CSF) examination is done in patients with suspected symptomatic neurosyphilis and is also desirable in other patients with syphilis greater than 1 year's duration, to exclude asymptomatic neurosyphilis. In late syphilis, no treatment can repair structural damage that has already occurred.

The *Jarisch–Herxheimer reaction* is a reaction appearing within hours after therapy is initiated for syphilis, particularly in the secondary stage. It consists of transient fever and flulike symptoms of malaise, chills, headache, and myalgia that subside within 24 hours. The reaction is thought to be due to the sudden release of large amounts of treponema antigen with subsequent antigen–antibody reaction in the patient. It managed with bed rest, aspirin, and reassurance..

Nursing Interventions

Chancres contain large numbers of spirochetes and are contagious through direct contact. Body discharge precautions should be employed. The patient treated with penicillin is monitored for 30 minutes after the injection to watch for a possible reaction. The following are important preventive and patient education factors:

- Patients exposed to infectious syphilis within the preceding 3 months should be treated as for early syphilis.
- All patients with early syphilis should return for repeat follow-up testing. Follow-up should include evaluation and treatment of sexual partners. Patients with syphilis of more than 1 year's duration should, in addition, have a serologic test 24 months after treatment.

- Assure the patient infected with primary syphilis that, with proper treatment and follow-up, the chancre will disappear (within a week or two) and the blood test should (but not always) become nonreactive within a year. Those with secondary syphilis will see the rapid disappearance of their rash, and the blood test will become nonreactive within 2 years.
- Instruct the patient to refrain from sexual contact with previous partners not under treatment.
- A program of sex education and epidemiologic screening should be ongoing. Mass screening of special groups with a known high incidence of sexually transmitted diseases should be conducted.

▶ Nursing Process
The Patient With a Sexually Transmitted Disease

▷ Assessment

A sexual history is taken, including dates of exposure, symptoms, location of lesions, discharges, past history of STD, and self-treatment. Although there are a variety of clinical manifestations, depending on the disease, the most common are dysuria and urethral or vaginal discharge. At the time the patient enters the health care system, every effort is made to learn the names of the patient's sexual partners so they can be brought in for treatment.

In order to help the patient, the nurse must confront her own anxiety about sexual matters and approach the patient with honesty and sensitivity. Because the patient may be fearful of the health professional, it is important to listen patiently and carefully without passing judgment or moralizing so that the person is not placed on the defensive about life-style and does not feel that it is necessary to "cover up" important diagnostic information.

Confidentiality is very important when sexual issues are involved. Privacy is assured during information-getting sessions, and interruptions are avoided. To avoid confusion and negative implications, use terms that the patient understands, and refer to "sex partner" when asking open-ended questions.

While performing the physical examination, look at the skin for signs of irritation and itching and for burrows from scabies. Inspect the body and pubic hair for lice. In addition, evaluate the skin for rashes, lesions, drainage, and trauma. Inspect the mouth and throat for signs of infection, and palpate the inguinal nodes for size and consistency.

Gloves, of course, are worn while the genitalia are examined. Any discharge, secretion, or pus is considered to be potentially infectious. The body fluids and tissues of patients with systemic STDs (AIDS, hepatitis B, cytomegalovirus infection, syphilis, disseminated gonorrhea) are regarded as potentially infectious.

The genitalia are examined for redness, swelling, lesions, rashes, warts, and drainage. The urethra in both sexes and the vagina are inspected for mucopurulent discharge. (Is there an odor? Any itching?) The patient can be requested to point to the exact area of perineal discomfort. The presence of vaginal discharge and uterine tenderness suggest pelvic infection. The rectal area is examined for tenderness, discharge, signs of trauma, *etc.*

When a digital vaginal and rectal examination is carried out in a woman with a suspected STD, gloves should be changed after the vaginal examination, to prevent the transmission of gonococci, chlamydiae, or herpes simplex virus from the cervix or vagina to the rectum.

▷ *Nursing Diagnoses*

Based on the assessment data, the patient's major nursing diagnoses may include the following:

- Anxiety related to embarrassment and fear
- Noncompliance with treatment related to the stigmatizing nature of the disease and lack of understanding
- Knowledge deficit of the nature of the disease and potential for recurrence
- Potential for reinfection

Other nursing diagnoses could include social isolation and altered self-image related to the nature of the disease.

▷ *Planning and Implementation*

▷ *Goals:* The major goals of the patient may include achievement of reduction in anxiety, compliance with the treatment program, acquisition of knowledge of the nature and treatment of the disease, and prevention of recurrence and complications.

Nursing Interventions

Reducing Anxiety. The patient may fail to seek treatment owing to anxiety, embarrassment, or the hope that the infection will "go away." Anxiety may also cause the patient to withhold information, thereby interfering with understanding and hence compliance with treatment. A vaginal or urethral discharge can cause increased anxiety and a poor self-image.

Comfort and privacy without interruption as well as verbal and nonverbal assurances of confidentiality are essential in establishing and maintaining rapport. Allow the patient to air frustrations and feelings; talking itself helps to relieve anxiety and gain insight into problems.

Patient Education. The treatment schedule for most STDs is made as simple as possible to ensure compliance. Gently inform the patient of the consequences, especially to personal health and the health of the partner, if the condition is not properly treated.

The patient is taught how the disease is transmitted, how to recognize the major signs and symptoms, how long the infectious period lasts, how the disease is cured, and how to prevent its spread. The importance of taking the prescribed medication is emphasized. The patient is advised to continue taking the medication, even after the symptoms disappear. The possible adverse effects of the medicaton are discussed. The patient is advised to abstain from sexual activity until posttreatment examinations verify a cure.

The control of the spread of a sexually transmitted disease requires considerable patient involvement, education, and compliance. The following are important points to stress:

- An STD is acquired by sexual contact (vaginal sexual intercourse, anal intercourse, oral intercourse) and by close and direct contact with an infected person.
- A person who thinks that he or she may have an STD or who has been exposed to someone who might be infected should have a checkup. Immediate treatment should be sought if symptoms develop.
- Anyone who is sexually active with a number of sexual partners should have regular checkups.
- Washing the sex organs (before and after sexual contact) and the use of a condom may give limited protection.
- Birth control pills and IUDs give no protection against STDs.
- Gonorrhea and syphilis are different diseases, caused by different germs; they attack the body in different ways but are spread in the same manner. A person may have both gonorrhea and syphilis as well as other sexually transmitted diseases at the same time.
- There appears to be no natural or acquired immunity to gonorrhea and syphilis. A person can get gonorrhea and syphilis again and again.
- A pregnant woman with syphilis may pass the infection to her unborn child. A pregnant woman with gonorrhea may pass it to her baby during the birthing process.
- Bacteria from gonorrhea may enter the bloodstream and affect joints, joint linings, heart valves, *etc.*
- The VD National Hotline (1-800-227-8922 [nationwide]; 1-800-982-5883 [California]) provides toll-free information and referral services for sexually transmitted diseases.

Preventing Recurrence and Complications. The patient is encouraged to persuade his or her partner or partners to be examined and tested promptly (usually within 24–48 hours). Reinfection can often be traced to the person who was the source of the original infection. Preventing recurrences includes modification of sexual activity. This may mean practicing monogamy (having sexual relations with only one person) or reducing the number of sex partners, avoiding partners known to have multiple partners, and questioning and inspecting partners before having sex. Avoiding certain types of sexual practices (anorectal intercourse; oral–anal and digital–anal activity) will reduce the likelihood of infection. The use of the barrier methods of contraception (condoms) protects the partner from contact with semen, urethral discharge, or penile lesions, and vaginal spermicides may chemically inactivate some infectious agents.

▷ *Evaluation*

▷ *Expected Outcomes*

1. Patient demonstrates a less anxious demeanor.
2. Complies with treatment.
   a. Achieves a cure.
   b. Reports for follow-up examination.
3. Acquires knowledge and understanding of STDs.
   a. Recalls signs and symptoms of the most common STDs.
   b. Inspects self for lesions, rashes, discharge, *etc.*
4. Participates in a program to prevent recurrence of disease.

a. Identifies sexual partners for examination and treatment.
b. Recalls risk factors for recurrence.

Specific Bacterial Infections

Nosocomial (Hospital-Associated) Infections

A nosocomial infection is an infection acquired during hospitalization. Usually the patient has no infection at the time of admission unless it is related to a previous hospitalization. Nosocomial infections occur in approximately 5% to 6% of all hospital patients in the United States, accounting for an incidence of two million hospital-acquired infections per year. These infections prolong the hospital stay (an average of 13 days for one infection) and represent a direct economic liability of 5 to 10 billion dollars annually. Nosocomial infections are a significant cause of death among hospitalized patients.

The major cause of these infections is gram-negative bacteria. (For the particular species, see the following section on septic shock). Such infections arise from the patient's own flora or from opportunistic organisms that gain access to the patient during hospitalization or that are acquired from other sources. The syndrome of septic shock is a complication of gram-negative bacteremia (bacteria in the bloodstream).

Host Susceptibility

Most gram-negative bacilli are not invasive in normal hosts but become invasive in hospitalized patients who have underlying disease and altered host defenses.

The risk of developing nosocomial infection parallels the severity of the underlying disease. Gram-negative infections occur in the very young; the elderly; patients with impaired immune systems, blood dyscrasias, burns, trauma, or poorly controlled diabetes; those underoing prolonged procedures that result in extensive tissue damage; or those in whom a foreign body has been implanted. Any procedure involving the insertion of a tube into a normally sterile site (catheter into bladder; intravenous cannula into vein) may cause infection by allowing organisms to enter the sterile site through either the lumen or the outer surface of the tube or catheter. Potent immunosuppressive and cytotoxic drugs, steroids, and radiation, further diminish the patient's defense mechanisms. Antibiotics add to the problem by altering the patient's normal flora and encouraging overgrowth of hospital pathogens that are resistant to antibiotics. New pathogens continue to emerge as nosocomial opportunists. In fact, almost any organism can become a nosocomial pathogen, especially in an immunocompromised person.

Thus, the susceptible patient who is exposed to invasive diagnostic and monitoring equipment is predisposed to develop a gram-negative infection. However, in some patients the original source of bacteremia cannot be identified.

Prevention

Awareness of the possible risk of infection among hospitalized patients is the first step in preventing such infections.

- Fundamental to the control of infection are correct hand washing procedures and strict aseptic technique applied to all diagnostic and therapeutic procedures involving the use of catheters, cardiac pacing, intravenous therapy, endotracheal and tracheostomy tubes, tube drainage, and wound care.
- Catheter-associated urinary tract infections are the leading cause of hospital-associated infections and are the most common predisposing factors in fatal gram-negative sepsis in hospitals. As indicated so many times throughout this text, an indwelling catheter should be used only when absolutely necessary. A patient can be infected with his own bowel flora, by cross contamination with other patients or hospital flora, or by exposure to contaminated solutions or nonsterile equipment. If possible, avoid the use of indwelling catheters; use an alternate form of drainage, such as condom drainage, suprapubic catheterization, or intermittent catheterization. If an indwelling catheter must be used, it should be removed promptly when no longer needed.
- Pulmonary infections account for approximately 15% of all hospital-acquired infections. Endotracheal and tracheostomy tubes bypass normal defense mechanisms, allowing organisms to enter the lungs. A grave problem with ventilator-related respiratory infections is aspiration around the tube. Great care must be exercised in using and sterilizing respiratory therapy equipment. Every precaution should be taken to reduce the possibility of aspiration.
- Prolonged intravenous therapy should be avoided; when used, the intravenous catheter should be securely anchored to prevent it from moving in the vein. Scrupulous attention should be paid to inserting the needle properly, protecting the needle site, and observing and caring for the intravenous setup. Evidence indicates that most septicemias from intravascular devices originate from the patient's own flora or from the hands of the person inserting the device.
- Wound infections are more apt to occur in operations lasting over 2 hours, in abdominal operations, in contaminated or "dirty operations" (those involving gross spillage from the gastrointestinal tract or perforated viscera), or in patients with several diagnoses. Most wound infections are caused by endogenous organisms, for example, the bacteria being spread to the wound from the flora of the patient's own skin, nose, perineum, or gastrointestinal tract. Thus host factors play a predominant role. The nurse must be aware of those patients who may be at risk.
- Every hospital should have infection control personnel, including an infection control nurse, to monitor infection control procedures. Every health care provider should use all surveillance and preventive methods known to provide the safest possible environment for patients, personnel, and visitors.

Gram-Negative Bacteremia and Septic Shock

Gram-negative bacteremia (invasion of the bloodstream by a variety of bacterial species) may cause a life-threatening state of inadequate tissue perfusion called septic shock. (The terms *septic shock, gram-negative shock,* and *endotoxin shock* are used interchangeably.) Most cases occur when the body's normal protective mechanical barriers are disrupted or when the person's defenses against infection are impaired. The organisms most frequently associated with gram-negative bacteremia and septic shock are *Escherichia coli, Klebsiella-Enterobacter-Serratia* species, *Pseudomonas aeruginosa, Proteus* species, *Neisseria meningitidis,* and *Bacteroides fragilis.* Gram-positive bacteria (*Staphylococcus aureus; Streptococcus pneumoniae*) have also been incriminated in septic shock.

Pathophysiology

The pathophysiology of septic shock is complex and poorly understood. It is thought that when gram-negative organisms invade the bloodstream, shock results in reaction to an endotoxin that initiates a number of events: cell injury, extracellular release of lysosomal enzymes from leukocytes, changes and interactions among the coagulation and fibrinolytic systems, and metabolic injury due to tissue anoxia.

Septic shock produces arteriolar and venous spasm leading to pooling of blood in the pulmonary, splanchnic, renal, and peripheral tissues, resulting in anoxia and acidosis of these tissues. The intense vasoconstriction increases peripheral resistance, decreases cardiac output, and diminishes blood flow to major organs.

Gram-negative bacilli or their endotoxins can activate Hageman factor (Factor XII) of the intrinsic coagulation system, which in turn can result in intravascular coagulation, fibrinolysis, and shock.

Clinical Manifestations

The onset of septic shock may be abrupt with a shaking chill and rapid rise in temperature. (Temperature elevation may be blunted in the elderly or those receiving corticosteroids.) The patient has warm dry skin. Respirations are increased secondary to anoxia and increased lactic acid (respiratory alkalosis). Hypotension is present.

As the blood pressure falls, tissues and organs are inadequately perfused with oxygenated blood. When shock develops, the patient experiences tachypnea, tachycardia, profound hypotension, cool extremities, mental obtundation (depression of cerebral function), and oliguria. Various abnormalities of intravascular coagulation (DIC, thrombocytopenia) are frequently observed. A variety of skin lesions may be encountered.

Gerontologic Considerations. In the elderly patient, septic shock may be manifested in atypical or confusing clinical signs. Septic shock should be suspected in any elderly person who develops an unexplained acute confused state, tachypnea, or hypotension.

Diagnostic Evaluation

The patient is examined to identify the source of sepsis. The etiologic agent is isolated and identified through blood cultures. Other smears and cultures are taken from any possible site of infection. Urinalysis is done to detect the presence of pyuria, hematuria, casts, and bacteria.

Management

Usually, the patient is too ill to await the result of culture and sensitivity tests. Therapy is usually started immediately with agents effective against a broad spectrum of bacteria and with consideration given to the prevalence of resistant strains of bacteria in the hospital. Antibiotics are usually given intravenously to provide high levels of the drug in the blood, tissue, and body cavity fluids. Serum levels of antibiotics are monitored to assure adequate doses and to prevent toxicity.

Any possible source of infection such as an intravenous or urinary catheter is removed. Surgical drainage of localized infection (abscess) and debridement of necrotic tissue are undertaken.

Aggressive fluid volume replacement with intravenous fluids is a priority to ensure perfusion of vital organs and to correct fluid and electrolyte disturbances. Shock is treated by fluid replacement and vasoactive drugs (to alter the capacity of the vessels to overcome abnormalities of blood flow). Oxygen is administered to keep arterial PO_2 at the desired level, although additional respiratory support with intubation and assisted ventilation may be necessary when arterial hypoxemia complicates shock. Sodium bicarbonate may be given for severe acidosis. Heart failure is treated with pharmacologic agents: dopamine or isoproterenol, digitalis, diuretics.

▶ Nursing Process
The Patient With Septic Shock

▷ Assessment

The patient's nursing history may indicate the nature of his problem (previous use of urinary catheter, cytotoxic therapy or immunotherapy, *etc.*). In addition to almost constant blood pressure monitoring, the nurse observes the patient for hyperventilation, apprehension, prostration, vomiting, and diarrhea. Reduced blood flow to cerebral vessels impairs mental status and causes the patient to be confused. The skin may be dry and warm or moist and pale, depending on the type of circulatory derangement. The urinary output is monitored; oliguria is evidence of circulatory insufficiency. Hemodynamic monitoring (pulmonary wedge pressure or central venous pressure, cardiac output) is part of assessment because respiratory failure and cardiac failure are important causes of death in patients with septic shock.

▷ Nursing Diagnoses

Based on all assessment data, the patient's major nursing diagnoses may include the following:

- Alteration in tissue perfusion (cerebral, renal, peripheral) related to vasoconstriction from septic shock
- Ineffective breathing pattern (tachypnea, hyperpnea) related to pulmonary complications
- Alteration in urinary elimination (oliguria) related to decrease in circulating blood volume

Potential complications include disseminated intravascular coagulation, respiratory failure, cardiac failure, renal failure, and metabolic acidosis.

▷ Planning and Implementation

▷ *Goals:* The major goals of the patient may include achievement of tissue perfusion, normalization of breathing, attainment of adequate urinary output, avoidance/management of complications, and reduction of fever.

Nursing Interventions

Enhancing Tissue Perfusion. The nurse monitors those parameters that relate to tissue perfusion: state of responsiveness, skin temperature, moisture, color and turgor, appearance of mucous membranes and nails, respiratory rate, pulse, blood pressure, heart and lung sounds, peripheral pulses, intake, and urinary output. The assessment focuses on *trends* and *patterns of change.*

The intravenous catheter sites are monitored. Central venous pressure measurements provide a gauge for the rate and amount of volume replacement. The Swan-Ganz catheter measures pulmonary wedge pressure, which is an estimate of left ventricular–end diastolic pressure. The nurse keeps in mind that fluid deficits also occur from fever, vomiting, and diarrhea and uses appropriate interventions. (See Nursing Care Plan 59-1.)

The lung fields are auscultated when fluid is being administered to detect inspiratory and expiratory wheezes, moist fine crackles, and rhonchi, which may indicate impending pulmonary edema.

Promoting Adequate Breathing Patterns. Blood gas and *p*H measurements are monitored to determine if the patient needs assisted ventilation, because inadequate respiratory exchange is a frequent cause of death. (Severe shock and metabolic acidosis require correction with bicarbonate because severe hypoxemia does not respond well to oxygen administration.) These measures represent a collaborative function with the physician. Nursing interventions for the patient requiring assisted ventilation are found in Chapter 22.

The patient is instructed to cough frequently and may need to be suctioned when a productive cough is present. Turning and changing position reduce the potential for retention of secretions and infection.

Assuring Adequate Urinary Output. Urinary output is monitored because kidney function deteriorates with septic shock. The specific gravity of urine is measured at prescribed intervals. Urinary specific gravity increases when oliguria is present. An increase in urine output (greater than 30 ml/hr) usually indicates that tissue perfusion and hence renal perfusion are improving.

Managing Complications. When shock occurs in the course of bacteremia, there is an immediate threat to life,

with a 30% to 60% mortality rate in the elderly. Nursing support requires continuing patient assessment and strict adherence to hand washing and aseptic techniques. The nursing management for disseminated intravascular coagulation, respiratory failure, cardiac failure, and renal failure are found in the appropriate sections of this book.

▷ Evaluation

▷ *Expected Outcomes*

1. Patient achieves adequate tissue perfusion.
   a. Shows progressive increase in blood pressure to normal range.
   b. Reveals warm skin, normal skin color.
   c. Has normal mentation.
   d. Responds to volume replacement by increasing urinary output.
2. Has normal breathing pattern.
   a. Shows no evidence of tachypnea after infection has improved.
   b. Has respiratory rate within normal limits.
   c. Demonstrates arterial blood gas measurements within normal limits.
3. Attains adequate urinary output (greater than 30 ml/hr).
4. Absence of complications.
   a. No evidence of shock.
   b. Vital signs within normal range.
5. Attains normal body temperature.
   a. Shows progressive decline in fever.
   b. Has negative blood cultures.

Staphylococcal Infections

Staphylococci are widely distributed in nature, with humans serving as the predominant reservoir. These bacteria constitute a good part of the common body flora and are found on the skin surface and in the mouth, nose, and throat. It is estimated that 30% to 40% of healthy adults carry *Staphylococcus aureus* in their noses. Transmission is by contact with a person who is an asymptomatic carrier or who has a draining lesion. Food may become contaminated by a carrier who is a food handler. Staphylococci are also transmitted through the air (thereby contaminating a wound during dressing changes), by way of contaminated needles, and through animal sources.

When the continuity of the skin has been disrupted or bypassed (abrasions, wounds, surgical incisions, burns, cutaneous viral infections), the patient is susceptible to infection by staphylococci.

Staphylococci are responsible for most human skin infections. The furuncle, or common boil, is almost always a staphylococcal abscess, and the carbuncle on the back of the neck represents a coalition of staphylococcal abscesses. Most staphylococcal abscesses are located in superficial subcutaneous tissues and do not extend beyond the original site. Eventually, their purulent contents, under mounting pressure, perforate the overlying skin and are evacuated externally, leaving the empty cavities to fill in with granulation tissue, close over, and heal.

Systemic Staphylococcal Infections

If the peripheral defenses are unable to contain the staphylococcus, the infection may spread or invade the bloodstream, attended by profound toxemia.. Invasion of the lymphatics may result in axillary, cervical, mediastinal, retroperitoneal, or subdiaphragmatic abscesses. Bloodstream invasion may produce acute bacterial endocarditis, staphylococcal pneumonia, empyema, perinephric abscess, hepatic abscess, staphylococcal enteritis, pyogenic arthritis, meningitis, osteomyelitis, or generalized sepsis. Constitutional symptoms are severe.

Irrespective of location, staphylococcal lesions possess many characteristics in common, including varying degrees of necrosis, a tendency to localize, and a tendency to persist, despite intensive chemotherapy, until the exudate finds an escape route or is evacuated.

Its resistance to therapy is explained in part by the extraordinary ability of the staphylococcus to adapt itself to an unfavorable environment. Resistance to the commonly used antibiotics is frequently observed in strains of staphylococci. Thus, responsiveness to antibiotic chemotherapy, however gratifying at the onset, may diminish to the point of true refractoriness.

Management

Control Measures and Prevention. The major means by which staphylococci are transmitted within the hospital is through person-to-person transmission. The prevention of hospital staphylococcosis requires a working infection control committee, excellent hand washing and aseptic techniques, and immediate isolation of patients with staphylococcal infections.

Treatment. Treatment for severe staphylococcal infection is an antistaphylococcal antibiotic (penicillinase-resistant penicillin). An alternative antimicrobial agent (*e.g.*, cephalosporin) is considered if the patient has a penicillin allergy. Intravenous administration is the route usually selected when large doses are required. Serious staphylococcal infections may require prolonged treatment to prevent infection of the heart valves.

Nursing Interventions. The nurse monitors the patient's response to the prescribed therapy. If the patient experiences continuing or recurring fever, the cause may be a drug resistance, drug allergy, or superinfection (infection with a second organism resistant to the antibiotic in use).

Careful observations are made of the patient because fatal complications may develop during the early period of antimicrobial therapy. The promotion of comfort in the patient with fever is discussed in Nursing Care Plan 59-1, pages 1652–1653.

Streptococcal Infections

There are many strains of hemolytic streptococci, but group A streptococci account for the majority of pathogenic infections in humans. Included in this group are the beta hemolytic streptococci, which gain entrance to the body primarily through the upper respiratory tract from persons with streptococcal infections or those who are asymptomatic carriers. Included in these infections are streptococcal pharyngitis, scarlet fever, sinusitis, otitis media, peritonsillar abscess, pericarditis, pneumonia and empyema, and various wound and skin infections—impetigo, puerperal infections, and erysipelas. Rheumatic fever and acute glomerulonephritis may occur as a sequel to group A streptococci infection.

Streptococcal Pharyngitis

The most common type of streptococcal infection is streptococcal pharyngitis (strep throat) caused by group A streptococcus. Transmission occurs by way of droplets from respiratory secretions of infected persons or from healthy carriers.

Clinical Manifestations. The organism establishes itself in the lymphoid tissues and produces an abrupt onset of illness, with sore throat, fever (38.2°C [101°F]), chills, and headache. The patient may complain of throat pain that is aggravated by swallowing or even turning the head.

Upon inspection, the pharynx shows varying degrees of redness and edema and may be covered with an exudate. The presence of tender anterior cervical lymph nodes is a significant finding. Although these are the usual symptoms associated with streptococcal pharyngitis, most patients have some, but not all, of these symptoms.

In a few persons, a rash appears, starting over the neck and chest and spreading over the skin of the abdomen and extremities. If the rash becomes pronounced, the patient has scarlet fever. This presentation of group A streptococcus is uncommon today.

Diagnostic Evaluation. The presence of an exudate suggests streptococcal pharyngitis. A throat culture is taken to confirm the presence of streptococcus. (See Fig. 20-3, page 387.)

Management

Penicillin, in a variety of forms, is the drug of choice for treating streptococcal infections (except for enterococcal group D infections). If the patient is sensitive to penicillin, a course of erythromycin may be used. Therapy is continued for at least 10 days to eliminate the organisms, prevent relapses, reduce the frequency of suppurative complications, and prevent the majority of cases of rheumatic fever. Unfortunately, the risk of developing acute glomerulonephritis, which is also a complication of streptococcal pharyngitis, has not been shown to be altered by treatment of the initial infection.

Patient Education

The patient must understand the importance of *completing the course of antibiotic treatment* in order to prevent the development of complications, namely, rheumatic fever and suppurative complications: otitis media, sinusitis, peritonsillar abscess, and cervical adenitis.

During the course of febrile illness, the patient is encouraged to rest at home. He should be noncontagious to others 24 to 48 hours after treatment is started. A liberal fluid intake is important, especially if the patient has fever. Oral hygiene will add greatly to his comfort and aid in preventing the development of fissures of the lips. Warm saline gargles may relieve some of the throat soreness. The intermittent application of an ice collar is soothing to the throat. The patient is advised to monitor his temperature and is familiarized with the symptoms of possible complications.

Prevention. Ongoing health education programs are needed to emphasize the relationship of streptococcal infections to heart disease and glomerulonephritis. Persons with these conditions, especially rheumatic heart disease, are at risk and may require long-term prophylaxis with penicillin. Hospitalized patients who are at risk—and this includes the obstetrical patient—must be protected from personnel or visitors with respiratory or skin infections. For the health of the public at large, food handlers should be instructed about hygienic procedures and closely monitored to assure compliance.

Pulmonary Tuberculosis

Tuberculosis is an infectious disease caused by *Mycobacterium tuberculosis*, and rarely by *Mycobacterium bovis* or *Mycobacterium avium*. It usually involves the lungs, but it may spread to almost any part of the body, including the meninges, kidneys, bones, and lymph nodes. The term *Mycobacterium* is descriptive of the organism, which is a bacterium that resembles a fungus. The organisms multiply slowly and are characterized as acid-fast aerobic organisms that can be killed by heat, sunshine, drying, and ultraviolet light.

In contrast with the majority of infectious agents, the bacillus of tuberculosis, once it has gained a foothold in the body, is likely to remain there, quiescent, for years after the forces of immunity have controlled the original infection. If, during this quiescent period, the immunity of the host is diminished as a result of malnutrition, immunosuppression, *etc.*, the organisms at once begin to multiply, causing any one of several tuberculous diseases. If the patient's body proves able to recover from this illness, the tubercle bacilli again become dormant.

Transmission and Risk Factors

Tuberculosis is transmitted from a person with active pulmonary disease who expels the organisms while talking, coughing, sneezing, or singing. A susceptible person inhales the droplets and becomes infected.

Persons at high risk for acquiring the infection are as follows:

- Those who have been previously infected
- Those who harbor live though dormant tuberculous bacilli
- Those in close contact with someone who has infectious tuberculosis
- Those whose tuberculin skin tests have recently "converted" to show a significant reaction
- Those with lowered resistance because of factors such as alcoholism

- Elderly persons who live in nursing homes and have healed dormant infections, diabetes, or malignancy, or who are on corticosteroid therapy
- Persons receiving corticosteroid or immunosuppressive therapy
- Patients with chronic renal failure undergoing maintenance hemodialysis
- Patients who have had intestinal bypass surgery for obesity
- Those with silicosis or diabetes mellitus or who are in a postgastrectomy state

The vast majority of cases arise from the already infected minority of the population.

Crowded living conditions, low income, substandard housing, and inadequate health care contribute to the spread of tuberculosis. Tuberculosis is a common infectious disease throughout the world, since most of the world lives in poverty. In the United States, newly arrived immigrants, refugees, and migrant workers constitute a large number of persons with tuberculosis. The homeless ("street people") are another infection-prone group. There appears to be an increased incidence of patients infected with both human immunodeficiency virus (HIV) and tuberculosis.

Pathophysiology

Once inhaled by a susceptible host, the tuberculosis bacilli, in the form of droplet nuclei, pass through the airways and are deposited on the alveolar surface where they begin to multiply.

Tuberculosis is one of the so-called *granulomatous* diseases; that is, when the organism invades normal tissues, the response is the formation of new tissue masses, which are called *infectious granulomas*.

Another more diffuse and equally characteristic tissue reaction also occurs in response to the tuberculosis bacillus. The bacilli, swept along by the lymph and bloodstream, lodge in susceptible tissues in small clumps, or *tubercles*. The neighboring tissue cells quickly accumulate around each of these clumps, forming a protective wall that checks their further spread. If immunity is successful, after a long time the germs die, and the tubercle becomes transformed into a tiny mass of fibrous tissue. On the other hand, the tissue of the tubercle may become necrotic and transformed into a cheesy mass, a process known as *caseation*. If this occurs, the germs are liberated from the imprisonment and lymph sweeps them into the surrounding tissues, which respond by enclosing these freed germs in new tubercles. In this way, the original miliary (like millet seeds) tubercle grows into larger and larger irregular masses.

The fate of the patient depends on which of these two processes prevails. If the tissue barriers survive, the imprisoned tubercle bacilli cease to multiply and may die. Lime salts from the blood are deposited in the dead caseous material, and scar tissue forms around the infected area, which remains throughout life as a healed, calcified mass. However, if the germs survive and are freed from the tubercle, they multiply and are swept along by the lymph stream into the neighboring tissues, and by the bloodstream into other organs, where they lodge and repeat the same process.

Host Defense Mechanisms. Individuals who have experienced a primary tuberculous infection are sensitized or allergic to the chemical constituents of the organism. Henceforth, contact with the bacillus, whether it is alive or killed, produces an acute local tissue inflammation. This is the basis of the tuberculin test, in which a suspension of ground-up killed tuberculosis bacilli obtained from a culture is injected into the skin. If the patient is allergic—that is, has at one time had a tuberculous infection—a local skin reaction results, whereas if there is no allergy, no reaction is obtained.

A similar inflammatory reaction develops in the lung of a person who has been sensitized previously to the tubercle bacillus if this lung is invaded later by more organisms than the immune processes can handle at the time. In contrast with the relatively bland, silent, primary type of pulmonary tuberculosis, the course of the reinfection type is complicated by necrosis, with resulting ulceration of the infected lung tissue. Clusters of tubercles, as in the primary type of tuberculosis, form at once around the nest of organisms, but now, due to the tissue sensitivity, these become surrounded by zones of inflammatory reaction. The alveoli in the area become filled with exudate; in other words, a tuberculous bronchopneumonia develops. The tuberculous tissue in this area gradually becomes caseous and ulcerates into a bronchus, causing a cavity. At the same time, as the ulcerations heal, considerable scar tissue forms locally, especially around the cavities. The pleura over the infected lobe, more often an upper lobe, becomes inflamed, then thickened and retracted by scar tissue.

This cycle of inflammatory bronchopneumonia proceeds to ulceration with cavitation, followed by scarring. Unless the process can be arrested, it spreads slowly downward toward the hilum and later extends into adjacent lobes. The activity of the process may be very prolonged and characterized by long remissions, when the disease may appear to be arrested, only to be followed by periods of renewed activity.

Clinical Manifestations

Chronic pulmonary tuberculosis is insidious in its onset and course. The majority of patients present with fever, loss of strength, cough productive of mucopurulent sputum, and weight loss. If the patient does not seek treatment until late in the disease, constitutional symptoms are marked—daily recurring fever with chills, weight loss, anemia, hemoptysis, and large numbers of bacilli in the sputum.

Gerontological Considerations. Tuberculosis may have atypical manifestations in the elderly, such as changes in behavior or mentation, organ dysfunction or fever, anorexia, and weight loss. It is being increasingly encountered in the nursing home population.

Diagnostic Evaluation

The initial diagnostic evaluation includes a tuberculin skin test, examination of a sputum sample (smear and culture), and an x-ray evaluation of the chest.

The majority of new cases of active tuberculosis arise from previously quiescent lesions that have become activated. Tuberculin testing serves to identify the group at greatest risk of developing active disease.

Tuberculin Skin Test. The intracutaneous test (Mantoux test) is the standard test used to identify the infected person. Tubercle bacillus extract (tuberculin) is inoculated into the intradermal layer of the inner aspect of the forearm. Intermediate strength of purified protein derivative (PPD) is usually used. The tuberculin syringe should be held close to the skin, so that the hub of the needle (26 or 27 gauge) touches it as the needle is introduced, bevel up. This reduces the needle angle at the skin surface and facilitates the injection of tuberculin just beneath the surface of the skin, to form a wheal (Fig. 59-3). The test is read 48 to 72 hours after injection; since tuberculin skin tests are tests of delayed hypersensitivity, this is when the induration (hardening or thickening of tissues) is the most evident.

Test reactions should be read in a good light, with the forearm slightly flexed at the elbow. After the area is inspected for the presence of induration, it is lightly palpated across the injection site, from the area of normal skin to the margins of induration. A pencil mark is made where the area of induration is felt. Then the diameter of the induration (*not erythema*) is measured in millimeters, at its widest part (Fig. 59-4). Erythema or redness without induration is generally considered to be of no significance. The size of the induration is documented, as well as the antigen strength, the date the testing was conducted, the date when the reading was taken, and the lot number used, if available.

Interpretation of Skin Test. An area of induration measuring 10 mm or more in diameter is interpreted as significant.

Doubtful reactions measure 5 mm through 9 mm and require that the test be repeated at a different site. (Individuals who are close contacts of persons with active tuberculosis and who have reactions in the 5-mm through 9-mm range should be considered significant reactors and should receive preventive treatment.) Usually, an induration of 0 mm to 4 mm is not considered significant. This shows either a lack of

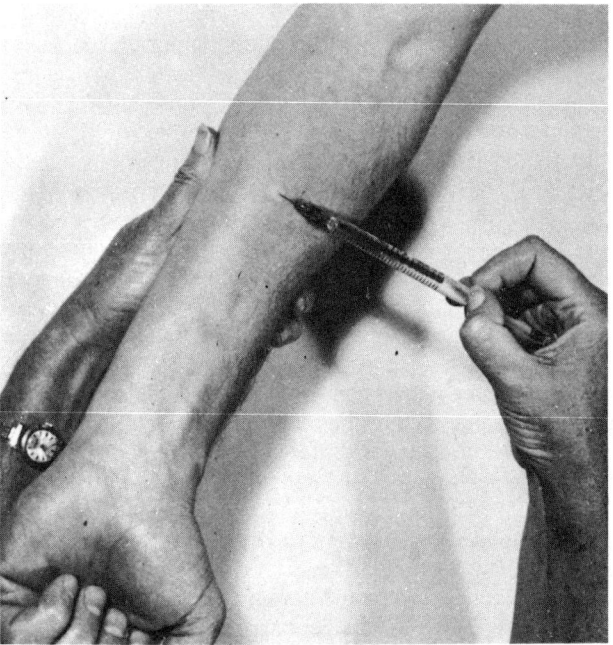

Figure 59-3
The Mantoux intracutaneous test. A tuberculin syringe and a subcutaneous needle, with the bevel up, are used to inject tubercle bacillus extract into the skin of the forearm to form a wheal. (American Lung Association.)

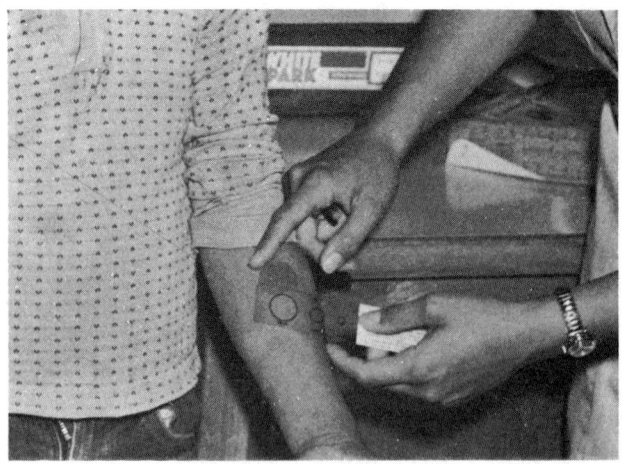

Figure 59-4
Interpretation of Mantoux test. The area of induration is measured most accurately with the aid of a plastic ruler containing concentric circles of specific diameters. (American Lung Association.)

tuberculin sensitivity or low-grade sensitivity that probably is not caused by *M. tuberculosis.*

- *A significant reaction indicates that a patient has been exposed to Mycobacterium tuberculosis recently or in the past. It does not necessarily mean that active disease is present in the body.* The vast majority (more than 90%) of people who are tuberculin-significant reactors will *not* develop clinical tuberculosis. (However, all significant reactors are candidates for active tuberculosis.)

In general, the more intense the reaction, the greater the likelihood of an active infection. A nonsignificant (negative) skin test does not exclude tuberculous infection or disease.

A *tuberculin converter* is a person whose tuberculin reaction changes from less than 10 mm in diameter to more than 10 mm in diameter, with the increase measuring at least 6 mm. (This usually indicates recent infection.)

Other Skin Tests. Multiple-puncture skin tests are used for surveying and screening large groups and are not intended to establish positive diagnosis, since there is no way to standardize the amount of tuberculin introduced. The test introduces tuberculin into the skin either by puncturing with a device with points coated with dried tuberculin or by puncturing through a film of liquid tuberculin. The test is read 48 to 72 hours after administration. If the reaction is in the form of papules, the diameter of the largest single papule or the largest diameter of coalescent induration is measured. If vesiculation is present, the person is sensitive to the tuberculin and is termed a ''reactor.'' However, not all reactors are infected with tuberculosis. All reactors should be retested with the Mantoux test and should have a chest x-ray.

Sputum Testing. Diagnosis is also confirmed by finding the acid-fast bacilli in smears of sputum. Sputum can be coughed up directly or induced by inhaling aerosols, which irritate the trachea and produce coughing. Bronchoscopic aspiration using a fiberoptic bronchoscope or transtracheal aspiration are other possible means of obtaining a sputum specimen. An early-morning specimen has pooled overnight

secretions and is more apt to be productive and less contaminated. If the patient is unable to expectorate but has swallowed sputum, then a gastric specimen may be obtained by means of a nasogastric tube to permit study of swallowed sputum. Tubercle bacilli may also be obtained and cultured from ascitic fluid, pleural fluid, cerebrospinal fluid, urine, and pus that has been aspirated or drained from abscesses. Tissue such as liver, bone marrow, and lymph nodes may also be cultured.

Chest X-ray. Tuberculosis is a possibility in anyone with an abnormal chest x-ray. Certain patterns, such as patchy infiltrates, are suggestive of tuberculosis.

Management

The goals of management are (1) to relieve pulmonary and systemic symptoms by eliminating all viable tubercle bacilli; (2) to return the patient to health, work, and family life as quickly as possible; and (3) to prevent transmission of the infection.

- Every active case of tuberculosis must be reported to the local health department so that close contacts may be examined and followed. Contacts are usually placed on preventive therapy (usually isoniazid) to prevent the development of active disease.

Chemotherapy. Active tuberculosis is usually treated with simultaneous administration of a combination of drugs to which the organisms are susceptible. Such therapy is carried out until the disease is brought under control. Multiple drug regimens are used to destroy as many viable microbial organisms as quickly as possible and to minimize the emergence of organisms resistant to the various antituberculosis drugs. Although the tubercle bacillus is susceptible to several drugs, there are no drugs to which it cannot develop resistance. Such resistance results from genetic mutations of the organism. The use of a variety of drugs enables one agent to destroy those mutants that are resistant to the initial drug.

In the United States, a 9-month regimen consisting of isoniazid and rifampin is frequently used. Ethambutol or streptomycin is added for an initial 2 to 8 weeks. Other accepted regimens include isoniazid (INH) combined with one or more of the following: rifampin, streptomycin, ethambutol, and pyrazinamide. (See Table 59-3 for further information about these drugs.)

The patient is instructed to have a sputum examination every 2 to 4 weeks until two successive cultures are free of bacilli, verifying the patient's noninfectious state.

Surgical Treatment. Since the advent of chemotherapy, surgical intervention is rarely necessary for tuberculosis. Pulmonary resection may be performed when the possibility of cancer coexists. It may also be carried out for the purpose of eliminating lesions that have ceased to decrease in size after several months of therapy. Surgical procedures may also be done for thoracic drainage of empyema, decompression of constrictive pericarditis, or drainage of a paravertebral abscess.

Preventive Treatment. Eradicating tuberculosis depends on prevention, detection, health education, and improved standards of living. Most cases of tuberculosis occur in persons known to be significant tuberculin reactors. These patients are the reservoir from which more than 90% of active

TABLE 59-3
Treatment of Mycobacterial Disease in Adults and Children

Commonly Used Agents	Most Common Side-Effects*	Tests for Side-Effects*	Drug Interactions†	Remarks*
Isoniazid	Peripheral neuritis, hepatitis, hypersensitivity	SGOT/SGPT (not as a routine).	Phenytoin—synergistic Antabuse	Bactericidal to both extracellular and intracellular organisms. Pyridoxine 10 mg as prophylaxis for neuritis; 50 to 100 mg as treatment.
Rifampin	Hepatitis, febrile reaction, purpura (rare)	SGOT/SGPT (not as a routine).	Rifampin inhibits the effect of oral contraceptives, quinidine, corticosteroids, Coumarin drugs and methadone, digoxin, oral hypoglycemics; PAS may interfere with absorption of rifampin.	Bactericidal to all populations of organisms. Orange urine and other body secretions. Discoloring of contact lens.
Streptomycin	8th nerve damage, nephrotoxicity	Vestibular function, audiograms;‡ BUN and creatinine	Neuromuscular blocking agents—may be potentiated to cause prolonged paralysis	Bactericidal to extracellular organisms. Use with caution in older patients or those with renal disease.
Pyrazinamide	Hyperuricemia, hepatotoxicity	Uric acid, SGOT/SGPT		Bacteriostatic to intracellular organisms. Combination with an aminoglycoside is bactericidal.
Ethambutol	Optic neuritis (reversible with discontinuation of drug; very rare at 15 mg/kg), skin rash	Red-green color discrimination and visual acuity.‡ Difficult to test in a child under 3 years.		Bacteriostatic to both intracellular and extracellular organisms, primarily used to inhibit development of resistant mutants. Use with caution with renal disease or when eye testing is not feasible.

*Check product labeling for detailed information on dose, contraindications, drug interaction, adverse reactions, and monitoring.
† Reference should be made to current literature, particularly on rifampin, because it induces hepatic microenzymes and therefore interacts with many drugs.
‡ Initial examination should be done at start of treatment.
(Modified from American Thoracic Society. Treatment of tuberculosis and other mycobacterial diseases. Am Rev Respir Dis 1983 June; 127[6]:791. Used with permission.)

disease develops. Infected persons must be identified, and preventive therapy (isoniazid prophylaxis) given to those at risk of developing disease and becoming transmitters. The following groups may benefit from preventive therapy with isoniazid:

- Contacts of newly discovered cases of tuberculosis
- Newly infected persons
- Tuberculin reactors with radiographic abnormalities
- Tuberculin reactors with certain clinical problems (*e.g.,* certain neoplasms, silicosis, chronic renal insufficiency)
- Tuberculin-positive persons age 35 years and younger with no other factors that increase risk

Isoniazid, for preventive therapy, is given in a single daily dose for 1 year. The most significant adverse reaction is hepatitis; this risk is increased if the person drinks alcohol on a daily basis. All persons taking isoniazid for preventive therapy should be seen in a health care facility on a regular basis to allow for detection of reactions to the medication and to provide personnel with an opportunity to encourage compliance with medication.

BCG Vaccine. Another means of prevention is the vaccine BCG (bacille Calmette-Guérin), which is used in areas of high tuberculosis outside the United States. BCG does not prevent initial infection with *M. tuberculosis,* but it does alter the host defense mechanisms if such an infection occurs. Its use is restricted to persons who have negative reactions to the tuberculin skin test, because it does not benefit those who are already infected. Also, BCG vaccinations will convert a negative tuberculin reactor to a positive reactor, which makes subsequent skin tests invalid.

In the developing countries, whose limited resources must be concentrated on the detection and treatment of patients with sputum-positive disease, it has been found that BCG gives substantial protection against tuberculosis. BCG vaccination has been a major tool of the World Health Organization's efforts to control tuberculosis in countries with high rates of transmission. The vaccine is infrequently used in the United States, because the medical and socioeconomic conditions are better here than in some other parts of the world, and there are better methods of control and treatment.

▶ Nursing Process
The Patient With Tuberculosis

▷ Assessment

The nursing history and nursing observation focus on the patient's fatigue, cough, sputum expectoration, weight loss, chills, and fever. It is important to determine if the patient has experienced hemoptysis. The patient's educational level, emotional readiness to learn, and perceptions and understanding of tuberculosis are evaluated. Since therapy may be prolonged, his social support system is assessed.

The results of the physical and laboratory evaluations are reviewed.

▷ Nursing Diagnoses

Based on the assessment data, the patient's major nursing diagnoses may include the following:

- Knowledge deficit of disease, medications, and self-care techniques
- Potential for infection (spread of infection to others)
- Noncompliance with treatment regimen related to possible disorganized life-style, alcoholism, or distrust of authority

▷ Planning and Implementation

▷ *Goals:* The major goals of the patient may include acquisition of knowledge and understanding of the disease and its treatment, prevention of spread of infection to others, and compliance with the treatment regimen.

Nursing Interventions

Prevention and Patient Education. There is evidence that patients probably forget at least 50% of what they are told, especially when anxiety levels are high. The role of the nurse is pivotal in building a trusting relationship so that the patient education will be an ongoing process and behavioral changes will be made.

Although tuberculosis is a communicable disease, effective chemotherapy is the most effective means of preventing transmission. This fact bears frequent repetition.

- *A major reason for treatment failure is that patients do not take their medications regularly and for the period of time prescribed.* One of the teaching functions of the community health nurse is to stress the importance of taking the medicine faithfully and exactly as prescribed.

All details of drug therapy are carefully explained. Watch the patient's reactions and determine if he understands and agrees with the instructions. The American Lung Association has an array of patient teaching aids that can be used to reinforce teaching and learning.

The patient is usually treated at home except in rare instances where social circumstances or drug-resistant organisms pose a threat to the community. In the home-treated patient, respiratory isolation is usually not necessary since the hazard to the family already occurred before the disease was diagnosed. The patient is instructed to cover his mouth and nose with double-ply tissue when he coughs or sneezes; these can be discarded in a paper bag and burned. (Covering the mouth with the bare hand does not stop small droplets.) Hand washing is demonstrated and stressed.

The patient and family should be instructed carefully about possible complications, including hemorrhage, pleurisy, and other untoward symptoms, that are indicative of a possible recurrence of tuberculous activity. Chronic alcoholism is a troublesome complication that makes ambulatory treatment difficult. This patient should be referred to an alcoholic clinic or appropriate health agency.

Usually, the patient can return to his former employment. However, he should avoid exposure to excessive amounts of silicone (dusty jobs in foundry, rock quarry, sand blasting), since silicone dioxide dust may be harmful to the lungs.

In the hospitalized patient, tuberculosis isolation is used if the sputum smear is positive or if the chest x-ray film strongly suggests active tuberculosis. To protect the patient's privacy, the instruction card posted on the patient's door reads "AFB Isolation" (AFB = acid-fast bacilli). This category of isolation requires a private room with special ventilation and the door kept closed. Masks are indicated only if the patient is coughing and does not reliably cover his mouth. Gowns are indicated only if needed to prevent gross contamination of clothing. *Hands must be washed after touching the patient or potentially contaminated articles and before taking care of other patients.*

Minimizing Noncompliance. Tuberculosis is often seen in patients who are economically and socially deprived. A significant percentage of these patients fail to take their medication as prescribed or abandon treatment altogether. Their lives may be marked by social upheaval and alcoholism. Many are poorly motivated to participate in their treatment. Those patients who are noncompliant should receive their medications under direct supervision.

Most patients with tuberculosis, however, will report to the health care facility as outpatients. They will require time, support, and, as previously mentioned, education. Try to fit the medication regimen into the patient's routine or life-style, since new habits are difficult to establish. Link the time of medication to some daily habit (*e.g.*, morning cup of coffee). Uncomfortable side-effects of a drug may be a reason the patient discontinues the treatment. Find out if the prescribed medication is causing problems and discuss these with the physician to see if a change or adjustment of medication is in order. If the patient has adequate literacy skills, providing written instructions is valuable when starting a program of treatment.

An ongoing supportive relationship is built not on dependency, but on valuing the patient's beliefs and strengthening his self-confidence in order to change his health behaviors in a positive manner.

▷ *Evaluation*

▷ *Expected Outcomes*

1. Patient acquires knowledge and understanding of tuberculosis.
   a. Answers questions about tuberculosis correctly.
   b. Knows names of medications he is receiving and schedule for taking them.
   c. Can name expected side-effects of medications.
2. Prevents spread of infection to others.
   a. Remains on drug therapy.
   b. Uses tissues correctly when coughing, sneezing, *etc.*
   c. Reports for sputum monitoring.
   d. Encourages persons who are close contacts to report for examination.
3. Complies with treatment regimen.
   a. Keeps appointments.
   b. Takes medications exactly as prescribed.

Miliary Tuberculosis

Miliary tuberculosis is the result of bloodstream invasion by the tubercle bacillus. It is usually a consequence of late reactivation of dormant infection in the lung or elsewhere, with blood-borne dissemination to multiple organs. It is the most serious form of tuberculosis. The origin of the bacilli that flood the bloodstream is either some chronic focus that has ulcerated into a blood vessel, or multitudes of miliary tubercles

lining the inner surface of the thoracic duct. The germs, poured from these foci into the bloodstream, are carried throughout the body and locate throughout all tissues, with myriads of tiny miliary tubercles developing in the lungs, spleen, liver, kidneys, meninges, and other organs.

The clinical course of miliary tuberculosis may vary from an acute, rapidly progressive infection with high fever to an indolent process with low grade fever, anemia, and debility. At first there may be no localizing signs except for an enlarged spleen and a reduced number of leukocytes. Within a few weeks, however, a roentgenogram of the chest reveals small densities scattered diffusely throughout both lung fields; these are the miliary tubercles, which gradually increase in size. Very few physical signs may be elicited on physical examination of the chest, but at this stage the patient suffers from a severe harassing cough, dyspnea, and cyanosis. Treatment is the same as that described for pulmonary tuberculosis.

Atypical Mycobacteria

It is now recognized that some bacteria which give a staining reaction similar to that of *M. tuberculosis,* but which have distinctly different growth and culture characteristics, may produce pulmonary disease clinically similar to tuberculosis. When tuberculosis was a much more common disease than at present, and when more sophisticated bacteriologic techniques were not used, these infections were overlooked or the organisms discarded as contaminants. Today, these strains of mycobacteria are classified more precisely. They are transmitted from the environment to humans by mechanisms not well understood. *Mycobacterium kansasii* and *Mycobacterium avium-intracellulare* are thought to cause the majority of pulmonary infections. Most of these species are found in a variety of environmental sources, including house dust, tap water, fresh and coastal waters, soil, and milk. They have become more prominent since tuberculosis has declined. There is no evidence of person-to-person transmission.

These mycobacteria are usually partially or totally resistant to antituberculosis drugs. Therapy usually involves the use of multiple drugs (4 to 5 drug regimens). Surgical resection of the diseased lung tissue may be carried out.

The nursing management is similar to that of the patient with tuberculosis, except that respiratory isolation is not required.

Legionnaires' Disease

Legionnaires' disease is an acute respiratory infection from a gram-negative bacterium, *Legionella pneumophila.* It is named after an outbreak of the disease that occurred in Philadelphia, in 1976, among people attending the state convention of the American Legion.

Epidemiological evidence indicates that Legonnaires' disease is transmitted by inhalation of organisms in an aerosol form of infected water from environmental sources. Legionellae are ubiquitous (everywhere) in water, and the organisms have been found in plumbing fixtures, drinking water, and air conditioning systems in hotels and hospitals.

It is proposed that one way in which the aerobic gram-negative bacillus finds its way into humans is through the cooling towers and evaporative condensers of large air conditioners, where the bacteria multiply and are discharged as an infectious aerosol through fans and exhaust vents. The disease is not considered highly communicable. Persons at risk are middle-aged and older men, especially those who smoke, consume alcohol, work in or near construction sites, or are immunosuppressed from disease or medications that affect cellular immunity.

Pathophysiology. Autopsy specimens from tissues of patients with Legionnaires' disease have shown different amounts of lung consolidation in varying distributions. The histologic pattern has been that of an acute fibrinopurulent pneumonia, which resembles a stage of lobar pneumonia. An exudate containing neutrophils, macrophages, and fibrin is found in the alveolar spaces.

Clinical Manifestations. The target organ appears to be the lungs. The earliest symptoms are profound malaise, myalgias, mild headache, and a dry cough. Within a day, the patient experiences a rapidly rising fever and chills. The fever remains high and unremitting, 39°C–41°C (102°F–105°F), until specific therapy is started. Occasionally, diarrhea precedes other symptoms. Associated manifestations include pleuritic pain, confusion, and impaired renal function. A chest x-ray will document evidence of pneumonia. Tachypnea and dyspnea may reflect the extent of the pneumonic process. There may be clinical and laboratory evidence of abnormalities of the gastrointestinal, musculoskeletal, hepatic, renal, and central nervous systems. The diagnosis is made on the basis of an increase in specific serum antibodies and by culture of the organisms on appropriate culture media.

Management. Erythromycin (administered early) is the drug of choice in treatment. These patients may be seriously ill. Death may occur from intractable shock and hemodynamic collapse.

Nursing Interventions. The nursing management is that described for the patient with pneumonia (see p. 465–467). Respiratory isolation is recommended for persons whose illness is strongly suspicious of Legionnaires' disease.

Salmonella Infections (Salmonellosis)

Salmonellosis is infection caused by bacteria of the genus *Salmonella*. Clinically, salmonellosis is seen in four forms: gastroenteritis (the most common form), enteric fever (such as typhoid and paratyphoid disease), bacteremia with and without focal extraintestinal infection, and asymptomatic carrier state. Infection caused by *Salmonella typhi* (typhoid fever) is discussed on page 1679. Although approximately 2000 serotypes are known, *Salmonella typhimurium* is the most commonly reported in the United States. In this country salmonellae are implicated in 3% of cases of gastroenteritis; they cause 3% to 5% of infectious diarrheas in developing countries.

Salmonella organisms may penetrate the epithelial cells of the small intestine and colon, producing an intestinal inflammatory response. The diseases resulting from these infections are quite similar clinically, and the infecting organisms are spread in exactly the same manner as the typhoid bacillus. The patient is infected by ingesting the organism in food contaminated by infected human or animal feces, in whole eggs and egg products, in meat and meat products, in poultry (especially turkey), and in pharmaceuticals of animal origin. It has been proposed that large numbers of eggs and chickens on the market are contaminated by salmonella microorganisms. Common foods causing salmonella infections include commercially processed meat pies, poultry, sausages, foods containing eggs or egg products, and unpasteurized milk and other dairy products.

Clinical Manifestations. Symptoms usually develop within 8 to 48 hours after ingestion of contaminated food. The patient experiences headache, abdominal discomfort, low-grade fever, and watery diarrhea that may contain blood and mucus. Some patients have only a headache and occasional loose stools. The infectious agent may localize and cause necrosis in any body tissue, producing abscesses, cholecystitis, arthritis, endocarditis, meningitis, pericarditis, pneumonia, and pyelonephritis. Petechiae, splenomegaly, and leukopenia may also be manifested. Salmonella infection complicated by bacteremia is seen in the very old who have other underlying disease.

Diagnosis of salmonella infection is made by finding the organism in feces and blood. Later, after acute infection subsides, serologic agglutination tests are useful in establishing the diagnosis.

Management. Rehydration of the patient with fluids and essential salts is the foundation of treatment. Oral intake of fluids is sufficient in the majority of patients. Fruit juices and soft drinks are effective even in severe diarrhea. (Glucose is absorbed in the small intestine.) The patient should avoid beverages with caffeine, which causes increased intestinal motility.

Antimotility drugs (anticholinergics, paregoric) may be counterproductive, since a slowed peristaltic activity may extend the period of infection by interfering with an effective cleansing mechanism.

Patients with moderate to severe illness (those requiring hospitalization) may be treated with trimethoprim-sulfamethoxazole or chloramphenicol. Enteric precautions are indicated.

Prevention and Patient Education. There is no active or passive immunization. Raw eggs or egg drinks should not be eaten, nor should dirty or cracked eggs be used, since salmonellae can penetrate cracked eggs. All foods from animal sources, especially poultry, egg products, and meat should be *thoroughly cooked*. Food service workers should be instructed about food-borne illnesses and given guidelines on avoiding food contamination, storing and preparing food, cleaning food preparation and service areas (contaminated countertops can serve as a means of transmission), and practicing good personal hygiene. Foods should be refrigerated during storage and protected against insects and rodents. Chickens, ducks, and turtles (as well as other domestic pets) are sources of infection.

The patient must wash his hands after going to the bathroom, particularly during illness and carrier state (several months) to prevent transmission of infection to others.

Shigellosis (Bacillary Dysentery)

Shigellosis is an acute bacterial disease of the intestinal tract. There are approximately 40 serotypes of shigellae, divided into four groups or species: *Shigella sonnei* (most common serotype isolated in industrialized countries), *Shigella dysen-*

teriae, Shigella flexneri, and *Shigella boydii.* The source of infection is feces from an infected person, with the route of spread being fecal–oral. *Shigella* species are gaining prevalence as agents of sexually transmitted disease (see p. 1651). Shigellosis may be passed through toilet paper onto the fingers. The bacilli have also been recovered from milk, eggs, cheese, and shrimp.

While encountered in all countries, bacillary dysentery is endemic in the tropics, where serious epidemics are frequent. It continues to pose a very substantial problem for people in the United States, especially those with a substandard environment and those living in a closed-group population—day care centers, military installations, nursing homes, and other resident care centers.

Pathogenesis. The pathology of shigellosis, in severe cases, consists of organisms reaching the small intestine, where they multiply and release a toxin that initiates secretion of water and electrolytes from the jejunal area. The shigellae are thought to invade the distal ileum and colon, where they establish themselves in epithelial cells, multiply, spread to adjacent cells, and destroy them. The invading pathogens are capable of initiating an intense inflammatory response in the mucosa, followed by small patches of ulceration, which may coalesce to form large ulcers.

Clinical Manifestations. Initially there is fever, cramping, and abdominal pain. Watery diarrhea soon appears, often followed by frank dysentery, with the passage of varying amounts of blood, mucus, and pus. There may be high fever. At the height of the active infection, the symptoms are severe and the prostration is quite profound. The patient has a constant desire to defecate, and the straining is severe during the attempts. The disease is usually self-limited in healthy adults, and improvement is noted in about 1 week. Some cases last 2 or 3 weeks, and chronic cases last several months, or even years, unless adequately treated. In severe cases, shock, volume depletion, and electrolyte imbalance may supervene.

Management. The objectives of treatment are to maintain fluid and electrolyte balance and to eliminate the spread of shigellosis to the patient's contacts (*e.g.*, eliminate the carrier state). To eliminate the spread of shigellosis, every patient is questioned about travel to underdeveloped countries, exposure to crowded institutions, swimming in contaminated water, and oral–anal sexual activity. Inquiries are made concerning water supplies and food eaten at home and in restaurants. Local and state authorities are notified.

The organism may be recovered from the stool; sensitivity tests are done in order to determine the appropriate antibiotic, since the organism may be resistant to certain drugs. Treatment of shigellosis with antibiotics is important in shortening the period of fecal excretion and in aborting the course of illness. Antibiotics that are absorbed from the intestinal tract and to which the shigellae are sensitive (ampicillin, trimethoprim-sulfamethoxazole) may shorten the clinical course and decrease the period of intestinal shedding of the organisms, thus decreasing the period fo communicability. The use of antimotility drugs (*e.g.*, Lomotil) to control diarrhea prolongs the symptoms and the presence of the organism in the intestines, and is therefore not recommended.

Intravenous fluids are administered to maintain the electrolyte balance and prevent profound dehydration due to an excessively large loss of water and electrolytes (sodium, potassium, chloride, bicarbonate) in the diarrheic stools. The patient may require supplemental potassium.

Nursing Interventions. The patient is assessed for weight loss, skin turgor, and dryness of mucous membranes, and his vital signs and urinary volume are monitored. Clear fluids are offered by mouth during the acute stage.

Prevention and Patient Education. Dysentery bacilli are spread by drinking water polluted by infected human excreta, by sexual transmission, and by food handled carelessly by shigella carriers, some of whom have the active disease, others being entirely asymptomatic. Thus, the same precautions must be observed, and the same control of water sources and food handling enforced, in the prevention of shigellosis as of typhoid fever. This includes proper hand washing, effective sanitation, adequate sewage disposal, a program of fly control, and the detection of carriers. Untreated sexual partners, particularly those of homosexual men, may reinfect the patient.

Typhoid Fever

Typhoid fever is an acute systemic bacterial disease resulting from infection with *Salmonella typhi.* The organism gains access to the body through ingestion of food or water that has been contaminated by infected feces or urine. In the United States it is spread chiefly by carriers, patients who have recovered from the disease but whose stools or urine may spread the bacilli for years. Since it is eliminated in the stools and urine of patients, the organism can find its way into food and water through sewage, flies, and the hands of carriers handling raw fruits, vegetables, and other food. Another source of infection is the ingestion of oysters and shellfish harvested from polluted waters. Typhoid fever, although rare in the United States, is a serious public health problem in regions of the world where there is neither a safe water supply nor adequate sewage disposal.

Pathophysiology. The organism enters the body by way of the mouth and invades the walls of the gastrointestinal tract. There, multiplying rapidly, it gives rise to a massive bacteremia that continues for about 10 days. The chief localization of the organism is in the mesenteric lymph nodes and the masses of lymphatic tissue in the mucous membrane of the intestinal wall, which are called *Peyer's patches,* and in small solitary lymph follicles, numerous in the ileum and the colon. The blood vessels of the Peyer's patches become thrombosed, and the swollen mass of lymphatic tissue dies and sloughs away, leaving clean ulcers in the mucous membrane, the floor of which may be the muscularis, or even the peritoneum. If the latter, they may perforate, causing peritonitis.

Clinical Manifestations. The onset of typhoid fever is gradual, with headache, fever, malaise, somnolence, and abdominal pain. The patient may not seek health care at this time since these are nonspecific symptoms. At the end of the first week, rose spots (a cluster of pink lesions that initially blanch with pressure) may be found on the chest and abdomen. Without therapy, the temperature rises steadily, reaching its highest level—usually 40°C to 41°C (104°F–105°F)—in from 3 to 7 days. During this period of rising temperature, most patients suffer with a severe headache and a nonproductive cough. During the second week, if the patient is not treated, the temperature remains consistently high. During the third week, however, it becomes more and more remittent, a little lower each morning and not quite so elevated each afternoon. The pulse rate may be relatively slow in spite of high fever. Other clinical manifestations are an enlarged liver and spleen, delirium, and intestinal bleeding.

Diagnostic Evaluation. The diagnosis is made by recovery of the causative agent from blood samples, bone marrow aspirate, rose spot aspirate, or stool.

Management

Chloramphenicol, ampicillin, amoxicillin, or trimethoprim-sulfamethoxazole is used in the treatment of typhoid fever. The fever usually subsides in 3 to 5 days following initiation of antibiotic therapy. However, bacteriologic cure is not achieved in all patients. Relapses have occurred and positive stool cultures have been obtained after one course, and even repeated courses, of antibiotic therapy. Thus, while chloramphenicol has reduced the fatality rate of typhoid fever significantly and has curtailed the excretion of typhoid bacilli during convalescence, it has not reduced the frequency of complications or the incidence of the chronic carrier state following typhoid fever.

Nursing Interventions

The goals of nursing management are to give supportive care and to monitor for complications.

Delirium is common in the severe form of the disease, and the patient will require special support during this period. He may be drowsy, indifferent to his surroundings, and incontinent of urine and feces. Enteric precautions are used while the patient is ill, and he should be awakened for administration of medications, fluids, and nourishment, and for position changes.

Tepid water fever sponges are given for temperatures over 40°C (104°F). A high fluid intake is encouraged to prevent dehydration from fluid losses due to fever, perspiration, and poor oral intake.

Watch for bladder distention, since the patient may lose the urge to void during the toxic state. Retention of feces may also pose a problem. Enemas, if indicated, are given *under low pressure* to diminish the chance of intestinal perforation.

Monitoring for Complications. Many structures may become infected in the course of typhoid fever, including the lungs, the pleura, the pericardium, the heart, the kidneys, and the bones. However, the most common of the dangerous complications are intestinal hemorrhage and perforation of the bowel, with resultant peritonitis.

Intestinal hemorrhages, secondary to bacterial invasion of the Peyer's patches which leads to necrosis, ulceration, and erosion of blood vessels, occur in 4% to 7% of patients, usually during the third week. Signs of hemorrhage include apprehension, sweating, pallor, weak, rapid pulse, hypotension, and bloody or tarry stools. Hemorrhage is generally managed by supportive measures, including blood transfusions. Operative intervention (bowel resection) is sometimes necessary.

Intestinal perforation, the most serious complication, may happen at any time, but most often occurs during the third week. The perforation usually takes place in the lower ileum. It occurs when the ulcer causing the slough involves the entire thickness of the bowel wall. The intestinal contents pour into the abdominal cavity at once causing peritonitis. The patient usually experiences acute abdominal pain. There is associated abdominal tenderness and rigidity and a silent abdomen. However, the pain may last only a few seconds and then stop, with the patient falling sound asleep within a few minutes. If such signs occur, a nasogastric tube is passed and intravenous fluids started to correct fluid and electrolyte imbalance. Surgical closure of perforation is usually carried out.

Other complications of typhoid fever may occur when the typhoid bacilli localize in specific tissues, causing hepatitis, meningitis, cholecystitis, pneumonitis, and pericarditis. During the course of the disease, the gallbladder and bile ducts are routinely infected.

Patient Education. Since typhoid fever is a very serious disease, the process of recovery may be slow. Once a patient has recovered, stools must be checked to see if he has become a carrier, because approximately 3% of treated typhoid patients become chronic carriers. Carriers harbor the organism and excrete it in their urine and stools. The presence of Vi-agglutinins in the blood of suspected carriers has strong predictive value for the carrier state. A positive stool or urine culture for a year or more indicates a carrier state. Carriers may be given ampicillin or amoxicillin with probenecid in an attempt to abolish the carrier state.

Public health agencies maintain surveillance of carriers, because the occurrence of typhoid fever in the United States is almost always traceable to a known or undetected carrier. These persons must not become food or milk handlers.

Prevention. There is no substitute for good sanitation. The eradication of typhoid fever depends upon the availability of safe water and sewer systems. The detection of carriers and restriction of their occupations is also essential. Typhoid fever patients, convalescents, and carriers must wash their hands after defecation. All persons handling food should use proper hand washing techniques. Flies must be controlled by screening and spraying, and their breeding controlled by adequate collection and disposal of garbage. Shellfish should be obtained from an approved source. Scrupulous cleanliness in the preparation and storage of food is vital.

Typhoid vaccination is no longer recommended for people in the United States. It is, however, recommended for those living with chronic typhoid carriers and is considered for persons traveling to countries where typhoid is common. On the basis of the above recommendation, adults may be given typhoid vaccine subcutaneously on two occasions separated by 4 or more weeks. Oral live attenuated vaccine (TY21a) is being used successfully in areas of endemic disease.

Meningococcal Meningitis (Bacterial Meningitis)

Meningitis is inflammation of the membranes surrounding the brain and spinal cord and is caused by a variety of bacteria, viruses, protozoa, or fungi. The most important form is bacterial.

The bacteria most frequently encountered in acute bacterial meningitis are *Neisseria meningitidis, Streptococcus pneumoniae* (in adults), and *Haemophilus influenzae* (in children and young adults). The mode of transmission is by direct contact, including droplets and discharges from the nose and throat of carriers (most often) or infected persons. Of those exposed to it, the great majority do not develop the infection but become carriers. There has been an increased incidence of meningitis caused by enteric gram-negative bacteria in persons over 60 as well as in those who have had neurosurgery or who have a compromised immune response.

Meningococcal disease is endemic in the United States and throughout the world, and occurs most frequently in the winter and spring months. Epidemics are most apt to occur in people who live in crowded quarters, notably in cities, crowded institutions, military installations, or prisons, but the disease also occurs in rural regions.

Bacterial meningitis starts as an infection of the oropharynx and is followed by meningococcal septicemia, which extends to the meninges of the brain and upper region of the spinal cord. There are several distinct immunologic strains of the meningococcus, but groups A, B, C, and Y cause the majority of cases of bacterial meningitis. It can be one of the most fulminating of all diseases (*i.e.,* coming on suddenly with severity).

Pathophysiology

Predisposing factors include upper respiratory tract infections, otitis media, mastoiditis, sickle cell anemia and other hemoglobinopathies, recent neurosurgical procedures, head trauma, and immunologic defects. The venous channels serving the posterior nasopharynx, middle ear, and mastoid drain toward the brain and are near the veins draining the meninges; these channels favor bacterial proliferation.

The meningococci enter the bloodstream and cause an inflammatory reaction in the meninges and underlying cortex, which may result in vasculitis with thromboses and reduced cerebral blood flow. The cerebral tissue is metabolically impaired from the presence of meningeal exudate, vasculitis and underperfusion, and cerebral edema. A purulent exudate may spread over the base of the brain and spinal cord. The inflammation spreads also to the membrane lining the cerebral ventricles. Bacterial meningitis is associated with profound alterations in intracranial physiology, including increased permeability of the blood–brain barrier, cerebral edema, and raised intracranial pressure.

In acute infections, however, the patient dies from the toxin of the bacteria before meningitis develops. In these patients, meningococcemia is overwhelming, with adrenal damage, circulatory collapse, and associated widespread hemorrhages (Waterhouse-Friderichsen syndrome) occurring as a result of endothelial damage and vascular necrosis caused by the meningococci.

Clinical Manifestations

The symptoms of meningitis result from infection and increased intracranial pressure. Usually the patient experiences a sudden onset of severe headache, myalgia, back pain, photophobia, fever, and neck pain and stiffness (from spasm of the extensor muscles due to meningeal irritation). Frequently,

aggressive and almost maniacal behavior is displayed. Another striking feature is a rash ranging from petechiae (small red spots) to a combination of petechiae and ecchymoses (large bruise-like areas) occurring in about two thirds of patients with meningococcal disease.

Upon physical examination there is resistance to neck flexion. Other signs of meningeal irritation include

- *Positive Kernig's sign:* When the patient is lying with his thigh flexed on the abdomen, he cannot completely extend his leg.
- *Positive Brudzinski's sign:* When the patient's neck is flexed, flexion of the knees and hips is produced; when passive flexion of the lower extremity of one side is made, a similar movement is seen for the opposite extremity.

In approximately 10% of patients, a fulminating infection occurs, with signs of overwhelming septicemia: an abrupt onset of high fever, extensive purpuric lesions (over face and extremities), shock, and signs of intravascular coagulation. Death may occur within a few hours after onset.

The infecting organisms can usually be identified through a smear and culture of the cerebrospinal fluid and blood. Counter immunoelectrophoresis is widely used to detect bacterial antigens in body fluids, particularly cerebrospinal fluid and urine.

Management

Successful management depends on the administration of an antibiotic that crosses the blood–brain barrier into the subarachnoid space in sufficient concentration to halt the multiplication of bacteria. When the CSF and blood cultures are obtained, antimicrobial therapy is immediately started. Penicillin, ampicillin, or chloramphenicol, or one of the cephalosporins may be used. Other antibiotics may be used if resistant strains of bacteria are identified. The patient is maintained on large intravenous doses of the appropriate antibiotic.

Dehydration or shock is treated with fluid volume expansion. Seizures, which may occur in the early course of the disease, are controlled with diazepam or phenytoin. An osmotic diuretic (*e.g.,* mannitol) may be used to treat cerebral edema.

Nursing Interventions

The patient's outcome may depend on the supportive care given. The patient is very ill, and the combination of fever, dehydration, alkalosis, and cerebral edema may predispose to seizures. Airway obstruction, respiratory arrest, or cardiac dysrhythmias may follow. Thus, some of the nursing interventions are collaborative with those of the physician.

- In meningitis of all causes, the patient's clinical status and vital signs are constantly assessed, since altered consciousness may lead to airway obstruction. Arterial blood gas determinations, insertion of a cuffed endotracheal tube (or tracheostomy), and mechanical ventilation may be prescribed. Oxygen may be given to maintain the arterial Po_2 at desired levels.
- The central venous pressure is monitored to assess for incipient shock, which precedes cardiac or respiratory

failure. Generalized vasoconstriction, circumoral cyanosis, and cold extremities may be noted. The high fever must be reduced to decrease the load on the heart and the brain's oxygen demand. See Nursing Care Plan 59-1, page 1652, for appropriate nursing interventions.

- Rapid intravenous fluid replacement may be prescribed, but care is taken not to overhydrate the patient because of risk of cerebral edema.
- The body weight, serum electrolytes, urine volume and specific gravity, and osmolality of urine are closely monitored, especially if inappropriate ADH secretion is suspected.
- Continuing nursing management requires ongoing assessment of the patient's clinical status, attention to skin and oral hygiene, promotion of comfort, and protection during seizures (p. 1489) and while comatose.
- Discharges from the nose and mouth are considered infectious. Respiratory isolation is advised for 24 hours after the start of antibiotic therapy.

Prevention and Patient Education. Persons having close contact with the patient should be considered candidates for antimicrobial prophylaxis (rifampin). Close contacts are observed and immediately examined if fever or other signs and symptoms of meningitis develop.

The meningococcal vaccine currently licensed in this country includes the polysaccharides of groups A, C, W135, and Y, and is used primarily in military recruits. Vaccine may be of benefit for some travelers visiting countries that are experiencing epidemic meningococcal disease. Vaccination should also be considered as an adjunct to antibiotic chemoprophylaxis for anyone living with a patient who has meningococcal disease.

A polysaccharide vaccine (Haemophilus b Polysaccharide Vaccine) against invasive *Haemophilus influenzae* type b has recently been licensed in the United States.

Tetanus (Lockjaw)

Tetanus is an acute disease caused by the tetanus bacillus, *Clostridium tetani*, whose spores are introduced into the body when an injury is contaminated with soil, street dust, or animal and human feces. The bacillus is an anaerobe (it cannot live in the presence of oxygen). It is found most commonly in wounds with small external openings, and is also seen in drug addicts. It may occur in any deep wound that is contaminated with soil or that harbors foreign bodies. Frequently, the presumed site of infection is a "minor wound." Not infrequently, the wound entrance is so insignificant that it cannot be found. Wounds may be minor injuries, scratches, bee stings, lacerations, frostbite, animal injuries, abortions, circumcision, surgery, and dental and orofacial trauma. The incidence is greater among low-income groups (who often have not been immunized), among women, and among the elderly who never were immunized as children or have lost their immunity.

In the developing countries, tetanus is a common and serious disease. The majority of cases are caused by contamination of a wound, of a newborn's umbilical stump, or of the puerperal uterus.

Pathophysiology

Tissues with low oxygen tension (due to infection or foreign material, or damaged blood supply) provide conditions in which the spores become vegetative forms, multiply, and produce toxins. *C. tetani* is known to produce three exotoxins: tetanospasmin, which is a neurotoxin with a special affinity for nervous tissue, especially in the spinal cord and cranial nerves, and which produces intense and severe muscle spasms; nonconvulsive neurotoxin; and tetanolysin, which may have hemolytic and cardiotoxic effects. These neurotoxins are absorbed by the peripheral nerves and carried to the spinal cord, where they produce a reaction that amounts to a stimulation of the nervous tissue. The sensory nerves become sensitive to the slightest stimuli, and the hypersensitive motor nerves carry impulses that produce spasms of the muscles that they supply.

Clinical Manifestations

Early symptoms include irritability, restlessness, headache, low-grade-fever, and muscle rigidity. The jaw muscles are the first group affected, making it difficult to open the mouth because of spasms of the masticatory muscles (trismus). This characteristic symptom has given the disease the common name *lockjaw*. The spasms of the facial muscles produce a distorted grin (risus sardonicus), which is quite characteristic of the disease and persists even during convalescence.

The spasm rapidly involves other groups of muscles until the whole body is affected, with tightness of the chest and rigidity of the abdominal wall, back, and extremities. The spasm is continuous, but the least stimulus—a door banging or a loud voice—may cause a generalized convulsion, with every muscle in violent contraction. In fact, fractures of the vertebral bodies can occur during severe spasms. Because the extensor muscles are stronger than the flexors, the head is retracted, the feet are extended fully, and the back is arched, so that during a convulsion the whole body may be supported on the back of the head and the feet. This condition is called *opisthotonos*. The patient is alert and in pain from muscle spasms. Death may occur from asphyxia, due to spasms of the respiratory muscles, and from pneumonia.

Management

The goals of management are to provide an airway to prevent respiratory and cardiovascular complications and to neutralize the residual circulating toxins.

The patient with established tetanus is immediately given tetanus immune globulin (TIG) 1 to 2 hours before wound debridement so that the neurotoxin released into the circulation during debridement cannot attach to nerve endings. Active immunization with tetanus toxoid is also started at the beginning of the treatment since even severe tetanus produces no immunity. When tetanus toxoid and TIG are given concurrently, separate syringes and separate sites should be used.

The wound is debrided because necrotic tissue favors the growth of tetanus bacillus. The wound is irrigated copiously to wash out tissue fragments and foreign bodies; it may be left open and drainage instituted.

Immune globulin may also be infiltrated into the wound site. Usually, penicillin G (or an alternate antibiotic) is given intravenously or intramuscularly in high doses to eradicate persisting *C. tetani* and other pathogens from the wound.

Diazepam is used to reduce restlessness and apprehension (which can induce spasm), for its amnesic effect, and to provide muscle relaxation to treat spasm. Neuromuscular blocking agents (metocurine iodide [Metubine]) is given for treatment of severe tetanus.

The overactivity of the sympathetic nervous system may lead to "sympathetic crisis" and death. Isolated tachycardia, temporary hypertension, premature ventricular contractions, and sweating require aggressive physiologic monitoring and pharmacologic treatment. Propranolol may be given to control tachycardia while phentolamine is administered to control hypertensive episodes.

Nursing Interventions

In severe tetanus infection, one of the most important nursing objectives and priorities is constant supportive care of the patient to assure respiratory function. Convulsive paroxysms, especially those involving the respiratory muscles, impair pulmonary gas exchange by preventing normal swallowing and by obstructing the airway. Tetanic spasms of the larynx, pharynx, and respiratory muscles usually occur during convulsions and can lead to asphyxiation and death. Rigidity and spasm of the trunk muscles also contribute to ventilatory failure. In fact, ventilation ceases during a tetanus convulsion.

The patient requires expert respiratory management in an intensive care unit, with early endotracheal intubation and mechanical ventilation. Oral secretions are usually constant and profuse, requiring frequent suctioning. The nursing management of the patient with convulsions is discussed on page 1489. See Chapter 22 for the management of the patient requiring respiratory intensive care.

Overactivity of the sympathetic nervous system, as manifested by tachycardia, dysrhythmias, labile blood pressure, hyperpyrexia, and excessive sweating and salivation, may eventually lead to circulatory failure and death. A significant increase in the heart rate and mean arterial blood pressure may indicate a need for an adrenergic blocking agent (propranolol) to lessen the possibility of catecholamine-induced myocardial damage. Therefore, cardiac monitoring is essential.

Since the slightest stimulation may trigger paroxysmal spasm, sudden stimuli and light must be avoided. The patient is placed in a quiet, semidark environment to avoid stimulating reflex spasms. Nursing activities are carried out during the periods when sedation has its maximum effect so that the patient is disturbed as little as possible, since tactile stimulation often provokes spasms. Usually, a vein is kept open for emergency situations, such as cardiac or respiratory arrest, and for infusions to maintain careful fluid and electrolyte balance. Insensible fluid losses in the form of sweat and saliva are high and result in dehydration, which, in the presence of impaired cardiovascular control and overactivity of the sympathetic nervous system, can predispose to deep vein thrombosis and pulmonary embolism. Parenteral nutrition may be required, since aspiration pneumonia during oral food intake is a hazard.

Constant attention is given to the eyes, mouth, skin, and bladder and bowels. The patient is monitored for signs of infection (skin, urinary tract, aspiration pneumonia).

Watch the patient for urinary retention, which occurs when perineal muscles are affected. Pressure sores and contractures can be the outcome of prolonged immobility; therefore, preventive nursing interventions are necessary (see Chap. 14). Even with expert care, the mortality rate of tetanus may be 50% or higher.

Prevention and Patient Education. Tetanus can be prevented through proper immunization programs; immunization establishes basal immunity before exposure to the risk of tetanus. For primary immunization of adults, three doses of adult-type tetanus and diphtheria toxoids (Td) are given, followed by a booster dose every 10 years to maintain adequate immunity. About two thirds of the tetanus cases in the United States occur in persons over age 50; these persons are least likely to have been immunized as children.

- The most important step in the prevention of tetanus is the thorough washing and cleaning of the wound, with removal of all foreign material and devitalized tissue. This helps eliminate tetanus bacilli from wounds and removes the material that forms a focus in which tetanus spores can develop.
- Every break in the skin must be considered a potential portal of entry for *C. tetani*.

Following injury, the immunization status of the patient will determine whether or not to provide active immunization with tetanus toxoid and passive immunization with tetanus immune globulin. The nature and age of the wound, the conditions under which it was incurred, and the treatment are considered on an individual basis. Encourage the patient to keep an up-to-date record of his immunization status.

Clostridial Myonecrosis (Gas Gangrene)

Gas gangrene is a severe infection of skeletal muscle caused by several species of gram-positive clostridia that may complicate trauma, compound fractures, contusions, or lacerated wounds by producing exotoxins that destroy tissue. These organisms (*Clostridium perfringens, Clostridium novyi, Clostridium septicum* and others) may produce gas gangrene. They are anaerobes and spore-formers, and are found normally in the intestinal tract of humans and in soils. Their growth occurs primarily in deep wounds where the oxygen supply is reduced, a situation enhanced by the presence of foreign bodies or necrotic tissue, which leads to further reduction of oxygen tension in wounds.

In contaminated wounds in which the vascular supply may be impaired, the environment is suited for the growth of spores and the production of exotoxins that adversely affect the blood and cause vessel thrombosis and damage to the myocardium, liver, and kidneys.

Spores formed by anaerobic bacilli are highly resistant to heat, cold, sunlight, drying, and many chemical agents. Because the gas bacillus is an inhabitant of the human intestinal tract, it is likely to be the infecting organism in thigh wounds following amputations, especially if the patient is incontinent. Patients with chronic arterial disease and diabetes mellitus are at risk of developing gas gangrene following amputation of the leg because these conditions favor the development of local tissue anoxia necessary for the development of gas gangrene.

Clinical Manifestations

The onset of gas gangrene is usually attended by sudden, severe pain at the site of injury, which is caused by gas and edema in the tissues, usually occurring 1 to 4 days following the injury. The wound is very tender. The surrounding skin initially appears normal, or white and tense, but later becomes bronzed, brown, or even black in color. Vesicles filled with red, watery fluid appear, and crepitus (crackling) produced by gas in the tissue may be felt. Frothy fluid with a foul, sweetish odor may escape from the wound. The gas and edema fluid increase local pressure and impair the blood supply and drainage. The involved muscles become black or reddish purple (necrotic). Amputation of an affected extremity is sometimes necessary. The infection may spread quickly, resulting in systemic toxicity.

The patient is pale, prostrated, and apprehensive, but usually quite alert. Pulse and respirations are rapid, but the temperature usually does not exceed 38.3°C (101°F). Anorexia, diarrhea, vomiting, and vascular collapse may occur. Death from toxemia is frequent.

Management

Prevention. Gas gangrene may be prevented if all devitalized and infected tissue is excised and debrided, using wide incisions made to render the wound unsuitable for the growth of clostridium.

Treatment. Treatment usually involves surgery, antibiotics, and sometimes hyperbaric oxygen. Once infection has developed, extensive incisions in the affected part allow air to inhibit the growth of anaerobic organisms. Antibiotic therapy is combined with prompt surgical debridement of the wound.

Hyperbaric oxygen (oxygen administered under pressure greater than atmospheric) has proven extremely effective in treating gas gangrene. This increases the dissolved oxygen in the arterial system by increasing the partial pressure of oxygen breathed by the patient. With hyperbaric oxen therapy, it may not be necessary to amputate the extremity.

Nursing Interventions

The nursing functions are collaborative with the surgeon. The patient is very ill, since the infection produces an intense toxemia. The pulmonary capillary wedge pressures, central venous pressures, and urinary output are closely monitored. Intravenous fluids are administered as prescribed to support the cardiovascular system and to maintain fluid and electrolyte balance. Transfusions may be necessary and are prescribed to maintain adequate hematocrit levels. Hemolysis and tissue destruction can lead to hyperkalemia; thus, potassium levels are also evaluated. Enteral nutrition is critical in establishing nutritional balance.

Botulism

Botulism is a type of food poisoning that affects the central nervous system. It is caused by eating food in which the bacterium *Clostridium botulinum* has grown and produced toxins. These toxins are extremely potent and are rapidly ab-

sorbed by the GI tract, becoming bound to neural tissue and producing a neuroparalytic syndrome. Toxic effects usually follow ingestion of contaminated foods: home-canned, dried, or smoked foods or poorly processed foods.

Of the seven immunologically distinct types of *C. botulinum,* types A, B, E, and F have accounted for the documented cases of human botulism, although types G and D have been reported recently. Local, state, and federal public health officials are notified when a case of botulism is diagnosed.

Clinical Manifestations. The symptoms appear 12 to 36 hours after ingestion of the contaminated food. If the symptoms appear in less than 24 hours after ingestion, a more severe illness and a higher fatality rate are usually encountered. Gastrointestinal symptoms (nausea and vomiting) may occur within hours after ingestion of contaminated food. The toxin causes paralysis of skeletal muscles, interfering with release of acetylcholine.

Cranial nerve symptoms include diplopia, ptosis and blurred vision (extraocular muscle involvement), dysphagia and pharyngeal pain (involvement of pharynx), and dysphonia (involvement of larynx). Paralysis then occurs, slowly descending through the body and affecting all muscle groups, usually in a symmetrical fashion. Throughout the ordeal, the patient's mind remains clear. Almost three fourths of the patients have respiratory problems.

Diagnostic Evaluation. The diagnosis is confirmed by finding the toxin in the serum, gastric contents, stools, and incriminated food. There are also characteristic electrophysiologic abnormalities in clinically involved muscle groups.

Management. A botulinal antitoxin to neutralize any toxin that may be in the circulation is available from the Centers for Disease Control. Ventilatory equipment and emergency drugs should be readily available in the event of a life-threatening reaction.

Organisms and unabsorbed toxin are eliminated from the gastrointestinal tract by means of gastric lavage, cathartics, and enemas. In instances of respiratory paralysis or an ileus, these procedures may not be prescribed.

Nursing Interventions. Since the neurotoxins produced by *C. botulinum* may result in neuroparalytic syndromes, the patient is given respiratory care and support as the basic management to prevent the pulmonary complications that are responsible for most fatalities due to botulism. The patient is prepared for endotracheal intubation and mechanical ventilation. (The respiratory care of the paralyzed patient is discussed in detail in Chap. 22.)

The patient's heart is monitored in order to detect immediately any signs of cardiac arrest. Skin care and positioning are also important facets of management to prevent pressure sores and musculoskeletal complications. The patient is monitored for urinary retention; if this occurs, an indwelling catheter is usually necessary and is prescribed by the physician. The appearance of fever usually indicates a nosocomial infection.

Following the acute phase of illness, there is a high prevalence of persistent symptoms (tiredness, weakness, dyspnea) that may last a year or more. The patient and family are informed of the need for rest periods throughout the day, energy-saving techniques, and the importance of follow-up care.

Prevention and Patient Education. Home-processed foods pose a serious danger of *C. botulinum*, because this germ is a spore-bearer and is not killed rapidly at boiling temperature. (Reliable commercial packing houses sterilize their products at 120°C [248°F], which kills all the spores.) Preserved foods in which this germ has been growing often look soft, contain gas bubbles, and give off an odor of decay; however, contaminated food items may have a normal appearance and taste. Canned foods should be heated at temperatures over 80°C (176°F) for 30 minutes or boiled for 10 minutes, as the toxins are heat-labile and destroyed by proper cooking of food. Vegetables, including mushrooms, beans, tomatoes, beets, okra, peppers, corn, and asparagus, have been implicated; meats, fish, and poultry have also accounted for some outbreaks.

Home canners should be advised to take care in preparing food for canning at high altitudes, where it is difficult to provide a temperature high enough to destroy the spores of *C. botulinum.* The use of the pressure cooker method of canning at high altitudes is advised.

Persons are also cautioned not to use punctured and swollen cans or jars with defective seals. Canned commercial products that are damaged or swollen should not be used.

Leprosy (Hansen's Disease)

Leprosy is a chronic infectious disease caused by *Mycobacterium leprae,* a bacillus that produces lesions in the skin tissues and peripheral nerves. This organism resembles the tubercle bacillus in many respects. It is not known exactly how leprosy bacilli enter the body, but it is known that a higher percentage of people living with leprosy patients have the disease. Large numbers of organisms are disseminated when a person with leprosy sneezes. It is possible that the organism gains entrance through the upper respiratory tract or through broken skin.

As the bacilli multiply, they invade adjoining skin areas and find their way into the axis cylinders of nerves by way of the axon-plasma filaments (*i.e.,* the ultimate terminals of the nerves supplying the skin). As the infection spreads, organisms break out of the nerves at various points in the skin to produce macules and papules. These are painless, since the bacilli that caused them to form have already destroyed the nerve supply.

Incidence. An estimated 12 million people throughout the world suffer from this ancient, feared, and disfiguring disease. It is most prevalent in third world countries, which have inadequate human and financial resources to cope with leprosy. In the United States, the influx of immigrants and increasing world travel by U.S. citizens is a factor in its occurrence. It is endemic in California, Hawaii, Texas, Florida, Louisiana, Puerto Rico, and New York City.

Clinical Manifestations. Leprosy chiefly affects the skin and peripheral nerves. The earliest manifestation is a skin lesion, located anywhere on the body. The lesions are either tuberculoid, lepromatous, or borderline. In the tuberculoid type, the lesions are colorless or reddish brown. The earliest sign is usually a loss of feeling in a small area of the skin, as a result of damage to the dermal nerves. Nerve involvement can lead to damage of muscles and bones. In the lepromatous form, the bacillus grows unchecked, with skin lesions (macules, papules, nodules, or plaques) appearing over most of the body. These nodules, resembling skin tumors

and sores, may appear anywhere on the body. When the face is involved, the nodules, together with the loss of the eyebrows and eyelashes, give the face a typical leonine appearance. Because the nodules are easily infected, giving rise to deep ulcers that heal slowly, scars deform the face. This process often dissects the nose, fingers, and toes, and destroys sight.

In borderline leprosy, the lesions are variable, falling between the tuberculoid and lepromatous range of the disease.

Diagnostic Evaluation. Diagnosis is made on the basis of the appearance of the lesions and the discovery of the leprosy bacilli, obtained from slit-scrape smears of the skin lesions and smears from nasal mucosa.

Management. The goals of management are to give specific chemotherapy until cure is attained and to prevent and treat deformities. Leprosy is best treated with dapsone (DDS) plus one or two additional drugs (rifampin, clofazimine) to prevent the emergence of resistant mutant strains.

Mucosal lesions respond most readily, disappearing within a few months, resulting in relief of nasal obstruction and clearing of laryngeal lesions. The smaller nodular lesions in the skin shrink and are absorbed, leaving only pigment spots. Larger lesions disperse, with eventual scar formation. However, bacilli can persist following treatment, resulting in relapse at a later date.

Reconstructive surgery and rehabilitation to restore damaged hands, feet, face, *etc.* require the services of reconstructive and plastic surgeons, physical therapists, orthopedists, and others. Because the disfigurement of leprosy is such a stigma, surgery is absolutely necessary if the patient is to return to society.

To counter the crippling effects of the disease, the patient must realize the importance of maintaining mobility of the affected extremities and preventing fixed deformities. The principles are similar to those stressed in patient education for rheumatoid arthritis. The patient is encouraged to inspect sites of potential injury (eyes, hands, feet) daily, as these areas are not sensitive and injuries can be neglected. The skin is kept hydrated and an emollient applied to maintain suppleness and pliancy.

The Public Health Service maintains a hospital in Carville, Louisana (National Hansen's Disease Center), that serves as a treatment, research, and training facility. Research is still being conducted in the hope of finding a specific skin test for leprosy. Investigators have succeeded in infecting armadillos with leprosy and are using the microorganisms to produce a vaccine. No isolation precautions are required, since the infection declines rapidly under chemotherapy. Segregation is no longer required in any state of the United States.

Ornithosis (Psittacosis)

Ornithosis is an infectious and atypical form of pneumonia or systemic febrile illness transmitted to humans by infected birds. The agents responsible for ornithosis belong to the genus *Chlamydia* (intracellular organisms that were formerly considered viruses but are now classed as bacteria). The chlamydiae cause trachoma, lymphogranuloma venereum, and ornithosis; they are found in nasal secretions and in the feathers, feces, and blood of sick birds. The organisms, *Chlamydia psittaci,* are transmitted to humans inhaling the etiologic agent from dried droppings of infected birds, or directly from infected birds (*i.e.*, workers in food processing plants), or rarely from person to person. Birds of the parrot family (parakeets, parrots, cockatoos, budgerigars), as well as many other species of birds (canaries, sparrows, pigeons, turkeys), may be infected.

Clinical Manifestations. The illness may appear as a transient, influenzalike illness or a severe pneumonia, or it may be asymptomatic. After an incubation period lasting 4 to 15 days (it may be as long as 6 weeks in humans, 6 months in parrots), the disease begins abruptly, with malaise, headache, photophobia, and chills. Its course is characterized by high fever, great weakness, marked depression, and delirium, with surprisingly slow pulse and respiration. Cough is a prominent symptom. The lungs become involved, with edema, mononuclear cells, and lymphocytes appearing in the alveoli and interstitial areas. Chest x-ray may reveal an interstitial pneumonitis. Convalescence is apt to be prolonged.

Management. Ornithosis responds to the tetracyclines. Supportive therapy includes bed rest, oxygen (when necessary), and measures to reduce the fever. Relapses are common.

Prevention. Persons at risk are those who work in pet shops or around poultry and pigeons, bird fanciers, workers who may handle infected birds in the food processing and marketing business, and veterinarians. Care should be taken to avoid dust from feathers and bird-cage contents. Infected birds should be treated or destroyed. No protective vaccination is available.

Spirochetal Infections

Syphilis

See page 1663.

Lyme Disease

Lyme disease is a multisystem inflammatory disorder caused by the recently recognized spirochete, *Borrelia burgdorferi*. It is transmitted by the bite of Ixodid ticks, which have a wide range of hosts including sheep, cattle, deer, and mice. In the United States it is endemic along the east coast from Massachusetts to Virginia, and in Wisconsin, Minnesota, California, and Oregon.

Clinical Manifestations. The early manifestations occur in spring through late fall. The most characteristic finding is an expanding skin lesion, erythema chronicum migrans (ECM), that may be accompanied by flulike symptoms. The skin manifestations generally appear 4 to 20 days after a tick bite and may be located anywhere on the body. The skin lesion at the site of the tick bite starts as a red macule or papule and expands to become an annular erythema. The skin manifestations may be followed weeks to months later by central nervous system abnormalities (aseptic meningitis, encephalitis), heart abnormalities (AV block), and joint abnormalities (arthritis). Serologic tests show a rise in antibodies directed against the spirochete.

Management. Tetracycline or penicillin given as early as possible shortens the duration and prevents recurrence of the skin manifestations. High-dose penicillin administered intravenously is the treatment for other organ involvement.

Prevention and Patient Education. See Rocky Mountain spotted fever, page 1690.

Viral Infections

Influenza

Influenza is an acute infectious disease caused by an RNA-containing myxovirus. It is characterized by respiratory and constitutional symptoms. It sweeps through the entire world approximately every 20 years, attacking as many as 40% of the people in the affected areas. The striking features of these epidemics have been the speed with which the disease has spread and an extremely high attack rate.

Typical epidemics of influenza have been characterized by three successive waves, separated by brief intermissions. The first wave lasts from 3 to 6 weeks and is explosive in outbreak, widespread, and mild in form in the majority of cases, with few complications. The second wave also is widespread, but lasts longer; the cases are more severe, and the complications are serious. The third wave lasts still longer (from 8 to 10 weeks) and involves fewer persons, but the complications are quite severe. During the years succeeding a major epidemic, there follow scattered local waves of decreasing severity, with sporadic cases of influenza occurring during the intervals.

Etiology. The primary factor in the etiology of influenza is a filtrable virus, of which three major strains have been isolated, designated as types A, B, and C. Types A and B have been associated with epidemics. The numerous variants within a given type are called subtypes.

It is difficult to control influenza because the surface antigens of the virus have the capacity to change. Major changes in these viruses and new influenza strains arise from time to time. Therefore, previously acquired antibodies against earlier influenza strains may not be effective against the newly emerging strain, depending on the extent of the surface change. It has been observed that when a new influenza virus strain becomes prevalent throughout the country, the old virus strain disappears.

Transmission is by close contact or by droplets from the respiratory tract of an infected person. The virus is airborne and multiplies in the upper respiratory tract, invading the nasal, tracheal, and bronchial mucosal cells.

Clinical Manifestations. In the majority of patients, influenza begins after a short incubation period (24–72 hours) with an abrupt onset of chills, fever, headache, backache, and malaise. Respiratory features include a dry cough, sore throat, and nasal obstruction and discharge. Other patients start with acute sinusitis, bronchitis, pleurisy, or bronchopneumonia. These symptoms are always abrupt in onset, and prostrating. In still another group, there are gastrointestinal symptoms of nausea, vomiting, abdominal pain, and diarrhea; and finally, in each epidemic, cases develop without local symptoms but with chills or a continuous fever. The patient usually recovers within a week if there are no complications.

Complications. Persons at risk of developing the complications of influenza are those over 65, persons with chronic pulmonary or cardiac disease (especially rheumatic valve disease), and those with diabetes or other chronic metabolic disorders or chronic renal disease. The influenza virus damages the ciliated epithelium of the tracheobronchial tree, rendering the patient vulnerable to the development of secondary invaders such as pneumococci or staphylococci, *H. influenzae,* various streptococci, and other organisms.

Dyspnea early in the course of the disease points to bronchopneumonia, which is potentially life-threatening. This pneumonia may be viral, mixed viral, or bacterial in origin. Significant mortality occurs not only as a result of pneumonia but also from cardiopulmonary or other chronic diseases that are exacerbated during influenza infection. Other complications include myocarditis, myositis, and meningoencephalitis.

Management

The goals of management are to relieve symptoms and to prevent and treat complications.

The troublesome symptom of cough is treated with an expectorant–antitussive combination. The patient may be advised to take acetaminophen for headache and myalgias. (Children and teenagers are not given aspirin because of its apparent association with Reye's syndrome.) Antiviral therapy (amantadine hydrochloride), if given early, can shorten the course of illness and reduce the titer of virus excreted.

The patient is encouraged to rest at home, not only to relieve malaise and headache but also to reduce spread of the infection. Transmission of infection to others is most apt to occur early in the illness.

A liberal fluid intake (water, juices, carbonated beverages) is advised to thin secretions and help reduce fever. A vaporizer will increase air humidity and reduce irritation of the respiratory mucosa. Advise the patient to avoid respiratory irritants, particularly smoking, since smoking interferes with clearance of secretions by impairing ciliary function. Alcoholic beverages are discouraged since they can increase viscosity of secretions.

If acetaminophen is prescribed, the patient is advised to take it regularly to avoid marked swings of temperature with sweating and chills, which can lead to dehydration and exhaustion.

Prevention and Patient Education

The Immunization Practices Advisory Committee of the Public Health Service recommends annual influenza vaccination ("flu shots") for adults with chronic cardiovascular and pulmonary disorders that are severe enough to require regular medical follow-up or that have required hospitalization during the previous year. In addition, residents of nursing homes and other chronic care facilities, as well as health care personnel who have extensive contact with high-risk patients (*e.g.,* staff of intensive care units) are encouraged to have annual flu shots. The composition of the vaccine is changed yearly to match any new antigenic variation of the virus. It is recommended that influenza vaccine be administered in October or November.

The risk of developing influenza is related to crowding and close contact of groups of individuals. Therefore, visiting privileges within health care facilities and nursing homes should be restricted during epidemics to minimize any chance

of introducing influenza. Elective admissions and surgery are avoided as much as possible during an influenza outbreak.

Amantadine, an antiviral drug, can prevent clinical infection with influenza A virus. (It blocks an early step in the replication of this virus.) It is given only to certain high-risk patients, since most patients exposed to influenza require no prophylaxis. Amantadine does not protect against endemic influenza or influenza B. Amantadine is also given for the treatment of symptomatic influenza A infection and may shorten the duration and diminish the severity of illness. Adverse effects, occurring mainly in the elderly, include central nervous system toxicity, confusion, dizziness, slurred speech, headache, sleep disturbances, and visual hallucinations. To be effective, amantadine should be given prior to, and for the duration of, exposure to type A influenza virus.

Infectious Mononucleosis

Infectious mononucleosis ("mono") is an acute infectious disease of the lymphatic system caused by the Epstein-Barr virus (EBV), a DNA virus of the herpesvirus group. Another virus, cytomegalovirus, can cause virtually identical symptoms. A third infecting organism, *Toxoplasma* (a protozoan), can also produce a similar clinical picture.

The basic pathology is an intense proliferative response of the lymphoid tissue and organs (lymph nodes, spleen, tonsils), but all organs can be affected. Infectious mononucleosis is usually self-limited, but in rare instances complications and even death do occur.

Epidemiology. Infectious mononucleosis is encountered most frequently in the 15 to 25 age group. It has been shown that when natural primary infection with EBV develops in childhood, a mild and nonspecific or inapparent illness occurs, and the child has immunity for many years. Infectious mononucleosis occurs only in individuals without antibody to EBV. If natural primary infection does not take place in childhood and a susceptible person (adolescent/young adult) acquires the infection, this event will lead to clinical manifestations of infectious mononucleosis in about 50% of patients. Thus, infectious mononucleosis is more frequently encountered in countries with a high standard of living; in developing countries or among deprived socioeconomic groups, primary infection almost always occurs in early childhood, so that the disease is virtually unknown in adults. In this country, in persons of college age the rate of clinical attack is three to five times that of the population at large.

Transmission of infectious mononucleosis is by oral contact. The virus may persist in the pharynx for weeks or months. This suggests that a large number of young adults are probably convalescent carriers of this disease. The virus can also be spread by blood transfusion. The incubation period ranges from 30 to 50 days.

Clinical Manifestations. The early clinical manifestations are usually vague and masquerade as those of streptococcal sore throat, leukemia, and hepatitis. The triad of fever, sore throat, and cervical lymph node enlargement suggests infectious mononucleosis. A typical attack begins with fever and chills, anorexia, sore throat, and myalgia. Headache and diarrhea are often seen. On the second or third day, the lymph nodes begin to swell and become tender, usually the posterior cervical group first, and then the anterior groups.

This causes pain in the neck. Generalized lymphadenopathy may occur. Early in the course of the disease, supraorbital edema occurs and the spleen enlarges in the majority of patients. Although hepatomegaly occurs in less than 25% of patients, the majority of patients have abnormal liver function tests. A faint erythematous or maculopapular eruption may appear on the trunk and proximal extremities in the early stage of the disease.

There is evidence that the clinical syndrome of chronic Epstein-Barr virus infection does occur. These patients complain of chronic fatigue, recurrent sore throat, and nonspecific symptoms (swollen glands, musculoskeletal pains, headaches, difficulty with concentration).

Diagnostic Evaluation.   The diagnosis is made on the basis of the typical picture of clinical illness, as well as such laboratory findings as lymphocytosis with many atypical lymphoctyes, detection of heterophile antibodies, and positive EBV-specific antibody test results. The slide agglutination "spot test" is widely used to screen for heterophile antibodies. A few drops of the patient's blood are added to a specially prepared slide on which there are preserved red blood cells from horses. If heterophile antibodies are present, agglutination (clumping) of the animal cells will occur. This test requires just a few minutes to perform and can be done in the physician's office. Spot tests are generally accurate but they can give false-positive or false-negative results.

Management.   The treatment is symptomatic and supportive. The patient is encouraged to remain on bed rest while fever lasts and to rest at intervals during recovery. Aspirin or acetaminophen is given for headache and muscle pains. Constipation (which leads to straining and sudden increase in portal venous pressure, which in turn can contribute to splenic rupture) is to be avoided. Steroids may be used when severe or life-threatening complications develop, such as marked hepatic dysfunction, neurologic manifestations, thrombocytopenia, hemolytic anemia, and airway obstruction. Most patients recover in 1 to 3 weeks, although illness may be prolonged in some, with complaints of fatigue, poor exercise tolerance, and depression predominating for as long as 1 year.

Patient Education.   The patient is advised of the need for additional rest and sleep for a period of time. Strenuous physical activity and competitive sports are discouraged until recovery is complete because the enlarged spleen of the patient with infectious mononucleosis is vulnerable to injury and may rupture if subjected to relatively mild trauma. For the athlete, this may mean up to 6 months. However, the exact length of time is uncertain, since the spleen may rupture even after clinical, hematologic, and serologic evidence reveals recovery.

Rabies (Hydrophobia)

Rabies is a severe viral infection of the central nervous system, communicated to humans from the saliva of infected animals, and commonly transmitted by a bite or by contact of the animal's saliva with mucous membranes or open wounds such as cuts, scratches, or abrasions. In the United States the disease occurs mainly among wildlife: skunks, raccoons, foxes, and bats. The number of rabid dogs has decreased markedly as a result of organized canine rabies vaccination and leash laws.

The etiologic agent is an ultramicroscopic virus (rhabdovirus) present in the saliva and the central nervous system of rabid animals. Negri bodies (round objects about one quarter the size of red blood corpuscles) are found in the brain tissues so consistently in this disease that their presence is sufficient for diagnosis. In humans the virus is spread from the wound to the local muscle cells and then invades the peripheral nerves, spreading to the central nervous system, where rabies viral encephalitis ensues.

Management of the Biting Animal.   The animal inflicting the bite is captured (if possible) and kept under surveillance by veterinarians or animal control personnel. This may enable the bitten person to avoid undergoing unnecessary rabies vaccination. If the animal remains healthy for about 10 days, it is assumed that it was not infective.

Early signs of rabies in animals include an altered disposition and behavior, fever, loss of appetitite, and a change in the tone of bark (in dogs). If the animal becomes sick, the health department is notified. The animal is humanely killed, and its head is shipped, under refrigeration, to a qualified laboratory where the brain is examined for the characteristic Negri bodies. A wild animal that bites a person without provocation is killed at once, and the brain is sent for examination. If the brain of the animal is negative for rabies, it is assumed that the saliva contained no virus and that the bitten person need not be treated.

Prophylactic Management of the Patient

Local Treatment of the Wound.   Animal bites on the face, neck, and hands present the highest risk because of the rich nerve supply in these regions. The bite wounds should be cleansed immediately with thorough and prolonged washing with soap and water to remove the saliva, to dilute viral exposure, and for the virucidal benefits of soap. The patient is then taken immediately for emergency treatment, at which time the wound is again flushed and cleansed. The patient is given tetanus prophylaxis and antimicrobial therapy as indicated to counter any other possible infection transmitted by the animal.

Postexposure Prophylaxis.   Postexposure prophylaxis is designed to prevent the development of rabies illness in an exposed person. The decision to give postexposure treatment is made on an individual basis and depends on the type of animal involved (skunk, bat, fox, raccoon), the circumstances surrounding the exposure incident, whether or not the animal was captured, the vaccination status of the animal, and the presence of rabies in the region.

A combination of passive and active immunization is recommended when postexposure treatment is deemed necessary. Two types of immunizing products are used concurrently: (1) globulin, providing rapid protection; and (2) vaccine, which induces an active immune response that develops more slowly. As soon as possible, rabies immune globulin (RIG), which is made from the serum of immunized donors and is free of the danger of animal antiserum, is administered. (Part of the RIG dose is infiltrated around the wound, and the rest is administered intramuscularly in the patient's gluteus muscle.) At the same time the single dose of RIG is given, human diploid cell rabies vaccine (HDCV) is given intramuscularly in a separate site using a separate syringe, followed by four more vaccine doses given on days 3, 7, 14, and 28 after the first dose. (The product information sheet will provide drug data, schedule, and precautions, as well as instructions for persons who have been immunized previously.)

HDCV appears to produce immunity more quickly than previous rabies vaccines and causes substanially fewer side-effects. After the completion of the series of inoculations, a serum specimen for rabies antibody testing is drawn to assure that active immunity has been achieved. Serum antibody testing is arranged through the state health department.

Development of Rabies in Humans

Diagnostic Evaluation. The diagnosis of rabies is made on the basis of the history of exposure (the patient was bitten or exposed to animal saliva), the development of characteristic symptoms, and the demonstration of rabies antibodies in the patient's blood, along with the characteristic Negri bodies in samples of brain tissue taken from the infected animal.

Clinical Course in Humans. The incubation period in humans is extremely variable, depending on the location and severity of the wound and the length of the nerve over which the virus must travel before it reaches the brain. The incubation period may be only 10 days to several weeks for bites around the face, or from 60 to 90 days and up to a year for a bite in another part of the body.

There are several clinical phases of rabies in humans. During the prodromal phase of the illness, there are abnormal sensations around the site of infection, and the individual experiences an uneasy feeling and general anxiety, accompanied by depression and irritability. Headache, nausea, sore throat, and loss of appetite may occur, or unusual sensitivity to sound, light, and changes in temperature may be noted.

Then follows the stage of excitement. There are episodes of irrational excitement alternating with periods of alert calm. During this stage, convulsions occur. Attempting to swallow or even looking at liquids induces such severe and painful spasms of the muscles of swallowing and respiration that the patient writhes, and the ensuing choking may produce apnea. (Hence, the older name for rabies is *hydrophobia*, or fear of water.) Death usually occurs in this stage from cardiac or respiratory failure.

If the patient survives this stage, the muscle spasms and agitation cease. The paralytic phase is one of usually progessive ascending paralysis terminating in coma and death.

Management

There is no specific treatment for rabies, and the care of the patient is supportive. The patient is placed in the intensive care unit and receives continuing cardiac and pulmonary monitoring. The room should be quiet and darkened. The outcome is usually fatal.

- Bear in mind that the rabies virus is contained in the saliva of patients with this disease, constituting a distinct hazard to personnel caring for him. All personnel must be on guard against being bitten by such a patient or allowing saliva to contaminate a skin abrasion. If this

occurs, personnel must receive postexposure prophylactic treatment.

Rickettsial Infection: Rocky Mountain Spotted Fever

Rocky Mountain spotted fever (tick-borne typhus fever) is characterized by a continuous fever. It is caused by the bite of an infected tick, by an infected tick being crushed on the skin, or by the conjunctiva becoming contaminated with infected tick secretions. The organism responsible is *Rickettsia rickettsii*. The most common vectors for transmitting the disease to humans are the wood tick (*Dermacentor andersoni*) and the dog tick (*Dermacentor variabilis*). The incidence of infections increases in April and reaches its highest level in May and June.

Pathophysiology and Clinical Manifestations

During infection in humans, *R. rickettsii* organisms invade both the endothelial and smooth muscle cells of blood vessels, causing a generalized vasculitis. Cell damage may lead to alterations in capillary permeability, thrombosis, and hemorrhage. This generalized vasculitis accounts for the manifestations of the disease, both the cutaneous lesions and visceral disturbances. It may involve virtually every organ.

Early symptoms, appearing several days after an infected tick bite, are severe headache, malaise, anorexia, photophobia, slight fever, and muscle and joint pain. Within a few days, the fever, rash, and edema are quite pronounced. The rash is the most specific manifestation of the infection and consists of rose-colored macules (nonelevated discolorations) of variable size that appear on the wrists, ankles, soles, and palms, gradually spreading over the entire body. The rash becomes papular, (consisting of solid elevated lesions) darker red, and slightly dusky, and after a few days has a petechial or purpuric character (Fig. 59-5). In some cases, however, the rash appears in the terminal stages of illness or not at all. Large subcutaneous hemorrhages may appear. In severe forms of the disease, areas of skin necrosis appear as a result of endarteritis (inflammatory blockage of arterioles). This necrosis may involve the ear lobes, fingers, toes, and scrotum—those areas at the extreme periphery of the vascular system. There may be marked thrombocytopenia due to inflammation of the vessels communicating with the bone marrow. As a result of generalized vascular involvement and resulting escape of serum, generalized edema occurs.

Restlessness, insomnia, and hyperesthesias are distressing symptoms of this disease. Neurological manifestations, generally attributed to the effects of vasculitis on brain tissue, include altered mental status (confusion, delirium), headache, and stiff neck. The spleen is large and tender. Gastrointestinal symptoms include abdominal tenderness, pain, and muscular rigidity. Pneumonia may occur. Mental confusion, deafness, and visual disturbances are common and may last for weeks.

Diagnostic Evaluation

Early diagnosis is important and is almost always made on a high suspicion for the disease during tick season and on

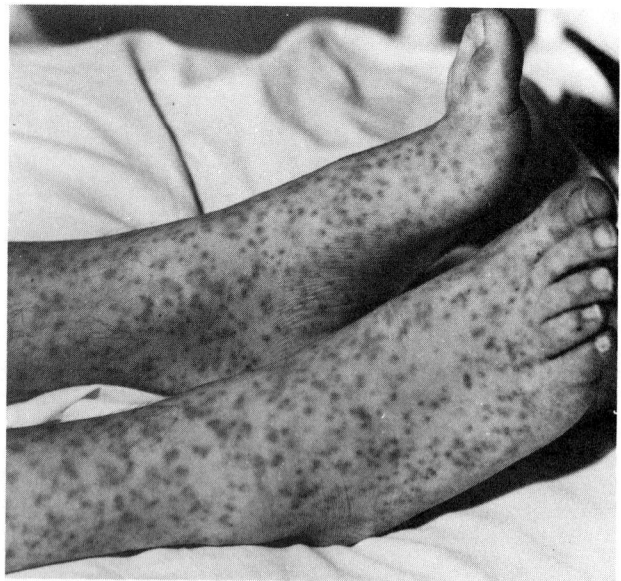

Figure 59-5
The rash of Rocky Mountain spotted fever. (Armed Forces Institute of Pathology photograph, Neg. No. N-67987-3.)

clinical grounds. Laboratory confirmation of Rocky Mountain spotted fever is made by serologic or other methods.

Management

One of the tetracyclines or chloramphenicol are both specific rickettsiostatic drugs if administered in the *early stages* of the disease. Rocky Mountain spotted fever can run a rapid and fulminating course, but the majority of patients recover if treated early.

Because Rocky Mountain spotted fever is an infectious vasculitis, the patient may display marked physiologic disturbances, including circulatory collapse, hypotension, oliguria, hypoproteinemia, and edema. Central venous pressure measurements are used to guide fluid and electrolyte replacement. The patient may be given transfusions of packed red blood cells and platelets. Severe coagulation disturbances may be treated with heparin.

Nursing Interventions

Supportive nursing measures are used to combat fever, restlessness, and pain, and to promote comfort (see Nursing Care Plan 59-1, p 1652). The patient is positioned carefully since he may have severe edema and necrosis from vasculitis. The circumferences of the abdomen, arms, and legs are measured at prescribed intervals to determine the extent of the edema. Intake and output records are kept and evaluated to assess for oliguria, since the patient may develop renal failure because of poor tissue perfusion from vascular degeneration.

Prevention and Patient Education. Rocky Mountain spotted fever is the most commonly reported rickettsial infection in the United States, with the majority of cases occurring in the southern Atlantic and western south-central states. The disease has almost vanished from its original home in the Rockies.

As increasing numbers of Americans participate in backpacking and other camping activities, more people will be exposed to this disease. Important aspects of prevention are wearing protective clothing and conscientiously searching for and removing ticks. Persons living in tick-infested areas or visiting such places should examine their scalp, skin, and clothing two to three times daily for ticks. This is important, as an infected tick must usually be attached and feeding several hours before it can transmit the disease. Tick repellent should be applied to the exposed parts of the body and clothing, especially socks and trouser cuffs and any openings in the clothing (neck, top of pants, button areas).

Ticks may be removed from the body by grasping the tick with tweezers as close to the point of attachment as possible and pulling slowly and steadily. Fingers, protected with facial tissue, may be used when tweezers are not available. Other means of removing a tick are to touch it with gasoline or cover it with a thick ointment to lessen the tick's hold on the skin. Care should be taken not to crush the tick, thus avoiding contamination of the broken skin with infectious tick secretions. Disinfect the tick bite immediately, and wash the hands immediately after tick removal.

Household pets should be examined for ticks on a regular basis.

Protozoan Infections

Malaria

Malaria is an acute infectious disease caused by protozoa, which are transmitted by way of an intermediate host, the bite of an infective female *Anopheles* mosquito. Malaria has also been transmitted through blood transfusions and from the needles and syringes shared by drug addicts.

Incidence. Malaria affects an estimated 300 million people in the world annually. It is claimed that in Africa, one fourth of all adults suffer from malarial fever at one time or other. It causes more disability and a heavier economic burden than any other parasitic disease. International travel and the recent influx of Asian and Middle Eastern immigrants have been responsible for a resurgence of malaria in many nontropical countries. In addition, more than 20 species of anopheline mosquitoes have become resistant to commonly used insecticides.

Types of Malaria. There are four species of malarial parasites, grouped under the generic name *Plasmodium*, each causing a different type of malaria: *Plasmodium falciparum* (which poses the greatest danger), *Plasmodium vivax, Plasmodium malariae*, and *Plasmodium ovale*. Each malarial parasite lives within a red blood corpuscle, using the hemoglobin as food. When full grown, it divides (segments) into 10 to 20 small, young parasites, called *hyalines* (segments), which burst the cell; this bursting of cells causes chills in the patient. The majority of these hyalines die, but a few find their way into new red cells, and the process is repeated.

Clinical Manifestations. The majority of patients present with paroxysms of chills, fever and sweating. Nausea, fatigue, and dizziness are present, along with intense headache and muscle pains. Paroxysms of chills and fever may last about 12 hours, after which the cycle may be repeated daily, every other day, or every third day.

Complications occur most frequently with *P. falciparum*. Patients with severe malaria of any form may become comatose and die (pernicious malaria); they may develop renal failure (due to the precipitation of free hemoglobin in the kidney tubule), a serious gastrointestinal disturbance, or cerebral symptoms (due to an accumulation of the parasites in the blood vessels of the affected organ).

Diagnostic Evaluation. The patient should be asked about travel outside the United States, since the majority of cases in this country are brought in by travelers. Travel or residence in an area where malaria is endemic is an important diagnostic clue. The diagnosis is confirmed by the finding of the parasites in stained peripheral blood smears. The blood should be examined as soon as the patient seeks treatment. More than one blood examination may be required, since the diagnosis can be missed on a routine smear.

Management

The goal of treatment is to destroy the blood trophozoites and schizonts of *Plasmodium* that cause the clinical manifestations and the pathologic effects that characterize the disease.

The use of antimalarial drugs depends on the stage of the life cycle of the parasite. The species of parasite infecting the patient is determined by means of a blood smear.

Chloroquine is given for infections caused by *P. vivax*, *P. ovale*, and *P. malariae*, followed by a course of primaquine to eliminate the hepatic form of these species. Quinine is given with pyrimethamine-sulfadoxine (Fansidar) to patients with malaria in areas known to be resistant to chloroquine or for malaria due to *P. falciparum* strains.

Cerebral malaria, which occurs in about 2% of patients with acute falciparum malaria, is the most feared complication. It produces changes in consciousness, behavioral changes, seizures, and cerebral edema. Patients with acute *P. falciparum* malaria are critically ill and must be hospitalized because the infection can be so overwhelming. In fact, acute malaria of this type is considered a medical emergency. Intravenous quinine is administered intermittently. Because neurologic toxicity can occur from the quinine infusion, the patient is monitored for twitching, delirium, confusion, convulsions, and coma. Oxygen is administered to counter tissue anoxia. The patient may have jaundice as a result of the density of malarial parasites in the blood and abnormalities in hepatic function. The degree of anemia present is related to the severity of the infection. Abnormal bleeding (nosebleeds, oozing of blood from venipuncture sites, passage of blood in the stool) may occur as a result of either decreased production of clotting factors by a damaged liver or disseminated intravascular coagulation (DIC).

Blood precautions are used during the patient's hospitalization. A screened room is required for the patient who is ill in a tropical climate.

Prevention and Patient Education. The essence of malaria control is the eradication of malaria as an endemic disease. In several areas of the world, this goal has been achieved. To escape malaria, one must avoid *Anopheles* mosquitoes that have fed on the blood of patients with malaria

about 3 weeks previously. This includes remaining in well-screened areas, using mosquito nets, and wearing clothes that cover most of the body. The application of mosquito repellant to exposed skin decreases the chance of being bitten. Travelers should be advised to try to reduce contact with mosquitos between dusk and dawn since malarial transmission occurs primarily in these hours due to nocturnal feeding habits.

The Centers for Disease Control (CDC) publishes *Health Information for International Travel*, which lists the areas of the world where there is risk of infection with malaria, and also the areas with strains of *P. falciparum* that are resistant to chloroquine. Persons planning a visit to endemic malarious areas are advised to seek the most recent prophylactic recommendations, usually chloroquine which is taken before entry into the area and continued for a specified time after returning to the United States. In areas where there is chloroquine resistance, advice from the CDC should be sought.

The traveler is also advised that regardless of the prophylactic regimen used, it is still possible to contract malaria. The onset of fever, chills, and headache should not be attributed to "flu," and medical advice should be *promptly* sought. Travelers to malarious areas should not donate blood for up to 3 years.

Giardiasis

Giardiasis is a protozoan infection of the small intestine caused by the flagellate *Giardia lamblia*. This water-borne parasite is found in two forms: cysts and trophozoites. Transmission depends on the ingestion of cysts that are excreted in the feces of a human or animal host. It is transmitted to humans by inadequately treated water, animal excretion into water (beaver colonies), and person to person.

Giardiasis is the cause of traveler's diarrhea in many countries, both underdeveloped and modern, usually associated with inadequately treated drinking water. In this country outbreaks have occurred in mountainous regions (Rockies, Appalachians, Pacific Northwest) where the pathogen affects campers, hikers, and mountainous communities drinking water from streams or rivers without a water filtration system. Person-to-person transmission occurs by hand-to-mouth transfer or cysts from the feces of an infected person and is responsible for outbreaks in day care centers, nursing homes, and other institutions. The incidence is high among homosexual men, particularly those practicing oral–anal sexual activity.

Clinical Manifestations. Patients with a mild infection report only a constant bloated feeling or abdominal pain without diarrhea. Other patients have persistent diarrhea with loose, watery, foul-smelling stools, abdominal cramping, and weight loss. Malabsorption of fats and fat-soluble vitamins may occur. The disease is usually self-limiting, lasting 2 to 6 weeks, but may recur intermittently and persist for months or even years.

Giardiasis is diagnosed by finding *Giardia lamblia* in feces. The trophozoites may be found in duodenal fluid obtained by having the patient swallow a weighted nylon string which passes to the bowel and is later withdrawn (enterotest). Alternatively, a sample of mucosa may be obtained by small intestine biopsy.

Management.   The treatment of giardiasis for adults is either quinacrine or metronidazole.

Prevention and Patient Education.   Travelers and hikers should boil water or treat it with commercially available iodine compound. Raw, unpeeled fruits and vegetable should not be eaten in areas where giardiasis is endemic. Control of person-to-person transmission requires personal cleanliness, careful hand washing, and sanitary disposal of feces.

Amebiasis (Amebic Dysentery)

Amebae are protozoa, larger than leukocytes, that move by ameboid action. Only a few amebae infect humans. One of the most important of these is *Entamoeba histolytica*, the cause of amebic dysentery. These amebae survive outside the body in resistant encysted forms.

Amebiasis is a worldwide parasite disease of the large intestine. It is acquired through the ingestion of the cyst stage of *E. histolytica* in food or water contaminated by infected human feces, flies, or the hands of infected food handlers who may be symptomless or convalescent carriers. The infection may also be transmitted through oral–anal or oral–genital sexual contact (both heterosexual and homosexual).

It is estimated that 10% of the world's population is infected, and in some tropical countries the infection rate may exceed 30%. In the United States it is becoming more common as a result of increased numbers of carriers. Persons at risk in this country are immigrants and visitors from developing countries, travelers returning from these areas, sexually active male homosexuals, and family contacts of infected persons living in poor sanitary conditions.

Pathophysiology.   The amebae burrow their way into the intestinal mucosa, where they feed mainly on bacteria. Pus pockets may form, with only a small orifice opening into the bowel from which numerous burrows extend for considerable distances in all directions under the mucous membrane. Here the amebae live. Abscesses form in the mucous membrane, and eventually slough off, exposing an underlying ulcer that may enlarge to sizes of 1 cm to 2 cm in diameter. The large bowel may be so covered by such ulcers that very little normal mucous membrane is left. Usually, the floor of these ulcers is the muscle wall of the bowel, but they may perforate its entire wall and cause fatal peritonitis.

In the small intestine, the organism may erode intestinal mucosa, invade the bloodstream, and gain access to the liver through the portal vein.

Clinical Manifestations and Course.   The majority of infected individuals are asymptomatic. The clinical manifestations depend on the site of involvement. Amebiasis may present as an intestinal or extraintestinal disease. When the amebae become invasive in the intestines, the chief symptom is diarrhea, with abdominal cramping and pain. Diarrhea may be mild, with loose stools, or there may be severe dysentery with stools containing considerable amounts of blood, exudate, and mucus, the latter swarming with amebae. Persons with chronic disease usually have associated weight loss and anemia. Amebiasis may mimic irritable bowel syndrome. The illness may present as appendicitis, abdominal mass, or partial intestinal obstruction.

The two important features of this disease are its chronicity (one attack of acute dysentery following another, separated by periods of constipation that last for months) and the tendency of the infection to cause liver abscess, as a result of dissemination to the liver by way of the portal vein. Complications include peritonitis, abscess formation, hemorrhage, and extraintestinal disease.

Diagnostic Evaluation

The diagnosis is made by finding trophozoites or cysts in a freshly purged stool specimen, in a nonpurged, warm stool specimen, or in proctosigmoidoscopic material or abscess contents. (Moving trophozoites disintegrate at room temperature, and false negative tests can occur.) Rectal biopsy may reveal the organism. There are serologic tests (indirect hemagglutination test and indirect fluorescent antibody test) to diagnosis amebiasis.

Management

The objectives of treatment are to eradicate the organism, to give symptomatic relief, to prevent spread of amebae to other tissues, and to replace fluids and electrolytes.

There is uncertainty about what constitutes the best treatment, and a significant number of patients require multiple courses of therapy. Usually two drugs are used: one to rid the intestines of the trophozoites and the other to dispose of the cysts. Metronidazole (Flagyl) followed by iodoquinol (active against the cyst form) is a standard form of treatment. Alternative therapies are available. Excretion precautions are observed.

To support the patient's general condition, intravenous infusions are given as required to correct fluid and electrolyte imbalance resulting from severe diarrhea. If diarrhea is acute, the patient remains on bed rest and is offered low-residue, bland foods. Follow-up study of the stools are necessary, since relapses are common.

Control and Patient Education

Transmission of *E. histolytica* is principally by ingestion of contaminated food or water. Methods of control include sanitary disposal of human feces, protection of the public water supply, raising and preparing food free of contamination, and an ongoing program of health education, including emphasis on meticulous hand washing after defecation and before preparing and eating food. In areas of high prevalence, fresh fruits and vegetables that cannot be peeled may be a source of contamination. Contacts of recently diagnosed patients should be examined. Patients should abstain from oral–anal and oral–genital sexual practices while they are under treatment. Sexual partners of infected patients should have a stool examination.

Amebic Liver Abscess

Amebic liver abscess represents the most common extraintestinal complication of amebiasis. It occurs when the amebae invade the liver tissue and form abscesses that increase in size, progressively damaging the liver.

In most patients, the right lobe of the liver is involved, and the abscess may be single or multiple. The major complaints are pain in the right upper abdomen (caused by the liver's rapid enlargement and stretching of its capsule), right upper chest pain (due to the liver's enlarging in an upward direction), fever, anorexia, and loss of weight. Physical examination reveals an enlarged, tender liver (due to hepatic abscess) and auscultatory abnormalities of the right lung field (from direct extension or rupture of a contiguous liver abscess). If the abscess is in the left lobe of the liver, a tender epigastric mass is noted. There is also sweating, weight loss, and pallor. A CT scan of the liver suggests the diagnosis and is useful in identifying the site, size, and number of lesions as well as in following the resolution of the abscess. Ultrasonography is used. Immunologic techniques, mainly serologic methods, are also used in diagnosis. One point to be emphasized is that not infrequently the abscesses are found unexpectedly in patients who have had few or no symptoms suggesting amebiasis.

Usually, the patient responds promptly to amebicidal therapy. Metronidazole (Flagyl) has generally been successful, and it may be combined with other drugs. Needle drainage of the abscess may be necessary if there is concern that the abscess may rupture and cause peritonitis, or after rupture to reduce further spread of infection, or when clinical illness persists after adequate drug therapy. The supportive treatment is that outlined for amebiasis.

Systemic Mycotic Infections (Fungal Infections)

Fungi are primitive organisms that take their nourishment from living plants and animals and decaying organic material. Fungi have the ability to exist as yeasts or as molds and may alternate between the yeast and mold form. The fungi present difficult problems in control because they are so widespread in nature—in soil, decaying vegetation, and bird excreta. Although there are thousands of known species of fungi, 100 or more species are generally recognized as pathogens to humans. The three main types of mycoses (fungal infections), as determined by the tissue level at which the fungus settles, are as follows:

1. Systemic or deep mycoses involving primarily the internal organs, with a primary focus in the lungs.
2. Subcutaneous mycoses that involve the skin, subcutaneous tissue, and sometimes the bone.
3. Superficial or cutaneous mycoses that grow in the outer layer of skin (epidermis), the hair, and the nails.

Systemic infections are usually acquired by accidental inhalation (spores carried on wind currents), occasionally by traumatic implantation (from contaminated soil or plant materials), or by the pathologic takeover of a normal inhabitant when the resistance of the host is lowered. The responsible fungi commonly spread to other organs by either the hematogenous or, less frequently, the lymphatic route. These infections are not transmitted from person to person.

Persons at Risk. The systemic mycoses are occurring more frequently, since they are more common in patients with impaired immunologic resistance and in patients receiving immunosuppressive agents (steroids, antilymphocyte serum, chemotherapy for cancer). Many patients who are receiving such treatment, or who are debilitated or severely ill and have reduced defenses, become prey to invasion by fungi that they could ordinarily withstand.

In addition to those receiving immunosuppressive agents, patients at risk for invasive fungal infections are those with certain immunologic deficiencies, those with advanced malignancies, kidney or other organ-transplant patients, open heart surgery patients, severely burned patients, patients receiving prolonged intravenous feedings, and those with renal failure and diabetes.

Histoplasmosis

Histoplasmosis is a chronic systemic fungus infection caused by a spore-bearing mold, *Histoplasma capsulatum*. This highly infectious mycosis is transmitted by airborne dust that contains *H. capsulatum* spores. Partially decayed droppings of pigeons, chickens, bats, and birds offer an excellent medium for growth of this fungus.

Clinical Manifestations. The patient may have no detectable illness or he may have signs and symptoms of a mild respiratory disease: fever, malaise, headache, myalgias, and anorexia. If the infection is more severe, signs and symptoms will resemble those of pulmonary tuberculosis; fever, cough, dyspnea, anorexia, and loss of weight and strength. Fungal infections mimic symptoms of other diseases, and the patient may present findings of malignant lymphoma, including anemia, thrombocytopenia, splenomegaly, and hepatomegaly.

Management. Most patients do not require treatment, since a mild self-limited course is the rule. Patients are followed clinically and radiologically to determine the course of the disease. Amphotericin B has traditionally been the mainstay of treatment for disseminated or acute pulmonary disease, since it has a wide spectrum of activity against fungal infections. It is given intravenously and is reserved for serious infections, because this agent has significant toxicity. Severe toxic reactions include nausea, vomiting, chills, fever, diarrhea, hypokalemia, and phlebitis.

Ketoconazole is an antifungal angent that is orally absorbable and effective against the etiologic agents of systemic mycoses. It has been associated with hepatic toxicity requiring close patient monitoring.

Health Education. Avoid stirring up dust by raking and sweeping around bird roosting sites. Exposure to dust in a contained, enclosed environment (chicken coop) should be minimized. Spraying the area with water will reduce dust.

Helminthic Infestations

Major helminthic (worm) infections are among the most prevalent of the human infectious diseases. They are global in distribution, and have profound effects on the nutritional status of humans and animals, and on the physical and mental development of children. There are three major groups of helminths that are intestinal parasites in humans: the nematodes (roundworms), the cestides (tapeworms), and the trematodes (flukes).

Trichinosis (Trichinellosis)

Trichinosis is infestation by the parasite *Trichinella spiralis*, one of the roundworms. It is acquired by consuming infected meat, usually pork.

Clinical Manifestations and Course. Trichinosis is a disease of pigs in the continental United States and of bears in Alaska. Tiny embryos of *T. spiralis* become encysted in the muscle fibers of an infected pig. These calcifed cysts, barely visible to the naked eye, appear in the meat like tiny grains of sand. If such pork is insufficiently cooked and then eaten, the embryos are set free by the gastric juice and develop in the intestine during the following week into adult worms, about 3 to 4 mm in length. These worms make their way into the mucous membrane and there produce myriad embryos. The intestinal phase starts about 24 hours after larval ingestion, causing symptoms of gastrointestinal disturbance: nausea, vomiting, diarrhea, and abdominal pain.

The embryos, carried by the bloodstream and by their own activity, migrate to all parts of the body. The patient's symptoms, arising from muscle invasion (due to an inflammatory process in the muscles), include edema of the eyelids, scleral hemorrhages, pain on eye motion, and generalized pain and soreness of muscles. Trichinosis causes high fever. Peripheral eosinophilia is a constant finding. Occasional heart irregularities (due to trichinae in the heart muscle) may be seen and may be fatal. Difficulties in breathing, masticating, swallowing, or speaking may also occur.

Diagnostic Evaluation. A biopsy specimen taken from a painful muscle (deltoid, biceps, gastrocnemius) reveals the larvae. Serologic tests may be positive, with demonstrable titers 3 to 4 weeks after the infection. Usually, the eosinophil count begins to rise in the second week. A skin test based on an extract of trichinae as the test antigen becomes positive after 16 to 20 days and may be positive for years afterward.

Management. The treatment of trichinosis is symptomatic. Mebendazole (Vermox) is used in both the intestinal and muscular stages of infection. The patient is advised to rest and is given analgesics to relieve muscle pain. Corticosteroids may be given to critically ill patients during the acute phase.

Electrocardiograms are taken for evidence of myocarditis.

Prevention and Patient Education. The public should be educated about the importance of thoroughly cooking all pork and pork products, especially sausage. There should be no trace of pink in cooked pork. Cooking pork in a microwave oven may fail to kill larvae. Smoking, pickling, seasoning, or spicing does not make pork safe unless it is cooked. Beef hamburger may be contaminated by a meat grinder that has been used for pork.

Garbage intended for hogs should be cooked. Finally, pork should be inspected by regular meat inspectors to determine if the disease is present.

Hookworm Disease (Ancylostomiasis)

Hookworm disease is the result of infestation of the small intestine by one or two quite similar roundworms about 1.2 cm (½ inch) long. Two species are parasitic in the human intestinal tract: *Necator americanus* (predominant U.S. species) and *Ancylostoma duodenale*. The infection is usually acquired by walking barefoot, whereby infected larvae of the worms penetrate the skin.

Incidence. Approximately 700 to 900 million persons are infected with hookworm. It is found mainly in tropical and subtropical regions, notably Asia, the Mediterranean area, South America, Africa, and in most of the western hemisphere. In the U.S., hookworm infections are more prevalent in the southeastern states.

Pathology and Clinical Course. The embryos of this worm, hatched from eggs passed in human feces onto the ground, live in dirt, sand, and clay, and easily infest humans. They enter by mouth when food is eaten with dirty hands, or they bore through the skin of bare feet, causing itching and burning followed by vesicular eruption (ground itch). Having gained access to the blood or lymph vessels, they are carried by the bloodstream to the lungs, and migrate from the pulmonary capillaries into the alveolar sacs. The larvae migrate up the bronchi and trachea, pass over the epiglottis and down the esophagus, and into the bowel. The worms attach themselves to the intestinal mucosa and suck the blood of the host. The effect of the blood-sucking and hemorrhages at the attachment sites is iron-deficiency anemia. A patient with heavy infection and with inadequate dietary iron may develop profound anemia. He presents with lassitude, dyspnea, anorexia, and pedal edema. Severe anemia may cause cardiac symptoms. Maturation of the worms in the intestine may cause diarrhea and other gastrointestinal symptoms. A dry cough and dyspnea develop when the larve rupture through the capillary bed and are spread throughout the bronchial tree.

Management. Mebendazole or pyrantel pamoate (Antiminth) are both effective for hookworm disease. The patient should be placed on a nutritious diet, since hookworm disease occurs in persons suffering from malnutrition. Protein and iron supplementation is administered to aid in the correction of the anemia.

Prevention. The prevention of hookworm disease depends on sanitary disposal of human excreta, proper hand washing, and the wearing of shoes. Night soil (human excrement) and sewage effluents should not be used for fertilizer.

Ascariasis (Roundworm Infestation)

Ascariasis is an infection by the nematode *Ascaris lumbricoides* (intestinal roundworm). This is the most common worm parasitizing the human intestine, with an estimated 1 billion infections worldwide. In the U.S., ascariasis is more common in the southeastern states.

This disease is usually found in overcrowded areas with poor sanitation. Contamination of the soil by human feces is a factor in its spread. Indiscriminate defecation in the fields, streets, and doorways provide a major source of infective eggs. Humans are infected by ingestion of the eggs in contaminated raw vegetables and drinking water. Infection may be contracted from eating raw vegetables when night soil is used for fertilizer. Water pollution may cause water transmission.

Life Cycle and Clinical Features. The eggs are swallowed and pass into the intestine, where they hatch as larvae. The larvae enter the bloodstream and pass through the pulmonary circulation, migrate through the lungs, and return to the gastrointestinal tract, where they grow, mature, and mate. Large numbers of worms may migrate into various organs of the body and cause obstruction to the trachea, bronchi, bile duct, appendix, and pancreatic duct. Masses of worms in the intestine cause gastointestinal discomfort, severe abdominal pain, and vomiting. Fever, chills, dyspnea, cough, and pneumonia may develop from invasion of the lungs by large numbers of larvae. Adult worms may migrate into the ampulla of Vater and then to the pancreatic or biliary ducts, causing acute and agonizing pain.

Ascariasis is diagnosed by detecting ova or worms in the feces.

Management. Mebendazole (Vermox) given twice daily for 3 days is currently the drug of choice. Piperazine (Antepar) and pyrantel pamoate (Antiminth) are also effective drugs. No isolation or precautions are required.

Prevention. Preventive measures include providing adequate toilet facilities and teaching the importance of personal hygiene. All patients with the infestation should be treated.

Bibilography

Books

Benenson AS (ed). Control of Communicable Diseases in Man, 14th ed. Washington, D.C., American Public Health Association, 1985.

Berquist LM. Changing Patterns of Infectious Disease. Philadelphia, Lea & Febiger, 1984.

Braude AI, Davis CE and Fierer J. Infectious Diseases and Medical Microbiology, 2nd ed. Philadelphia, WB Saunders, 1986.

Brettle RP and Thomson M. Infection and Communicable Diseases. London, William Heinemann Medical Books, 1984.

Centers for Diseases Control. CDC Guideline for Handwashing and Hospital Environmental Control, 1985. Springfield, Virginia, National Technical Information Service, 1985.

Centers for Disease Control. CDC Guideline for Prevention of Surgical Wound Infections, 1985. Springfield, Virginia, National Technical Information Service, 1985.

Cheng TC. General Parasitology. New York, Academic Press, 1986.

DeVita VT Jr, Hellman S and Rosenberg SA. AIDS. Etiology, Diagnosis, Treatment, and Prevention. Philadelphia, JB Lippincott, 1985.

Dick G. Practical Immunization. Boston, MTP Press Limited, 1986.

Doak CC, Doak LG and Root J. Teaching Patients with Low Literacy Skills. Philadelphia, JB Lippincott, 1985.

Felman, YM. Sexually Transmitted Diseases. New York, Churchill Livingstone, 1986.

Fields BN (ed). Virology. New York, Raven Press, 1985.

Fox RA, Immunology and Infection in the Elderly. New York, Churchill Livingstone, 1984.

Holmes KK et al. Sexually Transmitted Diseases. New York, McGraw-Hill, 1984.

Holt JG (ed). Bergey's Manual of Systematic Bacteriology. Baltimore, Williams & Wilkins, 1984.

Kaplan C, Turner GS and Warrell DA. Rabies. New York, Oxford University Press, 1986.

Kass EH and Platt R. Current Therapy in Infectious Disease 1983–1984. St Louis, CV Mosby, 1983.

Ledger WJ. Infection in the Female, 2nd ed. Philadelphia, Lea & Febiger, 1986.

Ma P and Armstrong D. The Acquired Immune Deficiency Syndrome and Infections of Homosexual Men. New York, Yorke Medical Books, 1984.

Mandell GL, Douglas RC Jr and Bennett JE. Principles and Practice of Infectious Diseases. New York, John Wiley & Sons, 1985.

Mandell LA and Ralph ED (eds). Essentials of Infectious Diseases. Boston, Blackwell Scientific Publications, 1985.

Marquardt WC and Demaree RS Jr. Parasitology. New York, Macmillan, 1985.

Noble RC. Sexually Transmitted Diseases, 3rd ed. New Hyde Park, New York, Medical Examination Publishing, 1985.

Pickering LK and DuPont HL. Infectious Diseases of Children and Adults. Menlo Park, California, Addison-Wesley, 1986.

Report of a WHO Study Group. Epidemiology of Leprosy in Relation to Control. Technical Report Series 716. Geneva, World Health Organization, 1985.

Roberts RB. Infectious Diseases: Pathogenesis, Diagnosis, and Therapy. Chicago, Year Book Medical Publishers, 1986.

Rytel MW and Mogabgab WJ. Clinical Manual of Infectious Diseases. Chicago, Year Book Medical Publishers, 1984.

Sherris JC (ed). Medical Microbiology. An Introduction to Infectious Diseases. New York, Elsevier, 1984.

Sweet RL and Gibbs RS. Infectious Diseases of the Female Genital Tract. Baltimore, Williams & Wilkins, 1985.

Taylor-Robinson D (ed). Clinical Problems in Sexually Transmitted Diseases. Boston, Martinus Nijhoff Publishers, 1985.

Valanis B. Epidemiology in Nursing and Health Care. Norwalk, Appleton-Century-Crofts, 1986.

Waldman RH and Kluge RM. Textbook of Infectious Diseases. New Hyde Park, New York, Medical Examination Publishing, 1984.

Youmans GP, Paterson PY and Sommers HM. The Biologic and Clinical Basis of Infectious Diseases. Philadelphia, WB Saunders, 1985.

Articles

Bacterial Infections

Ayliffe GA. Nosocomial infection—the irreducible minimum. Infect Control 1986 Feb; 7(2 Suppl):92–95.

Baohong JI. Drug resistance in leprosy—a review. Lepr Rev 1985 Dec; 56(4):265–278.

Besch CL and Sanders CV. Managing sepsis—a common cause of geriatric death. Geriatrics 1986 Apr; 41(4):55–66.

Butler T et al. Typhoid fever complicated by intestinal perforation: A persisting fatal disease requiring surgical management. Rev Infect Dis 1985 Mar/Apr; 7(2):244–256.

Davis CE et al. Tuberculosis. Chest 1985 Nov; 88(5):726–729.

Dutt AK, Moers D and Stead WW. Short-course chemotherapy for extrapulmonary tuberculosis. Ann Intern Med 1986 Jan; 104(1):7–12.

Edelstein PH and Meyer RD. Legionnaires' disease: A review. Chest 1984 Jan; 85(1):114–120.

Fallon RJ. The Legionellaceae. Med Lab Sci 1986 Jan; 43(1):64–71.

Gottlieb LS. Current patterns of pulmonary tuberculosis. Am Fam Physician 1985 June; 31(6):113–117.

Haley RW et al. The efficacy of infection surveillance and control programs in preventing nosocomial infections in US populations. Am J Epidemiol 1985 Feb; 121(2):182–205.

Hornick RB. Selective primary health care. Strategies for control of disease in the developing world. XX. Typhoid fever. Rev Infect Dis 1985 July/Aug; 7(4):536–546.

Iseman MD and Sbarbaro JA. National ACCP Consensus Conference on Tuberculosis. Chest 1985 Feb; 87(2 Suppl):115S–149S.

Joint Statement of American Thoracic Society and Centers for Disease Control. Treatment of tuberculosis and other mycobacterial diseases. Am Rev Respir Dis 1983 June; 127(6):790–796.

Krebs B, Moller BN & Jensen BH. Gas-producing infections after lower-limb amputation because of ischemia. Arch Orthop Trauma Surg 1986; 104(6):374–376.

Kunin CM. Genitourinary infections in the patient at risk: Extrinsic risk factors. Am J Med 1984 May 15; 76(5A):131–139.

Lefrock JL. Drugs of choice for bacterial meningitis. Am Fam Physician 1986 Feb; 33(2):285–291.

Mandel JH. Pharyngeal infections. Postgrad Med 1985 Feb 15; 77(3): 187–199.

Mayer G and Kang R. Gas gangrene, diabetes, and cholecystitis. Am J Emerg Med 1985 Jan; 3(1):42–45.

McGowan JE Jr. Changing etiology of nosocomial bacteremia and fungemia and other hospital-acquired infections. Rev Infect Dis 1985 July/Aug; 7(Suppl 3):S357–S370.

Meyer RD. Legionnaire's disease. Am J Med 1984 Apr; 76(4):657–663.

Nagami P and Yoshikawa TT. Management of tuberculosis in elderly persons. Compr Ther 1984 July; 10(7):57–62.

Neu HC (ed). Proceedings of a symposium: Emergency prospectives in management and prevention of infectious diseases. Am J Med 1985 June 28; 78(6B):1–236.

Palmer DL. Microbiology of pneumonia in the patient at risk. Am J Med 1984 May 15; 76(5A):53–60.

Phillips KF and Hailey FJ. The use of furoxone: A perspective. J Int Med Res 1986; 14(1):19–29.

Quinn TC, Bender BS, and Bartlett JG. New developments in infectious diarrhea. DM 1986 Apr; 32(4):174–244.

Sande MA, Smith AL and Root RK. Bacterial meningitis. Contemp Issues Infect Dis 1985; 3:1–264.

Sbarbaro JA. Strategies to improve compliance with therapy. Am J Med 1985 Dec 20; 79(6A):34–37.

Schofield F. Selective primary health care: Strategies for control of disease in the developing world. XXII. Tetanus: A preventable problem. Rev Infect Dis 1986 Jan/Feb; 8(1):144–156.

Sellin LC. Botulism—an update. Milit Med 1984 Jan; 149(1):12–16.

Snider DE Jr, Caras GJ and Koplan JP. Preventive therapy with isoniazid. JAMA 1986 Mar 28; 255(12):1579–1583.

Stead WW et al. Tuberculosis as an endemic and nosocomial infection among the elderly in nursing homes. N Engl J Med 1985 June 6; 312(23):1483–1487.

Weinstein L. Bacterial meningitis. Med Clin North Am 1985 Mar; 69(2): 219–229.

Werry DG and Meek RN. Clostridial gas gangrene complicating Colles' fracture. J Trauma 1986 Mar; 26(3):280–283.

West TE and Apicella MA. Microbial factors in the pathogenesis of sepsis. Contemp Issues Infect Dis 1985; 4:27–40.

Winn WC Jr. Legionella and Legionnaires' disease: A review with emphasis on environmental studies and laboratory diagnosis. CRC Crit Rev Clin Lab Sci 1985; 21(4):323–381.

Infection Control

Amin NM. Adult immunizations. Am Fam Physician 1986 June; 33(6): 89–104.

Ashworth P. Infection control and the nursing process—making the best use of resources. J Hosp Infect 1984 Dec; 5(Suppl A): 35–44.

Garner JS and Favero MS. CDC guideline for handwashing and environmental control, 1985. Infect Control 1986 Apr; 7(4):231–243.

Garner JS and Simmons BP. CDC guideline for isolation precautions in hospitals. Infect Control 1983 July/Aug; 4(4):248–325.

Haley WR, Garner JS and Simmons BP. A new approach to the isolation of hospitalized patients with infectious diseases: Alternative systems. J Hosp Infect 1985 June; 6(2):128–139.

Poland GA, Rosborough TK and Love KR. Immunizing the adult. Postgrad Med 1986 Mar; 79(4):133–138.

Recommendations of the Immunization Practices Advisory Committee: Polysaccharide vaccine for prevention of *Haemophilus influenzae* Type b disease. MMWR 1985 Apr 19; 34(15):201–205.

Tafuro P and Gurevich I (eds). Symposium on infections in the compromised host. Nurs Clin North Am 1985 Mar; 20(1):143–260.

Williams WW. CDC guideline for infection control in hospital personnel. Infect Control 1983 July/Aug; 4(4):329–349.

Protozoan Infections

Brooks JL and Kozarek RM. Amebic colitis. Postgrad Med 1985 July; 78(1):267–274.

Feldman YM and Nikitas JA. Giardiasis. Cutis 1985 Apr; 35(4):305–306.

Gorski ED. Management of giardiasis. Am Fam Physician 1985 Nov; 32(5): 157–164.

Knight R. Hepatic amebiasis. Semin Liver Dis 1984 Nov; 4(4):277–292.

Pearson RD, Hewlett EL and Guerrant RL. Tropical diseases in North America. DM 1984 Mar; 30(6):7–68.

Revised recommendations for preventing malaria in travelers to areas with chloroquine-resistant *Plasmodium falciparum*. MMWR 1985 Apr 12; 34(14):185–195.

Smith PD. Pathophysiology and immunology of giardiasis. Annu Rev Med 1985; 36:295–307.

Stevens DP. Selective primary health care: Strategies for control of disease in the developing world. XIX. Giardiasis. Rev Infect Dis 1985 July/Aug; 7(4):530–535.

Wilson ME and Pearson RD. Parasitic disease of normal hosts in North America. Hosp Pract 1986 Apr 15; 21(4):164A–164D.

Rickettsial Infections

Massey EW et al. Neurologic complications of Rocky Mountain spotted fever. South Med J 1985 Nov; 78(11):1288–1290.

McHugh TP et al. Rocky Mountain spotted fever. Ann Emerg Med 1984 Dec; 13(12):1132–1136.

Sexton DJ. Rocky Mountain spotted fever. Arch Intern Med 1985 Dec; 145(12):2173.

Sexually Transmitted Diseases

Bardin E and Berger RE. Sexually transmitted diseases in men. Primary Care 1985 Dec; 12(4):761–785.

Bell TA and Grayston JT. Centers for Disease Control guidelines for prevention and control of *Chlamydia trachomatis* infections. Ann Intern Med 1986 Apr; 104(4):524–526.

Buntin DM. Cutaneous features of sexually transmitted diseases. Postgrad Med 1985 Nov; 78(7):121–128.

Cates W et al. Adolescents and sexually transmitted diseases: An expanding problem. J Adolesc Health Care 1985 Sept; 6(5):257–323.

Centers for Disease Control. 1985 STD treatment guidelines. 1985 Oct 18; 34(4S):75S–108S.

Cooney TG and Ward TT (eds). AIDS and other medical problems in the male homosexual. Med Clin North Am 1986 May; 70(3):499–720 (entire volume).

Crissey JT and Denenholz DA. Syphilis. Clin Dermatol 1985 Jan/Mar; 2(1):1–166.

Fiumara NJ. Treatment of primary and secondary syphilis: Serologic response. J Am Acad Dermatol 1986 Mar; 14(3):487–491.

Hart G. Syphilis tests in diagnostic and therapeutic decision making. Ann Intern Med 1986 Mar; 104(3):368–376.

Lutz R. Stopping the spread of sexually transmitted diseases. Nursing '86 1986 Mar; 16(3):47–50.

Perine PL. Epidemiology of the sexually transmitted disease. Annu Rev Public Health 1985; 6:85–106.

Romanowski B and Harris JRW. Sexually transmitted diseases. Clin Symp 1984; 36(1):2–32.

Schoonover-Smith L and Lauver D. Assessment and management of vaginitis and cervicitis. Nurs Pract 1984 June; 9(6):34, 39–47.

Stone KM, Grimes DA and Magder LS. Primary prevention of sexually transmitted diseases. JAMA 1986 Apr 4; 255(13):1763–1766.

Treatment of sexually transmitted diseases. Med Lett Drug Ther 1986 Feb 28; 28(708):23–28.

Valle S-L. Current views on sexually transmitted diseases. Ann Clin Res 1985; 17(2):43–44.

Spirochetal Diseases

Malawista SE and Steere AC. Lyme disease: Infectious in origin, rheumatic in expression. Adv Intern Med 1986; 31:147–166.

Mertz LE et al. Ticks, spirochetes, and new diagnostic tests for Lyme disease. Mayo Clin Proc 1985 June; 60(6):402–406.

Williams CL et al. Lyme disease: Epidemiologic characteristics of an outbreak in Westchester County, NY. Am J Public Health 1986 Jan; 76(1):62–65.

Viral Diseases

Bean B. Antiviral therapy. Postgrad Med 1986 July; 80(1):109–120.

Chronic Epstein-Barr Virus Disease: A workshop held by the National Institute of Allergy and Infectious Diseases. Ann Intern Med 1985 Dec; 103(6, Pt 1):951–953.

Mandel JH. Pharyngeal infections. Postgrad Med 1985 Feb 15; 73(3): 187–199.

McSherry JA. Diagnosing infectious mononucleosis. Am Fam Physician 1985 Oct; 32(4):129–132.

Niederman JC. Chronicity of Epstein-Barr virus infection. Ann Intern Med 1985 Jan; 102(1):119–121.

Recommendation by the Immunization Practices Advisory Committee. Prevention and control of influenza. MMWR 1985 May 17; 34(19): 261–275.

Sumaya CV. Serologic testing for Epstein-Barr virus—developments in interpretation. J Infect Dis 1985 June; 151(6):984–987.

Volpi A and Rocchi G. Natural history, diagnosis and management of Epstein-Barr virus infection. Ala J Med Sci 1985 Apr; 22(2):157–159.

Other Infections

Davis A. Chemotherapy of gastrointestinal helminths. Introduction. Handbook Exp Pharmacol 1985; 77:1–5.

Drugs for treatment of systemic fungal infections. Med Lett Drug Ther 1986 Apr 11; 28(711):41–44.

Agencies

International

World Health Organization (Regional Office for the Americas), Pan American Health Organization, 525 23rd Street, NW, Washington, D.C. 20037.

World Health Organization, Avenue Appia, CH 1211 Geneva 27, Switzerland.

Governmental

Centers for Disease Control (Center for Prevention Services, Center for Environmental Health, Center for Health Promotion and Education, Center for Infectious Diseases), Atlanta, Georgia 30333.

National Institute of Allergy and Infectious Diseases, National Institutes of Health, Bethesda, Maryland 20892.

US Department of Health and Human Services, Public Health Service, 200 Independence Ave., SW, Washington, DC 20201.

Voluntary

American Lung Association, 1740 Broadway, New York, New York 10019.

American Public Health Association, 1015 Fifteenth Street, NW, Washington DC 20005.

American Social Health Association, VD National Hotline, 260 Sheridan Ave., Suite 307, Palo Alto, California 94306.

American Venereal Disease Association, Box 22349, San Diego, CA 92122.

National Foundation for Infectious Diseases, P.O. Box 42022, Washington, D.C. 20015.

Chapter 60

Emergency Nursing

Nursing in Emergency Conditions

The term *emergency management* has traditionally referred to the care given to patients with urgent and critical needs. However, hospital emergency departments and emergency clinics are increasingly being used for nonurgent problems, and the philosophy of emergency care has broadened to include the concept that an emergency is whatever the patient or his family considers it to be. The staff have an obligation to treat the patient with understanding and to respect the anxiety that he undoubtedly feels. If they downgrade his complaint, the therapeutic process may very well be impaired.

A large number of people seek emergency help for serious life-threatening cardiac conditions, such as myocardial infarction, acute congestive failure and pulmonary edema, and cardiac dysrhythmias. The priorities of management of such cardiac conditions, as well as the ECG patterns evoked by the dysrhythmias, are discussed in Chapters 25 and 26. This chapter deals mainly with the emergency management of trauma and other conditions not found elsewhere in this book. *It is assumed that treatment is given under the direction of a physician.*

The Nursing Process in the Emergency Department

The nursing process provides a logical framework for problem solving in the time-limited and pressured environment of the emergency department. The nurse in the emergency department, through specialized education, training, and experience, has expertise in assessing and identifying patients' health care problems in crisis situations, establishing priorities, monitoring acutely ill and injured patients, supporting and attending to families, supervising allied health personnel, and teaching patients and families. Nursing interventions are also accomplished interdependently with consultation or direction from the physician. The strengths of nursing and medicine are especially complementary in an emergency situation. The nurse anticipates appropriate nursing and medical interventions based on the assessment data and works as a team member in performing the high-tech, high-touch skills necessary in the care of emergency patients.

Patients in the emergency department have a wide variety of actual or potential problems. The patient's condition may change from minute to minute, and nursing assessment is ongoing. Thus the nursing diagnoses change just as rapidly. Although a patient may have several diagnoses at a given point of time, the following discussions focus on the most immediate and assume both independent and interdependent nursing interventions.

Gerontological Considerations

The elderly are major consumers of health care in the emergency department, accounting for 20% to 35% of visits to urban emergency facilities. Most of these are nonurgent visits, with skin, cardiovascular, and abdominal problems predominating. Elderly clients have multifaceted problems and often arrive in the emergency department with one or more presenting conditions that, while not considered urgent in the younger person, can readily become life-threatening in the aged if untreated. Acute illness may be manifested in the aging person by nonspecific signs such as weakness and fatigue, falling episodes, incontinence, and change in mental status.

Some type of social service support may need to be initiated during the visit to the emergency department. The aged client may perceive the "emergency" as a crisis, since it may signal the end of an independent life-style or even result in death.

Psychological Management of Patients and Families in Emergencies and Crisis Situations

Approach to the Patient

Body trauma is an insult to both physiologic and psychological homeostasis and requires both physiologic and psychological healing.

An assessment of the patient's psychological functioning includes evaluation of his emotional expression, degree of anxiety, and cognitive functioning (oriented to time, place, person). In addition, a rapid physical examination, focusing on the clinical problem that caused the patient to seek help, is carried out. The nursing diagnoses may include anxiety related to the uncertain potential outcomes of trauma and ineffective individual coping related to acute situational crisis. The first major goal is reduction of anxiety, which is a prerequisite to recovering the ability to cope.

Interventions

Patients experiencing sudden injury or illness are often overwhelmed by anxiety, since they have not had time to mobilize their resources to adapt to the crisis. They experience real and terrifying fear—of death, mutilation, immobilization, and other assaults on their personal identity and body integrity. Those caring for the patient should act confidently and competently to help relieve his excessive anxiety. Personalizing the situation as much as possible and speaking, reacting, and responding to the patient in a warm manner contributes to a sense of security. In addition, explanations should be given on a level that the patient can grasp; an informed patient is able to cope more positively with psychological and physical stress. Ongoing human contact helps reduce the panic of the severely injured person, and reassuring words aid in dispelling fear of the unknown. The emotionally distressed patient and family can more effectively mobilize their own psychological resources when the emergency department staff conveys optimism and concern for the welfare of the patient in a calm and reassuring manner.

If the patient is unconscious, he should be treated as if he were conscious: by touching him, calling him by name, and explaining every procedure that is being done. As soon as the patient regains consciousness, a primary concern is to orient him by stating his name, the date, and the place. If necessary, this basic information should be repeated over and over. The patient is brought back to reality in a calm, reassuring way.

Approach to the Family

In the admitting area, the family is told where the patient is and that he is receiving expert care. When crises of trauma, severe disfigurement, and sudden death are confronted, the family goes through several stages, beginning with "unbearable anxiety" and progressing through denial, remorse, grief, anger, and reconciliation. (In addition to anxiety, the nursing diagnoses may include grieving and alterations in family processes related to acute situational crisis.)

The family members are encouraged to recognize and talk about their feelings of anxiety. The approach is to tune into the family's thinking and to deal with reality as gently and as quickly as possible. Although denial is an ego-defense mechanism that protects one from recognizing painful and disturbing aspects of reality, prolonged denial cannot be encouraged or supported, since the family must be prepared for the reality of what has happened (and not for what they wish it could be) and for what may come.

Expressions of remorse and guilt are frequently heard, with family members accusing themselves (or each other) of negligence or minor omissions. The nursing approach is to allow expressions of remorse, over and over if need be, until the family members realize that there was probably little that they could have done to prevent the accident or illness.

Expressions of anger are common in crisis situations; they are a way of handling the anxiety. The anger is frequently directed at the patient, but it is also often expressed toward the physician, the nurse, or the admitting officer. Without condemnation or rejection, the therapeutic approach is to allow the anger to be ventilated in order to help the family identify their feelings of frustration.

Grief is a complex emotional response to anticipated or actual loss. In this stage, the nursing intervention is to help family members work through their grief and to support their usual coping mechanisms, letting them know that it is normal and acceptable for them to cry and feel this way.

The following are guidelines for helping a family deal with sudden death in the emergency department:

- Take the family to a private place.
- Talk to the family together, so that they can mourn together.
- Assure the family that everything possible was done; inform them of the treatment rendered.
- Avoid using euphemisms such as "passed on," *etc.* Show the family that you care by touching, offering coffee, *etc.*
- Allow family members to talk about the deceased and what he meant to them; this permits ventilation of feelings of loss. Encourage the family to talk about events preceding admission to the emergency department.
- Encourage family members to support each other and to express emotions freely (grief, loss, anger, helplessness, tears, disbelief).
- Avoid volunteering unnecessary information (patient was drinking, *etc.*).
- Avoid giving sedation to family members; this may mask or delay the grieving process, which is necessary to achieve emotional equilibrium and prevent prolonged depression.
- Encourage the family to view the body if they wish to do so; this action helps to integrate the loss. Cover mutilated areas before the family sees the body. Go with the family to see the body. Show acceptance of the body by touching, to give the family "permission" to touch, talk to the body, *etc.*
- Spend a few minutes with the family, listening to them.

Posttraumatic Stress Disorder

Posttraumatic stress disorder is the development of characteristic symptoms after a psychologically stressful event that is generally outside the range of human experience (rape, combat, car accident, natural catastrophe). The symptoms of this disorder include intrusive thoughts and dreams, phobic-avoidance reaction (avoidance of activities that arouse recollection of the traumatic event), heightened vigilance and exaggerated startle reaction, generalized anxiety, and social withdrawal. Posttraumatic stress disorder may be acute, chronic, or delayed.

Assessment includes an evaluation of the patient's pretrauma history, the trauma itself, and posttrauma functioning.

Interventions

The patient's goal is to organize and begin to integrate his experience in order to return to his pretrauma level of functioning as soon as possible. The nurse carries out a wide range of interventions involving crisis intervention strategies, establishing a trusting and sharing relationship, and educating the patient and family about stress management and support services available in the community.

Priorities and Principles of Emergency Management

Priorities of Emergency Management

When care is being given to a patient in an emergency situation, many crucial decisions must be made. Such decisions require sound judgment based on an understanding of the condition that produced the emergency and its effect on the person.

The major goals of emergency medical treatment are (1) to preserve life, (2) to prevent deterioration before more definitive treatment can be given, and (3) to restore the patient to useful living.

When the patient is first received into the emergency department, the goal is to determine the extent of injury or illness and to establish priorities for the initiation of treatment. These priorities are determined by the comparative threat to the person's life. Injuries or conditions interfering with vital physiologic function (obstructed airway, massive bleeding) take precedence. Usually, injuries of the face, neck, and chest that impair respiration are the highest priorities. Every member of the emergency team is alert to the total problem of the patient since the body cannot be isolated into parts.

Principles of Emergency Management

The following principles are applicable to the emergency management of any patient:

1. Maintain a patent airway and provide adequate ventilation, employing resuscitation measures when necessary. Assess for chest injuries with subsequent airway obstruction.
2. Control hemorrhage and its consequences.
3. Evaluate and restore cardiac output.
4. Prevent and treat shock; maintain or restore effective circulation.
5. Carry out a rapid initial and ongoing physical examination; the clinical course of the injured or seriously ill patient is not static.
6. Assess whether or not the patient can follow commands; evaluate the size and reactivity of the pupils and motor responses.
7. Start ECG monitoring if appropriate.
8. Splint suspected fractures, including fractures of the cervical spine in patients with head injuries.
9. Protect wounds with sterile dressings.
10. Check to see if the patient has a Medic Alert tag or similar identification designating allergies, *etc.*
11. Start a flow sheet of the patient's vital signs, blood pressure, neurologic status, *etc.*, to guide decision making.

Obtaining Data From the Patient

If possible, a brief history of the accident or illness is taken from the patient or the person accompanying him to the emergency department. As part of the history, the following questions should be answered:

1. What were the circumstances, forces, location, and time of the injury?
2. When did the symptoms appear?
3. Was the patient unconscious after the accident?
4. How did the patient reach the hospital?
5. What was the health status of the patient before the accident or illness?
6. Is there a past history of illness? of admissions to the hospital?
7. Is the patient currently taking any medications, especially hormones, insulin, digitalis, anticoagulants?
8. Does the patient have any allergies?
9. Does the patient have any bleeding tendencies?
10. When was the last meal eaten? (Important if an anesthetic is to be given.)
11. Is the patient under a physician's care? name of physician?
12. What was the date of the patient's most recent tetanus immunization?

Recording of Data

Consent to examine and treat the patient is part of the emergency department record. More sophisticated procedures (angiography, lumbar puncture) should be specifically consented to by the patient. If the patient is unconscious and brought to the emergency department without family or friends, this fact should be documented. Following treatment, a notation is made on the record about the patient's condition on discharge or transfer and the patient education instructions that are given for follow-up care.

Emergency Resuscitation Measures

The first priority in the treatment of any emergency condition is the establishment of the airway. If the airway is obstructed, the ensuing hypoxia will produce permanent brain damage or death within 3 to 5 minutes, depending on the age of the patient.

- *Complete airway obstruction* is readily recognized: the patient suddenly stops breathing, becomes cyanotic, and falls unconscious for no apparent reason.
- *Partial airway obstruction* that interferes with air flow will produce an apprehensive look, inspiratory and expiratory stridor, labored use of accessory muscles (suprasternal and intercostal retraction), flaring nostrils, and progressive anxiety, restlessness, and confusion. Cyanosis of the earlobes and nail beds may be a late sign. Partial obstruction of the airway can produce progressive hypoxia and hypercarbia and can lead to respiratory and cardiac arrest.

Emergency Management of Airway Obstruction

1. Gently shake the victim and shout, "Are you O.K.?" to prevent injury from attempted resuscitation of a person who is not truly unconscious.
2. Place the patient supine on a firm, flat surface; if he is lying face down, turn his body as a unit so that the head, shoulders, and torso move simultaneously with no twisting.
3. Methods for opening the airway
   a. Head-tilt/chin-lift maneuver
      (1) Place one hand on the victim's forehead and apply firm backward pressure with the palm to tilt the head back.
      (2) Place the fingers of the other hand under the bony part of the lower jaw near the chin and lift, bringing the chin forward and the teeth almost to occlusion, thus supporting the jaw and helping to tilt the head back.
   b. Jaw-thrust maneuver: Grasp the angles of the victim's lower jaw and lift with both hands (one on each side), displacing the mandible forward while tilting the head backward. (This is a safe approach to opening the airway of a victim with suspected neck injury, because it can usually be accomplished without extending the neck.)
4. Remove any foreign body obstructing the airway.
5. Start cardiopulmonary resuscitation (CPR) immediately (pp. 592–593) to provide oxygen to the brain, heart, and other vital organs until definitive medical treatment can restore normal heart and ventilatory action. (CPR consists of establishing an effective airway and providing artificial ventilation by external cardiac compression.)

Airway management is discussed in detail in Chapter 22.

Management of Foreign Body Upper Airway Obstruction

Obstruction of the upper airway by food ("café coronary") is a cause of unconsciousness and cardiopulmonary arrest. Foreign bodies may cause either partial or complete airway obstruction. In adults, a piece of meat is the most common cause of obstruction. Factors associated with choking on food include large, poorly chewed pieces of food, alcohol consumption, and upper or lower dentures.

Assessment reveals that the victim is unable to speak, breathe, or cough. He may clutch his neck between the thumb and fingers (universal distress signal). Ask if he is choking.

Gerontological Considerations

In extended care facilities, sedatives and hypnotic drugs as well as diseases affecting motor coordination (Parkinson's disease) and mental functioning (senility, mental retardation) are risk factors for asphyxiation by food.

Chart 60-1
Guidelines: Management of Foreign Body Airway Obstruction

Action	*Rationale/Amplification*
Assessment for Airway Obstruction Victim may clutch his neck between his thumb and fingers. Weak, ineffective cough; high-pitched noises on inspiration. Increased respiratory distress. Inability to speak, breathe, or cough. Collapse.	Air movement is absent in the presence of *complete airway obstruction.* Oxygen saturation in the blood will decrease rapidly because the obstructed airway prevents entry of air into the lungs. Thus, oxygen deficit occurs in the brain, resulting in unconsiousness with death following rapidly. The term *Heimlich maneuver* is employed for the sake of uniformity. The terms *subdiaphragmatic abdominal thrusts* and *abdominal thrusts* are used interchangeably, depending on the circumstances.
Heimlich Maneuver (subdiaphragmatic abdominal thrusts) **For Standing or Sitting Conscious Patient** 1. Stand behind the patient; wrap your arms around his waist and proceed as follows: 2. Make a fist with one hand, placing the thumb side of the fist against the patient's abdomen, in the midline slightly above the navel and well below the xiphoid process. Grasp the fist with the other hand. 3. Press your fist into the patient's abdomen with a quick upward thrust. Each new thrust should be a separate and distinct maneuver. **With Patient Lying (Unconscious)** 1. Position patient on his back. 2. Kneel astride the patient's thighs, facing his head. 3. Place the heel of one hand against the patient's abdomen, in the midline slightly above the navel and well below the tip of the xiphoid; place the second hand directly on top of the first. 4. Press into the abdomen with a quick upward thrust.	A subdiaphragmatic abdominal thrust, by elevating the diaphragm, can force air from the lungs to creat an artificial cough intended to move and expel an obstructing foreign body in the airway.

(continued)

Emergency Management

For Partial Obstruction (if patient is breathing and able to cough spontaneously)
1. Encourage the victim to cough forcefully; there may be some wheezing between coughs.
2. Continue to encourage victim to persist with spontaneous coughing and breathing efforts as long as good air exchange persists.
3. If patient demonstrates a weak, ineffective cough, high-pitched noise while inhaling, increased respiratory difficulty, and possibly cyanosis, he is managed as if it were complete airway obstruction (see below).

For Complete Obstruction
See Chart 60-1 for management of foreign body airway obstruction.

Methods for Providing a Patent Airway
Insertion of an Oropharyngeal Airway

An oropharyngeal airway is a semicircular-shaped tube or tubelike device of plastic or rubber that is inserted into the lower posterior pharynx over the back of the tongue in a spontaneously breathing, unconscious patient in order to keep the tongue from falling back against the posterior pharynx and obstructing the airway and to permit suctioning of secretions.

Guidelines for Insertion of an Oropharyngeal Airway

1. Extend the patient's head by placing one hand beneath the neck close to the occiput and gently lifting the neck; simultaneously, with the other hand, tilt the head backward by applying pressure on the forehead.

Chart 60-1 (continued)

Action	*Rationale/Amplification*
Finger Sweep	
1. Open patient's mouth by grasping both the tongue and lower jaw between the thumb and fingers and lifting the mandible (tongue–jaw lift)	This manuever is to be used only in the unconscious patient. This action draws the tongue away from the back of the throat and away from the foreign body that may be lodged there.
2. Insert the index finger of the other hand down along the inside of the cheek and deeply into the throat to the base of the tongue.	
3. Use a hooking action to dislodge the foreign body and maneuver it into the mouth for removal.	Use care not to force the object deeper into the throat.
Chest Thrusts With Conscious Patient Standing or Sitting	
1. Stand behind patient with arms under patient's axillae to encircle patient's waist.	This technique is to be used only in the advanced stages of pregnancy or in the markedly obese person.
2. Place thumb side of your fist on middle of patient's sternum, taking care to avoid xiphoid process and margins of rib cage.	
3. Grasp your fist with the other hand and perform backward thrusts until the foreign body is expelled or patient becomes unconscious.	Each thrust should be administered with the intent of relieving the obstruction.
Chest Thrust With Patient Lying (Unconscious)	
1. Place the patient on his back and kneel close to the side of his body.	This maneuver is used only in the advanced stages of pregnancy when the rescuer cannot apply the Heimlich maneuver effectively to the unconscious, markedly obese person.
2. Place the heel of your hand on the lower half of the sternum.	
3. Deliver each chest thrust slowly and distinctly with the intent of relieving the obstruction.	

(Adapted from Standards and Guidelines for Cardiopulmonary Resuscitation [CPR] and Emergency Cardiac Care [ECC]. Part II. Adult Basic Life Support. JAMA 1986 June; 255[21]:2915–2932)

2. Open the patient's mouth.
3. Insert the oropharyngeal airway with the tip facing up towards the roof of the mouth until it passes the uvula; then rotate the tip 180° so that the tip is pointed down toward the pharynx (Fig. 60-1).
4. The distal end of the oropharyngeal airway will be in the hypopharynx, and the flange will be approximately at the patient's lips; make sure that the tongue has not been pushed into the airway.

Insertion of an Esophageal Obturator Airway (EOA)

The esophageal obturator airway (EOA) is a ventilatory device used in respiratory emergencies for resuscitation. It consists of (1) a face mask to seal off the nose and mouth and anchor the airway; (2) a flexible tube with openings at the level of the pharynx to permit ventilation of the lungs; and (3) a balloon on the distal end of the tube to block the esophagus, thus reducing the possibility of aspirating gastric contents. The purpose of the EOA is to ventilate the apneic, unconscious patient when endotracheal intubation is not possible.

The tube is inserted through the mouth and advanced into the esophagus just below the bifurcation of the trachea. The proximal part of the tube has air holes at the level of the pharynx through which air or oxygen is blown into the lungs.

The esophageal gastric tube airway (EGTA) is a modification of the esophageal airway (Fig. 60-2). It has a central lumen that permits passage of a nasogastric tube so that suctioning of the stomach can be accomplished without interfering with ventilation.

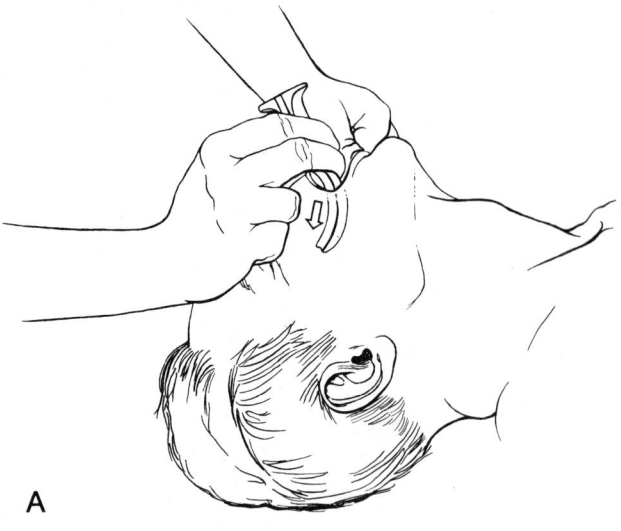

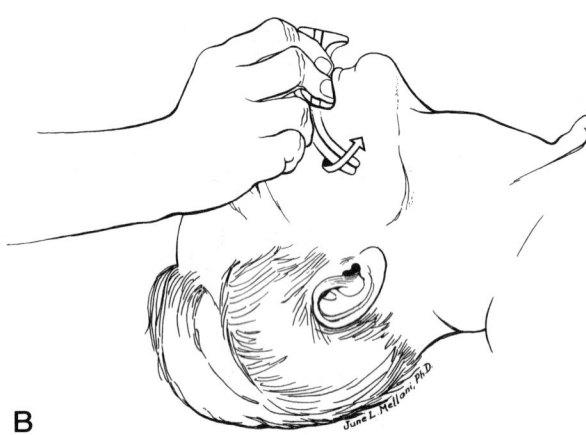

Figure 60-1
Insertion of an oropharyngeal airway. (*A*) Place the airway in the mouth of the unconscious patient with the tip pointing up. (*B*) Rotate the airway 180°, pointing the tip down toward the pharynx. This displaces the tongue anteriorly, and the patient then breathes through and around the airway.

Guidelines for Insertion of an EOA

Equipment
Esophageal obturator airway (EOA)
50-ml syringe
Water-soluble gel
Bag and mask unit

Procedure
1. Lubricate the tube and attach the face mask to the tube by the snap lock.
2. Place the patient's head in a neutral position.
3. Using the left hand, insert the thumb as deeply as possible over the back of the patient's tongue, pulling on it while using the fingers to lift the jaw upward and away from the posterior pharyngeal wall.

4. Insert the EOA tip into the mouth, carefully guiding the tube over the tongue and past the pharynx; rotate the tube 180 degrees into the esophagus.
5. Stop advancing the tube when the mask reaches the face; press the mask firmly against the face.
6. Ventilate the patient by blowing a few breaths through the tube or by attaching a bag mask to it. IF THE TUBE IS IN THE ESOPHAGUS, THE CHEST WILL RISE.
7. If the chest does not rise or no breath sounds are heard, the airway is possibly blocking the trachea; remove airway. Continue ventilating the patient (by bag-mask ventilation) and prepare for and proceed with second attempt at insertion.
8. Auscultate over both lung fields to check that *both* lungs are receiving adequate ventilation and that the airway is in the esophagus and *not* in the trachea.
9. Inflate the cuff (balloon) with approximately 20 ml of air. Inflating the cuff results in occlusion of the esophagus, minimizes the incidence of regurgitation, and prevents air leakage.
10. Connect the end of the esophageal obturator to a bag-mask or mechanical ventilator, or continue mouth-to-tube ventilation.
11. Do not remove the EOA until the patient regains consciousness or has a gag reflex, *or* until the endotracheal intubation has been accomplished. The EOA tube must be deflated before it is removed. If the tube is taken out prematurely, regurgitation and aspiration are almost inevitable.
12. To remove the tube: Have suction available. Turn the patient's head to the side; deflate the cuff and remove the tube.

- This procedure is contraindicated in conscious or semiconscious patients and in those with corrosive poisoning, esophageal disease, or a foreign body in the trachea.

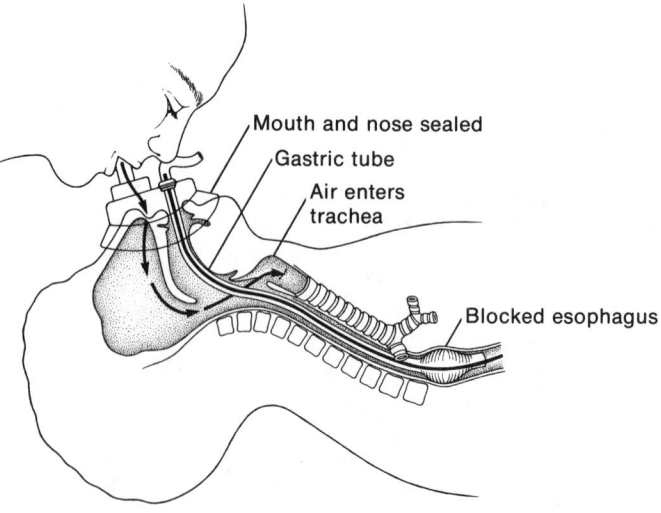

Figure 60-2
The esophageal gastric tube airway (EGTA), a modification of the esophageal obturator airway. (Courtesy of Brunswick Mfg. Co., Inc; redrawn.)

Emergency Endotracheal Procedures

Emergency Endotracheal Intubation

The purpose of endotracheal intubation is to establish and maintain the airway in patients with respiratory insufficiency or hypoxia. Endotracheal intubation is indicated for the following reasons: (1) to establish an airway for patients who cannot be adequately ventilated with an oropharyngeal airway, (2) to bypass an upper airway obstruction, (3) to prevent aspiration, (4) to permit connection of the patient to a resuscitation bag or mechanical ventilator, and (5) to facilitate the removal of tracheobronchial secretions.

Because the procedure requires skill, endotracheal intubation should be done only by those who have had intensive training in which they have practiced the technique on a mannequin. It should be done under expert clinical supervision.

Details for emergency endotracheal intubation are outlined in Chart 60-2, p. 1706. Also, see Figure 60-3.

Cricothyroidotomy (Cricothyroid Membrane Puncture)

Cricothyroidotomy is the puncture or incision of the cricothyroid membrane to establish an airway. This procedure is used in certain emergency situations when endotracheal intubation or tracheostomy are either not possible or contraindicated, as in airway obstruction from extensive maxillofacial trauma, cervical spine injuries, laryngospasm, laryngeal edema (following allergic reaction), hemorrhage into neck tissue, or obstruction of the larynx.

Emergency Medical Management

1. With the patient in a supine position, extend the neck so that the cricothyroid membrane can be palpated readily. Place a towel roll beneath the shoulders.

2. Identify the prominent thyroid cartilage (Adam's apple) as shown in Fig. 60-4, p. 1708, and allow your finger to descend in the midline to the depression between the lower border of the thyroid cartilage and the upper border of the cricoid cartilage. This depression represents the cricothyroid membrane.

3. Insert a needle or any sharp instrument at a 10- to 20-degree caudal direction in the midline just above the upper part of the cricoid cartilage.
   a. Listen for air passing back and forth through the needle synchronous with the patient's respiration.
   b. Direct the needle downward and posteriorly.
   c. Tape the needle with adhesive for stability.

4. An alternate method is to make a transverse incision overlying the cricothyroid membrane and a similar incision through the membrane itself. The membrane incision is spread and a tracheotomy tube is advanced caudally into the trachea.

5. Prepare for endotracheal intubation. This procedure is usually followed by elective tracheostomy.

6. Monitor for potential complications: vocal cord injury, subcutaneous emphysema, bleeding.

Special Resuscitation Situation: Near-Drowning

Near-drowning is survival for at least some period of time after suffocation from submersion in water.

Drowning is one of the three leading causes of accidental death; an estimated 9,000 fatalities from drowning and 80,000 near-drownings occur yearly in the United States. Factors associated with drowning and near-drowning include alcohol ingestion, inability to swim, diving injuries, hypothermia, and exhaustion. Efforts to save the victim should not be abandoned too soon, since successful resuscitation with full neu-

(Text continues on p. 1708)

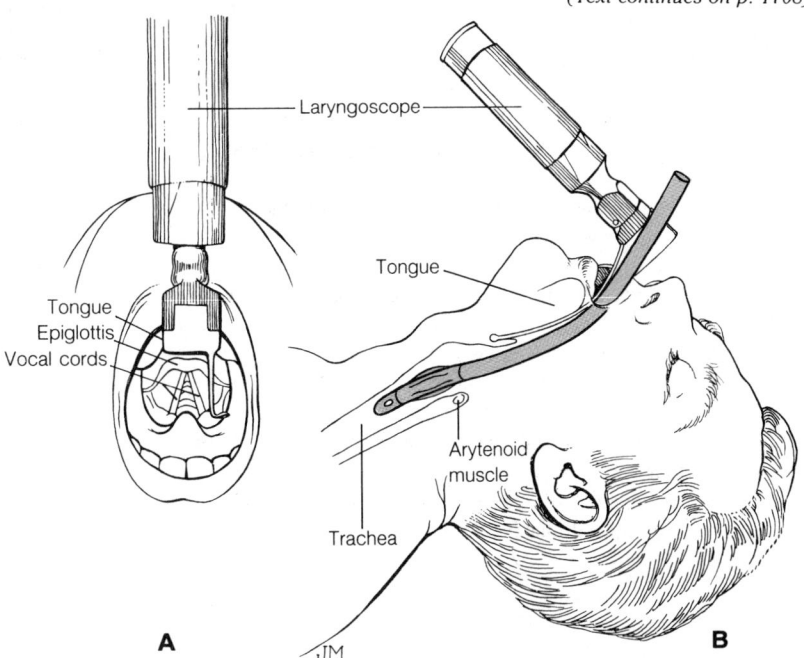

Figure 60-3
Endotracheal intubation. (*A*) The primary glottic landmarks for tracheal intubation as visualized with proper placement of the laryngoscope. (*B*) Positioning the endotube. (Brunner LS and Suddarth DS. The Lippincott Manual of Nursing Practice, 4th ed. Philadelphia, JB Lippincott, 1986.)

A

B

Chart 60-2
Assisting With Emergency Endotracheal Intubation

Clinical Signs for Intubation

1. Respiratory arrest
2. Respiratory insufficiency—marked respiratory effort, substernal retraction, nostril flaring, increasing or decreasing pulse rate, increasing or decreasing respiratory rate, changing color (*cyanosis is a late sign*)
3. Airway obstruction (asphyxia)

Equipment

1. Laryngoscope with curved and straight blades and working light source (Check batteries and bulb periodically)
2. Endotracheal tubes with low-pressure cuffs (to seal airway) and adapter (to connect tube to ventilator or bag)
3. Stylet to guide endotracheal tube
4. Oral airway (assorted sizes), or bite block (to keep patient from biting into and occluding endotracheal tube)
5. Adhesive tape or tube fixation system
6. Sterile anesthetic lubricant jelly (water-soluble)
7. Syringe
8. Suction source
9. Resuscitation bag and mask connected to oxygen source
10. Anesthetic spray
11. Sterile towel

Action	*Rationale/Amplification*
1. Remove the patient's dental bridgework and plates.	1. May interfere with insertion; will not be able to remove easily once patient is intubated.
2. Remove headboard of bed (optional)	
3. Prepare equipment.	
a. Ensure function of resuscitation bag and mask, and suction.	a. Patient may require ventilatory assistance during procedure. Suction should be functional, since gagging and emesis may occur during procedure.
b. Assemble the laryngoscope; make sure the lightbulb is tightly attached and functional.	
c. Select an endotracheal tube of the appropriate size (6.0–9.0 mm for average adult).	
d. Place the endotracheal tube on a sterile towel.	d. Although the tube will pass through the contaminated mouth or nose, the airway below the vocal cords is sterile, and efforts must be made to prevent iatrogenic contamination of the distal end of the tube and cuff. The proximal end of the tube may be handled, since it will reside in the upper airway.
e. Inflate the cuff to make sure it assumes a symmetrical shape and holds volume without leakage. Then deflate maximally.	e. Malfunction of the cuff must be ascertained before tube placement occurs.
f. Lubricate the distal end of tube liberally with the sterile anesthetic water-soluble jelly.	f. Aids in insertion.
g. Insert the stylet into the tube (if oral intubation is planned; nasal intubation does not employ use of the stylet).	g. Stiffens the soft tube, allowing it to be more easily directed into the trachea.
4. Assist the physician with the following:	
a. If cervical spine is not injured, for oral intubation place head in a "sniffing" position: flexed at the junction of the neck and thorax and extended at the junction of the spine and skull.	a. Upper airway is open maximally in this position and mouth of the unconscious patient will often open.
b. Spray the back of the patient's throat with an anesthetic spray if time is available.	b. This will decrease gagging.

(continued)

Chart 60-2 *(continued)*

Action	*Rationale/Amplification*
c. Ventilate and oxygenate the patient with the resuscitation bag and mask before intubation.	c. This decreases the likelihood of cardiac dysrhythmias or respiratory distress secondary to hypoxemia.
d. Hold the handle of the laryngoscope in the left hand and hold the patient's mouth open with the right hand by placing crossed fingers on the teeth.	d. Leverage is improved by crossing the thumb and index fingers when opening the patient's mouth (scissor-twist technique).
e. Insert the curved blade of the laryngoscope along the right side of the tongue, push the tongue to the left, and use right thumb and index finger to pull patient's lower lip away from lower teeth.	e. Rolling the lip away from teeth prevents injury by being caught between teeth and blade.
f. Lift laryngoscope forward (toward ceiling) to expose the epiglottis.	f. Do not use teeth as a fulcrum, which could lead to dental damage.
g. Lift laryngoscope upward and forward at a 45-degree angle to expose glottis and visualize vocal cords.	g. This stretches the hypoepiglottis ligament, folding the epiglottis upward and exposing the glottis.
h. As the epiglottis is lifted forward (toward ceiling), the vertical opening of the larynx between the vocal cords will come into view.	h. Do not use wrist; use shoulder and arm to lift epiglottis.
i. Once vocal cords are visualized, insert tube into the right corner of the mouth and pass the tube—guided by blade, but keeping vocal cords in constant view.	i. Make sure you do not insert tube into esophagus; the esophageal mucosa is pink and the opening is horizontal rather than vertical.
j. Gently push the tube through the triangular space formed by the vocal cords and back wall of trachea.	j. If the vocal cords are in spasm (closed), wait a few seconds before passing tube.
k. Stop insertion just after the tube cuff has disappeared from view beyond the cords.	k. Advancing tube further may lead to its entry into a main-stem bronchus (usually the right bronchus), causing collapse of the unventilated lung.
l. Withdraw laryngoscope while holding endotracheal tube in place. Disassemble mask from resuscitation bag and ventilate the patient.	
m. Inflate cuff with the minimal amount of air required to occlude the trachea.	m. The amount of air used for cuff inflation depends on the size of the cuff and the diameter of the patient's trachea. Occlusion occurs when no air is felt or heard passing through the patient's nose or mouth.
n. Insert oral airway or bite block if necessary.	n. This keeps patient from biting down on the tube and obstructing the airway.
o. Ascertain expansion of both sides of the chest by observation and auscultation of breath sounds.	o. Observation and auscultation help in determining that tube remains in position and has not slipped into the right main stem bronchus.
p. Mark proximal end of tube with marking pen or tape at the point where the tube reaches the corner of the patient's mouth.	p. This will allow for detection of any later change in tube position.
q. Secure tube to the patient's face with adhesive tape or apply a commercially available endotracheal tube stabilization device.	q. The tube must be fixed securely to ensure that it will not be dislodged. Dislodgement of a tube with an inflated cuff may result in damage to the vocal cords.
r. Obtain chest x-ray to verify tube position.	
s. Measure cuff pressure with manometer; adjust pressure. Make adjustment in tube placement on the basis of chest x-ray results.	s. The tube may be advanced or removed several centimeters for proper placement on the basis of the chest x-ray result.
t. Record tube type and size, cuff pressure, and patient tolerance of the procedure. Auscultate breath sounds every 1 to 2 hours or if signs and symptoms of respiratory distress occur. Assess arterial blood gases after intubation if requested by physician.	t. Arterial blood gases may be prescribed to ensure adequacy of ventilation and respiration. Tube displacement outward may result in extubation (cuff above vocal cords). Tube displacement forward may result in tube touching carina (causing paroxysmal coughing) or intubation of a main stem bronchus (resulting in collapse of the unventilated lung).

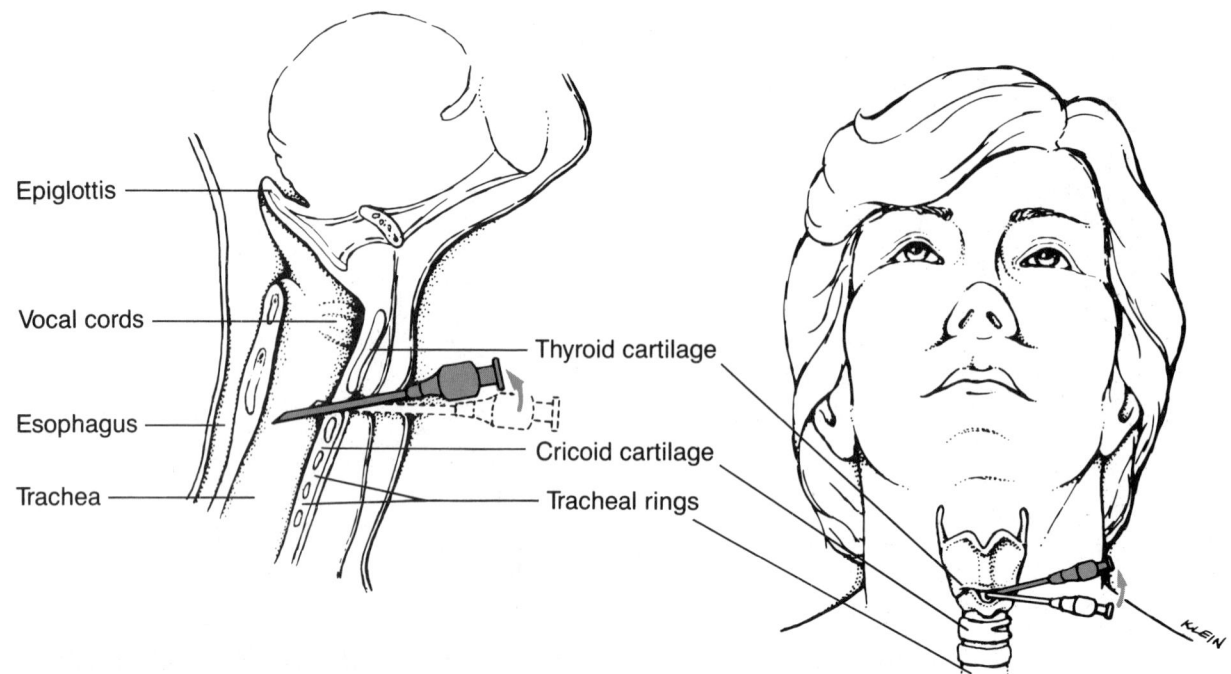

Figure 60-4
Cricothyroidotomy (cricothyroid membrane puncture) is the puncture or incision of the cricothyroid membrane to establish an emergency airway. The needle is inserted at a 10- to 30-degree angle, caudal direction, in the midline just above the upper part of the cricoid cartilage. The cricothyroid membrane is an accessible route for the establishment of an emergency airway in a minimal amount of time. This procedure is generally reserved for patients in whom intubation cannot be safely accomplished.

rologic recovery has occurred in near-drowning victims with prolonged submersion in cold water.

Following resuscitation, the primary problems of a victim who has nearly drowned are hypoxia and acidosis, which will require immediate intervention in the emergency department. The resultant pathophysiologic changes and pulmonary injury depend on the type of fluid (fresh water or salt water) and the volume of aspiration. When water has been aspirated, alterations of pulmonary function may be anticipated. After a person has survived immersion, secondary drowning (acute adult respiratory distress syndrome) with hypoxia, hypercarbia, and respiratory or metabolic acidosis can occur.

Emergency Management in the Emergency Department

Therapy is aimed at maintaining cerebral perfusion and adequate oxygenation to prevent further damage to vital organs.

1. Ensure adequacy of the airway, respiration, and peripheral perfusion.
   a. Use a rectal probe to determine the degree of hypothermia if the patient has been submerged in cold water.
   b. Start rewarming procedures during resuscitation (extracorporeal warming, warmed peritoneal dialysis, inhalation of warm aerosolized oxygen, surface warming); the choice is determined by the severity and duration of hypothermia and available resources.

2. Draw arterial blood to evaluate oxygen and carbon dioxide tensions, *p*H, and bicarbonate levels; these parameters will determine the type of ventilatory support required and the subsequent dosage of sodium bicarbonate to be given.

   - Hypotension and impaired tissue perfusion are managed by intravascular volume expansion and inotropic agents.

3. Improve ventilation and oxygenation. Initiate endotracheal intubation with positive pressure ventilation (with PEEP) to improve oxygenation, to keep alveoli patent, and to correct intrapulmonary shunting and ventilation–perfusion abnormalities (caused by aspiration of water). Continue with supplemental oxygen by way of a mask (if patient is breathing spontaneously) or with an endotracheal tube (if patient is not breathing spontaneously).

   - Respiratory acidosis is managed by improving ventilation.

4. Initiate ECG monitoring, because dysrhythmias occur frequently.
5. Assist with nasogastric intubation to empty the stomach, to prevent the patient from regurgitating gastric contents.
6. Continue to monitor the patient closely: vital signs, serial arterial blood gas values, *p*H, ECG, intracranial pressure, serum electrolytes, serial chest x-rays.

7. Insert an indwelling catheter to determine urinary output; metabolic acidosis may compromise renal function.
8. Admit the patient to a hospital/ICU; the appearance of the patient may be deceptive. Complications of near-drowning that can lead to death include the following:
   a. Hypoxic/ischemic cerebral injury.
   b. Acute respiratory distress syndrome and pulmonary damage secondary to aspiration.
   c. Cardiac arrest.

Control of Hemorrhage Due to Trauma

One of the primary causes of shock is the reduction in circulating blood volume. Only a few conditions, such as obstructed airway or a sucking wound of the chest, take precedence over the immediate control of hemorrhage. "Stop the bleeding" is fundamental to the care and the survival of patients in an emergency or a disaster situation. However, minor bleeding will usually stop spontaneously unless the patient has a bleeding disorder. Most of this type of blood loss will be venous.

Assess the patient for cool, moist skin (resulting from poor peripheral perfusion), falling blood pressure, increasing heart rate, and decreasing urine volume. The nursing diagnoses may include actual fluid volume deficit related to bleeding. The goals of emergency management are to control the bleeding, maintain an adequately circulating blood volume for tissue oxygenation, and prevent shock. The nursing interventions are carried out interdependently with other members of the health care team.

Emergency Management

1. Cut the patient's clothing away quickly to identify the area of hemorrhage, and carry out a rapid physical assessment.
2. Apply direct, firm pressure over the bleeding area or the artery involved (Fig. 60-5). Almost all bleeding can be stopped by direct pressure (except when a major artery has been severed). Unchecked arterial bleeding produces death.
3. Apply a firm pressure dressing. Elevate the injured part to stop venous and capillary bleeding. Immobilize an injured extremity to control blood loss.

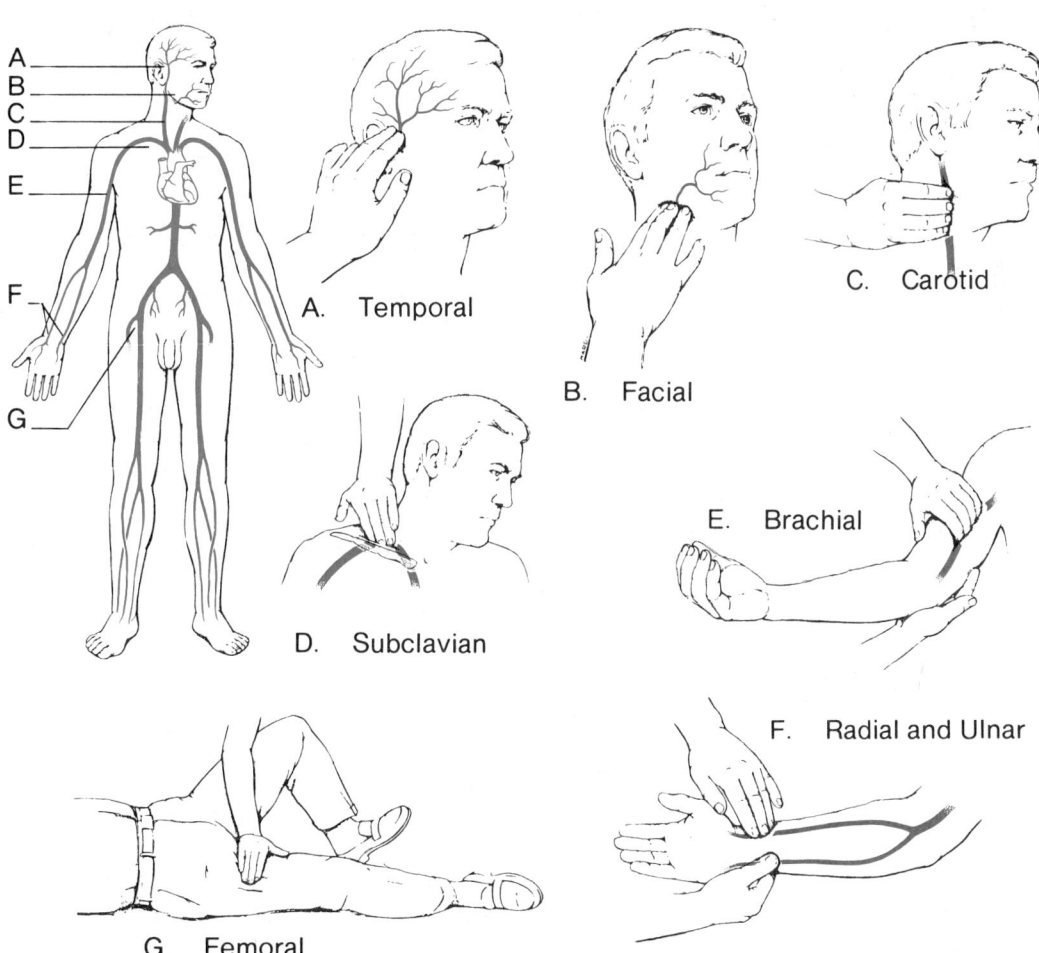

A. Temporal
B. Facial
C. Carotid
D. Subclavian
E. Brachial
F. Radial and Ulnar
G. Femoral

Figure 60-5
Pressure points for control of hemorrhage.

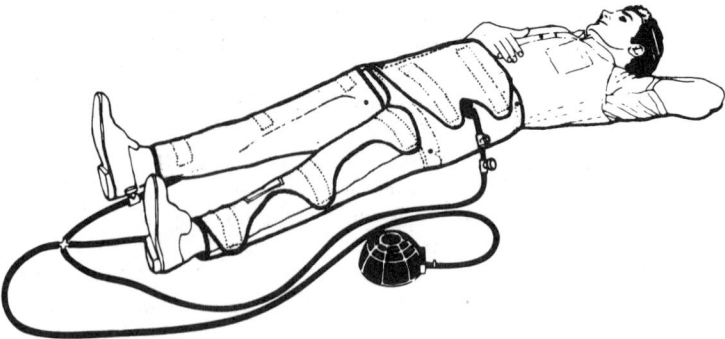

Figure 60-6
The Medical Anti-Shock Trouser (MAST) is a garment designed to correct internal bleeding and hypovolemia by the application of counter pressure around the legs and abdomen. This creates an artificial peripheral resistance and helps sustain coronary perfusion. It should be applied as soon as possible after injury, preferably before the patient is transferred to the emergency department. (Courtesy of David Clark Co., Inc., 360 Franklin Street, Worcester, MA 01604.)

4. Insert an intravenous cannula to provide a means of blood replacement.
   a. Withdraw blood samples for analysis, typing, and cross-matching.
   b. Give replacement fluids, including isotonic electrolyte solutions, plasma or plasma protein fractions, or blood (depending on clinical estimates of the type and volume of fluid lost).
      (1) Fresh blood is infused when there is massive blood loss.
      (2) Additional platelets and clotting factors are given when large amounts of blood are needed, since replacement blood is deficient in clotting factors.
      (3) The blood is warmed, using a commercial warmer or basin of warm water (massive blood replacement has a cooling effect that can cause cardiac arrest).
   The rate of infusion depends on the severity of blood loss and clinical evidence of hypovolemia.
5. Take the following steps for internal bleeding:
   a. Suspect internal bleeding in patients with hypovolemic shock with no external signs of bleeding: rising pulse rate; falling blood pressure; thirst, apprehension; cool, moist skin.
   b. Give whole blood or plasma expanders at the rate of blood loss.
   c. Apply an antishock garment (pneumatic counter-pressure device), if available, to control internal bleeding and to facilitate the blood flow to vital areas (Fig. 60-6). (Its primary use is for hypovolemic shock secondary to bleeding in the lower part of the body.)
   d. Prepare the patient immediately for surgical intervention.
   e. Monitor the patient's hemodynamic responses.
   f. Obtain arterial blood for blood gas determination; establish central venous pressure monitoring as an index of the amount of fluid the patient can tolerate.
   g. Maintain patient in supine position until hemodynamic/circulatory parameters improve.
6. Apply a tourniquet on an extremity only as a *last resort,* when the hemorrhage cannot be controlled by any other method. Anticipate loss of an extremity if a tourniquet is applied.
   a. Apply the tourniquet just proximal to the wound; tie it tightly enough to control the arterial blood flow.
   b. Tag the patient with a skin-marking pencil or on ad-

hesive tape on his forehead with a "T," stating the location of the tourniquet and the time applied.
   c. Loosen the tourniquet as directed to prevent irreparable vascular or neurologic damage if the patient is in an emergency facility. If there is no arterial bleeding, remove the tourniquet and again try a pressure dressing.
   d. In the event of a traumatic amputation, leave the tourniquet applied until the patient is in the operating room.
7. Watch for cardiac arrest; patients who hemorrhage are candidates for cardiac arrest caused by hypovolemia with secondary anoxia.
8. See page 367 for further discussion of hemorrhage.

Control of Hypovolemic Shock

Shock is a condition in which there is loss of effective circulating blood volume. Inadequate organ and tissue perfusion result, ultimately causing cellular metabolic derangements. In any emergency situation, it is wise to anticipate shock before it develops. Any injured person should be assessed immediately to determine the presence of shock. Its underlying cause must be discovered (hypovolemic, cardiogenic, neurogenic, or septic shock). Hypovolemia is the most common cause of shock (see also pages 362–367).

Assess for the following signs and symptoms, which in varying combinations indicate that the patient is in some degree of hypovolemic shock: decreasing arterial pressure; increasing pulse rate; cold, moist skin; pallor; thirst; diaphoresis; decreased sensorium; oliguria; metabolic acidosis; and hyperpnea. Of these, the most dependable criterion is the level of arterial blood pressure.

The nursing diagnoses may include alteration in tissue perfusion related to failing circulation; impaired gas exchange related to ventilation–perfusion imbalance; and alteration in urinary elimination (oliguria/anuria) related to decreased renal perfusion.

The goals of treatment are to restore and maintain tissue perfusion and to correct physiologic abnormalities.

Emergency Management

1. Ensure a patent airway and maintain breathing and circulation. Give additional ventilatory assistance as required.
2. Restore the circulating blood volume with rapid fluid

and blood replacement to optimize cardiac preload, correct hypotension, and maintain tissue perfusion.

   a. Insert a central venous pressure catheter in or near the right atrium to serve as a guide for fluid replacement. Continuing central venous pressure (CVP) readings give the direction and degree of change from baseline readings; the catheter also is a vehicle for emergency fluid volume replacement.

   b. Insert large-gauge intravenous needles or catheters into peripheral vein(s). Two or more catheters may be necessary for rapid replacement and reversal of hemodynamic instability; the emphasis is on volume replacement.

     (1) Establish IV lines in both upper and lower extremities if there is suspicion that a major vessel in the chest or abdomen has been disrupted.

     (2) Withdraw blood for specimens: arterial blood gases (arterial blood), chemistry studies, typing and cross-matching and hematocrit.

3. Start intravenous infusion at a rapid rate until CVP rises to a satisfactory level above the baseline measurement or until there is improvement in the patient's clinical condition.

   a. Infusion of lactated Ringer's solution is useful initially, since it approximates plasma electrolyte composition and osmolality, allows time for blood typing and cross matching, restores circulation, and serves as an adjunct to whole blood.

   b. Start transfusion of blood component therapy, especially when blood loss has been severe or when the patient continues to hemorrhage.

   c. Control hemorrhage; hemorrhage will compound the shock state. Carry out serial hematocrit examinations if continued bleeding is suspected.

   d. Maintain the systolic blood pressure at a satisfactory level by administering fluids and blood.

4. Insert an indwelling urinary catheter; record urinary output every 15 to 30 minutes. (Urinary volume reveals adequacy of kidney perfusion.)

5. Carry out a rapid physical assessment to determine the cause of shock.

6. Maintain ongoing nursing surveillance of the *total patient*—blood pressure, heart and respiratory rates, skin temperature, color, CVP, arterial blood gases, ECG, hematocrit, hemoglobin, coagulation profile, electrolytes, and urinary output—to assess patient response to treatment. Keep a flow sheet of these parameters; trend analysis reveals improvement or deterioration of patient.

7. Elevate the feet slightly to improve cerebral circulation and promote return of venous blood to the heart. (*This position is contraindicated in patients with head injuries.*) Avoid unnecessary movement.

8. Give specific pharmacologic agents (inotropic drugs such as dopamine, *etc.*) to improve cardiovascular performance.

9. Support the defense mechanisms of the body.

   a. Reassure and comfort the patient; sedation may be necessary to relieve apprehension.

   b. Relieve pain by *cautious* use of analgesics or narcotics.

   c. Maintain the body temperature.

     (1) Too much heat produces vasodilatation, which counteracts the body's compensatory mechanism of vasoconstriction and also increases fluid loss by perspiration.

     (2) A patient who is in septic shock should be kept cool, since high fever will increase the cellular metabolic effects of shock.

Wounds

Wounds (injury to tissues) vary from minor lacerations to severe crushing injuries. Life-threatening problems, such as airway obstruction, hemorrhage, and shock, must be dealt with before the wound is treated.

Assessment

1. Ask the patient *when* as well as *how* the wound occurred; a delay over 3 hours in treatment increases the risk of infection.

2. Inspect the wound, using aseptic technique, to determine the extent of damage to underlying structures.

3. Assess for sensory, motor, or vascular complications.

   The nursing diagnoses may include alteration in skin integrity (puncture wound, laceration) related to injury and potential for infection.

   The patient's goal is restoration of the physical integrity and function of the injured tissue without the development of infection and with minimal scarring.

Emergency Management

1. Clip hairs or shave around the wound (with the exception of eyebrows) only if directed (this is done when it is anticipated that hairs will interfere with wound closure).

2. Cleanse around the wound with prescribed agent. Do not allow the cleansing solution to get into the wound, since it may be injurious to exposed tissues.

3. Infiltrate with a local anesthetic intradermally through the wound margins or by regional block. (Patients with soft tissue injuries usually have pain localized at the site of injury.)

4. Cleanse and debride the wound.

   a. Irrigate gently and copiously with isotonic sterile saline to remove surface dirt.

   b. Remove devitalized tissue and foreign matter, which impairs the wound's ability to resist infection.

   c. Clamp and tie small bleeding vessels, or achieve hemostasis with a cautery.

5. Suture the wound (usually done by physician) if primary closure is indicated. (This depends on the nature of the wound, the length of time since the injury was sustained, the degree of contamination, and the vascularity of tissues.)

   a. Subcutaneous fat is approximated loosely with a few sutures to close off the dead space.

   b. The subcuticular layer is then closed.

   c. The epidermis is closed; sutures are placed close to the wound edge with the skin edges leveled carefully to promote optimum healing.

   d. Sterile strips of reinforced microporous tape may be used to close clean, superficial wounds.

6. Apply nonadherent dressing to protect the wound. (The dressing may serve as a splint and as a reminder to the patient that he has sustained an injury.)
7. For delayed primary closure:
   a. A thin layer of gauze (to ensure drainage and prevent pooling of exudate) covered by an occlusive dressing may be used, or split-thickness cadaver or porcine xenografts may be used since they simulate the function of epithelium.
   b. Splint the wound in a position of rest to prevent motion.
   c. Close the wound (using local anesthesia) when there are no signs of suppuration.
8. Give antimicrobial treatment as directed. (This depends on how the injury occurred, the age of the wound, the presence of soil-infection potential, *etc.*)
9. Immobilize the site if the wound is contaminated; elevate the site to limit accumulation of fluid in wound interstitial spaces.
10. Give tetanus prophylaxis as indicated, based on the condition of the wound and the patient's immunization status.
11. Inform the patient to contact the physician/clinic if there is sudden or persistent pain, fever or chills, bleeding, rapid swelling, foul odor, drainage, or redness surrounding the wound.

Intra-abdominal Injuries

Penetrating Abdominal Injuries

Penetrating abdominal injuries (gunshot wounds, stab wounds) are serious and usually require surgery. In penetrating injuries, the most important factor is the velocity with which the missile entered the body. High-velocity missiles (bullets) create extensive tissue damage. Almost all gunshot wounds require surgical exploration. Stab wounds may be managed more conservatively.

Assessment for Abdominal Injuries

- Obtain a history of the mechanism of the injury: Penetrating force (gunshot, stab)? Blunt force (blow)?
- Inspect the abdomen for obvious signs of injury: Penetrating injuries, bruises, *etc.*
- Auscultate for the presence or absence of bowel sounds and record baseline data so changes can be noted. (Absence of bowel sounds is an early sign of intraperitoneal involvement; if signs of peritoneal irritation are present, an immediate exploratory *celiotomy* [surgical incision into abdominal cavity] is usually performed.)
- Assess the patient for progression of distention, involuntary guarding, tenderness, pain, muscular rigidity or rebound tenderness, diminished bowel sounds, hypotension and shock.
- Look for chest injuries, which frequently accompany intra-abdominal injuries; look for associated injuries.
- Record all physical signs as patient is examined.

The nursing diagnoses may include actual impairment of skin integrity related to penetrating injuries. The goals of the patient may include control of bleeding, maintenance of blood volume, and prevention of infection of wounds that disrupt the gastrointestinal tract.

Emergency Management

1. Start resuscitation procedures (restoration of airway, breathing, circulation).
2. Keep the patient on the stretcher, since movement may cause fragmentation of a clot in a large vessel and produce massive hemorrhage.
   a. Ensure patency of the airway and stability of the respiratory, circulatory, and nervous systems.
   b. Cut the clothing away from the wound.
   c. Tabulate the number of wounds.
   d. Look for entrance and exit wounds.
   e. If the patient is comatose, splint the neck until after cervical films are made.
3. Assess for signs and symptoms of hemorrhage. *Hemorrhage frequently accompanies abdominal injury*, especially if the liver and spleen have been traumatized.
4. Control the bleeding and maintain the blood volume until surgery can be performed.
   a. Apply compression to external bleeding wounds and occlusion of chest wounds.
   b. Insert indwelling intravenous catheter(s) for rapid fluid replacement to restore circulatory dynamics.
   c. Watch for the occurrence of shock after an initial response to transfusion therapy; this is often the first sign of internal hemorrhage.
5. Aspirate the stomach contents with a nasogastric tube. This procedure also helps detect gastric wounds, lessens contamination of the peritoneal cavity, and prevents lung complications due to aspiration.
6. Cover protruding abdominal viscera with sterile, moist saline dressings to prevent the viscera from drying.
   a. Flex the patient's knees, because this position will prevent further protrusion.
   b. Withhold oral fluids to prevent increased peristalsis and vomiting.
7. Insert an indwelling urethral catheter to ascertain the presence of hematuria and to monitor the urinary output.
8. Keep an ongoing flow sheet of the patient's vital signs, urinary output, central venous pressure readings (when indicated), hematocrit values, and neurologic status.
9. Prepare for paracentesis or peritoneal lavage (Chart 60-3) when there is uncertainty about intraperitoneal bleeding.
10. For stab wounds, prepare for sinography to determine whether there is peritoneal penetration.
    a. A purse-string suture is placed around the wound.
    b. A small catheter is introduced through the wound.
    c. A contrast medium is introduced through the catheter; x-rays are made and will reveal whether or not peritoneal penetration has taken place.
11. Carry out tetanus prophylaxis as directed.
12. Give a broad-spectrum antibiotic to prevent infection, since trauma predisposes to infection (by disruption of mechanical barriers; by exogenous bacteria from the environment at time of accident; by diagnostic and therapeutic maneuvers [nosocomial infection]).

13. Prepare the patient for surgery if he shows continuing evidence of shock, blood loss, free air, evisceration, hematuria, *etc.*

Blunt Abdominal Trauma

Blunt trauma to the abdomen may result from automobile accidents, falls, and blows to the abdomen. Patients with blunt trauma are a challenge because of potential hidden injuries that may be difficult to detect. The incidence of delayed trauma-related complications is greater than that associated with penetrating injuries. This is especially true of blunt injuries involving the liver, kidneys, spleen, or blood vessels, which can lead to substantial blood loss into the peritoneal cavity. Blunt abdominal trauma is frequently associated with extra-abdominal injuries to the chest, head, or extremities, and the evaluation and treatment of these injuries may take precedence over the abdominal problem.

Assessment

1. Take a detailed history (although this is frequently unobtainable, inaccurate, or misleading). Obtain all possible data about the following:
   a. Method of injury.
   b. Time of onset of symptoms.
   c. Passenger location if in an automobile accident (driver frequently sustains rupture of the spleen/liver).
   d. Time of last food/fluid intake.
   e. Bleeding tendencies.
   f. Concurrent disease/medications.
   g. Immunization history, with attention to tetanus.
   h. Allergies.
2. Make a rapid examination of the entire patient to detect life-threatening problems.

The clinical manifestations of blunt abdominal trauma include pain (especially on movement), rebound and maximal point tenderness (may indicate peritoneal irritation from blood or gastrointestinal fluid), muscle guarding, and diminishing or absent bowel sounds.

Emergency Management

1. Begin resuscitation procedures and evaluation of the patient simultaneously.
2. Carry out ongoing physical assessment: inspection, palpation, auscultation, and percussion of the abdomen. The changes noted in subsequent examinations may reveal an undetected abdominal injury.
   a. Avoid moving the patient until the initial assessment is done. Movement may fragment a clot in a large vessel and produce massive hemorrhage.
   b. Expect a wide variety of signs and symptoms resulting from blood loss, bruising and tearing of solid organs, and leaking of secretions from hollow abdominal viscera.
   c. Look for chest injuries, especially for fractures of the lower ribs.
   d. Inspect the front, flanks, and back for bluish discoloration, asymmetry, abrasion, and contusion.
   e. Evaluate for signs and symptoms of hemorrhage, which frequently accompanies abdominal injury, especially if the liver and spleen have been traumatized. Massive intraperitoneal bleeding is associated with shock.
   f. Note tenderness, rebound tenderness, guarding, rigidity, and spasm.
      (1) Press the area of maximal tenderness (let the patient point to the area).
      (2) Remove the fingers quickly; pain at the suspected point indicates peritoneal irritation.
   g. Look for increasing abdominal distention. Measure the abdominal girth at the umbilical level upon admission; this serves as a baseline from which changes can be determined.
   h. Ask about referred pain. (This is helpful in detecting intraperitoneal injury. Pain in the left shoulder may be encountered in a patient bleeding from a ruptured spleen; pain in the right shoulder can result from laceration of the liver.)
   i. Auscultate for bowel sounds. (Silent abdomen accompanies peritoneal irritation.)
   j. Note loss of dullness over the solid organs (liver or spleen)—indicates presence of free air. Dullness over regions normally containing gas indicates presence of blood.)
3. Assist with rectal or vaginal examination for diagnosis of injury to the pelvis, bladder, and intestinal wall.
4. Avoid giving narcotics during the observation period, since this may mask the clinical picture.
5. Monitor vital signs frequently and carefully. This may be the only clue to intra-abdominal bleeding.
6. Prepare the patient for diagnostic procedures.
   a. Laboratory studies
      (1) Urinalysis: as a guide to possible urinary tract injury (hematuria) and to monitor urinary output.
      (2) Serial hematocrit levels: trend reflects presence or absence of bleeding.
      (3) CBC: white blood cell count is elevated with trauma in general.
      (4) Serum amylase determinations: rising level may indicate pancreatic injury or perforations of gastrointestinal tract.
   b. X-ray studies
      (1) Computed tomography scans: permit detailed evaluation of abdominal contents and retroperitoneal examination.
      (2) Abdominal and chest x-rays: may reveal free air beneath diaphragm, indicating a ruptured hollow viscus (a large interior organ).
7. Prepare for peritoneal lavage to test for intraperitoneal bleeding (see Chart 60-3); organ laceration or bleeding may be diagnosed by gross and microscopic examination of fluid returned after peritoneal lavage.
8. Assist with insertion of a nasogastric tube to prevent vomiting and subsequent aspiration. It is also helpful in decompressing (removing fluid/air from) the gastrointestinal tract.
9. The patient may be admitted for observation or exploratory laparotomy.

Chart 60-3
Assisting With Peritoneal Lavage

Peritoneal lavage is a technique of irrigation of the peritoneum and examination of the irrigating fluid in order to evaluate the effects of trauma to the abdomen.

Purposes

1. To test for intra-abdominal bleeding following trauma
2. To look for injuries requiring surgical treatment
3. To test patients with equivocal abdominal findings
4. To avoid unnecessary operation, especially in patients with altered states of consciousness (from head injuries, drugs, alcohol) and when physical findings are unreliable (spinal cord injuries)

Equipment

Peritoneal dialysis tray (or alternate method may be used)
Sterile solution (lactated Ringer's solution, normal saline)
IV tubing, IV pole
Peritoneal dialysis catheter (multiple perforations)
Local skin anesthetic, sterile gloves

Procedure

Nursing Action	Rationale/Amplification
Preparatory Phase	
1. Explain the procedure to the patient; see that the consent form has been signed.	
2. Empty the bladder (by catheter if necessary)	2. To prevent puncture of the urinary bladder.
3. Pass a nasogastric tube as directed.	3. To decompress the stomach.
4. Prepare the abdomen as for surgery.	4. To minimize or eliminate surface bacteria and decrease the possibility of wound contamination and infection.
5. Fill the IV tubing with solution, using aseptic technique.	
Performance Phase (by the Physician)	
1. The skin is infiltrated 2 to 3 cm (0.7–1.2 inches) below the umbilicus in the midline with local anesthetic.	1. The midline area is relatively avascular.
2. A vertical incision is made down to the linea alba.	
3. Local pressure is applied to suppress capillary leakage. Bleeding vessels are carefully ligated.	3. Ligation of vessels helps avoid a false-positive lavage.
4. The peritoneum is opened under direct vision, and a peritoneal dialysis catheter is inserted into the peritoneal cavity.	

(continued)

10. *Complications*
    a. *Immediate:* hemorrhage, shock and associated injuries
    b. *Delayed:* infectious complications

- Paralysis of a part
- Erythema and blistering of skin
- Damaged part (usually an extremity): becomes swollen, tense, and hard
- Renal dysfunction (prolonged hypotension causes kidney damage and acute renal insufficiency)

Crush Injuries

Crush injuries occur when a person is crushed beneath debris, run over, or compressed by machinery.

Assessment

Observe for the following:

- Oligemic shock due to extravasation of blood and plasma into injured tissues after compression has been released

Emergency Management

1. Control shock.
2. Observe carefully for acute renal insufficiency. Injury to the back may cause severe kidney damage.
3. Splint major soft tissue injuries to control bleeding and pain early.

Chart 60-3 *(continued)*

Procedure

Nursing Action	*Rationale/Amplification*
Performance Phase (by the Physician)	
5. A syringe is attached to the catheter, and the peritoneal cavity is aspirated.	5. If gross blood is obtained (or bile or intestinal contents), the tap shows positive findings and the patient is prepared for immediate celiotomy (incision into the abdominal cavity).
6. If no blood is present, the catheter is attached to the IV tubing; 500 to 1000 ml of solution is infused into the peritoneal cavity through the intravenous tubing attached to the dialysis catheter.	6. If not contraindicated by the patient's condition, he may be turned from side to side to mix the peritoneal contents with the solution.
7. After the solution is infused, remove the empty IV bag from the pole and lower it below the abdominal level (near the floor).	7. Lowering the bottle creates a siphon effect to drain the excess fluid. As much of the fluid as possible is siphoned out of the peritoneal cavity by gravity.
8. The peritoneal dialysis catheter is removed and the wound is closed (unless laparotomy is necessary).	
9. The fluid recovered from the peritoneal cavity is examined visually and is usually sent to the laboratory for cell counts and microscopic inspection of a spun-down sediment.	
Interpretation of Lavage Fluid	
1. *Gross examination (visual):* Inability to read newsprint through the intravenous tubing usually means that the amount of blood is sufficient to indicate a laparotomy.	1. If the test results are positive, a laparotomy is usually done. If the test results are negative, the catheter is removed and the wound closed.
2. *Laboratory evaluation (positive tests):* Free aspiration of blood/grossly bloody fluid. RBC greater than 100,000/mm³ WBC greater than 500/mm³ Bacteria—pathologic when present Bile—pathologic when present	2. If the test results are questionable, the catheter may be left in place and the lavage repeated. If the test results are weakly positive, the patient may have echography and arteriography if his condition is stable.
Follow-up Phase	
1. Assess the patient for complications.	1. Complications include wound problems, visceral injury, and inadequate fluid return.
2. Watch the patient closely for any type of deterioration.	2. Repeated physical examinations of the abdomen should be carried out when intra-abdominal injury is suspected.

4. Elevate the extremity. Incise fascia if the blood supply is blocked to relieve the pressure of extravasated fluid.
5. Administer medication for pain and anxiety.

Multiple Injuries

The patient with multiple injuries requires a team approach, with one person responsible for coordinating the treatment. Multiple trauma potentially affects every body system.

Assessment

Evidence of gross trauma may be slight or absent. The injury regarded as the least significant may be the most lethal. Following trauma, there may be general depression of body functions leading to such complications as reduced blood pressure, oxygen deficiency in the bloodstream and primary organ systems, dysrhythmias, and respiratory and heart failure. It is thought that the defense mechanism of the body becomes depressed, contributing to total organ failure. Mortality in patients with multiple injuries is related to the severity of the injuries and the number of systems and organs involved.

Emergency Management

The goals of treatment are to determine the extent of injuries and to establish priorities of treatment. Any injury interfering with a vital physiologic function (airway, breathing, circulation, *etc.*) is an immediate threat to life and has the highest

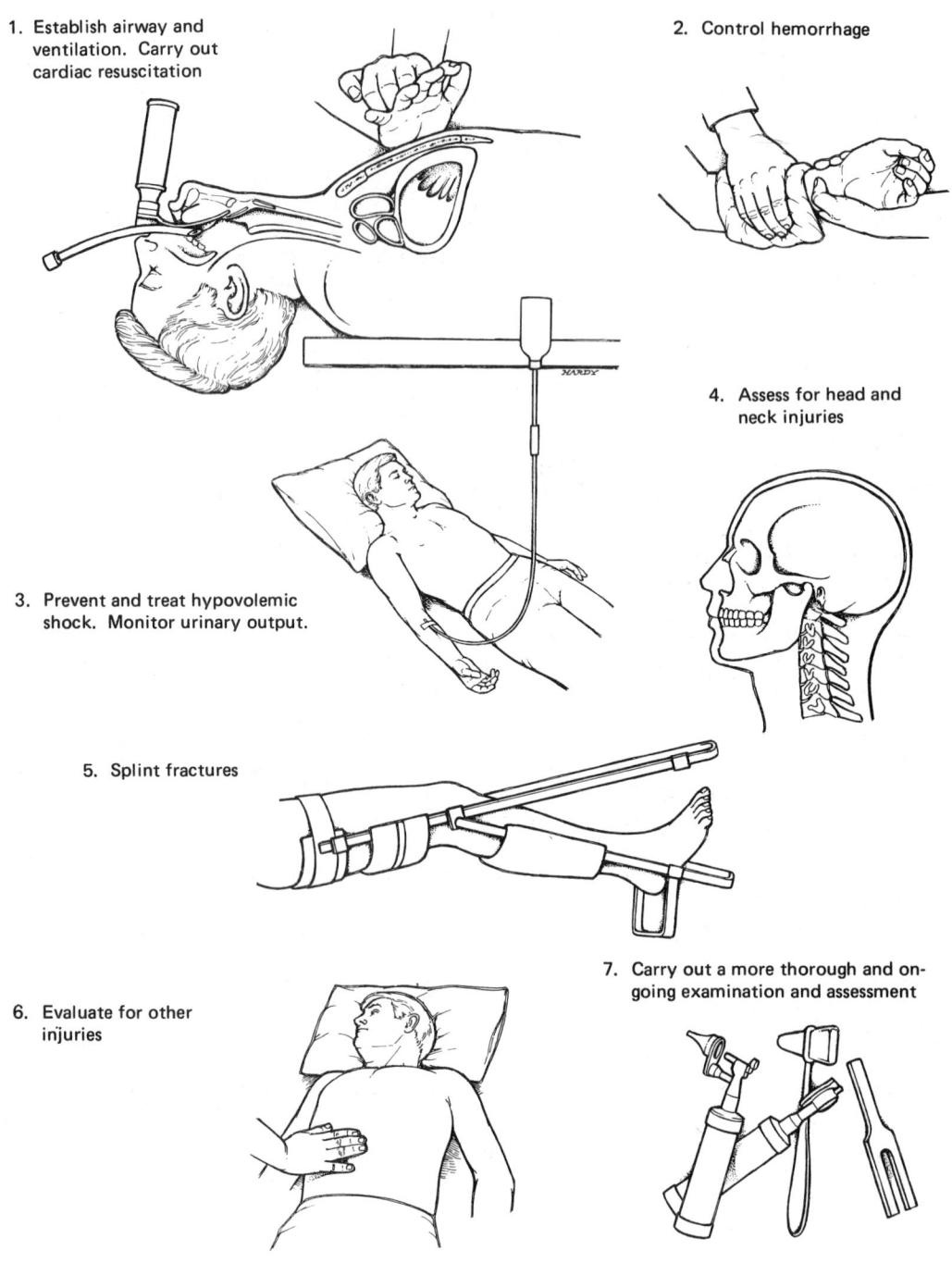

1. Establish airway and ventilation. Carry out cardiac resuscitation

2. Control hemorrhage

3. Prevent and treat hypovolemic shock. Monitor urinary output.

4. Assess for head and neck injuries

5. Splint fractures

6. Evaluate for other injuries

7. Carry out a more thorough and on-going examination and assessment

Figure 60-7
Management of the patient with multiple injuries.

priority for immediate treatment. *Imperative lifesaving procedures are performed simultaneously by the emergency team.* As soon as the patient is resuscitated, the clothes are usually cut off and a rapid physical assessment is done. Critically traumatized patients should not be moved off the stretcher until they are stable. Treatment in a trauma center is appropriate for major trauma patients.

Treatment priorities are as follows (see also Fig. 60-7):

1. Carry out a *rapid* physical examination to determine if the patient is breathing, bleeding, or in shock; deter-

mine the status of his responsiveness and if he has severe wounds or fracture deformities.*

2. Start resuscitation procedures (airway breathing, circulation, *etc.*) simultaneously while another team member is conducting physical assessment.*

   a. Note the character and symmetry of chest wall motion and the pattern of breathing. Auscultate the chest.

* Imperative lifesaving procedures are performed simultaneously by the emergency team.

b. Ask the conscious patient if he is having difficulty breathing. Ask if he has chest pain.

c. Apply suction to clear the trachea and bronchial tree.

d. Insert an oropharyngeal airway to prevent occlusion by the tongue.

e. Ventilate the patient (bag-mask system) to alleviate hypoxia.

f. Prepare for endotracheal intubation if an adequate airway cannot be maintained.

g. Suspect serious intrathoracic injuries if respiratory distress continues after an adequate airway has been established. See pages 496–500 for management of chest injuries.

3. Assess cardiac function and treat cardiac arrest; hypoxia, metabolic acidosis, and chest trauma may precipitate cardiac arrest.*

a. For cardiac arrest, start closed chest compression and ventilation (see pp. 592–593).

b. If the chest wall is unstable (flail chest), emergency thoracotomy and manual compression may be necessary.

c. Give sodium bicarbonate (IV) to compensate for acidosis if indicated; severely traumatized patients with respiratory and circulatory embarrassment will have some degree of metabolic acidosis.

4. Control hemorrhage.*

a. Apply pressure over bleeding points if hemorrhage is overt.

b. Expect significant blood loss in the patient with a fracture of the shaft of the femur, with multiple fractures, or with major pelvic trauma.

c. Use tourniquet(s) for massive arterial bleeding from extremities that cannot be halted with pressure.

d. Prepare for immediate surgical intervention if the patient is bleeding internally.

5. Prevent and treat hypovolemic shock.

a. Insert at least two (sometimes four) IV lines: one above the diaphragm and one below. Use venous cutdown if necessary.

b. Draw blood for laboratory studies as directed (typing and cross matching, baseline CBC, electrolytes, blood urea nitrogen, glucose, prothrombin time).

c. Introduce a central venous catheter to monitor the patient's response to fluid infusion, to prevent fluid overload, and as a route for fluid infusion.

d. Start intravenous infusions.

(1) Lactated Ringer's solution is usually given for volume replacement until blood is available.

(2) Give intravenous infusions rapidly enough to keep central venous pressure readings at 5 to 15 cm H_2O; monitor the rate and direction of change (important parameters).

e. Give blood as directed. Massive transfusions have a cooling effect that can cause cardiac irritability and arrest; blood should be warmed.

f. Insert an indwelling urethral catheter and monitor urinary output to aid in diagnosis of shock, and monitor effectiveness of therapy. Do not force the catheter, because the patient may have a ruptured urethra.

g. Monitor the ECG to detect changes.

h. Carry out ongoing clinical evaluation to observe for improvement or deterioration; improvement in the level of responsiveness, skin warmth, speed of capillary filling, *etc.,* shows a reversal of the shock state.

i. Prepare for immediate surgical intervention if the patient does not respond to fluids or blood. Inability to restore blood pressure and circulatory volume in the patient usually indicates major internal bleeding.

6. Assess for head and neck injuries.

a. Make definite statements about the baseline neurologic status of the patient: level of responsiveness, size and reactivity of pupils, motor power, reflexes.

b. Neck (and chest) films may be taken; apply rigid cervical collar until x-rays preclude the possibility of cervical spine injury.

c. Intracranial pressure monitoring may be instituted.

7. Administer dexamethasone as directed; corticosteroids appear to protect pulmonary function in patients with multiple injuries and help prevent posttraumatic pulmonary insufficiency. (However, this is considered a controversial issue.)

8. Splint fractures to prevent further trauma to soft tissues and blood vessels and to relieve pain; note the presence or absence of pulses in fractured extremities.

9. Assess the patient for gastrointestinal injuries.

a. Examine the patient repeatedly for abdominal pain, muscular rigidity, tenderness, rebound tenderness, diminished bowel sounds, hypotension, and shock.

b. Prepare for peritoneal lavage to assess for intraperitoneal bleeding.

c. Assist with insertion of a nasogastric tube if upper gastrointestinal bleeding is suspected or if gaseous distention of the stomach develops; this will decrease the incidence of vomiting and aspiration.

d. Prepare for laparotomy if the patient shows continuing signs of hemorrhage and deterioration.

10. Continue to monitor urinary output hourly; urinary output reflects cardiac output and state of perfusion of visceral organs.

a. Assess for hematuria and oliguria.

b. Record measurements on a flow sheet.

11. Evaluate patient for other injuries and institute appropriate treatment, including tetanus immunization.

12. Carry out a more thorough physical examination after resuscitation and management of the above priorities.

Fractures

The immediate management of a fracture may determine the patient's outcome and make the difference between recovery and disability. In examining for fracture, handle the part gently and as little as possible. Cut off clothing to minimize trauma to the part. Evaluate for pain over or near a bone, swelling (from blood, lymph, and exudate infiltrating the tissue), and circulatory disturbance. Look for ecchymosis, tenderness, and crepitation. *Keep in mind that the patient may have multiple fractures accompanied by head, chest, and other serious injuries.*

Emergency Management

1. Give immediate attention to the patient's general condition. If there is any question of multiple injury, the patient needs to be completely undressed, draped, and examined periodically.
   a. Evaluate for respiratory difficulties from edema due to facial and neck injuries, accumulation of secretions in the respiratory tract, *etc.*
      (1) Examine the chest for evidence of sucking chest wounds, pneumothorax, flail chest, *etc.*
      (2) Prepare for tracheal intubation or emergency tracheostomy.
   b. Control hemorrhage.
      (1) Control venous bleeding by applying direct pressure along with digital pressure over the artery nearest to the bleeding area.
      (2) Suspect internal hemorrhage (pleural, pericardial, or abdominal) in the event of continuing shock and in the presence of injuries to the chest and abdomen.
   c. Treat for shock, which is usually the result of blood loss in patients with fractures.
      (1) Assess for falling blood pressure; cold, clammy skin; and rapid, thready pulse.
      (2) Keep in mind that a large amount of blood loss may accompany fractures of the femur and pelvis.
      (3) Maintain the blood pressure with intravenous infusions, plasma, or plasma expanders.
      (4) Give blood transfusion(s) or blood component therapy as soon as blood is available.
      (5) Administer oxygen, since cardiopulmonary embarrassment causes a decreased oxygen supply to the tissues and circulatory collapse.
      (6) Give an analgesic to control pain. (Splinting the extremity and controlling pain are essential in treating shock accompanying fractures.)
      (7) Look for evidence of head, chest, and other injuries.
2. Inspect the fractured part(s).
   a. Observe the entire body using a methodical head-to-toe physical examination; inspect for lacerations, swelling, and deformities.
   b. Look for *angulation* (bending), *shortening*, and *rotation*.
   c. Feel the pulse distal to the extremity fracture. Check all peripheral pulses.
   d. Assess for coolness, blanching, decreased sensation and motor function, and diminished or absent pulses; these indicate injury to nerves or the blood supply.
   e. Handle the part gently and as little as possible.
3. Apply the splint before the patient is moved; splinting relieves pain, improves circulation, prevents further tissue injury, and prevents a closed fracture from becoming an open one.
   a. Immobilize the joint above and below the fracture. Place one hand distal to the fracture and apply some traction while placing the other hand beneath the fracture for support.
   b. Extend the splints well beyond the joints adjacent to the fracture.
      (1) Use the patient's clothing for padding (shirt, tie) if nothing else is available.
      (2) Use newspapers, magazines, pillows, tree limbs, or boards for splints if nothing else is available. Specialized splints and traction are available on ambulances and in hospitals.
      (3) Splint joints in functional positions.
   c. Check the vascular status of the extremity after splinting; check color, temperature, pulse, blanching of nail bed.
   d. Evaluate for neurologic deficits caused by the fracture.
   e. Apply a sterile dressing if the fracture is an open one.
4. Investigate any complaint of pain or pressure.
5. Transport the patient carefully and gently.
6. See pages 1583 to 1601 for a complete discussion of the treatment of fractures at specific sites.

Temperature Emergencies

Heat Stroke

Heat stroke is an acute medical emergency caused by failure of the heat-regulating mechanisms of the body during extended heat waves, especially with high humidity. Persons at risk are those not acclimatized to heat exposure, those with advanced age, those who are unable to care for themselves, those with chronic and debilitating diseases, and those who are taking certain medications (major tranquilizers, anticholinergics, diuretics, propranolol). Another form of heat stroke, *exertional heat stroke*, is a leading cause of death in athletes in this country.

   Gerontological Considerations.   The majority of heat-related deaths occur in the aged, because their circulatory systems are unable to compensate for the stress imposed by heat.

Assessment

Heat stroke causes thermal injury at the cellular level and resulting widespread damage to the heart, liver, kidney, and blood coagulation systems. When assessing the patient, note the following: profound central nervous system dysfunction (manifested by confusion, delirium, bizarre behavior, coma); elevated body temperature (40.6°C [105°F] or more); hot, dry skin; and usually anhidrosis (absence of sweating).

   The nursing diagnoses may include ineffective thermoregulation related to inability of body's homeostatic mechanisms to maintain normal body temperature. The patient's goal is reduction of the high temperature as quickly as possible. (Mortality is directly related to the duration of hyperthermia.)

Emergency Management

1. Remove the patient's clothing.
2. Reduce the core (internal) temperature to 39°C

(102°F) as rapidly as possible. Use one or more of the following as directed:
   a. Immerse the patient in an ice water bath or tepid water.
   b. Use cool sheets and towels or continuous sponging with cool water.
   c. Apply ice to the skin while spraying with tepid water.
   d. Use cooling blankets.
   e. Iced saline lavage of stomach or colon may be done if temperature does not come down.
3. Massage the patient, especially the torso to neck and extremities, to promote circulation and maintain cutaneous vasodilation during the cooling procedure.
4. Place an electric fan so that it blows on the patient to augment heat dissipation by convection and evaporation.
5. Monitor the patient's temperature constantly by a thermistor probe in the rectum or esophagus (monitors core temperature) to avoid hypothermia.
6. Monitor the patient carefully; vital signs, ECG, CVP, and level of responsiveness change with rapid alterations in body temperature.
7. Administer oxygen to supply tissue needs exaggerated by the hypermetabolic condition. Intubate the patient with a cuffed endotracheal tube and attach to a ventilator if necessary to support failing cardiorespiratory systems.
8. Start intravenous infusion as directed to replace fluid losses and maintain adequate circulation; give slowly because of the danger of myocardial injury from high body temperature or poor renal function.
9. Give supportive care as directed:
   a. Dialysis for renal failure.
   b. Diuretics (mannitol) to promote diuresis. (Monitor the blood pressure carefully, as hypotension may be precipitated.)
   c. Anticonvulsant agents to control seizures.
   d. Potassium for hypokalemia and sodium bicarbonate to correct metabolic acidosis, depending on laboratory results.
10. Measure urinary output; acute tubular necrosis is a complication of heat stroke.
11. Continue to monitor ECG for possible ischemia or occult myocardial infarction.
12. Carry out serial testing for bleeding diatheses (disseminated intravascular coagulation) and serum enzymes to estimate thermal hypoxic injury to the liver and muscle.
13. Admit the patient to the intensive care unit; permanent liver, cardiac, and central nervous system damage may occur.

Patient Education

1. Advise the patient to avoid immediate re-exposure to high temperatures; he may remain hypersensitive to high temperatures for a considerable length of time.
2. Emphasize the importance of maintaining an adequate fluid intake, wearing loose clothing, and reducing activity in hot weather.

3. Advise athletes to monitor fluid losses, replace fluids, and use a gradual approach to physical conditioning, allowing sufficient time for acclimatization.
4. Direct the frail elderly living in urban settings with high environmental temperatures to centers where air conditioning is available (shopping mall, library, church).

Cold Injuries

Frostbite

Frostbite is trauma from exposure to freezing temperatures that causes actual freezing of the tissue fluids in the cell and intracellular spaces, resulting in vascular damage. The body parts most frequently affected by frostbite are the feet, hands, nose, and ears. A frozen extremity may be hard, cold, and insensitive to touch and appear white or mottled blue-white. The extent of injury from exposure to cold is not always known when the patient is seen initially.

Emergency Management

The goal of management is to restore normal body temperature.

1. Do not allow the patient to walk if the lower extremities are involved.
2. Remove all constricting clothing.
3. Rewarm the extremity by controlled and rapid rewarming, 38°C to 42°C (100°F to 108°F), usually in a whirlpool, until the tips of the injured part flush (about 30 to 45 minutes); flush indicates that circulatory flow is reestablished. Early thawing appears to decrease the amount of tissue loss.
   a. Administer an analgesic for pain; the thawing process may be very painful.
   b. Handle the part gently to avoid further mechanical injury.
   c. Protect the thawed part; do not rupture blebs, which develop from 1 hour to a few days after rewarming.
   d. Place sterile gauze or cotton between affected fingers or toes to prevent maceration.
   e. Elevate the part to help control swelling.
   f. Use a foot cradle to prevent contact with bedclothes if the feet are involved.
4. Carry out physical assessment to look for concomitant injury (soft tissue injury, dehydration, alcohol coma, fat embolism).
5. Restore electrolyte balance; dehydration and hypovolemia occur frequently in frostbite victims.
6. Use strict aseptic technique during dressing changes; frostbite injuries make the patient susceptible to infection.
7. Give tetanus prophylaxis if indicated by associated trauma.
8. The following may be carried out when appropriate:
   a. Whirlpool bath (with disinfectant) for the affected extremity to aid circulation, débride dead tissue, and help prevent infection.

b. Escharotomy (incision through the eschar) to prevent further tissue damage, allow for normal circulation, and permit joint motion.

c. Fasciotomy (incision in fascia to release pressure on the muscles, nerves, blood vessels) to treat compartment syndrome.

9. Encourage hourly active motion of the affected digits to promote maximum restoration of function and to prevent contractures.
10. Advise patient not to use tobacco because of its vasoconstrictive effect.

Accidental Hypothermia

Accidental hypothermia is a condition in which the core (internal) temperature is 35°C (95°F) or below as a result of exposure to cold. *Urban hypothermia* (extreme exposure to cold in an urban setting) is associated with a high mortality rate; elderly people and infants are particularly susceptible.

In assessing the patient, the following factors are kept in mind. Hypothermia leads to physiologic changes in all organ systems. There is progressive deterioration with apathy, poor judgment, ataxia, dysarthria, drowsiness, and eventually coma. Shivering may be suppressed below a temperature of 32.2°C (90°F). Below this temperature, the body's self-warming mechanisms become ineffective. The heartbeat and the blood pressure may be so weak that the peripheral pulsation becomes undetectable. Cardiac irregularities also may occur. Other physiologic abnormalities include hypoxemia and acidosis.

Emergency Management

Management consists of continuing monitoring, rewarming, and supportive care.

1. Monitor the patient: vital signs, CVP, urinary output, arterial blood gases, blood chemistry determinations (BUN, creatinine, glucose, electrolytes), chest x-ray.
   a. Monitor body temperature with an esophageal or rectal thermistor probe.
   b. Employ continuous ECG monitoring; cold-induced myocardial irritability leads to conduction disturbances, especially ventricular fibrillation.
   c. Maintain an arterial line for recording blood pressure and to facilitate blood sampling.
2. Rewarm the patient. Rewarming methods include active core (internal) rewarming, active external rewarming, and passive or spontaneous rewarming. The optimal method has not been determined.
3. Supportive care during rewarming includes the following:
   a. External cardiac compression if indicated.
   b. Electrical cardioversion of ventricular fibrillation.
   c. Mechanical ventilation with PEEP and heated humidified oxygen, to maintain tissue oxygenation.
   d. IV fluids (warmed) to correct hypotension and maintain urinary output.
   e. Sodium bicarbonate to correct metabolic acidosis.
   f. Antiarrhythmic drugs as necessary.
   g. Indwelling urethral catheter to monitor fluid status.
   h. Prophylactic antibiotics. (A large percentage of hypothermic patients have serious infections.)

Anaphylactic Reaction

An anaphylactic reaction is an acute systemic hypersensitivity reaction that occurs within seconds to minutes after exposure to a variety of foreign substances, for example, drugs (penicillin, iodinated contrast material) and stinging insects (*Hymenoptera* [bee, wasp, yellow jacket, hornet]). Repeated administration of parenteral or oral therapeutic agents also may precipitate an anaphylactic reaction.

An anaphylactic reaction is the result of an antigen–antibody interaction in a sensitized individual who, as a consequence of previous exposure, has developed a special type of antibody (immunoglobulin) that is specific for this particular allergen. The antibody immunoglobulin IgE is responsible for the great majority of the immediate type of human allergic responses: the individual becomes sensitive to a particular antigen after production of IgE to this antigen.

Assessment

Anaphylactic reaction produces a wide range of clinical manifestations.

- *Respiratory signs* include (1) nasal congestion, itching, sneezing and coughing; (2) possible respiratory distress that progresses rapidly and is caused by bronchospasm or edema of the larynx; (3) tightness of the chest; and (4) other respiratory difficulties, such as wheezing, dyspnea, and cyanosis.
- *Skin manifestations* appear in the form of flushing with a sense of warmth and diffuse erythema. *Generalized itching over the entire body indicates that a general systemic reaction is developing.* Urticaria (hives) may also appear. When massive facial angioedema develops, upper respiratory edema may occur.
- *Cardiovascular manifestations* include tachycardia or bradycardia and peripheral vascular collapse as indicated by pallor, imperceptible pulse, falling blood pressure, and circulatory failure, leading to coma and death.
- *Gastrointestinal discomforts* may occur, such as nausea, vomiting, and colicky abdominal pains or diarrhea.

Emergency Management

1. Establish an airway. (This is done while another person administers epinephrine.)
   a. Turn the face to one side; support the angles of the mandible.
   b. Insert an oropharyngeal or endotracheal tube; apply oropharyngeal suction for excessive secretions.
   c. Employ resuscitative measures (especially for patients with stridor and progressive pulmonary edema).
   d. If glottic edema is present, an incision through the cricothyroid membrane will provide an airway.
   e. Use positive pressure oxygen therapy by mask and compression bag.
   f. Use closed chest cardiac massage if necessary.
2. Give aqueous epinephrine as directed to provide rapid relief of hypersensitivity reaction. (This should be done simultaneously while another person is establishing the airway.) Epinephrine may be repeated if necessary as prescribed. Use judgment in choosing the route of administration for epinephrine:

a. Subcutaneous injection for mild, generalized symptoms.

b. Intramuscular or sublingual injection when the reaction is more severe and progressive, and when there is concern that vascular collapse will inhibit absorption.

c. Intravenous route (aqueous epinephrine diluted in saline and given *slowly*), used in rare instances in which there is complete loss of consciousness and severe cardiovascular collapse. This method may precipitate cardiac dysrhythmias; *monitor ECG and have defibrillator available.*

3. Apply a tourniquet above the injection site if an anaphylactic reaction followed the injection or insect sting, to retard antigen absorption.

a. Infiltrate the injection site with epinephrine as directed.

b. Loosen the tourniquet at regular intervals to allow adequate circulation to the extremity.

4. Start an intravenous infusion of saline for emergency access to a vein and for hypotension.

Additional Treatment as Indicated

5. Give antihistamine drugs, for example, diphenhydramine hydrochloride (Benadryl, IM) to block further histamine binding at target cells.

6. Give aminophylline IV *slowly* over a period of time for patients with severe bronchospasm and wheezing that is refractory to treatment. Monitor vital signs.

7. Treat prolonged hypotension with crystalloids or colloids and possibly vasopressors; monitor blood pressure. A patient with reduced cardiac output may respond to an infusion of isoproterenol or dopamine.

8. Administer oxygen if significant respiratory or cardiovascular deficits are present.

9. Watch for dysrhythmias and cardiorespiratory arrest.

10. If the patient is convulsing, give an IV injection of short-acting barbiturate or diazepam over a period of several minutes.

11. Administer corticosteroids if the patient is having a prolonged reaction and persistent hypotension or bronchospasm.

12. The patient is usually admitted to the hospital after the symptoms abate.

Preventive Measures/Patient Education

1. Be aware of the danger of anaphylactic reactions and the early signs of anaphylaxis.

2. Ask about the patient's previous allergies to medications; if positive, do not give medication or injection.

3. Question the patient before giving a foreign serum or other types of antigenic agents to determine whether he has had it at some earlier time.

4. Question the patient about previous allergic reactions to food or pollen.

5. Avoid giving drugs to patients with hay fever, asthma, and other allergic disorders unless absolutely necessary.

6. Avoid giving parenteral medications unless absolutely necessary. Anaphylactic reactions are more likely to occur when the agent is given parenterally.

7. Do skin testing before administration of certain materials known to produce anaphylactic reactions, such as horse serum. Skin testing can precipitate anaphylaxis in highly sensitive individuals.

a. A negative skin test does not always indicate safety.

b. Have epinephrine, IV infusions, and intubation and tracheostomy equipment available as precautionary measures.

8. If the patient is being treated as an outpatient, keep him in the office, hospital, or clinic at least 30 minutes after injection of any agent. Caution the patient to return if symptoms develop.

9. Caution patients who are sensitive to insect bites to carry kits equipped to treat insect stings (tourniquet, epinephrine).

10. Encourage allergic persons to wear identification tags or bracelets.

Poisoning

A poison is any substance that, when ingested, inhaled, absorbed, applied to the skin, or produced within the body in relatively small amounts, causes injury to the body by its chemical action. Poisoning from inhalation and ingestion of toxic materials, both accidental and by design, constitutes a major health hazard. The problem is one of real magnitude; approximately 7% of all emergency department visits are the direct result of toxic problems.

Ingested (Swallowed) Poisons

The goals of emergency treatment are (1) to remove or inactivate the poison before it is absorbed, (2) to give supportive care to maintain vital organ systems, (3) to use the specific antidote to neutralize the poison, and (4) to give treatment to hasten the elimination of the absorbed poison.

General Management*

1. Attain control of the airway, ventilation, and oxygenation; in the absence of cerebral or renal damage, the patient's prognosis depends largely on successful management of respiratory and circulatory systems.

a. Assess adequacy of ventilation by observing ventilatory effort, through blood gas analysis, or by the use of Wright's spirometer.

b. Assess cardiovascular function by measurement of pulse, blood pressure, central venous pressure, and temperature (core and peripheral).

c. Give artificial respiration if respiration is depressed. Positive expiratory pressure applied to the airway (bag-mask) may help keep the alveoli inflated.

d. Administer oxygen for respiratory depression, unconsciousness, cyanosis, and shock.

e. Prevent aspiration of gastric contents by positioning (on side with head down), use of oropharyngeal airway, and suctioning.

* Many of these measures are done simultaneously by the emergency department team.

f. Stabilize cardiovascular function. Take ECG.

g. Insert an indwelling urinary catheter to monitor kidney function.

h. Obtain blood to test for concentration of drug or poison.

i. Monitor neurologic status (including mentation); monitor the course of vital signs and neurologic status over time.

j. Conduct a rapid physical examination.

2. Try to determine the product taken, amount, time since ingestion, symptoms, age and weight of the patient, and pertinent health history. Call the poison control center in the area if an unknown toxic agent has been taken, or if it is necessary to identify an antidote for a known toxic agent.

3. Treat shock appropriately; it may be due to cardiodepressant action of the drug ingested, venous pooling in lower extremities, or a reduction in circulating blood volume due to increased capillary permeability.

4. Remove the toxin or decrease its absorption. Consider gastric emptying procedures; the following may be used:

a. Induction of emesis with syrup of ipecac for the alert patient.

- *Do not induce emesis after ingestions of caustic substance or petroleum distillates.*

b. Gastric lavage (Fig. 60-8, Chart 60-4) for the obtunded patient. (Save gastric aspirate for toxicology screens.)

c. Activated charcoal administration if poison is one that is absorbed by charcoal.

d. Cathartic, when appropriate.

5. Give specific therapy. Administer the specific chemical antagonist or physiologic antagonist as early as possible to reverse or diminish effects of the toxin.

6. Support the patient having convulsions; many poisons excite the central nervous system, or the patient may convulse from oxygen deprivation.

7. Assist in carrying out procedures to enhance the removal of the ingested substance if the above are not effective:

a. Diuresis for agents excreted by renal route.

b. Dialysis.

c. Hemoperfusion (process of passing blood through an extracorporeal circuit and a cartridge containing an adsorbent [such as charcoal or resins], after which the detoxified blood is returned to patient).

d. Multiple doses of charcoal.

8. Monitor central venous pressure as indicated.

9. Monitor for fluid and electrolyte imbalance.

10. Reduce elevated temperature.

11. Give analgesics for pain cautiously; severe pain causes vasomotor collapse and reflex inhibition of normal physiologic functions.

12. Assist in securing specimens of blood, urine, stomach contents, and vomitus.

13. Provide constant nursing surveillance and attention to the patient in a coma; coma from poisoning results from interference with brain cell function or metabolism.

14. Monitor and treat for complications such as hypotension, cardiac dysrhythmias, and seizures.

15. If the patient is discharged, give written instructions of signs and symptoms of potential problems and procedures for call-back or return.

a. Refer patient for psychiatric evaluation if poisoning was a suicide attempt.

b. Give poison prevention and home poison-proofing instructions to a patient with accidental ingestion.

Corrosive Poisons

Corrosive poisons include alkaline and acid agents that can cause tissue destruction after coming in contact with mucous membranes.

- *Alkaline products:* Lye, drain cleaners, toilet bowl cleaners, bleach, nonphosphate detergents, oven cleaners, button batteries (batteries used to power watches, calculators, cameras), Clinitest tablets
- *Acid products:* Toilet bowl cleaners, swimming pool cleaners, metal cleaners, rust removers, battery acid

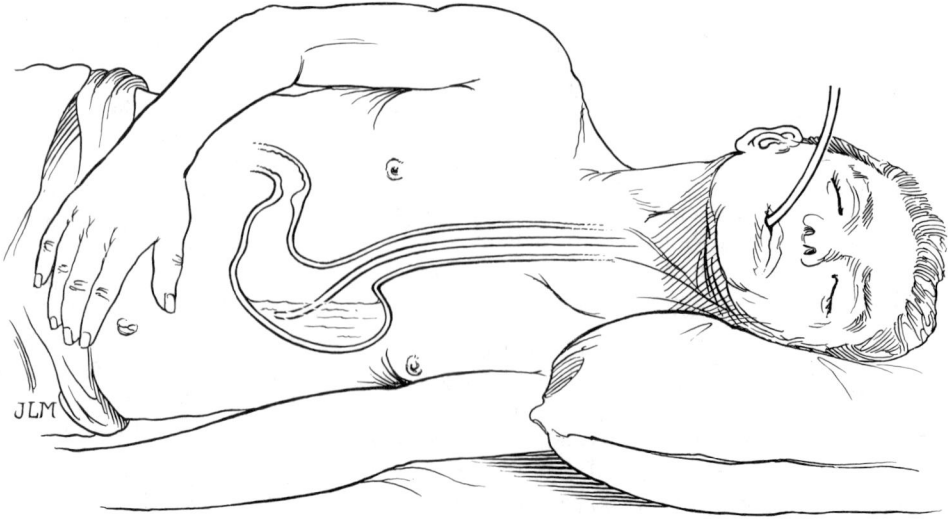

Figure 60-8
Gastric lavage. During gastric lavage the patient is positioned on his left side to allow pooling of the gastric contents and decrease the passage of fluid into the duodenum during lavage.

Assessment

1. Obtain history of type and quantity of agent ingested.
2. Assess for severe pain and burning sensations in mouth and throat, pain on swallowing, inability to swallow, vomiting, drooling, hematuria.

The nursing diagnoses may include alteration in mucous membranes related to swallowing corrosive poison, and self-directed violence.

Emergency Management

1. Give water (or milk) to drink for dilution.

   - Dilution is *not* attempted if patient has acute airway swelling or obstruction or if there is clinical evidence of esophageal, gastric, or intestinal perforation.
   - *Do not induce vomiting if the patient has consumed a strong acid, alkali, or other corrosive substance.*

2. The patient is usually admitted to the hospital for observation and elective endoscopy to evaluate for the presence of burns and deep ulceration.
3. Refer the patient for psychiatric evaluation if poisoning was a suicide attempt.

Inhalation Exposure

General Management

1. Carry the patient to fresh air immediately; open all doors and windows.
2. Loosen all tight clothing.
3. Apply artificial respiration if required.
4. Prevent chilling; wrap the patient in blankets.
5. Keep the patient as quiet as possible.
6. Do not give alcohol in any form.

Carbon Monoxide Poisoning

Carbon monoxide (CO) poisoning may occur as an industrial or household accident or as an attempted suicide. It causes more deaths than any other toxic agent except alcohol. Carbon monoxide exerts its toxic effect by binding to circulating hemoglobin to reduce the oxygen-carrying capacity of the blood. Hemoglobin absorbs CO more than 200 times more readily than oxygen. Carbon monoxide-bound hemoglobin, called *carboxyhemoglobin*, is unavailable to transport oxygen.

Clinical Manifestations/Assessment

The central nervous system has a critical need of oxygen and will show signs of carbon monoxide toxicity. A person suffering from carbon monoxide poisoning will appear intoxicated (from cerebral hypoxia). Other symptoms and signs include headache, muscular weakness, palpitation, dizziness, and mental confusion, which can progress rapidly to coma. The skin color is not a reliable sign; the skin may be pink, cherry red, or cyanotic and pale. History of exposure to carbon monoxide justifies immediate treatment.

Emergency Management

The goals of management are to reverse cerebral and myocardial hypoxia and to hasten carbon monoxide elimination.

1. Give 100% oxygen at atmospheric or hyperbaric pressures to reverse hypoxia and accelerate the elimination of carbon monoxide.
2. Draw blood for carboxyhemoglobin levels; oxygen is administered until the carboxyhemoglobin level is less than 5%.
3. Observe the patient constantly. Psychoses, spastic paralysis, ataxia, visual disturbances, and deterioration of personality may persist following resuscitation and may be symptoms of permanent central nervous system damage.
4. When unintentional carbon monoxide poisoning occurs, the health department should be contacted and the dwelling or building in question should be inspected.

Skin Contamination Poisons (Chemical Burns)

Injuries from exposure to chemicals are challenging, because there are a large number of offending agents with diverse actions and metabolic effects. The severity of a chemical burn is determined by the mechanism of action, penetrating strength and concentration, and amount and duration of exposure of the chemical to the skin.

Emergency Management

1. Drench the skin with running water from a shower, hose, or faucet.
2. Continue to apply a stream of water to the skin while removing the clothing; health care personnel should be appropriately garbed if the burn is extensive or the agent significantly toxic.
3. Apply *prolonged* lavage with tepid water in copious amounts.
4. Try to determine the identity and characteristics of the chemical agent for appropriate future treatment.
5. Give the standard burn treatment appropriate for the size and location of the wound (antimicrobial treatment, tetanus prophylaxis).
6. Instruct the patient to have the affected area reexamined at 24 and 72 hours and 7 days; there is a significant risk of underestimating these types of injuries.

Injected Poisons: Stinging Insects (Bees, Hornets, Yellow Jackets, Wasps)

A person may have an extreme sensitivity to the venoms of the *Hymenoptera* (the stings of bees, hornets, yellow jackets, and wasps). It is thought that venom allergy is an IgE-mediated reaction; this constitutes an acute emergency. Stings of the head and neck are especially serious, although stings in any area of the body can result in anaphylaxis.

The clinical response may range from generalized urticaria, itching, malaise, and anxiety to laryngeal edema, severe bronchospasm, shock, and death. In general, the shorter the time between the sting and the onset of severe symptoms, the worse the prognosis.

Chart 60-4
Assisting With Gastric Lavage

Gastric lavage is the aspiration of the stomach contents and washing out of the stomach by means of a gastric tube. Gastric lavage may be dangerous after acid or alkali ingestion, in the presence of convulsions, or after ingestion of hydrocarbons or petroleum distillates. It is dangerous after ingestion of strong corrosive agents.

Purposes

1. For urgent removal of ingested substance in order to decrease systemic absorption
2. To cleanse the stomach before endoscopic procedures
3. To diagnose gastric hemorrhage and to arrest hemorrhage

Equipment

Large-bore/orogastric tubes or large-bore Ewald tube
Large irrigating syringe with adapter
Large plastic funnel with adapter to fit stomach tube
Water-soluble lubricant
Tap water or appropriate antidote (milk, saline solution, sodium bicarbonate solution, fruit juice, activated charcoal)
Bucket for aspirate
Mouth gag, nasotracheal or endotracheal tubes with inflatable cuffs
Containers for specimens

Procedure

Action	Rationale/Amplification
1. Remove dental appliances and inspect the oral cavity for loose teeth.	1. This will prevent accidental aspiration.
2. Measure the distance between the bridge of the nose and the xiphoid process. Mark the tube with indelible pencil or tape.	2. This distance is a rule-of-thumb measurement of the distance the tube is passed to reach the stomach. This avoids curling and kinking of excess tubing in the stomach.
3. Lubricate the tube with water-soluble lubricant.	
4. If comatose, the patient is intubated with a cuffed nasotracheal or endotracheal tube.	4. A cuffed endotracheal tube prevents aspiration of gastric contents.
5. Place the patient in a left lateral position with the head lowered approximately 15° downward.	5. This position decreases passage of gastric contents into the duodenum during lavage and minimizes the possibility of aspiration into the lungs.

(continued)

Emergency Management

1. Give epinephrine (aqueous) as directed. Massage the site to hasten absorption. If the sting is on an extremity, apply a tourniquet with sufficient compression to occlude venous and lymphatic flow.
2. See page 1720 for treatment of anaphylactic shock.
3. Counsel all persons known to be sensitive to *Hymenoptera* venom to carry a commercially available self-treatment kit containing a tourniquet, injectable and inhalant forms of epinephrine, an oral antihistamine, and written instructions; the kit is available on prescription. Instruct the patient to do the following if he is stung:
   a. Inject himself with epinephrine immediately.
   b. Remove the stinger with one quick scrape of the fingernail. Do not squeeze the venom sac; this may cause additional venom to be injected.
   c. Cleanse the area with soapy water and apply ice.
   d. Apply a tourniquet proximal to the sting.
   e. Report to the nearest health care facility for further examination.
4. All allergic individuals should wear medical warning bracelets indicating hypersensitivity.
5. Hyposensitization therapy should be given to persons who have had systemic or large local reactions.

Patient Education

Instruct the patient to limit exposure to stinging insects by the following measures:

· Avoiding locales with stinging insects (camp and picnic sites).
· Staying away from insect feeding areas (flower beds, ripe fruit orchards, garbage, fields of clover).

Chart 60-4 (continued)

Procedure

Action	*Rationale/Amplification*
6. Pass the tube by the oral route while keeping the head in a neutral position. Pass the tube to the adhesive marking or about 50 cm (20 inches). After the lavage tube is passed, the head of the table is lowered. Have standby suction available.	6. The depth of insertion of the tube will vary with the height of the patient. If the tube enters the trachea instead of the esophagus, the patient will experience coughing, dyspnea, stridor, and cyanosis.
7. Submerge the free end of the tube below water level at the moment of the patient's exhalation, or auscultate the stomach during injection of air with a syringe to confirm gastric location.	7. If the tube is inadvertently in the lungs, the water will bubble with each exhalation.
8. Aspirate the stomach contents with the syringe attached to the tube before instilling water or an antidote. Save the specimen for analysis.	8. Aspiration is carried out to remove the stomach contents.
9. Remove the syringe. Attach the funnel to the stomach tube, or use a 50-ml syringe to put lavage solution in the gastric tube. The volume of fluid placed in the stomach should be small.	9. Overfilling the stomach may cause regurgitation and aspiration or force the stomach contents through the pylorus.
10. Elevate the funnel above the patient's head and pour approximately 150 to 200 ml of solution into the funnel.	
11. Lower the funnel and siphon the gastric contents into the bucket.	11. The fluid should flow in freely and drain by gravity.
12. Save samples of the first two washings.	12. Keep the first washing sample isolated from other washings for toxicological analysis.
13. Repeat the lavage procedure until the returns are relatively clear and no particulate matter is seen.	13. This usually requires a total volume of at least 2 liters; some clinicians advocate the use of 5 to 20 liters.

14. At the completion of lavage:
   a. The stomach may be left empty.
   b. An adsorbent (powder form of activated charcoal mixed with water to form slurry, the consistency of thick soup) may be instilled in the tube and allowed to remain in the stomach.
   c. A saline cathartic may be instilled in the tube.
	
	   b. Activated charcoal reduces absorption by absorbing (attaching to its surface) a wide range of substances; it renders the poison inaccessible to the circulation, thereby reducing its toxicity.
	   c. A cathartic may be given to hasten the elimination of remaining ingested material.

15. Pinch off the tube during removal or maintain suction while the tube is being withdrawn.	15. Pinching off the tube prevents aspiration and the initiation of the gag reflex. Keeping the patient's head lower than the body also gives this protection.
16. Warn the patient that his stools will turn black from the charcoal.	

- Not going barefoot outdoors (yellow jackets may nest on the ground).
- Avoiding perfumes, scented soaps, and bright colors, which attract bees.
- Keeping car windows closed.
- Spraying garbage cans with rapid-acting insecticide.
- Securing a professional exterminator to dispose of wasp and hornet nests or bee hives in the home area.
- Remaining motionless if an insect buzzes around him. (Motion, especially running, increases the likelihood of being stung.)
- Learning self-injection of epinephrine.

Food Poisoning

Food poisoning is a sudden, explosive illness that may occur after ingestion of contaminated food or drink. Botulism, a serious form of food poisoning, is discussed on page 1684, since the treatment differs and the patient requires continuing surveillance.

Emergency Management

1. Determine the source and type of food poisoning.
   a. Have the family bring the suspected food to the medical facility.
   b. Take the history:
      (1) How soon after eating did the symptoms occur? (Immediate onset suggests chemical, plant, or animal poisoning.)
      (2) What was eaten in the previous meal? Did the food have any unusual odor or taste? (Most foods causing bacterial poisoning do not have unusual odor or taste.)

(3) Did anyone else become ill from eating the same food?

(4) Did vomiting occur? What was the appearance of the vomitus?

(5) Did diarrhea occur? (Diarrhea is usually absent with botulism and with shellfish or other fish poisoning.)

(6) Are any neurologic symptoms present? (These occur in botulism and in chemical, plant, and animal poisoning.)

(7) Does the patient have a fever? (Fever is seen in salmonella, favism [ingestion of fava beans], and some fish poisoning.)

(8) What is the patient's appearance?

2. Collect food, gastric contents, vomitus, serum, and feces for examination.

3. Monitor vital signs on a continuing basis.

a. Assess respiration, blood pressure, sensorium, CVP (if indicated), and muscular activity.

b. Weigh the patient for future comparisons.

4. Support the respiratory system. Death from respiratory paralysis can occur with botulism, fish poisoning, *etc.*

5. Maintain fluid and electrolyte balance. Severe vomiting produces alkalosis, and severe diarrhea produces acidosis; large amounts of electrolytes and water are lost by vomiting and diarrhea.

a. Watch for oligemic shock from severe fluid and electrolyte losses.

b. Evaluate for apathy, rapid pulse, fever, oliguria, anuria, hypotension, and delirium.

c. Carry out blood electrolyte studies.

6. Correct and control hypoglycemia.

7. Control the nausea.

a. Give an antiemetic drug parenterally if the patient cannot tolerate fluids or medications by mouth.

b. Give sips of weak tea, carbonated drinks, or tap water for mild nausea.

c. Give clear liquids 12 to 24 hours after nausea and vomiting subside.

d. Graduate to a low-residue, bland diet.

Substance Abuse

Substance abuse is the misuse of specific substances to alter mood or behavior.

Drug Abuse

Drug abuse is the use of drugs for other than legitimate medical purposes. The clinical manifestations may vary with the drug used, but the underlying principles of management are essentially the same. Table 60-1 notes the most commonly abused drugs, listing their clinical manifestations and therapeutic management.

Drug users tend to take a variety of drugs simultaneously (*e.g.*, alcohol, barbiturates, narcotics, and tranquilizers) that may have additive effects. Intravenous drug abusers are at increase risk for acquired immunodeficiency syndrome and infectious hepatitis, and are the most frequent victims of tetanus in the United States.

The treatment goals for a patient suffering from drug intoxication are to support the respiratory and cardiovascular functions and to enhance the clearance of the agent.

Emergency Management of Acute Drug Reaction

1. Assess the presence and adequacy of respirations. Attain control of the airway, ventilation, and oxygenation.

a. Use a cuffed endotracheal tube and provide assisted ventilation in a severely depressed patient with absent gag or cough reflexes.

b. Measure arterial blood gases for hypoxia due to hypoventilation and acid–base derangements.

c. Administer oxygen.

2. Stabilize the cardiovascular system. (This is done simultaneously with airway management.)

a. Begin external cardiac compression and ventilation in the absence of heartbeat.

b. Start ECG monitoring.

c. Draw blood samples for testing glucose, electrolytes, BUN, creatinine, and appropriate toxicologic screen.

d. Start intravenous fluids.

3. Give a specific drug antagonist if the drug is known. Naloxone hydrochloride (Narcan) is frequently used; 50% dextrose in water is also used (for hypoglycemia).

4. Remove the drug from the stomach as soon as possible.

a. Induce vomiting if the patient is seen early after ingestion; save the vomitus for toxicologic study.

b. Use gastric lavage if the patient is unconscious or if there is no way to determine when the drug was ingested.

• In patients with absent gag or cough reflexes, carry out this procedure only after intubation with a cuffed endotracheal tube to prevent aspiration of the stomach contents.

c. Activated charcoal may be a useful adjunct to therapy and is used after emesis or lavage.

d. Save gastric aspirate for toxicologic analysis.

5. Give supportive care.

a. Take rectal temperature; extremes of thermoregulation (hyperthermia/hypothermia) must be recognized and treated.

b. Treat convulsions.

c. Assist with hemodialysis/peritoneal dialysis for potentially lethal poisoning.

d. Try to maintain a free urine flow since the drug or metabolites are excreted by the urine.

6. Do a thorough physical examination to rule out insulin shock, meningitis, subdural hematoma, stroke, *etc.*

a. Look for needle marks and external evidence of trauma.

b. Carry out a rapid neurologic survey (level of responsiveness, pupil size and reaction, reflexes, focal neurologic findings).

c. Keep in mind that many drug users take multiple drugs simultaneously.

d. Be aware that there is a high incidence of infectious hepatitis among drug users, which is thought to be the result of communal use of unsterile needles and syringes.

(Text continues on p. 1730)

TABLE 60-1
Emergency Management of Drug Abuse Patients

Drug	Clinical Manifestations	Therapeutic Management
Narcotics		
Cocaine: Intranasally ("snorting"): inhaled into nostrils through straws By smoking ("freebasing"): cocaine hydrochloride dissolved in ether to yield a pure cocaine alkaloid base (called "crack"); smoking in a small pipe delivers large quantities of cocaine to lungs Intravenously	Cocaine is a CNS simulant that can increase heart rate and blood pressure and cause hyperpyrexia, seizures, and ventricular dysrhythmias. It produces intense euphoria, then anxiety, sadness, insomnia, and sexual indifference; cocaine hallucinosis with delusions; psychosis with extreme paranoia with ideas of persecution; and hypervigilance. Chronic psychotic symptoms may persist.	1. Correct the most fundamental problem during depressive phase (ensure airway and ventilation). 2. Control seizures. 3. Monitor cardiovascular effects; have lidocaine and defibrillator available. 4. Treat for hyperthermia. 5. Refer for psychiatric evaluation and treatment in an inpatient unit that eliminates access to the drug.
Heroin Opium or paregoric Morphine, codeine, synthetic derivatives (methadone, meperidine)	Acute intoxication (overdose) Pinpoint pupils (may be dilated with severe hypoxia) Marked respiratory depression Stupor → coma Fresh needle marks along course of any superficial vein; skin abscesses	1. Support respiratory and cardiovascular functions. 2. Establish an IV line; withdraw blood for chemical and toxicologic analysis. Patient may be given bolus of glucose to eliminate possibility of hypoglycemia 3. Give narcotic antagonist (naloxone hydrochloride [Narcan]) to reverse severe respiratory depression and coma. 4. Continue to monitor level of responsiveness and respirations, pulse, and BP. Duration of action of naloxone hydrochloride is shorter than that of heroin; repeated dosages may be necessary. 5. Send urine for analysis; opiates can be detected in urine. 6. Secure an ECG. 7. Do not leave patient unattended; he may lapse back into coma rapidly. Clinical status may change from minute to minute. Hemodialysis may be indicated for severe drug intoxication. 8. Monitor for pulmonary edema, which is frequently seen in patients who abuse/overdose on narcotics. 9. Send patient for psychiatric evaluation prior to discharge.
Barbiturates		

Pentobarbital (Nembutal)
 	
Secobarbital (Seconal)
 	
Amobarbital (Amytal)
	Acute intoxication (may mimic alcohol intoxication):
	Flushed face
	Decreased pulse rate
	Increasing nystagmus
	Depressed tendon reflexes
	Decreasing mental alertness
	Difficulty in speaking
	Poor motor coordination
	Coma, death
		1. Maintain airway and give respiratory support.
		2. Consider endotracheal intubation or tracheostomy if there is any doubt about the adequacy of airway exchange.
		  a. Check airway frequently.
		  b. Perform *regular* suctioning.
		3. Support cardiovascular and respiratory functions; most deaths result from respiratory depression or shock.

(continued)

TABLE 60-1 *(continued)*

Drug	Clinical Manifestations	Therapeutic Management
Barbituates		

(Barbituates — Therapeutic Management continued)

4. Start intravenous infusion through large-gauge needle or intravenous catheter to support blood pressure; coma and dehydration result in hypotension and respond to infusion of intravenous fluids with elevation of blood pressure. Sodium bicarbonate may be given to alkalinize urine; it promotes excretion of barbiturates.
5. Evacuate stomach contents or lavage as soon as possible to prevent absorption; repeated doses of activated charcoal may be administered.
6. Assist with hemodialysis for severely overdosed patient.
7. Maintain neurologic and vital sign flow sheet.
8. Patient awakening from overdose may demonstrate hostility; this can stimulate automatic angry response by health care personnel.
9. Refer for psychiatric consultation to evaluate suicide potential and drug abuse.

Amphetamine-Type Drugs (Pep Pills, "Uppers," "Speed")

Drug	Clinical Manifestations	Therapeutic Management
Amphetamine (Benzedrine) Dextroamphetamine (Dexedrine) Methamphetamine (Desoxyn)	Nausea, vomiting, palpitations, anxiety, nervousness Repetitive or stereotyped behavior Irritability, insomnia Visual misperceptions, auditory hallucinations Fearful anxiety/depression, cold, distant hostility Hyperactivity, rapid speech, euphoria	1. Provide airway support, ventilation, cardiac monitoring; insert IV line. 2. Employ gastrointestinal decontamination in cases of oral overdose; activated charcoal, gastric lavage. 3. Keep in calm, quiet environment; elevated temperature potentiates amphetamine toxicity. 4. Use small doses of diazepam (IV) for CNS and muscular hyperactivity. 5. Employ appropriate pharmacologic therapy for severe hypertension and ventricular dysrhythmias. 6. Try to communicate with patient if delusions, hallucinations, *etc.* are present 7. Place in a protective environment (preferably psychiatric security room with video monitoring) to observe for suicide attempt. 8. Refer for psychiatric evaluation.

Hallucinogens or Psychedelic-Type Drugs

Drug	Clinical Manifestations	Therapeutic Management
Lysergic acid diethylamide (LSD) Phencyclidine HCl (PCP, "angel dust") Mescaline, psilocybin Jimson weed seeds	Nystagmus, mild hypertension Marked confusion bordering on panic Incoherence, hyperactivity Hazardous behavior: delirium, mania, self-injury Hallucinations, body image distortion *Flashback*: recurrence of LSD-like state without having taken the drug; may occur weeks or months after drug was taken	*Emergency Management* 1. Evaluate and maintain patient's airway, breathing, and circulation. 2. Determine whether the patient has ingested hallucinogenic drug or has a toxic psychosis. 3. Try to communicate with the patient; use "vocal anesthesia" to reassure him, except for PCP abusers.

(continued)

TABLE 60-1 *(continued)*

Drug	Clinical Manifestations	Therapeutic Management
Hallucinogens or Psychedelic-Type Drugs		
	Convulsions, coma, circulatory collapse, death	a. "Talking down" involves understanding the process through which the patient is proceeding and helping him overcome his fears while establishing contact with reality. b. Remind the patient that fear is common with this problem. c. Reassure the patient that he is not losing his mind—that he is experiencing effect of drugs and that this will wear off. d. Instruct the patient to keep his eyes open; this reduces intensity of reaction. e. *Reduce sensory stimuli*: minimize noise, lights, movement, tactile stimulation. f. Do not leave the patient alone. 4. Sedate the patient if his hyperactivity cannot be controlled; diazepam (Valium) or a barbiturate may be given. 5. Search for evidences of trauma; hallucinogen users have a tendency to "act out" their hallucinations. 6. Manage convulsions; place patient in ICU. 7. Watch patient closely; his behavior may become hazardous. 8. Monitor for hypertensive crisis if patient has prolonged psychosis due to drug ingestion. 9. Place patient in a protected environment under proper medical supervision to prevent self-inflicted bodily harm. *Management for Phencyclidine Abusers* 1. Place patient in a calm, supportive environment to minimize stimuli; protect from self-injury. 2. Avoid "talking down." 3. Do not leave patient unobserved. Treat symptoms as they occur. a. Drug effects are unpredictable and prolonged. b. Symptoms are likely to exacerbate; patient becomes out of control. 4. Refer patient for psychiatric evaluation.
Drugs Producing Sedation, Intoxication, Psychological and Physical Dependence (Nonbarbiturate Sedatives)		
Diazepam (Valium) Chlordiazepoxide (Librium) Oxazepam (Serax) Lorazepam (Ativan)	Acute intoxication: Decreasing mental alertness Confusion Slurred speech Ataxia Pulmonary edema Coma, death	*Management* 1. Insert endotracheal tube as a precaution; use assisted ventilation to stabilize and correct respiratory depression. Watch for sudden apnea and laryngeal spasm (especially in patients habituated to glutethimide [Doriden]).

(continued)

TABLE 60-1 *(continued)*

Drug	Clinical Manifestations	Therapeutic Management
Drugs Producing Sedation, Intoxication, Psychological and Physical Dependence (Nonbarbiturate Sedatives)		

		2. Assess for hypotension.
		  a. Insert indwelling catheter for comatose patient; decreased urinary volume is an index of reduced renal flow associated with reduced intravascular volume or vascular collapse.
		  b. Start volume expansion with saline or dextrose as required.
		3. Evacuate stomach contents; emesis; lavage; activated charcoal; cathartic.
		4. Start ECG monitoring. Watch for dysrhythmias.

Salicylate Poisoning		
Aspirin (present in compound analgesic tablets)	Restlessness, tinnitus, deafness, blurring of vision Hyperpnea, hyperpyrexia, sweating Epigastric pain, vomiting, dehydration Respiratory and metabolic acidosis Disorientation, coma, cardiovascular collapse	1. Treat respiratory depression. 2. Induce gastric emptying: emesis or lavage. 3. Give activated charcoal to adsorb aspirin; a cathartic may be administered with charcoal to help assure intestinal cleansing. 4. Support patient with intravenous infusions to establish hydration and correct electrolyte imbalances. 5. Enhance elimination of salicylates by forced diuresis, alkalinization of urine or peritoneal dialysis, or hemodialysis, according to severity of intoxication. 6. Monitor serum salicylate level for efficacy of treatment 7. Give specific pharmacologic agent for bleeding, *etc.*

   e. Examine the patient's breath for the characteristic odor of alcohol, acetone, *etc.*

7. Try to obtain a history of the drug experience (from the person accompanying the patient or the patient himself).
  a. Adapt a supportive and realistic relationship with the patient.
  b. Do not leave the patient alone; there is a potential for the patient to harm himself or emergency department staff.

8. Admit the patient to ICU if he remains unconscious; if the patient has deliberately overdosed, psychiatric consultation is necessary.

9. Make every effort to enroll the patient in a drug treatment program (detoxication and rehabilitation) to intervene in a life-style that fosters addiction.

Alcohol Abuse

Acute Alcohol Intoxication

Alcohol is a psychotropic drug affecting mood, judgment, behavior, concentration, and consciousness. A significant number of heavy drinkers are over 60 years of age. There is a high prevalence of alcoholism in emergency patients. Because alcoholic patients return frequently to the emergency department, they are often exasperating, taxing the endurance of the health professionals caring for them. Thus, their management requires patience as well as thoughtful and correct treatment.

Assessment

Ethanol (alcohol) is a direct multisystem toxin and central nervous system depressant that causes drowsiness, incoordination, slurring of speech, sudden mood changes, aggression, belligerency, grandiosity, and uninhibited behavior. It can cause stupor and coma and even death if taken in excessive amounts.

    The patient should be assessed for head injury, hypoglycemia (which mimics intoxication), and other health problems. The nursing diagnosis may include potential for violence (self-directed or directed at others) related to severe intoxication from alcohol.

Emergency Management of the Acutely Intoxicated Patient

The treatment involves (1) detoxification of the acute poisoning; (2) recovery, or "drying out"; and (3) rehabilitation.

1. Approach the patient in a nonjudgmental manner, without condemnation or reproach.
   a. Expect the patient to use mechanisms of denial and defensiveness.
   b. Adapt a firm, consistent, accepting, and reasonable attitude.
   c. Speak calmly and slowly; alcohol interferes with thought processes.
   d. If the patient appears intoxicated, he is probably drunk even though he denies alcohol intake.
2. Take a blood alcohol test as directed.
3. Allow the drowsy patient to "sleep off" the state of alcoholic intoxication.
   a. Observe for symptoms of central nervous system depression; keep the patient under observation.
   b. Protect the airway.
   c. Undress the patient and cover him with a blanket.
4. Sedate the noisy, belligerent patient as directed.
   a. *Monitor the patient carefully;* watch for hypotension and decreased level of consciousness.
   b. Check vital signs and monitor heart rate and blood pressure.
5. Examine the patient for injuries and organic disease, which can easily be masked by alcoholic intoxication. (Persons with alcoholism suffer more injuries than the general population.)
   a. Assess neurologic status; look for symptoms of head injury.
   b. Assess for alcoholic coma, which is a medical emergency.
   c. Monitor carefully for alcoholic convulsions.
   d. Evaluate for pulmonary infection.
      (1) Pulmonary infections are more common in patients with alcoholism owing to respiratory depression, an impaired defense system, and a tendency toward gastric aspiration.
      (2) The patient may show little increase in temperature or white blood cell count.
   d. Watch for hypoglycemia.
6. Hospitalize the patient if necessary or admit him to a detoxification center; an effort should be made to examine the problems underlying the substance abuse.

Delirium Tremens (Alcoholic Hallucinosis)

Delirium tremens is an acute toxic state that follows a prolonged bout of steady drinking or sudden withdrawal from prolonged intake of alcohol. It may be precipitated by acute injury or infection (pneumonia, pancreatitis, hepatitis).

Clinical Manifestations/Assessment

Patients suspected of delirium tremens will show signs of anxiety, uncontrollable fear, tremor, irritability, agitation, insomnia, and incontinence. They will be talkative and preoccupied, and will experience visual, tactile, olfactory, and auditory hallucinations that are frequently terrifying. Autonomic overactivity will occur and is evidenced by tachycardia, dilated pupils, and profuse perspiration. Usually, all vital signs are elevated in the alcoholic toxic state. Delirium tremens is life-threatening and carries a high mortality rate.

Emergency Management

The goals of management are to give proper sedation and support to enable the patient to rest and recover without danger of injury or peripheral vascular collapse.

1. Take the blood pressure, since the patient's subsequent medication may depend on blood pressure readings.
2. Carry out a physical examination to identify preexisting or contributing illnesses or injuries (head injury, pneumonia, *etc.*).
3. Obtain a drug history (difficult) to elicit information that may facilitate adjustment of sedative requirement.
4. Sedate the patient with a sufficient dosage of medication to establish and maintain sedation to reduce agitation, prevent exhaustion, and promote sleep.
   a. A variety of drugs and combinations of drugs are used, for example, chlordiazepoxide, diazepam, paraldehyde. Haloperidol may be given for severe acute alcoholic hallucinosis.
   b. The dosage is adjusted according to the patient's symptoms (agitation, anxiety) and blood pressure response.
4. Place the patient in a private room and observe closely.
   a. Keep the room lighted to minimize potential for illusions and hallucinations.
   b. Close closet and bathroom doors to eliminate shadows.
   c. Keep the environment calm and nonstressful.
   d. Observe the patient closely; homicidal or suicidal responses may result from hallucinations.
   e. Have someone stay with the patient as much as possible; the presence of another person has a reassuring and quieting effect and helps the patient maintain contact with reality.
   f. Explain visual misrepresentations (illusions) to strengthen the link with reality.
   g. Explain in detail every procedure being done to the patient.
   h. Shut out loud noises.
   i. Call the patient by name.
   j. Take the patient to the bathroom if permitted.
   k. Use restraints if necessary, if the patient is not under direct and constant observation.
5. Maintain electrolyte balance and hydration by way of the oral or intravenous route; fluid losses may be present from gastrointestinal losses (diarrhea) and profuse perspiration, and from the respiratory tract (hyperventilation). Or the patient may be overhydrated related to the effect of alcohol on antidiuretic hormone (ADH).
6. Record temperature, pulse, respiration, and blood pressure frequently (every 30 minutes in severe forms of delirium) in anticipation of peripheral circulatory collapse or hyperthermia (the two most lethal complications).
7. Administer phenytoin (Dilantin) or other anticonvulsant drugs as prescribed to prevent or control repeated withdrawal seizures.
8. Assess the respiratory, hepatic, and cardiovascular status; infections (pneumonia), trauma, hepatic failure, hypoglycemia, and cardiovascular problems are complications.

a. Hypoglycemia may accompany alcoholic withdrawal, because alcohol depletes liver glycogen stores and impairs gluconeogenesis; also, many patients with alcoholism suffer from malnutrition.

b. Administer parenteral dextrose if the liver glycogen is depleted. Give orange juice, Gatorade, or other carbohydrates to stabilize the blood sugar and to counteract tremulousness.

9. Give supplemental vitamin therapy and a high-protein diet; these patients are usually vitamin deficient.

10. Refer the patient to an alcoholic treatment center for subsequent follow-up and rehabilitation.

Psychiatric Emergencies

A psychiatric emergency is an urgent, serious disturbance of behavior, affect, or thought that makes the patient unable to cope with life situations and interpersonal relationships. A patient presenting with a psychiatric emergency may be (1) overactive or violent, (2) underactive or depressed, or (3) suicidal.

The most important concern of the emergency department personnel is whether the patient is likely to cause personal harm or injury to others. In general, the aim is to try to maintain the patient's self-esteem (and life, if necessary) while carrying out assessment and management. The patient is asked if he is currently under psychiatric treatment.

Overactive Patients

Patients in the overactive category will display disturbed, uncooperative, and paranoid behavior, as well as anxiety and paniclike feelings. They may be prone to assaultive and destructive impulses and abnormal social behavior. Intense nervousness, depression, and crying are also evident in some patients. Their disturbed and noisy behavior may be compounded by alcohol or drug intoxication.

Emergency Management

1. Determine from the family or another reliable source the events that led up to the crisis; whether the patient has had past mental illness, hospitalizations, injuries, or serious illnesses; uses alcohol or drugs; or has experienced crises in interpersonal relationships or intrapsychic conflicts.
    a. Be aware that abnormal thought and behavior may be a manifestation of an underlying physical disorder, such as hypoglycemia, stroke, epilepsy, and drug toxicity, including alcohol toxicity.
    b. Carry out a physical examination when feasible.
2. Try to gain control of the situation.
    a. Approach the patient with a calm, confident, and firm manner; this attitude is therapeutic and will have a calming effect.
    b. Introduce yourself by name.
    c. Tell him, "I am here to help you."
    d. Repeat the patient's name from time to time.
    e. Speak in one-thought sentences. Be consistent.
    f. Give the patient space. Let him slow down by himself and allow him to become compliant.

g. Be interested in and listen to the patient; encourage him to talk of his thoughts and *feelings*.

h. Offer appropriate explanations. Tell the truth.

3. Administer a psychotropic agent for emergency management of functional psychosis when appropriate. Chlorpromazine (Thorazine) or haloperidol (Haldol) act specifically against psychotic symptoms of thought fragmentation and perceptual and behavioral aberrations.
    a. The initial dosage depends on the patient's body weight and the severity of the symptoms.
    b. Observe the patient for 1 hour after the initial dose to determine the degree of change in psychotic behavior.
    c. Subsequent dosages depend on the patient's reaction.
    d. If the behavior is caused by hallucinogens (*e.g.,* LSD), psychotropic drugs (exerting an effect on the mind) are not used.
4. Use restraints only as a last resort.
5. Admit the patient to a psychiatric unit or arrange for psychiatric outpatient treatment.

Violent Patients

Violent and aggressive behavior is usually episodic and is a means of expressing feelings of anger, fear, or hopelessness about a situation. Usually, the patient has a history of outbursts of rage, temper tantrums, or generally impulsive behavior. Persons with a tendency to violence frequently lose control when intoxicated with alcohol or drugs. Family members are the most frequent victims of their aggression. Patients with a propensity for violence include those intoxicated by drugs or alcohol; those going through drug or alcohol withdrawal; and those with acute paranoid schizophrenic state, acute organic brain syndrome, acute psychosis, a paranoid character, a borderline personality, or an antisocial personality.

A specially designated room with at least two exits should be used for the interview. No objects that could be used as weapons should be in sight. If the interviewer feels anxious or uneasy about the patient's response, security staff, a family member, or another health care worker should be asked to remain in the hall nearby in the event that additional help is needed.

The nursing diagnoses could include potential for violence (self-directed or directed at others) related to acute paranoid schizophrenic state. The patient's goal is to bring his violence under control.

Emergency Management

1. Keep the door of the room open and be in clear view of the staff. You should be between the patient and the door. Do not block the patient's exit to the door; the patient may feel closed in and threatened.
2. Help the patient bring his violence under control.
    a. Give the patient space. Do not make any sudden movement.
    b. If the patient is carrying a weapon, ask him to surrender it.
    c. If the patient is unwilling to surrender his weapon, call the security staff; they may seek assistance from the local police department.

3. Do not leave the patient alone; this can be interpreted as rejection, or the patient may try to harm himself.
4. Adopt a calm, noncritical approach and remain in control of the situation. External calm and structure may help the patient to gain control.
5. Talk and listen to the patient.
   a. Crisis intervention is best done with an attitude of interest in the patient's well-being and with an attempt to "tune in" to the patient while at the same time remaining firm.
   b. Acknowledge the patient's state of agitation, for example, "I want to work with you to relieve your distress."
   c. Give the patient the opportunity to ventilate his anger verbally; avoid challenging the delusional state.
   d. Try to hear wht the patient is saying.
   e. Convey an expectation of appropriate behavior and make him aware that help is available for him to gain control.
      (1) Let the patient know that his behavior may be frightening to those around him and that violence is not acceptable.
      (2) Describe the help available in crisis situations: clinic, emergency department, mental health facility.
      (3) Offer the patient something to eat or drink if talking does not defuse the situation.
6. Allow the security personnel/police to intervene if the patient does not become calm.
   a. Offer protection of hospitalization; this is usually welcomed by the patient who fears losing control or harming himself or others.
   b. If the above fails to attenuate the patient's tension, offer medication (rapid tranquilization with haloperidol, diazepam, or chlorpromazine) to reduce tension, anxiety, and hyperactivity.
   c. Use restraints when necessary but with a minimum of force.
      (1) Use restraints with verbal intervention to calm the patient and make him more compliant.
      (2) Have enough personnel available when applying restraints.
7. Refer the patient for further mental health treatment after combativeness, agitation, and fear have cooled.

Depressed Patients

In the emergency department, depression may be seen as the primary condition bringing the patient to the health care facility, or depression may be masked by anxiety and somatic complaints.

The depressed person will have some sort of mood disturbance. Assessment includes observing for sadness, apathy, feelings of worthlessness, self-blame, suicidal thoughts, desire to escape, avoidance of simple problems, anorexia and weight loss, lessened interest in sex, sleeplessness, and reduction in activity or ceaseless activity.

The agitated depressed individual may exhibit motor restlessness and severe anxiety.

Emergency Management

1. Listen to the patient in a calm, unhurried manner.
   a. The patient will benefit from ventilation of feelings.
   b. Give the patient an opportunity to talk about his problems.
   c. Anticipate that the patient may be suicidal.
   d. Attempt to find out if the patient has thought about or attempted suicide: "Have you ever thought about taking your own life?" The patient is generally relieved because of the opportunity to discuss his feelings.
   e. Find out if there is an illness, perceived or real.
   f. Assess whether there has been sudden worsening of depression.
   g. Notify relatives about a seriously depressed patient. Do not leave the patient alone, since suicide is usually committed in solitude.
2. Give antidepressant and antianxiety agents as prescribed.
3. Point out to the patient that depression is treatable.
4. Be aware of crisis and supportive services in the community: mental health center, telephone counseling and referral, suicide prevention centers, group therapy, marital and family counseling, befriending programs.
5. Refer the patient for psychiatric consultation or to a psychiatric unit.

Suicidal Patients

Suicide is an act that stems from depression (the loss of a loved one, the loss of body integrity or status, poor self-image) and can be viewed as a cry for help and intervention. Those at risk include older people; males; young adults; people who are enduring unusual loss or stress; those who are unemployed, divorced, widowed, or living alone; those who are showing significant depression (weight loss, sleep disturbances, somatic complaints, suicidal preoccupation); and those who have a history of previous suicidal attempt or completed suicide(s) in the family, or who have a psychiatric illness.

Prevention

1. Be aware of persons at risk.
2. Determine whether a person has communicated *suicidal intent*, such as preoccupation with death or talking of someone else's suicide:
   "I'm tired of living."
   "I've put my affairs in order."
   "I'm better off dead."
   "I'm a burden to my family."
3. Determine whether he has ever attempted suicide; the risk is much greater in these cases.
4. Is there a family history of suicide?
5. Was there loss of a parent at an early age?
6. Does he have a specific plan for suicide? A means to carry out the plan?

Emergency Management

1. Treat the consequences of the suicide attempt (gunshot wound, drug overdose, *etc.*).
2. Prevent further self-injury; a patient who has made a suicidal gesture may do so again.
3. Employ crisis intervention (a form of brief psychotherapy) to determine suicidal potential; discover areas of depression and conflict; find out about the patient's

support system; and determine whether hospitalization, psychiatric referral, *etc.*, are warranted.
4. Admit the patient to ICU (if condition warrants), arrange follow-up care, or admit him to the psychiatric unit, depending on the assessment of suicide potential.

Sexual Assault

Legally, *rape* is defined as carnal knowledge of a female by force or the threat of force against her will. It is one of the fastest growing crimes of violence. The feminist movement has focused on the rights and care of rape victims, and law enforcement agencies are becoming increasingly sensitive and aggressive in the management of these crimes. Rape crisis centers offer extensive support and education of victims and help them through the subsequent courtroom experience.

The manner in which the patient is received and treated in the emergency department is important to her future psychological well-being. Crisis intervention should begin when the patient enters the health facility. She should be seen immediately upon entrance into the emergency department. Most hospitals have a written protocol that reflects consideration for the victim's physical and emotional needs as well as concern for meeting requirements for subsequent legal proceedings.

The patient's reaction to rape has been termed the "rape trauma syndrome" and is seen as an acute stress reaction to a life-threatening situation. The nurse performing the assessment is aware that the patient may go through several phases of psychological reactions:

1. An acute disorganization phase that may be manifested in two ways:

   - Expressed state, in which shock, disbelief, fear, guilt, humiliation, anger, *etc.*, are encountered.
   - Controlled state, in which feelings are masked or hidden and the victim appears composed.

2. A phase of denial and unwillingness to talk about the incident, followed by a phase of heightened anxiety, fear, flashbacks, sleep disturbances, hyper-alertness, and psychosomatic reactions.
3. A phase of reorganization, in which the incident is put into perspective. Some victims never fully recover and develop chronic stress disorders and phobias.

The nursing diagnosis may include rape trauma syndrome related to a life-threatening situation. The patient's goal is to regain control over her life.

Emergency Management

The goals of management are to give sympathetic support, to reduce the emotional trauma of the patient, and to gather available evidence for possible legal proceedings.

1. Respect the privacy and sensitivity of the patient; be kind and supportive.
   a. Reassure the patient that anxiety is natural and that appropriate support is available from professional and community resources.

   b. Accept the emotional reactions of the patient (hysteria, stoicism, overwhelmed feeling, *etc.*).
   c. Do not leave the patient alone.
2. Assist with the physical examination.
   a. Secure written, witnessed informed consent from the patient (or parent/guardian if the patient is a minor) for examination and for taking of photographs if necessary, and for release of findings to police.
   b. Take a history only if the patient has not already talked to a police officer, social worker, or crisis intervention worker. Do not ask the patient to repeat the history. Record the history of the event in the patient's own words.
   c. Ask if the patient has bathed, douched, brushed teeth, changed clothes, urinated, or defecated since the attack; this may alter interpretation of subsequent findings.
   d. Record the time of admission, time of examination, date and time of alleged rape, and general appearance of the patient.
      (1) Document any evidence of trauma: discoloration, bruises, lacerations, secretions, torn and bloody clothing.
      (2) Record emotional state.
   e. Assist the patient to undress; drape properly.
      (1) Ask the patient to place each item of clothing in a separate paper bag. (Plastic bags promote moisture retention, which may lead to formation of mold and mildew that can destroy evidence.)
      (2) Label bags appropriately; give to appropriate law enforcement authorities.
   f. Examine the patient (from head to toe) for injuries, especially to the head, neck, breasts, thighs, back, and buttocks.
      (1) Assess for external evidence of trauma (bruises, contusions, lacerations, stab wounds).
      (2) Assess for dried semen stains (appearing as crusted, flaking areas) on the patient's body.
      (3) Inspect fingers for broken nails and tissue and foreign materials under nails.
      (4) Assist in conducting oral examination. Secure a specimen of saliva; take prescribed cultures of gum and tooth areas.
      (5) Document evidence of trauma with body diagrams and photographs.
3. Assist with pelvic and rectal examinations.
   a. Advise the patient of the nature and necessity of each procedure; give the rationale for each question asked.
      (1) Examine perineum (and other areas) with a Woods lamp or other filtered ultraviolet light; areas that are found to fluoresce may indicate semen stains.
      (2) Note color and consistency of any discharge present.
      (3) Use a water-moistened vaginal speculum for examination; do not use lubricant, which contains chemicals that may interfere with later forensic testing of specimens and acid phosphatase determinations.

b. Assist with securing laboratory specimens.
   (1) Collect vaginal aspirate, which is examined for presence or absence of motile and nonmotile sperm.
   (2) Use a sterile swab to draw secretions from the vaginal pool for acid phosphatase, blood group antigen of semen, and precipitin test against human sperm and blood.
   (3) Obtain separate smears from the oral, vaginal, and anal areas.
   (4) Obtain culture of body orifices for gonorrhea.
   (5) Obtain blood serum for syphilis; a sample of serum may be frozen and saved for future testing.
   (6) Conduct a test for pregnancy if there is a possibility that the patient may be pregnant.
   (7) Collect foreign material (leaves, grass, dirt) and place in a clean envelope.
   (8) Comb the pubic hairs with a prepackaged clean comb. Trim areas of pubic hair suspected of containing semen. Obtain several pubic hairs with follicles; place in separate containers and identify these as patient's pubic hairs.
   (9) Examine rectum for signs of trauma, blood, semen stains.
   (10) Label each specimen with name of patient, date, time of collection, body area from which specimen was obtained, and names of personnel collecting specimens to preserve chain of evidence; give to designated person (*e.g.,* crime laboratory) and obtain an itemized receipt.
   (11) Photographs are taken by designated person.

4. Treat associated injuries as indicated. Give the patient the option of prophylaxis against sexually transmitted disease.
  a. Give probenecid orally as prescribed, followed in 30 minutes by IM penicillin.
  b. A patient with an allergy to penicillin may receive alternate therapy that may not be effective in the treatment of incubating syphilis; the patient should have a serology check in 6 weeks.

5. Antipregnancy measures may be considered if the patient is of childbearing age, is using no contraceptives, and is at high risk in her menstrual cycle.
  a. Postcoital contraceptive drugs may be given after a pregnancy test: ethinyl estradiol (Estinyl) or conjugated estrogens (Premarin).
  b. An antiemetic may be given to decrease discomfort from side-effects.
  c. Inform the patient that if she misses a menstrual period she has the option of having menstrual extraction or abortion.

6. Offer cleansing douche, mouthwash, and fresh clothing.

7. Provide for follow-up services:
  a. Make an appointment for follow-up surveillance for pregnancy and sexually transmitted disease.
  b. Inform the patient of counseling services to prevent long-term psychological effects; counseling services should be made available to the family.

c. Encourage the patient to return to the previous level of functioning as soon as possible.
d. The patient should be accompanied by a family member or friend when leaving the health care facility.

Bibliography

Books

Abel EL. A Dictionary of Drug Abuse Terms and Terminology. Westport, Greenwood Press, 1984.

Abels L. Critical Care Nursing. St Louis, CV Mosby, 1986.

Aguilera DC and Messick JM. Crisis Intervention. St Louis, CV Mosby, 1986.

Bassuk EL and Birk AW. Emergency Psychiatry. New York, Plenum Press, 1984.

Cain HD (ed). Flint's Emergency Treatment and Management, 7th ed. Philadelphia, WB Saunders, 1985.

Cosgriff JH Jr and Anderson DL. The Practice of Emergency Care, 2nd ed. Philadelphia, JB Lippincott, 1984.

Edlich RF, Spyker DA and Haury BB. Current Emergency Therapy '85. Rockville, Maryland, Aspen Systems, 1985.

Etheredge EE. Management Techniques in Surgery. New York, John Wiley & Sons, 1986.

Eubanks DH and Bone RC. Comprehensive Respiratory Care. St Louis, CV Mosby, 1985.

Figley CR (ed). Trauma and Its Wake. New York, Brunner/Mazel, 1985.

Foley TS and Davies MA. Rape: Nursing Care of Victims. St Louis, CV Mosby, 1983.

Fought SG and Throwe AN. Psychosocial Nursing Care of the Emergency Patient. New York, John Wiley & Sons, 1984.

Gardner LB. Textbook of Acute Internal Medicine. New Hyde Park, New York, Medical Examination Publishing, 1986.

Goldfrank LR et al. Goldfrank's Toxicologic Emergencies, 3rd ed. East Norwalk, Connecticut, Appleton-Century-Crofts, 1986.

Harmon AR. Nursing Care of the Adult Trauma Patient. New York, John Wiley & Sons, 1985.

Hoffer HP (ed). Emergency Problems in the Elderly. Oradell, New Jersey, Medical Economics Books, 1985.

Holloway NM. Nursing the Critically Ill Adult. Menlo Park, California, Addison-Wesley, 1984.

Hyman SE. Manual of Psychiatric Emergencies. Boston, Little, Brown & Co, 1984.

Johanson BC et al. Standards for Critical Care, 2nd ed. St Louis, CV Mosby, 1985.

Kreis DJ Jr and Baue AE. Clinical Management of Shock. Baltimore, University Park Press, 1984.

Krueger DW. Emotional Rehabilitation of Physical Trauma and Disability. New York, SP Medical & Scientific Books, 1984.

May HL (ed). Emergency Medicine. New York, John Wiley & Sons, 1984.

Mills J et al. Current Emergency Diagnosis and Treatment, 2nd ed. Los Altos, California, Lange Medical Publications, 1985.

Moore EE, Eiseman B and Van Way CW. Critical Decisions in Trauma. St Louis, CV Mosby, 1984.

Nurse's Reference Library. Emergencies. Springhouse, Pennsylvania, Springhouse Corp, 1985.

O'Boyle CM et al. Emergency Care: The First 24 Hours. Norwalk, Connecticut, Appleton-Century-Crofts, 1985.

Parker JG. Emergency Nursing. New York, John Wiley & Sons, 1984.

Rippe JM et al (eds). Intensive Care Medicine. Boston, Little, Brown & Co, 1985.

Roberts JR and Hedges JR. Clinical Procedures in Emergency Medicine. Philadelphia, WB Saunders, 1985.

Roberts SL. Physiological Concepts and the Critically Ill Patient. Englewood Cliffs, New Jersey, Prentice-Hall, 1985.

Roberts SL. Behavioral Concepts and the Critically Ill Patient, 2nd ed. Norwalk, Connecticut, Appleton-Century-Crofts, 1986.

Schwartz RG et al (eds). Principles and Practice of Emergency Medicine, Vol 1 and 2, 2nd ed. Philadelphia, WB Saunders, 1986.

Sheehy SB and Barber J. Emergency Nursing: Principles and Practice, 2nd ed. St Louis, CV Mosby, 1985.

Shires GT. Principles of Trauma Care. New York, McGraw-Hill, 1985.

Tintinalli JE, Rothstein RJ and Krome RL. Emergency Medicine. New York, McGraw-Hill, 1985.

Vale JA and Meredith TJ. Concise Guide to Management of Poisoning, 3rd ed. New York, Churchill Livingstone, 1985.

Wilson LB, Simson SP and Baxter CR. Handbook of Geriatric Emergency Care. Baltimore, University Park Press, 1984.

Zuidema GD, Rutherford RB and Ballinger WF. The Management of Trauma, 4th ed. Philadelphia, WB Saunders, 1985.

Articles

(Asterisks indicate nursing research articles.)

Nursing Process in Emergency/Crisis Situations

Elliott FC. A nursing protocol for anxiety following catastrophic injury. Rehabil Nurs 1983 May/June; 8(3):18–20; 30.

Hickey M. Nursing diagnosis in the critical care unit. Dimens Crit Care Nurs 1984 Mar/Apr; 3(2):91–97.

Novotny-Dinsdale V. Implementation of nursing diagnosis in one emergency department. JEN 1985 May/June; 11(3):140–144.

Page RM, Wrye SW and Cole GE. The role of loneliness in health and wellness. Home Healthc Nurse 1986 Jan/Feb; 4(1):6–10.

Taylor H. Using the process in accident and emergency. Nurs Mirror 1984 Mar 28; 158(13):14–15.

Poisoning

Blye E, Lorch J and Cortell S. Extracorporeal therapy in the treatment of intoxication. Am J Kidney Dis 1984 Mar; 3(5):321–338.

Fitzpatrick KT and Moylan JA. Emergency care of chemical burns. Postgrad Med 1985 Oct; 78(5):189–194.

Goldberg MJ et al. An approach to the management of the poisoned patient. Arch Intern Med 1986 July; 146(7):1381–1385.

Hanson W Jr. Toxic emergencies. Clin Emerg Med 1984; 5:1–308.

Park GD et al. Expanded role of charcoal therapy in the poisoned and overdosed patient. Arch Intern Med 1986 May; 146(5):969–973.

Temple AR (ed). Symposium on medical toxicology. Emerg Med Clin North Am 1984 Feb; 2(1):3–197.

Temple AR and Culpit GO. Initial assessment and response. Clin Emerg Med 1984; 5:1–13.

Wason S. The emergency management of caustic ingestions. J Emerg Med 1985; 2(3):175–182.

Psychiatric Emergencies/Sexual Assault

Di Nitto D et al. After rape: Who should examine rape survivors. Am J Nurs 1986 May; 86(5):538–540.

Kobernick ME, Seifert S and Sanders AB. Emergency department management of the sexual assault victim. J Emerg Med 1985; 2(3):205–214.

*Lanza ML. Approaches to studying patient assault. West J Nurs Res 1986 Aug; 8(3):321–328.

Pellitier LR and Cousins A. Clinical assessment of the suicidal patient in the emergency department. JEN 1984 Jan/Feb; 10(1):40–43.

Rose DS. "Worse than death": Psychodynamics of rape victims and need for psychotherapy. Am J Psychiatry 1986 July; 143(7):817–824.

Tavani-Petrone C. Psychiatric emergencies. Primary Care 1986 Mar; 13(1):157–167.

Resuscitation

Hankins DG. Controversies in resuscitation. Postgrad Med 1986 May 15; 79(5):24–33.

McCabe CJ and Browne BJ. Esophageal obturator airway, ET tube and pharyngeal-tracheal lumen airway. Am J Emerg Med 1986 Jan; 4(1):64–71.

Narrod JA, Moore EE and Rosen P. Emergency cricothyrostomy—technique and anatomical considerations. J Emerg Med 1985; 2(6):443–446.

Neal JM. Near-drowning. J Emerg Med 1985; 3(1):41–52.

Ornato JP. The resuscitation of near-drowning victims. JAMA 1986 July 4; 256(1):75–77.

Pearn J. The management of near-drowning. Br Med J 1985 Nov 23; 291(6507):1447–1452.

Sarnaik AP and Vohra MP. Near drowning: Fresh, salt, and cold water immersion. Clin Sports Med 1986 Jan; 5(1):33–46.

Standards and guidelines for cardiopulmonary resuscitation (CPR) and emergency cardiac care (ECC). JAMA 1986 June 6; 255(21):2905–2954.

Substance Abuse

Abraham E, Shoemaker WC and McCartney SF. Cardiorespiratory patterns in severe delirium tremens. Arch Intern Med 1985 June; 145(6):1057–1059.

Gilmore GM. Behavioral management of the acutely intoxicated patient in the emergency department. JEN 1986 Jan/Feb; 12(1):13–17.

Lenehan GP, Gastfriend DR and Stetler C. Use of haloperidol in the management of agitated or violent, alcohol-intoxicated patients in the emergency department: A pilot study. JEN 1985 Mar/Apr; 11(2):72–79.

Rector CS and Foster ME. Assessment and care of the patient experiencing alcohol withdrawal syndrome. Crit Care Nurse 1984 July/Aug; 4(4):64–68.

Segar DL (ed). Substances of abuse. Top Emerg Med 1985 Oct; 7(3):1–54.

Temperature Emergencies

Caldroney RD. Heat-induced illness. Hosp Pract 1986 June 15; 21(6):48M–48T.

Edlich RF et al. Cold injuries and disorders. Curr Concepts Trauma Care 1986 Spr; 9(1):4–11.

Eisenman PA. Hot weather, exercise, old age, and the kidneys. Geriatrics 1986 May; 41(5):108–114.

Graham BS et al. Nonexertional heatstroke. Arch Intern Med 1986 Jan; 146(1):87–90.

Posey VM and Caruso CC. Life-threatening heat related emergencies. Dimens Crit Care Nurs 1986 July/Aug; 5(4):216–225.

Tucker LE et al. Classical heatstroke: Clinical and laboratory assessment. South Med J 1985 Jan; 78(1):20–25.

Weems C, Olson W and Nichols GR II. Risk factors for death during a heat wave. J Ky Med Assoc 1985 Sept; 83(9):475–478.

Trauma

Beckwith N and Carriere SR. Fluid resuscitation in trauma: An update. JEN 1985 Nov/Dec; 11(6):293–299.

Dellinger EP. The use of antibiotics in abdominal trauma. Curr Concepts Trauma Care 1985 Sum; 8(2):10–16.

Edlich RF. Current concepts of emergency wound management. Emerg Med Report 1984 Sum–Fall; Part 1: 5(22):165–172; Part 2: 5(23):173–180.

Feliciano DV. Managing penetrating abdominal trauma. Curr Concepts Trauma Care 1984 Sum; 7(2):4–11.

Flint CB. Nursing care of patients with abdominal trauma. Curr Concepts Trauma Care. 1984 Sum; 7(2):11–15.

Hall MM. Pros and cons of medical antishock trousers. JEN 1985 Jan/Feb; 11(1):22.

Kaback AR, Sanders AB and Meislin HW. MAST suit update. JAMA 1984 Nov 9; 252(18):2598–2603.

Long WB, Bachulis BL and Hynes GD. Accuracy and relationship of mechanisms of injury, trauma score, and injury severity score in identifying major trauma. Am J Surg 1986 May; 151(5):581–584.

Maher AB. An assessment tool for the patient with multi-system injuries. Dimens Crit Care Nurs 1984 Sept/Oct; 3(5):268–278.

Mucha P Jr. Changing attitudes toward the management of blunt splenic trauma in adults. Mayo Clin Proc 1986 June; 61(6):472–477.

Miscellaneous

*Brownell MJ. The concept of crisis: Its utility for nursing. ANS 1984 July; 6(4):10–21.

*Geissler EM. Crisis: What it is and is not. ANS 1984 July; 6(4):1–9.

Harrow JC. Systemic anaphylactic reactions. Med Times 1984 Mar; 112(3): 28–35.

Kolb LC. Treatment of chronic post-traumatic stress disorders. Curr Psychiatr Ther 1986; 23:119–127.

McDaniel E and McClelland P. Post-traumatic stress disorder. Am Fam Physician 1986 Aug; 34(2):180–189.

Modlin HC. Posttraumatic stress disorder. Postgrad Med 1986 Feb 15; 79(3):28–44.

Agencies and Sources of Information

Governmental

Food and Drug Administration, Poison Surveillance and Epidemiology Branch of the Division of Drug Experience, National Centers for Drugs and Biologics, 5600 Fishers Lane, Room 18B31, Rockville, Maryland 20857.

National Institute of Mental Health, National Center for the Prevention and Control of Rape, Parklawn Building, 5600 Fishers Lane, Rockville, Maryland 20857.

National Clearinghouse for Mental Health Information, National Rape Information Clearinghouse (above address).

National Institute on Alcohol Abuse and Alcoholism, National Clearinghouse for Alcohol Information (above address).

National Institute on Drug Abuse, National Clearinghouse for Drug Abuse Information (above address).

Voluntary

Alcoholics Anonymous World Services (AA), P.O. Box 459, Grand Central Station, New York, New York 10163.

American Red Cross, 17th and D Sts., NW., Washington, D.C. 20006.

National Council on Alcoholism, Inc., 12 W. 21st Street, New York, New York 10010.

National Safety Council, 444 North Michigan Ave., Chicago, Illinois 60611.

Appendix

Diagnostic Studies and Their Meaning

Abbreviations

kg = kilogram
gm = gram
mg = milligram
μg = microgram
$\mu\mu$g = micromicrogram
ng = nanogram
pg = picogram
dl = 100 milliliters
ml = milliliter
cu mm = cubic millimeter
fL = femtoliter
mM = millimole
nM = nanomole
mOsm = milliosmole
mm = millimeter
μ = micron or micrometer
mm Hg = millimeters of mercury
U = unit
mU = milliunit
μU = microunit
mEq = milliequivalent
IU = International Unit
mIU = milliInternational Unit

SI Units

g = gram
L = liter
d = day
h = hour
mol = mole
mmol = millimole
μmol = micromole
nmol = nanomole
pmol = picomole

*Reference Ranges—Hematology**

Determination	Reference Range		Clinical Significance
	Conventional Units	*SI Units*	
A₂ hemoglobin	1.5%–3.5% of total hemoglobin	Mass fraction: 0.015–0.035 of total hemoglobin	Increased in certain types of thalassemia
Bleeding time	2–8 min	2–8 min	Prolonged in thrombocytopenia, defective platelet function, and aspirin therapy
Factor V assay (proaccelerin factor)	60%–140%		
Factor VII assay (antihemophiliac factor)	50%–200%		Deficient in classical hemophilia
Factor IX assay (plasma thromboplastin component)	75%–125%		Deficient in Christmas disease (pseudohemophilia)
Factor X (Stuart factor)	60%–140%		Deficient in Stuart clotting defect
Fibrinogen	200–400 mg/dl	2–4 g/dl	Increased in pregnancy, in infections accompanied by leukocytosis, and in nephrosis. Decreased in severe liver disease and abruptio placentae
Fibrin split products	Less than 10 mg/liter	Less than 10 mg/L	Increased in disseminated intravascular coagulation
Fibrinolysins (whole blood clot lysis time)	No lysis in 24 hr		Increased activity associated with massive hemorrhage, extensive surgery, and transfusion reactions
Partial thromboplastin time (activated)	20–45 sec		Prolonged in deficiency of fibrinogen and of factors II, V, VIII, IX, X, XI, and XII, and in heparin therapy
Prothrombin consumption	Over 20 sec		Impaired in deficiency of factors VIII, IX, and X
Prothrombin time	9.5–12 sec		Prolonged by deficiency of factors I, II, V, VII, and X, fat malabsorption, severe liver disease, and coumarin-anticoagulant therapy
Erythrocyte count	Males: 4,600,000–6,200,000/cu mm	4.6–6.2×10^{12}/L	Increased in severe diarrhea and dehydration, polycythemia, acute poisoning, and pulmonary fibrosis
	Females: 4,200,000–5,400,000/cu mm	4.2–5.4×10^{12}/L	Decreased in all anemias, in leukemia, and after hemorrhage, when blood volume has been restored
Erythrocyte indices			
Mean corpuscular volume (MCV)	80–94 (cu μ)	80–94 fL	Increased in macrocytic anemias, decreased in microcytic anemia
Mean corpuscular hemoglobin (MCH)	27–32 $\mu\mu$g/cell	27–32 pg	Increased in macrocytic anemias, decreased in microcytic anemia
Mean corpuscular hemoglobin concentration (MCHC)	33%–38%	Concentration fraction: 0.33–0.38	Decreased in severe hypochromic anemia

* By radioimmunoassay
(Laboratory values vary acccording to the techniques used in different laboratories.)

(continued)

Reference Ranges—Hematology* (continued)

Determination	Reference Range Conventional Units	SI Units	Clinical Significance
Erythrocyte indices *(continued)* Reticulocytes	0.5%–1.5% of red cells	Number fraction: 0.005–0.015	Increased with any condition stimulating increase in bone marrow activity (*i.e.,* infection, blood loss [acute and chronic]); following iron therapy in iron deficiency anemia, polycythemia rubra vera Decreased with any condition depressing bone marrow activity, acute leukemia, late stage of severe anemias
Erythrocyte sedimentation rate (ESR)—Westergren method	Males under 50 yr: <15 mm/hr Males over 50 yr: <20 mm/hr Females under 50 yr: <20 mm/hr Females over 50 yr: <30 mm/hr	<15 mm/hr <20 mm/hr <20 mm/hr <30 mm/hr	Increased in tissue destruction, whether inflammatory or degenerative; during menstruation and pregnancy; and in acute febrile diseases
Erythrocyte sedimentation ratio—Zeta centrifuge	41%–54% in both sexes	Fraction: 0.41–0.54	Significance similar to ESR
Hematocrit	Males: 42%–50% Females: 40%–48%	Volume fraction: 0.42–0.5 Volume fraction: 0.4–0.48	Decreased in severe anemias, anemia of pregnancy, acute massive blood loss Increased in erythrocytosis of any cause, and in dehydration or hemoconcentration associated with shock
Hemoglobin	Males: 13–18 gm/dl Females: 12–16 gm/dl	2.02–2.79 mmol/L 1.86–2.48 mmol/L	Decreased in various anemias, pregnancy, severe or prolonged hemorrhage, and with excessive fluid intake Increased in polycythemia, chronic obstructive pulmonary diseases, failure of oxygenation because of congestive heart failure, and normally in people living at high altitudes
Hemoglobin F	Less than 2% of total hemoglobin	Mass fraction: <0.02	Increased in infants and children, and in thalassemia and many anemias
Leukocyte alkaline phosphatase	Score of 40–100		Increased in polycythemia vera, myelofibrosis, and infections; decreased in chronic granulocytic leukemia, paroxysmal nocturnal hemoglobinuria, hypoplastic marrow, and viral infections, particularly infectious mononucleosis

(continued)

*Reference Ranges—Hematology** (continued)

Determination	Reference Range		Clinical Significance
	Conventional Units	SI Units	
Leukocyte count	Total: 5,000–10,000/cu mm	$5–10 \times 10^9/L$	Elevated in acute infectious diseases, predominantly in the neutrophilic fraction with bacterial diseases, and in the lymphocytic and monocytic fractions in viral diseases
Neutrophils	60%–70%	Number fraction: 0.6–0.7	
Eosinophils	1%–4%	Number fraction: 0.01–0.04	
Basophils	0%–0.5%	Number fraction: 0.00–0.05	
Lymphocytes	20%–30%	Number fraction: 0.2–0.3	
Monocytes	2%–6%	Number fraction: 0.02–0.06	Elevated in acute leukemia, following menstruation, and following surgery or trauma
			Depressed in aplastic anemia, agranulocytosis, and by toxic agents, such as chemotherapeutic agents used in treating malignancy
			Eosinophils elevated in collagen diseases, allergy, intestinal parasitosis
Osmotic fragility of red cells	Increased if hemolysis occurs in over 0.5% NaCl Decreased if hemolysis is incomplete in 0.3% NaCl		Increased in congenital spherocytosis, idiopathic acquired hemolytic anemia, isoimmune hemolytic disease, ABO hemolytic disease of newborn Decreased in sickle cell anemia, thalassemia
Platelet count	100,000–400,000/cu mm	$0.1–0.4 \times 10^{12}/L$	Increased in malignancy, myeloproliferative disease, rheumatoid arthritis, and postoperatively; about 50% of patients with unexpected increase of platelet count will be found to have a malignancy Decreased in thrombocytopenic purpura, acute leukemic aplastic anemia, and during cancer chemotherapy, infections, and drug reactions

Reference Ranges—Serum, Plasma, Whole Blood Chemistries

Determination	Normal Adult Reference Range		Clinical Significance	
	Conventional Units	SI Units	Increased	Decreased
Acetoacetate	0.2–1.0 mg/dl	19.6–98 μmol/L	Diabetic acidosis Fasting	
Acetone	0.3–2.0 mg/dl	51.6–344.0 μmol/L	Toxemia of pregnancy Carbohydrate-free diet High-fat diet	
Adrenocortico-tropic hormone (ACTH)— plasma, RIA*	Less than 50 pg/ml	Less than 50 mg/L	Pituitary-dependent Cushing's syndrome Ectopic ACTH syndrome Primary adrenal atrophy	Adrenocortical tumor Adrenal insufficiency secondary to hypopituitarism

* By radioimmunoassay

Reference Ranges—Serum, Plasma, Whole Blood Chemistries (continued)

Determination	Normal Adult Reference Range		Clinical Significance	
	Conventional Units	SI Units	Increased	Decreased
Aldolase	3–8 Sibley-Lehninger U/dl at 37°C	22–59 mU/L at 37°C	Hepatic necrosis Granulocytic leukemia Myocardial infarction Skeletal muscle disease	
Aldosterone—plasma, RIA	Supine: 3–10 ng/dl Upright: 5–30 ng/dl Adrenal vein: 200–800 ng/dl	0.08–0.30 nmol/L 0.14–0.90 nmol/L 5.54–22.16 nmol/L	Primary aldosteronism (Conn's syndrome) Secondary aldosteronism	Addison's disease
Alpha-1-antitrypsin	200–400 mg/dl	2–4 g/L		Certain forms of chronic lung and liver disease in young adults
Alpha-1-fetoprotein	None detected		Hepatocarcinoma Metastatic carcinoma of liver Germinal cell carcinoma of the testis or ovary Premature fetal neural tube defects due to elevation in maternal serum	
Alpha-hydroxy-butyric dehydrogenase	Up to 140 U/ml	Up to 140 U/L	Myocardial infarction Granulocytic leukemia Hemolytic anemias Muscular dystrophy	
Ammonia (plasma)	40–80 μg/dl (enzymatic method); varies considerably with method	22.2–44.3 μmol/L	Severe liver disease Hepatic decompensation	
Amylase	60–160 Somogyi U/dl	111–296 U/L	Acute pancreatitis Mumps Duodenal ulcer Carcinoma of head of pancreas Prolonged elevation with pseudocyst of pancreas Increased by drugs that constrict pancreatic duct sphincters: morphine, codeine, cholinergics	Chronic pancreatitis Pancreatic fibrosis and atrophy Cirrhosis of liver Pregnancy (second and third trimesters)
Arsenic	6–20 μg/dl; if 50 μg/dl, suspect toxicity	0.78–2.6 μmol/L	Accidental or intentional poisoning Excessive occupational exposure	
Ascorbic acid (vitamin C)	0.4–1.5 mg/dl	23–85 μmol/L	Large doses of ascorbic acid as a prophylactic against the common cold	

(continued)

Reference Ranges—Serum, Plasma, Whole Blood Chemistries (continued)

Determination	Normal Adult Reference Range		Clinical Significance	
	Conventional Units	SI Units	Increased	Decreased
Bilirubin	Total: 0.1–1.2 mg/dl	1.7–20.5 μmol/L	Hemolytic anemia (indirect)	
	Direct: 0.1–0.2 mg/dl	1.7–3.4 μmol/L	Biliary obstruction and disease	
	Indirect: 0.1–1 mg/dl	1.7–17.1 μmol/L	Hepatocellular damage (hepatitis)	
			Pernicious anemia	
			Hemolytic disease of newborn	
Blood gases				
Oxygen, arterial (whole blood):				Anemia
				Cardiac obstruction
Partial pressure (PaO$_2$)	95–100 mm Hg	12.64–13.30 kPa	Polycythemia	Chronic
			Anhydremia	Anemia
Saturation (SaO$_2$)	94%–100%	Volume fraction: 0.94–1		Cardiac obstruction
				Chronic obstructive pulmonary disease
Carbon dioxide, arterial (whole blood): partial pressure (PaCO$_2$)	35–45 mm Hg	4.66–5.99 kPA	Respiratory acidosis	Respiratory alkalosis
			Metabolic alkalosis	Metabolic acidosis
pH (whole blood, arterial)	7.35–7.45	7.35–7.45	Vomiting	Uremia
			Hyperpnea	Diabetic acidosis
			Fever	Hemorrhage
			Intestinal obstruction	Nephritis
Calcitonin	Basal: Nondetectable 400 pg/ml	400 ng/L	Medullary carcinoma of the thyroid	
			Some nonthyroid tumors	
			Zollinger-Ellison syndrome	
Calcium	8.5–10.5 mg/dl	2.125–2.625 mmol/L	Tumor or hyperplasia of parathyroid	Hypoparathyroidism
			Hypervitaminosis D	Diarrhea
			Multiple myeloma	Celiac disease
			Nephritis with uremia	Vitamin D deficiency
			Malignant tumors	Acute pancreatitis
			Sarcoidosis	Nephrosis
			Hyperthyroidism	After parathyroidectomy
			Skeletal immobilization	
			Excess calcium intake: milk-alkali syndrome	
CO$_2$	Adults: 24–32 mEq/L	24–32 mmol/L	Tetany	Acidosis
	Infants: 18–24 mEq/L (venous)	18–24 mmol/L	Respiratory disease	Nephritis
			Intestinal obstruction	Eclampsia
			Vomiting	Diarrhea
				Anesthesia

(continued)

Reference Ranges—Serum, Plasma, Whole Blood Chemistries (continued)

Determination	Normal Adult Reference Range		Clinical Significance	
	Conventional Units	SI Units	Increased	Decreased
Carcinoembryonic antigen (CEA) RIA	0–2.5 ng/ml	0–2.5 µg/L	The repeatedly high incidence of this antigen in cancers of the colon, rectum, pancreas, and stomach suggest that CEA levels may be a useful adjunct in the diagnosis of these conditions and therapeutic monitoring.	
Catecholamines—plasma, RIA	Epinephrine, random up to 90 pg/ml Norepinephrine, random 100–550 pg/ml Dopamine, random up to 130 pg/ml	Up to 490 pmol/L 590–3240 pmol/L Up to 850 pmol/L	Pheochromocytoma	
Ceruloplasmin	30–80 mg/dl	300–800 mg/L		Wilson's disease (hepatolenticular degeneration)
Chloride	95–105 mEq/L	95–105 mmol/L	Nephrosis Nephritis Urinary obstruction Cardiac decompensation Anemia	Diabetes Diarrhea Vomiting Pneumonia Heavy metal poisoning Cushing's syndrome Burns Intestinal obstruction Febrile conditions
Cholesterol	150–250 mg/dl	3.9–6.5 mmol/L	Lipemia Obstructive jaundice Diabetes Hypothyroidism	Pernicious anemia Hemolytic anemia Hyperthyroidism Severe infection Terminal states of debilitating disease
Cholesterol esters	60%–70% of total	Fraction of total cholesterol 0.6–0.7		The esterified fraction decreases in liver diseases
Cholinesterase	Serum: 0.6–1.6 delta pH Red cells: 0.6–1 delta pH	0.6–1.6 U 0.6–1 U	Nephrosis Exercise	Nerve gas intoxication (greater effect on red cell activity) Insecticides, organic phosphates (greater effect on plasma activity)
Chorionic gonadotropin, beta subunit—RIA	0–5 IU/L	0–5 IU/L	Pregnancy Hydatidiform mole Choriocarcinoma	
Complement, human C_3	Males: 88–252 mg/dl Females: 88–206 mg/dl	880–2520 mg/L	Some inflammatory diseases	Acute glomerulonephritis Disseminated lupus erythematosus with renal involvement

(continued)

Reference Ranges—Serum, Plasma, Whole Blood Chemistries (continued)

Determination	Normal Adult Reference Range		Clinical Significance	
	Conventional Units	SI Units	Increased	Decreased
Complement C₄	14–51 mg/dl	140–510 mg/L	Some inflammatory diseases	Often decreased in immunologic disease, especially with active SLE Hereditary angioneurotic edema
Complement total (hemolytic)	90%–94% complement		Some inflammatory diseases	Acute glomerulonephritis Epidemic meningitis Subacute bacterial endocarditis
Copper	70–165 μg/dl	11–25.9 μmol/L	Cirrhosis of liver Pregnancy	Wilson's disease
Cortisol—RIA	8 AM: 7–25 μg/dl 4 PM: 2–9 μg/dl	193–690 nmol/L 55–248 nmol/L	Stress: infectious disease, surgery, burns, *etc.* Pregnancy Cushing's syndrome Pancreatitis Eclampsia	Addison's disease Anterior pituitary hypofunction
C-peptide reactivity	1.5–10 ng/ml	1.5–10 μg/L	Insulinoma	Diabetes
Creatine	0.2–0.8 mg/ml	15.3–61 μmol/L	Pregnancy Skeletal muscle necrosis or atrophy Starvation Hyperthyroidism	
Creatine phosphokinase (CPK)	Males: 50–325 mU/ml Females: 50–250 mU/ml	50–325 U/L 50–250 U/L	Myocardial infarction Skeletal muscle diseases Intramuscular injections Crush syndrome Hypothyroidism Delirium tremens Alcoholic myopathy Cerebrovascular disease	
Creatine phosphokinase isoenzymes	MM band present (skeletal muscle); MB band absent (heart muscle)		MB band increased in myocardial infarction, ischemia	
Creatinine	0.7–1.4 mg/dl	62–124 μmol/L	Nephritis Chronic renal disease	Kidney diseases
Creatinine clearance	100–150 ml of blood cleared of creatinine per minute	1.67–2.5 ml/s		
Cryoglobulins, qualitative	Negative		Multiple myeloma Chronic lymphocytic leukemia Lymphosarcoma Systemic lupus erythematosus Rheumatoid arthritis Subacute bacterial endocarditis Some malignancies Scleroderma	

(continued)

Reference Ranges—Serum, Plasma, Whole Blood Chemistries (continued)

Determination	Normal Adult Reference Range		Clinical Significance	
	Conventional Units	SI Units	Increased	Decreased
11-Deoxycortisol	1 μg/dl	<0.029 μmol/L	Hypertensive form of virilizing adrenal hyperplasia due to an 11-β-hydroxylase defect	
Dibucaine number	Normal: 70%–85% inhibition Heterozygote: 50%–65% inhibition Homozygote: 16%–25% inhibition			Important in detecting carriers of abnormal cholinesterase activity who are susceptible to succinyldicholine anesthetic shock
Dihydrotestosterone	Males: 50–210 ng/dl Females: None detectable	1.72–7.22 nmol/L		Testicular feminization syndrome
Estradiol—RIA	Females: Follicular: 10–90 pg/ml Midcycle: 100–500 pg/ml Luteal: 50–240 pg/ml Follicular phase: 2–20 ng/dl Midcycle: 12–40 ng/dl Luteal phase: 10–30 ng/dl Postmenopausal: 1–5 ng/dl Males: 0.5–5 ng/dl	37–370 pmol/L 367–1835 pmol/L 184–881 pmol/L	Pregnancy	Depressed or failure to peak: ovarian failure
Estriol—RIA	Nonpregnant females: <0.5 ng/ml Pregnant females: 1st trimester: up to 1 ng/ml 2nd trimester: 0.8–7 ng/ml 3rd trimester: 5–25 ng/ml	<1.75 nmol/L Up to 3.5 nmol/L 2.8–24.3 nmol/L 17.4–86.8 nmol/L	Pregnancy	Depressed or failure to peak: ovarian failure
Estrogens, total—RIA	Females cycle days: Day 1–10: 61–394 pg/ml Day 11–20: 122–437 pg/ml Day 21–30: 156–350 pg/ml Males: 40–115 pg/ml	61–394 ng/L 122–437 ng/L 156–350 ng/L 40–115 ng/L	Pregnancy Measured on a daily basis, can be used to evaluate response of hypogonadotrophic, hypoestrogenic women to human menopausal or pituitary gonadotropin	Fetal distress Ovarian failure

(continued)

Reference Ranges—Serum, Plasma, Whole Blood Chemistries (continued)

Determination	Normal Adult Reference Range		Clinical Significance	
	Conventional Units	SI Units	Increased	Decreased

Estrone—RIA	Females:
	Day 1–10:
	    4.3–18 ng/dl
	Day 11–20:
	    7.5–19.6 ng/dl
	Day 21–30:
	    13–20 ng/dl
	Males: 2.5–7.5 ng/dl
		
		15.9–66.6 pmol/L
		
		27.8–72.5 pmol/L
		
		48.1–74 pmol/L
		9.3–27.8 pmol/L
			Pregnancy	Depressed or failure to peak-ovarian failure

Ferritin—RIA	Males: 10–270 ng/ml Females: 5–100 ng/ml	10–270 μg/L 5–100 μg/L	Nephritis Hemochromatosis Certain neoplastic diseases Acute myelogenous leukemia Multiple myeloma	Iron deficiency
Folic acid—RIA	4–16 ng/ml	9.1–36.3 nmol/L		Megaloblastic anemias of infancy and pregnancy Inadequate diet Liver disease Malabsorption syndrome Severe hemolytic anemia

Follicle stimulating hormone (FSH)—RIA	Females:
	Follicular phase:
	    5–20 mIU/ml
	Peak of middle cycle:
	    12–30 mIU/ml
	Luteinic phase:
	    5–15 mIU/ml
	Menopausal females:
	    40–200 mIU/ml
		
		5–20 IU/L
		
		12–30 IU/L
		
		5–15 IU/L
		
		40–200 IU/L
			Menopause and primary ovarian failure	Pituitary failure

Galactose	<5 mg/dl	<0.28 mmol/L		Galactosemia
Gamma glutamyl transpeptidase	Males: <45 IU/L Females: <30 IU/L	45 U/L 30 U/L	Hepatobiliary disease Anicteric alcoholics Drug therapy damage Myocardial infarction Renal infarction	

Gastrin—RIA	Fasting: 50–155 pg/ml
	Postprandial:
	    80–170 pg/ml
	Zollinger-Ellison
	    syndrome: 200–over
	    2000 pg/ml
	Pernicious anemia:
	    130–2260 pg/ml
	    (mean 912)
		50–155 ng/L
		
		80–170 ng/L
		
		200–over 2000 ng/L
		
		130–2260 ng/L
		    (mean 912)
			Zollinger-Ellison syndrome
			Peptic ulceration of the duodenum
			Pernicious anemia	

Glucose	Fasting: 60–110 mg/dl Postprandial (2 hr): 65–140 mg/dl	3.3–6.05 mmol/L 3.58–7.7 mmol/L	Diabetes Nephritis Hyperthyroidism Early hyperpituitarism Cerebral lesions Infections Pregnancy Uremia	Hyperinsulinism Hypothyroidism Late hyperpituitarism Pernicious vomiting Addison's disease Extensive hepatic damage

(continued)

Reference Ranges—Serum, Plasma, Whole Blood Chemistries (continued)

Determination	Normal Adult Reference Range		Clinical Significance	
	Conventional Units	SI Units	Increased	Decreased
Glucose tolerance (oral)	Features of a normal response: 1. Normal fasting between 60–110 mg/dl 2. No sugar in urine 3. Upper limits of normal are: Fasting–125 1 hour–190 2 hours–140 3 hours–125	3.3–6.05 mmol/L 6.88 mmol/L 10.45 mmol/L 7.70 mmol/L 6.88 mmol/L	(Flat or inverted curve) Hyperinsulinism Adrenal cortical insufficiency (Addison's disease) Anterior pituitary hypofunction Hypothyroidism Sprue and celiac diseases	(High or prolonged curve) Diabetes Hyperthyroidism Primary adrenal cortical tumor or hyperplasia Severe anemia Certain central nervous system disorders
Glucose-6-phosphate dehydrogenase (red cells)	Screening: Decolorization in 20–100 min Quantitative: 1.86–2.5 IU/ml RBC	1860–2500 U/L		Drug-induced hemolytic anemia Hemolytic disease of newborn
Glycoprotein (alpha-1 acid)	40–110 mg/dl	400–1100 mg/L	Neoplasm Tuberculosis Diabetes complicated by degenerative vascular disease Pregnancy Rheumatoid arthritis Rheumatic fever Infectious liver disease Lupus erythematosus	
Growth hormone—RIA	<10 ng/ml	<10 mg/L	Acromegaly	Failure to stimulate with argrine or insulin— hypopituitarism
Haptoglobin	50–250 mg/dl	0.5–2.5 g/L	Pregnancy Estrogen therapy Chronic infections Various inflammatory conditions	Hemolytic anemia Hemolytic blood transfusion reaction
Hemoglobin (plasma)	0.5–5 mg/dl	5–50 mg/L	Transfusion reactions Paroxysmal nocturnal hemoglobinuria Intravascular hemolysis	
Hexosaminidase, total	Controls: 333–375 nM/ml/hr Heterozygotes: 288–644 nM/ml/hr Tay-Sachs disease: 284–1232 nM/ml/hr Diabetics: 567–3560 nM/ml/hr	333–375 μmol/L/h 288–644 μmol/L/h 284–1232 μmol/L/h 567–3560 μmol/L/h	Diabetes Tay-Sachs disease	

(continued)

Reference Ranges—Serum, Plasma, Whole Blood Chemistries (continued)

| Determination | Normal Adult Reference Range | | Clinical Significance | |
	Conventional Units	SI Units	Increased	Decreased
Hexosaminidase A	Controls: 49%–68% of total Heterozygotes: 26%–45% of total Tay-Sachs disease: 0%–4% of total Diabetics: 39%–59% of total	Fraction of total: 0.49–0.68 0.26–0.45 0–0.04 0.39–0.59		Tay-Sachs disease and heterozygotes

High-density lipoprotein cholesterol (HDL cholesterol)

Age (yr)	Males (mg/dl)	Females (mg/dl)	Males (mmol/L)	Females (mmol/L)
0–19	30–65	30–70	0.78–1.68	0.78–1.81
20–29	35–70	35–75	0.91–1.81	0.91–1.94
30–39	30–65	35–80	0.78–1.68	0.91–2.07
40–49	30–65	40–85	0.78–1.68	1.04–2.2
50–59	30–65	35–85	0.78–1.68	0.91–2.2
60–69	30–65	35–85	0.78–1.68	0.91–2.2

Clinical Significance, Decreased: It has been claimed that HDL cholesterol is lower in patients with increased risk for coronary heart disease; this, however, has not been universally accepted.

Determination	Conventional Units	SI Units	Increased	Decreased
17-Hydroxy-progesterone—RIA	Males: 0.4–4 ng/ml Females: 0.1–3.3 ng/ml Children: 0.1–0.5 ng/ml	1.2–12 nmol/L 0.3–10 nmol/L 0.3–1.5 nmol/L	Congenital adrenal hyperplasia Pregnancy Some cases of adrenal or ovarian adenomas	
Immunoglobulin A	Adults: 50–300 mg/dl (in children the normals are lower and vary with age)	0.5–3 g/L	Gamma A myeloma Wiskott-Aldrich syndrome Autoimmune disease Hepatic cirrhosis	Ataxia telangiectasis Agammaglobulinemia Hypogammaglobulinemia, transient Dysgammaglobulinemia Protein-losing enteropathies
Immunoglobulin D	0–30 mg/dl	0–300 mg/L	IgD multiple myeloma Some patients with chronic infectious diseases	
Immunoglobulin E	20–740 ng/ml	20–740 μg/L	Allergic patients and those with parasitic infestations	
Immunoglobulin G	Adults: 635–1400 mg/dl	6.35–14 g/L	IgG myeloma Following hyperimmunization Autoimmune disease states Chronic infections	Congenital and acquired hypogammaglobulinemia IgA myelomas, Waldenstrom's (IgM) macroglobulinemia Some malabsorption syndromes Extensive protein loss
Immunoglobulin M	Adults: 40–280 mg/dl	0.4–2.8 g/L	Waldenstrom's macroglobulinemia Parasitic infections Hepatitis	Agammaglobulinemias Some IgG and IgA myelomas Chronic lymphatic leukemia
Insulin—RIA	5–25 μU/ml	0.2–1 μg/L	Insulinoma Acromegaly	Diabetes mellitus
Iodine, butanol extractable	3.5–6.5 mg/dl	0.28–0.51 μmol/L	Hyperthyroidism	Hypothyroidism
Iodine, protein-bound	4–8 μg/dl	0.32–0.63 μmol/L	Hyperthyroidism	Hypothyroidism

(continued)

Reference Ranges—Serum, Plasma, Whole Blood Chemistries (continued)

Determination	Normal Adult Reference Range		Clinical Significance	
	Conventional Units	SI Units	Increased	Decreased
Iron	65–170 μg/dl	11.6–30.4 μmol/L	Pernicious anemia Aplastic anemia Hemolytic anemia Hepatitis Hemochromatosis	Iron deficiency anemia
Iron-binding capacity	IBC: 150–235 μg/dl TIBC: 250–420 μg/dl % Saturation: 20–50	26.9–42.1 μmol/L 44.8–75.2 μmol/L Fraction of total iron-binding capacity: 0.2–0.5	Iron deficiency anemia Acute and chronic blood loss Hepatitis	Chronic infectious diseases Cirrhosis
Isocitric dehydrogenase	50–180 U	0.83–3 U/L	Hepatitis: cirrhosis Obstructive jaundice Metastatic carcinoma of the liver Megaloblastic anemia	
Lactic acid (whole blood)	Venous: 5–20 mg/dl Arterial: 3–7 mg/dl	0.6–2.2 mmol/L 0.3–0.8 mmol/L	Increased muscular activity Congestive heart failure Hemorrhage Shock Some varieties of metabolic acidosis Some febrile infections May be increased in severe liver disease	
Lactic dehydrogenase (LDH)	100–225 mU/ml	100–225 U/L	Untreated pernicious anemia Myocardial infarction Pulmonary infarction Liver disease	

Lactic dehydrogenase isoenzymes
  Total lactic dehydrogenase
  LDH-1
  LDH-2
  LDH-3
  LDH-4
  LDH-5
	100–225 mU/ml
	
	20%–35%
	25–40%
	20–30%
	0–20%
	0–25%
		100–225 U/L
		Fraction of total LDH:
		0.2–0.35
		0.25–0.4
		0.2–0.3
		0–0.2
		0–0.25
			LDH-1 and LDH-2 are increased in myocardial infarction, megaloblastic anemia, and hemolytic anemia
			LDH-4 and LDH-5 are increased in pulmonary infarction, congestive heart failure, and liver disease	

Lead (whole blood)	Up to 40 μg/dl	Up to 2 μmol/L	Lead poisoning	
Leucine aminopeptidase	80–200 U/ml	19.2–48 U/L	Liver or biliary tract diseases Pancreatic disease Metastatic carcinoma of liver and pancreas Biliary obstruction	
Lipase	0.2–1.5 U/ml	55–417 U/L	Acute and chronic pancreatitis Biliary obstruction Cirrhosis Hepatitis Peptic ulcer	

(continued)

Reference Ranges—Serum, Plasma, Whole Blood Chemistries (continued)

Determination	Normal Adult Reference Range		Clinical Significance	
	Conventional Units	*SI Units*	*Increased*	*Decreased*
Lipids, total	400–1000 mg/dl	4–10 g/L	Hypothyroidism Diabetes Nephrosis Glomerulonephritis Hyperlipoproteinemias	Hyperthyroidism

Lipoprotein phenotype

Summary of Findings in the Primary Hyperlipoproteinemias

Type	Frequency	Appearance	Triglyceride	Cholesterol	Lipoprotein Staining				Secondary Causes
					Beta	*Pre-Beta*	*Alpha*	*Chylomicrons*	
Normal		Clear	Normal	Normal	Moderate	Zero to moderate	Moderate	Weak	
I	Very rare	Creamy	Markedly increased	Normal to moderately increased	Weak	Weak	Weak	Markedly increased	Dysglobulinemia
II	Common	Clear	Normal to slightly increased	Slightly to markedly increased	Strong	Zero to strong	Moderate	Weak	Hypothyroidism, myeloma, hepatic syndrome, macroglobulinemia, and high dietary cholesterol
III	Uncommon	Clear, cloudy, or milky	Increased	Increased	Broad intense band	Extends into beta	Moderate	Weak	
IV	Very common	Clear, cloudy, or milky	Slightly to markedly increased	Normal to slightly increased	Weak to moderate	Moderate to strong	Weak to Moderate	Weak	Hypothyroidism, diabetes mellitus, pancreatitis, glycogen storage diseases, nephrotic syndrome, myeloma, pregnancy, and oral contraceptives
V	Rare	Cloudy to creamy	Markedly increased	Increased	Weak	Moderate	Weak	Strong	Diabetes mellitus, pancreatitis, and alcoholism

Types I and II are fat induced: types III and IV are carbohydrate induced; type V is fat and carbohydrate induced.

Reference Ranges—Serum, Plasma, Whole Blood Chemistries (continued)

Determination	Normal Adult Reference Range		Clinical Significance	
	Conventional Units	*SI Units*	*Increased*	*Decreased*
Lithium	Usual maintenance level: 0.5–1 mEq/L	0.5–1 mmol/L		
Low-density lipoprotein cholesterol (LDL cholesterol)	Age (yr) mg/dl 0–19 50–170 20–29 60–170 30–39 70–190 40–49 80–190 50–59 80–210	mmol/L 1.30–4.40 1.55–4.40 1.80–4.92 2.07–4.92 2.07–5.44	LDL cholesterol is claimed to be higher in patients with increased risk for coronary heart disease. This claim, however, is not universally accepted.	

(continued)

Reference Ranges—Serum, Plasma, Whole Blood Chemistries (continued)

Determination	Normal Adult Reference Range		Clinical Significance	
	Conventional Units	*SI Units*	*Increased*	*Decreased*

Luteinizing hormone—RIA	Males: 6–30 mIU/ml
	Females:
	  Follicular phase:
	    2–3 mIU/ml
	  Ovulatory peak:
	    40–200 mIU/ml
	  Luteal phase:
	    0–20 mIU/ml
	  Postmenopausal:
	    35–120 mIU/ml
		1.4–6.9 mg/L
		
		0.5–6.9 mg/L
		
		9.2–46 mg/L
		
		0–5 mg/L
		
		8–27.5 mg/L
			Pituitary tumor
			Ovarian failure
				Depressed or failure to
				  peak—pituitary failure

Lysozyme (muramidase)	2.8–8 μg/ml	2.8–8 mg	Certain types of leukemia
			  (acute monocytic
			  leukemia)
			Inflammatory states and
			  infections
				Acute lymphocytic leukemia

Magnesium	1.3–2.4 mEq/L	0.7–1.2 mmol/L	Excess ingestion of
			  magnesium-containing
			  antacids
				Chronic alcoholism
				Severe renal disease,
				  diarrhea
				Defective growth

Manganese	0.04–1.4 μg/dl	72.9–255 nmol/L		
Mercury	Up to 10 μg/dl	Up to 0.5 μmol/L	Mercury poisoning	
Myoglobin—RIA	Up to 85 ng/ml	Up to 85 μg/ml	Myocardial infarction Muscle necrosis	
Nonprotein nitrogen	20–35 mg/dl	14.3–25 mmol/L	Acute nephritis Polycystic kidneys Obstructive uropathy Peritonitis Congestive heart failure Pregnancy	
5′ Nucleotidase	3.2–11.6 IU/L	3.2–11.6 U/L	Hepatobiliary disease	

Osmolality	280–300 mOsm/kg	280–300 mmol/L	Useful in the study of
			  electrolyte and water
			  balance
				Inappropriate secretion of
				  antidiuretic hormone

Parathyroid hormone	160–350	160–350 ng/L	Hyperparathyroidism	
Phenylalanine	1.2–3.5 mg/dl 1st week 0.7–3.5 mg/dl thereafter	0.07–0.21 mmol/L 0.04–0.21 mmol/L	Phenylketonuria	
Phosphatase, acid, total	0–11 IU/L	0–NU/L	Carcinoma of prostate Advanced Paget's disease Hyperparathyroidism Gaucher's disease	
Phosphatase, acid, prostatic—RIA	0–10 ng/ml Borderline: 2.5–3.3 IU/L	0–10 μg/L	Carcinoma of prostate	

Phosphatase, alkaline	Adults: 30–115 mU/ml	30–115 μ/L	Conditions reflecting
			  increased osteoblastic
			  activity of bone
			Rickets
			Hyperparathyroidism
			Liver disease	

(continued)

Reference Ranges—Serum, Plasma, Whole Blood Chemistries (continued)

Determination	Normal Adult Reference Range		Clinical Significance	
	Conventional Units	SI Units	Increased	Decreased
Phosphatase, alkaline, thermostable fraction	Thermostable fraction greater than 35%: hepatic disease and combined disease with predominant hepatic component Thermostable fraction between 25% and 35%: combined hepatic and skeletal disease Thermostable fraction <25%: skeletal disease with increased osteoblastic activity		Hepatic disease	
Phosphohexose isomerase	20–90 IU/L	20–90 U/L	Malignancy Disease of heart, liver, and skeletal muscles	
Phospholipids	125–300 mg/dl	1.25–3 g/L	Diabetes Nephritis	
Phosphorus, inorganic	2.5–4.5 mg/dl	0.8–1.45 mmol/L	Chronic nephritis Hypoparathyroidism	Hyperparathyroidism Vitamin D deficiency
Potassium	3.8–5 mEq/L	3.8–5 mmol/L	Addison's disease Oliguria Anuria Tissue breakdown or hemolysis	Diabetic acidosis Diarrhea Vomiting
Progesterone—RIA	Follicular phase: up to 0.8 ng/ml Luteal phase: 10–20 ng/ml End of cycle: <ng/ml Pregnant: up to 50 ng/ml in 20th week	2.5 nmol/L 31.8–63.6 nmol/L <3 nmol/L Up to 160 nmol/L	Useful in evaluation of menstrual disorders and infertility and in the evaluation of placental function during pregnancies complicated by toxemia, diabetes mellitus, or threatened miscarriage	
Prolactin—RIA	6–24 ng/ml	6–24 µg/L	Pregnancy Functional or structural disorders of the hypothalamus Pituitary stalk section Pituitary tumors	
Protein, total Albumin Globulin	6–8 gm/dl 3.5–5 gm/dl 1.5–3 gm/dl	60–80 g/L 35–50 g/L 15–30 g/L	Hemoconcentration Shock Multiple myeloma (globulin fraction) Chronic infections (globulin fraction) Liver disease (globulin)	Malnutrition Hemorrhage Loss of plasma from burns Proteinuria

(continued)

Reference Ranges—Serum, Plasma, Whole Blood Chemistries (continued)

Determination	Normal Adult Reference Range		Clinical Significance	
	Conventional Units	SI Units	Increased	Decreased
Electrophoresis (cellulose acetate)				
Albumin	3.5–5 gm/dl	35–50 g/L		
Alpha-1 globulin	0.2–0.4 gm/dl	2–4 g/L		
Alpha-2 globulin	0.6–1 gm/dl	6–10 g/L		
Beta globulin	0.6–1.2 gm/dl	6–12 g/L		
Gamma globulin	0.7–1.5 gm/dl	7–15 g/L		
Protoporphyrin erythrocyte (whole blood)	15–100 μg/dl	0.27–1.80 μmol/L	Lead toxicity Erythropoietic porphyria	
Pyridoxine	3.6–18 ng/ml			A wide spectrum of clinical conditions such as mental depression, peripheral neuropathy, anemia, neonatal seizures, and reactions to certain drug therapies
Pyruvic acid (whole blood)	0.3–0.7 mg/dl	34–80 μmol/L	Diabetes Severe thiamine deficiency Acute phase of some infections, possibly secondary to increased glycogenolysis and glycolysis	
Renin (plasma)—RIA	Normal diet: Supine: 0.3–1.9 ng/ml/hr Upright: 0.6–3.6 ng/ml/hr Low salt diet: Supine: 0.9–4.5 ng/ml/hr Upright: 4.1–9.1 ng/ml/hr	0.3–1.9 μg/h/L-1-1 0.6–3.6 μg/h/1L-1 0.9–4.5 μg/L-1L 4.1–9.1 μg/L-1.L-1	Renovascular hypertension Malignant hypertension Untreated Addison's disease Primary salt-losing nephropathy Low-salt diet Diuretic therapy Hemorrhage	Frank primary aldosteronism Increased salt intake Salt-retaining steroid therapy Antidiuretic hormone therapy Blood transfusion
Sodium	135–145 mEq/L	135–145 mmol/L	Hemoconcentration Nephritis Pyloric obstruction	Alkali deficit Addison's disease Myxedema
Sulfate (inorganic)	0.5–1.5 mg/dl	0.05–0.15 mmol/L	Nephritis Nitrogen retention	
Testosterone—RIA	Females: 25–100 ng/dl Males: 300–800 ng/dl	0.9–3.5 nmol/L 10.5–28 nmol/L	Females: Polycystic ovary Virilizing tumors	Males: Orchidectomy for neoplastic disease of the prostate or breast Estrogen therapy Klinefelter's syndrome Hypopituitarism Hypogonadism Hepatic cirrhosis
T_3 (triiodothyronine) uptake	25%–35%	Relative uptake fraction: 0.25–0.35	Hyperthyroidism TBG deficiency Androgens and anabolic steroids	Hypothyroidism Pregnancy TBG excess Estrogens and antiovulatory drugs

(continued)

Reference Ranges—Serum, Plasma, Whole Blood Chemistries (continued)

Determination	Normal Adult Reference Range		Clinical Significance	
	Conventional Units	SI Units	Increased	Decreased
T_3, total circulating—RIA	75–200 ng/dl	1.15–3.1 nmol/L	Pregnancy Hyperthyroidism	Hypothyroidism
T_4 (thyroxine)—RIA	4.5–11.5 µg/dl	58.5–150 nmol/L	Hyperthyroidism Thyroiditis Elevated thyroxine-binding proteins caused by oral contraceptives Pregnancy	Primary and pituitary hypothyroidism Idiopathic involvement Cases of diminished thyroxine-binding proteins caused by androgenic and anabolic steroids Hypoproteinemia Nephrotic syndrome
T_4, free	1–2.2 ng/dl	13–30 pmol/L	Euthyroid patients with normal free thyroxine levels may have abnormal T_3 and T_4 levels caused by drug preparations	
Thyroid stimulating hormone (TSH)—RIA	0–10 µIU/ml	0-10-3 IU/L	Primary hypothyroidism	
Thyroid-binding globulin	10–26 µg/dl	100–260 µg/L	Hypothyroidism Pregnancy Estrogen therapy Oral contraceptives Genetic and idiopathic	Androgens and anabolic steroids Nephrotic syndrome Marked hypoproteinemia Hepatic disease
Transaminase, serum glutamic-oxaloacetate (SGOT, aspartate aminotransferase)	7–40 U/ml	4–20 U/L	Myocardial infarction Skeletal muscle disease Liver disease	
Transaminase, serum glutamic-oxaloacetate (SGPT, alanine aminotransferase)	10–40 U/ml	5–20 U/L	Same conditions as SGOT, but increase is more marked in liver disease than SGOT	
Transferrin	230–320 mg/dl	2.3–3.2 g/L	Pregnancy Iron-deficiency anemia due to hemorrhaging Acute hepatitis Polycythemia Oral contraceptives	Pernicious anemia in relapse Thalassemic and sickle cell anemia Chromatosis Neoplastic and hepatic diseases
Triglycerides	10–150 mg/dl	0.10–1.65 mmol/L	See lipoprotein phenotype	
Tryptophan	1.4–3 mg/dl	68.6–147 nmol/L		Tryptophan-specific malabsorption syndrome
Tyrosine	0.5–4 mg/dl	27.6–220.8 mmol/L	Tyrosinosis	
Urea nitrogen (BUN)	10–20 mg/dl	3.6–7.2 mmol/L	Acute glomerulonephritis Obstructive uropathy Mercury poisoning Nephrotic syndrome	Severe hepatic failure Pregnancy
Uric acid	2.5–8 mg/dl	0.15–0.5 mmol/L	Gouty arthritis Acute leukemia Lymphomas treated by chemotherapy Toxemia of pregnancy	Xanthinuria Defective tubular reabsorption

(continued)

Reference Ranges—Serum, Plasma, Whole Blood Chemistries (continued)

Determination	Normal Adult Reference Range		Clinical Significance	
	Conventional Units	*SI Units*	*Increased*	*Decreased*
Viscosity	1.4–1.8 relative to water at 37°C (98.6°F)		Patients with marked increased of the gamma globulins	
Vitamin A	50–220 μg/dl	1.75–7.7 μmol/L	Hypervitaminosis A	Vitamin A deficiency Celiac disease Sprue Obstructive jaundice Giardiasis Parenchymal hepatic disease
Vitamin B₁ (thiamine)	1.6–4 μg/dl	47.4–135.7 nmol/L		Anorexia Beriberi Polyneuropathy Cardiomyopathies
Vitamin B₆ (pyridoxal phosphate)	3.6–18 ng/ml	14.6–72.8 nmol/L		Chronic alcoholism Malnutrition Uremia Neonatal seizures Malabsorption, such as celiac syndrome
Vitamin B₁₂—RIA	130–785 pg/ml	100–580 pmol/L	Hepatic cell damage and in association with the myeloproliferative disorders (the highest levels are encountered in myeloid leukemia)	Strict vegetarianism Alcoholism Pernicious anemia Total or partial gastrectomy Ileal resection Sprue and celiac disease Fish tapeworm infestation
Vitamin E	0.5–2 mg/dl	11.6–46.4 μmol/L		Vitamin E deficiency
Xylose absorption test	2 hr, 30–50 mg/dl	2–3.35 mmol/L		Malabsorption syndrome
Zinc	55–150 μg/dl	7.65–22.95 μmol/L	Zinc is essential for the growth and propagation of cell cultures and the functioning of several enzymes	

Reference Ranges—Urine Chemistry

Determination	Normal Adult Reference Range		Clinical Significance	
	Conventional Units	*SI Units*	*Increased*	*Decreased*
Acetone and acetoacetate	Zero		Uncontrolled diabetes Starvation	
Acid mucopolysaccharides	Negative		Hurler's syndrome Marfan's syndrome Morquio-Ulrich disease	

Aldosterone	Normal salt:
	 Normal:
	  4–20 μg/24 hr
	 Renovascular:
	  10–40 μg/24 hr
	 Tumor:
	  20–100 μg/24 hr
		
		11.1–55.5 nmol/24 hr
		
		27.7–111 nmol/24 hr
		
		55.4–277 nmol/24 hr
			Primary aldosteronism (adrenocortical tumor)
			Secondary aldosteronism
			Salt depletion
			Potassium loading
			ACTH in large doses
			Cardiac failure	

(continued)

Reference Ranges—Urine Chemistry (continued)

Determination	Normal Adult Reference Range		Clinical Significance	
	Conventional Units	*SI Units*	*Increased*	*Decreased*
			Cirrhosis with ascites formation Nephrosis Pregnancy	
Alpha amino nitrogen	50–200 mg/24 hr	3.6–14.3 mmol/24 hr	Leukemia Diabetes Phenylketonuria Other metabolic diseases	
Amylase	35–260 units excreted per hour	6.5–48.1 U/hr	Acute pancreatitis	
Arylsulfatase A	Greater than 2.4 U/ml			Metachromatic leukodystrophy
Bence-Jones protein	None detected		Myeloma	
Calcium	<150 mg/24 hr	<3.75 mmol/24 hr	Hyperparathyroidism Vitamin D intoxication Fanconi syndrome	Hypoparathyroidism Vitamin D deficiency
Catecholamines	Total: 0–275 μg/24 hr Epinephrine: 10%–40% Norepinephrine: 60%–90%	0–275 μg/24 hr Fraction total: 0.10–8.4 Fraction total: 0.60–0.90	Pheochromocytoma Neuroblastoma	
Chorionic gonadotrophin, qualitative (pregnancy test)	Negative		Pregnancy Chorionepithelioma Hydatidiform mole	
Copper	20–70 μg/24 hr	0.32–1.12 μmol/24 hr	Wilson's disease Cirrhosis Nephrosis	
Coproporphyrin	50–300 μg/24 hr	0.075–0.45 μmol/24 hr	Poliomyelitis Lead poisoning Porphyria hepatica Porphyria erythropoietica Porphyria cutanea tarda	
Cortisol, free	20–90 μg/24 hr	55.2–248.4 nmol/d	Cushing's syndrome	
Creatine	0–200 mg/24 hr	0–1.52 mmol/24 hr	Muscular dystrophy Fever Carcinoma of liver Pregnancy Hyperthyroidism Myositis	
Creatinine	0.8–2 gm/24 hr	7–17.6 mmol/24 hr	Typhoid fever Salmonella infections Tetanus	Muscular atrophy Anemia Advanced degeneration of kidneys Leukemia
Creatinine clearance	100–150 ml. of blood cleared of creatinine per minute	1.67–2.50 ml/s		Measures glomerular filtration rate Renal diseases
Cystine and cysteine	10–100 mg/24 hr	0.08–0.83 mmol/24 hr	Cystinuria	

(continued)

Reference Ranges—Urine Chemistry (continued)

| Determination | Normal Adult Reference Range | | Clinical Significance | |
	Conventional Units	SI Units	Increased	Decreased
Delta aminolevulinic acid	0–0.54 mg/dl	0–40 μmol/L	Lead poisoning Porphyria hepatica Hepatitis Hepatic carcinoma	
11-Desoxycortisol	20–100 μg/24 hr	0.6–2.9 μmol/d	Hypertensive form of virilizing adrenal hyperplasia due to an 11-beta hydroxylase defect	
Estriol (placental)	*Weeks of pregnancy* *μm/24 hr* 12 <1 16 2–7 20 4–9 24 6–13 28 8–22 32 12–43 36 14–45 40 19–46	<3.5 nmol/24 hr 7–24.5 nmol/24 hr 14–32 nmol/24 hr 21–45.5 nmol/24 hr 28–77 nmol/24 hr 42–150 nmol/24 hr 49–158 nmol/24 hr 66.5–160 nmol/24 hr		Decreased values occur with fetal distress of many conditions, including preeclampsia, placental insufficiency, and poorly controlled diabetes mellitus

Estrogens, total (fluorometric)	Females:
	  Onset of menstruation:
	    4–25 μg/24 hr
	  Ovulation peak:
	    28 μg/24 hr
	  Luteal peak:
	    22–105 μg/24 hr
	  Menopausal:
	    1.4–19.6 μg/24 hr
	Males: 5–18 μg/24 hr
		4–25 μg/24 hr
		28 μg/24 hr
		22–105 μg/24 hr
		1.4–19.6 μg/24 hr
		5–18 μg/24 hr
			Hyperestrogenism due to gonadal or adrenal neoplasm	Primary or secondary amenorrhea

Etiocholanolone	Males: 1.9–6 mg/24 hr Females: 0.5–4 mg/24 hr	6.5–20.6 μmol/24 hr 1.7–13.8 μmol/24 hr	Adrenogenital syndrome Idiopathic hirsutism	

Follicle-stimulating hormone—RIA	Females:
	  Follicular:
	    5–20 IU/24 hr
	  Luteal:
	    5–15 IU/24 hr
	  Midcycle:
	    15–60 IU/24 hr
	  Menopausal:
	    50–100 IU/24 hr
	Males: 5–25 IU/24 hr
		5–20 IU/d
		5–15 IU/d
		15–60 IU/d
		50–100 IU/d
		5–25 IU/d
			Menopause and primary ovarian failure	Pituitary failure

Glucose	Negative		Diabetes mellitus Pituitary disorders Intracranial pressure Lesion in floor of 4th ventricle	
Hemoglobin and myoglobin	Negative		Extensive burns Transfusion of incompatible blood Myoglobin increased in severe crushing injuries to muscles	

(continued)

Reference Ranges—Urine Chemistry (continued)

Determination	Normal Adult Reference Range		Clinical Significance	
	Conventional Units	SI Units	Increased	Decreased
Homogentisic acid, qualitative	Negative		Alkaptonuria Ochronosis	
Homovanillic acid	Up to 15 mg/24 hr	Up to 82 μmol/d	Neuroblastoma	
17-hydroxycorti-costeroids	2–10 mg/24 hr	5.5–27.5 μmol/d	Cushing's disease	Addison's disease Anterior pituitary hypofunction
5-Hydroxyindoleacetic acid, qualitative	Negative		Malignant carcinoid tumors	
Hydroxyproline	15–43 mg/24 hr	0.11–0.33 μmol/d	Paget's disease Fibrous dysplasia Osteomalacia Neoplastic bone disease Hyperparathyroidism	
17-ketosteroids, total	Males: 10–22 mg/24 hr Females: 6–16 mg/24 hr	35–76 μmol/d 21–55 μmol/d	Interstitial cell tumor of testes Simple hirsutism, occasionally Adrenal hyperplasia Cushing's syndrome Adrenal cancer, virilism Arrhenoblastoma	Thyrotoxicosis Female hypogonadism Diabetes mellitus Hypertension Debilitating disease of mild to moderate severity Eunuchoidism Addison's disease Panhypopituitarism Myxedema Nephrosis
Lead	Up to 150 μg/24 hr	Up to 60 μmol/24 hr	Lead poisoning	
Luteinizing hormone	Males: 5–18 IU/24 hr Females: Follicular phase: 2–25 IU/24 hr Ovulatory peak: 30–95 IU/24 hr Luteal phase: 2–20 IU/24 hr Postmenopausal: 40–110 IU/24 hr	2–25 IU/d 30–95 IU/d 2–20 IU/d 40–110 IU/d	Pituitary tumor Ovarian failure	Depressed or failure to peak—pituitary failure
Metanephrines, total	Less than 1.3 mg/24 hr	Less than 6.5 μmol/d	Pheochromocytoma; a few patients with pheochromocytoma may have elevated urinary metanephrines but normal catecholamines and VMA	
Osmolality	Males: 390–1090 mM/kg Females: 300–1090 mM/kg	390–1090 mmol/kg 300–1090 mmol/kg	Useful in the study of electrolyte and water balance	
Oxalate	Up to 40 mg/24 hr	Up to 456 μmol/d	Primary hyperoxaluria	
Phenylpyruvic acid qualitative	Negative		Phenylketonuria	

(continued)

Reference Ranges—Urine Chemistry (continued)

Determination	Normal Adult Reference Range		Clinical Significance	
	Conventional Units	SI Units	Increased	Decreased
Phosphorus, inorganic	0.8–1.3 gm/24 hr	26–42 mmol/24 hr	Hyperparathyroidism Vitamin D intoxication Paget's disease Metastatic neoplasm to bone	Hypoparathyroidism Vitamin D deficiency
Porphobilinogen, qualitative	Negative		Chronic lead poisoning Acute porphyria Liver disease	
Porphobilinogen, quantitative	0–1 mg/24 hr	0–4.4 μmol/24 hr	Acute porphyria Liver disease	
Porphyrins, qualitative	Negative		See porphyrins, quantitative	
Porphyrins, **quantitative** (coproporphyrin and uroporphyrin)	Coproporphyrin: 50–160 μg/24 hr Uroporphyrin: up to 50 μg/24 hr	0.075–0.24 μmol/24 hr Up to 0.06 μmol/24 hr	Porphyria hepatica Porphyria erythropoietica Porphyria cutanea tarda Lead poisoning (only coproporphyrin increased)	
Potassium	40–65 mEq/24 hr	40–65 mmol/24 hr	Hemolysis	
Pregnanediol	Females: Proliferative phase: 0.5–1.5 mg/24 hr Luteal phase: 2–7 mg/24 hr Menopause: 0.2–1 mg/24 hr Pregnancy:	 1.6–4.8 μmol/24 hr 6–22 μmol/24 hr 0.6–3.1 μmol/24 hr	Corpus luteum cysts When placental tissue remains in the uterus following parturition Some cases of adrenocortical tumors	Placental dysfunction Threatened abortion Intrauterine death
	Weeks of gestation *mg/24 hr* 10–12 5–15 12–18 5–25 18–24 15–33 24–28 20–42 28–32 27–47	 15.6–47 μmol/24 hr 15.6–78.0 μmol/24 hr 47.0–103.0 μmol/24 hr 62.4–131.0 μmol/24 hr 84.2–146.6 μmol/24 hr		
	Males: 0.1–2	0.3–6.2 μmol/24 hr		
Pregnanetriol	0.4–2.4 mg/24 hr	1.2–7.1 μmol/24 hr	Congenital adrenal androgenic hyperplasia	
Protein	Up to 100 mg/24 hr	Up to 100 mg/24 hr	Nephritis Cardiac failure Mercury poisoning Bence-Jones protein in multiple myeloma Febrile states Hematuria	
Sodium	130–200 mEq/24 hr	130–200 mmol/24 hr	Useful in detecting gross changes in water and salt balance	
Titratable acidity	20–40 mEq/24 hr	20–40 mmol/24 hr	Metabolic acidosis	Metabolic alkalosis
Urea nitrogen	9–16 gm/24 hr	0.32–0.57 mol/L	Excessive protein catabolism	Impaired kidney function

(continued)

Reference Ranges—Urine Chemistry (continued)

Determination	Normal Adult Reference Range		Clinical Significance	
	Conventional Units	SI Units	Increased	Decreased
Uric acid	250–750 mg/24 hr	1.48–4.43 mmol/24 hr	Gout	Nephritis
Urobilinogen	Random urine: <0.25 mg/dl	<0.42 mol/24 hr	Liver and biliary tract disease	Complete or nearly complete biliary obstruction
	24-hour urine: up to 4 mg/24 hr	Up to 6.76 μmol/24 hr	Hemolytic anemias	Diarrhea
				Renal insufficiency
Uroporphyrins	Up to 50 μg/24 hr	Up to 0.06 μmol/24 hr	Porphyria	
Vanillylmandelic acid (VMA)	0.7–6.8 mg/24 hr	3.5–34.3 μmol/24 hr	Pheochromocytoma Neuroblastoma Coffee, tea, aspirin, bananas, and several different drugs	
Xylose absorption test (5 hour)	16%–33% of ingested xylose	Fraction absorbed: 0.16–0.33		Malabsorption syndromes
Zinc	0.15–1.2 mg/24 hr	2.3–18.4 μmol/24 hr	Zinc is an essential nutritional element	

Reference Ranges—Cerebrospinal Fluid

Determination	Normal Adult Reference Range		Clinical Significance	
	Conventional Units	SI Units	Increased	Decreased
Albumin	15–30 mg/dl	150–300 mg/L	Certain neurologic disorders Lesion in the choroid plexus or blockage of the flow of CSF Damage to the blood-CNS barrier	
Cell count	0–5 mononuclear cells per cu/mm	$0–5 \times 10^6$/L	Bacterial meningitis Neurosyphilis Anterior poliomyelitis Encephalitis lethargica	
Chloride	100–130 mEq/L	100–300 mmol/L	Uremia	Acute generalized meningitis Tuberculous meningitis
Glucose	50–75 mg/dl	2.75–4.13 mmol/L	Diabetes mellitus Diabetic coma Epidemic encephalitis Uremia	Acute meningitides Tuberculous meningitis Insulin shock
Glutamine	6–15 mg/dl	0.41–1 mmol/L	Hepatic encephalopathies, including Reye's syndrome Hepatic coma Cirrhosis	
IgG	0–6.6 mg/dl	0–66 mg/L	Damage to the blood-CNS barrier Multiple sclerosis Neurosyphilis Subacute sclerosing panencephalitis Chronic phases of CNS infections	

(continued)

Reference Ranges—Cerebrospinal Fluid (continued)

	Normal Adult Reference Range		Clinical Significance	
Determination	Conventional Units	SI Units	Increased	Decreased
Lactic acid	Less than 24 mg/dl	Less than 2.7 mmol/L	Bacterial meningitis Hypocapnia Hydrocephalus Brain abscesses Cerebral ischemia	
Lactic dehydrogenase	One-tenth that of serum	Activity fraction: 0.1 of serum	CNS disease	

Protein:
  Lumbar
  Cisternal
  Ventricular
	
	15–45 mg/dl
	15–25 mg/dl
	5–15 mg/dl
		
		150–450 mg/L
		150–250 mg/L
		50–150 mg/L
			Acute meningitides
			Tubercular meningitis
			Neurosyphilis
			Poliomyelitis
			Guillain-Barre syndrome	

Protein electrophoresis (cellulose acetate)
  Prealbumin
  Albumin
  Alpha$_1$ globulin
  Alpha$_2$ globulin
  Beta globulin
  Gamma globulin
	% of total
	
	3–7
	56–74
	2–6.5
	3–12
	8–18.5
	4–14
		Fraction:
		
		0.03–0.07
		0.56–0.74
		0.02–0.065
		0.03–0.12
		0.08–0.185
		0.04–0.14
			An increase in the level of albumin alone can be the result of a lesion in the choroid plexus or a blockage of the flow of CSF. An elevated gamma globulin value with a normal albumin level has been reported in multiple sclerosis, neurosyphilis, subacute sclerosing panencephalitis, and the chronic phase of CNS infections. If the blood–CNS barrier has been severely damaged during the course of these diseases, the CSF albumin level may also be elevated.	

Miscellaneous Values

Determinations	Normal Value	Clinical Significance (Conventional Units)	SI Units
Acetaminophen	Zero	Therapeutic level = 10–20 μg/ml	10–20 mg/L
Aminophylline (theophylline)	Zero	Therapeutic level = 10–20 μg/ml	10–20 mg/L
Bromide	Zero	Therapeutic level = 5–50 mg/dl	50–500 mg/L
Carbon monoxide	0%–2%	Symptoms with over 20% saturation	
Chlordiazepoxide	Zero	Therapeutic level = 1–3 μg/ml	1–3 mg/L
Diazepam	Zero	Therapeutic level = 0.5–2.5 μg/dl	5–25 μg/L
Digitoxin	Zero	Therapeutic level = 5–30 ng/ml	5–30 μg/L
Digoxin	Zero	Therapeutic level = 0.5–2 ng/ml	0.5–2 μg/L
Ethanol	0%–0.01%	Legal intoxication level = 0.10% or above 0.3%–0.4% = marked intoxication 0.4%–0.5% = alcoholic stupor	

(continued)

Miscellaneous Values (continued)

Determinations	Normal Value	Clinical Significance (Conventional Units)	SI Units
Gentamicin	Zero	Therapeutic level = 4–10 μg/ml	4–10 mg/L
Methanol	Zero	May be fatal in concentration as low as 10 mg/dl	100 mg/L
Phenobarbital	Zero	Therapeutic level = 15–40 μg/ml	10–20 mg/L
Phenytoin	Zero	Therapeutic level = 10–20 μg/ml	10–20 mg/L
Primidone	Zero	Therapeutic level = 5–12 μg/ml	5–12 mg/L
Quinidine	Zero	Therapeutic level = 0.2–0.5 mg/dl	2–5 mg/L
Salicylate	Zero	Therapeutic level = 2–25 mg/dl Toxic level = over 30 mg/dl	20–250 mg/L 300 mg/L
Sulfonamide	Zero	Therapeutic levels: Sulfadiazine 8–15 mg/dl Sulfaguanidine 3–5 mg/dl Sulfamerazine 10–15 mg/dl Sulfanilamide 10–15 mg/dl	 80–150 mg/L 30–50 mg/L 100–150 mg/L 100–150 mg/L

Gastric Analysis

Determination	Normal Adult Reference Range		Clinical Significance	
	Conventional Units	SI Units	Increased	Decreased
pH	<2	<2		Pernicious anemia
Basal acid output	0–6 mEq/hr	0–6 mmol/h	Peptic ulcer	Gastric carcinoma
Maximum acid	5–40 mEq/hr	5–40 mmol/h	Zollinger-Ellison syndrome	Chronic atrophic gastritis Decreased normally with age

INDEX

The letter *f* following a page number indicates a figure; the letter *t* following a page number indicates a table.

whole, 694
normal chemistry of, 1741–1750
Blood clot, 666
Blood coagulation, 666–667, 666t, 667f
Blood data, interpretation of, 72t
Blood disorders. *See also* Hematologic system, disorders of
problems of patients with, 669t
therapeutic measures in, 693–698
Blood flow, through cardiovascular system, 624
Blood gas(es), arterial
changes due to shock, 365
studies of, 419–420, 422f
systemic assessment of, 124
Blood glucose, self-monitoring of, 914–915
Blood glucose tests, for diabetes, 904–905
Blood plasma, 667–668
Blood pool scanning, 533–534
Blood pressure
in cardiac patient, 520–521, 521f
changes due to shock, 365
classification of, 642t
diastolic, 520
elevated, 538
postural changes in, 521
regulation of, mechanisms of, 85–86
systolic, 520
Blood transfusion, 693–698
assessment of procedure, 696
complications of, 694
diseases transmitted by, 697–698
donor interviewing for, 693–694
nursing interventions in reaction to, 698
nursing management, 696–698
technique of, 695–696
Blood urea nitrogen (BUN)
in cardiac patient, 528
reference ranges in, 1755, 1760
Blood vessel(s). *See also* Artery(ies); Vein(s)
alterations in, 625
in homeostasis, 102
Body, ringworm of, 1265
Body contouring surgery, 1289
Body fluid(s)
amount and composition of, 100, 100t
disturbances in, 103–106
electrolytes in, 100, 100t, 101t
in preoperative patient, 309
regulation of, 100–101, 101f
routes of gains and losses of, 101, 101t
Body image
altered, continuous ambulatory peritoneal dialysis and, 1024
in cancer patient
changes of, 289
improved, 293
concept of, 173–174
fear of destruction of, 308
sexuality and, 203–204
social adjustments to, 174
threats to, 173
Body louse, 1266–1267
Body movement(s)
as guide to patient status, 62–63
turning and active, 313, 315t

Body organ systems. *See also specific body system*
review of, 54–55, 56t–57t
Body temperature
as guide to patient status, 63
maintenance of
in burn victim, 1303
following cardiovascular surgery, 618
postoperative, 349
Body weight
ideal, 66t
loss of, 71, 71f
Body wrap ventilator(s), 435
Bone
avascular necrosis of, following fracture, 1583
formation of, 1535
healing of, 1575–1576, 1576t
health promotion for, 149
maintenance of, 1535
metastatic cancer in, 1629, 1630
pain, 1542
tumors, 1626–1629, 1631. *See also specific type of tumor*
Bone marrow, 664, 1535
aspiration of, 668, 670, 671f
transplantation of, 698
Bone matrix, 1535
Bone scan, 1539
Botulism, 1684–1685
Bouchard's nodes, 1232, 1232f
Boutonniere's deformity, 1222
Bowel
elimination from, postoperative resumption of, 350–351
large. *See also* Colon; Rectum
obstruction of, 831
small, 828–831
Bowel patterns, nasoenteric tube feedings and, 761–762
Bowel sounds, 64
in assessment of myocardial infarction, 546
Bowel training
to overcome incontinence, 238–239
for paraplegics, 1512–1513
Brace(s), 1546, 1550–1551, 1551f
Brachial plexus block, 331
Brachioradialis reflex, 1404, 1405f
Bradycardia, sinus, 565, 566f
Bradypnea, 413
Brain. *See also* Intracranial pressure
abscess of, 1470–1471
anatomy of, 1394–1396, 1395f
cerebral cortex of, 1395, 1395f
cerebrospinal fluid of, 1396
examination of
air studies in, 1409
angiography in, 1407–1408
electroencephalography in, 1409–1410
electromyography in, 1410
imaging procedures in, 1406–1407
lumbar puncture in, 1410–1411
radionuclide imaging studies in, 1408
sonography and echoencephalography in, 1408–1409
hypothalamus of, 1399

injury to, 1496–1497
internal capsule, pons, amd medulla of, 1395–1396
interpretation of stimuli in, 90–91, 91f
pathophysiology of, 1396–1401
sensory pathways in, 1399
thalamus of, 1398–1399
tumors of, 1465–1468
acoustic neuroma, 1466–1467
angiomas, 1466
classification of, 1465–1466, 1466t
clinical manifestations of, 1467
diagnostic evaluation of, 1467
gliomas, 1466
incurable, 1468–1470
management of, 1467–1468
pituitary adenomas, 1466
Brain stem, 1394
Breast, 1127–1148
biopsy of, aspiration cytology, 1130, 1132
cancer of
adjuvant chemotherapy for, 1136
advanced
care of patient with, 1141, 1142t–1144t
treatment modalities for, 1145t–1147t
assessment of patient with, 1136
clinical manifestations of, 1134
clinical staging of, 1134, 1135f, 1135t
etiology of, 1133–1134
high risk for, 1132t
hormonal therapy for, 1136
incidence of, 1132t, 1133
management of, 1134–1136
pathophysiology of, 1133, 1134f
postoperative nursing interventions in, 1137–1139, 1138f, 1139t, 1140t
preoperative nursing interventions in, 1137
prognosis of, 1134
radiotherapy for, 1136
surgical management of, 1134–1135. *See also* Mastectomy
cystic disease of, 1132–1133
development of, 1127–1128
disease of, incidence of, 1128
examination of, 1128–1130, 1129f
fibroadenoma of, 1133
hypertrophy of, 1141
infection of, 1132
inspection of, 1128
male, 1129
diseases of, 1147–1148
operations to enlarge or uplift, 1141, 1144
Paget's disease of, 1132
palpation of, 1128–1129, 1129f
reconstruction of, 1144, 1147, 1148f–1149f
self-examination of, 1129–1130, 1131t
Breathing
Cheyne-Stokes, 408
diaphragmatic, 314t, 430
Kussmaul, 921
pursed-lip, 430–431
segmental, 431
Breathing ability, assessment of, 413
Breathing disorders, during sleep, 492
Breathing exercises, 430